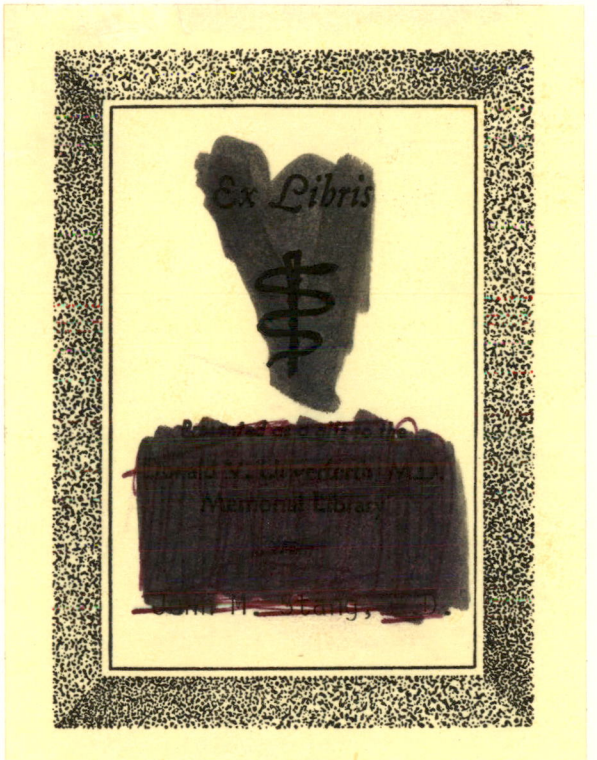
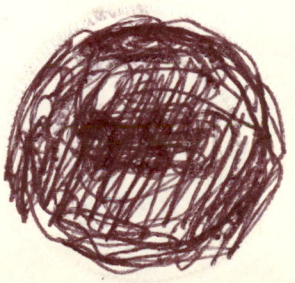

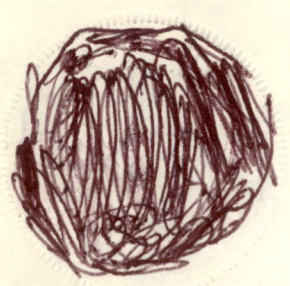

INTERNAL MEDICINE
FOR DENTISTRY

INTERNAL MEDICINE FOR DENTISTRY

LOUIS F. ROSE, D.D.S., M.D.

Professor of Periodontics,
University of Pennsylvania, School of Dental Medicine;
Professor of Medicine and Surgery,
Chief, Division of Dental Medicine,
The Medical College of Pennsylvania,
Philadelphia, Pennsylvania

DONALD KAYE, M.D.

Professor and Chairman, Department of Medicine,
The Medical College of Pennsylvania,
Philadelphia, Pennsylvania

SECOND EDITION
with **275** illustrations

The C. V. Mosby Company

ST. LOUIS • BALTIMORE • PHILADELPHIA • TORONTO   1990

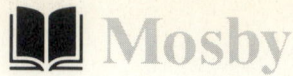

Editor: Robert W. Reinhardt
Assistant editor: Melba Steube
Editorial assistant: Cathy Laird
Editing supervisor: Trish Tannian
Manuscript editor: Kathy Lumpkin
Book and cover design: Gail Morey Hudson

SECOND EDITION

The C.V. Mosby Company
11830 Westline Industrial Drive, St. Louis, Missouri 63146

Library of Congress Cataloging in Publication Data

Internal medicine for dentistry/[edited by] Louis F. Rose, Donald Kaye.—2nd ed.
    p.   cm.
    Includes bibliographical references.
    ISBN 0-8016-4301-5
    1. Internal medicine. 2. Dentists. I. Rose, Louis F., 1942-
II. Kay, Donald, 1931-
    [DNLM: 1. Internal Medicine. 2. Oral Manifestations.   WB 115
I607]
RC46.I524 1990
616′.00246176—dc20
DNLM/DLC
for Library of Congress

89-13392
CIP

GW/VH/VH 9 8 7 6 5 4 3 2 1

SECTION EDITORS

DORIS G. BARTUSKA, M.D.

Professor of Medicine and Chief, Division of Endocrinology and Metabolism, The Medical College of Pennsylvania, Philadelphia, Pennsylvania

ROSALIE A. BURNS, M.D.

Professor and Chairman, Department of Neurology, The Medical College of Pennsylvania, Philadelphia, Pennsylvania

TOBY R. ENGEL, M.D.

Professor of Medicine, and Chief, Division of Cardiology, University of Nebraska, College of Medicine, Omaha, Nebraska

ROSALINE R. JOSEPH, M.D.

Professor of Medicine and Chief, Division of Hematology and Oncology, The Medical College of Pennsylvania, Philadelphia, Pennsylvania

WARREN A. KATZ, M.D.

Chairman, Department of Medicine and Chief, Division of Rheumatology, Presbyterian Medical Center of Philadelphia; Clinical Professor of Medicine, University of Pennsylvania, School of Medicine, Philadelphia, Pennsylvania

DONALD KAYE, M.D.

Professor and Chairman, Department of Medicine, The Medical College of Pennsylvania; Chief of Medicine, The Hospital of the Medical College of Pennsylvania, Philadelphia, Pennsylvania

BERNARD A. KIRSHBAUM, M.D.

Clinical Professor of Medicine and Chief, Division of Dermatology, The Medical College of Pennsylvania, Philadelphia, Pennsylvania

SANDRA P. LEVISON, M.D.

Professor of Medicine and Chief, Division of Nephrology and Hypertension, The Medical College of Pennsylvania, Philadelphia, Pennsylvania

WILLIAM L. MORRISSEY, M.D.

Professor of Medicine, The Medical College of Pennsylvania; Director, Department of Medicine, Frankford Hospital, Philadelphia, Pennsylvania

DONNA M. MURASKO, Ph.D.

Professor of Microbiology and Immunology, Professor of Medicine, The Medical College of Pennsylvania, Philadelphia, Pennsylvania

LOUIS F. ROSE, D.D.S., M.D.

Professor of Periodontics, University of Pennsylvania, School of Dental Medicine; Professor of Medicine and Surgery, Chief of Dental Medicine, The Medical College of Pennsylvania, Philadelphia, Pennsylvania

WALTER RUBIN, M.D.

Professor of Medicine and Anatomy and Chief, Division of Gastroenterology, The Medical College of Pennsylvania, Philadelphia, Pennsylvania

ASSOCIATE EDITORS FOR DENTAL MEDICINE

MARTIN S. GREENBERG, D.D.S.

Professor of Oral Medicine, University of Pennsylvania, School of Dental Medicine; Chairman, Department of Dental Medicine, Hospital of the University of Pennsylvania, Philadelphia, Pennsylvania

PETER D. QUINN, D.M.D., M.D.

Chairman, Department of Oral and Maxillofacial Surgery, University of Pennsylvania, School of Dental Medicine; Chief, Oral and Maxillofacial Surgery, Hospital of the University of Pennsylvania, Philadelphia, Pennsylvania

CONTRIBUTORS

JANET L. ABRAHM, M.D.

Associate Professor, Department of Medicine, University of Pennsylvania, School of Medicine; Chief, Hematology/Oncology Section, Philadelphia Veterans Administration Medical Center, Philadelphia, Pennsylvania

ELIAS ABRUTYN, M.D.

Professor of Medicine and Associate Chairman, Department of Medicine, The Medical College of Pennsylvania; Chief, Infectious Diseases and Associate Chief, Medical Service, Philadelphia Veterans Administration Medical Center, Philadelphia, Pennsylvania

BRAJESH N. AGARWAL, M.D.

Professor of Medicine, Jefferson Medical College; Chief of Medicine, Veterans Administration Medical Center, Wilmington, Delaware

PASHA AGARWAL, M.D.

Consultant Pathologist, Smith, Kline and French Laboratories, Norristown, Pennsylvania

STANLEY L. ALTSCHULER, M.D.

Clinical Assistant Professor of Medicine, The Medical College of Pennsylvania, Philadelphia, Pennsylvania

KARL E. ANDERSON, M.D.

Professor of Preventive Medicine and Community Health, Division of Human Nutrition, University of Texas Medical Branch, Galveston, Texas

ALLAN M. ARBETER, M.D.

Associate Professor of Pediatrics, Temple University School of Medicine, Philadelphia, Pennsylvania

ROBERT N. ARM, D.M.D.

Chairman, Department of Dentistry and Director, General Practice Residency, The Medical Center of Delaware, Wilmington, Delaware; Clinical Professor, Department of Oral Medicine, Temple University School of Dentistry, Philadelphia, Pennsylvania; Consultant and Educational Coordinator, Delaware State Hospital, Dental Clinic, New Castle, Delaware

BALU H. ATHREYA, M.D.

Director, Pediatric Rheumatology, Children's Seashore House/Children's Hospital of Philadelphia, Philadelphia, Pennsylvania

ROBERT R. ATKINS, M.D.

Former Assistant Professor of Medicine, The Medical College of Pennsylvania, Philadelphia, Pennsylvania

DANIEL G. BAKER, M.D.

Associate Professor of Medicine, The Medical College of Pennsylvania; Rheumatology Immunology Center, Philadelphia Veterans Administration Medical Center, Philadelphia, Pennsylvania

FRANK J. BARCH, M.D.

Clinical Assistant Professor of Medicine, The Medical College of Pennsylvania, Philadelphia, Pennsylvania

MICHAEL J. BARRETT, M.D.

Clinical Associate Professor of Medicine, The Medical College of Pennsylvania, Philadelphia, Pennsylvania

WILLIAM E. BARRY, M.D.

Professor of Medicine and Director, Student Education, Department of Medicine, Temple University School of Medicine, Philadelphia, Pennsylvania

CHRISTINE P. BASTL, M.D.

Professor of Medicine, Temple University School of Medicine, Philadelphia, Pennsylvania

ROBERT W. BEIDEMAN, D.M.D.

Associate Professor, Director of Radiology, University of Pennsylvania, School of Dental Medicine, Philadelphia, Pennsylvania

ANTHONY V. BENEDETTO, D.O.

Clinical Assistant Professor of Medicine (Dermatology), The Medical College of Pennsylvania, Philadelphia, Pennsylvania

NANCY E. BENNET, M.D.

Assistant Professor of Medicine, University of Massachusetts Medical School, Worchester, Massachusetts

JOHN E. BENNETT, M.D.

Head, Clinical Mycology Section, National Institutes of Health, Bethesda, Maryland

EMANNUEL C. BESA, M.D.

Associate Professor of Medicine, Department of Medicine, Hematology-Oncology Division, The Medical College of Pennsylvania, Philadelphia, Pennsylvania

IAIN F. S. BLACK, M.D.

Visiting Professor of Pediatrics, The Medical College of Pennsylvania; Acting Chairman and Professor, Department of Pediatrics, Temple University School of Medicine, Philadelphia, Pennsylvania

RANDOLPH C. BLODGETT, Jr., M.D.

Clinical Professor of Medicine, The Medical College of Pennsylvania, Philadelphia, Pennsylvania

JEROME A. BOSCIA, M.D., F.A.C.P.

Clinical Associate Professor of Medicine, The Medical College of Pennsylvania, Philadelphia, Pennsylvania

GEOFFREY L. BRADEN, M.D.

Clinical Associate Professor of Medicine, The Medical College of Pennsylvania, Philadelphia, Pennsylvania

MICHAEL N. BRAFFMAN, M.D.

Assistant Professor of Clinical Medicine, University of Pennsylvania, School of Medicine; Associate Physician, Infectious Diseases Section, Pennsylvania Hospital, Philadelphia, Pennsylvania

JEROME I. BRODY, M.D.

Professor of Medicine, Hematology-Oncology Division, The Medical College of Pennsylvania, Philadelphia, Pennsylvania

R. MICHAEL BUCKLEY, M.D.

Associate Professor of Clinical Medicine, University of Pennsylvania, School of Medicine; Associate Physician, Chief, Infectious Diseases Section, Pennsylvania Hospital, Philadelphia, Pennsylvania

WILLIAM J. BURTIS, M.D., Ph.D.

Research Associate, West Haven Veterans Administration Medical Center, West Haven, Connecticut; Assistant Professor of Medicine, Yale University School of Medicine, New Haven, Connecticut

CHARLES A. BUSH, M.D.

Professor of Internal Medicine, Assistant Director of Clinical Affairs, Division of Cardiology, Ohio State University, College of Medicine, Columbus, Ohio

†JOHN J. CALABRO, M.D., F.A.C.P.

Former Professor of Medicine and Pediatrics, University of Massachusetts Medical School; Former Director of Rheumatology, Saint Vincent Hospital, Worcester, Massachusetts

DAVID M. CAPUZZI, M.D., Ph.D.

Professor of Medicine and Professor of Physiology/Biochemistry (Biochemistry), The Medical College of Pennsylvania, Philadelphia, Pennsylvania

JAIME CARRIZOSA, M.D.

Infection Control Consultant, Florida Hospital, Orlando, Florida

HUGH J. CARROLL, M.D.

Professor of Medicine and Director, Electrolyte and Hypertension Division, State University of New York, Downstate Medical Center, Brooklyn, New York

PATRICIA M. CATALANO, M.D.

Associate Professor of Medicine, The Medical College of Pennsylvania, Philadelphia, Pennsylvania

HARRIS R. CLEARFIELD, M.D.

Professor of Medicine and Chief of Gastroenterology, Department of Medicine, Hahnemann University, Philadelphia, Pennsylvania

RAPHAEL COHEN, M.D.

Clinical Assistant Professor of Medicine, University of Pennsylvania, School of Medicine; Section of Nephrology, Graduate Hospital, Philadelphia, Pennsylvania

S. GARY COHEN, D.M.D.

Clinical Assistant Professor of Oral Medicine; University of Pennsylvania, School of Dental Medicine; Attendant Staff Dentist, Department of Dental Medicine, Hospital of the University of Pennsylvania, Philadelphia, Pennsylvania

JOSE de la ROSA, M.D.

Former Assistant Professor of Medicine, The Medical College of Pennsylvania; Medical Director of Dialysis, Mercy Hospital, Cadillac, Michigan

SANDEEP DHAND, M.D.

Clinical Associate Professor of Medicine, The Medical College of Pennsylvania, Philadelphia, Pennsylvania

NIKOLAY V. DIMITROV, M.D.

Professor of Medicine, Department of Medicine, Michigan State University, College of Human Medicine, East Lansing, Michigan

MARDA E. DONNER, M.D.

Clinical Instructor in Medicine, The Medical College of Pennsylvania, Philadelphia, Pennsylvania

GERALD L. DONOWITZ, M.D.

Associate Professor, Infectious Disease, University of Virginia School of Medicine, Charlottesville, Virginia

MARY B. DRATMAN, M.D.

Professor of Medicine, The Medical College of Pennsylvania; Veterans Administration Medical Center, Philadelphia, Pennsylvania

W. BRUCE DUNKMAN, M.D.

Associate Professor of Medicine, University of Pennsylvania, School of Medicine, Philadelphia, Pennsylvania

ROGER DUVOISIN, M.D.

Professor and Chairman, Department of Neurology, University of Medicine and Dentistry of New Jersey, Robert Wood Johnson Medical School, New Brunswick, New Jersey

JOEL B. EPSTEIN, D.M.D., M.S.D.

Medical/Dental Staff, Cancer Control Agency of British Columbia; Head, Division of Oral Medicine and Clinical Dentistry, Vancouver General Hospital; Clinical Professor, Department of Oral Medical and Surgical Sciences, University of British Columbia, Faculty of Dentistry, Vancouver, British Columbia, Canada; Research Associate, Department of Oral Medicine, University of Washington, School of Dentistry, Seattle, Washington

NORMAN H. ERTEL, M.D.

Chief, Medical Service, Veterans Administration Medical Center, East Orange, New Jersey; Professor and Vice-Chairman, Department of Medicine, University of Medicine and Dentistry of New Jersey, New Jersey Medical School, Newark, New Jersey

GERALD H. ESCOVITZ, M.D.

Professor of Medicine, The Medical College of Pennsylvania, Philadelphia, Pennsylvania

CALVIN EZRIN, M.D.

Clinical Professor of Medicine, University of California, Los Angeles; Attending Physician, Cedars-Sinai Medical Center, Los Angeles, California

ANTHONY S. FAUCI, M.D.

Chief, Laboratory of Immunoregulation, National Institute of Allergy and Infectious Diseases, National Institutes of Health, Bethesda, Maryland

HELEN FEIT, M.D.

Assistant Professor of Medicine, The Medical College of Pennsylvania; Chief of Endocrinology, Philadelphia Geriatric Center, Philadelphia, Pennsylvania

---

† Deceased

PEDRO C. FERNANDEZ, M.D.

Professor of Medicine, The Medical College of Pennsylvania; Adjunct Associate Professor, University of Pennsylvania School of Medicine, Philadelphia, Pennsylvania

JOSEPH A. FRANCIOSA, M.D.

Director, Cardiorenal Drugs, ICI Pharmaceutical Group, Wilmington, Delaware

WILLIAM O. FRANK, M.D.

Clinical Assistant Professor of Medicine, The Medical College of Pennsylvania, Philadelphia, Pennsylvania; Smith, Kline and French Laboratories, Norristown, Pennsylvania

HARVEY M. FRIEDMAN, M.D.

Associate Professor of Medicine, University of Pennsylvania, School of Medicine; Medical Director, Clinical Virology Laboratory, Children's Hospital of Philadelphia, Philadelphia, Pennsylvania

JUNE M. FRY, M.D., Ph.D.

Associate Professor of Neurology and Chief, Division of Somnology, The Medical College of Pennsylvania, Philadelphia, Pennsylvania

FRANK H. GARDNER, M.D.

Professor of Medicine, Department of Internal Medicine, Division of Hematology/Oncology, University of Texas Medical Branch, Galveston, Texas

ROBERT E. GERHARDT, M.D.

Physician to the Hospital, Pennsylvania Hospital; Clinical Professor of Medicine, University of Pennsylvania, School of Medicine, Philadelphia, Pennsylvania

ELAINE GERMAN, M.D.

Director of Medical Education, United Hospitals Medical Center; Clinical Professor of Medicine, University of Medicine and Dentistry of New Jersey, Newark, New Jersey

LEONARD S. GIRSH, M.D.

Director of Allergy and Clinical Immunology, Associate Professor of Internal Medicine, The Medical College of Pennsylvania, Philadelphia, Pennsylvania

MICHAEL GLICK, D.M.D.

Director of Infectious Disease Center, Assistant Professor of Oral Medicine, Temple University School of Dentistry, Philadelphia, Pennsylvania

STEPHEN J. GLUCKMAN, M.D.

Cooper Hospital/University Medical Center; Head, Division of General Internal Medicine, University of Medicine and Dentistry of New Jersey, Robert Wood Johnson Medical School of Medicine, Camden, New Jersey

†ERNEST M. GOLD, M.D.

Former Executive Associate Dean, Professor of Internal Medicine, University of California—Davis School of Medicine, Davis, California

BURTON H. GOLDSTEIN, D.M.D.

Private Practice, Vancouver, British Columbia, Canada

FRANCISCO GONZALEZ-SCARANO, M.D.

Associate Professor, Departments of Neurology and Microbiology, University of Pennsylvania, School of Medicine, Philadelphia, Pennsylvania

---

† Deceased

ROBERT H. GORDON, M.D.

Assistant Professor of Medicine, The Medical College of Pennsylvania; Philadelphia Geriatric Center, Philadelphia, Pennsylvania

HARRY GOTTLIEB, M.D.

Clinical Professor of Medicine, Subsection of Diabetes and Metabolic Diseases, The Medical College of Pennsylvania, Philadelphia, Pennsylvania

MARTIN S. GREENBERG, D.D.S.

Professor of Oral Medicine, University of Pennsylvania, School of Dental Medicine; Chairman, Department of Dental Medicine, Hospital of the University of Pennsylvania, Philadelphia, Pennsylvania

LEE W. GREENSPON, M.D.

Chief, Division of Pulmonary and Critical Care Medicine and Associate Professor of Medicine, The Medical College of Pennsylvania, Philadelphia, Pennsylvania

ROBERT L. GRISSOM, M.D.

Professor of Internal Medicine, Section of Cardiology, University of Nebraska College of Medicine, Omaha, Nebraska

ROBERT A. GROSSMAN, M.D.

Associate Professor of Medicine and Surgery, Renal Section, Department of Medicine, Hospital of the University of Pennsylvania, Philadelphia, Pennsylvania

BENJAMIN F. HAMMOND, D.D.S., Ph.D.

Professor of Microbiology, Associate Dean for Academic Affairs, University of Pennsylvania, School of Dental Medicine, Philadelphia, Pennsylvania

RICHARD N. HARNER, M.D.

Professor and Vice-Chairman, Department of Neurology, The Medical College of Pennsylvania, Philadelphia, Pennsylvania

BARRY H. HENDLER, D.D.S., M.D.

Clinical Professor of Oral and Maxillofacial Surgery, Director of Postgraduate Oral and Maxillofacial Surgery Program, University of Pennsylvania, School of Dental Medicine; Clinical Professor of Medicine and Surgery, Director of Oral and Maxillofacial Surgery, The Medical College of Pennsylvania, Philadelphia, Pennsylvania

DAVID J. HENSON, M.D.

Assistant Professor of Medicine, The Medical College of Pennsylvania; Associate Chief, Pulmonary Section, Veterans Administration Medical Center, Philadelphia, Pennsylvania

MARGARET TREXLER HESSEN, M.D.

Assistant Professor of Medicine, The Medical College of Pennsylvania, Philadelphia, Pennsylvania

LINDA B. HINER, M.D.

Associate Professor of Pediatrics, The Medical College of Pennsylvania, Philadelphia, Pennsylvania

BRUCE I. HOFFMAN, M.D.

Associate Professor of Medicine, The Medical College of Pennsylvania, Philadelphia, Pennsylvania

STUART M. HOMER, M.D.

Attending Physician, Puritan Bay Medical Center, Perth Amboy, New Jersey and John F. Kennedy Hospital, Edison Bay, New Jersey; Clinical Assistant Professor of Medicine, University of Medicine and Dentistry of New Jersey, Robert Wood Johnson Medical School, New Brunswick, New Jersey

WILLIAM A. HORTON, M.D.

Associate Professor, Department of Pediatrics and Director, Medical Genetics Program, The University of Texas Health Science Center at Houston, Houston, Texas

LEONORE C. HUPPERT, M.D.

Assistant Professor of Obstetrics and Gynecology, University of Pennsylvania College of Medicine; Associate Physician, Pennsylvania Hospital, Philadelphia, Pennsylvania

MARK J. INGERMAN, M.D.

Clinical Assistant Professor of Medicine, The Medical College of Pennsylvania, Philadelphia, Pennsylvania

ROY A. JACKEL, M.D.

Assistant Professor of Neurology, The Medical College of Pennsylvania, Philadelphia, Pennsylvania

GRAHAM H. JEFFRIES, M.B., Ch.B., D.Phil.

Professor of Medicine, Department of Medicine, The Pennsylvania State University College of Medicine, Hershey, Pennsylvania

SERGIO A. JIMINEZ, M.D.

Professor of Medicine and Professor of Biochemistry and Molecular Biology; Director, Rheumatology Research, Jefferson Medical College of Thomas Jefferson University; Director, Scleroderma Center, Thomas Jefferson University Hospital, Philadelphia, Pennsylvania

ADAM J. JONAS, M.D.

Associate Professor, Department of Pediatrics, Harbor/University of California, Los Angeles Medical Center, Torrance, California

THOMAS C. JONES, M.D.

Clinical Research, Head, Allergy and Infectious Diseases, Sandoz Ltd., Basle, Switzerland

LESTER J. KARAFIN, M.D.

Professor of Surgery and Chief of Urology, The Medical College of Pennsylvania; Professor of Urology, Temple University Medical Center, Philadelphia, Pennsylvania

JOHN H. KARAM, M.D.

Professor of Medicine and Chief, Clinical Endocrinology, University of California—San Francisco Medical Center, San Francisco, California

JULIAN KATZ, M.D.

Clinical Professor of Medicine, The Medical College of Pennsylvania, Philadelphia, Pennsylvania

LOIS ANNE KATZ, M.D.

Associate Chief, Nephrology, New York Veterans Administration Medical Center; Associate Professor of Clinical Medicine, New York University School of Medicine, New York, New York

PAUL KATZ, M.D.

Associate Professor and Vice-Chairman, Department of Medicine and Chief, Division of Rheumatology, Immunology and Allergy, Georgetown University School of Medicine, Washington, D.C.

DONALD KAYE, M.D.

Professor and Chairman, Department of Medicine, The Medical College of Pennsylvania, Philadelphia, Pennsylvania

JANET M. KAYE, Ph.D.

Associate Professor of Psychiatry and Medicine, The Medical College of Pennsylvania, Philadelphia, Pennsylvania

JUNE F. KLINGHOFFER, M.D.

Professor of Medicine, The Medical College of Pennsylvania, Philadelphia, Pennsylvania

OKSANA M. KORZENIOWSKI, M.D.

Associate Professor of Medicine, Division of Infectious Diseases, The Medical College of Pennsylvania, Philadelphia, Pennsylvania

PAUL J. KOVNAT, M.D.

Clinical Professor of Medicine, The University of New Mexico School of Medicine, Santa Fe, New Mexico

SAMUEL T. KUNA, M.D.

Assistant Professor of Medicine, Pulmonary Division, University of Texas Medical Branch, Galveston, Texas

†ELIZABETH A. LABOVITZ, M.D.

Former Associate Professor of Medicine, Division of Nephrology and Hypertension, The Medical College of Pennsylvania, Philadelphia, Pennsylvania

SALLY D. LANE, M.D.

Clinical Associate Professor of Medicine, The Medical College of Pennsylvania, Philadelphia, Pennsylvania

ROBERT L. LAVINE, M.D.

Physician, Division of Endocrinology and Metabolism, The Medical Center Clinic and West Florida Regional Medical Center, Pensacola, Florida

HARVEY B. LEFTON, M.D.

Clinical Professor of Medicine, The Medical College of Pennsylvania, Philadelphia, Pennsylvania

CARL V. LEIER, M.D.

Director, Division of Cardiology, Professor of Medicine and Pharmacology, Ohio State University Medical Center, Columbus, Ohio

SANFORD LEVINE, M.D.

Professor of Medicine, The Medical College of Pennsylvania; Chief, Pulmonary Section, Veterans Administration Medical Center, Philadelphia, Pennsylvania

MATTHEW E. LEVISON, M.D.

Professor of Medicine and Chief, Division of Infectious Diseases, The Medical College of Pennsylvania, Philadelphia, Pennsylvania

SHARON F. LEVY, M.D.

Assistant Professor of Medicine, The Medical College of Pennsylvania, Philadelphia, Pennsylvania

HARVEY M. LICHT, M.D.

Associate Professor of Medicine, The Medical College of Pennsylvania, Philadelphia, Pennsylvania

DONALD H. LIEBERMAN, M.D., F.A.C.P.

Clinical Assistant Professor of Medicine, The Medical College of Pennsylvania; Section Head, Department of Rheumatology, Frankford Hospital, Philadelphia, Pennsylvania

JOHN J. LIPUMA, M.D.

Assistant Professor of Pediatrics, Research Assistant Professor of Microbiology and Immunology, The Medical College of Pennsylvania, Philadelphia, Pennsylvania

---

† Deceased

STEVEN D. LONDON, D.D.S., Ph.D.

Research Associate, Department of Microbiology and Immunology, Washington University School of Medicine, St. Louis, Missouri

ROBERT J. LUCHI, M.D.

Professor of Medicine and Chief, Geriatrics Section, Baylor College of Medicine, Houston, Texas

JERRY C. LUCK, M.D.

Associate Professor of Medicine, Pennsylvania State University College of Medicine, Hershey, Pennsylvania

DAVID T. LUSH, M.D.

Associate Professor of Medicine and Chief, Division of General Medicine, The Medical College of Pennsylvania, Philadelphia, Pennsylvania

MALCOLM W. MacNAB, M.D., Ph.D.

Executive Director, Clinical Research, Ciba-Geigy Corporation, Summit, New Jersey; Assistant Professor of Medicine and Visiting Assistant Professor of Pharmacology, The Medical College of Pennsylvania, Philadelphia, Pennsylvania

GERALD L. MANDELL, M.D.

Professor of Medicine, Owen R. Cheatham Professor of the Sciences, and Head, Division of Infectious Diseases, University of Virginia School of Medicine, Charlottesville, Virginia

DEBORAH MAYER, R.N., M.S.N., O.C.N.

Oncology Clinical Specialist, Massachusetts General Hospital, Boston, Massachusetts

BRUCE M. McMANUS, M.D.

Professor, Departments of Pathology and Internal Medicine, University of Nebraska Medical Center, Omaha, Nebraska

MARIAN F. McNAMARA, M.D.

Vice-Chief, Division of Vascular Surgery, Harper Hospital; Associate Professor, Department of Surgery, Wayne State University, School of Medicine, Detroit, Michigan

STEVEN G. MEISTER, M.D.

Professor of Medicine, The Medical College of Pennsylvania, Philadelphia, Pennsylvania

DAVID G. MEYERS, M.D., F.A.C.C., F.A.C.P.

Assistant Professor of Medicine, Department of Internal Medicine, Section of Cardiology, University of Nebraska College of Medicine, Omaha, Nebraska

HIROSHI MITSUMOTO, M.D.

Director, Department of Neurology, Neuromuscular Program, The Cleveland Clinic, Cleveland, Ohio

MICHAEL T. MONTGOMERY, D.D.S.

Assistant Professor, Department of General Practice, University of Texas Health Science Center, San Antonio, Texas

THEODORE L. MUNSAT, M.D.

Professor of Neurology and Director, Neuromuscular Unit, Tufts—New England Medical Center, Boston, Massachusetts

DAVID M. F. MURPHY, M.D.

Chief, Department of Pulmonary Diseases, Deborah Heart and Lung Center, Browns Mills, New Jersey

RALPH M. MYERSON, M.D.

Clinical Professor of Medicine, The Medical College of Pennsylvania, Philadelphia, Pennsylvania

ROBERT G. NARINS, M.D.

Professor of Medicine and Chief, Section of Nephrology, Temple University Health Sciences Center, Philadelphia, Pennsylvania

THOMAS F. NIKOLAI, M.D.

Clinical Associate Professor of Medicine, University of Wisconsin Medical School; Staff Physician, Department of Internal Medicine, Section of Endocrinology, Marshfield Clinic, Marshfield, Wisconsin

MAN S. OH, M.D.

Associate Professor of Medicine and Co-Director, Electolyte and Hypertension Division, State University of New York Downstate Medical Center, Brooklyn, New York

SUNG HEE OH, M.D.

Department of Pediatrics, Hanyang University Hospital, Seoul, Korea

GEORGE A. OMURA, M.D.

Professor of Medicine, University of Alabama at Birmingham, Birmingham, Alabama

OLIVER E. OWEN, M.D.

Professor and Chairman, Department of Internal Medicine, Southern Illinois University, School of Medicine, Springfield, Illinois

GEORGE PAULSON, M.D.

Professor and Chairman of Neurology, Ohio State University, College of Medicine, Columbus, Ohio

STEVEN J. PEITZMAN, M.D.

Associate Professor of Medicine, The Medical College of Pennsylvania, Philadelphia, Pennsylvania

LEWIS PERELMUTTER, Ph.D.

Cooper Hospital/University Medical Center; Assistant Professor, University of Medicine and Dentistry of New Jersey; Professor, Department of Medicine, Thomas Jefferson University, Philadelphia, Pennsylvania

MICHAEL E. PLISKIN, D.D.S., Ph.D.

Acting Assistant Dean for Clinical Affairs, Chairman and Associate Professor, Department of Oral Medicine, Temple University School of Dentistry, Philadelphia, Pennsylvania

GEORGE A. POPORAD, M.D.

Clinical Assistant Professor of Medicine, The Medical College of Pennsylvania, Philadelphia, Pennsylvania

CRAIG M. PRATT, M.D.

Associate Professor of Medicine, Section of Cardiology, Baylor College of Medicine, Houston, Texas

PETER D. QUINN, D.M.D., M.D.

Chairman, Department of Oral and Maxillofacial Surgery, University of Pennsylvania, School of Dental Medicine; Chief, Oral and Maxillofacial Surgery, Hospital of the University of Pennsylvania, Philadelphia, Pennsylvania

HOWARD RASMUSSEN, M.D., Ph.D.

Professor of Medicine, Departments of Physiology and Cell Biology, Yale University School of Medicine, New Haven, Connecticut

GARY REA, M.D., Ph.D.

Associate Professor of Neurosurgery, Ohio State University, College of Medicine, Columbus, Ohio

SPENCER W. REDDING, D.D.S., M.Ed.

Associate Professor, Department of General Practice, Associate Dean of Advanced Education and Hospital Affairs, University of Texas Health Science Center, San Antonio, Texas

MICHAEL F. REIN, M.D.

Associate Professor of Medicine, Division of Infectious Diseases, University of Virginia Health Science Center, Charlottesville, Virginia

LOUIS J. RILEY, Jr., M.D.

Assistant Professor of Medicine and Director, Dialysis Unit, Temple University Health Sciences Center, Philadelphia, Pennsylvania

LARY A. ROBINSON, M.D.

Associate Professor of Surgery (Cardiothoracic) and Associate Professor of Pharmacology, University of Nebraska Medical Center, Omaha, Nebraska

LESLIE I. ROSE, M.D.

Professor of Medicine, Hahnemann Medical College and Hospital, Philadelphia, Pennsylvania

LOUIS F. ROSE, D.D.S., M.D.

Professor of Periodontics, University of Pennsylvania, School of Dental Medicine; Professor of Medicine and Surgery, Chief, Division of Dental Medicine, The Medical College of Pennsylvania, Philadelphia, Pennsylvania

MORTON RUBENSTEIN, M.D.

Clinical Assistant Professor of Medicine, Pennsylvania State University College of Medicine, Hershey, Pennsylvania

DONALD H. RUBIN, M.D.

Associate Professor of Medicine and Microbiology, University of Pennsylvania, School of Medicine; Research Associate, Veterans Administration Medical Center, Philadelphia, Pennsylvania

MICHAEL R. RUDNICK, M.D.

Clinical Associate Professor of Medicine, University of Pennsylvania, School of Medicine; Chief, Section of Nephrology, Graduate Hospital, Philadelphia, Pennsylvania

MERLE A. SANDE, M.D.

Professor and Vice-Chairman, Department of Medicine, University of California, San Francisco School of Medicine; Chief, Medical Service, San Francisco General Hospital, San Francisco, California

JEROME SANTORO, M.D.

Clinical Associate Professor of Medicine, Thomas Jefferson University Medical School, Philadelphia, Pennsylvania

W. MICHAEL SCHELD, M.D.

Professor, Departments of Internal Medicine (Infectious Diseases) and Neurosurgery, University of Virginia School of Medicine, Charlottesville, Virginia

STANLEY R. SCHIFF, M.D., Ph.D.

Former Assistant Professor of Medicine, Department of Neurology, The Medical College of Pennsylvania, Philadelphia, Pennsylvania

PAUL L. SCHRAEDER, M.D.

Professor of Medicine and Neurology, University of Medicine and Dentistry of New Jersey, Robert Wood Johnson Medical School; Head, Division of Neurology, Cooper Hospital University, Medical Center, Camden, New Jersey

SHELLEY S. SCHULER, M.D.

Assistant Professor of Medicine (Dermatology), The Medical College of Pennsylvania, Philadelphia, Pennsylvania

H. RALPH SCHUMACHER, Jr., M.D.

Professor of Medicine, University of Pennsylvania, School of Medicine; Adjunct Professor of Medicine, The Medical College of Pennsylvania; Director, Arthritis-Immunology Center, Philadelphia Veterans Administration Medical Center, Philadelphia, Pennsylvania

I. ROBERT SCHWARTZ, M.D.

Senior Attending and Division Head, Albert Einstein Medical Center, Northern Division; Clinical Professor of Medicine, Temple University School of Medicine, Philadelphia, Pennsylvania

TOBY SHAWE, M.D.

Resident, Internal Medicine, Hahnemann University Medical Center, Philadelphia, Pennsylvania

CHARLES R. SHUMAN, M.D.

Professor of Medicine, Department of Metabolism, Temple University School of Medicine, Philadelphia, Pennsylvania

PAUL D. SIEGEL, M.D.

Clinical Professor of Medicine, The Medical College of Pennsylvania, Philadelphia, Pennsylvania

SOL SILVERMAN, Jr., M.A., D.D.S.

Professor and Chairman, Division of Oral Medicine, University of California, School of Dentistry, San Francisco, California

GREGORY W. SISKIND, M.D.

Professor of Medicine and Head, Division of Allergy and Immunology, The New York Hospital—Cornell Medical Center, New York, New York

RICHARD V. SMALLEY, M.D.

Professor of Human Oncology, University of Wisconsin School of Medicine, Madison, Wisconsin

RICHARD SNEPAR, M.D.

Clinical Assistant Professor of Medicine, University of Medicine and Dentistry of New Jersey, Robert Wood Johnson Medical School, New Brunswick, New Jersey

ALEXIS B. SOKIL, M.D.

Assistant Professor of Medicine, The Medical College of Pennsylvania, Philadelphia, Pennsylvania

ROGER D. SOLOWAY, M.D.

Professor of Medicine and Chief, Division of Gastroenterology, University of Texas Medical Branch, Galveston, Texas

PHILIP S. SPRINGER, D.M.D.

Clinical Assistant Professor of Oral Medicine, University of Pennsylvania, School of Dental Medicine, Philadelphia, Pennsylvania

JOHN M. STANG, M.D.

Associate Professor of Internal Medicine, Division of Cardiology and Assistant Director for Educational Affairs, Ohio State University College of Medicine, Columbus, Ohio

STUART E. STARR, M.D.

Associate Professor of Pediatrics, University of Pennsylvania, School of Medicine; Division of Infectious Diseases, Children's Hospital of Pennsylvania, Philadelphia, Pennsylvania

BARBARA J. STEINBERG, D.D.S.

Professor of Medicine (Dental Medicine) and Associate Professor of Surgery, The Medical College of Pennsylvania; Clinical Associate Professor of Oral Medicine, University of Pennsylvania, School of Dental Medicine, Philadelphia, Pennsylvania

FRANCIS H. STERLING, M.D.

Professor of Medicine, University of Pennsylvania, School of Medicine; Adjunct Professor of Medicine, The Medical College of Pennsylvania; Chief of Endocrinology, Philadelphia Veterans Administration Medical Center, Philadelphia, Pennsylvania

MARY CATHERINE STOM, M.D.

Associate Professor of Medicine, University of Medicine and Dentistry of New Jersey, Robert Wood Johnson Medical School, New Brunswick, New Jersey; Head, Division of Nephrology, Cooper Hospital/University Medical Center, Camden, New Jersey

TERRENCE L. STULL, M.D.

Associate Professor of Pediatrics and Research Assistant Professor of Microbiology and Immunology, The Medical College of Pennsylvania, Philadelphia, Pennsylvania

NEIL M. SUSSMAN, M.D.

Associate Professor of Neurology, The Medical College of Pennsylvania, Philadelphia, Pennsylvania

GEZA T. TEREZHALMY, D.D.S., M.A.

Acting Dean and Professor of Oral Diagnosis, Radiology, and Oral Medicine; Chairman, Department of Oral Diagnosis and Radiology, Case Western Reserve University School of Dentistry, Cleveland, Ohio

JOSEPH U. TOGLIA, M.D.

Professor of Neurology, Temple University Medical School, Philadelphia, Pennsylvania

KATHLEEN E. TOOMEY, M.D., J.D.

Chief, Section of Medical Genetics, St. Christopher's Hospital for Children; Assistant Professor of Pediatrics, Temple University College of Medicine, Philadelphia, Pennsylvania

WALLACE W. TOURTELLOTTE, M.D., Ph.D.

Chief of Neurology, Veterans Administration Wadsworth Hospital; Professor and Vice-Chairman, Department of Neurology, University of California—Los Angeles, School of Medicine, Los Angeles, California

JAY H. TUREEN, M.D.

Assistant Clinical Professor, Department of Pediatrics, University of California, San Francisco School of Medicine, San Francisco, California

JOHN VARGA, M.D.

Assistant Professor of Medicine, Jefferson Medical College of Thomas Jefferson University; Associate Director, Scleroderma Center, Thomas Jefferson University Hospital, Philadelphia, Pennsylvania

MICHAEL J. WALSH, M.B., B.Ch.

Former Assistant Professor, Department of Neurology, University of California Los Angeles School of Medicine, Los Angeles, California

ARTHUR S. WALTERS, M.D.

Assistant Professor, Department of Neurology, University of Medicine and Dentistry of New Jersey, Robert Wood Johnson Medical School, New Brunswick, New Jersey; Staff Physician, Neurology Service, Lyons Veterans Administration Medical Center, Lyons, New Jersey

PAUL B. WEISBERG, M.D.

Clinical Assistant Professor of Medicine, The Medical College of Pennsylvania, Philadelphia, Pennsylvania

GARY B. WEISS, M.D., Ph.D.

Clinical Associate Professor of Medicine, Department of Internal Medicine, Division of Hematology/Oncology, University of Texas Medical Branch, Galveston, Texas

WILLIAM WEISS, M.D.

Emeritus Professor of Medicine, Hahnemann Medical Center College and Hospital, Philadelphia, Pennsylvania

CHARLES J. WOLF, M.D.

Physician to the Hospital, Pennsylvania Hospital; Clinical Professor of Medicine, University of Pennsylvania, School of Medicine, Philadelphia, Pennsylvania

NELSON M. WOLF, M.D.

Professor of Medicine, Cardiology Division and Director, Cardiac Catheterization Laboratory, The Medical College of Pennsylvania, Philadelphia, Pennsylvania

CLINTON W. YOUNG, M.D.

Associate Clinical Professor of Medicine, University of California, San Francisco Medical School; Associate Professor of Medical Education and Director, Medical Clinics, Presbyterian Hospital, San Francisco, California

JAMES B. YOUNG, M.D.

Associate Professor of Medicine, Section of Cardiology, Baylor College of Medicine, Houston, Texas

To my wife
Claire
my children
David and **Michael**
and my parents and grandmother
with love
L.F.R.

To my wife
Janet
my children
Kenneth, Karen, Kendra, and **Keith**
and my parents
with love
D.K.

PREFACE

Dental education has been remiss in adequately preparing the dentist to evaluate the general health status of a patient. Today, more than ever before, when one considers the revolutionary advances that are occurring in medicine and the fact that a rapidly growing segment of the population consists of geriatric and medically compromised patients, the importance of medicine and its relationship to dental practice becomes clear. One area of special neglect is the failure to correlate internal medicine to dental practice. Unfortunately, many of the concepts of medical management of the dental patient are lost once the student is thrust into an intensive course in the technical principles of dentistry.

Recent dental graduates, although far more sophisticated in many ways than their predecessors, may not possess a sufficient understanding of the mechanisms of the disease processes to deal intelligently with the dental problems of such patients. *Internal Medicine for Dentistry* has been written for both the dental student and the dental practitioner.

This textbook describes the basic mechanisms involved in the various disease processes included in internal medicine, the symptoms they produce, and the manner in which they are diagnosed and managed. The information available in the field of internal medicine is enormous, and we believed that a complete yet concise textbook specifically designed for dentistry was needed. We have attempted to organize and present dental considerations in a succinct fashion at the end of each organ system. The exceptions to this format are microbial diseases, skin diseases and manifestations of systemic diseases, and genetics and metabolism. In these sections, the dental information is an integral part of the body of the medical text. The book provides all the necessary information relevant to internal med-

icine, but even more important to the dental professional, it discusses, where appropriate, the oral manifestations and dental management of patients with medical disorders.

Among the changes in this edition are a thorough update of cardiology with the latest procedures in angioplasty; contemporary treatment of gastrointestinal disorders and urologic infections reflecting the latest drugs; coverage of AIDS, Lyme disease, and other disorders of new or renewed interest; and the dental correlations have been strengthened with details newly linking periodontal pathogens and systemic disease.

The textbook has been arranged by organ systems with a description of the disease entities affecting each system. To minimize repetition, it was necessary to arbitrarily classify a disease within a specific system. For example, gout is discussed in the section "Rheumatic and Granulomatous Diseases," but it could just as properly have been classified as a metabolic or renal disease. When such multisystem diseases are described primarily under one system, cross-references to the major description are included.

We would like to thank our wives, Claire Rose and Janet Kaye, and our children, David and Michael Rose and Kenneth, Karen, Kendra, and Keith Kaye, for their patience. Those who have never taken part in a project such as this cannot possibly appreciate the enormity of the task and the many hundreds of hours required that we might otherwise have spent with our families. Special thanks are due the section editors, who took much of the load off our shoulders and without whom we could never have completed this book.

Louis F. Rose
Donald Kaye

CONTENTS

SECTION SIX

NEOPLASTIC DISEASES

Edited by **Rosaline R. Joseph**

SECTION SEVEN

CARDIOVASCULAR DISEASES

Edited by **Toby R. Engel**

SECTION TWELVE

SKIN DISEASES AND THEIR ORAL MANIFESTATIONS

Edited by **Bernard A. Kirshbaum** and **Robert N. Arm**

156   Congenital diseases, 771

Bernard A. Kirshbaum and **Robert N. Arm**

157   Endocrine and metabolic disorders, 782

Anthony V. Benedetto and **Robert N. Arm**

158   Gastrointestinal disorders with cutaneous lesions, 788

Shelley S. Schuler and **Robert N. Arm**

159   Liver disorders, 794

Shelley S. Schuler

160   Renal disorders, 795

Shelley S. Schuler and **Robert N. Arm**

161   Hematologic disorders, 796

Shelley S. Schuler and **Robert N. Arm**

INTERNAL MEDICINE
FOR DENTISTRY

APPROACH TO EVALUATION OF THE PATIENT

Edited by **Donald Kaye**

INTRODUCTION

David T. Lush, Louis F. Rose, *and* **Barbara J. Steinberg**

The history and physical examination produce a comprehensive evaluation of the patient's medical status. A standard method of performing and recording this evaluation has evolved.

Although the history and physical examination are appropriately treated in this section in mechanical fashion, the examiner must remember that these are significant events for most patients, and the examiner must display a personal as well as a professional attitude for the proper rapport to develop. Enlisting the patient's cooperation is an important aspect of an accurate, comprehensive examination.

Every practicing dentist and the auxiliary staff are responsible for identifying any patient who may be a potential medical risk by performing a comprehensive pretreatment physical evaluation.

In their article on the significance of physical diagnosis, patient history, data, and medical screening in the dental office, Little and King summarize the reasons for physical evaluation as follows:

1. To identify patients with undetected systemic disease that could be a serious threat to the life of the patient or that could be complicated by dental treatment
2. To identify patients who are taking drugs or medication that could be potentiated by drugs prescribed by the dentist, that would complicate dental therapy, or that may serve as a clue to an underlying systemic disease that the patient has omitted from the history
3. To allow the dentist to modify the treatment plan in light of any systemic disease the patient may have or any drugs he may be taking
4. To protect the patient and the dentist from any malpractice (or allegations thereof)
5. To enable the dentist to select and confer with a medical consultant about a patient's possible systemic problems
6. To help establish a good patient/doctor relationship by showing the patients that the dentist is interested in them as individuals and that the dentist is concerned about their overall well-being

In fact, the data obtained from a history and physical examination may even prevent a medical emergency. A well-conceived total physical evaluation involves (1) medical history, (2) physical examination, (3) laboratory studies (if indicated), and (4) medical/dental consultation or referral.

Two basic methods for obtaining a medical history are the questionnaire and the personal dialogue interview. A personal history elicited by dialogue allows the dentist to observe the patient's reactions to questions and to evaluate the patient's mental status in a nonthreatening atmosphere. The patient who is uninterested or evasive may respond quite differently from one who is anxious to provide complete information. The questionnaire is a legitimate method of securing data if used in conjunction with a dialogue. It may help a patient recall frequently used medications or various symptoms of disease.

The questionnaire component (Fig. 1) also can assist the dentist in ascertaining which areas in the dialogue history to emphasize and explore further. More importantly, a completed and dated form, signed by the patient, may be used as evidence in any possible malpractice litigation.

Obviously, a dialogue medical history (Fig. 2) helps the dentist evaluate the patient's present health status, medical history, allergies, medications, and the like. Here the focus shifts from one of intensive diagnostic effort to a procedure that must effectively determine the patient's physical and emotional ability to tolerate dental treatment. Although evaluation in an outpatient setting may be somewhat less detailed, the information obtained should adequately identify any condition that might compromise the patient's well-being during therapy. In essence, an abbreviated outpatient evaluation must assure the dentist that treatment may be carried out with relative safety; if this is not the case, medical consultation must be obtained before instituting any treatment.

It is evident that any total physical evaluation actually can be elicited in two ways. The first is a systemic approach to history and physical examination suitable for contact with the hospital inpatient, and the second is a physical evaluation of the patient in an ambulatory care facility, such as the dental office. All practitioners must know and use the more comprehensive format as a basis for the less comprehensive second approach. The text that follows offers the essential information required in performing the most comprehensive and diagnostic type of inpatient history and physical examination.

1·HISTORY

David T. Lush

PATIENT IDENTIFICATION

Before recording the examination, note the patient's full name, age and date of birth, sex, race, and marital status. When pertinent, occupation, place of birth, or religion should be included; otherwise, they may be considered later as part of the social history.

MEDICAL HISTORY

Date _____

Name _____   Address _____

      Last   First   Middle   Number & Street

_____

City   State   Zip Code   Home Phone   Business Phone

Date of Birth _____ Sex _____ Height _____ Weight _____ Occupation _____

Social Security No. _____ Single _____ Married _____ Name of Spouse _____

Closest Relative _____ Phone _____

If you are completing this form for another person, what is your relationship to that person? _____

Referred By: _____

In the following questions, circle yes or no, whichever applies. Your answers are for our records only and will be considered confidential.

1. Are you in good health?	YES	NO
2. Has there been any change in your general health within the past year?	YES	NO
3. My last physical examination was on _____		
4. Are you now under the care of a physician?	YES	NO
a. If so, what is the condition being treated? _____		
5. The name and address of my physician is _____		
6. Have you had any serious illness or operation?	YES	NO
a. If so, what was the illness or operation? _____		
7. Have you been hospitalized or had a serious illness within the past five (5) years?	YES	NO
a. If so, what was the problem? _____		
8. Do you have or have you had any of the following diseases or problems?		
a. Damaged heart valves or artificial heart valves	YES	NO
b. Congenital heart lesions	YES	NO
c. Cardiovascular disease (heart trouble, heart attack, coronary insufficiency, coronary occlusion, high blood pressure, arteriosclerosis, stroke)	YES	NO
1) Do you have pain in chest upon exertion?	YES	NO
2) Are you ever short of breath after mild exercise?	YES	NO
3) Do your ankles swell?	YES	NO
4) Do you get short of breath when you lie down, or do you require extra pillows when you sleep?	YES	NO
5) Do you have a cardiac pacemaker?	YES	NO
d. Allergy	YES	NO
e. Sinus trouble	YES	NO
f. Asthma or hay fever	YES	NO
g. Hives or a skin rash	YES	NO
h. Fainting spells or seizures	YES	NO
i. Diabetes	YES	NO
1) Do you have to urinate (pass water) more than six times a day?	YES	NO
2) Are you thirsty much of the time?	YES	NO
3) Does your mouth frequently become dry?	YES	NO
j. Hepatitis, jaundice or liver disease	YES	NO
k. Arthritis	YES	NO
l. Inflammatory rheumatism (painful swollen joints)	YES	NO
m. Stomach ulcers	YES	NO
n. Kidney trouble	YES	NO
o. Tuberculosis	YES	NO
p. Do you have a persistent cough or cough up blood?	YES	NO
q. Low blood pressure	YES	NO
r. Veneral disease	YES	NO
s. Other _____ _____ _____		

Fig. 1 Dental health questionnaire.

9. Have you had abdominal bleeding associated with previous extractions, surgery, or trauma? .... YES   NO
   a. Do you bruise easily .... YES   NO
   b. Have you ever required a blood transfusion? .... YES   NO
      If so, explain the circumstances _____

10. Do you have any blood disorder such as anemia? .... YES   NO

11. Have you had surgery or x-ray treatment for a tumor, growth, or other condition of your head or neck? .... YES   NO

12. Are you taking any drug or medicine? .... YES   NO

13. Are you taking any of the following:
   a. Antibiotics or sulfa drugs .... YES   NO
   b. Anticoagulants (blood thinners) .... YES   NO
   c. Medicine for high blood pressure .... YES   NO
   d. Cortisone (steroids) .... YES   NO
   e. Tranquilizers .... YES   NO
   f. Antihistamines .... YES   NO
   g. Aspirin .... YES   NO
   h. Insulin, tolbutamide (Orinase) or similar drug .... YES   NO
   i. Digitalis or drugs for heart trouble .... YES   NO
   j. Nitroglycerin .... YES   NO
   k. Oral contraceptive or other hormonal therapy .... YES   NO
   l. Other _____

14. Are you allergic or have you reacted adversely to:
   a. Local anesthetics .... YES   NO
   b. Penicillin or other antibiotics .... YES   NO
   c. Sulfa drugs .... YES   NO
   d. Barbiturates, sedatives, or sleeping pills .... YES   NO
   e. Aspirin .... YES   NO
   f. Iodine .... YES   NO
   g. Codeine or other narcotics .... YES   NO
   h. Other _____

15. Have you had any serious trouble associated with any previous dental treatment? .... YES   NO
    If so, explain _____
    _____

16. Do you have any disease, condition, or problem not listed above that you think I should know about .... YES   NO
    If so, explain _____
    _____

17. Are you employed in any situation which exposes you regularly to x-rays or other ionizing radiation? .... YES   NO

18. Are you wearing contact lenses? .... YES   NO

19. Have you been in contact with any one at risk for the following: YES   NO
       a. Herpes   b. Hepatitis
       c. Tuberculosis   d. AIDS

WOMEN

20. Are you pregnant? .... YES   NO

21. Do you have any problems associated with your menstrual period? .... YES   NO

22. Are you nursing? .... YES   NO

CHIEF DENTAL COMPLAINT:

_____

	SIGNATURE OF PATIENT
ADJA American Dental Association	
	SIGNATURE OF DENTIST

Fig. 1, *cont'd*

SOURCE OF INFORMATION

Be sure to include the sources of information used in compiling the history. The patient, a friend or relative, previous medical charts, or a referral letter from a physician or institution are usual sources. Include also an assessment of the reliability of this information.

CHIEF COMPLAINT

Ascertain the principal reason the patient is seeking medical attention. This is best recorded as a simple phrase stating the complaint and its duration. The patient's own words need not be used, although they may be enlightening.

For example, a typical chief complaint may be written as follows:

1. Abdominal pain for 1 month
2. Vomiting blood for 1 day

PRESENT ILLNESS

Question the patient in detail about his complaints, and record the history in chronologic order. Unlike the chief com-

---

HOSPITAL OF THE MEDICAL COLLEGE OF PENNSYLVANIA
DEPARTMENT OF DENTAL MEDICINE

DENTAL HISTORY:

CHIEF COMPLAINT:

HISTORY OF PRESENT ILLNESS:

PAST DENTAL HISTORY:

MEDICAL HISTORY

Physician _____ Clinic _____ Last C. Ph. Exam. _____

PRESENT HEALTH STATUS:

HOSPITALIZATIONS:

ILLNESSES: _____

ALLERGIES: _____ A.S.A. _____ L.A. _____ ANBT. _____

MEDS. _____ O.C. _____

REVIEW OF SYSTEMS

Skin _____

EENT _____

Respiratory _____

Cardiac _____ RhF _____ RhHD _____ M _____

Gastro-intestinal _____

Genito-urinary _____

Menstrual Hx. _____ Pregnancy _____ Children _____

Endocrine _____ Diabetes _____

Extremities _____

Nervous _____ Psychiatric _____

Hematopoietic _____

FAMILY HISTORY

Diabetes _____ Hypertension _____ Cardiac _____

Epilepsy _____ Other _____

SOCIAL HISTORY

Occupation _____ Smoking _____ Alcohol _____ Other _____

MEDICAL SUMMARY:

Fig. 2   Comprehensive dialogue medical history.

plaint, the description of the present illness should be written in paragraph form. Inquire about all the symptoms in the system that you believe to be the site of the chief complaint. Ask also about the presence or absence of symptoms classically associated with diseases known to cause similar complaints. *Pertinent negatives* are a fundamental part of this portion of the history. Laboratory tests performed during the course of the present illness workup and the results of previous attempts at therapy likewise should be included. The patient's current medications should be reviewed completely.

PAST HISTORY

Check the following areas in this section:

1. General: previous illnesses and response to therapy, known active medical problems, previous hospitalizations and surgery, history of chronically abnormal laboratory tests, particularly elevated lipids
2. Medication allergies: drugs, contrast media
3. Immunizations: tetanus, diphtheria, pneumonia, influenza, poliomyelitis, measles, rubella, mumps, hepatitis
4. Trauma: significant injuries, blood transfusions

REVIEW OF SYSTEMS

When reviewing the systems as part of the medical history, present each major symptom to the patient and ask if he is experiencing or has experienced it. The purpose is to uncover symptoms that may aid in identifying the process responsible for the patient's chief complaint and to identify any possible unrelated coexisting disease. At the same time, asking about previous symptoms serves as a check on the accuracy and completeness of the patient's past history.

When symptoms pertinent to the present illness are discovered during the review of systems, they are, of course, incorporated into the present illness portion of the history when the examination is put into writing. Most examiners then record only positives and related pertinent negatives in the review of systems.

Following is a list of the symptoms reviewed in this section of the history:

1. General: fever, chills, perspiration, weakness, fatigue, weight change
2. Skin: lesions or moles, rash, itch, pigmentation, bruising, scars; *nails*—change in shape, brittleness, pitting; *hair*—excessive loss, change in texture or distribution
3. Head: headache, trauma
4. Eyes: double vision, blurry vision, transient or permanent loss of vision, spots, pain, redness, tearing, discharge, sensitivity to light, use of glasses or contact lenses, cataracts, most recent examination for glaucoma
5. Ears: hearing loss, ringing, dizzy spells (with or without a sensation of motion), pain, discharge
6. Nose and sinuses: bleeding, discharge, obstruction, colds, change in sense of smell, facial pain
7. Mouth: pain, lesions, dryness; *tongue*—soreness, taste; *teeth*—pain, extractions, most recent dental examination; *gums*—bleeding, lesions, discoloration; *throat*—frequent sore throats or tonsillitis, hoarseness, problems with swallowing
8. Neck: pain, stiffness, swelling, lumps, limitation of motion, thyroid enlargement
9. Breasts: lumps, tenderness, discharge, change in nipple, changes in self-examination
10. Respiratory system: cough, sputum, coughing up blood, night sweats, shortness of breath, wheezing, pain with breathing, exposure to tuberculosis (TB), most recent TB skin test and chest roentgenogram
11. Heart: chest pain, shortness of breath with exertion or when lying down, swelling in legs or feet, chest pounding, irregular or rapid heartbeats, heart murmur, high blood pressure
12. Vascular system: foot pain, lower extremity pain with exertion, leg cramps, blood clots, varicose veins, coldness or change in color of extremity
13. Gastrointestinal tract: poor appetite, food intolerance, regurgitation, chest pain or burning after eating or when lying down, pain or problems with swallowing, belching, nausea, vomiting, vomiting blood, abdominal pain, diarrhea, constipation, change in bowel habits or in color or character of stool, hemorrhoids, anal itch, gallstones, yellow color to eyes or skin, abdominal swelling, liver disease or hepatitis, hernia
14. Urinary tract: pain on urination; frequent, urgent, repeated, or nocturnal need to void; bloody urine; loss of urine on clothes or bed; difficulty starting or stopping stream; change in size of stream or color of urine; kidney stones; infections; flank pain
15. Genitoreproductive system
    a. Female: *menses*—age of onset, frequency, duration, pain or other associated symptoms, amount of flow, presence of clots, bleeding between periods, date of most recent period; *menopause*—age, hot flashes, vaginal dryness, bleeding since menopause; *pregnancy*—number, outcome, use of diethylstilbestrol by patient or mother; *general*—vaginal pain, itch, discharge, or odor; date of most recent pelvic examination and Pap smear; contraceptive history, sexual history, venereal diseases
    b. Male: penile lesions, discharge, and pain; ability to achieve and maintain erection; scrotal or testicular pain, swelling, and lumps; venereal diseases, sexual history
16. Joints: pain, redness, warmth, swelling, stiffness, limitation of motion, deformities
17. Lymph nodes: enlargement, pain, tenderness
18. Blood: anemia, easy bruising or bleeding, blood transfusions
19. Endocrine system: thyroid enlargement or malfunction; heat or cold intolerance; change in skin or hair texture; diabetes; excessive eating, drinking, or urinating; change in skin pigmentation or hair distribution
20. Allergies: hives, hay fever, allergic rashes, asthma, nonmedication allergies
21. Neurology: *cerebral*—seizures, loss of consciousness, fainting, memory loss, confusion, speech impairment; *cranial nerves* (covered in review of head and neck systems); *motor*—loss of strength, local paralysis, involuntary movements, loss of coordination; *sensory*—numbness, tingling, pain
22. Psychiatric considerations: depression; anxiety; worries; problems with family, friends, job, or financial matters; difficulty in sleeping

The review of body systems is actually the main component of the interview approach to history taking. Fig. 1-1 is an abbreviated form that can be used in the dental office.

SOCIAL HISTORY

Developing the social history involves the patient's interactions in three major areas:

1. Environment: present and previous residences, occupations, and climatic exposures
2. Society: education; religion; marital status; living arrangements; financial situation; hours of work, sleep, and daily exercise
3. Drugs: coffee, tea, alcohol, cigarettes, illegal drugs

FAMILY HISTORY

Inquire about the age, medical problems, and, if applicable, cause of death of parents, spouse, siblings, and children. Then ask specifically about the presence in the family of cancer, high blood pressure, heart disease, diabetes, tuberculosis, anemia,

---

REVIEW OF SYSTEMS

1. **Skin:** itching, rash, ulcers, excessive dryness, pigmentary change, changes in hair or nails, hair loss.
2. **Eyes:** vision, inflammation, diplopia, blurring.
3. **Ears, Nose, Throat:** hearing, earache, epistasix, sore throat, hoarseness, sinus pain.
4. **Respiratory:** cough, sputum (describe quantity, color, odor, blood), wheezing, infections, exposure to tuberculosis, prior chest x-ray.
5. **Cardiac:** chest pain on exertion, palpitation, dyspnea, orthopnea, swelling of ankles, history of rheumatic fever, rheumatic heart disease, "heart attack", high blood pressure, murmur.
6. **Gastro-intestinal:** appetite, nausea, vomiting, dysphagia, heartburn, indigestion, food intolerance, abdominal pain, jaundice, hepatitis.
7. **Genito-urinary:** dysuria, nocturia, polyuria, hematuria, frequency, difficulty starting stream; sexually transmitted diseases, kidney infection.

   For women:
   a. menstrual history: last menstrual period and previous menstrual period; dysmennorrhea
   b. menopause: age of occurrence, hot flushes
   c. obstretrical history: pregnancies, miscarriages, living children
8. **Extremities:**
   a. vascular: varicose veins, phlebitis
   b. joints: pain, stiffness, swelling of joints
   c. muscles: weakness, pain, tenderness, cramps
9. **Endocrine System:** thyroid enlargement or malfunction: heat or cold intolerance; diabetes; excessive eating, drinking or urinating.
10. **Nervous System:** syncope, convulsions, headache, vertigo, tremor, paralysis, paresthesias, anesthesias.
11. **Hematopoietic:** bleeding tendency, excessive bruising, anemia, known exposure to radiation or toxic agents.
12. **Psychiatric:** "nervousness", irritability, depressions, history of previous "nervous breakdown"

Fig. 1-1   Information that should be obtained regarding each body system.

bleeding disorders, migraine headaches, seizures, kidney disease, psychiatric problems, allergies, alcoholism, glaucoma, blindness, arthritis, ulcers, or strokes.

2·PHYSICAL EXAMINATION

David T. Lush

The areas covered in the physical examination of the patient are presented in this chapter, and the methods of performing specific parts of the examination are described where appropriate. The material is listed in a systems approach. Some parts of one system may be best examined in the supine position, whereas other parts of the same system may require the sitting or standing position for adequate analysis. Therefore, in the interests of efficiency for the examiner and convenience for the patient, the examination is not performed in a strictly systems manner. The examiner must be prepared to perform the examination with minimal position change of the patient. This is especially important with the incapacitated patient.

METHODS

Four methods of examination are available.

INSPECTION. This involves observing the whole patient and then visualizing various areas of the body more closely. It is performed with the patient at rest and during certain maneuvers.

PALPATION. This method involves using the fingertips for touch, the metacarpophalangeal area of the palms for vibration, and the dorsal aspect of the hand for temperature.

PERCUSSION. Indirect percussion consists of striking the distal interphalangeal joint of the middle finger of one hand with the tip of the middle finger of the other hand. This is used

to define the position of certain organs and to analyze the density of tissues. The examiner must be able to distinguish tympany (stomach bubble), hyperresonance (emphysematous lung), resonance (normal lung), dullness (normal liver), and flatness (normal thigh). Direct percussion—tapping the patient directly with the finger—is used much less frequently.

AUSCULTATION. In most instances, auscultation involves listening through the stethoscope. High-pitched sounds are best heard with the diaphragm, and low-pitched sounds with the bellpiece.

PRELIMINARIES

For the purpose of standardization, the examiner should consistently use the patient's right side in performing the examination.

The recording of the physical examination should begin with a brief description of the patient's overall appearance, including references to his general state of health and nutrition and to any distress. Gross abnormalities of posture, facial expression, personal hygiene, and mental status should be noted. This description might be stated as follows: Mr. Jones is a well-developed but moderately obese white male who appears to be in no distress.

SPECIFIC AREAS

VITAL SIGNS. Check blood pressure, pulse, respiration rate, and temperature, and record height and weight.

SKIN. Observe turgor, texture (rough, smooth), color, pigmentation, lesions (distribution, configuration, morphology), scars, hair distribution, and nails. Measure turgor by squeezing some skin between the thumb and index finger. When released, the skin should return promptly to its usual place. This customarily is done over the sternum.

HEAD. Check size, shape, lumps, depressions, and hair distribution.

EYES. Examine position, color vision, and visual acuity. Check vision with standard pocket or wall charts.

Visual fields. Position yourself facing the patient at a distance of about 50 cm. Have the patient stare into your left eye with his right eye. Both of you should close the other eye. Bring a target object in from the periphery at different angles, and have the patient tell you when it comes into view. Compare his performance with your own. Lateral vision must be tested by bringing the object in from behind the patient rather than from a distance because even distant objects should be detectable laterally.

Lids. Check motion, swelling, and lesions.

Sclera and conjunctiva. Examine for injection, hemorrhage, or icterus.

Cornea and lens. Check for arcus senilis and for abrasions or opacities.

Pupils. Check size, equality, roundness, reaction to light (direct and consensual), and accommodation. Shine a light obliquely into a pupil. Observe for constriction in the same (direct) and opposite (consensual) pupil. Repeat on the other pupil. With the patient looking into the distance, test accommodation by having him change his focus to your finger, which is held about 5 cm from his nose. The normal response is convergence of the eyes and pupillary constriction.

Extraocular movements. Have the patient fixate on your finger as it traces an "H" in the air.

Nystagmus. Observe the eyes in primary position and with some lateral gaze for repetitive movements.

Ophthalmoscopic examination (Fig. 2-1). Check pupil and lens (red reflex, opacities), disc (margins, size of physiologic cup), vessels (size, crossing changes), retina (hemorrhage, exudate), and macula (hemorrhage, exudate). With the ophthalmoscopic lens set at 0 diopters, darken the room and have the patient stare straight into the distance. Examine the patient's right eye with your right eye and with your right hand on the ophthalmoscope, reversing the procedure for his left eye. Beginning at a distance of about 30 cm, find the red reflex, and move slowly closer to the patient's eye. Then adjust the lens setting until the retinal structures come into focus. Find the optic disc. The margins should be distinct, although there may be slight blurring medially. The physiologic cup is a pale area within the disc but on its lateral side. Note its size in relation to the disc as a whole. Next, follow the course of each major vessel from its emergence in the disc, through the disc margin (it should remain in focus), then distally as far as possible. An artery and vein should run together, the vein being larger and darker red. Compare the relative size of the vessels, and record this as vein to artery ratio (usually about 5:4). Note any focal vessel spasm. Inspect the arteriovenous crossings for any humping, banking, tapering, or nicking. As you follow the course of the vessels, also notice any hemorrhages or exudates in that area of the retina. The location and size of any abnormalities observed can most conveniently be expressed in terms of disc diameters. The macula is located about 2 to 3 disc diameters lateral to the disc. It appears as a small, dark red spot with a central point light reflex. Always examine this area for hemorrhages and exudates. If opacities are noted on initial viewing of the red reflex, the lens can be examined by changing the ophthalmoscope to the short focal-length settings, usually about +12 diopters.

EARS

External. Check for deformities and pain with movement.

Otoscopic examination. Check the canal for cerumen, discharge, swelling, redness, masses, or foreign bodies. Examine the middle ear area (Fig. 2-2) for light reflex, malleus, drum perforation, bulging, or retraction. When examining the patient's right ear, hold the otoscope in your right hand. With your left hand gently pull the auricle upward and backward. Use the largest speculum the patient's canal will accommodate comfortably, and insert it at a slightly anterior and downward angle. It eventually will be necessary to tilt or rotate the speculum slightly to see as much of the drum and middle ear structures as possible.

Hearing tests. *Spoken and whispered voice:* Test each ear separately, occluding the other with your finger or the patient's. Test hearing using high-pitch (whisper—512-cycle-per-second [cps] tuning fork) and low-pitch (spoken voice) sounds. Note that the 512-cps fork is used in the ear examination, and the

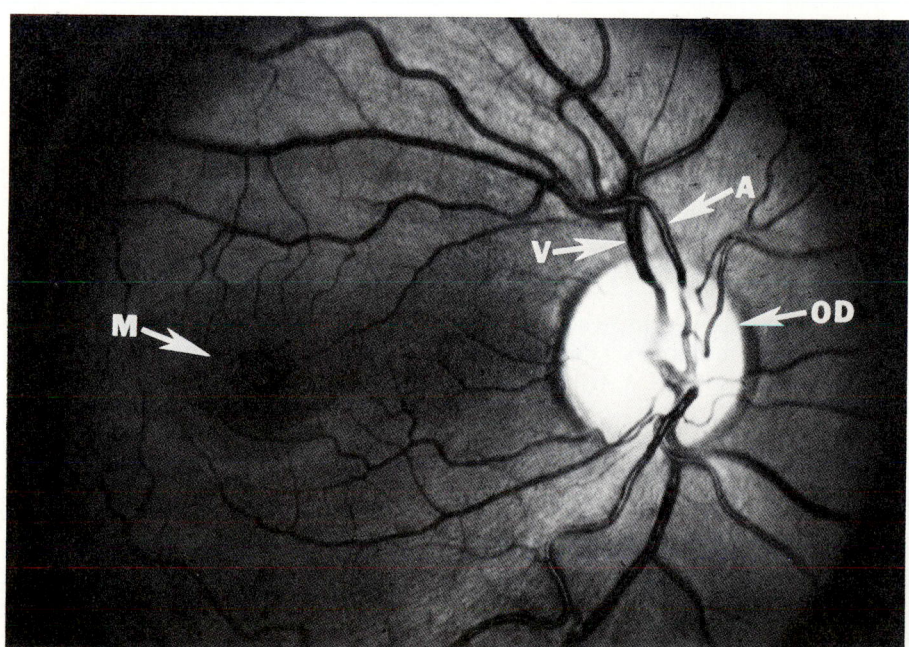

Fig. 2-1   Retina. Note optic disc, *OD*, artery, *A*, vein, *V*, and macula, *M*. Fovea centralis can be seen in center of macula. (Courtesy of W Tasman, MD.)

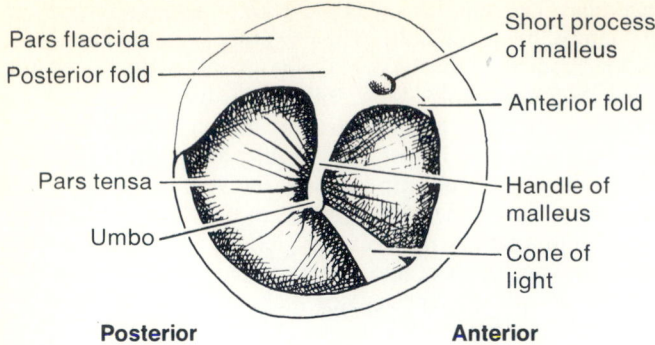

Fig. 2-2   Otoscopic view of tympanic membrane and middle ear structures.

125-cps fork is used to test vibration sense. *Weber's test:* Touch the handle of the vibrating tuning fork against the patient's forehead. The sound should be heard with equal intensity in both ears. *Rinne test:* Touch the handle of the vibrating tuning fork to the patient's mastoid process. When the patient no longer can hear this sound, hold the vibrating end near the ear. This air-conducted sound should still be audible, although the bone-conducted sound is not.

NOSE. Check deformities and patency of nostrils. Note mucosal color or swelling, septal deviation or perforation, and turbinate swelling or polyps. Compress each nostril, and have the patient breathe through the other. The internal structures of the nose are best examined with a nasal speculum, but an otoscope with a short, wide nasal attachment can be used.

MOUTH

Lips. Check color and lesions.

Teeth. Examine for missing or loose teeth, caries, and fillings, and check shape and tenderness.

Gums. Note any retraction, discoloration, bleeding, swelling, or inflammation.

Buccal mucosa. Assess color, lesions, and duct openings.

Tongue (dorsum and undersurface). Check color, size, papilla, coating, tremors, lesions, and masses.

Palate. Note color, masses, and petechiae.

Tonsils. Examine pillars, size, and exudate.

Pharynx. Check color, exudate, masses, and gag reflex.

Procedure. Dentures should be removed to allow complete examination of the mouth. Examine the undersurface of the tongue with special care. Have the patient raise his tongue against the roof of his mouth while you inspect anteriorly. Then, with his tongue behind his lower teeth, insert a tongue blade between the lower teeth and push the tongue medially, inspecting this gutter area as far back as the tonsillar pillar.

NECK. Check position, symmetry, and masses.

Muscles. Examine for hypertrophy, atrophy, and tenderness.

Nodes. Assess size, mobility, and tenderness (Fig. 2-3). Stand facing the seated patient with your fingertips on the upper sternomastoid muscle bilaterally. Palpate over and behind the muscle from above downward. Repeat this sequence from above downward further and further posteriorly to the sternomastoid muscle. Pay special attention to areas where node groups are known to occur (Fig. 2-3). Next examine the areas posterior to and then anterior to the ears. Step to the right side of the patient and palpate upward with your right thumb along the anterior portion of the right sternomastoid and with your second and third fingers along the anterior portion of the left sternomastoid. Examine along the base of the mandible in the same manner.

Trachea. Check position.

Thyroid gland. Note size, shape, symmetry, nodules, tenderness, and bruits (Fig. 2-4). With the thumb and index finger, begin at the base of the thyroid cartilage and palpate downward until the thyroid isthmus is detected. Ask the patient to swallow, and feel the thyroid rise against your fingers. Move your thumb laterally along the upper portion of the right lobe of the thyroid, and move your second and third fingertips laterally along the upper portion of the left lobe of the thyroid. Again, have the patient swallow, and feel the gland rise against your fingers. Then face the patient with your index and middle fingers behind the sternomastoid muscle and your thumb anterior to it. With the thumb of your opposite hand, push the thyroid cartilage toward the side being examined as the patient swallows.

Jugular venous distention. Observe the external jugular vessels as the patient's position is changed from the sitting to the supine position. Stop at the point where the venous column is visible a few centimeters above the clavicle. The internal jugular pulse is even more reliable but is clinically more difficult to evaluate. The central venous pressure is the distance from the top of the venous column to the right atrium, which is estimated to be 6 cm below the sternal angle.

BREASTS. Assess size, symmetry, venous pattern, tenderness, and masses. With the patient sitting, observe the breasts for retraction or asymmetry, both at rest and while she performs specific maneuvers. Have the patient raise her arms above her head, push her hands firmly against her hips, and lean forward. Then have the patient assume the supine position, with the hand on the side of the breast to be examined behind the head. Examine each quadrant by pressing the breast against the chest wall with the tips of the fingers. It may be necessary to place one hand on the lateral side of the breast for stabilization. Then repeat the examination, this time squeezing the breast between your thumb and index finger. Use your other hand to support the remainder of the breast during this procedure.

Nipple and areola. Check color, lesions, retraction, discharge, and fissures. Squeeze the nipples, and observe for discharge.

AXILLAE. Note any lesions, lumps, or nodes. Examine the patient's right axilla with your right hand, controlling the patient's arm position with your left hand on the patient's right wrist. Push your hand deep into the axilla, and then let the patient's arm drop lightly over your hand. Use your fingertips to compress the axillary contents against the ribs.

THORAX. Assess chest size and shape, rib deformities, and any tenderness.

LUNGS

Inspection. Check respiratory rate and rhythm, retraction of interspaces with inspiration, accessory muscles of respiration, and respiratory excursions.

Palpation. Examine for tactile fremitus. The patient should be in the sitting position. Since vibration is being measured, use the metacarpophalangeal area of the palm. Ask the patient to repeat the words "ninety-nine." Using only one hand, begin at the top and compare symmetric areas of the chest as you descend.

Percussion. Check lung resonance, lower borders, and diaphragmatic movement. Percuss symmetric areas of the chest, and compare the sounds.

Auscultation. *Breath sounds*—note intensity and inspiratory to expiratory ratio. *Adventitious sounds*—note location, timing, pitch, and persistence after coughing. *Voice sounds*—note loudness, distinctness, and symmetry. Listen to the breath sounds as the patient breathes deeply through his mouth. The

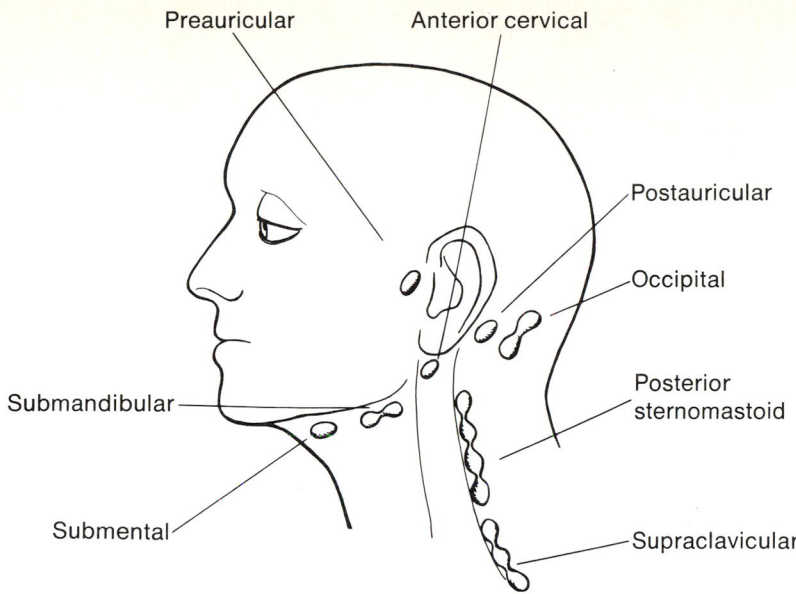

Fig. 2-3 Superficial lymph nodes of neck. (Redrawn from DeGowin EL and DeGowin RL: Bedside diagnostic examination, ed 2, New York, 1969, Macmillan, Inc.)

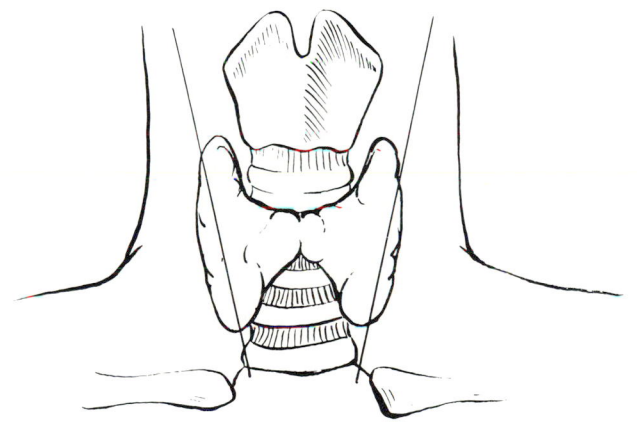

Fig. 2-4 Thyroid gland.

inspiratory phase normally is longer than the expiratory phase, except in the area over the manubrium and in the upper interscapular region, where the two phases may be about equal. Again, ask the patient to repeat the words "ninety-nine," comparing this time the sounds heard through the stethoscope. Test with both spoken and whispered voice. The sounds should be equal bilaterally and very indistinct. Some abnormalities, such as consolidation, may make these sounds more distinct, while others, such as pleural effusion, make the sounds more distant.

HEART

Inspection. Check apical impulse and other impulses. With the patient in the supine position, look for the apical impulse. This is visibly present in about one fifth of the normal population and usually is located about 1 cm medial to the midclavicular line on the left side on the fifth intercostal space. Then inspect the remainder of the chest wall for other impulses. Impulses medial to the apical impulse in the third to fifth intercostal spaces are from the right ventricle. Note whether the impulse is visible only in the interspaces or if the lower sternum also moves.

Palpation. Note apical impulse, abnormal impulses, pal-

pable heart sounds, rubs, and thrills. Use the metacarpophalangeal area of the palms to palpate over the heart, since findings through vibration more than through touch are being sought. Palpate over visible impulses first. The normal location of the apical impulse, described earlier, often is palpable despite not being visible in most people. Then palpate over the remainder of the precordium. The presence of the right ventricular impulse (location already described) is abnormal, as are pulsations over the base of the heart. Note the difference between pulsations and vibrations. Vibrations representing palpable murmurs are called thrills. Note their timing by comparing them to the apical impulse or carotid pulse.

Auscultation. Check rate, rhythm, heart sounds, gallops, and murmurs. Auscultation of the heart also is usually performed with the patient in the supine position; changing to other positions brings out specific abnormalities, such as sitting and leaning forward to check for aortic disorders and assuming the left lateral decubitus position for mitral disorders. Listen first over the apex for rate and rhythm. Then sequentially auscultate over the entire precordium for normal heart sounds, then extra heart sounds, and finally murmurs. Move the stethoscope in short steps, beginning in the aortic area (right second intercostal space), moving toward the pulmonic area (left second intercostal space), Erb's point (third intercostal space at left sternal border), mitral area (left fifth intercostal space in midclavicular line), and finally toward the axilla. Repeat this procedure as necessary, evaluating each sound or murmur individually. The apical impulse or the carotid pulse can be used to identify which of the sounds is the first heart sound. Note especially the splitting of the second sound with inspiration in the second left intercostal space. Clearly identify the heart sounds before pursuing other sounds. Distinguish between extra heart sounds (S_3, S_4, click) and murmurs or rubs. Note the timing, location, and pitch of extra sounds. Evaluate murmurs for timing, location, pattern (decrescendo, crescendo, diamond shaped), pitch, quality (blowing, rumbling), radiation, and effect of position change (standing, squatting), and Valsalva maneuver. Intensity is graded on a scale of 1 to 6. The subjectivity of this scale can be minimized by following these guidelines:

Grade 1—very faint and heard only when paying close attention

Grade 2—faint, but unmistakably present

Grade 3—clearly louder than "faint" but not associated with a thrill

Grade 4—loud and associated with a thrill

Grade 5—very loud but requiring the stethoscope partly on the chest

Grade 6—able to be heard with the stethoscope off the chest

ABDOMEN

Inspection. Check contour, pulsations, venous dilation, peristalsis, scars, and masses. With the patient in the supine position, inspect the abdomen from the side, your head at a level only slightly above that of the abdominal surface.

Auscultation. Assess bowel sounds, bruits, and friction rubs. Note that in the abdominal examination, auscultation should precede palpation and percussion.

Palpation. Examine for muscle spasm, tenderness, normal organs, organomegaly, masses, and aorta. Using the fingertips of the right hand, press lightly over all regions of the abdomen. This will help relax the anxious patient and localize tender areas. Then repeat the examination using deeper palpation. Examine from lower to upper abdomen to avoid missing the liver or spleen edge. Examine the left side first unless it has a history of pain or is tender on light palpation. The quadrant where symptoms are located should be examined last, because if palpation there causes pain, it will be difficult for the patient to relax for palpation of the other abdominal areas. If tenderness is elicited, check for rebound tenderness by pushing in slowly and then quickly letting go.

Since the spleen should not be palpated on routine deep palpation, pull up on the patient's left lower thorax with the left hand while pushing the right hand under his lower ribs on the left as the patient inspires deeply. If the spleen is not palpated, feel for the spleen on deep inspiration, with the patient in the right lateral decubitus position with his left knee bent and his right leg straight. Examine the middle upper abdomen for the aortic pulse. Assess the aortic diameter by simultaneously feeling the aorta's left border with the left hand and its right border with the right hand. Put the left hand under the patient at the level of the lower right ribs, and pull lightly while the right hand is pressed under the lower right ribs just lateral to the rectus muscles. As the patient inspires deeply, the liver will descend toward the examining hand. Masses should be evaluated for location, size, shape, consistency, mobility, pulsations, and tenderness.

Percussion. Estimate liver size. Note that liver palpation does not provide any information regarding the location of the upper border of the liver; therefore percussion is essential to estimate liver size. Percuss the right chest in the midclavicular line from the upper part downward. Identify the site of liver dullness in expiration, and mark the chest. Then percuss upward from the right lower quadrant, also in the midclavicular line, making sure to start in an area of unequivocal tympany. Identify the lower border of liver dullness in expiration. The liver normally measures 6 to 12 cm along the midclavicular line.

MALE GENITALIA

Gloves should be worn for the genital exam.

Penis. Examine circumcision status, lesions, urethral orifice, and any discharge. Be sure to retract foreskin if the patient is uncircumcised. Squeeze the tip of the penis to try to express discharge.

Scrotum. Check skin lesions, testicular size, tenderness or lumps, nontesticular masses, and hernia. Lift the scrotal sac away from the thighs so that the entire surface can be visu-

alized. Then palpate each testicle. The normal adult testicle measures about 5 cm in diameter. If masses are detected, touch your penlight to the posterior surface of the scrotum and observe for transillumination. Follow the course of the spermatic cord superiorly, checking for masses along its path. Have the patient stand, and instruct him to bear down. Observe the inguinal area for any bulges. Push the index finger of the right hand through the scrotal skin posterior to the testicle into the right inguinal ring area. Have the patient bear down, and note any masses descending to touch the finger. Examine the left side with the left hand.

RECTAL AREA. Check for hemorrhoids, lesions, sphincter tone, anal and rectal wall masses, tenderness, and induration. Also examine prostate size, consistency, or lumps; stool color; and occult blood.

In the male patient the rectal examination usually is performed with the patient in the left lateral decubitus position with his hips flexed. The examination also can be performed with the patient standing and resting his chest on the examining table. The disadvantage of these positions is that abdominal masses tend to fall away from the examining finger; these positions should not be used if there is any reason to suspect an abdominal mass. The supine position is best for detecting abdominal masses. With the patient in the left lateral decubitus position, use the left hand to push up on the right buttock to allow visualization of the anal area. Lubricate the palmar surface of the right index fingertip, and make initial penetration with this portion of the finger. Then flex the finger slightly so that the palmar surface is facing posteriorly. Insert the finger fully, and examine 90 degrees in each direction. Rotate position so that the flexor surface of the finger faces anteriorly. Identify the median furrow of the prostate gland, which separates the lateral lobes. Palpate the entire surface of the gland.

In the female patient the rectal examination usually is performed in the supine position as part of the pelvic examination, which is not discussed here.

PULSES. Check for the presence of carotid, radial, femoral, dorsalis pedis, and posterior tibial pulses. Examine their equality, contour, and rhythm, and check for volume changes and bruits. Grading the strength of pulses is necessarily arbitrary. This is most simply done by designating them normal, diminished, or absent. Examine the carotid pulse in the lower half of the neck so as not to stimulate the carotid sinus.

EXTREMITIES. Check venous pattern, lesions, hair distribution, nails, redness, cyanosis, edema, temperature, and nodes. Check the patient's lower extremities for edema by pressing the thumb firmly over the dorsum of the foot and over the tibia at midankle. If edema is found, check at higher levels as well. If the patient has been supine, check also over the sacrum. Estimate the depth of pitting in millimeters.

SPINE. Examine for kyphosis, scoliosis, and lordosis; check range of motion, spinal process tenderness, and local muscle spasm. Test cervical range of motion by observing the patient's ability to extend his neck and to touch ear to shoulder, chin to shoulder, and chin to chest. Evaluate the thoracic spine with trunk rotation and lateral bending. Have the patient attempt to touch his toes to assess lumbar spine motion.

PERIPHERAL JOINTS. Check for redness, swelling, active range of motion, deformity, local muscle atrophy, tenderness, passive range of motion, warmth, and crepitation. Examine each joint individually.

NEUROLOGY

Cranial nerves. Note that the evaluation of the cranial nerves involves many maneuvers already described. Evaluate these nerves by assessing the following functions related to the separate nerves:

I—smell
II—visual acuity, color vision, visual fields
III, IV, VI—extraocular movements, pupil reactions
V—motor; masseter muscle strength, lip tremor (Have the patient bite down while you palpate the masseter muscle for strength and symmetry.)
V—sensory; sensation over face; corneal reflex (Touching the cornea with a piece of gauze should cause blinking.)
VII—motor; asymmetry, tics (Have the patient perform several facial movements, such as exposing the teeth, puffing the cheeks, closing the eyes tightly, and raising the eyebrows, and check for asymmetry.)
VII—sensory; taste
VIII—cochlear; hearing
VIII—vestibular; nystagmus
IX, X—uvula movement, gag reflex
XI—trapezius and sternocleidomastoid strength (Have the patient force his head from the side toward the midline against the resistance of your hand. Note the force generated, and use your other hand to feel the tension in the sternocleidomastoid muscle.)
XII—tongue movement, tremor, atrophy

Motor nerves. Check for atrophy, symmetry, and abnormal movements. Assess strength of proximal and distal muscle groups of upper and lower extremities. Strength is measured using an arbitrary scale of 0 to 5:

0—no motion or muscle contraction
1—slight muscle contraction but no joint motion
2—motion without gravity
3—motion against gravity
4—motion against some resistance
5—motion against significant resistance (normal)

Screen for proximal muscle weakness by having the patient hold his arm straight out laterally from the shoulder while you attempt to push his arm down. With the patient lying down, have him flex and then extend his hip against the resistance of your hand. Screen distal muscle strength by having the patient squeeze your hands. Have him flex and then extend his feet against the resistance of your hand.

Sensory nerves. Assess superficial pain, touch, proprioception, vibration, and stereognosis. *Superficial pain*—test ability to distinguish the sharp from the dull end of a safety pin in symmetrical areas. *Touch*—check ability to detect cotton stimulation. *Proprioception*—holding a finger or toe by its sides (to avoid stimulating pressure sensation), see if the patient can differentiate the flexed from the extended position. *Vibration*—using a 125-cps fork, compare symmetry and sensation (by comparison with yourself) of vibratory sense over superficial bones. *Stereognosis*—place common small objects in the patient's hand (coin, keys, pen), and have him identify them by touch alone.

Deep tendon reflexes. Routine testing should include biceps, triceps, knee, and ankle reflexes. Reflexes can be arbitrarily graded as:

0—no response
1—decreased
2—normal
3—increased
4—clonus

Superficial reflexes. Check abdominal and cremasteric (male) reflexes. *Abdominal reflex*—with the patient in the supine position, stroke his abdomen with a moderately sharp object, such as a key or a reflex hammer handle, from the lateral side toward the midline. There should normally be abdominal muscle contraction on the side of the stimulation, with movement of the umbilicus toward the stimulus. Test both sides, above and below the umbilicus. This reflex may be difficult to elicit in obese patients.

Pathologic reflexes. Test Babinski's sign also with the patient in the supine position and using a moderately sharp stimulus. Lightly stroke the lateral aspect of the sole of the foot vertically from heel to the base of the toes. As you approach the toes, change the course of the stimulation to a medially directed path along the base of the toes toward the great toe. The normal response is plantar flexion of the toes. Be careful not to confuse an abnormal response (dorsiflexion of the great toe, fanning of the other toes, dorsiflexion of the ankle, flexing of the knee and thigh) with a simple withdrawal response.

Brainstem reflexes. Test with the cranial nerves.

Coordination. Observe the patient's gait and his ability to perform rapid alternating movements.

MENTAL STATUS. Assess by noting the following:
Appearance—dress, grooming
Motor behavior—facial expression, posture, poise
Verbal behavior—voice (pitch, intensity), relevance, vocabulary
Mood—emotion, tones
Thought processes—delusions, hallucinations
Cognitive functions—orientation (person, place, time), memory (immediate, distant), general knowledge (name of presidents, large cities), abstraction (proverb interpretation, similarities), calculations (serial sevens), judgment (test questions)

BIBLIOGRAPHY FOR SECTION ONE

Bates B: A guide to physical examination, ed 4, Philadelphia, 1987, JB Lippincott Co.
DeGowin EL and DeGowin RL: Bedside diagnostic examination, ed 2, New York, 1969, Macmillan Publishing Co.
Delp MH and Manning RT: Physical diagnosis, ed 8, Philadelphia, 1975, WB Saunders Co.
Little JW and King OR: The significance of physical diagnosis, patient history, data, and medical screening in the dental office, Ann Dent 3:31, Fall 1972.

SECTION TWO

IMMUNOLOGIC AND ALLERGIC DISEASES

Edited by **Donna M. Murasko and Donald Kaye**

3 · IMMUNOLOGIC PRINCIPLES

Donald Kaye *and* **Donna M. Murasko**

Immunologic reactions are the result of cells of the immune system recognizing and responding to foreign stimuli called antigens. This system is characterized by two features, specificity and memory. Specificity means that the immune cells initiating the reaction recognize and generate a response against the antigen in question but against none other. Memory is demonstrated by the fact that on second and subsequent exposure to the same antigen, the immune response is generated both more quickly and more vigorously.

The immune system has two major divisions: humoral and cellular. The humoral arm is characterized by the immune reactions mediated by antibodies, whereas reactions of the cellular arm are mediated by lymphocytes and macrophages. The classic example of cell-mediated immunity is skin test reactivity to antigens such as tuberculoprotein. In either humoral or cellular immunity, the clinical manifestation can be positive (humoral: protection from bacterial infections; cellular: recovery from viral infections) or negative (humoral: hay fever; cellular: poison ivy). Although one arm of the immune response is usually the major mediator of the clinical outcome, it is rare for either arm to be induced independently.

The elements of the immune system include the lymphocytic, the phagocytic, and the complement systems. This chapter describes these systems, along with various immunoglobulins and immunologic reactions.

LYMPHOCYTIC SYSTEM

Lymphocytes are derived from the pluripotent bone marrow stem cell and develop into two major cell types. One type originates in the bone marrow but leaves the marrow for the thymus, where it completes its development. After maturing in the thymus under the influence of the thymic environment and thymic hormones such as thymopoietin and thymosin, the thymus-derived lymphocyte, or *T-cell,* disseminates throughout the body. The other major type of lymphocyte also originates in the marrow; it matures in the marrow and perhaps in other sites and is called a *B cell.*

T lymphocytes mediate cellular immunity, which is important in defense against mycobacteria, viruses, and fungi and is responsible for tumor immunity and graft rejection. For T-cell activation to occur, antigen-presenting cells (APCs) (for example, macrophages) must first interact with the antigen. These APCs serve a dual role in T-cell responses: (1) they present antigen to T lymphocytes possessing receptors specific

Table 3-1 Some of the lymphokines produced by activated T lymphocytes

Lymphokines	Function
Interleukin 2 (IL 2)	Induces the proliferation of activated T cells
Interferon gamma (IFN g)	Increases class II MHC antigen expression; activates macrophages; limits viral infections
Migration inhibitory factor	Inhibits movement of macrophages from the site of the reaction
B-cell stimulating factor-1 (BSF-1; IL 4)	Stimulates proliferation of antigen activated B cells
B-cell differentiation factor (BCDF)	Stimulates differentiation of B cells
Chemotactic factors	Attracts macrophages, non-antigen specific lymphocytes, and other inflammatory cells to the area
Colony stimulating factors	Stimulates growth of immature lymphocytes, monocytes, and granulocytes

for the antigen, and (2) they produce a substance called interleukin 1 (IL 1), which results in activation of the T cells. Both antigen and IL 1 are needed for initiation of T-cell-mediated responses. T-cell activation is characterized by macromolecular synthesis (DNA, RNA, and protein synthesis). Activated T cells produce substances called lymphokines, which are responsible for continued proliferation of the T cells (that is, interleukin 2 [IL 2]) and for amplification of the response that has been initiated. Some of the lymphokines involved in amplification of the immune response are listed below (Table 3-1). During this activation process, T cells also differentiate into cells that have distinct functions: (1) cytotoxic T cells (TK) that can recognize cell-associated antigens (such as a tumor), antigens expressed by malignant cells, or a cell expressing viral antigens and that can destroy the target cell; (2) helper-T cells (TH) that can release lymphokines that together with antigen can affect B lymphocytes and other T lymphocytes and cause them to proliferate and differentiate; (3) T cells that mediate delayed type hypersensitivity reactions (TD) by releasing factors that kill target cells or that activate other effectors (for example, macrophages); (4) suppressor T cells (TS) that down-regulate the immune response and can decrease the response of both T and B lymphocytes. These T-cell subpopulations are defined not only by their different functions but also by reagents called monoclonal antibodies that can be used to identify each of them (Table 3-2).

For an antigen to stimulate T-cell-mediated responses, it must be presented to the T cell as a complex with (or at least

13

Table 3-2   Identification of lymphocytes with monoclonal antibodies

Monoclonal antibody*	Reacts with
OKT6, Leu 1	Thymocytes
OKT3, Leu 4	All mature circulating T cells
OKT11, Leu 5	All mature circulating and resident T cells (SRBC receptor)
OKT4, Leu 3a	Helper-inducer T cells
OKT8, Leu 2a	Suppressor-cytotoxic T cells
Leu 2a and Leu15	Suppressor T cells
Leu 2a, but not Leu 15	Cytotoxic T cells
Leu 15	Suppressor T cells and natural killer (NK) cells (also monocytes and granulocytes)
Leu 11	NK and lymphokine-activated killer (LAK) cells (also granulocytes)
OKB5, CR2	Mature B cells
Leu 12	Immature B cells

*Names are designations of manufacturers

in close proximity to) surface molecules on APCs that are encoded by genes in the major histocompatibility complex (MHC). The MHC is a group of closely linked genetic loci that are usually inherited as one unit. In humans this complex is found on chromosome 6. Some of the proteins coded for by this complex are referred to as HLA antigens; the antigens coded by the A, B, and C loci are called the class I antigens. These antigens are found on most cells of the body, the primary exception being the cells of the nervous system. TK cells recognize antigens in the context of class I MHC antigens. The D loci, of which there are at least four, code for the proteins called the class II antigens. These antigens have a more limited distribution in the body, being found on B lymphocytes, macrophages, epidermal cells, and sperm. TH and TD cells require the recognition of class II antigens in addition to the foreign antigen in order to initiate an immune response.

B cells are responsible for humoral immunity mediated by antibodies produced by these cells. For B cells to react to an antigen, the antigen usually must be "processed" by APCs that interact with TH cells. When lymphokines released by the TH cells (for example, B-cell stimulating factor 1 [IL 4] and B-cell differentiation factor [BCDF]) and antigen interact with mature B cells that have specific surface receptors for the antigen, the B cells are stimulated to differentiate and multiply to yield an expanded clone of specific B cells, some of which further differentiate into plasma cells that produce large amounts of antibody specific for the immunogen. The responses to different antigens vary in their degree of requirement for helper-T-cell activity. Thus some antigens are referred to as thymic (T-cell) dependent and others as thymic independent. These should be understood to be relative rather than absolute distinctions. Antibodies may act in a variety of ways. They may neutralize an antigen, such as a virus; they may coat the antigen to promote phagocytosis (opsonization); or they may bind complement, markedly augmenting phagocytosis. Binding of complement may also lyse cells expressing the antigen. Furthermore, the interaction with complement generates a cascade phenomenon that produces pharmacologically active fragments of complement that dilate blood vessels, increase vascular permeability, and attract polymorphonuclear leukocytes.

In this way an acute inflammatory reaction is produced, and the killing of bacteria proceeds efficiently.

B and T cells cannot be distinguished microscopically. However, B cells, which constitute 10% to 15% of the circulating lymphocyte population, have immunoglobulin on their surfaces and possess receptors for the Fc portion of immunoglobulin of the IgG class and for C3b, a fragment of one of the elements of the complement system. T cells, which form about 85% of the circulating lymphocyte population, have no demonstrable surface membrane immunoglobulin. Although the ability to form rosettes with sheep red blood cells was once a useful distinguishing tool, the availability of monoclonal antibodies reactive either with all T cells or with subpopulations of T cells have decreased the diagnostic value of this marker.

In addition to cell surface markers, B and T cells react differently during in vitro tests. Both cell populations have the ability to proliferate in vitro when exposed to antigens or to substances from plants and bacteria called mitogens. Although the antigens only induce the proliferation of the small number of cells that have specific receptors for that antigen, the mitogens stimulate proliferation in large populations of cells. Phytohemagglutinin (PHA) and concanavalin A (ConA) stimulate T lymphocytes, whereas pokeweed mitogen primarily stimulates B cells. The in vitro blastogenic responses to these stimulants and to specific antigens are useful in assessing the functional integrity of immune responses.

Lymphocytes that have no immunoglobulin on their surface and that do not react with anti-pan T-cell monoclonal antibodies (anti-OKT3) were formerly called *null cells*. Although this was once thought to be a single population of cells constituting about 5% of peripheral blood lymphocytes, it is now known to be a very heterogenous population. In this population are NK (natural killer) cells, K (killer) cells, and LAK (lymphokine-activated killer) cells. Currently these subpopulations of cells are identified only by functional activity. NK cells directly kill a limited panel of virus-infected or tumor cells. The basis of their selective reactivity is unknown. Their activity is present throughout life and is increased by interferon. LAK cells are similar to NK cells, except that they have a wider range of activity and are only demonstrable after activation by lymphokines. Neither NK nor LAK cells require recognition of MHC antigens for effector function. K cells mediate antibody-dependent cellular cytotoxicity (ADCC). These cells do not react independently with any target cell. However, once a specific antibody is attached to a target cell, the K cell can bind to the antibody via a receptor for the Fc fragment of the antibody and then lyse the target cell.

IMMUNOGLOBULINS

The immunoglobulins produced by plasma cells may be divided into five major classes: IgG, IgM, IgA, IgD, and IgE. IgG can be further divided into four subclasses: IgG1, IgG2, IgG3, and IgG4. There are two heavy (H) polypeptide chains and two light (L) polypeptide chains, which are held together by disulfide bonds. The H chain is about twice as long as the L chain. One end of the H and L chains (Fab) is highly variable in amino acid sequence and combines with antigen. The extreme variability in structure undoubtedly accounts for the ability to respond with specific immunoglobulin production to an enormous number of different antigens. The other end of the chains (Fc) is constant in structure and does not directly participate in antigen binding; rather it participates in attachment of the antigen-antibody complex to the cell membrane, complement activation, and transfer across the placenta. Light chains are of two types: κ and λ. The heavy chains are specific for the five immunoglobulin classes. The four-chain basic structure can be split enzymatically into one Fc and two Fab fragments. The Fab fragments contain the antigen-combining sites, and the Fc fragment is active in complement fixation and binding to cell membranes.

IgG (and probably IgD and IgE) appears as a four-chain molecule and is a 7S protein. IgM also has a basic four-chain structure and is polymerized into a macroglobulin of five such four-chain units, forming a 19S protein. IgA is either a four-chain 7S molecule or a polymer of larger size. Polymerized immunoglobulins are held together with J chains. IgG crosses the placenta, whereas IgM and IgA do not.

IgG constitutes about 75% of the serum immunoglobulins. It is the only immunoglobulin that crosses the placenta. It can fix complement, and the Fc fragment of IgG will bind to phagocytic cells. It is a major defense against invading organisms by virtue of its opsonizing and complement-fixing activities.

IgM accounts for about 10% of serum immunoglobulins. It is extremely efficient in fixing complement. IgM production predominates early in response to antigenic stimulation. Later, IgG production predominates. This difference in host response is often helpful in distinguishing recent from more distant infection. IgM is a major defense against invading microorganisms and is also an important cell surface antigen receptor on B lymphocytes. Anti-A or anti-B blood group antibody is IgM. It has been suggested that IgG antibody inhibits formation of IgM through mechanisms not yet clearly defined.

IgA constitutes about 15% of serum immunoglobulins. It is the predominant antibody in secretions, consisting of two four-chain units and attached to a protein called secretory component, which is produced by epithelial cells. It probably coats viruses and bacteria and prevents attachment to mucosal surfaces so that penetration cannot occur.

IgD is found in serum only in small amounts, representing 0.2% of immunoglobulins. This immunoglobulin is found on the surface of many immature B lymphocytes and may be important as an antigen receptor.

IgE, called reagin, is also found in serum in only trace amounts. It binds to tissue mast cells and basophils. When mast cell–bound IgE combines with an antigen, the mast cell releases histamine and other vasoactive substances. This mechanism is responsible for many allergic reactions. Both IgA and IgE are synthesized locally in tissues.

PHAGOCYTIC SYSTEM

The phagocytic system includes polymorphonuclear leukocytes and the monocyte-macrophage system. These cells mobilize to the site of injury or microbial invasion, then ingest and degrade or destroy antigen. Fixed macrophages in the liver, spleen, lung, and other sites (the reticuloendothelial system) are also part of the phagocytic system.

Macrophages are major components of the host defense system both for their nonspecific phagocytic ability and for their participation in specific immune responses. The substances they release are recognized as important mediators of cell interactions. IL 1 not only activates T cells that have encountered antigen but is also the substance formerly known as "endogenous pyrogen," inducing fever in the host. IL 1 can induce release of prostaglandins, alter glycolysis, and stimulate bone resorption. Tumor necrosis factor (TNF) is also produced by macrophages. Originally defined by its ability to

kill tumor cells, this substance can inhibit lipase activity (formerly known as cachectin) and can increase class I antigen expression on cells. Both IL 1 and TNF are induced by bacterial cell products (endotoxin) as well as by lymphokines (interferon).

COMPLEMENT SYSTEM

The complement system is composed of circulating blood proteins (C1 to C9) that react in a specific sequence, or cascade, when activated. Activation of the complement system can result in direct destruction of cells (bacteria, viruses, erythrocytes), attraction of white blood cells (chemotaxis), release of histamine (anaphylatoxin activity), and kinin activity, which causes increased vascular permeability and smooth muscle contraction.

There are two pathways by which the complement system can be activated: the *classic pathway* and the *alternative pathway*, or properdin pathway. The two pathways differ in the sequence leading to activation of C3; thereafter the sequence is the same (Fig. 3-1).

The classic pathway is activated by antigen-antibody (IgG1, IgG2, IgG3, or IgM) complexes, trypsinlike enzymes, and staphylococcal protein A. Activation of C1, composed of the three proteins C1q, C1r, and C1s, results in the formation of serine esterase, an enzyme that acts on C2 and C4 to form a complex proteolytic enzyme, $\overline{C1,4,2}$ (the bar indicates enzymatic activity), that adheres to the cell membrane. $\overline{C1,4,2}$ then cleaves C3 and C3a and C3b; the latter forms enzyme $\overline{C1,4,2,3b}$ on the membrane. C3b has an affinity for receptors on phagocytes.

The alternative pathway may be activated by IgA, possibly IgE, and occasionally IgG. It can also be activated by trypsinlike enzymes, polysaccharides, lipopolysaccharides (endotoxin, part of the cell wall of gram-negative bacilli), and cobra venom. In this pathway C3 is activated directly to C3b, some of which complexes with proteins (different from those in the classic pathway) and is fixed on the cell membrane. This complex then activates more C3 (amplification system).

The next step in both pathways is activation of C5. C5 is cleaved by $\overline{C1,4,2,3b}$ (the classic pathway) or the C3b complex (the alternative pathway), resulting in formation of C5a and C5b. C5b binds C6 and C7, forming $\overline{C5b,6,7}$. Thereafter C8 and C9 are bound, resulting in $\overline{C5b,6,7,8,9}$, which lyses the membrane.

Natural inhibitors of activation exist at many stages of the cascade, such as C1 esterase inhibitor and C3b inactivator. The well-known C1 esterase inhibitor is absent in patients with hereditary angioedema.

C3a and C5a are products of the reaction sequence and cause release of histamine from mast cells (anaphylatoxin activity). C3a has kinin activity; C5a causes release of enzymes from lysosomes; and C5a has chemotactic activity, attracting leukocytes, particularly polymorphonuclear ones. $\overline{C5b,6,7}$ also has chemotactic activity.

TYPES OF IMMUNOLOGIC REACTIONS

According to the Gell and Coombs classification, there are four types of immunologic tissue damage. This classification, although useful, is somewhat arbitrary. In most situations complex combinations of mechanisms are operative.

Type I reactions

Type I reactions, also called immediate anaphylactic hypersensitivity reactions, occur within minutes after exposure to an

THE COMPLEMENT SYSTEM

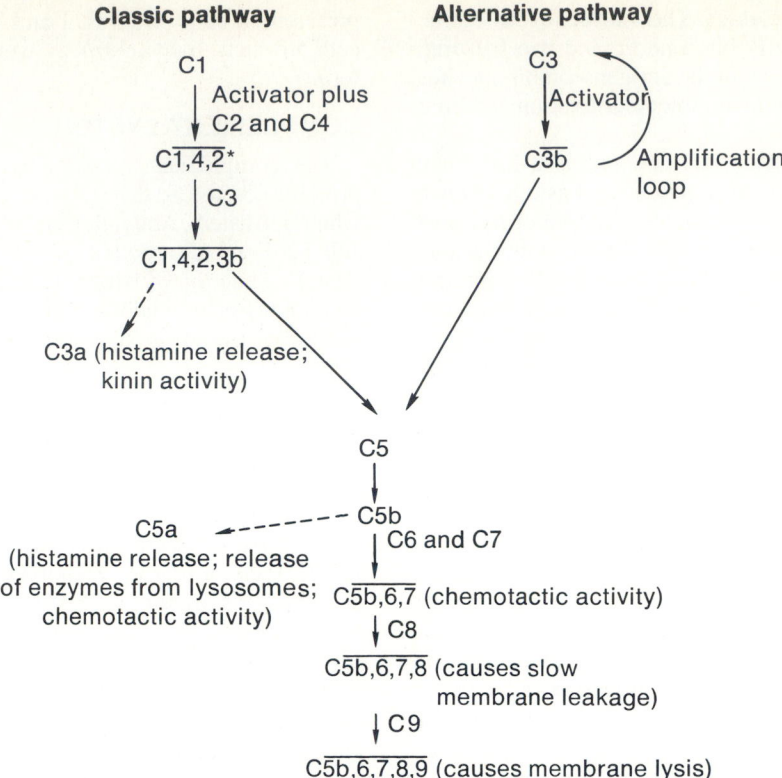

Fig. 3-1 Complement system can be activated by classic pathway or alternative pathway (see text). *Bar indicates activated substance with enzymatic activity.

allergen. Allergic rhinitis, hay fever, asthma, urticaria, and generalized anaphylaxis fall into this group. In this reaction antibodies (usually IgE) become fixed to basophils and tissue mast cells by the Fc fragment. When the antibodies combine with antigen, these cells release chemical mediators, which cause the clinical manifestations. The allergic reaction follows combination of the cell-associated or cytotropic IgE (reagin) with the specific allergen (for example, ragweed pollen). Some of the mediators released are histamine, serotonin, kinins, eosinophil chemotactic factor, slow-reacting substance of anaphylaxis (SRS-A), and platelet activating factor. These mediators act on the shock organs, producing the clinical manifestations. There is evidence that eosinophils, which are attracted to sites of IgE-mediated reactions by eosinophil chemotactic factor released from mast cells, serve to down-regulate the reaction. Thus eosinophils release histaminase that destroys histamine, arylsulfatase that destroys SRS-A, and phospholipase that destroys platelet activating factor.

Type II reactions

Type II reactions, or cytotoxic reactions, involve combination of IgG or IgM antibody with antigenic constituents on cell membranes, either as a part of the cell membrane or as an antigen fixed to the cell. Cytotoxicity may be mediated either via complement fixation (with destruction of the cell) or via phagocytosis (when leukocytes become bound to the Fc portion of the antibody). Examples of type II reactions are immune

hemolytic anemias, idiopathic thrombocytopenia, and acute kidney graft rejection.

Type III reactions

Type III reactions result from localization of antigen-antibody complexes in vessels or tissues, causing vasculitis or other tissue damage. Complement is fixed and phagocytes are attracted. There is release of vasoactive amines, an increase of vascular permeability, and release of lysosomal enzymes from leukocytes, all resulting in tissue damage. Examples of type III reactions include types of immune-complex reactions, such as the Arthus reaction (local swelling at the site of antigen injection occurring several hours later), serum sickness, autoimmune glomerulonephritis, and lupus nephritis. In these conditions antibody combines with an often unknown antigen intravascularly and the immune complex is deposited in blood vessels, provoking the inflammatory reaction and tissue injury.

Type IV reactions

Type IV reactions, or delayed type hypersensitivity reactions, occur when T cells and macrophages produce cellular injury. Neither antibody nor complement is involved. Type IV reactions include contact dermatitis and graft rejection. In such reactions, antigen present on the surface of cells expressing appropriate MHC antigens interacts with T cells possessing receptors specific for the antigen-MHC complex. After T-cell activation, lymphokines are produced by the T cells that induce proliferation of T cells (IL 2), attract macrophages to the area (chemotactic factors), and activate the macrophages as evidenced by increased phagocytosis, enhanced class II MHC antigen expression, and increased production of enzymes (interferon). The result is inflammation and tissue injury at the site of the antigen. The clinical reaction is "delayed" compared to antibody-mediated reactions; reactions slowly develop over 24 to 48 hours.

Sensitive patients may exhibit any combination of the four types of reactions. For example, immunologic reactions to penicillin can produce anaphylaxis (type I), hemolytic anemia (type II), a serum sickness–like illness (type III), and delayed hypersensitivity (type IV).

• • •

Other reactions that do not produce tissue damage occur when antibodies interact with hormones or other biologically active molecules or with receptors for these molecules and either activate or block a process. Examples include long-acting thyroid stimulator (LATS), which is an antibody to the thyrotropin receptor in thyroid disease; antibodies to intrinsic factor in pernicious anemia; anti–acetylcholine receptor antibody in myasthenia gravis; antiinsulin antibody or antibodies to the insulin receptor in some diabetics; antibodies to the β-adrenergic receptor in some patients with asthma; and blocking antibodies that inhibit the interaction of the antigen with antibodies of a different class (for example, IgG antibody blocking IgE interaction with an allergen).

AUTOIMMUNITY

Some people develop antibodies against autologous antigens. These antibodies may cause little or no observable injury or may result in disease. Some examples of autoantibodies are antiplatelet antibody in idiopathic thrombocytopenic purpura, anti–red cell antibody in acquired hemolytic anemia, anti–acetylcholine receptor antibody in myasthenia gravis, antithyroid antibody in Hashimoto's disease, anti-γ-globulin antibody (rheumatoid factor) in rheumatoid arthritis, and anti-DNA and antinuclear antibodies in systemic lupus erythematosus. Autoimmune diseases affect mainly young adults, with a preponderance of women. This is in contrast to the incidence of autoantibodies, which increases in the aged in the absence of apparent autoimmune disease. Thus the diagnostic significance of detecting auto-antibodies is very different in old and young subjects. It must be emphasized that the mere presence of autoantibodies does not mean that they are causing pathologic consequences such as autoimmune disease.

IMMUNE-COMPLEX DISEASE

Deposition of antibody-antigen complexes in blood vessels produces a type III reaction in the organ. This is the main mechanism of disease production in lupus nephritis and poststreptococcal glomerulonephritis. Many of the manifestations of infective endocarditis are thought to occur on an immune-complex basis, such as glomerulonephritis, petechiae, and arthritis. Patients who have persistent antigenemia with the surface antigen of hepatitis B virus may develop a polyarteritis-like syndrome related to circulating immune complexes.

GRAFT-VERSUS-HOST DISEASE

Graft-versus-host disease occurs when immunocompetent foreign lymphoid cells are transplanted into a genetically dis-similar immunoincompetent host. This syndrome may occur in persons who have received bone marrow grafts or in immunodeficient patients who have received transfusions of fresh blood. Skin lesions (ulceration, thickening, and loss of hair), edema, cardiac disease, hepatic lesions, joint lesions, and hemolytic anemia have all been described in relation to this disease.

BIBLIOGRAPHY

Bellanti JA: Immunology, III, Philadelphia, 1985, WB Saunders Co.
Fudenberg HH and others, editors: Basic and clinical immunology, ed 5, Los Altos, Calif, 1984, Lange Medical Publications.
Sell S: Basic immunology, New York, 1987, Elsevier.

4 · ATOPIC DISEASE
Gregory W. Siskind

The term "atopy" refers to a predisposition to develop IgE-mediated allergic reactions to environmental antigens (often referred to as allergens). This predisposition to allergies affects roughly 15% of the population and appears to have a genetic basis, although no simple inheritance pattern has been identified. The tendency to manufacture IgE in response to environmental allergens is most often manifested clinically as rhinitis (hay fever), asthma, or urticaria. The nature of the manifestation (that is, asthma or hay fever) also appears to be influenced by genetic factors, since familial clustering of symptom patterns has been described. IgE-mediated allergic reactions are clearly not the only cause of rhinitis, asthma, and urticaria; they are the sole etiologic factor in only a minority of cases. When IgE-mediated allergic reactions are involved, the mechanism for generating symptoms is the type I reaction described in Chapter 3. It must be remembered that other immunologic mechanisms can also cause urticaria and asthma.

Childhood (atopic) eczema is a characteristic feature of the atopic state. Nearly half the children with atopic eczema have asthma with or without other allergies as they grow older. Many atopic adults have a history of eczema in infancy and childhood. Children with atopic eczema have high serum IgE levels and often have multiple food allergies. In addition, several metabolic abnormalities have been demonstrated in these patients. Elimination of foods to which a patient appears to be allergic results in improvement of symptoms in childhood atopic eczema. However, the condition is usually not completely controlled by rigorous dietary regulation. As the child grows older, he is often able to tolerate foods to which he previously appeared to be allergic. The mechanism for this change in clinical sensitivity is unknown, but it may be related to changes in absorption or digestion of foods. The relationship between atopic eczema and the IgE-mediated manifestations of the atopic state is not fully understood, but the association is unequivocal. In the adult there is no convincing evidence that eczema is caused by an IgE-mediated mechanism.

The predisposition to produce IgE antibodies manifested by atopic persons appears to be related mainly to antigens presented repeatedly, usually in relatively low concentration, across a mucosal membrane (nasal, tracheobronchial, or gastrointestinal). It is not clear whether such patients have an increased tendency to produce IgE antibodies to parenterally administered allergens. Observations have suggested that atopic persons are no more likely to develop IgE antibodies to penicillin than are nonatopic persons.

RHINITIS

CLINICAL MANIFESTATIONS, CLASSIFICATION, AND PATHOGENESIS. Rhinitis is characterized by nasal congestion and rhinorrhea. The patients complain of stuffiness or running of the rose. Rhinitis may be associated with sneezing; itching of the nose and sometimes also of the eyes, throat, and ears; conjunctivitis that is usually mild; postnasal drip; and signs and symptoms of sinusitis. The physical findings include swollen nasal mucosa that may be pale, grayish, or inflamed and increased nasal secretions that vary from clear and watery to frankly purulent. Rhinitis can be classified as allergic, vasomotor, infectious, or medicamentosum.

Allergic rhinitis. In allergic rhinitis the pathogenetic mechanism is a type I, IgE-mediated, immunologic reaction to inhaled organic substances (see Chapter 3). The allergens commonly involved are animal danders (epithelial flakes), tree, grass, weed, or other pollens, and mold spores. The severity of the symptoms presumably depends on a large number of poorly understood factors including the concentration and affinity of the allergen-specific IgE, IgG, and IgA antibodies, the extent of transport of antibodies of different isotypes (classes) from serum to nasal secretions, the concentration and isotype of locally produced antibodies, the number of allergens to which the patient has IgE antibodies and to which the patient is simultaneously exposed, the structure of the nasal passages as it influences airflow patterns, the permeability of the nasal mucosa, the baseline rate of production and the consistency of the nasal secretions, and the physiologic state (responsiveness to stimuli) of the nasal vasculature and mucus-secreting cells. Other factors affecting the severity of symptoms include the concentration of allergens to which the patient is exposed, which is influenced by both the concentration of allergens in the environment and the patient's breathing pattern; the number of allergens to which the patient is exposed simultaneously; the frequency of exposure to an allergen; and simultaneous exposure to an allergen and any of numerous irritants such as perfume, smoke, or organic solvents. With frequent exposure, as occurs during a normal pollen season, the patient's sensitivity changes and the concentration of allergen required to elicit a given degree of symptoms decreases.

Vasomotor rhinitis. Vasomotor rhinitis occurs in a large group of patients whose symptoms appear to reflect hyperresponsiveness of their nasal mucosa to a wide variety of chemical and physical irritants. Sudden changes in temperature (as occur when going from the cold outdoors into a heated room) and numerous irritants such as dust, perfumes, smoke, strong odors, organic solvents, gas vapors, soap powders, and ammonia bring on nasal congestion, paroxysmal sneezing, and watery nasal discharge. The symptoms may be essentially continuous with exacerbation following exposure to irritants, or they may occur only after exposure to irritants. Vasomotor rhinitis appears to represent an unusually vigorous response of a normal host defense mechanism, aimed at removing a noxious agent or preventing it from entering the nasal passages. At a high enough concentration most substances that elicit vasomotor rhinitis cause the same symptoms in all persons. Patients who manifest vasomotor rhinitis appear to have a more vigorous response to these substances, which occurs at concentrations of the irritant that are too low to affect the average person. In some cases the release of mediators from mast cells by poorly understood nonallergic mechanisms appears to underlie the generation of symptoms.

Infectious rhinitis. In infectious rhinitis patients have hyperplastic sinusitis, purulent nasal secretions, infiltrates of neutrophils in their nasal mucosa, and a variety of organisms (most often staphylococci, streptococci, or pneumococci) detected in culture specimens of their nasal membranes and sinuses. It has been suggested that rhinitis in these patients is caused by a chronic bacterial infection of the nasal membranes, perhaps complicated by an allergic reaction to products of the infecting bacteria. There is, however, no adequate evidence to support this concept. Autogenous and stock bacterial vaccines have not been shown to be efficacious in treatment of these patients, and the role of infection in causing chronic rhinitis is still unclear.

Rhinitis medicamentosum. Rhinitis medicamentosum results from the irritant effects of nasal medications, usually nose drops. It is most often seen in patients who have had rhinitis of allergic, vasomotor, or infectious origin and have treated it with nose drops. The palliative effect of the nose drops is often followed by a rebound in which greater congestion occurs, the patient uses more nose drops, and a vicious circle of increasing symptoms and increasing use of nose drops is established.

DIAGNOSIS. The diagnosis of rhinitis is based primarily on a detailed history of the conditions associated with the symptoms. A seasonal history or symptoms occurring after exposure to a particular species of animal such as a cat or dog suggest an allergic basis. The seasonal distribution of symptoms provides clues as to the probable offending allergen (such as ragweed hay fever in the fall). The time of appearance of different pollens and the nature of the dominant allergenic pollens vary from place to place. Sneezing, conjunctival symptoms, and itching of the nose, throat, and eyes occur more commonly in allergic rhinitis. Patients with allergic rhinitis have a greater incidence of other allergic manifestations such as food allergies and childhood eczema. A family history of allergies is also useful in diagnosing allergic rhinitis. Perennial symptoms, without seasonal exacerbation, and an association of symptoms with exposure to the types of irritants previously noted suggest vasomotor rhinitis. However, certain allergens such as dog dander may be present throughout the year and can therefore induce perennial symptoms. Rhinitis medicamentosum is diagnosed on the basis of a history of nose drop abuse or habitual use of some other local medication or drug. Infectious rhinitis is suggested by the presence of an inflamed nasal mucosa and purulent nasal secretions.

LABORATORY FINDINGS. Laboratory tests are of limited value in confirming the diagnosis of rhinitis. Moderate eosinophilia and an abundance of eosinophils in the nasal secretions suggest an allergic basis. However, similar findings are often present in vasomotor rhinitis. An elevated serum IgE level suggests that the patient is atopic and makes an allergic basis for the rhinitis more likely but does not prove that the symptoms have an allergic origin. In many patients with rhinitis, multiple mechanisms are involved in the generation of symptoms. For example, a patient with perennial vasomotor rhinitis may have an exacerbation of symptoms in the spring or fall because of a superimposed allergic reaction to pollens.

If allergic rhinitis is suggested by the patient's history, the specific allergens involved can be identified by skin tests or by the radioallergosorbent test (RAST). Other types of tests are sometimes employed, including scratch, prick, and provocative intranasal challenge; since the overall significance of these procedures is similar to that of the more common intradermal skin test, they are not discussed here. Skin testing is most often performed by injecting approximately 0.02 ml of a low concentration of the suspected allergen intradermally, generally into the outer aspect of the upper arm. After 15 to 20 minutes the diameter of any wheal formed at the site of injection is measured. A wheal 5 mm or greater in diameter is generally regarded as a positive reaction. A positive skin test indicates the presence of IgE antibodies specific for antigens in the skin test preparation. It should be emphasized that positive results of a skin test can be seen in persons who have no symptoms after exposure to the allergen in question. Therefore, the presence of IgE antibodies does not in itself mean that symptoms will occur following exposure to the allergen under the usual conditions. This is why the diagnosis of a specific allergy is based on the patient's history rather than on skin test results. Skin tests should be regarded as merely confirmatory and not diagnostic. Their primary importance is in patients who are candidates for immunotherapy (hyposensitization) (see "Management"), and patients who are not being considered for immunotherapy should not be subjected to extensive skin testing. When the history does not provide a definitive diagnosis, especially in patients who seem to have combined vasomotor and allergic rhinitis, skin tests may be helpful diagnostically because multiple positive reactions make an allergic origin more likely.

The RAST, a radioimmunoassay for specific IgE antibodies, has recently become popular. The significance of a positive assay is essentially identical to that of a positive skin test; the RAST provides no more diagnostic information than does a skin test. The advantages of the RAST over the routine skin test are the following:

1. *Ease of performance.* The RAST requires no technical skill because it is performed by a commercial laboratory on a serum sample.
2. *Patient comfort.* Multiple intradermal injections are unnecessary, which is especially important with young children.
3. *Special patient problems.* The RAST is useful for patients with disseminated skin lesions who lack sites for intradermal testing and for patients whose skin fails to form a wheal in response to histamine. (These patients can be identified during skin testing because they have a negative reaction to a skin test with histamine; this occurs very rarely and many such patients have normal skin reactions to specific allergens.)
4. *Safety.* There is an extremely small possibility of an anaphylactic reaction in response to the intradermally injected allergen.

The advantages of the skin test over the RAST are the following:

1. *Sensitivity.* The skin test is more sensitive than the RAST, which more often yields false negative results.
2. *Specificity.* Available allergen preparations are generally crude extracts that vary quantitatively from lot to lot. A positive result of a skin test indicates that the patient has antibody to an allergen in the preparation used, whereas a positive RAST indicates that the patient has antibody to something in the laboratory's preparation but does not indicate if that allergen is actually present in significant amounts in the skin test preparation. This could have negative implications for immunotherapy if the skin test preparation is used.
3. *Cost.* If multiple tests are to be performed, skin testing is significantly less expensive.

It is probable that the best test is an inhalation challenge with an appropriate allergen preparation and observation for the appearance of symptoms, but to perform such challenges properly is difficult, time consuming, and expensive. They are therefore rarely used except for research purposes. Skin testing is preferred in all but a few cases.

Some comment should be made regarding tests for food allergies, even though such allergies are more germane to a discussion of urticaria (see Chapter 5). Skin tests for food allergies have proved unreliable; there is a high incidence of false positive reactions, and perhaps false negative reactions

also occur. The false positive reactions may be caused by the presence of nonspecific irritants in the crude extracts used for testing or to the presence of IgE antibodies in the patient that are not clinically significant. The false negative results probably occur when extracts used for testing do not contain the same allergens the patient absorbs after cooking and digesting food.

Cytotoxicity testing, which involves observing a change in the microscopic morphology of leukocytes following exposure to an allergen, has not proved to be a reproducible procedure.

MANAGEMENT

Allergic rhinitis. Eliminating or reducing the concentration of the offending allergen leads to marked improvement, but this approach is often not practical.

The primary treatment of allergic rhinitis is antihistamine medication. The main side effect of these medications is sedation. Although some generalizations can be made (for example, diphenhydramine [Benadryl] is highly sedative, whereas chlorpheniramine maleate [Chlor-Trimeton] causes little sedation), individual responses differ widely; a trial with a variety of antihistamines ultimately determines the best one for a given patient. Some patients are effectively treated with occasional use of antihistamines when their symptoms are severe; however, most patients seem to do best with continuous use of antihistamines throughout their "allergy season."

Corticosteroids are highly effective in eliminating symptoms of allergic rhinitis. The serious side effects of these medications, when administered systemically, make their use in this relatively benign disease undesirable. However, when symptoms are extremely severe and of short duration, such as 1 month, a brief course of systemic steroids can occasionally be justified. Administration of steroids locally by nasal spray (for example, Turbinaire Decadron) is also effective and reduces some of the complications of systemic steroids. Steroids are, however, absorbed across the nasal mucosa and can have systemic effects. Recently steroid preparations that are absorbed to a lesser extent or are degraded rapidly after absorption have become available for nasal administration.

Immunotherapy (also referred to as hyposensitization) is useful for patients whose symptoms are severe and cannot be controlled by antihistamines. The procedure involves weekly injections of allergen in increasing doses. After a high dosage is achieved, the interval between injections is extended gradually until treatment is given once a month. If improvement is to occur, it usually does so within 2 years. However, some patients do not improve for up to 4 to 5 years. Therapy is discontinued after improvement followed by 3 years of minimal or no symptoms or after 5 years with no improvement. Following successful immunotherapy, symptoms often do not recur or recur only mildly, and no further treatment is required. If symptoms return and are severe enough to warrant therapy, immunotherapy can be reinstituted. Double-blind studies have documented the efficacy of immunotherapy in the treatment of allergies to pollens. The degree of improvement varies, and rarely are symptoms totally eliminated. There is currently no way of predicting which patients will benefit. Immunotherapy is ineffective in the treatment of food allergies. Allergies to the dander (epithelial flakes) of household pets are a common problem. Immunotherapy for this condition has not generally proved effective in improving symptoms, probably because the concentration of allergen in the home environment is so high.

The mechanism of hyposensitization has been extensively studied but is still incompletely understood. At least two factors appear to be involved: (1) the stimulation of specific suppressor T cells that depress the IgE response to the offending allergen, and (2) the stimulation of production of IgG antibodies specific for the offending allergen. These so-called blocking antibodies appear to act by two mechanisms: (1) they compete with IgE antibodies on mast cells for available antigen, thereby preventing the elicitation of symptoms, and (2) they bind antigen, thus blocking it from stimulating further IgE antibody production and preventing the usual seasonal boost in specific IgE antibodies.

Eliminating the allergen from the environment or reducing its concentration is generally the most effective method of alleviating symptoms. Often, however, this is not a practical approach. Drug therapy with antihistamines and steroids is next in order of effectiveness. Immunotherapy is, in general, the least effective of the routinely employed approaches to the treatment of allergic rhinitis.

Vasomotor rhinitis. The treatment of vasomotor rhinitis generally relies on antihistamines and avoidance, if possible, of the inciting irritants. In view of the chronicity of the symptoms, systemic steroids should usually not be administered, although the use of local steroids may at times be justified. Similarly, the use of nose drops should usually be avoided since, although they provide temporary relief, their habitual use tends to be locally irritating, thereby exacerbating the problem.

Infectious rhinitis. The approach to infectious rhinitis is similar to that used for allergic rhinitis, but antibiotic therapy is often administered in addition. The effectiveness of the antibiotics has been difficult to evaluate.

Rhinitis medicamentosum. Rhinitis medicamentosum is treated by terminating the regular use of nose drops. A short course (7 to 10 days) of local steroid treatment is useful to control symptoms while nose drops are being discontinued.

ASTHMA OF ALLERGIC ETIOLOGY

Asthma is a common disorder, affecting nearly 5% of the population. The term "asthma" refers to a group of diseases characterized by wheezing, coughing, and dyspnea. The cause is narrowing of the air passages as a consequence of bronchoconstriction, mucosal edema, increased thick bronchial secretions, or some combination of these factors. A number of different etiologic factors and pathogenic mechanisms can lead to airway narrowing with signs and symptoms of asthma.

CLINICAL MANIFESTATIONS, CLASSIFICATION, AND PATHOGENESIS. The major symptom of asthma is wheezing. In addition, the patient may complain of a heaviness in the chest, shortness of breath, especially on exertion, cough with or without sputum production, and a sense of anxiety or air hunger. A conventional but not completely satisfactory classification of asthma divides it into intrinsic and extrinsic forms. Extrinsic asthma is considered to be IgE mediated and caused purely by allergic reactions to substances in the environment. Intrinsic asthma includes asthma caused by all other (nonallergic) mechanisms and is discussed in Chapter 130. The majority of patients with asthma appear to have multiple etiologic factors combining to cause symptoms. Factors that may be involved include allergies, infection (bronchitis), hyperresponsiveness of bronchi to nonspecific irritants or to cold, increased vagal tone, relative β-adrenergic blockade, alterations in the cyclic AMP system, and psychologic factors. Allergic factors appear to predominate in a relatively small proportion of asthma patients, although they may contribute to the disease process in a somewhat larger group. Immunologic mechanisms also play major causative roles in occupational asthma, hypersensitivity pneumonitis, and bronchopulmonary aspergillosis. These conditions are discussed in Chapters 130 and 132.

The pathogenesis of allergic asthma is a type I mechanism similar to that of allergic rhinitis except that the site of reaction is the bronchi and bronchioles.

Some patients exhibit symptoms only during exercise or have symptoms exacerbated by exercise. This exercise-induced asthma most commonly occurs in children and young adults. It may be present as an isolated finding or may complicate asthma caused by other factors. This symptom reflects a hyperreactivity of the bronchi to cooling. With exercise, an increase in airflow causes an increased evaporation of water from the mucosa of the tracheobronchial tree leading to cooling and reflex bronchoconstriction. It is important to note that not all forms of exercise (at equivalent levels of work performed) have the same tendency to induce asthma in susceptible individuals. Swimming is far better tolerated than are other forms of exercise because the ambient air during swimming is saturated with water vapor; evaporation from mucous membranes is reduced and cooling does not occur.

Psychologic factors appear to contribute to the generation of symptoms in many asthmatic patients. However, they are unlikely to be the sole etiologic factor in the disease. Often the patients are aware of a relationship between exacerbation of their symptoms and acute stress. More complex psychosomatic theories of asthma have thus far not been supported by unambiguous evidence. The efficacy of psychotherapy in the treatment of asthma has not yet been adequately documented, and in a disease such as asthma that is characterized by remissions and exacerbations, such documentation is extremely difficult to obtain. A patient who is unaware of a relationship between acute stress and the onset or exacerbation of symptoms should not be told that his disease is due to psychologic factors, since such a conclusion would likely be incorrect.

A clinical triad of asthma (generally intrinsic), nasal polyps, and aspirin sensitivity has been described. It is important to be aware of this relationship because aspirin ingestion by these patients may lead to marked exacerbation of asthmatic symptoms. This sensitivity to aspirin can be thought of as an idiosyncratic drug reaction. It is clearly not IgE mediated. Aspirin-sensitive patients are often also sensitive to aminopyrine, mefenamic acid, dextropropoxyphene, pentazocine, indomethacin, and some other nonsteroidal anti-inflammatory drugs. A small percentage of aspirin-sensitive patients also react to tartrazine dyes, which are common additives in foods and medications. Aspirin-sensitive patients can generally tolerate sodium salicylate, acetaminophen, and propoxyphene. Aspirin-induced asthma is believed to be related to the effects of the incriminated drugs on prostaglandin production because these drugs are inhibitors of the cyclo-oxygenase pathway of prostaglandin synthesis.

DIAGNOSIS. The diagnosis of asthma is based primarily on a detailed patient's history. Allergic (extrinsic) asthma is distinguished from other forms of asthma by a tendency for onset at an earlier age (usually in childhood); association of symptoms with exposure to some allergen; a tendency for patients to have other allergic manifestations such as childhood eczema, food allergies, or hay fever; a family history of allergy; complete absence of symptoms when the patient is not exposed to the allergen; and absence of a chronic cough or the production of purulent sputum. Allergies to pollens may induce seasonal symptoms, and allergies to household pets may induce perennial symptoms. The role of allergies to dust or mold spores must also be considered.

Physical findings during an attack include a prolongation of the expiratory phase of the respiratory cycle and wheezing that is usually more pronounced during expiration. Rhonchi may be present as a result of increased mucus secretion. The chest may be hyperresonant, and the diaphragms may be low. In severe cases breath sounds may be markedly decreased and the patient uses the accessory muscles of respiration. The patient may be cyanotic, mainly as a consequence of a ventilation-perfusion imbalance caused by mucus plugging of small airways and airway narrowing caused by bronchoconstriction.

Laboratory studies are useful in diagnosis. Moderate eosinophilia is somewhat more common in extrinsic asthma, although marked eosinophilia is sometimes seen in intrinsic asthma, especially in aspirin-sensitive patients. Elevated serum IgE levels and positive results of IgE-mediated skin tests to environmental allergens suggest an allergic cause. If a patient is atopic and has multiple allergies, an allergic cause for the asthma is more likely. Pulmonary function studies are of value in confirming the diagnosis of asthma and documenting its course but are of no help in establishing its cause. It is important to determine whether the airway obstruction is improved with bronchodilators. Irreversibility suggests that factors other than or in addition to bronchoconstriction are involved, including excessive mucus production, thick viscous mucus, or infection (bronchitis). Details of pulmonary function testing are discussed in Chapter 158. Studies of patients after an acute asthmatic attack have shown that symptoms clear first but physical findings of bronchoconstriction often persist for several weeks after symptoms disappear. Careful testing may show that pulmonary function abnormalities persist for weeks. It appears that after an acute attack of asthma the bronchi are particularly sensitive to both allergens and irritants for a relatively prolonged period. This provides the rationale for continuing therapy after symptoms subside. During an acute attack of asthma, arterial blood gas studies (PO_2, PCO_2, and pH) may be useful for evaluating the severity of the attack. A low PO_2 and a normal or low PCO_2 are commonly observed. An increased PCO_2 is a particularly ominous sign.

It should be pointed out that many patients with asthma, both intrinsic and extrinsic, have "hyperirritable" bronchi. That is, in response to agents such as methacholine that cause bronchoconstriction in all persons, their bronchi constrict at concentrations that are considerably lower than those required to induce bronchoconstriction in nonasthmatic subjects. This bronchial hyperreactivity may play an important role in both intrinsic and extrinsic asthma. Many asthmatic patients find their symptoms exacerbated by exposure to smoke, dust, paint fumes, and other irritants. These reactions are generally not allergic but rather reflect the hyperreactivity of these subjects' bronchi to a variety of irritants.

MANAGEMENT. In general the medical treatment of allergic asthma is similar to the treatment of asthma of other causes. β-Adrenergic agonists and theophylline derivatives are the mainstay for management of the routine case of asthma (see Chapter 166).

In severe cases corticosteroids are extremely valuable. Inhaled steroid preparations can be used to minimize the undesirable systemic side effects of long-term steroid therapy, but inhaled steroids are ineffective in acutely ill patients. Therefore therapy is usually initiated with parenteral or oral medication, and after symptoms are controlled, inhaled steroids are initiated. The dosage of oral steroids is then gradually decreased if possible, and the patient is maintained with inhaled steroids. The majority of patients with asthma can be treated successfully without the use of steroids.

As noted previously, for several months after an acute asthmatic attack a patient may be particularly prone to the triggering

of bronchoconstriction by irritants, allergens, or other factors. This leads to the common clinical situation of a patient whose asthmatic attack is treated in the emergency room and who is discharged symptom free without medication only to return a day or two later with repeated attacks of increasing severity. When such a pattern is observed, more prolonged therapy should be undertaken even though the patient is symptom free. When a patient has had frequent severe asthmatic attacks, it is therefore logical to maintain steroid therapy for a long time and then reduce the dosage slowly to a level sufficient to maintain the patient without signs and symptoms. In some cases, after symptoms are controlled, the patient can be given alternate-day steroid therapy or inhaled steroids to minimize systemic side effects. After the patient has done well for several months, steroid therapy should be terminated if possible.

Cromolyn sodium has been used by inhalation with considerable success in some patients (particularly children) with asthma. The drug acts locally to inhibit the release of pharmacologically active mediators from mast cells. It is generally recommended for patients with extrinsic asthma. However, since some patients with intrinsic asthma may benefit from cromolyn, a trial of this drug in these patients is reasonable if their disease is not otherwise controlled. In some severe cases its use permits the reduction of steroid dosage required for maintenance. It should be emphasized that cromolyn is used only prophylactically. It is not a bronchodilator and has no efficacy in treating an acute asthmatic attack. Cromolyn is particularly useful in preventing exercise-induced asthma.

Several aspects of therapy are specifically related to allergic asthma. (1) Environmental manipulation is directed toward eliminating environmental substances to which the patient is allergic, including removal of pets from the home, extensive cleaning to remove dust, redecorating to eliminate dust-promoting factors such as rugs and draperies, use of electrostatic air filters, use of foam rubber rather than feather pillows, and use of mattress and blanket covers. A cold water humidifier is sometimes helpful, but it must be cleaned meticulously every day to prevent the growth of molds that in themselves can be a significant cause of allergic asthma. (2) In patients who have symptoms that can be attributed to specific allergens on the basis of the history and skin test findings, immunotherapy (hyposensitization) appears appropriate. Although the efficacy of immunotherapy in asthma has not been definitely established, its use in *clearly* allergic patients with severe disease seems reasonable in view of the low toxicity of the therapy, the logic of the therapy, and the existence of data suggesting its beneficial effects. A trial of 3 to 5 years seems appropriate. After that time the physician should discontinue therapy and attempt a clinical judgment as to whether the therapy was beneficial. If the patient's symptoms seem worse without therapy, injections can be reinstituted. It should be emphasized that, as in the treatment of allergic rhinitis, immunotherapy is generally ineffective in treating asthma caused by allergic reactions to the dander of household pets.

BIBLIOGRAPHY

Bellanti JA: Immunology, ed 2, Philadelphia, 1978, WB Saunders Co.

Middleton E, Reed C, and Ellis E, editors: Allergy: principles and practice (2 vols), St. Louis, 1978, The CV Mosby Co.

Norins AL: Atopic dermatitis, Pediatr Clin North Am 18:801, 1971.

Patterson R, editor: Allergic diseases: diagnosis and management, Philadelphia, 1972, JB Lippincott Co.

Patterson R: Rhinitis, Med Clin North Am 58:43, 1974.

Sheldon JM, Lovell RG, and Mathews KP: A manual of clinical allergy, ed 2, Philadelphia, 1967, WB Saunders Co.

5·URTICARIA AND ANGIOEDEMA

Leonard S. Girsh *and* **Lewis Perelmutter**

Urticaria, a very common disease with an estimated incidence of 20%, and angioedema, often associated with urticaria, are type I allergic reactions that develop when the skin is the organ system involved. These reactions may be acute or chronic (recurrent). Urticaria (hives) is characterized by elevated, erythematous wheals that are intensely pruritic. Angioedema (angioneurotic edema) is the allergic swelling of an entire anatomic part, such as the thumb, hand, lip, eyelid, or buttock; it is not painful or pruritic. Angioedema is urticaria involving the subcutaneous or submucosal tissues rather than the skin.

ETIOLOGY AND PATHOGENESIS. Allergic urticaria and allergic angioedema are most commonly produced by foods or drugs against which the patient has IgE antibodies. Eggs, fish, condiments, spices, cheese, pork, seafood, and nuts are among the foods most often implicated in IgE-mediated allergic reactions manifested as urticaria or angioedema. Some cases of food-induced urticaria may not be caused by an IgE mediated reaction, but by substances in some foods (such as strawberries) that act directly on mast cells to release histamine and other mediators. Penicillin is the agent most often implicated in IgE-mediated allergic reactions to drugs. Sulfonamides and aspirin are often associated with urticaria, but in the case of aspirin, the mechanisms involved are not well understood. The combination of circulating antigen with IgE fixed to mast cells in the skin results in hives (urticaria) or more extensive subcutaneous or submucosal edema (angioedema). Lesions can also occur from infection with parasites, bacteria, fungi, and viruses as a result of Hymenoptera stings and in patients with neoplasms (especially lymphoma) or autoimmune diseases. The interaction of antigen and IgE directed against the antigen results in the release of mediators such as histamine, kinins, and slow-reacting substance of anaphylaxis (SRS-A) from mast cells. This results in capillary leakage, edema, and formation of urticaria or angioedema. The onset of lesions usually occurs within minutes after exposure to the allergen.

Immune mechanisms are most commonly of the IgE-mediated type, but occasionally the activation of complement as C3a, C5a, and C4a anaphylotoxins, which are very potent histamine releasers, occurs. Complement activation could result in urticaria associated with cryoglobulinemia, systemic lupus erythematosus, and rare drug reactions associated with lidocaine and procarbazine. Rare cases of impaired breakdown of anaphylotoxin and bradykinin are associated with deficiency of carboxy peptidase, an enzyme that inactivates anaphylotoxin; the deficiency results in urticaria.

When urticaria occurs on an apparently nonimmunologic basis, the mediators of the reaction are probably the same—histamine, kinins, and SRS-A. Some of the nonimmunologic causes are heat; emotions and exercise, which cause vasodilation (cholinergic mechanisms may also be involved); physical factors such as cold; and drugs that can cause nonimmunologic release of mediators by direct action on mast cells (for example, morphine, hydralazine, quinine, and organic iodides). Cold urticaria may also occur in underlying diseases such as syphilis and cryoglobulinemia.

Recurrent (chronic if more than 6 weeks duration) urticaria occasionally may be caused or triggered by drug or food allergy, but in most cases is not deemed to be of allergic origin.

Malignancy (especially lymphoma), thyroid disease, the collagen-vascular group of diseases, vasculitis, and circulating antigen-antibody complexes are all associated with chronic urticaria. However, in the majority of cases no underlying cause can be identified.

CLINICAL MANIFESTATIONS. The urticarial lesion is usually a 1 to 5 cm irregular wheal with a pale center surrounded by erythema. Lesions are often intensely pruritic and usually appear and fade rapidly. They tend to occur at pressure points. Urticaria is most often disseminated.

Angioedema is a painless, usually nonpruritic swelling of an area (for instance, the finger, hand, foot, lip, eyelid, or penis) that tends to last for several days. There is a syndrome of angioedema, asthma, and nasal polyps that is associated with aspirin ingestion. Laryngeal involvement is an uncommon but severe complication of allergic angioedema.

PREVENTION AND MANAGEMENT. Avoidance of the identified etiologic agents is the key to prevention. Allergic urticaria or angioedema is treated with antihistamines, such as 50 mg diphenhydramine hydrochloride or 25 to 100 mg hydroxyzine four times daily. If the patient is acutely ill, epinephrine in a dose of 0.3 ml of a 1 : 1000 solution administered subcutaneously usually gives relief. Prednisone (40 to 60 mg day) is reserved for severe cases. A small number of patients obtain relief of urticaria after the addition of an antihistaminic that blocks H_2 receptors, such as Cimetidine (300 mg four times daily) or ranitidine HCl (150 mg two times daily).

Patients with chronic recurrent urticaria should be evaluated for underlying diseases, such as malignancies or connective tissue disease. Chronic urticaria frequently responds to hydroxyzine therapy. After prolonged treatment, the drug can often be gradually discontinued without a recurrence of symptoms.

Dietary causes of urticaria may be apparent to the patient; when not apparent, a dietary trial of 3 to 4 weeks may be helpful. Foods of high allergic potential (listed in the previous section on etiology and pathogenesis), as well as dyes, preservatives, and antioxidants (bisulfite in lettuce, shrimp, or wines), are eliminated from the diet. One new food is then added every 5 to 7 days to determine which is the exciting agent.

The treatment of food allergies is strictly dependent on avoiding the offending allergen. Skin testing and the radioallergosorbent test (RAST) have a high incidence of false positive and false negative reactions and therefore may not be helpful.

Urticaria pigmentosa (systemic mastocytosis)

Urticaria pigmentosa consists of benign mast cell tumors; it is associated with hyperpigmentation in spots that represent mast cell infiltrates. When these frecklelike lesions are stroked, histamine is released and an urticarial lesion develops.

Papular urticaria

This is a multiple, delayed, type IV, nodular allergic reaction to flea bites. Insecticides applied to the family pet are required to prevent future reactions.

Hereditary angioedema

Patients with a hereditary defect of $C\bar{1}$ esterase inhibitor are prone to develop recurrent attacks of nonpruritic angioedema on a nonimmunologic basis. The skin, viscera, and laynrx are often involved. In the absence or during dysfunction of $C\bar{1}$ esterase inhibitor, the $C\bar{1}$ molecule tends to autoactivate and initiate the complement cascade.

Most patients are young women. Patients may complain of

either episodes of angioedema (often involving the face) or a nonspecific gastrointestinal disturbance including abdominal pain, nausea, vomiting, and diarrhea with onset often precipitated by trauma or a surgical procedure. Death commonly occurs as a result of laryngeal edema. The disease has two forms: one in which no C1 esterase inhibitor is produced, and one that is less common in which an inactive C1 esterase inhibitor protein is present. The two forms are clinically identical and are treated in the same manner. However, the usual assay for C1 esterase inhibitor, which measures the protein immunologically, gives a false normal value in patients who have the functionally inactive protein. Thus if a normal test result is obtained for a patient with a history suggestive of the disease, more sophisticated assays of inhibitor activity are needed. The low C4 level during quiescent periods is evidence of the ongoing complement turnover.

Hereditary angioedema usually responds poorly to antihistamines, epinephrine, and steroids. Administration of nonmasculinizing androgens such as danazol (200 mg three times daily) has resulted in increased levels of C1 esterase inhibitor in serum and marked clinical improvement.

BIBLIOGRAPHY

Fudenberg HH and others, editors: Basic and clinical immunology, ed 3, Los Altos, Calif, 1980, Lange Medical Publications.

Gelfand JA and others: Treatment of hereditary angioedema with danazol: reversal of clinical and biochemical abnormalities, N Engl J Med 295:1444, 1976.

Lockey F and Bukantz C: Principles of immunology and allergy, Philadelphia, 1987, WB Saunders Company.

Mathews P: The urticarias: current concepts in pathogenesis and treatment, Drugs 30:552, 1985.

NIAD Task Force Report: Asthma and the other allergic diseases, NIH Pub No 79-387, Washington, DC, 1979, US Department of Health and Human Services, US Public Health Service.

6 · SERUM SICKNESS

Leonard S. Girsh and **Lewis Perelmutter**

The serum sickness syndrome (a type III and perhaps type I immunologic reaction) refers to the syndrome that occurs as a hypersensitivity reaction following the injection of foreign serum. A similar syndrome, if not identical to classic serum sickness, can be produced by nonprotein drug allergy, although the precise mechanism may be somewhat different. It is thought that the nonprotein drug acts as a haptone, binding and coupling with body protein, and then functioning as an allergen. The disease is characterized by fevers, arthralgia or arthritis, and urticaria or other rashes. Lymphadenopathy may be present.

ETIOLOGY AND EPIDEMIOLOGY. Before the development of antibiotics, several types of bacterial infections in humans were prevented or treated by injecting patients with a large volume of antiserum prepared in horses or rabbits. Heterologous antisera are now used much less in medicine; for example, tetanus antitoxin is mainly derived from human instead of horse serum. Currently, serum sickness–like reactions most commonly occur as allergic reactions to penicillin or other drugs.

Historically, serum sickness has occurred in about 5% of those receiving equine tetanus antitoxin and in 15% of those receiving equine rabies antitoxin. Other causes include bee venoms, intraarterial streptokinase, equine antibotulinal antitoxin, equine antivenom for black widow spider bites, and antitoxin for gas gangrene and diptheria.

The probability of an individual experiencing serum sickness is increased with larger volumes of serum; and increased antibody content volumes approaching 100 ml have nearly a 100% incidence of serum sickness. Incidence and severity are greater in adults than in children.

PATHOGENESIS. Serum sickness is a generalized allergic reaction thought to be caused by deposition of antigen-antibody complexes in blood vessels. The induction or incubation period for serum sickness is dependent on the period of sensitization, usually 3 to 12 days. During this incubation period, heterologous serum (or the drug) continues to circulate as the host becomes sensitized to the foreign material and produces antibody. The allergic reaction occurs when circulating antibody combines with circulating antigen to produce antigen-antibody complexes. These complexes are deposited in the walls of blood vessels at various sites. IgG and IgM complexes fix complement and attract polymorphonuclear leukocytes, producing injury that may result in thrombosis and hemorrhage. IgE complexes cause release of vasoactive substances from mast cells, such as histamine, kinins, serotonin, and the slow-reacting substance of anaphylaxis, with production of edema (for example, urticaria). Facilitated by IgE-dependent release of vasoactive substances, these immune complexes diffuse into the vascular walls with resultant fixation and activation of complement.

Drugs causing serum sickness usually must combine with host protein to produce a protein-drug antigen (the drug is a hapten) against which the antibody is produced. In rabbits, renal disease (immune complex nephritis) is common, but this manifestation is rare in humans.

Removal of the immune complexes by the mononuclear phagocytes and reticuloendothelial system cells ultimately ends the disease. However, as long as circulating antibody remains, readministration of the antigen reproduces manifestations of the disease with a shorter incubation period.

CLINICAL MANIFESTATIONS. Serum sickness includes four symptom complexes: fever; enlarged lymph nodes, enlarged spleen, or both; erythematous, petechial, or urticarial rashes; and arthralgia or arthritis. The disease may be self-limited with avoidance of allergen and subsides within a few days to weeks. Other manifestations include abdominal pain, carditis, and neurologic disease.

LABORATORY FINDINGS. Eosinophilia is uncommon and the erythrocyte sedimentation rate is often normal. ECG abnormalities may be seen. Antibodies against sheep erythrocytes may be present. Guinea pig tissue absorption studies help in differential diagnosis of infectious mononucleosis.

Evidence for circulating immune complexes can be detected by various techniques not commonly available except in specialized reference laboratories; these techniques include C1Q binding assay and Raji cell tests.

Serum complement levels are decreased. Occasionally, circulating plasma cells are seen. Elevated plasma levels of C3a anaphylotoxin have been found.

MANAGEMENT. Antihistamines are used in mild forms of serum sickness, but corticosteroids are required in severe cases. Response to steroids is prompt; a dosage of 40 to 60 mg of prednisone daily for 4 to 5 days, then tapered and stopped, is usually sufficient.

PREVENTION. Prevention depends on the maintenance of active immunization when possible to prevent the need for passive immunization. Human serum products rather than foreign serum should be used when possible. Currently in the United States, it is rarely, if ever, necessary to use horse serum.

BIBLIOGRAPHY

Erffmeyer JE: Serum sickness, Ann Allergy 56:105, 1986.

7·CONTACT DERMATITIS

Leonard S. Girsh *and* Lewis Perelmutter

Contact dermatitis, typified by poison ivy, is a type IV (cell-mediated) reaction. Specific T cells interact with the antigen and secrete a series of pharmacologically active protein mediators (lymphokines) that collectively bring about local changes characteristic of a chronic inflammatory reaction. This reaction occurs 24 to 48 hours after contactant exposure. Other incitants include soap, detergents in fabrics, nickel and dyes that may cross-react with sulfonamides, benzocaine local anesthetics, and paraben preservatives. Rubber products containing antioxidants and accelerators, as well as drugs such as penicillin, neomycin, sulfonamides, and ethylene diamine stabilizer in ointments, may act as contactant haptens.

Substances that cause contact sensitivity reactions are generally chemically reactive haptens that combine with host proteins to yield complete antigens. Primary irritant chemicals and seborrheic or atopic dermatitis must be excluded in the differential diagnosis.

The skin lesions are erythematous with vesicles. The presence of lesions on exposed areas is characteristic of contact dermatitis. Lesions limited to clothed areas suggest a reaction to laundry detergents or to a particular fabric. The diagnosis is usually based on a patient's history and patch tests with common allergens. Avoidance is the primary approach to prevention.

Poison ivy is a self-limited disease, and mild cases do not require treatment. In severe cases local or systemic steroids, given in moderate doses for 7 to 10 days, are usually effective in eliminating symptoms. When large areas of skin are involved, systemic steroids are probably preferable because they are more convenient to use and are usually more effective. Furthermore, when local steroids are applied to large areas of inflamed skin, a sufficient amount is absorbed to produce systemic effects, thus eliminating one of the major advantages of local application.

Prophylactic measures include patient education regarding techniques of avoidance. Prophylactic hyposensitization has been found useful by some clinicians in the prevention of contact dermatitis caused by poison ivy. This therapeutic efficacy has been documented by cautious, repeated patch testing after the hyposensitization course is completed. Acquired tolerance to former patch testing with increasing concentrations of poison ivy extract may be observed after a desensitization treatment course.

BIBLIOGRAPHY

Fisher AA: Contact dermatitis, Philadelphia, 1974, Lea & Febiger.
Lockey RF and Bukantz C: Principles of immunology and allergy, Philadelphia, 1987, WB Saunders Company.
Strauss M: Personal communication.

8·DRUG ALLERGY

Leonard S. Girsh *and* Lewis Perelmutter

"Drug allergy" refers to a reaction to a drug that is mediated by an immunologic mechanism. The term does not include toxic, pharmacologic, or idiosyncratic reactions to drugs that are not immunologic in origin, such as tremor and syncope with the use of epinephrine or diarrhea with the use of tetra-cycline. Drug allergy does not include idiosyncratic reactions that have no immune basis, such as aplastic anemia from chloramphenicol, which is probably related to pecularities of drug metabolism in the individual. Similarly, the organic iodides, such as contrast media, may cause an idiosyncratic release of mediators from mast cells, producing an anaphylactoid reaction that is clinically indistinguishable from an IgE-mediated anaphylactic reaction, although it is not immunologically mediated.

ETIOLOGY AND EPIDEMIOLOGY. Any drug may produce an allergic reaction; drugs may be of high or low allergic potential. Drugs of high allergic potential include penicillins and cephalosporins, which may cross-react with one another. Drugs of low allergic potential include erythromycin, tetracycline, lidocaine (free of the parabens), digitalis derivatives, and acetaminophen. Sulfonamides, dyes, and other para-aminobenzenes such as the "caine" drugs couple with body protein and act as an allergen in this fashion. Narcotics often cause drug reactions believed to be caused by histamine or other mediator release. However, the precise mechanisms are uncertain in most cases.

The risk of drug allergy depends not only on the composition of the drug but also on the degree of exposure, route of administration, and patient susceptibility. Intermittent exposure seems to heighten the risk of developing an allergic reaction. Topical application also increases the risk, whereas oral administration lessens the risk. The risk of drug reaction is greater in adults than in children. Drug hypersensitivity reactions are probably more common in patients with prior drug reactions. Disease states characterized by hyperactive immune responses, such as lupus erythematosus, are commonly associated with an increased risk of drug reaction.

PATHOGENESIS. Allergic drug reactions occur as a result of sensitization, particularly after repeated exposure to drugs of high allergic potential, whether administered topically, orally, or by injection. The allergen in drug allergy is usually composed of a protein-drug complex (a bond is formed between the low-molecular-weight drug or metabolic degradative product of the drug and plasma or tissue protein). The drug or a product derived from it acts as a hapten, and the host protein is the carrier. Drugs, or their metabolites, that readily form covalent bonds with proteins are most apt to cause drug allergy. All types of immunologic tissue damage may result from drugs. A type I reaction results when a drug-protein complex reacts with IgE antibody bound to mast cells. This interaction causes release of mediators from the mast cells and can result in generalized anaphylaxis or localized urticaria (see Chapter 5). Type II reactions occur when the drug binds to a host cell such as a red blood cell or a platelet. IgG or IgM antibodies interact with the drug bound to the host cell and cause rapid destruction of the cell, leading to anemia or thrombocytopenia. Complement may or may not be bound to the antibody-drug-cell complex. This mechanism of tissue damage is most often seen when large doses of a drug are being administered. Serum sickness–like reactions (type III mechanism) can also result from drugs (see Chapter 6).

Local application of drugs can result in a type IV reaction following interaction of drug-protein complexes with sensitized T lymphocytes. This delayed hypersensitivity reaction produces contact dermatitis (see Chapter 7).

CLINICAL MANIFESTATIONS. Although a drug reaction may be seen as pure urticaria or serum sickness, many reactions have mixed features. The nature of the drug reaction depends on many factors such as drug dose, specificity of the antibodies produced, class (isotype) and subclass of the antibodies produced, distribution of the drug, and its interaction with different host constituents.

Generalized anaphylaxis. Generalized anaphylaxis (a type I reaction) is the systemic reaction generally resulting from release of vasoactive mediators, such as histamine and slow-reacting substance of anaphylaxis from mast cells following an antigen-IgE reaction. Alternatively, the complement system may be activated through a variety of mechanisms that release C3a and C5a, both of which have anaphylatoxin activity; however, the complement system does not appear to be a common mechanism in human anaphylaxis. The result is vasodilation, increased vascular permeability, and contraction of smooth muscle. Multiple organ systems are involved simultaneously, and death may ensue. Although drugs are the most common cause of generalized anaphylaxis, foods and insect stings are also causes.

Shortly after exposure to an allergen, one or more of the following systems are involved: cardiovascular, respiratory, skin, and gastrointestinal. Shock may be a secondary result to generalized vasodilation and increased vascular permeability leading to decreased blood volume from leakage of plasma into extravascular sites. Nasal obstruction, rhinorrhea, laryngeal edema, and bronchospasm can occur. Urticaria, angioedema, and severe pruritus can affect the skin. Gastrointestinal involvement can cause abdominal pain, vomiting, and diarrhea. There is evidence that cardiac arrhythmias can occur. A severe anaphylactic reaction can lead to death within a few minutes.

Drug fever. Fever, which can be high and accompanied by shaking chills, may be the only manifestation of a drug reaction or may be accompanied by arthralgia, arthritis, rash, or eosinophilia. Relative bradycardia is frequent in a patient who otherwise appears well. The fever probably has an immunologic origin and generally disappears within several days after stopping the drug.

Allergic rash. Rashes, most of which are probably caused by hypersensitivity vasculitis, may be maculopapular and erythematous (measleslike), urticarial, eczematoid (contact dermatitis), petechial, or even exfoliative. Erythema nodosum or erythema multiforme may occur.

Erythema nodosum. Erythema nodosum is often associated with drug reactions, especially involving penicillins and sulfonamides, but other common causes are sarcoidosis, streptococcal pharyngitis, and acute coccidioidomycosis. It also occurs in patients with tuberculosis, leprosy, viral infections, other fungal infections, and inflammatory bowel disease. The rash usually appears as bilateral tender erythematous nodules on the pretibial area and occasionally on the extensor surfaces of the arms. It is associated with fever and arthralgia or arthritis. It usually lasts several weeks, and relapses may occur.

Erythema multiforme. Erythema multiforme is a rash consisting of erythematous patches that tend to be sharply outlined and have central clearing. These evolve into concentric rings, the so-called target lesion. Although drugs are a common cause, the rash can occur with viral or mycoplasmal infection or malignancy. It can occur without apparent cause. The rash may be accompanied by high fever and extensive bullous lesions. In its most severe form, in which there is mucosal involvement, it is called the Stevens-Johnson syndrome. There are ulcerations in the mouth, vagina, conjunctivae, and gastrointestinal tract. Pneumonia and nephritis may also occur.

Photosensitivity. Certain drugs (for instance, tetracycline derivatives, sulfonamides, and thiazides) can increase the tendency for hyperreaction to sun on the exposed parts of the body, resulting in hypersensitivity dermatitis. Some of these reactions may be allergic.

Disseminated vasculitis. As part of a drug reaction, vasculitis can involve essentially any organ. For example, a polyarteritis nodosa–like syndrome may be produced by sulfonamides. Penicillins, especially methicillin, may produce nephritis, commonly associated with hematuria, rash, and eosinophilia.

The most common dermal vasculitis that may result is a palpable granular sharply circumscribed purpuric dermatitis (immune-complex depositions) involving the lower extremities. Procainamide, hydralazine, and other agents can cause a syndrome similar to systemic lupus erythematosus. The liver, central nervous system, and gastrointestinal tract can be involved in the vasculitis from drug allergy.

Hematologic disorders. Drugs may produce hemolytic anemia (for instance, penicillins and methyldopa) and thrombocytopenia (for instance, penicillins, quinine, and quinidine) on an immunologic basis. Leukopenia (produced by penicillins, cephalosporins, and sulfonamides) and eosinophilia may appear without other manifestations or with rash or fever.

DIAGNOSIS. Any unexpected occurrence in a patient receiving a drug should suggest a drug reaction. Any drug may be responsible, including aspirin, cathartics, sleeping pills, and any other self-medication the patient may be taking. Patients must be questioned carefully as to drug history; this is important for both diagnosis and prevention of reactions.

There is no certain way of proving that a reaction is caused by a drug other than administering the drug and observing the same reaction (that is, rechallenging). Occult reactions, such as drug fever, are virtually impossible to prove as a drug reaction without rechallenge. However, rechallenge is often unwise and unnecessary and may be dangerous. Although eosinophilia may suggest a drug reaction, it is often absent. Furthermore, eosinophilia per se does not indicate that the observed reaction is caused by the drug. Many patients who are prone to allergies normally have eosinophilia or may develop eosinophilia as a secondary reaction to drugs with no other clinical manifestations.

MANAGEMENT. Discontinuation of the causative agent is the major approach to treating drug reactions. However, it is also important to recognize that environmental contamination with drugs is common (for example, traces of penicillin in milk products).

Generalized anaphylaxis is a medical emergency, with a mortality risk when severe; it requires immediate therapy. The drug of choice is 0.2 to 0.5 ml of 1:1000 aqueous epinephrine subcutaneously, repeated every 15 minutes as required. The cardiac rate and blood pressure level must be monitored. If anaphylaxis occurs after injection of a drug, a tourniquet should be placed proximal to the site of injection and 0.2 ml of 1:1000 aqueous epinephrine introduced at the drug injection site to slow absorption of the drug. The shock seen in anaphylaxis is due to hypovolemia. Therefore a slow response to epinephrine indicates the need for expansion of blood volume with saline or other volume expanders. Although steroids and antihistamines are often administered, these agents (at least initially) are clearly of secondary importance to the immediate therapeutic effect of epinephrine and volume replacement. Vasopressors, such as levarterenol bitartrate, are sometimes used when shock does not respond sufficiently to other measures; however, these vasopressors tend to be ineffective if the blood volume is not expanded and are unnecessary once an adequate intravascular volume is achieved with appropriate volume expanders. An endotracheal tube may be necessary.

PREVENTIVE MANAGEMENT. To screen out drug allergy, carefully detailed histories are imperative. When drug allergy, such as to penicillin, is suspected, cautious skin testing is helpful. It is also helpful to selectively choose drugs of low allergic potential when therapeutically feasible (for example, erythromycin instead of penicillin).

Antihistamines, such as 50 mg diphenhydramine hydrochloride or 25 to 100 mg hydroxyzine four times daily, may be used in milder allergic reactions involving the skin. More severe reactions, such as the Stevens-Johnson syndrome and severe disseminated vasculitis, should be treated with 60 mg prednisone daily, with rapid tapering after control of the reaction.

BIBLIOGRAPHY

Austen KF: Systemic anaphylaxis in the human being, N Engl J Med 29:661, 1974.

Cunha BA: Drug fever, Postgrad Med 80:123, 1986.

Dash CH and Jones HEH: Mechanisms in drug allergy, Baltimore, 1972, The Williams & Wilkins Co.

Girsh LS and Perelmutter LL: The diagnosis of drug allergies utilizing in vitro mast cell test and IgE inhibition test, Immunol Allergy Pract 3:158, 1981.

Lieberman P: Hypersensitivity reactions to drugs, Clin Rev Allergy 4:143, 1986.

Parker CW: Drug therapy. I. Drug allergy, N Engl J Med 292:511, 1975.

Parker CW: Drug therapy. II. Drug allergy, N Engl J Med 292:732, 1975.

Parker CW: Drug therapy. III. Drug allergy, N Engl J Med 292:957, 1975.

Dental correlations

Martin S. Greenberg

The field of allergy has direct application to dental practice in two major circumstances: the differential diagnosis of a patient presenting with ulcerative or vesiculobullous lesions of the oral mucosa, and the evaluation of a patient with a history of allergy to medication or materials used by a dentist. Many patients, as well as some clinicians, use the term "allergy" to describe all adverse reactions. This broad, unfortunate use of the term causes difficulty for the patient and the dentist. All too frequently, patients who feel dizzy or nauseous or who have heart palpitations from a psychic or toxic reaction after a local anesthetic injection are labeled "allergic." Such patients then inform each succeeding dentist and physician of the "allergy," unnecessarily complicating treatment. It is the dentist's responsibility to use the term "allergic reaction" carefully so that the patient is not denied the use of a medication or a material that will be helpful for successful management. It is important to be capable of distinguishing between true allergic reactions and toxic or psychic reactions. When a true allergic reaction occurs to a local anesthetic, the dentist should inform the patient regarding the class of local anesthetic that caused the allergic reaction. For example, patients allergic to the amide group may frequently be able to take the paraaminobenzoic acid group safely.

CLINICAL MANIFESTATIONS. Anaphylactic (type I) allergic reactions or cell-mediated (type IV) allergic reactions have been ascribed to a wide variety of substances used in dental practice. Contact allergy to dental amalgam is most frequently caused by mercury released during condensation. Dermatitis and stomatitis developing from mercury have been described. Investigations have demonstrated an increasing level of allergy to mercury in a group of dental students as they progressed through school. At the beginning of the freshman year 2% of the dental students had a positive reaction to mercury. This is consistent with the level of mercury allergy in the general population. During their senior year, 11% of the students had positive reactions to mercury. All reactions were from mercury itself and not to condensed amalgam, which is a much less common cause of allergy. Although allergy to properly condensed amalgam is rare, several proven cases of true allergy requiring removal of amalgams have been reported.

Incorrect information has led some dentists to recommend patch testing for mercury "allergy" in patients with nonspecific symptoms such as chronic fatigue, gastrointestinal complaints, depression, or headache. Positive results, according to this theory, indicate that amalgam fillings must be replaced with other materials. Since there is no evidence that amalgam hypersensitivity causes nonspecific symptoms, this form of testing has no rational basis and cannot be justified.

Most reactions to acrylic are caused by contact with the free monomer. The number of allergic reactions to acrylic can be greatly reduced by avoiding use of uncured acrylic directly in the mouth. There have been reported cases of severe allergic dermatitis, stomatitis, and bronchospasm occurring after contact with a bench-cured acrylic temporary bridge. An erythema multiforme reaction after contact with uncured acrylic has been noted. The lesions resolved after the acrylic bridge was heat cured to remove the free monomer. An allergic reaction to heat-cured acrylic is rare. There have also been occasional reports of allergic reactions to composite resin, nickel in chrome, cobalt prostheses, cinnamon oil in chewing gum, and epimine-containing impression materials.

Eugenol, which is widely used in temporary fillings and periodontal dressings, has also been reported as a rare cause of contact allergy. A case of an anaphylactic reaction to eugenol has been reported.

Hypersensitivity reactions not caused by dental materials may also affect the oral region. One major example is angioneurotic edema of the lips or tongue. This is a type I allergic reaction caused by IgE bound to mast cells, which release mediators such as histamine, causing edema. This disfiguring disorder may be life-threatening if it compromises the airway by involving the posterior tongue or larynx.

Erythema multiforme is a symptom complex involving the skin and mucous membranes; it may be caused by reactions to microorganisms, food, drugs, radiotherapy, or malignancy. The drugs most commonly related to an erythema multiforme reaction are antibiotics, barbiturates, phenylbutazone, and carbamazepine (Tegretol). Particularly interesting are the reports of erythema multiforme related to recurrent herpes labialis. Shelly reported that 15% of the cases of recurrent erythema multiforme have a preceding recurrent herpes simplex infection as the precipitating factor. The majority of cases of erythema multiforme have no related allergy to disease and are labeled idiopathic. Erythema multiforme most frequently occurs in children and young adults and has an acute onset. The most common cutaneous lesions are found on the hands, feet, and extensor surfaces of the elbows and knees. The face and neck are also commonly involved but only severe cases affect the trunk. Oral lesions appear along with the cutaneous manifestations, but in some cases the oral lesions are the predominant or only sign of the disease. The skin lesions may take many forms, but the target lesion is the pathognomonic sign and should be searched for in each case. The target lesion consists of a central bulla surrounded by edema with concentric bands of erythema. The oral lesions begin as bullae on an erythematous base, but these break rapidly into large irregular lesions. In full-blown cases the lips are extensively eroded and large portions of the oral mucosa are denuded of epithelium. Treatment of erythema multiforme consists of supportive care for mild cases. In severe cases, systemic corticosteroids should be used.

DENTAL MANAGEMENT. Treatment of contact or type IV allergic reactions of the oral mucosa can be treated successfully by eliminating the allergen and using topical corticosteroids and diphenhydramine (Benadryl). Anaphylactic or type I reaction can be treated with 0.5 ml of 1:1000 epinephrine subcutaneously when a life-threatening reaction occurs. Hives are not life threatening and can be treated successfully with Benadryl.

BIBLIOGRAPHY

Barkin ME, Boyd JP, and Cohen S: Acute allergic reaction to eugenol, Oral Surg 57:441, 1984.

Catsakis LH and Sulica VI: Allergy to silver amalgams, Oral Surg 46:371, 1978.

Duxbury AJ, Turner EP, and Watts DC: Hypersensitivity to epimine containing dental materials, Br Dent J 147:331, 1979.

Eversole LR: Allergic stomatitides, J Oral Med 34:93, 1979.

Fisher AA: The misuse of the patch test to determine "hypersensitivity" to mercury amalgam dental fillings, Cutis 35:110, 1985.

Mackert JR; Hypersensitivity to mercury from dental amalgams, J Amer Acad Dermatol 12:877, 1986.

Nathanson D and Lockhart P: Delayed extraoral hypersensitivity to dental composite material, Oral Surg 47:329, 1979.

Rickles NH: Allergy in surface lesions of the oral mucosa, Oral Surg 33:744, 1972.

Sturgis TL and Fink JN: Hypersensitivity to acrylic resin, J Prosthet Dent 22:425, 1969.

White RR and Brandt RL: Development of mercury hypersensitivity among dental students, J Am Dent Assoc 92:1204, 1976.

Wood JFL: Mucosal reaction to cobalt-chromium alloy, Br Dent J 136:423, 1974.

9 • IMMUNODEFICIENCY DISEASES

Donna M. Murasko *and* **Donald Kaye**

Immunodeficiency diseases are characterized by increased susceptibility of patients to infection; the types of infection may suggest the type of deficiency. These patients may also have an increased tendency to develop malignancies, particularly lymphomas. The defects may be severe or mild and may involve the phagocytic system, the complement system, or the immunologic system itself (B lymphocytes, T lymphocytes, or both). Clinical manifestations thus vary in nature and severity.

DISORDERS OF B LYMPHOCYTES

Patients with disorders of the B-lymphocyte arm have a defect in antibody production, ranging from a complete absence of all immunoglobulins to a selective deficiency of one immunoglobulin class. The extent of the symptoms observed in patients is related to the severity of the deficiency; for example, many individuals exhibiting selective IgA deficiency demonstrate no apparent dysfunction. In situations where clinical symptoms are observed, recurrent bacterial infections, particularly caused by encapsulated organisms that require antibody for efficient phagocytosis by monocytes or granulocytes, are common. The primary pathogenic organisms are *Streptococcus pneumoniae* and *Haemophilus influenzae*. Other organisms sometimes implicated are group A β-hemolytic streptococci and meningococci. The types of infection commonly seen are recurrent pneumonia, sinusitis, otitis media, bacteremia, and meningitis. *Giardia lamblia* infections are common in patients with no IgA in intestinal secretions.

DISORDERS OF T LYMPHOCYTES

Patients with disorders of the T-lymphocyte arm have decreased cellular immunity. The infections noted most often are those caused by intracellular parasites. In particular, these patients are more likely to develop the following infections and have a more severe form: bacterial infections (tuberculosis, *Listeria monocytogenes* infections), herpesvirus infection (herpes simplex, herpes zoster with dissemination, cytomegalovirus infection), fungal infections (cryptococcal meningitis, mucocutaneous and/or disseminated *Candida* infection), and protozoan infections (*Pneumocystis carinii* pneumonia, severe toxoplasmosis). Graft-versus-host reactions can occur following blood transfusion because of the survival of donor lymphocytes.

Patients with T-lymphocyte abnormalities also may have variable defects in antibody production, which result from the loss of the normal modulating effect of T cells on antibody production.

DISORDERS OF POLYMORPHONUCLEAR LEUKOCYTES

In patients with neutropenia, infections are most often caused by gram-negative bacilli (*Escherichia coli, Klebsiella-Enterobacter, Proteus, Pseudomonas*) and *Staphylococcus aureus*. For polymorphonuclear and other phagocytic cells to function normally in host defense, they must be capable of three distinct processes: (1) directed movement toward the site of the foreign organism (chemotaxis); (2) binding and internalizing the foreign organism (phagocytosis); and (3) performing a series of chemical reactions that generate substances toxic for the foreign organism. Defects in all three of these essential functions have been described and can be responsible for an increased susceptibility to the infections just listed.

DEFECTS IN THE COMPLEMENT SYSTEM

Defects in the complement system have also been associated with increased susceptibility to bacterial infection. C3 deficiency or low C3 secondary to absent C3b inactivator (resulting in consumption of C3) predisposes to *S. aureus* and gram-negative bacillary infections. Deficiencies of C6, C7, and C8 have been associated with recurrent meningococcal and gonococcal bacteremia.

Complement deficiencies have been associated with autoimmune disease, particularly a syndrome resembling systemic lupus erythematosus.

The basis of hereditary angioedema is a deficiency of $\overline{\text{C1}}$ esterase inhibitor.

EVALUATION OF IMMUNITY

Evaluation of the status of the immune system involves a careful history and a series of laboratory tests. The types of infection may suggest whether the defect is one of antibody production, cellular immunity, phagocytic function, or the complement system. A number of tests can be performed to evaluate defense mechanisms. Many of these tests are widely available, but others require specialized laboratories.

B-cell function

Measurement of serum immunoglobulins determines if immunoglobulins are present in sufficient concentrations. Lower limits of the normal range for adults are 550 mg/dl for IgG,

45 mg/dl for IgM, and 60 mg/dl for IgA. If borderline values are found or if there is a question about the ability to make antibodies, existing or induced antibodies can be measured. Measurement of anti-A and anti-B blood group antibodies and determination of antibodies against influenza virus after influenza vaccination are particularly helpful. However, a patient suspected of an immunodeficiency should never be immunized with a live attentuated microorganism since this procedure may result in disseminated disease. Other studies requiring special laboratories include determination of IgA in secretions, measurement of the four IgG subclasses, staining and enumeration of blood lymphocytes for surface immunoglobulins, and in vitro induction of B-cell proliferation or immunoglobulin secretion by pokeweed or other mitogens. Although lymph node biopsies have been recommended in the past for identification of B lymphocytes by histology and immunocytochemistry, the newer diagnostic tools make this invasive procedure unnecessary except in the most difficult cases.

T-cell function

Delayed hypersensitivity skin tests such as *Candida,* mumps, and *Trichophyton,* which are positive in a large proportion of the normal population, are helpful in screening for defects. The ability to develop delayed hypersensitivity to a new antigen can be determined by using an effective sensitizing antigen, dinitrochlorobenzene. A sensitizing dose is applied to the skin and a patch test is applied 2 weeks later at another site. Other studies requiring specialized laboratory procedures are enumeration of circulating T cells and T-cell subpopulations using specific monoclonal antibodies, in vitro stimulation of T cells by phytohemagglutinin, concanavalin A, or antigens such as purified protein derivative (of tuberculin) (PPD), and measurement of the production of lymphokines by activated T cells.

Complement

Assay of total hemolytic complement, C2, C4, $C\bar{1}$ esterase inhibitor protein, and C3 are available in most hospital laboratories. Measurement of the other components is available only in specialized laboratories.

Leukocytes

A white blood cell count and differential smear can determine whether adequate mature polymorphonuclear leukocytes are present or if abnormal forms can be detected (such as the giant granules of Chédiak-Higashi syndrome). Studies for leukocyte function, such as reduction of nitroblue tetrazolium (for chronic granulomatous disease), chemotactic response, and phagocytic, metabolic, and bactericidal activity, are available only in specialized laboratories.

CLASSIFICATION

Immunodeficiency diseases may be primary or secondary to an underlying disease. The primary diseases are discussed in this chapter. The diseases that secondarily produce immunodeficiencies are discussed in the appropriate chapters. Examples of secondary immune deficiencies include the following: defects in antibody production in chronic lymphatic leukemia, in multiple myeloma, and in protein-losing enteropathies; defects in cellular immunity in Hodgkin's disease and in acquired immunodeficiency syndrome (AIDS); and defects caused by use of radiation therapy or immunosuppressive drugs. Corticosteroids decrease adherence and migration of phagocytic cells and interfere with cellular immunity.

The primary immunodeficiency diseases are usually congenital and are classified by whether or not the defect involves B-cell function (antibody production), T-cell function (cellular immunity), or both. In fact, most T-cell immunodeficiency diseases also affect B-cell function, and an apparent B-cell defect may actually be related to abnormalities in T cells (helper or suppressor function).

To appreciate the basis of immunodeficiencies and the rationale for the various therapeutic approaches being employed for the different immunodeficiency diseases, a thorough understanding of the immune system from the development of the system to the function of the mature effector cells is required.

Defects in B-cell function (antibody production)

X-LINKED AGAMMAGLOBULINEMIA (BRUTON TYPE). Bruton-type X-linked agammaglobulinemia (or hypogammaglobulinemia) represents an inherited failure in the development of the pre–B cell to a mature B cell, resulting in the absence of most circulating B cells and of plasma cells. Affected patients show an isolated defect in humoral immunity, having no immunoglobulin of any class in the serum, and an inability to produce antibody even when stimulated with a strong antigen. This disorder is transmitted as an X-linked recessive trait and occurs almost exclusively in males. Because of the transplacental transfer of maternal IgG antibodies, affected individuals do not become symptomatic until about 6 months of age. They develop severe and recurrent infections caused by pyogenic bacteria. The lack of intestinal IgA also permits *Giardia lamblia* to cause chronic diarrhea. In addition, there is a particular risk of vaccine-associated poliomyelitis. Unlike most viral infections that are limited by T-cell immunity, picornavirus infections (for example, polio) do not induce cell-surface viral antigens and are only limited by neutralizing antibodies. Management of this immunodeficiency disease consists of prompt therapy of bacterial infections with antibiotics and replacement therapy with γ-globulin. Although γ-globulin is usually administered every 2 weeks to maintain adequate levels of circulating immunoglobulin, the treatment schedule should be individually designed. The time interval between administration should be based on effective control of infections rather than on the level of immunoglobulin in the serum.

X-LINKED IMMUNODEFICIENCY WITH HYPER-IgM. In this defect the IgM level is elevated, and serum IgG and IgA levels are decreased. Infections and management are similar to those for X-linked agammaglobulinemia. Lack of IgG or IgA is thought to be due to the inability of the B lymphocyte to "switch" its genetic information from production of the IgM class (the first immunoglobulin produced in both a primary immune response and during ontogeny) to other immunoglobulin classes.

SELECTIVE DEFICIENCIES OF IMMUNOGLOBULIN

IgA deficiency. The most common immunoglobulin deficiency is that of IgA, involving both serum and secretory IgA and affecting 1 in every 600 people. The cause of the defect is not known. However, since normal numbers of B cells demonstrate surface IgA, it appears that the defect may involve differentiation of the B cell to a plasma cell or of synthesis or release of antibody. About half of the individuals with this disease are symptomatic, and symptoms may not appear until late in life.

IgA deficiency is often observed after treatment with phenytoin or penicillamine. Cessation of drug therapy sometimes results in restoration of the normal level of IgA. Recurrent "low-grade" respiratory infections are common. Severe infections such as those seen in agammaglobulinemia are uncommon. Patients have an increased tendency to develop an allergic diathesis (such as asthma and other atopic diseases), chronic diarrhea, and autoimmune disorders and connective tissue diseases (particularly rheumatoid arthritis and systemic lupus erythematosus). *G. lamblia* infection is common in IgA-deficient patients.

Patients may develop anaphylaxis from blood transfusions, since they are capable of developing antibody against IgA. No treatment is available for IgA deficiency. Administration of γ-globulin is contraindicated for two reasons: it is not effective and patients with selective IgA deficiency have a tendency to develop high titers of anti-IgA antibodies. Whether these antibodies are autoantibodies or the result of exposure to breast milk or bovine immunoglobulins is not clear. The IgA present in the γ-globulin or in blood transfusions may therefore stimulate allergic reactions. Transfusions, if required, should be from IgA-deficient donors.

Other isotype deficiencies. Isolated deficiency of IgM or of one or more of the IgG subclasses has rarely been reported. Infections and management are similar to those for X-linked agammaglobulinemia.

COMMON VARIABLE (UNCLASSIFIABLE) IMMUNODE-FICIENCY (ACQUIRED AGAMMAGLOBULINEMIA). Common variable immunodeficiency is a mixed group of defects (familial or acquired) with the common manifestation of agammaglobulinemia. It is not linked to sex, and symptoms usually do not appear until after age 15.

Since this classification represents a group of diseases, elucidation of the mechanism of the defect is difficult. However, the presence of normal numbers of B cells and reports of increased suppressor T-cell and decreased helper-T-cell activities suggest that the defect probably involves activation of the B cells, differentiation of the B cells, or both. Sinopulmonary infections and infections caused by pneumococci and *Hemophilus influenzae* are common. Autoimmune diseases and diarrhea with malabsorption are frequent manifestations. Lymphoid nodular hyperplasia and splenomegaly are common in acquired agammaglobulinemia but are absent in X-linked agammaglobulinemia.

Plasma cells are absent in lymph nodes, and there is little or no antibody response. Cell-mediated immunity is usually normal. However, patients should be sequentially evaluated for T-cell function, since many patients demonstrate progressive loss of T-cell function with time. Therapy is the same as for X-linked agammaglobulinemia.

Defects in T-cell function (cellular immunity)

DiGEORGE SYNDROME. DiGeorge syndrome is a developmental abnormality that results from a failure in the embryologic development of the third and fourth pharyngeal pouches. As a result, both the parathyroid glands and the thymus fail to develop; the T-lymphoid system is thus deficient. It does not appear to have a hereditary basis. Hypocalcemia often occurs in the first 24 hours after birth. Cardiac defects are also common and are diagnosed during the early neonatal period. Children who survive the early neonatal period commonly experience recurrent infections with viruses, fungi, protozoa, and certain bacteria. Immunoglobin levels may be normal or selectively decreased. Patients usually do not survive beyond age 2 without transplantation of fetal thymus. With transplantation, prolonged survival has been reported.

CHRONIC MUCOCUTANEOUS CANDIDIASIS. Recurrent, protracted superficial *Candida* infections may involve the skin, nails, and oral and vaginal mucous membranes. Hypoparathyroidism and hypoadrenalism can occur. The immune defect is usually limited to T-cell responses specific for *Candida* infec-

tions. T-cell lymphoproliferative responses to mitogens and to allogeneic cells are usually normal. Patients with the defect produce normal quantities of antibodies to all antigens, including *Candida*. Except for the skin infection, serious infection is uncommon. Administration of agents active against *Candida* is the major approach to therapy. Extracts of *Candida*-immune T lymphocytes, called transfer factor, have been successful in adoptively transferring skin test reactivity to some patients. Oral ketoconazole is the drug of choice in control of this disease.

Defects in both B- and T-cell function

SEVERE COMBINED IMMUNODEFICIENCY DISEASE. Combined immunodeficiency disease represents the most severe form of immunodeficiency. Although the cause of the disease is not proven, it is postulated that lack of differentiation of lymphocyte stem cells is responsible for the disease. Affected infants show marked impairment in development of both the B- and T-lymphoid systems. Autosomal recessive, X-linked (Swiss-type agammaglobulinemia), and sporadic types have been described. Clinical manifestations usually appear shortly after birth as profound failure in normal growth and development. Severe recurrent infections with bacteria, viruses, fungi, and parasites occur. Diarrhea and generalized unremitting dermatitis are present. Survival beyond age 2 is rare. There have been reports of successful bone marrow transplants with restoration of immunity. Some patients have been successfully treated with bone marrow, fetal liver, or fetal thymus transplants.

WISKOTT-ALDRICH SYNDROME. Wiskott-Aldrich syndrome, an X-linked recessive disease, is characterized by eczema, thrombocytopenia, and recurrent infections caused by pneumococci, *H. influenzae*, meningococci, and viral organisms. Affected individuals show a low concentration of IgM, normal IgG concentrations, and high IgA and IgE concentrations. There is a poor response to polysaccharide antigens. Although T-cell function seems to be intact at the time of diagnosis, T-cell reactivity appears to decrease with time. Patients are predisposed to develop lymphoproliferative neoplasms. The major approach to therapy is prompt treatment of infections. Bone marrow transplantation has been successful in a few patients; however, successful treatment of the immunodeficiency is difficult and infrequent.

IMMUNODEFICIENCY WITH THYMOMA. Patients with agammaglobulinemia may have a thymoma. Myasthenia gravis, aplastic anemia, granulocytopenia, and thrombocytopenia may also be present. Some patients have deficient T-cell function. Removal of the thymoma does not result in improvement of the immunodeficiency.

Replacement therapy with γ-globulin is often successful in limiting recurrent bacterial infections; however, death resulting from secondary bacterial infections is not uncommon.

ATAXIA TELANGIECTASIA. Ataxia telangiectasia, an autosomal recessive inherited disease, is characterized by progressive degeneration of the cerebellum with ataxia, cutaneous and ocular telangiectasia, recurrent sinopulmonary infections, and immunologic deficiencies. Ataxia begins in infancy and is progressive; patients also show an increased susceptibility to lymphomas. The abnormalities in the immune compartment are variable. Numbers of B cells are usually normal, whereas numbers of T cells may be normal or decreased. T-cell responses as measured by mitogen-induced lymphoproliferation or skin test reactivity may be normal or decreased, even when T-cell numbers are normal. Serum IgA levels are low or absent in about 40% of patients. Decreased IgE and IgG levels have also been observed. Diagnosis is often difficult. It is the association of the ataxia and telangiectasia with decreased IgA levels that usually confirms the diagnosis. Aggressive treatment of bacterial and fungal infections with antibodies is essential. Fetal thymus transplant or γ-globulin therapy has been effective in controlling the disease in a limited number of patients.

MANAGEMENT

Therapy for the immunodeficiency diseases mainly involves replacement of γ-globulins in patients with agammaglobulinemia and use of bone marrow, fetal liver, or fetal thymus transplants in those with T-cell defects. γ-Globulin is contraindicated in patients with selective IgA deficiency. Prompt therapy of infection and proper bronchopulmonary care, chest physiotherapy, and postural drainage in patients with chronic pulmonary infections are essential.

BIBLIOGRAPHY

Rosen FR, Cooper MD, and Wedgwood RJP: The primary immunodeficiencies, N Eng J Med 311:235 and 300, 1984.
Stites DP, Stobo JD, and Wells JV: Basic and clinical immunology, ed 6, Norwalk, Conn, 1987, Lange Medical Publications.

Dental correlations

Martin S. Greenberg *and* **Philip S. Springer**

CLINICAL MANIFESTATION. Oral signs are common in patients with T-lymphocyte disorders. The most prominent oral sign in this group of patients is chronic oral candidiasis. These lesions are widespread and deep seated. They are not easily scraped off the mucosa, and biopsies demonstrate yeast deep into the epithelium. The dentist should consider the possibility of impaired T-lymphocyte function in patients with chronic oral candidiasis that does not respond permanently to standard antifungal medication.

Herpes simplex virus infections are often commonly seen in patients with T-lymphocyte disorders. The patients may have severe primary herpes infections that may become disseminated. More frequently they develop extensive recurrent herpes infections involving the lips and intraoral mucosa.

Recently, there has been significant interest in the relationship of the immune response to periodontal disease, oral ulcers, and dental caries. A recent study evaluated 23 patients with primary immune deficiencies and compared them with normal controls. The patients with immune deficiencies had decreased gingival inflammation resulting from a decreased inflammatory response, but there was no difference noted in the extent of periodontal breakdown. Also noted was a decreased caries rate in the immune-deficient group.

DENTAL MANAGEMENT. Patients with T-lymphocyte abnormalities have a decrease in the levels of circulating immunoglobulins. Dental treatment should not be performed on these patients unless the γ-globulin level is at least 20 mg/dl. When oral surgery is necessary, an extra dose of γ-globulin should be administered the day before surgery at a dose between 100 and 200 mg/kg body weight. This dose should be administered intramuscularly rather than intravenously to decrease the risk of transfusion reaction.

Transfusion reactions are common in patients with the primary immunodeficiency diseases since the missing immunoglobulin is a foreign protein and may cause an allergic response. Therefore patients with a selective immunoglobulin deficiency must be given blood with the missing immunoglobulin depleted. A second problem that may occur in patients with primary immunodeficiency is a development of graft-versus-host disease. The lymphocytes in the transfused blood react against the tissues of the immunodeficient recipient. Only fresh blood in which the immunocompetent lymphocytes have been destroyed can be used.

BIBLIOGRAPHY

Barreckman RW and others: Gingivitis in hypogammaglobulinemia, J Periodontol 44:171, 1973.
Robert WR and Walker DM: The periodontal management of a patient with a profound immunodeficiency disorder, J Clin Periodontol 3:186, 1976.
Robertson PB and others: Periodontal status of patients with abnormalities of the immune system, J Periodont Res 13:37, 1978.

RHEUMATIC AND GRANULOMATOUS DISEASES

Edited by **Warren A. Katz**

Rheumatic diseases are extremely common in medical practice. More than 35 million Americans suffer from one or more rheumatic diseases, and another 75 million experience chronic or recurrent low back pain.

Few subspecialties of internal medicine have engendered more confusing terminology than the field of rheumatology. For example, arthritis in its narrowest sense implies inflammation of the joint, yet the term "arthritis" is usually interpreted more broadly. Arthritis is sometimes used interchangeably with rheumatoid arthritis or osteoarthritis. It has been used to describe forms of nonarticular rheumatism, such as fibromyalgia, even when the joints are not involved.

Arthritis is often confused with the term "rheumatic disease" when used to describe any acute or chronic affliction of joints or other parts of the musculoskeletal system, with the exception of fractures or congenital abnormalities. Arthritis is only one type of rheumatic disease. Connective tissue disorders refer to those diseases that affect not only the musculoskeletal system but the skin and internal organs of the body as well. These disorders tend to be more severe than most primary forms of arthritis and cause immune phenomena that may be fatal. Major connective tissue diseases include rheumatoid arthritis, rheumatic fever, systemic lupus erythematosus, systemic sclerosis (scleroderma), dermatomyositis or polymyositis, vasculitis, and Sjögren's syndrome. Some features from two or more of these entities may coexist in the same patient in a variety of ways. Under these circumstances the terms "overlap," "undifferentiated," or "mixed" connective tissue disease are applied. Noninfectious granulomatous diseases, such as sarcoidosis, share the tendency toward multiorgan involvement, musculoskeletal system manifestations, and a variety of immunologic phenomena.

Fibromyalgia and other forms of nonarticular rheumatism are the most common rheumatic diseases seen in office practice. Osteoarthritis is the most prevalent type of arthritis; almost all people over 60 years of age display at least roentgenographic evidence of the disease. Some types of arthritis are peculiar to certain age groups: rheumatic fever is basically a disease of children; gonococcal arthritis is most apt to be found in young adults; and rheumatoid arthritis is primarily a disease of young to middle-aged women. Gout usually strikes middle-aged and older men, whereas polymyalgia rheumatica and pseudogout almost always occur in the elderly.

Patients with rheumatoid arthritis and other joint diseases complain of pain as the major symptom. Stiffness, muscle weakness, disability, swelling, tenderness, redness, heat, and deformity are other clinical features of rheumatic disease. Several rheumatic disorders affect the head and neck, and many cause primary arthritis of the temporomandibular joint. Still others exhibit nonarticular features in the mouth and teeth. A variety of biochemical and immunologic blood studies, as well as various roentgenographic procedures, provide more precise diagnosis, but these ancillary features alone are rarely diagnostic. Few forms of rheumatic diseases are curable, but most can be treated to the point that the patient is relatively asymptomatic. In some instances precise therapy is lifesaving. As with all diseases, proper management depends on proper diagnosis; therefore the development of a basic understanding of the various arthritic, connective tissue, and granulomatous diseases is a requisite for sound medical practice.

10·RHEUMATOID ARTHRITIS
Warren A. Katz

Although rheumatoid arthritis is a prototype of chronic destructive joint disease, the inflammatory process extends not only to the articular and tendon synovium but to many organs of the body. Rheumatoid arthritis is a protean disease: some patients exhibit mild evanescent arthritis, with 25% having one or more remissions, whereas others experience unrelenting joint inflammation with ultimate crippling that confines them to bed. Most patients, even those with early remissions, develop slowly progressive, moderately painful polyarthritis. However, patients with rehumatoid arthritis usually manage to function, although with difficulty.

Rheumatoid arthritis appears to be a disease of modern times, with no descriptions of it apparent in the literature before the 1800s. Innumerable research studies and new medical technical advances have not brought a cure but have enabled physicians to render most patients relatively symptom free and functional.

PATHOGENESIS AND PATHOLOGY. The cause of rheumatoid arthritis is unknown, but many investigators have suspected infections and genetic and endocrine factors. The current theory proposes that the genetically predisposed host (a locus related to HLA-DR4) subjected to a foreign, offensive agent, such as infection or trauma, undergoes unique immunologic changes that result in a perpetuating inflammatory process within the joints. Normally, in response to insult, the body mobilizes its immune defenses. IgG antibodies form in re-

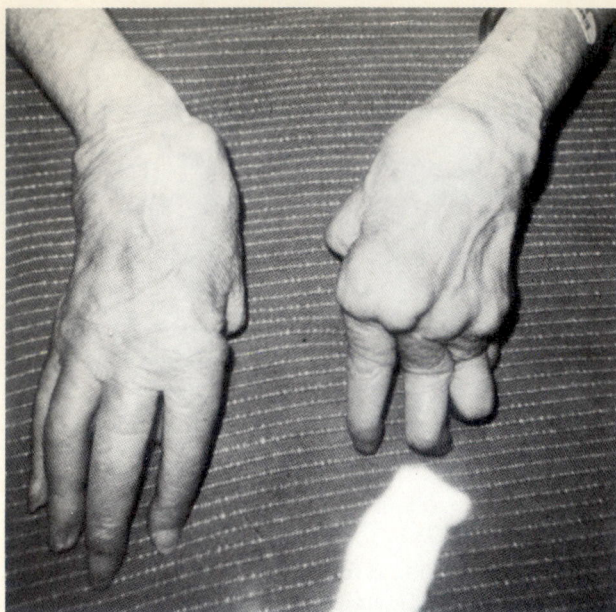

Fig. 10-1   Swan-neck deformity, ulnar deviation, dorsal interosseous muscle atrophy, and swelling of wrist—characteristics of rheumatoid arthritis.

sponse to antigenic stimulation but somehow become altered or aggregated in patients with rheumatoid arthritis so that the body no longer recognizes IgG as "self." Rheumatoid factor (RF) is an antibody against this altered IgG antibody, and molecules of RF can link together to form *self-associated rheumatoid factor complexes* that in effect generate inflammation. One theory contends that the offending agents in rheumatoid arthritis act as a chronic immunogenic stimulus. Furthermore, once destructive change in the joints occurs, altered cartilage components (proteoglycans) evoke additional immune responses, perpetuating inflammation. In the process the complement cascade is activated, and polymorphonuclear leukocytes are attracted and ingest immune complexes. These eventually trigger the release of multiple mediators of inflammation that include prostaglandins, elaboration of leukotrienes, oxygen free radicals, hydrolytic enzymes, and collagenase, all of which aid in joint destruction by the chronic rheumatoid granulomatous response referred to as *pannus*. How and why the rheumatoid process is self-propagating are poorly understood, but the ensuing antigen-antibody reaction begets more inflammation that further degrades IgG. The synovial immune response includes immune dysregulation, B lymphocyte proliferation, elaboration of rheumatoid factor, and immune complex formation.

CLINICAL MANIFESTATIONS. Rheumatoid arthritis can strike at any age, but bimodal distribution peaks are usually seen at 40 and 60 years of age. Women are two and a half times more likely than men to develop the disease. In some cases emotional stress, trauma, and exposure to infections seem to predispose to rheumatoid arthritis.

Onset. Rheumatoid arthritis may develop at any time and in many ways. The usual mode of onset is that of indolent polyarthralgias, sometimes preceded by fatigue and muscle aches. The hands, feet, elbows, shoulders, and knees may, in additive fashion, become involved. Prolonged morning stiffness and clumsiness may be relatively early symptoms. Within weeks symmetric polyarthritis characterized by tenderness and swelling becomes apparent. Less frequently, arthritis begins episodically in only one joint or causes excessive morning stiffness

without appreciable joint pain. In other cases a marked systemic component is present, characterized by low-grade fever, malaise, anorexia, and weight loss. Rarely, explosive polyarthritis may be associated with high fever. Occasionally, relatively asymptomatic progressive swelling of the joints occurs, particularly in the knees. Generalized weakness may accompany any presentation of arthritis.

Joint manifestations. Physical findings may be sparse in early rheumatoid arthritis. Ultimately, well-established patterns of involvement are noted, usually characterized by tenderness, swelling, and heat. Redness, except in very acute forms, is usually absent. Metacarpophalangeal joints, proximal interphalangeal joints, metatarsophalangeal joints, wrists, knees, shoulders, hips, elbows, ankles, tarsal joints, cervical spine, and temporomandibular joints are all prone to arthritis. The lower spine and distal interphalangeal joints are usually spared. The following is the distribution of joint involvement in adult rheumatoid arthritis:

Usual
  Ankles
  Cervical spine
  Elbows
  Hips
  Knees
  Metacarpophalangeal joints
  Metatarsophalangeal joints
  Proximal interphalangeal joints
  Shoulders
  Tarsal joints
  Temporomandibular joints
  Wrists
Unusual
  Carpometacarpal joints
  Cricoarytenoid joints
  Sacroiliac joints
  Sternoclavicular joints
Rare
  Distal interphalangeal joints
  Dorsal spine
  Lumbar spine

Painless tenosynovitis, particularly of the extensor carpi ulnaris tendon, may be one of the earliest signs of rheumatoid arthritis. Often a cystic swelling at the distal ulna is noted (double-hump sign). There is evidence of autonomic dysfunction in the hands and feet, such as palmar erythema, increased swelling, generalized edema, and a mottled appearance to the skin.

The changes of rheumatoid arthritis most useful for diagnosis are noted in the hands and wrists. Dorsal interosseous muscle atrophy frequently occurs. Swan-neck or boutonniére deformities of the hands are subsequent findings (Fig. 10-1). The metacarpophalangeal joints may be subluxated and deviated in an ulnar direction. Elbows become swollen and contracted. Limitation of motion is noted at the shoulders; with chronic progressive disease, the distal clavicles may erode and resorb.

One of the most ominous of all rheumatoid changes is subluxation of the first cervical vertebra on the second, which is caused by weakening of the transverse ligament. Although most patients with a C1-2 subluxation have no neurologic symptoms, occipital headaches, weakness, and digital paresthesias should alert the physician to the diagnosis. Sudden snapping of the neck or undue mobilization during anesthetic or dental procedures may cause further dislocation if caution is not taken.

Temporomandibular arthritis is not uncommon in the rheumatoid process. Jaw pain, especially when chewing, is the major symptom. Overt inflammation may be noted just anterior to the ear. Opening the mouth may cause a snap or click. Occasionally, crepitus and hypermobility of the jaw develop. Extensive resorption of the mandibular condyles may cause recession of the chin.

Extra-articular manifestations. In about one third of the patients with progressive rheumatoid arthritis, several extraarticular manifestations may be noted. These include subcutaneous rheumatoid nodules in areas of pressure, cardiac lesions (endocarditis, myocarditis, pericarditis), pulmonary lesions (pleuritis, parenchymal lung infiltration, rheumatoid nodules), peripheral neuritis, vasculitis, skin ulcerations, myositis, lymphadenopathy, and osteoporosis. Felty's syndrome is a complex of chronic rheumatoid arthritis, splenomegaly, anemia, thrombocytopenia, and neutropenia. Infections, leg ulcerations, and cutaneous pigmentation may be present with this disease.

Sjögren's syndrome

Sjögren's syndrome, seen predominantly in women, is a chronic inflammation of the salivary, lacrimal, and other secreting glands characterized primarily by keratoconjunctivitis sicca and xerostomia. Although a separate entity, it is often associated with rheumatoid arthritis. Dryness of the mouth, nose, eyes, tracheobronchial tree, rectum, and vagina may be profound. Patients complain of the tongue sticking to the roof of the mouth. The tongue is characteristically cracked, dry, and red. Salivary glands may be enlarged. Salivary flow rates are diminished or absent, and radioisotopic scintigraphy studies reveal glandular dysfunction. Diagnosis is confirmed by a lip biopsy. Renal tubular acidosis, nonthrombocytopenic purpura, polymyopathy, neuritis, chronic liver disease, lymphoma, interstitial lung disease, hyperviscosity, and other plasma cell dyscrasias may be noted. A variety of antibodies are associated with Sjögren's syndrome.

LABORATORY FINDINGS

Laboratory studies. None of the multiple blood, synovial fluid, and biopsy studies in rheumatoid arthritis is specific for the disease. Almost all patients exhibit an elevated erythrocyte sedimentation rate during active phases, but this is nonspecific.

Yet, a normal sedimentation rate should cause the physician to look on the diagnosis with some degree of suspicion. About 25% of patients with rheumatoid arthritis have some degree of anemia. This is usually a result of failure of iron utilization rather than direct iron loss through gastrointestinal blood loss.

Antinuclear antibody (ANA) is detectable in more than 50% of patients with rheumatoid arthritis but has no diagnostic specificity because many other connective tissue diseases are characterized by high titers of ANA.

About 80% of patients with classic or definite rheumatoid arthritis exhibit significant elevations of RF, which are not, however, diagnostic. The higher the titer of RF, the more likely the presence of rheumatoid arthritis, particularly when the titers are greater than 1:1280. The physician should bear in mind that RF does not parallel disease activity, although it is more likely to be present in high levels in patients with more advanced stages of the disease. High titers of RF, particularly when they appear early, seem to serve as indicators of a poor prognosis.

Rheumatoid synovial fluid is cloudy and often tinged green (Fig. 10-2). It forms a poor clot when acetic acid is added (Ropes test). The white cell counts may vary from 5000 to 60,000; the cells are predominantly polymorphonuclear leukocytes. White cells that have engulfed immune complexes are sometimes noted in rheumatoid synovial fluid in high numbers. These cytoplasmic inclusions in leukocytes are called *ragocytes*. Rheumatoid fluid is watery because of the breakdown of viscous protein hyaluronate. Glucose in rheumatoid synovial fluid and pleural fluid is appreciably lower than in serum. Rheumatoid nodules often give a characteristic pathologic picture on biopsy, but histologic evaluation of synovium, muscle, or other tissue mainly serves to rule out other confusing diseases.

Roentgenographic findings. Soft tissue swelling, subchondral osteopenia, marginal erosions, and joint space narrowing and deformity are the most common rheumatoid changes on roentgenograms, especially when symmetric (Fig. 10-3). Cervical spine roentgenograms may indicate a C1-2 subluxation that is recognized on the flexion-extension views as a widening of the interval between the odontoid process and the anterior

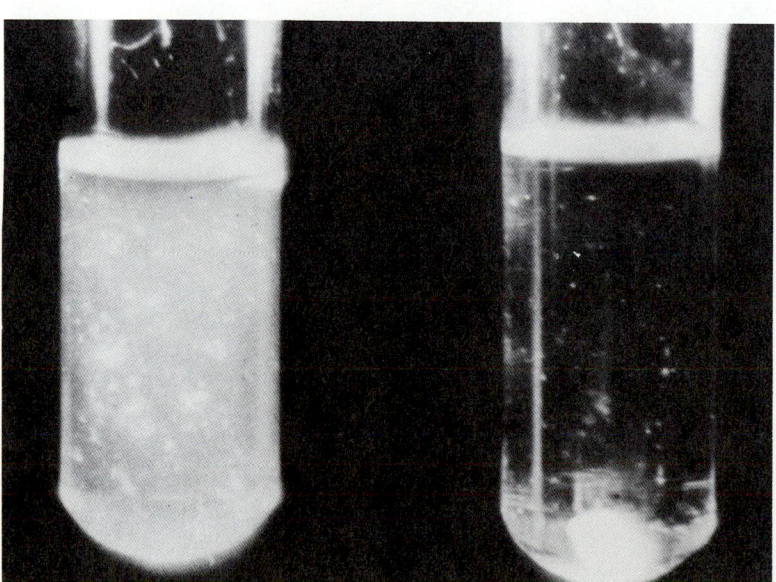

Fig. 10-2   Rheumatoid synovial fluid is cloudy and exhibits poor clotting when acetic acid is added *(left)*, compared to the tight clump formed in osteoarthritic fluid *(right)*. (From the Revised Clinical Slide Collection on the Rheumatic Diseases. Copyright 1981 by the Arthritis Foundation.)

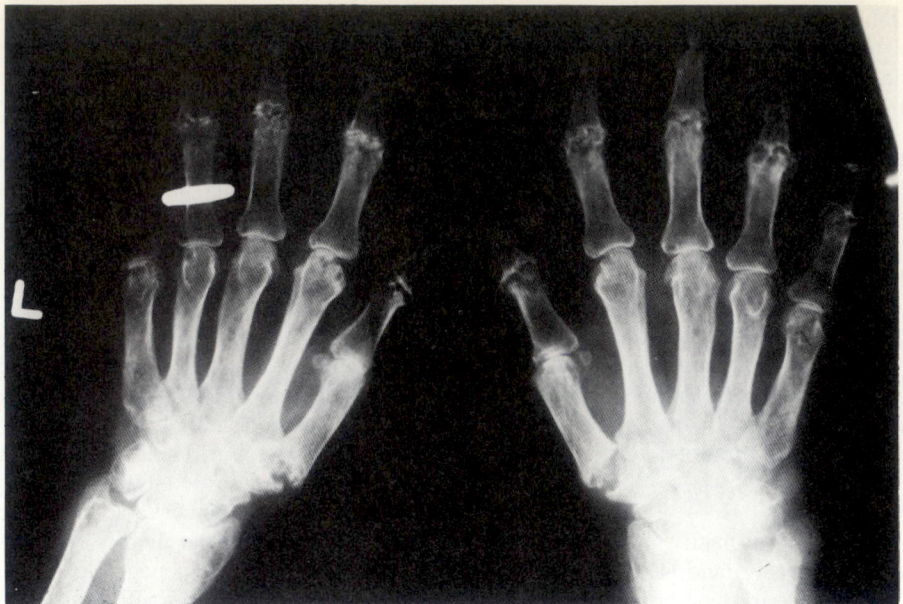

Fig. 10-3   Typical roentgenographic changes in hands of patient with rheumatoid arthritis. Note osteopenia, joint-space narrowing, and erosions. (From Katz WA: Rheumatic diseases: diagnosis and management, Philadelphia, 1977, JB Lippincott Co.)

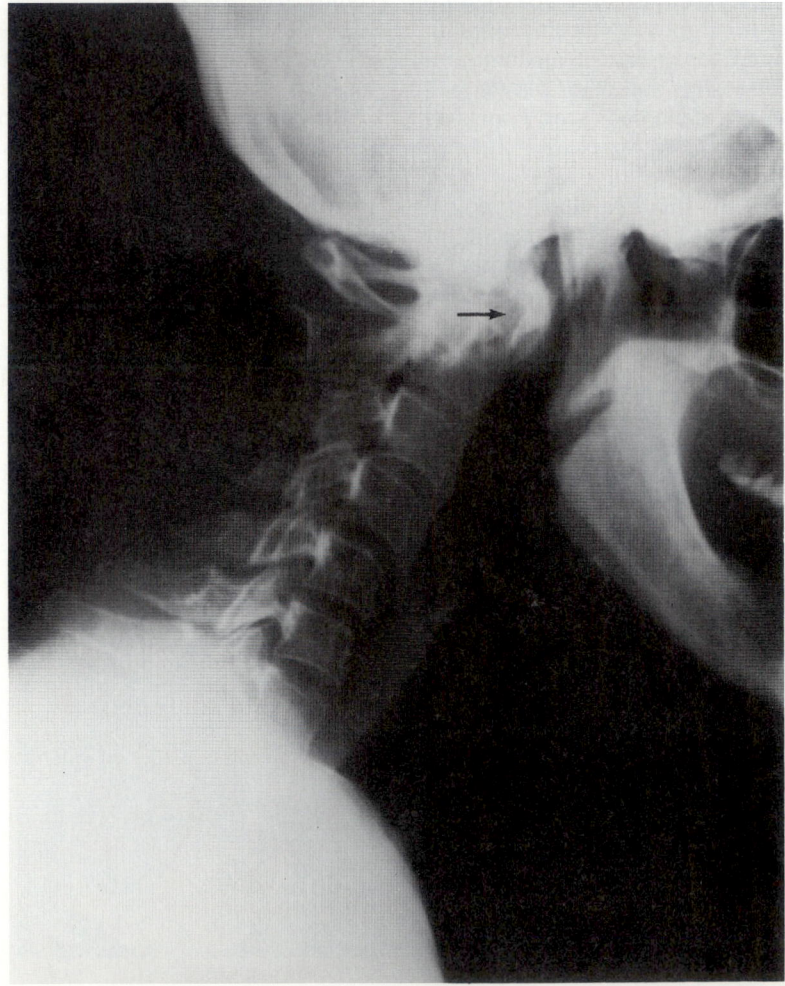

Fig. 10-4   C1-2 subluxation in rheumatoid arthritis. Arrow points to space between odontoid process and anterior arch of atlas.

Table 10-1 Nonsteroidal antiinflammatory drugs used in the treatment of rheumatoid arthritis.

Drug	Usual daily dose
Piroxicam	20 mg o.d.
Sulindac	150-200 mg b.i.d.
Naproxen	250-500mg b.i.d.
Salsalate	1000-1500 mg b.i.d.
Choline magnesium trisalicylate	1000-1500 mg b.i.d.
Diolofenae	25-75 mg b.i.d.
Flurbiprofen	100 mg b.i.d. or t.i.d.
Meclofenamic acid	50-100 mg t.i.d.
Ketoprofen	50-75 mg t.i.d.
Ibuprofen	400-800 mg t.i.d. or q.i.d.
Indomethacin	75 mg (SR) b.i.d.
	50-100 mg t.i.d. or q.i.d.
Aspirin	900 mg q.i.d.
Tolmetin	200-400 mg q.i.d.
Fenoprofen	300-600 mg q.i.d.

Table 10-2 Remittive drugs used in the treatment of rheumatoid arthritis

Drug	Usual dose
Antimalarials (chloroquine, 250 mg, or hydroxychloroquine, 200 mg)	One tablet b.i.d., then o.d.
Gold parenterally (sodium aurothiomalate or a urothioglucose)	Test dose 10 mg, then 25-50 mg weekly for 4-6 mo, then every 2 wk, then every 3 wk; maintenance dose 50 mg monthly as tolerated
Gold orally (auranofin, 3 mg)	One tablet b.i.d.
Methotrexate orally (2.5 mg)	One tablet t.i.d. once or twice *weekly*
Penicillamine (125-250 mg)	Initial dose 250 mg daily, raised by 125-mg increments every 6-8 wk as tolerated if active arthritis persists; maximal daily dose 1500 mg

ramus of the atlas (Fig. 10-4). Subluxation with a "staircase" appearance may be noted in lower cervical vertebrae.

Temporomandibular joint narrowing, erosion, subluxation, limitation of motion, and flattening of the condylar heads are apparent rheumatoid findings. Tomography, computed tomography scanning, or magnetic resonance is sometimes indicated to detect these changes.

DIAGNOSIS. The diagnosis of rheumatoid arthritis is based on a carefully obtained history, a diligent physical examination to uncover subtle signs of inflammation, and appropriate use of ancillary studies. By the time advanced deformities have taken place, the diagnosis is clear cut. The art of medicine in rheumatoid arthritis is to detect the disease as early as possible in an effort to prevent crippling changes.

The American Rheumatism Association's diagnostic criteria aid in clinical diagnosis but were primarily designed for research and literary purposes (see box on pp. 36 and 37).

Differential diagnosis includes ankylosing spondylitis, psoriatic arthritis, Reiter's syndrome, arthritis of chronic inflammatory bowel disease, infectious arthritis, chronic tophaceous gout, pseudogout, polytendinitis, osteoarthritis, reflex sympathetic dystrophy, sarcoidosis, and hypertrophic arthropathy. Other connective tissue diseases, such as systemic lupus erythematosus, polymyositis, and systemic sclerosis, may mimic the disease. In older people polymyalgia rheumatica, characterized by symmetric polyarthralgias in association with a markedly elevated erythrocyte sedimentation rate, poses a formidable differential diagnosis. Fibromyalgia syndrome is a relatively benign condition in terms of crippling; patients have multiple joint pain but no constitutional symptoms. The erythrocyte sedimentation rate is normal, and the test for RF is usually negative. Roentgenograms of the involved joints are normal. Some of these patients complain of jaw pain and clicking that may imitate arthritis of the temporomandibular joint.

MANAGEMENT. Clearly the success of managing rheumatoid arthritis lies in a comprehensive, multidisciplinary approach. Systemically administered drugs, local injections of corticosteroids, physical therapy, occupational therapy, psychosocial support, patient education, family involvement, surgical intervention, and vocational rehabilitation are all part of the daily management program of patients with rheumatoid arthritis.

In general patients should be fully and honestly indoctrinated concerning their disease and the advantages of proper therapy and should be assured of a favorable outcome in terms of crippling if the management program is followed. Families are frequently helpful in motivating patients, aiding them in taking their medications, and assisting in physical and occupational therapy. Patients with rheumatoid arthritis require a balance of rest and exercise. Although certain vitamins and diets appear to be effective in some patients with rheumatoid arthritis, none has been proved to be better than the expected placebo response. More investigation is certainly required before diet and vitamin therapy can be recommended to the exclusion of other modalities of therapy.

Drugs. The pharmaceutical agents used against rheumatoid arthritis include analgesics, nonsteroidal anti-inflammatory drugs (NSAIDs), corticosteroids, disease-modifying antirheumatic drugs, and immunosuppressive drugs. NSAIDs (Table 10-1), whether aspirin or the more potent, more expensive drugs, reduce inflammation and then pain. Because of significant differences in patient response to the NSAIDs, each patient should be given an adequate trial before abandoning this type of therapy. These drugs as a general class tend to cause gastrointestinal irritation and fluid retention. Skin rash and mouth ulcers may occur.

Systemic corticosteroids usually are reserved for certain cases of rheumatoid arthritis when other forms of therapy fail to stem a progressive, disabling, consumptive course. In all instances the dose of prednisone should be minimized.

On the other hand, local injections of corticosteroids, particularly after aspiration of one or two inflamed joints, may be extremely valuable and render the disease in some instances completely asymptomatic. At the very least, corticosteroid injections are adjunctive to systemic agents.

Available disease-modifying antirheumatic drugs include parenterally or orally administered gold, antimalarial drugs, methotrexate, and penicillamine (Table 10-2). With long-term administration these drugs stand the best chance of inducing remission or at least effecting a long-term suppression of symptoms. None of these drugs works well in all patients with rheumatoid arthritis, but those who respond tend to respond well. Significant alleviation of symptoms, however, is not to be expected before 6 weeks. The dose of penicillamine is gradually increased over several months. Major toxicity to parenteral gold consists of mouth ulcerations and skin rashes, but usually the drug can be recontinued after the side effects have cleared. Auranofin (orally administered gold) infrequently induces diarrhea. Antimalarial agents may cause gastrointestinal upset and changes in vision. Penicillamine may precipitate

---

AMERICAN RHEUMATISM ASSOCIATION CRITERIA FOR THE DIAGNOSIS OF RHEUMATOID ARTHRITIS

A. *Classical rheumatoid arthritis*
This diagnosis requires seven of the following criteria. In criteria 1 through 5 the joint signs or symptoms must be continuous for at least 6 weeks. (Any one of the features listed under "Exclusions" will exclude a patient from this and all categories.)
1. Morning stiffness.
2. Pain on motion or tenderness in at least one joint (observed by a physician).
3. Swelling (soft tissue thickening or fluid, not bony overgrowth alone) in at least one joint (observed by a physician).
4. Swelling (observed by a physician) of at least one other joint (any interval free of joint symptoms between the two joint involvements may not be more than 3 months).
5. Symmetrical joint swelling (observed by a physician) with simultaneous involvement of the same joint on both sides of the body (bilateral involvement of proximal interphalangeal, metacarpophalangeal, or metatarsophalangeal joints is acceptable without absolute symmetry). Terminal phalangeal joint involvement will not satisfy this criterion.
6. Subcutaneous nodules (observed by a physician) over bony prominences, on extensor surfaces, or in juxta-articular regions.
7. Roentgenographic changes typical of rheumatoid arthritis (which must include at least bony decalcification localized to or most marked adjacent to the involved joints and not just degenerative changes). Degenerative changes do not exclude patients from any group classified as rheumatoid arthritis.

8. Positive agglutination test—demonstration of the "rheumatoid factor" by any method which, in two laboratories, has been positive in not over 5% of normal controls—or positive streptococcal agglutination test. (The latter is now obsolete.)
9. Poor mucin precipitate from synovial fluid (with shreds and cloudy solution).
10. Characteristic histologic changes in synovium with three or more of the following: marked villous hypertrophy; proliferation of superficial synovial cells, often with palisading; marked infiltration of chronic inflammatory cells (lymphocytes or plasma cells predominating) with tendency to form "lymphoid nodules"; deposition of compact fibrin either on surface or interstitially; foci of necrosis.
11. Characteristic histologic changes in nodules show granulomatous foci with central zones of cell necrosis, surrounded by a palisade of proliferated macrophages, and peripheral fibrosis and chronic inflammatory cell infiltration, predominantly perivascular.

B. *Definite rheumatoid arthritis*
This diagnosis requires five of the above criteria. In criteria 1 through 5 the joint signs or symptoms must be continuous for at least 6 weeks.

C. *Probably rheumatoid arthritis*
This diagnosis requires three of the above criteria. In at least one of 1 through 5 the joint signs or symptoms must be continuous for at least 6 weeks.

D. *Possible rheumatoid arthritis*
This diagnosis requires two of the following criteria and total duration of joint symptoms must be at least 3 weeks.
1. Morning stiffness.
2. Tenderness or pain on motion (observed by a physician) with history of recurrence or persistence for 3 weeks.

---

mouth ulcers, renal toxicity, and gastrointestinal upset; some patients may note a rash. Bone marrow suppression may occur. A peculiar side effect is loss of taste, although smell usually remains intact. Azathioprine, another drug for the treatment of chronic, recalcitrant forms of rheumatoid arthritis is less frequently used.

Methotrexate was approved by the FDA in 1988 for administration to patients with resistant rheumatoid arthritis. It is used when NSAIDs and at least one disease-modifying antirheumatic drug have been ineffective or caused intolerable side effects. The majority of patients show improvement within several weeks to months of initiation of therapy, although clear-cut reduction in the incidence of erosion formation and deforming changes has not yet been demonstrated. The toxic effects of methotrexate can be reduced appreciably from those occurring in cancer patients who are treated with this drug by keeping the dose low (7.5 to 15 mg weekly) by either the oral or parenteral route. Nonetheless the physician usually observes for mouth ulcers, alopecia, liver toxicity, and bone marrow suppression.

Tranquilizers, antidepressants, and muscle relaxants may be prescribed for certain patients with rheumatoid arthritis. The physician must bear in mind that other illnesses that call for specific therapy may affect a rheumatoid patient beneficially.

Physical and occupational therapy. Pain relief and reduction of inflammation can be achieved through applications of heat and ice; the form used is a matter of personal preference. Range-of-motion exercises to all joints help prevent restriction of joints. Fitness and aerobic exercise programs seem to have a salutory effect on many patients. Splints of various types help immobilize the joint, reduce inflammation, and alleviate the pain.

Surgery. Various operations are now performed on patients with rheumatoid arthritis. Persistent synovitis, despite conservative but intensive medical therapy, may call for a synovectomy. In most cases, by the time surgery is performed, moderate to marked destructive changes are noted so that the surgeon is required to perform an arthroplasty in addition to a synovectomy. When the joint space is destroyed and the patient is rendered either disabled or in severe pain because of joint destruction, total joint replacement, such as a total knee or total hip arthroplasty, is considered.

Psychosocial-sexual problems. Psychologic ramifications of rheumatoid arthritis are unlimited. Some cases of rheumatoid arthritis arise from stressful situations; in others the rheumatoid arthritis itself creates the stress. It is almost impossible to treat patients with chronic rheumatoid arthritis without dealing with their problems of stress and other psychologic situations. Rheumatoid arthritis, by causing persistent pain and limitation of motion in key joints, presents sexual difficulties. When social or occupational difficulties arise, families, friends, and employers are often drawn into the therapeutic interaction.

Hospitalization. Most patients with rheumatoid arthritis do not require hospitalization, but removing the patient from his usual environment often fosters a remission of disease activity. Other advantages of hospitalization include facilitation of the indoctrination period when onset of rheumatoid arthritis is recent, intensive physical and occupational therapy, assurance that medication and other therapies are carried out, administration of potent drugs that need monitoring, and joint surgery in the setting of a comprehensive team approach.

PROGNOSIS. In most patients rheumatoid arthritis becomes chronic, but progressive disabling deformities are not inevitable. Most patients have flare-ups and exacerbations for many years, yet with proper management and encouragement they can work and function well in activities of daily living.

The prognosis is worse in females, when onset is insidious, and when active arthritis persists. The presence of multiple effusions, early constitutional symptoms, rheumatoid nodules, and high levels of RF in serum adversely affect the prognosis.

BIBLIOGRAPHY

Anderson PA and others: Weekly pulse methotrexate in rheumatoid arthritis, Ann Intern Med 103:489, 1985.
Bennett JC: The infectious etiology of rheumatoid arthritis: new considerations, Arthritis Rheum 21:531, 1978.
Bluestone R and Bacon PA: Extraarticular manifestations of rheumatoid arthritis, Clin Rheum Dis 3:385, 1973.
Bunch TW and O'Duffy JD: Disease-modifying drugs for progressive rheumatoid arthritis, Mayo Clin Proc 55:161, 1980.
Garber EK, Fan PT, and Bluestone R: Realistic guidelines of corticosteroid therapy in rheumatic disease, Semin Arthritis Rheum 11:231, 1981.
Harris ED Jr: Recent insights into the pathogenesis of the proliferative lesion in rheumatoid arthritis, Arthritis Rheum 19:68, 1966.
Jaffe IA: D-Penicillamine, Bull Rheum Dis 28:948, 1977–1978.
Johnson PM and Faulk WP: Rheumatoid factor: its nature, specificity, and production in rheumatoid arthritis, Clin Immunol Immunopathol 6:414, 1976.
Katz WA and others: The efficacy and safety of auranofin compared to placebo in rheumatoid arthritis, J Rheumatol [Suppl] 9:173, 1984.
Mason M and Currey HLF: Clinical rheumatology, Philadelphia, 1970, JB Lippincott Co.
McMichael AJ and others: Increased frequency of HLA-Cw3 and HLA-D24 in rheumatoid arthritis, Arthritis Rheum 20:1037, 1980.
Mowat AG and Huskisson EC: D-Penicillamine in rheumatoid arthritis, Clin Rheum Dis 1:319, 1975.
Short CL: Rheumatoid arthritis: types of courses and prognosis, Med Clin North Am 52:549, 1968.
Wolfe F and Hawley DJ: Remission in rheumatoid arthritis, J Rheumatol 12:245, 1985.
Yoshimo S and Uchida S: Sexual problems of women with rheumatoid arthritis, Arch Phys Med Rehabil 62:122, 1981.

11·JUVENILE RHEUMATOID ARTHRITIS

Balu H. Athreya

Juvenile rheumatoid arthritis (JRA) is a disease characterized by chronic synovitis, with or without extra-articular manifestations. It is also known as Still's disease, juvenile chronic polyarthritis, and chronic childhood arthritis; the preferred term in the United States is JRA.

There are approximately 100,000 to 200,000 children with JRA in the United States. The ratio of JRA compared with adult rheumatoid arthritis is approximately 1:20. JRA has been reported from tropical, subtropical, and temperate climates.

JRA is not a single disease; it is probably a group of diseases. There are at least five recognized subgroups, each with a fairly characteristic clinical course and prognosis. Whether splitting JRA into subgroups will lead to better understanding of the cause or pathogenesis remains to be seen.

JRA is a *chronic* disease. Since there are no diagnostic laboratory tests, it is diagnosed *clinically* after *exclusion* of other diseases.

ETIOLOGY. The etiology of JRA is unknown. A history of recent systemic infection or trauma is obtained in many patients with JRA. Exacerbations of the disease may follow intercurrent infections, trauma, or psychologic stress. Usually there is no family history of rheumatoid arthritis. Most of the subtypes occur more commonly in girls than in boys, suggesting an endocrine influence. Genetic factors may also play a part, as shown by the association between HLA (histocompatibility) antigens and various subtypes of JRA. For example, HLA-B35 has been associated with the systemic type and HLA-DR5 with the pauciarticular variety. HLA-DR4 is associated with rheumatoid factor–positive (seropositive) JRA, as in adults with seropositive rheumatoid arthritis.

The proposed etiologic mechanisms and pathology are similar to those in adults, but there are many differences in the clinical syndromes (Chapter 10). Even rheumatoid factor (RF), which is present in over 80% of adults with rheumatoid arthritis, is found in less than 20% of children with JRA. It is also interesting to note that, in children with agammaglobulinemia and IgA deficiency, chronic polyarthritis indistinguishable from JRA may develop.

CLINICAL MANIFESTATIONS OF VARIOUS SUBTYPES (TABLE 11-1). JRA is classified into various subgroups according to the mode of *onset*, as systemic, polyarticular, or pauciarticular (Table 11-1). The onset period is defined as the first 6 months after the start of the illness. A recent follow-up study showed that the *course* after the first 6 months is as important to the outcome as the onset.

Polyarticular (RF-positive) JRA. Polyarticular (RF-positive) JRA occurs in approximately 10% of children with JRA. As the name implies, these children have RF in the serum, and the disease course resembles adult-onset arthritis. Girls are more often affected. The onset is usually in the preadolescent age group and is characterized by symmetric and polyarticular

involvement of both large and small joints. Characteristic swelling of small joints of the fingers is common (Fig. 11-1). The cervical spine is involved in approximately 30% of the children, as evidenced by neck pain, torticollis, and limitation of range of movement of the neck. Subluxation of the atlantoaxial joint is a serious consequence of cervical spine involvement. This is an important point to remember, since careless manipulation of the neck during anesthesia in the presence of atlantoaxial subluxation may be fatal.

Temporomandibular joint (TMJ) involvement is also common in this group. The involvement may be unilateral or bilateral, with such symptoms as pain at the joint, ear pain, pain during eating, and inability to open the mouth. Micrognathia (Fig. 11-2) is also a common feature in children with severe polyarticular disease.

Other findings include low-grade fever, loss of weight, anemia, and growth retardation. Morning stiffness is very common and often disabling. Rheumatoid nodules occur most commonly in this group and are seen often over the extensor aspect of the joints and behind the ear. Sjögren's syndrome and rheumatoid vasculitis may also develop in this age group. All these patients have RF in the serum, and almost 75% have antinuclear antibody (ANA).

Polyarticular (RF-negative) JRA. Polyarticular (RF-negative) JRA occurs in almost 30% of patients with JRA. It affects mostly girls, and the clinical characteristics are similar to those of polyarticular (RF-positive) disease. The major differences are that (1) RF is absent in the serum; (2) onset is common at any age; (3) prognosis is more favorable (Table 11-1); (4) rheumatoid vasculitis does not occur; and (5) erosions are less common. About 5% of these patients have ANA in the serum. Approximately 30% of children with polyarticular JRA enter remission, although only half of this group maintains this remission. The majority of the children, particularly those with seropositive disease, follow a polyarticular course.

Pauciarticular JRA (type 1). Pauciarticular JRA (type 1) with chronic iridocyclitis occurs predominantly in girls under

Table 11-1 Subgroups of JRA

Subgroup	Sex ratio	Age at onset	Joints affected	Serologic and genetic tests*	Extra-articular manifestations	Prognosis
RF positive, polyarticular	80% girls	Late childhood	Any joints	ANA 75% RF 100%	Low-grade fever, anemia, malaise, rheumatoid nodules	>50% severe arthritis
RF negative, polyarticular	90% girls	Any age	Any joints	ANA 5% RF negative	Low-grade fever, mild anemia, malaise, growth retardation	10%-15% severe arthritis
Pauciarticular (type 1)	80% girls	Early childhood	A few large joints (hips and sacroiliac joints spared)	ANA 50% RF negative	Few constitutional complaints, chronic iridocyclitis in 50%	Severe arthritis uncommon, 10%-20% ocular damage from iridocyclitis
Pauciarticular (type 2)	90% boys	Late childhood	A few large joints (hip and sacroiliac involvement common)	ANA negative RF negative HLA-B27 75%	Few constitutional complaints, acute iridocyclitis in 5%-10% during childhood	Some have ankylosing spondylitis at follow-up
Systemic onset	60% boys	Any age	Any joints	ANA negative RF negative	High fever, rash, organomegaly, polyserositis, leukocytosis, growth retardation	25% severe arthritis

Modified from Schaller JG: The spectrum of juvenile rheumatoid arthritis. In Franklin EC, editor: Clinical immunology update, New York, 1979, Elsevier Publishing Co.
*ANA, antinuclear antibody; RF, rheumatoid factor; HLA-B27, histocompatibility antigen-B27.

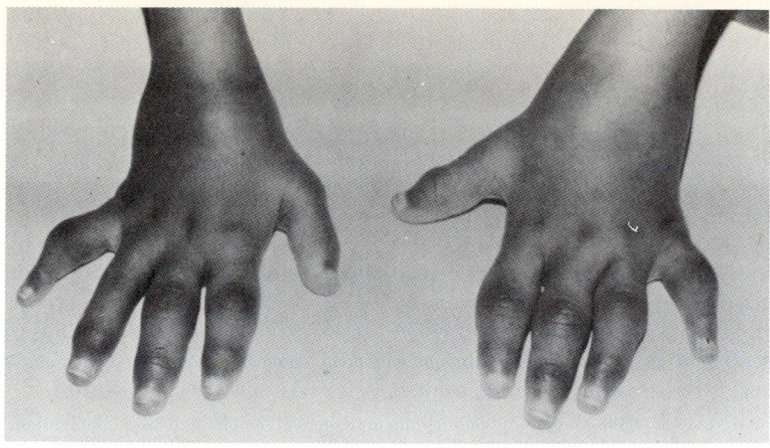

Fig. 11-1   Hands of child with severe JRA. Note bilateral involvement of wrists and small joints of fingers.

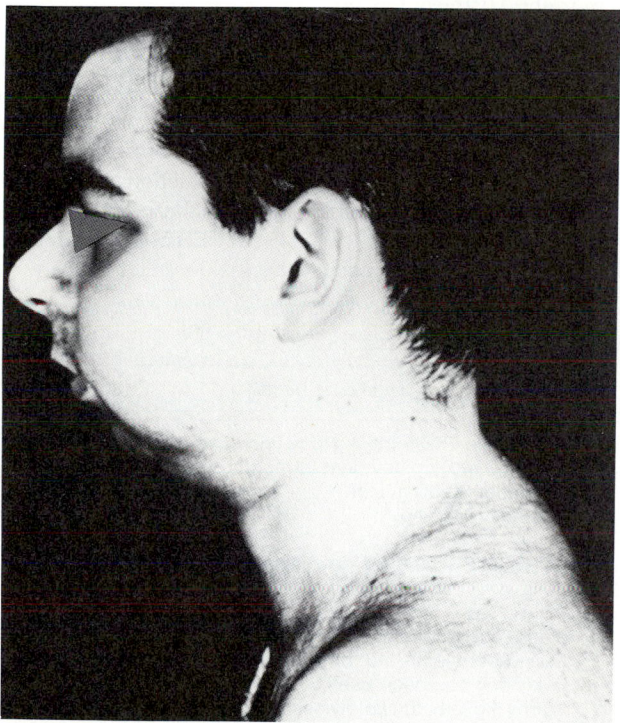

Fig. 11-2   Micrognathia of JRA. (From the Revised Clinical Slide Collection on the Rheumatic Diseases. Copyright 1981 by the Arthritis Foundation.)

5 years of age. It accounts for almost 25% of patients with JRA. The term "pauciarticular" denotes that these children have four or less joints affected during the first 6 months of the disease. Usually large joints are affected, although not to the exclusion of the temporomandibular joints, cervical spine, and small joints of the fingers. Even though these children may have chronic or recurrent bouts of arthritis, serious disability rarely occurs.

Children in this particular group, however, are at high risk for chronic iridocyclitis. The iridocyclitis can occur before, during, or after the onset of arthritis. It is usually unilateral and insidious in onset (unlike acute iridocyclitis of ankylosing spondylitis). Occasionally, patients complain of watering from the eyes and photophobia. Routine slit-lamp examination, even in asymptomatic patients, may show early evidence of irido-

cyclitis. Therefore it is advisable to repeat the procedure every 3 months. If not detected and treated early, the iridocyclitis may progress to corneal opacity, posterior synechiae, secondary glaucoma, cataracts, and phthisis bulbi.

About half of the children in this group (pauciarticular type 1) have ANA in the serum, and these are the children at high risk for iridocyclitis.

Pauciarticular JRA (type 2). Pauciarticular JRA (type 2) is seen in almost 15% of children with JRA. These are mostly preadolescent boys. They do not have RF or ANA in the serum. Although they are classified clinically as having JRA at the time of diagnosis, the condition of many will probably evolve into ankylosing spondylitis or Reiter's syndrome. About 75% of the children in this group carry HLA-B27 antigen. They are more likely to have acute than chronic iridocyclitis. The remission rate in the entire pauciarticular group is about 15% to 20%. Only half of these maintain the remission. The majority of the children follow an oligoarticular course. A small percentage of this group who are also seropositive for rheumatoid factor have a polyarticular course with erosive arthritis.

Systemic-onset JRA. Systemic-onset JRA, also known as the febrile form or Still's disease, occurs in 20% of children with JRA. This is most common in children under age 5, although it is now being recognized later in life as adult-onset Still's disease. It occurs in both boys and girls. The onset is characterized by high fevers, up to 104° F (40° C), which should initially alert physicians to exclude various infectious diseases. These children get an evanescent, macular pink rash that appears during the height of fever. It is seen mostly on the trunk and upper arm and is nonpruritic. Generalized lymphadenopathy and hepatosplenomegaly are common; therefore leukemia and neuroblastoma have to be considered in the differential diagnosis and excluded. Pleuritis and pericarditis may be heralded by chest pain. In the early stages these children may have arthralgia, muscle spasm, and morning stiffness but no true synovitis. After 1 or 2 years, febrile episodes subside, but polyarticular arthritis remains as the major problem. RF or ANA are not detected in the serum.

Fever and the other systemic manifestations of systemic-onset JRA usually subside in 2 to 5 years. Remission is seen in about 50% of children with this onset type. Those who enter remission seem to maintain the remission. Others follow either a polyarticular or an oligoarticular pattern.

LABORATORY FINDINGS. Mild to moderate anemia and leukocytosis (up to $50,000/mm^3$) are common, particularly in systemic JRA. Platelet counts, when elevated in the systemic and polyarticular varieties, often indicate poor prognosis for full recovery. Urinalysis findings are normal. Acute phase reactants, such as erythrocyte sedimentation rate (ESR), C-reactive protein, haptoglobin, and C3 complement, are elevated, even in the pauciarticular variety. Serum proteins are often abnormal with elevated α_2-globulins and γ-globulins. RF factor ($>1:40$) is demonstrated in the serum of all patients with the special RF-positive subtype described earlier, but it is present in only 10% to 20% of the entire group. ANA may be present in the sera of patients with polyarticular arthritis (both types) and pauciarticular arthritis (type 1) but not in pauciarticular arthritis (type 2) and systemic forms.

Synovial fluid analysis is often essential in the diagnosis of pauciarticular arthritis. The fluid appears cloudy, with an increased number of cells (up to $100,000/mm^3$), most of which are polymorphonuclear. Glucose levels are normal, cultures are negative, and levels of C3 and C4 may be low.

Early roentgenographic findings of affected joints include swelling of soft tissue, effusion, and periostitis. Later, osteoporosis and accelerated bone growth may be seen. In longstanding arthritis, subchondral erosions, narrowing of joint space, bone destruction, and fusion may develop. In roentgenograms of the temporomandibular joint, erosion, flattening, and rarefaction of the condyle are seen. The glenoid fossa is often shallow.

DIFFERENTIAL DIAGNOSIS. Since JRA is a diagnosis of exclusion and there are many subgroups, the differential di-

Table 11-2   Drug treatment of JRA

Drug	Initial dose range	Side effects
Acetylsalicylic acid (aspirin, ASA)	Initial dose 75-90 mg/kg/day, increase gradually to 120 mg/kg/day, aim for serum salicylate level of 20-30 mg/dl	Gastric irritation, hepatotoxicity, hyperpnea, platelet problems, Reye's syndrome
Nonsteroidal antiinflammatory drugs (NSAIDs)	Alternative to aspirin	
Tolmetin (Tolectin), FDA approved for pediatric use	Initial dose 15 mg/kg/day, increase to 30 mg/kg/day, maximal dose 1800 mg/day	Gastric irritation, headache, hematuria
Indomethacin (Indocin), not approved by FDA	Initial dose 0.5 mg/kg/day, increase gradually to 2.5 mg/kg/day or a maximal of 100 mg/day	Gastric irritation, headache, hematuria
Ibuprofen (Motrin), not approved by FDA	Dose not established for children, up to 40 mg/kg/day has been used	Transient rash, gastric irritation, thrombocytopenia, hematuria
Naproxen (Naprosyn)	10 mg/kg/day in two divided doses	Gastric irritation, rash, headache
Slow-acting antirheumatic drugs (SAARDs)	Administered with aspirin or one of the NSAID	
Gold parenterally (Myochrysine or Solganal)	Weekly injections for 20-24 wk; test dose is 2 mg for infants, 5 mg for older children, 10 mg for adolescents, intramuscular If no anaphylactoid reaction to test dose, increase weekly dose gradually, with 0.25 mg/kg on wk 1, 0.5 mg/kg on wk 2, 0.75 mg/kg on wk 3; maintain on 1 mg/kg/wk with maximal single weekly dose of 25 mg for older children and 50 mg for adolescents; after 20-24 wk, if no response, discontinue; with response, continue at same dose but only once monthly	Rash, bone marrow depression, renal toxicity
Gold orally (Ridaura)	0.1-0.2 mg/kg/day in two divided doses; maximal 6 mg/day	Diarrhea, rash Anemia, hematuria
Chloroquine (Aralen)	4-5 mg/kg/day, maximal 250 mg/day	Toxicity to retina, corneal deposits, bleaching of hair, light sensitivity
Hydrochloroquine (Plaquenil)	7-8 mg/kg/day, maximal 400 mg/day	
Penicillamine (Cuprimine, Depen)	Initial dose 3 mg/kg/day, after 1 mo increase to 6 mg/kg/day, after 3 mo increase to 9 mg/kg/day	Skin rash, renal toxicity, bone marrow depression
Corticosteroids	Use sparingly and for as short a time as possible; intraarticular corticosteroids for persistently active single joint disease, topical use for iridocyclitis	Many side effects include growth retardation, osteoporosis, hypertension

agnostic process should continue throughout follow-up. A male child with pauciarticular arthritis may have clinical features of seronegative spondyloarthropathies in later life. A child with the systemic type of JRA may later show features of systemic lupus erythematosus.

In the systemic form, infections, leukemia, and neuroblastoma have to be ruled out. In the monoarticular variety, however, local causes of joint disease, such as infectious arthritis, aseptic necrosis, and pigmented villonodular synovitis, must be considered. In the differential diagnosis of early stages of polyarticular arthritis, the following diseases have to be considered: acute rheumatic fever, systemic lupus erythematosus, gonococcal arthritis-dermatitis syndrome, and scleroderma. The differential diagnosis of pauciarticular arthritis includes ankylosing spondylitis, Reiter's syndrome, arthritis of inflammatory bowel disease, and Lyme disease.

MANAGEMENT. Since JRA carries a reasonably good prognosis and is not life threatening, the goals of treatment should be (1) to treat with drugs less dangerous than the disease, (2) to preserve joint function, and (3) to educate the family and the child so that the child is encouraged to lead as normal a life as possible. This requires a comprehensive management program supervised by a primary physician. Teamwork involving the primary physician, rheumatologist, child, family, orthopedic surgeon, physical therapist, occupational therapist, school teacher, school gym teacher, and orthodontist is ideal.

Bed rest is not of proven value, particularly in the pediatric age group, except in the presence of pericarditis. Local rest, best provided with a splint, is indicated for severely inflamed joints. Proper nutrition is obviously needed. A list of drugs commonly used in this disease is given in Table 11-2. Of these drugs, acetylsalicylic acid (aspirin, ASA) is the safest, simplest, and most economic and is adequate to control the disease in over 80% of cases. One of the other nonsteroidal anti-inflammatory drugs (NSAIDs) may be used in the place of ASA, but none of them is more effective than ASA. One of these drugs is used when the child is allergic to ASA or has gastric or hepatic complications with ASA. After a trial with one of these drugs (ASA or NSAID) for 6 to 12 weeks in adequate dosages with no response, one of the drugs from the slow-acting antirheumatic group (SAARD), such as gold, is added to the treatment program. Steroids are used only for pericarditis, severe systemic forms of JRA unresponsive to therapy, or severe iridocyclitis. Local steroids are used for less severe eye disease and for intra-articular injections of single joints with severe inflammation.

Simple measures to alleviate morning stiffness include sleeping in a sleeping bag and taking warm tub baths in the morning. Physical therapy and occupational therapy programs should be tailored to the child's age and developmental needs and the family's problems. Simple activities such as tricycling, bicycling, and swimming are more likely to be followed than formal therapy programs. Children with severe deformities and active disease may need intensive therapy programs.

Children with severe TMJ pain may have to be fed liquids with a straw to maintain nutrition. Fortunately, this is needed for only 1 or 2 days during an acute flare-up. The best physical therapy program for TMJ, in my experience, is chewing gum.

In the pediatric age group, orthopedic surgery is infrequently indicated. Soft tissue surgery to release contractures is likely to be needed more often than synovectomy or joint replacement. Total hip replacements, however, have been performed successfully in teenagers.

Iridocyclitis needs urgent, expert care. All children with JRA require yearly slit-lamp examinations. Children with pauciar-

ticular arthritis (type 1) should have their eyes checked every 3 months during the active stage of the disease and every 6 months for 4 to 5 years after the arthritis is controlled or until the child reaches 17 years of age.

PROGNOSIS. With proper total care, most children with JRA should be able to lead active lives. Although there is no "cure" for this disease, it is not a "killing disease," and prognosis is good for most patients. About 15% of these patients have mild to moderate deformities. Less than 5% are left with severe deformities. The mortality rate is less than 1%. The prognosis is worse for children with systemic and polyarticular (RF-positive) varieties of JRA. For children with pauciarticular (type 1) JRA, the major problems are related to the eyes.

BIBLIOGRAPHY

Brewer EJ, Giannini EH, and Person DA: Juvenile rheumatoid arthritis. Vol VI. Major problems in clinical pediatrics, ed 2, Philadelphia, 1982, WB Saunders Co.

Calabro JJ et al: Juvenile rheumatoid arthritis: a general review and report of 100 patients observed for 15 years, Semin Arthritis Rheum 5:257, 1976.

Cassidy JT et al: A study of classification criteria for a diagnosis of juvenile rheumatoid arthritis, Arthritis Rheum 29:274, 1986.

Howard JF, Sigsbee A, and Glass DN: HLA genetics and inherited predisposition to JRA: an editorial, J Rheum 12:7, 1985.

Proceedings of the ARA conference on the rheumatic diseases of childhood, Arthritis Rheum 20(suppl 2):1, 1977.

Schaller JG: The spectrum of juvenile rheumatoid arthritis. In Franklin EC, editor: Clinical immunology update, New York, 1979, Elsevier Publishing Co.

12·ANKYLOSING SPONDYLITIS

John J. Calabro

Ankylosing spondylitis (AS) is a heterogeneous rheumatic disorder characterized by inflammation of the sacroiliac and the spinal (axial) and large peripheral joints, as well as a host of systemic manifestations. It affects 3 million Americans and is the third most prevalent form of arthritis, following osteoarthritis (16 million) and rheumatoid arthritis (8 million).

EPIDEMIOLOGY. AS is three times more frequent in men than in women and begins most often between 20 and 40 years of age. Familial clustering and the higher than expected frequency of the HLA-B27 tissue antigen among patients support a genetic basis for this disease, although environmental factors also appear to be operative. Based on two American surveys, one of B27-positive blood donors and another of B27-positive tissue donors, it has been calculated that the risk for development of spondylitis in individuals having the B27 antigen may be as high as 20%.

CLINICAL MANIFESTATIONS. The early diagnosis of AS rests on the recognition of three distinct modes of onset: back pain, peripheral arthritis, and uveitis. The subsequent course of disease is highly variable and unpredictable, as is the occurrence of systemic manifestations.

SIGNS AND SYMPTOMS. Although back pain is the most frequent initial symptom, AS can begin atypically in peripheral joints, especially in children and women, and even with acute iritis (anterior uveitis), although this is rare. Whatever the mode of onset, recurrent back pain that is often nocturnal and of varing intensity is an eventual complaint, as is early morning stiffness that is characteristically relieved by activity. Patients automatically ease back pain and paraspinal muscle spasm by adopting a flexed or bent-over posture. Consequently, in untreated persons some degree of kyphosis is a common sequela. Another early sign is diminished chest expansion that results from diffuse costovertebral involvement. Additional early symptoms are fever, fatigue, anorexia, weight loss, and anemia.

SYSTEMIC MANIFESTATIONS. Systemic findings include recurrent attacks of acute iritis that affect a third of patients but are usually self-limiting. Only rarely are bouts of iritis protracted and severe enough to impair vision. Neurologic signs result from compression radiculitis or sciatica, vertebral fracture or subluxation, and the cauda equina syndrome. The last produces impotency, nocturnal incontinence of urine, diminished bladder and rectal sensation, and absence of ankle jerks. Cardiovascular manifestations include angina, pericarditis, electrocardiographic conduction abnormalities, and rarely aortic insufficiency. A rare pulmonary finding is upper lobe fibrosis, occasionally with cavitations that may be mistaken for tuberculosis and complicated by infection with *Aspergillus* organisms.

LABORATORY FINDINGS. The Westergren erythrocyte sedimentation rate (ESR) is elevated in most patients with active disease, as are other acute phase reactants, such as serum IgA levels. Notably negative are tests for both IgM rheumatoid factor (latex fixation) and antinuclear antibodies. A positive test for the HLA-B27 antigen is the best single laboratory clue. Its absence, however, does not preclude a diagnosis of AS.

ROENTGENOGRAPHIC FINDINGS. Diagnosis must be confirmed by roentgen-ray examination. The earliest abnormalities occur in the sacroiliac joints and include pseudowidening or narrowing of these articulations from subchondral erosions and sclerosis. Early changes in the spine are diffuse vertebral squaring and demineralization, as well as spotty ligamentous calcification and one or two evolving syndesmophytes. The classic "bamboo spine," with its prominent syndesmophytes and diffuse paraspinal ligamentous calcification (the usual textbook illustration), is not useful for early diagnosis. In fact, such advanced changes occur in only 10% of patients and take an average of 10 years to develop.

DIFFERENTIAL DIAGNOSIS. One of the most important disorders from which AS must be differentiated is a herniated intervertebral disc. This condition is limited to the spine, has no systemic manifestations such as fatigue, anorexia, or weight loss, and does not produce laboratory test abnormalities, even of the ESR. The only certain way to diagnose a herniated disc is to confirm the defect by myelography or a computerized tomography (CT) scan.

A more difficult diagnosis to rule out is the diffuse idiopathic skeletal hyperostosis (DISH) syndrome. It occurs primarily in men over 50 years of age and may resemble AS both clinically and roentgenographically. Patients with the DISH syndrome may have spinal pain, stiffness, and loss of spine motion that develops insidiously. Findings on roentgen-ray examination include ligamentous calcification, which most often affects the cervical and lower thoracic spine. However, in the DISH syndrome the sacroiliac and spinal apophyseal joints are not involved. Moreover, the ESR is normal, and the DISH syndrome is not linked to the B27 antigen.

MANAGEMENT. Effective management demands both immediate and long-term objectives. The physician must first relieve the patient's joint discomfort with antirheumatic drugs and then begin long-range planning to prevent, delay, or correct deformity. Consequently, daily exercises and other supportive measures are vital to promote proper posture and joint motion. The objective of all supportive measures, whether they be postural training or therapeutic exercise, is to build up muscle groups that oppose the direction of potential deformities and thus to strengthen extensor rather than flexor muscle groups.

Finally, the psychosocial and rehabilitative needs of the patient require careful attention in long-range planning.

Drug therapy

Nonsteroidal antiinflammatory drugs. By suppressing articular inflammation, pain, and spasm, the nonsteroidal antiinflammatory drugs (NSAIDs) facilitate exercise and other supportive measures. The drugs listed in Table 12-1 should be considered first, since these are of proven value in AS. Although aspirin or other salicylates may be tried first, they are seldom adequate and in no way comparable to the effectiveness of other drugs, such as phenylbutazone, indomethacin, sulindac, or naproxen.

The task of selecting the most appropriate drug is often influenced more by tolerance or potential toxic risks than by marginal differences in efficacy. Regardless of the choice, patients should be monitored and warned of potential adverse reactions. Moreover, patients receiving phenylbutazone should be routinely screened for rare but serious renal or hematopoietic adverse reactions, including fatal aplastic anemia. Consequently, complete blood and platelet counts as well as a urinalysis must be performed weekly for the initial 2 months and then monthly thereafter.

The average daily dosage and range of approved drugs are listed in Table 12-1. Every effort should be made to reduce the daily dose to the lowest possible. Complete drug withdrawal should be attempted only slowly and after all systemic and articular signs of active disease have been suppressed for several months.

Orally administered corticosteroids have limited therapeutic value in management. In fact, their long-term use may be risky, predisposing patients to steroid-induced compression fractures of the spine or ischemic necrosis of the femoral head. For acute iritis, topically administered steroids (and mydriatric agents) are usually adequate, so oral administration of steroids is rarely indicated. The use of intraarticular steroids may prove beneficial, particularly when one or two peripheral joints are more severely inflamed than others, thereby compromising exercise and rehabilitation.

Miscellaneous drugs. The slow-acting (remittive) drugs used in rheumatoid arthritis, such as orally or intramuscularly administered gold, have never been shown to be effective in AS and are therefore not recommended. All narcotic drugs, strict analgesic agents, and muscle relaxants lack the antiinflammatory property required for effective disease suppression. Consequently, except when prescribed for short periods to control severe back pain and spasm, they should be avoided.

Radiation. Radiotherapy to the spine, although an effective form of therapy, should be recommended only as a last resort. Unfortunately, patients receiving irradiation have a twofold risk of subsequent development of acute myelogenous leukemia.

Physical therapy

Postural training. To prevent the tendency to stoop, the patient must always consciously stand as erect as possible and walk "tall." Even when picking up objects from the floor, the patient should not bend over but should "squat erect." The patient must always sit erect, preferably on a chair with a hard, straight back and seat. Suitable braces may help to maintain good posture, but most patients do as well without them.

Therapeutic exercise. Prescribed by a physician or a qualified associate, exercise must become an intrinsic part of the patient's daily life (Fig. 12-1). The use of heat to alleviate stiffness and discomfort, particularly a warm shower on arising, helps to enhance exercise and activity. Therapeutic exercise must be tailored not only to the degree of spine involvement but also to the patient's age, strength, and capacity to

Table 12-1   Chronologic listing of nonsteroidal antiinflammatory drugs for ankylosing spondylitis*

Drug (U.S. marketing)	Average daily dosage (range) for adults	Major adverse reactions
Acetylsalicyclic acid (1915)†	4 g (3-6 g)	Tinnitus, deafness, gastric distress, ulcer
Phenylbutazone (1952)‡	300 mg (100-400 mg)	Gastric distress, ulcer, stomatitis, nephrotoxicity, suppression of hematopoiesis§
Indomethacin (1965)	100 mg (25-200 mg)	Headache, drowsiness, gastric distress, ulcer
Naproxen (1976)†	750 mg (250-1000 mg)	Gastric distress, ulcer
Sulindac (1978)	300 mg (100-400 mg)	Gastric distress, ulcer
Sustained-release indomethacin (1982)	75 mg (75-150 mg)	Headache, drowsiness, gastric distress, ulcer

*Only nonsteroidal antiinflammatory drugs with U.S. Food and Drug Administration (FDA) approval for ankylosing spondylitis are included.

†Of those listed, only salicylates and naproxen have FDA approval for children under 15 years of age. For children the average daily dosage of acetylsalicylic acid is 80 mg/kg and that of naproxen, 10-15 mg/kg.

‡Currently recommended only after other drugs have been tried first.

§Including anemia, leukopenia, agranulocytosis, thrombocytopenia, and aplastic anemia.

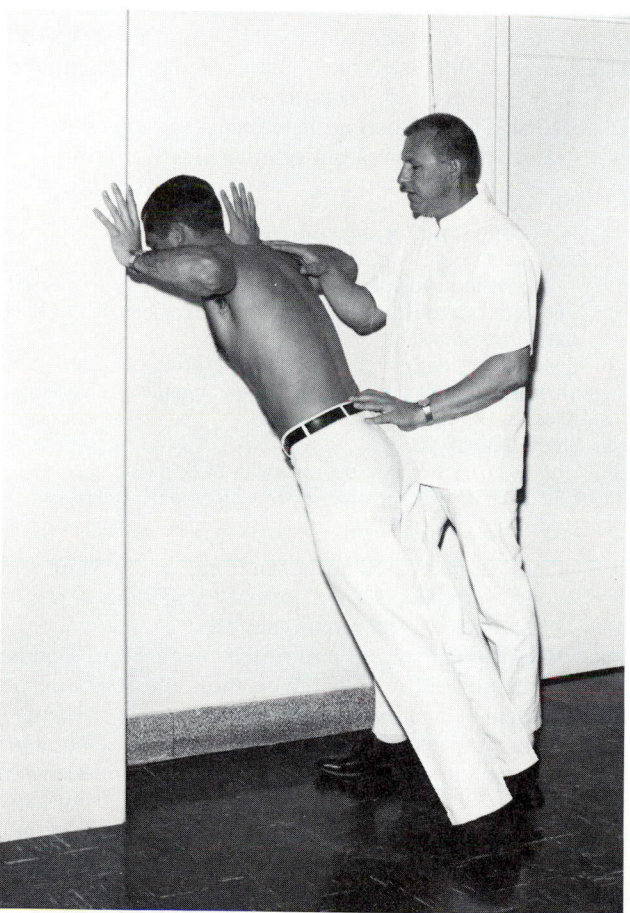

Fig. 12-1   Exercise combining spinal extension and chest expansion. Patient faces corner of room and touches opposite walls at shoulder height. Patient bends elbows and leans forward, extending neck and inhaling as deeply as possible. Patient returns to original upright position and repeats exercise 20 times.

cooperate. Moreover, exercises must be performed daily and should be reevaluated periodically as part of the patient's regular follow-up.

Surgical intervention. Reconstructive surgery should be contemplated only after all conservative measures have failed. Even though the techniques of lumbar osteotomy are constantly improving, it is still an extensive and delicate procedure that also requires prolonged postoperative care.

Total hip replacement may also provide dramatic results initially, but the subsequent development of bony ankylosis

above the prosthesis may result in failure. Whereas spine, hip, or other reconstructive procedures are a last resort, correction of a vertebral fracture or dislocation is an urgent problem because of the potential for nerve root injury or compression of the spinal cord.

Course of disease and prognosis

The course of disease is usually characterized by mild or moderate flares of active spondylitis, alternating with periods when disease is almost or totally inactive, so that with proper treatment, minimal or no disability results. Rarely is the course severe and progressive so that patients end up with pronounced deformities that largely incapacitate them. The prognosis may be bleak for patients with refractory iritis and for the rare patient who develops secondary amyloidosis.

With early diagnosis, comprehensive management, and patient compliance, a satisfactory functional capacity is maintained in most patients, who can lead full and productive lives.

BIBLIOGRAPHY

Calabro JJ: The seronegative spondyloarthropathies, Postgrad Med 80:173, 1986.

Calin A and Fries JF: Striking prevalence of ankylosing spondylitis in "healthy" w27 positive males and females, N Engl J Med 293:835, 1975.

Khan MA, Kushner I, and Braun WE: Comparison of clinical features in HLA-B27 positive and negative patients with ankylosing spondylitis, Arthritis Rheum 20:909, 1977.

13·PSORIATIC ARTHRITIS

Warren A. Katz

Various types of arthritis may be found in patients with psoriasis—a fairly common, chronic, erythematous, scaling lesion of the skin. Psoriasis tends to appear over the elbows, knees, and scalp but may be found on any part of the body. The silver-scaled lesions sometimes cover all cutaneous surfaces; at other times they must be sought as minute, localized plaques hidden in the navel, creases of the buttocks, or scalp. Nail changes in psoriasis consist of pitting, hyperkeratosis, brownish discoloration, or even total destruction. It was once thought that joint inflammation in association with psoriasis was really rheumatoid arthritis; however, now there are enough distinctive features to recognize psoriatic arthritis as a separate entity. The cause of psoriasis or psoriatic arthritis is generally not known, but a hereditary predisposition is apparent in some families. The incidence of the histocompatibility antigen HLA-

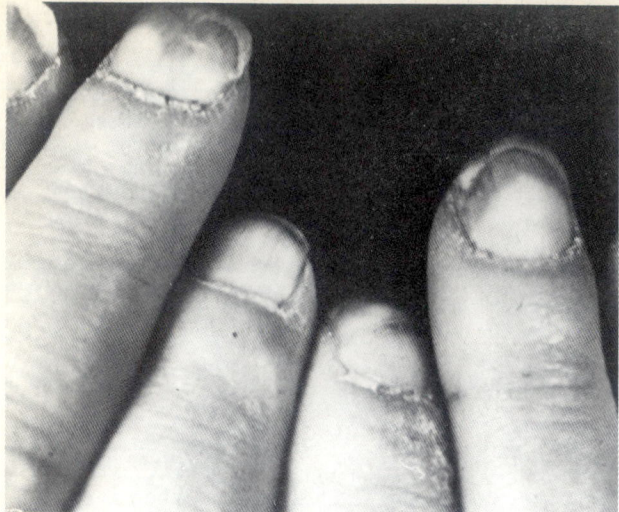

Fig. 13-1. Distal interphalangeal involvement and nail and skin changes in psoriatic arthritis.

B27 is especially high in psoriatic spondylitis (arthritis of the spine).

CLINICAL MANIFESTATIONS. In about 75% of patients with psoriatic arthritis, the most common presentation is asymmetric oligoarthritis, with one or a few joints involved at a time. Characteristically, a sausagelike swelling of either the fingers or toes is found and may herald the disease, even in an asymptomatic patient. Most patients, however, complain of pain of varying degrees; sometimes there is tenderness, redness, and heat. Few joints are spared, but the feet, knees, hands, and (in contrast to rheumatoid arthritis) the distal interphalangeal (DIP) joints are frequently involved (Fig. 13-1). Digital flexor tenosynovitis, often painful, may dominate the arthritis picture. Attacks of psoriatic arthritis tend to appear more abruptly and disappear more rapidly than those of rheumatoid arthritis. Despite having active arthritis, most patients are able to function.

Less often, psoriatic arthritis is confined to the DIP joints. Signs of inflammation may be subtle. Multiple DIP joint involvement with simultaneous nail psoriasis is a striking picture. About 15% of all patients have symmetric polyarthritis that is similar to rheumatoid arthritis. These patients, however, are seronegative for rheumatoid factor (RF); the types of deformities developed are identical to those of rheumatoid arthritis. Actually, extensive destruction to the point of resorption of the joint is more common in psoriatic arthritis. The telescoping digit has been referred to as *main en lorgnette* (opera-glass hand); fortunately, this catastrophe is uncommon.

Sacroiliac joint and spinal inflammation may be similar to that of ankylosing spondylitis. In contrast, unilateral sacroiliitis is more common in psoriasis. The patient with HLA-B27 antigen is predisposed to both ankylosing and psoriatic spondylosis. An acute monarticular presentation of psoriatic arthritis resembles gout. A search for urate crystals in synovial fluid should differentiate the two.

In some cases psoriasis and arthritis flare concomitantly; however, in most patients skin manifestations antedate those of joints by many years. In the few cases in which the arthritis precedes the psoriatic skin lesions, diagnosis is a challenge. Psoriatic arthritis occasionally has been associated with Sjögren's syndrome.

LABORATORY FINDINGS. Since there are no characteristic laboratory tests for psoriatic arthritis, diagnosis is based on clinical grounds. The erythrocyte sedimentation rate (ESR) is elevated during flare-ups of the disease and tends to fall to normal between episodes. This is in contrast to rheumatoid arthritis, in which the ESR may remain elevated even though the patient feels better. Tests for RF are normal. Synovial fluid analysis usually shows the same changes as in rheumatoid arthritis.

Roentgenograms of patients with psoriatic arthritis, although rarely diagnostic, may provide important clues in advanced cases. The characteristic sausagelike soft tissue swelling may be evident. Marginal erosions along the phalangeal shaft may produce a scalloped appearance despite the maintenance of the joint space. The distal phalanx of both fingers and toes may become whittled and actually resorbed. There may be bone overgrowth at the site of the tendon insertions, producing a pencil-in-cup deformity. The tendency for the DIP joints to be involved is evident on the roentgenogram. Sometimes periostitis is present along the shafts of the metatarsal bones. Less common findings are calcification of the nails, ankylosis of the interphalangeal joints, arthritis mutilans, and paravertebral calcification in patients with psoriatic spondylitis.

DIAGNOSIS. The following are features that suggest psoriatic arthritis rather than rheumatoid or other types of arthritis:

1. Psoriasis, with the tendency for nail lesions
2. A predisposition for the DIP joints
3. Sausagelike swelling of fingers and toes
4. Asymmetric pauciarticular arthritis
5. Unilateral sacroiliitis with "skip" involvement of the lumbar and dorsal spine
6. Concomitant flaring of arthritis and psoriasis
7. More abrupt exacerbations and more complete remissions
8. Absence of subcutaneous nodules
9. Seronegativity for RF
10. HLA-B27 in psoriatic patients with back pain
11. Characteristic resorptive roentgenographic changes with periostitis

Rheumatoid arthritis, Reiter's syndrome, ankylosing spondylitis, gout, sarcoidosis, and primary generalized osteoarthritis are the major differential diagnoses.

MANAGEMENT. Psoriatic arthritis is managed in a manner similar to rheumatoid arthritis, with the same focus on drug therapy, patient education, physical modalities, and surgery. Patients with psoriatic arthritis usually respond well to nonsteroidal antiinflammatory agents. Some with psoriatic arthritis react exceedingly well to small doses of systemic corticosteroids. There seems to be little justification for the prolonged use of high-dose corticosteroids. Periodic local corticosteroids may be all that is needed to treat periodic pauciarticular psoriatic arthritis. Remittive agents, such as gold, have been used successfully in patients with psoriatic arthritis.

Immunosuppressive drugs, notably methotrexate, have been used with outstanding success in many patients with extensive psoriatic skin lesions and arthritis. Because there is a moderate incidence of hepatotoxicity and hematologic abnormalities, careful follow-up is essential. Liver biopsy may be necessary to assess the adverse effects of methotrexate if administered for a long time; stomatitis may be profound.

It is not surprising that pain, extensive joint destruction, and unsightly skin changes may produce emotional problems in some patients with the disease. The physician plays an important role in implementing a psychosocial program.

BIBLIOGRAPHY

Baker H, Golding DM, and Thompson M: Psoriasis and arthritis, Ann Intern Med 58:909, 1963.
Eastmond CJ and Woodrow JC: The HLA system and the arthropathies associated with psoriasis, Ann Rheum Dis 36:112, 1977.

Lassus A and Karvonen J: Reactive arthritis, Reiter's disease, and psoriatic arthritis, Clin Rheum 3:281, 1977.
Moll JMH and Wright V: Psoriatic arthritis, Semin Arthritis Rheum 3:55, 1973.
Richter MB, Kinsella P, and Corbet M: Gold in psoriatic arthropathy, Ann Rheum Dis 39:279, 1980.
Wright V: Seronegative polyarthritis: a unified concept, Arthritis Rheum 21:619, 1978.

14 • REITER'S SYNDROME AND REACTIVE ARTHRITIS

Warren A. Katz

Reiter's syndrome, classically referred to as the triad of polyarthritis, conjunctivitis, and urethritis, has now been expanded to include mucosal ulcerations, keratoderma blennorrhagica, and balanitis circinata. In addition, involvement of the heart and central nervous system may occur infrequently

PATHOGENESIS AND PATHOLOGY. The etiology of Reiter's syndrome is unknown, but the nature of the illness, with occasionally apparent venereal transmission, suggests an infectious cause. *Mycoplasma* and *Chlamydia* organisms have been suspected as etiologic agents. The finding of HLA-B27 tissue type in more than 75% of patients with Reiter's syndrome suggests a hereditary predisposition. Some or all of its manifestations can be seen in genetically predisposed persons after infections with *Yersinia* and *Shigella* organisms and other agents. These manifestations have been referred to as reactive arthritis. Pathologic examination of the involved synovial membrane shows hyperemia without the pannus found in rheumatoid arthritis. There may be osteolysis late in the course of the disease.

CLINICAL MANIFESTATIONS. Reiter's syndrome almost always affects young men, and it may affect women more often than believed, often going undetected. It frequently begins with nongonococcal urethritis after sexual intercourse. Arthritis, conjunctivitis, and other signs may then develop sequentially or simultaneously. Most patients are not seriously ill, although considerable fatigue, weight loss, hectic fever, lymphadenopathy, or splenomegaly has been seen. Arthritis is generally acute, asymmetric, and pauciarticular. The small joints of the feet, ankles, and knees and the saroiliac joints may be involved. Reiter's syndrome infrequently resembles ankylosing spondylitis clinically. Achilles tendinitis and heel tenderness secondary to calcaneal bursitis ("lover's heel") may be striking. Residual joint deformity resembling rheumatoid arthritis is unusual.

Conjunctivitis is the most common ocular manifestation of Reiter's syndrome, occurring in at least one third of cases. Iritis is more apt to develop later in the disease than during the first attack. Urethritis produces a frankly purulent or watery discharge. Digital prostatic massage may yield pus in otherwise asymptomatic patients. Keratoderma blennorrhagica is a peculiar skin lesion suggested by macular hyperkeratotic lesions on the hands and soles of the feet. Subungual lesions resembling psoriasis may occur with the other skin manifestations or as an isolated finding. Weeping or dry ulcerations and scaling of the penis (balanitis) may be noted in some patients with Reiter's syndrome. Asymptomatic mucosal ulcerations of the buccal or palatal mucosa are found in approximately 10% of patients. If these lesions are painful, another diagnosis should be sought.

With a marked systemic component to Reiter's syndrome, initial bed rest is indicated. Patients should be educated as to the nature of the disease and the generally favorable prognosis, since chronic disability resulting from destructive, deforming

changes in the joints is unusual. Some patients have recurrent acute or subacute polyarthritis for several years.

ENTERIC AND REACTIVE ARTHRITIDES

Reactive arthritis that follows certain enteric bacterial infections in genetically predisposed hosts represents one of the most obvious associations between specific microbial organisms and HLA antigens. A syndrome resembling Reiter's syndrome may follow infection with *Yersinia*, *Campylobacter*, *Salmonella*, and *Shigella* organisms in patients positive for HLA-B27. The knee, ankle, and wrist are most frequently involved, and a migratory pattern is common. The term "reactive arthritis" has been used for these arthritides and for arthritis associated with ulcerative colitis, regional enteritis, and intestinal bypass surgery in the broad category of enteric arthropathy.

Patients with ulcerative colitis or regional enteritis may have subacute asymmetric polyarthritis or spondylitis either alone or with flare-ups of diarrhea, mucous stools, and abdominal pain. Erythema nodosum and oral ulcerations are other extraintestinal manifestations. Most patients with enteric spondylitis have a detectable HLA-B27 antigen.

Arthritis and arthralgias complicate jejunocolic bypass surgery in 20% to 30% of patients. Joint symptoms usually remit spontaneously over several weeks, but chronic, recurrent cases have been reported.

It is clear that ankylosing spondylitis is the prototype of a group of seronegative spondyloarthropathies that also include psoriatic arthritis, Reiter's syndrome, and enteric arthritis. common to each is (1) a negative test for rheumatoid factor, (2) absence of rheumatoid nodules, (3) inflammatory peripheral arthritis, (4) roentgenographic sacroiliitis with or without spondylitis, (5) mucocutaneous, ocular, genital, or gastrointestinal manifestations, (6) association with HLA-B27, and (7) tendency for familial clustering.

BIBLIOGRAPHY

Amor B: Reiter's syndrome and reactive arthritis, Clin Rheumatol 2:315, 1983.
Calin A: HLA-B27 in 1982: reappraisal of a clinical test, Ann Intern Med 96:114, 1982 (editorial).
Calin A and Fries JF: An experimental epidemic of Reiter's syndrome revisited: follow-up evidence on genetic and environmental factors, Ann Intern Med 84:564, 1976.
Good AE: Reiter's disease: a review with special attention to cardiovascular and neurologic sequelae, Semin Arthritis Rheum 3:253, 1974.
Kosunen TU et al: Arthritis associated with *Campylobacter jejuni* enteritis, Scand J Rheumatol 10:77, 1981.
Leirisalo M et al: Follow-up study on patients with Reiter's syndrome and reactive arthritis with special reference to HLA-B27, Arthritis Rheum 25:249, 1982.
Martin DH et al: *Chlamydia trachomatis* infections in men with Reiter's syndrome, Ann Intern Med 100:207, 1984.
McEwen C et al: Ankylosing spondylitis and spondylitis accompanying ulcerative colitis, regional enteritis, psoriasis and Reiter's syndrome: a comparative study, Arthritis Rheum 14:291, 1971.
Wilkens RF et al: Reiter's syndrome: evaluation of preliminary criteria for definite disease, Arthritis Rheum 24:844, 1981.

15 • INTERMITTENT RHEUMATIC DISEASES

Randolph C. Blodgett, Jr.

The four entities discussed in this section have in common an episodic pattern of clinical symptoms and therefore tend to be classified together. Their major theme is the recurrent nature of their symptoms with intervals devoid of apparent rheumatic disease. Although several of the common rheumatic disorders such as gout may be episodic or paroxysmal in their clinical activity, their natural history follows an established and predictable course.

The customary term for regular recurrences of a disease is "periodic"; a disease with irregular intervals between episodes is "intermittent." The actual terminology is not precise in describing some of these disorders.

INTERMITTENT HYDRARTHROSIS

Intermittent hydrarthrosis is an uncommon clinical entity of obscure origin characterized by episodes of joint effusion usually lasting 2 to 5 days. These generally occur in a predictable pattern with 2 to 4 weeks of normal health between episodes. The term "intermittent" is traditional, even though the symptoms occur regularly and it thus could be classified as a periodic entity.

Episodes of intermittent hydrarthrosis occur predominantly in women and most commonly affect the knee. An abrupt effusion may produce discomfort from distention of the joint capsule but without the classic signs of inflammation (pain, tenderness, warmth). Repetitive effusions generally involve the same joint(s). Although the knee is usually involved, other large joints such as hip, ankle, or elbow may be affected. The small joints are characteristically not affected.

These recurrent episodes commonly begin in adolescence and may resolve spontaneously—or last indefinitely. Pregnancy may ameliorate the course of this disorder.

There are no diagnostic laboratory findings. Aspiration of synovial fluid has demonstrated 500 to 6500 cells/mm³. The erythrocyte sedimentation rate (ESR) is generally normal or unchanged during the attack. The rheumatoid factor (RF) is characteristically nonreactive. Synovial biopsy shows only a mild, nonspecific inflammatory reaction with occasional infiltration of lymphocytes. There are no characteristic roentgenographic abnormalities.

Specific or other satisfactory therapy is lacking, but spontaneous resolution of the effusion is anticipated. Pain of an acutely distended joint capsule may be transiently relieved by synovial fluid aspiration.

PALINDROMIC RHEUMATISM

Palindromic rheumatism is an uncommon disease of unknown origin characterized by attacks of acutely inflamed joints at irregular intervals. Some cases of rheumatoid arthritis begin in a palindromic fashion.

An episode of palindromic rheumatism usually involves one to a few joints and may vary in location from attack to attack. Intense synovitis displaying all the cardinal signs of inflammation may last a few hours to several days but seldom more than a week. The asymptomatic intervals may vary from a few days to several months. Occasionally, an episode may begin while a previous one is resolving.

The most common site of the synovitis is the knee; less often it may involve the wrists or the metacarpophalangeal or proximal interphalangeal joints. Involvement of the metatarsophalangeal joints resembles gout.

It should be emphasized that this is an active synovitis, not just arthralgia. The inflammation may also involve paraarticular structures, including fingerpads, heels, and ankles, as well as tender swelling along the flexor and extensor surfaces of the forearm and hand. Transient subcutaneous nodules may occur at sites typical of rheumatoid arthritis.

Nonspecific inflammatory changes may be visible in the synovial biopsy. It is remarkable that the fluid withdrawn from an intensely inflamed joint should exhibit evidence of only mild inflammation. Synovial fluid analysis is usually noninflammatory. The ESR may be elevated at the time of an attack but promptly remits during asymptomatic periods. RF may occasionally be found in elevated titers, especially in those patients whose disease ultimately evolves into rheumatoid arthritis.

Roentgenograms of the joints are almost always normal. Exceptional joints that bear the brunt of numerous attacks reveal some rheumatoid stigmata, such as osteopenia and erosions. These usually occur in those patients destined to develop more overt rheumatoid arthritis.

The diagnosis is based on the peculiar pattern of signs and symptoms. The painful synovitis differentiates it from the painless effusion of intermittent hydrarthrosis. Lack of crystals in the microscopic examination of the synovial fluid helps to rule out a crystal-induced arthropathy.

Treatment is generally unsatisfactory. Gold therapy has induced remissions in some cases. Although it is difficult to evaluate therapeutic efficacy when symptoms disappear in 2 to 5 days, the nonsteroidal antiinflammatory agents may modify the attacks. The degree of pain in some patients mandates short-term use of more potent analgesics. Rest, splints, ice, and assistive devices should be considered.

There are three usual patterns to palindromic rheumatism: (1) complete resolution or spontaneous remission after a few months or years, (2) evolution into rheumatoid arthritis in 30% to 50% of patients, or (3) a chronic pattern of episodic synovitis with complete resolution of symptoms between attacks.

FAMILIAL MEDITERRANEAN FEVER

Familial Mediterranean fever (FMF), or *periodic disease,* is an inherited disorder of unknown origin characterized by an irregular pattern of attacks of arthritis, serositis, and fever. Thus, by strict definition, periodic disease really occurs intermittently. The majority of cases occur in the Middle East, primarily but not exclusively in patients with Arabic, Sephardic Jewish, Armenian, or other Mediterranean backgrounds. The gene is apparently autosomal recessive.

The illness usually becomes symptomatic in patients between 5 and 15 years of age. The frequency of attacks may vary greatly in the same patient, ranging from once or twice per week to once yearly. The usual asymptomatic interval is 2 to 4 weeks, and the duration of the acute attack ranges from 24 hours to 1 or 2 weeks.

Fever is the universal symptom, occurring during most attacks. Abdominal pain simulating peritonitis is commonly present, with pleuritic or pericardial pain occurring less commonly. Transient, painful, erythematous swelling may be noted around the ankle, distinct from the arthritis that occurs in 50% to 75% of patients.

There is no established pattern of joint involvement, which runs the gamut from transient arthralgia to acute oligoarthritis involving primarily the large joints, particularly the knees. Less commonly, protracted episodes of joint pain with effusion may last up to a year. Generally, FMF does not leave residual joint damage, but destructive hip disease sometimes develops.

Amyloid, which involves the kidneys, spleen, and adrenal glands but spares the liver and heart, may develop. This complication is common in Israel but rare in the United States.

There are no specific laboratory tests, although the ESR may be elevated during the attack. Roentgenographic findings include nonspecific juxtaarticular osteoporosis that may return to normal between attacks.

The diagnosis may be difficult in the sporadic or atypical

patient; however, a family history, intermittent symptoms, and typical signs should suggest the diagnosis. There is the hazard of performing an unnecessary exploratory laparotomy when the undiagnosed patient has severe abdominal pain.

Treatment should provide symptomatic and supportive measures. Colchicine has been of value in some patients, even in protection from amyloidosis, but this use of the drug is considered investigational. Another approach is long-term prophylaxis, but chronic therapy requires periodic observation for mild steatorrhea or other adverse effects.

The prognosis is generally good except for patients who develop amyloidosis and secondary renal failure.

BEHÇET'S SYNDROME

Behçet's syndrome is a disorder of undetermined origin characterized by recurrent multisystem signs and symptoms involving the skin, mucous membranes, vessels, and joints. This syndrome is more commonly recognized in Japan, Turkey, and Mideastern countries than in North America.

The typical features of Behçet's syndrome include the following:

1. Recurrent, painful, aphthouslike ulcerations of the oral mucosa, lips, and pharynx
2. Painful ulcerations of the male genitalia or painless ulcerations of the female vulva and vaginal mucosa
3. Iritis, often associated with other signs of ocular inflammation (conjunctivitis, episcleritis, retinal changes)
4. Neurologic manifestations such as organic confusional states, encephalitis, meningitis, and hemiparesis
5. A variety of lesions including vasculitis, migrating thrombophlebitis, pyoderma, colitis, seronegative arthritis, erythema nodosum, or pustule formation at the site of a needle puncture

Whereas arthralgia is the most common musculoskeletal symptom, synovitis may occur in two thirds of patients, involving primarily the large joints, such as the knee and ankle. The small joints are much less commonly affected. The arthritis tends to remain an irregular episodic acute arthritis, although it may become chronic.

The ESR may be elevated during the attack. There is no diagnostic test. The clinical course of Behçet's syndrome is variable. Generally the oral ulcers and ocular lesions occur first, followed by the genital lesions and skin and joint manifestations.

Behçet's syndrome must be differentiated from Reiter's syndrome, which may appear similar even though the orogenital ulcerations are not painful. The painful oral ulcerations of Stevens-Johnson syndrome and systemic lupus erythematosus should be differentiated by the history and findings.

Fibrinolytic agents, immunosuppressive agents, steroids, whole blood transfusions, and transfer factor have all been used therapeutically with varying response. However, evaluation of the treatment of Behçet's syndrome is difficult because of the pattern of exacerbations and remissions.

BIBLIOGRAPHY

Benamour S et al: La maladie de Behçet, a propos de soixante cas, Sem Hop Paris 62:1317, 1986.

Chajek T and Fairnaru M: Behçet's disease: report of 41 cases and review of the literature, Medicine 54:179, 1975.

Sohar E, Pras M, and Gafni J: Familial Mediterranean fever and its articular manifestations, Clin Rheum Dis 1:195, 1975.

Wong R, Ellis C, and Diaz L: Behçet's disease, Int J Dermatol 23:25, 1984.

Wright DG et al: Efficacy of intermittent colchicine therapy in familial Mediterranean fever, Ann Intern Med 86:162, 1977.

Zemer D et al: Colchicine in the prevention and treatment of the amyloidosis of familial Mediterranean fever, N Engl J Med 314:1001, 1986.

16·SYSTEMIC LUPUS ERYTHEMATOSUS

June F. Klinghoffer

Systemic lupus erythematosus (SLE) is a chronic, inflammatory, multisystem disease that occurs predominantly in young women. Because of the numerous autoantibodies found in patients, SLE is regarded as the prototype of autoimmune disease. It may more aptly be termed an "immune-complex disease," since tissue damage is secondary to the deposition of immune complexes formed by the autoantibodies and host antigens. The clinical picture may be exceedingly varied, but the most common manifestations are skin rashes, joint pain, fever, pleurisy, and nephritis.

Before 1948, SLE was considered a rare and grave disease. The recognition of the lupus erythematosus (LE) cell phenomenon by Hargraves in that year provided the first specific diagnostic test for SLE and ushered in a new era of understanding concerning the disease and immunologic mechanisms. A marked apparent increase in incidence of SLE has occurred in the past 30 years; the availability of more sensitive diagnostic tests has led to the recognition of earlier and milder cases, and SLE is now considered fairly common and compatible with long survival.

A recent epidemiologic study in a large prepaid health clinic in San Francisco found the incidence of new cases of SLE to be 7.6 per 100,000 persons. The overall prevalence was 1 case in 1969 persons; in women aged 15 to 64 it was 1 in 700; and in black women of the same age it was 1 in 245.

Women are affected 5 to 10 times more frequently than men, and blacks are affected more frequently than whites. Onset of symptoms is most frequent between the ages of 15 and 40, but the disease may occur in both children and the elderly.

ETIOLOGY AND PATHOGENESIS. The serologic hallmark of SLE is the presence of multiple autoantibodies. Those antibodies directed against nuclear material are known as antinuclear antibodies (ANA). Other autoantibodies to cytoplasmic material, blood proteins, and cell membranes may be present. Some of these latter antibodies may have a direct pathogenetic role in such manifestations as hemolytic anemia, leukopenia, or thrombocytopenia. The major pathologic effects, however, are mediated via immune complex formation and deposition in such sites as blood vessel walls, glomerular basement membrane, skin, and other areas. These complexes are formed by nuclear antigens and ANA, especially DNA/anti-DNA. The complexes activate the complement system, causing the release of chemotactic factors and subsequent release of lysosmal enzymes that directly attack and damage the various tissue sites.

The basic etiologic or initiating factors are not known. Evidence pointing to the importance of genetic factors includes the increased incidence of clinical SLE or serologic positivity in family members, increased concordance of SLE in identical twins, increased incidence in persons with congenital deficiency of certain components of complement (especially C2), increased frequency of certain HLA antigens (DR2 and DR3), and spontaneous appearance of a lupuslike disease in the NZB/NZW hybrid strain mouse.

Exogenous factors, such as sun exposure, infections, and drug ingestion, appear operative in some patients. The possible role of a specific infectious agent such as a virus is speculative at this time. C-type RNA virus has been found in the NZB/NZW mouse, as well as in certain colonies of dogs with SLE. Suggestive evidence in human SLE includes the presence of antibodies to double-stranded RNA and elevated titers of measles antibodies.

Endocrine factors have long been suspected because of the strikingly high female-to-male ratio of incidence. Recent studies have found evidence of altered hormonal metabolism with increased hydroxylation products of estrone in both female and male patients. Several factors may thus be involved in the pathogenesis of SLE, including (1) genetic predisposition, (2) abnormal host immune reaction, (3) endocrine factors, and (4) latent viral infection or other environmental agents.

PATHOLOGY. Few characteristic lesions are seen grossly or by routine light microscopy. Fibrinoid deposits may be seen on serosal surfaces and in blood vessel walls. Vasculitis involves the small arteries. "Onion-skin" lesions and concentric perivascular fibrosis are seen in the spleen; nonbacterial vegetations are occasionally seen on the heart valves. The kidneys may show focal glomerulitis, diffuse proliferative nephritis, or membranous nephritis. Thickening of the basement membrane of the glomeruli may produce the characteristic "wire-loop" lesion. Hematoxylin bodies, similar in appearance to the inclusions within LE cells, are infrequently seen in the various tissues but are considered pathognomonic. The mesangial lesion, present in all patients with SLE, is characterized by proliferation of glomerular mesangial cells and deposition of immune complexes that may be detected by immunofluorescence.

During acute SLE of the skin, histologic examination of skin shows hyperkeratosis of the epidermis and follicular plugging. More chronic events include hypertrophy of the periphery of the lesion and central fibrosis. Immunofluorescent staining is demonstrated at the dermal-epidermal junction (lupus band test). Even clinically uninvolved skin may show a positive band test in SLE.

CLINICAL MANIFESTIONS. The clinical picture may range from a mild, indolent disorder manifested chiefly by recurrent arthralgias or skin rash to a fulminant life-threatening illness with renal failure. Onset may be abrupt but more usually is insidious. The course is most often one of exacerbations and remissions over many years. The initial complaints are usually joint pain or skin rash. Constitutional symptoms such as fatigue, malaise, and fever are common.

Musculoskeletal manifestations. Almost all patients have joint involvement at some time during the disease, often at the onset. They may have polyarthralgias or actual arthritis with objective signs of swelling and inflammation. The small joints of the fingers, hands, and wrists are most frequently involved, but knees, ankles, and elbows are also affected. Swelling of the proximal interphalangeal and metacarpophalangeal joints may be highly suggestive of rheumatoid arthritis. Minor deformities such as swan-neck fingers may develop; these appear to be caused by soft tissue laxity. No bone erosions are seen on roentgenograms.

Avascular necrosis of bone develops in a small percent of patients, especially those receiving prolonged high-dose corticosteroid therapy. The femoral head is most frequently involved.

Proximal muscle pain or weakness is occasionally seen and reflects accompanying myositis.

Mucocutaneous manifestations. Between 75% and 85% of patients have signs or symptoms involving the skin, mucous membranes, or hair. The classic butterfly rash over the cheeks and bridge of the nose is seen in about 50% of patients and ranges from a faint malar flush to a more extensive scaly, maculopapular, erythematous rash (Fig. 16-1). About one third exhibit photosensitivity, with the rash appearing only after sun exposure. Skin rashes are most common on the face, neck,

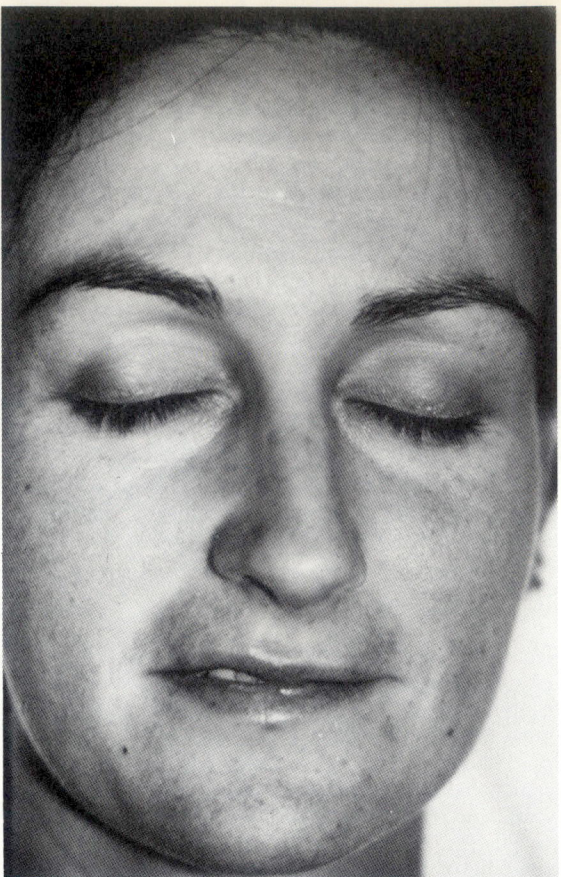

Fig. 16-1   Facial rash over bridge of nose, upper lip, and chin in patient with active SLE.

and upper chest but may appear elsewhere, especially on sun-exposed areas such as the extremities and scalp. Vasculitic lesions are commonly seen on the palms of the hands and on the distal finger pads. Raynaud's phenomenon occurs in about 20% of patients. Telangiectasia, livedo reticularis, periungual erythema, petechiae, purpura, bullae, and urticaria have all been described. Areas of hyperpigmentation and vitiligo are quite common.

Mucosal ulcerative lesions occur in approximately 40% of patients. Since these ulcers are frequently painless, they must be actively sought through the history and examination. The ulcers characteristically occur on the hard or soft palate but may also involve the buccal and gingival mucosa and resemble the common aphthous ulcer (Fig. 16-2). They occur most frequently in those patients with active skin lesions or during flare-ups of SLE. Ulcers may also involve the nasal mucosa and may lead to septal perforation.

Alopecia is an important but frequently overlooked diagnostic sign. The hair loss may be diffuse or patchy; the patient may merely be aware of the hair thinning or of an unusual amount of hair coming out on combing. Alopecia often signals a flare-up in the disease and is reversible.

Serositis. Pleurisy or painless pleural effusion is common. Less frequently, pulmonary infiltrates or patchy areas of atelectasis may be seen on roentgenograms. Pericarditis with or without effusion is also fairly common. Nonbacterial verrucous endocarditis (Libman-Sacks endocarditis) may be seen at autopsy but is not commonly recognized clinically. Sterile peritonitis occasionally occurs.

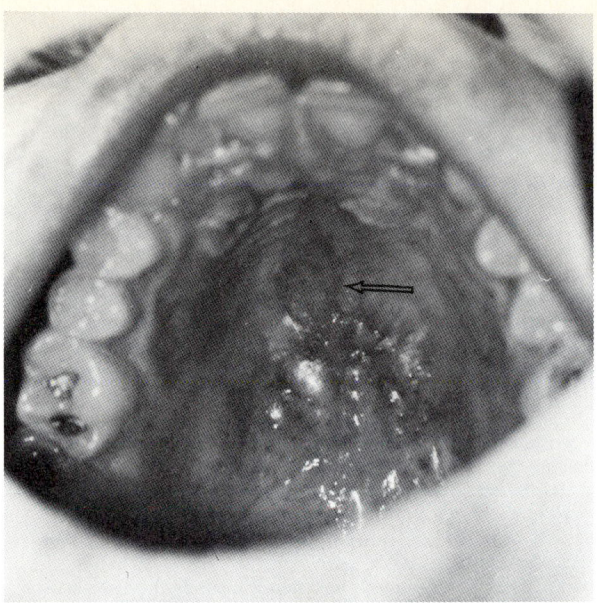

Fig. 16-2 Palatal mouth ulcer *(arrow)* in acutely ill patient.

Renal disease. More than 50% of patients show evidence of renal involvement. This may be clinically expressed as the nephrotic syndrome with marked proteinuria and edema, or a nephritis with hematuria, hypertension, and progressive impairment of renal function with eventual uremia. This is the most serious complication of SLE and is the leading cause of death. Fortunately, most patients show only a mild to moderate proteinuria. A rising blood urea nitrogen (BUN) and creatinine is an ominous sign. Renal biopsy with immunofluorescence may help to assess the presence and extent of renal changes.

Nervous system. There has been increasing recognition of the significant incidence of both neurologic and psychiatric manifestations. Seizures, psychosis, and organic brain syndrome are the major manifestations. Also seen are coma, hemiparesis, chorea, cranial nerve palsies, aphasia, and peripheral neuropathy. It is often difficult to differentiate between organic psychosis secondary to the disease and steroid psychosis. Depression and anxiety are common. A brain scan may show a diffuse abnormality.

Other manifestations. Lymph nodes may be enlarged but are not tender. Splenomegaly may occur in 10% to 15% of cases but is usually of a slight degree. The liver is normal in size. Abdominal pain may be secondary to peritonitis, pancreatitis, mesenteric lymphadenopathy, or mesenteric arteritis. Parotid gland enlargement may occur and sometimes reflects an accompanying Sjögren's syndrome. "Cotton wool" exudates or "cytoid bodies" may be seen on the retina.

LABORATORY FINDINGS. Mild to moderate normochromic anemia is common. The Coombs' test may be positive, with or without accompanying hemolytic anemia. Leukopenia occurs in 50% of patients, usually with significant lymphopenia. Thrombocytopenia is usually of a mild degree and in most cases not clinically significant; occasionally frank thrombocytopenic purpura may be the initial manifestation of SLE. A circulating anticoagulant may be present and is detected by a prolonged partial thromboplastin time. The erythrocyte sedimentation rate is rapid. With renal involvement, the urine may show protein, red and white blood cells, and casts.

Immunologic abnormalities abound. The most significant from the standpoint of diagnosis and monitoring response to therapy are positive LE cell test (70% to 80% of patients),

ANA (95% to 100%), antibody to native DNA (70%), antibody to Sm nuclear antigen (30%), rheumatoid factor (20%), false positive serologic test for syphilis (20%), increased γ-globulin, and decreased serum complement.

A positive LE cell test previously represented one of the major diagnostic criteria (see discussion of diagnosis). For screening purposes now, however, it has been superseded by the far more sensitive and less time-consuming fluorescent test for ANA (FANA).

A positive FANA is found in virtually all cases, and thus a negative test weighs against the diagnosis of SLE. A positive test is not diagnostic, since it occurs in rheumatoid arthritis and other connective tissue diseases. Four patterns of fluorescent staining are recognized: (1) homogeneous, or diffuse; (2) peripheral, or rim; (3) speckled; and (4) nucleolar. The diffuse pattern is produced by antibody binding to nucleoprotein (the LE factor); the peripheral pattern results from antibody binding to DNA and is more specific, especially if in high titer. Rising titer of anti-DNA antibody and decreasing levels of serum complement are indicative of acute activity and highly suggestive of lupus nephritis. Serum complement may be profoundly depressed with active SLE. Cryoglobulins indicate the presence of circulating immune complexes.

Identification of individual antinuclear antibodies has led to increased diagnostic specificity and has also suggested the possibility of a causal relationship between specific antibodies and certain clinical manifestations of lupus. Thus antibody to the Sm nuclear antigen is now recognized to be a specific marker for SLE. The circulating anticoagulant factor is associated with an increased incidence of venous and arterial thrombosis, and the related anticardiolipin antibody appears to be associated with an increased incidence of spontaneous abortions and intrauterine fetal death. The Ro/SS-A antibody may play a pathogenetic role in neonatal lupus; this antibody has been identified in both the maternal and fetal blood in infants born with congenital heart block, with or without SLE skin lesions.

DIAGNOSIS. The following 11 manifestations represent the 1982 revised criteria for SLE proposed by the American Rheumatism Association. The presence of any four of these either serially or simultaneously is considered sufficient to identify the patient with SLE:

1. Malar rash
2. Discoid rash
3. Photosensitivity
4. Oral ulcers
5. Arthritis (nonerosive)
6. Serositis: pleuritis or pericarditis
7. Renal disorder: persistent proteinuria or cellular casts
8. Neurologic disorder: seizures or psychosis
9. Hematologic disorder: hemolytic anemia or leukopenia or lymphopenia or thrombocytopenia
10. Immunologic disorder: positive LE cell preparation or anti-DNA or anti-Sm or false positive VDRL
11. Antinuclear antibody

Differential diagnostic problems are most apt to occur with rheumatoid arthritis, with the overlap syndromes, and in those cases with a single manifestation, such as convulsions or pericarditis. The diagnosis must always be considered in women in their childbearing years, especially when symptoms appear in the early postpartum period or after unusual sun exposure.

The most sensitive diagnostic screening test is the FANA. The most specific diagnostic findings are a high titer of anti-DNA antibodies and decreased serum complement levels.

PROGNOSIS. Survival figures have shown dramatic improvement. Five-year survival now approximates 95% and 10-

year survival 85%. The chief causes of death are intercurrent infection, renal failure, and central nervous system (CNS) involvement.

MANAGEMENT. Many patients do well on simple supportive measures. All should be advised to avoid sun exposure, guard against infections, avoid drugs, such as sulfonamides or oral contraceptives, that often precipitate exacerbations of SLE, and avoid overfatigue. Topical sunscreen preparations are useful in patients with marked photosensitivity.

Arthralgias and arthritis usually respond well to salicylates or one of the nonsteroidal antiinflammatory drugs. Hydroxychloroquine, an antimalarial drug, is effective in controlling skin lesions and arthritis at a dose of 200 mg daily. Periodic ophthalmologic evaluations every 6 months are necessary when this drug is used because of the danger of retinal damage. Topical corticosteroids are effective for cutaneous lesions. Sunscreens may prevent them.

Systemic corticosteroid therapy is indicated for renal and CNS disease, pericarditis, pulmonary disease, and hematologic complications, such as hemolytic anemia or thrombocytopenia. Such therapy may also be required in patients with fever, arthritis, and skin lesions that do not respond to other measures. Dosage varies widely. Renal and CNS disease may require 100 to 200 mg of prednisone daily. Other manifestations will usually respond to a dose of 40 to 60 mg daily. Dosage is tapered as early as possible to avoid complications, such as avascular necrosis of bone, osteoporosis, and fluid retention. Alternate day therapy is used when possible. "Pulse therapy," consisting of intravenous bolus doses of 1 g of methylprednisolone daily for 3 days, is often used for acute renal disease or other serious manifestations of lupus activity that have not responded to orally administered prednisone. Immunosuppressive drugs, such as azathioprine or cyclophosphamide, are often used in addition to corticosteroids in the management of lupus nephritis. When cyclophosphamide is administered intravenously as a "pulse," it is effective and diminishes the toxicity of the drug.

DRUG-INDUCED CONNECTIVE TISSUE DISEASE (DRUG-INDUCED LUPUS)

Many drugs are capable of triggering exacerbations of SLE. Others are capable of inducing the formation of ANA, including the LE cell. A smaller group of drugs produces a clinical lupuslike syndrome. Procainamide, a drug widely used in the treatment of cardiac arrhythmias, is the major cause of drug-induced connective tissue disease. Three fourths of patients receiving the drug develop ANA and LE cells; a much smaller percentage develop the clinical syndrome.

Characteristics of drug-induced connective tissue disease are increased incidence in males and older patients, absence of renal and CNS involvement, normal serum complement, and absence of antibodies to native DNA. The most frequent manifestations are arthralgias, fever, and pleural and pericardial effusions. Symptoms usually disappear when the drug is stopped, but FANA may persist for months to several years.

Other implicated drugs are hydralazine, isoniazid, the anticonvulsants, thiouracils, phenothiazine compounds, penicillamine, sulfonamides, and oral contraceptives.

CHRONIC DISCOID LUPUS ERYTHEMATOSUS

Skin lesions of chronic discoid lupus erythematosus (CDLE) may occur in a small percentage of patients with SLE but generally represent an independent entity. The typical CDLE lesion starts as a papular eruption that spreads and yields to erythema, edema, induration, and ultimately fibrosis with central atrophy and depression. The lesions are usually found on the scalp and face. Hair loss and loss of pigmentation may ensue.

BIBLIOGRAPHY

Baldwin DS and others: Lupus nephritis, Am J Med 62:12, 1977.
Cathcart ES and others: Beneficial effects of methylprednisolone "pulse" therapy in diffuse proliferative nephritis, lancet 1:163, 1976.
Feinglass EJ, Arnett FC, and Dorsch CA: Neuropsychiatric manifestations of systemic lupus erythematosus, Medicine 55:323, 1976.
Feldson DT and Anderson J: Evidence for the superiority of immunosuppressive drugs and prednisone over prednisone alone in lupus nephritis, N Engl J Med 311:1582, 1984.
Fessel WJ: Systemic lupus erythematosus in the community, Arch Intern Med 134:1027, 1974.
Fries JF and Holman HR: Systemic lupus erythematosus: a clinical analysis. In Smith LH, editor: Major problems in internal medicine, vol VI, Philadelphia, 1975, WB Saunders Co.
Lahita RG: Systemic lupus erythematosus, New York, 1987, John Wiley & Sons.
Lee SL and Chase HP: Drug-induced lupus erythematosus: a critical review, Semin Arthritis Rheum 5:83, 1975.
Phillips PE: The virus hypothesis in systemic lupus erythematosus, Ann Intern Med 83:709, 1975.
Rothfield NF: Systemic lupus erythematosus. In McCarty DJ, editor: Arthritis and allied conditions, ed 10, Philadelphia, 1985, Lea & Febiger.
Schur PH: The clinical management of systemic lupus erythematosus, New York, 1983, Grune & Stratton.
Urman JD: Oral mucosal ulceration in systemic lupus erythematosus, Arthritis Rheum 21:58, 1978.
Wallace DJ and Dubois EL: Dubois' lupus erythematosus, ed 3, Philadelphia, 1987, Lea & Febiger.

17·SYSTEMIC SCLEROSIS

Sergio Jimenez and **John Varga**

Systemic sclerosis is a disease of unknown origin characterized by excessive deposition of collagen and other connective tissue components in skin and multiple internal organs. It is associated with prominent and often severe alterations in the microvasculature and the autonomic nervous system. Because immunologic abnormalities frequently are present, systemic sclerosis has been included in the group of autoimmune diseases.

The disease is relatively uncommon; it has been stated that four to 12 new cases per 1 million population are diagnosed in the United States each year, but this probably is an underestimation. Systemic sclerosis affects women three to four times more frequently than men, and there is no racial predilection. The initial symptoms usually appear in the third to fifth decade of life, although the disease has been described in children and the elderly. Systemic sclerosis is a complex and clinically heterogeneous disease with clinical forms ranging from localized skin involvement with minimal systemic alterations (limited scleroderma) to forms with severe internal organ disease and a fulminant course (diffuse scleroderma).

In many cases skin involvement is confined to the digits and the dorsum of the hands and feet (acrosclerosis), and progression of the sclerotic process is relatively slow. This form of disease frequently is associated with calcinosis, long-standing Raynaud's phenomenon, esophageal dysmotility, sclerodactyly, and telangiectasia and has been termed CREST syndrome. Although the distinction between CREST syndrome and more fulminant visceral scleroderma often is clear-cut, in many instances it is difficult to make a distinct separation because the clinical manifestations frequently overlap.

In another group of patients classic clinical features of systemic sclerosis overlap manifestations of the other connective tissue diseases, such as systemic lupus erythematosus and dermatomyositis/polymyositis. One subgroup of these patients, with a more specific entity called *mixed connective tissue disease* (see later in this chapter), has been identified based on the presence of a specific antiribonucleoprotein antibody in their sera.

Other syndromes resembling systemic sclerosis include chemically induced sclerosis, graft-versus-host disease of bone marrow transplants, the scleroderma-like chronic illness that has followed consumption of adulterated cooking oil in Spain, and the severe fasciitis associated with eosinophilia. Pseudoscleroderma embraces a variety of genetic and acquired diseases that should be excluded whenever the possibility of systemic scleroderma is considered.

PATHOGENESIS. Although the exact pathogenetic mechanisms in systemic sclerosis are not understood, it is clear that many of the clinical manifestations of the disease, as already stated, are caused by the accumulation of excessive collagen and other connective tissue components in the affected organs. Experimental evidence has indicated a marked increase in the rate of collagen synthesis by scleroderma fibroblasts. Rather than a primary event, this probably represents only the final pathway of a variety of mechanisms. Cutaneous cellular infiltrates consisting predominantly of lymphocytes and macrophages have been noted in patients with early systemic sclerosis. Such cells have been shown to elaborate soluble factors (lymphokines and monokines) capable of stimulating fibroblast chemotaxis, proliferation, and extracellular matrix protein synthesis. Because alterations in the microvasculature frequently are found in scleroderma and in many instances precede clinical manifestations, it has been suggested that they may be responsible for increased fibroblast activity.

PATHOLOGY. The pathologic changes in systemic sclerosis represent variable stages of progression and development of at least three major processes occurring in the affected tissues:

1. Connective tissue alterations, with fibroblast proliferation, fibrosis, and increased ground substance
2. Inflammation, occurring predominantly in the early stages of disease and characterized by infiltration with mononuclear cells, predominantly lymphocytes
3. Vascular disease, characterized by intimal proliferation, concentric subendothelial deposition of collagen and mucinous material, and narrowing of the vessel lumen and thrombosis

Some less frequent pathologic changes include classic vasculitic lesions, with necrotic disruption and inflammatory infiltration of vessel walls, and deposition of calcific material in the subcutaneous and periarticular tissues.

Progression of the vascular and fibrotic reactions and decrease in the inflammatory component lead to the final stage of atrophic changes in the affected organs. Skin changes include a marked decrease in the thickness of the epidermis, flattening of the rete pegs, and replacement of sebaceous and sweat glands, as well as hair follicles, by dense fibrous tissue. Fibrotic infiltration of the alveolocapillary membrane occurs in the lungs, with atrophy of the alveolar lining, and finally, complete disruption of the lungs' architecture. In the heart and other areas replacement with dense connective tissue, cellular atrophy, and tissue fibrosis occur.

CLINICAL MANIFESTATIONS. The most impressive clinical features of systemic sclerosis are related to the generalized thickening and fibrosis of the skin, but some degree of multiple

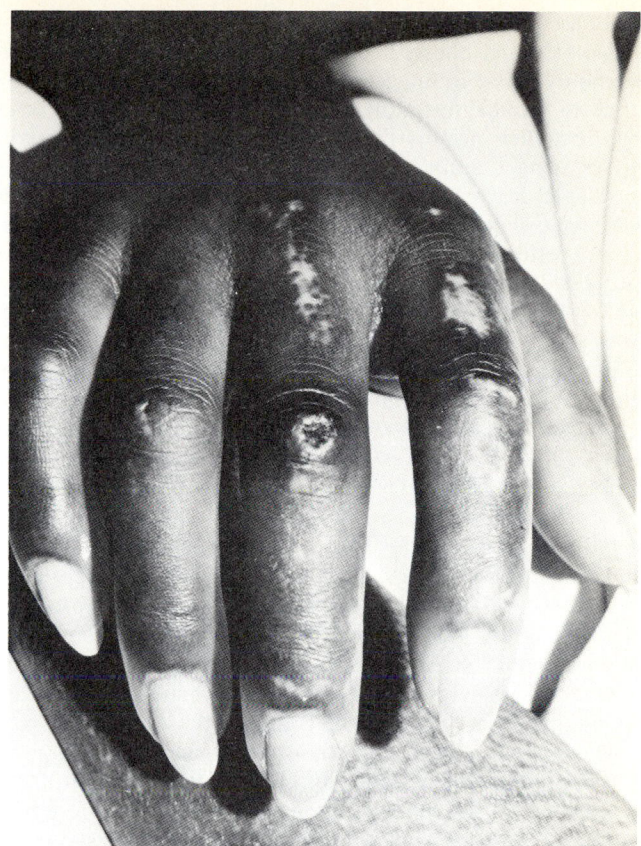

Fig. 17-1 Hand of 29-year-old woman with systemic sclerosis demonstrating digital sclerosis, pigmentary changes, cutaneous ulcers, and joint flexion contractures.

organ involvement almost always is present. The skin is almost always affected, but in rare cases classic visceral involvement can be demonstrated without clinical evidence of skin disease.

Comparison of a clinical with a pathologic study has shown that the incidence of internal organ involvement is much more frequent in the autopsy series, particularly involvement of lungs, heart, and kidneys.

Skin. Sclerosis and thickening of the skin are present in almost all patients. The affected areas are firmly matted and bound to the subcutaneous tissue. Because of the marked dermal infiltration with collagen, the skin thickness is almost always increased. Subsequently, atrophy of the normal cutaneous structures occurs, with disappearance of hair follicles and sweat glands. The skin over the hands is most frequently affected, but as the disease progresses, the sclerotic changes extend to the entire upper extremities, face, neck, trunk, and abdomen. The lower extremities, however, sometimes are spared the infiltrative process.

Skin ulceration, usually localized to fingertips or areas of pressure, is present in about 30% of cases (Fig. 17-1). Ulceration of nostrils and ear lobes is less common.

Pigmentary changes are frequent and characterized by diffuse darkening associated with localized areas of depigmentation that often assume a punctate appearance (Fig. 17-1). Intense pruritus may precede pigmentary changes. Nonpitting edema localized to hands and feet usually is an early manifestation.

The telangiectases, present in about 20% of cases, commonly are periungual or mucosal, although they can occur on the palms, face, chest, neck, or elsewhere. Calcinosis, most commonly found in fingertips and periarticular tissues, can be a clue to the diagnosis of systemic sclerosis. In many cases large, calcified masses promote ulceration of the skin, with development of draining sinus tracts.

Vessels. Raynaud's phenomenon is the second most common manifestation of systemic sclerosis, present in more than 85% of patients. It usually appears simultaneously with other manifestations but may antedate them by several years. Raynaud's phenomenon usually is triggered by cold exposure and occasionally by stressful circumstances. Episodes often are painful and are characterized by a triphasic reaction involving fingers, toes, and occasionally the face. Initial vasoconstriction and blanching are followed by a dusky cyanosis. With return of blood flow, reactive erythema occurs. In many patients the number of skin capillary loops decreases, which is readily demonstrated by capillaroscopy at the nail folds and in the skin over the distal phalanges. Marked dilation and distortion of the remaining capillaries often are observed. In some cases larger blood vessels are affected, and luminal narrowing and occlusion, which may be demonstrated by angiographic studies, can result in ischemic necrosis of the extremities or internal organs. Patients who do not manifest Raynaud's phenomenon either at the onset or during the course of the disease may have a higher risk of a rapidly progressive course.

Musculoskeletal system. Musculoskeletal symptoms, present in about 45% of patients, often are the initial manifestations of disease. Symptoms vary from mild polyarthralgias to severe arthritis sometimes indistinguishable from that of rheumatoid arthritis. Severe flexion contractures result from thickening and induration of periarticular tissues. Distal phalangeal atrophy and resorption of digital tufts may lead to total disappearance of the phalanx. An early sign of the disease is the presence of a leathery rub heard on movement of various tendons. Many patients frequently complain of myalgia and weakness; at times muscle tenderness and objective weakness may be present, but more often physical examination is negative. Determination of serum enzymes, particularly aldolase, or electromyographic or histologic examination may be necessary to document the presence of muscle involvement. These techniques can reveal a mild myopathy in most patients with scleroderma. Synovitis with effusion may be found; characteristically, the aspirated synovial fluid is mildly inflammatory.

Gastrointestinal tract. The gastrointestinal tract is the most common internal organ system involved in scleroderma. Esophageal symptoms are present in approximately 40% of patients and may antedate the appearance of skin involvement. When sensitive methods such as cineradiography and manometric study are used, esophageal abnormalities can be detected in about 90% of cases. Early symptoms are characterized by midchest pain, fullness, heartburn, and regurgitation of food, especially in the recumbent position. In severe cases chronic peptic esophagitis can lead to stricture and dysphagia. Poor gastric emptying and involvement of the small intestine may cause abdominal distention, bloating, nausea, and pain. In many cases bacterial overgrowth with deconjugation of bile salts and secondary vitamin deficiency, malabsorption, diarrhea, and weight loss have been described. Occasionally obstipation associated with abnormalities in colonic motility can occur.

Lungs. The most prominent symptoms in the lungs are tachypnea and exertional dyspnea, usually secondary to pulmonary fibrosis. Less often a chronic nonproductive cough and pleuritic chest pain are present. Many patients remain asymptomatic despite evidence of fibrotic involvement of the parenchyma. Dry, basilar "crackling" rales may be found. In some cases, particularly in patients with the CREST syndrome, fulminant pulmonary hypertension can lead to rapid death.

Heart. Pericardial involvement may appear as acute or chronic pericarditis but usually is asymptomatic. Pericardial effusions, however, are found by echocardiography or autopsy examination in about half of patients. Anginal pain, arrhythmias (including various degrees of heart block), myocardiopathy with left ventricular or biventricular insufficiency, and cor pulmonale may be found in patients with systemic sclerosis.

Kidneys. Renal disease is the most serious internal organ involvement in systemic sclerosis, and it is responsible for most deaths in patients with this disorder. It typically is characterized by abrupt development of highly malignant arterial hypertension and progressive renal insufficiency.

In most cases renal disease appears in patients with rapidly progressive systemic sclerosis and only rarely in individuals with the CREST syndrome. The development of hypertension often is heralded by severe headache, visual symptoms resulting from severe hypertensive retinopathy, seizures and other central nervous system symptoms, or sudden left ventricular failure. In these patients renal function often deteriorates rapidly. In rare cases the blood pressure remains within normal limits, but severe hypertension associated with extremely high plasma renin levels is the rule. In the past patients died 3 to 6 months after the onset of this most feared complication, but a more aggressive approach has improved the prognosis.

Nervous system. Peripheral neuropathy and trigeminal neuralgia have been reported but rarely are apparent clinically. In contrast to direct involvement of the nervous system, entrapment neuropathies are relatively common, especially carpal tunnel syndrome, which can be an early and self-limited manifestation of the disease.

Liver. Primary disease of the liver is unusual in systemic sclerosis, but the occurrence of primary biliary cirrhosis in a number of patients with the CREST syndrome has been documented. In these patients jaundice, pruritus, and hepatomegaly develop, and laboratory tests show marked elevation of serum alkaline phosphatase and high titers of antimitochondrial antibodies.

Miscellaneous manifestations. Functional thyroid abnormalities occur in up to 30% of patients with systemic sclerosis. These abnormalities include Hashimoto's thyroiditis with elevated levels of thyroid auto-antibodies, clinical and subclinical hypothyroidism, and the "euthyroid sick" state. Male impotence caused by erectile failure may be a significant early feature of systemic sclerosis, and some degree of erectile dysfunction ultimately develops in a third of male patients. The simultaneous onset of Raynaud's phenomenon and impotence in some patients suggests penile microvascular involvement as a cause of impotence. Occasionally female gonadal fibrosis can develop in systemic sclerosis, and fertility is reduced. Pregnancy can be complicated by hypertension and preeclampsia, but fetal outcome appears to be relatively unaffected by maternal scleroderma. Patients may develop the sicca syndrome (keratoconjunctivitis sicca and xerostomia) or a complete Sjögren's syndrome caused by fibrosis and lymphocytic infiltration of the salivary and lacrimal glands. Several recent studies have shown an association between systemic sclerosis and cancer. An increased rate of breast cancer has been found in a subset of women at or near the time of onset of scleroderma. Lung cancer also occurs more frequently in patients with scleroderma, especially in those with disease of many years' duration. Lung cancer occurs in the setting of chronic interstitial pulmonary fibrosis. Although alveolar cell carcinoma is considered to be often associated with long-standing scleroderma lung fibrosis, malignant lung tumors of any type of cell may develop.

Uncommon manifestations. Unusual clinical manifestations include visceral perforation caused by vasculitic necrosis, pneumatosis cystoides intestinalis with pneumoperitoneum, hoarseness from vocal cord involvement, and microangiopathic hemolytic anemia, which usualy accompanies or precedes renal crisis.

LABORATORY FINDINGS. Hematologic studies show mild anemia, usually normochromic and normocytic, in one third of patients. Elevation of the erythrocyte sedimentation rate (ESR) is not common; when present it usually is related to rapid disease activity or is the result of intercurrent infection, malignancy, or other overlapping inflammatory disease.

Antinuclear antibodies (ANA) are found in almost all cases of scleroderma and often have a speckled or nucleolar pattern. The nucleolar pattern, although less common, seems relatively specific for diffuse scleroderma. Two distinctive autoantibodies have been recognized in scleroderma. Antibodies to the Scl-70 antigen (identified as topoisomerase I) are found in up to a third of patients with scleroderma and appear to be highly specific for the diffuse form of the disease. Antibodies directed against the kinetochore of mitotic chromosomes (anticentromere) appear selective for the subgroup of patients with the CREST syndrome.

Some laboratory tests may provide a clue to involvement of different organ systems. Proteinuria or azotemia almost invariably precedes the development of severe renal disease; elevated creatinine phosphokinase and aldolase levels indicate the presence of myositis; elevations in lactic acid dehydrogenase and glutamic oxaloacetic transaminase levels may result from both muscular and pulmonary involvement.

The most common abnormality found on musculoskeletal roentgenographic examination is erosion and resorption of the tufts of the terminal digital phalanges, frequently accompanied by periarticular and subcutaneous calcinosis. Alterations in the joints generally are confined to thickening of the periarticular soft tissues and juxtaarticular osteoporosis. These features help differentiate the articular involvement in systemic sclerosis from that of other inflammatory arthritides, particularly rheumatoid arthritis.

Roentgenographic examination of the gastrointestinal tract shows the characteristic findings of hypomotility and dilation of the distal esophagus; gastroesophageal reflux and frequently diaphragmatic hernias occur even in asymptomatic patients. Other findings include gastric dilation and poor emptying, small intestinal dilation (especially of the duodenum), slow transit time throughout the bowel, and distinctive widemouthed sacculations of the colon. Chest roentgenograms are an insensitive indicator of early lung involvement in scleroderma. When abnormalities are present, the classic finding is fine, fibronodular interstitial fibrosis, most prominent at the lung bases. Pleural effusions occasionally are seen. In advanced cases fine honeycombing can be seen, and even changes suggestive of bibasilar emphysema have been described.

Manometric determinations to detect lower-third esophageal dysfunction are even more sensitive than cineradiographs, showing abnormalities in about 90% of patients with systemic sclerosis. The classic findings are decreased or absent peristalsis in the lower esophagus and decreased lower esophageal sphincter pressure. The upper esophagus is normal in systemic sclerosis, a feature that helps differentiate the disorder from polymyositis/dermatomyositis.

Pulmonary function tests usually show decreased diffusing capacity early in the disease, even in the absence of any clinical or roentgenographic findings. Somewhat later a restrictive picture resulting from interstitial, pleural, and chest wall fibrosis can be found.

Lung scans with gallium may be helpful in the early detection of pulmonary involvement in systemic sclerosis. Recently, cytologic analysis of bronchoalveolar lavage fluid has been used to detect early lung involvement.

Electrocardiograms, Holter monitoring, and echocardiography usually show evidence of rhythm abnormalities, cardiac hypertrophy, pericardial effusion, pulmonary hypertension, and conduction defects.

DIAGNOSIS. The American Rheumatism Association has established preliminary criteria for the diagnosis and classification of systemic sclerosis. These criteria are useful for epidemiologic investigational studies and for moderately advanced cases. Skin sclerosis, involving parts of the body proximal to the metacarpophalangeal or metatarsophalangeal joints or truncal and facial skin, constitutes the single major criterion for systemic sclerosis. Minor criteria are sclerodactyly, digital pitting, scars of fingertips or loss of substance of the distal finger pads, and bibasilar pulmonary fibrosis. The major or two minor criteria were found in 97% of patients with definite systemic sclerosis but in only 2% of patients with systemic lupus erythematosus, polymyositis/dermatomyositis, or Raynaud's phenomenon not associated with connective tissue disease.

The diagnosis of systemic sclerosis is not as difficult in patients with Raynaud's phenomenon and characteristic hidebound skin as in those with Raynaud's phenomenon alone. Raynaud's phenomenon may be present in other rheumatic diseases, in cryoglobulinemia and serum hyperviscosity syndromes, in association with obliterative vascular disorders, and with occupational use of vibrating instruments. It is important to search for evidence of visceral scleroderma, such as esophageal hypomotility, abnormalities in pulmonary function tests, and the presence of autoantibodies; these serve as clues even in asymptomatic patients.

A number of diseases with cutaneous features resembling the skin involvement in systemic sclerosis should be considered in the differential diagnosis.

MANAGEMENT. At present no specific treatment exists for systemic sclerosis. Steroids, immunosuppressive drugs, and cytotoxic agents have proved remarkably ineffective in the treatment of this disease. Because excessive collagen deposition causes many of the clinical manifestations, drugs capable of inhibiting collagen accumulation hold the best promise of halting the progression of fibrosis in cases of early scleroderma. Penicillamine prevents the formation of stable collagen crosslinks and thus interferes with collagen maturation. The drug has been shown to reduce skin thickening, to slow the rate of development of new organ involvement, and most importantly, to prevent the development of renal involvement in some patients. In a recent retrospective study patients treated with penicillamine had an improved 5-year survival rate compared to untreated patients. However, these observations must be interpreted with caution; severe toxic reactions may develop during penicillamine treatment, and patients treated with this drug require close follow-up.

Colchicine, which stimulates synthesis of collagenase and decreases collagen secretion by fibroblasts, has a low risk of toxic reaction with long-term administration and therefore may be considered in the treatment of scleroderma, although its beneficial effect remains unproved.

The treatment of Raynaud's phenomenon often is disappointing. Vasodilating agents, particularly the calcium channel blockers and prazosin, often are useful in reducing the frequency and severity of episodes of Raynaud's phenomenon. For optimal response the maximum tolerated dose of these drugs should be used. However, side effects, including headache, postural hypotension, and exacerbation of gastroesophageal reflux, sometimes limit their usefulness. Other vasoactive agents, such as reserpine, methyldopa, and guanethidine, appear much less effective. Preganglionic sympathectomy no longer should be performed for Raynaud's phenomenon associated with scleroderma because of the generally poor response to this procedure. In severe attacks of Raynaud's phenomenon with impending tissue necrosis, which do not respond to optimal oral vasodilating drugs, intraarterial injection of reserpine or infusion of prostaglandin via a central venous catheter may produce improvement.

Since exposure to cold is an important factor in determining the persistence and frequency of vasospastic episodes, patients should be advised to avoid exposure to cold, to dress warmly, and to wear heavy gloves, especially during winter. When peripheral gangrene and occlusion of medium-sized and small vessels have been documented by arteriographic studies, intravascular platelet thrombosis may contribute to the symptoms; therefore antiplatelet therapy may be beneficial. In severe cases dipyridamole can be used to potentiate the antiplatelet effect of aspirin.

Symptomatic esophageal hypomotility must be managed aggressively. Supportive and pharmacologic measures must be instituted early and followed vigorously to prevent formation of esophageal stricture. Avoiding the recumbent position after meals, elevating the head of the bed, and using antacid preparations are helpful in the treatment of peptic esophagitis. Cimetidine and ranitidine have been used effectively to decrease gastric acid production. Metoclopramide may be effective in improving esophageal sphincter pressure. Patients with Barrett's esophagus need periodic endoscopy and esophageal biopsy to detect the development of carcinoma. Symptoms of intestinal bacterial overgrowth can be ameliorated with the cyclic use of broad-spectrum antibiotics such as tetracycline. Occasionally, medium-chain triglyceride food may be necessary. In severe cases of generalized gastrointestinal atony, intravenous hyperalimentation may be required.

Arthritis and arthralgia often require treatment with high doses of aspirin or other antiinflammatory agents. The myopathy of scleroderma does not require corticosteroid therapy unless laboratory findings demonstrate severe muscle inflammation. Severe and painful calcinosis is difficult to treat, but it may respond to treatment with warfarin or probenecid. Although established pulmonary fibrosis does not respond to corticosteroid treatment, patients with inflammatory interstitial lung disease demonstrated by biopsy, gallium scanning, or bronchoalveolar lavage may be treated with prednisone. In two recent studies prolonged therapy with penicillamine was associated with improved lung-diffusing capacity in patients with scleroderma. Vasodilating drugs used in the treatment of pulmonary hypertension have produced inconsistent results and have been associated with adverse side effects. General measures for management of pulmonary involvement include low-flow oxygen (which may improve pulmonary vasoconstriction) prophylaxis with pneumococcal and influenza vaccines, prompt antibiotic treatment of pulmonary infection, prevention of as-

piration episodes, and chest expansion exercises. Cigarette smoking should be strongly discouraged. Patients with pulmonary involvement should have yearly chest roentgenographic examinations. Treatment of sclerodermatous and hypertensive cardiomyopathy is difficult, since patients are extremely prone to digitalis toxicity. These patients should be carefully managed with digitalis therapy, salt restriction, and diuretics. If pericardial constriction occurs, surgical decompression should be performed.

Kidney involvement is the most significant and serious complication of progressive scleroderma and usually appears abruptly. It previously was thought that development of kidney disease in scleroderma was irreversible and often fatal; however, it has been shown that a combination of aggressive antihypertensive therapy with chronic hemodialysis can prolong survival in these patients, especially if instituted early. The prognosis of patients with systemic sclerosis who have renal involvement has improved in the past several years. Recognition of the crucial role that the renin-angiotensin axis plays in the development of hypertension and scleroderma renal crisis prompted the use of specific angiotensin converting enzyme (ACE) inhibitors. Unlike other antihypertensive agents, ACE inhibitors may prevent progression of renal disease. Early recognition and aggressive control of hypertension is crucial. Uremia can be managed effectively with long-term hemodialysis, and occasionally patients may recover glomerular functions during dialysis.

PROGNOSIS. The prognosis of systemic sclerosis and its variants is as heterogeneous as the clinical manifestations; it depends on the type and extent of internal organ involvement and on the rapidity and progression of visceral and skin changes. A recent study correlated the rate of development of specific organ failure with prognosis employing life-table analysis. In this series the 5-year cumulative survival rate for patients with systemic sclerosis was 77% from the onset of symptoms. However, in a group of patients with rapidly progressive disease, the 5-year survival rate was only 20%. Most of the patients with this fulminant course of systemic sclerosis had no evidence of renal, cardiac, or pulmonary involvement at the time of initial medical evaluation. Thus the absence of demonstrable abnormalities in these organs at the time of diagnosis is no assurance that the patient will have a slowly progressive course. Careful observation during the first 8 to 12 months is necessary to identify patients who may undergo rapid disease progression.

Although systemic sclerosis is a systemic and occasionally lethal disease, recent advances in diagnosis and treatment have improved the outlook and quality of life for most of these patients. Early recognition and management of renal and pulmonary involvement may retard the progressive deterioration of function. Histamine-receptor blockers can prevent the development of esophagitis and its complications. Identification of patients who have the fulminant form of the disease helps determine those patients most likely to benefit from drugs aimed at preventing progressive fibrosis. However, physicians must emphasize to their patients that systemic sclerosis can not be cured with the therapeutic measures currently available. Many patients have a tendency to search from doctor to doctor for a miraculous cure, and they may receive unapproved treatments that sometimes result in severe complications. The role of physicians in counseling the patient and his family, explaining the complications and prognosis of scleroderma, and attempting to convey a clear understanding of the goals in management of systemic sclerosis is of paramount importance.

BIBLIOGRAPHY

Black CM and Myers AR: Systemic sclerosis (scleroderma), New York, 1985, Gower Medical Publishing Ltd.

D'Angelo WA and others: Pathologic observation in systemic sclerosis (scleroderma), Am J Med 46:428, 1969.

Jimenez SA: General management and prognosis of scleroderma, Gastroenterology 79:163, 1980.

Lally EV, Jimenez SA, and Kaplan SR: Progressive systemic sclerosis: mode of presentation, rapidly progressive disease course, and mortality based on an analysis of 91 patients, Semin Arthritis Rheum, 1988.

Rodman GP: Progressive systemic sclerosis, Clin Rheum Dis 5:49, 1979.

Varga J, Lally EV, and Jimenez SA: Endocrinology and other visceral organ involvement in progressive systemic sclerosis. In Jayson MIV and Black CM, editors: Systemic sclerosis, London, 1988, John Wiley & Sons.

18 · RAYNAUD'S PHENOMENON

Warren A. Katz

Raynaud's phenomenon is characterized by periodic attacks of bilateral digital pallor followed by cyanosis, usually on exposure to cold. Raynaud's phenomenon most often begins in women between 18 and 40 years of age. The ischemic changes in the fingers and toes are caused by vasoconstriction of the digital and palmar or plantar arteries. Early in the attack the small cutaneous vessels are constricted, causing pallor; later the capillaries and venules dilate, and the slow blood flow causes cyanosis. Following relief of vasoconstriction, the blood supply increases considerably and a red color (rubor) develops. Pathologically, the vessels are normal in the early stages of Raynaud's phenomenon, but later intimal proliferation of the vessel wall and hypertrophy of the muscle layer become evident. If the vessels thrombose, focal gangrene of the tips of the fingers and toes develops.

CLINICAL MANIFESTATIONS. Clinical manifestations in the typical patient with Raynaud's phenomenon consist of pain, paresthesias, and stiffness in the fingers and toes on exposure to refrigerator air, cold wind, air-conditioning, or other low-temperature settings. Three sequential stages of Raynaud's phenomenon are recognized: pallor (vasoconstriction), cyanosis (poorly oxygenated blood in dilated capillaries and venules), and rubor (reactive hyperemia). The digits are cold and numb during vasoconstriction and painful during hyperemia. Not all stages may be prominent during each attack of Raynaud's phenomenon. In addition to the fingers and toes, the earlobes, nose, cheeks, and chin may exhibit ischemic changes. Besides exposure to cold, emotional tension and trauma may precipitate Raynaud's phenomenon.

Most cases are accompanied by one or more of a variety of conditions. Raynaud's phenomenon often heralds rheumatic disorders such as systemic sclerosis (particularly the CREST variety) and mixed connective tissue disease by months or several years. Systemic lupus erythematosus, polymyositis, and rheumatoid arthritis are less often associated with Raynaud's phenomenon. The condition is rare in polyarteritis and giant cell arteritis. Raynaud's phenomenon may be associated with the following factors:

Connective tissue disorders
    Systemic sclerosis
    Mixed connective tissue disease
    Systemic lupus erythematosus
    Rheumatoid arthritis
    Dermatomyositis and polymyositis
Peripheral arterial disease
    Thromboangiitis obliterans (Buerger's disease)
    Arteriosclerosis obliterans
    Arteritis
Neurovascular compression syndromes
    Thoracic outlet syndrome
Hematologic abnormalities
    Cryoproteinemia
    Paraproteinemia
    Polycythemia vera
Occupational exposures
    Vibratory tool workers (pneumatic hammer operators)
    Percussion instrument workers (pianists, typists)
    Acroosteolysis (resorption of digital tips) caused by polyvinyl-chloride
    Traumatic occlusive arterial disease
Drugs and toxins
    Ergot compounds
    β-Adrenergic blockers
    Sympathomimetic drugs
    Oral contraceptives
    Methysergide
    Heavy metals

Raynaud's disease is the term applied if no associated conditions are apparent after at least 2 years of observation. In contrast to Raynaud's phenomenon, Raynaud's disease usually is not attended by digital necrosis, cutaneous atrophy, or calcinosis. Angiography generally reveals no structural changes in the vessels. Laboratory evaluations for connective tissue and other diseases are unremarkable.

The course of Raynaud's phenomenon is variable. It may recur at irregular intervals but usually is worse in the winter. Some patients improve spontaneously, but most have recurring mild to severe symptoms. With long-standing Raynaud's phenomenon, atrophic changes of the fingers, characterized by tapering and flattening of the digital pulp, may develop. Sometimes the skin over the proximal interphalangeal joints becomes taut and shiny (sclerodactyly).

DIAGNOSIS. Raynaud's phenomenon is suspected when pain, paresthesias, pallor, or cyanosis of the fingers and toes develops following the patient's exposure to cold. The workup is designed to differentiate Raynaud's phenomenon from Raynaud's disease and also to establish any of the usual causes of Raynaud's phenomenon listed previously. It must be recognized, however, that Raynaud's phenomenon may precede any of the associated diseases. The minimal ancillary evaluation includes a complete blood count, erythrocyte sedimentation rate, rheumatoid factor, antinuclear antibody, cryoglobulins, serum protein electrophoresis, and muscle enzyme determinations. Raynaud's phenomenon may be differentiated from acrocyanosis (persistent cyanosis aggravated by exposure to cold) and occlusive vascular disease by the sequential color changes, intermittency, and localization of gangrene to the digital tips in Raynaud's phenomenon.

MANAGEMENT. Proper management of Raynaud's phenomenon usually diminishes digital ischemia, alleviates symptoms once they develop, and prevents dystrophic alterations in the extremities. Because emotional stress in itself may trigger Raynaud's phenomenon, patients generally respond to the reassurance that the overall prognosis is good and that, although there is no cure, the condition can be treated. As with other forms of peripheral vascular disease, patients with Raynaud's phenomenon should be discouraged from smoking. The hands must be kept warm during the winter months by avoiding cold when possible and wearing heavy gloves and outerwear when such exposure cannot be avoided. Patients should be careful about touching cold doorknobs, reaching into the refrigerator for cold bottles, and swimming in cold pools. Sores and ulcers, once having developed, may be slow to heal, so whenever possible patients should wear protective gloves while indulging in activities such as gardening or carpentry that may cause trauma to the hands. Seemingly, keeping the hands well lubricated will prevent chafing and cracking.

Drug therapy may decrease peripheral vasoconstriction. Reserpine (0.25 to 0.5 mg/day), guanethidine (10 to 40 mg/day), methyldopa (1.5 to 2 g/day), nifedipine (10 to 60 mg/day), and prazosin (1 to 12 mg/day) may be partially successful in relieving or preventing Raynaud's phenomenon.

Sympathectomy to eliminate vasoconstricting impulses is successful in some cases of Raynaud's phenomenon. The procedure is of no benefit in patients with scleroderma. Treating the underlying cause of Raynaud's phenomenon may be the most important aspect of therapy when such treatment is available.

BIBLIOGRAPHY

Belch J and Sturrock R: Raynaud's syndrome, Current trends, Br J Rheumatol 22:50, 1983.

Blunt RJ and Porter JM: Raynaud syndrome, Semin Arthritis Rheum 10:282, 1982.

Fitzgerald O, Hess EV, and Spencer-Green G: Markers of progression to systemic illness in Raynaud phenomenon, Arthritis Rheum 28:S81, 1985.

Harper FE and others: A prospective study of Raynaud phenomenon and early connective tissue disease, Am J Med 72:883, 1982.

19 · POLYMYOSITIS AND DERMATOMYOSITIS

Donald H. Lieberman

Polymyositis is an inflammatory disorder of striated muscle associated with symmetric proximal weakness and atrophy. When accompanied by characteristic skin lesions, the disease is referred to as dermatomyositis. The cause is unknown, but recent evidence incriminates abnormalities in cellular immunity. It is more common in women (2:1) and has a peak incidence in the sixth and seventh decades. The childhood disease resembles the adult form but has distinct characteristics that are discussed separately. The following classification provides a useful framework for discussion:

Type I—polymyositis in adults
Type II—typical dermatomyositis in adults
Type III—inflammatory myositis associated with malignant disease
Type IV—childhood myositis
Type V—myositis associated with an overlap syndrome (for example, scleroderma or systemic lupus erythematosus)

"Pure" polymyositis and dermatomyositis (types I and II) constitute more than half of the cases in this classification.

Polymyositis may be mimicked by other connective tissue diseases or muscular dystrophy.

CLINICAL MANIFESTATIONS. The constant feature in all types of polymyositis regardless of other associations is weakness of proximal muscles. The onset of the disease is variable, and the initial diagnosis may be missed when the disease has an insidious onset. Muscle weakness rarely occurs acutely, and patients often have symptoms for 3 to 6 months before seeing a physician. The pelvic and shoulder girdles seem to be affected most often. Patients may complain of difficulty ascending stairs, getting on a bus, or rising from a chair. Later they may find it difficult to reach overhead. The flexors of the neck and the pharyngeal muscles often become involved. Severe dysphagia and dysphonia can result. If the respiratory muscles become involved in a rapidly progressive or advanced case, the patient may have a life-threatening or fatal respiratory insufficiency.

Skin. When the myositis is accompanied by a rash, the disease is referred to as dermatomyositis. The rash consists of a purplish, dusky, erythematous eruption chiefly involving the face, neck, upper arms, and trunk. A violaceous discoloration of the eyelids has been called a "heliotrope" rash and is a characteristic sign of dermatomyositis. A rash also may be seen on the extensor surfaces of the forearms, knees, elbows, and knuckles. These lesions may become scaly and plaquelike as the disease progresses.

Raynaud's phenomenon. Raynaud's phenomenon is relatively uncommon unless patients have an overlap with another connective tissue disease, most commonly scleroderma or systemic lupus erythematosus. When it does occur, it usually is mild and does not result in digital ulceration or necrosis.

Other clinical manifestations. When patients do not have an overlap form of myositis, involvement outside the skeletal muscle is uncommon. Mild arthralgias or arthritis can occur and may be accompanied by joint effusions. Joint destruction is rare, and the arthritis responds well to corticosteroid therapy. Pulmonary involvement as a primary finding (as opposed to that caused by aspiration) is uncommon. When it occurs, interstitial pneumonitis with a nonproductive cough, dyspnea, and hypoxemia characterize the clinical picture. The chest roentgenogram demonstrates interstitial infiltrates with a predilection for the lung bases. Most cases respond favorably to corticosteroids. When cardiac muscle is involved, conduction abnormalities and nonspecific electrocardiographic changes result. Purely neurologic symptoms do not occur. The other clinical features seen with overlap forms are characteristic of the disease in concert with the myositis. Periorbital edema may develop.

ASSOCIATION WITH MALIGNANCY. The association of malignancy with polymyositis and dermatomyositis remains a controversial subject. Some studies suggest an association with malignancy in 6% to 35% of cases of polymyositis. The male to female ratio for disease associated with malignancy is almost equal; however, the average age for these patients is higher than for those without malignancy. The tumors most commonly are found in the breast, lung, ovary, stomach, colon, and uterus. No clinical manifestations seem to be specifically associated with patients with malignancy. Most tumors are discovered within 1 year of the onset of myopathy; conversely, when myositis develops after the discovery of the malignancy, it usually does so within 1 year. There are anecdotal reports of amelioration of myositis after treatment of the associated malignancy, but the improvement usually is only temporary, and the patients eventually die as a result of the malignancy.

DERMATOMYOSITIS OF CHILDHOOD. When myositis occurs in childhood, the rash of dermatomyositis is seen in most patients. The other features resemble those seen in adults. Proximal muscle weakness predominates. Some children have a benign course, whereas others have severe atrophy and muscle shortening with resultant crippling contractures. The erythematous patches seen over the knuckles in some adults are particularly characteristic of the disease in childhood. Abdominal pain, sometimes accompanied by gastrointestinal bleeding, is a feature unique to the disease in the young. Vasculitis involving the gastrointestinal tract is responsible for this severe complication. Vasculitis also may be present in the skeletal muscles, and in many children marked subcutaneous calcifications develop when dermatomyositis is long standing.

LABORATORY FINDINGS. Routine "connective tissue screening" tests are not very helpful in the diagnosis of polymyositis. The erythrocyte sedimentation rate may be elevated, but this is an inconsistent finding; it may be normal even in the presence of active disease. Tests for antinuclear antibodies, rheumatoid factor, and alteration of the erythrocyte sedimentation rate lend little help in diagnosis. These tests are useful, however, in assessing the possibility of disease overlap with the other connective tissue disorders.

Muscle enzymes. Necrosis of muscle during the course of myositis results in the release of enzymes into the serum. Evaluation of the enzyme levels is helpful not only diagnostically but also prognostically as a guide to therapy. Determination of creatine phosphokinase (CPK), aldolase, and lactic dehydrogenase levels is of greatest use, since the levels of these enzymes decline rapidly with treatment. However, these enzymes are not elevated in every patient, and not every patient has elevations of all three enzymes simultaneously. CPK is the enzyme elevated most frequently.

Precipitating antibodies. Precipitating antibodies to antigens in calf thymus nuclear extracts have been observed in most patients with polymyositis; notably, Jo-1 occurs in 18% to 23% of cases (includes overlap syndromes). There is an association between the presence of anti-Jo-1 antibody and pulmonary fibrosis.

Electromyogram. The triad of spontaneous fibrillation, polyphasic action potentials, and pseudomyotonic discharges is said to be almost pathognomonic of polymyositis.

Pulmonary function tests. Early evaluation of pulmonary function is helpful in detecting intercostal muscle involvement, which is especially prevalent in children. Defects in vital capacity and oxygen diffusion may exist.

Muscle biopsy. Proximal muscles are preferred for biopsy. The electromyogram (EMG) may be helpful in the selection of a biopsy site. A common practice is to obtain the biopsy from the side of the body opposite that in which the EMG was done to avoid changes caused by needle insertion. The classic biopsy shows widespread degeneration of muscle fibers, basophilia with central positioning of nuclei (evidence of regeneration), a chronic inflammatory cell infiltrate (especially lymphocytes), variation in cross-sectional fiber diameter (partial regeneration), and fibrosis.

MANAGEMENT. It is now accepted that all patients with polymyositis or dermatomyositis should be treated with corticosteroids. The usual starting dose is 60 mg/day of prednisone. Response to steroids means increased muscle strength but not necessarily a decrease in enzyme levels, which may precede a return of strength or may occur with little or no clinical improvement in some cases. Once strength returns, the dose of steroids should be slowly tapered and increased if any "flare-up" is detected. Rarely patients can be completely weaned from corticosteroids, but most patients require persistent maintenance therapy with doses of 7.5 to 20 mg/day.

It must be kept in mind that no carefully controlled study has been done to determine if steroids have an influence on ultimate mortality in this disease. One investigation found that, although morbidity was greatly improved, corticosteroids did not appear to affect the eventual outcome. In patients in whom the response is poor or the disease becomes life threatening, immunosuppressive agents such as methotrexate have been used with reported success.

PROGNOSIS. When not accompanied by a malignancy, polymyositis and dermatomyositis have a good prognosis. The most dramatic factors negatively influencing survival are age, dysphagia, and acute progressive onset. Most patients have an impressive return of muscle strength and live fairly normal lives.

BIBLIOGRAPHY

Barnes BE: Dermatomyositis and malignancy: a review of the literature, Ann Intern Med 84:68, 1976.

Benbassat J: Prognostic factors in polymyositis/dermatomyositis: a computer assisted analysis of ninety-two cases, Arthritis Rheum 28:249, 1985.

Bohan A: A computerized analysis of 153 patients with polymyositis and dermatomyositis, Medicine 56:255, 1977.

Hochberg MC, Feldman D, and Stevens MB: adult onset polymyositis/dermatomyositis: an analysis of clinical and laboratory features and survival in 76 patients with a review of the literature, Semin Arthritis Rheum 15:168, 1986.

Kagen LJ, Kimball AC, and Christian CL: Serologic evidence of toxoplasmosis among patients with polymyositis, Am J Med 56:186, 1974.

Manchul LA and others: the frequency of malignant neoplasm in patients with polymyositis-dermatomyositis: a controlled study, Arch Intern Med 145:1835, 1985.

Schumacher HR and others: Articular manifestations of polymyositis and dermatomyositis, Am J Med 67:287, 1979.

Schwarz MI and others: Interstitial lung disease in polymyositis and dermatomyositis: analysis of six cases and a review of the literature, Medicine 55:89, 1976.

Winkleman RK and others: Course of dermatomyositis-polymyositis: comparison of untreated and cortisone treated patients, Mayo Clin Proc 43:545, 1968.

Wolfe JF, Adelstein E, and Sharp GC: Antinuclear antibody with distinct specificity for polymyositis, J Clin Invest 59:176, 1976.

20 · VASCULITIS

Paul Katz and **Anthony S. Fauci**

Vasculitis encompasses a broad range of heterogeneous syndromes characterized by inflammation and necrosis of blood vessels. This clinicopathologic process may be the primary manifestation of a particular disease, or it may exist merely as an accessory finding of another underlying disease. A major problem in discussing the vasculitides is proper delineation of specific disease syndromes. Previous attempts at classification have resulted in the oversimplification of complicated processes or the creation of cumbersome and often artificial categories with little allowance for disease overlap. We propose the following revised scheme for classification of the vasculitides:

Polyarteritis nodosa group of systemic necrotizing vasculitis
  Classic polyarteritis nodosa
  Allergic angiitis and granulomatosis
  Systemic necrotizing vasculitis—"overlap syndrome"
Hypersensitivity vasculitis
  Serum sickness and serum sickness–like reactions
  Schönlein-Henoch purpura
  Essential mixed cryoglobulinemia with vasculitis
  Vasculitis associated with malignancies
  Vasculitis associated with other primary disorders
Wegener's granulomatosis
Lymphomatoid granulomatosis
Giant cell arteritides
  Temporal arteritis
  Takayasu's arteritis
Miscellaneous vasculitides
  Thromboangiitis obliterans (Buerger's disease)
  Mucocutaneous lymph node syndrome

From this basic outline we direct our attention to the pathogenesis, immunologic mechanisms, clinical manifestations, and therapeutic approach to this heterogeneous group of disorders as a whole and to certain specific disease states.

PATHOGENESIS. It has become increasingly apparent that most if not all of the vasculitides are initiated by immunopathogenic mechanisms. Although in most cases a definite offending agent or antigen cannot be identified, the histologic and clinical aspects of the vasculitides suggest that they are mediated by immunologic events. Currently the predominant theory is that these disorders are initiated by the deposition of immune complexes in blood vessel walls. Experimental data suggest that, after exposure to antigen, soluble antigen-antibody complexes in a state of antigen excess are formed in the circulation. If these are not cleared by the reticuloendothelial system, they are deposited in blood vessel walls. This deposition is aided by increased vascular permeability caused by the release of vasoactive amines from platelets and basophils. The deposited complexes activate the complement cascade, resulting in the generation of factors chemotactic for neutrophils. After migration into the vessel wall, these cells release their lysosomal enzymes, which damage and eventually cause necrosis of the involved blood vessel. Secondarily, thrombosis, occlusion, hemorrhage, and tissue ischemic changes may ensue. Even in such situations with presumed immune-complex origins, circulating or tissue antigen-antibody complexes often are not demonstrable. In all likelihood the lack of detectable circulating complexes is caused by rapid clearance from the circulation. Furthermore, in animals tissue immune complexes have been shown to disappear from tissue sites 24 to 48 hours following deposition.

Besides immune-complex mediation, cell-mediated immune reactions may play a role in the development of vascular damage.

CLINICAL MANIFESTATIONS. The original description of systemic vasculitis involved a case of classic polyarteritis nodosa noted by Kussmaul and Maier in 1866. Subsequently, as additional cases of similar but not identical systemic vasculitides appeared, they were grouped into the single category of polyarteritis nodosa. As it became apparent that further categorization of these processes was needed, numerous and often oversimplified classifications appeared. We have devised a classification of the systemic vasculitides based on the etiologic, pathologic, clinical, and therapeutic differences within this group (see the preceding outline). Although certain of these disorders have distinct clinicopathologic features that render them easily distinguishable, others lack this clarity. With this in mind we have found this classification to be useful not as an artificial separator of often similar syndromes but rather as a guide to the systematic approach to these disorders.

Systemic necrotizing vasculitis. Systemic necrotizing vasculitis is a rather large group encompassing classic polyarteritis nodosa, allergic angiitis and granulomatosis, and what we refer to as the overlap syndrome.

Classic polyarteritis nodosa as originally described is a systemic necrotizing vasculitis of small and medium-sized arteries. Vessel involvement tends to be segmental with a propensity for bifurcations and branches. Vascular lesions in all stages of development may be seen, and the type and degree of clinical findings reflect the location and severity of vessel involvement. The following are typical findings of classic polyarteritis nodosa:

Necrotizing vasculitis of small and medium-sized muscular arteries
Eosinophilia and granulomata not characteristic
Allergic history uncommon
Renal involvement
   Related to vasculitis (80%)
   Glomerulitis (30%)
Hypertension
Gastrointestinal—infarction of viscera
Hepatic—subclinical disease caused by chronic active hepatitis in

patients with hepatitis B antigenemia; liver disease related to vasculitis (up to 50%)
Coronary arteritis—particularly in children
Neurologic—mononeuritis multiplex
Lung and spleen characteristically uninvolved
Cutaneous—uncommon; usually subcutaneous nodules, livedo reticularis
Genitourinary—testes, bladder, epididymis, ovary involved
Arthralgias common; arthritis rare

These features are important to remember, since they aid in distinguishing classic polyarteritis nodosa from other syndromes in the systemic necrotizing vasculitis group.

Allergic angiitis and granulomatosis is a disorder similar in many respects to classic polyarteritis nodosa, except that the hallmark of this disease is pulmonary involvement. It frequently is characterized by a history of asthma and allergies. The exact incidence of allergic granulomatosis is uncertain, but it appears to be relatively rare. Pulmonary symptoms, usually in the form of asthma, dominate the clinical picture. Granulomatous tissue reactions with eosinophilic infiltration typically are seen, and peripheral eosinophilia is seen in half of patients. With the exception of the pulmonary manifestations, the clinical characteristics of allergic angiitis and granulomatosis may be virtually identical to those of classic polyarteritis nodosa.

We refer to the third syndrome in this group as the overlap syndrome, since it is manifested by features of both classic polyarteritis nodosa and allergic angiitis and granulomatosis. This is a multisystem vasculitis with variable clinical manifestations. Patients may or may not have atopic histories, peripheral eosinophilia, eosinophilic tissue infiltration, granulomatous inflammation, and lung involvement accompanying necrotizing vasculitis of the small vessels (arterioles, capillaries, and venules) and small and medium-sized arteries.

Hypersensitivity vasculitis. Hypersensitivity vasculitis is a large, heterogeneous group comprising syndromes with predominantly small vessel involvement. The term evolved from the fact that in many cases this syndrome could be traced to offending antigens such as drugs or microorganisms. Recently it has been shown that endogenous "self"-antigens such as autologous proteins or tumor antigens could incite antibody production. Other predisposing associated conditions include "classic" connective tissue diseases, cryoglobulinemia, serum sickness, and malignancies. Immune complexes have been postulated as the pathogenetic bases for these syndromes. Typically the skin is the most frequently involved system, usually in the form of leukocytoclastic vasculitis of the postcapillary venules. Skin lesions may be present as palpable purpura, papules, nodules, vesicles, bullae, or ulcers. Although virtually any organ system may be involved in varying degrees, the cutaneous involvement dominates the clinical picture. In this regard this group differs from the systemic necrotizing vasculitides, in which extracutaneous disease generally prevails. This large group of disorders comprises many distinct identifiable syndromes.

Lymphomatoid granulomatosis. Lymphomatoid granulomatosis is an unusual form of vasculitis hallmarked by angiotrophic and angiodestructive tissue infiltration with atypical cells in combination with a granulomatous reaction. Cellular infiltrates in this disease are polymorphic and composed of normal lymphoid cells with atypical lymphocytoid, plasmacytoid, and reticuloendothelial cells. These cells often have mitotic figures, giving them the appearance of a lymphoproliferative disease. In the past this disorder often was confused with Wegener's granulomatosis because of the presence of granulomatous vasculitis. However, in lymphomatoid granulomatosis granulomata are fewer in number and less distinct and the "vasculitis" is characterized by an infiltration of blood vessels of various sizes with atypical mononuclear cells. Of the patients in whom the disease is left untreated and who survive the acute illness, at least 50% develop a lymphoproliferative disorder.

Giant cell arteritides. The giant cell arteritides are temporal arteritis and Takayasu's arteritis (Table 20-1). Both disorders are panarteritides with involvement of medium-sized and large arteries, although they differ in the age of onset, location of vessel involvement, and response to therapy. Their causes are uncertain, but immunologic mechanisms are postulated for both.

Temporal arteritis often is accompanied by the polymyalgia rheumatica syndrome of stiffness and pain of the neck, shoulder, lower back, hip, and thigh muscles (see Chapter 23). The clinical picture of temporal arteritis usually is well circumscribed. It consists of fever, anemia, headache, myalgias, and a high erythrocyte sedimentation rate in older people. Although seen in only 10% to 20% of patients, jaw claudication (that is, pain with mastication) is an extremely specific sign of this process. The diagnosis is confirmed by the finding of panarteritis in temporal artery biopsy specimens. One of the most serious complications of temporal arteritis is sudden blindness caused by ophthalmic arteritis. It is important to be attentive to symptoms in this disorder (which are described later), since ocular involvement usually can be prevented by corticosteroid therapy.

Takayasu's arteritis, or pulseless disease, is a less common disorder with characteristics clearly different from those of temporal arteritis (Table 20-1). This disease may have complex and varied symptoms ranging from generalized, nonspecific complaints to local signs caused by compromised blood flow to the extremities or other organs. Most commonly, this is manifested as absent pulses or bruits. Clinically the course of this disease is variable, but generally a gradual deterioration is seen. Because of this variability with a tendency toward remissions and exacerbations, evaluation of appropriate therapy has been difficult. However, compared to temporal arteritis, Takayasu's arteritis is much less responsive to corticosteroid

therapy. Death usually is caused by congestive heart failure or a cerebrovascular accident.

Other vasculitides. Other, less common vasculitic syndromes include thromboangiitis obliterans (Buerger's disease) and the mucocutaneous lymph node syndrome (Kawasaki disease).

Thromboangiitis obliterans. Thromboangiitis obliterans is an inflammatory occlusive peripheral vascular disease of arteries and veins. It is more common among men, and the age of onset usually is 20 to 40 years. The vasculitis segmentally involves veins and small to medium-sized arteries. The inflammatory stage of the disease almost always is associated with a thrombus. The cause of Buerger's disease is unknown, but almost uniformly it is associated with heavy smoking. Evidence implying immunologic mediation is lacking. Patients show signs of vascular insufficiency in the extremities. The disease follows an indolent course characterized by recurrences and leading finally to amputation unless interrupted by the therapy of choice, cessation of tobacco use.

Mucocutaneous lymph node syndrome. The mucocutaneous lymph node syndrome (Kawasaki syndrome) is an acute febrile illness of children and young adults characterized by nonsuppurative cervical lymphadenopathy, erythema of the oropharynx, desquamative skin rash, and unresponsiveness to antibiotics. Although it usually is self-limited, a small number of patients (approximately 2%) die suddenly from coronary arteritis. This syndrome first was believed to be restricted to Japan, but cases have now been well documented throughout the continental United States. The cause of the disease is uncertain, and intravenous gamma globulin may be of value in preventing coronary artery involvement.

MANAGEMENT. Much of the difficulty in developing treatment protocols for the vasculitides has been related to problems with their classification. Using the categories described in this chapter, we have developed a therapeutic approach. The prototype disorder for our pharmacologic regimen is Wegener's granulomatosis. Because this disease is uniformly fatal and usually fails to respond to corticosteroids, cyclophosphamide has been used.

Because of the regimen's success with Wegener's granulomatosis, it has been used to treat lymphomatoid granulomatosis

Table 20-1 Characteristics of the giant cell arteritides

	Temporal arteritis	Takayasu's arteritis
Patients	Disease of the elderly; more women than men	More prevalent in young women; more common in the Orient but neither racially nor geographically restricted
Blood vessels	Characteristically involves branches of carotid artery (temporal artery) but is a systemic arteritis and may involve any medium-sized or large artery	Large and medium-sized arteries with predilection for aortic arch and its branches; may involve pulmonary artery
Histopathology	Panarteritis; inflammatory mononuclear cell infiltrates; frequent giant cell formation within vessel wall; fragmentation of internal elastic lamina; proliferation of intima	Panarteritis; inflammatory mononuclear cell infiltrates; intimal proliferation and fibrosis; scarring and vascularization of media; disruption and degeneration of elastic lamina
Manifestations	Classic complex of fever, anemia, high erythrocyte sedimentation rate, muscle aches in an elderly person; headache may be present; strongly associated with polymyalgia rheumatica syndrome	Generalized systemic symptoms; local signs and symptoms related to involved vessels; occlusive phase
Complications	Ocular (sudden blindness)	Related to distribution of involved vessels; death usually occurs from congestive heart failure or cerebrovascular accident
Diagnosis	Temporal artery biopsy; lesions may be segmental; multiple sections, arteriography, and bilateral biopsy may aid in diagnosis	Arteriography; biopsy of involved vessel
Treatment	Coricosteroids highly effective	Corticosteroids not of proven efficacy; cytotoxic agents untried

Adapted from Fauci AS, Haynes BF, and Katz P: Ann Intern Med 89:660, 1978.

and systemic necrotizing vasculitis. Patients with lymphomatoid granulomatosis, if left untreated, have a fulminant, usually fatal course often characterized by the development of an aggressive lymphoproliferative disorder. Similarly, without therapy patients with systemic necrotizing vasculitis have a poor prognosis. Thus in the past both diseases had a dismal prognosis even with the use of various cytotoxic regimens. Using cyclophosphamide alone or in combination with corticosteroids, in the same manner as in Wegener's granulomatosis, we have seen a significant reduction in the morbidity and mortality from these two diseases. It is imperative, however, that therapy be instituted early in the course of these disorders, before irreversible end-organ damage has occurred.

In the hypersensitivity vasculitides in which an offending antigen or an underlying disorder can be identified, therapy is aimed at removal of the antigen or treatment of the primary illness. When such causes are suspected but cannot be proved or when the process appears to be self-limited, a brief course of corticosteroids may be warranted to hasten resolution of the process.

As described previously, giant cell arteritis usually is extremely responsive to corticosteroids. Initial high-dose therapy of 40 to 60 mg/day of prednisone is gradually tapered to a daily maintenance dose of 7.5 to 10 mg. Therapy probably should be continued for 1 to 2 years. With this regimen, the prognosis generally is good and complete remission usually is attained. In Takayasu's arteritis corticosteroid therapy has proved to be of variable efficacy, but it does not appear that these agents prolong life. Experience with cytotoxic agents in this disease is at present only anecdotal, and no firm conclusions can yet be drawn regarding the efficacy of these agents.

In all types of vasculitis treatment of underlying or associated conditions, such as connective tissue disease or infection, is imperative. Management depends in large part on which organs are primarily involved (for example, myocardial infarction, ischemic bowel, or digital gangrene).

BIBLIOGRAPHY

Churg J and Strauss L: Allergic granulomatosis, allergic angiitis, and periarteritis nodosa, Am J Pathol 27:227, 1951.

Cupps TR and Fauci AS: The vasculitides, 1981, Philadelphia, WB Saunders Co.

Fauci AS: Granulomatous vasculitis: distinct but related, Ann Intern Med 87:782, 1977.

Fauci AS and Wolff SM: Wegener's granulomatosis: studies in eighteen patients and a review of the literature, Medicine 52:535, 1973.

Fauci AS, Haynes BF, and Katz P: The spectrum of vasculitis: clinical, pathologic, immunologic, and therapeutic consideration, Ann Intern Med 89:660, 1978.

Fauci AS and others: Cyclophosphamide therapy of severe systemic necrotizing vasculitis, N Engl J Med 301:235, 1979.

Rose GA and Spencer H: Polyarteritis nodosa, Q J Med 26:43, 1957.

21 · SCHÖNLEIN-HENOCH PURPURA

Warren A. Katz

Schönlein-Henoch purpura is a vasculitic syndrome closely related to hypersensitivity angiitis. It usually follows streptococcal infections in children, but occasionally it may be caused by a drug or food allergy. Most typically it consists of a clinical tetrad of purpura, arthralgias, abdominal pain, and glomerulonephritis. Cutaneous manifestations are invariable and consist of raised purpuric or ecchymotic lesions, most often on the extensor surface of the lower extremities. The lesions may appear hemorrhagic or urticarial. The rash may involve the face.

Rheumatic manifestations include polyarthralgia and sometimes overt arthritis, particularly of the knees and ankles. Deformities do not develop. Hemorrhage within the gastrointestinal wall may cause colicky abdominal pain, hematemesis, and melena. Hematuria is the most common manifestation of glomerulonephritis; some patients have chronic nephritis with uremia. The most characteristic finding is a leukocytoclastic angiitis seen on skin biopsy with IgG and C3 deposits on immunofluorescence studies.

The disease is usualy self-limited, particularly in young people. Systemic administration of corticosteroids may be required for acutely ill patients.

BIBLIOGRAPHY

Cream JJ, Gumpel JM, and Peachey RD: Schönlein-Henoch purpura in the adult: a study of 77 adults with anaphylactoid or Schönlein-Henoch purpura, Q J Med 34:461, 1970.

22 · WEGENER'S GRANULOMATOSIS AND MIDLINE GRANULOMA

Paul Katz and **Anthony S. Fauci**

Wegener's granulomatosis (WG) and midline granuloma (MLG) are uncommon diseases of unknown cause. Although these disorders are clinically distinct, they may be misdiagnosed because of their propensity to involve the upper airways. WG is a systemic disease with glomerulonephritis and necrotizing granulomatous vasculitis of the upper and lower respiratory tracts. Upper airway disease in WG rarely causes the palatal perforation and facial erosion characteristic of MLG. Conversely, MLG is a localized process of the nasal and oropharyngeal area that infrequently manifests true vasculitis. Additionally, these diseases differ in their response to cytotoxic therapy. The following discussion highlights the important points of both diseases and compares and contrasts the clinical, pathologic, and therapeutic aspects of each.

WEGENER'S GRANULOMATOSIS

WG is a disseminated granulomatous necrotizing vasculitis of the small vessels of the upper and lower respiratory tracts. In the generalized form, glomerulonephritis is an important component of the disease process. Although a localized, limited form confined to the airways has been described, this likely represents an early stage of generalized disease before the development of detectable renal disease.

PATHOGENESIS. The immunopathogenic mechanisms responsible for the development of WG remain largely unknown. Circulating and tissue immune-complex–like material are demonstrable in some individuals with this disease. Theoretically these complexes could activate the complement cascade, with the resultant generation of factors chemotactic for neutrophils. Sensitized lymphocytes likewise could react with the offending antigen(s), which cause the release of lymphokines important in the initiation of granulomatous inflammation. Furthermore, immune complexes potentially can directly trigger monocyte-macrophages to form granulomata. It must be emphasized that in many patients immune-complex mediation can only be assumed and not conclusively proved. The identity and nature of the antigen or antigens that initiate the inflammatory processes are unknown.

PATHOLOGY. The histologic features characteristic of WG include necrotizing vasculitis of small arteries and veins with coexistent granuloma formation. Disease of the upper airway is manifested by paranasal sinus and nasopharyngeal necrotizing granulomata in the presence or absence of vasculitis. This may be accompanied by pansinusitis, bony erosion, septal perforation, and in some cases saddle nose deformity. Lung lesions usually are present roentgenographically as multiple, bilateral nodular infiltrates with a tendency to cavitate. Histologically, involved lung tissue manifests the classic necrotizing vasculitis and associated granulomata. Renal disease in WG is characterized by focal and segmental glomerulonephritis with accompanying crescent formation. Depending on the stage of kidney involvement at the time of biopsy, renal disease may range from mild focal glomerulitis to fulminant proliferative glomerulonephritis to fibrosed and sclerosed end-stage glomeruli. Organ systems other than the lungs and kidneys may display vasculitis or granulomata or both.

CLINICAL MANIFESTATIONS. The mean age at onset of WG is 40 years, and the male to female ratio is 3:2. Early in the disease the clinical picture is dominated by upper respiratory tract signs, including rhinorrhea, paranasal sinus pain, sinusitis, nasal ulcerations, purulent or bloody nasal discharge, septal perforation, saddle nose deformity, and otitis media. However, virtually any manifestation of the disease may be seen at the time of presentation. Nonspecific pulmonary complaints may include cough, hemoptysis, chest discomfort, and shortness of breath. It is not uncommon for asymptomatic pulmonary infiltrates to be seen on roentgenograms of the chest.

Renal disease as the sole presenting manifestation of WG is rare without demonstrable airway disease. The development of renal disease may be insidious, with only smoldering low-level activity, or it may be acute and rapidly progressive, with ultimate progression to end-stage kidney failure.

Virtually any organ system may be involved in WG, but these manifestations usually are less dramatic in comparison to the respiratory tract and renal disease (Table 22-1). However, certain important manifestations are worth mentioning. Peripheral or central nervous system disease occurs in 25% to 50% of the patients, with peripheral involvement more common. Neuropathy induced by vasculitis of the vasa nervorum is manifested as cranial neuritis or mononeuritis multiplex. The rarer central nervous system involvement is caused by cerebral vasculitis or space-occupying granulomata that directly extend from paranasal sinuses or form in situ. Cardiac disease is seen as pericarditis or coronary artery vasculitis in one third of the patients. Skin disease results from vasculitis with or without granuloma formation and is manifested in up to 50% of the patients as petechiae, palpable purpura, papules, vesicles, ulcerations, or subcutaneous nodules. Oral and other mucosal membrane ulcerations also can occur (Fig. 22-1). Half of the patients have eye disease ranging from mild conjunctivitis to episcleritis, sclerouveitis, or scleromalacia perforans. Vasculitic compromise of the optic nerve may lead to sudden blindness, and retroorbital granuloma formation may cause proptosis.

LABORATORY FINDINGS. No specific laboratory tests are diagnostic of WG. However, there are several nonspecific laboratory abnormalities, including the invariably elevated erythrocyte sedimentation rate, mild anemia, leukocytosis, and thrombocytosis. Low-titer rheumatoid factor, mild elevations of serum immunoglobulins, particularly IgA, and positive tests

Table 22-1 Characteristic features of organ system involvement in Wegener's granulomatosis

Organ system	Approximate frequency (%)	Typical features
Nasopharynx	75	Necrotizing granuloma with mucosal ulceration; saddle nose deformity
Paranasal sinuses	90	Pansinusitis; necrotizing granuloma; secondary bacterial infection
Eyes	60	Keratoconjunctivitis; granulomatous sclerouveitis
Ears	35	Serous otitis media; secondary bacterial infection
Lungs	95	Multiple nodular cavitary infiltrates; necrotizing granulomatous vasculitis
Kidneys	85	Focal and segmental glomerulitis; necrotizing glomerulonephritis later in course
Heart	15	Coronary vasculitis; pericarditis
Nervous system	20	Mononeuritis multiplex; cranial neuritis
Skin	40	Dermal vasculitis with secondary ulcerations
Joints	50	Polyarthralgias

Adapted from Fauci AS, Haynes BF, and Katz P: Ann Intern Med 89:660, 1978.

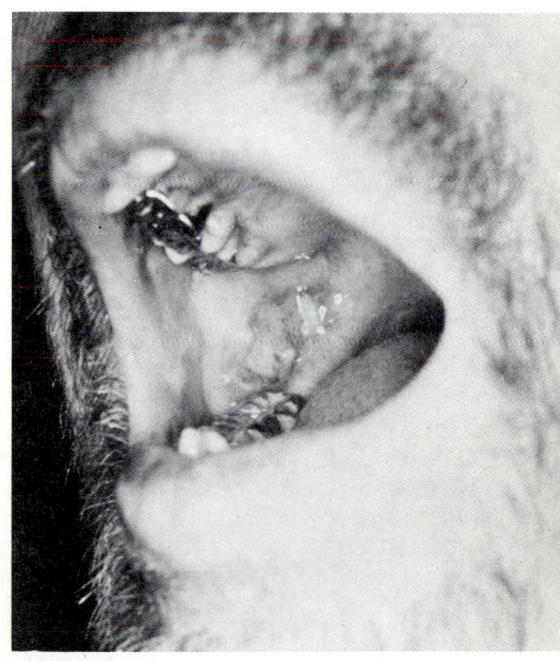

Fig. 22-1 Oral mucosal membrane ulcerations in patient with Wegener's granulomatosis.

for circulating immune complexes are frequently seen. HLA-B8, a histocompatibility antigen often associated with autoimmune diseases, occurs with increased frequency in these patients.

Recent evidence suggests that up to 96% of patients with WG have anti–neutrophil cytoplasm antibodies. Also, titers appear to correlate with disease activity.

DIAGNOSIS. The diagnosis of WG can be clinically suspected in an individual with the classic triad of upper and lower respiratory tract disease and coexistent renal involvement. Histologic diagnosis is mandatory and can be confirmed by the presence of necrotizing granulomatous vasculitis in involved tissue. Lung parenchyma is the source with the highest yield and is usually best approached via open thoracotomy. Percutaneous renal biopsy is advisable not only to confirm the diagnosis but also to assess the extent of involvement.

The clinical triad in combination with the characteristic histopathologic findings usually makes the diagnosis reasonably straightforward. Included in the differential diagnosis are the other vasculitides, infectious and noninfectious granulomatous diseases, collagen vascular diseases, and neoplasms of the upper and lower airways. Goodpasture's syndrome may be differentiated by the presence of circulating or tissue anti–glomerular basement membrane antibody. The distinction from idiopathic midline granuloma, which is discussed later in the chapter, can be made on the basis of clinical and pathologic criteria.

Lymphomatoid granulomatosis (see Chapter 20) is a type of vasculitis with many characteristics of a lymphoma involving the skin, lungs, kidney, and central nervous system. The vasculitis is unlike WG in that there is angiocentric and angiodestructive inflammation with atypical lymphocytoid and plasmacytoid cells. Additionally, renal involvement in lymphomatoid granulomatosis is caused by nodular infiltration with clusters of these atypical cells rather than a true glomerulonephritis.

MANAGEMENT AND PROGNOSIS. Before the advent of cytotoxic therapy, WG was uniformly fatal within several months following the onset of renal involvement. Corticosteroids produced a transient clinical improvement but alone were ineffective in prolonging life. Approximately 10 years ago we began a treatment protocol with cyclophosphamide in an oral dose of 1 to 2 mg/kg/day. Therapy in fulminant cases may be initiated with 4 to 5 mg/kg/day of the drug intravenously for 3 to 4 days followed by conversion to the lower oral maintenance dose. After therapy is begun, the dose is carefully adjusted to maintain the total leukocyte count in a range of 3000 to 4000 cells/mm^3 with an absolute neutrophil count of 1000 to 1500 cells/mm^3. In this range life-threatening infection resulting from neutropenia is avoided. In subjects unable or unwilling to take cyclophosphamide because of leukopenia, hemorrhagic cystitis, or potential gonadal damage, azathioprine in similar doses may be substituted. It should be remembered, however, that this agent is clearly less effective in inducing remissions than cyclophosphamide.

Corticosteroids, usually 1 mg/kg/day of prednisone, are used early in the course of the disease until cyclophosphamide becomes effective; that is, about 2 to 3 weeks. At that time prednisone is converted to an alternate-day regimen, then tapered, and finally discontinued. Longer courses of daily or alternate-day prednisone should be reserved for patients with ocular disease, central nervous system involvement, or symptomatic serosal inflammation. The erythrocyte sedimentation rate is the most sensitive indicator of disease activity and should be normal for at least 1 year before cyclophosphamide is tapered and ultimately discontinued. With this treatment protocol several patients have had prolonged remissions following cessation of cytotoxic therapy.

Besides drugs, maintenance of a patent airway by tracheostomy, if required, control of complicating infection, monitoring of fluids and electrolytes, and advice regarding activities of daily living are important features of the management program.

MIDLINE GRANULOMA

Midline granuloma (MLG) is a locally destructive, progressive process of the nose, paranasal sinuses, and palate, often with erosion through the face and orbit. An uncommon disease, it can occur in all age groups, although most patients are in the fifth and sixth decades of life. There is a slight female predominance.

PATHOGENESIS AND PATHOLOGY. The cause of idiopathic MLG is unknown. Because of the presence of granulomatous inflammation suggestive of a hypersensitivity or cell-mediated immune reaction, it has been postulated that the disease represents a localized hypersensitivity reaction to unidentified antigen(s). It may be that certain susceptible individuals hyperreact to this antigenic stimulus, resulting in the chronic inflammation characteristic of this entity. Certain tumors can produce a clinical and histologic picture so similar to MLG as to camouflage the underlying neoplastic process. Likewise, certain infectious processes can induce similar upper airway destruction. However, in true idiopathic MLG no underlying neoplasm or microbial agent can be identified even with careful histologic study of multiple tissue specimens, meticulous culturing of involved tissue, and searches for disease outside the facial area.

The histologic diagnosis of MLG is complicated by the nonspecificity of the pathologic changes. The usual features include necrosis accompanying acute and chronic inflammation. The tissue is infiltrated with neutrophils, lymphocytes, monocytes, plasma cells, and in some cases eosinophils. As indicated by its name, MLG is characterized by granuloma formation (with or without Langhans' giant cells), although in many cases this may be obscured by the massive amounts of tissue necrosis. Vascular involvement in the form of small vessel thrombosis and perivascular cellular infiltration may occur, but true vasculitis is rare.

CLINICAL MANIFESTATIONS. Although the presentation is variable, most patients develop rhinorrhea and nasal congestion early in the course of the disease. These symptoms become progressive, and the nasal discharge may become purulent because of infection. Nonhealing ulcerations and perforation of the nasal septum frequently occur. Disease initially confined to the oropharynx may be present as ulcerations of the buccal mucosa, gums, and hard and soft palates. Occasionally ocular complaints develop first. Regardless of location the disease process is always progressive, with destruction of soft tissue, cartilage, and bone. In most patients destructive lesions of the palate, the nasal septum, and in some cases the entire nose eventually develop. With erosion and mutilation of the facial architecture, necrotic tissue frequently becomes superinfected, usually with *Staphylococcus aureus*. In addition to the idiopathic form in which no underlying or neoplastic process can be identified, MLG may occur as a manifestation of a local upper airway neoplasm. These localized neoplasms usually can be diagnosed through a careful study of adequate histologic sections and a complete search for sites of tumor involvement elsewhere.

LABORATORY FINDINGS. There are no characteristic laboratory features of MLG that aid in its diagnosis. With chronic inflammation, leukocytosis, an elevated erythrocyte sedimentation rate, mild anemia caused by chronic disease, and hypergammaglobulinemia may be observed. Laboratory evidence of disease activity outside the upper airways necessitates the search for a different disease. Roentgenography of the sinuses reveals pansinusitis with varying degrees of destruction of bone and cartilage.

Table 22-2 Differences between Wegener's granulomatosis and midline granuloma

	Wegener's granulomatosis	Midline granuloma
Organ systems involved	Systemic disease with upper and lower respiratory tracts and kidneys primarily involved	Local disease of upper respiratory tract exclusively
Nature of upper airway lesions	Palatal perforation and facial erosion virtually never occur	Palatal perforation and facial erosion common
Pathologic findings	Necrotizing granulomatous vasculitis	Nonspecific inflammation with or without granulomata
Response to cytotoxic agents	Good	Poor

Fauci AS, Johnson RE, and Wolff SM: Radiation therapy of midline granuloma, Ann Intern Med 84:140, 1976.

Fauci AS and Wolff SM: Wegener's granulomatosis: studies in eighteen patients and a review of the literature, Medicine 52:535, 1973.

Fauci AS and others: Wegener's granulomatosis: prospective clinical and therapeutic experience with 85 patients for 21 years, Ann Intern Med 98:76, 1983.

Friedman I: Midline granuloma, Proc R Soc Med 57:289, 1964.

Savage COS and others: Prospective study of radioimmunoassay for antibodies against neutrophil cytoplasm in diagnosis of systemic vasculitis, Lancet 1:1389, 1987.

Stewart JP: Progressive lethal granulomatous ulceration of the nose, J Laryngol Otol 48:657, 1933.

Wolff SM and others: Wegener's granulomatosis, Ann Intern Med 81:513, 1974.

23 · POLYMYALGIA RHEUMATICA AND TEMPORAL ARTERITIS

June F. Klinghoffer

DIAGNOSIS. The diagnosis rests on the histopathologic findings in concert with a compatible clinical picture. It cannot be emphasized too strongly that other diseases with similar presentations and features must be ruled out before the diagnosis of idiopathic MLG is made. The most difficult distinction is between idiopathic MLG and neoplasms of the upper airways, particularly midline malignant reticulosis and certain lymphomas. This difficulty in diagnosis is caused by the similarity in inflammatory and destructive histopathologic changes that can obscure the true malignant character of the underlying tumor. It is therefore imperative in all cases of suspected idiopathic MLG that a meticulous search for disseminated malignancy be made. This should be combined with a careful microscopic review of adequate biopsy specimens. Infectious diseases included in the differential diagnosis are syphilis, tuberculosis, histoplasmosis, lepromatous leprosy, blastomycosis, coccidioidomycosis, mucocutaneous leishmaniasis, rhinoscleroma caused by *Klebsiella rhinoscleromatis*, and orbital pseudotumor. Wegener's granulomatosis can cause similar upper airway findings. The distinction can be made on the basis of the clinical and pathologic findings listed in Table 22-2.

MANAGEMENT AND PROGNOSIS. Although the course may vary in the rapidity of its progression, the disease is uniformly fatal if untreated. Death usually results from systemic infection, inanition, erosion into blood vessels with exsanguination, or erosion into the central nervous system.

Earlier attempts at surgical therapy of idiopathic MLG often resulted in an acceleration of the disease process without effecting a beneficial response. Corticosteroids and cytotoxic agents likewise have proved to be of little benefit unless the disease was misdiagnosed. We have had success with local, high-dose (5000 rad) radiation in the involved areas. With this therapy a remission rate of greater than 70% has been achieved, often with remissions lasting 10 years or more. The side effects and complications of therapy may be profound, but they obviously are worth the risk considering the otherwise fatal outcome. Once remission has been achieved, reconstructive plastic surgery and prosthetic placement can be performed to correct much of the disfigurement.

BIBLIOGRAPHY

Fauci AS, Haynes BF, and Katz P: The spectrum of vasculitis: clinical, pathologic, immunologic, and therapeutic considerations, Ann Intern Med 89:660, 1978.

Polymyalgia rheumatica (PMR) is a clinical syndrome of unknown cause seen primarily in older patients. It is characterized by pain and stiffness in the muscles of the shoulder, neck, low back, and pelvic girdle and by a rapid erythrocyte sedimentation rate.

Giant cell arteritis is a granulomatous form of arteritis that involves large and medium-sized arteries. The cause is unknown. The major branches coming off the aortic arch, especially the cranial arteries, are most characteristically involved. By common usage the term "temporal arteritis" includes giant cell arteritis of any of the cranial arteries, such as the temporal, facial, ophthalmic, and occipital arteries.

PMR and temporal arteritis are closely associated. The myalgic syndrome often precedes or appears simultaneously with evidence of temporal arteritis. Conversely, clinical or histologic evidence of temporal arteritis is found in 20% to 40% of cases of PMR. Thus it is not clear whether PMR is a distinct, separate entity or always a clinical manifestation of underlying vasculitis.

EPIDEMIOLOGY. Some authors have estimated the prevalence of PMR to be similar or equal to that of gout or systemic lupus erythematosus. It occurs primarily in people over 55 years of age and is rare in those under 50 years of age. Women are affected somewhat more frequently than men; the disorder is uncommon in blacks.

CLINICAL MANIFESTATIONS. The onset of PMR may be insidious or acute. Many patients can give a specific date on which their illness began. They may describe a flulike syndrome at the onset or refer to waking sore and stiff one morning as if they had engaged in vigorous physical exertion the previous day. There is muscle pain and stiffness involving the shoulders, upper arms, and neck. Patients may complain of inability to lift the arms and difficulty in combing the hair or dressing. Pain also may be present in the hips, buttocks, groin, and thighs, and patients may have difficulty walking up stairs or getting up from a chair.

The limitation of movement may be misinterpreted as weakness, but physical examination rules out both muscle weakness and joint disease. Muscle atrophy usually is not seen, although there may be some muscle tenderness. Morning stiffness often is so severe that the patient requires help getting out of bed. Nocturnal discomfort interferes with sleep.

Constitutional symptoms are frequent, including low-grade

fever, night sweats, fatigue, malaise, anorexia, weight loss, and depression. The clinical presentation, especially with associated arteritis, may be solely fever of unknown origin.

The classic presenting symptom in temporal arteritis is unilateral or bilateral temporal headache, most often associated with tenderness over the temporal artery and thickening or nodularity of the artery with diminished or absent pulsation. Visual disturbances or blindness may occur with the localized headache; in rare cases this may be the presenting clinical manifestation. Scalp tenderness is frequent. Jaw pain on chewing or talking (masseter claudication) is occasionally seen and is considered a pathognomonic sign of giant cell arteritis. Other less common manifestations are trismus caused by masseter spasm, difficulty in swallowing, recurrent blanching or gangrene of the tongue, facial pain, earache, toothache, and loss of the sense of taste.

LABORATORY FINDINGS. The most striking finding is a very rapid erythrocyte sedimentation rate—almost always over 50 mm/hr (Westergren method) and often in the range of 80 to 120 mm/hr. A mild hypochromic or normochromic anemia is common. Alpha-2 globulin and fibrinogen may be elevated. Recent reports document a high incidence of elevated alkaline phosphatase and occasional elevations of the other liver enzymes.

Other laboratory studies, including muscle enzymes, are normal. The muscle biopsy usually is normal, as are electromyographic studies. Tests for rheumatoid factor, antinuclear antibodies, and complement are normal.

Biopsy of the superficial temporal artery may reveal the classic picture of giant cell arteritis, but false negative results are possible because of the patchy nature of the vascular involvement.

DIAGNOSIS. A detailed clinical history is most important for diagnosis. Proximal symmetric muscle pain and stiffness in older patients, a rapid sedimentation rate, absence of intrinsic muscle weakness or objective arthropathy, normal muscle enzymes, and the presence of constitutional symptoms constitute the classic clinical picture. Symptoms suggestive of associated temporal arteritis must be actively sought.

The diagnosis of temporal arteritis can be confirmed by positive biopsy result of the temporal artery; it cannot be excluded on the basis of a negative biopsy because of the segmental nature of giant cell arteritis. Diagnoses to be excluded are polymyositis, rheumatoid arthritis, fibrositis, occult neoplasms (especially multiple myeloma), and occult infection. The diagnosis is confirmed by a therapeutic test with small doses of prednisone.

COURSE AND PROGNOSIS. PMR is considered a self-limited illness that runs its course in 1 to 5 years. In the absence of associated giant cell arteritis there is no increase in mortality, but severe incapacity may occur if the disease goes untreated. In the presence of arteritis the gravest threat is blindness, and early adequate therapy is essential. Complications arising from systemic giant cell arteritis such as cerebrovascular accident, myocardial infarction, claudication of the extremities, and other ischemic manifestations occasionally are seen.

MANAGEMENT. Few if any illnesses show as rapid and gratifying a response to low-dose steroids as PMR. Complete relief of symptoms occurs within 4 or 5 days (often within 1 to 2 days) with a dose of 10 to 20 mg/day of prednisone. This experience has enabled some physicians to use a 10-day trial of corticosteroids as a diagnostic aid. The sedimentation rate falls to normal, and the anemia is corrected within 2 weeks. The prednisone dosage is tapered, using the patient's clinical status and sedimentation rate as guides. The average patient

can be maintained without symptoms with 5 to 7.5 mg/day of prednisone for 1 to 2 years. Alternate-day corticosteroid therapy is ineffective.

In the presence of clinical or histologic evidence of temporal arteritis, higher prednisone dosage is necessary; 60 mg/day should be started immediately. Tapering of the dosage usually can begin after approximately 1 to 3 months. Recurrences have been noted even several years after therapy was discontinued.

BIBLIOGRAPHY

Allen NB and Studenski SA: Polymyalgia rheumatica and temporal arteritis, Med Clin North Am 70:369, 1986.
Chuang T and others: Polymyalgia rheumatica: a 10-year epidemiologic and clinical study, Ann Intern Med 97:672, 1982.
Healey LA and Wilske KR: The systemic manifestations of temporal arteritis, New York, 1978, Grune & Stratton, Inc.
Healey LA and Wilske KR: Presentation of occult giant cell arteritis, Arthritis Rheum 23:641, 1980.

24 · SARCOIDOSIS

Warren A. Katz

Sarcoidosis is a systemic disease of unknown cause that is characterized pathologically by the presence of noncaseating giant cell granulomata in multiple organs. Granulomatous lesions are found in lymph nodes, lungs, liver, skin, and synovial membrane. Bones, subcutaneous tissues, muscle, bursae, tendon sheaths, eyes, and the viscera may be sites of sarcoid infiltration.

PATHOGENESIS AND PATHOLOGY. Although the cause of sarcoidosis is unknown, various organisms have been said to cause the disease, including mycobacteria and viruses. The occurrence of sarcoidosis in family lines suggests a mode of inheritance in some people. Indeed, a high incidence of HLA-B8 tissue type has been noted in patients who have sarcoidosis with erythema nodosum and arthritis. Pine cone pollen, clay dust, peanut dust, and pine pitch all have been implicated in the etiology. Foreign body reactions to beryllium, talc, silica, zirconium, and fungi form sarcoidlike noncaseating granulomata. One theory of the pathogenesis of sarcoidosis presupposes that an antigenic insult triggers a T-cell and B-cell immunologic response and that through a variety of possible mechanisms, including transformation, inhibition, and cell interaction, T cells become depleted. This theory explains the depressed delayed reactivity to skin tests and depressed lymphocyte transformation observed in sarcoidosis. Unopposed B-cell lymphoproliferation results in an increase in circulating immunoglobulins and histologically in granuloma formation, both seen in sarcoidosis. In addition, circulating immune complexes may be present in erythema nodosum with hilar adenopathy in sarcoidosis. Histologically, the granulomata are composed of discrete hyperplastic tubercles consisting primarily of epithelioid cells containing Langhans'-type giant cells with cytoplasmic inclusions.

CLINICAL MANIFESTATIONS. Two types of sarcoidosis are apparent, with differences in onset, physical manifestations, ancillary phenomena, prognosis, and treatment. The acute (or abortive) form is more common than the chronic form worldwide (Table 24-1).

Chronic sarcoidosis. Chronic sarcoidosis is the more common form of sarcoidosis recognized in the United States. It is mainly a disease of blacks. Although it frequently begins in young adults, it often is not detected until after 40 years of age.

Chronic sarcoidosis is characterized by respiratory symp-

Table 24-1   Differentiation between acute and chronic sarcoidosis

Parameter	Acute	Chronic
Onset	Abrupt	Insidious
Age	Under 40 years	Over 40 years
Race	Predominantly whites	Predominantly blacks
Erythema nodosum	Usually present	Usually absent
Respiratory symptoms	Usually absent	Usually present
Duration of arthritis	Transient	Persistent
Distribution in joints	Polyarthritis	Pauciarthritis
Periarthritis of ankles	Usually present	Absent
Digital swelling	Usually absent	Often present
Joint deformity	Never	Sometimes
Roentgenograms of joints	Soft tissue swelling	Bone lesions sometimes
Synovial biopsy	Mild, nonspecific inflammation	Noncaseating granuloma
Roentgenogram of chest	Bilateral hilar adenopathy	Hilar adenopathy and parenchymal infiltration
Hypercalcemia	Usually absent	Sometimes present
Angiotensin-converting enzyme	Increased	Increased unless burned out
Urinary hydroxyproline	Increased	Normal
Spontaneous remission	Usual	Unusual

toms, manifestations of extrathoracic involvement, and constitutional symptoms of fever, malaise, and weight loss; or it may be seen as asymptomatic bilateral hilar adenopathy detected on chest roentgenography. Pulmonary symptoms usually include dyspnea, cough, nonpleuritic chest pain, or in rare cases hemoptysis. Even though only 60% of patients with chronic sarcoidosis actually have a respiratory presentation, some abnormality on the chest roentgenogram is present in 92%. Early in the course of the disease the chest roentgenogram is negative, but later mediastinal adenopathy becomes apparent. With advancing disease, pulmonary parenchymal infiltrates may appear on the roentgenogram as discrete fluffy nodules, confluent infiltrates, or linear interstitial fibrosis. At this stage dyspnea becomes apparent with even mild exercise. Patients with pulmonary parenchymal disease usually do not have subsequent hilar adenopathy, although the reverse may be true. In the later stages there is extensive parenchymal involvement with marked fibrosis characterized clinically by chronic dyspnea even at rest. Bronchiectasis may result from compression of the bronchi.

Hemoptysis, sometimes massive, may be associated with bronchiectasis. Pulmonary function studies correlate with the degree of pulmonary involvement. The diffusion capacity, vital capacity, and maximal midexpiratory flow rate are markedly diminished. The defect in gas exchange is the first abnormality to be detected on pulmonary function studies.

Granulomatous lesions of the nose, nasopharynx, and larynx occasionally may develop. This presentation is far more common in women than in men and occurs particularly in the third decade of life. The degree of destruction may resemble that of midline granuloma.

Sarcoid skin lesions may be of several types, including maculopapular rashes, plaques, subcutaneous nodules, and scars. When biopsied most of these lesions show a typical sarcoid reaction.

Uveitis can be detected in 25% of the patients with chronic sarcoidosis; in addition, conjunctival lesions, keratoconjunctivitis, scleral plaques, retinal vasculitis, papilledema, and even cataracts may be present. Glaucoma may result from ocular sarcoidosis. Heerfordt's disease consists of uveitis in association with parotid gland enlargement, seventh nerve palsy, and fever. Salivary gland enlargement, unilateral or bilateral, may be present, as sometimes is Sjögren's syndrome, consisting of keratoconjunctivitis sicca.

Chronic sarcoidosis also may cause hepatosplenomegaly, peripheral and central nervous system lesions (including diabetes insipidus), cardiomyopathy, and renal disease. Peripheral lymphadenopathy may be evident in any part of the body, notably the supraclavicular fossa.

Chronic sarcoidosis of bone is most often characterized by pain in the hands or feet caused by "punched-out" bony lesions or destruction of the joint surfaces. Multiple joints may be painful and swollen, because the synovium is infiltrated with noncaseating granulomata. Ankles, knees, elbows, wrists, and the small joints of the hand most commonly are affected. Flexion contractures of the fingers may develop, but these pose minimal discomfort to the patient. Tenosynovitis of the wrist may occur, and the fingers may become irregularly swollen and deformed, taking on a rheumatoid appearance. Usually, however, chronic sarcoid arthritis is nondestructive. Granulomata may infiltrate muscle, causing proximal muscle weakness and pain.

Abortive or acute sarcoidosis. Acute sarcoidosis most commonly manifests itself as the so-called Löfgren's syndrome, characterized by polyarthritis, erythema nodosum, and bilateral hilar adenopathy. The disease is abrupt in onset, generally strikes people under 40 years of age, and is most prevalent in Sweden. It develops mostly in the spring and summer. Most patients seek medical attention because of articular manifestations, but constitutional symptoms of fatigue, malaise, weakness, anorexia, weight loss, minor chills, and low-grade fever may antedate arthritis by several weeks. Acute transient sarcoid arthritis does not cause symptoms secondary to sarcoid involvement of the joint. Rather, the synovitis is nonspecific. Lymph node enlargement, including bilateral hilar adenopathy, erythema nodosum, sarcoid skin lesions, skin lesions, uveitis, and even sialadenitis may be evident; however, bone cysts and chronic arthritis are not seen in this form of the disease.

Articular manifestations of acute sarcoidosis may be profound, characterized by stiffness and pain in several joints. Initially arthralgias are migratory, but then overt inflammation persists in one or more joints. The most dramatic articular finding is inflammation, predominantly in tissues around the ankle (periarthritis); the joint seems to move well with minimal pain on motion, but there is marked periarticular tenderness, redness, and swelling (Fig. 24-1). Periarthritis, commonly mistaken for gout, is a manifestation of erythema nodosum.

LABORATORY FINDINGS. Whether sarcoidosis is acute or chronic, the diagnosis can be established by histologic exam-

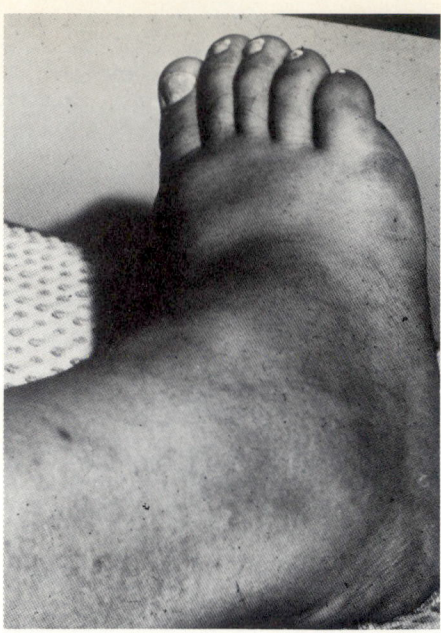

Fig. 24-1 Swelling of ankle in patient with acute sarcoidosis. Darkened skin areas are sites of erythema.

ination of affected tissue, notably the skin, lymph nodes, and liver. To be certain of the diagnosis, it is useful to demonstrate sarcoid lesions in at least two separate organs. Liver biopsy helps detect sarcoidosis in the liver (about 70% positive). Sarcoidosis is the most common cause of hepatic granulomata. Bronchial or lung tissue obtained through a fiberoptic bronchoscope is positive for granulomata in 80% of the cases, particularly if hilar adenopathy is present. Gastrocnemius biopsy may show granulomata even in the absence of muscle symptoms. The Kveim-Siltzbach skin test, positive in 80% to 90% of patients with acute or chronic sarcoidosis, currently is not used often. In abortive sarcoidosis, synovium, periarticular tissues of the ankle, and the lesions of erythema nodosum fail to show noncaseating granulomata.

In both forms of the disease, the erythrocyte sedimentation rate is elevated and the latex fixation test for rheumatoid factor may be positive in low titer. Purified protein derivative (PPD) anergy is the rule.

The serum angiotensin converting enzyme (ACE) is elevated in most patients with active disease but is normal in burned-out sarcoidosis, lymphoma, leukemia, and other pulmonary conditions that mimic sarcoidosis, such as tuberculosis. Increased levels of urine hydroxyproline may be found in patients with acute sarcoidosis. On the other hand, hypercalcemia and increased alkaline phosphatase are peculiar to the chronic type, appearing in 15% of patients. Broncho-alveolar lavage of patients with pulmonary sarcoidosis reveals an increase of helper-T cells, alveolar macrophages, nonspecific IgG secreting cells, and alveolar ACE, a more sensitive marker than serum ACE.

Roentgenograms of the chest are valuable in the diagnosis of both forms. Almost all patients exhibit bilateral hilar adenopathy either before or after the onset of other manifestations of sarcoidosis. In the chronic form pulmonary infiltration predominates, and pleural effusions are rare. Roentgenograms of bones and joints in chronic sarcoidosis show mottled radiolucent areas and "punched-out" lesions, usually in the phalanges. No changes such as these are noted in the abortive form.

DIAGNOSIS. Polyarthritis, periarticular inflammation of the ankles, erythema nodosum, and bilateral hilar adenopathy (Löfgren's syndrome) constitute a symptom complex so distinctive that the diagnosis of acute (abortive) sarcoidosis should not be difficult. Indeed, any young person with polyarthritis and erythema nodosum should be suspected of having sarcoidosis, which can be confirmed by sequential chest roentgenograms. Elevations of serum ACE and hydroxyprolinuria provide additional ancillary evidence. There usually is concern that hilar adenopathy may represent lymphoma, but erythema nodosum coexisting with asymptomatic bilateral adenopathy is extremely strong evidence against a malignancy.

The chronic forms of sarcoidosis may present difficulties in diagnosis. The presence of pulmonary findings with multiple-system disease, particularly if the eyes are involved, should raise suspicion. Sarcoidosis can be distinguished from other granulomatous diseases by appropriate biopsies.

Articular manifestations of sarcoidosis may mimic rheumatoid arthritis, rheumatic fever, lymphoma, gout, psoriatic arthritis, infection, and a variety of other conditions.

MANAGEMENT AND PROGNOSIS. Mild sarcoidosis, particularly of the abortive type, may be managed by salicylates. Colchicine has been shown to be effective in some cases of acute sarcoid arthritis, and small doses of corticosteroids (such as prednisone, 5 mg/day) may be administered if fatigue is profound. Articular manifestations disappear within several weeks with or without treatment. Higher doses (such as prednisone, 40 to 60 mg/day) may be needed for chronic sarcoidosis, especially if uveitis, progression of pulmonary manifestations, marked hypercalciuria, extremely disfiguring skin lesions, progressive arthritis, and hypersplenism are present. If corticosteroids fail, azathioprine has been shown to be useful in certain cases.

Acute sarcoidosis usually resolves within several weeks except for adenopathy, which may last up to 1 year. In the chronic type, lifelong disease, particularly pulmonary fibrosis, can be expected in many cases. Fortunately, mortality is low; death usually results from respiratory failure, myocarditis, or renal failure caused by nephrocalcinosis.

BIBLIOGRAPHY

Greening AP: Bronchoalveolar lavage, Br Med J 284:1896, 1982.
Lieberman J: Serum angiotensin-converting enzyme and sarcoidosis, Am J Med 59:365, 1975.
Siltzbach LE, editor: Seventh International Conference on Sarcoidosis and Other Granulomatous Disorders, Ann NY Acad Sci 278:1, 1976.
Spilberg I, Siltzbach LE, and McEwen C: The arthritis of sarcoidosis, Arthritis Rheum 12:126, 1969.
Williams WJ: Sarcoidosis and other granulomatous disorders, Philadelphia, 1985, WB Saunders Co.
Winterbauer RH, Belic N, and Moores KD: A clinical interpretation of bilateral hilar adenopathy, Ann Intern Med 78:65, 1973.

25 · WEBER-CHRISTIAN DISEASE AND RELATED SUBCUTANEOUS FAT DISORDERS

Robert H. Gordon and **Bruce I. Hoffman**

Weber-Christian disease (nodular nonsuppurative panniculitis) is characterized by an acute, febrile, recurrent, nodular inflammation of adipose tissue involving the subcutaneous fat and, less often, adipose tissue elsewhere in the body (systemic Weber-Christian disease).

EPIDEMIOLOGY. The term "Weber-Christian disease" in the

past encompassed a heterogeneous group of disorders. It now is applied only when panniculitis is the primary pathologic finding and after other underlying diseases have been ruled out. This disorder is uncommon and generally affects adults of either sex between the ages of 20 and 60, although cases in children as young as newborns have been reported. It does not appear to have any distinct familial, racial, or geographic associations.

PATHOGENESIS AND PATHOLOGY. The cause of Weber-Christian disease is unknown. Local pressure and trauma sometimes play a role. Hypersensitivity to drugs such as bromides, iodides, and some antibiotics or to bacterial and viral antigens following infection or immunization has been implicated. Cultures of the lesions are sterile. Other suggested causes have included disordered fat metabolism, α-1-antitrypsin deficiency, and autoimmunity. Immunoglobulins have not been identified in the lesions. One case report described an infant who had a remission of his disease when T lymphocytes were depleted. This finding raised the possibility of altered cellular immunity. Pancreatic enzymes have been elevated in some patients.

The histopathologic picture is nonspecific; it can occur in any condition causing acute panniculitis. Three stages have been noted: (1) infiltration of fat lobules by polymorphonuclear cells, often accompanied by fat cell degeneration, (2) mononuclear and histiocytic infiltration of the panniculus with variable fat cell necrosis and phagocystosis of fatty debris with formation of lipophages, and (3) fibroblastic proliferation with subsequent fibrosis. The inflammatory process usually spares the epidermis and dermis. Blood vessels are affected by circumferential spread only.

CLINICAL MANIFESTATIONS. The characteristic finding of nodules in Weber-Christian disease is important in establishing the diagnosis. These can be few or many in number and located in one area or all over the body. The legs, thighs, buttocks, abdomen, and breasts may be particularly affected. The nodules range in size from 0.5 to 8 cm. They are tender and occasionally erythematous, and some may suppurate, draining an oily material. At first they are slightly mobile, but later they become adherent to the skin; this results in cutaneous dimpling or a central depression.

The systemic features depend on the sites of involvement. The lungs (parenchymal infiltrates, effusions), heart (pericarditis), liver (hepatomegaly), spleen (splenomegaly), kidneys, gastrointestinal tract (abdominal pain, perforation), retroperitoneum, mediastinum, and even the bone marrow can be involved. Musculoskeletal complaints include arthralgias, myalgias, and occasional joint effusions. Retroperitoneal and mediastinal fibrosis have been associated with Weber-Christian disease.

LABORATORY FINDINGS. No laboratory tests are diagnostic. The sedimentation rate may be elevated. Anemia, leukocytosis, and in rare cases eosinophilia have been reported. Serum, urine, or tissue levels of amylase and lipase sometimes are elevated without documentable pancreatic disease. Cryoglobulinemia and normal serum complement also are reported.

DIAGNOSIS. Weber-Christian disease should be considered in the evaluation of subcutaneous nodules that show evidence of recent or healed panniculitis on biopsy. Neither finding is pathognomonic for the disease, however; therefore patients need a thorough evaluation to rule out other underlying conditions.

Erythema nodosum is one of the most common disorders giving rise to painful subcutaneous nodules on the legs and occasionally on the arms and face. The nodules are limited to subcutaneous tissue and are not found elsewhere. This syndrome is associated with many nonrelated diseases and is believed to be a hypersensitivity response. Polyarteritis, erythema induratum, morphea, and a rare syndrome called subcutaneous fat necrosis of the newborn also must be considered. Lupus profundus is a lesion of subcutaneous fat occurring in 2% to 3% of patients with systemic lupus erythematosus. Management with systemic corticosteroids and antimalarials often proves effective. Nodular liquifying panniculitis (metastatic fat necrosis) is associated with pancreatitis or pancreatic carcinoma. Painful lesions may occur anywhere except on the face. They may coalesce and drain. There is no effective therapy. Other conditions resembling panniculitis include Sweet's syndrome, multicentric reticulocytosis, mastocytosis, and Fabry's disease. However, in an effort to diagnose exotic disease, common causes of painful panniculitis should not be overlooked. These include trauma, infection, bites, local fat atrophy from insulin injections, drug abuse, and self-inflicted wounds.

MANAGEMENT. Many treatments have been tried through the years, including potassium iodide, antibiotics, antituberculous drugs, antihistamines, antimalarials, hormones, vitamins, sulphones, heavy metals, antirheumatics, blood transfusions, and even radiation therapy. None of these has proved successful. Corticosteroids offer the best symptomatic relief, but the basic pathologic process may continue.

COURSE AND PROGNOSIS. The course is variable. Although each nodule may last between 2 and 6 weeks, the disease itself may persist for 8 months to several years. Morbidity and mortality are related to visceral complications.

BIBLIOGRAPHY

Forstrum L and Wilkleman RK: Acute panniculitis: a clinical and histopathologic study of 34 cases, Arch Dermatol 113:909, 1977.

Ginsburg WW and O'Duffy JD: Multicentric reticulohistiocytosis. In Kelley WN and others, editors: Textbook of rheumatology, Philadelphia, 1985, WB Saunders Co.

Gunnawardena OA, Gunawardena R, and Ratnayzka RMRS: The clinical spectrum of Sweet's syndrome (acute febrile neutrophilic dermatosis): a report on 18 cases, Br J Dermatol 92:363, 1975.

Khat JA: Fabry's disease. Alpha galactosidase deficiency, Science 167:1268, 1970.

Korenblat PE and others: Systemic mastocytosis, Arch Intern Med 144:2249, 1984.

Milner RDG and Mitchinson MJ: Systemic Weber-Christian disease, J Clin Pathol 18:150, 1965.

26 · INFECTIOUS ARTHRITIS

Bruce I. Hoffman

Infectious arthritis occurs when microbial agents (bacteria, mycobacteria, fungi, or viruses) are introduced into the synovium, overwhelm the normal clearance mechanisms, and multiply. In most instances organisms are introduced hematogenously from an extraarticular focus. However, infection may be caused by direct introduction from trauma, intraarticular injection, surgery, or a paraarticular focus. Infectious arthritis may be classified as (1) pyogenic arthritis (gonococcal and nongonococcal septic arthritis), (2) tuberculous and fungal arthritis, (3) arthritis caused by viruses, and (4) arthritis caused by spirochetes. The presentation, course, and therapy are sufficiently different that each syndrome will be discussed separately.

PYOGENIC ARTHRITIS

Pyogenic infections are those caused by gonococcal or nongonococcal bacteria. The bacteria that cause septic arthritis tend to differ with the age and condition of the patient. Gram-positive organisms, particularly *Staphylococcus aureus*, are most important in the causation of septic arthritis in all ages except adolescence and young adulthood. Of particular importance is the vast predominance of *Neisseria gonorrhoeae* in adolescents and young adults. In infants *Haemophilus influenzae* causes a significant number of injections of the joints, as it does at other sites. A minority of cases are produced by gram-negative bacilli; however, this number has increased, particularly in older, debilitated adults. In general, septic arthritis produces joints that are more painful than in any other entity except gout.

Gonococcal arthritis

See discussion of "Gonococcal infections" in Chapter 46.

Nongonococcal septic arthritis

Septic arthritis caused by pyogenic bacteria other than *N. gonorrhoeae* is uncommon, but its potential for rapid joint destruction and mortality gives it an important position in the differential diagnosis of acute monarticular and pauciarticular arthritis.

PATHOGENESIS. Gram-positive organisms, particularly *S. aureus*, *Streptococcus pyogenes*, and *S. pneumoniae*, predominate as causes of nongonococcal septic arthritis. In adults gram-negative enteric bacillary infections have become more prevalent, especially after urinary tract operative procedures. A wide variety of other bacteria have caused septic arthritis less frequently.

PATHOLOGY. After organisms become established and multiply, an intense inflammatory response is provoked. Enzymes that cause the degradation of articular cartilage are released. It appears that the bacteria can cause an immunogenic arthritis that can continue after the organisms have been eradicated. As infection progresses, bone is invaded and osteomyelitis ensues. It is not known why joints are damaged so rapidly in comparison to noninfectious diseases such as gout in which an equally intense response occurs.

CLINICAL MANIFESTATIONS. Nongonococcal septic arthritis (NGSA) rapidly progresses to severe pain, swelling, warmth, and erythema over 24 to 72 hours. It generally is a monarticular disease, but patients may have two to five joints simultaneously involved. Fever, tachypnea, and rigors may be intense. Infection is most common in large joints, including in order of frequency the knees, hips, shoulders, elbows, wrists, and ankles. Small joints such as the sternoclavicular or sacroiliac joints may be affected.

Factors that predispose individuals to the development of septic arthritis include (1) an extraarticular focus, (2) debilitating illness, (3) immunosuppressive therapy, (4) previous joint damage, and (5) intravenous drug abuse. Not surprisingly, in many patients an extraarticular focus in the skin, lungs, genitourinary system, or gastrointestinal tract can be identified. Unlike gonococcal arthritis, in which the hosts are otherwise healthy, NGSA tends to strike debilitated individuals. Patients often have diabetes mellitus, malignancies, or cirrhosis. They may be receiving immunosuppressive drugs or corticosteroids. Perhaps most importantly, NGSA affects previously damaged joints. Patients with rheumatoid arthritis comprise as much as 30% of those with NGSA. The propensity to joint infections is related to impaired local defenses against infections and intraarticular injection of corticosteroids. In intravenous drug abusers septic arthritis develops in unusual locations such as sternoclavicular and sacroiliac joints and with unusual organisms such as *Pseudomonas aeruginosa* and *Serratia marcescens*.

LABORATORY FINDINGS. Patients with NGSA generally have peripheral leukocytosis. Synovial fluid examination usually shows 80,000 to 100,000 white blood cells/mm^3, of which greater than 90% are polymorphonuclear leukocytes. The synovial fluid glucose level is less than 40 mg/dl. Gram stain of the synovial fluid is positive in 50% to 80%, whereas a culture nearly always is positive unless antibiotics have been administered previously. Organisms grow in blood cultures in approximately 50% of the patients.

Early in the course the joint appears normal on roentgenographic examination. Osteoporosis subsequently develops, and the joint space narrows as cartilage is eroded. Ultimately, total joint destruction, fusion, and osteomyelitis may be seen.

DIAGNOSIS. NGSA is rare in young or middle-aged healthy adults. In the usual older age range of NGSA, gout and pseudogout are the most common entities associated with acute inflammatory monarticular arthritis. Monarticular inflammation in a patient with preexisting rheumatoid arthritis often signals a flare of the disease but also may indicate pyogenic arthritis. In patients with rheumatoid arthritis any joint involved out of proportion to the others should be aspirated and cultured.

MANAGEMENT. The principles of treatment are the same as those in any closed-space infection. They include adequate antibiotics, drainage, and physical measures to protect the joint and preserve function.

When the identity and sensitivity of the infecting organism are known, parenteral administration of high doses of minimally toxic bactericidal agents is indicated. Treatment should not be delayed while awaiting cultures and should be based on Gram stain (Table 26-1). Therapy is continued for 2 to 4 weeks.

Involved joints should be drained by arthrocentesis at least daily. If there is no response in 5 to 7 days (that is, there is continued fever, failure to sterilize the joint, purulent exudate, or development of joint destruction), surgical drainage procedures are advised. Surgery also is indicated in all septic hips and when adequate drainage cannot be accomplished with a needle.

Joints should be splinted until inflammation subsides. They

Table 26-1. Treatment of pyogenic arthritis based on Gram stain

Gram stain finding	Therapy	
	First choice	**Alternative**
Gram-positive cocci		
Clusters, single cocci, or diplo-cocci	Penicillinase-resistant penicillin or cephalo-sporin for *S. aureus*	Vancomycin
Chains	Penicillin G for strepto-cocci	Erythromycin
Gram-negative cocci	See Chapter 46 for *N. gonorrhoeae*	
Gram-negative bacilli	Carbenicillin or ticarcillin plus gentamicin or to-bramycin	
Gram-negative coccobacilli	Ampicillin for *H. influenzae*	Chloramphenicol
Gram stain negative		
In young patients	Treatment for gonococcal infection	
In older or debilitated patients	Penicillinase-resistant penicillin and amino-glycoside	

should be put through a passive range of motion several times a day as soon as pain permits.

PROGNOSIS. Even with appropriate therapy the outcome of NGSA is unsatisfactory. The most important factor is early diagnosis, because patients treated less than 7 days from the beginning of symptoms fare better. The outcome is poor, as shown by ankylosis, recurrence, osteomyelitis, or death in 50% of *S. aureus* infections, 20% of streptococcal infections, 5% of pneumococcal infections, and 75% of gram-negative bacillary infections. Younger, healthier patients have a better prognosis.

Septic bursitis

Infection in the olecranon or prepatellar bursa is not uncommon. Almost all episodes represent traumatic inoculation of the bursa, and in more than 90% of cases *S. aureus* is the etiologic agent. The bursa becomes swollen, with palpable effusion, and is erythematous and tender. Often surrounding cellulitis is present. Diagnosis is made by aspiration, gram stain, and culture of bursal fluid. The white cell counts of the synovial fluid often are lower than those seen in septic arthritis. Differential diagnosis requires consideration of other causes of bursitis in these areas, including trauma, gout, and rheumatoid arthritis.

Treatment involves repeated aspiration and administration of appropriate antibiotics. Virtually all episodes resolve without residua, although occasionally the bursa must be surgically excised.

TUBERCULOUS AND FUNGAL ARTHRITIS
Arthritis caused by *Mycobacterium tuberculosis*

The incidence of tuberculosis in the United States has declined dramatically over the past 40 years. Arthritis caused by *M. tuberculosis,* never common, is now rare. The diagnosis of bone and joint infection often is delayed. During primary dissemination foci of infection develop by direct extension or secondary hematogenous spread, and they later reactivate. At the time of presentation 10% to 50% of the patients have active pulmonary disease. Commonly there is no evidence of previous tuberculosis.

CLINICAL MANIFESTATIONS. Bone and joint tuberculosis takes two general forms: osteomyelitis and synovitis. Tuberculous osteomyelitis classically affects the thoracic spine (Pott's disease). The infection destroys the disc space and occasionally the vertebral bodies. The patients have back pain, spasm, and root pain. Complications include kyphosis from collapse of the disc space or vertebral body, cold (tuberculous) abscesses, and neurologic sequelae from cord compression. Other sites of involvement are the ribs and sacroiliac joints.

Tuberculosis of the joints generally occurs as a monarticular arthritis. The hip and knee are involved most frequently, but other joints and tendon sheaths also are affected. The patients have slowly progressive pain, stiffness, and swelling.

LABORATORY FINDINGS. The synovial fluid white cell count has a wide range, generally 10,000 to 20,000/mm³ — most are polymorphonuclear leukocytes. The glucose level often is reduced. Roentgenograms may be normal initially, but later show osteoporosis, marginal erosions, and finally joint destruction with little reactive bone. When concurrent osteomyelitis occurs, oval lucencies are seen beneath the articular cartilage.

DIAGNOSIS. An intermediate-strength purified protein derivative (PPD) skin test should be performed. The results are positive except with advanced disease and in debilitated or immunosuppressed hosts. Synovial fluid cultures are positive in 80% of the cases. Biopsy of the synovium should be done in every suspected case. The histologic finding is granulomatous synovitis. The combination of histology and culture permits a precise diagnosis in more than 90% of patients.

MANAGEMENT. Efffective therapy requires adequate chemotherapy and occasionally surgery (see Chapter 49). Surgery is performed for debridement of osteomyelitis, synovectomy, or joint fusion. Successful total hip replacement is performed routinely in previously affected hips once the infection is controlled. Fusion of spinal lesions occasionally is performed.

Arthritis caused by other mycobacteria

Mycobacteria other than *M. tuberculosis* can cause bone and joint infection, sometimes involving multiple joints. Infections cause by *M. kansasii, M. marinum, M. intracellularis,* and *M. scrofulaceum* have been reported. These infections often are more difficult to treat (see "Nontuberculous mycobacterial infections" in Chapter 51).

Arthritis caused by fungi

Arthritis caused by mycotic infection is rare. Coccidioidomycosis is most prevalent in the southwestern United States. The primary infection usually is a self-limited pulmonary disease. During this phase arthritis is accompanied by erythema nodosum. With disseminated disease, monarthritis of the knee, ankle, or other joints and tenosynovitis may occur. Joint destruction eventually may occur. Osteomyelitis with multiple lytic lesions is a complication. The diagnosis is by culture; synovial biopsy shows granulomata. The therapy is with amphotericin B.

Sporotrichosis occurs after skin inoculation and usually is limited. When it is disseminated, a monarticular or pauciarticular arthritis may occur. The diagnosis is by culture, and the treatment is with amphotericin B.

Arthritis may follow transient candidemia; it rarely is seen with blastomycosis, histoplasmosis, or cryptococcosis.

Arthritis caused by viruses

Viruses frequently cause self-limited arthritis and perhaps are involved in the pathogenesis of rheumatoid arthritis and systemic lupus erythematosus.

Hepatitis B is associated with arthralgia and arthritis during the incubation period in approximately 50% of the cases. Patients have a variety of skin lesions, usually urticarial. The arthritis is polyarticular and symmetric. It generally subsides with the onset of jaundice. These manifestions probably are caused by circulating immune complexes. The diagnosis is made by demonstration of hepatitis B surface antigen in the blood. The treatment is symptomatic with salicylates.

Rubella (German measles) is associated with a symmetric polyarthritis lasting 1 to 7 days and usually associated with the rash. It is much more common in adults than in children. Rubella vaccination also has been associated with arthritis, again much more frequently in adults.

Clinicians often witness transient monarthritis or polyarthritis as part of an obvious viral clinical picture, but specific diagnoses rarely are made. Treatment of the various viral arthritides is supportive only.

A reactive arthritis has been noted in some patients with acquired immunodeficiency syndrome (AIDS).

Arthritis caused by spirochetes

Arthritis and tenosynovitis may occur in secondary syphilis. Lyme disease is an arthropod-borne infection caused by *Bor-*

relia burgdorfori. The tick vector, *Ixodes dammini*, is found in an expanding area that includes parts of New England, New York, the East Coast from New Jersey through the Carolinas, southeastern Pennsylvania, Wisconsin, and the West Coast.

The initial lesion occurs at the site of the bite and develops into an expanding erythematous ring with central clearing and at times satellite lesions. The skin lesion is termed erythema chronicum migrans. After an interval generally of several weeks 20% of patients develop either central nervous system or cardiac involvement. Later approximately 50% of patients develop an oligoarthritis predominently affecting the knees and characterized by spontaneous remissions and exacerbations. This eventually resolves in all but 10% of patients, in whom chronic knee arthritis ensues.

Diagnosis is by specific antibody test for the spirochete, although results may be negative at the time of the initial skin lesion. Approximately 40% of patients do not have a history of erythema chronicum migrans.

BIBLIOGRAPHY

Berney S, Goldstein M, and Bisko F: Clinical and diagnostic features of tuberculous arthritis, Am J Med 53:36, 1972.

Brandt RD, Cathcart ES, and Cohen AS: Gonococcal arthritis: clinical features correlated with blood, synovial fluid and genitourinary cultures, Arthritis Rheum 17:503, 1974.

Goldberg DL and Cohen AS: Acute infectious arthritis: a review of patients with non-gonococcal joint infections (with emphasis on therapy and prognosis), Am J Med 60:369, 1976.

Handsfield HH, Wiesner PJ, and Holmes KK: Treatment of the gonococcal arthritis-dermatitis syndrome, Ann Intern Med 84:661, 1976.

Rosenthal J, Bole GG, and Robinson WD: Acute nongonococcal infectious arthritis: evaluation of risk factors, therapy and outcome, Arthritis Rheum 23:889, 1980.

Schmid FR: Bacterial arthritis. In Katz WA, editor: Diagnosis and management of rheumatic diseases, Philadelphia, 1988, JB Lippincott Co.

27·OSTEOMYELITIS

Bruce I. Hoffman

Osteomyelitis is infection of bone by microorganisms. Usually these are bacterial infections; however, mycobacteria and fungi also cause osteomyelitis when they invade the skeleton.

EPIDEMIOLOGY. Osteomyelitis is more common in men than in women and usually is confined to bones of the lower extremities. Several factors predispose an individual to the development of osteomyelitis: diabetes with vascular insufficiency of the lower extremities, genitourinary infection, neoplasms, intravenous drug abuse, and sickle cell anemia.

PATHOLOGY. Bone becomes infected by three routes: hematogenously, by contiguous infection, or directly, as during surgery. These types of infection often are caused by different bacteria and have a different clinical spectrum.

Before puberty infection occurs at the metaphysis of long bones because of slow blood flow in this area and the absence of phagocytic cells. When infection is established in children or adults, regardless of route, pus spreads along haversian and Volkmann's canals until it reaches the periosteum. As pressure increases, ischemic necrosis of bone forms a sequestrum of necrotic bone. At this point the infection is considered chronic.

CLINICAL MANIFESTATIONS. The clinical picture and causative bacteria vary according to the route and site of infection and the patient's age. Acute hematogenous osteomyelitis usually seeds the long bones of children or vertebral body of adults. Most cases are caused by *Staphylococcus aureus* in

both children and adults, but the incidence of gram-negative bacillary infection increases in adults. In drug abusers *Pseudomonas aeruginosa* is particularly important. Patients with sickle cell hemoglobinopathy have a propensity for *Salmonella osteomyelitis*.

Children generally have high fever and local symptoms at the site of infection. In adults symptoms usually are insidious in onset, with low-grade fever, and the diagnosis often is delayed.

Infection from a contiguous focus is a sequela of surgery, soft tissue infections, or oral infections. The infections often are polybacterial, although *S. aureus* still predominates. Fever with local pain, erythema, and swelling is the characteristic finding in osteomyelitis.

Vascular insufficiency, especially caused by diabetes mellitus, is particularly important in the development of osteomyelitis in the older age group. Most commonly osteomyelitis occurs in the feet at the site of a diabetic ulcer and is polybacterial. Often there is a neuropathy with the plantar ulceration but few systemic symptoms.

Once osteomyelitis is established and bone necrosis develops, the disease becomes chronic and difficult to treat and tends to recur.

LABORATORY FINDINGS AND DIAGNOSIS. Early in the course osteomyelitis may be difficult to diagnose. The only useful laboratory study is the erythrocyte sedimentation rate, which almost always is elevated. An important exception is sickle cell anemia, in which the sedimentation rate may be normal.

Roentgenographic findings are most specific. First the periosteum is elevated, followed by development of a lucent area in the underlying bone, and then by formation of a sequestrum. These findings often are delayed. Bone scanning offers an opportunity to make an early diagnosis. Technetium or gallium scanning usually is positive within the first few days.

Magnetic resonance imaging may become a more sensitive and specific means of visualizing affected areas, particularly in the spine.

The definitive diagnosis is by bone biopsy, which allows the infecting organism to be clearly identified. Cultures of sinus drainage are less exact, because the sinus tract may contain organisms not found in the bone. Blood cultures are positive in 50% of those with hematogenously spread disease.

MANAGEMENT. Osteomyelitis is treated with antibiotics appropriate to the infecting organism. This treatment should be prolonged, often for months. Therapy is given by the parenteral route usually for 4 to 6 weeks and then continued with orally administered agents. When chronic osteomyelitis ensues, surgical debridement often is essential.

COURSE AND PROGNOSIS. The prognosis of acute osteomyelitis is excellent when treatment starts within the first few days. When osteomyelitis becomes chronic, the prognosis is much worse; patients often are left with recurring draining sinuses. In some patients generalized amyloidosis develops in response to chronic osteomyelitis.

BIBLIOGRAPHY

Norden CW: Osteomyelitis. In Mandell GL, Douglas RG, Jr, and Bennett JE, editors: Principles and practice of infectious diseases, New York, 1979, John Wiley & Sons, Inc.

Waldvogel FA, Modoff G, and Swartz MN: Osteomyelitis: a review of clinical features, therapeutic considerations and unusual aspects, I, N Engl J Med 282:198, 1970.

Waldvogel FA, Modoff G, and Swartz MN: Osteomyelitis: a review of clinical features, therapeutic considerations and unusual aspects, II, N Engl J Med 282:260, 1970.

Waldvogel FA, Modoff G, and Swartz MN: Osteomyelitis: a review of clinical

features, therapeutic considerations and unusual aspects, III. Osteomyelitis associated with vascular insufficiency, N Engl J Med 282:316, 1970.
Waldvogel FA and Vasey H: Osteomyelitis: the past decade, N Engl J Med 303:360, 1980.

28 · OSTEOARTHRITIS

Daniel G. Baker *and* **H. Ralph Schumacher, Jr.**

Osteoarthritis (OA) is the most common cause of rheumatic complaints. OA also is known as "degenerative joint disease" or "osteoarthrosis," terms that emphasize the noninflammatory nature of the disease. It has become clear, however, that low-grade inflammation may be a contributing factor, although probably not the primary cause, in many cases of OA. Although the incidence of OA increases with age, it should not necessarily be considered a natural consequence of aging. OA is not a disease only of the elderly; one survey found radiologic evidence of OA in the hands and feet of 40 million Americans. The disorder is one of the primary causes of disability in the United States. Racial differences in distribution of OA have been described, but whether these are genetic or environmental differences is unknown.

OA is classified as either primary or secondary. Primary OA shows no apparent predisposing factors such as trauma or malalignment of joints. The tissue breakdown is assumed to be caused by still undefined intrinsic factors. Secondary OA has an underlying cause such as trauma, surgery, or previous infection.

In primary osteoarthritis the most frequently involved joints are the distal interphalangeal (DIP) joints, with enlargement resulting from bony proliferation and subsequent spur formation. Such findings in the DIP joints are called Heberden's nodes. The term "generalized osteoarthritis" is used when numerous joints are involved, most frequently the proximal interphalangeal (PIP) joints, DIP joints, first carpometacarpal joint, hips, knees, first metatarsophalangeal joint, cervical spine, and lumbar spine. Other joints seem to be spared in primary osteoarthritis; if they are involved, causes for secondary OA should be sought.

PATHOGENESIS. The pathogenesis of osteoarthritis has not been defined fully. Heberden's nodes accompanied by generalized OA appear to have a genetic predisposition determined by a single autosomal gene that is dominant in women and recessive in men. Whether obesity leads to the development of OA is controversial, although obesity clearly aggravates the disorder once it has been established. Exactly how such factors lead to disease is unclear. Proteoglycans are depleted and altered, allowing cartilage fibrillation and erosion. Both altered production and increased breakdown of cartilage matrix can occur. The development of OA may best be considered a physiologic imbalance between the amount of stress applied to a joint and the ability of the joint tissue to deal with that stress.

CLINICAL MANIFESTATIONS. The clinical findings in OA depend on the joints involved and the severity of the involvement. Classically the pain is a dull ache localized to the involved joints that worsens during and after use and weight bearing. In several diseases there may be pain at rest, and patients frequently complain of pain at night. Morning stiffness and swelling are common but usually last only for several minutes and are localized to the involved joints. Limitation of motion can develop secondary to chronic muscle spasm, flexion contractures from capsular fibrosis, intraarticular loose bodies,

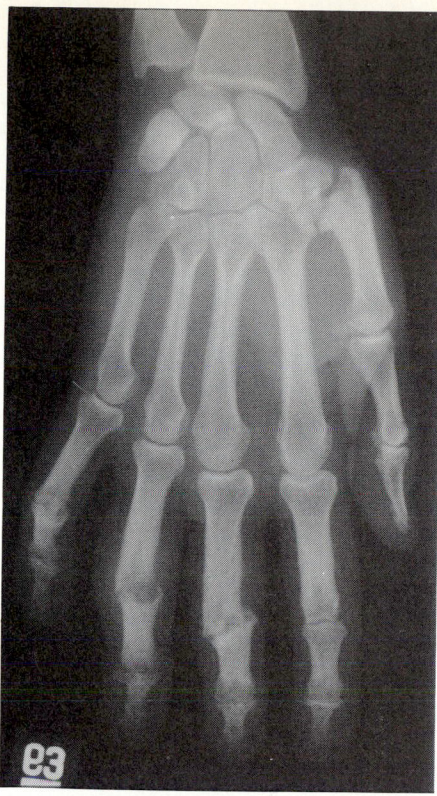

Fig. 28-1 Joint space narrowing, sclerosis, and osteophayte formation of distal and proximal interphalangeal joints in patient with osteoarthritis of hands.

or large osteophytes. Occasionally large amounts of synovial fluid can accumulate and limit motion.

On physical examination the involved joints may be tender. Localized areas may be specifically painful, such as the medial tibial plateau in OA of the knee. The joints frequently are warm but usually not erythematous. Commonly there is bony enlargement of the joints, especially in the hands. Crepitus is common. Loss of motion with flexion contractures also is a frequent finding in advanced OA. Eventually, gross deformities can occur.

LABORATORY FINDINGS. There are no specific laboratory findings in OA. The erythrocyte sedimentation rate generally is normal, as are complete blood count levels, urinalyses, and serum chemistries. Synovial fluid classically is noninflammatory with fewer than 2000 white blood cells/mm³. However, synovial fluid frequently contains calcium-containing crystals such as calcium hydroxyapatite or calcium pyrophosphate dihydrate. The role of these crystals in the pathogenesis of OA remains unclear.

The roentgenogram is the most useful diagnostic tool available. Typical features are narrowing of joint space, new bone (spur) formation, and bony sclerosis (Fig. 28-1). It should be emphasized, however, that symptoms typically occur before changes become apparent in roentgenographic examinations. In addition, it cannot be assumed that the changes seen on the roentgenogram are always the cause of the pain.

CLINICAL FINDINGS AT SPECIFIC SITES

Hips. The hips commonly are involved in OA, although men show a preponderance for hip involvement. The condition most often is unilateral, but 20% of patients with unilateral degeneration eventually develop contralateral involvement. Although hip involvement occurs most often in older individuals, there is frequent predisposition by congenital or developmental abnormalities such as slipped capital epiphysis. Hip pain usually is located in the groin area, but occasionally it is localized to the gluteal area or laterally over the trochanter. More common, and frequently confusing, is referral of the pain to the knee. Hip pain usually is reproduced by range of motion. Range of motion commonly is reduced, with rotation usually limited first.

Knees. OA of the knee is characterized by pain on weight bearing or motion; frequently it is relieved by rest. There can be isolated involvement of the medial or lateral compartments or of the patellofemoral compartment. In severe cases all three compartments are affected. There is bony enlargement with localized tenderness, especially of the medial tibial plateau. Effusions usually are small but can be quite large. Crepitus is common on range of motion. Eventually, gross deformity can occur, such as extreme varus or valgus.

Spine. OA of the apophyseal joints commonly is accompanied by degeneration of the intervertebral discs. Usually osteophytes develop anterolaterally and posteriorly. When posterior these osteophytes can impinge on the nerve roots or the spinal column. The most common areas of involvement are the cervical spine and the lumbar spine. Patients generally complain of localized pain in the involved area or of radicular pain involving the arm or leg if there is nerve-root impingement.

OA may narrow the cervical spine, or more often the lumbar spine, to cause spinal stenosis. Although patients with this condition often are asymptomatic, many walk with a forward flexed back and have an urgent need to rest after walking just a short distance.

In rare cases the spinal cord itself can become compressed. When this happens in the cervical spine, signs and symptoms can occur involving the attendant upper motor neuron. In addition, severe hypertrophic new bone formation in the cervical spine can cause compression of the vertebrobasilar system, with subsequent insufficiency resulting in headaches, dizziness, ataxia, and visual disturbances.

Hands. The most common finding of OA of the hands is Heberden's nodes. These nodes are 10 times more common in women than in men. They may go unnoticed and be asymptomatic, but they also can be quite painful and become inflamed. These nodes may involve one finger at the onset but eventually can be found on all DIP joints. PIP joints also can be affected, and such nodes are called Bouchard's nodes. When the condition is severe, the fingers may be deviated laterally, with loss of range-of-motion and marked bony changes on roentgenograms.

OA infrequently involves the metacarpophalangeal (MCP) joints; the distribution of the involvement is helpful in distinguishing OA from rheumatoid arthritis (RA), which commonly affects the MCP joints but rarely the DIP joints. The other commonly involved joint in the hand in OA but not RA is the first carpometacarpal (CMC) joint. Clinically pain, swelling, and tenderness of the base of the thumb may be present. The thumb may become adducted. When adduction is accompanied by subluxation, the appearance is one of squaring at the base of the thumb.

Metatarsophalangeal joint. The first metatarsophalangeal (MTP) joint is an extremely common site of OA. There is bony enlargement of the joint and frequent bursal swelling overlying the medial aspect of the joint, called a bunion.

MANAGEMENT. Treatment of OA must be tailored to the individual patient and to the joints affected. For example, development of Heberden's nodes, although often asymptomatic, may provoke anxiety. In these cases education, range-of-motion exercises, and reassurance that the patient does not have a progressive crippling disorder may be all that are necessary.

Stress should be placed on lessening mechanical factors contributing to symptoms in patients with OA. Weight loss should be encouraged if appropriate as a way of reducing both symptoms and the rate of further joint deterioration. The use of a cane, walker, or other assistive devices should be encouraged in severe OA as a means of decreasing the amount of weight bearing necessary for the involved joint. Instruction in other joint conservation techniques is also useful in non-weight-bearing joints. Exercise aimed at preserving range-of-motion and strengthening muscles also is helpful; non-weight-bearing exercises such as swimming and bicycling are the best.

A wide variety of pharmacologic agents are available for the therapy of OA. The use of analgesic and nonsteroidal antiinflammatory drugs clearly gives symptomatic relief, although there is no evidence that drugs can alter the course of OA. In fact, there is some evidence that the roentgenograms of patients using analgesics actually may show more damage than those of patients who are not administered these drugs. Nonetheless, aspirin, acetaminophen, and other nonsteroidal antiinflammatory agents remain staples in the therapy of OA. Acetaminophen probably is underused as an analgesic in OA, since it is effective and has little toxicity. The usual starting dose of acetaminophen is 650 mg four times a day, but this can be increased to slightly higher doses if necessary.

Antiinflammatory effects can be aided by the use of aspirin or any of the other nonsteroidal agents. The use of nonsteroidals other than aspirin may improve compliance and reduce side effects. Aspirin therapy has the advantage of being more economical.

Local injection of corticosteroids is controversial. There is little doubt that some patients get relief for long periods of time. Whether this relief is mostly from the medication or from the effects of arthrocentesis and the removal of fluid and debris from the joint space is unclear. Regardless, local injections should not be performed frequently on the same joint, since corticosteroids may damage cartilage. Oral steroids are ineffective and contraindicated in OA.

Minor surgical procedures have shown some promise. Some centers have reported excellent results from arthroscopic debridement of knees in certain cases. Total joint arthroplasty has offered relief to many patients with severe hip or knee OA with marked joint destruction.

VARIANTS OF OSTEOARTHRITIS
Diffuse idiopathic skeletal hyperostosis (DISH)

Also known as Forrestier's disease, diffuse idiopathic skeletal hyperostosis (DISH) chiefly occurs in men over 50 years of age. It can cause back pain and stiffness and has characteristic roentgenographic changes that must be differentiated from ankylosing spondylitis. Roentgenograms show exuberant flowing spinal osteophytes that span four or more vertebral bodies. However, in contrast to OA, the intervertebral disc spaces are not reduced, and there are no vacuum signs and no sclerosis of the vertebral end-plates. Sacroiliac joints are not eroded or sclerotic, although osteophytes may be present. Ligamentous calcifications can be quite exuberant and involve extraspinal sites. The greatest ossification of the spine generally is in the lower thoracic area, but it can be found in any area. Dysphagia can occur with prolific cervical ossification, causing esophageal compression.

Clinically most patients are asymptomatic, but some can have pain and stiffness, often with a remarkable lack of restriction of motion. Extraspinal involvement may be expressed as recurrent tendinitis and large osseous spurs where tendons or ligaments attach.

The etiologic factors of DISH are unknown. Many patients are obese and exhibit glucose intolerance, although the association with diabetes is not clear. There is no predominance of any human lymphocyte antigen haplotype. Ossification does seem to appear in response to surgery in patient with DISH, but the significance of this is unknown.

Therapy is similar to simple OA, involving local care, nonsteroidal antiinflammatory drugs, and exercises where appropriate. No measures effective in preventing ossification are yet available.

Neuropathic arthropathy

Also known as Charcot's joints, this type of arthropathy occurs in patients who experience loss of pain or propriosensation. This usually is associated with syphilis, diabetes mellitus, syringomyelia, or other chronic neurologic diseases resulting in sensory deficits. Physical examination reveals a large, distorted joint that is not painful. These changes develop slowly, resulting in marked destruction of the articular structures and striking roentgenographic abnormalities. The joints can be braced and immobilized, but a more effective therapy does not exist.

BIBLIOGRAPHY

Moskowitz RW: Cartilage and osteoarthritis: current concepts, J Rheumatol 4:329, 1977.
Moskowitz RW and others: Osteoarthritis: diagnosis and management, Philadelphia, 1984, WB Saunders Co.
Peyrove JG: Epidemiologic and etiologic approach to osteoarthritis, Semin Arthritis Rheum 8:288, 1979.
Resnick D and others: Diffuse idiopathic skeletal hyperostosis (DISH), Semin Arthritis Rheum 7:153, 1978.

29 • PAGET'S DISEASE (OSTEITIS DEFORMANS)

Donald H. Lieberman

Paget's disease of bone is a common chronic disease characterized by excessive osteoblastic and osteoclastic activity that results in poorly mineralized, distorted bones. Most cases are clinically inapparent. Pagetic bones usually produce typical roentgenographic changes, and the diagnosis often is made when roentgenograms are taken during the workup of another problem. The incidence of disease rises with age, and men have a slight predominance. There are some reports of familial clustering.

ETIOLOGY. The cause of Paget's disease is unknown. Recently a "slow viral" origin has been proposed. The intranuclear inclusions seen in slow viral disease such as subacute sclerosing panencephalitis (SSPE) resemble intranuclear inclusions described in the osteoclasts in Paget's disease. No virus has been isolated to date; even if isolation is achieved, it remains to be established whether the virus is responsible for the pathologic changes or is merely an innocent bystander. Other possible causes of Paget's disease are hormonal deficiency or excess, neoplasm, autoimmune disease, inherited abnormality of connective tissue, and vascular disturbance.

CLINICAL MANIFESTATIONS. Pain is the most common complaint in symptomatic Paget's disease. It may be present before roentgenographic changes, and the diagnosis at that time often is missed. The pain is aggravated by weight bearing if the lower extremity or spine is involved.

Headaches, dizziness, and reduced hearing may result from disease in the skull. Cranial enlargement may develop over many years. With marked involvement of the skull, patients may have cranial nerve compression. Other skeletal deformities can include distortion of the clavicles, multiple compression fractures of pagetic vertebrae resulting in severe kyphosis, bowing and elongation of the tibia and fibula, and unsuspected pathologic fractures.

Radionuclide bone scanning has added much to the delineation of the disease, and the following anatomic distribution has been reported: pelvis, 78%; spine, 63%; skull 48%; femur, 48%; scapula, 37%; tibia, 22%; humerus, 17%; and lesser amounts in other bones. Patients who have one third or more of the skeleton involved can have increased cardiac output owing to increased vascularity of the bone lesions. This can lead to congestive heart failure.

On physical examination bowing of one or both lower extremities may be observed. The tibia generally is more involved than the femur. Shortening of the involved leg occurs, and painful osteoarthritis may develop in the opposite limb as it bears more stress. Juxtalesional joints, especially the hip and knee, may show marked degenerative arthritis with loss of range of motion. Because of the increased vascularity of bone often found, the skin over the involved area may be much warmer than the contralateral side.

Angioid streaks may be seen around the optic discs; these appear as gray "cracks" in the retina. Angioid streaks are not pathognomonic signs of Paget's disease.

DIAGNOSIS AND ROENTGENOGRAPHIC FINDINGS. Roentgenographic evaluation of the skull and long bones remains the primary means of diagnosing Paget's disease (Fig. 29-1). The roentgenographic appearance includes a mottled increase in bone density, incomplete fractures or pseudofractures, localized areas of demineralization of the skull (osteoporosis circumscripta), thickening of the cortex, and coarse trabeculae. In some instances advanced Paget's disease is difficult to distinguish from metastatic disease. The use of bone scanning has enhanced the ability to make an earlier diagnosis. It is employed when pain is present without roentgenographic change and is also helpful in determining whether particular lesions are active.

LABORATORY FINDINGS. Both serum alkaline phosphatase and urinary hydroxyproline excretion are elevated. The latter is most helpful diagnostically when other concomitant disease may elevate the alkaline phosphatase. Serum calcium and phosphorus usually are normal. Occasionally patients who are immobilized may have elevated calcium levels. If patients have an unusual presenting location and the diagnosis is in question, a bone biopsy is useful. Findings on the specimen depend on the stage of disease present and require an experienced pathologist. Biopsy also is used to diagnose the rare complication of osteogenic sarcoma.

The typical roentgenographic findings and an elevated serum alkaline phophatase usually are sufficient for diagnosis. Major concerns in differential diagnosis are the presence of osteosarcoma or carcinoma that has metastasized to bone, especially from the prostate. Bone biopsy may be needed for confirmation, particularly if pain has been a salient feature. The acid phosphatase usually is elevated in prostatic carcinoma.

MANAGEMENT. Only patients with symptomatic disease require treatment. Mildly symptomatic disease can be treated

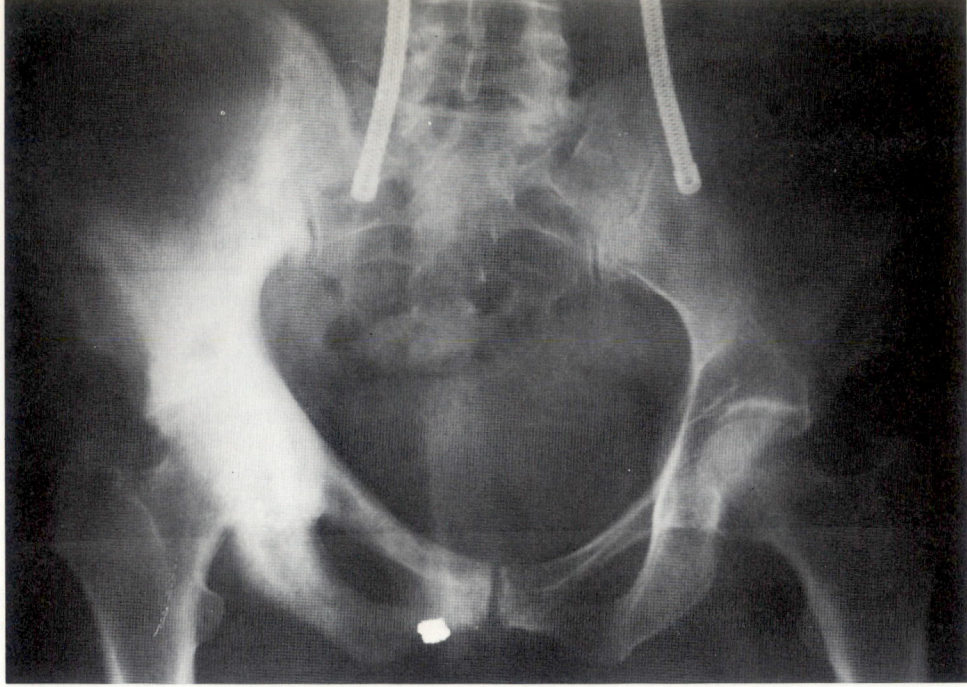

Fig. 29-1   Paget's disease of right pelvis and femur. Note thickening of bone and coarse trabecular pattern.

with analgesics or antiinflammatory drugs. With more severe disease therapeutic decisions become more difficult. The following criteria for more vigorous treatment of Paget's disease have been proposed:

1. Disabling pain unrelieved by analgesics and antiinflammatory agents
2. Progression of the skeletal aspects of the disease as indicated by increasing deformity, increased head or appendicular bone enlargement, frequent fractures, vertebral compression, or acetabular protrusion
3. Neurologic complications
4. Rapidly increasing deafness
5. High-output congestive heart failure
6. A greatly increased serum alkaline phosphatase and/or urinary hydroxyproline excretion (four or more times the normal in symptomatic patients)

The most promising drugs now employed in the treatment of Paget's disease are the calcitonins and diphosphonates. Calcitonin inhibits bone resorption. The patient response is extremely variable. The recommended dosage is 50 to 100 MRC units per day or every other day, either subcutaneously or intramuscularly. If no improvement is noted after 3 months, the drug usually is stopped. The side effects include nausea, malaise, flushing and a metallic taste. The treatment need not be discontinued because of the side effects, which usually decrease with continued therapy.

Salmon calcitonin is the species of hormone approved for use in the United States. Porcine and human calcitonin are used in other countries. In more than 50% of patients antibodies appear in the circulation that can inactivate the calcitonin.

Diphosphonates are the newest class of drugs available for treatment of Paget's disease. Etidronate disodium is the agent most frequently used. The current recommended dosage is 5 mg/kg/day, although higher doses have been used with more severe disease. This medicine is taken orally and is active in suppressing both osteoblastic and osteoclastic activity. The diphosphonates produce a more sustained control of bone turn-

over than does calcitonin. Larger dosages used to control very active disease may cause defective bone mineralization and result in pathologic fractures. Combination therapy using etidronate disodium and calcitonin in conventional dosage seems to have an additive effect and may be indicated for more active disease.

Intraarticular injection of steroids in the knee and hip has been helpful in local disease. When severe hip disease is present, total joint replacement may become necessary.

BIBLIOGRAPHY

Altman RD: Paget's disease of bone (osteitis deformans), Bull Rheum Dis 34(3), 1984.

Hoskins DJ: Paget's disease of bone: an update on management, Drugs 30:156, 1985.

Nagant de Deuxchaisnes C and Krane SM: Paget's disease of bone: clinical and metabolic observations, Medicine 43:233, 1964.

Shirazi PH, Ryan WG, Fordham EW: Bone scanning in evaluation of Paget's disease of bone, CRC Crit Rev Clin Radiol Nucl Med 5:523, 1974.

Wallach S and others: Paget's disease of bone, Phoenix, Ariz, 1979, Armour Pharmaceutical Co.

30 · OSTEOPOROSIS

Donald H. Lieberman

Osteoporosis is the most common metabolic bone disorder and the most common cause of osteopenia in the elderly. It represents a disease state of skeletal metabolism in which the rate of bone matrix formation is depressed and unable to compensate for the excessive resorption. Ossification is normal, but there is inadequate matrix to ossify. It is known that loss of bone mass accompanies normal physiologic aging, but in osteoporosis the rate of atrophy is accelerated well beyond the usual 1% per year. Clinical osteoporosis, characterized by bone pain and pathologic fractures, develops when 30% or more of the bone mass is lost. The rate of loss determines the age at which the disease is clinically apparent. Osteoporosis must be differentiated from osteomalacia, a condition involving failure to mineralize the organic matrix of bone. In osteoporosis the ratio of mineralized bone to unmineralized matrix is normal, but the mass per unit volume of bone is decreased.

Osteoporosis is a major public health problem, because bone loss can lead to fractures even with minimal trauma. Estimates of the number of hip fractures in the United States range as high as 200,000 annually. As many as 25% of these patients die of complications, and another 20% require institutionalization.

Although osteoporosis is primarily associated with aging, the presence of underlying disease must be evaluated. The following is a useful classification:

Association with aging
  Postmenopausal
  Senile
Association with endocrine disturbances (not necessarily causative)
  Hypogonadism
  Thyrotoxicosis
  Hyperadrenocorticism
  Diabetes mellitus
  Acromegaly
Nutritional deficiency
  General malnutrition
  Calcium deficiency
  Scurvy
  Malabsorption syndrome
Heritable disorders
  Ehlers-Danlos syndrome
  Osteogenesis imperfecta
  Marfan's syndrome
States involving chronic inanition
  Rheumatoid arthritis and related disorders
  Malignant tumors
  Alcoholism
  Epilepsy
  Chronic obstructive pulmonary disease
Iatrogenic conditions
  Immobilization
  Prolonged heparin use
  Excessive antacid intake
  Prolonged corticosteroid therapy
Miscellaneous
  Idiopathic osteoporosis of children and adults
  Trauma

In many of these disease states a pathophysiologic explanation exists for the decreased skeletal mass. Many of the conditions, however, have a higher incidence of osteoporosis without explanation.

Osteoporosis is uncommon in black women and extremely rare in black men. Among whites it occurs more frequently in women.

CLINICAL MANIFESTATIONS. Osteoporosis is a generalized disorder that affects trabecular bone more commonly than cortical bone. The vertebrae and ends of long bones are therefore more likely to become involved. Mild trauma may result in fractures, with the midthoracic, low thoracic, and lumbar spine and the femoral neck most commonly involved. Patients may relate the sudden onset of pain to minor stress such as lifting a child. The pain of a vertebral fracture may follow a segmental distribution corresponding to the distribution of the affected nerve rootlets. Finding a comfortable position becomes extremely difficult; coughing and sneezing can produce severe pain. Weeks to months may pass before the symptoms subside. Some patients continue to have pain even after the

bone heals. Many patients have several similar episodes. Fortunately, cord compression is rare. Decrease of body height may ensue, with forward bending leading to dorsal kyphosis. As height continues to diminish with successive fractures, skinfolds may develop along the base of the thoracic cage, and in some patients there is virtually no distance between the pelvis and rib cage.

ANCILLARY FINDINGS. Routine roentgenographic examinations are of little value in detecting early osteoporosis because the skeletal mass must be reduced by 30% before the loss is apparent roentgenographically. Most findings on the plain film are nonspecific. The vertebral bodies may become biconcave because of the pressure of the intervertebral discs. This produces the so-called codfish vertebrae. Localized disc herniations into softened vertebrae are called Schmorl's nodes. Fractures of end-plates and flattening of vertebral bodies are seen most prominently in the anterior portion. Loss of striation and decrease in cortical thickness may be noted in the proximal femur. If destructive lesions or cortical discontinuity is detected, an underlying disorder should be sought.

Serum and urinary calcium and phosphorus determinations usually are normal in primary osteoporosis. Alkaline phosphorus is not elevated.

Newer noninvasive methods are now more widely used to measure bone density. These methods include radiogrammetry, computed tomography (CT) scanning, photon absorptiometry, and neutron activation. Because of its low cost and low radiation exposure, dual-photon absorptiometry has become the most widely used procedure for diagnosis of spinal osteoporosis. However, according to recent studies, mass screening in asymptomatic people probably is not economical, and it is not recommended.

MANAGEMENT. The most important therapeutic consideration is not to miss another disorder underlying or mimicking osteoporosis. A careful review of the patient's record often is helpful in considering differential diagnoses. Secondary forms of osteoporosis should be sought so they can be optimally treated.

Once the diagnosis of senile osteoporosis is fairly certain, the physician must decide which therapeutic course to follow. Analgesics help relieve the pain of vertebral fractures. Some patients may require narcotics, but habituation is common and must be avoided. Braces are poorly tolerated by most patients, but they provide comfort to some. Although initial bed rest is required following acute vertebral fracture, excessive inactivity promotes osteopenia.

DRUG THERAPY. Many drugs have been used in the treatment of osteoporosis. The role of fluoride, anabolic steroids, calcitonin, and vitamin D metabolites remains unclear. Although the role of calcium is controversial, some studies have shown a small positive correlation between lower calcium intake and lower bone mass. Supplements of 1000 mg/day of elemental calcium in premenopausal women and 1500 mg/day in postmenopausal women are the current recommended dosages.

There is evidence that estrogens prevent age-related bone atrophy in women who take them after menopause. The usual dosage has been 0.625 to 1.25 mg/day of conjugated estrogen. Recent studies have suggested that 0.625 mg/day is adequate; higher dosages show no significant advantage yet increase the risks of endometrial hyperplasia or cancer. It is still unclear whether progesterone and estrogen should be cyclically administered. Used in this way, they appear to decrease the risk of endometrial cancer, but their long-term effects are unknown. The Food and Drug Administration has approved the use of estradiol patches. Although they may represent a more physiologic approach to replacement therapy, their role in slowing bone loss is unknown.

PHYSICAL THERAPY. Exercise is an important component in the management of osteoporosis and may help maintain skeletal mass. A good regimen promotes flexibility, gradual muscle strengthening, and aerobics. Unfortunately, exercise may be difficult for the elderly, the group at greatest risk for bone loss and fracture. Conversely, after injury, immobilization should be minimized and exercise programs begun as soon as possible.

BIBLIOGRAPHY

Avioli AV: Osteoporosis: pathogenesis and therapy. In Avioli LV, Krane SM, editors: Metabolic bone disease, vol 1, New York, 1977, Academic Press, Inc.

Bauwens SF, Drinka PJ, and Boh LE: Pathogenesis and management of primary osteoporosis, Clin Pharm 5:639, 1986.

Howell DS: Metabolic bone disease. In McCarty DJ, editor: Arthritis and allied conditions, Philadelphia, 1979, Lea & Febiger.

Wallach S: Management of osteoporosis, Hosp Practice 13:91, 1978.

Woolf AD, Dixon A St J: Osteoporosis: an update on management, Drugs 28:565, 1984.

31 · GOUT AND PSEUDOGOUT

Warren A. Katz

GOUT

Gout is a metabolic disorder characterized by hyperuricemia, recurrent attacks of acute arthritis, deposition of sodium urate in and around joints, and formation of urinary uric acid calculi in some cases. The hereditary nature of gout has been recognized since earliest times. The reported family prevalence varies from 40% to 60%. Gout rarely occurs in females. It previously was thought that gout was a disease of the wealthy or of geniuses, but current knowledge has altered the significance of the social status of gout, even though some reports find elevated levels of uric acid in college professors, business executives, and other high achievers. Stress has been suggested as a contributing factor to hyperuricemia.

Secondary gout refers to gout developing in lymphoproliferative and myeloproliferative diseases, starvation, and hypertriglyceridemia and following administration of certain drugs.

PATHOGENESIS AND PATHOLOGY. The pathogenesis of gout is conveniently described in three phases: hyperuricemia, urate deposition, and inflammation induced by urate crystals.

Hyperuricemia. Uric acid is the major end product of urine metabolism. Normal serum urate levels vary from one laboratory to another. The upper limits of normal levels are 6 to 8.8 mg/dl, depending on the testing method used. Women have slightly lower values that by menopause approach the levels found in men. Hyperuricemia may be defined as excessive levels of uric acid in serum. Not all patients with hyperuricemia develop gout. More than 5% of the normal adult population have hyperuricemia, yet gout develops in only a small minority of these. Although not all patients with bona fide gout have hyperuricemia, all those with untreated gout have excess quantities of urate in the extracellular tissues. The average patient with gout has a serum urate level of 9 to 10 mg/dl; the value is considerably higher in secondary forms of gout caused by blood dyscrasias.

Normally, uric acid is a breakdown product of purine that is formed de novo in the biosynthesis of nucleic acids. Some purines are derived from the diet, and others may be traced to tissue breakdown. Adenine and guanine are the usual sources of uric acid through a complicated metabolic pathway. Uric acid in the form of monosodium urate exists in most body fluids that are slighly alkaline. About two thirds of uric acid formed is eliminated through the kidneys and the remainder through the gastrointestinal tract. Because uric acid is degraded by intestinal bacteria, only minimal amounts of it may be found in the feces. All the uric acid that is presented to the kidneys is filtered through the glomerulus, and almost all of it is immediately reabsorbed in the proximal tubules. The amount of uric acid found in urine depends on several factors, including the rate of de novo synthesis, the degree of tissue breakdown, the amount of ingested purine, and renal function.

Hyperuricemia usually results from excessive de novo synthesis, failure of renal elimination of uric acid, or a combination of these factors. Some mechanisms of primary hyperuricemia have been clearly defined, and they usually result from specific enzyme defects.

Renal factors. Uric acid excretion by the kidneys involves glomerular filtration, tubular reabsorption, and tubular secretion. About 99% of the filtered urate is reabsorbed by the renal tubules. The filtered urate that escapes reabsorption accounts for less than 20% of the uric acid excretion in the urine, the major portion deriving from the tubular secretion. In most cases of gout expected increased urinary excretion of uric acid does not occur.

A variety of drugs, especially the thiazide diuretics, and certain metabolites (lactic acid) diminish urate clearance in the kidneys and may be responsible for hyperuricemia in some patients with gout.

Urate deposition. In most patients with hyperuricemia, gout or uric acid stones never develop. The higher the serum uric acid levels and the longer it persists, the more likely that the predisposed patient will have clinical manifestations of gout.

Despite a recent focus of attention on the urate deposition phenomenon, its cause is still unknown. Several theories involving urate concentration, sodium flux, avascularity, and diminished permeability of urate in the synovium have been proposed to explain urate crystallization in the joint.

Urates tend to be deposited in the articular cartilage of patients with gout, but they also may be found in tendon sheaths, synovium, synovial fluid, and subcutaneous tissues. Urates rarely are found in parenchymal organs such as the brain, liver, or spleen. It has been proposed that urates have an affinity for connective tissue proteoglycans. One theory for urate deposition is that proteoglycans entrap urate molecules, rendering them supersaturated in hyperuricemic subjects and therefore preventing the deposition of urates. When the normal metabolic turnover of connective tissue is accelerated under the influence of lysosomal and other proteolytic enzymes, the proteoglycans so digested no longer can solubilize urates. Therefore urate deposition results just as crystallization would take place from supersaturated solutions of proteoglycans with urate if similar enzymes were added. Indeed, the breakdown products of proteoglycans (glycosaminoglycans) is found to be elevated in serum of most patients with proven gout but not in normal individuals or hyperuricemic individuals without gout. Selective nocturnal water resorption from traumatic joint effusions may lead to increased urate concentrations. Once deposited, urates induce local necrosis and subsequent fibrosis. Cartilage degeneration ensues, and bone destruction follows.

Acute gouty attack. Monosodium urate is sparingly soluble in plasma and other body fluids. Once urates are deposited, for whatever reason, they may or may not be phagocytized to set off an intense inflammatory reaction, including activation of factor XII (Hageman factor), kinin release, complement pathway activity, leukotriene formation, and release of lysosomal enzymes. Neither the initial mechanism of urate crystallization nor the mechanism of the initial urate inflammatory stimulating effect is known. Microcrystals of monosodium urate are coated with plasma proteins, including immunoglobulins. The presence of IgG is believed to promote phagocytosis by polymorphonuclear leukocytes that carry immunoglobulin (Fc) receptor sites on their surfaces. Phagocytosis having been achieved, the microcrystals become incorporated into phagolysosomes, leading to the formation of chemotactic factor that mobilizes additional leukocytes. Almost immediately after crystal phagocytosis, rapid degranulation and disintegration of the cells occurs, with the release of more lysosomal enzymes and superoxide ion, which induce inflammation. In addition, lysosomal enzymes degrade articular cartilage and ultimately destroy it (Fig. 31-1).

CLINICAL MANIFESTATIONS

Acute gouty arthritis. Acute arthritis is the major clinical expression of gout. Podagra, or involvement of the first metatarsophalangeal joint, occurs during the first attack in about 75% of the cases (Fig. 31-2). Sydenham's initial description in 1683 is so clear and dramatic that it remains the classic description of acute gouty arthritis:

The victim goes to bed and sleeps in good health. About two o'clock in the morning he is awakened by severe pain in the great toe; more rarely in the heel, ankle or instep. This pain is like that of a dislocation, and yet the parts feel as if cold water were poured over them. Then follows chills and shivers, and a little fever. The pain, which was at first moderate, becomes more intense. With its intensity, the chills and shivers increase. After a time, this comes to its height, accommodating itself to the bones and ligaments of the tarsus and metatarsus. Now it is a violent stretching and tearing of the ligaments—now it is a gnawing pain, and now a pressure and tightening. So exquisite and lively meanwhile is the part affected, that it cannot bear the weight of the bed clothes nor the jar of a person walking in the room. Night is passed in torture, sleeplessness, turning of the part affected, and perpetual change of posture.

Examination shows the toe or adjacent area to be swollen, shiny, and red or sometimes even violaceous. The overlying skin frequently becomes desquamated as the attack resolves. If untreated a gouty attack lasts for several days but may persist longer. Complete resolution is the rule.

The other small joints of the feet and the ankles, knees, elbows, and wrists frequently are involved with acute gouty arthritis. Less commonly the finger joints and in rare cases the shoulders, hips, and sacroiliac joints are affected.

Acute arthritis of one joint is most typical, but polyarthritis may be seen even during the first attack. Under these circumstances the joint distribution is asymmetric and confined mostly to the lower extremities.

Acute gouty attacks tend to recur in unpredictable and episodic fashion. About 60% of those with gout have a second attack within a year, especially if they are untreated. Many patients report minor attacks of joint inflammation even in the absence of the more florid typical attacks.

Polyarticular gouty arthritis is noted in about one third of patients, particularly those in whom monoarticular involvement is poorly controlled. Most of these patients suffer from concomitant, complex medical problems such a hypertension, congestive heart failure, chronic renal disease, or alcoholism.

It is not always clear what precipitates the acute attack of gout in the predisposed hyperuricemic patient or for that matter in the nonhyperuricemic patient. The association with wine and gluttony dates back to ancient times. Indeed, about half of the patients with gout are significantly overweight, and about 75% have hypertriglyceridemia. It is possible, but not proven, that excessive caloric intake, particularly of certain foods, makes uric acid precursors such as phosphoribosyl pyrophosphate more readily available and thus stimulates the metabolic pathway. Heavy alcoholic intake may raise the concentration of blood lactate to a point at which it interferes with the renal excretion of urates so that a rapid rise in uric acid concentration results. Dramatic fluctuations in serum urate induced by fasting, heavy consumption of alcoholic beverages, and certain foods often are followed by flares in gouty arthritis. Identical swings may be noted during treatment with uric acid–lowering drugs such as allopurinol or probenecid or with drugs that affect renal handling of uric acid such as the thiazide diuretics. Trauma, surgery, and associated illnesses may predispose an individual to gouty arthritis.

Hematologic diseases, neoplastic diseases, hypertension, coronary artery disease, diabetes mellitus, glycogen storage disease, lead intoxication (saturnine gout), and intrinsic renal disease are all associated with gout and hyperuricemia. Hyperuricemia also may be induced by ethacrynic acid, furosemide, acetazolamide, pyrazinamide, low-dose salicylates, and certain other drugs.

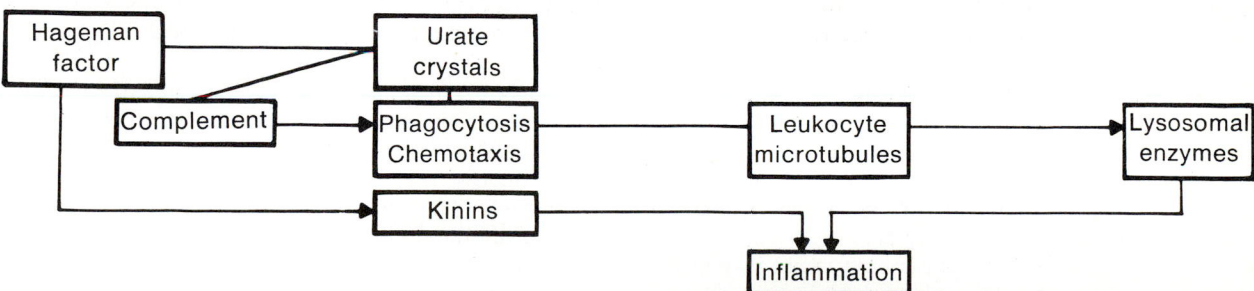

Fig. 31-1. Postulated schema for urate crystal-induced inflammation in gout. Once deposited in joint, urate crystals evoke foreign body-like reaction that causes chemotaxis of leukocytes and then phagocytosis of crystals through leukocyte microtubule mechanism. Hageman factor, complement, and kinins are released, and these factors plus lysosomal enzymes released from leukocytes immediately after phagocytosis produce inflammatory reaction. (Modified from Katz WA: Diagnosis and management of rheumatic diseases, Philadelphia, 1977, JB Lippincott Co.)

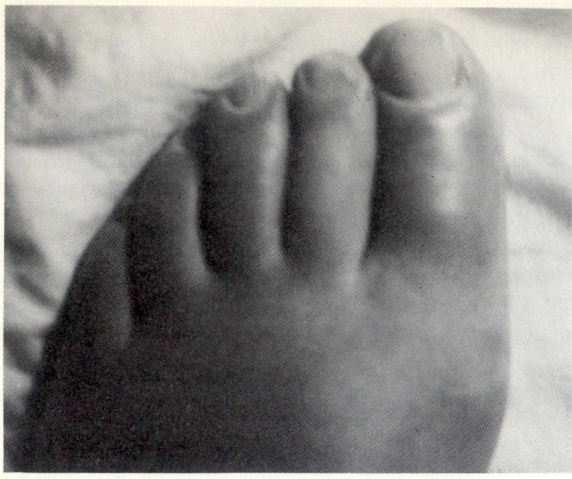

Fig. 31-2. Typical inflamed first metatarsophalangeal joint and adjacent tissues during acute gout. Note sheen of dorsum toe and loss of normal wrinkles.

Secondary hyperuricemia and gout occur in leukemia, myeloproliferative diseases, lymphomas, and polycythemia. Aggressive treatment of these conditions produces accelerated turnover of purine nucleotide and nucleic acids, thereby inducing even greater incidence of gout.

Chronic tophaceous gout. Early in the course of gout, asymptomatic intervals usually are prolonged. As attacks become more frequent, symptom-free periods become shorter; ultimately, in the untreated individual, tophaceous deposits with secondary degenerative changes will leave permanent arthralgias and stiffness. Extensive tophaceous gout may be just as disabling and crippling as advanced rheumatoid arthritis. Tophi may cause similar deformity, entrap nerves, and cause draining, infected sinus tracts.

Tophi usually are seen in the first metatarsophalangeal joint, olecranon, articular synovium, and tendon sheaths of the hand. The development of tophi in predisposed individuals is directly related to the duration and degree of hyperuricemia.

Uric acid lithiasis. In the general population 10% of all renal stones are composed of uric acid. Nephrolithiasis develops in about 20% to 25% of the patients with primary gout, as compared with about 50% of those with secondary gout. In more than one third of the patients with primary gout, renal lithiasis precedes the first attack of acute gouty arthritis. The prevalence of uric acid lithiasis is related to the serum and urinary uric acid output. This association, however, it not as strong as once thought.

LABORATORY FINDINGS. Most, but not all, patients with gout exhibit hyperuricemia either during or after the acute attack. However, the serum uric acid level cannot be used as a diagnostic tool, because hyperuricemia is so variable, fluctuates from day to day, is not universal in patients with gout, and affects so many otherwise healthy people.

Estimation of the 24-hour urine uric acid is not diagnostic either; however, it does help to predict whether a patient is a candidate for uric acid stones. Extremely high levels of urine uric acid, especially when greater than 1 g/day, make the patient with gout particularly vulnerable to nephrolithiasis.

The identification, under the light of a polarized microscope, of monosodium urate crystals in the synovial fluid from an acute gouty joint definitely establishes the diagnosis. The needlelike crystals frequently may be found piercing the leukocytes during an acute attack. Monosodium urate crystals also can be detected in aspirates from tophi or biopsy material.

Roentgenographic findings. It is unusual to find roentgenographic abnormalities during the first attack of gout. However, some patients have gouty episodes of such low-grade intensity that they may be missed, yet many years later characteristic tophaceous lesions may be found in the joints, notably in the feet. For this reason roentgenograms of the feet should be obtained when there is a diagnostic dilemma. Typical lesions are sharply defined. Marginal erosions of subchondral bone may appear at the periphery as a thin shell with an overhanging edge. These changes are seen particularly at the first metatarsophalangeal joint; although they are highly suggestive, they are not diagnostic of gout.

DIAGNOSIS. In the typical case of acute podagra developing in a susceptible patient, the diagnosis of gout usually is correctly suspected. Nonetheless, synovial fluid analysis for urate crystals is a necessary confirmatory test. Since gout rarely develops in premenopausal women, in this age group other causes of acute arthritis should be sought. Uric acid crystals are not always obtainable from joint fluid. Under these circumstances the diagnosis must rely heavily on a history of repeated attacks of acute arthritis that peak within 1 day and are associated with redness and exquisite tenderness, particularly in the first metatarsophalangeal joint. In the early stages (first 24 to 48 hours) of acute gouty arthritis, colchicine given orally or intravenously induces a dramatic therapeutic response not usually seen in other rheumatic diseases.

The differential diagnosis of gout includes pseudogout, rheumatoid arthritis, rheumatoid variants, osteoarthritis, sarcoid arthritis, psoriatic arthritis, infectious arthritis, palindromic rheumatism, cellulitis, acute bursitis, acute rheumatic fever, and local trauma.

MANAGEMENT. With the development of highly effective drugs, dietary restriction of purines and alcohol is not as important in treating gout as it once was. However, in patients whose gout is difficult to control, a diet relatively free of purines may be recommended at least temporarily. A well-balanced diet somewhat lower in calories and proteins is desirable. Obese patients should make every attempt to lose weight gradually, since starvation usually causes ketone-induced hyperuricemia and susceptibility to the acute gouty attack.

The management of acute gouty arthritis is fairly standard, although treatment of asymptomatic hyperuricemia, intercritical gout (asymptomatic intervals), and tophaceous gout remains somewhat controversial.

Acute gouty arthritis. Acute attacks of gout can be treated with colchicine, nonsteroidal antiinflammatory drugs, adrenocorticotropic hormone (ACTH), and local injections of corticosteroids.

Because of colchicine's effectiveness and relative specificity, it has the advantage of facilitating the diagnosis of gout. The sooner colchicine is administered during the acute attack, the more effective it is. Colchicine is effective in about 75% of the patients. Gastrointestinal toxic reactions in the form of cramps, diarrhea, and nausea may appear within 12 hours of initiating therapy. Colchicine can be administered intravenously to avoid gastrointestinal side effects. The major risk of intravenous administration of colchicine is extravasation of the drug with local tissue damage.

Phenylbutazone, oxyphenbutazone, indomethacin, sulindac, and a number of other nonsteroidal antiinflammatory drugs have been advocated in the treatment of acute gout. Each is effective and may be continued during the first few days of therapy until the attack subsides completely.

Aspiration of crystals from the joint, local administration of corticosteroids, or parenteral administration of ACTH also is advocated for patients who cannot take drugs by mouth or who are intolerant of the agents usually given to treat the acute attack of gout. Warm soaks, ice application, immobilization, and hydration provide additional nondrug therapy.

Asymptomatic hyperuricemia. Few patients with asymptomatic hyperuricemia require treatment. Most such patients have uric acid levels just a milligram or two greater than normal and therefore are at minimal risk of ever having an acute attack of gout. Patients with significantly higher levels of uric acid might be at greater risk of having gouty arthritis and even uric acid stones, but the incidence and ultimate morbidity would be so small that prophylactic treatment is unwise. There is no strong evidence to indicate that significant, irreversible renal damage develops in patients with asymptomatic hyperuricemia.

Intercritical gout. No drug therapy is needed for patients whose attacks of arthritis occur at wide intervals, but they should be assessed periodically. If gouty episodes are becoming frequent and prolonged, colchicine will prevent almost all attacks regardless of serum uric acid levels. If the patient cannot tolerate higher levels of colchicine, if recurrent attacks develop during colchicine therapy, or if roentgenographic changes are taking place, uric acid–lowering drugs should be introduced slowly.

Chronic tophaceous gout. A very large tophus may be removed surgically providing it has not become an integral part of bone mass. Most patients with chronic tophaceous gout are treated with uric acid–lowering drugs such as uricosuric agents (probenecid or sulfinpyrazone) or allopurinol, a xanthine oxidase inhibitor.

Uric acid stones. Whether or not uric acid stones occur in association with gouty arthritis, a large daily fluid intake is required to prevent stone formation. In most instances alkalinization of the urine with sodium citrate or bicarbonate to maintain a pH greater than 6 is desired. This increases the solubility of urates. Allopurinol is a more specific method of preventing uric acid stones.

PSEUDOGOUT

Pseudogout is a crystal-induced disease characterized by acute arthritis that mimics gout caused by urate crystals. Chronic joint inflammation may develop, mimicking rheumatoid arthritis and osteoarthritis. Pseudogout has been referred to as chondrocalcinosis, pyrophosphate arthropathy, and calcium pyrophosphate crystal disease. The disorder represents a distinct clinical entity caused by the deposition of calcium pyrophosphate dihydrate (CPPD) crystals in joints. Pseudogout is the clinical state, whereas "chondrocalcinosis" merely refers to calcification of cartilage whether or not the patient is symptomatic. Although many cases of pseudogout undoubtedly are missed diagnostically, gout is still a much more common disease. Familial aggregations of pseudogout have been noted in Czechoslovakia and Chile; a dominant pattern of transmission is suggested.

PATHOLOGY AND PATHOGENESIS. The metabolic basis for CPPD deposition is unknown. Deficiency of pyrophosphatases in cartilage and other connective tissues has been considered. The initial site of CPPD crystal formation is most likely in the articular cartilage, and indeed CPPD crystals frequently are found in these sites. It is not clear how the crystals precipitate. Somehow they are shed into the joint space and evoke acute inflammation similar to that of gout. The role of trauma, metabolic disorders, and concomitant medical illnesses remains to be clarified. The degree of degenerative change in the joint, resembling osteoarthritis, varies from quite mild to marked destruction akin to that of Charcot's joints.

CLINICAL MANIFESTATIONS. Pseudogout has several presentations. Acute inflammation of one or a few joints is the hallmark of the disease. The inflammation is intense and sometimes associated with low-grade fever. Pseudogout is slightly more prevalent in women than in men. Most patients are in their sixties during the first attack. Those in a younger age group usually inherit the disease. Larger joints, especially the knees, are most prone to involvement. Wrists, elbows, ankles, and even shoulders and hips frequently are affected. Smaller joints of the fingers and toes are less likely to be inflamed. Involvement of the temporomandibular joint has been noted. The first metatarsophalangeal joint usually is not involved in pseudogout.

The duration of the acute attack of pseudogout varies from several days to several weeks, certainly lasting longer than the typical untreated attack of gout. As in gout the joint becomes red, hot, swollen, and limited in motion. Attacks tend to cluster in a given extremity. The intercritical period is variable and may last from days to years.

McCarty lists the following primary types of pseudogout:

1. In type A, pseudogout, there are typical intermittent acute attacks with asymptomatic intervals.
2. In type B, pseudorheumatoid arthritis, patients may have multiple-joint involvement with subacute attacks lasting for several weeks to months. Because of prolonged morning stiffness, fatigue, and synovial thickening with an elevated erythrocyte sedimentation rate, these patients often are thought to have rheumatoid arthritis.
3. In types C and D, pseudo-osteoarthritis, progressive degeneration of multiple joints occurs. In contrast to typical osteoarthritis, the wrists, metatarsophalangeal joints, shoulders, elbows, and ankles frequently are involved. Patients with type C have superimposed acute attacks, whereas those with type D have no apparent inflammatory component.
4. Type E is lanthanic (asymptomatic CPPD crystal deposition).
5. In type F, pseudoneuropathic joints, patients have Charcot's arthropathy, sometimes without neurologic deficit but with evidence of chondrocalcinosis.

Associated disease. A true association exists between CPPD crystal deposition disease and hyperparathyroidism, hemochromatosis, hemosiderosis, hypophosphatasia, hypomagnesemia, hypothyroidism, gout, neuropathic joints, and aging. A less clear-cut association is noted between CPPD and hyperthyroidism, calcium renal stones, ankylosing hyperostosis, ochronosis, Wilson's disease, and hemophilic arthropathy. Despite previous statements to the contrary, it is unlikely that there is a true association with diabetes mellitus, hypertension, mild azotemia, hyperuricemia, gynecomastia, inflammatory bowel disease, rheumatoid arthritis, Paget's disease, and acromegaly.

LABORATORY FINDINGS. Synovial fluid analysis provides the most important diagnostic determination of pseudogout. A single drop is all that is needed to detect the typical crystals, which vary in morphology but generally are irregular, rhomboid, or parallelepiped. During an acute attack crystals usually are seen in leukocytes. They also may be rod shaped, and as such they resemble urate crystals except that the ends are blunted. The cell counts in synovial fluid may be very high as in infectious arthritis, but cell counts of 21,000/mm^3 are the average.

Synovial biopsy may be necessary to establish the disease if synovial fluid is unavailable for diagnosis. High-power microscopy and sometimes electron microscopy are required for identification of crystals.

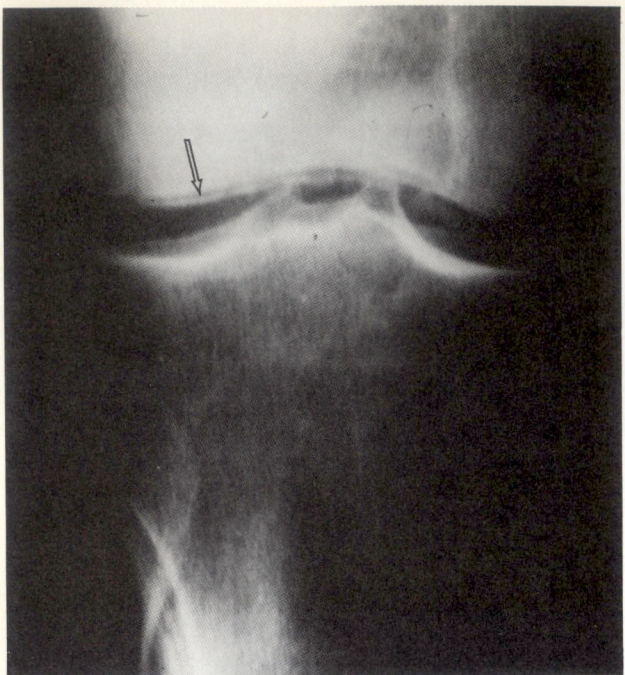

Fig. 31-3. Linear calcification of cartilage of knee (chondrocalcinosis) in patient with pseudogout.

Roentgenographically, CPPD crystal deposition is noted in fibrocartilaginous structures, articular cartilage, ligaments, and joint capsules. The radiodensity may be linear or punctate, particularly in the meniscus and articular cartilage of the knees (Fig. 31-3). The articular disc of the distal radial ulnar joint, the symphysis pubis, the acetabular and glenoid fossae, and the anulus fibrosus of the intervertebral disc may calcify.

DIAGNOSIS. Pseudogout is suspected whenever acute or pauciarticular arthritis develops in an elderly person, especially if concomitant associated diseases are present. Discovery of the characteristic CPPD crystals when phagocytized in synovial fluid and the typical linear calcifications on the roentgenogram are additional evidence for the existence of this disease. Septic arthritis, gouty arthritis, palindromic rheumatism, intermittent hydrarthrosis, osteoarthritis, and rheumatoid arthritis are the usual differential diagnoses.

MANAGEMENT. Acute attacks of pseudogout are treated by thorough aspiration and perhaps even lavage of the involved joint, followed by local instillation of corticosteroids. Phenylbutazone, indomethacin, and other nonsteroidal antiinflammatory drugs usually are effective. Colchicine seems to abort some attacks of pseudogout, but its effectiveness is unpredictable. There is no reliable way of preventing pseudogout.

OTHER CRYSTAL DEPOSITION DISEASE

Calcium hydroxyapatite crystals have been seen in calcific periarthritis for many years. These crystals also have been detected in synovial fluid from patients with previously undiagnosed acute arthritis and exacerbations of osteoarthritis. Calcium hydroxyapatite crystals may induce synovitis similar to that caused by urate crystals in gout and pyrophosphate crystals in pseudogout. Detection of these crystals by light microscopy is difficult. Purple-staining cytoplasmic inclusions or extracellular globules may suggest clumps of calcium crystals, but electron microscopic and roentgenographic differential techniques, not readily available in most laboratories are needed to confirm their presence.

A peculiar type of hydroxyapatite crystal–induced arthritis

may affect the shoulders in the elderly, usually women (Milwaukee shoulder). The joints may become acutely or subacutely painful and swollen. Shoulder motion is limited. Rotator cuff tears usually can be demonstrated by arthroscopy. These patients usually have osteoarthritis and chondrocalcinosis in other joints. Temporary relief can be obtained from aspiration of the joint, instillation of corticosteroids, nonsteroidal antiinflammatory drugs, rest, and range-of-motion exercises.

BIBLIOGRAPHY

Fessel WJ: Renal outcomes of gout and hyperuricemia, Am J Med 67:74, 1979.

Gatter R: Pseudogout. In Katz WA, editor: Diagnosis and management of rheumatic diseases, Philadelphia, 1988, JB Lippincott Co.

Kelley WN and Weiner IM: Uric acid: handbook of experimental pharmacology, Berlin, 1978, Springer-Verlag.

McCarty DJ: Calcium pyrophosphate crystal deposition disease (pseudogout; articular chondrocalcinosis). In McCarty DJ: Arthritis and allied conditions, Philadelphia, 1979, Lea & Febiger.

McCarty DJ and others: "Milwaukee shoulder"—association of microspheroids containing hydroxyapatite crystals, active collagenase, and neutral protease with rotator cuff defects. I. Clinical aspects, Arthritis Rheum 24:464, 1981.

Schumacher HR Jr and others: Arthritis associated with apatite crystals, Ann Intern Med 87:411, 1977.

Wyngaarden JB and Kelley WN: Gout and hyperuricemia, New York, 1976, Grune & Stratton, Inc.

Yu TF: Milestones in the treatment of gout, Am J Med 56:767, 1974.

Yu TF: The efficacy of colchicine prophylaxis in articular gout. A reappraisal after 20 years, Semin Arthritis Rheum 12:255, 1982.

Yu TF: Gout. In Katz WA, editor: Diagnosis and management of rheumatic diseases, Philadelphia, 1988, JB Lippincott Co.

32 · NONARTICULAR RHEUMATISM

Robert H. Gordon

The term "nonarticular (soft tissue) rheumatism" encompasses a variety of musculoskeletal complaints that do not arise directly from disease in the joints. Pain in these conditions is attributed to dysfunction or inflammation of connective tissues such as muscle, tendons, ligaments, and bursae. In some conditions the intercellular matrix, the supporting ground substance of connective tissue, may be involved, although the exact nature of the involvement is unknown.

Some of the disorders of nonarticular rheumatism have signs and symptoms that are well localized and quite specific. For these, successful treatment can be offered. However, other forms are marked by vague complaints of diffuse pain that the physician cannot easily attribute to local pathology. These conditions are distressing for both the patient and the physician because the diagnosis is difficult, and the results of treatment sometimes are less than satisfactory.

Laboratory studies usually are of little help in making or supporting these diagnoses. The erythrocyte sedimentation rate most often is normal despite the intensity of symptoms. Other routine blood studies also are normal or, when not, should suggest the presence of other underlying disease. The correct diagnosis therefore usually is made on the basis of the clinical history and physical findings.

FIBROSITIS

Fibrositis is known by a number of names, including myofascitis, fibromyositis, and fibromyalgia. Although these terms frequently are used to describe pain complaints that fail to fit other diagnoses, recent studies have done much to define the syndrome.

PATHOGENESIS. Attempts to define the disease by muscle biopsy or electromyography results have been unsuccessful. Changes in neurogenic amine metabolism and immune mechanisms have been described.

Sleep studies have focused on the relationshp between non–rapid eye movement (non–REM) sleep disturbances and fibrositis complaints. Some fibrositic patients showed abnormal electroencephalograms characterized by non–REM sleep disturbances. Normal subjects whose sleep was interrupted during the same non–REM phase also complained of morning fatigue and other musculoskeletal symptoms suggestive of fibrositis. Further studies tested the effects of chlorpromazine, a drug that had been reported to facilitate slow-wave non–REM sleep, and amelioration of symptoms was noted. Tricyclic antidepressants also may be of benefit by inducing a similar normalization of this stage of sleep.

CLINICAL MANIFESTATIONS. Two types of fibrositis are described. Primary fibrositis has no known underlying disease. Secondary fibrositis is associated with a wide array of systemic diseases, including rheumatic disorders (most commonly rheumatoid arthritis) and infectious, endocrine, and neoplastic diseases. The two types of fibrositis have similar presentations.

Pain, the chief complaint, is diffuse, aching, and especially pronounced about the neck, shoulders, low back, and pelvis. The trunk and extremities also may be involved. When present, stiffness and fatigue often are worse on wakening, typically after a restless sleep. Muscle strength generally is maintained. Some patients think that their muscles are swollen, but the apparent enlargement usually represents muscle spasm. Headaches, dysesthesias, and irritable bowel syndrome are quite common nonrheumatic complaints.

Tension, anxiety, cold, fatigue, and prolonged immobility exacerbate the condition, whereas heat, relaxation, and gentle exercises tend to alleviate it. The onset of the disease often is dated to a stressful situation, family upheaval, or accident.

The physical examination initially may appear to be normal. Muscle strength is preserved, and the patient seems to be in good health. However, more detailed evaluation elicits trigger points, specific sites of tenderness that reproduce the pain when palpated. Patients frequently are unaware of these areas and often are relieved to know that the physician is able to find the source of their pain. Fourteen characteristic sites have been described (Fig. 32-1). It is important to appreciate that these areas often are tender in normal individuals. It is the *degree* of the tenderness that marks the patient with fibrositis. Excessive cutaneous blanching followed by hyperemia often is noted after these areas are palpated. The muscles may be in spasm.

LABORATORY FINDINGS. Roentgenographic and laboratory studies are of no help in diagnosing primary fibrositis. Despite extreme muscle tenderness, muscle enzymes and the sedimentation rate are normal. Other laboratory studies, including tests for rheumatoid factor and autoantibodies, are negative. The muscle biopsy is normal. If any of these are abnormal, other diseases or conditions associated with secondary fibrositis should be considered.

DIAGNOSIS. Several criteria have been proposed to support the diagnosis of fibrositis. These include (1) widespread aching of more than 3 months' duration, (2) local tenderness at 12 of the 14 sites (Fig. 32-1), (3) diffuse tenderness in the upper scapular region, (4) disturbed sleep with morning fatigue and stiffness, and (5) normal sedimentation rate, rheumatoid factor, antinuclear antibody, muscle enzymes, and other laboratory studies. The last criterion is necessary in ruling out conditions

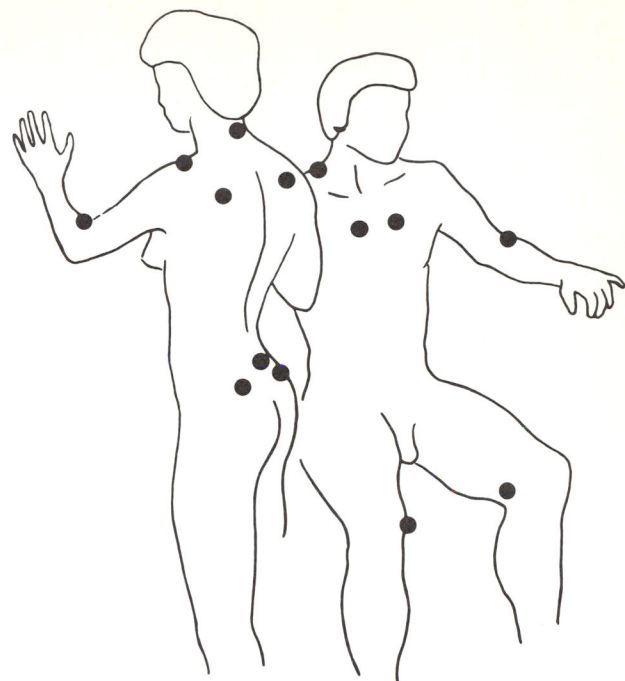

Fig. 32-1   Location of 14 sites of deep tenderness in fibrositis. (From Smythe HA and Moldofsky H: Bull Rheum Dis 28:928, 1977-1978.)

that can mimic fibrositis but have different causes and treatment.

MANAGEMENT. It is important to assure the patient that the disease is not crippling, that the prognosis is good, that significant disability is rare, and that a productive lifestyle can be maintained. Patients should be encouraged to maintain good muscle tone through graded programs of exercise, but overexercise can worsen symptoms. Back or neck supports may be helpful. Rest and relaxation are important and should be encouraged for overanxious or overworked individuals. Physical therapy using heat packs, ultrasound, massage, and whirlpool is beneficial. Antiinflammatory drugs, including aspirin and other nonsteroidal agents, can be tried, but their efficacy has not been determined by controlled tests. Sometimes injections of local anesthetics are helpful for specific trigger points; whether local injections of corticosteroids provide additional benefits is a moot point. The disturbed sleep pattern may be helped by small to moderate doses of tricyclic antidepressant medications (such as imipramine, 25 to 100 mg) before bedtime. Counseling regarding marital, occupational, or other problems is critical to successful therapy in some fibrositic patients.

REGIONAL AND LOCAL NONARTICULAR SYNDROMES
Myofascial syndromes

HEAD AND NECK. Several specific myofascial pain syndromes can be identified in the head and neck on careful evaluation (Fig. 32-2). Tenderness and spasm can be detected over trigger points in one or more of the following muscles: temporalis, masseter, external pterygoid (Fig. 32-3), internal pterygoid, sternocleidomastoid, and splenius capitis. Treatment of these myofascial pain syndromes is identical to that in other areas of the body.

SHOULDER, UPPER ARMS, AND CHEST. As in the head and neck, several important muscle syndromes can cause sig-

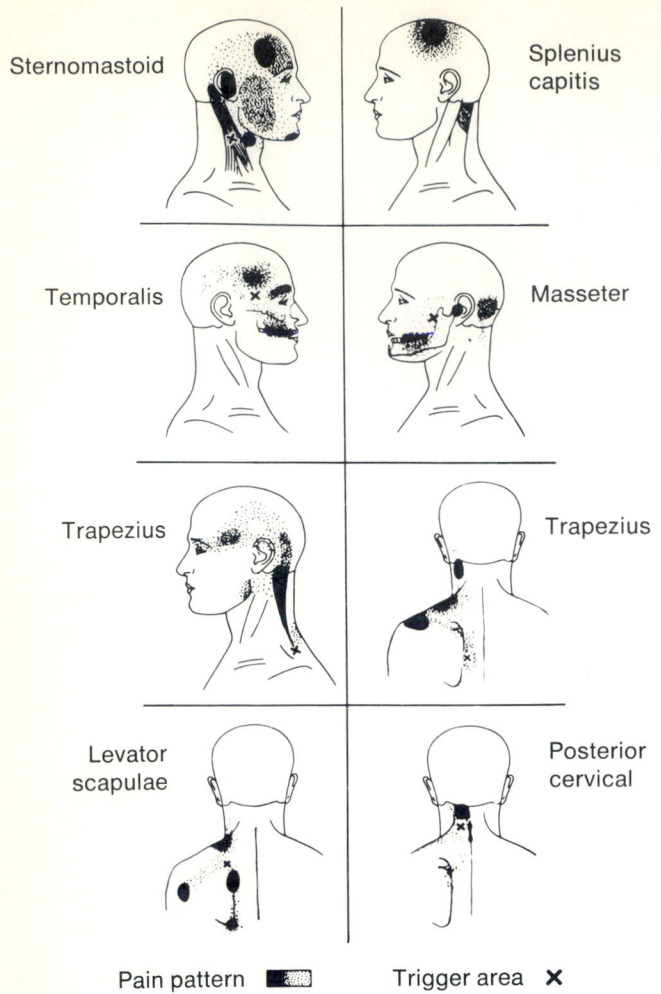

Pain pattern ▬   Trigger area ✕

Fig. 32-2 Myofascial syndromes of head and neck. (From Travell J and Rinzler SH: Postgrad Med 11:425, 1952.)

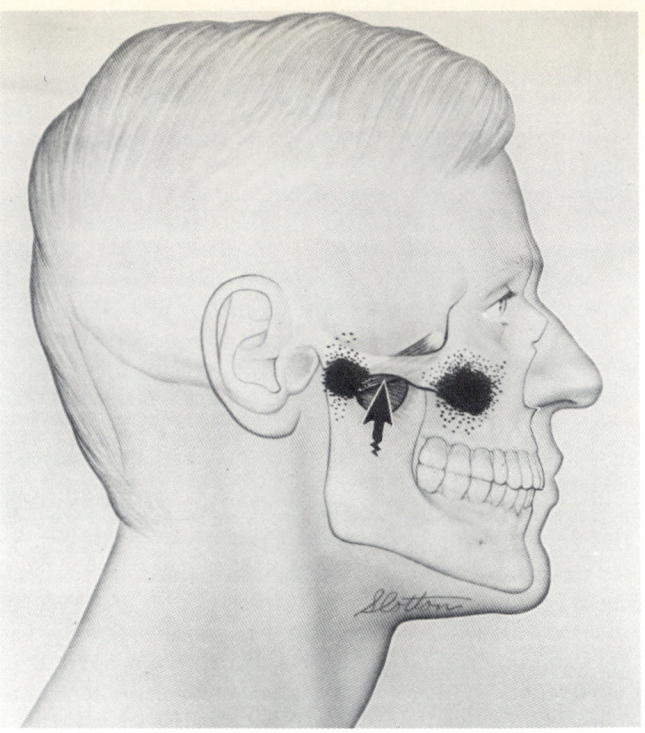

Fig. 32-3 External pterygoid trigger point. (From Shaber EP: Considerations in the treatment of muscle spasm. In Morgan DH, Hall WP, and Vamvas SJ: Diseases of the temporomandibular apparatus, St Louis, 1977, The CV Mosby Co.)

nificant pain and disability in the shoulder, upper arm, and chest. The *supraspinatus muscle* frequently causes radiation of pain from the muscle body into the deltoid and upper outer portions of the upper arm. The *subscapularis muscle* can give rise to pain felt maximally at the posterior aspect of the shoulder and over the scapula. Other not infrequent syndromes involve the *infraspinatus, scaleni, deltoid, trapezius,* and *pectoral muscles.*

BACK AND LEG. Specific muscle pain syndromes can be found on examination of the painful back or leg. Frequently these can mimic lumbar disc disease with radicular pain, and their identification may save the patient from unnecessary diagnostic or therapeutic procedures. Spasm of the gluteus medius and minimus muscles is particularly likely to be misdiagnosed as true sciatica.

Nerve entrapments

CARPAL TUNNEL SYNDROME. Carpal tunnel syndrome is the most common cause of pain and paresthesia in the first three fingers of the hand. Occasionally the pain radiates proximally into the forearm and even into the shoulder. The symptoms are caused by compression of the median nerve at the proximal volar wrist underneath the tight transverse carpal ligament. Patients frequently complain of waking during the night with a numb and painful hand that is relieved only by vigorous shaking. The condition may be worsened by prolonged wrist flexion (Phalen's sign) or by tapping the nerve at the wrist (Tinel's sign). The syndrome is seen in any condition that causes pressure on the nerve, such as trauma, tenosynovitis, and connective tissue diseases (for example, rheumatoid arthritis). Diabetes mellitus, pregnancy, myxedema, acromegaly, and amyloidosis are other associated conditions. Nerve conduction studies document median nerve injury. Treating the primary disease may relieve the compression. Wrist splints to hold the wrist in slight extension, corticosteroid injections, or surgical release of the nerve may be necessary.

MERALGIA PARESTHETICA. Meralgia paresthetica is a syndrome produced by compression of the lateral femoral cutaneous nerve beneath the inguinal ligament medial to the iliac spine. Paresthesias are noted in the lateral thigh. Pregnancy, obesity, or a tightly fitted corset may be associated factors. Gradual weight loss and proper posture usually are corrective. Local injections of corticosteroids may be tried. Transcutaneous electrical nerve stimulators have been helpful for this and other localized pain syndromes.

TARSAL TUNNEL SYNDROME. Tarsal tunnel syndrome is produced by entrapment of the posterior tibial nerve as it passes beneath the medial malleolus. It is associated with a burning pain and numbness of the toes and sole of the foot. It can be traumatic in origin, although it also has been associated with rheumatoid arthritis, ankylosing spondylitis, and leprosy. Neuromas and ganglia in the area also may entrap the nerve. The treatment is similar to that for carpal tunnel syndrome.

Bursitis

SUBDELTOID BURSITIS. Subdeltoid bursitis (Fig. 32-4) causes pain that in many instances is difficult to distinguish

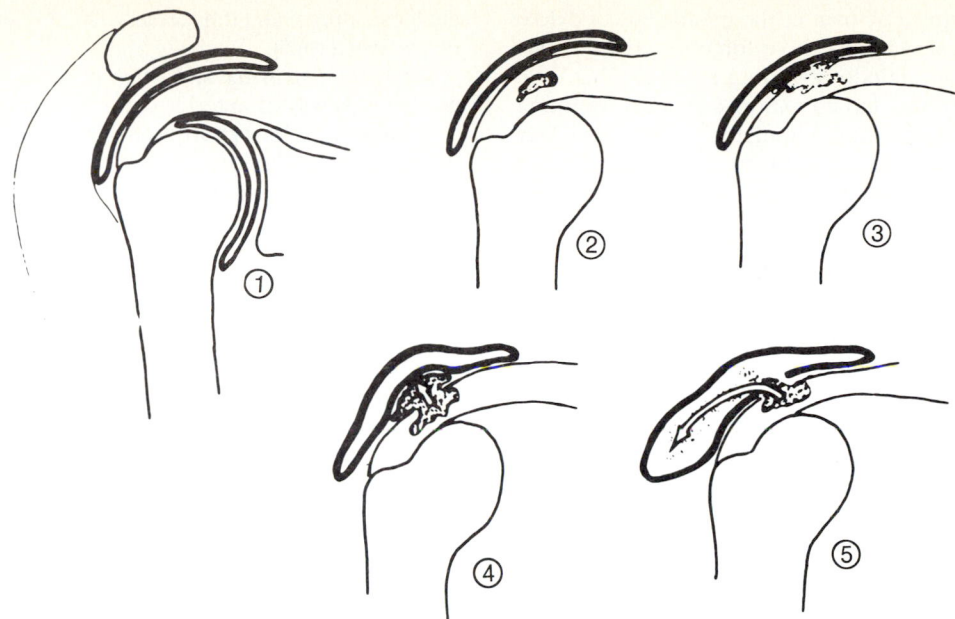

Fig. 32-4   Subdeltoid bursitis. Sequential changes showing deposition of calcium *(2)*, rupture through rotator cuff *(3)*, pressure on overlying bursa *(4)*, and rupture into bursa *(5)*. (From Cailliet R: Neck and arm pain, Philadelphia, 1964, FA Davis Co.)

from that of rotator cuff injuries (discussed later in the chapter). Pain is felt about the shoulder and down the upper third of the arm. Pain is usually most severe on abduction of the arm to 90° when the bursa or rotator cuff is impinged on by the acromion, hence the term "impingement syndrome." This condition often coexists with rotator cuff injuries. The treatment involves rest, physical therapy, analgesics, and antiinflammatory agents. Aspiration of calcified material and local injection of corticosteroids are helpful in acute episodes.

OLECRANON BURSITIS. Olecranon bursitis is an inflammatory condition of the bursa overlying the olecranon at the tip of the elbow. The bursa is swollen, usually warm, and tender, although occasionally remarkably asymptomatic. Causes include trauma, infections, and systemic disease such as rheumatoid arthritis and gout. The treatment is by oral antiinflammatory drugs along with aspiration of the bursa and local injection of corticosteroids. Antibiotics are used when appropriate.

BURSITIS IN THE LOWER EXTREMITIES. Bursitis is a common cause of pain in the leg. *Ischial gluteal bursitis* is an inflammation of the bursa that separates the gluteus maximus muscle from the ischial tuberosity. It is exposed and irritated when the patient is in a sitting position, and thus this condition sometimes is called weaver's bottom. Chronic inflammation in this area may be associated with calcification seen on roentgenographic examination. *Trochanteric bursitis* frequently causes pain over the lateral aspect of the thigh with radiation down the leg. Pressure over the greater trochanter will reproduce the patient's pain. *Prepatellar bursitis,* or what was once called housemaid's knee, is a tender, usually warm swelling just over the patella. It most commonly is caused by repeated local trauma, as occurs in carpet layers. *Anserine bursitis,* an inflammation of the sartorius bursa located inferomedial to the patella, frequently is misdiagnosed as an intraarticular pathologic condition. Injection therapy, antiinflammatory agents, and physical therapy as described for subdeltoid bursitis are helpful.

Tendinitis

CALCIFIC TENDINITIS. Calcific tendinitis is marked by tendon inflammation with calcium deposits seen on roentgenogram. The supraspinatus tendon most frequently is involved. Many cases are related to degenerative changes within the tendon from trauma or arthritis, but others have no known predisposing cause. The treatment involves rest, physical therapy, analgesics, antiinflammatory agents, and local injection of corticosteroids.

BICIPITAL TENDINITIS. Bicipital tendinitis is a common condition caused by inflammation of the tendon sheath as it passes through the bicipital groove of the humeral head. Pain is felt at the anterior aspect of the shoulder and is produced by forced supination of the hand with the elbow flexed. Bicipital tendinitis also may be associated with rotator cuff injuries (discussed later in the chapter). The therapy is as for calcific tendinitis.

FLEXOR TENOSYNOVITIS. Flexor tenosynovitis (trigger fingers) refers to inflammation of the flexor tendon sheaths of the hand. Free movement of the tendons within the sheaths is impeded. The patient feels a snapping sensation in the palm when the fingers are flexed and may be unable to reextend the fingers. Deep massage to break adhesions and local injection of corticosteroids are useful. Surgical release of the tendon may be needed.

DeQUERVAIN'S DISEASE. DeQuervain's disease is a tenosynovitis of the extensor pollicis brevis and abductor pollicis longus tendons at the radial wrist below the base of the thumb. It is more common in women and may be related to trauma, although the cause usually is unknown. The treatment is with antiinflammatory drugs, injections, splinting, and occasionally surgical tendon release.

LATERAL EPICONDYLITIS. "Tennis elbow" is the common term for inflammation of the wrist extensor tendons at their origins on the lateral epicondyle. The condition is induced by forceful wrist extensions. It is often seen in tennis players, although any activity requiring repetitive wrist extension may cause it. Similarly, pain at the medial epicondyle of the elbow may be related to repetitive forceful wrist flexions. The treatment for both includes avoiding activities that exacerbate the pain until the inflammation subsides, splinting, local application of heat, antiinflammatory drugs, and local corticosteroid injections. Exercise to strengthen the forearm extensor and flexor muscles is helpful in preventing recurrence.

Miscellaneous nonarticular syndromes
DISORDERS OF THE HEAD AND NECK

Tension headache and cervical tension state. The most common cause of cephalic pain is the common tension headache. The pain is described as a tight or pressurelike sensation, usually bilateral, localizing in the frontal or occipital-nuchal area. It can be unrelenting, lasting several days, and is noted even when the patient wakes briefly during the night.

The causes are numerous. All tend to produce prolonged voluntary or involuntary spasm of the cranial and cervical musculature. Anxiety and chronic tension states are frequent culprits. Poor posture, osteoarthritis of the cervical spine with intervertebral disc degeneration or herniation, spur formation, and apophyseal joint disease all may play a role by inducing secondary muscle spasm or nerve root irritation. Intracranial lesions, visual problems, severe hypertension, and metabolic and other disorders also must be considered.

Temporomandibular joint syndrome (Costen's syndrome). Pain in the area of the temporomandibular joint can be caused by abnormal joint mechanics with secondary muscle strain and spasm or actual damage within the joint. Patients often complain of a clicking sensation on opening the mouth and pain radiating into the scalp. Crepitation and local muscle tenderness often are elicited. The treatment consists of alleviating the underlying condition, exercises to help coordinate joint motion, intraarticular injections, reassurance, and, infrequently, surgical correction.

DISORDERS OF THE SHOULDER, UPPER ARM, AND CHEST

Reflex sympathetic dystrophy (shoulder-hand syndrome). In reflex sympathetic dystrophy, also known as causalgia, the shoulder is painful and motion is limited. The extremity may be edematous, cool, and tender. Patients complain of painful paresthesias. Causative factors include fracture, nerve injury, cerebrovascular accident, heart attack, cervical osteoarthritis, and some drugs. In one third of patients the syndrome develops without a known cause. Most of those affected are over 50 years of age. This syndrome can affect the legs. Without treatment the shoulder and hand become stiff, atrophied, and contracted. Roentgenograms may show patchy demineralization. Once this syndrome is recognized, it should be treated promptly. Physical therapy with remobilization exercises and local application of heat is extremely helpful. Orally administered or locally injected corticosteroids and nerve blocks also may be used.

Costochondritis or Tietze's syndrome. Costochondritis, or Tietze's syndrome, is a painful nodular tenderness at the costochondral junctions of the anterior ribs that is worsened by pressure or motion of the chest. It can involve any of the costochondral junctions, but most frequently the second and third are affected. Local inflammatory signs such as redness or heat are rare. Swelling is caused by cartilaginous hypertrophy and can be palpated easily. The cause is unknown, but local trauma may play a role. The treatment first includes reassurance that the pain is not cardiac in origin, then local application of heat, oral administration of antiinflammatory or analgesic drugs, and if necessary, local injections of anesthetics or corticosteroids.

Intercostal neuritis and *intercostal myalgia* are additional common causes of anterior chest discomfort.

Thoracic outlet syndromes. The term "thoracic outlet syndromes" is used to describe several neurovascular syndromes that produce symptoms in the shoulder and upper arm. The thoracic outlet is the region through which the neurovascular supply of the arm leaves the neck and thorax to enter the axilla. It represents an area of narrowed and fixed passages, and thus the exiting structures are subject to compression. The symptoms are variable and intermittent and may be felt as a burning or ache associated with numbness and paresthesia in the shoulder and down the arm into the fingers. The physical examination may show weakness or muscle atrophy. Depending on the structures involved, neural or vascular, there may be diminished sensation or changes in color and temperature. Raynaud's phenomenon and edema in the involved extremities also may be found.

The *scalenus anticus syndrome* is caused by a change from normal in the size, shape, or insertion of the scalenus anticus muscle (Fig. 32-5). Spasm may be a contributing cause. Compression of the subclavian artery or vein and the brachial plexus can occur between the muscle and first rib. Pain radiates into the arm and hand, usually on the ulnar side. The symptoms depend on relative neural, arterial, or venous impairment. Procedures useful in making the diagnosis include applying direct pressure to the muscle or using the Adson maneuver, which is performed by palpating the radial pulse on the side of involvement while the patient takes a deep breath, holds it, and extends and turns the head to the involved side. In positive test results the pulse is lost and the patient experiences a reproduction of the symptoms. This test is useful but not diagnostic. A systolic bruit can be heard below the midclavicle during the maneuver in some patients.

Cervical ribs, which rise from the seventh cervical vertebra, are present in less than 1% of the population. The symptoms are caused by compression of neurovascular structures between the rib and the scalenus anticus muscle. The diagnosis is supported by roentgenographic findings.

The *costoclavicular syndrome* results from compression of the vein, artery, and nerve between the clavicle and first rib when the shoulders are braced backward and downward. As in the scalenus anticus syndrome, the radial pulse may be decreased and a subclavian bruit may be heard. Backpackers whose backpack straps place excessive weight on the shoulders can have this syndrome.

The *hyperabduction* or *pectoralis minor syndrome* results from neurovascular compression between the pectoralis minor muscle, coracoid process, clavicle, and first rib. The symptoms are brought in by abducting and externally rotating the arms above the head. This can occur during sleep when the arms are folded under the head or as an occupational hazard in auto mechanics, painters, and ballet dancers.

Therapy of the thoracic outlet syndromes is directed at relieving the obstruction. If muscle spasm is present, deep heat as by ultrasound or local anesthetic injection can be tried. Exercises are helpful, but persistent symptoms may indicate the need for surgical resection of the first rib or scalenus anticus muscle.

Rotator cuff injury. The *rotator cuff* at the shoulder represents a conjoining of the tendons from the supraspinatus, infraspinatus, teres minor, and subscapularis muscles. Tears of the rotator cuff are common, especially on the dominant side. The lesions are divided into partial and complete tears. Both

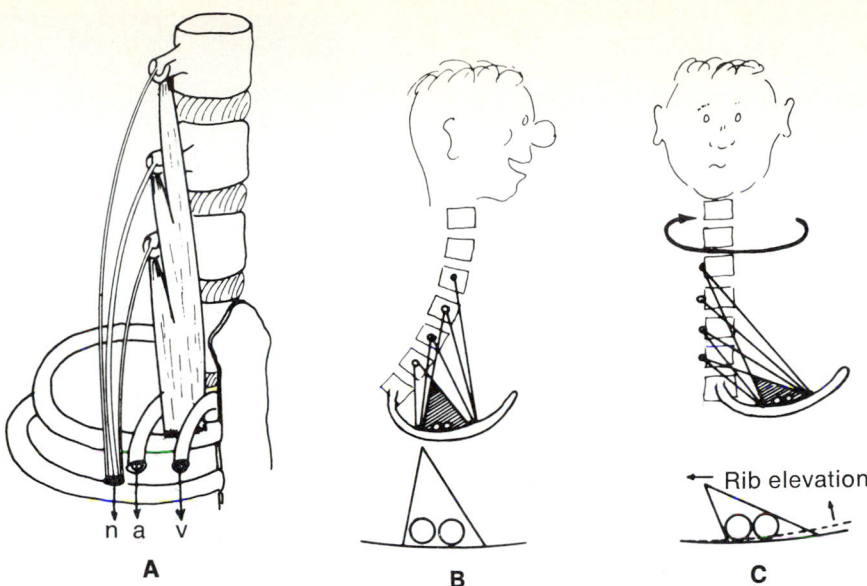

Fig. 32-5 **A,** Scalenus anticus syndrome. *n,* Brachial plexus; *a,* subclavian artery; *v,* subclavian vein. Scalenus anterior muscle lies between subclavian artery and vein. **B** and **C,** Rotating head and neck can place pressure on nerve, artery, or vein. Additionally, rib elevation as occurs by scalene action in deep inspiration can further compress neurovascular bundle. (From Cailliet R: Neck and arm pain, Philadelphia, 1964, FA Davis Co.)

may produce acute pain and inability to fully abduct the arms, but patients with complete tears are demonstrably weak on abduction even when the pain is controlled. The treatment includes rest, physical therapy, analgesics, and antiinflammatory drugs. Exercise is important once the inflammation has subsided. Surgery may be indicated for some complete tears.

Adhesive capsulitis. Adhesive capsulitis or *frozen shoulder* refers to shoulder pain that follows immobilization resulting from a fracture, wearing a cast, or other conditions facilitating disuse. The treatment is directed at remobilizing the shoulder through exercises that stretch the shoulder capsule. Intracapsular corticosteroid-anesthetic injections and antiinflammatory drugs may be needed.

DISORDERS OF THE ELBOW, WRIST, AND HAND
Dupuytren's contracture. Dupuytren's contracture refers to a tightening and contracture of the palmar fascia. The cause is unknown. The condition is more common in men past the fourth decade and can affect the plantar fascia. Occasionally it has been associated with diseases such as diabetes mellitus and alcoholism. The fourth and fifth fingers are particularly affected and may become permanently flexed into the palm. The treatment for advanced contracture is surgery.

Synovial cysts. Synovial cysts or *ganglia* are cystic swellings containing a thick mucinous material that are found along tendon sheaths or joint capsules. They are especially common at the dorsum of the wrist, are usually slow growing, and are not painful. Simple aspiration of the cyst and injection of corticosteroids may be effective, although some require excision.

DISORDERS OF THE BACK AND LEGS
Chronic low back pain. Back pain affects more than 10% of the population. It may be acute or chronic; often it is related to low back strain or injury. More than 85% of cases are related to the soft tissues rather than to arthritis, discogenic disease, tumors, fractures, or infections. Low back pain may radiate to the buttocks and thighs without radiculopathy. Physical ex-

amination shows diffuse or localized tenderness and muscle spasm of the lower back. An index of suspicion for other diseases must be held for patients with severe intractable pain (especially at night), with pain radiation to the legs with neurologic findings, or who appear systematically ill. Treatment of nonspecific low back pain consists of initial bed rest, physical therapy, antiinflammatory drugs, and injection of tripper points.

Fibrofatty nodules. Fibrofatty nodules may occur in subcutaneous tissue along the iliac crest and over the sacroiliac joints. They appear to be herniated adipose tissue and can be very tender. Biopsy shows mild cellular infiltration about blood vessels. The treatment is by injection of corticosteroids or surgical excision.

Shin splints. "Shin splints" is the common term for pain felt usually over the distal third of the tibia. Jogging is a common cause. Muscle-strengthening exercises may be helpful in relieving the problem.

DISORDERS OF THE FOOT AND ANKLE
Calcaneal spurs (plantar fasciitis). Calcaneal spurs are common causes of pain in the sole of the foot. Spurs may form at the origin of the plantar fascia as a result of constant strain applied to the calcaneus. These conditions often are traumatic in origin, and athletes frequently are affected. Connective tissue diseases such as ankylosing spondylitis, psoriatic arthritis, and Reiter's syndrome can cause spur formation. The treatment is aimed at reducing local pressure by supplying well-fitted shoes, heel cups, and sometimes strapping. Ultrasound and local injections of corticosteroids are useful.

Heel neuromas. Heel neuromas can form just below the calcaneus and cause a great deal of pain on walking. Orthoses are helpful in alleviating local pressure.

Pes planus. Pes planus, or flat feet, may be associated with an aching discomfort in the lower legs. This condition may be the result of peroneal muscle spasm, improper shoes, overweight, or most commonly a developmental abnormality. It is often corrected by properly fitted shoes.

BIBLIOGRAPHY

Cailliet R: Soft tissue pain and disability, Philadelphia, 1977, FA Davis Co.

Hench PK: Nonarticular rheumatism. In Katz WA, editor, Diagnosis and management of rheumatic diseases, Philadelphia, 1988, JB Lippincott Co.

Moldofsky H and Scarisbrick P: Induction of neurasthenic musculoskeletal pain syndrome by selective sleep stage deprivation, Psychosom Med 38:35, 1976.

Moldofsky H and others: Musculoskeletal symptoms and non-REM sleep disturbance in patients with "fibrositis syndrome" and healthy subjects, Psychosom Med 37:341, 1975.

Norris CW and Eakins K: Head and neck pain: temporomandibular joint syndrome, Laryngoscope 84:1466, 1974.

Simons DG: Muscle pain syndromes. I. Am J Phys Med 54:289, 1975.

Simons, DG: Muscle pain syndromes. II. Am J Phys Med 55:15, 1976.

Wolfe F, Cathey MA, and Kleinheksel SM: Fibrositis (fibromyalgia) in rheumatoid arthritis, J Rheumatol 11:814, 1984.

Yunus M and others: Primary fibromyalgia (fibrositis): clinical study of 50 patients with matched normal controls, Semin Arthritis Rheum 11:151, 1981.

33 · MISCELLANEOUS RHEUMATIC DISORDERS

Warren A. Katz

RELAPSING POLYCHONDRITIS

Relapsing polychondritis is an uncommon disorder characterized by inflammation of cartilage and other tissues such as the joints, ears, nose, and trachea that contain large amounts of proteoglycans. In about one third of the cases the disease may coexist with other rheumatic and immunologic diseases. There may be inflammation of the synovium and eyes, auditory disturbance, cardiovascular abnormalities, and fever. The disease tends to remit for varying periods of time lasting up to several years. Most patients are between 20 and 60 years of age, although infants and the elderly also may be affected.

PATHOGENESIS AND PATHOLOGY. The cause of relapsing polychondritis is unknown; however, the disease is thought to be immunologically mediated because delayed hypersensitivity and antibodies to cartilage have been demonstrated in many patients. Examination of diseased cartilage shows aggregates of plasma cells and lymphocytes. Toluidine blue staining, specifically used for connective tissues, demonstrates a loss of proteoglycans (proteinpolysaccharide), most likely as a result of lysosomal hydrolytic action. With progressive destruction of cartilage, granulation tissue develops but the cartilage does not show evidence of regeneration. Similar changes are noted in the aorta.

CLINICAL MANIFESTATIONS. Usually one or both ears suddenly become inflamed (Fig. 33-1). One of the clinical hallmarks of the disease is thickened, floppy ears. They are red, hot, and swollen, although the noncartilaginous portions such as the lobe are spared. A saddle nose deformity is a sign of septal involvement. Arthralgias, sometimes intense, generally are evident; occasionally overt arthritis is present. Most often, like other aspects of the disease, the arthritis is migratory and intermittently acute. Infrequently the destructive changes are so severe that peripheral arthritis closely resembles rheumatoid arthritis or spinal involvement resembles ankylosing spondylitis. Chest pain may result from costochondritis.

Less often, neck pain caused by laryngotracheitis may be detected. The larynx and trachea are tender. Some patients complain of cough and dyspnea when the cartilaginous tracheal rings collapse. Cartilage destruction in the nose may lead to a saddle deformity.

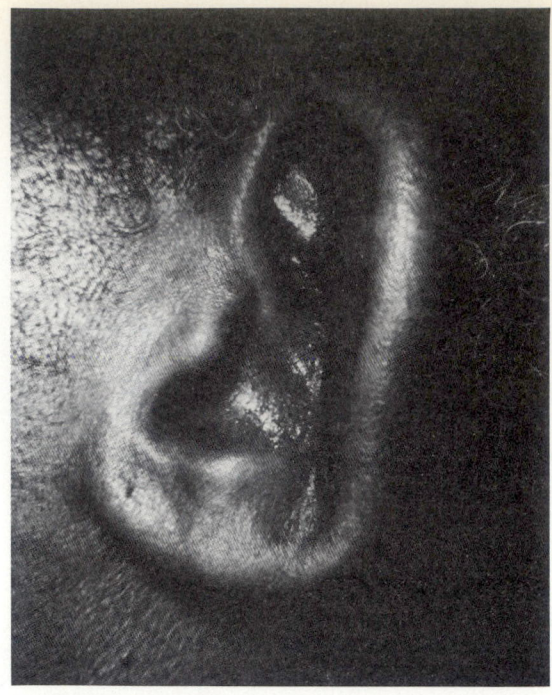

Fig. 33-1 Redness and swelling of entire ear in patient with relapsing polychondritis. (Courtesy of June F. Klinghoffer, M.D.)

Ocular inflammation usually is in the form of episcleritis, but iritis, conjunctivitis, keratitis, keratoconjunctivitis sicca, exophthalmos, ophthalmoplegia, and retinal exudation may be apparent. Narrowing of the external auditory meatus by edematous tissues may cause hearing defects.

About 25% of the patients with relapsing polychondritis exhibit some cardiovascular manifestations, including valvular insufficiency caused by a prolapsed mitral valve or involvement of the aortic ring, aneurysmal dilation of the thoracic or abdominal aorta and its branches (occasionally with dissection and rupture), conduction defects, and cardiomegaly.

LABORATORY FINDINGS. Cartilage biopsy is the most definitive procedure in diagnosing relapsing polychrondritis. When affected, the ear, is the most accessible cartilaginous tissue. Detection of anticartilage antibodies in serum may be helpful, but this is still investigational. The erythrocyte sedimentation rate is elevated during the acute attack and tends to return to normal with remission. Roentgenographic evaluation, especially computed tomography (CT) scanning, may demonstrate collapse of tracheal cartilage and calcification of the ears.

DIAGNOSIS. When relapsing polychondritis appears with two or more cartilaginous sites involved, the diagnosis is relatively easy. When arthritis is extensive, rheumatoid arthritis should be suspected; however, ear, nose, and laryngotracheal cartilaginous involvement are not expected with rheumatoid arthritis. Chondrodynia costosternalis, a variant of Tietze's syndrome, can resemble relapsing polychondritis but tends to be isolated to the anterior aspect of the chest. Wegener's granulomatosis, midline granuloma, sarcoidosis, syphilis, and tuberculosis may cause destructive changes of the nose. Aural calcification may be caused by Addison's disease, hypervitaminosis A, hypoparathyroidism, and trauma. The diagnosis of relapsing polychondritis becomes most difficult when it is associated with other rheumatoid diseases such as systemic lupus erythematosus, rheumatoid arthritis, vasculitis, ankylosing spondylitis, ulcerative colitis with arthritis, Reiter's syndrome, and Sjögren's syndrome.

MANAGEMENT AND PROGNOSIS. The treatment of relapsing polychondritis depends on systemic administration of corticosteroids, usually in relatively large doses (for example, prednisone, 30 to 60 mg/day). The clinical manifestations usually are rapidly suppressed; however, if protracted therapy is needed, corticosteroids should slowly be reduced to a minimum. Nonsteroidal antiinflammatory drugs such as indomethacin have been found useful by some observers and probably will exert a corticosteroid-sparing effect. Immunosuppressive agents such as azathioprine or cyclophosphamide may be helpful when corticosteroids are not.

Tracheostomy, if tracheal collapse is imminent or has recently taken place, and aspiration of secretions may be lifesaving. Replacement of the aortic and mitral valves may be necessary, and aneurysmal dilations of the aorta may require repair. Most deaths result from cardiovascular or pulmonary complications such as infection or vasculitis.

HYPERTROPHIC OSTEOARTHROPATHY

Hypertrophic osteoarthropathy is a syndrome characterized by digital clubbing of the fingers and toes, periostitis of distal long bones, polyarthritis, and evidence of autonomic disturbance such as profuse sweating, flushing, and blanching of the hands and feet. The syndrome usually is associated with pulmonary neoplasms—hence the name hypertrophic pulmonary osteoarthropathy (HPO). However, osteoarthropathy may be associated with other types of malignancies and diseases. In addition, it may be hereditary or may occur without any apparent association.

The cause of HPO is unknown. Postulated mechanisms include autonomic reflex stimulation, excessive arteriolar pulse pressure, toxins or osteoblastic-stimulating agents released by tumors, pulmonary arteriovenous shunts, and growth hormone production by tumors.

The typical pathologic changes are found at the distal ends of the metacarpals, metatarsals, and long bones of the legs and arms. Other bones may be involved with advanced disease. Histologic changes are nonspecific and are characterized by round cell infiltration and periosteal edema. The synovial membrane, articular capsule, and surrounding periarticular structures are similarly affected. In acute cases pannuslike arthritis may result in cartilage destruction, matrix loss, and bony ankylosis.

Secondary hypertrophic osteoarthropathy may be associated with pulmonary neoplasms but also with diseases such as bronchiectasis, pulmonary abscess, cystic fibrosis, biliary cirrhosis, inflammatory bowel disease, sprue syndromes, and cardiac disorders such as subacute bacterial endocarditis, cyanotic heart disease, and atrial myxoma. Thyroacropachy is a form of osteoarthropathy associated with thyroid dysfunction. Aneurysms of the aorta or its branches may cause unilateral clubbing of the fingers and toes, injury to the median nerve, sarcoidosis, and tophaceous gout.

Patients may have an aching pain in the fingers aggravated by dependency of the limb. The clubbing that develops insidiously consists of widening of the distal fingers and toes, much like a drumstick. A loss of the normal 15-degree angle between the dorsal surface of the phalanx and the proximal portion of the nail is an early sign of clubbing. In addition, the base of the nail may be reduced by compression. Arthralgia and synovial thickening may precede the clubbing or pulmonary symptoms. Noninflammatory joint effusions may develop.

Autonomic dysfunction is evidenced by excessive sweating of the hands and feet and warmth of the fingertips. Gynecomastia may occur in some patients. The symptoms of hypertrophic osteoarthropathy may develop insidiously over months to years, but development may be markedly progressive in the presence of a malignancy.

The erythrocyte sedimentation rate may be elevated. Other laboratory tests are unremarkable. Roentgenograms of involved joints may show symmetric subperiosteal new bone formation, typically at the distal diaphyseal regions of long bones.

The treatment of pulmonary hyperosteoarthropathy is directed toward removal of the primary causative factor, if possible. In the interim patients can be treated with salicylates and other nonsteroidal antiinflammatory drugs, local injections of corticosteroids, and if required, systemic administration of corticosteroids. The prognosis of the disease varies with the primary cause.

FIBROUS DYSPLASIA

Fibrous dysplasia is a developmental disease of bone mesenchyme characterized by replacement of bone by cellular fibrous tissue. Histologically, numerous immature bone spicules resembling those of osteitis fibrosa are visible on roentgenographic examination. However, islands of cartilage are seen in fibrous dysplasia but not in osteitis fibrosa.

Although fibrous dysplasia generally is a localized disease, widespread involvement may be seen. Almost all cases involve insidious invasion of bone, often beginning in infancy but not becoming clinically apparent until 5 or 10 years of age, when deformities such as bowing or pathologic fractures develop. At that time roentgenograms indicate the diagnosis. Typically they show cystlike lesions of the metaphysis with an expansion of adjacent cortex. Sometimes the bone architecture is destroyed. Areas of increased density may give way to a ground-glass appearance over a period of years. Serum calcium and phosphorus levels are normal; with severe disease the alkaline phosphatase may be variably elevated.

In some young women fibrous dysplasia is associated with precocious puberty and a brownish pigmentation of the skin (Albright's syndrome). With extensive invasions of the skull, neurologic symptoms may appear because of nerve impingement. Some patients have concomitant osteomalacia, vitamin D–resistant rickets, or myositis ossificans.

There is no specific treatment for fibrous dysplasia. Calcitonin therapy has been tried but needs further investigation. Supportive measures such as splints, braces, and exercises may be suited to individual cases.

AVASCULAR NECROSIS

Avascular necrosis (osteonecrosis) is a consequence of disrupted blood supply to bone (most commonly the femoral head) with resultant pain and disability. Pathologically, necrosis of cancellous subarticular bone is followed by softening of bone and eventual collapse. In a effort to repair the process, new bone formation develops but is outstripped by bone dissolution. Trauma from dislocation, fracture, or occasionally, thermal injury or radiation is the usual cause. Avascular necrosis may be associated with a variety of hematologic disorders, including hypercoagulability states, polycythemia vera, and hemoglobinopathies. Caisson disease is avascular necrosis caused by a nitrogen embolus in divers who fail to decompress themselves adequately. Sometimes avascular necrosis is seen in association with systemic lupus erythematosus, prolonged adrenocorticosteroid therapy, renal transplantation, hepatic cirrhosis, pancreatitis, alcoholism, hyperuricemia, and Gaucher's disease. In many instances, such as avascular necrosis in the femoral head in children (Legg-Calvé-Perthes disease), there is no associated cause. Similar types of osteonecrosis may be noted in other joints.

Pain and dysfunction resulting from involvement of a specific joint are the major complaints. The joint may be swollen. Roentgenograms characteristically show areas of bone resorption adjacent to areas of increased bone density with fragmentation. The surface of the joint becomes flattened, and the hip shows an area of radiolucency just below the joint surface, giving a thin eggshell appearance in early cases. Radioisotopic scanning may show increased uptake over affected joints, sometimes before roentgenographic changes appear.

Management depends on the specific joint involved, the patient's age, and the underlying disorder. In most instances treatment consists of rest, physical therapy, and avoiding overuse or misuse of the joint by means of canes, crutches, and other assistive weight-bearing devices. Analgesic agents and nonsteroidal antiinflammatory drugs may be beneficial. In the early cases, before destructive changes have taken place, intramedullary bone grafting can be performed. Later, however, total joint replacement is the treatment of choice.

HEMARTHROSIS

Hemarthosis, bloody effusion into one or more joints, may be caused by a variety of situations. Most often blunt trauma with or without associated fracture will result in pain, swelling, and, if the blood remains in the joint for a long enough time, even synovitis with heat and redness. Hemophilia, an inherited sex-linked recessive disorder of coagulation resulting from a deficiency of clotting factor VIII or IX, is responsible in some cases. Repeated hemorrhage into the joint causes arthritis of varying severity, depending on the adequacy of treatment, the number of bleeding episodes, and the duration of the blood in the joint. Villous hypertrophy of the synovium similar to that in rheumatoid arthritis may develop because of the irritant effect of blood on the synovium. Cartilage exposed to blood may be destroyed. Furthermore, bleeding within muscles surrounding joints causes "pseudotumors" because of the expanding hematomas. Patients with hemophilia have a great deal of joint pain and dysfunction. The disability may be profound and may result in a wheelchair- or bed-bound existence.

Intraarticular bleeding infrequently follows anticoagulation therapy. Hemorrhagic synovial fluid also may be found in association with pigmented villonodular synovitis, synovioma, neuropathic arthropathy, hemangioma, Ehlers-Danlos syndrome, and scurvy.

Initially, roentgenograms show soft-tissue swelling indicative of the effusion. Later, large cyst formation, irregularity of the joint surface resulting from cartilage destruction, and even complete obliteration of the joint space may be found with repeated hemarthroses.

Management is directed toward aspiration of blood from the joint and elimination of the precipitating factors if possible. Initial mobilization of the involved joints and assistive walking devices also are necessary. In more advanced cases, particularly of hemophilic arthropathy, extensive physical rehabilitation is required and in some instances even total joint arthroplasty is performed. Replacement of clotting factors is a requisite in the mangement of hemophilic arthropathy.

BIBLIOGRAPHY

Arnold WD and Hildpartner MW: Hemophilic arthropathy: current concept of pathogenesis and management, J Bone Joint Surg 59:287, 1977.

Bauer GG: Osteonecrosis of the knee, Clin Orthop 130:210, 1978.

Firat D and Strutzman L: Fibrous dysplasia of the bone, Am J Med 44:421, 1968.

Hammarstein JF and O'Leary J: The features and significance of hypertrophic osteoarthropathy, Arch Intern Med 99:431, 1957.

McAdam LP and others: Relapsing polychondritis: prospective study of 23 patients and a review of the literature, Medicine 55:193, 1976.

Michet DJ and others: Relapsing polychondritis—survival and predictive role of early disease manifestations, Ann Intern Med 104:74, 1986.

Schumacher HR: Articular manifestations of hypertrophic osteoarthropathy in bronchogenic carcinoma: a clinical and pathologic study, Arthritis Rheum 19:629, 1976.

34 · FIBROSING SYNDROMES

Margaret Trexler Hessen *and* **Jerome A. Boscia**

The fibrosing syndromes are a group of rare disorders characterized by anatomic areas of chronic low-grade inflammatory processes progressing to scar tissue, which causes clinical manifestations by encasing, constricting, and limiting the movement of nearby structures. Usually these syndromes are reported as separate disease entities and are either idiopathic or caused by an underlying insult. Occasionally two or more of these conditions have been observed in the same individual, suggesting a common process with multiple-system involvement, which has been termed multifocal fibrosclerosis.

Retroperitoneal fibrosis is idiopatic in about 70% of the cases. Another 20% are associated with methysergide therapy or malignancy. The disorder most commonly affects men in their sixth decade who have low back pain and may develop obstructive uropathy. An intravenous pyelogram reveals hydroureteronephrosis and medial displacement of the ureters. Laparotomy usually is indicated to relieve ureteral obstruction by ureterolysis and to exclude malignancy. Steroid therapy is controversial as an adjuvant to surgery, but it is worthwhile for patients who are not surgical candidates or who have recurrences. The prognosis is good if there is no associated malignancy.

Fibrosing mediastinitis usually is a result of granulomatous disease, particularly histoplasmosis, but it may be idiopathic. The clinical manifestations include cough, wheezing, and hemoptysis resulting from bronchial involvement. Obstruction of the superior vena cava usually progresses slowly, allowing collateral circulation to develop and therefore causing minimal morbidity and mortality. Mediastinoscopy or mediastinotomy may be required to establish the diagnosis and exclude malignancy. Antibiotic therapy probably is indicated for any underlying infectious process, but has had only limited success. Corticosteroids may also be helpful, but their use in this setting has not been well evaluated. Surgical therapy is difficult and hazardous.

Sclerosing cholangitis may be associated with ulcerative colitis, but usually the cause is unknown. Patients have jaundice, pruritus, and occasionally right upper quadrant discomfort. Liver function tests are compatible with extrahepatic biliary tract obstruction. Endoscopic retrograde cholangiography usually reveals the lesion, and laparotomy confirms the diagnosis and excludes malignancy. Prolonged T-tube or internal biliary tract drainage appears palliative. Liver transplantation has been successful in some cases and may become the treatment of choice. Steroids rarely seem useful. The prognosis is determined by the development of secondary biliary cirrhosis and its complications.

Practolol peritonitis is fibrotic encasement of the small intestine caused by the β-adrenergic blocking drug practolol. The disease is manifested by small bowel obstruction, for which surgery is indicated. *Riedel's thyroiditis* is a fibrotic process of the thyroid and surrounding structures. Surgery is required to exclude malignancy and may be necessary to relieve pressure symptoms. Other fibrosing lesions include *Peyronie's disease,* which affects the corpora cavernosa of the penis, and *pseudotumor of the orbit,* which causes exophthalmos and must be differentiated from malignancy.

BIBLIOGRAPHY

Alberti-Flor JJ, Avant GR, and Dunn GD: Primary sclerosing cholangitis, South Med J 78:173, 1985.

Dines DE and others: Mediastinal granuloma and fibrosing mediastinitis, Chest 75:320, 1979.

Srinivas V and Dow D: Retroperitoneal fibrosis, Can J Surg 27:111, 1984.

Dental correlations

RHEUMATOID ARTHRITIS
Martin S. Greenberg

Involvement of the temporomandibular joint (TMJ) in rheumatoid arthritis results from granulomatous involvement of the articular surface of the synovial membrane leading to destruction of the underlying bone. The literature is inconsistent regarding the incidence of TMJ involvement in patients with rheumatoid arthritis because of the varied criteria used by investigators to diagnose arthritis of the joint. Most patients with rheumatoid arthritis have involvement of the temporomandibular joint sometime during the course of their disease, but only a small percentage of these patients will experience permanent, serious disability. A recent study analyzed 50 adults both clinically and roentgenographically for TMJ involvement. Thirty-one of these patients had symptoms of TMJ disease, with 21 having positive roentgenographic signs. Signs of rheumatoid arthritis of the temporomandibular joint appeared in 21 of the 28 patients who had had rheumatoid arthritis for longer than 10 years. In another study TMJ involvement was studied in 62 patients with rheumatoid arthritis. Sixty-one percent of these patients had clinical evidence of TMJ disease, and 79% had roentgenographic changes.

CLINICAL MANIFESTATIONS. Common symptoms of rheumatoid arthritis of the temporomandibular joint include bilateral stiffness, crepitus, tenderness, and swelling over the region of the joints. Pain appears to be present only in the acute phase of the disorder, although destruction often causes permanent limitation of opening. This decrease in mandibular opening, while apparent on clinical examination, is not clinically significant in many cases. Patients with juvenile rheumatoid arthritis appear to have a higher incidence of TMJ involvement. When these changes occur during growth, micrognathia, anteriorly opened bite, and other occlusal changes result. Yet even in juvenile rheumatoid arthritis, severe damage that is dramatically demonstrated on roentgenograms may have no clinical signs. In rare cases ankylosis requiring surgery is seen in patients with juvenile rheumatoid arthritis.

Roentgenographic changes noted include narrowed joint space, flattened condyles, erosions, subchondral cysts, and osteoporosis.

DENTAL MANAGEMENT. Arthritis itself usually does not interfere with dental treatment unless fibrosis or ankylosis of the temporomandibular joint causes a decreased oral opening. One exception occurs in patients with Felty's syndrome. These patients may have neutropenia or thrombocytopenia. When treating a patient with a history of rheumatoid arthritis, the dentist should determine whether the disease process is affecting the hematologic system.

Although arthritis rarely is a contraindication to dental treatment, the medications used to treat arthritis are a more common cause of complications. The dentist treating a patient with a history of arthritis must take a careful drug history. Some patients are taking high doses of aspirin, resulting in disorders of platelet function. Therefore the dentist should consider evaluation of platelet function before extensive surgical procedures. The template bleeding time is a good screening test for platelet function.

Other patients with arthritis may be taking gold salts or phenylbutazone. Either of these medications may cause blood dyscrasias, including neutropenia or aplastic anemia. Patients taking these medications should have a routine complete blood count every other week. Indomethacin or ibuprofen is a rare cause of thrombocytopenia or granulocytopenia.

Since the discovery of nonsteroidal antiinflammatory agents, the use of long-term systemic corticosteroids for the treatment of rheumatoid arthritis has decreased dramatically. However, some patients with severe forms of rheumatoid arthritis that do not respond to nonsteroidal antiinflammatory agents or gold still are treated with systemic corticosteroids. The dentist must consider the possibility of adrenocortical suppression and increased susceptibility to infection.

Treatment depends on the severity of the signs and symptoms observed. Since patients with rheumatoid arthritis rarely have involvement of the temporomandibular joint alone, they usually are given antiinflammatory drugs, which effectively treat all involved joints. During acute exacerbation the patient should be restricted to a soft diet. In the past intermaxillary fixation has been used to manage patients experiencing acute exacerbations. This should be avoided because of the risk of fibrous ankylosis. The patient should begin an exercise program as soon as possible after the acute symptoms subside. Intraarticular steroids have been used successfully to relieve severe pain, but this therapy should be employed sparingly, since localized osteoporosis and articular erosion may result, increasing the chance of ankylosis. The dentist should replace missing posterior teeth to decrease stress on the joint, since some evidence indicates that destructive joint changes occur more frequently in edentulous patients.

TMJ surgery should be considered only for patients with severe pain that does not respond to conservative therapy or to restore significant loss of function. Orthognathic surgery also is helpful in cases with secondary occlusal or cosmetic deformity.

BIBLIOGRAPHY

Chalmers IM and Blair GW: Rheumatoid arthritis of the temporomandibular joint, QJ Med 42:369, 1973.

Kent JN, Carlton DM, and Zide ME: Rheumatoid disease and related arthropathies, Oral Surg 61:423, 1986.

Kreutziger KL and Mahan PL: Temporomandibular degenerative joint disease. I. Anatomy, Pathophysiology and clinical description, Oral Surg 40:165, 1975.

Kreutziger KL and Mahan PL: Temporomandibular degenerative joint disease. II. Diagnostic procedure and comprehensive management, Oral Surg 40:297, 1975.

Larheim TA, Haannaes HR, and Ruud AS: Mandibular growth, temporomandibular joint changes and dental occlusion in juvenile rheumatoid arthritis, Scand J Rheumatol 10:225, 1981.

Ogus H: Rheumatoid arthritis of the temporomandibular joint, Br J Oral Surg 12:275, 1975.

Trenwith JA and Beale G: Rheumatoid arthritis in the temporomandibular joint, NZ Dent J 72:195, 1977.

Zide MF, Carlton DM, and Kent JN: Rheumatoid disease and related arthropathies, Oral Surg 61:119, 1986.

PSORIATIC ARTHRITIS OF THE TEMPOROMANDIBULAR JOINT
Martin S. Greenberg

Psoriatic arthritis is a rare cause of TMJ disease. When it occurs, patients have symptoms similar to those seen in rheumatoid arthritis but the pain is most frequently unilateral. Symptoms include pain on opening the jaw, limitation of movement, deviation to the side of the pain, and tenderness directly over the joint. Roentgenographic findings are not specific and are similar to those seen in rheumatoid arthritis, including erosion of the condyle surface, flattening of the condyle, and proliferative changes. Diagnosis is based on arthritis occurring in a patient who has psoriasis and a negative rheumatoid factor. Case reports of psoriatic arthritis of the temporomandibular joint have noted improvement with conservative treatment, including diathermy, physical therapy, exercise, and salicylates. The occlusal abnormalities associated with rheumatoid arthritis do not occur.

BIBLIOGRAPHY

Blair GS: Psoriatic arthritis and the temporomandibular joint, J Dent 4:123, 1976.

Franks AST: Temporomandibular joint arthrosis associated with psoriasis, Oral Surg 19:301, 1965.

Lowry JC: Psoriatic arthritis involving the temporomandibular joint, J Oral Surg 33:206, 1975.

Rasmussen DC and Bakk EM: Psoriatic arthritis of temporomandibular joint, Oral Surg 53:351, 1982.

Sanders B and Halliday R: Psoriasis and rheumatoid arthritis: their relationship in temporomandibular joint ankylosis, J Oral Med 34:4, 1979.

OSTEOARTHRITIS OF THE TEMPOROMANDIBULAR JOINT
Martin S. Greenberg

The most common intracapsular disorder of the temporomandibular joint is degenerative joint disease. The evaluation of the temporomandibular joints from 400 cadavers revealed degenerative changes in 40% of the joints from patients over 40 years of age. These changes, however, usually were seen in individuals who had no history of complaints relative to TMJ disease. Therefore clinicians must be careful when evaluating the cause of facial pain. Degenerative changes in the temporomandibular joint found on roentgenographic examination may be an incidental finding and not responsible for the symptoms. When one considers degenerative joint disease as a cause of pain in the region of the temporomandibular joint, the incidence of the disorder decreases dramatically. In another study 1500 patients with pain around the area of the temporomandibular joint were evaluated: The incidence of degenerative joint disease was found to be only 8%.

Some divide degenerative joint disease into primary and secondary arthritis. Primary arthritis refers to asymptomatic osteoarthritis of unknown cause, whereas secondary osteoarthritis results from trauma, infection, or other forms of stress placed on the joint. Patients with generalized degenerative joint disease rarely have involvement of the temporomandibular joint as an important clinical finding. In one study 39 patients with a diagnosis of primary degenerative joint disease and 44 control patients were evaluated clinically and with circular tomography

of the joint. No significant difference was found in the incidence of TMJ involvement between the two groups, and researchers concluded that primary osteoarthritis does not affect the temporomandibular joint.

CLINICAL MANIFESTATIONS. Major symptoms of degenerative joint disease of the temporomandibular joint include unilateral pain directly over the condyle; decreased range-of-motion of the mandible, particularly limitation of opening, crepitus, and a feeling of stiffness after a period of inactivity. Examination reveals pain on palpation with deviation of the jaw toward the affected side. This is in contrast to myofascial pain dysfunction syndrome, in which the jaw deviates to the side opposite the pain because of spasm of the lateral pterygoid muscle.

Roentgenographic findings in osteoarthritis include loss of lamina dura of the condyle, particularly at the point of articular contact, narrowing of the joint space, irregular joint space, flattening of the articular surface, osteophyte formation, marginal lipping, and so-called elys cysts. In distinguishing roentgenographic changes found in degenerative joint disease from those changes noted in rheumatoid arthritis, one researcher noted that in degenerative joint disease degenerative changes begin at the center of the condyle, causing flattening, whereas in rheumatoid arthritis the joint destruction begins in the periphery, causing a spike.

DENTAL MANAGEMENT. Degenerative joint diseases of the temporomandibular joint can be managed conservatively in most cases. Toller noted a significant improvement of many cases after 9 months and also noted a burning out of many cases by the end of 1 year. It seems prudent to manage a patient conservatively for a year before considering surgery. Conservative management includes soft diet, treatment of secondary myofascial pain dysfunction syndrome, and use of nonsteroidal antiinflammatory drugs. Intraarticular steroids can be used once a year during acute episodes, but repeated injections may cause degenerative bony changes. Ankylosis is rare in degenerative joint disease, but in some cases the pain and disability are so severe that surgery may be indicated. In the case of localized osteophyte formation in areas easily accessible to surgery, shaving of the condyle may help to relieve the symptoms. In other cases in which involvement is more generalized, a high condylotomy should be performed.

BIBLIOGRAPHY

Blackwood HJJ: Arthritis of the mandibular joint, Br Dent J 115:317, 1963.

Chalmers IM and Blair GS: Is the temporomandibular joint involved in primary osteoarthrosis? Oral Surg 38:75, 1974.

Hecker R and others: Symptomatic osteoarthritis of the temporomandibular joint: report of a case, J Oral Surg 33:780, 1975.

Kopp S: Subjective symptoms in temporomandibular joint osteoarthrosis, Acta Odontol Scand 35:207, 1977.

Nickerson JW, Grafft ML, and Sasima HJ: Bilateral coronoid process enlargement: report of case, J Oral Surg 27:885, 1969.

Rowe NL: Bilateral development hyperplasia of the mandibular coronoid process: report of two cases, Br J Oral Surg 1:90, 1963.

Toller PA: Osteoarthrosis of the mandibular condyle, Br Dent J 134:223, 1973.

SYNOVIAL CHONDROMATOSIS OF THE TEMPOROMANDIBULAR JOINT (CHONDROMETAPLASIA)
Martin S. Greenberg

Synovial chondromatosis is metaplasia of the synovial membrane resulting in the formation of small foci of hyaline cartilage. In this disorder cartilage develops from the connective in the synovial membrane. Pieces of the cartilage are pinched off and released into the joint space, causing a secondary degenerative joint disease. The most common joint involved with synovial chondromatosis is the knee, but several cases of this disorder in the temporomandibular joint have been reported. In one case a 61-year-old woman had been complaining of swelling and crepitus in the temporomandibular joint region. Initially this swelling was confused with a parotid tumor. Roentgenograms showed calcified nodules in the joint. Several cases have been reported from the Mayo Clinic. The patients ranged in age from 40 to 60 years of age, and women had a higher incidence. Symptoms included pain, limitation of opening, deviation to the affected side, crepitus, and swelling. The presence of swelling helps to distinguish the disorder from degenerative joint disease. Roentgenographic findings include an irregular joint surface and loose calcified cartilage in the region of the joint. In addition, sclerosis of the glenoid fossa and mandibular condyle has been reported. Proper treatment of this disorder is surgical removal of the metaplastic tissue.

BIBLIOGRAPHY

Brooke RI: Secondary osteoarthrosis (osteoarthritis) of the temporomandibular joint, Dent J 43:325, 1977.

Guralnick W and others: Temporomandibular joint afflictions, N Engl J Med 298:1263, 1978.

Marbach JJ: Arthritis of the temporomandibular joints and facial pain, Bull Rheum Dis 27:918, 1976.

Miller AS, Harwick RD, and Daley DJ: Temporomandibular joint synovial chondromatosis: report of case, J Oral Surg 36:467, 1978.

Noyek AM and others: The radiologic findings in synovial chondromatosis of the temporomandibular joint. J Otolaryngol 6:45, 1977.

Ronald JB, Keller EE, and Welland JL: Synovial chondromatosis of the temporomandibular joint, J Oral Surg 36:13, 1978.

Rosen PS and others: Synovial chondromatosis affecting the temporomandibular joint: case report and literature review, Arthritis Rheum 20:736, 1977.

SEPTIC ARTHRITIS OF THE TEMPOROMANDIBULAR JOINT
Martin S. Greenberg

Septic arthritis of the temporomandibular joint most commonly results from blood-borne bacterial infection but also may result from trauma directly to the joint or extension of infection from adjacent sites such as the middle ear, maxillary molars, and parotid gland. Gonococci cause most cases of septic arthritis of the temporomandibular joint. Other bacterial infections that have been reported include those with streptococci, staphylococci, and pneumococci. Cases have been reported of temporomandibular joint arthritis resulting from infection with viruses, particularly measles and influenza.

CLINICAL MANIFESTATIONS. Symptoms of septic arthritis of the temporomandibular joint include severe pain on movement and an inability to occlude the teeth because of infection in the joint space. Examination reveals redness and swelling in the region of the involved joint. Large, tender cervical nodes frequently are present on the side of the infection. This helps to distinguish septic arthritis from more common types of temporomandibular joint disorders. In some cases the swelling may be fluctuent and extend well beyond the region of the joint. Septic arthritis of the temporomandibular joint may result in serious sequelae, including ankylosis or involvement of growth centers in children, resulting in facial asymmetry. In a review of 185 cases of ankylosis of the temporomandibular joint, 73 of the 185 cases resulted from infection. The most common sites of origin of the infections were the middle ear, teeth, and hematologic spread of gonorrhea. Evaluation of patients with suspected septic arthritis must include an evaluation for signs and symptoms of gonorrhea such as purulent urethral discharge or dysuria. The affected temporomandibular joint should be aspirated and fluid gram stained and cultured. If gram-negative diplococci are seen in the Gram stain or clinical symptoms and signs indicate the possibility of gonorrhea, cultures for *Neisseria gonorrhoeae* should be obtained on special media and placed in an atmosphere containing carbon dioxide.

DENTAL MANAGEMENT. Treatment consists of surgical drainage and appropriate antibiotic coverage. Occasionally immobilization may be temporarily performed during the acute stage when severe pain is present, but physical therapy should be started as soon as the acute symptoms subside. Surgical management of the ankylosis may be necessary.

BIBLIOGRAPHY

Bradley P: Actinomycosis of the temporomandibular joint, Br J Oral Surg 9:54, 1971.

Chue PW: Gonococcal arthritis of the temporomandibular joint, Oral Surg 39:592, 1975.

Keffer CS and Spink WW: Gonococcal arthritis: pathogenesis, mechanism of recovery and treatment, JAMA 109:1448, 1937.

Seymoor RA and Summersgill GB: *Haemophilus influenzae* pyarthrosis in a young adult with subsequent temporomandibular joint involvement, Br J Oral Surg 20:260, 1982.

Shapiro L and Gorlin RJ: Disorders of the temporomandibular joint. In Gorlin RJ and Goldman HM, editors: Thoma's oral pathology, vol 2, St. Louis, 1970, The CV Mosby Co.

Winters SE: Staphylococcus infection of the temporomandibular joint, Oral Surg 8:148, 1955.

GOUT AND PSEUDOGOUT OF THE TEMPOROMANDIBULAR JOINT
Martin S. Greenberg

Reports of gouty arthritis involving the temporomandibular joint have been rare in the American and European literature. Some authors have suggested that gout does not affect the temporomandibular joint. Three cases have been reported of pain in the TMJ region occurring during periods of hyperuricemia. The pain resolved with antigout medications, but no attempt was made to confirm the diagnosis by aspirating monosodium urate crystals from the synovial fluid of the temporomandibular joint. It has been suggested that clinicians should suspect gouty arthritis as a cause of TMJ pain in Filipinos, Chinese, and Japanese, who are said to be susceptible to this condition.

Pseudogout, which is more accurately called calcium pyrophosphate dihydrate (CPPD) arthropathy, is caused by deposition of CPPD crystals in the synovial membranes and joint cartilages. Accurate diagnosis is made by identification of CPPD crystals in synovial fluid using roentgenographic diffraction. Only a few cases of significant temporomandibular joint involvement have been reported.

BIBLIOGRAPHY

Cacioppi JT, Morrissey JB, and Bacon AS: Condyle destruction concomitant with advanced gout and rheumatoid arthritis, Oral Surg 25:919, 1968.

Chun H: Temporomandibular joint gout, JAMA 226:353, 1973.

DeVos RAI and others: Calcium pyrophosphate dihydrate arthropathy of the temporomandibular joint, Oral Surg 51:497, 1981.

Kleinman HZ and Eubank RL: Gout of the temporomandibular joint, Oral Surg 27:281, 1969.

MYOFASCIAL PAIN DYSFUNCTION SYNDROME OF THE TEMPOROMANDIBULAR JOINT
Martin S. Greenberg

Significant confusion exists in both the medical and dental literatures, as well as among clinicians, regarding temporomandibular joint disorders. Most complaints centering around the area of the temporomandibular joint do not originate from the joint itself but are caused by spasm of the muscles of mastication around the joint. Tenderness, spasm, and dysfunction of these muscles in known as myofascial pain dysfunction syndrome (MPD). Schwartz, in his pioneering work, was the first investigator to distinguish myofascial pain from other causes of discomfort in the region of the temporomandibular joint. Schwartz's work also was important in determining that malocclusion was not the most important cause of this disease. Studies by Laskin and others have confirmed and enlarged on much of Schwartz's work.

Most cases of myofascial pain dysfunction are caused by oral habits such as clenching or grinding the teeth, which can be precipitated by stress. Patients with myofascial pain dysfunction have been shown to have difficulties in interpersonal relationships and social adjustment and increased anxiety levels. These habits may appear in otherwise normal individuals going through periods of stress as well as in patients with severe psychiatric disturbances.

The symptoms of myofascial pain dysfunction are related to the severity of the spasm and the muscles of mastication involved. Common symptoms include pain in the temporal, preauricular, and masseteric regions that is worsened by eating or speaking, limitation of mandibular movement, deviation of the mandible on opening, and clicking or popping sounds in the temporomandibular joint. Patients with spasm of the muscles of mastication also may have pain and spasm of other muscles, most commonly the trapezius and sternocleidomastoid muscles. This has led some clinicians to speculate that back pain is caused by disorders of the temporomandibular joint. No evidence exists, however, to substantiate this theory. It is reasonable to assume that patients with spasm in one group of muscles are more prone to a similar problem in another group.

CLINICAL MANIFESTATIONS. Careful questioning often will reveal a patient with a history of habitual clenching or grinding of the teeth. If the patient clenches during sleep, the most severe pain will be experienced in the morning. If the habit is the result of activities of daily living, the patient may awake asymptomatic but experience increased symptoms as the day progresses.

Examination of patients with suspected myofascial pain dysfunction must include careful palpation of each of the muscles of mastication. The muscles most commonly involved are the lateral pterygoid and masseter muscles. Pain and spasm of the lateral pterygoid muscle often are referred to the region of the joint itself and mistaken for evidence of temporomandibular joint disease. Spasm of the temporalis muscle also may occur either at its attachment on the skull or on the coronoid process, which must be palpated intraorally. Tenderness and spasm of the medial pterygoid muscle are observed less frequently. Other signs include decreased interincisal opening, which can be measured easily on a millimeter ruler, and deviation of the jaw on opening. Deviation is caused by muscle spasm, causing the patient to appear to have an abnormal occlusion. This sign of the disease has led some clinicians to regard occlusion as the primary cause and attempt treatment by adjusting the occlusion either with grinding or with prosthetics.

DENTAL MANAGEMENT. Treatment of myofascial pain dysfunction must be individualized according to the underlying cause and severity of the symptoms. Some patients require nothing more than counseling consisting of an explanation of the cause of their pain and a method to help them decrease the clenching of their teeth.

Patients with acute myospasm can be treated with a combination of nonsteroidal antiinflammatory agents, analgesics, and physical therapy techniques. Use of refrigerant spray on the skin overlying the affected masticatory muscles followed by passive stretching often is effective for interrupting the pain-spasm cycle. Severe cases may be treated with injection of a local anesthetic into the area of spasm followed by passive stretch. If nocturnal bruxism is an important feature of the disorder, temporary use of a mild tranquilizer at bedtime may be helpful in some cases.

Use of an occlusal appliance is helpful in treating chronic myospasm. Much has been written regarding the relative merits of various styles of occlusal appliances. When treating myospasm the clinician should choose an appliance that is unlikely to cause the complication of extrusion or movement of teeth. Coordinating this management with an experienced physical therapist frequently is beneficial. Patients who do not respond to conservative treatment often have difficulty managing anxiety. Muscle relaxation techniques or psychiatric consultation may be necessary for successful management in these cases.

BIBLIOGRAPHY

Cohen ES and Hillis RE: The use of hypnosis in treating the temporomandibular joint pain dysfunction syndrome, Oral Surg 48:193, 1979.

Kotani H and others: Quantitative electromyographic diagnosis of myofascial pain-dysfunction syndrome, J Prosthet Dent 43:450, 1980.

Kydd W: Psychosomatic aspects of temporomandibular joint pain, J Am Dent Assoc 59:31, 1959.

Laskin DM: Etiology of the pain-dysfunction syndrome, J Am Dent Assoc 79:147, 1969.

Schwartz L: Pain associated with the temporomandibular joint, J Am Dent Assoc 51:594, 1955.

Weinberg LA: The etiology, diagnosis, and treatment of temporomandibular joint dysfunction-pain syndrome. II. Differential diagnosis, J Prosthet Dent 43:58, 1980.

Weinberg LA: The etiology, diagnosis, and treatment of temporomandibular joint dysfunction-pain syndrome. III. Treatment, J Prosthet Dent 43:186, 1980.

REITER'S SYNDROME

Philip Springer

CLINICAL MANIFESTATIONS. The reported incidence of oral lesions associated with Reiter's syndrome has been variable. As many as 85% of the patients diagnosed as having Reiter's syndrome may exhibit oral changes. The oral lesions may not be noted consistently, because they are painless.

The oral lesions in Reiter's syndrome may affect the palate, tongue, gingiva, buccal mucosa, lips, tonsillar pillars, and pharynx. Involvement of the buccal mucosa, gingiva, and lips has been described as red, papular lesions measuring 1 mm to 1 cm in diameter and surrounded by a whitish circinate line. Frank ulcerations may develop. The tongue lesions appear similar to geographic tongue and are characterized by areas of superficial erosion. Several small, bright red macules that later blend to form a darker area may be apparent when the palate is affected. Small opaque vesicles and areas of glistening erythema with a granular surface also have been reported as oral manifestations of Reiter's syndrome.

Histologically, these oral lesions exhibit parakeratosis, acanthosis, and elongation of the rete pegs. Intraepithelial microabscesses with a polymorphonuclear leukocyte infiltration may be apparent. A mixed inflammatory cell infiltrate usually is discernible in the connective tissue.

Striking clinical and histopathologic similarities have been noted between the oral lesions seen in Reiter's syndrome and those found in intraoral psoriasis, benign migratory glossitis, and "ectopic geographic tongue" of the buccal mucosa. These lesions have been grouped together and called psoriatiform; however, it is unknown whether these conditions are related.

Erythema multiforme and Behçet's syndrome must be included in the differential diagnosis of the intraoral lesions of Reiter's syndrome. Erythema multiforme is characterized by greater involvement of the lips and by target lesions on the skin. The lesions of Behçet's syndrome are painful aphthous ulcerations. The histocompatibility antigen HLA-B27 has been identified in most patients with Reiter's syndrome.

DENTAL MANAGEMENT. Because they are painless and self-limiting, the oral lesions associated with Reiter's syndrome usually do not require treatment. If the lesions cause significant discomfort, topical analgesic mouth rinses are beneficial. Recent studies have shown that an 8-week regimen of the immunosuppressive drug azathioprine may decrease the symptoms associated with Reiter's syndrome.

BIBLIOGRAPHY

Arnet GF: Reiter's syndrome: report of a case, J Oral Surg 38(5):382, 1976.
Calin A: A placebo controlled crossover study of Azathioprine in Reiter's syndrome, Ann Rheum Dis 45(8):653, 1986.
McClusky OE, Lordon RB, and Arnett FC: HL-A 27 in Reiter's syndrome and psoriatic arthritis: a genetic factor in disease susceptibility and expression, J Rheumatol 1:263, 1974.
Pindborg JJ, Gorlin RJ, and Ashoc-Hansen G: Reiter's syndrome, Oral Surg 16:551, 1963.
Weathers DR and others: Psoriasiform lesions of the oral mucosa (with emphasis on "ectopic geographic tongue"), Oral Surg 37(6):872, 1974.

BEHÇET'S SYNDROME
Martin S. Greenberg

CLINICAL MANIFESTATIONS. Behçet's syndrome is a disease of unknown cause that has been classically described as a triad of oral ulcers, genital ulcers, and inflammatory disease of the eye. Vasculitis is the predominant pathologic lesion, and involvement of several organ systems, including the joints, the blood vessels, and the gastrointestinal tract, have been reported frequently. The incidence of the disease is highest in Japan and the Middle East, but cases have been found worldwide, including in Great Britain and North America.

The involvement of several organ systems has let to confusion regarding the diagnosis of Behçet's syndrome, particularly since no diagnostic laboratory tests exist. To alleviate this confusion, Mason and Barnes have listed the major and minor manifestations of the disease. The major manifestations include oral ulcerations, genital ulcerations, and ocular involvement. Minor manifestations include arthritis, thrombophlebitis, and gastrointestinal lesions. Diagnosis is based on the presence of three major manifestations or two major and two minor manifestations.

The most common site involved in Behçet's syndrome is the oral mucosa, with 90% of the patients reporting recurring oral ulcerations. The severity of the oral involvement varies considerably from patient to patient and may resemble the small lesions of recurring aphthous stomatitis or the large, scarring, disabling lesions of major aphthous ulcers (Sutton's disease). The characteristic skin lesion is erythema nodosum or a pustule that may occur spontaneously or be precipitated by trauma. One diagnostic feature of the disease is the formation within 1 day of a lesion resembling a delayed hypersensitivity reaction at the site of a needle stick; the lesion is caused by exaggerated dermographia.

Involvement of the eye may take many forms. The lesions may include conjunctivitis or uveitis, involvement of the retinal vessels, or glaucoma. These lesions may be reversible or lead to permanent blindness.

Arthritis, which occurs in more than 50% of patients, most frequently involves the large joints, which clinically appear red and swollen. The arthritis is reversible and rarely leads to permanent disability. Ulcerative colitis may appear as a manifestation of the disease, and involvement of the blood vessels can cause thrombophlebitis, arterial occlusion, aneurysms, or gangrene. A particularly distressing sign of Behçet's syndrome is the involvement of the central nervous system, which can include cranial nerve damage, spinal cord involvement, meningeal and spinal encephalitis leading to paralysis, psychiatric disease, and death. Central nervous system involvement occurs in approximately 25% of patients and has a poor prognosis.

Diagnosis is based on clinical signs. Laboratory testing will demonstrate an elevated erythrocyte sedimentation rate, circulating immune complexes, and an increased serum concentration of Cq.

DENTAL MANAGEMENT. Treatment of Behçet's syndrome depends on the severity of the disease. Minor oral ulcers may be treated with topical or intralesional corticosteroids. Severe disease is most frequently treated with a combination of systemic corticosteroids and immunosuppressive drug therapy. Recent reports regarding the use of colchinine for the treatment of Behçet's syndrome have been encouraging. Colchinine, the commonly used antigout medication, inhibits the function of leukocytes, particularly the adhesiveness, motility, and hemotaxis of polymorphonuclear leukocytes. The best results appear to be on mucosal lesions, with less effect on neurologic, vascular, and gastrointestinal problems.

BIBLIOGRAPHY

Hazen PG and Michel B: Management of necrotizing vasculitis with colchicine, Arch Dermatol 115:1303, 1979.
James DW, Walker JR, and Smith MJH: Abnormal polymorpholeucocyte chemotaxis in Behçet's syndrome, Ann Rheum Dis 38:219, 1979.
Jorizzo JL and others: Behçet's syndrome: immune regulation, circulating immune complexes, neutrophil function, and colchicine therapy, J Am Acad Dermatol 10:205, 1984.
Ketch LL and Buerk CA: Surgical implications of Behçet's disease Arch Surg 115:759, 1980.
Mason RM and Barnes CG: Behçet's syndrome with arthritis, Ann Rheum Dis 28:95, 1969.
Sandler HJ and Randle HW: Use of colchicine in Behçet's syndrome, Cutis 37:344, 1986.

LUPUS ERYTHEMATOSUS
Philip S. Springer

CLINICAL MANIFESTATIONS
Chronic discoid lupus erythematosus. Oral manifestations of chronic discoid lupus erythematosus are apparent in approximately 25% of patients. The buccal mucosa, gingiva, labial mucosa, and vermilion border of the lips are common sites of involvement.

Lip lesions initially are erythematous but gradually become keratotic and scaly. An atrophic, red area or crusted ulcer surrounded by a keratotic border ultimately develops.

The lesion of chronic discoid lupus affecting the oral mucosa typically appears as a central red, slightly depressed atrophic area surrounded by a 2 to 4 mm wide white elevated zone of keratinization. A hyperemic area often is observed encircling the keratotic zone. Unlike lesions that form on the skin and at the vermilion border of the lips, scale formation rarely occurs in lesions of the oral mucosa. The central area may ulcerate, causing the lesion to become painful, especially when eating hot or spicy foods or during toothbrushing. In most cases, however, the lesions remain asymptomatic.

Discoid lupus involvement of the tongue is characterized by atrophy of the papillae and occasional deep fissuring. The palatal and gingival tissues also are commonly affected. Ulcerated areas tend to heal by scar formation.

Lichen planus is clinically and histologically similar to chronic discoid lupus erythematosus (CDLE), and it often is difficult to differentiate between them, especially with early lesions. The most significant differences are the sawtooth configuration of the rete pegs in lichen planus and the pseudo-epitheliomatous hyperplasia alternating with atrophy seen in chronic discoid lupus. Direct and indirect immunofluorescence may be helpful in diagnosing oral lesions of both chronic discoid and systemic lupus erythematosus.

Systemic lupus erythematosus. Three types of oral lesions may be associated with systemic lupus erythematosus (SLE): (1) discoidlike, (2) erythematous, and (3) ulcerative. The typical oral lesion of systemic lupus erythematosus, as in chronic discoid lupus erythematosus, is a central atrophic area surrounded by a keratotic border. These are apparent in 20% to 40% of patients. Increased hyperemia, edema, and peripheral spreading are seen in the oral lesions of systemic as compared to chronic discoid lupus erythematosus. The lesions also have a greater tendency to ulcerate and bleed with the systemic disorder. Lesions may involve the lips, hard palate, buccal mucosa, and tongue. The erythematous and ulcerative oral lesions of SLE are relatively nonspecific and may be difficult to clinically distinguish from the lesions of lichen planus, erythema multiforme, or pemphigus. An increase in oral lesions is observed during exacerbations of the systemic disease.

Other oral manifestations include petechiae, especially evident on the hard palate, and small superficial ulcerations surrounded by a red halo. The petechiae may be attributable to the thrombocytopenia associated with the disease.

Patients with SLE commonly display signs of salivary gland disease, including reduced salivary flow and increased concentrations of sodium, protein, and carbohydrates. Sicca syndrome (Sjögren's syndrome) may be evident in these individuals.

Temporomandibular joint dysfunction, with flattening and erosion of the condyles, has been associated with SLE.

DENTAL MANAGEMENT

Chronic discoid lupus erythematosus. If the oral lesions of chronic discoid lupus erythematosus are painful, they can be treated by topical steroids under an occlusive dressing. Intralesional or systemic administration of steroids also is beneficial. Cryosurgery and conventional surgery can be used when lesions are well demarcated. Patients who have chronic lip lesions should avoid direct sun exposure and use sunscreen. Schiodt has recommended that patients with oral discoid lesions be examined at least yearly, because the onset of ulceration of these lesions may help predict the development of SLE.

Systemic lupus erythematosus. The dental management of patients with systemic lupus erythematosus must take into consideration the systemic complications associated with the disease process and problems attributable to steroid therapy.

Basic laboratory tests can aid the dentist in assessing the severity of systemic involvement. These tests include a complete blood count with differential to determine the extent of hemolytic anemia and leukopenia; a platelet count to determine the possibility of thrombocytopenia; and blood urea nitrogen and creatinine levels to evaluate kidney function.

The leukopenia, the decreased phagocytic ability of leukocytes, and the immunosuppressive action of high-dose systemic steroid therapy cause patients with SLE to be more susceptible to infection. It therefore is advantageous to prophylactically administer antibiotics before an oral surgery procedure. Some clinicians advocate the administration of prophylactic antibiotics to all patients with SLE before any dental procedure that might induce a bacteremia because of the high incidence of valvular lesions (Libman-Sacks endocarditis) in these individuals.

Systemic steroid therapy may lead to adrenal suppression.

To prevent stress crisis, the steroid dosage may need to be supplemented for oral surgery and other stress-producing dental procedures.

Bleeding problems usually are related to a thrombocytopenia. If more than 50,000 platelets/mm^3 are present, routine dental procedures, including extractions, usually can be performed safely. Other problems with hemostasis in SLE can result from abnormal platelet function, acquired von Willebrand's disease, and the presence of antibodies to the coagulation factor proteins.

BIBLIOGRAPHY

Andreasen JO: Oral manifestations in discoid and systemic lupus erythematosus—clinical investigation, Acta Odontol Scand 22(3):295, 1964.

Jonsson R, Bratthall D, and Nyberg G: Histologic and sialochemical findings indicating sicca syndrome in patients with systemic lupus erythematosus, Oral Surg Oral Med Oral Pathol 54(6):635-639, 1982.

Mesa M: Oral discoid lupus erythematosus—a case report and review of the literature, J Periodontol 50(2):90, 1974.

Nisengard RJ and others: Diagnostic importance of immunofluorescence in oral bullous diseases and lupus erythematosus, Oral Surg 40(3):365, 1975.

Samuelson SJ, Friedlander AH, and Swerdloff M: Systemic lupus erythematosus, J Am Dent Assoc 100:553, 1980.

Schiodt M and Pindborg JJ: Histologic differential diagnostic problems for oral discoid lupus erythematosus, Int J Oral Surg 5(5):250, 1976.

Schiodt M: Oral manifestations of lupus erythematosus, Int J Oral Surg 13(2):101, 1984.

M: Oral discoid lupus erythematosus. III. A histopathologic study of sixty-six patients, Oral Surg Oral Med Oral Pathol 57(3):281, 1984.

Schwartz S and Esseltine DW: Post-extraction hemorrhage in a young male patient with systemic lupus erythematosus, Oral Surg Oral Med Oral Pathol 57(3):254, 1984.

Zysset MK and others: Systemic lupus erythematosus. A consideration for antimicrobial prophylaxis, Oral Surg Oral Med Oral Pathol 64(1):30, 1987.

SYSTEMIC SCLEROSIS
Philip S. Springer

CLINICAL MANIFESTATIONS. The most common dental findings in systemic sclerosis are rigidity and thinness of the lips. Besides contributing to the masklike, expressionless appearance of patients with the disease, the circumoral fibrosis causes puckering and pallor when an attempt is made to open the mouth wide. The collagenization may progress to produce a microstomia. The patient's inability to open his mouth may hinder oral hygiene, mastication, speech, and placement of prostheses.

In his study Eversole observed prominent lingual and buccal mucosal crenations and loss of tongue mobility with fibrotic induration in 25% of the patients with systemic sclerosis. The mucous membrane may become ulcerated by the teeth as pressure intensifies. Eversole also noted foci of severe gingival recession caused by fibrous strictures and attached gingiva stripping in patients with advanced disease. Inhibition of the reparative process following trauma to the oral mucosa has been reported. The diffuse hyperpigmentation of the skin commonly seen in systemic sclerosis rarely involves the oral mucous membrane.

A roentgenographic finding that has been classically associated with systemic sclerosis is widening of the periodontal ligament spaces, usually in posterior teeth. This finding, however, appears to be highly variable. One report noted thickening of the periodontal ligament in only 7% of 127 cases, whereas another found it in 37% of 35 patients studied. The investigators in the latter study theorized that the much higher incidence they noted may have resulted from the use of different criteria or the increased severity of the disease process in the patient population they studied. The first study also noted a decrease in the lamina dura of affected teeth, whereas the second usually did not. Teeth in patients with systemic sclerosis tend to remain firm, although these patients showed thickening of the periodontal ligament.

Additional roentgenographic changes that have been reported include resorption of the angle of the mandible, the condyle, and the coronoid process. These osseous changes apparently are related to pressure atrophy or ischemia and are associated with the advanced stages of systemic sclerosis. Pathologic fractures of the mandible may result from progression of the osseous resorption.

Telangiectasias, a common manifestation of several forms of systemic sclerosis, often are found on the lips and in the mouth. They are histologically identical to the lesions of hereditary hemorrhagic telangiectasia. A distinction usually can be made by the additional presence of Raynaud's phenomenon and a lack of family history.

MANAGEMENT. The most common complication encountered in attempting to perform routine dentistry on patients with systemic sclerosis is the lack of access to the oral cavity because of microstomia; therefore an attempt should be made to improve the patient's oral hygiene to prevent oral problems. The inability to open, however, may limit even basic oral cleansing.

Techniques have been devised using a sectional tray technique to permit the taking of impressions for oral prostheses.

Nonsurgical treatment of microstomia includes facial grimacing exercises and oral augmentation. In the latter technique tongue blades are progressively inserted between the teeth to stretch sclerotic facial skin and musculature. A bilateral commissurotomy should be considered when the overall disease process appears controlled and the limitation of opening significantly interferes with mastication, speech, or insertion of oral prostheses.

Practitioners performing surgical procedures should be cognizant of the serious bleeding problem that can occur when oral telangiectasias are inadvertently involved.

BIBLIOGRAPHY

Brown AE: The CRST syndrome (calcinosis, Raynaud's phenomenon, sclerodactly and telangiectasias), Br J Oral Surg 14(2):137, 1976.

Caplan HI and Benny RA: Total osteolysis of the mandibular condyle in progressive systemic sclerosis, Oral Surg 46(3):362, 1978.

Eversole LR, Jacobsen PL, and Stone CE: Oral and gingival changes in systemic sclerosis (scleroderma), J Periodontol 55(3):175, 1984.

Green DL: Scleroderma and its oral manifestation, Oral Surg 15:1312, 1962.

Naylor WP: Oral management of the scleroderma patient, J Am Dent Assoc 105(5):814, 1982.

Naylor WP, Douglass CW, and Mix E: The non-surgical treatment of microstomia in scleroderma: a pilot study, Oral Surg 57(5):508, 1984.

Sanders B, McKelvy B, and Cruickshank G: Correction of microstomia secondary to sclerodermatomyositis, J Oral Surg 35:57, 1977.

Seifert MH, Stergerwald JC, and Cliff MM: Bone resorption of the mandible in progressive systemic sclerosis, Arthritis Rheum 18:507, 1975.

Smith DB: Scleroderma: its oral manifestations, Oral Surg 11:865, 1958.

Stafne EC and Austin LT: A characteristic dental finding in acrosclerosis and diffuse scleroderma, Am J Orthod 30:25, 1944.

Uthman AA, Winkler S, and Scott DJ: The scleroderma patient, J Oral Med 33(2):65, 1978.

White SC and others: Oral radiographic changes in patients with progressive systemic sclerosis, J Am Dent Assoc 94:1178, 1977.

POLYMYOSITIS-DERMATOMYOSITIS
Philip S. Springer

CLINICAL MANIFESTATIONS. In one study of patients with polymyositis-dermatomyositis, 55% had signs or symptoms associated with the head and neck. These signs include facial rash or pigmentary changes or both, facial swelling, dysphagia, oral lesions, vocal changes, and facial weakness. Weakness of the posterior pharyngeal muscles and tongue may cause dysphagia, dysphonia, and occasionally dysarthria. In addition, weakness of facial muscles and muscles of mastication can cause difficulty in chewing.

The periorbital region is involved most frequently when facial swelling occurs in polymyositis-dermatomyositis. Swelling of the lips also may be noted. These areas of swelling may mimic dental and sinus infections and need to be distinguished from them.

A generalized stomatitis, including a gingivitis and glossitis, has been observed in dermatomyositis in approximately one third of patients. A diffuse erythema of the mucous membranes with occasional telangiectasias has been reported. The tongue sometimes appears denuded of papillae. Vesicles surrounded by an erythematous halo, similar to aphthous ulcerations, may be seen involving the palate, gingiva, and tongue. The lips and palate may be affected by erosive areas that heal by scar formation. Eating and swallowing may become increasingly difficult in dermatomyositis when the painful stomatitis occurs in patients already complaining of dysphagia related to muscle weakness.

Delay in exfoliation of the primary dentition and eruption of the permanent teeth, caused by a lack of primary root resorption, has been reported in children with dermatomyositis. Children also are more likely to show manifestations of soft tissue calcification, including the tongue, floor of the mouth, salivary glands, buccal mucosa, and muscles of mastication.

DENTAL MANAGEMENT. Adrenal suppression secondary to steroid therapy is the primary complication that must be considered before treating a patient with dermatomyositis. Augmentation of the steroid dose may be required for stress-producing oral surgery and dental procedures. An increased risk of infection also must be given attention in cases in which cytotoxic agents such as methotrexate are administered. In children with dermatomyositis, primary teeth may need to be extracted to permit eruption of the permanent dentition.

BIBLIOGRAPHY

Cunningham JD Jr and Lowry LD: Head and neck manifestations of dermatomyositis-polymyositis, Otolaryngol Head Neck Surg 93(5):673, 1985.

Fridrich KL, Taylor RW, and Olson RAJ: Dermatomyositis presenting with Ludwig's angina, Oral Surg Oral Med Oral Pathol 63(1):21, 1987.

Hamlin C and Shelton JE: Management of oral findings in a child with an advanced case of dermatomyositis: clinical report, Pediatr Dent 6(1):46, 1984.

Keil H: The manifestations in the skin and mucous membranes in dermatomyositis with special reference to the differential diagnosis from systemic lupus erythematosus, Ann Intern Med 16:828, 1942.

Metheny JA: Dermatomyositis: a vocal and swallowing disease entity, Laryngoscope 88:147, 1978.

Pearson DM and Bohan A: The spectrum of polymyositis and dermatomyositis, Med Clin North Am 61(2):439, 1977.

WEGENER'S GRANULOMATOSIS
Philip S. Springer

The oral lesions commonly associated with Wegener's granulomatosis may be the initial manifestation of the disorder before several organs become involved. The most characteristic oral complication is a hyperplastic gingivitis often referred to as "strawberry gums." The gingiva appears red to purplish in color with a granular surface texture. Biopsy of these gingival lesions reveals pseudoepitheliomatous hyperplasia with hemorrhage, necrosis, and acute and chronic inflammation of subepithelial tissues. The gingivitis tends to diminish following treatment for the disorder with cyclophosphamide in responsive patients.

Extensive inflammation and ulceration of the oral mucosa also have been associated with Wegener's granulomatosis. Alveolar bone loss, with tooth mobility and failure of extraction sites to heal, has been reported.

The dentist may play an important role in the early detection of Wegener's granulomatosis by associating the oral manifestations with the systemic changes of mild anemia, leukocytosis, thrombocytosis, and elevated erythrocyte sedimentation rate.

BIBLIOGRAPHY

Handlers JP and others: Oral features of Wegener's granulomatosis, Arch Otolaryngol 111(4):267, 1985.

Hansen LS and others: Limited Wegener's granulomatosis, Oral Surg Oral Med Oral Pathol 60(5):524, 1985.

Horan RF and others: Recent onset of gingival enlargement, Arch Dermatol 122(12):1435, 1438, 1986.

Israelson H, Binnie WH, and Hurt WC: The hyperplastic gingivitis of Wegener's granulomatosis, J Periodontol 52(2):81, 1981.

Kakehasi S and others: Wegener's granulomatosis—report of a case involving the gingiva, Oral Surg 19:120, 1965.

Raustia AM, Harmainen HI, and Knuuttila MLE: Ultrastructural findings and clinical follow-up of "strawberry gums" in Wegener's granulomatosis, J Oral Pathol 14(7):581, 1985.

Scoth J and Finch LD: Wegener's granulomatosis presenting as gingivitis: review of the clinical and pathologic features and report of a case, Oral Surg 34:920, 1972.

MIDLINE GRANULOMA

Philip S. Springer

The term "midline nonhealing granuloma" has been used to describe collectively certain destructive lesions of the upper airway. These include idiopathic midline granuloma, polymorphic reticulosis, and extranodal lymphoma. It currently is believed that these lesions actually may be different stages of the same malignant process. Idiopathic midline granuloma is characterized by nonspecific acute and chronic inflammation and necrosis. It is clinically similar to the upper airway lymphoproliferative neoplasms but histologically appears to be inflammatory in nature with no recognizable malignant cell type. A novel T-cell phenotype commonly found in peripheral T-cell lymphoma recently has been identified in some cases of idiopathic midline granuloma.

The oral presentation of midline granuloma has been described as a progressive ulceration and sloughing of soft tissue with osseous destruction. A fetid odor is characteristic, and pain usually is not a major complaint. The nonhealing granulomatosis frequently involves the hard palate as the lesion spreads from the maxillary sinus or floor of the nose.

Cases of midline granuloma have been first recognized following tooth extraction. This may be related to an apparent acceleration of the lesion's destructive process after trauma or surgery.

Untreated midline granuloma is fatal as a result of infection or hemorrhage or both. Chemotherapy, steroids, and surgery usually are ineffective and may be detrimental. Radiation therapy has provided the most successful treatment for the disorder.

BIBLIOGRAPHY

Batsakes JG: Wegener's granulomatosis and midline (nonhealing) granuloma, Head Neck Surg 1:213, 1979.

Fechner RE and Lamppin DW: Midline malignant reticulosis: a clinicopathologic entity, Arch Otolaryngol 95:467, 1972.

Jarrett JE and Lehman RH: Lethal midline granuloma: a review of the literature, Rocky Mt Med J 68:40, 1971.

Kornblut AD and Fanci AS: Idiopathic midline granuloma, Otolaryngol Clin North Am 15(3):685, 1982.

Lippmann SM, Grogan TM, and Spier DM: Lethal midline granuloma with a novel T-cell phenotype as found in peripheral T-cell lymphoma, Cancer 59(5):936, 1987.

MacKinnon DM: Lethal midline granuloma of the face and larynx, J Laryngol Otol 84:1193, 1970.

Nelson JF and others: Midline nonhealing granuloma, Oral Surg Oral Med Oral Pathol 58(5):554, 1984.

SARCOIDOSIS

Philip S. Springer

CLINICAL MANIFESTATIONS. The most commonly reported involvement of structures associated with the oral cavity in patients with sarcoidosis are asymptomatic cervical lymphadenopathy and parotid gland enlargement. In a postmortem study of 31 confirmed cases of sarcoidosis, cervical lymphadenopathy was evident in 78% and unilateral or bilateral parotid gland swelling existed in 35% of the subjects.

Parotid gland enlargement, uveitis, seventh nerve palsy, malaise, and fever delineate the clinical picture of sarcoidosis associated with Heerfordt's syndrome. The granulomatous lesions in salivary glands may lead to xerostomia.

Intraoral sarcoid lesions generally are considered rare. However, some investigators believe that these lesions are not uncommon but that they remain undiagnosed and unreported. The distinction between oral lesions that are simply isolated local sarcoid reactions and those that are associated with systemic sarcoidosis has been stressed by some researchers, who have emphasized that corroborative clinical, roentgenographic, and laboratory studies are required before a diagnosis of systemic sarcoidosis can be made.

The lesions of the gingiva, tongue, and oral mucosa have been described as nodular, papular, ulcerated with elevated margins, plaquelike, or scaly. Involvement of the tongue may lead to gross enlargement, pain, and difficulty in speech and swallowing. Sarcoidosis should be considered in the differential diagnosis when lingual swelling with induration is evident.

Sarcoid involvement of the maxilla and mandible also has been reported. Punched-out radiolucencies have been noted roentgenographically. Increased tooth mobility and failure of extraction sites to heal have been attributed to intrabony sarcoid lesions.

Biopsy of normal-appearing oral tissue as an aid in confirming the diagnosis of sarcoidosis has been recommended. Cahn and his associates performed punch biopsies of normal-appearing palatal tissue. In 10 of the 23 samples they noted the characteristic nodules of sarcoid and in 56% of the cases a degenerative change was noted in the minor salivary glands. Tarpley and coworkers similarly biopsied the normal-appearing mucosal surface of the lower lip and noted changes in the minor salivary glands in three of five samples consistent with sarcoidosis. Fine-needle aspiration biopsies of enlarged salivary glands and cervical lymph nodes have been useful, inexpensive, and rapid techniques for diagnosing head and neck sarcoidosis. Gallium scintigraphy also has been demonstrated to be an effective means of detecting sarcoid involvement of parotid and submandibular glands.

DENTAL MANAGEMENT. Dental management of patients with sarcoidosis usually is unremarkable. Adrenal suppression may need to be assessed in patients being treated with steroids. A saliva substitute or a sialogogue such as pilocarpine may be beneficial in cases of xerostomia related to sarcoid involvement of the salivary glands. Intraoral lesions usually are excised, especially if they interfere with speech, mastication, or deglutition.

BIBLIOGRAPHY

Cahn LR and others: Biopsies of normal appearing palates in patients with known sarcoidosis, Oral Surg 18:342, 1964.

DeLuke DM and Sciubba JJ: Oral manifestations of sarcoidosis: report of a case masquerading as a neoplasm, Oral Surg Oral Med Oral Pathol 59(2):184, 1985.

Frable MS and Frabel WJ: Fine-needle aspiration biopsy: efficacy in the diagnosis of head and neck sarcoidosis, Laryngoscope 94(10):1281, 1984.

Gold RS and Sager E: Oral sarcoidosis: review of the literature, J Oral Surg 34:237, 1976.

Greer RO and Sanger RG: Primary intraoral sarcoidosis, J Oral Surg 35:507, 1977.

Hamner JE and Scofield HJ: Cervical lymphadenopathy and parotid gland swelling in sarcoidosis: a study of 31 cases, J Am Dent Assoc 74(5):1224, 1977.

Hoggins GJ and Allan D: Sarcoidosis of the maxillary region, Oral Surg 28:623, 1969.

Lubat E and Kramer EL: Gallium-67 citrate accumulation in parotid and submandibular glands in sarcoidosis, Clin Nucl Med 10(8):593, 1985.

Macleod RI, Snow MH, and Hawkesford JE: Sarcoidosis of the tongue—a case report, Br J Oral Maxillofac Surg 23(4):243, 1985.

Makus GP and Stoller NH: Rapidly advancing periodontitis in a patient with sarcoidosis. A case report, J Periodontol 54(11):690, 1983.

Orlian AI and Birnbaum M: Intraoral localized sarcoid lesion, Oral Surg 49(4):341, 1980.

Rohatgi PK, Singh R, and Vieras F: Extrapulmonary localization of gallium in sarcoidosis, Clin Nucl Med 12(1):9, 1987.

Tarpley TM and others: Minor salivary gland involvement in sarcoidosis: report of 3 cases with positive lip biopsies, Oral Surg 33:755, 1972.

Thomas RF, Merkow L, and White NS: Sarcoidosis with involvement of the mandibular condyle, J Oral Surg 34:1026, 1976.

Tillman HH: Sarcoidosis with unsuspected oral manifestations: report of a case, Oral Surg 18:130, 1964.

Tillman HH, Taylor RG, and Carchidi JE: Sarcoidosis of the tongue: report of a case, Oral Surg 21:190, 1966.

Watts KD: Sarcoid of the gingivae: a case report, Br J Oral Surg 6:108, 1968.

PAGET'S DISEASE OF THE JAWS

Philip S. Springer

CLINICAL MANIFESTATIONS. Jaw involvement is common in Paget's disease. In a review of 138 patients with polyostotic osteitis deformans, 23 cases, a 16.6% incidence, displayed associated jaw lesions. Of the 23 cases 20 occurred in the maxilla and three in the mandible. The greater frequency of the disease in the maxilla has been confirmed by other investigators. Jaw involvement usually is symmetric, but unilateral lesions have been reported. Although the etiology of Paget's disease of bone remains unclear, increasing evidence indicates that a slow virus infection of the osteoclasts may be involved.

The primary oral manifestation of Paget's disease of the jaws is a gradual enlargement of the maxilla, the mandible, or both. This osseous enlargement in the edentulous patient often causes an inability to wear existing dentures. In patients with teeth jaw expansion causes spreading and flaring of the dentition and an abnormal occlusal pattern. The palate typically appears flattened. Teeth may be moderately mobile in early phases of the disease and become ankylosed in later stages.

The characteristic osteolytic, osteoblastic, and combined phases are evident in Paget's disease of the jaws. The initial demineralization is reflected by a ground-glass appearance of bone. Radiolucent, ill-defined demineralized areas also may be apparent. The osteoblastic and combined phases produce the well-known cotton-wool appearance associated with the disease. The new bone that is laid down during the osteoblastic stage is soft and extremely vascular. The overlying mucosa in affected areas tends to feel warmer than in normal regions because of extensive arteriovenous communications. Bone during the final "burnt-out" stage is extremely dense and radiopaque.

Paget's bone gradually may encroach on the teeth. Roentgenographic changes include a gradual loss of lamina dura, hypercementosis, and occasional calcification of pulp chambers. Increased periapical radiopacities have been associated with involved teeth, with little or no differentiation between tooth and bone. A case of Paget's disease of the mandible has been reported in which three teeth required extraction because of progressive resorption of the roots by the disease process.

DENTAL MANAGEMENT. Most cases of Paget's disease of the jaws require no treatment. Surgical alveolectomy may be performed to recontour the expanded jaws in selected cases. Bleeding is the most important complication encountered in performing oral surgery during the early stage of Paget's disease. Nonhealing extraction sites, bone exposure, and osteomyelitis commonly occur during the late stages of the disease. The use of antibiotics before, during, and after surgical procedures has been advocated to minimize the risk of osteomyelitis. Excision has been recommended if sequestration should occur.

An interesting observation has been made that enlargement of the jaws appears to be inhibited when the freeway space becomes obliterated. It has been hypothesized that accurate dentures, worn all the time, may be able to contain jaw expansion.

High dose salicylates and nonsteroidal antiinflammatory drugs have been used to control pain and decrease collagen synthesis in mild cases of Paget's disease of bone. In severe cases chemotherapeutic agents such as calcitonin, diphosphonates, and mithramycin have been used to suppress the increased metabolic activity of bone.

BIBLIOGRAPHY

Akin RK, Barton K, and Walters PJ: Paget's disease of bone: a case report, Oral Surg 39(5):707, 1975.

Kirby JW and Robinson ME: Osteitis deformans of the maxilla: report of atypical case, J Oral Surg 31:64, 1973.

McGowan DA: Clinical problems in Paget's disease affecting the jaws, Br J Oral Surg 11:230, 1974.

Murphy JB, Segelman A, and Doku C: Osteitis deformans: report of a long-standing case with extensive oral involvement, Oral Surg:46:(6)765, 1978.

Otis LL, Terezhalmy GT, and Glass BJ: Paget's disease of bone: etiological theories and report of a case, J Oral Med 41(4):214, 273, 1986.

Ripp GA: A complication after extractions in a patient with advanced Paget's disease, Oral Surg 33:35, 1972.

Shatz A, Calderon S, and Amavi Y: Monostotic Paget's disease of the mandible, J Oral Med 41:(3):164, 209, 1986.

Smith NHH: Monostotic Paget's disease of the mandible presenting with progressive resorption of the teeth, Oral Surg 46(2):247, 1978.

Spika CJ and Callahan KR: A review of the differential diagnosis of the oral manifestations in early osteitis deformans, Oral Surg 11:809, 1958.

Stafne EC and Austin LT: A study of dental roentgenograms in cases of Paget's disease (osteitis deformans), osteitis fibrosa, cystica, and osteoma, J Am Dent Assoc 25:1202, 1938.

Tillman HH: Paget's disease of bone: a clinical radiographic and histopathologic study of twenty-four cases involving the jaws, Oral Surg 15:1225, 1962.

OSTEOPOROSIS

Philip S. Springer

CLINICAL MANIFESTATIONS. The mandible, in addition to the long bones and vertebrae, may exhibit changes related to generalized osteoporosis. Osteoporosis most commonly is found in postmenopausal women in whom a decrease in estrogen often is combined with a decrease in calcium intake. Although most patients with osteoporosis do not suffer from an underlying systemic disease, certain disorders cause a decrease in mineral density that may become apparent in the mandible and alveolar bone. For this reason changes in the mandible and alveolar bone can be an important means of recognizing disease states.

Osteoporosis of the mandible usually is manifested by a decrease in trabeculation. However, a decrease in mineral content of 30% to 50% is required before diminished bone density becomes apparent on dental roentgenograms.

It has been shown that the densities of the mandible and radius are similarly affected by age; both show a comparable decrease in mineral density with increasing age. Lack of calcium intake, lack of calcium absorption, lactose deficiency, lack of blood circulation, and low estrogen all may contribute to increasing osteoporosis with age.

Most of the systemic disorders causing secondary osteoporosis produce in the mandible, as in other bones, a decrease in trabeculation. This may be observed in Cushing's disease and hyperthyroidism. The demineralization associated with hyperparathyroidism may cause a ground-glass appearance of bone and a loss of lamina dura.

The effect of osteoporosis on alveolar bone has been investigated. Ward and Manson noted no correlation between the amount of alveolar bone loss and the extent of osteoporosis as measured by the metacarpal index. In contrast, an experimentally induced osteoporosis using a diet high in protein and low in calcium caused a significant increase in mandibular bone resorption in rats. Dreizen and associates found that steroid-induced osteoporosis involved the alveolar bone as well as the vertebral and appendicular skeleton.

DENTAL MANAGEMENT. Periodic, routine dental roentgenograms provide a means to compare density changes in the mandible over a period of time. It is believed that osteoporosis of the mandible, as in the long bones and vertebrae, can be prevented by taking 1000 to 1200 mg/day of oral calcium. Estrogen supplements, when indicated, also may be beneficial. Further investigation is required when precipitous osteoporosis occurs that cannot be correlated with the aging process. A detailed review of systems is essential in following up on suspicious changes. A complete blood count with differential and serum calcium, phosphorus, and alkaline phosphatase levels should be determined to rule out endocrine, metabolic, or hematologic disorders. A bone biopsy may be helpful.

BIBLIOGRAPHY

Carranza FA and others: Histometric analysis of interradicular bone in protein deficient animals, J Periodont Res 4:292, 1969.

Dreizen S, Levy B, and Bernick S: Studies on the biology of the periodontium of marmosets: cortisone induced periodontal and skeletal changes in adult cotton top marmosets, J Periodontol 42:217, 1971.

Hemikson P and Wallenius K: The mandible and osteoporosis, J Oral 1:67, 1974.

Kribbs PJ, Smith DE, and Chestnut CH: Oral findings in osteoporosis. I. Measurement of mandibular bone density, J Prosthet Dent 50(4):576, 1983.

Kribbs PJ, Smith DE, and Chestnut CH: Oral findings in osteoporosis. II. Relationship between residual ridge and alveolar bone resorption and generalized skeletal osteopenia, J Prosthet Dent 50(5):719, 1983.

Massler M: Nutritional deficiencies and oral tissues, Gerodontology, 3(4):251, 1984.

Renner RP, Baucher LJ, and Kaufman HW: Osteoporosis in post-menopausal women, J Prosthet Dent 52(4):581, 1984.

Shapiro S and others: Postmenopausal osteoporosis: dental patients at risk, Gerodontics, 1(5):220, 1985.

Sones AD, Wolinsky LE, and Dratochvil FJ: Osteoporosis and mandibular bone resorption: a prosthodontic perspective, J Prosthet Dent 56(6):732, 1986.

FIBROUS DYSPLASIA OF THE JAWS
Martin S. Greenberg

CLINICAL MANIFESTATIONS. Fibrous dysplasia involving the jaws long has been a controversial topic, and many conflicting classification systems exist because of various theories of causation. The major reason for controversy is the fact that lesions may originate from dental and periodontal structures as well as from bone. Fibroosseous lesions of the jaw have been divided into two categories: those originating from the periodontal membrane and those originating from medullary bone. Periodontal membrane lesions include cementoma and ossifying fibroma. Medullary bone lesions include cherubism, giant cell tumor, Paget's disease of bone, and fibrous dysplasia.

The clinical presentation of fibrous dysplasia of the jaws varies greatly. Lesions occur more frequently in the maxilla than in the mandible. Most mandibular lesions occur in the angle of the jaw. Monostotic fibrous dysplasia lesions occur 20 times more frequently in the jaws than the polyostotic form of the disease. Clinical signs are related to a slow expansion of the jaw, usually on the buccal surface. Lesions may cause movement of teeth and resorption of roots. Approximately 1% of fibrous dysplasia lesions undergo malignant transformation. This is significantly higher if the lesion was treated with radiation.

Roentgenographic findings depend on the proportion of fibrous tissue to osseous tissue in the particular lesion encountered. Therefore roentgenographic findings may range from a cystlike appearance to diffuse sclerotic bone. Many lesions have a mixture of both radiolucency and radiopacity. Diagnosis is based on a combination of clinical, roentgenographic, and histologic findings. Suspected lesions of fibrous dysplasia should be biopsied.

Treatment of fibrous dysplasia of the jaw varies according to the severity. If deformity is minimal, no treatment is indicated, since the lesion may regress after puberty. In the case of deforming lesions, surgery is indicated. The type of surgery will depend on the histologic stage of the lesion. Curettage is indicated for osteolytic lesions, whereas a superficial cosmetic recontouring or "shave" usually is performed for the solid osseous lesions. Radiation therapy is contraindicated because of the increased incidence of malignant transformation.

DENTAL MANAGEMENT. Dental management of patients with monostotic fibrous dysplasia provides no particular problem for restorative dentistry. However, the dentist should contact the patient's physician in cases of polyostotic dysplasia, since this form of the disease may be associated with endocrinopathies, particularly hyperthyroidism or Cushing's syndrome.

BIBLIOGRAPHY

El Deeb M and others: Fibrous dysplasia of the jaws: report of five cases, Oral Surg 47:312, 1979.

El Deeb M, Waite DE, and Gorlin RJ: Congenital monostotic fibrous dysplasia—a new possibly autosomal recessive disorder, J Oral Surg 37:520, 1979.

Hamner JE, Scofield HH, and Cornyn J: Benign fibro-osseous jaw lesions of periodontal membrane origin: an analysis of 249 cases, Cancer 22:861, 1968.

Obisesan AA and others: The radiologic features of fibrous dysplasia of the craniofacial bone, Oral Surg 44:949, 1977.

Waldon CA and Giansanti JS: Benign fibro-osseous lesions of the jaws: a clinical-radiologic-histologic review of sixty-five cases. II. Benign fibro-osseous lesions of periodontal ligament origin. Oral Surg 35:340, 1973.

Zimmerman DC, Dahlen DC and Stafne EC: Fibrous dysplasia of the maxilla and mandible, Oral Surg 11:55, 1958.

OSTEOMYELITIS OF THE JAWS
Philip S. Springer

The inflammation of bone and marrow associated with osteomyelitis of the jaws usually occurs secondary to a bacterial dental infection. *Staphylococcus aureus, S. albus,* and varieties of *Streptococcus* are the microorganisms most commonly isolated from the involved bone. Both the maxilla and the mandible can be affected by osteomyelitis, but the mandible is more susceptible because of its discrete blood supply.

Osteomyelitis may be acute or chronic and may produce suppurative, sclerosing, or proliferative responses in the jaws. The response that is seen depends on the pathogenicity of the organism, the extent of the infection, and the resistance of the patient.

Although osteomyelitis of the maxilla and mandible usually occurs in otherwise healthy individuals, certain patients may be more prone to its occurrence. Individuals with sickle cell disease, diabetes, and the bone disorders of osteopetrosis and Paget's disease are more susceptible. In addition, patients who have undergone radiation therapy for head and neck malignancies increasingly risk the occurrence of osteomyelitis of the mandible because of the severely compromised blood supply. Steroids and immunosuppressive drugs also may increase susceptibility to osteomyelitis by decreasing the body's ability to limit infection.

The acute suppurative form of osteomyelitis of the mandible and maxilla usually is accompanied by severe pain, increased body temperature, soft tissue swelling, cervical lymphadenopathy, and an increase in white blood cells. Paresthesia of the area innervated by the mental nerve is a common finding in acute osteomyelitis of the mandible. The paresthesia probably is caused by compression of the neurovascular bundle.

Chronic varieties of osteomyelitis usually are associated with milder symptoms or may be totally asymptomatic. Scintigraphy with technetium has proved useful in detecting osteomyelitis when the clinical presentation and roentgenograms are inconclusive.

Dental Management. Treatment of acute osteomyelitis of the jaws usually involves drainage, debridement of necrotic bone when indicated, and antibiotic therapy. Cephalosporins have become popular in the treatment of osteomyelitis because of their broad-spectrum coverage and excellent penetrance. Antibiotics usually are continued for at least 4 to 6 weeks after the patient becomes asymptomatic.

Hyperbaric oxygen therapy used in conjunction with antibiotics and sequestrectomy has proved extremely beneficial in treating chronic cases of osteomyelitis of the mandible and maxilla. Several patients who had chronic, diffuse, sclerosing osteomyelitis were treated with prednisone and achieved excellent resolution of symptoms. A new method for treatment of chronic sclerosing osteomyelitis of the mandible involves the radical removal of the avascular core and immediate reconstruction with particulate hydroxyapatite. When a major resection of the mandible is necessary, an iliac osteocutaneous flap transferred by microsurgical technique has improved rehabilitation.

BIBLIOGRAPHY

Austin G, Deasy M, and Walsh RF: Osteomyelitis associated with routine endodontic and periodontal therapy: a case report, J Oral Med 33(4):120, 1978.

Barnard JD: Osteomyelitis of the jaws as a sequel to dental local anesthetic injections, Br J Oral Surg 13(3):264, 1976.

Block MS, Zide MF, and Kent JN: Excision of sclerosing osteomyelitis and reconstruction with particulate hydroxyapatite, J Oral Maxillofac Surg 44(3):244, 1986.

Ellis DJ, Winslow JR, and Indovina AA: Garre's osteomyelitis of the mandible: report of a case, Oral Surg 44(2):183, 1977.

Gallo WJ, Shapiro DN, and Moss M: Suppurative candidiosis: review of the literature and report of case, J Am Dent Assoc 1976.

Girasole RV and Lyon ED: Sickle cell osteomyelitis of the mandible: report of three cases, J Oral Surg 35:231, 1977.

Goldstein BH, Byrne JE, and Miller AS: Chronic sclerosing osteomyelitis. I., J Oral Surg 37:52, 1979.

Goldstein BH, Byrne JE, and Miller AS: Chronic sclerosing osteomyelitis. II., J Oral Surg 37:101, 1979.

Goupil MT and others: Hyperbaric oxygen in the adjunctive treatment of chronic osteomyelitis of the mandible: report of a case, J Oral Surg 36(2):138, 1978.

Grodecki EZ: Mandibular osteomyelitis secondary to infarcts associated with sickle cell anemia, Spec Care Dentist 5(5):217, 1985.

Head MD and others: Bilateral microvascular free iliac graft for mandibular reconstruction in intractable osteomyelitis: report of a case, J Oral Maxillofac Surg 44(9):724, 1986.

Jacobsson S: Diffuse sclerosing osteomyelitis of the mandible, Int J Oral Surg 13(5):363, 1984.

Jacobsson S and Hollender L: Treatment and prognosis of diffuse sclerosing osteomyelitis (DSO) of the mandible, Oral Surg 49(1):7, 1980.

Jacobsson S and others: Chronic sclerosing osteomyelitis of the mandible, Oral Surg 45(2):167, 1978.

McWalter GM and Shaberg SJ: Garre's osteomyelitis of the mandible resolved by endodontic treatment, J Am Dent Assoc 108(2):193, 1984.

Nakajima T and others: Surgical treatment of chronic osteomyelitis of the mandible resistant to intraarterial infusion of antibiotics: report of a case, J Oral Surg 35:823, 1977.

Triplett RG and others: Experimental mandibular osteomyelitis therapeutic trials with hyperbaric oxygen, J Oral Maxillofac Surg 40(10):640, 1982.

Van Merkesteyn JPR and others: Hyperbaric oxygen treatment of chronic osteomyelitis of the jaws, Int J Oral Surg 13(5):386, 1984.

MICROBIAL DISEASES

Edited by **Donald Kaye**

35 · INTRODUCTION TO MICROBIAL DISEASES

Donald Kaye

Infections can be categorized both by type of organism producing the infection (for example, virus, bacteria, protozoa) and by site of infection (for example, pneumonia, meningitis, urinary tract infection). This section uses both a microorganism and a site of infection approach.

FEVER AND CHILLS

Fever is the most common manifestation of infection, but fever can be produced by many other conditions such as vascular events (for example, pulmonary embolus and myocardial infarction), diseases of immunity (for example, drug fever and connective tissue disorders), neoplasms (especially lymphomas and solid tumors), trauma, and metabolic diseases (for example, thyroid crisis and an acute gouty attack).

Shaking chills occur with wide swings in temperature and precede the rises in temperature. Chills occur more often in bacterial than viral infections, but they also occur in fevers unrelated to infection. Aspirin and other antipyretics tend to precipitate chills by causing a sudden drop in temperature, which is followed by a sudden rise in temperature. Fever can be accompanied by symptoms such as myalgias or arthralgias, or it can be asymptomatic and go unnoticed by the patient.

Fever is ordinarily harmless to the patient and does not require therapy. Exceptions are temperatures over 106° F (41° C), fever in patients with borderline cardiac compensation, fever that causes delirium, fever in patients with thrombocytopenia, and fever that produces seizures. In these circumstances the body temperature should be reduced by using cool body baths, a cooling blanket, antipyretics such as aspirin, or, if necessary, corticosteroids. Antipyretics and corticosteroids must be used cautiously in the presence of very high fever, since the rapid drop in temperature can cause hypotension.

Fever can be of several different types: sustained (seen in typhoid fever and pneumococcal pneumonia); intermittent or spiking, in which the temperature fluctuates between febrile and normal each day (seen in abscesses and miliary tuberculosis); remittent, in which the temperature returns toward normal but does not reach normal each day (seen in many febrile illnesses); and relapsing, in which the temperature becomes normal for 1 or more days between episodes of fever (seen in malaria, tick- or louse-borne relapsing fever, and Pel-Ebstein fever in Hodgkin's disease).

Patients with infection can be afebrile or even hypothermic. Chronic or indolent infections may not be associated with fever. Shock and hypothermia can be seen in patients with acute life-threatening infections (for example, bacteremia caused by gram-negative bacilli); these are most likely to occur in infants, the elderly, and the immunocompromised host. Patients with renal failure tend to be hypothermic. Although the temperature rises with infection, it may not reach febrile levels.

DIAGNOSIS OF MICROBIAL DISEASES

The history and physical examination usually lead to a presumptive diagnosis. For example, cough, rales, and signs of pulmonic consolidation together suggest pneumonia. However, laboratory studies are needed to confirm the diagnosis (by direct isolation or by indirect demonstration of the presence of the pathogen) and at times can be the only clues to diagnosis (for example, positive blood cultures in fever from infective endocarditis with no abnormal physical findings).

LABORATORY EVALUATION

Some of the laboratory tests commonly available for diagnosis of microbial infections are listed below:

1. Complete blood count with examination of the smear
2. Erythrocyte sedimentation rate
3. Urinalysis with Gram stain
4. Microscopic examination with cell counts and/or smears of any exudate, effusions, indicated body fluid, lesion, or stool; biopsies occasionally necessary; Smears: unstained as for *Treponema pallidum* (darkfield), Gram stained for bacteria, acid-fast stained for mycobacteria, stained with fluorescent antibody, or stained with other special stains
5. Cultures of blood, exudate, lesion, effusion, indicated body fluids, or occasionally mucosal surface (for example, group A streptococcal pharyngitis or gonorrhea); biopsies occasionally necessary for material to culture
6. Acute and convalescent serum specimens for study for a change in antibody titer to suspected infecting organisms; serologic test for syphilis
7. Antigen detection by counter immunoelectrophoresis or other techniques (for example, for *Haemophilus influenzae*, pneumococci, meningococci, or cryptococci in spinal fluid)
8. Skin tests (for example, tuberculosis)
9. Chest roentgenogram and any other roentgenography and scans (radioactive, ultrasound, computed tomography, magnetic resonance imaging) as determined by localized findings
10. Liver chemistries

The use of these tests should be directed by the findings on the history and physical examination and by the course of the disease. The tests and their interpretation are discussed in the appropriate sections. However, some general comments are made here.

A blood count can be helpful in suggesting bacterial, viral, or helminthic infection. Leukocytosis with a shift to the left of the white cell series suggests bacterial infection; the presence of atypical lymphocytes suggests viral infection; and eosinophilia suggests helminthic infection. However, the white count may be normal (or there may even be leukopenia) in bacterial infection, and leukocytosis can occur in viral infections. The blood smear can show parasites in red cells (malaria) or bacteria in white cells (overwhelming meningococcemia or pneumococcemia). The erythrocyte sedimentation rate (ESR) serves as a screening test for inflammation; it is usually elevated in bacterial infections and often normal in viral illnesses. However, a normal ESR does not rule out bacterial infection nor does an elevated ESR rule out viral illness.

The major laboratory tools are microscopic examination of smears, cultures, and serologic studies for the etiologic agent. Exudates, effusions, lesions, body fluids, and so forth are studied as determined by the history and physical findings (for example, examination of sputum in a patient with cough or examination of fluid from a vesicle in a patient with vesicles). It is best to obtain specimens for smear and culture from closed spaces such as a joint or deep abscess rather than from an open surface where contamination is likely.

Appropriate media must be used for culture; special media and culture techniques are required for many bacteria (for example, chocolate agar with increased CO_2 for *Neisseria gonorrhoeae*). Urine should be cultured quantitatively. Anaerobic cultures should not be obtained on specimens that have been in contact with mucosal, skin, or sinus tract surfaces (for example, a draining sinus of osteomyelitis), because these surfaces can contain large numbers of anaerobes. For example, transtracheal or sheathed bronchoscopic aspirates rather than sputum and cul de sac puncture specimens rather than vaginal specimens should be submitted for anaerobic cultures. In general, anaerobic bacteria play an important role in infections in the abdomen and pelvis, in areas contiguous with the mucosa of the mouth and nose, and in aspiration pneumonia.

Testing of serologic specimens must be directed at specific diseases. It is inappropriate to ask for "viral antibody studies," since the laboratory must know which viruses to test for. The expense and quantity of serum necessary to test for antibodies to all viruses are prohibitive. A two-dilution (fourfold or greater) rise in titer early in the disease or an equivalent fall in titer late in the disease is strongly suggestive of infection with that agent. However, usually at least 1 to 2 weeks must elapse between titers, and by that time most patients have recovered spontaneously or have been treated.

Isolation of an organism or demonstration of a high titer of antibody to that organism does *not* unequivocally indicate that the agent was responsible for the observed clinical syndrome. The laboratory findings must be interpreted in light of the history, physical findings, and course of the disease. For example, the organism isolated can be part of the patient's normal flora or can be a contaminant, and a single high titer can reflect past infection.

Skin tests can be useful for determining past exposure to an antigen but are useless in determining the presence of infection. A negative test is not evidence against present or past infection. Skin tests for mumps and *Trichophyton* and *Candida* organisms are positive in most normal hosts and are therefore useful in evaluating for anergy.

MANAGEMENT

Many microbial diseases (for example, most viral illnesses) are self-limited, and therapy is often not indicated. In some infections (for example, chronic osteomyelitis and asymptomatic urinary tract infection) therapy should await specific bacteriologic diagnosis. However, life-threatening infections such as pneumonia, meningitis, or bacteremia should be treated before a specific diagnosis is made. The general rule is to direct therapy at the likely pathogens based on the history, physical examination, and laboratory tests that are immediately available (for example, Gram stains and chest roentgenograms).

FEVER OF UNKNOWN ORIGIN

When the temperature reaches at least 101° F (38.3° C) for at least 2 to 3 weeks and no diagnosis is obvious after an initial hospital evaluation, the patient is considered to have a fever of unknown origin (FUO). The use of these criteria will eliminate most viral illnesses and many infections such as pneumonia and urinary tract infection) that are diagnosable by history, physical examination, simple roentgenograms, and laboratory examinations. The most common cause of febrile illness is viral infection. Since these infections are usually self-limited and the expense and morbidity of an FUO evaluation are great, the above criteria should be met to exclude common viral illnesses before embarking on an FUO workup. The usual course of such illnesses is less than 2 weeks of fever; exceptions are infectious mononucleosis, cytomegalovirus infection, and hepatitis.

Many of the causes of FUO are listed below:

1. Infections
   a. Miliary tuberculosis
   b. Intraabdominal and pelvic bacterial infections
   c. Bacteremias, including bacterial endocarditis, brucellosis, meningococcemia, and salmonella bacteremia
   d. Viral infections such as hepatitis, infectious mononucleosis, and cytomegalovirus infections
   e. Rickettsial infections such as Q fever and psittacosis
   f. Parasitic infections such as trichinosis, visceral larva migrans, strongyloidiasis, malaria, and amebiasis
2. Neoplasms
   a. Solid tumors such as those of kidney, liver, and pancreas
   b. Metastatic tumors
   c. Lymphomas, sarcomas, and leukemias
   d. Atrial myxoma
3. Connective tissue disorders such as polyarteritis, lupus erythematosus, and giant cell arteritis
4. Inflammatory bowel disease such as regional enteritis and ulcerative colitis
5. Granulomatous hepatitis
6. Sarcoidosis
7. Multiple pulmonary emboli
8. Familial Mediterranean fever and other periodic fevers
9. Diseases of the central nervous system such as tumor, cerebrovascular accident, and hypothalamic disease
10. Drug fever
11. Factitious fever

The vast majority of FUOs are caused by infections (the most common are miliary tuberculosis and intraabdominal or pelvic infections), neoplasms (most commonly lymphomas), and connective tissue disorders. Drug and factitious fevers must always be excluded.

The evaluation of an FUO involves (1) a systematic evaluation beginning with a careful history and physical examination (including a pelvic and rectal examination) followed by progressive laboratory evaluation for the statistically most likely causes and (2) a directed approach when a localized finding suggests a direct route to diagnosis. Noninvasive tests are generally performed first and invasive tests reserved for later. For example, a history of potential exposure to an infectious disease (such as skinning a rabbit [tularemia] or working as a butcher or farmer [brucellosis or Q fever]) would suggest specific studies for these infections; a very high ESR plus tenderness over a temporal artery would suggest early biopsy of the artery to diagnose giant cell arteritis; abnormal liver chemistries would suggest early liver biopsy to attempt a histologic diagnosis.

LABORATORY APPROACH

Some of the tests that might be required either to reach a diagnosis or to suggest a localized area of disease that could be studied further include the following:

Initial studies

1. Complete blood count with examination of the smear
2. Urinalysis
3. Microscopic examination and cultures of exudates, effusions, and indicated body fluids, and excreta; blood cultures
4. Erythrocyte sedimentation rate
5. Liver chemistries
6. Serologic studies for possible infectious diseases (for example, infectious mononucleosis, cytomegalovirus infection, toxoplasmosis, brucellosis) and for connective tissue disorders (for example, antinuclear antibody and rheumatoid factor)
7. Chest roentgenogram
8. Ultrasound of the abdomen and heart valves
9. Liver-spleen scan
10. Skin tests for presence or absence of delayed hypersensitivity (for example, to PPD, *Tricophyton* or *Candida* spp.)
11. Stool examination for occult blood

Subsequent studies

1. Computed tomography or magnetic resonance imaging of the abdomen, lung, and brain
2. Roentgenograms—intravenous pyelogram, cholecystogram, barium enema, upper gastrointestinal and small bowel roentgenograms, bone roentgenograms

3. Sigmoidoscopy
4. Scans—bone scan, gallium scan, lung scan, renal scan
5. Biopsies (with cultures where indicated)—liver, bone marrow, lymph node (preferably not an inguinal node), skin and muscle, any abnormal mass or lesion, and temporal artery (only in the elderly)

Other studies

1. Abdominal aortography
2. Lymphangiogram
3. Exploratory laparotomy with biopsies and cultures

The recent availability of computed tomography of the abdomen has often helped define intraabdominal lesions early in a workup, leading to a direct surgical approach and eliminating the need for many of the tests in the preceding outline. Blind exploratory laparotomy with no localizing findings is usually not rewarding and is no longer considered a reasonable approach to diagnosis of FUO.

Therapeutic trials are never definite. Lysis of fever can be fortuitous and unrelated to the drug administered. However, therapeutic trials may be justified when no diagnosis can be made or when the patient is moribund and therapy cannot await a diagnosis. Regimens should be as specific as possible for the suspected pathogen. Examples are the administration of isoniazid and ethambutol to patients who may have occult tuberculosis or the administration of penicillin plus gentamicin when endocarditis is suspected.

After a complete evaluation, up to 10% of patients with FUO remain undiagnosed. Some of these patients recover spontaneously, and others continue to be febrile without a diagnosis. In some who continue to have fever, an explanation is found on subsequent evaluation or at autopsy; others remain undiagnosed even by autopsy.

BIBLIOGRAPHY

Larson EG, Featherstone HJ, and Petersdorf RG: Fever of undetermined origin: diagnosis and follow-up of 105 cases, 1970-1980, Medicine 61:269, 1982.
Mandell GL, Douglas RG, and Bennett JE: Principles and practice of infectious diseases, ed 3, New York, 1990, Churchill Livingstone.
Petersdorf RG and Beeson PB: Fever of unexplained origin: report of 100 cases, Medicine 40:1, 1961.

UNIT A • VIRAL DISEASES

36 · INTRODUCTION, CLASSIFICATION, AND LABORATORY DIAGNOSIS

Harvey M. Friedman

Viruses are among the most common infecting organisms of humans. They range in size from 17 nm to over 300 nm and contain DNA or RNA but not both. The nucleic acid is surrounded by a protein shell termed a *capsid* that is arranged in either icosahedral (cubic) or helical symmetry. Those with cubic symmetry assume the shape of regular polyhedrons with 20 triangular surfaces and 12 corners. All viruses with helical symmetry are surrounded by a lipid *envelope*, whereas some viruses with cubic symmetry are enveloped but most are *naked*. The envelope is derived in part from host cells but also contains virus-specific proteins composing both the inner membrane layer and the glycoprotein spikes that protrude from the surface. Viruses multiply only within living cells and have sufficient nucleic acid to code from 2 to approximately 50 proteins. Several steps occur preceding replication, including attachment of viruses to host cells, penetration into the cells, and uncoating to expose the viral nucleic acid. For DNA viruses the nucleic acid serves as a template for production of messenger RNA, whereas for RNA viruses the RNA serves as the template or functions as its own messenger. RNA retroviruses and the DNA hepatitis B virus contain reverse transcriptase, an enzyme capable of catalyzing synthesis of DNA from an RNA template. Once formed, messenger RNA codes for viral protein using host cell polysomes. Generally, synthesis of host cell proteins is suppressed to a variable degree during viral replication. Synthesis of viral daughter nucleic acid from parental templates occurs after early viral protein synthesis. Intact *virions* are then assembled and released from the cell by lysis or by budding. During extrusion, a lipid membrane may envelop the virus and form its outer coat.

Some viruses have the ability to remain latent within host cells following infection and subsequently reappear. An example is varicella virus, which is manifested as chickenpox during the primary infection and as shingles during a recurrence. Similarly, relapsing herpes lip and genital lesions represent latent infection with exacerbations of herpes simplex virus. The mechanisms of initiating and maintaining viral latency are incompletely understood but involve complex interactions among the virus, the infected host cells, and the immune system.

Transmission of viral infections may occur by aerosol spread, direct contact, fecal-oral contamination, foodborne and waterborne routes, and insect or animal bites. Once introduced, viruses spread to different organs by contiguous spread, by dissemination in blood or lymphatics, or by ascension in neural tissue. For some viruses (for example, cytomegalovirus) subclinical infection is the rule, whereas for others (for example, chickenpox and measles viruses), clinical illness is the usual result. The type of virus, the titer of the inoculum, the previous immune experience of the host, and the adequacy of the immune response are all determinants of the eventual outcome of the infection.

The immune system is beneficial to the host in terminating viral infections and preventing reinfections; however, in some circumstances the immune response can also be detrimental. For example, some chronic carriers of hepatitis B virus surface antigen have circulating immune complexes composed of surface antigen and antibody to this antigen. These complexes can be deposited in glomeruli, dermal vessels, and medium-sized arteries, producing glomerulonephritis and vasculitis.

A detailed discussion of the role of the immune response to viral infections is beyond the scope of this chapter. It is likely that a complex interaction of many components of the immune system is involved in control of most if not all viral infections. For some viruses, such as enteroviruses, humoral immunity appears to be of major importance for control of infection; whereas for others, including those in the herpes family, termination of viral shedding correlates closely with the development of cellular immunity. Interferon production in vesicle fluid appears to be important in preventing dissemination of varicella-zoster virus in patients with lymphoma. In addition, several viruses have been noted to activate the complement sequence in the absence of antibody, an event that can be an important early host response to the invading virus.

Over 300 antigenically distinct viruses causing at least 50 different clinical syndromes in humans have been identified. Viruses can be classified by chemical and physical characteristics or by the diseases they produce. For the clinician the latter is probably more useful. A classification of viruses commonly associated with various types of infections is shown in Table 36-1, and a classification based on viral nucleic acid content is presented in Table 36-2. The virology chapters in this book are prepared from a clinical perspective, discussing disease syndromes and the viruses that produce them.

Attempts at specific viral diagnosis are performed for a variety of reasons, ranging from etiologic diagnosis of an acute illness to retrospective serologic surveys. In some instances the diagnosis can influence patient management; in others the

Table 36-1   Viruses associated with various types of infections

Type of infection	Common viral causes
RESPIRATORY TRACT	
Upper respiratory infection	Rhinoviruses
	Coronaviruses
	Respiratory syncytial virus
	Adenoviruses
	Parainfluenza viruses types 1-3
	Influenza viruses types A and B
Croup, bronchiolitis	Respiratory syncytial virus
	Parainfluenza viruses types 1-3
Pneumonia (adults)	Influenza viruses types A and B
	Cytomegalovirus
	Adenoviruses
Pneumonia (children)	Respiratory syncytial virus
	Parainfluenza viruses types 1-3
	Influenza viruses types A and B
EYE	
Conjunctivitis	Adenoviruses
	Herpes simplex virus
	Enterovirus 7
CENTRAL NERVOUS SYSTEM	
Aseptic meningitis	Enteroviruses
	Mumps virus
	Human immunodeficiency virus 1
Encephalitis	St. Louis encephalitis virus
	California encephalitis virus
	Western equine encephalitis virus
	Eastern equine encephalitis virus
	Herpes simplex viruses types 1 and 2
	Mumps virus
	Human immunodeficiency virus 1
SKIN AND MUCOUS MEMBRANE	
Mouth ulcers	Herpes simplex virus type 1
	Group A coxsackieviruses
Genital ulcers	Herpes simplex virus type 2
Maculopapular rash	Measles virus
	Rubella virus
	Enteroviruses
Vesicular rash	Herpes simplex viruses types 1 and 2
	Varicella-zoster virus
GASTROINTESTINAL TRACT	
Gastroenteritis	Rotaviruses
	Norwalk agent group
Hepatitis	Hepatitis A, B, and non A/B
	Epstein-Barr virus
	Cytomegalovirus
CONGENITAL INFECTION	
Microcephaly, hepatospleno-megaly	Cytomegalovirus
	Rubella virus
	Herpes simplex viruses
OPPORTUNISTIC INFECTION	
Acquired immunodeficiency syndrome	Human immunodeficiency viruses types 1 and 2

ultimate benefit can be to the community at large. In recent years technical improvements have permitted the emergence of methods for rapid viral diagnosis, which have become particularly important with the advent of antiviral chemotherapies.

The four major methods for the diagnosis of viral infections include (1) microscopy of tissues or exfoliated cells, examining

Table 36-2   Classification and common clinical manifestations of viruses

Virus group	Members	Common clinical manifestations
DNA VIRUSES		
Adenoviruses	Types 1-31	Pharyngitis, pharyngoconjunctival fever, pneumonia
Herpesviruses	Herpes simplex types 1 and 2	Gingivostomatitis (type 1), vulvovaginitis (type 2), recurrent mucocutaneous eruption (types 1, 2), keratoconjunctivitis, generalized infection of newborn, encephalitis, esophagitis
	Varicella-zoster	Chickenpox, localized and disseminated zoster
	Cytomegalovirus	Congenital infection, mononucleosis syndrome, prolonged fever, and pneumonia in immunosuppressed patients
	Epstein-Barr virus	Infectious mononucleosis, encephalomyelitis, Guillian-Barré syndrome
Poxviruses	Smallpox (variola)	Smallpox
	Vaccinia	Complications of vaccination including disseminated vaccinia and encephalitis
	Cowpox, orf	Skin lesions in humans who handle infected cows (cowpox) or sheep (orf)
	Molluscum contagiosum	Pearly white 2-mm skin nodules
Papovaviruses	Papillomavirus	Human warts
	SV40, JC virus	Progressive multifocal leukoencephalopathy
	BK virus	Undetermined
Hepadnaviruses	Hepatitis B virus	Acute or chronic hepatitis, hepatocellular carcinoma
RNA VIRUSES		
Orthomyxoviruses	Influenza A, B, C	Influenza
Paramyxoviruses	Parainfluenza 1-4	Upper respiratory infections, pharyngitis, croup, laryngitis, pneumonia
	Mumps	Mumps, aseptic meningitis, encephalitis
	Measles	Measles, encephalitis
	Respiratory syncytial virus	Bronchiolitis, pneumonia, upper respiratory infections
Picornaviruses	Rhinoviruses, over 100 types	Upper respiratory infections

	Enteroviruses
	    Polioviruses 1-3
	    Coxsackieviruses A 1-24 and B 1-6
	    Echoviruses 1-34
	    Enteroviruses 68-72
		Aseptic meningitis, myocarditis, herpangina, fever with or without maculopapular rash, paralysis (poliomyelitis), hepatitis A (enterovirus 72)

Rhabdovirus	Rabies	Rabies
Coronaviruses	229E, OC43, B814, OC16, OC37, OC48	Upper respiratory infections
Togaviruses	Rubella	Rubella, congenital infection
	Alphavirus, flavivirus (formerly arboviruses)	Encephalitis, yellow fever, dengue, hemorrhagic fever
Arenaviruses	Lymphocytic choriomeningitis	Aseptic meningitis
	Lassa fever	Lassa fever
	Junin, Machupo	Hemorrhagic fever
Reoviruses	Reovirus	Undetermined
	Orbivirus	Colorado tick fever
	Rotaviruses	Gastroenteritis
Retroviruses	Human immunodeficiency viruses types 1 and 2	Acquired immunodeficiency syndrome, encephalopathy
	Human T-cell lymphotrophic viruses types 1 and 2	T-cell lymphoma, leukemia, tropical spastic paralysis
Bunyaviruses	California encephalitis virus Hantaan virus Crimean hemorrhagic Fever virus	Encephalitis, hemorrhagic fevers, acute febrile illnesses

for viral inclusions or other changes characteristic of certain viruses; (2) isolation and identification of viruses from infected tissues; (3) serologic studies to measure virus-specific antibodies in a patient's serum; and (4) tests to detect viruses or viral antigens directly in clinical specimens without requiring cultivation of the agents in the laboratory.

Microscopic examination of fixed and stained tissues or of exfoliated cells is usually performed by pathology or cytology laboratories. These methods are rapid and useful for establishing with high probability that a particular illness is caused by a virus. However, they do not permit specific identification of the agent involved. Many different organisms can demonstrate viral inclusions. In particular, the characteristic changes produced in the brain by herpes simplex and rabies viruses, in skin vesicles by varicella-zoster and herpes simplex, in cervical cells by herpes simplex, and in lung tissue by cytomegalovirus are valuable diagnostic aids.

The isolation of viruses requires living host systems and is the cornerstone of diagnostic virology. Growth and identification of viruses usually take longer than their counterparts in bacteriology, ranging from 1 day to 6 weeks. A wide variety of host systems can be used for viral isolation, including embryonated eggs, tissue culture cells, and animals. Since many of these require expensive equipment and facilities, the range of methods available depends in part on the size of the laboratory. The most widely used method involves tissue culture isolation, in which clinical specimens are inoculated into cell cultures that are then observed for changes indicative of viral growth.

Deciding which specimens to select for viral cultures depends in part on which organs are involved and which viral agents are suspected. Some suggested specimens for viral isolation are shown in Table 36-3. In general, specimens taken from diseased organs are most useful, for example, spinal fluid

Table 36-3 Selection of specimens for viral isolation

Clinical syndrome	Type of specimen
Upper respiratory infection, laryngitis, croup, pneumonia	Nasopharyngeal aspirate, throat swab, or sputum
Meningitis	Cerebrospinal fluid, throat swab, stool or rectal swab
Congenital infection	Throat swab, urine
Vesicular lesions including oral and genital ulcers	Swab of base of lesion
Maculopapular rash	Throat or nasopharyngeal swab
Opportunistic infection, acquired immunodeficiency syndrome	Buffy coat (leukocytes)

in meningitis cases or respiratory secretions from patients with pneumonia. Several aspects of specimen collection require emphasis:

1. All swabs must be kept moist (in transport media).
2. Body fluids such as urine, pleural fluid, and spinal fluid can be transported to the laboratory without any special transport medium.
3. A specimen should be transported to the laboratory quickly, since most viruses have a short survival time once outside the body.
4. While waiting for transport, specimens keep best if stored at 39° F (4° C).

Specimens that are commonly contaminated with bacteria such as stool, urine, or respiratory secretions are treated with broad-spectrum antibiotics before inoculation onto tissue culture monolayers. To indicate the presence of a virus, cultures are observed for alterations in cell morphology (cytopathic effect [CPE]). Alternatively some viruses can be detected by attachment of erythrocytes to infected cells in monolayers (hemadsorption) or by the interference with growth of other viruses in the infected monolayers. Based on the changes noted in the cell monolayer, a presumptive identification of the type of virus can be made. Specific immunologic methods are needed to identify definitively the isolated agent. A wide variety of tests are available for definitive identification, all of which employ antisera of known titer and specificity.

Isolation of a virus indicates that the patient is infected with that agent. Whether the virus is also causing the clinical illness requires consideraton of several factors. It is important to realize that viruses often cause asymptomatic infection and that some viruses persist for extended periods in the body after infection. The site from which an isolate is obtained and the recognized capacity of the virus isolated to cause disease are important considerations in assigning significance to a particular isolate. Failure to recover virus from a patient does not mean that the illness is not caused by a virus, since some human viruses are noncultivatable. More commonly, a negative result reflects improper collection methods, the obtaining of specimens too late in the illness, poor transport, or incorrect storage of the specimens.

Serologic studies are useful to define, retrospectively, the incidence of viral infections in communities; to elucidate the need for, and efficacy of, immunization programs; and to monitor for recent infection. For the last, generally two serum samples are required, one in the acute phase taken as early as possible after the onset of illness and the other in the convalescent period drawn 1 to 3 weeks later. By comparing antibody titers in the two sera, which must be tested simultaneously, a diagnosis of recent infection can be established if the convalescent serum shows a fourfold or greater rise in antibody titers.

High antibody titers alone are not a reliable guide to recent infection, but often experience permits a presumptive diagnosis to be made on the basis of a single high titer in convalescent-phase serum. A more confident diagnosis can be made by measuring virus-specific IgM antibodies in convalescent-phase serum. However, at present few clinical laboratories can measure IgM responses to a wide variety of viruses.

For antibody testing, serum is the correct sample to obtain. Blood should not be frozen, since the ensuing red blood cell lysis interferes with serologic testing. Whole blood or the separated serum can be transported to the laboratory at room temperature; however, if there is a lag between collection and transport, the sample should be refrigerated at 39° F (4° C).

A wide variety of serologic assays are available. The complement fixation (CF) test is widely used because of its applicability to the vast majority of viruses and because reagents are commercially available. Other common assay methods include hemagglutination, neutralization, immunofluorescence, enzyme immunoassay, and radioimmunoassay. A serologic diagnosis requires the use of known viral antigens and therefore cannot supplant virus isolation as a means of discovering new viruses.

Detection of viral antigens in clinical specimens before inoculation of tissue culture monolayers has received wide attention in recent years. This permits rapid diagnosis of infection but requires viral antigens to be present in relatively high concentrations. Electron microscopy using negative staining methods is useful for detecting viruses in stool specimens (hepatitis A, rotavirus, Norwalk agent virus), in vesicle fluids (chickenpox, herpes simplex viruses), and in urine (cytomegalovirus). Immunologic assays using ^{125}I-radiolabeled or enzyme-labeled immunoglobulins have been successfully used to detect hepatitis B surface antigen in serum. Recently viral antigens in stool, respiratory secretions, and urine have been detected using enzyme immunoassays. A widely used technique for rapid viral diagnosis is immunofluorescence. Cells from infected tissues are spread on glass slides and examined for virus by direct or indirect immunofluorescence using virus-specific immune reagents.

Clinical laboratories skilled in diagnostic virology are becoming more numerous. At university hospitals, the spectrum of services offered varies from testing antibodies to a select group of viruses, to broad-scale serologic and isolation studies. The current acquired immunodeficiency syndrome (AIDS) epidemic and the advent of effective antiviral agents for certain viruses have placed renewed emphasis on the need for accurate, rapid, and specific viral diagnosis. Clinicians involved in the care of acutely ill patients find themselves requesting viral studies with increasing frequency.

BIBLIOGRAPHY

Drew WL: Basic virology: classification and general concepts. In Drew WL, editor: Viral infections: a clinical approach, Philadelphia, 1976, FA Davis Co.

Gardner PS and McQuillin J, editors: Rapid virus diagnosis: application of immunofluorescence, ed 2, Woburn Mass, 1980, Butterworth, Inc.

Hawkes RA: General principles underlying laboratory diagnosis of viral infections. In Lennette EH and Schmidt NJ, editors: Diagnostic procedures for viral, rickettsial and chlamydial infections, Washington, DC, 1979, American Public Health Association.

Herrmann EC Jr and Herrmann JA: Laboratory diagnosis of viral disease. In Drew WL, editor: Viral infections: a clinical approach, Philadelphia, 1976, FA Davis Co.

Melnick JL: Taxonomy of viruses, Prog Med Virol 25:160, 1979.

Menegus MA and Douglas RG Jr: Viruses, rickettsiae, chlamydiae and mycoplasmas. In Mandel GL, Douglas RG Jr, and Bennett JE, editors: Principles and practice of infectious diseases, ed 2, New York, 1985, John Wiley & Sons, Inc.

37 · DISEASES CAUSED BY VIRUSES

Viral infections of the fetus and newborn

Sung Hee Oh *and* **Stuart E. Starr**

Possible consequences of viral infections of the fetus include abortions, stillbirths, and congenital malformations. Symptomatic live-born infants can die within the first few months of life, and survivors of infection are frequently left with neurologic and other sequelae. Infected neonates who appear undamaged at birth may later develop deficits of varying severity. The spectrum of viral infections acquired at the time of birth ranges from asymptomatic to severe and life threatening.

DEFINITION. A congenital infection is one that is present at the time of birth. Natal infections are acquired at the time of birth, most commonly from maternal cervicovaginal or stool flora, whereas postnatal infections are acquired after birth. The term "perinatal infection" is inclusive, designating infections occurring before, during, or shortly after the time of birth.

ETIOLOGY. Several viruses can cause infection of the fetus and newborn. Those most commonly responsible are cytomegalovirus, herpes simplex types 1 and 2, rubella, coxsackievirus B, hepatitis B, varicella-zoster, and human immunodeficiency virus (HIV).

EPIDEMIOLOGY. Congenital rubella may occur in epidemic fashion; the last outbreak in the United States took place in 1964 and was associated with an estimated 20,000 cases. Currently in the United States perinatal HIV infection occurs primarily in cases involving maternal intravenous drug abuse or sexual exposure to infected bisexual or drug-abusing males. Other viruses that commonly affect the fetus or newborn are endemic in human populations. Postnatal infections can be acquired as a result of exposure to breast milk or blood products or as a result of contact with infected individuals, including health personnel. Seasonal variation has been noted only for coxsackievirus B infections, which tend to occur during summer months.

PATHOGENESIS. Congenital infection is thought to occur usually as a result of maternal viremia and transplacental spread of the virus to the fetus. Several effects of virus infection, including inhibition of cell division, tissue necrosis, and vasculitis, can result in fetal damage. In the congenital rubella syndrome and rarely with varicella-zoster and herpes simplex infections, pathologic changes can cause congenital malformations. The timing of the maternal infection appears to be crucial in that damage tends to be more severe when the fetus is infected during the first trimester. Possible late manifestations of tissue damage include fibrosis and calcification. Persistent infection with rubella or cytomegalovirus during the first few years of life can result in further damage to certain organs.

Possible portals of entry for natal and postnatal virus infections include the skin, eyes, and gastrointestinal tract. Acquired infections can remain localized or can disseminate to involve multiple organs. The relative immaturity of neonatal immune defense mechanisms can contribute to the severity of some infections.

CLINICAL MANIFESTATIONS

Cytomegalovirus. From 0.5% to 2.5% of all newborns are congenitally infected with cytomegalovirus, making this virus the most common known cause of congenital infection. Congenital infections that occur after primary maternal infections can be associated with fetal damage and subsequent sequelae, whereas congenital infections that occur after maternal reactivation infections are rarely associated with sequelae.

Only around 5% of congenitally infected neonates are symptomatic at the time of birth. Possible manifestations include intrauterine growth retardation, jaundice, hepatosplenomegaly, petechial skin rash, chorioretinitis, and intracranial calcifications. Microcephaly can be present at birth or develop during the first year of life. Most infants who have clinically apparent disease during the neonatal period survive, but they are left with sequelae that can include mental retardation, spasticity, seizure disorders, and visual or hearing deficits. Hearing deficits can be detected in 15% to 20% of congenitally infected neonates who are asymptomatic at the time of birth, making cytomegalovirus an important cause of deafness.

Cytomegalovirus infection can also be acquired at the time of birth from maternal cervical secretions. Neonates infected in this fashion begin to excrete the virus at 3 to 12 weeks of age. These infections are usually asymptomatic, but occasionally infants have an interstitial pneumonitis that can take several weeks to resolve. Asymptomatic postnatal infection can also occur as a result of ingestion of breast milk containing cytomegalovirus. In premature infants who acquire infection as a result of blood transfusions, encephalitis, pneumonitis, hepatosplenomegaly, and thrombocytopenia can develop.

Herpes simplex virus. The incidence of neonatal herpetic infection is estimated at 1 per 2000 of 10,000 live births. The infection is generally acquired at the time of birth from the maternal genital tract and usually results from herpes simplex type 2, the virus type responsible for most genital herpetic infections. In most instances the maternal herpetic infection is not diagnosed because of the absence of specific findings. Vesicular skin lesions usually appear 2 to 12 days after birth; however, in around 20% of the cases of neonatal herpes, cutaneous lesions do not appear and the diagnosis is unsuspected. Infants are rarely born with herpetic lesions as a result of ascending or transplacental infection. In approximately 30% of the cases of neonatal herpes, infection remains localized to the skin or eyes. Isolated encephalitis occurs in 30% of the cases; in 40% of the cases disseminated infection develops with involvement of the liver, adrenal glands, lungs, and other organs. Possible clinical manifestations include vesicular skin rash, keratoconjunctivitis, hepatosplenomegaly, chorioretinitis, seizures, and bleeding caused by disseminated intravascular coagulation. Before antiviral therapy was available, disseminated infections were fatal 80% to 90% of the time. Two thirds of neonates with localized encephalitis died, and around half of those that survived had neurologic damage. Neonates with infection limited to the skin had a better prognosis, but some of them also had neurologic sequelae, presumably as a result of undetected encephalitis.

Rubella virus (German measles). Congenital rubella has become uncommon in the United States since the introduction of rubella vaccine. Clinical findings in neonates with congenital rubella include jaundice, hepatosplenomegaly, thrombocytopenic purpura, glaucoma, cataracts, bone lesions consisting of areas of radiolucency in the metaphyses of long bones, and congenital heart disease. The most common cardiac lesions are patent ductus arteriosus, pulmonary artery stenosis, and pulmonary valvular stenosis. Deafness is the most common consequence of congenital rubella and may occur in the absence of other symptoms. Possible neurologic sequelae include mental retardation, behavioral disorders, and autism. Other possible late manifestations are agammaglobulinemia, diabetes, and progressive panencephalitis.

Hepatitis B virus. Neonates are at highest risk of acquiring hepatitis B infection if their mothers are actively infected with the virus at the time of birth. Neonates whose mothers are chronic carriers of hepatitis B virus can also acquire infection. Carrier mothers who are e antigen positive are more likely to transmit the virus to their offspring. Most neonates who become infected remain asymptomatic, but some become chronic carriers of the virus. Mild elevations of liver enzymes and pathologic changes in liver biopsy specimens have been detected in some of these infants. Occasionally acute icteric hepatitis occurs at around 3 to 4 months of age. Fulminant hepatitis leading to early death from cirrhosis has rarely been observed.

Coxsackievirus B. In neonates with coxsackievirus B infection, symptoms usually develop 3 to 5 days after birth. Clinical findings often mimic those of bacterial sepsis, meningitis, or both and include pneumonitis, seizures, hepatosplenomegaly, myocarditis, and heart failure. Neonates with severe infections can die, whereas less severely involved neonates usually recover completely.

Varicella-zoster virus (chickenpox). Transmission of varicella-zoster infection to the fetus is uncommon, since most pregnant women are immune. A rare syndrome of congenital varicella has occurred following first-trimester maternal varicella. Possible manifestations include hypoplastic extremities, atrophic digits, chorioretinitis, cataracts, optic atrophy, encephalitis, and severe psychomotor retardation.

Neonatal varicella can occur if varicella develops in a pregnant woman around the time of delivery. If maternal varicella appears within 5 days before or 2 days after delivery, the neonate can have typical vesicular skin lesions 5 to 10 days after birth. Fatal disseminated infection with pneumonitis, hepatitis, and encephalitis can develop. If maternal infection appears more than 5 days before delivery, neonatal varicella tends to be mild.

Human immunodeficiency virus. Routes of transmission of human immunodeficiency virus (HIV) from pregnant women to their offspring have not been defined. Recent recognition of a dysmorphic syndrome in some children with acquired immunodeficiency syndrome (AIDS) suggests that infection may occur in utero. Infection may also be acquired perinatally or postnatally. Neonates destined to develop pediatric AIDS are asymptomatic at birth. Symptoms appear at 1 to 24 months of age with mean onset at 5.5 months. The most common manifestations include failure to thrive, developmental delay, small for gestational age, microcephaly, lymphocytic interstitial pneumonitis, hepatosplenomegaly, generalized adenopathy, thrombocytopenia, salivary gland enlargement, encephalopathy, chronic diarrhea, and oral candidiasis. Less common findings include hepatitis, cardiomyopathy, and nephrotic syndrome. In contrast to the incidence in adults with AIDS, Kaposi's sarcoma is rare. Patients with pediatric AIDS frequently develop infections with common pathogens such as *Streptococcus pneumoniae* and *Haemophilus influenzae*. Infections with opportunistic pathogens, such as *Pneumocystis carinii* and nontuberculous mycobacteria, occur less commonly than in adults with AIDS. Increased susceptibility to infection is a consequence of the severe immunodeficiency resulting from HIV infection. Early in the clinical course agammaglobulinemia is usually found, but ability to make specific antibodies is impaired. As the disease progresses there is a loss of T-lymphocyte function accompanied by inversion of the helper-T cell:suppressor-T cell ratio. Most children with severe AIDS eventually

die. Children with asymptomatic infection or with less severe symptoms have also been described. The natural history of infection in such children remains to be determined.

LABORATORY FINDINGS. Routine laboratory tests are useful to define the extent and follow the course of perinatal infections. Hemolytic anemia and thrombocytopenia are commonly detected. Elevations of direct bilirubin and liver enzymes indicate liver involvement. Cerebrospinal fluid pleocytosis and elevated protein content can be detected if encephalitis is present. Elevated levels of IgM in cord blood or sera collected during the first few days of life suggest congenital infection, since maternal IgM does not usually cross the placenta and the fetus does not produce IgM unless it is antigenically stimulated. Not all congenitally infected neonates, however, have elevated IgM levels. Possible roentgenographic findings include abnormalities in the metaphyses of long bones, pneumonitis, and calcifications of brain or liver.

DIAGNOSIS. Perinatal virus infection cannot be diagnosed on the basis of clinical findings and routine laboratory studies alone. Bacterial or fungal infections, toxoplasmosis, and noninfectious conditions such as erythroblastosis fetalis and autoimmune thrombocytopenia may be initially seen with similar findings. Certain manifestations do suggest a viral origin; for example, the presence of skin vesicles or keratoconjunctivitis suggests herpes simplex infection, whereas congenital cytomegalovirus infection should be suspected when periventricular intracranial calcifications are detected. An appropriate epidemiologic history and the presence of typical clinical manifestations suggest the diagnosis of pediatric AIDS.

Viral infections can be identified on the basis of morphologic, virologic, and serologic findings. Characteristic histopathologic changes may be found in autopsy or biopsy specimens. Inclusion-bearing cells can be found in the urine of about 30% of neonates with symptomatic cytomegalovirus infection. Scrapings of skin or conjunctival lesions of neonates with herpes simplex or varicella-zoster infections frequently reveal multinucleated giant cells with intranuclear inclusions. In congenital cytomegalovirus infection, virus particles can be detected in the urine by electron microscopy. Definitive diagnosis is accomplished by isolation of virus from throat, nasopharyngeal, urine, stool, skin, eye, buffy coat, or cerebrospinal fluid specimens.

Serologic tests are also available for the diagnosis of neonatal infections but must be interpreted with caution. The detection of antibodies in a neonate's serum may only reflect transplacental passage of maternal antibodies. The presence of IgM antibodies to a particular virus suggests congenital infection, since IgM antibodies do not usually cross the placenta; however, reliable tests for specific IgM antibodies are either not available or available in only a few laboratories. The serologic diagnosis of congenital infection can also be based on the persistence of specific antibodies in an infant, since transplacentally acquired maternal antibodies decline with time. The results of serologic testing of parents may support the diagnosis of pediatric AIDS.

MANAGEMENT. Appropriate isolation procedures should be instituted whenever perinatal virus infection is suspected. Neonates with possible herpes simplex or varicella-zoster infections should be strictly isolated, and those with possible cytomegalovirus or rubella infections should be kept away from pregnant women. Blood precautions should be instituted for neonates exposed to maternal hepatitis B or HIV infection.

For symptomatic neonates, supportive measures such as blood and platelet transfusions, anticonvulsant therapy, and ventilatory assistance may be required. Parenterally administered acyclovir and vidarabine are equally effective in reducing morbidity and mortality associated with neonatal herpes. Periodic administration of intravenous γ-globulin can protect children with AIDS from bacterial infections. Children who survive perinatal virus infections should receive careful follow-up study, including tests for hearing, vision, and neurologic function. Clinicians caring for such children must be alert for possible late manifestations.

PREVENTION. Prevention of perinatal viral infections is highly desirable in view of the associated morbidity and mortality. Congenital rubella is theoretically completely preventable with the availability of rubella vaccine. In fact, since the introduction of rubella vaccine, the number of cases in the United States has fallen markedly. The Centers for Disease Control has recommended that women infected with HIV defer pregnancy until further information becomes available about transmission and risk to the fetus and newborn. When primary infection with rubella or cytomegalovirus or infection with HIV is detected in a pregnant woman, termination of the pregnancy to prevent possible congenital infection is an option.

Other possible preventive measures for pregnant women include avoidance of close contact with patients who are known to be infected with rubella or cytomegalovirus. Pregnant women should also avoid sexual intercourse with individuals known to be infected with HIV. The use of condoms should be encouraged if sexual partners belong to groups at high risk for developing AIDS. Intravenous drug abusers should avoid needle sharing. Insofar as possible, blood transfusions should be avoided in pregnant women, since cytomegalovirus and possibly other viruses can be transmitted in this fashion. Delivery by cesarean section is advised to prevent neonatal herpes when active genital herpes is documented in a pregnant woman close to the time of delivery.

Passive immunization of neonates can prevent varicella. It is currently recommended that zoster immune globulin be given to neonates in whose mothers varicella developed less than 5 days before or 2 days after delivery. Neonates whose mothers either are actively infected with hepatitis B or are chronic carriers of this virus should be given hepatitis B immune globulin and hepatitis B vaccine at birth followed by additional doses of hepatitis B vaccine at 1 and 6 months of age. Transfusion-acquired cytomegalovirus infection in premature infants can be avoided by use of blood obtained from seronegative donors or frozen blood obtained from random donors. The screening of blood donors has almost completely abolished the transmission of HIV and hepatitis B virus by blood products.

BIBLIOGRAPHY

Hanshaw JB, Dudgeon JA, and Marshall WC: Viral diseases of the fetus and newborn, ed 2, Philadelphia, 1985, WB Saunders Co.

Overall JC Jr: Viral infections of the fetus and neonate. In Feigin RD and Cherry JD, editors: Textbook of pediatric infectious diseases, ed 2, Philadelphia, 1987, WB Saunders Co.

Remington JS and Klein JO: Infectious diseases of the fetus and newborn infant, ed 2, Philadelphia, 1983, WB Saunders Co.

Rubinstein A: Pediatric AIDS, Curr Probl Pediatr 16:361, 1986.

Herpesviruses

John J. LiPuma *and* Terrence L. Stull

There are four members of the human herpesvirus family: herpes simplex virus (HSV or herpesvirus hominis), varicella-zoster virus (VZV or herpesvirus varicellae), cytomegalovirus (CMV), and Epstein-Barr virus (EBV). These relatively large viruses are comprised of a DNA core, an icosahedral protein capsid, and an outer lipid envelope. They are worldwide in distribution and produce disease at any age from the fetal period to the geriatric years. The infections vary in severity from trivial to fatal, with the most serious infections occurring in the immunocompromised host. Following the primary infection, a persistent viral carrier state is established.

Each of the herpesviruses is discussed individually. Infections in the fetus and newborn are described in the preceding section.

HERPES SIMPLEX VIRUS

EPIDEMIOLOGY. There are two subtypes of herpes simplex virus (HSV) that differ in their antigenicity and anatomic distribution. HSV-1 more frequently causes oral lesions, and HSV-2 is usually isolated from the genital area. However, both subtypes can cause genital and oral lesions. Both subtypes cause infections throughout the world; however, although small outbreaks are seen, large-scale epidemics do not occur.

The initial infection with HSV is asymptomatic in 80% to 90% of the patients. Serologic surveys have established antibody prevalence rates of 50% to 100% among adults, depending on socioeconomic status. In children the majority of infections are caused by HSV-1, which is transmitted nonvenereally. HSV-2 is increasingly common after puberty, primarily as a result of spread by the genital route. HSV infections are frequently seen in patients with acquired immunodeficiency syndrome (AIDS).

PATHOGENESIS. After inoculation at the primary site on the skin or mucosa, HSV replicates locally. In the intact host viremia has been infrequently observed; however, despite an immune response, the virus spreads to local ganglion cells via ascension along the neurons. Humoral antibodies achieve detectable levels in 1 to 3 weeks, and cell-mediated immunity can be demonstrated concurrently. Various local and systemic insults such as trauma or fever can reactivate the latent virus.

Pathologically, the lesions of HSV are characterized by intranuclear inclusions and multinucleated giant cells. Degeneration of epithelial cells leads to interstitial edema and vesicle formation. Subsequently, polymorphonuclear leukocytes invade the area.

In the severely malnourished or immunocompromised host, viremia may result in visceral dissemination. Characteristic lesions, as described previously, are seen in the involved organs.

CLINICAL MANIFESTATIONS. The incubation period ranges from 2 to 20 days, with the average being 1 week. Primary infections produce clinically apparent lesions on the skin or mucosa in only 10% to 20% of cases. Acute gingivostomatitis is the most common manifestation in childhood, and it is increasingly seen among young seronegative adults with lower socioeconomic backgrounds. The illness begins with fever and inflammation of the oral mucosa. Over the next 1 to 2 days painful vesicular lesions appear in the mouth, usually anteriorly. These painful lesions can involve the facial area, as well as the hard palate, soft palate, gingiva, tongue, and lips. The regional lymph nodes swell and become tender. Ulceration of the vesicles occurs rapidly, but complete resolution requires up to 14 days.

Primary infections also occur at sites of cutaneous trauma. In athletes this manifestation is referred to as herpes gladiatorum. Patients with extensive atopic dermatitis are susceptible to widespread skin involvement (eczema herpeticum). Herpetic whitlow, an infection of the fingers often seen in healthcare personnel, can be misdiagnosed as a pyogenic bacterial infection. Prompt diagnosis of this condition is necessary to avoid transmission to patients. The eye is rarely the site of a primary infection. Primary genital infections have become increasingly prevalent. In some venereal disease clinics herpes simplex is the most common cause of genital ulcerations. There are two clinical syndromes of primary infection in the central nervous system. A benign aseptic meningitis is associated with HSV-2, and an extremely severe encephalitis is associated with HSV-1 (see discussion of "Viral infections of the central nervous system").

Recurrent infections are more common than primary infections, particularly in patients over 30 years of age. Herpes labialis is the most frequent and well-known manifestation, but vesicles can reappear at any site of initial infection. Chronic mucocutaneous herpes and herpetic esophagitis are opportunistic infections commonly seen in patients with AIDS.

LABORATORY FINDINGS. There are no characteristic laboratory findings with skin or mucous membrane infection. A mononuclear pleocytosis in the cerebrospinal fluid (CSF) generally accompanies central nervous system (CNS) involvement. Encephalitis caused by HSV is manifested as a focal lesion by radionuclide scanning, computed tomography (CT), or electroencephalogram (EEG).

DIAGNOSIS. Histologic evidence of intranuclear inclusions and multinucleated giant cells at the base of a vesicle or in tissue is suggestive of an HSV infection. Immunofluorescent staining of brain biopsy specimens has proved useful clinically. A definitive diagnosis is made by isolation of the virus. Inoculation of tissue cultures produces cytopathic changes rapidly, often in 48 hours. Acute and convalescent sera can be tested for antibodies using a complement fixation, immunofluorescent, or neutralization assay. A fourfold rise in titer points to a recent infection.

The differential diagnosis of gingivostomatitis includes herpangina as a result of group A coxsackieviruses (see discussion of "Exanthems of viral or presumed viral origin") and thrush caused by *Candida* species. The lesions in herpes simplex are located predominantly in the anterior portion of the mouth, whereas those resulting from coxsackievirus typically are seen in the posterior oropharynx. In addition, the duration of illness is longer with herpes simplex virus. Genital herpetic lesions can be confused with chancroid or syphilis. Herpes encephalitis can be initially seen as a mass lesion or resemble disease caused by the arboviruses.

COURSE. In the normal host, primary herpetic infections resolve spontaneously in 1 to 2 weeks. Persistence should prompt an investigation for immunodeficiency. Gingivostomatitis can lead to dehydration as a result of limitation of oral intake because of painful mouth lesions. Bacterial superinfection occurs occasionally. The widespread cutaneous disease seen with extensive disruption of the integument has a more complicated course and can be fatal. Recurrent infections are generally mild and of short duration.

Immunocompromised patients have more frequent and longer lasting mucocutaneous infections than the general population. However, visceral dissemination is reported only rarely.

MANAGEMENT. The treatment of gingivostomatitis is supportive. Topical anesthetics and systemic analgesics provide some relief from pain; young children occasionally require intravenous hydration.

Ocular involvement mandates ophthalmologic consultation. Topical vidarabine, idoxuridine, and acyclovir are beneficial, whereas steroids are contraindicated. Intravenous acyclovir (10 mg/kg every 8 hours for 10 days) has been shown to be superior to vidarabine in the treatment of HSV encephalitis. Oral acyclovir (200 mg five times per day) has some benefit in the treatment of primary and recurrent episodes of genital infections, and long-term prophylactic use of acyclovir (400 to 1000 mg/day) reduces the frequency of recurrent disease in patients with frequent genital infections.

PREVENTION. Patients who have extensive skin disease or who are immunocompromised should avoid contact with patients who have active skin lesions. Sexual contact should be avoided during the active phase of genital herpes. In Scandinavian countries the use of condoms has markedly reduced the incidence of primary genital herpes infection. Attempts at prevention with passive immunization have been ineffective, but trials of active immunization using a subunit herpes simplex vaccine are in progress.

VARICELLA-ZOSTER VIRUS

EPIDEMIOLOGY. Herpesvirus varicellae, the cause of both zoster (shingles) and varicella (chickenpox), has a worldwide distribution. Varicella is endemic in industrialized countries and occurs in epidemics among clustered subgroups of susceptible children in settings such as classrooms or hospital wards. This disease is most prevalent during the winter and spring.

Varicella occurs predominantly in children between 2 and 10 years of age. Although transplacental passage of antibodies has been demonstrated, they do not confer protection against infection with the same reliability observed in many other childhood diseases. Thus cases occasionally are seen in the first few months of life. Sporadic episodes also occur in susceptible adults. Most adults are seropositive from childhood exposures, since the attack rate within households is 90%. Seroepidemiologic surveys using the complement fixation technique have detected antibodies in 70% of the 10- to 20-year-old population in the United States; however, this is an underestimate of immunity, since these antibodies frequently decline to undetectable levels, with patients still being protected against infection.

Transmission is by airborne droplets and direct contact with infectious lesions. An individual is considered contagious from 1 to 2 days before the eruption until all the lesions are crusted, usually 6 to 7 days after eruption. However, infectivity decreases markedly after the first 3 days of illness.

In contrast to varicella, zoster occurs predominantly in older adults. More than 60% of episodes are in individuals over 45 years of age, although the disease is seen occasionally in childhood. There is an increased incidence of zoster in immunocompromised hosts, for example those with Hodgkin's disease or AIDS.

Since a reactivation of latent virus is the antecedent of the eruption in zoster, an individual does not acquire this disease from an exogenous source. However, in a susceptible person exposed to zoster lesions, varicella can develop. Viral shedding occurs until all lesions are crusted, usually after 7 to 10 days in the normal host.

PATHOGENESIS. Entry of the virus, probably through the oropharynx, is followed in the susceptible host first by local replication and then by dissemination via the blood or lymphatics. Viremia occurs before the onset of the exanthem. Specific humoral and cellular immune responses terminate the viremic stage, but enlargement of cutaneous lesions continues for several days. These intraepidermal vesicles become pustular after invasion by polymorphonuclear leukocytes. Multinucleated giant cells are located at the base of the vesicles.

It is postulated that during an episode of varicella, virus invades sensory nerve endings and ascends along the nerve fibers to the dorsal root ganglion where it becomes latent.

Zoster is the reactivation of this latent virus. The virus then migrates along the nerve to the skin, resulting in eruptions typically confined to a single dermatome. Vesicle formation outside a dermatome occurs occasionally in 25% of healthy individuals with zoster, probably caused by viremia. In immunocompromised patients extensive disease can occur outside a dermatome and virus can be isolated from the blood.

CLINICAL MANIFESTATIONS. In the normal individual the incubation period of varicella is 10 to 21 days, with an average of 14 days. A mild 1- to 3-day prodrome of fever and malaise frequently precedes the exanthem; however, the presence of the rash is often the first sign of illness. In children the fever seldom exceeds 103.1° F (39.5° C) and accompanies the rash for 2 to 3 days. The fever and malaise are more pronounced in adults.

The exanthem appears initially on the trunk or face and spreads centripetally. The individual lesions are pruritic and evolve from erythematous macules and papules to vesicles and then pustules. This transition can occur rapidly over 6 or 8 hours. Early vesicles are 2 to 4 mm in diameter and have a "dewdroplike" appearance. Successive crops of new lesions erupt for 2 to 4 days and involve the mucosa of the oropharynx and vagina. Resolution occurs by rupture of the pustules and crusting. Characteristically there are lesions at all stages in any one area of the body. The severity of the cutaneous involvement in varicella is quite variable; the total number of lesions may vary from one or two to several hundred.

Fever may or may not be present with zoster. The eruptions are often preceded by neuralgia, which is generally more severe in adults. Aside from confinement to a single dermatome in zoster, the appearance and evolution of the lesions are identical in both zoster and varicella. Regional lymph nodes are generally enlarged. Visceral involvement with pneumonitis, meningoencephalitis, and hepatitis is seen in immunocompromised patients with malignancies but has not been reported in AIDS patients.

LABORATORY FINDINGS. There are no significant laboratory findings in uncomplicated varicella or zoster. In most cases the white blood cell count is within the normal range. If dissemination occurs, there can be leukocytosis, marked elevation of liver enzymes, pleocytosis in the cerebrospinal fluid, and infiltrates on the chest roentgenogram.

DIAGNOSIS. The typical case of varicella or zoster is diagnosed on the basis of clinical features, but laboratory confirmation is available. A Giemsa-stained smear from the base of a vesicle shows multinucleated giant cells. Varicella virus can be isolated from vesicular fluid obtained early in the course. Serologic tests include complement fixation (CF), fluorescent antibody to membrane antigen (FAMA), immune adherence hemagglutination (IAHA), and neutralization.

The differential diagnosis of varicella includes eczema herpeticum, insect bites, scabies, and impetigo. Zoster can be confused at times with herpes simplex. In the preeruptive phase the pain can resemble that of pleural, cardiac, or peritoneal origin.

COURSE. In the normal host varicella is a mild disease, although adults often experience more pronounced malaise. The lesions develop crusts by the end of a week and resolve in another 4 to 7 days. Secondary bacterial infection of the skin with staphylococci or streptococci is the most common complication and rarely can lead to distant septic foci. CNS complications occur in approximately 1:2500 cases and vary from mild aseptic meningitis to fulminating encephalitis. Cerebellar ataxia, the most common manifestation of CNS involvement, is typically seen towards the end of the first week after the onset of the rash. From 20% to 30% of cases of Reye's syndrome follow varicella. Transverse myelitis and Guillain-Barré syndrome have also been described as neurologic complications of varicella. Pneumonia occurs mainly in adults. Other rare complications include myocarditis, hepatitis, uveitis, orchitis, glomerulonephritis, arthritis, and hemorrhagic diathesis.

In immunosuppressed patients, particularly with lymphoreticular malignancies, varicella is a serious infection. In addition to the complications just listed, visceral dissemination occurs in 25% to 33% of the cases. The lungs, liver, and CNS are frequently involved, leading to a mortality rate of 5% to 10%.

The eruption in zoster follows a course similar to that of varicella, but the duration of lesions and time for healing are often slightly longer. Postherpetic neuralgia and secondary bacterial infection can follow zoster in any location. The former is more frequent in adults. Other complications depend on the segmental localization. Ocular lesions occur in up to 50% of trigeminal nerve cases and can lead to visual impairment. Zoster of the seventh cranial nerve can produce facial palsy (Hunt's syndrome), and with involvement of cervical ganglia, diaphragmatic paralysis. Zoster can also disseminate viscerally in the immunocompromised patient, but this is not a frequent occurrence. As in varicella, the organs involved include the liver, lungs, and brain. Cutaneous dissemination can occur with or without visceral disease.

MANAGEMENT. In the normal host with varicella or zoster, symptomatic treatment alone is provided in the form of analgesics and antipruritics. Ocular involvement in zoster demands the attention of an ophthalmologist and can require the instillation of topical steroids and antibiotics.

Varicella or zoster infection in an immunocompromised host should be treated with parenteral antiviral chemotherapy. Acyclovir (500 mg/m² administered intravenously every 8 hours) has been shown to be superior to vidarabine for such patients and is currently regarded as the treatment of choice.

PREVENTION. Epidemiologic measures, as well as both passive and active immunization, play a role in the prevention of varicella. Patients with lesions are isolated until crusting occurs, and susceptible individuals exposed to the disease should be excluded from critical areas such as hospitals from 10 to 21 days after the onset of the rash in the index patient. Varicella-zoster immune globulin (VZIG), a γ-globulin preparation with a high titer of antibodies to varicella-zoster virus, has been demonstrated to be effective in preventing the disease if administered within 72 hours of exposure. This therapy is indicated in patients with neoplasms or primary immunodeficiency and those undergoing immunosuppressive therapy, but not the normal host. A vaccine containing attenuated live virus has been shown to be effective in preventing varicella in both children with leukemia and healthy children. The long-term safety and protective efficacy of the vaccine continue to be evaluated.

CYTOMEGALOVIRUS

EPIDEMIOLOGY. Cytomegalovirus (CMV) has a worldwide distribution. It is found endemically and has no seasonal pattern. Of infants in the United States 1% to 2% acquire this infection perinatally and another 10% during the first 3 months of life. By 10 years of age approximately 33% of children have seroconverted, and by the age of 70 years 80% to 90% of the population is seropositive.

The mode of acquisition of CMV remains to be definitively established, but it appears that direct contact is necessary for the spread of natural infection. Transmission of CMV among children in day-care settings has been described. Both blood transfusions and organ transplantation can also transmit CMV. Following a primary infection, the virus persists in a latent state. Conditions such as neoplasia and pregnancy or the use of immunosuppressive medications often induce a reactivation of endogenous infection leading to excretion of virus.

In the normal host the vast majority of illnesses caused by CMV after the newborn period are asymptomatic. Serious, often fatal, infections do occur with frequency in patients with AIDS and other immunodeficiencies.

PATHOGENESIS. The pathogenesis of postnatally acquired CMV in humans remains uncertain. Viremia has been demonstrated during primary infection. Almost any organ system can be affected during this phase. The liver, kidneys, and salivary glands are frequently involved. A primary CMV infection evokes both humoral and cell-mediated immune responses that contain the infection. Histologically, CMV disease is characterized by enlarged cells that contain intranuclear inclusions. Focal areas of necrosis occur, and there is an infiltration of mononuclear cells.

CLINICAL MANIFESTATIONS. The incubation period of naturally acquired CMV is unknown; however, symptoms begin 3 weeks after the transfusion of infected blood and a mean of 6 weeks after renal transplantation. The majority of immunologically normal children and adults with antibody to CMV remain asymptomatic or have a mild, nonspecific illness. In probably 1% or fewer an infectious mononucleosis–like (IM-like) syndrome, hepatitis, or pneumonia develops. The IM-like syndrome is characterized by 2 to 6 weeks of fever, mild adenopathy, minimal pharyngitis, and hepatitis. This syndrome has been observed in 10% of patients following open heart surgery with extracorporeal circulation. Hepatitis caused by CMV is generally mild. Neurologic syndromes described in association with this virus include encephalitis and the Guillain-Barré syndrome.

Both primary infection and reactivation of latent virus represent a serious threat to the immunocompromised host. A syndrome of severe respiratory distress and hepatomegaly during early infancy has been described. In childhood leukemia up to 25% of the patients excrete CMV when followed longitudinally, and pathologic evidence of disseminated disease is seen in 2% to 3% at autopsy. CMV infection occurs in as many as 90% of renal allograft recipients. Approximately half are asymptomatic. The rest have prolonged fever, leukopenia, thrombocytopenia, pneumonia, or hepatitis. CMV pneumonia occurs in 30% of individuals receiving bone marrow transplants.

Active CMV infection is common in AIDS patients. Dissemination to lungs, gastrointestinal tract, and CNS produces significant morbidity and mortality in this population. Retinitis caused by CMV is the leading cause of blindness in AIDS patients.

LABORATORY FINDINGS. In CMV mononucleosis and the postperfusion syndrome there is significant lymphocytosis. As many as 25% of the mononuclear cells can be atypical. Although mild to moderate elevation of the liver enzymes occurs frequently, significant hyperbilirubinemia is rare.

DIAGNOSIS. The diagnosis of CMV infection may be suggested pathologically by the presence of intranuclear inclusions in biopsy material or in exfoliated cells in the urine. They are present in less than half of the confirmed cases. The virus can be routinely cultured from the urine of infants and young children with infection, and viral excretion can continue for years in congenitally infected children. CMV can be isolated from greater than 90% of AIDS patients from sites including throat,

urine, and blood. Serologic testing is available by many methods including CF, indirect immunofluorescence, and neutralization. It is often difficult, however, to distinguish a primary infection from reactivation, even with specific serology and recovery of the virus, unless a preillness serum sample has no measurable antibodies. A fluorescent test to detect an IgM response and measurement of antibodies to early antigens currently suffers from technical difficulties and limited availability.

The differential diagnosis of acquired CMV includes hepatitis, toxoplasmosis, and other IM-like syndromes (see discussion of "Epstein-Barr virus").

COURSE. Most infections with CMV, whether asymptomatic or clinically evident, resolve without complications in the immunologically intact host beyond the neonatal period. Immunocompromised patients experience more severe infections with this virus. CMV infections requiring hospitalization occur frequently in renal transplant recipients. The rate of graft rejection is significantly increased in these patients. In patients receiving bone marrow transplants CMV is the most commonly identified cause of interstitial pneumonia and has a fatality rate of 60% to 90%. Overwhelming CMV infection is believed to be a major contributing factor to the high mortality among AIDS patients.

Effective therapy for CMV infections has not been demonstrated. However, the combination of acyclovir and vidarabine inhibits viral replication in vitro, and a new agent, dihydroxy-propoxy-methyl guanine (DHPG), has shown promise in preliminary clinical trials among AIDS patients.

PREVENTION. In a double-blind, placebo-controlled prophylactic trial, human leukocyte interferon delayed, but did not prevent, viral excretion in renal transplant recipients. Trials of passive immunization with high-titer CMV immunoglobulin are currently under way in high-risk patients. A live attenuated vaccine with demonstrated safety and immunogenicity in normal individuals and renal transplant patients has been developed. Studies of vaccine efficacy are now being conducted.

EPSTEIN-BARR VIRUS

EPIDEMIOLOGY. The Epstein-Barr virus (EBV) causes infectious mononucleosis (IM) and is etiologically associated with Burkitt's lymphoma (BL) and nasopharyngeal carcinoma (NPC). Infections with EBV have been detected serologically in all parts of the world. Based on these antibody surveys, primary EBV infection generally occurs in early childhood in underdeveloped countries under conditions of crowding and poor hygiene. Infants in the first 6 months of life are spared because of protection by maternal antibodies. A survey in Ghana, Africa, found a seroconversion rate of 85% by age 2 years. In economically advanced countries, however, nearly half of the more affluent individuals escape infection until late adolescence. Among college students, there is then a seroconversion rate of 10% to 15% yearly. In contrast to young infants (who remain asymptomatic) 33% to 50% of adolescents and young adults undergoing a primary EBV infection manifest the clinical picture of infectious mononucleosis. In school-age children there are sporadic cases of IM, but the majority of EBV infections are thought to be asymptomatic. Occasionally episodes of clinical disease are described in adults even in the seventh and eighth decades. In the United States 90% of the population have antibodies at age 30 years.

Intimate salivary contact appears to be the most frequent mode of transmission of EBV. This has led to the name "kissing disease." Although airborne spread has been postulated as an explanation for one outbreak of IM, there is not an increased

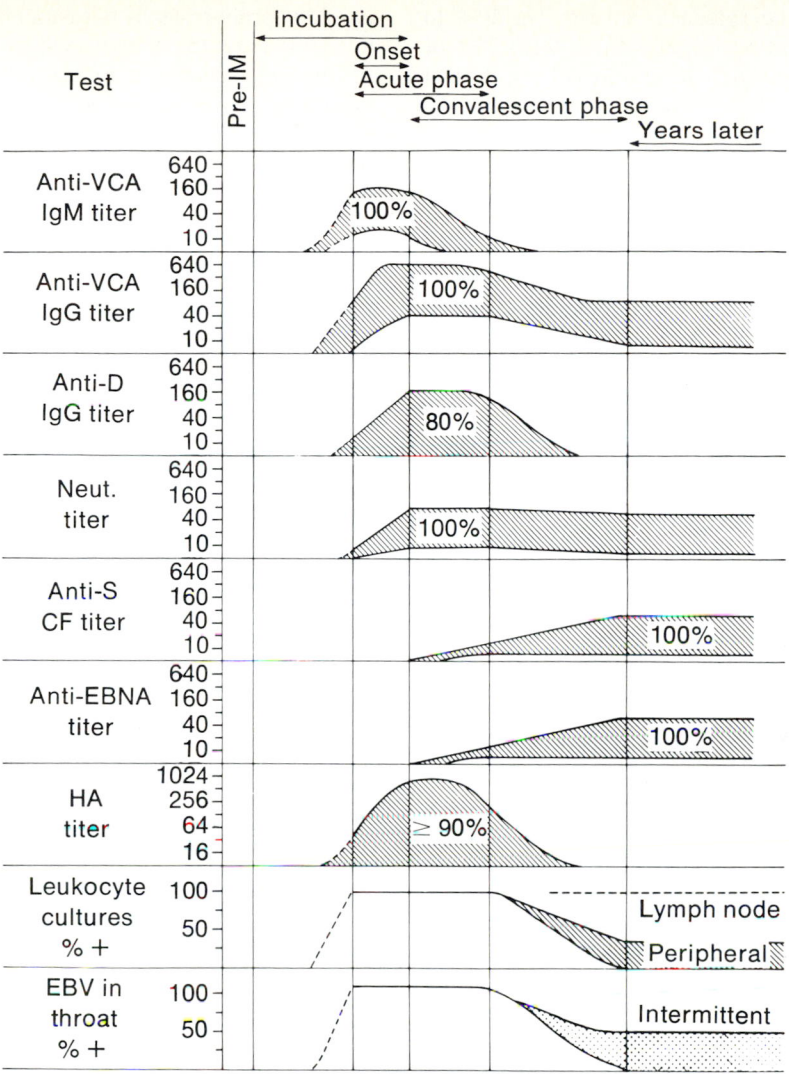

Fig. 37-1   Scheme of antibody response, leukocyte cultures, and EBV assays in throat washings during course of infectious mononucleosis. *IM*, Infectious mononucleosis; *Anit-VCA*, antibody against viral capsid antigen; *Anti-D*, antibody against diffuse component of early antigen complex; *Neut.*, neutralizing; *Anti-S*, antibody against soluble antigen; *Anti-EBNA*, antibody against EB virus–associated nuclear antigens; *HA*, hemagglutination antibody; *EBV*, EB virus. (From Henle W, Henle G, and Horwitz CA: Hum Pathol 5:551, 1974.)

incidence of disease among college roommates or classmates of clinically ill individuals.

EBV, in addition to causing IM, has been linked with two forms of cancer, BL and NPC. EBV was initially discovered in a lymphocyte culture from a child with BL. This lymphoma occurs predominantly in Africa, and virtually all African children with BL have very high titers of antibodies to EBV. Additionally, EBV genomes have been demonstrated in BL cells. NPC occurs frequently in southern China and northern Africa. Again, there are high titers of antibodies to EBV almost universally, and the genome is found in the tumor cells. However, in other parts of the world many cases are not EBV associated. Although several lines of evidence implicate EBV as a causal agent, other environmental or host factors are important, since the vast majority of infected individuals remain free of these neoplasms.

PATHOGENESIS. The pathogenesis of IM remains speculative. The virus enters via the oropharynx, invading and replicating in epithelial cells. Although the infection can be somewhat contained in asymptomatic cases, spread to circulating B lymphocytes and lymph nodes occurs in symptomatic IM. Both

an antibody and a cellular immune response develop to the virus. The atypical lymphocytes seen on peripheral smear are primarily suppressor-T cells responding to neoantigens on transformed B lymphocytes.

There is extensive hyperplasia of the lymphoid tissues in IM. The lymph nodes retain their follicular appearance, but the sinuses are invaded by macrophages and atypical lymphocytes. Infiltration of mononuclear cells may be noted in almost every organ.

CLINICAL MANIFESTATIONS. Following an incubation period of 4 to 6 weeks, the usual patient with IM has the triad of fever, sore throat, and extensive adenopathy. Malaise is a prominent early symptom that can persist for several months. The fever varies but can be as high as 102° to 104° F (39° to 40° C) and remain elevated 3 or 4 weeks. The pharynx is usually intensively inflamed, at times with exudate. Lymph nodes in any region may enlarge. Although anterior cervical adenopathy accompanies pharyngitis of any cause, posterior cervical involvement is very suggestive of IM. Nodal enlargement in the inguinal and axillary areas is common. Mediastinal widening has been described in patients with IM as a result of lymphoid hyperplasia at the hilum. The spleen is enlarged in 50% to 60% of the cases, and the liver is enlarged in 10% to 20% of the cases. Additional findings include periorbital edema and an occasional maculopapular rash. Petechiae may occur at the junction of the hard and soft palates.

EBV-specific serologic alterations have been associated with Reye's syndrome, Kawasaki disease, lymphoma of the CNS, hemophagocytosis, and chronic fatigue; the possible role of EBV in these conditions is not clear.

LABORATORY FINDINGS. The white blood cell count in most cases is 10,000 to 15,000/mm^3, but a leukocytosis of up to 30,000/mm^3 is not unusual. There is an absolute lymphocytosis, frequently 70% to 80%, and many of the lymphocytes appear atypical. Heterophil antibodies to sheep or horse red blood cells are detectable in 90% of adolescents but less frequently in younger children by routine assays. If followed serially, liver enzymes are significantly elevated in over 95% of the patients. Hyperbilirubinemia, however, is minimal and less frequent. Anemia and thrombocytopenia occur at times.

DIAGNOSIS. Usually the diagnosis of IM is made on the basis of the clinical and hematologic features in association with a significantly elevated heterophil antibody titer. As mentioned, these antibodies to sheep or horse red cells appear in 90% of the cases among adolescents. The specificity of the heterophil antibody response can be established by differential absorption with beef red cells and guinea pig kidney. The IM-specific antibodies are absorbed by the former but not by the latter.

In heterophil-negative IM or in atypical EBV infections the diagnosis is made by assay of virus-specific antibodies. Antibodies are directed against viral capsid antigen (VCA), early antigens (EA), and EBV-associated nuclear antigen (EBNA). Each of these antibodies has a different chronology in relation to the time of EBV infection (Fig. 37-1). The IgM anti-VCA and IgG anti-VCA appear early in the course. Whereas the IgM response disappears in 4 to 6 weeks, the IgG anti-VCA response merely declines to lower levels that persist for life. About 80% of the patients with IM show a transient response to the diffuse (D) component of the early antigen complex, whereas antibodies to the restricted (R) component often develop in individuals with asymptomatic infections. In contrast to the antibodies just mentioned, those to EBNA appear, with few exceptions, weeks to months after the onset of illness. Viral culture is not a useful diagnostic tool, since it does not distinguish between past infection and recent infection. During the course of a primary EBV infection, the presence of virus can be demonstrated in oropharyngeal secretions (Fig. 37-1). The addition of this material to cord blood lmyphocytes produces transformation in a large percentage of cases. However, there is intermittent excretion of virus in the oropharynx for many years after the primary infection.

Several organisms produce an IM-like syndrome and thus enter into the differential diagnosis. Those most frequently responsible include cytomegalovirus and *Toxoplasma*. Serum sickness and drug reactions can lead to a similar clinical picture.

COURSE. Most infections with EBV are asymptomatic, and these generally resolve without complications. Occasionally IM is a brief illness, but the usual course is 4 to 6 weeks. Lymphadenopathy may persist for 3 months or longer. A subgroup of patients with recurrent episodes of fever and malaise may have chronic IM.

Complications, although infrequent, can involve almost any organ in both symptomatic and asymptomatic infections. Lym-phoid hyperplasia leads occasionally to significant respiratory obstruction by the tonsils and stretches the capsule of the spleen, predisposing it to rupture with even minor trauma. Neurologic involvement includes encephalitis, Guillain-Barré syndrome, and peripheral neuropathy. Hemolytic anemia and thrombocytopenia are at times clinically significant. Uveitis, myocarditis, pneumonia, nephritis, and Reye's syndrome have all been reported in association with IM. Unlike the other herpesviruses, EBV does not cause particularly severe disease in immunosuppressed patients other than those with X-linked immunoproliferative syndrome; however, the interactions of infections caused by EBV and human immunodeficiency virus (HIV) are an area of active investigation.

MANAGEMENT. No specific antiviral therapy is available. The treatment is directed at alleviation of the symptoms. The malaise and fatigue mandate a period of decreased activity, the duration being determined by the severity of the illness. Because of the potential for splenic rupture, the patient should be cautioned to avoid contact sports for at least 6 weeks. Aspirin or acetaminophen is frequently sufficient for analgesia, but orally administered corticosteroids (up to 60 mg prednisone each day) can be necessary for patients with a more toxic condition. The lympholytic property of the steroids also makes them useful in the therapy of complications clearly resulting from lymphoid hyperplasia such as airway obstruction by large tonsils. Occasionally a patient requires hospitalization and intravenous hydration.

PREVENTION. The patient with IM should avoid intimate oral contact with others while virus excretion in the saliva is heaviest during the period of clinical illness. However, no isolation measures are indicated. Neither passive nor active immunization has been studied in humans. However, viral antigens have been purified as the first step in the preparation of a vaccine.

BIBLIOGRAPHY
Herpes simplex virus

Corey L and Spear PG: Infections with herpes simplex viruses. I. N Engl J Med 314:686, 1986.

Corey L and Spear PG: Infections with herpes simplex virus. II. N Engl J Med 314:749, 1986.

Glezen WP, Fernald GW, and Cohn JN: Acute respiratory disease of university students with special reference to the etiologic role of herpesvirus hominis, Am J Epidemiol 101:111, 1975.

Rawls WE and others: Measurement of antibodies to herpesvirus types 1 and 2 in human sera, J Immunol 117:728, 1976.

Whitley RJ and others: Vidarabine versus acyclovir therapy in herpes simplex encephalitis, N Engl J Med 314:144, 1986.

Douglas JM and others: A double-blind study of oral acyclovir for suppression of recurrences of genital herpes simplex virus infection, N Engl J Med 310:1551, 1984.

Varicella-zoster virus

Gershon AA: The success of varicella vaccine, Pediatr Infect Dis 3:500, 1984.

Gershon AA and Krugman S: Seroepidemiologic survey of varicella: value of specific fluorescent antibody test, Pediatrics 56:1005, 1975.

Preblud SR, Orenstein WA, and Bart KJ: Varicella: clinical manifestations, epidemiology and health impact in children, Pediatr Infect Dis 3:505, 1984.

Shepp DH, Dandliker PS, and Meyers JD: Treatment of varicella-zoster virus infection in severely immunocompromised patients, N Engl J Med 314:208, 1986.

Weller TH: Varicella and herpes zoster. I. N Engl J Med 309:1362, 1983.

Weller TH: Varicella and herpes zoster. II. N Engl J Med 309:1434, 1983.

Cytomegalovirus

Glenn J: Cytomegalovirus infections following renal transplantation, Rev Infect Dis 3:1151, 1981.

Machen AM and others: Death in the AIDS patient: role of cytomegalovirus, N Engl J Med 309:1454, 1983.

Masur H and others: Effect of 9-(1,3-dihydroxy-2-propoxy methyl)guanine on serious cytomegalovirus disease in 8 immunosuppressed homosexual men, Ann Intern Med 104:41, 1986.

Murph JR and others: Cytomegalovirus transmission in a Midwest day-care center: possible relationship to child care practices, J Pediatr 109:35, 1986.

Yow MD and others: Acquisition of cytomegalovirus infection from birth to 10 years: a longitudinal serologic study, J Pediatr 110:37, 1987.

Epstein-Barr virus

Andiman AA: Epstein-Barr virus-associated syndromes: a critical reexamination, Pediatr Infect Dis 3:198, 1984.

Henle W and Henle GE: Seroepidemiology to the virus. In Epstein M and Achang B, editors: The Epstein-Barr virus, Berlin, 1979, Springer-Verlag.

Henle W, Henle GE, and Horwitz CA: Epstein-Barr virus specific diagnostic tests in infectious mononucleosis, Hum Pathol 5:551, 1974.

Rinaldo CR and others: Association of HTLV-III with Epstein-Barr virus infection and abnormalities of T lymphocytes in homosexual men, J Infect Dis 154:556, 1986.

Straus SE and others: Persisting illness and fatigue in adults with evidence of Epstein-Barr virus infection, Ann Intern Med 102:7, 1985.

Viral infections of the central nervous system

Stephen Gluckman

(See also Chapter 151.)

Acute viral infections of the central nervous system (CNS) are more frequent than reported data would indicate. Some diagnosed infections are unreported, many more presumed viral infections are unproven, and probably still more are not even suspected. Recent statistics compiled by the Centers for Disease Control in Atlanta, Georgia, describe about 4500 cases of acute viral CNS infections each year in the United States. About one third are encephalitis, and the remainder are aseptic meningitis. A discussion of the major causes of acute viral CNS infections is included here. A relatively recent addition to the list is the human immunodeficiency virus (HIV). It must be stressed at the outset that the clinical syndromes and cerebrospinal fluid (CSF) findings are rarely specific for viral infections; therefore nonviral causes that are often treatable must be considered and recognized.

DEFINITIONS. The distinction between aseptic meningitis and encephalitis is determined by clinical features, although the syndromes can overlap. Although some organisms are more likely to cause one syndrome than the other, in general, infection with an organism may produce either syndrome. Aseptic meningitis implies meningeal inflammation. Patients may be lethargic, but their CNS function remains normal. In encephalitis CNS functional impairment can manifest as altered mental status, motor or sensory deficits, or movement disorders. In most patients with encephalitis there are also findings of meningeal inflammation, and hence the term "meningoencephalitis" is properly used.

Encephalitis can be either primary or postinfectious. In the former there is invasion of the CNS by the pathogen. Histologically, neuronal involvement is found. The virus can often be cultured from the tissue, and inclusion bodies on light microscopy or viral particles on electron microscopy may be seen. In postinfectious encephalitis the virus cannot be seen or recovered and the neurons are spared; however, perivascular infiltrates and demyelination are present. It occurs after an infectious illness or the administration of certain vaccines. The pathogenesis of this disease has not been clearly established, but it is presumed to have a hypersensitivity basis. Infections with certain viruses may result in either syndrome.

ETIOLOGY. The following are major causes of aseptic meningitis and encephalitis in the United States:

Primary infections

Herpes simplex viruses types 1 and 2
Enteroviruses
 Coxsackievirus A
 Coxsackievirus B
 Echovirus
 Poliovirus
Arboviruses
 California encephalitis virus
 Eastern equine encephalitis virus
 Western equine encephalitis virus
 St. Louis encephalitis virus
 Venezuelan equine encephalitis virus
Childhood infections
 Mumps virus
 Measles virus
 Varicella-zoster virus
HIV
Other
 Cytomegaloviruses
 Epstein-Barr virus
 Lymphocytic choriomeningitis virus
 Adenoviruses
 Rabies virus
 Influenza virus

Postinfectious

Measles, mumps, varicella, rubella, influenza
Vaccine associated: vaccinia, yellow fever, rabies (duck embryo vaccine), pertussis

Several generalizations can help in approaching the specific origin of viral CNS infections. Of the proven causes of aseptic meningitis, the vast majority are associated with enteroviruses or with mumps; the former occur primarily in the summer and fall and the latter in the winter and spring. Other causes are rarely found. Similarly, the majority of proven encephalitis cases are caused by arboviruses, childhood infections, herpes simplex type 1, or HIV. Arboviruses predominate in the summer and fall. Childhood infections are most common in the winter and spring but like herpes virus can occur throughout the year. By merely using these few facts, most of the provable cases can be identified. The most common causes of aseptic meningitis and encephalitis where a cause is defined are as follows:

 Aseptic meningitis
 Summer-fall: enteroviruses
 Winter-spring: mumps
 Encephalitis
 Summer-fall: arboviruses
 Winter-spring: mumps
 Throughout year: herpes simplex, HIV

CLINICAL MANIFESTATIONS. The clinical presentation of aseptic meningitis is generally nonspecific, with fever and headache. Physical examination usually detects signs of meningeal irritation, but unless there are findings related to the specific virus (for example, swollen parotid glands with mumps, skin rash with enteroviruses), there are no other abnormalities. Encephalitis can have a similar presentation, but in addition, there is altered mental status ranging from a subtle inability to calculate to complete unresponsiveness. Seizures are common, and focal abnormalities such as hemiparesis can develop. Hypothalamic involvement can result in either diabetes insipidus or the syndrome of inappropriate antidiuretic hormone (ADH) secretion. In the encephalitis of herpes simplex there are characteristically bizarre behavior, olfactory hallucinations, and aphasia, suggesting temporal lobe localization.

Examination of the CSF, although not diagnostic, confirms the presence of CNS disease. The CSF protein is generally elevated; usually this is only to modestly high levels (that is, less than 150 mg/dl). The CSF glucose level is usually normal (greater than 50% of the simultaneous blood glucose). However, infections with herpes simplex type 1, mumps, some enteroviruses, and lymphocytic choriomeningitis can result in hypoglycorrhachia. The CSF glucose is usually not at the extremely low levels seen with pyogenic bacteria, but such values should raise the possibility of other diagnoses, including tuberculosis, cryptococcosis, or meningeal spread of tumor. The CSF white blood cell count is typically elevated. However, levels of greater than 1000/mm³ are unusual and should prompt concern for other, nonviral causes. In general, lymphocytes predominate, but early in the course there can be a predominance of polymorphonuclear leukocytes. A repeat CSF cell count in 8 hours should show a clear shift from polymorphonuclear leukocytes to lymphocytes in 90% of those with viral disease.

In a patient with viral encephalitis the presence of red blood cells in the CSF that are not the result of a traumatic lumbar puncture should suggest herpes simplex.

HERPES SIMPLEX

Herpes simplex type 2 is traditionally associated with genital infections. It can, however, produce CNS disease. In newborns it is responsible for severe, usually fatal disseminated disease with encephalitis. In adults, however, the illness is characteristically an aseptic meningitis rather than encephalitis.

In contrast to type 2, herpes simplex type 1 CNS infections in adults usually result in encephalitis. Specific diagnosis is established only if brain tissue is obtained for viral studies by biopsy. Untreated, biopsy-proven cases have a mortality of about 70%, and over 50% of the survivors are left with significant sequelae. The availability of antiviral therapy with acyclovir has changed these statistics as discussed in the following and in Chapter 38.

The disease can occur with primary infection or with reactivation of the latent organism. There is no seasonal predilection, and it is not associated with community outbreaks. It can affect persons of any age. Of the encephalitides, herpes simplex seems most likely to result in focal disease. On pathologic examination extensive necrosis with hemorrhage is characteristic. Cowdry type A intranuclear inclusions are often seen in the neurons.

CLINICAL MANIFESTATIONS. The onset can be acute or have a vague, subacute prodrome consisting of frontal headache and malaise lasting several days or weeks. Changes in mentation are often the first indication that the CNS is involved. When initially seen, herpes simplex encephalitis may not be distinguishable from other causes, but certain features if present are characteristic. Evidence of focal disease, particularly that of temporal lobe involvement, is typical. Symptoms of bizarre behavior, speech disorders, and gustatory or olfactory hallucinations are particularly suggestive of herpes simplex infection.

The focal involvement can occasionally occur elsewhere in the CNS, including the brainstem. Ninety percent of patients have fever, often as high as 103° to 106° F (39.4° to 41.1° C). During the course of untreated illness in biopsy-proven cases, 85% of patients become comatose, 20% have aphasia, and 40% to 60% have seizures. Cutaneous herpes is seen in less than 10% of the cases. Furthermore, the appearance of herpetic skin lesions can be a nonspecific concomitant of many febrile illnesses. Therefore the presence or absence of cutaneous herpes is of no diagnostic importance.

Standard laboratory tests are of limited value in diagnosis.

CNS findings are nonspecific, although when present the findings of several hundred red cells and a low glucose level should suggest herpes simplex. The electroencephalogram (EEG), brain scan, and computed tomography (CT) scan are useful in confirming the locality of the disease and especially in confirming temporal lobe involvement if present. However, none of these tests establishes a specific etiologic diagnosis. Because of the localized illness, space-occupying lesions, such as a brain abscess, tumor, or intracerebral bleeding, are frequent differential diagnostic considerations.

In the laboratory, herpes encephalitis can be confirmed only by examination of brain tissue. Immunofluorescent staining of the tissue with fluorescein-labeled anti–herpes simplex antibody is sensitive (about 75% to 85%) and specific and can be performed in a few hours. Demonstration of typical Cowdry type A intranuclear inclusions by histologic stains is strongly suggestive of herpes simplex in acute encephalitis. The virus can usually be grown from brain tissue in 1 to 5 days. However, it has been cultured from lumbar CSF on only a few occasions. Serologic tests demonstrating significant antibody titer rises in serum are not specific for CNS disease, since they may reflect active virus infection elsewhere in the body (for example, reactivation of mouth lesions). A recent study suggests that the ratio of CSF antibodies to serum antibodies can be useful in diagnosis, but these changes develop fairly late after the onset of infection and are of little value in establishing an early diagnosis. Acyclovir is the most effective drug for the treatment of HSV encephalitis. The dosage is 10 mg/kg given intravenously every 8 hours for 10 days. Both the mortality and the long-term residua can be significantly reduced when this drug is instituted before there is a major alteration in the patient's level of consciousness; treating a patient who is already comatose is of no benefit.

The exact role of brain biopsy versus empiric therapy in approaching suspected herpes encephalitis has been a source of recent debate. These factors should be considered (1) herpes simplex is a devastating illness; (2) acyclovir is moderately effective if used early in the disease; (3) diagnosis of herpes encephalitis cannot be established by clinical evaluation or basic laboratory tests but requires brain biopsy; (4) there is the possibility of finding an alternative treatable diagnosis with a biopsy. At present, early biopsy rather than empiric therapy appears to be the best approach.

ENTEROVIRUSES

Although enteroviruses can be associated with a variety of neurologic syndromes, symptomatic CNS infections with these agents generally are manifested as aseptic meningitis. The enteroviruses are 20- to 30-nm icosahedral RNA viruses; they include over 70 serotypes that are grouped into the echoviruses, group A and B coxsackieviruses, and polioviruses. Many of the different viral serotypes can be responsible for CNS illness. Most frequently implicated are echoviruses 4, 6, 9, 11, 16, and 30; group A coxsackieviruses 7 and 9; and group B coxsackieviruses 1 to 5. These organisms are widespread and highly contagious. Serologic studies have revealed that infections in household contacts are frequent, although often asymptomatic. Infections with enteroviruses may result in a variety of different illnesses including febrile exanthems, herpangina, pleurodynia, myopericarditis, orchitis, and respiratory tract infections. The presence of these types of illnesses in the household or community of a patient with CNS infection is a useful epidemiologic suggestion that the causative agent is an enterovirus. Infections peak in the summer and fall, and most occur in children or young adults. They are spread via the fecal-oral route.

CLINICAL MANIFESTATIONS. Although aseptic meningitis is most frequent, neurologic illness can be manifested in a variety of less common ways, including encephalitis, cerebellar ataxia, radiculitis, and muscle weakness or paralysis such as that classically described in poliomyelitis. After an incubation period of 2 to 12 days, the onset may be subacute or acute, with increased temperatures, chilliness, myalgias, and headache being the predominant symptoms. Nausea and vomiting may occur. Meningeal signs are present on physical examination, and occasionally an erythematous maculopapular rash suggestive of an enterovirus can be seen. On occasion the disease is diphasic, beginning with a nonspecific febrile illness that lasts a few days. This is followed by 2 to 10 days of improvement that is terminated by the reappearance of fever, this time accompanied by meningeal signs. Patients who have had several remissions or relapses of enterovirus aseptic meningitis have been described.

Poliomyelitis infections are usually subclinical; however, an estimated 0.1% result in paralysis as a result of damage to anterior horn cells of the spinal cord or to motor nuclei of the pons and medulla. Poliomyelitis has a usual incubation period of 9 to 12 days. Some patients have a nonspecific prodromal "minor illness" (fever, headache, sore throat) lasting 1 to 3 days, followed by a 2- to 5-day period of well-being. There is then an onset of typical aseptic meningitis "major illness" (fever, headache, malaise, and meningeal signs). In some patients this is followed by muscle stiffness, pain, and progressive asymmetric paralysis, most often involving the lower extremities, that develops over a period of days. Transient fasciculations may be noted in the involved muscles. There is no sensory loss. Bulbar palsy, often affecting the ninth and tenth cranial nerves, and autonomic dysfunction (hypertension, excessive sweating, urinary retention) can occur. Recovery of muscle strength can be noted for up to 1 year after the illness.

With enterovirus infection, routine laboratory test findings are usually normal. CSF findings are abnormal but nonspecific. The CSF cell count generally ranges from 5 to 300/mm^3, with a predominance of lymphocytes. (As described previously, polymorphonuclear leukocytes can be seen early in the illness.) The CSF glucose is generally normal, and the protein is normal or mildly elevated.

Specific virologic diagnosis can be achieved by viral isolation from the CSF and by serologic testing. Coxsackievirus and echovirus can often be recovered from the CSF during the first several days of the illness. Throat and rectal swabs have a higher yield than CSF cultures, and the virus persists for a longer time, but isolation from these areas can only suggest the etiologic agent because of the possibility of asymptomatic carriage of the enterovirus. This is especially likely in an epidemic. There is no group-specific serologic test. Because there are many enteroviruses, serologic screening is impractical. However, the clinical significance of a throat or rectal isolate can be confirmed by demonstrating a fourfold or greater rise in serotype-specific antibody titer to that isolate.

Treatment for all enteroviral infections is symptomatic, since there is no specific therapy. In fact, in epidemic situations when a patient is not severely ill and has a typical history, hospitalization may not be necessary. The prognosis for most enteroviral CNS infections is excellent, with the exception of paralytic poliomyelitis and infections in infants during the first year of life. Other than poliovirus vaccines, there are no specific preventive measures. Enteric precautions are suggested in hospitalized patients.

ARBOVIRUSES

Arboviruses are a heterogeneous group of organisms that have in common a primary mode of transmission by arthropod vectors. In the United States the most common arboviruses causing CNS disease are the California encephalitis (CE) group and the togaviruses—western equine encephalitis (WEE), eastern equine encephalitis (EEE), and St. Louis encephalitis (SLE). Venezuelan equine encephalitis (VEE) has also been responsible for several small epidemics in Florida, Louisiana, and Texas. Although the spectrum of illness caused by these viruses includes asymptomatic infection and aseptic meningitis, the majority of proven cases are encephalitic. In the last decade in the United States, there have been approximately 100 to 200 cases per year. Most have been SLE or CE. There are epidemiologic features that characterize each of these viruses; however, since the syndromes are clinically indistinguishable, the clinical manifestations can be considered together.

CLINICAL MANIFESTATIONS. Illnesses resulting from infection with any of the arbobiruses can be variable both in the type of symptoms and in severity. The incidence peaks in the summer, corresponding to the presence of the mosquito vectors. Place of residence, vocation, and recreational activities, as they are related to mosquito exposure, are obviously important in historical inquiries. The onset may be abrupt or subacute and includes the nonspecific symptoms of fever, headache, nausea, and vomiting. CNS manifestations usually develop on the second or third day. Changes in mental status can vary from minimal difficulty elicited only with specific testing to total unresponsiveness. Virtually any CNS abnormality can be seen, including hemiparesis, tremors, seizures, and cranial nerve palsies. General laboratory tests are not particularly helpful in the diagnosis; both leukocytosis and leukopenia have been observed. CSF examination usually reveals normal glucose, slightly to moderately increased protein, and several hundred white blood cells. As with the other viral CSF infections, polymorphonuclear leukocytes may predominate early, but by several days of illness there is a clear shift to mononuclear cells. EEG abnormalities are nonspecific and can be focal or diffuse.

California encephalitis group

Despite the name, CE viruses are found throughout the world. Although the exact zoonotic cycle has not been proved, small mammals and various species of *Aedes* mosquito appear to be involved. Transmission to humans occurs through the bite of an infected female mosquito. School-age children are the most commonly affected group.

Eastern equine encephalitis

EEE has its natural reservoir in various species of birds. The mosquito *Culiseta melanura* is the principal vector. The virus generally is limited to the Atlantic coast states in the United States, and illness is particularly associated with exposure to freshwater swamps. The disease has a bimodal distribution, with most illness in either infants or the elderly. Human encephalitis is often associated with epizootics in horses and birds.

Western equine encephalitis

The most common vector of WEE virus is *Culex tarsalis*. As with EEE, birds are the principal reservoir. Most illness is in children under 10 years of age; almost 25% of patients are less than 1 year old. Although the virus is concentrated west of the Mississippi, sporadic cases have been reported throughout the United States.

Table 37-1   Epidemiologic features of encephalitis caused by arboviruses in the Americas

Encephalitides	Age	Distribution	Mortality (%)	Reservoir
CE	Childhood	United States	<1	Small mammals
EEE	Very young and very old	Eastern United States, Canada, and Central America	70	Birds
SLE	Over 50	United States and South America	8	Birds
VEE	Any	Florida, Texas, Louisiana, South America, and Mexico	<1	Horses and rodents
WEE	Less than 10 years	Western United States and Canada	2-3	Birds

St. Louis encephalitis

SLE is the most frequently identified arbovirus encephalitis in the United States. It, too, has a wild bird reservoir. Several species of *Culex* mosquito serve as vector. Clinical infection is most frequent in persons over 50 years of age.

Venezuelan equine encephalitis

VEE is a 3- to 5-day illness with fever, headache, vomiting, diarrhea, and rarely encephalitis. It is rare. It has been responsible for epidemics in South and Central America. The virus activity has been limited to Texas, Florida, and Louisiana in the United States. Horses serve as reservoirs during epidemics, whereas rodents appear to be a more important group in maintaining endemic cycles. Many species of mosquito can act as vectors. Unlike the other viruses, infection with VE can be contagious from person to person via the aerosol route. This necessitates respiratory isolation of patients and particular care with specimens in the laboratory.

• • •

The main epidemiologic features of arboviruses are summarized in Table 37-1.

Arbovirus infections are generally diagnosed by serologic tests with acute and convalescent sera. Cultures of blood, CSF, and material other than brain tissue are generally negative (VEE is an exception with frequently positive blood and throat cultures).

There is no specific treatment for any of these viruses. Mortality depends on the organism and the age of the patient. The approximate mortality figures are CE, less than 1%; WEE, 2% to 3%; SLE, 8%; EEE, 70%, and VEE, 3%. The extremes of age are overrepresented in these mortality figures. The extent of residual damage depends, in a similar fashion, on the specific organism and the age of the patient.

Prevention of arbovirus encephalitis is primarily a matter of mosquito control. Experimental vaccines for VEE, WEE, and EEE are available for epidemics. VEE vaccine can occasionally be appropriate for laboratory personnel who work with this organism, since it is contagious by aerosol.

MUMPS

Despite the introduction of live attenuated vaccine in 1967, mumps virus continues to be a commonly diagnosed viral cause of CNS disease reported in the United States. Since the 1960s the incidence has decreased. However, mumps virus is still responsible for about 10% of encephalitis cases and 6% of aseptic meningitis cases for which an etiologic agent is determined.

CLINICAL MANIFESTATIONS. Mumps infections occur most frequently in the winter and spring months. These are seasons in which arboviral and enteroviral activity is virtually absent. Because of the contagious nature of mumps, the physician who suspects this infection should ask whether the patient has been exposed to parotitis.

CNS disease is the most common extrasalivary manifestation of mumps. Typically, CNS infection results in aseptic meningitis or encephalitis; rare cases of transverse myelitis, Guillain-Barré syndrome, facial palsy, cerebellar ataxia, and a poliomyelitis-like paralysis have been reported in association with mumps virus. In addition, deafness that is usually transient has been associated with mumps virus infection. Abnormalities of the CSF have been found in up to half of the patients with mumps parotitis. Clinical CNS disease, however, occurs in approximately 1%. On the other hand, at least one third of patients with proven mumps CNS infection do not have parotitis. If both parotitis and CNS disease do occur, the CNS symptoms can be seen before, during, or up to 2 weeks after the parotid gland swelling.

Mumps meningitis or encephalitis is clinically indistinguishable from those caused by other viruses unless parotitis is present. However, the CSF leukocyte count is often particularly elevated for viral infection (occasionally greater than 1000/mm^3), and the shift from polymorphonuclear leukocytes to lymphocytes can be delayed for several days. In addition, a mild hypoglycorrhachia can occur. These findings make the consideration of other causes of the illness such as bacterial, mycobacterial, or fungal infection more urgent.

The diagnosis cannot be made with certainty on clinical grounds. However, in a susceptible person a history of exposure suggests the disease, and associated parotitis makes mumps quite likely. The diagnosis can be confirmed both by culture and by serology. Mumps virus can be grown from the pharynx and CSF for several days after the onset of illness and from the urine for several weeks. Complement-fixing antibodies directed against the soluble (S) antigen appear early in the illness and stay elevated for several months, whereas those directed against the viral (V) antigen appear after 2 to 4 weeks and stay elevated for years. Therefore a diagnosis of recent infection can be made from a single serum specimen if the titers are increased to S antigen and negative or increased to V antigen. Past infection is suggested by a negative S but an increased V titer.

There is no specific treatment. Complete recovery is the rule, although sequelae of mental retardation, permanent deafness, and seizure disorders can occur. The live virus vaccine is quite effective in preventing mumps (see Chapter 38). It is usually administered to children at 15 months of age as part of the measles-mumps-rubella (MMR) vaccine. Postexposure passive prophylaxis with immune serum globulin (ISG) or hyperimmune globulin has not been proved effective.

OTHER CHILDHOOD INFECTIONS
Measles

Encephalitis is a relatively common complication of measles, occurring in about 1 in 1000 cases. Typically, the initial symptoms are fever, headache, and altered mental status seen 1 to 2 weeks after the appearance of the rash. The pathogenetic mechanism, primary or postinfectious, has not been clearly delineated.

Measles encephalitis can range from mild to severe, but generally is it a serious illness with a mortality rate of 10% and with permanent neurologic sequelae in 10% to 60%

of the cases. Subacute sclerosing panencephalitis (SSPE), a late CNS complication of measles, is not included in these numbers.

Although the virus can be cultured, isolation procedures are difficult. Therefore measles is generally confirmed by demonstrating a fourfold or greater rise in serum antibody titers. Because the diagnosis can usually be suspected clinically, antibody measurement is often unnecessary.

There is no specific therapy. The live attenuated vaccine is very effective in preventing measles and is usually given at age 15 months along with mumps and rubella. ISG can be given as postexposure prophylaxis but is indicated only for susceptible persons at high risk of serious disease, that is, immunocompromised hosts.

Varicella-zoster

CNS disease can be a complication of varicella infections. It generally develops toward the end of the first week of the exanthem, although there have been cases in which the CNS involvement preceded the rash. The most frequent manifestation is a self-limited, acute cerebellar ataxia. Aseptic meningitis, encephalitis, transverse myelitis, and Guillain-Barré syndrome have all been reported.

CNS involvement can also be associated with zoster infection. Encephalitis can occur without cutaneous dissemination and with cutaneous involvement limited to noncranial dermatomes. As with varicella, symptoms usually appear toward the end of the first week of the rash and are more likely to develop in the immunocompromised host. Guillain-Barré syndrome, transverse myelitis, Bell's plasy, and Hunt's syndrome have all been associated with zoster infections. Finally, 7% of patients with Reye's syndrome have had a preceding varicella infection.

The diagnosis is suspected based on clinical features and can be confirmed by vesicular culture or by immunofluorescent staining of material scraped from the vesicular base. Histologic stains of such material can demonstrate herpesvirus inclusions and syncytial formation but do not permit distinction between herpes simplex and varicella-zoster viruses. There is no effective treatment once encephalitis has developed. Acyclovir can be beneficial in preventing dissemination of zoster infections in immunologically impaired patients (see Chapter 38). In similar patients zoster immune globulin is effective in attenuating varicella and preventing serious sequelae if given to susceptible individuals within 3 days of exposure.

EPSTEIN-BARR VIRUS

Infection with Epstein-Barr virus (EBV) can produce a number of neurological syndromes including aseptic meningitis and encephalitis. These can occur in association with the typical mononucleosis syndrome, or CNS disease can be the only manifestation of infection. In the latter situation there is nothing characteristic about the neurologic disease or the routine laboratory tests that would suggest the diagnosis. Monospot test results are often negative. The diagnosis is proved serologically by finding the pattern of EBV antibodies that are specific for acute EBV infection. There is no specific therapy. The disease generally resolves without sequelae.

LYMPHOCYTIC CHORIOMENINGITIS VIRUS

Lymphocytic choriomeningitis virus (LCM) is an arenavirus that is endemic in small rodents. Infections in humans occur in persons with close exposure to such animals as hamsters and mice. Most cases are reported in laboratory workers or during the winter months when rodents move indoors. The

illness is generally a self-limited aseptic meningitis, but fatal cases have been reported. This virus has been associated with relatively low CSF sugar levels and high CSF cell counts. The early predominance of polymorphonuclear leukocytes in the CSF can persist longer than most viral infections. Thus the CSF findings occasionally mimic those of bacterial meningitis. The diagnosis is made by serologic testing and is generally suspected only in persons with a history of contact with rodents. There is no specific therapy.

RABIES

Rabies in humans has decreased to fewer than five cases per year in the United States. Cases in domestic animals have similarly decreased. Wild animals have taken on a proportionately larger role as a source of infection in humans. Skunks, bats, foxes, and raccoons are the most frequently infected animals.

After an incubation period (usually 2 weeks to 2 months), half or more of the patients complain of pain or paresthesias at the site of the bite. However, initial symptoms can be nonspecific. Furthermore, early intubation and artificial ventilation can obscure the characteristic signs of hydrophobia and periods of hyperactivity interrupted by intervals of lucidity. Therefore the clinical diagnosis can be overlooked. It is important to consider the diagnosis of rabies in every undiagnosed case of encephalitis because of the potential public health implications. Diagnosis can be established by immunofluorescent staining of corneal impression smears, skin biopsies from the back of the neck or brain tissue, and assay for rabies antibody. There is no specific therapy. The disease is generally fatal. Considerations as to who should receive postexposure prophylaxis with rabies vaccine are discussed in Chapter 38.

HUMAN IMMUNODEFICIENCY VIRUS

Neurologic abnormalities are frequent in patients infected with human immunodeficiency virus (HIV). Although many abnormalities are due to opportunistic infections or lymphoma, the most frequent etiologic agent is the virus itself. Several peripheral and CNS syndromes have been associated with HIV. CNS problems include acute aseptic meningitis, subacute encephalitis, and subacute encephalopathy. Neurologic abnormalities can occur in the absence of other manifestations of HIV infection.

An acute aseptic meningitis can be the initial manifestation of HIV disease. It is usually clinically indistinguishable from other aseptic meningitides, and as with other viral CNS infections there can be alterations in mental status indicative of a meningoencephalitis. Aseptic meningitis caused by HIV can be associated with other manifestations of acute HIV disease such as sore throat, acute adenopathy, and diffuse rash. It may appear similar to mononucleosis. Acquired immunodeficiency syndrome (AIDS) is not seen at this stage of the infection. There is no specific therapy. Symptoms resolve spontaneously but can recur. The diagnosis can be established by demonstrating a seroconversion to HIV antibodies. Findings from serologic studies for HIV are usually negative during the acute illness and turn positive weeks to months after recovery.

A more common manifestation of HIV infection of the CNS is subacute encephalopathy. In this syndrome there is a gradual deterioration in CNS function that begins with subtle cognitive abnormalities and may progress to a totally withdrawn profound psychomotor retardation; paranoid ideas are also often observed. The typical CSF reveals only mildly elevated protein levels, although a mild pleocytosis can be seen. The glucose level is invariably normal. CT demonstrates a characteristic diffuse atrophy. The diagnosis is generally established by the absence of other causes of CNS disease and is supported by the characteristic CT scan. HIV can be recovered from brain biopsy specimens and from CSF, though techniques for isolation are available only in specialized laboratories. Patients with HIV encephalopathy have shown dramatic responses to therapy with Zidovudine.

TREATABLE CAUSES OF "ASEPTIC MENINGOENCEPHALITIS"

With the exception of herpes simplex type I encephalitis, no viral infections of the CNS are treatable with specific agents. Because of this, because the clinical presentations are usually relatively nonspecific, and because the CSF findings are not diagnostic, possible nonviral causes for the patient's illness must always be kept in mind. Generally, these causes have specific therapies. A partial list of diseases that may mimic CSF findings in viral meningitis and encephalitis follows:

Tuberculosis
Fungal infection (cryptococcosis, coccidioidomycosis)
Listeriosis
Partially treated bacterial meningitis
Falciparum malaria
Syphilis
Amoeba infection
Toxoplasmosis
Parameningeal infection (brain abscess, epidural and subdural infections)
Rocky Mountain spotted fever
Vasculitis
Behçet's disease
Sarcoidosis
Carcinomatous and lymphomatous meningitis
Nonsteroidal antiinflammatory drugs
Leptospirosis

EVALUATION OF THE PATIENT WITH ASEPTIC MENINGITIS OR VIRAL ENCEPHALITIS

After deciding that a viral CNS infection is most likely, the physician is confronted with the problem of proving which agent is responsible. The approach to this problem should include the following steps:

1. Consider the age of the patient and the season of the year.
2. Obtain travel and exposure history.
3. Look for clues associated with specific viruses during the general physical examination.
4. Obtain viral cultures. Culture the CSF for enteroviruses, herpesviruses, and mumps; culture the throat for enteroviruses and mumps; and culture the stool for enteroviruses. Consider CSF culture for HIV.
5. Obtain serologic tests. A single specimen may be employed to diagnose mumps and Epstein-Barr virus infection. Paired sera are required for other viruses. HIV antibody can be negative with acute infection and should be repeated.
6. If the clinical situation suggests herpes simplex, consider a brain biopsy and acyclovir therapy.
7. Always consider nonviral causes and obtain appropriate studies to evaluate these diseases.

BIBLIOGRAPHY

Barza M and Pauker SG: The decision to biopsy, treat or wait in suspected herpes simplex encephalitis, Ann Intern Med 92:641, 1980.
Centers for Disease Control: Aseptic meningitis surveillance, Annual Summary, Atlanta, 1976.
Centers for Disease Control: Encephalitis surveillance, Atlanta, 1977.
Ehrenkranz NH and Ventura AK: Venezuelan equine encephalitis virus infection in man, Annu Rev Med 25:9, 1974.
Feigin RD and Shackleford PG: Value of repeat lumbar puncture in the differential diagnosis of meningitis, N Engl J Med 289:571, 1973.
Hollander H and Levy JA: Neurologic abnormalities and recovery of human immunodeficiency virus from cerebrospinal fluid, Ann Intern Med 106:692, 1987.
Levine, DP, Lauter CV and Lerner AM: Simultaneous serum and cerebrospinal fluid antibodies in herpes simplex virus encephalitis, JAMA 240:356, 1978.
Levy RM and others: Neurological manifestations of the acquired immunodeficiency syndrome (AIDS): experience at UCSF and review of the literature, J Neurosurg 62:475, 1985.
Plotkin SA and Koprowski H: Phobia of hydrophobia justified, N Engl J Med 300:620, 1979.
Southern PM Jr. and others: Clinical and laboratory features of epidemic St. Louis encephalitis, Ann Intern Med 71:681, 1969.
Vanzee BE and others: Lymphocytic choriomeningitis in university hospital personnel, Am J Med 58:803, 1975.
Whitley R and others: Adenine arabinoside therapy of biopsy-proved herpes simplex encephalitis: National Institute of Allergy and Infectious Diseases collaborative antiviral study, N Engl J Med 297:289, 1977.
Young DJ: California encephalitis virus report of 3 cases and review of the literature, Ann Intern Med 65:419, 1966.

Mumps

Donald Kaye

Mumps is an RNA virus that infects only humans. Most cases occur between 5 and 15 years of age. Transmission is by direct contact or by contact with droplets of saliva that contain virus several days before and up to 1 week after swelling of the parotid gland appears. Organs involved include the salivary glands, pancreas, testes, and central nervous system (see discussion of "Viral infections of the central nervous system"). Inapparent infection is common and results in lifetime immunity.

After an incubation period of 14 to 21 days, fever develops and is accompanied by swelling and tenderness of one or both parotid glands. Infection of other salivary glands, one or both testicles (rare before puberty), and meningoencephalitis can occur. The last can develop in patients who do not have parotitis. Clinical pancreatitis is uncommon.

The diagnosis is proved by isolation of the virus from saliva or by serologic means (see discussion of "Viral infections of the central nervous system"). There is no specific therapy. Analgesics and corticosteroids have been used to relieve the pain of orchitis, but they do not prevent atrophy. However, sterility is a rare consequence of mumps orchitis.

BIBLIOGRAPHY

Mandell GL, Douglas RG, and Bennett JR: Principles and practice of infectious diseases, ed 3, New York, 1990, Churchill Livingstone.

Viral respiratory infections

R. Michael Buckley, Jr., *and* Michael N. Braffman

Over 60,000 deaths annually in the United States are attributable to respiratory illness, and over half the visits to primary care physicians are related to respiratory infections. An estimated 80% of acute respiratory illnesses are viral in origin, indicating the major importance of respiratory viruses to clinician and investigator alike. More than 150 viruses have been associated with respiratory illnesses; however, distinct clinical features often permit a presumptive etiologic diagnosis and enable viral illnesses to be distinguished from bacterial infections. This latter point is important, since antibacterial antibodies are of no benefit in the treatment of viral diseases. However, with the recent availability of effective antiviral agents such as ribavirin and acyclovir, the rapid diagnosis of viral respiratory diseases is growing increasingly important. The concentration here is on the clinical characteristics of the common viral respiratory pathogens that are listed below:

Influenza viruses
Respiratory syncytial virus
Parainfluenza viruses
Adenoviruses
Picornaviruses
    Rhinoviruses
    Enteroviruses
Other viruses
    Coronaviruses
    Cytomegalovirus
    Herpes simplex virus
    Varicella-zoster virus
    Measles virus

INFLUENZA

Influenza is an acute respiratory tract infection caused by influenza viruses. It occurs in localized outbreaks, epidemics, or pandemics (that is, epidemics of worldwide scope) and is associated with high morbidity and occasionally high mortality. Since 1580, 31 pandemics have been described, the greatest being the swine influenza pandemic of 1918-1919, which accounted for 21 million deaths worldwide and over 500,000 in the United States.

Three distinct types of influenza viruses exists: types A, B, and C. Minor outbreaks and epidemics have been associated with types A and B virus infections, as have pandemics (such as the influenza B pandemic of 1985-6). Type C rarely causes detectable disease, although serologic surveys indicate that a large proportion of the population have evidence of past infection. The success of the influenza virus as a major respiratory pathogen is primarily related to two properties of the virus. The first is the highly contagious nature of the virus, enabling it to spread through communities. The second is related to changes in viral antigenicity. Strains of influenza A virus and, to a lesser extent, influenza B virus have the remarkable ability to change their genetic composition radically. Minor changes in influenza A strain (antigen drifts) generally occur every 1 to 4 years, whereas major changes (antigen shifts) develop approximately every 10 to 15 years (since 1918). To date, only antigen drifts have been detected in influenza B strains. The effect of these changes is that individuals who may have been immune to a previous influenza strain are not partially or totally susceptible to the new virus strain.

ETIOLOGY. Influenza viruses are 90-nm RNA viruses; they have helical symmetry and an envelope coat. Spikes composed to two antigenically and anatomically distinct glycoproteins protrude from the lipid envelope. These are the viral hemagglutinin and neuraminidase. Antibodies against hemagglutinin assume a central role in protection against infection, whereas antibodies against neuraminidase appear less protective.

These viruses are typed A, B, or C according to their nucleocapsid proteins. All type A strains share a common nucleocapsid antigen that is distinct from the common antigens shared by B viruses or C viruses. Within each type (A, B, and C), strain differences are detected by antigenic variations in the hemagglutinin and neuraminidase. The present nomenclature of influenza viruses takes into account the viral type, the geographic location where the virus was first isolated, the strain number, the year when the virus was first isolated, and the antigenic composition of the hemagglutinin and neuraminidase. Thus one of the influenza A viruses isolated in England in the 1972 epidemic was termed A/England/42/72 (H3N2).

EPIDEMIOLOGY. Influenza viruses are spread by transmission of respiratory secretions, predominantly in the form of small-particle (<10 µm) aerosols.

The age-related attack rate of influenza tends to vary from one epidemic to another; however, generally the highest incidence occurs in children 5 to 9 years of age, whereas the most severe manifestations occur in elderly patients or those with complicating underlying disease. A typical outbreak of influenza is characterized by an abrupt onset, a high attack rate in the population (often up to 30% to 50%), and rapid spread. Outbreaks often peak in 3 to 4 weeks and then subside over the next month. The severity of disease in a given outbreak depends on many factors, including strain virulence and prior immunity in the population.

The severity of an outbreak can be estimated from the increased incidence of school absenteeism, emergency room visits for respiratory illnesses, and deaths caused by pneumonia.

PATHOGENESIS AND PATHOLOGY. The influenza virus hemagglutinin probably attaches to receptors on the surface of ciliated respiratory epithelial cells. Virus penetration and replication then follow, leading to degeneration and desquamation of respiratory cells and a mononuclear infiltrate. The alveolar walls become thickened, and hyaline membrane formation can occur.

CLINICAL MANIFESTATIONS. The clinical syndromes of influenza A and B viruses are usually indistinguishable and classically consist of fever, dry cough, myalgias, and headache after an incubation period of 1 to 3 days. Often chills, nasal discharge, and painful eyes are also present. While fever need not be high, prostration can be marked. Nausea and vomiting may be present initially, but a predominance of these symptoms should lead to a different diagnosis. Fever lasts approximately 3 days, butthe cough, nasal discharge, and malaise often persist for 1 to 2 weeks. Infection with influenza C does not produce this syndrome; rather, it causes afebrile common colds.

On physical examination the patient appears ill, and the temperature is generally elevated to 100° to 104° F (38° to 40° C). Expiratory wheezes and rhonchi can be detected even if the chest roentgenogram is normal. Clear nasal discharge, conjunctivitis, and injected throat can be present.

Laboratory parameters are nonspecific. The white blood cell count is often elevated initially and then falls, with a predominance of lymphocytes. Liver function studies are usually normal. The electrocardiogram can show some nonspecific T-wave changes but usually shows only a persistent tachycardia. An abnormal chest roentgenogram indicates either influenzal lower respiratory tract infection or secondary bacterial pneumonia. The former is usually a patchy, often diffuse, interstitial infiltrate, and the latter is more consolidated. Gram stain of expectorated sputum examined for polymorphonuclear leukocytes and bacteria is particularly helpful in distinguishing between the two.

The major cause of excess mortality is development of pulmonary complications. Patients with underlying diseases such as chronic obstructive pulmonary disease, mitral stenosis, and other cardiovascular diseases are particularly prone to pneumonia, either primary influenza viral pneumonia (a high-mortality disease), which usually develops shortly after the onset of infection, or secondary bacterial pneumonia, which typically begins in the second week after a period of improvement from the initial symptoms. The bacteria most commonly associated with this entity are the pneumococcus, *Staphylococcus aureus,* and *Haemophilus influenzae.* Less common but potentially serious complications of influenza include myocarditis, encephalopathy, and Reye's syndrome. The last has been described chiefly in children and more often follows influenza B infection. The pathogenesis of this syndrome is unknown. Recent reports suggest a higher frequency of Reye's syndrome in children who receive aspirin during the acute infection. The syndrome is characterized by nausea and vomiting and progression to lethargy, coma, and seizures. Laboratory tests reveal abnormal liver function tests, hypoglycemia, and, most commonly, an increase in blood ammonia. The mortality rate is approximately 20% to 40%. Minor complications of influenza include otitis media and sinusitis.

DIAGNOSIS. Once influenza virus has been isolated in the community, the diagnosis can generally be made based on the clinical syndrome. Some laboratories can perform immunofluroescence for rapid identification of the virus in respiratory secretions. The diagnosis can be established by viral isolation from respiratory secretions; although this can take 7-14 days. A fourfold rise in antibody titer from the acute to the convalescent specimen also confirms the diagnosis of recent influenza infection.

MANAGEMENT AND PREVENTION. In uncomplicated influenza, antipyretics, analgesics, rest, and oral fluids help to relieve symptoms. Most authorities recommend avoiding salicylates (aspirin) because of the possible association with Reye's Syndrome. Acetaminophen (Tylenol) is a suitable alternative. Antibiotics are not indicated. If pneumonia develops, Gram stains of expectorated sputum are important to distinguish viral from bacterial infection. Antibiotics should be used to treat otitis media, sinusitis, or bacterial pneumonia. Amantadine hydrochloride (Symmetrel) is useful against type A influenza viruses, mainly as a prophylactic drug but also as a therapeutic agent, especially if given within the first 24 to 48 hours of symptoms (see Chapter 38). A dose of 200 mg/day is generally well tolerated. Yearly vaccination with inactivated virus is essential for high-risk patients. For vaccines see Chapter 38.

RESPIRATORY SYNCYTIAL VIRUS

Respiratory syncytial virus (RSV) is a major cause of life-threatening lower respiratory infection in infants and an important pathogen worldwide. So effective is its spread that essentially all humans become infected by a young age. Unfortunately, immunity is incomplete and reinfections are common. Although RSV is primarily a pathogen of children, it causes upper respiratory infections in adults and can cause severe lower respiratory illness in aged indivduals and immunocompromised hosts. RSV is easily and rapidly transmitted within pediatric hospitals and is a major cause of severe nosocomial pneumonia among children with chronic lung and heart disease.

ETIOLOGY. RSV is a member of the paramyxovirus group, along with mumps, parainfluenza, and measles. It has an RNA-containing nucleocapsid, and in contrast to influenza only one antigenic variety is known. The virus derives its name from the fact that it forms large syncytia on primary inoculation of certain cell monolayers.

EPIDEMIOLOGY. The virus is probably transmitted by the airborne route or by contact with infected secretions. Its spread is rapid and extensive and occurs predominantly in midwinter and early spring. Outbreaks develop yearly, mainly affecting infants and children under 5 years of age.

PATHOGENESIS. After inoculation into the eye, nose, or mouth, the virus incubates for 2 to 8 days, with a mean of 5 days. Infection is generally confined to the respiratory tract. In bronchiolitis a lymphocytic peribronchiolar infiltrate develops with subsequent necrosis of bronchiolar epithelium. The

small airway lumina become obstructed, airflow is impeded, and hyperinflation and air trapping ensue. Some patients have pneumonia characterized by mononuclear infiltrates, edema, and necrosis. Recovery is generally complete; however, morphologic alteration may persist indefinitely.

The mechanisms by which RSV induces these pathologic changes are unclear. Circulating humoral and cellular immunity is not totally protective; moreover, immunologic mechanisms may actually contribute to the pathogenesis of disease. This observation is supported by the severity of RSV infection in young infants in the presence of passive maternal antibody. In addition, children with high levels of humoral and cellular immunity induced by inactivated RSV vaccine can have severe disease on reinfection.

CLINICAL MANIFESTATIONS. The clinical syndrome of RSV infection are somewhat age dependent. Infants and children under 5 years of age have a higher incidence of pneumonia, bronchiolitis, and otitis media than older children, in whom upper respiratory tract infection or tracheobronchitis is common. Adults and older children have a "common cold" syndrome with a prolonged course compared with common colds of other causes. RSV can produce an acute exacerbation of bronchitis, and in immunosuppressed individuals bronchopneumonia may appear.

The typical patient with bronchiolitis is a child less than 1 year old who has a febrile upper respiratory infection and a cough, mucus production, expiratory wheezing, dyspnea, rib retraction, poor oral intake, and air hunger. On the chest roentgenogram diffuse hyperaeration and scattered infiltrates are seen. The infiltrates are caused by atelectasis but can be difficult to distinguish from changes seen in pneumonia. In the child or adult with bronchopneumonia, rales can be heard on examination of the chest. The roentgenogram shows patchy or consolidated infiltrate, and the sputum is nonpurulent. The upper respiratory syndrome is nonspecific, with fever, cough, rhinitis, and mild pharyngitis.

DIAGNOSIS. In children the diagnosis is often suspected based on the seasonal presentation of a typical syndrome, bronchiolitis, or bronchopneumonia. Specific virologic diagnosis can best be made by culturing the virus fron respiratory secretions, especially nasopharyngeal aspirates. However, it can take up to 14 days to isolate the virus. More rapid diagnostic methods, primarily by enzyme-linked immunosorbent assays (ELISA) and immunofluorescence, are sensitive and specific and are being used more widely.

MANAGEMENT. A new antiviral agent, ribavirin, has been shown to be effective when administered as an aerosol to sick infants with RSV pneumonia. Antibiotics should be used only for treatment of suspected or proven bacterial superinfections such as otitis media or pneumonia.

PREVENTION. Attempts to prevent or ameliorate symptoms with vaccine have so far proved unsuccessful.

PARAINFLUENZA VIRUSES

Parainfluenza viruses are a subgroup of the paramyxoviruses and are second only to respiratory syncytial virus as a cause of respiratory disease in infants and young children. They are the major identifiable cause of the croup syndrome. Like RSV, however, they cause a spectrum of disease ranging from a mild upper respiratory infection to pneumonia. Immunity after parainfluenza infection is incomplete, and most infections in older children and adults represent reinfection.

ETIOLOGY. Parainfluenza viruses are pleomorphic, contain a single-stranded RNA nucleocapsid, and possess an outer membrane with a hemagglutinin on the surface. Four antigenic types (1, 2, 3, 4), which have remained antigenically stable, have been identified. Typing is based on complement-fixing and hemagglutinating antigens.

EPIDEMIOLOGY. The distribution of all four types is worldwide. The virus is capable of rapid spread, especially among children in large confined groups. Like most respiratory viruses, an increase is often noted in the fall and winter months, although some disease activity occurs throughout the year. The clinical syndromes caused by the parainfluenza viruses are somewhat type specific. Type 4 virus appears to cause subclinical or mild clinical illness, which is not particularly well characterized yet. Types 1 and 2 are the most frequent causes of croup, accounting for about one third of the cases. Type 3 predominantly causes lower respiratory infections, including bronchiolitis and pneumonia, in very young infants. Although types 1 and 2 often alternate year to year as causes of respiratory illness in a given community, the level of type 3 activity remains relatively constant.

PATHOGENESIS. Parainfluenza viruses are transmitted from person to person quite readily, probably by direct contact and large droplet aerosols. The target cells of the respiratory tract seem to be ciliated epithelial cells. The mechanism for the subglottic involvement in laryngotracheobronchitis (the croup syndrome) is not understood.

CLINICAL MANIFESTATIONS. The spectrum of clinical illness caused by parainfluenza viruses ranges from the common cold to life-threatening lower respiratory infections. The syndromes are best discussed in relation to the age of those affected.

In children there are three major syndromes. The mildest is a typical respiratory infection with a sore throat, nasal discharge, and low-grade fever. The best-recognized childhood illness caused by parainfluenza viruses is the croup syndrome. This begins as a febrile upper respiratory infection and progresses to a characteristic barking spasmodic cough, hoarseness, and in severe cases inspiratory stridor. The last finding appears to be more common in children less than 4 years of age, and croup in general appears to be more severe when caused by parainfluenza viruses in contrast to other viral causes. Despite the stridor observed in some cases, the epiglottis is normal. The third syndrome usually associated in children with type 3 infection is lower respiratory infection, in which bronchitis, bronciolitis, or pneumonia can occur. It is difficult to distinguish lower respiratory infections caused by parainfluenza viruses from those caused by respiratory syncytial virus except that the former are usually less severe. Bacterial superinfection is also less common after parainfluenza virus infections.

In adults the disease is commonly manifested as a mild upper respiratory infection. However, occasionally prostration may be severe, suggesting influenza infection. Parainfluenza virus infections in older children and adults are frequently accompanied by hoarseness, moderately severe sore throat, and low-grade fever. As with other viral respiratory infections, immunocompromised patients can have a more severe course.

DIAGNOSIS. The diagnosis is suspected in a child with croup or an adult with an upper respiratory infection if hoarseness is prominent. Viral isolation establishes the diagnosis, but like many respiratory viruses, this can take 7 to 14 days. Rapid immunofluorescent techniques can be used to identify parainfluenza viruses in respiratory secretions. A fourfold rise in complement-fixing or hemagglutinating antibody is also diagnostic, retrospectively, of recent infection.

MANAGEMENT. There is no specific antiviral chemotherapy. Symptomatic therapy is sufficient for upper respiratory illness. In mild cases management of the croup syndrome includes sedation and humidified air. If laryngeal obstruction supervenes, this constitutes a medical emergency. Intubation or tracheostomy can occasionally be required, but fortunately this is infrequent following parainfluenza infections. There is no convincing evidence that steroids are effective in croup.

PREVENTION. Reinfection with parainfluenza viruses is common even in the presence of antibody. Nevertheless, it has been observed that reinfection, especially in the presence of high antibody titer, is clinically milder than primary infection, and viral shedding occurs for a shorter period. Therefore there is great interest in the future development of vaccines against parainfluenza viruses.

ADENOVIRUSES

Adenoviruses are clinically important causes of conjunctivitis and acute respiratory infections. As with most respiratory viruses, they have diverse clinical manifestations. Although there is overlap, the clinical syndromes are somewhat type specific.

ETIOLOGY. Adenoviruses contain double-stranded DNA and have a protein or capsid coat. Over 30 types have been detected, certain ones of which are associated with common disease syndromes.

EPIDEMIOLOGY. Adenoviruses are worldwide in distribution. Infection spreads by aerosol and occurs with increasing frequency if crowding exists. In contrast to respiratory syncytial virus, infection before the age of 6 months is unusual; however, most children have been infected by age 10. Infection becomes uncommon after age 15 except in the military. The type of adenovirus causing infection and the resulting clinical syndrome are somewhat age dependent.

Types 1, 2, 5, and 6 are frequently isolated from tonsils and adenoids of children with upper respiratory tract infections. Types 3, 4, and 7 are often isolated from young adults with upper and lower respiratory tract diseases. Type 8 has frequently been isolated from the conjunctiva in adults. Type 4 has caused an acute respiratory disease in military recruits.

PATHOGENESIS. Adenoviruses can produce persistent or latent infection of tonsilar lymphoid tissue, lytic infection of respiratory epithelium, and oncogenic transformation of several in vitro cell strains. Most acute respiratory infections caused by adenoviruses are probably the result of host cell lysis produced during viral replication.

CLINICAL MANIFESTATIONS. The illnesses produced by adenoviruses are generally age related and fall into five major clinical syndromes: a mild upper respiratory infection, acute respiratory disease, pneumonia, pharyngoconjunctival fever, and keratoconjunctivitis. The last occurs in epidemics or as sporadic cases, usually involves adults, and consists of conjunctivitis of 1 to 4 weeks' duration, preauricular adenopathy, and keratitis that appears as the conjunctivitis wanes. The age-related syndromes are discussed in the following.

In contrast to RSV and parainfluenza viruses, infants are usually asymptomatic following adenovirus infections or have a mild coryza and pharyngitis. A fulminant bronchiolitis or pneumonia can rarely be seen. Children generally have either pharyngoconjunctival fever or an upper respiratory infection with a mild tracheitis indistinguishable from other viral infections. The former occurs predominantly in school-age children, most often in the summer, and is characterized by conjunctivitis that is usually unilateral, pharyngitis, rhinitis, cervical adenitis, and fever. The infection is abrupt in onset and lasts 3 to 5 days. Bacterial superinfection or eye damage is rare. Adenovirus has also been isolated from children in association with whooping cough, but its precise role in this syndrome is not well defined.

In young adults, especially military recruits, the major syndromes are acute respiratory disease (ARD) and pneumonia, the latter being clinically indistinguishable from other viral pneumonias except on an epidemiologic basis. ARD is an epidemic disease of military recruits with cough, fever, pharyngitis, and rhinorrhea. Viral pneumonia appears to complicate ARD in approximately 10% of recruits. The morbidity is significant, but the mortality is low.

Adenoviruses can cause hemorrhagic cystitis in children (usually girls).

DIAGNOSIS. The diagnosis is often made clinically by recognizing one of the characteristic syndromes, such as ARD in military recruits. The virus can be isolated from respiratory secretions within 5 to 7 days or demonstrated by immunofluorescent staining of exfoliated cells. Serologic testing can be helpful in some cases.

MANAGEMENT AND PREVENTION. There is no specific chemotherapy currently available. Oral vaccines consisting of live type 4 and 7 viruses in enteric-coated capsules have been developed for use in military recruits. These are not attenuated viruses but do not produce disease when introduced by the gastrointestinal route. They have been effective in reducing the frequency of ARD in recruits.

PICORNAVIRUSES

The picornavirus group of RNA viruses has two major subgroups, the rhinoviruses and the enteroviruses. This is the largest group of viruses causing respiratory disease, although the respiratory illnesses are for the most part quite mild. The rhinoviruses are associated with the common cold syndrome, and the enteroviruses are associated with multiorgan disease, including infection of the respiratory tract.

RHINOVIRUSES

ETIOLOGY. There are more than 90 serotypes of rhinoviruses currently known. Since they do not share a common antigen, immunity appears to be largely type specific. The virus is small, has an RNA core, and exhibits cubic symmetry.

EPIDEMIOLOGY. The rhinoviruses are worldwide in distribution, infect adults more often than children, and occur year round but mainly in autumn and spring. They account for 30% of adult respiratory infections. Transmission may be by hand transfer and by the airborne route.

CLINICAL MANIFESTATIONS. The common cold caused by rhinovirus is an afebrile upper respiratory infection with nasal stuffiness, sneezing, and a scratchy throat. Often an inflamed nasopharynx and a postnasal drip that leads to a cough is present. There is an extremely low conplication rate. The incubation period is 1 to 3 days.

DIAGNOSIS, MANAGEMENT, AND PREVENTION. The diagnosis is easily suspected by the clinical syndrome. Although isolation of the virus and serologic confirmation are possible, the mild nature of the illness makes them impractical other than in research settings. Intranasally administered interferon has been shown to reduce the symptoms and the frequency of acquisition of rhinovirus infection. The benefit, however, may be outweighed by local irritation of nasal mucosa. The common cold is caused by many antigenically unrelated viruses. Prevention by vaccination would therefore be difficult.

ENTEROVIRUSES

The enteroviruses include polioviruses, coxsackieviruses, and echoviruses. Certain coxsackieviruses and echoviruses cause a small percentage of respiratory infections, especially in the summer and fall months. They are, however, better known as causes of meningitis (see discussion of "Viral infections of the central nervous system"), myopericarditis, and febrile illnesses with or without exanthems (see discussion of "Exanthems of viral or presumed viral origin").

CLINICAL MANIFESTATIONS. Herpangina, caused by group A coxsackieviruses, is characterized by fever, sore throat, and generally two to six papular lesions that progress to painful ulcers of the soft palate, tonsillar pillars, tonsils, pharynx, or tongue. Groups A and B coxsackieviruses also cause lymphonodular pharyngitis.

Group B coxsackieviruses cause epidemic pleurodynia (devil's grippe), which is characterized by the abrupt onset of pleuritic or abdominal pain, often paroxysmal and spasmodic, ranging from mild to severe. Cough is notably absent. The illness lasts approximately 5 days, and the pain gradually lessens over this period of time.

Echoviruses are occasionally isolated from children with fevers and sore throats. Bronchiolitis has been reported with echoviruses, and rarely lower respiratory infections can occur.

DIAGNOSIS. Presumptive diagnosis is made on the basis of the clinical syndrome, but definitive diagnosis requires isolation of the virus from respiratory secretions, stool, or spinal fluid (in cases of aseptic meningitis).

MANAGEMENT AND PREVENTION. There is no specific therapy. Poliomyelitis prevention is discussed in Chapter 38. The large number of serotypes and the generally mild illnesses make the development of vaccines unlikely.

OTHER RESPIRATORY VIRUSES
Coronavirus

Coronaviruses are RNA viruses. They cause clinical illnesses in adults and children and most often are responsible for common cold syndromes similar to those of rhinoviruses. Specific diagnosis is difficult, either clinically or by viral isolation.

Cytomegalovirus

Like other herpesviruses, cytomegalovirus (CMV) is often an opportunistic pathogen. Although it usually causes a mild mononucleosis-like illness in healthy patients, it can cause life-threatening pneumonia in immunocompromised patients such as transplant recipients. It is emerging as a major respiratory pathogen in patients with AIDS. The drug dihydroxy-propoxy-methyl-guanine (DHPG), an acyclovir analogue, has been less effective for CMV pneumonia than for CMV in other sites. Rapid diagnosis using immunofluorescence of respiratory secretions or lung tissue is a recent advance that makes the technique far superior to viral isolation, which can take up to 4 to 6 weeks.

Herpes simplex virus

Herpes simplex virus (HSV) has been reported as a cause of both upper and lower respiratory tract disease. Pneumonia can be seen in immunocompromised patients. Diagnosis by viral isolation is simple and fast. Acyclovir is an effective drug for HSV infections and can be administered orally or intravenously.

Varicella-zoster virus

Varicella (chicken pox) can cause pneumonia in older children and adults. In immunocompromised patients, zoster (shingles) can disseminate, involving the lung as well as other organs. Intravenous acyclovir is useful both in preventing dissemination of zoster in immunocompromised patients and in treating complications of varicella.

Table 37-2 Common viral causes of various respiratory illnesses

Clinical syndromes	Common viral causes
UPPER RESPIRATORY INFECTIONS	
Common cold	Rhinoviruses, coronaviruses, respiratory syncytial virus, parainfluenza viruses
Tonsillitis, pharyngitis	Adenoviruses, Epstein-Barr virus, influenza viruses, parainfluenza viruses, respiratory syncytial virus, enteroviruses
LOWER RESPIRATORY INFECTIONS	
Croup (hoarseness, barking cough, inspiratory stridor)	Parainfluenza viruses, respiratory syncytial virus
Tracheobronchitis (cough, rhonchi)	Respiratory syncytial virus, influenza viruses, parainfluenza viruses
Bronchiolitis (air trapping, expiratory wheezing)	Respiratory syncytial virus, parainfluenza viruses
Pneumonia (rales, infiltrate on roentgenogram)	Respiratory syncytial virus, influenza viruses, adenoviruses, parainfluenza viruses, cytomegalovirus, varicella-zoster virus, herpes simplex virus

Rubeola (measles)

Typical measles in childhood, with its characteristic rash and conjunctivits, is often associated with cough. However, young adults who received the inactivated vaccine in 1964-1967 can have an atypical measles syndrome, with an unusual rash, fever, and interstitial pulmonary infiltrates. No specific therapy is available. Vaccination of healthy toddlers with live attenuated vaccine prevents measles.

Many other viruses can involve the respiratory tract. Epstein-Barr virus usually causes pharyngitis; rubella can cause upper respiratory tract symptoms before the onset of the rash; and mumps can cause upper respiratory tract infection with or without the usual parotitis.

● ● ●

A large number of viruses cause acute respiratory illness. The more common causes of isolated respiratory illnesses are shown in Table 37-2.

It is important to remember that most upper respiratory infections are caused by viruses, with group A β-hemolytic streptococci being the only cause of acute pharyngitis and tonsillitis requiring antibiotics. On clinical grounds it is often difficult to distinguish group A streptococcal infection from viral pharyngitis, and a bacterial throat culture is required. With lower respiratory illness the distinction between viral and bacterial infection can be even more difficult. The clinical syndrome, seasonal occurrence, and, if available, examination of expectorated sputum by Gram stain are useful distinguishing features. The presence of polymorphonuclear leukocytes favors a bacterial cause. As antiviral therapy continues to improve and expand, the diagnosis, and in particular the rapid diagnosis, of viral infections will assume much greater practical clinical importance. An awareness of the different viral respiratory illnesses reviewed here permits earlier recognition and therefore more effective therapy for these patients.

BIBLIOGRAPHY

Anderson LJ and others: Viral respiratory illnesses, Med Clin N Am 67:1009, 1983.

Burrows B, Knudson RJ, and Lebowitz MD: The relationship of childhood respiratory illness to adult obstructive airway disease, Am Rev Respir Dis 115:751, 1977.

Douglas RM and others: Prophylactic efficacy of intranasal alpha-2-interferon against rhinovirus infections in the family setting, N Engl J Med 314:65, 1986.

Fiala M and Guze LB: The rhinoviruses of man, Calif Med 112:1, 1970.

Glezen WP: Viral pneumonia as a cause and result of hospitalization, J Infect Dis 147:765, 1983.

Glezen WP: Respiratory viruses and mycoplasma pneumonia. In Drew WL, editor: Viral infections: a clinical approach, Philadelphia 1976, FA Davis Co.

Glezen WP and Denny FW: Epidemiology of acute respiratory diseases in children, N Engl J Med 288:498, 1973.

Hall CB and others: Aerosolized ribavirin treatment of infants with respiratory syncytial virus infection, N Engl J Med 308:1443, 1983.

Hayden FG and others: Prevention of natural colds by contact prophylaxis with intranasal alpha-2-interferon, N Engl J Med 314:71, 1986.

Jackson GG and Muldoon RL: Viruses causing common respiratory infections in man. I. J Infect Dis 127:328, 1973.

Jackson GG and Muldoon RL: Viruses causing common respiratory infections in man. II. Enteroviruses and paramyxoviruses, J Infect Dis 128:387, 1973.

Jackson GG and Muldoon RL: Viruses causing common respiratory infections in man. III. Respiratory syncytial viruses and coronaviruses, J Infect Dis 128:674, 1973.

Jackson GG and Muldoon RL: Viruses causing common respiratory infections in man. IV. Reoviruses and adenoviruses, J Infect Dis 128:811, 1973.

Knight V, editor: Viral and mycoplasma infections of the respiratory tract, Philadelphia, 1973, Lea & Febiger.

Knight V and others: Amantadine therapy of epidemic influenza A2 (Hong Kong), Infect Immun 1:220, 1970.

Koretz SH and others: Treatment of serious cytomegalovirus infections with 9-(1,3-dihydroxy-2-propoxymethyl) guanine in patients with AIDS and other immunodeficiencies, N Engl J Med 314:801, 1986.

Mandell GL, Douglas RG, and Bennett JE, editors: Principles and practice of infectious diseases, New York: 1984, John Wiley & Sons, Inc.

Ramsey PG: Herpes simplex virus pneumonia, Ann Intern Med 97:813, 1982.

Waldman RJ and others: Aspirin as a risk factor in Reye's syndrome, JAMA 247:3089, 1982.

Exanthems of viral or presumed viral origin

Allan M. Arbeter

MEASLES (RUBEOLA)

Measles is an acute respiratory infection associated with a 3- to 5-day prodrome and a characteristic maculopapular rash that lasts 5 to 7 days.

Measles virus is an enveloped RNA paramyxovirus with a diameter of 120 to 350 nm. The envelope contains surface hemagglutinin and hemolysin antigens. Antibody against the hemagglutinins correlates with protection against reinfection.

Measles occurs in young and school-age children worldwide. In countries where the vaccine for measles is in use, the number of cases in young children has declined daramtically but an increased incidence of the disease has occurred in older children and teenagers. The number of cases in a current "epidemic" year is less than 1% of the cases that occurred in the prevaccine era.

Measles virus initially infects the respiratory epithelium and is followed by viremia within leukocytes. Infection develops within reticuloendothelial cells, virus is released and reinvades leukocytes, and a secondary viremia occurs. During this phase extensive respiratory mucosal and skin infection develops. Respiratory manifestations consist of cough, coryza, bronchopneumonia, and croup. The rash coincides with the development of an immune response and appears to be mediated by a delayed hypersensitivity reaction to the virus in the skin.

The incubation period is 10 to 14 days in children but may be as long as 21 days in adults. This is followed by a 3- to 5-day prodrome of increasing severity, consisting of cough, conjunctivitis, fever, malaise, loss of appetite, and coryza. At this time the disease may be indistinguishable from other severe upper respiratory illnesses except for the presence of Koplik's spots. These are multiple 0.25- to 1-mm whitish blue spots on a red base found in clusters on the buccal mucosa, usually opposite the second molars. These lesions represent sites of virus replication. A characteristic intense maculopapular rash then develops on the face and neck and spreads in a descending pattern to reach the hands and feet 3 to 5 days later. As the rash spreads, areas of earlier involvement become confluent. Desquamation may occur. Complications of measles include viral pneumonia, secondary bacterial pneumonia, otitis media, laryngotracheal bronchitis, and encephalitis. The encephalitis may be fatal or leave the patient with permanent neurologic sequelae. Subacute sclerosing panencephalitis is a rare chronic sequelae of measles virus infection when measles occurs early in life.

Unusual forms of measles include *modified measles* and *atypical measles*. Modified measles, which is mild measles, occurs when the patient has received γ-globulin within 3 days of exposure. Modified measles has also been described in patients who previously had vaccine-induced immunity. Atypical measles is a distinct clinical syndrome occurring in patients previously immunized with killed measles vaccine; it rarely occurs after natural virus exposure in an individual who received live attenuated vaccine. The illness includes high fever, maculopapular or purpuric rash of the extremities, and severe pneumonitis. The illness can resemble Rocky Mountain spotted fever or meningococcemia. When measles occurs in patients with deficiencies in cellular immunity, a severe giant cell pneumonia (Heckt's pneumonia) without rash can occur. This disease is frequently fatal in immunosuppressed patients, especially leukemic children undergoing chemotherapy.

Measles can be diagnosed by examination of mucosal cells, virus isolation, and antibody tests. Scraped cells from the conjunctiva, nasopharynx, or Koplik's spots demonstrate multinucleated giant cells and cells containing eosinophilic cytoplasmic inclusions. Direct immunofluorescent staining of exfoliated cells or skin biopsy material with measles virus–specific antisera can demonstrate viral antigen. Because the virus is difficult to grow in the laboratory, the diagnosis is usually made by serologic testing using either a complement fixation, enzyme immunoabsorbent, or a hemagglutination inhibition assay. When paired sera samples are tested, a fourfold or greater antibody rise is diagnostic of recent infection.

There is no specific therapy for measles virus infection.

Active immunization with live attenuated measles vaccine has been highly successful in reducing measles infection. When given at or after 15 months of age, the immunization is expected to produce lifelong immunity. Live measles vaccine should not be given to immunosuppressed patients. Measles can be modified and sometimes prevented by giving 0.5 ml/kg of immune serum globulin. However, this does not provide permanent immunity.

RUBELLA (GERMAN MEASLES)

Rubella is a mild respiratory virus infection associated with an exanthem. Of major importance is the fetal damage that develops following transplacental infection (see discussion of "Viral infections of the fetus and newborn"). Infection occurring before 12 weeks' gestation may lead to abortions; severe birth defects, including microcephaly; and cardiac anomalies. Infection later in pregnancy can lead to hepatitis, jaundice, thrombocytopenia, lymphadenopathy, and pneumonitis. Some infected infants are born without anomalies but can have progressive mental retardation and spastic diplegia.

Rubella virus contains an RNA nucleoprotein and a lipid envelope, has a diameter of 60 nm, and is classified as a togavirus. Serologic tests are for antibody against nucleoprotein (complement fixation), envelope antigens (hemagglutinin), and total virus (enzyme immunoassay).

Rubella occurs predominantly in the spring and early summer. The agent is highly contagious by the respiratory route. The incidence of rubella has decreased since the introduction of vaccine. Since introduction of the combination measles, mumps, and rubella vaccine, outbreaks have become rare.

The virus is spread by respiratory secretions. Although heaviest viral shedding occurs at the time of the rash, rubella virus can be isolated several days before and after the onset of the eruption. As with measles, primary and secondary viremia develop. The rash occurs at the end of the secondary viremia and coincides with the development of the immune response, suggesting that immune mechanisms may participate in the pathogenesis of the rash.

Postnatally acquired rubella is generally a benign disease in children and adults. The incubation period is 14 to 21 days. The rash can occur in a typical pattern or be nonspecific. The typical rash appears as a maculopapular eruption on the face and neck and is preceded by or associated with posterior cervical adenopathy. The rash descends from head to foot over 2 to 3 days, fades above as it appears below, and does not become confluent. An enanthem can develop simultaneously with the rash and consists chiefly of petechial lesions on the soft palate (Forscheimer spots). Fever is present for 1 to 2 days at the onset of the rash. In 30% to 40% of adult women with rubella, arthritis or arthralgias of the fingers, wrists, and knees develop.

A severe postinfectious encephalitis can occur with rubella but is uncommon. In several patients with congenital rubella a subacute sclerosing panencephalitis–like illness has developed in subsequent years.

The manifestations of rubella may be sufficiently mild (for example, nonspecific or absent rash) so that many cases go undiagnosed. In addition, several other viruses can produce similar-appearing rashes. Therefore a clinical history of rubella cannot be relied on to indicate immunity. In nonvaccinated women of childbearing age the immune status should be evaluated by antibody testing.

Specific diagnosis of rubella is made by virus isolation or serologic tests. The virus can be cultured from throat samples and from urine in infants with congenital infection. The most widely used antibody tests are the hemagglutination inhibition and enzyme immunoassays. Detecting recent infection is particularly important in pregnant women, since a positive result could lead to a termination of pregnancy. In paired serum samples a fourfold or greater rise in rubella antibody is diagnostic of recent infection. If only a convalescent serum sample is available, a rubella-specific IgM antibody assay can be performed; this is a useful diagnostic aid during pregnancy.

There is no treatment for rubella.

Since 1969, live attenuated rubella vaccines have been available. The currently available strain is RA 27/3, which is given subcutaneously. Although fetal damage from inadvertent immunization during gestation is rare or even absent, populations for immunization remain limited to prepubertal children and seronegative nonpregnant women.

Immune serum globulin is ineffective in preventing viremia and intrauterine infection, although it can modify the clinical illness.

ROSEOLA (EXANTHEMA SUBITUM)

Roseola is an acute illness of undefined origin. The diagnosis is established by the characteristic clinical syndrome. The disease occurs predominantly in infants and young children between 6 months and 3 years of age. It does not recur, suggesting that it is caused by a single serotype with persistent immunity. Illness occurs year round with a springtime peak. Secondary cases are usually limited to children of similar age rather than to siblings. The incubation period is 10 to 15 days.

The disease usually begins without a prodrome. There is a sudden onset of high temperature, commonly 104° F (40° C), malaise, irritability, and anorexia. The pharynx can be injected, anterior and posterior cervical adenopathy is often present, and on days 3 to 5 a maculopapular rash develops. The rash characteristically appears as the fever is declining or has disappeared. Rash is rarely found on the face or extremities but is located on the chest, abdomen, and neck and lasts 6 hours to 2 days. The diagnosis is made by the typical clinical manifestations. Laboratory tests are not helpful. The white blood cell count can be decreased, normal, or elevated.

Febrile convulsions can occur because of the rapid onset of fever in young children. Since a rash is not present at the onset of fever, a lumbar spinal puncture for suspected meningitis is performed in many children. The cerebrospinal fluid (CSF) is normal.

There is no specific therapy for this illness. Temperature control is recommended to prevent seizures. Since the etiologic agent has not been identified, no vaccine is available.

ERYTHEMA INFECTIOSUM (FIFTH DISEASE)

Erythema infectiosum has been associated with human parvovirus infection. The disease is categorized as an infection, probably viral, because of the seasonal occurrence (predominantly winter) and the clustering of cases separated by a 5- to 10-day incubation period. It most often affects children and is unusual in adults.

The clinical manifestations of erythema infectiosum are variable. The rash may be preceded by a mild prodrome of fever and coryza lasting 1 to 2 days. A marked erythema of the cheeks (so-called slapped cheeks) follows. Either simultaneously or shortly therafter a red macular rash develops on the extremities, sparing the palms and soles. The rash, involving the face and extremities, is frequently sufficiently characteristic to enable a diagnosis. Circumoral pallor is common. On the extremities the rash has been described as lacy and includes a pattern of red blotches, some of which are confluent, circular, or annular. The rash can fade and reappear for several weeks. Additional features include high fever, pharyngitis, vomiting and diarrhea, adenopathy, and joint complaints. In adults there are more frequent complaints of arthritis.

The diagnosis of erythema infectiosum is based on the constellation of clinical features. When the clinical pattern is unusual, other illnesses must be considered, including erythema multiforme, infectious mononucleosis, Lyme disease, rubella, and measles. There are no laboratory tests that confirm the diagnosis, and no specific treatments or preventive therapies available.

KAWASAKI DISEASE

Kawasaki disease, also termed mucocutaneous lymph node syndrome, is an acute febrile disease of children with a reported 1% to 2% fatality rate, worldwide distribution, and unknown origin. The disease was originally described in Japan, where over 10,000 cases have been recorded, but has been diagnosed throughout North America as well. Several etiologic agents have been associated with specific outbreaks or individual cases, including rickettsiae, streptococci, and respiratory viruses. However, a specific etiologic agent for this syndrome has not been confirmed.

Fever occurs in almost 100% of cases and lasts for a minimum of 1 week but can persist for 2 to 4 weeks, reaching daily spikes of 102° to 104° F (39° to 40° C). During the first week conjunctivitis, stomatitis, diffuse adenopathy, and a rash of the trunk and extremities develop. The conjunctivitis is predominantly bulbar and can be mild or severe. The discharge is thin and white, if present. The lips are bright red, fissured, and painful. The tongue is frequently desquamated, exposing the papillae and resembling the strawberry tongue of scarlet fever. The extremity rash can include a papular eruption of the arms and legs, but most striking are the edema and redness of the palms and soles. This blanching erythema can continue for 1 to 2 weeks before desquamation of the skin of the hands occurs. Desquamation occurs in sheets, taking several days. In mild cases the peeling occurs only on the edges of the nails. The truncal rash can be a nonspecific papular rash reminiscent of measles, scarlet fever, or infectious mononucleosis. Nonsuppurative adenopathy, which is usually cervical but occasionally diffuse, can occur. Other clinical manifestations include gastrointestinal complaints, joint symptoms, and aseptic meningitis.

The major complication of Kawasaki disease is coronary arteritis early in the course and eventuating as coronary artery aneurysms. In addition, there can be a carditis affecting the conduction system and papillary muscles. Death as a result of arrhythmias, coronary artery obstruction, and rupture or thrombosis of a coronary artery aneurysm can occur suddenly at any time from the acute illness to years later. The carditis is similar to that described as infantile polyarteritis nodosa, which may be the same disease.

Laboratory studies may support the clinical diagnosis. Findings include a leukocytosis with a shift toward immature forms, a marked thrombocytosis, sometimes exceeding 10^6 platelets/mm^3, and an elevated erythrocyte sedimentation rate. Serum IgE is elevated in the majority of cases. The electrocardiogram may show abnormalities in conduction and repolarization. If heart disease is suspected, further evaluation for carditis and aneurysms is indicated.

Therapy with an initial high-dose of aspirin followed by a maintenance low-dosage of aspirin appears to decrease the severity of coronary artery disease.

ADENOVIRUS EXANTHEMS

The adenoviruses are 70-nm double-stranded DNA viruses that cause frequent infections in humans. The diseases produced include conjunctivitis, pharyngitis, laryngitis, laryngotracheal bronchitis, pneumonitis, adenitis, and hemorrhagic cystitis (see discussion of "Viral respiratory infections"). Any of the clinical syndromes of adenovirus infection may be accompanied by rash. Although over 30 serotypes of adenoviruses exist, disease is most commonly produced by types 1 to 8.

The rash is nonspecific. It may vary from a very diffuse macular disease to a heavy, confluent maculopapular disease with involvement of the face, neck, trunk, and extremities. The rash may be present for 1 day or mimic measles, occurring after a prodrome and remaining for 5 to 7 days. The rash rarely becomes vesicular. The nonspecific nature of the rash makes diagnosis more difficult; however, the presence of conjunctivitis, pharyngitis, and adenitis indicates a probable adenovirus infection.

The results of routine laboratory studies are nonspecific. Adenoviruses can be isolated on tissue culture cells. Viral serology, using the complement fixation method, confirms recent infection if a fourfold or greater rise in antibody is observed.

There is no specific therapy for adenovirus infections. Prevention has been demonstrated after inoculation with live virus and inactivated vaccines. However, these vaccines are not in general use.

ENTEROVIRUS EXANTHEMS

The enteroviruses are members of the picornavirus family. These small RNA viruses lack a lipoprotein envelope. Those that cause exanthems include group A and B coxsackieviruses and the echoviruses. These viruses cause disease worldwide in infants, children, and adults. More than 70 serologically different enteroviruses have been detected.

Enterovirus infections result in a large number of clinical syndromes. Illnesses include nonspecific febrile diseases, stomatitis, tonsillitis, pharyngitis, aseptic meningitis, encephalitis, gastroenteritis, pneumonitis, pleurodynia, pericarditis, myocarditis, and exanthems.

The exanthems may be of a specific character (hand-foot-and-mouth disease) or of a variety of nonspecific types. The nonspecific rashes can include manifestations and clinical syndromes similar to measles, rubella, roseola, erythema infectiosum, and herpes simplex. The eruptions can occur with fever alone or in combination with any of the other enteroviral syndromes.

One of the characteristic exanthems of enteroviruses is hand-foot-and-mouth disease. This mild illness includes fever and oral vesicles followed by vesicles on the hands, feet, fingers, toes, soles, palms, and extensor surfaces of the arms and legs. These papulovesicular lesions can be painful and can last over 1 week. Virus can be isolated from the lesions. Coxsackieviruses A5, A10, A16, B2, and B5 have all been associated with hand-foot-and-mouth disease.

An additional characteristic exanthem is caused by coxsackievirus A9. This virus produces a papulovesicular rash that occurs with the onset of fever. Like chickenpox, the rash is heaviest on the trunk, neck, and head, but it differs because the lesion remains vesicular without pustulating or crusting. There is usually no enanthem.

Enteroviruses, particularly group A coxsackieviruses, can cause a vesicular enanthem of the fauces and soft palate termed herpangina. Fever, sore throat, and pain on swallowing are frequent symptoms. The throat is erythematous, and the tonsils may contain a mild exudate. Two to six, but rarely more, painful lesions are located on the soft palate, frequently at the free-hanging margin between the tonsils and uvula. Occasionally the tonsils, posterior pharyngeal wall, or buccal mucosa is involved. Lesions begin as small macules and over 24 hours evolve into 2- to 4-mm erythematous papules, which then centrally vesiculate. Fever lasts 2 to 4 days, and mouth lesions persist for up to 1 week.

Since enteroviral disease usually appears in epidemic form during the summer or fall months, the diagnosis is aided by knowledge of the local epidemiology.

Standard laboratory tests are generally not helpful. Cultures of throat and stool for viral isolation are the main methods for establishing a specific diagnosis. Group B coxsackieviruses and echoviruses will grow on cell culture, but group A coxsackieviruses may require suckling mouse inoculation for isolation. Serologic confirmation of enterovirus infection is not routinely done unless a specific enterovirus is suspected. The lack of a group-specific antigen common to all serotypes limits the use of antibody testing.

No specific antiviral treatment is available for enterovirus infections. An inactivated parenteral vaccine and an attenuated oral vaccine have been prepared for polioviruses (see Chapter 38); however, vaccines for other enteroviruses are not available.

For exanthems associated with herpesviruses see the discussion "Herpesviruses."

BIBLIOGRAPHY

Cherry JD: Newer viral exanthems, Adv Pediatr 16:233, 1969.
Evans AS: Viral infections of humans: epidemiology and control, New York, 1976, Plenum Publishing Corp.
Feign R and Cherry J: Textbook of pediatric infectious diseases, Philadelphia, 1987, WB Saunders Co.
Krugman S and Katz SL: Infectious diseases of children, ed 7, St. Louis, 1980, The CV Mosby Co.
Mandell GL, Douglas RG, and Bennett JE: Principles and practice of infectious diseases, New York, 1985, John Wiley & Sons, Inc.
Morens DM, Anderson LJ, and Hurwitz ES: National surveillance of Kawasaki's disease, Pediatrics 65:21, 1980.
Vaughan VC III, McKay RJ, and Behrman R: Nelson's textbook of pediatrics, ed 11, Philadelphia, 1979, WB Saunders Co.

Viral gastroenteritis

Steven D. London and **Donald H. Rubin**

Acute gastroenteritis resulting from viral infection is a major cause of morbidity and can be life threatening for young children, the elderly, and debilitated individuals. Mortality is significant in underdeveloped countries where adequate medical care is not available. Symptoms of gastroenteritis can include a combination of the following: abdominal pain, nausea, vomiting, diarrhea, and fever.

Traditionally, picornaviruses (poliovirus, echovirus, and coxsackievirus) have been considered "enteric" viruses, yet only certain echovirus serotypes are believed to be associated with enteritis. Most picornaviruses enter through the intestine, and produce their major impact in organs outside the gastrointestinal tract, especially the central nervous system (CNS). These viral agents are considered elsewhere in more detail (see discussions of "Viral infections of the central nervous system" and "Exanthems of viral or presumed viral origin"). In the early 1970s, the techniques of immune electron microscopy (IEM) of stool samples and electron microscopy (EM) of infected intestinal mucosa from individuals with nonbacterial gastroenteritis identified two major viral groups as causative agents: the rotaviruses and the Norwalk-like (or 27-nm) agents. Other viruses can also cause gastroenteritis, yet they are responsible for far fewer cases than rotavirus or Norwalk-like viruses (Table 37-3). Rotavirus and Norwalk-like

Table 37-3 Agents thought to be responsible for gastroenteritis in humans

Virus	Known serotypes or classifications	Diagnostic tests for viral detection
Rotavirus	Group A (strains 1-4), group B, group C	EM, IEM, ELISA, tissue culture, dot blotting
Norwalk-like agents	Various isolates	IEM
Adenovirus	Enteric strains 40,41	IEM, IF
Coronavirus	Enteric strains (?)	IEM, IF
Picornavirus	Echovirus type 4,11,14,18,19	Tissue culture
Astrovirus	5 strains	IEM
Calicivirus	4-5 types	IEM
Minireovirus	?	IEM

agents are considered separately, since they produce unique syndromes.

ROTAVIRUSES

The rotaviruses are the most common agents causing sporadic and epidemic outbreaks of enteritis in infants and young children worldwide. In temperate climates 50% of pediatric hospitalizations resulting from gastroenteritis are caused by rotaviruses. Symptomatic disease occurs primarily in the 6- to 24-month age-group. On occasion, neonates and adults can develop symptomatic illness, but subclinical infection is more common. When symptoms occur in adults, they tend to be milder than in children. The incidence of symptomatic infection peaks during the winter months. Transmission is by the fecal-oral route. Nosocomial spread in pediatric wards has occurred.

The major symptom of rotavirus gastroenteritis is diarrhea; dehydration is the main cause for admission to pediatric wards. Death is a rare sequela and occurs when dehydration is inadequately treated. The incubation period is 24 to 48 hours, and symptoms peak in the following 1 to 3 days. When it occurs, vomiting develops early. Fever is present in 75% of the patients.

Five groups of rotavirus exist (A-E) based on unique immunodeterminants present on the inner viral protein VP6. Group A serotypes 1-4 are the major human pathogens predominantly infecting young children. Recently, analysis of clinical isolates in neonates has demonstrated unique, potentially less virulent strains of group A rotavirus infecting this age-group. In addition, epidemic outbreaks of diarrhea among adults in China have been identified with group B rotavirus. Group C rotavirus has also been isolated from humans in Australia and Brazil.

The pathogenesis of rotavirus-induced gastroenteritis is incompletely understood. The virus appears primarily in the small bowel and is visualized in intestinal epithelial cells within the villi tips. Villi are shortened, crypts are hyperplastic, and an inflammatory cell infiltrate appears in the lamina propria. Impaired D-xylose absorption has been observed, and some patients have depressed levels of disaccharidases. Adenyl cyclase activity appears normal in experimental animal model systems.

Diagnosis of rotavirus gastroenteritis was initially made by IEM; however, conventional EM is adequate for the morphologic identification of rotavirus obtained from stool or rectal swab specimens. Radioimmunoassay (RIA) or en-

zyme-linked immunosorbent assay (ELISA) can also be used for the detection of rotavirus particles. Dot blot hybridization assays are capable of detecting rotavirus from stool or rectal swab specimens. The serologic response to rotavirus infection can also be examined by several assays (complement fixation, IEM, ELISA, RIA, and hemagglutination inhibition).

27-NM NORWALK-LIKE AGENTS

Norwalk-like agents are responsible for epidemic outbreaks of gastroenteritis among older children and adults. Symptoms include vomiting and diarrhea of varying severity; these are generally milder than rotavirus-induced symptoms. Other symptoms are abdominal cramps, headache, malaise, nausea, myalgia, and low-grade fever. Symptoms usually start within 24 hours after exposure to virus and last 1 to 2 days.

The pathologic lesions caused by the Norwalk-like agents are similar to those described for rotaviruses. In the small intestine, villi become shortened and blunted, and crypt hyperplasia occurs. Although the intestinal mucosa is intact, there is an inflammatory infiltrate of polymorphonuclear leukocytes and monocytes in the lamina propria. Virus particles have not been seen on EM examination of the small intestine. Alterations in fat and carbohydrate absorption occur. Vomiting is thought to be caused by delayed gastric emptying, possibly resulting from abnormal gastric motor function. Adenyl cyclase activity appears normal in infected patients, and the exact mechanism for diarrhea is still unclear.

The 27-nm Norwalk-like agents have not been successfully adapted to tissue culture nor do they produce disease in animals. IEM is the method of choice for the definitive identification of Norwalk-like agents from specimens of infected individuals. RIA can be used to detect virus or virus antigens and a serum antibody response.

OTHER AGENTS

Other viruses have been described as causes of symptomatic gastroenteritis. Two enteric noncultivatable adenovirus strains (40 and 41) that seem to be an important cause of acute gastrointestinal disease in young children have recently been identified. These viruses have been visualized by EM and have been detected by serologic methods. The coronaviruses are likely to be a cause of enteritis, since they are recognized causes of severe enteritis in numerous animal species. Coronavirus particles, visualized by EM, can exist in the stool of persons who are suffering from gastroenteritis. However, a causal relation has been difficult to define because coronavirus particles are frequently found in the stool of healthy individuals. Recently, two strains of human coronaviruses have been characterized from infants who are suffering from acute gastroenteritis. Further studies of these strains are necessary to define their role in the pathogenesis and epidemiology of coronavirus-induced gastroenteritis in humans. A number of echovirus types (especially 4, 11, 14, 18, and 19) have been implicated in gastroenteritis in humans.

Astroviruses have been associated with mild gastroenteritis in all age-groups. Although studies using astrovirus inoculation of human volunteers have shown that most recipients produce infectious virus in their stool, few of these subjects developed diarrhea. Calicivirus-like particles have been associated with gastroenteritis of infants and young children in epidemics, nosocomial outbreaks, and isolated cases. These two virus groups can be identified by their unique morphology in IEM preparations and RIA assays. Minireoviruses have been detected in both pediatric patients with nosocomial gastroenteritis and in sporadic cases.

Although these groups of viruses can be associated with acute gastroenteritis, they do not appear to be an important cause of gastroenteritis in humans.

DIAGNOSIS. The diagnosis of viral gastroenteritis depends in part on eliminating other known causes of gastroenteritis, especially bacterial agents. Specific viral diagnosis is indicated in severely ill patients. If available, EM is the procedure of choice, since it is rapid and sensitive. When available for particular viruses, ELISA, RIA, or immunofluorescence (IF) assays can also be used to detect viral antigens. Serologic diagnostic procedures can confirm a diagnostic impression but do not yield positive results during the acute illness.

MANAGEMENT. The treatment of viral enteritis is symptomatic. Dehydration is a major concern, especially in young children, the elderly, or debilitated patients. Oral rehydration therapy with a glucose- and electrolyte-rich solution is the treatment of choice. Adding glucose to the rehydration solution enhances fluid absorption because the sodium and glucose transport mechanisms are linked, and the net transport of fluids is enhanced when both substrates are present. The WHO oral glucose-electrolyte formula is 3.5 g NaCl, 2.5 g NaHCO$_3$, 1.5 g KCl, and 20 g glucose per liter of water. Commercial preparations are also available. Oral administration of bismuth subsalicylate (Pepto-bismol) after the onset of symptoms in Norwalk-like virus illness can significantly reduce the severity and duration of abdominal cramps but is of little value in treating acute diarrhea. Because of the association of Reye's syndrome with certain viral infections (most notably influenza and varicella-zoster viruses, although others have been implicated) and treatment with salicylates, care should be exercised when administering these compounds to children and adolescents. In extreme cases, hospitalization may be required in dehydrated patients with severe vomiting or diarrhea to monitor fluid and electrolyte balance.

BIBLIOGRAPHY

Battaglia M, Passarani N, De Matteo A, and Gerna G: Human enteric coronaviruses: further characterization and immunoblotting of viral proteins, J Infect Dis 155:140, 1987.

Bridger JC, Pedley S, and McCrae MA: Group C rotaviruses in humans, J Clin Microbiol 23:760, 1986.

Chen GM, Hung T, Bridger JC, and McCrae MA: Chinese adult rotavirus is a group B rotavirus, Lancet 8464:1123, 1985.

De Jong JC and others: Candidate adenoviruses 40 and 41: fastidious adenoviruses from human infant stool, J Med Virol 11:215, 1983.

Dolin R, Treanor JJ, and Madore HP: Novel agents of viral enteritis in humans, J Infect Dis 155:365, 1987.

Flores J and others: Conservation of the fourth gene among rotaviruses recovered from asymptomatic newborn infants and its possible role in attenuation, J Virol 60:972, 1986.

Kibrick S: Current status of coxsackie and ECHO viruses in human disease, Prog Med Virol 6:27, 1964.

Wolf JL and Schreiber DS: Viral gastroenteritis, Med Clin N Am 66:575, 1982.

Acquired immunodeficiency syndrome

Oksana M. Korzeniowski

DEFINITION. Acquired immunodeficiency syndrome (AIDS) is a clinical syndrome characterized by opportunistic infections and unusual malignancies occurring as a result of profound deficiency of the helper-T$_4$ lymphocytes (CD$_4$ lymphocytes) induced by infection with the human immunodeficiency viruses (HIVs).

ETIOLOGY AND PATHOGENESIS. Presently at least two human retroviruses (HIV-1, or human T lymphotropic virus type III [HTLV-III]/lymphadenopathy-associated virus type I [LAV-I], and HIV-2, or lymphadenopathy-associated virus type II [LAV-II]) have been recognized as etiologic agents for the development of AIDS. Retroviruses are RNA viruses that possess a reverse transciptase enzyme and thus are capable of synthesizing a DNA copy of the viral genome through subversion of the host's synthetic machinery. Cells with CD$_4$ receptors, such as T$_4$ lymphocytes, are most susceptible to infection, but macrophages and cells of neural origin also permit viral replication. HIVs appear to be related to the simian lymphotrophic retroviruses and pathogenically resemble the visna virus of sheep.

In the host cell the DNA copy of the viral genome is inserted into the host's genomic material; there, it can remain quiescent or can induce synthesis of new viral particles, a process that results in eventual cell death. The stimulus for viral replication has not been defined but probably consists of any antigen capable of inducing the terminal differentiation of the host cell. The initial host response is a nonspecific stimulation of B cells followed by a rise in the number of suppressor- and killer-T cells (CD$_8$) and a concurrent decline in the number of helper-T cells (CD$_4$). Abnormal B-cell function occurs as shown by the presence of polyclonal gammopathy and immune thrombocytopenias; however, the predominant immunologic defect is a severe deficiency of the cellular immune system. Sequential isolates of virus from an infected individual show genomic variability. Although neutralizing antibodies have been demonstrated, no effective containment or eradication of virus occurs. Reconstitution of the helper-T cells does not occur; however, partial improvement has been documented with zidovudine (Azidothymidine).

EPIDEMIOLOGY. Although HIV infection is now recognized throughout the world, it appears to be a new pathogen. The virus was first isolated in 1983; however, retrospective serologic studies have identified infected blood in African samples obtained in the 1960s. The highest incidence of infection occurs in the United States, Haiti, and Central African countries.

HIV has been isolated from blood, semen, saliva, cerebrospinal fluid (CSF), milk, and from major organs such as the brain. Viral titers are highest in individuals who are asymptomatically infected and in individuals with profound CD$_4$ lymphocyte depletion in whom reactivation of viremia has occured. Transmission of virus occurs through intimate sexual contact (particularly receptive anal intercourse and contact with multiple partners) and through exposure to blood or blood products. In the United States individuals at risk of infection are primarily homosexual males, intravenous drug users, prostitutes, heterosexual partners of infected individuals, and children of infected women (transmission can occur in utero or post partum). The male to female ratio is 9:1. Before 1985, recipients of contaminated blood products constituted a significant risk group. The risk has been diminished but not totally eliminated through testing of donated blood for HIV antibody; occasionally seronegative but infected transfusions can transmit virus. Heat treatment of clotting factors has eliminated virus from factor VIII and reduced the rate of infection among hemophiliacs. Findings from epidemiologic studies of AIDS in Europe, Asia, and South America parallel findings in the United States. In Haiti and Central African countries transmission appears to be primarily through sexual contact (male to female ratio 1 to 2:1), although blood transfusion and the use of contaminated needles in medical practice are also implicated. Health-care workers with parenteral exposure to infected blood (via needle sticks or surface contamination of broken skin) are at risk of HIV infection, but the efficiency of viral transmission is low. Fomite and arthropod transmission have not been demonstrated; thus nonsexual household contacts of HIV-infected individuals have a negligible risk of infection.

CLINICAL MANIFESTATIONS. Primary exposure to HIV results in a mononucleosis-like illness occurring 2 weeks after infection. Acquisition of HIV can also be asymptomatic. Antigen can be detected for several months until IgG antibody formation is induced. Seroconversion occurs 2 to 4 months after exposure, but seropositive individuals remain infectious. An infected individual can remain asymptomatic and immunologically intact, or he can develop any of the clinical syndromes associated with progressive immunologic compromise. Although the period of risk for disease progression is as yet unclear, a 10- to 15-year mean incubation period for AIDS has been estimated. In fact, infected individuals may face a lifetime risk for AIDS. Presently there are no definitive predictors for disease progression, but persistent symptoms of fever and malaise, appearance of thrush, lack of in vitro responsiveness of CD_4 lymphocytes to phytohemagglutinin and reduction of total CD_4 lymphocyte count below $200/mm^3$ and reappearance of p24 antigen (HIV core protein) in the serum appear to be indicators of poor prognosis. In cohort studies of homosexual or hemophiliac patients who test positive for HIV, 10% to 35% develop AIDS or AIDS-related complex (ARC) within a period of 5 years. ARC is characterized by nonspecific, persistent (longer than 3 months) complaints of fever, malaise, diarrhea, lymphadenopathy, oral thrush, and weight loss, as well as with laboratory studies that include a reduced number of CD_4 cells, cutaneous anergy, and hematologic abnormalities including leukopenia, lymphopenia, thrombocytopenia, or anemia. Symptoms associated with ARC can persist chronically, or patients can develop AIDS. The diagnosis of AIDS is based on the presence of opportunistic infections, manifestations of unusual malignancies (for example, Kaposi's sarcoma), or both, in an individual who has tested positive for HIV and has no other causes for cellular immunodeficiency. Typically, infections in AIDS are characterized by an insidious onset, high tissue titers of the infecting organisms, poor host tissue response, the simultaneous presence of multiple pathogens, and a very high relapse rate after treatment. Malignancies are poorly differentiated and occur in atypical sites (that is, the central nervous system). In general, the appearance of infections is indicative of more profound immunodeficiency, whereas malignant lesions can be associated with types of human lymphocyte antigen (HLA) and coinfections.

Although both infections and malignancies can be quite variable, the clinical presentations of patients with suspected AIDS fall into several common patterns. Dyspnea occurs in approximately 60% of patients with AIDS and is most commonly associated with *Pneumocystis carinii* pneumonia, although *Mycobacterium tuberculosis*, cytomegalovirus (CMV), Epstein-Barr virus (EBV), *Cryptococcus neoformans, Histoplasma capsulatum*, and Kaposi's sarcoma can be present concurrently.

Nonhealing skin ulcers in the perioral or perirectal area are most frequently caused by herpes simplex viruses. Raised violaceous nodules, particularly along skin folds and on palms and soles, suggest Kaposi's sarcoma, which occurs in 20% of males with AIDS. Disseminated fungal infection, especially with *Cryptococcus, Candida,* or *Histoplasma* spp., must also be ruled out.

Dysphagia is a common complaint and in the presence of thrush is most likely indicative of *Candida esophagitis;* however, herpes simplex infection must also be considered. Diar-

rhea, particularly fulminant diarrhea with profound weight loss and malabsorption may be due to common intestinal pathogens such as *Campylobacter jejuni* or *Salmonella* spp.; however, unusual protozoa such as *Cryptosporidium* organisms and *Isospora belli* have been isolated in homosexual AIDS populations. In addition, the gastrointestinal tract can be diffusely involved with *Mycobacterium-avium intracellulare* (MAI) or CMV, and diagnosis may require biopsy.

The onset of visual disturbance is usually associated with CMV retinochondritis and can progress rapidly to total blindness.

Diffuse lymphadenopathy is common in individuals with ARC and AIDS and is usually a nonspecific immunologic response to HIV infection. However, biopsy should be performed to exclude disseminated mycobacterial infections (both tuberculosis and MAI), fungal infection, toxoplasmosis, lymphoma, and Kaposi's sarcoma.

Neurologic symptoms in AIDS are also quite variable and present a particularly difficult diagnostic differential. Primary HIV involvement of the brain can occur in as many as 60% of the individuals with AIDS, and symptoms can antedate the diagnosis of AIDS. Dementia and paranoia are the most commonly described symptoms, but peripheral neuropathies, meningitis, and encephalopathy can also occur. HIV infection must be differentiated from underlying primary psychiatric problems, opportunistic infections, and malignancies. Encephalitis with focal neurologic signs and seizures is most commonly caused by *Toxoplasma gondii;* however, herpes simplex infection and lymphoma must be excluded. *C. neoformans* is the most common cause of meningitis, but other opportunistic fungi (*M. tuberculosis,* lymphoma, and *Listeria monocytogenes*) have also been implicated.

DIAGNOSIS. HIV infection is probable when antibodies to viral core (p24) and envelope (gp41) proteins are detected by the ELISA test. A positive Western blot test result is confirmatory. Individuals infected with LAV-II can have borderline or negative ELISA test results. Virus can be isolated from blood, CSF, or other body fluids, but specialized tissue culture techniques are necessary. An ELISA test for the detection of HIV antigen has been developed and is available commercially.

The immune status may be estimated by cutaneous anergy tests, total CD_4 lymphocyte counts, CD_4/CD_8 ratios, and lymphocyte stimulations tests; however, the diagnoses of ARC and AIDS are based on clinical grounds and demonstration of an infectious agent or a malignancy.

PROGNOSIS AND COURSE. AIDS is a uniformly fatal disease. The course is dictated by the clinical manifestations. In general, individuals who have Kaposi's sarcoma have a longer median survival (18 to 24 months) than individuals with an opportunistic infection (6 to 8 months). Infants who acquire the infection in utero have a more rapid onset of AIDS and a more rapid demise, presumably because of the underlying immaturity of their immune systems.

The recent introduction of zidovudine has modified the inexorable deterioration of individuals with AIDS. Although a cure is not achieved, inhibition of viral replication (by measurement of reverse transcriptase in serum) has reduced mortality (at least during the study period of 1 year) and the frequency of infections and malignancies. In a few patients, skin reactivity to antigens was again detected. Furthermore, CNS dysfunction caused by HIV is less severe. Toxicities, primarily anemia, with this drug are considerable, and its long-term usefulness is as yet undetermined.

MANAGEMENT. Blood and needle precautions should be taken for hospitalized patients with HIV seropositive test results. Antimicrobial therapy is directed at the bacterial, viral, or fungal pathogens that have been identified. Similarly, radiotherapy or chemotherapy can be indicated for the treatment of associated malignancies. Because of the high relapse rate of infections in individuals with AIDS, long-term prophylactic administration of antimicrobial agents may be necessary. Adverse effects (marrow suppression and allergic rashes) are frequently encountered with the extended use of sulfonamides. Individuals with documented *Pneumocystic carinii* pneumonia, with a total CD_4 lymphocyte count below $200/mm^3$, or both are eligible for treatment with zidovudine and can receive it indefinitely. Patients can also qualify for enrollment in clinical trials with investigational antiviral agents and with immunomodulators that are currently underway.

PREVENTION. Currently, prevention of AIDS can only be accomplished through prevention of infection with HIV. Control measures are based on avoidance of exposure to HIV contaminated blood and of intimate sexual contact with infected individuals. Barrier methods, such as gloves or condoms, provide a limited measure of safety but do not eliminate all potential routes of exposure. The efficacy of barrier methods is further enhanced by spermicides and antiseptics such as Na perchlorate (Chlorox), which readily kills extracorporeal HIV. Circumspect sexual practices such as monogamy; avoidance of prostitutes, intravenous drug abusers, and other high-risk individuals; and avoidance of receptive anal intercourse have been shown to reduce the risk of infection.

Because of the high risk of maternal transmission of HIV to the fetus, prevention or interruption of pregnancy in HIV seropositive women has also been recommended. Antiviral agents currently in use or under investigation suppress viral replication but have not eradicated virus from HIV-infected individuals. A vaccine has not yet been developed.

BIBLIOGRAPHY

Archibald DW and others: Antibodies to human T lymphotropic virus type III (HTLV-III) in saliva of acquired immunodeficiency syndrome (AIDS) patients and in persons at risk for AIDS, Blood 67:831, 1986.
Biggar RJ: The AIDS problem in Africa, Lancet 1:79, 1986.
Broder S: AIDS: Modern concepts and therapeutic challenges, New York, 1987, Marcel Dekker.
Centers for Disease Control: Revision of the case definition of acquired immunodeficiency syndrome for national reporting—United States, MMWR 34:373, 1985.
Centers for Disease Control: Summary: recommendations for preventing transmission of infection with human T lymphotropic virus type III/lymphadenopathy-associated virus in the workplace, MMWR 34:681, 1985.
Cooper DA and others: Acute AIDS retrovirus infection, Lancet 1:537, 1985.
Friedland GH and others: Lack of transmission of HTLV-III/LAV infection to household contact of patients with AIDS or AIDS-related complex with oral candidiasis, N Engl J Med 314:344, 1986.
Gallo RC: The AIDS virus, Sci 26:46, 1987. Acheson ED: AIDS: a challenge for the public health, Lancet 1:662, 1986.
Ho DD and others: Infection of monocyte/macrophages by human T lymphotropic virus type III, J Clin Invest 77:1712, 1986.
Koenig S and others: Detection of AIDS virus in macrophages in brain tissue from AIDS patients with encephalopathy, Science 233:1089, 1986.
Lane HC and others: Correlation between immunologic function and clinical subpopulations of patients with the acquired immune deficiency syndrome, Am J Med 78:417, 1985.
Levy JA and others: Isolation of AIDS-associated retroviruses from cerebrospinal fluid and brain of patients with neurological symptoms, Lancet 1:586, 1985.
Levy RM and others: Neurological manifestations of the acquired immunodeficiency syndrome (AIDS): experience at UCSF and review of the literature, J Neurosurg 62:475, 1985.
Lifson JD and others: AIDS retrovirus induced cytopathology: Giant cell formation and involvement of CD_4 antigen, Science 232:1123, 1986.
Oleske J and others: Immune deficiency syndrome in children, JAMA 249:2345, 1983.
Quinn TC and others: Serologic and immunologic studies in patients with AIDS in North America and Africa, JAMA 257:2617, 1987.
Yarchoan R and others: Response of human immunodeficiency virus associated neurological disease to 3'-azido-3'-deoxythymidine, Lancet 1:132, 1987.

38 · PREVENTION AND TREATMENT WITH VACCINES AND ANTIVIRAL AGENTS

Harvey M. Friedman

VIRAL VACCINES IN GENERAL USE
Poliovirus

Both inactivated and live attenuated poliovirus vaccines have been effective in controlling paralytic poliomyelitis. Since 1969 trivalent oral poliovirus vaccine has been used almost exclusively in the United States. However, in countries such as Holland, Finland, and Sweden, which have used inactivated poliomyelitis vaccines, the decline in paralytic poliomyelitis has paralleled the response in the United States. The principal disadvantages of the inactivated vaccine are the need for multiple injections and boosters, the stringent production controls to ensure complete inactivation, and in some vaccine lots inadequate antigenic potency. The main disadvantage of live poliovirus vaccines is the risk of paralytic infection in vaccines or their contacts. The risk is highest for unimmunized young adults who are household contacts of vaccinated children, for immunodeficient children, and for adults undergoing initial vaccination. Approximately 5 to 10 cases of vaccine-related poliomyelitis occur annually in the United States.

The currently recommended immunization schedule for infants is three doses of trivalent oral poliovirus vaccine given at 6 to 12 weeks of age, 2 months later, and at 8 to 12 months of age. Because of the risk of vaccine-associated paralysis, live vaccine is not routinely recommended for previously unimmunized adults. Unimmunized adults at increased risk of acquiring poliomyelitis, such as some health-care workers, persons traveling to endemic areas, and those living in an epidemic focus, should receive immunization. If a rapid immune response is required, trivalent live vaccine is recommended, whereas if time permits, a series of inactivated vaccinations is preferred. The inactivated vaccine is also recommended for immunodeficient children.

In the United States 95% of children entering kindergarten and first grade have received three or more doses of polio vaccine. The live virus trivalent vaccine confers substantial immunity in even a single dose, and nonvaccinated persons may become immunized by contact infection. The almost total elimination of poliomyelitis from the United States argues strongly for the efficacy of the live vaccine.

Rubella virus

Live attenuated rubella vaccine was licensed in the United States in 1969. The rationale for its use is to prevent congenital rubella infection. The vaccine is recommended mainly for children and susceptible postpubertal females. Vaccination of children protects them against rubella and prevents them from spreading infection to susceptible females, and vaccination of postpubertal females confers individual protection against rubella-induced fetal injury. The vaccine, given as a single subcutaneous injection, is produced in monovalent form and in combinations: measles-rubella or measles-mumps-rubella.

The vaccine is recommended for use at 12 months of age unless given with measles vaccine, in which case it is administered at 15 months or older. The vaccine includes antibodies in approximately 95% of susceptible persons. Reinfection without illness can occur in individuals with low levels of naturally acquired or vaccine-induced antibody. However, viremia and significant pharyngeal excretion have not been detected after reinfection, which therefore poses little risk to susceptible contacts and fetuses.

Since the vaccine may cause viremia and can cross the placenta, women of childbearing age should receive vaccine only if they are not pregnant and they should not become pregnant for 3 months after vaccination. No infant has had the congenital rubella syndrome because of vaccination during pregnancy; however, virus has been isolated from fetal tissue and placenta after vaccination inadvertently given during pregnancy. Complications of vaccination are more common in adults than in children and are most common in women over 25 years of age. Side effects including rash, adenopathy, arthralgias, and occasionally arthritis occur in up to 40% of adults. Joint symptoms generally begin 2 to 10 weeks after vaccination and persist for 1 to 3 days. Vaccination of children whose mothers are pregnant and susceptible to rubella does not pose a significant risk to the fetus.

Measles virus

Live and killed measles virus vaccines were licensed in the United States in 1963. The killed vaccine was withdrawn in 1968 because atypical measles infections occurred in vaccine recipients after exposure to natural virus (see "Exanthems of viral or presumed viral origin" in Chapter 37). The initial live virus vaccine (Edmonston B strain) was associated with a high incidence of side effects. To modify this, the vaccine was often administered with immune serum globulin. The development of better attenuated vaccines has reduced the incidence of reactions, and concomitant administration of immune serum globulin is no longer indicated. Passive immunization with immune serum globulin (0.5 mg/kg intramuscularly and 0.25 mg/kg below 1 year of age) is recommended for susceptible individuals who have been exposed and are at high risk of severe or fatal measles. These include children less than 1 year of age and children and adults with malignant diseases or defects in cellular immunity. To be effective, passive immunization should be given within 3 days of exposure.

It is currently recommended that live measles vaccine be given to all healthy children at 15 months of age. Approximately 95% manifest an antibody response. Children immunized before 12 months of age, with killed vaccine, or with concomitant administration of immune serum globulin should be reimmunized with live measles vaccine. Measles epidemics have occurred in previously immunized individuals. Therefore reimmunization on entering primary or secondary schools is now recommended. No deleterious effects of reimmunization have been noted. The vaccine should not be used in pregnant women or in patients with defects in cellular immunity.

Mumps virus

Live attenuated mumps virus vaccine became available in the United States in 1967. A single subcutaneous inoculation produces mumps antibody in more than 95% of vaccines. Adverse reactions to the vaccine are uncommon. The vaccine should be administered to all children over the age of 12 months. If given with measles vaccine, it should be administered at 15 months. Immunization can also be given to susceptible male adolescents and adults, especially medical personnel, to prevent orchitis, which occasionally is complicated by sterility. The vaccine is contraindicated in pregnancy and should not be given to patients undergoing immunosuppressive therapy or those with malignancies or immunodeficiency states.

VIRAL VACCINES FOR SPECIAL CIRCUMSTANCES
Influenza viruses

Inactivated influenza virus vaccines were first used in the United States in the 1940s. The composition of the vaccines varies from year to year, but generally they contain both influenza A and B viruses of types isolated during the previous influenza season. The viruses are grown in allantoic fluid of embryonated hen's eggs, are formalin inactivated, and are purified to remove egg proteins. Most preparations in the United States are treated with lipid solvents to produce split-product or subunit vaccines, which are less likely to cause febrile reactions in children. Minor discomfort at the inoculation site occurs in approximately 25% of vaccines within 24 hours of vaccination. Myalgias and fever develop in only 1% to 2% of adults but in a large percentage of children. During the 1976 national immunization program against swine influenza, an excess rate of Guillain-Barré syndrome occurred 2 to 6 weeks after vaccination. The estimated risk of neurologic disease was 1 in 100,000. Approximately 5% of these patients died, and an additional 5% to 10% had residual neurologic abnormalities. Since 1976 no increased incidence of Guillain-Barré syndrome has been detected among recipients of influenza vaccines.

The preferred route of administration of the vaccine is intramuscular, usually in the deltoid muscle of adults and anterolateral thigh of children. Adults requiring vaccination (see the following paragraph) should receive yearly injections. Children who have not been previously vaccinated require two doses separated by at least 1 month.

High-priority groups for vaccination have been identified. These include adults and children with chronic disorders of the cardiovascular or pulmonary systems; residents of nursing homes and other chronic care facilities; those at moderate risk for influenza-related complications, such as individuals over 65 years of age, patients with chronic metabolic diseases, and children receiving long-term aspirin treatment, who appear to be at increased risk of Reye's syndrome after influenza infection. The vaccine is also indicated for medical personnel and other health-care providers who may transmit influenza to high-risk patients. The vaccine is considered safe in pregnancy and can be administered to pregnant women at high risk for complications of influenza. Vaccine should not be administered to people with an anaphylactic sensitivity to eggs.

Hepatitis B virus

Hepatitis B virus causes acute and chronic hepatitis, cirrhosis, and primary hepatocellular carcinoma. A safe and effective plasma-derived vaccine has been available since 1982. In 1986 a recombinant vaccine produced in yeast by DNA technology became available. The two vaccine preparations appear to be of equal efficacy, although experience with the recombinant vaccine is still limited. Antibody titers are generally higher in recipients of the plasma-derived vaccine, whereas the recombinant vaccine has the theoretic advantage of being free of contaminating agents found in blood. Both vaccines have excellent safety records; in particular, no increased incidence of HIV infection has been detected in recipients of the plasma-derived vaccine. Side effects occur in approximately 15% of recipients and consist of soreness at the injection site and mild systemic reactions (fever, headache, fatigue, nausea). No severe side effects or significant allergic reactions have been recorded.

Vaccination programs are aimed primarily at three risk groups: health-care workers who are exposed to blood, staff and patients at institutions for the developmentally disabled, and staff and patients in hemodialysis units. Vaccine use in these settings has been modest (20% to 45% of those recommended for vaccination) but is increasing. Despite the availability of vaccine, the incidence of hepatitis B infection is rising in the United States. Currently the majority of acute hepatitis B cases occur in homosexual men, parenteral drug abusers, and sexually active heterosexual individuals. To reduce hepatitis B infection, physicians must increase efforts to reach all high-risk populations.

Preexposure hepatitis B vaccine is recommended for health-care workers with potential blood or needle stick exposure, persons in institutions for the developmentally disabled, patients receiving hemodialysis, homosexually active men, intravenous drug abusers, recipients of certain blood products, and household members and sexual contacts of hepatitis B virus carriers. In addition, vaccine should be considered for inmates at correctional facilities, heterosexually active persons with multiple sexual partners, and international travelers to endemic areas of hepatitis B virus.

Postexposure prophylaxis should be administered to infants born to hepatitis B virus–positive mothers, and to persons who have needle stick exposure to human blood. The first dose of vaccine given to infants should be combined with a single injection of hepatitis B immune globulin. Vaccination of persons with needle stick exposure to known hepatitis B virus–positive blood should also include administration of hepatitis B immune globulin.

Vaccine is administered in a series of three doses over 6 months (time 0, 1, and 6 months). Older children and adults should be vaccinated in the deltoid muscle, and infants in the anterolateral thigh muscle. Pregnancy is not a contraindication for vaccination. Antibody responses (anti-HBs) occur in more than 90% of healthy persons. Testing for antibody response is recommended only for those receiving vaccine in an inappropriate site (such as the buttock) or immunosuppressed patients (such as patients receiving dialysis). Booster doses are not recommended for persons with normal immune status. Dialysis patients should have antibody tests at 6-month intervals and booster doses given if antibody levels decline to less than 10 ImU/ml.

Rabies virus

POSTEXPOSURE PROPHYLAXIS. Deciding which patients should receive prophylactic vaccination against rabies requires consideration of the species of the biting animal, the type of exposure, and the circumstances of the biting incident. Carnivorous wild animals such as skunks, raccoons, foxes, coyotes, and bobcats are much more likely to be infected with rabies virus than rodents such as squirrels, hamsters, guinea pigs, gerbils, chipmunks, rats, mice, rabbits, and hares. Prophylaxis should be initiated after the bite of or salivary exposure to a carnivorous animal unless it is tested and shown not to be rabid, whereas rodent bites rarely call for antirabies prophylaxis. The likelihood of rabies in dogs and cats varies from region to region. In many cases the state or local health department should be consulted before postexposure prophylaxis is initiated.

Rabies is transmitted by introducing the virus into open wounds or mucous membranes. Rarely, transmission to laboratory personnel has occurred by aerosols. Any bite penetration of skin and any contamination of scratches, wounds, or mucous membranes by saliva or other potentially infectious material (such as brain) should be considered significant exposure. An unprovoked attack is more likely to indicate that the animal is rabid than a provoked attack. Wild animals and stray dogs or cats that bite or scratch should be killed, and the head should be removed and tested for rabies antigen by immunofluorescence at the local or state health department. Domestic dogs and cats should be confined and observed for illness for 10 days. Any illness should be evaluated by a veterinarian, and if signs suggest rabies, the animal should be killed and the brain evaluated for rabies.

The essential components of postexposure prophylaxis are thorough washing of all bites, wounds, and scratches with soap and water and initiation of immunization as soon as possible. Immunization is both passive and active and includes human rabies immune globulin (20 units/kg), or if unavailable, equine antirabies serum (40 units/kg), which is given with the first dose of killed virus vaccine. Up to half the dose of rabies immune globulin should be infiltrated in the areas around the wound, and the rest is administered intramuscularly. The human diploid cell vaccine is now the vaccine of choice. Five doses, the first given with immune globulin, are administered intramuscularly in the deltoid muscle on days 0 (the day treatment begins), 3, 7, 14, and 28. Antibody levels should be checked only in immunosuppressed patients at the time of the last immunization. If the human diploid vaccine is unavailable, duck embryo vaccine should be given subcutaneously in 21 doses over 14 to 21 days, followed by doses 10 and 20 days after the twenty-first dose. Antibodies should be checked at the time of the last dose, and if no antibodies are present, three doses of the human diploid cell vaccine are given.

PREEXPOSURE IMMUNIZATION. Preexposure vaccination should be considered in certain high-risk groups such as veterinarians, animal handlers, some laboratory workers, and people living in countries where rabies is a constant threat. Although preexposure vaccination does not eliminate the need for additional therapy after rabies exposure, it does eliminate the need for globulin and decrease the number of vaccine doses required. The human diploid cell vaccine is preferred and should be given intramuscularly or intradermally on days 0 (first day of treatment), 7, and 28. Routine serologic testing after vaccination is not recommended. Individuals working with live rabies virus should have antibody titers determined every 6 months; booster doses of vaccine should be administered as required. Other workers at lower risk should receive a booster every 2 years or have serum titers checked and shown to be adequate. When a person with previously demonstrated rabies antibody is exposed to rabies, two doses of the human diploid cell vaccine (days 0 and 3) or five daily doses of duck embryo vaccine followed by a booster dose 20 days later are indicated.

Smallpox virus

With the recent global eradication of smallpox, vaccination is no longer recommended.

Yellow fever

Vaccination against yellow fever is indicated before travel to infected areas, currently parts of Africa and South America. In addition, a few countries require evidence of vaccination from all entering travelers, and some countries require proof of vaccination from travelers arriving from infected areas. It is best to check with the state health department or the embassy or local consulate of the country in question before traveling. A single 0.5 ml dose is administered as the primary vaccination, and a booster dose every 10 years is recommended.

ANTIVIRAL AGENTS

For many years the replication of viruses and the functioning of host cells were thought to require identical metabolic machinery. However, intracellular molecular events unique to virus replication are now recognized and can be used in defining virus-specific targets for new antiviral drugs. Rapid viral diagnosis is of major importance as a guide to the proper use of antiviral agents, since the toxic manifestations and narrow spectrum of the drugs indicate the need for cautious administration.

Amantadine

Amantadine was initially licensed for prophylactic use against Asian influenza (H2N2) infections in 1966. In 1976 it was licensed for use against all strains of influenza A viruses. It is ineffective against influenza B viruses. Although the mechanism of action is not fully known, the drug may interfere with the virus's ability to penetrate the cell. It blocks uncoating of the virus and subsequent release of nucleic acid from the virus into the cell. The drug is rapidly absorbed after oral administration, it has a serum half-life of 9 to 37 hours (mean of 24 hours), and 90% is excreted unchanged in urine. Dose adjustments should be made in renal failure and in persons over 65 years of age. Approximately 5% of healthy adults have side effects consisting of confusion, light-headedness, hallucinations, anxiety, and insomnia. These usually occur shortly after the start of therapy, are reversible if the drug is discontinued, and often cease even if therapy is continued.

Controlled trials of amantadine as a prophylactic agent indicate protection against clinical illness in 70% to 90% of patients and protection against subclinical infection (measured by seroconversion) in about 50%. For optimal results the drug must be taken for the full period of the epidemic (usually 6 to 12 weeks). Amantadine is not a substitute for vaccination. It is recommended for prophylaxis under the following conditions: in presumed influenza A outbreaks in institutions housing high-risk persons; as an adjunct to immunization once influenza A has appeared in the community (to provide protection while awaiting an immune response to the vaccine); to offer increased protection to immunosuppressed patients who may have a poor antibody response to vaccine; for persons allergic to vaccine; and in circumstances where a virulent strain of influenza A not included in the vaccine preparation emerges.

Amantadine used to treat influenza in the same dosage has caused an approximate 50% reduction in fever duration and a shortened course of illness. The drug should be administered within 24 to 48 hours of the onset of illness and continued 48 hours after the resolution of symptoms. Its value for influenza pneumonia or other complications of influenza remains to be established.

Vidarabine (adenine arabinoside)

Initially vidarabine was developed as a potential anticancer agent. However, several human herpesviruses were found to be sensitive to it, and its therapeutic/toxic ratio was better than those noted for previous purine and pyrimidine analogs such as idoxuridine and cytosine arabinoside. Vidarabine inhibits DNA synthesis, with a preferential effect on viral, rather than cellular, DNA synthesis.

Vidarabine has been shown to be effective therapy for herpes simplex virus encephalitis, neonatal herpes infection, varicella

infection in immunocompromised children, and herpes zoster in immunocompromised adults. However, acyclovir has largely replaced vidarabine for the treatment of herpes simplex and varicella-zoster infections because of lower toxicity and greater efficacy.

Acyclovir (acycloguanosine)

Acyclovir is a purine analog and has an acyclic side chain that replaces the normal cyclic sugar moiety. It has in vitro activity against herpes simplex virus types 1 and 2 (HSV-1 and HSV-2), varicella-zoster virus, and to a limited extent cytomegalovirus and Epstein-Barr virus. In vivo efficacy is restricted to HSV-1, HSV-2, and varicella-zoster. In cells infected with these viruses, acyclovir is converted into acyclovir monophosphate through the action of the viral-encoded enzyme thymidine kinase. Cellular enzymes then convert the monophosphate form of acyclovir to a triphosphate. This is the active form of the drug, which blocks the synthesis of viral DNA by competitively inhibiting the enzyme viral DNA polymerase. The drug also acts as a terminator of DNA elongation when incorporated into DNA.

Resistance to acyclovir can develop in viruses that mutate their thymidine kinase or DNA polymerase genes. The frequency of these mutations arising during therapy in vivo appears to be low. In addition, most mutants demonstrate decreased virulence in animal model studies.

Acyclovir has a serum half-life of 2.9 hours. Approximately 80% is excreted as unmetabolized drug in the urine. Dosage modifications are required in patients with renal failure. After intravenous infusion, peak serum levels at 1 hour are 10 to 100 times greater than 50% of the minimal inhibitory concentration (MIC_{50}) for HSV-1 and HSV-2. The bioavailability of orally administered drug is much less (15% to 30%); therefore peak serum levels exceed the MIC_{50} by a smaller margin, generally 2 to 5 times. The MIC_{50} for HSV-2 is approximately twice as high as for HSV-1, and the MIC_{50} for varicella-zoster virus is 5 to 10 times higher than for HSV-1. Therefore oral therapy for varicella-zoster requires higher dosages of acyclovir.

Acyclovir is well tolerated. Toxic effects are uncommon and are dose dependent. They include phlebitis at the intravenous site, crystalluria, rising creatinine level, lethargy, tremors, seizures, and nausea.

Acyclovir therapy is indicated for a variety of HSV-1 and HSV-2 infections, including neonatal HSV infection, HSV encephalitis, HSV keratitis, HSV in immunocompromised patients, and genital HSV. Prolonged continuous oral therapy for genital HSV has been shown to reduce or eliminate outbreaks in most patients while they are receiving therapy. However, therapy with acyclovir does not eliminate viral latency, so patients usually have relapses once the drug is stopped. Prolonged therapy is recommended only for patients who have frequent recurrences or are greatly disabled (mentally or physically) by their disease. The drug can be administered safely for up to 18 months. Acyclovir's efficacy for orolabial HSV in a normal host has not been demonstrated.

Acyclovir is also indicated for treatment of varicella or zoster in immunocompromised patients. Zoster in a normal host heals more rapidly when treated with acyclovir, but the drug has not been shown to reduce the incidence or severity of postzoster neuralgia. Large oral doses of acyclovir are required to exceed the MIC of the virus, which makes oral therapy expensive and inconvenient. Therefore a valuable role for acyclovir in a normal host has yet to be established. An exception to this statement is zoster involving the ophthalmic division of the fifth cranial nerve. The incidence and severity of eye complications are reduced by acyclovir treatment. The optimal dosage of oral acyclovir for this indication has not been established.

Zidovudine

Zidovudine, formerly known as azidodeoxythymidine (AZT), is an antiviral drug with in vitro activity against the human immunodeficiency virus (HIV) type 1. It is available for oral administration and is currently the only drug approved by the Food and Drug Administration (FDA) for treatment of HIV infection. The drug is a thymidine analog that inhibits the viral enzyme reverse transcriptase, which is required for viral nucleic acid replication. Zidovudine also acts as a chain terminator if it is incorporated into the growing DNA chain.

When zidovudine is added to cultures in vitro, it inhibits viral replication at low drug concentrations, well within the therapeutic range of achievable blood levels. However, when it is added to chronically infected cultures, much higher drug levels are required for inhibition. The latter situation probably more closely mimics conditions in vivo.

The bioavailability of orally administered zidovudine is excellent (approximately 65%). However, it has a short serum half-life (1 hour), which necessitates administration every 4 hours to maintain adequate blood levels. The drug is excreted in the urine, and dosage modifications are required in renal failure.

Drug toxicity is a major problem. Toxic effects include severe headache, nausea, insomnia, myalgia, and the most troublesome effects, granulocytopenia and anemia, each of which occurs in 25% to 50% of patients. These adverse effects usually necessitate dose modifications or cessation of therapy.

Zidovudine has proven efficacy, established by controlled clinical trials, for treating HIV-infected patients who have recovered from *Pneumocystis carinii* pneumonia or who have symptoms of the AIDS-related complex. Treated patients had longer survival than control subjects receiving placebo. They also had fewer opportunistic infections, higher T_4 lymphocyte blood levels, better mentation, less weight loss, and less deterioration in performance on standardized tests. The duration of benefits from treatment is unknown, but positive effects appear to wane by approximately 6 months. Treatment does not eradicate the virus and therefore is not a cure for the disease.

Ribavirin

Ribavirin is a guanosine analog that inhibits in vitro replication of many DNA and RNA viruses. The mechanism of action of this drug is not fully understood but is related in part to inhibition of messenger RNA synthesis. The pharmacology of orally administered or aerosolized ribavirin is complex and incompletely elucidated. Oral ribavirin may result in elevated serum bilirubin, uric acid, and iron levels. The aerosolized drug is well tolerated but may cause mild conjunctivitis.

Aerosolized ribavirin reduces the severity of bronchiolitis in infants with respiratory syncytial virus infection. The aerosolized drug also shortens the course of respiratory syncytial virus pneumonia, but the manufacturer's instructions must be followed to avoid blockage of respirators if infants are receiving respiratory support. The aerosolized drug is also effective therapy for influenza A and B virus infections when administered early in the illness. Studies comparing ribavirin to amantadine have not been performed.

Ganciclovir

Ganciclovir, also known as DHPG, is 9-(1,3-dihydroxy-2-propoxymethyl) guanine. It is an acyclic analog of thymidine, and like acyclovir it is a prodrug that must be converted to an active form by cellular enzymes. Once phosphorylated to the triphosphate form, it is a potent inhibitor of DNA polymerase by competing with guanine nucleotides. It is effective in vitro and in vivo against cytomegalovirus, although the exact mechanism of action has not been determined.

As initial therapy ganciclovir is administered intravenously in doses of 2.5 mg/kg every 8 hours or 5 mg/kg every 12 hours. Long-term maintenance therapy at 5 to 6 mg/kg/day is often required to retard relapses. A dose of 2.5 mg/kg results in a peak serum titer of 18 to 24 μmol/L which is 5 to 10 times the dose required to inhibit 50% of cytomegalovirus isolates. The drug is excreted unchanged in urine, so dosage modification is indicated in renal failure.

The most common serious toxic effect is neutropenia, which may be severe enough to warrant discontinuation of therapy. Thrombocytopenia, hepatitis, and phlebitis are less common side effects. Azospermia occurs in laboratory animals, but its incidence in humans is unknown.

The widest experience using ganciclovir therapy is for cytomegalovirus infection in AIDS patients. In most patients with retinitis the disorder stabilizes during treatment. However, relapse eventually occurs despite prolonged maintenance therapy. Cytomegalovirus esophagitis and colitis also respond to ganciclovir, although relapses are common. A response to ganciclovir in patients with cytomegalovirus pneumonia has not been established.

Interferons

Interferons are not specific for a single virus but are capable of inhibiting a variety of DNA and RNA viruses. Interferons are experimental drugs and are not licensed for therapy by the FDA. α-Interferon has been used in most clinical trials. Interferons act by inhibiting the translation of viral messenger RNA into viral proteins and by modulating the immune response, thus enhancing the activity of natural killer cells and macrophages.

Clinical trials in immunocompromised patients with herpes zoster have shown that interferon decreased cutaneous spread, prevented dissemination, diminished the acute pain and severity of postherpetic neuralgia, and decreased visceral complications compared with placebo-treated controls. Treatment with interferon also diminished the visceral spread of virus following chickenpox infection in children with neoplasia.

Interferon has been evaluated as a prophylactic agent. Renal transplant recipients were treated twice weekly for 6 weeks in an attempt to prevent cytomegalovirus infection. Excretion of cytomegalovirus was delayed but not prevented, and cytomegalovirus viremia was reduced in the interferon group compared with controls. The prophylactic effects of interferon on herpes simplex infection have also been studied in patients undergoing microsurgical decompression of the trigeminal sensory root for treatment of trigeminal neuralgia. The incidence of herpesvirus shedding and herpes labialis was reduced in interferon recipients compared with controls. Interferon was also found effective in preventing rhinovirus (common cold) infections. The eventual importance of interferons as antiviral agents remains to be determined.

BIBLIOGRAPHY

Hayden RC and Douglas RG Jr: Antiviral agents. In Mandel GL, Douglas RG Jr, and Bennett JE, editors: Principles and practice of infectious diseases, New York, 1985, John Wiley & Sons, Inc.

Prevention and control of influenza, MMWR 36:24, 1987.

Report of the Committee on Infectious Diseases. In Red Book, Elk Grove Village, Ill, 1986, American Academy of Pediatrics.

Update on hepatitis B prevention, MMWR 36:23, 1987.

UNIT B • BACTERIAL DISEASES

39 · USE OF ANTIMICROBIAL AGENTS

Donald Kaye

About one third of all hospitalized patients receive antimicrobial agents, and over half of these are treated improperly (wrong agent or dosage). Appropriate use of antimicrobial agents is critical in the patient who is seriously ill with an infection. Using unnecessary agents exposes patients to unnecessary side effects (allergic and toxic reactions) and the risk of superinfection and encourages the emergence of resistant organisms.

Appropriate use of antimicrobial agents requires a bacteriologic diagnosis (either tentative or proven); knowledge of the susceptibility patterns of the likely infecting organism (that is, the antimicrobial spectra of different antimicrobial agents); knowledge of the pharmacology of the agents (absorption, distribution, levels, protein binding, sites and rate of excretion or metabolism, and toxicity); knowledge of how to alter doses when excretion is impaired; and knowledge of drug interactions with other agents. Cost also is a major consideration when choosing an antimicrobial agent. Before describing specific agents, certain of these principles of antimicrobial therapy are discussed.

DETERMINATION OF SUSCEPTIBILITY OF MICROORGANISMS

Some organisms are uniformly susceptible to certain antimicrobial agents. For example, virtually all group A streptococci and meningococci are susceptible to penicillin G. However, these observations may not necessarily be true in the future, since susceptibility patterns are continually changing. For example, pneumococci (Streptococcus pneumoniae) were uniformly highly susceptible to penicillin G until resistant strains appeared in recent years. In many infections the infecting microorganisms are not uniformly susceptible to any single antimicrobial agent. Therefore it often is necessary to choose the agent or agents most likely to be active and to perform susceptibility tests as soon as the organism is isolated. The usual pattern of activity of an antimicrobial agent against microorganisms is known as its *spectrum of activity*.

The major methods of testing antimicrobial susceptibility are *agar diffusion* and *broth* or *agar dilution* methods, and these have been applied primarily to testing of bacteria. In the agar diffusion method a paper disk containing a standard amount of antimicrobial agent is placed on an agar plate containing a standardized inoculum of the microorganism. After incubation for 24 hours the zone size of inhibition is measured and results are reported as susceptible, resistant, or intermediate. An intermediate-size zone indicates the need for high doses of the antimicrobial agent unless the therapy is for urinary tract infection (since very high concentrations of drug usually are achieved in urine). The zone size is inversely proportional to the minimal inhibitory concentration (MIC) of antimicrobial, that is, the minimal amount required to prevent growth.

The broth and agar dilution methods require dilution of the antimicrobial agent in broth or agar, addition of a standard inoculum of the microorganism, and incubation (for 24 hours with most bacteria). The MIC is the lowest concentration of antimicrobial agent that prevents growth in broth or agar.

Broth dilution methods allow determination of bactericidal activity of antimicrobial agents. After incubation for 24 hours the number of organisms remaining is determined by streaking on a plate. A 99.9% kill (1000-fold decrease in the number of organisms) is considered to be the criterion for bactericidal activity. The minimal concentration of antimicrobial required to achieve a bactericidal effect (99.9% kill) is the minimal bactericidal concentration (MBC).

SIGNIFICANCE OF BACTERIOSTATIC VERSUS BACTERICIDAL ACTIVITY

Agents may be divided into those that are bactericidal at or near the MIC and those that have an MBC much higher (for example, 16-fold or greater) than the MIC. The former are considered bactericidal and the latter bacteriostatic. Penicillins, cephalosporins, vancomycin, aminoglycosides, and polymyxins generally are considered bactericidal, whereas erythromycin, tetracyclines, chloramphenicol, clindamycin, lincomycin, and sulfonamides generally are bacteriostatic. However, this division is not absolute, since bactericidal agents may be bacteriostatic against certain microorganisms and vice versa. For example, chloramphenicol is bactericidal against pneumococci, and penicillin has poor bactericidal activity against enterococci.

In certain infections bactericidal activity is necessary for a high cure rate. It appears that in these infections host defense mechanisms are at least partially lacking, either at the local site or systemically. These infections are endocarditis, meningitis, serious staphylococcal infection, and perhaps serious gram-negative bacillary infection in the leukopenic patient. In such infections better results are obtained with agents that result in bactericidal activity than with those that have bacteriostatic activity. The outcome in endocarditis treated with bacteriostatic agents such as erythromycin, clindamycin, tetracycline, or chloramphenicol is poor. Penicillin, a bactericidal drug, usually does not cure enterococcal endocarditis unless an aminoglycoside is added to achieve a greater bactericidal effect. Chloramphenicol results in high cure rates in *Haemophilus influenzae* and meningococcal and pneumococcal meningitis; it is bactericidal against these organisms. However, the failure rate is high in *Escherichia coli* meningitis despite bacteriostatic spinal fluid levels; chloramphenicol is not bactericidal against *E. coli*. The failure rate in *Staphylococcus aureus* pneumonia or bacteremia treated with bacteriostatic agents is high. Much better results are achieved with penicillins, cephalosporins, and vancomycin. The leukopenic patient with serious gram-negative bacillary infection also seems to fare better with bactericidal therapy such as penicillins, cephalosporins, and/or aminoglycosides.

In most infections, including pneumococcal pneumonia and urinary tract infection, there seems to be no advantage to using bactericidal over bacteriostatic agents.

Combinations of antimicrobial agents often are necessary in serious infections before the infecting organism's antimicrobial susceptibility pattern is known in order to guarantee antimicrobial activity against the organism. Combinations also are frequently required in mixed infections. When antimicrobial agents are used in combination, certain in vitro observations can be made. In comparison to the effect of one of the agents alone, there may be more rapid or more complete bactericidal activity *(synergism)*, no change in bactericidal activity *(indifference)*, or less bactericidal activity *(antagonism)*.

In general, combinations of bactericidal agents produce synergism, combinations of bacteriostatic agents produce indifference, and combinations of a bacteriostatic agent with a bactericidal agent produces antagonism. However, these interactions are not totally predictable, and in vitro testing is necessary to determine the true interaction.

Antagonism has been shown to be of clinical significance in very few situations. Pneumococcal meningitis has a higher mortality rate when treated with penicillin (a bactericidal agent) plus tetracycline (a bacteriostatic agent) than when treated with penicillin alone. If bacteriostatic agent were added to a bactericidal agent in treating endocarditis, the results probably would also be poor. In these infections host defenses at the site of infection are poor, and antimicrobial agent must sterilize the site.

Synergism also has been shown to be of importance in relatively few infections. One such infection is enterococcal endocarditis, in which an aminoglycoside must be added to penicillin to produce good in vitro bactericidal activity. Without the addition of an aminoglycoside, the relapse rate is very high. Synergism probably is also important in leukopenic patients with serious *Pseudomonas aeruginosa* infection, since in these patients an aminoglycoside such as tobramycin plus a penicillin such as ticarcillin may give better results than either agent alone.

ACTIVITY OF AGENT AT SITE OF INFECTION

The results of therapy will not be satisfactory unless the antimicrobial agent is present in effective concentrations at the site of infection. It is important to remember in this regard that bacteremia is a manifestation of tissue infection, with organisms secondarily found in the blood; therapy *must* be directed at the tissue site.

In considering the site of infection, the local conditions and the penetration, protein binding, and blood levels of the antimicrobial agent must be taken into account. In general, all agents other than the polymyxins penetrate well into inflamed joints and other body cavities such as the pleural and peritoneal spaces, but not necessarily into the cerebrospinal fluid (CSF). Therefore there is no advantage in instilling these agents into body cavities.

Less agent will reach an area with a poor blood supply such as necrotic tissue. Many agents, including penicillins, pass through the blood-brain barrier poorly, resulting in low CSF concentrations as compared to serum concentrations, although higher CSF concentrations usually are achieved in the presence of inflammation. Therefore high doses of penicillins are required in meningitis. Some agents such as chloramphenicol, sulfonamides, and rifampin achieve adequate CSF levels with normal doses. The vegetation of endocarditis also is probably an area where penetration of some antimicrobials is impaired; therefore large doses are required. In contrast, urinary levels of most antibiotics are very high in patients with normal renal function. Since the results of therapy in urinary tract infections are related to urinary levels of antimicrobial agent, relatively low doses can be used. Most agents also achieve therapeutic levels in bile. However, with obstruction of the biliary or urinary tracts, levels are low in bile and urine.

The pH at the local site can have a major effect on therapy. For example, aminoglycosides and erythromycin are much less active at an acid pH (as in an abscess or infected body fluid) or the usual pH of urine. Sulfonamides are relatively inactive in abscesses because of the presence of large concentrations of paraaminobenzoic acid. Drainage of pus and removal of foreign bodies are essential for cure or even response in many infections. In addition to the low pH and poor blood supply of an abscess or a foreign body, there are other local factors. These areas are anaerobic, and aminoglycosides are not active against anaerobically metabolizing bacteria. Host defenses seem not to operate well at these sites. Furthermore, the bacteria may be metabolically altered so that even if effective concentrations of agents are reached, they may not be antimicrobial.

Protein binding may be important in determining tissue concentrations of an agent. Concentrations of free agent determine antibacterial activity. Although binding is reversible, with highly protein-bound agents, relatively small concentrations may be available for diffusion to a tissue site. In general, with agents having protein binding of less than 75%, impairment of diffusion is not a major factor. Such agents include penicillin G, methicillin, cephalothin, cephalexin, chloramphenicol, and aminoglycosides. With agents having higher protein binding, such as nafcillin, oxacillin, cloxacillin, and dicloxacillin, doses large enough to compensate for protein binding must be given.

The goal of antimicrobial therapy is to deliver to the site of infection an amount of free antimicrobial agent that exceeds the MIC of the infecting organism, taking local conditions into consideration. This concentration must be achieved often enough to prevent microorganisms from multiplying between doses.

PHARMACOLOGY
Route of administration

The drug must be administered in such a way as to ensure antimicrobial activity at the site of infection. Some agents such as the third-generation cephalosporins, aminoglycosides, and vancomycin are not absorbed orally, and some such as methicillin are destroyed by gastric acid. For systemic infections these agents must be given by injection. Some agents (for example, cephalexin, doxycycline, chloramphenicol, and rifampin) are absorbed as well orally as by injection. However, with all oral agents there is the possibility of food or drugs binding to or in some other way interfering with absorption of the agent. It is prudent to give oral agents when the patient is in the fasting state, preferably 1 to 2 hours before meals. The intramuscular injection of some agents (such as penicillin G in large doses, tetracycline, and erythromycin) is painful, and these agents must be given intravenously when injection is required.

With serious infections the effort usually is to achieve free antibacterial concentrations in serum (see discussion of protein binding under "Activity of agent at site of infection") that are active against the infecting organism. In infective endocarditis serum bactericidal activity generally must be achieved at a one-eighth dilution of serum (see discussion of "Infective endocarditis" in Chapter 40). In meningitis, serum concentrations must be high enough to guarantee adequate CSF concentrations. In urinary tract infection without bacteremia, serum concentrations are not important; only urinary concentrations are significant. This explains why agents such as nitrofurantoin are effective in urinary tract infection without achieving antibacterial activity in serum.

Plasma (serum) concentrations

The plasma concentration after the initial dose is determined by rate of absorption, rate of administration if given intravenously, size of dose, size of the individual, body habitus (that is, obese or lean), rate of excretion or inactivation, and volume of distribution in the body.

Volume of distribution refers to the body compartments in which the drug is distributed. The major compartments are the intravascular or plasma, the interstitial fluid, and the intracellular fluid compartments. Some antimicrobial agents are distributed mainly in the intravascular space, some in intravascular and interstitial spaces, and some even intracellularly. Some agents may be sequestered in various tissues (such as nafcillin in the liver).

With rapid intravenous injection of an agent, the drug initially is found mostly in the plasma compartment. After about 30 minutes intravascular drug equilibrates with the concentrations in the extravascular compartments. Subsequently, most drugs are eliminated from the body as a first-order process (that is, at a constant rate). With slow intravenous infusion, intramuscular injection, or oral administration, equilibration (and also excretion) takes place simultaneously with absorption. Therefore peak plasma levels are higher with rapid intravenous injection than with the other routes of administration.

If not all the agent is eliminated before the next dose is given, the drug accumulates, giving higher plasma levels until a steady state eventually is reached. In general, accumulation does not occur if the maintenance dose is given every 3 to 4 plasma half-lives (see the following).

In serious infections agents should be given intravenously or intramuscularly to guarantee rapid achievement of effective serum levels. With hypotension the intravenous route must be used, since poor perfusion at the site of injection may slow absorption from the muscle. Sufficiently large doses should be given to guarantee adequate serum concentrations. Doses of toxic agents such as the aminoglycosides usually are given on the basis of milligrams per kilogram of body weight. Dosage based on body surface area is an alternative method commonly used in pediatrics. With relatively nontoxic agents such as the penicillins and cephalosporins, standard dosages can be used in adults.

Body habitus is important when administering the aminoglycosides. Aminoglycosides are not lipid soluble, and little reaches the adipose tissue. Therefore dosage should be based on lean body weight to avoid overdosage.

Excretion or inactivation

The rate of excretion or inactivation of an agent helps determine its duration of activity in serum and at other sites and its peak serum concentrations with repeated doses. (With retention of the agent, each dose adds to existing levels.) The excretion or inactivation rate also plays a role in determining the serum concentration with the initial dose when the antimicrobial agent is absorbed relatively slowly, as with oral, intramuscular, or slow intravenous routes.

Most antimicrobial agents, including most penicillins, cephalosporins, aminoglycosides, tetracyclines, vancomycin, and polymyxins, are excreted by the kidneys. Many penicillins and cephalosporins are excreted by tubular secretion and glomerular filtration; probenecid has a marked effect in reducing the rate of excretion of these drugs by blocking tubular secretion. The aminoglycosides, most tetracyclines, vancomycin, sulfonamides, and polymyxins are excreted mainly by glomerular filtration. Erythromycin, lincomycin, clindamycin, rifampin, nafcillin (a penicillin), and cefoperazone (a cephalosporin) are excreted mainly in the bile. Doxycycline is excreted mainly in the stool. Some agents are inactivated before excretion; ceph-

alothin and certain other cephalosporins are deacetylated, chloramphenicol is conjugated by glucuronyl transferase, and isoniazid is acetylated in the liver. The rate of acetylation of isoniazid varies according to genetic composition; individuals may be rapid or slow acetylators.

A useful concept for describing the duration of antimicrobial activity in the blood is the plasma (or serum) half-life. This is the time required for the blood plasma level to fall by half. The rate of fall is constant after equilibrium has been reached with the different fluid compartments. Elimination of a drug is virtually complete (90% or more) after 3 to 4 half-lives.

MODIFICATION OF DOSAGES

When excretion of an agent is impaired, plasma levels may be higher or more prolonged than desired. In this situation, following a normal loading dose, subsequent doses must be decreased or the time between the doses increased.

Renal or hepatic function must be monitored in patients receiving antimicrobial agents that are excreted or inactivated by the kidney or liver. When renal function is impaired, it is essential to modify dosage regimens of aminoglycosides, vancomycin, polymyxins, tetracyclines (other than doxycycline), sulfonamides, and flucytosine. When large doses of penicillins or cephalosporins are being used, it also is prudent to lower the dosage. With impairment of liver function doses of erythromycin, lincomycin, clindamycin, chloramphenicol, and nafcillin may need to be decreased.

Although nomograms are available for modifying dosage regimens in cases of renal insufficiency, they are not reliable. Determinations of serum concentrations are required for dosage modification, especially when toxic agents such as the aminoglycosides are used.

DURATION OF THERAPY

The recommended duration of therapy for most infections is empiric. Most infections are treated for 7 to 14 days. Enterococcal endocarditis and serious staphylococcal infections usually require at least 4 weeks of treatment. With suppuration (lung abscess, liver abscess, and so on) and osteomyelitis, longer therapy usually is needed. Mycobacterial and deep fungal disease may require a year or more of therapy. Specific recommendations are discussed under the disease entities.

TOXICITY OF ANTIMICROBIAL AGENTS

All agents have side effects. The side effects may be local reactions such as pain or phlebitis at the site of administration, allergic reactions such as rash or anaphylaxis, metabolic reactions such as sodium loading and hypokalemic alkalosis from carbenicillin, or organ toxicity such as nephrotoxicity from aminoglycosides. Allergic reactions are not dose related, whereas metabolic reactions and organ toxicity are.

Toxicity may be related to the patient's age, renal function, or pregnancy or to interaction with another drug. For example, nephrotoxic and ototoxic agents such as aminoglycosides are more likely to cause toxic reactions in the elderly and in patients with renal insufficiency. Tetracyclines can cause damage to the teeth in the fetus when used in pregnancy or in the child when taken before age 8. Sulfonamides can cause kernicterus in the newborn by displacement of bilirubin from serum albumin, and chloramphenicol can cause the lethal "gray syndrome" in the newborn. Side effects are discussed with the specific agents.

FAILURE OF THERAPY WITH ANTIMICROBIAL AGENTS

Therapy may fail for many reasons.

Delay of therapy

All serious infections have a point of no return beyond which therapy is not effective. This is true even in infections with organisms that are highly susceptible to antibiotics (such as pneumococcal pneumonia). Therapy must be started promptly in the seriously ill patient.

Incorrect diagnosis

If the patient does not have an infection, antimicrobial agents cannot be expected to have an effect.

Microbial resistance

An antimicrobial agent is not effective when the organism is resistant. This can occur from lack of recognition of the infecting organism (for example, treatment of an intraabdominal abscess containing aerobes and anaerobes with antibiotics active only against the aerobes). Resistance can be present and not recognized unless special tests are used. Such tests may include incubation at reduced temperatures such as 86° F (30° C) or use of a large inoculum for *S. aureus* resistant to methicillin. Resistance can develop in vivo as the patient is being treated, or superinfection with a new resistant organism can occur.

Failure to deliver the agent to the site of infection in antimicrobial concentrations

If an obstruction (such as a biliary or urinary one) is present, effective antimicrobial levels may not be achieved in urine or bile. Many agents (for example, clindamycin and aminoglycosides) when given parenterally do not reach sufficient concentrations in the central nervous system (CNS) to be effective. Many agents do not reach adequate concentrations in necrotic tissue or in an abscess. High blood levels of an agent are required for diffusion into a vegetation in infective endocarditis.

Adverse conditions at the site of infection

Antimicrobial agents do not work well in an area of necrosis, foreign body, or pus. For example, aminoglycosides are not very active at an acid pH as in pus or acid urine, and penicillin will not kill bacteria that are not multiplying, as in pus. Pus and necrotic tissue must be drained and foreign bodies removed.

Infection in the immunocompromised host

In the severely immunocompromised patient (such as one with severe leukopenia) the results of therapy are not as good as in the nonimmunocompromised patient. Even with optimal bactericidal therapy, host defense mechanisms are important.

Apparent failure related to drug fever

Fever caused by the antimicrobial agent may develop after the initial response. This is most likely to occur with penicillins, cephalosporins, vancomycin, and amphotericin B. If the drug is critically important, it should be continued despite the fever. However, other causes of fever such as microbial resistance or superinfection should be sought. If the drug is not critical, discontinuance with or without substitution of another agent elucidates the problem, since the fever usually disappears over a period of 1 to 3 days.

SPECIFIC ANTIMICROBIAL AGENTS

The important antibacterial agents are reviewed in this section. Table 39-1 lists the usual doses in adults with normal renal function and dosage regimens with creatinine clearances of less than 10 ml/min, 30 to 50 ml/min, and 75 ml/min. Table 39-2 lists some important infecting organisms and the appropriate antimicrobial agents used in therapy. Agents used in the treatment of tuberculosis (isoniazid, rifampin, ethambutol, and so on) are reviewed in the discussion of "Antituberculosis drugs" in Chapter 50. Agents used in the treatment of fungal diseases (such as amphotericin B and flucytosine) are reviewed in Chapter 53.

Penicillins

Penicillins are bactericidal antibiotics that work by inhibiting bacterial cell wall synthesis. The penicillins are relatively nontoxic, and to ensure adequate therapy, they generally are given in doses considerably larger than needed.

PENICILLINASE-SENSITIVE PENICILLINS. Penicillin G (benzyl penicillin) is active in relatively low concentrations against essentially all gram-positive cocci and bacilli (including anaerobes) with the exception of penicillinase-producing *S. aureus*, methicillin-resistant *S. aureus*, many strains of *S. epidermidis*, and rare strains of pneumococci. All meningococci and many gonococci are susceptible to relatively low concentrations of penicillin G.

Although penicillin G is active in much higher concentrations against many strains of *H. influenzae*, *E. coli*, *Proteus mirabilis*, and *Salmonella*, the tendency is to use "broad-spectrum" penicillins such as ampicillin for infections caused by these organisms. In high concentrations penicillin G also is active against many anaerobic gram-negative bacilli. Penicillin G is available as aqueous penicillin G, procaine penicillin G, and benzathine penicillin G.

Aqueous penicillin G usually is given intravenously because intramuscular injection is painful. The intravenous form is used when high serum concentrations are required and large amounts must be given, as in meningitis or endocarditis. The standard dosage in adults is 5 to 20 million units each day either by continuous intravenous drip or in divided doses every 2 to 4 hours, since the half-life in the blood is only 30 minutes.

Procaine penicillin G is well tolerated intramuscularly but provides relatively low serum concentrations of penicillin. Because of slow release from the muscle, blood levels are prolonged and doses can be given every 6 to 24 hours. Procaine penicillin G is used in therapy for pneumococcal and group A streptococcal infections other than meningitis and in gonorrhea, syphilis, and endocarditis caused by highly susceptible organisms. The dosage is 600,000 to 1.2 million units intramuscularly every 12 to 24 hours. In endocarditis 1.2 million units every 6 hours is used.

Benzathine penicillin G is used intramuscularly and is released over a period of weeks. It provides very low blood levels of penicillin G that are adequate only for treatment of pneumococcal and group A streptococcal infections (excluding meningitis and endocarditis) and syphilis and for prophylaxis of rheumatic fever. One injection of 1.2 million units provides therapy for pneumococcal or streptococcal infection. For prophylaxis of rheumatic fever, monthly injections are given. The regimen in syphilis depends on the stage (see discussion of "Syphilis" in Chapter 51).

Penicillin G can be used orally, but it is unstable in the presence of gastric acid and absorption is unreliable. Therefore

Table 39-1   Doses of some commonly used antimicrobial agents

Agent	Usual total daily dose in adults	Dose interval	Route	Daily dose with creatinine clearance (ml/min) <10	Daily dose with creatinine clearance (ml/min) 30-50	Daily dose with creatinine clearance (ml/min) ≥75
Penicillinase-sensitive penicillins						
Aqueous penicillin G	5-20 million units	Continuous IV or q2-4h	IM, IV	1-2 million units q6h	NC*	NC
Procaine penicillin G	600,000-4.8 million units	q6-24h	IM	NC	NC	NC
Benzathine penicillin G	600,000-2.4 million units	Every 4 wk	IM	NC	NC	NC
Phenoxymethyl penicillin (penicillin V)	1-2 g	q6h	PO	250 mg q6h	NC	NC
Broad-spectrum penicillins						
Amoxicillin, amoxicillin-clavulanic acid (in doses of amoxicillin)	0.75-3 g (0.75-1.5 g for amoxicillin-clavulanic acid)	q8h	PO	500 mg q12h	NC	NC
Ampicillin	1-4 g	q6h	PO	500 mg q12h	NC	NC
Ampicillin, ampicillin-subactam (in doses of ampicillin)	4-12 g	q4-6h	IM, IV	1 g q8h	NC	NC
Carbenicillin (in serious infection)	500 mg/kg	q4h	IV	2 g q8h	2.5 g q4h	NC
Carbenicillin indanyl sodium	2-4 g	q6h	PO	Avoid use	NC	NC
Ticarcillin, mezlocillin, piperacillin, azlocillin, ticarcillin-clavulanic acid (in doses of ticarcillin)	250 mg/kg	q4h	IV	1 g q6h	1 g q4h	NC
Penicillinase-resistant penicillins						
Cloxacillin	1-2 g	q6h	PO	NC	NC	NC
Dicloxacillin	1-2 g	q6h	PO	NC	NC	NC
Methicillin, nafcillin, oxacillin	6-12 g	q4h	IM, IV	1 g q4h	NC	NC
Cephalosporins						
Cephalothin, cephapirin	6-12 g	q4h	IV	1 g q8h	1 g q4-6h	NC
Cefazolin	2-6 g	q6-8h	IM, IV	0.5 g/day	0.5 g q6-12h	NC
Cefamandole, cefoxitin	6-12 g	q4h	IV	0.5 g q8h	1 g q6h	NC
Cefotetan	2-4 g	q12h	IM, IV	1 g q24h	NC	NC
Cefuroxime	2.25-9 g	q8h	IM, IV	1.5 g q24h	NC	NC
Cefuroxime	0.5-1g	q12h	PO	NC	NC	NC
Cephalexin, cephradine	1-2 g	q6h	PO	0.25 g/day	0.25 g q6h	NC
Cefaclor	750 mg-1.5 g	q8h	PO	NC	NC	NC
Cefotaxime	4-12 g	q4-6h	IM, IV	2 g q12h	NC	NC
Ceftizoxime	3-8 g	q6-8h	IM, IV	1 g q24h	1 g q12h	NC
Ceftriaxone	1-4 g	q12-24h	IM, IV	1 g q24h	NC	NC
Moxalactam	1-8 g	q8-12h	IM, IV	1 g q24h	2 g q12h	NC
Cefoperazone	3-12 g	q8-12h	IM, IV	NC	NC	NC
Ceftazidime	2-6 g	q8-12h	IM, IV	1 g q24h	1 g q12h	NC
Imipenem	2-4 g	q6h	IV	0.5 g q12h	1 g q12h	NC
Aztreonam	2-8 g	q6-8h	IV	0.5 g q12h	1 g q8h	NC
Aminoglycosides						
Amikacin	15 mg/kg	q12h	IM, IV	See text—measurement of serum levels is essential		NC
Gentamicin, tobramycin, netilmicin	5 mg/kg	q8h	IM, IV	See text—measurement of serum levels is essential		NC
Streptomycin	1-2 g	q12h	IM	0.5 g q3days	0.25 g q12-24h	NC
Vancomycin	2 g	q6h	IV	See text—measurement of serum levels is essential		NC
Vancomycin	1-2 g	q6h	PO	NC	NC	NC
Erythromycin	1-4 g	q6h	PO, IV	NC	NC	NC
Clindamycin	0.6-2.4 g	q6-8h	PO, IM, IV	NC	NC	NC
Tetracyclines						
Tetracycline	1-2 g	q6h	PO	Avoid use	Avoid use	NC
Tetracycline	1 g	q12h	IV	Avoid use	Avoid use	NC
Doxycycline	200 mg	q12h	PO, IV	NC	NC	NC
Chloramphenicol	50-100 mg/kg	q6h	PO, IV	NC	NC	NC
Sulfonamides						
Sulfisoxazole	4 g	q6h	PO	Avoid use	1 g q12h	NC
Sulfamethoxazole	2 g	q12h	PO	Avoid use	0.5 g q12h	NC
Trimethoprim-sulfamethoxazole†	320 mg trimethoprim and 1.6 g sulfamethoxazole (2 tablets q12h)	q12h	PO	Avoid use	1 tablet q12h	NC
Trimethoprim	200 mg	q12h	PO	Avoid use	50 mg q12h	NC
Metronidazole	750 mg-2.25 g	q6-8h	PO	NC	NC	NC
Metronidazole	30 mg/kg	q6h	IV	NC	NC	NC
Klitrofurantion	200-400 mg	q6h	PO	Avoid use	Avoid use	NC
Quinolones						
Nalidixic acid	4 g	q6h	PO	Avoid use	NC	NC
Oxolinic acid	1.5 g	q12h	PO	Avoid use	NC	NC
Norfloxacin	800 mg	q12h	PO	400 mg q24h	400 mg q24h	NC
Ciprofloxacin	500 mg-1.5g	q12h	PO	250 mg q24h	0.5 g q12h	NC
Methenamine mandelate	4 g	q6h	PO	Avoid use	Avoid use	NC
Methenamine hippurate	2 g	q12h	PO	Avoid use	Avoid use	NC

*NC, no change from usual total daily dose.

†For *Pneumocystis carinii,* 20 mg/kg trimethoprim and 100 mg/kg sulfamethoxazole daily IV or PO in divided doses q6h.

Table 39-2   Commonly used antibiotic regimens for selected infections (adult doses)

Bacteria	Infection	Regimen for adult patients with normal renal function
Mycoplasma pneumoniae	Pneumonia	Erythromycin or tetracycline, 500 mg PO q.i.d. × 7 days
Chlamydia trachomatis	Urethritis, cervicitis, salpingitis, proctitis, epididymitis	Tetracycline, 500 mg PO q.i.d. × 7 days
Streptococcus pneumoniae (pneumococcus)	Pneumonia	Procaine penicillin G, 600,000 units q12h × 7 days[1,2]
	Meningitis	Aqueous penicillin G, 20 million units/day IV × 10 days[3]
	Endocarditis	Aqueous penicillin G, 20 million units/day IV × 4 wk[2,4]
Group A *Streptococcus*	Pharyngitis	Penicillin V, 250 mg PO q.i.d. × 10 days[1]
	Cellulitis	Procaine penicillin G, 600,000 units/day IM × 10 days or as for pharyngitis[1]
Staphylococcus aureus	Soft tissue infection	Cloxacillin or cephalexin, 500 mg PO q.i.d. × 10 days, or nafcillin, 1.5 g IV q4h × 10 days
	Pneumonia	Nafcillin, 1.5 g IV q4h × 14 days[2,4]
	Bacteremia or endocarditis	Nafcillin, 1.5 g IV q4h × 4-6 wk[2,4]
Neisseria gonorrhoeae	Urethritis, cervicitis, proctitis, pharyngitis	Procaine penicillin G, 4.8 million units IM, plus probenecid, 1 g PO; or tetracycline, 0.5 g PO q.i.d. × 7 days; or ampicillin, 3.5 g PO, plus probenecid, 1 g PO; or spectinomycin, 2 g IM (ampicillin and spectinomycin not effective in gonococcal pharyngitis); or ceftriaxone, 250 mg IM
	Arthritis, bacteremia with skin lesions	Aqueous penicillin G, 10 million units/day IV until improvement, then ampicillin, 0.5 g PO q.i.d. × 7 days; or ceftriaxone, 1g IV or IM q.d. × 7 days
	Salpingitis	Aqueous penicillin G, 20 million units/day IV until improvement, then ampicillin, 0.5 g PO q.i.d. × 10 days; or ceftriaxone, 1g IV or IM q.d. × 10 days
Neisseria meningitidis	Meningitis	Aqueous penicillin G, 20 million units/day IV × 10 days[3]
Haemophilus influenzae	Bronchitis in patient with chronic obstructive pulmonary disease	Ampicillin, 1 g PO q.i.d.; or amoxicillin, 0.5 g PO t.i.d.; or tetracycline, 250 mg PO q.i.d.; or amoxicillin-clavulanic acid 0.5 g (amoxicillin) PO t.i.d.; or trimethoprim-sulfamethoxazole, 1 double-strength tablet b.i.d.; all × 3-7 days
	Pneumonia	Cefotaxime 2 g IV q6h; ceftizoxime 2 g IV q8h; ceftriaxone 1 g IV q12h; or ampicillin (if susceptible) 2 g IV q4h; all × 7-10 days
	Meningitis	Cefotaxime 2 g IV q4h; ceftriaxone 2 g IV q12h; chloramphenicol 12.5 mg/kg IV q6h; or ampicillin (if susceptible) 50 mg/kg IV q4h; all × 7-10 days
Escherichia coli	Urinary tract infection without bacteremia	Lower tract: Oral therapy with one dose of 3 g amoxicillin or 320 mg trimethoprim plus 1.6 g sulfamethoxazole; or 1-3 days of sulfisoxazole, 1 g q.i.d., ampicillin, 500 mg q.i.d., cephalexin, 500 mg q.i.d., tetracycline, 250 mg q.i.d., nitrofurantoin, 50-100 mg q.i.d.; or norfloxacin, 400 mg, or ciprofloxacin, 250 mg PO b.i.d. Upper tract: Two weeks of oral therapy with sulfisoxazole, 1 g q.i.d., ampicillin, 500 mg q.i.d., amoxicillin, 500 mg t.i.d., cephalexin, 500 mg q.i.d., tetracycline, 250 mg q.i.d., trimethoprim-sulfamethoxazole (160 mg and 800 mg respectively) q12h, or norfloxacin, 400 mg, or ciprofloxacin, 500 mg PO b.i.d.
	Bacteremia	Ampicillin, 2 g q4h IV, or cephalothin or cefazolin,[2] and/or gentamicin or tobramycin, 1.7 mg/kg q8h IM or IV, all × 7-10 days[5-7]
Klebsiella pneumoniae	Urinary tract infection without bacteremia	Lower tract: Cephalexin, 500 mg q.i.d. or norfloxacin, 400 mg, or ciprofloxacin, 250 mg PO b.i.d. × 1-3 days Upper tract: Cephalexin, 500 mg q.i.d. or norfloxacin, 400 mg, or ciprofloxacin, 500 mg PO b.i.d. × 14 days
	Pneumonia, bacteremia	Cephalothin, 2 g IV q4h, or cefazolin, 1-2 g IV or IM q6-8h, and/or gentamicin or tobramycin, 1.7 mg/kg IM or IV q8h × 14 days for pneumonia and 7-10 days for bacteremia[5-7]

[1]When penicillin cannot be used, erythromycin, 500 mg q.i.d., can be substituted.

[2]Cephalothin, 2 g IV q4h, or cefazolin, 1-2 g IM or IV q6-8h, can be administered.

[3]When penicillin cannot be used, chloramphenicol, 12.5-25 mg/kg IV q6h, can be given.

[4]Vancomycin, 500 mg IV q6h, should be used when a penicillin or cephalosporin cannot be given.

[5]If organism is resistant to gentamicin or tobramycin, amikacin, 7.5 mg/kg IM or IV q12h, can be administered.

[6]Cefotaxime, 2 g IV q6h, or other third-generation cephalosporins may be used alone.

[7]Ampicillin, a cephalosporin, carbenicillin, ticarcillin, mezlocillin, or piperacillin often is used with gentamicin or tobramycin in serious gram-negative bacillary infection.

acid-stable analogs such as *phenoxymethyl penicillin (penicillin V)* have been developed. This agent is useful only in the treatment of nonserious gram-positive coccal infections such as pneumococcal pneumonia after response to parenteral penicillin or group A streptococcal pharyngitis. The usual therapeutic dose is 250 to 500 mg four times a day.

BROAD-SPECTRUM PENICILLINS. *Ampicillin* has the same spectrum as penicillin G (it also is destroyed by staphylococcal penicillinase) but is more active against *H. influenzae*, *E. coli*, *P. mirabilis*, *Salmonella*, and *Shigella*. The injectable form can be used intramuscularly or intravenously. In serious infections the usual dosage is 12 g daily intravenously in divided doses every 4 to 6 hours. The oral form is useful in urinary tract infection, shigellosis, and respiratory tract infections in a dose of 250 mg to 1 g every 6 hours. In gonococcal urethritis a single dose of 3.5 g together with 1 g of probenecid is administered. *Bacampicillin* is an oral ester of ampicillin that gives ampicillin levels in blood over twice those achieved

Table 39-2 Commonly used antibiotic regimens for selected infections (adult doses)—cont'd

Bacteria	Infection	Regimen for adult patients with normal renal function
Enterobacter species	Urinary tract infection without bacteremia	Lower tract: Carbenicillin indanyl sodium, 1 g PO q.i.d. or norfloxacin, 400 mg PO b.i.d., or ciprofloxacin, 500 mg b.i.d. × 1-3 days Upper tract: Carbenicillin indanyl sodium, 1 g PO q.i.d. or norfloxacin, 400 mg PO b.i.d., or ciprofloxacin, 500 mg b.i.d. × 14 days
	Bacteremia	Ticarcillin, mezlocillin, or piperacillin 40 mg/kg IV q4h and/or gentamicin or tobramycin 1.7 mg/kg IM or IV q8h; or cefotaxime, 2 g IV q6h, ceftizoxime, 2 g IV q8h, or ceftriaxone, 1 g IV q12h
Proteus mirabilis	Urinary tract infection without bacteremia	Lower tract: One dose of 3 g amoxicillin PO or ampicillin, 500 mg PO q.i.d. × 1-3 days, or cephalexin, 500 mg PO q.i.d. × 1-3 days Upper tract: Two weeks of oral therapy with ampicillin, 500 mg q.i.d., amoxicillin, 500 mg t.i.d., or cephalexin, 500 mg q.i.d.
	Bacteremia	As for *E. coli* bacteremia
Indole-positive *Proteus*	Urinary tract infection without bacteremia	Lower tract: As for *Enterobacter* urinary tract infection Upper tract: As for *Enterobacter* urinary tract infection
	Bacteremia	As for *Enterobacter* bacteremia
Pseudomonas aeruginosa	Urinary tract infection	Lower tract: As for *Enterobacter* urinary tract infection Upper tract: As for *Enterobacter* urinary tract infection
	Bacteremia	Ticarcillin, mezlocillin, or piperacillin 40 mg/kg IV q4h; or ceftazidime 2 g IV q8h; or imipenem 1 g IV q6h; all plus gentamicin or tobramycin 1.7 mg/kg IM or IV q8h
Bacteroides fragilis	Abscess or bacteremia	Clindamycin, 600 mg IV q6-8h, or chloramphenicol, 12.5 mg/kg IV q6h, or metronidazole, 7.5 mg/kg IV q6h as long as necessary[8]
Salmonella species	Typhoid fever	Ampicillin, 1 g IV q4h × 14 days, or chloramphenicol, 12.5 mg/kg PO or IV q6h × 14 days
	Bacteremia	Ampicillin, 2 g IV q4h × 2-4 wk, or chloramphenicol, 12.5 mg/kg PO or IV q6h × 2-4 wk
Shigella species	Colitis	Tetracycline 2.5 g PO in one dose, or ampicillin, 0.5-1 g PO q.i.d., or trimethoprim-sulfamethoxazole (160 mg and 800 mg, respectively) b.i.d. × 5 days; norfloxacin, 400 mg PO b.i.d., or ciprofloxacin, 500 mg b.i.d. is also effective

[8]Abscesses must be surgically drained. Aerobes often are present in abscesses, and appropriate therapy must be included. Clindamycin cannot be used in CNS infection.

with oral ampicillin. *Hetacillin,* another preparation, has no advantages over ampicillin.

Amoxicillin is very similar to ampicillin but is given only orally. It is absorbed much better than ampicillin, producing serum levels that are at least double. It can be substituted for ampicillin except in shigellosis, against which it is less effective.

Carbenicillin and *ticarcillin* have a spectrum of activity similar to that of ampicillin. They have less activity against gram-positive cocci, equivalent activity against the gram-negative bacilli *E. coli* and *P. mirabilis,* and much greater activity against other gram-negative bacilli. They are also active against *Enterobacter* species, *P. aeruginosa,* and indole-positive *Proteus* spp. (that is, those other than *P. mirabilis*). *Klebsiella* and *Serratia* spp. are resistant to these agents. In general they should be reserved for use in proven or suspected *P. aeruginosa* or to a lesser degree in *Enterobacter* or indole-positive *Proteus* infections, since there is a potential problem of the emergence of resistant *P. aeruginosa.*

Minimal inhibitory concentrations of carbenicillin required to inhibit a majority of *P. aeruginosa* are 75 to 150 μg/ml. Therefore very high serum concentrations requiring high doses are needed to achieve therapeutic efficacy in serious infections. The dosage of carbenicillin in serious infections is 500 mg/kg body weight/day in divided doses every 4 hours by the intravenous route. Ticarcillin is twice as active as carbenicillin against *P. aeruginosa* and can be used in a dosage of 250 mg/kg/day in divided doses every 4 hours. Carbenicillin indanyl sodium, an oral form of carbenicillin, is useful only in urinary tract infection and chronic bacterial prostatitis. The dosage is 0.5 to 1 g every 6 hours. *Piperacillin, azlocillin,* and *mezlocillin,* the newer broad-spectrum penicillins, have greater activity than ticarcillin against many gram-negative bacilli. In

addition, they are active against *Klebsiella* and *Serratia* spp. They are used in the same doses as ticarcillin.

PENICILLINASE-RESISTANT PENICILLINS. *Methicillin, nafcillin,* and *oxacillin* parenterally and *cloxacillin* and *dicloxacillin* orally are the pencillins resistant to degradation by staphylococcal penicillinase. These agents have a narrow spectrum and are used primarily for the treatment of *S. aureus* infection. However, they also constitute adequate treatment for pneumococcal, group A streptococcal, and susceptible *S. epidermidis* infections. Injectable forms (methicillin, nafcillin, and oxacillin) must be used in serious infection and are given intravenously, 6 to 12 g/day in divided doses every 4 hours.

The oral agents cloxacillin and dicloxacillin are used in the treatment of nonserious *S. auerus* infection, such as soft tissue infections, in doses of 250 to 500 mg every 6 hours.

PENICILLINS COMBINED WITH PENICILLINASE INHIBITORS. *Amoxicillin* combined with *clavulanic acid* (a β-lactamase inhibitor) for oral use and *ampicillin* combined with *sulbactum* (a β-lactamase inhibitor) for intravenous or intramuscular use have the antibacterial activity of *amoxicillin* or *ampicillin* plus an added spectrum. They have activity against gram-positive cocci other than methicillin-resistant staphylococci, against gram-negative cocci including penicillinase-producing gonococci, against *E. coli, Klebsiella* spp., *Proteus* spp., and penicillinase-producing *H. influenzae,* and against gram-positive and gram-negative anaerobes. They are particularly useful for infections with aerobes and anaerobes such as human bite infections and intraabdominal and pelvic infections. The doses are the same as for amoxicillin and ampicillin. *Ticarcillin* combined with *clavulanic acid* for intravenous use has the antibacterial activity of ticarcillin, plus an added spectrum. It is active against most aerobic and anaerobic gram-positive and gram-negative cocci and bacilli with the exception of methicillin-resistant staphylococci. It is particularly useful in hospital-acquired mixed infections with aerobes and anaerobes such as hospital-acquired pneumonia and hospital-acquired intraabdominal infections.

EXCRETION AND SIDE EFFECTS. All the penicillins except nafcillin are excreted primarily by the kidneys, both by tubular secretion and by glomerular filtration. Nafcillin is excreted mainly by the liver. Although it is advisable to decrease the doses of penicillins administered to patients with renal insufficiency, these modifications are often not critical.

All penicillins can cause hypersensitivity reactions, and there is cross-sensitivity among the different penicillins. The two types of reaction are (1) immediate, including anaphylaxis, urticaria, and angioneurotic edema, and (2) delayed, including morbilliform eruption and serum sickness. About 5% of patients given penicillins have hypersensitivity reactions, the most common being morbilliform rash. Drug fever also may be caused by hypersensitivity. Ampicillin causes a rash in most patients with infectious mononucleosis; however, this rash is not related to hypersensitivity and has no negative implications for future use of the drug.

All penicillins can cause nephritis as the result of an immune reaction, but methicillin is most likely to cause this syndrome. All penicillins can cause leukopenia, but nafcillin is the most likely to produce this side effect. Coombs'-positive hemolytic anemia and thrombocytopenia may result from the use of any penicillin.

With very high doses of penicillins (as used in meningitis), especially in the presence of renal insufficiency, myoclonus and generalized seizures may be observed. Carbenicillin and ticarcillin in high doses, especially in patients with renal insufficiency, interfere with platelet function and can contribute to a bleeding diathesis.

Potassium penicillin G contains 1.6 mEq of potassium per 1 million units, and carbenicillin and ticarcillin contain about 5 mEq of sodium per gram. Large doses of these compounds in patients with renal insufficiency or heart failure, respectively, can cause a significant ion overload. In addition, hypokalemia and alkalosis may result from the use of carbenicillin or ticarcillin.

Cephalosporins

The cephalosporins are bactericidal agents with both a gram-positive and a gram-negative spectrum of activity. They work by inhibiting bacterial cell wall synthesis. They are relatively nontoxic, and to ensure adequate therapy, they generally are given in doses considerably larger than needed.

FIRST-GENERATION CEPHALOSPORINS. *Cephalothin,* a parenterally administered cephalosporin, is active against most gram-positive cocci and bacilli (including anaerobes). However, enterococci are resistant. Cephalothin also is active against *E. coli, Klebsiella* organisms, and *P. mirabilis. Enterobacter* sp., indole-positive *Proteus* sp., *Pseudomonas* sp., and many anaerobic gram-negative bacilli (especially *Bacteroides fragilis)* are resistant. In serious infections a dose of 2 g is given every 4 hours intravenously. *Cephapirin* can be used interchangeably with cephalothin.

Cefazolin, a parenterally administered cephalosporin, has activity similar to that of cephalothin but does not cause as much pain when given intramuscularly. It provides higher blood levels that persist longer. The usual dose in serious infections is 1 to 2 g every 6 to 8 hours intramuscularly or intravenously.

The orally administered cephalosporins have a spectrum of activity similar to cephalothin and are used in urinary tract infection, soft tissue infection, and other non-life-threatening infections.

Cephalexin and *cephradine* are the most commonly used oral cephalosporins and are given in doses of 250 to 500 mg every 6 hours.

SECOND-GENERATION CEPHALOSPORINS. *Cefamandole* and *cefoxitin* are parenterally administered cephalosporins with an antimicrobial spectrum somewhat greater than that of cephalothin. Besides having the spectrum of cephalothin, cefamandole has better activity against *H. influenzae* and some *Enterobacter* strains, and cefoxitin has much better activity against indole-positive *Proteus* strains, *Serratia* spp., anaerobic gram-negative bacilli (including *B. fragilis),* and some *E. coli, Klebsiella* organisms, and *P. mirabilis* strains that are resistant to cephalothin. In serious infections a dose of 2 g is given intravenously every 4 hours. Neither of these agents is active against *P. aeruginosa.* They are more expensive than cephalothin and cefazolin and should be used only in the relatively few situations where they have a real advantage.

Cefuroxime and *cefonicid* resemble cefamandole in activity. Cefuroxime is used in doses of 0.75 to 3 g every 8 hours intravenously or intramuscularly and is useful in pneumococcal, meningococcal and *H. influenzae* meningitis. Cefonicid is given in doses of 0.5 to 2 g intramuscularly or intravenously every 24 hours. *Cefotetan* resembles cefoxitin in activity and is used in doses of 1 to 2 g intramuscularly or intravenously every 12 hours. Orally administered *cefuroxime* (1 g every 12 hours) and *cefaclor* (1.5 g every 8 hours) have better activity against *H. influenzae* than the other oral cephalosporins and are used in otitis media and other infections caused by *H. influenzae.*

THIRD-GENERATION CEPHALOSPORINS. The available third-generation cephalosporins are *cefotaxime, ceftizoxime, ceftriaxone, moxalactam, cefoperazone,* and *ceftazidime.* All are more active against *H. influenzae, E. coli, Klebsiella* organisms, *Enterobacter, P. mirabilis,* indole-positive *Proteus* organisms, and *Serratia* spp. and gram-negative cocci than the older cephalosporins. Cefotaxime, ceftizoxime, and ceftriaxone have equivalent excellent activity against these gram-negative organisms and reasonably good activity against gram-positive cocci (except for enterococci). Moxalactam and cefoperazone have excellent activity against these gram-negative cocci and bacilli but much poorer activity against gram-positive cocci.

Ceftazidime has an excellent spectrum against gram-negative bacilli and cocci but is not as active as cefotaxime, ceftizoxime, or ceftriaxone against gram-positive cocci. Ceftazidime is the only cephalosporin with good activity against *P. aeruginosa.* Cefotaxime, ceftizoxime, ceftriaxone, moxalactam, and ceftazidime are effective in gram-negative bacillary and coccal meningitis.

The usual doses are: cefotaxime, 1 to 2 g every 4 to 6 hours; ceftizoxime, 1 to 2 g every 8 hours; ceftriaxone, 1 to 2 g every 12 to 24 hours; moxalactam, 1 to 2 g every 8 hours; cefoperazone, 2 g every 8 to 12 hours; and ceftazidime, 1 to 2 g every 8 hours. All are given intravenously or intramuscularly. These agents are expensive and should be reserved for serious infections.

Imipenem

Imipenem, a β-lactam antibiotic, has excellent activity against gram-positive cocci, including enterococci, gram-negative cocci, gram-negative bacilli (including *P. aeruginosa),* and anaerobic bacteria. The dose is 500 mg to 1 g every 6 hours intravenously. Imipenem is expensive and should be reserved for serious infections.

Aztreonam

Aztreonam, a monobactam, has excellent activity against gram-negative bacilli, including *P. aeruginosa,* but is not active against gram-positive cocci and anaerobic bacteria. The dose is 1 to 2 g intravenously every 8 hours. It may be less prone than the cephalosporins to cause an allergic reaction in a penicillin-sensitive patient. Aztreonam is expensive and should be reserved for serious infections.

EXCRETION AND SIDE EFFECTS. The cephalosporins are relatively nontoxic. As with the penicillins, the doses used generally are much larger than needed. Most of the cephalosporins are excreted primarily in the urine, by glomerular filtration and some also by tubular secretion. Cefoperazone is excreted mainly by the liver. Although it is advisable to decrease doses in the presence of renal insufficiency, such decreases often are not of critical importance.

Hypersensitivity reactions (rash, urticaria, and anaphylaxis) occur less commonly with cephalosporins than with penicillins. Cross-sensitivity between penicillins and cephalosporins probably is uncommon. Cephalosporins can be administered cautiously to a patient with a history of a delayed hypersensitivity reaction to penicillins. However, they should not be used if the patient has a history of an immediate reaction to a penicillin. Drug fever probably occurs as frequently with cephalosporins as with penicillins.

Thrombophlebitis is common with intravenous use of cephalothin, cephapirin, and some of the other cephalosporins. A positive Coombs' test, thrombocytopenia, and leukopenia may be seen following the use of cephalosporins.

Some of the cephalosporins such as cefamandole, cefotetan, moxalactam, and cefoperazone have a disulfiram-like effect (causing nausea and vomiting with ingestion of alcohol) and can cause elevations in the prothrombin time and partial thromboplastin time, requiring vitamin K therapy. Moxalactam tends to cause irreversible inactivation of platelets and bleeding.

Aminoglycosides

The aminoglycosides are bactericidal and work by binding to the 30S ribosome and thus inhibiting bacterial protein synthesis. They include streptomycin, neomycin, kanamycin, gentamicin, tobramycin, netilmicin, and amikacin, none of which is absorbed orally. With the exception of streptomycin, which has a limited antimicrobial spectrum, all have good activity against gram-negative aerobic bacilli but lack activity against anaerobes. Neomycin and kanamycin are not active against *P. aeruginosa,* whereas gentamicin, tobramycin, netilmicin, and amikacin have good activity against these organisms. The aminoglycosides are active against staphylococci but are not active against streptococci, including pneumococci.

Streptomycin has specific, limited uses because many bacteria develop a resistance to it. It is used as a companion drug with isoniazid or rifampin in the treatment of tuberculosis and with penicillin or vancomycin in the treatment or prophylaxis of streptococcal endocarditis. It also is used in the therapy for brucellosis, tularemia, and plague. The usual adult dose is 0.5 to 1 g every 12 hours intramuscularly. In tuberculosis 1 g usually is given once daily for several months and thereafter three times a week.

Neomycin and *kanamycin* at one time were used parenterally. Currently their use should be limited to oral or topical (eye,

ear) application because of toxicity and the development of bacterial resistance. These agents are active against most *E. coli, Klebsiella, Enterobacter,* and *Proteus* strains but not active against *P. aeruginosa.* When they are used for bowel preparation before surgery or in the treatment of hepatic coma to reduce bacterial populations and therefore absorption of ammonia, the oral dosage is 4 to 8 g/day in divided doses every 6 hours. Topical use should be restricted to small amounts in small areas, since absorption and toxicity can occur. Use on skin generally is not of value.

Gentamicin and *tobramycin* should be used only in the treatment of serious gram-negative bacillary infection. Gentamicin also can be used as a companion drug with a penicillin or vancomycin in the treatment of enterococcal or *S. aureus* endocarditis or in prophylaxis of enterococcal endocarditis. These two agents are very similar in antimicrobial activity with only two significant differences. Tobramycin is about four times as active as gentamicin against *P. aeruginosa,* and gentamicin is more active than tobramycin against *S. marcescens.* The dosage of gentamicin or tobramycin in patients with normal renal function and serious infection is 5 mg/kg/day in divided doses every 8 hours intravenously (by slow infusion over at least 20 to 30 minutes) or intramuscularly.

Resistance of gram-negative bacilli to gentamicin and tobramycin has occurred in some hospitals, and hospital-acquired infections in those institutions cannot be treated with these agents. The resistance is most commonly caused by a plasmid-mediated enzymatic alteration of the aminoglycoside.

Netilmicin has the same spectrum of activity as gentamicin and tobramycin but is somewhat less susceptible to enzymatic inactivation. The dosage in serious infections is 6.5 mg/kg/day in divided doses every 8 hours intravenously.

Amikacin has the same spectrum of activity as gentamicin and tobramycin but is much less susceptible to enzymatic inactivation. Therefore amikacin has great value in the management of serious infections caused by gram-negative bacilli that are resistant to gentamicin and tobramycin. Amikacin should be reserved for use in these infections or in gram-negative bacillary infections acquired in hospitals where organisms are known to be commonly resistant to gentamicin and tobramycin.

In patients with normal renal function the dosage of amikacin is 7.5 mg/kg body weight by slow intravenous infusion over at least 20 to 30 minutes or intramuscularly every 12 hours. Some use 5 mg/kg every 8 hours. Amikacin must be given in higher doses (15 mg/kg/day) than gentamicin, tobramycin, or netilmicin (peaks of about 20 μg/ml for amikacin as compared to about 6 μg/ml for the other agents) to produce the higher concentrations of amikacin required to inhibit gram-negative bacilli.

EXCRETION AND SIDE EFFECTS. All aminoglycosides are excreted by glomerular filtration. They are toxic agents, and toxicity increases as blood levels increase. Therefore the principle in using these agents is to give doses large enough to yield therapeutic levels but no larger.

It is important to be cautious even in the topical use of the aminoglycosides, since they are absorbed from areas of denuded skin such as burns. They are absorbed well from the peritoneum, pleural cavity, and joints and should never be instilled in these cavities. Furthermore, there is no need to inject aminoglycosides into these spaces, since therapeutic levels are easily achieved following parenteral administration. However, intrathecal injection (5 mg of gentamicin every 24 hours) is necessary in gram-negative bacillary meningitis because penetration into the CSF is poor.

Some aminoglycosides are slowly inactivated by high concentrations of carbenicillin and ticarcillin (and probably other penicillins and cephalosporins as well), and these agents should never be mixed with aminoglycosides in infusion bottles. Inactivation can occur in patients with renal failure when blood levels of carbenicillin or ticarcillin are high and the aminoglycoside is given with long intervals between doses.

All aminoglycosides are nephrotoxic and ototoxic. Neomycin and kanamycin, which should no longer be used parenterally, probably are more toxic than the other aminoglycosides discussed here. Streptomycin has very little nephrotoxicity. Gentamicin probably is more nephrotoxic than tobramycin and amikacin. Nephrotoxicity is reversible and is more likely to occur with larger doses, higher blood levels, or longer duration of therapy and in elderly patients, those with preexisting renal disease, and those receiving furosemide, ethacrynic acid, or possibly cephalothin.

Streptomycin and gentamicin are more likely to produce vestibular damage than hearing loss, whereas tobramycin and amikacin are more likely to produce hearing loss than vestibular damage. The eighth nerve toxicity often is irreversible. It is more likely to occur with larger doses, higher blood levels, or longer duration of therapy and in elderly patients, those with renal insufficiency, and those receiving ethacrynic acid.

To minimize the possibility of ototoxic and nephrotoxic reactions, doses should be decreased in patients with impaired renal function. Following a normal loading dose (1.7 mg/kg body weight for gentamicin, tobramycin, or 7.5 mg/kg for amikacin), smaller doses can be given at the customary intervals or normal doses can be given at longer intervals. It is best to give smaller doses at normal or somewhat longer intervals to avoid long periods of time with subtherapeutic blood levels. Although nomograms are available to calculate doses based on serum creatinine or creatinine clearance values, they are inaccurate, and with changing renal function they are absolutely worthless. When a nomogram must be used, the simplest method is to give the loading dose and then as a maintenance dose to give the loading dose divided by the serum creatinine value (assuming a stable creatinine) at the usual intervals. Another way to calculate the maintenance dose is to multiply the loading dose by the creatinine clearance, express this amount as a percentage, and add 5% to 10%. For example, with a creatinine clearance of 20 ml/min, give 25% to 30% of the loading dose at the usual intervals.

The best approach is to give a normal loading dose and then a second dose estimated on the basis of a nomogram. Serum concentrations should be measured just before ("trough") and 60 minutes after the second and subsequent intramuscular doses or 30 minutes after the second and subsequent 30-minute infusions of drug. The level 60 minutes after an intramuscular injection is the "peak" and is equivalent to the level 30 minutes after a 30-minute infusion. Doses are adjusted to give serum peak levels of 4 to 8 µg/ml for gentamicin, tobramycin, and netilmicin, and 16 to 25 µg/ml for amikacin. Troughs above 2 µg/ml for gentamicin and tobramycin and above 5 µg/ml for amikacin indicate retention of drug and a greater chance of toxicity. However, therapy must be aimed at achieving adequate peak levels every 8 hours for gentamicin and tobramycin and every 12 hours for amikacin. Netilmicin is managed like gentamicin. When doses are adjusted and levels are stable, levels can be measured once a day or once every other day.

Intravenous injections of aminoglycosides should never be rapid, and these agents should never be instilled into a body cavity, since neuromuscular blockade with respiratory arrest can occur. This is especially likely in patients with myasthenia gravis or in those receiving curare-like drugs. It is reversible with neostigmine or intravenous administration of calcium. Paresthesias and peripheral neuropathy may occur in rare cases. Hypersensitivity reactions occasionally may be observed.

Vancomycin

Vancomycin is a bactericidal agent that acts by inhibiting cell well synthesis. It is active against all gram-positive cocci and bacilli, including *S. aureus* and *S. epidermidis* strains that are resistant to all penicillins and cephalosporins. It is the agent of choice in treating serious infections caused by these organisms, as well as serious staphylococcal infection and endocarditis caused by *viridans* streptococci or enterococci when penicillins or cephalosporins cannot be used because of drug allergy. All gram-negative bacilli are resistant to vancomycin.

Vancomycin is not absorbed orally and must be given intravenously to treat systemic illness. The dose is 500 mg intravenously every 6 hours or 1 g every 12 hours in a slow infusion lasting over an hour.

Vancomycin is used orally in the treatment of *Clostridium difficile* colitis (antibiotic-associated colitis). The dose is 125 to 250 mg every 6 hours.

EXCRETION AND SIDE EFFECTS. Common side effects with vancomycin are phlebitis and chills and fever during the infusion. Rash may be seen. Nephrotoxicity occurs occasionally, and deafness may be associated with very high blood levels, usually in patients with renal insufficiency. Since vancomycin is excreted by glomerular filtration, it is retained in the presence of renal insufficiency. Therefore serum concentrations must be measured and doses are accordingly reduced in patients with decreased renal function. The absence of excretion in patients with renal failure can be used to advantage in treating infection in patients requiring dialysis, since 0.5 to 1 g of vancomycin given every 7 days provides therapeutic serum levels.

Erythromycin, lincomycin, and clindamycin

Erythromycin, lincomycin, and clindamycin are primarily bacteriostatic agents that work by binding to the 50S ribosome and thus inhibiting bacterial protein synthesis. These agents have a similar spectrum of activity against bacteria and are absorbed when given orally; they also can be administered parenterally.

Erythromycin is active against gram-positive cocci (including anaerobes) with the exception of enterococci. However, many *S. aureus* strains are now resistant to erythromycin. It is also active against *Mycoplasma pneumoniae*, *Chlamydia trachomatis*, the bacillus of Legionnaires' disease (*Legionella pneumophila*) and related organisms, *Corynebacterium diphtheriae*, and *Treponema pallidum*. It is the substitute of choice in group A streptococcal and pneumococcal infections (except meningitis) when penicillin cannot be used. It is the drug of choice in *M. pneumoniae* and *L. pneumophila* (and related organism) infection and in *C. diptheriae* carriers. Erythromycin should not be used in serious *S. aureus* infection. Although erythromycin is active against anaerobic gram-negative bacilli, it is much less active than clindamycin. It has, however, been used orally in combination with an oral aminoglycoside as a bowel preparation before gastrointestinal tract surgery.

Erythromycin base, estolate, proprinate, and stearate all can be given orally in doses of 250 mg to 1 g every 6 hours. Parenteral therapy rarely is required, but when necessary (as in severe *Legionella* infection), the intravenous route should be used.

Lincomycin is similar to clindamycin. It has no advantages over clindamycin, which is more active in vitro, is better absorbed orally, and therefore is a preferable drug.

Clindamycin has a spectrum of activity similar to erythromycin except that its activity against *Mycoplasma* is poor. As with erythromycin, clindamycin is not a reliable drug in serious *S. aureus* infection. The major advantage of clindamycin over erythromycin is its much greater activity against anaerobic bacteria, especially *Bacteroides* species (including *B. fragilis*), which often are resistant to penicillins and cephalosporins. The principal use of clindamycin is in serious infections caused by anaerobic microorganisms, particularly when *B. fragilis* is likely to be present. However, clindamycin cannot be used in CNS infection because penetration through the blood-brain barrier is poor.

The usual dose is 150 to 300 mg every 6 hours orally or 300 to 600 mg every 6 to 8 hours intramuscularly or intravenously.

EXCRETION AND SIDE EFFECTS. Erythromycin, lincomycin, and clindamycin are excreted mainly in the bile, and little if any adjustment in dosage is required in the presence of renal insufficiency.

Common side effects of erythromycin are gastrointestinal tract disturbances, including nausea, vomiting, and diarrhea. Cholestatic jaundice can occur with the use of erythromycin estolate (and to a lesser degree other erythromycins); it usually appears after 10 days of therapy but can occur earlier if the agent has been given previously. Erythromycin cannot be used intramuscularly because of pain on administration, and it causes severe phlebitis when used intravenously. Hypersensitivity reactions are rare.

Oral and parenteral administration of clindamycin and lincomycin can cause diarrhea, which sometimes is severe. Pseudomembranous colitis may result. It has been recognized that the type of colitis caused by lincomycin and clindamycin also can result from administration of many other antibiotics such as ampicillin and cephalosporins. The cause of colitis is *C. difficile*, which produces a toxin in the colon. The colitis responds to treatment with oral vancomycin or metronidazole. Hypersensitivity reactions may occur with lincomycin and clindamycin.

Tetracyclines

The tetracyclines are bacteriostatic agents that work by binding to the 30S ribosome and thus inhibiting bacterial protein synthesis. These agents are active against *Rickettsia, Mycoplasma*, and *Chlamydia* organisms, *T. pallidum*, and many gram-positive and gram-negative bacteria. However, many bacteria formerly sensitive to the tetracyclines have become resistant. Over 5% of pneumococci, more than 20% of group A streptococci, most *S. aureus*, and many strains of gram-negative bacilli currently are resistant to tetracyclines.

At present the primary uses for the tetracyclines are in treating urinary tract infection, rickettsial infections, chlamydial infections, *Mycoplasma* infections, chronic bronchitis, shigellosis, brucellosis, granuloma inguinale, and chancroid and as alternative therapy to penicillin in gonorrhea and syphilis.

Tetracycline and *oxytetracycline* are equivalent, but tetracycline is by far the more commonly used. It usually is given orally in doses of 250 to 500 mg every 6 hours. Intramuscular administration is too painful, but tetracycline can be given intravenously in doses of 0.5 g (in rare cases 1 g) every 12 hours.

Demethylchlortetracycline (demeclocycline), methacycline, doxycycline, and *minocycline* are long-acting tetracyclines for oral use. Their excretion is very slow, therefore they can be given every 12 to 24 hours. They have no therapeutic advantages except the need for fewer daily doses. The disadvantages are higher price, lower urine levels (in fact, they may be subtherapeutic in some urinary tract infections), and more toxicity (see "Excretion and side effects" below).

In patients with renal insufficiency, doxycycline is the only tetracycline that can be used without accumulation and higher blood levels; however, circumstances in which a tetracycline must be used in the presence of renal insufficiency are rare. The dose is 100 mg every 12 hours.

Minocycline is one of three agents (the others are rifampin and sulfonamides) that can eradicate meningococci from the nasopharynx. Presumably this is because of its high concentration owing to high lipid solubility. However, because of minocycline's tendency to cause vertigo, rifampin or a sulfonamide (if the meningococcus is susceptible to sulfonamides) is preferred.

EXCRETION AND SIDE EFFECTS. All the tetracyclines except doxycycline are excreted primarily in the urine by glomerular filtration, and in the presence of renal insufficiency blood levels increase with all tetracyclines other than doxycycline. All tetracyclines produce gastrointestinal side effects such as nausea, vomiting, and diarrhea with oral use and thrombophlebitis with intravenous use. Staining of teeth, hypoplasia of dental enamel, and abnormal bone growth can occur in the fetuses of pregnant women given tetracyclines or in children under 8 years of age given these agents. In infants, pseudotumor cerebri with increased intracranial pressure and bulging fontanelles may develop.

All tetracyclines have an antimetabolic effect and increase protein breakdown. In patients with renal insufficiency this can result in worsening of the uremic state by increasing the urea and acid load to the kidney. Outdated tetracyclines can degenerate and cause Fanconi's syndrome.

With excessive blood levels resulting from large doses, intravenous use, or renal insufficiency, fatal acute fatty degeneration of the liver may occur. This is especially likely during pregnancy.

The long-acting tetracyclines (especially demethylchlortetracycline) cause photosensitivity. Demethylchlortetracycline also can cause nephrogenic diabetes insipidus. Minocycline commonly causes vertigo.

Chloramphenicol

Chloramphenicol is bacteriostatic and works by binding to the 50S ribosome and thus inhibiting bacterial protein synthesis. It has a wide spectrum of activity against gram-positive and gram-negative cocci and bacilli (including anaerobes), as well as *Rickettsia, Mycoplasma,* and *Chlamydia* organisms. The major reason for restricting its use is the rare but lethal complication of aplastic anemia.

Chloramphenicol is the drug (or one of the drugs) of choice in the following infections: (1) typhoid fever and other serious *Salmonella* infections; (2) meningitis caused by *H. influenzae* resistant to ampicillin or when ampicillin cannot be used with sensitive strains; (3) meningococcal or pneumococcal meningitis when a penicillin cannot be used; (4) serious infection caused by *B. fragilis* (including CNS infection); and (5) rickettsial infection not responding to tetracycline or in which tetracycline cannot be used. Chloramphenicol is well absorbed orally. The usual dosage is 50 mg/kg/day in four evenly divided doses; 100 mg/kg/day has often been used in CNS infection. It is not absorbed well intramuscularly, and parenteral therapy should be by the intravenous route in the same dose regimen as orally.

EXCRETION AND SIDE EFFECTS. Chloramphenicol is metabolized by the liver, and therefore doses are not altered by renal insufficiency.

Two types of bone marrow depression may be caused by chloramphenicol: a dose-related reversible interference with iron metabolism and an irreversible idiosyncratic form of aplastic anemia. The reversible form occurs during therapy, particularly with high doses or a prolonged course and especially in patients with liver disease. It is manifested by increased serum iron, increased saturation of iron-binding capacity, decreased reticulocytes, vacuolization of red cell precursors, anemia, leukopenia, and thrombocytopenia.

Irreversible idiosyncratic aplastic anemia occurs less often than 1 in 25,000 patients given chloramphenicol. The onset may be delayed until after therapy has been discontinued.

The "gray syndrome" (pallor and listlessness), which often is fatal, can occur in neonates given chloramphenicol. The syndrome is related to very high blood levels resulting from the immature liver's inability to metabolize chloramphenicol. Optic neuritis and peripheral neuropathy may be seen with prolonged use of chloramphenicol.

Polymyxins

Polymyxin B and *polymyxin E (colistin)* are polypeptide antibiotics that are bactericidal against most gram-negative bacilli (including *P. aeruginosa*) except *Proteus* spp. They work by disrupting the bacterial cell membrane. They are not absorbed orally. Their major use has been in the treatment of *P. aeruginosa* infection. However, because the aminoglycosides are less toxic and probably more effective, they are used more frequently by the parenteral route for this purpose than the polymyxins. Polymyxin B is used topically for ear and eye infections.

When given parenterally, polymyxin B is administered intramuscularly every 8 hours or by continuous intravenous infusion in doses up to 2.5 mg/kg/day. Colistin is given in the form of colistimethate sodium, 3 to 5 mg/kg/day intramuscularly or intravenously in divided doses every 6 hours.

EXCRETION AND TOXICITY. The polymyxins are excreted by glomerular filtration. Higher blood levels are associated with increased toxicity, and therefore doses must be reduced in patients with impaired renal function.

The major toxic side effects are nephrotoxicity, which usually is reversible, and neurotoxicity. Nonserious neurotoxicity in the form of circumoral and fingertip paresthesias is common. With toxic blood levels, respiratory paralysis may occur; this is reversible with intravenously administered calcium but not with neostigmine. Hypersensitivity reactions also may be seen.

Sulfonamides

The sulfonamides are bacteriostatic and work by competitive inhibition of paraaminobenzoic acid. They are well absorbed orally. Sulfonamides currently are used in very few circumstances. These are (1) urinary tract infection (especially caused by *E. coli*); (2) nocardiosis when they are the agents of choice; (3) in combination with pyrimethamine in the treatment of toxoplasmosis; (4) as a substitute for penicillin in prophylaxis of rheumatic fever; (5) as prophylaxis against susceptible meningococcal strains; (6) in the form of sulfasalazine in ulcerative colitis; (7) in the form of silver sulfadiazine or mafenide in burns; (8) in chloroquine-resistant *Plasmodium falciparum* infection; (9) dermatitis herpetiformis; and (10) in combination with trimethoprim for certain indications (see "Trimethoprim-sulfamethoxazole" in the following).

Sulfisoxazole and *sulfamethaxozole* are the major agents used for urinary tract infection. *Sulfadiazine* rarely is used because of the danger of crystalluria. Combinations of three sulfonamides (trisulfapyrimidines) also are used because of their great solubility and low danger of crystalluria. The dosages usually are 1 g four times a day for sulfisoxazole and 1 g every 12 hours for sulfamethoxazole.

Long-acting sulfonamides are more toxic than shorter-acting sulfonamides and should not be used.

EXCRETION AND SIDE EFFECTS. The sulfonamides are excreted by glomerular filtration. They should not be used in the presence of renal insufficiency. One side effect is crystalluria, which can result in urinary obstruction or renal tubular necrosis. It is unlikely to occur with sulfisoxazole or sulfamethoxazole, and the risk can be diminished with the other sulfonamides by increasing fluid intake and by alkalinizing the urine to increase the drugs' solubility. Hypersensitivity reactions with fever and rash are common; vasculitis may occur. Activation of quiescent lupus erythematosus has been reported. Photosensitivity, hepatitis, and aplastic anemia all are complications of sulfonamide therapy. Administration of sulfonamides to the mother at term or to the newborn can cause kernicterus in the newborn by displacement of bilirubin from albumin. When patients with glucose-6-phosphate dehydrogenase deficiency are given sulfonamides, hemolytic anemia may result. Long-acting sulfonamides are more likely to cause Stevens-Johnson syndrome or myocarditis than the short-acting preparations.

Trimethoprim-sulfamethoxazole

Trimethoprim-sulfamethoxazole (co-trimoxazole) is a fixed combination of trimethoprim and sulfamethoxazole. Both drugs act to block the folic acid metabolism cycle of bacteria, and they often are much more active together than either agent alone would be. Sulfonamides competitively inhibit the incorporation of paraaminobenzoic acid, and trimethoprim prevents the reduction of dihydrofolate to tetrahydrofolate. The combined agent is bacteriostatic.

Trimethoprim-sulfamethoxazole is active in urinary tract infections. It will cure a minority of patients with chronic bacterial prostatitis caused by susceptible bacteria when given for 12 weeks. It also is effective in the prophylaxis of urinary tract infection in women who have multiple reinfections. Trimethoprim-sulfamethoxazole is the drug of choice for treatment of *Pneumocystis carinii* pneumonia and also is effective in prophylaxis of this infection in children with malignancies. It is effective for the treatment of typhoid fever when ampicillin and chloramphenicol cannot be used. It is effective in shigellosis, otitis media, gonorrhea, and acute exacerbations of chronic bronchitis.

The usual dose is two tablets (160 mg trimethoprim and 800 mg sulfamethoxazole) twice a day. Much higher doses (20 mg/kg/day trimethoprim and 100 mg/kg/day sulfamethoxazole in four divided doses) are used in the treatment of *P. carinii* pneumonia. Much lower doses (40 mg trimethoprim and 200 mg sulfamethoxazole each night) are used in the prophylaxis of urinary tract infection.

EXCRETION AND SIDE EFFECTS. Both trimethoprim and sulfamethoxazole are excreted in the urine. The side effects are those already listed for sulfonamides. Trimethoprim is less likely to cause side effects but can cause nausea, vomiting, rash, and folate deficiency resulting in macrocytic anemia. Nephrotoxicity can occur in patients with impaired renal function.

Trimethoprim

Trimethoprim alone is available for patients allergic to sulfonamides. It has been used mainly in the treatment of chronic bacterial prostatitis and urinary tract infection and the prophylaxis of urinary tract infection. The dose is 100 mg every 12 hours. The side effects are listed under "Trimethoprim-sulfamethoxazole."

Spectinomycin

Spectinomycin is a bactericidal antibiotic that works by binding to the 30S ribosome and thus inhibiting bacterial protein synthesis. It is approved for and used only in the treatment of gonococcal infections. It should be reserved for patients allergic to penicillin, for the treatment of infections caused by *N. gonorrhoeae* that produce penicillinase, and for patients who fail to respond to therapy with penicillin, ampicillin, or tetracycline. Spectinomycin is not effective in gonococcal pharyngitis.

A single dose of 2 g is given intramuscularly for gonococcal urethritis, cervicitis, and proctitis.

EXCRETION AND SIDE EFFECTS. Spectinomycin is excreted by glomerular filtration. Side effects other than hypersensitivity reactions and fever are rare with the dose used.

Metronidazole

Metronidazole is a microbicidal agent that has activity only against strictly anaerobic bacteria and protozoa, such as *Giardia lamblia, Entamoeba histolytica,* and *Trichomonas vaginalis.* It is not active against aerobic or even microaerophilic bacteria. Its major use is in the treatment of protozoal infections and serious infections caused by anaerobes, particularly when *B. fragilis* is likely to be present (since this is the anaerobe most likely to be resistant to penicillins and cephalosporins). The major use in infections caused by anaerobes, therefore, is in intraabdominal and pelvic infections. Because of poor activity against microaerophilic gram-positive cocci, it is not very effective in lung abscess when these organisms play an important role. Metronidazole penetrates the CSF in high concentrations, making it an effective drug in the treatment of meningitis or brain abscess caused by susceptible anaerobes. It is effective in the treatment of *C. difficile* colitis. It has also been used for prophylaxis of infections associated with bowel surgery.

Metronidazole is absorbed well when given orally. The dose is 250 mg three times a day for 10 days in *Trichomonas* or *Giardia* infection and 750 mg three times a day for 5 to 10 days in amebiasis. A single 2 g dose also is effective in trichomoniasis. In serious infections caused by anaerobes, the agent should be given intravenously in a dose of 15 mg/kg body weight followed by 7.5 mg/kg every 6 hours. A dose of 500 mg every 6 hours can be given orally when the infection is less serious. A dose of 500 mg four times a day for 10 days is used for *C. difficile* colitis.

EXCRETION AND SIDE EFFECTS. Metronidazole is metabolized, and the metabolites and some unmetabolized metronidazole are excreted mainly in the urine. The side effects are nausea, vomiting, headache, seizures, syncope, other CNS reactions, and peripheral neuropathy. Rash, fever, and reversible neutropenia have been reported. Metronidazole has caused cancer in mice and rats, but the risk to humans is unknown. A disulfiram-like reaction may occur if alcohol is ingested.

Nitrofurantoin

Nitrofurantoin is used orally, and the only indication is the treatment or prophylaxis of urinary tract infection. It is active against *E. coli* and *Klebsiella-Enterobacter* spp., *Pseudomonas* organisms and many strains of *Proteus* are resistant. The dose is 50 to 100 mg four times a day for the treatment of urinary tract infection and 50 to 100 mg each night for prophylaxis in

women who have multiple reinfections. Emergence of resistant organisms is not a major problem. Nitrofurantoin is excreted in the urine; it does not give antibacterial blood levels, but urinary levels are high.

Nitrofurantoin is contraindicated in the presence of renal insufficiency, since serious toxicity is possible. Its side effects are nausea and vomiting, which are less likely with the macrocystalline form (Macrodantin). Hypersensitivity reactions, including fever, rash, and hypersensitivity pneumonitis, may be observed. In addition, progressive pulmonary interstitial fibrosis may occur. Paresthesias, followed by a severe polyneuropathy if the drug is not discontinued, can result, especially when serum levels rise as in renal failure. Hemolytic anemia can occur in patients with glucose-6-phosphate dehydrogenase deficiency. Leukopenia and hepatotoxicity have also been reported.

Quinolones (nalidixic acid, norfloxacin, ciprofloxacin)

Nalidixic acid is an oral antimicrobial agent used only in the treatment of urinary tract infection. It is active against *E. coli, Klebsiella-Enterobacter,* and *Proteus* but not *Pseudomonas* organisms. However, bacteria tend to become rapidly resistant. Nalidixic acid is excreted in the urine, giving very low blood levels but antibacterial urinary concentrations. It should not be used in the presence of renal insufficiency.

The dose is 1 g four times a day. The side effects are nausea, vomiting, rash, fever, headache, psychosis, and seizures. Papilledema may occur with the headache in children. Another very similar agent is *oxolinic acid.*

Norfloxacin is an oral agent approved for treatment of urinary tract infection. It is also effective in the treatment of gonorrhea and many types of bacterial gastroenteritis and probably in the treatment of acute and chronic bacterial prostatitis. It is active against virtually all gram-negative aerobic bacilli, including *E. coli, P. aeruginosa,* and *Klebsiella-Enterobacter, Proteus, Salmonella, Shigella, Campylobacter, Vibrio,* and *Yersinia* organisms. It is moderately active against gram-positive cocci and is not active against anaerobes. Blood levels are not adequate to treat systemic infections. The dose is 400 mg twice a day.

Ciprofloxacin has the same spectrum of activity as norfloxacin, is more active, and achieves blood levels with oral dosage adequate to treat systemic gram-negative bacillary infection. The dosage is 250 to 750 mg every 12 hours orally.

The major side effects of norfloxacin and ciprofloxacin are CNS toxicity, including lightheadedness and seizures.

Methenamine mandelate and methenamine hippurate

Methenamine mandelate and methenamine hippurate are oral agents used only for the suppression or prophylaxis of urinary tract infection. They are excreted into the urine in high concentrations. At a pH of 5.5 or less, mandelic and hippuric acids are antibacterial and methenamine is converted to formaldehyde, which is antibacterial. These agents are active against *E. coli* and to a lesser extent against other bacilli.

To reduce the urinary pH to 5.5 or less, an acidifying agent such as methionine or ascorbic acid often must be added. When *Proteus* infections occur, these agents usually are not helpful because *Proteus* organisms produce urease and alkalinize the urine.

The usual dose is 1 g of methenamine mandelate four times a day and 1 g of the hippurate twice a day. The side effects are nausea, vomiting, rash, dysuria (especially with high doses), and metabolic acidosis, especially with the addition of acidifying agents in the presence of renal insufficiency. These agents should not be used in cases of renal insufficiency.

BIBLIOGRAPHY

Goodman LS and Gilman A: The pharmacological basis of therapeutics, ed 6, New York, 1980, Macmillan, Inc.

Handbood of antimicrobial therapy. The Medical Letter on Drugs and Therapeutics (revised ed), New Rochelle, NY, 1988.

Mandell GL, Douglas RG, and Bennett JE: Principles and practice of infectious diseases, ed 3, New York, 1990, Churchill Livingstone.

Sanford JP: Guide to antimicrobial therapy, West Bethesda, Md, 1989, Antimicrobial Therapy, Inc.

40·INFECTIONS OF SPECIFIC ANATOMIC SITES

Bacterial pneumonia

Gerald R. Donowitz and **Gerald L. Mandell**

Pneumonia may be defined as parenchymal infection of the lung. Identifying the etiologic agent is of the utmost importance; the dangers and expense of "broad-spectrum," shotgun therapy and the impossibility of including all possible causes of pneumonia with empiric therapy make presumptive or, preferably, specific etiologic diagnosis a prerequisite for proper therapy. The following are the major etiologic agents of pneumonia:

I. Bacterial
  A. Common
    1. *Streptococcus pneumoniae*
    2. *Staphylococcus aureus*
    3. *Haemophilus influenzae*
    4. Mixed anaerobic bacteria (aspiration)
    5. Enterobacteriaceae
      (a) *Escherichia coli*
      (b) *Klebsiella pneumoniae*
      (c) *Enterobacter* spp.
      (d) *Serratia* spp.
    6. *Legionella* sp. (*L. pneumophila, L. micdadei*)
    7. *Mycoplasma pneumoniae*
    8. *Chlamydia* spp. (*C. psittaci, C. trachomatis*, and TWAR)
    9. *Mycobacterium tuberculosis*
    10. *Pneumocystis carinii* (usually in patients with AIDS)
    11. *Pseudomonas aeruginosa*
  B. Uncommon
    1. *Acinetobacter* var. *anitratus*
    2. *Actinomyces* and *Arachnia* spp.
    3. *Aeromonas hydrophilia*
    4. *Bacillus anthracis*
    5. *Branhamella catarrhalis*
    6. *Campylobacter fetus*
    7. *Eikenella corodens*
    8. *Francisella tularensis*
    9. *Neisseria meningitidis*
    10. *Nocardia* spp.
    11. *Pasteurella multocida*
    12. *Proteus* spp.
    13. *Pseudomonas pseudomallei*
    14. *Salmonella* spp.
    15. *Enterococcus faecalis*
    16. *Streptococcus pyogenes*

PATHOGENESIS. Defense mechanisms exist throughout the respiratory tract, and in the absence of disease they serve to maintain essentially sterile infralaryngeal airways and lung parenchyma. Lung defense mechanisms important in preventing infection include (1) filtration and humidification of inspired air through the upper airways; (2) intact reflexes, including epiglottic and cough reflexes; (3) tracheobronchial secretions containing antibacterial substances such as α-1-antitrypsin, lysozyme, and lactoferrin; (4) mucociliary transport via the ciliated epithelium; (5) cell-mediated immunity (alveolar macrophages, T lymphocytes); (6) humoral immunity (B lymphocytes, immunoglobulin, complement); and (7) polymorphonuclear leukocytes. The development of pneumonia implies a defect in normal lung defense mechanisms, a challenge by a particularly virulent organism, or an overwhelming inoculation. Inhalation of aerosolized material and aspiration of oropharyngeal contents are the most common means by which pathogens enter the lung. Less commonly, pneumonia may result from hematogenous spread of bacteria to the lung from reactivation of a dormant infection such as cytomegalovirus or perhaps *Pneumocystis carinii*.

PNEUMONIA SYNDROMES

Because of the wide variety of organisms involved in causing pneumonia, recognizing pneumonia syndromes and their likely causes aids in guiding diagnostic maneuvers and selecting specific antimicrobial therapy (Table 40-1). The major pneumonia syndromes caused by bacteria are reviewed here.

Syndrome of acute community-acquired pneumonia

Most patients with acute community-acquired pneumonia are in the sixth decade of life or older and have one or more chronic underlying diseases such as chronic obstructive pulmonary disease, cardiovascular disease, diabetes, or alcoholism. The disease usually occurs in midwinter or early spring. The onset of pneumonia is acute and may be marked by the development of a sudden chill. Sustained temperature elevations of approximately 104° F (40° C), a cough that produces mucopurulent sputum, and pleuritic chest pain follow. On physical examination the patient is febrile, tachycardic, and tachypneic. Localized pulmonary abnormalities are present, with rales noted early in the disease. There may be increased transmission of breath sounds, dullness to percussion, whispered pectoriloquy, and "E to A" changes. In the presence of a pleural effusion, dullness to percussion and decreased breath sounds may be noted.

White blood cell (WBC) counts are in the range of 15,000 to 35,000 cells/mm³ with an increased number of juvenile forms. The hematocrit usually is normal, suggesting an acute rather than a chronic process. Chest roentgenography reveals areas of parenchymal involvement, either in a bronchopneumonic pattern or less frequently in a dense lobar consolidation (Fig. 40-1). Arterial blood gas studies reveal moderate degrees of hypoxemia caused by ventilation-perfusion abnormalities. Many polymorphonuclear (PMN) leukocytes may be present in the sputum, and the causative organism may be identified by Gram stain and culture of expectorated sputum, transtracheal aspirate, pleural fluid, or blood.

In most areas most cases of community-acquired pneumonia (70% to 90%) are caused by *S. pneumoniae, S. aureus,* and *H. influenzae*. Although some studies have indicated a marked rise in the incidence of community-acquired pneumonia caused by *Legionella* spp., this does not appear to be a generalized phenomenon. In areas with large numbers of patients with the acquired immunodeficiency syndrome (AIDS), *Pneumocystis carinii* pneumonia has become an important etiologic agent of community-acquired pneumonia. Because the signs and symp-

Table 40-1   Pneumonia syndromes

Syndrome	Onset	Clinical manifestations	Laboratory findings	Roentgenographic findings	Etiologic agent
Community-acquired pneumonia	Acute (hours)	Fever, chills, pleuritic chest pain, productive cough, localized pulmonary findings	WBC elevated; sputum Gram stain shows many PMNs with predominant organism	Bronchopneumonia or lobar consolidation	*Streptococcus pneumoniae, Staphylococcus aureus, Haemophilus influenzae, Legionella* and *Enterobacteriaeae* spp.
Nosocomial gram-negative bacillus pneumonia	Acute (hours)	Fever, chills, pleuritic chest pain, productive cough, localized pulmonary findings	WBC elevated; sputum Gram stain shows many PMNs with predominant organism	Lower lobe most commonly involved; pleural effusion and cavities may be seen	*Pseudomonas* and *Klebsiella* spp., *Escherichia coli*
Atypical pneumonia	Subacute (3-4 days)	Predominantly constitutional symptoms; variably productive cough; pleuritic chest pains uncommon; respiratory findings minimal (different for AIDS patients; see text)	WBC normal; sputum Gram stain shows few organisms or PMNs	Patchy, diffuse infiltrates in lower lobes; consolidation rare	*Mycoplasma pneumoniae, Legionella pneumophila, Coxiella burnetii* (Q fever), *Chlamydia* (psittacosis, TWAR) *Pneumocystis carinii*
Aspiration pneumonia	Acute (hours) or indolent (weeks-months)	Fever, weight loss, productive cough, foul-smelling sputum	WBC elevated; foul sputum; Gram stain shows many PMNs with mixed population of microbes	Necrotizing pneumonia, lung abscess, empyema	Mixed aerobic-anaerobic pathogens, including *Bacteroides*, streptococci, and *Fusobacterium* spp.

toms of *Pneumocystis* infection are different from those of acute bacterial infection, they are discussed in the section on "Atypical pneumonia syndrome."

PNEUMOCOCCAL PNEUMONIA

Etiology. The pneumococcus *(S. pneumoniae)* is a gram-positive, lancet-shaped coccus usually appearing as paired diplococci but occasionally appearing as short chains or single cocci. Virulent strains of the organism are encapsulated, which inhibits phagocytosis by host neutrophils and thereby increases the organism's pathogenicity.

Epidemiology. The pneumococcus may be found in the oropharynx of normal individuals. Carriage rates have been shown to be highest in children (29% to 35%) and in adults who have preschool-age children in their families (18%). Patients with a history of chronic bronchitis have a higher incidence of upper airway colonization with the pneumococcus. These organisms may serve as a reservoir for exacerbation of chronic bronchitis and development of pneumonia.

Clinical manifestations. There is little to differentiate the onset of pneumococcal pneumonia from that of pneumonia caused by other pathogens. As noted previously, the sudden onset of chills followed by fever, pleuritic chest pain, and productive cough, which marks the onset of bacterial pneumonia in general, is characteristic of pneumococcal pneumonia.

Bacteremia occurs in 25% to 30% of patients and has been associated with an increased mortality. Pleural effusion, which occurs in approximately 25% of the patients, is the most common complication of pneumococcal pneumonia. Usually the effusions are exudative, with no demonstrable organisms on Gram stain or culture. True empyema is noted in about 1% of patients. Lung abscess and pericarditis have occurred in association with pneumococcal pneumonia, but they are rare.

Diagnosis. The examination and culture of expectorated sputum remain the most valuable tools in the diagnosis of pneumococcal pneumonia. Using strict criteria for sputum Gram-stain positivity (that is, a predominant flora, more than 10 gram-positive lancet-shaped diplococci per oil immersion field, or both) the specificity of the Gram stain has been shown to be 85% with a sensitivity of 62%.

The diagnostic yield of sputum culture may be enhanced by rapid processing and by examining only those sputum samples with minimal oropharyngeal contamination (fewer than 10 epithelial cells per low-power field [×100], more than 25 neutrophils per low-power field, or both).

Blood cultures should be obtained in patients ill enough to be hospitalized, since positive test findings provide a definitive diagnosis. Although various methods of detecting antigens in sputum and urine have been developed, they are not commonly used in adults. Similarly, more invasive procedures such as bronchoscopy, percutaneous biopsy, and open lung biopsy have no real role in diagnosing the common community-acquired pneumonias.

Course. With adequate therapy fever usually resolves promptly. This may occur as quickly as 24 hours after therapy begins, or it may take several days. The normalization of physical findings and roentgenographic changes may be much slower. Abnormal physical findings may persist for a week or more. Roentgenographic changes may persist for 4 to 6 weeks. Failure to respond suggests focal complications such as lung abscess, empyema, or pericarditis.

Patients with sickle cell disease or splenectomy may have a more accelerated disease course and a rapidly fatal outcome. Patients with agammaglobulinemia, lymphoma, myeloma, or lymphocytic leukemia also are at risk of more severe disease.

Management. Penicillin G remains the antibiotic of choice for pneumococcal pneumonia in patients who are not allergic to penicillin. Patients with uncomplicated pneumococcal pneumonia should be treated with aqueous procaine penicillin G, 600,000 units given intramuscularly twice a day for 7 to 10 days. In pneumonia complicated by empyema, intravenous administration of 20 million units of penicillin daily is indicated, as well as drainage of the fluid. The decision to treat a patient with pneumonia as an outpatient involves assessment of the severity of the disease, the patient's clinical stability, and the potential for close clinical monitoring. In these cases intramuscular administration of 600,000 units of procaine penicillin G may be followed by penicillin V in doses of 500 mg orally four times a day for 10 days. Erythromycin or a ceph-

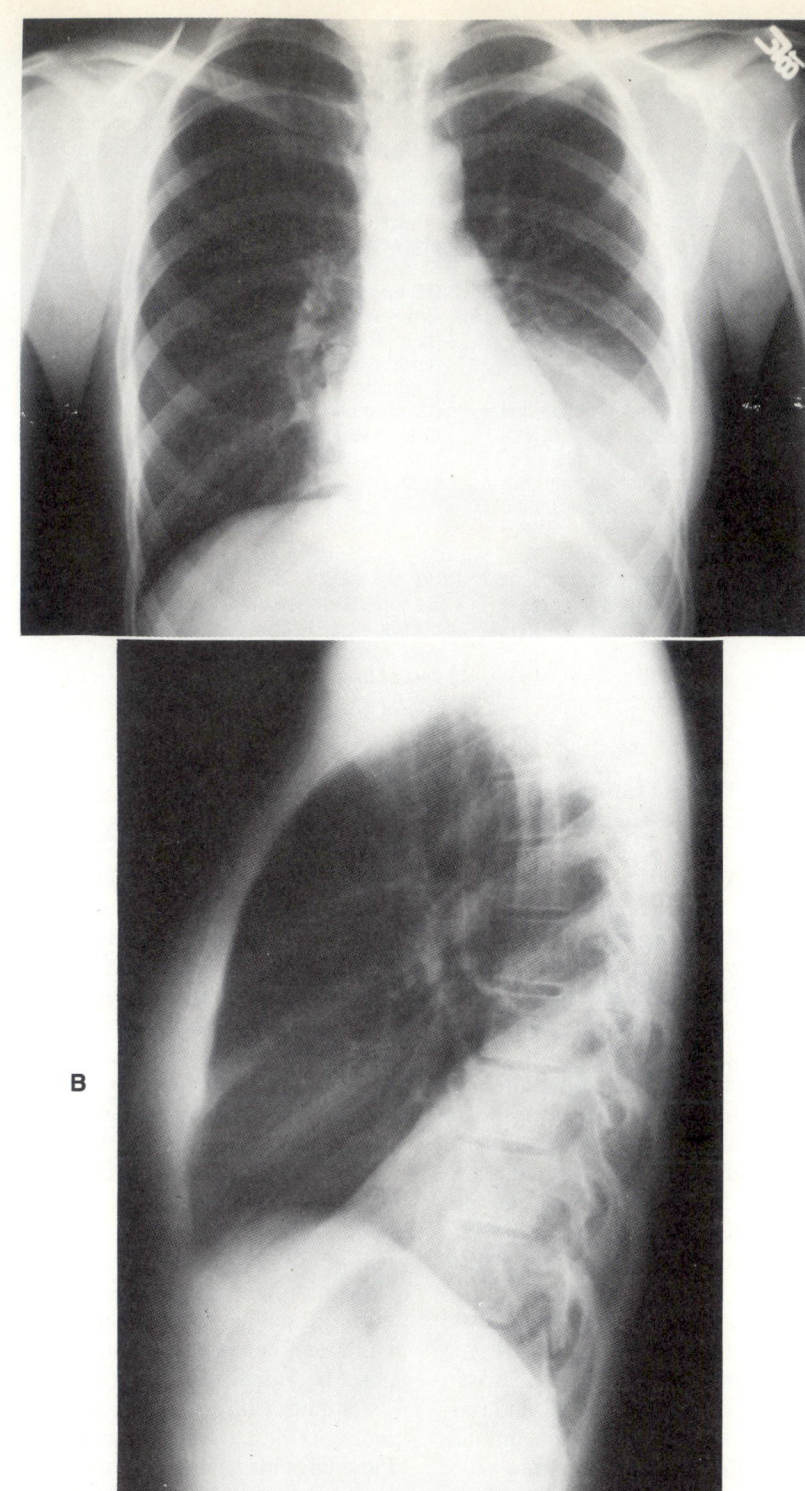

Fig. 40-1 **A,** PA and, **B,** lateral roentgenograms of patient with pneumococcal pneumonia. Dense lobar consolidation in left lower lobe is consistent with diagnosis but is less commonly seen than bronchopneumonic pattern. (From Mandell GL, Douglas RG, Jr, and Bennett JE, editors: Principles and practice of infectious disease, New York, 1979, John Wiley & Sons, Inc.)

alosporin may be used in patients who are allergic to penicillin. Although penicillin-resistant strains of pneumococci have been noted elsewhere in the world, they are rare in the United States.

Prevention. A polyvalent antipneumococcal vaccine has been developed, although data concerning its efficacy are controversial. Patients with underlying chronic renal, pulmonary, or cardiovascular disease, patients with diabetes, elderly pa-

tients in general, and patients over 2 years of age with splenectomy (either functional or actual) should receive the vaccine. Children under 2 years of age do not respond as well to the vaccine as those in older age groups.

STAPHYLOCOCCUS AUREUS PNEUMONIA

Epidemiology. S. aureus pneumonia accounts for less than 5% of all community-acquired pneumonia. Infants, patients with cystic fibrosis, immunosuppressed patients, and those with or recovering from influenza are at particular risk. The importance of staphylococcal pneumonia in adults during outbreaks of influenza should be stressed. Although streptococcal (*S. pneumoniae*) pneumonia still accounts for most cases of postinfluenzal pneumonia, staphylococcal pneumonia is seen in about 25% of cases. Hematogenous spread of staphylococci to the lungs may occur in patients with endocarditis or other diseases associated with staphylococcal bacteremia.

Clinical manifestations. Patients with staphylococcal pneumonia usually are toxic with fever, multiple chills, and a cough that produces markedly purulent sputum. Localized signs of consolidation usually are found on lung examination. Roentgenographically, early abscess formation, pleural effusions, or empyema is characteristic. Thin-walled cavities (pneumatoceles) are seen more often in children but may be seen in adults.

In patients with postinfluenzal staphylococcal pneumonia, symptoms of influenza initially appear to resolve. After a variable time period, usually 2 to 14 days, respiratory symptoms and systemic toxicity suddenly reappear.

Diagnosis. An elevated white blood cell count with a marked shift to the left may be noted. Staphylococcal pneumonia may be diagnosed by culturing the organism from sputum, blood, or pleural fluid. Sputum Gram stain reveals numerous neutrophils and gram-positive cocci in clumps.

Course. Even with adequate therapy, response is slow, and the case fatality rate is 15% to 20%. A 3- to 4-week convalescent period is not unusual.

Management. The therapy of choice for staphylococcal pneumonia is a parenterally administered, penicillinase-resistant penicillin such as nafcillin, 1.5 g intravenously every 4 hours usually for 14 days. A cephalosporin or vancomycin may be used in patients who are allergic to penicillin; vancomycin should be used when methicillin-resistant *S. aureus* is are suspected.

HAEMOPHILUS INFLUENZAE PNEUMONIA
Etiology. *Haemophilus* species are small, gram-negative rods that may appear as coccobacillary forms on Gram stain of clinical material. *H. influenzae* is a somewhat fastidious organism, requiring the presence of two blood-associated factors (X and V) for growth.

Epidemiology. *H. influenzae* pneumonia usually occurs in the setting of chronic disease, most commonly chronic obstructive pulmonary disease, cardiovascular disease, and alcoholism. The upper airways of patients with chronic pulmonary disease frequently are colonized with this organism, and this may serve as a source of lower respiratory tract infections. Encapsulated type B organisms are responsible for most cases of pneumonia with bacteremia.

Clinical manifestations. The onset of *H. influenzae* pneumonia is similar to that of pneumonia caused by the other common bacterial pathogens. Pleural involvement with either demonstrable pleural fluid or pleuritic chest pain may be seen in up to 50% of the patients. Lower lobe involvement is noted most commonly, with more than one lobe involved in over two thirds of patients.

Diagnosis. Definitive diagnosis of *H. influenzae* pneumonia is difficult. In cases of bacteremic pneumonia, sputum culture has been found positive in only 50% to 75% of the patients. Sputum Gram stains often may be misread, and the presence of *H. influenzae* may be overlooked. Since the organism may colonize the upper airways, its presence in sputum does not necessarily indicate that it is the cause of pneumonia.

Management. Ampicillin is the therapy of choice for pneumonia caused by sensitive strains of *H. influenzae*. Ampicillin-resistant strains of *H. influenzae* have been isolated from clinical material with variable frequency (5% to 30%). Cefuroxime or a third-generation cephalosporin may be used for suspected ampicillin-resistant *H. influenzae* infections. Trimethoprim-sulfamethoxazole or chloramphenicol are alternate regimens for patients who are allergic to penicillin; these drugs also are useful against ampicillin-resistant organisms.

LEGIONNAIRES' DISEASE
Etiology. The *Legionella* spp. are facultative gram-negative bacilli that primarily cause pneumonia. *Legionella pneumophila* is the organism most commonly involved in human disease; *Legionella micdadei* causes disease primarily in immunosuppressed patients. Only small numbers of patients have been reported with infections caused by other *Legionella* spp. *Legionella* are water-related organisms that have been cultured from air-conditioner reservoirs, water towers, and water taps.

Epidemiology. Legionnaires' disease has been described in all age groups. Most commonly patients with the disease are in their midfifties and have chronic underlying diseases such as chronic obstructive pulmonary disease, cardiovascular disease, alcoholism, or diabetes. Epidemics most often occur in the summer months, although sporadic cases of disease have been noted to occur throughout the year. The disease is spread via the airborne route. Epidemics have been associated with contaminated air-conditioning and air treatment systems. Recently disturbed soil and excavation and construction sites have been suspected as sources of the organism. Person-to-person transmission of the disease has not been proved.

Pathogenesis. *Legionella* organisms can grow in human monocytes. Infection causes a fibrinopurulent pneumonia, often with diffuse alveolar damage. Bronchi appear to be spared. The inflammatory exudate consists of neutrophils and large numbers of macrophages. Focal necrosis appears to be more extensive than that noted in more common bacterial pneumonias.

Clinical manifestations. Pneumonia caused by *Legionella* spp. often is clinically indistinguishable from pneumonia caused by other bacteria. A prodrome of malaise, myalgia, and headache often is described. Within 48 hours fever and chills develop. Nausea, vomiting, and diarrhea may be seen in the early stages of the disease. Cough generally develops several days after the onset of symptoms and usually is nonproductive, although hemoptysis may occur. Pleuritic chest pain is seen in 30% to 40% of the patients. Confusion and delirium may develop out of proportion to the degree of fever. The leukocyte count usually is moderately elevated with a shift to the left. Microscopic hematuria, proteinuria, elevations of liver transaminases, hypophosphatemia, and hyponatremia have been described. With progression of disease, hypoxemia develops. Gram stain of expectorated sputum or transtracheal aspirates is unrevealing. Chest roentgenograms most commonly show either a patchy infiltrate or consolidation. Although most patients initially have unilateral involvement, bilateral, multilobar involvement usually develops. Rapid development of clinical toxicity and roentgenographic changes is a hallmark of pneumonia caused by *Legionella* spp. Cavitation has not been reported, and pleural effusions are uncommon.

L. pneumophila also may be responsible for nonpneumonic disease. Diagnostic rises in antibody titer have been associated with a mild, febrile illness without signs of pneumonia (Pontiac fever).

L. micdadei commonly causes disease in compromised hosts, having a predilection for renal homograph recipients receiving high-dose steroid therapy. The clinical manifestations of disease are similar to those of *L. pneumophila*, although in some series 25% of patients had symptoms suggestive of pulmonary emboli with fever, dyspnea, and pleuritic chest pain.

Diagnosis. Legionnaires' disease is difficult to distinguish from other causes of community-acquired pneumonia. The prodromal symptoms of diarrhea, confusion out of proportion to fever, nonproductive cough, and lack of pathogens noted on Gram stains of sputum or transtracheal aspirates should suggest this diagnosis.

The diagnosis of Legionnaires' disease can be made by culturing the organisms from lung tissue, pleural fluid, or sputum and by demonstrating the presence of the organisms in lung tissue with fluorescent antibody staining or the Dieterle silver stain. Detection of rising antibody titers also has been used to diagnose *Legionella* pneumonia. In most centers, however, the time delay involved makes the test unhelpful for the acutely ill patient. Given the specialized nature of these diagnostic techniques, presumptive diagnosis usually is made on clinical grounds and therapy is started before the presence of *Legionella* infection is definitely documented.

Course. Without therapy Legionnaires' disease often runs a fulminant course. A 15% mortality is noted with a rapid progression of disease over 5 to 6 days. Respiratory failure and shock usually are terminal events. In nonpneumonic disease gradual spontaneous clearing of symptoms occurs.

Management. Erythromycin in doses of 0.5 to 1 g every 6 hours for 3 weeks is the therapy of choice. Intravenous therapy should be used until clinical stabilization is achieved, with the remainder of the treatment given orally. Rifampin may be added to erythromycin in patients who are not responding, but the combination has not been proved more effective than erythromycin alone. Trimethoprim-sulfamethoxazole has been used successfully to treat *L. micdadei* infections that are unresponsive to erythromycin therapy.

Nosocomial gram-negative bacillus pneumonia syndrome

EPIDEMIOLOGY. Unlike *S. pneumoniae* and *H. influenzae*, gram-negative enteric organisms are relatively uncommon causes of community-acquired pneumonia. When gram-negative bacillus pneumonia does occur, chronic obstructive pulmonary disease, chronic cardiovascular disease, and alcoholism are important underlying factors.

Gram-negative organisms are important etiologic agents of pneumonia in hospitalized patients and immunosuppressed hosts. Within 24 to 48 hours after admission, colonization of the upper respiratory tract by enteric gram-negative rods has been shown to occur in patients in intensive care units. An increased incidence of gram-negative bacillus pneumonia has been associated with this colonization. Contaminated nebulizers have been demonstrated to be an important cause of hospital-acquired gram-negative bacillus pneumonia. Gram-negative rod pneumonia accounts for 21% of infectious episodes in patients with leukemia. Furthermore, the lungs serve as a source for bacteremia in over 60% of these patients. Tracheostomy sites frequently become infected with gram-negative bacilli.

CLINICAL MANIFESTATIONS. Patients frequently have severe underlying disease and often are on respirators. The signs and symptoms of gram-negative bacillus pneumonia are not distinctive. Fever, chills, and productive cough usually are seen.

Lower lobe disease is most common, with multilobar involvement occurring in 40% of the patients. Cavitation, microabscesses, and pleural effusion may occur. There is no char-

acteristic roentgenographic picture that can differentiate one gram-negative organism from another.

DIAGNOSIS. Pleural fluid, sputum, and blood should be examined and cultured to establish a cause. Since upper airway colonization takes place in hospitalized patients, transtracheal aspiration is of help in differentiating upper airway colonization from lower airway infection, provided no tracheal tube is in place. In immunosuppressed hosts pneumonic infiltrates often are assumed to be caused by gram-negative rods and are treated accordingly until a definitive diagnosis is made.

COURSE. Even with appropriate antibiotic therapy, the mortality from gram-negative bacillus pneumonia is about 50%. The debilitated condition of the host accounts for this high figure. Even with adequate therapy, signs and symptoms may persist for weeks.

MANAGEMENT. The treatment for gram-negative bacillus pneumonia depends on the antimicrobial sensitivities of the specific etiologic agent. Dual drug regimens have been used in certain instances to achieve antibiotic synergy. Recommended regimens of therapy include a cephalosporin plus an aminoglycoside for *Klebsiella* pneumonia and an aminoglycoside plus an extended-spectrum penicillin for *Pseudomonas* pneumonia. If multiply resistant organisms are suspected, a third-generation cephalosporin or imipenem should be used.

Atypical pneumonia syndrome

The atypical pneumonia syndrome is a symptom complex associated most commonly with *Mycoplasma pneumoniae* (see Chapter 44). Unlike the acute bacterial pneumonias described previously, atypical pneumonias develop over a 3- to 4-day period. Constitutional symptoms predominate over specific respiratory symptoms. Fever, malaise, coryza, headache, and cough are the major symptoms. Pleuritic chest pain and respiratory distress are not usually seen. Sputum production is variable, and although sputum is purulent in one third of the patients, polymorphonuclear leukocytes are absent in most patients, and Gram stain and culture usually reveal only sparse normal flora. Roentgenographic findings most commonly include a patchy or diffuse infiltrate without lobar consolidation. WBC counts usually are less than 10,000/mm³. Other etiologic agents that may cause the atypical pneumonia syndrome include parainfluenza virus. Epstein-Barr virus, respiratory syncytial virus, and adenovirus. Q fever and psittacosis are rare causes of atypical pneumonia. Recently a new strain of chlamydia, TWAR, has been shown to cause respiratory disease, including pneumonia. Up to 12% of young adults and 6% of other patients with pneumonia may demonstrate serologic or culture evidence of infection with this organism. *Legionella* organisms also may cause severe atypical pneumonia.

Pneumocystis carinii pneumonia

Although *P. carinii* is a protozoan and not a bacteria, it has become an important part of the differential diagnosis of atypical pneumonias and therefore warrants discussion.

EPIDEMIOLOGY. Before 1981 *P. carinii* pneumonia was a relatively uncommon disease that usually affected debilitated infants or immune-compromised hosts. With the onset of the AIDS epidemic, the disease has begun to play a much greater role as a pulmonary pathogen. Of patients with AIDS, over 80% will have significant pulmonary disease sometime during their course. *P. carinii* will be involved in 50% to 80% of those cases, either alone or in association with other pathogens.

ETIOLOGY. *P. carinii* is a protozoan that may occur as a cyst or as a trophozoite (extracystic form). The cyst forms usually contain intracystic cells or sporozoites. Both forms can be identified in infected lungs.

CLINICAL MANIFESTATIONS. In patients who do not have AIDS, the onset of *P. carinii* infection usually is acute or subacute with development of symptoms over several days. The common symptoms include fever (temperature over 100° F [38° C]), shortness of breath, cough, and hypoxia. Other signs and symptoms commonly associated with pneumonia occur less commonly in patients with *P. carinii* infections; sputum production and chest pain are uncommon, and localized rales are noted in only about one third of patients. Although extrapulmonary infections have been described, they are unusual. Roentgenograms of the chest are abnormal in more than 90% of patients. Initially perihilar haziness is noted, which rapidly progresses to diffuse, bilateral, interstitial or alveolar infiltrates. In severe or untreated cases complete opacification of the lungs may occur. Pleural reaction, hilar adenopathy, and cavitation are extremely rare roentgenographic manifestations of *P. carinii* infection, and their presence suggests an alternate diagnosis.

Patients with AIDS have a more subacute or a chronic onset. Symptoms may develop over weeks to months. Patients with AIDS who have *P. carinii* pneumonia may be less febrile, less tachypneic, and less hypoxemic. Initial chest roentgenograms may be normal.

DIAGNOSIS. *P. carinii* pneumonia is diagnosed by demonstrating the organism in lung material or respiratory tract secretions. Open lung biopsy is the definitive means of making a diagnosis, especially in patients who do not have AIDS. In patients with AIDS, bronchoscopy with brushing, bronchoalveolar lavage, transbronchial biopsy, or a combination of these provides a diagnosis in more than 85% of patients.

THERAPY. Trimethoprim-sulfamethoxazole (15 to 20 mg/kg/day of trimethoprim intravenously or orally) and pentamidine isethionate (4 mg/kg/day intravenously or intramuscularly) are the accepted drug regimens for treatment of *P. carinii* infections. They are equally effective, but both are associated with a high incidence of toxicity (40% to 50%). While other therapeutic programs have been used (for example, dapsone plus trimethoprim), they remain experimental. Response rates of approximately 85% have been noted with the two accepted regimens. In patients with AIDS, relapses commonly occur with both regimens.

Aspiration (anaerobic organism) pneumonia syndrome

ETIOLOGY. Anaerobic organism pneumonia is most commonly associated with organisms of the oropharynx. Pneumonia may be caused by anaerobic bacteria alone (45% to 58% of the cases) or by anaerobes in conjunction with aerobic organisms (41% to 46% of the cases). The most commonly isolated anaerobes include the anaerobic or microaerophilic streptococci, *Fusobacterium,* and *Bacteroides* spp. (*melaninogenicus, fragilis,* and *oralis*). In its chronic form anaerobic organism pneumonia often is classified as lung abscess.

EPIDEMIOLOGY. Anaerobic infections of the lung most commonly occur when oropharyngeal contents have been aspirated. Conditions that compromise the normal gag and cough reflexes such as sedative overdose, seizures, alcoholism, or loss of consciousness predispose patients to aspiration and the development of anaerobic organism pneumonia. Lung damage from other causes such as tumor or bronchiectasis may create conditions in which anaerobic organisms can flourish. Poor dentition plays a major role in providing a source of anaerobes.

Periodontal disease, heavy tartar deposition, and carious teeth commonly are found in patients with anaerobic organism disease. Anaerobic organism infection is uncommon in edentulous patients.

CLINICAL MANIFESTATIONS. The three major syndromes recognized as a consequence of aspiration are chemical pneumonitis, bronchial obstruction caused by aspiration of particulate matter, and bacterial aspiration pneumonia. Chemical pneumonitis and mechanical obstruction usually cause acute symptoms. In contrast, bacterial aspiration pneumonia is more insidious. Symptoms develop gradually several days to weeks after the initial episode of aspiration. Pneumonitis, necrotizing pneumonia, abscess, and empyema are the most common manifestations of anaerobic organism pneumonia. Symptoms of fever, weight loss, and productive cough may be present for several weeks before the patient seeks medical care. Putrid sputum is produced in 50% of the cases. Anemia and elevated white blood cell counts frequently are associated findings. Anemia suggests the presence of a chronic disease rather than the sudden change of health noted in the community-acquired pneumonia syndrome. Roentgenographic changes include necrotizing pneumonia, cavitation, or pleural effusion or empyema. Aspiration pneumonia most commonly involves either the posterior segment of the upper lobe or the superior or basilar segment of the lower lobe, depending on whether aspiration occurs in the reclining or upright position. Chronic aspiration most frequently results in a bilateral lower lobe pneumonia, although one side may be more involved than the other.

DIAGNOSIS. Foul-smelling sputum in a patient with necrotizing or cavitary pneumonia suggests aspiration pneumonia. The isolation of anaerobic organisms from blood or pleural fluid requires special processing of samples. Cultural confirmation rarely is necessary, but if sputum is cultured, transtracheal aspiration should be carried out to bypass the oral anaerobic flora. Gram-stained empyema fluid, sputum samples, or transtracheal aspirates reveal numerous polymorphonuclear leukocytes with a mixed population of organisms.

COURSE. Even with the appropriate therapy, symptoms commonly resolve slowly with anaerobic lung infection. Residual pulmonary disease with bronchiectasis, pulmonary fibrosis, or chronic effusions occurs in 10% of the patients. A mortality rate of 15% to 19% has been noted.

MANAGEMENT. Penicillin or clindamycin are considered the therapies of choice for infections caused by mixed aerobic-anaerobic bacteria. Either intravenous administration of 20 million units of penicillin daily or 600 mg of clindamycin intravenously every 6 hours can provide effective initial therapy. Lung abscesses may require up to 6 weeks of therapy. If empyema exists, adequate drainage is mandatory. For cavitary lung disease appropriate postural drainage is important.

BIBLIOGRAPHY

Bartlett JG and Finegold SM: Anaerobic pleuropulmonary infections, Medicine 51:413, 1972.

Bartlett JG and Finegold SM: Anaerobic infections of the lung and pleural space, Am Rev Respir Dis 110:56, 1974.

Chang HY and others: Causes of death in adults with acute leukemia, Medicine 55:259, 1976.

Fekety FR and others: Bacteria, viruses, and mycoplasmas in acute pneumonia in adults, Am Rev Respir Dis 104:449, 1971.

Grayston IT and others: A new *Chlamydia Psittaci* strain, TWAR, isolated in acute respiratory tract infection, N Engl J Med 315:161, 1986.

Hendley JO and others: Spread of *Streptococcus pneumoniae* in families. I. Carriage rates and distribution of types, J Infect Dis 132:55, 1975.

Johanson WG and others: Nosocomial respiratory infections with gram negative bacilli: the significance of colonization of the respiratory tract, Ann Intern Med 77:701, 1972.

Kovacs JA and others: *Pneumocystis carinii* pneumonia: A comparison between patients with the acquired immunodeficiency syndrome and patients with other immunodeficiencies, Ann Intern Med 100:663, 1984.

Merrill C and others: Rapid identification of pneumococci, N Engl J Med 288:510, 1973.

Mills J: *Pneumocystis carinii* and *Toxoplasma gondii* infections in patients with AIDS, Rev Infect Dis 8:1001, 1986.

Newhouse M, Sanchis J, and Bienenstock J: Lung defense mechanisms, N Engl J Med 295:990, 1976.

Rein MF and others: Accuracy of the Gram stain in identifying pneumococci in sputum, JAMA 230:2671, 1978.

Schwarzmann SW and others: Bacterial pneumonia during the Hong Kong influenza epidemic of 1968-1969, Arch Intern Med 127:1037, 1971.

Sprunt S: Infection in chronic lung disease, Bull NY Acad Med 48:698, 1972.

Swartz MN: Clinical aspects of Legionnaires' disease, Ann Intern Med 90:492, 1979.

Unger JD, Rose HD, and Unger GF: Gram-negative pneumonia, Radiology 107:283, 1973.

Wharton JM and others: Trimethoprim-sulamethoxazole or pentamidine for *Pneumocystis carinii* pneumonia in the acquired immunodeficiency syndrome, Ann Intern Med 105:37, 1986.

Infective endocarditis

Donald Kaye

DEFINITION. Infective endocarditis is an infection on the endocardium; it may involve a heart valve, a septal defect, or mural endocardium. It may be classified into acute and subacute disease. Acute endocarditis is most frequently caused by *Staphylococcus aureus;* it often occurs on a normal heart valve and results in rapid, severe destruction. Metastatic foci of infection are common. If untreated the infection will kill in days to weeks.

Subacute endocarditis usually is caused by streptococci of the viridans group and occurs on already damaged valves, producing additional damage slowly. Metastatic foci of infection are rare. Without therapy the infection takes 6 or more weeks or even years to kill. However, streptococci of the viridans group occasionally can cause endocarditis with an acute course on a normal valve, and *S. aureus* can cause subacute disease.

It is more important to classify endocarditis by infecting organism (for example, enterococcal endocarditis). The identity of the organism has implications for the course (that is, acute or subacute), but more importantly, it has therapeutic implications for the antimicrobial regimen.

Endarteritis, infection in an artery (for example, on a coarctation of the aorta), produces a syndrome indistinguishable from endocarditis.

ETIOLOGY. Almost any species of bacteria is capable of producing infective endocarditis. However, streptococci and staphylococci account for the vast majority of cases.

Streptococci

Streptococci are the causative microorganisms in 40% to 80% of the cases of endocarditis. Viridans streptococci account for about 50% of the cases of streptococcal endocarditis, *S. bovis* cause about 25%, enterococci cause about 10%, and the remaining streptococci (microaerophilic and anaerobic streptococci, nonhemolytic streptococci, and group A β-hemolytic streptococci) are isolated in the remainder of the cases.

Enterococci and group A β-hemolytic streptococci can attack normal or previously damaged heart valves and may cause rapid destruction. The other streptococci are much more likely to produce endocarditis on already damaged heart valves and rarely cause rapid destruction.

Staphylococci

Staphylococci are the causative microorganisms in 10% to 30% of the cases of infective endocarditis. *S. aureus* is isolated much more frequently than *S. epidermidis*.

S. aureus attacks either normal or previously damaged heart valves and causes rapid destruction. The course often is fulminant, leading to death from overwhelming bacteremia within days or from heart failure within weeks. Abscesses are common at several sites (for example, kidneys, lungs, brain, and heart). *S. epidermidis* usually attacks abnormal heart valves without causing rapid destruction.

Other bacteria

Almost all species of bacteria are reported as occasionally causing endocarditis, including the enteric gram-negative bacilli, gonococci, pneumococci, *Salmonella, Bacteroides, Haemophilus,* and *Listeria* organisms, and even diphtheroids. Gram-negative bacilli account for less than 5% of the cases of endocarditis but are common causes in drug addicts and patients with prosthetic heart valves.

Fungi

Candida, Aspergillus, and *Histoplasma* spp. are the most common causes of fungal endocarditis, with *Candida* endocarditis occurring most frequently. Fungal endocarditis is common in narcotic addicts (*Candida* spp.) and in patients following cardiac surgery (*Candida* and *Aspergillus* spp.).

The course of fungal endocarditis usually is subacute. Large, friable vegetations are common and give rise to large emboli, often in the lower extremities. In patients with prosthetic cardiac valves, malfunction of the valve may occur because of the size of the vegetations.

Other microorganisms

Spirochetes (such as *Spirillum minus*), cell wall–deficient bacteria, rickettsiae *(Coxiella burnetii),* and the psittacosis agent all have been reported as rare causes of endocarditis.

EPIDEMIOLOGY. Mean ages of patients in most series range from the midforties to the midfifties. Endocarditis is uncommon in children. *Rheumatic valvular disease,* most often involving the mitral or aortic valves or both, is the underlying cardiac disease in about 25% to 40% of the patients with infective endocarditis, and the frequency seems to be decreasing.

Congenital heart disease is the underlying lesion in about 5% to 20% of the patients with endocarditis. Some predisposing lesions are patent ductus arteriosus, ventricular septal defect, tetralogy of Fallot, coarctation of the aorta, pulmonary stenosis, and bicuspid aortic valve. In contrast, atrial septal defects of the secundum type rarely serve as an underlying lesion.

Mitral valve prolapse is the underlying cardiac lesion in about 10% of the cases of endocarditis, and the frequency seems to be increasing.

Degenerative heart disease (for example, valves with degenerative changes and calcific aortic stenosis resulting from degenerative aortic valve disease or a bicuspid aortic valve) can be a predisposing cardiac lesion in endocarditis. Infective endocarditis has also been reported in patients with *asymmetric septal hypertrophy, Marfan's syndrome,* and *syphilitic aortic valve disease.*

A new and important cardiac lesion that serves as an underlying abnormality for production of endocarditis is the *prosthetic cardiac valve.* Similarly, intravascular sutures, pacemaker wires, and Teflon-Silastic tubes are predisposing factors to the devlopment of endocarditis or endarteritis. Arterioarterial or arteriovenous fistulas also predispose individuals to endocarditis. Up to 10% of the cases of endocarditis occur in people who abuse drugs intravenously.

In 20% to 40% of the patients with infective endocarditis, no underlying heart disease can be recognized.

PATHOGENESIS AND PATHOLOGY. The characteristic lesions of infective endocarditis are vegetations on the valve leaflets or elsewhere on the endocardium. The disease usually arises following localization of microorganisms on a sterile thrombotic vegetation (called nonbacterial thrombotic endocarditis). This may form as a result of trauma to the endothelial cells or over a subendothelial inflammatory reaction, as in acute rheumatic fever or myocardial infarction.

When bacteremia occurs, the surface of the vegetation can become secondarily infected and converted to the typical vegetation of infective endocarditis. This results from deposition of platelets and fibrin over the bacteria. The vegetation then becomes a "protected site," which phagocytic cells penetrate poorly.

Adherence of bacteria to valves, platelets, or fibrin seems to be important in the pathogenesis of endocarditis. For example, increased production of dextran by *Streptococcus sanguis* increases adherence of this organism in vitro and increases the ability to cause endocarditis in rabbits.

Hydrodynamic forces. The sites of involvement suggest an important role for hydrodynamic forces. Endocarditis occurs downstream from where blood flows through a narrow orifice at a high velocity from a high- to a low-pressure chamber. For example, endocarditis is found immediately distal to the constriction in coarctation of the aorta and on the pulmonary artery immediately beyond the junction with the ductus in patent ductus arteriosus.

Endocarditis does not usually occur when there is only a small pressure gradient, as in atrial septal defects. Valvular endocarditis occurs more frequently in valvular incompetence than in pure stenosis and is characteristically on the atrial side of the incompetent mitral valve and the ventricular surface of the incompetent aortic valve. A high-velocity stream of blood can produce satellite infected lesions at distant points of impact.

Invasion of circulation. Organisms must gain access to the circulation in sufficient numbers for a sufficient interval for endocarditis to result. Invasion of the bloodstream occurs in many infections (for example, pneumococcal pneumonia).

Transient bacteremia is common during traumatic procedures involving the epithelial surfaces normally laden with an indigenous bacterial flora (oropharynx, genitourinary and gastrointestinal tracts, and skin). Surgical incision of the skin, which ordinarily is inhabited by staphylococci and diphtheroids, often is associated with bacteremia, usually staphylococcal (with *S. aureus* or *S. epidermidis*). Bacteremia occurs in about 25% of patients after toothbrushing, chewing hard candy, or using an oral irrigation device. After trauma to the tissues of the mouth, streptococci of the viridans groups are the bacteria most commonly isolated from the blood, either alone or more often mixed with other bacteria. The frequency of bacteremia following dental procedures is related to the degree of periodontal disease and the amount of trauma.

Portal of entry. Although the portal of entry for the initiating episode of bacteremia in endocarditis often is inapparent, oral cavity infection or operative or manipulative dental procedures appear to be the most common clinically apparent portals of entry, especially in endocarditis caused by viridans streptococci. Endocarditis caused by viridans streptococci also has occurred in edentulous patients in association with oral ulcers from poorly fitting dentures.

Bacteremia occurs in up to one third of patients after trans-

urethral prostatic resection, cystoscopy, urethral dilation, and urethral catheterization. The organisms usually are enterococci and gram-negative bacilli.

Mechanisms of production of lesions. The pathogenesis of the manifestations of endocarditis is both a result of the vegetations themselves and an immune reaction to the infection. The vegetations may become so extensive, especially in fungal endocarditis, that the valve orifice is occluded. There may be rapid, massive destruction of tissue with consequent valvular insufficiency, especially in *S. aureus* endocarditis. Areas of healing may cause scar formation and consequent valvular stenosis or insufficiency. Infection may extend into the myocardium, producing burrowing abscesses. Conduction abnormalities, fistulas, or rupture of the chordae, a papillary muscle, or the ventricular septum may result.

The vegetations are friable, and pieces embolize to the heart itself and to the brain, kidneys, spleen, extremities, and lungs (in endocarditis of the right side of the heart). Infarcts and perhaps abscesses (with *S. aureus* endocarditis) result at these sites. Septic embolization to the vasa vasorum or direct bacterial invasion of the arterial wall may result in the formation of mycotic aneurysms that may rupture. They most often develop in the cerebral arteries, aorta, sinus of Valsalva, ligated ductus arteriosus, and superior mesenteric, splenic, coronary, and pulmonary arteries. Vessels in the head are involved in about 50% of the patients, vessels in the abdomen and chest in about 40%, and vessels in the limbs in about 10%.

In addition, vasculitis on an immunologic basis is thought to contribute to the findings. Patients with infective endocarditis usually have high circulating antibody titers against the infecting microorganism. This contributes to the formation of circulating immune complexes. Diffuse glomerulonephritis, focal embolic glomerulitis, Roth's spots, petechiae, and Osler's nodes are thought usually to be the result of allergic vasculitis caused by deposition of immune complexes. In contrast, Janeway's lesions are thought to have an embolic basis.

CLINICAL MANIFESTATIONS. A history of a dental procedure can be elicited in only 15% to 20% of the patients with endocarditis caused by streptococci of the viridans group. About 50% of the patients with enterococcal endocarditis have had a preceding urologic or genital tract procedure, and about 35% of the patients with staphylococcal endocarditis have a history of a preceding staphylococcal infection. Symptoms of endocarditis generally start within 2 or 3 weeks of the procedure. The onset usually is gradual, with mild fever and malaise in cases of endocarditis caused by streptococci of the viridans group and other organisms of low pathogenicity. With *S. aureus,* pneumococci, and other organisms of high pathogenicity, the onset often is acute with high fever.

Fever is present in almost all patients during the course of endocarditis. Most exceptions are elderly patients or patients with renal failure, congestive heart failure, or severe debility. The temperature usually is low grade (less than 103° F [39.4° C]) except with acute disease. *Cardiac murmurs* are almost always present except with acute endocarditis or in intravenous narcotic addicts. Addicts often have vegetations on the tricuspid valve, and murmurs frequently are absent. True changes in murmurs or the appearance of a new murmur is uncommon except in acute endocarditis, in which a new murmur (particularly aortic insufficiency) is a frequent occurrence.

Splenomegaly is present in about 30% of the reported cases of endocarditis and is most common in disease of long duration. *Petechiae* are present in 20% to 40% of patients, most commonly those with more prolonged illness. Petechiae are found most frequently in the conjunctivae, palate, buccal mucosa, and extremities.

Splinter hemorrhages are subungual, linear, dark red streaks that may appear in endocarditis but also are often the result of local trauma. What are commonly called *Roth's spots* are oval, retinal hemorrhages with a clear, pale center. These are seen in less than 5% of patients with endocarditis and may also occur in collagen vascular diseases and severe anemia. *Osler's nodes* are small, tender nodules most frequently found on the finger or toe pads that persist for hours to days. They are found in 10% to 25% of patients with endocarditis, but they also occur in other diseases such as typhoid fever and collagen vascular disease; they are uncommon in acute endocarditis. *Clubbing of the fingers* is present in some patients, usually those with long-standing disease. *Janeway's lesions* are nontender, macular, hemorrhagic areas on the palms and soles, most commonly seen in acute endocarditis.

Clinically apparent embolic episodes are recognized in about half of the patients with endocarditis and may occur as the first symptom or late (after successful therapy). *Mycotic aneurysms* occur in about 10% of the patients with infective endocarditis. These lesions can rupture at any time before, during, or even years after therapy for endocarditis.

Neurologic manifestations are present in about one third of the patients with endocarditis. Major cerebral emboli are not infrequent and usually involve the middle cerebral artery system. Mycotic aneurysms also most often involve this system. Toxic encephalopathy, personality changes, or both can occur in patients with endocarditis. Brain abscess and purulent meningitis are most common with *S. aureus* endocarditis.

Congestive heart failure is a frequent complication of endocarditis and may occur at any time during the course of the disease, including long after cure. Some factors that contribute to heart failure are valve destruction, myocarditis from vasculitis, coronary artery emboli with infarction, and myocardial abscesses.

Renal disease is present in most patients with infective endocarditis. Up to 50% of the patients with endocarditis have microscopic hematuria, and proteinuria is even more common. These findings may be the result of renal emboli, focal glomerulitis, or diffuse glomerulonephritis. Renal insufficiency may occur in diffuse glomerulonephritis but is rare as a consequence of emboli or focal glomerulitis.

SPECIAL SYNDROMES

Enterococcal endocarditis. Enterococci are streptococci that are normal inhabitants of the human gastrointestinal tract, the anterior urethra, and occasionally the mouth. All enterococci are in Lancefield's group D, although not all organisms in group D are enterococci.

The average age for men with enterococcal endocarditis is near 60 years, whereas in women it is just under 40 years. This age distribution probably is closely related to the suspected genitourinary tract portal of entry of the organism. About 50% of the patients give a history of recent genitourinary tract manipulation. For men this usually means instrumentation involving the prostate, thus explaining the older age in males. For women the genitourinary factors are abortion, pregnancy, cesarean section, and urethral catheterization, which occur mainly during the childbearing years. This explains the lower age of female patients.

Streptococcus bovis endocarditis. Two other group D streptococci, *S. bovis* and *S. equinus,* should be considered separately from the enterococci because endocarditis caused by these two species can be treated like endocarditis caused by viridans streptococci. For all practical purposes *S. bovis*

and *S. equinus* can be demonstrated not to be enterococci by the fact that they are highly susceptible to penicillin G (inhibited by 0.1 μg/ml), whereas enterococci are much more resistant. *S. bovis* endocarditis or bacteremia occurs in the elderly (80% over 60 years of age) and has a striking relationship to abnormalities in the gastrointestinal tract. One third to one half of the patients with this infection have gastrointestinal malignancies (usually of the colon) or villous adenomas or polyps of the colon.

Endocarditis in drug abusers. Infective endocarditis is a complication of parenteral narcotic addiction. *S. aureus* is responsible for over 50% of the cases, and fungi (mainly *Candida* organisms) and gram-negative bacilli (most of which are *Pseudomonas* species) cause most of the remaining cases. Viridans streptococci are uncommon infecting agents in endocarditis in addicts.

The tricuspid valve is infected in over 50% of addicts with endocarditis, the aortic valve in 25%, and the mitral valve in about 20%. There is a striking association of *S. aureus* endocarditis with tricuspid valve involvement; over 75% of the patients with *S. aureus* infection have endocarditis on the tricuspid valve.

Signs and symptoms of pulmonary emboli or pneumonia related to septic pulmonary emboli are common presentations in addicts with tricuspid valve endocarditis, and murmurs frequently are absent.

Prosthetic valve endocarditis. An intracardiac prosthesis predisposes a patient to the development of endocarditis and makes eradication of the infection extremely difficult. Endocarditis has been reported to occur in 1% to 3% of patients with prosthetic valves.

Prosthetic valve endocarditis usually is divided into early endocarditis (onset within 2 months of valve replacement) and late endocarditis (onset after 2 months). Early endocarditis is a consequence of contamination during the perioperative period, whereas late endocarditis is related to bacteremia from dental, skin, and genitourinary tract trauma.

About one third of both early and late endocarditis episodes are caused by staphylococci, with *S. epidermidis* occurring more frequently than *S. aureus*. Gram-negative bacilli cause up to 25% of the early cases and are less common in late endocarditis. Fungi (most commonly *Candida* organisms) are responsible for up to 10% of the early cases and are much less common in late endocarditis. Streptococci are the most frequent single causes of late endocarditis (about 40% of the cases) but are uncommon infecting organisms in early endocarditis. Diphtheroids have been the infecting organisms in up to 20% of the early cases and are less common in late endocarditis.

Early prosthetic valve endocarditis often is associated with valve dysfunction or dehiscence and a fulminant course. Although late endocarditis may have a similar clinical course, it commonly is characterized by a clinical syndrome indistinguishable from that occuring in patients without prosthetic valves.

LABORATORY FINDINGS. A normocytic and normochromic anemia usually is present in infective endocarditis except in acute cases. Most patients have normal white blood cell and differential counts. However, in acute disease leukocytosis may be present. Proteinuria, gross or microscopic hematuria, or both are present in most patients. The erythrocyte sedimentation rate is almost always elevated. In those with severe renal complications (usually diffuse glomerulonephritis), the blood urea nitrogen or serum creatinine may be elevated.

About 50% of the patients with endocarditis of at least several weeks' duration have a positive serum test for rheumatoid factor, and circulating immune complexes have been demonstrated in the sera of a great majority of patients with endocarditis. These tend to disappear with cure of endocarditis. The serum complement may be decreased, especially in patients with glomerulonephritis. Bacteria can be seen inside leukocytes in buffy coat preparations of blood in about 50% of the patients with bacterial endocarditis.

The single most important finding in patients with endocarditis is bacteremia or fungemia. Blood cultures should be obtained promptly in anyone with suspected endocarditis and are positive in over 90% of these patients. The bacteremia of endocarditis is constant; if any cultures are positive, all probably are positive.

In patients with subacute disease who have not received previous antimicrobial therapy, three blood cultures should be obtained over a period of 12 hours and therapy should be initiated. If previous therapy has been given, treatment may be expeditiously delayed in an attempt to obtain positive blood cultures. In general, in acute disease therapy should not be delayed for more than 2 to 3 hours while cultures are obtained. In selected patients (especially those who have received previous antimicrobial therapy), cultures in hypertonic media may be helpful in an attempt to isolate cell wall–deficient forms. The addition of pyridoxal hydrochloride or cysteine to the media improves the chances of isolating nutritionally variant streptococci.

Blood cultures usually have been negative in the rare cases of endocarditis caused by *Aspergillus* and *Histoplasma* organisms, and *Coxiella burnetti*. In fungal endocarditis large emboli to large arteries are common, necessitating embolectomy. Histologic examination and culture of the embolus may be diagnostic.

Echocardiograms may suggest the location of a vegetation. Serial phonocardiography and cineradiography are useful for evaluating valve dysfunction or dehiscence in patients with prosthetic valve endocarditis. The disappearance of an opening or closing click suggests a vegetation on the valve; this is especially likely to occur with large vegetations, as are seen in fungal endocarditis. Cineradiography of the valve shows abnormal motion if the sutures are pulling out.

DIFFERENTIAL DIAGNOSIS. Infective endocarditis should be suspected in any patient with a heart murmur and unexplained fever present for at least 1 week. A definitive diagnosis can be made only with positive blood cultures. In the small percentage of patients with sterile blood cultures, the differential diagnosis can be very difficult.

Two clinical entities that can exactly duplicate the syndrome of infective endocarditis (including fever, murmur, and emboli) are atrial myxoma and nonbacterial thrombotic endocarditis. Acute rheumatic fever, lupus erythematosus, and sickle cell disease also can produce fever and heart murmur. Fever related to another illness can develop in any patient with an existing heart murmur. Therefore in the absence of positive blood cultures, other causes of fever must be sought.

Even in the absence of fever, murmur, or other signs of endocarditis, sustained bacteremia with ordinarily nonpathogenic bacteria (such as viridans streptococci, coagulase-negative staphylococci, or diphtheroids) strongly suggests intravascular infection, usually endocarditis.

MANAGEMENT

Principles of therapy. To achieve cure of infective endocarditis, the vegetation must be sterilized. Therefore bactericidal drug regimens are required in the therapy of endocarditis, and treatment must be continued long enough to achieve sterilization of the vegetation. Available evidence indicates that if peak serum concentrations are bactericidal for the infecting microorganism at a 1:8 dilution in normal serum, therapy probably is adequate.

Specific antimicrobial regimens. The initial treatment of subacute infective endocarditis while awaiting culture results should be directed at the enterococcus. However, if the course is acute, the patient has an intracardiac foreign body, or the patient is a parenteral drug abuser, therapy for staphylococcal endocarditis must be added. Once the infecting organism is isolated, the regimen should promptly be altered.

Streptococcal endocarditis

STREPTOCOCCI INHIBITED BY 0.1 μg/ml PENICILLIN G. Streptococci inhibited by 0.1 μg/ml penicillin G are classified as penicillin susceptible and include over 90% of viridans streptococci but no enterococci. For these streptococci three regimens have been widely used: (1) penicillin G alone for 4 weeks in doses of 10 to 20 million units intravenously daily; (2) penicillin G, 10 to 20 million units intravenously daily, or procaine penicillin, 1.2 million units intramuscularly every 6 hours, plus streptomycin, 0.5 g intramuscularly every 12 hours or gentamicin, 1 mg/kg intravenously every 8 hours for 2 weeks; or (3) penicillin plus streptomycin or gentamicin for 2 weeks with penicillin therapy extended another 2 weeks. If penicillin is contraindicated because of hypersensitivity, cephalothin (2 g every 4 hours intravenously) or cefazolin, (1 g every 6 hours intravenously or intramuscularly) can be given for 4 weeks with or without streptomycin or gentamicin for the first 2 weeks. Patients who are hypersensitive to penicillin also may be hypersensitive to the cephalosporins. If neither penicillin nor a cephalosporin can be used, vancomycin can be given intravenously in a dose of 0.5 g every 6 hours for 4 weeks, with or without streptomycin or gentamicin for the first 2 weeks.

In these regimens streptomycin or gentamicin should be discontinued if vestibular toxic effects occur and should not be used if renal insufficiency is present.

STREPTOCOCCI RESISTANT TO 0.1 μg/ml PENICILLIN G. Streptococci resistant to 0.1 μg/ml penicillin G are classified as relatively resistant to penicillin and include all enterococci and 5% to 10% of viridans streptococci. Penicillin or ampicillin alone is inadequate therapy for enterococcal endocarditis. In vitro, streptomycin combined with penicillin provides a more rapid and complete bactericidal effect than penicillin alone against some strains of enterococci. Many strains of enterococci do not demonstrate this in vitro effect with penicillin and streptomycin but do with penicillin and gentamicin.

The therapy recommended for enterococcal endocarditis is aqueous penicillin G (20 million units/day intravenously) plus gentamicin (1 mg/kg intramuscularly or intravenously every 8 hours for 4 to 6 weeks). Four weeks of therapy probably are adequate for most cases. If the enterococcus is inhibited by 2000 μg/ml streptomycin, streptomycin (0.5 g every 12 hours intramuscularly) can be used instead of gentamicin.

In patients with renal insufficiency, serum levels of streptomycin or gentamicin should be measured and the doses adjusted to maintain streptomycin peak levels of 10 to 15 μg/ml and gentamicin peaks of 3 to 5 μg/ml.

Enterococci are highly resistant to cephalosporins in vitro, and the clinical results with these agents have been unsatisfactory. No alternative drug has been extensively tested for efficacy in the treatment of enterococcal endocarditis. Therefore an effort should be made to use penicillin in most patients who have a history of delayed skin rash to penicillin or in those who have minor reactions during the course of therapy.

Patients with a history of anaphylaxis to penicillin or those who have severe reactions can be treated with vancomycin in a dose of 0.5 g intravenously every 6 hours for 4 to 6 weeks. Streptomycin or gentamicin should be included in the therapeutic program.

Endocarditis caused by nonenterococcal streptococci that are relatively resistant, that is, not inhibited by 0.1 μg/ml penicillin G in vitro, should be managed with 20 million units penicillin intravenously daily for 4 weeks and 0.5 g streptomycin intramuscularly every 12 hours or gentamicin, 1 mg/kg intravenously every 8 hours for 2 to 4 weeks. Vancomycin should be substituted for penicillin in patients allergic to penicillin. However, with these nonenterococcal, relatively penicillin-resistant streptococci, a cephalosporin can often be used in patients allergic to penicillin, provided that adequate serum bactericidal activity is achieved.

Staphylococcal endocarditis. S. aureus endocarditis should be suspected when endocarditis occurs in narcotic addicts, after the insertion of prosthetic heart valves, or in the presence of the clinical syndrome of acute endocarditis. Only penicillinase-resistant penicillins (nafcillin, methicillin, or oxacillin) or cephalosporins may be relied on in the initial treatment of staphylococcal endocarditis. Therapy must be given for 4 to 6 weeks. The doses are 2 g of nafcillin, methicillin, oxacillin, or cephalothin intravenously every 4 hours or 1 to 2 g of cefazolin intramuscularly or intravenously every 6 hours. Only when staphylococci are inhibited by 0.1 μg/ml can penicillin G be used and then only in high doses (for example, 20 million units/day). If a penicillin or a cephalosporin cannot be used, vancomycin (0.5 g intravenously every 6 hours) is the drug of choice.

Penicillins and gentamicin have been shown in vitro and in animal studies to have a more rapid bactericidal effect against S. aureus than penicillins alone, and some investigators have recommended using the combination in endocarditis in humans. At present no evidence exists that the combination has any advantage over a penicillin or a cephalosporin alone. Rifampin (300 mg orally every 12 hours) has been added to penicillin, cephalosporin, or vancomycin in some reported cases when the clinical response was inadequate. The addition of rifampin resulted in an increase in serum bactericidal activity and a better clinical response in most reports.

Methicillin-resistant strains of S. aureus are resistant to other penicillinase-resistant penicillins and to the cephalosporins as well. Endocarditis caused by methicillin-resistant S. aureus requires vancomycin therapy.

S. epidermidis endocarditis, which often is associated with prosthetic valves, should be treated initially with vancomycin. These organisms often are resistant to methicillin. Endocarditis caused by methicillin-resistant strains of S. epidermidis requires therapy with vancomycin, since it may not respond well to therapy with cephalosporins despite apparent in vitro susceptibility. Many authorities are now adding rifampin (with or without gentamicin) to vancomycin because of unfavorable results with single-agent therapy. Endocarditis caused by methicillin-sensitive strains can be treated with a penicillinase-resistant penicillin with or without rifampin or gentamicin. If the organism is sensitive to penicillin G, this agent probably is the drug of choice.

Endocarditis caused by other organisms. Pneumococcal, gonococcal, and meningococcal endocarditis should be treated with 20 million units/day of penicillin G intravenously for 4 weeks.

The therapy for endocarditis caused by other organisms (including gram-negative bacilli) must consist of bactericidal an-

timicrobials, preferably a penicillin or cephalosporin with or without an aminoglycoside, and must be given in sufficient doses to achieve peak concentrations in the serum that are bactericidal for the infecting organism at a 1:8 dilution. If the organism is resistant to all penicillins and cephalosporins, vancomycin with (or without) an aminoglycoside should be used if in vitro studies indicate susceptibility. If the organism is resistant to penicillins, cephalosporins, and vancomycin, therapy probably will be unsuccessful. Under these circumstances treatment should be initiated with the bactericidal drug grouping that demonstrates the best activity in vitro; if the patient does not respond or if relapse occurs after 4 to 6 weeks of therapy, antimicrobial therapy plus cardiac surgery to remove the vegetation and replace the valve probably will be necessary.

Results of therapy of fungal endocarditis have been disappointing. Amphotericin B, the only fungicidal agent available for parenteral use, is very toxic and difficult to use. Another agent, flucytosine, is fungistatic but may increase the fungicidal activity of amphotericin B in vitro. Amphotericin B generally is administered intravenously in a dose of 0.5 mg/kg/day; flucytosine is given orally in a dose of 75 to 150 mg/kg/day. Although some cures have been reported with antifungal therapy alone, surgical intervention with valve replacement is usually necessary to achieve a cure.

Endocarditis with sterile blood cultures. Most experts favor treating patients with endocarditis and sterile blood cultures as they would patients with enterococcal endocarditis. If there is no clinical response to the penicillin-plus-aminoglycoside regimen within 3 to 5 days, the dose of penicillin should be doubled to 40 million units/day. When the course is acute and fulminant, antistaphylococcal therapy with a penicillinase-resistant penicillin or cephalosporin should be added.

Endocarditis on intracardiac prostheses or sutures. Patients with endocarditis on prostheses or sutures probably require longer courses of therapy than patients without intravascular foreign bodies. Treatment usually is continued for 4 to 6 weeks for streptococci inhibited by 0.1 μg/ml of penicillin and 6 to 8 weeks for all other microorganisms. With the exception of streptococcal endocarditis, results of medical therapy for prosthetic valve endocarditis have been poor. Therefore, in patients with endocarditis caused by organisms other than streptococci, valve replacement should be carefully considered.

Surgery in the management of endocarditis. When appropriate microbicidal therapy is unavailable and positive blood cultures continue during therapy or relapse occurs after therapy is discontinued, removal of the vegetation and replacement of the valve with a prosthesis should be considered. The surgical repair ideally should be performed after several days or more of the best available antimicrobial therapy. The therapy should be continued for 2 weeks or longer in the case of organisms that tend to produce metastatic foci. Immediate valve replacement (even after only hours of therapy) is essential if congestive heart failure develops as a result of severe valvular insufficiency.

Current evidence indicates that to achieve cure in fungal endocarditis, surgical intervention almost always is required in addition to treatment with antifungal agents.

Patients with prosthetic valve endocarditis often require valve replacement for cure. The indications for valve replacement are valve dysfunction, heart failure, myocardial abscess, continuation of embolization, organisms resistant to bactericidal antimicrobials, fungal infection, and continuing bacteremia during or relapses after an appropriate course of therapy. Surgery usually is required in early prosthetic valve endocarditis both because of the microorganisms involved and because of valve dysfunction. Surgery often is required in nonstreptococcal prosthetic valve endocarditis.

Response to therapy. Defervescence and an increased sense of well-being usually occur within several days to a week after the initiation of appropriate antimicrobial therapy. Persistent or recurrent fever may be associated with myocardial or metastatic abscess formation (especially in *S. aureus* endocarditis), but the most common cause of fever during therapy with an appropriate drug regimen is a reaction to the antimicrobial agents. Superinfection of a heart valve, although rare, is especially likely when intravascular plastic catheters are used for infusions.

Heart failure may occur at any time during or after therapy and is a poor prognostic sign. Heart failure is especially likely to develop in patients with aortic insufficiency, and these patients have a high mortality. In addition to valvular insufficiency, vegetations (especially in fungal endocarditis) may become large enough to cause obstruction of the valvular orifice.

The vast majority of relapses can be detected with blood cultures obtained 1, 2, and 4 weeks after discontinuation of therapy.

PROGNOSIS. The factors that tend to make the prognosis relatively unfavorable are (1) nonstreptococcal disease, (2) development of heart failure, (3) aortic valve involvement, (4) prosthetic valve, and (5) old age. The cure rate in streptococcal endocarditis is about 90%. Most failures are the result not of uncontrolled infection but of death from heart failure, an embolus, rupture of a mycotic aneurysm, or renal failure. The cure rate in nonaddicts with *S. aureus* endocarditis is about 50%, with most deaths caused by early overwhelming infection or heart failure. The cure rate in addicts with *S. aureus* endocarditis is much higher. Results in endocarditis caused by fungi and gram-negative bacilli have been poor. Early cardiac surgery for heart failure or for cases refractory to antimicrobial therapy should improve these results.

PREVENTION. An apparent portal of entry for the infecting organism can be demonstrated in only a minority of patients with infective endocarditis. However, it seems clear that the oropharynx serves as the site of origin for most patients, with the genitourinary tract next. Obviously, oral hygiene should be optimal in patients with underlying cardiac lesions that predispose them to endocarditis, especially those who are to have prosthetic cardiac valves implanted.

Although the risk of endocarditis is small and there is no proof of efficacy, antimicrobial prophylaxis is recommended for patients with predisposing cardiac lesions who are to undergo procedures known to result in transient bacteremia. The cardiac conditions for which prophylaxis is recommended are valvular or congenital heart disease (except for uncomplicated atrial septal defect), intracardiac prostheses, and a previous episode of infective endocarditis. The antimicrobial therapy is directed at the bacteria that lodge at an endocardial site and therefore is analogous to the treatment of very early endocarditis.

Dental manipulations and other procedures in the mouth, nose, or throat. Prophylaxis is directed against viridans streptococci and is recommended for all procedures likely to cause gingival bleeding and for tonsillectomy and bronchoscopy. The regimen recommended by the American Heart Association is penicillin V (2 g orally 1 hour before the procedure, then 1 g 6 hours later). For maximal protection (for example, for patients with prosthetic valves) the recommended regimen is 1 to 2 g of ampicillin (intramuscularly or intravenously) plus 1.5 mg/kg of gentamicin (intramuscularly or intravenously) 30 minutes before the procedure, followed by 1 g oral penicillin V or the parenteral regimen 8 hours later.

In patients allergic to penicillin, 1 g of erythromycin can be orally administered 1 hour before the procedure and 500 mg 6 hours later. For maximal protection in the patient allergic to penicillin, vancomycin is recommended (1 g intravenously starting 1 hour before the procedure and given over 1 hour).

Genitourinary and gastrointestinal tract procedures or surgery. Prophylaxis is directed against enterococci and is recommended for procedures that cause significant trauma to the genitourinary or gastrointestinal tracts (for example, urethral catheterization, prostatic surgery, and colonic or gallbladder surgery). The standard regimen recommended by the American Heart Association is ampicillin (2 g intramuscularly or intravenously) plus gentamicin (1.5 mg/kg intramuscularly or intravenously) given 30 minutes to 1 hour before the procedure; one follow-up dose may be given 8 hours later. In patients allergic to penicillin, vancomycin (1 g intravenously) is started 1 hour before the procedure and is given over 1 hour, together with gentamicin (1.5 mg/kg intramuscularly or intravenously); this regimen can be repeated once 8 to 12 hours later. An oral regimen recommended for minor or repetitive procedures in low-risk patients is 3 g of amoxicillin administered orally 1 hour before the procedure and 1.5 g given 6 hours later.

BIBLIOGRAPHY

Bisno AL and others: Antimicrobial treatment of infective endocarditis due to viridans streptococci, enterococci, and streptococci, JAMA 261:1471, 1989.

Karchmer AW, Archer GL, and Dismukes WE: *Staphylococcus epidermidis* causing prosthetic valve endocarditis: microbiologic and clinical observations as guides to therapy, Ann Intern Med 98:447, 1983.

Korzeniowski O, Sande MA, and The National Collaborative Endocarditis Study Group: Combination antimicrobial therapy for *Staphylococcus aureus* endocarditis in patients addicted to parenteral drugs and in non-addicts, Ann Intern Med 97:496, 1982.

Oikawa JH and Kaye D: Endocarditis epidemiology pathophysiology, management and prophylaxis, Cardiovasc Clin 16:335, 1986.

Sande MA, Kaye D, and Root RK, editors: Contemporary issues in infectious diseases, Vol 2, New York, 1984, Churchill Livingstone, Inc.

Scheld WM and Sande MA: Endocarditis and intravascular infections. In Mandell GL, Douglas RG, and Bennett JE, editors: Principles and practice of infectious diseases, ed 2, New York, 1985, John Wiley & Sons, Inc.

Schulman ST and others: Prevention of bacterial endocarditis, a statement for health professionals by the Committee on Rheumatic Fever and Infective Endocarditis of the Council on Cardiovascular Disease in the Young, Circulation 70:1123A, 1984.

Bacterial infections of the central nervous system

Merle A. Sande, Jay H. Tureen, *and* **W. Michael Scheld**

BACTERIAL MENINGITIS

DEFINITION AND PATHOLOGY. Bacterial meningitis is an infection involving the leptomeninges, the fine lining structures of the brain and spinal cord. These include the arachnoid, the pia mater, and the space between filled with the cerebrospinal fluid (CSF). The inflammatory process produces a purulent exudate that usually extends throughout the subarachnoid space, initially involving the basal cisterns, around the cerebellum, then over the cerebral hemispheres. Ventriculitis frequently is present. Usually, bacteria do not invade the brain tissue directly nor do abscesses form, but leukocytes occasionally are found in the outer cortical layers. Associated cortical thrombophlebitis and cortical edema with herniation and cranial nerve damage may occur.

ETIOLOGY AND PATHOGENESIS. The bacteria responsible for meningitis all possess important virulence factors that provide a selective advantage in gaining access to and surviving within the CSF. The exact mechanisms by which meningitis is produced are obscure, however. The disease appears to develop when several unique conditions occur simultaneously. These include (1) recent acquisition of or colonization with an encapsulated organism to which the patient lacks bactericidal antibody, (2) dissemination of the bacteria into the bloodstream, usually from the nasopharynx or lungs, and (3) penetration into the subarachnoid space through an area of damage in the blood-brain barrier. Invasion of the CSF also may occur directly from the nasopharynx through the cribriform plate or as a result of extension from suppurative sinusitis or mastoiditis. In the CSF the organisms initially must withstand phagocytosis, multiply, and induce an inflammatory response. Meningitis rarely is caused by bacteria when the host possesses specific bactericidal or opsonizing antibody. Thus to a great extent the age of the patient dictates the likely infecting pathogen (Table 40-2). Neonates have protective maternal antibodies against most common pathogens but may be traumatized and heavily colonized during normal delivery with pathogenic group B streptococci, *Escherichia coli,* or other enteric bacilli. For example, 70% of neonates born from mothers vaginally colonized with group B streptococci *(Streptococcus agalactiae)* acquire the organism during birth. In instances when meningitis occurred, neither mother nor child had opsonizing antibody to the typical type III capsular polysaccharide, the serotype that usually produces disease. Approximately 84% of *E. coli* strains that produce neonatal meningitis carry the K1 antigen (compared with 36% of strains that invade the bloodstream but do not produce meningitis). The K1 antigen is an acidic polysaccharide (one of more than 100 *E. coli* antigens) and is antigenically related to the capsular polysaccharides of group B *Neisseria meningitidis* and type III group B streptococci. The exact mechanism by which K1 antigen increases the propensity of these strains to produce meningitis is unknown, but it seems to be related to their ability to colonize the intestinal epithelium of the neonate and produce hematogenous dissemination. This important virulence characteristic has been confirmed in experimental infant animals fed *E. coli* with K1 antigen intragastrically.

The three most common etiologic agents of meningitis after the first month of age are *Haemophilus influenzae* (type b), *Neisseria mengingitidis,* and *Streptococcus pneumoniae.* All three possess polysaccharide capsules that protect them from phagocytosis. All are known to colonize the nasopharynx and produce disease in patients not possessing anticapsular antibody. The incidence of meningitis produced by *H. influenzae* falls dramatically after the first 6 years of life. This correlates with the appearance of antibody primarily directed against polyribose ribitol phosphate (PRP), the unique ribitol phosphate component of the type b polysaccharide capsule. These antibodies promote complement-mediated phagocytosis and bacteriolysis and are protective against type b disease in experimental animals and humans. The antibodies result from exposure not only to *H. influenzae* but also to other bacteria containing immunologically cross-reactive surface antigens. Other, less well-recognized protective antibodies that are directed against the so-called outer membrane (OM) antigens of *H. influenzae* also have been described.

The meningococcus produces meningitis in either epidemics or sporadic outbreaks, predominantly in children and young

Table 40-2   Approximate incidence, by age, of organisms causing bacterial meningitis

Organism	Age (%)		
	≤1 mo	1 mo-6 yr	≥6 yr
Haemophilus influenzae	0-1	40-50	5
Streptococcus pneumoniae	1-3	15-20	40-50
Neisseria meningitidis	0-1	25-30	30-40
Streptococcus agalactiae (group B)	30-40	1-4	1-5
Escherichia coli (and other gram-negative bacilli)	50-60	1-2	10
Listeria monocytogenes	2-10	1-2	5
Staphylococci	3-5	1-2	<5
Others plus unidentified	10	10	10

adults. The incidence of disease falls dramatically after the age of 40. The incidence is inversely proportional to the percentage of people with bactericidal antibody against the various capsular polysaccharides (see discussion of "Meningococcal infections" in Chapter 46).

The pneumococcus produces meningitis throughout life, a characteristic that may be related to the large number (84) of antigenically distinct capsular polysaccharide types and the prevalence of this organism as a respiratory tract pathogen. Specific opsonizing antibody develops following infection with each type and rarely after infection from selected cross-reacting types.

Listeria monocytogenes produces meningitis predominantly in patients with impaired cellular immunity such as very young patients (neonates), patients with Hodgkin's disease, or individuals receiving corticosteroids or other immunosuppressive therapy. *Staphylococcus aureus* occasionally produces a meningitis-cerebritis syndrome associated with an overwhelming staphylococcal infection, including endocarditis. Staphylococci and various gram-negative bacilli infect the meninges following accidental or neurosurgical traumatic disruption of the subarachnoid space. *Staphylococcus epidermidis* is the most common cause of meningitis complicating the insertion of intracranial foreign bodies (such as CSF shunts). Anaerobic bacteria can be isolated from CSF following rupture of a brain abscess into the ventricles or the subarachnoid space. Primary anaerobic organism meningitis is quite rare.

EPIDEMIOLOGY. The setting in which meningitis occurs may give significant clues as to the causative agent. Group B streptococcal and *E. coli* septicemia and meningitis frequently are associated with prematurity or follow maternal complications at delivery such as premature rupture of the membranes. The meningococcus has been a common cause of meningitis epidemics in military recruit camps, where crowding and introduction of new serogroups from widely disseminated regions occur. These outbreaks frequently follow spring epidemics of adenovirus infections and are preceded by a marked increase in the meningococcal carrier state. Susceptible close family contacts, especially sleeping partners of patients with either meningococcal or *H. influenzae* meningitis, are at increased risk of disease. *H. influenzae* meningitis also is frequently preceded by or accompanies an upper respiratory tract infection, especially otitis media or acute sinusitis.

Pneumococcal meningitis frequently is associated with acute otitis media and mastoiditis (30%), pneumonia (25%), and occasionally acute sinusitis. Significant head injury with or without skull fracture precedes pneumococcal meningitis in about 10% of the cases. The pneumococcus accounts for the vast majority of meningitis associated with a CSF leak (either otorrhea or rhinorrhea) and is by far the most common cause of recurrent episodes of meningitis. Meningitis occurring in the presence of immunodeficiency states (reduced levels of immunoglobulins), sickle cell disease, asplenism, or other conditions, including alcoholism, that reduce bacterial clearance from the bloodstream usually is caused by the pneumococcus. Meningococcal meningitis has been reported in complement deficiency states, especially when the terminal components of the complement cascade are absent.

CLINICAL MANIFESTATIONS. Early recognition of meningitis and prompt specific therapy are vital for survival in this disease. Thus it is critical to appreciate the setting and initial manifestations. The classic presentation of bacterial meningitis consists of the triad of fever, headache, and a stiff neck, usually in the setting of a preceding upper respiratory tract infection (rhinitis, sinusitis, otitis, or mastoiditis) and occasionally accompanied by pneumonia. Patients may have nausea and vomiting, especially when increased intracranial pressure is present. Generalized weakness and photophobia are common. With meningococcal disease severe myalgias, backache, and painful extremities (hyperalgesia) may occur. The level of consciousness nearly always is altered. Patients initially may be lethargic but can progress rapidly to coma. Seizures (either generalized or focal) accompany acute bacterial meningitis in 20% to 30% of the patients and cranial nerve palsies in 10% to 20%. The more rapid the onset of disease, the worse the prognosis. In approximately 10% of the patients symptoms leading to coma develop in less than 24 hours, and these patients have a mortality rate of at least 50%. Most patients have a more insidious onset, with symptoms developing over several days to a week. They have a mortality rate of less than 25%. Unfortunately, classic signs and symptoms frequently are obscure in neonates and the elderly. These patients may have only fever with irritability, lassitude, or confusion. Poor feeding in infants or an abrupt change in personality in the elderly may be the only manifestation of disease. In impaired hosts the presence of fever with confusion should suggest meningitis.

In most patients the physical examination reveals evidence of meningeal irritation (pain on flexion of the neck). A stiff neck may be absent very early in the disease, in neonates, or in obtunded elderly patients. Bulging fontanelles in infants are helpful diagnostically when present but usually are a late finding.

Cranial nerve abnormalities, especially of the third, fourth, sixth, and seventh cranial nerves, and focal cerebral signs including hemiparesis, dysphasia, and visual field abnormalities are not unusual early manifestations, especially in pneumococcal meningitis. Evidence of cerebral edema or increased intracranial pressure may accompany severe disease and should be recognized promptly. This may be manifested by third nerve dysfunction, corticospinal tract signs (abnormal reflexes), coma, hypertension, bradycardia, or abnormal respiration. Papilledema is unusual in bacterial meningitis, and when it is present, a mass lesion such as a brain abscess or epidural or subdural hematoma or abscess should be excluded before lumbar puncture.

The presence of rash (maculopapules, petechiae, or purpura) in a patient with meningeal signs usually indicates meningococcal sepsis and meningitis and occurs in approximately 50% of such cases. This clinical presentation also results in rare cases from echovirus (especially type 9) infection, in asplenic patients with pneumococcal or *H. influenzae* sepsis, and in meningitis in patients with endocarditis caused by *S. aureus*.

LABORATORY FINDINGS. Immediate CSF examination is important when meningitis is suspected. When the patient is severely ill, treatment should be initiated before or while lumbar puncture is being performed. The opening pressure is almost always elevated (average 200 to 300 mm H_2O), although extremely high pressures (such as 600 mm H_2O) may be seen, as with cerebral edema. A low pressure may indicate a CSF block.

CSF pleocytosis is the hallmark of bacterial meningitis, and leukocyte counts usually range from 100 to 10,000/mm^3 with an average of 500 to 2000. Very high counts (more than 50,000/mm^3) should alert the physician to the possibility of a ruptured intracranial abscess. Polymorphonuclear leukocytes predominate early in the disease (usually greater than 80%) with a gradual shift to mononuclear forms following successful therapy. Early in overwhelming bacterial meningitis, CSF white blood cell counts may be very low, even though the organism can be found on Gram stain of the CSF and cultures are positive.

CSF protein concentrations are elevated in over 90% of the cases, usually above 100 mg/dl. The CSF glucose is classically depressed to less than 40 mg/dl or less than 50% of simultaneous blood sugar (if the latter is less than 250 mg/dl). Hypoglycorrhachia is not diagnostic of bacterial infection, since a low CSF glucose also may be found in some cases of lymphocytic choriomeningitis virus infection, sarcoidosis, tuberculosis, fungal infection, meningeal carcinoma, or subarachnoid hemorrhage. In addition, patients with bacterial meningitis may have CSF glucose concentrations in the normal range.

The Gram stain of a spun specimen of CSF reveals the organism in up to 80% of the cases. However, errors in interpretation by inexperienced observers are common because overdecolorized pneumococci may look like *H. influenzae*, *H. influenzae* may demonstrate bipolar staining and be confused with pneumococci, stain artifact may resemble gram-positive cocci, and intracellular meningococci may be confused with nuclear debris. Concomitant use of the Quellung reaction (with omnisera) conclusively identifies the pneumococcus. Gram stains are positive in 60% of partially treated cases. Wayson stain, a variant of the methylene blue stain, may be more sensitive and positive in cases in which Gram stain was negative. When Gram stains are negative, cryptococci and mycobacteria always should be sought with india ink preparations and acid-fast (Ziehl-Neelsen) stains of CSF sediment. Cultures are positive in 70% to 90% of the cases of bacterial meningitis but may be negative if the patient has received prior antibiotic therapy. Cultures almost always remain positive in partially treated cases of *H. influenzae* meningitis.

New rapid techniques have become available to detect bacterial antigens in CSF. Until recently, the most widely used technique was the counterimmunoelectrophoresis (CIE) technique, which is positive in up to 80% of the cases of type b *H. influenzae*, meningococcal, or pneumococcal meningitis. Newer methods for antigen detection, including latex agglutination and staphylococcal coagglutination, are more sensitive, less expensive, and simpler than CIE and have largely supplanted it. Detection of CSF endotoxin by the Limulus lysate assay is possible in meningitis caused by gram-negative bacteria (including *H. influenzae* and the meningococcus). These methods are particularly helpful in cases in which the Gram stain is negative. Cryptococcal antigen detection in CSF is a sensitive and specific method for diagnosing cryptococcal meningitis. Elevated CSF lactate levels (greater than 35 mg/dl) may be of value in distinguishing purulent bacterial meningitis from aseptic meningitis.

Blood cultures always should be obtained, since they may

reveal the infecting organism when CSF cultures are negative. Blood cultures are positive in most patients with *H. influenzae* meningitis, in about half of those with pneumococcal meningitis, and in 40% of those with meningococcal meningitis. The serum sodium concentration should be measured because inappropriate antidiuretic hormone (SIADH) secretion may accompany meningitis and result in lethargy and seizures unless water is restricted during management. Clotting parameters may be abnormal, especially in meningococcal infection, in which disseminated intravascular coagulation may be a fatal complication. A peripheral leukocytosis with a shift to the left (early band forms) is common in bacterial meningitis and may be of value in distinguishing it from viral infections.

Roentgenographic evaluation of the chest, skull, mastoid processes, and sinuses is indicated early in the hospital course to elicit potentially inapparent areas of infection or fractures that may require medical or surgical attention. When evidence of elevated intracranial pressure is suspected during physical examination (and certainly if papilledema is present), a computed tomographic (CT) scan is necessary to exclude a mass lesion, that is, a brain abscess or subdural empyema.

DIAGNOSIS. The diagnosis of bacterial meningitis should be suspected in every patient with fever, alteration in mental status (lethargy, confusion, coma), headache, and a stiff neck. Initial evaluation should proceed immediately. If examination reveals no papilledema or focal neurologic signs that support the diagnosis of a mass lesion or impending herniation, a lumbar puncture should be performed. Antibiotic therapy should be initiated immediately after the lumbar puncture if the disease is acute (less than 24 hours' duration) or severe or if suspicion of meningitis is high. A meticulous examination of the CSF only wastes precious minutes. Therapy can be altered following such an examination.

If a mass is suspected, therapy should be initiated and a CT scan or other available procedures should be performed. In the vast majority of cases of bacterial meningitis, no evidence for a mass lesion is present and lumbar puncture can be performed safely.

If the presentation is subacute, careful evaluation of the CSF is indicated. Therapy should be instituted if any of the following are present: (1) a CSF pleocytosis with a predominance of polymorphonuclear leukocytes; (2) positive Gram stain; (3) hypoglycorrhachia (less than 50% of the blood sugar level without another obvious explanation); or (4) a positive CIE, latex agglutination, or limulus lysate assay.

Although the diagnosis usually is readily apparent in the typical case, it may be less obvious in elderly obtunded patients, confused alcoholics with delirium tremens or hepatic encephalopathy, and irritable neonates or infants that fail to thrive. In these cases there must be a low threshold for examination of the CSF.

DIFFERENTIAL DIAGNOSIS. Other conditions that can mimic bacterial meningitis include aseptic meningitis, parameningeal infections, tuberculous meningitis, fungal meningitis, and amebic meningitis.

Aseptic meningitis. Aseptic meningitis is caused predominantly by the enteroviruses. The presentation often is similar with fever, headache, and meningeal signs. These cases generally occur in clusters in the late summer or early fall, and they usually are not associated with peripheral leukocytosis. Although CSF examination may reveal pleocytosis with a predominance of polymorphonuclear leukocytes early in the disease, the degree of pleocytosis is typically low (fewer than 500 cells/mm^3) and the CSF glucose level is normal. Mumps meningitis may be associated with a CSF glucose in the 40 mg/dl

range but usually is associated with parotitis, orchitis, or pancreatitis. Other viral causes include lymphocytic choriomeningoencephalitis virus, herpes simplex virus, and adenovirus. Leptospirosis may also produce an aseptic meningitis syndrome with the same CSF findings as viral meningitis.

Parameningeal infections. Parameningeal infections, including brain abscess, epidural abscess, subdural empyema, and septic venous sinus phlebitis, may cause CSF pleocytosis and neurologic symptoms. These conditions should be considered when the neurologic manifestations precede the onset of meningeal signs and symptoms or when obvious suppurative infections are present in the sinuses, mastoid processes, or lungs.

Tuberculous meningitis. Tuberculous meningitis usually produces lymphocytic pleocytosis (generally fewer than 500 cells/mm^3) in the CSF and a subacute to chronic course. However, occasionally it is clinically indistinguishable from acute bacterial meningitis, with CSF pleocytosis consisting of predominantly polymorphonuclear leukocytes, hypoglycorrhachia, and a marked elevation in CSF protein. Careful examination of the CSF with Ziehl-Neelsen or fluorochrome stains may reveal the organism in up to 50% of the cases. The disease usually occurs in the course of miliary tuberculosis resulting from rupture of a leptomeningeal granuloma. Tuberculous foci of infection usually are evident elsewhere. This disease always should be considered when CSF pleocytosis is present and CSF glucose is depressed but Gram stains and cultures for routine bacteria are negative. CSF cultures are positive in 40% to 88% of the cases of tuberculous meningitis. Newer techniques, including the detection of adenosine deaminase or mycobacterial antigen in CSF, may suggest this diagnosis when acid-fast stains are negative and cultures are pending.

Fungal meningitis. Fungal meningitis usually is chronic but (like tuberculous disease) also may produce an acute form. *Cryptococcus neoformans* accounts for the vast majority of cases and should be suspected in patients with impaired cellular immune responses (as in those with Hodgkin's disease or acquired immunodeficiency syndrome [AIDS], or undergoing corticosteroid therapy). The CSF typically exhibits a mononuclear pleocytosis with fewer than 400 cells/mm^3, elevated protein, and usually a decreased CSF sugar. India ink preparations are positive in over 50% of the cases, and the yield is increased with multiple examinations and centrifugation of large volumes (for example, 10 to 20 ml) of CSF. Cryptococcal antigens can be detected in CSF or serum in up to 95% of cases. Coccidioidal meningitis should be considered in patients who have lived in or visited the southwestern United States. The diagnosis can be established by culture or detection of coccidioidal antigen (by complement fixation [CF] techniques) in CSF. *Candida* spp. occasionally produce meningitis in patients with disseminated candidiasis. Candidal meningitis may occur in patients receiving hyperalimentation and broad-spectrum antibiotics for prolonged periods of time.

Amebic meningitis. Amebic meningitis is a rare form of disease produced by free-living genera such as *Naegleria* and *Acanthamoeba*. Most patients give a history of swimming or diving in warm, shallow, freshwater lakes where these organisms may reach very high concentrations. They are motile and may be observed on wet mounts of unspun CSF.

Other forms. Other forms of culture-negative meningitis include meningeal carcinomatosis and sarcoidosis, which often are associated with marked hypoglycorrhachia; chemical meningitis from spinal anesthesics, roentgenographic contrast material, or other iatrogenically induced material; Behçet's syndrome, which is associated with recurrent oral and genital ulcers; Mollaret's recurrent meningitis (usually less acute and rare in the United States); systemic lupus erythematosus; and syphilitic meningitis.

MANAGEMENT. Bacterial meningitis constitutes a medical emergency, and antimicrobial treatment should be instituted promptly on recognition or suspicion. Since an etiologic agent frequently is not definitely established, selection must be aimed at the most likely possibilities based on available clinical clues such as age and setting (recruit camp, recent neurosurgical procedure, rash, and so forth). Ideal therapy includes the administration of bactericidal antibiotics in adequate dosages to achieve activity within the CSF. The following is suggested as initial therapy:

1. *Adults with suspected bacterial meningitis or with proven pneumococcal, or meningococcal meningitis.* Aqueous penicillin G (12 to 20 million units/day intravenously) either by constant infusion or in four to six divided doses. In patients with inflamed meninges this dose should ensure up to 1 µg/ml of penicillin in the CSF, which is bactericidal for all strains of meningococci and all but the rare penicillin-resistant strains of *S. pneumoniae*. Large (5 million units or more), rapid, intravenous bolus administration of penicillin should be avoided, since penicillin neurotoxicity (lethargy, multifocal myoclonus, and seizures) may occur when CSF concentrations exceed 10 µg/ml.

2. *Children with suspected bacterial meningitis.*
   (a) *Neonatal meningitis (less than 4 weeks of age).* Therapy must be directed against *E. coli*, group B streptococci, and *Listeria monocytogenes.* Therefore therapy should include ampicillin (50 mg/kg intravenously every 8 hours for neonates 7 days of age or younger or every 6 hours for neonates older than 7 days of age) and an aminoglycoside, usually gentamicin (1.5 mg/kg intravenously every 8 hours) or cefotaxime (50 mg/kg intravenously every 8 hours) if gram-negative meningitis is strongly suspected based on Gram stain. Currently, intrathecal administration of aminoglycosides is not recommended in neonatal *E. coli* meningitis, although it may be necessary if follow-up lumbar puncture reveals persistence of infection. Therapy for group B streptococcal meningitis should be continued for 14 days, therapy for gram-negative enteric meningitis for 21 days. Some authorities recommend a third-generation cephalosporin (for example, cefotaxime) plus ampicillin as empiric therapy in this age-group.
   (b) *Infants 1 to 3 months of age.* Therapy is directed against both neonatal pathogens and the more common pathogens of infancy (*H. influenzae* type b, *N. meningitidis, S. pneumoniae*). Intravenous therapy should include ampicillin (200 mg/kg/day in divided doses every 6 hours) plus cefotaxime (200 mg/kg/day in divided doses every 6 hours). The duration of therapy should be appropriate for the pathogen (see [a] and [c]).
   (c) *Children older than 3 months of age.* Therapy for this age group is aimed at *H. influenzae, N. meningitidis,* and *S. pneumoniae.* Initial therapy can be ampicillin (200 mg/kg/day in divided doses every 6 hours) plus choramphenicol (100 mg/kg/day in divided doses every 6 hours) until sensitivities are known or one of the newer third-generation cephalosporins (for example, cefotaxime, 200 mg/kg/day in divided doses every 6 hours; ceftriaxone, 100 mg/kg/day in divided doses every 12 hours). Therapy should continue for 7 to 10 days.

3. *Adults and children older than 3 months who are allergic to penicillin.* Several of the newer cephalosporins have proved effective in the treatment of meningitis in both children and adults. The risk of cross-allergenicity in patients allergic to penicillin appears to be small. Cefuroxime, a second-generation cephalosporin, and ceftriaxone, cefotaxime, and ceftizoxime,

third-generation cephalosporins, all are effective against meningitis caused by *S. pneumoniae, N. meningitidis,* and *H. influenzae*. The recommended intravenous dosages of these cephalosporins for adults are: cefuroxime, 1.5 to 3 g every 8 hours; cefotaxime and ceftizoxime, 2 g every 6 to 8 hours; ceftriaxone, 2 g every 12 to 24 hours. It should be remembered that these drugs are not active against *L. monocytogenes*. Chloramphenicol can be used in patients allergic to both penicillins and cephalosporins, and it often is recommended in patients with a history of anaphylaxis or laryngeal edema following penicillin administration, since a severe cross-reaction is possible in these patients.

4. *Gram-negative bacillary meningitis.* The third-generation cephalosporins listed above have significantly altered the therapy of gram-negative bacillary meningitis. Therapy with either cefotaxime, ceftizoxime (not yet approved for use in infants younger than 6 months of age), or ceftriaxone can be initiated and usually is active against most gram-negative bacilli except for *P. aeruginosa*. Recommended therapy for *P. aeruginosa* meningitis is parenteral administration of an antipseudomonal penicillin or ceftazidime in combination with an aminoglycoside (such as tobramycin) administered both parenterally (1.0 mg/kg every 8 hours) and intrathecally (up to 5 to 15 mg every 24 hours until cultures are sterile). In all cases final therapy should depend on in vitro sensitivity results after the infecting organism has been isolated.

5. *S. aureus meningitis-cerebritis syndrome.* Nafcillin or another penicillinase-resistant penicillin should be administered at a dosage of 9 g intravenously each day in four to six divided doses. In patients allergic to penicillin, vancomycin, given in a dosage of 500 mg every 6 hours or 1 g every 12 hours intravenously, can be used. In both instances CSF cultures should be monitored carefully, since intrathecal drug administration may be required in some cases. The penicillin, however, should not be given intrathecally.

COURSE. Therapy should be continued at full doses for at least 10 to 14 days or for 5 to 7 days after the patient becomes afebrile. Therapy generally is continued for 7 days for meningococcal meningitis, 10 days for *H. influenzae* disease, 14 days for pneumococcal meningitis, and 3 weeks for meningitis caused by aerobic gram-negative bacilli.

Repeated CSF examinations are not indicated for the common forms of meningitis unless the patient remains febrile or fever recurs. A single follow-up lumbar puncture obtained 3 to 4 days after therapy is initiated should reveal sterile CSF, a return toward a normal CSF glucose level, and a shift from a predominantly polymorphonuclear leukocyte pleocytosis to mononuclear cells. Prolonged fever may indicate persistent meningitis or subdural effusions, other areas of hidden infection (sinusitis, mastoiditis, empyema, and so on), sinus thrombosis, drug fever, phlebitis, or other nonbacterial diseases listed previously under "Differential diagnosis." Meningococcal disease may be associated with a syndrome of sterile polyserositis (pericarditis, arthritis), resulting in prolonged fever that initially appears 6 to 10 days following the onset of infection.

ADJUVANT THERAPY. Even with aggressive antimicrobial therapy, the mortality from bacterial meningitis remains at approximately 5% to 10% for *H. influenzae* or meningococcal meningitis and 25% for pneumococcal meningitis. Permanent neurologic sequelae may result in up to 30% of the children with *H. influenzae* meningitis. Many deaths that occur early in the course of disease are a result of cerebral edema and temporal lobe or cerebellar herniation. When cerebral edema is suspected, aggressive monitoring of intracranial pressure is indicated, and elevated pressures are treated with hyperventilation, intravenous administration of mannitol, high doses of dexamethasone, or all of these. Anticonvulsant therapy should be used when seizures occur. Patients with meningococcal disease and disseminated intravascular coagulation may require heparin therapy if bleeding occurs.

PREVENTION. Both chemoprophylaxis and immunization have been used to prevent bacterial meningitis. When proven cases of meningococcal meningitis are identified, chemoprophylaxis is recommended for intimate contacts of the index case. This includes close household family members or roommates and people with oral contact such as kissing or mouth-to-mouth resuscitation. Unless such intimate contact has occurred, prophylaxis usually is not recommended in groups such as classmates or hospital personnel. The drug of choice currently is rifampin (600 mg orally twice a day for 2 days for adults, 20 mg/kg/day in two divided doses for 2 days for children). Secondary cases of *H. influenzae* meningitis in close contacts also have been identified, and prophylaxis with rifampin (20 mg/kg/day in a single dose [not to exceed 600 mg] for 4 days) currently is recommended.

Immunization is available for meningococcal (serogroups A and C), pneumococcal (23 serotypes), and *H. influenzae* type b infections. The use of meningococcal vaccine has markedly reduced the incidence of epidemics in recruit camps and has effectively abated epidemics in Brazil and other areas. Patients entering highly endemic or epidemic areas of disease should be vaccinated. Pneumococcal vaccine is recommended for patients with a high risk of pneumococcal disease (that is, those with recurrent meningitis or CSF rhinorrhea, sickle cell disease, asplenism, or chronic debilitating diseases), but efficacy has not been conclusively shown in these clinical settings.

PARAMENINGEAL AND EPIDURAL INFECTIONS

Suppurative infections may be found within the cranial vault under specific clinical conditions in three locations: (1) within the brain parenchyma (brain abscess), (2) between the dura and the arachnoid membrane (subdural empyema), and (3) between the dura and the cranium (epidural or extradural abscess). Each process has unique predisposing conditions, pathogenesis, clinical presentation, and specific therapy. They must be recognized early and distinguished from each other, since each is associated with significant morbidity and mortality.

Brain abscess

DEFINITION. A brain abscess is a focal collection of pus within the parenchyma of the brain. It is approximately one sixth as common as bacterial meningitis.

ETIOLOGY AND PATHOGENESIS. The brain is remarkably resistant to infection, and it is impossible to produce an abscess in experimental animals unless there is associated tissue damage (infarction) or foreign material injected with the microorganism. In humans brain abscesses are produced either by contiguous spread from extracranial suppurative foci or by hematogenous dissemination from distant infections. Most brain abscesses result from extension of infection from chronic middle ear, mastoid, or sinus infections. The bacteria invade either directly through bone, dura mater, and across subdural and subarachnoid spaces to the brain or along venous channels by extension of a septic thrombophlebitis. Otic suppuration accounts for one third to one half of all brain abscesses and produces disease either in the ipsilateral cerebellar hemisphere (especially in children) or in the temporal lobe. Extension from frontal sinusitis may produce disease in the anteroinferior aspect of the frontal lobes. Sphenoidal sinusitis extends to the frontal or temporal lobes and ethmoid sinusitis to the frontal lobes. An exacerbation of otitis, mastoiditis, or sinusitis commonly precedes extension of the infection into the brain. Compound fractures, osteomyelitis of the skull, and penetrating head wounds also can lead to brain abscesses or hematogenous spread. Metastatic infections account for the minority of brain abscesses, and in most cases a primary suppurative focus can be found elsewhere. The most common site is the lung (bronchiectasis, lung abscess, empyema), but dental, tonsillar, and uterine sources also have been implicated. Endocarditis is a rare predisposing cause (2% to 5% of cases). Right-to-left cardiac shunts are a particularly common associated finding in patients with brain abscesses; these infections occur in approximately 2% of all patients with cyanotic congenital heart disease. It has been suggested that the polycythemia associated with these congenital defects leads to areas of brain ischemia and necrosis that are more susceptible to hematogenously disseminated bacteria. Shunting of venous-borne bacteria around the pulmonary clearance mechanisms may also deliver a higher inoculum (mostly anaerobic organisms) to the brain. Most hematogenous abscesses are multiple and tend to occur in the white matter, especially distally in areas perfused by the middle cerebral artery.

The organisms most commonly isolated from brain abscesses are anaerobic and microaerophilic streptococci, followed by the various *Bacteroides, Fusobacterium,* and *Veillonella* spp. These organisms are particularly common when the abscess is associated with suppurative infections of the lungs. *S. pneumoniae* is rarely found today, although it was common in the preantibiotic era. The anaerobic bacteria (especially *B. fragilis*) also may be found in combination with aerobic Enterobacteriaceae (*E. coli, Klebsiella,* and *Proteus* spp.), especially with otic infection. *S. aureus* is the isolate most frequently associated with penetrating wounds or endocarditis. Less commonly, *Actinomyces* spp. or *Nocardia asteroides* is found to be associated with pulmonary infections. Pulmonary infections with *Nocardia* organisms are uniquely prevalent in compromised hosts and patients with pulmonary alveolar proteinosis. Disseminated fungal infections, including aspergillosis, mucormycosis, and candidiasis, also may result in brain abscesses in patients with impaired host resistance.

PATHOLOGY. A brain abscess evolves through several pathologic steps in its maturation. Initially after bacterial implantation a localized but poorly demarcated area of cerebritis or encephalitis develops. This is characterized by local edema, leukocyte infiltration, hyperemia, and parenchymal softening. Within days to several weeks central liquefaction and necrosis occur. Intense fibroblastic activity results in formation of granulation tissue and collagen, leading to an abscess wall that matures over weeks to months into a thick capsule. The abscess may penetrate the white matter and rupture into the ventricles, usually with catastrophic results. Infiltration of the leptomeninges near the abscess with polymorphonuclear leukocytes is common and may lead to a low-grade CSF pleocytosis without abscess rupture.

CLINICAL MANIFESTATIONS. Brain abscess typically shows signs and symptoms of an expanding mass lesion of the brain. Systemic signs of infection are frequently absent. Fever is present in only 50% of the patients and is usually at least 101° F (38.3° C). One third of the patients never have fever. Since specific predisposing conditions are associated with brain abscesses, their presence should immediately suggest the disease. Severe headache is the most common single symptom, occurring in 70% or more of cases. Therefore, when an unexplained headache occurs in a patient with chronic otitis, sinusitis, mastoiditis, pulmonary infection, prior (even in the distant past) skull fractures or penetrating wound to the skull, or a right-to-left intracardiac shunt, a brain abscess should be considered. Alterations in the level of consciousness (lethargy, irritability, confusion, or coma) occur in most patients. Nausea and vomiting are present in at least half the patients and usually reflect increased intracranial pressure. Papilledema, however, often is a late finding and is reported in only one fourth of patients. Seizures, either generalized or focal, occur in 30%, and evidence of nuchal rigidity is present in 25%.

Focal neurologic signs are found in more than 50% of the patients and reflect the location of the abscess. Abscesses in the temporal lobes (approximately 30% of all brain abscesses) are manifested by a selective aphasia (inability to name objects, read, write, or understand the spoken word). In some patients visual field cuts (homonymous upper quadrantic or hemianopic defects) or occasionally weakness of the lower face develops. Cerebellar abscesses account for 15% to 20% of the total and usually run a rapid course. Patients typically have ataxia, nystagmus, incoordination of the extremities, and occasionally an intention tremor. Frontal lobe abscesses (30% of all brain abscesses) may be inapparent with absent neurologic signs except for drowsiness or mild impairment of mental function. Hemiparesis, dysphasia, and seizures may develop during the course. Parietal lobe abscesses are unusual and may result in typical parietal lobe signs (impaired two-point discrimination, altered position sense, and astereognosis with anterior involvement and homonymous hemianopia, visual inattention, and impaired opticokinetic nystagmus with posterior lesions).

LABORATORY FINDINGS. Routine blood tests are of little help in diagnosing brain abscess. Lumbar puncture is contraindicated when a brain abscess is suspected, since this procedure may precipitate herniation when intracranial pressure is elevated.

Roentgenograms of the skull, sinuses, mastoid processes, and chest are recommended to locate possible associated suppurative processes. Electroencephalograms locate the lesion in more than 50% of the cases, but this test is less sensitive than brain scan or CT scan. Radionuclide brain scan is a very accurate and sensitive technique for detecting brain abscesses 1 cm or larger. This test is positive in up to 95% of the cases. It is especially sensitive in the early cerebritis state when localized alterations in permeability of the blood-brain barrier may be visualized. CT scan is of greatest value when the abscesses are well formed and encapsulated, and it provides a more detailed view (for example, ventricular size, midline displacement) than the radionuclide scan. If the CT scan is negative, radionuclide scanning still should be performed if a high suspicion for brain abscess exists and symptoms are of short duration. Magnetic resonance imaging (MRI) may be more sensitive than CT scanning and when available can replace the CT scan.

Carotid arteriography is of value in locating temporal lobe abscesses, and posterior circulation angiography may be necessary to detect cerebellar abscesses. These invasive techniques usually are performed preoperatively.

DIAGNOSIS. With a demonstrated source of infection (ears, sinuses, lungs) or right-to-left cardiac shunt, evidence of increased intracranial pressure, focal neurologic signs, and consistent MRI results and CT or radionuclide scans, the diagnosis is easily established. When no signs of infection or other predisposing conditions are present, the differential diagnosis of an intracranial mass lesion includes neoplasm, hematoma, focal encephalitis, and subdural hematoma. When both the noninvasive and invasive techniques are inconclusive, surgical exploration must be performed to secure the diagnosis.

MANAGEMENT. Effective treatment usually requires a combination of antimicrobial agents and surgical drainage. The recommended antimicrobial regimen is a combination of penicillin G (20 million units/day intravenously) and either metronidazole (750 mg every 6 hours) or chloramphenicol (4 to 6 g/day intravenously). This provides wide antimicrobial coverage for most of the infecting organisms commonly implicated in brain abscess. However, if *S. aureus* is a serious consideration, as in endocarditis or a penetrating wound, a semisynthetic penicillinase-resistant penicillin such as nafcillin should be added.

The timing of surgical drainage is controversial. If the lesion is treated early with appropriate antibiotics while still in the cerebritis stage or if the abscess is small, surgery may be avoided and the patient should be followed carefully with serial CT scans. Some patients have responded to antibiotics alone. Antibiotics should be given for at least 6 weeks. Surgery is urgent when the level of consciousness deteriorates or neurologic deficits increase during therapy. Drainage may be accomplished with either aspiration or complete excision and evacuation, depending on the site of the lesion. The latter procedure is preferred if possible. Mannitol, corticosteroids, or both can be used to reduce brain edema temporarily before surgery. Regardless of the therapeutic approach, mortality remains significant, approaching 15% to 25% with residual neurologic deficits or seizures in 30% to 50% of the survivors.

Subdural empyema

DEFINITION AND PATHOLOGY. A subdural empyema is a collection of pus in the space between the dura and the arachnoid membrane. It varies in size from a few milliliters to over 200 ml and is restricted to one cerebral hemisphere in three fourths of the cases. The space is limited above by the falx, laterally by the tentorium, and inferiorly by the foramen magnum and the anterior spinal canal. The major collection usually is over the frontal hemisphere; the posterior fossa rarely is involved.

PATHOGENESIS AND ETIOLOGY. Approximately 50% to 80% of cases result from an extension of infection from the frontal or ethmoid sinuses, with an additional 10% to 20% arising from middle ear or mastoid foci of disease. The infection traverses the bone and dura either by direct extension (with osteomyelitis of the frontal bone or an epidural abscess; one or both of these associated infections occur in 50% of subdural empyemas) or by emissary veins directly into the subdural space. Occasionally (5% of cases) the infection may arise hematogenously, usually from the lung. Surgical or accidental trauma also may be complicated by a subdural empyema, and in rare cases a subdural hematoma becomes secondarily infected.

The bacteria responsible for subdural empyema include the same spectrum that produces brain abscess. Streptococci, either anaerobic or microaerophilic, are found in up to 50% of cases, *S. aureus* in 10% (again usually associated with penetrating wounds), and a wide variety of gram-negative bacilli make up the remainder.

CLINICAL MANIFESTATIONS. Subdural empyemas usually occur in adults, and males predominate. Most patients have chronic sinusitis or otitis, and subdural empyema typically occurs after a flare-up of the chronic disease (that is, an increase in purulent nasal or otic discharge and pain). The first signs of intracranial infection may be obscured by the underlying process, which produces erythema, swelling, and percussion tenderness. Headache, initially mild and localized, becomes generalized and severe. Fever usually is present and is associated with chills, nausea, and vomiting. Nuchal rigidity may be present. Approximately half of the patients manifest changes in mental status early in the disease and may pass rapidly from lethargy to obtundation or coma within 48 to 72 hours. Focal or generalized seizures occur in 50% of patients, and neurologic signs including hemiparesis, aphasia, sensory defects, or visual field cuts are common. Death caused by temporal lobe herniation usually occurs within 2 days following the onset of focal neurologic signs if the condition goes untreated. Since increased intracranial pressure occurs relatively late in the disease, papilledema develops in less than 50% of the patients. The neurologic signs and symptoms result either from the mass lesion effect with compression of a single cerebral hemisphere or from the commonly associated thrombosis and phlebitis of the cortical veins, with secondary ischemic necrosis of the superficial layers of the cortex.

DIAGNOSIS. The diagnosis of subdural empyema should be considered in any patient with meningeal signs and focal neurologic deficits that are particularly localized to one cerebral hemisphere, especially if chronic sinusitis is present. A lumbar puncture should not be performed if evidence of increased intracranial pressure is present.

Skull roentgenograms or CT scans show sinusitis, otitis, or mastoiditis in two thirds of the cases and may show a pineal shift. The diagnostic procedure of choice is either the CT scan, which shows a collection of pus, or cerebral arteriography, which demonstrates separation of cerebral vessels from the cranium. In some cases burr holes drilled through the skull are necessary for diagnosis.

MANAGEMENT. A subdural empyema constitutes a true neurosurgical emergency, since death usually occurs rapidly once neurologic findings have appeared. Mannitol, hyperventilation, or corticosteroids temporarily may reduce cerebral edema and allow time to organize a surgical procedure, but immediate surgical drainage is essential.

Antibiotic coverage should include penicillin G in high doses (20 million units/day intravenously) and chloramphenicol (4 to 6 g/day intravenously).

Epidural abscess

CEREBRAL EPIDURAL ABSCESS. A cerebral epidural abscess usually results from extension of infection from osteomyelitis of the skull or chronic infection of the ear or paranasal sinuses. Since the dura forms the intracranial periosteum of the skull, an abscess can develop only by stripping this membrane from bone. Thus an epidural abscess usually is well confined in extent. It is difficult to diagnose, since the features of the more external infection dominate the clinical picture. Patients are not as ill as with subdural empyema but usually have pain. As the abscess enlarges, neurologic signs may develop with evidence of increased intracranial pressure. The pathogenesis and bacteriologic findings are similar to those of subdural empyema, and these conditions may be viewed as a continuum. The diagnosis is best made with a CT scan. When detected, these abscesses should be surgically drained to prevent progression to a subdural empyema. Antibiotic therapy includes a combination of penicillin in high doses and chloramphenicol, as for subdural empyema and brain abscess.

SPINAL EPIDURAL ABSCESS

Definition. Within the spinal canal an epidural space that is filled with fat and vascular tissue separates the dura from the vertebral bodies. An infection that is established in this space encounters little resistance to longitudinal spread, and because outward expansion is rigidly limited by the vertebral column, small volumes of pus can produce serious spinal cord compression and necrosis.

Etiology and pathogenesis. The spinal epidural space can be infected via the hematogenous metastatic route from a distant site (most cases), by direct extension from vertebral osteomyelitis (less common except with tuberculosis), or by an invasion from a decubitus or perispinal abscess. Cases have been associated with back surgery, lumbar puncture, and epidural spinal anesthesia. Up to 30% of patients give a history of antecedent back trauma. Underlying conditions such as diabetes mellitus, intravenous drug use, and in rare cases pregnancy may predispose a patient to epidural abscesses.

S. aureus accounts for most (60% to 80%) cases. The most common concurrent infections are cutaneous furuncles, boils, ulcers, and wound infections. Respiratory tract and genitourinary tract infections also have been implicated. Streptococci (anaerobic and aerobic) account for approximately 20%, and gram-negative aerobic rods (*E. coli*, and *Pseudomonas*, *Salmonella*, and *Klebsiella* organisms, and others) cause approximately 10%. Ten percent of cultures are mixed. Tuberculosis is common in highly endemic areas. Various fungi also have been implicated in rare cases.

Pathology. Most abscesses are localized to the posterior portion of the spinal canal but spread to involve four to six vertebral bodies and occasionally the entire spine. The thoracic spine most commonly is involved (two thirds of cases), followed by lumbar areas (one fourth) and cervical areas (one fifth). Vertebral osteomyelitis is present in less than 20% of acute cases but in more than half of chronic cases.

Clinical manifestations. The clinical presentation of a spinal epidural abscess has been divided into four distinct phases. However, since this disease can present a very acute course, these artificial phases may fuse with each other. Initially there is focal pain or "spinal ache" and percussion tenderness over the involved area. Systemic symptoms (fever) usually are prominent, and spine stiffness and scoliosis may develop. The next phase is characterized by radicular or root pain. Meningeal signs become prominent, hyperalgesia or depressed reflexes may appear in the involved segments, and most patients have headache. The diagnosis may be readily made during this phase. Next, distinct neurologic deficits including motor loss (weakness), sensory loss (below the level of the lesion), or loss of sphincter tone (incontinence, urgency, retention) appear. Pain and nuchal rigidity become more severe. Within hours to several days paralysis that may be severe or even total occurs. If the lesion is not drained and paralysis remains for more than several hours, it usually is permanent.

The course is most rapid when hematogenous dissemination occurs and is accompanied by prominent systemic toxic effects and severe focal pain. When the abscess results from vertebral osteomyelitis, the initial phases may be prolonged (2 to 3 weeks); however, once radicular pain develops, the progression to paralysis often is rapid. Spinal epidural abscess can be mimicked by acute myelitis of various causes (although back pain usually is not as severe), progressive adhesive arachnoiditis, and in the chronic state malignant tumors, especially lymphomas.

Diagnosis. The diagnosis is still best established by myelogram, although CT scanning and MRI look promising. Lumbar puncture should be done with care, and the spinal needle should be inserted either above or below the suspected lesion. The needle is advanced slowly, and repeated aspirations are attempted. If pus is not located, the needle (with the stylet in) is advanced into the subarachnoid space, CSF is obtained, and a myelogram is performed. The CSF is characteristically xanthochromic with few leukocytes. The glucose level usually is normal, but the protein level may be quite elevated (200 to 2000 mg/dl).

Management. Immediate neurosurgical exploration and drainage are required. A semisynthetic penicillinase-resistant penicillin should be administered to cover *S. aureus* and the streptococci. This should be altered or expanded if the Gram stain of the surgical specimen demonstrates other pathogens such as gram-negative bacilli.

Transverse myelitis or myelopathy

Transverse myelitis is a rare clinical syndrome with several causes that produces impaired neurologic function below well-delineated spinal cord segments. Pathologically, the lesion is an area of destruction commonly affecting both white and gray matter and may be characterized by demyelination, necrosis, and occasionally an inflammatory reaction. The conditions associated with this unusual disease are numerous and include viral infections, particularly enterovirus, herpes zoster, and Epstein-Barr virus; rabies and B virus myelitis; inflammatory diseases of the meninges (syphilis, pyogenic infections, tuberculosis, parasitic or fungal infections, and chronic adhesive arachnoiditis); and various vascular and nutritional abnormalities. In many cases (acute multiple sclerosis, postinfectious or necrotizing myelitis) the cause is unknown.

The clinical course usually begins with abrupt onset, occasionally in a setting of viral illness or minor trauma. The neurologic findings are variable, as are the characteristics of the CSF. It is imperative to rule out a correctable lesion or one requiring treatment (such as an epidural abscess). Most patients improve with supportive care.

BIBLIOGRAPHY

American Academy of Pediatrics: Report of the Committee on Infectious Disease, ed 20, Elk Grove Village, Ill, 1986, The Academy.

Baker AS and others: Spinal epidural abscess, N Engl J Med 293:463, 1975.

Carpenter RR and Petersdorf RG: The clinical spectrum of bacterial meningitis, Am J Med 33:262, 1962.

Dacey RG Jr and Winn HR: Brain abscess and perimeningeal infections. In Stein JH, editor: Internal Medicine, ed 2, Boston, 1987, Little, Brown & Co, Inc.

Danner RL and Hartman BJ: Update on spinal epidural abscess: 35 cases and review of the literature, Rev Infect Dis 9:265, 1987.

deLouvois J: The bacteriology and chemotherapy of brain abscess, J Antimicrob Chemother 4:395, 1978.

Fothergill LD and Wright J: Influenza meningitis: the relation of age incidence to the bactericidal power of blood against the causal organism, J Immunol 24:273, 1933.

Kaufmann DM and others: Subdural empyema: analysis of 17 recent cases and review of the literature, Medicine 54:485, 1975.

Klein JO, Feigin RD, and McCracken GH Jr: Report of the task force on diagnosis and management of meningitis, Pediatrics 78:959, 1986.

McCracken GH Jr and others: Consensus report: antimicrobial therapy for bacterial meningitis in infants and children, Pediatr Infect Dis 6:501, 1987.

Meyer HM and others: Central nervous system syndromes of "viral" etiology: a study of 713 cases, Am J Med 29:334, 1960.

Quagliarello VJ and Scheld WM: Recent advances in the pathogenesis and pathophysiology of bacterial meningitis, Am J Med Sci 292:306, 1986.

Reinis CM, Shibl AM, and Sande MA: Pathophysiological processes of bacterial meningitis, Infections in Medicine 4:192, 1987.

Rosenblum ML and others: Nonoperative treatment of brain abscesses in selected high-risk patients, J Neurosurg 52:217, 1980.

Sande MA, Smith AL, and Root RK, editors: Bacterial meningitis. Contemporary issues in infectious diseases, vol 3, New York, 1985, Churchill Livingstone, Inc.

Scheld WM: Acute meningitis. In Stein JH, editor: Internal medicine, ed 2, Boston, 1987, Little, Brown & Co, Inc.

Swartz MN and Dodge PR: Bacterial meningitis: a review of selected aspects. I. General clinical features, special problems and unusual meningeal reactions mimicking bacterial meningitis, N Engl J Med 272:725, 779, 842, 898, 954, 1003, 1965.

Wispelwey B and Scheld WM: Brain abscess, Clin Neuropharmacol, 10:483, 1987 (in press).

Urinary tract infection and perinephric abscess

Donald Kaye

DEFINITIONS. *Significant bacteriuria* describes the numbers of bacteria in voided urine that exceed the numbers usually caused by contamination from the anterior urethra (that is, $\geq 10^5$ bacteria/ml). *Asymptomatic bacteriuria* refers to significant bacteriuria in a patient without symptoms. The term "cystitis" has been used to describe the syndrome involving dysuria, frequency, urgency, and occasionally suprapubic tenderness. However, these symptoms may be related to lower tract inflammation without bacterial infection and can be caused by urethritis (for example, gonorrhea or chlamydial urethritis). Furthermore, the presence of symptoms of lower tract infection without upper tract symptoms by no means excludes upper tract infection, which is also often present.

Acute pyelonephritis describes the clinical syndrome characterized by flank pain and tenderness and fever, often associated with dysuria, urgency, and frequency.

Urinary tract infection may occur de novo or may be a recurrent infection. Recurrences may be either *relapses* or *reinfections*. Relapse of bacteriuria refers to recurrence of bacteriuria with the *same* infecting microorganism that was present before therapy was started. This is caused by persistence of the organism in the urinary tract. Reinfection is a recurrence of bacteriuria with a microorganism different from the original infecting bacterium. It is a new infection. Occasionally reinfection may occur with the same microorganism, which may have persisted in the vagina or feces. This can be mistaken for a relapse.

The term "chronic pyelonephritis" means different things to different authors. To some, chronic pyelonephritis refers to pathologic changes in the kidney caused by infection only. However, identical pathologic alterations are found in several other entities such as chronic urinary tract obstruction, analgesic nephropathy, hypokalemic nephropathy, vascular disease, and uric acid nephropathy.

ETIOLOGY. *E. coli* causes most cases of urinary tract infection. In patients with recurrent infections, structural abnormalities of the urinary tract, or hospital-acquired infections the frequency of infection caused by *Proteus, Klebsiella-Enterobacter,* and *Pseudomonas* spp., enterococci, and staphylococci increases. Anaerobic organisms rarely cause urinary tract infection.

EPIDEMIOLOGY. Urinary tract infection is rare in men in the absence of instrumentation or structural abnormalities of the urinary tract. There is less than a 0.1% prevalence of infection in men until the age when prostatic disease occurs, at which time it increases to about 4%. The prevalence of bacteriuria is 1% to 3% in young adult women and rises with age (10% to 15% in elderly women). In the very old (men and women), the prevalence of bacteriuria is even higher. Each year bacteriuria clears in about 25% of bacteriuric women, and they are replaced by an equal number who have become infected (often women who have had urinary infection previously). At least 10% to 20% of the female population have a urinary tract infection at some time during their lives.

The prevalence of bacteriuria in pregnancy is 3% to 7% and increases with greater parity and a lower socioeconomic status. About 20% of the patients with bacteriuria early in gestation have acute pyelonephritis later in pregnancy. In contrast, less than 1% of the patients whose urine is uninfected early in gestation have acute infection. Over 75% of the cases of acute pyelonephritis can be prevented by eliminating asymptomatic bacteriuria in the early stages of pregnancy.

PATHOGENESIS. Although some renal infections occur via the hematogenous route (for example, staphylococcal abscesses resulting from staphylococcal bacteremia), classic urinary tract infection rarely if ever occurs this way. Most urinary tract infection occurs by the ascending route either spontaneously or following catheterization or instrumentation of the urinary tract. The vaginal introitus occasionally becomes colonized by gram-negative enteric bacilli, and this predisposes the woman to infection. The proximity of the vagina to the rectum and the short urethra of women undoubtedly increase the susceptibility of women to infection and help explain their much greater frequency of infection.

Obstruction, incomplete emptying of the bladder, and calculi all have been associated with infection. Vesicoureteral reflux tends to spread infection from the bladder to the kidney.

Certain virulence factors have been identified in bacteria (such as pili on *Proteus mirabilis* and *E. coli* and K antigen on *E. coli*).

CLINICAL MANIFESTATIONS. Most patients with either lower or upper urinary tract infection are asymptomatic. The symptoms of lower tract infection when present are dysuria, frequency, and urgency; fever usually is absent. However, up to 50% of the patients with these symptoms do not have significant bacteriuria. Some of these episodes (up to half) are associated with low titers of Enterobacteriaceae (for example, 1000/ml) in bladder urine. Others are caused by urethritis from trauma, gonorrhea, or *Chlamydia* organisms.

Symptoms of upper tract infection are flank pain, flank tenderness, and fever, which often are associated with lower tract symptoms.

DIAGNOSIS. Pyuria usually is present in symptomatic urinary infection but may be absent with asymptomatic bacteriuria. White cell casts in the urine indicate upper tract involvement. Many patients without infection have pyuria owing to other processes. Proteinuria is common in infection, and hematuria may occur.

Blood cultures occasionally are positive in patients with acute pyelonephritis. The most definitive diagnosis of urinary tract infection is based on finding $\geq 10^5$ bacteria/ml urine on a culture of a clean-catch, midstream urine specimen. One positive culture is adequate in the presence of symptoms, but two confirmatory cultures are necessary in asymptomatic patients. One positive culture gives only an 80% probability of infection in an asymptomatic patient; two positive cultures raise the probability to 95%. Visualization of more than one organism per $\times 400$ microscopic field in a midstream, Gram-stained, uncentrifuged urine specimen correlates highly with a titer of $\geq 10^5$ bacteria/ml. A titer of $\geq 10^5$ bacteria/ml of catheterized urine or any growth from a suprapubic aspirate of urine is highly suggestive of infection. Cultures containing gram-negative bacilli in titers of 10^4 to 10^5/ml should be repeated. Gram-positive cocci do not grow well in urine, and infections with these organisms may often give titers of 10^4 to 10^5/ml.

Many different techniques have been developed to localize the site of infection. Loss of ability to concentrate urine and production of circulating antibody have been found to correlate with upper tract infection. More reliable but invasive methods involve (1) direct catheterization of the ureters with quantitative cultures of urine or (2) washout of the bladder with a solution containing antibiotic and enzymes to sterilize the bladder, and then immediate collection and quantitative culture of newly formed urine. (Presumably if the bacteria are found, they come from the ureters.)

It has been determined that bacteria in urine of renal origin are coated with antibody. Thus the antibody-coated bacteria (ACB) test has been developed in which fluorescein-conjugated antihuman globulin added to bacteriuric urine is examined under a fluorescent microscope. Fluorescence indicates upper tract infection. False positive results may be observed in men with a prostatic focus of infection, and false negative results may occur in very early upper tract infection.

Patients at relatively high risk of urologic abnormalities (especially obstruction) should have an intravenous pyelogram and a postevacuation view of the bladder to evaluate for residual urine. This includes children, males of any age, patients who relapse after appropriate therapy, and those with bacteremia. It is unnecessary to obtain roentgenographic studies on adult women with their first urinary tract infection. After three or four reinfections evaluation may be indicated.

Vesicoureteral reflux is particularly important in preschool-age children and predisposes them to renal scarring. Therefore all preschool children with proven urinary tract infection probably should be evaluated with a voiding cystourethrogram to detect reflux. This procedure rarely is indicated in older children and adults.

COURSE. Bacteremia may occur with pyelonephritis (especially in the presence of obstruction) and can be fatal. With or without treatment, symptoms of infection are self-limited and subside. Many infections spontaneously disappear. Recurrence is common in the form of either relapse after treatment (infection never eradicated) or reinfection (new infection). Reinfections are common in women but unusual in men unless catheterized.

In children, especially in the presence of vesicoureteral reflux (which is common in young children), infection can seriously damage the kidneys. In adults, in the absence of obstruction it is questionable if urinary tract infection ever is the major factor leading to renal insufficiency. Similarly, there is no clear-cut relationship between urinary tract infection and hypertension.

There is a definite association between acute pyelonephritis of pregnancy and premature delivery. The rate of prematurity can be as high as 20% to 50%. Prematurity also seems to be increased in patients with asymptomatic bacteriuria. Because of the implications for both mother and fetus, screening for and treatment of bacteriuria at the first prenatal visit seem justified. Treatment of bacteriuria during pregnancy has little effect on the long-term course of the mother.

MANAGEMENT. Since the prognosis of urinary tract infection in nonpregnant adult women seems to be quite good and reinfection is common, therapy probably makes little contribution to the patient's well-being other than eradicating symptoms. Urinary tract infection is very common in the elderly, and a higher frequency of side effects from chemotherapy would be expected in the older age group because of preexisting renal, auditory, and other diseases. Considering the usual absence of progressive renal impairment, the large numbers of patients involved, and the fact that intensive antimicrobial therapy may lead to an unwarranted financial burden and the danger of drug toxicity, such treatment may do more harm than good in elderly patients.

In contrast, bacteriuria in preschool-age children with vesicoureteral reflux can result in stunted growth of the kidney, scar formation, and in rare cases renal failure. Bacteriuria in pregnancy also may have serious implications. Treatment of children and pregnant women is most likely to be beneficial. Furthermore, it is feasible to treat all of these patients, since the prevalence of bacteriuria is relatively low in these groups.

Symptomatic patients usually must be treated regardless of age, even when infection is likely to recur. Some patients have such frequent symptomatic episodes (either relapses or reinfections) that they are almost chronically incapacitated. In these patients it may be necessary to give prolonged therapy or prophylaxis to prevent recurrent symptoms.

Although there are theoretic reasons for (as well as against) forcing fluids in the management of urinary tract infection, these measures are not indicated in modern antimicrobial therapy. Urinary analgesics such as phenazopyridine hydrochloride (Pyridium) also have little place in the routine management of symptomatic infections. The dysuria of urinary tract infection usually responds rapidly to antibacterial therapy and requires no local analgesia.

Disappearance of bacteriuria is closely correlated with the sensitivity of the microorganism to the concentration of the antimicrobial agent achieved in the urine. Although blood levels of antimicrobials do not seem to be important in the treatment of urinary tract infection, they may be critical in patients with bacteremia.

In patients with renal insufficiency, dosage modifications are necessary for agents that are excreted primarily by the kidneys and cannot be cleared by any other mechanism. In renal failure the kidney may not be able to concentrate an antimicrobial agent in the urine, and difficulty in eradicating bacteriuria may occur.

There are four patterns of response of bacteriuria to antimicrobial therapy: cure, persistence, relapse, and reinfection. Quantitative bacterial counts in urine should decrease within 48 hours after initiation of an antimicrobial agent to which the microorganism is sensitive in vitro. If titers do not decrease within this time (*persistence*), the therapy being given will be unsuccessful.

Relapse usually occurs within 2 weeks after cessation of chemotherapy and often is associated with renal infection, structural abnormalities of the urinary tract, or chronic bacterial prostatitis. Relapse indicates that the infecting microorganism has persisted in the urinary tract during therapy. However, an apparent relapse can be related to reinfection (new infection) with the same microorganism.

After initial sterilization of the urine, *reinfection* may occur during administration of chemotherapy or at any time thereafter. Reinfection is easy to identify when there is a change in bacterial species. However, there may be reinfection with a different serotype of the same species (usually *E. coli*) or even the same serotype.

Symptomatic urinary tract infection. Most patients with symptomatic urinary tract infection are women, usually of childbearing age. The onset of symptoms frequently is related to sexual intercourse. Although no one chemotherapeutic agent is unequivocally the drug of choice, a short-acting oral sulfonamide such as sulfisoxazole (Gantrisin) (1 g four times a day in adults) has been used for many years. Other options are ampicillin, amoxicillin, cephalexin, cephradine, nitrofurantoin, tetracycline, and trimethoprim-sulfamethoxazole. The adult doses are ampicillin and amoxicillin, 500 mg to 1 g four times a day; cephalexin or cephradine, 250 to 500 mg four times a day; nitrofurantoin, 100 mg four times a day; tetracycline, 250 to 500 mg four times a day; trimethoprim-sulfamethoxazole, two tablets twice a day; amoxicillin-clavulanic acid, one tablet three times a day; norfloxacin, 400 mg twice a day; and ciprofloxacin, 250 mg twice a day.

In patients with lower tract infection, 1 day of therapy or, in fact, only one dose (for example, 3 g of amoxicillin or four tablets of trimethoprim-sulfamethoxazole) usually is sufficient for cure. It therefore seems reasonable to treat patients with lower tract symptoms only (that is, no fever, flank pain, or flank tenderness) with short-term therapy (that is, 1 to 3 days).

In contrast to lower tract infection, patients with upper tract infection require at least 2 weeks of treatment. In these patients, urine cultures or microscopic examination of the urine for significant bacteriuria should be obtained after 3 or 4 days of therapy. If bacteriologic response has not occurred, the therapy is changed to one of the alternative drugs on the basis of sensitivity tests.

If gram-negative bacillary bacteremia is suspected to be complicating urinary tract infection because of symptoms of high fever, shaking chills, and hypotension, chemotherapy should be directed at the life-threatening bacteremia.

A follow-up urine culture may be obtained 1 to 2 weeks after the discontinuance of therapy to detect relapses. In children additional follow-up cultures should be obtained at 6 weeks and 6 months to detect reinfections.

Asymptomatic bacteriuria. Most patients with asymptomatic bacteriuria are women, usually in the older age-group. Although cure may result following treatment, relapse and especially reinfection are common. Although all children should be treated, therapy of asymptomatic bacteriuria in adults is by no means mandatory in the absence of obstruction. If the infecting microorganism is resistant to all but toxic agents, treatment should not be instituted in nonobstructed, nonpregnant adults. It is reasonable to use short-course therapy as a first approach.

Relapsing urinary tract infection. A patient who suffers a relapse after short-course therapy should receive a standard 2-week course. A patient who relapses after a 2-week course most likely has (1) renal involvement, (2) a structural abnormality of the urinary tract (for example, calculi), or (3) chronic bacterial prostatitis.

Relapses, especially in the absence of structural abnormalities, may be related to renal infection that requires a longer duration of therapy (3 to 6 weeks or even longer). Urinary tract infection in the presence of obstruction is likely to be associated with renal involvement and a tendency for renal functional impairment and bacteremia. Calculi may be a cause of relapse of urinary tract infection. The ultimate success of chemotherapy depends on the removal of stones. Only carefully selected patients such as children, adults who have continuous symptoms, or adults who are at high risk of developing progressive renal damage (for example, those with obstruction not amenable to surgery) should be considered for long courses of therapy. Some of the agents that can be used for long-term therapy are ampicillin, amoxicillin, sulfisoxazole, cephalexin, cephradine, and trimethoprim-sulfamethoxazole in the usual doses already described; nitrofurantoin in full dosage for 1 week and then half the usual dose; nalidixic acid (1 g four times daily in adults); carbenicillin indanyl sodium (two tablets four times daily in adults); and methenamine mandelate (1 g four times daily in adults) with methionine or ascorbic acid to acidify the urine.

Patients receiving methenamine mandelate (or hippurate) are instructed to avoid alkalinizing foods such as milk, all fruit juices other than cranberry juice, and bicarbonate of soda. In addition, they are given nitrazine paper to test their urine several times a day to regulate the dosage of methionine or ascorbic acid so that the urinary pH is maintained at 5.5 or below. This increases the effectiveness of the antimicrobial agent. Urine cultures should be obtained at least monthly to determine the effectiveness of therapy.

Probably the most common cause of relapses of urinary tract

infection in males is *chronic bacterial prostatitis*. Patients with this entity usually have no symptoms or signs related to the prostate but have a nidus of infection in the gland. Rectal examination usually is unremarkable. Periodically, urinary tract infection occurs when enough bacteria reach the bladder to overwhelm its normal defense mechanisms. The diagnosis is proved by means of a quantitative bacterial localization technique.

This study should be done at a time when the patient does not have significant bacteriuria. If bacteriuria is present, ampicillin, cephalexin, or nitrofurantoin should be given for 2 to 3 days to sterilize the urine; these agents do not affect bacterial counts in the prostate in chronic bacterial prostatitis. Because bacteria present in the urethra can contaminate prostatic secretions obtained by prostatic massage, accurate diagnosis requires simultaneous quantitative cultures of (1) urethral or first-voided urine (VB_1); (2) midstream urine (VB_2); (3) prostatic secretions expressed by massage (EPS); and (4) the urine voided after massage (VB_3). An ejaculate probably is preferable to the EPS.

The specimens must be cultured immediately after collection, and methods of quantitating small numbers of bacteria must be used. If chronic bacterial prostatitis is present, the number of bacteria in the EPS or ejaculate will exceed those in VB_1 or VB_2 urine by at least 10-fold. If no EPS or ejaculate can be obtained, the bacterial counts in the VB_3 specimen should be at least 10-fold higher than the VB_1 or VB_2 samples.

Trimethoprim-sulfamethoxazole appears to be an effective therapy available for chronic bacterial prostatitis. Approximately one third of patients can be cured with prolonged therapy with this agent (that is, two tablets given twice daily for 12 weeks). Oral carbenicillin indanyl sodium also may be useful when given for long periods. Norfloxacin and ciprofloxacin also seem to be effective. If cure is not obtained, the patient should be managed either with treatment of acute exacerbations of urinary tract infection or with long-term suppressive therapy using low daily doses (for example, half normal doses) of an antimicrobial agent.

Reinfection of the urinary tract. Patients with reinfection generally can be divided into two groups: (1) those who have relatively infrequent reinfections, perhaps only once every 2 or 3 years to several times a year, and (2) those who have frequent reinfections. With infrequent reinfections, each episode can be approached with a course of therapy as if it were a new episode of either symptomatic or asymptomatic infection.

Many patients with frequent reinfections after therapy are middle-aged or elderly women in whom infection is limited to the lower urinary tract. Most asymptomatic reinfections in this group should not be treated because the frequent use of antimicrobial agents is apt to result in toxic side effects and because progressive destruction of the kidneys is rare. If, however, the episodes are symptomatic or the likelihood of renal damage is increased, these patients should be treated.

Occasionally patients of any age have symptomatic reinfection so frequently that they can be incapacitated. In some women these symptomatic reinfections are associated with sexual activity. Voiding immediately after intercourse may help prevent reinfection. However, single-dose prophylactic chemotherapy taken after sexual intercourse is a more effective method of decreasing episodes.

In other patients with frequent symptomatic reinfections, no precipitating event is apparent; in these patients, long-term chemoprophylaxis may be instituted when symptoms are severe. Although these courses seem to decrease the incidence of reinfections and symptoms in most patients, it is impossible to prevent reinfection completely in many patients. When reinfection occurs during chemoprophylaxis, the prophylactic agent must be changed.

Long-term chemoprophylaxis should be considered for asymptomatic patients who are reinfected frequently and are at risk of developing renal parenchymal damage with each reinfection (for example, young children with vesicoureteral reflux and children and adults with obstructive uropathy). Keeping patients in these groups abacteriuric helps protect the kidneys. Trimethoprim-sulfamethoxazole and nitrofurantoin are particularly useful for long-term prophylaxis because these drugs are unlikely to allow the emergence of antimicrobial-resistant bacteria with prolonged use. One 100 mg tablet of nitrofurantoin or half a tablet of trimethoprim-sulfamethoxazole nightly will suffice.

Patients receiving long-term prophylaxis should be followed closely, with urine cultures performed at least monthly or more often if interim symptomatic episodes develop. Therapy is continued with the same agent as long as patients remain abacteriuric. If bacteriuria persists or recurs during administration of an antimicrobial agent, therapy is altered using the response of bacteriuria as a parameter of adequacy of therapy. Long-term prophylaxis can be undertaken only if urine cultures are obtained frequently, and therapy is altered if bacteriuria recurs.

PREVENTION. Catheterization of the urinary bladder should be avoided if possible. The risk of infection after a single catheterization is about 1% but is higher in elderly or debilitated patients, patients with urologic abnormalities, and pregnant women. Individuals with indwelling catheters have a much greater risk of infection. Essentially all patients with an open drainage system develop infection within 4 days. The use of a triple-lumen catheter with a neomycin-plus-polymyxin B continuous rinse or the use of a sterile drainage system delays the development of bacteriuria to beyond 10 days in most patients.

PERINEPHRIC ABSCESS

Perinephric abscess is an uncommon complication of urinary tract infection. It usually occurs as a result of obstruction of an infected kidney or calyx or occasionally as a result of bacteremia. The infecting bacteria are usually gram-negative enteric bacilli and occasionally gram-positive cocci when the infection is of hematogenous origin.

The patients have a syndrome suggestive of acute pyelonephritis with fever, abdominal and flank pain (usually unilateral), and often symptoms of lower urinary tract infection. The patients have often been ill for 2 or more weeks. The diagnosis of perinephric abscess should be strongly considered in any patient with a febrile illness and unilateral flank pain who does not respond to therapy for acute pyelonephritis. A palpable mass may or may not be present. About half of the patients have an abnormal plain film of the abdomen (such as abdominal mass, a calculus, or a poorly defined renal shadow), and most have abnormal intravenous pyelograms.

Perinephric abscess is treated with surgical drainage after first starting parenteral antimicrobial therapy directed against the infecting organism isolated from the urine.

BIBLIOGRAPHY

Andriole VT: Advances in the treatment of urinary infections, J Antimicrob Chemother 9(suppl A):163, 1982.

Meares EM: Long-term therapy of chronic bacterial prostatitis with trimethoprim-sulfamethoxazole, Can Med Assoc J 112:225, 1975.

Romano JM and Kaye D: UTI in the elderly: common yet atypical, Geriatrics 36:113, 1981.

Sobel JD and Kaye D: Urinary tract infections. In Mandell GL, Douglas RG

Jr, and Bennett JE, editors: Principles and practice of infectious diseases, New York, 1990, Churchill Livingstone.

Souney P and Polk BF: Single antimicrobial therapy for urinary tract infections in women, Rev Infect Dis 4:29, 1982.

Stamey TA and others: Serum versus urinary antimicrobial concentrations in cure of urinary tract infections, N Engl J Med 291:1159, 1974.

Stamm WE: Guidelines for prevention of catheter-associated urinary tract infections, Ann Intern Med 82:386, 1975.

Stamm WE and others: Antimicrobial prophylaxis of recurrent urinary tract infections, Ann Intern Med 92:770, 1980.

Stamm WE and others: Causes of the acute urethral syndrome in women, N Engl J Med 303:409, 1980.

Stamm WE and others: Treatment of the acute urethral syndrome, N Engl J Med 304:956, 1981.

Thomas VL and Forland M: Antibody coated bacteria in urinary tract infections, Kidney Int 21:1, 1982.

41 · DISEASES SPREAD THROUGH FOOD AND WATER

Matthew E. Levison

DEFINITION. An ingested substance in the form of food or water can produce illness by being toxic itself or by being contaminated with (1) chemical toxins (Table 41-1) or (2) infectious agents (Tables 41-2 to 41-4). Two types of microbial waterborne or foodborne illness are recognized: (1) intoxications following the ingestion of a preformed microbial toxin, examples of which are given in Table 41-2 (botulism, an example of this type of disease, is described in more detail in a subsequent section); and (2) true infections following the ingestion of viable microorganisms (Tables 41-2 to 41-4). Some of these intestinal pathogens only superficially colonize the mucosal surface, for example, enterotoxigenic *Escherichia coli* or *Vibrio cholerae* (Table 41-2). In these cases disease results from elaboration of various enterotoxins once mucosal colonization is established. Cholera, an example of this type of infection, is described in more detail in a subsequent section. Other intestinal pathogens invade the bowel wall, and disease results from the subsequent inflammatory reaction and in some cases from the additional elaboration of enterotoxins (Tables 41-3 and 41-4).

DIAGNOSIS. The types of food ingested frequently can suggest the diagnosis. For example, foodborne outbreaks caused by chemical toxins usually involve fish, mushrooms, Chinese food, and beverages (Table 41-1), whereas foodborne outbreaks caused by bacteria involve beef, poultry, ham, desserts, and salads. Exceptions are smoked fish and mushrooms, which have caused botulism, and Chinese food, which has caused *Bacillus cereus* intoxication.

An intoxication, either from the food itself or from chemical or microbial contaminants, is suggested by an incubation period of less than several hours' duration (with the exception of botulism and some types of mushroom poisoning, which may have longer incubation periods).

Slightly longer incubation periods (hours to a few days) are associated with (1) diseases that require an initial bacterial proliferation in the intestinal tract and subsequent invasion, as listed in Table 41-3, and (2) diseases resulting from intraluminal production of an exterotoxin following colonization of the small bowel, as listed under "Endogenously produced toxins" in Table 41-2. Parasitic infections and illnesses caused by certain viruses become clinically manifest days to weeks following exposure (Table 41-4).

The presence of neurologic signs suggests chemical intoxication or botulism. An elevated temperature indicates tissue invasion caused by the organisms in Tables 41-3 and 41-4.

A search for fecal leukocytes, using methylene blue stain, should be done in any patient with fever or bloody diarrhea. Fecal polymorphonuclear leukocytes in such a patient indicate invasive colonic disease, as in Table 41-3. (Note that fecal leukocytes are present in *Clostridium difficile* colitis but may be sparse or absent in *Salmonella* gastroenteritis and amebic colitis). The presence of fecal leukocytes, moderate to severe diarrhea (6 or more unformed stools) or fever is an indication for performing a stool culture or other laboratory tests to establish an etiologic diagnosis.

PROGNOSIS. Fortunately, most waterborne and foodborne illnesses are acute and self-limited and require only symptomatic therapy such as oral electrolyte and fluid therapy. In cases of giardiasis, amebiasis, shigellosis, typhoid fever, and *Salmonella* bacteremia and localized infection, specific antibiotic therapy is indicated. Antimicrobial therapy may be helpful in *Yersinia* or *Campylobacter* infections and other causes of infectious diarrhea. The fluorinated quinolones (for example, norfloxacin and ciprofloxacin) have proved useful in treating acute infectious diarrheal illness caused by a variety of intestinal pathogens, including *Campylobacter*, *Salmonella*, and *Shigella* organisms and *E. coli*. Although not approved as yet in the United States for this purpose, these oral agents may become the drugs of choice for febrile or inflammatory diarrheas, especially when used empirically (that is, when cultures cannot be done or have not as yet yielded answers). However, these agents are not active against *C. difficile* or the protozoas. These diseases are fatal only in patients with chronic, debilitating diseases, in those at the extremes of age, or in those with severe chemical food poisoning or botulism.

BOTULISM

Botulism is an acute intoxication following ingestion of food containing a heat-labile neurotoxin elaborated by *Clostridium botulinum*. Neuromuscular disturbances occur. Similar manifestations can be seen when the neurotoxin is released in wounds infected with *C. botulinum* (wound botulism) or when exotoxin is released within the bowel lumen colonized by *C. botulinum* (infant botulism).

ETIOLOGY. *C. botulinum*, a sporeforming, gram-positive, anaerobic rod, can produce one of seven antigenically different types of neurotoxin, A to G. Disease usually is caused by types A, B, or E.

EPIDEMIOLOGY. The spores of *C. botulinum* are highly heat resistant; in water their destruction requires 5 hours at 212° F (100° C) or 6 minutes at 248° F (120° C). In improperly prepared food, spores may germinate and neurotoxin may be released when the food is preserved in an anaerobic environment (canned or vacuum-packed foods). Heating the food at 176° F (80° C) for 30 minutes or boiling for 10 minutes readily destroys the neurotoxin, but eating the food without prior cooking sufficient to destroy the neurotoxin may result in botulism. Since multiplication of *C. botulinum* is inhibited in acid media, alkaline-preserved foods most commonly are involved. These include home-preserved or commercially preserved vegetables such as mushrooms, string beans, or corn; canned fruits; smoked fish; or pork and beef products. Widespread illness occurs as a result of national distribution of commercially prepared food, which may be marketed under several different brand names. Recent outbreaks have involved canned tuna, canned vichyssoise, and vacuum-packed smoked whitefish. Type E frequently is found in fish from the Great Lakes. Type E spores are relatively heat sensitive but survive smoking or light cooking.

Table 41-1   Chemical food poisoning

Etiology	Incriminated foods	Incubation period	Clinical features	Duration of illness	Diagnosis	Therapy
Ciguatera fish poisoning: heat-stable ciguatoxin	Liver, other viscera, and muscle of large fish such as barracuda, red snapper, amberjack, and grouper (Hawaii and Florida)	1-6 hours	Paresthesias of lips, tongue, and throat, visual disturbances, vomiting, watery diarrhea; in more severe cases, sinus bradycardia, respiratory paralysis, hypotension	Few days-weeks	Detection of ciguatoxin in food	Symptomatic: cleansing of GI tract to remove unabsorbed toxin; ventilatory assistance
Scombroid fish poisoning: bacterial decomposition of fish flesh	Tuna, mackerel, bonito, shipjack	Few minutes-1 hour	Flushing, headache, abdominal cramps, nausea, vomiting, diarrhea, urticaria, and pruritus (symptoms are those of a histamine reaction); in more severe cases, bronchospasm	Few hours	Detection of toxic levels of histamine in food	Symptomatic—antihistamines, bronchodilators
Paralytic shellfish poisoning: ingestion of toxic heat-stable neurotoxin of dinoflagellates by shellfish	Bivalve mollusks: mussels, clams, oysters, scallops (June-October) (Pacific Coast and New England)	<30 minutes	Paresthesias of mouth, lips, face, and extremities, visual disturbances, nausea, vomiting, diarrhea; in more severe cases, respiratory paralysis, muscle weakness, and paralysis	Few hours-days	Detection of toxin in shellfish; detection of dinoflagellates in water where shellfish were gathered	Symptomatic; cleansing of GI tract; ventilatory assistance
Neurotoxic shellfish poisoning ingestion of toxic dinoflagellates by shellfish	Shellfish (Florida)	Few minutes-few hours	Paresthesias, nausea, vomiting, diarrhea, ataxia	Hours-days		Symptomatic
Heavy metal: tin, copper, zinc	Acidic liquids—fruit juices, carbonated beverages stored in metal containers	≤1 hour	Nausea, vomiting, diarrhea, abdominal cramping	Hours-days	Detection of metal in food	Symptomatic
Chinese restaurant syndrome	Chinese foods	≤1 hour	Paresthesias, headache	≤2 hours	High concentration of monosodium glutamate in food	Symptomatic
Mushroom poisoning Mushroom species containing ibotenic acid and muscimol	Mushrooms	2-3 hours	Abdominal cramps, sweating, salivation, miosis, and bradycardia	Hours-few days	Detection of toxin in food	Symptomatic: remove unabsorbed toxin from GI tract; atropine
Mushroom species containing amatoxins	Mushrooms	6-12 hours	Abdominal pain, vomiting, diarrhea, confusion, paralysis, hepatic and renal failure	Days-weeks	Detection of toxin in food	Symptomatic

PATHOGENESIS. Once ingested, even in extremely small amounts, the neurotoxin, which is resistant to gastric acidity, rapidly is absorbed from the intestinal tract. The toxin blocks neural conduction by preventing acetylcholine release.

CLINICAL MANIFESTATIONS. After an incubation period of 12 to 36 hours (range of 4 hours to 8 days), symptoms of weakness, blurred or double vision, difficulty swallowing and speaking, and dry mouth appear, accompanied by nausea, vomiting, and abdominal distention in some patients. Weakness spreads to involve the neck, trunk, and proximal limb muscle groups and the muscles of respiration. Nasal regurgitation and aspiration pneumonia may occur. Urinary retention and constipation are common. Sensory function, deep tendon reflexes, and level of consciousness are unimpaired.

DIAGNOSIS. The clinical manifestations may suggest botulism, but the diagnosis may not be obvious unless several patients are seen simultaneously with characteristic manifestations following ingestion of the same meal. Confirmation is obtained by demonstration of the toxin or *C. botulinum* in the suspected food and occasionally by the demonstration of the toxin in the blood and feces of the patient. Electromyography (EMG) may show diminished response to a single stimulus but facilitation of action potentials with repeated nerve stimulation.

PROGNOSIS. Mortality may be as high as 70% for type A, 10% to 30% for type B, and 30% to 50% for type E botulism. Death usually results from respiratory paralysis and aspiration pneumonia. In those who survive, recovery is complete but may be slow. If patients are supported by assisted ventilation during the acute phase of the illness, mortality should be reduced considerably.

Table 41-2   Waterborne and foodborne illnesses not usually accompanied by fever

Etiology	Incriminated foods	Incubation period	Clinical features	Duration of illness	Diagnosis	Therapy
Preformed toxins						
Staphylococcus aureus	Meat, dairy products	1-6 hours	Afebrile, nausea, vomiting, retching, abdominal cramping, diarrhea	6-8 hours	Detection of toxin or organism in food	Symptomatic
Clostridium botulinum	Vegetables (usually home-processed)	12-36 hours	Afebrile, dry mouth, pharyngeal pain, cranial nerve palsies, respiratory paralysis, nausea, vomiting, abdominal distention	Weeks	Detection by mouse inoculation of toxin in serum, stool, food*; culture of food for *C. botulinum*	Cleanse GI tract, administer trivalent (ABE) antitoxin*†; supportive care; measure vital capacity; guanidine HCl, 50 mg/kg/day‡
Bacillus cereus (emetic form)	Fried rice	1-6 hours	Vomiting, abdominal cramping	8-10 hours	Isolation of 10^5 organisms/g of food	Symptomatic
Colonization of upper small bowel						
Giardia lamblia	Water, vegetables, or fruit	9-15 days	Abdominal distention, flatulence, and diarrhea	Days-months	Identification of cyst in stool or trophozoite in stool or duodenal aspirate	Metronidazole** 250 mg PO t.i.d. × 10 days, or quinacrine, 100 mg PO t.i.d. × 7 days
Cryptosporidium spp.		?	Abdominal distention, flatulence, diarrhea, malabsorption	1-10 days in immunocompetent; months in AIDS patients	Oocysts in stool (acid-fast positive) or organisms along microvillus border in small bowel biopsy	None
Superficial invasion of small bowel						
Isospora belli	Human fecal contaminated food or water	?	Abdominal distention, flatulence, diarrhea, malabsorption, and eosinophilia	Months in AIDS patients	Oocyst in stool or intracellular organisms on small bowel biopsy	Two double-strength trimethoprim-sulfamethoxazole, 320 mg-1600 mg PO q.i.d. × 10 days, then b.i.d. × 3 weeks
Colonization of upper small bowel and endogenous production of enterotoxin						
Clostridium perfringens, type A	Reheated meat dishes	8-24 hours	Diarrhea, abdominal cramping	<24 hours	Isolation of organism from food, stool	Symptomatic
Enterotoxigenic *Escherichia coli* (major cause of traveler's diarrhea)	Raw vegetables, water	8-14 hours	Watery diarrhea, abdominal cramping	48 hours	Detection of enterotoxin-producing strain in stool	Symptomatic, Pepto-Bismol, 30 ml or 1 tab PO q ½h × 8 doses PO; severe illness may be treated like shigellosis

*Obtain from Centers for Disease Control, Atlanta, Ga. 30333; 404-639-3670 or 404-639-3356 (24 hr a day) or call Atlanta Information 404-555-1212.
†Initial skin test for horse serum sensitivity.
‡Investigational.
**This use of metronidazole is not listed in the manufacturer's official directive. Metronidazole has teratogenic potential and should be avoided in pregnancy.

Continued.

Table 41-2 Waterborne and foodborne illnesses not usually accompanied by fever—cont'd

Etiology	Incriminated foods	Incubation period	Clinical features	Duration of illness	Diagnosis	Therapy
Vibrio cholerae	Water, fruit, vegetables	1-6 days	Watery diarrhea, vomiting, muscle cramps	1-7 days	Isolation of *V. cholerae* from stool—use TCBS agar	Symptomatic; volume replacement; tetracycline, 40 mg/kd/day PO × 2 days
Bacillus cereus (diarrheal form)	Meat, vegetables	6-14 hours	Watery diarrhea, abdominal cramps	24-36 hours	Isolation of *B. cereus* from food	Symptomatic
Infant botulism	Honey	?	Constipation, cranial nerve palsies, generalized weakness, especially of neck muscles—"floppy infants"		Isolation of *C. botulinum* from feces; demonstration of toxin in stool; EMG	Supportive

Colonization of the large bowel and endogenous production of cytotoxin

Escherichia coli Serotype O 157:H7	Fast-food hamburgers	1-5 days	Afebrile, bloody stool	7 days	Detection of cytotoxin in stool	Antibiotic

MANAGEMENT. Specific horse antitoxin probably is most efficacious in type E botulism but is used for all types because of the possibility of the continued presence of circulating toxin. Multivalent antitoxin is used unless the type of botulism is definitely known. After testing for sensitivity to horse serum, two vials of trivalent (A, B, and E) serum are given intravenously and repeated in 2 to 4 hours. Guanidine (15 to 50 mg/kg/day via nasogastric tube) may improve nerve conduction. Catharsis may aid elimination of the toxin from the intestinal tract.

Measures to support respiration are most important in the treatment of botulism. Respiratory paralysis is best treated by using a cuffed tracheostomy and mechanically assisted ventilation.

PREVENTION. Prevention depends on proper home and commercial preservation of food and adequate heating of food before serving.

CHOLERA

DEFINITION. Cholera is an acute intoxication of the small bowel mucosa caused by an enterotoxin produced by *Vibrio cholerae,* which have colonized the epithelial surface of the small bowel. Profuse, watery diarrhea occurs and is accompanied by muscle cramps, dehydration, circulatory collapse, and renal failure.

ETIOLOGY. *V. cholerae* are short, motile, slightly curved, gram-negative bacilli. Two biotypes exist, the classic biotype and the El Tor variety. El Tor is distinguished by resistance to polymyxin B.

EPIDEMIOLOGY. Cholera has been endemic in the delta regions of the Ganges (Calcutta) and Brahmaputra rivers, from which the disease has spread sporadically to become worldwide. The latest pandemic reached peak levels in 1971. In endemic areas cholera is a disease of children, but in epidemics people of all ages are affected.

PATHOGENESIS. Humans are the only known reservoir of infection. Vibrios are passed in the stool during the illness, for a variable period (usually for less than 1 month) during convalescence, in asymptomatic transient carriers, and perhaps in a small number of chronic gallbladder carriers. Cholera is spread by ingestion of water contaminated by feces, improperly

prepared shellfish from contaminated seawater, or food directly contaminated with infected stool or night soil.

When large numbers (10^{10}) of relatively acid-susceptible vibrios are ingested, some may survive gastric acidity to colonize the mucosal surface of the small bowel and elaborate an enterotoxin. This toxin irreversibly binds to the epithelial surface and stimulates adenyl cyclase production. As a result, rapid excretion of isotonic alkaline fluid into the small bowel lumen occurs. Structural damage or inflammation in the bowel is not present.

CLINICAL MANIFESTATIONS. The disease starts, after an incubation period of about 1 to 6 days, with an abrupt onset of a variable amount of watery stool. Up to 1 L of stool is lost per hour during the first 24 hours with loss of spincter control. There is no fever, severe abdominal cramping, or tenesmus. In severe cases muscle cramps and prostration develop. Stools that resemble rice water may be produced. If fluid loss is sufficiently severe and is not replaced rapidly enough, hypovolemic shock, metabolic acidosis, and renal failure develop. In children neurologic complications (seizures and decreased level of consciousness) may be seen.

DIAGNOSIS. Cholera should be suspected in an afebrile patient with an acute onset of painless, voluminous, watery diarrhea in an epidemic or endemic area. A similar illness also may be produced by other enterotoxin-producing organisms such as *Escherichia coli* or *Bacillus cereus,* and if fluid loss is equally severe, these illnesses require similar therapy. Examination of stool reveals no blood or pus (which are characteristic of dysentery produced by *Shigella* or invasive strains of *E. coli*). The vibrios may be isolated from stool by cultivation on thiosulfate citrate bile salts sucrose (TCBS) agar and produce opaque yellow colonies in 18 hours.

MANAGEMENT. Rapid replacement of fluid and electrolytes is the most important means of treatment. A solution that is prepared by the addition of 4 g of sodium chloride, 6.5 g of sodium acetate, 1 g of potassium chloride, and 10 g of glucose to 1 L of sterile distilled water or lactated Ringer's solution may be given intravenously at a rate equal to gastrointestinal losses or to maintain a strong pulse and normal skin turgor. Oral replacement with a solution that contains 20 g of glucose, 3.5 g of sodium chloride, 2.5 g of sodium bicarbonate, and

Table 41-3 Waterborne and foodborne bacterial illnesses that may be accompanied by fever

Etiology	Incriminated foods	Incubation period	Clinical features	Duration of illness	Diagnosis	Therapy
Invasion of distal small bowel and large bowel						
Shigella	Water, poultry, dairy products	1-4 days	Watery diarrhea followed at times by dysentery with headache, nausea, abdominal pain, tenesmus	1-2 weeks	Isolation of *Shigella* from stool	Ampicillin, 2 g/day PO × 5 days or tetracycline, 2.5 g as a single dose in adults; symptomatic Ciprofloxacin, 500 mg b.i.d.; norfloxacin, 400 mg b.i.d.; trimethoprim, 2.5 mg/kg-sulfamethoxazole, 12.5 mg/kg b.i.d. PO × 5 days
Escherichia coli	Water	8-24 hours	Same as shigellosis	1-2 weeks	Isolation of invasive *E. coli* from stool	Symptomatic—may treat like shigellosis
Salmonella Gastroenteritis	Water, poultry, eggs	8-48 hours	Nausea, vomiting, abdominal pain, diarrhea	2-5 days	Isolation of nontyphoid *Salmonella* from stool	Symptomatic; severe illness may be treated like shigellosis, especially in infants < 12 wks and immunocompromised patients
Enteric (typhoid) fever	Water food	1-2 weeks	Headache, cough, abdominal pain, constipation or diarrhea	3-4 weeks	Isolation from blood, stool, urine	Chloramphenicol, ampicillin, or ciprofloxacin
Bacteremia	Same as *Salmonella* gastroenteritis	?	Fever, chills, no intestinal symptoms—metastatic foci	Weeks	Isolation of organism from blood	Same as typhoid fever
Vibrio parahaemolyticus	Seafoods	12-24 hours	Nausea, vomiting, abdominal pain, diarrhea	2-5 days	Isolation of organism from stool or vomitus, peptone water enrichment medium with 3% NaCl; TCBS agar	Symptomatic; severe illness may be treated like shigellosis
Yersinia enterocolitica	Dairy products	?	Abdominal pain, tenderness, diarrhea, erythema nodosum, polyarthritis	Days to weeks	Serologic response (*Yersinia* agglutinins); isolation of organism from stool (cold enrichment of fecal specimens)	Symptomatic; severe illness may be treated like shigellosis
Campylobacter jejuni	Poultry, water	2-11 days	Abdominal pain, diarrhea, dysentery, or metastatic foci	10-14 days	Isolation from stool and/or blood	Supportive; may be treated like shigellosis, except trimethoprim-sulfamethoxazole not effective against *C. jejuni*
Aeromonas hydrophila	Untreated water	?	Diarrhea, cramps, fever	Days-months	Isolation from stool	Antibiotics; may be treated like shigellosis
Plesiomonas shigelloides	Uncooked shellfish, travel to Mexico	?	Diarrhea with blood-streaked mucus, abdominal cramps, fever	7-14 days	Isolation from stool	Antibiotics
Entamoeba histolytica	Water, raw vegetables	1 week	Diarrhea with blood-streaked mucus, abdominal pain	Weeks to months	Trophozoites and cysts in stool, serology	Metronidazole*, 750 mg PO t.i.d. × 5-10 days, with or without diiodohydroxyquin, 650 mg PO t.i.d. × 21 days

*Metronidazole has teratogenic potential and should be avoided in pregnancy.

Continued.

Table 41-3 Waterborne and foodborne bacterial illnesses that may be accompanied by fever—cont'd.

Etiology	Incriminated foods	Incubation period	Clinical features	Duration of illness	Diagnosis	Therapy
Colonization of upper small bowel and loss of villus tips						
Rotavirus (Reovirus)	?	?	Diarrhea, vomiting, fever during winter in patients 6 mo to 2 yr old	2-4 days	Virus detection in stool by ELISA (Rotazyme test)	Symptomatic
Parovirus (Norwalk agent)	Water	1-2 days	Nausea, vomiting, diarrhea, abdominal cramps during winter in adults	1-2 days	Virus detection by immunoelection microscopy	Symptomatic
Colonization of the large bowel and endogenous production of cytotoxin						
Clostridium difficile	?	≥4 days after starting antibiotic	Diarrhea, blood, abdominal pain, pseudomembranous colitis on sigmoidoscopy	7-10 days after stopping inciting antibiotic or starting specific antibiotic therapy	Detection of cytotoxin in stool	Vancomycin, 125-500 mg PO 6h × 7-10 days or metronidazole*, 250-500 mg PO or IV q6h × 7-10 days

*Metronidazole has teratogenic potential and should be avoided in pregnancy.

Table 41-4 Miscellaneous waterborne and foodborne illnesses

Etiology	Incriminated foods	Incubation period	Clinical features	Duration of illness	Diagnosis	Therapy
Trichinella spiralis	Undercooked meats, mainly pork	7-14 days	Diarrhea followed by fever, myalgias, periorbital edema, subungual hemorrhages, encephalopathy, urticarial rash, myocarditis, and pneumonitis	4-8 weeks	Serology (bentonite flocculation and immunofluorescent test); demonstration of larvae in muscle biopsy after 2 wk of illness; eosinophilia (up to 70%)	Symptomatic; bed rest; analgesics; corticosteroids if signs of CNS, pulmonary, or cardiac involvement are present; thiabendazole, 50 mg/kg/day in two divided doses × 5-7 days
Hepatitis A virus	Improperly cooked shellfish, water	15-40 days	Fever, myalgias, headache, abdominal pain, nausea, anorexia, jaundice, tender hepatomegaly, adenopathy	2-3 weeks	Liver function abnormalities; hepatitis A antibody	Symptomatic

1.5 g of potassium chloride per liter of drinking water can be given in mild cholera or after initial intravenous correction of hypovolemia. Tetracycline (40 mg/kg/day for 2 days orally) can eradicate vibrios from stool and decrease the duration and volume of the diarrhea.

PROGNOSIS. In inadequately treated patients the mortality can exceed 50%, but almost all properly treated patients should survive.

PREVENTION. Immunization against cholera with either toxoid or killed bacterial vaccine confers only about 70% protection, which lasts for 3 to 6 months. The best protection in endemic or epidemic regions is the use of boiled water for drinking and the avoidance of uncooked vegetables or unpeeled, uncooked fruits. Eating improperly cooked shellfish from the Gulf of Mexico has posed a problem in the United States recently.

SHIGELLOSIS

DEFINITION. Shigellosis is an acute superficial infection of the distal large bowel caused by *Shigella*. Patients have frequent passage of stools containing blood, pus, and mucus, accompanied by abdominal cramps, tenesmus, and fever.

ETIOLOGY. Shigellae are members of the Enterobacteriaceae family. They are nonmotile, gram-negative bacilli that usually do not ferment lactose and do not produce gas when grown anaerobically. There are four species—*S. sonnei, S. flexneri, S. dysenteriae,* and *S. boydii*—and 39 serotypes. The frequency of isolation of the different species of shigellae varies geographically. *S. sonnei* and, to a lesser extent, *S. flexneri* produce disease in the United States. In other countries *S. dysenteriae* (Central America) and *S. boydii* are more frequent isolates, and these species may be imported into the United States by travelers from endemic areas.

EPIDEMIOLOGY. Man is the only known reservoir of infection. The source is the stool of infected individuals during illness or during a variable time in the convalescent period. There is no known chronic intestinal carriage of these bacteria. Because of the relatively few organisms sufficient to produce illness after ingestion (100 shigellae are sufficient to cause disease in 50% of exposed individuals), the disease is produced not only by contaminated food or water but also by direct person-to-person spread via the fecal-oral route. The conditions for person-to-person transmission are primarily related to poor personal hygiene and are most evident in the young, in the institutionalized retarded, and among the poor in crowded urban ghettos and underdeveloped countries. Shigellosis may be seen more frequently in homosexual men because of oral-anal sexual contact.

PATHOGENESIS. The few relatively acid-resistant shigellae ingested may survive gastric acidity and pass into the colon, where the organisms attach and colonize the epithelial surface (about 10^6 to 10^{10}/g of stool). They then invade epithelial cells to cause superficial ulcerations in the tips of the villi, which are covered by an exudate of polymorphonuclear leukocytes. An acute inflammatory reaction occurs in the lamina propria. Bacteremia and metastatic infection are rare. Certain strains produce an enterotoxin of unknown clinical significance that experimentally results in fluid and electrolyte loss from the small bowel.

CLINICAL MANIFESTATIONS. Shigellae may cause asymptomatic infection, or after an incubation period of 1 to 4 days, may produce a febrile illness of varying severity with either watery diarrhea or dysentery (tenesmus and frequent passage of blood, pus, and mucus in small-volume stools). A biphasic illness with watery diarrhea followed by dysentery may occur. Neurologic findings (irritability, lethargy, nuchal rigidity, or convulsions) are rare in adults but quite common in children 1 to 4 years of age. Symptoms may take up to 1 to 2 weeks to subside. In rare cases nonseptic arthritis may complicate the illness in the convalescent period in patients with histocompatibility antigen HLA = B27.

DIAGNOSIS. Diarrheal illness accompanied by fever, tenesmus, and frequent passage of stools with mucus, blood, and pus can be presumed to be shigellosis. Other pathogens that produce a similar illness include *Campylobacter jejuni*, enteroinvasive *E. coli*, and *Yersinia enterocolitica*. Organisms that produce enterotoxin (*E. coli* or *V. cholerae*) cause an illness characterized by watery diarrhea and by the absence of fever or fecal purulence. *E. coli* 0157:H7, which produces a cytotoxin, causes hemorrhagic colin that is characterized by afebrile illness with bloody stool. This illness may be complicated by the hemolytic-uremia syndrome, as may shigellosis in rare cases. Illness produced by more deeply invasive microorganisms such as salmonellae is characterized by fever but is unaccompanied by markedly purulent stool (although a moderate number of polymorphonuclear leukocytes may be seen in stool specimens). Sigmoidoscopy in salmonellosis reveals diffuse erythema and edema without the superficial ulcerations of the mucosa seen in shigellosis. The definitive diagnosis depends on isolation of shigellae from stool but may require more than one specimen to yield a positive culture if fresh stool is not cultured, because shigella survive for only a short time in stool specimens.

MANAGEMENT. Correction of fluid and electrolyte losses may be critical, especially in the type of watery diarrheal illness with signs of severe volume and electrolyte depletion that occurs in the very young and very old.

The use of agents that decrease bowel motility has been associated with more prolonged fever, diarrhea, and fecal excretion of shigellae and therefore should be avoided. Appropriate antimicrobial therapy shortens the illness and duration of excretion of shigellae. Shigellosis can be treated with ciprofloxacin (500 mg) or norfloxacin (400 mg) twice daily for 5 days in adults, ampicillin, administered in oral doses of 500 mg four times daily in adults (100 mg/kg/day in four divided doses in children) for 5 days; tetracycline, given in a single dose of 2.5 to 3 g in adults; or trimethoprim-sulfamethoxazole double strength, given as one tablet four times daily for 5 days, depending on antimicrobial susceptibility of strains. Although active in vitro, amoxicillin and aminoglycosides are not as effective clinically.

PROGNOSIS. *S. dysenteriae* produces the most severe infections, associated with mortality of 10% to 20% in untreated individuals, although adequate supportive and specific antimicrobial therapy undoubtedly would lower these rates. *S. sonnei* usually produces mild illness with a mortality of less than 1%.

PREVENTION. Good personal hygiene and the avoidance of potentially contaminated food and water are important in the prevention of shigellosis. Patients should avoid preparing food until three stool cultures are negative on consecutive days after discontinuation of antimicrobial therapy.

SALMONELLOSES

Salmonellae are Enterobacteriaceae that can cause asymptomatic infection or several different types of diseases: enteric fever, gastroenteritis, bacteremia, and localized metastatic infection at any site. There are more than 1700 serotypes of salmonellae.

Salmonella gastroenteritis

DEFINITION. *Salmonella* gastroenteritis is an acute gastroenteritis of variable severity that follows ingestion of food or water contaminated with salmonellae.

ETIOLOGY. *S. typhimurium* is the most common species isolated in cases of *Salmonella* gastroenteritis. Other common isolates are *S. newport*, *S. enteritidis*, and *S. heidelberg*.

EPIDEMIOLOGY. Salmonellae are found in many domestic animals (poultry, cattle, pigs, sheep). Salmonellae in meats may contaminate equipment in the processing plant, market, or kitchen and be carelessly transferred to other food from these items. If the contaminated food is allowed to stand at room temperature or is only minimally rewarmed before serving, it may become heavily contaminated as a result of growth of salmonellae. Cooking may not always eliminate these organisms. For example, cooking temperatures in the center of a stuffed turkey may be just right for optimal proliferation rather than for sterilization of the salmonellae. Other sources of food contamination include household pets such as dogs, cats, birds, and even turtles that are fed contaminated products of the meat processing industry.

Because enormous numbers of the relatively acid-sensitive salmonellae must be ingested for a few to survive gastric acidity and result in gastroenteritis, usually food in which the salmonellae have proliferated acts as the source for infection. Person-to-person spread is unusual except in especially susceptible individuals such as infants, the very elderly, those with achlorhydria, and homosexuals who have direct oral-anal contact. Homosexuals with oral-anal contact have been similarly shown to be at risk of other infections spread by the fecal-oral route such as giardiasis, shigellosis, hepatitis A, and amebiasis.

PATHOGENESIS. A few of the large numbers of ingested

salmonellae survive gastric acidity, enter the small bowel, invade the lamina propria of the mucosa, and produce a deep inflammatory reaction, at times associated with transient bacteremia. There is little superficial ulceration.

CLINICAL MANIFESTATIONS. After an incubation period of ½ to 2 days, there is abrupt onset with chills, fever up to 105° F (40.5° C), headache, and myalgias accompanied by nausea, vomiting, abdominal cramps, and diarrhea of variable severity. This usually lasts from 2 to 5 days, and recovery generally is complete. Rarely do patients have metastatic infection from the early, transient bacteremia. Metastatic infection usually is seen in patients with hemolytic states such as sickle hemoglobinopathies, malaria, or bartonellosis. In sickle hemoglobinopathies salmonellae usually infect bone infarcts and result in septic arthritis or osteomyelitis.

DIAGNOSIS. If the illness develops in a group of patients who become ill at about the same time, a single exposure to a certain food usually can be defined by a careful food history. The food usually involves poultry products that have been improperly prepared. The food, if still available, may appear normal but may grow salmonellae on culture. The stool of patients contains only moderate numbers of pus cells, but salmonellae can be grown from the stool during the illness and may persist in stool for several weeks after the illness. Blood cultures taken during the acute illness rarely grow the organism, except in infants. Agglutination tests (febrile agglutinins) are too nonspecific to be of diagnostic importance.

PROGNOSIS. The illness usually is transient and is rarely (less than 1%) severe enough to cause death except in infants, the very elderly, or the severely debilitated, who die as a result of dehydration.

MANAGEMENT. Replacement of fluid and electrolyte losses should be instituted. Agents that slow bowel motility theoretically are not indicated, but they have been commonly used in the past to relieve abdominal discomfort without reported untoward effects. Although other antimicrobials do not alleviate *Salmonella* gastroenteritis clinically or bacteriologically, and in fact, when these agents are given during the illness, they may prolong fecal shedding of the organism during convalescence; ciprofloxacin and norfloxacin may shorten the course of the illness somewhat and in some patients eradicate fecal shedding during convalescence.

PREVENTION. Prevention of *Salmonella* gastroenteritis involves care in the processing of food, especially food known to be frequently contaminated, such as poultry products. Professional food handlers may shed salmonellae on occasion in their stool as a result of constant occupational exposure. Attention to proper handwashing is essential in this group. Patients with acute illness should be isolated, and convalescent carriers should not prepare food for others unless three consecutive stool cultures obtained when the patient is not taking antibiotics are negative for salmonellae.

Enteric (typhoid) fever

DEFINITION AND ETIOLOGY. Enteric fever is an acute generalized infection caused by *S. typhi* and characterized by fever, prostration, relative bradycardia, a rose-colored exanthem, abdominal pain, hypoactive bowel sounds, and splenomegaly. A similar illness, although milder, can be produced by other salmonellae, usually *S. paratyphi* A or B. Of more than 1700 serotypes of *Salmonella,* only *S. typhi* is a pathogen restricted to humans.

EPIDEMIOLOGY. The source of infection is feces or urine from patients and asymptomatic carriers. (Two percent to 5% of patients may become chronic carriers, that is, have positive stool cultures for more than 1 year after illness.) Water or food becomes contaminated from these infectious materials. In the United States about 500 cases occur each year either in recent travelers from endemic areas or in those who have eaten food contaminated by a human carrier. Chronic carriers, when discovered, are registered with health authorities.

PATHOGENESIS. Following ingestion of large numbers of salmonellae, those that survive gastric acidity enter the small bowel, penetrate the mucosa, then invade the mesenteric nodes and subsequently the bloodstream. *S. typhi* parasitize mononuclear macrophages of the reticuloendothelial system. The macrophages fail to kill these organisms, which multiply and then are discharged into the bloodstream. Hypertrophy of the reticuloendothelial system occurs in the liver (micronodular areas of necrosis surrounded by macrophages and lymphocytes), spleen, and Peyer's patches in the gut. Enlarged lymphoid tissue in the terminal ilium and cecum may erode a blood vessel, resulting in intestinal hemorrhage, or may rupture into the bowel lumen, resulting in areas predisposed to perforation.

CLINICAL MANIFESTATIONS. The incubation period is 1 to 2 weeks, depending to some extent on the number of organisms ingested. There is a gradual onset of increasingly higher fever, chills, malaise, headache, myalgias, and abdominal pain, usually in the right lower quadrant. This is accompanied by constipation and cough or sore throat. After about 1 week the fever becomes sustained between 103° F (39.4° C) and 105° F (40.6° C) and diarrhea develops. Physical examination frequently reveals relative bradycardia, rose-colored exanthem ("rose spots") on the anterior trunk, splenomegaly, abdominal distention, and hypoactive bowel sounds. Because of the sustained fever, patients may become severely debilitated. In some patients the temperature may remain around 106° F (41.1° C) with delirium. Intestinal hemorrhage of varying severity or perforation may complicate the illness in the second to third weeks. Gradual recovery begins to occur in the fourth week of illness in untreated individuals. Granulocytopenia, thrombocytopenia, and anemia are commonly noted. Metastatic infection may occur in the lungs, kidneys, bones, joints, and gallbladder. In rare cases alopecia, myocarditis, parotitis, and peripheral neuritis occur. Some patients, usually older women with preexisting gallbladder disease, become lifetime (chronic) gallbladder carriers. The infected bile in these patients discharges large numbers of salmonellae into the bowel lumen without local or systemic symptoms.

DIAGNOSIS. The diagnosis depends on the cultivation of the typhoid bacillus. Blood cultures are positive for *S. typhi* in the first week of illness in most patients; stool cultures and, in some patients, blood cultures are positive in the second week of illness; and urine and stool cultures are positive in the third week of illness. Because of frequent nonspecific rises in titer of agglutinins against O and H antigens of *S. typhi* (Widal's test), a diagnosis based on these tests alone is not dependable.

PROGNOSIS. Relapse occurs in about 10% of untreated cases and 20% of treated cases, and the frequency of relapse has been noted to be greater with early institution of antibiotic therapy. Untreated individuals have a mortality of 10% to 15%. Death occurs in less than 1% of antibiotic-treated patients. Severe intestinal hemorrhage or perforation carries about a 25% mortality and is the usual cause of death in typhoid fever.

MANAGEMENT. Typhoid fever can be treated with either chloramphenicol (50 mg/kg/day intravenously or orally), ampicillin (200 mg/kg/day intravenously), or perhaps ciprofloxacin (750 mg twice daily orally), if the organism is susceptible in vitro. Antimicrobial therapy is given for 2 weeks. In areas where plasmid-mediated resistance (R factor) to chloramphenicol and ampicillin is a problem, trimethoprim-sulfamethoxazole is the drug of choice. Relapse may be successfully treated by another 2-week course of the same drug that was used initially. Corticosteroids may be given for severe toxicity, and the dose can be rapidly tapered in 3 to 4 days. Antipyretics and ice blankets cause chilling, which may make the patient more uncomfortable. A too rapid fall in temperature may be associated with hypotension. Intestinal perforation is managed by nasogastric suction, antibiotics, and, only if necessary, surgery.

About half to two thirds of chronic gallbladder carriers (primarily those without gallstones) can be cured with 1.5 g ampicillin and 500 mg probenecid given every 6 hours orally for 6 weeks. In those who fail to respond to this regimen (especially those with cholelithiasis), cholecystectomy may be considered, but this procedure carries an operative risk and may not cure about 15% of the patients.

PREVENTION. Chronic carriers should avoid preparation of food for others, and travelers should avoid drinking unboiled water or eating uncooked vegetables and unpeeled fruits in areas where sanitation is not optimal. Hospitalized patients should be treated with enteric precautions. Vaccination against *S. typhi* prevents typhoid fever from developing in about 70% of those vaccinated and should be repeated every 3 years for travelers in endemic regions. Because the immunity afforded by vaccination can be overcome by ingestion of large numbers of *S. typhi,* the best protection for travelers is to avoid potentially contaminated food and beverages. Vaccine against *S. paratyphi* A or B is of no value.

Salmonella bacteremia and localized infection

DEFINITION. A clinical syndrome identical to bacteremia produced by other facultative gram-negative bacilli is also produced by salmonellae and is characterized by repeated episodes of shaking chills, hectic fever followed by drenching sweats, and, in some patients, signs of localized infection.

ETIOLOGY. Although almost any serotype is capable of producing bacteremia or metastatic localized infection, *S. choleraesuis* and *S. typhimurium* are the most common causes.

EPIDEMIOLOGY AND PATHOGENESIS. About one third to half of patients with *Salmonella* bacteremia have a severe underlying illness, for example, cancer, cirrhosis, systemic lupus erythematosus, or hemolytic conditions such as sickle cell anemia, bartonellosis, or malaria. In addition, persistent *Salmonella* bacteremia has been described in patients with schistosomiasis, probably as a result of salmonellal parasitism of the schistosome.

Bacteremia results from invasion of the intestinal tract after ingestion of a sufficient number of organisms. Some bacteremias may be associated with an initial phase of gastroenteritis, but more commonly there is no history of gastroenteritis.

Salmonellae tend to localize at sites of preexisting disease such as bone infarcts in patients with sickle hemoglobinopathies, areas of degenerative arthritis, tumors, hematomas, or atherosclerotic aneurysms. In fact, salmonellae rather than *Staphylococcus aureus* are the most common cause of osteomyelitis in patients with sickle hemoglobinopathies.

CLINICAL MANIFESTATIONS. Patients with *Salmonella* bacteremia have hectic fever. Unlike those with enteric fever, they do not have sustained fever, cough, rose spots, splenomegaly, and hypoactive bowel sounds. Localized infection may occur at almost any site and result in pneumonia, empyema, endarteritis, endocarditis, pyelonephritis, osteomyelitis, arthritis, or meningitis.

DIAGNOSIS. Diagnosis depends on isolation of the salmo-nellae from blood or pus in localized infections. Agglutination reactions ("febrile agglutinins") are too nonspecific to be of diagnostic importance.

MANAGEMENT. Chloramphenicol (50 mg/kg/day in four divided doses) or ampicillin (12 g intravenously each day for at least 2 weeks) is the drug of choice for *Salmonella* bacteremia or localized infection, except for *Salmonella* endarteritis or endocarditis. Surgical drainage and a more prolonged course of antibiotic therapy (4 to 6 weeks) may be necessary for localized infection. In endarteritis or endocarditis bactericidal therapy is essential for cure, and ampicillin is the drug of choice if the *Salmonella* strain is susceptible. Ampicillin also is preferred for more prolonged courses of antibiotic therapy because of problems with reversible bone marrow suppression seen with chloramphenicol. Some non-*typhi* salmonellae, however, are resistant to ampicillin.

PROGNOSIS. The morbidity of localized infection may be considerable, and the mortality rate of *S. choleraesuis* bacteremia may approach 20%. Therefore when these infections are suspected, they should be treated early and appropriately, especially in patients at greater risk of *Salmonella* bacteremia and metastatic infection (for example, in those with sickle hemoglobinopathies).

BIBLIOGRAPHY

Black RE and others: Epidemic *Yersinia enterocolitica* infection due to contaminated chocolate milk, N Engl J Med 298:76, 1978.

Blaser MJ and Reller LB: *Campylobacter* enteritis, N Engl J Med 305:1444, 1981.

Bolen JL, Zamiska SA, and Greenough WB III: Clinical features in enteritis due to *Vibrio parahemolyticus,* Am J Med 57:638, 1974.

Bradford WD, Noce PS, and Gutman LT: Pathologic features of enteric infection with *Yersinia enterocolitica,* Arch Pathol 98:17, 1974.

Davidson GP and others: Importance of a new virus in acute sporadic enteritis in children, Lancet 1:242, 1975.

Ericsson CD and others: Bismuth subsalicylate inhibits activity of crude toxins of *Escherichia coli* and *Vibrio cholerae,* J Infect Dis 136:693, 1977.

Finch MJ and Blake PA: Foodborne outbreaks of campylobacteriosis: The United States experience, 1980-1982, Am J Epidemiol 122:262, 1985.

George WL and others: *Aeromonas*-related diarrhea in adults, Arch Intern Med 145:2207, 1985.

Gorbach SL and others: Traveler's diarrhea and toxigenic *E. coli,* N Engl J Med 292:933, 1975.

Guerrant RL and others: Campylobacteriosis in man: pathogenic mechanisms and review of 91 bloodstream infections, Am J Med 65:584, 1978.

Gurwith J and others: A prospective study of rotavirus infection in infants and children, J Infect Dis 144:218, 1981.

Holmberg SD and Farmer JJ III: *Aeromonas hydrophila* and *Plesiomonas shigelloides* as causes of intestinal infections, Rev Infect Dis 6:633, 1984.

Hughes JM and Merson MH: Current concepts: fish and shellfish poisoning, N Engl J Med 295:1117, 1976.

Hughes JM and others: Foodborne disease outbreaks of chemical etiology in the United States, 1970-1974, Am J Epidemiol 105:233, 1977.

Kumar S and others: Non-01 *Vibrio cholerae* gastroenteritis in Northern California, West J Med 140:783, 1984.

Loewenstein MS: Epidemiology of *Clostridium perfringens* food poisoning, N Engl J Med 286:1026, 1972.

Levine MM and Edelman R: Enteropathogenic *Escherichia coli* of classic serotypes associated with infant diarrhea: Epidemiology and pathogenesis, Epidemiol Rev 6:31, 1984.

Pai CH and others: Sporadic cases of hemorrhagic colitis associated with *Escherichia coli* 0157:H7, Ann Intern Med 10:738, 1984.

Rosenberg ML and others: Epidemic diarrhea at Crater Lake from enterotoxigenic *Escherichia coli:* a large, waterborne outbreak, Ann Intern Med 86:714, 1977.

Terranova W and Blake PA: *Bacillus cereus* food poisoning, N Engl J Med 298:143, 1978.

Wolfe MS: Current concepts in parasitology: giardiasis, N Engl J Med 298:319, 1978.

Botulism

Koenig MG and others: Clinical and laboratory observations on type E botulism in man, Medicine 43:517, 1964.

Koenig MG and others: Type B botulism in man, Am J Med 42:208, 1967.

Merson MH and Dowell VR: Epidemiologic, clinical and laboratory aspects of wound botulism, N Engl J Med 289:1005, 1973.

Pickett J and others: Syndrome of botulism in infancy: clinical and electrophysiologic study, N Engl J Med 295:770, 1976.

Cholera

Barua D and Burrows W, editors: Cholera, Philadelphia, 1975, WB Saunders Co.

Woodward WE and Mosley WH: The spectrum of cholera in rural Bangladesh. II. Comparison of El Tor, Ogawa and classical Inaba infection, Am J Epidemiol 96:342, 1971.

Shigellosis

DuPont H and Hornick R: Adverse effects of Lomotil therapy in shigellosis, JAMA 226:1525, 1973.

DuPont H and Hornick R: Clinical approach to infectious diarrheas, Medicine 52:265, 1973.

DuPont H and others: The response of man to virulent *Shigella flexneri* 2a, J Infect Dis 119:296, 1969.

Nelson JD and others: Trimethoprim sulfamethoxazole therapy of shigellosis, JAMA 235:1239, 1976.

Pickering LK, DuPont HL, and Olarte J: Single-dose tetracycline therapy for shigellosis in adults, JAMA 239:853, 1978.

Salmonelloses

Bennett IL Jr and Hook EW: Infectious disease (some aspects of salmonellosis), Annu Rev Med 10:1, 1957.

Black PH, Kunz LJ, and Swartz MN: Salmonellosis—a review of some unusual aspects, N Engl J Med 262:811, 864, 921, 1960.

Hoffman TA and others: Waterborne typhoid fever in Dade County, Florida: clinical and therapeutic evaluation of 105 bacteremic patients, Am J Med 59:481, 1975.

Hornick RB and others: Typhoid fever: pathogenesis and immunologic control, N Engl J Med 283:686, 739, 1970.

Mandal BK and Mani V: Colonic involvement in salmonellosis, Lancet 1:887, 1976.

Rubin RH and Weinstein L: Salmonellosis: microbiologic, pathologic and clinical features, New York, 1977, Thieme Medical Publishers Inc.

Saphria I and Wasserman M: *Salmonella choleraesuis:* a clinical and epidemiological evaluation of 329 infections identified between 1940 and 1954 in the New York Salmonella Center, Am J Med Sci 228:525, 1954.

Saphria I and Winter JW: Clinical manifestations of salmonellosis in man: an evaluation of 7779 human infections identified at the New York Salmonella Center, N Engl J Med 256:1128, 1957.

Stuart BM and Pullen RL: Typhoid: clinical analysis of three hundred and sixty cases, Arch Intern Med 78:629, 1946.

Walker W: The Aberdeen typhoid outbreak of 1964, Scott Med J 10:466, 1965.

42 · DISEASES CAUSED BY RICKETTSIAE

Oksana M. Korzeniowski

DEFINITION. Rickettsial diseases of humans include a variety of clinical entities caused by intracellular bacteria of the family Rickettsiaceae. With the exception of Q fever (caused by *Coxiella burnetii),* all share common clinical and pathologic features and require an insect vector for the transmission of infection to man.

ETIOLOGY. Rickettsiae are small, pleomorphic coccobacilli approximately 0.3 μm in diameter and 1 to 2 μm in length. They stain poorly with aniline dyes and are best demonstrated in tissues by Giemsa or Gimenez stains. All rickettsiae are obligate intracellular parasites. They are clearly bacterial in origin and possess independent metabolic activity and well-defined multilamellar cell walls. With the exception of *C. burnetii,* rickettsiae survive only briefly outside the host. Isolation can be achieved by infection of tissue culture monolayers, by subculture of host monocytes, by passage in embryonated eggs, or by animal inoculation. However, such methods are hazardous and should be performed only in reference laboratories skilled in handling rickettsiae.

The family of Rickettsiaceae contains *Rickettsia* and *Coxiella.* The members of the genus *Rickettsia* have been broadly divided into the spotted fever and typhus groups on the basis of antigenic similarities and intracellular growth characteristics. The spotted fever group includes *R. rickettsii* (Rocky Mountain spotted fever), *R. conorii* (boutonneuse fever), *R. australis* (Queensland tick typhus), *R. sibirica* (North Asian tick typhus), and *R. akari* (rickettsialpox). The typhus group consists of *R. prowazekii* (epidemic and recrudescent typhus or Brill-Zinsser disease), *R. typhi* (murine typhus), and *R. tsutsugamushi* (scrub typhus). The genus *Coxiella* contains only one species, *C. burnetii.* This organism is unique in its resistance to desiccation, heat, and sunlight and its transmissibility by the airborne route without need for an intermediate vector.

EPIDEMIOLOGY. Rickettsiae are maintained in nature in reservoirs involving mammals and arthropod vectors. Each of the rickettsiae pathogenic for humans is capable of multiplying in one or more arthropods and in several mammals, usually small rodents or cattle. Except for louse-borne typhus, in which man is the principal reservoir, man is an incidental host and is not needed to propagate the organism.

Rickettsial diseases are found in all areas of the world. In the United States, Rocky Mountain spotted fever (RMSF), murine typhus, and Q fever are endemic; rickettsialpox occurs but is recognized infrequently. Brill-Zinsser disease (recrudescent typhus) still occurs, predominantly in post–World War II Eastern European immigrants.

PATHOGENESIS. Infection with rickettsiae occurs through the skin or the respiratory tract. Ticks and mites, which transmit agents of the spotted fever group and scrub typhus, inoculate rickettsiae directly into the skin. Local lesions at the site of entry of rickettsiae appear with regularity only in scrub typhus, rickettsialpox, and spotted fevers of the Eastern Hemisphere. The louse and flea, vectors of epidemic typhus, trench fever, and murine typhus, deposit infected feces on the skin. Infection occurs when organisms are rubbed into the puncture wound produced by the arthropod. Inhalation of infected dust in Q fever deposits the rickettsial organisms in the lungs and results in pneumonitis.

Rickettsiae of the spotted fever and typhus groups invade endothelial cells of small arteries, veins, and capillaries, causing swelling, proliferation, and degeneration of involved endothelium. Fibrin-platelet thrombi may form. Perivascular cuffing with mononuclear cell infiltration is characteristic. Such foci of infection involve primarily skin but also brain, lungs, heart, and kidneys and can account for the clinical and pathophysiologic abnormalities seen in these infections, that is, rash, edema, increased extravascular fluid space, hypotension, gangrene, and clotting abnormalities.

CLINICAL MANIFESTATIONS AND LABORATORY FINDINGS. At the onset the signs and symptoms of rickettsial diseases are those common to many acute infectious processes. Exposure history in an endemic area is critical to early consideration of the diagnosis. In classic form rickettsial diseases display many common clinical features that vary in degree and detail: fever, cough, headache, prostration, rash, altered mental state, and hypotension.

Laboratory features are nonspecific and include a low to normal white blood cell count, hyponatremia, renal insufficiency, and thrombocytopenia with or without other parameters of disseminated intravascular clotting.

DIAGNOSIS. Because isolation techniques for rickettsiae are cumbersome and hazardous, diagnosis is confirmed most often by serologic means. The Weil-Felix reaction, based on the agglutination of suspensions of rough strains of *Proteus* species (OX-2, OX-19, and OX-K) by serum from patients with spotted fever and typhus infections, has been widely applied. Complement fixation (CF) tests are more specific and can differentiate infections with rickettsia producing similar Weil-Felix reactions; however, titer rises can be delayed and depressed by early antimicrobial therapy. Several newer serologic tests currently entering use—primarily, indirect hemagglutination (IHA) and indirect fluorescent antibody (IFA) tests—are more sensitive, are immunoglobulin specific, and are unaffected by treatment. Direct immunofluorescent skin tests have been developed for Rocky Mountain spotted fever, Q fever, and the typhus group rickettsioses.

COURSE. The course and outcome of rickettsial infections depend on the infecting organism, the inoculum, and the institution of appropriate therapy. Rickettsialpox is a mild, uniformly nonfatal disorder, whereas untreated RMSF and epidemic typhus can result in high mortality. Relapses can occur even with appropriate antimicrobial therapy.

MANAGEMENT. Tetracycline and chloramphenicol are the antimicrobial agents of choice for the treatment of rickettsial diseases. Both drugs shorten the duration of symptoms and reduce mortality virtually to zero except in complicated cases. Since neither drug is rickettsicidal, ultimate clinical response and freedom from relapse depend on an adequate immune response of the patient. Both oral (tetracycline, 25 to 50 mg/kg/day in four divided doses; chloramphenicol, 50 to 75 mg/kg/day in four divided doses) and parenteral (tetracycline, 0.5 g every 6 hours intravenously; chloramphenicol succinate, 1 g every 8 to 12 hours intravenously) routes are effective. Antibiotics should be administered until the patient is afebrile and 10 to 14 days have elapsed from the onset of illness.

ROCKY MOUNTAIN SPOTTED FEVER

DEFINITION. RMSF, or tick-borne typhus, caused by *R. rickettsii,* is characterized by fever, headache, and rash originating on the extremities. Ticks capable of transmitting the disease to man are limited to the Western Hemisphere (United States, Mexico, Brazil).

ETIOLOGY. *R. rickettsii* shares group antigens with other members of the spotted fever group. It is unique in its ability to penetrate and multiply in the cytoplasm and nucleus of the host cell. An exotoxin has been identified, but its role in the pathogenesis of the disease is unclear. Although other species of spotted fever rickettsiae have been isolated from ticks in the United States, they have not been implicated in infections of man.

EPIDEMIOLOGY. The main vectors for transmission of *R. rickettsii* to man are hard (Ixodidae) ticks: *Dermacentor variabilis,* the dog tick, primarily distributed in the southern United States, and *D. andersoni,* the wood tick, found in the western United States. Other species serve as vectors in Central and South America. Rickettsiae multiply in salivary glands of infected ticks without causing vector death and are transmitted transovarially to all progeny. The reservoir for *R. rickettsii* in nature is a zoonotic cycle between infected ticks and small mammals, principally rodents. Illness is produced only in man, a dead-end host who intrudes into the zoonotic cycle by occupational or recreational exposure to tick-infested wooded areas or dogs. All ages are susceptible, but the disease is most common in children under age 15. The peak incidence of RMSF in the United States, from mid-April to mid-September, corresponds to the peak feeding and reproductive season of ticks.

PATHOGENESIS. Rickettsiae are inoculated directly into skin by a tick bite. Tick attachment of 4 to 6 hours appears critical. Ocular contamination with infected tick blood may also result in illness. A transient rickettsemia deposits the organism in vascular endothelial cells and produces a systemic angiitis. The virulence of *R. rickettsii* resides in its capacity to penetrate cells beyond the endothelium, thus producing pronounced thrombosis and necrosis of muscular layers of involved vessels. Microinfarction of organs such as skin, brain, heart, and kidneys is characteristic. Rickettsial action on tissue cell membranes produces a pronounced shift of water and electrolytes from intracellular to extracellular spaces.

CLINICAL MANIFESTATIONS. A history of tick exposure may be obtained from most patients, but the site of the tick bite frequently is inapparent. The incubation period depends on the inoculum of rickettsiae and may range from 1 to 10 or more days (median 5.5 days). Clinical presentation is more severe after short incubation periods.

The onset usually is sudden with a severe frontal headache, chills, fever of 102.2° to 104° F (39° to 40° C), myalgia (especially in the legs), conjunctival injection, photophobia, periorbital edema, nausea, and prostration. The characteristic rash appears on the third to fifth day but occasionally may be present as early as the first day of illness. Of confirmed cases between 1977 and 1980, 12% did not develop a rash.

The initial lesions are macular and blanching, 1 to 4 mm in diameter, and distributed primarily over the ankles and wrists. Rapid spread involves the palms, soles, trunk, face, and occasionally mucous membranes. In the absence of treatment the lesions become petechial, then purpuric, and finally coalesce. In fulminant or untreated cases shock, azotemia, peripheral gangrene, and skin infarction and gastrointestinal hemorrhage may occur. Adult respiratory distress syndrome may supervene. Central nervous system involvement manifested by delirium and stupor is common. Coma, focal neurologic findings, and seizures may ensue. Splenomegaly occurs in about 20% of patients.

LABORATORY FINDINGS. The total white blood cell count frequently is normal or slightly depressed. Thrombocytopenia and disturbed clotting parameters may indicate disseminated intravascular coagulation. Hyponatremia from increased production of antidiuretic hormone is particularly common in children. Oliguria and azotemia are common in severe cases. The cerebrospinal fluid usually is normal but may contain a few mononuclear cells and elevated protein levels.

DIAGNOSIS. An acute febrile illness accompanied by a rash occurring during the appropriate season in a person with a history of exposure to ticks should alert the physician to the possibility of RMSF. Serologic confirmation by the Weil-Felix reaction (elevated serum antibody titers to *Proteus* OX-2 and OX-19) or CF test rarely yields results early enough for efficient management. Antibody rises are first detected 7 to 14 days after infection and may be delayed by antimicrobial treatment. The most useful early diagnostic technique is direct immunofluorescent detection of rickettsiae in skin biopsies. An IgM-specific immunofluorescence assay detects serologic responses within the first week of illness.

COURSE AND MANAGEMENT. Overall mortality for RMSF remains between 3% and 10% (20% in untreated cases). Prognosis depends in part on the severity of the infection and the host's age. The single most critical factor is early institution of appropriate antirickettsial treatment with tetracycline or chloramphenicol. In uncomplicated cases treated before the fifth day of illness, the residual morbidity and mortality are nil. In severe or complicated cases defervescence is by slow lysis and convalescence may take months. Death in nonfulminant cases usually occurs because atypical initial symptoms and late appearance of rash result in delay in diagnosis and treatment and cardiac and respiratory failure ensue.

PREVENTION. Prophylactic measures are aimed primarily at prevention of tick attachment or early tick removal. Effective vaccines are still in the experimental phase. Chemoprophylaxis only delays the onset of the disease.

RICKETTSIALPOX

DEFINITION. Rickettsialpox is a mild, self-limited rickettsial disease transmitted by rodent mites. It is characterized by an initial eschar and a papulovesicular rash.

ETIOLOGY. The agent of rickettsialpox is *R. akari,* a member of the spotted fever group.

EPIDEMIOLOGY. *R. akari,* isolated in the United States, Soviet Union, and Korea, is maintained in nature in a zoonotic cycle involving house mice, voles, and the rodent mite *Allodermanyssus sanguineus.* Transovarial transmission of rickettsiae occurs in mites. Man is an incidental host parasitized by mites distributed by rodents proliferating in urban areas.

PATHOLOGY. Infection with *R. akari* produces the vascular lesions typical of other rickettsial infections; however, such lesions are limited to the epidermis and do not result in frank arteritis or hemorrhage. Necrosis of the superficial epithelium in the skin leads to formation of fluid-filled vesicles.

CLINICAL MANIFESTATIONS. An eschar develops at the site of rickettsial inoculation 7 to 10 days after a painless mite bite. The lesion progresses from an erythematous papule to a vesicle to a black encrusted lesion 1 to 2 cm in diameter that heals with scarring. Regional lymphadenopathy is common. Constitutional symptoms appear suddenly 1 week after the initial skin lesion develops and consist of intermittent fever, chills, headache, lassitude, myalgia, and photophobia. A sparse, generalized vesicular eruption, sparing the palms and soles, appears 1 to 4 days after the onset of fever.

LABORATORY FINDINGS AND DIAGNOSIS. Diagnosis is made primarily on clinical grounds; chickenpox must be excluded. Laboratory findings are not distinctive. Complement-fixing antibody titers peak 2 to 4 weeks after infection, but the Weil-Felix reaction is negative. The immunofluorescent antibody test appears more sensitive.

COURSE AND MANAGEMENT. In the absence of specific therapy the course of rickettsialpox remains benign; defervescence occurs in 1 week and the vesicles heal by desquamation without scarring. No deaths have been recorded. Antimicrobial therapy reduces the severity and duration of illness. Tetracycline is most effective.

PREVENTION. No vaccines are available. Rodent control is the definitive preventive measure, but effective miticides exist.

LOUSE-BORNE (EPIDEMIC) TYPHUS FEVER

DEFINITION. Classic typhus fever, a man-adapted acute rickettsial infection, is transmitted in epidemics by the human body louse. It is characterized by a sustained high fever, altered mental state, and a macular rash. Brill-Zinsser disease is a generally milder recurrent or recrudescent form of primary typhus.

ETIOLOGY. *R. prowazekii* has been isolated from patients with primary and recrudescent typhus. It is related antigenically to the agent of murine typhus.

EPIDEMIOLOGY. Louse-borne typhus occurs wherever living conditions predispose to the transfer of body lice among people. Rickettsiae from a person with primary or recrudescent typhus are ingested during a blood meal and multiply in the midgut of the body louse. Before its death from intestinal obstruction, the insect vector excretes large numbers of rickettsiae in its feces; there is no transovarian infection. Human disease is acquired by contamination of the louse bite site with crushed infective lice or lice feces or by inhalation of airborne infective lice feces. Primary louse-borne typhus no longer occurs in the United States. The recrudescent form of the illness continues to surface in European immigrants who acquired the primary disease during World War II; such individuals could initiate new epidemics if body lice were prevalent. Sporadic *R. prowazekii* infections have been confirmed in 33 patients in the eastern United States since 1976. A nonhuman reservoir appears to be present in eastern flying squirrels (*Glaucomys volans*). Transmission of rickettsiae to humans from squirrels has not been proved but is highly suggested on epidemiologic grounds. The mechanism of transmission has not been defined, but infections tend to occur in winter months, when squirrels nest in attics.

PATHOGENESIS. Histopathologically, classic typhus produces the systemic vasculitis of small vessels and capillaries typical of other rickettsial diseases. Skin, heart, muscle, brain, and kidneys are primary sites of involvement. Virulent, unmodified *R. prowazekii* can survive in tissues of an immune host for months to years. Rickettsemic recrudescence is believed to result from waning immunity.

CLINICAL MANIFESTATIONS. Abrupt onset of fever, chills, severe headache, myalgias, and mental clouding occurs 7 to 12 days after an inapparent louse bite. Photophobia, deafness, tinnitus, and vertigo are prominent features. Relative bradycardia and a nonproductive cough with minimal physical findings are present in most patients. On approximately the fifth day a maculopapular rash begins on the trunk and in axillary folds and spreads to involve the extremities. The face, palms, and soles are spared. In severe cases the rash may become petechial and varying degrees of skin necrosis may occur. In classic untreated typhus hypotension, cyanosis, azotemia, progressive neurologic dysfunction with selective cranial nerve involvement and hemiplegia from vascular thrombosis, and gangrene of extremities may develop. Bacterial superinfection is common.

DIAGNOSIS. The Weil-Felix reaction yields positive results against *Proteus* OX-2 and OX-19 but does not distinguish among primary typhus, RMSF, and murine typhus. CF tests exclude RMSF. Indirect immunofluorescent techniques using serum selectively absorbed with *R. prowazekii* or *R. typhi* (murine typhus) can differentiate classic and murine typhus. The Weil-Felix reaction is negative in Brill-Zinsser disease. Detection of complement-fixing antibody of the IgG class separates recrudescent from primary (IgM) typhus.

COURSE. Death or recovery in primary classic typhus occurs between the ninth and the eighteenth days of illness. Mortality in untreated cases has ranged from 10% to 60%. Poor prognostic factors include advanced age, poor nutrition, concurrent diseases, hypotension, and deep coma. Antimicrobial treatment with tetracycline before the moribund state virtually eliminates fatal illness, but relapse may occur if treatment is begun very early after the onset of symptoms. Patients with squirrel-associated epidemic typhus respond rapidly to appropriate antimicrobial therapy; however, to date no patient has died regardless of treatment. Mortality is negligible in patients with prior vaccination or recrudescent disease.

PREVENTION. A formalin-killed vaccine is available and attenuates the severity and mortality of the disease. Decontamination and delousing of the infected patient and those at risk are of paramount importance in epidemic situations. Quarantine measures are unnecessary.

MURINE (FLEA-BORNE) TYPHUS FEVER

DEFINITION. Murine typhus, a sporadic rickettsial disease transmitted from rodent hosts to man by a rat-flea vector, resembles a mild form of classic epidemic typhus.

ETIOLOGY. *R. typhi* (formerly *R. mooseri*) closely resembles the agent of classic typhus and confers cross-immunity after infection but not after vaccination.

EPIDEMIOLOGY. Murine typhus is found all over the world; recently a clustering of cases was documented in southern Texas. The disorder usually is transmitted to man by contamination of flea bites with infective flea feces, but inhaling dried flea feces or contact with conjunctivae also may result in infection. There is no seasonal predilection, although the disease is more prevalent in urban areas during summer and fall months.

The fleas normally coexist with rats and other small mammals, the amplifying hosts and reservoirs for murine typhus in nature. Rickettsiae multiply in and are shed from the guts of infected fleas without injuring the host.

PATHOLOGY. The lesions of murine typhus resemble those of louse-borne typhus.

COURSE AND DIAGNOSIS. Clinically, murine typhus closely resembles louse-borne typhus, but the manifestations are milder, the duration is shorter, and complication and mortality (less than 5%) are lower. Deaths usually occur only in the elderly and the debilitated. Response to antirickettsial therapy is prompt. Serologic differentiation from classic typhus is based on indirect immunofluorescent techniques.

PREVENTION. Preventive measures are aimed at control of rodent and flea populations and prevention of flea infestation by repellent treatment of clothing.

Q FEVER

DEFINITION. Q fever is a rickettsial disease of man with three unique features: (1) it is acquired by inhalation and requires no arthropod vector, (2) it usually produces a granulomatous hepatitis, and (3) it very infrequently produces a rash.

ETIOLOGY. *C. burnetii*, the agent of Q fever, is resistant to desiccation and can survive for prolonged periods in dust and soil, on clothing, and in animal hides, possibly as a result of sporelike structures. In the host it multiplies in cytoplasmic vacuoles of endothelial cells and serosal cells. Two antigenic phases have been identified: phase I, or host-adapted, organisms are obtained from tissues of infected animals; phase II, or egg-adapted, organisms are recovered after serial passage in embryonated eggs.

EPIDEMIOLOGY. The true incidence of Q fever in man is unknown. Worldwide serologic evidence of animal and human exposure to *C. burnetii* suggests frequent occurrence of inapparent infections that remain undiagnosed.

Two major patterns of transmission are known: a first cycle involves wild animals, in which rickettsiae are transmitted by a tick vector, and a second cycle involves domesticated ungulates (cattle, sheep, goats), rabbits, and cats, in which the principal mode of transmission is by an infectious aerosol of rickettsiae. Human beings acquire the disease by inhalation of dust contaminated by rickettsiae derived from birth tissues or excreta of infected animals, by processing infected animal products, or by ingestion of contaminated milk.

PATHOGENESIS. Pulmonary involvement in Q fever resembles a viral or chlamydial pneumonia, with alveolar and bronchial necrosis and mononuclear cell infiltration. Granulomata (particularly lipoid granulomas with fibrin rings) and/ or inflammatory foci showing hepatocellular necrosis with macrophage infiltration are present in liver biopsy specimens. Myocarditis, pericarditis, or subacute endocarditis may complicate the course of this disease.

CLINICAL MANIFESTATIONS AND COURSE. In patients with overt acute infections, severe headache, fever, chills, drenching sweats, myalgias, headache, and prostration develop abruptly after an incubation period of 9 to 28 days. The frequency of clinical and roentgenographic pneumonitis varies (10% to 90%). A macular trunkal rash has been reported infrequently (3% to 4%). Anicteric hepatitis with hepatomegaly and abnormalities of hepatic function is common. Defervescence usually occurs in 2 to 3 weeks, although fever occasionally may persist for several months. Convalescence is prolonged, and relapse may occur. Mortality is less than 1%, even in untreated patients. In rare cases chronic disease in the form of micronodular cirrhosis or subacute endocarditis may appear years after the acute attack. Endocarditis usually occurs in patients who already have valvular disease or who have prosthetic valves.

DIAGNOSIS. The diagnosis is based on epidemiologic data and on serologic methods. The indirect immunofluorescence antibody test currently is the method of choice for Q fever laboratory diagnosis, since it permits the detection of IgG-, IgM-, and IgA-specific antibodies against the two phases of *C. burnetii* in a single serum specimen. CF tests are based on fourfold antibody rises in serial serum samples. In acute Q fever the major antibody response is directed against the phase 2 antigen and is present in the IgM, IgG, and IgA fractions. In chronic Q fever endocarditis the serologic pattern shows an absence of IgM antibody and high levels of antibody (particularly IgA-specific antibody) to phase 1 antigen.

MANAGEMENT. Q fever is less clinically responsive to antimicrobial treatment than are the other rickettsioses. Tetracycline shortens the course of the acute disease only if administered within the first 3 days of illness. Q fever endocarditis is particularly resistant to antibiotics and requires prolonged drug therapy (usually with tetracycline and trimethoprim-sulfamethoxazole) and possible valve replacement to effect a cure.

PREVENTION. Commercial vaccines are not available, although in recent trials in Australia a formalin-inactivated phase 1 vaccine conferred protection with minimal adverse reactions. Current control measures are limited to pasteurization of milk and prompt destruction of infected placentas.

EHRLICHIOSIS

DEFINITION. Ehrlichia are tick-borne rickettsial organisms that cause disease in animals and that recently have been recognized as human pathogens.

ETIOLOGY. Ehrlichia are obligate, intracellular bacterial members of the family Rickettsiaceae that infect the circulating leukocytes of domestic and wild animals. Five species are recognized (*Ehrlichia canis, E. risticii, E. equi, E. phagocytophila,* and *E. sennetsu*), which cause natural infections in dogs, horses, sheep, cattle, and bison.

EPIDEMIOLOGY. *E. sennetsu* has been associated with a mononucleosis-like illness confined to western Japan and Malaysia. *E. canis* infection has been recognized as the cause of tropical canine pancytopenia. In the United States seroprevalence of antibody to *E. canis* in dogs ranges from 11% to

58% (highest rates in southern states). The brown dog tick (*Rhipicephalus sanguineus*) is the vector. Human infections have been recognized only recently in individuals exposed to ticks and in patients with AIDS. Limited serologic surveys suggest that infection may not be uncommon.

PATHOGENESIS. Data on pathogenesis are derived from experimental infections in dogs. Extensive plasmacyte infiltration and perivascular cuffing occurs in the lungs, meninges, kidneys and spleen. Increased mononuclear cell adherence to vascular endothelium is noted in association with the presence of *E. canis* in the endothelial vessels. Pneumonitis, vasculitis, phlebitis, and glomerulonephritis are observed. In one well-documented human infection peripheral blood smears revealed inclusion bodies (identified as rickettsiae of the genus *Ehrlichia*) in lymphocytes, neutrophils, and monocytes. The frequency of parasitemia was 1 to 2 infected cells per 100 white cells. Bone marrow biopsies reveal hypocellularity and non-caseating granulomas.

CLINICAL MANIFESTATIONS. All patients have reported tick exposure. After an incubation period of 10 to 14 days, an acute illness resembling Rocky Mountain spotted fever develops; fever is accompanied by headache, encephalopathy, nausea, and vomiting. Leukopenia, lymphocytopenia, and thrombocytopenia are striking during the first week of illness. Mild liver function test abnormalities with hyperbilirubinemia are common. A rash does not occur. Renal tubular necrosis and anemia also may develop.

DIAGNOSIS. The presence of rickettsia-like intraleukocytic organisms provides a clue to the pathogenic organism. In the absence of this finding, ehrlichial infection must be considered in a patient with a febrile illness but no rash who has been exposed to ticks. Serologic rises against *E. canis* can be detected by an indirect fluorescent antibody test.

MANAGEMENT AND COURSE. Defervescence and normalization of pancytopenia occur promptly after treatment with tetracycline or its analogs.

PREVENTION. The epidemiology of *E. canis* infections in man is not fully defined. Avoiding tick attachment seems prudent.

BIBLIOGRAPHY
Rocky Mountain spotted fever

Ascher MS and others: Initial clinical evaluation of Rocky Mountain spotted fever vaccine of tissue culture origin, J Infect Dis 138:217, 1978.
Helmick CG and others: Rocky Mountain spotted fever: clinical, laboratory, epidemiologic features of 262 cases, J Infect Dis 150:480, 1984.
Kaplan JE and Schonberger LB: The sensitivity of various serologic tests in the diagnosis of Rocky Mountain spotted fever, Am J Trop Med Hyg 35:840, 1986.
Miller JO and Price TR: Involvement of the brain in Rocky Mountain spotted fever: identification of rickettsiae in skin tissues, J Infect Dis 65:437, 1972.
Wilfert CM and others: Epidemiology of Rocky Mountain spotted fever as determined by active surveillance, J Infect Dis 150:469, 1984.
Wilson LB and Chowning WM: Studies on pyroplasmosis hominis: "spotted fever" or "tick fever" of the Rocky Mountains, Rev Infect Dis 1:540, 1979.
Woodward TE and others: Prompt confirmation of Rocky Mountain spotted fever: identification of rickettsiae in skin tissues, J Infect Dis 134:297, 1976.

Rickettsialpox

Brettman LR and others: Rickettsialpox: report of an outbreak and a contemporary review, Medicine 60:363, 1981.

Louse-borne (epidemic) typhus fever

Duma RJ and others: Epidemic typhus in the United States associated with flying squirrels, JAMA 245:2318, 1981.
Murray ES and others: Briss's disease. I. Clinical and laboratory diagnosis, JAMA 142:1059, 1950.

Woodward TE: Rickettsial diseases in the United States, Med Clin North Am 43:1507, 1959.

Murine (flea-borne) typhus fever

Murine typhus: clinical conference at the Johns Hopkins Hospital, Johns Hopkins Med J 141:303, 1977.
Taylor JP and others: Epidemiology of murine typhus in Texas, 1980 through 1984, JAMA 255:2173, 1986.

Q fever

Clark WH and others: Q fever in California, Arch Intern Med 88:155, 1951.
Derrick EH: The course of infection with *Coxiella burnetii*, Med J Aust 1:1051, 1973.
Marmion BP and others: Vaccine prophylaxis of abattoir-associated Q fever, Lancet 2:1411, 1984.
McCaul TF and Williams JC: Developmental cycle of *Coxiella burnetii's* structure and morphogenesis of vegetative and sporogenic differentiation, J Bacteriol 147:1063, 1981.
Peacock MG and others: Serologic evaluation of Q fever in humans, enhanced phase-1 titer to immunoglobulin G and A are diagnostic for Q fever endocarditis, Infect Immun 41:1089, 1983.
Spelman DW: Q fever: a study of 111 consecutive cases, Med J Aust 1:547, 1982.

Ehrlichiosis

Fishbein DB and others: Unexplained febrile illness after exposure to ticks. Infection with *Ehrlichia*? JAMA 257:3100, 1987.
Maeda K and others: Human infection with *Ehrlichia canis*, a leukocytic rickettsia, N Engl J Med 316:853, 1987.

43 · DISEASES CAUSED BY CHLAMYDIAE

Michael F. Rein

Chlamydiae were described in the first decade of the twentieth century and have been known by a variety of names, including *Bedsonia, Miyagawanella*, psittacosis-lymphogranuloma-trachoma (PLT) agents, and trachoma-inclusion conjunctivitis (TRIC) agents. They have a biphasic life cycle. Elementary bodies are nonreproducing, infectious, 300 nm particles that are taken up by host cells. They then differentiate into reticulate bodies, approximately 1000 nm in size, which divide by binary fission through several generations and form one or more cytoplasmic inclusions that may displace the nucleus of the host cell. Each inclusion is actually a microcolony of reticulate bodies that change back into elementary bodies and burst forth from the cell to infect their neighbors. The reproductive cycle requires approximately 24 hours and depends on the host cell's ability to generate metabolic energy. Because they are obligate intracellular parasites, chlamydiae have been confused with viruses and can only be isolated in tissue culture systems. Recently, direct immunofluorescence and enzyme-linked immunosorbent assay (ELISA) techniques have become available for identifying chlamydiae in clinical specimens. Unlike the viruses, chlamydiae reproduce by binary fission rather than subunit assembly, possess both DNA and RNA, and most importantly from the clinical standpoint, are susceptible to a variety of antimicrobial agents. They cause disease in a number of birds and mammals, but only three species are pathogenic for man: *Chlamydia trachomatis, Chlamydia psittaci*, and the newly described TWAR agent.

CHLAMYDIA TRACHOMATIS

C. trachomatis is characterized by its sensitivity to sulfonamides, tetracyclines, and erythromycins and its limited sensitivity to β-lactams. Intracellular inclusions stain with iodine.

infections and their complications; and L$_1$ to L$_3$, which cause lymphogranuloma venereum (LGV).

Trachoma

The major single cause of blindness worldwide, trachoma is most prevalent in the Middle East and North Africa. In the 1950s there was a recrudescence of cases among Indians in the southwestern United States. Chlamydiae are thought to reach the conjunctiva by personal contact or on the feet of flies. The disease may begin abruptly with inflammation of the conjunctiva. Within a few weeks the patient develops hypertrophic follicles on the palpebral conjunctiva and microscopic ulcerations on the cornea. It is believed that initial infections may heal spontaneously at this point without significantly impairing vision. In endemic areas, however, reinfection is common, and experimental evidence indicates that with each reinfection the disease becomes more severe, suggesting that an immune response may contribute to pathogenesis. Patients have vascularization of the cornea and scarring of the conjunctiva that result in a turning in of the lid and chronic irritation of the cornea by the lashes. Intercurrent bacterial infections also may be a problem. Typical chlamydial inclusions can be demonstrated by Giemsa stain or direct immunofluorescence of conjunctival scrapings, and chlamydial antibody is detectable in tears. Oral therapy with a sulfonamide, tetracycline, or erythromycin can eradicate the infection, but surgery may be required to correct scarring.

Genital infections and complications

Men who have urethritis not caused by *Neisseria gonorrhoeae* are said to have nongonococcal urethritis (NGU). *C. trachomatis* causes 30% to 50% of such infections. The agents responsible for chlamydiae-negative NGU have not been completely identified but include *Ureaplasma urealyticum*. Chlamydial urethritis tends to manifest somewhat differently from gonococcal urethritis, but there is considerable clinical overlap. The incubation period for chlamydial urethritis typically is described as lasting 7 to 14 days, but in one study almost 50% of the infected men had urethral symptoms within 4 days of infection. The urethral discharge is purulent in about one third of men with chlamydial infection and mucopurulent in about half. A completely clear discharge may be seen in 10% of infected men. Dysuria is noted by 50% to 75% of patients with chlamydial urethritis and generally is less severe than with gonococcal infection. The symptoms of chlamydial urethritis may increase gradually over several days and may even resolve for brief periods. In women symptoms of urethritis include dysuria, frequency, urgency, and nocturia, thus resembling those of cystitis. Frank urethral discharge is noticed by relatively few women. Symptomatic women with pyuria whose urine cultures fail to reveal standard bacterial pathogens are said to have the urethral syndrome; some of these cases are clearly chlamydial urethritis and respond to treatment with tetracycline. Sexual partners must be treated simultaneously.

So great are the clinical overlaps between chlamydial and gonococcal urethritis that differential diagnosis should not be made on clinical grounds alone. Initial management should include examination of a Gram-stained smear of urethral discharge. The smear reveals typical, gram-negative diplococci in about 95% of cases of gonococcal urethritis. The observation of gram-negative diplococci lying between the cells predicts gonorrhea correctly only about 25% to 75% of the time. Urethral smears from patients with chlamydial urethritis generally show polymorphonuclear neutrophils and normal urethral flora. Patients with smears diagnostic of gonorrhea should be treated

for that infection. Patients with smears suggesting NGU should be cultured for gonococci, because the smear will miss 5% of gonococcal infections, but such patients may be started immediately on therapy directed against chlamydiae. Doxycycline (100 mg orally two times daily for at least 7 days) is the treatment of choice for uncomplicated genital infection in men and nonpregnant women. Erythromycin stearate, ethylsuccinate, or a base in the same doses is an effective alternative in pregnancy; this avoids the risk of staining or dysplasia of fetal bones and teeth with tetracycline.

Chlamydia can be carried in the urethras of asymptomatic men. Many of these men have urethral inflammation manifested as polymorphonuclear neutrophils observed on a Gram-stained smear of material recovered from within the urethra.

Direct proximal extension of urethral infection can involve the epididymis. *C. trachomatis* is a major cause of acute epididymitis in young, sexually active men. About 75% of such patients have a urethral discharge, and a similar number note inguinal pain. Scrotal edema and erythema are more suggestive of other causes.

Chlamydiae may be transferred from the genitalia to the conjunctiva on the fingers to cause an oculogenital syndrome. Ocular findings resemble those of early trachoma, with hypertrophy of conjunctival follicles. Chlamydial urethritis apparently can incite Reiter's syndrome, consisting of NGU, conjunctivitis, arthritis, and dermatitis, but in this case the multiple-system involvement results from an altered immune response rather than disseminated infection.

Chlamydiae have been recovered from the pharynx and have recently been associated with pharyngitis. They also are cultured from the rectum, and although most of this carriage is asymptomatic, they may cause infectious proctitis in homosexual men who practice receptive anal intercourse.

N. gonorrhoeae and *C. trachomatis* are sometimes acquired from the same sexual exposure. In this setting symptoms of gonococcal urethritis usually appear first. If the patient is treated with a β-lactam antibiotic, his gonorrhea will be cured and he may feel better for several days before a recurrence of milder urethral symptoms is seen. This syndrome of postgonococcal urethritis reflects the generally longer incubation period and relative resistance to penicillins of chlamydial infection. The physician must rule out the possibilities of reinfection with gonorrhea or true treatment failure. Postgonococcal urethritis is treated like NGU. So frequently are patients with gonorrhea also infected with chlamydiae that the physician initially should consider treating patients for gonorrhea with a single dose of a β-lactam antibiotic followed by a week of a tetracycline to cover occult coincident chlamydial infection.

C. trachomatis can be recovered from the endocervix of 60% to 90% of the sexual partners of men with chlamydial NGU. Although such women usually are asymptomatic, the organism is far from benign, and the sexual contacts of infected men should be routinely treated. Cervical abnormalities, often mild, are seen in 80% of chlamydial carriers attending venereal disease clinics. *N. gonorrhoeae* and herpes simplex also can cause cervicitis and are part of the differential diagnosis. Chlamydial infection has been associated with mucopurulent cervicitis, manifesting as a purulent or mucopurulent cervical discharge and cervical erythema. After appropriate treatment with a tetracycline, the purulent discharge and congested appearance resolve.

Chlamydiae can spread from the endocervix to the fallopian tubes, resulting in nongonococcal pelvic inflammatory disease (PID). The frequency with which PID follows chlamydial infection of the cervix has yet to be defined. Clinical features of chlamydial and gonococcal PID are similar—principally, lower abdominal pain that may be accompanied by vaginal discharge, dysuria, and fever. The pain often is dull or occasionally cramping, and it frequently begins or is exacerbated at the time of menstruation. Mild vaginal discharge occurs in more than half of infected women, and menstrual irregularities are described by about a third. Adnexal tenderness is detected in about 90% of such women, and pain on movement of the cervix is common. Peritonitis and perihepatitis may complicate chlamydial PID. Optimal antibiotic therapy is not defined.

Cervical infection frequently is transmitted to the newborn during the birth process. Up to 70% of infants vaginally delivered of infected women are colonized with chlamydiae at the conjunctiva, pharynx, or rectum. In 40% to 50% of such infants, chlamydial ophthalmia neonatorum will develop, and silver nitrate prophylaxis seems to have less effect on the incidence of this disease than it does on gonococcal conjunctivitis. Symptoms generally develop at about 8 days and include conjunctival injection, edema of the lids, and purulent discharge. Conjunctival follicular hypertrophy, characteristic of infection in adults, is not observed in neonates. Once again, the clinical overlap with gonococcal disease is extensive; differential diagnosis cannot be made on clinical grounds alone but must depend on microscopic examination and culture of the conjunctival discharge. Infected children should be treated with systemic antibiotics, such as erythromycin, which would also eliminate organisms from extraocular sites of colonization. Tetracyclines should be avoided in children under 8 years of age, because they may cause staining and dysplasia of bones and teeth.

Nasopharyngeal carriage of chlamydia has been associated with the subsequent development of pneumonia. Symptoms appear between 2 and 12 weeks of age and consist of paroxysms of coughing without the inspiratory whoop of the pertussis syndrome. Affected babies usually are afebrile, although they may become significantly hypoxic. About 50% have an accompanying or preceding conjunctivitis, and 75% manifest circulating eosinophilia. Chest roentgenograms reveal diffuse infiltrates and usually some degree of hyperinflation. Treatment with erythromycin ameliorates the condition.

Lymphogranuloma venereum

Fewer than 500 cases of lymphogranuloma venereum (LGV) are reported annually in the United States, but the disease is considerably more prevalent in Southeast Asia and parts of Africa and South America. LGV is acquired principally through sexual contact, and the incubation period ranges from 3 days to 3 weeks. The initial genital lesion—a small, soft papule that may ulcerate—goes unnoticed by 70% to 95% of patients. Inguinal adenopathy is the most common initial complaint. It is unilateral in 70% of cases and often is initially noted as stiffness or aching in the groin 2 to 6 weeks after the infecting sexual contact. The nodes become matted and attached to the overlying skin, which sometimes develops a purplish color. Involved nodes often are painful and frequently suppurate and rupture; chronic lymphadenopathy develops in about 5% of patients. Inguinal adenopathy above and below Poupart's ligament often looks like a single lymphoid mass bisected by a groove. This phenomenon is observed in only 15% to 30% of patients with LGV but is highly suggestive of the diagnosis.

Primary inoculation into the oral or conjunctival mucosa has been reported. In these cases anterior and posterior cervical and preauricular adenopathy may result.

Fever, chills, headache, meningismus, anorexia, and myalgias are common. An acute proctocolitis syndrome with a bloody, purulent discharge sometimes follows direct inoculation of organisms into patients practicing receptive anal intercourse. Late involvement of the rectum may result from direct inoculation of patients practicing receptive anal intercourse or possibly by extension along lymphatics from a primary genital source. A colitis syndrome with a bloody, purulent discharge sometimes occurs, and stenosis, fissuring, and even perforation of the colon may result. Rectal complications can develop a decade after the initial manifestations of disease. Obstructive scarring of the regional lymphatics occasionally causes lymphedema of the genitalia or lower extremities.

Diagnosis is best made by culturing chlamydiae from tissue but also may be made presumptively by CF or microimmunofluorescent tests. A significant rise in antibody titer is observed in 95% of cases but also may occur in patients with other chlamydial infections.

LGV can be treated with tetracycline (500 mg); erythromycin (500 mg); or sulfisoxazole (1 g); each administered orally four times daily for 3 weeks.

CHLAMYDIA PSITTACI

C. psittaci differs from C. trachomatis in that its intracellular inclusions do not contain glycogen. The organism is resistant to sulfonamides but is sensitive to tetracyclines and erythromycin. An economically important cause of illness in a variety of birds, it is transmitted to man following inhalation of dust contaminated with droppings. Sporadic cases have been associated with psittacine birds (parrots) but also with canaries, ducks, and pigeons. Psittacosis is also referred to as ornithosis, recognizing its acquisition from nonpsittacine birds. Recent epidemics have followed occupational exposure to turkeys, and rare acquisition from mammals also has been described. About 50 human cases are reported each year, and the decline in human incidence may be related to incorporation of tetracycline into animal feeds.

Psittacosis

After an incubation period of 7 to 14 days, psittacosis usually starts abruptly with fever. The pulse rate may be slower than expected, but this pulse-temperature deficit occurs in a variety of other infections, including mycoplasmal pneumonia. About 50% of infected patients complain of a persistent and usually nonproductive cough, although small amounts of mucoid sputum, sometimes blood-tinged, may be seen; about 25% of those infected describe chills, headache, chest pain, or myalgias. In rare cases patients have meningitic manifestations or fever in the absence of any localizing symptoms.

Examination reveals rales but usually not consolidation. Roentgenographic changes often are considerably more extensive than expected on the basis of physical examination. Splenomegaly has been reported in up to 75% of infected patients, a finding suggestive of psittacosis.

The diagnosis generally is suspected on clinical grounds but may be confirmed using the chlamydial serologic tests already described. Major differential diagnoses include mycoplasmal pneumonia in young people and Legionnaires' disease in older people. Treatment with tetracycline, 500 mg orally four times daily for 21 days, is effective.

TWAR

A newly described chlamydial agent causing acute, community-acquired pneumonia, the organism derives its unusual name from the first two isolates, TW-183 and AR-39. Clinical disease usually is mild and does not distinctly differ from other commonly acquired pneumonias. Tetracycline (500 mg orally four times daily for 14 days) apparently is effective therapy.

BIBLIOGRAPHY

Alexander ER: *Chlamydia:* the organism and neonatal infection, Hosp Practice, July 1979.

Brunham RC and others: Mucopurulent cervicitis—the ignored counterpart in women of urethritis in men, N Engl J Med 311:1, 1984.

Holmes KK: The *Chlamydia* epidemic, JAMA 245:1718, 1981.

Jacobs NF and Kraus SJ: Gonococcal and nongonococcal urethritis in men: clinical and laboratory differentiation, Ann Intern Med 82:712, 1975.

Marrie TJ and others: Pneumonia associated with the TWAR strain of *Chlamydia,* Ann Intern Med 106:507, 1987.

Hobson D and Holmes KK, editors: Nongonococcal urethritis and related infections, Washington, DC, 1977, American Society of Microbiology.

Schachter J: Chlamydial infections, N Engl J Med 298:428, 490, 540, 1978.

Schachter J and Dawson CR: Human chlamydial infections, Littleton, Mass, 1978, PSG Publishing Co, Inc.

44 · DISEASES CAUSED BY MYCOPLASMAS

Gerald R. Donowitz *and* Gerald L. Mandell

Mycoplasmas are bacteria-like organisms that lack cell walls. They may exist as intracellular parasites or as saprophytes. Three species of mycoplasma cause disease in man. *Mycoplasma pneumoniae* causes a range of respiratory illnesses, including atypical pneumonia, tracheobronchitis, pharyngitis, otitis media, and bullous myringitis. The organism has been suspected of playing an etiologic role in pericarditis, myocarditis, arthritis, and erythema multiforme. *Ureaplasma urealyticum* (T-strain mycoplasma) and *Mycoplasma hominis* cause urogenital infections. *U. urealyticum* may cause nongonococcal urethritis, salpingitis, and chorioamnionitis and may be associated with increased perinatal morbidity and mortality. *M. hominis* has been more clearly associated with pelvic inflammatory disease and has been implicated in puerperal sepsis and postpartum fever. *M. hominis* recently has also been implicated in bacteremia in a small number of trauma patients.

MYCOPLASMAL PNEUMONIA

EPIDEMIOLOGY. Mycoplasmal pneumonia occurs in only 3% to 10% of patients infected with *M. pneumoniae,* but it may account for up to 20% of community-acquired pneumonias. Infections occur throughout the year, with a relative increase in disease in late summer and early fall. The disease affects older children, adolescents, and young adults. Patients with sickle cell disease or immunodeficient states may be at greater risk of developing disease. An increased incidence of the disease and true epidemics have been noted in enclosed populations, such as military bases, colleges, and boarding schools.

PATHOGENESIS. *M. pneumoniae* organisms appear to adhere to the surface epithelium of the respiratory tract and remain extracellular. Disease is thought to be caused by both local effects of the organism and the host immune response to the organism.

Infections are associated with disruption of ciliary function and bronchial and bronchiolar epithelial cells. Mycoplasma organisms have been isolated from a variety of extrapulmonary sites. The role of direct invasion versus autoimmune phenomenon in the pathogenesis of extrapulmonary disease remains unclear.

CLINICAL MANIFESTATIONS. Constitutional symptoms usually predominate initially, with fever, malaise, and headache

being major features. Cough develops several days later and becomes a prominent symptom. Specific respiratory tract signs and symptoms—shortness of breath, pleuritic chest pain, and splinting—usually are absent. Rhonchi, wheezing, or rales may be heard on physical examination, although evidence of consolidation is unusual. Sputum production is quite variable; purulent sputum has been noted in approximately one third of cases. Skin rash, pharyngitis, tender cervical lymphadenopathy, and myringitis may be associated findings. White blood cell counts are usually less than 10,000 cells/mm^3, with higher counts noted in only 20% of patients. Chest roentgenograms often reveal more extensive disease than would have been expected from the history or physical examination. Patchy infiltrates are most common, usually involving the lower lobes in a bronchial or peribronchial distribution. Upper lobe involvement and pleural effusions have been described but are unusual. Gram stain and culture of sputum, if any is present, reveal sparse mouth flora only. There are few polymorphonuclear leukocytes in the sputum smear.

COURSE. The course of mycoplasmal pneumonia is usually benign. Without therapy, symptoms may persist for several weeks, with gradual normalization. Recurrences and progression of infiltrates, even with appropriate therapy, may occur. Rare complications include intravascular hemolysis, Raynaud's phenomenon, disseminated intravascular coagulation, meningoencephalitis, cerebellar ataxia, Guillain-Barré syndrome, myocarditis, pericarditis, Stevens-Johnson syndrome, hepatitis, arthritis, and pancreatitis.

DIAGNOSIS. While the definitive diagnosis of mycoplasmal pneumonia requires isolation of the organism, this may take several weeks, which greatly minimizes its clinical usefulness. Serologic diagnosis may be made in approximately 80% of the cases by demonstration of a significant rise of antibodies via complement fixation, enzyme-linked immunosorbent assay (ELISA), or indirect immunofluorescence.

MANAGEMENT. The therapy of choice for mycoplasmal pneumonia is oral erythromycin (500 mg every 6 to 8 hours,) or tetracycline (250 mg every 6 hours) for 2 to 3 weeks.

OTHER SYNDROMES

Tracheobronchitis and pharyngitis. Tracheobronchitis and pharyngitis may occur with mycoplasmal pneumonia or may appear as the sole manifestation of disease. Tracheobronchitis is the most common clinical manifestation of *M. pneumoniae* infection. The clinical presentation is much like that of mycoplasmal pneumonia, with constitutional symptoms predominating. Chest roentgenograms are normal. Pharyngitis caused by mycoplasma is indistinguishable from that caused by *Streptococcus pyogenes* or respiratory viruses. An erythematous palate and posterior pharyngeal and tonsillar exudates are noted, along with tender cervical adenopathy. In both tracheobronchitis and pharyngitis, definitive diagnosis requires the isolation of the organism or a rise in specific antibody titer. No specific therapy is recommended, since the disease is self-limited.

Bullous myringitis and otitis. Bullous myringitis, otitis externa, and otitis media occur in association with mycoplasmal pneumonia and as isolated disease entities. Drainage of any fluid behind the tympanic membrane together with 7 to 10 days of erythromycin or tetracycline therapy is recommended.

GENITAL MYCOPLASMAS

M. hominis and *U. urealyticum* are known as the genital mycoplasmas and cause disease in both males and females.

EPIDEMIOLOGY. Both of these mycoplasmas have been isolated frequently from the genitourinary tract of sexually active men and women. In most cases patients with a positive culture have been asymptomatic, indicating a high rate of colonization but a rather low predilection for true infection. Lower socioeconomic status and increased sexual activity have been associated with a higher frequency of carriage. Infants may be colonized with genital mycoplasmas as they pass through an infected or colonized birth canal.

PATHOGENESIS. The genital mycoplasmas are associated with the epithelial lining of the genitourinary tract. The mechanism of cell destruction and the means by which disease symptoms are caused are not known. The production of toxins by the organisms has been postulated but not proved.

CLINICAL MANIFESTATIONS

Nongonococcal urethritis. Nongonococcal urethritis (NGU) is a symptom complex of dysuria, frequency, urgency, and urethral discharge. The discharge associated with NGU usually is mucopurulent and may contain relatively few polymorphonuclear leukocytes with no gonorrhea-like organisms on Gram stain. Postgonococcal urethritis is a related syndrome in which symptoms of urethritis persist after adequate therapy for proven gonorrhea. Chlamydiae are the cause of most cases of nongonococcal and postgonococcal urethritis. Although *U. urealyticum* may cause NGU, its incidence remains unclear.

Pelvic inflammatory disease. Both *M. hominis* and *U. urealyticum* have been isolated from patients with salpingitis, tuboovarian abscesses, and pelvic abscesses. In most cases fever, lower abdominal pain, and a cervix that is tender on palpation and movement have been characteristic features. In one series genital mycoplasmas were isolated via laparoscopy from the fallopian tubes in approximately 10% of cases of salpingitis. *M. hominis* has been more commonly associated with this syndrome than *U. urealyticum*.

Septic abortion and puerperal infections. *M. hominis* has been isolated from the blood in 7.8% of women undergoing febrile abortions. In one series 50% of women showed a rise in antibody titers to one or more strains of *M. hominis*. *U. urealyticum* has only rarely been associated with this syndrome. Postpartum fever without abdominal signs has also been associated with the isolation of both organisms.

Infertility, spontaneous abortion, perinatal morbidity. The role of the genital mycoplasma in causing infertility remains controversial. Data suggest an association of *Ureaplasma urealyticum* and infertility in couples when male factors for fertility problems have been identified. Although clear cause and effect have not been demonstrated, therapy of males with tetracycline has led to an increased incidence of posttherapy pregnancies. Isolation of genital mycoplasmas has been associated with spontaneous abortion and increased perinatal mortality.

DIAGNOSIS. The genital mycoplasmas are difficult to culture and are not routinely sought by most microbiologic laboratories. The clinical picture is therefore of great importance in making a diagnosis.

MANAGEMENT. Tetracycline, (250 mg orally every 6 hours for 7 to 10 days) is the therapy of choice for disease caused by the genital mycoplasmas. *M. hominis* is resistant to erythromycin, although *U. urealyticum* is not. Specific therapy for septic abortion and puerperal infections associated with *M. hominis* has not been shown to be effective.

BIBLIOGRAPHY

George RB and others: Roentgenographic appearance of viral and mycoplasma pneumonias, Am Rev Respir Dis 96:1144, 1967.
Jacobs NF and Kraus SJ: Gonococcal and nongonococcal urethritis in men: clinical and laboratory differentiations, Ann Intern Med 82:712, 1975.
Kundsin RB and others: Association of ureaplasma urealyticum in the placenta with perinatal morbidity and mortality, N Engl J Med 310:941, 1984.

Levine DP and Lerner AM: The clinical spectrum of mycoplasma pneumonia infection, Med Clin North Am 62:961, 1978.
McCormack WM, Braun P, and Lee YH: The genital mycoplasmas, N Engl J Med 288:78, 1973.
Murray HW and others: The protean manifestations of mycoplasma pneumonia in adults, Am J Med 58:229, 1975.
Robinson DT and McCormack WM: The genital mycoplasmas, N Engl J Med 302:1003, 1980.

45 · DISEASES CAUSED BY GRAM-POSITIVE COCCI

Staphylococcal infections

Gerald R. Donowitz *and* Gerald L. Mandell

Staphylococci cause a wide variety of diseases that affect all age-groups. Three staphylococcal species are important in man: *Staphylococcus aureus* causes most infections; *Staphylococcus epidermidis* plays an important role in infections of intravenous lines, vascular shunts, and prosthetic implants; and *Staphylococcus saprophyticus* is a pathogen in urinary tract infections.

ETIOLOGY. Staphylococci are gram-positive cocci that occur in grapelike clusters in clinical and culture material. *S. aureus* can be separated from the other staphylococci by its production of coagulase and its positive reaction for deoxyribonuclease (DNase). The organism produces an array of extracellular products that may serve as virulence factors. These include *catalase*, which breaks down H_2O_2 produced by phagocytes as an important component of their antibacterial defense; *hyaluronidase*, which hydrolyzes mucopolysaccharides in connective tissue, allowing for easier spread of the organism; *toxins* (α, β, γ, δ) and *leukocidin*, which are cytotoxic to red cells, white cells, and fibroblasts; *enterotoxins*, which cause food poisoning; *exfoliative toxin*, which produces the symptoms of scalded skin syndrome; and *toxic shock syndrome toxin*, which produces the manifestations of toxic shock syndrome.

EPIDEMIOLOGY. Intermittent colonization and subsequent autoinfection or spread to other people directly or via fomites is the characteristic epidemiology of staphylococcal infections. Twenty percent to 40% of adults are colonized with *S. aureus*, usually in the anterior nares. Approximately 10% of women are colonized vaginally. In newborns, the umbilicus, perineum, and stool are the major sites of colonization. Health-care workers, insulin-dependent diabetics, and intravenous drug users have higher rates of colonization than the general population. Although previously healthy people may be infected with staphylococci, patients with severe underlying disease and with abnormal host defense mechanisms represent specific groups at high risk. The presence of foreign bodies, such as intravenous catheters, vascular or cerebrospinal fluid shunts, and prosthetic devices, also represents a major risk factor.

CLINICAL SYNDROMES (OTHER THAN OSTEOMYELITIS)

Skin and soft tissue infections. The major skin and soft tissue infections associated with *S. aureus* are reviewed in Table 45-1. All ages are at risk of both superficial and deep infections.

Infections associated with major skin manifestations. Staphylococcal infections may produce major skin manifestations without direct invasion. Staphylococcal scalded skin syndrome and toxic shock syndrome are examples that are discussed later.

Staphylococcal scalded skin syndrome. The staphylococcal

Table 45-1   Skin diseases caused by *Staphylococcus aureus*

Disease	Age	Clinical characteristics	Other	Therapy
Bullous impetigo	Newborns, children	Localized form of scalded skin syndrome		Systemic antibiotics with penicillinase-resistant penicillin
Carbuncles	All ages	Resembling furuncles but more extensive Lesions may coalesce with multiple draining sinuses May become necrotic Bacteremia in 25% of patients	May be associated with underlying disease, especially diabetes or uremia	Incision, drainage Systemic antibiotics with penicillinase-resistant penicillin
Cellulitis	All ages	May be confused clinically with erysipelas, with well-delineated margins Induration, inflammation over affected site Fever, chills Lymphangitis may be present	Disease underlying cellulitis (infectious arthritis, osteomyelitis) to be considered	Systemic antibiotics with penicillinase-resistant penicillin
Furuncles	All ages	Infection around hair follicles Appears as nodule with fluctuant center Neck, thigh, buttocks affected in males Axillae, perineum affected in females	Associated with nasal or perineal carriage of *S. aureus*	Local therapy—moist heat Incision, drainage Identification, treatment of carrier state
Impetigo	Preschool age	Slowly evolving pustular eruption, usually on face Thick, yellow crust; weeping lesions	Often associated with streptococcal impetigo	Erythromycin Oral penicillinase-resistant penicillin
Scalded skin syndrome	Newborns, children under age 5, occasionally adults	Painful rash with formation of flaccid blisters Occurs over face, groin, axillae first, then becomes generalized	*S. aureus,* phage group 2 associated with toxin production Disease may be associated with *S. aureus* infection elsewhere	Systemic antibiotics with penicillinase-resistant penicillin
Hydradenitis suppurativa	All ages	Recurrent furuncles in the axilla and perineal area associated with chronic draining sinuses	Represents infection of the apocrine sweat glands	Oral penicillinase-resistant penicillin, local therapy, incision, and drainage as needed
Pyomyositis	All ages	Primary infection of skeletal muscle involving subacute onset of pain and swelling, tenderness, and "woody" duration	Most commonly occurs in the tropics	Drainage, parenteral penicillinase-resistant penicillin

scalded skin syndrome represents a form of toxic epidermal necrolysis associated with toxin production by staphylococci of phage group 2. The infection usually is not located where the skin lesions appear.

Although isolated cases have been reported in adults, most cases occur in children under 5 years of age. The disease is caused by an epidermolysin that cleaves the epidermis beneath the stratum granulosum. The central area of the face, neck, axillae, and groin most commonly are affected. Cutaneous tenderness and demonstration of Nikolsky's sign (normal skin that easily separates from the deeper layers if rubbed) are characteristic findings. Within 24 to 48 hours after the onset of symptoms, a progression from a scarlatiniform rash to generalized spontaneous skin separation occurs, resulting in the formation of large, flaccid bullae. Recovery occurs in 5 to 7 days and is associated with a generalized postinflammatory desquamation. Although recovery is common, sepsis, cellulitis, and pneumonia may occur, especially in newborns. Increased morbidity and mortality have been described in patients treated with steroids.

Toxic shock syndrome. Toxic shock syndrome (TSS) is a multiple-system disorder caused by toxin-producing *S. aureus.* The strict case definition of TSS involves fever (over 102° F [38.9° C]), hypotension (blood pressure under 90 mm Hg or demonstration of orthostatic hypotension); rash, usually diffuse and macular with subsequent desquamation, especially on the palms and soles; and involvement of at least three of the following: gastrointestinal tract, mucous membranes, musculoskeletal system, kidneys, liver, blood, or nervous system. Cultures must be negative for organisms other than staphylococci, and serologic titers must be negative for leptospirosis, rubeola, and Rocky Mountain spotted fever. Cases of probable TSS that don't meet the strict case definition have been described, suggesting a broad range of clinical presentations. The syndrome is caused by a toxin (toxic shock syndrome toxin-1 [TSST-1]) elaborated by certain strains of *S. aureus* that act in part by stimulating the production of interleukin 1.

Most cases of TSS have involved women who became ill during their menstrual period. In these cases toxin is elaborated by staphylococci colonizing the vagina. Use of tampons, especially superabsorbent tampons, is a major risk factor, although the exact mechanism involved remains unclear. TSS cases involving nonmenstruating women and males have been reported. In these cases toxin is elaborated by staphylococci colonizing or infecting a variety of sites. Most recently TSS has been described in patients with influenza or influenza-like illnesses whose respiratory tracts were colonized with staphylococci.

Therapy involves aggressive supportive care, especially fluid resuscitation for hypotension and specific antistaphylococcal therapy with penicillinase-resistant penicillins. Removal of tampons or other involved foreign material (for example, surgical packing) and local care for infected wounds are important interventions. Steroids may be helpful when used early in the course of the disease, although definitive studies are lacking. Most patients recover, although a 3% mortality has been observed.

Gastrointestinal syndromes. *S. aureus* causes two major syndromes involving the gastrointestinal tract: acute food poisoning and enterocolitis.

Staphylococcal food poisoning. Staphylococcal food poisoning is caused by the ingestion of a heat-stable, acid-stable toxin. High-protein foods that have been allowed to remain at temperatures that permit bacterial growth and elaboration of toxin most commonly are involved. These include beef, pork, milk products, mayonnaise, and potato salad. Approximately 17% of confirmed cases of food poisoning are caused by staphylococcal enterotoxin.

The clinical presentation of staphylococcal food poisoning is quite characteristic. Anorexia, malaise, increased salivation, nausea, and vomiting develop, usually 2 to 7 hours after eating. In some cases diarrhea and abdominal distention may be present without any other symptoms. In more severe cases diarrhea accompanies nausea and vomiting. Fever is usually absent but may occur with more severe forms of the disease. Hypotension and electrolyte imbalances may follow more fulminant presentations.

Staphylococcal food poisoning is self-limited, with gradual resolution of symptoms over 24 to 48 hours. The disease is diagnosed by finding more than 100,000 staphylococci per gram of food in the proper epidemiologic setting. Therapy involves supportive measures only.

Staphylococcal enterocolitis. Staphylococcal enterocolitis is a rare syndrome resembling pseudomembranous colitis caused by *Clostridium difficile*. It was seen in the early days of broad-spectrum antibiotic therapy but has virtually disappeared. Many investigators believe that this entity was unrecognized *C. difficile* colitis with overgrowth of *S. aureus*. The use of broad-spectrum antibiotics, usually before abdominal surgery, was the most common predisposing factor. Diarrhea was the most common symptom, with profuse, watery, foul-smelling stool. Fever commonly was noted. Hypotension, shock, and renal failure occurred as a result of marked volume depletion.

The diagnosis was made by the presence of large numbers of gram-positive cocci on stool Gram stain and stool cultures positive for staphylococci. Therapy consists of oral vancomycin with or without a parenteral penicillinase-resistant penicillin. Supportive fluid and electrolyte therapy also may be indicated.

Staphylococcal bacteremia. Staphylococcal bacteremia may occur with any localized staphylococcal infection but most commonly is associated with skin infections, infected intravenous catheters, intravascular shunts and prosthetic devices, postoperative wound infections, endocarditis, and osteomyelitis. Neonates, the immunosuppressed, the chronically ill, and the elderly are particularly at high risk. Spiking fevers, multiple rigors, arthralgias, and marked systemic toxicity are characteristic clinical findings. Occasionally, disseminated intravascular coagulation is present, and the clinical picture resembles that of acute meningococcemia. Depending on the source and duration of bacteremia, metastatic foci of infection may develop in the kidneys, lungs, bones, brain, skin, and heart. Even when treated appropriately, staphylococcal bacteremia may be associated with a 40% mortality.

The development of metastatic foci, especially on heart valves, is the most serious complication. Controversy exists concerning the frequency of endocarditis following *S. aureus* bacteremia and the optimal duration of therapy. Fifteen percent

to 25% of patients with *S. aureus* bacteremia may have endocarditis. The percentage is higher if underlying cardiac lesions are present. The risk of endocarditis appears lower when an identifiable and removable source of infection is noted, when the disease is nosocomially acquired, and when no metastatic foci are found. In such patients 2 weeks of intravenous therapy with a penicillinase-resistant penicillin, cephalosporin, or vancomycin may be adequate therapy, although this remains controversial. In patients with underlying cardiac disease, or when bacteremia is community acquired or unassociated with an obvious primary focus, or when metastatic foci are noted, the risk of endocarditis is high, and 4 to 6 weeks of therapy should be given. Although teichoic acid antibodies may be elevated in patients with endocarditis, the sensitivity and specificity of the assays available remain too low to be reliable.

MANAGEMENT (OTHER THAN FOR OSTEOMYELITIS). Minor staphylococcal skin infections such as furuncles are treated with incision and drainage with or without oral antibiotics. More extensive skin disease or skin disease associated with signs of systemic toxicity requires systemic antibiotics for 5 to 10 days. Impetigo may be treated with oral antibiotics, but severe cellulitis and scalded skin syndrome require parenteral drugs. The presence of systemic staphylococcal disease such as bacteremia, endocarditis, pneumonia, and enterocolitis requires therapy with parenteral antibiotics.

Over 90% of staphylococcal infections are caused by organisms that produce penicillinase and are therefore resistant to penicillin. Penicillinase-resistant penicillins such as nafcillin, methicillin, or oxacillin are the parenteral drugs of choice and should be used for serious infections. Our preference is nafcillin (1.5 g intravenously every 4 hours). For oral therapy of minor infections, available penicillinase-resistant penicillins include oxacillin, cloxacillin, and dicloxacillin; our preference is cloxacillin (500 mg every 6 hours). For the patient allergic to penicillin who needs intravenous therapy, cephalosporins (which should be used with caution because of cross-sensitivity) and vancomycin are suitable alternatives. Cephalosporins should not be given to patients who have had a recent immediate-type adverse reaction (anaphylaxis, hives, bronchospasm) to a penicillin. Strains of *S. aureus* resistant to penicillinase-resistant penicillins have been noted with increasing frequency in the United States since 1982 (methicillin-resistant strains). Vancomycin is the therapy of choice in these cases; cephalosporins are not effective even when in vitro susceptibility data indicate that they may be used.

Tolerant staphylococci are those strains inhibited by usual levels of β-lactam antibiotics but that require very high levels of drug for bactericidal effect. The demonstration of tolerance greatly depends on the laboratory techniques used, and its clinical significance remains unclear.

STAPHYLOCOCCAL OSTEOMYELITIS

S. aureus is the most common cause of acute osteomyelitis in both pediatric and adult patients.

PATHOGENESIS. Three basic mechanisms spread disease to bone. By far the most common is hematogenous spread. Bacteremia often is produced by an inapparent infection; bacteria are carried to the metaphyseal area of long bones, where blood flow is slow and phagocytic cells are few. Since the blood supply in these areas is nonanastomotic, obstruction to flow via thrombosis or bacterial plugging allows for microinfarction, devitalization of bone, and production of an excellent area for bacterial growth. In children rapidly growing long bones are most commonly involved, with bones of the lower extremity (tibia, femur) predominating. In adults the vertebrae often are involved, an anatomic predilection that remains unexplained. Lumbar vertebrae are more commonly involved than thoracic vertebrae, and cervical vertebrae are least commonly involved. The body of the vertebrae is the part usually infected. Disease spreads easily to adjacent vertebrae via venous anastomoses, and at the time the patient is seen two vertebrae usually are simultaneously involved. Patients with a history of intravenous drug abuse may develop osteomyelitis of the clavicle.

The second mechanism by which staphylococci reach bone is by spread from a contiguous focus of infection. This occurs most commonly postoperatively or with soft tissue infection. Osteomyelitis of the skull may occur after craniotomy or in association with infection of the sinuses and mastoid processes. Osteomyelitis of the fingers and toes usually is secondary to contiguous soft tissue infection. Osteomyelitis of the mandible has been associated with dental infections. Severe peripheral vascular disease predisposes to osteomyelitis of the toes and small bones of the foot.

Osteomyelitis resulting from traumatic contamination of bone is the third pathogenic mechanism and occurs when organisms are driven into bone or tissue close to the bone. Organisms involved tend to represent those found on the skin, including *S. aureus*.

CLINICAL MANIFESTATIONS. In acute hematogenous osteomyelitis in children, localized pain, swelling, and limitation of movement occur in the infected limb and are accompanied by fever, rigors, and marked systemic toxicity. A history of trauma may be elicited in up to 30% of patients, although the etiologic importance of this finding is not clear. In adults symptoms may be confined to the infected limb. Draining sinus tracts are uncommon in acute osteomyelitis.

The onset of vertebral osteomyelitis usually is insidious, with a gradual development of back or neck pain that is slowly progressive over several weeks to months. Limitation of movement of the involved vertebrae with spasm of the paravertebral muscles commonly is noted, but spiking fevers, rigors, and systemic toxicity are uncommon.

Chronic osteomyelitis is not usually associated with systemic toxicity. Development of draining sinus tracts in the area of involvement may be the major manifestation of disease.

The earliest roentgenographic signs of osteomyelitis are localized areas of deep, soft tissue swelling in the metaphyseal area of infected long bones. This may occur as early as 3 days after onset of symptoms. Swelling of muscles and obliteration of radiolucent planes between muscles appear next. Bone changes consistent with osteomyelitis may not be seen for at least 10 days after the onset of symptoms and may be delayed for up to 1 month. Lytic bone lesions are not roentgenographically visible until 30% to 50% of bone is demineralized. Periosteal elevation usually occurs at the same time that lytic lesions are seen. Bone sclerosis and new bone formation usually are noted later, and their presence on a roentgenogram suggests that the disease has been present for longer than 1 month. In addition to lytic lesions, periosteal elevation, and new bone formation, cortical irregularity and sequestrum formation are other roentgenographic signs of osteomyelitis. In vertebral osteomyelitis, disc space narrowing, erosion of vertebrae, and new bone formation bridging vertebral disc spaces are characteristic roentgenographic signs.

The use of technetium bone scans and gallium scans may aid in the diagnosis of osteomyelitis. Positive bone scans indicate an increased blood supply or increased bone turnover in the involved area. Gallium collects in the area of inflammation or tumor. Scans have been shown to be positive as early as 3 days after the onset of symptoms, often before any roentgenographic changes occur.

Establishing a specific microbiologic etiology for osteomyelitis depends on isolation of the offending organism from blood, bone, or joint fluid. Cultures of draining sinus tracts in chronic osteomyelitis do not reflect the true etiologic agents of bone disease except when *S. aureus* or mycobacteria are isolated. In most cases bone biopsy for culture and a histologic examination are needed for definitive diagnosis.

COURSE. If acute osteomyelitis is treated appropriately and quickly, usually within 3 to 5 days after the onset of symptoms, most cases resolve without sequelae. Delay in diagnosis and improper therapy with an inadequate drug or inadequate duration of therapy may allow the development of chronic osteomyelitis. Once chronic osteomyelitis occurs, therapy becomes much more difficult, requiring both surgical and medical intervention. Even with such intervention, a failure rate of 23% to 42% has been noted. In vertebral osteomyelitis, spinal compression, meningitis, and paravertebral abscess may occur. Cervical osteomyelitis may lead to retropharyngeal abscess. Osteomyelitis of the thoracic vertebrae may cause mediastinitis or mediastinal abscess. Secondary amyloidosis and nephrotic syndrome have been described as rare complications of chronic osteomyelitis.

MANAGEMENT. A major goal in the management of acute osteomyelitis is to prevent chronic osteomyelitis. In children less than 3 weeks of therapy is associated with an unacceptably high failure rate; 4 weeks of therapy with parenteral penicillins or cephalosporins is the therapy of choice. In adults 6 weeks of therapy with parenteral penicillins or cephalosporins is recommended because the onset is usually less acute. See "Management (other than for osteomyelitis)" earlier in this chapter for doses and agents. Therapy for chronic osteomyelitis should include a combined medical and surgical approach consisting of 6 weeks of parenteral antibiotics in association with surgical removal of devitalized bone. In addition, oral antibiotic therapy is given for another 2 to 6 months.

COAGULASE-NEGATIVE STAPHYLOCOCCI

CLINICAL SYNDROMES. *Staphylococcus epidermidis* has been recognized only recently as an important human pathogen rather than a commensal or contaminant. In general, infections with this organism have been associated with prosthetic implants (heart valves, orthopedic devices), central nervous system shunts, dialysis catheters, intravenous and intraarterial catheters, and peritoneal dialysis catheters. The very young, the elderly, and the immunosuppressed are patient groups most often infected. In the absence of prosthetic devices, virtually all *S. epidermidis* infections are nosocomial. Although acute presentations have been well described, the usual clinical picture is that of an indolent infection with few distinguishing clinical or laboratory characteristics. The isolation of *S. epidermidis* from a single culture may be regarded as a contaminant; however, the possibility of a true infection must be considered when prosthetic devices or vascular catheters are present. Most blood cultures that are positive for *S. epidermidis* represent contaminants. Organisms growing in both aerobic and anaerobic cultures, rapid growth of organisms, and repeatedly positive cultures suggest true bacteremia. Corroborative clinical evidence (fever, elevated white blood cell count, blood pressure changes) should be used in helping to distinguish contamination from infection.

Most strains of *S. epidermidis* are resistant to β-lactam antibiotics, including the penicillinase-resistant penicillins and cephalosporins. Vancomycin is the therapy of choice. In severe infections such as prosthetic valve endocarditis, vancomycin plus rifampin, gentamicin, or both should be used. In addition to antibiotics, removal of any prosthetic device, shunt, or vascular catheter should be considered.

Staphylococcus *saprophyticus* is a coagulase-negative staphylococcus that causes urinary tract infections. In several studies this organism was second only to *Escherichia coli* in causing such infections in young women. Signs and symptoms of infection are indistinguishable from those of other urinary tract pathogens. The organism is susceptible to most of the antibiotics commonly used for therapy of urinary tract infections, although relatively high resistance rates have been noted for tetracycline and the organism has absolute resistance to nalidixic acid. Recurrent infections have been observed in up to 10% of patients.

BIBLIOGRAPHY

Bayer AS and others: Staphylococcus aureus bacteremia: clinical, serologic, and echocardiographic findings in patients with and without endocarditis, Arch Intern Med 147:457, 1987.
Beaty HN: Staphylococcus aureus bacteremia. In Remington JS and Swartz MN, editors: Current clinical topics in infectious diseases, New York, 1980, McGraw-Hill, Inc.
Capitanio MA and Kirkpatrick JA: Early roentgen observations in acute osteomyelitis, Am J Roentgenol Radium Ther Nucl Med 108:488, 1970.
Causey WA: Staphylococcal and streptococcal infection of the skin, Primary Care 6:127, 1979.
Dearing WH and Needham GM: Hospitalized patients with Staphylococcus aureus in the intestine, JAMA 174:125, 1960.
Dich VQ, Nelson JD, and Haltalin KC: Osteomyelitis in infants and children, Am J Dis Child 129:1273, 1975.
Elias PM, Fritsch P, and Epstein EH: Staphylococcal scalded skin syndrome, Arch Dermatol 113:207, 1977.
Horwitz MA: Specific diagnosis of food borne disease, Gastroenterology 73:375, 1977.
Latham RH, Running K, and Stamm WE: Urinary tract infections in young adult women caused by Staphylococcus saprophyticus, JAMA 250:3003, 1983.
Mackowiak PA, Jones SR, and Smith JW: Diagnostic value of sinus-tract cultures in chronic osteomyelitis, JAMA 239:2772, 1978.
Sheagren JN: Staphylococcus aureus: The persistent pathogen, N Engl J Med 310:1368, 1437, 1984.
Smith CB and Jacobson JA: Toxic shock syndrome, Dis A Month 32:82, 1986.
Waldvogel FA, Medoff G, and Swartz MN: Osteomyelitis: a review of clinical features, therapeutic considerations, and unusual aspects. I. N Engl J Med 282:198, 1970.
Waldvogel FA, Medoff G, and Swartz MN: Osteomyelitis: a review of clinical features, therapeutic considerations, and unusual aspects. II. N Engl J Med 282:260, 1970.
Waldvogel FA, Medoff G, and Swartz MN: Osteomyelitis: a review of clinical features, therapeutic considerations, and unusual aspects. Osteomyelitis associated with vascular insufficiency. III. N Engl J Med 282:316, 1970.
West WF, Kelly PJ, and Martin WJ: Chronic osteomyelitis. I. Factors affecting the results of treatment in 186 patients, JAMA 213:1837, 1970.

Streptococcal infections and rheumatic fever

Jerome Santoro *and* Mark J. Ingerman

The streptococci constitute a large group of gram-positive bacteria that are among the most frequent microbial pathogens infecting man. They cause several disease syndromes, including pharyngeal infections, skin infections, bacteremia, neonatal infections, puerperal sepsis, urinary tract infections, endocarditis, and others. In addition to causing serious bacterial infection, *Streptococcus pyogenes*, the most important pathogen in the group, is responsible for the so-called nonsuppurative sequelae of acute glomerulonephritis and rheumatic fever.

CLASSIFICATION. The streptococci are widely found in nature and also are among the normal bacterial flora of humans. The organisms are catalase-negative, nonsporeforming gram-positive cocci that are facultatively anaerobic or in some instances strictly anaerobic. Streptococci are classified by either the pattern of hemolysis they produce when forming 1 to 2 mm nonpigmented colonies on blood agar or the antigenic composition of their cell wall carbohydrate. Three types of hemolytic reactions are noted: (1) α, or partial, hemolysis produces a greenish pigment around the colonies. Organisms that produce greening reactions are frequently designated viridans streptococci or *Streptococcus viridans;* these organisms tend to be less invasive and are part of the upper respiratory tract flora. (2) β, or complete, hemolysis refers to total clearing of the blood agar. Strains that produce β hemolysis often are among the more virulent pathogens for humans, such as *S. pyogenes* and *Streptococcus agalactiae.* (3) γ-Hemolytic streptococci are nonhemolytic.

A more precise method of classifying streptococci originally described by Lancefield is based on the antigenic differences in their cell wall carbohydrates. Identification is made by precipitin reactions with group-specific antiserum. By this method organisms are designated group A to H or K to T. Most β-hemolytic streptococci, which tend to be more virulent pathogens, belong to groups A through D, F, and G. Some but not all α- and γ-streptococci have group antigens. Group D organisms, which can be β-hemolytic but frequently show α or γ reactions, are important pathogens for humans.

Anaerobic and microaerophilic streptococci, including peptostreptococci, exhibit variable hemolysis and are classified separately. These organisms are part of the normal flora of the upper respiratory, gastrointestinal, and female genital tracts.

GROUP A STREPTOCOCCI

ETIOLOGY. The group A β-hemolytic streptococcus, *S. pyogenes,* is one of the most important bacterial pathogens for man. This organism is identified by its β reaction and the inhibition of its growth by low concentrations of bacitracin impregnated in a paper disk (A disk). Alternatively, the group carbohydrate can be identified using a fluorescent antibody technique.

S. pyogenes is a structurally complicated organism. There is a hyaluronic acid capsule that is not antigenic because of the similarity to the hyaluronic acid found in humans. The cell wall has three components: the group-specific carbohydrate, structural proteins, and mucopeptides. The group-specific carbohydrate is a polymer of rhamnose and *N*-acetyl glucosamine. The most important of the cell wall proteins is the *M protein*. The M protein resists phagocytosis by polymorphonuclear leukocytes and is thus an important virulence factor; strains that produce more abundant M protein tend to be more virulent. Antibodies to the M protein promote opsonization and are protective. However, more than 70 M types are known, so repeated group A streptococcal infections may occur. Two other structural proteins, R and T, are important for epidemiologic purposes but are not virulence factors. The mucopeptide, which consists of alternating units of *N*-acetyl glucosamine and *N*-acetyl muramic acid, can produce carditis in rabbits, but its importance in the pathogenesis of rheumatic fever remains unclear. The cell membrane of group A streptococci has antigens that cross-react with human cardiac muscle, but the importance of this phenomenon also is unknown. Lipoteichoic acid (LTA), another component of the cell wall found in other streptococci and staphylococci as well, is important for adherence to host mucosal cells.

As group A streptococci grow, they produce a number of extracellular products. *Erythrogenic toxin* is responsible for the rash of scarlet fever. A particular strain of *S. pyogenes* acquires the ability to produce erythrogenic toxin via lysogeny with a bacteriophage. Streptolysin O, which is inhibited by oxygen and thus induces subsurface hemolysis on blood agar plates, is produced by all group A organisms as well by some group C and G organisms. This substance is highly immunogenic, and detection of antibody to streptolysin O (ASO titer) is an important laboratory tool used to detect recent streptococcal infection. Streptolysin S is responsible for surface hemolysis on blood agar plates but does not evoke an antibody response. However, both toxins are thought to be damaging to host cells. Other extracellular products, which may act by liquefying pus (streptokinase, deoxyribonucleases [DNases] A to D), facilitating spread of infection through tissue planes (hyaluronidase), or interfering with leukocytes (nicotinamide-adenine dinucleotidase [NADase]), also can promote antibody responses that may be useful in retrospective diagnosis.

EPIDEMIOLOGY. Streptococcal pharyngitis and pyoderma (impetigo) are quantitatively the most common infections caused by group A organisms. However, these two infections have very different epidemiologic factors. Upper respiratory tract infections from streptococci occur most frequently among children 5 to 15 years of age in the winter in colder climates. The major mode of spread is by droplet nuclei, but foodborne epidemics (from milk) have been described. Children with streptococcal pharyngitis are highly infectious and can transmit disease within a household to most siblings and even to some adults. Streptococcal carriers are not nearly as infectious as individuals with disease. Organisms that cause pharyngitis tend to be low M types (such as 1 to 24).

In contrast, impetigo most often is seen during the summer or in tropical climates among preschool children. Under these circumstances the skin of the extremities and other areas of the body is likely to be exposed and subjected to minor trauma, such as scratches or insect bites. Presumably, these breaks in the skin barrier predispose to secondary invasion by bacteria. However, infection of normal skin probably occurs. Once impetigo is established, it can be spread from one part of the body to another by autoinoculation or to other individuals. Strains causing pyoderma frequently are high M types or nontypable. With both pharyngitis and pyoderma, epidemics occur when person-to-person spread is likely because of crowded conditions, as among lower socioeconomic groups or in the military. Other streptococcal skin infections, such as erysipelas, are acquired much like pyoderma. Nosocomial streptococcal skin infections also are recognized. These infections can occur post partum or postoperatively. Rectal or vaginal carriage of group A organisms by hospital personnel has been implicated in some institutional outbreaks.

Acute streptococcal pharyngitis

The pharynx and tonsillar regions are the most common sites of streptococcal infection in man. However, the accurate diagnosis of "strep throat" in the nonepidemic setting can be difficult. In the winter pharyngeal carriage of *S. pyogenes* in children can exceed 30%; many go on to develop pharyngitis, but only about 50% exhibit a significant rise in streptococcal antibodies. If one assumes that antibody production distinguishes infection from carriage, the isolation of group A

β-hemolytic streptococci from a child with pharyngitis can have a false positive rate of infection that approaches 50%.

The patient's clinical picture, although suggestive, also can be misleading. In a typical case (observed in the older child or adult) there is an incubation period of 2 to 4 days, followed by the sudden onset of fever (greater than 101° F [38.3° C]), headache, and severe sore throat with dysphagia. Anorexia and occasionally abdominal pain with nausea and vomiting (in younger children) may be present. On physical examination a beef-red pharynx with or without exudate and tender cervical adenopathy is seen. Cough, coryza, and hoarseness are not characteristic of streptococcal infection except in infants and should suggest a different diagnosis. It has been shown that most of these signs and symptoms are nonspecific, and viral illnesses such as that caused by adenovirus can reproduce them exactly. The only totally reliable sign is the presence of the rash of scarlet fever (see next section), which is encountered relatively infrequently. The presence of cervical adenopathy seems to be somewhat helpful but is found in only about 50% of cases. In adults, however, the correlation of signs and symptoms with true infection is much better but by no means absolute. Infants with streptococcal upper respiratory tract infection do not have pharyngitis. In fact, pharyngitis in children under 3 years of age is rarely streptococcal in origin. Infants display low-grade fever, rhinorrhea, and excoriation of the anterior nares. The illness in infants tends to be protracted, as opposed to 3 to 5 days' duration in older individuals.

The best approach to diagnosis is to combine clinical, epidemiologic, and bacteriologic information. In patients with equivocal findings, it is best to withhold therapy until culture results are available. If the epidemiologic data dictate, as with an infected sibling or a community epidemic, or in an adult with impressive findings, therapy can be started immediately.

Throat cultures are not difficult to obtain and can be performed in the office. Patients with bona fide streptococcal pharyngitis generally harbor large numbers of organisms in the throat, and this is reflected by heavy growth on the agar plate. On the other hand, the isolation of a few β-hemolytic colonies is more characteristic of the carrier state. Recently kits that immunologically and rapidly detect group A antigen have become available; within minutes these kits can provide an accurate diagnosis of streptococcal pharyngitis in the office setting. These tests are quite specific but less sensitive than throat cultures when a small number of bacteria are present; however, it is usually the carrier state rather than infection that is missed. Thus rapid testing in the office allows diagnosis of most cases of group A streptococcal pharyngitis. Streptococcal pharyngitis can be diagnosed retrospectively by measuring the host's antibody response to the organisms' extracellular products, such as streptolysin O, DNase, and hyaluronidase. However, such tests are much more helpful in establishing preexistent infection in a patient who is suspected of having poststreptococcal glomerulonephritis or rheumatic fever and lend little to the everyday management of streptococcal disease.

The differential diagnosis of acute streptococcal pharyngitis includes diphtheria, Vincent's angina, and viral pharyngitides, especially those caused by Epstein-Barr virus and adenovirus. The latter can appear identical to streptococcal pharyngitis and can be differentiated accurately only with the use of throat cultures.

COMPLICATIONS. The complications of streptococcal pharyngitis include scarlet fever and suppurative and nonsuppurative sequelae.

The incidence of scarlet fever has declined dramatically since the antibiotic era began. The initial symptoms of scarlet fever are identical to those of uncomplicated streptococcal pharyngitis. Within 1 to 5 days a characteristic fine "sandpaper" eruption appears, beginning on the chest and then spreading to other parts of the body. The tongue and buccal mucosa usually are involved, but the perioral area tends to be spared (circumoral pallor). The tongue initially is coated with bright-red papillae protruding through a white coating (strawberry tongue). Later the coating disappears and a beef-red tongue is noted (raspberry tongue). The rash is caused by capillary damage produced by erythrogenic toxin. In areas of trauma, such as the antecubital fossae, petechial hemorrhages called Pastia's lines are seen. These reflect the overall capillary fragility, which can be further demonstrated by the application of a tourniquet to the arm for 5 minutes (Rumpel-Leede sign). The latter maneuver produces extensive petechiae distal to the occlusion. Following recovery, desquamation is common.

The suppurative complications of streptococcal pharyngitis include peritonsillar abscess (quinsy), otitis media, sinusitis, acute cervical adenitis, and impetigo. Most of these entities are unusual in the antibiotic era and frequently occur (with the exception of peritonsillar abscess) in untreated preschool children.

Peritonsillar abscess begins with abrupt onset of increased soreness and swelling on the involved side. Initially, the tonsils and the involved anterior pillar are edematous, and the tonsil moves toward the midline of the throat. The involved cervical lymph nodes also enlarge and become more tender. A large, fluctuant mass eventually results. Infection may spread through tissue planes in the neck, or suppurative thrombophlebitis may occur. Interestingly, the organisms cultured from a peritonsillar abscess are not usually group A streptococci but the anaerobic flora of the upper respiratory tract. It is thought that the initial streptococcal infection somehow allows the normal upper airway bacteria to invade the pharyngeal lymphoid tissue.

Direct spread of hemolytic streptococci from the throat to the sinuses, mastoid processes, middle ear, and cervical lymph glands is responsible for infection of these organs. The clinical presentation of these syndromes is identical to those produced by other organisms infecting these structures. Streptococci can be found in the throat of many children with clinical evidence of skin infection. However, obvious pharyngitis is the exception rather than the rule, and these organisms probably reach the pharynx after the skin is colonized.

Bacteremia with metastatic infection to such areas as bones, joints, and meninges is now a practically unheard-of occurrence. Treatment of the suppurative complications of streptococcal pharyngitis consists of antimicrobial therapy (see next section) and surgical drainage when indicated.

The nonsuppurative complications are acute rheumatic fever and acute glomerulonephritis; both may follow all types of respiratory tract infections caused by group A β-hemolytic streptococci. Rheumatic fever (discussed later in this chapter) can occur in up to 3% of cases of severe epidemic pharyngitis, but the incidence in routine outbreaks is less than 0.1%. Glomerulonephritis occurs in 10% to 15% of patients when the infecting strain is nephritogenic. Unlike glomerulonephritis following impetigo (discussed later), penicillin treatment of pharyngitis dramatically reduces the incidence of rheumatic fever. The diagnosis of rheumatic fever and poststreptococcal glomerulonephritis is based on the presence of a compatible clinical picture and the demonstration of recent antecedent streptococcal infection by the use of serum antibody studies. It is important to remember that antibody response varies with the type of infection. For example, ASO and anti-NADase titers may not rise at all or be only weakly positive after impetigo. Since a history of previous infection cannot always be obtained, a combination of tests may be necessary (ASO, anti-DNase B, antihyaluronidase). The "streptozyme" test combines several streptococcal antigens fixed to red blood cells but has a higher false positive rate than a battery of individual antibody determinations. However, this test is very sensitive and, when negative, recent antecedent streptococcal infection can be considered unlikely.

MANAGEMENT. Previously it was thought that treatment had little effect on the course of pharyngitis per se. However, recent studies have shown that early antimicrobial therapy given to children with streptococcal pharyngitis does substantially alter the course of disease and rapidly results in negative throat cultures. Thus with the aid of rapid diagnostic tests available in the office, children quickly can be rendered asymptomatic and return to school. The other major reasons for treating "strep throat" are to reduce the incidence of nonsuppurative complications, especially rheumatic fever, and perhaps to prevent other problems, such as otitis media or peritonsillar abscess. Rheumatic fever can be prevented even if therapy is begun as long as 9 days after infection, so there is no harm in waiting for culture results to begin therapy. However, to consistently eradicate *S. pyogenes* from the throat, penicillin levels must be present in pharyngeal secretions for at least 10 days. This can be accomplished in two ways: penicillin V in doses of 250 mg orally twice a day for 10 days; or benzathine penicillin in one dose of 300,000 to 600,000 units for infants and children less than 66 pounds, (30 kg), 900,000 units for older children, and 1.2 million units for adults intramuscularly. The latter mode of therapy may be much more effective among lower socioeconomic groups in which patient compliance is a factor. Patients allergic to penicillin should receive erythromycin (30 to 50 mg/kg/day in three or four divided doses). These dosage regimens can be applied to cases of streptococcal otitis media and sinusitis, but benzathine penicillin should be avoided. Peritonsillar abscesses can be treated with either intramuscular procaine penicillin G or intravenous penicillin G, 2 to 4 million units daily. Streptococci are variably resistant to tetracyclines, and these drugs should be avoided in all streptococcal infections.

Streptococcal skin infections

PYODERMA (IMPETIGO). The lesions of streptococcal impetigo begin as small papules that are rapidly transformed into 2 to 3 mm serous fluid–filled vesicles surrounded by a thin, erythematous margin. Fluid aspirated from these vesicles frequently will grow group A streptococci in pure culture. However, the vesicular phase is transient and easily missed. Lesions quickly become pustules, which rupture and form thick, amber-colored crusts. At this point cultures of lesions may yield both *S. pyogenes* and *S. aureus*. *S. aureus* has thus been implicated in the origin of this type of pyoderma. However, prospective studies have shown that group A streptococci are the primary pathogens responsible for most cases of *nonbullous* pyoderma, which is characterized by thick, amber crusts. *S. aureus*, on the other hand, plays a secondary, noninfectious role of colonization under these circumstances. This concept is further supported by the changing over time of the phage type of *S. aureus* isolates as serial cultures are obtained. Whereas streptococcal pyoderma is characterized by small vesicles, persistent, often large bullae are seen with staphylococcal impetigo. Crusting occurs with staphylococcal disease, but the crusts are thin and white to gray in color. When there is difficulty distinguishing streptococcal and staphylococcal impetigo, a Gram stain of vesicular or bullous fluid may aid in differentiating the two entities.

In contrast to streptococcal pharyngitis, impetigo is a slowly developing, insidious disease that is rarely if ever accompanied by fever, erythema, pain, or constitutional symptoms. Also in contradistinction to pharyngeal infection, rheumatic fever is *not* a sequela of pyoderma. However, when nephritogenic strains cause impetigo, acute glomerulonephritis can develop in as many as 15% of cases. Because the infection involves only the most superficial dermis, scarring does not occur.

Untreated streptococcal impetigo is a mild, indolent, and occasionally self-limited illness. Local measures, such as the removal of crusts and washing with antiseptic soap, seem to promote healing of lesions. However, impetigo not treated with antimicrobial agents can lead to local and distant foci of infection. Antimicrobial therapy thus can be justified to prevent such complications. There is no good evidence to indicate that treatment prevents glomerulonephritis following impetigo, as is the case for rheumatic fever following pharyngitis and perhaps for glomerulonephritis following pharyngitis.

Thus the proper treatment of streptococcal impetigo consists of the use of local measures and either local or systemic antimicrobial agents. Gentle but thorough debridement and removal of crusts are accomplished by washing with warm soap and water several times a day. If the lesions are well localized and few in number, bacitracin ointment can be tried. Mupirocin, an antibiotic derived from *Pseudomonas fluorescens*, has been used topically in impetigo in recent studies. Its efficacy is said to equal that of systemic antibiotics. There is no systemic absorption and local side effects are minimal. Oral or parenteral penicillin therapy generally is more efficacious than bacitracin and should always be used when lesions are extensive. Benzathine penicillin (300,000 to 600,000 units for infants and children less than 66 pounds [30 kg], 900,000 units for older children, and 1.2 million units for adults) can be given intramuscularly as one dose. Intramuscular penicillin circumvents the problem of patient compliance, but nonsuppurative complications are not as great a consideration in this instance; an oral penicillin preparation such as penicillin V (125 to 250 mg every 6 hours for 7 to 10 days) is quite acceptable. In patients allergic to penicillin, erythromycin (30 to 50 mg/kg/day in three or four divided doses) is the alternative agent of choice. It should be pointed out that during epidemics of pyoderma, prophylactic intramuscular benzathine penicillin reduces the number of new cases. Measures of this type become important when the infecting strain is nephritogenic and glomerulonephritis is occurring in epidemic proportions.

OTHER STREPTOCOCCAL SKIN INFECTIONS. Streptococci can invade lacerations, burns, and surgical wounds. When wounds and lacerations are involved, infection may remain localized or result in cellulitis as well (see next section). Infected burns appear inflamed and edematous and are characterized by marked weeping. In this situation severe systemic symptoms may be present. Lacerations sometimes can be managed with local measures, such as debridement and antibiotic ointment, and in some instances with oral antibiotics. Infected burns and wounds require parenteral therapy.

Streptococcal cellulitis (erysipelas) frequently follows minor, often unnoticed trauma. It also is common among patients with chronic dermatitis or venous stasis. A typical case involves intense erythema, warmth, and brawny thickening of the skin clearly demarcated from the as yet uninvolved dermis. This border advances rapidly as infection spreads, and on occasion streptococci can be isolated from the advancing margin; lymphangitis and bullae may be seen. Lymphangitis is character-

ized by red linear streaks emanating from the origin of infection to the regional lymph nodes, which become tender and enlarged. Lymphangitis may occur in the absence of cellulitis and can be accompanied by bacteremia.

Erysipelas of the face once was a common infection but now is encountered infrequently. It characteristically begins near the nose and spreads laterally to involve the face in a "butterfly" distribution. On resolution of cellulitis of all types, desquamation is common.

Cellulitis often is a serious disease that can cause high fever, toxicity, and prostration; bacteremia is not uncommon, and shock can occur. Erysipelas of the face tends to cause milder systemic signs and symptoms. Cellulitis can spread rapidly. For these reasons treatment must be prompt. In cases in which more than just a small area of skin is involved and systemic symptoms and toxicity are present, parenteral administration of antibiotics and hospitalization often are indicated.

Staphylococci can produce cellulitis similar to streptococcal disease. However, the area of involvement tends to remain more localized, and lymphangitis is less common. Because of the difficulty in delineating these two entities, cellulitis should be treated with a parenteral penicillinase-resistant semisynthetic penicillin or cephalosporin, such as intramuscular or intravenous cefazolin (2 to 4 g/day in three or four divided doses); or intravenous nafcillin, oxacillin, or cephalothin (6 to 12 g/day in four to six divided doses). When neither a penicillin nor a cephalosporin can be administered, vancomycin (2 g/day intravenously in four divided doses) is the drug of choice.

Streptococcal cellulitis has the propensity to become recurrent and involve the same areas of the body. Recently, recurrent cellulitis at the site of saphenous vein donation for coronary artery bypass grafting has been described. Prophylactic antimicrobials have been advocated for recurrent cellulitis, but their efficacy has not been proved.

Other group A streptococcal infections

BACTEREMIA. Group A strepcococcal bacteremia usually occurs as a result of skin and soft tissue infection. Uncomplicated pharyngeal infection rarely causes bacteremia. Septic arthritis, osteomyelitis, meningitis, and endocarditis are potential complications of bacteremia. The clinical course of streptococcal septicemia may be fulminant, with shock, disseminated intravascular coagulation, and high mortality.

PNEUMONIA. Bacterial pneumonia caused by group A streptococci is uncommon. It is seen most often after pertussis and viral respiratory infections, such as influenza, measles, and varicella. It also occurs in epidemic form in the military. Streptococcal pneumonia is characterized by a 60% incidence of pleural involvement with bloody empyema. Treatment consists of penicillin therapy (4 to 6 million units every 24 hours) and drainage of the pleural space by either thoracentesis or chest tube.

BONE AND JOINT INFECTION. *S. pyogenes* is a relatively common cause of osteomyelitis and septic arthritis. These infections are clinically similar to bone and joint infections caused by other bacteria.

PUERPERAL INFECTION. Puerperal infection (childbed fever) occurs when streptococci invade the endometrium. The abrupt onset of fever, chills, and toxicity, with abdominal or pelvic pain, usually occurs within 24 to 48 hours after delivery. Serosanguineous, odorless vaginal discharge is noted. If not treated quickly, infection may result in pelvic cellulitis, septic pelvic thrombophlebitis, peritonitis, and pelvic abscess. A similar syndrome may be caused by group B streptococci and anerobic streptococci as well (see next section).

GROUP B STREPTOCOCCI

S. agalactiae was first recognized in association with bovine mastitis. However, these organisms now are clearly recognized as important pathogens for humans. Most group B streptococci exhibit β hemolysis and are resistant to bacitracin. They can be further distinguished from group A organisms by their ability to hydrolyse sodium hippurate. Group B organisms are divided into five antigenic subgroups: Ia, Ib, Ic, II, and III.

Group B streptococci have emerged as an extremely important cause of neonatal sepsis, and the incidence of group B infection rivals that of *E. coli* as the most common organism. The bacteria colonize the birth canal, and neonates can acquire infection at the time of delivery. Alternatively, nosocomial transmission occurs in nurseries. The incidence of maternal carriage may be as high as 25%, and transmission to the neonate also may be quite high. Fortunately, the incidence of disease is low, about 2 cases for every 1000 births. This may be related to some degree, especially for type III organisms, to the transmission of maternal antibody to the neonate. Antibiotics have not been successful in eliminating maternal carriage.

Two syndromes of neonatal infection have been described, early-onset and late-onset infection. Early-onset infection begins in the first 10 days of life. The neonate acquires the organisms from vaginal colonization and infection. This condition is more common with prematurity and prolonged rupture of the membranes. However, infection can occur after uncomplicated term deliveries as well. The syndrome consists of fulminating bacteremia and shock. Pneumonia, meningitis, or both are found in almost 50% of cases; despite antimicrobial therapy the mortality rate exceeds 50%. The late-onset syndrome, appearing after 10 days of life is acquired nosocomially, is not correlated with obstetric complications, and most often is seen as meningitis. The prognosis for the late-onset syndrome is somewhat better, with a mortality of less than 30%. Whereas all subtypes of group B organisms may be encountered in the early syndrome, type III dominates with the late-onset presentation.

Group B streptococci cause a broad range of infections in adults. Patients frequently are women of childbearing age who develop infection in conjunction with delivery of gynecologic disorders. Elderly patients with genitourinary problems, diabetes, or other chronic diseases also are prone to these infections. In fact, about 2% of all bacteremias and about 8% of all streptococcal bacteremias in adults are caused by group B organisms. Infections caused by group B streptococci include pyelonephritis, peritonitis, endometritis, meningitis, endocarditis, bacteremia, pulmonary infections, and soft tissue infections (gangrene and cellulitis in patients with diabetes).

Group B streptococci are sensitive to penicillin, but the minimum inhibitory concentrations (MIC) are somewhat higher when compared to *S. pyogenes*. Cephalosporins, erythromycin, clindamycin, and vancomycin also are active agents. Antimicrobial therapy for adults with serious infections from group B streptococci consists of high-dose intravenous penicillin (10 to 20 million units every 24 hours).

GROUP C AND G STREPTOCOCCI

Group C and G streptococci are less commonly isolated in human streptococcal disease than group A organisms, with which they have many features in common. For example, most strains are β-hemolytic and some are even sensitive to bacitracin. Both groups also produce similar enzymes and toxins to those of group A streptococci, such as streptolysin O, streptokinase, DNase, NADase, hyaluronidase, and erythrogenic toxin. The group C carbohydrate also is similar to that of group A, and cross-reacting cell-membrane antigens can be demonstrated among groups A, C, and G. Two outbreaks of group C disease linked to dairy products were associated with acute glomerulonephritis.

These organisms are recognized as part of the normal throat, skin, and genitourinary flora. However, they also have been implicated as a cause of skin and wound infections, puerperal sepsis, bacteremia, and endocarditis. Purulent pharyngitis also sometimes occurs with scarlatiniform eruptions. Following these infections, elevations of the ASO titer and other antibodies to other extracellular products frequently can be demonstrated. Both group C and G organisms are sensitive to penicillin and erythromycin, and treatment regimens for group A streptococci can be employed for similar clinical situations.

GROUP D STREPTOCOCCI

Group D streptococci are divided into two major groups. Organisms that grow on bile and in 6.5% NaCl are designated *enterococci*, which include *Streptococcus faecalis* and other species. These organisms can be α-, β-, or γ-hemolytic. Organisms that grow on bile but not in 6.5% NaCl and that are nearly always α-hemolytic are called *nonenterococcal* group D streptococci and include *Streptococcus bovis* and *Streptococcus equinus*. Both groups are part of the normal gastrointestinal and genitourinary flora and frequently are isolated from patients with infections involving these areas. Both groups also are commonly the cause of bacterial endocarditis, and in this light their differences become important. Enterococci are the only members of the streptococci family that are consistently resistant to penicillin. Although ampicillin may be sufficient for urinary tract infections or other minor infections caused by these organisms, therapy for more serious processes, such as bacteremia or endocarditis, requires the synergistic combination of penicillin and an aminoglycoside (see Chapter 40). The patient who is allergic to penicillin often requires vancomycin with an aminoglycoside or penicillin desensitization. Enterococci are resistant to cephalosporins, which should not be used.

S. equinus rarely causes infections in people. On the other hand, *S. bovis* is a very common cause of endocarditis. *S. bovis* is sensitive to penicillin, and treatment of endocarditis caused by this organism is similar to endovascular infection from *S. viridans*. Perhaps more importantly, an association between *S. bovis* bacteremia and endocarditis with colon carcinoma and perhaps other gastrointestinal tumors has been elucidated. Thus any patient with *S. bovis* isolated from the blood requires a thorough search for gastrointestinal (especially colon) neoplasia.

VIRIDANS STREPTOCOCCI

Viridans streptococci (by definition α-hemolytic) are members of the normal upper respiratory tract flora. They are still the most common cause of subacute bacterial endocarditis. Their classification is confusing in that some species are groupable and others are not. Five major species have been described: *Streptococcus salivarius, Streptococcus mitior, Streptococcus milleri, Streptococcus sanguis,* and *Streptococcus mutans*. *S. mutans* has been implicated in the development of dental caries. These organisms produce substances that are important in plaque formation. For the most part viridans streptococci are noninvasive and cause infection on damaged heart valves after transient bacteremia. However, *S. milleri* can cause serious pyogenic processes such as brain abscess, empyema, liver abscess, and peritonitis. *S. milleri* frequently is classified as microaerophilic; its behavior is similar to that of the anaerobic streptococci (see next section). Metastatic infection also is more likely to occur when *S. milleri* causes endocarditis when compared to other viridans streptococci.

These organisms are sensitive to penicillin but not to the degree that group A streptococci are. Parenteral penicillin therapy, sometimes with an aminoglycoside, is required for viridans streptococcal endocarditis (see Chapter 40).

ANAEROBIC STREPTOCOCCI

Anaerobic and microaerophilic streptococcal species reside in the pharynx, gastrointestinal tract, and genitourinary tract. These organisms can cause several types of infection, including necrotizing pneumonia, lung abscess, empyema, sinusitis, brain abscess, and skin and wound infections. They often are found along with other anaerobic or aerobic bacteria. Foul-smelling pus and gas in the soft tissues are characteristic of these infections. The anaerobic streptococci are sensitive to penicillin. High-dose parenteral therapy generally is required.

ACUTE RHEUMATIC FEVER

EPIDEMIOLOGY. Because the diagnosis of acute rheumatic fever (ARF) is largely clinical and there is no specific diagnostic test, the exact incidence of this disorder is unknown. ARF seems to be much less common now than years ago, probably because of better living conditions, the advent of antimicrobial agents, and perhaps decreased "rheumatogenicity" of the streptococci themselves. Nevertheless, outbreaks of ARF continue to be described in the United States. When it occurs, ARF most commonly is seen in patients of lower socioeconomic strata between 5 and 16 years of age. During epidemics of severe streptococcal pharyngitis in closed groups such as the military, the incidence of ARF may approach 2% to 3% among the untreated. On the other hand, with milder sporadic pharyngitis, the incidence is much lower. Other factors that seem to be related to the attack rate of ARF are the duration of carriage of group A streptococci in the throat and the magnitude of the individual's immune response to streptococcal antigens. Patients who have suffered one attack of rheumatic fever are clearly at high risk for recurrence following subsequent group A streptococcal upper respiratory tract infections.

PATHOGENESIS. The exact mechanism by which group A streptococci precipitate tissue damage still is unproved. However, much experimental work and various clinical observations have provoked many theories in this regard. It appears both host and bacterial factors play important roles. For instance, since pyoderma does not precipitate ARF, investigators postulate that access to the rich lymphoid tissues of the pharynx that have connections with the heart may be needed to produce the disease. Other differences between strains that produce only pharyngitis and those that produce both pyoderma and pharyngitis have been pointed out. For example, strains producing pyoderma evoke a weak ASO response. These strains also are less "rheumatogenic"—they differ from those streptococcal strains that lack a serum opacity factor (SOF-negative) and that seem to elicit high antibody levels as well as being capable of causing ARF. Certain streptococcal products such as streptolysin O have been shown to have direct cardiotoxic effects in animals. Some streptococcal antigens seem to have common components with cardiac tissue. In this regard, antibodies directed at the streptococcal antigens could cross-react with heart tissue and cause damage. Circulating heart antibodies have been demonstrated in high titers in the sera of patients with rheumatic fever. However, it is unclear whether these antibod-

ies are the cause of the damage or the result of previous heart tissue destruction from some other insult. Another theory, which also emphasizes the role of humoral immunity, is the possibility of immune-complex deposition causing the disease. Some experimental evidence also links streptococcal antigens to a nonspecific mitogenic response of delayed hypersensitivity. The latter would then precipitate T-cell cytotoxicity to cardiac cells. Recent studies have associated certain human histocompatability leukocyte antigens with the development of ARF and carditis, which supports the concept of a genetically determined susceptibility to ARF and rheumatic heart disease.

CLINICAL MANIFESTATIONS. The severity of ARF tends to differ with the patient's age. In young children carditis seems to predominate, whereas in older children and adults joint manifestations are most prominent.

ARF has five major clinical features. *Acute migratory arthritis* occurs early in about 70% to 80% of cases and involves the large joints of the extremities. Arthralgia is seen in most of the remaining patients. The rash of ARF, *erythema marginatum,* is a nonpainful, nonpruritic, evanescent eruption that appears on the trunk and extremities. The rash is salmon colored with serpiginous borders (smoke-ring–like). Lesions enlarge with central pallor and then disappear. Erythema marginatum is found in fewer than 5% of cases. *Sydenham's chorea* (St. Vitus' dance) also is a relatively uncommon feature of ARF. It is seen several months after the streptococcal infection, which usually has occurred without subsequent arthritic symptoms. Chorea is characterized by purposeless, involuntary movements that disappear with sleep, slurred speech, and emotional lability. The disorder usually clears without residual effects. Freely movable, painless *subcutaneous nodules* are found on extensor surfaces over tendons and over bony prominences such as the occiput. Nodules are found in severe disease, frequently with serious carditis. All of the manifestations just mentioned are seen only in ARF, and no permanent damage occurs. The one exception is Jaccoud's arthritis, which is seen in patients with repeated episodes of rheumatic fever. It is characterized by ulnar deviation and flexion of the metacarpophalangeal joints without pain.

The most important manifestation of ARF is *carditis*. It is the only manifestation that has the potential for causing long-term disability or death. Heart involvement in ARF can be pancarditis, causing endocarditis, myocarditis, and pericarditis. No cardiac involvement or any combination of cardiac lesions may be present in the patient with ARF. In the absence of pericarditis or congestive heart failure, carditis may be silent. The clinical signs of carditis may include new heart murmur(s) (such as mitral or aortic regurgitation, but not stenosis), cardiac enlargement, congestive heart failure, and pericardial friction rub. Prolongation of the PR interval frequently is found but is not diagnostic of ARF.

DIAGNOSIS. Because there is no specific laboratory test for rheumatic fever and the clinical features are so diverse, accurate diagnosis of ARF may be difficult. Obviously, the need for a precise diagnosis is critical to prevent subsequent attacks.

To avoid misdiagnosis, the modified Jones' criteria have been used (Table 45-2). However, this system is not foolproof, especially when arthritis is the sole major manifestation. Thus in addition to satisfying Jones' criteria, one must be able to verify that there has been a recent streptococcal infection. The latter is best documented either by a history of scarlet fever or by antibody evidence of recent injection with group A streptococci, such as elevated ASO, DNase, antihyaluronidase, or positive streptozyme test. A history of recent pharyngitis or a positive throat culture, while suggestive, is not specific. Many

Table 45-2   Revised Jones' criteria* for diagnosis of ARF

Major manifestations	Minor manifestations	Supporting evidence
Carditis	Clinical	Elevated streptococcal antibodies
Polyarthritis	Previous rheumatic fever or rheumatic heart disease	Recent scarlet fever
Chorea	Arthralgia	Positive throat culture for group A streptococcus
Erythema marginatum	Fever	
Subcutaneous nodules	Laboratory	
	Elevated erythrocyte sedimentation rate	
	C-reactive protein	
	Leukocytosis	
	Prolonged PR interval	

Adapted from the recommendations of the Rheumatic Fever Committee of The American Heart Association (Circulation 69:204A, 1984).
*The presence of two major criteria, or one major and two minor criteria with supporting evidence of recent group A streptococcal infection, indicates high probability of rheumatic fever. The absence of the latter makes the diagnosis doubtful, except in instances of a long period of latency between infection and symptoms, as with Sydenham's chorea or low-grade carditis.

patients with ARF give no history of recent sore throat, and the incidence of streptococcal carriage in the general population can be quite high.

COURSE. Acute disease usually subsides within a few weeks, and in most patients evidence of active inflammation is gone in 90 days. Less than 5% of patients may remain ill for 6 months or more. Valvular lesions may heal completely or may progress. In the preantibiotic era, more than 50% of patients had at least one recurrence and the risk of permanent valvular damage became more likely with each new attack. However, if carditis was absent during the initial bout, it was unlikely carditis would develop with recurrences.

MANAGEMENT. The goals of therapy in ARF are to decrease fever and toxicity, alleviate inflammation, and control congestive heart failure. The cornerstones of treatment are salicylates and corticosteroids. However, neither of these agents prevent or modify the development of chronic rheumatic heart disease. Patients with joint manifestations and mild carditis (not congestive heart failure) can be managed with aspirin (90 to 100 mg/kg/day) with modification of dosage to achieve a therapeutic salicylate level. Although the use of steroids remains somewhat controversial, most experts use steroids (the equivalent of 40 to 60 mg/day of prednisone orally or intravenously) when heart failure is present. The treatment of heart failure does not differ from the management of failure caused by other forms of organic heart disease. Bed rest for 3 weeks is recommended when carditis is absent. The period is extended to 1 month after subsidence of symptoms in mild cases of carditis, and longer periods are recommended when heart failure and cardiac enlargement are present. If streptococci are detected in throat cultures, therapy as for streptococcal pharyngitis should be undertaken.

PREVENTION. Primary prevention consists of eradicating streptococci from the pharynx when the initial infection is detected. Prevention of subsequent bouts of rheumatic fever requires the use of antimicrobial prophylaxis. Clinical studies have indicated that monthly intramuscular benzathine penicillin (1.2 million units) is the most effective method. Alternate, but less reliable, methods include the use of oral penicillin G (125 mg twice daily) or sulfisoxazole (1 g/day or 500 mg/day for small children). When carefully adhered to, antimicrobial prophylaxis is extremely effective in protecting against acquisition of group A streptococci and therefore against rheumatic fever. At one time it was recommended that prophylaxis be continued for life. However, many experts now believe that it is safe to discontinue prophylaxis in adults who do not have intimate contact with school-age children and who have not had an attack of rheumatic fever since childhood.

BIBLIOGRAPHY

American Heart Association: Jones criteria (revised) for guidance in the diagnosis of rheumatic fever, Circulation 69:204A, 1984.

American Heart Association Committee on Rheumatic Fever and Bacterial Endocarditis: Prevention of rheumatic fever, Circulation 70:1118A, 1984.

Auckenthaler R and others: Group G streptococcal bacteremia: clinical study and review of the literature, Rev Infect Dis 5:196, 1983.

Ayoub EM and others: Association of class II human histocompatibility leukocyte antigens with rheumatic fever, J Clin Invest 77:2019, 1986.

Baddour LM and Bisno AL: Recurrent cellulitis after coronary bypass surgery: association with superficial fungal infection in saphenous venectomy limbs, JAMA 251:1049, 1984.

Baker CJ: Group B streptococcal infections, Adv Intern Med 25:475, 1980.

Barnham M and others: Nephritis caused by *Streptococcus zooepidemicus* (Lancefield group C), Lancet 1:945, 1983.

Bass JW: Treatment of streptococcal pharyngitis revisited, JAMA 256:740, 1986.

Bisno AL and Ofek I: Serologic diagnosis of streptococcal infection: comparison of a rapid hemagglutination technique with conventional antibody tests, Am J Dis Child 127:676, 1974.

Brennan RO and Durack DT: The viridans streptococci in perspective. In Remington JS and Swartz MN, editors: Current clinical topics in infectious diseases, New York, 1984, McGraw-Hill, Inc.

Centor RM and others: Throat culture and rapid tests for diagnosis of group A streptococcal pharyngitis, Ann Intern Med 105:892, 1986.

Gallagher PG and Watanakunakorn C: Group B streptococcal bacteremia in a community teaching hospital, Am J Med 78:795, 1985.

Kaplan EL and others: Diagnosis of streptococcal pharyngitis: differentiation of active infection from the carrier state in the symptomatic child, J Infect Dis 123:490, 1971.

Klein RS and others: *Streptococcus bovis* septicemia and carcinoma of the colon, Ann Intern Med 91:560, 1979.

McDanald EC and Weisman MH: Articular manifestations of rheumatic fever in adults, Ann Intern Med 89:917, 1978.

Murray HW and others: Serious infections caused by *Streptococcus milleri*, Am J Med 64:759, 1978.

Reinarz JA and Sanford JP: Human infections caused by nongroup A streptococci, Medicine 44:81, 1965.

Veasy LG and others: Resurgence of acute rheumatic fever in the intermountain areas of the United States, N Engl J Med 316:421, 1987.

46 · DISEASES CAUSED BY GRAM-NEGATIVE COCCI

Gonococcal infections

Donald Kaye

DEFINITION AND ETIOLOGY. Gonorrhea is an infection of the mucous membranes of the urethra and genital tract caused by *Neisseria gonorrhoeae*. The pharynx and anal canal commonly are involved. Infection is almost always the result of sexual contact. After invasion of mucosal sites, gonococci may spread and cause infections such as arthritis, tenosynovitis, perihepatitis, endocarditis, and meningitis.

Primary isolation of the gonococcus is difficult. Chocolate agar or special commercial media must be used. Most strains require an atmosphere of 2% to 10% carbon dioxide.

Thayer-Martin selective medium, containing a mixture of antimicrobials, permits growth of *Neisseria meningitidis* and *N. gonorrhoeae* but inhibits growth of many other bacteria frequently found in specimens from the urethra, cervix, anal canal, and pharynx.

EPIDEMIOLOGY. Although gonorrhea almost always is acquired from sexual contact, exceptions are gonococcal conjunctivitis, which occurs primarily in infants, and vulvovaginitis. Conjunctivitis results either from passage of the infant through an infected genital tract (ophthalmia neonatorum) or from contamination after birth. Vulvovaginitis is an infection of the genital tract of infants and preadolescent girls that results from direct contact with infected adults or in rare cases from contact with contaminated towels or linens.

Repeated attacks of gonorrhea are common; therefore individual attacks seem to confer little or no immunity. After an episode of acute gonorrhea, *N. gonorrhoeae* may remain in the genital tract for months. Chronic asymptomatic carriers of the gonococcus are an important epidemiologic factor of gonorrhea, because they are difficult to detect and therefore are rarely treated. Most women with gonorrhea are relatively asymptomatic, and 5% to 10% of males with urethral gonorrhea are asymptomatic. It has been estimated that more than 2 million new cases of gonorrhea occur annually in the United States. Many patients with a gonococcal infection also have a chlamydial infection.

PATHOGENESIS AND PATHOLOGY. In males the urethra is attacked first, resulting in purulent urethritis and involvement of the urethral glands. Direct spread of infection may result in prostatitis, epididymitis, or seminal vesiculitis (all rare). During healing, stricture formation may occur. Gonococcal proctitis in the male almost always is the result of rectal intercourse.

In the female urethritis is mild and transient. Bartholin's and Skene's glands and glands of the cervix may become infected with or without involvement of the urethra. Contiguous spread of infection can cause acute salpingitis, which occurs in about 10% of women. Proctitis may result from contiguous spread or rectal intercourse. Gonococcal salpingitis usually is bilateral and may cause pyosalpinx and formation of a tuboovarian abscess. The inflammation tends to heal with fibrosis and adhesions that may produce obstruction of the fallopian tubes and sterility.

Gonococcal infection of the pharynx is common and results from orogenital contact. Gonococcal pharyngeal infection has been demonstrated in up to 20% of homosexual men and 20% of women practicing fellatio who had gonococcal infection at any site.

Occasionally invasion of the blood occurs, and *N. gonorrhoeae* desseminate and produce infection at distant foci in about 1% to 3% of infections. Joints are the most frequent extragenital sites of localization, but tenosynovitis, endocarditis, meningitis, skin lesions, and infection at other foci also may occur.

Dissemination of gonococcal infection is more common in women than in men and more common in homosexual males than in heterosexual males. The source for dissemination may be the genital tract, rectum, or pharynx.

CLINICAL MANIFESTATIONS

Gonorrhea in the male. The incubation period of gonococcal urethritis in the male usually is 2 to 8 days. There is sudden onset of dysuria, urgency, and frequency associated with mucoid urethral discharge that rapidly becomes purulent and profuse. Gonococcal urethritis usually does not cause fever.

Gonorrhea in the female. The disease may begin in the female with dysuria, urgency, and frequency after an incubation period of 2 to 8 days. However, the urethritis frequently is of short duration and often is mild or completely asymptomatic. Cervicitis gives rise to a mucopurulent discharge. Involvement of Skene's ducts or Bartholin's glands is common. Gonococci can be isolated from the anal canal in 20% to 50% of women with gonorrhea and occasionally can produce symptomatic proctitis. In 5% of women with gonococcal infection only the anorectal culture contains gonococci.

Salpingitis is manifested by acute onset of fever and lower abdominal pain. Physical examination usually reveals lower abdominal tenderness, pain on movement of the cervix, and tenderness of the adnexa (with or without palpable masses).

Extragenital gonococcal infection

Proctitis. Gonococcal proctitis usually is asymptomatic but may be manifested by anal discharge, burning rectal pain, blood and pus in the stools, and pain on defecation.

Pharyngitis. Gonococcal infection in the oropharynx probably can cause symptomatic pharyngitis, tonsillitis, and gingivitis but is usually asymptomatic.

Arthritis. Arthritis, the most common form of clinically recognized disseminated gonococcal infection, usually occurs within 1 to 3 weeks after initial infection in the genital tract or may follow pharyngeal or rectal infection. Onset may be gradual, with migratory polyarthralgias leading to frank arthritis in one or more joints, or it may be sudden, with hot, swollen, and extremely painful joints. Fever and leukocytosis usually are present. More than 75% of patients have polyarthritis. The joints most commonly involved are the knees, ankles, and wrists, but any joint may be affected. *Tenosynovitis*, which rarely is observed in other types of pyogenic arthritis, is common in gonococcal arthritis and most often occurs around the wrists and ankles. The skin lesions associated with gonococcal bacteremia also are frequently present. *N. gonorrhoeae* can be isolated from joint fluid in only 25% to 50% of cases. The fluid ranges from serous to frankly purulent, has the protein content of an exudate, and usually contains increased numbers of leukocytes that are mainly polymorphonuclear.

Gonococcal bacteremia. Gonococcal bacteremia can produce a syndrome with recurrent episodes of fever, skin lesions, tenosynovitis, arthralgia or arthritis, and intermittently positive blood cultures. This syndrome occurs with infection in the genital tract, anal canal, or pharynx, and, if untreated, can recur over months or even years. The rash usually appears during the first day of symptoms and may recur with each episode of fever. The rash is found on the distal part of the extremities and consists of scanty, pinpoint erythematous macules that rapidly become maculopapular, vesiculopustular, and frequently hemorrhagic. Gram-negative cocci often can be seen in stains of fluid from the lesions, but cultures for *N. gonorrhoeae* usually are negative. Immunofluorescent studies on the exudate from the pustules demonstrate *N. gonorrhoeae* in a high percentage of patients.

Perihepatitis (Fitz-Hugh–Curtis syndrome). Perihepatitis, a rare complication in women with gonococcal pelvic inflammatory disease, results from direct spread of gonococci from the pelvis to the upper abdomen. It is manifested by fever, upper quadrant pain (usually right), tenderness and spasm of the abdominal wall, and occasionally a friction rub over the liver. *N. gonorrhoeae* frequently can be found in the cervical or vaginal discharge.

The untreated disease subsides after 1 to 4 weeks, leaving "violin-string" adhesions between the anterior surface of the liver and the anterior abdominal wall. Perihepatitis also can result from *Chlamydia trachomatis* infection.

DIAGNOSIS. In the male the presence of intracellular gram-negative diplococci in smears of exudate from the urethra is strongly indicative of gonorrhea. Confirmation is obtained by culture or, if available, fluorescent antibody studies. Cultures of the anal canal should be obtained in homosexual males.

In a routine screening cervical cultures detect most females with asymptomatic gonorrhea. In the female with suspected gonorrhea, cultures of exudate from the cervix and anal canal should be obtained.

Pharyngeal cultures of *N. gonorrhoeae* should be obtained from homosexual males and females practicing fellatio. In all patients with suspected disseminated gonococcal infections, cultures of the pharynx and anal canal should be obtained in addition to genital tract cultures.

Exudates should be inoculated as soon as possible on Thayer-Martin medium or on a suitable transport medium for *N. gonorrhoeae*.

A substantial portion of the cases of urethritis in men in the United States today are nongonococcal. Many of these are caused by *C. trachomatis* and probably by *Ureaplasma urealyticum*.

Salpingitis. Acute salpingitis must be differentiated from appendicitis and tubal pregnancy. The presence of bilateral tenderness in the adnexa, a history of recent sexual intercourse followed by urethritis or vaginal discharge, and demonstration of gonococci in the cervical exudate are strongly suggestive of gonococcal salpingitis.

Arthritis; bloodborne lesions. Isolation of *N. gonorrhoeae* from the genital tract, rectum, or pharynx is supportive evidence in a patient with suspected disseminated gonococcal infection, and demonstration of gonococci in skin lesions, blood, or joint fluid is confirmatory.

When stains and cultures of joint fluid are negative for gonococci, as found in 50% to 75% of cases, it frequently is difficult to differentiate gonococcal arthritis from Reiter's syndrome (nonbacterial urethritis, conjunctivitis, and arthritis). Urethritis and arthritis in a female suggest gonococcal arthritis, because this disease is more common in females, whereas Reiter's syndrome is rare in females. The presence of tenosynovitis and response to antimicrobial therapy strongly imply gonococcal arthritis.

MANAGEMENT
Uncomplicated gonorrhea. The recommendations of the Division of Sexually Transmitted Diseases of the Centers for Disease Control for treatment of uncomplicated gonorrhea (urethral, cervical, or anal canal) or for patients with known exposure to gonorrhea are directed at both gonorrhea with presumptive coexisting infection with chlamydia, which often is present. The regimens for gonorrhea are amoxicillin (3 g) or ampicillin (3.5 g) orally in a single dose; or aqueous procaine penicillin G (4.8 million units intramuscularly [at two sites]) or ceftriaxone (250 mg intramuscularly). If amoxicillin, ampicillin, or procaine penicillin is used, probenecid (1 g orally) must be given simultaneously. Ceftriaxone has become routine therapy in many parts of the United States because of the spread of penicillinase-producing gonococci that are resistant to the penicillins and often to the tetracyclines. The regimen for chlamydia, immediately following the regimen for gonorrhea, is tetracycline (500 mg orally four times daily); doxycycline (100 mg orally twice daily); or (if these agents are not tolerated or

in pregnancy), erythromycin base or stearate (500 mg orally four times daily for 7 days).

If the patient is allergic to penicillin and cephalosporins, the tetracycline or doxycycline regimen can be used for both gonorrhea and chlamydial infection. When patients who are allergic to penicillin cannot tolerate tetracycline, spectinomycin (2 g intramuscularly) can be used for gonorrhea followed by erythromycin for chlamydia.

Although all of the above regimens are effective for rectal gonococcal infection in women, homosexual men with rectal infection should be treated only with the single-dose procaine penicillin or ceftriaxone regimen. Spectinomycin (2 g intramuscularly) should be used in those who are allergic to penicillin. In the homosexual male with gonorrhea, it is not necessary to give tetracycline or doxycycline, as coexisting infection with chlamydia is less likely.

The procaine penicillin, tetracycline, and ceftriaxone regimens are the only ones effective in pharyngeal gonococcal infection.

All of the regimens used for gonorrhea or chlamydia are likely to cure incubating (seronegative) syphilis except spectinomycin alone.

Follow-up cultures for gonococci should be obtained from the infected site 4 to 7 days after completion of therapy. Rectal follow-up cultures should be obtained from all women. Treatment failures are treated with spectinomycin or ceftriaxone.

Patients in whom treatment has failed and those with uncomplicated gonorrhea known or suspected to be caused by a penicillinase-producing gonococcus should be treated with the spectinomycin or ceftriaxone regimens followed by therapy for chlamydia. However, spectinomycin is not effective for pharyngeal infection, and if ceftriaxone cannot be used for penicillinase producers in the pharynx, the alternative is nine tablets of trimethoprim-sulfamethoxazole (trimethoprim, 720 mg, and sulfamethoxazole, 3600 mg) per day in one daily dose for 5 days.

Epididymitis, arthritis, bacteremia, and pelvic inflammatory disease. Gonococcal epididymitis is treated with a single-dose regimen for gonorrhea followed by a 10-day regimen for chlamydia.

Gonococcal arthritis or the bacteremia syndrome is treated with aqueous penicillin G (10 million units intravenously daily for at least 3 days) followed by amoxicillin or ampicillin (500 mg orally four times daily to complete at least 7 days of therapy). Oral therapy can be given with amoxicillin (3 g) or ampicillin (3.5 g) plus probenecid (1 g) followed by amoxicillin or ampicillin (500 mg four times a day for at least 7 days). Cefoxitin in a dosage of 1 g or cefotaxime in a dosage of 500 mg intravenously four times daily or ceftriaxone (1 g intravenously once daily for 7 days) also can be used and is the regimen of choice for penicillinase-producing strains. Tetracycline or doxycycline should be given for 7 days for possible chlamydial infection after completion of the regimen for gonococcal infection.

The recommendations of the Centers for Disease Control for treatment of acute pelvic inflammatory disease are directed at gonococci, chlamydia, and the aerobic and anaerobic bacteria that often are present. For ambulatory patients the recommendation is cefoxitin (2 g intramuscularly), amoxicillin (3 g orally), ampicillin (3.5 g orally), procaine penicillin (4.8 million units intramuscularly), or ceftriaxone (250 mg intramuscularly). Each is given with probenecid (1 g orally) except for ceftriaxone. This single-dose therapy for gonorrhea is followed by doxycycline (100 mg orally twice a day for 10 to 14 days).

For hospitalized patients doxycycline (100 mg intravenously twice a day) plus cefoxitin (2 g intravenously four times daily) is preferred. After four days of therapy (at least 48 hours after improvement), doxycycline alone can be continued orally to complete 10 to 14 days of total therapy. Another regimen recommended for hospitalized patients is clindamycin (600 mg four times daily intravenously) plus gentamicin (2 mg/kg intravenously followed by 1.5 mg/kg three times daily). After 4 days (at least 48 hours after improvement), clindamycin (450 mg orally four times daily) is continued to complete 10 to 14 days of total therapy.

In gonococcal arthritis, pus should be aspirated by needle when possible. With the exception of the hip, open drainage of the joint rarely is necessary. Injection of penicillin into the joint is not indicated.

Serologic tests for syphilis should be performed before initiation of therapy in all patients treated for gonococcal infections. If the serologic test is positive, therapy for syphilis must be initiated.

PREVENTION. Use of a condom provides a high degree of protection for the uninfected partner. Sexual partners of patients with gonorrhea should be identified and treated as quickly as possible to prevent further spread of disease.

The instillation of 1% silver nitrate or an antimicrobial drug into the eyes of the newborn has largely eradicated gonococcal ophthalmia neonatorum.

BIBLIOGRAPHY

Barnes RC and Holmes KK: Epidemiology of gonorrhea; current perspectives, Epidemiol Rev 6:1, 1984.

Eschenbach DA and others: Polymicrobial etiology of acute pelvic inflammatory disease, N Engl J Med 293:166, 1975.

Handsfield HH: Recent developments in gonorrhea and pelvic inflammatory disease, J Med 14:281, 1983.

Hansfield HH, Wiesner PJ, and Holmes KK: Treatment of the gonococcal arthritis-dermatitis syndrome, Ann Intern Med 84:661, 1976.

Hook EW and Holmes KK: Gonococcal infections, Ann Intern Med 102:229, 1985.

Hutt DM and Judson FN: Epidemiology and treatment of oropharyngeal gonorrhea, Ann Intern Med 104:655, 1986.

Judson FN: Treatment of uncomplicated gonorrhea with ceftriaxone: a review, Sex Transm Dis 13:199, 1986.

Klein EJ and others: Anorectal gonococcal infection, Ann Intern Med 86:340, 1977.

Morbidity and Mortality Weekly Reports Supplement 34:4S, 1985.

Wiesner PJ and others: Gonococcal diseases, DM 26:1, 1980.

Meningococcal infections

Merle A. Sande and W. Michael Scheld

DEFINITION. The meningococcus is a virulent organism that has been responsible for some of the most notorious epidemics in modern history. Recent studies have advanced our understanding of the spread, immunity, and pathophysiology of the diseases produced by this organism. However, identification of an isolated case of meningococcal disease in the community continues to elicit considerable alarm among medical and lay people.

Neisseria meningitidis is a gram-negative coccus that characteristically is found in diplococcus form, with flattened adjacent edges producing the so-called biscuit shape. It is easily grown on media enriched with 10% blood or serum and grows best at 95° to 98.6° F (35° to 37° C) in a 5% to 10% CO_2 environment. Chocolate agar in a candle jar serves as an excellent culture environment. This organism is very susceptible to drying or chilling. It is definitively identified by various sugar fermentation steps and a positive "oxidase" reaction.

Meningococci are divided into distinct serogroups on the basis of chemical and antigenic differences in their polysaccharide capsules. The most common currently recognized types are A, B, C, D, X, Y, Z, W-135, and 29E. A, B, C, and Y account for most human disease.

EPIDEMIOLOGY. The only known reservoir for meningococcus is the human nasopharynx, and carrier rates vary from 2% to 15% in a normal population but increase to 40% when sporadic cases are identified and up to approximately 100% during epidemics. The carrier state lasts for weeks to months; one series had a median of 9.6 months.

The organism probably spreads by the respiratory droplet route, and spread is maximized in crowded environments. Most disease occurs during the late winter and early spring and may follow outbreaks of other respiratory viral infections. Attack rates are highest in children over 6 months of age, with a second peak occurring in adolescence. Close household contacts of index cases have a high attack rate of between 2.5% and 4%. Military recruits were particularly susceptible to epidemics, but in recent years civilian populations in Brazil, Finland, and Alaska have been similarly affected. Alcoholics, especially those living in unhealthy conditions, seem to be especially susceptible.

Historically, most epidemics have been produced by serogroup A; however, in 1963 serogroup B emerged as a predominant pathogen, and in 1969 to 1972 serogroup C was the prevalent epidemic-producing strain. In recent years a shift back toward serogroup B predominance and outbreaks of serogroup Y (mostly of pneumonia) have occurred. The epidemic in Brazil in 1971 began as predominantly group C but changed to group A in 1973 and finally faded out in 1976 after a massive immunization program.

PATHOGENESIS AND IMMUNITY. Meningococcal disease apparently occurs when the organism disseminates from the nasopharynx, producing generalized meningococcemia or metastatic infections in the meninges, joints, heart, pericardium, or skin. The factors that produce dissemination are not understood, but there is no doubt that the presence of bactericidal antibody is a strong deterrent. The peak attack rate of disease occurs in children between 6 and 12 months of age, when antibody titers are at the nadir. In a prospective study of military recruits, it was found that only 3 of 54 subjects who developed meningococcal disease had preexisting type-specific bactericidal serum antibody compared to 440 of 550 matched controls who did not develop disease during an epidemic; 38.5% of recruits without antibody who acquired the epidemic strain developed meningococcal disease. These and other studies formed the basis for development of a vaccine containing type A and C polysaccharide, which has successfully aborted epidemics worldwide and recently has nearly eliminated these serogroups from vaccinated military recruits in the United States. Antibody develops naturally approximately 2 weeks following acquisition of the organism in the nasopharynx, and protective cross-reacting antibodies appear following colonization with avirulent, nongroupable *Neisseria* and other related species.

Following dissemination, the organism may produce a number of clinical syndromes, ranging from a transient benign bacteremia to overwhelming meningococcemia with shock. The meningococcus primarily affects blood vessels, with endothelial damage, inflammation, necrosis, thrombosis, and hemorrhage. Thus most involved organs exhibit evidence of vasculitis. The mediator of these pathologic changes is primarily the lipopolysaccharide endotoxin, similar to that found in gram-negative bacilli. Endotoxin also may directly produce disseminated intravascular coagulation (DIC) by activation of the clotting cascade. It also may be directly responsible for the pathologic changes in the adrenal glands and kidneys seen in the Waterhouse-Friderichsen syndrome. This process resembles that found in an experimentally induced, generalized Swartzman reaction.

CLINICAL MANIFESTATIONS. Infection confined to the nasopharynx is the most common and usually is asymptomatic, although many patients with meningococcal disease report antecedent nasopharyngitis.

Meningococcemia without meningitis. A mild form of meningococcemia is the most common form of illness. Following a nondescript prodrome with cough, headache, and sore throat, the patient typically develops spiking fever and chills associated with arthralgias and occasionally frank arthritis. Severe muscle pains are common in the back and lower extremities. At least 75% of patients develop rash. Early in the disease the rash may have a pink, macular appearance that disappears within 2 days. Most patients develop the typical petechial rash, which varies in presentation from a few crops, often located on the conjunctiva, wrists, or ankles, to a generalized rash spreading across the trunk and lower body. Ecchymosis may develop and in severe cases can lead to extensive subcutaneous hemorrhage. Vesicular or pustular lesions may appear on a hemorrhagic base. Purpuric lesions with irregular borders also have been described. Gram stains of scrapings of the petechial lesions may reveal the causative organism in 50% to 70% of cases.

Symptoms may regress, remit, or persist as the disease progresses. Diagnosis is definitively established by identification of the organisms on smear or culture from petechiae or blood cultures. Some patients with mild disease spontaneously recover in several weeks.

Approximately 10% to 20% of patients with meningococcemia develop acute fulminant meningococcemia (Waterhouse-Friderichsen syndrome). This condition usually is more abrupt in onset than the milder form and proceeds to severe prostration within hours. Typically, the patient exhibits shaking chills, severe headache, and dizziness associated with severe orthostatic hypotension; shock rapidly supervenes. Patients usually are vasoconstricted, cyanotic, and pale with cold extremities but may be lucid. Most exhibit extreme evidence of subcutaneous ecchymosis and bleeding indicative of DIC. Bleeding around needle puncture sites may be profuse. Untreated, the patients rapidly progress to vascular collapse, with decreased cardiac output, oliguria, congestive heart failure, coma, and death.

Laboratory studies during the course of fulminant meningococcemia may reveal either leukocytosis or leukopenia, and organisms frequently can be seen within polymorphonuclear leukocytes in the peripheral blood (an indication of the high level of bacteremia). A metabolic acidosis with hypoxemia usually is present, and lactate levels are elevated in severe forms of the disease. Measurements of central venous or pulmonary wedge pressures usually reflect a low filling pressure initially, indicative of a decreased effective blood volume. As myocardial failure ensues, the filling pressure rises without a concomitant increase in cardiac output. Pulmonary edema secondary to cardiac failure or the adult respiratory distress syndrome from endotoxemia or shock frequently can be detected clinically or by roentgenographic examination. Evidence of DIC with an elevated prothrombin time, partial thromboplastin time, and fibrin-split products with a reduced platelet count are common.

Therapy is aimed at correction of the metabolic, electrolyte, cardiovascular, pulmonary, and clotting abnormalities while eliminating the infection with penicillin (20 million units intravenously daily). Meticulous attention to correction of each abnormality and close continuous monitoring is paramount to success in these extremely ill patients. Shifts in electrolyte and fluid balance occur quickly as the acid-base abnormalities develop, and abnormalities in cardiac function occur. Cardiotonic drugs such as dopamine frequently are necessary to maintain output. Acidosis must be corrected with sodium bicarbonate, which also increases the sodium load. Oxygen should be administered. Heparin may be indicated with fulminant DIC and clinical bleeding, but complications are common. The role of corticosteroids remains controversial. Even with the best of care, mortality is high and necrosis of limbs with gangrene is common in patients who survive.

Meningitis. More than 50% of patients with documented meningococcemia develop infection within the cerebrospinal fluid. The features of meningococcal meningitis are described under "Bacterial infections of the central nervous system" in Chapter 40.

Pneumonia. The meningococcus has been recognized as a potential lower respiratory tract pathogen for many years but only in the last decade has the importance of this disease been recognized. Most cases are produced by serogroup Y, and most reported series have originated from military camps. Presentation of the disease is similar to that seen with pneumococcal pneumonia, and since it responds well to penicillin, most cases probably go unrecognized. It is estimated that 1% to 2% of all cases of community-acquired pneumonia may be caused by the meningococcus. There are no typical clinical features that allow distinction between pneumonia caused by *Streptococcus pneumoniae* and that caused by the meningococcus.

COMPLICATIONS

Arthritis. Up to 10% of patients with meningococcemia develop monarticular or polyarticular arthritis. This may be a late occurrence, following the onset of bacteremia by 1 to 2 weeks. Cultures of the synovial fluid usually are sterile, and the pathogenesis of the disease may in part be an immunologic reaction to the organism. The development of arthritis may cause a persistent low-grade fever in the patient who has been adequately treated for his infection. These patients usually respond to recurrent aspirations of the affected joint and treatment with antiinflammatory drugs.

Pericarditis. Between 5% to 20% of patients with meningococcemia develop a friction rub and/or ECG evidence of pericarditis late in the course of the disease (up to 20 days after bacteremia). The typical clinical features of pericarditis may be present, with sharp anterior chest pain that changes with the position of the patient. This complication has led to cardiac tamponade.

Myocarditis. Myocarditis develops in most fatal cases of overwhelming meningococcemia and usually occurs within the first or second day of disease. It is manifested by the appearance of cardiomegaly, tachycardia, an S_3 gallop, and increased pulmonary wedge pressure; these may result in congestive heart failure. Although the pathogenesis is unclear, myocarditis probably results from the endotoxemia or associated vasculitis.

MANAGEMENT AND PREVENTION. Therapy and prevention of meningococcal meningitis are discussed under "Bacterial infections of the central nervous system" in Chapter 40.

BIBLIOGRAPHY

Ansari BM and others: A comparative study of adverse factors in meningococcemia and meningococcal meningitis, Postgrad Med J 55:780, 1979.
Feldman HA: Meningococcal infections, Adv Intern Med 18:177, 1972.
Goldschneider I and others: Human immunity to the meningococcus. I. The role of humoral antibody, J Exp Med 129:1307, 1969.

Koppes GM and others: Group Y meningococcal disease in United States Air Force recruits, Am J Med 62:661, 1977.

Peltola H: Meningococcal disease—still with us, Rev Infect Dis 5:71, 1983.

Peltola H and others: Clinical efficacy of meningococcus group A capsular polysaccharide vaccine in children three months to five years of age, N Engl J Med 297:686, 1977.

Pierce I and Cooper E: Meningococcal pericarditis: clinical features and therapy in five patients, Arch Intern Med 129:918, 1972.

47 · DISEASES CAUSED BY GRAM-NEGATIVE BACILLI

Haemophilus influenzae infections

Mark J. Ingerman and Jerome Santoro

DEFINITION. *Haemophilus influenzae* is a small, facultative gram-negative rod that is pathogenic only for humans. The organism is an important cause of respiratory and systemic infections in preschool children and has become a more common cause of systemic disease in adults during the past several decades.

ETIOLOGY. *H. influenzae* is distinguished from other *Haemophilus* species by its aerobic growth requirements for heat-labile nicotinamide-adenine dinucleotide (NAD) (V factor) and heat-stable hematin (X factor). Growth of the organism is accelerated by facilitating the release of these factors from red blood cells in the medium by either using chocolate agar or culturing the organism with *Staphylococcus aureus* (satellism). Growth also is promoted under 10% CO_2 (candle jar). Organisms obtained from agar plates examined by Gram stain are small, uniform gram-negative coccobacilli. However, in smears of clinical specimens the morphology of *H. influenzae* can vary from typical organisms to filamentous forms and even chains. In addition, organisms in stained clinical material may not take up dye properly and may be missed.

H. influenzae are found among the upper respiratory tract flora of up to 80% of individuals. Most of these strains are nonencapsulated. Six encapsulated species (A to F) have been recognized. Type B is the most commonly isolated encapsulated strain and is responsible for virtually all cases of serious disease. The capsular polymer of type B contains polyribose ribitol phosphate (PRP), which is antigenically cross-reactive with the cell wall and capsular constituents of certain gram-positive organisms and enteric bacilli.

EPIDEMIOLOGY. Disease caused by *H. influenzae* is worldwide and is endemic among children 3 months to 5 years of age. Epidemiologic data seem to indicate that *H. influenzae* infections are occurring more frequently. Serious infections tend to be more common in certain families and among poor rural populations. Patients with splenectomy, sickle cell anemia, agammaglobulinemia, treated Hodgkin's lymphoma, and alcoholism also are more susceptible to infection.

PATHOGENESIS AND IMMUNITY. *H. influenzae*, usually unencapsulated strains, can cause disease by contiguous spread to respiratory tract structures such as the paranasal sinuses, middle ear, and bronchial tree (as in chronic obstructive pulmonary disease). The events that change asymptomatic infection, or carriage, into disease are not precisely known, but experimental evidence exists supporting a synergistic role for respiratory tract viruses. Unencapsulated strains also occasionally produce pneumonia with subsequent seeding of the bloodstream. Bacteremia and deep tissue infections (pneumonia, cellulitis, epiglottitis) are more commonly caused by

encapsulated strains that are almost always type B. In this regard the capsule of the organism is thought to protect it from phagocytosis by polymorphonuclear leukocytes, explaining why patients with defects in nonspecific opsonizing ability (splenectomy, sickle cell disease) are prone to infection with type B. However, the reason why type B and not other encapsulated strains tends to cause infection is unknown.

The antibody response to naturally acquired *H. influenzae* infection is complex and variable. Factors such as age, genetic makeup, and type of infection influence the production of one or several antibodies directed against components of the organism, such as PRP, outer membrane antigens, and lipopolysaccharides. These antibodies alone or in combination provide protection against further infection unless events in later life (chemotherapy, splenectomy, or aging per se) again place the individual at risk.

CLINICAL MANIFESTATIONS. Nonencapsulated strains of *H. influenzae* are a relatively frequent cause of otitis media in preschool children and sinusitis and bronchitis in all age groups. The clinical manifestations of these infections are not unique and mimic similar syndromes caused by other bacteria.

Type B organisms are responsible for more serious infections, of which *meningitis* is the most common, and *H. influenzae* is the most frequent cause of bacterial meningitis between the ages of 9 months and 4 years. The clinical picture is that of typical bacterial meningitis (see discussion of "Bacterial infections of the central nervous system" in Chapter 40), but very young children may have nonspecific symptoms such as fever, lethargy, and poor feeding. The mortality, despite therapy, is about 5% to 10%, and more than one third of survivors develop significant neurologic residua. Meningitis may be seen in adults with basilar skull defects, alcoholism, and altered immunocompetence.

Epiglottitis is an extremely serious manifestation of *H. influenzae* infection. The disease begins with fever, malaise, and severe dysphagia, frequently without obvious pharyngitis or external swelling. This is followed by anxiety, evidence of upper airway obstruction, and drooling from inability to swallow oral secretions. Direct visualization of the epiglottis, which should only be done in the process of placing an airway, reveals a swollen and inflamed "cherry-red" structure.

Pneumonia caused by *H. influenzae* may be bronchial or lobar. Children with haemophilus pneumonia may develop empyema or pericarditis. *H. influenzae* is being recognized with greater frequency as a cause of pneumonia in elderly adults who may have underlying pulmonary disease or alcoholism.

H. influenzae cellulitis in children usually occurs on the cheek or the periorbital area and is characterized by a bluish hue. *H. influenzae* bacteremia may complicate pneumonia, epiglottitis, and cellulitis or occur without an obvious source in compromised individuals. Presumably, transient bacteremia (either symptomatic or asymptomatic) can lead to *septic arthritis* and less commonly *osteomyelitis*, as well as *bacterial endocarditis*.

DIAGNOSIS. Diagnosis of *H. influenzae* infection is most readily established with the acquisition of body fluids (spinal, pleural, joint) for Gram stain and subsequent cultures. Obviously isolation of the organism from blood also is diagnostic. Epiglottitis and facial cellulitis are distinctive enough to be diagnosed without culture confirmation. However, blood cultures may be positive in these two entities, and organisms sometimes can be isolated from an aspirate of the cellulitic margin. When Gram stains are negative or equivocal, the detection of PRP in cerebrospinal fluid, blood, and urine by counterimmunoelectrophoresis (CIE), enzyme-linked immunosorbent assay (ELISA), or latex agglutination has proven useful in early diagnosis of haemophilus disease. However, as previously mentioned, PRP may cross-react with other bacterial antigens and false positive results, although infrequent, may occur. The diagnosis of *H. influenzae* pneumonia in adults without bacteremia may depend on the sputum Gram stain, since the presence or absence of organisms in the sputum culture is not helpful.

MANAGEMENT. The treatment of serious systemic *H. influenzae* infection has been complicated in recent years by the emergence of strains that produce β-lactamase and are thereby resistant to ampicillin. The incidence of resistance varies geographically and approaches 5% to 25% in some areas. Until the etiologic organism is shown to be sensitive to ampicillin, serious systemic illness in children caused by *H. influenzae* should be treated with chloramphenicol (100 mg/kg/day intravenously in four divided doses at 6-hour intervals) and ampicillin (200 to 400 mg/kg/day intravenously in six divided doses at 4-hour intervals). When the infecting strain is found to be sensitive to ampicillin, chloramphenicol is discontinued and ampicillin is continued. Chloramphenicol is used alone for a full course when the patient is allergic to penicillin. Owing to their excellent activity against β-lactamase-producing strains of *H. influenzae,* the new broad-spectrum cephalosporins such as cefuroxime, cefotaxime, ceftizoxime, and ceftriaxone have been widely accepted for use in treating deep-seated infections, including meningitis. Treatment is continued for 10 to 14 days when meningitis is present. The length of therapy for other syndromes is dictated by the clinical response or the disease process; for example, longer courses are required for endocarditis or osteomyelitis. Oral ampicillin, amoxicillin, Augmentin (amoxicillin plus clavulanic acid, an irreversible inhibitor of β-lactamase) or trimethoprim-sulfamethoxazole is used for ambulatory therapy of less serious disease. Because of the problem of β-lactamase production, it is reasonable to use trimethoprim-sulfamethoxazole or Augmentin as initial therapy. Other measures, such as drainage of empyema fluid, arthrocentesis for joint infection, maintenance of a patent airway in epiglottitis, and supportive care for patients with meningitis, are of obvious but paramount importance.

PREVENTION. Attempts at preventing *H. influenzae* infection with a vaccine composed of PRP have not been successful in children less than 18 months of age—those most frequently affected by these infections. In the United States, *H. influenzae* type B polysaccharide vaccine is recommended for all children 24 to 59 months of age. The Advisory Committee on Immunization Practices also advises immunization of children 18 to 23 months of age considered at increased risk of disease (for example, children attending day-care centers). Adults at risk of invasive *H. influenzae* disease also should be considered for vaccination. Recently, rifampin has been recommended prophylactically for close contacts of individuals with *H. influenzae* infections. Dosages are similar to those used in meningococcal prophylaxis.

Pertussis (whooping cough)

Mark J. Ingerman *and* **Jerome Santoro**

DEFINITION. Whooping cough is an acute respiratory tract infection that is seen primarily in infants and young children. The illness is characterized by paroxysms of cough followed by prolonged inspiratory stridor.

ETIOLOGY. The genus *Bordetella* is made up of three species: *Bordetella pertussis, Bordetella parapertussis,* and *Bor-*

detella bronchiseptica. B. bronchiseptica causes infection in animals but rarely in humans. *B. pertussis* and *B. parapertussis* are minute, gram-negative coccobacilli that have complex growth requirements that are met by Bordet-Gengou culture medium. These organisms were at one time classified with *Haemophilus* species, but the *Bordetella* group has no strict requirement for X and V factors and is antigenically distinct. Primary isolates of *B. pertussis* do not grow on conventional media, are designated phase I or S organisms, and are virulent. With passage, organisms can be induced to grow on standard media and change through phases II, III, and IV or R. Each phase is less virulent and only killed phase I organisms can be used as immunizing agents. *B. parapertussis* occasionally causes disease in humans that is generally milder than that caused by *B. pertussis.*

EPIDEMIOLOGY. Pertussis is a disease of infants and young children with worldwide distribution. It is spread by droplet nuclei and has an attack rate of 70% to 90%. Among nonimmune groups, neither disease nor immunization produces lifelong protection and disease can be seen in adults. The incidence of pertussis, about 3000 cases a year in the United States, has fallen greatly because of several factors, such as improved living conditions and, most importantly, vaccination. The mortality also has dropped, probably as a result of better supportive care. Most deaths (about 70%) occur in individuals less than 1 year of age, and most of these are children less than 6 months of age.

PATHOLOGY AND PATHOGENESIS. Killed phase I organisms cause encephalomyelitis, lymphocytosis, histamine and serotonin sensitivity, increased susceptibility to anaphylaxis, and other effects when injected into animals. The significance of these properties is not clear in human carriers of the disease. *B. pertussis* attaches to the epithelium of the bronchi and bronchioles, where it multiplies but does not invade the lung tissue or blood. Local bronchial and peribronchial inflammation with inspissation of mucus and debris results in atelectasis, localized emphysema, and interstitial pneumonitis. These effects can be devastating in infants and children because of their small airways. Proposed mechanisms for the neurologic manifestations of pertussis are hypoxia from respiratory disease or the action of a bacterial neurotoxin.

CLINICAL MANIFESTATIONS. Illness begins after an incubation period of 7 to 10 days. Pertussis classically has been divided into three clinical phases: catarrhal, paroxysmal, and convalescent.

The catarrhal stage is characterized by nonspecific symptoms resembling a typical viral upper respiratory infection. Symptoms include malaise, anorexia, rhinorrhea and sneezing, conjunctivitis, and sometimes mild fever. During this stage the disease is highly contagious. Late in the catarrhal stage, a nonproductive cough appears and a lymphocytosis is first noted.

After 1 to 2 weeks the paroxysmal stage begins. At this time the illness is characterized by as many as 40 to 50 periods of severe coughing daily. During paroxysms there may be venous engorgement and even cyanosis. The paroxysm is terminated by air drawn in forcibly through the glottis—the whoop. The whoop often is followed by vomiting, which is said to aid in the removal of the thick, tenacious mucus. Between paroxysms the patient is quiet but apprehensive. Fever is absent but lymphocytic leukocytosis is present, with counts as high as 100,000 consisting almost totally of small, typical lymphocytes. When fever and polymorphonuclear leukocytosis are present, bacterial superinfection should be suspected.

The convalescent stage begins within 4 weeks, when the

frequency and severity of paroxysms decrease. Interestingly, patients experiencing respiratory tract infections several months after a bout of pertussis may again have symptoms similar to whooping cough.

The possible complications of pertussis are legion. Small children develop dehydration, malnutrition, and electrolyte and acid-base disturbances from vomiting and inability to eat or drink. In rare cases cerebral complications such as seizures and hemorrhage can result from anoxia or perhaps from elevated venous pressure. Epistaxis, petechiae, and scleral and conjunctival hemorrhages with periorbital edema are common. In the lung atelectasis and localized emphysema are frequently found; pneumothorax and pneumomediastinum are less commonly seen. Secondary bacterial otitis media occasionally occurs. The major causes of death in pertussis are bacterial superinfection of the lung and probably neurologic complications. Residual bronchiectasis is now less common, perhaps because of the availability of effective antimicrobial agents.

LABORATORY FINDINGS AND DIAGNOSIS. Unfortunately, because of the nonspecific findings, pertussis is very difficult to diagnose in the catarrhal stage, when it is most contagious and when the pending paroxysmal phase could possibly be modified. The differential diagnosis of whooping cough in the paroxysmal stage includes viral tracheobronchitis, *Mycoplasma pneumoniae* infection, and in infants, chlamydial pneumonia. A syndrome caused by adenovirus that is very similar to pertussis has been described. When present, the marked lymphocytosis previously described is helpful in differentiating these syndromes.

B. pertussis and *B. parapertussis* can be cultured by immediately plating material obtained by nasopharyngeal swab onto Bordet-Gengou medium containing penicillin. The yield is 80% to 90% during the catarrhal stage but 50% or less in the paroxysmal stage. Cough plates have been abandoned because the yield is too low. A fluorescent antibody test can detect *B. pertussis* in nasopharyngeal smears but has a very high false positive rate. The test is perhaps more helpful in rapidly identifying organisms already isolated.

In patients with negative cultures, the ELISA can be used to detect IgM, IgA, and IgG antibodies in serum. IgA antibodies can be detected in nasopharyngeal secretions by ELISA beginning in the second or third week of illness. This antibody is induced by infection, not vaccination.

MANAGEMENT. Treatment of pertussis with antimicrobial agents in the catarrhal stage can decrease the severity of and shorten the paroxysmal stage. However, initiation of therapy in the paroxysmal stage has no effect. Nevertheless, antimicrobial therapy is justified to prevent spread of infection. The drug of choice is erythromycin (50 mg/kg/day in children and 2 g/day in adults in four divided doses for 5 to 10 days). Corticosteroids equivalent to hydrocortisone (30 mg/kg/24 hours for 2 days) have been shown to shorten the duration and decrease the severity of the illness even when begun in the paroxysmal state. However, it probably is wise to reserve this therapy for severe cases. Hyperimmune human globulin is available but is not recommended routinely. Its use in severely ill infants and small children remains controversial.

Supportive therapy in the form of good nursing care, proper fluid and electrolyte balance, maintenance of adequate nutrition, and antimicrobial therapy of superinfection is of paramount importance, especially among the very young.

PREVENTION. Susceptible individuals who are exposed to pertussis should be vaccinated to prevent disease and treated with erythromycin to prevent infection and transmission. Before the pertussis vaccine became available, this infectious disease caused as many deaths in the United States as all other contagious diseases of children combined. The vaccine is composed of a chemical extract of bacterial cells. This vaccine is now mixed with tetanus and diphtheria toxoids for convenience and enhancement of antibody response. It is administered five times during the first 6 years of life with three doses being given at 2-month intervals beginning at 8 weeks of age.

The pertussis vaccine has proved to be 70% to 80% effective in preventing disease among intimately exposed children. Vaccine does not confer complete or prolonged immunity, and after 10 years most individuals are again susceptible to disease. Pertussis vaccine provokes local reactions in 50% of recipients. Side effects such as neurologic complications, including uncontrollable screaming fits, convulsions, and encephalopathy are rare sequelae. Since the risk of neurologic events after routine vaccination is very small, the Immunization Practices Advisory Committee continues to advocate immunization. In children with a history of seizures, pertussis vaccination should be deferred.

BIBLIOGRAPHY
Haemophilus influenzae infections

American Adademy of Pediatrics Committee on Infectious Diseases: Ampicillin-resistant strains of *Hemophilus influenzae* type B, Pediatrics 55:145, 1975.
Hirshmann JV and Everett ED: *Haemophilus influenzae* infections in adults: report of nine cases and a review of the literature, Medicine 58:80, 1979.
Todd JK and Bruhn FW: Severe *Haemophilus influenzae* infections, Am J Dis Child 129:607, 1975.

Pertussis

Bassili WR and Stewart GT: Epidemiological evaluation of immunization and other factors in the control of whooping cough, Lancet 1:471, 1976.
Olson LC: Pertussis, Medicine 54:427, 1975.

Donovanosis (granuloma inguinale)

Michael F. Rein

Donovanosis, also referred to as granuloma inguinale, is a sexually transmitted infection caused by *Calymmatobacterium granulomatis*, a gram-negative bacterium possibly related to *Klebsiella* spp. that can be cultured only with great difficulty. Fewer than 50 infections are reported annually in the United States, but the disease is prevalent in New Guinea, India, and parts of Australia, Africa, and South America. Infectivity is low, and prolonged or repeated contact may be necessary for transmission of the infection. About 50% of patients have symptoms within 4 weeks of infection, but incubation periods of 3 months have been reported. The initial lesion is a papule, which erodes to form a gradually enlarging ulcer, usually in the genital area. A typical lesion has a heaped-up edge and a base consisting of beefy granulation tissue that becomes exuberantly hypertrophic in about 20% of patients. Extensive destruction of involved sites may result if treatment is delayed. Lesions have occurred in the mouth following orogenital contact. Infection may spread by autoinoculation, via the lymphatics to form subcutaneous granulomas in the groin, or in rare cases via the bloodstream to bone or the liver. The organism multiplies within host macrophages. Biopsy shows an infiltrate with polymorphonuclear neutrophils and macrophages and the capillary proliferation typical of granulation tissue. Diagnosis is best made by crushing a small biopsy specimen between glass slides. Wright's stain reveals macrophages loaded with the organisms (Donovan's bodies) in about 80% of cases, but the usual H and E sections are positive less than 10% of the time. Oral treatment with tetracycline (500 mg four times a day) generally is successful, and gentamicin, chloramphenicol, or trimethoprim-sulfamethoxazole also has been used. Some studies have suggested an association between donovanosis and the subsequent development of genital carcinoma.

Chancroid

Michael F. Rein

Chancroid is a sexually transmitted infection caused by *Haemophilus ducreyi*. Localized outbreaks have occurred in North America, but the disease is much more prevalent in the Far East. Although the incubation period may range from 24 hours to 3 weeks, symptoms generally develop about 7 days after infection. Symptomatic infections are 10 times more common in men than in women. The initial lesion is a papule, which becomes pustular and then ulcerated and painful. About 70% of patients have a single ulcer at the time they seek medical attention, but multiple ulcerations are characteristic of untreated disease. These ulcers may vary considerably in size, which differentiates them from those of herpes genitalis, which usually are rather uniform. The ulcers are ragged with an undermined edge and a necrotic base. They have an erythematous border, but induration is unusual and should suggest a diagnosis of syphilis. Lesions may develop on the thighs by autoinoculation from lesions on the penis. Within 1 week following the appearance of skin lesions, 25% to 60% of patients develop tender inguinal adenopathy, usually unilateral, with periadenitis and some erythema of the overlying skin. If untreated, these nodes become fluctuant and may rupture. The disease usually is diagnosed clinically, but care should be taken to avoid confusion with herpes simplex genitalis infections or syphilis, which are many times more common in the United States and also are seen as multiple, painful, genital ulcerations. A smear from the undermined edge of a lesion may reveal chains of gram-negative streptobacilli but is negative in at least 30% of cases. The organism is cultured with difficulty from a lesion or an aspirate of the enlarged inguinal nodes. *H. ducreyi* has become resistant to several standard treatments in many parts of the world. Treatment should consist of erythromycin (500 mg orally four times a day for 7 days) or ceftriaxone (250 mg intramuscularly as a single dose).

BIBLIOGRAPHY
Donovanosis

Coovadia YM, Steinberg JL, and Kharsany A: Granuloma inguinale (donovanosis) of the oral cavity, S Afr Med J 68:815, 1985.
Sehgal VN and Shyam Prasad AL: Donovanosis: current concepts, Int J Dermatol 25:8, 1986.

Chancroid

Ronald AR: Chancroid: recent advances in treatment and control, Int J Dermatol 25:31, 1986.

Gram-negative bacillary bacteremia

Margaret Trexler-Hessen *and* Jerome A. Boscia

Bacteremia caused by gram-negative bacilli has been found with increasing frequency in the adult hospital population and accounts for many hospital-acquired (nosocomial) infections. It also is seen as a complication of community-acquired infection, for example, pyelonephritis. Bacteremia may be asymptomatic or may cause a syndrome of sepsis in which the patient appears toxic, generally with fever and rigors. Shock occurs in 20% to 40% of cases, with an associated mortality of 30% to 70%.

ETIOLOGY. In both nosocomial and outpatient settings, the genitourinary tract is the most common source of gram-negative bacillary (GNB) bacteremia (60% of patients). Common predisposing factors are urinary tract obstruction, instrumentation, surgery, and an indwelling urinary catheter. The female genital tract can be a source following delivery, abortion, or gynecologic surgery. In approximately 25% of cases of GNB bacteremia, the gastrointestinal tract is implicated as the source, usually in patients who have had some insult to bowel integrity or who are neutropenic. Common predisposing factors are surgery, bowel obstruction or infarction, and neoplasms. Acute intraabdominal infections such as diverticulitis, appendicitis, cholecystitis, and infection following penetrating abdominal wounds also are common clinical settings. In 5% of cases the skin appears to be the source of GNB bacteremia. Common predisposing factors are operative wound infections, indwelling vascular catheters, and extensive damage to the skin, as in burns or exfoliative dermatitis. The respiratory tract is not a common source of GNB bacteremia. However, in cases of pneumonia secondary to contaminated aerosols or in patients with infected tracheostomies, GNB bacteremia may occur. In about 10% of cases the source of bacteremia is unidentified.

Certain systemic diseases are associated with bacteremia. Patients with hematologic malignancies (leukemia, lymphoma, multiple myeloma) or agranulocytosis and patients receiving corticosteroids have altered host defense mechanisms, predisposing them to the development of GNB bacteremia. Patients with diabetes mellitus and severe liver disease also appear to have significant predisposition to GNB bacteremia.

The most common organisms responsible for GNB bacteremia belong to the family Enterobacteriaceae. This is expected because this group of organisms is an important constituent of the bowel flora and is the major cause of urinary tract infections. *Escherichia coli* accounts for about 40% of the infections. *Klebsiella*, *Enterobacter*, and *Proteus* spp. follow in importance. *Bacteroides fragilis*, a gram-negative anaerobic rod and a predominant organism in bowel flora, is becoming increasingly important as a cause of bacteremia. Bacteremia caused by *Pseudomonas aeruginosa* has increased because of increasing numbers of neutropenic patients. *P. aeruginosa* bacteremia occurs most frequently in the presence of neutropenia (fewer than 1000 mature polymorphonuclear leukocytes/mm^3), or denudation of the skin, as in burns or exfoliative dermatitis.

PATHOGENESIS OF SEPTIC SHOCK. The pathophysiology of shock resulting from GNB bacteremia is not completely understood. The basic phenomena seen in bacteremia and subsequent shock appear to be related to the toxic effects of endotoxin, a complex lipopolysaccharide that is part of the bacterial cell wall of gram-negative bacilli. However, gram-positive organisms and fungi that lack endotoxin also can produce the septic shock syndrome; therefore other mechanisms play a role in infections with these organisms. The shock syndrome associated with GNB sepsis classically is divided into two stages, "warm" and "cold" shock. Warm shock is characterized by normal or slightly low blood pressure, normal or high cardiac output, and peripheral arterial dilation resulting in warm but dry extremities. This phase is thought to be initiated by activation of factor XII (Hageman factor of the clotting cascade) by endotoxin, a component of the GNB cell wall. Activated Hageman factor in turn activates the coagulation, fibrinolytic, complement, and bradykinin systems. Activation of both the clotting and fibrinolytic cascades results in the uncoordinated coagulation and clot lysis that characterize the clinical syndrome of disseminated intravascular coagulation (DIC) with associated microangiopathy and tissue ischemia. Vasodilators, anaphylotoxins, and leukocyte chemotactic factors are released through the complement and bradykinin pathways, resulting in generalized tissue inflammation and capillary leakage. Leukocyte aggregation, capillary leakage, and DIC all contribute to the development of the adult respiratory distress syndrome (ARDS), which may complicate GNB sepsis.

Cold shock is characterized by a decrease in cardiac output with compensatory peripheral arterial constriction. Blood flow to the extremities, kidneys, brain, and other organs may be insufficient to maintain normal function, with resulting cool, clammy extremities, oliguria, and altered mental status. This phase occurs as a result of venous pooling and reduced venous blood return to the heart. As cardiac output and tissue blood flow are reduced, the tissues convert from aerobic to anaerobic metabolism and lactic acidosis occurs. Acidosis causes further depression of cardiac function. The contribution of an ill-defined "myocardial depressant factor" remains unproven.

DIAGNOSIS. GNB bacteremia is a clinical diagnosis that should be considered in febrile patients with a known predisposing condition.

Classically, the onset of bacteremia is manifested by a shaking chill preceding the fever spike. The temperature usually ranges from 101° to 105° F (37.2° to 40.5° C). Some patients, especially the elderly or debilitated, may not have fever. Patients receiving steroids, patients with renal failure, and those who are in severe shock may be hypothermic. Patients with the syndrome of sepsis generally are restless, apprehensive, disoriented, tachypneic, and tachycardic. When the initial manifestation is warm shock, progression to cold shock follows unless therapy is initiated. When shock progresses, increasing mental confusion, oliguria or anuria, and respiratory distress with cyanosis develop.

Laboratory abnormalities include leukopenia or leukocytosis with neutrophilia. Continuing leukopenia may be associated with overwhelming sepsis. Initially, arterial blood gases demonstrate a respiratory alkalosis associated with tachypnea and hyperventilation. Subsequently, metabolic acidosis and hypoxia occur. No roentgenographic changes in the chest are seen in initial stages of shock, but in the later stages a pattern typical of pulmonary edema (ARDS) may develop. In patients suspected of having GNB bacteremia, blood cultures (both aerobic and anaerobic) and other appropriate cultures (for example, urine) should be obtained.

Neutropenic patients with GNB bacteremia, particularly with *P. aeruginosa* infection, may develop the skin lesions of ecthyma gangrenosum. This is a tender vesicle that ulcerates and becomes necrotic. The pathogenesis is bacterial invasion of blood vessel walls with thrombosis. Gram stain of material from the lesions may reveal organisms, and culture of the material usually is positive.

MANAGEMENT. Monitoring the state of consciousness, blood pressure, and hourly urine output allows proper assessment of perfusion to vital organs. An alert sensorium, a stable blood pressure, and a urine output of 30 ml an hour indicate adequate perfusion. Measurements of central venous or pulmonary wedge pressures permit assessment of intravascular volume and cardiac performance. Arterial blood gases are necessary to evaluate the patient's respiratory and metabolic status. Determinations of serum creatinine measure renal function. Evaluation of possible coagulation abnormalities includes measurements of the platelet count, prothrombin time, partial thromboplastin time, fibrinogen level, and fibrin-split products.

The first priority in the treatment of septic shock is the restoration and expansion of the blood volume. This is accomplished by the rapid infusion of blood, normal saline, dextran, or any other volume expander to raise the blood pressure and increase tissue perfusion. Rapid volume expansion should be continued until the central venous pressure reaches 12 cm H_2O or the pulmonary wedge pressure rises to 18 mm Hg. If these pressures rise or are elevated from the start and hypotension persists, a pressor agent such as dopamine is indicated.

Administration of dopamine results in increases in cardiac output, blood pressure, and urine output. Infusion of dopamine is titrated upward until the desired hemodynamic and renal responses are obtained. It is recommended that low infusion rates (2 to 5 µg/kg/min intravenously) be used as initial therapy in patients with moderate hypotension and oliguria. In patients with more severe degrees of shock, it may be necessary to start at higher initial doses. Most patients, however, respond to rates less than 20 µg/kg min. Doses greater than 40 µg/kg/min produce vasoconstriction and are to be avoided if possible. Since dopamine and other sympathomimetic drugs do not exert their full effect in the presence of acidosis, hypoxia and acidosis must be corrected.

Specific empiric antibiotic therapy depends on evaluation for the most likely source of infection and etiologic microorganism. Often these can be determined by examining the patient and reviewing the initial laboratory studies. Traditionally, empiric antimicrobial therapy for GNB bacteremia has included an aminoglycoside such as gentamicin combined with a first-generation cephalosporin (for example, cefazolin). However, with the advent of extended-spectrum cell-wall-active antimicrobial agents such as the third-generation cephalosporins (cefotaxime), ureidopenicillins (piperacillin), monobactams (aztreonam) and carbapenems (imipenem), some authorities currently favor empiric treatment of GNB bacteremia with one of these agents alone or in combination with an aminoglycoside.

When an intraabdominal or pelvic source is likely, coverage for anaerobic gram-negative bacilli such as *B. fragilis* is necessary and the addition of metronidazole or clindamycin is recommended. In patients with significant neutropenia (fewer than 1000 mature polymorphonuclear leukocytes/mm³) or extensive burns, *P. aeruginosa* bacteremia should be suspected and an antipseudomonal penicillin such as piperacillin plus an aminoglycoside such as gentamicin should be used. Alternatively, ceftazidime, a third-generation cephalosporin with excellent activity against *P. aeruginosa,* may be used in place of the antipseudomonal penicillin.

Following identification and sensitivity studies of the pathogen, antibiotic coverage is appropriately tailored and continued for at least 10 to 14 days.

Although it seems logical that antiinflammatory agents such as steroids might be helpful in preventing many of the manifestations of septic shock, this issue remains controversial. Some studies in animals and humans have shown a beneficial effect from the use of steroids, but other, more recent studies have demonstrated decreased survival with the use of steroids. Currently, administration of steroids for GNB sepsis cannot be advocated.

Presumably, endogenous opiates (endorphins) are released during the stress of bacteremia and may contribute to hypotension. Recently naloxone, an opiate antagonist, has been shown to increase systolic blood pressure transiently in animal models of sepsis and in some human trials. However, not all studies are confirmatory, and the value of naloxone in treating septic shock remains unproven.

Leukocyte transfusions may be helpful in neutropenic patients with documented bacteremia not responding to antibiotic therapy. However, severe pulmonary side effects may be encountered when amphotericin B is given concurrently to these patients.

A recent study produced encouraging results in the adjunctive use of antiserum against certain strains of *E. coli* in the treatment of GNB bacteremia; however, this approach remains experimental.

PROGNOSIS. The prognosis is related to the infecting organism (for example, the mortality is higher with *P. aeruginosa* than with *E. coli*), whether shock develops, and the underlying disease. With rapidly fatal diseases such as acute leukemia the mortality is much higher than with nonfatal diseases such as bacteremia after prostatectomy.

PREVENTION. In view of the high mortality associated with GNB bacteremia, special consideration should be given to its prevention. Handwashing remains the most important measure in preventing widespread colonization of patients with nosocomial pathogens. Other potential causes of infection are the urinary catheter, the intravenous catheter, and contaminated respiratory equipment. Indwelling urinary catheters should be avoided if possible, and if they are necessary, sterile drainage systems should be used. Intravascular catheters also should be avoided; if they are essential, they should be handled aseptically and removed as soon as possible. Respiratory equipment should be cleaned daily and nebulization reservoirs sterilized each day.

In the past several years much interest has been focused on antibiotic prophylaxis of patients at risk of GNB bacteremia, such as patients with neutropenia. However, this approach has not been routinely adopted, because studies have demonstrated conflicting results with regard to efficacy, and adverse reactions to the antibiotics have been a concern.

BIBLIOGRAPHY

Berringer R and Harwood-Nuss A: Septic shock, J Emerg Med 3:475, 1985 and 4:49, 1986.

Jacobs ER and Bone RC: Clinical indicators in sepsis and septic adult respiratory distress syndrome, Med Clin North Am 70:921, 1986.

Karakusis PH: Considerations in the therapy of septic shock, Med Clin North Am 70:933, 1986.

Parker MM and Parrillo JE: Septic shock: hemodynamics and pathogenesis, JAMA 250:3324, 1983.

Young LS: Gram-negative sepsis. In Mandell GL, Douglas RG, and Bennett JE, editors: Principles and practice of infectious diseases, New York, 1985, John Wiley & Sons, Inc.

Ziegler EJ and others: Treatment of gram-negative bacteremia and shock with human antiserum to a mutant *Escherichia coli*, N Engl J Med 307:1225, 1982.

Plague

Elias Abrutyn

DEFINITION. The plague bacillus causes a zoonosis that is occasionally transmitted to humans. In humans, bubonic plague is seen most commonly, but bacteremia, meningitis, and pneumonia also occur.

ETIOLOGY. *Yersinia pestis,* formerly *Pasteurella pestis,* is a pleomorphic, aerobic, nonmotile, nonsporeforming gram-negative rod that grows well but slowly on most culture media. The characteristic bipolar or safety-pin appearance is best demonstrated with Wayson's or Giemsa stain. Virulence appears partially related to an endotoxin and a capsular antigen that inhibits phagocytosis. Other factors important to virulence or pathogenesis have been described. Some of these are plasmid-mediated.

EPIDEMIOLOGY. Infected wild rodents and mammals (sylvatic plague) forms a large, usually inapparent natural reservoir

of infection. Transmission is maintained primarily by fleas, and spread of infected fleas to the domestic rat (urban or rat plague) establishes the setting for transmission to humans and epidemics. Humans also may acquire disease by direct contact with contaminated animal tissues. Nonreservoir hosts such as dogs, cats, and other carnivores have been implicated as the source for human infection. Asymptomatic human infection has been described, but its role in transmission is unknown.

In the United States animal plague is prevalent in the 15 Western States, and human plague is reported most frequently in Arizona, Colorado, New Mexico, California, and Oregon. During the summer, cases usually are related to fleas, whereas a seasonal pattern related to hunting and direct contact is less apparent, since these activities are undertaken throughout the year. Rat plague has been virtually eliminated in the United States. In recent years an average of 19 cases per year have been reported; 40 cases were identified in 1983.

PATHOGENESIS AND PATHOLOGY. During feeding, fleas whose foregut has been blocked by a mass of organisms regurgitate thousands of bacteria into the host. The bacilli travel via the lymphatics to the regional lymph nodes, where they multiply. The nodes become hyperplastic, necrotic, and contain masses of bacteria; edema with or without hemorrhage surrounds the involved nodes. Although polymorphonuclear leukocytes ingest and kill the bacteria, the organisms survive in monocytes and elaborate a capsule that enables them to resist further phagocytosis. Bacteremia occurs commonly and can result in metastatic infection, including involvement of the meninges and lungs.

CLINICAL MANIFESTATIONS. The incubation period for bubonic plague is 2 to 6 days. Fever, constitutional symptoms, and excruciatingly painful lymphadenopathy (bubo) are characteristic. In descending order of frequency, the nodes involved are the inguinal-femoral, axillary, cervical, and epitrochlear; multiple areas of nodal involvement occasionally occur. In rare cases a pustule or papule develops at the flea bite site. Septicemic plague differs from bubonic plague in that nodal involvement is inapparent. Bacteremia, which can complicate either form, may result in meningitis or pneumonia (secondary plague pneumonia). The latter complication has special public health significance, because such infected people may be the source for airborne spread of pneumonia to contacts (primary plague pneumonia), resulting in a highly contagious, fulminant, often fatal disease. Untreated patients may develop shock, convulsions, and DIC with bleeding or necrosis of peripheral tissues. In rare cases plague has been associated with acute pharyngitis.

DIAGNOSIS. The disease must be differentiated from other causes of regional lymphadenitis, and a diagnosis is made most readily in people who have had known contact with infected animals or their ectoparasites. Fluid from buboes, blood, and other body fluids should be stained, examined microscopically, and cultured. Material stained using the fluorescent antibody technique may provide a rapid presumptive diagnosis to be verified by culture and other means. Specific antibody may be detected in convalescent-phase serum, but serologic tests are not useful for diagnosis during the acute phase.

MANAGEMENT. Streptomycin (30 mg/kg/day in two divided doses for 7 to 10 days in adults) is preferred. Tetracycline (30 to 50 mg/kg/day in four divided doses) also is effective. Chloramphenicol is active and may be used to treat meningitis and pregnant women. Gentamicin is used by some. Trimethoprim-sulfamethoxazole, kanamycin, and sulfonamides have been reported effective, but experience with these is limited.

PROGNOSIS. When treated, bubonic plague has an excellent prognosis. The other forms respond well if recognized and treated early, but positive blood cultures or bacilli on blood smears are bad prognostic signs.

PREVENTION. Control measures include education of people in endemic areas, surveillance for plague activity in reservoir animals or carnivores, rat control, and immunization of people at high risk of exposure. Chemoprophylaxis may be indicated for contacts of patients with plague pneumonia and for household contacts of cases acquired from fleas; this consists of tetracycline (1 g/day), trimethoprim-sulfamethoxazole, or a sulfonamide for 5 to 7 days. Quarantine may be necessary, and strict isolation procedures are mandatory for hospitalized patients for the first 48 hours of chemotherapy.

BIBLIOGRAPHY

Butler T: Plague and other *Yersinia* infections. In Grunough WE and Merigan TC, editors: Current topics infectious disease, New York, 1983, Plenum Publishing Corp.

Centers for Disease Control. Plague in the United States, 1983 by AM Barnes and JD Poland. 1984: 33 (No. 1SS) 15SS-21SS.

Ell SR: Immunity as a factor in the epidemiology of medieval plague, Rev Infect Dis 6:866, 1984.

Ganem DE: Plasmids and pestilence—biological and clinical aspects of bubonic plague—medical staff conference, University of California, San Francisco, West J Med 144:447, 1986.

Hull HF, Montes JM, and Mann JM: Septicemic plague in New Mexico, J Infect Dis 155:113, 1987.

Palmer DL: Plague and other *Yersinia* infections. In Braunwald E and others, editors: Harrison's principles of internal medicine, ed 11, New York, 1987, McGraw-Hill, Inc.

Poland JD: Plague. In Hoeprich PD, editor: Infectious diseases, ed 3, Hagerstown, Maryland, 1983, Harper & Row Publishers, Inc.

Reed WP and others: Bubonic plague in the Southwestern United States: a review of recent experience, Medicine 49:465, 1970.

Welty TK and others: Nineteen cases of plague in Arizona—a spectrum including ecthyma gangrenosum due to plague and plague in pregnancy, West J Med 142:641, 1985.

Welty TK: Plague, Am Fam Physician 33:159, 1986.

Tularemia

Oksana M. Korzeniowski

DEFINITION. Tularemia is a zoonotic bacterial infection acquired by humans from mammals or arthropods. The various portals of entry determine the clinical variant of the disease.

ETIOLOGY. *Francisella tularensis* is a nonmotile, pleomorphic gram-negative rod. It does not grow on routine culture media, but aerobic cultivation on agar that contains cystine yields colonies in 2 to 4 days. Two antigenically identical variants differing in a few biochemical reactions have been identified. Type A strains cause 5% to 7% mortality among untreated cases and commonly are associated with rabbits and tick vectors. Type B strains are less virulent and are associated primarily with rodents.

EPIDEMIOLOGY. Tularemia occurs in the Northern Hemisphere: America, Europe, and Asia. Type B strains occur worldwide, but type A strains are found only in North America. Many species of wild and domestic mammals, birds, amphibians, and arthropods harbor the organism. In the United States the main reservoirs are rabbits, hares, and ticks found in Arkansas, Illinois, Tennessee, Missouri, Texas, and Virginia. A bimodal distribution of cases occurs, with tick-associated disease peaking in the summer and rabbit-associated disease peaking in the winter. Humans are highly susceptible to infection and acquire the disease through skin contact with tissues or body fluids of infected animals, arthropod bites, inhalation of infectious aerosols, or ingestion of contaminated water or inadequately cooked meat of infected animals. Ten to 50 bacilli

inhaled or inoculated into minimally abraded skin can produce disease, but 100 million organisms are needed to produce disease following oral challenge.

PATHOGENESIS. An ulcerated lesion develops at the site of bacterial inoculation in 60% to 75% of patients. Bacteremia results in entrapment of the organism within macrophages of the reticuloendothelial system, where it may survive for prolonged periods. The early lesions in affected organs (lymph nodes, liver, spleen, lung) demonstrate focal necrosis surrounded by polymorphonuclear leukocytes and macrophages. Later, granulomas with central caseation or small local abscesses can be found.

CLINICAL MANIFESTATIONS. The incubation period is 2 to 10 days. Constitutional symptoms of fever, malaise, and headache, frequently preceded by rigor, are nonspecific. Splenomegaly, meningitis, pericarditis, and hepatomegaly may be present. A skin rash may occur in up to 20% of cases, usually after the onset of other symptoms. Lesions are quite variable and may include erythema nodosum.

Ulceroglandular tularemia acquired by skin inoculation is the most common variant, occurring in 60% to 85% of reported cases. A reddish papule that ulcerates is usually located on the fingers, hands, lower extremities, or perineal region. Painful regional lymph node enlargement progresses to fluctuation. Early incision of fluctuant nodes produces bacteremia and toxemia. Pneumonic tularemia, found in 20% to 30% of cases, can result from inhalation or from hematogenous spread of organisms. Laboratory accidents are the most common cause of primary pulmonary involvement. Symptoms include cough, which may be productive of mucoid or bloody sputum, substernal tightness, pleuritic chest pain, and respiratory distress. Physical findings of consolidation are scant, but pleural effusions are common. Roentgenographs demonstrate patchy, ill-defined infiltrates and hilar node enlargement. Typhoidal tularemia, occurring in 5% to 15% of patients, results from ingestion of organisms or from intradermal or respiratory challenge and may resemble typhoid fever; abdominal pain, weight loss, prostration, and fever are predominant symptoms; lymph node enlargement is uncommon. Mortality is two to three times higher than in other forms of tularemia. Oropharyngeal tularemia occurs after ingestion of inadequately cooked meat or contaminated water. Clinical features include exudative or membranous pharyngitis with cervical adenitis.

Oculoglandular tularemia, found in less than 1% of patients, is a unilateral, painful purulent conjunctivitis with ulceration of the conjunctivae or cornea; it occurs after contamination of the eye with infected animal or tick fluids. Preauricular or cervical lymph nodes are enlarged. Loss of vision may occur in untreated cases.

DIAGNOSIS. Gram stains of sputum or exudates frequently do not demonstrate presence of the organism. Cultivation of the bacillus usually is not attempted in hospital laboratories because of the hazard of aerosolization. Diagnosis most frequently is made serologically. A rise in agglutins may be detected 8 to 10 days after the onset of illness. An intradermal test of the delayed sensitivity type that uses a purified killed suspension of *F. tularensis* is highly specific and becomes positive in the first week of illness; however, the antigen is not commercially available.

COURSE. Untreated tularemia may produce significant prolonged morbidity and a mortality of 5% to 30%. Antimicrobial therapy results in prompt defervescence and constitutional improvement. Lifelong immunity usually develops, although a few reinfections have been documented.

MANAGEMENT. Streptomycin (15 to 20 mg/kg/day for 7

to 10 days) is the preferred antimicrobial agent for the treatment of tularemia. Gentamicin (5 mg/kg/day) appears to be an acceptable alternative. Chloramphenicol and tetracycline are effective in producing a clinical response, but they may fail to eradicate the organism, and relapse may occur.

PREVENTION. The risks of acquiring tularemia may be minimized by wearing gloves when processing potentially infected animals, by thoroughly cooking suspected meat, and by avoiding tick infestation. A vaccine prepared from an attenuated strain of *F. tularensis* provides partial protection and is available for laboratory workers and others who may be frequently exposed to infected animals.

BIBLIOGRAPHY

Evans ME and others: Tularemia: a 30 year experience with 88 cases, Medicine 64:251, 1985.
Francis E: Tularemia, landmark article, JAMA 250:3216, 1983.
Jacobs RF and others: Tularemia in adults and children: a changing presentation, Pediatrics 70:818, 1975.
Miller RP and Bates JH: Pleuropulmonary tularemia: a review of 29 patients, Am Rev Respir Dis 99:31, 1967.
Pullen RL and Stuart BM: Tularemia: analysis of 225 cases, JAMA 129:495, 1945.

Brucellosis

Mark J. Ingerman *and* **Jerome Santoro**

DEFINITION. Brucellosis is an infectious disease characterized by fever, malaise, and weight loss that is caused by bacteria of the genus *Brucella*. It is acquired by humans from infected animals through either occupational or food contact.

ETIOLOGY. The brucellae are small, nonmotile, nonspore-forming, aerobic gram-negative bacilli. Three of the six recognized species—*Brucella abortus* (cattle), *Brucella suis* (hogs), and *Brucella melitensis* (goats)—are responsible for the majority of human infections. *Brucella canis* (dogs) occasionally has caused illness in humans. Human infection occurs through contact of infected animal tissues with breaks in the skin or less commonly via conjunctival contact and inhalation. Infection from ingestion of contaminated milk, cheese, or meat is now less frequent because of pasteurization and refrigeration. *B. abortus* strain 19, an attenuated strain used to vaccinate animals, causes infections among veterinarians.

EPIDEMIOLOGY. Brucellosis in the United States is chiefly an occupational disease of abattoir workers, livestock raisers, farmers, and veterinarians. About 200 to 300 cases are reported each year. *B. melitensis* is the most common cause of disease worldwide, but in the United States *B. suis* and *B. abortus* are isolated most frequently. Most cases are seen in recent slaughterhouse employees and younger veterinarians, which implies that immunity is acquired through long-term exposure. Studies have confirmed the existence of brucella antibodies in chronically exposed individuals. Interestingly, most of these have no history of clinical illness, illustrating that asymptomatic infection is more common than overt disease.

PATHOGENESIS. After invasion of epithelial cells of the oropharynx or skin, brucellae are taken up by cells in the reticuloendothelial system (lymph nodes, liver, spleen, bone marrow). At this time the infection presumably can be controlled by the killing of bacteria by macrophages. Alternatively, organisms may multiply intracellularly; in response the host forms epithelioid granulomas. Eventually bacteria escape from their intracellular habitat and enter the bloodstream. If this process is allowed to continue, infection can occur in virtually any organ in the body, including bones, joints, lungs, the genitourinary tract, and the cardiovascular system. Granulomas eventually coalesce and may suppurate in any organ or tissue

affected. *B. suis* and *B. melitensis* tend to be more virulent and cause more severe infection than *B. abortus;* strain 19 disease tends to be quite mild.

CLINICAL MANIFESTATIONS AND COURSE. After an incubation period of 1 to 3 weeks the illness begins either insidiously or, less commonly, acutely (chills, fever, prostration). The signs and symptoms of brucellosis for the most part are nonspecific. Often such diseases as influenza, typhoid fever, infectious mononucleosis, endocarditis, and nonspecific viral illnesses are suspected until a history of animal exposure is elicited. Most patients typically have fever, sweating, weakness, and malaise, and more than 50% have anorexia, weight loss, and headache. The physical examination usually is not helpful. Findings such as lymphadenopathy, hepatosplenomegaly, and orchitis are seen in severe and often long-standing forms of the disease.

The complications of brucellosis are many. Infection may develop in various tissues and organ systems, such as bones and joints (especially the vertebrae), the genitourinary system (orchitis, epididymitis, cystitis, pyelitis), lungs, pleural spaces, heart valves, and the gallbladder. Abscesses can be found in liver, spleen, kidneys, and other areas. Sometimes there are nervous system and ophthalmic manifestations that cannot always be explained by invasion of the organism, such as aseptic meningitis, encephalitis, retinitis, optic neuritis, keratitis, and uveitis. Enlargement of the spleen and perhaps chronic infection involving the bone marrow may result in pancytopenia. In short, brucellosis can resemble other chronic granulomatous infections caused by such organisms as mycobacteria and various fungi.

In the preantibiotic era most patients attained permanent remission within 3 to 6 months after the initial symptoms. A small percentage of patients may relapse even with therapy. Chronic brucellosis is defined as ill health for more than 1 year following onset of disease. There is no doubt that a minority of patients can develop bacteriologically proven disease that lasts for years. However, many patients with nonspecific neuropsychiatric complaints have a diagnosis of chronic brucellosis made on the basis of meager evidence, such as a skin test or misinterpreted agglutinin test (see next section) or may actually have reinfection.

Most individuals, asymptomatic or symptomatic, who acquire brucellosis probably are at least partially protected from further infection, but reinfections surely occur. Veterinarians previously exposed to brucella organisms sometimes develop an acute local inflammatory response accompanied by high fever and malaise in response to skin contact with infected material or vaccine; the latter quickly responds to corticosteroids.

DIAGNOSIS AND LABORATORY FINDINGS. Routine laboratory studies, including white blood cell count, erythrocyte sedimentation rate, and urinalysis, are not helpful in making a precise diagnosis of brucellosis. The diagnosis is best secured by the isolation of the organism. Blood cultures, which may take up to 3 weeks of incubation for growth, are positive early in the illness in more than 50% of cases. Later, cultures of lymph nodes, liver, and especially bone marrow may be more fruitful than blood cultures. However, most cases of brucellosis in the United States are not diagnosed by isolation of the organism but by the *Brucella agglutination test,* which measures both IgG and IgM antibodies. Early in primary disease, from weeks 1 to 3, IgM antibody is detected, and later, both IgG and IgM are found. Thus the demonstration of a fourfold or greater rise in agglutinin titer is good evidence for brucellosis, provided infectious diseases caused by agents with cross-reacting antibodies are not being considered, such as *Vibrio* species, *Yersinia* species, and *Francisella tularensis*. In addition, when high titers of antibody circulate, blocking antibodies may be formed and titers may be falsely negative. This problem, called "prozone," can be ruled out if all tests are carried out to high dilution, greater than or equal to 1:1280. As infection resolves, IgG antibody disappears, but IgM may continue to circulate. With persistent, relapsing, or new infection IgG titers remain elevated or again rise. Therefore a simple positive agglutinin test may not be accurate for diagnosis in the latter situations because of possible persistence of IgM antibody. This problem can be circumvented by measuring IgG antibody alone, after mercaptoethanol precipitation of IgM. Titers of 1:160 or greater are said to make active or ongoing disease likely. Conversely, a "negative" test in a patient with prolonged symptoms makes the possibility of active brucellosis remote.

The *Brucella* skin test has no diagnostic worth and should not be used because of interference with serologic studies.

MANAGEMENT. The course of brucellosis is shortened and complications are prevented by antimicrobial therapy. Tetracycline (500 mg orally four times daily for at least 3 weeks in adults) is the best single agent and has the lowest relapse rate. The addition of streptomycin (500 mg intramuscularly every 12 hours for the first 2 weeks) further reduces the risk of relapse. Patients with severe disease usually should receive both drugs. Most relapses occur within 3 months of terminating therapy. For patients who are extremely debilitated with severe anorexia, adrenocorticosteroids such as prednisone (40 to 60 mg/day for 72 hours) can be used.

PREVENTION. The most important aspect of prevention of brucellosis is the ongoing surveillance, prevention (vaccine), and elimination of the disease in domestic animals. No vaccine for humans is available in the United States. Individuals at risk should carefully cover lacerated skin and wear gloves, wear protective goggles to avoid splashes, and avoid unpasteurized milk.

BIBLIOGRAPHY

Buchanan TM and others: Brucellosis in the United States, 1960-1972: an abattoir-associated disease, Medicine 53:403, 1974.

Fox M and Kaufman AF: Brucellosis in the United States, 1965-1974, J Infect Dis 136:312, 1977.

48 · DISEASES CAUSED BY GRAM-POSITIVE BACILLI

Anthrax

Elias Abrutyn

DEFINITION. Anthrax is a disease of animals occasionally transmitted to humans; it occurs as a cutaneous, pulmonary, or gastrointestinal illness. Bacteremia and meningitis may complicate any form.

ETIOLOGY. *Bacillus anthracis* is a large, gram-positive, aerobic, nonmotile, sporeforming organism. In clinical specimens the organism occurs singly or in chains of two or three square-ended bacilli. The organism is surrounded by a capsule (poly D-glutamic acid) that has antiphagocytic properties. A toxin with three elements—protective antigen, lethal factor, and edema factor—is produced. Both virulence factors—capsule formation and toxin production—appear plasmid-mediated.

EPIDEMIOLOGY. In the United States anthrax occurs primarily after industrial exposure to imported contaminated animal products, such as hides, goat hair, wool, and bone, and to a lesser extent after agricultural exposure to diseased animals, such as horses and cattle. Over the last two decades up to seven cases have been reported annually.

PATHOLOGY AND PATHOGENESIS. Cutaneous and gastrointestinal anthrax follow dermal inoculation or ingestion of spores, respectively. In inhalation anthrax spores are deposited in the lung and are transported to the mediastinal lymph nodes, where they germinate and multiply. Histologically, edema, necrosis, hemorrhage, and inflammatory cells are seen.

CLINICAL MANIFESTATIONS. Cutaneous anthrax (malignant pustule), the most common form, frequently involves exposed areas, particularly the arms or head and neck. The lesion begins as a papule that becomes vesicular and then ulcerates. Eventually, the characteristic black eschar is formed. Nonpitting edema that surrounds the lesion may be quite prominent. Pain is rare, but pruritus occurs. Constitutional symptoms are infrequent. Pharyngeal anthrax has been reported but is exceedingly rare.

In inhalation anthrax (wool-sorter's disease), an initial stage resembling mild respiratory illness is followed by hemorrhagic mediastinitis and respiratory distress. Disseminated disease, including hemorrhagic meningitis, also may occur. Gastrointestinal anthrax is characterized by anorexia, nausea, vomiting, acute abdominal pain, bloody diarrhea, toxemia, and shock.

DIAGNOSIS. Anthrax is most readily diagnosed in humans with occupational exposure to infected animals or their products. Gram smears and cultures of fluid from skin and other body fluids usually are positive. Serologic tests are useful for confirmation but not in the diagnosis of acute disease.

PROGNOSIS. Cutaneous anthrax has an excellent prognosis, but inhalation and gastrointestinal forms of the disease usually are fatal.

MANAGEMENT. For cutaneous anthrax, parenteral penicillin (procaine penicillin, 600,000 units every 12 hours, or penicillin G, 2 million units every 6 hours) may be given until the edema subsides. Oral penicillin then may be given for a total of 7 to 10 days. Inhalation and gastrointestinal anthrax require high-dose intravenous penicillin (18 to 24 million units daily). Tetracycline, erythromycin, and chloramphenicol are effective alternatives.

PREVENTION. Control depends on proper handling of infected animals and their products. Vaccination is recommended for those with a high risk of exposure.

BIBLIOGRAPHY

Brachman P: Anthrax. In Evans AS and Feldman HA, editors: Bacterial infections of humans: epidemiology and control, New York, 1982, Plenum Publishing Corp.

Doyle RJ, Keller KF, and Ezzell JW: Bacillus. In Lennette EH and others, editors: Manual of clinical microbiology, ed 4, Washington, DC, 1985, American Society for Microbiology.

Gold H: Treatment of anthrax, Fed Proc 67:1563, 1967.

Kaye D and Petersdorf RG: Anthrax. In Braunwald E and others, editors: Harrison's principles of internal medicine, ed 11, New York, 1987, McGraw-Hill, Inc.

Knudson GB: Treatment of anthrax in man: history and current concepts, Milit Med 151:71, 1986.

Nalin DR and others: Survival of a patient with gastrointestinal anthrax, Am J Med 62:130, 1977.

Plotkin SA and others: An epidemic of inhalation anthrax: the first in the twentieth century, Am J Med 29:992, 1960.

Listeriosis

Jaime Carrizosa

Listeriosis is an infectious disease caused by *Listeria monocytogenes*, a gram-positive, nonsporeforming, aerobic bacillus.

The organism, found worldwide, causes infection in humans and domestic animals. The infection may be acquired by direct contact, inhalation, or ingestion. Transmission from pregnant women to their offspring also occurs.

Listeriosis is primarily a disease of infants, immunocompromised hosts, and the elderly. The disease recently has been reported with increasing frequency in healthy individuals.

Several clinical pictures are associated with the disease. Meningitis, the most common clinical presentation, appears abruptly or may have an insidious course. Its clinical manifestations include headache, fever, nausea, vomiting, and nuchal rigidity. Cranial nerve involvement and other focal findings, as well as a diffuse encephalitic syndrome, also may be seen. The cerebrospinal fluid shows a cellular response that initially is mainly granulocytes but later can become predominantly mononuclear cells. The protein is high, and the sugar is low.

In the neonate the disease ranges from meningitis to a disseminated infection with a papular skin rash, hepatosplenomegaly, respiratory distress syndrome, and circulatory collapse. Diffuse organ involvement characterized by development of microabscesses and granulomatous formation resembling miliary tuberculosis may be found. Disseminated listeriosis has also been seen in children and adults, particularly in patients with cancer or debilitating diseases or in those receiving steroids or immunosuppressive agents.

Other clinical presentations include pharyngitis associated with diffuse lymphadenopathy, endocarditis, and a purulent conjunctivitis also associated with lymphadenopathy.

The diagnosis of listeriosis is based on the isolation and identification of the organism from cultures. Since the isolation of a gram-positive bacillus usually receives the label of a diphtheroid, special measures should be taken to provide appropriate identification. Serologic tests to detect agglutinins have low specificity and are not diagnostic. Leukocytosis with neutrophilia is common in all acute forms of the disease; monocytosis is uncommon.

L. monocytogenes is sensitive to many antibiotics in vitro, including penicillin, erythromycin, tetracyclines, chloramphenicol, and sulfonamides. The drug of choice for the treatment of meningitis, endocarditis, or disseminated disease is intravenous penicillin G or ampicillin. Penicillin G (20 million units intravenously in adults daily and 200,000 units/kg/day in children in divided doses every 4 hours) is recommended. In severe disseminated disease the addition of an aminoglycoside has been suggested because of the synergistic activity of this combination. Pharyngitis or conjunctivitis can be treated with oral erythromycin (500 mg every 6 hours or 30 mg/kg/day in four divided doses for 2 weeks).

The prognosis of appropriately treated *Listeria* infections is good. However, meningitis may be associated with residual damage or with normal pressure hydrocephalus that may require decompression. Severe cases of disseminated listeriosis carry a significant mortality.

Erysipeloid

Jaime Carrizosa

Erysipeloid is an infection caused by a gram-positive, non-sporeforming aerobic bacillus, *Erysipelothrix rhusiopathiae*. The infection usually is acquired by contact through a break in the skin and usually is restricted to individuals who handle dead animals or animal products. It has a worldwide distribution.

The clinical manifestations of the disease are a severely edematous but relatively nontender violaceous lesion of the hand or fingers resembling severe cellulitis; the lesion is not accompanied by suppurative lymphangitis or satellite adenopathy. It rarely extends above the wrist. The adjacent joints may be stiff and moderately painful. The area of involvement has a slow progression, primarily in a proximal direction. The disease heals spontaneously in about 3 to 4 weeks, but relapses are frequent. Systemic symptoms and signs such as fever are uncommon.

The infection occasionally progresses to a generalized form characterized by polyarthritis and additional skin lesions with erythema, swelling, and pruritus. The most serious form of the disease is *Erysipelothrix* endocarditis. The organism affects normal as well as previously damaged valves. Most patients are young men with a typical occupational history and classical manifestations of endocarditis.

The diagnosis of erysipeloid is made on the basis of the clinical picture and the isolation of the organism from a skin biopsy at the margin of the lesion, body fluids, or blood cultures.

The organism is susceptible to many antibiotics, such as penicillin, tetracycline, erythromycin, clindamycin, cephalosporins, and chloramphenicol. The drug of choice is benzathine penicillin G in a single intramuscular dose of 1.2 million units. Systemic infection is treated with 20 million units of penicillin G intravenously each day for 4 to 6 weeks.

BIBLIOGRAPHY
Listeriosis

Nieman RE and Lorber B: Listeriosis in adults. A changing pattern. Report of eight cases and review of the literature 1968-1978, Rev Infect Dis 2:207, 1980.

Erysipeloid

Borchardt KA: *Erysipelothrix rhusiopathiae* endocarditis, West J Med 127:149, 1977.
Nelson E: Five hundred cases of erysipeloid, Rocky Mt Med J 52:40, 1955.

Actinomycosis

John E. Bennett

Actinomycosis is the name of a clinical syndrome caused by a closely related group of organisms that are all anaerobic or microaerophilic branching higher bacteria. *Actinomyces israelii* is the most common microbe. All the etiologic agents are normal inhabitants of the human mouth and gastrointestinal tract. The microbes grow in tissue as tightly packed clusters called sulfur granules. These pale yellow, firm granules (a few millimeters in diameter) are found in the pus of abscesses or draining sinuses caused by the infection. Resected tonsils sometimes show a sulfur granule in a tonsillar crypt that does not cause disease. Illness comes when the microbe penetrates deeper tissue. Infection usually begins in the cervicofacial, thoracic, or ileocecal area. The portal of entry for cervicofacial infection may be dental caries, dental abscesses, tooth extraction, or penetrating trauma. An indolent indurated mass forms in the submandibular area, cheek, or anterior cervical triangle. Tenderness may be only slight; fever typically is absent. Draining sinuses intermittently discharge pus.

Pulmonary actinomycosis presumably results from aspiration of normal oral flora. A chronic pneumonia results and tends to extend to contiguous structures, such as the chest wall and thoracic spine. Abdominal actinomycosis most often originates in the appendix. Draining sinuses may extend outside the abdominal wall. Pelvic actinomycosis may result from long-term use of an intrauterine contraceptive device. Hematogenous dissemination can result from any site, with resulting abscesses in liver, brain, bone, or other organs.

Diagnosis of actinomycosis depends heavily on the demonstration of sulfur granules in pus. Granules may be found by examining the dressing covering a wound or by close inspection of pus in aspirates or biopsied tissue. Suspected sulfur granules should be Gram stained to demonstrate the branching, gram-positive hyphae. Washing the granules in sterile saline before culture may diminish the number of associated bacteria in the pus. Reliance on histologic section to demonstrate sulfur granules is unwise because the granules are present only in scattered areas. Culture of *A. israelii* from the mouth, stool, or sputum is of no diagnostic value.

Antibiotic therapy of actinomycosis often must be prolonged for 6 to 12 months to prevent relapse. Milder cases may be treated with tetracycline (2 g/day), oral penicillin V (3 to 4 g/day), or erythromycin (1 to 2 g/day). More severe cases may require initial therapy with intravenous penicillin (20 million units each day).

Nocardiosis

John E. Bennett

Nocardia are aerobic, branching, higher bacteria that normally live in soil. When introduced into subcutaneous tissue by minor trauma, they grow in pus as grains, causing mycetoma (see Chapter 54). When no grains are formed, the infection is called nocardiosis. Nocardiosis usually begins as pneumonia but has a marked tendency to spread hematogenously to the brain and other organs. Therapy with adrenal corticosteroids, the presence of Cushing's disease, and hematologic malignancies predispose to nocardiosis. Diagnosis is suspected by the demonstration of gram-positive, weakly acid-fast, branching bacteria in pus or sputum. Confirmation of the diagnosis is by culture.

Infection may be subacute or chronic, but fatal progression occurs in the absence of appropriate therapy. The therapy of choice usually is trimethoprim (10 to 20 mg/kg/day) in combination with sulfamethoxazole (50 to 100 mg/kg/day). Sulfonamides also can be used alone or in combination with ampicillin. Minocycline has been used successfully in a few patients who are allergic to sulfonamides.

BIBLIOGRAPHY
Actinomycosis

Bennhoff DF: Actinomycosis: diagnostic and therapeutic considerations and a review of 32 cases, Laryngoscope 94:1198, 1984.

Nocardiosis

Smego RA, Moeller MB, and Gallis HA: Trimethoprim-sulfamethoxazole therapy for Nocardia infections, Arch Intern Med 143:711, 1983.

Diphtheria

Oksana M. Korzeniowski

DEFINITION. Diphtheria, caused by *Corynebacterium diphtheriae,* is an acute infectious disease that may be symptomless or may be seen as a rapidly fatal hypertoxic disease characterized by a local inflammatory lesion in the upper airway or skin and by remote effects produced by an exotoxin elaborated by the organism.

ETIOLOGY. *C. diphtheriae* is an aerobic, gram-positive, pleomorphic, nonsporeforming, nonmotile organism. In stained preparations it appears club shaped, contains metachromatic granules, and aligns in palisades resembling Chinese characters. Media containing tellurite promote growth and impart a characteristic black pigment to the isolates. The diphtheria bacillus has been classified by in vitro characteristics into three stable types: gravis, intermedius, and mitis. Each type can cause epidemic diphtheria. Virulence depends on the production of an exotoxin (conferred by lysogeny with a β-prophage) and of other biologically active extracellular products such as spreading factor (hyaluronidase). Spreading factor promotes tissue invasion and may account for the occurrence of diphtheria in well-immunized individuals or in individuals infected with nontoxigenic strains.

EPIDEMIOLOGY. Diphtheria is primarily a disease of nonimmunized low-income urban populations living in crowded conditions. It is worldwide in distribution, and epidemics still occur in the United States. Intimate contact is required for spread of diphtheria. Transmission occurs by infected droplets generated from nasopharyngeal secretions or by exudates from infected skin lesions; fomites, milk, and dust may have a minor role. Asymptomatic carriers harboring toxin-producing strains in the nasopharynx or skin constitute the reservoir from which disease spreads to susceptible individuals. Immunity against diphtheria does not prevent nasopharyngeal carriage or the development of local disease but does attenuate or abort the distant toxic effects. The highest attack rates, morbidity, and mortality in diphtheria occur in nonimmunized children under 14 years of age. Highly contagious skin infections may be important in maintaining the endemicity of diphtheria by increasing the rates of acquisition and transmission of the organism and thus expanding the potential reservoir.

PATHOGENESIS. The membrane, the primary local manifestation of diphtheria, is composed of bacteria, necrotic epithelium, fibrin, and phagocytes. The painless, thick, leathery, blue-white membrane usually is located in the upper airway, where it firmly adheres to underlying tissues. Other sites, such as conjunctivae, vagina, or ear, also may be involved. Forcible removal of the membrane causes bleeding.

Exotoxin is elaborated and absorbed at the primary lesion. Rapidly distributed hematogenously, it binds to specific receptors on susceptible cells (primarily nerve, myocardium, and kidney) and penetrates into the cytoplasm, where it inactivates the "elongation factor," a critical protein moiety required for the translocation of transfer RNA during protein synthesis. Arrest of protein synthesis results in fatty degeneration of muscle and of medullary sheets of motor nerves (and to a lesser degree of sensory nerves), as well as enlargement and cloudy swelling of the kidney.

CLINICAL MANIFESTATIONS. The primary determinants of the clinical manifestation of diphtheria are the patient's immune status, the virulence and toxigenicity of the infecting strain, and the anatomic location of infection. Strains that do not produce toxin cause only local disease.

The incubation period is 2 to 6 days. A copious, thick, serosanguineous discharge in nasal diphtheria produces local irritation but rarely results in intoxication. Pharyngeal diphtheria confined to the tonsils may cause only local discomfort (pharyngitis) and mild systemic symptoms of fever and headache. Spread of the membrane to the uvula, soft palate, and pharyngeal wall enlarges the surface area for toxin absorption; signs of toxemia, such as listlessness, tachycardia, and weakness, are common. Local edema of submandibular areas and the anterior neck imparts a characteristic "bull-neck" appearance. Airway occlusion, as well as severe toxic manifestations, occurs in laryngeal, tracheal, and bronchial diphtheria. Cutaneous diphtheria, which occurs primarily in the tropics but has caused epidemic outbreaks in North America, develops as a shallow, nonhealing ulcer covered by a grayish membrane.

Conduction abnormalities and arrhythmias appearing in the first or second week of illness are indicative of diphtheritic myocarditis. Circulatory collapse is an ominous sign. Cranial and peripheral motor nerve palsies develop after 2 to 6 weeks. Respiratory insufficiency may result from paralysis of the diaphragm. Encephalitis is a rare toxic complication.

DIAGNOSIS. A provisional diagnosis of diphtheria should be made on clinical grounds and treatment instituted immediately. Specific diagnosis by bacteriologic confirmation, strain identification, and detection of toxin elaboration by precipitin reactions with antiserum (Elek test) is important for epidemiologic reasons but should not delay therapy.

COURSE. Nontoxic diphtheria is a self-limited disease, although chronic carriage of the bacillus may ensue. Before the use of antitoxin, diphtheria of moderate severity (that is, accompanied by toxemia) and laryngeal diphtheria carried mortality rates of 35% and 90%, respectively. Currently, overall mortality in the United States remains between 4% and 10%. Myocarditis, paralysis, and death occur primarily in nonimmunized, very young, or very old people. Myocardial damage (fibrosis) and neurologic deficits may persist in survivors.

MANAGEMENT. Patients with diphtheria require isolation and strict bed rest. Early use of diphtheria horse serum antitoxin, 20,000 to 100,000 units, depending on the extent of the disease, is the most important specific treatment for the prevention of toxic complications. Rapid binding of the toxin to susceptible tissue sites may render antitoxin ineffective if it is administered more than 48 hours after the onset of illness. Sensitivity to horse serum must be determined, with desensitization performed if necessary. Antibiotics are used to terminate the carrier state. Erythromycin (500 mg four times a day for 7 days) is the drug of choice, but procaine penicillin is an effective alternative. Control of epidemic outbreaks requires early treatment of carriers and active immunization of susceptible individuals. Since diphtheria infection may not confer immunity, active immunization should be instituted at the time of recovery from illness.

PREVENTION. Diphtheria is preventable with active immunization. Diphtheria-pertussis-tetanus (DPT) vaccines should be administered in three (in infants) and two (in children) doses of 0.5 ml each at 4- to 6-week intervals. Boosters should be given after 1 year and just before starting school. Adult primary immunization follows the same schedule, but adult-type diphtheria-tetanus (dT) vaccine, which contains less diphtheria toxoid, should be used. Recent serosurveys indicate that the proportion of the population lacking protective levels of circulating antitoxin against diphtheria increases with increasing age and that at least 40% of people 60 years of age or older lack protective antitoxin levels. To ensure continued adequate protection in patients, booster doses of dT should be administered every 10 years. An intradermal injection of highly purified diphtheria toxin (Schick test) may be useful in determining immune status. A local reaction indicates lack of antibody and therefore lack of immunity.

BIBLIOGRAPHY

McCloskey RW and others: The 1970 epidemic of diphtheria in San Antonio, Ann Intern Med 75:495, 1971.

Chen RT and others: Diphtheria in the United States, Am J Public Health 75:1393, 1985.

Pappenheimer AJ: Diphtheria toxin, Ann Rev Biochem 46:69, 1977.

Hewlett EL: Selective primary health care: strategies for the control of disease

in the developing world. XVIII. Pertussis and diphtheria, Rev Infect Dis 7:426, 1985.

Centers for Disease Control: Diphtheria, tetanus and pertussis: guidelines for vaccine prophylaxis and other preventive measures, leads from MMWR, JAMA 254:895, 1985.

Scheid W: Diphtherial paralysis, J Nerv Ment Dis 116:1095, 1952.

49 · DISEASES CAUSED BY ANAEROBIC BACTERIA

Infections caused by nonsporeforming anaerobes

Matthew E. Levison

DEFINITION. Obligate anaerobic bacteria are those that require an anaerobic environment for survival and growth.

Sporeforming obligate anaerobes are called clostridia. Pathogenic sporeless obligate anaerobes are either species of *Fusobacterium* or *Bacteroides* (gram-negative bacilli); *Propionibacterium, Lactobacillus, Actinomyces, Bifidobacterium,* or *Eubacterium* (gram-positive bacilli); *Peptococcus* or *Peptostreptococcus* (gram-positive cocci); or *Veillonella* or *Acidaminococcus* (gram-negative cocci). The obligate anaerobes are the predominant members of the normal microflora on the skin and adjacent mucous membranes, that is, gingival crevice, lower intestinal tract, vagina, or distal third of the urethra. In the gingival crevice and colon there are 10 billion to 100 billion organisms/ml, and in the vagina there are 100 million to 1 billion/ml. Each site has a characteristic flora composed of a distinctive number of species, including more than 100 in the gingival crevice or colon but only about five in the vagina, and a distinctive type of species, such as *Bacteroides melaninogenicus* in the gingival crevice, *Bacteroides thetaiotaomicron* and *Bacteroides fragilis* in the colon, and *Lactobacillus* organisms and anaerobic gram-positive cocci in the vagina.

PATHOGENESIS. Infections caused by anaerobes usually are endogenous in origin; they are caused by the microflora on the skin and mucous membranes. These infections depend primarily on defects in local host defense mechanisms (defects in the mucosal barrier and presence of necrotic tissue as a consequence of trauma, neoplasia, or ischemia) at sites that normally have a microflora. Most intraabdominal and pelvic infections and infections in and about the mouth are due to anaerobes. However, of the numerous species found in the microflora, only a few are frequently isolated from clinical specimens. Of the anaerobic species involved, the more commonly found are those containing virulence factors, such as polysaccharide capsules (*B. fragilis, Bacteroides asaccharolyticus*), or endotoxin (*Fusobacterium nucleatum*). Other virulence factors include production of proteolytic enzymes, gas, or heparinase, which promote further tissue necrosis, local spread, or hematogenous dissemination. In addition, the anaerobes isolated from clinical specimens tend to be characteristic of the microflora normally found at that site, such as *B. fragilis* if the infection is colonic in origin or *B. asaccharolyticus* if it is oral in origin. These infections characteristically are polymicrobial; about five species (range 3 to 10) usually are isolated. The anaerobes are at times mixed with aerobic or facultative species. The aerobic or facultative component of these polymicrobial infections also reflects the microflora at the site of the defect in host defenses, such as *Escherichia coli* or enterococci if the infection is colonic in origin or various streptococci if it is oral in origin. Alterations of the microflora on the skin or mucosal surface caused by a primary disease process also are reflected in the type of pathogens isolated from the clinical specimen. For example, the vaginal microflora after a normal delivery, abortion, gynecologic surgery, or in the presence of trichomoniasis may be composed of colonic-type microorganisms, such as *B. fragilis, E. coli*, or enterococci, and infections in these situations reflect the change in microflora.

CLINICAL MANIFESTATIONS. Certain findings suggest an anaerobic bacterial origin. Anaerobic infections usually are located at or near sites that contain a predominantly anaerobic microflora. There usually is associated tumor, vascular obstruction (such as that caused by atherosclerosis or diabetes mellitus), or trauma that has resulted in tissue necrosis. The obstruction of a paranasal sinus or of the lower respiratory airway by a tumor or foreign body may be associated with anaerobic infection in the poorly ventilated and poorly drained areas. The aspiration of the contents of the oral cavity into the lower respiratory tract may result in anaerobic pleuropulmonary infection. Anaerobic bacteria usually produce a foul odor in purulent material, unlike most aerobic or facultative pathogens; the absence of such an odor, however, does not exclude the presence of anaerobic pathogens. Gas frequently is produced in tissues, resulting in crepitation. Anaerobic infection in the female genital tract may be complicated by suppurative thrombophlebitis of the pelvic veins, with septic embolization to the lung; anaerobic infection in the intestinal tract may be complicated by thrombophlebitis in the portal system, with septic embolization to the liver. Bacteremia may also result in endocarditis or metastatic infection in any organ, such as the brain, bones, joints, spleen, and liver.

Infection by the anaerobic microflora also may result from an animal or human bite or accidental subcutaneous or intravenous self-inoculation of saliva or feces.

DIAGNOSIS. The presence of anaerobes should be suspected in the appropriate clinical setting as described previously. Gram stain is important in identifying the anaerobes that may have a characteristic morphology such as *Actinomyces* organisms and in detecting the presence of a polymicrobial infection. Bacteriologic confirmation depends on avoiding contamination, even by minute amounts of secretions that contain skin or mucosal microflora, such as upper respiratory tract, intestinal, vaginal, or urethral secretions. These secretions contain enormous numbers of microorganisms that may or may not be identical to the organisms causing the disease.

To obtain lower respiratory tract material for anaerobic culture, an invasive procedure such as transtracheal aspiration or percutaneous lung puncture is involved. Frequently, these invasive and risky procedures are not performed if the clinical diagnostic features (for example, community-acquired putrid lung abscess) are sufficiently apparent. Blood and pleural, synovial, or peritoneal fluid should be obtained for anaerobic culture depending on the clinical situation.

Anaerobes frequently are fastidious and do not grow at optimal rates when handled by methods that are routinely used for facultative organisms. These organisms must be transported to the laboratory as quickly as possible in an anaerobic environment (for example, aspirated purulent material transported to the laboratory in a "corked" syringe) and placed on enriched solid and liquid media as soon as they arrive in the laboratory. The media should then be incubated in an anaerobic environment for at least 48 to 72 hours before being discarded. If the Gram stain of the purulent material initially revealed a polymicrobial infection but few of the organisms or only the facultative organism were recovered on culture, the more fastid-

ious anaerobes can be presumed to have been lost in the laboratory processing.

MANAGEMENT. Surgery is the primary mode of therapy, except for lung abscess or endometritis. The aims of surgery are (1) to stop further contamination; (2) to remove all gross foreign material, such as necrotic tissue, feces, and blood, since virulence is enhanced by the presence of these substances; (3) to eliminate anaerobic conditions; (4) to reduce the bacterial count to a minimum; and (5) to provide drainage of purulent material. In some patients percutaneous aspiration of an abscess by means of needle and syringe under ultrasound or computerized tomographic guidance, when feasible, may replace surgery. At times drainage alone may be all that is necessary for a well-localized abscess, such as a surgical wound abscess.

The role of antimicrobial therapy in the outcome of infection caused by anaerobes is extremely difficult to assess. This is primarily because of the often dramatic response to surgical drainage and debridement alone in cases of localized infection. Nevertheless, appropriate antimicrobial therapy has been shown to significantly reduce mortality among patients with bacteremic infections caused by Bacteroidaceae or Enterobacteriaceae. Antimicrobial drugs are expected to control bacteremia and early metastatic foci of infection, to reduce suppurative complications if administered early, and to prevent local spread of existing infection. However, once suppuration has occurred, unless abscesses are quite small, antimicrobial drugs without percutaneous aspiration by needle and syringe or surgical drainage and debridement cannot be expected to eliminate the infection.

Antimicrobial therapy should be started immediately after appropriate specimens such as blood and purulent material are obtained for culture. This means that antimicrobial therapy often is started before completion of in vitro antimicrobial sensitivity testing of the specific facultative pathogens. Rapid isolation and identification of anaerobes, in contrast to the testing of facultative pathogens, often are not possible in many community hospitals. In addition, in vitro sensitivity testing by the conventional disk diffusion technique has not been standardized for anaerobes. Therefore initial chemotherapy usually is empiric, based on the most reliable and least toxic antimicrobial agents for the most probable anaerobic and facultative pathogens.

Because these infections commonly are polymicrobial, a broad spectrum of antimicrobial activity is required. Drugs active against anaerobic bacteria may be quite inactive against the accompanying aerobic or facultative pathogens in the mixed infections and vice versa. For this reason combinations of usually two or three drugs may have to be used. These combinations are selected for their activity against most of the more virulent pathogens expected to be present in the infective mixture (such as in infection caused by colonic microflora, the Enterobacteriaceae and *B. fragilis*).

Infection caused by oral anaerobes cannot be reliably treated with β-lactamase-sensitive penicillins, because oral microflora, especially *B. melaninogenicus*, produce β-lactamase. Since Enterobacteriaceae usually are not involved in these infections unless the infection is hospital-acquired, effective therapy includes: (1) clindamycin alone, or possibly (2) metronidazole plus penicillin G or V, (3) amoxicillin/clavulanate, (4) ampicillin/sulbactum, or (5) cefoxitin. Because of its poor activity against microaerophilic gram-positive cocci (for example, *Streptococcus milleri*), metronidazole must be combined with a β-lactam antibiotic such as penicillin.

Infection caused by colonic microflora (intraabdominal, pelvic, or perineal organisms) or hospital-acquired oral microflora can best be initially treated with the following:

1. Chloramphenicol, 50 to 100 mg/kg/day orally or intravenously in four divided doses and gentamicin (or tobramycin), 1.7 mg/kg intravenously or intramuscularly every 8 hours (if renal function is normal)
2. Clindamycin, 600 mg intravenously or intramuscularly every 6 to 8 hours and gentamicin (or tobramycin)
3. Metronidazole, 15 mg/kg intravenously followed by 7.5 mg/kg intravenously or orally every 6 hours, gentamicin (or tobramycin), and a penicillin or cephalosporin (Some physicians use ampicillin in these first three regimens because of the frequent presence of enterococci, but this antibiotic does not always seem to be necessary despite the presence of this organism. If multiple, antibiotic-resistant, enteric, gram-negative bacilli are suspected or known to be involved [as in hospital-acquired infection], a third-generation cephalosporin antibiotic such as cefotaxime, cetizoxime, or ceftriaxone [or if *Pseudomonas aeruginosa* is known or suspected to be involved, ceftazidime] may be used with metronidazole.)
4. Imipenem alone, 500 mg intravenously every 6 hours (imipenem is active against almost all anaerobes and all aerobes, including *P. aeruginosa* and multiple, antibiotic-resistant, enteric, gram-negative bacilli. Amikacin is the aminoglycoside of choice if gentamicin-resistant gram-negative facultative bacilli are suspected.)

Clavulanic acid and sulbactam, β-lactams that have poor antimicrobial activity, irreversibly binds to and inactivates certain β-lactamases. When clavulanic acid is combined with either amoxillin (Augmentin; an oral agent), ticarcillin (Timentin; a parenteral agent), or ampicillin with sulbactam (Unasyn, a parenteral agent), the β-lactamase inhibitor allows amoxicillin, ticarcillin, or ampicillin to be active against otherwise resistant β-lactamase-producing anaerobes such as *B. fragilis* and presumably *B. melaninogenicus*. Ticarcillin–clavulanic acid has a spectrum sufficient for almost all aerobes and anaerobes, the exceptions being those gram-negative bacillary organisms that produce inducible β-lactamase (that is, *Enterobacter cloacae*, *Serratia marcescens*, and *Pseudomonas aeruginosa*. Amoxicillin–clavulanic acid and ampicillin-sulbactam are similarly active against *E. coli* and *Klebsiella* and *Proteus* organisms but have significantly less activity against other Enterobacteriaceae and no activity against *Pseudomonas* organisms. Therefore ticarcillin–clavulanic acid may prove useful in serious anaerobic infections involving colonic flora or hospital-acquired oral microflora. Amoxicillin–clavulanic acid and ampicillin and sulbactam may prove useful in treating anaerobic infections involving oral anaerobes in the ambulatory patient (for example, in human bite infections).

An appropriate β-lactam antibiotic such as a cephalosporin or penicillin should subsequently be substituted for the aminoglycoside if indicated by results of in vitro disk susceptibility tests on the facultative isolates. No reliable disk sensitivity tests are available for anaerobes. The duration of therapy usually is prolonged to prevent relapse, because host defenses cannot be relied on to completely eradicate the pathogens from sequestered areas of extensive tissue necrosis and abscess formation, many of which are not accessible to adequate surgical drainage. Antibiotic therapy should be given before, during, and after surgery to ensure tissue and blood levels that will combat local and metastatic spread of the infection.

PROGNOSIS. Morbidity is unusually prolonged in patients with anaerobic infection. The presence of residual infection as a result of inadequate surgical management (more common in patients with multiple abscesses); extensive tissue necrosis caused by malignancy, ischemia, or trauma; or continued contamination is associated with significantly greater morbidity or mortality.

PREVENTION. Anaerobic infection can be prevented by adequate management of conditions that predispose to invasion by surface microflora. For example, prevention of postoperative wound infection and peritonitis requires avoiding contamination of the peritoneum with gastrointestinal or vaginal secretions during abdominal or pelvic surgery. In addition to good surgical technique, the complex gastrointestinal or vaginal flora can be reduced before surgery. Mechanical cleansing of the bowel with a low-residue diet followed by a liquid diet, cathartics, and enemas can reduce the total fecal mass. Preoperative oral antibiotics to reduce the bacterial concentration in the colon also are commonly used.

Parenteral antibiotics also have been used in gastrointestinal and gynecologic surgery prophylactically when there is a chance of contamination with normal microflora at the operative site ("clean, contaminated surgery"). These types of operations involve, for example, cutting through the large bowel without significant spillage; compromising the blood supply of the large bowel; cutting through the stomach or small bowel when there is anticipated intraluminal bacterial overgrowth; appendectomy for appendicitis without rupture; penetrating wounds of the abdomen; gallbladder surgery in the elderly; cesarean section following rupture of the membranes and labor; vaginal hysterectomy in the premenopausal woman; and radical pelvic surgery for gynecologic malignancy. Several studies have shown significant reduction in the frequency of postoperative infection from about 20% to 30% to about 4% to 8% following prophylactic antibiotics in clean, contaminated surgery.

The basic principle of antibiotic prophylaxis is to provide adequate tissue levels at the site of contamination and adequate blood levels during the procedure and for about 24 hours following the procedure. Prophylaxis is started within 1 to 2 hours before the procedure and continued for about 24 hours. Early treatment of a primary infection also can reduce the rate of postoperative infection. For example, in one study the rate of postoperative wound infection in patients with a perforated appendix was greater than 50% if no chemotherapy was used and 15% in the group given appropriate antibiotic therapy.

Clostridial infection

Matthew E. Levison

Clostridia are anaerobic sporeforming gram-positive (occasionally gram-negative) bacilli normally found in the intestinal tract of humans and animals and in the soil. Most disease is produced by *Clostridium perfringens*, but other pathogenic species include *Clostridium novyi*, *Clostridium septicum*, *Clostridium sordellii*, *Clostridium histolyticum*, and *Clostridium difficile*. These organisms produce a variety of diseases that are found worldwide, including wound infection, spreading cellulitis, myonecrosis, transient bacteremia, septicemia, metastatic infection (as in the lung, pleura, and meninges), enterotoxigenic enteritis or colitis, tetanus, and botulism.

TETANUS

DEFINITION. Tetanus is an acute infectious disease characterized by tonic spasm of voluntary muscles with episodic tonic convulsions and autonomic nervous dysfunction, caused by a potent neurotoxin elaborated in tissues by *Clostridium tetani*.

ETIOLOGY. Tetanus is caused by an exotoxin produced by

C. tetani, a motile gram-positive anaerobic sporeforming bacillus. Terminal spores, larger in diameter than the width of the vegetative cell, distend the ends of the rod (drumstick shape). The spores are found in soil and in human and animal feces; they survive for many years in dried earth.

EPIDEMIOLOGY. Spores may contaminate wounds caused by nail punctures, hypodermic injections of addicts, gunshots, compound fractures, and accidents to agricultural or construction workers. Occasionally, the postpartum uterus or umbilical cord is contaminated. Because spores may remain dormant in wounds for prolonged periods, the site of entry may not be obvious.

PATHOGENESIS. The presence in the wound of calcium salts, tissue anoxia, or increased acidity caused by infection with other soil bacteria (and the activity of granulocytes) facilitate germination of *C. tetani* spores. Subsequently, a potent neurotoxin is produced that acts on motor end-plates and also on the anterior horn cells of the spinal cord and brainstem, causing spasm. Generalized tonic spasticity occurs with intermittent tonic convulsions.

CLINICAL MANIFESTATIONS. There are three forms of tetanus: localized, cephalic, and generalized.

The localized form is characterized by spasticity of a group of muscles close to the site of injury. The spasticity may persist for several months and usually resolves gradually without residual findings. Some patients, however, may develop generalized tetanus.

Cephalic tetanus usually occurs 1 or 2 days following injury to the head or otitis media. It is characterized by involvement of the cranial motor nerves, primarily the seventh cranial nerve, and has a poor prognosis.

Generalized tetanus usually affects the body in a descending manner, beginning with trismus and ultimately involving the extremities. Less than 1 week between the occurrence of the wound and the first symptoms of generalized tetanus and less than 48 hours between the first symptoms and the first generalized spasm is associated with more severe disease. The initial complaint is stiffness of the jaw, followed by difficulty swallowing and opening the jaw (trismus), spasm of the facial muscles (risus sardonicus), and rigidity and painful spasms of the anterior abdominal wall and of neck and back muscles (opisthotonos). There is usually diffuse sweating. Painful tonic convulsions are precipitated by minor stimulation. Other findings include a moderate fever, rapid shallow respirations, rapid pulse rate, and widely fluctuating blood pressure. Hyperpyrexia may occur in the absence of infection, a result of continuous heat production from muscle contractions and cutaneous vasoconstriction. Because of spasm of the glottis and respiratory muscles, the patient may develop respiratory insufficiency. Difficulty in swallowing secretions may result in aspiration. Constipation and urinary retention result from spasm of the respective sphincters.

DIAGNOSIS. The history and clinical findings suggest the diagnosis. Tetanus must be differentiated from trismus caused by dental infections, nuchal rigidity caused by meningitis (in which trismus is absent), and strychnine or phenothiazine intoxication.

PROGNOSIS. Mortality may exceed 50% with inadequate treatment. In severe cases the prognosis is related to the ability to support the patient's respirations and to prevent dehydration and aspiration pneumonia for up to 2 weeks. In patients who survive, recovery is complete except for some muscle stiffness that may persist for months.

MANAGEMENT. Human antitoxin (3000 to 6000 units intramuscularly) should be administered as early as possible, and before exploration of the wound, to inactivate toxin released during surgery. The wound, if present, should be incised, foreign bodies should be removed, and the wound thoroughly cleansed. Penicillin (10 million units intravenously daily for 10 days) or tetracycline should be administered to eradicate vegetative clostridia present in wounds.

An attack of tetanus does not confer immunity, since a fatal dose of toxin is probably less than that required to stimulate an immune response. Therefore patients should be immunized with adsorbed toxoid, the full course being completed during the recovery period (for example, three doses of toxoid no less than 1 month apart).

To minimize respiratory problems in patients with difficulty swallowing secretions or with laryngeal spasm, tracheal intubation with a cuffed tube should be initiated, followed by elective tracheostomy with a cuffed tube. Muscle spasms can be controlled to some extent with diazepam (10 mg every 4 hours orally or parenterally). Muscle spasms complicated by drug-induced sedation may lead to hypoventilation; patients may then require total muscle paralysis with curare and mechanically assisted ventilation. After 1 to 4 weeks of therapy in severely affected patients, curare and diazepam requirements gradually decrease.

As a result of excessive sweating and increased insensible fluid loss, dehydration may occur if intravenous fluid replacement is not carefully maintained.

Marked muscle spasms, cyanosis, cardiac arrhythmias, and hypertension may occur as a result of stimulation such as tracheal suction. β-Adrenergic blocking agents such as propranolol have been used to control some of these problems, which are thought to result from sympathetic autonomic overreactivity.

PREVENTION. Active immunization should be given to children as part of a mixed diphtheria-pertussis-tetanus (DPT) vaccine program in infancy, on entry to school, and subsequently at 10-year intervals. Booster injections should be administered after injury if the last injection was given more than 5 to 10 years previously, depending on the type of wound; in addition, human tetanus antitoxin (250-500 units intramuscularly) is recommended for dirty wounds untreated for more than 24 hours.

CLOSTRIDIAL SOFT TISSUE INFECTION (GAS GANGRENE AND CLOSTRIDIAL CELLULITIS)

DEFINITION. Clostridial soft tissue infection is a rapidly spreading infection of soft tissue caused by *Clostridium* organisms, usually *C. perfringens.* If myonecrosis, or gas gangrene, occurs as a result of bacterial exotoxins, the disease is accompanied by toxemia and prostration.

ETIOLOGY. Several species of *Clostridium* may be associated with gas gangrene or clostridial cellulitis. The most commonly encountered are *C. histolyticum, C. perfringens, C. novyi,* and *C. septicum.* Each alone can cause the disease, but wounds may often contain two or more species. *C. perfringens* is a large, gram-positive or gram-negative rod, frequently surrounded by a capsule. Abundant gas and volatile organic acid production during fermentation is typical of many clostridia.

EPIDEMIOLOGY AND PATHOGENESIS. Infection usually is the result of contamination of a wound with clostridia or their spores. Severe wounds acquired in military combat, automobile or industrial accidents, criminal abortions, surgery or hypodermic injections in the hip or thigh, or any wounds grossly contaminated with soil or fecal matter are particularly likely to contain clostridial spores. Severity of infection may vary from simple contamination or mild cellulitis to gas gangrene. Conditions that facilitate germination of clostridial spores are the low redox potential and acidity of devitalized tissue and concomitant growth of facultative organisms inoculated into the wound at the same time as the clostridia. As a result, the clostridia proliferate and elaborate potent exotoxins that cause further tissue necrosis. The exotoxins of *C. perfringens* include α toxin (a lecithinase and hemolysin), collagenase, hyaluronidase, and deoxyribonuclease. Since lecithin is present in membranes of many different kinds of cells, the α toxin can cause extensive damage. The resulting edema and gas (hydrogen and carbon dioxide) in tissues and fascial sheaths tend to spread the infection and increase tissue pressure, further impairing blood supply. Gas gangrene is accompanied by severe prostration and terminal shock. Clostridia may also be found in localized collections of foul-smelling pus in wounds (Welch's abscess).

CLINICAL MANIFESTATIONS. The incubation period for clostridial cellulitis usually is more than 3 days after wounding. Its onset is gradual with only slight toxicity and little local pain, swelling, or change in skin color. A dark, thin, foul-smelling discharge is produced, showing short, wide, gram-positive rods and a variable number of polymorphonuclear leukocytes on Gram stain. Extensive gas production is characteristic and causes spreading crepitus; muscles are not involved. A similar clinical presentation also is caused by other organisms, usually a mixed flora consisting of *Bacteroides* organisms, anaerobic gram-positive cocci, and Enterobacteriaceae.

In contrast to clostridial cellulitis, gas gangrene is characterized by an incubation of less than 3 days, sudden onset, severe local pain, and swelling. Initially blanched, the skin becomes dark. Blebs appear and are filled with a dark, thin fluid containing many clostridia and few polymorphonuclear leukocytes. Gas production is usually not extensive and may be obscured by the edema. Exploration of the wound reveals necrotic muscle that fails to contract on stimulation. Although patients with gas gangrene are severely toxic, the syndrome of *C. perfringens* septicemia (hemolytic anemia, hemoglobinemia, and hemoglobinuria) rarely is seen in gas gangrene unless the uterus is involved.

Clostridial uterine myonecrosis is characterized by fever, bacteremia, rapidly developing severe intravascular hemolysis, hemoglobinuria and hemoglobinemia, shock, and renal failure. Gas may be evident in the uterine wall on roentgenograms and at surgery.

After penetrating wounds, clostridia can infect the traumatized organ (for example, the brain, lung, or eye) or cause hematogenous infection (for example, of the pleura, endocardium, or meninges). Clostridia also may cause cholecystitis or transient, benign bacteremia.

DIAGNOSIS. Gas gangrene is evident by clinical presentation, by roentgenography (which may show gas bubbles in muscle), and by the presence of myonecrosis on surgical exploration. Blood cultures generally are negative unless the uterus is involved. Myonecrosis caused by anaerobic gram-positive cocci develops insidiously 3 to 4 days after wounding, with swelling and a purulent exudate in which many polymorphonuclear leukocytes and chains of gram-positive cocci are found; pain follows. This disease has been seen in addicts who self-administer drugs intramuscularly.

PROGNOSIS AND MANAGEMENT. Gas gangrene is a uniformly fatal disease if not treated early and aggressively. Clostridial cellulitis has a lower mortality. All necrotic tissue and foreign bodies—materials conducive to growth of clostridia—must be removed in both clostridial cellulitis and gas gangrene. Amputation of an involved extremity or hysterectomy may be

necessary in myonecrosis. The incised area is left open with drains in place to allow free drainage and to increase the partial pressure of oxygen locally.

Hyperbaric oxygen at 3 atm has been used in therapy of gas gangrene. In this treatment, a patient breathes oxygen at a markedly increased P_{O_2}, thus raising arterial P_{O_2} and potentially increasing tissue oxygen. The reports of use of hyperbaric oxygen in clostridial myonecrosis seem promising. Therefore, if adequate hyperbaric oxygen facilities are available (hyperbaric chambers large enough for medical personnel to attend the patient), the patient with clostridial myonecrosis should be transported immediately to these facilities. Hyperbaric oxygen *does not* eliminate the need for surgical removal of necrotic muscle or treatment with antimicrobial agents. Both cellulitis and myonecrosis are treated with penicillin (20 million units intravenously daily) or cephalothin (12 g/day intravenously). Antimicrobial therapy for gas gangrene can be administered in hyperbaric chambers.

The efficacy of clostridial polyvalent antitoxin for clostridial myonecrosis or bacteremia is unclear, and anaphylaxis and serum sickness are complications of its use.

PREVENTION. Careful and prompt cleansing and surgical care of dirty wounds to remove all devitalized tissue and foreign material is essential; vascular obstruction from tight casts or tourniquets should be avoided.

BIBLIOGRAPHY
Infections caused by nonsporeforming anaerobes

Attebery HR, Sutter VL, and Finegold SM: Effect of a partially chemically defined diet on normal human fecal flora, Am J Clin Nutr 25:1391, 1972.
Finegold SM: Anaerobic bacteria in human disease, New York, 1977, Academic Press, Inc.
Levison ME and others: Clindamycin compared with penicillin for the treatment of anaerobic lung abscess, Ann Intern Med 98:466, 1983.
Rosenblatt JE, Fallon A, and Finegold SM: Comparison of methods for isolation of anaerobic bacteria from clinical specimens, Appl Microbiol 25:77, 1973.
Tally FP and others: Oxygen tolerance of fresh clinical anaerobic bacteria, J Clin Microbiol 1:161, 1975.

Tetanus

Buchanan TM and others: Tetanus in the United States, 1968 and 1969, J Infect Dis 122:564, 1970.
Faust RA, Vickers OR, and Cohn I: Tetanus: 2449 cases in 68 years at Charity Hospital, J Trauma 16:704, 1976.
Kanarek DJ, Kaufman B, and Zwi S: Severe sympathetic hyperactivity associated with tetanus, Arch Intern Med 132:602, 1973.
Weinstein L: Tetanus, N Engl J Med 289:1293, 1973.

Clostridial soft tissue infection

Altemeier WA and Culbertson WR: Acute non-clostridial crepitant cellulitis, Surg Gynecol Obstet 87:206, 1948.
Finegold SM: Anaerobic bacteria in human disease, New York, 1977, Academic Press, Inc.
MacLennan JD: The histotoxic clostridial infections of man, Bacteriol Rev 26:232, 1962.

50·MISCELLANEOUS BACTERIAL INFECTIONS

Allan M. Arbeter

Cat-scratch disease

Cat-scratch disease is a bacterial infection contracted from cats. The presumed etiologic agent is a small pleomorphic bacillus that has been observed in infected tissues. It is best stained by the Warthin-Starry silver stain. The disease has been reported in temperate climates but may occur worldwide. Most cases occur in the autumn and early winter, predominantly in young adults and children. A history of exposure to cats is present in almost all the individuals, but demonstrable cat scratches may be lacking at the time of clinical illness.

The initial lesion usually is at the site of a scratch and occurs from 1 to 4 weeks after the scratch. A 0.5 to 1 cm nodular erythematous lesion develops that pustulates directly from the nodule. Lesions heal within 2 weeks. At that time regional lymph node involvement appears, but the onset may be as late as 2 to 3 months after the primary lesion. Lymphadenopathy is predominantly regional and often axillary but may include cervical or groin nodes. The usual clinical course is self-limited, with the nodes regressing spontaneously in 2 months. The lymph nodes may suppurate, requiring needle aspiration or excision. Malaise and fever occur in 30% to 60% of the patients. Other evidence of systemic involvement includes a nonspecific maculopapular rash, pneumonitis, headache, encephalitis, hepatosplenomegaly, thrombocytopenia, and osteolytic bone lesions. Occasionally a preauricular node enlarges, confusing the diagnosis with mumps or streptococcal pharyngitis.

The diagnosis usually is made on clinical grounds. Histologic examination of a resected lymph node may show one or more features consistent with the diagnosis. These include hyperplastic elements, granulomatous areas, and suppuration. If all three are present, the diagnosis is reasonably certain. The organism may be seen on stains.

Skin test material can be prepared from an inactivated filtrate of the pus from another individual's lesion. The skin test (which is intradermal and read at 48 hours) is positive in 90% of patients and about 20% of family members. However, the skin test reagent is not commercially available. Because of concern about possible extraneous infectious or oncogenic agents, the skin test is indicated only in extremely ill patients when confirmation of the diagnosis is essential. Antimicrobial therapy has not proved effective and is not recommended.

BIBLIOGRAPHY

Wear DJ and others: Cat scratch disease: a bacterial infection, Science 221:1403, 1983.

51 · DISEASES CAUSED BY MYCOBACTERIA

Elias Abrutyn

TUBERCULOSIS

DEFINITION. Tuberculosis is a chronic bacterial infection of the lungs and other organs caused by the tubercle bacilli, *Mycobacterium tuberculosis* and *Mycobacterium bovis*. In the United States disease caused by *M. bovis* is rare.

ETIOLOGY. *M. tuberculosis* is a nonmotile, nonsporeforming bacillus approximately 1 to 4 μm in length and 0.3 to 0.5 μm in width. The organism, perhaps related to lipid constituents, is acid fast, that is, it resists decolorization with acid-alcohol solution. Although this characteristic is typical of *M. tuberculosis,* it is nonspecific.

M. tuberculosis is an obligate aerobe, growing best in oxygen concentrations approximating that found in alveolar air (140 mm Hg). This may account for the frequent appearance of infection in organs with a high oxygen content (kidneys, bones, and the apices of the lungs). Because the doubling time

is long, about 12 to 18 hours, growth in cultures is slow, and colonies, which have a rough appearance, first become visible after 3 to 4 weeks. The organism has a distinctive spiral-like pattern of growth that produces colonies with an appearance resembling cords. This characteristic is related to a lipid called cording factor. The presence of colonies demonstrating cording permits presumptive identification of an isolate as *M. tuberculosis*. Other characteristics useful in identifying *M. tuberculosis* include optimal growth at 95° to 102° F (35° to 39° C), absence of pigment production, ability to synthesize niacin and reduce nitrates, and loss of catalase activity at 154° F (68° C).

EPIDEMIOLOGY. Compared to the early 1900s the case and death rates for tuberculosis have declined dramatically, changes attributed in part to an improved standard of living. These declines have been accelerated further by the introduction of effective chemotherapy. Yet despite the decreases, tuberculosis remains a common problem. For example, in 1985 22,201 cases and 1729 deaths were recorded in the United States. Provisional data for 1986 indicated a total of 22,575 cases, an increase of 374. This is the first increase in tuberculosis morbidity in the United States since national reporting began in 1953. The increase may be related to patients concurrently infected with human immunodeficiency virus, to cases among the homeless and minorities, or to both.

An increase in the age at first infection has occurred. In the early 1900s infection at a young age was common; today infection among school-age children is rare. For the population in general the annual estimated incidence of new infection is 1 per 5000 to 10,000, an attack rate so low as to be difficult to measure. The risk of infection is highest in those in close contact (such as household contact) with people with untreated, sputum-positive tuberculosis. The risk of clinical disease is highest in the first 5 years after infection but remains present lifelong. In the United States the case rates are higher in the elderly, in males, in races other than white, in large cities, in the Southeast, and along the Mexican border.

PATHOGENESIS AND PATHOLOGY. Tuberculosis is almost always acquired by inhalation of airborne droplet nuclei containing tubercle bacilli; inoculation and ingestion also occur but are rare. Droplet nuclei are small (1 to 5 μm) particles that are generated and dispersed by people with active respiratory tract disease during coughing, sneezing, singing, or talking. Their small size imparts two characteristics important in the acquisition and spread of tuberculosis: they remain suspended in air for long periods, and they are small enough to escape deposition on the nasal hairs or mucociliary blanket and to enter the terminal airways, respiratory bronchioles, alveolar ducts, and alveoli. These particles are commonly deposited in the lower portions of the lung, where ventilation is best. After deposition the bacteria multiply, and a nonspecific inflammatory response occurs. Despite the presence of phagocytes, multiplication continues, and the bacteria spread via the lymphatic system to the regional lymph nodes and then into the bloodstream. The invasion of the blood leads to widespread dissemination throughout the body, including other parts of the lung, and is the critical factor responsible for later development of pulmonary or extrapulmonary disease. After several weeks specific cell-mediated immunity develops, which affects localization and control of the infection, and the characteristic tissue reaction, the granuloma, forms. The granuloma is characterized by epithelioid cells, Langhans' giant cells, lymphocytes, and a particular form of necrosis called caseation necrosis, a name derived from the macroscopic appearance, which resembles cheese. Cavities formed after liquefaction and drainage of the caseous material into the bronchial tree are particularly important, because they are associated with large populations of bacteria and thus are associated with a high likelihood of spread to others.

In most patients cell-mediated immunity controls the infection and the lesions heal by resolution, fibrosis, and calcification; bacilli, however, may survive in a dormant state in the lung or other sites, providing a nidus for possible reactivation at a later date. In other patients the cell-mediated immune responses fail to arrest the infection and progressive disease occurs (progressive primary tuberculosis).

The sequence of events—(1) primary pulmonary infection; (2) lymphohematogenous spread; and (3) host response (producing usually dormant infection)—must be understood to comprehend the varied clinical presentations of tuberculosis. These events explain clinical disease developing in the lung or at other sites with the initial infection or disease developing in any of these sites at a later date after reactivation of a focus that has been quiescent.

CLINICAL MANIFESTATIONS. Recent initial infection most often produces no symptoms. When present, the symptoms are nonspecific and can include fever, cough, and malaise. With the development of cell-mediated immunity, they usually subside. In rare cases the initial pulmonary infection is uncontrolled and infection progresses, producing progressive primary pulmonary tuberculosis. Infection at sites infected during the bacteremia also is usually controlled by cell-mediated immunity, but occasionally infection progresses, producing clinical disease. For example, the bacteremia may result in tuberculous meningitis or in a debilitating generalized acute infection called miliary tuberculosis, because the appearance of the lesions resembles millet seeds. The bacteremia also may result in tuberculous pleurisy or lymphadenitis. In young children enlarged hilar nodes may produce bronchial obstruction and collapse of a portion of the lung, or they may become necrotic and discharge bacilli into the lung, producing tuberculous pneumonia, a diffuse, particularly severe form of pneumonia. Occasionally the initial infection is accompanied by allergic manifestations such as erythema nodosum. The risk of certain manifestations appears to depend partly on age; miliary and meningeal forms of tuberculosis are common in young children, and progressive primary disease and pleural disease are common in young adults.

Pulmonary tuberculosis. Pulmonary tuberculosis may evolve either from the initial infection or after a variable period by reactivation of a dormant focus, usually in the lung apex.

The onset usually is insidious. Nonspecific constitutional symptoms are common and include fever, fatigue, malaise, weakness, anorexia, and weight loss. The temperature may rise in the afternoon or evening and fall at night; drenching perspiration (night sweats) may accompany the fall in temperature. Cough occurs and may be accompanied by production of sputum that occasionally is blood streaked; massive hemoptysis occurs in rare cases. Chest pain may be present if the infection extends to the pleura. Wheezing, shortness of breath, and shaking chills are rare.

The physical examination often underestimates the extent of disease demonstrable roentgenographically, and the two must be correlated. Rales may be heard over diseased areas, particularly when a full expiration and then a cough precede a full inspiration (posttussive rales). Dullness, increased fremitus, and other signs of consolidation may be present but are uncommon. The destructive and reparative processes producing cavitation and fibrosis may lead to a variety of findings, including tracheal deviation, decreased mobility and volume of the affected hemithorax, apical dullness, and bronchial breath sounds. Extrapulmonary findings that suggest previous tuberculous infection but are insignificant in gauging activity of disease include choroid tubercles in the retina and nodules in the epididymis. Erythema nodosum suggests active disease.

Pulmonary tuberculosis may lead to involvement of the pleura, bronchi, trachea, and larynx. Inflammation of the pleura overlying a parenchymal lesion may give rise to pleuritic chest pain, so-called dry pleurisy. Erosion of a parenchymal lesion through the pleura and discharge of the caseous material into the pleural space evokes a vigorous inflammatory response and formation of large amounts of pleural fluid (tuberculous pleural effusion). Such effusions are usually unilateral and may be accompanied by fever, cough, pleuritic pain, and shortness of breath. The fluid is exudative in character. It contains protein in excess of 3 g/dl, an elevated lactic dehydrogenase, and between 300 and 3000 white blood cells/mm^3, predominantly lymphocytes. The glucose concentration may be decreased. The diagnosis of pulmonary tuberculosis should be considered strongly in young adults with an unexplained pleural effusion. The diagnosis must occasionally be made on clinical grounds because the confirmatory tests can be negative. Pleural biopsy can be helpful. Tuberculous empyema, a rare, occasionally fatal complication resulting from massive contamination, can be differentiated from tuberculous pleural effusion because the fluid more closely resembles pus, and smears usually are positive for the organisms. Pneumothorax and bronchopleural fistula also may complicate pulmonary tuberculosis.

The bronchial mucosa bathed in secretions from tuberculous lesions may become infected. Endobronchial tuberculosis almost always appears near cavitary lesions, because such lesions have a high bacterial population. Endobronchial spread also may be responsible for the development of lesions remote from the main area of active infection such as in dependent regions or the contralateral lung. The lesions are ulcerative and may bleed, producing blood-streaked sputum; massive hemoptysis results from erosion of a branch of the pulmonary artery. Large endobronchial lesions, particularly in the prechemotherapy era, produce bronchial obstruction and collapse of a segment or lobe. Bronchial distortion often occurs in areas involved in the tuberculous process. Bronchiectatic lesions in the upper lobes rarely are of consequence, but secondary bacterial infection of lesions in the lower lobes can cause chronic cough and sputum production. Tuberculosis of the larynx may develop through direct contamination with infected bronchial secretions, or it may result from bloodborne spread of tubercle bacilli. Hoarseness and pain are common symptoms. Laryngeal tuberculosis, although rare, is of special importance, because contagiousness is high owing to ready generation of contaminated aerosols by the vibrating vocal cords.

Tuberculosis in other organs. Tuberculosis in organs other than the lungs may be accompanied by concurrent active pulmonary disease. Whenever extrapulmonary tuberculosis is found, an evaluation for active pulmonary tuberculosis is required.

Cervical nodes (scrofula). Tuberculosis may involve the cervical nodes as well as the hilar nodes. The spread usually is hematogenous, but it may result from lymphatic drainage of a primary pulmonary focus or in rare cases from direct cervical lymphatic drainage of a local oropharyngeal infection. Clinically, there usually is unilateral, painless enlargement without signs of acute inflammation. The nodes are soft, and systemic manifestations commonly are absent. Untreated, the nodes may rupture and discharge caseous material. The response to therapy is excellent. Bacteriologic confirmation is required, because scrofula commonly is caused by other mycobacteria that are more resistant to drugs and require surgery for cure. Control of bovine tuberculosis and pasteurization of milk have made disease caused by *M. bovis* rare.

Pericardium. The pericardium becomes involved by spread of organisms from a contiguous focus in the lymph node or the lung or in rare cases by hematogenous dissemination. As in the pleura and other serosal surfaces, infection stimulates an intense inflammatory reaction and accumulation of fluid with characteristics of an exudate; with resolution there may be fibrosis. During the exudative phase the clinical picture is that of fever and chest pain with or without cardiac tamponade. Dyspnea, cough, ankle swelling, cervical venous distention, and apparent cardiac enlargement may be present. With fibrosis the findings are those of constrictive pericarditis.

Peritoneum. The peritoneum also may become involved directly as a consequence of hematogenous dissemination or indirectly by spread from an adjacent focus. Fever, abdominal pain, and unexplained ascites may be present, accompanied by weight loss, anorexia, and night sweats. Abdominal tenderness may occur, but rebound may be absent. A "doughy" abdomen is now a rare finding. Recognition in cirrhotic patients who have ascites may be difficult.

Kidneys. The kidneys become infected by hematogenous spread of tubercle bacilli early in the primary pulmonary infection. Clinical disease usually develops after reactivation of dormant foci that undergo caseation, form cavities, and discharge bacilli into the collecting ducts, the ureters, and the bladder. Because spread is bloodborne, both kidneys usually are infected, although disease may be evident on only one side.

Symptoms are highly variable and may be absent. Common symptoms are frequency, dysuria, nocturia, urgency, and hematuria. Fever and other signs common to acute bacterial infection of the kidneys may be absent. The diagnosis should be suspected when pyuria with or without hematuria is noted in a patient who has negative urine cultures by standard techniques (sterile pyuria). Intravenous pyelography and cystoscopy may reveal parenchymal calcification or cavitation, papillary necrosis, calyceal dilation, ureteral strictures, and structural defects of the ureteral orifices.

Male genitalia. The prostate, epididymis, vas deferens, seminal vesicles, and rarely the testes may become involved, either from hematogenous spread or from active or previously active renal tuberculosis. Epididymitis, a common form of male genital tuberculosis, appears as a painless nodule or as a tender mass that may drain. Tenderness and swelling also may be found with active infection in the other genital organs.

Female genitalia. Female genital tuberculosis begins in the fallopian tube after hematogenous dissemination and spreads to the ovary, the peritoneum, the endometrium, or rarely the cervix. The symptoms are mild and include abdominal pain, vaginal discharge, and menstrual disorders. Constitutional signs often are absent, but a tubal mass may be found. Tubal scarring may lead to infertility or ectopic pregnancy.

Bones and joints. In children infection of the skeleton results from hematogenous spread and commonly involves the long bones and vertebrae. In adults infection also results from hematogenous seeding or by spread from adjacent infected paravertebral lymph nodes and commonly involves the anterior portion of the lower thoracic and lumbar vertebrae (Pott's disease). Pain with or without limitation of motion or constitutional symptoms may be found. Roentgenographically, the earliest finding is narrowing of the intravertebral disc space. Later, destruction is evident in both vertebrae adjacent to the involved disc. Severe destruction leads to scoliosis and kyphosis, which when marked cause severe anterior flexion of the spine with protrusion of the spine posteriorly (hunchback deformity or gibbus formation).

Tuberculous arthritis occurs as a chronic monarticular arthritis involving the hips, knees, elbows, shoulders, and other joints. Tuberculosis also may involve the costochondral junctions of the ribs or the bursae.

Meningitis. Tuberculous meningitis occurs by extension from an adjacent focus, or it can complicate miliary tuberculosis. The onset usually is subacute but may be more abrupt or slow, and the clinical findings are nonspecific, resembling those found in meningitis from any cause. The spinal fluid pressure is elevated, and the cerebrospinal fluid typically contains an elevated protein content, depressed sugar concentration, and a cell count below $1000/mm^3$ with a predominance of lymphocytes. A cerebrospinal fluid containing predominantly lymphocytes and a low glucose concentration always should lead to consideration of this diagnosis, even though other conditions can produce the same findings. The complications are related to the inflammatory process and the thick exudate at the base of the brain and include cranial nerve palsies, hydrocephalus, blindness, and optic atrophy. Therapy should be instituted promptly when the diagnosis of tuberculous meningitis is considered highly likely, because death is almost inevitable if the condition is untreated and bacteriologic confirmation, even if positive, requires several weeks.

Disseminated (miliary) tuberculosis. Miliary tuberculosis results from widespread bloodborne dissemination of the tubercle bacillus from a focus in the lungs or other organs, causing infection in many organs throughout the body. This complication, dreaded because of the high mortality it produces if untreated, may occur during the initial infection or years later after reactivation of a dormant focus. The disease may be acute and overwhelming or chronic in nature. The acute form appears as a severe, prostrating illness with fever, night sweats, anorexia, and headache. There may be abdominal pain with or without peritonitis, pleuritis, and meningitis. The presence of "miliary" lesions on chest roentgenogram should suggest the diagnosis, but they may be absent. The chronic form is similar but more indolent. Destructive lesions may be identified in bones, kidneys, or other organs. The nonspecific protean nature of the findings mandates consideration of this diagnosis whenever a persistent, unexplained febrile illness is present.

Rare forms of tuberculosis. Gastrointestinal tuberculosis occurs as a complication of pulmonary disease or from ingestion of contaminated milk. Tuberculosis may involve the oropharynx, esophagus, small and large intestines, and rectum. The lesions are ulcerative or hyperplastic or both and may lead to bleeding, obstruction, or perforation. The diagnosis usually is made at surgery. Addison's disease resulting from tuberculosis is now rare. Involvement of other organs including the eye, ear, thyroid, pancreas, and breast occasionally occurs.

DIAGNOSIS AND LABORATORY FINDINGS

Tuberculin skin test. The preferred test is the Mantoux (intracutaneous) test employing 5 tuberculin units (TU) of purified protein derivative (PPD), the intermediate-strength PPD. Forty-eight to 72 hours after injecting the antigen (0.1 ml) into the dermis of the forearm, the diameter of induration around the injection site is measured; erythema is disregarded. A positive test, that is, induration of 10 mm or more, denotes previous infection with *M. tuberculosis*. A doubtful reaction, 5 to 9 mm, signifies probable prior infection with other related mycobacteria, but previous infection with *M. tuberculosis* also is possible. A negative test, 0 to 4 mm, means that previous tuberculous infection or infection with other organisms is unlikely.

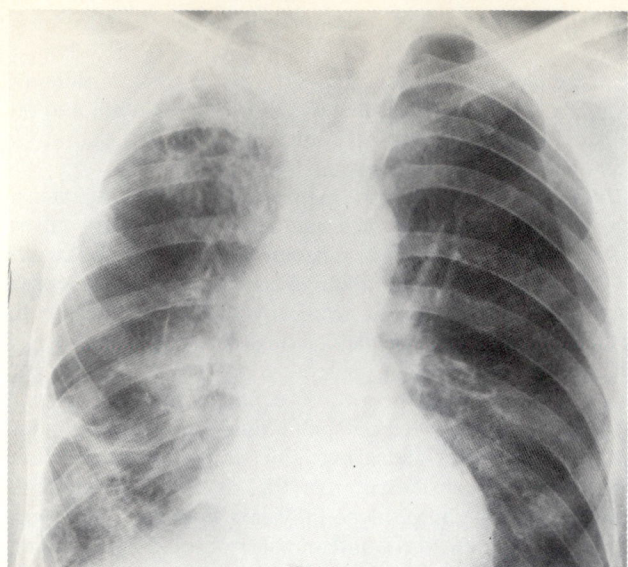

Fig. 51-1.   Pulmonary tuberculosis with right upper lobe cavity and spillage of disease to middle and lower lobes.

If the "intermediate" skin test is negative and tuberculosis remains a likely possibility, repeat testing with 250 TU (second-strength PPD) is indicated. Other skin test antigens (*Candida,* mumps, *Trichophyton,* and so forth) frequently are applied simultaneously to determine whether the patient is anergic. A negative response to all skin test antigens means that the person is anergic and that tuberculosis should remain a diagnostic possibility. A positive second-strength test irrespective of the other tests means that infection with either *M. tuberculosis* or other mycobacteria has occurred and that the patient is not anergic. A negative second-strength test in a person responding to at least one other antigen means that anergy is not present and prior infection with *M. tuberculosis* is most unlikely.

A first-strength skin test employing 1 TU as antigen as available for use in patients likely to develop large necrotic lesions at the injection site, but it rarely is used.

Roentgenography. The chest roentgenogram never provides an etiologic diagnosis, but the findings often are sufficient to make the diagnosis highly likely. The chest film also is useful in monitoring response to therapy. The initial lesions appear as a parenchymal infiltrate in any portion of the lung in association with hilar adenopathy. With healing, these lesions may calcify and remain identifiable as the "Ghon complex." In reactivation tuberculosis involving the lung, the type most commonly found in adults, the roentgenogram usually shows parenchymal infiltrates with or without cavitation or fibrosis in the apical-posterior area(s) of the upper lobe(s) (Fig. 51-1). Occasionally the predominant lesion is found in the superior segment of the lower lobe. In contrast to lung abscess, cavities in tuberculosis usually contain no fluid. Discrete, fluffy infiltrates in other areas of the lungs indicate bronchogenic spread. Healed inactive disease may appear as apical pleural scars, fibrosis with loss of volume in affected areas, or calcified areas. Tuberculous pneumonia resembles other bacterial pneumonias, and in miliary tuberculosis fine, discrete nodules may be found distributed throughout both lungs. Evidence of pleural or pericardial effusion also may be found. Other roentgenographic studies such as intravenous pyelography and bone roentgenograms may be useful in demonstrating destructive or fibrotic lesions consistent with tuberculosis.

Bacteriology. Definitive diagnosis requires isolation and speciation of the organism from body fluids or tissue, a process that takes several weeks because the organism grows slowly. A presumptive diagnosis can be made, however, when smears stained for examination by fluorescent microscopy or by conventional methods (Ziehl-Neelsen or Kinyoun stain) are positive.

Sputum is the material most frequently examined. Multiple specimens, preferably those obtained in the early morning, should be examined. If the patient fails to produce sputum spontaneously, sputum production can be induced by having the patient breathe an aerosol of heated saline. Occasionally sputum is obtained by bronchial washing and brushing during bronchoscopy; postbronchoscopy sputum specimens may be positive when other specimens are negative. Gastric aspiration to obtain swallowed bronchial secretions sometimes is helpful. Although cultures of this material may be positive, smears are unreliable because nontuberculous mycobacteria frequently are present. Urine smears are unreliable for the same reason. Smears of other body fluids (pleural, pericardial, peritoneal, cerebrospinal, synovial, and pus) should always be performed, because a positive result is highly suggestive, but the yield usually is low.

Histology. A presumptive diagnosis also may be made when granulomas with or without caseation or organisms are seen in histologic secretions, although granuloma formation is not specific for tuberculosis. Histologic examination of tissue is particularly useful when the pleural, pericardial, peritoneal, or synovial membranes appear involved, because cultures of the respective body fluids and tissues themselves often are negative. Examination of biopsy material from the liver and bone marrow is helpful in miliary tuberculosis, and biopsy may be useful in diagnosing disease in other sites, including the lymph nodes and the genital tract.

Other laboratory tests. Routine laboratory tests are of little value. The hemoglobin and hematocrit may be normal or show anemia of chronic disease. The white cell count may be normal, but a leukemoid reaction occasionally is seen. The serum sodium may be low from inappropriate secretion of antidiuretic hormone or in rare cases from Addison's disease. Hypercalcemia secondary to enhanced formation of 1,25-dihydroxy-vitamin D_3 has been seen. Sterile pyuria or hematuria suggests renal involvement. Exudative pleural, peritoneal, pericardial, or synovial effusion, with lymphocytes as the predominant cell type, should suggest tuberculosis, as should lymphocytosis in the cerebrospinal fluid. Methods to detect mycobacterial antigen(s) in the serum have been developed and are being evaluated for their value as a diagnostic test.

MANAGEMENT. The treatment of tuberculosis no longer requires institutionalization, prolonged bed rest, or deforming chest surgery, but it does require prolonged antituberculous chemotherapy. Hospitalization, although not required, facilitates performance of diagnostic procedures and permits evaluation of the response to and tolerance of chemotherapy.

The treatment of tuberculosis necessitates rigid adherence to certain principles. First, bactericidal drugs are preferred, and at least one should be included in the therapeutic regimen if possible. Second, two drugs active against the infecting organism should always be used to treat active disease, because resistance is likely to emerge during therapy when only one drug is employed. Third, chemotherapy should be continued sufficiently long to eradicate the organism; a major reason for failure of therapy is noncompliance with the prescribed regimen. Fourth, retreatment requires a regimen containing two drugs not previously used in the therapy or at least two drugs known to be active. Last, chemotherapy should not be withheld from ill people pending culture results, because the morbidity and mortality rates of untreated disease are high. Rather, treatment should be begun when the results of clinical findings and diagnostic tests (smears, roentgenograms, histologic tests, and so on) indicate that tuberculosis is the most likely diagnosis.

Antituberculosis drugs. The major drugs used in treatment are isoniazid, rifampin, pyrazinamide, ethambutol, and streptomycin. Supplemental drugs include ethionamide, cycloserine, paraaminosalicylic acid, capreomycin, kanamycin, and amikacin.

Isoniazid. Isoniazid (INH), the most useful chemotherapeutic agent, is tuberculocidal, effective when given orally, inexpensive, and relatively nontoxic. The prevalence of INH resistance among untreated cases in the United States is low. In the Far East INH resistance is common. In adults the daily dose is usually 5 to 10 mg/kg or 300 mg once daily orally; the twice weekly dose is 15 mg/kg (maximum 900 mg) each session. The drug diffuses into tissues well. It is acetylated in the liver and excreted by the kidneys. Individuals vary in their ability to acetylate INH, but the response to chemotherapy with the regimens in common use is not altered because of this. The toxic effects include peripheral neuritis, which can be prevented or treated with pyridoxine; hypersensitivity reactions; and liver damage. About 10% of the patients have transient elevations in serum transaminase levels, which often resolve despite continued administration of the drug. A more severe, occasionally fatal form of hepatitis with nausea, vomiting, and jaundice also occurs. The frequency is low but is increased in older age groups; alcohol use may be a factor. Treatment requires stopping INH; resolution usually follows. When INH is given with phenytoin, the serum levels of both may be elevated. Pyridoxine (50 mg/day) often is given to prevent neuropathy and is recommended when the daily dose of INH exceeds 300 mg.

Rifampin. The introduction of rifampin (RIF) has revolutionized the treatment of tuberculosis by permitting the development of regimens requiring shorter courses of therapy. The drug is bactericidal, absorbed from the gastrointestinal tract, widely distributed in tissues, and of low toxicity, but it is more expensive than INH. In adults the dose of 10 mg/kg or 600 mg is administered once daily. The dose administered twice weekly also is 10 mg/kg to a maximum of 600 mg. RIF causes hepatitis, gastrointestinal reactions, rashes, and hypersensitivity reactions, including flulike syndrome, hemolytic anemia, thrombocytopenia, and renal failure. When high doses are given intermittently, hypersensitivity reactions are common, but with doses of 450 to 600 mg, they are rare. RIF induces microsomal enzymes in the liver and thereby decreases the effectiveness of warfarin sodium, corticosteroids, birth control pills, and many other drugs by increasing metabolism. The potential for drug interaction should be considered in all patients receiving this drug. RIF turns the urine, tears, and possibly contact lenses orange-red.

Pyrazinamide. Pyrazinamide (PZA), a drug used for retreatment until recently, now has special importance, because it is a component of a recommended 6-month short-course treatment regimen. It is bactericidal at low pH (such as found in macrophages), and it is considered to have significant sterilizing activity, particularly early in treatment. Hepatotoxicity, the major side effect, does not appear enhanced when administered with INH and RIF as recommended. Hyperuricemia occurs; acute gout is rare. The daily adult dose is 15 to 30 mg/kg to a maximum of 2 g; 50 to 70 mg/kg (3 to 3.5 g) is used twice weekly.

Ethambutol. Ethambutol (EMB) is a bacteriostatic agent widely used as a companion drug in conventional long-term treatment regimens, as substitution therapy when resistance or a toxic reaction to another drug develops, and as a component of some short-course treatment regimens. The dose of 15 to 25 mg/kg is administered once daily orally and is well tolerated; 50 mg/kg is used for twice weekly dose. Optic toxicity manifested by changes in visual acuity, color vision, and visual fields is dose dependent and usually reversible. Hyperuricemia has been reported.

Streptomycin. Streptomycin (SM), an aminoglycoside antibiotic that inhibits protein synthesis, is administered parenterally. It is bactericidal in an alkaline milieu. It is used in some long- and short-course treatment regimens and for those unable to ingest medication. It also is used for poorly compliant patients in intermittent treatment regimens fully supervised by medical personnel. The dosage of SM during the first few months is 15 mg/kg/day (maximum 1 g) intramuscularly in one injection. A lower dose (10 mg/kg or 750 mg) should be considered for the elderly. The dose twice weekly is 25 to 30 mg/kg. Eighth cranial nerve toxicity may occur, usually in the form of vertigo; nephrotoxicity is extremely rare. Dose reduction is appropriate for people with renal failure and for the elderly.

Ethionamide. Ethionamide (ETH), related in structure to INH but less effective, is used primarily in retreatment, especially when multiple drug resistance is present. Gastrointestinal intolerance (manifested by metallic taste, anorexia, and vomiting) or liver injury limits use. The dosage is 15 to 20 mg/kg/day to a maximum of 1 g, given as three or four oral doses after meals.

Cycloserine. Cycloserine (CS), a toxic, relatively ineffective agent that inhibits cell wall synthesis, is used in retreatment. Seizures, depression, psychotic behavior, and other central nervous system symptoms occur; the drug is contraindicated in epileptic patients and patients with psychosis. The dosage is 15 to 20 mg/kg/day to a maximum of 1 g, given orally as two equally divided doses.

Paraaminosalicylic acid. Paraaminosalicylic acid (PAS) is rarely used today; previously it was a major drug. Gastrointestinal intolerance is frequent, and hypersensitivity reactions occur. PAS preparations with bentonite as the excipient may inhibit the absorption of RIF. The usual daily dosage of 150 mg/kg to a maximum of 12 g is given orally in three or four equally divided portions.

Capreomycin. Capreomycin (CM) resembles streptomycin in activity, dosage, and side effects. It is used intramuscularly in retreatment.

Kanamycin. Kanamycin (KM), a nephrotoxic and ototoxic aminoglycoside antibiotic, is primarily reserved for retreatment regimens. It is given intramuscularly.

Amikacin. Amikacin resembles kanamycin.

Choice of regimen. Short-course chemotherapy has become the preferred mode of therapy for newly diagnosed cases of pulmonary tuberculosis. Two regimens have been recommended, each consisting of an initial treatment phase of daily therapy and a second phase of either daily or twice weekly intermittent, supervised therapy. Twice weekly therapy is of particular value for patients likely to be noncompliant. The 6-month short-course regimen consists of an initial treatment phase of at least 2 months of daily INH, RIF, and PZA followed by daily or twice weekly INH and RIF to a total of 6 months. The 9-month regimen employs INH and RIF daily for 1 to 2 months followed by either daily or intermittent supervised therapy with INH and RIF for a minimum of 9 months and for at least 6 months after sputum conversion to negative. When drug resistance is likely, EMB should be added pending the results of susceptibility tests. These regimens are likely to be effective also in treatment of extrapulmonary disease. After pretreatment baseline tests have been obtained, (complete blood count, platelet count, blood urea nitrogen or creatinine, and liver function tests), patients should be informed of potential adverse reactions and should be followed clinically for occurrence of these reactions. Patients should be seen monthly, but routine laboratory monitoring is not advised. Supervised intermittent regimens should be used for patients who cannot or will not comply with daily regimens. When one of the short-course regimens cannot be used, INH and EMB can be given for 18 months.

Retreatment of patients given inadequate initial therapy, those failing to complete a prescribed regimen, or those with relapse after apparently successful therapy requires great skill, and expert advice should be sought. In such cases drug susceptibility testing is mandatory, and if treatment is begun before the results are available, the regimen must include at least two drugs not used previously.

Additional measures. Corticosteroids occasionally are used in the treatment of patients seriously ill or moribund from overwhelming disease. They have been employed in tuberculous meningitis, pericarditis, and pleuritis. Their efficacy in preventing or retarding the development of residual fibrosis and the complications thereof remains unproven. Routine use of corticosteroids is not advised, but when they are used, concurrent chemotherapy is mandatory.

Surgery is now used infrequently, because chemotherapy is effective. Surgery may be required for massive hemoptysis, bronchopleural fistula, pneumothorax, tuberculous empyema, bronchiectasis, pericardial tamponade, constrictive pericarditis, intestinal obstruction, ureteral obstruction, or abscess. In cases of spinal tuberculosis, surgery or immobilization with casts is rarely if ever necessary.

PREVENTION AND CONTROL

Preventive chemotherapy. The risk of reactivating dormant tuberculosis can be reduced by administering INH at a dose of 300 mg (10 mg/kg in children, not to exceed 300 mg) once daily for 6 to 12 months. Patients with stable, previously untreated, inactive parenchymal lesions should be treated for 12 months. In recommending preventive therapy, the risk of disease must be balanced against the risk of INH hepatitis.

Household and other close contacts of patients with newly discovered tuberculosis are at special risk and should be examined for active disease, which if present should receive therapy. Contacts with a positive skin test, that is, a 5 mm or greater reaction to PPD intermediate, without active disease should receive preventive therapy. Contacts whose skin tests are negative also may be started on INH (children are always treated), but they should have a repeat skin test at 3 months. If the repeat test is positive, therapy is either continued or started; if the test is negative, no further treatment is required unless exposure to an active case continues.

Other candidates for preventive therapy are: (1) patients with positive skin tests, and clinical and chest roentgenographic findings consistent with nonprogressive "inactive" tuberculosis; (2) patients with a history of tuberculosis never treated adequately with chemotherapy; (3) newly infected people, that is, those whose skin test has converted within the previous 2 years; and (4) patients with special conditions associated with a high risk of reactivation, including prolonged steroid therapy (appraised at 15 mg of prednisone or equivalent for more than 2 to 3 weeks), immunosuppressive therapy, malignancy such as

Hodgkin's disease, acquired immunodeficiency syndrome or human immunodeficiency virus infection (vide infra), diabetes mellitus, silicosis and situations associated with severe weight loss or chronic malnutrition such as intestinal bypass surgery, the postgastrectomy syndrome, and oropharyngeal or upper gastrointestinal tumors preventing adequate nutrition. Finally, tuberculin reactors under 35 years of age should be considered for therapy even in the absence of risk factors associated with reactivation. Those over 35 years of age should be considered only if they are contacts of converters or have a special condition enhancing the risk for reactivation, because their risk of INH hepatitis is high. Preventive therapy for pregnant patients generally is begun after delivery.

Vaccination. Bacille Calmette Guérin (BCG) is a live attenuated strain of *M. bovis* used as a vaccine. Vaccination may not reduce the risk of infection but does reduce the risk of serious forms of the disease such as miliary tuberculosis or meningitis. The efficacy of vaccination remains a controversial issue, and in the United States use is restricted to uninfected people who have repeated exposure to infectious cases and who could not obtain or accept treatment if they were to become ill. Adverse reactions include severe or prolonged ulceration at the vaccination site, lymphadenitis, osteomyelitis, disseminated infection, and death. Pregnancy and impaired immunity preclude vaccination.

PROGNOSIS. With adequate chemotherapy, the prognosis of tuberculosis is excellent.

NONTUBERCULOUS MYCOBACTERIAL INFECTIONS

DEFINITION. Many mycobacteria other than *Mycobacterium tuberculosis* and *Mycobacterium leprae* have been identified, some of which cause disease. In the past these organisms were called atypical or anonymous mycobacteria or mycobacteria other than tuberculosis, but today they are best referred to by the specific species name.

ETIOLOGY. In 1959 Runyon grouped the mycobacteria according to colonial morphology, pigmentation, and rate of growth, but exceptions to these groupings occur, and their utility is decreased. The relationship between the Runyon classification and the various species is as follows. The group I organisms, the photochromogens, grow slowly, produce pigment only after exposure to light, and include *Mycobacterium kansasii*, *Mycobacterium marinum*, and *Mycobacterium simiae*. Group II organisms, the scotochromogens, also grow slowly and produce pigment in the dark; *Mycobacterium scrofulaceum* and *Mycobacterium szulgai* are in this group. Group III, the nonchromogens, grow slowly, produce no pigment, and include the *Mycobacterium avium-intracellulare* complex, *Mycobacterium xenopi*, and *Mycobacterium ulcerans*. Group IV, the rapid growers, grow quickly, produce no pigment, and include *Mycobacterium chelonei* and *Mycobacterium fortuitum*. In the United States *M. kansasii*, the *M. avium-intracellulare* complex, and *M. scrofulaceum* are the predominant agents of human disease. Other species also have been identified that occasionally cause disease.

EPIDEMIOLOGY. Disease caused by the nontuberculous mycobacteria occurs worldwide. Several species are present in the environment, and isolates of some have ben recovered from food, water, animals, soil, and house dust. They also have been recovered from people without recognizable evidence of disease. Multiple cases in families are rare, and evidence of person-to-person transmission is lacking.

Results of skin tests with antigens from several species reveal that there is wide cross-reactivity among the various species and to *M. tuberculosis,* that skin tests are not generally helpful in diagnosing infection in the individual patient, and that many healthy individuals have had infection with these organisms.

PATHOGENESIS AND PATHOLOGY. The exact mode of transmission is unknown, but inhalation, ingestion, and inoculation may account for pulmonary disease, cervical lymphadenitis, and dermal infection, respectively. Histologically, the lesions are granulomatous, resembling tuberculosis, but suppuration occasionally is present.

CLINICAL MANIFESTATIONS

Pulmonary disease. Pulmonary disease clinically indistinguishable from tuberculosis may be caused by *M. kansasii,* the *M. avium-intracellulare* complex, and, less commonly, other species. Chronic obstructive pulmonary disease frequently is present. The diagnosis requires isolation of the organism from multiple specimens because these mycobacteria may occur as saprophytes. Antibiotic susceptibility testing is required because susceptibility varies among the different species and resistance is common. *M. kansasii* generally responds well to a combination of isoniazid, rifampin, and ethambutol given for 2 years in the same doses as for tuberculosis. The other species are more resistant, and four or more antituberculosis drugs often are used in initial therapy. Surgery occasionally is required.

Lymphadenitis. Painless, unilateral cervical lymphadenitis may be seen, particularly in children. *M. scrofulaceum* frequently is isolated, but other species also may be incriminated. Total excision of the involved nodes is required for cure.

Skin and subcutaneous infection. *M. marinum,* the cause of "swimming pool granuloma," has been isolated from swimming pools, fish tanks, and natural bodies of water. After entering the skin through abrasions or cuts, the organism produces verrucous or ulcerating lesions that remain localized because the organism grows poorly, if at all, at body temperature, Rifampin and ethambutol given for 6 weeks or more in the same doses as for tuberculosis are effective; tetracycline (500 mg every 6 hours) or minocycline (100 mg twice a day) may also be useful.

M. ulcerans produces deep, mutilating ulceration involving the skin, subcutaneous tissue, and muscle. The disease occurs in tropical areas. Surgery usually is required.

Other infections. Local abscess after injection with contaminated needles, bone and joint disease, genitourinary infection, sternal wound infection after cardiac surgery, and eye infection have occurred. Disseminated disease, particularly in immunosuppressed hosts, and endocarditis also have been described. Surgery may be required for cure.

MYCOBACTERIAL AND HUMAN IMMUNODEFICIENCY VIRUS COINFECTION

Mycobacterial infections occur frequently in patients who are also infected with human immunodeficiency virus (HIV), and the features are sufficiently noteworthy to warrant separate discussion. The common etiologic agents are *Mycobacterium tuberculosis* and *Mycobacterium avium-intracellulare.* Disease caused by *M. tuberculosis* may predate the diagnosis of acquired immunodeficiency syndrome (AIDS); recovery of *M. avium-intracellulare* represents on occasion the initial opportunistic infection in patients classified consequently as having AIDS. Clinically, mycobacterial disease in patients coinfected with HIV can resemble that in normal hosts, but pulmonary involvement may appear less pronounced or absent even on chest roentgenogram; extrapulmonary disease, especially lymphatic or disseminated disease, is more likely; and anergy is found frequently but not predictably. A negative skin test can-

not be used to rule out tuberculosis. When apparent, pulmonary involvement may effect any area in the lung and can be associated with hilar and/or mediastinal lymphadenopathy. Cavitation is rare. Central nervous system involvement occurs. Histologically, granuloma formation may be poor or absent, and all specimens from patients suspected of coinfection should be examined for acid-fast bacilli. Similarly, all tissue specimens submitted for bacteriologic studies should be evaluated by smear, when appropriate, and culture for mycobacteria; importantly, blood cultures may be positive. The response to chemotherapy of patients with disease from *M. tuberculosis* appears good, but relapse rates and the need for maintenance therapy remain to be defined. Effective therapy for disease caused by *M. avium-intracellulare* also remains to be defined; clofazimine and rifabutin (ansamycin) are included in the multidrug regimens used by some, but clear proof of efficacy is lacking. Initial therapy of presumptive mycobacterial infection in individuals infected with HIV should include three drugs effective against *M. tuberculosis,* in part because the public health risk of that infection is greater. Details of therapy can be found in the recommendations of the Centers for Disease Control. All with known HIV infection should have a tuberculin skin test and patients with positive skin tests should receive preventive chemotherapy with isoniazid; HIV testing should be offered to all patients at high risk of AIDS who have tuberculosis, especially extrapulmonary disease.

LEPROSY

DEFINITION. Leprosy is a chronic granulomatous disease affecting the skin and preipheral nerves. The disease is highly variable, and different forms with prognostic and therapeutic significance have been defined. The major types, listed in order from limited to widespread disease, are tuberculoid, borderline, and lepromatous leprosy. An indeterminate form that may evolve into one of the other forms is also seen.

ETIOLOGY. *M. leprae* is an intracellular, acid-fast bacillus that has never been grown in vitro. A relationship to other mycobacteria has been established on the basis of the presence of mycolic acids, multiple cross-reacting antigens, and similar filamentous surface structures. *M. leprae* can be readily transmitted to animals. In the mouse foot pad it produces a distinctive growth curve with an unusually slow generation time of 11 to 13 days, and in armadillos it causes a lepromatous leprosy–like illness. These animal models have provided a means to study immunotherapy and chemotherapy and sufficient antigen for biochemical and metabolic analyses and for vaccine development. Recently, monkeys have been found that are infected naturally, promising a better understanding of leprosy through study of a natural infection. The ability of *M. leprae* to infect peripheral nerves is unique, providing a marker distinct for this disease. Temperature may be an important factor in growth, since disease occurs in cooler areas of the skin.

The lepromin skin test uses heat-killed *M. leprae* from tissues of lepromatous patients or armadillos as an antigen. Intradermal injection may elict a tuberculin-like reaction (Fernandez reaction) at 48 hours or a papular reaction (Mitsuda reaction) at 3 to 4 weeks. The latter reaction aids in classifying patients, because it is negative in lepromatous leprosy and positive in tuberculoid leprosy. However, the skin test is not useful in diagnosis, because normal adults frequently are positive.

EPIDEMIOLOGY. Leprosy affects 10 to 20 million people worldwide and is found in most tropical and temperate regions. In the United States the disease is reported frequently from

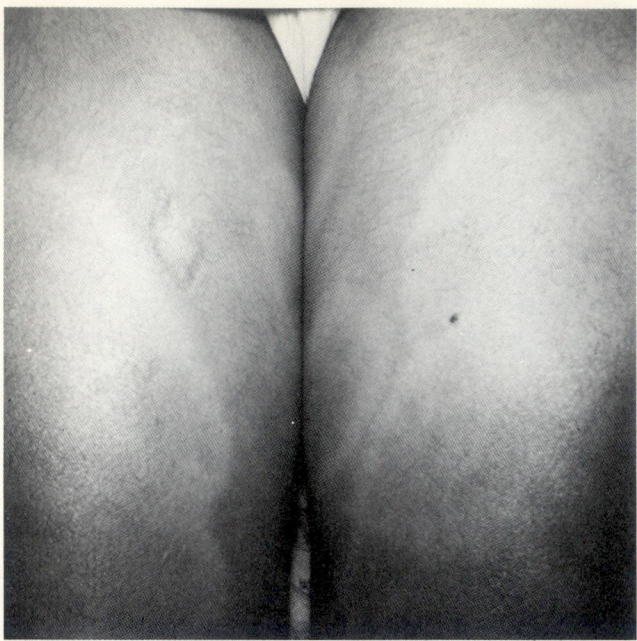

Fig. 51-2. Tuberculoid leprosy showing two large, well-demarcated plaques on thighs with hypopigmented centers.

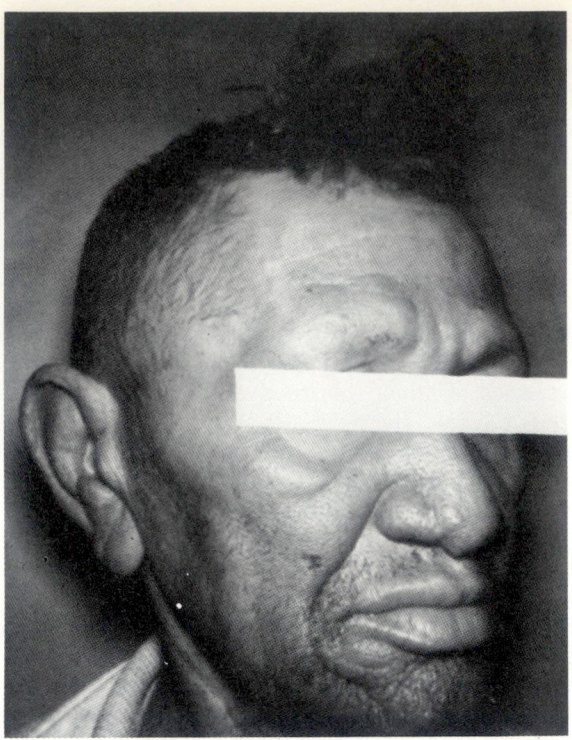

Fig. 51-3. Lepromatous leprosy showing loss of eyebrows, pendulous earlobes, and leonine facies with prominence of eyebrow ridge.

Florida, Texas, California, Hawaii, Louisiana, New York, and Puerto Rico. Although many cases are indigenous, most are imported, often from Mexico, the Philippines, and American Samoa. The recent increase in new cases is related to cases among immigrants.

The mode of transmission is unknown but had been assumed to be direct skin-to-skin contact. Recently the respiratory route has been considered the likely major mode of transmission, because the number of organisms shed from the skin is low and in untreated lepromatous individuals shedding from the nose is high. Contagiousness appears to be related to the number of viable bacilli shed from the nose and is highest in lepromatous leprosy; tuberculoid leprosy probably is not contagious. Study of transmission is most difficult because of the long incubation period, estimated to average 3 to 5 years. Prolonged contact appears to be important in the acquisition of disease; casual contacts are at low risk.

PATHOLOGY AND PATHOGENESIS. The pathogenesis is poorly understood, but bacteremia is thought to be important in the development and perhaps the progression of the disease. Defects in cellular immunity in all types of leprosy have been described and are most severe in the more generalized forms. The ability of the host to generate an immune response to *M. leprae* after infection may determine the subsequent course of the disease. Human lymphocyte antigen (HLA) tissue type may be important.

Histologically, the lesions in tuberculoid leprosy are characterized by epithelioid cells, lymphocytes, giant cells, and rare bacilli. In lepromatous leprosy foamy histiocytes, occasional lymphocytes, and many intracellular bacilli are seen. Borderline lesions have features of both types. nerve involvement is found in all forms of the disease and is most severe in tuberculoid leprosy.

CLINICAL MANIFESTATIONS. In tuberculoid leprosy one (occasionally two or three) large, well-demarcated plaque is formed that has a raised erythematous edge and a flat, hypopigmented, hairless, dry center (Fig. 51-2). Nerves (commonly the ulnar, radial, median, great auricular, or superficial pero-

neal) in the area of the plaque often are visibly or palpably enlarged. The area is anesthetic and therefore susceptible to infection or trauma. Muscle atrophy and contractures may occur as complications.

The lesions of lepromatous leprosy are bilaterally symmetric, diffuse, and poorly demarcated. They appear as macules, nodules, or plaques commonly involving the face, wrists, buttocks, knees, or skin over other bony prominences, but they can occur anywhere on the body. Nasal involvement producing complaints of nasal "stuffiness" occurs early, and lesions involving the gums, buccal mucosa, tongue, palate, tonsillar pillars, and posterior pharyngeal wall may be seen. Infiltration and thickening of the skin progress slowly and can produce loss of eyebrows, the classic leonine facies, or pendulous earlobes (Fig. 51-3). Septal and palatal perforation, nasal collapse, atrophy of the maxillary alveolar process, laryngitis, blindness, gynecomastia, and sterility may occur late in the course. Nerve involvement, although diffuse, is less severe than in tuberculoid disease. nerve thickening is not marked, and sensory loss is patchy.

The course of patients with leprosy may be complicated by a variety of acute episodes called reactions. Erythema nodosum leprosum (ENL), one reaction form, occurs in lepromatous leprosy, often during the first year of therapy. Tender, inflamed, subcutaneous nodules appear. Histologically, the lesions resemble an Arthus reaction, and bacterial viability may be reduced. There may also be fever, arthritis, lymphadenopathy, iridocyclitis, and glomerulonephritis. Reversal reactions occur in borderline cases; existing lesions become erythematous and indurated, and new lesions may occur. The histologic findings may shift toward either the tuberculoid or the lepromatous type.

DIAGNOSIS. The peripheral nerve involvement in leprosy distinguishes it from other skin diseases with a similar appearance. The diagnosis is best confirmed by skin biopsy. The finding of acid-fast bacilli in smears of material obtained by scraping the cut surface of a fresh skin incision is highly suggestive.

MANAGEMENT. Dapsone is the drug of choice, but use of just one drug cannot be recommended because of drug resistance. The regimens employed by the G.W. Long Hansen's Center in the United States follow. Patients with paucibacillary disease (indeterminate, tuberculoid, and borderline tuberculoid) and dapsone-sensitive organisms receive dapsone (100 mg/day for 4 to 7 years) plus rifampin (600 mg/day for 6 months). Multibacillary disease with dapsone-sensitive organisms is treated with dapsone (100 mg/day for life) plus rifampin (600 mg/day for the first 3 years). Clofazimine, which may cause skin discoloration, is used in place of dapsone in patients with dapsone-resistant organisms. The World Health Organization's (WHO) regimens differ in duration of therapy, the inclusion of clofazimine on a daily and intermittant basis for multibacillary disease, and the intermittant use of rifampin. Successful results with the shorter WHO regimens have been reported, but more data is probably needed before recommending widespread use. ENL and reversal reactions may require antipyretics, antiinflammatory agents, or steroids. Thalidomide, a teratogenic compound contraindicated in pregnancy, is remarkably effective in ENL but not in reversal reactions. The dose is 300 mg/day tapered to 100 mg/day. Immunotherapy remains experimental. In addition to specific chemotherapy, plastic surgery, vocational training, education, and physiotherapy are important.

PREVENTION. New cases of leprosy should be reported to public health authorities, and household contacts should be examined for active disease. Preventive chemotherapy and periodic examinations may be indicated for some contacts, and guidance in these matters should be sought from experts. The efficacy of BCG in preventing cases has been evaluated, but the results are variable. The U.S. Public Health Service, which has a mandate to maintain facilities for treating leprosy, can provide assistance.

PROGNOSIS. Patients with indeterminate or tuberculoid leprosy may undergo spontaneous cure, but progressive disease is common with the other types. Amyloidosis is a late complication. With therapy, the prognosis is excellent, but relapses occur.

BIBLIOGRAPHY
Tuberculosis

American Thoracic Society/Centers for Disease Control: Treatment of tuberculosis and tuberculosis infection in adults and children, Am Rev Respir Dis 134:355, 1986.

Baciewicz AM, Self TH, and Bekemeyer WB: Update on rifampin interactions, Arch Intern Med 147:565, 1987.

British Thoracic Society, Research Committee: Short course chemotherapy for tuberculosis of lymph nodes. A controlled trial, Br Med J 290:1106, 1985.

Centers for Disease Control: Tuberculosis and human immunodeficiency virus infection; recommendations of the Advisory Committee for the Elimination of Tuberculosis, MMWR 38:236, 1989.

Daniel TM: Tuberculosis. In Braunwald E and others, editors: Harrison's principles of internal medicine, ed 11, New York, 1987, McGraw-Hill, Inc.

Dutt AK, Moers D, and Stead WW: Short-course chemotherapy for extrapulmonary tuberculosis: nine years' experience, Ann Intern Med 104:7, 1986.

Dutt AK, Moers D, and Stead WW: Short-course chemotherapy for pleural tuberculosis: nine years' experience in routine treatment service, Chest 90:112, 1986.

Edwards D and Kirkpatrick CH: The immunology of mycobacterial diseases, Am Rev Respir Dis 134:1062, 1986.

International Union against Tuberculosis, Committee on Prophylaxis: Efficacy of various durations of isoniazid preventive therapy for tuberculosis: 5 years follow-up in the IUAT trial, Bull WHO 60:555, 1982.

Johnston RF and Wildrick KH: The impact of chemotherapy on the care of patients with tuberculosis, Am Rev Respir Dis 109:636, 1974.

Ninth Report of the Medical Research Council Working party on Tuberculosis of the Spine: A 10-year assessment of controlled trials of inpatient and outpatient treatment of plaster-of-paris jackets for tuberculosis of the spine in children on standard chemotherapy: studies in Massan and Pusan, Korea, J Bone Joint Surg 67:102, 1985.

Pitchenik AE and Rubinson HA: The radiographic appearance of tuberculosis in patients with the acquired immunodeficiency syndrome (AIDS) and pre-AIDS, Am Rev Respir Dis 131:393, 1985.

Pitchenik AE and others: Tuberculosis, atypical mycobacteriosis, and the acquired immunodeficiency syndrome among Haitian and non-Haitian patients in south Florida, Ann Intern Med 101:641, 1984.

Runyon EH: Anonymous mycobacteria in pulmonary disease, Med Clin N Am 43:273, 1959,

Sheller JR and Des Prez RM: CNS tuberculosis, Neurol Clin 4:143, 1986.

Snider D: Tuberculosis and gastrectomy, Chest 87:414, 1985.

Stead WW and Dutt AK, editors: Tuberculosis, Clin chest Med, 1:165, 1980.

Tuberculosis prevention trial: trial of BCG vaccines in south India for tuberculosis prevention: first report, Bull WHO 57:819, 1979.

Wolinsky E: Tuberculosis. In Wyngaarden JB and Smith LH Jr, editors: Cecil textbook of medicine, ed 17, Philadelphia, 1985, WB Saunders Co.

Nontuberculous mycobacterial infections

Donta ST and others: Therapy of *Mycobacterium marinum* infections: use of tetracyclines vs rifampin, Arch Intern Med 146:902, 1986.

Good RC: Opportunistic pathogens in the genus *Mycobacterium*, Annu Rev Microbiol 39:347, 1985.

Horsburgh CR Jr and others: Disseminated infection with *Mycobacterium avium-intracellulare;* a report of 13 cases and a review of the literature, Medicine 64:36, 1985.

Horsburgh CR Jr and others: Response to therapy of pulmonary *Mycobacterium avium-intracellulare* infection correlates with results of in vitro susceptibility testing, Am Rev Respir Dis 135:418, 1987.

Masur H and others: Effect of combined clofazimine and ansamycin therapy on *Mycobacterium avium-Mycobacterium intracellulare* bacteremia in patients with AIDS, J Infect Dis 155:127, 1987.

Wolinsky E: Non-tuberculous mycobacteria and associated diseases, Am Rev Respir Dis 119:107, 1979.

Woods GL and Washington JA III: Mycobacteria other than *Mycobacterium tuberculosis:* review of microbiologic and clinical aspects, Rev Infect Dis 9:275, 1987.

Leprosy

Girdhar BK and Deskian KV: A clinical study of the mouth in untreated lepromatous patients, Lepr Rev 50:25, 1979.

Jacobson RR: Antibiotic therapy for leprosy. In Peterson PK and Verhoef J, editors: The antimicrobial agents annual 2, New York, 1987, Elsevier Science Publishing Co, Inc.

Kaplan G and Cohn Z: The immunobiology of leprosy, Int Rev Exp Pathol 28:45, 1986.

Levis WR: Treatment of leprosy in the United States, Bull NY Acad Med 60:696, 1984.

Report of a WHO Study Group: Chemotherapy of leprosy for control programmes, World Health Organization Tech Rep Series 675, 1982.

52 · DISEASES CAUSED BY SPIROCHETES

Syphilis

Michael F. Rein

Syphilis is a specific infection with the spirochete *Treponema pallidum*. The disease is chronic with subacute symptomatic periods and asymptomatic intervals during which the diagnosis can be made only serologically. Because of its ability to involve all organ systems and the variability of its clinical presentations, syphilis has been called "the great imitator." The infection is acquired almost entirely by sexual contact, although it must be recognized that this term encompasses far more than coitus.

ETIOLOGY. The genus *Treponema* includes at least three

species pathogenic for man: *Treponema carateum,* the agent of pinta; *Treponema pertenue,* the agent of yaws; and *T. pallidum,* the agent of syphilis. Bejel, a nonvenereal infection, is caused by an organism that is indistinguishable from *T. pallidum* and is usually referred to as a subspecies. Some believe that *T. pallidum* evolved as the cause of venereal syphilis from the older organisms responsible for the nonvenereal treponematoses. Infection with any of these agents elicits reactive serologic test results for syphilis.

T. pallidum is a fine spiral organism approximately 0.15 μm wide and 6 to 15 μm long. The organism is poorly visualized with routine microbiologic and histologic stains, but it can be seen in tissue with a variety of silver stains and is identified by darkfield microscopy in fluid recovered from lesions or lymph nodes. When observed in the living state, the organism displays 6 to 14 regular spirals that are maintained during its movements. *T. pallidum* has a characteristic motility that helps the observer to differentiate it from other spirochetes. The organism is seen to rotate in corkscrew fashion around the long axis of the cylinder formed by its spirals. it moves forward and backward along this axis and is sometimes observed to bend at its midpoint.

T. pallidum has a trilaminar outer membrane similar to that seen in gram-negative bacteria. Unlike these, however, *T. pallidum* has not been shown to possess a biologically active endotoxin.

The spirochete is microaerophilic and survives poorly in atmospheric oxygen. This, in addition to its sensitivity to drying and to extremes of temperature, explains in part its almost exclusively venereal mode of transmission. It undergoes limited replication in tissue culture systems, and its viability and virulence can be maintained only by serial passage in susceptible animals, principally rabbits. The inability to culture the organism has increased our dependence on clinical, microscopic, and serologic diagnosis.

Fortunately, *T. pallidum* has remained sensitive to most antibiotics used for the treatment of syphilis. The organism appears to be killed with first-order kinetics; a maximal rate of killings occurs at 0.1 μg/ml of penicillin. Exposing organisms to higher concentrations of penicillin does not increase the rate at which they are killed. Thus syphilis can be cured by treatments that present the spirochete with very low levels of penicillin. On the other hand, a relatively long course of therapy is required to eradicate the infecting organisms, since the rate of killing is for the most part uninfluenced by increasing the dose of antibiotic administered.

EPIDEMIOLOGY. The venereal nature of syphilis is clearly established and was recognized in its earliest descriptions. As one would expect, the disease is prevalent among the sexual partners of infected patients. Syphilis appears to develop in 30% to 50% of these people, but some have had many exposures to the infected partner, whereas others have had only a single sexual contact. Thus, although the 30% to 50% figure represents an average prevalence, the risks to an individual cannot be quantitated. There is no estimate of the risk of acquiring syphilis from a single sexual exposure to an infected partner; this clearly depends on the type of exposure and the specific condition of the active lesions. The risk to sexual partners, however, is considered sufficiently high to indicate a need for "epidemiologic treatment." Persons who within the past 90 days have been the sexual partners of patients with infectious syphilis should be treated even before their infections have been confirmed in the laboratory. This approach undoubtedly results in the treatment of uninfected people, but it eliminates the risk of failing to treat some infected individuals who

will not return for their test results, prevents the development of infectious lesions and further spread of disease, and often prevents the development of seroreactivity. Epidemiologic treatment has been a cornerstone of syphilis control in the United States.

Syphilis is most prevalent in sexually active populations and age-groups. The highest age-adjusted rates for early syphilis reported in the United States are found in 20- to 24-year-old men and women. Syphilis is also particularly prevalent among 24- to 34-year-old men. Interestingly, syphilis is prevalent in a somewhat older age group than gonorrhea. As with other sexually transmitted diseases, syphilis is more common in larger cities. The prevalence of infection is also increased in homosexual men; more than half of the cases in larger cities are reported in homosexual populations. More than one third of infected men are exclusively homosexual or bisexual, and overall the disease is three times more common in men than in women. Recently, however, the incidence of syphilis has decreased in some homosexual populations, as the sexual behavior of these groups has modified in response to the threat of acquired immunodeficiency syndrome (AIDS).

Other sexually transmitted diseases are prevalent among patients with syphilis, although the exact coincidence figures probably vary markedly among populations. In 1946, for example, gonorrhea was found in 23% of the patients with early syphilis, and syphilis was diagnosed in 8.4% of the patients with gonorrhea. The frequency with which gonorrhea and incubating syphilis occur in the same patient today is unknown but probably very low. This possibility previously served as one of the bases for regarding aqueous procaine penicillin G as the treatment of choice for uncomplicated gonococcal infection, for such treatment would also presumably abort the incubating syphilis. Although this therapeutic consideration may no longer be valid because the prevalence of syphilis among patients with gonorrhea is now low, patients with syphilis should still be carefully screened for other sexually transmitted diseases.

About 80,000 cases of syphilis in all stages are reported annually among American civilians. Of these some 30,000 are early syphilis, so defined because the disease is still potentially contagious. The number of reported cases of syphilis diminished rapidly after the introduction of penicillin in the late 1940s and reached a nadir in 1955. Although the prevalence of late syphilis has continued to decrease dramatically since the introduction of penicillin, the incidence of early syphilis initially rose and since the early 1960s had been relatively stable. The number of cases of early syphilis actually declined each year between 1981 and 1986, but during the first 3 months of 1987, the reported incidence increased by 22% compared to the same period in 1986. This increase is the largest reported in 10 years, and the resurgence occurred primarily among heterosexuals principally in association with drug abuse.

About one fifth of the patients with primary and secondary syphilis are identified serologically. Another two thirds of these patients present themselves for examination because they have noticed symptoms of illness or because they have been advised by sexual partners to seek medical attention. Finally, about one sixth of these patients are brought to treatment through the efforts of public health workers performing careful contact tracing. It is this last category that makes it particularly important to report cases of syphilis to the appropriate public health facility so that individuals with unsuspected infection can be diagnosed and treated.

Nonvenereal transmission. Syphilis can be spread by kissing a syphilitic individual with active oral lesions. Digital chancres have occasionally been noted to develop in dentists coming in contact with such lesions. Acquisition by transfusion is no longer a significant problem because serologic tests for syphilis are routinely performed on donated blood and because *T. pallidum* does not survive some of the current methods of prolonged blood storage. The disease has been acquired from contaminated needles, but this is an extraordinarily rare occurrence.

Syphilis can be contracted from intimate but nonvenereal contact with an infected person. Cases of children acquiring syphilis by sharing a bed with an infected parent have been reported. However, acquired syphilis in a child should raise the question of child abuse in the mind of the examiner, and the possibility should be discreetly but thoroughly investigated.

The most important nonvenereal mode of acquisition occurs in utero. Congenital infection begins with maternal spirochetemia, which usually occurs early in infection. Thus the risk of congenital syphilis is increased if syphilis is acquired during pregnancy. Penicillin administered to pregnant women in doses appropriate to cure their syphilis also eradicates the infection in the fetus. Babies vaginally delivered of mothers with active genital lesions can acquire syphilis during the birth process, and a typical primary chancre can develop.

PATHOGENESIS. *T. pallidum* can penetrate intact mucous membranes or infect via tiny cuts or abrasions in cornified epithelium. The minimal infecting dose in experimental syphilis is two spirochetes injected intradermally. The organism divides every 30 to 33 hours, and lesions appear when the organisms have attained a concentration of approximately $10^7/$g of tissue. Very early in infection, well before the first lesion appears or the blood test becomes reactive, spirochetes enter the blood and lymphatic systems and widely disseminate.

Two relatively nonspecific pathologic lesions characterize syphilis. The first is an obliterative endarteritis manifested as endothelial proliferation and perivascular infiltration primarily with mononuclear cells. This process can impair blood flow. Involvement of blood vessels in the central nervous system (CNS) gives rise to many of the neurologic sequelae of late syphilis, and involvement of the vasa vasorum can damage large blood vessels and lead to the syndromes of cardiovascular syphilis.

The second characteristic lesion of syphilis is a granulomatous reaction called a gumma. The granuloma is nonspecific and invites confusion with other chronic infections and granulomatous diseases of unknown origin including sarcoidosis and Crohn's disease. Gummas can occur in any organ, and when they involve the skin, they give rise to the characteristic lesions of late "benign" syphilis.

Immunologic processes contribute to the pathogenesis. Work with experimental human syphilis suggests that the gumma is a manifestation of delayed hypersensitivity in the immune host. For many years it was believed that a fetus of less than 16 weeks' gestation would not be invaded by spirochetes. This conclusion was based on the consistent lack of pathologic evidence of congenital syphilis in early abortuses. Recent work, however, has shown that spirochetes do indeed cross the placenta early in gestation but that before 16 weeks the fetus fails to mount an inflammatory reaction to the microorganisms, and the infection remains clinically inapparent. Thus immune processes appear to be of great significance in the pathogenesis of congenital syphilis.

Antigen-antibody complexes have been detected in the blood of patients with secondary syphilis. These complexes are responsible for the glomerulonephritis and nephrotic syndrome that occasionally accompany this stage. Treatment of primary

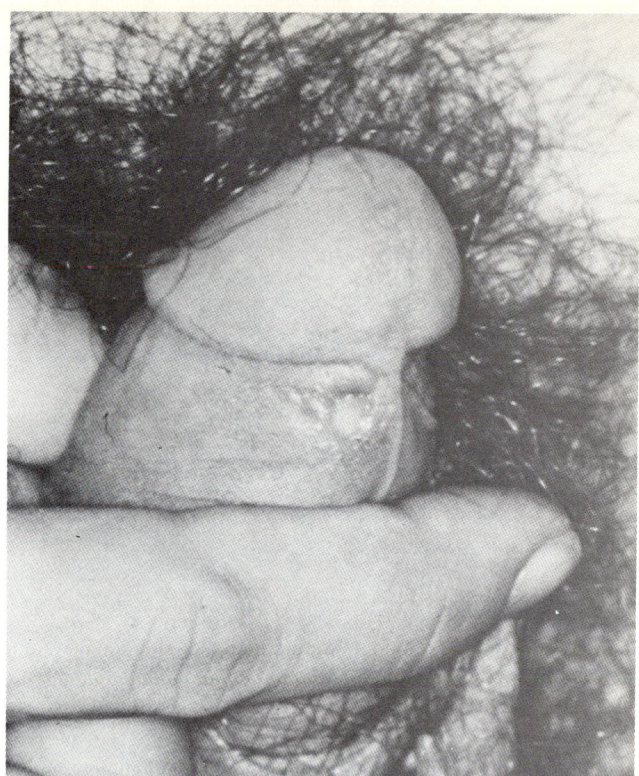

Fig. 52-1   Penile chancre.

or secondary syphilis often results in an acute, febrile response known as the Jarisch-Herxheimer reaction. Although the pathogenesis of this reaction remains incompletely defined, one attractive explanation is that it results from the rapid lysis of spirochetes with the subsequent release of bacterial antigen and exacerbation of immune-complex disease.

Patients with syphilis develop antibodies directed against a variety of lipids. These antibodies are detected by the standard nontreponemal tests for syphilis. Lipids cross-reacting with these antibodies are found in the liver, heart, brain, and mitochondria and raise the possibility that some manifestations of syphilis may have an autoimmune basis. The pathogenetic role of such antibodies, however, is speculative at present.

CLINICAL MANIFESTATIONS. In the early nineteenth century the natural history of syphilis was divided into stages. After acquiring the organism but before clinical or serologic manifestations develop, patients are said to have incubating syphilis. Spirochetemia occurs early, and such patients may be able to transmit syphilis via blood transfusion or transplacentally.

Primary syphilis. The incubation period for syphilis can range from 10 to 90 days but generally lasts about 3 weeks. At that time a lesion, the chancre, develops at the point of initial inoculation of the spirochete. The chancre typically begins as a papule that subsequently erodes to form a gradually enlarging ulcer with a clean base and an indurated edge (Fig. 52-1). The chancre can be slightly tender, but severe pain is extremely rare. Although the classic chancre of primary syphilis is a single lesion, in recent series almost half of the patients with proven primary syphilis had more than one penile ulcer. If the infected patient's normal skin comes in contact with the chancre, autoinoculation can produce additional lesions. Although most chancres appear on the genitalia, the clinician must always bear in mind the possible syphilitic origin of sores on other parts of the body. Chancres of the gum, throat and tonsil, lip, nipple, hand, and a variety of other anatomic sites have been well described.

The appearance of chancres is highly variable, and the differential diagnosis of uncerative lesions of the genitalia can be difficult. Herpes simplex genital infection usually occurs initially as grouped, umbilicated vesicles on an erythematous base that subsequently ulcerate to form groups of painful lesions. Chancroid produces one or more painful ulcers that are usually ragged and have necrotic bases. Lymphogranuloma venereum often produces a tiny primary ulceration that goes unnoticed by 70% of the infected men and almost all infected women. Tularemia and Behçet's syndrome are discussed in Chapters 47 and 15, respectively.

Relatively painless, usually bilateral, inguinal adenopathy (satellite bubo) appears in 50% to 70% of the patients with primary syphilis of the genitalia. Since the cervix and the proximal portion of the vagina are drained by deep inguinal nodes, satellite bubo does not occur in women with chancres at these sites. Regional adenopathy can, however, accompany primary inoculation at other sites. The patient with an oral, gingival, tonsillar, or pharyngeal chancre often manifests anterior cervical adenopathy. Sometimes the chancre can go completely unnoticed, and the patient appears to have isolated adenopathy. Affected nodes generally become enlarged about 7 days after the appearance of the chancre. They usually occur as a chain and are discrete, firm, and freely movable.

Primary syphilis can go unnoticed by the patient, particularly if the chancre develops in an area not routinely examined. Subcurative doses of antibiotics can modify or almost entirely eliminate the chancre. Primary syphilis per se does not occur in patients with congenital syphilis in which organisms are introduced directly into the bloodstream.

Even without treatment, the chancre heals completely within about 4 to 6 weeks, and the regional adenopathy resolves.

Secondary syphilis. In 2 to 8 weeks after the appearance of the chancre, the manifestations of secondary syphilis can develop. The course is highly variable and can range from 2 weeks to 6 months. In most cases the chancre already has healed by the time secondary syphilis appears, but sometimes primary and secondary syphilis overlap. Secondary syphilis is a generalized illness that often begins as a syndrome suggesting a viral infection. Headache, sore throat, and low-grade fever are common, and some health-care workers have described a nasal discharge as part of the syndrome. Mild leukocytosis with a relative lymphocytosis frequently occurs, but atypical lymphocytes are not seen, a feature that can help to differentiate the syndrome from infectious mononucleosis.

The hallmarks of secondary syphilis are lymphadenopathy and lesions of the skin and mucous membranes. Adenopathy, often generalized, is described in 75% of the affected patients. The nodal groups most commonly involved are the inguinal, suboccipital, posterior auricular, and cervical, particularly the posterior cervical chains. Epitrochlear adenopathy is seen frequently and should raise suspicions of secondary syphilis, although it also occurs with other conditions causing generalized lymphadenopathy, particularly infectious mononucleosis, sarcoidosis, and lymphoma. Affected nodes are usually discrete, relatively nontender, firm, and freely movable. Suppuration is extremely uncommon, and periadenitis and lymphangitis are rare.

Skin lesions are found in 80% of the infected patients, but they are highly variable, and diligent examination is often required. The lesions are protean and have contributed much

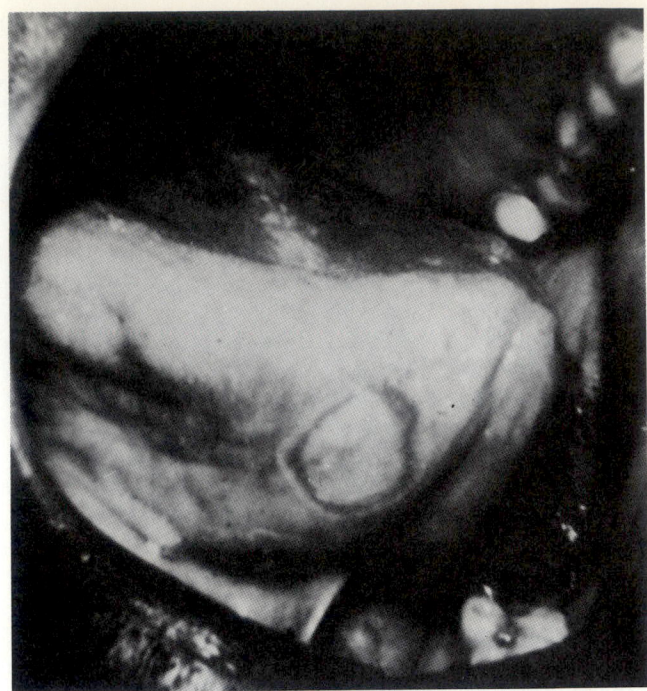

Fig. 52-2   Mucous patch in patient with secondary syphilis. (Courtesy of Department of Health and Human Services, Centers for Disease Control, Atlanta, Ga.)

to the status of syphilis as the great imitator. Macular lesions are seen in about one third of the patients, primarily over the flanks, abdomen, shoulders, and back. They are generally bilaterally symmetric, tend to follow lines of skin cleavage, and have a coppery or boiled ham color. The lesions are only mildly if at all pruritic, and severe pruritus argues against a diagnosis of secondary syphilis. The rash almost invariably involves the genitalia, and when generalized it is frequently prominent on the palms and soles, a distribution highly suggestive of syphilis. Maculopapular lesions are also commonly seen, and follicular lesions can be particularly prevalent on the back and extensor surfaces of the extremities. Somewhat less common skin lesions include annular lesions appearing principally around the face and pustular lesions, which are seen in only about 2% of the patients. Vesicles or bullae are rare in secondary syphilis in adults, although they may be seen in congenital syphilis.

The mucous membranes are involved in more than half of the cases of secondary syphilis. Here again, however, the lesions can be sufficiently subtle to avoid detection by casual examination. It is important to use a tongue blade and to examine the buccal mucosa and the undersurface of the tongue completely. Mucous patches develop in about one third of the patients. These are painless, oval ulcerations usually covered with a grayish or yellowish membrane (Fig. 52-2). Split papules may be observed at the corners of the mouth.

Condylomata lata are flat, hypertrophic lesions resembling warts and develop in moist areas. They are frequently found around the anus or vagina and occasionally in the axilla or under the breasts. They do not reflect areas of inoculation with *T. pallidum* but are manifestations of hematogenous dissemination.

The moist lesions of secondary syphilis (mucous patches, condylomata lata) contain large numbers of spirochetes and must be considered potentially contagious. Dry lesions can reveal spirochetes if vigorously abraded, but their potential for spreading infection is considerably lower. This discrepancy further supports the venereal nature of syphilis.

Patchy, nonpruritic alopecia can involve the scalp, the beard, or even the eyebrows and suggests secondary syphilis.

The degree of clinical overlap between secondary syphilis and a variety of other dermatologic and generalized diseases is very high. Therefore the clinician should have a low threshold of suspicion for secondary syphilis and should be willing to order nontreponemal tests (such as the Venereal Disease Research Laboratories [VDRL] or Rapid Plasma Reagin [RPR] tests) to confirm or rule out the diagnosis. It is important to remember that about one fifth of men and almost half of women with secondary syphilis do not give a history of a specific primary lesion.

Although CNS symptoms accompany only about 2% of the cases of secondary syphilis, asymptomatic involvement of the CNS occurs in about one third of the patients and can be manifested by pleocytosis, elevated protein, and reactive nontreponemal tests for syphilis in the cerebrospinal fluid (CSF). It has long been thought that such asymptomatic CNS involvement does not require special therapy and responds to standard treatments for secondary syphilis. Recent preliminary data have called this concept into question, and physicians are advised to consult current guidelines regarding the possible need for initial or follow-up examination of CSF in patients being treated for early syphilis. Symptomatic involvement of the CNS occurs in approximately 2% of the affected patients, and in many of these, acute syphilitic meningitis develops. In such a case the CSF can contain 500 white cells/mm^3, principally mononuclear cells. CSF protein is frequently in excess of 100 mg/ml. The symptoms are those of basilar meningitis, with meningeal signs and cranial nerve involvement in more than half of the patients. Such patients should probably be treated with penicillin intravenously in the high doses that are effective for pneumococcal and meningococcal meningitis as well.

Hepatitis is occasionally described in secondary syphilis, but splenomegaly is quite rare. Nephritis and even a nephrotic syndrome develop in some patients because of antigen-antibody complex deposition in the glomeruli. Uveitis and osteitis are occasionally observed.

Secondary syphilis usually resolves within 2 to 6 weeks even in the absence of therapy, although some of the lesions may heal with scarring.

Latent syphilis. With the disappearance of the stigmata of secondary syphilis, patients enter a stage of latency in which the diagnosis can be made only serologically. This stage is usually divided into early latency (within 1 to 2 years of infection) and late latency (thereafter). The distinction is important because during early latency at least 25% of the patients have one or more mucocutaneous relapses during which the dermatologic and systemic manifestations of secondary syphilis reappear. At these times patients once again become infectious to sexual partners and, if pregnant, can transmit infection to the fetus. Most of these relapses occur within the first year following the acquisition of syphilis, and they are extremely rare after 4 years of latency. Thus after 4 years patients are no longer public health hazards.

About one third of the patients who enter latency are spontaneously cured of their disease with a gradual return of nontreponemal serologic tests to nonreactive. Another one-third of the patients remain seroreactive and presumably infected but never have further clinical manifestations of disease. Late syphilis develops in the remaining one third of the patients. Thus latent syphilis is likely to lead to significant clinical disease in a sizable minority of affected patients. Attempts to detect unsuspected latent syphilis by serologic screening constitute the majority of the millions of serologic tests for syphilis performed in the United States annually.

Late syphilis. Late benign syphilis is the term applied to granulomatous (gummatous) involvement, which may affect about 15% of untreated syphilitic individuals and appears many years after acquisition of the disease. The granulomata destroy surrounding tissue, but their rate of progression and the degree of inflammation can be low. Gummas of the skin display a variety of clinical features. Small numbers of solitary or grouped lesions, distributed asymmetrically about the body, are often indurated and indolent. An arciform configuration with the borders of lesions forming segments of circles is suggestive of syphilis. Lesions can be serpiginous, healing in one area while advancing in another area. Active lesions usually have a sharp margin, and ulcers can have a punched-out appearance with peripheral hyperpigmentation. Gummas often heal with atrophic, superficial scarring, but their destructive clinical picture can erroneously suggest malignancy. The biopsy is nonspecific, revealing granulomata. Organisms are rarely seen.

Gummas can also involve the viscera, resulting in gastrointestinal or hepatic disease. Bones are frequently involved, with periostitis characterized by thickening and with localized increases in bone density and destructive lesions surrounded by sclerosis. The tibia is involved in about half of the patients and the clavicle, skull, or fibula in about one fourth each.

In about 10% of persons with untreated syphilis, late cardiovascular manifestations develop. The mean age at diagnosis is 65 years, and the disease is almost twice as common in men as in women. These observations have led to the theory that prolonged cardiac strain, perhaps related to a lifetime of manual labor, or diastolic hypertension might contribute to the pathogenesis. *T. pallidum* can directly affect the aortic endothelium, and the involved aorta shows a characteristic irregularity of the intima reminiscent of tree bark. The aortic valve cusps themselves can be involved, with rolling and thickening leading to aortic insufficiency, to which weakening and dilation of the aortic valve ring can contribute. Aortic insufficiency decreases coronary perfusion, and the coronary arteries themselves can be directly involved in the endarteritic process leading to coronary occlusion. Endarteritis of the vasa vasora causes ischemia and weakening of the aortic media, and an aortic aneurysm that is more commonly saccular than fusiform can then develop. About half of syphilitic aneurysms occur in the aortic arch, and another 40% involve other parts of the thoracic aorta. The abdominal aorta is involved in only 10% of syphilitic aneurysms.

Patients with cardiovascular syphilis can be asymptomatic for long periods of time. Early clues to the diagnosis include the observation of localized aortic bulging on chest roentgenogram; an altered aortic second sound, sometimes described as having a tambour quality; an aortic diastolic murmur in a young person, and precordial chest pain in a young person without other predisposing factors. Clinical or serologic evidence of syphilis of course supports the diagnosis. Later, symptoms of aortic insufficiency develop. Symptoms of congestive heart failure or angina generally develop, but dissection of an aortic aneurysm is uncommon. The value of antisyphilitic therapy remains controversial; treatment certainly does not reverse existing cardiac damage. There is some suggestion, however, that appropriate therapy can slow the progression of the disease.

In about 8% of untreated persons, late syphilis affects the CNS. CNS involvement has been detected in 15% to 40% of the patients with cardiovascular syphilis, although in this setting it is usually mild. CNS involvement is initially asymptomatic and in this stage can be detected only by examination of the CSF. Thus CSF should be examined in all patients being treated for syphilis of more than 1 year's duration or whose disease is of unknown duration. The CSF should also be examined in patients who have had a suboptimal serologic response to therapy for early syphilis, since unsuspected, asymptomatic neurosyphilis may account for a small percentage of "treatment failures."

In untreated persons symptoms of neurosyphilis can develop. Meningovascular syphilis results from syphilitic endarteritis and is usually manifested as seizures or cerebrovascular accident. Symptoms can develop 5 to 10 years after the acquisition of syphilis, and a cerebrovascular accident in a young person with no history of hypertension should prompt evaluation for meningovascular syphilis. In a few patients meningeal signs predominate, and syptoms suggesting a basilar meningitis can develop. These patients usually have a lymphocytic pleocytosis and increased protein in the CSF. The VDRL test of spinal fluid (see "Serologic tests") is almost always positive and should be regarded as diagnostic of this form of syphilis because false positive reactions in the CSF are rare.

Spirochetes also involve the substance of the brain directly. Within 15 to 20 years after acquiring syphilis, general paresis may develop, usually as a disorder of higher cerebral functions. The patients may suffer personality changes and dementia. Delusional states are common and have been frequently portrayed in song and story. Sometimes the patients have the Argyll Roberston pupil, which is small and further constricts with accommodation but does not react to light, a finding highly suggestive of neurosyphilis. Some series suggest that the CSF is always abnormal, and the serologic tests for syphilis on serum and CSF are invariably reactive. The concept is misleading, however, and depends on the fact that since dementia has multiple causes, the diagnosis of paresis is usually dependent on positive serologic tests.

Tabes dorsalis resulting from involvement of the posterior columns and dorsal roots of the spinal cord usually develops somewhat later, often 30 years after acquiring syphilis. Affected individuals often manifest loss of vibration sense and proprioception resulting in a characteristic broad-based gait. Patients also complain of severe, sharp pains (lightning pains) that can affect any part of the body. Impotence and bladder dysfunction are relatively common. Optic atrophy can be seen in one fourth of the affected patients, and Argyll Robertson pupils are more common than in paresis. The syndrome of tabes dorsalis accounts for somewhat less than half of all cases of neurosyphilis. It is considered sufficiently characteristic that it can be diagnosed clinically. Thus it is not surprising that some patients with tabes have normal CSF and some have nonreactive nontreponemal tests for syphilis on serum and CSF.

Congenital syphilis. Spirochetemia during pregnancy can result in syphilitic placentitis and subsequent infusion of spirochetes into the fetus via the umbilical vein. Babies with congenital syphilis can be completely normal at birth but often have highly suggestive stigmata. Disseminated lesions of the skin and mucous membranes can develop in affected children. The nasal mucous membranes are particularly susceptible, and syphilitic involvement results in snuffles, a persistent, mucopurulent nasal discharge containing large numbers of spirochetes. Hemorrhagic rhinitis eventuates in severe cases and is almost pathognomonic of congenital syphilis. Condylomata

lata, which are frequently seen in secondary syphilis in adults, occur in moist areas, often around the anus or vagina in babies, and contain large numbers of spirochetes. Roentgenographic evidence of bone involvement is seen in almost all babies with congenital syphilis. The long bones show a characteristic area of provisional calcification at the epiphysis that surmounts an area of rarefaction. Proximally, there is moth-eaten calcification of the metaphysis with tongues of calcium protruding into the area of rarefaction. Periostitis can result in concentric layers of subperiosteal bone formation, giving a layered appearance to the shafts of long bones. Wimberger's sign (bilateral rarefaction of the medial tibial metaphyses) is highly suggestive of congenital syphilis. Skeletal involvement can create pain on movement resulting in voluntary splinting of an extremity, the pseudoparalysis of Parrot.

Many other signs are relatively common in congenital syphilis but are less specific. Neonatal hepatosplenomegaly and jaundice are seen in about one fifth of the infected patients. Skin lesions can be diffuse and involve the palms and soles. They are often, however, associated with a diaper rash distribution. The lesions can closely resemble those of secondary syphilis in adults, but bullous lesions are considerably more common in congenital syphilis.

Approximately 75% to 90% of cases of congenital syphilis are diagnosed in patients over 10 years old. This distressing finding indicates the flaws in the neonatal health care delivery system and also suggests the need for clinicians to be aware of the late manifestations of congenital syphilis. The hutchinsonian triad is traditionally associated with late congenital syphilis. One element, Hutchinson's teeth, is generally recognized only after the eruption of the permanent central and lateral incisors at 7 years of age (Fig. 52-3). The affected teeth are shorter and narrower than normal. The middle third of the tooth is most severely affected, resulting in the appearance of a semilunar notch in the center of the edge. The central third of the tooth can also be discolored because of an incomplete enamel covering. Hutchinson's teeth have been diagnosed before eruption on the basis of dental roentgenograms. The six-year molar can also be affected, with distortion of the cusps yielding a mulberry-like appearance. A second element of the triad is interstitial keratitis, usually appearing between 5 and 20 years of age. The inflammation is manifested by photophobia, eye pain, blurred vision, and tearing; it can be chronic. Spirochetes are not found in the eye in this setting, and the mechanism is incompletely understood. Nerve deafness completes the triad. Characteristic fissures around the mouth and anus, called rhagades, are rare, and the mechanism is unknown. Skeletal lesions can be hypertrophic, with new-bone formation resulting in anterior bowing of the tibia (saber shins) or enlargement of the medial end of the clavicle. Erosive lesions occasionally result in perforation of the palate, and syphilis was once its most common cause. Collapse of the nasal bones can produce a saddle nose deformity.

LABORATORY FINDINGS. Syphilis is most convincingly diagnosed by demonstrating typically motile spirochetes in a lesion. Because of its small size and poor staining characteristics, *T. pallidum* is best observed by darkfield microscopy, in which the organisms are visualized with reflected rather than transmitted light. Chancres, mucous patches, and condylomata lata usually test positive for the organism, but differentiating *T. pallidum* from normal spirochetal flora of the mouth or vagina can be difficult. Dry skin lesions of secondary syphilis are occasionally darkfield positive. Proper preparation of the lesion is crucial and involves cleaning its surface and lightly abrading it so that relatively blood-free tissue fluid can be

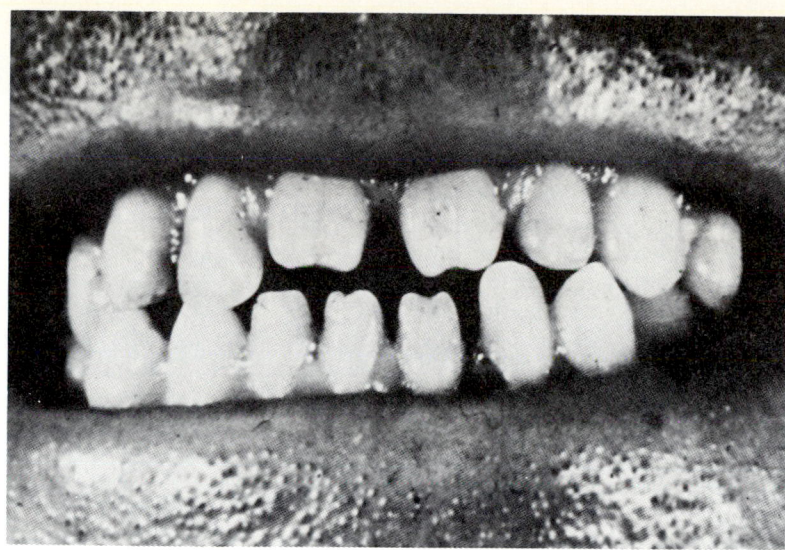

Fig. 52-3 Hutchinson's teeth in patient with late congenital syphilis. (Courtesy of Department of Health and Human Services, Centers for Disease Control, Atlanta, Ga.)

collected and examined as a wet mount. Darkfield diagnosis can be difficult and is best left to clinicians with previous experience.

Serologic tests. Patients with syphilis usually have antibodies directed against a poorly defined lipid that may be a component of the spirochete. Cross-reacting lipids are found in a variety of normal tissues and serve as the basis for the nontreponemal tests for syphilis, which employ a lipid extracted from beef heart (cardiolipin) as an antigen. The antigen is mixed with patient's serum, and clumping of the antigen particles is detected by a variety of techniques that vary among the tests. Nontreponemal tests are inexpensive and technically easy to perform. Many such tests have been developed in the past, but those commonly in use today are the VDRL test, the RPR test, and the Automated Reagin Test (ART). Any of these tests can be positive in a variety of other conditions, including acute viral illnesses such as varicella, hepatitis, and infectious mononucleosis; bacterial infections such as leprosy, tuberculosis, and leptospirosis; and disorders associated with the formation of unusual immunoglobulins such as intravenous drug abuse and collagen vascular diseases.

Nontreponemal tests can be quantitated, and the results are usually expressed as the highest dilution of serum yielding a positive reaction. The clinician should be cautioned, however, that the RPR and ART can yield titers twofold to eightfold higher than those obtained with the VDRL on the same serum. Since rising or falling titers can have great clinical significance, patients observed over a period of time should be studied with the same nontreponemal test.

Patients with syphilis also have antitreponemal antibodies that can be detected by a variety of procedures using *T. pallidum* as the antigen. The fluorescent treponemal antibody absorption (FTA-ABS) test detects antitreponemal antibody by an indirect fluorescence method using spirochetes attached to a slide. Although the FTA-ABS test requires a fluorescence microscope and is more technically demanding than the nontreponemal tests, it is the current standard for the diagnosis of syphilis. The microhemagglutination test for *T. pallidum* (MHA-TP) uses treponemal antigens attached to the surface of erythrocytes, which will agglutinate when mixed with the serum from patients with syphilis. This test is considerably easier

to perform than the FTA-ABS test and is now in common use. It is, however, slightly less sensitive than the FTA-ABS test. Treponemal tests are generally used to confirm the diagnosis of syphilis in patients with reactive nontreponemal tests.

The interpretation of serologic tests for syphilis has resulted in some confusion. Certain facts should be borne in mind. Both the treponemal and nontreponemal tests can be nonreactive in the patient who has just developed a chancre. Thus a nonreactive test for syphilis does not rule out the diagnosis in the patient whose lesion has just appeared. Of such patients, about 10% have a nonreactive nontreponemal test but a reactive treponemal test for syphilis. In secondary syphilis essentially all of the serologic tests are reactive. This is particularly useful because the clinical diagnosis of secondary syphilis can be difficult. Thus a negative quantitative (that is, serially diluted) nontreponemal serologic test for syphilis essentially rules out secondary syphilis. Unfortunately, nontreponemal tests for syphilis frequently become nonreactive in patients with late syphilis. Fully 50% of patients diagnosed as having tabes dorsalis have a nonreactive nontreponemal test for syphilis. Patients being evaluated for late syphilis should have a treponemal test performed even if the nontreponemal tests are nonreactive because many of these patients can be diagnosed only by the more sensitive treponemal tests. Following adequate treatment of syphilis, the titer of the nontreponemal tests should drop at least fourfold (for example, from 1:32 before treatment to 1:8 or less after treatment), but such reductions usually require about 3 months. Within 2 years of adequate treatment, the VDRL returns to nonreactive in about 95% of the patients with primary syphilis and 75% of those with secondary syphilis. Patients with syphilis of longer than 2 years' duration can have a persistently positive nontreponemal test for syphilis. The treponemal tests remain positive for many years (possibly for life) even after adequate treatment of syphilis. Thus a persistently positive treponemal test is not an indication for retreating patients with a prior history of adequate therapy. A rise in titer of the nontreponemal tests, however, can indicate relapse or reinfection and indeed can indicate a need for retreating patients previously thought to have been adequately treated.

Serodiagnosis of neonatal congenital syphilis poses special problems because it can be difficult to differentiate fetal antibody synthesized in response to in utero infection from trans-placentally acquired maternal antibody. Tests based on the identification of IgM antibody that does not cross the placenta are beset by an apparent lack of sensitivity and specificity.

MANAGEMENT. Penicillin G remains the treatment of choice for all stages of syphilis in patients who are not hypersensitive to the drug. Duration of therapy is important, and treatment for early syphilis is usually based on the administration of benzathine penicillin G, which produces very low serum levels persisting for 3 weeks following a single intramuscular injection. Early syphilis (up to 1 year) can be adequately treated with a single administration of 2.4 million units of benzathine penicillin G. Syphilis of more than 1 year's duration, with the possible exception of neurosyphilis, can be adequately treated with three or four weekly injections of the same dose of benzathine penicillin G. The therapy for neurosyphilis remains somewhat controversial because of the relatively poor penetration of penicillin into the CSF. Therefore syphilis of the CNS might better be treated with regimens producing considerably higher levels, such as aqueous penicillin G by continuous intravenous administration at a rate of 20 million units a day for at least 10 days. Congenital syphilis that has spared the CNS can be treated with benzathine penicillin G, but if the CNS is involved, a penicillin regimen yielding higher serum levels should be used.

Patients allergic to penicillin can be treated with doxycycline (100 mg orally twice daily) or tetracycline (500 mg orally every 6 hours) to which the spirochete is sensitive. These regimens generally involve taking the medication for 2 weeks for syphilis of less than 1 year's duration and for 4 weeks in all other circumstances. They require considerable patient compliance. The overall efficacy of drugs other than penicillin in the treatment of syphilis has been less well established, and the history of penicillin allergy should be carefully investigated in patients requiring treatment for syphilis. Recent observations indicate that some isolates of *T. pallidum* are resistant to erythromycin.

The management of syphilis in patients infected with human immunodeficiency virus (HIV) remains controversial. Symptomatic involvement of the CNS appears to occur earlier among patients with the acquired immunodeficiency syndrome than it does in normal hosts. All patients with syphilis should be tested for HIV infection, and patients with dual infections should be treated with high-dose regimens effective for CNS syphilis.

More than half of the patients treated for early syphilis with penicillin have a Jarisch-Herxheimer reaction, usually beginning within 6 hours of treatment. The reaction consists of fever, a transient exacerbation of skin lesions or adenopathy, occasional arthralgias, and, rarely, transient hypotension. The reaction is usually mild and abates in less than 24 hours. It can be managed with aspirin and reassurance.

BIBLIOGRAPHY

Brown ST and others: Serological response to syphilis treatment: a new analysis of old data, JAMA 253:1296, 1985.
Chapel TA: The variability of syphilitic chancres, Sex Transm Dis 5:68, 1978.
Chapel TA: The signs and symptoms of secondary syphilis, Sex Transm Dis 7:161, 1980.
Crissey JT and Denenholz DA: Syphilis, Clin Dermatol 2:1, 1984.
Hart G: Syphilis tests in diagnostic and therapeutic decision making, Ann Intern Med 104:368, 1986.
Jaffe HW: The laboratory diagnosis of syphilis: new concepts, Ann Intern Med 83:846, 1975.
Kampmeier RH: The late manifestations of syphilis: skeletal, visceral, and cardiovascular, Med Clin North Am 48:667, 1964.
Krolls SO and others: Oral manifestations of syphilis, Hosp Med 8:14, 1972.
Sparling PF: Diagnosis and treatment of syphilis, N Engl J Med 284:642, 1971.
Stokes JH, Beerman H, and Ingraham NR: Modern clinical syphilology, Philadelphia, 1944, WB Saunders Co.
Syphilis: a synopsis, Washington, DC, 1968, USPHS Pub no 1660.
Syphilotherapy 1976: position papers for the current USPHS recommendation, J Am Vener Dis Assoc 3:98, 1976.

Rat-bite fever

Merle A. Sande

"Rat-bite fever" is a term used to describe two distinct types of febrile illnesses that usually follow the bite of a rat, mouse, or other rodent. The more common in the United States is caused by *Streptobacillus moniliformis* and has become predominantly a disease of laboratory workers. The second is caused by a spirochete, *Spirillum minus*.

STREPTOBACILLARY RAT-BITE FEVER

S. moniliformis is a pleomorphic, gram-negative bacillus found in the oropharynx of over 50% of healthy rats. It can cause pneumonia, conjunctivitis, or other infections in rats, mice, turkeys, and guinea pigs. It usually causes disease in humans following an animal bite, but contact with dead rodents and ingestion of contaminated milk (Haverhill fever) have been implicated in human outbreaks. Disease occurs most commonly in persons having contact with rats (laboratory workers, children, slum dwellers) and has a worldwide distribution.

CLINICAL MANIFESTATIONS. Usually within 10 days following the animal bite, fever and shaking chills; headache; severe myalgias, especially in the back; weakness; and vomiting develop. These symptoms are followed in several days by arthralgias and frank arthritis usually involving multiple large joints, especially the wrists and elbows. On the third day of illness a morbilliform or petechial rash appears in over 90% of cases. The initial bite heals well. Symptoms typically remit after 2 to 5 days but can relapse at irregular intervals for weeks to months. Endocarditis and pericarditis have been reported and can lead to death.

LABORATORY FINDINGS. Leukocytosis is common, with white blood cell counts ranging from 6000 to 30,000/mm³. Biologically false serologic tests for syphilis have been reported in 25% of cases. The diagnosis is established by isolating the bacteria from blood or joint fluid. The organism grows well in ordinary nutrient media (trypticase soy broth or agar), particularly when supplemented with 20% horse serum and incubated in 5% to 10% CO_2. Growth can be slow, and cultures should be held for several weeks if this diagnosis is suspected.

DIFFERENTIAL DIAGNOSIS. Streptobacillary fever should be considered in any patient (especially a laboratory worker) who has been exposed to rats and has fever, arthritis, and rash. Other infections that should be ruled out include several viral diseases (rubella, hepatitis B, dengue, and the various arboviruses), Rocky Mountain spotted fever, disseminated gonococcal disease, meningococcemia, and leptospirosis.

MANAGEMENT. Either penicillin V or tetracycline administered orally (500 mg every 6 hours) or procaine penicillin (600,000 units intramuscularly every 12 hours for 10 days) is effective in reducing the duration of fever. The organism is also sensitive to many other antimicrobial drugs.

SPIRILLARY RAT-BITE FEVER

S. minus is a thick, tightly coiled, flagellated, gram-negative spirochete that is 2 to 5 µm in length and contains two to five spirals. It can be recognized in wet mounts of infected tissue by its rapid, darting motion. The organism produces an ocular infection in rats.

The disease in humans usually occurs at least 10 days after a rat bite. The primary site initially heals but then becomes inflamed, suppurates, and may ulcerate. Fever and regional adenitis develop and last for 3 to 5 days. An urticarial rash can occur but is usually less prominent than that seen in strepto-bacillary fever. Arthritis is rare. Recurrence of symptoms in several days is common.

The diagnosis is established by darkfield examination of aspirated material from the primary infected site or an involved lymph node. The organism has not been cultured. Treatment with either penicillin or streptomycin is effective.

Leptospirosis

Merle A. Sande

ETIOLOGY AND EPIDEMIOLOGY. "Leptospirosis" is a term used to identify several clinical entities caused by a single species of spirochete, *Leptospira interrogans*. Although documented relatively rarely (fewer than 100 cases per year reported in the United States), it probably accounts for a much higher number of cases of undiagnosed aseptic meningitis. *L. interrogans* is a primary pathogen for wild animals (foxes, skunks, opposums, rats) and domestic animals (cattle, dogs, cats) throughout the United States. It occasionally causes disease in animals. The organism commonly invades the renal tubules, where it can be asymptomatically excreted in the urine for years. Under optimal conditions it remains viable in soil or water for weeks. Humans are usually infected following contact with the contaminated environment. The spirochete penetrates mucous membranes or abrasions in the skin and rapidly and widely disseminates hematogenously. Most cases occur in the summer and fall, and the disease affects predominantly children, teenagers, and housewives. It also has been found in farmers, abbatoir workers, veterinarians, coal miners, sewer workers, and people who have swum in rivers or freshwater ponds. Since cross-infection between wild and domestic animal species can occur, household pets (even though vaccinated) can acquire and secrete the organism in their urine. Rats are the most common source of disease throughout the world except in the United States, where transmission is usually from dogs, livestock, and cats.

Over 130 serotypes have been identified and grouped into 16 serogroups. Some of the more common of these are *Leptospira pomona*, *Leptospira canicola*, *Leptospira icterohaemorrhagiae*, *Leptospira autumnalis*, and *Leptospira grippotyphosa*. There seems to be little relationship between these serogroups and the clinical syndrome, although historically *Leptospira icterohaemorrhagiae* has been associated with the severe form of the disease (Weil's disease).

CLINICAL MANIFESTATIONS. Most cases of leptospirosis are probably asymptomatic, as judged by the relatively high rate of seropositivity in persons with a high exposure to animals. In addition, over 90% of those with clinical disease have a relatively mild form. The typical illness is characterized by a biphasic pattern. Following a 1- to 2-week incubation period, the first or septicemic phase begins abruptly with high fever (102° F [39° C]), chills, frontal or generalized headache, severe muscle pains, malaise, prostration, conjunctival suffusion, and frequently cough or chest pain. Nausea, vomiting, and abdominal pain are common, and diarrhea can also occur. A rash can be present on the trunk. During this phase, which usually last

4 to 7 days, spirochetes can be isolated from the blood and cerebrospinal fluid (CSF). Symptoms then disappear as the leptospires are cleared from the bloodstream, and in many instances this signals the end of the illness.

The second or immune phase, which begins after 1 to 3 symptom-free days, can simulate the first phase except fever is usually mild and short lived or absent. Myalgias again dominate the clinical picture and are typically localized to the back and calves. The frontal or bitemporal headache is usually severe and constant and signifies the presence of aseptic meningitis. Nausea, vomiting, and abdominal pain are usually present. Examination of the CSF reveals pleocytosis (fewer than 1000 white blood cells/mm^3), mainly with lymphocytes, although polymorphonuclear leukocytes can predominate in the early phases. The CSF protein is elevated, and the glucose is normal. This disease is self-limited and almost never fatal. Mild delirium can occur, but other signs of CNS dysfunction are rare.

A small proportion (5% to 10%) of patients have the severe form of disease (Weil's disease), which is characterized by jaundice of the intrahepatic obstructive type without significant hepatic destruction and by renal failure with acute tubular necrosis and associated azotemia, proteinuria, pyuria, and hematuria. Alterations in mental function usually follow. Vascular collapse, severe hemorrhage, and death occur in 5% to 10% of these cases. Mortality is significantly increased in the older age-group. Myocarditis is common in the fatal disease. Leukocytosis is usually present, and hemolytic anemia and thrombocytopenia can occur. The initial stages of Weil's disease are similar to the less severe forms of leptospirosis, but high persistent fever, sometimes lasting several weeks, generally accompanies the second phase of the disease. The resolution of disease is usually complete, with occasional mild residual impairment of renal function.

DIAGNOSIS. The diagnosis is usually established retrospectively by serologic methods. The macroscopic slide agglutination is an excellent screening test, and the microscopic agglutination is more specific and used for confirmation. Antibodies against the *Leptospira* antigens usually appear during the second week of illness and reach peak titers in the third or fourth week. A fourfold rise in agglutinating antibody is diagnostic of leptospirosis. A single titer of greater than 1:100 by the microscopic agglutination test or a positive slide agglutination test is presumptive evidence when combined with a compatible clinical course. Patients rarely remain seronegative.

During the first or septicemic phase of illness (first week) organisms can be cultured from blood and CSF, and they then can be found in the urine for months following the clinical disease. Whole blood or CSF should be cultured on a semisolid medium such as the Fletcher medium or the Tween 80-albumin medium. Organisms also survive up to 11 days in noncitrated anticoagulated blood. Blood can then be sent to either state laboratories or the Centers for Disease Control for culture of the organisms if local facilities are unavailable.

Most cases of leptospirosis undoubtedly go undiagnosed because of the physician's failure to consider this organism in the differential diagnosis. it should be at least considered in any patient with a history of contact with animals who has a high fever and severe muscle pains, conjunctival suffusion, clinical symptoms of a biphasic temporal character, aseptic meningitis, or an ill-defined febrile illness.

MANAGEMENT. The efficacy of antimicrobial therapy for leptospirosis is open to question. Some studies suggest that either penicillin G or tetracycline can shorten the duration of fever or reduce the incidence of complications but only if given before the fifth day of illness. Thus in the vast majority of diagnosed cases the therapy is probably instituted after any benefit could be expected.

BIBLIOGRAPHY
Rat-bite fever

Cole JS, Stoll RW, and Bulger RJ: Rat bite fever: report of three cases, Ann Intern Med 71:979, 1969.

Murray HW: *Spirillum minor* (rat bite fever). In Mandell GL, Douglas RG Jr, and Bennett JE, editors: Principles and practice of infectious diseases, ed 2, New York, 1985, John Wiley & Sons, Inc.

Murray HW: *Streptobacillus moniliformis* (rat bite fever): In Mandell GL, Douglas RG Jr, and Bennett JE, editors: Principles and practice of infectious diseases, ed 2, New York, 1985, John Wiley & Sons, Inc.

Roughgarden JW: Antimicrobial therapy of rat bite fever, Arch Intern Med 116:39, 1965.

Leptospirosis

Farrar WE: *Leptospira* species. In Mandell GL, Douglas RG Jr, and Bennett JE, editors: Principles and practice of infectious diseases, ed 2, New York, 1985, John Wiley & Sons, Inc.

Feigin RD and Anderson D: Human leptospirosis, CRC Crit Rev Clin Lab Sci 5:413, 1975.

Lyme disease

George A. Poporad *and* Donald Kaye

Lyme disease (named for Lyme, Connecticut) is a syndrome that includes a characteristic skin rash, monarticular or oligoarticular arthritis, and neurologic and cardiac abnormalities.

EPIDEMIOLOGY AND ETIOLOGY. Cases have been described along the northeast shore of the United States from Long Island to Virginia, in the Midwest (Wisconsin, Minnesota), and in the West (California, Oregon). The disease is caused by a newly recognized spirochete named *Borrelia burgdorferi*. The spirochete is transmitted by a tick vector, usually *Ixodes dammini* in the United States or related *Ixodes* ticks. Disease manifestations are probably caused by both direct tissue invasion by the spirochete and the host's immunologic response.

CLINICAL MANIFESTATIONS. Lyme disease typically occurs in summer or fall. Initially the patient has a characteristic skin lesion called erythema chronicum migrans, which begins as an erythematous papule and develops into an expanding, red, flat, annular lesion usually with partial central clearing (Fig. 52-4). The lesion (occasionally multiple) is often on the proximal part of an extremity or on the trunk and can grow to be as large as 20 to 50 cm in diameter. It can itch or burn. Malaise, fatigue, fever, vomiting, headache, stiff neck, malar rash, sore throat, lymphadenopathy, and splenomegaly can occur with the rash or precede it by a few days. Some patients recall being bitten by a tick 4 days to 3 weeks before the onset of the rash. Typically the rash lasts 1 to 5 weeks, but evanescent lesions can recur.

Arthritis can appear within days of the onset of the rash or in some instances more than 2 years later. Intermittent, recurrent attacks of arthritis in several large joints, particularly the knee, are characteristic. Occasionally chronic arthritis develops. Fever, myalgias, headache, stiff neck, and the rash can occur with or precede the attacks of arthritis.

A small percentage of patients have neurologic abnormalities that appear while the rash is still present or 1 to 6 months later. The usual pattern is one of recurrent attacks of meningoencephalitis with superimposed cranial and peripheral radiculoneuropathy. The patient has weeks of illness alternating with weeks of well-being. Neurologic abnormalities such as facial paralysis, oculomotor weakness, peripheral motor weakness,

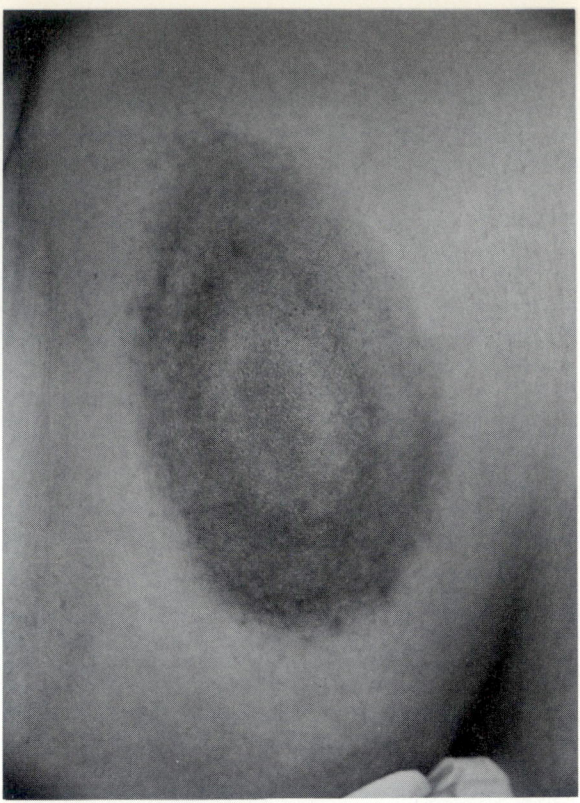

Fig. 52-4   Erythema chronicum migrans on chest wall and breast. Note its large size, ring pattern, and central clearing. (Courtesy of Joseph A Witkowski, MD.).

radicular pain, cerebellar ataxia, and chorea have been reported. Recovery generally occurs in 2 to 8 months.

Rarely, cardiac abnormalities develop from 4 days to several months after the onset of erythema chronicum migrans. Most commonly these are fluctuating degrees of arteriovenous (AV) block, but ST-T wave changes or pericarditis can also occur.

LABORATORY FINDINGS. The white blood cell count can be slightly elevated with a mild left shift of the differential count. The erythrocyte sedimentation rate is usually elevated. Patients can have elevated serum transaminase levels (SGOT and SGPT) or lactate dehydrogenase (LDH). A spinal fluid lymphocytic pleocytosis of up to 450 cells/mm³ with elevated protein and normal glucose can occur in patients with neurologic involvement. Patients with arthritis can have a joint fluid white cell count of 20,000 to 75,000/mm³, mainly granulocytes.

DIAGNOSIS. Skin, joint, and presumably nervous system or cardiac involvement can occur separately. Without the classic rash or a history of tick bite, the diagnosis of Lyme disease is extremely difficult. Onset in summer and occurrence in a geographic area where erythema chronicum migrans has been reported are important clues to the diagnosis. Culture of *B. burgdorferi* from blood, cerebrospinal fluid (CSF), or joint fluid is presently a low yield procedure. Determination of specific antibody titers by indirect immunofluorescence or enzyme-linked immunosorbent assay is the most helpful diagnostic tool. IgM titers reach a peak 3 to 6 weeks after disease onset. IgG titers rise slowly and are highest months later when arthritis, carditis, or neuritis is present. There may be cross-reactivity of these antibody tests in patients with syphilis. Patients with mild illness who receive treatment early may not have elevated IgM or IgG antibody levels.

MANAGEMENT. Oral tetracycline (250 mg four times daily) or phenoxymethyl penicillin (500 mg four times daily) for 10 to 20 days, depending on symptom resolution, shortens duration of the rash when used early in the illness. This antibiotic therapy can also prevent subsequent development of major cardiac, neurologic, and arthritic complications (myocarditis, meningoencephalitis, recurrent arthritis). Up to 10% of patients may experience a Jarisch-Herxheimer reaction (fever and chills) during the first 24 hours of therapy. Patients with neurologic abnormalities, chronic arthritis, or both respond to high dose penicillin (20 million units/day intravenously). Treatment of cardiac complications is less clear, and presently it is unknown if antimicrobials or steroids are beneficial.

BIBLIOGRAPHY

Steere AC and others: Erythema chronicum migrans and Lyme arthritis: the enlarging clinical spectrum, Ann Intern Med 86:685, 1977.

Steere AC and others: Neurologic abnormalities of Lyme disease: successful treatment with high dose intravenous penicillin, Ann Intern Med 98:767, 1983.

Steere AC and others: The spirochetal etiology of Lyme disease, N Engl J Med 308:733, 1983.

Steere AC and others: Treatment of the early manifestations of Lyme disease, Ann Intern Med 99:22, 1983.

UNIT C • FUNGAL DISEASES

53·DISEASES CAUSED BY FUNGI

John E. Bennett

HISTOPLASMOSIS

Histoplasmosis is the infection caused by *Histoplasma capsulatum*. This fungus is encountered in many parts of the world, living in bat guano and in rich, moist soil, particularly soil enriched with bird droppings. The fungus grows as a mold in nature, and its spores reach the lung by inhalation. In the lung the fungus changes to a small budding yeast. The resulting pneumonia is usually self-limited and causes only a few days of fever, dry cough, and chest ache. These mild cases are detectable as persistent positive skin test reactivity to histoplasmin. In highly endemic areas of the central and mid-Atlantic United States, up to 80% of the adults have positive skin test results. Patients with more severe cases (also usually self-limited) can have up to 2 weeks of high fever, cyanosis, and prostration. Chest roentgenography reveals one or more areas of infiltration. Death is rare, but the disease can leave one or numerous areas of calcification in the lung and hilar nodes. Enlarged hilar nodes can cause bronchial compression and atelectasis. The slowly resolving pulmonary granuloma can resemble carcinoma roentgenographically and may lead to an unnecessary thoracotomy.

More serious complications occur in less than 1% of infections and are usually not preceded by severe primary pneumonia. Chronic fibrocavitary pulmonary infection, closely resembling tuberculosis, tends to occur in 30- to 50-year-old men who have a long history of cigarette smoking. The illness progresses insidiously and variably, but the untreated disease usually leads to death by bacterial pulmonary superinfection or cor pulmonale within several years.

Dissemination beyond the lung and hilar nodes can occur in self-limited primary pulmonary infection. Progressive extrapulmonary dissemination is a rare but highly lethal form of the disease. Many patients are either young children or immunosuppressed adults, but previously normal adults can also acquire the disease. The clinical manifestations are extremely variable, depending on which organs are involved. Hepatomegaly, splenomegaly, lymphadenopathy, chronic meningitis, endocarditis, adrenal insufficiency, pancytopenia, or granulomatous hepatitis can develop. Ulcerations of the upper airway occur in one fourth of the adults with disseminated histoplasmosis. Methenamine silver stain of the biopsy shows numerous small yeast cells in the submucosa.

H. capsulatum can be cultured from the sputum of patients with chronic fibrocavitary disease and from the mucosal lesions, blood, bone marrow, liver, lymph nodes, or urine of many patients with disseminated disease.

A complement fixation or agar gel diffusion test can be used to detect serum antibody to the fungus. Conversion from positive to negative in one of these tests can confirm the diagnosis of acute pulmonary histoplasmosis. In other clinical forms, serologic tests can suggest the possibility of infection but are too insensitive and nonspecific to make or exclude the diagnosis. Skin testing is not helpful in diagnosis except when conversion from negative to positive is observed in acute infection.

Intravenous administration of amphotericin B is very effective in curing fibrocavitary pulmonary or progressive disseminated infection. The drug is too toxic to warrant its use in self-limited pulmonary disease. Ketoconazole is a useful alternative to amphotericin B in patients who are not immunosuppressed, have nonmeningeal infection, are not severely ill, will take oral medications reliably, and have no contraindication to the use of ketoconazole. The usual dose for adults is 400 to 800 mg/day, given for 6 to 12 months.

COCCIDIOIDOMYCOSIS

Coccidioidomycosis is the infection caused by *Coccidioides immitis*. The fungus lives as a mold in the soil of certain hot, dry portions of the southwestern United States, Mexico, and Central and South America. Spores of this fungus are very resistant to heat and desiccation. When airborne, they can be inhaled into the lung and cause pneumonia. The resulting infection can pass unnoticed or be a self-limited influenza-like illness with cough, fever, and chest pain. Within the lung the fungus is transformed into a rounded form (spherule) that does not bud like a yeast but reproduces by endosporulation. Tiny spores form inside a "mother" cell that ruptures, releasing them. Each spore grows into a mature spherule, and the process is repeated. Depending on the stage of maturation, the structures can be much smaller than a human erythrocyte or several times that size.

Initial pulmonary infection can be associated with arthralgia, erythema nodosum, or erythema multiforme. Mild eosinophilia is common. The fever often subsides within 2 weeks, but roentgenographic resolution of the pneumonia is slow. Easy fatigability can persist for many weeks. The diagnosis can be suspected when there has been exposure to desert dust, as in construction, rock collecting, or digging for archeologic artifacts. Seroconversion of the complement fixation or agar gel test for *Coccidioides* organisms is helpful for diagnosis but can require several weeks from the onset of illness.

The resolving pulmonary infiltrate can be rounded and suggest carcinoma. The round lesion can cavitate and persist as a thin-walled cavity for months or years. Such cavities can be a source of hemoptysis.

Dissemination beyond the lung and hilar nodes is a rare but frequently lethal complication. This complication is more likely when the patient is black, Filipino, pregnant, or immunosuppressed. Dissemination can be manifested by chronic meningitis, one or more areas of indolent osteomyelitis, skin lesions, or subcutaneous abscesses. Spread beyond the lung is most likely to be recognized at the time of primary infection rather than years later. Clues to dissemination include continuation beyond the initial illness of the fever, elevated erythrocyte sedimentation rate, and eosinophilia, as well as a negative skin test with coccidioidin and elevation of the complement fixation titer to *Coccidioides* antigen beyond a level of roughly 1:16. The fungus can be recovered from pus, urine, cerebrospinal fluid (CSF), or, rarely, blood.

Amphotericin B provides amelioration of the infection, although relapse of disseminated infection is usual. Ketoconazole has resulted in improvement in some patients with chronic disseminated coccidioidomycosis. Persistent thin-walled cavities are best treated by observation or lobectomy.

BLASTOMYCOSIS

Blastomycosis is the infection caused by *Blastomyces dermatitidis*. The majority of cases occur in the United States and Canada, but occasional cases occur in Mexico, Africa, Central America, and northern South America. The portal of entry is the lung. A few cases of acute, self-limited pneumonitis have been recognized, but most cases occur as pneumonia of indolent onset and slow progression. Hematogenous dissemination to the skin occurs in about half the cases, forming chronic verrucous or crusted lesions. Spread to bone, prostate, epididymis, or other sites is less common. Painless nodular or plaquelike lesions rarely occur in the mouth, larynx, or nose. The fungus can be seen as a budding yeast in methenamine silver–stained biopsy tissue or can be cultured from sputum, pus, urine, or tissue samples from infected sites. Skin tests and serologic tests are not helpful. Either ketoconazole or intravenous amphotericin B can be used for treatment.

CRYPTOCOCCOSIS

Cryptococcosis is the mycosis caused by *Cryptococcus neoformans*, an encapsulated, budding, yeastlike fungus. The infection is infrequent but worldwide. It is rare in children but more common in patients with corticosteroid therapy, lymphoma, or sarcoidosis. The portal of entry is the lungs. The most common presentation is as chronic meningitis, with headache, nausea, vomiting, and unsteady gait. The CSF may demonstrate decreased glucose, lymphocytic pleocytosis, and elevated protein. If untreated, the infection is fatal in a few weeks to a year. Less commonly infection is seen as a chronic pneumonia or lesions in the skin, bones, or other organs. The diagnosis can be made by culturing the fungus from CSF, blood, urine, or pus. In about half the cases of meningitis the fungus can be seen in an India ink stain of CSF. Latex agglutination tests of serum and CSF detect the capsular antigen in about 94% of the patients with meningitis and in the serum of a lesser proportion of nonmeningeal cases. The treatment of choice is intravenously administered amphotericin B given either alone or in combination with oral flucytosine.

PARACOCCIDIOIDOMYCOSIS

Paracoccidioidomycosis, also called South American blastomycosis, is infection caused by the fungus *Paracoccidioides brasiliensis*. The disease is confined to South and Central America, but indolent infection can be first recognized years after the patient has left the endemic area. The patient has lesions in the mucous membranes of the mouth, nose, or gastrointestinal tract or in the skin, lymph nodes, or liver. A chronic, patchy pulmonary infiltrate is usually present but rarely symptomatic. Fever can be absent, and the oral or nasal lesions can be mistaken for leishmaniasis or squamous cell carcinoma. The diagnosis can be made by demonstrating the distinctive yeastlike fungus in methenamine silver stains of infected tissue. The fungus can also be cultured readily from infected tissue or oral ulcers. Oral ketoconazole is effective therapy (200 to 400 mg/day for at least 1 year). Severely ill patients should receive intravenous amphotericin B initially, followed by a prolonged course of ketoconazole.

SPOROTRICHOSIS

Sporotrichosis is the mycosis caused by *Sporothrix schenckii*. The infection occurs worldwide but infrequently. The fungus lives on certain plants and enters the skin following minor injury, such as by rose thorns. Within subcutaneous tissue the fungus grows in a budding, yeastlike form. A small, slightly tender pimple forms and may discharge small amounts of pus intermittently. The lesion persists, and over the ensuing weeks other nodules form in the same extremity along proximal lymphatic channels. Infection beginning in the skin is chronic but not life threatening. Uncommonly, infection begins in the lung. Hematogenous dissemination to bones and joints can occur, albeit rarely, from the lung or from an occult portal of entry. The diagnosis is best made by culturing the fungus from pus. The fungus can be difficult to see or identify in histologic section. Cutaneous disease responds well to oral administration of saturated potassium iodide. The adult dosage is 2 ml three times a day with meals, increasing gradually as tolerated to 3 to 4 ml three times a day. Hematogenously disseminated disease requires therapy with amphotericin B.

CANDIDIASIS

Candidiasis, also called moniliasis or candidosis, is an infection by species of *Candida,* a yeastlike fungus. By far the most common species is *Candida albicans,* a normal inhabitant of the human mouth, vagina, and intestinal tract. Superficial invasion of the mucous membranes and skin by *Candida* sp. is called thrush. In the mouth thrush most commonly occurs as a white, adherent plaque on the buccal mucosa. Scraping up an edge of the leathery plaque reveals a bleeding base. Plaques also can be present on the inner aspect of the lips or on the gums, palate, or tongue. Thrush under an upper denture can be erythematous without a distinct membrane. Oral thrush is relatively painless except for fissuring at the corners of the mouth (angular cheilitis), which is usually painful.

Vaginal thrush causes discharge, burning, and dyspareunia. Cutaneous thrush occurs as erythema of moist areas, such as diaper rash and rash under pendulous breasts and in intergluteal clefts of obese patients. Perianal thrush can cause pruritus ani. Onychomycosis can occur when hands are exposed frequently to water, as in cannery workers or bartenders.

Systemic factors also contribute to thrush. Newborn infants are prone to this condition, as are patients with the acquired immunodeficiency syndrome (AIDS), diabetes mellitus, or those receiving adrenal corticosteroids or broad-spectrum antibiotics. Women taking oral contraceptives or in the third trimester of pregnancy are predisposed to vaginal thrush. Children with certain immunodeficiency states and adults with thymoma can acquire chronic mucocutaneous candidiasis. These patients have heaped-up skin lesions in addition to thrush of the mouth, vagina, and nails.

The diagnosis of thrush is best made by demonstrating pseudohyphae in wet smears of scrapings from the lesions. Gram stain is less helpful. Culture can confirm the diagnosis but is not diagnostic alone because *Candida* organisms are frequent commensals in the same sites.

Oral thrush can be treated with either nystatin suspension or clotrimazole troches. Vaginal thrush appears to respond somewhat better to creams or suppositories of either clotrimazole or miconazole than to nystatin. Thrush of moist intertriginous lesions is improved by keeping the area clean and dry. Topical creams, such as miconazole, are also beneficial in intertriginous areas but are ineffective in the verrucous lesions of chronic mucocutaneous candidiasis. Oral ketoconazole is the drug of choice for this latter condition.

Disseminated candidiasis results from a break in the integument when there is either a foreign body (such as an intravascular catheter) at the site or impaired host defense. Patients receiving hyperalimentation are particularly prone to *Candida* sepsis. The fungus passes from the skin to a deep vein along the plastic intravenous catheter. Patients with neutropenia resulting from acute leukemia and its treatment are at special risk of gastrointestinal candidiasis, which then can disseminate. The most common sign of disseminated candidiasis is fever. Focal findings are often absent but include symptoms and signs of endophthalmitis, endocarditis, renal abscess, hepatitis, meningitis, embolic skin lesions, and osteomyelitis. The diagnosis can be made by culture of blood, CSF, or biopsy material. Appearance of the fungus in methenamine silver–stained tissue is also diagnostic. Serologic tests are not of proven value. The treatment is with intravenously administered amphotericin B, with or without orally administered flucytosine.

ASPERGILLOSIS

As currently used, aspergillosis is a broad term referring to infection, allergy, or colonization with species of *Aspergillus*. This extremely common mold lives on decaying vegetation and grain the world over. Most normal individuals are highly resistant to infection. Infection occurs in patients who are severely immunosuppressed, particularly those with acute leukemia. Infection begins as a dense pneumonia that is prone to hematogenous dissemination. Vascular invasion by fungal hyphae leads to infarction of tissue. Positive sputum cultures are not usually helpful, since they do not necessarily indicate tissue invasion. The diagnosis is made by demonstrating the narrow, septate hyphae in biopsied tissue. Death often occurs within 2 weeks of onset. Patients whose immunosuppression is lessened dramatically may respond to intravenous administration of amphotericin B.

Patients with chronic lung disease and impaired bronchopulmonary clearance mechanisms can have *Aspergillus* organisms growing in their bronchi. Plugs of fungal hyphae may be expectorated. Preexisting cavities or cysts in the lung can fill with hyphae, creating a so-called fungus ball. No tissue invasion occurs under most circumstances. Repeated hemoptysis demonstrated to be from a fungus ball can require surgical excision. Antifungal therapy is ineffective.

Allergic bronchopulmonary aspergillosis is a syndrome in which patients exhibit asthma, IgE and frequently IgG antibody to *Aspergillus* sp., and intermittent bronchial plugging. Eosinophilia and elevated serum IgE are usual.

MUCORMYCOSIS

Mucormycosis is infection caused by fungi of the order Mucorales. Zygomycosis is a broader term that includes not only mucormycosis but also infections caused by related fungi. Most of the fungi causing mucormycosis are common saprophytes in nature. There are two principal forms of the disease: craniofacial infection in patients with diabetes mellitus and pneumonia in patients with immunosuppression. Craniofacial mucormycosis, which is caused most often by species of *Rhizopus*, usually begins in the maxillary sinus. The symptoms resemble those of bacterial sinusitis for the first few days, but the infection progresses to contiguous structures such as the orbit, nose, hard palate, face, and eventually the brain. The fungus invades blood vessels, causing infarction and necrosis of tissue. Proptosis, ophthalmoplegia, coma, and necrotic lesions of the palate or nasal mucous membranes are common findings. The diagnosis is made by demonstrating the distinctive hyphae in biopsied tissue. If mucormycosis is untreated, death ensues in a week or two. Approximately half the patients are cured by rigorous control of the diabetes mellitus, radical surgical exenteration of infected tissue, and intravenous administration of amphotericin B.

Pulmonary mucormycosis is most often caused by species of *Mucor*. Infection occurs in patients with severe immunosuppression. They are usually severely neutropenic and are also receiving adrenal corticosteroids or cytotoxic drugs. The infection is seen most often as a rapidly fatal pneumonia. The diagnosis requires demonstrating the broad nonseptate fungi in lung biopsy specimens. Amphotericin B is the drug of choice, but recovery is rare.

MYCETOMA

Mycetoma, or maduromycosis, is a chronic, suppurative infection of the subcutaneous tissue. The causative agent can be any one of a large number of fungi or aerobic higher bacteria called actinomycetes. These organisms live in soil or vegetation in many tropical and subtropical areas of the world and enter the feet or other unprotected areas of the body through minor trauma. The microbe lives in pus as a colony or grain a few millimeters in diameter. Extensive fibrosis, swelling, draining sinuses, destruction of underlying bone, and extension to contiguous soft tissues mark the slow progression of the lesion. Antibiotic therapy benefits actinomycete mycetoma. Fungal mycetoma usually requires amputation.

CHROMOMYCOSIS

Chromomycosis is a chronic mycotic infection of the skin and subcutaneous tissue. Certain fungi growing on soil or vegetation enter the skin during minor trauma. These fungi grow in the subcutaneous tissue as brownish round cells. One or more verrucous plaques form during the ensuing months or years and can become papillary. There is no pain or bony destruction. The diagnosis is made by culture and histologic examination of the lesion. Excision of small lesions and oral flucytosine therapy are helpful. For extensive chronic lesions, intravenously administered amphotericin B plus oral flucytosine may be preferable because drug resistance tends to develop with flucytosine alone.

BIBLIOGRAPHY
Histoplasmosis

Goodwin RA, Loyd JE, and Des Prez RM: Histoplasmosis in normal hosts, Medicine 60:231, 1981.
Wheat LJ, Slama TG, and Zeckel ML: Histoplasmosis in the acquired immune deficiency syndrome, Am J Med 78:203, 1985.

Coccidioidomycosis

Drutz DJ and Catanzaro A: State of the art. Coccidioidomycosis, Am Rev Respir Dis 117:559, 1978.
Drutz DJ: Amphotericin B in the treatment of coccidioidomycosis, Drugs 26:337, 1983.

Blastomycosis

Dismukes WE and others: Treatment of blastomycosis and histoplasmosis with ketoconazole, Ann Intern Med 103:861, 1985.

Cryptococcosis

Stockstill MT and Kauffman CA: Comparison of cryptococcal and tuberculous meningitis, Arch Neurol 40:81, 1983.
Zuger A and others: Cryptococcal disease in patients with the acquired immunodeficiency syndrome, Ann Intern Med 104:234, 1986.

Candidiasis

Epstein JB, Truelove EL, and Izutzu KT: Oral candidiasis: pathogenesis and host defense, Rev Infect Dis 6:96, 1984.
Solomkin JS, Flohr AM, and Simmons RL: Indications for therapy for fungemia in postoperative patients, Arch Surg 117:1272, 1982.
Scherr SA and others: Chronic candidiasis of the oral cavity and esophagus, Laryngoscope 40:769, 1980.
Jones JM: The recognition and management of candida esophagitis, Hosp Pract 16:64, 1981.

Aspergillosis

Rinaldi MG: Invasive aspergillosis, Rev Infect Dis 5:1061, 1983.

Mucormycosis

Maniglia AJ, Mintz DH, and Novak S: Cephalic phycomycosis: a report of eight cases, Laryngoscope 92:755, 1982.
Rangel-Geurra R, Martinez HR, and Saenz C: Mucormycosis: report of 11 cases, Arch Neurol 42:578, 1985.

54 · AGENTS USED IN TREATMENT OF MYCOTIC INFECTIONS

Donald Kaye

TREATMENT OF DEEP MYCOSES

Amphotericin B is the primary agent used in the therapy of systemic fungal infections. It is degraded in the body, and serum levels are unaffected by renal or hepatic failure.

Amphotericin B is a very toxic drug and must be given intravenously. It regularly produces nephrotoxicity, some of which is irreversible. It results in hypokalemia (caused by renal loss of potassium) and a normocytic, normochromic anemia. Patients frequently have fever, chills, nausea, and vomiting during amphotericin B treatment, and phlebitis is common.

The dose usually is 0.3 to 0.5 mg/kg intravenously daily or 1 mg/kg every other day. Doses are given over 2 to 4 hours in 5% glucose in water. When therapy is started, a test dose of 1 mg is given to assess its pyrogenicity in the patient. Gradually increasing doses over 3 to 4 days are then given, followed by full dosage. In a critically ill patient, 1 mg, 10 mg, 20 mg, and so on can be given 8 hours apart, followed by full dosage. Therapy continues for 6 to 12 weeks for most systemic fungal infections.

Cryptococcal meningitis can be treated with intravenous administration of amphotericin B for 10 weeks. With the addition of orally administered *flucytosine* (150 mg/kg/day in four divided doses), doses of amphotericin B should be decreased to 0.3 mg/kg/day and therapy for 6 weeks often is adequate. Flucytosine may be synergistic or additive in action with amphotericin B against other fungi such as *Candida* and *Aspergillus* organisms, but clinical trials are inconclusive. Although relatively nontoxic in patients with normal renal function, flucytosine has bone marrow toxicity when excessive blood levels are achieved. This occurs in the presence of renal insufficiency. Flucytosine also may demonstrate a dose-related gastrointestinal toxicity with nausea, abdominal pain, and diarrhea. Abnormal liver chemistries and rash may also occur.

In meningitis caused by *Coccidioides* fungus, in addition to parenteral therapy, amphotericin B is given intrathecally in doses of 0.5 mg three times a week. Therapy usually is prolonged for months.

Miconazole and *ketoconazole* are imidazoles that are active in vitro against many fungi. Miconazole is not absorbed orally and is given intravenously for deep mycotic infections. However, effective blood levels are difficult to maintain. Ketoconazole is absorbed orally, and effective blood levels are more easily achieved and maintained. Both agents are metabolized in the body and are relatively nontoxic. The doses are not changed in patients with renal insufficiency.

Miconazole is given intravenously in a dose of 200 mg to 1.2 g (usually 1 g) every 8 hours over a 1- to 2-hour period. Therapy is continued for weeks to months, depending on the infection. Miconazole does not penetrate well into the cerebrospinal fluid (CSF) nor are effective urinary levels achieved; intrathecal or bladder instillation is necessary for infections at these sites. Side effects are rash, phlebitis, pruritus, nausea, vomiting, fever, hyponatremia, and hyperlipidemia (from the infusion fluid). The dose is not altered with renal insufficiency. Miconazole does not seem to be the therapy of choice for any deep mycosis, and it is rarely indicated.

Ketoconazole is given orally in a recommended dose of 200 to 400 mg once daily. Gastric acid must be present for absorption. Ketoconazole is effective in chronic mucocutaneous candidiasis, in which it is the drug of choice. It also is effective in griseofulvin-resistant dermatomycoses. It is effective in paracoccidioidomycosis, histoplasmosis, blastomycosis, and some cases of coccidioidomycosis. Therapy is continued for weeks to months, depending on the infection (at least 6 months for systemic mycoses). Chronic mucocutaneous candidiasis requires maintenance therapy. Ketoconazole does not penetrate well into the CSF. Side effects include nausea, vomiting, abdominal pain, pruritus, rash, headache, somnolence, gynecomastia, decreased libido, menstrual irregularity, and abnormal liver chemistries.

TREATMENT OF SUPERFICIAL MYCOSES

(See the discussion of fungal and yeast infections in Chapter 167.)

A number of agents are useful by local application for the treatment of superficial mycoses.

Nystatin is available for local use in oral and vaginal candidiasis. *Miconazole*, *clotrimazole* , and *econazole* are imidazoles that are effective against *Candida* fungi and dermatophytes (*Trichophyton*, *Microsporum*, and *Epidermophyton* organisms) that cause tinea infections.

Undecylenic acid, haloprogin, and *tolnaftate* are topical antifungal agents that are active against dermatophytes but not *Candida* organisms. They are not as effective as the imidazoles.

Griseofulvin is an oral agent that is active against the dermatophytes but not *Candida* spp. The dose is 500 mg once a day for 4 weeks; for infection of the nail treatment lasts 4 to 6 months. Griseofulvin is not effective against deep mycoses, and it should not be used in patients with porphyria. Side effects are photosensitivity and hypersensitivity reactions, nausea, vomiting, diarrhea, headache, fatigue, confusion, and leukopenia. It can cause a disulfiram-like reaction when taken with alcohol. It also necessitates increases in the dosage of coumarin drugs needed for anticoagulation.

BIBLIOGRAPHY

Goodman LS and Gilman A: The pharmacological basis of therapeutics, ed 6, New York, 1980, Macmillan, Inc.
Handbook of antimicrobial therapy. The Medical Letter on Drugs and Therapeutics (revised ed), New Rochelle, NY, 1988.
Mandell GL, Douglas RG, and Bennett JE; Principles and practice of infectious diseases, ed 3, New York, 1990, Churchill Livingstone.
Sanford JP: Guide to antimicrobial therapy, West Bethesda, MD, 1989, Antimicrobial Therapy, Inc.

UNIT D • PROTOZOAL DISEASES

55 · DISEASES CAUSED BY PROTOZOA

Thomas C. Jones

Protozoa are single-cell eukaryotic microbes. They form a diverse group of organisms that are divided on the basis of morphologic and functional characteristics into flagellates, amebae, sporozoa, and ciliates. Protozoa such as the trypanosomes or the malaria parasites reside primarily in the tissue, whereas those such as trichomonads, *Giardia* organisms, or amebae reside on the mucosal surfaces. Some protozoa such as amebae and *Giardia* organisms are transmitted to humans by ingestion of food or water contaminated with human feces. Other protozoa are transmitted to humans by insect vectors of disease such as those that transmit malaria and leishmaniasis.

This chapter emphasizes seven protozoal diseases of humans: malaria, amebiasis, giardiasis, cryptosporidiosis, toxoplasmosis, trichomoniasis, and leishmaniasis. In addition, the diseases African trypanosomiasis, South American trypanosomiasis, pneumocytosis, and babesiosis are discussed. The diagnosis of protozoal diseases depends on smears of body secretions when the protozoa are lumen-dwelling microbes such as those causing amebiasis, giardiasis, cryptosporidiosis, and trichomoniasis; smears of peripheral blood in cases of malaria, babesiosis, and trypanosomiasis; smears of tissue specimens from affected areas in leishmaniasis and pneumocytosis; and serologic antibody testing in cases of toxoplasmosis, hepatic amebiasis, and South American trypanosomiasis.

Protozoal infections are sufficiently distinct from one another that the commonly used phrase "rule out parasitic disease" is both unhelpful and unnecessary. The following descriptions of each of the protozoal diseases should provide the background for making a clinical diagnosis and supporting that diagnosis by appropriate laboratory testing.

MALARIA

Malaria in nonimmune individuals is an acute febrile illness associated with vigorous shaking chills, prostration, splenomegaly, and anemia. In partially immune patients who live in an area endemic for malaria, the illness is characterized by splenomegaly, anemia, intermittent fever, and occasionally immune-complex glomerulonephritis.

EPIDEMIOLOGY. Malaria occurs throughout the tropics and subtropics and even in temperate climates where treatment of patients with malaria and control of the mosquito vectors are inadequate. The incidence of malaria is increasing throughout Africa, Asia, and Central and South America. Approximately 100 million cases of malaria occur each year. The mortality associated with malaria varies, depending on the *Plasmodium* sp. prevalent in the area, the availability of medical care, and the level of immunity in the population. Mortality may be over 10% in areas where *Plasmodium falciparum* occurs.

LIFE CYCLE OF THE ORGANISM. The protozoa plasmodia are part of the subphylum Sporozoa. This class of microbes has two cycles: a sexual cycle, termed "sporogony," which occurs in the female *Anopheles* mosquito vector, and an asexual cycle, termed "schizogony," which occurs in the human host. For a human to be infected during the mosquito bite, the mosquito must have taken up the blood of an infected human 2 weeks previously. The blood meal contains the male and female gametocytes, which are necessary for initiation of the sexual cycle in the mosquito. After ingestion of the blood meal, the gametocytes are liberated in the stomach of the mosquito, the male gametocyte fertilizes the female, and a zygote is formed. This transforms into a motile ookinete that migrates through the stomach wall, encysts in the tissue of the stomach wall, and replicates. The cyst then ruptures, releasing sporozoites that migrate to the salivary gland of the mosquito, where they remain until the mosquito next feeds. At the time of the bite the sporozoites in the mosquito's salivary juices are inoculated into the vascular system of the human host. The sporozoites circulate for less than half an hour and then enter the cells of the liver. At this point they are said to initiate the preerythrocytic stage of malaria infection. After a period lasting from 5 to 16 days, depending on the species of *Plasmodium*, the parasites rupture the hepatic cells, enter the vascular system, and, now termed "merozoites," enter circulating red blood cells (RBCs). This initiates the erythrocytic cycle of malaria. During this cycle they replicate in the RBCs by the process termed "schizogony" and are called "schizonts." After 48 to 72 hours, depending on the species, the cycle is complete and the RBCs rupture, releasing the merozoites to infect additional RBCs. During this process some of the merozoites become male and female gametocytes. These then circulate along with the schizonts of malaria, awaiting ingestion with the next blood meal of a mosquito and the continuation of the cycle. Patients also can be infected by transfusions or communal use of a needle as occurs among drug addicts. Although there are more than

100 different species of *Plasmodium* that can infect various mammals, birds, and reptiles, only four of these species—*P. falciparum, Plasmodium vivax, Plasmodium ovale,* and *Plasmodium malariae*—infect humans.

PATHOLOGY. The pathologic changes seen in malaria occur at the time the merozoites enter and replicate within the RBCs. During this process RBCs are changed dramatically. Under the electron microscope, for example, the membranes of erythrocytes appear to have electron-dense knoblike projections; the cells take on unusual shapes and are no longer as deformable as RBCs from uninfected people. Most importantly, they become adhesive to vascular endothelium and to each other, and they demonstrate an increase in osmotic fragility. As a result of these changes and the rupture of RBCs during the cycle of schizogony, the patient demonstrates changes of intravascular hemolysis, progressive anemia, and occlusion of blood vessels. This leads to generalized tissue anoxia, which is noted in falciparum malaria most prominently as cerebral and renal anoxia. Patients with severe forms of malaria also may have hepatitis and pulmonary edema. Patients also have evidence of bone marrow impairment and the syndrome of disseminated intravascular coagulation. Some patients have such impressive hemolysis that they are described as having "blackwater fever," a complication of malaria caused by rapid hemolysis with hemoglobin damage to the kidneys, resulting in acute renal failure. Patients with more prolonged malaria may have immune-complex damage to the glomeruli of the kidney, resulting in a nephrotic syndrome. Others with chronic malaria may demonstrate the syndrome of tropical splenomegaly caused by repeated malaria attacks and an exaggerated immune response. Some patients are resistant to malaria because of hemoglobinopathies that interfere with replication of the malaria parasite in the RBC. For example, *P. falciparum* multiplies poorly in RBCs containing sickle hemoglobin. Some patients are resistant because they lack the blood groups on the surface of the RBC that are necessary for attachment of the malaria parasite, a requirement for entry into the cells. For example, one of the blood group substances called the Duffy blood group is essential for the attachment of *P. vivax* to RBCs. Patients without the Duffy blood group substance are resistant to vivax malaria. Blacks frequently lack Duffy substance.

CLINICAL MANIFESTATIONS. Patients with malaria have shaking chills, fever, headache, and myalgias. During the early stages of the infection the fever may occur daily, but within a few days a synchronous pattern emerges. This has been referred to as tertian or quartan malaria, depending on whether the malaria fevers are occurring at 48- or 72-hour intervals. With *P. vivax* and *P. ovale*, fever occurs every 48 hours; with *P. malariae*, fever occurs every 72 hours; and with *P. falciparum*, fever tends to be continuous or irregular. A characteristic attack is preceded by a shaking chill, and then the temperature increases to 104° F (40° C). This is followed by malaise and headache lasting several hours. The attack is terminated by profuse sweating and a fall in the patient's temperature. The patient may then feel well for 1 to 2 days before the fever recurs. Malaria is associated with a number of nonspecific symptoms such as cough, abdominal pains, nausea, vomiting, and diarrhea. These symptoms mislead physicians to make other diagnoses such as upper respiratory tract illness or gastroenteritis. Occasionally liver dysfunction is a prominent feature of malaria, and the disease may be misdiagnosed as hepatitis. Enlargement of the spleen is common in vivax and ovale malaria but is seen less frequently during the early stages of falciparum malaria. Laboratory tests reveal the anemia and thrombocytopenia associated with malaria. Eosinophilia is not a feature of malaria. Liver dysfunction often is evidenced by elevated serum transaminase levels and bile in the urine. The complications of malaria are those associated with severe anoxia to the brain, kidneys, and lungs and severe hemolytic anemia.

DIAGNOSIS. The diagnosis of malaria is made by first suspecting the disease in any symptomatic patient who has been to a malarious area, has received a blood transfusion, or is a drug addict. The clinical suspicion of malaria is confirmed by taking thin and thick smears of the patient's blood, staining them with Giemsa stain, and examining them microscopically for evidence of RBCs infected with *Plasmodium* organisms. The falciparum malaria parasite appears as a delicate ring of blue cytoplasm with a purple dot, which resembles a signet ring. This is called the "ring form" of malaria. The RBCs are normal in size, and the erythrocyte has no red dots characteristic of other forms of malaria. Since the maturation of this form of malaria does not occur in the peripheral blood, mature-stage schizogony is not seen in *P. falciparum* infection. In contrast to other types of malaria, parasitemia may reach high levels (over 10%). The gametocyte of *P. falciparum* is characteristic and is shaped like a banana or crescent. *P. vivax* readily can be distinguished from falciparum ring forms. Unlike other types of malaria, the RBCs are larger than uninfected RBCs and contain red dots referred to as Schuffner's dots. In addition, the blue cytoplasm of *P. vivax* is much larger and more diffusely distributed throughout the RBC. Since vivax malaria parasites mature in the peripheral blood (unlike *P. falciparum*), developmental forms of schizogony, including the mature schizont that contains 12 to 24 chromatin dots, can be seen. *P. malariae* and *P. ovale* also mature in the peripheral blood. *P. malariae* may be recognized by the band form in which the mature schizont stretches in a band across the red cell. Malaria parasites are present in the peripheral blood throughout the period of malaria infection, although they may be present in larger numbers a few hours after the patient's chills and fever begin. Antibodies appear in the peripheral blood; however, serologic tests are not useful in diagnosing the acute illness. They are of value for screening blood donors when transfusion malaria has occurred and for determining the prevalence of malaria in the population.

MANAGEMENT. The therapy of malaria is directed at eradicating *Plasmodium* organisms during the erythrocytic stage of the infection. This is done primarily by the use of chloroquine, which interferes with nucleic acid synthesis of the developing parasite. Over a period of 2 days 1.5 g of base is given (600 mg base initially followed by 300 mg base at 6, 24, and 48 hours). Administration is oral or if necessary parenteral. When patients are infected with species of *Plasmodium* such as vivax and ovale that have prolonged hepatic stages of infection, primaquine must be added to eradicate the tissue phase. Primaquine is given orally as one tablet (15 mg of base) daily for 14 days.

In some parts of the world, such as Southeast Asia, East Africa, and the central regions of South America, *P. falciparum* malaria is resistant to chloroquine. Malaria acquired in these regions requires use of the time-honored drug against malaria, quinine, in combination with pyrimethamine and a sulfa drug such as sulfadiazine. The quinine is given in a dose of 650 mg every 8 hours for 7 days, and the pyrimethamine (50 mg each day) and sulfa (for example, sulfadiazine, 1 g every 6 hours) are given for 3 and 5 days, respectively. This combination eradicates parasitemia and prevents the recrudescence of the malaria. The patient with severe malaria must be provided with important supportive therapy, such as management of coma when the patient is unconscious, to prevent aspiration pneumonia and pressure ulcerations. In addition, acute renal failure may require dialysis, and anemia may necessitate the transfusion of RBCs.

PREVENTION. Malaria can be prevented only by decreasing the contact with infected mosquitos through appropriate use of mosquito netting and insect repellents and by taking drugs prophylactically against the erythrocytic stage. Chloroquine (300 mg base orally once a week for adults) is used in areas where the malaria is still sensitive to the drug. This treatment should be started 1 week before arriving in the endemic area and should be continued during the stay and for at least 6 weeks after leaving the endemic area. In areas where chloroquine resistance occurs, a tablet combining pyrimethamine and sulfadoxine is taken in a similar fashion once a week, together with chloroquine or doxycycline once a day. When patients return from areas heavily infected with vivax or ovale, they should be given a 2 week course of primaquine (15 mg base daily orally) to prevent relapse of their malaria. Currently, no vaccine is available for preventing malaria; however, active investigation in this area makes it a likely possibility in the near future. Control of malaria in a community depends primarily on controlling the insect vector by draining areas of insect development and residual insecticide spraying.

DISEASES CAUSED BY AMEBAE
Amebiasis

Amebiasis is an infection of the human colon yielding a spectrum of illness from asymptomatic to severe invasive inflammatory bowel disease. In addition, it may cause extraintestinal disease, particularly liver abscess. The infection is acquired by the ingestion of water or food contaminated with human feces.

EPIDEMIOLOGY. The pathogenic organism that causes amebiasis, *Entamoeba histolytica,* is distributed widely throughout the tropics, subtropics, and temperate climates. It is most common where proper disposal of human feces is not provided, including all of the developing countries of the world, and where fecal contamination is common for sociologic reasons, as among the homosexual community. In many areas of the tropics over 40% of the population is infected. Epidemics of amebiasis have occurred where ameba-contaminated stool has gained access to water supply systems. The disease associated with amebiasis appears to be more severe in some parts of the world than in others. This may be associated with variations in strains of *E. histolytica.*

LIFE CYCLE OF THE ORGANISM. *E. histolytica* exists in two stages: an encysted stage, in which the organism can persist in nature for long periods of time, and a trophozoite stage, in which the organism exists in the human bowel under appropriate environmental conditions. An infected person may pass either the cyst or the trophozoite in the stool. However, the trophozoite must encyst shortly after passage to survive in the conditions outside the human gastrointestinal tract. During conversion of the trophozoite to the cyst, the trophozoite first develops a wall around itself, then a glycogen vacuole and a chromatoid body. The nuclear material of the newly encysted trophozoite then divides twice, forming a cyst containing four nuclei. This encysted structure can persist in water or moist soil for weeks to months. When this form is ingested, the organism can successfully pass the low pH of the stomach and then emerge from the cyst in the environment of the upper small intestine. If conditions are proper in the colon, it may persist in the lumen for long periods or invade the mucosa of the bowel. Trophozoites are facultative anaerobes and can survive and replicate only under complex conditions, such as the presence of other bacteria in the environment, low oxygen tension, and the availability of carbohydrates. These conditions determine the degree of virulence of the ameba and also lead to the wide spectrum of symptoms seen in patients infected with the same ameba. Some patients, for example, are completely asymptomatic, with infection documented only by the identification of the ameba in the stool. Others may have a progressive, even fatal, disease associated with the invasion of the ameba into tissue.

PATHOLOGY. The ameba gains access to the submucosa of the large bowel by excreting a material that allows it to pass between the mucosal cells. Once in the submucosal environment, the organism releases substances that contribute to tissue anoxia, necrosis, and changes in the environment that render it ideal for replication of the ameba. The ameba then ingests host tissue, particularly RBCs, to maintain its growth. During this process an ulcer is formed in the submucosa. Since the ulcer is much larger at the base of the submucosa than at the mucosal surface, it appears flask shaped. Depending on the degree of inflammatory changes in the bowel, a few punctate lesions may be associated with the bowel infection or there may be generalized and marked inflammatory changes. Marked inflammation often follows loss of mucosal integrity after significant submucosal tissue destruction by the ameba. This then leads to secondary bacterial infection. Ulceration of the bowel may extend through the serosal surface and lead to peritonitis.

During the submucosal infection two other complications may result. The first is a local marked inflammatory reaction to the combination of amebae and bacteria. This causes an intestinal mass called an ameboma. The second and most common complication of amebiasis is invasion of the vascular system of the bowel, which allows amebae to be transported to the liver. Amebic infection of the liver results in progressive necrosis of liver substance in the region where amebae are replicating. This appears pathologically as a gradually expanding necrotic lesion referred to as amebic liver abscess. The central region of the abscess is filled with debris and the end products of liver necrosis. The liquid has a reddish brown, anchovy paste–like appearance. Under the microscope the amebae are seen at the periphery of the abscess at the edge of normal liver tissue. It should be pointed out that this lesion, although referred to as an abscess, is not a typical inflammatory abscess that requires surgical drainage but rather an area of liver necrosis. Occasionally this enlarging area of liver necrosis may rupture into the peritoneum, through the diaphragm into the pleural cavity, or into the pericardial space. This rupture is a serious and often fatal complication of amebiasis. In rare cases amebae may gain access to other sites such as the brain or skin.

CLINICAL MANIFESTATIONS. Amebiasis can be divided into two distinct clinical entities: intestinal amebiasis and extraintestinal amebiasis. Patients with intestinal amebiasis show signs and symptoms of colonic irritation, including abdominal pain with mucus and occasionally blood in the stools. When the colonic involvement becomes severe, the patient may have all the signs and symptoms of an acute abdominal condition, including abdominal distention, absence of bowel sounds, and vomiting. A patient with an ameboma may have subtle clinical manifestations, and the ameboma may be identified during barium enema examination. It is often confused with a colonic carcinoma. A distinguishing feature is that the serologic test for amebae is positive if the lesion is caused by ameboma. Some patients have a chronic irritative bowel syndrome associated with amebic colitis, which may be indistinguishable from that of ulcerative colitis.

Extraintestinal amebiasis may be present without any history of or association with gastrointestinal signs or symptoms. The patient with hepatic amebiasis usually has fever, pain in the right upper quadrant and epigastrium, right shoulder pain caused by irritation of the diaphragm, and a palpable liver. The patient may have a history of rapid weight loss of 20 to 30 pounds over several weeks. The hepatic lesions of amebiasis are more often in the right lobe of the liver. Point tenderness over that part of the chest and abdomen is an important sign in identifying amebic liver abscess. Laboratory testing in amebic abscess reveals anemia, leukocytosis without eosinophilia, an elevated diaphragm on chest roentgenogram, and abnormal liver function tests. The leukocytosis associated with amebic liver abscess may lead some physicians to consider a diagnosis of pyogenic infection of the liver, but leukocytosis is a common feature of amebiasis. Jaundice may or may not be present. When rupture of amebic abscess occurs, it is a catastrophic illness causing severe impairment in function at the site of the rupture. If the rupture occurs, for instance, into the pleural space, pulmonary signs and symptoms are prominent; with rupture into the pericardial space, cardiac tamponade may be an impressive feature of the illness.

DIAGNOSIS. Intestinal amebiasis is diagnosed by identifying the ameba, *E. histolytica,* in microscopic examination of stool specimens. The diagnosis is confirmed by finding either trophozoites or cysts. The physician can do this during sigmoidoscopy by placing a small aspirate of liquid from a colonic lesion on a glass slide and looking for the characteristic motility of the ameba. When specimens are sent to the laboratory, the technician examines a specimen directly and then a concentration of the stool looking for cysts. Some laboratories culture the fluid for the ameba. Since the shedding of amebae in mild infections may be intermittent, several stools over a period of days may be necessary to exclude the diagnosis of amebiasis. In addition, purging to obtain multiple stool samples has been suggested as a means for diagnosis of amebiasis. Serologic tests are of limited value in the diagnosis of intestinal amebiasis. However, they should be obtained because of the possibility of invasive disease such as ameboma and amebic liver abscess. The diagnosis of extraintestinal amebiasis relies on demonstrating antibodies against the ameba in the peripheral blood and on obtaining tissue from the site of the inflamed bowel or fluid from an amebic liver abscess. Findings that are characteristic of amebic liver abscess include elevation of the right diaphragm on chest roentgenogram, leukocytosis, and liver function abnormalities. Radioisotopic scanning and computed tomography of the liver are helpful in the diagnosis of amebic liver abscess. The stool examination shows amebae in only one third of those cases with documented amebic abscess of the liver. The clinical signs and symptoms of extraintestinal amebiasis resolve promptly after therapy against amebiasis is initiated, and this has been suggested as a reasonable and noninvasive diagnostic test.

MANAGEMENT. The treatment of amebiasis varies, depending on whether the site of the inflammation is in the colon or the liver. The treatment of intestinal amebiasis depends on whether it is asymptomatic or evidence of invasive disease is present. If there is no evidence of invasive disease, drugs directed at the luminal phase of the infection are used. These include paromomycin, diiodohydroxyquin, and diloxanide fu-

roate (available from the Centers for Disease Control*). The nitroimidazoles are the most effective drugs against the invasive form of the disease. Metronidazole is the only drug in this group available in the United States. The dosage is 2.25 g/day in three divided doses for 5 to 10 days. Metronidazole may cause some side effects such as nausea and abdominal discomfort. In addition, drinking alcohol during treatment with this drug may make the patient very ill.

Extraintestinal amebiasis also is treated with metronidazole in the same doses. Some physicians add chloroquine (500 mg/day) as an adjunct to the therapy of amebic liver abscess. If a patient with amebic liver abscess does not respond during the first few days of metronidazole therapy, aspiration of the abscess site is indicated. This can be done either by needle aspiration or by open drainage, depending on the patient's clinical course. If amebic peritonitis is a complication of intestinal amebiasis, laparotomy should be avoided if possible because the bowel is almost impossible to resuture. Supportive measures such as maintaining fluid and electrolyte balance are essential when patients with amebic liver abscess and peritonitis are seriously ill.

PREVENTION. Amebiasis is prevented by interrupting the contamination of food and water with human feces. The most commonly contaminated foods are vegetables grown near the ground such as lettuce, celery, tomatoes, and cucumbers. In addition, water is a frequent vehicle for the transmission of amebiasis. Both fresh, uncooked food and water should be avoided in any developing country because of the danger of contamination with amebae. Chlorine treatment is not completely effective in preventing infection by amebae. Boiling water for 10 minutes, on the other hand, kills both trophozoites and cysts. Improvement in waste disposal and water purification is the most important factor in ultimately reducing the risk of acquiring amebic disease.

Diseases caused by free-living amebae

There are free-living amebae that live in fresh water and the soil as well as in the oral cavity of humans. Recently one genus, *Naegleria,* has been associated with amebic meningoencephalitis in humans. This disease occurs when amebae in fresh water are forced under pressure through the nasal mucosa covering the cribriform plate and into the brain tissue. This occurs during diving and water-skiing in contaminated freshwater lakes. Another ameba, *Acanthamoeba,* has been found as a normal inhabitant of the human mouth. It has been associated recently with progressive inflammatory lesions of the cornea and granulomatous lesions in the brain. There is no known disease of the oral cavity associated with the *Acanthamoeba.* Treatment is ineffective in both of these illnesses, although amphotericin B has been successful in two cases in the treatment of *Naegleria* meningoencephalitis. The infection of the eye with *Acanthamoeba* organisms usually is associated with other organisms that contribute to the ulcerative lesion.

GIARDIASIS

Giardia lamblia is a flagellate that resides in the lumen of the upper gastrointestinal tract and may cause inflammatory changes in the mucosa leading to enteritis and malabsorption.

EPIDEMIOLOGY. *Giardia* organisms are distributed throughout the world in both temperate and tropical climates. Because of the resistance of the cyst stage of the organism in water,

---

*Parasitic Disease Drug Service, Center for Infectious Diseases, Centers for Disease Control, Atlanta, Ga. 30333. Telephone: days, 404-329-3670.

the occurrence of giardiasis is one of the first signs of a break in the water purification system. The disease is both endemic and epidemic. For example, in Colorado there is a high prevalence of infection among citizens in rural towns, and the disease has occurred in epidemics among skiers at ski lodges during the winter months. These epidemics undoubtedly result from overtaxing of waste disposal and water purification facilities by large numbers of people. The organism is a common cause of infection throughout the developing countries because of incomplete management of human waste disposal. Recently strains of *Giardia* that can infect humans have been identified in animal reservoirs such as beavers, further complicating the epidemiology and efforts to control the spread of infection. Immunodeficient patients have a much higher prevalence of giardiasis than normal individuals even though they have not traveled to recognized endemic areas.

LIFE CYCLE OF THE ORGANISM. *Giardia* organisms exist in two stages: the cyst and the trophozoite. The cyst stage is the mechanism by which the organism can persist in water for long periods. The cyst is oval shaped, approximately 14 μm long and 8 μm wide. It has two to four nuclei and a characteristic central rodlike structure called an axostyle. When the cyst is ingested, it can pass through the stomach to the upper duodenum, where excystation occurs. The second stage is the trophozoite. This organism has two nuclei and four pairs of flagella that contribute to its active motility. The trophozoite resides on the mucosal surface of the upper intestinal tract. For unknown reasons this association produces impaired absorption and changes leading to the signs and symptoms of giardiasis.

CLINICAL MANIFESTATIONS. The main symptoms of giardiasis include abdominal pain, distention, increased sensations of bowel activity, nausea, and intermittent watery diarrhea. During chronic infections anorexia, intolerance of certain foods, and weight loss are characteristic. The diagnosis is made by identifying either the cysts or the trophozoites of *Giardia* on microscopic examination of stool specimens. Occasionally the presence of *Giardia* organisms cannot be detected in the stool, and the organism must be sought in specimens from the upper intestinal tract. This is done by microscopic examination of a string that has been passed into the upper intestinal tract. An aspirate of duodenal contents can also reveal the organisms.

MANAGEMENT. Treatment of giardiasis is accomplished by one of two drugs: quinacrine (100 mg three times a day for 7 days) or metronidazole (one tablet [250 mg] three times a day for 5 to 10 days). Either will eradicate the infection in most patients. If patients have a recurrence of their illness, retreatment is indicated.

PREVENTION. Giardiasis is prevented only by ensuring that water purification systems are complete. The cysts are resistant to chlorination alone; therefore purification systems that rely entirely on this mechanism are not safe. Boiling water for 10 to 15 minutes and sophisticated water purification systems such as aeration, sedimentation, filtration, and chlorination will prevent spread of the infection.

CRYPTOSPORIDIOSIS

Cryptosporidium organisms are coccidian protozoa that recently have been demonstrated to cause serious, progressive gastrointestinal disease in immunocompromised patients, particularly those with acquired immunodeficiency syndrome (AIDS), and to be a relatively common cause of transient illness in immune-competent humans. The infection is transmitted to humans from animals such as lambs, goats, calves, pigs, rodents, puppies, cats, and poultry, and from human to human by fecal-oral contamination.

EPIDEMIOLOGY. Two of the 17 recognized species of *Cryptosporidium* have been documented to infect mammals, *Cryptosporidium parrum* and *Cryptosporidium muris*. These organisms commonly infect young farm and domestic animals, putting veterinarians and other animal handlers at high risk of infection. In addition, spread has occurred via human to human transmission in families, day-care centers and among homosexual males. Waterborne spread has occurred in travelers. Organisms are excreted in feces during episodes of diarrhea, but asymptomatic infected animals and humans may allow spread of the infection.

LIFE CYCLE OF THE ORGANISM. The life cycle includes ingestion of infectious oocysts, invasion (to an intracellular, extracytoplasmic position) of microvilli of the intestinal tract by sporozoites released from the oocyst, replication, and reinvasion of other cells to initiate the male and female gametes of the sexual cycle (sporogony). Oocysts are then formed that can release organisms within the intestine, leading to an autoinfection, or that can be passed in the stool. The microvillus border becomes lined with the developing organisms, which are 2 to 4 μm in size. Organisms may appear as artifacts on routine microscopy because of their tiny size; electron microscopy may be necessary to visualize them.

The pathologic changes in the intestine include loss of epithelium, villus atrophy, and inflammation of the adjacent lamina propria. The organism has been found associated with the mucosal surface in the entire intestinal tract, including the pharynx, as well as the biliary ducts, gallbladder, and bronchi.

CLINICAL MANIFESTATIONS. Clinical manifestations of the infection appear to be governed almost entirely by the immunologic competence of the infected individual. In immunocompetent humans the disease includes transient diarrhea with watery stools lasting 1 to 2 weeks, abdominal cramps, and occasionally fever and nausea. The symptoms and shedding of oocysts stop spontaneously. Some individuals remain completely asymptomatic during the infection. In a recent study using serologic evaluation, 86% of those tested were infected without recognized disease. In the immunocompromised human, the infection may be prolonged, associated with marked signs of malabsorption, fluid and electrolyte loss, continuous identification of large numbers of oocysts in the feces, and unresponsiveness to therapy. The first cases of severe infection were associated with immunoglobulin deficiencies, but recently severe infection has been observed primarily in patients with AIDS. In these patients symptoms may persist for months and contribute to death of the patient. Cryptosporidial cholecystitis has been documented in these patients as well.

DIAGNOSIS. The diagnosis of cryptosporidiosis is made by identifying oocysts in the stool and by careful examination of small bowel biopsy specimens. The stool examination requires special testing, including such techniques as iodine and acid-fast staining of fecal specimens (*Cryptosporidium* organisms are iodine negative and acid-fast positive) and special sugar flotation technique (Sheather sugar flotation) for concentrating the oocysts.

MANAGEMENT. Since there is no effective therapy, attention to fluid and electrolyte management, parenteral nutrition, and reversal of immunosuppressive factors are the important steps in altering morbidity and mortality from the disease. A few patients have been said to respond to spiramycin (3 gm/day for 3 days), and in some patients α-difluorimethylornithine has been partially effective.

PREVENTION. Preventing cryptosporidial infection requires avoiding all potential sources of contamination from animal and human feces. Reversing immunodeficient states prevents progression of the disease.

TOXOPLASMOSIS

Infection with the protozoan *Toxoplasma gondii* is common in all mammals and birds. Human infection often occurs without symptoms; however, there may be transient lymphadenopathy and fever in immunologically normal adults and a severe progressive disease in individuals with impaired immune responsiveness. Recurrent inflammatory disease of the eye also is a manifestation of toxoplasmosis. The organism is acquired by ingesting undercooked meat that contains the viable organisms or by ingestion of the infectious oocyst stage in the feces of cats.

EPIDEMIOLOGY. *T. gondii* is the most common single species that infects all mammals. Its prevalence rate is extremely high in some parts of the world, such as Tahiti and some Caribbean islands, where infection approaches 100% in humans. In most parts of the world the prevalence ranges from 30% to 60%, depending on the disposal facilities for cat feces and the propensity of the population to eat undercooked meats such as mutton, pork, or beef. Only in very dry or extremely cold areas in the world is the infection of low prevalence. A few islands in the Pacific where cats have never been introduced remain free of toxoplasmosis. The most common means of the spread of disease among humans in the United States is by ingesting meat contaminated with *Toxoplasma* cysts. Because of this, 1% of the 15- to 50-year-old population is infected each year. Once infected, a person remains infected for life, although symptoms of the infection may be absent or only transient in nature.

LIFE CYCLE OF THE ORGANISM. When a mammal eats meat containing the cyst, the cyst passes into the intestine and liberates hundreds or thousands of trophozoites, the obligate intracellular form. The trophozoites, which are 7 μm long and 3 to 4 μm wide, enter the mucosal cells of the gastrointestinal tract. They then divide with a generation time of 5 to 10 hours, rupture the cells, and infect adjacent cells. During this process they enter cells that gain access to the vascular system and are distributed throughout the body. During the immune response the generation time of the parasite lengthens, and a firm wall forms around the *Toxoplasma* organism. The encysted parasite persists in muscle and brain tissue throughout the lifetime of the host. When another mammal ingests this tissue, the life cycle is continued. This is referred to as the asexual cycle of toxoplasmosis.

When a cat ingests the infectious form of the *Toxoplasma* organism, an additional process occurs. A sexual cycle is initiated in the intestinal mucosa of members of the feline family. The penetrating trophozoites develop into macrogametocytes or microgametocytes. After cross-fertilization a zygote is formed and matures into an infective oocyst. The excreted cat feces containing the infective oocysts then contaminate the environment. Cattle, sheep, and pigs usually are infected by ingesting these oocysts. These two mechanisms are responsible for the high prevalence of infection in nature.

PATHOLOGY. After the *Toxoplasma* organism has entered the cell, divided, and caused the rupture of the cell, an acute inflammatory response occurs in the presence of this progressive tissue necrosis. If the human has no immune responsiveness, as in a fetus, a progressive severe necrotic process results throughout the body. However, in immunologically normal adults an immune response against the organism occurs. This is first manifested by fever and enlargement of lymph nodes. At this time the invasion of muscle tissue by *Toxoplasma* or-

ganisms leads to limited myositis. If the immune response is complete, the encysted *Toxoplasma* organism causes no further damage to the infected tissue after the initial invasion period. Intermittently, a cyst may rupture and is then rapidly controlled by an intense delayed hypersensitivity inflammatory response to the organism. This prevents spread of the infection once the patient is immune, even though living organisms persist in the tissue for life. In very sensitive areas, such as the retina of the eye, this well-localized inflammatory reaction can cause signs and symptoms such as retinochoroiditis. If an illness associated with immunosuppression develops, toxoplasmosis can reactivate and lead to progressive necrosis. This often occurs in the central nervous system (CNS), and the patient exhibits signs of encephalitis.

CLINICAL MANIFESTATIONS. Toxoplasmosis can be divided into four clinical patterns of disease: acquired lymphatic toxoplasmosis, congenital toxoplasmosis, toxoplasmic retinochoroiditis, and the syndrome of toxoplasmosis in the altered host. Those with acquired toxoplasmosis, when symptomatic, usually have lymph node enlargement, most commonly of the cervical lymph nodes. Approximately half of these patients also have fever, myalgias, malaise, and fatigue. The lymph nodes usually are nontender and rubbery in consistency. These symptoms last for 1 to 2 weeks; however, in most patients the lymphadenopathy persists for months. In rare cases symptoms of severe myocarditis or myositis occur at the time of acute infection in an otherwise healthy adult. Laboratory tests of patients with acquired toxoplasmosis demonstrate a slight monocytosis or lymphocytosis. Atypical lymphocytes, which are seen in infectious mononucleosis, are not present in large numbers. There may be slight changes in liver function tests during the first few days or weeks of the illness. The blood cell counts usually are normal. Biopsy of the lymph node shows a typical pattern of hyperplasia of histiocytes.

Neonates with congenital toxoplasmosis have severe inflammatory changes in the organs. The manifestations may be microphthalmia, hydrocephalus, hepatosplenomegaly, pneumonitis, and fever. The brain lesions may lead to calcification that can be identified roentgenographically several months after infection. Some neonates may not show the full picture of congenital toxoplasmosis at birth, and there may be a progressive inflammatory disease during the first months of life. In addition, some infants infected late in the pregnancy may have only mild signs or symptoms at birth but may demonstrate subtle changes in the CNS such as seizures or retinochoroiditis later in life.

The onset of toxoplasmic retinochoroiditis most often occurs during the second or third decade of life, even though infection commonly occurs during intrauterine life. This is therefore a later sequela of infection associated with a hypersensitivity response to the organisms. This illness often is recurrent with intermittent episodes of loss of vision and pain in the eye and resulting scar formation. Systemic signs of *T. gondii* infection are not present during this local inflammatory reaction.

Toxoplasmosis usually occurs as a disseminated disease in patients with altered cellular immune responsiveness such as those with AIDS or Hodgkin's disease. Patients often have fever and signs of encephalitis. Disseminated signs and symptoms such as those seen in congenital toxoplasmosis also may be present. Patients with less severe immunosuppression may have recurrent lymphadenopathic toxoplasmosis or progressive polymyositis as evidence of impaired ability to control the replication of the *Toxoplasma* organisms.

DIAGNOSIS. The diagnosis of toxoplasmosis rests on three standard procedures: first, the isolation of the protozoan from infected tissue; second, histopathologic identification of the organism in tissue; and third, interpretation of the changing serologic pattern associated with infection.

Since the organism is an obligate intracellular parasite, isolation techniques require the use of animal inoculation or cell culture systems. In most laboratories animal inoculation is used. The tissue for examination is made into a suspension and inoculated into the peritoneal cavity of mice. Several weeks after the inoculation the mice are examined for the presence of developing *Toxoplasma* organisms. *Toxoplasma* organisms can be identified in tissue by routine staining procedures. It must be recognized that identification of *Toxoplasma* cysts in muscle or brain tissue may have no pathologic significance, because these are present in the tissue of any person with antibodies against the organism. On the other hand, identification of clusters of organisms in muscle or brain associated with inflammatory cells is good evidence for an association of the pathologic process and the microbe.

Usually the diagnosis of toxoplasmosis rests on noninvasive testing such as serologic evaluation. Four different serologic tests are used in toxoplasmosis. The classic test, the Sabin-Feldman dye test, is one of the most specific antibody tests in medicine; a positive test indicates previous infection. However, since infection with *T. gondii* is so common, it may not be helpful in distinguishing the recently infected, diseased patient from the patient infected many years before. The indirect fluorescent antibody (IFA) test measures the same antibody as the Sabin-Feldman dye test and can be substituted for that test, since it is simpler to perform and less expensive. Laboratories using the IFA test must be aware that it depends on appropriate standardization of the reagents. To document recent exposure to *T. gondii,* the IgM-fluorescent antibody test, the double sandwich IgM–enzyme-linked immunosorbent assay (IgM-ELISA) test, and the soluble-antigen complement fixation test are available. High or changing antibody titers of these tests are consistent with recent infection. A hemagglutination test also is used in toxoplasmosis. Like the Sabin-Feldman dye test, it is helpful in documenting past *Toxoplasma* infection; however, it is unreliable for determining recent infection. In patients with AIDS, serologic tests alone usually are not helpful in diagnosis of reactivated toxoplasmosis. Brain scan and brain biopsy are necessary in this setting.

The four main clinical presentations of toxoplasmosis have separate differential diagnoses. Adult-acquired toxoplasmosis must be distinguished from infectious mononucleosis and lymphoma. Congenital toxoplasmosis must be distinguished from cytomegalovirus infection, viral encephalitis, and the rubella syndrome. Toxoplasmic retinochoroiditis must be distinguished from other causes of inflammation of the retina such as tuberculosis, histoplasmosis, and sarcoidosis. Toxoplasmosis in the altered host requires differentiation from the other disseminated infectious diseases occurring in immunosuppressed patients. These include viral encephalitis, cryptococcosis, and progression of the underlying disease.

MANAGEMENT. Toxoplasmosis is treated with a combination of drugs directed at inhibiting folate metabolism. The most effective combination currently is a combination of pyrimethamine and sulfadiazine. Pyrimethamine is given in doses of 75 mg the first day and 25 mg each day thereafter for 1 to 2 months, depending on the illness. Sulfadiazine is given as 4 g/day in four divided doses. Folinic acid is administered intramuscularly along with these medicines to prevent bone marrow toxicity.

Patients with mild forms of adult-acquired toxoplasmosis do not require therapy. However, those with severe toxoplasmosis, toxoplasmic retinochoroiditis, and congenital toxoplasmosis may benefit from therapy against *Toxoplasma* organisms. In addition, retinochoroiditis is treated with corticosteroids to inhibit the inflammatory response that leads to much of the eye damage.

PREVENTION. Toxoplasmosis is prevented by appropriate cooking of all meats. This means that meat should be cooked to a temperature of at least 140° F (60° C) throughout for 15 minutes. Exposure to oocysts from cat feces can be limited by having little contact with scavenger cats and their environment, changing cat litter boxes daily, and using gloves for gardening and work in sandboxes. Pregnant women and immunosuppressed patients should be particularly cautious and should avoid exposure to either of the two means of acquiring toxoplasmosis. Prophylactic use of antifolate drugs in patients with AIDS to prevent pneumocystis also may delay reactivation of toxoplasmosis.

TRICHOMONIASIS

One of the most common protozoal infections in temperate climates is caused by the venereally spread protozoan *Trichomonas vaginalis*. The organism is a flagellate, 10 to 20 μm in size with a single nucleus, a central structure called an axostyle, and an undulating membrane. It moves in exudative material by a jerky, rotating motion. Unlike *Giardia* organisms or amebae, the trichomonad has no vegetative stage, and infection requires direct contact with infected surfaces. The organism may persist for long periods in endocervical or urethral glands and less commonly in other sites of the genitourinary system without causing inflammation. It is sensitive to pH changes and does not survive well at a pH below 5. Under ideal conditions for protozoal replication, it induces marked inflammation of the mucosal surfaces of the vagina, urethra, urinary bladder, or prostate. Patients usually have symptoms of vaginal itching, burning, and a yellow, blood-tinged discharge. If the urethra is involved, the symptoms of inflammation include dysuria and frequency of urination.

The diagnosis is made by observing the motile organisms in fresh vaginal or urethral material. A drop of the material is mixed with saline and a small amount of methylene blue and examined under the low or medium power of the microscope. Culture of *Trichomonas* organisms also is possible.

Treatment of *T. vaginalis* is accomplished by a single dose of metronidazole. Either 1 or 2 g has been recommended. If this is ineffective, the more traditional, longer duration therapy with 250 mg three times a day for 10 days can be used. The most important point in the management of trichomoniasis is that all sexual partners must be treated to prevent reinfection. In rare cases the infection can be transmitted to infants during birth and among individuals in institutions where personal hygiene is poor.

Two other *Trichomonas* species, *Trichomonas tenax* and *Trichomonas hominis,* exist in humans but are considered nonpathogens.

LEISHMANIASIS

Leishmaniasis refers to several different diseases caused by species of the genus *Leishmania*. The disease can be subdivided into three primary disease processes: visceral leishmaniasis (kala-azar), cutaneous leishmaniasis (also referred to as Old World leishmaniasis), and mucocutaneous leishmaniasis.

EPIDEMIOLOGY. Visceral leishmaniasis is caused by the organism *Leishmania donovani*. It is distributed throughout the world but occurs primarily in tropical climates. However, one form of visceral leishmaniasis occurs in temperate climates extending from the Mediterranean region to China. The organism is maintained in nature in several animal reservoirs including dogs and rodents, as well as humans. The sandfly, *Phlebotomus,* is responsible for transmitting the disease from one mammalian host to another.

Cutaneous leishmaniasis is seen in the Near and Middle East and in Africa. The organism causing this disease is *Leishmania tropica*. Animal reservoirs also are important in the persistence of this disease in nature.

Mucocutaneous leishmaniasis is caused by a complex of *Leishmania* organisms, but most disease of a mucosal type is caused by members of the group *Leishmania braziliensis*. These diseases occur primarily in Central and South America.

LIFE CYCLE OF THE ORGANISM. *Leishmania* organisms are single-cell obligate intracellular parasites that parasitize phagocytic cells of the mammalian host. As the name implies, visceral *Leishmania* organisms tend to survive well at mammalian host temperature and to parasitize the reticuloendothelial cells of the liver, spleen, and bone marrow. The cutaneous and mucocutaneous forms of leishmaniasis are confined primarily to the skin and mucosal membranes. At these sites the amastigote or nonflagellated form persists. When an appropriate species of sandfly bites an infected person, the sandfly becomes infected and the promastigote or flagellated form of the *Leishmania* parasite develops in the gut of the fly. After an appropriate period of development, during biting a regurgitation of the intestinal material allows infection of another mammalian host.

PATHOLOGY. The pathology of the lesion, whether in the visceral or the cutaneous form of the disease, includes replication of the *Leishmania* organisms in the histiocytes and a chronic inflammatory reaction at the site of microbe replication. In some of the cutaneous forms of the infection and in the visceral form, the immune reaction appears ineffective and large numbers of organisms can be identified. In the mucosal disease, however, there is a marked inflammatory reaction but very few organisms can be identified. In the mucosal disease there is progressive destruction of the cartilage and supporting structures of the oral and nasal cavities. This leads to marked deformity in late stages of the disease.

CLINICAL MANIFESTATIONS. In visceral leishmaniasis the organism replaces bone marrow function and normal spleen. Visceral leishmaniasis often occurs in young children and is manifested by signs of fever, splenomegaly, leukopenia, anemia, and thrombocytopenia. The complications leading to death in this illness are associated with bleeding and septicemia.

Cutaneous leishmaniasis occurs as an ulcer on the skin at the site of the *Phlebotomus* bite. This ulcer, which may persist as long as 1 to 2 years, is a flat, buttonlike lesion with erythematous raised edges. The lesion often is secondarily infected. In most patients this lesion heals spontaneously; however, in rare cases a diffuse, nonhealing form of the disease is present.

The clinical manifestations of mucocutaneous leishmaniasis are more complex. The illness usually begins as cutaneous leishmaniasis with a slowly healing ulcer at the site of the *Phlebotomus* bite on the extremities or face. Metastatic lesions occasionally occur years after healing of this lesion and produce a progressive inflammatory lesion of the nasal or oral cavity. This may be manifested by signs of nasal stuffiness or a progressive mass lesion of the palate, larynx, or other sites in the oral cavity. This lesion may be confused with the lesions of midline granuloma or paracoccidioidomycosis. If the lesion goes untreated, secondary problems such as aspiration pneumonia and dietary insufficiency develop. The diagnosis of

leishmaniasis depends on isolation of the parasite from appropriate tissue, such as spleen, bone marrow, skin, or the mucosal lesion. Antibodies can be detected in the circulation of most patients with leishmaniasis. A skin test called the Montenegro test has been useful in identifying patients with leishmaniasis, even early in the illness. In patients with disseminated disease this test may be negative.

MANAGEMENT. Patients with all varieties of leishmaniasis can be treated with antimony preparations. Sodium stibogluconate (available from the Centers for Disease Control*) is the drug of choice. However, recently some patients with visceral or mucocutaneous leishmaniasis have shown inadequate response to this drug, and for these patients amphotericin B must be used.

PREVENTION. Leishmaniasis is prevented only by decreasing exposure to the infected sandfly vectors. Fine-mesh mosquito netting and careful application of insect repellents are necessary to avoid contact with these vectors.

TRYPANOSOMIASIS

There are two main types of trypanosomes that infect humans. The first is organisms in the *Trypanosoma brucei* complex, which cause Africa trypanosomiasis. The second is *Trypanosoma cruzi*, the cause of American trypanosomiasis. These two diseases are distinct clinically and geographically. Their geographic distribution is determined by their different vectors. African trypanosomiasis, also called sleeping sickness, is transmitted from person to person or animal to human by the tsetse fly. American trypanosomiasis is transmitted during the feeding of the reduviid bug.

African trypanosomiasis, because of the distribution of the vector, is confined to tropical regions of Africa. The pathologic response during African trypanosomiasis includes an initial immune response with lymph node and spleen enlargement while the flagellated protozoa are circulating in the peripheral blood. Following the vascular phase, invasion of the CNS occurs, causing CNS vasculitis and encephalitis. The cellular response includes infiltration of mononuclear cells around the blood vessels of the brain. During the immune response to trypanosomiasis large amounts of IgM antibody are produced. Continued variation in the antigens on the surface of the trypanosome is believed to allow persistence of the organism in the host until death occurs. The clinical features of African trypanosomiasis include high fever and lymphadenopathy in the early phase of the illness. During CNS invasion there is initially a phase of sleeplessness, then a progression to somnolence and coma. In this phase the lack of attention to proper eating and aspiration leads to death of the patient as a result of malnutrition and secondary infection. The diagnosis is made by identifying the flagellated protozoa in the peripheral blood or CNS. Serologic tests may be helpful in confirming the diagnosis. The treatment is complex and includes the use of arsenicals and the polysulfated drug suramin. Prevention of the infection depends mainly on avoiding the bite of an infected tsetse fly. Chemoprophylaxis is not recommended.

American trypanosomiasis, or Chagas' disease, occurs throughout South America. Durirng the bite of the reduviid bug, which feeds at night while the subject is sleeping, the contaminated feces of the bug are inoculated into the wound. At this site a trypanosomal chancre occurs, and if it is in the eye, a unilateral conjunctivitis referred to as Romaña's sign is seen. Shortly after inoculation of the protozoa there is a period

---

*CDC Drug Service Center for Infectious Diseases, Centers for Disease Control, Atlanta, Ga. 30333. Telephone: 404-329-3670.

of parasitemia. The microbes then enter the muscle cells of the myocardium and also induce damage in the parasympathetic ganglia (particularly Auerbach's plexus in the esophagus). Damage to these organs produces the late complications of Chagas' disease, including dysfunction of the myocardium and abnormal function of the intestinal tract. The clinical presentation of Chagas' disease includes an initial acute-phase illness and a subsequent chronic phase. The acute illness is characterized by high fever and myocarditis. The initial illness may have as a hallmark the appearance of a skin lesion at the inoculation site or unilateral conjunctivitis. Some patients are asymptomatic during this initial infection. The diagnosis is made by observation of parasitemia. Many years later persistence of the organism in the myocardium and nerve tissue leads to signs of congestive myocardiopathy and/or the so-called mega-syndromes, that is, megaesophagus caused by dysfunction of esophageal motility or megacolon caused by dysfunction of the colon. A patient with congestive myocardiopathy also may have complications of intermittent arrhythmias and thrombi on the inner surface of the myocardium. Pulmonary emboli or fatal arrhythmias are the common causes of death in Chagas' heart disease. The diagnosis in this chronic phase is made by serologic tests or xenodiagnosis. The acute phase of the illness is treated with nifurtimox (available from the Centers for Disease Control*). The chronic form of the disease does not respond to antiprotozoal therapy, and careful management of arrhythmias and thrombotic complications is indicated. Prevention of the disease is accomplished only by avoiding the bite of the reduviid bug, which resides especially in and around houses constructed of mud and sticks. In addition, the disease may be transmitted by the transfusion of improperly treated blood.

PNEUMOCYSTOSIS

Pneumocystosis is an acute infection of the lungs characterized by fever, shortness of breath, and cyanosis. It occurs in patients who are immunodeficient as a result of malnutrition, malignancy, AIDS, or immunosuppressive therapy. The causative organism, *Pneumocystis* sp. is of uncertain classification but is probably a protozoan. It is presumed to cause frequent but asymptomatic infection in healthy mammalian hosts.

EPIDEMIOLOGY. Different species of *Pneumocystis* are widely distributed throughout the animal kingdom. However, pneumocystosis is not a zoonosis because the organisms are species specific. Therefore humans are infected only from other human reservoirs, not from other animals. It is thought that the disease is spread by respiratory droplet spray from an infected individual. The epidemiologic data suggest that the organism is quite infectious but of low pathogenicity. The disease occurs most commonly in patients who have AIDS, who are agammaglobulinemic, or who are receiving corticosteroids or antimetabolites.

LIFE CYCLE OF THE ORGANISM. *Pneumocystis* organisms occur in two stages in the lung of the infected host. The first stage is referred to as the trophozoite. In the second stage the trophozoite evolves into a cyst, apparently by converting an inner membrane into a germinal surface from which oval bodies called sporozoites develop. Six to eight sporozoites develop within the cyst, which is surrounded by a thick, polysaccharide-containing wall. The cyst then ruptures, releasing sporozoites to initiate other cysts. After release the sporozoites are termed

trophozoites. It is also believed that some form of division of trophozoites can lead to a trophozoite-trophozoite cycle. The trophozoite forms can be stained with Giemsa stain; however, the cyst requires staining with special stains for the cyst wall such as the Gram-Weigert and methenamine silver stains.

PATHOLOGY. When patients are immunosuppressed, the *Pneumocystis* organisms divide in the alveolar spaces of the lung. This initiates an inflammatory response characterized by mononuclear cells, in some cases including plasma cells. The alveoli become filled with a proteinaceous material and clumps of *Pneumocystis* organisms. The interstitial spaces of the alveoli are filled with inflammatory cells. This process leads to decreased oxygen exchange and the signs and symptoms of respiratory insufficiency.

CLINICAL MANIFESTATIONS. The major symptoms of pneumocystosis are shortness of breath and a nonproductive cough. Fever may be present. In some patients the symptoms are insidious in onset, whereas in others they are more rapid. The patient may progress to a moribund state caused by the anoxia resulting from poor oxygen exchange. Physical examination indicates respiratory distress and cyanosis. The lungs may reveal diffuse scattered rales and rhonchi. Diagnostic laboratory tests detect abnormalities in blood gas exchange, and chest roentgenography shows diffuse alveolar and interstitial pneumonitis.

DIAGNOSIS. The diagnosis of pneumocystosis is made by bronchial lavage or biopsy of infected lungs and appropriate staining for the cysts. An immunofluorescent antibody test also is available; however, it should not be relied on for definite diagnosis, since it may not always be positive in immunosuppressed patients.

MANAGEMENT. Pneumocystosis is treated with the combination drug trimethoprim-sulfamethoxazole (20 mg/kg/day of trimethoprim and 100 mg/kg/day of sulfamethoxazole in four divided doses orally or intravenously) or with pentamidine for several weeks. This therapy has reduced mortality from nearly 100% to below 50%. Supportive therapy for respiration is essential. In addition, reduction in doses of corticosteroids should be attempted. However, the symptoms may require a transient increase in the dose.

PREVENTION. Pneumocystosis can be prevented by interfering with the transmission of the organism among immunosuppressed patients. Therefore patients with the disease should be managed with respiratory precautions. In addition, crowding among patients who are potentially immunosuppressed, as in wards devoted to patients with malignancies or in clinics, should be avoided. Early detection, rapid treatment, and isolation of infected patients can also diminish the spread of the disease.

Prophylaxis of pneumocystosis has been achieved in selected high-risk populations (such as patients with acute lymphocytic leukemia or with AIDS) by giving maintenance trimethoprim-sulfamethoxazole.

BABESIOSIS

Babesiosis is an acute febrile disease characterized by fever, myalgias, and hemolytic anemia. It is caused by the intraerythrocytic protozoan microbe *Babesia,* which is transmitted to humans by infected ticks.

EPIDEMIOLOGY. *Babesia* organisms are distributed widely throughout nature and infect numerous animals, including cattle, dogs, horses, and rodents. In the past, infection of humans was confined to those who were immunosuppressed, such as by splenectomy, and who had exposure to farm animals infected with *Babesia* organisms. Recently, however, epidemics have occurred on the northeastern coast of the United States,

---

*CDC Drug Service Center for Infectious Diseases, Centers for Disease Control, Atlanta, Ga. 30333. Telephone: 404-329-3670.

where transmission of *Babesia microti* from rodents to humans has occurred.

PATHOLOGY. In human infection with *Babesia* spp. the organism enters and destroys RBCs, which leads to hemolytic anemia and obstruction of capillary blood flow with secondary tissue anoxia. The infection usually is controlled by immune responses in the normal host. However, infection with *B. microti* occurs in patients over the age of 45 years who are immunologically normal. Patients who have had splenectomy are susceptible to severe and progressive disease.

CLINICAL MANIFESTATIONS. The clinical manifestations of babesiosis include high fever, drenching sweats, and chills, as well as marked lethargy and muscle discomfort. The illness usually begins 1 to 6 weeks after the tick bite transmits the infection to the patient. The patient may appear very toxic. In addition, nausea, vomiting, and abdominal pain have been reported. Laboratory tests demonstrae thrombocytopenia, anemia, and proteinuria. Liver function may be slightly abnormal. The diagnosis of babesiosis is made by examination of a blood smear stained with Giemsa or Wright's stain, which demonstrates the intracellular *Babesia* organisms in 1% to 10% of RBCs. The diagnosis can be confirmed by inoculating the patient's blood into animals and performing serologic tests for the presence of *Babesia* organisms.

MANAGEMENT. The treatment is with clindamycin (600 mg four times a day) and quinine (650 mg three times a day for 7 days) both orally. In some patients exchange transfusion has been necessary to reverse progressive deterioration. Some patients can be managed successfully with analgesics alone.

PREVENTION. Babesiosis is prevented by avoiding tick-infested areas and using appropriate tick repellents. Splenectomized patients should not vacation or work during the summer months in areas of heavy tick infestation.

BIBLIOGRAPHY
General references

Beaver PC, Jung RC, and Cupp EW: Clinical parasitology, ed 4, Philadelphia, 1984, Lea & Febiger.
Drugs for parasitic infections, Med Lett Drugs Ther 28:9, 1986.
Manson-Bahr DEC: Manson's tropical diseases, ed 18, London, 1982, Baillière Tindall.

Malaria

Hall AP: The treatment of malaria, Br Med J 1:323, 1976.
Jeffrey GM: Malaria control in the twentieth century, Am J Trop Med Hyg 25:361, 1976.
Maegraith B and Fletcher A: The pathogenesis of mammalian malaria, Adv Parasitol 10:49, 1972.
Neva FA and others: Malaria: host-defense mechanisms and complications, Ann Intern Med 73:295, 1970.
World Health Organization: Chemotherapy of malaria and resistance to antimalarials, WHO Tech Rep Ser No 529, p 1, 1973.

Amebiasis

Adams EB and MacLeod IN: Invasive amebiasis. I. Amebic dysentery and its complications, Medicine 56:315, 1977.
Adams EB and MacLeod IN: Invasive amebiasis. II. Amebic liver abscess and its complications, Medicine 56:325, 1977.
Barbour GL and Juniper K Jr: A clinical comparison of amebic and pyogenic abscess of the liver in sixty-six patients, Am J Med 53:323, 1972.

Elsdon-Dew R: The epidemiology of amoebiasis, Adv Parasitol 1:62, 1968.
Kean BH: The treatment of amebiasis, JAMA 235:501, 1976.
Powell SJ and Elsdon-Dew R: Some new nitroimidazole derivatives: clinical trials in amebic liver abscess, Am J Trop Med Hyg 21:518, 1972.
Nagington J and others: Amoebic infection of the eye, Lancet 2:1537, 1974.
Neva FA: Amebic meningoencephalitis: a new disease, N Engl J Med 282:450, 1970.
Wang SS and Feldman HA: Isolation of *Hartmanella* species from human throats, N Engl J Med 277:1174, 1967.

Giardiasis

Hoskins LC and others: Clinical giardiasis and intestinal malabsorption, Gastroenterology 53:265, 1967.
Knight R: Giardiasis, isosporiasis, and balantidiasis, Clin Gastroenterol 7:31, 1978.
Yardley JH, Takano J, and Hendrix TB: Epithelial and other mucosal lesions of the jejunum in giardiasis: jejunal biopsy studies, Bull Hopkins Hosp 115:389, 1964.

Cryptosporidiosis

Current WL and others: Human cryptosporidiosis in immunocompetent and immunodeficient individuals. Studies of an outbreak and experimental transmission, N Engl J Med 308:1252, 1983.
Soave R and Armstrong D: *Cryptosporidium* and cryptosporidiosis, Rev Infect Dis 8:1012, 1986.

Toxoplasmosis

Beverley JKA: Toxoplasmosis, Br Med J 2:475, 1973.
Frenkel JK: Toxoplasma in and around us, Bio Science 26:343, 1973.
Remington JS: Toxoplasmosis: recent developments, Annu Rev Med 21:201, 1970.
Ruskin J and Remington JS: Toxoplasmosis in the compromised host, Ann Intern Med 84:193, 1976.
Welch PC and others: The serologic diagnosis of acute lymphadenopathic toxoplasmosis, J Infect Dis 142:256, 1980.

Trichomoniasis

Dykers JR: Single dose metronidazole for trichomonal vaginitis: a follow-up, N Engl J Med 295:395, 1976.
Trussell RE: *Trichomonas vaginalis* and trichomoniasis, Springfield, Ill, 1947, Charles C Thomas, Publisher.

Leishmaniasis

Marsden PD and Nonata RR: Mucocutaneous leishmaniasis: a review of clinical aspects, Rev Soc Bras Med Trop 9:309, 1975.
Winslow DJ: Visceral leishmaniasis. In Marcial-Rojas RA: editor: Pathology of rickettsial and helminthic disease, Baltimore, 1971, The Williams & Wilkins Co.

Trypanosomiasis

American trypanosomiasis research, PAHO Scientific Publication 318, 1975.
Andrade Z and Andrade SG: Chagas' disease (American trypanosomiasis). In Marcial-Rojas RA, editor: Pathology of protozoal and helminthic diseases, Baltimore, 1971, The Williams & Wilkins Co.

Pneumocystosis

Burke BA and Good RA: *Pneumocystis carinii* infection, Medicine 52:23, 1973.
Mills J: *Pneumocystis carinii* and *Toxoplasma gondii* infections in patients with AIDS, Rev Infect Dis 8:1001, 1986.
Walzer PD and others: *Pneumocystis carinii* pneumonia in the United States: epidemiologic, diagnostic, and clinical features, Ann Intern Med 80:83, 1974.

Babesiosis

Healy GR, Spielman A, and Gleason N: Human babesiosis: reservoir of infection on Nantucket Island, Science 192:479, 1976.
Ruebush RK II and others: Human babesiosis on Nantucket Island, Ann Intern Med 86:6, 1977.

UNIT E • HELMINTHIC DISEASES

The parasitic worms that infect humans can be divided into the nematodes (roundworms), cestodes (tapeworms), and trematodes (flukes). All helminthic infections can produce eosinophilia. The more invasive the worm or the stage of the disease, the higher the eosinophilia. Large worm burdens in close contact with tissue such as occur in strongyloidiasis, visceral larva migrans, and trichinosis are particularly prone to cause high eosinophilia. Eosinophilia caused by parasitic infection must be differentiated from that occurring in polyarteritis nodosa, eosinophilic leukemia, lymphoma, and allergic conditions.

56 · DISEASES CAUSED BY NEMATODES (ROUNDWORMS)

Donald Kaye

ENTEROBIASIS

Enterobius vermicularis (pinworm) is found worldwide in all socioeconomic groups and infects mainly children. The adult female is about 10 mm long and lives with the smaller male in the large bowel. At night the females migrate to the anus, where they deposit eggs. The eggs and the migrating females cause pruritus ani. The eggs can be transmitted to the mouth via the hands or can contaminate the bedclothes and then be carried to the mouth on the hands. If swallowed, the eggs can develop into adult worms and perpetuate the infection. Appendicitis and vaginitis are occasional complications related to migration of the worms.

The diagnosis is best made by demonstrating eggs in the perianal area. On arising in the morning, before washing, the patient folds cellophane tape sticky side out over the finger or a tongue depressor and applies it against the anal margins. The tape is then folded on itself or stuck on a slide and examined for the characteristic eggs, which are 50 μm long and flattened on one side. Adult worms occasionally may be found in the feces or in the perianal area. Examination of the stool for ova is not a reliable way to make the diagnosis of pinworm. It is common for more than one member of the family to be affected, and all should be examined. Eosinophilia is rare.

Therapy is achieved with one 100 mg tablet of mebendazole, which should be repeated in 2 weeks. All bedclothes and undergarments should be cleaned during the 2 weeks between treatments.

TRICHURIASIS

Trichuris trichura (whipworm) is found all over the world but most frequently in the tropics. The worms are 30 to 50 mm long with a thin anterior (the whip) buried in the mucosa of the colon and a thicker posterior (the whip handle) projecting into the colon. Eggs passed in the feces become infective after 3 weeks in the soil and are ingested following contamination of food and water. Adult worms develop and survive in the large bowel for at least 3 years.

Although most patients are asymptomatic, heavy worm loads may cause colic, diarrhea, bleeding, and iron deficiency anemia. Large rectal worm loads can cause rectal prolapse (coconut cake rectum). Migrating worms can result in appendicitis. Eosinophilia is mild if present.

The diagnosis is made by finding the characteristic eggs, which are 50 μm long with bipolar plugs, in the feces. The treatment is with mebendazole (100 mg twice a day for 3 days). Prevention depends on sanitary disposal of human feces and avoidance of fecal contamination of food.

CAPILLARIASIS

Capillaria phillippinensis, found in the Philippines, is a 4 mm worm that infects the small intestine. It can produce colic, diarrhea, malabsorption, protein-losing enteropathy, edema, wasting, and death. The eggs found in the feces have bipolar plugs but are smaller than those of *T. trichura*. The treatment is with mebendazole (100 to 400 mg/day for 10 to 30 days).

ASCARIASIS

Ascaris lumbricoides is found worldwide but most often in the tropics. The adult is 15 to 30 cm long and lives in the small intestine. The worms stay in place by bridging themselves across the lumen of the gut. The life span of *A. lumbricoides* is 1 to 2 years.

Eggs passed in the feces become infective after about 10 days. After ingestion the eggs hatch in the small intestine, and larvae penetrate the intestinal mucosa. They are borne in the lymphatic system and bloodstream to the lung, where they rupture into the airways, are carried up the respiratory passages via ciliated epithelium, and are reswallowed. The adult worms then develop in the small intestine.

Light infections usually are asymptomatic. During the pulmonary phase of larval migration, fever, cough, bronchospasm, and hemoptysis may occur. There may be peripheral and sputum eosinophilia. Intestinal infection with the large, muscular worms may result in colic, perforation with peritonitis, obstruction (from large masses of worms) or appendicitis, bile duct obstruction, or pancreatic duct obstruction (from migration of the worms). Worms may be vomited up and aspirated.

The diagnosis is made by finding the characteristic eggs, which are rough and 50 μm long, in the feces. The worms may be seen after a barium meal, since barium appears in the *A. lumbricoides* intestine.

The therapy is mebendazole (100 mg twice a day for 3 days). Prevention depends on sanitary disposal of human feces and avoidance of fecal contamination of food.

VISCERAL LARVAE MIGRANS

Visceral larva migrans, an infection primarily of children, results from human infection with the dog or cat *Ascaris* organisms and is found all over the world. *Toxocara canis* (dog *Ascaris*) and *Toxocara cati* (cat *Ascaris*) eggs become infective 2 weeks after being passed in the feces of the host animal (usually a puppy). If ingested by humans, larvae penetrate the wall of the intestine as in *A. lumbricoides* infection. However, the cycle is not completed, and the larvae migrate to the liver and other organs such as the eye, where they become trapped.

The symptoms are fever and high eosinophila (50% or more). Tender hepatomegaly, endophthalmitis, pneumonitis, cerebritis, myositis, and other manifestations of local organ involvement can result. Symptoms can persist for over a year.

Isoagglutinin titers (anti-A and anti-B) usually are elevated in visceral larva migrans, as are other antibody titers (for example, indirect hemagglutination or precipitins against the worm), but these are nonspecific. The diagnosis may be suggested by serologic tests, but biopsy of an affected organ showing larvae is the only definitive method of diagnosis.

Diethylcarbamazine, thiabendazole, and steroids have all been used in therapy. Thiabendazole (50 mg/kg/day for 1 to 2 weeks) probably is the treatment of choice. In life-threatening infections 20 to 40 mg/day of prednisone is added. Prevention depends on worming pets and teaching children to wash their hands before putting them in their mouths.

ANISAKIASIS

Anisakiasis is caused by larvae of *Anisakis marina,* an ascarid of sea mammals (porpoises, dolphins, seals, and whales). The disease occurs in humans when the 2- to 4-cm-long larval form is ingested while eating raw or pickled squid, cod, salmon, or most often herring. The larvae may be vomited up, or they can burrow into the mucosa of the stomach or intestine and produce eosinophilic granulomatous tumors. The lesion can be mistaken for carcinoma or inflammatory bowel disease. The larvae also can penetrate the bowel wall and cause lesions in other organs.

There may be an acute syndrome in which epigastric pain and vomiting occur within a few hours of ingesting the larvae; these are caused by larvae penetrating the wall of the stomach. In another syndrome the small intestine most often is involved, and there may be an acute abdominal condition with fever, pain, and tenderness, requiring surgery. This usually is more delayed and occurs 1 week or longer after the larvae have been ingested.

Eosinophilia may or may not occur. The diagnosis can be made only by seeing larvae through an endoscope or by histologic means in tissue. Removal through an endoscope often is possible. Therapy is conservative unless surgery for intestinal perforation or obstruction becomes necessary. The larvae can be killed by cooking fish or storing it at $-4°$ F ($-20°$ C) for 24 hours. Thiabendazole (22 mg/kg twice a day for 3 days) may be helpful.

HOOKWORM DISEASE

Ancylostoma duodenale and *Necator americanus* are the two hookworms that infect humans. They are found all over the world, mainly in warm climates. The worms are about 1 cm long and live in the small intestine, where they attach and suck blood.

The eggs are passed in the feces and hatch into rhabditiform larvae that molt into filariform larvae. Filariform larvae can survive in warm soil for months and can rapidly penetrate intact skin. After they penetrate the skin, the cycle is much like that of *A. lumbricoides.* Larvae travel in the lymphatic system and the bloodstream to the lungs where they break out into the airways. They are carried up the trachea by ciliated epithelium, are swallowed, and develop into adults in the small intestine.

Light infection is asymptomatic. A pruritic rash may develop at the site of entry of the larva. As with *A. lumbricoides* infection, eosinophila and pulmonary symptoms may occur during the pulmonary phase. With a heavy worm load, iron deficiency anemia and associated symptoms of anemia may develop.

The diagnosis is made by demonstrating characteristic eggs in the stool; they are 60 μm by 40 μm and have a clear shell.

Mebendazole (100 mg twice a day for 3 days) is the treatment of choice. The anemia should be treated with ferrous sulfate. Prevention depends on sanitary disposal of human feces and wearing of shoes.

CUTANEOUS LARVA MIGRANS

The usual cause of cutaneous larva migrans (creeping eruption) is *Ancylostoma braziliiense,* a hookworm of dogs and cats. The disease is found in warm climates (including the southern United States) where the soil supports development of the larvae.

The larvae of *A. braziliense* develop in soil and penetrate the skin in a fashion similar to hookworms. However, the cycle is not completed, and the larvae migrate in the skin at a speed of 1 to 2 cm per day. They produce an erythematous, serpiginous, intensely pruritic burrow in the skin. The burrowing can continue for up to a year.

The treatment is with thiabendazole (25 mg/kg body weight twice a day for 2 days). Wearing of shoes helps prevent the infection.

STRONGYLOIDIASIS

Strongyloides stercoralis is about 2 mm long and lives in the mucosa of the small intestine. It is found worldwide but is most common in tropical climates.

The eggs produced by the worms hatch into larvae in the intestine and can (1) invade the bowel mucosa directly; (2) invade soiled perianal skin after defecation; or (3) invade skin that contacts larvae deposited in the soil. A free-living form that develops in the soil can keep soil infected for long periods of time.

After invasion of the skin or mucosa, the cycle is similar to the *Ascaris* spp. and hookworm cycles. Larvae are carried to the lungs and up the airways. They are then swallowed and develop in the small intestine, where they burrow into the mucosa.

A puritic, urticarial rash may occur at the site of invasion (often on the buttocks). The pulmonary phase may be associated with cough, hemoptysis, pneumonia, or bronchospasm. The infection is often asymptomatic, but because of the possibility of unchecked autoinfection, the potential for lethal overwhelming infection exists. The potentially lethal hyperinfective syndrome tends to occur in patients who are debilitated or receiving corticosteroids or immunosuppressive agents.

The hyperinfective syndrome may result in intensely inflamed bowel mucosa, intestinal hemorrhage, and malabsorption. Larvae become trapped in the liver, lungs, and other organs. *Escherichia coli* bacteremia may occur because of bowel ulceration.

Abdominal pain, tenderness, diarrhea, and vomiting occur with marked intestinal involvement. With the hyperinfective syndrome, marked eosinophilia is usually present and symptoms can result from multiple-organ involvement. Bacterial infection frequently contributes to death. Unexplained eosinophilia should suggest the possibility of strongyloidiasis. On the other hand, eosinophilia may not occur even with heavy infections in immunosuppressed patients. The diagnosis is made by finding larvae in fresh stool or a duodenal aspirate. A serologic test may be helpful in making the diagnosis.

All patients with *S. stercoralis* infection should be treated with thiabendazole (25 mg/kg body weight twice daily for 3 days). Prevention depends on sanitary disposal of human feces and wearing of shoes.

TRICHINOSIS

Trichinosis is found all over the world among meat-eating populations. *Trichinella spiralis* infection is acquired when infected meat of a carnivorous animal (such as a pig or bear) is ingested. The larvae develop into adults within a week in the small intestine. The adult females release larvae for 4 to 8 weeks. The larvae penetrate the mucosa and are carried to organs all over the body. They encyst in striated muscle, where they persist. In other organs such as the heart, brain, and eye the larvae degenerate, provoking an inflammatory reaction such as myocarditis, cerebritis, or retinitis.

Many patients with trichinosis are asymptomatic. With heavy infection there may be mild intestinal symptoms during the first week while the adult worms develop. Subsequently there are fever, high eosinophilia (over 50%), muscle pain, and periorbital edema lasting 4 to 8 weeks. Myocarditis may cause heart failure, and cerebritis may lead to coma. Death may result.

The diagnosis of trichinosis should be suspected when there is high eosinophilia. Muscle pain and tenderness with elevated serum muscle enzymes in a patient with eosinophilia are suggestive. Although serologic tests may be helpful, a muscle biopsy demonstrating larvae in the deltoid or gastrocnemius muscle is the preferred diagnostic test.

Severe infection should be treated with corticosteroids and thiabendazole (25 mg/kg body weight twice daily for 5 days). Prevention depends on adequately cooking the meat of pigs and other carnivorous animals.

ANGIOSTRONGYLIASIS

Angiostrongylus cantonensis (rat lungworm) is found mainly in the Far East, Hawaii, and other Pacific areas. The infection is acquired by ingesting larvae in slugs, snails, crabs, or freshwater prawns or larvae deposited by an intermediate host on food.

In humans the larvae migrate to the brain and produce eosinophilic meningoencephalitis. There are fever, signs of meningitis, and an eosinophilic response in the cerebrospinal fluid (CSF). The illness continues for weeks and then resolves spontaneously. No therapy has been sufficiently evaluated in this disease. Prevention involves avoidance of raw crabs, prawns, and snails.

BANCROFTIAN AND MALAYAN FILARIASIS

Wuchereria bancroft and *Brugia malayi* are filariae found in Africa, Asia, and South America. The adult worms are 5 to 10 cm long and live for many years in the lymphatic system (often in the inguinal region). The females release microfilariae (larval forms) found in the peripheral circulation, often only at night. The infection is acquired by the bite of a mosquito, which injects larval forms. The mosquito becomes infected by aspirating microfilariae when drinking a blood meal.

Light infections usually are asymptomatic. Inflammation and fibrosis in the lymphatic system may lead to lymphadenopathy, lymphatic obstruction, and edema.

In rare cases, marked edema of the lower extremities, scrotum, or arms may occur. The end result may be gigantic, deformed, hyperkeratotic limbs (elephantiasis). Lymphatic obstruction may result in chyluria from either the kidneys or the urinary bladder. Streptococcal cellulitis is common in edematous areas and may make the edema worse by damaging the lymphatic system.

The diagnosis is made by observing microfilariae on a blood smear (usually at night). microfilariae usually are absent in late stages of the disease. Eosinophilia is generally low grade or absent. A positive complement-fixing antibody test indicates only infection with one of the filarial group but is suggestive of *W. bancrofti* or *B. malayi* infection in a patient with unexplained edema.

Lymphangiograms demonstrate the extent of lymphatic obstruction, and roentgenograms may reveal dead calcified worms. Involved lymph nodes should not be resected, since this may further compromise lymphatic drainage.

The treatment of choice is diethylcarbamazine (6 mg/kg body weight orally in three divided doses [after meals] each day for 21 days).

LOIASIS

Loa loa is a filaria found only in Africa. The adults are about 5 cm long and live in the subcutaneous tissue, where they migrate continuously. Female adults deposit microfilariae, which are found in the blood. The infection is spread by the bite of the deer fly *(Chrysops)*.

Although usually asymptomatic, *Loa loa* infection can produce 10 cm or larger, hot, erythematous, painful swellings (Calabar swellings) that subside in several days. They occur at the location of a worm. Worms occasionally can be seen crossing the eye beneath the conjunctivae.

The diagnosis is made by finding microfilariae in blood, usually during the day. The group filarial complement fixation test is usually positive.

Treatment is with diethylcarbamazine, as described for onchocerciasis.

ONCHOCERCIASIS

Onchocerca volvulus, the cause of river blindness, is found in Africa and Central and South America. The threadlike adult filarial worms are found in nodules in subcutaneous tissues. The females produce microfilariae that migrate in the skin. They are not found in blood. The adults live for many years.

Infection is spread by the bite of the black fly *(Simulium)*, which acquires infection when biting an infected person. *Simulium* usually are found along rivers. In Africa they tend to bite on the legs, and in the Americas they usually bite on the head, leading to a different distribution of nodules.

The major manifestations of the disease are pruritic skin lesions and blindness. The skin lesions initially are papular and later become nodular. Microfilariae can migrate into the tissues of the eye, producing keratitis, iritis, or chorioretinitis. The diagnosis is proved by shaving skin sections and putting them in saline. Within an hour microfilariae are seen in the saline.

The nodules should be excised. Suramin (available from the Centers for Disease Control*) in a dose of 1 g intravenously weekly for 5 weeks kills the adult worms, and diethylcarbamazine kills microfilariae. Small doses of diethylcarbamazine should be used initially, since a dose-related exacerbation of skin and eye lesions occurs with therapy. The initial dosage is 0.25 mg/kg body weight daily in three divided doses, increasing to 6 mg/kg/day in three divided doses (after meals). Full dosage is continued for 3 weeks. Eye reactions are controlled with local administration of corticosteroids, and generalized

---

*Parasitic Disease Drug Service, Center for Infectious Diseases, Centers for Disease Control, Atlanta, Ga. 30333. Telephone 404-329-3670.

reactions are managed with systemically administered corticosteroids.

DRACUNCULIASIS

Dracunculus medinensis (guinea worm) is found only in the tropics. The adult worm is a meter in length and lives in the subcutaneous tissues.

Infection occurs when water fleas *(Cyclops)* bearing larvae are ingested. The larvae penetrate the wall of the intestine and enter the subcutaneous tissues. After the female reaches maturity, which takes about a year, her head emerges from a blister formed on the skin and ruptures on contact with water. Larvae are extruded and complete the cycle by infecting *Cyclops*. The blister usually forms on the lower leg, about the urethra, or, with water carriers, on the back. Bacterial cellulitis is common at the site of the blister.

Worms are removed surgically or by turning them on a matchstick a few centimeters each day. If a worm breaks during attempted removal, a marked inflammatory reaction may occur. Metronidazole (250 to 500 mg three times a day for 1 week) is given therapeutically. Thiabendazole also is used. Prevention consists of boiling drinking water that may contain *Cyclops*.

BIBLIOGRAPHY

Beaver PC, Jung RC, and Cupp EW: Clinical parasitology, ed 4, Philadelphia, 1984, Lea & Febiger.
Handbook of antimicrobial therapy, New Rochelle, NY, 1988, The Medical Letter on Drugs and Therapeutics.
Manson-Bahr DEC: Manson's tropical diseases, ed 18, London, 1982, Baillière Tindall.
Sanford JP: Guide to antimicrobial therapy, West Bethesda, MD, 1989, Antimicrobial Therapy, Inc.

57·DISEASES CAUSED BY CESTODES (TAPEWORMS)

Jaime Carrizosa

The cestodes are flatworms that in their adult stage live in the gastrointestinal tract of vertebrates. The infected vertebrate becomes the definitive host of the parasite. The adult tapeworm is composed of a scolex or head that possesses organs that allow attachment to the intestinal mucosa; the neck; and the strobila composed of many segments or proglottids, each containing one or more sets of reproductive organs. A proglottid can copulate with itself or with other proglottids of the same or other worms. After fertilization the gravid proglottid, full of eggs, reaches the end of the strobila, detaches, and passes into the feces or disintegrates, releasing eggs that may be visualized in the stool. When eggs are ingested by an intermediate host, they hatch and larvae are released. The larva penetrates the gut wall and develops into the cysticercus, which is the head of the future tapeworm in a cyst. Development of the larva varies in the different species, and this leads to different clinical syndromes. Ingestion of larvae in uncooked meat results in digestion of the cyst wall, release of the head, and maturation into an adult worm. The ingestion of eggs leads to the development of cysticercosis.

TAENIASIS SAGINATA

Infection with *Taenia saginata*, the beef tapeworm, is acquired by the ingestion of cysticercus forms in poorly cooked or raw beef. Humans are the definitive hosts of the worm. The worm matures in about 2 months, reaching lengths of 5 to 10 m with over 1000 proglottids. The scolex is characterized by the presence of four suckers and has no hooklets. Proglottids, which can be passed intact, contain over 12 uterine branches. This distinguishes them from the proglottids of *Taenia solium*, the pork tapeworm. Eggs found in the stool have a thick, brown, radially striated shell and contain a full embryo. When the eggs are ingested by cattle or other herbivores, the embryo released in the intestine traverses the intestinal wall and is carried by the circulation into the muscles of the limbs, diaphragm, and tongue. In striated muscles the embryo develops into a cysticercus that remains viable for 1 to 3 years.

The infection is found all over the world. However, it is most frequent in the Middle East, Kenya, Ethiopia, and Yugoslavia. The clinical manifestations are mild, nonspecific abdominal pain and diarrhea. Mild eosinophilia may be present. There may be passage of motile proglottids through the anal sphincter. The diagnosis of *T. saginata* infection is made by identification of the proglottids or the eggs in the stool. Thorough cooking of beef prevents the infection.

TAENIASIS SOLIUM

Infection with *Taenia solium*, the pork tapeworm, is acquired by ingestion of pork containing cysticercus forms. As with *T. saginata*, humans are the definitive hosts of the worm. However, unlike *T. saginata*, cysticercosis, the intermediate form of the infection, also can develop in humans.

After ingestion the cysticercus is digested and the worm is released in the small bowel, where it establishes habitat and matures to a full size of 2 to 4 m. *T. solium* is differentiated from *T. saginata* by the presence of four suckers and two rows of hooklets on the scolex and fewer than 12 uterine branches in the gravid proglottid. The eggs of *T. solium* and *T. saginata* are indistinguishable. The infection is found all over the world but is most frequent in Eastern Europe, Central and South America, Spain, and Portugal.

The clinical manifestations of *T. solium* infection are similar to those of *T. saginata* infection. The diagnosis is made by examining the feces for the proglottids and eggs of *T. solium*. When the scolex is available, the diagnosis is more reliable. Mild eosinophilia may be seen in both *T. saginata* and *T. solium* infection. Thorough cooking of pork prevents the infection.

HUMAN CYSTICERCOSIS

Human infection caused by the ingestion of eggs of *T. solium* is known as cysticercosis. After ingestion the larva penetrates the intestinal wall and invades the tissues. Commonly involved organs are the subcutaneous tissue, central nervous system (CNS), muscle, heart, liver, and lung. Infection of the brain is associated with headaches, signs of increased intracranial pressure and seizures. The disease is particularly common in Mexico. The diagnosis of cysticercosis is based on the identification of multiple space-occupying lesions by radioisotope scan, computed tomography, arteriography, and skull roentgenographic films, since the cysticercus calcifies after its death. However, the diagnosis is made frequently by identification of the cyst at surgery. A serologic test, indirect hemagglutination, detects the presence of antibodies and is useful in the confirmation of the diagnosis.

The treatment of cysticercosis usually is surgical. Symptomatic treatment consists of anticonvulsants and steroids to reduce edema. Praziquantel, a pyrazino-isoquinoline drug, has been shown to induce regression or improvement of cystic lesions and other symptoms such as headaches and seizures. Further controlled studies are needed to evaluate the efficacy of this agent. Mebendazole has shown in vitro activity against the larvae, but its effectiveness in vivo has not been established.

DIPHYLLOBOTHRIASIS

Infection with *Diphyllobothrium latum,* the fish tapeworm, is acquired by eating raw or undercooked fish. Humans are the definitive hosts of the tapeworm, but other fish-eating animals also serve as final hosts. The adult worm is the largest tapeworm, reaching lengths of up to 10 to 15 m. Eggs released from an infected host reach the water, embryonate and release a ciliated larva (coracidium). The coracidium, when eaten by a freshwater flea, develops into a procercoid. In turn, when the flea is eaten by a fresh-water fish, the procercoid further develops into a plerocercoid. When infected raw fish is eaten by a human or a fish-eating mammal, the plerocercoid develops into an adult worm. The infection is common in the Scandinavian countries, the Baltic Sea area, Canada, Alaska, the nothern United States, and Florida. The clinical manifestations of the disease are minimal, but complications of the infection produce important symptoms. The tapeworm splits vitamin B_{12} from its complex with intrinsic factor and utilizes it, resulting in vitamin B_{12} deficiency with megaloblastic anemia and associated neurologic symptoms.

The diagnosis of *D. latum* infection is made by the identification of the eggs in the stool. The eggs, usually found in large numbers, are yellowish and operculated. The infection is prevented by thorough cooking of fresh fish; freezing for more than 24 hours also kills the larvae.

TREATMENT OF *TAENIA SAGINATA, TAENIA SOLIUM,* AND *DIPHYLLOBOTHRIUM LATUM* INFECTION

Niclosamide is the drug of choice in the treatment of *T. saginata, T. solium,* and *D. latum* infections. One oral dose of 2 g (four tablets) kills the worm on contact; during expulsion the worm is digested, and it is not possible to identify it in the stool. The stool should be examined at 3 and 6 months to verify the effectiveness of the treatment. Quinacrine (Atabrine), paromomycin (Humatin), and praziquantel have been used as alternative therapies.

ECHINOCOCCOSIS (HYDATID DISEASE)

Echinococcosis is an infection produced by the larvae of *Echinococcus granulosus* or *Echinococcus multilocularis,* tapeworms that have as definitive hosts the dog and other canines such as the wolf, the fox, and the jackal. Humans and other mammals such as sheep and cattle serve as intermediate hosts. When eggs of *Echinococcus* are ingested, they hatch and release embryos that penetrate the small bowel wall and enter the portal circulation. They lodge primarily in the liver and lung but may reach other organs such as the brain, kidney, or bone. By a very slow process of growth, the larva (oncosphere) develops into a cystic structure that can reach the size of a human head and is lined by an outer hard layer and an inner germinal layer. The latter gives origin to the daughter cysts, each filled with scolices, that produce infection when eaten by the definitive host. Residua from the cyst layers and released scolices from cyst sediment are known as hydatid sand.

Hydatid disease can occur anywhere but is seen more frequently in countries with predominant sheep- and cattle-raising economies such as Australia, New Zealand, Argentina, and Wales. Most of the infections diagnosed in the United States have been contracted outside the country.

The clinical manifestations of the infection result from pro-

gressive enlargement of the hydatid cyst, and many cases are diagnosed during routine examinations of asymptomatic individuals. The most common location of hydatid cysts is the right lobe of the liver. The enlarging cyst causes diffuse pain, cholestasis, and atrophy of the adjacent tissues. Occasionally the cyst ruptures, causing acute complications. Rupture or just leakage of the fluid may cause anaphylactic reactions and seeding of the peritoneal cavity with formation of new cysts; moreover, the cysts may become secondarily infected and produce a liver or lung abscess. Rupture of a lung cyst may cause chest pain, bronchospasm, and hemoptysis. Rupture into the biliary tract may resemble acute cholecystitis. Hydatid cysts of the brain present symptoms of space-occupying lesions, those in the kidney cause hematuria and flank pain, and those in bone result in a destructive process with the development of a pathologic fracture. The diagnosis is established by the demonstration of the cysts with ultrasonic scanning, radioisotope scanning, computed tomography, and arteriography. On roentgenograms of the abdomen, the cysts may show a small rim of calcification, which suggests the diagnosis. Several serologic tests are available to detect antibodies against the *Echinococcus* organisms. The indirect hemagglutination test and the bentonite flocculation test frequently are used. Casoni's test, a skin test that uses cyst fluid, usually is positive in cases of echinococcosis, but it has not been standardized and thus is unreliable. Eosinophilia may occur.

Surgery with complete removal of the intact cyst is the preferred treatment. When the cyst cannot be removed, marsupialization and sterilization of the cyst with a solution of 10% formalin, 1% iodine, or hypertonic (30%) saline should be attempted. Aspiration of the cyst should never be attempted because of the danger of rupture and spillage of the cyst fluid. A new method of treatment using high doses of mebendazole has been tried in patients in whom surgery cannot be performed. Although therapeutic trials have shown good results, more information is necessary before the treatment is accepted. High doses of the drug may cause bone marrow depression.

The disease can be prevented by avoiding contamination with feces of infected animals and by proper disposal of organs containing cysts from infected sheep and cattle to prevent the disease in the definitive hosts.

BIBLIOGRAPHY

Conlon CP and Ellis CJ: Praziquantel, J Antimicrob Chemother 15:1, 1985.
Jones TC: Cestodes, Clin Gastroenterol 7:105, 1978.
Katz AM and Pan C: *Echinococcus* disease in the United States, Am J Med 25:759, 1958.
Most H: Drug therapy: common parasitic infections of man, N Engl J Med 287:495, 1972.
Pawlowski Z and Schultz ME: Taeniasis and cysticercosis *(Taenia saginata),* Adv Parasitol 10:296, 1972.
Williams JF and others: Current prevalence and distribution of hydatidosis with special reference to the Americas, Am J Trop Med Hyg 20:224, 1971.

58 · DISEASES CAUSED BY TREMATODES (FLUKES)

Jaime Carrizosa

SCHISTOSOMIASIS (BILHARZIASIS)

Schistosomiasis is a chronic infection caused by three different trematodes (flukes), *Schistosoma mansoni, Schistosoma haematobium,* and *Schistosoma japonicum.* The disease affects people living in tropical and subtropical areas of the world.

The infection is acquired by repeated immersion in fresh water contaminated with cercariae, the infecting forms of the schistosome, which penetrate the skin, develop into adult worms in the circulatory system, and settle into a permanent habitat in the veins of the intestine or the urinary bladder. The disease is produced by the severe inflammatory reaction resulting from the presence of ova released by mature parasites into the adjacent tissues or the bloodstream. The characteristics of schistosomiasis depend on the type of infecting schistosome, the specific organ involved, the degree of infestation, and the duration of the illness.

ETIOLOGY. As just discussed, three species of schistosomes are known to parasitize humans. The males of these species are shorter than the females and have a ventral longitudinal groove, the gynecophoral canal, where the female resides. The worms absorb metabolites through the intestine and integument and have a rapid metabolic rate dependent on energy obtained from the anaerobic oxidation of carbohydrates. The adult worms live in the veins that drain organs of the abdominal cavity. Each species has specific preferences: *S. haematobium* lives in the veins of the urinary bladder plexus, *S. mansoni* lives in the veins of the colon, and *S. japonicum* lives primarily in the veins of the small intestine. The eggs are distinctive for each species. The egg of *S. haematobium* is ellipsoidal with a terminal spine, the egg of *S. mansoni* is ellipsoidal but has a lateral spine, and the egg of *S. japonicum* is oval, almost spherical, with only a rudimentary spine. Once the eggs are laid, some traverse the venule wall and pass through the tissues, producing significant inflammatory reaction, until they reach the bladder or gut lumen and are excreted from the body in the urine or stool. Many eggs never reach the lumen but remain in the tissues or bloodstream and are carried to other organs such as the liver or lungs.

The life cycle of the schistosome begins when the eggs hatch following exposure to fresh water. The miracidium develops and emerges from the egg to seek its snail host. It then penetrates the snail and develops into a sporocyst. Two weeks later the mother sporocyst gives birth to daughter sporocysts that migrate to the organs of the snail. In 2 to 3 weeks the snail begins to shed fork-tailed cercariae into the water, where they remain alive for 1 to 3 days but lose their infectivity by 20 hours. When they come in contact with the skin of a prospective host, they attach to and penetrate the epidermis, losing their tails in the process. Within 24 hours after penetration, the altered cercariae, now called schistosomula, enter the peripheral circulation and reach the pulmonary vessels, where they remain several days before they enter the systemic circulation and are carried into the liver. After reaching maturity in the liver, the worms migrate to their final organ of infestation, where they copulate and begin producing eggs, thus completing the life cycle. The life span of a schistosome is 5 to 10 years.

EPIDEMIOLOGY. It is estimated that schistosomiasis affects more than 200 million people in tropical and subtropical areas of the world. The disease is not found in the continental United States, owing to the lack of the appropriate snail, but it is endemic in Puerto Rico.

In the Western Hemisphere infection is caused by species of *S. mansoni*, most probably brought to America by African slaves. The infection is found in Brazil, Venezuela, Surinam, and some Caribbean islands (Dominican Republic, Martinique, St. Lucia, Antigua, Guadeloupe, and Puerto Rico). Infection with both *S. mansoni* and *S. haematobium* is widespread in Africa. *S. japonicum* is endemic in the Orient (Japan, China, the Philippines, and Southeast Asia).

The single most important epidemilogic factor in schistosomiasis is the deposition of human waste in water containing the appropriate intermediate snail host. The species of snail prevalent in the area determines the specific infecting schistosome. The disease frequently occurs in children who bathe, wade, or play in water contaminated with cercariae. Reinfection occurs every time there is contact with contaminated water. The best measures for the control of schistosomiasis are based on the proper disposal of excreta, appropriate provision of water supplies, education of the population concering the methods of acquisition of the infection, and availability of treatment programs. Programs for extermination of the intermediary hosts (snails) have not been highly successful.

PATHOGENESIS AND CLINICAL MANIFESTATIONS. The characteristics of schistosomiasis depend on the degree of infection and the species of schistosome. Initial manifestations of the infection occur within 1 day following the penetration of the cercariae and are characterized by a papular, pruritic rash known as swimmers' itch. The rash develops as a result of the death of some of the cercariae following penetration of the skin. All cercariae of schistosomes nonpathogenic to humans die after penetration, causing the most severe rashes. The dermatitis appears to be a sensitization phenomenon characterized by infiltration of the dermis and epidermis with round cells as seen in delayed hypersensitivity reactions.

Katayama fever. Katayama fever is a syndrome of schistosomiasis characterized by fever, chills, profuse diaphoresis, cough, wheezing, headache, and diarrhea associated with hepatosplenomegaly, lymphadenopathy, and urticaria. The clinical picture most frequently is seen 20 to 60 days after infection with *S. japonicum,* but it can occur with very heavy infestations of *S. mansoni.* The syndrome may last up to 12 weeks, and occasional deaths have been reported. The symptoms are caused by a severe hypersensitivity reaction to a large antigenic load of ova and parasites.

Intermediate phase of schistosomiasis. The changes seen in the intermediate phase of the disease result from the deposition of a large number of eggs in the venules of the infected organs. Eggs may be finally excreted in the stool or urine, may be carried in the bloodstream to the liver or lungs, or may remain in the adjacent tissues. At this stage the infection is characterized by a severe tissue reaction to the deposited eggs. Manifestations of bowel invasion range from mild diarrhea and congestion to fibrosis, ulceration, bleeding, or formation of inflammatory polyps. Manifestations of bladder invasion are ulceration, fibrosis, hematuria, polyps, and calcification.

Hepatosplenic schistosomiasis. Deposition of eggs in the liver initiates a granulomatous reaction that results in intrahepatic blocking of portal blood flow with subsequent development of portal hypertension, usually over a period of many years. The clinical manifestations are hepatosplenomegaly, development of collateral circulation, esophageal varices, and hematemesis. Patients with hepatic schistosomiasis have relatively normal liver function, and hepatic insufficiency is rarely seen. Bacteremia caused by *Salmonella* organisms and *Escherichia coli* is a frequent complication of hepatic schistosomiasis. Other manifestations of the disease are anemia, moderate eosinophilia, and pancytopenia resulting from hypersplenism.

Pulmonary schistosomiasis. Schistosomal eggs reach the pulmonary capillaries through collateral veins developed because of portal hypertension or by passage of eggs from the vesical plexus into the inferior vena cava. The presence of eggs in the pulmonary capillaries produces marked inflammation and fibrosis with development of pulmonary hypertension and cor pulmonale.

Urinary tract schistosomiasis. Urinary tract involvement in *S. haematobium* infection is initially manifested by hematuria and ureteral obstruction caused by granuloma formation. Bladder involvement results in fibrosis and calcification. Obstructive uropathy and renal insufficiency may complicate the infection. In countries with a high prevalence of urinary schistosomiasis, a significant association with bladder carcinoma and urinary carriage of *Salmonella* organisms has been noted.

Central nervous system schistosomiasis. Schistosomal eggs carried into the CNS can result in seizure activity and in focal damage suggestive of space-occupying lesions. Spinal cord lesions such as transverse myelitis have been reported in cases of *S. mansoni* and *S. haematobium* infection.

DIAGNOSIS AND LABORATORY FINDINGS. The diagnosis of schistosomiasis is established by the presence of ova in the stool, urine, or biopsy specimens. Concentration techniques may be necessary to establish the presence of eggs in the stool. The Kato thick smear provides a method to estimate egg output and severity of the infection. Determination of eggs in urine specimens is made by examining the sediment in samples obtained at noon. Rectal biopsy is one of the preferred methods in cases of *S. mansoni* or *S. japonicum* infection. Several specimens are taken from the valves of Houston, pressed between glass slides, and examined for eggs under the microscope. Since dead eggs may persist in the tissues for prolonged periods of time, a hatching test performed by incubating eggs in water and observing them for the emergence of miracidia is necessary to rule out burned-out or successfully treated disease. Eosinophilia is characteristic of schistosomiasis, and its presence provides additional laboratory support. Radioimmunoassays and enzyme-linked immunosorbent assays (ELISA) using antigens from eggs and worms are being used in research and epidemiologic studies. The intradermal skin test for schistosomiasis has epidemiologic value but should not be used as a diagnostic tool.

In cases of *S. mansoni* and *S. japonicum* infection, liver biopsy and roentgenographic evaluation of the gastrointestinal tract are helpful in determining the extent of the disease. In *S. haematobium* infection, cystoscopy and an intravenous pyelogram may help confirm the diagnosis.

MANAGEMENT. Schistosomal dermatitis is treated symptomatically. Specific treatment is not available. In recent years praziquantel has become the drug of choice. It is used in a dose of 20 mg/kg three times a day for 1 day.

Patients with severe hepatosplenic schistomiasis have portal hypertension and frequently bleeding from esophageal varices. Surgical treatment is not recommended unless there are repeated episodes of bleeding, because patients have good hepatic function, and hepatic encephalopathy rarely develops. If shunting is necessary, splenorenal shunt is preferred and antiscistosomal treatment is recommended to prevent passage of the eggs into the caval circulation with seeding of the lungs and development of pulmonary complications.

PROGNOSIS. Many patients with schistosomiasis are asymptomatic; only patients with heavy infections have symptoms and complications and may die of the disease. Treatment results in symptomatic improvement, prevention of organ damage, and perhaps even gradual regression of lesions. The overall prognosis of the disease is good.

OTHER TREMATODE INFECTIONS (HERMAPHRODITIC FLUKES)

The hermaphroditic flukes are flat, leaflike worms each having both sets of sex organs, which frequently results in self-fertilization. Hatched eggs produce a motile miracidium that penetrates a snail host leading to the development of cercariae in a cycle similar to that of the schistosomes. However, unlike schistosomes the hermaphroditic flukes need a second intermediate host. In the second host—fish, crab, or plant—the metacercariae or infection forms develop. When ingested by humans this form hatches, producing a fluke that migrates to the target tissues and matures into an adult worm.

Clonorchiasis

Clonorchiasis is an infection of the biliary tract produced by *Clonorchis sinensis*. The infection is acquired by eating raw fish infected with metacercariae and is endemic in Japan, Korea, Southeast Asia, and China. Humans and some animals (dogs, cats, pigs, and rats) serve as hosts for the parasite. When the metacercariae are ingested, abdominal pain, anorexia, malaise, hepatomegaly, and eosinophilia develop. Light infections generally are asymptomatic. Mature worms lodge in the biliary duct and induce inflammation and fibrosis. The clinical manifestations result from obstruction caused by dead flukes or formation of biliary stones. The most common complications are cholangitis, biliary cirrhosis, and pancreatitis. *Salmonella typhi* carriage is associated with the presence of stones, and cholangiocarcinoma is known to occur in patients with long-standing infection.

The diagnosis of clonorchiasis is established by the presence of eggs in the stool. Stones present in the biliary ducts may be visualized on roentgenograms of the abdomen.

Asymptomatic patients are not treated. In symptomatic infection the drug of choice is praziquantel at a dose of 75 mg/kg given in three divided doses in 1 day. Chloroquine base (300 mg three times a day for 3 to 6 weeks) is the alternative treatment. Surgery may be required in cases of biliary obstruction. The infection is prevented by avoiding the ingestion of uncooked fish.

Opisthorchiasis

Opisthorchiasis is an infection of the biliary tract caused by *Opisthorchis felineus* or *Opisthorchis viverrini*. The former is epidemic in the Philippines, India, Japan, the Soviet Union, and Southeast Asia, and the latter is common in Thailand, Laos, and Cambodia. The life cycle of the fluke is similar to that of *Clonorchis* organisms. The disease is also acquired by eating raw infected fish or infected vegetables. The clinical manifestations are indistinguishable from those of clonorchiasis. As in chlonorchiasis praziquantel is the drug of choice.

Fascioliasis

Fascioliasis, like clonorchiasis, is an infection of the biliary tract caused by the fluke *Fasciola hepatica*. The usual final host of *F. hepatica* is the sheep. The disease is generally acquired by ingestion of infected watercress containing metacercariae and is found worldwide where wild watercress is eaten. The clinical manifestations of the disease are similar to those of clonorchiasis; the fluke easily causes biliary obstruction because of its size (2 to 3 cm in length and 1 cm in breadth). The patients usually have epigastric pain, jaundice, pruritus, eosinophilia, and diarrhea. An unusual manifestation of the disease called halzoun produces severe pharyngeal inflammation with respiratory distress and dysphagia. The syndrome is caused when organisms ingested in raw liver parasitize the pharynx. The treatment of fascioliasis is praziquantel as indicated for the treatment of *Chlonorchis* infections. Alternative treatments are hexylresorcinol (1 g in adults) or tetrachloroethylene (0.1 ml/kg) in single oral doses.

Fasciolopsiasis

Fasciolopsiasis is an infection of the upper gastrointestinal tract caused by *Fasciolopsis buski*. The infection is acquired by humans after eating water chestnuts or other aquatic vegetables infected with metacercariae. The final host of the infection is the pig. It is endemic in the Far East, China, and India. As in all trematode infections, the disease usually is asymptomatic except in cases of heavy infection. The clinical manifestations are abdominal pain, diarrhea, and sometimes intestinal obstruction. The diagnosis is established by finding the eggs in the feces. Fasciolopsiasis also is treated with praziquantel.

Paragonimiasis

Paragonimiasis is an infection of the lung caused by the trematode *Paragonimus westermani* and other related species. The disease is acquired by eating crayfish or crabs infected with metacercariae. The organisms penetrate the intestinal wall and peritoneal cavity and later migrate into the lung. They also are found in tissues of the dog, cat, pig, and other carnivores. The clinical manifestations of the disease are cough and hemoptysis. Other manifestations are bronchiectasis, pulmonary nodules or infiltrates, and sometimes cavities. Eosinophilia is common. The diagnosis is established by identification of the eggs in expectorated sputum or in feces when the eggs excreted in the sputum are swallowed. A skin test is available for epidemiologic studies. Praziquantel is the drug of choice for the treatment of paragonimiasis. The dosage is the same as that given for chlonorchiasis. Alternative treatment is bithionol (30 to 40 mg/kg every other day for 10 to 14 doses) (available from the Centers for Disease Control*).

BIBLIOGRAPHY

Jones EA and others: Massive infection with *Fasciola hepatica* in man, Am J Med 63:842, 1977.

Jong EC and others: Praziquantel for the treatment of chlonorchis/opisthorchis infections: report of a double blind placebo controlled trial, J Infect Dis 152:637, 1985.

Mahmoud AA: Curent concepts—schistosomiasis, N Engl J Med 297:1329, 1977.

Pearson RD and Guerrant RL: Praziquantel: a major advance in antihelmintic therapy, Ann Intern Med 99:195, 1983.

Sadum EH and Buck AA: Paragonimiasis in South Korea: immunodiagnostic, epidemiologic, clinical, roentgenologic and therapeutic studies, Am J Trop Med Hyg 9:562, 1960.

Seah SKK: Digenetic trematodes, Clin Gastroenterol 7:871, 1978.

Strauss WG: Clinical manifestations of clonorchiasis: a control study of 105 cases, Am J Trop Med Hyg 11:625, 1962.

Dental correlations

Peter D. Quinn, Louise F. Rose, Sol Silverman, Jr., Michael Glick, *and* Benjamin Hammond

VIRAL INFECTION
Herpes simplex

Acute herpetic gingivostomatitis is a common primary infection with herpes simplex virus, usually type 1 but occasionally type 2. The renewed interest in this disease arises from the recognition that it attacks not only infants and young children but also adults in their second and third decades. Primary herpetic gingivostomatitis is the most acute form of oral herpetic infection. Usually 90% of the population is infected before puberty, but most people do not develop noticeable lesions.

Approximately 10% of adults, as shown by seroepidemiologic study, either do not become infected in childhood or have not developed adequate antibodies; therefore this infection is not limited to children. Adult infections of primary herpetic gingivostomatitis usually are more severe than the childhood form. Both forms can be mistaken for more severe diseases such as erythema multiforme, infectious mononucleosis, blood dyscrasias, and pemphigus.

Individuals who are immunosuppressed (for example, those with acquired immunodeficiency syndrome [AIDS] or cancer or who are transplant patients) have an increased risk for developing a primary herpetic stomatitis. Under these conditions lesions may manifest as an atypical ulcerative stomatitis and also may be recurrent.

ORAL MANIFESTATIONS. The oral manifestations are dominated by small vesicles that rupture easily and lead to the formation of shallow ulcers with smooth margins surrounded by a red halo. The lesions occur on all areas of the mouth, with the most dramatic signs on the lips and gingivae. The lip ulcers, which penetrate into the subepithelium, induce bleeding with formation of crusts. The gingiva shows signs of acute inflammaton caused by the viral infection, which is further aggravated by accumulation of dental plaque resulting from poor oral hygiene and the interruption of masticatory function. Superinfection by the normal oral flora may further complicate the picture. Ulcers develop on the gingival tissues, and bleeding from the marginal gingiva is not uncommon. Severe pain with marked difficulty in chewing, talking, and swallowing is the chief complaint of patients with primary herpetic gingivostomatitis and as a direct result, saliva drooling is apparent. In infants lack of food and fluid ingestion may result in dehydration, requiring hospitalization and parenteral fluid administration. Swollen, tender regional lymph nodes frequently are observed. The ulcerations heal in approximately 14 days, although the gingival inflammation may take longer to resolve. Herpesvirus sialadenitis is rare, although the virus has been cultured from saliva and gingival crevicular fluid.

A clue to the diagnosis may be obtained rapidly by cytologic examination of material from the base of the vesicle or ulcer, which shows multinucleated cells with nuclear inclusion bodies and ballooning of the nucleus. Definitive diagnosis is by isolation of the virus from the vesicular fluid and culture of the virus in tissue cell culture systems. Both vesicles and oral secretions yield positive cultures in the acute symptomatic phase and for several weeks after the acute disease. A fourfold rise in antibody titer comparing acute and convalescent sera points to a recent infection but is not helpful in the initial clinical presentation. When primary herpetic gingivostomatitis occurs during the first trimester of pregnancy as a result of viremia, the herpes virus may cross the placental barrier and infect the fetus, resulting in severe congenital malformations. If the oral infection is diagnosed close to delivery, a pelvic examination is indicated and if vaginal or cervical involvement coexists a cesarean section must be considered. Both primary and reactivation herpetic oral lesions in immunocompromised hosts are characterized by their severity and intensity of local complications.

DENTAL MANAGEMENT. Treatment of acute herpetic gingivostomatitis is mainly supportive, to alleviate the pain and reduce the chance of secondary infection. Mouth rinses with a 2% lidocaine viscous solution are beneficial and facilitate drinking, eating of soft foods, and oral hygiene. A milder anesthetic action may be obtained by the use of a 5% aqueous diphenhydramine (Benadryl) solution. An ice cube containing

---

1 ml may be held in the mouth; it should not be swallowed but rather spit out as it melts. Abundant bicarbonate or saline solution mouthwashes provide mechanical cleansing. Antibiotics are of no benefit. In severe cases, secondary monilial infection occurs and is treated with antimycotic agents such as nystatin suspension (100,000 U/ml) or amphotericin B lozenges, four to six times a day. When severity dictates, systemic acyclovir is effective. However, the dosage (minimum of 1 g/day) and expense limits usage. Preventive use of acyclovir has not been adequately studied. Therefore an empirical approach, with which any patient gets the best result, is still indicated.

Recurrent herpes simplex virus infection

Herpesvirus in a latent form may continuously infect sensory ganglia in patients who recover from the primary infection. Following infection in the oral and circumoral areas, the latent virus may be cultured from the trigeminal ganglia.

Recurrent herpes labialis (the common coldsore or fever blister) is not the only form of recurrent oral infection; it may also be present in an intraoral form. The latter develops as small but painful vesicles and ulcers on heavily keratinized mucosa. They appear in clusters, have regular borders, are shallow (intraepithelial vesicles), and are surrounded by an inflammatory halo. Intraoral herpesvirus infection has to be differentiated from recurrent aphthous ulcerations, a condition that is nonviral in origin.

Herpes simplex labialis develops on the vermilion border, which is considered a "locus minoris resistentiae." The lesions then spread to the adjacent skin, and clusters of deep-seated vesicles form. The surrounding lip tissue is swollen as with an allergic reaction. An itching sensation generally precedes the appearance of the lesions, and experienced patients easily can predict a new attack. This endogenous infection is reactivated by stimuli such as fever, sunlight, stressful situations, hormonal imbalance, or surgical resection of the trigeminal ganglion in cases of trigeminal neuralgia.

In healthy people the treatment of recurrent herpes infections of the lip is palliative. In patients with debilitating diseases, topical or systemic acyclovir may be indicated.

Cytomegalovirus

Few instances of intraoral manifestations of cytomegalovirus (CMV) infections have been documented, despite the prevalence of antibodies to CMV in the general population (50% to 80% have such antibodies). In healthy individuals initial CMV infection usually is asymptomatic, but as in all herpesvirus infections, it can remain latent in several sites, including lymphocytes and monocytes. Young people shed the virus from the oropharynx for many years; white adults with CMV mononucleosis remain contagious for months. The most important routes of transmission are via saliva and urine. However, venereal transmission also may occur.

In CMV infections, cytopathology shows enlarged cells with pathognomonic intranuclear and cytoplasmic inclusions in cells of salivary glands. Except for congenital CMV infection, expression of the virus in the oral cavity is only associated with immunocompromised or otherwise debilitated individuals. The lips, tongue, buccal mucosa, pharyngeal mucosa, and palatal gingiva show painful, edematous ulcerations with indurated borders surrounded by an erythematous zone. The oral mucosa exhibits petechiae-like lesions when leukoplasia and thrombocytopenia are present. Congenital CMV infections are associated with a generalized yellowish discoloration of the primary dentition. Soft, opaque enamel can be removed easily from the dentinal base. Treatment of oral involvement of CMV

infections is symptomatc, but in severe disseminated cases, systemic administration of gancyclovir has a good response.

Differential diagnosis of oral manifestations of CMV infections includes erythema multiforme, allergic stomatitis, recurrent aphthous stomatitis, coxsackievirus infection, and varicella-zoster virus infection.

Epstein-Barr virus

Antibodies to Epstein-Barr virus (EBV) are acquired early in life, with 90% to 95% of most populations being seropositive by adulthood. Up to 20% of EBV seropositive individuals excrete EBV at any one time. The oropharynx is the site of viral replication, and viral transmission is most likely to occur via saliva during the close contact typical of "deep kissing." Blood transmission also is possible.

The incubation period of EBV varies from 30 to 60 days following initial infection. Primary infection with EBV often is asymptomatic in young children but causes infectious mononucleosis in adolescents and adults. Classic or typical infectious mononucleosis is an acute illness characterized clinically by a sore throat, fever of 103° to 105° F (39.4° to 40.6° C) and lymphadenopathy with an injected pharynx. Tonsillar enlargement and ulceration of the pharyngeal mucosa with pseudomembranous formation also may be present. Intraoral manifestations occasionally include palatal petechiae and mucosal ulcerations when a reduced polymorphonuclear leukocyte count is present, as well as acute stomatitis and gingivitis. EBV also has been implicated in various malignancies such as Burkitt's lymphoma, recurrent parotitis, midline lethal granuloma, and oral hairy leukoplakia. Laboratory values show an increase in heterophile antibody, an increased number of atypical lymphocytes, and a positive Paul-Bunnell test. Included in the differential diagnosis are coxsackievirus infections and herpes simplex virus infections.

Varicella-zoster virus

The presence of varicella-zoster virus (VZV) in children produces what is clinically known as chicken pox (varicella). Vesicular eruptions on the skin, characterized by inflammation of the corium and edema of epidermal cells, heal by crusting and may leave hypopigmentation and scarring. Small blisterlike eruptions involving the mucosa of the oral cavity and the pharynx often appear with occasional ulcer formations.

An exfoliative cytologic examination reveals inclusion bodies and multinucleated giant cells similar to those in herpes zoster and herpes simplex virus. After initial infection, VZV nucleic acids are found in the dorsal root ganglion cell, where they become latent. When reactivated the virus descends along sensory axons to the skin and mucosa of the dermatome, where the characteristic unilateral zoster develops. Reactivation can occur by dental injections inside the oral cavity. Cranial nerves are involved in 25% of all zoster cases, with the ophthalmic branch of the trigeminal nerve being the most common. Zoster involvement of the maxillary and mandibular divisions of the trigeminal nerve causes oral ulcerations and occasional ipsilateral or orofacial pain. Zoster infection in older children has caused devitalization and partial occlusion of pulp chambers and root canals. Tooth abnormalities such as shortened, irregular roots with normal crowns and disturbed eruptions and sequence also have been reported. Local neurovascular changes can explain these abnormalities, as well as the case of necrosis of the alveolar bone found unilaterally in a child.

Zoster is more common in elderly and immunocompromised patients. These individuals show high morbidity, significant tissue destruction, scarring, and occasional dissemination of the virus. At times the lesions are accompanied by severe pain. If the pain persists for 6 to 8 weeks after resolution of the lesions, the condition represents postherpetic neuralgia. The pain may persist for months or years. Pain also can occur without eruption in cases of zoster sine herpete. This zoster has to be part of a differential diagnosis involving pain of one dermatome.

Cytologic findings are similar to those in herpes simplex virus infections and include multinucleated giant cells and nuclear ballooning and degeneration. Disseminated VZV in immunocompromised patients is treated with vidarabine (ARA-A) and acyclovir. In elderly patients good results have been reported with corticosteroid therapy.

Papilloma virus

HUMAN PAPILLOMA VIRUS. Human papilloma virus (HPV) can be transmitted via oral-oral, oral-cutaneous, and oral-genital routes. Only a few of the approximately 50 different types of HPV actually cause oral manifestations. HPV has been implicated in numerous clinical lesions, including laryngeal papilloma, condylomata accuminatum, focal epithelial hyperplasia, verruca vulgaris and plana, multiple and single papillomas, and malignancies.

HPV-1, -2, -4, -6, -11, -13, and -18 are not found in healthy oral mucosa, whereas HPV-16–related virus is found in over 40% of intact oral mucosa. The presence of HPV in nonpathologic oral mucosa implies a possibly innocent role of the virus, but HPV may be an etiologic agent in oral squamous papillomas and warts (HPV-6, -11, -16), focal epithelial hyperplasia (HPV-13, -31), oral lichen planus (HPV-11, -16, -16–related) and oral leukoplakia (HPV-16–related). An increased number of intraoral papillomatous lesions have been observed in patients with human immunodeficiency virus.

Microscopically, stratified squamous epithelium extending above the mucosa in long fingerlike projections that sometimes exhibit hyperkeratosis can be observed.

Enterovirus

COXSACKIEVIRUS. The coxsackievirus has been divided into two types, group A and group B. Although each group has subtypes and characteristic clinical manifestations, some overlap does exists. Coxsackievirus group A causes myositis and necrosis of voluntary muscles and is subdivided into 24 types. Coxsackievirus group B affects the brain, pancreas, and myocardium and is subdivided into six types. The virus is transmitted either by direct contact or by ingested droplets. An initial stage of replication occurs in the gut, after which the virus spreads to target organs such as mucosal membranes, skin, muscles, and pericardium. At the target site additional multiplication occurs, causing the characteristic signs and symptoms of the disease.

The oral involvement in coxsackievirus group A infection represents herpangina and hand-foot-and-mouth (HFM) disease. Both diseases are characterized by a short incubation period of 5 days from contact to vesicle formation. Along with fever of up to 104° F (40° C) small vesicles are formed in the pharynx, fauces, tonsils, and soft palate. The vesicles rupture within 3 to 4 days, leaving a shallow ulcer 2 to 3 mm in diameter with a grayish base and erythematous margin. These ulcerative manifestations can be differentiated from herpes simplex virus infection by being absent from the anterior part of the oral cavity and by occuring seasonally around May to October in epidemics. In hand-foot-and-mouth disease, additional vesicle formations are present on the palms and the soles of the feet. Coxsackievirus group types 2, 4, 5, 6, 8, and 10

are implicated in herpangina, whereas types 5, 10, and 16 are more common in hand-foot-and-mouth disease. Coxsackievirus group B rarely affects the mouth, although it may play a role in hand-foot-and-mouth disease.

Apart from vesiculoulcerative lesions, a report of palatal paralysis also has been attributed to coxsackievirus group A infection. Cytologically, no multinucleated giant cells or nuclear balloon degeneration is present, thus differentiating coxsackievirus infection from herpes simplex virus infections.

Paramyxovirus

MEASLES (RUBEOLA). The most common childhood disease is acute measles infection. This disease is widespread and highly contagious, being transmitted by propret infection. The virus has an affinity for the respiratory epithelium, where it replicates and causes flulike symptoms. From there the virus disseminates via the circulatory system to stratified squamous epithelium, where a characteristic skin rash develops. Before the cutaneous manifestations appear, a rash may develop in the buccal mucosa, causing the appearance of Koplik's spots. These are white, plaquelike, and oval to round in contour. Only one lesion of less than 10 mm may appear, or there may be several small lesions on bilateral mucosal surfaces. The skin rash appears 1 to 2 days later.

MUMPS. This paramyxovirus is transmitted by droplets from the saliva and respiratory tract. It multiplies in the upper respiratory tract and local lymph nodes and can cause severe lymphadenopathy. A salivary gland infection occurs 16 to 18 days after exposure, and ensuing acute parotitis may develop. A painful swelling of one or both parotid glands is common, together with fever. Clinically, the earlobe on the affected side is laterally displaced when viewed from behind. The saliva contains infectious virus 6 days before clinical manifestations of the disease and 9 days after reduction of the glandular swelling.

Severe complications from mumps are more common in adults, in whom orchitis, meningitis, pancreatitis, and oophoritis may occur.

Rubivirus

RUBELLA (GERMAN MEASLES). Rubella virus infection is spread by droplets shed from the respiratory secretions of infected people. Infants born with congenital rubella shed large quantities of the virus from body secretions for many months. Acquired rubella virus infection can manifest in the oral cavity as small petechiae like spots of the soft palate. The defects of congenital infection from an infected mother are more severe. Enamel defects include hypoplasa, pitting, and abnormal tooth morphology. Partial or total aplasia of the primary dentition can occur. Apart from morphologic defects, irregular eruption patterns also occur. Maternal rubella infection also can cause cleft lip and palate in the neonate, as well as facial paralysis.

Cat-scratch disease

Children with cervical lymphadenopathy suspected of having cat-scratch disease are referred for dental examination to exclude oral infection as the reason for the lymph node involvement. Shklar described one patient with laboratory confirmation of cat-scratch disease in whom oral vesicular lesions appeared and ruptured to form ulcers.

BIBLIOGRAPHY
Herpesvirus

Check WA: Acyclovir for herpes: no clinical payoff yet (news), JAMA 244:2021, 1980.

Cooper JC: Tooth exfoliation and osteonecrosis of the jaw following herpes zoster, Br Dent J 143:297, 1977.

Guinan ME and others: Topical ether and herpes simplex labialis, JAMA 243:1059, 1980.

Morgan DG and others: Site of Epstein-Barr virus replication in the oropharynx, Lancet 2:1154, 1979.

O'Meara A and others: Acyclovir for treatment of mucocutaneous herpes infection in a child with leukemia (letter), Lancet 2(8153):1196, 1979.

Human papilloma virus

Scully C and others: Papillomaviruses: the current status in relation to oral disease, Oral Surg 65:526, 1988.

Coxsackievirus

Bell EJ and others: Enterovirus infections, Update 26:967, 1983.

Conway SP: Coxsackie B2 virus causing simultaneous hand, foot and mouth disease and or cephalitis, J Infect Dis 15:91, 1987.

Couch RG and others: Airborne transmission of respiratory infection with coxsackie virus A type 21, Am J Epidemol 91:78, 1970.

Lindenbaum JE, VanDyck PC, and Allen RG: Hand food and mouth disease associated with coxsackie group B, Scand J Infect Dis 7:161, 1975.

Nussey AM: Paralysis of the palate in a child, Br Med J 2:165, 1977.

Rubella

Gullikson JS: Tooth morphology in rubella syndrome children, J Dent Child 42:479.

Cytomegalovirus

Kanas RJ and others: Oral mucosal cytomegalovirus as a manifestation of the acquired immune deficiency syndrome, Oral Surg 64:183, 1987.

Stagno S and others: Cytomegalovirus infection: epidemiology, diagnosis and clinical outcome with particular reference to oral pathology. In Hooks J and Jordon G, editors: Viral infections in oral medicine, Amsterdam, 1982, Elsevier Science Publishing Co, Inc.

Whitley RJ: Ganciclovir—have we established clinical value in the treatment of cytomegalovirus infections? Ann Intern Med 108(3):452, 1988.

Epstein-Barr virus

Evans AS: The transmission of EB viral infections. In Hooks J and Jordan G, editors: Viral infections in oral medicine, Amsterdam, 1982 Elsevier Science Publishing Co, Inc.

Niederman JC and others: Infectious mononucleosis: EBV shedding in saliva and the oropharynx, N Engl J Med 294:1353, 1976.

Vilde JL and others: Association of Epstein-Barr virus with lethal midline granuloma, N Engl J Med 313:1161, 1985.

Wolf H and Seibl R: Benign and malignant disease caused by EBV, J Invest Dermatol 83:885, 1983.

Varicella-zoster virus

Atterbury RA: Facial herpes zoster, J Oral Surg 35:151, 1977.

Chenitz JE: Herpes zoster in Hodgkin's disease: unusual oral sequelae, J Dent Child 43:184, 1976.

Easton HG: Zoster sine herpete causing acute trigeminal neuralgia, Lancet 3:1065, 1970.

Eisenburg E: Intraoral isolated herpes zoster, Oral Surg 45:214, 1978.

Hill PA and Lamey PJ: Oral herpes zoster with contralateral skin involvement, Br Dent J 161:217, 1986.

Loeser JD: Herpes zoster and postherpetic neuralgia, Pain 25:149, 1986.

Mandal BK: Herpes zoster and the immunocompromised, J Infect 14:1, 1987.

Smith S, Ross JR, and Scully C: An unusual oral complication of herpes zoster infection, Oral Surg 57:388, 1984.

Straus SE and others: Varicella zoster virus infections, Ann Intern Med 108:221, 1988.

ORAL MANIFESTATIOINS OF HUMAN IMMUNODEFICIENCY VIRUS INFECTION

Once the acquired human immunodeficiency virus (HIV) infects a person, that person will be infected with the virus for life. Eventually the virus induces an irreversible and progressive immunosuppression that renders the person susceptible to a variety of opportunistic infections and malignancies. This leads to innumerable oral manifestations that involve the dental profession in both diagnosis and treatment.

Kaposi's sarcoma

Kaposi's sarcoma (KS) is the most common malignancy of acquired immunodeficiency syndrome (AIDS). KS appears orally in about half of the patients, most often as a mild malignancy of the skin. Intraorally, early lesions appear as flat, purplish-red lesions that vary in size and usually are asymptomatic. As the disorder progresses, the lesions become more nodular and symptomatic (Fig. 1).

Diagnosis is confirmed by biopsy, which shows a classic pattern of atypical vascular proliferation, malignant-appearing endothelial cells, and extravasation of red blood cells. The most common treatment when the lesions are not widespread is by low-dose radiation therapy, using daily doses of approximately 150 cGy for approximately 10 to 15 days. In some situations surgery with the carbon dioxide laser and chemotherapy with vinblastine have been useful.

Candidiasis

The most common opportunistic infection of patients with HIV infection is candidiasis (Fig. 2). Diagnosis and treatment (discussed previously) are important because of the symptoms and because of the possibility that the candidal organisms could further suppress the immune system and serve as a focus for spread to other sites such as the esophagus. Management becomes difficult because of the tendency of candidiasis to recur. Therefore combinations of mouth rinses, systemic antifungals, and topical medications must be used.

Hairy leukoplakia

Hairy leukoplakia derived its name from its somewhat corrugated or hairy appearance; it is white in color (Fig. 3). It almost always occurs either unilaterally or bilaterally on the lateral tongue and occasionally on other mucosal surfaces. The diagnosis is confirmed by biopsy, which reveals little connective tissue inflammation, epithelial hyperplasia, immature surface keratin, and vacuolated epithelial cells. The vacuolated cells are associated with a herpes family virus, the Epstein-Barr virus.

This lesion is significant, because it may be the first sign of HIV infection. Most individuals with these lesions are infectious and in time probably will develop AIDS. Since these lesions often are asymptomatic, treatment is not necessary. There is no evidence that removing the lesions has any bearing on the prognosis and eventual progressive immunosuppression.

HIV-associated periodontal disease

A large number of those infected with the AIDS virus show a clinical gingivitis and roentgenographic evidence of bone loss. This periodontal condition is progressive and related to alterations in the subgingival microbial flora. Treatment is conventional, with home and office care supplemented with effective mouth rinses such as chlorhexidine. When young, high-risk individuals demonstrate periodontal disease, immunosuppression and HIV infection should be suspected.

Other relatively common manifestions of HIV infection, high-risk activity, and immunosuppression include initial and/or increased severity and frequency of attacks involving herpes simplex virus; recurrent aphthous stomatitis, often occurring as major aphthae; venereal warts (condyloma acuminatum) associated with human papilloma viruses; lichenoid reactions, reflecting increased hypersensitivities; idiopathic salivary gland swellings associated with sialadenitis; and nonspecific oral infections associated with organisms that usually do not inhabit the oral cavity. Management in these high-risk individuals in-

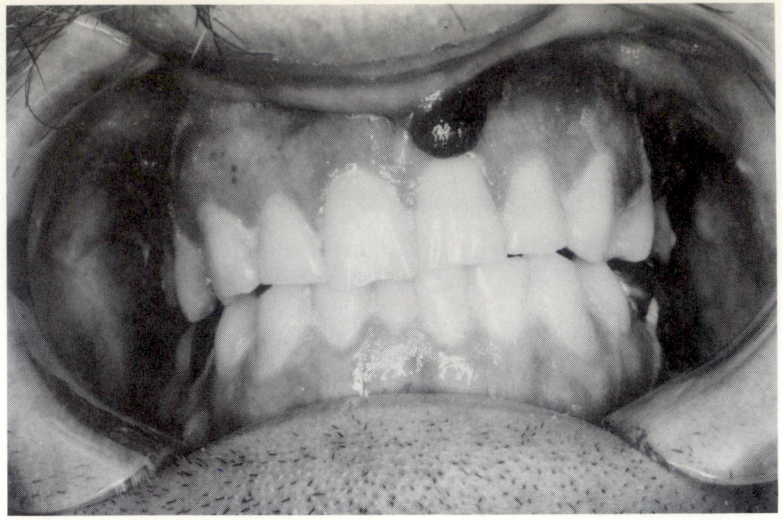

Fig. 1 Kaposi's sarcoma.

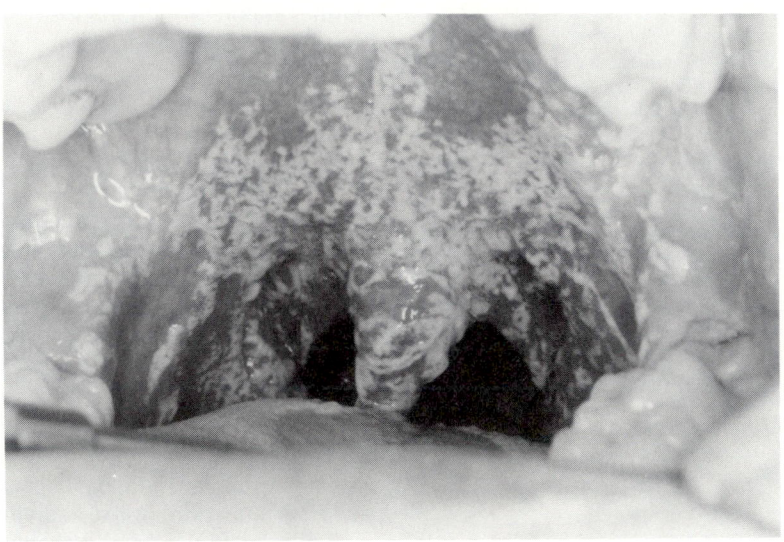

Fig. 2 Oral candidasis.

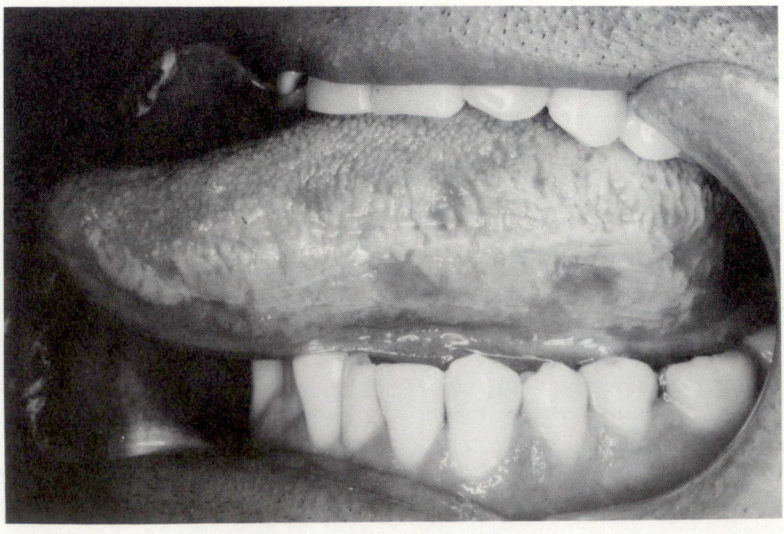

Fig. 3 Oral hairy leukoplakia.

clude a differential diagnosis, definitive diagnosis, and referral for treatment, counseling, and staging.

BACTERIAL INFECTIONS
Periodontal disease

MICROBIAL ENVIRONMENT OF THE GINGIVAL CREVICE IN HEALTH AND DISEASE. Several generalizations can be made about the crevicular microbiota in the absence of disease. First, the amount of adherent plaque is of minimal thickness (about one to 20 cells). Second, most of the organisms are gram-positive facultative/anaerobic cocci and rods, particularly *Streptococcus sanguis* and species of *Actinomyces*, both members of the indigenous flora and presumed to be initial colonizers of the tooth surface. Third, although there is not a great deal of plaque, the total microscopic counts reported by Socransky have indicated that there are over 2×10^{11} organisms/gm wet weight of crevicular material. Included in this number are many other species of gram-negative bacteria, particularly the anaerobic rods, primarily the *Bacteroides* and *Fusobacteria* organisms. Therefore, even in healthy people the crevicular area accommodates a large and diverse population. However, this population has a discernible profile, composed mostly of gram-positive facultative streptococci and actinomycetes.

MARGINAL GINGIVITIS. Gingivitis, the most common form of periodontal disease, is an inflammatory condition confined to the gingiva. If not treated, it may develop into periodontitis with destruction or involvement of the periodontal membrane and alveolar bone. Plaque accumulation at the gingival margin results in the release of toxic bacterial metabolic products followed by changes in the vessels subadjacent to the junctional epithelium (vasculitis). There is an increased flow of gingival exudate (crevicular fluid) and the concomitant migration of leukocytes from the lamina propria into the crevicular epithelium. Changes in the gingival color, tissue texture, and surface anatomy occur later in the development of the gingivitis lesion.

The bacterial flora associated with gingivitis, like most forms of periodontal disease, has a characteristic population profile, described in the following:

Specific microbiotas associated with periodontal disease

1. *Gingivitis.* Gram-positive facultative and microaerophilic cocci and rods with a predominance of *Actinomyces* and *Streptococcus* spp.
2. *Acute necrotizing ulcerative gingivitis* (ANUG, Vincent's infection, trench mouth). Gram-negative anaerobes. *Bacteroides intermedius, Fusobacterium nucleatum,* spirochetes (*Treponema* spp. and selenomonads).
3. *Periodontitis* (advancing periodontitis, adult periodontitis). Heterogeneity of microbial types but predominance of gram-negative asaccharolytic anaerobic bacteria; many are motile. *Bacteroides gingivalis, Bacteroides intermedius, Eikenella corrodens, Wolinella recta, Actinobacillus actinomycetem-comitans,* spirochetes, *Bacteroides forsythus, Peptostreptococcus micros.*
4. *Juvenile periodontitis* (localized juvenile periodontitis [LJP] periodontosis). Gram-negative, CO_2 requiring (capnophilic rods). *Actinobacillus actinomycetem-comitans* (most important agent), *Capnocytophaga* spp. (juvenile diabetes).

Unlike the normal crevicular plaque, the gingivitis (especially chronic) is quite thick, with some layers more than 100 cells thick. Most of the cultivable flora in early gingivitis are gram-positive with *Actinomyces* spp. (*Actinomyces naeslundii* and *Actinomyces odontolyticus*) and streptococci (*Streptococcus anginosus*) predominating. Recent studies have indicated that the actinomycetes and streptococci alone usually do not pro-

duce experimental gingivitis in humans but probably require the participation of other organisms, including *Fusobacterium nucleatum, Treponema* and *Selenomonas* spp., and other gram-negative organisms. There is also reason to believe that the microbiota associated with gingivitis in children is different than in adult gingivitis, with greater proportions of *Leptotrichia, Capnocytophaga, Selenomonas,* and certain *Bacteroides* spp. The therapy for gingivitis almost always is removal of plaque and maintenance of proper oral hygiene. Antibiotics are not indicated.

ACUTE NECROTIZING ULCERATIVE GINGIVITIS (ANUG, VINCENT'S INFECTION, TRENCH MOUTH). As the name indicates, this disease is an inflammatory periodontal disease with characteristic clinical signs and symptoms, that is, a fulminating inflammation of the gingivae that leads to macroscopic ulceration and necrosis of the soft tissues. Clinical criteria used to diagnose ANUG include (1) interproximal soft tissue craters, (2) spontaneous gingival bleeding, often occurring during mastication or toothbrushing, (3) presence of a gray pseudomembrane separated from the gingival mucosa by a pronounced linear erythema, (4) fetor oris, (5) pain, and (6) a history of sudden onset.

Early studies of the cause of ANUG were mostly morphologic and ultrastructural and did not critically evaluate the contributions of all the strict anaerobes to the microflora. It now is clear that three major anaerobic populations are routinely associated wth ANUG: (1) motile spirochetes, including *Treponema* spp. (of the intermediate type, having more than six axial fibrils originating from each end) and selenomonads; (2) *Bacteroides intermedius;* and (3) *Fusobacterium nucleatum* (see the previous outline). The disease was often called "fusospirochetal disease," but closer analysis of the flora has demonstrated convincingly that *B. intermedius* probably is more prominent (24% versus 3% of the total cultivable microflora). Loesche and others have hypothesized that these particular anaerobic species predominate because of the availability of host-derived nutrients in individuals who have undergone certain physiologic and psychologic stresses. A related study showed that the levels of *B. intermedius* in pregnancy gingivitis strongly correlated with plasma levels of estrogen and progesterone. Both of these hormones can substitute for menadione as an essential growth factor for *B. intermedius*. In addition, spirochetes routinely are seen in the gingival tissue up to 300 μm from the crevicular surface, indicating the invasive potential of these organisms under conditions in which host resistance and other local factors are predisposing.

The diagnosis of ANUG usually is made on clinical grounds; microscopic validation of a fusospirochetal flora in a phase contrast or darkfield wet mount preparation is helpful. Serologic tests or culturing are not indicated.

Although a number of predisposing factors (for instance, poor oral hygiene, tobacco, localized trauma, acute emotional stress) must be dealt with, the therapy for ANUG almost always is the administration of antibiotics. Penicillin and metronidazole have been used with great success.

PERIODONTITIS. Periodontitis is characterized as an inflammatory lesion in which the loss of alveolar bone is accompanied by a loss of gingival attachment with the appearance of the pathognomonic "periodontal pocket." Histologically, there is destruction of the collagen fiber network below the cementoenamel junction and an apical shift of the epithelial attachment. With the creation of the pocket any number of destructive changes may occur affecting the epithelium, underlying connective tissue, and alveolar bone. (Some of these are discussed later under mechanisms of pathogenicity.)

The microbiota associated with periodontitis vary, and identification depends on whether the lesion is actually breaking down or quiescent. The one general feature common to most studies is the predominance of nonsaccharolytic (non-sugar-using) anaerobic, gram-negative rods, many of which are motile (see the previous outline). Among the organisms most commonly described as disease-associated are *Bacteroides gingivalis, Bacteroides intermedius, Wolinella recta, Eikenella corrodens, Actinobacillus actinomycetem-comitans, Bacteroides forsythus,* fusobacteria, and spirochetes. *Peptostreptococcus micros,* a gram-positive, proteolytic coccus, also has been identified as an important disease-associated organism. The evidence implicating *B. gingivalis* is particularly impressive and satisfies the most stringent criteria for establishing the specific etiologic agents of a periodontal disease. However, it should be remembered that good longitudinal studies on microbial changes in active or quiescent lesions are not sufficiently precise at this time to rule out the possibility that other microbes (listed above) acting alone or in concert may play major roles in pathogenesis at different times. Therapy for periodontitis depends on the extent of tissue or bone destruction. In addition to debridement and curettage, it often requires surgical intervention and antibiotics. Tetracycline has been used with apparent success, not only because of its antibacterial properties but because it is concentrated in the crevicular fluid and indirectly inhibits tissue collagenases.

LOCALIZED JUVENILE PERIODONTITIS ("MOLAR-INCISOR PERIODONTOSIS," LJP). Localized juvenile periodontitis is a relatively rare disease in most western countries. It is a rapidly advancing disease seen in adolescents who often have basically good oral hygiene with minimal supragingival plaque but with deep pockets and considerable bone loss. A single etiologic agent, *Actinobacillus actinomycetem-comitans* has been identified for most LJP cases. (In juvenile diabetes, *Capnocytophaga* spp. appear to have the dominant etiologic role.) The data implicating *A. actinomycetem-comitans* as the prime etiologic agent are excellent and include host response studies (elevated antibody levels in patients), microbiologic culture surveys (*A. actinomycetem-comitans* is regularly isolable from subgingival plaques in patients), and experimental animal studies showing the pathogenic potential of the organism and its products. Morever, recent studies have shown that *A. actinomycetem-comitans* actually invades the gingival tissues and has an array of virulence factors (collagenase, leukotoxin, endotoxin, immunosuppressive factors, inhibitors of fibroblasts, and epithelial cell growth), which could explain the severity and fulminating character of the clinical disease. For example, the lysis of polymorphonuclear leukocytes (PMNs) by the leukotoxin would result in the release of numerous lysosomal enzymes known to destroy periodontal tissue. Similarly, the destruction of PMNs by the leukotoxin also would represent the loss of one of the host's first lines of defense (PMN phagocytosis).

Antibiotics, primarily tetracycline, have been used with success in therapy for the disease, that is, the destructive processes are stopped and the organism is eliminated from the tissues for the most part. However, debridement and surgical intervention often are necessary as well.

LABORATORY DIAGNOSIS. Periodontal diseases usually are diagnosed using various clinical criteria (for instance, roentgenograms, pocket depth, and bleeding on probing). However, with the compelling evidence of bacteriologic specificity in the causes of these diseases, it is possible to adopt the methods of the infectious disease laboratory to aid in diagnosis. If there is a characteristic microbial complex or a single etiologic agent with chemically definable effector macromolecules, then the putative pathogen(s) can be isolated from clinical samples (subgingival plaque) and specific antibodies can be sought in patients' sera. Various laboratories have been developed recently that perform such services, providing the referring dentist with data on the microbial composition of crevicular samples, the antibiotic sensitivities of the isolates, and antibody levels to suspected pathogens. Considerable effort has been expended in this regard for LJP because of the clear association of *A. actinomycetem-comitans* with the disease and the well-known immunogenic potential of the organism in humans with the disease. In the future, with the advent of simple but more sophisticated technologic advances, such as DNA hybridization probes, dentists may perform some of these services routinely in the dental office. Some dentists already are using phase contrast or darkfield microscopy of subgingival plaque samples in evaluating disease status and monitoring effectiveness of therapy. (A nonmotile coccal flora is more indicative of a healthy periodontium than a flora dominated by motile rods.) Similar approaches (darkfield examination of oral smears) also have been used for ANUG diagnosis.

BIBLIOGRAPHY

Hammond BF: The microbiology of periodontal diseases with emphasis on localized juvenile periodontitis, Alpha Omegan 76:27, 1983.

Loesche W and others: The bacteriology of acute necrotizing gingivitis, J Periodontol 53:223, 1982.

Moore WEC and others: Bacteriology of experimental gingivitis in young adult humans, Infect Immun 38:651, 1982.

Moore WEC and others: Bacteriology of experimental gingivitis in children, Infect Immun 46:1, 1984.

Socransky SS: Relationship of bacteria to the etiology of periodontal disease, J Dent Res 49:203, 1970.

Dental caries

Dental caries results from a chronic bacterial infection that affects more than 95% of people in the United States. Acid-producing microorganisms demineralize the inorganic portion and destroy the organic structure of the tooth, causing carious lesions. As in all bacterial infections, three factors must interact to cause a reaction. In dental caries, the agent (the cariogenic microorganism) acts on the host (the tooth) in a suitable environment (appropriate foodstuff that can be metabolized by the microorganism).

AGENT. Because of the diverse oral flora and the ideal temperature and humidity of the oral cavity, numerous bacteria have been identified as causative agents of dental caries. A layer of salivary proteins, mucin, and desquamative epithelial cells immediately coat a newly cleaned tooth. This layer, or acquired pellicle, serves as a matrix for colonization of microorganisms. The process takes 24 to 48 hours. *Streptococcus sanguis* is the first microorganism to colonize the acquired pellicle. *Streptococcus mutans* produces glucan from available carbohydrates, enhancing the colonization and accumulation of other species. If the tooth is not cleaned, a soft, nonmineralized mass consisting of microorganisms, the bacterial plaque, will form. The plaque restricts saliva, with its high buffering capacity, from reaching the acid-producing bacteria.

Numerous streptococci, lactobacilli, and actinomycetes in the oral flora have the characteristics of a cariogenic microorganism, that is, the ability to colonize, metabolize carbohydrates, and produce acid with a sufficiently low pH to demineralize enamel. Streptococci are believed to be the primary etiologic agents, including *Streptococcus salivarius, Streptococcus sanguis,* and *Streptococcus faecalis.* Other microorganisms such as *Lactobacillus casei, Actinomyces viscosus, Actinomyces naeslundii,* and *Actinomyces israelii* also have been implicated in pit and fissure, smooth surface, and root surface caries.

HOST. The structure and composition of enamel and dentin, as well as the spacing between teeth, may explain similar caries susceptibility in families. Family dietary regimens also play a part. The saliva composition, with its high buffering capacity and potential bacteriostatic components, may be genetically determined. No direct genetic predisposition to caries has been determined. An increased incidence of caries has been noted in people with xerostomia. Patients born without salivary glands or those whose glands have been removed surgically and patients with irradiated glands, Sjögren's syndrome, or graft-versus-host disease may have rampant caries. Partial xerostomia also can be a side effect of certain drugs.

ENVIRONMENTAL FACTORS. Fluoride has been shown to be effective against caries. Fluoride ion replaces the hydroxy group in the hydroxyapatite crystal, thereby strengthening the enamel. Fluoride released from the enamel and dentin favorably influences some remineralization of tooth structure destroyed by cariogenic microorganisms. Systemic fluoride also may have antibacterial action. The addition of fluoride, one part per million, to communal drinking water has been shown to reduce the incidence of caries by up to 60%.

Carbohydrates must be present for any carious activity to occur. The longer and the more frequently the dentition is exposed to simple carbohydrates in the presence of acidogenic bacteria, the higher the incidence of caries.

Gonococcal stomatitis

Gonococcal infection of the oral cavity is uncommon and occurs mainly in adults. The incubation period of *Neisseria gonorrhoeae* in the oral cavity varies from 1 day to 2 weeks. Oral lesions in adults result from orogenital contact or contamination through the hands. In newborns, gonococcal stomatitis is acquired during contact with the mother's vaginal mucosa.

The appearance of oral lesions is nonspecific. Superficial ulcers with a yellow-white slough or pseudomembrane may develop on the gingiva, tongue, and soft palate. The gingivae generally are inflamed and resemble necrotizing ulcerative gingivitis. If the stomatitis becomes generalized, the entire oral mucosa appears red or inflamed. Alternatively and most commonly, infection is asymptomatic or present as pharyngitis. Gonococci also can invade the salivary glands and lead to parotitis.

Therapy of gonococcal lesions of the oral mucosa, although similar to that of genital gonorrhea, differs in that antibiotic failures have been seen with ampicillin and tetracycline, hence parenteral procaine penicillin is the method of choice.

Lymphogranuloma venereum (LGV)

In rare cases lymphogranuloma venereum may involve the oropharynx and occur as a result of orogenital sex.

In oral infection with *Chlamydia trachomatis,* the tongue most often is affected and a blisterlike lesion develops. The lesion is painless, and the tongue is involved with areas of acute inflammation and depapillation, leading to sensitivity to spicy foods. The tongue generally shows signs of inflammation for long periods of time. Prominent submandibular lymphadenopathy develops that may progress to fluctuant buboes.

Syphilis

Oral manifestations of syphilis are found in both congenital and acquired syphilis and continue to be seen in the primary and secondary stages of active syphilis.

In primary syphilis a chancre can develop on the lips (ver-

milion border or commissural area), the tip of the tongue, the tonsils, or the gingiva. Significant regional lymphadenopathy is observed unilaterally and facilitates the diagnosis. The chancre, as well as the lymph nodes, abound with *Treponema pallidum.* Intraoral chancres tend to be infected by other commensal oral spirochetes as well. Accordingly, darkfield examination of intraoral syphilitic lesions may be unreliable.

In secondary syphilis the oral lesions are protean in nature, including the characteristic intraoral mucous patches that resemble the macular and maculopapular skin lesions of secondary syphilis. The mucous patches are raised on the mucosal surface and appear inflamed with an area of central erosion covered by a grayish white membrane. Upon removal of the membrane a clear, flat, erythematous base is seen. The patches are found on the tongue, buccal mucosa, oropharynx, and the inner aspect of the lips but rarely are seen on the gingival surface. Syphilitic, mucous patches are highly contagious, and during this phase infected saliva droplets can easily transmit the disease.

Maculopapular lesions may develop on the palate. When present at the corners of the mouth, they are called "split papules." They form a painless fissure between the upper and lower lip. These lesions must be differentiated from angular cheilosis such as caused by riboflavin deficiency. Papular lesions of the hard or soft palate may break down, resulting in snail-track ulcers.

Relapses of oropharyngeal mucosal involvement may interrupt the early latent stage of syphilis.

Gummatous infiltration of oral tissue and diffuse glossitis are manifestations of tertiary syphilis. Gummas are painless granulomas that become necrotic. They develop on the lips, oral mucosa, salivary glands, palate, and jawbone. Proliferative changes and necrosis accompany the pathologic process, leading to the formation of punched-out ulcers. Involvement of the palate eventually is followed by its perforation. Gummas on the tongue produce lingua lobulata. Ulcerations and fibrosis induce surface irregularities of the tongue.

Clinical and histologic diagnosis is difficult, since such lesions are similar to those found in tuberculosis, leishmaniasis, sarcoidosis, or leprosy or mycotic granulomas. Malignancy of the tongue cannot be ruled out without a biopsy.

Atrophy of the tongue secondary to the resulting ischemia is the next stage, together with a smooth surface and shrinkage in the musculature. Leukoplakia often accompanies these changes, which result from the chronic irritation of depapillated, unprotected tongue surface. This leukoplakic area may undergo malignant changes.

The hutchinsonian triad is a result of spirochetemia during the development of the embryo. The dental deformities are caused by hypoplasia following spirochetemia. The timing of hypoplasia corresponds with the attack on the middle mamelon of the central incisors, resulting in an increased anteroposterior diameter, with a narrow incisal dimension. Only the permanent teeth are affected, and among them only those in which the calcification started in the first year of life, for example, upper central incisors and all first molars. The first molars have a narrow crown with multiple small, underdeveloped cusps and are called "mulberry molars." It was estimated that about 45% of patients with congenital syphilis had typical syphilitic incisors, and 22% had characteristic syphilitic molars. These dental changes can be prevented if appropriate antimicrobial therapy is initiated before the fourth month of fetal development. Perioral rhagades are present in perhaps 15% of patients with congenital syphilis. These linear lesions are found around the oral and anal orifices and are the result of luetic skin involvement. The rhagades appear at first as red or copper-colored linear areas covered with a crust. They are radially arranged, as if starting from the vermilion border. These cracks are considered pathognomonic for congenital syphilis.

Bacterial infections of the central nervous system

Oral and dental infections may be complicated by acute bacterial infections of the brain and meninges, often with fatal outcome. Microorganisms isolated from these infections include *Fusobacterium* species and anaerobic gram-positive cocci. Although dental infection may spread spontaneously, not infrequently complications follow extraction of infected teeth.

The propagated infection from dental foci may take a direct route via openings in the cranial bones, such openings being found mostly in the temporal bone. Another route may be the venous system via emissary veins connecting the extracranial and intracranial venous systems. The most important of these emissary veins is the one leading from the facial to the ophthalmic vein. The ophthalmic vein directly communicates with the cavernous sinus.

Cavernous sinus thrombosis is a rare but grave complication of dental infection. The common clinical picture of this condition presents with unilateral or bilateral proptosis, periorbital and conjunctival edema, ophthalmoplegia, and fever. The involved teeth are sensitive to percussion and in most of the cases roentgenographic evidence is present as radiolucent areas of chronic dental infection. Nerve involvement of the trigeminal nerve, ophthalmic division, and trochlear and abducens nerves can be observed, resulting in paralysis, ptosis, dilated pupils, and abolition of corneal reflexes. The antibiotic treatment is directed at streptococcal, staphylococcal, and anaerobic organisms. Massive doses of parenteral penicillin, chloramiphenicol, and a penicillinase-resistant β-lactam antibiotic are recommended. In the presence of a fluctuating oral abscess, incision and drainage should be undertaken and extraction of the involved tooth should be considered.

Meningitis, encephalitis, and brain abscesses are discussed in the chapter on bacterial infections of the central nervous system.

Tuberculosis

Tubercular infection of oral tissues may arise from either an exogenous or an endogenous source of microorganisms. It appears that direct primary infection of oral tissues is rarer than seeding of tuberculous microorganisms via hematogenous or lymphatic routes. The prevalence of oral tuberculosis, according to the literature, ranges from 0.05% to 1.44%.

ORAL MANIFESTATIONS

Tuberculous ulceration. Tuberculous ulceration is irregular with a typically undermined border. The ulcer base is covered with a purulent exudate; the surrounding tissue is indurated. Tuberculous proliferative lesions may be seen singly or concomitantly with ulcerative ones.

Tuberculous granulomas. Tuberculous granulomas have been misdiagnosed as periapical dental lesions when seen roentgenographically. The only clinical manifestation is increased mobility of the involved teeth.

Orofacial tuberculosis. Oral mucosal tuberculous lesions typically are found near the mucocutaneous junction. In addition, the tongue, bucal mucosa, palate, or gingiva may be the site of infection. Lesions result from autoinoculation of tubercle bacilli emanating from underlying advanced pulmonary tuberculosis, although occasionally they may represent the primary lesion.

Tubercular lesions of the lips usually begin as swellings that later develop into ulcers. The ulcers are extremely painful and characterized by prolonged healing time that may take months to complete. The adjacent facial skin may exhibit various manifestations, including plaquelike verrucous and nodular lesions. Occasionally, tuberculous erythematous nodular gingivitis occurs. The organisms may enter the alveolar bone through the teeth and form a periapical granuloma or even osteomyelitis.

Tuberculous osteomyelitis of the jaws. Although rare, tuberculous osteomyelitis of the mandibular and maxillary bones has been encountered. In tuberculous lesions of the jaw bones, some swelling occurs over the involved area as a result of subperiosteal new bone formation. Bone destruction is characteristic, and sequestra develop. With time, the swelling ruptures and secreting fistulas are evident.

The roentgenographic picture of tuberculous osteomyelitis reveals blurring of bone detail and erosion of the cortical plate. When tuberculosis affects the periodontal tissues, the roentgenographic signs may be the same as those of destructive periodontal disease.

Tuberculosis of the salivary glands. Fewer than 100 cases of tuberculosis of the salivary glands have been described in the literature. Tuberculosis mainly affects the parotid glands of young adults. Two types of lesions were described including a chronic encapsulated form and an acute diffuse inflammatory process. The chronic lesions are present as small swellings that usually are freely movable when palpated.

Tuberculous cervical lymphadenitis (scrofulosis). Enlargement of the submandibular and cervical lymph nodes is not always present in association with oral mucosal tuberculous disease and often is only the consequence of secondary bacterial infection. Nevertheless, the presenting manifestation of oral tuberculosis includes progressive enlargement of regional lymph nodes.

Tuberculous cervical lymphadenitis also may occur in the absence of visible oropharyngeal tuberculosis. Formerly a common disease in children, it has become infrequent. It usually represents breakdown of prior cervical node tuberculosis, either acquired by ingestion of infected milk (bovine tuberculosis) or more commonly by lymphohematogenous spread of infection from a primary pulmonary focus. In the United States scrofula in young children is now most frequently caused by atypical mycobacteria, particularly *Mycobacterium scrofulaceum*.

Treatment. In cases of oral involvement in tuberculosis, the systemic treatment is supplemented with local palliative measures. Causes of trauma, such as sharp broken teeth, ill-fitted dentures, or massive dental calculus, should be eliminated. Mouth rinses should be instituted in copious amounts to prevent secondary infection of the existing specific ulcers.

BIBLIOGRAPHY

De Lathouwer, L and others: A rare and complex case of multifocal mucocutaneous lupus tuberculosis with isolated lesion of the tongue, Oral Surg 39(2):211, 1975.

Fujibayashi T and others: Tuberculosis of the tongue: a case report with immunologic study, Oral Surg 47(5):427, 1979.

Garber HT and others: Tuberculous osteomyelitis of the mandible with pathologic fracture, J Oral Surg 36(2):144, 1978.

Prabhu SR and others: Tuberculous ulcer of the tongue: report of a case, J Oral Surg 36(5):384, 1978.

Rauch MD and others: Systemic tuberculosis initially seen as an oral ulceration: report of a case, J Oral Surg 36:384, 1978.

Turbiner S and others: Orificial tuberculosis of the lip, J Oral Surg 33(6):443, 1975.

Leprosy

Facial and oral manifestations of leprosy continue to be seen, particularly in endemic areas in both hemispheres. The clinical manifestations depend on both the histopathologic type and the duration of leprosy.

Facial involvement results in a "leonine" facies, including loss of eyebrows and sagging of facial skin. Deformity of the ears is common, and lesions of the oral mucosa and tongue have been reported in 20% to 60% of these patients. Early manifestations of oral leprosy include the formation of nodules or lepromas which may be yellowish red, soft or hard, sessile, and often ulcerated. Healing tissues usually are fibrotic, which tends to add to the physical disfigurement. Although all oral structures may be involved, the incisive papilla, premaxilla, hard and soft palate, uvula, and tongue most commonly are involved. Granulomatous bone involvement leads to destruction of the premaxilla and loss of the front teeth. Chronic gingivitis and periodontitis with loss of alveolar bone, although frequently observed, are not specific for leprosy.

Dental changes are described as odontodysplasia leprosa. Tooth diameters are concentrically reduced and roots are shortened and tapered. Enamel and cement hypoplasia has been found in osteoarcheologic material.

Both sensory and motor peripheral nerve fibers of the cranial nerves commonly are involved. Hence bilateral facial nerve paralysis occurs in about 25% of patients with tuberculoid leprosy and trigeminal neuralgia may develop, the most commonly affected branch being the maxillary division.

BIBLIOGRAPHY

Reichart P: Facial and oral manifestations in leprosy: an evaluation of seventy cases. Oral Surg 41(3):385, 1976.

Actinomycosis

CERVICOFACIAL MANIFESTATIONS. *Actinomyces israelii,* a normal inhabitant of the oral cavity, has been isolated from dental plaque, calculus, salivary calculus, necrotic dental pulps, and tonsils. In spite of its prevalence, clinical infection from *Actinomyces* organisms is relatively rare.

Poor oral hygiene is one of the contributory factors in oral actinomycosis. The infection extends from the necrotic tooth pulp to the periapical area and alveolar bone and penetrates through the periosteum into the muscles. The infection becomes apparent as sinus tracts on the skin. Cases have been described in which the infection ascended along the mandibular ramus and penetrated the middle cranial fossa, causing intracranial infection.

In typical cases, the mandibular area is involved, a condition known as "lumpy jaw." Involvement of the gums, oral mucosa, floor of the mouth, and palate may follow localized infection. Ascending infection of the salivary glands is possible through their ducts. Further spread of the disease may involve the muscles of mastication, resulting in severe trismus.

Actinomycosis of the tongue is rare. It involves the anterior third of the tongue as an indurated nodule that is deep seated, painful to palpation, and adherent to the musculature. The absence of regional lymphadenopathy is a striking feature.

The prognosis of cervicofacial actinomycosis is relatively good, except in the presence of chronic osteomyelitis. Therapy consists of prolonged parenteral penicillin administration.

BIBLIOGRAPHY

Kuepper RS and Harrigan WT: Actinomycosis of the tongue: report of case, J Oral Surg 37(2):123, 1979.

Tularemia

Sporadic cases of oral involvement by *Francisella tularensis* has been reported. Solitary, painful necrotic ulcers of the labial, lingual, and palatal mucosa are described. The ulcers are covered with a whitish pseudomembrane, and in rare cases generalized stomatitis has been reported. Oral manifestations are invariably accompanied by other typical clinical manifestations, including conjunctivitis, regional lymphadenopathy, headache, chills, and fever.

Diphtheria

The recent literature has few reports of diphtheritic involvement of the oral tissues. This is the direct result of effective worldwide immunization; however, sporadic cases still are seen in many countries when immunization is absent or incomplete.

Diphtheria pseudomembrane may cover the entire oral mucosa. Involvement of the lower lip, the gums around erupting primary teeth, and the corners of the mouth and tongue have been reported in young children. Lowender and Squires described a case of diphthertic involvement of the lip following the extraction of two loosened anterior teeth. Cultures obtained from the sockets indicated the presence of the diphtheria bacillus, most likely as a result of direct infection or contamination from the saliva.

Cervial lymphadenopathy accompanies oral and pharyngeal lesions.

BIBLIOGRAPHY

Diphtheritic involvement of the lips with absence of signs in the nose and throat, JAMA 111:915, 1938.

Anthrax

Infection with *Bacillus anthracis* limited to the oral cavity is an uncommon condition. A typical case was described by Burnett and associates as being caused by a toothbrush contaminated with anthrax spores. The hard palate first was involved, was severely swollen, and discharged a "straw-colored" fluid. The infectious process spread to the bone, destroying the palate and alveolar bone. Overeruption of the teeth was apparent. On the mucosal surface pustules with bright-red bases appeared and developed into vesicles that broke, scabbed, and later healed. The treatment recommended in this case was antianthrax serum.

The perioral and intraoral types of anthrax are particularly dangerous because of the possibility that they may spread to the oropharynx. Edema of the glottis also is possible. Involvement of the lips and tongue has been encountered in workers from industries involving a risk of exposure to anthrax. This anthrax infection is most frequently the edematous type, characterized by cinnabar to black-red edema of doughy consistency. The tongue, lips, and eyelids become severely enlarged. Anthrax of the face, mouth, or throat has a much graver prognosis than that of the skin.

BIBLIOGRAPHY

Anthrax of the oral cavity, J Am Dent Assoc 36:119, 1948.

Staphylococcal oral lesions

In large population studies staphylococci frequently were found in the oral cavity. In the gingival sulcus they constituted 2% of the viable count and about 6.5% on the dorsum of the tongue. However, they rarely were found in dental plaque.

Staphylococcus aureus was found in low counts in saliva of about half of the subjects examined. However, the proportion of carriers increased to about three quarters when the nose, throat, and mouth were cultured. Despite the prevalence of this organism, oral mucosal lesions caused by *S. aureus* are rare. In toxic epidermal necrolysis induced by this organism, bullae are formed, involving the lips and oral mucosa, followed by desquamation of the epithelium.

FURUNCLES. Furuncles resulting from staphylococcal infection of the face and mainly of the upper lip may present a serious danger to the patient because of possible spread of the infection from the facial region. The most common pathway involves the superior labial veins to the external nasal veins and subsequently to angular veins to the inferior and superior ophthalmic veins, reaching the cavernous sinus. The infection may result in cavernous sinus thrombosis, meningitis, and encephalitis.

Gram-negative oral lesions
ORAL MANIFESTATIONS
Pseudomonas aeruginosa infections. *Pseudomonas* spp. were cultured in more than 50% of patients with acute leukemia. The infections observed were mainly septicemia and cellulitis. Oral lesions developed in the perioral skin, lips, and mucosa. The lesions were characterized by a central black area of necrosis surrounded by a red halo. There was no pus formation or exudate present, and the lesions were dry and gangrenous.

Patients complained of discomfort when eating, drinking, or talking.

Serratia. Patients with hematologic malignancies develop infections with *Serratia* spp. following the use of broad-spectrum antibiotics. The oral lesions are white, well-circumscribed papules that become darker and ulcerate. They are observed at the commissures of the lips and other sites of tissue trauma.

Klebsiella. *Klebsiella* spp. infection are common in patients with acute leukemia. *Klebsiella* organisms constitute a substantial percentage of fatal infection.

The intraoral lesions are "creamy white," raised, glistening, spreading, and superficially erosive on the reddened base. They are painful, and a lack of pus is frequently observed. Lesions occur on the gingiva, lips, tongue, and palatal mucosa. The gingival lesions must be differentiated from those found in acute necrotizing gingivitis.

Enterobacter. Oral lesions with *Enterobacter* organisms present as peritonsillar abscess, tongue ulcers, and diffuse involvement of the oral mucosa. Their clinical appearance is similar to that of *Klebsiella* infection. They are extremely painful, erosive, and ulcerative. The gingival lesions resemble acute necrotizing gingivitis.

Escherichia coli and Proteus spp. Oral infections caused by *Escherichia coli* and *Proteus* spp. in patients with acute leukemia are manifested as gingivitis, mucositis, and osteomyelitis. The oral mucosal lesions are grayish white or yellow with a slight exudate and surrounded by a red halo. They vary in size from 2 to 5 mm in diameter. Pain is the chief complaint of patients with *E. coli* infection of the tongue.

DENTAL MANAGEMENT. Early diagnosis and treatment of oral lesions produced by gram-negative bacilli are imperative because of the precipitous course following these infections in leukemic patients. Antibiotic therapy administered according to sensitivity studies must be initiated immediately.

The importance of aggressive treatment of even innocent-looking gram-negative oral lesions cannot be overemphasized. Carbenicillin plus aminoglycosides are indicated for *Pseudomonas* infections, and cephalosporins and gentamicin are effective in eliminating the infection of the remaining gram-negative organisms.

BIBLIOGRAPHY
Palank EA and others: Fatal acute bacterial endocarditis after dentoalveolar abscess, Am J Cardiol 43(6):1238, 1979.
Pyrexia of dental origin (editorial), Lancet 1(8179):1175, 1980.
Sanchez CS and others: Occurrence of staphylococcus in periodontal pockets of diabetic and nondiabetic adults, J Periodontal 50:109, 1979.
Stenhouse D and others: Staphylococcal submandibular lymphadenitis in childhood, Br J Oral Surg 16:73, 1978.
Those venerable notions (editorial), N Engl J Med 301(16:):888, 1979.

FUNGAL INFECTIONS
Candidiasis (moniliasis, thrush)

Candida albicans is a normal oral flora resident in about 30% to 40% of the population. For reasons not always clearly understood, the fungi can become overpopulated and produce clincial signs and symptoms. Most frequently oral candidal infections are associated with:

1. Prematurity in infants
2. Debilitation
   a. Postoperative, multiple trauma
   b. Underlying malignancy
   c. Stress-induced conditions such as necrotizing ulcerative gingivitis
3. Immunosuppression
   a. Hematologic disease (acute leukemia and advanced lymphoma, granulocytopenia)
   b. Drug-induced (for example, corticosteroids agathioprim) chemotherapy or neoplasia
4. Radiotherapy of head and neck
5. Prolonged antibiotic treatment
6. Diabetes (brittle, insulin-dependent)
7. Oral contraceptives
8. Endocrinopathy, hypoparathyroidism, hypoadrenalism
9. Chronic irritants
   a. Denture stomatitis (combined with poor oral hygiene)
   b. Heavy smoking
10. Xerostomia secondary to salivary gland disease

Different species of *Candida* have been cultured from the mouths of patients who are considered asymptomatic carriers and from patients with frank oral candidiasis. *C. albicans* is the most commonly isolated fungal pathogen in oral thrush. *Candida* yeast frequently are found as normal oral inhabitants in the general population and are considered noncontagious and of low virulence. The above-mentioned predisposing factors have to be present to permit or facilitate overgrowth of *Candida* organisms and the development of symptomatic disease. Hence oral candidiasis is considered an opportunistic infection. Furthermore, in severely immunocompromised patients, the dangers of oral candidiasis are not limited to the local disease manifestations; in addition, candidemia and systemic metastatic dissemination of fungi occur, resulting in life-threatening sequelae, including *Candida* endophthalmitis, meningitis, osteomyelitis, and renal abscesses.

CHRONIC MUCOCUTANEOUS CANDIDIASIS. This rare congenital syndrome is characterized by chronic and relapsing *Candida* infection of the oral mucosa, lips, perioral skin, and nails. In vitro studies have identified a specific defect in cell-mediated immunity (CMI) in relation to *Candida* antigen while T-cell function in response to other antigens is normal. The clinical manifestations tend to be severe, unrelenting, and hypertrophic or atrophic in nature, yet systemic manifestations and visceral spread are rare.

Another clinical syndrome characterized by chronic oral *Candida* yeast infection has been noted to be associated with familial hypoparathyroidism, mental retardation, and often additional hypoadrenalism. The finding of chronic or recurrent oral *Candida* infections in otherwise healthy patients should alert the dental practitioner to the possibility of undiagnosed endocrinopathy or defective immunity, justifying further investigation.

ASYMPTOMATIC CARRIERS. In healthy dentate adult subjects the prevalence of oral carriers of *C. albicans* varies from 29.6% to 44.4%, depending on the culture method used. Smokers have higher rates than nonsmokers, and women are more frequent carriers than men. The highest frequency of *C. albicans* isolation occurs from the posterior half of the tongue. As such the tongue is considered a primary reservoir from which the rest of the oral tissues are colonized. It follows therefore that, in the absence of typical mucosal lesions showing yeast and pseudohyphae on Gram stain, the finding of *Candida* organisms on oral or pharyngeal cultures does not prove complicity in causing symptoms.

DIAGNOSIS. Oral candidiasis often is recognized by complaints of generalized mouth discomfort, including pain, burning, bad taste, and halitosis. It may be acute or chronic. Although examination frequently reveals the typical surface creamy white fungal colonies, often the manifestation is that of irregular or widespread erythema. Occasionally there are erosive changes. Angular cheilitis is a common finding.

Since the clinical appearance often is only suggestive, smears or cultures (to observe pseudomycelia and spores) may be required to confirm the diagnosis. If biopsies are obtained, special staining with the periodic acid-Schiff (PAS) method may show the fungus, which grows in the most superficial epithelial stratum.

TREATMENT. The first step in treatment is to rule out underlying identifiable factors and then to stabilize the patient as well as possible. Hydrogen peroxide–saline mouth rinses (3% H_2O_2 diluted with equal parts warm saline) are helpful. Chlorhexidine gluconate (Peridex) and Listerine also have been shown to have antifungal properties. Specific treatment includes orally dissolving mystatin vaginal troches (100,000 units three or four times daily). Dystatin suspension is not as effective, since the contact time with the oral mucosa is much shorter. Clotrimazole tablets (10 mg dissolved orally five times daily) appear to be equally effective. Recent trials with ketoconazole taken systemically (200 to 400 mg/day with food) appear to offer an alternative to oral dissolution. Systemic administration often promotes improved compliance. The angular cheilitis is most effectively treated with nystatin and triamcinolone acetonide ointment (Mycolog cream).

Mucormycosis

Oral infection with Mucorales fungi is rare but its outcome may be fatal. Patients at risk include those with diabetes (who are prone to ketoacidosis), leukemia, granulocytopenia, and uremia.

The involved mucosa, whether palatal or nasal, becomes dark, magenta-black colored, and necrotic. Ulceration of these areas eventually is followed by perforation. Ipsilateral facial and other cranial nerve palsy develops with intracerebral mucormycosis. Anesthesia of the areas supplied by the ophthalmic and maxillary branches of the trigeminal nerve is a common finding.

BIBLIOGRAPHY

Arondor TM and Walker DM: The prevalence and intraoral distribution of *Candida albicans* in man, Arch Oral Biol 25:1, 1980.

Kirkpatrick CH and Alling DW: Treatment of chronic oral candidiasis with clotrimazole troches: a controlled clinical trial, N Engl J Med 299:1201, 1978.

Neisel P and Taylor DS: Chronic mucocutaneous candidiasis: treatment of the oral lesion with miconazole, Br J Oral Surg 18:51, 1980.

Pisanty S and Garfunkel A: Familial hypoparathyroidism with candidiasis and mental retardation, Oral Surg 44:374, 1977.

Histoplasmosis

About one third of patients with progressive disseminated histoplasmosis develop oral lesions. Ulcers and granulomas are the dominant manifestations in the oral cavity. Cases have been described in which primary lesions were diagnosed in the mouth.

Extreme destruction of the palate, pharynx, and nasal septum is known to follow the infection of these respective areas. Histoplasmosis of the jawbone induces mobility of the teeth in the area and possible oroantral fistulas. Roentgenograms show diffuse osteolysis of the alveolus without subperiosteal new bone formation.

The diagnostic process requires a biopsy and culture. Microscopic examination reveals a granuloma with enlarged histiocytes containing spores of *Histoplasma* organisms.

As in the case of systemic histoplasmosis, the treatment of choice for oral involvement is amphotericin B. Miconazole has been used with varying success.

BIBLIOGRAPHY

Daramola JO and others: Maxillary African histoplasmosis mimicking malignant jaw tumour, Br J Oral Surg 16(3):241, 1979.

Mace MC: Oral African histoplasmosis resembling Burkitt's lymphoma, Oral Sug 46(3):407, 1978.

Yusuf H and others: Disseminated histoplasmosis presenting with oral lesions: report of a case, Br J Oral Surg 16(3):234, 1979.

BIBLIOGRAPHY OF SECTION FOUR

Altman EG: Rational use of metromidazole, Aust Dent J 25:135, 1980.

Brown LR and others: Comparison of the plaque microflora in immunodeficient and immunocompetent dental patients, J Dent Res 58:2344, 1979.

Burnett GW and Schester GS: Oral microbiology and infectious disease, Baltimore, 1978, The Williams & Wilkins Co.

Gorlin RJ and Goldman HM: Thoma's oral pathology, ed 6, St. Louis, 1970, The CV Mosby Co.

Greenberg RN and others: Microbiologic and antibiotic aspects of infections in the oral and maxillofacial region, J Oral Surg 37:873, 1979.

Levinson SL and others: Occult dental infection as a cause of fever of obscure origin, Am J Med 66:463, 1979.

Lynch MA: Burket's oral medicine: diagnosis and treatment, ed 7, Philadelphia, 1977, JB Lippincott Co.

McCarthy PL and Shklar G: Disease of the oral mucosa, ed 2, Philadelphia, 1980, Lea & Febiger.

Van Palenstein-Helderman WH: Longitudinal microbial changes in developing human supragingival and subgingival dental plaque, Arch Oral Biol 26:7, 1980.

SECTION FIVE

HEMATOLOGIC DISORDERS

Edited by **Rosaline R. Joseph**

59 · INTRODUCTION TO HEMATOLOGIC DISORDERS

Rosaline R. Joseph

A wide variety of diseases are considered within the realm of hematology, including not only disturbances of the hematopoietic organs and the cellular elements of the peripheral blood but also abnormalities of the lymphoreticular and hemostatic mechanisms. The latter represents a complex interaction among the blood vessels, the platelets, and the plasma coagulation factors.

The cardinal symptoms and signs associated with hematologic disease are those resulting from underproduction or overproduction of red blood cells (anemia or erythrocytosis), leukocytes (leukopenia or leukocytosis), or platelets (thrombocytopenia or thrombocytosis); defective hemostasis (hemorrhage or intravascular coagulation); or neoplasia of the lymphoreticular system (lymphomas, reticuloendothelioses, or plasma cell dyscrasias). The disturbance in hematologic parameters may represent a primary hematologic disorder or may be caused by an underlying disease. However, in both situations the signs and symptoms are the same. It is extremely important to differentiate between primary and secondary disorders. Anemia caused by bleeding from a gastrointestinal neoplasm, leukocytosis caused by an infection, bleeding tendency resulting from a vitamin K deficiency caused by biliary obstruction, or splenomegaly resulting from malaria is of vastly different significance from a morphologically similar anemia associated with a thalassemia trait, a similar degree of leukocytosis from chronic granulocytic leukemia, bleeding caused by a congenital factor deficiency, or splenomegaly from Hodgkin's disease. Frequently it is the careful evaluation of an apparent hematologic abnormality that leads to the diagnosis of a previously unsuspected primary disorder.

Proper laboratory investigation of hematologic abnormalities should follow a logical sequence. Often a few simple, inexpensive, but crucial studies provide more information than a whole battery of more costly, frequently unnecessary or inappropriate tests. For instance, a reticulocyte count can generally distinguish the anemias associated with marrow dysfunction from the hemolytic anemias associated with increased red blood cell destruction. Careful attention to red blood cell morphology on a well-stained peripheral blood smear can yield a wealth of data on the pathophysiologic basis of an anemia. Assessment of the size (microcytic, normocytic, or macrocytic) and degree of hemoglobinization (hypochromic, normochro-

mic) of the red blood cell is important in narrowing the diagnostic possibilities in a given case. The degree of variability in size (anisocytosis) and shape (poikilocytosis) provides a measure of the severity of the process. Finally, discovery of specific red blood cell morphologic abnormalities, such as sickle cells, target cells, teardrop cells, and basophilic stippling, on the peripheral smear is of major diagnostic importance. Differential white blood counts and examination of white cell morphology on the peripheral smear give invaluable information in evaluating leukocytic disorders.

In the investigation of bleeding disorders, an initial screening consisting of prothrombin time, partial thromboplastin time, platelet count, and bleeding time will categorize the abnormalities into intrinsic, extrinsic, common pathway, or platelet-vascular disorders. Further studies may then be directed to the specific pathway or pathways concerned. For the diagnosis of hematologic malignancy, examination of tissue in essential. Bone marrow aspiration, biopsy, or both are imperative in all cases of unexplained leukopenia, leukocytosis, anemia, or thrombocytopenia. A diagnosis of lymphoma cannot be made without histologic examination of an involved area, most often a lymph node. In all of these situations further studies may be necessary to pinpoint the exact diagnosis, but expense and inconvenience to the patient are minimized by appropriate initial screening.

The treatment of hematologic disorders should, whenever possible, be directed to the correction of a specific defect. Proper evaluation of a hypochromic microcytic anemia will avoid unnecessary, prolonged, and even harmful iron therapy for situations other than iron deficiency. Indiscriminate use of "shotgun" hematinic combinations should be condemned, and cyanocobalamin should not be administered unless a vitamin B_{12} deficiency has been documented. Use of corticosteroids should be confined to situations in which there is a rational indication for their use, such as autoimmune hemolytic anemia. Use of specific blood components for specific clinical needs should be emphasized. This practice not only maximizes the efficient use of whole blood but also minimizes the risks to the patient of unnecessary transfusion. The availability of factor VIII concentrates has vastly improved the lot of the patient with classic hemophilia, and patients who require repeated platelet transfusions can receive HLA-typed, matched platelets.

The treatment of hematologic malignancies is an area of constant change and improvement. In no branch of medicine has there been greater progress recently in treating heretofore fatal disease. The availability of successful chemotherapy and radiation therapy together with sophisticated support systems has changed the outlook for many patients with acute leukemia or lymphoma.

UNIT A • DISORDERS OF RED BLOOD CELL PRODUCTION AND IRON METABOLISM

60 · INTRODUCTION TO ANEMIA AND APPROACH TO PATIENTS WITH ANEMIA

Emmanuel C. Besa

Anemia is usually discovered accidentally, since this clinical condition has vague, nonspecific symptoms and commonly occurs in such a slow, chronic fashion that the patient may not realize that he or she is unwell. However, once the anemia is discovered, the physician should determine the underlying disease process. There is no correlation between the degree of anemia and the severity of the underlying disease. A patient often needs several uncomfortable and expensive laboratory tests to find the cause of the anemia. Thus the physician must decide when these tests are necessary to rule out a serious disorder such as an early occult malignancy. However, the physician should practice restraint in subjecting a young woman with iron deficiency probably caused by menstrual loss to unnecessary testing.

Anemia is usually defined as a significant decrease in red corpuscles or hemoglobin. The laboratory measurements that are generally used to determine the presence or the absence of anemia are the packed red blood cell (RBC) volume or the hematocrit and the hemoglobin concentration of the peripheral blood.

Any hemoglobin or hematocrit value that is below the lower limits of normal is worthy of investigation. The normal hemoglobin value in men is 15.5 g/dl of blood with a range from 13.3 to 17.7 g/dl. In women the average is 13.7 g/dl of blood with a range from 11.7 to 15.7 g/dl. A drop in hemoglobin is suspicious even if the level is still within the normal range.

The normal value for the hematocrit in men is 46 ml/dl of blood with a range of 39.8 to 52.2 ml/dl. In women the normal value is 40.9 ml/dl of blood with a range of 34.9 to 46.9 ml/dl. These measurements merely reflect the ratio of RBCs to plasma. The degree or severity of an anemia may be accentuated or masked by conditions that alter the plasma volume. For example, dehydration increases the hematocrit by decreasing the plasma volume, whereas abnormal serum proteins, such as those in multiple myeloma, expand the plasma volume, producing the opposite effect and accentuating a mild anemia. Acute bleeding with equal amounts of erythrocyte and plasma loss may not change the hematocrit for the first 12 to 24 hours even when it is severe. Because the more accurate blood volume measurements are often not readily available, the physician must depend on hematocrit and hemoglobin measurements. These tests are adequate for evaluation of the anemia if the physician understands the limitations of the measurements and correlates them with the clinical picture. The plasma volume is altered by fluid depletion, electrolyte imbalances, and abnormal serum proteins. The presence of any of these conditions should influence the interpretations of the laboratory results and aid in the evaluation of the severity of the anemia.

NORMAL RED BLOOD CELL PRODUCTION AND PATHOLOGY (FIG. 60-1)

The normal RBC survival time is approximately 120 days. Old RBCs are removed from the circulation by the reticuloendothelial cells in the spleen and liver. The old cells are replaced by reticulated young RBCs called reticulocytes, which are released from the bone marrow. A sensitive oxygen sensor in the kidney informs the bone marrow to increase or decrease the rate of maturation of young RBCs. The amount of oxygen delivered to the kidney is altered by changes in oxygen diffusion from the lung, the amount of hemoglobin available, the affinity or ability of the hemoglobin to release the oxygen to the cells, and the adequacy of the circulation of the kidney. Any hypoxic stimulus systemically or locally in the kidney results in the release of erythropoietin from the kidney and perhaps from the liver. This hormone induces proliferation of the RBC precursors in the bone marrow and shortens the time of maturation so that more RBCs can be released more quickly into the circulation.

Anemia may result from any disturbance or breakdown in the normal mechanism of RBC production. The causes of anemia fall into the following groups: (1) decreased RBC production owing to bone marrow failure or deficiency of "building blocks," (2) increased RBC destruction or blood loss, and (3) low erythropoietin levels in severe renal failure.

One or more of these categories are generally involved in the pathophysiology of the usual forms of anemia. Decreased RBC production owing to bone marrow failure or aplasia may also produce defective erythrocytes that do not survive long enough to be released into the circulation. This is referred to as "ineffective erythropoiesis."

APPROACH TO THE ANEMIC PATIENT

HISTORY AND PHYSICAL EXAMINATION. After detection of the anemia, the physician may benefit by reviewing the history and physical examination as a check for information that was missed during the initial evaluation or inquiring about a family history of anemia, jaundice, splenectomy, bleeding, and abnormal hemoglobin. The patient may have had occupational exposure to chemicals, drugs, or radiation.

The patient frequently neglects to mention taking aspirin or other nonsteroidal antiinflammatory agents that can give rise to gastric mucosal damage and gastrointestinal bleeding. The patient should be asked specifically about the use of these agents. The dietary history is often omitted and may be deliberately hidden from the physician owing to the patient's embarrassment.

Although iron deficiency is rarely due to dietary deficiency in adults, it remains a fairly common cause in infants, especially premature infants. The possibility of an underlying chronic disease should be explored by a meticulous review of systems. A careful examination should be performed with special attention to adenopathy, organ enlargement, bleeding in the skin and mucous membranes, nail changes, and neurologic abnormalities. An important component of the examination is the rectal examination and a test of the stool for occult blood. The importance of a carefully done and complete physical

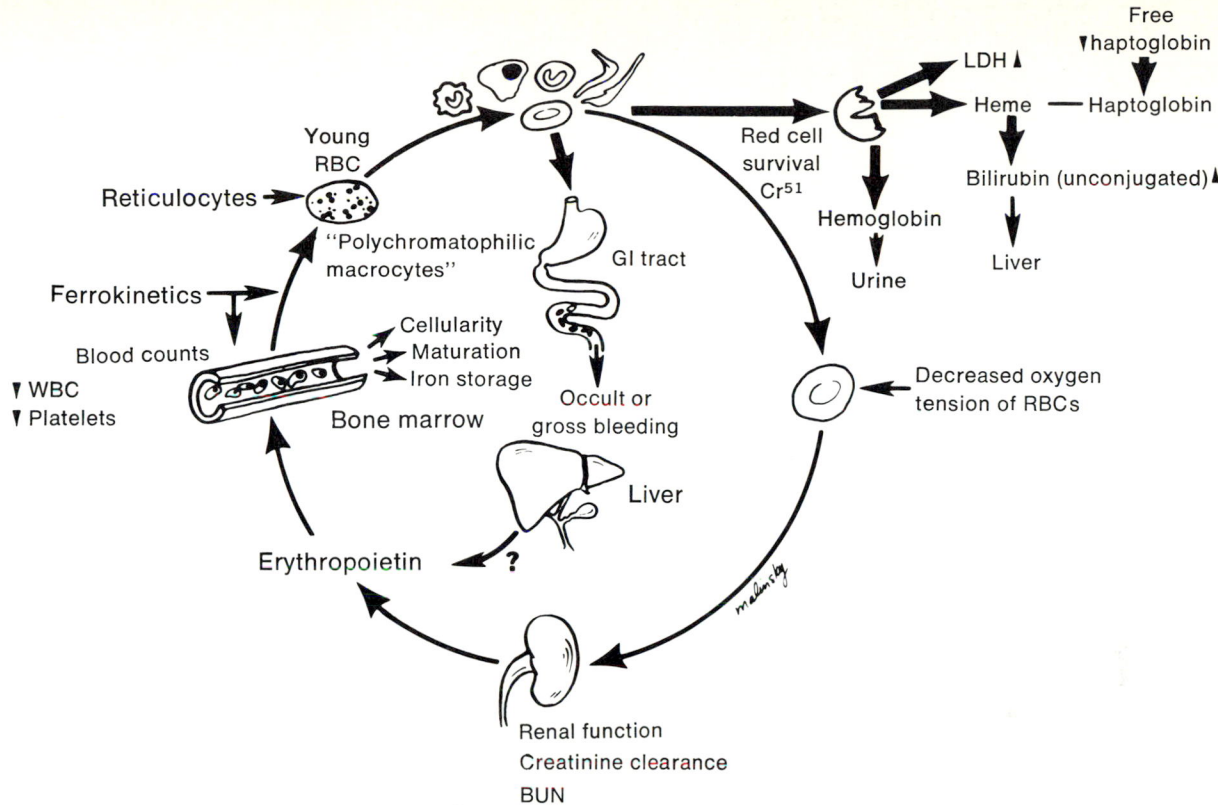

Fig. 60-1   Different tests used in defining cause of anemia are shown in relation to normal mechanism of red blood cell production. Evaluation of blood smear is direct study of finished product in which defective red cells are most likely to be uncovered. Testing stools for blood is used to search for obscure bleeding source. Increased blood levels of LDH, free hemoglobin, or decreased haptoglobin reflect hemolysis. Hemoglobin may eventually be excreted in urine or increase unconjugated bilirubin in serum. Severe renal dysfunction eventually affects ability of kidney to release regulatory hormone erythropoietin and excrete waste products inhibitory to bone marrow function. Liver may be another source of erythropoietin but is unable to compensate for diseased kidney. Finally, source of cells may be involved and can be studied either by direct examination of bone marrow or its ability to compensate for anemia by rate of release of young red cells or reticulocytes. Cellular marrow with red cell precursors may be unable to produce viable RBCs (called ineffectve erythropoiesis). Rate of red cell production and release can be studied by tracing radioactive iron as it is taken up by bone marrow and its appearance in circulation (called ferrokinetics). Presence or absence of iron or cells in bone marrow reflects nature of functional failure of blood production.

examination in the evaluation of a patient's anemia cannot be overemphasized.

DIAGNOSTIC PROCEDURES. A logical and orderly approach to a patient with anemia is shown in Fig. 60-2. With the advent of electronic counting devices, values used for computing the indices have become more consistent and reproducible. Most reports of blood counts include computer values for the RBC indices. The physician, however, cannot rely on the technician's ability to interpret peripheral blood smears and should examine the blood smear to avoid missing valuable clues and information.

Normal RBC indicies (Coulter counter) are as follows:

RBC indices	Formula	Normal values
Mean corpuscular or cell volume (MCV)	$\dfrac{Hct}{RBC}$	$92 \pm 10\ \mu m^3$
Mean corpuscular or cell hemoglobin (MCH)	$\dfrac{Hgb}{RBC}$	30 ± 3 pg
Mean corpuscular or cell hemoglobin concentration (MCHC)	$\dfrac{Hgb}{Hct}$	33 ± 2 g/dl or %

EXAMINATION OF THE SMEAR. Certain changes in the size or shape of the RBCs and the presence of certain inclusion

bodies may give the physician information to pursue the diagnosis in a more systematic fashion. Table 60-1 lists these changes and the particular conditions in which they are frequently observed. The morphologic RBC changes may reflect the pathophysiology of the underlying disease or cause of the anemia. Examination of the smears also gives the physician an opportunity to observe abnormalities in the white blood cells and platelets, which are often affected when the bone marrow is involved in the disease process.

Reticulocyte count. The reticulocyte count is one of the most neglected parts of the blood count. Since this test is done using in vivo staining with methylene blue, fresh blood is necessary; fixed smears of the peripheral blood cannot be used. The test is inexpensive and can be performed as an office procedure. Because the counts are reported in a percentage as the number of reticulated cells per 100 RBCs, the degree of anemia may falsely elevate a low or normal reticulocyte count. The correction factor is calculated as follows:

Corrected reticulocyte count =

$$\frac{\text{Reported reticulocyte count (\%)} \times \text{Hct (\%)}}{\text{Normal Hct (40\%-45\%)}}$$

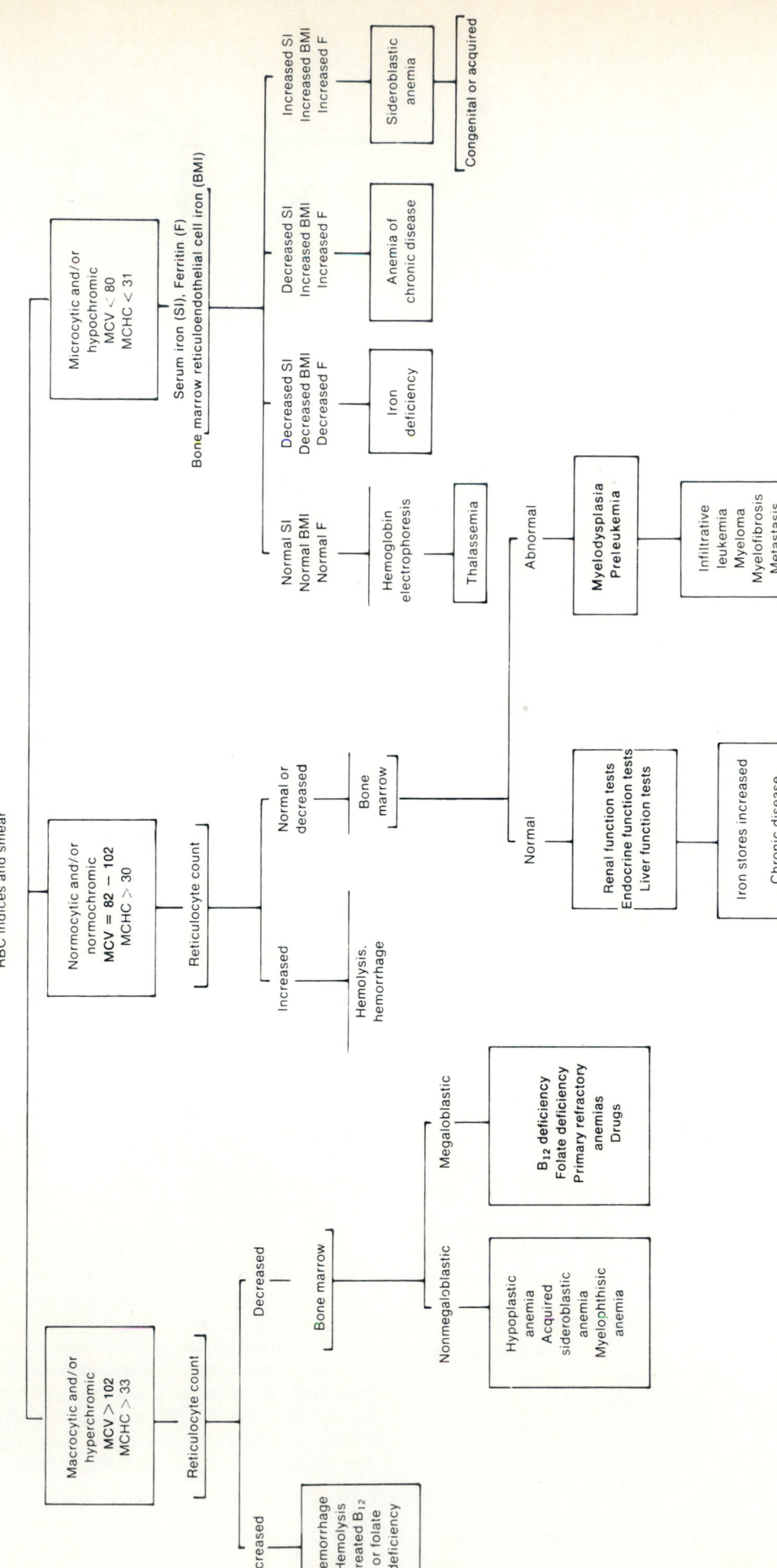

Fig. 60-2 Logical and systematic decision tree illustrates successive steps in differential diagnosis of anemia. Good history, physical examination, blood smear examination, and determination of red cell indices may make subsequent steps unnecessary in some cases. (From Besa EC: Current topics, vol 2, Philadelphia, 1978, Medical College of Pennsylvania.)

Table 60-1 Evaluation of RBCs in the examination of the blood smear

Name of cell or inclusion	Description	Disease entity
Abnormal shapes		
Acanthocyte ("spur cells" or "burr cells")	Spicules on cell	Abetalipoproteinemia, cirrhosis and other liver diseases, uremia
Dacryocyte	Teardrop shape	Most commonly myelofibrosis but also Heinz body anemia, thalassemia, hemolytic anemia
Drepanocyte	Sickle shape	Sickle cell anemia (trait after deoxygenation), other rare hemoglobinopathies
Schistocyte	Helmet form, RBC fragments	Intravascular coagulation, fibrin deposits in blood vessels, vascular or valve prostheses, malignant hypertension
Spherocyte	Spheroid	Hereditary or acquired hemolytic anemia
Stomatocyte	Slitlike area of central pallor	Hereditary or acquired hemolytic anemia
Target cell	Target form	Hemoglobin C or E, liver disease, obstructive jaundice, thalassemia, postsplenectomy
Inclusion bodies		
Nucleated RBCs	Pyknotic nucleus	Acute hemorrhage, acute anoxemia with congestive heart failure, severe hemolytic anemia, leukemia, myelofibrosis, bone marrow metastasis, normal asplenic individuals
Basophilic stippling	Punctate basophilia	Lead intoxication, sideroblastic anemias, disordered erythropoiesis associated with myeloproliferative syndrome
Howell-Jolly bodies	Small round bodies	Most commonly asplenic individuals or functional asplenia but also hemolytic anemias
Cabot rings	Rings or figures-of-eight	Severe anemias, dyserythropoiesis

A normal value is 0.5% to 1.5%. Elevation of the reticulocyte count indicates that the bone marrow is producing more RBCs than in the normal steady state and thus usually implies a hemorrhagic episode, a hemolytic process, or a response to an appropriately treated anemia. An elevation in the reticulocyte count also indicates the bone marrow's ability to respond to erythropoietin. Low counts often reflect bone marrow hypoplasia or dysplasia, or failure of the kidney to release erythropoietin. The information provided by the reticulocyte count may not be very specific but often leads to a systematic evaluation of an obscure anemia.

Serum chemistries. Other helpful serologic tests and findings include (1) elevated lactate dehydrogenase (LDH), low haptoglobin, and increased unconjugated bilirubin levels, which reflect RBC hemolysis (Fig. 60-1); (2) serum iron, iron-binding capacity, and percentage of saturation of iron-binding protein (to detect iron deficiency); serum vitamin B_{12} and folate levels to detect vitamin deficiency; (3) liver, endocrine, and renal function tests where indicated (may reflect other system dysfunction); and (4) serum ferritin levels, which have recently been advocated to replace bone marrow in the evaluation of iron stores. The serum ferritin seems to correlate well with iron stores; that is, when ferritin levels are low or absent, iron stores are low, and when the serum ferritin level is markedly elevated, iron stores are increased. However, normal serum ferritin levels may be found in some patients with iron deficiency who also have liver damage. This test needs further evaluation to determine its clinical applicability.

Special procedures. A bone marrow aspiration is indicated to evaluate the marrow cellular elements, evalute iron stores, evalute maturation of cellular elements, and look for the presence of abnormal cells or infection. Bone marrow biopsy is indicated to judge accurately the cellularity of the marrow, to look for malignancies or granulomas, and when aspiration is "dry" or inadequate, for evaluation.

Other special procedures such as RBC survival and ferrokinetics are performed in complicated and mixed-type anemias. The patient's RBCs are tagged with ^{51}Cr to determine how long they stay in the circulation. Information about splenic sequestration or occult intermittent gastrointestinal bleeding may be gathered by scanning the spleen and measuring radioactivity

of ^{51}Cr in the stools, respectively. In patients with refractory anemia the alterations in RBC production may be elucidated by ferrokinetic studies. ^{59}Fe is given intravenously, and the time for the patient to clear the ^{59}Fe from the plasma indicates the activity of the bone marrow. Patients with iron deficiency and hemolytic anemias have a rapid clearance, whereas in aplastic anemia and other bone marrow failure states that plasma ^{59}Fe clearance is prolonged. The true measure of effective erythrocyte production is ^{59}Fe incorporation into the circulating RBCs; 80% to 100% of the radioactive dose is incorporated 10 to 14 days after administration in normal individuals. In patients with bone marrow failure or ineffective erythropoiesis this value is decreased below normal depending on the severity of the anemia.

Electrophoretic analysis of the patient's hemoglobin is indicated in characterizing the different hemoglobinopathies and their combinations. It is also used in the differential diagnosis of hypochromic, microcytic anemia when iron deficiency has been ruled out (Fig. 60-2).

Patients with occult iron deficiency anemia should receive a thorough gastrointestinal workup including a barium enema, an upper gastrointestinal series, and sigmoidoscopy.

MANAGEMENT. There are numerous specific therapies for different types of anemia (once the cause is identified by the physician) that are discussed in subsequent chapters. However, supportive therapy such as blood transfusion is often erroneously given, modifying the clinical picture so that establishment of the diagnosis becomes more difficult.

Emergency blood transfusions are indicated only in life-threatening situations such as when anemia is accompanied by severe coronary artery disease, congestive heart failure, or severe hypoxia. The physician should try to obtain most of the diagnostic tests before transfusion. Freezing serum samples and keeping unstained smears for examination at a later date are always good practices.

Most chronic anemias are compensated by increments of RBC 2,3-diphosphoglycerate, which increases the ability of hemoglobin to release oxygen to the tissue. Most anemic patients with normal cardiac function and deficiency anemia can tolerate a hematologic workup and recover by replacement therapy without needing a blood transfusion. Circulatory overload and pulmonary edema are risks of transfusion in severely anemic patients with borderline or poor cardiac function. Transfusion of packed RBCs and the use of rapid-acting diuretics are often necessary in this situation.

The use of hematinic drugs containing combinations of iron, folate, vitamin B_{12}, and other vitamins and minerals without first identifying the type and cause of the anemia should be condemned. This type of therapy should be differentiated from properly supervised therapeutic trials, which may be necessary when mixed types of anemia complicate the clinical and laboratory picture. Under these circumstances baseline studies of the blood counts are performed and repeated at intervals to determine a response. The drugs or vitamins are prescribed individually, using optimal doses so that the response can be identified. "Shotgun" therapy or indiscriminate use of these drugs without careful follow-up should be conscientiously avoided.

61 · MEGALOBLASTIC ANEMIA

Emmanuel C. Besa

DEFINITIONS. The term "megaloblast" describes the large erythroid precursors, which have morphologically immature nuclei associated with normally hemoglobinized cytoplasm. This dissociation of maturation between nuclei and cytoplasm is not limited to the erythoroid precursors but may be observed in all cell lines in the bone marrow. Macrocytosis, the presence of large red blood cells (RBCs) in the peripheral blood, is characterized by an increased mean corpuscular volume (MCV). Mild to moderate degrees of macrocytosis may be seen with an increase in reticulocytes or in liver disease without a megaloblastic bone marrow. Macrocytosis greater than 10% (MCV of 115 μm^3 or greater) even in the absence of anemia should be pursued, since early vitamin B_{12} or folate deficiency, liver disease, or neoplasm may be found.

ETIOLOGY. A state of unbalanced growth in the hematopoietic cells of the bone marrow is due to abnormal DNA synthesis with a delay in nuclear maturation while protein synthesis in the cytoplasm proceeds at a normal rate. This "cytonuclear dissociation" results from impairment of conversion of deoxyuridylate to thymidilate, which is necessary for DNA synthesis. The exact mechanism of the resulting anemia is unclear, but evidence points to an early destruction of the hematopoietic cells before their release into the circulation. The ineffective erythropoiesis is not confined to RBCs but involves all cell lines in hematopoiesis and other cells with a rapid cellular turnover rate such as those of the intestinal mucosa.

In the majority of patients megaloblastic anemia is due to folate or vitamin B_{12} deficiency. A small number of cases may be caused by a disturbance in hematopoiesis unrelated to either deficiency, for example, erythroleukemia, Lesch-Nyhan syndrome, or congenital abnormalities such as orotic aciduria.

Vitamin B_{12} and folate are closely interrelated, as evidenced by clinical and biochemical studies. High doses of folate can correct the anemia of vitamin B_{12} deficiency but exacerbate the neurologic symptoms, and high doses of vitamin B_{12} can cause reticulocytosis in folate deficiency. Serum levels of folate are reduced in vitamin B_{12} deficiency, and depressed vitamin B_{12} serum levels accompany folate deficiency. The urinary excretion of formiminoglutamic acid (FIGLU) is increased in both folate and vitamin B_{12} deficiency.

FOLATE METABOLISM. Folates are widely distributed in a variety of foods, and the normal daily diet contains 600 to 700 μg of folate. Since folates are water soluble and heat labile, excessive heating or boiling of food substantially decreases dietary folate content. This loss of folate may be important in patients with malabsorption or with increased requirement for the vitamin as in pregnancy or hemolytic anemia. Folate is best absorbed in the proximal jejunum and duodenum. Approximately 50 to 100 μg is required daily to balance the fecal and urinary losses. Liver and other tissues store small amounts (5 to 20 mg) of folate. This usually takes 5 weeks to 4 months to exhaust in the absence of dietary folate intake.

FOLATE DEFICIENCY. The following are some clinical causes of folate deficiency:

Dietary deficiency
    Water and toast diet
Malabsorption
    Sprue
    Jejunal resection
Drugs
    Alcohol
    Phenytoin
    Methotrexate
    Triamterene
    Trimethoprim
Increased requirement
    Pregnancy
    Chronic hemolytic anemia
    Hyperthyroidism
    Neoplasms
    Exfoliative dermatitis
    Long-term hemodialysis

A dietary lack of folate leads to megaloblastic anemia in a few months. Lack of absorption caused by diseases involving the proximal small intestine such as celiac disease (gluten enteropathy) frequently results in a deficient state. Increased DNA synthesis, as in pregnancy, hemolysis, hyperthyroidism, malignancies, agnogenic myeloid metaplasia, and chronic exfoliative dermatitis, increases the folate requirement and may cause mild to moderate folate deficieny. Folate and other dialyzable vitamins must be replaced in patients undergoing long-term hemodialysis.

One common cause of folate deficiency is alcoholism. The anemia of alcoholism is due to diverse etiologic mechanisms of which folate deficiency is only one. Drugs such as phenytoin, methotrexate, triamteren, and trimethoprim have been associated with folate deficiency anemia. The mechanisms implicated in this relationship are poor absorption owing to drug effects on intestinal cells, competitive interaction between folate coenzymes and the drug, increased catabolism of folate by the liver induced by the drug, and displacement of folate from serum binding proteins.

VITAMIN B_{12} METABOLISM. The main source of vitamin B_{12} in the human diet is bacterially synthesized vitamin B_{12} in animal tissues. In vegetarians a mild megaloblastic anemia may eventually develop. The average diet contains 5 to 30 μg of vitamin B_{12}. The daily requirement is 1 to 3 μg. Since large amounts (2 to 4 mg) of the vitamin are stored in the liver, malabsorption of vitamin B_{12} does not cause megaloblastic anemia until 2 to 5 years after the effective absorption of the vitamin ceases.

Only about 1% of vitamin B_{12} is absorbed throughout the small intestine by the passive route. Vitamin B_{12} is actively absorbed in the distal ileum. Active absorption of the vitamin depends on the presence of a glycoprotein, intrinsic factor (IF), secreted by the parietal cells in the fundus of the stomach. IF has a molecular weight of about 60,000 with two polypeptide chains that bind vitamin B_{12} and protect it from proteolytic digestion and from utilization by intestinal bacteria. The IF-B_{12} complex passes through the ileal mucosal cell, and vitamin B_{12} reaches the portal circulation bound to a specific transport protein called transcobalamin II (TC II). The other binding protein, TC I, is present intracellularly and is used mainly for storage.

VITAMIN B_{12} DEFICIENCY (PERNICIOUS ANEMIA). The causes of vitamin B_{12} deficiency include the following:

    Lack of intrinsic factor
        Pernicious anemia
        Gastrectomy
    Dietary deficiency
        Strict vegetarian diet
    Biologic competition
        Small bowel bacterial overgrowth
            Diverticulosis
            Anastomosis and fistulas
            Blind loops and strictures
            Scleroderma
        Fish tapeworm
    Impaired absorption
        Regional ileitis, ileal resection
        Sprue (tropical)
        Drugs such as alcohol, neomycin, colchicine, and para-aminosalicylic acid

The most common and classic form of vitamin B_{12} deficiency is pernicious anemia (PA) caused by malabsorption owing to the absence of IF secretion. This usually occurs in middle-aged and elderly persons with an associated genetic susceptibility and age-related chronic atrophic gastritis. PA has been described most frequently in patients of Northern European ancestry. Recent studies in the United States demonstrate that PA is found with equal frequency in the black population and in white patients of all origins. PA occurs at a younger age in black women and is associated with a greater prevalence of circulating antibodies against IF.

The origin of the impairment in the production of IF in PA is poorly understood. An autoimmune process has been implicated, since most patients with PA have antibodies directed against IF and parietal cells in the serum and gastric juice.

The association of PA and other autoimmune disorders such as Hasimoto's thyroiditis and Graves' disease has strengthened the concept that PA is an autoimmune disease. A cause-and-effect relationship between the antibodies and the disease process has not been proved, and current evidence suggests that a cell-mediated immune mechanism, rather than the abnormal circulating antibodies, may be responsible for the atrophic gastritis in PA.

Dietary deficiency of vitamin B_{12} is rare and is limited to strict vegetarians who do not eat dairy products.

Poor absorption of vitamin B_{12} can result from the destruction of the absorption site at the distal ileum or of the vitamin B_{12} en route to the ileum. The mucosa of the distal ileum may be damaged in diseases such as regional ileitis or by drugs such as alcohol, neomycin, colchicine, or paraaminosalicylic acid. The vitamin B_{12} may not reach the ileum because of utilization by bacteria in intestinal diverticula or in "blind loops." The fish tapeworm *(Diphyllobothrium latum)*, frequently found in Scandinavian countries, also utilizes vitamin B_{12}.

CLINICAL MANIFESTATIONS. The history and physical examination often provide important clues for differentiating folate deficiency and vitamin B_{12} deficiency, the two most common causes of megaloblastic anemia. A positive family history may be found in a third of the cases of PA. The dietary history is essential and usually is normal in PA. Vegetarians who do not eat any food of animal origin may become vitamin B_{12} deficient. Folate deficiency is usually due to a poor or bizarre diet. Knowledge of previous gastric or intestinal resection and symptoms of malabsorption may help identify a patient's particular deficiency. Information concerning medications and drugs is essential in the history of patients with megaloblastic anemia.

Neurologic abnormalities are associated mainly with vitamin B_{12} deficiency (see Chapter 185). Paresthesias, abnormalities in gait and fine coordination, and overt psychoses (megaloblastic madness) are often described as part of PA. Neurologic abnormalities referable to subacute combined degeneration involving the posterior and lateral columns of the spinal cord are manifested by impairment of vibratory and position sense, increases in deep tendon reflexes, ataxic or spastic gait, and impairment of bowel and bladder functions. These changes may occur in PA without anemia in 1 of 500 cases, usually in patients taking folates or in vegetarians eating a high-folate diet. A recent study of patients with severe folate deficiency in a general hospital revealed a significant increase in organic brain syndrome and pyramidal tract damage. These findings were independent of the degree of anemia or presence of alcoholism, suggesting that severe folate deficiency per se may cause neurologic deficits.

Physical findings include a smooth tongue with absent papillation, pallor, mild icterus, and minimal splenomegaly. Weight loss, anorexia, and bowel disturbances indicate megaloblastic changes in the gastrointestinal tract. Palmar hyperpigmentation has been observed in black patients with PA. This finding is reversed with vitamin B_{12} therapy.

LABORATORY FINDINGS. Macrocytosis can easily be identified with the use of electronic erythrocyte sizing equipment. When the MCV is 115 μm^3 or greater, the chances of having a deficiency of folate or vitamin B_{12} or both are significant. The peripheral blood smear confirms the presence of large RBCs and poikilocytosis. The platelets may be large, and the polymorphonuclear leukocytes are hyypersegmented. Hypersegmentation refers to the presence of six or more lobes in a significant number of neutrophils. Varying degrees of anemia, thrombocytopenia, neutropenia, or pancytopenia may be found.

The bone marrow is usually hypercellular with an increase in mitotic figures. The typical cytonuclear dissociation is manifested morphologically in all the hematopoietic cell lines. The RBC precursors demonstrate an immature, nonpyknotic nucleus with open chromatin material and a normally hemoglobinized cytoplasm. The myeloid series shows large metamyelocytes and bands with huge "horse-shoe" nuclei and hypersegmented neutrophils. Megakaryocyte nuclei have been described to be multilobulated with an absence of normal connections between the lobes. The increase in cellularity may be confused with a malignant or preleukemic state.

The diagnostic tests differentiating the cause of the megaloblastic anemia are the measurements of the serum and RBC folate levels and the serum vitamin B_{12} level. The serum levels of folate vitamin B_{12} can be determined by microbiologic methods or by radioimmunoassay. The advantages of the latter technique are rapidity in obtaining the results and lack of influence by drugs such as folate antagonists or antibiotics.

Once a deficiency of vitamin B_{12} is found in the serum, the Schilling test or vitamin B_{12} absorption test is performed to differentiate PA from vitamin B_{12} malabsorption of intestinal origin.

Gastric achlorhydria is present in virtually all patients with

PA. They do not demonstrate any response when maximally stimulated with histamine.

In therapeutic trials with vitamin B$_{12}$ or folate given in physiologic doses for 10 days, the patient is observed for a reticulocyte response, which should occur within 7 days. The physiologic dose is 2 μg of vitamin B$_{12}$ intramuscularly or 100 μg of folate orally or intramuscularly each day; higher doses should not be used in a therapeutic trial. The diet during the therapeutic trial must be low in vitamin B$_{12}$ and folate. The demonstration of circulating antibodies to IF is strong evidence in favor of PA.

MANAGEMENT. Patients with documented folate deficiency respond well to small doses of folic acid given orally even in the presence of small bowel disease. Since most of the larger doses of folate are lost in the urine and such doses may exacerbate the neurologic symptoms in PA, the maximal recommended dose of folate is 1 mg of folic acid a day. After the body stores are replenished in 2 weeks, lower doses of 0.1 to 0.15 mg daily can be given as maintenance or supplements. Alcoholic patients respond to these doses even if they continue to imbibe alcohol. Folate therapy can be given during anticonvulsant therapy without the need to withdraw the anticonvulsant. Preventive or prophylactic doses are required in pregnancy, hemolytic anemias, tropical sprue, and patients undergoing hemodialysis.

Vitamin B$_{12}$ deficiency often requires parenteral administration of cyanocobalamin, except perhaps in vegetarians, who can be given oral preparations. Hydroxycobalamin, the preferred preparation, is given intramuscularly on a schedule of six weekly doses of 1000 μg to build body stores of about 3 mg. Then a maintenance dose of 1000 μg every 3 months should provide adequate vitamin B$_{12}$ levels. The widespread use of vitamin B$_{12}$ shots as a tonic or placebo is deplorable.

Blood transfusions are not required unless the patient is elderly or critically ill. Packed RBCs given slowly with or without diuretics may be necessary to prevent the precipitation of congestive heart failure.

BIBLIOGRAPHY

Carmel R and Johnson CS: Racial patterns in pernicious anemia: early age at onset and increased frequency of intrinsic-factor antibody in black women, N Engl J Med 298:647, 1978.

Doscherholmen A and Ripley D: Plasma absorption of cyanocobalamin Co 57: diagnostic value in vitamin B$_{12}$ malabsorption sites, Arch Intern Med 134:1019, 1974.

Erbe RW: Inborn errors of folate metabolism, N Engl J Med 293:753, 1975.

Goldberg LS and others: Human autoimmunity, with pernicious anemia as a model, Ann Intern Med 81:372, 1974.

Lindenbaum J, Pezzimenti JF, and Shea N: Small-intestinal function in vitamin B$_{12}$ deficiency, Ann Intern Med 80:326, 1974.

McPhedran P and others: Interpretation of electronically determined macrocytosis, Ann Intern Med 78:677, 1973.

62 · BONE MARROW FAILURE, SIDEROBLASTIC ANEMIA, AND MYELOPHTHISIC ANEMIA

Emmanuel C. Besa

Bone marrow failure may occur with a reduction in one, two, or all three formed elements of the blood—the red cells, leukocytes, and platelets. The mechanisms involved are not fully understood. The following conditions lead to bone marrow failure:

Hypoplasia or aplasia of marrow
  Aplastic anemia, idiopathic or caused by drugs, chemicals, ionizing radiation, or viral infections
  Fanconi's constitutional anemia, Diamond-Blackfan anemia
  Paroxysmal nocturnal hemoglobinuria
  Immune mechansims
Normocellular or hypercellular states of marrow
  Myelodysplastic syndromes
  Refractory anemia, preleukemia
  Sideroblastic anemia
Infiltrating lesions in marrow
  Myelophthisic anemia
  Primary myelofibrosis, myelosclerosis
  Agnogenic myeloid metaplasia

Direct injury to the marrow by toxins and drugs or infiltration and destruction by malignant tissue with reactive fibrosis will result in a decrease in marrow cellularity. In such instances the bone marrow study is diagnostic. However, since some patients with peripheral cytopenia may have a normal or hypercellular marrow, peripheral sequestration or destruction of cells in a hypertrophied and overreactive reticuloendothelial system must be considered as a type of "marrow failure." Ineffective hematopoiesis has been inferred in patients with pancytopenia and normal or hypercellular marrows, indicating formation of defective cells that are rapidly removed from the circulation or death within the marrow. Patients with no obvious cause for bone marrow failure should be investigated for marrow cellularity and extent of cytopenia. Some individual clinical syndromes reflecting these mechanisms, such as aplastic anemia, the primary refractory anemias (preleukemic syndromes), sideroblastic anemia, and myelophthisic anemia, are discussed in this chapter.

APLASTIC ANEMIA

The term "aplastic anemia" usually refers to a condition characterized by abnormally low red blood cell (RBC), neutrophil, and platelet counts in the peripheral blood and by a hypocellular or aplastic bone marrow. Since a single bone marrow aspiration may not represent the total marrow cellularity, it is often difficult to classify patients with one study if a cellular marrow was obtained. Repeat bone marrow aspirations performed at others sites often confirm the overall hypocellularity of the marrow despite the fact that localized areas of the marrow may remain cellular. Patients with pancytopenia and a hypercellular marrow fall into the broad category of primary refractory anemia. Even if the term "aplastic anemia" is restricted to the hypocellular marrow group, it has become evident that aplastic or hypoplastic anemia is not a single clinical entity.

ETIOLOGY. The following factors may be involved in aplastic anemia:

Genetic factors
  Fanconi's anemia, Diamond-Blackfan anemia
  Chloramphenicol sensitivity
Agents
  Drugs (antineoplastic, chemotherapeutic, chloramphenicol)
  Chemicals (benzene)
  Ionizing irradiation
  Viral infection (hepatitis)
Immune mechanisms
  Pure red cell aplasia
  Systemic lupus erythematosus
Paroxysmal nocturnal hemoglobinura

Most cases can be divided into two general groups: those

associated with exposure to some toxic agent and those that develop with no identifiable bone marrow insult, that is, idiopathic aplastic anemia (IAA).

The toxic agents can be divided into those that regularly induce bone marrow suppression and those that cause "idiosyncratic" reactions in a few patients. Chemotherapeutic drugs used in cancer treatment produce a predictable dose-related marrow suppression that is usually followed by recovery after withdrawal of the drug. However, a drug such as chloramphenicol may cause either of the two types of bone marrow toxicity. Current evidence indicates a lack of relationship between the reversible suppression and the irreversible aplastic anemia associated with chloramphenicol. The reversible bone marrow suppression is due to mitochondrial injury with profound inhibition of protein synthesis, whereas the aplastic anemia induced by chloramphenicol may be due to a genetic predisposition, as evidenced by studies of DNA synthesis in marrows from patients and their relatives.

Transient bone marrow failure may occur during a viral infection. This may lead to mild depression of blood counts with no clinical consequences. In patients with sickle cell anemia and other hereditary hemolytic anemias, a viral infection may induce an aplastic crisis needing supportive care during this transient period. These patients ultimately recover. The aplastic anemia developing after viral hepatitis, however, is a more severe form of bone marrow failure and is often fatal.

PATHOGENESIS. The current concept of hematopoiesis proposes that blood cells originate from pluripotential stem cells that give rise to unipotential committed cells and differentiate into the mature cellular blood elements under the influence or presence of appropriate stimulating substances, among which erythropoietin is the best characterized. These cells have been studied in vitro and defined by their ability to form colonies of mature cells. Bone marrow culture studies in both humans and animals have suggested several possible pathologic sites in aplastic anemia.

The defect in aplastic anemia may be quantitative or qualitative abnormalities of hematopoietic stem cells, abnormal humoral or cellular control of hematopoiesis, or abnormal or hostile hematopoietic microenvironment such as "stromal" abnormalities and immune suppression of hematopoiesis.

The majority of cases represent a stem cell defect with low colony growth from the bone marrow and successful therapy by transplanting normal marrow from an identical twin or HLA-compatible donor. Providing normal hematopoietic stem cells to these patients may correct the hematologic defect.

It appears that aplastic anemia will prove to be several diseases that share common clinical and morphologic features. With greater use of bone marrow culture techniques, it may be possible to differentiate subgroups of patients and help determine the best possible therapy for each group.

CLINICAL MANIFESTATIONS. The usual symptoms of anemia may bring the patient to a physician, but in most instances, the clinical course is insidious. When pancytopenia occurs, the patient has symptoms of bleeding, fever, and severe infection (often gram-negative bacillary bacteremia). It may be difficult to distinguish between disseminated intravascular coagulopathy and the underlying thrombocytopenia as the cause of hemorrhage. Petechiae, purpura, or gum bleeding sometimes occurs. The physical examination may be unremarkable except for pallor and petechiae. The spleen is not usually enlarged but may become palpable in the final stages of the disease. It is unusual for hepatomegaly or lymphadenopathy to be present in these patients. Patients who have had multiple transfusions

may have had signs and symptoms of hemosiderosis or hemochromatosis.

LABORATORY FINDINGS. Pancytopenia is an invariable finding in aplastic anemia, with varying degrees of severity in the individual erythrocyte, leukocyte, and platelet counts. The anemia is usually normochromic and normocytic but may occasionally be macrocytic. Reticulocytopenia is usually found, but counts may vary from none to 5%. The total granulocyte count is low and is responsible for the leukopenia, but the absolute lymphocyte count is often decreased as well. Coagulation tests are normal except for the increased bleeding time and poor clot retraction, which reflect the underlying thrombocytopenia. The plasma iron level is normal or slightly increased with a normal iron-binding capacity. Erythropoietin levels are increased in proportion to the degree of anemia, and the fetal hemoglobin level may be elevated in some patients.

The bone marrow may be cellular or markedly hypocellular. When it is cellular, another site is chosen for aspiration and biopsy, since focal areas of hyperplasia may occur and may not reflect the total marrow activity. Marked hypocellularity causes bone marrow aspiration to be "dry," indicating the importance of performing a core biopsy. The biopsy may also reveal other causes, for example, granulomas or malignancy such as metastatic carcinoma or aleukemic leukemia. Iron stores are usually increased unless there was a chronic bleeding problem before the onset of the disease.

It is essential to rule out the other possible causes of pancytopenia listed on p. 280.

COURSE AND PROGNOSIS. The course of aplastic anemia may be short and rapidly fatal, evolving in a few months, or chronic and prolonged, lasting for many years.

The prognosis appears to be better when a bone marrow toxin is evident than in the idiopathic type. Aplastic anemia after viral hepatitis carries a poor prognosis in most instances. When the disease process demonstrates a steady progression, it is invariably fatal. Of patients with a protracted course, a third may go into remission, another third will continue to have a tolerable but low platelet (and sometimes leukocyte) count, and the remaining third will continue to depend on steroids or androgens.

MANAGEMENT. Supportive therapy is necessary to maintain patients with aplastic anemia, and recent developments in blood component separation have made it possible to administer specific cells as required. An ambulatory, asymptomatic patient should be maintained without transfusions, since serious complications such as iron overload, development of platelet antibodies, and serum hepatitis often accompany multiple, long-term transfusions. The value of granulocyte transfusions is still questionable, and they should be reserved for serious infection with a poor response to antibiotic therapy. Iron overload may be prevented by the early administration of desferrioxamine. HLA-matched platelets may benefit patients who are sensitized to previous random-donor platelet transfusions. Specific antibiotics are indicated for different types of infections. Splenectomy is of questionable value and should be avoided unless there is evidence of shortened RBC or platelet survival owing to hypersplenism.

Androgen therapy alone or with corticosteroids may be of value in some patients. A 50% response rate has been observed, but this has been questioned because there are a significant number of spontaneous remissions. The recommended forms of androgen are nandrolone decanoate (3 mg/kg/week intramuscularly), xymetholone (2 to 4 mg/kg/day orally), or testosterone enanthate (3 to 5 mg/kg/week intramuscularly). The oral forms of androgen have a high incidence of liver toxicity, and all these preparations are virilizing. The grave prognosis of aplastic anemia, however, merits a clinical trial of androgens for 3 months.

In the severe type of aplastic anemia, patients less than 25 years of age and their relatives should have tissue typing. If an identical twin or HLA-compatible donor is available, bone marrow transplantation in a center where there are existing facilities and expertise should be attempted. An 82% probability of survival at 10 years has been reported in patients who received successful grafts in a major medical center.

MYELODYSPLASTIC SYNDROMES (PRELEUKEMIA, PRIMARY REFRACTORY ANEMIA)

The myelodysplastic syndromes (MDSs) are a heterogeneous group of disorders of the bone marrow hematopoietic stem cells. They are characterized by varying degrees of anemia, leukopenia, and thrombocytopenia. These manifestations of bone marrow failure are associated with a normal to increased cellularity, which distinguishes the syndrome from aplastic anemia. The exclusion of disorders resulting in increased peripheral destruction, known nutritional deficiencies, and acute leukemias is required. The term "refractory" refers to the usual unresponsive course of these syndromes to vitamins, iron, or hormonal therapy.

Several descriptive names such as megaloblastic refractory anemia, aregenerative anemia, chronic smoldering leukemia, and preleukemia have been used and interpretation of the literature on this subject has been complicated by the lack of a universally accepted system of nomenclature. The classification proposed by the French-American-British (FAB) group is an excellent first step and is used in this chapter.

ETIOLOGY. The majority of patients with MDS are elderly (median age 66 years) without obvious etiologic factors. However, MDSs occurring in younger person exposed to ionizing radiation, cytotoxic drugs (alkylating agents), or both indicate a cause-and-effect relationship even though the latter may occur 2 to 10 years later. The only known environmental or occupational hazard that has been closely linked with leukemia and MDS is benzene. Patients with MDS secondary to this agent have multiple chromosomal abnormalities and a higher incidence of transformation to acute leukemia. Other chemicals implicated are solents, insecticides, and petroleum products or their combustion agents.

PATHOGENESIS. The initial genetic insult causes an irreversible change in the structure and function of the hematopoietic stem cell's DNA, which results in an expansion of an abnormal cell population with a growth advantage over the normal cells. The abnormalities in growth and differentiation of this clone of cells lead to ineffective hematopoiesis and cytopenia. Further insults can cause other mutations to a more aggressive form and transformation into acute leukemia. The basic mechanisms of the role of growth factors, receptors, cytoplasmic mediators, and gene mapping of their locations in the chromosomes, as well as the role of oncogenes, in the pathogenesis of these disorders is under investigation.

CLINICAL MANIFESTATIONS. There are no specific symptoms or signs other than those of bone marrow failure similar to aplastic anemia, but patients may have a decrease in one or two cell lines rather than pancytopenia. About 50% of patients are asymptomatic at the time of diagnosis, which is often based on a routine blood cell count. Splenomegaly is found in about 20% of cases.

LABORATORY FINDINGS. The anemia in this disorder is usually normocytic or macrocytic with RBCs demonstrating anisopoikilocytosis. Reticulocyte levels are often decreased, and neutropenia is common. Neutrophils demonstrate poor granulation with abnormalities in segmentation (Pelger-Huet-like anomaly) characterized by unsegmented round or bilobed nuclei. Elevated white blood cell levels with monocytosis may occur. Platelet counts may vary from normal to severe thrombocytopenia with abnormally large platelets that have poor granulation.

The bone marrow is often cellular to hypercellular, and maturational defects are seen in all cell lines. "Megaloblastoid" changes in the RBC precursors with occasional binucleated and trinucleated cells, vacuolated erythroblasts, and ringed sideroblasts are seen. The myeloid cells show nuclear and cytoplasmic dissociation of maturation with abnormal granule formation. The myeloid cells expand at the myelocyte and metamyelocyte stages with varying percentage of myeloblasts. Levels of megakaryocytes may be decreased or increased with predominance of small immature forms that have single or bilobed nuclei.

The FAB group classifies MDSs according to the percentages of myeloblasts and promyelocytes, presence of sideroblasts, and peripheral monocytosis. Patients with less than 5% blast cells are said to have refractory anemia (RA), 5% to 20% blast cells indicates RA with excess blasts (RAEB), and 20% to 30% blasts cells is RAEB in transformation (RAEB-T). The presence of bone marrow similar to that in RA with a significant number of ringed sideroblasts (more than 15%) is classified as RA with ringed sideroblasts (RARS). The presence of marrow resembling that in RAEB, an elevated monocyte level of 500 to 1000 cells/mm^3, and an elevated serum lysozyme level with or without splenomegaly is classified as chronic myelomonocytic leukemia (CMML).

Chromosone abnormalities are observed in 45% to 50% of patients with primary MDS and 80% to 100% of those with secondary MDS.

DIAGNOSIS. Unexplained and persistent anemia with macrocytosis, leukopenia, monocytosis, or thrombocytopenia in a patient over 50 years of age should be investigated for MDS. Cellular marrow with maturational defects on all cell lines is often the basis for diagnosis. Serum folate and vitamin B$_{12}$ studies may be necessary to rule out nutritional deficiency anemia. A trial of pyridoxine for 1 to 3 months should exclude familial sideroblastic anemia. Chromosome studies to rule out chronic myelocytic leukemia (CML) with the Philadelphia chromosome in patients with elevated leukocyte levels and splenomegaly may be important.

CLINICAL COURSE. The duration of the hematologic disorder before the development of an acute or fatal type of leukemia is generally a few months to 2 years; a few patients have a prolonged course of up to 20 years. Patients with RAEB and CMML usually have shorter survival than those with RA or RARS. Patients in transformation usually survive less than 6 months. Patients with normal chromosomes or a single chromosomal abnormality survive longer than those with multiple abnormalities or a single 7 chromosome, which are associated with a higher rate of transformation to acute leukemia. Secondary MDS usually has a bad prognosis. The overall incidence of acute leukemia is about 45% to 50%. Patients with prolonged survival frequently die from other illness such as congestive heart failure or from the complications of the cytopenia.

MANAGEMENT. The treatment of MDS remains difficult, since supportive care with periodic blood transfusions gives only temporary relief and is associated with iron overload, hepatitis, and other transfusion-related complications. Attempts to stimulate the bone marrow with cyanocobalamin, folate, pyridoxine, pyridoxal phosphate, androgens, and corticosteroids have been of limited success. Splenectomy is usually ineffective, although occasionally a patient shows a decrease in neutropenia or thrombocytopenia. Aggressive antileukemic therapy has not been shown to be of benefit until an overt form of leukemia becomes evident and then is poorly tolerated and may produce only a short remission.

Abnormal MDS cells can be induced to differentiate by agents such as low doses of cytosine arabinoside, retinoic acid, and cholecalciferol growth factors. These drugs are being investigated in vitro and by clinical trials and may provide a future approach to this disorder.

SIDEROBLASTIC ANEMIA

Sideroblastic anemia is another form of bone marrow failure. Anemia, the most prominent feature, is associated with an increase in RBC precursors called ringed sideroblasts that contain excess stainable iron granules around the cell nucleus. Electron microscopy of these cells demonstrates the abnormal accumulation of iron in the mitochondira. This hematologic disorder may be either hereditary or acquired and is observed in association with a heterogeneous etiologic background.

ETIOLOGY. Familiar forms of sideroblastic anemia may or may not respond to high doses of pyridoxine and may have an X-linked or autosomal form of inheritance (see Chapter 65). The acquired form of this syndrome may be idiopathic or secondary to a toxin. Drugs such as chloramphenicol, pyrazinamide, and isoniazid and toxins such as alcohol and lead have been observed to cause a reversible form of sideroblastic anemia that responds favorably to the administration of pyridoxine and the withdrawal of the causative agent. The idiopathic refractory form does not respond to such treatment and carries a risk of leukemic transformation. The syndrome may be another form or manifestation of a hematopoietic stem cell mutation similar to preleukemia. An immunologic cause has been implicated in some cases, and association with lupus erythematosus, autoimmune hemolytic anemia, and monoclonal gammopathy with lymphoma has been reported. An IgG antibody–mediated acquired sideroblastic anemia has been shown to respond to immunsuppressive therapy.

PATHOGENESIS. The basic defect in sideroblastic anemia is an impairment of the heme biosynthetic pathway at the iron and protoporphyrin step, resulting in the accumulation of mitochondrial iron and lack of heme synthesis. Deficiency or abnormalities in the enzyme activities of aminolevulinic acid (ALA) synthetase, uroporphyrinogen decarboxylase, or heme synthetase have been observed in these patients. A deficiency in pyridoxine or a defect in the conversion of pyridoxine to pyridoxal-5-phosphate, the active moiety for the ALA synthetase, may lead to sideroblastic anemia. These abnormalities lead to lack of protoporphyrin and iron accumulation in the mitochondria. Iron loading of the mitochondria eventually causes peroxidation of the lipids, swelling and disintegration of these organelles, and cell death, resulting in ineffective erythropoiesis.

CLINICAL MANIFESTATIONS. Idiopathic refractory sideroblastic anemia occurs equally in men and women in their sixth decade. Most of these patients have symptoms referable to the anemia. Skin and mucosal pallor is the most prominent physical finding. Less than half of the patients have hepatosplenomegaly.

LABORATORY FINDINGS. The acquired idiopathic type of sideroblastic anemia is usually associated with a macrocytic, hypochromic type of anemia. The reticulocyte count is usually normal or increased, and the peripheral blood smear shows a dimorphic population with both normal-appearing RBCs and large hypochromic cells with basophilic stippling. The white blood cell and platelet counts are usually normal. The bone marrow is hypercellular with a characteristic erythroid hyperplasia and increased iron stores. Ringed sideroblasts may occur in 20% to 60% of the nucleated RBC precursors. Megaloblastic changes are also observed in these cells. Chromosomal aberrations similar to those described in preleukemia have been observed.

DIAGNOSIS. The important diagnostic feature is the demonstration of characteristic ringed sideroblasts in the bone marrow. Although the RBC indices indicate hypochromia, the peripheral RBCs tend to be macrocytic rather than microcytic, in contrast to iron deficiency, thalassemia, and the pyridoxine-responsive sideroblastic anemias. It is important to eliminate secondary causes in the history; occasionally serum lead levels may reveal an occult lead poisoning. Megaloblastic changes in the RBC precursor may also require differentiation from disorders of vitamin B_{12} and folate metabolism. Differentiation from the preleukemic state can be the most difficult problem. It is suggested that chromosomal aberration and the presence of elevated levels of hemoglobin F indicate a poor prognosis whereas thrombocytosis may indicate a benign course. The appearance of sideroblasts in the bone marrow of patients taking alkylating agents usually indicates an early stage of leukemic transformation.

COURSE. Hereditary forms of sideroblastic anemia are heterogeneous and may or may not respond to pyridoxine. The pyridoxine-responsive anemias require maintenance therapy. The acquired idiopathic form may have a chronic, protracted course or may terminate in acute leukemia. Reports have suggested that half of the patients are preleukemic or at an early state of Di Guglielmo's syndrome. However, a recent larger study indicates that the majority of patients have a prolonged course with a median survival of 10 years and that only about 7% to 10% undergo leukemic transformation. Hemosiderosis usually complicates the course when long-term transfusion therapy is required. Most patients die of other diseases to which the elderly are susceptible.

MANAGEMENT. Sideroblastic anemia is refractory to all forms of therapy, and most patients require maintenance transfusions. The use of iron chelators may be necessary to avoid iron overload. Every patient should have a therapeutic trial of pyridoxine (100 to 300 mg orally each day for 3 months) and folic acid. Steroids and androgens for 3 months may reduce the transfusion requirement in a few patients. Immunosuppression by cyclophosphamide has been successful in documented immune-mediated sideroblastic anemia. Aggressive chemotherapy may be indicated at the time of leukemic transformation, but the outcome is usually unfavorable.

MYELOPHTHISIS AND SECONDARY FORMS OF MYELOFIBROSIS

The term "myelophthisis" refers to the association of marrow invasion or injury by abnormal cells and/or fibrosis with characteristic "leukoerythroblastic" peripheral blood changes.

ETIOLOGY. The following are some causes of myelophthisic anemia:

> Hematologic neoplasm
>> Leukemia
>>> Chronic myelocytic leukemia
>>> Acute myeloblastic leukemia
>> Multiple myeloma
>> Hodgkin's disease
>> Lymphosarcoma

Reticulum cell sarcoma
Other tumors
  Prostatic carcinoma
  Breast carcinoma
  Stomach adenocarcinoma
  Lung carcinoma, primarily oat cell carcinoma
Infection
  Tuberculosis
  Osteomyelitis (focal fibrosis)
Other diseases
  Agnogenic myeloid metaplasia, polycythemia vera
  Marble bone disease
  Paget's disease
  Gaucher's disease
  Amyloidosis

The majority of the hematologic malignancies such as leukemias, lymphomas, and multiple myeloma involve infiltration of the marrow by abnormal cells, resulting in failure of normal hematopoiesis. Malignant tumors from other organs such as the prostate, breast, and lungs often metastasize to the marrow. Tuberculosis and fungal infections may involve the marrow and cause myelophthisic anemia. Inherited enzymatic defects such as Gaucher's disease may be associated with abnormal cells in the bone marrow, but the hematologic abnormality in these diseases usually results from hypersplenism.

PATHOGENESIS. The marrow is usually replaced by tumor cells and myelofibrosis. The mechanism involved in the resulting cytopenia, release of the hematopoietic precursor cells into the circulation, and myelofibrosis is unknown. Tumor cells are not always demonstrated in the marrow with myelofibrosis, but reversal of the fibrosis is associated with response of the primary disease to antitumor therapy in Hodgkin's disease and carcinomas of the prostate and breast.

CLINICAL MANIFESTATIONS AND LABORATORY FINDINGS. The most striking findings in this entity or syndrome are the laboratory test results. The clinical manifestations are attributable to the primary disease but occasionally include symptoms referable to the pancytopenia such as infection, bleeding, or severe anemia. Hepatosplenomegaly is prominent if hypersplenism is present. The leukoerythroblastic blood picture consists of nucleated RBCs and the presence of myeloid precursor cells.

Bone marrow aspiration and biopsy are usually the basis for diagnosis of the primary disease if performed in the involved area. The bone scan may be helpful in determining which iliac crest should be the biopsy site if the marrow is involved in localized areas. In disseminated metastasis or miliary tuberculosis the marrow examination can be performed in any of the usual sites of bone marrow examination.

MANAGEMENT. Myelophthisis is managed with supportive therapy for the hematologic abnormalities and specific treatment of the underlying disease.

BIBLIOGRAPHY

Anasetti C and others: Marrow transplantation for severe aplastic anemia: long-term outcome in fifty "untransfused" patients, Ann Intern Med 104:461, 1986.
Camitta, BM and others: A prospective study of androgens and bone marrow transplantation for treatment of severe aplastic anemia, Blood 53:504, 1979.
Chang DS, Kushner JP, and Wintrobe MM: Idiopathic refractory sideroblastic anemia: incidence and risk factors for leukemic transformation, Cancer 44:724, 1979.
Fichen JH and Klein MJ: Recent developments in understanding the pathogenesis of aplastic anemia, Am J Hematol 5:365, 1978.
Linman JW and Saarni MI: The preleukemic syndrome, Semin Hematol 11:93, 1974.
Nowell PC and others: Chromosome studies in preleukemic states, V. Prog-
nostic significance of single versus multiple abnormalities, Cancer 58:2571, 1986.
Speck B and others: Immunologic aspects of aplasia, Transplant Proc 10:131, 1978.
Wintrobe MM and others: Clinical hematology, ed 8, Philadelphia, 1981, Lea & Febiger.

63 · ACUTE POSTHEMORRHAGIC ANEMIA

William E. Barry

Acute posthemorrhagic anemia results from the rapid loss of whole blood. It may occur from trauma (including surgery), rupture or erosion of blood vessels, or defects in hemostasis. It is usually apparent, except when it occurs in body tissues (muscle, retroperitoneal space), body cavities (pleural, pericardial, or peritoneal), or transiently in the gastrointestinal tract.

CLINICAL MANIFESTATIONS. The clinical manifestations vary with the amount, rate, and location of the hemorrhage, as well as with the patient's general state of health and the presence of disease in critical organ systems. The early effects of hemorrhage involve changes in blood volume and organ perfusion. Following cessation of hemorrhage, compensatory or reparative functions related to red blood cell (RBC) production become apparent. In the healthy young adult the rapid loss of 500 to 1000 ml of blood (10% to 20% of blood volume) is usually tolerated without symptoms. Some, however, have weakness, sweating, nausea, bradycardia, hypotension, and syncope. The rapid loss of 1000 to 1500 ml of blood (20% to 30% of blood volume) may cause symptoms only in the upright position or with exertion. The rapid loss of 1500 to 2000 ml (30% to 40% of blood volume) usually results in hypovolemic shock, which may be irreversible if the blood loss exceeds 2000 to 2500 ml (40% to 50% of blood volume).

LABORATORY FINDINGS. After hemorrhage there is no immediate change in the hemoglobin or hematocrit level, since plasma and RBCs are lost proportionately. Within hours an increase in white blood cells and platelets is seen. The restoration of plasma volume begins quickly, but its magnitude is such that dilutional changes in the hemoglobin and hematocrit continue for 2 to 3 days. Thus the magnitude of the blood loss cannot be appreciated in the first few hours, perhaps not even for 24 hours, by which time the maximal rate of plasma volume restoration is achieved. Decline in the hemoglobin and hematocrit levels continues slowly over the next 48 to 72 hours but is less significant than the decline at 24 hours.

Evidence of active RBC regeneration, manifest as an increase in reticulocytes, begins after about 3 days, reaching a maximum (rarely higher than 15%) in 5 to 10 days. Thus acute blood loss in the presence of normal iron sources does not usually result in a hypochromic anemia. Chronic blood loss with exhaustion of iron stores is necessary to produce the hypochromic anemia of iron deficiency.

MANAGEMENT. The immediate treatment of posthemorrhagic anemia is directed toward restoration of blood volume, preferably with whole blood. If whole blood is not immediately available, albumin, plasma, plasma volume expanders, or even saline solution can be given intravenously.

BIBLIOGRAPHY

Wintrobe MM and others: Clinical hematology, ed 8, Philadelphia, 1981, Lea & Febiger.

64 • IRON DEFICIENCY ANEMIA

William E. Barry

On a worldwide basis, iron deficiency is the most common cause of anemia encountered in epidemiologic studies and clinical practice. About 10% to 15% of women in the reproductive years have been noted to have iron deficiency anemia. Even in women without overt anemia, body iron depletion, that is, absent or diminished iron stores, is common. Pregnancy, infancy, and adolescence are other periods of life when body iron deficiency and iron deficiency anemia are frequent. The importance of iron deficiency anemia can scarcely be overestimated, not only because it is such a common health problem but also because of the tragic implications for the patient whose iron deficiency anemia is caused by blood loss from an unrecognized and hence neglected gastrointestinal neoplasm.

ETIOLOGY. The most important cause of iron deficiency anemia in adults is *blood loss*. Most often this is due to gastrointestinal tract lesions such as peptic ulcer, hemorrhoids, colonic neoplasms, gastritis from long-term aspirin ingestion, hiatus hernia, and diverticulosis.

In women menstrual blood loss accounts for most instances of iron deficiency anemia. Rare causes in both sexes include mechanical hemolytic anemia with persistent urinary hemoglobin loss, excessive blood donation, idiopathic pulmonary hemosiderosis, and hereditary hemorrhagic telangiectasia.

Dietary lack of iron is an important cause of iron deficiency anemia *only* in children under 3 years of age. This is especially true when body iron stores are deficient at birth, as in premature infants, twins, and those with late clamping of the umbilical cord. A prolonged milk diet in infancy, containing little iron, is perhaps the most frequent cause of iron deficiency anemia in such children. The early introduction of solid foods and iron fortification of infant formulas reduce the frequency of this problem. Even in this age group gastrointestinal blood loss from a Meckel's diverticulum or from mucosal bleeding caused by milk intolerance occasionally occurs. The growth spurt of adolescence, although less rapid than in the first year of life, may cause a transient discrepancy between iron supply and body iron requirements, resulting in iron deficiency but rarely in overt iron deficiency anemia.

Pregnancy causes a net iron loss of about 680 mg to the mother and a temporary "loss" of another 450 mg to her expanded red blood cell (RBC) mass. This exceeds a woman's usual iron stores. Most of the iron drain occurs in the last trimester and cannot be made up rapidly enough from dietary sources despite increased absorption of iron from food. Hence, iron supplementation is needed to prevent overt iron deficiency anemia in most pregnant women. The problem is aggravated if a woman enters pregnancy with depleted or absent iron stores owing to menstrual blood loss.

PATHOGENESIS. Iron deficiency anemia results, ultimately, from an inadequate supply of iron for normal hemoglobin synthesis in developing erythroid cells in the bone marrow. Understanding how this comes about requires an appreciation of certain aspects of normal iron metabolism.

CLINICAL MANIFESTATIONS. The symptoms of iron deficiency anemia vary in severity, depending on the degree of anemia, the rapidity of its onset, and the presence of disease in other organ systems. In older patients symptoms of dyspnea, palpitations, or angina pectoris may occur, reflecting the frequency of coexisting organic heart disease. In younger patients the symptoms may be vague and nonspecific and may include fatigue, lassitude, and anorexia.

Physical findings include pallor of the skin and mucous membranes. Loss of papillae on the lateral aspect of the tongue frequently occurs, and occasionally cracking at the corners of the mouth is seen. Hemic (flow) murmurs are commonly heard. A palpable spleen has been reported in up to 10% of the patients. Rarely, retinal hemorrhages and even papilledema are seen with severe anemia. Spoon-shaped nails are characteristic but not pathognomonic of severe iron deficiency anemia.

LABORATORY FINDINGS. A hypochromic microcytic anemia is characteristic of iron deficiency anemia. In cases where the anemia is only slight, the RBC indices may be normal. The serum iron level is low, and the total iron-binding capacity is usually increased. A variety of abnormal RBC shapes may be seen in the stained blood smear. The reticulocyte count is normal or low, and the platelet count may be increased.

The bone marrow is usually cellular. Erythroid hyperplasia is sometimes seen. The nucleated RBCs are hemoglobin poor, with scanty cytoplasm. No stainable iron is visible in the marrow fragment or the nucleated erythroid cells. The serum ferritin level is low. The level of protoporphyrin in mature RBCs is elevated.

DIAGNOSIS. The diagnosis of iron deficiency anemia is made by finding the characteristic hypochromic microcytic RBC indices with a low serum ferritin level (less than 20 pg/ ml), a low serum iron level, and elevated total iron-binding capacity. In doubtful cases the diagnosis of iron deficiency is confirmed by lack of stainable marrow iron.

Iron deficiency anemia can be confused with the thalassemia trait, and the two occasionally coexist. The β-thalassemia trait is associated with an elevated percentage of hemoglobin A_2. Patients with the α-thalassemia trait have normal levels of hemoglobin A_2, and family studies are needed to establish the diagnosis.

Anemia of chronic disease usually has normocytic normochromic RBC indices, but occasionally the RBCs are hypochromic. In this disorder the serum iron level is low, similar to iron deficiency, but the total iron-binding capacity is low rather than high. In addition, stainable iron is present in the marrow in reticuloendothelial cells. Rarely, iron deficiency coexists with anemia of chronic disease and defies precise diagnosis.

When iron deficiency anemia is confirmed, it is imperative to determine the cause, which almost always is blood loss. Excluding a gastrointestinal neoplasm by appropriate studies is particularly important.

COURSE. Iron deficiency anemia often pursues an insidious course owing to adaptive mechanisms that limit the impact on the patient despite significantly low levels of hemoglobin. These adaptive mechanisms include an increase in RBC production and an increase in the level of 2,3-diphosphoglycerate (2,3-DPG) in the mature erythrocyte. The increase in 2,3-DPG, a product of glycolysis, causes a shift in the oxygen dissociation curve of hemoglobin, enabling oxygen to be more readily released to tissues. Despite these adaptive mechanisms, and possibly because iron deficiency may affect intracellular enzyme function in a way not yet clearly defined, the symptoms eventually assume proportions sufficient to cause the patient to seek help. Alternatively, the asymptomatic state may prevail, and the diagnosis is made by a routine blood cell count in the course of evaluating an unrelated disorder.

Once the diagnosis is defined accurately, treatment with iron usually results in a satisfactory improvement in the symptoms and the hemoglobin level. Anemia may recur if the cause is not permanently removed. Thus any source of chronic blood loss may be an important cause of the failure to correct, completely or permanently, iron deficiency anemia despite appropriate therapy.

MANAGEMENT. The treatment of iron deficiency anemia is usually simple, effective, and inexpensive. Ferrous sulfate (300 mg orally three times a day) is the treatment of choice. About 10% of the patients complain of unacceptable gastrointestinal intolerance and may require parenteral therapy. Delayed-release forms of orally administered iron, although well tolerated, may be ineffective owing to relatively poor absorption of iron beyond the duodenum.

In an otherwise uncomplicated case a complete response is achieved by 4 to 8 weeks. If a response is not achieved by that time, reevaluation is indicated regarding accuracy of the diagnosis, patient compliance with the prescribed dose of iron, continued blood loss, or (rarely) malabsorption of orally administered iron.

BIBLIOGRAPHY

Cook JD: Clinical evaluation of iron deficiency, Semin Hematol 19:6, 1982.
Finch CA and others: Ferrokinetics in man, Medicine 49:17, 1970.
Hallberg L, Harwerth HG, and Vannotti A, editors: Iron deficiency: pathogenesis, clinical aspects, therapy, New York, 1970, Academic Press, Inc.
Hillman RS and Finch CA: Red cell manual, Philadelphia, 1974, FA Davis Co.

65 • OTHER HYPOCHROMIC MICROCYTIC ANEMIAS

William E. Barry

In addition to iron deficiency, other disorders may result in inadequate hemoglobin synthesis in erythrocytes. Three principal mechanisms usually account for this: inadequate porphyrin synthesis, a defect in the coupling of iron to protoporphyrin to form heme, and a defect in globin synthesis. Compared with iron deficiency, these disorders are rare.

Inadequate porphyrin synthesis occurs in *pyridoxine-responsive anemia*. Pyridoxal phosphate is required as a cofactor in the first step in porphyrin synthesis, the formation of δ-aminolevulinic acid from glycine and coenzyme A. Since large amounts of pyridoxine are necessary for therapy, it appears that the anemia is not due to an absolute deficiency of pyridoxine. A similar anemia may occur if drugs such as isoniazid interfere with pyridoxine activity. Lead poisoning interferes with porphyrin synthesis at several steps, resulting in a net deficiency of hemoglobin, among other effects of lead on protein synthesis and membrane function. Lead poisoning characteristically causes basophilic stippling in erythrocytes. Other laboratory features of lead poisoning include elevated blood and urine lead levels and increased excretion of porphyrins in urine. Defects in enzymatic coupling of iron to protoporphyrin to form heme have been implicated rarely as a cause of hypochromic anemia.

"Ringed" sideroblasts, resulting from the perinuclear mitochondrial accumulation of iron not utilized in heme synthesis, may be seen in these hypochromic anemias. The presence of ringed sideroblasts is characteristic of the sideroblastic anemias, some of which result from identifiable defects in heme synthesis as just noted. In others (the hereditary or acquired "idiopathic" types), the exact mechanisms have not been defined. These are discussed in Chapter 62.

The thalassemias are examples of inadequate synthesis of α- or β-globin chains. Since heme synthesis is unaffected, ringed sideroblasts do not occur.

A rare cause of hypochromic anemia is atransferrinemia, wherein iron cannot be transported to the erythroblasts but is deposited in excess amounts in other organs. A rare disorder has also been described in which transferrin iron, although present in increased amount, cannot enter erythroblasts, possibly because of an abnormality in the transferrin receptor site on the erythroblast membrane.

BIBLIOGRAPHY

Anemias characterized by deficient hemoglobin synthesis and impaired iron metabolism. In Wintrobe MM and others, editors: Clinical hematology, ed 8, Philadelphia, 1981, Lea & Febiger.

66 • ANEMIA OF CHRONIC DISEASE

William E. Barry

DEFINITION. The anemia of chronic disease is the most common anemia seen in hospitalized patients. A variety of terms, such as "anemia of infection," "anemia of malignancy," and "simple chronic anemia," have been used to describe this disorder.

ETIOLOGY. Systemic illnesses, especially those characterized by chronic inflammation, frequently are associated with the anemia of chronic disease. These include lung abscess, osteomyelitis, pneumonia, bacterial endocarditis, and a variety of other chronic inflammatory processes. Rheumatoid arthritis and metastatic malignancy are other typical diseases characterized by this secondary form of anemia. The anemia is not confined to these illnesses, however, and occasionally is found in the absence of any identifiable underlying disease.

PATHOGENESIS. The anemia of chronic disease is characterized by a hemolytic component manifest as a slight shortening of red blood cell (RBC) survival, inadequate marrow compensatory response to this shortened RBC survival, and low serum iron level and decreased total iron-binding capacity.

The mechanism of the shortened RBC survival has not been clearly defined. Immunoglobulins are not detected on the erythrocyte membrane, nor are there identified abnormalities of the cell itself. It has been suggested that the phagocytic function of the reticuloendothelial (RE) system is "hyperactive" for both circulating RBCs and developing erythroblasts in the marrow.

The mechanism for the functional marrow inadequacy has been the subject of recent investigation. The evidence is conflicting, but it appears that an inappropriately low synthesis of erythropoietin or a defect in marrow response to erythropoietin is the most likely explanation. Whether the inadequate marrow response is related to an insufficient usable marrow supply of iron has not been definitely proved. Nevertheless, the characteristically low serum iron level is an essential marker of the anemia and is related to a block in RE cell release of iron to plasma transferrin. It has been suggested that the RE cell, during the processing of hemoglobin from senescent RBCs, shunts iron preferentially into ferritin within the cell rather than dispersing it rapidly out of the cell to plasma transferrin, resulting in a low serum iron level.

CLINICAL MANIFESTATIONS. The anemia of chronic disease is usually of little clinical consequence. The underlying disease responsible for the anemia dominates the clinical picture. Occasionally, however, the anemia is severe enough to cause symptoms and may require erythrocyte transfusions.

The anemia develops slowly as a rule, only occasionally occurring in illnesses lasting less than 3 to 6 weeks. Thus acute infections are not usually associated with anemia unless additional mechanisms, such as an autoimmune hemolytic process, or an underlying illness is already present.

LABORATORY FINDINGS. The anemia of chronic disease, with hemoglobin levels between 9 and 11 g/dl, is typically normochromic and normocytic, but on occasion a hypochromic picture is noted. The reticulocyte count is low. The most characteristic feature is a low serum iron level accompanied (unlike iron deficiency) by a low total iron-binding capacity. The serum ferritin level is usually modestly elevated.

Bone marrow examination discloses no morphologic abnormalities, except for the iron stain, which shows stainable iron in RE cells but reduced iron in developing RBCs.

DIAGNOSIS. The finding of a mild normocytic normochromic anemia in a patient with a chronic illness, accompanied by a low serum iron level and a low total iron-binding capacity, is enough to establish a diagnosis of anemia of chronic disease. The most important differential diagnosis is between mild iron deficiency anemia and anemia of chronic disease. When the serum iron changes are equivocal, determination of the serum ferritin level or, more reliably, a sample of bone marrow stained for iron is necessary to distinguish between the two disorders.

COURSE AND MANAGEMENT. The course of anemia of chronic disease varies with the progress of the underlying illness. No useful treatment is available for the anemia, which responds only to successful treatment of the underlying disease. Packed RBC transfusions are sometimes of temporary benefit if the anemia is severe or compromises cardiovascular function. Iron therapy is ineffective.

BIBLIOGRAPHY

Cartwright G: The anemia of chronic disorders, Semin Hematol 3:351, 1966.
Lee GR: The anemia of chronic disease, Semin Hematol 20:61, 1983.

67 • ANEMIAS CAUSED BY RED BLOOD CELL DESTRUCTION

Jerome I. Brody

Hemolytic anemia is the clinical state or condition in which there is a reduction in the life span (normally about 120 days) of the circulating red blood cell (RBC) associated with failure of the bone marrow to restore completely the quantity of erythrocytes prematurely eliminated from the peripheral blood. Normally, erythropoiesis maintains a dynamic state in which the rate of RBC production equals the rate of destruction. These processes are balanced, so that in a 70 kg person 1% of the total RBC mass or 25 ml of RBCs is replaced daily. If RBC destruction exceeds the bone marrow's capacity to increase output (the usual maximum is six to eight times normal), the hemolysis is uncompensated and anemia results. On the other hand, if the marrow can meet the peripheral demands, hemolysis may be ongoing but is compensated and anemia does not occur.

There are certain similarities and differences between the events of normal RBC clearance and those sequences occurring during inappropriate hemolysis. Whereas gross RBC membrane injury, such as that caused by a mismatched transfusion, may lead to intravascular hemolysis, the alterations associated with erythrocyte aging are more delicate. Physiologic erythrocyte removal takes place within the reticuloendothelial system, especially the spleen and liver, and less importantly in the bone marrow and lungs. Most abnormal and excessive RBC destruction also occurs extravascularly.

The exact signal that identifies the effete RBC and the precise and detailed mechanism for its removal are unknown. Conceivably, subtle changes in shape and biophysical characteristics indicate senescence and recognition for elimination. Because of its microanatomy and vascular structure, the spleen is admirably suited to mechanical trapping of RBCs as they course through the splenic arterioles into the sinuses of the red pulp. Approximately 1% to 2% of the RBCs enter the blind, narrow splenic cords that are connected to the sinuses by openings measuring 3 μm in diameter. Movement through these apertures is especially difficult for erythrocytes. It is in this area that erythrostasis, glucose deprivation, and local acidosis occur. The liver also participates in erythrocyte removal but clears those having comparatively more severe biochemical, physical, and immunogenic injury or abnormalities.

Within the reticuloendothelial macrophages, erythrocyte hemoglobin degradation begins by cleavage of heme protoporphyrin to produce biliverdin, which is promptly reduced to bilirubin. After conjugation in the liver the bilirubin is excreted into the bile and reduced in the colon to urobilinogen by anaerobic bacteria. In a healthy, 70 kg person, the 6.25 g of hemoglobin derived daily from the 25 ml of aged erythrocytes is metabolized easily by the liver. Unconjugated hyperbilirubinemia may occur if there is a twofold increase in bilirubin turnover or a 50% reduction in hepatic bilirubin clearance. Such changes result in a doubling of the plasma bilirubin concentration. However, even when the maximal daily rate of bilirubin production of 40 mg/kg, about eight times the upper limit of normal, is reached, such overproduction elevates the plasma unconjugated bilirubin concentration no higher than 3.5 to 4 mg/dl. Therefore a plasma unconjugated bilirubin concentration persistently in excess of 4 mg/dl implies abnormal hepatic function irrespective of hemolysis.

If intravascular hemolysis rather than extravascular RBC removal occurs, hemoglobinemia and hemoglobinuria may be detected. When the plasma haptoglobin binding capacity for hemoglobin of 125 to 150 mg/dl and the proximal renal tubular reabsorption ability of 25 mg/dl are exceeded, free hemoglobin passes into the glomerular filtrate, resulting in hemoglobinuria. The hemoglobin may be absorbed by the renal tubular cells, degraded to hemosiderin in situ by heme oxygenase, and later excreted, resulting in hemosiderinuria. A portion of the intravascular hemoglobin may also be oxidized to methemoglobin, which then dissociates to free hemin and globin. Free plasma hemin is bound by the β-globulin hemopexin, which may also be removed as a complex by the liver cells. Finally, in the absence of hemopexin, free hemin may attach to albumin forming methemalbumin, a useful indicator of recent hemolysis because of its relatively slow plasma clearance.

The diagnosis of hemolytic anemia may be suspected because of the ethnic, racial, and familial background of the patient; prior anemia; ingestion of drugs known to cause hemolysis; presence of certain systemic disorders; special events such as previous surgery for valvular heart disease; and specific patient complaints involving organ systems frequently associated with excessive RBC destruction.

The symptoms of hemolytic anemia are those of anemia in general. Their severity depends on how low the hemoglobin and packed cell volume levels are, the rate at which these levels have been reached, the degree of shift in the oxygen dissociation curve, the compensatory capacity of the cardiovascular and pulmonary systems, and, finally, whether the anemia is stable, progressive, or episodic. General complaints therefore may be variable and may include early fatigue, lassitude, decreased exercise tolerance, palpitations, dyspnea, tachypnea, dizziness, headache, and tinnitus. Some symptoms may be more specific and directed toward a particular organ system. Physical findings depend on the specific disease present and may include pallor, tachycardia, icterus, lymphadenopathy, hepatomegaly, splenomegaly, bony tenderness, and neurologic abnormalities.

The following outline classifies the causes of hemolytic anemia:

I. Congenital hemolytic anemias
  A. Membrane defects
    1. Hereditary spherocytosis
    2. Hereditary elliptocytosis
    3. Hereditary stomatocytosis
    4. Lipid abnormalities
  B. Enzyme deficiencies
    1. Defects of the Embden-Meyerhof pathway
    2. Deficiencies in the hexose monophosphate shunt and glutathione metabolism
    3. Other enzyme defects
  C. Disorders of hemoglobin
    1. Single amino acid substitutions
      a. β-Chain (hemoglobins S, C, D, and so on)
      b. α-Chain
      c. γ-Chain
      d. δ-Chain
    2. Two amino acid substitutions in the subunit (hemoglobin C$_{Harlem}$)
    3. Unbalanced subunit synthesis (quantitatively deficient globin chain synthesis)
      a. β-Thalassemia
      b. α-Thalassemia and so on
    4. Errors in subunit termination (nucleoside base substitution in terminal codon)
      a. α-Chain (hemoglobin Constant Spring)
      b. β-Chain (hemoglobin Tak)
    5. Fusion hemoglobins (hemoglobins Lepore, Miyada, Kenya)
    6. Amino acid deletions (many unstable hemoglobins)
    7. Frame shift mutation (deletion of one or two codon nucleoside bases; hemoglobin Wayne)
    8. Other abnormal hemoglobins
II. Acquired hemolytic anemias
  A. Immunohemolytic anemias
    1. Alloimmune
      a. Incompatible blood transfusions
      b. Hemolytic disease of the newborn
    2. Autoimmune
      a. Warm-reacting antibodies
      b. Cold-reacting antibodies
  B. Traumatic hemolytic anemia
    1. Prosthetic valves and other vascular abnormalities
    2. Microangiopathic hemolysis
    3. March hemoglobinuria
  C. Paroxysmal nocturnal hemoglobinuria (PNH; membrane dysplasia)
  D. Drug-induced anemia
    1. Immunocytolytic
    2. Nonimmune
      a. Enzyme deficiencies
      b. Unstable hemoglobins
      c. Others
  E. Hemolysis owing to other causes
    1. Chemical and physical agents
    2. Metabolic defects
    3. Infectious agents
  F. Sequestration hemolysis
    1. Hypersplenism
    2. Reticuloendothelioses

The degree of anemia and reticulocytosis may be inconstant. The level of reticulocytosis is a function of the bone marrow's attempt to compensate for the reduced peripheral erythrocyte mass. Reticulocytosis should be comparatively higher as the anemia becomes more severe, providing the bone marrow is competent and sufficient hematinic agents are available. Depending on the dynamics, degree, and type of the anemia, methemoglobinemia, hemoglobinemia, hemoglobinuria, and hemosiderinuria may or may not be present.

The definitive diagnostic test for excessive erythrocyte destruction is the evaluation of the RBC life span. For clinical purposes this is usually done by labeling RBCs with ^{51}Cr and calculating their survival from the radioactivity in sequential blood samples using the dilution principle. Normal survival as measured by this method is 60 rather than 120 days, with results expressed as the chromium activity half-life ($T_{1/2}$). Normally this is 28 to 32 days. If gastrointestinal bleeding is a clinical consideration in addition to hemolysis, simultaneous assay of fecal radioactivity is necessary to avoid misinterpretation of the data provided by this technique.

CONGENITAL HEMOLYTIC ANEMIAS
Membrane defects

Inherited or acquired structural abnormalities of the RBC membrane form the pathogenetic basis for several hemolytic anemias. The RBC membrane is composed of a phospholipid and cholesterol lipid bilayer associated with three types of functional proteins. The first type is on the external surface of the RBC and is exemplified by blood group antigens or receptors. The next category of proteins, glycophorins A, B, and C and protein 3, span the RBC membrane and are attached to the underlying cytoskeleton. The cytoskeleton incorporates the third and last protein group: α- and β-spectrin, protein 4.1, and F-actin. Spectrin is a heterodimer associated head to head with itself to form a tetramer. Ankyrin fastens spectrin to protein 3, which extends across the lipid bilayer. Protein 4.1 facilitates association of spectrin with actin. The mechanisms by which cytoskeletal defects result in alteration of RBC shape, decreased deformability, and reduced survival are not completely defined.

HEREDITARY SPHEROCYTOSIS

Definition and pathogenesis. Hereditary spherocytosis (HS), also called congenital hemolytic jaundice, is a congenital hemolytic anemia transmitted as an autosomal dominant trait. There are multiple RBC membrane abnormalities in HS. These consist of deficient binding of spectrin to protein 4.1 and actin, quantitative abnormalities of protein 4.1 itself, and abnormal glycophorins. Such changes are partially responsible for the morphologic and physical distortions produced by metabolic stress and resulting RBC fragmentation.

The membrane changes lead to a gradual loss of surface area during the life span of the erythrocyte, so that instead of remaining a flexible biconcave disk it becomes a tight sphere. The defect increases the glycolytic rate, augments the entry of sodium and water into the cell, and alters the shape of the cell. The reduced cell deformability is pivotal for the spleen, with its low-velocity blood flow and acidic environment, to become the selective and focal organ of RBC sequestration and destruction.

Epidemiology and clinical manifestations. HS occurs worldwide but most commonly in people of Northern European ancestry. It is the most frequently observed congenital hemolytic anemia in whites.

The clinical manifestations of HS are remarkably diverse and may vary from one patient to another and from family to family. Its mode of presentation may be age dependent. It can be mild and go completely unnoticed in childhood until a systemic infection intervenes, provoking either an aplastic or a hemolytic crisis. In adults HS may surface first as cholelithiasis or cholecystitis, found in 43% to 80% of the patients. Physical findings may include intermittent, variable jaundice. The spleen is commonly enlarged, and usually palpable. Hypersplenism may occur, especially during active infection. Chronic leg ulcerations are present in 10% to 15% of the patients.

Laboratory findings. The anemia may be variable with hemoglobin levels usually at 9 to 12 g/dl. Depending on the marrow's ability to increase erythropoiesis, compensation for hemolysis may be complete or partial. During a crisis the hemoglobin may fall rapidly and leukocytosis may occur. Lymphocytosis and basophilia have been described with chronic, steady anemia. A reticulocyte count of 5% to 20% is common, and during hemolytic crises it may rise as high as 50% to 90%. Reticulocytopenia may follow aplastic episodes.

The peripheral blood smear may show the characteristic small, dark, spheroidal RBCs without a central area of pallor. Polychromasia and nucleated RBCs also may be present. There is inconstant indirect hyperbilirubinemia (bilirubin level 1 to 4 mg/dl), the haptoglobin level may be low even though the hemolysis is mainly extravascular, the fecal urobilinogen level may be elevated, and thrombocytopenia with or without leukopenia and caused by hypersplenism may be detected. The bone marrow shows erythroid hyperplasia; however, during an aplastic crisis, compensation is transiently interrupted, which produces erythroid hypoplasia and bone marrow failure.

Diagnosis. HS should be suspected when the mean corpuscular hemoglobin concentration (MCHC) rises above 36% in association with the preceding clinical and laboratory data. The diagnosis is confirmed by the osmotic fragility test in which RBCs are suspended in saline solutions of varying tonicity, producing a greater hemoglobin leak in spherocytes than in normal, control RBCs. The concentration of hemoglobin appearing in the suspension supernatants can be measured spectrophotometrically, and a curve can be plotted using these values. For the test to be positive, at least 1% to 2% of the erythrocyte population must be spherocytic. Therefore in mild disease this assay may be normal. The occult RBC defect is uncovered by the incubated osmotic fragility test in which whole blood is held at 98.6° F (37° C) for 24 hours and then the procedure just described is repeated. Another examination is the autohemolysis test performed by suspending RBCs in a glucose-free medium, which results in 10% to 50% spontaneous hemolysis of spherocytes. Coombs' test is negative in HS.

Management. The treatment is by splenectomy when the disease is active. This increases the RBC survival almost but not quite to normal because the primary RBC defect persists. Splenectomy markedly increases susceptibility to infections caused by pneumococci, meningococci, and *Haemophilus influenzae*. Since susceptibility is greatest below 6 years of age, it is best to postpone surgery until the patient is older. Immunization with the pneumococcal vaccine before surgery seems prudent.

Blood transfusions are rarely necessary except in aplastic crises, which are sometimes due to folate deficiency, occur most frequently in childhood, and are usually provoked by infection. Because of the ongoing hemolysis and increased hematinic needs, 1 mg of folic acid daily probably should be administered.

Enzyme deficiencies
DEFICIENCIES WITHIN THE HEXOSE MONOPHOSPHATE (HMP) SHUNT

Glucose-6-phosphate dehydrogenase deficiency. The HMP shunt forms pentose from glucose and, more important, serves as the sole mechanism that prevents oxidative denaturation of intracellular and membrane components of the erythrocyte. Glucose-6-phosphate dehydrogenase (G6PD) is a crucial enzyme because it initiates the first reaction in the shunt pathway and generates nicotinamide-adenine dinucleotide phosphate (NADPH) required as a cofactor in the maintenance of glutathione (GSH) (Fig. 67-1). The latter compound protects hemoglobin sulfhydryls (—SH) and —SH-containing enzymes against oxidation and destruction. In the face of G6PD deficiency the NADPH reductive processes and maintenance of GSH are impaired, leading to deleterious biochemical and physical changes in the RBC and its premature removal from the circulation.

G6PD deficiency causes a hereditary, sex-linked hemolytic anemia apparent mainly during certain stressful situations. The defect is due to a coded gene on the X chromosome and is completely expressed in male hemizygotes, observed in rare female homozygotes, and minimally overt in female heterozygotes. The deficiency has been shown to have a worldwide distribution but is most common among people living in tropical and subtropical areas. About 10% of American blacks and 8% to 20% of West African blacks harbor the deficiency.

Although over 100 forms of G6PD already have been discovered, the majority are mainly of theoretic and biochemical interest. Only a few require special mention. The genotypic symbol for the enzyme is Gd. The normal enzyme, designated GdB +, represents the comparative enzyme standard, with the plus sign indicating full-level enzyme activity. It is the most commonly observed form in all population groups, being present in almost all whites and approximately 70% of normal blacks. GdA +, another normal variant, is prevalent in 30% of normal blacks. On electrophoresis this form migrates more rapidly than GdB +. The next type, GdA −, is the most frequent, clinically significant abnormal form in blacks. The minus sign denotes enzyme activity reduced to less than 25% of the normal counterpart, GdA +. Electrophoretic migration of GdA − is identical to that of GdA +, but the former is less active, possibly because it is relatively unstable and its activity diminishes as the RBC ages.

The most common abnormal variant in white people is Gd Mediterranean. The intracellular enzyme concentration is less than 1% of normal, in contrast to the usual 5% to 15% enzyme level observed in the GdA − form. Mild subclinical hemolysis with a minimal reduction of the erythrocyte life span is always present in the RBCs with Gd Mediterranean deficiency. The defect is not restricted to RBCs, as with GdA −, but extends to the leukocytes and platelets as well.

Hemolysis in G6PD deficiency is overt only under the following circumstances.

Drug-induced hemolysis. These compounds induce hemolysis in persons with G6PD deficiency:

Antibacterials
  Chloramphenicol*
  Isoniazid
  Paraaminosalicylic acid
  Nalidixic acid
Antipyretics and analgesics
  Acetanilid
  Aspirin
  Acetophenetidin (phenacetin)

Antipyrine
Aminopyrine
Antimalarials
  Chloroquine
  Primaquine
  Pamaquine
  Pentaquine
  Quinocide
  Quinacrine (Atabrine)
  Quinine
Sulfonamides
  Sulfanilamide
  Sulfapyridine
  Salicylazosulfapyridine (Azulfidine)
  Sulfamethoxypyridazine (Kynex)
  Sulfacetamide
  N_2-Acetylsulfanilamide
  2-Amino-5-sulfanilythiazole
  Sulfisoxazole (Gantrisin)‡
Sulfones
  Thiazolsulfone (Promizole)
  Diaminodiphenylsulfone (DDS)
  Sulfoxone (dapsone)‡
Nitrofurans
  Nitrofurantoin (Furadantin)
  Furazolidone (Furoxone)
  Nitrofurazone (Furacin)
Miscellaneous compounds
  Naphthalene (mothballs)
  Probenecid (Benemid)
  Vitamin K (water-soluble analogs)
  Phenylhydrazine
  Trinitrotoluene
  Methylene blue‡
  Dimercaprol (BAL)
  Quinidine*
  Fava beans*
  Ascorbic acid†

The mechanism by which these drugs produce oxidative degradation of hemoglobin is not entirely clear. These agents, or their active derivatives, interact with oxyhemoglobin, resulting in either the formation of free radicals or the generation of hydrogen peroxide, which oxidizes and precipitates globin recognizable as Heinz bodies after incubation with supravital stains. These damaged erythrocytes are removed by the spleen.

The typical hemolytic episode may occur from 1 to 3 days after drug administration and may last 7 to 12 days. With GdA−, hemolysis usually occurs 24 to 36 hours after exposure. Hemoglobinemia, hemoglobinuria, and jaundice are usual; the resultant anemia is moderate with the hemoglobin level rarely less than 8 g/dl. Hemolysis is self-limited, and the anemia reaches its nadir at 8 to 12 days. Recovery occurs even during continued drug administration because the younger cells leaving the bone marrow contain the more active enzyme resistant to oxidant stress. In the Gd Mediterranean defect hemolysis may occur earlier, within 3 to 24 hours of drug ingestion. Hemoglobinuria and jaundice are constant concurrents, hemolysis may not be self-limited, and the hemoglobin may drop to an extremely low level. Because massive intravascular hemolysis can cause severe hypotension and renal failure, these episodes may be fatal. Usually, however, clinical recovery is the rule, and the hemoglobin and hematocrit levels return to normal by approximately 5 weeks.

Infection. Hemolysis also may be induced during viral or bacterial infection, perhaps by hydrogen peroxide evolving during phagocytosis by neutrophils. The vulnerability of the erythrocyte to destruction in this case is analogous to that produced by drug contact. Anemia caused by infection is mild, and jaundice usually is absent. Reticulocytosis may not be observed because infection per se may suppress erythropoiesis. Recovery from the anemia therefore may be delayed until the infection has disappeared. The mechanism of injury, in addition to peroxide generation, also may be attributed to the infectious organism itself and its toxic metabolic products. Shock, hypotension, decreased renal function, and death have been described in the Gd Mediterranean form of deficiency when hemolysis has been associated with the hepatitis virus. RBC destruction may be massive, jaundice extreme, and hyperbilirubinemia striking.

Favism. Hemolysis is induced by fresh or dried fava beans only in those with the Gd Mediterranean defect and may be sudden, occurring within a few hours after plant pollen inhalation or within 2 days after the vegetable is eaten. It is produced mainly, but not solely, in male children between the ages of 2 and 5 years. The resultant anemia may reach hemoglobin levels of 2 g/dl with lethal clinical consequences. Favism is not to be taken lightly as a clinical entity. Not all G6PD-deficient patients have hemolysis when exposed to fava beans, suggesting that additional, possibly nonenzymatic factors may provoke susceptibility. On the other hand, favism affects only individuals who are G6PD deficient.

Neonatal jaundice. The premature, white, G6PD-deficient infant is especially prone to excessive hemolysis, jaundice, and hyperbilirubinemia without evidence of immunologic incompatibility and unrelated to drugs given to either the mother or her infant. This syndrome occurs in babies with the Gd Mediterranean variant and is rare among black infants with GdA− deficiency. The jaundice that follows may be severe enough to require exchange transfusions to prevent kernicterus.

Hereditary nonspherocytic hemolytic anemia. Hemolysis without drug ingestion occurs in certain rare types of G6PD deficiency, usually when the enzyme is unstable or its level is very low. This form of anemia generally is observed in whites, may begin in early infancy, and is mild, with limited or negligible transfusion needs. Exacerbations may be caused by fever, infection, and drugs. Splenomegaly is common. Rarely, when the anemia is severe, splenectomy has been clinically helpful in treatment.

Other causes. In addition to hereditary nonspherocytic hemolytic anemia, hemolysis may be provoked without drug contact in the presence of acidosis, renal disease, uremia, and diabetic coma. The features of erythrocyte destruction in these instances resemble those of infection-related hemolysis.

• • •

The erythrocyte in G6PD deficiency usually looks normal on the peripheral blood smear between hemolytic episodes. During active hemolysis, however, polychromasia, spherocytes, schistocytes, and Heinz bodies may appear. The level of the reticulocytosis depends on the severity of the stress. Hyperbilirubinemia of varying levels may be observed.

The diagnosis of G6PD deficiency depends on the demonstration of enzyme deficiency through either screening tests or quantitative enzyme assay. The former methods are visual, more easily available, and sufficient for clinical purposes. They include the ascorbate-cyanide test and the reduction of certain

---

*Hemolytic in persons with G6PD Mediterranean deficiency.
‡Slightly hemolytic in large doses only in GdA− persons.
§Hemolytic in whites, not in GdA− persons.
‖Hemolytic in massive doses.

dyes such as brilliant cresyle blue (BCB) or methylene blue (MB). Actual spectrophotometric, quantitative measurement of enzyme activity in RBC hemolysates is rarely necessary but may be useful when the Gd variant is unusual or escapes detection by simpler means. Since hemolysis induced by drugs may occur in the presence of unstable hemoglobins, tests for these hemoglobin forms also should be considered.

Usually no active treatment is needed for G6PD deficiency other than the avoidance of drugs known to initiate hemolysis. When RBC destruction is particularly severe, as with the Gd Mediterranean defect (especially when associated with viral hepatitis), the episode should be treated like any other hemolytic anemia in which renal failure and anuria are potential sequelae.

Disorders of hemoglobin

Abnormalities of hemoglobin may be classified as caused either by departures from the usual structural organization of this iron-containing protein or by the absence or reduced synthesis of one or more of the normal globin polypeptides necessary for complete integrity of the hemoglobin molecule. "Hemoglobinopathy" is the term applied to the former category, and the thalassemias represent the latter group.

In adults there are three physiologic hemoglobins. The first is hemoglobin A (Hb A), constituting approximately 97% of the total hemoglobin complement. It consists of four polypeptide chains, two α-chains, each with 141 amino acids, and two β-chains, each with 146 amino acids. The whole molecule is designated $\alpha_2\beta_2$. An iron-containing heme group is attached to each polypeptide. This tetrameric structure provides for cooperative binding of four oxygen molecules and establishes normal hemoglobin's affinity for oxygen. A minor adult component is hemoglobin A_2 (Hb A_2), consisting of two α- and two δ-chains ($\alpha_2\delta_2$). The final normal adult component is hemoglobin F (Hb F), fetal hemoglobin, which is present in concentrations of less than 1%, is composed of two pairs of α- and two pairs of γ-polypeptides, and is designated $\alpha_2\gamma_2$. Hemoglobin F is the major fetal and newborn hemoglobin component. During the neonatal period a switch occurs to Hb A synthesis, and γ-chain production is considerably reduced.

The capability of hemoglobin to function as a respiratory protein depends on its inherent molecular structure and three major interdependent properties. The first is oxygen affinity, generally expressed in terms of oxygen tension when the hemoglobin is 50% saturated (P_{50}). Oxygen affinity of normal hemoglobin rises with its increasing saturation. Oxygen affinity is influenced by and inversely proportional to the intracellular concentration of 2,3-DPG. The presence of 2,3-DPG facilitates oxygen unloading to the tissues by shifting the oxygen dissociation curve to the right. This is a major advantage under circumstances such as anemia, high altitude, and chronic hypoxia.

The next important characteristic of hemoglobin is its cooperative interactions, which produce a sigmoid-shaped oxygen dissociation curve. The sigmoidal oxygen dissociation curve reflects the successive binding of oxygen to each of the four iron atoms within the hemoglobin molecule and progressive affinity for this gas. The physiologic benefit of this curve form is obvious. For example, at the plateau portion of the curve, PO_2 levels from 70 to 100 mm Hg all result in nearly complete hemoglobin saturation, even at the lower oxygen partial pressures. Therefore maximal oxygen delivery occurs with a minimal change in oxygen tension.

The final salient feature of hemoglobin is the Bohr effect, the change in oxygen affinity with altered pH. As acidity increases, oxygen affinity is reduced, so that oxygen release is enhanced in the tissues with dropping pH and rising carbon dioxide or lactate levels. Conversely, within the lungs the increased pH that follows carbon dioxide excretion increases oxygen affinity and uptake.

In addition to the genetically determined, hereditary disorders of hemoglobin, analogous abnormalities also may be acquired. These deviations are hemoglobin A_1, a glycosylated, posttranslation hemoglobin observed in poorly controlled diabetes mellitus, iron deficiency, and azotemia, in which a hexose is bound to the amino terminal valine of the β-chains; increased Hb F in pregnancy, leukemia, aplastic anemia, and certain of the myeloproliferative disorders; elevated Hb A_2 in megaloblastic anemias; and lowered Hb A_2 in iron deficiency. Finally, hemoglobin H, a β-tetramer (β_4), may rise progressively during the evolution of erythroleukemia.

HEMOGLOBINOPATHIES. Hemoglobinopathies, of which sickle cell anemia is the first and prime example, are inherited as autosomal codominants. Heterozygotes called carriers have a proportionately greater concentration of normal hemoglobin but also have the abnormal hemoglobin present in each RBC. The simplest example of this is sickle cell trait, designated Hb AS. Since the genes that determine the structure of each hemoglobin polypeptide chain are alleles, a patient with sickle cell–Hb C disease, to cite another instance, acquires the sickle hemoglobin gene from one parent and the gene for Hb C from the other. The genotype for Hb S-C, then, would be written $\alpha^A\beta^S/\alpha^A\beta^C$, recognizing that both Hb S and Hb C are β-chain abnormalities. This is a double form of heterozygosity. A mixed heterozygote is one in which different, rather than the same, polypeptide chains are abnormal.

Sickle cell anemia

Definition and pathogenesis. Sickle cell anemia (SCA) is a homozygous, genetically determined hemolytic anemia caused by a mutation at a single point in the DNA codon that results in an mRNA coding for valine rather than the glutamic acid usually placed in the sixth position of the β-globin polypeptide. This genetic change leads to the synthesis of Hb S. The amino acid substitution forms the molecular basis for sickling observed when, at a PO_2 of 50 to 60 mm Hg, deoxyhemoglobin S first begins to undergo molecular alignment into spirally arranged, insoluble, fibrillar polymers, also called tactoids, that cause the hemoglobin to gel. This hemoglobin rearrangement distorts the RBC shape, increases cellular rigidity, and causes membrane damage with potentially irreversible sickling.

Such a sequence provokes a vicious circle of sickling, erythrostais, increased blood viscosity, reduced blood flow velocity, hypoxia, and further sickling. These events are compounded by the inherent diminished oxygen affinity of deoxyhemoglobin S, which itself augments sickling, and the local change to an acid pH, which also lowers oxygen affinity. All of these further advance gelation and sickling. The ability of the sickled RBC to pass through the microvasculature is impaired, producing vasocclusion, the protean manifestations of SCA, and its long-term and widespread organ damage. The recent demonstration that the sickled erythrocyte is more adherent than normal RBCs to the vascular endothelium suggests an additional mechanism for vascular obstruction.

Epidemiology and clinical manifestations. In Africa the Hb S gene is distributed in a broad equatorial belt and may reach an incidence of 40% in some mid-African tribes. In the United States the homozygous state producing a hemolytic anemia occurs in 1 of 600 blacks. The characteristic clinical features of SCA are the crises, which are acute, episodic manifestations superimposed on a chronic hemolytic state. These incidents add a new series of usually transient signs and symptoms. Crises may be classified as follows.

The first and most common is the *symptomatic, vasocclusive, or infarctive crisis*. This usually begins de novo or occasionally, as in children, may be provoked by an upper respiratory tract or other type of infection. It is the clinical outcome of the sickling phenomenon previously described and results from blood vessel obstruction by the rigid, tangled, sickled RBCs. The major symptom is pain, sometimes excruciating to the point of immobility. The patient may be jaundiced with fever, tachycardia, tachypnea, occasional hypertension, and abdominal tenderness with or without rigidity.

The next and less frequent crisis is the *hematopoietic crisis*, which may be *hemolytic* or *aplastic*. The former may be associated fortuitously with G6PD deficiency, may be provoked by infection, and may lead to active intravascular RBC destruction with all the clinical and laboratory features of abrupt diminution in the RBC mass. The aplastic or hypoplastic crisis is marked by sudden cessation of marrow function, worsening of the anemia, and reticulocytopenia.

The last type of crisis is the *sequestration syndrome*, occurring mainly in children and expressed as sudden, massive, painful enlargement of the liver and spleen and an acute fall in the hemoglobin level. This is a serious complication with a high morbidity and mortality.

Although not actually considered a form of crisis, in children a singular abnormality called the hand-foot syndrome or sickle cell dactylitis may develop, with painful, swollen, hot, tender hands and feet. It may be associated with fever, leukocytosis, and roentgenographic evidence of periostitis and osteolysis.

Symptoms of SCA usually begin during the second half of the first year of life as the amount of hemoglobin F progressively is reduced and supplanted by Hb S. SCA truly is a systemic disease. There is scarcely an organ system or body focus that is not touched by this hemoglobinopathy.

The central nervous system is damaged by thromboses that occur in the capillaries and the small and large arteries and veins can produce hemiplegia, convulsions, decreased consciousness, and visual disturbances. Intracranial and subarachnoid hemorrhage and spinal cord infarctions also occur. Conjunctival vessel tortuosity, vitreous hemorrhages, retinal detachment, microaneurysms, and chorioretinal infarction all may appear as ocular sequelae.

Cardiovascular involvement manifested as dyspnea, palpitations, and decreased exercise tolerance is not unusual. Precordial murmurs are heard frequently and may mimic those of mitral valve disease. These physical findings are in accord with roentgenographically demonstrable biventricular enlargement, prominence of the pulmonary artery conus, and electrocardiographic evidence of abnormalities in the right and left ventricles. Congestive heart failure may occur with aging.

Significant pulmonary disease and pulmonary hypertension evolve mainly because of infarction resulting from vasocclusion. Infection caused by the pneumococcus is common. Infarction and infection may occur separately or in combination and at times are hard to differentiate from one another, especially during a symptomatic crisis when patients are febrile and complain of chest pain. Gas exchange may be abnormal, and there may be ventilation-perfusion disparity as a result of intrapulmonary shunting.

Episodic abdominal pain is common and is related to microinfarction of the gastrointestinal tract. Gallbladder disease is often present in patients with SCA; 30% to 60% of the patients have cholelithiasis with radiolucent stones, but only 10% to 15% have signs and symptoms related to this abnormality. Elective cholecystectomy is not recommended, but the possibility of cholecystitis should always be considered in patients with SCA who enter the hospital with abdominal pain.

Hepatomegaly and liver dysfunction are extremely common. Liver enlargement is moderate and is seen in about 55% of the patients. Elevated liver enzymes, alkaline phosphatase, and bilirubin levels reflect the microinfarction, destruction, and regeneration of the hepatic parenchyma. These events actually are continuous even when the patients are in the supposed stable state without an overt crisis. Hepatitis and hemosiderosis, which may follow repeated blood transfusion, also contribute to liver damage.

Splenomegaly, sometimes with tenderness, is seen in 50% of the younger patients and is particularly prominent in the childhood sequestration crises described previously. As the disease continues, repetitive infarction and thrombosis diminish the size of the spleen, and it ultimately atrophies. Splenic hypofunction is not uncommon in adolescents and adults with SCA, as demonstrated by the presence of Howell-Jolly bodies in the peripheral blood. A consequence of reduced splenic activity is an increased tendency toward infection. In febrile adolescents and young adults an impalpable spleen may suddenly become enlarged, suggesting the presence of bacteremia and sepsis.

Renal disease has diverse presentations in SCA. These include hyposthenuria (the most common renal defect) hematuria, papillary necrosis, renal infarcts, the nephrotic syndrome, occasionally renal vein thrombosis, and inability to acidify the urine. The frequency of pyelonephritis may also be increased. In spite of functional impairment, end-stage renal failure is an unusual cause of death.

An additional urinary tract abnormality is priapism resulting from engorgement of the corpora cavernosa. Repeated microthromboses leading to fibrosis of the arteriovenous mechanism of penile erection may prevent detumescence.

Leg ulcerations, most commonly around the medial malleolus, are observed in 10% to 12% of the patients, mainly those who are younger. Lymphadenopathy occurs in a large proportion of patients with SCA and may be detected by careful examination.

Joint abnormalities in SCA include hemarthroses with or without hemosiderosis, gout, and avascular (aseptic) necrosis of the humerus and femur. Finger clubbing resulting from chronic anemia occurs in approximately 8% of the individuals with SCA. Bony infarcts caused by vascular obstruction are largely responsible for the pain in the symptomatic crises. The infarcts may be demonstrated by roentgenograms or radionuclide tracer studies. Bone marrow erythroid hyperplasia eventuates in widening of the diploë, frontal bossing, occasional maxillary overgrowth, and compression of the vertebrae with a central concavity leading to the fish-mouth appearance.

Pregnancy and SCA may interact. During the last trimester and the immediate postpartum period, congestive heart failure, thrombophlebitis, and pulmonary infarction or infection all may be observed. There is an increased incidence of toxemia, endometritis, spontaneous abortions, stillbirths, prematurity, and decreased infant viability.

Laboratory findings. The hemoglobin level ranges from 5 to 13 g/dl and does not change in the usual symptomatic crisis. The anemia is mainly normocytic and normochromic, but the mean corpuscular volume (MCV) may be diminished. During infection and aplasia the anemia may become more severe. The peripheral smear may show marked and diverse morphologic distortions. Basophilic stippling, nucleated RBCs, polychromasia, Howell-Jolly bodies, Cabot's rings, and Pappenheimer bodies (granules of hemosiderin) may be present. Reticulocytosis usually is sustained, and the reticulocyte count averages 5% to 10%. Reticulocytopenia may develop during infection or sepsis associated with an aplastic crisis. A constant leukocytosis of 12,000 to 15,000 cells/mm³ is common; this increases during a crisis to above 20,000 cells/mm³. The platelet level is often elevated; however, immediately before crises it may decrease. The bone marrow shows marked erythroid hyperplasia. Megaloblastosis also may appear because of an increased need for folic acid.

Diagnosis. SCA may be suspected in anemic patients with the proper racial background and sickled cells seen in the peripheral blood smear. The presumption should be supported by a screening test using sodium metabisulfite or the newer commercially available reagents. The definitive identification of the abnormal hemoglobin is made by hemoglobin electrophoresis.

Management and prognosis. Since there is no specific treatment for SCA, major attention should be given to managing the many complications of each organ injury, such as congestive heart failure. Anticoagulants are not routinely recommended for pulmonary infarcts. Infections in SCA should be treated aggressively with appropriate antibiotics based on bacteriologic culture data. Regardless of the number of times a patient has been admitted for what appears to be a febrile symptomatic crisis, a search for infection must never be neglected. Organisms producing disease with special frequency in SCA are *Streptococcus pneumoniae,* perhaps resulting from decreased serum opsonins and defective alternate complement pathway, and *Salmonella* organisms. The most common infections are bacteremia, pneumonia, meningitis, and osteomyelitis. *Salmonella* organisms are the most common cause of osteomyelitis in SCA.

Unfortunately, the treatment of acute crises still remains symptomatic, with pain controlled by the judicious use of narcotics. Patients given this type of therapy are potential drug addicts. Ordinary hydration to maintain adequate fluid balance and administration of oxygen are appropriate during crises. Folic acid, (1 mg daily) particularly in children, may prevent worsening of the anemia but does not raise the hemoglobin level beyond that dictated by the genetic code. Pneumococcal vaccine should be given as prophylaxis. Regular and continuing blood transfusions, as employed in thalassemia major, usually are not required. When a symptomatic crisis is extended, narcotic requirements are rising, or pain relief does not occur, limited isovolemic exchange transfusion usually terminates a particular episode. Although previously patients with sickle cell disease often died in childhood, they are currently living longer.

Newer approaches to the management of SCA are directed toward modifying the pathophysiology of intracellular sickling and the secondary changes occurring in the RBC membrane. Compounds such as Cetiedil, a peripheral vasodilator and relaxer of smooth muscle, may reduce potassium loss in adenosine triphosphate–depleted (ATP-depleted) and deoxygenated sickled RBCs. Cetiedil increases intracellular sodium and water, reduces calcium uptake, and lowers the concentration of hemoglobin S. Despite the speculated benefits of Cetiedil, its place in clinical treatment is unclear. Hydroxyurea (Hydrea) has been used in clinical trials because it raises the amount of fetal hemoglobin in the RBC and diminishes its sickling tendency. Calcium channel blockers and zinc salts also have been used prophylactically to treat SCA.

Sickle cell trait. Individuals heterozygous for Hb S have sickle cell trait. They have inherited one gene for the abnormal Hb S β-polypeptide and one determinant for the normal Hb A

β-chain. Heterozygosity is seen in 8% to 10% of blacks in the Western Hemisphere. This carrier state is innocuous except in the following circumstances. With marked reductions in oxygen tension, as may occur in the renal medulla, in vivo sickling of trait erythrocytes occurs. This may explain the renal abnormalities of hyposthenuria, spontaneous hematuria, and renal papillary necrosis. Most recently, von Willebrand's disease has been discovered in some of these patients and has been suggested as an auxiliary basis for their hematuria. Asymptomatic bacteriuria seems to be more frequent in women with sickle cell trait than in the general population. Aseptic necrosis rarely occurs in patients with sickle cell trait.

Sickle cell–hemoglobin C disease. Sickle cell–hemoglobin C or Hb S-C disease is a doubly heterozygous state in which the RBCs contain a mixture of Hb S and Hb C resulting from the inheritance of the S gene from one parent and the C gene from the other. The disease may be so mild as to be virtually asymptomatic and may be discovered only during routine screening procedures or physical examination. On the other hand, the presentation may be that of a mild form of SCA. In about half of the patients with symptoms the disease is detected during childhood, and in the remainder the disease is diagnosed as growth and development proceed through adolescence into adulthood.

General physical and sexual development is nearly normal. The most common complaint is focal or diffuse bone pain, with any portion of the skeleton involved. Of particular importance is the development of aseptic necrosis of the femoral head in a high proportion of these patients. Splenomegaly is detected in approximately two thirds of adults and may result in splenic infarction and the sequestration syndrome. Hepatomegaly, usually without clinical evidence of jaundice, is present in 40% of the cases. Proliferative retinal vascular disease and acute pulmonary infarction are frequently observed. Leg ulceration in 20% of the patients and hematuria also occur.

The hemoglobin level rarely is less than 10 g/dl, and reticulocytosis is modest. The RBCs generally are normocytic and normochromic, but the peripheral smear contains many target cells, rare sickle cells, and a variety of bizarrely shaped erythrocytes. The diagnosis is based on hemoglobin electrophoresis.

Hemoglobin C disease. In the Hb C defect, lysine replaces glutamic acid in the sixth position of the β-chain polypeptide. About 1 in 6000 American blacks has Hb C disease. Patients may be completely asymptomatic or complain of mild, intermittent abdominal pain and occasional arthralgia with periodic mild jaundice and occasional hematuria. Splenomegaly is fairly common. Cholelithiasis is not unusual. The hemoglobin level in Hb C disease may vary from 8 to 12 g/dl. Reticulocytosis, marrow erythroid hyperplasia, and a modest reduction in the erythrocyte life span all are part of the clinical complex. The peripheral RBCs are strikingly abnormal with a large proportion of target cells, microspherocytes, and occasional cells with intraerythrocytic crystals. Specific therapy is neither available nor required.

Thalassemias. The thalassemic syndromes are a group of hereditary hemoglobin disorders in which synthesis of one or more of the normal hemoglobin polypeptides is absent or reduced, causing decreased hemoglobinization of the erythrocytes, microcythemia, and hypochromia. Continued unbalanced synthesis of the normal globin chain, however, leads to its intracellular precipitation, altered flow characteristics of the RBCs, and their premature destruction. The last provides a significant hemolytic component to this group of erythrocyte abnormalities.

The thalassemias are classified according to the type of globin chain that is absent or present in decreased amount. Each thalassemia may occur in the homozygous or heterozygous form. The thalassemias and their principal features are listed in Tables 67-1 and 67-2.

β-thalassemias

Homozygous β-thalassemia. The homozygous β-thalassemia syndromes are observed most frequently within the Mediterrean basin, Middle East, Southeast Asia, India, Pakistan, and foci in West and North Africa. Actually, however, their distribution is worldwide, and they may appear sporadically in all racial groups, including whites of Northern European ancestry. The symbol β° in Table 67-1 denotes that protein synthesis from this affected genetic locus is totally absent, so that there is no Hb A in these patients' RBCs. Erythropoiesis is ineffective, leading to the severe disease known as Cooley's anemia or thalassemia major. Infants appear normal at birth, but anemia occurs during the first few months of life and becomes progressively severe. Physical growth and development are impaired. The physical features of prominent frontal bossing and cheekbones, maxillary overgrowth, and mongoloid facies all appear with time. Gallstones, leg ulcers, and skin pigmentation also are frequent complications. In addition to delayed sexual maturation, other endocrine disturbances such as hypoparathyroidism and hypoadrenalism develop. Later, diabetes mellitus and pigmentary infiltration of the myocardium and pericardium occur, resembling the changes of hemochromatosis. Intellectual development is not retarded.

Anemia is severe, with the hemoglobin level falling as low as 2 to 3 g/dl. The peripheral blood smear shows anisopoikilocytosis, target cells, microcythemia, hypochromia, polychromasia, and basophilic stippling. Poorly hemoglobinized normoblasts are seen in the peripheral blood with their number increasing markedly after splenectomy. Even when the anemia is severe, the reticulocyte count may not be very high because of ineffective erythropoiesis and massive intramedullary erythrocyte death. The bone marrow is very hypercellular with marked erythroid hyperplasia. Poorly hemoglobinized normoblasts appear as micronormoblasts. Occasionally, storage cells resembling Gaucher's cells are observed. If the bone marrow is examined under phase microscopy or stained with methyl violet, α-chain aggregates are visible as inclusion bodies in normoblasts. This may be used as a diagnostic test for homozygous β-thalassemia. Increased indirect hyperbilirubinemia and other evidence of hemolysis may be present. The total white blood cell and platelet counts may be mildly elevated unless hypersplenism has intervened. The hemoglobin pattern is described in Table 67-1.

In vitro data relative to the pathophysiology of β-thalassemia show that α-chain synthesis alone exceeds that of β, γ, and δ together. This leads to polypeptide imbalance and excess free α-chains that are present as inclusion bodies and are responsible for altered membrane behavior. Heme synthesis also is defective, probably as a result of diminished globin formation. Consequently, increased amounts of intracellular and mitochondrial iron are deposited, suppressing ATP regeneration. All the foregoing factors compound the ineffective erythropoiesis. There is an attempt to raise the hemoglobin level by the compensatory γ-chain synthesis, but this is never quite sufficient. The Hb F thus produced is distributed heterogeneously in the RBCs. In addition to inherently increased iron absorption, tissue iron storage is augmented further by autologous iron recycling resulting from hemolysis and by the repeated blood transfusions that are the mainstay of therapy in patients with thalassemia.

Roentgenographic changes consist of widening of the diploë, the "hair-on-end" appearance of the cranial vault, and increased trabeculation of the long bones and phalanges. All of these reflect medullary expansion that may lead to bony fractures. Additional complicating aspects of this disease are extramedullary hematopoiesis occurring as paraspinal or mediastinal masses, splenomegaly leading ultimately to hypersplenism, and bleeding, occasionally uncontrollable, resulting from hepatic dysfunction. Finally, deposition of iron in the myocar-

Table 67-1   Classification of the more common β-thalassemias*

Type of thalassemia	Parental genotype	Hemoglobin findings	Clinical designation and features
HOMOZYGOUS			
β°-Thalassemia	Both β°/β	Hb F, 10%-95% Hb A$_2$, variable	Thalassemia major (Cooley's anemia); pallor, jaundice, bony deformities, abnormal facies, hepatosplenomegaly; transfusion dependent; severe anemia with markedly abnormal RBC morphology
β⁺-Thalassemia	Both β⁺/β	Hb A, present but reduced; Hb F, 46%-80%; Hb A$_2$, variable	Thalassemia major (Cooley's anemia); pallor, hepatosplenomegaly, jaundice, anemia, and morphologic changes moderate; transfusions usually not required; in blacks may be less severe and resemble thalassemia intermedia
δβ-Thalassemia (high F)	Both δβ°/δβ	Absent Hb A and Hb A$_2$; Hb F, 100%	Thalassemia intermedia; mild jaundice, hepatosplenomegaly, anemia mild to moderate; moderate morphologic distortions; usually survival without transfusion
Hb Lepore	Both Hb Lepore/β	Absent Hb A and Hb A$_2$; Hb F, 75%; Hb Lepore, 25%	Thalassemia major (Cooley's anemia)
HETEROZYGOUS			
β°-Thalassemia	β°/β, normal	Hb A$_2$, 3.5%-7.5%; Hb F, 1%-6%	Ordinary or high Hb A$_2$ thalassemia (thalassemia minor); most common type; perhaps mild icterus and splenomegaly; anemia mild to moderate; microcythemia and hypochromia
β⁺-Thalassemia	β⁺/β, normal	As above	Thalassemia minor; physical findings usually absent; anemia absent to mild; microcythemia and hypochromia
δβ°-Thalassemia	δβ°/δβ, normal	Hb A$_2$, normal or low; Hb F, 5%-20%	Thalassemia minor; physical findings usually absent; anemia absent to mild; microcythemia and hypochromia
Hb Lepore	Hb Lepore/β, normal	Hb A, low or normal; Hb F, slightly elevated; Hb Lepore, 6%-15%	Thalassemia minor; resembles ordinary high Hb A$_2$ thalassemia

*Molecular defect complex.

Table 67-2   Classification of α-thalassemias

Type of thalassemia	Parental genotype	Hemoglobin findings	Molecular defects	Clinical designation and features
Homozygous α-thalassemia	Both α-thalassemia₁	Hb Bart's, 80%; rest Hb H and Hb Portland (an embryonic hemoglobin)	All α genes deleted	Lethal hydrops fetalis; hepatosplenomegaly, heart failure, stillbirth, or death within 24 hours; RBC hypochromia, anisopoikilocytosis, severe anemia
Hb H disease	α-Thalassemia trait/ silent carrier	Hb H, 4%-30% in adults; Hb Bart's, 25% in cord blood	Three of four genes gone, marked deficiency of α-chain synthesis	Variable severity; thalassemia intermedia; microcythemia and hypochromia
	α-Thalassemia trait/Hb CS heterozygote	When CS gene present, 2%-3% Hb Cs	Two of four genes gone; one normal, one Hb CS gene	
Heterozygous α-thalassemia 1	α-Thalassemia trait/ normal	Normal in adults; Hb Bart's, 5%-15% in newborn	Two of four genes gone on same chromosome*	Clinically mild; very mild in blacks†
Heterozygous α-thalassemia 2	Silent carrier/normal	Normal in adults; Hb Bart's, 1%-2% in newborn	One of four genes gone	Neither anemia nor RBC morphologic abnormalities
Heterozygous Hb CS	Hb CS heterozygote/ normal	Hb CS, 1%	Three of four genes present; one Hb CS gene	Silent

Hb CS, Hemoglobin Constant Spring.
*See text.

dium and pericardium, which ultimately leads to congestive cardiomyopathy and heart failure, plays a major role in the decreased longevity of these patients.

Another form of homozygous thalassemia is designated in Table 67-1 by the symbol β +. This denotes that, in contrast to the previously described thalassemia in which β-chain production is totally absent, some synthesis of β-polypeptides does occur in this form of thalassemia. The capacity for β-chain synthesis is stable within families but shows a family-to-family variation. Thus the molecular defect in β + -thalassemia demonstrates considerable heterogeneity. The clinical expression of β + -thalassemia is somewhat less severe than classic thalassemia major or Cooley's anemia, but it may nevertheless resemble the latter. β + -Thalassemia may be appreciably less destructive in blacks than in whites and may be considered a form of thalassemia intermedia. The features of this syndrome are shown in Table 67-1.

Heterozygous thalassemias. Table 67-1 indicates that the thalassemias also may be present in the heterozygous form. This occurs when only a single β-thalassemia mutation is inherited, resulting clinically in the thalassemic trait or thalassemia minor. In this instance hemoglobin synthesis depends largely on the compensatory capacity of the normal β-globin gene in the trans position, that is, on the noninvolved, opposite chromosome. Usually it is capable of a limited, increased output of β-chains, and developing RBCs accumulate approximately 75% of the normal amount of Hb A. However, the marrow responds to this reduction in Hb A synthesis by producing a larger number of smaller-than-normal RBCs. This is observed as the classic hypochromia and microcythemia of the β-thalassemia trait. Since δ-chain synthesis also is relatively, and sometimes absolutely, increased, the percentage of Hb A₂ is elevated unless the gene is deleted or otherwise abnormal.

Complications and the management of the thalassemias. The thalassemic syndromes are preventable by genetic counseling of documented heterozygous prospective parents and antenatal study of fetuses. Active treatment is necessary mainly in homozygous and severe heterozygous forms and is basically supportive, since specific therapy does not exist.

One line of therapy is regular blood transfusion to produce hematocrit levels between 33% and 35%, which helps normalize patient growth and development, suppresses ineffective erythropoiesis, reduces iron absorption, and helps prevent bony abnormalities. However, this therapy has the disadvantage of organ iron loading, which is only partially ameliorated by desferrioxamine chelation. Repeated blood transfusions also may produce bleeding syndromes caused by hepatic dysfunction, endocrinopathies, and progressive splenomegaly with hypersplenism. Increasing splenic enlargement may aggravate the anemia, actually augment the transfusion requirements by causing sequestration of transfused RBCs, and produce pancytopenia. Splenectomy may eliminate these adverse transfusion effects. Because splenectomy promotes the hazard of infection, particularly in young children, it is prudent to delay this operation at least until the patient is older than 5 years of age. The availability of the pneumococcal vaccine makes this surgery somewhat less worrisome.

Hereditary persistence of fetal hemoglobin. In hereditary persistence of fetal hemoglobin (HPFH) the synthesis of relatively large amounts of fetal hemoglobin persists into adult life without major hematologic abnormalities. HPFH is a heterogeneous entity expressing itself with some diversity in several ethnic groups. It is inherited as a single autosomal codominant, closely linked or allelic to the gene determining the structure of the β-chain itself in the β-thalassemia gene. In black homozygotes who are clinically well, 100% of the hemoglobin is Hb F, distributed homogeneously in the small, poorly hemoglobinized peripheral erythrocyte, with total absence of β- and δ-polypeptide synthesis. In black heterozygotes Hb F ranges from 20% to 35%. Additional patterns are observed in the Greek, Swiss, and English variants.

HEMOLYSIS CAUSED BY ACQUIRED ABNORMALITIES
Immunohemolytic anemias

Erythrocyte destruction in the immunohemolytic anemias is immunogenic. If the anemia is caused by specific RBC antibodies, as occurs in transfusion reactions and hemolytic disease of the newborn (HDN), it is called *isoimmune* or *alloimmune*. If the anemia is due to the selective deposition of certain self-produced immunoglobulins and complement on the RBC, the anemia is considered autoimmune. Transfusion reactions are discussed in Chapter 70.

HEMOLYTIC DISEASE OF THE NEWBORN

Definition and pathogenesis. HDN is caused by the transplacental entry of IgG antibodies into the fetal circulation following isoimmunization of the mother against the infant's RBCs, which contain an antigen foreign to her. This results in the coating of the fetal erythrocytes with antibody and thereby hemolysis in the infant. In Rh hemolytic disease the most common offender is the Rh_0 (D) antigen. Incompatibilities provoked by C, E, and Kell antigens also occur. Immunization by the ABO antigen group, although more common than Rh hemolytic disease of the newborn, is not as important clinically because it results in disease of far less severity.

Initial maternal immunization takes place most commonly during the last half of pregnancy and at delivery as small numbers of fetal RBCs escape through the placenta and enter the mother's bloodstream. A prior blood transfusion with Rh-positive RBCs or an abortion may serve the same immunizing purpose. A later challenge as small as 0.1 ml of RBCs produces anamnestic antibody that becomes available to react against fetal erythrocytes during subsequent gestations.

Clinical manifestations. Hepatosplenomegaly, jaundice, generalized edema (hydrops fetalis), congestive heart failure, bone marrow erythroid hyperplasia, the release of nucleated RBCs into the peripheral blood, and progressive anemia if destruction exceeds marrow compensation all may occur, depending on the level of maternal immunization. However, the principal danger to the live-born neonate lies in the accumulation of unconjugated bilirubin, which occurs because the protective effect of the placenta, the organ responsible for removing excess bilirubin, is no longer present. The neonatal liver is not able to conjugate and excrete bilirubin effectively. When the amount of unconjugated bilirubin exceeds the albumin-binding capacity, the unbound, unconjugated bilirubin diffuses into the central nervous system. Kernicterus that often is fatal or produces permanent brain damage results.

Laboratory findings. Babies with HDN look well at birth when the cord hemoglobin level may be only at the lower limits of normal (14 g/dl). Icterus usually develops during the first 24 hours of life. Bilirubin levels of 4 mg/dl suggest severe disease, and levels up to 40 to 50 mg/dl may be reached. The hemoglobin level begins to fall during the first 24 hours of life and thereafter may drop at a rate of 3 g/day. Microcythemia and polychromasia are marked. Spherocytosis is found only in ABO-related HDN and not in that caused by anti-Rh antibodies. The reticulocyte count may be as high as 60%. There is a great increase in peripheral blood nucleated RBCs, hence the term "erythroblastosis." Leukocytosis may be pronounced, and counts in excess of 30,000 cells/mm³, especially in severely affected infants, have been reported. The platelet level is usually normal but may be depressed in severe disease.

Diagnosis. Laboratory investigation of suspected HDN should begin with antenatal titers of the mother's blood for anti-Rh antibodies. A baseline titer should be measured at 16 weeks' gestation, followed by a second titer at 28 to 32 weeks, and subsequent assays at intervals of 1 to 4 weeks, depending on the rate of increase. If the titer rise shows evidence of possible HDN in utero, the suspicion may be verified by antenatal examination of the amniotic fluid spectrophotometrically for levels of bilirubin-like catabolic products.

The immediate diagnosis of anti-Rh HDN at birth is by a positive direct Coombs' test of cord RBCs using an anti-IgG reagent. Most infants also show a positive indirect Coombs' reaction.

Management. If there is risk of hydrops fetalis, the standard procedure is intrauterine and intraperitoneal transfusions followed by induced labor at 34 weeks. For a baby with documented and overt HDN, exchange transfusion using blood compatible with the mother's serum is the proper treatment. Guidelines for this are a hemoglobin level of 13 g/dl or less and a serum bilirubin level higher than 4 mg/dl. An alternative form of management, especially in ABO incompatibility, is phototherapy using a blue light that converts indirect bilirubin into water-soluble products excreted in the bile and urine. Finally, IgG anti-D antibody should be given at delivery to Rh-negative mothers who deliver Rh-positive infants and to all Rh-negative women who have abortions unless the father of the fetus is known to be Rh negative.

AUTOIMMUNE HEMOLYTIC ANEMIAS. The autoimmune hemolytic anemias (AIHA) may be divided into those caused by warm-reacting antibodies, usually involving IgG (and sometimes complement), and those caused by cold-reacting antibodies, invariably mediated by IgM and complement.

Warm-reacting autoimmune hemolytic anemia

Etiology and pathogenesis. Incomplete antibodies of many different specificities, functional at 98.6° F (37° C) or close to this physiologic thermal point, have been incriminated in the pathogenesis of warm-reacting AIHA. Erythrocyte destruction is the hallmark of this disease. Premature RBC removal may be generated, in part, by the attachment of the IgG to the RBC. This occurs with the Fc portion of the immunoglobulin molecule protruding outward from the cell surface, an arrangement permitting the splenic and the liver macrophage to hold the coated RBC and ultimately to destroy it. Complement (C3) probably also is present on the red RBC perimeter and may be a stronger attractant for the monocyte and macrophage receptor than the IgG itself.

This form of hemolytic anemia is recognized under three primary circumstances. First is its de novo occurrence in approximately 25% to 30% of the patients, especially young women, without any obvious predisposing cause. The second and more common presentation (about 50% of instances) results from the lymphoproliferative disorders, mainly chronic lymphocytic leukemia. The remaining patients with warm-reacting AIHA are those with the connective tissue disorders, especially systemic lupus erythematosus. AIHA may also be found associated with immunodeficiency disorders, drug reactions, other malignant tumors, inflammatory bowel syndromes, and liver diseases.

Clinical manifestations. The clinical characteristics depend on the underlying disease provoking the inappropriate, mainly extravascular RBC destruction and the level of anemia. Jaundice and pallor may be evident on physical examination. Splenomegaly occurs in more than half of the patients, and hepatomegaly also may occur.

Laboratory findings and diagnosis. The degree of anemia and reticulocytosis is variable. The peripheral smear shows macrocytes, polychromasia, anisopoikilocytosis, microspherocytes, and nucleated RBCs in differing proportions and combinations. A mild leukocytosis also may be observed. There is predominantly indirect hyperbilirubinemia with levels between 2.5 and 5 mg/dl. Although the hemolysis is mainly extravascular, the serum haptoglobin level may be depressed. The bone marrow demonstrates erythroid hyperplasia.

The diagnosis is made by a positive direct Coombs' reaction obtained first with broad-spectrum screening and thereafter with a more specific reagent. The immunoreactant coating the RBC may reflect the primary disease with which the anemia is associated. The differing disorders produce certain characteristic serologic reactivity patterns. Coombs' test in idiopathic AIHA and that caused by the lymphoproliferative disorders is positive for IgG with or without complement and rarely for complement alone. On the other hand, Coombs' test in systemic lupus erythematosus is never positive only against IgG but is reactive with complement alone or combined with the immunoglobulin.

Management. Warm-reacting AIHA is treated first with 1 mg/kg prednisone in three or four divided daily doses because single doses are ineffective under acute circumstances. Initial improvement, signaled by reduced reticulocytosis and a rising hemoglobin level, occurs within the first 2 weeks in approximately 50% of the patients with de novo or connective tissue–related hemolysis. After 3 to 4 weeks the steroids are reduced gradually over a similar period to avoid recurrence. Treatment of a specific disease is an obvious concurrent necessity. Transfusions are used during the acute hemolytic episode only in a life-threatening emergency because of the difficulty in obtaining complete cross-match compatibility.

Patients who do not show a respone to prednisone and do not have a treatable underlying disease are considered for splenectomy. If surgery also is unsuccessful, immunosuppressive agents such as azathioprine or cyclophosphamide may be tried. However, these drugs are teratogenic and oncogenic, and their efficacy is erratic and unpredictable.

Cold-reacting autoimmune hemolytic anemia. Immunohemolytic anemias caused by cold-reacting antibodies are those in which the humoral reactants are characterized by their ability to coat RBCs at temperatures below 98.6° F (37° C), their dissociation from the binding site when the temperature rises to that of the body, and their production of agglutination and/ or hemolysis. Cold agglutinins cause two major clinical disorders, the cold agglutinin syndrome and paroxysmal cold hemoglobinuria.

Cold agglutinin syndromes. Cold agglutinins originate in association with certain infections, most commonly those caused by *Mycoplasma pneumoniae,* cytomegalovirus, and Epstein-Barr virus. These antibodies are polyclonal, most frequently of the IgM and rarely of the IgA or IgG class, with specificity directed against the I-i and Pr groups of RBC antigens. Monoclonal cold agglutinins with I-i specificity may be found in patients with malignant diseases such as the lymphoproliferative disorders and gastric and ovarian carcinomas. Finally, IgM monoclonal cold agglutinins may arise de novo without obvious cause, leading to the chronic, idiopathic cold agglutinin syndrome.

Cold agglutinins do not react with RBCs at temperatures of 89.7° F (32° C) or higher but may induce injury within the range of 50° to 89.7° F (10° to 32° C). Subsequent RBC destruction may evolve in more than one way. The first occurs when the IgM antibody attaches to the RBC at lower temperatures and simultaneously fixes complement (C) to the cell membrane. At higher temperatures, which the erythrocyte meets as it comes from distal body sites (nose, fingers, and toes) and enters the core circulation, IgM is disengaged and C fixation occurs with potential activation of the complement attack unit (C5 through C9). If this sequence is completed and there is enough complement on the RBC surface, intravascular hemolysis follows. Usually this does not occur, because there is complement adequate only for RBC sequestration via the C3b receptor in the reticuloendothelial system. This produces rapid removal by Kupffer's cells and the extravascular means for reduction of RBC longevity. RBCs also are phagocytosed by the spleen.

The RBC, however, may be held only transiently by the macrophage and released by serum C3 inactivator. This protects the RBC mass from progressive destruction and additional phagocytosis. These immunologic features partially explain the comparative benignity of the cold agglutinins.

CLINICAL MANIFESTATIONS. The signs and symptoms frequently are those of the underlying disease. With infection, clinically overt hemolysis is most unusual despite the high cold agglutinin titers that peak at about 2 to 3 weeks after the onset of the illness. Cold-related hemolysis is not ordinarily a major manifestation of lymphoid neoplasms.

Chronic idiopathic cold agglutinin disease produces a chronic hemolytic anemia that occurs predominantly in the sixth through the eighth decades, although it may occur in patients in their twenties and thirties. The disorder is accompanied by mild hepatosplenomegaly, milk jaundice, and, predominantly, circulatory changes of acrocyanosis. This phenomenon is caused by intravascular RBC agglutination taking place in the cooler distal body parts. These may turn purple and be painful, with rapid reversion to normal on rewarming. Repetitive episodes may lead to local tissue destruction and necrosis. With sudden exposure to severe chilling, fever, chills, hemoglobinemia, hemoglobinuria, and renal failure may occur.

LABORATORY FINDINGS. The degree of anemia varies, with hemoglobin levels infrequently below 7 g/dl. The total serum bilirubin rarely exceeds 3 g/dl. Serum complement may be decreased, especially if hemolysis is acute and severe. Serum cold agglutinin titers, which normally are measurable up to a 1:64 dilution, may vary from 1:1000 to 1:1,000,000. Coombs' test specific for complement components is positive.

MANAGEMENT. Treatment of acute cold agglutinin disease rarely is necessary, since the disease is usually self-limited. Occasionally, with excessive hemolysis, transfusions with washed RBCs are needed. Problems in typing and cross-matching may be encountered. In unusual situations when hemolysis is fulminant, exchange transfusion is applied.

Splenectomy and the administration of adrenal corticosteroids have little value. Alkylating agents, theoretically the most rational approach to suppress antibody synthesis, have been successful mainly during the treatment of lymphoid malignancies. Idiopathic chronic cold agglutinin disease is treated primarily by avoiding exposure to low temperatures.

Paroxysmal cold hemoglobinuria. The rarest form of immunohemolytic anemia, paroxysmal cold hemoglobinuria (PCH), is characterized by sudden, episodic hemoglobinuria occurring after local or general body exposure to the cold. The cause of this syndrome is the Donath-Landsteiner (D-L) antibody identified as an IgG antibody, which acts as an extremely potent hemolysin, sometimes even in relatively low concentrations. It is frequently directed against the P antigen held by nearly all RBCs. The antibody is described classically as biphasic because it unites avidly with RBCs at lower temperatures (32° to 59° F [0° to 15° C]), and then hemolyzes them when the temperature of the reacting mixture moves closer to or reaches that of the body. The hemolytic sequence in the peripheral circulation consists of sensitization of the RBC with IgG and complement at low temperature, elution of IgG on warming, and hemolysis following activation of the entire complement cascade. Initially, the IgG also may cause RBC agglutination.

Previously the disease was thought to be associated primarily with congenital or tertiary syphilis, but this seems rare nowadays. More commonly, it occurs during the course of acute viral infections, especially in children with measles or mumps, or may arise without any apparent preceding disease or event.

CLINICAL MANIFESTATIONS. The syndrome, usually mild,

may be life threatening, particularly in children after viral infections. There is striking passage of dark-brown or black urine after local or general exposure to cold. Lethargy, pallor, and fatigue may follow the acute attack, and icterus may be clinically apparent. Hepatosplenomegaly also may be present. The disease may become chronic in patients who are continually exposed to cold, and a persistent hemolytic anemia may evolve thereafter.

LABORATORY FINDINGS AND DIAGNOSIS. A massive hemolytic episode may cause hemoglobinuria and hemoglobinemia. Other pigments resulting from intravascular hemolysis, such as met-hemalbumin, and moderate, indirect hyperbilirubinemia also may be detectable. The RBCs appear normal on peripheral blood smear. Occasionally, erythrophagocytosis and immature leukocytes are visible in the peripheral blood.

During an acute attack the direct Coombs' test with a complement-specific reagent is positive. The diagnosis is established by demonstrating supernatant hemolysis in RBC suspensions that have been chilled in ice and subsequently warmed to 98.6° F (37° C).

MANAGEMENT. Aside from treating syphilis, specific therapy is unavailable. Acute hemolytic episodes during infections are self-limited. In chronic PCH, avoidance of exposure to cold is the most prudent and practical approach. Adrenal corticosteroids have not been beneficial, and immunosuppressive agents are both toxic and relatively untried.

Traumatic hemolytic anemias and red blood cell fragmentation syndromes

When RBCs are subjected to excessive physical trauma within the cardiovascular system, they may undergo premature fragmentation and lysis because undue shear stress is placed on them and the elastic limits of their membranes are exceeded. In an abnormal environment progressive membrane deformation leads to eventual membrane rupture. Syndromes produced as the result of these events are fragmentation hemolysis associated with abnormalities of the heart and great vessels and RBC destruction related to small-vessel disease, so-called microangiopathic hemolytic anemia.

CARDIOVASCULAR ANOMALIES. Hemolysis may be produced by many types of valvular prostheses; valvular heart disease per se, especially aortic valve abnormalities; arteriovenous fistulas; and aortic coarctation. Early erythrocyte death is due mainly to turbulence and secondarily to direct trauma to the erythrocyte caused by impact on an abnormal natural or artificial vascular structure. Hemolysis rises as patient activity and the cardiac output increase. A vicious circle of greater hemolysis, more severe anemia, augmented cardiac hyperkinesis, and progressive anemia is the outcome.

The severity of the anemia varies. The peripheral RBCs usually are normocytic and normochromic, although microcythemia and polychromasia with brisk reticulocytosis may be seen if the hemolysis is active. Morphologic evidence of trauma with a variety of bizarre RBC forms also may be observed. With prolonged hemolysis, hemosiderinuria and hypochromia resulting from iron deficiency may develop. Elevations of bilirubin, lactate dehydrogenase (LDH), and methemalbumin and decreased serum haptoglobin also are found.

If the anemia is stable and tolerated by the patient and the bone marrow provides an acceptable degree of compensation, the treatment may be with iron and other hematinic agents such as folic acid. Otherwise, management may require valve replacement or other appropriate operative procedures, since these syndromes usually do not improve spontaneously. Rarely hypersplenism develops, and splenectomy may be necessary.

MICROANGIOPATHIC HEMOLYSIS. Hemolysis resulting from irregularities in the microcirculation is associated with thrombotic thrombocytopenic purpura (TTP); the hemolytic-uremic syndrome; disseminated intravascular coagulation (DIC); pregnancy with eclampsia, preeclampsia, and the postpartum hemolytic syndrome; immunogenic vasculitides, as are present in the collagen disorders; renal homograft rejection and glomerulonephritis; vascular anomalies such as the giant cavernous hemangiomas (Kasabach-Merritt syndrome); disseminated carcinomatosis; oral contraceptives; and malignant hypertension.

The adverse effects in microangiopathic hemolytic anemia are related to changes in the RBCs as they course through a fibrin mesh network under applied pressure, which leads to their incisional sectioning and ultimate fragmentation. Release of abnormally shaped residual elements follows. A second mechanism operates when there is a direct vascular lesion. RBC fragmentation then is thought to result from shearing stress applied to the erythrocytes by the forceful column of arterial blood as it moves past RBCs attached to an inflamed, proliferative, and distorted endothelium.

The manifestations of and suspicion for a microangiopathic hemolytic anemia depend on the underlying process responsible for the patient's clinical presentation. Diagnostic support is provided by demonstrating schistocytes and other RBC irregularities in the peripheral blood. The treatment depends largely on the management of the basic disease.

MARCH HEMOGLOBINURIA. March hemoglobinuria is a hemolytic disorder caused by injury to normal RBCs within the microcirculation of certain body parts as they forcefully strike hard surfaces. It is detected in marathon runners, karate experts, pelota players, bongo drummers, and patients who hit their heads repeatedly during unusual emotional behavior. It is most probably due to mechanical disruption of the circulating RBCs, producing intravascular hemolysis and resulting hemoglobinuria.

The clinical findings usually are insignificant. Transient hemoglobinuria after exertion is the only complaint. Mild jaundice may be present. Nausea and muscle aching may occur early in the episode.

Anemia is very uncommon. The peripheral blood smear shows only polychromasia with a mild reticulocytosis. The serum bilirubin level does not exceed 2 mg/dl, although the serum LDH level may be elevated. Albuminuria and abnormalities of the urinary sediment occasionally have been noted, but chronic renal disease is rare. The disorder occurs most commonly at the beginning of an exercise program and often remits spontaneously despite continuation of activity.

Paroxysmal nocturnal hemoglobinuria

DEFINITION. Paroxysmal nocturnal hemoglobinuria (PNH; Marchiafava-Micheli syndrome) is an uncommon, acquired intrinsic disorder of the erythrocyte membrane characterized by chronic hemolysis, intermittent but persistent hemoglobinuria and hemosiderinuria, thrombotic phenomena, and bone marrow hypoplasia.

ETIOLOGY AND PATHOGENESIS. The disease supposedly evolves from a defective bone marrow stem cell clone producing several RBC populations that vary in their sensitivity to activated complement components. This diverse vulnerability permits division of the disease into three clinical subgroups, with progressive severity depending on the inherent hemolytic features of the erythrocyte. Increased complement susceptibility, greatest among the youngest circulating erythrocytes, occurs via the classic, antibody-activated, C1-

dependent pathway, as well as through the alternate, properdin-dependent complement route in an acidified medium. The RBCs are deficient in a membrane regulator protein known as decay-accelerating factor, which modulates the severity of hemolysis.

CLINICAL MANIFESTATIONS. PNH may be benign or aggressive and debilitating. In its classic form it is a hemolytic anemia of insidious onset without racial, familial, or sexual predilection, most frequently surfacing in the third and fourth decades but occasionally manifesting first during childhood. Rather than beginning abruptly with nocturnal hemoglobinuria, the disease may initially be indicated by general signs and symptoms of anemia. Episodic hemoglobinuria actually occurs in only 25% of instances. It is sleep related, since the hemolytic pattern is reversible if the patient sleeps by day rather than during the night. The nocturnal exacerbations, followed by morning excretion of dark urine, may be related to mild reduction in blood pH. Hemolysis, however, also may follow infection, strenuous exercise, or other events such as surgery, menstruation, blood transfusion, and therapeutic ingestion of iron. Symptoms that may be associated with hemolysis are bone and muscle aching, malaise, and fever.

The tendency toward spontaneous intravascular thromboses, perhaps caused by the release of RBC thromboplastins, may produce abdominal pain with obstruction of the mesenteric, portal, or hepatic veins. Obstruction in the last site, which is especially frequent, is associated with sudden hepatomegaly and ascites and may be fatal. Headache caused by cerebrovascular occlusions is a common complaint. Infections are relatively frequent and may be ascribed to qualitative and quantitative neutrophil abnormalities. Additional findings during the patient's clinical course are pallor, jaundice, bronzing of the skin, and splenomegaly.

PNH or a variant may be associated with aplastic anemia, preleukemia, myeloproliferative disorders, and overt leukemia. These combinations support the perception that PNH is one of several myelodysplastic syndromes.

LABORATORY FINDINGS. The anemia may be severe with hemoglobin levels of 6 g/dl or less. Anisocytosis is observed with hypochromia and microcythemia caused by prolonged hemosiderinuria. A relative reticulocytosis, which actually is low in absolute terms, may be present. The bone marrow most often is hyperplastic, but hypoplasia and even aplasia evolve during some stage of the disease. Leukopenia, low levels of leukocyte alkaline phosphatase, and thrombocytopenia all may be found. Coombs' test is negative. The serum LDH level may be elevated, and the haptoglobin level may be reduced. Hemosiderinuria is detected easily, a process that leads to renal tubular iron deposition and proximal tubular dysfunction.

DIAGNOSIS. The diagnosis, which should be considered in any patient with a puzzling hemolytic anemia, iron deficiency, pancytopenia, splenomegaly, and thrombotic episodes, is based on special tests that challenge the RBCs' resistance to small amounts of complement.

MANAGEMENT. Since there is no specific treatment, management is directed toward the symptoms. If blood transfusions become necessary, saline-washed or, better still, thawed frozen deglycerolized packed RBCs should be used, since fresh donor plasma may accelerate hemolysis. Therapeutic administration of iron may precipitate hemolysis by causing membrane peroxidation or the release of young, susceptible RBCs into the circulation. It should be given after transfusion-suppressed erythropoiesis. Androgens also have been recommended. Heparin and the coumarin-type anticoagulants may be useful on a limited, short-term basis during surgery, parturition, or acute

episodes when progressive, diffuse hepatic thrombosis is suspected. Adrenal corticosteroids have modified hemolysis in a few patients, particularly in those rare instances associated with a positive Coombs' test. They should be given to patients with otherwise unmanageable signs and symptoms. Splenectomy carries a high morbidity and postoperative mortality. Bone marrow transplantation may become an option in the future.

Hemolytic anemias caused by drugs

IMMUNE HEMOLYSIS. Drug-related immune hemolytic anemias fall into three categories. In the first type the drugs act as antigens only when bound to plasma proteins and stimulate antibodies mainly of the IgM class. Antigen-antibody (immune) complexes form and adsorb to the RBC surface while simultaneously fixing and activating complement. Drugs frequently associated with this innocent bystander reaction are quinidine, quinine, thorazine, phenacetin, chlorpropamide, para-aminosalicylic acid, and stibophen. The patient need take only a small quantity of the drug for acute intravascular hemolysis, hemoglobinemia, hemoglobinuria, and renal failure to occur. Thrombocytopenia may also be observed occasionally. The direct Coombs' test is positive as a result of the presence of surface complement components. The immune complex does not bind very firmly to the RBCs, usually dissociates, and becomes free to react with other cells and extend hemolysis.

In the second form of drug-related hemolysis, caused mainly by penicillin, the drug forms a hapten with the RBC itself, resulting in elaboration of a high-titer IgG antibody directed against the erythrocyte-penicillin complex. Typically, hemolysis develops only in patients receiving very large intravenous doses of penicillin, at least 10 million units daily, for more than 1 week. The anemia commonly is less acute in onset than that caused by drugs of the prior group, RBC destruction is mainly extravascular, and complement is not a major, active ingredient. Although this form of anemia is comparatively benign, it may be lethal if the hemolytic episode goes unrecognized and drug administration is continued. The direct gamma (IgG) Coombs' test is strongly positive. Complete recovery usually follows drug withdrawal, but hemolysis of decreasing severity may persist for several weeks thereafter.

The third type of drug-related hemolytic anemia involves an IgG antibody resembling that of warm-reacting autoimmune hemolytic anemias. The direct IgG Coombs' test is positive in 5% to 15% of the patients taking methyldopa (Aldomet), with the highest incidence in whites, lower frequency in Asians, and the reaction almost absent in blacks. The anemia appears after 3 to 6 months of treatment, with the positive Coombs' test showing dose dependence. Approximately three times more patients taking more than 2 g of the drug daily have a positive Coombs' test compared with patients receiving less than 1 g. Similar antibodies have been observed in patients taking levodopa and mefenamic acid. Splenomegaly may occur. The frequency of overt hemolysis in those receiving methyldopa varies from none to 5%, with the general average approximately 0.8%. The hemolysis is usually extravascular but may be intravascular if RBC sensitization is especially great. Occasional fatalities have been described in this anemia. The anemia resolves spontaneously after the drug is discontinued. Coombs' test may remain positive for up to a year after the drug is discontinued and during resolution of the anemia and hemolysis.

NONIMMUNE HEMOLYSIS. In addition to hemolysis generated by oxidant and immune injury and hemoglobin dissociation, as described earlier, certain substances may be toxic by membrane injury or destruction. These include alcohols, steroids, general anesthetics, nonionic detergents, antihistamines, antimalarials, tranquilizers, neuroleptics, antidepressants, local anesthetics, organic and acidic compounds such as phenytoin, barbiturates, and fatty acids. They may produce stomatocytes and acanthocytes.

Anemias related to antineoplastic agents. Anemias associated with or caused by compounds used to treat malignancies may be grouped as follows:

1. *Microangiopathic hemolytic anemias.* These are caused by mitomycin, cisplatin (Platinol), bleomycin, and the vinca alkaloids. The drugs damage the vascular endothelium, which causes injury to the RBCs and ultimately hemolysis.
2. *Immunohemolytic anemias.* This type of anemia occurs with chlorambucil and other alkylating drugs, 5-fluorouracil, teniposide, methotrexate, and cisplatin. Anemia and accelerated RBC destruction may depend on IgG- or IgM-sensitizing antibodies with or without the presence of complement coating the erythrocyte surface.
3. *Other anemias.* Hemolysis with daunorubicin, augmented by G6PD deficiency, occurs as a result of the generation of reactive oxygen compounds and methemoglobin. Hemolysis observed with pentostatin (deoxycoformycin) can be acute and may be dependent on reduced erythrocyte ATP levels.

Hemolysis resulting from other causes

TOXINS, CHEMICALS, AND POISONS. Phospholipase in snake and spider venoms may cause hemolysis by releasing membrane phospholipids. Heavy metals such as copper may produce the hemolytic anemia in Wilson's disease by binding to sulfhydryl membrane groups. Zinc and chloramines also have been implicated in hemolysis.

METABOLIC AND RELATED ABNORMALITIES. Hemolysis may occur in liver failure and with alcoholism. The latter may result from the altered membrane cholesterol/phospholipid ratio, as in spur cell anemia. Premature RBC destruction may also be observed in renal failure and in hypophosphatemia. Low serum phosphate levels may reduce erythrocyte ATP synthesis and cause increased membrane rigidity.

INFECTIONS. RBC injury and removal from the circulation may follow infection caused by microorganisms such as gram-positive cocci, gram-negative bacilli, clostridia, and protozoa (plasmodia, *Babesia, Leishmania,* and *Toxoplasma*). The effects are probably caused by direct membrane injury.

BIBLIOGRAPHY
Congenital hemolytic anemias

Beutler E: Red cell enzyme defects as nondiseases and diseases, Blood 54:1, 1979.
Brody JI, Levison SP, and Jung CJ: Sickle cell trait and hematuria associated with von Willebrand syndromes, Ann Intern Med 86:529, 1977.
Brody JI and others: Sickle cell crisis treated by limited exchange transfusion, Ann Intern Med 72:327, 1970.
Dean J and Schechter AN: Sickle cell anemia: molecular and cellular basis of therapeutic approaches, N Engl J Med 299:752, 804, 863, 1978.
Elgsaeter A, Stokke BT, Mikkelsen A, and Branton B: The molecular basis of erythrocyte shape, Science 234:1217, 1986.
Higgs DR and others: The interaction of alpha-thalassemia and homozygous sickle-cell disease, N Engl J Med 306:1441, 1982.
Huisman THJ: Sickle cell anemia as a syndrome: a review of diagnostic features, Am J Hematol 6:173, 1979.
Huntsman RG and Lehmann H: Treatment of sickle-cell disease, Br J Haematol 25:437, 1974.
Miwa S: Significance of the determination of red cell enzyme activities, Am J Hematol 6:163, 1979.
Nicholson-Weller A, Spicer DB, and Austen FA: Deficiency of the complement regulatory protein, "decay-accelerating factor," on membranes of granulocytes, monocytes and platelets in paroxysmal nocturnal hemoglobinuria, N Engl J Med 312:1091, 1985.

Nienhuis AW, Anagnow NP, and Ley TJ: Advances in thalassemia research, Blood 63:738, 1984.
Valentine WN: The Stratton lecture: hemolytic anemia and inborn errors of metabolism, Blood 54:549, 1979.

Hemolysis caused by acquired abnormalities

Brown DL: The immune interaction between red cells and leukocytes and the pathogenesis of spherocytosis, Br J Haematol 25:691, 1973.
Doll DC and Weiss RB: Hemolytic anemia associated with antineoplastic agents, Cancer Treat Rep 69:777, 1985.
Engelfriet CP: Autoantibodies in hematological disorders, Clin Immunobiol 3:345, 1976.
Frank MM, Atkinson JP, and Gadek J: Cold agglutinins and cold-agglutinin disease, Annu Rev Med 28:291, 1977.
Frank MM and others: Pathophysiology of immune hemolytic anemia, Ann Intern Med 87:210, 1977.
Garratty G and Petz LD: Drug-induced immune hemolytic anemia, Am J med 58:398, 1975.

68 · ABNORMAL HEMOGLOBIN PIGMENTS

Jerome I. Brody

METHEMOGLOBINEMIA

Methemoglobinemia is a clinical condition in which greater than normal 1% level of methemoglobin, an oxidation product of hemoglobin, is present in the circulation. It may be acquired or hereditary.

Acquired methemoglobinemia

Various therapeutic agents, industrial compounds, materials used in the home, food, and well water can cause methemoglobinemia when they either oxidize circulating hemoglobin directly or facilitate its coupled oxidation by molecular oxygen. Although methemoglobin is constantly present in vivo, its excess formation is prevented by a hemoglobin conversion system in the red blood cell (RBC) with the major pathway involving nucleotide adenine dinucleotide (NADH)–methemoglobin reductase (diaphorase). This enzyme catalyzes methemoglobin reduction via cytochrome b_5, using NADH as a hydrogen donor. The reduced cytochrome reduces methemoglobin to hemoglobin.

The symptoms of methemoglobinemia vary in intensity depending on the offending compound's rate of entry into the circulation, its metabolism and conversion to various intermediate forms, its excretion, and the capacity of the erythrocyte to reduce the oxidized pigment. Generally, a 10% to 25% methemoglobin level produces cyanosis but is tolerated without illness. At a 35% to 40% methemoglobin level, slight exertional dyspnea, headache, fatigue, vertigo, and tachycardia may be observed. However, if methemoglobinemia develops quickly, symptoms may occur at the somewhat lower concentration of 20% to 30%. At a 55% to 60% level of methemoglobin, lethargy and stupor result. The 70% methemoglobin level is lethal. Levels above 50% do not occur in hereditary methemoglobinemia (see following discussion), and toxic symptoms are most uncommon in this form of pigment disorder. Symptoms are caused largely by the inability of methemoglobin to transport oxygen and by increased oxygen affinity of the residual unaltered hemoglobin.

The diagnosis should be suspected if the clinical situation warrants it and the presence of cyanosis defies a common explanation. The specific diagnosis is confirmed spectrophotometrically by the presence of a hemolysate absorption band

Table 68-1 Hemoglobin M variants

Hemoglobin	Amino acid change
Hb M$_{Boston}$	($\alpha_2$58 His → Tyrβ_2)
Hb M$_{Iwate}$	($\alpha_2$87 His → Tyrβ_2)
Hb M$_{Saskatoon}$	($\alpha_2\beta_2$63 His → Tyr)
Hb M$_{Hyde Park}$	($\alpha_2\beta_2$92 His → Tyr)
Hb M$_{Milwaukee_1}$	($\alpha_2\beta_2$ Val → Glu)

at 502 and 632 nm that disappears on the addition of cyanide. If the oxidant stress is especially severe, supravital dye staining may show Heinz bodies in the peripheral blood, and overt hemolysis may take place.

Methemoglobinemia with levels of 20% to 30% disappears spontaneously 24 to 72 hours after the inducing agent is removed, and therefore treatment usually is unnecessary. When exposure has been great and signs and symptoms are severe, treatment with methylene blue is appropriate. A 1% solution in a dosage of 1 mg/kg may be injected intravenously over a 5-minute period. This promptly activates the hexose monophosphate shunt, and conversion of methemoglobin begins. If cyanosis has not disppeared within the hour, a second dose of 2 mg/kg may be given. It is unwise to exceed a total dose of 7 mg/kg because methylene blue itself is toxic.

Hereditary methemoglobinemias

Hereditary methemoglobinemias are caused by structurally altered hemoglobins and also by an enzyme variant. The precise location and nature of the abnormal amino acid substitutions in the altered hemoglobins are shown in Table 68-1. The miscoded amino acid replacements in the primary hemoglobin structure lead to an increased oxidation tendency of the heme iron or prevent reduction of methemoglobin. Only heterozygotes have been identified, since the homozygous condition probably is incompatible with life. The concentration of the abnormal hemoglobin does not exceed 25% to 30%, the hemoglobin M is heterogeneously distributed among the erythrocytes, and the older RBCs contain comparatively more of the abnormal pigment. Hemoglobin M$_{Iwate}$ probably is the most important hemoglobinopathy in Japan and is called hereditary nigremia because of the peculiar color of the blood pigment.

A second form of hereditary methemoglobinemia is due to NADH–methemoglobin reductase (diaphorase) deficiency. In homozygotes the enzyme is completely absent. No clinical or laboratory abnormality is detectable in heterozygotes because the RBC's reducing capability exceeds its oxidizing capacity by 250 times.

Cyanosis usually is the sole clinical manifestation in patients with the M hemoglobins. The diagnosis may be suspected clinically and confirmed by spectrophotometric examination of acid methemoglobin hemolysates at wavelengths between 500 and 600 nm and also by electrophoresis.

Patients with the enzyme defect are not ill. The most striking clinical feature is their cyanotic slate-gray, gray-brown, or violet skin color, with these changes particularly conspicuous on the lips, oral mucous membranes, tongue, palate, nose, and ears. Clubbing and other evidence of cardiopulmonary disease are absent.

Methemoglobin is present at a level of 20% to 50%. Most of the methemoglobin is in the minor, aging RBC population, possibly because the protection provided by ancillary (glutathione) pathways is reduced as the RBC becomes senescent. The decreased oxygen-carrying capacity of the abnormal pig-

ment may inconstantly lead to mild erythrocytosis. The RBC life span is normal. The initial diagnosis of the enzyme disorder may be made with a rapid screening test using the disappearance of fluorescence during formation of NADH as an endpoint. Treatment is not required for the hemoglobin variants, and it is given for the enzyme deficiency only for cosmetic reasons. Methylene blue (100 to 300 mg a day orally) to reduce the methemoglobin concentration to 10%, has been recommended. A less effective alternative is oral ascorbic acid.

OTHER PIGMENTS
Sulfhemoglobinemia

Sulfhemoglobin (SH) is an irreversibly denatured, further oxidized form of hemoglobin defined by its solubility and its spectral absorption band at 620 nm, which does not disappear with the addition of cyanide. SH is associated with drugs similar to those producing methemoglobinemia. Why methemoglobin develops in certain patients and SH in others under identical circumstances is unclear. The clinical symptoms resemble those of methemoglobinemia. Since sulfhemoglobin cannot be reconverted to hemoglobin, there is no treatment other than waiting for the abnormal RBCs to disappear.

Carboxyhemoglobinemia

Carbon monoxide (CO) binds reversibly to hemoglobin when the iron is in the reduced state to produce carboxyhemoglobin. Its adverse effects are negligible at the normal endogenous level of 0.3% to 0.7%. The toxicity of CO is related to its high affinity for heme, which is 210 times greater than that of oxygen. At a 20% concentration of carboxyhemoglobin a healthy person complains of headache, nausea, vomiting, and loss of manual dexterity. When a 50% carboxyhemoglobin level is reached in normal persons, convulsions and coma occur. The lethal level of this pigment is 70%. Patients with heart disease may be symptomatic at lower CO concentrations.

After acute CO exposure the gas remains tightly bound to hemoglobin for 4 hours, causing a left shift of the oxygen dissociation curve and relative homogeneous RBC distribution of CO. The treatment of choice remains exposure to the highest possible concentration of inspired oxygen. The half-life of carboxyhemoglobin while the subject is breathing room air is approximately 240 minutes. At 100% oxygen ventilation the half-life decreases to 40 minutes.

BIBLIOGRAPHY
Jackson DL and Menges H: Accidental carbon monoxide poisoning. JAMA 243:772, 1980.

69 · HEMOCHROMATOSIS
William E. Barry

DEFINITION. Hemochromatosis is a syndrome characterized by increased deposition of iron in body tissues, frequently accompanied by organ damage.

ETIOLOGY. Body iron overload occurs in several disorders. Refractory anemia with multiple transfusions (100 or more), prolonged excess dietary iron (as in Bantu siderosis) or medicinal iron, and other environmental sources of iron such as certain forms of alcoholic beverages consumed by patients with alcoholic cirrhosis cause typical varieties of "secondary" hemochromatosis. In the absence of an underlying disease or an identifiable source of excess iron, hemochromatosis is termed "primary" or "idiopathic." There is compelling evidence that idiopathic hemochromatosis is a genetically determined disorder of iron absorption.

PATHOGENESIS. The amount of iron absorbed from the diet is controlled within narrow limits by poorly understood mechanisms and normally amounts to about 1 mg a day. Physiologic iron loss exactly balances absorption but cannot be increased significantly; hence, increments in total body iron reflect changes in absorption. Since there are limits to iron absorption even when intake is high, it takes many years to accumulate the enormous amounts of body iron found in hemochromatosis, unless the iron excess occurs by blood transfusions or parenteral administration of iron. An excess of only 2 mg of absorbed iron daily over 60 years results in more than 40 g of excess body iron, an amount commonly found in patients with hemochromatosis.

It is not difficult to understand how excess environmental iron over many years can lead to large increases in total body iron. When there is no increase in environmental iron, as in idiopathic hemochromatosis, it seems clear that the iron absorption process is enhanced. The precise defect has not yet been established. Genetic determination is supported by the familial occurrence of the disease and the recently noted association with certain HLA markers.

The mechanism of organ damage associated with iron overload is not well understood. The liver parenchyma is most commonly involved by iron overload in primary hemochromatosis; eventually fibrosis occurs with cirrhosis as the result. Iron deposition in advanced disease also occurs frequently in the pancreas, endocrine glands, and myocardium. Skin pigmentation commonly results from increased melanin deposition; iron in skin is often lacking or present in only small amounts.

Parenteral iron, or iron derived from multiple transfusions, is deposited initially in reticuloendothelial cells and does not appear to result in organ damage. Redistribution to parenchymal cells eventually occurs, however, and the clinical and pathologic features of primary hemochromatosis may be seen in some patients with secondary hemochromatosis.

CLINICAL MANIFESTATIONS. Hemochromatosis is found most commonly in men and postmenopausal women. The classic clinical findings of increased skin pigmentation, cirrhosis, and diabetes occur in advanced disease. There is much variation in individual patients. Skin pigmentation may be minimal or lacking, and diabetes mellitus may or may not be present. Family members of patients with hemochromatosis and diabetes have a higher incidence of diabetes than the general population. Congestive heart failure is not confined to older patients but seems to be less common than in earlier reports.

Cirrhosis of the liver is the dominating clinical feature, with the usual findings of spider angiomas, palmar erythema, gynecomastia, and testicular atrophy. The liver is usually enlarged, and splenomegaly may be present. Hepatoma is said to be a more frequent complication in hemochromatosis than in alcoholic cirrhosis.

Arthritis is present in many patients at some time in the course of their disease. Chondrocalcinosis is common, and occasionally iron deposits are found in synovial membranes.

LABORATORY FINDINGS. Anemia is not a typical feature of hemochromatosis but may occur as a manifestation of the accompanying cirrhosis or dietary folate deficiency. Liver function abnormalities may be relatively mild. The most consistent laboratory feature is an elevated serum iron level, often with near saturation of transferrin. An increased serum ferritin level

is seen. Depending on the extent of other organ dysfunction, abnormalities in the blood sugar, hormone levels, or electrocardiogram may be found.

DIAGNOSIS. The diagnosis is not difficult when the clinical triad of increased skin pigmentation, diabetes mellitus, and hepatic cirrhosis is present. Confirmation is best made by liver biopsy, which demonstrates iron overload accompanying the histologic features of cirrhosis. Support for a diagnosis of idiopathic hemochromatosis rests on (1) excluding a source of excess iron and (2) family studies documenting idiopathic iron overload. HLA typing may prove a useful means of identifying family members who warrant particular attention. Simpler measures such as the determination of serum iron and ferritin levels are readily available screening tests for family members, especially those in younger age-groups, who may have only moderate degrees of iron overload and hepatic damage. Family studies, although tedious and time consuming, are important to identify members in the precirrhotic stage, who may clearly benefit from the removal of excess iron by periodic phlebotomies.

COURSE. Improvement in overall survival since the institution of phlebotomy therapy in hemochromatosis has been documented. The most common causes of death are hepatoma, liver failure, and congestive heart failure. Improvement in liver function and decreased insulin requirements in the diabetic may follow successful phlebotomy therapy, but such therapy may not prevent the development of hepatoma nor the severity of the arthritis that may accompany hemochromatosis.

MANAGEMENT. The treatment of choice in primary hemochromatosis is phlebotomy therapy to eliminate iron overload. This can often be done at weekly intervals and is surprisingly well tolerated. Since each 500 ml of blood removed by phlebotomy contains about 250 mg of iron, it may take several years to remove the often enormous amounts of iron (40 to 60 g) present. Iron-chelating agents are not generally used owing to their relative inefficiency compared with phlebotomy, the need for parenteral injection, their cost, and their uncertain long-term adverse effects.

In secondary hemochromatosis resulting from transfusions for refractory anemia, phlebotomies have little place. In these patients iron-chelating agents may prove beneficial, but experience with this therapy is still limited.

BIBLIOGRAPHY

Crosby WH: Hemochromatosis: the unsolved problems, Semin Hematol 14:135, 1977.
Fairbanks VF, Fahey JL, and Beutler E: Hemosiderosis and hemochromatosis. In Fairbanks VE, Fahey JL, and Beutler E, editors: Clinical disorders of iron metabolism, ed 2, New York, 1971, Grune & Stratton, Inc.
Finch SC and Finch CA: Idiopathic hemochromatosis: an iron storage disease, Medicine 34:381, 1955.
Jacobs A: Iron overload: clinical and pathologic aspects, Semin Hematol 14:89, 1977.

70·PRINCIPLES OF BLOOD BANKING AND TRANSFUSION THERAPY

I. Robert Schwartz

Much of the recent progress in medicine and surgery would not have been possible without concurrent advances in blood transfusion therapy. Blood transfusions now exceed 5 million a year in the United States alone and tend to be regarded as commonplace and routine. However, as with many boons to mankind, blood transfusion is fraught with dangers and pitfalls. Those whose job it is to prescribe blood for transfusions must have adequate knowledge of this complex subject to maximize benefits while minimizing risks. The amount of information, with its detailed specifics, has become so voluminous that only a specialist in this field can hope to maintain scientific and clinical mastery. Physicians who order blood should at least be conversant with the principles of transfusion therapy, so that they can provide rational therapy for their patients and cooperate intelligently with those in the blood transfusion service. All involved should be committed to safety in transfusion therapy. The work of the blood bank extends to every aspect of transfusion therapy, and a discussion of its activities serves as a framework for the introduction of the essential principles and practice of transfusion therapy.

PROCUREMENT AND COLLECTION

Improvements in the technique for the collection of blood have led to increased versatility and flexibility in its use. The most noteworthy advances include the use of plastic containers rather than glass bottles, the use of improved anticoagulant storage solutions, the development of automated blood cell separators, and the permanent storage of frozen glycerolized red blood cells (RBCs).

Plastic containers provide ease in transferring plasma and other components to satellite bags without breaking sterility. Thus blood can readily be fractionated into its component parts: plasma, RBCs, platelet concentrates, and cryoprecipitates. Unwanted components such as white blood cells (WBCs) can be removed. This has led to the present era of component therapy, in which only the specific component required is transfused. An additional benefit, the salvage of the remaining components of whole blood, makes the system efficient in the conservation of this valuable resource.

Automated cell separators are machines that instantly separate blood into its component parts as it flows from the donor and strikes the wall of a spinning centrifuge bowl. These machines are of two types. In the continuous flow method the separator operates continuously from beginning to end of the donation, simultaneously returning the RBCs to the donor. The intermittent flow method accomplishes the same purpose, with short interruptions of flow for the return of RBCs to the donor. Large quantities of plasma (plasmapheresis), WBCs (leukapheresis), or platelets (plateletpheresis) may be removed from a donor very rapidly. Fractionation may also be carried out without the benefit of an automated separator by drawing whole blood into a plastic container, centrifuging it, separating the plasma, WBCs, or platelets, and then returning the RBCs to the donor. This method does not require expensive equipment, but it is tedious and time consuming and exposes the donor to the risk of receiving the wrong RBCs in return. In certain diseases plasma exchange has been shown to be useful in the removal of undesirable constituents from the blood. The removed plasma is replaced partially with saline solution and partially with normal plasma, serum albumin, or plasma protein fraction.

Cell separators can be used for plasma exchange to correct the hyperviscosity syndrome seen in Waldenström's macroglobulinemia. Immune-complex disease and diseases of excessive antibody formation are also being treated experimentally in this way. Examples of such diseases are systemic lupus erythematosus, Goodpasture's syndrome, and myasthenia gravis. Cell separators are also used to collect single-donor

platelets and WBCs for transfusion. However, most platelet concentrates ae made from whole blood drawn into plastic bags and then centrifuged gently to produce platelet-rich plasma. This then is transferred to a satellite bag and centrifuged rapidly, yielding a platelet concentrate and a supernatant of platelet-poor plasma. The platelet-poor plasma is removed to be used for fresh-frozen plasma or for the production of cryoprecipitate. Patients requiring platelet transfusions generally receive 6 to 10 such preparations at one time, each concentrate coming from a different donor. Antibodies against foreign platelets develop within several weeks of such transfusions, and transfusions of random platelets are then useless because of the rapid destruction of the platelets by alloantibodies. However, the platelets of a donor who has the same HLA antigens as the patient may survive normally in the patient's circulation. The problem is to obtain a yield of platelets from the single matched donor equal to the amount derived from 6 to 10 random donors. The cell separator can do this efficiently, and it is in such instances that it finds its best present-day use in the area of platelet transfusion. WBC transfusions are still somewhat controversial, but most authorities agree that such transfusions are useful as part of the total care of children with a temporary marrow aplasia.

Cell processors can produce WBCs fairly efficiently if hydroxyethyl starch (an RBC sedimenting agent) is used to facilitate cell separation and if corticosteroids are given to raise the donor's granulocyte count. All processors can achieve clinically significant yields (about 10^{10} WBCs).

The freezing of blood for prolonged storage has become a practical reality. However, because of the relatively high cost of the process (about two to three times the cost of storage in the liquid form), it has not become routine. Its best application is in the stockpiling of bloods of rare types for use in patients who have antibodies against most donor RBCs. This provides rapid availability of blood for such patients, avoiding the search for suitable ambulatory donors on short notice. In addition, nonanemic patients with rare antibodies may donate their own blood for storage in the frozen state in anticipation of future transfusion needs (autologous transfusion). Glycerol is added to the blood before freezing, and the blood is stored at $-136°$ F ($-80°$ C) or lower. After thawing but before transfusion, the glycerol must be removed from the RBCs or hemolysis will occur on contact with plasma. A continuous automated method for deglycerolization using wash solutions during centrifugation simplifies the procedure. Since only laboratories equipped for cryopreservation can provide the services necessary, frozen blood is generally available onlyin hospitals with such facilities or through a community blood center. Frozen blood cells are virtually free of plasma, WBCs, and platelets as a result of the deglycerolizing process. Therefore thawed cells for transfusion are useful in avoiding sensitization to leukocyte transplantation antigens in patients who are to have organ transplants.

Frozen RBCs have some important specialized applications but are unsuitable for routine use because of two factors, the high cost and the need to use them within 24 hours of thawing to avoid bacterial contamination. Although it was once believed that serum hepatitis from blood transfusion might be eliminated by using frozen blood, more recent experience has not borne this out.

FITNESS AND SAFETY

The safe use of blood transfusions depends on the quality of the blood itself, as well as its compatibility with the recipient's blood.

Transmissible diseases

Certain diseases may be transmitted by blood transfusions. The most significant of these are hepatitis, syphilis, malaria, and acquired immunodeficiency syndrome (AIDS). Exclusion of these diseases from blood depends in large part on careful donor selection. Each donor must be asked a series of questions to uncover possible infection or exposure to these diseases. Blood obtained from voluntary donors is far less frequently involved in the transmission of disease from blood from paid donors. This is especially true of serum hepatitis, which is transmitted about 10 times more frequently by blood drawn from paid donors than by blood from voluntary donors. The use of blood from paid donors should be avoided whenever possible. The reasons for the difference are unknown but probably have to do with the reliability of the donor history and the increased prevalence of hepatitis in the less affluent paid donor population. Tests for hepatitis-associated antigen are now mandatory for every unit of blood for transfusion. The most common method for detecting the hepatitis B surface antigen (Hb$_s$Ag) is the radioimmunoassay. This procedure has dramatically reduced the transmission of hepatitis B. There is still considerable transmission of non A/non B hepatitis, for which there is not yet a reliable test, but so-called surrogate testing has begun employing tests for serum alanine transferase (ALT) levels and for antibody to hepatitis B core (anti-Hbc). These are not specific for the virus, but they do have predictive value.

Even when all precautions have been taken, a significant, unavoidable risk of transmitting hepatitis remains. Therefore the administration of blood and all of its products capable of transmitting hepatitis should be regarded as potentially harmful and life threatening. No transfusion should be ordered without good justification. Blood should be used to correct the adverse effects of anemia when there is no other way to accomplish this. It should never be used capriciously, cosmetically, or carelessly.

AIDS is a sexually transmitted disease, but it can also be spread by inoculation of contaminated blood. U.S. blood supply is now well protected, but there have been reports of transfusion-transmitted AIDS, especially in patients with hemophilia. Most of these incidents happened before the advent of heat-treated antihemophilic blood products and before the universal testing of blood donors for antibodies against the human immunodeficiency virus (anti-HIV). This test is effective in screening out donors with AIDS-transmitting potential, except for those who may still be in the incubation period and have not yet produced antibodies. Blood collection facilities therefore continue to ask all donor candidates to exclude themselves if they belong to any of the identified high-risk groups. Nevertheless, AIDS is spreading rapidly through intravenous drug use and sexual transmission, and it is creating serious concerns for blood transfusion safety.

Transfusion-transmitted syphilis is now rare with serologic testing and refrigeration of blood, which in most cases destroys the spirochete in about 3 days.

Blood containing malarial parasites may remain infective after a week of refrigerated storage. Donors who may have malaria must be screened by a careful history, which should include the donor's past involvement with malaria, recent malarial attacks, antimalarial medication, and sojourn or travel in a malarial area. Definite rules for blood donation and donor rejection are prescribed for these conditions.

Cytomegalovirus infection may occur after the transfusion of large amounts of blood, especially after heart surgery. This produces a disorder resembling infectious mononucleosis, with fever, splenomegaly, and leukopenia (postperfusion syndrome). Infectious mononucleosis may occasionally be transmitted by blood transfusions. Other diseases reported to be transmitted in this manner are brucellosis, Chagas' disease, sleeping sickness (trypanosomiasis), kala azar (leishmaniasis), filariasis, and possibly toxoplasmosis.

The medical and lay communities are aware of the serious risks associated with blood transfusion. As a result, autologous blood use is becoming common. This is the use of the patient's own blood to replace blood lost during surgery. There are two methods of autologous blood transfusion, predeposit and intraoperative. In the former procedure a qualified patient undergoing elective surgery donates blood in advance, which is then stored until needed. In the latter, shed blood is collected and reinfused during surgery. Barrring accidental transfusion of the wrong blood, autologous transfusion safeguards against transfusion reactions and disease transmission. It is as close to risk free as possible.

Compatibility

Before blood can be safely transfused into a patient, the possibility of immunologic incompatibility between donor and recipient must be investigated. Such an incompatibility may result in the rapid destruction of the transfused RBCs with immediate consequences to the recipient or in the delayed sensitization of the recipient to donor cells with production of antibodies. Sensitization may jeopardize the safety of future transfusions or pregnancies. When blood is transfused, the greatest potential mischief lies in the donor RBCs, which contain antigens foreign to the recipient. The donor plasma is far less likely to produce serious problems, since plasma antibodies usually are rendered harmless by dilution in the recipient's plasma before they can interact with the recipient's cells. Exceptions to this are the transfusion of massive amounts of plasma and also of plasma with very high titers of antibody. Occasionally anaphylactoid reactions develop in IgA-deficient recipients after transfusions as a result of the action of the recipient's antibodies (anti-IgA) against IgA immunoglobulins in the donor plasma.

There are more than 20 known blood group systems and 389 red cell antigens, and it is impossible to test for donor-recipient compatibility in all of these systems. Fortunately, it is unnecessary to do so, since not all blood groups are of equal clinical importance.

The most important systems by far are the ABO and Rh systems because (1) almost everyone (AB individuals excepted) has naturally occurring alloantibodies against blood group antigens A or B; (2) 15% of the population is Rh negative and 70% of these produce antibodies if the Rh antigen is introduced into their blood; and (3) all of these antibodies are capable of producing severe hemolytic reactions. The rest of the blood group systems are of lesser importance, some being very rarely involved in transfusion reactions.

Most RBC antibodies are formed in response to the transfusion or injection of RBCs or as a result of pregnancy with the fetus carrying the sensitizing antigen. When antibodies form without sensitizing antigenic exposure, they are said to be naturally occurring. In the ABO system the absence of an antigen from an individual's phenotype is always associated with the development of naturally occurfjing antibodies against that antigen. In some other blood group systems naturally occurring antibodies sometimes form, and in still others antibodies never occur naturally but only in response to specific antigenic exposure via transfusions or pregnancy.

The discovery of the ABO system opened the way to the

clinical use of blood transfusions. For each phenotypic antigen, A, B, and O, there is a corresponding gene, *A, B,* and *O*. Each individual inherits one gene from each parent, resulting in the following possible combinations.

Genotype	Phenotype	Antigen present A	B
AA	A	+	−
AO	A	+	−
BB	B	−	+
BO	B	−	+
OO	O	−	−
AB	AB	+	+

It can be seen that there is no recognizable antigen as a result of having *O* genes. Individuals produce antibodies against A and B antigens when they are lacking. Therefore antibodies are formed as follows:

Phenotype of red cell	Alloantibody in the plasma
A	Anti-B
B	Anti-A
O	Anti-A and anti-B
AB	None

The prevalence of the various phenotypes in the American population is as follows:

Phenotype	West European descent	African descent
A	45%	29%
B	8%	17%
O	43%	50%
AB	4%	4%

With the use of antiserum known to be specific against A or B antigen, the presence of these phenotypes can be detected in donor and recipient blood. Naturally occurring antibodies against A or B are of the IgM type and agglutinate RBCs in a saline medium at room temperature. They are complete antibodies and do not require incubation or special techniques to produce agglutination. Further confirmation of the blood group is carried out by reverse grouping, which employs RBCs of known blood groups. The test serum is checked against these RBCs to see whether it contains the corroborative antibodies.

When the patient's blood group is known, donor blood of the same group is chosen for further testing. When group-specific blood is unavailable, group-compatible blood may be used. Compatible blood contains no RBC antigens for which there are specific antibodies in the recipient plasma but may contain antibodies against the recipient's RBCs. Therefore, when many units of nonidentical blood are to be given, it is important to use blood with the plasma removed (packed RBCs) or whole blood with a low titer of antibody in the plasma. The following are examples of group-compatible blood:

Recipient's group	Compatible donor group
A	O
B	O
O	—
AB	O, A, B

In an immunologic reaction resulting from direct exposure to RBCs of group A or B, a different class of antibodies is formed. These are of the IgG type and are termed "hyperimmune." They may cross the placenta to produce erythroblastosis. They are also incomplete antibodies and can be distinguished in the laboratory from naturally occurring antibodies.

When choosing blood for cross-matching purposes, both the ABO and the Rh systems are taken into account. In the Rh system the blood is specifically tested for the antigen called Rh$_o$ or D. It is by far the most immunogenic of the Rh antigens and is therefore the most significant clinically. Because it is so immunogenic, the donor and recipient should be matched for it whenever possible, but occasionally it is necessary to give Rh-positive blood to an Rh$_o$-negative recipient when there is a life-threatening emergency and no Rh-negative blood can be obtained. This can be done only if the recipient has no anti-Rh$_o$ antibodies. Rh-positive transfusions expose the recipient to Rh$_o$ sensitization and may affect the recipient's future transfusability with Rh-positive blood. Transfusions of Rh-positive blood in young Rh-negative patients, especially girls and women of childbearing age, should be avoided because of the danger of Rh sensitization with possible future hemolytic disease of the newborn. Rh-negative women who have been pregnant may have formed antibodies against Rh$_o$ as a result of fetal sensitization. These patients would almost certainly have a severe hemolytic transfusion reaction if given a transfusion of Rh-positive blood by error. Rh sensitization may be prevented in most cases if adequate amounts of anti-D (Rh$_o$) immune globulin are administered shortly after exposure to the Rh$_o$ antigen as a result of either childbirth or the transfusion of Rh-positive blood. The administered Rh immune globulin combines with the Rh$_o$ antigen, rendering it nonimmunogenic. Maternal sensitization may therefore be avoided and transfusions of unmatched blood (by mistake or intention) may be made harmless if treated promptly.

About 15% of whites and 2% of blacks are Rh negative. This low frequency sometimes leads to the problem of short supply of Rh-negative blood for transfusions. Testing for the other antigens in the Rh system (C, c, E, e) is not routinely performed because they cause sensitization much less frequently. This also holds true for all other blood group antigens. Nevertheless, anyone of these antigens may be a potential source of trouble in a given case. The solution to this problem is to depend on the cross-match test between the recipient's serum and the donor's cells. If an incompatibility is found, attempts should be made to identify the irregular antibody or antibodies present. This may be done by the use of a "panel" of test cells that has been carefully constructed to yield a specific reaction pattern for each antigen included in the panel. According to the pattern of reactions produced by a given antibody, the corresponding antigen can be identified. It then becomes a matter of screening many units of blood with the specific antiserum to find compatible units that lack the antigen in question and therefore are not reactive with the recipient's serum.

In emergency transfusions there may not be time to identify an antibody causing incompatible cross-matches. In this case many units of blood are cross matched in the hope of finding a sufficient number of compatible units by chance alone. The decision to use such "compatible" blood must be based on the relative risk of waiting for proper antibody identification versus the risk of proceeding with transfusion in the face of an unidentified antibody or antibodies. In such circumstances reliance on the cross-match alone for donor selection is risky. Although the amount of antibody present in the recipient's serum may be sufficient to detect incompatible donor units with RBCs homozygous for the offending antigen, it may be insufficient to detect units with heterozygous RBCs. The final decision must be made by the attending physician in consultation with the director of the transfusion service.

Compatibility testing is the foundation of the blood bank's safety procedure. It is the final common pathway of the blood bank's activities leading to the release of blood for transfusion. It is the last in a series of steps to find possible immunologic discrepancies, the ultimate check for possible technical errors previously committed, and the final seal of approval placed on the blood by those performing the testing. Nevertheless, in rare instances cross-matching will be unable to detect certain problems such as potential delayed transfusion reactions.

Cross-matching or compatibility testing is carried out by mixing donor RBCs with patient serum to detect antibodies against donor RBC antigens as manifested by RBC agglutination or hemolysis.

PRINCIPLES OF TRANSFUSION THERAPY

Blood transfusion should be used only when other, less dangerous methods of correcting anemia are not applicable. Whenever a timely and safe correction can be achieved by using hematinic agents such as iron or cyanocobalamin, this course is preferable. However, at times these alternatives are ineffective or take too long to be useful and safe. Some example are refractory chronic anemias, anemia in patients with ischemic heart disease, anemia severe enough to be life threatening, and anemia in a patient being prepared for nonelective surgery. With today's availability of component therapy, the deficiencies that need to be corrected in any given case should be determined, and only the required components should be used. The practice of using whole blood for blood transfusion has been largely overcome through educational efforts and by making whole blood much less available than it was previously. Most large regional blood centers remove the plasma from the majority of blood drawn. This plasma is used for the preparation of other blood components and derivatives such as fresh-frozen plasma, cryoprecipitates, serum albumin, and clotting factor concentrates. RBCs have several advantages over whole blood in transfusion therapy: less fluid volume, less citrate, less storage waste products such as potassium and ammonia, and less donor antibodies. The major advantage is volume reduction, which may be essential for safe transfusions in patients with actual or borderline cardiac decompensation. In massive transfusion the advantages of less citrate and less storage waste products take on considerably more importance. Since it is now more difficult to obtain whole blood than RBCs, the clinician is forced to think of RBCs as the routine way to use blood and must have indications for selecting whole blood. Most authorities agree that these indications are few.

Most transfusions are used to correct the inadequate oxygen-carrying power of the blood resulting from anemia, and RBCs are needed for this purpose. The problem arises in the treatment of shock and massive hemorrhage, when the circulatory volume must be restored. However, even under these circumstances whole blood should be used sparingly and not in every case. A number of plasma substitutes, used alone or in conjunction with RBCs, provide optimal management of such patients. These plasma substitutes are colloid solutions of dextran and starch, albumin, and plasma protein derivative. Also, plasma itself may be used as a separate component to provide the volume of fluid to be replaced. In the initial treatment of shock, crystalloids (saline solution, Ringer's lactate solution, and so forth) have been found useful and can be administered immediately without waiting for preparation of blood, thawing of plasma, or reconstitution of powdered materials. In cases of massive hemorrhage, blood can be replaced with RBCs, adding additional volume in the form of colloids or solutions of plasma proteins as required. When the amount of blood loss exceeds 40% of the patient's blood volume, whole blood transfusion can justifiably be employed. Even under these circumstances it is probably best to alternate each unit of whole blood

with 1 unit of RBCs. If additional fluid volume is required (as judged by the central venous pressure), it can be given in the form of colloids or plasma protein solution. There is no need for whole blood during routine blood replacement at surgery. The blood volume, as judged by the vital signs, may be maintained easily with intravenous solutions, and the oxygen-carrying capacity may be maintained with RBC transfusions based on estimated blood loss.

Massive blood loss requires massive replacement transfusion, which may produce problems of its own. Stored blood undergoes changes that generally do not cause clinical problems if transfusions are given in usual amounts over suitable periods of time. However, these abnormalities may become significant when massive transfusions (more than 10 units in 24 hours) are given. The transfused blood is cold and acidic; has no ionized calcium but a high sodium and potassium content; has decreased ability to deliver oxygen to tissues (low 2,3-diphosphoglycerate level); contains potential microemboli in the form of microaggregates of platelets, leukocytes, and fibrinogen; and has low levels of labile coagulation factors. Furthermore, the blood contains large amounts of citrate, which if given rapidly may produce serious toxic effects such as cardiac arrhythmias because of a reduction in the ionized calcium level. This may require correction with intravenous calcium solution. Impaired liver function makes the patient much more susceptible to citrate toxicity. Patients with advanced liver disease present a special problem, since they are more likely to have clinical emergencies requiring massive transfusions, such as esophageal varices, peptic ulcer, and coagulation defects. Ice-cold blood may also produce cardiac arrhythmias when given rapidly. Blood should be prewarmed when rapid transfusion is required. In posttransfusion studies of patients receiving massive amounts of blood, it was found that the serum sodium level did not rise, and the serum potassium level actually fell despite high levels in the transfused blood. A suggested explanation was the loss of potassium through hemorrhage. In some cases it was even necessary to administer additional potassium after massive transfusions. Microaggregates may be filtered out using special micropore filters, but these may reduce the maximal rate at which blood can be administered. Furthermore, there is no definite proof that these microaggregates are capable of causing pulmonary insufficiency, and there is no consensus favoring the usefulness of the filters. Platelet transfusions may be given if the posttransfusion platelet count falls to levels (below $20,000/mm^3$) that may give rise to spontaneous bleeding or cause a perpetuation of preexisting bleeding. Fresh-frozen plasma is useful to correct deficiencies of labile clotting factors. An acceptable routine to be employed for massive blood replacement is to (1) use a blood warmer after the administration of 3 units of bank blood; (2) administer one ampule of sodium bicarbonate (44.6 mEq) for every 5 units of blood transfused; and (3) give 2 units of fresh-frozen plasma for every 10 units of blood transfused. If RBCs are being transfused, the serum albumin level should be checked and electrolyte administration should be carefully monitored. When liver function is impaired, evidence of citrate toxicity should be sought, and if present it should be treated with judicious amounts of intravenous calcium. Electrocardiographic monitoring should be a part of the total care of these patients whenever possible.

TRANSFUSION REACTIONS

Blood group incompatibilities cause the most serious transfusion reactions, usually producing intravascular hemolysis.

This should be a rare event, but it may occur when procedure is not followed. Errors in the blood bank laboratory may come from attempting to set up more than one cross-match at a time or from careless labeling of cross-matched blood. There is greater danger in patient care areas because many more people are involved, responsibility is more diffuse, and constant supervision is nearly impossible. The major concern is the incorrect identification of the patient or the patient's blood specimen. The blood bank cannot detect an erroneously labeled specimen from a patient new to the blood bank. If previous records are available in the blood bank, they must be consulted every time a new specimen is received. When no records exist, the patient receives whatever blood is compatible with the blood in the submitted specimen tube. Some safeguards can be taken. It may be advisable at the bedside to recheck the recipient's blood type on a fresh specimen before starting a new transfusion. This is especially useful in the operating and delivery rooms, where signs of blood transfusion reactions are likely to be masked as a result of general anesthesia. Emphasis on rigid identification procedures can prevent possible labeling errors when specimens are drawn for typing and cross-matching and when blood transfusions are started. Although such procedures may be tedious and difficult to follow at times, uncompromising insistence on adherence to exact performance is the only effective safeguard against errors in identification.

If a hemolytic transfusion reaction should occur, it is usually heralded by chills, fever, and back pain. The patient should be warned to signal for help immediately if any of these symptoms appears. On discovery of such a reaction, the first step is to stop the blood transfusion and to keep the needle open with a saline drip. An immediate check for a possible error in identification should be made. Specimens of blood and urine should be sent to the laboratory for immediate examination, including tests for free hemoglobin, retyping, re-cross-matching, evidence of antigen-antibody reactions, and bacterial contamination. The blood bag, even if empty, should also be returned to the blood bank.

The patient should be observed carefully for decreased urinary output and evidence of hemolysis. If either is present, mannitol or furosemide should be given intravenously to promote urinary flow. A nephrology consultation should be obtained as soon as possible. Hypovolemic shock should be treated promptly with appropriate solutions. After a cross-match for compatibility, type O RBCs may be used in cases of severe anemia. The patient should be observed for possible intravascular coagulation. Urinary output must be monitored hourly for the next several days. In the case of persistent uremia, renal dialysis is necessary. Other reactions to blood may be dealt with according to their specific nature. Initially they may mimic hemolytic transfusion reactions.

Allergic reactions are fairly common and not often serious. They may be controlled with parenteral administration of antihistamines or corticosteroids. Severe reactions such as anaphylactoid reactions or angioneurotic edema may require epinephrine. Whether to continue the blood transfusion cautiously is a decision that must be individualized in each case. Premedication may prevent subsequent allergic reactions in many instances.

Antileukocyte antibodies arising from previous transfusions or pregnancies sometimes cause febrile transfusion reactions. Such reactions may be prevented by removing leukocytes from the donor blood. This may be done by filtration, centrifugation, batch washing, the addition of sedimenting agents, or a combination of these procedures. Also, frozen and thawed RBCs are leukocyte free and may be used for transfusion in this case.

Bacterial contamination of donor blood is extremely uncommon, but if sepsis is produced in this way, it should be treated promptly with appropriate antibiotics.

Antibodies against IgA are occasionally found in blood recipients who are IgA deficient, and these may incite anaphylactic reactions to plasma protein. These reactions can be severe even with the administration of very small amounts (2 to 3 ml) of plasma. Prompt and vigorous treatment for anaphylaxis should be given immediately after the transfusion has been stopped. Future transfusions should be taken from donors with IgA deficiency, or transmembrane-washed RBCs (as in deglycerolizing) should be used. A small amount of blood should be injected as a test dose before further blood transfusion is given after a previous reaction.

BIBLIOGRAPHY

Greenwalt TJ: General principles of blood transfusion, ed 3, Chicago, 1977, American Medical Association.

Issitt PD and Issitt CH: Applied blood group serology, Oxnard, Calif, 1975, Spectra Biologicals.

Mollison PL: Blood transfusion in clinical medicine, Oxford, Eng, 1983, Blackwell Scientific Publications.

Race RR and Sanger R: Blood groups in man, Oxford, Eng, 1975, Blackwell Scientific Publications.

Technical manual of the American Association of Blood Banks, ed 9, Philadelphia, 1985, The Association.

71 · POLYCYTHEMIA

Frank H. Gardner *and* Gary B. Weiss

The diagnosis of polycythemia (defined as an increased number of circulating red blood cells [RBCs]) used to be made by an interpretation of peripheral blood measurements reflecting changes in the RBC, hemoglobin, and hematocrit values. With accurate isotopic measurements of RBC and plasma volumes, it can now be appreciated that the peripheral blood measurement might be misinterpreted, since a reduced plasma volume elevates the hematocrit and hemoglobin values. Although polycythemia vera is the classic disorder that initiated the study of erythrocytosis, the most common form of elevated hemoglobin is *stress polycythemia* or erythrocythemia. This is 10 times more frequent than polycythemia vera.

The rate of RBC production in the normal individual is carefully regulated and involves the response of the committed stem cell compartment to the predominantly kidney-elaborated hormone erythropoietin. It is believed that minimal changes in oxygen diffusion activate the release of erythropoietin from the kidney. The hormone, depending on the concentration, interacts with the committed erythroid stem cell to increase RBC maturation. When there is a marked increase in erythropoietin that can react with the committed stem cell, production of RBCs increases with concurrent elevation of the peripheral hematocrit and hemoglobin values. Hence, any stimulus that increases erythropoietin production eventually could elevate the total RBC volume. Such changes in *secondary polycythemia* have been noted with the physiologic adaptation to hypoxia and with inappropriate erythropoietin production by kidney, liver, and lung tumors. A classification of the various types of polycythemia follows:

I. Polycythemia vera (decreased erythropoietin)
II. Secondary polycythemia (increased erythropoietin)
A.   Generalized hypoxia

1. High altitude
2. Chronic obstructive pulmonary disease
3. Cardiovascular shunt (right to left)
4. Pickwickian syndrome (massive obesity)
5. High–oxygen affinity hemoglobin
6. Smoking
B. Localized hypoxia
  1. Renal cysts
  2. Hydronephrosis
  3. Renal artery stenosis
C. Autonomous erythropoietin production
  1. Tumor
    a. Renal carcinoma
    b. Hepatoma
    c. Cerebellar hemangioblastoma
    d. Uterine fibroid tumors
    e. Miscellaneous
  2. Recessive familial polycythemia
III. Relative polycythemia
  A. Acute
  B. Chronic (stress)

POLYCYTHEMIA VERA

Polycythemia vera is a relatively uncommon disorder most frequently diagnosed after 50 years of age. The disease occurs slightly more frequently in men and is seen more often in Jews of Eastern European ancestry; it is rare in blacks and Latin Americans. It traditionally has been classified as a myeloproliferative disorder, implying that there is autonomous production of all cell lines, erythrocytes, granulocytes, and platelets, with a rare chance of transformation into myelofibrosis or acute leukemia.

Polycythemia vera is a specific clonal proliferation of a marrow population. When the various stem cell components can be identified by glucose-6-phosphate dehydrogenase (G6PD) enzyme classification (in women heterozygous for G6PD enzymes), there is evidence that all of the proliferating cells observed in polycythemia vera have only a single enzyme component. This demonstrates transformation to a generalized proliferation of a single clone of cells. A second (normal) clone of cells remains relatively inactive in the marrow and is overshadowed by the transformed polycythemia vera clone. The autonomous abnormal clone has no response in vitro to erythropoietin. Serum concentrations of erythropoietin are usually low in the untreated patient owing to inhibition of its production by erythrocytosis.

CLINICAL MANIFESTATIONS. Polycythemia vera may be an insidious clinical illness that goes undiagnosed for years. Patients may ignore the predominant symptoms of headache, weakness, dizziness, and sweating for a long time. The diagnosis is often considered because of physical findings of plethora (67%), conjunctival engorgement (59%), splenomegaly (70%), and hepatomegaly (40%). However, most often the diagnosis begins with identification of an elevated hematocrit and/or hemoglobin level. A hemoglobin value greater than 17.5 g/dl for men or 16 g/dl for women (hematocrit of 55% and 50% at sea level, respectively) is abnormal and requires further diagnostic study.

As noted, early measurement of the RBC mass is most critical for diagnosis, and this procedure is usually carried out by labeling a known amount of RBCs with ^{51}Cr and determining the radioactivity in the blood samples after reinjection. Some laboratories also simultaneously perform a plasma volume determination by injecting ^{131}I-labeled albumin. An RBC mass greater than 36 ml/kg for men or 32 ml/kg for women is abnormal and can be considered diagnostic of polycythemia.

Bone marrow studies, if performed, show hyperplasia of all precursors with a decreased amount of marrow fat. A variety of abnormal chromosome patterns have been described in these patients before therapy. However, in the past decade these abnormalities have not been helpful in defining the response to therapy or determining survival. Bone marrow studies may be useful for this type of data collection but do not contribute to the diagnosis.

The first steps in the study of these patients are to obtain a careful medical history and to perform a physical examination to note if the findings just listed are present. Careful attention must be paid to the history of smoking, symptoms of pulmonary disease, and the presence or absence of a palpable spleen. Clues to secondary polycythemia in the history or physical examination may shorten the laboratory workup and allow an earlier diagnosis. Secondary polycythemia must be excluded before a diagnosis of polycythemia vera can be made. This can be done through measurement of serum erythropoietin levels; accurate commercial measurements are only now becoming available. Until they are, a systematic search for other causes remains necessary.

The causes of secondary polycythemeia include high-altitude acclimatization, pulmonary disease, cardiovascular disease with arteriovenous shunts, alveolar hypoventilation, defective oxygen transport, and elevated carbon monoxide levels in tobacco smokers. In essence, this group of causes for secondary polycythemia represents a physiologic response to hypoxia with an elevation of erythropoietin. The remaining causes of secondary polycythemia are also related to increased production of erythropoietin and include erythrocytosis resulting from renal vascular impairment, renal cyst, or hydronephrosis. Other sources of abnormal erythropoietin production are hypernephromas, uterine myomas, cerebellar hemangiomas, hepatomas, and endocrine disorders associated with increased androgen production. A small but important group of patients have a rare hereditary overproduction of erythropoietin associated with erythrocytosis from early childhood. Because of the rarity of some of these diagnoses, many hematologists limit the screening laboratory tests to arterial blood oxygen saturation, hemoglobin electrophoresis or determination of the hemoglobin-oxygen dissociation curve, and intravenous pyelogram. The type of secondary polycythemia usually can be identified on the basis of the results of these tests.

In the absence of a cause for secondary polycythemia, the Polycythemia Vera Study Group (PVSG) has established the following widely accepted criteria for the diagnosis of polycythemia vera: an increased RBC mass, a normal arterial oxygen saturation (greater than or equal to 92%), and splenomegaly. In the absence of splenomegaly, two of the following abnormalities must be present: thrombocytosis (platelet count greater than 400,000/mm^3); leukocytosis (WBC count greater than 12,000 cells/mm^3 in the absence of fever or infection); elevated leukocyte alkaline phosphatase score (greater than 100 in the absence of fever or infection); and elevated serum vitamin B$_{12}$ level (greater than 900 pg/ml) or an unbound vitamin B$_{12}$–binding capacity greater than 2200 pg/ml.

Patients with polycythemia vera have an increased tendency toward thrombotic episodes (such as cerebrovascular thrombosis) and bleeding (such as gastrointestinal hemorrhage). Both tendencies generally become normal after correction of the hematocrit to normal. Patients with polycythemia vera also have an increased risk of acute myeloblastic leukemia.

MANAGEMENT. The PVSG has been evaluating treatment programs for the past 20 years. The cooperative group has noted a marked increase in the transition to acute myeloblastic leukemia in patients receiving alkylating drugs such as chlorambucil. The more accepted therapy with radioactive phosphorus (^{32}P) has about half the incidence of leukemia, and a regular program of phlebotomies has the lowest incidence of leukemia. In the initial years of treatment with phlebotomy this therapy carried an increased risk of cerebrovascular accident. This has made optimal choice of therapies complicated. The hematocrit should be maintained at levels between 40% to 42% for ideal control of the disease. The addition of aspirin (325 mg/day) has been suggested. Studies to assess the efficacy of hydroxyurea are under way. Radioactive phosphorus has been suggested as the treatment of choice in the elderly. Falsely high microhematocrit values may be observed when the spun hematocrit is compared with that derived from calculations using the RBC count and the mean corpuscular volume (MCV). Therefore, in patients with polycythemia vera, hematocrit values should be determined with automated equipment and hemoglobin levels should be determined spectrophotometrically. Bleeding problems, especially at surgery, are common in untreated persons with polycythemia. All elective surgery, including dental extractions, should be delayed until treatment has normalized the hematocrit.

SECONDARY POLYCYTHEMIA
Hypoxia

The majority of patients with secondary polycythemia have an increased RBC mass attributable to hypoxia. Significant elevations of RBC mass do not occur unless the arterial oxygen saturation falls below 92% and the Po$_2$ is less than 65 mm Hg. Polycythemia may be present in patients with chronic hypoxemia even in the absence of dyspnea, and it is not rare for polycythemia rather than dyspnea to be the abnormality that first brings the hypoxemic patient to medical attention. It must be emphasized that the peripheral blood values are not always as elevated as would be expected for the degree of hypoxia because of an inappropriate response of the marrow to erythropoietin in the presence of a persistent pulmonary infection (chronic bronchitis).

All types of cardiac shunts that allow mixing of venous with arterial blood result in decreased oxygen saturation and secondary polycythemia. The patient with severe cardiac disease may have an hematocrit of 75% to 85%. This is associated with a marked increase in the red cell mass and a very diminished plasma volume. These patients must be protected from dehydration at all times, since enhanced viscosity from fever may cause sludging and infarction in the cerebral circulation. Patients with cyanotic secondary polycythemia may also have thrombocytopenia. The cause of the low platelet count has not been defined completely but may be related to decreased plasma volume or low-grade disseminated intravascular coagulopathy.

MANAGEMENT. There is no agreement on a specific therapy program. Treatment, if possible, should be aimed at the cause. Many patients have felt better when the hematocrit was lowered to about 60% by a regular phlebotomy program, but relief of symptoms is more important than laboratory values, and each patient must be titrated to obtain optimal results. Some clinics reinfuse equal amounts of colloid or plasma substitutes to replace the volume of blood removed. Patients with cardiac disease have improved exercise tolerance and variable increments in the platelet count, probably as a result of expansion of the plasma volume with the phlebotomy program. The patients are iron depleted by the frequent phlebotomies. If there are symptoms of glossitis, skin irritation, or fatigue, small doses of iron may be given orally with subjective improvement. Oral folate should be prescribed if there is any doubt about adequate dietary intake. At all times the physiologic abnormalities require attention, such as correction of pulmonary infection or surgical repair of an arteriovenous shunt. Many patients are unable to have surgical procedures, and a phlebotomy program must be continued indefinitely.

Familial polycythemia

The clinical measurement of erythropoietin has defined a small group of patients who have an increased RBC mass resulting from elevated serum erythropoietin levels caused by a genetic abnormality. The onset of erythrocytosis is in childhood. Hematocrit values vary in the range of 70% to 80%. The diagnosis is more likely if the patient had elevated hematocrit values in childhood. The diagnosis must be related to the exclusion of other forms of secondary polycythemia that also have elevated erythropoietin values, the presence of elevated hematocrit values in other family members, usually siblings, and measurements of erythropoietin. There is no specific therapy other than phlebotomy to reduce the hematocrit to 60% or less and to obtain maximal subjective improvement, as in hypoxic polycythemia.

Polycythemia related to abnormal hemoglobin

A variety of abnormal hemoglobins associated with erythrocytosis have been reported in the past 25 years. The erythrocytosis is related to a shift in the oxygen dissociation curve to the left of the normal pattern. This shift causes a slower release of oxygen for tissue utilization and thus mild hypoxia. Since the initial description of hemoglobin Chesapeake, many other abnormal hemoglobins with high oxygen affinity have been described. The inherited abnormality is ascribed to deranged function of oxygen release from the heme molecule. The increased affinity of oxygen to the heme molecule induces impaired oxygen release to varying degrees. There is a wide spectrum of oxygen dissociation curves with these hemoglobin mutants, and a determination of the dissociation curve may be required in the patient's evaluation. Again, we emphasize that these patients have only the expected response to erythropoietin, namely erythroid hyperplasia but no leukocytosis, thrombocytosis, or splenomegaly.

Polycythemia related to tumor

Some tumors have been found to excrete erythropoietin, resulting in polycythemia. This is most common with renal (hypernephroma), liver (hepatoma), and cerebellar tumors but can occur with other tumors as well. Treatment of the malignancy, if possible, may control the polycythemia.

Polycythemia related to local hypoxia

The kidney is the normal site of erythropoietin production. When the oxygen supply to one kidney is decreased by renal arterial stenosis, a cyst, or ureteral obstruction, polycythemia can develop. These conditions are amenable to surgical therapy.

RELATIVE POLYCYTHEMIA

A decreased plasma volume may be the reason for increased hemoglobin and hematocrit values in patients whose RBC mass is not elevated, as determined by isotopic measurements. This condition is called relative polycythemia. Although such a decreased plasma volume may rarely be associated with the use of a diuretic, vomiting, diarrhea, excessive sweating, or high capillary pressure (increased catecholamines or heart failure), these causes usually are easily recognized.

The chronic form of relative polycythemia has been called *spurious polycythemia, pseudopolycythemia, stress polycythe-*

mia, benign polycythemia, or *Gaisböck's syndrome.* Most patients with this disorder are middle-aged white men, often tense or under physiologic stress, mildly overweight, hypertensive, and frequently heavy smokers. Indeed, almost all of the studies refer to smoking as a contributory cause or do not report the smoking data.

An estimated 3% of the 50 million adults who smoke have an elevated hematocrit value. The inhalation of carbon monoxide by smokers may elevate carboxyhemoglobin levels 4% to 30% with a mean of 10%. Since most of these patients have the same clinical manifestations as those with stress polycythemia, we have included smokers' polycythemia under the general classification of stress polycythemia, although it is actually a form of secondary polycythemia.

Aside from the elevated hematocrit and hemoglobin values and decreased plasma volume levels in stress polycythemia, laboratory findings are generally normal, although an increased incidence of elevated serum uric acid and lipid levels has been noted. The cause of the decreased plasma volume is unknown, but altered venous tone from increased catecholamine secretion induced by carbon monoxide has been suggested as an explanation. Although this disorder has been considered a benign form of polycythemia and does not represent a hematologic malignancy, stress polycythemia carries a poor prognosis. Studies have demonstrated an increased incidence of cardiovascular accidents in these patients. Since stress polycythemia represents the most common cause of elevated hematocrit and hemoglobin, its detection is most important.

MANAGEMENT. The major goal of treatment of stress polycythemia is to lower the elevated level of carboxyhemoglobin that causes inefficient oxygen transport. Smoking should not be permitted. The patient should also initiate a weight reduction program to an ideal body weight. If hypertension is present, treatment should preferably be with minimal use of diuretics, which might reduce the plasma volume. The results of treatment can be impressive, with the hematocrit returning to the normal range in 6 to 8 months after weight reduction and cessation of smoking.

Treatment may be much more important for these patients than for those with polycythemia vera. The patients were previously looked on as having only an abnormal laboratory measurement, and until recent years reassurance was the main therapy, with occasional participation in regular phlebotomy programs. Patients with stress and/or smokers' polycythemia require the most careful supervision, since both morbidity and mortality are high.

BIBLIOGRAPHY

Berk PD and others: Therapeutic recommendations in polycythemia based on Polycythemia Vera Study Group protocols, Semin Hematol 23:132, 1986.

Burge PS, Johnson WS, and Prankerd TAJ: Morbidity and mortality in pseudopolycythemia, Lancet 1:1266, 1975.

Harrison BDW and Stokes TC: Secondary polycythemia: its causes, effects and treatment, Br J Dis Chest 76:313, 1982.

Smith JR and Landaw SA: Smokers' polycythemia, N Engl J Med 298:6, 1978.

UNIT B • WHITE BLOOD CELL DISORDERS

72 · QUALITATIVE AND QUANTITATIVE NEUTROPHIL DISORDERS

Janet L. Abrahm

NEUTROPHIL KINETICS

The production of mature polymorphonuclear neutrophils or neutrophilic granulocytes represents an orderly process wherein various stem cell compartments provide a continuous supply of precursor cells in the bone marrow. Such stem cells have not been recognized morphologically but have been assayed by various experimental techniques. From transplantation studies in animals, it is clear that virtually all hematopoietic cells arise from a common pluripotential stem cell that is responsible for erythroid, granulocytic, and megakaryocytic production. This cell appears to differentiate into three classes of committed stem cells, each of which is restricted to a single line of differentiation, that is, erythroid, granulocytic, monocytic, or megakaryocytic. These committed stem cells seem to respond to humoral stimuli that induce the further growth and maturation of specific precursor cells in the marrow. It is well established that erythropoietin is a humoral substance responsible for erythroblast maturation; however, thrombopoietic control mechanisms are less well defined.

Recent in vivo and in vitro studies have identified other humoral stimuli, a family of glycoproteins termed "colony-stimulating factors" (CSFs). These include factors that stimulate only granulocyte or macrophage development, granulocyte-CSF (G-CSF) and macrophage-CSF (M-CSF [or CSF-1]), as well as the pluripoietins granulocyte-monocyte CSF (GM-CSF) and interleukin 3, which stimulate the formation of granulocytes, monocytes, eosinophils, megakaryocytes, and, with the addition of erythropoietin, erythroid cells. The genes for GM-CSF and M-CSF are located on chromosome 5.

GM-CSF is made by activated macrophages and T lymphocytes. The stimulated macrophages also produce tumor necrosis factor-α and interleukin 1, which stimulate endothelial cells and fibroblasts to produce G-CSF, GM-CSF, and M-CSF. Lithium enhances CSF production, and most patients receiving lithium have granulocytosis. Hydrocortisone also enhances CSF production by endothelial cells.

GM-CSF not only stimulates production of new cells but also has many actions on mature effector cells. GM-CSF activates neutrophils, inhibits them from migrating from the site of CSF production, and enhances the ability of granulocytes and monocytes to phagocytose bacteria and yeast. It is possible, however, that inappropriate, continued CSF production and activation of effectors have harmful consequences. CSF has been found in joint effusions and may contribute to the tissue damage occurring in chronic inflammatory states, such as rheumatoid arthritis.

Recently, infusions of recombinant human G-CSF and GM-CSF have confirmed the physiologic capabilities of these substances. Animals given either product showed sustained granulocytosis of normally functioning cells, and the factors significantly shortened the granulocytopenia induced by chemotherapy or irradiation. In the future the factors may be used to minimize such granulocytopenias occurring in patients.

Several inhibitors of the production of CSF or of its effects on the committed stem cells have been identified. Their role in the physiologic regulation of hematopoiesis is uncertain. Acidic isoferritins inhibit CSF release. Prostaglandin E_2 produced by macrophages, γ-interferon produced by activated T cells, and lymphotoxin (also called tumor necrosis factor-β) produced by B cells all inhibit the proliferation of granulocyte and monocyte committed stem cells despite the presence of CSF. Interferon and lymphotoxin may play a role in the neutropenias found in some patients with viral infections.

The committed stem cells that form colonies of granulocytes and monocytes in vitro represent about 0.1% of the total marrow cells. They are not morphologically identifiable.

The identifiable granulocytic precursor cells in the marrow are classified as (1) the proliferative compartment, which includes myeloblasts, promyelocytes, and myelocytes, and (2) a maturation and storage pool of nonproliferative metamyelocytes, band cells, and segmented neutrophils. These cells are readily identified by the appearance of granules seen only in the neutrophilic series. Large red-purple (on Wright stain) or primary granules that contain myeloperoxidase and other enzymes initially develop in the promyelocyte. Specific or secondary granules form in the myelocyte stage. Both types of granules persist throughout development to the mature neutrophil, where they function in the process of bacterial killing.

Transit through the bone marrow requires about 9 to 12 days, of which 4 to 6 days are spent in the proliferative compartment. The storage pool of band and segmented cells is approximately 10 times the size of the peripheral blood granulocyte pool and can be readily mobilized in response to peripheral demand. In times of increased need, as with severe infection, band cells and mature neutrophils are immediately released from the marrow into the circulation. The release appears to result from the action of another serum factor termed "neutrophil-releasing factor," which is rapidly produced in response to bacterial endotoxins. This material is believed to be responsible for the early neutrophilia seen with infection but probably is not involved in the basal level of granulocyte production. A similar response is noted after injection of etiocholanolone or corticosteroids, which are the basis of experimental tests for neutrophil reserves in patients with various types of neutropenia.

Once released into the circulation, mature neutrophils are equally divided between the circulating and marginal pools. The latter consists of cells loosely adherent to the blood vessels in the lungs, spleen, and elsewhere, which are immediately available in response to stress. Injection of epinephrine causes a transitory increase in the neutrophil count owing to rapid demargination of these cells. This stress reaction probably explains the neutrophilia seen in acutely agitated patients, particularly in the pediatric age-group. In some instances infusion of epinephrine may be used to document neutropenic syndromes that are characterized by excessive sequestration rather than destruction of neutrophils.

The half-life of circulating neutrophils is a relatively short 6 to 7 hours. The intravascular life span is frequently shortened to several hours in the neutropenic state and prolonged with neutrophilia. For instance, neutrophils in patients with uncontrolled chronic myelogenous leukemia may circulate for up to 3 days; half-lives return to normal values with appropriate therapy. The short intravascular life span limits the use of therapeutic white blood cell transfusions in the treatment of acute infections in patients with reversible agranulocytosis.

Neutrophils leave the circulation by traversing the endothelium of capillaries, usually in response to chemotactic factors generated by bacterial growth. Materials such as endotoxin, bradykinin, activated components of complement, and antigen-antibody complexes induce a positive stimulus for neutrophil migration into the tissues. It is believed that the extravascular life span may exceed the time in the circulation by several days. Eventual loss occurs by destruction in the reticuloendothelial system, shedding into the respiratory, genital, or gastrointestinal tracts, or more likely by cell dissolution after phagocytosis and bacterial killing.

NEUTROPHIL DYSFUNCTION SYNDROMES

In response to chemotactic stimuli, neutrophils migrate to the site of infection where they ingest bacteria by phagocytosis. This process is augmented in the presence of opsonizing materials such as immunoglobulins and complement components, which coat the bacterial cell wall. The opsonized bacteria are engulfed and carried to the interior of the cell in a phagocytic vacuole, which is lined by the invaginated cell membrane. This process leads to a sequence of events that includes degranulation with discharge of granule contents into the vacuole and a series of metabolic events termed the respiratory burst. Oxygen consumption rises, and oxygen is converted to superoxide and then to hydrogen peroxide. This is accompanied by a marked increase in activity of the hexose monophosphate shunt.

Although superoxide and hydrogen peroxide have modest bactericidal properties, the major degree of cell killing requires interaction with chloride or other halide ions. Myeloperoxidase released from primary granules catalyzes the reaction of chloride ion with hydrogen peroxide to form hypochlorite, which directly kills the invading organisms.

A number of defects in bacterial killing by neutrophils have been described. The most common serious defect is neutropenia or a lack of neutrophils (see "Neutropenia and agranulocytosis"). There may also be defects in chemotaxis, phagocytosis, and microbicidal activity.

Defects in chemotaxis

Neutropenia results in inadequate accumulation of leukocytes in areas of inflammation. In addition, alcohol and corticosteroids interfere with adherence of neutrophils to endothelial cells, which impairs mobilization to the site of injury. Defects in the complement system can interfere with the production of chemotactic factors, resulting in poor chemotaxis. These may be seen in newborns, on a congenital basis, and acquired by diabetic patients. A cellular defect in chemotaxis has been described in newborns and patients with diabetes, rheumatoid arthritis, hypophosphatemia, Chédiak-Higashi disease, Job's syndrome, and the lazy leukocyte syndrome.

Job's syndrome is characterized by recurrent indolent staphylococcal skin abscesses, eczema, and high serum IgE levels. The neutrophils manifest a cellular defect in chemotaxis.

The *lazy leukocyte syndrome* is a syndrome of neutropenia in association with recurrent episodes of gingivitis, stomatitis, and otitis media. There is a cellular defect in chemotaxis.

Defects in phagocytosis

Defects in phagocytosis can result from agammaglobulinemia or from poor opsonization of microorganisms as a result of congenital or acquired defects in the complement system. Patients with chronic lymphocytic leukemia, myeloma, and acquired hypoglobulinemia have decreased γ-globulin levels. Opsonins are defective in some newborns and in some patients with lupus erythematosus and cirrhosis. The lack of opsonins for pneumococci may contribute to the association of sickle cell anemia with severe pneumococcal infections.

Cellular defects in phagocytosis have been described in some patients with diabetes, rheumatoid arthritis, systemic lupus erythematosus, hypophosphatemia, immune complex disease, thermal burns, and sarcoid.

Defects in microbicidal activity

A number of syndromes associated with known defects in neutrophil microbicidal activity have been described.

CHRONIC GRANULOMATOUS DISEASE. The best-characterized disorder of neutrophil (and monocyte) microbicidal function is a condition termed "chronic granulomatous disease" (CGD), in which infants have repeated severe pyogenic infections with *Staphylococcus aureus* and gram-negative bacteria. The infections are slow to heal and invariably lead to multiple granulomatous abscesses. The most common form is X linked, with male inheritance and an asymptomatic carrier state in females.

Patients with CGD have normal or elevated neutrophil counts, immunoglobulin levels, and delayed hypersensitivity. The chemotatic and phagocytic responses are normal. CGD results from an inability of the neutrophil to produce hydrogen peroxide, which is necessary for cell killing. The deficient enzyme is usually nicotinamide adenine dinucleotide phosphate oxidase, but other enzymes may be deficient in variants of CGD. CGD neutrophils can effectively kill those organisms such as streptococci and pneumococci that provide hydrogen peroxide, the substrate for the myeloperoxidase reaction.

The diagnosis is readily established by documenting an impaired respiratory burst activity in response to bacterial exposure. One common test employs the ability of normal neutrophils to reduce nitroblue tetrazolium (NBT) dye to blue formazan. All neutrophils of patients with CGD and a portion of the neutrophils of female carriers are unable to reduce NBT dye. Another in vitro test involves measurement of the rate at which neutrophils kill *S. aureus;* CGD neutrophils kill at a much slower rate than normal neutrophils, and CGD carriers have neutrophils of a mixed population that kill at an intermediate rate.

Chronic lymphadenitis with extensive and diffuse lymphadenopathy is the most common feature of the disease. Severe eczematoid dermatitis, pneumonitis, and hepatosplenomegaly are regularly observed. Subphrenic abscesses, osteomyelitis, and perianal abscesses are frequent features. Thus far, treatment is confined to antibiotic therapy and surgical drainage of the abscesses. Continuous prophylactic antibiotic therapy may be of use in some patients; granulocyte transfusions may be required in severe, life-threatening infection.

CHÉDIAK-HIGASHI DISEASE. Chédiak-Higashi disease is an autosomal recessive disorder that is usually discovered during childhood and consists of partial albinism, increased susceptibility to infection, and morphologic and functional abnormalities of leukocytes. The cytoplasm of the neutrophils, monocytes, and lymphocytes contains giant granules readily seen on routine Wright-Giemsa stains. Functional abnormalities of the neutrophils include decreased chemotaxis and slow degranulation resulting in delayed microbial killing. An "accelerated phase" with pancytopenia; lymphohistiocytic infiltration in the liver, spleen, and bone marrow; unexplained fever; peripheral neuropathy; and frequent bacterial and viral infection is usually fatal.

The treatment consists of appropriate antibiotic therapy. Corticosteroids and vincristine have been used in the treatment of the accelerated phase, but results have been inconsistent.

OTHER DISORDERS. Neutrophil dysfunction and increased susceptibility to infection have been seen in severe glucose-6-phosphate deficiency, myeloperoxidase deficiency, and lipochrome histiocytosis.

NEUTROPENIA AND AGRANULOCYTOSIS

Blood leukocyte counts normally range between 5000 and 10,000 cells/mm³ with a predominance of neutrophils. Although a reduction in circulating neutrophils usually leads to a decline in the total leukocyte count, such values are not meaningful unless a differential count is performed and the absolute numbers of each cell type are calculated. In healthy individuals total neutrophil counts range between 1800 and 7200 cells/mm³, with slightly lower values in the black population. Thus neutropenia is defined as a decrease in the neutrophil count below 1800 cells/mm³, with the reservation that certain blacks may have values as low as 1200 to 1500 cells/mm³ with no detectable disease process.

Neutropenia may occur as an isolated finding or may be associated with a variety of underlying disorders, which may cause anemia and thrombocytopenia as well. In general, neutropenia associated with some definable disease process results from marrow production defects or excessive cellular destruction.

Production defects

APLASIA OR HYPOPLASIA. The most common form of reversible bone marrow hypoplasia results from the use of cytotoxic drug regimens for the treatment of neoplastic disease. Many of the combination therapies include alkylating agents, which induce acute neutropenia and thrombocytopenia that persist 1 to 2 weeks. Exceptions are noted with the nitrosourea agents, which generally manifest a delayed reaction with variable degrees of neutropenia 3 to 4 weeks after therapy.

Ionizing irradiation in doses of 2000 to 4000 rad causes a near total ablation of myelopoiesis in the areas of irradiated bone marrow. The injury is biphasic, with a transient loss of cell production resulting from ablation of the hematopoietic stem cells. Cellularity returns for several months but eventually ceases owing to a permanent defect in the microcirculation. If the extent of the irradiation field is sufficiently wide, some patients may have a permanent depression in cell production with borderline neutrophil counts. In evaluating neutropenia in this situation, it is important to obtain bone marrow samples outside the previous treatment field, since irradiated sites show severe degrees of aplasia.

Severe acquired aplastic anemia usually affects all three major cell lines, resulting in neutropenia, thrombocytopenia, and severe anemia. The disease generally has an abrupt onset owing to infection or widespread mucosal bleeding caused by low numbers of platelets. In most instances this disorder is thought to result from a quantitative reduction in hematopoietic stem cells, since marrow aspirates and biopsy specimens show only scattered foci of lymphocytes and plasma cells. However, a small percentage of cases may be due to immunologic suppression of the marrow or to a basic defect in the marrow stroma.

Paroxysmal nocturnal hemoglobinuria may represent a variant form of bone marrow aplasia. It is believed that spontaneous recovery from aplasia may result in an aberrant stem cell that yields mature cells with abnormal membrane characteristics. The red cells are unduly sensitive to pH change, which is the basis for the acid hemolysis test. Recently membrane abnormalities have been detected in the neutrophils and platelets as well. This disorder is characterized primarily by hemolysis, iron deficiency, venous thrombosis, thrombocytopenia, and neutropenia. In some cases further stem cell mutation may occur with conversion to acute myeloblastic leukemia.

INFILTRATIVE DISORDERS OF THE BONE MARROW. Infiltration of the marrow with foreign cells may result in a myelophthisic process with a disruption of the usual orderly release of mature cells. The peripheral blood may show leukopenia, thrombocytopenia, and anemia with a leukoerythroblastic picture (variable numbers of myelocytes, metamyelocytes, and nucleated red cell precursors). This often results from hematologic neoplasms such as the leukemias, non-Hodgkin's lymphomas, and multiple myeloma. The presence of bone pain or the finding of marked bony tenderness over the involved areas may be the major clue to the diagnosis.

A variety of carcinomas may also diffusely infiltrate the marrow cavity and produce a similar clinical picture. The neoplasms that most commonly "seed" in the marrow arise from the breast, lung, kidney, prostate, and thyroid. At times the primary tumor may be undetectable, and multiple diagnostic tests may be required to document the site of origin. The marrow may also be infiltrated or largely replaced by fibroblasts, granulomas, or storage cells. Idiopathic myelofibrosis may be suggested by the presence of marked hepatosplenomegaly and numerous teardrop poikilocytes in the peripheral blood smear. Attempts at bone marrow aspiration usually result in a "dry tap"; core biopsy of the marrow reveals a dense collagen fibrosis. On occasion, diffuse hematogenous spread of tuberculosis mimics the picture of idiopathic myelofibrosis with hepatosplenomegaly, anemia, thrombocytopenia, and variable changes in neutrophil counts. The diagnosis of tuberculosis or other granulomatous processes may be established by biopsy of the bone marrow or the liver.

Various types of lipid storage abnormalities are characterized by lipid-filled macrophages throughout the reticuloendothelial system. Infants with Gaucher's, Tay-Sachs, or Niemann-Pick disease may have variable degrees of neutropenia as a result of the marrow infiltration. In contrast, the adult form of Gaucher's disease is usually characterized by hypersplenic destruction of platelets and neutrophils with some improvement following splenectomy.

METABOLIC DISORDERS. Deficiencies of vitamin B_{12} and folic acid may cause decreases in neutrophil counts in addition to megaloblastic anemias. These deficiencies are characterized by glossitis, gastrointestinal disturbances, mild hyperbilirubinemia, and, in pernicious anemia, associated neurologic defects. Peripheral blood smears show macrocytosis with oval cells, high red blood cell mean corpuscular volumes, and numerous hypersegmented neutrophils. Although five-lobed neutrophils may be seen occasionally in the normal smear, the finding of six- or seven-lobed cells is virtually diagnostic of a megaloblastic process. Marrow aspirates are hypercellular with increased numbers of granulocytic precursors, many of which are twice the normal size. This form of neutropenia is characterized by excessive intramedullary destruction of the precursor cells. Neutrophil counts promptly return to normal levels with appropriate therapy.

INFECTIOUS DISEASES. Acute viral infections such as influenza and infectious mononucleosis are often associated with modest degrees of neutropenia. Although most bacterial infections lead to neutrophilia, typhoid fever is frequently associated with a depression in circulating neutrophils. The exact mechanism has not been defined, but with many viral infections there is a related depression in platelet counts and red blood cell production, particularly in patients with severe chronic

hemolytic anemias. It seems likely that these changes result from an acute suppression of bone marrow function. The neutropenia is of modest degree, with recovery of normal counts within 1 to 2 weeks of diagnosis.

This form of neutropenia must be distinguished from that seen in acute overwhelming bacterial infections. Occasional patients with extensive pneumonitis, diffuse skin infections resulting from exfoliative dermatitis, or severe sepsis have virtually no circulating neutrophils. Bone marrow aspirates show increased numbers of proliferative cells but few metamyelocyte, band, or segmented neutrophils. This is due to depletion of the marrow storage pool with exudation of the cells into the site of infection. Such patients require vigorous therapy with bactericidal antibiotics, since 4 to 5 days may elapse before a new wave of mature cells is generated.

OTHER HEMATOLOGIC DISEASE

Neutropenia is a common feature of the acute leukemias that are discussed in Chapter 73 and of the myelodysplastic syndromes that are discussed in Chapter 62. It has also been associated with both malignant and benign expansions of T-suppressor cells or large granular lymphocytes.

Destructive defects

Increased neutrophil destruction may result from hypersplenism or from the presence of antibodies directed against mature neutrophils.

HYPERSPLENISM. Hypersplenism is suggested by the finding of variable degrees of neutropenia, thrombocytopenia, and a mild hemolytic anemia in association with splenomegaly. In the peripheral blood smear the ratio of band to segmented cells is increased, and marrow aspirates show hyperplasia of proliferative cells. The marrow storage pool is reduced as a reflection of the increased rate of cellular release into the peripheral blood. Although the exact mechanism has not been defined, it seems likely that the hyperplastic reticuloendothelial cells of the splenic sinusoids are responsible for the neutrophil destruction.

Hypersplenism usually results from congestive splenomegaly that accompanies long-standing hepatic cirrhosis, but it may be seen with portal vein thrombosis, with chronic infections involving the reticuloendothelial system (such as brucellosis), or occasionally with chronic lymphocytic leukemia. Splenectomy usually resolves the neutropenia but is rarely indicated.

Rheumatoid arthritis may lead to the development of splenomegaly and neutropenia (Felty's syndrome). This usually occurs in patients with long-standing disease with rheumatoid nodules and high rheumatoid factor titers. Frequently the arthritis is relatively inactive; indeed, the major problem may be that of indolent leg ulcers. It is assumed that Felty's syndrome is due to splenic sequestration or to antineutrophil antibodies; however, multiple mechanisms may be operative. Some patients show increased neutrophil production, whereas others have an associated marrow defect. Splenectomy has been variably successful but should be attempted only in patients with repeated episodes of infection.

ANTINEUTROPHIL ANTIBODIES. Certain neonatal forms of neutropenia are due to transplacental passage of leukoagglutinins from the mother to the fetus. This results from maternal immunization to specific neutrophil antigens of the fetus by virtue of previous pregnancies or prior blood transfusions. The disorder persists for several months until the maternal antibody is gradually consumed.

Only a few cases of autoimmune neutropenia have been

described in adults. It is likely that this mechanism occurs in association with rheumatoid arthritis, systemic lupus erythematosus, and other connective tissue diseases; however, documentation has been hampered by the difficulties inherent in the antibody assays. Leukoagglutinins occur in the sera of many individuals without a corresponding abnormality in leukocyte production. Serum inhibitors have been detected by the colony-forming assays, but such determinations are often plagued by nonspecific inhibitory materials, particularly when assayed against bone marrows from unrelated donors. In the absence of a specific assay system, autoimmune neutropenia can be inferred only by the absence of splenomegaly and the finding of granulocytic hyperplasia of the marrow in the appropriate clinical setting. Therapy with corticosteroids may occasionally reduce the accelerated cell destruction and increase the numbers of circulating neutrophils. Such treatment may also be somewhat hazardous, since corticosteroids block the egress of neutrophils into inflammatory exudates.

Congenital neutropenia

Various forms of congenital neutropenia have been defined. Many show a dominant inheritance pattern, but the mechanisms of neutropenia are widely disparate. Granulocytic stem cells have been increased in some types, reduced in others, and virtually absent from the marrow in one variant. In most instances the defect is mild, with neutrophil counts in the range of 500 to 1000 cells/mm^3 and only modest infections. Some patients with severe neutropenia may show a compensatory increase in monocytes, which appears to reduce the likelihood of infections.

Chronic idiopathic neutropenic syndromes

After appropriate evaluation to exclude other causes, there remains a group of adult patients with variable degrees of neutropenia and normal myeloid cellularity in the bone marrow. In one series of 41 patients studied over a 6-year period, infection occurred in 27%. The majority of these had fewer than 500 circulating neutrophils/mm^3. Most patients had normal or increased numbers of granulocytic stem cells in the marrow and appeared to respond to the neutropenic stress with an increased proportion of these colony-forming cells in DNA synthesis. The defect that has been identified in this group is a reduction in CSF production by marrow cells themselves, suggesting that this form of neutropenia may result from insufficient medullary production of this regulator of granulopoiesis.

T lymphocyte–mediated granulocytopenia has also been described. In 25 of 93 patients studied, removal of the T cells or incubation with corticosteroids restored the in vitro marrow growth of granulopoietic committed stem cells. Clinical neutropenia resolved in 24 of the 25 after steroid therapy. There was no clinical response to steroids in the 68 other patients whose granulocyte growth did not improve in response to steroids. Hemopoietic inhibitory T cells disappeared in steroid-responsive patients during therapy but persisted in steroid-resistant patients.

Some patients with chronic neutropenia have a period of oscillatory cell production. This "cyclic neutropenia" does not represent a distinct clinical syndrome but rather reflects a markedly reduced pluripotential stem cell compartment. Neutrophil counts vary cyclically from none to approximately 2000 cells/mm^3 every 2 to 3 weeks, with frequent infections during the severely neutropenic intervals. The reticulocyte and platelet counts frequently oscillate out of cycle with the neutrophils, which suggests that stem cell competition may be responsible for this unique phenomenon. On occasion the oscillation may disappear with normalization of the blood counts later in life.

Drug-induced neutropenia

Aside from the cytotoxic drugs used in cancer chemotherapy, a wide variety of agents can cause a severe reversible neutropenia. This symptom complex, which has been termed "agranulocytosis," arises as an idiosyncratic reaction, usually within 4 to 8 weeks of instituting therapy. The most severe reactions produce fever, pharyngitis with gray, necrotic oral ulcers, and a virtual absence of circulating neutrophils. Without prompt recognition and therapy the course is complicated by hyperpyrexia, stupor, and generalized sepsis, which may lead to death. The mortality rate has been about 20% in the past decade, but it can be reduced to less than 5% with proper therapy.

The reaction to aminopyrine and its derivative dipyrone, available in some over-the-counter preparations, is characterized by the development of drug-dependent antibodies and acute neutropenia caused by rapid destruction of circulating neutrophils. The initial reaction leads to agranulocytosis, fever, and infection, with increased numbers of neutrophil precursors such as myeloblasts, promyelocytes, and myelocytes in the marrow. Discontinuation of the offending drug usually leads to recovery in 5 to 6 days. On reexposure the patient has shaking chills and a disappearance of circulating neutrophils within hours of drug ingestion. In volunteers who receive an infusion of the patient's plasma, a similar immediate neutropenia develops after a single drug exposure.

In contrast, the antibiotic agents, one of the major causes of drug-induced neutropenia, probably act by directly suppressing marrow production of granulocytes, although antibody reactions have been described. Similarly, drugs of the phenothiazine group produce agranulocytosis by inhibiting cell production. In patients with the severe, idiosyncratic reaction, the bone marrow is characterized by selective granulocyte aplasia, leading to a prolonged agranulocytosis for intervals of up to 2 weeks. Modest quantities of chlorpromazine inhibit normal cell growth in vitro, whereas even minute doses of this agent are inhibitory to granulocyte colonies from susceptible individuals. Idiosyncratic reactions to phenothiazines are relatively uncommon, but a mild stable neutropenia develops in many patients during the course of therapy with chlorpromazine. Bone marrow studies show only a slight generalized reduction in granulocytic cells. If necessary, drug therapy may be continued, since most such patients do not have the severe idiosyncratic suppression of granulopoiesis. The lower doses of those phenothiazines used for the treatment of nausea and vomiting are rarely if ever associated with neutropenia.

Most of the other agents in the following outline appear to act by inhibiting cell production, although occasional reports have suggested that antithyroid compounds, gold salts, phenylbutazone, and sulfonamides may also serve as haptens to induce drug-dependent antibodies:

Analgesics
　　Aminopyrine, dipyrone*
Antibiotics
　　Cephalosporins*
　　Chloramphenicol
　　Semisynthetic penicillins*
　　Sulfonamides*

---

*Most frequent or most severe.

Anticonvulsants
  Phenytoin
Antihistamines
  Cimetidine
Antihypertensives
  Captopril
Antiinflammatory agents
  Phenylbutazone*
  Gold
  Indomethacin
Antithyroid agents
  Methimazole*
  Propylthiouracil*
Cardiovascular antiarrythmics
  Procainamide
Phenothiazines
  Chlorpromazine*
Miscellaneous agents
  Allopurinol
  Ethanol
  Levamisole
  Penicillamine

General approach to the neutropenic patient

Frequently a careful history reveals drug ingestion, toxin exposure, a recent viral illness, or symptoms suggestive of a generalized disorder associated with neutropenia. The findings of adenopathy and splenomegaly may indicate an underlying lymphoproliferative disease or infectious mononucleosis. Splenomegaly alone may suggest either primary myelofibrosis or myelofibrosis from tumor infiltration of the marrow. Petechiae and sternal tenderness raise the suspicion of acute leukemia. In most cases careful study of the peripheral blood and bone marrow is sufficient to establish the diagnosis.

In general, a reduction in circulating neutrophils to 500 to 1000 cells/mm³ is associated with a modest increase in the risk of infection. Values below 500 cells/mm³ frequently lead to life-threatening sepsis. However, it must be emphasized that these generalizations are derived from patients with severe production defects such as those with acute leukemia or aplastic anemia. Occasional individuals with severe hypersplenism or Felty's syndrome tolerate circulating neutrophil levels of 100 to 200 cells/mm³ without an increased frequency or severity of infection. In all likelihood such patients have a redistribution phenomenon with an increase in marginated cells. Thus the marginal blood granulocyte pool may exceed circulating levels by threefold to fivefold and may be readily mobilized on demand.

Infection prevention and treatment

For patients with acute granulocytopenia, however, several interventions can minimize the risk of infection. The integrity of the mucous membranes and skin should be maintained by avoiding unnecessary venipunctures or operative procedures and by prohibiting the taking of rectal temperatures. The risk of infection from the patient's skin or the hands of personnel coming in contact with the patient can be minimized by washing with a preparation that decreases *S. aureus* colonization. Proper dental care before chemotherapy can significantly reduce the septicemias resulting from mouth organisms in adult patients treated for acute leukemia. (This is discussed in detail in the "Dental Correlations" portion of this section.)

Half the cases of septicemia are caused by hospital-acquired organisms. The most aggressive of these are the gram-negative bacteria *Pseudomonas aeruginosa* and *Klebsiella pneumoniae*,

---

*Most frequent or most severe.

but fungi can also be acquired if patients are exposed to areas of the hospital under construction. Standard hospital protective isolation measures are no more effective than simple hand-washing and are not recommended. More complex and expensive approaches employ laminar airflow rooms and orally administered, nonabsorbable antibiotics in an attempt to eliminate the patient's own intestinal organisms. There has been no consistent demonstration of improved survival with these regimens. Newer studies have been done of orally absorbed prophylactic antibiotics, which preserve anaerobic intestinal organisms that prevent colonization by the virulent gram-negative organisms mentioned previously. These also have failed to increase survival.

Optimal nutrition is needed to maintain the functioning of T cells. Protein-calorie malnutrition and deficiencies of folate, zinc, iron, or vitamin B₆ cause defective T-cell function, which exacerbates the infectious risk in a neutropenic patient.

If a fever develops, aggressive diagnostic and therapeutic measures are required. A thorough physical examination to elucidate the source of the infection must be performed, with special attention to the skin, eyes, nose, mouth, and anal area. Diagnostic efforts are often hampered by the masking of the usual manifestations of bacterial infections in neutropenic patients. Without polymorphonuclear granulocytes, no pus forms, and instead of the usual fluctuance and exudate, pain and erythema may be the only signs of the infection. Specimens for culture must be taken from blood, urine, sputum, and any suspected site. Empiric therapy should be started with broad-spectrum antibiotics that have demonstrated efficacy against organisms endogenous to the patient or likely to have been acquired by the patient in the hospital. If fever persists after 2 to 3 days of therapy, infusions of white blood cells may be started. They do not increase the circulating neutrophil count but do improve survival in patients such as those with acute leukemia who have acute, reversible neutropenia.

The reversal of the neutropenia depends largely on the causative factor. Aplastic anemia may be cured by transplantation with HLA-compatible bone marrow or in some instances by treatment with antithymocyte globulin or cyclosporine, since recent evidence suggests an immune origin in a small proportion of cases. Although androgens and corticosteroids are widely used in the treatment of bone marrow failure, most controlled studies show no substantial benefit. Leukemia, lymphoma, myeloma, other responsive neoplasms, and collagen-vascular diseases are best managed by appropriate drug regimens. Splenectomy is rarely indicated in patients with hypersplenism, except those with Felty's syndrome. In patients with drug-induced neutropenia, immediate cessation of the drug is crucial. Therapy is supportive through the period of neutropenia. Lithium therapy may shorten the neutropenic interval after chemotherapy but has no substantial benefit in patients with stable neutropenic disorders. Infusion of CSF may be a therapeutic option in the future.

LEUKEMOID REACTIONS

The term "leukemoid reaction" usually refers to a marked increase in circulating mature neutrophils, whereas specific designations such as lymphocytosis, monocytosis, or eosinophilia are used to describe marked elevations in other normal cell types. Leukemoid reactions are characterized by a marked elevation in the total leukocyte count, frequently in excess of 50,000 cells/mm³, with a predominance of mature neutrophils. The cells appear relatively normal but may show increased azurophilic granules (toxic granulation) or pale blue inclusions in the cytoplasm (Döhle's bodies).

Leukemoid reactions can be acute or chronic. Acute leukemoid reactions occur in response to hypoxia, stress, violent exercise, severe pain, or administration of drugs such as epinephrine or corticosteroids. They can be seen in severe bacterial infection, presumably secondary to endotoxin and other mediators released during the infection, and can persist several days after anesthesia or surgery.

Chronic leukemoid reactions are found in patients with chronic blood loss, heavy smoking, emotional disturbance, chronic inflammatory diseases such as rheumatoid arthritis, chronic infection, splenectomy, or tumor, especially in those with cancers of the lung, kidney, or genitourinary tract. Tumor neutrophilia may be due to CSF production, as has been demonstrated, for example, in isolated cases of lung and bladder carcinomas. Patients receiving steroids or lithium also often have mild elevations of the neutrophil count, as do 20% of women in the third trimester of pregnancy.

Occasionally a person has a stable chronic neutrophilia for years without detection of an underlying cause or other hematologic abnormality. This condition has been termed chronic idiopathic leukocytosis. It probably represents a mild aberration in normal feedback control mechanisms.

Leukemoid reactions are differentiated from myeloproliferative syndromes or leukemia by the absence of red blood cell or platelet abnormalities, the absence of organ infiltration, and the finding of a high neutrophil alkaline phosphatase level. Bone marrow samples are hypercellular with increased granulocytic precursors but are not diagnostic of this condition. Leukemoid reactions may mimic chronic myelogenous leukemia (CML) but can be differentiated from this condition by the absence of splenomegaly, anemia, and thrombocytosis. Furthermore, leukemoid reactions are not associated with the Philadelphia chromosome in marrow cells nor with a depression in neutrophil alkaline phosphatase, both of which characterize CML.

Leukemoid reactions should also be differentiated from a distinctly unusual myeloproliferative syndrome known as *chronic neutrophilic leukemia*. This disease is characterized by splenomegaly and marked neutrophilia but differs from CML in that the cells are mature, platelet counts ae normal, neutrophil alkaline phosphatase values are high, and the Philadelphia chromosome is lacking. This form of neutrophilic leukemia is characterized by extensive infiltration of the liver, spleen, and lymph nodes with mature neutrophils and by a bleeding tendency.

MONOCYTES AND MONOCYTOSIS

Monocytes constitute 1% to 9% of blood leukocytes. They are produced in the bone marrow by the action of a specific "macrophage" subclass of CSF or by one of the other CSFs, which act on stem cells with bipotential capabilities for either granulocyte or macrophage differentiation. The cells pass through the monoblast and promonocyte stage to emerge into the peripheral blood as mature monocytes. The differentiation pathway is more rapid than that of the granulocytic series. This explains the early monocytosis, which, after granulocytic aplasia, frequently precedes neutrophil recovery by 48 to 72 hours. Monocytes leave the blood with a half-life of 8 hours and lodge in the liver, spleen, bone marrow, and lung to mature into tissue macrophages. These cells, which are an integral part of the reticuloendothelial system, may persist for many weeks in the tissues.

Both monocytes and macrophages actively phagocytose bacteria and fungi, but they have a predilection for dealing with intracellular organisms such as mycobacteria and *Brucella*.

Monocytes also play an important role in the immunologic response to infection in both production and activation of granulocytes and T cells. As discussed previously, they produce CSF and stimulate other cells to produce it. Furthermore, they present antigen to T cells and produce the interleukin 1 required for T-cell activation.

Monocytopenia occurs, in general, in conditions that cause granulocytopenia. Total absence of monocytes is characteristic of the syndrome of hairy cell leukemia.

Monocytosis is a frequent finding in patients with malignant tumors and myelodysplastic syndromes. In one study 62% of patients with solid tumors had greater than 500 monocytes/mm³. Monocytosis also occurs in patients with lymphoma and is seen in 25% of patients with Hodgkin's disease. Additional disease processes that are believed to be autoimmune in nature, such as rheumatoid arthritis, systemic lupus erythematosus, regional enteritis, and ulcerative colitis, account for approximately 15% of all patients with monocytosis. Infections such as tuberculosis, brucellosis, and subacute bacterial endocarditis may also produce this blood picture. On occasion, extensive carcinomas and widely disseminated tuberculosis may be associated with extreme monocytosis with counts as high as 100,000 cells/mm³. These marked reactions have often been termed monocytic leukemoid reactions. Gradual improvement of the monocytic reaction generally occurs with effective treatment of the underlying condition.

EOSINOPHILS

Eosinophils are produced in the bone marrow in much the same way as neutrophilic granulocytes. A separate stem cell is acted on by a specific eosinophilic type of CSF to induce cellular differentiation. Eosinophilic precursors are first recognizable at the promyelocyte stage by the presence of large orange-red granules in the cytoplasm. Over a period of approximately 9 days, the precursor cells differentiate into eosinophils, and these mature cells are released into the blood where they disappear rapidly with a half-life of less than 1 hour. The life span of eosinophils in the tissues is relatively long, with some mature cells persisting for 7 to 10 days. Surveys have yielded different values for normal blood eosinophil counts, with ranges of none to 450 cells/mm³ in one study and none to 700 cells/mm³ in another.

Eosinophilia is observed in patients with certain neoplasms, collagen-vascular diseases, parasitic infections, allergic diseases, drug reactions, and dermatoses such as pemphigus, pemphigoid, and atopic dermatitis (see Chapter 74). These conditions and the eosinophilic pulmonary syndromes are discussed in later chapters.

BIBLIOGRAPHY

Abrahm JL: Management of the immunocompromised host, Med Clin North Am 68:617, 1984.
Babior BM: Oxygen-dependent killing by phagocytes, N Engl J Med 298:659, 721, 1978.
Bagby, GC Jr and others: T lymphocyte–mediated granulopoietic failure, N Engl J Med 309:1073, 1983.
Blume RS and Wolff SM: The Chediak-Higashi syndrome: studies in four patients and a review of the literature, Medicine 51:247, 1972.
Boggs DR: The kinetics of neutrophilic leukocytes in health and disease, Semin Hematol 4:359, 1967.
Boxer LA and others: Autoimmune neutropenia, N Engl J Med 293:748, 1975.
Burlington H and others: Colony stimulating activity in cultures of granulocytosis-inducing tumor, Proc Soc Exp Biol Med 154:86, 1977.
Cassileth PA: Monocytosis. In Williams WJ, editor: Hematology, ed 3, New York, 1983, McGraw-Hill Book Co.
Dale DC and others: Chronic neutropenia, Medicine 58:128, 1979.

Finch SC: Neutropenia. In Williams WJ, editor: Hematology, ed 3, New York, 1983, McGraw-Hill Book Co.

Greenberg PL and others: The chronic idiopathic neutropenia syndrome: correlation of clinical features with in vitro parameters of granulocytopoiesis, Blood 55:915, 1980.

Metcalf D: The granulocyte-macrophage colony-stimulating factors, Science 229:16, 1985.

Ward PCJ: The myeloid leukocytoses, Postgrad Med 67:219, 1980.

73 • THE LEUKEMIAS

George A. Omura

The leukemias are cancers of the hematopoietic tissues characterized by infiltration of peripheral blood, bone marrow, and other tissues by cells of a particular line, usually lymphoid or myeloid. The involved cells may be immature in appearance, in which case the process is called "acute," or they may be mature looking, in which case the process is "chronic." Originally the morphologic distinction correlated well with the prognosis, but progress in the treatment of acute leukemia has been so great, especially relative to the chronic leukemias, that the terms "acute" and "chronic" have become less meaningful. Although the leukemias have much in common, there are sufficient differences regarding symptoms, physical examination, hematologic findings, prognosis, and response to various treatments that acute leukemia, chronic myelogenous (or granulocytic) leukemia (CML), and chronic lymphocytic leukemia (CLL) should be considered separately. Hairy cell leukemia and adult T-cell leukemia-lymphoma are mentioned in this chapter because of special features. There are other uncommon varieties of acute and chronic leukemias that are not included here because of their rarity, lack of effective treatment, and failure to illustrate principles not otherwise covered.

There are about 26,000 new cases of leukemia each year in the United States, with a slightly higher incidence in males. Almost half of the cases are acute, about 30% CLL, 20% CML, and the rest uncommon types of leukemia.

There are marked variations with age: acute lymphoblastic leukemia (ALL) comprises about 80% of childhood leukemias, whereas acute myelogenous leukemia (AML) is the usual type of adult acute leukemia. In children CML is uncommon and CLL virtually unknown.

Progress in understanding the cause and treatment of leukemia has had and will have relevance to the management of other types of cancer. Parallel with the goal of cure is the need to identify minimal residual disease. Minute amounts of residual leukemia may represent thousands, millions, or billions of malignant cells remaining after treatment, more than enough to reproduce the disease. Thus a breakthrough in treatment may not be recognized with confidence until a breakthrough also occurs in identifying, with immunologic, biochemical, or other techniques, minimal residual disease. Progress in diagnosis, treatment, and supportive care is occurring in a stepwise fashion, although progress is sometimes hard to recognize without time-consuming, large-scale clinical trials and lengthy follow-up.

ACUTE LEUKEMIAS

DEFINITION. Acute leukemias are cancers of the blood-forming organs causing marrow failure and infiltration of various organs and tissues by blast cells. If the disease is untreated, death ensues in a few weeks to several months.

ETIOLOGY. The cause of human acute leukemia remains uncertain, but of the many possible causes that have been suggested, ionizing irradiation, certain chemicals, and viruses have received the most attention. Radiation exposure from atomic bomb blasts, radiation therapy, or inadequate shielding of radiologists has been associated with an increased incidence of AML and CML. Chronic benzene exposure, chloramphenicol, and certain anticancer drugs such as alkylating agents have also been implicated. Viruses may cause some human leukemias. Circumstantial evidence includes the observation that animal leukemias, including some in primates, are of viral causation. RNA-dependent DNA polymerase characteristic of certain RNA tumor viruses has been found in some human leukemias. Moreover, a viral cause of adult T-cell leukemia-lymphoma is now widely accepted. Patients with Down's syndrome (trisomy 21) or Fanconi's anemia and the identical twins of leukemic children have an increased incidence of leukemia, suggesting a role for genetic and hereditary factors.

PATHOGENESIS. Once the leukemic process is initiated, there is a progressive, but not necessarily rapid, expansion of the leukemic cell population. In particular, there is an increase in the population of leukemic stem cells (that is, cells that retain their ability to multiply in the future). This process is associated with a maturation defect (the acute leukemic cells mature very little beyond the blast stage), so that mature functional cells capable of fighting infection (and having a limited life span) are not produced. Although leukemic, the abnormal cells may respond at least partially to normal regulatory mechanisms. For example, there is a decrease in "growth fraction" with increase in population density, as in normal tissues. The presence of leukemic cells in the marrow inhibits production of normal blood cells; this seems to be caused not only by the space-occupying effect of the leukemic infiltrate but also by inhibitory effects on normal cell growth at population densities that would not be expected to interfere on a physical or mechanical basis. Although maturation is not typical of acute leukemia cells, some laboratory evidence and a few case reports indicate that under certain circumstances leukemic blast cells can be made to differentiate. In cases where a marker of the acute leukemic clone is present (such as an abnormal karyotype), this marker is not detectable during remission and reappears in relapse, indicating that the leukemic population is in fact a separate clone and that normal marrow elements persist that are capable of repopulating the marrow. This is in contrast to CML in which the marker chromosome seldom disappears during "remission."

CLINICAL MANIFESTATIONS. The signs and symptoms of acute leukemia are caused by marrow failure (anemia, granulocytopenia, and thrombocytopenia from decreased production) and by infiltration of the blood and other organs and tissues by leukemic cells. The severity of manifestations is quite variable, as is the duration of symptoms before diagnosis; symptoms may have been present for less than a week or for many months. Easy fatigability, dyspnea, palpitations, and other symptoms of anemia may be present. Fever with or without demonstrable infection is common. Bleeding or easy bruising or both may occur. Bone or joint pain may be prominent, especially in children. The physical examination may be normal or may show fever, pallor, petechiae or purpura, enlargement of cervical and other peripheral lymph nodes, splenomegaly, and sometimes hepatomegaly. Signs of an infection may be present, although typical findings of a purulent infection or inflammatory response may be muted in patients with severe granulocytopenia. Other signs of tissue and organ infiltration by the leukemia may include striking gum hypertrophy, especially in monocytic variants of AML; a mediastinal mass in T-cell ALL; tonsillar enlargement; or skin infiltrates. Discrete tumor masses (chloromas) may occur in various tissues in AML. Tenderness over the sternum or other marrow-containing bones is frequently present. If the circulating blast count is markedly elevated (blast crisis), the patient may be obtunded, short of breath, or both from impaired cerebral or pulmonary circulation. A variety of neurologic signs and symptoms may occur during the course of the disease, especially meningeal leukemia, but these are not usually overt at the time of initial diagnosis.

LABORATORY FINDINGS. Anemia of variable severity is almost always present and is usually normochromic and normocytic. The reticulocyte count may be normal but is inappropriately low in relation to the anemia, indicating decreased production of erythrocytes. The platelet count is usually low; when it is extremely low (5000 to 10,000), especially in conjunction with generalized bleeding, the possibility of disseminated intravascular clotting (DIC), usually associated with the promyelocytic variant of AML, should be considered. A high platelet count raises the possibility that the patient had a previously undiagnosed "chronic myeloproliferative disorder" that has now transformed into an acute leukemic phase.

Although the term "leukemia" was originally coined to emphasize the elevated white blood count, normal or low counts are not uncommon. The terms "subleukemic" and "aleukemic" leukemia have been used, but the disease process is basically the same; in fact, cases with high white blood cell counts might be viewed as very advanced stage disease. The differential count in the peripheral blood includes a variable percentage, usually reduced in absolute number, of mature neutrophils. In most cases at least a few abnormal cells circulate; these are usually blast forms with large nuclei, one or more nucleoli, and no cytoplasmic inclusions. Additional features and special stains (discussed later) may indicate that they are lymphoblasts or myeloblasts. In some cases monocytes (in AML) or lymphocytes of varying maturity may be part or most of the leukemic population. Abnormal promyelocytes may be seen in AML, but it is unusual for granulocytes of intermediate differentiation (myelocytes and metamyelocytes) to be part of the blood picture; this gives rise to the "hiatus leukemicus" or gap (mature and immature cells, but not intermediate forms) seen in the differential count in acute leukemia as distinct from the complete spectrum of maturation seen in CML. The two major types of acute leukemia should be distinguished whenever possible, since management and prognosis differ substantially.

In ALL on routine staining, lymphoblasts have a relatively large round or oval nucleus that occupies most of the cell. Only one or two nucleoli are usually seen, although this may vary with the stain. Cytoplasmic granules are rare or absent; Auer rods (discussed later) are not expected. The periodic acid–Schiff (PAS) stain is positive, whereas Sudan black and peroxidase stains are negative. Although the "common" case shows a very uniform population of cells in size and appearance, some patients have more pleomorphic populations, and a few patients have large cells with striking cytoplasmic vacuoles (B-cell ALL). Immunologic studies may be helpful. Cases may thus be identified as T-cell, B-cell, pre-B-cell and so on. Some patients react with a "common" ALL antigen; in addition, many such patients show immunoglobulin gene rearrangements, reflecting B-cell lineage. Another distinctive feature of many lymphoblasts is the presence of large amounts of terminal deoxynucleotidyltransferase, an enzyme not expected in myeloblasts.

Although ALL may have several subtypes, AML is even more heterogeneous. Included in this group are myeloblastic, promyelocytic, myelomonocytic, monocytic, and erythroleukemic variants. The myeloblast tends to be larger than the lymphoblast with more abundant cytoplasm. Multiple nucleoli and a finely granular nuclear chromatin pattern are frequent, although the stain may modify these details. Cytoplasmic granules may be present; distinctive inclusions known as Auer rods are sometimes seen. These needlelike structures apparently represent the abnormal development of lysosomal granules and are virtually pathognomonic of AML. Some patients have a mixed population of blasts plus promyelocytes, blasts plus monocytes, or blasts plus megaloblastoid erythroid precursors. Myeloblasts usually give positive reactions with peroxidase and Sudan black stains but not with PAS. Esterase stains may be helpful in identifying monocytes. Lysozyme (muramidase) may be increased in the serum and urine in monocytic leukemia. Anti–myeloid monoclonal antibodies have been developed recently and may be helpful in distinguishing AML from ALL.

On chromosome analysis abnormalities are seen in many patients both with AML and with ALL, but there is no consistent finding except in promyelocytic leukemia, in which a 15 to 17 translocation is found, and in B-cell ALL, which has been associated with an abnormal number 14 chromosome (t8;14). In AML the prognosis varies according to the type of chromosome abnormality found. Occasional patients with ALL, especially adults, have the Philadelphia chromosome, a poor prognostic sign.

The bone marrow aspirate is usually hypercellular with a profusion of leukemic cells. Normal marrow elements are moderately to markedly depleted. In ALL virtually all the cells are abnormal, giving a monotonous appearance, whereas in AML less complete replacement of the marrow is common, giving a more pleomorphic appearance.

Some cases of acute leukemia are not readily or consistently classified by the preceding techniques and may be referred to as acute undifferentiated leukemia. In addition, there are rare cases in which another cell line is involved in the abnormal proliferation.

Sometimes no marrow can be aspirated (dry tap) because the marrow cavity is "packed" with leukemic cells. This can be misinterpreted as an empty marrow (that is, aplastic anemia), but the confusion is quickly resolved by a needle biopsy of the marrow; "touch" preparations are made from the core of marrow to visualize cellular detail, and sections of the biopsy show diffuse infiltration of the marrow with primitive round cells. Occasionally the marrow in AML is surprisingly hypocellular despite a predominance of blasts; this raises the possibilities that the leukemia has developed in the setting of a previously undiagnosed aplastic anemia or that the process will behave in a somewhat indolent fashion (smoldering leukemia).

DIAGNOSIS. Although the diagnosis is not difficult in the average case and major progress has been made in treatment, the diagnosis of acute leukemia is still a devastating one that should not be made in haste. On occasion other disorders including benign ones can cause confusion. Most patients can be maintained with supportive measures for a few days while any residual doubt is resolved. Two exceptions occur when the process represents a medical emergency: the patient with disseminated intravascular clotting complicating the leukemia and the leukostasis syndrome in which the cerebral or pulmonary circulation is compromised. In those situations correct diagnosis and treatment must be rendered on an urgent basis.

One of the most troubling problems in morphologic diagnosis

is the regenerating marrow after a toxic injury, the cause of which may be readily apparent or quite obscure. For example, a normal recovering marrow, after a large dose of cytotoxic chemotherapy, may transiently show a relatively homogenous population of immature blast cells indistinguishable from acute leukemia. Within a few days to a week at least some of the cells mature, the blood cell counts normalize, and the confusion resolves.

A patient with anemia, thrombocytopenia, granulocytopenia, and a profusion of blast forms infiltrating the blood and marrow usually presents little difficulty in diagnosis, even though subclassification may be a problem. However, when the patient first comes to medical attention, the various signs and symptoms may suggest an upper respiratory tract infection, mononucleosis or other viral syndromes, a bleeding disorder, or even rheumatic fever. Once the blood cell counts are known, aplastic anemia, lymphoma, carcinoma or fibrosis in the marrow, or megaloblastic anemias (pernicious anemia or folate deficiency) may be suspected if pancytopenia is present. If the white blood cell count is high, the possibility of a leukemoid reaction is raised. However, leukemoid reactions with a predominance of blast cells are uncommon; severe anemia and thrombocytopenia are not expected as features, and an underlying process (for example, severe infection or metastatic carcinoma) should be demonstrable. Finally, splenomegaly or other evidence of tissue infiltration from the leukemoid reaction is not expected. Depending on the morphology and extent of maturation of leukemic cells, confusion with the chronic leukemias may occur, but this is not usually troublesome. There are instances in which the acute phase of CML is seen without an antecedent chronic phase or in which a preexisting hematologic disorder may cause confusion.

MANAGEMENT. In the late 1940s drugs that had striking, albeit temporary, effects on acute leukemia began to be available; a patient on the brink of death from infectious or bleeding complications might have a complete resolution of signs, symptoms, and laboratory evidence of leukemia, yet within a few months full relapse of the disease was apparent. Considerable progress has been made in preventing relapse, so that relapse is now infrequent in the common type of childhood ALL; a small number of adults with AML also remain in prolonged remission.

Before discussing treatment, it is appropriate to define remission and comment on the "arithmetic" of leukemia. A complete remission exists when there is no evidence of leukemia by current testing capabilities. Symptoms of the disease should disappear; splenomegaly, adenopathy, and other evidence of tissue infiltration should resolve; the blood counts should become normal; and the bone marrow should appear normal. When the patient is in complete remission, the quality of life should be excellent; at the point there might be no remaining leukemic cells in the body (cure) or there might be as many as several billion. (In a mouse leukemia model, one transplanted leukemic cell can reproduce the disease.)

These billions of cells may not be recognized because it is normal to have a few (0.3% to 5%) blast cells in a healthy marrow and because the leukemic cells are usually insufficiently distinctive to be recognizable in the midst of normal marrow elements. If the normal marrow weights 500 to 1000 g and a million cells (10^6) weigh roughly 1 mg, 1% blast cells in the marrow would represent 5 to 10 billion cells throughout the body. With a trillion cells (10^{12}) present at the time of diagnosis, a 3 log reduction (to 10^9) produces a complete remission. If the generation time is 5 days, 10 doublings increase the leukemic population from 10^9 back to 10^{12} in 50 days. It should not be surprising that a partial remission is significantly inferior to a complete remission in prolonging survival, since the "cell kill" is apt to be far less.

A treatment strategy has evolved in which the first step is remission induction with a follow-up phase (or phases) of cytoreduction to reduce the leukemic cell burden still further below the level currently detectable as residual disease. This second step is frequently divided into an earlier phase of consolidation of the remission and then remission maintenance, although some regimens emphasize a lengthy consolidation phase whereas others use an intensive maintenance program. The point is that the leukemic cells develop resistance to particular classes of anticancer drugs, which is frequently relative rather than absolute; moreover, sanctuaries exist where adequate drug concentrations are not achieved after systemic administration. The latter finding has led to a major advance in the management of ALL, prophylactic central nervous system therapy (intrathecal administration of methotrexate with or without cranial irradiation) to irradicate occult foci of leukemia that are not adequately treated by systemic drugs.

Drug dosages are not given here because dose and drug regimens are still evolving, and the use of these regimens should be restricted to specialists.

Childhood acute lymphoblastic leukemia. At least eight classes of drugs have activity in childhood ALL, including corticosteroids (prednisone), the plant alkaloid vincristine, folic acid analogs (methotrexate), purine analogs (6-mercaptopurine, thioguanine), alkylating agents (cyclophosphamide), the enzyme asparaginase, the pyrimidine nucleoside analog arabinosyl cytosine, and the anthracycline antibiotics (daunorubicin, doxorubicin). Mitoxantrone, amsacrine, and the epipodophyllotoxins also have some activity. Remission can be accomplished in about 90% of children with a combination of vincristine and prednisone (VP). Some programs also include asparaginase, an anthracycline, or methotrexate.

In contrast to the temporary enhancement of marrow failure caused by the type of induction therapy required in AML, VP does not exacerbate marrow dysfunction. It rapidly causes regression of lymphoblastic leukemia so that in 1 or 2 weeks the hematologic status is usually improved, and by 3 or 4 weeks many patients are in remission. If VP is continued on a long-term basis, however, not only are steroid side effects and neurotoxicity from vincristine increasingly troublesome, but resistance rapidly develops leading to early relapse. Thus there is a need in the postremission cytoreductive phase to change to other active drugs, usually in combinations designed to reduce the likelihood of resistance while attacking multiple biochemical sites in the leukemic cells. Long-term administration of two or three drugs such as 6-mercaptopurine and methotrexate with or without cyclophosphamide has been used as has a rapidly rotating schedule of multiple drugs. Increasing the number of drugs may, however, increase the frequency of severe or life-threatening immunosuppressive complications. Periodic reinforcement or inducer doses of VP are sometimes used, although the need for them is disputed. Early in remission a series of intrathecal injections of methotrexate is given; this is frequently coupled with a fractionated course of supravoltage irradiation of the cranial contents designed to encompass all the extensions of the meninges. Late effects of irradiation on mentation in long-term survivors have been reported; thus long-term intrathecal methotrexate maintenance therapy without cranial irradiation has its proponents. The optimal duration of combination chemotherapy is unclear; up to 3 years of treatment has been given in some trials, in the hope of eradicating leukemic cells that may be in a prolonged resting phase in which they are less sensitive to chemotherapy than actively growing cells. Late relapse in the testis is an occasional problem. Although very late hematologic relapses (or possible reinduction of the disease by the causative agent) may occur, comprehensive treatment cures at least half the patients with childhood ALL.

Treatment is still evolving, partly to reduce the short and long-term toxicity of these complex regimens in the highly responsive "common" ALL and partly to develop more intensive regimens for less responsive patients such as those with T-cell ALL.

In patients who have had relapses, remission can frequently be reinduced, but sustained second remissions are rare; remission duration tends to become shorter and shorter with retreatment to the point at which neither standard nor investigational drugs are effective and fatal infections or bleeding supervene.

Adult acute lymphoblastic leukemia. Adults with ALL have a lower remission rate and shorter remission duration and survival than do children given the same treatment. Three-drug induction regimens are usually successful in inducing remission (80% overall, 90% in teenagers); multidrug consolidation and maintenance are used in an effort to improve remission duration. Central nervous system (CNS) prophylaxis has decreased the incident of overt CNS leukemia. It is likely that some of the adult ALLs actually are poorly differentiated lymphomas. Current clinical trials are attempting to identify, by immunologic, cytogenetic, and biochemical means, subsets of patients who are curable with current treatment and those whose disease requires new approaches.

Adult acute myelogenous leukemia. In contrast to ALL the spectrum of drugs useful in systemic treatment of AML is limited; only two classes of drugs have significant activity: cytidine analogs, especially arabinosyl cytosine (cytosine arabinoside, ara-C) and anthracycline antibiotics such as daunorubicin and doxorubicin. The other classes of drugs previously noted have only marginal activity. Regimens including daunorubicin or doxorubicin (Adriamycin) plus ara-C with or without other drugs are capable of inducing complete remission in at least half of AML patients; with careful selection and skillful management, most younger adults can achieve remission. Older patients tend to fare poorly, but this may be largely because of the multisystem diseases to which they are prone rather than an intrinsic difference in the disease. On the other hand, some older adults have atypical features to their leukemia and may have an indolent course without specific treatment. Special care should be used in selecting them for antileukemic treatment.

With three doses of an anthracycline and a 7-day infusion of ara-C, the peripheral blood blast count usually falls dramatically; by the end of the infusion about 85% of the patients have severely hypocellular or aplastic marrows. Over the next 2 or 3 weeks normal precursors appear in the marrow, the peripheral platelet count and reticulocyte count rise, and granulocytes reappear in the blood. Some patients require repeated courses of treatment to achieve remission, whereas a few are completely refractory to current drugs. Until remission occurs, intensive supportive care is essential.

The optimal postremission strategy is unclear but may involve one or both of the highly active agents in combination with other drugs. The intensity and duration of consolidation treatment are somewhat limited by the restriction on total accumulated dose of anthracyclines, which are cardiotoxic; by the isoimmunization that frequently develops to transfused platelets and thus interferes with supportive care; by the reduced tolerance of the normal marrow to chemotherapy while normal marrow elements are rapidly regenerating; by the physical toll of sustained therapy, repeated courses of nephrotoxic antibiotics, and malnutrition, which is sometimes correctable only by hyperalimentation; and by the psychologic burden of prolonged hospitalization. Despite all these problems, it may be possible to give three or more courses of combined therapy, for example, with cytosine arabinoside and daunorubicin over a 3-month period. Although early relapses occur, the majority of patients remain in remission through the consolidation period.

It is customary to continue treatment beyond the consolidation phase. Repeated courses of ara-C combinations are usually employed. Unfortunately, the value of maintenance regimens is not routinely tested by comparison with no maintenance.

Childhood acute myelogenous leukemia. About 15% of children with acute leukemia have AML; the complete remission rate (56% to 66%) and remission duration (10 to 21 months) in various series are markedly inferior to results in ALL. The spectrum of active drugs appears to be broader than in adult AML. The strategy for treatment of these children continues to evolve.

Immunotherapy. Spontaneous remissions of acute leukemia occur on rare occasions, suggesting that host factors may be important in combating the disease. Moreover, some studies have indicated a correlation between immunocompetence and prognosis. Several clinical trials have been carried out using active nonspecific stimulation of the immune system with agents such as bacille Calmette-Guérin as an adjunct to chemotherapy for acute leukemia. The results have been disappointing.

Transplantation. Young patients who have a healthy identical twin should undergo marrow transplantation. Others who have an HLA-compatible sibling should be considered for transplantation once they are in chemotherapy-induced remission, since the interim results of this procedure appear superior in remission duration and survival to what was been accomplished so far with chemotherapy. Many problems are encountered in transplant patients, such as graft-versus-host disease and interstitial pneumonitis. Despite preparation of the patient with total body irradiation and high-dose chemotherapy, the leukemia recurs in some cases.

COMPLICATIONS AND SUPPORTIVE CARE. Infections are a major and recurrent problem while the acute leukemia is in relapse and are the usual cause of death. Because of leukopenia, the usual infecting organisms are gram-negative bacilli and *Staphylococcus aureus*. Gram-negative bacillary pneumonias and septicemias, especially caused by *Pseudomonas* organisms and *Escherichia coli*, are particularly common as are perirectal abscesses and urinary tract infections. Dental infections and thrush may be troublesome. Systemic fungal infections are not common early but become more likely later in the course. Fevers usually result from infection that, because of neutropenia, rapidly becomes fulminant despite only minimal signs and symptoms. Prompt broad-spectrum antibiotic coverage (along with appropriate diagnostic studies) is essential. *Pneumocystis carinii* infections require specific treatment with trimethoprim-sulfamethoxazole (see Chapter 54). Strict reverse isolation techniques may be helpful in reducing the incidence of infections but interfere with frequent examination of the patient and incur a psychologic burden; use of a private room, limiting the traffic in the room, and handwashing before touching the patient may be an acceptable compromise. Prophylaxis with trimethoprim-sulfamethoxazole during consolidation has been advocated. Granulocyte transfusions may be a useful adjunct for documented infections occurring while the patient is severely leukopenic.

Cutaneous, gingival, and nasal bleeding are common. Gastrointestinal and pulmonary bleeding are life threatening; intracranial bleeding is usually progressive and fatal. Prophylactic platelet transfusions are given when the platelet count is falling precipitously or is less than 20,000. Menses should be suppressed with a progestin while a young female patient is in relapse, since endometrial bleeding is occasionally uncontrollable. Heparin and replacement of consumable clotting factors may be helpful if DIC is demonstrated. Extreme elevation of the peripheral blast count may result in occlusion and perivascular infiltration of cerebral and pulmonary vessels; cerebral hemorrhage is a common sequela. In addition to urgent initiation of chemotherapy, the use of hydroxyurea, leukapheresis, or both may be helpful in promptly reducing the cell count.

The rapid breakdown of tumor tissue can elevate serum uric acid and result in acute renal failure from marked deposition of urate in the kidneys or ureters. The use of allopurinol prophylactically for the first 2 or 3 weeks of treatment is indicated, and vigorous hydration for the first few days, within the patient's tolerance, should also be used.

Leukemic meningitis occurs in the majority of children and increasing numbers of adults with ALL if the CNS is not specifically treated. Since this process, once overt, is very difficult to eradicate and is a source of reseeding the marrow with leukemic cells, prophylaxis is indicated. This complication is not sufficiently common at present in adult AML to warrant prophylaxis, but the incidence may increase as more patients achieve prolonged hematologic remission.

Anemia should be at least partially corrected with packed red blood cell transfusions to relieve symptoms and to provide a margin in the event of sudden hemorrhage.

PROGNOSIS. Without treatment or if treatment does not result in a complete remission, the median survival for acute leukemia is about 3 months. On the other hand, half of the properly treated children with ALL survive without evidence of recurrent leukemia and are cured. The prognosis for adult ALL is much less favorable; in one series the median remission duration was 19 months and survival 26 months for adult ALL patients receiving CNS prophylaxis. In selected series 20% or more of adult ALL patients have been cured. In adult AML a median remission duration of 8 to 14 months and median survival of about 2 years have been observed for patients in complete remission. Sustained remissions are seen in a few cases; the percentage may be increasing in recent trials. Promyelocytic leukemia patients may have a longer survival and monocytic leukemia patients a shorter survival. Thus, although still one of the most feared diseases, acute leukemia is no longer invariably hopeless, and depending on the specific type, cure may be a realistic goal of current management.

CHRONIC MYELOGENOUS LEUKEMIA

DEFINITION. CML or granulocytic leukemia is a disorder of the bone marrow, spleen, and other blood-forming organs in which marrow elements, especially granulocytes and sometimes megakaryocytes and erythroid precursors, proliferate inappropriately. After a variable period of time ranging from months to years, most cases terminate in a refractory acute leukemic process.

ETIOLOGY. In most instances the cause is unclear, but ionizing irradiation or long-term benzene exposure has been associated with some cases.

PATHOGENESIS. Proliferation kinetic studies show increased production as well as longer survival of granulocytes in CML. There is also an appreciable spontaneous death rate of the leukemic cells. There is usually an increased number of colony-forming cells in the marrow and a marked increase in these cells in the circulation as shown by in vitro agar culture techniques. There is an active exchange of leukemic cells among the bone marrow, blood, and spleen. In some cases spontaneous oscillations of the white blood cell count occur, suggesting some residual feedback control.

CLINICAL MANIFESTATIONS. CML is typically a disease of young to middle-aged adults but can occur at any age. Fatigue, sweating, indigestion, and left upper quadrant discomfort are common early complaints, but sometimes there are no symptoms. Occasionally, abdominal pain (from splenic infarction), symptoms of anemia, an attack of secondary gout, or bleeding manifestations (related to platelet dysfunction) after a dental procedure first bring the patient to medical attention. Moderate to marked splenomegaly is usually present, but adenopathy is not expected in the chronic phase; if present, adenopathy may indicate that the blastic phase (see later discussion) has already started or that a second disorder exists. It should be kept in mind that granulocytic infiltration of lymph nodes may be mistaken on biopsy for lymphoma. Hepatomegaly and bone tenderness may be present. Fever is uncommon.

LABORATORY FINDINGS. The peripheral white blood cell count is usually 50,000 and may reach several hundred thousand. There is a profusion of neutrophils, band cells, metamyelocytes, and myelocytes, with relatively few promyelocytes and blasts in the chronic phase. Eosinophils and basophils are increased, sometimes so strikingly as to jusify calling a case eosinophilic leukemia or basophilic leukemia. The platelet count may be high, low, or normal. In some cases thrombocytosis is the most significant management problem, causing bleeding or clotting complications. The hematocrit value may be normal, slightly increased, or decreased. Anemia if present is usually normochromic and normocytic. The bone marrow is hypercellular with a spectrum of granulocytic elements; megakaryocytes may be strikingly increased as well. A marrow biopsy may show variable amounts of fibrous tissue. A characteristic finding demonstrable in about 85% of cases in marrow preparations and in immature granulocytes from peripheral blood is the Philadelphia chromosome, a deletion of one of the long arms of a number 22 chromosome. The missing arm is usually translocated to a number 9 chromosome.

Recently it was found that this translocation results in a hybrid gene (bcr-abl) and an abnormal protein product, which may play a role in pathogenesis. Although present in granulocytes, erythroid precursors, and megakaryocytes, this translocation is not found in skin fibroblasts, or buccal mucosa cells, indicating that it is an acquired rather than inherited abnormality. Curiously, patients who have CML without this abnormality tend to fare worse. Another distinctive finding in most patients with CML is a low or zero leukocyte (neutrophil) alkaline phosphatase (LAP) score. With treatment or with secondary infections the LAP score in CML may increase into the normal range; old neutrophils tend to have less enzyme than young ones. The pretreatment serum uric acid is frequently increased as is the serum vitamin B_{12} level, the latter as a consequence of an increase in transcobhalamin I, one of the vitamin B_{12}–binding proteins. These increases result from the increased turnover of white blood cells in this disorder. In contrast to acute leukemia and CLL, the leukemic cells in CML are functional, thus accounting for the low incidence of infection and the relatively benign course of the chronic phase.

DIAGNOSIS. In the typical middle-aged patient with splenomegaly, a white blood cell count of 200,000, including a spectrum of mature and immature granulocytes, and a low LAP score, the diagnosis is not difficult. Nevertheless, a chromosome analysis should be performed, since it is of diagnostic (if positive) and prognostic (if negative) value.

A bone marrow biopsy may be helpful in demonstrating extreme hyperplasia and fibrosis. The major sources of confusion are myelofibrosis with myeloid metaplasia (MMM) and leukemoid reactions. Rarely, polycythemia vera and other myeloproliferative disorders are troublesome. Patients with MMM tend to have lower white blood cell counts but truly massive splenomegaly, more extensive marrow fibrosis, and higher LAP scores; no consistent chromosome abnormalities are found. A leukemoid reaction should be in response to some underlying process such as an infection or a carcinoma, does not itself produce organomegaly or marrow changes other than hyperplasia, and should be associated with a normal chromosome analysis and a high LAP score. Occasionally none of the initial findings is clear-cut, in which case careful observation rather than a hasty diagnosis is appropriate.

COURSE AND PROGNOSIS. The typical patient responds well to intermittent therapy for 3 or 4 years, at which point it becomes increasingly difficult to control the white blood cell count, platelet count, or recurrent left upper quadrant pain (splenic infarctions). Serial karyotypes may become increasingly bizarre. Fever, skin infiltrates, or adenopathy may herald the onset of the blastic phase, which is largely indistinguishable from acute leukemia except that it is usually refractory to treatment. The acute phase lasts weeks or months. A fulminating "blastic crisis" with extreme leukocytosis, cerebrovascular accident, or pulmonary insufficiency is much less common than a gradual metamorphosis or transformation evolving over several months. A few patients die of marrow failure with extensive marrow fibrosis, of drug toxic effects, or of other causes without entering an acute phase, but most patients have a blastic transformation sooner or later.

MANAGEMENT. Drug dosages are not given because dose and drug regimens are still evolving, and the use of these regimens should be restricted to specialists.

Alkylating agents, especially busulfan (Myleran), have been the treatment of choice for CML. The chronic phase of CML may be managed with deceptive ease through use of busulfan. Even patients who denied having symptoms often feel better after treatment is started. Nevertheless, patients should be undertreated with this drug. On a short-term basis, busulfan is treacherous because of its prolonged marrow toxicity; the hematologic toxic effect may be slow in onset (weeks or months) but once established may be life threatening and is slow to resolve. During the period of daily treatment, frequent reduction of dose is essential as the patient responds; treatment should be stopped before the blood cell counts reach normal so as not to overshoot and cause marrow aplasia. On a long-term basis, pulmonary fibrosis, cytologic atyia (? carcinogenesis), and an addisonian-like syndrome of weakness, hypotension, and hyperpigmentation may occur. More important, survival is not significantly prolonged, although the quality of life is frequently improved. Intermittent treatment with busulfan when leukocytosis and splenomegaly recur is recommended in most cases; only in selected instances or later in the course is long-term maintenance therapy indicated. Hydroxyurea has a rapid effect that is also rapidly dissipated; this is useful in quickly lowering blood cell counts but requires frequent monitoring to adjust the dose. Thioguanine is occasionally useful.

Splenic irradiation may cause a hematologic remission by an "abscopal" or remote effect that is not well understood. Intravenous radioactive phosphorus has also been used. Even though the blood cell counts, marrow hypercellularity, and splenomegaly may be dramatically improved by treatment, repeat chromosome analysis of the marrow in Philadelphia chromosome–positive cases shows this leukemic cell marker in abundance; thus the magnitude of leukemic cell kill has been minimal (from 10^{12} to perhaps 10^{11}) despite the appearance of remission, which might better be called pseudoremission. Moreover, the onset of the blastic or "malignant" phase is not delayed. Since a true complete remission is not achieved and the accelerated phase is unaltered, it is not surprising that survival has not been lengthened.

Recently α-interferon was shown to produce both hematologic and cytogenetic improvement in some patients. Whether it prolongs survival remains to be determined. When a suitable donor is available, bone marrow transplantation should be considered, since prolonged remissions with a normal karyotype have been achieved.

Once the patient is in the blastic phase, the leukemia is usually quite resistant to the type of therapy used in AML. A minority of patients, however, show a temporary response to prednisone and vincristine combinations. This largely corresponds to the curious observation that about 30% of blastic CMLs have cell characteristics (surface markers, terminal transferase, corticoid receptors, morphologic or staining characteristics) of lymphoblasts rather than myeloblasts. Presumably the leukemic transformation in these cases is occurring in primitive cells that antedate differentiation into myeloid and lymphoid lines. Splenectomy in the blastic phase (for cytopenia or recurrent splenic infarcts) is occasionally useful but has a high complication rate in some series. There is controversy about its value in the chronic phase.

CHRONIC LYMPHOCYTIC LEUKEMIA

DEFINITION. CLL is a monoclonal proliferation of mature-looking, long-lived lymphocytes that accumulate in the bone marrow, blood, and lymphoid tissues of some older adults. It usually, but not invariably, shortens life expectancy. Less than 30% of leukemias in the United States are of this type.

ETIOLOGY. The cause of CLL is unknown. In contrast to the myeloid leukemias, neither ionizing irradiation nor chemicals have been implicated. A viral causation has not been shown. Familial ocurrence has been reported but is rare. Immune defects may play a role.

PATHOLOGY. A profusion of lymphocytes may be seen infiltrating the marrow, nodes, spleen, and liver, but the extent of infiltration at the time of diagnosis is variable. Other tissues may be affected, but virtually never the CNS. The histologic appearance is that of a well-differentiated lymphocytic lymphoma.

CLINICAL MANIFESTATIONS. The typical patient is a 60-year-old man complaining of fatigue and perhaps painless lumps in the neck, armpits, or groin. On examination, symmetrically enlarged, firm, nontender lymph nodes are usually felt in most or all node-bearing areas. The spleen is frequently enlarged, but not massively. The liver may also be enlarged. A few patients have no signs or symptoms, and the disease is recognized by an absolute lymphocytosis found at the time of a routine blood cell count. Occasionally symptoms of anemia, bleeding, or recurrent infection bring the patient to medical attention. Fever if present is rarely attributable to the disease process; secondary infection is usually the cause. Skin lesions of specific (infiltrative) and nonspecific types are sometimes seen.

Infections with encapsulated bacteria (pneumococci, *Haemophilus influenzae,* and group A streptococci) are common, presumably because of the patient's inability to produce antibody.

LABORATORY FINDINGS. In a normal adult the absolute lymphocyte count (percentage of lymphocytes × total white blood cell count) is less than 4500. When the lymphocyte count is 100,000 to 200,000, the abnormality is readily apparent, but minimal elevations, for example, a white blood cell count of 10,000 with 60% lymphocytes, are troublesome unless the monoclonal nature of the lymphocyte population or tissue infiltration can be shown. The percentage of mature neutrophils in the differential cell count is often very low, but the absolute neutrophil count may be normal except in advanced disease or as a result of treatment. The platelet count is usually normal or slightly decreased; severe anemia may result from an associated autoimmune (Coombs'-positive) hemolysis, bleeding, or very advanced disease. The serum uric acid concentration is usually normal before treatment but may increase significantly with treatment. Bone marrow examination is largely confirmatory rather than essential for diagnosis; a profusion of lymphocytes, mostly mature looking, is seen. Marrow cellularity may be normal but is sometimes "packed" with a lymphocytic infiltrate. The pattern of marrow infiltration has prognostic value. Serum immunoglobulin levels are frequently low and the circulating antibody response to vaccines is impaired, but delayed hypersensitivity reactions to recall antigens are usually intact. In vitro lymphocyte transformation after stimulation with mitogens is impaired. Most patients have cell surface characteristics of a single clone of B lymphocytes. Patients with T-lymphocyte characteristics have also been described. Hilar, mediastinal, or retroperitoneal adenopathy may be demonstrated with appropriate roentgenograms and scans. An abnormal serum paraprotein or cryoglobulin may be found.

DIAGNOSIS. An adult with a markedly elevated lymphocyte count, especially in association with generalized adnopathy and splenomegaly, usually presents no problem in diagnosis. Other causes of lymphocytosis such as pertussis, infectious mononucleosis, and infectious lymphocytosis occur largely in childhood or adolescence. A slight lymphocytosis may occur in tuberculosis, thyrotoxicosis, and Addison's disease, but the associated features should be distinctive. In all of these non-neoplastic disorders the lymphocyte proliferation should be polyclonal. When there is uncertainty, especially with a modest lymphocytosis, lymphocyte typing should be done. Confusion may arise in differentiating CLL from a well-differentiated lymphocytic lymphoma when there is a minimal increase in circulating lymphocytes, but current management is similar. Variants of CLL such as chronic lymphosarcoma cell leukemia and prolymphocytic leukemia have been described.

MANAGEMENT. Several treatments of modest value are available, including corticosteroids, alkylating agents such as chlorambucil, and ionizing irradiation. There is considerable controversy about whether asymptomatic patients should be treated, since they often have a benign course over months or years, treatment may have side effects and complications, and survival is not predictably improved. A popular clinical staging system ranging from stage 0 to stage IV is as follows: stage 0 is lymphocytosis alone; stage I is lymphocytosis plus adenopathy; stage II adds splenomegaly and/or hepatomegaly; in stage III anemia is present; and in stage IV thrombocytopenia occurs. There is a significant difference in survival of early- and late-

stage patients. Current efforts are focused on treating advanced disease, since the prognosis for such cases with casual treatment is relatively poor. It is possible, using chlorambucil plus prednisone, to achieve a response in most patients. Unfortunately, responses are seldom complete when assessed by immunologic as well as hematologic parameters, and survival is not predictably prolonged by a partial response. Bulky masses of nodes may regress dramatically after localized radiation therapy when the response to systemic treatment is inadequate. A variety of dosage schedules of chlorambucil and prednisone have been advocated; typically, chlorambucil is given on a long-term daily basis, but a fortnightly bolus of the drug can be used. Several intermittent schedules of prednisone are currently used; it is important to avoid a daily dose if possible because of the well-known complications of long-term steroid therapy, especially in a group of patients who already have multiple defects of immunocompetence. At present, treatment is not recommended for early-stage, asymptomatic patients. High lymphocyte counts are not associated per se with the acute leukostasis problem occurring in acute leukemia, but extreme leukocytosis (several hundred thousand cells per cubic millimeter) may be an indication for treatment. Patients with progressive, symptomatic, or advanced-stage disease should have a trial of systemic therapy for at least 6 months. The maximal response may require many months. The optimal duration of treatment is unclear, but indefinite therapy must be tempered by the potential carcinogenic effects of alkylating agent treatment. Patients whose leukemia progresses after an unmaintained remission may respond again, although resistance to standard agents ultimately develops. Other drugs have generally been disappointing after failure with chlorambucil and prednisone. Pentostatin (deoxycoformycin) and interferons are being evaluated.

SUPPORTIVE CARE. Before treatment is started, allopurinol and vigorous hydration should be used to decrease the risk of uric acid nephropathy. Fever should always be assumed to result from infection rather than the leukemia, although other causes such as drugs may be apparent. Prompt diagnosis and treatment of infections are essential. Prophylactic antibiotics or γ-globulin injections have been advocated but are not recommended for routine use. Splenectomy may be useful for autoimmune hemolysis or thrombocytopenia unresponsive to steroids and for "hypersplenism."

COURSE AND PROGNOSIS. CLL may be indolent or progress rapidly over a matter of several months with hematologic deterioration and recurrent, ultimately fatal infections. Blastic transformation has been reported but is rare. The incidence of second malignancies is increased.

The prognosis depends on the stage of the disease and the quality of the response to treatment. Longevity may range from 19 months in stage IV to over 12 years in stage 0.

HAIRY CELL LEUKEMIA

Hairy cell leukemia is an intriguing disorder that is briefly described because, although it is uncommon, notable progress has been made in treatment. This hematologic malignancy, usually of older men, is typically manifest as splenomegaly, pancytopenia, and abnormal hairy cells in the blood and bone marrow. These cells contain a tartrate-resistant acid phosphatase and usually have B-lymphoid markers. The customary treatment for severe cytopenias has been splenectomy, which may be of major although temporary benefit. Chlorambucil has been less helpful. Recently, significant responses have been observed with α-interferon and with an investigational agent, pentostatin (deoxycoformycin). The optimal use of these agents, alone or in combination, is being assessed.

BIBLIOGRAPHY
Acute leukemias

Champlin R and Gale RP: Bone marrow transplantation for acute leukemia: recent advances and comparison with alternative therapies, Semin Hematol 24:55, 1987.

Gale RP and Hoffbrand AV: Acute leukaemia, Clin Haematol 15:3, 1986.

Omura GA and Raney M: Long term survival in adult acute lymphoblastic leukemia: follow-up of a Southeastern Cancer Study Group Trial, J Clin Oncol 3:1053, 1985.

Chronic myelogenous leukemia

Champlin RD and Golde DW: Chronic myelogenous leukemia: recent advances, Blood 65:1039, 1985.

Molecular biology and chronic granulocytic leukaemia (editorial), Lancet 2:666, 1986.

Chronic lymphocytic leukemia

Gale RP and Foon KA: Chronic lymphocytic leukemia: recent advances in biology and treatment, Ann Intern Med 103:101, 1985.

Hairy cell leukemia

Ratain MJ, Vardiman JW, and Golomb HM: The role of interferon in the treatment of hairy cell leukemia, Semin Oncol 13(suppl 2):21, 1986.

74 · THE EOSINOPHIL AND EOSINOPHILIC SYNDROMES

Richard Snepar and **Donald Kaye**

The finding of increased numbers of eosinophils in the peripheral blood is abnormal and may represent one of a number of diverse pathologic conditions. Blood eosinophilia rarely occurs as an isolated event and is usually associated with other sites of organ infiltration.

Eosinophils are produced in the bone marrow, but their cell of origin remains unknown. In the peripheral blood "normal" ranges for eosinophils vary depending on how they are expressed. As a percentage of the total leukocyte count, up to 4% is considered normal. A more accurate expression is the number of eosinophils per cubic millimeter. Counted in this manner, the range of normal is approximately 0 to 700 cells/mm^3, with a mean normal value of 120 cells/mm^3 in adults.

The eosinophil is distinct from other leukocytes; most have bilobed nuclei, and the granules stain orange to deep red with Wright or Giemsa stains. The granules elaborate numerous enzymes. The role of the eosinophil in the host response is probably to modulate the inflammatory reaction and to aid in the defense against multicellular parasites (worms).

Certain conditions are frequently associated with a rise in the level of circulating eosinophils. Parasitic infection is a prominent cause. Although most helminthic infections can cause a mild rise in circulating eosinophils, those associated with tissue invasion cause the most marked elevations. *Trichinella, Strongyloides,* and *Toxocara canis* and *cati* are notorious causes of high peripheral blood eosinophil counts. Protozoan infections (other than *(Pneumocystis carinii)* rarely cause a significant eosinophilia.

The eosinophilic pulmonary syndromes (see Chapter 168) are (1) *Löffler syndrome,* a 3- to 4-week illness consisting of peripheral blood eosinophilia, eosinophils in the sputum, and transient fluffy pulmonary infiltrates, which is often caused by drugs, inhaled antigens, or parasitic infections and is responsive to steroid therapy; (2) *pulmonary infiltrates with eosino-philia* (PIE), an illness of longer duration characterized by peripheral and apical pulmonary infiltration, fever, and dyspnea often caused by drugs, parasites, connective tissue disorders, or neoplasms and frequently responsive to steroids; and (3) *tropical pulmonary eosinophilia,* a syndrome of fever, pulmonary infiltrates, and bronchospasm caused by occult microfilarial infection. The last usually responds to diethylcarbamazine.

The *hypereosinophilic syndrome* represents a group of conditions characterized by persistent marked eosinophilia and diffuse organ infiltration with eosinophils. These conditions lack evidence of a known cause of eosinophilia. They range from prolonged benign eosinophilia to eosinophilic leukemia. The cardiovascular system is nearly always involved, generally in the form of myocarditis and endocardial fibrosis with congestive heart failure (presumably caused by a direct effect of the eosinophil), and marrow eosinophilia and leukocytosis are consistently noted. The lung (interstitial infiltrates), skin (rash), kidney, central nervous system, and liver are frequently involved.

Eosinophilia is also seen in association with asthma, polyarteritis nodosa, allergic rhinitis, drug allergy, and skin diseases, notably pemphigus and pemphigoid. Less frequently, eosinophilia may be associated with lymphoma and disseminated carcinoma, immune deficiency states, graft-versus-host reactions, and inflammatory bowel disease.

There is a group of pathologic conditions involving specific organ infiltration with eosinophils with or without blood eosinophilia. Eosinophilic gastroenteritis is characterized by eosinophilic infiltration of the stomach and small intestine (see Chapter 125). Eosinophilic fasciitis refers to eosinophilic infiltration and thickening of the fascia clinically resembling dermatomyositis (see Chapter 17). Eosinophilic cholecystitis, cystitis, and prostatitis have also been described. Eosinophilic granulomas, aggregates of histiocytes and eosinophils, may be found in bone or soft tissues (see Chapter 78). Corticosteroids are often useful in these conditions.

BIBLIOGRAPHY

Fauci AS and others: The idiopathic hypereosinophilic syndrome: clinical pathophysiologic and therapeutic considerations, Ann Intern Med 97:78, 1982.

Glelch GJ and Luegeung DA: Immunobiology of eosinophils, Ann Rev Immunol 2:429, 1984.

75 · MYELOPROLIFERATIVE DISORDERS

Frank H. Gardner and **Gary B. Weiss**

The term "myeloproliferative disorders" has been used to characterize a group of clinical neoplastic proliferations of all bone marrow precursor elements. The encompassing term has been useful in emphasizing that proliferation of pluripotent stem cells can have an abnormal response in any of the committed cell compartments. Fig. 75-1 outlines a schematic concept regarding the overlapping definitions of these various disorders. The proliferation of committed stem cells is self-perpetuating and in this regard appears to be a neoplastic disease. Indeed, the transition may be a preneoplastic disorder for years or through the lifetime observation of the patient. In this group of diseases we include chronic granulocytic leukemia, polycythemia vera, agnogenic myeloid metaplasia with myelofibrosis, and essential thrombocythemia. A schematic relation-

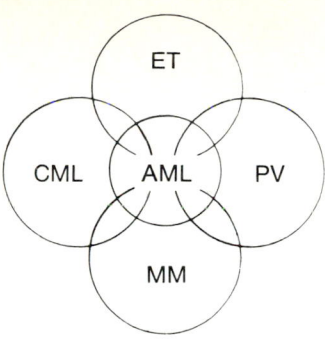

Fig. 75-1 Schematic concept of interaction of different types of myeloproliferative disease. Lower overlaps of circles indicate relationship of myeloid mataplasia, *MM*, with chronic granulocytic leukemia. *CML*, and polycythemia vera, *PV*. Upper overlaps of circles reflect transitions of essential thrombocythemia, *ET*, into CML and PV. In a small number of patients any of these disorders can evolve into acute myeloblastic leukemia, *AML*.

ship of the transition among these different types of proliferative disorders is represented in Fig. 75-1.

Since the 1982 French-American-British (FAB) classification of myelodysplastic syndromes (refractory anemia, acquired idiopathic sideroblastic anemia, refractory anemia with excess blasts, and chronic myelomonocytic leukemia), intense investigation of these preleukemic states has been undertaken. Their interrelationships with the other myeloproliferative disorders is being discovered, and cytogenetic studies show frequent abnormalities. These are discussed in Chapter 62.

In all instances the stimulation of one committed stem cell is associated with a generalized marrow hyperplasia, implying general activation of all the committed stem cell compartments. With this proliferative activity, reticulin fibers are increased, which suggests that bone marrow fibroblasts also have increased activity.

CHRONIC GRANULOCYTIC LEUKEMIA

As with polycythemia vera, current data that show that chronic granulocytic leukemia or chronic myelogenous leukemia (CML) is an abnormal clonal malignancy. CML is discussed in Chapter 73, and polycythemia vera is discussed in Chapter 71.

ESSENTIAL THROMBOCYTHEMIA

Essential thrombocythemia is defined as an elevation of the platelet count above 600,000/mm³, associated with a bone marrow megakaryocytic hyperplasia and a mild neutrophilic leukocytosis without marrow fibrosis, an increased red blood cell mass, iron deficiency, or evidence of another cause for thrombocytosis. Glucose-6-phosphate dehydrogenase (G6PD) isoenzyme studies have shown clonal involvement of platelets as well as neutrophils, red blood cells, and B lymphocytes as occurs in polycythemia vera. Essential thrombocythemia is seen most commonly in middle-aged women. The disease usually is diagnosed because of spontaneous subcutaneous bleeding that may occur for months or years. It is characterized by frequent gastrointestinal bleeding with associated hypochromic iron deficiency anemia. On physical examination the patient may have evidence of superficial phlebitis, and splenomegaly is found in more than three fourths of the patients.

Laboratory examination may establish the diagnosis. The platelet count ranges from 600,000 to several million; the platelets are enlarged and found in large clumps on examination of the peripheral blood smear. In many instances the abnormal platelet morphology is associated with impaired platelet function as measured by platelet aggregation techniques and a prolonged bleeding time.

The presence of thrombocytosis should alert the physician to associated myeloproliferative disorders. Platelet counts are usually not as high in chronic leukemia, myeloid metaplasia, or polycythemia vera.

The disease is not treated unless the patient is symptomatic or elderly. If there is evidence of bleeding as demonstrated by ecchymoses or abnormal venous coagulation with thrombophlebitis or by hypochromic anemia with chronic gastrointestinal bleeding, the patient should be treated with either an alkylating agent (busulfan or L-phenylalanine mustard) or radioactive phosphorus. From current observations both alkylating agents work more rapidly than radioactive phosphorous. Both modalities are associated with an increased frequency of acute leukemia if therapy is continued over many years. Hence it is the usual policy to treat the patient only until the platelet count is 200,000 to 400,000/mm³. Thereafter, retreatment is not planned until there is evidence of abnormal platelet function with symptoms.

AGNOGENIC MYELOID METAPLASIA (MYELOFIBROSIS WITH MYELOID METAPLASIA)

DEFINITION. The term "agnogenic myeloid metaplasia" has been used to describe a group of middle-agd patients (50 to 70 years predominantly) who have fibrosis of the bone marrow (myelofibrosis) and bone marrow precursors circulating in the blood and found outside sites of normal adult marrow, especially in the liver and spleen. Since the fibrosis is the predominant pathologic finding without explanation, the term "agnogenic," for an unknown mechanism, has been preferred.

It is thought that myelofibrosis is the end stage of polycythemia vera in possibly 10% of such patients. In past years there have been repeated references to myelofibrosis associated with toxicity from solvents, especially benzene. This was much more frequent 30 years ago, especially in the shoe industry with the use of rubber cement, than it is today. After the atomic bomb episode in Japan, increased myeloid metaplasia was described, suggesting that ionizing irradiation also may be a factor. Although estrogens may induce an alteration like myelofibrosis in many animals, no correlation has been made in humans. The disorder is associated with abnormal chromosomes in the hematopoietic cells of 40% to 50% of the patients, but the bone marrow fibroblasts do not have the same chromosome abnormality. Similarly, studies of G6PD isoenzymes demonstrate the clonal involvement of hematopoietic cells but not marrow fibroblasts.

PATHOGENESIS. With the abnormal proliferation of bone marrow–committed stem cells in extramedullary areas, there is progressive enlargment of the spleen and liver and ultimately the lymph nodes, as well as increased fibrosis in the marrow cavity. There is a concurrent osteosclerosis. Transition to an acute leukemic process may occur as with other myeloproliferative disorders, and a blastic crisis develops in 5% to 10% of patients with myeloid metaplasia.

CLINICAL MANIFESTATIONS. Although the disease is primarily one of middle to old age (over 95%), with men affected slightly more frequently than women, it occurs in a small number of patients between 20 and 40 years of age, who have a tendency for a more rapid progression and complications. The clinical manifestations are protean and vary from the asymptomatic patient who is discovered to have splenomegaly on routine examination, with evidence of a mild leukocytosis and a rare normoblast on the peripheral blood smear, to other patients who have numerous symptoms. Seventy-five percent of patients complain of marked fatigue, which may or may not be associated with anemia. In over half of the patients there is a weight loss, which has been attributed to an increased metabolic rate and to distortion of the alimentary tract with impaired nutrition because of the massive splenomegaly. Indeed, some patients may be seen in a terminal cachectic state related to the weight loss. Abnormal abdominal pressure and signs of distention because of the splenomegaly are noted in 90% of the patients. About 65% have hepatomegaly.

It should be emphasized that over half of the patients may have prolonged intervals of low-grade fever associated with the organ enlargement. Often it is difficult to distinguish this fever from infection. About one fourth of the patients have bone pain, which can be a diagnostic problem to the physician and the patient. Usually such patients have roentgenographic evidence of osteosclerosis (Fig. 75-2). The pain has a chronic aching pattern, characteristically in the humeri and femora. In some instances the patient may have swollen joints suggestive of rheumatoid arthritis. Indeed, with marked hyperuricemia, the physician may interpret this to be a gouty attack.

Often there are complications of impaired platelet function. Patients may initially have symptoms similar to those of essential thrombocythemia because of platelet abnormalities.

Although the spleen is usually grossly enlarged, in a few instances the splenomegaly may not be palpable and may be demonstrable only by radioisotope scanning. There is some correlation between the duration of the disease and the size of the spleen.

LABORATORY FINDINGS. The peripheral blood smear in myeloid metaplasia characteristically contains tear-shaped red blood cells. Polychromatophilia, stippling, and nucleated red blood cells are required by some clinicians for a well-defined diagnosis. Reticulocytosis usually is insignificant and ranges from 2% to 7% in the classic case. The leukoerythroblastic response demonstrates all stages of granulocyte precursors with variable numbers of myeloblasts (2% to 20%) and nucleated red blood cells. The morphology of the red blood cells may be helpful in distinguishing the disease from chronic granulocytic leukemia.

The degree of anemia varies somewhat with the duration and severity of the disease. Leukocyte counts can range from normal to values above 80,000/mm^3. Platelet counts exceeding 1 million with abnormal platelet morphology and function are seen, but most often the platelet count is 200,000 to 400,000/mm^3. Leukocyte alkaline phosphatase (LAP) scores are not helpful except in excluding chronic granulocytic leukemia. In all instances the scores are higher than in CML. Hyperuricemia with occasional gouty attacks occurs in 25% to 50% of the cases. About one fourth of the patients have abnormal serum protein electrophoretic patterns of either a monoclonal or a polyclonal type. With the elevated levels of early granulocytes, the histamine blood levels are always elevated.

In recent years the cytogenetic abnormalities on bone marrow study have been of special interest in myeloid metaplasia, since about half of the patients have a variety of duplications or translocations, most frequently in the C group. There is no evidence that the Philadelphia chromosome is found in this disorder.

Roentgenographic studies demonstrate the generalized increase in bone density with a mottled appearance of the bones, especially vertebrae and long bones. Bone marrow biopsy is the most important diagnostic study in demonstrating the increased thickness of trabecular patterns along with marrow fibrosis. These changess are best demonstrated by 2 to 3 cm long cores obtained from the posterior iliac crest. The degree of fibrosis varies markedly from only increased reticulin fibers

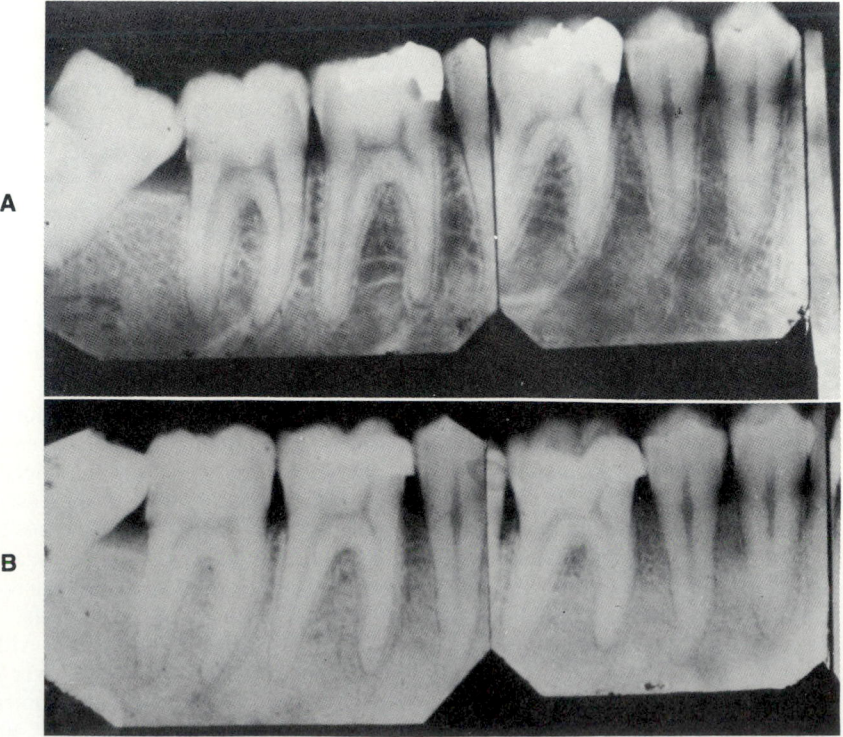

Fig. 75-2 Roentgenograms of 26-year-old man with myeloid metaplasia. He complained of diffuse aching of entire mandible. Radiologic studies, B, revealed osteosclerosis with distinct loss of alveolar bone with crestal deficiency reaching level of molar bifurcation. Similar view taken 2 years previously, A, was available to show progressive osteosclerosis, B, from normal pattern.

to more than two thirds of the marrow replaced by collagen. In the early stages of the fibrotic phase, megakaryocytes appear to be increased, but there has not been an exact way to quantitate them. Aspirations are often unsuccessful (dry tap).

There is an increased frequency of complications from needle aspiration biopsies of the liver in this disorder, and in most instances it should not be performed. Gastrointestinal roentgenograms may reveal an increased incidence of asymptomatic esophageal varices, possibly related to the disproportion of blood flow from the enlarged spleen into the portal circulation. A few patients have had serious bleeding complications requiring a portacaval shunt. Radioisotope scanning techniques may demonstrate large areas of opacity in the spleen from repeated splenic infarcts.

PROGNOSIS. Patients with myeloid metaplasia usually survive 4 to 5 years from the time of diagnosis. The major causes of death are hemorrhage and infection. Leukemic transformation probably occurs in 10% of the cases. Current data suggest that patients with myeloid metaplasia who have an abnormal chromosome have a shorter survival than patients without a cytogenetic abnormality. A rare variety called acute myelofibrosis is characterized by a rapidly fatal course with pancytopenia and diffuse marrow fibrosis. This may be a transitional form of acute myeloblastic leukemia.

MANAGEMENT. There is no available literature that demonstrates an improvement in survival with the various therapies currently available. Androgens in high doses (testosterone or nandrolone [200 to 400 mg weekly]) have increased hemoglobin levels and red blood cell mass and decreased the need for red blood cell transfusions. Patients with abnormal chromosome patterns have not responded satisfactorily to any type of androgen treatment. Androgen therapy is well tolerated by men but is distressful to women because of masculinization. It should be emphasized that all androgens used orally to treat these disorders are associated with abnormal results of liver function tests.

Patients with excessive hemolysis, thrombocytopenia, or painful massive spleens have tolerated splenectomy with marked improvement. Large painful spleens become intolerable to some patients. Patients with high white blood cell counts and no significant anemia may tolerate irradiation of the spleen to decrease the size and to improve alimentary nutrition. Some patients who have marked leukocytosis may benefit from judicious use of alkylating agents such as L-phenylalanine mustard or busulfan, and some investigators have recently suggested that this be used more frequently. Patients with massive splenomegaly and thrombocytosis who receive splenectomy have been treated with cytosine arabinoside or hydroxyurea to decrease platelet counts in the postsplenectomy period. Some patients with massive hemolysis have responded to corticosteroids, but the therapy for the most part is distressing because of the complications of adrenal steroids and is therefore not advised unless necessary. In rare patients with acute myelofibrosis, bone marrow transplantation has been successfully employed.

BIBLIOGRAPHY

Buzaid AC, Garewal HS, and Greenberg BR: Management of myelodysplastic syndromes, Am J Med 80:1149, 1986.

Murphy S and others: Essential thrombocythemia: an interim report from the Polycythemia Vera Study Group, Semin Hematol 23:177, 1986.

Smith RE, Chelmowski MK, and Szabo EJ: Myelofibrosis: a concise review of clinical and pathologic features and treatment, Am J Hematol 29:174, 1988.

Varki A and others: The syndrome of idiopathic myelofibrosis: a clinicopathologic review with emphasis on the prognostic variables predicting survival, Medicine 62:353, 1983.

76 · PLASMA CELL DISORDERS

Nikolay V. Dimitrov

The immune system includes two major components, cellular immunity and humoral immunity. These components develop along separate but interrelated pathways of differentiation. The lymphocyte is considered to be the central cell involved in the physiology and pathophysiology of the immune system. Studies of various membrane markers of lymphocytes and their functional activities have provided tools for identification of two major populations of lymphocytes. Thymus-derived cells (T cells) are responsible for cell-mediated immune responses. Bone marrow–derived cells (B cells) are the precursors of the plasma cell line and are responsible for antibody production. B cells can be readily identified by immunoglobulin determinants present on their surface. These cells constitute about 30% to 40% of the circulating lymphocytes and have relatively short life spans. They are found in the lymphoid follicles and medullary cords of lymph nodes, in the peripheral white pulp and red pulp of the spleen, and in the lymphoid follicles adjacent to the mucosa of the gastrointestinal and respiratory tracts. Although the circulating antibodies are produced by lymphocytes and plasma cells, which are progeny of B cells, the participation of suppressor-T and helper-T cells in regulation of the antibody response is essential (Fig. 76-1). This chapter discusses disorders of plasma cells and B lymphocytes that share the common characteristics of production of excessive or abnormal monoclonal immunoglobulins. This occurs as a result of uncontrolled proliferation of cells normally involved in antibody production. Thus the plasma cell disorders arise when a malignantly transformed B lymphocyte enters uncontrolled proliferation, forming a clone of abnormal cells. The growth of the malignant clone may be unrestrained, producing a systemic malignant disease as in multiple myeloma, Waldenström's macroglobulinemia, and some types of heavy-chain disease. In other disorders such as benign monoclonal gammopathy, the malignant clone may grow to a certain extent

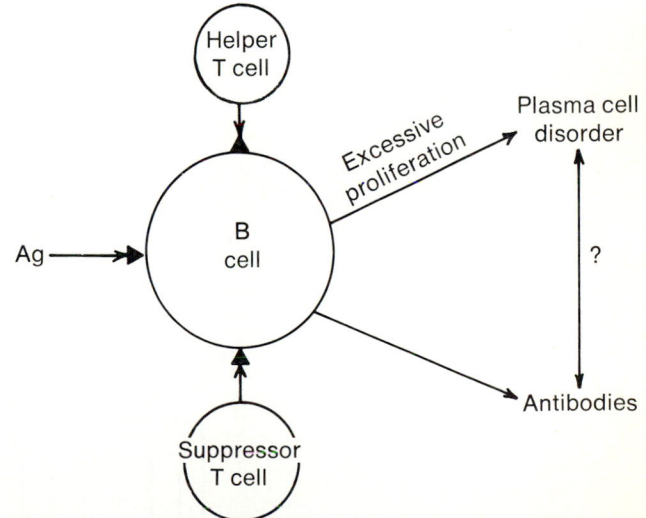

Fig. 76-1 Schematic presentation of factors affecting B-lymphocyte function. Antigen, *Ag,* interacts with B cells that proliferate to form plasma cells. B lymphocytes and plasma cells produce antibodies; antibody production is modulated by helper and suppressor T cells. Excessive proliferation of abnormal B cells and plasma cells leads to plasma cell malignancies. Relationship between normal production of antibodies and abnormal plasma cells is unclear.

and then become controlled with stabilization of the proliferation. Rarely in both instances the clone regresses.

Since plasma cell disorders are associated with anomalous production of proteins, the accurate diagnosis of these disorders requires identification and quantitation of the abnormal monoclonal immunoglobulins (IgG, IgA, IgM, IgD, IgE). Some authors use the term "M protein," which refers to the electrophoretically homogeneous components in the serum or urine and means "malignant," "myeloma," or more recently "monoclonal." "Monoclonal" should be used.

The structure of immunoglobulin molecules is a multichain assembly consisting of two heavy and two light polypeptide chains. The arrangements of IgG molecules are presented in Fig. 76-2. Various enzymes are capable of splitting the heavy chains, thus forming two fragments: the Fab fragment consisting of a light chain joined to a portion of the heavy chain and the Fc fragment consisting of portions of the two heavy chains (square portions on Fig. 76-2).

Protein electrophoresis is a routine test that in the majority of cases appears sufficient for detecting a monoclonal protein in the serum or urine (Fig. 76-3). For further identification of the monoclonal protein components, immunoelectrophoresis should be used. This method employs protein electrophoresis for separation of the major components and immunodiffusion using specific antisera for identification of the abnormal monoclonal immunoglobulin (Fig. 76-4). Quantitation of monoclonal immunoglobulin in the serum or of light chains in the urine provides a marker of malignant cell activity. Serial studies are useful as an evaluation procedure for changes that occur during the treatment or in the course of observation.

For practical purposes these three methods for identification and quantitation of monoclonal protein are sufficient. With the development of modern immunology many other methods for identification of numerous subclasses of immunoglobulins are available, but at this time their value lies mostly in research.

Although the information from the monoclonal protein studies appears quite specific, the approach to diagnosis and treatment of plasma cell disorders should rely on a combination of clinical, morphologic, and laboratory considerations.

MULTIPLE MYELOMA

Multiple myeloma is a malignant disorder of plasma cells with clinical manifestations characterized by the formation of a tumor, bone marrow dysfunction associated with marrow replacement by abnormal plasma cells, bony lesions, renal disease, and abnormal synthesis of immunoglobulins.

ETIOLOGY. Multiple myeloma shares some of the general aspects of the origin of the neoplastic diseases. The exact cause of multiple myeloma is unknown. Some clinical and experimental observations suggest that chronic stimulation of the reticuloendothelial system may play a role in the development of plasma cell disorders. This has been supported by the development of plasma cell tumors in mice after injections of mineral oil, Freund adjuvant, and plastics. In humans, plasma cell disorders have been found in association with chronic diseases such as tuberculosis, chronic osteomyelitis, pyelonephritis, chronic hepatitis, and rheumatoid arthritis. An association between high-dose radiation exposure and plasma cell myeloma among the survivors of the atomic bombs in Hiroshima and Nagasaki has been demonstrated. The standardized relative risk for individuals with air-dose exposure of more than 100 cGy was 4.7 times greater than that of control subjects.

A viral cause has been suggested by experiments in mice using transmissible viral agents that induce the development of plasmacytomas containing viruslike particles. This has been associated with the presence of monoclonal protein and excretion of Bence Jones proteins in some of the animals.

The importance of genetic factors has been suggested by observation of some familial aggregations of multiple myeloma, particularly those occurring in siblings.

PATHOGENESIS. The pathophysiologic manifestations in multiple myeloma are closely related to the abnormal proliferation of immature and mature plasma cells, bone marrow dysfunction, and protein abnormalities. The abnormal proliferation of plasma cells occurs in the bone marrow with the formation of solitary osseous tumors. Isolated extraskeletal myeloma tumors can be found occasionally. These pathologic findings are considered to be a cause for transient or permanent skeletal pain and diffuse or local skeletal demineralization. Extensive involvement of the skeleton frequently leads to pathologic fractures. Destruction of the bones may result in increased serum and urine calcium.

The abnormal proliferation of the plasma cells in the bone marrow appears to impair its function. The exact mechanism for the decreased bone marrow function is unknown, but the

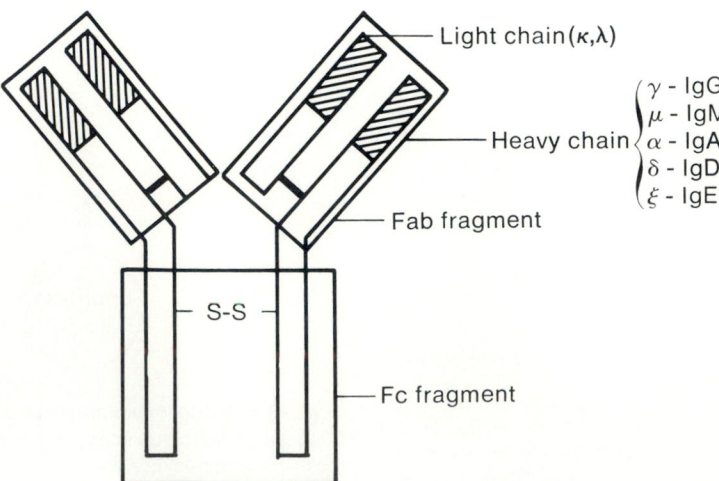

Fig. 76-2   Schematic representation of immunoglobulin molecule, showing two heavy (H) and two light (L) chains. Papain digestion cleaves molecule into Fc fragment (two portions of heavy chains) and two Fab fragments consisting of light chain and portion of heavy chain.

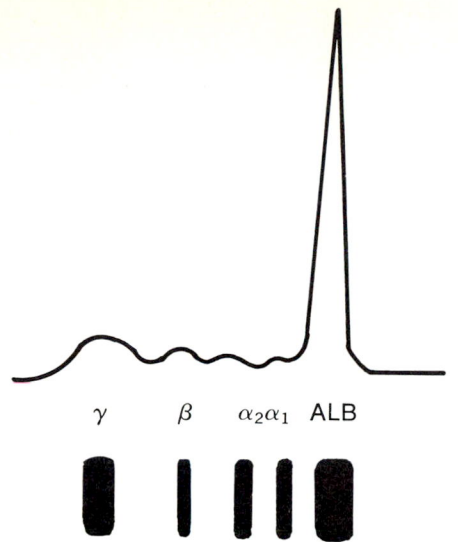

Fig. 76-3   Pattern of normal protein electrophoresis.

extent of the plasma cell infiltration seems to play an important role. Impairment of bone marrow function is usually proportional to the number of plasma cells in the marrow. Mainly the erythroid elements are affected, resulting in the development of anemia, but thrombopoietic and leukopoietic function may also be impaired with the development of thrombocytopenia and leukopenia.

Myeloma cells are responsible for the production of abnormal proteins found in the serum and urine of patients with the disease. These proteins play an important role in the diagnosis of multiple myeloma and related disorders. Most patients with plasma cell disorders have increased concentrations of homogeneous proteins called "M" (monoclonal) components in the serum. These components can be IgG, IgM, IgA, IgD, or IgE. In addition, either κ or λ light chains may be present in urine. In other cases free κ or λ light chains or fragments of heavy chains in the urine may be the only abnormality detected.

It has been generally accepted that the precipitation of the light-chain (Bence Jones) proteins in the renal tubule may result in a unique kidney disease, sometimes designated "myeloma kidney."

Although the γ-globulin level is increased, synthesis of antibodies appears to be defective. This, together with a decreased number of granulocytes, increased catabolism of γ-globulin, and the immunosuppressive effect of chemotherapy, leads to increased susceptibility to infection, which is the major problem in the management of this disorder. The infections are most commonly caused by encapsulated organisms (pneumo-

cocci, *Haemophilus influenzae,* and group A streptococci) and occur because of lack of antibody. There is also an increased incidence of herpes zoster, which is also more likely to generalize.

CLINICAL MANIFESTATIONS. Multiple myeloma is a disease predominantly of middle and old age. Almost 90% of the patients are over the age of 45. Men appear to be affected more often than women.

The onset may be preceded by an asymptomatic period that is variable in length. The most common presenting symptom is pain, which is related to bone involvement and pressure on the adjacent nerves. Pathologic fractures are a common complication that can lead to spinal cord or nerve root compression. Invasion of the nerve roots by myeloma cells or symmetric peripheral neuropathy unrelated to invasion has been reported. However, intracranial and cranial nerve involvement is considered a rare finding, even though the skull bones are a common site of myeloma lesions.

The roentgenographic abnormalities vary from patient to patient. The dominant pattern is generalized osteoporosis, occurring in 90% of the patients. Scattered osteolytic lesions may be found in about 75%. The most common sites of osteolytic lesions are the skull, mandible, ribs, clavicles, spine, pelvis, and sternum. The characteristic roentgenographic findings are described as "punched-out" lesions without osteoblastic reaction (Fig. 76-5). This indicates that roentgenograms are the method of choice for radiologic diagnosis of multiple myeloma. Bone scans have no practical value for the evaluation of patients with this disease. Solitary skeletal lesions can be found on roentgenograms in a small percentage of patients, mostly localized in the vertebra, pelvis, or femur. In such cases thorough investigation may reveal protein abnormalities or even distant bone marrow involvement. In a patient with solitary lesions disseminated disease usually develops after several months or years.

The presence of bone destruction frequently is associated with hypercalcemia. Patients with restricted physical activity are prone to hypercalcemia, which is aggravated by dehydration and oliguria. These patients have nausea, vomiting, drowsiness, and general weakness.

As a result of bone marrow impairment, anemia of variable severity is present in nearly all patients with multiple myeloma. In certain cases blood loss and shortened red blood cell survival may contribute to this abnormality. Most often anemia is moderate and has a normocytic and normochromic pattern. Examination of the peripheral blood smear shows formation of rouleaux, which is attributed to increased plasma protein concentration.

Abnormal bleeding can be a major problem for the clinician and surgeon. Besides thrombocytopenia, 2% to 5% of patients with multiple myeloma have hyperviscosity as a result of elevated serum levels of a monoclonal immunoglobulin. The

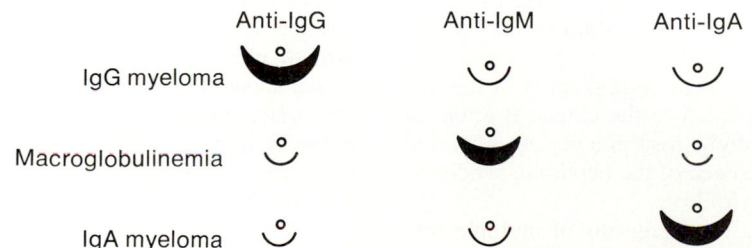

Fig. 76-4   Precipitation arcs resulting from exposure of patient's serum after electrophoresis to specific antisera. Patterns of IgG myeloma, IgA myeloma, and macroglobulinemia are illustrated.

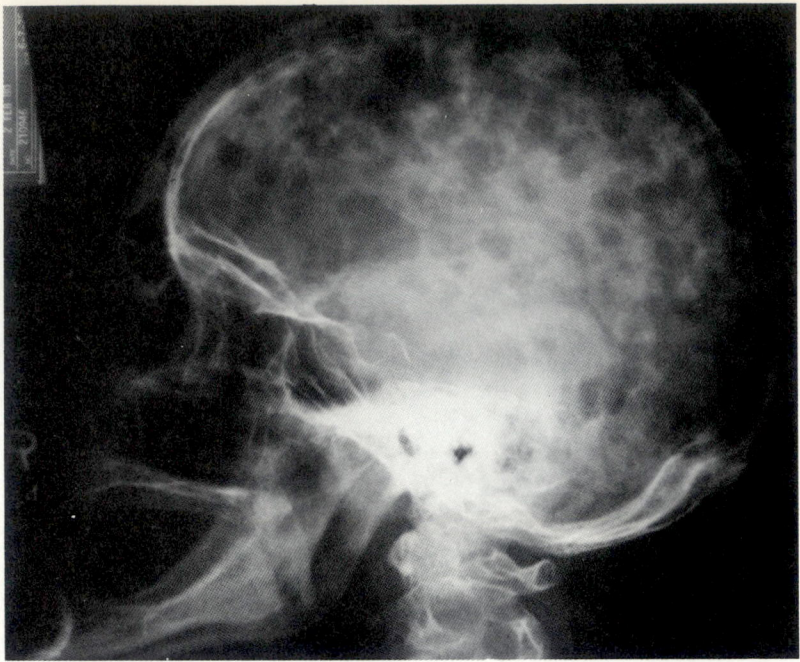

Fig. 76-5 Multiple myeloma. Roentgenogram of skull and mandible shows multiple lytic lesions ("punched-out" lesions).

Table 76-1 Some characteristics of immunoglobulins

Type	IgG	IgM	IgA	IgD	IgE
Molecular weight (approximate)	150,000	900,000	160,000	180,000	190,000
Serum concentration (mg/dl)	600-1600	50-150	60-330	2-5	0.01-0.04
Subclasses	$IgG_{1,2,3,4}$	$IgM_{1,2}$	$IgA_{1,2}$	—	—
Transport across placenta	+	—	—	—	—
Survival—$t_{1/2}$ (average days)	20	5	5	3	2

presence of this abnormal protein affects several of the coagulation factors and the function of the platelets, resulting in hemorrhagic disturbances such as epistaxis, gum bleeding, gastrointestinal bleeding, purpura, ecchymoses, and hemorrhage in the eye grounds. Patients with multiple myeloma who are scheduled for any kind of surgery, including tooth extraction, require a thorough hematologic evaluation. Hyperviscosity can interfere with blood circulation in the central nervous system, causing changing neurologic findings (paresis, impaired consciousness, and deafness). Heart failure and pulmonary insufficiency may also occur as a result of hyperviscosity.

The relationship between protein abnormalities in multiple myeloma and the formation of amyloid is well established. In some patients the occurrence of congestive heart failure, arthropathy, nephrotic syndrome, or peripheral neuropathy may be associated with amyloidosis. Occasionally patients with multiple myeloma may have increased cryoglobulins in the serum that can be responsible for aggravation of the clinical picture on exposure to cold.

Chronic renal failure is a frequent complication of the disease. The clinical picture is related to the extent of renal involvement and varies from slight insufficiency to advanced irreversible azotemia. The presence of the nephrotic syndrome is usually associated with amyloidosis.

LABORATORY FINDINGS. The diagnosis of multiple myeloma always requires thorough examination of the bone marrow. In most cases the aspirate is sufficient for diagnostic purposes, but if a dry aspiration is obtained because the marrow is packed with plasma cells, biopsy is indicated. Increased numbers of atypical plasma cells are present in almost all of the patients with multiple myeloma (Fig. 76-6). The number of such cells should exceed at least 15% of the total marrow cells. Plasmacytosis of bone marrow may be encountered in chronic infections and various neoplastic diseases. Plasma cells seen in multiple myeloma vary in size and shape, possess polychromasia, may contain a large nucleolus, and frequently have cytoplasmic and intranuclear inclusion bodies. The terms "Russell's bodies," "Mott cells," "morular cells," and "grape cells" refer to the presence of cytoplasmic spherules that appear to all be of the same origin. The increased numbers of plasma cells in the marrow usually suppress the erythroid, myeloid, and megakaryocyte function to a variable extent.

Protein abnormalities are the most important findings for documentation of the diagnosis. The serum globulin level is elevated in most cases. The exceptions are patients who overproduce only light chains that are lost in the urine. Serum protein electrophoresis typically shows a prominent monoclonal spike (Fig. 76-7). Immunoelectrophoresis identifies the involvement of specific immunoglobulin (Fig. 76-4). Quantitation is important for diagnosis and follow-up. Some characteristics of various types of immunoglobulins are presented in Table 76-1. Patients with plasma cells producing only κ or λ chains (light-chain disease) frequently have agammaglobulinemia.

Bence Jones proteins are found in the urine of most patients with multiple myeloma, with κ and λ chains being equally

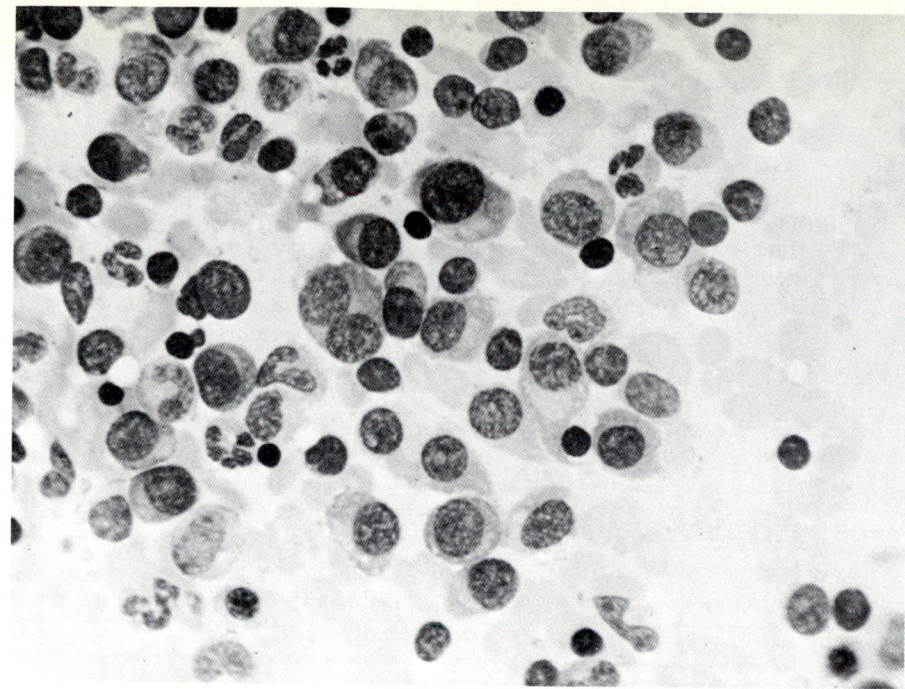

Fig. 76-6   Multiple myeloma. Bone marrow shows atypical mononuclear and binucleated plasma cells with pleomorphism.

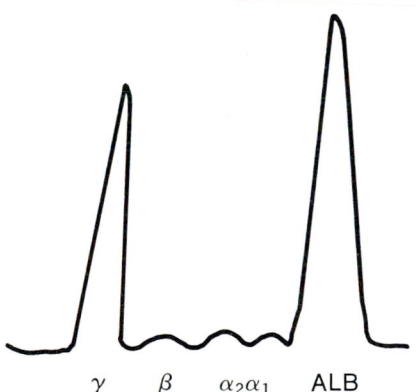

γ   β $\alpha_2\alpha_1$ ALB

Fig. 76-7   Electrophoretic pattern of serum protein from patient with multiple myeloma (IgG).

distributed. The detection of these proteins in the urine requires the presence of a protein concentration more than 0.1 to 0.2 g/dl.

Changes in the biochemical profile are related to the extent of the disease. Hypercalcemia is the most common complication that is frequently associated with hyperuricemia. If the kidneys are involved, elevated BUN and creatinine levels may be found. In some cases the serum alkaline phosphatase level is slightly elevated.

DIAGNOSIS. The clinical presentation does not have a characteristic pattern, and diagnosis requires the demonstration of uncontrolled growth of a plasma cell clone. This is provided by the invasion of normal tissues by plasma cells causing osteolytic bone lesions, extraskeletal plasma cell tumors, and a progressive increase in the amount of a serum M protein or light-chain proteinuria.

The following criteria are accepted for diagnosis of different forms of plasma cell neoplasms:

1. *Plasma cell myeloma.* The diagnostic triad is composed of bone marrow plasmacytosis (at least 10%), osteolytic bone lesions, and presence of serum or urinary M protein.
2. *Solitary skeletal plasmacytoma.* The diagnosis is confirmed by a biopsy demonstrating that the single lesion discovered on a roentgenogram is composed of plasma cells. Bone marrow should contain less than 5% plasma cells. If serum or urinary M protein is detectable, it should disappear after radiation therapy of the lesion.
3. *Extraskeletal plasma cell tumors.* These are usually located in the submucosal lymphoid tissue of the nasopharynx and paranasal sinuses. The diagnosis is confirmed by biopsy demonstrating plasma cells. Bone structures are preserved, but direct invasion into bones adjacent to the tumor may occur. Bone marrow usually contains less than 5% plasma cells.

COURSE. Multiple myeloma is a fatal disease with an average median survival of 3 years from the onset of symptoms. However, the survival may be prolonged, with repeated exacerbations and remissions. Kidney involvement is the most unfavorable factor influencing the prognosis. Recent developments in the management of myeloma patients, including supportive therapy, have contributed substantially to prolongation of their survival time.

MANAGEMENT. Severe pain is a common and almost permanent problem that must be addressed in the management of the patient with myeloma. Most of the time it is due to localized osteolytic lesions that usually respond well to radiation therapy. Orthopedic supports, physical therapy, and immobilization are additional approaches to the treatment of local pain.

Drugs are used to suppress plasma cell growth. Among them, alkylating agents (cyclophosphamide, L-phenylalanine mustard) and adrenocorticosteroids are the most commonly used. A variety of other antineoplastic agents have been used as well. New approaches to treatment using high doses of alkylating agents followed by autologous bone marrow transplantation or use of interferon appear to be promising.

Radiation therapy is a treatment of choice for a solitary skeletal plasmacytoma. Palliative irradiation of pathologic fractures and plasma cell tumors causing spinal cord or nerve root compression is beneficial.

A variety of androgenic steroids have been tried to stimulate erythropoiesis. In cases of extreme granulocytopenia and progressive infection, leukocyte transfusions are used as supportive therapy.

Physical therapy, anabolic steroids, fluoride, calcium, and vitamin D have been recommended to promote bone remineralization. However, their effects appear to be quite limited.

In cases of hypercalcemia, hydration and corticosteroids (prednisone) are usually sufficient. The use of mithramycin or chelation is reserved for resistant cases. Hyperuricemia requires hydration and administration of the xanthine oxidase inhibitor allopurinol for the reduction of serum and urinary uric acid levels. Hyperviscosity is best treated by plasmapheresis.

WALDENSTRÖM'S MACROGLOBULINEMIA

Increased concentrations of macroglobulins have been observed in a number of clinical conditions such as connective tissue disorders, chronic infections, viral infections, a variety of neoplastic diseases, and "benign monoclonal gammopathy," which is considered a stable serologic abnormality in the absence of other underlying disease. The levels of macroglobulins in these conditions are usually slightly to moderately elevated.

In Waldenström's macroglobulinemia there is lymphoid hyperplasia and marked elevation of serum macroglobulin levels. The origin and pathogenesis of this disorder do not differ from those described for multiple myeloma. The pathophysiologic mechanism involved in macroglobulinemia is related to the high intrinsic viscosity of the macroglobulins, resulting in serum hyperviscosity. This can cause impaired circulation in the central nervous system, resulting in vascular insufficiency syndromes (intermittent paresis, impaired consciousness, deafness, and so forth). Hyperviscosity can also produce heart failure and pulmonary insufficiency.

CLINICAL MANIFESTATIONS. Waldenström's macroglobulinemia is more common in men than in women and occurs mostly in patients over 50 years of age. In most cases the overt clinical picture is preceded by an asymptomatic or presymptomatic period of many years. The most common symptoms are fatigue, weakness, weight loss, bleeding, neurologic disturbances, visual disturbances, and sometimes cold sensitivity, cold urticaria, and Raynaud's phenomenon. The most frequent physical findings are hepatosplenomegaly, ocular changes (as described in the following paragraph), enlarged lymph nodes, neurologic abnormalities, purpura, and rarely symptoms of congestive heart failure. Mikulicz's syndrome (enlargement of salivary and lacrimal glands) may be observed in some patients. In most cases with gradual development of lymphadenopathy, splenomegaly, and hepatomegaly the clinical pattern closely resembles that of malignant lymphoma or chronic lymphocytic leukemia. In contrast to multiple myeloma, skeletal lesions, bone pain, and frequent infections are not prominent features of Waldenström's macroglobulinemia. Renal disease and amyloidosis may occur but are much less common than in multiple myeloma. Although osteoporosis has been frequently observed, no direct association with macroglobulinemia has been established.

The examination of the eye grounds reveals characteristic findings caused by hyperviscosity. The retinal veins present "sausage effects," consisting of alternating bulges and constrictions. This may be accompanied by exudates, hemorrhages, and visual impairment.

LABORATORY FINDINGS. A normocytic and normochromic anemia is the most common finding. In some cases the anemia may be profound with hemoglobin levels in the range of 6 to 8 g/dl. Several factors are responsible for this complication. The involvement of the bone marrow contributes to the decreased erythropoiesis, but hemolysis and blood loss may play a substantial role in the pathogenesis of anemia. The expanded plasma volume results in hemodilution, which contributes to the low hemoglobin concentration in patients with macroglobulinemia. Coating of the erythrocytes with IgM is considered a cause for erythrocyte rouleaux formation in the peripheral blood smear, positive Coombs' tests, autoagglutinins, and cross-matching problems encountered in many patients with this disease.

The patient may have neutropenia with a normal lymphocyte count. Eosinophilia is occasionally seen. In some cases lymphocytosis is observed. The morphologic characteristics of the lymphocytes in the peripheral blood may be changed in the terminal phase of the disease and resemble the lymphoid cells seen in the bone marrow. The circulating lymphocytes have monoclonal IgM on their surface, and some lymphocytes may show intracytoplasmic IgM.

Thrombocytopenia is present in about 10% of the patients and contributes to the bleeding diathesis, which is a result of several factors. Coating of the platelets with macroglobulins appears to interfere with their function and particularly with the release of platelet factor.

The pathogenesis of the bleeding diathesis includes changes of the vessels and slowing of the blood flow with increase of the lateral pressure in small vessels. This leads to dilation, tortuosity, and thrombosis with extravasation. This pattern is a result of the hyperviscosity in patients with macroglobulinemia. Formation of complexes between the macroglobulins and certain clotting factors also contributes to the bleeding diathesis.

The erythrocyte sedimentation rate is usually very high. The Sia test, which is based on the insolubility of the macroglobulins in water, is frequently positive. About 25% of patients with Waldenström's macroglobulinemia have Bence Jones proteins in the urine. Serum viscosity is elevated in the majority of the patients. In 49% of the patients the viscosity is above 4 (normal is 1.4 to 1.8).

Bone marrow examination reveals a preponderance of "plasmacytoid" cells that also possess the characteristics of the lymphocyte and the plasma cell. In addition, varying numbers of small lymphocytes, plasma cells, and reticulum cells are seen. Another characteristic feature of the bone marrow finding is an increased number of basophils and tissue mast cells. The cytologic picture of lymph node aspirates or imprints is similar to that described for the bone marrow.

The precise diagnosis of Waldenström's macroglobulinemia rests on the information obtained from protein studies. The serum electrophoresis reveals a homogeneous spike (M component) with mobility between β- and γ-fractions. This mobility suggests IgM protein, but immunoelectrophoresis is the definitive study that determines the IgM identity of the spike (Fig. 76-4). Ultracentrifugation of the serum demonstrates a homogeneous protein with a sedimentation coefficient of 19S. In addition to the macroglobulin, in about 40% of the patients serum cryoglobulins are demonstrated. This may precipitate symptoms of cold hypersensitivity, which is one of the clinical features of this disease (Raynaud's phenomenon).

DIAGNOSIS AND COURSE. The clinical presentation is dominated mostly by symptoms resulting from hyperviscosity, lymphadenopathy, hepatosplenomegaly, and anemia. The diagnosis is supported by bone marrow examination, revealing a proliferation of lymphocytic and plasma cell forms with many intermediate and transitional cell types. Hyperproteinemia with large quantities of monoclonal IgM confirms the diagnosis of Waldenström's macroglobulinemia. The presence of symptoms precipitated by cold is sustained by the demonstration of cryoglobulins.

The course of the disease varies from protracted in the majority of cases to fulminant in complicated cases. Uncontrolled hyperviscosity and severe hemorrhages are usually the causes for rapid deterioration of the patient's condition.

MANAGEMENT. The results of treatment of Waldenström's macroglobulinemia are erratic. Since the disease is relatively rare, organized randomized studies appear to be difficult. Treatment should be individualized. Asymptomatic patients and those with a mild clinical picture should not be treated but should be closely observed. Disease progression is an indication for therapeutic intervention.

The most effective drugs in the treatment of Waldenström's macroglobulinemia are the alkylating agents. Chlorambucil or possibly cyclophosphamide or L-phenylalanine mustard (melphalan) may produce objective responses in this disease. Addition of corticosteroids to the alkylating agent appears to be beneficial for some patients. In patients with a significant hyperviscosity syndrome the use of plasmapheresis should be considered as a temporary measure for control of symptoms. This procedure should be followed by chemotherapy. Use of chelating agents has also been of some benefit. These agents can reduce the disulfide bonds of the protein molecule, which may result in dissociation of macroglobulin aggregates. This treatment is also considered as an addition to chemotherapy.

Since the natural course of the disease varies substantially, the therapeutic response appears to follow similar patterns. Patients resistant to treatment will have a short survival time, whereas those who respond may survive a decade or longer.

HEAVY-CHAIN DISEASE

Heavy-chain diseases are proliferative disorders of B lymphocytes distinguished by the presence in the serum of a population of immunoglobulin molecules consisting of incomplete heavy chains belonging to a given class and devoid of light chains. Thus α, γ, or μ chain disease may be recognized by the presence of heavy chains from IgA, IgG, or IgM, respectively. The origin of this group of diseases is unknown, but there is an association with chronic infections, granulomas, autoimmune disorders, malignancies, and viral infections.

CLINICAL MANIFESTATIONS. More than 200 cases of heavy-chain disease with predominance of an α type have been reported since 1963. The disease affects young and old equally; the α type appears to have predilection for a younger age, including children. The majority of the patients with γ type are over 50 years of age. Type μ heavy-chain disease is the rarest among the three groups; only a few cases have been reported. Most of the cases of this type appear to have close association with long-standing underlying disease such as chronic lymphocytic leukemia or malignant lymphoma. The major clinical and laboratory features of the heavy-chain diseases are presented in Table 76-2.

The onset of the disease is gradual, but acute cases have been reported. The most common symptoms are generalized lymphadenopathy, fever, hepatosplenomegaly, and anemia. Palatal erythema and edema may result in respiratory difficulties of mechanical origin. This finding is considered to be a result of lymphadenopathy of the nodes composing Waldeyer's

ring. In patients with α-type heavy-chain disease, diarrhea and a malabsorption syndrome are characteristic clinical features. This is a result of massive infiltration of the intestine by plasma cells, lymphocytes, and reticulum cells. At a late stage, tumors may develop and cause intestinal obstruction. Occasionally pulmonary symptoms also develop. In some cases roentgenograms of the bones may reveal lesions similar to those seen in multiple myeloma. The suppressed immune system in these patients is a predisposing factor for repeated bacterial infections, which are the most common cause of death.

LABORATORY FINDINGS. All patients have normocytic and normochromic anemia. The majority have leukopenia with a decreased number of granulocytes and eosinophilia. Atypical lymphocytes or plasma cells may be present in the peripheral blood smear. The platelet count is decreased in half of the patients.

Bone marrow examination reveals an increased number of reticulum cells, plasma cells, lymphocytes, and eosinophils. Some of these cells possess neoplastic features. In patients with μ heavy-chain disease and chronic lymphocytic leukemia, the presence of vacuolated plasma cells in the marrow is a characteristic finding.

The serum protein level may be elevated, and an abnormal protein migrating from the β to γ region may be found on electrophoresis. The same protein may be detected in the urine. Immunochemical studies for detection of heavy-chain fragments in the serum are necessary for confirmation of the diagnosis.

In patients with α heavy-chain disease a small bowel biopsy reveals characteristic cellular infiltrates comprised of plasma cells, lymphocytes, and reticulum cells in the lamina propria of the intestine.

DIAGNOSIS AND COURSE. The diagnosis of heavy-chain disease is suggested by clinicopathologic and hematologic findings that resemble those of malignant lymphoma and is confirmed by immunochemical studies. Additional studies such as bone marrow examination and small bowel biopsy may be helpful.

The course of the disease depends on its extent, the frequency and type of infections, and the presence of underlying malignant disease. Survival varies from several months to several years. Various therapeutic attempts have failed to provide a successful treatment for these disorders.

BIBLIOGRAPHY

Azur HA and Potter M: Multiple myeloma and related disorders, vol 1, New York, 1973, Harper & Row Publishers, Inc.

Bergsagel DE and Rider WD: Plasma cell neoplasms. In DeVita VT and others, editors: Cancer, principles and practice of oncology, ed 2, Philadelphia, 1982.

Bloch KJ and Maki DG: Hyperviscosity syndromes associated with immunoglobulin abnormalities, Semin Hematol 10:113, 1973.

Frangione B and Franklin EC: Heavy chain disease: clinical features and molecular significance of the disordered immunoglobulin structure, Semin Hematol 10:35, 1973.

Franklin EC and Buxbaum J: Immunoglobulin structure, synthesis, secretion and relations to neoplasms of B cells, Clin Haematol 6:503, 1977.

Lackner H: Hemostatic abnormalities associated with dysproteinemias, Semin Hematol 10:125, 1973.

MacKenzie MR and Fudenberg HH: Macroglobulinemia: an analysis of forty patients, Blood 39:874, 1972.

Natvig JB and Kunkel HG: Human immunoglobulins: classes, subclasses, genetic variations and idiotypes, Adv Immunol 16:1, 1973.

Waldenström JG: Macroglobulinemia, Adv Metab Disord 2:115, 1965.

Waldenström JG: Benign monoclonal gammopathies. In Azur HA and Potter M, editors: Multiple myeloma and related disorders, vol 1, New York, 1973, Harper & Row, Publishers Inc.

Wintrobe MM: Clinical hematology; plasma cell dyscrasia: multiple myeloma, Philadelphia, 1974, Lea & Febiger.

Table 76-2   Features of heavy-chain disease

	γ	α	μ
Age (predilection)	Above 50	Below 40	Above 50
Underlying disease	—	—	Chronic lymphocytic leukemia, lymphoma
Palatal edema	Yes	—	—
Bowel lesions	—	Yes	—
Bony lesions	Rare	—	Rare
Hepatosplenomegaly	Yes	—	Yes
Peripheral lymphadenopathy	Yes	Rare	Yes
Bone marrow	Eosinophilia, plasmacytosis	—	Lymphocytosis
γ-Globulin	Reduced	Normal or reduced	Reduced
Urinary protein	γ Chain	α Chain	μ Chain

Amyloidosis

Malcolm W. MacNab

The term "amyloidosis" refers to amyloid, the extracellular tissue infiltrate that characterizes this group of diseases. Amyloid has a characteristic emerald-green birefringence as seen by polarized microscopy on Congo red–stained tissues. The deposition may be diffuse and is composed of proteinaceous fibrils of a β-pleated structure, a specific protein conformation not normally found in mammalian tissues. The nature of each specific protein is different and is used as a form of classification, but the unifying characteristic is the twisted β-pleated sheet fibrils of all amyloid deposits.

CLASSIFICATION. There is great diversity to amyloidosis, and it should not be considered one disease. The classification is based on differences in clinical syndromes and amyloid proteins. The types include primary amyloidosis in which there is no evidence of underlying systemic disease and the secondary form that occurs in association with chronic inflammation or infection such as rheumatoid arthritis and osteomyelitis.

Amyloid deposits are also associated with plasma cell dyscrasias and aging. There are heredofamilial amyloid syndromes, and amyloidosis is associated with familial Mediterranean fever. Localized deposition without evidence of systemic involvement has been reported. Since the clinical and pathologic syndrome of primary amyloidosis is similar to that associated with multiple myeloma and other plasma cell dyscrasias, it has been suggested that these amyloid diseases be classified together as "immunocyte dyscrasias with amyloidosis." Because the amyloid in these cases is actually "secondary" to the immunocyte abnormality, it may be best to discard the term "secondary amyloidosis." What was formerly called secondary amyloidosis (that is, secondary to other diseases such as tuberculosis) should now be called "reactive systemic amyloidosis" (Table 76-3).

PROTEINS. The fibril materials of primary and myeloma-associated amyloid (immunocyte dyscrasias with amyloidosis) have the same protein component, which is an N-terminal fragment of an immunoglobulin light chain termed AL (amyloid light chain). AL chains range from 5000 to 25,000 daltons. Primary and myeloma-associated amyloidosis is the most common type of the disease, and it is of interest that a plasma cell dyscrasia develops in some patients with this type.

In contrast, the amyloid protein of the secondary form (reactive systemic amyloidosis) and of familial Mediterranean fever is unrelated to any known immunoglobulin and is termed amyloid AA. It has a molecular weight of about 8500 daltons. The AA protein is a fragment of a normal serum component (SAA) whose function is unknown. SAA is an acute-phase reactant that is increased in infection, inflammation, cancer, all types of amyloidosis, multiple myeloma, lymphomas, and

pregnancy, making SAA measurement not very useful in differentiating the types of amyloidosis. The amyloidosis of familial Mediterranean fever results from the presence of AA protein, whereas the remaining heredofamilial types result from the presence of other proteins such as AFp, which is found in familial Portuguese polyneuropathy (type I).

Localized amyloid deposits have been associated with endocrine neoplasms. These amyloid fibrils are composed of peptide hormone fragments and are termed AE. An example is AEt, a fibril from medullary thyroid carcinoma with fragments of thyrocalcitonin. ASc represents the particular amyloid fibril of cardiac "senile" amyloidosis, and the ASb designation is used for an amyloid fibril formed in the brain. There are many other forms of local amyloidosis, but the nature of these amyloid fibrils has not been well defined (Table 76-3).

Fibrils are not the only components of the amyloid deposits. All types of amyloid also contain a pentagonal substance known as the P component. P component has an amino acid sequence different from that of amyloid fibrils and is found in normal serum with no relationship to the presence or absence of any type of amyloidosis. It is closely related to C-reactive protein. P component's role in the disease process is unclear, but it may act as a template for the amyloid-fibril proteins.

The pathogenesis of abnormal fibril production is unknown, but the destruction caused by the deposits can be significant, since the fibrils are nonimmunogenic and resist normal defense mechanisms. β-Pleated sheet fibrils have been produced in vitro from Bence Jones protein by proteolytic action. This may also occur in vivo by proteolytic cleavage of light chains. Similar proteolytic action producing AA fibrils may occur on SAA produced by the liver, on the surface of monocytes, or in phagocytic lysosomes.

CLINICAL MANIFESTATIONS. In primary or immunocyte dyscrasias with amyloidosis (AL amyloid fibrils) the sites of infiltration are widely dispersed. A restrictive cardiomyopathy is seen in this type of amyloidosis, but also in heredofamilial and "senile" types. There is direct infiltration of muscle, and macroglossia may result. Amyloid material in the glenohumeral joint results in the "shoulder-pad" sign of amyloidosis, and patients may have the carpal tunnel syndrome. In about 50% of patients with AL amyloidosis, renal disease and eventually the nephrotic syndrome develop. Gastrointestinal infiltration is also seen and may be manifest as diarrhea, malabsorption, or any one of multiple complaints. Sensory motor and autonomic neuropathies may occur. Dermatologic signs include purpura, waxy cutaneous papules, alopecia, and scleroderma-like infiltration. Small vessel infiltrates cause purpura, and bleeding may be aggravated by a deficiency of procoagulant factor X. Pulmonary tissue, as well as the liver and spleen, may be involved in primary immunocyte dyscrasias.

In secondary or reactive systemic amyloidosis (AA amyloid-

Table 76-3 Classification of amyloidosis

Classification	Disease	Fibril protein
ACQUIRED SYSTEMIC AMYLOIDOSIS		
Primary and myeloma associated or immunocyte dyscrasias with amyloidosis	Myeloma	AL
	Monoclonal gammopathy	AL
	Macroglobulinemia	AL
	Heavy-chain disease	AL
	Agammaglobulinemia	AL
Secondary or reactive systemic amyloidosis	Chronic infections (tuberculosis)	AA
	Chronic inflammation (rheumatoid arthritis)	AA
	Hodgkin's disease	AA
	Nonlymphoid tumors (hypernephroma)	X
Heredofamilial systemic amyloidosis	Neuropathic forms	
	Portuguese	AFp
	Japanese	AFj
	Icelandic	AFi
	Nonneuropathic forms	
	Familial Mediterranean fever	AA
Hemodialysis associated		AH
ORGAN LIMITED		
Cardiovascular (senile)		ASc_1/ASc_2
Brain (senile)		ASb_1
Cutaneous (lichenoid)		AD
Immunocyte derived	Respiratory tract, urinary tract, bone marrow, and lymphoid system	AL
LOCALIZED DEPOSITION		
Endocrine organ associated	Medullary carcinoma of the thyroid	AEt
	Insulinoma; pituitary, intestinal, and pancreatic tumors	X
Plasmacytoma		AL
Renal casts in "myeloma nephrosis"		AL
Nonlymphoid solid tumors, conjunctival, hereditary deposits, concretions (prostate, lung, liver)		X

Modified from Glenner G: N Engl J Med 302:1333, 1980; and Cohen AS and Connors LH: J Pathol 151:1, 1987.
X, Structure not confirmed.

fibril) the infiltrates are not as widely dispersed. Infiltration occurs primarily in the kidneys, spleen, liver, and adrenal glands and rarely in the cardiac, musculoskeletal, and gastrointestinal systems. The nephrotic syndrome develops in most patients with this form of amyloidosis. Hepatosplenomegaly may be marked. Carpal tunnel syndrome is uncommon, as are macroglossia, purpura, and peripheral neuropathies. Reactive amyloidosis is generally asymptomatic when it involves the gastrointestinal tract.

In several types of amyloidosis and localized amyloidosis the clinical presentation is limited to a specific organ. Lichenoid amyloid is a common local cutaneous type. This is a separate entity and should be distinguished from the lesions of systemic primary or immunocytic amyloidosis. Amyloid deposits are found in the cerebrum and heart of older people, with the incidence increasing with age. Amyloid deposits are frequently found in association with some of the microscopic lesions of Alzheimer's disease, especially the microangiopathic lesions.

DIAGNOSIS AND MANAGEMENT. The diagnosis requires histologic confirmation, with the biopsy site dependent on the clinical presentation. Material should be stained with Congo red and examined under a polarizing microscope. If a bone marrow biopsy is performed in the evaluation of an associated plasma cell dyscrasia, the diagnosis may be confirmed from the specimen, but if this examination is negative, a rectal biopsy should be performed, since 75% to 80% of patients with generalized amyloidosis show rectal deposition. It is important to include a small blood vessel because involvement is frequently limited to the vessels. A gingival biopsy may also be helpful, but a liver biopsy is contraindicated because of an increased risk of bleeding in the amyloid-involved liver.

There is no established treatment for amyloidosis, and therapeutic measures should be directed toward any associated diseases. Therapy has been unsatisfactory but includes cytotoxic agents, prednisone, colchicine, and dimethyl sulfoxide, an amyloid fibril denaturing agent. Cytotoxic drugs used in the treatment of monoclonal gammopathies have resulted in a decrease in levels of the immunoglobulin without changes in the amyloidosis. Colchicine therapy can decrease the febrile attacks of familial Mediterranean fever and prevent the progression of amyloidosis in this disease, but it has been ineffective in other types of amyloidosis.

BIBLIOGRAPHY

Cohen AS and Connors L: The pathogenesis and biochemistry of amyloidosis, J Pathol 151:1, 1987.

Glenner G: Amyloid deposits and amyloidosis: the beta-fibrilloses (in two parts), N Engl J Med 302:1283, 1333, 1980.

Glenner G, Costa P, and Frietas F, editors: Amyloid and amyloidosis: international congress series, vol 497, New York, 1980, Elsevier/Excerpta Medica.

77 · HODGKIN'S DISEASE AND NON-HODGKIN'S LYMPHOMA

Richard V. Smalley *and* Deborah Mayer

HODGKIN'S DISEASE

Hodgkin's disease, accounting for 40% of all lymphomas, has been recognized as a neoplastic entity since 1832. This disease, which was considered fatal two decades ago, now can

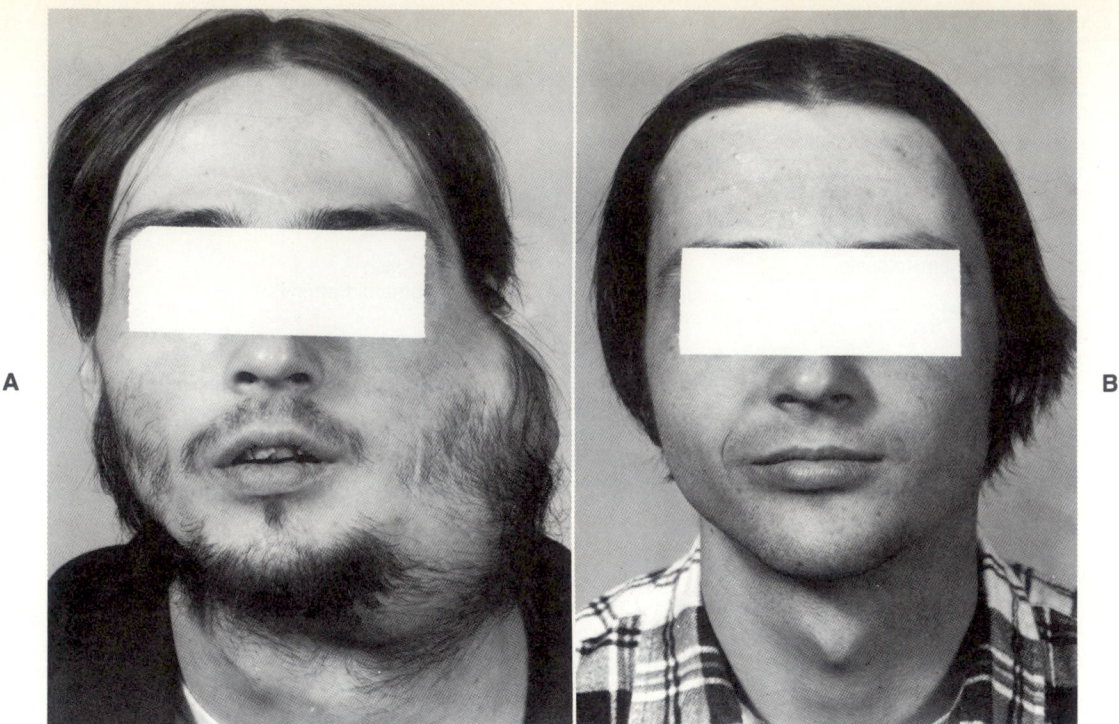

Fig. 77-1 **A,** Cervical lymphadenopathy in patient before treatment. **B,** Complete resolution after 6 months of combination chemotherapy.

be cured in a majority of patients. These significant advances are a result of a better understanding of the disease's biologic characteristics and clinical behavior and of interdisciplinary cooperation in disease management.

According to American Cancer Society estimates there were 7100 new cases and 1900 deaths from Hodgkin's disease in the United States in 1984, with an expected overall 5-year survival of 50% to 60%. A bimodal incidence has been noted with a peak in adolescence and young adulthood and a second sustained increase in later life. The characteristics vary depending on the age at onset. In younger patients there is an equal male/female ratio, a predominance of the nodular sclerosis histologic subtype, frequent mediastinal involvement, and in general a more benign clinical course. In older patients the mixed cellular histologic subtype, which is associated with a more aggressive clinical course, predominates. The overall male/female ratio is 1.4:1.

EPIDEMIOLOGY. There have been many studies exploring possible infectious, genetic, and environmental origins of this disease. Much effort has been placed in evaluating the occasional time-space case clusterings reported, but to date no lead has proved significant. There is the suggestion of an increased incidence of Hodgkin's disease after infectious mononucleosis, which raises the possibility of an association with the Epstein-Barr virus.

In developing countries the lower age peak of Hodgkin's disease occurs in adolescence, whereas in the United States it is during the twenties, proportional to the level of socioeconomic development. This pattern is similar to that of poliomyelitis. Although the cause of Hodgkin's disease remains unknown, both genetic and environmental factors appear to be involved.

IMMUNITY. The majority of patients with Hodgkin's disease have decreased or defective cellular immunity, and in most there is demonstrable cutaneous anergy. This decreased T-lymphocyte function may be due to increased suppressor cell

activity. The immunologic deficiency increases with both advancing disease and increasingly aggressive therapy, with the most pronounced effect noted in patients receiving both chemotherapy and radiation therapy. Because of their defective immune state, patients with Hodgkin's disease are at higher risk of infections caused by microorganisms and parasites that produce intracellular infection. These include bacteria such as *Mycobacterium tuberculosis* and *Listeria*, fungi such as *Cryptococcus*, viruses such as herpes zoster, and protozoa such as *Pneumocystis*.

CLINICAL MANIFESTATIONS. Patients with Hodgkin's disease generally have painless, asymmetric, "rubbery" lymphadenopathy, most commonly (60% to 80%) in the cervical area (Fig. 77-1). One fourth to one third of the patients also have associated symptoms of unexplained weight loss ($\geq$10% in 6 months), fever (>100.4° F [38° C]), and sweats. Malaise and pruritus may be present. Splenomegaly is noted in 50% to 70% of the patients, but despite being enlarged, the spleen may not be involved histologically. Other constitutional symptoms related to the site of nodal involvement include dry cough and dysphagia with mediastinal involvement and lower extremity edema or organ obstruction with abdominal involvement. It is said that rarely ingestion of alcohol causes pain at Hodgkin's disease sites. A mild normocytic and normochromic anemia with or without eosinophilia, neutrophilic leukocytosis, and autoimmune hemolytic anemia is present in 30% to 50% of the patients. The erythrocyte sedimentation rate and serum copper levels may be elevated and can be used as indicators of disease activity to monitor the effects of therapy.

Other disorders to be considered with this type of clinical presentation include infectious mononucleosis, phenytoin-reactive hyperplasia, and other infections that may cause reactive inflammatory changes. The diagnosis must be established by biopsy.

PATHOLOGY. The diagnosis and histologic subtype are established by pathologic examination of involved tissue, usually an enlarged lymph node. The Rye classification, established in 1966, is universally used by pathologists today. The presence of the Reed-Sternberg (R-S) cell, which has a macrophage derivation, is required but is not pathognomonic for the diagnosis of Hodgkin's disease. This cell has a large diameter, either a binucleated or a deeply indented lobate nucleus, one or more prominent acidophilic nucleoli, and a clear perinuclear area. Generally, the prognosis is worse when a large number of R-S cells are present. The following histologic subtypes are recognized.

Lymphocyte predominance. In lymphocyte predominance (LP), normal mature lymphocytes predominate with only an occasional R-S cell noted. As in all histologic subtypes, the normal lymph node architecture is destroyed by the cellular infiltrate. LP accounts for about 10% of all cases of Hodgkin's disease, and it occurs more commonly in younger patients. There is a slight male predominance. Patients with this subtype tend to have localized disease (75% are stage I or II) and therefore usually have an excellent prognosis.

Mixed cellularity. In mixed cellularity (MC) there is a pleomorphic infiltrate of normal-appearing plasma cells, eosinophils, neutrophils, and lymphocytes in addition to R-S cells. This subtype accounts for up to 35% to 40% of cases. Patients tend to have more extensive disease and are more commonly symptomatic (>50% stages III and IV). Therefore they have an intermediate prognosis.

Lymphocyte depletion. Lymphocyte depletion (LD) accounts for less than 5% of all cases, and patients with this subtype usually have the poorest prognosis. There generally are large numbers of R-S cells with few lymphocytes or other white cells. LD occurs more commonly in older patients and is usually extensive on initial examination (80% stages III and IV).

Nodular sclerosis. In nodular sclerosis (NS) the tumor infiltrate forms multiple nodules divided by bands of reticulin that are easily demonstrable, usually by hematoxylin-eosin stain and always by reticulin stain. The nodules generally are visible with the unassisted eye. In addition, "lacunar cells," atypical R-S cells with clear spaces surrounding the cytoplasm, are characteristically noted. This subtype is more predominant in women and in the younger age-group and carries almost as good a prognosis as LP because the patients usually have limited disease. It accounts for 50% to 60% of the cases.

DIAGNOSIS

Staging. Staging at the time of diagnosis is the single most important prognostic variable and the determinant of initial therapy. The Ann Arbor staging classification of patients with Hodgkin's and non-Hodgkin's lymphoma (below) was established in 1970 and is universally used by clinicians.

Stage	Definition
I	Involvement of a single lymph node region (I) or of a single extralymphatic* organ or site (I_E)
II	Involvement of two or more lymph node regions on the same side of the diaphragm (II) or involvement of a contiguous extralymphatic organ or site and one or more lymph node regions on the same side of the diaphragm (II_E)
III	Involvement of lymph nodes on both sides of the diaphragm (III), which may be accompanied by localized involvement of a contiguous extralymphatic organ or site (III_E), involvement of the spleen (III_S), or both (III_{SE})

---

*Extralymphatic may include sites in the lung, bone, bone marrow, liver, or brain. Each stage is subclassified by the presence (B) or absence (A) of one or more of the following unexplained symptoms: weight loss >10% over 6 months, fever >100.4° F (38° C), night sweats.

IV	Diffuse or disseminated involvement of one or more extralymphatic organs or tissue, with or without associated lymph node involvement

Hodgkin's disease most often arises as a single focus and spreads in a predictable manner from nodal group to contiguous nodal group. Parenchymal organ involvement may subsequently occur either by direct extension, that is, the lung contiguous to mediastinal involvement, or by hematogenous dissemination. The staging evaluation should be carried out in a logical manner, taking into account both "prior probabilities" (the probability of a patient having a greater or lesser clinical involvement as related to the histologic subtype) and benefit versus risk factors. Patients with Hodgkin's disease infrequently have extranodal disease (<5% with bone marrow, skeletal, liver, or brain involvement). Because of this, routine bone, brain, or liver scans should not be obtained unless there are specific clinical indications.

Initial staging begins with a thorough history and physical examination, with particular attention to weight loss, fever, sweats, lymphadenopathy, and abdominal organomegaly. The presence of any of the three so-called B symptoms (weight loss >10% of body weight, fever >100.4° F [38° C], and profuse night sweats) is associated with a poor prognosis. Patients with one or more of these symptoms are considered to be "symptomatic" according to the Ann Arbor classification and are subclassified "B." Patients without any of these symptoms have a better prognosis, are considered to be "asymptomatic" (regardless of other symptoms), and are classified "A."

Baseline blood studies include a complete blood cell count and biochemistry profile. A chest roentgenogram is adequate for demonstrating mediastinal or hilar adenopathy, which is present in 25% of the patients (Fig. 77-2). Occasionally, computed tomography (CT) of the thorax is helpful in further defining regional adenopathy. Obvious pulmonary parenchymal involvement is rare, although a relatively large percentage of patients probably have nondemonstrable contiguous pulmonary involvement in association with bulky mediastinal disease. CT of the abdomen and pelvis has generally supplanted ultrasonography, gallium scanning, and lymphangiography, although these latter procedures may be useful in certain isolated circumstances. A CT scan reveals involvement of nodes greater than 1.5 cm in size, whereas lymphangiography, which may be useful for documenting paraaortic and retroperitoneal involvement (Fig. 77-3), reveals involvement in normal-sized nodes. Lymphangiography is not useful in the evaluation of celiac, mesenteric, or splenic hilar nodes. Potential complications from this procedure include pulmonary dye embolism (especially in older patients with compromised pulmonary function) and cellulitis at the cutdown site.

Laparotomy. Despite the value of the procedures just described, surgical staging (laparotomy) is frequently indicated as a final definitive procedure. Patients with unequivocal stage IIIB or IV disease as determined by the preceding studies do not require laparotomy. Laparotomy may be useful in patients with clinical stage I to IIIA disease in whom positive laparotomy findings would change the therapeutic approach. Changes in staging occur after laparotomy in about one third of the patients. Morbidity and mortality from laparotomy are inversely proportional to the surgeon's expertise and are higher in older patients with more advanced disease. At laparotomy, after a general inspection of the abdomen, biopsy specimens are obtained from lymph nodes thought to be involved by radiographic studies, wedge resections and needle biopsies of the liver are carried out, and splenectomy is performed. A

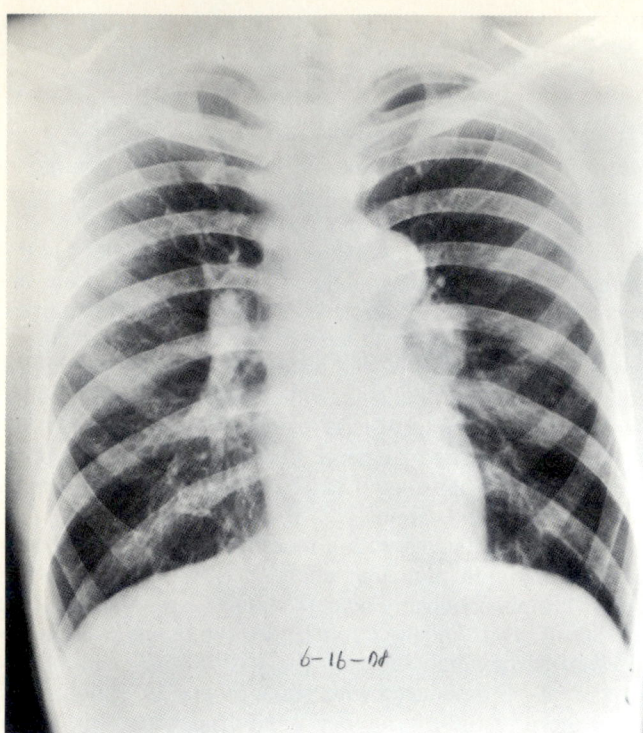

Fig. 77-2 Pronounced mediastinal and hilar adenopathy noted on chest roentgenogram of patient in Fig. 77-1.

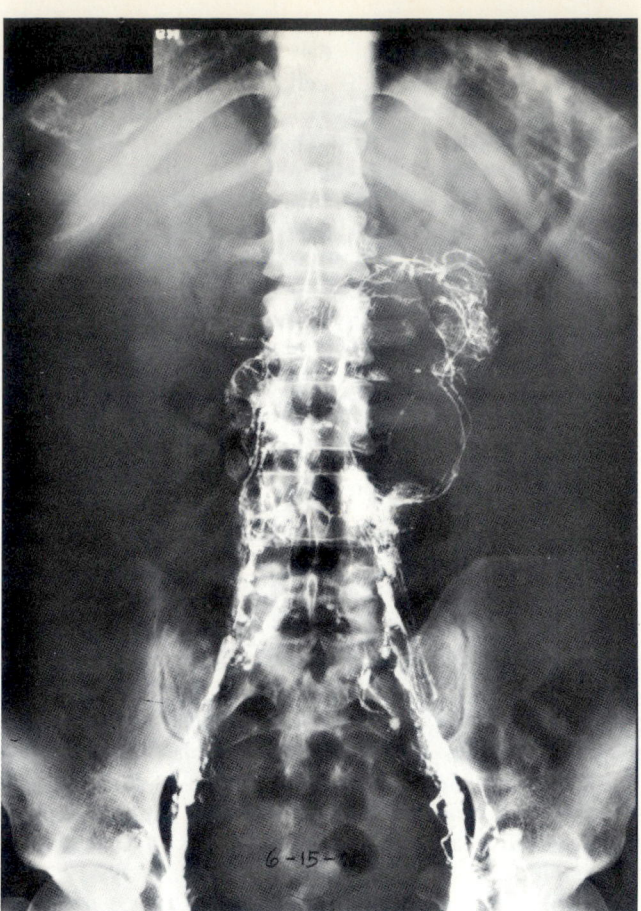

Fig. 77-3 Positive lymphangiogram with extensive para-aortic involvement. Wide deviation of left para-aortic lymphatics indicates collateral flow around enlarged nodes that have been replaced by tumor. Several right para-aortic nodes are also enlarged and foamy, suggestive of tumor involvement.

small percentage of patients (<10%) have splenic involvement as the only site of abdominal disease. The liver is almost never involved when the spleen is normal. When laparotomy is performed by an experienced surgeon, mortality from surgery is nil and complications are rare.

MANAGEMENT. The selection of treatment for patients with Hodgkin's disease is closely correlated with the stage of disease rather than the histologic subclassification. Hodgkin's disease is radiosensitive, and 4000 to 4500 rad given in 20 to 25 daily fractions effectively "sterilizes" and permanently controls nearly all disease within the treatment area. Patients with stage IA or IIA disease may thus anticipate a complete response and a prolonged disease-free survival after either involved field irradiation (treatment of disease-bearing areas only) or subtotal nodal irradiation (SNI). The latter technique delivers treatment to the mantle area (mediastinal, cervical, axillary, and supraclavicular areas bilaterally) and to the paraaortic nodes. It has not been adequately determined whether SNI is more valuable than involved field irradition. Several series have demonstrated a disease-free survival of at least 2½ to 10 years in 85% to 90% of pathologically staged IA or IIA patients after radiation therapy.

Patients with stage IIB disease (true stage IB disease may be nonexistent) may do well (85% to 90% prolonged survival) with a combined modality approach using either SNI or total nodal irradiation (TNI—treatment of all axial node-bearing areas), followed by 6 months of combination chemotherapy (Table 77-1). Recently, attempts have been made to define those patients with stage IIB disease who are most likely to benefit from this combined approach. Patients with a poor prognosis include those who have all three B symptoms and those with bulky mediastinal disease. Stage IIB patients with only one symptom and without bulky mediastinal adenopathy may do well with radiation therapy alone.

Therapy for patients with stage IIIA disease remains controversial. Most patients receive both radiation therapy and chemotherapy, initially undergoing TNI followed by 6 months of treatment with MOPP therapy (Table 77-1). As with stage IIB disease, 90% of patients with stage IIIA respond and maintain a complete response for years after combined therapy, whereas only 67% of the patients with stage IIIA disease receiving TNI alone achieve and maintain a prolonged disease-free status. However, since a course of chemotherapy administered to patients who ultimately have relapse after TNI may save a significant number of patients, some clinicians are reluctant to use combined therapy initially because of the increased toxicity.

Serious side effects of combined therapy include a second malignancy (primarily acute leukemia) in a small percentage and sterility in the majority of patients. Eighty percent of males and 60% of females receiving combined therapy are permanently sterilized. Newer approaches to chemotherapy, if they continue to prove successful, may circumvent these serious and disabling complications.

Patients with stage IIIB, IVA, or IVB disease are currently treated with combination chemotherapy. In 1965 investigators at the National Cancer Institute introduced the cytotoxic chemotherapy combination known as MOPP (Table 77-1), which established combination chemotherapy as a successful form of treatment in patients with malignancy and induced the first cures in what had been a uniformly fatal disease. This combination, now the most widely used chemotherapy regimen, has stood the test of 25 years. Seventy percent of patients with

Table 77-1 Cytotoxic combinations useful in treating Hodgkin's disease

MOPP (each cycle repeated every 28 days)

Nitrogen mustard (Mustargen)	6 mg/m² IV days 1, 8
Vincristine (Oncovin)	1.4 mg/m² IV days 1, 8 (max—2 mg)
Prednisone	100 mg/m² PO days 1-14
Procarbazine (Matulane)	100 mg/m² PO days 1-14

BCVPP (each cycle repeated every 28 days)

BCNU (carmustine)	100 mgsd/m² IV day 1
Cyclophosphamide (Cytoxan)	600 mg/m² IV day 1
Vinblastine (Velban)	5 mg/m² IV day 1
Procarbazine	100 mg/m² PO days 1-10
Prednisone	60 mg/m² PO days 1-10

ABVD (each cycle repeated every 28 days)

Doxorubicin (Adriamycin)	25 mg/m² IV days 1, 14
Bleomycin (Blenoxane)	10 mg/m² IV days 1, 14
Vinblastine	6 mg/m² IV days 1, 14
Imidazole carboxamide (DTIC, dacarbazine)	150 mg/m² IV days 1-5

Table 77-2 Working formulation and Rappaport classifications of non-Hodgkin's lymphoma

Working formulation	Rappaport classification
LOW GRADE	
Small lymphocytic	Diffuse lymphocytic well differentiated (DLWD)
Follicular small cleaved cell	Nodular lymphocytic poorly differentiated (NLPD)
Follicular mixed small cleaved and large cell	Nodular mixed (NM)
INTERMEDIATE GRADE	
Follicular large cell	Nodular histiocytic (NH)
Diffuse small cleaved cell	Diffuse lymphocytic poorly differentiated (DLPD)
Diffuse mixed small cleaved and large cell	Diffuse mixed (DM)
Diffuse large cell	Diffuse histiocytic (DH)
HIGH GRADE	
Large cell immunoblastic	Diffuse histiocytic (DH)
Lymphoblastic	Lymphoblastic
Small noncleaved cell	Diffuse undifferentiated lymphoma (DUL)
	Burkitt's and non-Burkitt's

stage IIIB, IVA, or IVB disease attain a complete response during a 6-month course of MOPP, and 75% of those have a sustained response of several years and apparent cure of their disease. Two other combination chemotherapy approaches (Table 77-1), one comprising BCNU, cyclophosphamide, vinblastine, procarbazine, and prednisone (BCVPP) and the other comprising Adriamycin, bleomycin, vinblastine, and DTIC (ABVD), give results comparable to or better than MOPP in appropriate circumstances. ABVD is not cross-resistant with MOPP and thus may be used in patients who have had relapses after MOPP therapy. Recent studies have demonstrated that the technique of alternating ABVD and MOPP over a 6-month period may induce more complete responses and an improved survival without additional toxic effect.

Toxic effects associated with combination chemotherapy include nausea and vomiting in 50% of the patients and alopecia in 25% to 33%. Late or long-term complications are pulmonary fibrosis after long-term administration of BCNU, congestive heart failure in patients receiving long-term administration of doxorubicin, secondary malignancies such as acute myelogenous leukemia and undifferentiated non-Hodgkin's lymphoma, and sterility. All of these occur more commonly in patients receiving combined modality therapy. There is thought to be a 2% to 4% risk of secondary malignancies after TNI and combination chemotherapy.

Relatively few prognostic criteria are available to aid in determining which patients will have a complete response or a prolonged disease-free survival. Age is a factor noted in many studies. Patients under 40 years of age are more likely than older patients to respond and remain free of disease. Other, minor favorable factors are white race, female gender, and high lymphocyte count (>1300 cells/mm³). A lesser stage and the absence of symptoms have also been noted to be beneficial. The histologic subtype, when corrected for stage, appears to have no influence on the prognosis.

Patients with advanced Hodgkin's disease (stage IIB or IV) who had a relapse after radiation therapy and are receiving salvage chemotherapy have a 75% or better chance of attaining a complete response. However, the likelihood of maintaining a disease-free state for a significant period is less in these patients than in those initially treated with chemotherapy. Only about a third maintain their disease-free state for up to 5 years after salvage chemotherapy.

NON-HODGKIN'S LYMPHOMA

Non-Hodgkin's lymphoma (NHL) is a heterogeneous group of malignant disorders of lymphoid derivation that range in biologic behavior from relatively indolent to very aggressive. This behavior can generally be predicted by and correlated with the histologic subclassification. NHL acounts for over two thirds of all lymphomas. Approximately 23,000 new cases and 12,400 deaths occurred in 1984, according to American Cancer Society estimates. Men predominate (1.7:1), and there is a peak incidence between 50 and 70 years of age. Irradiation and immune deficiencies have been implicated as possible etiologic factors. An increased incidence of NHL has been noted in Hiroshima survivors, kidney transplant patients undergoing immunosuppressive therapy, and patients with immune deficiency syndromes such as ataxia telangiectasia, Wiskott-Aldrich syndrome, and human T-lymphocyte immunodeficiency disorders including acquired immunodeficiency syndrome (AIDS). The overall 5-year survival of 30% to 40% is lower than that of patients with Hodgkin's disease, but survival is higher in certain histologic subclassifications. Common causes of death in patients with NHL are infection, organ failure, hemorrhage, and disseminated tumor.

HISTOLOGIC CLASSIFICATIONS. The classification originally defined by Rappaport in 1956 was until recently the most widely used and accepted. This system is based on lymph node architecture, cell type, and degree of cellular differentiation. As knowledge regarding different functions of the various types of lymphocytes emerged, new classifications, some correlating morphologic criteria with immunologic function, were developed. Several major classifications were evaluated in the early 1980s by an international panel that recommended separation of the histologic subtypes into low-, intermediate-, and high-grade lymphoma based on survival characteristics, using both morphologic and functional criteria. Table 77-2 shows the classification derived by the international panel, known as the Working Formulation, and the Rappaport equivalents.

These tumors develop in either a nodular (follicular) fashion (the tumor cells form nodules separated by reticulin and fibrous tissue) or a diffuse fashion (the tumor cells are diffusely distributed throughout the lymph node, effacing its normal architecture). There is roughly an equal distribution of each. It is generally believed that the tumor cell in nearly all patients with NHL is a malignant lymphocyte, in the majority of cases a B lymphocyte. Although the Rappaport classification, devised before the availability of current immunologic typing methods, refers to "lymphocytic," "histiocytic," and "mixed cell" lymphomas, all nodular (follicular) lymphomas are B-lymphocyte lymphomas. Diffuse lymphomas may have a B-lymphocyte, T-lymphocyte, null cell, or, rarely, truly histiocytic origin. In addition, the lymphocytic lymphomas are subclassified as either well or poorly differentiated by the Rappaport classification.

Follicular lymphomas (nodular lymphomas of Rappaport) are characterized by nodules of relatively uniform size without a well-defined lymphoid cuff. The malignant cells are either small atypical lymphocytes with scanty cytoplasm and an irregular cleaved nucleus (the small cleaved cell of the Working Formulation, or poorly differentiated cell of Rappaport) or cells two to three times larger with vesicular nuclei and two or three nucleoli (the large cell of the Working Formulation; generally referred to as a histiocyte by the Rappaport classification). Although these large cells resemble histiocytes morphologically, tests using immunologic markers have shown that both the small cleaved cell and the large cell are B lymphocytes. Nodules containing 75% to 80% small cleaved cells are classified as follicular small cleaved cell lymphomas (NPDL by Rappaport), and nodules consisting of 30% to 50% large cells are classified as follicular mixed, small cleaved and large cell, lymphoma (NM of Rappaport). Those with more than 50% large cells are classified as follicular large cell lymphoma (NH by Rappaport). Follicular lymphomas tend to progress histologically over the years to a more diffuse pattern with increasing numbers of large cells.

The diffuse lymphomas histologically are a heterogeneous group of diseases. Small lymphocytic lymphoma (DLWD of Rappaport) may be the same disease process as chronic lymphocytic leukemia and is characterized by morphologically normal-appearing lymphocytes (well differentiated according to Rappaport). Diffuse small cleaved cell lymphoma (DLPD of Rappaport) is characterized by a diffuse infiltration of small cleaved cells. It is possible that most patients with diffuse small cleaved cell lymphoma have gone through an asymptomatic follicular stage preceding their clinical manifestations. Diffuse mixed small cleaved and large cell lymphoma (DM of Rappaport) is a rare disorder characterized by a mixture of the two cells and probably also represents a histologic extension of the follicular variety. Finally, diffuse large cell lymphoma (one variety of DH of Rappaport) encompasses most of what was referred to as diffuse histiocytic lymphoma by the Rappaport classification. Follicular lymphomas and small cleaved cell lymphomas tend to be less aggressive than the diffuse and large cell variants. Gradation into low, medium, and high grade is based on the mix of these two variables. Although intermediate- and high-grade lymphomas are usually rapidly fatal if untreated, a significant number (more than 50% to as many as 90%) may be cured with aggressive chemotherapy. However, low-grade lymphomas, although initially responsive to chemotherapy and associated with a relatively long survival, frequently relapse during treatment and are rarely cured by it.

Large cell, immunoblastic lymphomas, as well as lymphoblastic lymphomas and small noncleaved cell lymphomas (the latter perhaps a confusing misnomer because these cells are small only compared with lymphoblastic and immunoblastic types of lymphomas), are characterized by a diffuse proliferation of very large cells with vesicular nuclei and prominent nucleoli that may differ morphologically from each other and from those in the low- and intermediate-grade lymphomas. They are undifferentiated cell lymphomas with a relatively poor prognosis. These tumors are heterogeneous and morphologically represent the undifferentiated state of a number of functionally different cells. Biochemical, enzymatic, and surface marker studies reveal that slightly more than half of these high-risk tumors are of B-lymphocyte origin, a small number are of T-lymphocyte origin, an even smaller number are of histiocytic origin, and about a third are unclassifiable or null cell in origin. These lymphomas frequently develop in extranodal sites. Three clinically and morphologically distinctive variants of high-grade lymphoma are Burkitt's lymphoma, lymphoblastic lymphoma (histologically akin to T-cell acute lymphocytic leukemia), and immunoblastic sarcoma. These variants are characterized by a proliferation of undifferentiated large cells with relatively distinctive morphologic and clinical features.

CLINICAL MANIFESTATIONS. The clinical presentation of NHL is similar to that of Hodgkin's disease, although patients with NHL more commonly have stage III or IV disease on initial examination. However, the extent of disease on presentation varies depending on the histologic classification. Nearly 80% of patients with nodular lymphocytic lymphoma have stage IV disease, whereas less than 10% have stage I or II disease. Slightly less than a third of patients with diffuse large cell lymphoma of either intermediate- or high-grade classification have generalized stage IV disease at initial examination. Follicular small cleaved cell lymphoma and diffuse large cell lymphoma are the most common histologic variants of NHL. In general, follicular small cleaved cell lymphoma occurs in older patients, whereas 35% of patients with diffuse large cell lymphoma are less than 40 years of age. Bulky abdominal disease, B symptoms, advanced age, and advanced clinical stage are negative prognostic factors, but histologic subtype is the single most predictive factor. Although the majority of patients are asymptomatic initially, 10% to 20% have weight loss, fever, or night sweats. Roughly one fourth of patients have extranodal disease. Unlike Hodgkin's disease, in NHL the cellular immunologic system generally remains intact until the late stages of the disease.

STAGING. The reasons for staging a tumor in any patient are to obtain prognostic information, aid in therapeutic decision making, standardize a system for comparison of results, and provide an accepted descriptive system to facilitate communication. Although the Ann Arbor staging classification fulfills all four needs for patients with Hodgkin's disease, it fulfills only the latter two for patients with NHL. When compared with histologic subclassification, clinical staging plays a relatively minor role in influencing therapeutic decisions and almost no role in determining prognosis.

Staging procedures include a complete history and physical examination, chest roentgenogram, CT scan of the abdomen and pelvis, and bone marrow biopsy. Rarely, lymphangiography or bone scan is indicated. The advantage of lymphangiography over CT is in its usefulness in demonstrating involvement of normal-sized lymph nodes. This is rarely helpful clinically, however. Liver function studies (alkaline phosphatase, aspartate aminotransferase, lactate dehydrogenase) are occasionally helpful in evaluating the liver. Bone marrow aspiration or biopsy reveals marrow involvement in 30% to 60% of the patients, most commonly those with nodular lymphomas.

It is the rare patient who requires extensive staging procedures. Treatment is determined by histologic subtyping and rarely if ever by clinical staging. Recent studies have dem-

Table 77-3 Cytotoxic combinations useful in treating non-Hodgkin's lymphoma

COP (cycle repeated every 21 days)

Cyclophosphamide (Cytoxan)	400 mg/m² PO days 1-5
Vincristine (Oncovin)	1.4 mg/m² IV day 1 (max—2 mg)
Prednisone	100 mg/m² PO days 1-5

CHOP (cycle repeated every 21 days)

Cyclophosphamide	750 mg/m² IV day 1
Doxorubicin (Adriamycin)	50 mg/m² IV day 1
Vincristine (Oncovin)	1.4 mg/m² IV day 1 (max—2 mg)
Prednisone	100 mg/m² PO days 1-5

C-MOPP (cycle repeated every 28 days)

Cyclophosphamide	650 mg/m² IV days 1, 8
Vincristine (Oncovin)	1.4 mg/m² IV days 1, 8 (max—2 mg)
Procarbazine (Matulane)	100 mg/m² PO days 1-14
Prednisone	40 mg/m² PO days 1-14

Table 77-4 Aggressive cytotoxic combination approaches under investigation

MACOP-B (12-week total duration of treatment)

Methotrexate	400 mg/m² IV weeks 2, 6, 10
Doxorubicin	50 mg/m² IV odd weeks
Cyclophosphamide	350 mg/m² IV odd weeks
Vincristine	1.4 mg/m² IV even weeks
Bleomycin	10 units/m² IV weeks 4, 8, 12
Prednisone	75 mg PO daily

proMACE (cycle repeated every 28 days for 6 to 9 months)

Etoposide	120 mg/m² IV days 1,8
Cyclophosphamide	650 mg/m² IV days 1,8
Doxorubicin	25 mg/m² IV days 1,8
Methotrexate	1.5 gm/m² IV day 15
Leucovorin	50 mg/m² IV every 6 hours × 5 (start 24 hours after methotrexate)
Prednisone	60 mg/m² PO days 1-15

M-BACoD (cycle repeated every 21 days for 6 to 9 months)

Bleomycin	4 mg/m² IV day 1
Doxorubicin	45 mg/m² IV day 1
Cyclophosphamide	600 mg/m² IV day 1
Vincristine	1 mg/m² IV day 1 (maximum dose 2 mg)
Dexamethasone	6 mg/m² PO days 1-5
Methotrexate	200 mg/m² IV days 8,15
Leucovorin	10 mg/m² PO every 6 hours × 6 (start 24 hours after methotrexate)

onstrated that most patients with intermediate- or high-grade histologic subtypes respond adequately to aggressive chemotherapy administered with curative intent; such an aggressive chemotherapeutic approach is indicated in patients with high-grade lymphomas regardless of stage. Radiation therapy adds little to the overall therapeutic benefit in these patients. This obviates the need for extensive staging procedures in patients with clinically limited disease.

MANAGEMENT. The treatment of patients with NHL is dictated primarily by their histologic subclassification. Patients with low-grade lymphomas should be managed with nonaggressive treatment. Some believe that asymptomatic patients with these subtypes require no treatment at all, since they may remain asymptomatic for 2 to 3 years after diagnosis. With or without immediate treatment, such patients may anticipate a relatively long survival, with the majority surviving more than 10 years after diagnosis. A variety of treatments, including total nodal irradiation; a chemotherapeutic combination of cyclophosphamide, vincristine (Oncovin), and prednisone (COP; Table 77-3); or even single-agent chemotherapy with cyclophosphamide, may induce a complete response in three fourths of these patients. Despite this high complete response rate, survival is not significantly improved because all patients subsequently have relapse (15% to 20% annually) and require additional therapy. Treatment for this group of patients therefore is palliative and directed toward symptom and disease control. Follicular mixed (small cleaved and large cell) lymphoma may represent an exception to the preceding general dictum regarding treatment for low-grade lymphomas. Some investigators have indicated that aggressive cytotoxic chemotherapy in this histologic subtype is curative. Currently, this remains controversial.

Most intermediate- or high-grade lymphomas require an aggressive therapeutic approach. Many patients with these so-called poor prognostic types of lymphomas can be cured with aggressive chemotherapy, a phenomenon that does not occur with the low-grade lymphomas. Diffuse small cleaved cell lymphoma is an exception; patients are subject to early and continuous relapse similar to the course with follicular small cleaved cell lymphoma, and there is little indication that a significant number of these patients achieve a long-term disease-free survival. However, patients whose tumors are predominantly large cell respond to aggressive chemotherapy, and a large percentage are cured.

A variety of combination chemotherapeutic approaches

have evolved over the past 10 years. Initially, trials with three similar combination approaches—CHOP, a combination of cyclophosphamide, doxorubicin (Adriamycin), vincristine (Oncovin), and prednisone; C-MOPP, a combination of cyclophosphamide, vincristine, prednisone, and procarbazine (Matulane); and BACOP, a combination of cyclophosphamide, doxorubicin, vincristine, and prednisone plus bleomycin (Blenoxane)—have been used for 10 or more years and can be expected to induce a complete response in 40% to 60% of patients with intermediate- or high-grade lymphoma, about half of whom may anticipate a long-term disease-free survival and probable cure. Recently, more aggressive cytotoxic combination approaches have been used including M-BACoD, a combination of cyclophosphamide, doxorubicin, vincristine, prednisone, and bleomycin with the addition of intermittently administered moderate- or high-dose methotrexate with leucovorin rescue; MACOP-B, a similar combination including cyclophosphamide, doxorubicin, vincristine, prednisone, and bleomycin and moderate-dose methotrexate all administered in an interspersed fashion with treatment given each week for a relatively short total treatment time of 12 weeks; and proMACE, a combination of cyclophosphamide, doxorubicin, prednisone, etoposide, and high-dose methotrexate with leucovorin rescue (Table 77-4). These combinations are undergoing intensive clinical study. They are significantly more aggressive than the original CHOP combination, have greater toxicity, and may be associated with an occasional fatality from therapy. However, this approach may induce a significantly greater number of complete responses. It remains to be determined whether this increased complete response rate will translate into an overall improvement in survival and a greater number of cures. Perhaps the most intriguing of the recent approaches is the MACOP-B regimen, in which treatment is administered intensively for only 12 weeks. In all other approaches, treatment is administered for the first week to 10 days of every 21- to 28-day period over a total treatment period of 6 to 9 months.

Other approaches under investigation include the use of autologous bone marrow transplantation after aggressive chemotherapy or radiation therapy in patients who have relapse after primary treatment and biologic response modifiers such as α-interferon. The α-interferons may prove useful in patients with follicular lymphomas.

A substantial number (20% to 25%) of patients have localized (stage I or II) disease when initially examined. As in patients with stage III or IV disease, the histologic subtype plays a significant prognostic role. Recent clinical studies have demonstrated that aggressive chemotherapy over a relatively short period can cure patients with stage I or stage II, intermediate- or high-grade NHL. This obviates the need for extensive staging procedures. Patients with stage I or II follicular small cleaved cell lymphoma have a better prognosis than patients with stage III or stage IV disease, but it is unlikely that the former, who are few in number, will require treatment.

Extranodal disease

Extranodal disease occurs in 25% of patients with NHL. The two most common sites are the stomach and the head and neck. Less commonly the disease may involve bone, skin, testis, or the central nervous system. Of cases with apparent localized extranodal involvement of the head and neck, nearly three fourths involve Waldeyer's ring and one fourth involve the paranasal sinuses. The symptoms vary depending on the site of the primary lesion. It is unclear whether the biologic behavior of extranodal lymphomatous disease differs from or is similar to that of nodal disease, but correlations between survival and histologic features resemble those in patients with nodal presentations. Lymphoma in the gastrointestinal tract most commonly involves the stomach, is more frequently of the diffuse large cell subtype, and if localized has a relatively good prognosis. The treatment is frequently surgical and, provided there is no serosal penetration or lymph node involvement, induces a disease-free 5-year survival in 50% of the patients. Radiation therapy is also effective.

BIBLIOGRAPHY

Anderson T and others: Malignant lymphoma. I. The histology and staging of 473 patients at the National Cancer Institute, Cancer 50:2699, 1982.
Bonadonna G: Chemotherapy of malignant lymphoma, Semin Oncol 12:1, 1985.
Bonadonna G, Valagussa P, and Santoro A: Alternating noncross resistant combination chemotherapy or MOPP in stage IV Hodgkin's disease, Ann Intern Med 104:739, 1986.
Coleman M: Chemotherapy for large cell lymphoma: optimism and caution, Ann Intern Med 103:140, 1985.
Cornbleet MA and others: Pathologic stages IA and IIA Hodgkin's disease: results of treatment with radiotherapy alone (1968-1980), J Clin Oncol 3:758, 1985.
Desforges JF, Rutherford CJ, and Piro A: Hodgkin's disease, N Engl J Med 301:1212, 1979.
Hoppe RT: The role of radiation therapy in the management of the non-Hodgkin's lymphoma, Cancer 55:2716, 1985.
Koletsky AJ and others: Second neoplasms in patients with Hodgkin's disease following combined modality therapy—the Yale experience, J Clin Oncol 4:311, 1986.
Leslie NT, Mauch PM, and Hellman S: Stage IA to IIB supradiaphragmatic Hodgkin's disease: long-term survival and relapse frequency, Cancer 55:2072, 1985.
Longo DL and others: Twenty years of MOPP therapy for Hodgkin's disease, J Clin Oncol 4:1295, 1986.
Lukes RJ: The immunologic approach to the pathology of malignant lymphomas, Am J Clin Pathol 72:657, 1979.
Matis LA, Young RC, and Longo DL: Nodular lymphomas: current concepts, CRC Crit Rev Oncol Hematol 5:171, 1986.
Non-Hodgkin's Lymphoma Pathologic Classification Project: National Cancer Institute sponsored study of classifications of non-Hodgkin's lymphomas: summary and description of a working formulation for clinical usage, Cancer 49:2112, 1982.
Rosenberg SA: The low-grade non-Hodgkin's lymphomas: challenges and opportunities, J Clin Oncol 3:299, 1985.
Rudders RA, Ross ME, and DeLellis RA: Primary extranodal lymphoma, Cancer 42:406, 1978.

78 · DISEASES OF THE SPLEEN AND RETICULOENDOTHELIAL SYSTEM

Sally D. Lane

The spleen is an organ that operates directly or indirectly in a number of critical body functions. It is the chief organ of the reticuloendothelial system (RES). Along with the liver, lymph nodes, bone marrow, and specialized reticuloendothelial (RE) cells throughout the body (circulating monocytes and fixed tissue macrophages), it participates in the phagocytic and immunologic activities that form one of the body's chief defenses against infection. Destruction of various intravascular particles (including senescent or deformed red blood cells, infectious organisms, and cellular breakdown products) and metabolic processing of their components are additional functions of the RES. Finally, the RES includes multipotential stem cells capable of differentiation along a number of cell lines: hematopoietic, histiocytic (phagocytic and nonphagocytic), and fibroblastic. Because of its highly vascular nature, the spleen may also be implicated in disorders of the circulatory system, particularly the portal circulation. As such, it may be indirectly affected by portal hypertension (particularly in association with liver disease) and by vascular events such as splenic vein thrombosis.

EVALUATION OF THE PATIENT WITH SPLENOMEGALY

Determination of the cause of splenomegaly presents a diagnostic challenge to the physician. Although it is often difficult to isolate a specific cause for splenomegaly via noninvasive procedures, a number of clinical guidelines exist.

A finding of a palpable or roentgenographically enlarged spleen generally connotes a pathologic condition. The spleen, along with the other lymphoid tissues of the body, enlarges promptly in response to any infectious insult in children, and occasionally lymphatic hyperplasia occurs in healthy adults as well. One series demonstrated the finding of palpable spleens in 3% of healthy college freshmen. Of these, a large number can probably be related to prior infection with delayed or incomplete resolution. Furthermore, the presence of emphysema or a low diaphragm may make a normal-sized spleen palpable.

Nonetheless, a definitely enlarged spleen should prompt an evaluation for the more likely benign and malignant causes of splenomegaly. The chief malignant causes of splenomegaly, lymphomas and leukemias (particularly chronic granulocytic and chronic lymphocytic leukemia), are discussed in Chapters 73 and 77. Enlargement of the spleen is seen in a majority of patients with myeloproliferative disorders. Among nonmalignant causes of splenomegaly, hemolysis, infections, collagen-vascular disorders, hypersensitivity states, vascular congestion, and proliferative and infiltrative diseases of the RES are perhaps most common. The last two of these are discussed in this section. The reader is referred to the appropriate sections of this text for consideration of splenomegaly in association with other disease states.

A finding of massive splenomegaly should suggest portal

hypertension, myeloproliferative disorders, the sphingolipidoses (especially Gaucher's disease), malaria, or occasionally splenic cysts. Among patients in whom no cause for splenomegaly can be identified clinically ("idiopathic splenomegaly"), lymphoma will be ultimately identified in a small percentage.

FUNCTIONAL DISORDERS
Hyposplenism

DEFINITION AND PATHOGENESIS. The functional capacity of the spleen is defined primarily by its activity in clearing microorganisms (especially poorly opsonized bacteria), in filtering and processing blood cells, and in synthesizing both immunoglobulin M (IgM) and opsonizing proteins. Thus hyposplenism can be thought of as a state in which any or all of these functions are disrupted. However, it is usually defined by its specific origin. Clearly, absence of the spleen, either congenital or after splenectomy, produces the extreme manifestations of this state. A severe degree of hyposplenism occurs in sickle cell anemia, in which repeated infarctions lead to atrophy and a condition known as autosplenectomy. The organ may be enlarged in young children but does not function normally. It shrinks with repeated infarctions and is rarely palpable in older children. Other disorders that are frequently associated with hyposplenism include ulcerative colitis (in which splenic function can wax and wane with the activity of the colitis), celiac sprue, and dermatitis herpetiformis.

CLINICAL MANIFESTATIONS AND LABORATORY FINDINGS. Hyposplenism is frequently recognized by the findings of abnormal red blood cell forms in the peripheral blood. Howell-Jolly bodies (nuclear remnants) and target cells are the hallmarks of a hypofunctional or absent spleen; acanthocytes and siderocytes may also be seen.

Typical laboratory changes follow surgical removal of the spleen. Granulocytosis occurs immediately after splenectomy but is replaced within several weeks by sustained lymphocytosis and monocytosis. Transient thrombocytosis (usually less than 2 weeks in duration) also occurs after splenectomy. This is generally of little clinical significance unless there is an underlying myeloproliferative disorder, in which sustained platelet counts in excess of 1 million/mm³ may predispose the patient to bleeding or thrombosis or both. Infrequently, the typical postsplenectomy rise in white blood cell count or platelet count may persist for months or even years.

The most devastating clinical manifestation of hyposplenism is vulnerability to overwhelming infection, particularly pneumococcemia. This most frequently occurs in sickle cell anemia and in young children who have undergone splenectomy, especially within the first 2 years after surgery. The risk of postsplenectomy sepsis may as high as 20% in patients with underlying RES disorders such as thalassemia major, histiocytosis, and Wiskott-Aldrich syndrome. In normal adults undergoing incidental splenectomy for trauma, the risk appears low. However, case reports of fatal sepsis in such situations continue to appear, and there is controversy in the literature as to the magnitude of risk in this group. The fatality rate from overwhelming postsplenectomy infection has been reported to be as high as 50%. *Streptococcus pneumoniae* is responsible for most cases, but other encapsulated bacteria, such as *Haemophilus influenzae,* may be the infectious agents. Extraordinarily high numbers of microorganisms are found in the blood; shock and disseminated intravascular coagulation are frequent accompaniments. The disorder is believed to be related to loss of phagocytic activity of the spleen, decreased IgM levels, changes in the alternative pathway of complement activation, decreased levels of opsonizing proteins, and possibly alteration of lymphocytic function.

MANAGEMENT. The functional capacity of an absent or atrophied spleen clearly cannot be replaced. The most significant therapeutic interventions that can be made include avoidance of unnecessary splenectomy, bacterial (particularly pneumococcal) vaccines for patients with hyposplenism or absent spleens, and in selected situations prophylactic penicillin. Unfortunately, the value of pneumococcal vaccine in patients who have already undergone splenectomy and in those with hematologic disorders that alter immunity has not been established. The treatment of undiagnosed fevers or documented sepsis in hyposplenic patients is an emergency and requires prompt institution of antibiotics and supportive measures.

Hypersplenism

DEFINITION. Hyperfunction of the spleen is characterized by splenomegaly, reduction in any or all of the formed blood elements (red blood cells, white blood cells, and platelets), compensatory bone marrow hyperplasia, and response to splenectomy. An enlarged spleen does not necessarily lead to hypersplenism and may be asymptomatic or produce mechanical disturbances without functional alteration.

PATHOGENESIS. Increased sequestration of blood cells appears to be the primary mechanism for hypersplenism. Normally about 20 to 30 ml of erythrocytes, roughly 30% of the peripheral pool of platelets, and a small fraction of the granulocytes are located in the spleen. In states of splenic enlargement, increased pooling of these cells causes a reduction in peripheral blood cell counts. Red blood cell survival is usually shortened in proportion to the size of the spleen. The degree of anemia, if any, that results depends on the compensatory response of the bone marrow. The dilutional effect of increased plasma volume, which typically results from splenic enlargement, may also contribute to anemia. When increased platelet pooling in the spleen occurs, the bone marrow appears to respond more to the total body platelet mass than to the circulating platelet pool. Leukopenia associated with simple sequestration is frequently "balanced," with a normal differential cell count. Disorders associated with increased RES activity, such as Gaucher's disease, renal transplantation, and Felty's syndrome (rheumatoid arthritis, neutropenia, and splenomegaly), may produce a more severe degree of leukopenia.

CLINICAL MANIFESTATIONS. Hypersplenism may be entirely asymptomatic, or it may produce symptoms resulting from the depression of blood elements. Hemolysis may produce symptomatic anemia. The degree of anemia depends on bone marrow response (often suboptimal in patients with systemic illnesses associated with splenomegaly) and on the presence of other diseases, such as coronary artery disease or pulmonary insufficiency, that alter the patient's tolerance to anemia. When splenic enlargement occurs as a result of work hypertrophy from hemolytic anemia (for example, hereditary spherocytosis, thalassemia), a vicious circle often occurs in which increasing hemolysis produces increasing splenomegaly and vice versa. Platelets sequestered in an enlarged spleen can be mobilized in response to hemorrhage and appear to function normally; thus significant bleeding is infrequently associated with hypersplenic thrombocytopenia. This may not be the case, however, when a qualitative platelet defect exists, as in some myeloproliferative disorders. Furthermore, in Banti's syndrome (chronic congestive splenomegaly with pancytopenia and portal hypertension), significant bleeding can occur, particularly from esophageal varices. In general the mild granulocytopenia that occurs with splenomegaly is of little clinical concern; however, the leukopenia occurring in Felty's syndrome is associated with a significant risk of infection. Immune destruction of granulocytes may play a role in this disorder.

LABORATORY FINDINGS AND DIAGNOSIS. The salient laboratory feature of hypersplenism is the reduction of the affected blood element(s). Reticulocytosis is routinely found unless severe bone marrow dysfunction exists. Examination of the bone marrow in hypersplenism shows compensatory hyperplasia, particularly in the erythroid series. Quantitation of splenic hyperfunction can be made by measuring the survival of transfused ^{51}Cr-labeled red blood cells with scanning over the spleen. Radioisotope labeling has also been used to study platelet survival.

COURSE AND MANAGEMENT. The clinical course of hypersplenic states may be benign or progressive, depending in large part on the underlying disease. Certain acute infectious causes such as miliary tuberculosis, viral hepatitis, infectious mononucleosis, and subacute bacterial endocarditis may be self-limited or responsive to antimocrobial therapy. When hypersplenism is progressive or severe, splenectomy or splenic irradiation may be indicated.

Extramedullary hematopoiesis

All organs of the RES retain an inherent capacity for hematopoietic function. This function is normally active in the fetus. The liver is the primary hematopoietic organ from the second through sixth months of gestation and remains active until shortly before birth. Lesser contributions are made during the middle third of fetal life by the spleen, lymph nodes, and thymus. From birth onward, the bone marrow is the sole organ of normal hematopoiesis. However, under circumstances of increased stress and particularly in disease states characterized by bone marrow replacement or fibrosis, the organs of the RES (chiefly the liver and spleen) can again become active in blood formation. This syndrome is characterized by splenomegaly, hepatomegaly, and the finding of immature red and white blood cell precursors in the peripheral blood. A more detailed discussion of this entity is presented in Chapter 75.

Infiltrative disorders

A number of inherited disorders are characterized by abnormal accumulation of materials in phagocytic cells with resultant enlargement of RE organs. Most often the defect is related to the absence of a critical enzyme.

Gaucher's disease

Gaucher's disease is the most common of the lysosomal storage diseases. The metabolic defect is a deficiency of the enzyme glucocerebrosidase, resulting in the accumulation of glucocerebroside (ceramide glucose). This material, one of the sphingolipids, is a metabolic breakdown product of neutrophils and erythrocytes. The enzyme deficiency is inherited as an autosomal recessive trait and in the most common forms shows a predilection for Ashkenazic Jews.

Three clinical forms of Gaucher's disease exist. The most severe is the infantile (acute neuronopathic) form, characterized by rapid progression and commonly death before 2 years of age. The hallmark of the disorder is severe neurologic dysfunction consisting of cranial nerve abnormalities, extrapyramidal signs, hypertonicity, hyperreflexia, and hyperextension of the neck. Splenomegaly and hepatomegaly are usually present, as is pancytopenia. Death frequently results from pulmonary infection.

In the juvenile (subacute neuronopathic) form onset usually

occurs between 1 and 8 years of age. Neurologic defects are often present but are more variable. Hepatosplenomegaly is usually rapidly progressive, and thrombocytopenia may produce symptomatic bruising. Bone destruction is common and may be painful. The disease is often fatal but always at a later age than in the infantile form.

The adult (chronic nonneuronopathic) form is the most common. As the name suggests, neurologic findings are absent. The diagnosis may be made at any age from adolescence to late middle age (and rarely in the elderly). Splenomegaly is usually the presenting manifestation; occasionally abnormal bleeding from thrombocytopenia heralds the diagnosis. Often the disease is asymptomatic, but usually some degree of pancytopenia is present. The major difficulties result from splenomegaly and bone lesions.

The sine qua non of Gaucher's disease is the finding of Gaucher's cells in the spleen, liver, bone marrow, and sometimes lymph nodes. These are large cells (20 to 80 μm in diameter) with small eccentric nuclei and coarsely clumped cytoplasm having the appearance of wrinkled tissue paper. They are phagocytic cells filled with glucocerebroside. The other laboratory hallmark is elevated levels of serum acid phosphatase (tartrate resistant, in contrast to prostatic acid phosphatase).

As noted previously, anemia, leukopenia, and thrombocytopenia are present to some degree (usually greater in the more severe forms). The anemia is hypochromic and normocytic. Hypersplenism is believed to contribute to leukopenia and thrombocytopenia in the juvenile and adult forms, but decreased red blood cell survival is not prominent.

The combination of the clinical findings with identification of Gaucher's cells in the RES establishes the diagnosis. "Gaucher-like" cells may be seen in leukemia, especially chronic granulocytic leukemia, in which increased breakdown of granulocytes probably results in accumulation of a glucocerebroside precursor.

Niemann-Pick disease

Niemann-Pick disease is a somewhat more heterogeneous group of disorders, all distinguished by hepatosplenomegaly and the finding of characteristic foamy RE cells. Like Gaucher's disease, it is most common in Jews. The metabolic defect in most if not all forms appears to be a deficiency of sphingomyelinase, with accumulation of sphingomyelin. However, abnormal accumulation of cholesterol also occurs and may predominate. Mental impairment and death within the first 3 years of life are characteristic but not universal. At least four clinical subtypes have been identified, based on rapidity of progression and relative importance of hepatosplenomegaly versus central nervous system involvement.

Anemia and thrombocytopenia are much less common than in Gaucher's disease, and the serum acid phosphatase level is normal. The pathognomonic storage cell is as large as the Gaucher's cell but contains a foamy rather than wrinkled-appearing, blue-green cytoplasm when stained with Wright-Giemsa stain.

Chédiak-Higashi disease

Chédiak-Higashi disease is an uncommon inherited lysosomal storage disease characterized by striking reddish purple inclusion bodies in many cells. These are most commonly seen in neutrophils and lymphocytes of the peripheral blood but are also identified in tissues such as the skin, hair, and nervous system. They appear to represent abnormal fusion of lysosomal precursors. They are acid phosphatase positive, but other cytochemical stains vary with the specific cell. Some have classified this syndrome as a lipidosis.

Clinically, Chédiak-Higashi disease is characterized by increased susceptibility to infection (particularly caused by *S. aureus*) and by death in childhood. The chemotaxis of neutrophils is abnormal, and the large granules do not degranulate normally, leading to poor intracellular killing of some bacteria. Hepatosplenomegaly, anemia, and thrombocytopenia are common. An association with partial albinism and decreased retinal pigmentation is often found.

Other infiltrative disorders

A number of other inherited disorders of metabolism may produce splenomegaly on the basis of infiltration. Examples include the mucopolysaccharidoses (such as Hurler's and Hunter's syndromes) and some of the familial disorders of cholesterol metabolism and storage (for example, Tangier disease). At least one acquired infiltrative disorder, primary amyloidosis, is occasionally associated with a moderate degree of splenomegaly.

PROLIFERATIVE DISORDERS
Idiopathic histiocytosis

DEFINITION. The term "idiopathic histiocytosis" (or "histiocytosis X") includes a spectrum of disease processes ranging from focal to widely disseminated proliferation of lipid-laden histiocytes. These disorders were originally described as three separate entities: eosinophilic granuloma of bone (localized histiocytosis), Hand-Schüller-Christian disease (disseminated chronic histiocytosis), and Letterer-Siwe disease (disseminated acute histiocytosis). In 1953 Lichtenstein proposed the concept of a single category, histiocytosis X, to encompass all three, based on similarities in histologic features and on the possible identification of intermediate forms and transition between the subtypes. This concept has been widely debated in the subsequent literature, however, and many authors prefer to maintain the distinction between localized and disseminated forms.

ETIOLOGY AND PATHOGENESIS. The cause of idiopathic histiocytosis remains unknown. Occasional reports suggesting either infectious or genetic factors have appeared, but there are no consistent data to support a particular origin. In its most aggressive forms the disease may take on the features of a neoplastic process. The clinical features are an expression of the location and extent of proliferation of abnormal histiocytes.

CLINICAL MANIFESTATIONS. The most localized and benign form of histiocytosis, eosinophilic granuloma, is characterized by solitary or multifocal lesions of bone, usually in children or young adults. The lesions most often appear osteolytic on roentgenogram, may stimulate periosteal reaction, and occur most commonly in the skull, ribs, pelvis, and scapulae. Pathologically, they are composed of histiocytes with abundant eosinophilic cytoplasm and many polymorphonuclear cells, largely eosinophils. Localized pain is the usual presenting symptom, and systemic manifestations are rare. The disease generally has a benign course and responds well to local excision or radiation therapy.

The chronic disseminated form of histiocytosis is a rare condition of childhood, in which bone lesions similar to those just described are found in association with other manifestations such as diabetes insipidus, exophthalmos, chronic otitis media or externa, or skin infiltration. Involvement of visceral organs such as lymph nodes, liver, spleen, or lung may occur but is not usually prominent. The course is more variable than in the localized form but usually has a good prognosis. In about half the patients the disease eventually burns out, leaving fi-

brotic lesions at the sites of involvement but no clinical residual. It may be fatal in up to 15% of the cases.

Of the three subtypes, the acute disseminated form is most readily differentiated from the other two. This is an acute, fulminant disease of infants that generally leads to death within the first few years of life. Bone tumors, hepatosplenomegaly, lymphadenopathy, fever, anemia, and bleeding are prominent features. The prognosis is poorer at an earlier age of onset.

MANAGEMENT. Localized tumors are readily treated by surgery or radiation therapy. In the disseminated forms a number of systemic agents have been used with some reports of success. The most experience has been with corticosteroids and vinca alkaloids (especially vinblastine), although a variety of alkylating agents, antimetabolites, and cytotoxic antibiotics have been used as well.

Histiocytic medullary reticulosis (malignant histiocytosis)

Histiocytic medullary reticulosis is a rare malignant disorder of RE tissues that is believed by some to be a variant of the true "histiocytic" lymphomas. It affects all ages and may occur in the first decade of life. The principal clinical features are fever, wasting, purpura, generalized adenopathy, hepatosplenomegaly, severe pancytopenia, and a rapid downhill course. Infiltration of other organs, including the skin, bone, and gastrointestinal tract, may occur. Histologically it is characterized by the proliferation of large, atypical histiocytes in the bone marrow, medullary portions of lymph nodes, and other involved organs. Phagocytosis of blood elements, especially erythrocytes, is a hallmark of the disease and is believed to be largely responsible for the pancytopenia. Although the anemia shows many features of a hemolytic process, there is usually inadequate reticulocytosis, and Coombs' test is typically negative. Histiocytes are infrequently found in the peripheral blood. When the disease occurs in early childhood, the distinction from Letterer-Siwe disease can be difficult but is usually possible on histologic grounds. Malignant histiocytosis is generally unresponsive to radiation therapy or chemotherapy, but occasional long-term responses to combination chemotherapy have been described.

MISCELLANEOUS DISORDERS

Splenic infarction may result from hemoglobinopathies, leukocytic infiltration (as in the chronic leukemias), or large vessel thrombosis. Rupture of the spleen may occur as a result of blunt trauma to the abdomen or "spontaneously" in disorders in which the spleen is abnormal, such as leukemia, infectious mononucleosis, malaria, or typhoid fever.

Space-occupying lesions of the spleen include abscesses, cysts, and tumors. Abscesses may result from bacteremia, extension from a perforated or diseased neighboring abdominal organ, or secondary infection of a sterile infarct. The characteristic signs are fever, chills, abdominal pain, and irritation of either the pleural or peritoneal surface, depending on the location.

Splenic cysts are rare. They may result from parasitic infestation (especially echinococcosis) or from benign neoplasms such as dermoid cysts, cystic lymphangiomas, or cavernous hemangiomas. Primary malignant tumors of the spleen are uncommon. Sarcomas, such as hemangiosarcomas or fibrosarcomas, can originate in the spleen. Isolated splenic lymphoma is rare; less than 1% of non-Hodgkin's lymphomas are localized to the spleen. In almost all cases in which splenomegaly is the initial finding, there is evidence of widespread involvement. Metastatic tumor to the spleen occurs in less than

10% of patients with cancer. Breast and lung cancers are the most common primary sites; melanomas and cancers of the prostate, colon, pancreas, and stomach may also spread to the spleen. The involvement may vary from large nodular deposits to diffuse infiltration, and extensively involved spleens may attain enormous sizes.

BIBLIOGRAPHY

Case records of the Massachusetts General Hospital (Case 15-1982), N Engl J Med 306:918, 1982.

Eichner ER: Splenic function: normal, too much and too little, Am J Med 66:311, 1979.

Frederickson DS and Sloan HR: Glucosyl ceramide lipidoses: Gaucher's disease. Sphingomyelin lipidoses: Niemann-Pick disease. In Stanberry JB and others, editors: The metabolic bases of inherited diseases, ed 4, New York, 1978, McGraw-Hill Inc.

Krivit W: Overwhelming post-splenectomy infection, Am J Hematol 2:193, 1977.

Miale JB: Laboratory medicine: hematology, ed 6, St Louis, 1982, CV Mosby Co.

Schwartz PE and others: Postsplenectomy sepsis and mortality in adults, JAMA 248:2279, 1982.

Videbaek A, Christensen BE, and Jonsson V: The spleen in health and disease, Chicago, 1982, Year Book Medical Publishers Inc.

Vogel JM and Vogel P: Idiopathic histiocytosis: a discussion of eosinophilic granuloma, the Hand-Schüller-Christian syndrome, and the Letterer-Siwe syndrome, Semin Hematol 9:349, 1972.

Warnke RA, Kim H, and Dorfman RF: Malignant histiocytosis (histiocytic medullary reticulosis), Cancer 35:215, 1975.

UNIT C • HEMOSTATIC DISORDERS

79 · INTRODUCTION TO HEMOSTASIS

Patricia M. Catalano

Evaluation of the patient with a history of bruising and bleeding is a common clinical problem. The accurate diagnosis and appropriate management of such patients depend on a thorough understanding of the normal hemostatic mechanisms and the tests of these mechanisms.

It is convenient to consider the normal sequence of events that leads to hemostasis as occurring in two phases. The first phase involves the immediate control mechanisms related to the vasculature and the formation of a platelet plug at the site of vessel injury. The long-term control mechanisms constitute the second phase and consist of a biochemical chain of events that involve the humoral coagulation factors, platelet factors, and calcium, resulting in the formation of a fibrin clot. As understanding of the hemostatic mechanism increases, so does the realization of the complexity of the interactions among the vascular, platelet, and humoral components of the system. Nonetheless, an astute clinician usually is able to determine from the history and initial physical and laboratory findings approximately where the abnormality in an individual patient is most likely to be found and to direct the subsequent evaluation accordingly.

Several aspects of the history of a patient with a suspected bleeding disorder should be emphasized. The nature and severity of the bleeding episodes should be determined. A defect of the immediate control mechanisms is usually manifest as mucous membrane bleeding, with epistaxis, menorrhagia, and gingival bleeding prominent features. Disorders of coagulation factors, on the other hand, are more often associated with massive bleeding after trauma or surgery. Spontaneous hemarthroses are a prominent feature of severe hemophilia, a disorder of coagulation factors.

It is important to ascertain whether the disorder is congenital or acquired, and the family history may be extremely valuable. Family members may have a known disorder; when the bleeding tendency is familial but the diagnosis is unknown, its mode of inheritance may be helpful.

Often the most difficult patients to assess are those who are to undergo a surgical procedure and who have only a history of increased bruising but no previous major surgery or family history of bleeding. The significance of the bleeding tendency can often be elucidated in such patients by a careful dental history. The extraction of a permanent tooth is a significant stress to the hemostatic mechanisms and one the patient seldom thinks to mention if not questioned directly. Any excessive bleeding after dental procedures deserves evaluation, even in an otherwise asymptomatic patient. This history may provide the only clue to a serious bleeding disorder, and the diagnosis of such a disorder before surgery is of course extremely important.

A careful drug history is always important in evaluating a patient for a bleeding disorder. This history may uncover the origin of the bleeding, and it is also important to determine whether the patient has taken any drugs that may interfere with the evaluation tests, such as aspirin that will prolong the bleeding time.

The physical examination may provide further clues to the nature of the defect. For example, petechiae are almost exclusively a manifestation of thrombocytopenia. Arthropathy of the large joints is a common complication of the repeated hemarthroses of severe hemophilia.

The ultimate diagnosis of a bleeding disorder must of course be made in the laboratory. A routine coagulation survey consisting of a platelet count, partial thromboplastin time, prothrombin time, and bleeding time serves as the first screen of the platelet, intrinsic, and extrinsic coagulation pathways. More elaborate tests of platelet function or specific factor assays may in rare instances be important even when such a screen is normal.

80 · PLATELET AND VASCULAR DISORDERS

Patricia M. Catalano

Platelets are disk-shaped blood cells 3 to 4 μm in diameter, normally present in whole blood in a concentration of 200,000 to 400,000/mm^3. Structurally they consist of a bilipid membrane and cytoplasm that contains a variety of granules, a few mitochondria, and no nucleus. Within the granules are stored calcium, adenosine diphosphate (ADP), serotonin, platelet factor 4, fibrinogen, von Willebrand's factor, fibronectin, and a host of other functionally important proteins. Platelets are formed in the bone marrow from precursor cells called mega-karyocytes and circulate with an average life span of 7 to 9 days.

Platelets adhere to a variety of substances, most notably collagen, which is exposed when a blood vessel is interrupted. The adherence of platelets at the site of vessel injury is rapidly followed by the aggregation of large numbers of platelets to form a platelet plug. Interaction of these activated platelets with the coagulation system then leads to the sequence of events that results in fibrin clot formation.

The ability of platelets to adhere normally has proved to be a difficult function to quantitate. The most readily available test of adherence in vitro is the retention of platelets in a glass bead column. In spite of the relatively crude nature of this test, it has been useful in documenting that this function in some way depends on the presence of the "von Willebrand factor" activity of the coagulation protein factor VIII. Because it is subject to technical variability, this and other tests of adhesion are not in widespread clinical use.

Platelet aggregation, on the other hand, has been extensively studied in vitro. The addition of a variety of stimulating agents, such as ADP or epinephrine, to a stirred solution of platelet-rich plasma results in a characteristic response for the particular agent used. Aggregation stimulated by these agents usually proceeds in two phases, a primary reversible aggregation and a second wave of aggregation that is irreversible. The primary wave of aggregation is associated with the binding of fibrinogen to the membrane glycoprotein IIb IIIa. The development of a second wave of aggregation is, at least in part, mediated by the platelet prostaglandin pathway. Arachidonic acid is released from the platelet membrane during aggregation and is metab-olized by the enzyme cyclooxygenase to a variety of prosta-glandins, cyclic endoperoxides, and thromboxanes. Throm-boxane A_2 produced by this pathway is a potent stimulus to aggregation. When thromboxane production is blocked by as-pirin, which inhibits cyclooxygenase, secondary aggregation does not occur. This inhibition can, however, be overcome by potent aggregating agents such as thrombin. Therefore an al-ternative pathway, perhaps mediated by platelet-activating fac-tor (PAF), must also exist.

The second phase of aggregation is also accompanied by the phenomenon known as the release reaction, during which the contents of the platelet granules are secreted, further enhancing the aggregation. A special form of aggregation stimulated by the antibiotic ristocetin is also dependent on factor VIII.

Although these methods of studying adherence and aggre-gation have been invaluable in the development of the under-standing of platelet physiology, it is often difficult to interpret subtle abnormalities and the techniques are subject to numerous artifacts. It is therefore extremely important that they be per-formed by someone experienced in their interpretation.

A bleeding tendency can be the result of an abnormality at any stage of the events just described. Abnormalities of the vasculature, platelet number, and platelet function have all been well documented, and the evaluation of a patient with a bleed-ing tendency must take all these aspects of the initial coagu-lation mechanism into consideration.

THROMBOCYTOPENIA

DEFINITION. Thrombocytopenia of clinical significance ex-ists when the whole blood platelet count is less than 150,000/mm³, although the precise limits for normal vary slightly among laboratories. Because of the potential for laboratory error or artifact, the finding of a low platelet count should always be confirmed by examination of the peripheral blood smear.

ETIOLOGY AND PATHOGENESIS. The origins of the thrombocytopenic disorders are many and varied and are often poorly understood. Thrombocytopenia is probably most commonly drug induced (see outline below), but primary bone marrow disorders, infections, and immunologic and in-herited disorders have all been associated with thrombocyto-penia.

Drugs commonly implicated in thrombocytopenia

I. Marrow suppressive agents
 A. Chemotherapeutic agents
  1. Doxorubicin
  2. Cytosine arabinoside
  3. Cyclophosphamide
  4. Nitrogen mustard
  5. Nitrosoureas
  6. Busulfan
  7. Methotrexate
  8. VP-16
 B. Other marrow suppressive agents
  1. Chloramphenicol
  2. Phenylbutazone
  3. Thiazide diuretics
  4. Alcohol
  5. Estrogens
II. Immunologic (proven and suspected)
 A. Quinidine
 B. Quinine
 C. Heparin
 D. Aspirin
 E. Sulfonamides
 F. Rifampin
 G. Aminosalicylic acid
 H. Thiazides
 I. Methyldopa
 J. Gold salts

Studies using isotopically labeled platelets for the determina-tion of platelet life span have greatly enhanced the understand-ing of platelet kinetics. Such studies support the intuitive con-cept that thrombocytopenia results from either decreased pro-duction or increased destruction, although thrombocytopenia as a result of abnormal distribution has also been described. Because the mechanism by which the thrombocytopenia occurs has important clinical and therapeutic implications, it is useful to consider the specific disorders that result in thrombocyto-penia grouped on the basis of their platelet kinetics.

Thrombocytopenias caused by decreased platelet production

The disorders that cause decreased platelet production have varied origins. The clinical manifestations of the thrombocy-topenia that results from these disorders are similar, regardless of the cause. Consequently, these aspects are discussed after a review of the individual disorders.

Iatrogenic bone marrow suppression. With the advent of successful chemotherapy and radiation therapy for a variety of malignancies, bone marrow suppression has become an ac-cepted consequence of such therapy. Both ionizing irradiation and a wide variety of myelosuppressive chemotherapeutic agents cause a fairly predictable decrease in platelet count, with granulocytopenia often the major manifestation. The se-verity and duration of the suppression are drug and dose related.

Increasingly, chemotherapeutic regimens are being designed

as pulses of multiple agents that result in a transient, often severe marrow suppression with its nadir 10 to 14 days after treatment. Rapid recovery usually occurs thereafter. However, long-term continuous treatment or even repeated aggressive pulse therapies may result in a prolonged suppression. Prolonged platelet suppression is commonly seen after aggressive or prolonged treatment with busulfan and has also been noted with nitrosoureas.

Drug-related bone marrow suppression. Other drugs that inadvertently or idiosyncratically suppress the bone marrow have been described. Chloramphenicol, sulfonamides, and phenylbutazone (Butazolidin) are well known for their aplastic effect, with thrombocytopenia a part of this aplasia. Alcohol is a frequent bone marrow suppressant. Thiazide diuretics are among the most common causes of drug-induced thrombocytopenia. Decreased megakaryocytes have been noted in the bone marrow of some of these patients, making marrow suppression one possible mechanism. In other cases, however, an immunlogic mechanism seems likely. Estrogens have been described to lower platelet levels, and variations in platelet count during the menstrual cycle have been noted in some women. It is postulated that this phenomenon is the result of marrow suppression, but the mechanism is uncertain.

Bone marrow infiltration. Bone marrow infiltration is frequently associated with cytopenias. When the disease is diffuse, as with the leukemias or myelofibrosis, the mechanism for the cytopenias appears to be marrow replacement. However, spotty infiltration with nests of tumor cells has also been associated with cytopenias and occasionally isolated thrombocytopenia. In these instances it appears that the presence of the foreign cells is toxic or suppressive to normal marrow elements in a manner that is poorly understood. This phenomenon has also been noted in nonmalignant invasive disorders such as granulomatous diseases and in Gaucher's disease.

Congenital disorders. Congenital disorders that result in decreased marrow production are rare but well documented. In addition to the congenital aplastic anemia known as Fanconi's syndrome, a form of congenital aplastic anemia specifically associated with the megakaryocyte is sometimes seen. This may occur with other somatic anomalies, most often in the form of a syndrome of thrombocytopenia with absence of the radii.

Other. Viral infections, rubella vaccination, and megaloblastic anemia are all variably associated with thrombocytopenia resulting from decreased production.

CLINICAL MANIFESTATIONS. The clinical manifestations of this group of disorders of course vary with the underlying disease. The manifestation of the thrombocytopenia per se, however, depends largely on its severity. Between the limits of 20,000 and 100,000 platelets/mm³, an inverse correlation has been observed between platelet count and bleeding time. Clinically, platelet counts of 50,000 to 100,000/mm³ are seldom symptomatic unless the patient is subjected to surgical or traumatic stress. Platelet counts of 20,000 to 50,000/mm³ may be manifest as an increased bruising tendency, and platelet counts of fewer than 20,000/mm³ are often associated with petechiae, bruises, and bleeding from the mucous membranes. Despite these observations, it should be remembered that even a mildly thrombocytopenic patient can have significant bleeding. Such bleeding can be life threatening when it involves intracranial or visceral organs. In addition, the tendency for a thrombocytopenic patient to bleed is aggravated by a variety of conditions. Medications that interfere with platelet function, for example, may greatly increase this tendency and should be studiously avoided. The presence of concomitant infection (a common problem in leukemic patients) is another condition that predisposes to bleeding seemingly out of proportion to the degree of thrombocytopenia.

LABORATORY FINDINGS. The laboratory findings common to all these disorders are a decreased platelet count and decreased numbers of megakaryocytes in the bone marrow. This may be apparent on the bone marrow smear, but often a marrow biopsy gives a better estimate of cellularity and megakaryocyte number. If an isotopic study of platelet life span can be performed, it will be normal. Associated findings depend entirely on the origin of the marrow suppression. For example, the presence of nucleated red blood cells and immature myeloid elements may suggest bone marrow invasion by tumor or fibrosis; hypersegmented neutrophils may be a manifestation of vitamin B$_{12}$ or folate deficiency or an effect of chemotherapy with antimetabolites.

DIAGNOSIS. The diagnosis of decreased platelet production depends on the findings of thrombocytopenia with decreased numbers of megakaryocytes in the bone marrow. The history of the circumstances surrounding the development of thrombocytopenia is critical in the assessment of such patients. A specific drug history or associated illness may in a few circumstances obviate the need for further investigation. The history may raise the suspicion of tumor, in which case a bone marrow biopsy and aspiration are extremely important.

Differentiating marrow suppression from platelet destruction is occasionally a difficult clinical problem. Unfortunately, current techniques for evaluating platelet survival are cumbersome and not widely available. It is therefore occasionally useful diagnostically to determine whether a patient is responsive to platelet transfusions as evidence that there is not a large element of platelet destruction contributing to the thrombocytopenia.

COURSE. The course of the illness also depends on the cause. Drug-induced thrombocytopenias, particularly chemotherapeutically induced, usually respond to withdrawal of the drug over a period of 7 to 14 days. Occasionally there is prolonged or even irreversible damage, especially in the idiosyncratically induced aplasias. The resolution of thrombocytopenia associated with marrow replacement or invasion depends on the success of the treatment of the underlying disorder. Congenital disorders generally persist without improvement.

MANAGEMENT. Management of the patient who is thrombocytopenic because of marrow failure is entirely supportive. In conditions in which the underlying disease can be treated (leukemias and lymphomas) and a finite period of thrombocytopenia is anticipated, prophylactic platelet transfusions are used to maintain the platelet count over 20,000/mm³. When there is no effective treatment for the underlying disorder, the decision to use platelet transfusions is more complex because the patient may become sensitized to the transfusions with the result that their efficacy decreases with time. In these circumstances it is often necessary to give transfusions only for bleeding episodes. Rare reports of responses to androgenic steroids, especially in aplastic states, make a trial of their administration (if not precluded by the underlying disorder) useful in some cases of prolonged hypoplasia (see Chapter 62).

Thrombocytopenias caused by increased platelet destruction

IDIOPATHIC THROMBOCYTOPENIC PURPURA

Definition. Idiopathic thrombocytopenic purpura (ITP) is a relatively common disorder in which isolated thrombocytopenia occurs in otherwise healthy individuals. Two clinical forms of the disease are recognized: acute and chronic. Acute ITP is seen most frequently in children but may occur at any age. The onset is usually sudden, with thrombocytopenia manifested by bruising, bleeding, and petechiae a few days to several weeks after an otherwise uneventful viral illness. Acute ITP is a self-limited disease that generally remits permanently without sequelae.

Chronic ITP is usually a disease of adults and can be sudden or insidious in onset. It is three times more frequent in women than in men, and the course is characterized by remissions and exacerbations. In both acute and chronic ITP, thrombocytopenia and its manifestations are the only physical or laboratory abnormalities.

Etiology and pathogenesis. Although the cause of ITP is unknown, the pathophysiologic mechanism is well documented to be the peripheral destruction of platelets. It has long been believed that this destruction has an immunologic basis, and now a large body of evidence supports this. The presence of a humoral factor that can cross the placenta is shown by the fact that infants born to mothers with ITP are also thrombocytopenic but recover over a period of 1 to 3 months. Also, infusion of plasma from patients with ITP into normal individuals has been documented to induce thrombocytopenia in the recipients. In vitro antiplatelet activity has been found in the 7S globulin fraction of plasma, and ITP platelets have increased surface IgG. Further circumstantial evidence is the occurrence of ITP-like syndromes in association with other immunologically mediated diseases such as systemic lupus erythematosus and autoimmune hemolytic anemia.

Clinical manifestations. Patients with ITP often manifest severe thrombocytopenia and may have significant bruising and bleeding as a result. Surprisingly, however, they often have less bleeding than would be anticipated for the degree of thrombocytopenia. A patient with fewer than 10,000 platelets/mm^3 may have only a few dependent petechiae and be otherwise asymptomatic. At the other end of the spectrum, some patients have a remarkably acute and devastating course, and 1% of the patients have intracranial bleeding.

It must be emphasized that ITP is a disorder of platelets only, and the presence of any other abnormality should put the diagnosis in question. Occasionally, patients have a concomitant iron deficiency anemia owing to blood loss, but any other hematologic abnormality is inconsistent with straightforward ITP. There are no abnormal physical findings in ITP other than petechiae and ecchymoses. The presence of splenomegaly or lymphadenopathy should raise the possibility that an underlying infectious, lymphoproliferative, or autoimmune disorder is the cause of the thrombocytopenia.

Diagnosis and laboratory findings. Despite the volume of evidence for the presence of the antiplatelet antibodies in ITP, efforts to develop tests specifically for the antibody have met with only variable success, and consequently the diagnosis of ITP must still be made on clinical grounds. The presence of isolated thrombocytopenia accompanied by plentiful bone marrow megakaryocytes is the significant finding. It must be emphasized that these findings constitute evidence of increased platelet destruction. The diagnosis of ITP remains one of exclusion. Lack of historical, physical, or laboratory evidence of associated disorders or drugs that could result in platelet destruction is confirmatory. An accurate diagnosis is critical. Other disorders that result in platelet destruction, such as disseminated intravascular coagulation or thrombotic thrombocytopenic purpura, require specific management, and misdiagnosis could have devastating consequences.

Some authors have emphasized that the platelets in ITP may be larger than normal, primarily because these platelets are very young. The usefulness of assessment of platelet size on peripheral smear varies with the experience of the examiner. The application of the isotopic platelet survival test in this disorder is limited by its availability. In most instances the destructive mechanism of the thrombocytopenia is apparent, but in occasional therapeutic dilemmas it is appropriate to refer patients to a center where a study to document the decreased platelet life span can be performed.

Course and management. Corticosteroids and splenectomy are the mainstays of therapy for ITP. Steroids apparently diminish antibody production and inhibit phagocytosis of platelets. Splenectomy also results in diminished antibody production and in removal of the major site of platelet destruction. Childhood ITP usually remits spontaneously, and many clinicians choose not to treat these patients. Most treat all adult patients, and some treat children with severe manifestations. The initiation of prednisone (1 mg/kg) induces a response in the majority of patients, often with a gratifyingly rapid increase in platelet count and resolution of symptoms. Once a response has occurred, management must be individualized. The ideal goal of therapy is normalization of the platelet count without medication. In a small percentage of adult patients the steroids can be tapered and the platelet count will remain normal. More frequently, however, the platelets decrease with decreasing steroid dosages, or a relapse occurs after prednisone has been discontinued. In such patients splenectomy usually results in a permanent remission.

If a remission does not occur or cannot be maintained with less than 10 mg/day of prednisone after a trial of 3 months, a splenectomy should be considered. Patients usually have at least a partial response to splenectomy, and in approximately 50%, splenectomy induces a permanent remission. Some patients with no apparent response to splenectomy become responsive to steroid therapy after the procedure.

There remains a small percentage of patients who do not respond to steroids or splenectomy, and it is in this population that immunosuppressive agents such as cyclophosphamide, azathioprine, or vincristine may be useful.

Danazol, an attenuated androgen, is occasionally useful. High-dose, intravenously administered γ-globulin has recently been found to be highly effective. Unfortunately, the effect is usually transient, and each treatment is extraordinarily expensive. It is therefore usually reserved for emergency treatment in refractory patients.

None of the therapies used in this disease is without risk, and the goals of therapy must be assessed for each patient and tempered with reason. The ultimate purpose of therapy is to prevent bleeding, and it may not be necessary to have a completely normal platelet count to achieve this end. The risk of bleeding in an individual patient must be weighed against the risk of therapy. For example, many patients with ITP are relatively symptom free with 50,000 platelets/mm^3, so it may be reasonable in such a patient to postpone additional therapy until the clinical situation merits it.

Syndromes resembling idiopathic thrombocytopenic purpura. A number of disorders can be accompanied by ITP-like syndromes. The lymphoproliferative disorders, chronic lymphocytic leukemia, Hodgkin's disease, and non-Hodgkin's lymphomas all have a small but significant incidence of peripheral platelet destruction. Systemic lupus erythematosus is surprisingly frequently accompanied by an apparently immunologically mediated thrombocytopenia. Autoimmune hemolytic anemia is also occasionally associated with ITP (Evans' syndrome), as is infectious mononucleosis. An ITP-like picture may be the initial symptom in any of these disorders. It is therefore important in the process of diagnostic exclusion to ascertain that the ITP is not simply the initial symptom of another disorder, since the treatment of an underlying lymphoproliferative disorder, for instance, may be critical to the patient. The management of thrombocytopenia in these disorders is similar to that for straightforward ITP, with steroids and splenectomy.

An immunologic thrombocytopenia clinically indistinguishable from ITP is being seen with increasing frequency in patients exposed to the human immunodeficiency virus (HIV). With the increasing incidence of heterosexual transmission of this virus, a high index of suspicion must be maintained even in patients without an obvious history of high-risk behavior. The treatment of the thrombocytopenia is identical to that of classic ITP, but the implications of HIV seropositivity are so great that appropriate medical follow-up and counseling must be arranged for such a patient.

Drug-related platelet destruction. Among the drugs reported to cause thrombocytopenia, many are suspected to do so via immunologically mediated peripheral platelet destruction. Quinine, quinidine, and their derivatives are the classic examples of drugs that are documented to cause immunologic thrombocytopenia. In susceptible individuals the responsible drug apparently induces an antibody that, in the presence of the drug, has antiplatelet activity. This effect can be demonstrated in vitro. The patient's plasma, in combination with the drug, lyses platelets in an isotopic release assay, whereas the plasma or drug alone does not. The analogous in vivo counterpart is the observation that the platelet destruction ceases as soon after the drug is stopped as it takes for the drug to be cleared from the plasma. These patients are therefore managed simply by discontinuation of the responsible drug, which should result in a prompt rise in the platelet count.

A number of the drugs that have been reported to cause thrombocytopenia by this mechanism are listed on p. 347. It is an important point in the management of patients susceptible to quinine-induced thrombocytopenia that this susceptibility does not extend to quinidine and vice versa. A patient sensitive to one may be treated with the other without adverse effect.

Gold-induced thrombocytopenia is an interesting example of drug-related platelet destruction. Because gold salts are excreted slowly, the duration of the thrombocytopenia is prolonged. Steroid treatment is frequently required in these patients to maintain an acceptable platelet count until the drug is cleared—often a matter of months.

Thrombotic thrombocytopenic purpura. Thrombotic thrombocytopenic purpura (TTP) is a clinical syndrome in which thrombocytopenia, microangiopathic hemolytic anemia, and neurologic abnormalities occur. There are also often fever and renal failure. The origin is unknown, but the pathogenesis is related to the presence of deposits of hyaline material and platelet thrombi in the capillaries and arterioles. Which of these lesions is causative remains obscure. The disorder usually runs a fulminant course, with mortality ranging in different series from 50% to 90%. A chronic form is now also recognized. The clinical picture varies with renal, neurologic, or hematologic manifestations; the most prominent feature depends on the site of the vascular occlusions. Gum biopsy is a useful diagnostic procedure in some situations. It is likely that TTP in adults and the so-called hemolytic-uremic syndrome in children are the same disorder, although the vascular lesions in the latter are confined to the kidneys.

The therapies that have been proposed are difficult to assess because the disease is uncommon and published series are small. Steroids, splenectomy, and antiplatelet agents such as aspirin or dipyridamole have been tried and reported to have some effect. More recently, encouraging reports of responses to plasma exchange, either alone or in combination with antiplatelet agents, have generated enthusiasm for this approach.

Posttransfusion purpura. In a small number of patients severe thrombocytopenia has been found to develop approximately 1 week after blood transfusion. Patients in whom this occurs almost always lack the platelet-associated antigen PL^{A1}, which is present in 98% of the population. Apparently the transfusion induces the development of anti-PL^{A1} antibodies, and the patient's platelets are destroyed as innocent bystanders. Exchange transfusion and plasmapheresis have been reported to result in successful resolution. The same antibody is responsible for isoimmune neonatal purpura.

Disseminated intravascular coagulation. Disseminated intravascular coagulation (DIC) is a disorder in which coagulation factors and platelets are consumed by the formation of fibrin clots. The process is discussed in detail in Chapter 81. DIC is most frequently associated with overwhelming infections and with obstetric complications such as abruptio placentae and toxemia. It must always be considered in a patient with unexplained platelet destruction, particularly if bleeding is out of proportion to the degree of thrombocytopenia.

Disorders of distribution

Splenomegaly, which is usually associated with some degree of increased platelet turnover, has been reported to be associated with thrombocytopenia and a normal platelet survival. In these instances the thrombocytopenia probably results from altered distribution, with pooling in the large vascular bed of the spleen.

THROMBOCYTOSIS

Thrombocytosis exists when the whole blood platelet count is above 400,000/mm³. It may be either primary (the result of a myeloproliferative disorder) or secondary (reactive to a variety of nonhematologic disorders).

Primary thrombocytosis

Primary thrombocytosis occurs as part of the spectrum of myeloproliferative diseases. It may be the only manifestation of myeloproliferation (essential thrombocythemia) or be part of one of the other myeloproliferative disorders, most frequently polycythemia vera. Occasionally, myelofibrosis or chronic granulocytic leukemia has an associated thrombocytosis. The origin is unknown. Presumably thrombocytosis results from overproduction by an abnormal clone of stem cells or megakaryocytes.

The clinical manifestations of primary thrombocytosis are extremely variable, ranging from the asymptomatic to the life threatening. Thrombotic complications may develop, or in patients with abnormal platelet function, bleeding may occur.

The laboratory findings include an increased number of platelets, which are often morphologically abnormal. There may be spurious hyperkalemia. For the most part laboratory findings are related to the underlying myeloproliferative disorder. For example, there may be an elevated serum vitamin B$_{12}$ or leukocyte alkaline phosphatase level. On physical examination some degree of splenomegaly is usually found. Isolated essential thrombocythemia may be difficult to differentiate from reactive thrombocytosis; in these cases the diagnosis is made when evidence of an associated myeloproliferation can be demonstrated. The presence of platelet function abnormalities strongly suggests a myeloproliferative disorder.

Functionally normal platelets are the rule in secondary thrombocytosis.

The course and treatment of the disease vary with symptoms and with the underlying myeloproliferative disorder, but generally busulfan, radioactive phosphorus (^{32}P), or more recently hydroxyurea and uracil mustard have been used to decrease the platelet count. In acutely symptomatic patients, plateletpheresis may be necessary.

Secondary thrombocytosis

For unknown reasons platelet counts greater than 400,000/mm^3 are associated with a wide variety of disorders. A transient thrombocytosis almost invariably occurs after splenectomy. Patients with severe iron deficiency occasionally have significant thrombocytosis, and in chronic hemolytic states the platelet count may be elevated. A variety of inflammatory and stressful situations have been described as predisposing factors in reactive thrombocytosis. Among the most common causes are tumors of any origin. Patients are almost invariably asymptomatic, and platelet function is normal. The occurrence of abnormal platelet function strongly suggests a myeloproliferative disorder rather than a reactive thrombocytosis. Thrombotic events, although rare, occur, especially if the thrombocytosis persists for a prolonged period. This is more common in patients with hemolytic disease who have persistent hemolysis after splenectomy. The laboratory findings are usually thrombocytosis and those of the underlying disorder. Spurious hyperkalemia may be noted. The platelets are morphologically normal.

The diagnosis is one of exclusion of a myeloproliferative disorder. The documentation of an underlying disorder associated with reactive thrombocytosis is important. The course and treatment are those of the primary disorder, and the thrombocytosis resolves with the underlying cause. In cases of prolonged or extraordinary thrombocytosis (>1 million cells/mm^3) many clinicians employ drugs that inhibit platelet function, such as aspirin or dipyridamole, and most avoid the use of cytotoxic agents. The merits of heparin or warfarin are uncertain, but they may be indicated for other reasons, as in a bedridden patient who is at high risk of thromboembolic disease.

QUALITATIVE PLATELET ABNORMALITIES

Platelet function defects can be congenital or acquired. In either case disorders of any facet of platelet function are possible, and it is useful to categorize these disorders according to the specific physiologic defect. Congenital defects are rare, but acquired defects are surprisingly common, especially when drug-induced platelet function defects are included.

Congenital disorders of platelet function

BERNARD-SOULIER SYNDROME. Bernard-Soulier syndrome is an autosomal recessive disorder of platelet adhesion. It is characterized by giant platelets that do not aggregate when stimulated with the antibiotic ristocetin. Unlike the similar phenomenon in von Willebrand's disease, this inability to aggregate is not corrected by factor VIII replacement. In fact, all the factor VIII activities are normal in the plasma of these patients. The defect is an intrinsic abnormality of the platelet membrane, which has been shown to have decreased amounts of glycoprotein Ib. Glycoprotein Ib is a receptor for factor VIII–related ristocetin cofactor activity.

In addition to this functional defect, which results in a prolonged bleeding time, patients may have a mild thrombocytopenia. The bleeding may be severe, with epistaxis, menor-

rhagia, and bruising, and may require treatment with platelet transfusions.

THROMBASTHENIA. Thrombasthenia is also an autosomal recessive disease characterized by a prolonged bleeding time, but unlike the Bernard-Soulier syndrome, platelet adhesion is normal and there is diminished or absent aggregation to almost all stimuli. The platelet count is normal. An abnormality of the membrane glycoprotein IIb IIIa complex is the apparent cause. The patients have symptoms similar to those of the Bernard-Soulier syndrome, and platelet transfusions are the therapy for bleeding episodes.

STORAGE-POOL DISEASE. Storage-pool disease is an inherited disorder of variable transmission sometimes associated with albinism. It is caused by a deficiency of the dense platelet granules containing the "storage pool" of the adenine nucleotides adenosine diphosphate (ADP) and adenosine triphosphate (ATP), which are normally secreted during the release reaction. This deficiency results in a selective absence of second-wave aggregation. Platelet transfusion may be necessary to treat bleeding episodes in these patients, but treatment with corticosteroids has also been reported to be of benefit.

Acquired disorders of platelet function

DRUG-INDUCED DISORDERS. By far the most frequent platelet function abnormalities today are drug induced. The importance of recognizing this effect of many commonly used drugs cannot be overemphasized. Drugs have been found to inhibit all phases of platelet function. Coating of the cell membrane is reported to be the mechanism by which dextran interferes with platelet adhesion. Phosphodiesterase inhibitors such as dipyridamole increase platelet cyclic adenosine monophosphate (cyclic AMP) and consequently inhibit aggregation. The agents that most commonly inhibit platelet function are the nonsteroidal antiinflammatory agents, which inhibit the platelet prostaglandin pathway and therefore second-wave aggregation. The most extensively studied of these agents is aspirin, which irreversibly acetylates the enzyme cyclooxygenase, inhibiting the production of thromboxane A$_2$ for the duration of the life of the platelet. This means that platelet function is still abnormal several days after even a single dose of aspirin. Other nonsteroidal antiinflammatory agents such as indomethacin also act by inhibition of cyclooxygenase but do so in a manner that is of a shorter duration. The following is a list of commonly used agents that have been documented to inhibit platelet function:

Nonsteroidal antiinflammatory agents (cyclooxygenase inhibitors)
  Aspirin
  Indomethacin
  Sulfinpyrazone
  Naproxen (Naprosyn)
  Ibuprofen
Phosphodiesterase inhibitors
  Dipyridamole
  Theophylline
Unknown mechanism
  Penicillins
  Clofibrate
  Dextran

Many other drugs have been described to inhibit platelet function in vitro, but the clinical significance of an isolated in vitro effect is uncertain.

Laboratory findings in patients taking these drugs vary but can include a prolonged bleeding time, abnormal platelet aggregation, and, in laboratories where it can be measured, decreased thromboxane production.

The clinical result is not a severe bleeding disorder but one that can exaggerate bleeding after surgery, particularly if the drugs are continued. Most normal individuals can tolerate a minor surgical procedure after aspirin, but it is especially important to avoid such medications in patients with underlying bleeding disorders. In these patients significant bleeding may occur.

Aspirin is ubiquitous in commercially available remedies, and the current interest in the role of platelet inhibition in the prevention of arteriosclerotic vascular disease further encourages the use of drugs that inhibit platelet function. These drugs are often useful, and the physician need not be afraid to administer them appropriately. Patient and physician awareness is the most important aspect of management. Should bleeding occur, a decision regarding discontinuation of the drug must be made.

MYELOPROLIFERATIVE DISORDERS. All of the myeloproliferative disorders can be complicated by the development of a platelet function abnormality. These are most likely intrinsic defects resulting from the production of abnormal cells by the diseased clone. Thrombocytosis has been associated with prolonged bleeding time, aggregation abnormalities, and even abnormalities of arachidonic acid metabolism. Similarly, patients with myeloid metaplasia often have large, functionally abnormal platelets. Patients with acute myelogenous leukemia or preleukemia may have functionally abnormal platelets, although this is less conspicuous because the patients are often dramatically thrombocytopenic. Support with platelet transfusions is the treatment for bleeding episodes.

UREMIA. Bruising and bleeding are frequent complications of uncontrolled uremia, and the fact that the bleeding time is often prolonged in these patients suggests a platelet function abnormality. The exact nature of the abnormality is uncertain, but it appears to be an extrinsic defect, since it improves when the patients are dialyzed.

VASCULAR PURPURAS

A variety of disorders of the vasculature can result in clinically significant bruising and bleeding in the presence of an otherwise normal coagulation system. Although most are relatively uncommon, they are important to recognize and differentiate from disorders of the coagulation system per se, since management will be entirely different.

Cushing's syndrome

Purpura associated with Cushing's syndrome or more frequently with exogenously administered corticosteroids is a common finding. Petechiae are uncommon. The cause of this purpura is unknown, but it appears to be related to decreased vascular support in the skin with spontaneous or minimally induced bruising.

Amyloidosis

Amyloidosis is a relatively uncommon disorder that can result in vascular infiltration with fibrous amyloid protein. This may or may not be associated with increased vascular fragility. An associated defect in coagulation factor function may, however, complicate this picture.

Vitamin C deficiency

Scurvy is fortunately now a rare disease but may be found in indigent and alcoholic populations. Unless it is recognized

and treated, a syndrome of petechiae and perifollicular hemorrhages may occur in the advanced state and present a diagnostic dilemma. Connective tissue and endothelial abnormalities as a result of the vitamin deficiency appear to be the cause. Bleeding gums are common, and subperiosteal hemorrhages occur in children. The vascular abnormality reverses with the administration of vitamin C.

Autoerythrocyte sensitization

Autoerythrocyte sensitization is a disorder predominantly of young women in whom spontaneous, inflammatory ecchymoses occur. The lesions usually appear at times of stress and can masquerade as a bleeding or thrombotic event. There is no apparent underlying coagulation abnormality. When the patients are tested by the intradermal injection of their own red blood cells, red blood cell membrane, or hemoglobin, the lesions can be reproduced. An important differentiating point is the inflammatory nature of the lesions. Steroids and antihistamines, however, have little effect. There is a strong psychologic element, and the therapy is treatment of the underlying depression or hysteria.

Schönlein-Henoch purpura

Schönlein-Henoch purpura is an allergic vasculitis that occurs most often in children 1 to 3 weeks after an upper respiratory tract infection. It has been postulated to represent a hypersensitivity to streptococci, but evidence for this is controversial.

The skin lesions, which occur predominantly over the extensor surfaces of the lower extremities, are the result of an aseptic vasculitis. They commence as urticarial lesions and then evolve into hemorrhagic lesions. Complement, IgA, and IgG have all been reported to be deposited in the skin capillary bed. Polyarthralgias and abdominal pain may occur, and there is an associated glomerulonephritis. Steroids and immunosuppressive therapy have been tried but are of uncertain benefit. Relapse occurs in 50% of the patients, and some progress to chronic renal failure.

Osler-Weber-Rendu syndrome

Osler-Weber-Rendu syndrome is an inherited disorder in which telangiectasias occur on the mucous membranes. The lesions become more numerous with time, and hemorrhage from these vessels frequently occurs. The size of the lesions and their hemorrhagic tendencies vary. Occasionally lesions are large and result in significant arteriovenous shunting. The bleeding that occurs can be life threatening. Nosebleeds are frequent and often difficult to control. Bleeding from the gastrointestinal tract can be the greatest management problem, often requiring repeated resections to remove the vascular lesions. About 20% of the patients have pulmonary arteriovenous fistulas. There is no specific treatment. Estrogens have been suggested, but they are of questionable benefit.

Various connective tissue disorders

Several congenital connective tissue disorders, including the Ehlers-Danlos syndrome, pseudoxanthoma elasticum, and osteogenesis imperfecta, can result in increased bruising and bleeding.

Other purpuric disorders

Purpura simplex is a syndrome of easy bruisability unassociated with a specific pathologic condition. It may represent a mixture of underdiagnosed mild platelet and coagulation abnormalities. Cryoglobulinemia and a variety of other γ-globulin abnormalities may be associated with purpura. Many vasculitides are manifest as a mild increased bruising tendency.

VON WILLEBRAND'S DISEASE

Von Willebrand's disease is an inherited disorder of the portion of factor VIII complex necessary to support normal platelet function. As a result, the disease is manifest as a platelet function abnormality. It is a surprisingly common disorder, and it has provided a natural model for the understanding of the relationship between platelet function and the coagulation mechanism. It is discussed in detail in Chapter 81.

BIBLIOGRAPHY

Thrombocytopenia

Aster RN: Thrombocytopenia due to enhanced platelet destruction. In Williams WJ and others, editors: Hematology, ed 3, New York, 1983, McGraw-Hill Inc.

Bolton FG and Young RV: Observations on cases of thrombocytopenic purpura due to quinine, sulphamezathine and quinidine, J Clin Pathol 6:320, 1953.

Harker LA and Slichter SJ: The bleeding time as a screening test for evaluation of platelet function, N Engl J Med 238:155, 1972.

Kelton JG: Advances in the diagnosis and management of ITP, Hosp Pract 19:95, 1983.

Walsh CM, Nardi MS, and Karpatkin MD: On the mechanism of thrombocytopenic purpura in sexually active homosexual men, N Engl J Med 311:635, 1984.

Thrombocytosis

Hirsh J and Dacie JV: Persistent post-splenectomy thrombocytosis and thromboembolism: a consequence of continuing anaemia, Br J Haematol 12:44, 1966.

Murphy S: Thrombocytosis and thrombocythaemia, Clin Haematol 12:89, 1983.

Qualitative platelet abnormalities

Rao AK and Walsh PN: Acquired qualitative platelet disorders, Clin Haematol 12:201, 1983.

Shattil SJ and Bennett JS: Platelets and their membranes in hemostasis: physiology and pathophysiology, Ann Intern Med 94:108, 1981.

Vascular purpuras

Gottlieb AJ: Nonthrombocytopenic purpuras. In Williams WJ and others, editors: Hematology, ed 3, New York, 1983, McGraw-Hill Inc.

McKusick VA: Heritable disorders of connective tissue, ed 4, St Louis, 1972, CV Mosby Co.

81 · DISORDERS OF THE COAGULATION MECHANISM

Patricia Catalano

The biochemical events that lead to clot formation are complex and can be initiated by a variety of stimuli. The coagulation cascade is illustrated in Fig. 81-1. Abnormalities can of course occur at any point in this cascade. Defining the exact problem requires a fairly sophisticated laboratory, especially for individual factor assays. However, the location of the abnormality can usually be approximated with relatively few, simple screening tests. These basic tests include prothrombin time (PT), which measures the activity of the extrinsic and common pathways, partial thromboplastin time (PTT), which detects abnormalities in the intrinsic and common pathways, and thrombin time (TT), which is a measure of the formation of fibrin from fibrinogen. A quantitative fibrinogen study, platelet count, and bleeding time complete the evaluation in conjunction with an accurate history. Specific factor assays can

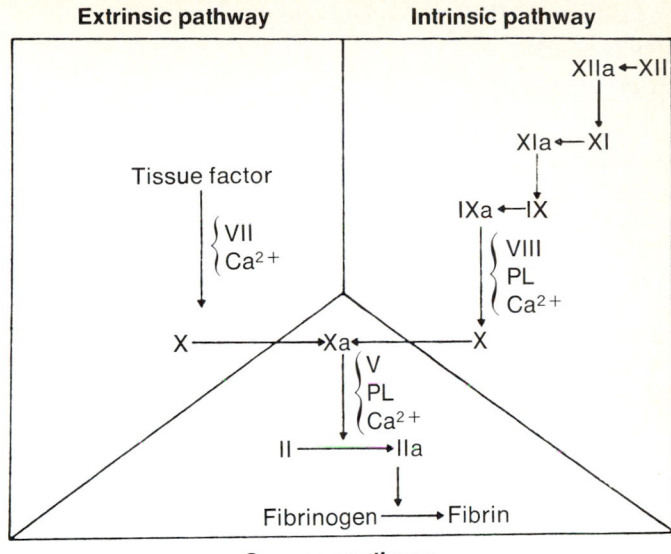

Fig. 81-1 Extrinsic and intrinsic pathways to factor X activation and fibrin formation. In presence of calcium, inactive plasma procoagulants are activated in cascade mechanism to convert inactive factor X to activated Xa. This is intrinsic mechanism. Tissue factor and factor VII in presence of calcium also act on X, converting ti to Xa. After this, Xa in presence of factor V, platelets, and calcium converts factor II (prothrombin) to IIa (thrombin), which in turn converts fibrinogen to fibrin. *a,* Activated; Ca^{2+} calcium; *PL,* platelets. (From Esneuf, M.P.: Br. Med. Bull. 33:213, 1977.)

then be obtained selectively based on the information gained through the initial screening.

INHERITED DISORDERS OF COAGULATION

Congenital deficiencies of virtually every clotting factor have been reported. By far the most common disorders, however, are those of factor VIII: hemophilia A and von Willebrand's disease. A detailed discussion of the biochemistry of coagulation factors is beyond the scope of this text, but a conceptual understanding of factor VIII is singularly important to understanding these diseases.

Factor VIII is a high-molecular-weight glycoprotein synthesized primarily in the endothelial cell. It is actually a complex of two distinct components. The first, the procoagulant portion, is usually referred to as VIIIc. This is the portion of the complex that participates in the coagulation cascade and corrects the abnormality in hemophilia A. The majority of the complex is composed of von Willebrand's factor (VIIIvonW). This is the part of factor VIII that binds to glycoprotein Ib on the platelet and supports the normal platelet function of adhesion. It also serves as a carrier protein for VIIIc. VIIIvonW can be quantitated by a variety of immunologic techniques and may be referred to in this context as VIIIag. (It should be noted that the contribution of VIIIc to the total antigenic activity of the complex is so minimal that its presence is not detected by these techniques unless specific antibodies are used.) VIIIvonW is necessary to support the aggregation of platelets by ristocetin. The ristocetin cofactor (VIIIrcof) activity is the measure of this function. The in vivo test of VIIIvonW activity is of course the bleeding time.

Agarose gel electrophoresis reveals that factor VIII is composed of a series of subunits called multimers. High-, intermediate-, and low-molecular-weight bands can readily be identified. Factor VIII is also present on platelets, where its multimeric distribution is usually similar to that in plasma.

HEMOPHILIA A

Hemophilia A is a congenital deficiency of the VIIIc portion of the factor VIII complex. The severe form, in which patients have less than 1% of the normal VIIIc level, is the most common. Moderate disease, in which patients have 2% to 5% of the normal VIIIc, also occurs, as does a mild form, in which the VIIIc level may be as high as 20% to 25%.

ETIOLOGY AND PATHOGENESIS. Since VIIIc is coded for on the X chromosome, hemophilia A is a sex-linked disease. Hemophilia occurs in approximately 1 in 10,000 live male births, and the vast majority of cases are hemophilia A. Up to 30% of cases have been estimated to be spontaneous mutations, accounting for the fairly consistent incidence over the centuries. DNA probe analysis provides evidence to suggest that the mutation may be unique in each family. Daughters of hemophiliac men are of course obligatory carriers of the gene. Half of the offspring of a carrier inherit the gene. If they are male, they have hemophilia, but females (with few exceptions) are phenotypically normal whether they are carriers or not. The ability to detect carriers is critical in being able to offer genetic counseling to relatives of persons with hemophilia. Similarities in the location of the mutations make DNA probe analysis a useful tool for carrier testing and prenatal diagnosis.

CLINICAL MANIFESTATIONS. Severe hemophilia is a lifelong, crippling disease. Although few neonates have bleeding episodes, the diagnosis almost invariably comes to light within the first year even if there is no family history to suggest it. Patients bleed spontaneously into joints and sometimes soft tissue, and minor trauma can be associated with life-threatening bleeding. The most common site of bleeding is into the joints, especially elbows and knees, although any joint can be affected. These hemarthroses are painful even before physical findings are apparent, and a patient complaining of bleeding deserves prompt treatment regardless of the physical findings. The sequela of repeated hemarthroses is a severe arthropathy characterized by bony overgrowth, spur formation, limited range of motion, and chronic pain. Soft tissue bleeding can result in neurologic compromise from peripheral nerve compression. Spontaneous intracranial bleeding, hematuria, and retroperitoneal bleeding can also occur.

Patients with mild disease rarely have bleeding episodes except with surgery or trauma, and probably the biggest threat to such patients is when their problem has not been diagnosed before such an episode occurs. In moderate hemophilia spontaneous bleeding may occur rarely, and minor trauma may require treatment several times a year.

One complication occurring in approximately 15% of patients is the development of an inhibitor to factor VIIIc. When this occurs, the clinical manifestations of the disease seldom worsen, but treatment becomes much more difficult.

LABORATORY FINDINGS AND DIAGNOSIS. The diagnosis of hemophilia is straightforward. The PTT is prolonged, and specific factor assays confirm the diagnosis. VIIIag level, VIIIrcof level, and bleeding time are normal, but especially in mild disease these parameters should be checked at initial diagnosis to avoid overlooking a severe form of von Willebrand's disease.

Carrier detection has traditionally relied on the theory that a woman with one abnormal X chromosome should have an VIIIc level that is 50% of normal and a normal VIIIag level. Now that DNA probe analysis is possible, it is rapidly becoming the diagnostic test of choice. It has the added advantage of being applicable to early prenatal diagnosis.

COURSE AND MANAGEMENT. Replacement therapy is the mainstay of treatment in hemophilia. The development of cryoprecipitate and of lyophilized factor concentrates has dramatically altered the course of this disease as demonstrated by the marked increase in life expectancy that accompanied these developments. Clinicians now have the luxury of titrating the level of factor VIII to accommodate the needs in an individual situation.

Potentially life-threatening bleeding is usually treated with 100% replacement. The half-life of factor VIII is approximately 10 to 12 hours, so 50% replacement given at 12-hour intervals maintains the level between 50% and 100%. Less threatening bleeding such as spontaneous hemarthroses is treated with 50% replacement or less if the patient is able to self-administer the product immediately. The management of bleeding episodes must be individualized.

Most patients with severe hemophilia are taught to treat themselves at home with lyophilized concentrates. This dramatically improved the quality of patients' lives and decreased the number of days spent in the hospital. Minimal restrictions on physical activity, such as the avoidance of contact sports or specific recommendations for some patients with arthropathy, are now the only limitations necessary to impose on patients with hemophilia. Routine medical procedures, such as aggressive dental care, should no longer be neglected for fear of inducing bleeding.

Advances in hemophilia treatment have not come without cost. The threat of hepatitis and its sequelae must always be considered in patients receiving multiple transfusions. Approximately 95% of patients with severe hemophilia have antibodies to hepatitis B. Probably a similar exposure rate is the case for non-A, non-B hepatitis. The recent human immunodeficiency virus (HIV) epidemic has similarly exposed many patients with severe hemophilia to HIV. The incidence of HIV seropositivity in hemophiliac patients is estimated to be approximately 85%, and acquired immunodeficiency syndrome (AIDS) is rapidly becoming the biggest threat to these patients. Because of the frequency of these viral infections, all patients with hemophilia regardless of HIV serologic findings should be managed as if they were seropositive. Counseling and support must be made available to these patients, and appropriate precautions taken when exposure to blood or body fluids is likely.

The management of mild hemophilia is somewhat different. When major trauma occurs or surgery is anticipated, the transfusion requirements are approximately the same as for severe patients in terms of VIIIc units. In mild hemophilia, however, cryoprecipitate has been the traditional treatment of choice because of the significantly lower risk of hepatitis from this product, which is made from blood from a limited number of donors. Unfortunately, fresh blood products still carry a small risk of viral contamination, including HIV, and this risk must be considered when choosing therapy for infrequently or previously untransfused patients. All lyophilized concentrates are now viral inactivated by a variety of means, including pasteurization and chromatographic or monoclonal purification. As a result, these products are considered by some hematologists to be the treatment of choice, especially in areas of the country where fresh blood products are very likely to be virus contaminated. This therapeutic decision remains a controversial and difficult one.

Fortunately, 1-deamino (8-D-arginine) vasopressin (DDAVP)

is now available for the treatment of mild factor VIII deficiency. This synthetic vasopressin analog appears to work by stimulating the release of stores of factor VIII in the patient's endothelial cells. A significant level may be achieved in patients with some reserve—usually those with greater than 5% VIIIc. Treatment with DDAVP can therefore help avoid any exposure to blood products in some patients. A part of the comprehensive evaluation of a patient with mild disease should include a challenge with DDAVP to ascertain responsiveness, especially if the patient's baseline level is 5% to 10%.

Patients with inhibitors to factor VIII are significantly more difficult to treat. In some instances a low-titer antibody can be overwhelmed by use of large doses of factor VIII. More frequently, an alternative must be found. For reasons that are not clear, prothrombin complex concentrate in high doses stops the bleeding in approximately 50% of episodes. Activated factor concentrates are also available, but their significantly greater expense and arguable clinical advantages cause most hematologists to reserve them for situations when a patient is unresponsive to standard preparations. Porcine factor VIII concentrate is a newly available alternative that has a number of possible advantages.

There are many additional concerns in the management of hemophilia. Aspirin and other drugs that inhibit platelet function must be avoided, which makes pain management of arthropathy difficult. Hepatitis B immunization should be accomplished in patients who have newly diagnosed hemophilia or are hepatitis B seronegative. The judicious use of ε-aminocaproic acid (EACA) may decrease the transfusion requirements after dental procedures in both mild and severe hemophilia. The safety profile of factor concentrates continues to be of concern. Recombinant factor VIII preparations are now in clinical trials and, if proved safe, should eliminate the risk of viral contamination.

The psychosocial impact of hemophilia has always been great, and the financial burden can be overwhelming. The medical threats are obvious. For these reasons patients with hemophilia should be treated by physicians and support personnel familiar with the disease and its management. State and federal hemophilia centers that specialize in comprehensive care are located throughout the United States, and if possible patients with hemophilia should be treated in such centers.

VON WILLEBRAND'S DISEASE

DEFINITION. Von Willebrand's disease is a common inherited disorder in which a prolonged bleeding time is associated with abnormalities of factor VIII. It is a disease of great interest, both because of its frequency and because it illustrates the complex relationship between the platelet and the intrinsic coagulation system.

ETIOLOGY AND PATHOGENESIS. Von Willebrand's disease is actually a group of disorders of the autosomally controlled portion of the factor VIII complex. We now know that the subunit protein for von Willebrand's factor is coded for on chromosome 12, but the complex way in which this protein is processed and assembled into multimers is not fully understood. Clearly there is potential for a wide variety of abnormalities, and many have been described. Von Willebrand's disease is classified based on factor VIIIvonW multimer distribution. The basic types are summarized in Table 81-1 and represent the great majority of cases.

Fundamental to understanding the dynamics of factor VIII–platelet interaction is the fact that factor VIIIvonW is present both on the platelet and in the plasma, and the multimeric composition of the two pools is not necessarily the same. Normally, high-, intermediate-, and low-molecular-weight multimers are present in a continuum with distinct bands, and the spectrum of distribution is similar on the platelets and in the plasma. In von Willebrand's disease, however, the multimers are diminished or have abnormal distribution on the platelets or in the plasma.

In type I all the multimers are diminished or absent from plasma, whereas those on the platelet are essentially normal.

Type II is characterized by a loss of the high-molecular-weight multimers from the plasma. In the IIa subtype neither the highest- nor the intermediate-weight multimers are found on platelets or in plasma. In the IIb subtype, however, the highest-molecular-weight multimers are missing from the plasma but can be found on the platelets. The abnormal VIIIvonW in type IIb has an increased avidity for platelets, which "sponge" the highest-molecular-weight multimers from the plasma. This also results in an increased sensitivity to aggregation with ristocetin. The clinical implications of this rare but important subtype are discussed later in the chapter.

Type III von Willebrand's disease represents the most severe form of the disease, in which all multimers are absent both in the plasma and on the platelets.

CLINICAL MANIFESTATIONS. The clinical severity of von Willebrand's disease is variable. Patients with the classic severe form (type III) usually have a lifelong history of spontaneous bruising and episodes of bleeding from mucous membranes. Bleeding after dental cleaning is common, and epistaxis may be a problem. Menorrhagia is common in women and may require hormonal manipulation to stop excessive blood loss. For unknown reasons factor VIII–related activities usually increase during pregnancy and with the use of oral contraceptive agents. Although postpartum hemorrhage does occur in patients with severe disease, it is rare in patients with milder variants.

Patients with milder disease (usually type IIa) may have only easy bruisability or a history of excessive blood loss after a dental extraction. During evaluation of patients with this kind of history, a high index of suspicion is invaluable.

LABORATORY FINDINGS AND DIAGNOSIS. Unfortunately, although von Willebrand's disease must be considered in terms of platelet and plasma multimers, few laboratories are equipped to provide this analysis. It is therefore necessary to translate the previous discussion into terms of factors VIIIc, VIIIag, and VIIIrcof. It is important to realize that the VIIIag measures all multimers and does not differentiate between loss of high-molecular-weight multimers and a decrease in all multimers. Nonetheless, the physician can make a diagnosis of von Willebrand's disease and choose an appropriate plan of management in most instances.

In the severe form of the disease (types III and I) the bleeding time is long and all the above-noted factor VIII–related activities are diminished. Type II disease may be more difficult to diagnose because, although the high-molecular-weight multimers may be decreased, the smaller multimers may actually be increased. Therefore the total antigen may not be significantly decreased. The other studies may be borderline normal as well, although the VIIIrcof and bleeding times are usually abnormal. In addition, the physician must be certain that such patients do not have the IIb variant because treatment would be different. In this situation the use of ristocetin aggregation is invaluable for diagnosis. Platelet-rich plasma from patients with the IIb variant not only responds to ristocetin but is more sensitive than normal to its aggregating effects. Patients with the IIb variant may also have mild to moderate

Table 81-1 Von Willebrand's disease classification based on factor VIII multimer distribution

Type	Plasma	Platelets
I	↓ All multimers	Normal multimers
IIa	↓ High- and intermediate-molecular-weight multimers	↓ High- and intermediate-molecular-weight multimers
IIb	↓ High-molecular-weight multimers	Normal multimers
IIc	Abnormal multimer structure	Abnormal multimer structure
III	↓ All multimers	↓ All multimers

thrombocytopenia, presumably because of in vivo aggregation induced by spontaneous binding of the abnormal VIIIvonW to platelets.

COURSE AND MANAGEMENT. Because of the variability in clinical manifestations, the treatment must be individualized. Only in the most severe cases does spontaneous bleeding occur. Most treatment is aimed at preventing bleeding during surgical or dental procedures or after trauma. Fortunately DDAVP is now available and is extremely useful for many patients. As discussed in relation to mild hemophilia, its apparent mechanism of action is to stimulate the release of factor VIII reserves from the endothelial cells. In type I disease, in which all multimers are being made (as evidenced by the platelet pool) but are not present in plasma, a release of reserves is the ideal treatment. In type IIa disease the only multimers available are the low-molecular-weight ones, which are not significantly active in supporting platelet function. In most cases more of these would not correct the disorder, but this group of patients is heterogeneous, and a therapeutic trial is justifiable. The alternative is treatment with cryoprecipitate, and the risks of hepatitis or HIV infection from this blood product are far greater than the risks of a trial of DDAVP. This is not the case in IIb disease, where the release of more high-avidity factor VIII could actually threaten the patient. Cryoprecipitate is the treatment of choice for this and for type III disease, in which there are no significant reserves.

The judicious use of EACA after dental procedures may help prevent the necessity for transfusion. As in all bleeding disorders, drugs that interfere with platelet function must be avoided.

HEMOPHILIA B

DEFINITION. Hemophilia B, or Christmas disease, is an inherited bleeding disorder characterized by the deficiency of functional factor IX.

ETIOLOGY AND PATHOGENESIS. As in hemophilia A, the gene for factor IX is on the X chromosome, making this a sex-linked disease. The coagulant function of factor IX is missing in this disease, but unlike in factor VIII deficiency, in many cases the protein antigen is not detectable. Factor IX is a much smaller glycoprotein than factor VIII, and its sequence has been well documented. Many variants of the disease have been described, initially based on the presence or absence of antigenic properties and now further characterized at the molecular level.

CLINICAL FINDINGS. The manifestations of Christmas disease are identical to those of hemophilia A, with the same musculoskeletal problems and the same complications from chronic transfusion therapy. Interestingly, although the incidence of HIV seropositivity is high in factor IX–deficient patients, it is somewhat less than in factor VIII–deficient patients. Nonetheless, this is a high-risk population, and all patients in it must be handled with appropriate precautions and receive counseling.

LABORATORY FINDINGS. The diagnosis of factor IX de-ficiency is straightforward. The PTT is prolonged, the PT and bleeding times are normal, and specific factor assays confirm the diagnosis. In the past, the variability in antigenic activity in different kindreds made carrier detection extremely difficult. The development of DNA probe analysis has now made carrier detection and prenatal diagnosis possible in the majority of kindreds.

COURSE AND MANAGEMENT. Principles of therapy for hemophilia B are basically the same as for hemophilia A. A variety of lyophilized blood products for factor IX replacement are available, and home therapy is the mainstay of patients with severe disease. In patients with a mild deficiency or newly diagnosed disease, fresh-frozen plasma is the blood product of choice. When calculating a transfusion regimen the physician must remember that the half-life of factor IX is longer than that of factor VIII, approximately 24 hours. DDAVP is not a useful alternative in these patients. An aggressive home therapy program with a comprehensive care center for support can afford these patients a nearly normal life-style.

OTHER INHERITED DISORDERS OF COAGULATION
Factor XI deficiency

Factor XI deficiency is an uncommon autosomal recessive disorder occurring most frequently in patients of Jewish ancestry. The bleeding disorder is quite mild and may be manifest only after surgical or dental procedures. Although heterozygotes may have factor XI levels as low as 10% to 20% of normal, this is not usually associated with bleeding. Treatment consists of replacement therapy with fresh-frozen plasma.

Factor XII deficiency

Factor XII deficiency is an inherited abnormality that can prolong the PTT but is not associated with a bleeding disorder. Similar findings occur in Fletcher factor (prekallikrein) and Fitzgerald factor (high-molecular-weight kininogen) deficiencies.

Factors V, VII, and X prothrombin deficiencies

Deficiencies of factors V, VII, and X and prothrombin are associated with mild to moderate bleeding disorders. Replacement therapy with fresh-frozen plasma is occasionally necessary. Rarely, prothrombin complex concentrate is needed.

Fibrinogen deficiency

Hypofibrinogenemias and a variety of inherited dysfibrinogenemias have been described. They can be associated with bleeding and may need treatment with cryoprecipitate. Severe hypofibrinogenemia is associated with a prolonged bleeding time, since normal platelet function requires at least small amounts of fibrinogen.

Factor XIII deficiency

Factor XIII effects cross-linking of fibrinogen and thus its stabilization. Factor XIII is not measured in coagulation screening, but a deficiency can cause a significant bleeding disorder. It is therefore important to think of factor XIII deficiency as a possibility when a patient has a suggestive history and to test for it specifically. Therapy consists of transfusion with small amounts of fresh-frozen plasma or cryoprecipitate.

ACQUIRED DISORDERS OF COAGULATION
Vitamin K deficiency

Vitamin K is a fat-soluble vitamin that is necessary for the γ-carboxylation of factors II, VII, IX, and X. Without the addition of carboxylic acid these coagulation factors cannot bind calcium and are functionally inert.

Malabsorption and liver disease are the most frequent causes of vitamin K deficiency if anticoagulation with vitamin K antagonists is excluded. Because it is a fat-soluble vitamin, such conditions as steatorrhea, celiac disease, or biliary obstruction greatly diminish its absorption.

Broad-spectrum antibiotic therapy can also result in vitamin K deficiency by eliminating intestinal flora that are normally a source of vitamin K_2. Postoperative patients who are receiving antibiotics and have diminished dietary intake are especially susceptible to vitamin K deficiency for this reason.

Insufficient dietary intake combined with immaturity of the hepatic mechanism for synthesis of vitamin K–dependent factors can result in a severe bleeding disorder in neonates.

The clinical manifestations of vitamin K deficiency can vary from mild bruising to life-threatening bleeding. The diagnosis should be suspected based on a prolonged PT and the appropriate clinical data. Occasionally the PTT is prolonged as well. The diagnosis is confirmed if the administration of vitamin K completely corrects the abnormality. Fortunately, the presence of inactive precursors of the affected factors means that replacement therapy results in prompt reversal of the condition. Vitamin K can be administered intramuscularly or intravenously depending on the urgency of the situation. Fresh-frozen plasma is indicated for immediate correction in the face of life-threatening bleeding.

Liver disease

The liver is the site of synthesis of the majority of coagulation factors, as well as the source of the carboxylase necessary for γ-carboxylation of vitamin K–dependent factors. In addition, activated coagulation factors and plasminogen activator are normally cleared from the circulation by the liver. Therefore it is not surprising that the coagulopathy of liver disease is usually multifactorial. Its severity generally correlates with the severity of the underlying liver disease, and it can be a management problem.

Hepatocellular disease results in decreased production of essentially all the coagulation factors except factor VIII, which as discussed previously is made primarily in the endothelial cells. Hypofibrinogenemia can result from decreased production or increased consumption in severe liver disease, but a characteristic dysfibrinogenemia is even more common. The decreased clearance of plasminogen activator can result in a fibrinolytic state, and the presence of activated factors can in severe cases result in disseminated intravascular coagulation (DIC). Thrombocytopenia can be the result of splenic sequestration or consumption, and platelet function abnormalities have been described.

Because of the variety of possible abnormalities, laboratory screening tests should include a platelet count, PT, PTT, and thrombin time. If DIC or significant fibrinolysis is suspected, fibrin split products may prove useful. The level of factor V (which is not a vitamin K–dependent factor) may also prove useful in differentiating the effects of vitamin K deficiency from those of parenchymal liver disease. The factor VIII concentration, which is not usually depressed in liver disease, may be a useful monitor of consumption.

Except for a trial of vitamin K, it is usually inappropriate to attempt therapy on the strength of abnormal laboratory tests alone. However, support during bleeding episodes or in anticipation of surgical procedures is necessary. Fresh-frozen plasma and platelets as needed provide the appropriate factors, but volume considerations are often limiting. Cryoprecipitate can provide significant amounts of fibrinogen in a small volume but is of no advantage for other factors. Use of prothrombin complex concentrates is generally ill advised because activated factors in these preparations are not cleared and DIC may be induced. Some clinicians believe that this risk is justified in desperate situations.

Acquired anticoagulants

Acquired inhibitors of coagulation, although rare, can present challenging management problems. These anticoagulants are actually immunoglobulins with antibody activity against one or more coagulation factors. Most common are those directed against factor VIII, which result in a bleeding disorder of variable severity. The condition can occur in a variety of circumstances including autoimmune disease, post partum, after penicillin administration, and in otherwise well individuals, especially the elderly.

The diagnosis is suggested when a prolonged PTT is not corrected by the addition of normal plasma. Specific factor assays may then define the antibody specificity.

Treatment depends in part on the clinical presentation. Acute, life-threatening bleeding may require transfusion; depending on the titer of antibody, overwhelming it may be possible, or prothrombin complex concentrates may be required. Ultimately, therapy aimed at decreasing the antibody is desirable but not uniformly successful. Treatment with steroids, cyclophosphamide, or other immunosuppressants may be useful. Spontaneous remissions also occur.

One relatively common antibody of particular interest is the lupus anticoagulant. This antibody is not directed against coagulation factors but prolongs the PTT and sometimes the PT by virtue of its activity against phospholipids, especially cardiolipin. It is usually detected on a routine coagulation screen and is generally not associated with a bleeding disorder. In fact, patients with the lupus anticoagulant are more likely to have thrombotic events. Recurrent spontaneous abortion is another clinical problem associated with this anticoagulant.

Although the lupus anticoagulant can be seen in systemic lupus erythematosus (SLE), it may be the only evidence of autoimmune phenomena in a given patient. It is important to remember that prolongation of the PTT in patients with SLE can also be due to anticoagulants with factor specificity and a resultant bleeding disorder. Therefore a thorough laboratory investigation is always important in these patients. Therapy with steroids is often useful.

Disseminated intravascular coagulation

DIC is an acquired consumptive coagulopathy that results from pathologic activation of the coagulation system. It is invariably the consequence of an underlying disease process and should always be evaluated in the context of that disease.

A wide spectrum of disease has been associated with DIC, and various pathogenic mechanisms have been postulated for the different causative disorders. Overwhelming infection, usually with a gram-negative organism, is probably the most common pathogenesis of the acute, fulminant form of DIC in the United States. Activation of the coagulation system in infection is usually attributed to endotoxins, but even viral illness can be associated with DIC, with endothelial cell damage as the postulated mechanism.

Activation of platelets by antigen-antibody complexes may play a role in initiating consumption in hemolytic transfusion reactions, autoimmune phenomena, or graft rejection. Release of proteolytic enzymes in malignant diseases such as promyelocytic leukemia is another mechanism. Damage to tissues rich in thromboplastin probably activates the coagulation system in obstetric conditions such as abruptio placentae, amniotic fluid embolism, or preeclampsia. Snake venoms act as direct activators at various points in the coagulation cascade, a fact that is exploited in certain laboratory tests. In some parts of the world, snake bite is a common cause of DIC.

Whatever the precipitating cause, the result of the initial activation of platelets is intravascular deposition of fibrin. Mechanical damage to red blood cells as a result of fibrin strands leads to microangiopathic hemolytic anemia, and secondary fibrinolysis is stimulated. Platelets and coagulation factors are consumed in the process. Organ damage as a result of fibrin thrombi can occur anywhere, but the most common sites are the kidneys, gastrointestinal (GI) tract, and central nervous system (CNS). The dominant clinical manifestation, however, is the bleeding diathesis, which results from the consumption of platelets and coagulation factors, fibrinolysis, and the anticoagulant properties of some of the fibrin degradation products themselves.

Typically a seriously ill patient with sepsis or an obstetric patient suddenly has oozing from venipuncture sites and mucous membranes. Spontaneous GI bleeding or CNS symptoms may occur. The spectrum of clinical presentations is wide, and the manifestations in some cases may be so mild that the laboratory abnormalities are more striking than the clinical manifestations.

A chronic form of DIC, usually the result of malignancy or vascular disorders, is often associated with a milder bleeding tendency. When the tempo of the disease is slower, consumption can be compensated to some degree and the bleeding disorder is proportionately less severe. A localized site of consumption, such as a dissecting aortic aneurysm, giant cavernous hemangioma, or renal allograft can also result in this picture.

The diagnosis is based on the combination of laboratory abnormalities and the clinical setting. Depending on the rate of consumption, some or all of the parameters may be abnormal. Examination of the peripheral blood smear for evidence of microangiopathic changes is critical. Platelet count, PT, PTT, and thrombin time may all be affected and should be evaluated. Thrombin time and quantitative fibrinogen assay are also helpful and may be used in monitoring the success of replacement therapy. The demonstration of fibrin degradation products is critical. Specific factor assays, especially factors V and VIII, may prove helpful in differentiating consumption from other contributing factors such as vitamin K deficiency or liver disease in a patient with numerous, simultaneous disease processes.

The definitive treatment of DIC is elimination of the underlying cause. Replacement therapy in the form of platelet concentrates, fresh-frozen plasma, or even cryoprecipitate may be necessary to support the patient during treatment of the underlying process. Heparin, frequently used in the past to interrupt the consumption cycle, is now rarely thought necessary and may actually contribute to bleeding in some cases.

Occasional patients with chronic DIC may benefit from heparin, however, and it may also be necessary in patients in whom the thrombotic manifestations predominate. Patients with promyelocytic leukemia are commonly treated with heparin as prophylaxis, since DIC often develops with the onset of cell lysis shortly after chemotherapy is begun. The necessity for heparin even in these patients is now being questioned.

ANTICOAGULANT THERAPY

HEPARIN. Heparin is an organic acid derived from porcine intestine or bovine lung. It is a powerful anticoagulant that inhibits the effect of thrombin and activated factors IX, X, and XII. It does so by binding to and enhancing the effect of naturally occurring inhibitors of coagulation, primarily antithrombin III (ATIII). The effect of heparin is best measured with the activated partial thromboplastin time, which tests the intrinsic and common pathways. Given intravenously, heparin is immediately effective, and its effect is readily reversible by the use of protamine sulfate. It is therefore an ideal agent when immediate anticoagulation is necessary or when immediate termination of anticoagulation is important, as in hemodialysis.

The principal use of heparin is for the treatment and prevention of thromboembolic disease. The usual regimen for established thrombosis is an intravenous bolus followed by a continuous infusion sufficient to keep the PTT at 1½ times normal. Therapy is usually continued for 7 to 10 days, after which the patient is switched to oral anticoagulants. Smaller doses given subcutaneously are adequate for prophylactic treatment in certain surgical and bedridden patients. Significant resistance to anticoagulation with heparin should alert the clinician to the possibility of ATIII deficiency.

The use of frequent heparin flushes of peripheral and central catheters can occasionally result in significant anticoagulation. It is important to be alert to this possibility in a hospitalized patient with a complicated disease picture. The thrombin time is sensitive to the effects of heparin and may prove revealing in this situation.

The major adverse effect of heparin therapy is untoward bleeding. Administration by continuous infusion avoids wide swings in anticoagulant effect and therefore reduces the likelihood of excessive anticoagulation, but bleeding can occur even in appropriately controlled patients. Heparin occasionally induces significant thrombocytopenia, which can augment the bleeding problem. This is not an infrequent complication, and platelet counts must be monitored closely. Heparin also can induce platelet function abnormalities, which can contribute to the likelihood of bleeding. Newer preparations of heparin that may dissociate the antithrombotic from the untoward effects are being investigated. Long-term administration of heparin has been associated with bone demineralization.

COUMARIN DRUGS. The coumarin anticoagulants (warfarin, dicumarol) are vitamin K antagonists that act by interfering with γ-carboxylation of vitamin K–dependent factors. The result is the production of essentially nonfunctional factors II, VII, IX, and X. This effect is most readily measured by PT.

Unlike heparin's effects, those of the coumarins are not immediate and depend on the half-life of the factors in the circulation when the drug is administered. Since factor VII has the shortest half-life of the vitamin K–dependent factors, it is the first to be functionally depressed. This may prolong the PT, but adequate anticoagulation is not achieved until all the factors are depressed, usually after 3 to 4 days. The daily dose is then adjusted to maintain the PT at 2 to 2½ times control.

The major use of the coumarins is long-term oral anticoagulation as treatment or prophylaxis for thromboembolic disease. Patients treated initially with heparin must continue to receive it for the 3 to 4 days needed for coumarin to be effective. Therapy is then usually continued for 4 to 6 months or longer, depending on the indication. The PT should be monitored at regular intervals, and both physician and patient should be aware of the potential for concomitant medications or conditions to alter the drug's effect. For example, oral antibiotics may interfere with vitamin K absorption, thus potentiating the effect. Similarly, cholestyramine and other bile salt binders may decrease absorption. Barbiturates may accelerate drug metabolism, and chloral hydrate and diazoxide displace the drug from its plasma protein binding sites, potentiating its effects. Even seemingly innocuous over-the-counter drugs such as acetaminophen have been implicated. Use of aspirin and other platelet function inhibitors should also be avoided during systemic anticoagulation.

The major untoward effect of coumarin is bleeding. The effects of the drug decline gradually after it is withdrawn as active factors are produced. The effect can be reversed by the oral, intramuscular, or intravenous administration of vitamin K. In more urgent situations, transfusion with fresh-frozen plasma may be required. Coumarins cross the placenta, and a high incidence of abortion is associated with these agents when they are used in the difficult situation of thrombophelbitis in pregnancy; alternative treatment should therefore be considered.

A rare complication of coumarins can occur when the drug is given to patients who are deficient in the naturally occurring anticoagulant protein C. This and its cofactor protein S are both also vitamin K–dependent factors, and a deficiency of either results in a lifelong tendency to thrombus formation. Vitamin K antagonists may actually initially make the deficiency worse, and rather than an anticoagulant effect, a paradoxic thrombotic effect occurs. Coumarin necrosis is the dermatologic manifestation of this. It is a characteristic skin lesion, usually on the lower extremities or abdominal wall, that progresses to a full-thickness skin necrosis. Such an event should alert the clinician to the possibility of protein C deficiency.

Surreptitious coumarin ingestion occasionally occurs and should be considered when vitamin K deficiency seems to be the explanation of a mysterious acquired bleeding disorder, especially in medical personnel or persons with access to the drug.

THROMBOLYTIC THERAPY. Whereas the goal of systemic anticoagulation is to inhibit the propagation of an established thrombus, the goal of thrombolytic therapy is to dissolve such a thrombus. The currently available thrombolytic agents are streptokinase and urokinase. Both work by activating the normal fibrinolytic mechanism. Urokinase is an enzyme that directly converts plasminogen to plasmin. Streptokinase acts by forming a complex with plasminogen. This complex converts uncomplexed plasminogen to plasmin, the serine protease that degrades fibrin in the normal fibrinolytic mechanism.

Patients selected for thrombolytic therapy should have well-documented thrombotic or thromboembolic disease of recent onset, usually less than 7 days. Absolute contraindications include active internal bleeding and severe cerebrovascular disease. Relative contraindications include major surgery or trauma within 10 days, severe hypertension, coagulopathy, and pregnancy.

The usual regimen for administering either agent is to give a loading dose followed by a continuous infusion for 24 hours in pulmonary embolus and up to 72 hours in deep venous thrombosis. This is followed by continuous-infusion heparin therapy for 5 to 10 days and then oral anticoagulants.

Unlike anticoagulant therapy, thrombolytic therapy is not titrated based on laboratory tests. A coagulation screen before therapy is advisable to exclude a coagulopathy. Three to 4 hours after beginning therapy the establishment of a lytic state is documented by a thrombin time or euglobulin lysis time. The degree to which these studies are affected does not alter therapy as long as it is clear that fibrinolysis is occurring. This is especially important for streptokinase therapy because the presence of preexisting streptococcal antibodies might neutralize the effect of the streptokinase.

Bleeding is the most frequent complication of thrombolytic therapy. Although it is usually in the form of oozing at the sites of venipuncture or invasive procedures, a small but significant incidence of intracranial bleeding does occur, often with catastrophic consequences. Discontinuation of the drug rapidly diminishes its lytic effect, but fresh-frozen plasma or cryoprecipitate can be used in more urgent situations. ε-Aminocaproic acid also reverses the effect but is rarely necessary.

Other adverse reactions include fever and allergic reactions, especially in patients treated with streptokinase.

Recombinant DNA technology has recently resulted in the availability of tissue plasminogen activator (TPA) for investigational purposes. TPA has the significant advantage of being fibrin specific. It binds to plasminogen, which is bound to fibrin, and the result is a lytic effect at the site of the clot but no significant activation of circulating plasminogen. Therefore a generalized fibrinolytic state does not occur, and the likelihood of bleeding should be less. The majority of trials have been in patients with myocardial infarction, but wider application is anticipated.

Thrombolytic therapy is generally underused. Encouraging data have shown that thrombolytic therapy results in more rapid normalization of diffusion capacity after pulmonary embolus than when heparin is used. Also, the incidence of postthrombotic syndrome is decreased when thrombolytic therapy is used. Therefore thrombolytic therapy should be considered for carefully selected patients. TPA or other fibrin-specific thrombolytic agents under investigation may prove to be safe and effective alternatives in the foreseeable future.

BIBLIOGRAPHY
Inherited disorders of coagulation

Hoyer LW: The factor VIII complex: structure and function, Blood 58:1, 1981.

Hoyer LW and others: Von Willebrand factor multimer patterns in von Willebrand's disease, Br J Haematol 55:493, 1983.

Richardson DW and Robinson AG: Desmopressin, Ann Intern Med 103:228, 1985.

Acquired disorders of coagulation

Prentice CRM: Acquired coagulation disorders, Clin Haematol 14:413, 1985.

Shapiro SS: Disorders of hemostasis—acquired disorders of blood coagulation. In Williams WJ and others, editors: Hematology, ed 3, New York, 1983, McGraw-Hill Inc.

Anticoagulant therapy

Verstraete M and Collen D: Thrombolytic therapy in the eighties, Blood 67:1529, 1986.

Wessler S and Gitel SN: Warfarin, from bedside to bench, N Engl J Med 311:645, 1984.

Williams WJ: Thrombosis. In Williams WJ and others, editors: Hematology, ed 3, New York, 1983, McGraw-Hill Inc.

Dental correlations

ANEMIAS AND DEFICIENCY STATES
Pernicious anemia
S. Gary Cohen *and* **Michael Glick**

The onset of pernicious anemia (PA) is usually insidious and progressive. The diverse clinical presentation results in an average period of almost 1½ years between onset of symptoms and the correct diagnosis.

ORAL MANIFESTATIONS. The mucosa may appear pale or icteric. Erythematous macules with irregular borders involving any of the mucosal surfaces may be an early sign of pernicious anemia. The tongue undergoes atrophic or fissural changes in 50% to 60% of these patients. Atrophy of the filiform and later fungiform papillae imparts the classic "beefy red" appearance to the tongue. Lingual paresthesia, burning, or itching may develop but resolve with therapy. Distortions in taste may accompany the thinned epithelium. Increased susceptibility to irritation and trauma results from the oral epithelium becoming parakeratinized or nonkeratinized.

In long-standing, undiagnosed cases, ulcers appear in areas of severe atrophy. These lesions cause significant discomfort, particularly when a patient wears a dental prosthesis. The dentist may be the first clinician to examine the patient and should remember to rule out pernicious anemia in cases of nonspecific stomatitis. If lesions appear in a patient with known pernicious anemia, the practitioner should suspect relapse secondary to cessation of vitamin B_{12} therapy. Megaloblastic anemia, including the oral symptoms, can also occur as a consequence of gastric bypass surgery. This causes the impaired absorption of vitamin B_{12}. The symptoms may be delayed significantly because of adequate body stores of vitamin B_{12}. Therefore the key to diagnosis lies in a thorough medical history and confirmation by the use of blood tests, including complete blood cell and differential cell counts, serum iron level, total iron binding capacity, measurements of specific vitamin levels, and the Schilling test.

DENTAL MANAGEMENT. The oral lesions heal rapidly when vitamin B_{12} therapy is initiated. There are no contraindications to dental treatment in a patient taking vitamin B_{12} for pernicious anemia. However, patients who have vitamin B_{12} deficiency should not be given nitrous oxide analgesia because it has been shown to interfere with vitamin B_{12} metabolism and may precipitate moderate to severe neuropathy.

Folic acid deficiency
S. Gary Cohen *and* **Michael Glick**

The clinical presentation of a folic acid deficiency is similar to vitamin B_{12} deficiency except that central nervous system symptoms are rare. Individuals with an increased incidence of folic acid deficiency anemia include alcoholics, hemodialysis patients (folic acid is dialyzable), patients taking phenytoin (Dilantin) or oral contraceptives, and those being treated with folic acid inhibitors such as methotrexate.

ORAL MANIFESTATIONS. The most common presentation is a red, sore tongue with varying degrees of papillary atrophy, which progresses until the tongue is smooth and shiny. Angular cheilitis is seen and often becomes secondarily infected with bacteria and fungi. Candidal infections of the mouth and at times the entire gastrointestinal tract can be found. In some cases ulcerative stomatitis is present.

On histologic examination the epithelium shows an increased nuclear size similar to that seen in vitamin B_{12} deficiency. The cells of the prickle and granular layers of the oral epithelium are enlarged and ballooning. The cytoplasm is lightly stained, and nuclear chromatin is clumped in a manner similar to the megaloblastic changes noted in pernicious anemia. Decreased keratinization and extensive shallow ulcerations are also described.

Glossitis may be a symptom of both folic acid deficiency and pernicious anemia. In both disorders the pain disappears as soon as 48 hours after appropriate therapy. If pernicious anemia is inadvertently treated with pharmacologic doses of folic acid, the macrocytic anemia may temporarily be corrected but the neurologic degeneration progresses.

Congenital hypoplastic anemia (Diamond-Blackfan anemia)
S. Gary Cohen *and* **Michael Glick**

ORAL MANIFESTATIONS. Diamond-Blackfan anemia has been associated with severe gingivitis, multiple carious lesions, and poor healing of recent extraction sites. An unexplained radiographic finding of nearly total obliteration of the coronal pulp chambers of the erupted dentition, with the teeth having normal color and crown morphology and no excessive attrition, has been reported.

DENTAL MANAGEMENT. Medically management includes either corticosteroids or transfusions. Adrenal insufficiency should be considered. Human immunodeficiency virus (HIV) and hepatitis precautions should be instituted.

Aplastic anemia
S. Gary Cohen *and* **Michael Glick**

The clinical picture of aplastic anemia combines the signs and symptoms of severe anemia with those of neutropenia and thrombocytopenia. These patients may have the mucosal pallor of anemia, but glossitis, glossopyrosis, and papillary atrophy are rare.

One cause of aplastic anemia is the injudicious use of chloromycetin. This antibiotic should be prescribed only when other antibiotics are ineffective.

ORAL MANIFESTATIONS. The purpura and spontaneous gingival bleeding of thrombocytopenia may be seen in aplastic anemia. These patients are often advised by the dentist to discontinue oral hygiene measures to prevent gingival bleeding, but the accumulation of plaque can intensify gingival ulceration and bleeding. Some oral hygiene measures should be taken to prevent this additional problem.

A severe ulcerative stomatitis or pharyngitis is common in all neutropenic patients. These ulcers are necrotic and foul smelling and may reach several centimeters in diameter. Because of the lack of neutrophils, purulence is absent. Another manifestation is cervical and submandibular lymphadenopathy.

DENTAL MANAGEMENT. A thorough dental evaluation reveals any source of chronic or potential infection. The elimination of the source improves the long-term prognosis by decreasing the incidence of septicemia during the neutropenic state (less than 500 cells/mm³). In chronic or recurrent cases proper patient management should include an oral hygiene program. Patients should use a soft toothbrush, further softened by hot water and dental tape, which causes less gingival trauma than floss. This technique has been effective in treating patients even with platelet counts less than 10,000/mm³. Gingival ulceration and bleeding may be reduced by decreasing plaque accumulation. This results in fewer transfusions and a decreased potential for septicemia.

If emergency dental treatment is necessary during periods

of severe bone marrow suppression, use of platelet and neutrophil transfusions should be discussed with the hematologist.

The associated ulcerative stomatitis can be severe enough to prevent eating, drinking, and swallowing medication. The management is usually palliative. Good oral hygiene must be maintained, and saline and sodium bicarbonate mouth rinses are recommended to cleanse the surfaces of the ulcers. Use of topical anesthetics improves comfort during eating. Diphenhydramine (Benadryl) and 0.5% dyclonine (Dyclone) mixed with kaolin/pectin or milk of magnesia has been effective for this purpose.

Antibacterial agents can be used on the ulcers to reduce secondary infection. Use of a vacuformed splint to hold topical medications is recommended. The splint is lined with a 10% neomycin and 1% bacitracin ointment. After the patient wears the splint for 2 hours, it is removed and rinsed and a nystatin (Mycostatin) ointment (10,000 units/g) is applied for the next 2 hours. These alternating medications are used until improvement is noticed. Aqueous chlorhexidine (0.12%) solution (Peridet) is also used with good results.

Partial or full dentures should be removed to reduce the chance of ulcers caused by friction. When not in use, dentures should be soaked in a nystatin solution (10 ml of a 500,000 units/ml solution in 6 oz water). Orthodontic appliances should be removed because they hamper oral hygiene and can be a source of irritation.

The most serious complication of dental treatment for neutropenic patients is life-threatening infection. Only necessary dental procedures should be performed. If the neutrophil count is less than 2500 cells/mm^3, the patient should receive prophylactic parenteral, broad-spectrum antibiotic coverage. If oral infection develops, surface specimens of the infected tissue should be submitted for culture and sensitivity testing. While awaiting the results the patient should begin receiving a broad-spectrum antibiotic or combination of antibiotics.

Another consideration is bleeding secondary to a decreased platelet count. To ensure adequate clotting, a bleeding profile, including a platelet count, should be obtained before any dental treatment. If the platelet count is less than 50,000/mm^3, posterosuperior and inferoalveolar block injections are dangerous because of the potential for hematoma formation and therefore should be avoided (see section on dental management in thrombocytopenia).

Medical management often includes transfusions and steroids and must be considered during dental treatment. Viral hepatitis is a potential hazard with blood transfusions. Therefore sterilization precautions should be taken (see section on hepatitis). The acquisition of HIV can be another consequence of frequent blood transfusions. Corticosteroid therapy at adrenosuppressive levels increases susceptibility to shock (see chapter on "The adrenal cortex").

Specific dental treatment is limited to infection control and palliation until the patient's blood cell counts improve. If an acute infection develops and extraction is necessary, a bleeding profile should be obtained. In addition, a culture and sensitivity test of the areas to be treated is necessary to determine whether unusual oral organisms are present. If the patient is thrombocytopenic, platelet transfusions may be indicated.

Iron deficiency anemia
S. Gary Cohen *and* Michael Glick

The clinical manifestations of iron deficiency anemia generally appear in relatively severe disease and may be discovered during a routine history and examination by a dentist. The signs and symptoms include pallor of the skin and nail beds, progressive fingernail concavity resulting in a spooning effect (koilonychia), a tendency of the nails to crack and split, fatigue, anorexia, headache, and neurologic disturbances. The patient may crave unusual or toxic substances such as paint, starches, or ice.

ORAL MANIFESTATIONS. Gingival and mucosal pallor may be evident along with atrophy of the lingual papillae. Atrophy of the filiform and fungiform papillae continues until the dorsal surface of the tongue becomes totally smooth and its color changes from pale pink to red. The tip and lateral borders are usually affected first, resulting in a patchy effect that may be confused with geographic tongue. However, unlike geographic tongue, these atrophic areas lack a white keratotic border and undergo a progressive increase in size rather than an alteration in distribution. All of these changes cause an increased susceptibility to irritation and traumatic ulceration. Symptoms of soreness and burning may result. Angular cheilitis or leukoplakia gradually develops in some cases. The buccal epithelium is significantly thinner than normal. The reduced thickness is due to a decrease in the thickness of the maturation compartment. Iron deficiency has been implicated as a cause of recurrent aphthous stomatitis. It has been suggested that the oral lesions are caused by a concurrent pyridoxine deficiency rather than the anemia. Salivary flow rates have been shown to be decreased in patients with iron deficiency when compared with normal subjects.

DENTAL MANAGEMENT. Wound healing may be prolonged, leading to delayed healing after tooth extraction or other oral surgical procedures. Elective dental procedures should not be performed until the hemoglobin level is more than 10 g/dl.

Treatment of iron deficiency anemia may include the use of liquid ferrous sulfate, which causes black stains of the teeth and tongue. This can be minimized by drinking the solution through a straw and rinsing the mouth after each dose.

Plummer-Vinson syndrome
S. Gary Cohen *and* Michael Glick

Plummer-Vinson syndrome (sideropenic dysphagia) is associated with stomatitis, pharyngoesophageal ulcerations, and dysphagia in addition to symptoms of severe anemia. It occurs almost exclusively in middle-aged women. Nail abnormalities in chronic disease include spooning, atrophy of the entire nail bed, and complete loss of the nail. The patient's facial expression and contraction of the lips of often create an appearance of primness or displeasure.

ORAL MANIFESTATIONS. Oral manifestations are similar to those of iron deficiency anemia, atrophic glossitis, angular cheilitis, and dysphagia. Xerostomia may also be present. Leukoplakia of the tongue is common, and biopsy shows dysplastic changes. Since the incidence of pharyngeal and oral squamous cell carcinoma is increased, biopsy of all suspicious lesions must be performed.

DENTAL MANAGEMENT. Patients being treated for Plummer-Vinson syndrome may undergo routine dental treatment as long as the hemoglobin levels are more than 10 g/dl. There has been a reported increased risk of infection associated with profound disturbances of iron metabolism. Also, as with all iron deficiency anemias, there may be delayed healing or poor tissue response after surgical procedures. Therefore these patients should be monitored closely after surgical procedures and maintained on a regular recall basis.

Sickle cell anemia

S. Gary Cohen *and* Michael Glick

The oral manifestations of sickle cell anemia are nonspecific. The most common signs are mucosal pallor caused by chronic anemia and jaundice caused by hemolysis.

Radiographic changes in the jaw occur in 79% to 100% of patients, in all age-groups, and in both the mandible and the maxillae. It has been suggested that dental radiographs show bony changes more dramatically than do other bone surveys because of the direct juxtaposition of the film to the bone, which results in finer detail and sharpness.

The bony abnormalities appear on radiographs as decreased radiodensity with a coarse trabecular pattern. These findings are attributed to erythroblastic hyperplasia and medullary hypertrophy with resultant loss of fine trabeculae and increased marrow spaces. This is most commonly visible as radiolucent areas between the apices of the teeth and the inferior border of the mandible. Another presentation, described as "stepladder" because of the characteristic horizontal trabecular arrangement, is most obvious when it occurs in the mandible between the root apices and the alveolar ridge. Some other changes attributed to bone marrow hyperplasia include thinning of the inferior border of the mandible, loss of the cortical layer along the alveolar ridge, interdental cuffing of interproximal bone, loss of alveolar bone height (especially in children under 10 years of age), and pronounced lamina dura.

The bony changes are classified into four groups: (1) bone marrow hyperplasia causing osteoporosis, loss of trabeculation, and cortical thinning; (2) thrombosis and infarction producing osteosclerosis; (3) changes subsequent to an infectious process where the bone shows areas of osteoporosis and erosion followed by osteosclerosis; and (4) generalized decreased bone growth caused by hypoxic effects on the growth centers.

These changes should not be considered definitive diagnostic criteria for sickle cell anemia. Similar changes occur in normal individuals, as well as in patients with other systemic disorders such as thalassemia, estrogen imbalance, hyperparathyroidism, Paget's disease, and metabolic bone disease. The diagnosis is made with a blood test utilizing a sickle cell preparation and hemoglobin electrophoresis.

Osteomyelitis of the jaws occurs with increased frequency in patients with sickle cell disease. The inherent vascular abnormalities cause vascular thrombosis and infarction, predisposing the patient to infection.

Multiple cases of osteomyelitis in the mandible of sickle cell patients have been reported in the literature. Long-standing infections secondary to carious teeth, periodontal disease, and sickle cell infarcts are considered to be causative agents. Since the initial manifestations of vascular infarction and osteomyelitis are similar, only clinical, laboratory, and histologic data can distinguish between the two.

Mental nerve neuropathy is another significant oral manifestation of sickle cell disease. Onset of this symptom is usually preceded by severe pain in the mandible. In several reports, pain in the mandible and lip paresthesia were associated with a sickle cell crisis. Mental nerve paresthesia is thought to be secondary to a vasoocclusive episode involving the inferior alveolar nerve at or near the mental foramen. Recovery of sensation may be slow, with the paresthesia lasting as long as 18 months.

The results of a cephalometric study noted that patients with sickle cell anemia had an increased angulation of the lower border of the mandible with a tendency toward mandibular retrusion. This may be attributed to the generalized bone growth retardation found in these patients.

Hypomineralization of the dentin and enamel and enamel staining occasionally occur. Thrombus formation resulting in an inadequate supply to the developing enamel organ is thought to be responsible for these changes.

Other head findings include spontaneous hematomas of unknown cause, headaches, and cranial nerve palsies secondary to cerebral thrombosis.

DENTAL MANAGEMENT. Preventive dental care is important, since oral infection may precipitate a sickle cell or aplastic crisis. Dental counseling should begin at an early age and be maintained throughout life. Preventive therapy includes fluoride application and frequent prophylaxis to prevent caries and periodontal disease.

Once detected, infections must be vigorously treated to prevent an extensive facial cellulitis. The infected area should be carefully debrided, culture and sensitivity tests performed, and the patient given appropriate antibiotic therapy. Attentive monitoring after the infection is required. Cellulitis may warrant hospitalization to administer high levels of intravenous antibiotics and provide close observation. Endodontics or extraction of the offending teeth should be accomplished. If a patient with sickle cell anemia has fever of unknown origin, a dental evaluation to rule out a possible dental etiology is recommended.

Routine dental treatment in a noncrisis period may be readily performed, but during a crisis therapy should be directed to palliation To drecrease the potential for transient septicemia secondary to dental treatment, which might seed necrotic infarcted tissue and cause osteomyelitis, prophylactic antibiotics should be used. A broad-spectrum antibiotic such as ampicillin should be used in a manner similar to the American Heart Association protocol before dental treatment. Elective oral surgical procedures should not be considered in these patients. However, extensive oral surgical procedures, including orthognathic surgery can be performed on patients with sickle cell trait. For teatment under general anesthesia, hemoglobin levels should be 7 to 10 mg/dl in adults and 10 to 12 mg/dl in children. Packed erythrocyte transfusions may be administered to obtain an acceptable hemoglobin level. Prophylactic broad-spectrum antibiotic coverage is suggested to minimize the incidence of postoperative wound infection.

If ataractic premedication is required, a non–respiratory depressant drug is recommended to minimize the possibility of potentiating a crisis. To prevent acidosis caused by suppression of central respiratory centers, barbiturates and narcotics should be avoided. High doses of salicylates impose an acid load and therefore should not be used. It is advisable to make morning appointments and to minimize the time for each sitting.

Local anesthesia with vasoconstrictors is a controversial issue. Some clinicians claim that vasoconstrictors may impair circulation locally to cause infarction, whereas others maintain that vasoconstriction has no effect on the local circulation despite the underlying hypovascularization.

The use of nitrous oxide–oxygen analgesia is another controversial issue. Hypoxia should be avoided with nitrous oxide–oxygen analgesia. A 50% oxygen concentration, high flow rate, and adequate ventilation should allow an adequate safety margin, but it has been proposed that the change in oxygen concentration may initiate sickle crisis.

General anesthetic techniques for patients with sickle cell anemia have been evaluated by many. The technical ability of the anesthesiologist is more important than the choice of anesthetic. Anesthetization of a patient with sickle cell anemia should be performed only in a hospital by a fully trained anesthesiologist.

The oral manifestations and dental management of the other hemoglobinopathies are similar to those described for sickle cell anemia.

Hemolytic disease of the newborn (erythroblastosis fetalis)
S. Gary Cohen and **Michael Glick**

A patient with hemolytic disease of the newborn (HDN) has discolorations of the crowns of all deciduous teeth that were developing during the period of severe hemolysis. The discoloration may appear yellow, green, blue-green, tan, deep gray, and even blue. It is caused by the bile pigments deposited in the enamel and dentin of the developing teeth. The color usually fades with time. Enamel hypoplasia has also been reported in association with HDN. When kernicterus follows hemolytic disease, enamel hypoplasia is present in 58% to 100% of cases reported. The lesion is most commonly in the enamel and corresponds to the 4½- to 7-month intrauterine period. The hypoplasia can be seen on radiographic examination before tooth eruption.

Since only the deciduous teeth are affected and these exfoliate, no modifications in dental treatment are needed.

Cold hemagglutinin disease
S. Gary Cohen and **Michael Glick**

Cold hemagglutinin disease is a form of autoimmune hemolytic anemia. Clinical manifestations occur only on exposure to cold. Mucosal purpura and mucosal changes that are associated with the hemolytic anemia may become evident during exacerbations of this disorder. When treating a patient with cold hemagglutinin disease, the practitioner must maintain the ambient temperature above the maximum at which the cold agglutinin reacts; this is known as the thermal amplitude. The extremities in particular should not be exposed to cold. If intravenous fluids are used for sedation, they should be warmed before administration.

Enzyme deficiency anemias
S. Gary Cohen and **Michael Glick**

The only reported manifestations of the Embden-Meyerhof pathway were reported in a case of hexokinase deficiency anemia. The teeth were narrow in the buccolingual dimension and had an abnormally large number of grooves and fissures. The central incisors were screwdriver shaped, with the incisal width narrower than the gingival width. This is similar to patients with thalassemia. Both disorders are caused by the hemolytic process occurring during enamel formation. Other oral signs that may be evident are pallor and jaundice of the mucosa.

Glucose 6-phosphate dehydrogenase deficiency
S. Gary Cohen and **Michael Glick**

Patients with glucose 6-phosphate dehydrogenase (G6PD) deficiency have no reported oral manifestations except for the pallor and jaundiced mucosa that occurs during a hemolytic episode. Such episodes can be triggered by dental infection, so prevention should be given a high priority. If infection does occur, vigorous treatment is indicated.

Drug sensitivity can also lead to hemolytic episodes. Sulfonamides and phenacetin have been implicated and therefore should be avoided.

The local anesthetic agent prilocaine (Citanet) in high doses (7 to 8 mg/kg) can induce life-threatening toxic methemoglobinemia. It is claimed that methemoglobin is not efficiently reduced in G6PD, but the evidence suggests that, when administered in normal doses (2 to 3 mg/kg), prilocaine is unlikely to result in methemoglobinemia.

Thalessemia
S. Gary Cohen and **Michael Glick**

The clinical manifestations of all thalessemias are associated with the reactive extramedullary hemopoietic nature of the disease and are more pronounced than in the hemolytic anemia of sickle cell disease. Unlike sickle cell anemia, painful crises do not occur, but bone pain has been reported at low hemoglobin concentrations secondary to marrow hyperplasia. These patients are usually small for their age and have typical facies (Cooley's facies), including separation of the eyes, depression of the bridge of the nose, high bulging cheeks, prominent frontal and parietal bones, and puffy eyes. The degree of cephalofacial deformities is closely related to the severity of the disease and the timing of therapy.

ORAL MANIFESTATIONS. Hypertrophy and remodeling of the maxilla often result in malocclusion. A severe overbite with either protruded and spaced or prominent but crowded maxillary anterior teeth may develop. The posterior segment may be buccally displaced with a concomitant expansion of the alveolar process.

The teeth occasionally show morphologic changes including reduced buccolingual diameters, diminutive premolars and second molars, and increased numbers of grooves, pits, and fissures. The enamel and dentin contain a higher iron concentration, which is related to the number of blood transfusions each year. Iron overload owing to an intensive blood transfusion regimen can cause a sicca syndrome, as well as pain and swelling of the parotid gland resulting from iron deposits in the serous glands.

Glossodynia and loss of papillae of the tongue, similar to those occurring in iron deficiency anemia and folic acid deficiency, are common complications of thalassemia minor.

The dental radiographic findings are similar to those in sickle cell disease. Osteoporosis, a widening of the trabecular spaces, or generalized rarefactions with a "honeycombed" trabecular appearance may be seen. Occasionally, circular radiolucencies at the root apex are mistaken for a pathologic lesion. Remaining trabeculae in rarefied areas appear prominent and have been referred to as compensatory lamellar striations. Also, the lamina dura may appear thin. These radiographic changes are caused by the persistent overgrowth of erythrocyte-forming marrow, which results in enlargements of the medullary cavities and thinning of the overlying cortex. Periosteal reactions and focal areas of ischemic necrosis do not occur with any frequency in thalassemia. The skull may show a notable cortical thickening and an unusual sunburst or "hair-on-end" appearance of the trabeculae at the cortex. Obliteration of the paranasal sinuses may occur as a result of the marrow hyperplasia, with only the ethmoid sinuses being spared.

DENTAL MANAGEMENT. Patients with β-thalassemia major require a recent complete blood count, including hemoglobin and hematocrit determinations, before any dental treatment. Only palliative care should be attempted if the hemoglobin level is less than 10 mg/dl. All routine dental treatment should be accomplished soon after regularly scheduled transfusions while all infection control precautions are observed. These patients are more susceptible to infection, and some clinicians advise prophylactic antibiotic coverage before dental treatment. This issue is controversial and should be discussed with the hematologist. A thorough dental evaluation is necessary to rule out an oral source of infection in any fever of unknown origin. Other considerations include increased risk of infection in thalassemic patients who have undergone splenectomy. It has been suggested that these patients receive prophylactic antibiotics, using the American Heart Association protocol, before dental treatment. Also, patients with thalessemia are at increased risk of human immunodeficiency virus and hepatitis because of the number of blood transfusions they receive. Therefore appropriate precautions should be taken when treating them.

Care should be exercised during surgical procedures to prevent pathologic fractures caused by the large marrow spaces. Orthodontic treatment can be undertaken to correct dental and cosmetic defects, particularly those of the maxillary anterior region.

Patients with thalassemia minor are usually asymptomatic, and in most cases dental treatment can be accomplished without special precautions.

Polycythemia vera
S. Gary Cohen and **Michael Glick**

Patients with polycythemia vera frequently have hypertension, clubbing of the fingernails, and neurologic manifestations such as headache, vertigo, visual disturbances, and paresthesias. These signs and symptoms resolve with therapy. The face may have a ruddy complexion, particularly around the ears, nose, and lips. The oral mucosa appears purplish red to crystal violet. The gingivae are congested and edematous and bleed spontaneously because of increased intravascular pressure and congestion of the vascular beds. Epistaxis is also seen with this disease. Excessive bleeding may follow oral surgical procedures or slight trauma. Petechiae, ecchymosis, and hematomas are occasionally noted, as are ulcerations of the oral mucosa, gingiva, and tongue.

Hemorrhage and thrombosis are major considerations in dental management. Before treatment a bleeding profile including complete blood cell count, platelet count, and bleeding time should be obtained. Most bleeding can be controlled with local measures such as pressure, topical thrombin, or microfibrillar collagen. ϵ-Aminocaproic acid (EACA) is contraindicated in these patients because of the risk of thrombosis.

BIBLIOGRAPHY

Alexander WN and Bechtold WA: Alpha thallassemia minor trait accompanied by clinical oral signs, Oral Surg 43:892, 1977.

Alexander WN and Ferguson RL: Beta thalassemia minor and cleidocranial dysplasia: a rare combination of genetic abnormalities in one family, Oral Surg 49:413, 1980.

Biderman PD: The orofacial manifestations of children with sickle cell anemia, Buffalo, 1973, Children's Hospital of Buffalo Press.

Daramola JO: Massive osteomyelitis of the mandible complicating sickle cell disease, J Oral Surg 39:144, 1981.

Dayal PK and Mani NJ: Clinical aspects of the tongue in anemia, Ann Dent 38:21, 1979.

Friedlander AH, Genswer L, and Swerdloff M: Mental nerve neuropathy: a complication of sickle-cell crisis, Oral Surg 79:15, 1980.

Garfunkel A and others: Iron concentration in teeth of patients with and without beta-thalassaemia major, Arch Oral Biol 24:829, 1979.

Garfunkel AA and others: Local therapeutic approach to agranulocytic oral ulcers, Pharm Ther Dent 4:21, 1979.

Girrasole RV and Lyons ED: Sickle cell osteomyelitis of the mandible: report of three cases, J Oral Surg 35:231, 1977.

Greenberg MS: Clinical and histologic changes of the oral mucosa in pernicious anemia, Oral Surg 39:320, 1981.

Halstead CL: Oral manifestations of hemoglobinopathies, Oral Surg 30:615, 1970.

Hjorting-Hansen E and Bertram V: Oral aspects of pernicious anemia, Br Dent J 125:266, 1968.

Holzman L and others: Anesthesia in patients with sickle cell disease, Anesth Analg 48:566, 1965.

Kinsey RW, Ballard JB, and Matukas VJ: Sickle cell hemoglobinopathies: a protocol for management, J Oral Surg 37:441, 1979.

Kirson LE and Tomaro AJ: Mental nerve paresthesia to sickle-cell crisis, Oral Surg 48:509, 1979.

Konutey-Ahulu FI: Mental-nerve neuropathy: a complication of sickle-cell crisis, Lancet 2:388, 1972.

Lasser SD, Camitta BM, and Needleman HG: Dental management of patients undergoing bone marrow transplantation for aplastic anemia, Oral Surg 43:181, 1977.

Menius JW and Webster WP: Dental management of mild hemophilia with polycythemia vera, Oral Surg 45:714, 1978.

Millard HD and Gobetti JP: Non specific stomatitis—a presenting sign in pernicious anemia, Oral Surg 39:562:1975.

Miller J and Forrester RM: Neonatal enamel hypoplasia associated with hemolytic disease and with prematurity, Br Dent J 106:93, 1959.

Mourshed F and Tuckson CR: A study of the radiographic features of the jaws in sickle cell anemia, Oral Surg 37:812, 1975.

Parkin SF: Dental treatment for children with thalassemia, Oral Surg 25:12, 1968.

Peterson DE and Overholser CD: Increased morbidity associated with oral infection in patients with acute nonlymphocytic leukemia, Oral Surg 51:390, 1981.

Poyton HG and Davey KW: Thalassemia: changes visible in radiographs used in dentistry, Oral Surg 25:561, 1968.

Richard PA: Pathophysiology of dental changes in sickle cell disease, J Conn St Dent Assoc 51:20, 1977.

Sanger RG and Bystrom EB: Radiographic bone changes in sickle cell anemia, J Oral Med 32:32, 1977.

Sanger RG, Greer RO, and Averbach RE: Differential diagnosis of some simple osseous lesions associated with sickle-cell anemia, Oral Surg 43:538, 1977.

Savide NL and Duperon DF: Hexokinase deficiency anemia with dental and other anomalies: report of case, J Dent Child 46:493, 1979.

Schofield IDF and Abbot WG: Review of aplastic anemia and report of a rare case (Fanconi type), J Can Dent Assoc 44:106, 1978.

Shepherd NJ and Samaras NG: Chloramphenicol-induced aplastic anemia, Oral Surg 29:689, 1970.

Silling G and Moss SJ: Cooley's anemia—orthodontic and surgical treatment, Am J Orthod 74:444, 1978.

Stamps JT: The role of oral hygiene in a patient with idiopathic aplastic anemia, J Am Dent Assoc 88:1025, 1974.

Tas I, Smith P, and Cohen T: Metric and morphologic characteristics of the dentition in beta thalassaemia major in man, Arch Oral Biol 21:583, 1976.

Walker JEG: Aphthous ulceration and vitamin B12 deficiency, Br J Oral Surg 11:165, 1973.

Winer HJ, McManon RE, and Olson RE: Palatal necrosis secondary to cytoxin therapy, J Am Dent Assoc 84:862, 1972.

NEUTROPHIL DYSFUNCTION SYNDROMES
Martin S. Greenberg

ORAL MANIFESTATIONS. Oral lesions are common and often severe in patients with neutrophil dysfunction syndromes. Three findings repeatedly reported are severe gingivitis, rapidly advancing periodontal disease, and oral ulcers. These oral findings are similar whether they are caused by Chédiak-Higashi syndrome, benign chronic neutropenia, or lazy leukocyte syndrome.

Since periodontal disease is caused by a chronic bacterial infection, it is not surprising that disorders of neutrophils are accompanied by an increased level of periodontal breakdown. This is a finding generally seen in patients with neutrophil dysfunction. Some investigators have suggested that juvenile periodontitis (periodontosis) may be caused by a neutrophil abnormality. There is evidence that individuals with juvenile peridontitis have neutrophils with reduced chemotactic function, decreasing their ability to phagocytose bacteria.

The lazy leukocyte syndrome is characterized by leukocytes that cannot be mobilized because of a defect in chemotactic function. Gingivitis and stomatitis are prominent manifestations of this disorder. Patients with Chédiak-Higashi syndrome have an inherited neutrophil disorder characterized by neutropenia, decreased chemotactic function of neutrophils, and decreased ability of neutrophils to destroy bacteria. This syndrome has prominent periodontal signs that have been described by several workers. In a study of four patients with Chédiak-Higashi syndrome, all four had a history of severe periodontal disease. Two patients had their teeth removed during childhood because of severe periodontal breakdown, and the other two patients had gingivitis, mobile teeth, deep periodontal pockets, and severe alveolar bone loss. Oral manifestations of benign neutropenia were reported, as well as severe gingivitis and rapidly advancing periodontal disease. The dentist should rule out neutropenia or neutrophil dysfunction syndrome in patients with severe oral ulcers or rapidly advancing periodontal disease that cannot be explained by local factors alone.

DENTAL MANAGEMENT. Patients with abnormal neutrophil function should be under the close supervision of a dentist to minimize local inflammatory factors causing periodontal disease, dental caries, and oral ulcers. Patients should follow a strict oral hygiene regimen and have periodic dental examinations. When extensive dental treatment is performed in susceptible patients, broad-spectrum antibiotic coverage should be considered. If surgical procedures are necessary or oral bacterial infection develops, granulocyte transfusions may be necessary.

BIBLIOGRAPHY

Cianciola LJ and others: Defective polymorphonuclear leukocyte function in a human periodontal disease, Nature 265:445, 1977.

Cohen DW and Morris AC: A periodontal manifestation of cycle neutropenia, J Periodontol 32:159, 1961.

Deasy MJ and others: Familial benign chronic neutropenia associated with periodontal disease: a case report, J Periodontol 51:206, 1980.

Kostman R: Infantile genetic agranulocytosis, Acta Paediatr Scand 64:362, 1975.

Kyle RA: Gingivitis and chronic idiopathic neutropenia; report of two cases, Mayo Clin Proc 45:494, 1970.

Lampert F and Fesseler A: Periodontal changes during chronic benign granulocytopenia in childhood: a case report, J Clin Periodontol 2:105, 1975.

Levine S: Chronic familial neutropenia with marked periodontal lesions: report of a case, Oral Surg 12:310, 1959.

Reichart PA and Dornon H: Gingivo-periodontal manifestations in chronic benign neutropenia, J Clin Periodontol 5:74, 1978.

Tempel TR and others: Host factors in periodontal disease: periodontal manifestations of Chediak Higashi syndrome, J Periodont Res 7:suppl 1026, 1972.

Weary PF and Bender AF: Chediak-Higashi syndrome with severe cutaneous involvement, Arch Intern Med 119:381, 1967.

LEUKEMIA

Martin S. Greenberg

ORAL MANIFESTATIONS. The most common sign of leukemia observed in a region routinely examined by a dentist is cervical lymphadenopathy caused by the infiltration of leukemic cells into the lymph nodes. Intraoral signs and symptoms of leukemia are related to the severity of the deficiency of the mature, normal white blood cells, red blood cells, and platelets. Other oral signs may be caused by infiltration of leukemic cells into the oral tissues and side effects of the chemotherapeutic drugs used to treat the disease.

Leukemia may cause a dramatic decrease in the number of normal red blood cells in a peripheral blood. Signs and symptoms noted in these patients are the same as for any other anemic patient, including complaints of dyspnea, heart palpitations, and dizziness. The oral mucosa shows a generalized pallor.

Thrombocytopenia also results from the replacement of normal marrow elements by the leukemic cells. When the platelet count falls below 25,000/mm³, spontaneous bleeding may occur that frequently includes petechiae and ecchymosis of the oral mucosa as well as gingival bleeding. The extent of the gingival bleeding depends on a combination of factors includ-

ing the severity of the platelet deficiency and the amount of local irritants causing gingival inflammation. Oral bleeding may also occur as a result of disseminated intravascular coagulation (DIC). This generalized pathologic coagulation of blood in the vessels causes hypofibrinoginemia, resulting in severe bleeding.

The most common cause of morbidity and fatality in patients with leukemia is infection. This increased susceptibility to infection may be the result of a decrease in normal white blood cells from the disease process itself or of the effects of the chemotherapeutic drugs used to treat the disease. In neutropenic leukemic patients, routine oral infections may lead to septicemia and death. Proper management of these infections may make the difference between the patient's dying of a generalized infection or successful remission induced by chemotherapy.

Diagnosis of periodontal abscesses or pericoronal infections may be difficult in patients with leukemia. Normal signs of infection are masked because of the dramatic decrease in normally functioning white blood cells. The usual degree of swelling and redness is often absent, leading clinicians inexperienced in examining oral tissues of patients with neutropenia to overlook potentially fatal infections. The dentist must carefully evaluate any clinical complaint in the oral cavity, remembering that a severe bacterial or fungal infection may be present with minimal clinical signs. It is also vital for the dentist to remember that oral infections in hospitalized leukemic patients are often caused by bacteria not considered common oral pathogens. Several investigators have shown that the oral flora of hospitalized leukemic patients has a greater number of aerobic gram-negative enteric bacilli. Organisms repeatedly reported as causing infection in patients with leukemia include *Pseudomonas, Klebsiella, Proteus,* and *Enterobacter* species and *Escherichia coli.* These organisms rarely cause infection in normal individuals but frequently cause infections in hospitalized immunosuppressed patients.

Oral mucosal ulcers are a common finding in patients with leukemia. These lesions may result from bacterial invasion owing to severe leukopenia or mucosal atrophy caused by the direct effect of the chemotherapeutic drugs on the epithelial cells. Minor trauma from a dental prosthesis or teeth may cause large, secondarily infected ulcers to progress to facial cellulitis or occasionally cancrum oris–like lesions, resulting in severe tissue destruction. In other instances, oral ulcers may result in septicemia.

Recent studies have demonstrated that the most common cause of oral ulceration in patients receiving chemotherapy for leukemia is recurrent herpes simplex infection. Reactivation of latent herpes simplex in otherwise normal patients causes recurrent herpes labialis and small clusters of lesions, but in immunocompromised patients, slowly enlarging ulcers result because of lack of normal lymphocyte function. The lesions often appear as craterlike ulcers with raised white margins. The lesions occur anywhere on the lips and intraoral mucosa and continue to enlarge until acyclovir treatment is initiated or the leukocyte count begins returning to normal levels.

Candidiasis is almost universally seen in hosptialized leukemic patients undergoing chemotherapy, but it is important to remember that infections with unusual organisms are common in this group of patients. Several cases of mucosal ulceration from gram-negative enteric bacilli such as *Pseudomonas* and *Klebsiella* have been reported. *Pseudomonas* infection of the oral mucosa appears as a raised, dry, nonpurulent, painless lesion that is sharply demarcated from the surrounding mucosa. Because of the frequency of unusual infections, these ulcers must be cultured to be certain that the patient is treated with the correct antibiotic. Routine treatment with penicillin is often inadequate. Fungal infections with *Aspergillus* or Phycomycetes may also occur. When these lesions are suspected, a biopsy must be performed in addition to a culture.

Oral signs may result from the presence of leukemic infiltrates. These are most frequently reported as gingival infiltrates in patients with acute myelomonoblastic leukemia or acute promyelocytic leukemia. Leukemic infiltrates involving the palate, alveolar bone, dental pulp, and fifth and sixth cranial nerves have also been noted. Disorders of the fifth and seventh cranial nerves in leukemic patients may be caused by vincristine, a commonly used chemotherapeutic drug.

DENTAL MANAGEMENT. The management of oral disease in patients with leukemia is a challenging aspect of dental care. Severe gingival bleeding resulting from thrombocytopenia is often managed successfully with localized treatment. The use of absorbable gelatin sponge with topical thrombin or placement of microfibrillar collagen is often sufficient. Some authors have reported successful management of gingival bleeding with oral rinses of antifibrinolytic agents. If these measures are not successful in stopping blood flow from an oral site, platelet transfusions are necessary. It is important, however, for the dentist to attempt local hemostasis before recommending platelet transfusions, which may lead to transfusion reactions or formation of antiplatelet antibodies. These antibodies reduce the usefulness of platelet transfusions during severe bleeding episodes that may follow.

Management of oral ulcers in leukemic patients should be directed toward preventing the spread of localized infection and bacteremia, promoting healing of the lesions, and decreasing pain.

Oral ulcers are a source of septicemia in patients with leukemia; therefore ulcer specimens must be cultured to determine the predominant microorganism. Topical antibacterial and antifungal medications should be used on leukemic patients. Chlorhexidine rinses are a valuable method of reducing oral bacteria and fungi. Acyclovir should be used to treat labial and intraoral herpes simplex infections. Povidone-iodine solution is a topical drug that can be placed directly over the lesion. Some practitioners have reported success in using chlortetracycline compresses over the ulcers. However, the use of topical antibiotics has the potential for increasing the incidence of *Candida* infection, as well as risking allergic reactions. Severe ulcers showing clinical signs of infection should be treated with a combination of topical medication and systemic antibiotics. The administration of multiple antibiotics is usually necessary to cover all the organisms commonly found in a group of leukemic patients. Candidiasis may be treated with topical nystatin or clotrimazole troches. In severe cases of infiltrating lesions of candidiasis or when the oral lesions are associated with esophageal lesions, systemic use of amphotericin B is recommended.

Every leukemic patient should have a dental evaluation to remove sources of infection before chemotherapy is begun. This should be done with adequate antibiotic coverage, preparation of the area for surgery with povidone-iodine solution, and, when necessary, preoperative use of platelets. When dental treatment is performed before chemotherapy, the rate of septicemia is significantly reduced.

BIBLIOGRAPHY

Carey JA and Chuote RR: Dental treatment for the child with acute lymphocytic leukemia, J Dent Child 42:191, 1975.
Cohen SG and Greenberg MS: Chronic oral herpes simplex infection in immunocompromised patients, Oral Surg 59:465, 1985.
Dreizen S, Bodey GP, and Brown LR: Opportunistic gram-negative bacillary infections in leukemia, Postgrad Med 55:135, 1974.
Ferguson MM and others: The presentation and management of oral lesions in leukemia, J Dent 6:201, 1978.
Goepferd SJ: Leukemia and its dental implications, J Dent Handicapped 4:44, 1979.
Goodstein DB and Himmelfarb R: Allopurinol-induced mandibular neuropathy, Oral Surg 39:51, 1975.
Greenberg MS and others: Oral flora as a source of septicemia in leukemia, Oral Surg 53:32, 1982.
Greenberg MS and others: Oral herpes simplex infections in patients with leukemia, J Am Dent Asoc 114:483, 1987.
Guggenheimer J and others: Clinicopathologic effects of cancer chemotherapeutic agents on human buccal mucosa, Oral Surg 44:58, 1977.
Lemongelli WA, Clark MS, and Williams AC: Nomalike lesions in a patient with chronic lymphocytic leukemia, Oral Surg 41:40, 1976.
Lynch MA and Ship II: Initial oral manifestations of leukemia, J Am Dent Assoc 75:932, 1967.
Montgomery MT, Redding SW, and LeMaietre CF: The incidence of oral herpes simplex virus infection in patients undergoing cancer chemotherapy, Oral Surg 61:238, 1986.
Segelman AE and Doku HC: Treatment of the oral complications of leukemia, J Oral Surg 35:469, 1977.
Smithe AC and Cowman SC: Pulp and periapical involvement in leukemia, NZ Dent J 65:32, 1969.
Weinstein RA, Choukas NC, and Wood WS: Cancrum oris–like lesion associated with acute myelogenous leukemia, Oral Surg 38:19, 1974.
Worth HM: Some significant abnormal radiologic appearances in young jaws, Oral Surg 21:609, 1966.

MULTIPLE MYELOMA
Martin S. Greenberg

ORAL MANIFESTATIONS. Lesions of the jaws are common in patients with multiple myeloma and may be the first clinical sign of disease. They may be manifest as generalized osteoporosis or as discrete, well-circumscribed, punched-out, radiolucent areas without surrounding bone reaction. Jaw lesions occur more frequently in the mandible than in the maxilla, with most lesions detected in the posterior portion of the mandible beneath the premolars or molars and in the ramus of the mandible. A study of 59 cases of multiple myeloma showed 17 with jaw lesions and seven with initial symptoms in the jaw. Another described the initial manifestation of multiple myeloma occurring in the mandibular condyle, affecting function of the temporomandibular joint. Extensive bony involvement has led to pathologic fracture of the mandible.

Some of the lesions of multiple myeloma are detected through symptoms of intraosseous expansion and compression such as paresthesia, pain, swelling, and pathologic fracture, whereas others are asymptomatic and are identified as a result of routine dental radiographs, particularly panoramic films. Lesions may involve the oral soft tissues and appear as a tumor of the gingiva, maxillary tuberosity, or alveolar mucosa. The punched-out lesions have been misdiagnosed as periapical lesions, leading to unnecessary endodontic therapy. Appearance of these lesions is nonspecific, and often they are not suspected until after the examination has been performed.

Occasionally an isolated plasma cell tumor is detected in the mouth or jaw without other radiologic or hematologic manifestations of multiple myeloma. In a majority of these patients, other signs of multiple myeloma eventually develop; they should be evaluated for a number of years with radiographs and blood studies.

Amyloidosis occurs in 5% to 15% of patients with multiple myeloma because of conversion of light chains by macrophage lysosomes. It may cause generalized infiltration of the muscles of the tongue leading to macroglossia or infiltration of the salivary glands, leading to enlargement and decreased salivary flow. In other cases, accumulations of amyloid result in the formation of discrete yellow nodules on the tongue, palate, or buccal and labial mucosa. In all patients with amyloidosis detected by oral biopsy the practitioner should rule out multiple myeloma as a cause.

DENTAL MANAGEMENT. The major concerns of a dentist treating a patient with multiple myeloma are bleeding and infection. The increased susceptibility to infection is caused by the effect of the disease on the bone marrow and the decreased levels of normal immunoglobulins. Bleeding tendencies result from thrombocytopenia and from the high levels of abnormal proteins, which interfere with normal coagulation. Renal failure may also result from the excessive serum proteins.

The dentist must carefully evaluate each patient with multiple myeloma before dental therapy to determine whether the patient has chronic renal failure or is receiving chemotherapy, radiotherapy, or adrenal steroids, which may affect the bone marrow or adrenal function. The results of a recent total and differential white blood cell count, as well as levels of normal immunoglobulin, should be determined to decide whether the patient requires antibiotic coverage to prevent infection. Elective dental procedures should be performed only for patients in remission who are not taking chemotherapy.

If surgery is necessary in a patient with multiple myeloma, the possibility of hemorrhage is a consideration. A careful history including the symptoms of epistaxis, gingival bleeding, gastrointestinal bleeding, petechiae, or ecchymoses should be obtained by the dentist. If there is suspicion of a bleeding problem, the results of a recent platelet count, prothrombin time, and partial thromboplastin time should be evaluated.

When hyperviscosity syndrome is present, patients occasionally have a bleeding problem although routine tests are normal. A hematology consultation before oral surgery is indicated in these cases.

BIBLIOGRAPHY

Bruce KW and Royer RQ: Multiple myeloma occurring in the jaws: a study of seventeen cases, Oral Surg 6:729, 1953.
Cataldo E and Meyer I: Solitary and multiple plasma-cell tumors of the jaws and oral cavity, Oral Surg 22:628, 1966.
Jagger RG, Helkimo M, and Carlsson GE: Multiple myeloma involving the temporomandibular joints, J Oral Surg 36:557, 1978.
Raubenheimer EJ and Dauth J: Multiple myeloma presenting with extensive oral and perioral amyloidosis, Oral Surg 61:492, 1986.
Senn JS and others: Multiple myeloma with initial presentation in the jaw: a clinical-pathologic discussion, J Oral Pathol 14:282, 1985.
Shawkat AH and Phillips JD: Multiple myeloma: report of a case, Oral Surg 37:969, 1974.
Tabachnick TT and Levine B: Multiple myeloma involving the jaws and oral soft tissues, J Oral Surg 34:931, 1976.

MACROGLOBULINEMIA
Martin S. Greenberg

ORAL MANIFESTATIONS. The major oral manifestation of Waldenström's macroglobulinemia is gingival and mucosal bleeding. It is not unusual for the initial complaint to be related to severe, spontaneous gingival bleeding or bleeding after dental extraction. A combination of factors contribute to the bleeding problem. The patient may have thrombocytopenia secondary to bone marrow infiltration with plasma cells and lymphocytes. In other cases the patient hemorrhages although the platelet count is normal. This is caused by hyperviscosity syndrome, wherein the abnormal serum proteins interfere with the normal function of platelets and coagulation factors.

Bone lesions are uncommon in patients with Waldenström's macroglobulinemia, although radiolucent lesions of the jaw have occasionally been noted. Oral mucosal ulcers related to the disease have been reported by some authors. Infiltration and enlargement of the salivary glands have also been de-scribed. This may be confused with Sjögren's syndrome.

DENTAL MANAGEMENT. Bleeding is the most common oral sign and also the most frequent complication of dental treatment. Before initiating dental care, the dentist should order a platelet count, prothrombin time, and partial thromboplastin time. If the patient has hyperviscosity syndrome, bleeding time should also be determined to evaluate platelet function.

If the patient has been recently treated with cancer chemotherapy, the dentist should determine the status of the immune and hematologic systems before proceeding with treatment. A complete blood cell count, including a total and differential white blood cell count, is helpful but does not reveal the level of immunoglobulins or lymphocyte function. A medical consultation is required in these cases.

BIBLIOGRAPHY

Gamble JW and Driscoll EJ: Oral manifestation of macroglubulinemia of Waldenstrom, Oral Surg 13:104, 1960.
Gorden RJ and Pindborg JJ: Macroglubulinemia of Waldenstrom. In Syndromes of the head and neck, New York, 1976, McGraw-Hill, Inc.
Shteyer A and Markitziun A: Lymphosarcoma of the mandible associated with macroglobulinemia of Waldenstrom, Int J Oral Surg 7:585, 1978.

AMYLOIDOSIS
Martin S. Greenberg

The most frequently described oral finding in patients with either primary or secondary amyloidosis is macroglossia. The tongue may have generalized, firm enlargement, often with indurations on the lateral border from the pressure of the teeth or with discrete yellow nodules. In a study of 236 cases of amyloidosis, 12% of the patients with primary amyloidosis and 26% of the patients with amyloidosis related to multiple myeloma had macroglossia. Nodular lesions underlying the palate or buccal and labial mucosa may also be seen. In patients with multiple myeloma, amyloidosis may cause tongue or mucosal nodules. Primary amyloidosis in the temporomandibular joint, which significantly limits mandibular movements, has been noted. Xerostomia may also result from amyloidosis involving the salivary glands.

The relative merit of gingival biopsy in the diagnosis of suspected cases of amyloidosis has been controversial. Gingival biopsy was the desired technique of diagnosis until 1962, when investigators demonstrated positive findings in 75% of rectal biopsies taken from patients with amyloidosis but in only 19% of gingival biopsies. Recent evidence, however, has caused a reevaluation of the efficacy of the oral biopsy in the diagnosis of amyloidosis. The oral biopsy taken from the mucobuccal fold region shows a high percentage of positive results in patients with amyloidosis. These results compare favorably to the rectal biopsy site. Using the mucobuccal fold is sensible, since amyloid is found most frequently around blood vessels and muscle tissue, which is found in the mucobuccal fold region and not in the region of the attached gingiva where most of the previous biopsy specimens were taken.

The following plan is recommended when a dentist is consulted regarding "gingival" biopsy to detect amyloidosis. The patient should first be carefully examined for nodules that may be consistent with amyloid deposits. Biopsies of any nodules noted should be performed. If nodular areas are not present, a biopsy should be performed in the mucobuccal fold. This biopsy site avoids some of the painful complications associated with rectal surgery, particularly in patients with cardiovascular disease.

BIBLIOGRAPHY

Babajews A: Occult multiple myeloma associated with amyloid of the tongue, Br J Oral Maxillofac Surg 23:298, 1985.

Flick WG and Lawrence FR: Oral amyloidosis as initial symptom of multiple myeloma, Oral Surg 49:18, 1980.

Kraut N and others: Amyloidosis associated with multiple myeloma, Oral Surg 43:63, 1977.

Kyle RA and Bayrd ED: Amyloidosis: review of 236 cases, Medicine 54:271, 1973.

Lehner T: Oral biopsy in the diagnosis of amyloidosis, Isr J Med Sci 4:1000, 1968.

Meyer I and others: Amyloidosis of the tongue secondary to multiple myeloma, J Oral Surg 36:459, 1978.

Schwartz HC and Olson DJ: Amyloidosis: a rational approach to diagnosis by intraoral biopsy, Oral Surg 39:837, 1975.

Schwartz Y and others: An unusual case of temporomandibular joint arthropathy in systemic primary amyloidosis, J Oral Med 34:40, 1979.

Smith A and Speculand B: Amyloidosis with oral involvement, Br J Oral Maxillofac Surg 23:435, 1985.

Timosca G and Gavritila L: Primary localized amyloidosis of the palate, Oral Surg 44:76, 1977.

LYMPHOMA

Martin S. Greenberg

ORAL MANIFESTATIONS. Dentists who examine the neck as part of their routine examination play a significant role in the early detection of lymphoma. The practitioner must be able to distinguish lymph node enlargement suggestive of lymphoma from old fibrotic nodes resulting from resolved infection. Suspicion of lymphoma should be increased when (1) the patient has a recent history of enlarged cervical nodes without localizing signs or symptoms of infection, (2) recently enlarged nodes are nontender and rubbery, (3) nodes are enlarged in more than one lymph node chain, and (4) enlargement of a lymph node 1 cm or more in diameter persists for more than 1 month. A patient whose history and examination suggest the possibility of lymphoma should be referred to an oncologist or surgeon for a thorough examination and lymph node biopsy.

Primary lesions of Hodgkin's disease rarely start in an extranodal site, but there are occasional reports of jaw lesions as the initial manifestation. Primary non-Hodgkin's lymphoma occurs wherever lymphoid tissue exists and is therefore much more frequently observed in extranodal sites. Approximately 50% of extranodal lymphomas in the head and neck region occur in the lymphoid tissue of Waldeyer's ring. Therefore biopsy to rule out lymphomas should be performed in all nontender enlargements of pharyngeal or lingual tonsillar tissue occurring in adults.

Several authors have reported non-Hodgkin's lymphoma of the palate. These lesions have been described as slow growing, painless, bluish, soft masses occurring in patients over 50 years of age. Because of their presence on the palate they have been often confused with minor salivary gland neoplasms.

Extranodal non-Hodgkin's lymphoma of the mouth mimics other lesions, such as localized gingival enlargements, radiolucent intraosseous lesions, or masses of the tongue. Lesions of the gingiva have been treated for months as infections such as periodontal abscesses or pericoronitis before a biopsy was performed and the proper diagnosis made. To avoid inappropriate dental treatment one should suspect lymphoma in patients over 50 years of age in the following circumstances: slow-growing palatal masses, isolated loose teeth, or paresthesia of the lip. Tissue from these sites should always be submitted for pathologic diagnosis, which can include cytologic study by use of a touch preparation. Extranodal lymphoma may also arise in the jaws of children. A majority of these are of the Burkitt's subtype.

Biopsy is the only proper method of diagnosing lymphoma. Lymphomas have been confused histologically with benign lymphoepithelial lesions or other benign lymphoproliferative disorders. When considering lymphoma one must be sure to take a representative tissue sample from the center of the lesion. Use of immunoperoxidase staining techniques is helpful in differentiating lymphoma from inflammatory lesions. This technique has determined that most extranodal oral lymphomas are of the B-cell type.

A patient with advanced Hodgkin's disease has decreased cellular immunity and an increased incidence of viral and fungal infection. Particularly significant in the oral region is the incidence of candidiasis and herpes zoster. Herpes zoster may affect the second and third divisions of the fifth cranial nerve, causing pain and unilateral facial and oral lesions along the course of the affected nerve.

DENTAL MANAGEMENT. Radiation therapy and chemotherapy are used to treat the lymphomas. The dose of radiation is much lower in lymphoma than in squamous cell carcinoma, significantly reducing the risk of osteoradionecrosis. The combination of radiation therapy and chemotherapy, however, depresses the bone marrow. Therefore, before providing dental care to a patient who has been recently treated for lymphoma, the dentist should order a complete blood cell count and evaluate the levels of leukocytes and platelets. Patients about to undergo chemotherapy for lymphoma should have a dental examination before treatment so that oral sources of infection can be eliminated.

BIBLIOGRAPHY

Bathard-Smith, PJ, Coonar HS, and Maskus AF: Hodgkin's disease presenting intra-orally, Br J Oral Surg 16:64, 1978.

Blok P, Van Delden L, and Van der Waal I: Non-Hodgkin's lymphoma of the hard palate, Oral Surg 47:445, 1979.

Cline RE and Stenger TG: Histiocytic lymphoma (reticulum-cell sarcoma), Oral Surg 43:422, 1977.

Handlers JP and others: Extranodal lymphoma. I. A morphologic and immunoperoxidase study of 34 cases, Oral Surg 61:362, 1986.

Eisenbug L and others: Oral presentation in non-Hodgkin's lymphoma: a review of thirty-one cases. I. Data analysis, Oral Surg 56:151, 1983.

Eisenbud L and others: Oral presentations in thirty-one cases of non-Hodgkin's lymphoma. II. Fourteen cases arising in bone, Oral Surg 57:272, 1984.

Lehrer B and Federman O: The presentation of malignant lymphoma in the oral cavity and pharynx, Oral Surg 41:441, 1976.

Mittelman D and Kaban LB: Recurrent "non-Hodgkin's lymphoma" presenting with gingival enlargement, Oral Surg 42:792, 1976.

Smith DB and others: Soft swelling of the hard palate, J Am Dent Assoc 102:199, 1981.

Steg RF and others: Malignant lymphoma of the mandible and maxillary region, Oral Surg 12:128, 1959.

Tomish CE and Shafter WG: Lymphoproliferative disease of the hard palate: a clinico-pathology entity: a study of twenty-one cases, Oral Surg 39:754, 1975.

Vickery LM and Midda M: Dental complications of cytotoxic therapy in Hodgkin's disease—a case report, Br J Oral Surg 13:282, 1976.

HISTIOCYTOSIS X (IDIOPATHIC HISTIOCYTOSIS)

Martin S. Greenberg

ORAL MANIFESTATIONS. Oral findings are present in all three subtypes of histiocytosis X. A review of 13 patients with Hand-Schüller-Christian disease demonstrated that approximately three quarters of the patients had oral manifestations at some point during the course of the disease. A recent study of tissue from patients with idiopathic histiocytosis of the jaws indicate that the primary tumor cells are derived from Langerhans' cells.

Rapid alveolar bone loss is a common oral manifestation of histiocytosis X and may be seen as an isolated loose tooth, early exfoliation of deciduous teeth, or multiple permanent teeth loosely retained in soft tissue. Dental radiographs of patients with extensive jaw involvement demonstrate bone destruction extending beyond the alveolus. The dentist must submit tissue for histopathologic examination when areas of apparent alveolar bone loss cannot be explained by local factors alone.

Although it is common for jaw lesions of histiocytosis X to appear as alveolar bone loss, nonspecific radiolucent lesions may occur. Histiocytosis X mimic many other intrabony lesions, and diagnosis of these cases cannot be made without biopsy.

DENTAL MANAGEMENT. See section on cancer chemotherapy.

BIBLIOGRAPHY

Blevins C and others: Oral and dental manifestations of histiocytosis X, Oral Surg 12:473, 1959.

Jones JC, Lilly G, and Martlette RH: Histiocytosis X, J Oral Surg 28:461, 1970.

Sedano HO and others: Histiocytosis X: clinical radiographic and histologic findings with special attention to oral manifestations, Oral Surg 27:760, 1969.

Stewart JCB and others: Immunohistochemical study of idiopathic histiocytosis of the mandible and maxilla, Oral Surg 61:48, 1986.

GAUCHER'S DISEASE
Martin S. Greenberg

ORAL MANIFESTATIONS. Intraosseous lesions of the jaw bone have been reported in patients with type I Gaucher's disease. The abnormal Gaucher cells, which are glucosylceramide-laden histiocytes, infiltrate bone, causing generalized osteoporosis, unilocular vacuoles, or pseudocysts.

In addition to generalized osteoporosis and specific radiolucencies, thinning of the mandibular cortex and resorption of root apices have been observed. Cases have been reported in which routine dental films with radiolucent areas in the mandible, generalized osteoporosis of the jaws, or widened marrow spaces led to the diagnosis of Gaucher's disease.

DENTAL MANAGEMENT. Infiltration of the marrow by abnormal cells and hypersplenism may cause leukopenia, anemia, or thrombocytopenia. Bleeding secondary to thrombocytopenia is the most frequent problem with dental treatment of patients with Gaucher's disease, particularly in patients who have not been splenectomized. A platelet count should be obtained in all cases before dental care, and if there is evidence of liver involvement a prothrombin time and a partial thromboplastin time should be determined as well. The dentist should know total and differential white blood cell count before dental treatment to determine whether the patient has an increased risk for postoperative infection. Jaw lesions may be difficult to manage because the lesions can cause bone infarction and osteomyelitis. The bony lesions have been successfully treated by extraction of the involved teeth and debridement of the bony lesion.

BIBLIOGRAPHY

Bender IB: Dental observations in Gaucher's disease, Oral Surg 112:546, 1959.

Bildman B and others: Gaucher's disease discovered by mandibular biopsy: report of a case, J Oral Surg 30:510, 1972.

Hall MB, Brown RW, and Baughman RA: Gaucher's disease affecting the mandible, J Oral Maxillofac Surg 43:210, 1985.

Michanowicz AE, Michanowicz JP, and Stein GM: Gaucher's disease: report of a case, Oral Surg 23:36, 1967.

Moch WS: Gaucher's disease with mandibular bone lesions, Oral Surg 6:1250, 1946.

Sela J and others: Involvement of the mandible in Gaucher's disease, Br J Oral Surg 9:246:1972.

Spiegel LH: Gaucher's disease, Oral Surg 10:158, 1950.

Weigler JM and others: Gaucher's disease involving the mandible: report of a case, J Oral Surg 25:158, 1967.

PLATELET AND VASCULAR DISORDERS
S. Gary Cohen and **Michael Glick**

Thrombocytopenia

ORAL MANIFESTATIONS. The oral manifestations of thrombocytopenia may represent its initial signs. Purpura, the most common oral sign, is defined as any escape of blood into subcutaneous tissues and includes petechiae, ecchymoses, hemorrhagic vesicles, and hematomas. These may appear on any mucosal surface and are often first seen on the tongue, lips, and occlusal line of the buccal mucosa secondary to minor trauma. Initially the color may be bright red, resembling vascular dilation. Purpura may be differentiated from vascular lesions by applying pressure directly to the area (diascopy). Purpuric lesions do not blanch and may be induced on the palate from the suction created by a full denture. Other oral signs include spontaneous gingival hemorrhage and prolonged bleeding following trauma, toothbrushing, extractions, or periodontal therapy. Similar purpuric findings are often seen on the skin. The patient may have a history of epistaxis, hematuria, melena, and increased menstrual bleeding. Initial manifestations of acute idiopathic thrombocytopenic purpura may be hemorrhagic bullae of the buccal and sublingual mucosa.

Gingival biopsy is helpful in the diagnosis of thrombotic thrombocytopenic purpura (TTP), since the gingiva is readily accessible, highly vascular, and amenable to hemostasis. However, gingival biopsy results are positive in only 40% to 45% of cases; in these cases platelet thrombus formations are seen.

DENTAL MANAGEMENT. Spontaneous gingival bleeding can usually be managed with oxidizing mouthwashes, but platelet transfusions may be required to stop the bleeding. Good oral hygiene and conservative periodontal therapy help to remove the plaque and calculus that potentiate the bleeding. Accidental trauma can be avoided by replacing ill-fitting prostheses and removing all orthodontic appliances. These patients should be cautioned not to sleep with any removable prosthesis in place.

Emergency care during severe thrombocytopenic episodes consists of endodontic therapy, antibiotics, and nonsalicylate analgesics. A stab incision and drainage may be performed, but blunt dissection of an abscessed area should be avoided. Definitive dental treatment should be delayed until normal platelet function returns. Platelet levels greater than 50,000/mm^3 are desirable before dental treatment, and further transfusions should be given as needed postoperatively to maintain hemostasis. Hepatitis and antiplatelet antibody formation are potential serious side effects of continued platelet transfusions. An alternative method, developed empirically by some clinicians, uses a single preoperative platelet transfusion given ½ hour before dental treatment. Postoperative hemorrhage is minimized by packing all bleeding sites with microfibrillar collagen. Clot integrity is ensured by giving ϵ-aminocaproic acid (EACA) in a 100 mg/kg loading dose, orally or intravenously, just before dental treatment, followed by 50 mg/kg every 6 hours for 8 days. EACA inhibits fibrinolysis after clot formation. Side effects, which include dizziness, diarrhea, nausea, and abdominal pain, may be bothersome but are usually not severe enough to warrant discontinuation of the EACA. EACA in the liquid form may make the required dosage more tolerable, particularly for children. EACA, 100 mg/kg every 6 hours for 8 days, and local measures may suffice when the platelet count is 20,000 to 50,000/mm^3. Platelet transfusions are used only when local measures fail.

Block injections should not be given when the platelet count is less than 30,000/mm³ because of the possibility of hematoma formation and airway obstruction. Infiltration or pericemental anesthesia is used instead. Intraligamentary anesthesia using a pressure syringe (Peri-Press syringe, Universal Dental Instruments, Inc.) may be helpful.

Aspirin-containing analgesics are contraindicated because they may potentiate bleeding. Use of any drug that has previously induced a thrombocytopenic episode should be avoided. Autoimmune thrombocytopenic purpura is treated with steroids or splenectomy. Patients with thrombocytopenia should be screened regularly for any source of dental infection. They may also have adrenal insufficiency.

REFERENCES

Karpatkin S: Auto-immune thrombocytopenic purpura, J Am Soc Hematol 56:329, 1980.
Kirshner JJ, Zamkoff KW, and Gottlieb AJ: Idiopathic thrombocytopenic purpura and Hodgkin's disease: report of two cases and a review of the literature, Am J Med Sci 280:21, 1980.
Nishioka GJ, Timmis DP, and Claire N: thrombotic thrombocytopenic purpura: report of case, J Oral Maxillofac Surg 4:740, 1986.

Thrombocytosis

A high platelet count can be paradoxically associated with oral bleeding, and therefore thrombocytosis should be included in the differential diagnosis of oral bleeding. The oral signs of thrombocytosis include gingival bleeding and mucosal ecchymosis. Petechiae rarely occur with this disorder.

The major dental concern is posttreatment bleeding. Dental treatment should be delayed only with rapidly rising platelet levels or counts greater than 800,000/mm³. Medical intervention may be required to return normal platelet function. The use of a local hemostatic agent, such as microfibrillar collagen, can significantly reduce postsurgical bleeding. Use of aspirin-containing analgesics should be avoided.

Thrombasthenia

The oral manifestations in Glanzmann's thrombasthenia, as well as in the other functional platelet disorders, are similar to those of thrombocytopenia. Bleeding is the main concern in providing dental care. Dental management is similar to that for patients with thrombocytopenia. The need for fewer platelet transfusions may occur with the use of EACA.

Bleeding secondary to aspirin

A thorough patient history should include the frequency with which aspirin products are used. Aspirin can potentiate prolonged bleeding in patients who have bleeding and clotting disorders, are taking anticoagulants, or have had recent surgery or trauma.

Aspirin use has been implicated in continued oral bleeding after dental extractions, periodontal surgery, and ultrasonic scaling. Bleeding may continue for 24 to 72 hours after discontinuation of aspirin. During this period local hemostatic agents are helpful, but occasionally platelet transfusions are required.

BIBLIOGRAPHY

Fox PC, Gordon RE, and Williams AC: Thrombotic thrombocytopenia purpura: report of case, J Oral Surg 35:921, 1977.
Lemkin SA and others: Aspirin induced oral bleeding: correction with platelet transfusion, Oral Surg 37:498, 1974.
McGaul T: Postoperative bleeding caused by aspirin, J Dent 6:207, 1979.
Nixon KC, Keys DW, and Brown G: Oral management of Glanzmann's thrombasthenia, J Periodontol 46:364, 1973.
Perkin RF, White GC, and Webster WP: Glanzmann's thrombasthenia: report of two oral surgical cases using a new microfibrillar collagen preparation and EACA for hemostasis, Oral Surg 47:36, 1979.
Pogrel MA: Thrombocythemia as a cause of oral hemorrhage, Oral Surg 44:535, 1977.
Sugar AW: The management of dental extractions in cases of thrombasthenia complicated by the development of iso-antibodies to donor platelets, Oral Surg 48:116, 1979.
Sugimura M and others: Tooth extraction in a patient with Glanzmann's thrombasthenia, Int J Oral Surg 4:130, 1975.
Weiss J: Thrombocytopenic purpura: the dentist's responsibility, J Am Dent Assoc 87:165, 1973.
Wood N: Management of extractions in a case of Glanzmann's disease, Br J Oral Surg 11:152, 1973.

HEREDITARY HEMORRHAGIC TELANGIECTASIA (RENDU-OSLER-WEBER SYNDROME)
S. Gary Cohen *and* **Michael Glick**

Identified as small venules, the telangiectasias occur as punctiform, spiderlike, or nodular lesions, are red to purple, and range in size from pinpoint to 3 cm in diameter. The lesions are nonpulsatile, blanch on pressure, and regain their original color on release. Lesions occur most often on the face and nasal mucosa. The lesions tend to bleed after slight trauma. Recurrent epistaxis and oral hemorrhage are frequently reported from these lesions.

ORAL MANIFESTATIONS. The lesions are found on the skin circumorally, and on the lips, tongue, gingiva, buccal mucosa, and less frequently the palate.

MANAGEMENT. Hemorrhage is usually controlled with local pressure, although hemostatic agents may be helpful. Removal of these lesions may become necessary in some periodontal or prosthetic treatments.

REFERENCES

Austin GB, Quart AM, and Novak B: Hereditary hemorrhagic telangiectasia with oral manifestations: report of periodontal treatment in two cases, J Oral Surg 51:245, 1981.
Bartolucci EG, Swan RH, and Hurt WC: Oral manifestations of hereditary hemorrhagic telangiectasia (Osler-Weber-Rendu disease): review and case report, J Periodontol 53:163, 1981.
Everett FG and Hahn CR: Hereditary hemorrhagic telangiectasia with gingival lesion: review and case reports, J Periodontol 47:295, 1976.
Olson JW and others: Hereditary hemorrhagic telangiectasia: prosthetic management and considerations, J Prosthet Dent 50:767, 1983.

VON WILLEBRAND'S DISEASE
S. Gary Cohen *and* **Michael Glick**

The oral manifestations of von Willebrand's disease include spontaneous gingival bleeding and prolonged bleeding after dental extractions or other surgical procedures. Ecchymosis and petechiae rarely occur. There is a significant variation severity among patients with this disorder, and treatment plans must be individualized to account for the degree of bleeding and the severity of the disorder in each patient.

Block anesthesia should be avoided to prevent possible hematoma formation. The use of a rubber dam to protect the soft tissues is recommended in routine restorative procedures. Mild oozing is to be expected at the injection site and around the teeth where the rubber dam clamp or matrix has been placed. This usually stops within 5 minutes with local application of pressure. Surgical hemostasis can be obtained with microfibrillar collagen and suturing.

In severe bleeding episodes or in patients with severe disease, cryoprecipitate should be used in dosages between 30 and 50 units/kg. This dosage should raise factor VIIIc levels and correct the bleeding time. Since the corrective effect on the latter is transient, lasting less than 12 hours, cryoprecipitates should be administered twice a day. In patients with mild disease who are undergoing dental treatment, the use of ε-aminocaproic acid (EACA) in association with or in lieu of cryoprecipitate, may reduce perioperative bleeding. EACA reduces the amount of plasma products that must be given and thereby decreases the possibility of antibody formation and the transmission of hepatitis and acquired immune deficiency syndrome (AIDS).

Tranexamic acid (AMCA), another systemic antifibrinolytic agent, is considered 7 to 10 times more potent than EACA. AMCA has fewer gastrointestinal side effects than EACA and therefore has largely replaced it. The recommended therapeutic dose of AMCA in conjunction with oral surgery is 15 to 25 mg/kg three times daily.

Another method of managing patients with von Willebrand's disease includes desmopressin (DDAVP), a synthetic analog of an antidiuretic pituitary hormone, vasopressin. A single intravenous infusion of DDAVP (0.3 to 0.4 mg/kg) induces a rapid increase (30 to 60 minutes) in the plasma level of factor VIII activity. Von Willebrand factor antigen, ristocetin cofactor, and plasminogen activator levels are also increased, presumably because of release from cellular compartments. DDAVP has been used effectively to treat von Willebrand's disease. However, it is without effect in the severe recessive form in which tissue stores of von Willebrand factor are markedly reduced or absent. DDAVP infusion should not be used in type IIb von Willebrand's disease because it can result in the immediate widespread platelet aggregation with marked thrombocytopenia. DDAVP can be used in conjunction with EACA or AMCA.

BIBLIOGRAPHY

Campbell HD and Payne RW: Dental extractions in a family with von Willebrand's disease, Br Dent J 142:402, 1977.

Cohen MP: Oral surgical complications with von Willebrand's disease: a case report, J Oral Med 30:115, 1975.

de la Fuente B and others: Response of patients with mild and moderate hemophilia A and von Willebrand's disease to treatment with desmopressin, Ann Intern Med 103:6, 1985.

Livingston RJ and others: Diagnosis and treatment of von Willebrand's disease, J Oral Surg 32:65, 1974.

Lorson EL and others: Von Willebrand's disease: current concepts and report of case, J Oral Surg 34:655, 1976.

McIvor EG: Von Willebrand's disease, NZ Dent J 66:252, 1970.

Pecoraro FJ, Kelner AM, and Deasy MJ: Periodontal therapy in von Willebrand's disease: a case report, J Oral Med 33:59, 1978.

Quast GL and Schoetlger JD: Von Willebrand's disease, J Oral Surg 32:840, 1974.

Sydney SB and Ross R: Periodontal surgery in a patient with von Willebrand's disease, J Am Dent Assoc 102:660, 1981.

Takahashi H: Replacement therapy in platelet-type von Willebrand's disease, Am J Hematol 18:351, 1985.

Takahashi H and others: DDAVP in acquired von Willebrand's syndrome associated with multiple myeloma, Am J Hematol 22:421, 1986.

Vierrou AM and others: DDAVP (desmopressin) in the dental management of patients with mild or moderate hemophilia and von Willebrand's disease, Pediatr Dent 7:297, 1985.

Wallack M: Periodontal therapy for a patient with von Willebrand's disease: a case report, J Periodontol 43:495, 1972.

Westwood RM and others: A new approach to the surgical management of patients with von Willebrand's disease, J Oral Surg 31:483, 1973.

Zakrzewska J: Gingival bleeding as a manifestation of von Willebrand's disease, Br Dent J 155:157, 1983.

FACTOR DEFICIENCIES
Hemophilia A—factor VIII deficiency
S. Gary Cohen and Michael Glick

The high incidence of dental problems among patients with hemophilia is the result of neglect and fear of bleeding during treatment. These patients benefit from a comprehensive multidisciplinary treatment plan. A history should include type and severity of the disorder, presence of inhibitors, medications used for pain, replacement therapy, and previous dental treatment. The dentist should be aware of a factoring period so required dental treatment can be accomplished at that time.

ORAL MANIFESTATIONS. Episodic prolonged bleeding, either spontaneous or traumatic, is the most common oral presentation. Bleeding from the nose, mouth, and lips may be severe. Hemarthroses, which may lead to ankylosis and erosion of the joint surface, are incapacitating and painful. Temporomandibular joint hemarthrosis, although rare, does occur.

Pseudotumors of hemophilia are an uncommon oral manifestation. The hemophilic pseudotumor is a progressive cystic swelling produced by recurrent hemorrhage and may be accompanied by roentgenographic evidence of bone involvement. Pain may be the only early symptom. Early diagnosis can often be made with computed tomographic scanning. Management involves curettage of the lesion after adequate factor replacement therapy.

DENTAL MANAGEMENT. Dental management should be directed toward prevention. Good oral hygiene helps in the reduction of gingival bleeding. There has never been a reported case of significant bleeding from proper brushing or flossing.

Oral prophylasis can generaly be accomplished without factor replacement. Bleeding caused by supragingival ultrasonic scaling or rubber cup prophylaxis is controlled by the platelets. However, deep scaling can cause serious hemorrhage in patients who have not had factor replacement.

Hematomas can be prevented by taking care during x-ray film placement, when using high-speed vacuum and saliva ejectors, and in all oral tissue management. Foam rubber—tipped or gauze-padded instruments can minimize hematoma formation.

The administration of local anesthetics is a major concern in dental treatment. Dissecting hematomas, airway obstruction, and death are known complications of block anesthesia in hemophiliac patients. The injections should not be given unless the patient has a plasma factor level of 50% or greater. Additional plasma factors are required if blood is aspirated, a hematoma develops, or other symptoms of bleeding such as pain in the area of injection occur. In severe hemophilia (2%) replacement therapy should precede any anesthetic technique. Local anesthesia may be accomplished by infiltration or pericemental injections with an interligamentary injection syringe (see section on thrombocytopenia). Intramuscular injections are also contraindicated because of the potential for hematoma formation.

Most restorative treatment can be performed without factor replacement. A rubber dam should be used to protect the oral tissues against accidental lacerations. Wedges should be placed before any interproximal preparations to both protect and retract the papilla.

Endodontic treatment is preferable to extraction. Pulpal bleeding is readily controlled in any conventional manner. Overinstrumentation and overfilling should be avoided.

Periodontal therapy, including surgery, is not contraindicated. Periodontal surgery should be performed only if the anticipated therapeutic benefits outweigh the possibility of severe postoperative complications. No factor replacement is needed for probing and careful supragingival scaling. Replacement is recommended before deep scaling, curettage, and surgery.

Orthodontic treatment can be performed in a well-motivated patient. Care should be exercised in the placement of bands. Minor intraoral bleeding caused by orthodontics responds to pressure within 5 minutes.

Primary teeth should be removed soon after they become loose. When radiographs reveal only soft tissue attachment, a vigorous oral hygiene program should be instituted for at least 2 days followed by tooth extraction. Initial bleeding can be controlled by pressure or with local hemostatic measures such as thrombin or microfibrillar collagen (Avitene). Antihemophilic factor as a topical agent to prevent postextraction bleeding has been reported to stop the bleeding within 12 hours. The extraction site need not be covered or protected. No replacement therapy is needed when using this technique.

Surgical treatment has often been avoided because of the potential for continued bleeding. Before any surgery, complete coagulation studies should be performed and factor levels and red blood cell type should be determined. The patient should be tested for inhibitors and replacement therapy should be available. One time-honored management protocol uses replacement therapy to achieve a plasma level of 100% 1 hour before the procedure. This is followed by maintaining a 60% level for 4 days and a 20% level for the next 4 days. A newer protocol consists of a single infusion to raise the plasma levels to 100% 1 hour before the procedure. In addition, a loading dose of EACA (100 mg/kg) or AMCA (20 mg/kg) is administered. All extraction sockets are packed with microfibrillar collagen, and postoperatively the patient receives EACA (50 mg/kg every 6 hours) or AMCA (10 to 20 mg/kg every 8 hours) for 7 days. Because of the amounts required, the liquid preparation is more acceptable to patients, especially children. Additional factor infusion should be instituted only when bleeding continues for longer than 24 hours. Levels should then be increased to 50%.

Another protocol uses desmopressin (DDAVP), a new therapeutic alternative, which causes a rise in factor VIII levels to provide normal hemostasis for most procedures. This occurs in most patients with mild to moderate hemophilia. Therefore they can be treated effectively without plasma derivatives, which are associated with a risk of hepatitis and other viral infections spread via plasma products.

Desmopressin (4 to 5 mg/kg) is given in 50 ml of isotonic saline by continuous intravenous infusion over 15 minutes. Peak levels are obtained 15 to 30 minutes after infusion. Thus dental procedures should be initiated immediately after the patient receives DDAVP. Desmopressin infusion cannot be assumed to be effective in every patient, and the response should be determined before therapeutic use if factor VIII assays are not possible during the procedure. Most patients who have dental work are given EACA or AMCA in addition. Therapy with these drugs is considered essential in that desmopressin tends to increase fibrinolysis, presumably by the release of plasminogen activator from vascular endothelium.

Inhibitors or circulating antibodies to the deficient factors further complicate dental management. Prevention of bleeding becomes paramount. Systemic replacement is not a reliable alternative for the patient. Topical measures along with the systemic use of EACA or AMCA must be employed to minimize bleeding.

All elective surgery should be avoided, since adequate hemostasis cannot be ensured. If surgery is necessary, one of the following regimens can be employed.

Infusion of sufficient amounts of factor may neutralize the antibody by saturating it and maintaining an antigen excess. The volume of preparation containing factor VIII is the major limiting factor in the saturation process. Therefore this technique is used only when inhibitor levels are low.

Alternatively, infusions of activated factor IX can be used in an attempt to bypass factor VIII antibodies. This activates the cascade at a point after the action of factor VIII. This method uses prothrombin complex concentrate (PCC) in doses of 50 to 100 units/kg every 12 hours until the bleeding is controlled. Prothrombin time (PT) and partial thromboplastin time (PTT) are determined before and after surgery to measure the effectiveness of the PCC. The patient is also given EACA (100 mg/kg every 6 hours) or AMCA (10 to 20 mg/kg every 8 hours) for 7 days. If bleeding is a problem, EACA can be given as a continuous intravenous drip.

One problem with PCC is its thrombogenicity; some researchers suggest avoiding use of antifibrinolytic agents when PCC is administered. Chemical cautery or electrosurgery should be avoided because of the possibility of tissue necrosis and secondary bleeding. Aspirin-containing analgesics should not be prescribed. All hemophiliac patients should be tested for hepatitis and AIDS because of the quantity of blood products and transfusions they have received (see section on hepatitis and AIDS). Dental treatments should be maximized while the patient is receiving replacement therapy.

BIBLIOGRAPHY

Berlocer WC and King DL: Considerations in the dental management of the factor VIII-deficient child with inhibitors, Pediatr Dent 1:188, 1979.

Bjorlin G and Nilsson IM: Tooth extractions in hemophiliacs after administration of a single dose of factor VIII or factor IX concentrate supplemented with AMCA, Oral Surg 36:482, 1973.

Chiono O: Pulpal therapy for the hemophiliac patient, J Acad Dent Handicapped, 1:23, 1975.

Cudziwowski L: Circulating antibodies in factor VIII deficiency hemophilia: report of case, J Dent Child 46:54, 1979.

Currier GF, Pabisco T, and McWilliams NB: Restorative dentistry in hemophiliac children, J Dent Handicapped 2:3, 1976.

Eastman JR, Nowakowski AR, and Triplett DA: DDAVP: review of indications for its use in the treatment of factor VIII deficiency and report of a case, Oral Surg 56:246, 1983.

Evans BE: Dental treatment for hemophiliacs: evaluation of dental program (1975-1976) at the Mt Sinai Hospital International Hemophilia Training Center, Mt Sinai J Med 44:409, 1977.

Hasson DM and others: The dental management of patients with spontaneous acquired factor VIII inhibitors, J Am Dent Assoc 113:633, 1986.

Larson CE and others: Anesthetic considerations for the oral surgery patient with hemophilia, J Oral Surg 38:516, 1980.

Mannucci PM and others: 1-Deamino-8-D-arginine vasopressive: a new pharmacological approach to the management of hemophilia and von Willebrand's disease, Lancet 1:869, 1977.

Mulkey TF: Hemophilic pseudotumors of the mandible, J Oral Surg 35:561, 1977.

Nakajima T and others: Topical application of antihemophilia factor after dental extractions in hemophilic patients, J Oral Surg 36:873, 1978.

Redding SW and Stiegler KE: Dental management of the classic hemophiliac with inhibitors, Oral Surg 56:145, 1983.

Shankar S and Lee R: DDAVP and tranexamic acid for dental extractions in a hemophiliac, Br Dent J 156:450, 1984.

Sharp HK, McIlveen LP, and Schumann NJ: Use of FEIBA and amicar in the operating room—dental treatment of a patient with hemophilia and high titer factor VIII inhibitors, Spec Care Dent, Sept-Oct, 1986, p 210.

Sindet-Pedersen S and Stenbjerg S: Effect of local antifibrinolytic treatment with tranexamic acid in hemophiliacs undergoing oral surgery, J Oral Maxillofac Surg 44:703, 1986.

Stajcic Z: The combined local/systemic use of antifibrinolytics in hemophiliacs undergoing dental extractions, Int J Oral Surg 14:339, 1985.

Storeman DW and Beierl CD: Pseudotumor of hemophilia in the mandible, Oral Surg 40:811, 1975.

Takeuchi M, Shikimori M, and Kandea M: Life-threatening sublingual hematoma in a severely hemophiliac patient with factor VIII inhibitor, J Oral Maxillofac Surg 44:401, 1986.

Wash PN and others: The therapeutic role of epsilon-aminocaproic acid (EACA) for dental extractions in hemophiliacs, Ann NY Acad Sci 240:267, 1975.

Hemophilia B—factor IX deficiency

Patients with factor IX deficiencies can be treated similarly to those with hemophilia A. Replacement therapy with concentrated factor IX is given before treatment. Bleeding should be minimal if factor IX levels can be kept above 30%.

Factor XI deficiency

Patients can be effectively managed with preoperative infusions of 10 to 20 ml/kg of fresh-frozen plasma or cryoprecipitate. This is followed by 5 ml/kg daily or 10 ml/kg every other day for 7 days postoperatively.

ε-Aminocaproic acid instead of postoperative infusions or in addition to a lesser volume of fresh-frozen plasma and cryoprecipitate has also been used. An alternative method involves the use of prothrombin complex concentrate, a factor XI–containing concentrate. Prothrombin complex concentrate has been associated with a high risk of transmitting hepatitis.

Factor V, VII, and X deficiency

Patients with deficiencies of factors V, VII, or X can be managed by any of the following methods: (1) no replacement therapy before dental treatment with only local hemostatic measures at the time of treatment and postoperatively, particularly if there is only a mild factor deficiency; (2) pretreatment infusion of fresh-frozen plasma if moderate to severe deficiency is present; or (2) local measures at the time of treatment along with the administration of ε-aminocaproic acid or tranexamic acid with or without preoperative factor infusions.

In mild to moderate factor VII and X deficiencies, use of prothrombin complex concentration (PCC) containing large amounts of factor VII and X is advisable. PCC can have severe side effects such as venous thrombosis, pulmonary embolism, myocardial infarction, and disseminated intravascular coagulation. Thus it must be administered with great care.

BIBLIOGRAPHY

Eastman JR, Triplett DA, and Nowakowski AR: Inherited factor X deficiency: presentation of a case with etiologic and treatment considerations, Oral Surg 56:461, 1983.
Sumi Y and others: Multiple extractions in a patient with factor VII deficiency, J Oral Maxillofac Surg 13:382, 1985.

Afibrinogenemia

The oral manifestations of afibrinogenemia are similar to those in mild hemophilia. These patients are unlikely to exhibit spontaneous bleeding but may have severe hemorrhage after injury or surgery.

DENTAL MANAGEMENT. Dental treatment is preceded by replacement therapy. Cryoprecipitate infusion 1 hour before treatment is the method of choice. Volume considerations usually preclude the use of plasma or whole blood as a source for fibrinogen replacement. The prothrombin time and partial thromboplastin time are used to follow the postinfusion hematologic profile. Once treatment is completed, the patient should receive daily cryoprecipitate infusions for 3 to 5 days. Most minor bleeding episodes respond to topical fibrinogen. The two major complications related to fibrinogen replacement therapy are hepatitis and antibody development. If antibodies are present, hemostasis may be achieved by saturating the antibodies with large volumes of cryoprecipitate.

BIBLIOGRAPHY

Bhoweer AL, Shirwatkar LG, and Desai AJ: Possible congenital deficiency of factor X (Stuart-Prower): a case report, Ann Dent 3:1, 1977.
Bick RL, Adams T, and Radlack K: Surgical hemostasis with a factor XI–containing concentrate, JAMA 229:163, 1974.
Blecker SM and Williams AC: Post-extraction bleeding in a patient with an acquired circulating anticoagulant against factor V, Oral Surg 32:538, 1971.
Evian CT and others: Complications of severe bleeding in a patient with undiagnosed afibrinogenemia—complications of supportive care, Pediatr Dent 3:42, 1981.
Murphy JB, Robinson K, and Segelman A: PTA deficiency (factor XI deficiency), Oral Surg 42:26, 1976.
Perhavec JC and Goldberg JS: Management of a patient with factor VII deficiency, Oral Surg 50:17, 1980.
Schwartz HC and Stowe JD: Hereditary factor XI deficiency, J Oral Surg 34:453, 1976.
Williams JL: Plasma thromboplastin antecedent deficiency, Br J Oral Surg 10:126, 1970.

Factor XIII

Factor XIII is responsible for the formation of a proper clot by the cross-linking of fibrin monomers into polymers. This produces increased clot strength and resistance to fibrinolysis. Findings of routine blood tests, such as prothrombin time, partial thromboplastin time, bleeding time, and platelet function, are normal.

Diagnosis is confirmed by dissolution of a recalcified plasma clot with either 5 M urea or 1% monochloroacetic acid. If factor XIII is present, the clot does not dissolve. Activity level is measured by solid-phase immunoradiometric assay and rocket immunoelectrophoresis.

ORAL MANIFESTATIONS. A tendency to bleed, particularly post-operatively, hematoma formation and delayed wound healing have been reported.

DENTAL MANAGEMENT. This factor has a long half-life (7 to 8½ days) and requires low concentrations (0.5% to 2%) to control superficial bleeding. Major bleeding episodes are presented by 30% to 50% of normal factor XIII levels. A single infusion of factor XIII concentrate (Fibrogammin) given 15 to 30 minutes before treatment controls bleeding. Fresh-frozen plasma may also be used. Utilizing either of these systemic measures along with topical/local measures allows most treatments to be carried out.

BIBLIOGRAPHY

Colin W and Needleman HL: Medical/dental management of a patient with a congenital factor XIII, Pediatr Dent 7:227, 1985.
Suzuki H and Kaneda T: Tooth extraction in two patients who had a congenital deficiency of factor XIII, J Oral Maxillofac Surg 43:221, 1985.

DISSEMINATED INTRAVASCULAR COAGULATION
S. Gary Cohen and Michael Glick

ORAL MANIFESTATIONS. The oral manifestations of disseminated intrasvasular coagulation (DIC) are similar to those in the hereditary coagulopathies. Bleeding is usually acute but may occur insidiously with petechiae, hematomas, or gingival bleeding. It is important to include DIC in the differential diagnosis of thromboses and/or hemorrhage in patients with no history of bleeding, especially patients with neoplastic tumors, leukemia, infections, systemic lupus erythematosus, splenectomy, or certain obstetric complications. Interestingly, there have been two reported cases of DIC after simple oral surgical procedures.

DENTAL MANAGEMENT. In a patient with DIC, all but palliative emergency care should be deferred until the condition is resolved because, like most disorders in which destruction of coagulation factors occurs, DIC may not be responsive to replacement therapy. If dental management is necessary, a bolus dose of heparin or its continuous infusion is most often used. The use of tranexamic acid and ε-aminocaproic acid is controversial because antiplasmin may precipitate or exacerbate organ insufficiency.

BIBLIOGRAPHY

Falace DA and Kelly DE: Disseminated intravascular coagulation and fibrinolysis as a cause of post-extraction hemorrhage, Oral Surg 41:718, 1976.
Kamel K and Hoerman KC: Disseminated intravascular coagulation, J Oral Surg 31:95, 1973.
Kazmier FJ and others: Treatment of intravascular coagulation and fibrinolysis (ICF) syndromes, Mayo Clin Proc 49:665, 1974.
Rawson DW and others: Clinical-pathological conference: disseminated intravascular coagulation, J Oral Surg 34:62, 1976.
Saito R and others: Disseminated intravascular coagulation associated with infection secondary to carcinoma of the maxillary sinus, J Oral Maxillofac Surg 44:917, 1986.
Shikimori and Oka T: Disseminated intravascular coagulation syndrome, Int J Oral Surg 14:451, 1985.

ANTICOAGULANT THERAPY

S. Gary Cohen and Michael Glick

Heparin

Patients undergoing heparin therapy should receive only emergency care. Patients who have postoperative hemorrhage while receiving continuous anticoagulant therapy can be treated with local hemostatic methods. The effects of heparin are reversed 6 hours after administration. An alternative method involves discontinuing the heparin 6 hours before treatment and then reinstituting therapy 6 to 12 hours postoperatively. In this way interruption of anticoagulant therapy is minimized. In each case the dentist should consult with the physician prescribing heparin to determine the risk of discontinuing anticoagulant therapy for a short period.

Coumarin

Dental treatment of patients receiving continuous anticoagulant therapy has been the subject of conflicting reports in both the dental and the medical literature. Many investigators have reported severe hemorrhage after extraction of single teeth. Some early investigators indicated the danger of thrombosis when anticoagulant therapy was suddenly interrupted before dental treatment. However, later studies concluded that this hypercoagulability does not actually occur, although upper airway obstruction caused by warfarin-induced sublingual hematoma has been reported.

One method used to treat patients while continuing their therapy involves monitoring the patients' prothrombin time (PT) and partial thromboplastin time (PTT) before treatment. If the PT is 2 to 2½ times the control value and the PTT is in a normal range, treatment can proceed with minimal postsurgical bleeding if adequate local hemostatic methods are employed. If the levels are above the proposed treatment range, the doses of anticoagulants can be reduced until this range is reached. Another method involves the use of a locally applied preparation of a coagulation-active substance consisting of fibrin, thrombin, and the patient's venous blood. This is formulated at the time of surgery and used for hemostasis.

These methods have been effective for all restorative treatment and simple surgical procedures. If extensive surgery is considered (or the patient is at great risk of thromboembolism), an alternative method should be considered. If it is determined that cessation of therapy is necessary, the period of time without anticoagulants must be as short as possible to decrease the patient's total exposure to risk of thromboembolism. This involves stopping the patient's coumarin for one dose before admission to the hospital and then initiating heparin therapy on admission. As soon as the PT has returned to normal, the patient is scheduled for the surgical procedure. Heparin therapy is discontinued 6 hours preoperatively. The PT and PTT are measured preoperatively, and if they are found to be in the normal range, the procedure is carried out. Heparin therapy is not resumed for 6 to 24 hours postoperatively, depending on the extent of the surgical procedure. Coumarin is reinstituted at that time, and a therapeutic level may be anticipated in 48 to 96 hours. Heparin therapy is then discontinued and the patient is discharged. In this way the patient remains without anticoagulants for 12 to 24 hours. If total cessation is deemed necessary, a 2-day hold period with reinstitution of therapy the night of the procedure is recommended.

BIBLIOGRAPHY

Bailey BMW and Fordyce AM: Complications of dental extraction in patients receiving warfarin anti-coagulant therapy, Br Dent J 155:308, 1983.

Benoliel R and others: Dental treatment for the patient on anti-coagulant therapy: prothrombin time value—what difference does it make? Oral Surg 62:149, 1986.

Duong TC, Burtch GD, and Shatney CH: Upper-airway obstruction as a complication of oral anti-coagulation therapy, Crit Care Med 14:830, 1986.

Greenberg MS, Miller MF, and Lynch MA: Partial thromboplastin time as a predictor of blood loss in oral surgery patients receiving coumarin anticoagulants, J Am Dent Assoc 84:583, 1972.

Kovacs KT and Kerenyi G: Post extraction hemostasis during coumarin anticoagulant therapy with locally applied coagulation-active substance, Int J Oral Surg 5:3, 1976.

Mashall J: Rebound phenomena after anticoagulant therapy in cerebrovascular disease, Circulation 28:329, 1963.

Michaels L: Incidence of thromboembolism after stopping anti-coagulation therapy: relationship to hemorrhage at the time of termination, JAMA 215:595, 1971.

Mulligan R: Response to anti-coagulant drug withdrawal, J Am Dent Assoc 115:435, 1987.

Poller L and Thomson J: Evidence for "rebound" hypercoagulability after stopping anticoagulants, Lancet 2:62, 1964.

Rooney TP: General dentistry during continuous anti-coagulation therapy, Oral Surg 56:252, 1983.

Roser SM and Rosenbloom B: Continued anticoagulation in oral surgery procedures, Oral Surg 40:4, 1975.

Vinckier F and Vermylen J: Blood loss following dental extractions in anti-coagulated rabbits: effect of tranexamic acid and socket packing, Oral Surg 59:2, 1985.

Ziffer AM and others: Profound bleeding after dental extractions during Dicumarol therapy, N Engl J Med 256:351, 1957.

SECTION SIX

NEOPLASTIC DISEASES

Edited by **Rosaline R. Joseph**

82 · INTRODUCTION TO MEDICAL ONCOLOGY

Rosaline R. Joseph

In perhaps no other field of medicine has there been such a rapid evolution of new attitudes, diagnostic tools, and therapeutic strategies as in the area of malignant neoplastic diseases. In contrast to the hopeless and despairing attitude with which physicians previously approached cancer patients, patients are now treated by a team of interested, hopeful medical professionals, who are concerned not only with specific therapy for the primary malignant disease but also with adequate control of symptoms, psychosocial support, and long-term rehabilitative efforts. Proper medical management of patients with cancer demands a multidisciplinary approach, with the treatment plan for each patient representing the optimal combination of surgery, radiotherapy, chemotherapy, experimental modalities, and support services. Advances in all these fields have resulted in potential curability of one of every two cancer patients diagnosed in 1989. In many of the remaining cases significant, long-term palliation can be achieved. Innovations in radiotherapeutic techniques, the discovery of new chemotherapeutic agents, and the introduction of new modalities occur with sufficient regularity to render oncology textbooks almost obsolete before they are published. As we constantly learn more about the existing modalities, improvements are made in therapeutic regimens. For this reason details such as dosages and schedules of chemotherapy and radiation have been selectively omitted in this section. The reader is referred to the most current oncologic literature for this information.

83 · AN OVERVIEW OF NEOPLASIA

Rosaline R. Joseph

Cancer, the second leading cause of death in the United States, can be defined as an abnormal proliferation of cells resulting in invasion of adjacent normal tissues, dissemination to distant organs (metastasis), or both. Cancer is not a single disease, since over 100 different forms of malignant neoplasia are recognized, each with different clinical and biologic characteristics. In 1987 over 483,000 Americans died of cancer and 965,000 new cases were diagnosed. It is estimated that one of four Americans will have cancer in his or her lifetime.

The magnitude and complexity of the cancer problem present a challenge to the entire medical community, from the laboratory researcher attempting to unravel the enigma of malignant change, to the physician who first suspects the diagnosis, to the multidisciplinary oncology team who assume responsibility of directing definitive therapy. Since malignant neoplasia occurs in every organ system, specific cancers are discussed in detail in the sections devoted to the respective systems. This section presents an overview of the current concepts of carcinogenesis; approaches to detection, diagnosis, and staging of malignant tumors; general aspects of their clinical behavior; and principles of treatment.

CARCINOGENESIS

Although the cause of human cancer is not yet fully understood, the past decade has seen a tremendous leap in unraveling the mystery of malignant transformation of normal cells, with the discovery of protooncogenes in normal mammalian cells. These protooncogenes are analogous to known viral genetic material and are capable of transforming, under multiple stimuli, into oncogenes. The exact mechanism by which oncogenes are involved in carcinogenesis is unclear, but it is believed that under the influence of such agents as viruses, radiation, or chemicals the protooncogene is deflected from its normal cell growth and development into an altered or inappropriate cancerous growth. As of 1987, over 20 oncogenes have been characterized at specific locations on chromosomes, and a few have been linked to human diseases, such as Burkitt's lymphoma. The ultimate role of these basic discoveries on the diagnosis and treatment of cancer is undetermined and is the subject of intense current investigation.

In the meantime, evidence implicating multiple factors in carcinogenesis continues to increase. It is probable that more than one event is necessary to produce a human cancer.

Environmental carcinogenesis

Exposure to carcinogens may be occupational or may result from substances widely distributed in our environment, such as food additives or dyes. Smoking, alcohol consumption, and other social or dietary customs account at least in part for a significant proportion of human cancers.

OCCUPATIONAL CARCINOGENESIS. The first causal relationship between an occupational exposure and the development of cancer was demonstrated in 1775 by Percivall Potts, who observed a high incidence of cancer of the skin and scrotum in chimney sweepers exposed to soot. We now know that the carcinogenic agents in soot are benzpyrene and polycyclic aromatic hydrocarbons.

The following are currently recognized occupational carcinogens and their associated neoplasms:

Substance	Site of neoplasm
Asbestos	Pleura, lungs, gastrointestinal tract
Chromium	Lung
Cadmium	Kidney, prostate
Nickel	Lungs, nasal sinuses
Arsenicals	Lungs, skin, liver
Benzene	Bone marrow (acute myelogenous leukemia)
Uranium	Lung
Vinyl chloride	Liver
Isopropyl oil	Nasal sinuses
Chloromethyl ethers	Lung

Many other industrial chemicals are suspected of being carcinogens, and the list is constantly growing. The magnitude of the problem of occupational cancer is illustrated by the fact that approximately 20% of all deaths in asbestos workers are caused by carcinoma of the lung; an additional 7% of the deaths are caused by pleural mesotheliomas, rare neoplasms in the general population. Gastrointestinal carcinoma has also been shown to be increased in these workers. The incidence of these neoplasms rises dramatically in exposed individuals who also smoke. Pleural mesothelioma has been reported in household members whose contact with asbestos was limited to the worker's clothing. The malignancies usually occur after at least a 20-year latent period. This prolonged period between exposure and development of malignancy is characteristic of many environmental carcinogens and necessitates careful history taking in all patients with carcinoma. Important associations may be missed if a complete occupational history is omitted.

GEOGRAPHIC AND SOCIAL FACTORS IN CARCINOGENESIS. Tobacco contains at least 15 identified carcinogens, and smokers have a marked increase in lung cancer. Cancers of the head, neck, esophagus, and bladder also occur more frequently in smokers. Chewing tobacco is associated with a high incidence of oral cancer, as is the chewing of betel nuts, a practice common in Central and Southeast Asia. Aflatoxin, a product of the fungus *Aspergillus flavus,* is a contaminant of certain foods such as peanuts. It is a potent carcinogen, resulting in liver cancer. Nitrates, widely used as food preservatives, have been implicated as a cause of stomach cancer. Carcinoma of the bladder occurs with increased frequency in patients infested with the parasite *Schistosoma haematobium.*

Epidemiologic studies that have not yet identified specific carcinogens nevertheless point to environmental factors as important in the etiology of some of the most common forms of cancer. These data show a wide geographic variance in the incidence of such cancers. Carcinomas of the lung, colon, breast, and prostate have a high incidence in the United States and western Europe, whereas carcinomas of the stomach and liver occur less frequently in these areas. In contrast, in Japan carcinomas of the stomach and liver are common, whereas carcinoma of the breast is relatively rare. Esophageal carcinoma is frequent in northeast Iran, and nasopharyngeal carcinoma is prevalent in southern China. Both of these cancers are rare in the Western countries. Evidence that these geographic concentrations of cancer are environmentally rather than genetically determined has come from studies of population migration. Daughters of Japanese immigrants to California have an incidence of breast carcinoma similar to the overall incidence in California rather than to the low incidence found in Japan. The change to a high-fat Western diet has been implicated in this phenomenon. On the other hand, the incidence of carcinoma of the stomach and liver in children of Japanese immigrants becomes similar to that of the United States, suggesting the removal of an environmental factor, possible a food preservative. Recently a multination study of the relative incidences of colon cancer revealed a higher incidence in countries whose diets contained a high percentage of meat and refined foods and lacked high-fiber foods.

DRUGS AS CARCINOGENIC AGENTS. Alkylating agents, which are themselves useful in the treatment of a wide variety of neoplasms, have been associated with an increased incidence of acute myelogenous leukemia. Immunosuppressive drugs, usually given to inhibit renal transplant rejection, have been linked to an extraordinary increase (200 times) in lymphoreticular malignancies in transplant patients.

Although synthetic estrogenic hormone administration has been suspected of contributing to the development of breast cancer, no statistically significant correlation has ever been established. However, administration of the synthetic estrogen diethylstilbestrol to pregnant women has definitely been associated with vaginal adenosis and clear-cell vaginal carcinoma in their daughters. An apparent increased risk for endometrial cancer in adults has been linked to the use of estrogen therapy.

Radiation has been implicated in the induction of many types of malignant neoplasia, including acute and chronic granulocytic leukemia in atomic bomb victims and acute leukemia in patients treated with radiation for ankylosing spondylitis. Thyroid cancer has been detected in large numbers of young people who had radiation therapy during childhood for thymic enlargement or acne. Lymphocytic lymphomas have been noted in patients exposed to radiation, and osteogenic sarcoma in radium dial painters.

Genetic predisposition

Only the following few, relatively rare neoplasms have been clearly shown to follow an autosomal pattern of inheritance:

Retinoblastoma
Nevoid basal cell carcinoma
Multiple endocrine adenomatosis
Polyposis coli
Gardner's syndrome (multiple colon polyps with extra-alimentary tumors)
Tylosis (palmar hyperkeratosis) with esophageal cancer.

A larger group of disorders with a variable inheritance pattern is associated with an increased risk of development of malignancy. This group, known as the preneoplastic or precancerous disorders, follows:

Hamartomas
  Neurofibromatosis
  Tuberous sclerosis
  Von Hippel-Lindau disease
  Multiple exostoses
  Peutz-Jeghers syndrome
Genodermatoses
  Xeroderma pigmentosum
  Albinism
  Polydysplastic epidermolysis bullosa
Chromosomal breakage syndromes
  Bloom's syndrome
  Fanconi's syndrome
Immunodeficiencies
  Ataxia-telangiectasia
  Wiskott-Aldrich syndrome
  Late-onset immunologic deficiencies
  X-linked agammaglobulinemia

Of particular interest within this latter group are the so-called chromosome breakage disorders, Bloom's syndrome and Fanconi's anemia, in which inherited chromosome abnormalities are associated with a high risk of leukemia, lymphoma, and other cancers. Patients with Down's syndrome, or trisomy 21, are subject to a 20- to 50-fold increase in the risk of acute leukemia.

Xeroderma pigmentosum is a rare disorder of special interest because of the clues it may give to the basic mechanism of carcinogenesis. It is an inherited skin disease in which the DNA repair mechanism is ineffective, resulting in a high percentage of multiple skin cancers.

Genetic factors probably play a much greater role in the cause of neoplasia than is evident in the rare malignancies just discussed. Genetic variation in susceptibility to cancer is suggested by the observation that cancer develops in only a small percentage of all people exposed to the same dose of a carcinogen in the same environment. This difference in susceptibility may be caused by hereditary variation in the enzymes necessary to process potential carcinogens. It has been suggested that elevated levels of arylhydrocarbon hydroxylase increase the risk of lung cancer in smokers.

Viral oncogenesis

Although viruses have been known to cause neoplasms in many mammalian species, until recently there was no human neoplasm that had been proved to be of viral origin. The isolation of the human T-cell leukemia–lymphoma virus (HTLVI) from patients with a characteristic T-cell lymphoproliferative disease has been the most consistent correlation yet seen and supports a viral etiology. Other neoplasms in which there have been significant viral associations are Burkitt's lymphoma and nasopharyngeal carcinoma with the Ebstein-Barr virus, carcinoma of the liver with the hepatitis B virus, and cervical carcinoma with herpes simplex type 2 virus.

Immune factors in carcinogenesis

In the 1950s Burnet and Thomas introduced the immune surveillance theory, which states that cancer arises as a result of a breakdown in the patient's natural immune mechanisms. The theory holds that neoplastic cells arise in everyone but do not become evident because they are destroyed by a normal immune system. When a breakdown occurs and the tumor cells are not recognized as "nonself," malignant proliferation takes place. Evidence supporting this theory includes the increased occurrence of lymphoreticular malignancies in the congenital immunodeficiency syndromes and the very high incidence of such malignancies in patients who have had long-term administration of immunosuppressive agents. The theory has been weakened by the inability to detect consistent signs of immunodepression in the vast majority of cancer patients, who do not fall into the special and limited categories previously mentioned. The role of immunity in carcinogenesis continues to be explored as new complexities in the human immune mechanism are uncovered.

DETECTION, DIAGNOSIS, AND STAGING OF CANCER
Detection

Early detection and diagnosis remain the most important factors in obtaining optimal cure rates in most cancers. A careful initial history of every new patient, regardless of complaint, with special attention to risk factors such as family history of cancer, occupational exposure, or smoking, will keep the physician's index of suspicion high and direct patients at risk to appropriate screening programs. For example, although annual mammography is not universally recommended for women under 50 years old, it should be performed regardless of age in women who have a family history of breast cancer. This procedure may detect small cancers before they are palpable. Detailed questioning as to recent changes in appetite, weight, digestion, bowel or bladder habits, voice, or appearance of a mole is of utmost importance in the early detection of cancer.

During the physical examination the clinician should pay particular attention to clues of possible occult malignancy. Inspection of the skin often provides the first such clue. Certain skin conditions, although not in themselves malignant, are so often associated with neoplasia as to arouse a high index of suspicion whenever they are found. Among these are herpes zoster, dermatomyositis, and acanthosis nigricans, a symmetric brownish black pigmentation in body folds. About 20% of cases of dermatomyositis coexist with a malignant tumor. Intradermal or subcutaneous nodules may be metastases from an occult tumor. Unfortunately, these lesions usually indicate advanced disease. Lymphadenopathy must always be explained. An enlarged, hard supraclavicular node on the left side (Virchow's or sentinel node) often points to an intraabdominal malignancy. Femoral (as opposed to inguinal) adenopathy is always significant and is highly suggestive of malignancy, as is the presence of a palpable mass in the umbilicus. Any mass, lump, or unexplained edema should be evaluated for malignancy.

Some parts of the physical examination most valuable in the early detection of cancer are frequently omitted. Careful examination of the oropharynx can identify premalignant or early malignant lesions. Digital rectal examination is invaluable for the detection of both rectal and prostatic carcinoma. Determination of occult blood in the stool is an important screening device for colon carcinoma, as is sigmoidoscopy. Early, asymptomatic gynecologic tumors can often be detected by pelvic examination. The use of Papanicolaou smears to identify abnormalities in cervical cytology has been an important factor in reducing deaths from cervical cancer.

Diagnosis

HISTOLOGIC CONFIRMATION AND CLASSIFICATION. The sine qua non for the diagnosis of cancer is histologic proof of malignancy. Tissue should be obtained by whatever means possible before any therapy is instituted. This rule is relaxed only in the case of suspected gliomas in critical areas of the brain. Besides confirming the presence of malignancy, histologic classification provides prognostic information and guidelines for therapy. The degree of differentiation of the tumor and the presence or absence of vascular invasion are important prognostic factors within each histologic type.

Accuracy in histologic classification is of utmost importance in bronchogenic carcinoma, lymphomas, acute leukemia, and testicular tumors. In all of these situations responses to therapy differ significantly according to cellular type. A most dramatic example of this phenomenon is small or oat cell carcinoma of the lung. Tumors of this cell type are highly sensitive to chemotherapy, whereas other types of bronchogenic carcinoma are much less responsive to available cytotoxic agents.

Malignancy is frequently diagnosed from a biopsy of an accessible metastatic site, such as liver or peripheral lymph node. Occasionally even the most careful search fails to reveal the primary lesion. In these situations procedures such as histochemical analysis or electron microscopy may be helpful in narrowing the list of possible primary sites. Determination of the primary tumor is of utmost importance in planning optimal therapy, since "metastatic" adenocarcinoma can arise from a lesion as resistant to therapy as pancreatic cancer or from one as sensitive as breast cancer.

TUMOR MARKERS. Despite emphasis on early detection, many cancer patients already have advanced disease at the time of diagnosis. Extensive research has been focused on attempts to identify a measurable substance or substances in body fluids that would signify the presence of cancer. This research has led to the discovery of a series of such tumor markers. Besides providing an early detection device, these markers can also be used as a chemical assay of tumor burden. Changes in their levels can serve as a measure of response to therapy or an indication of relapse. Unfortunately, the available markers are not specific for any particular tumor type and in many cases are present in normal individuals or in those with nonmalignant diseases, as well as in cancer patients. Nevertheless, in certain situations such as testicular carcinoma, initial measurement and constant monitoring of tumor markers have made a significant difference in the management of the disease.

Oncofetal antigens are products of gene expression during fetal life, which normally become repressed when tissue specialization and organization are completed. Malignant transformation of a cell is accompanied by derepression of these genes and reappearance of the fetal antigens.

Carcinoembryonic antigen (CEA), first described in 1965, is a glycoprotein that acts as a specific antigen for adenocarcinoma of the colon and digestive organs of human fetuses in the second to sixth months of gestation. It is also detectable in the feces of normal adults and in the secretion of the pancreatobiliary system and colon. Plasma levels of up to 2.5 ng/ml are detectable in healthy, nonsmoking individuals. Elevated levels have been found in 60% to 90% of patients with carcinoma of the gastrointestinal tract and lung and 50% of patients with advanced breast cancer. The frequency and degree of positivity increase with more extensive disease and more differentiated histology. The development of hepatic metastases is often accompanied by a rapid rise in the CEA level. Elevated CEA levels have also been found in alcoholic hepatitis, alcoholic pancreatitis, and biliary obstruction. There does not appear to be a specific level that separates benign from malignant disorders. Since CEA levels are so nonspecific, they cannot be used for detection or diagnosis of any cancer. The major usefulness of this determination is in monitoring the response to therapy or predicting relapse. Successful therapy should bring elevated CEA levels to normal within 1 month after treatment. A persistent elevation usually means residual disease. A return to normal CEA levels followed by recurrent elevation signifies recurrence of the disease.

α-Fetoprotein (AFP) has a molecular weight of 70,000 and is synthesized by the yolk sac, gastrointestinal tract, and liver of the human fetus. The normal adult level of 40 ng/ml is reached 6 to 12 months after birth. Elevated plasma levels of this protein occur in 70% to 90% of patients with hepatoma and about 70% of patients with nonseminomatous testicular carcinoma. Abnormally high levels also occur in a smaller percentage of patients with cancer of the pancreas, ovary, stomach, and lung, as well as in such benign conditions as viral and alcoholic hepatitis, ataxia-telangiectasia, and hereditary tyrosinemia. AFP determination is useful primarily as a monitor of therapeutic response.

Pancreatic oncofetal antigen (POA) is a glycoprotein found in fetal and malignant pancreatic tissue. Although it is not found in the normal adult pancreas, it is present in the serum of normal adults. Elevated levels have been found in some cases of lung, gastric, colon, and breast cancer, but the highest concentrations and greatest frequency of elevation occur in patients with pancreatic cancer.

CA-125 is a glycoprotein present during embryonic development that is expressed by many epithelial ovarian cancers. Levels are useful in monitoring treatment and in detection of such clinical recurrent disease.

Placental proteins may be increased in certain tumors. Human chorionic gonadotropin (HCG) is a glycoprotein normally secreted by the trophoblastic epithelium of the placental villi. It is composed of dissimilar α- and β-subunits. Radioimmunoassay can distinguish between the β-subunit of placental HCG and that of luteinizing hormone. Detectable levels of the β-subunit of HCG in a nonpregnant female or a male signal the presence of a tumor. Ectopic HCG has been found in 40% to 60% of patients with gonadal or extragonadal germ cell tumors and in a lesser percentage of patients with hepatoma and adenocarcinomas of the stomach, pancreas, and ovary. More than 50% of malignant insulinomas secrete HCG, whereas benign islet cell tumors do not. Measurement of HCG levels has been of particular importance in monitoring response to therapy and relapse in germ cell tumors.

Placental alkaline phosphatase (Regan isoenzyme) is synthesized in the trophoblast and can be distinguished from other alkaline phosphatases by heat stability, immunochemical specificity, and electrophoretic mobility. It is elevated in 5% to 15% of patients with cancer of the breast, lung, or female reproductive organs.

Ectopic polypeptides not usually produced by the cell of origin can be secreted by malignant tumors. This phenomenon of ectopic secretion has been explained by the hypothesis that all somatic cells contain a complete genetic complement and that with malignant transformation selective derepression for specific polypeptide production occurs. Elevated concentrations of these substances in body fluids can thus serve as tumor markers. Examples of such markers are adrenocorticotropic hormone (ACTH), antidiuretic hormone (ADH), and calcitonin secreted by small or oat cell carcinoma of the lung; ACTH, serotonin, and calcitonin by medullary thyroid cancer; and ACTH or serotonin by islet and germ cell tumors.

Other tumor markers include increased amounts of substances normally secreted by the cells of origin. Detection of this increased secretion may provide a diagnostic clue to the existence of tumors, and monitoring of secretion levels during the course of the disease and its treatment has prognostic and therapeutic significance. Among these substances are the paraproteins produced in the plasma cell dyscrasias, insulin in islet cell tumors, and tartrate-inhibitable acid phosphatase produced by prostatic acinar epithelium.

Staging of tumors

Determining the extent of involvement, or stage, of a tumor at the time of diagnosis is essential to the development of an optimal treatment program for patients with cancer. After a carefully planned series of studies, the patient's disease is classified according to one of several staging systems described later in this section.

Although the specific studies necessary for adequate staging vary with the type of tumor, certain techniques are widely applicable. Radionuclide scanning is useful in determining primary or metastatic tumor involvement of the bones, liver, and spleen. Bone scans generally detect metastatic lesions before they are evident roentgenographically, and they are particularly useful before definitive treatment of large (over 5 cm) breast cancers, since 25% of the patients with such cancers have been shown to have metastatic bone disease at the time of diagnosis. In breast tumors under 2 cm, the positive yield of preoperative bone scans is minimal. In cases of purely lytic lesions, such as those seen in multiple myeloma, the bone scan is usually negative and roentgenographic examination demonstrates the lesions. Liver scans reveal defects consistent with metastatic disease before either hepatomegaly or abnormal liver function tests are evident.

Computed tomography (CT) is invaluable in the diagnosis of primary and metastatic tumors of the brain. Abdominal CT scans are helpful in detecting mesenteric lymph nodes, liver metastases, retroperitoneal disease, and pelvic masses. Abnormalities in the pancreas, a notoriously difficult area in which to detect early disease, can also be revealed on the CT scan.

Ultrasonography is helpful in the detection of cardiac, pericardial, hepatic, pancreatic, renal, pelvic, and retroperitoneal lymph node abnormalities. Both CT and ultrasonography are valuable in guiding biopsies of tumor masses.

A newer technique, magnetic resonance imaging (MRI), does not entail ionizing radiation exposure and has the ability to obtain cross-sectional views in any plane. Specific advantages it may have over other imaging techniques are being evaluated. At present, it is clearly superior to CT for evaluation of tumors of the central nervous system, of the musculoskeletal system, and of the nasopharynx.

In certain well-defined situations it is necessary to go beyond the noninvasive studies just discussed to arrive at an adequate staging classification. This is the case when histologic evidence of involvement in a particular area would change the treatment plan for a patient. For example, involvement of mediastinal nodes may render a patient with lung carcinoma inoperable. Mediastinoscopy or exploratory thoracotomy may be required to prove such involvement. In Hodgkin's disease exploratory laparotomy with splenectomy and multiple liver and lymph node biopsies should be performed after clinical staging in cases in which the surgical findings might lead to a change in therapeutic approach.

Staging classifications help the physician estimate the prognosis, plan treatment, and evaluate results. Although a single system applicable to all tumors would seem to be ideal, attempts to establish one have not met with general acceptance. Differences in pathophysiology and natural history among malignant tumors make a single, universal staging classification unwieldy and impractical.

All classifications should be based on anatomic and histologic considerations. The following is a basic system useful for staging the anatomic extent of many solid tumors:

Stage I. Mass limited to organ of origin
Stage II. Local spread into surrounding tissue and first station lymph nodes
Stage III. Extensive primary lesions with fixation to deeper structures, bone invasion, and spread to lymph nodes
Stage IV. Evidence of distant metastases

A tumor-node-metastases (TNM) anatomic classification based on assessment of the primary tumor, lymph nodes, and distant metastases has been advocated by the American Joint Committee for Cancer Staging and Results Reporting. This system, which has been particularly valuable in classifying head and neck tumors, is as follows:

Tumor
  TX. Tumor cannot be assessed
  T0. No evidence of primary tumor
  TIS. Carcinoma in situ
  T1, T2, T3, T4. Progressive increase in tumor size and involvement

Nodes
  NX. Regional lymph nodes cannot be assessed clinically
  N0. Regional lymph nodes not demonstrably abnormal
  N1, N2, N3, N4. Increasing degrees of demonstable abnormality of regional lymph nodes
Metastases
  MX. Not assessed
  M0. No (known) distant metastasis
  M1. Distant metastasis present; specify sites of metastasis

Histologic staging is based on the degree of differentiation, with G1 being a well-differentiated tumor, G2 moderately well differentiated, G3 poorly differentiated, and G4 very poorly differentiated.

CLINICAL MANIFESTATIONS

The myriad clinical problems that may be encountered in patients with cancer are the result of the presence of a mass, of invasion or replacement of normal tissue, or of secretory products of the tumor. The specific symptoms depend on the sites of involvement or the particular substances produced.

Obstruction and compression

Obstructive and compressive symptoms caused by the presence of a mass are common in patients with gastrointestinal tract tumors. Dysphagia is the most frequent complaint of patients with carcinoma of the esophagus, pyloric obstruction occurs with carcinoma of the stomach, and intestinal obstruction is a common complication of carcinoma of the left side of the colon. Obstructive jaundice usually results from carcinoma of the pancreas or hepatobiliary tree or, less often, from pressure by malignant lymph nodes. External compression by such nodes also causes ureteral obstruction in carcinoma of the prostate or ovary and in lymphomas. Bronchogenic carcinomas obstruct bronchi and result in atelectasis. Compression of the spinal cord by epidural tumor produces radicular pain, bladder and bowel dysfunction, and sensory deficits. Progression to complete motor and sensory loss can occur if the compression is unrelieved. Lymphedema and effusions may result from the obstruction of lymphatic flow. Compression or invasion of the superior vena cava by bronchogenic carcinomas, lymphomas, or more rarely other tumors leads to facial swelling, distention of the cervical and upper chest wall veins, conjunctival injection, headache, and convulsions.

Loss or alteration of organ function

Invasion by cancer tissue often results in a loss or alteration of normal organ function. Bone marrow involvement with tumor leads to myelophthisic anemia characterized by the appearance of immature red and white cells in the peripheral blood. Thrombocytopenia is also occasionally seen. Diabetes insipidus, myxedema, or addisonism may arise with tumors involving the posterior pituitary gland, thyroid gland, or adrenal cortex, respectively. Steatorrhea may result from exocrine deficiency of the pancreas. Cardiac arrhythmias occur with invasion of the conduction system by tumor. Hypercalcemia is produced when tumors, most often metastatic carcinoma of the breast and multiple myeloma, invade bone.

Tumor secretion

(See Chapter 117.)

Some tumors are characterized by the production of an increased amount of a substance or substances that are normally produced by the cell of origin. In multiple myeloma many of the clinical manifestations result from the excessive secretion of a single or monoclonal immunoglobulin by the malignant plasma cells. Hyperviscosity syndrome, coagulation abnormalities, and renal damage in this disease are directly related to the presence of the malignant paraprotein. The β-cell tumor of the pancreas or insulinoma usually is manifested by hypoglycemia and tumors of the adrenal cortex by hypercortisolism. Carcinoid tumors may product diarrhea, colic, and malabsorption related to serotonin secretion or attacks of flushing from kallikrein release.

Other tumors are associated with the secretion of substances that are not normally produced by the cells of origin. Bronchogenic carcinomas are the tumors most frequently associated with ectopic hormonal secretion. Clinically apparent hypercortisolism occurs with many carcinomas, particularly small or oat cell carcinoma of the lung. Tumors of the thyroid gland, ovary, prostate, parotid gland, liver, and islet cells and pheochromocytomas also may produce this syndrome. Hypokalemia, weakness, and edema are more common in patients with ectopic ACTH production than in those with other types of Cushing's syndrome. Conversely, truncal obesity, cutaneous striae, and osteoporosis are uncommon in this situation.

Inappropriate secretion of ADH, usually by small or oat cell carcinoma of the lung, results in hyponatremia and excessive urinary sodium excretion. Usually the syndrome is suspected only because of abnormal laboratory values. Occasionally, however, confusion, convulsions, or coma results from profound hyponatremia. The diagnosis may be made by the finding of urine hypertonicity in relation to plasma, normal glomerular filtration rate, and normal adrenocortical function. ADH-like secretion indistinguishable from human pituitary ADH has been isolated from tumors of patients with this syndrome.

Some tumors produce a parathyroid hormone (PTH)–like substance resulting in hypercalcemia, lethargy, weakness, anorexia, nausea, and vomiting. The renal stones or bone disease associated with primary hyperparathyroidism is rarely seen in the ectopic syndrome. Squamous cell carcinomas of the lung and carcinomas of the ovary, kidney, uterus, pancreas, and colon have been associated with ectopic PTH secretion. Prostaglandins produced by tumors may also contribute to nonmetastatic hypercalcemia in cancer patients.

Other hormonal syndromes include hypoglycemia associated with large retroperitoneal or intrathoracic tumors, which may secrete an insulin-like substance, and gynecomastia resulting from gonadotropin secretions by lung, liver, or adrenal tumors.

Miscellaneous paraneoplastic syndromes

Besides the syndromes in which tumor secretion has been demonstrated, there is a heterogeneous group of disorders associated with malignancy for which no explanation has been found. It is presumed that they are effects of secretion of tumor substances, but no such substances have yet been isolated. These syndromes affect many systems and may provide the first clue to the presence of a neoplasm. The symptoms often abate or disappear with successful treatment of the primary tumor.

NEUROLOGIC SYNDROMES. Cerebellar degeneration and many types of peripheral neuropathy including pure sensory, lower motor neuron, and mixed varieties have been described in patients with malignant tumors in the absence of direct involvement of the nervous system. Necrotizing myelopathy, progressive multifocal leukoencephalopathy (probably a papovavirus disease), subacute myelitis, and a myasthenic syndrome (Eaton-Lambert syndrome) have also been observed. Carcinoma of the lung, breast, and ovaries and lymphomas are the tumors most commonly found with these syndromes (see Chapter 190).

RHEUMATIC SYNDROMES. Disorders of connective tissue, such as polymyositis, hypertrophic pulmonary osteoarthropathy, and rheumatoid-like arthropathies, are seen in patients with lung cancer, lymphoid malignancies, and less commonly other tumors. A malignancy is found in 20% of patients with dermatomyositis (see Chapter 19).

HEMATOLOGIC SYNDROMES. A variety of hematologic abnormalities unrelated to local tumor involvement are recognized in patients with cancer. Autoimmune hemolytic anemia not only occurs in leukemias or lymphomas, where it may be associated with an antibody produced by the tumor cells, but also is seen in certain cystic ovarian tumors in the absence of any detectable anti–red cell antibody. Pure red cell aplasia is often seen with thymomas. Conversely, erythrocytosis occurs with hypernephromas, carcinoma of the lung, prostate, and liver, and cerebellar hemangioblastoma. Erythropoietic activity has been detected in these tumors. Many types of cancer are associated with thrombocytosis and some with thrombocytopenia in the face of normal marrow megakaryocytic activity, pointing to an autoimmune phenomenon. Disseminated intravascular coagulation, particularly of the chronic type, is seen in a wide variety of neoplasms. It is postulated that intravascular coagulation may be initiated by thromboplastins derived from tumor cells, especially of the mucin-secreting types. Migratory thrombophlebitis is common in carcinoma of the lung and pancreas (see Chapter 201).

NEPHROTIC SYNDROME. The nephrotic syndrome has been reported in patients with malignant lymphomas and less frequently with other neoplasms. The mechanism is poorly understood but appears to be immunologic.

DERMATOLOGIC SYNDROMES. A wide variety of nonspecific dermatologic syndromes often herald or coexist with an internal malignancy. The most striking of these is acanthosis nigricans, which is most often seen with carcinoma of the stomach.

TUMOR CACHEXIA SYNDROME. A most puzzling accompaniment of malignancy is the marked cachexia seen in so many advanced cancers. Although anorexia with distortion of taste sensation and aversion to specific foods undoubtedly plays a role, cachexia is often out of proportion to the reduction in caloric intake. The mechanism responsible for this phenomenon is unknown.

COMPLICATIONS OF THERAPY

Antineoplastic therapy results in a host of clinical problems, some of which, such as infection, augment a tendency already present in a tumor-bearing host, and some of which are unique to a particular therapeutic modality. These are discussed in Chapter 84.

BIBLIOGRAPHY

American Joint Committee for Cancer Staging and End Results Reporting: Manual for staging of cancer, ed 3, Philadelphia, 1988, JB Lippincott.

Baxter SE and Longo DL: Use of serum tumor markers in cancer diagnosis and management, Semin Oncol 14:102, 1987.

Cline MJ, Slaman DJ, and Lipsick JS: Oncogenes: implications for the diagnosis and treatment of cancer, Ann Int Med 101:223, 1984.

Gallo RC and Wong-Staal F: Retroviruses as etiologic agents of some animal and human leukemias and lymphomas and as tools for elucidating the molecular mechanism of leukemogenesis, Blood 60:545, 1982.

Goepp CE: Cancer genetics: a Gordin knot, Semin Oncol 5:61, 1978.

Wynder EL and Rauscher FJ Jr, editors: The etiology of cancer, Semin Oncol 3:1, 1976.

Yarbro JE, editor: Oncologic emergencies, Semin Oncol 5:123, 1978.

84·PRINCIPLES OF SYSTEMIC CANCER THERAPY

Rosaline R. Joseph

The optimal management of patients with malignant tumors changes in response to continuing advances in both basic and clinical cancer research. Since details of therapeutic regimens might be outmoded by the time of publication, this chapter concentrates on principles of therapy. At present three major therapeutic modalities are available for the treatment of malignant tumors: surgery, radiation, and chemotherapy. The use of biologic response modifiers including interferon and monoclonal antibodies show clinical promise but are largely experimental at this time. Supportive and symptomatic therapy is all important in maintaining an optimal quality of life. Central to the construction of a treatment plan for each patient should be a consideration of the possible role of each of these modalities in that patient's case, and multidisciplinary consultation should be sought. Traditional roles for surgery, radiation therapy, and chemotherapy are changing, and it is necessary to have expert input in all of these fields. For example, surgery for metastatic disease is no longer always purely palliative. Removal of solitary pulmonary or intracranial metastatic lesions remaining after chemotherapy has resulted in long-term survival in some cancers. Chemotherapy is no longer a "last resort" but is employed before, concomitantly with, or immediately after local primary treatment modalities in an attempt to improve the cure rate in selected cancers.

The list of such "combined modality" approaches is long and represents a major advance in cancer therapy that has resulted in prolonged survival for many cancer patients and improved quality of life for others. Examples of this are discussed under "Management of specific malignancies."

TREATMENT OF LOCALIZED OR REGIONAL DISEASE

Surgery or radiation therapy is usually the treatment of choice in localized disease when careful pretreatment evaluation has revealed no evidence of metastases. If a tumor is accessible and amenable to complete surgical removal, this has traditionally been the recommended procedure. Radiation has been used as primary therapy in situations when surgery is contraindicated (mediastinal node involvement in lung cancer, poor medical condition of the patient) or will cause unacceptable loss of function (some tumors of the head and neck) or when the tumor is highly radiation sensitive (lymphomas). Radiation therapy following limited surgery (for instance, a lumpectomy) has been shown to be effective treatment for selected cases of early breast cancer. Chemotherapy is indicated as "adjuvant" to primary therapy of localized or regional disease when a patient group at high risk of recurrence can be identified and when an agent or agents exist that have demonstrated some level of efficacy in metastatic tumors of the type in question.

TREATMENT OF DISSEMINATED MALIGNANCIES

Effective treatment of disseminated malignant neoplasms is based primarily on the availability of chemotherapeutic agents that act systemically, killing tumor cells throughout the body. The theoretical potential for curing disseminated human tumors derives from the cell-kill hypotheses and an understanding of tumor cell kinetics. The cell-kill, or Skipper, hypotheses were originally based on the L-1210 mouse leukemia model but appear to hold true for malignant tumors in general. The major hypotheses state that (1) a single leukemia cell is capable of "cloning" enough cells to kill the host; (2) the life span of the host is inversely proportional to the numbers of clonogenic cells inoculated; (3) the life span of the host is inversely proportional to the number of clonogenic cells remaining at the end of therapy; and (4) first-order kinetics apply to leukemic cell kill by chemotherapy (a given dose of a given drug kills the same percentage, not the same number, of cells in populations varying widely in size). The chances of killing the last cell are calculable in populations that are homogeneous with respect to drug sensitivity.

Although these hypotheses have been useful in the construction of effective chemotherapeutic regimens, their practical value has been limited by the fact that in most human tumors the cells are not uniformly sensitive to chemotherapy. At any one time in any given tumor, only a portion of cells are undergoing division. This is the "growth fraction" of the tumor. The remaining cells are in a resting phase and are less sensitive to many chemotherapeutic agents. In the earliest stages of tumor development, growth is exponential, since there is a very large growth fraction. As the tumor enlarges, the growth fraction decreases, possibly because of decreased vascularization, and there is an increase in doubling time of the tumor. Human tumors vary widely in their growth fractions and doubling times.

Replication of the individual cell depends on the cell cycle, which consists of the G_1 or pre-DNA synthetic phase, which varies from 2 hours to infinity; the S phase of active DNA synthesis, which lasts from 6 to 23 hours; the G_2 or premitotic phase lasting 2 to 8 hours; and the M or mitotic phase lasting 0.5 to 2 hours. In addition to the actively dividing cells in the growth fraction, the tumors have a second population of cells that are not actively dividing but have the ability to do so. These are said to be in a G_0 (quiescent) or an extended G_1 phase. Finally, tumors contain a group of cells that are no longer capable of division and cannot reenter the cell cycle.

Many anticancer drugs exert their cytotoxic effects on the dividing cell and are inactive against the quiescent or permanently nondividing population. Accurate measurement of cell cycle times of individual cells or doubling times of individual tumors allows precise scheduling so that drugs can be given when the largest number of tumor cells are in the most vulnerable stage. Techniques permitting such measurements are becoming more widely available. Tumors with large growth fractions are generally sensitive to cytotoxic agents. In tumors with low growth fractions, toxicity to normal rapidly dividing cells, such as bone marrow and gastrointestinal mucosal cells, makes effective antitumor chemotherapy more difficult.

Recently the relevance of this kinetic model has been challenged. It does not adequately explain the varying response to therapy of patients with the same tumor type, nor does it explain developing resistance to drugs as the tumor volume diminishes after each course of treatment. The Goldie-Coldman hypothesis proposes that drug failure or resistance results from spontaneous, somatic mutations in tumor cell populations, which result in the production of resistant cells. These mutations may be secondary to intrinsic genetic instability as a property of cancer cells. According to this hypothesis, it is important to use as many drugs as possible in doses as high as possible, as soon as possible, to diminish maximally the number of mutations taking place. It is advisable to give full doses whenever possible rather than to reduce dosage in an attempt to prevent toxicity.

A major advance in the understanding of drug resistance resulted from the study of malignant cell lines resistant to multiple drugs, including colchicine, doxorubicin, vinblastine, and tactinomycin. This phenomenon is associated with an increase in the expression of a plasma-membrane glycoprotein, which appears to interfere with intracellular drug accumulation.

Despite these limitations, major advances in the treatment of disseminated malignancy have resulted from the successful use of the best available chemotherapeutic agents in the most effective manner. Some disseminated malignancies such as acute lymphoblastic leukemia of childhood, advanced Hodgkin's disease, diffuse histiocytic lymphoma, nodular mixed lymphoma, testicular tumors, ovarian carcinomas, choriocarcinomas of pregnancy, and Burkitt's lymphomas are curable by chemotherapy. Wilms' tumor, Ewing's sarcoma, and embryonal rhabdomyosarcoma are curable by multimodality therapy, of which chemotherapy is an integral part. In many other cancers the use of chemotherapy provides significant improvement in the quality and duration of life.

It must be emphasized that chemotherapy, although usually the mainstay of therapy for disseminated cancer, is not the only modality available for these patients. Judicious use of radiation therapy for such situations as bone pain and bronchial obstruction, as well as surgical relief of gastrointestinal obstruction, is invaluable and is further discussed in the section "Supportive care."

Chemotherapy

Compounds active in cancer treatment are usually cytotoxic. These agents exercise their effects on cell proliferation by interfering with DNA synthesis or transcription, damaging preformed DNA, blocking mitosis, or inhibiting RNA or protein biosynthesis. The following are the major types of chemotherapeutic agents:

I. Antimetabolites
  A. Folic acid antagonists
    1. Methotrexate
  B. Pyrimidine antagonists
    1. Cytosine arabinoside
    2. 5-Fluorouracil
  C. Purine antagonists
    1. 6-Mercaptopurine
    2. 6-Thioguanine
II. Natural products
  A. Antitumor antibiotics
    1. Dactinomycin
    2. Mithramycin
    3. Bleomycin
    4. Mitomycin C
    5. Doxorubicin
    6. Daunorubicin
  B. Vinca alkaloids
    1. Vinblastine
    2. Vincristine
  C. Enzymes
    1. Asparaginase
  D. Podophyllins
    1. Etoposide (VP 16)
III. Alkylating agents
  A. Mechlorethamine (nitrogen mustard)
  B. Cyclophosphamide
  C. Melphalan
  D. Chlorambucil
  E. Busulfan
  F. Nitrosoureas (BCNU, CCNU, methyl CCNU, streptozocin)
  G. DTIC (Dacarbazine)
IV. Miscellaneous agents
  A. Cisplatin
  B. Hydroxyurea
  C. Procarbazine

These agents are usually classified as cell cycle–specific and cell cycle–nonspecific agents. Cell cycle–specific agents are those that either are active at a specific point in the cell cycle (cycle-phase specific) or kill proliferating cells more effectively than resting cells. For example, cytosine arabinoside inhibits DNA synthesis in the S phase. Other agents that inhibit DNA synthesis, such as methotrexate and 6-mercaptopurine, also inhibit RNA and protein synthesis. These effects slow down the cell cycle and the number of cells entering the S phase, so that the action of these antimetabolites is somewhat self limited. The vinca alkaloids (vinblastine and vincristine) arrest mitosis in metaphase by interfering with the synthesis of proteins necessary for spindle formation. The cell cycle–nonspecific agents are those that interfere in various ways with the function of preformed DNA and are thus not dependent on the cell cycle for their effect. Among the mechanisms of action of these agents are cross-linkage (alkylating agents), depolymerization (procarbazine, dacarbazine or DTIC, cisplatin, nitrosoureas), intercalation with blockage of RNA synthesis (anthracycline antibiotics, actinomycin D, mitomycin C), and scission of DNA strands (bleomycin).

A brief summary of the important properties and toxicities of the most frequently used chemotherapeutic agents follows.

ANTIMETABOLITES

Folic acid antagonists. Methotrexate, the first antimetabolite used clinically as an antitumor agent, acts by inhibiting the enzyme dihydrofolate reductase, which catalyzes the reaction of dihydrofolate to tetrahydrofolate. The result of this inhibition is a block in the conversion of deoxyuridine to thymidylate and thus in DNA synthesis. RNA and protein synthesis are also inhibited by lack of tetrahydrofolate. Methotrexate is readily absorbed orally and is administered either by mouth or intravenously in various dosage schedules. Its plasma half-life is approximately 2 hours, and about half of it is bound to plasma proteins. It is excreted unchanged primarily through the urine.

These properties of methotrexate must be considered when determining dosage of the drug. Displacement from plasma albumin by simultaneous administration of salicylates, sulfonamide, tetracycline, chloramphenicol, or phenytoin can result in a significant increase in toxicity. Likewise, decreased renal function can result in dangerously prolonged blood levels.

Methotrexate in high doses with leucovorin (folinic acid) rescue has been used in the treatment of some malignant tumors in an effort to increase the inhibition of DNA synthesis. Leucovorin is given after the administration of high doses of methotrexate to rescue normal cells. Malignant cells seem less capable of being rescued.

The major toxic effects of methotrexate are myelosuppression, ulcerative mucositis, and alopecia. Rarer complications include interstitial pneumonitis and hepatic dysfunction that occasionally results in cirrhosis.

Pyrimidine antagonists. Cytosine arabinoside is an S phase inhibitor whose principle mode of action appears to be inhibition of DNA polymerase. It is rapidly deaminated to an inactive metabolite that is excreted in the urine. The drug may be administered intravenously or subcutaneously. Its most important toxic effect is severe bone marrow depression with megaloblastic changes. Stomatitis, gastrointestinal disturbances, hepatic dysfunction, dermatitis, and fever also occur.

5-Fluorouracil (5-FU) is an inhibitor of thymidylate synthetase and thus of DNA synthesis. It is degraded in the liver and excreted in the urine. 5-FU is usually administered intravenously, although there is significant absorption when administered orally. The compound is myelosuppressive and also causes stomatitis, nausea, vomiting, and diarrhea. Hyperpigmentation of the skin and nails and, more rarely, cerebellar ataxia may occur.

Purine antagonists. 6-Mercaptopurine, a hypoxanthine analog, interferes with de novo purine biosynthesis and interconversions. The drug is well absorbed from the gastrointestinal tract and is administered orally. It is metabolized to 6-thiouric acid and inorganic sulfate, which as excreted in the urine. Allopurinol, a xanthine oxidase inhibitor usually used to block uric acid formation, also blocks the metabolism of 6-mercaptopurine. When the two drugs are given simultaneously, the dose of 6-mercaptopurine must be reduced to prevent serious toxicity. The major toxic effect of 6-mercaptopurine is bone marrow suppression. Reversible cholestatic jaundice may develop in up to one third of adult patients taking the drug.

6-Thioguanine acts similarly to 6-mercaptopurine and is also usually given orally. It is currently used primarily in combination with other agents in the treatment of acute myelogenous leukemia.

NATURAL PRODUCTS

Antitumor antibiotics. Dactinomycin forms a complex with DNA, resulting in the inhibition of DNA-dependent RNA synthesis. It is administered intravenously and is caustic if extravasation occurs. It causes myelosuppression and gastrointestinal disturbances.

Mithramycin interferes with RNA synthesis and probably inhibits osteoclastic activity. It is administered intravenously and is more often used for its unique calcium-lowering effect than for its antineoplastic activity. The drug must be administered with great care because of the possibility of the development of a severe hemorrhagic diathesis resulting from a combination of thrombocytopenia, multiple coagulation abnormalities, and capillary damage. Other side effects are bone marrow suppression and gastrointestinal, renal, and hepatic abnormalities.

Bleomycin is a mixture of glycopeptide antibiotics that acts both by inhibition of DNA synthesis and by scission of DNA strands. It can be administered either intravenously or intramuscularly and is excreted by the kidneys. Preferential localization occurs in the lung and skin owing to failure of inactivation by the tissues of these organs. This phenomenon probably accounts for the peculiar toxicity of bleomycin. Serious pulmonary damage may occur, usually after a total dose of over 300 mg (units)/m². Pulmonary toxicity begins as pneumonitis and in 15% to 20% of cases progresses to fibrosis, which is fatal in about 1% of patients. Multiple dermatologic abnormalities such as ulceration, hyperkeratosis, and hyperpigmentation are common. Stomatitis, alopecia, and fever also sometimes occur. Because of reports of anaphylactoid reactions in patients with lymphomas receiving bleomycin, a test dose of 1 to 2 units is recommended before starting therapy.

Mitomycin C appears to form a cross-linkage with DNA after intracellular enzymatic reduction. It is administered intravenously, and extravasation may result in serious local tissue damage. Its toxic effect is primarily myelosuppression, with gastrointestinal, renal, pulmonary, and mucocutaneous effects also reported.

Doxorubicin and daunorubicin act by binding to DNA with untwisting of the helix to permit intercalation of the drug skeleton. Both these agents are administered intravenously and cause local tissue necrosis if even a small amount is extravasated. Metabolic degradation occurs in the liver, and severe toxicity can result if standard doses are given to patients with reduced liver function. Excretion of the drugs and their metabolites is primarily through the bile. Myelosuppression, nausea, vomiting, and alopecia are all major side effects of these agents. Patients should be warned that their urine will turn red for 1 to 2 days. The most serious toxic effect of these drugs is the development of cardiomyopathy. Two types of cardiotoxicity are recognized. The first or acute variety is characterized by ST-T wave changes, arrhythmias, and an acute reversible reduction in ejection fraction occurring 24 hours after a single dose. This reaction is usually brief and of no serious consequence. Chronic toxicity, however, is cumulative and dose related. It results in congestive heart failure, which is unresponsive to digitalis and carries a mortality rate of greater than 50%. The mechanism of the cardiomyopathy is unclear, but binding to cardiac DNA and oxidative damage have been implicated. Significant cardiotoxicity develops in 20% of patients taking doxorubicin at a total dose greater than 550 mg/m², with reports of toxicity at doses as low as 250 mg/m². For daunorubicin the critical dose appears to be 600 mg/m². Previous irradiation of the mediastinum, treatment with cyclophosphamide, and advanced age increase the risk of cardiotoxicity. No dependable predictive tests are generally available, and the onset of congestive heart failure is often delayed. Half of the cases occur longer than 6 months from the completion of therapy.

Vinca alkaloids. Vinca alkaloids are products of the periwinkle plant that interfere with the metaphase through spindle protein damage. Although there is great structural similarity between vinblastine and vincristine, the two alkaloids in current use, there are significant differences in cytotoxic action and little cross-resistance. The compounds are administered intravenously and cause local tissue damage if extravasated. They are cleared rapidly from the bloodstream and are excreted through the biliary tract.

Vinblastine is a bone marrow depressant, and gastrointestinal disturbances are common. Neurotoxicity and alopecia are only minor problems with vinblastine. Vincristine, unlike vinblastine, is not myelosuppressive. Its major toxic effect is neurologic, with paresthesias, loss of deep tendon reflexes, paresis, ptosis, and double vision. Severe constipation may occur, and all patients receiving vincristine should be given prophylactic stool softeners. Alopecia and inappropriate antidiuretic hormone secretion are other important side effects.

Etoposide. Etoposide (VP-16) is an epipodophyllotoxin that causes metaphase arrest but is not a spindle poison, such as the vinca alkaloids. It is active when administered either intravenously or orally. Toxicity is primarily hematologic. Alopecia, nausea, and vomiting also occur.

Asparaginase. Asparaginase, an enzyme prepared from *Escherichia coli*, catalyzes the hydrolysis of plasma asparagine to aspartic acid and ammonia. Although normal cells can synthesize asparagine, certain neoplastic cells lack asparagine synthetase and depend on exogenous asparagine. When malignant cells are exposed to asparaginase, they develop a selective nutritional deficiency. Although the drug has resulted in remission in up to 60% of children with acute lymphocytic leukemia, its usefulness is limited by anaphylactic and other allergic reactions. Resistance to the enzyme develops rapidly, and remissions are short lived. Other side effects of the inhibition of protein synthesis are mild decreases in hepatic, renal, pancreatic, and coagulation functions.

ALKYLATING AGENTS. The alkylating agents generate highly reactive electrophilic carbonium ions that alkylate with nucleophilic substances by forming covalent linkages. Cross-linkage of adjacent macromolecules may follow, with inhibition of mitosis resulting from prevention of separation of the DNA strands. Cell death may also occur during interphase when many targets, including RNA and protein, are damaged.

Mechlorethamine (nitrogen mustard) is very quickly bound to proteins or intracellular macromolecules. Almost none is excreted in the urine. Intravenous administration of nitrogen mustard must be very carefully performed, usually into the tubing of a rapidly flowing infusion, since thrombophlebitis may occur when high concentrations are in prolonged direct contact with the intima of the injected vein. The drug also has a local vesicant action. Nitrogen mustard may be instilled in body cavities for the control of malignant effusions. Its major toxic effects are myelosuppression, nausea, and vomiting. As with all alkylating agents, gonadal suppression often resulting in permanent sterility, particularly in males, is frequent. The patient should be informed of this possibility before starting any of these agents.

Cyclophosphamide is activated by hepatic microsomal enzymes, and therefore microsomal stimulators such as barbiturates increase its activity and toxicity. It can be administered either orally or intravenously. Bone marrow suppression and alopecia are important side effects. The accumulation of metabolites in concentrated urine causes a sterile hemorrhagic cystitis in about 5% of the patients. To avoid this complication, ample fluid intake and frequent voiding should be recommended to all patients taking cyclophosphamide. Occasional cases of pulmonary interstitial fibrosis attributed to cyclophosphamide have been reported.

Melphalan (L-phenylalanine mustard), chlorambucil, and busulfan are all alkylating agents that are well absorbed from the gastrointestinal tract. They are moderately myelosuppressive. Busulfan has been associated with pulmonary fibrosis.

The mechanism of action of the nitrosourea compounds is closely related to that of the alkylating agents. Active metabolites are probably responsible for their cytotoxic activity. An important feature of the nitrosoureas is their ability to cross the blood-brain barrier, with levels from 15% to 50% of plasma levels attainable in the cerebrospinal fluid. BCNU (carmustine) is administered intravenously through a running infusion. CCNU (lomustine) and methyl-CCNU (semustine) are well absorbed orally. Nausea, vomiting, and delayed bone marrow suppression are prominent side effects of this group of drugs, and pulmonary fibrosis has been reported. Streptozocin (streptozotocin), a naturally occurring nitrosourea, has a diabetogenic effect. Side effects include mild myelosuppression, nausea, and vomiting, hepatic damage, and severe proximal tubular renal toxicity.

Dacarbazine (dimethyltriazmo-imidazole carboxamide, DTIC) behaves like an alkylating agent. It is administered intravenously and activated in the liver. Myelosuppression and gastrointestinal disturbances are the major toxic effects. Fever, myalgias, malaise, alopecia, facial flushing, and hepatotoxicity have also been reported.

MISCELLANEOUS AGENTS. The platinum-coordinating complexes are capable of cross-linking with DNA. More than 90% of cisplatin (cis-diamminedichloroplatinum II) is protein bound and appears to be excreted primarily in the urine. Renal tubular toxicity is a major problem, and the drug should be cautiously administered with meticulous attention to concomitant administration of intravenous fluids. Mannitol with or without furosemide has been recommended as an additional safeguard to ensure adequate diuresis. Platinum is also myelotoxic and ototoxic. Baseline renal function should be assessed before instituting therapy.

Hydroxyurea is an S phase–specific agent that inhibits DNA synthesis. It is well absorbed orally and is largely excreted in the urine. The toxic effects include myelosuppression, gastrointestinal disturbances, and stomatitis. Occasionally alopecia, dermatitis, or neurologic manifestations occur.

Procarbazine, a compound whose basic mode of action is poorly understood, is capable of inhibiting DNA, RNA, and protein synthesis. It is absorbed from the gastrointestinal tract and metabolized by the liver. The metabolites are excreted in the urine. Bone marrow suppression and gastrointestinal disturbances are the major side effects. Because the drug is a weak monoamine oxidase inhibitor, sympathomimetics, tricyclic antidepressants, and other medications or foods with high tyramine content should not be taken concomitantly. Augmentation of the mild sedative effects of procarbazine has been seen with simultaneous use of central nervous system depressants, and ingestion of ethyl alcohol has resulted in an acetaldehyde syndrome resembling that produced by disulfiram.

PRINCIPLES OF COMBINATION CHEMOTHERAPY. In almost all situations, combination chemotherapy has proved more effective than single-agent regimens in the treatment of cancer. The principles of rational combinations are listed in the following:

1. Each drug must be individually active in the specific disease being treated.
2. Agents that produce different biochemical lesions should be combined, so that multiple sites of proliferation or function of cells may be attacked.
3. Agents having different toxicities should be selected, allowing a therapeutic dose of each to be employed with little or no increased risk.
4. Combining drugs whose toxicities occur at different times following administration also allows use of larger doses.
5. Agents in which there is a biochemical basis for suspecting synergism should be combined.

Hormonal manipulation

HORMONAL RECEPTORS. The growth of some tumors appears to depend on their hormonal environment, and many patients with carcinoma of the breast, prostate, and endometrium respond to endocrine manipulation. The mechanism of action of either additive or ablative procedures in carcinoma of the breast has recently been clarified, making the choice of therapy more rational than previously possible. It is known that the initial step in steroid hormone action is the binding of the hormone to highly specialized receptor proteins in the target cells. Cytoplasmic receptors have been identified for several steroid hormones. Binding of the hormone to the receptor initiates a series of steps, eventually leading to the characteristic hormonal effect on the target tissue. The presence of receptor protein appears to be necessary for hormonal responsiveness. Receptors for estrogen are present in about two thirds of primary breast cancers, with a somewhat lower rate of positivity in metastatic lesions. Tumors in premenopausal women are estrogen receptor (ER) positive in less than 50% of cases, and those in postmenopausal patients are positive in more than 50%. Objective responses to endocrine manipulation occur in 50% to 70% of patients whose tumors are ER positive, whereas only 5% to 10% of ER-negative patients respond. Progesterone receptors (PR) are found in about two thirds of ER-positive tumors and in about 5% of ER-negative tumors. The highest response rate to endocrine therapy (80%) is in tumors that are both ER positive and PR positive. It is of utmost importance to obtain receptor assays in all patients with breast cancer at the time of histologic diagnosis as a guide to future therapy. When metastatic disease occurs, it may involve a site inaccessible to biopsy, and a valuable tool in therapeutic planning is unavailable. The presence or absence of hormonal receptors also appears to have prognostic value. Estrogen receptor positivity seems to be correlated with a prolonged disease-free interval that is independent of other variables. Data relating ER status to response to chemotherapy are conflicting, and further studies are needed to resolve this issue.

Other steroid hormone receptors such as androgen and glucocorticoid receptors are found in some breast tumors. Their relevance in predicting therapeutic response has not been ascertained. Steroid receptors also exist in carcinoma of the prostate and endometrium and in malignant melanoma. The clinical significance in these tumors is uncertain.

SURGICAL ABLATION. Oophorectomy is useful in premenopausal women with metastatic or recurrent breast cancer whose tumors are ER positive, who have had a long disease-free interval, and whose metastatic sites are bone and soft tissues rather than viscera.

Previously common surgical ablative procedures designed to diminish estrogen effect, such as bilateral adrenalectomy and hypophysectomy, have largely been replaced by the use of aminoglutethimide, an inhibitor of the conversion to pregnenolone in the adrenal gland, and of the antiestrogen tamoxifen.

Orchiectomy for stage IV (distant metastases) prostatic carcinoma was first suggested by Charles B. Huggins in 1941. About 80% of the patients respond with reduction of bone pain and size of tumor mass. Occasionally, skeletal metastases show roentgenographic evidence of healing. Orchiectomy currently is the treatment of choice in men for whom estrogen administration is contraindicated.

HORMONE ADMINISTRATION. Estrogens such as diethylstilbestrol are useful in the management of metastatic breast cancer in postmenopausal women with ER-positive or unknown receptor status. Because of the troublesome side effects of estrogen (including nausea, vomiting, and edema), its use in breast cancer has largely been supplanted by the use of the antiestrogen tamoxifen, which appears to be equally effective with fewer side effects. Approximately 60% of patients with ER-positive breast cancer can be expected to respond to hormonal manipulation. Response is best when metastases are confined to bone or soft tissue.

Diethylstilbestrol, in doses of 3 mg/day, appears to be therapeutically effective in men with metastatic prostate cancer. Higher dosages lead to a high incidence of hypertension and cardiac complications without an increased therapeutic effect. In patients with preexisting cardiac disease, orchiectomy is the treatment of choice for metastatic prostate carcinoma.

Androgenic steroids are useful in premenopausal women with metastatic breast carcinoma who have previously had responses to hormonal manipulation. The masculinizing effects of these hormones, however, are often intolerable to patients, and their usefulness is severely limited.

Progestins have produced significant responses in about 30% of patients with metastatic endometrial carcinoma. There is evidence that some progestins act as antiestrogens and have proved useful in ER-positive metastatic breast cancer. Occasional improvement in metastatic renal cell carcinoma has been observed with progestational agents.

Prednisone is a cornerstone of therapy for the lymphoproliferative disorders. It causes lymphocyte lysis, presumably by inhibition of cellular protein synthesis. Specific receptors for corticosteroids have been found in acute lymphocytic leukemia. The beneficial effect of prednisone in carcinoma of the breast may be caused by suppression of adrenocortical estrogen production. Dexamethasone, which is used primarily to reduce edema surrounding brain tumors, may exert a direct antitumor effect against glioblastomas. Recent additions to the therapeutic armamentarium include luteinizing hormone-releasing hormone (LHRH) analogs and antiandrogens, which are useful in the management of metastatic prostate cancer.

Biologic response modifiers

The biologic response modifiers are agents that modify the host's biologic response to tumor cells with a resulting therapeutic benefit. They make up a heterogeneous group including cell products (for example, lymphokines), monoclonal antibodies, and external agents (for example, Bacillus Calmette-Guerin [BCG]). Basically, these agents act either by immunostimulation, cytotoxicity, or a combination of both.

Hundreds of products have been identified and are currently undergoing investigation; only a few have reached the stage of clinical trials.

INTERFERONS. Interferons are potent antiviral glycoproteins that also inhibit the multiplication of tumor cells in experimental systems. Currently, interferon (α) is indicated for the treatment of hairy cell leukemia and chronic myelogenous leukemia. Clinical trials have demonstrated some activity in melanoma, non-Hodgkin's lymphomas, renal cell carcinoma, and multiple myeloma. Monoclonal antibodies are produced by immunizing mice with a selected antigen (for example, tumor cells). Antibody-producing B cells are then harvested from the mouse spleen and fused with mouse myeloma cells. The resultant hybrid cells produce antibodies in unlimited quantities. Therapeutically these antibodies can be used alone or as part of a conjugate with a cytotoxic agent or radioactive isotope in an attempt to kill target tumor cells. Currently, therapeutic monoclonal antibodies are available only through clinical trials. Early results with nodular non-Hodgkin's lymphomas have been encouraging.

Interleukin 2 is a lymphokine that augments the cytotoxicity of several types of lymphocytes. It is currently in extensive clinical trials following early reports of its effectiveness in chemotherapy-resistant tumors, such as colon and renal cell carcinoma and melanoma. Growth factors for various hematoporetic cells (that is, granulocyte-monocyte colony stimulating factor [GM-CSF]) are being evaluated for their effectiveness in shortening the period of post-chemotherapy neutrogenia.

Supportive care

OBSTRUCTION AND COMPRESSION. The superior vena cava syndrome associated with malignancy is most effectively treated by radiation therapy. Diuretics and corticosteroids may offer some benefit but should not be relied on as definitive therapy. The degree of emergency in each case must be carefully evaluated. In patients for whom no previous histologic diagnosis is available, radiation therapy may render such a diagnosis difficult or impossible. When symptoms are mild, it is often possible to delay irradiation until tissue can be obtained. When there is evidence of significantly increased venous pressure, however, procedures such as mediastinoscopy or bronchoscopy may be hazardous. If a firm diagnosis of oat cell carcinoma has been established, chemotherapy alone may provide rapid relief of symptoms.

Bronchial airway obstruction resulting from direct tumor invasion or external compression by enlarged nodes and neoplastic obstruction of the esophagus should be treated with radiation therapy. Small bowel obstruction caused by malignancy is usually caused by extrinsic compression, whereas obstruction of the large bowel is usually the result of a primary colon tumor. In either case surgical removal of the obstructing lesion is the treatment of choice. When the primary tumor is a lymphoma or ovarian carcinoma, radiation may be effective in relieving the obstruction. Partial or complete obstruction of the biliary tree, usually from an infiltrating carcinoma of the head of the pancreas, is treated by surgical decompression. Ureteral obstruction can result from direct invasion by pelvic tumors or from extrinsic compression by enlarged lymph nodes. Uremia caused by ureteral obstruction is the major cause of death from cervical carcinoma. If the site of obstruction is identifiable and localized, radiation therapy may be effective. With more diffuse obstruction, diverting surgery may be necessary.

Epidural spinal cord compression should be treated as soon as it is recognized and the diagnosis is established by myelography. Irradiation may be used as initial therapy for patients with slowly progressing neurologic symptoms and signs and for those whose tumors are known to be radiation sensitive. Decompressive surgery is indicated for patients with rapidly progressive neurologic defects, especially if the tumor is radiation resistant. Peripheral nerve or plexus compression of recent onset may be relieved by radiation therapy, but the effects of long-standing compression are usually irreversible.

METABOLIC DERANGEMENT. *Hypercalcemia* of mild to moderate degree usually responds to ambulation, hydration with saline solutions, and diuresis. Severe or refractory hypercalcemia can be effectively treated with mithramycin, 25 μg/kg. Doses can be repeated at 3- to 7-day intervals. Calcitonin, corticosteroids, and prostaglandin inhibitors such as indomethacin are also useful in lowering serum calcium levels. Biphosphonates have recently been shown to be effective in lowering serum calcium in malignancy-induced hypercalcemia.

Hyponatremia resulting from inappropriate antidiuretic hormone (ADH) secretion can be corrected by water restriction. Demeclocycline, which inhibits the action of ADH on the kidneys, is effective in treating this syndrome. As in all ectopic hormonal syndromes, treatment of the primary tumor is the most effective way to eliminate the endocrine abnormalities.

MALIGNANT EFFUSIONS. Intrapleural instillation of sclerosing agents in an attempt to obliterate the pleural space is the standard therapy for recurrent pleural effusions in patients with cancer. Among the agents used have been chemotherapeutic drugs (nitrogen mustard, thioTEPA, 5-FU, bleomycin), quinacrine, talc, and tetracycline. If the effusion is caused by central lymphatic obstruction, irradiation of the mediastinum may be beneficial. Malignant pericardial effusions often require the surgical creation of a pleuropericardial window to prevent tamponade. Intrapericardial instillation of sclerosing agents has also successfully controlled such effusions.

Although intraperitoneal instillation of sclerosing agents has been used for intractable ascites in patients with cancer, it is rarely successful, and repeated paracenteses may be the only way to relieve this troublesome complication.

NUTRITIONAL PROBLEMS. Weight loss can seriously limit the cancer patient's quality of life and ability to tolerate intensive antineoplastic therapy. Since anorexia is often a prominent symptom, maintenance of adequate nutrition often requires the use of dietary supplements. These products supply calories in concentrated form. If it is impossible to achieve adequate nutrition orally, total parenteral nutrition (TPN) should be considered for patients in whom primary therapy for tumor control is possible. The solutions of 50% glucose, mixtures of essential amino acids, and vitamins used in TPN can provide up to 3000 calories a day. Gradual increases of glucose concentration usually prevent the hyperosmolar, nonketotic coma that has occasionally been associated with TPN.

PAIN. Half of all patients with cancer never experience disease-related pain, 30% have mild to moderate pain, and 20% have severe pain. With proper management, all patients with cancer can be rendered essentially pain free. A major stumbling block to achieving this goal has been the fear of addiction. In a patient with advanced cancer and pain that is unresponsive to local measures such as radiation therapy, adequate analgesics should be prescribed on a regular rather than "when necessary" basis. Attention should be paid to the frequency of medication. Meperidine has a short half-life (2 hours) and therefore is ineffective on an every-4-hour schedule. Morphine, hydromorphone, and levorphanol are better choices if narcotics are required.

Pain medication should be given orally whenever possible. The recent availability of morphine in both elixir and oral long-acting forms has led to greater flexibility and effectiveness of oral narcotic administration. If oral treatment is inadequate, administration of morphine by infusion pumps has proved effective. Morphine can be administered subcutaneously, intravenously, or intrathecally through the use of these devices. Some of the pumps include a mechanism for self-adjustment of dose, within limits prescribed by the physician.

Since all opiates are constipating, stool softeners should be prescribed routinely to patients receiving narcotics.

INFECTION. Infection is a frequent complication of malignant tumors and of antineoplastic therapy. Advanced cancer itself is often accompanied by a depressed immune response. Intensive chemotherapy and/or radiation therapy results in temporary immunosuppression and granulocytopenia, further increasing the already compromised patient's susceptibility to infection. Finally, local factors such as bronchial or ureteral obstruction make patients susceptible to infection in areas of poor drainage.

A particularly serious problem is the management of infection in the neutropenic, immunosuppressed host. Gram-negative bacteria are the most common pathogenic organisms in these patients, with *Pseudomonas aeruginosa, Escherichia coli,* and *Klebsiella-Enterobacter* organisms responsible for the largest number of infections. In many febrile episodes neither the source of infection nor the offending organism is identified despite aggressive diagnostic procedures. Since sepsis in the neutropenic patient can progress rapidly to a fatal conclusion, the physician should institute empiric combination antibiotic therapy while awaiting results of diagnostic studies. The most frequently recommended initial combination is an aminoglycoside with an antipseudomonal agent. This regimen should be appropriately modified when the pathogen is identified and sensitivity studies are completed. An increasing number of serious fungal infections are being recognized in cancer patients, with disseminated candidiasis, aspergillosis, and mucormycosis seen most often. Cryptococcosis is common in patients with lymphoma. The use of amphotericin B in febrile, neutropenic patients who have not responded to antibiotic therapy has been suggested by some. Neutropenic, immunsuppressed patients are particularly susceptible to infection by *Pneumocystis carinii*. If this diagnosis is suspected, the empiric use of trimethoprim-sulfamethoxazole is recommended.

Prophylaxis of infection in immunosuppressed patients should be vigorously pursued. Prolonged infusions, indwelling catheters, and endoscopies should be kept to a minimum. Careful attention should be paid to handwashing technique and frequent changes of intravenous infusion sites. Protective environments, such as laminar flow rooms and life islands, and the use of oral nonabsorbable antibiotics have resulted in decreased numbers of infections but not in increased overall survival in immunosuppressed patients.

HEMORRHAGE. The most frequent cause of hemorrhage in patients with cancer is thrombocytopenia, which may be a result of the cancer itself but more commonly is a side effect of cytoreductive therapy. Bleeding rarely occurs with platelet counts more than $20,000/mm^3$. For counts less than this level, prophylactic platelet transfusions should be administered. If repeated transfusions are anticipated, attempts should be made to obtain HLA-matched platelets to delay the appearance of antibodies and resistance to transfusion.

Disseminated intravascular coagulation (DIC) is occasionally responsible for bleeding in patients with cancer. The best treatment for DIC is treatment of the primary disease. Heparin is rarely indicated but may be lifesaving in the treatment of DIC in promyelocytic granulocytic leukemia.

TUMOR LYSIS SYNDROME. The rapid lysis of sensitive tumors following chemotherapy releases intracellular phosphate, resulting in hypocalcemia. Intracellular potassium is also released by lysing tumor cells. Potentially fatal cardiotoxicity from hypocalcemia and hyperpotassemia can be prevented by adequate hydration before chemotherapy. Hyperuricemia results from excessive uric acid production caused by tumor cell breakdown. Allopurinol should be administered whenever substantial tumor lysis is anticipated.

PSYCHOSOCIAL PROBLEMS. Perhaps the greatest challenge to the physician dealing with cancer patients is the management of the enormous emotional, social, and economic impact of the disease on patients and their families. Empathy, tact, and compassion are necessary from the time of diagnosis. It is generally agreed that it is preferable for patients to know the diagnosis, particularly if aggressive therapy is planned. They should be given an honest explanation of the illness and of the proposed treatment in terms thay can understand. Every allowable hope should be offered. If patients are not informed of the true nature of their disease, they will lose trust and confidence in their physicians and families as their condition deteriorates. Clergy, social workers, and oncology nurses all can contribute their own special skills in supporting the patient and family through the difficult postdiagnosis period. It is essential for the physician to keep the family informed throughout the course of the patient's illness and to be available to answer questions.

Vigorous attempts to keep the patient at home for as long as possible should be made, using all existing community agencies. It is often feasible to keep a patient at home with the help of a hospital bed, bedside commode, and a visiting nurse to give parenteral medication. If pain medication must be given frequently, a family member can be taught to administer it.

The hospice movement, emphasizing home care and comfortable homelike surroundings when inpatient care is necessary, is gaining momentum in the United States. The hospice concept allows unlimited family visits, including children and pets. Meticulous attention is paid to the control of pain, bowel disturbances, and other distressing symptoms of advanced cancer. A most important function of the hospice team is counseling of and continued contact with the bereaved family after the patient's death.

During the terminal period it is essential that the physician not withdraw from dying patients. Hospitalized patients should be seen daily. They should be given the opportunity to talk, and the physician should take the time to listen. Physical contact and continued attention to symptoms lessen the fears of abandonment and depersonalization characteristic of the last phases of a lingering, fatal disease.

MANAGEMENT OF SPECIFIC MALIGNANCIES
Carcinoma of the lung

Accurate histologic diagnosis is essential to planning proper management of lung cancers. Small cell or oat cell carcinoma, the most rapidly growing of all lung tumors, is usually disseminated by the time of diagnosis, and therefore surgery has no role in the primary management of this disease. The median survival of untreated persons with oat cell carcinoma is less than 4 months. Fortunately, this aggressive tumor is responsive to both radiation therapy and chemotherapy. Current drug combinations give response rates of 60% to 100%, with temporary complete response in 20% to 50% of cases. The most active agents in the treatment of small cell carcinoma are cyclophosphamide, doxorubicin, vincristine, cisplatin, and etoposide. Multimodality programs combining irradiation of the primary tumor and chemotherapy have produced somewhat higher response rates, but survival appears to be the same with or without radiation. The median survival for treated metastatic small cell carcinoma is approximately 8 to 10 months, and that for apparently limited disease is 12 to 15 months. Some patients are now surviving in a disease-free state for more than 2 years. Since 10% of patients have intracerebral metastases at the time of diagnosis and 30% have central nervous system involvement at autopsy, prophylactic cranial irradiation is now included in many treatment programs.

Epidermoid, or squamous cell, carcinoma, the most frequent lung cancer, is slower growing and has the lowest rate of distant metastases and a high frequency of local complications. Only 20% to 30% of patients have surgically resectable disease at diagnosis, since the disease has a long asymptomatic period. Even if no distant spread is obvious, involvement of mediastinal lymph nodes or proximity to the great vessels makes surgical removal inadvisable. Potentially curative radiation therapy should be considered as primary therapy for unresectable lesions confined to the hemithorax. The use of adjuvant chemotherapy following curative surgery or radiation therapy has not resulted in prolongation of the disease-free interval or survival and is not recommended except in an investigational setting. Chemotherapy for recurrent or metastatic epidermoid lung carcinoma has been only modestly effective. The best available agents are cisplatin, the vinca alkaloids, and etoposide. If possible, patients should be entered into randomized, controlled, prospective trials to attempt to improve the current 15% to 35% response rate.

Adenocarcinoma of the lung is intermediate between small cell and epidermoid carcinomas in its growth rate, speed of hematogenous spread, and resectability. Combination chemotherapy and multimodality trials are in progress in the management of metastatic disease.

Gastrointestinal cancer

CARCINOMA OF THE ESOPHAGUS. Primary treatment of squamous cell carcinoma of the esophagus involves surgery, radiation, or both. Long-term survival is rare, and, in an attempt to improve the generally dismal results, studies that use chemotherapy in an attempt to shrink the tumor before definitive local therapy is begun are under way. A regimen of bleomycin, vinblastine, and platinum has shown preliminary promise.

CARCINOMA OF THE STOMACH. Surgery is the treatment of choice for adenocarcinoma of the stomach. Even if there is extensive disease, resection of the lesion to prevent bleeding or obstruction should be performed. Of all alimentary tract carcinomas, gastric cancer is the most sensitive to chemotherapy.

A combination of 5-fluorouracil (5-FU), adriamycin, and mitomycin C (FAM) has proved beneficial in approximately 40% of cases of advanced or metastatic gastric cancers. Patients who respond show a modest prolongation of life. Locally recurrent or unresectable disease may benefit from a combined modality regimen of the same chemotherapy and radiation to the gastric bed. Research of adjuvant chemotherapy, with or without radiation therapy, following surgery with curative intent is under way.

COLORECTAL CANCER. Early diagnosis and surgical resection constitute the optimal primary management for colorectal cancers. The extent of surgery depends on the operative findings. If curative resection is impossible, the lesion should still be removed to prevent later bleeding or obstruction. The mainstay of medical therapy of metastatic colorectal cancer is 5-FU, administered intravenously in a variety of schedules. Despite initial enthusiastic reports of improved results with combinations of 5-FU and nitrosoureas, alkylating agents, vinca alkaloids, and other agents, these regimens appear to result in no greater survival than use of 5-FU alone. About 25% of treated patients have an objective response to this single agent. Repeated trials of postoperative adjuvant chemotherapy, with or without immunotherapy, have not resulted in any significant increase in 5-year survival, although all these studies have shown some slight benefit. At this time routine adjuvant chemotherapy for colorectal carcinoma is not recommended although early results of current randomized trials are encouraging.

Local symptoms of unresectable or recurrent rectal cancer, such as pain, tenesmus, and bleeding, can often be alleviated with palliative radiation therapy. Occasionally such radiation therapy may render a patient disease free. Since local recurrences account for 50% of relapses after complete resection of rectal cancer, preoperative or postoperative radiation has been employed in an attempt to prevent such recurrence.

PANCREATIC CANCER. Pancreatic cancer, whose incidence is increasing in the United States, has a negligible overall 5-year survival rate. Since only 5% of patients undergoing pancreatoduodenectomy are alive 5 years after the operation, the role of extensive surgery in the primary treatment of pancreatic carcinoma is controversial. Chemotherapy has been disappointing, although various combinations of 5-FU, mitomycin C, doxorubicin, and streptozocin produce objective responses in a minority of patients. External beam radiation, interstitial instillation of ^{125}I, and fast neutron radiation therapy are currently being evaluated in the treatment of pancreatic cancer.

Breast cancer

The traditional primary treatment of breast cancer has been radical or, more recently, modified radical mastectomy. The former removes the entire breast, all axillary nodes, and the pectoralis major muscle, whereas the latter preserves the pectoralis. Results of a large, cooperative, randomized study have demonstrated equally good results in early breast cancer from lesser surgery (lumpectomy or quadrantectomy) and axillary dissection followed by radiation therapy.

The single most important prognostic factor in predicting recurrence of breast cancer is the presence or absence of involvement of axillary lymph nodes at the time of primary therapy. Women with four or more positive nodes have an 80% chance of recurrence within 2 years, whereas those with negative axillary nodes have only a 20% chance of recurrence during the same period. Estrogen-receptor (ER) negativity has been demonstrated in a large proportion of women with negative nodes whose cancer does recur. Adjuvant use of systemic chemotherapy following surgery in premenopausal women with one to three positive axillary nodes significantly reduces the rate of recurrence up to 10 years after mastectomy. The most widely used regimen is 6 or 12 months of combination therapy with cyclophosphamide, methotrexate, and 5-FU. Other combinations and lengths of therapy are under investigation. Studies have failed to show a statistically significant advantage for postmenopausal women who have undergone adjuvant chemotherapy, but some data challenge these conclusions. Postmenopausal women with positive estrogen receptors benefit from the adjuvant use of the antiestrogen agent tamoxifen. Several large clinical trials have suggested an advantage for women with negative nodes through the use of adjuvant chemotherapy or hormonal treatment.

Therapy for advanced or recurrent breast cancer must be individualized depending on the sites of disease, menopausal status, and hormonal receptor status of each patient. Premenopausal women with positive estrogen receptors, a relatively long disease-free interval, and metastases limited to bone or soft tissue should have an oophorectomy or receive tamoxifen. Relapse following a good response to oophorectomy is usually followed by a second response to subsequent hormonal manipulation. ER-positive postmenopausal women with bone or soft tissue metastases should first be treated with estrogens or antiestrogens. In either of these groups, if there is no response to initial hormonal manipulation, if the disease-free interval is very short, or if there are visceral metastases, the patient should receive cytotoxic chemotherapy. Cytotoxic agents should be used as first-line therapy for all ER-negative tumors, since these patients have less than a 5% response rate after hormonal manipulation. Chemotherapeutic agents active against carcinoma of the breast are cyclophosphamide, doxorubicin, 5-FU, methotrexate, vincristine, and prednisone. Doxorubicin appears to be the single most effective agent.

Palliative radiation therapy for intracranial metastases and intractable bone pain is most important in achieving optimal quality of life for patients with advanced breast cancer.

Genitourinary tumors

RENAL CELL CARCINOMAS. Renal cell carcinomas should be surgically resected. Progestational agents or hydroxyurea has occasionally produced an objective decrease in the size of metastatic lesions, but both radiation therapy and chemotherapy have been generally disappointing in the treatment of renal cell tumors. There have been reports of regression of metastatic lesions following nephrectomy, and thus debulking of advanced tumors may be useful. Interferon and interleukin-2 have shown some benefit in 15% to 20% of cases in clinical trials.

CARCINOMA OF THE BLADDER. Low-grade transitional cell bladder cancers can be successfully treated by fulguration or transurethral resection followed by local instillation of cytotoxic agents. More aggressive tumors that invade the bladder wall require total cystectomy and radical radiation therapy. Response rates of 50% to 80% have been obtained in advanced bladder tumors with a regimen of methotrexate, vincristine, doxorubicin, and cisplatin.

CARCINOMA OF THE PROSTATE. Locally invasive tumors of the prostate may be treated by either radical prostatectomy or primary radiotherapy. Surgery is associated with a higher incidence of incontinence and impotence than is radiation. Symptomatic metastatic disease, especially painful bone lesions, should be treated with orchiectomy, diethylstilbestrol, or a lutenizing hormone-releasing hormone analog. Since cardiovascular complications are frequent with diethylstilbestrol, patients with a history of heart disease should have alternative treatment. The role of cytotoxic chemotherapy in advanced prostate cancer has not been firmly established, but there have been occasional responses to doxorubicin, cyclophosphamide, and 5-FU.

TESTICULAR CARCINOMA. Seminomas are exquisitely sensitive to both radiation therapy and chemotherapy. Almost all patients can be cured with radiation alone. If metastatic disease is present, single-agent chemotherapy is 90% effective.

Radical orchiectomy cures 75% to 80% of nonseminomatous tumors that are truly confined to the testes. The relative importance of lymphadenectomy and radiation therapy in the primary mangement of nonseminomatous tumors with nodal involvement is controversial. A major breakthrough resulting in potential curability of metastatic nonseminomatous testicular tumors has been the introduction of combination chemotherapy with vinblastine, bleomycin, and cisplatin. Other effective drugs are actinomycin, vincristine, cyclophosphamide, doxorubicin, and etoposide. The role of adjuvant chemotherapy in patients with paraaortic lymph node involvement at the time of initial surgery is uncertain. Since most of the patients at risk never have metastases because of adequate primary treatment, and since such an effective regimen for advanced disease is available, it may be more prudent to withhold chemotherapy until the appearance of metastases. These patients must be followed carefully with serum markers and frequent imaging studies.

Gynecologic cancers

CARCINOMA OF THE OVARY. Regardless of histologic type, the primary treatment of ovarian cancer is hysterectomy and bilateral salpingo-oophorectomy. Prophylactic partial omentectomy is often carried out because of the frequency of omental recurrence. Both single-drug and combination chemotherapy with alkylating agents, cisplatin, and doxorubicin achieve remission rates of up to 80%, with significant prolongation of life in patients who respond to chemotherapy. The exact role of radiation therapy in the overall management of ovarian carcinomas is under investigation as is the role of intraperitoneal chemotherapy.

ENDOMETRIAL CANCER. Endometrial tumors are most prevalent in obese, nulliparous women who often are diabetic or hypertensive or have a family history of this tumor. The primary treatment is surgery or radiotherapy, depending on the stage at presentation. Favorable responses are occasionally obtained in metastatic disease treated with progesterone, doxorubicin, and cyclophosphamide.

CARCINOMA OF THE CERVIX. Deaths from cervical carcinoma have dropped sharply following the introduction of Papanicolaou smears for early detection. A combined radiotherapeutic and surgical approach to therapy is recommended to achieve the best possible result for each patient. Chemotherapy has no proven value in the management of this disease.

Head and neck cancer

Squamous cell carcinomas constitute 90% of head and neck tumors. Lymphomas, adenocarcinomas, and salivary gland tumors account for the remaining neoplasms in this region. The most frequent primary sites are the lateral borders of the tongue, the floor of the mouth, gums, buccal mucosa, and lips. The majority of head and neck cancers occur in males, and there is a strong association with smoking and alcohol ingestion. Cancers in the oral cavity are often preceded by "premalignant" lesions such as leukoplakia or erythroplasia, so a thorough physical examination can serve as an extremely effective early detection device. Once they become invasive, these tumors spread locally and into regional lymph node chains. Distant metastases, most often to the lungs, are late and relatively uncommon. Head and neck cancers represent one of the most urgent indications for multimodality management. In early stages these lesions are often curable by appropriate surgical, radiotherapeutic, or combined therapy. Even if the tumor appears inoperable at the time of initial presentation, it is sometimes possible to convert it to operability by chemotherapy with a cisplatin containing regimen. Chemotherapy also can give dramatic, if short-lived, palliation in advanced local and metastatic disease.

Bone and soft tissue sarcomas

Osteogenic sarcoma, Ewing's sarcoma, and embryonal rhabdomyosarcoma are rapidly growing, early metastasizing tumors of young people. Appropriate multimodality treatment has resulted in prolonged survival and apparent cure in an increasing number of patients with these malignancies. In all cases as much of the tumor as possible should be removed, and postoperative irradiation of the tumor site should be considered. Systemic chemotherapy should be administered postoperatively even in the absence of detectable metastatic disease, since there is high risk of recurrence and effective chemotherapeutic agents are available.

Embryonal rhabdomyosarcoma responds to a combination of vincristine, dactinomycin, and cyclophosphamide, with 50% of patients enjoying a prolonged disease-free survival even in the face of metastatic disease. High-dose methotrexate with leukovorin rescue, doxorubicin, and cisplatin are effective as both adjuvant therapy and treatment of metastatic or recurrent osteogenic sarcoma. Isolated pulmonary metastases, apparently resistant to chemotherapy, can be resected with resultant long-term, disease-free survival. Ewing's sarcoma is highly radiation sensitive but has a tendency to metastasize widely. Local therapy should therefore be followed by adjuvant chemotherapy. Since central nervous system involvement is common, prophylactic cranial irradiation should be used.

Sarcomas in older adults are a heterogeneous group of diseases involving structures derived from the primitive mesenchyme. Their aggressivity depends largely on tumor grade, with grade 1 almost never metastasizing and grades 2 and 3 frequently metastasizing. Optimal management of these tumors is under investigation, but management now depends on a multimodality approach using surgery, radiation therapy, and chemotherapy in combinations depending on the location, extent, and grade of tumors.

MALIGNANT MELANOMA. Early diagnosis and adequate surgical resection remain the optimal therapeutic measures for malignant melanoma. Intralesional injection of Bacille Calmette-Guerin (BCG) may result in regression of tumor nodules but has no effect on visceral disease. Chemotherapy results have been disappointing, although DTIC shows some activity. Trials with α-interferon also have resulted in some responses.

Endocrine tumors

Islet cell tumors often grow slowly, so symptoms of hormone overproduction are more prominent than those caused either by the physical presence of a mass or by metastatic disease. Malignant insulinomas cause recurrent attacks of hypoglycemia that, if the tumor cannot be completely resected, may be managed by diet, corticosteroids, diazoxide, or phenytoin. In patients with unresectable gastrin-secreting tumors, the use of cimetidine results in healing of ulcers and relief of pain and diarrhea.

The most effective chemotherapeutic agent in the treatment of malignant islet cell tumors is streptozocin, which selectively destroys pancreatic β-cells. Objective antitumor and hormonal responses have been obtained in 40% of treated patients. 5-FU and doxorubicin also show some activity against these tumors.

Malignant carcinoid tumors produce symptoms related to serotonin and/or kallikrein secretion. Serotonin-related diarrhea, colic, and malabsorption usually respond to opiates and belladonna. If these symptoms are severe, serotonin antagonists such as cyproheptadine or methysergide provide effective palliation. Flushing attacks brought about by release of kallikrein are partially controlled with anti-α-adrenergic agents such as phenothiazines. More specific blockers including phentolamine and phenoxybenzamine are also useful. A recently released somatostatin analog is effective in the treatment of the acute carcinoid crisis and in chronic management of the syndrome. Antitumor responses have been obtained with streptozocin, 5-FU, alkylating agents, and doxorubicin.

BIBLIOGRAPHY

Chabner BA et al: Cancer chemotherapy: progress and expectations—1984, Cancer 54:2599, 1984.

DeVita FT, Young RC, and Canellos GP: Combination versus single-agent chemotherapy: a review of the basis for selection of drug treatment of cancer, Cancer 35:98, 1975.

Foley RM: The treatment of cancer pain, N Engl J Med 313:84, 1985.

Goepp CE and Hammond W: Supportive care of the cancer patient, Semin Oncol 2:283, 1975.

Goldie JH and Coldman AJ: Genetic instability in the development of drug resistance, Semin Oncol 13:222, 1985.

Legha SS, Davis HL, and Muggia FL: Hormonal therapy of breast cancers: new approaches and concepts, Ann Intern Med 88:69, 1978.

Oldham RK et al: Lymphokines, monoclonal antibodies and other biological response modifiers in the treatment of cancer, Cancer 54:2795, 1984.

Dental correlations

CHEMOTHERAPY
Spencer W. Redding

The goal of cancer chemotherapy is to destroy rapidly dividing cancer cells. The death of these cells is selective and caused by the drug's effect on cellular DNA itself or on the molecular events resulting in DNA synthesis and replication. Cells undergoing growth and division are more sensitive to the effects of chemotherapy than are resting cells. Unfortunately, normal cells that rapidly divide are also susceptible to these effects. These cells include bone marrow, gastrointestinal mucosa (including oral mucosa), reproductive cells, and hair. The effects on oral mucosa and bone marrow lead to the oral breakdown seen in patients receiving cancer chemotherapy. These manifestations include odontogenic infection, oral hemorrhage, and oral mucositis. Each year in the United States, approximately 250,000 patients have chemotherapy-induced oral complications.

Odontogenic infection in the cancer chemotherapy patient can lead to significant morbidity and even mortality. Bone marrow suppression secondary to chemotherapy leads to neutropenia (a reduction in neutrophils, the white blood cells that fight acute infection). Therefore a periapical, periodontal, or pericoronal infection that would normally be limited to the oral cavity in an otherwise healthy patient more commonly undergoes systemic spread in the chemotherapy patient. Oral organisms have been shown to be a significant cause of septicemia in this patient population. These patients become neutropenic approximately 7 days after chemotherapy is begun. Elimination of any potential sources of odontogenic infection before this time is critical.

Bone marrow toxicity also leads to a reduction in the production of megakaryocytes, the cells that break down to form platelets in the circulating blood. Patients receiving cancer chemotherapy often have significant reductions in circulating platelets (thrombocytopenia). This can lead to oral bleeding in the form of gingival hemorrhage or hematoma formation. Potential sources of oral hemorrhage, such as postoperative bleeding secondary to dental surgical procedures, which can be very difficult to control, must be eliminated before the initiation of chemotherapy.

Chemotherapy-induced oral mucositis (inflammation of oral mucosal tissues often with ulceration) can cause significant morbidity in patients. Generalized and localized ulcerations often occur and lead to severe oral pain. This pain can lead to reduction in oral intake and compromise the patient's nutritional status. In addition, these lesions can become secondarily infected and be a source for introduction of oral organisms into the bloodstream.

Oral mucositis is thought to be initiated by one of two mechanisms. First, chemotherapeutic agents can be toxic to the oral epithelium, resulting in thinning of the surface layer of mucosa. This leads to tissue sloughing and ulceration, which occur approximately 7 days after the initiation of chemotherapy (Fig. 1). Healing occurs 7 to 14 days later. Second, bone marrow suppression allows opportunistic oral organisms to initiate oral mucositis. These organisms include bacteria, fungae (particularly *Candida albicans*), and viruses (particularly herpes simplex).

Existing areas of chronic infection, such as periodontal lesions, or trauma may become secondarily infected by oral organisms. Since chemotherapy causes immunosuppression, such ulcerated lesions progress during the period of neutropenia. These lesions begin 12 to 16 days after the initiation of chemotherapy at the nadir (bottom) of the neutrophil count. Healing begins as the neutrophil count returns to normal.

C. albicans is an opportunistic fungal organism that initiates an oral soft tissue infection with immunosuppression. Patients' initial signs are usually white curdlike patches on any oral soft tissue (Fig. 2). When the white patches are removed, a red, inflamed surface is exposed. However, ulceration is uncommon.

Reactivation of herpes simplex virus (HSV) commonly leads

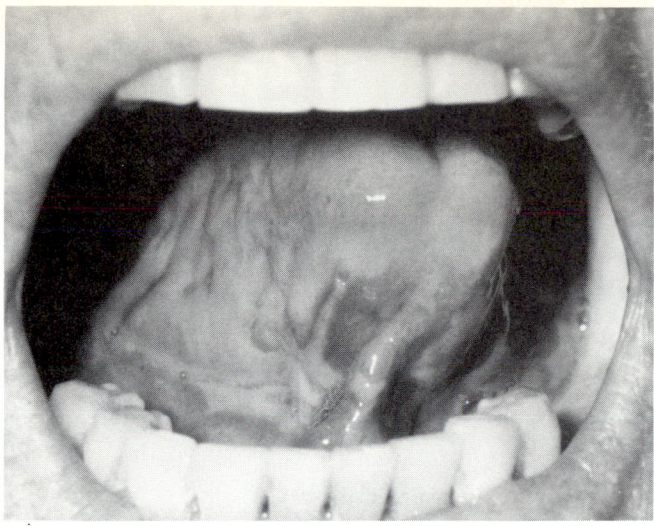

Fig. 1   Ulceration of ventral surface of tongue from direct effect of cancer chemotherapy.

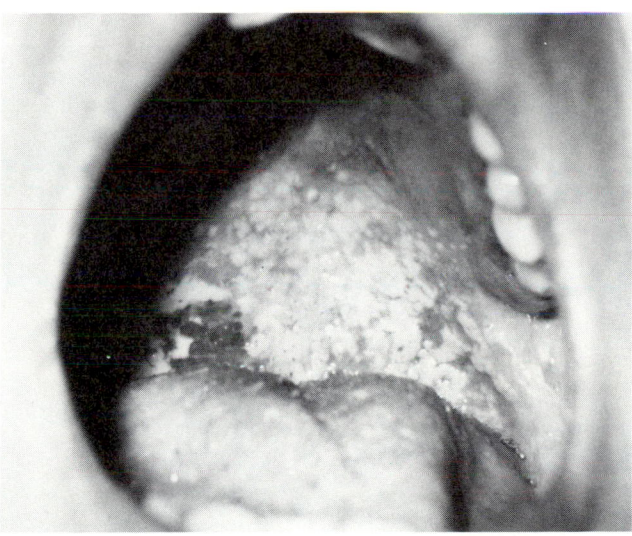

Fig. 2   Soft palate infection of *Candida albicans* in patient undergoing cancer chemotherapy.

to oral mucositis in the patient taking cancer chemotherapy. These ulcerated lesions tend to be severe in contrast to the small lesions that occur in otherwise healthy patients, and the lesions involve multiple intraoral sites in addition to the vermilion border of the lips (Fig. 3, *A* and *B*). Up to 40% of mucositis lesions in these patients have been found to have an HSV component.

Diagnosis of the cause of chemotherapy-induced oral mucositis is difficult. Clinical presentation of lesions is not a reliable criterion for diagnosis. Therefore each lesion should be evaluated for diagnosis before treatment (See discussion of "Management and treatment" in this chapter.).

A subset of chemotherapy patients, those receiving bone marrow transplantation, deserves special consideration. These patients receive high doses of chemotherapy and sometimes total-body radiation. Therefore oral manifestations of this therapy are even more severe than with conventional chemotherapy. Since more profound and longer-lasting immunosuppression occurs, the potential for systemic spread of oral infection increases. Oral mucositis tends to be more severe, and HSV plays a larger role in mucositis lesions that do occur (60% of

lesions in these patients have an HSV component). In addition, graft-versus-host disease (GVHD), which can result in a chronic oral mucositis and xerostomia, often develops in these patients.

Management and treatment

The dental management and treatment of patients who will be or are receiving chemotherapy are outlined in the following:

I. *Before chemotherapy*
   A. Perform thorough intraoral evaluation including radiographs. (Be especially careful to evaluate periodontal status, including pocket probing.)
   B. Aggressively eliminate any potential sources of odontogenic infection by extraction, root canal therapy, and oral prophylaxis. (Patients should have at least 50,000 platelets/mm³ and 500 neutrophils/mm³ neutrophils when treatment will involve the violation of oral epithelium.) Discuss the use of prophylactic antibiotics with the patient's oncologist when the patient is neutropenic (less than 2000 neutrophils).
   C. Restore any gross carious lesions in teeth that remain.
   D. Eliminate any rough or sharp edges from the remaining teeth.

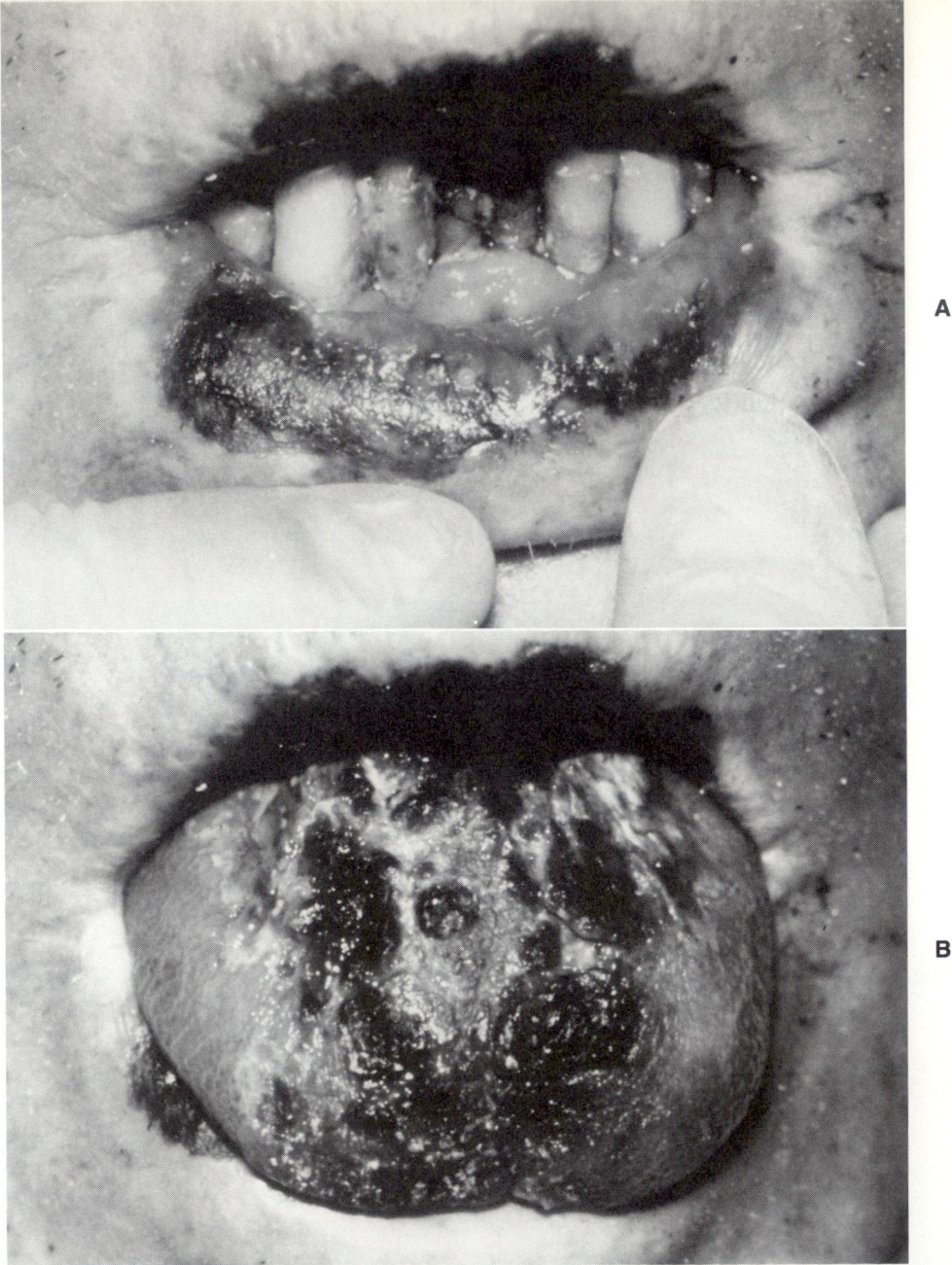

Fig. 3   **A,** Circumoral ulceration secondary to herpes simplex virus in patient undergoing cancer chemotherapy. **B,** Tongue involvement of same patient.

E. Institute oral hygiene instruction and reinforce during chemotherapy.

II. *During chemotherapy*

A. Consider prophylactic chlorhexidine oral rinses (see Table 1) to reduce the incidence and severity of mucositis and to reduce oral bacteria and *C. albicans* during chemotherapy.

B. *Odontogenic infection*

1. If neutrophil count is less than 500, a decision must be made whether to treat or wait until neutropenia resolves. This decision should be discussed with the oncologist.

2. Take a bacterial culture, if possible, to determine whether organisms are susceptible to broad-spectrum antibiotics the patient will be taking (usually a synthetic penicillin such as carbenicillin and an aminoglycoside such as gentamicin).

3. If a decision is made to treat, and extraction or periodontal scaling is necessary, attempt to achieve a platelet count of 50,000/mm³.

C. *Hemorrhage*

1. For localized gingival bleeding, apply pressure with topical thrombin–soaked gauze or apply microfibrillar collagen powder.

2. If generalized gingival bleeding occurs, apply microfibrillar collagen powder in custom oral carriers.

3. If bleeding does not respond to the above, consult with an oncologist to give a platelet transfusion.

D. *Mucositis*

1. All ulcerated lesions should be cultured for HSV and Gram stained, or placed on a slide with potassium hydroxide to determine whether *C. albicans* is present. A culture for

PRESCRIPTIONS FOR PATIENTS WITH ORAL COMPLICATIONS OF CANCER CHEMOTHERAPY

Ŗ Lidocaine (Xylocaine) Viscous 2%
Disp 450 ml bottle
Sig Rinse and expectorate every 2 hours with 1 tablespoonful for oral pain

Ŗ Dyclonine (Dyclone) 1% with milk of magnesia 50% mixture by volume
Disp 8 oz
Sig Rinse and expectorate every 2 hours with 1 teaspoonful for oral pain

Ŗ Nystatin (Mycostatin) oral suspension 100,000 units/ml
Disp 60 ml
Sig Rinse with 4 ml and swallow after 2 min 4 times per day

Ŗ Clotrimazole (Mycelex) 10 mg troches
Disp 70 troches
Sig Dissolve troche in mouth 5 times per day for 14 days

Ŗ Ketoconazole (Nizoral) 200 mg tabs
Disp 14 tabs
Sig Take 1 tab daily by mouth

Ŗ Acyclovir (Zovirax) sterile powder (treatment)*
Prepare with sterile water
Disp As needed
Sig 5 mg/kg every 8 hours for 7 days

Ŗ Acyclovir (Zovirax) 200 mg capsules (treatment)*
Disp 35 capsules
Sig Take 1 capsule by mouth 5 times per day for 7 days

Ŗ Chlorhexidine (Peridex) 0.12% rinse
Disp 16 oz
Sig Rinse vigorously with 15 ml and expectorate after 30 sec 3 times per day after meals. Continue during period of chemotherapy. (Warn patient that a transient change in taste sensation and tooth staining may occur. The above may be used for both treatment and prohylaxis.)

Ŗ Sodium fluoride 1% (Dental Gel Red)
Disp 2 oz bottle
Sig Apply 8 drops in custom oral trays for 5 minutes daily

*Acyclovir prophylaxis. All patients who are seropositive for HSV before bone marrow transplantation begin acyclovir, 200 mg capsules 3 times per day, 1 day before their transplant chemotherapy and continue for 6 weeks. If oral mucositis that precludes oral intake develops, intravenously administered acyclovir, 5 mg/kg every 8 hours, is begun. The patient resumes oral ingestion of acyclovir when it is no longer precluded.

Candida is not adequate, since many people have this organism as a normal part of their oral flora.)

2. If the lesions test positive for HSV, treat the patient with acyclovir (IV or oral capsules) (see Box).

3. If the lesions test positive for *C. albicans,* treat the patient with nystatin, clotrimazole, or ketoconazole (see Box).

4. If chlorhexidine is not used prophylactically, consider chlorhexidine oral rinses to treat mucositis by reducing oral bacteria and *C. albicans* (see Box).

5. For oral pain relief use topical anesthetics such as viscous lidocaine or dyclonine mixed with Milk of Magnesia (see Box).

6. If pain is too severe, switch to systemic pain medication after consultation with the patient's oncologist. (This care should be supervised by the oncologist.)

E. *Subset—bone marrow transplant*
   In addition to the preceding:
   1. Evaluate all patients before the procedure for antibodies to HSV; if a patient tests positive, consider prophylactic acyclovir (see Box).
   2. If the transplant is allogeneic, consider labial salivary gland biopsy after it to rule out GVHD.
   3. If GVHD develops, the patient must be followed closely for oral xerostomia, which should be treated with meticulous oral hygiene, frequent appointments for monitoring and daily topical fluoride treatment in custom fluoride carriers (see Box).
   4. If chronic oral mucositis occurs with GVHD, consider continuing chlorhexidine rinses during this period (see Box).

BIBLIOGRAPHY

Ferretti GA et al: Chlorhexidine for prophylaxis against oral infections and associated complications in patients receiving bone marrow transplants, J Am Dent Assoc 114:461, 1987.

Gold D and Corey L: Acyclovir prophylaxis for herpes simplex virus infection, Antimicrob Agents Chemother 31(3):361, 1987.

Greenberg MS et al: The oral flora as a source of systicemia in patients with acute leukemia, Oral Surg 53(1):32, 1982.

Montgomery MT, Redding SW, and LeMaistre CF: The incidence of oral herpes simplex virus infection in patients undergoing cancer chemotherapy, Oral Surg 61(3):238, 1986.

Overholser CD et al: Dental extractions in patients with acute nonlymphocytic leukemia, J Oral Maxillofac Surg 40(5):296, 1982.

Peterson D and Sonis L: Oral complications of cancer chemotherapy, Boston, 1983, Martinus Nijhoff.

Redding SW: Oral complications of cancer chemotherapy, Tex Dent J 103(6):18, 1986.

IRRADIATION

Michael T. Montgomery

Head and neck irradiation is a common form of therapy used to treat a variety of head and neck tumors. It is estimated that approximately 50% of all head and neck cancers are treated by radiation therapy alone or in conjunction with chemotherapy or surgery. The radiation combines with water within the tumor cells to form free radicals, which disrupt the nucleotide sequence in nuclear genetic material. This results in cell death. Because irradition acts on a genetic level (during the mitotic phase of cellular division), cells undergoing more rapid mitosis are more radiation sensitive. In addition, the presence of oxygen within the tumor cell facilities the lethal action of the free radicals; therefore oxygenated cells are more radiation sensitive. The lethal effects of the radiation, however, affect not only tumor cells but also adjacent oral tissues, especially tissues with a rapid turnover rate. Such oral tissues include epithelial cells and alveolar osteoblasts and osteocytes. Salivary gland acinar and ductal cells are also radiation sensitive, but this sensitivity cannot be attributed to rapid

Table 1   Impact of irradiation on oral tissues

Tissue impact	Manifestation
Burning of epithelium (mucous membrane and skin) and subepithelial layers	Mucositis; alopecia; tanning of skin
Destruction of taste buds	Dysgeusia
Acinar degeneration	Xerostomia and radiation caries
Endothelial necrosis, hyalinization, vascular thrombosis, periosteal fibrosis, death of osteocytes and osteoblasts, fibrosis of marrow spaces	Osteoradionecrosis
Ankylosis and myofibrosis	Trismus

cellular mitosis. Subsequent side effects of this insult on healthy tissues include mucositis, dysgeusia, glossodynia, xerostomia, radiation caries, and osteoradionecrosis. These side effects can significantly influence patient nutrition, and they determine the maximum irradiation dose tolerated by patients (see Table 1).

In providing dental care for radiation therapy patients, whether the dental care is before, during, or after radiation therapy, the dentist must be aware of essential diagnostic information that can be provided by the radiation oncologist. This information determines the type and scope of dental therapy offered to patients.

1. *Total dose*. The incidence of irradiation side effects increase as the total radiation dose increases. An average radiation dose for head and neck tumors is between 5000 and 7000 cGy (centigrays*), which is frequently divided into doses of 200 cGy per day given 5 days a week for 5 to 7 weeks. The dose is fractionated in this way to provide time for the oxygenation of tumor cells between treatments and thereby render them more radiation sensitive. Dosages greater than 7000 cGy are rare because of the severity of the side effects.
2. *Portals (radiation field)*. To determine the radiation field, it must be known which oral structures are within the radiation beam. Questions such as, "Were both parotid glands irradiated?" and "Is all of the mandible involved?" must be asked. Only structures within the radiation field are candidates for significant irradiation damage.
3. *Fractionation*. Most head and neck irradiation is fractionated in divided doses rather than delivered in a single large dose. However, if fractionation was not used, the amount of tissue destruction and, hence, the subsequent side effects should increase.
4. *External versus internal (implanted) radiation sources*. An internal radiation source is capable of delivering a higher radiation exposure to a smaller tissue area, thereby worsening local tissue side effects. In contrast, external radiation rersults in a wider area of tissue irradiation. However, the radiation dose per unit-area tends to be less.
5. *Radiation type*. Supervolt irradiation provides deeper tissue penetration and causes little skin necrosis, whereas ortho-radiation causes more superficial tissue damage. However, this distinction is artificial because the tissue-sparing advantage of supervolt irradiation allows higher doses of radiation to be used,

resulting in side effects equivalent to those produced with ortho-radiation.
6. *Patient sensitivity to irradiation*. After radiation therapy the radiation oncologist should have insight into a patient's relative tissue response.
7. *Patient's prognosis*. The poorer the patient's prognosis, the more the dental treatment is oriented toward the management of acute needs. The dentist should use the information gained from the radiation oncologist to determine the patient's expected complications. When this information is combined with various patient-related factors and with the timing of the dental treatment relative to the radiation therapy, an accurate individualized treatment plan is possible (Fig. 4).

Side effects
MUCOSAL CHANGES

Mucositis
Etiology. Mucositis is a result of the direct effects of radiation on the epithelial basal cell layer.

Signs. Signs include a whitish mucous membrane (epithelial sloughing), erythema, hyperemia, edema, ulcerations, and secondary infections such as fungal and viral infections.

Symptoms. Symptoms include pain, burning, hoarseness (dysphonia), sensitivity to spicy foods, and difficulty speaking and swallowing (dysphagia).

Onset. Signs and symptoms usually occur 2 weeks after the initiation of radiation therapy. Maturation of the basal cell layer takes 2 weeks, which accounts for this latency period between irradiation and the development of mucosal inflammation.

Duration. Mucositis usually lasts 2 to 3 weeks after the last irradiation treatment.

Reversibility. Radiation-induced mucositis is reversible. Recovery is complete, with mucosa returning to pretreatment status.

Radiation dose relationship. Mucositis can occur after a dose as low as 1000 cGy, with peak mucositis generally observed with dosages between 6000 to 7000 cGy.

Diagnosis. Diagnosis is made by clinical examination. However, dentists should be careful to rule out the presence of opportunistic fungal (*Candida*) and viral (herpes simplex) infections. Because of the degree of tissue damage caused by the radiation therapy and the location of the radiation beam, candidal and herpetic infections tend to be uncharacteristic in their appearance and location. Gram staining or potassium hydroxide wet preps can assist in the diagnosis of candidiasis, whereas cytology or culturing is suggested to diagnose herpes simplex.

Treatment. Treatment of mucositis is palliative and involves a combination of the following:

1. Alkaline rinses, such as peroxide 1 tbsp in 8 oz or bicarbonate ½ tsp in 8 oz
2. Analgesics
3. Topical anesthetics such as Dyclone plus milk of magnesia 1:1 concentration 1 tsp every 2 hours; 2% viscous lidocaine (1 tbsp every 2 hours); Benadryl and Kaopectate 1:1 concentration (hold 1 tbsp and expectorate after 1 minute every 2 hours); Colloidal silver solutions, or a variety of elixirs, which are comprised of various ratios of antibiotics; antifungal agents and corticosteriods in combination with topical anesthetics (see Chemotherapy section for prescriptions)
4. Modification of oral hygiene to include patient education in an effort to improve the patient's awareness of their responsibility in placating the problem. Have patients use toothettes, 2 × 2s,

---

*A gray (Gy) is the new standard unit describing absorbed radiation dose. This term replaces the term "rad," and 1 cGy (centigray) is equivalent to 1 rad.

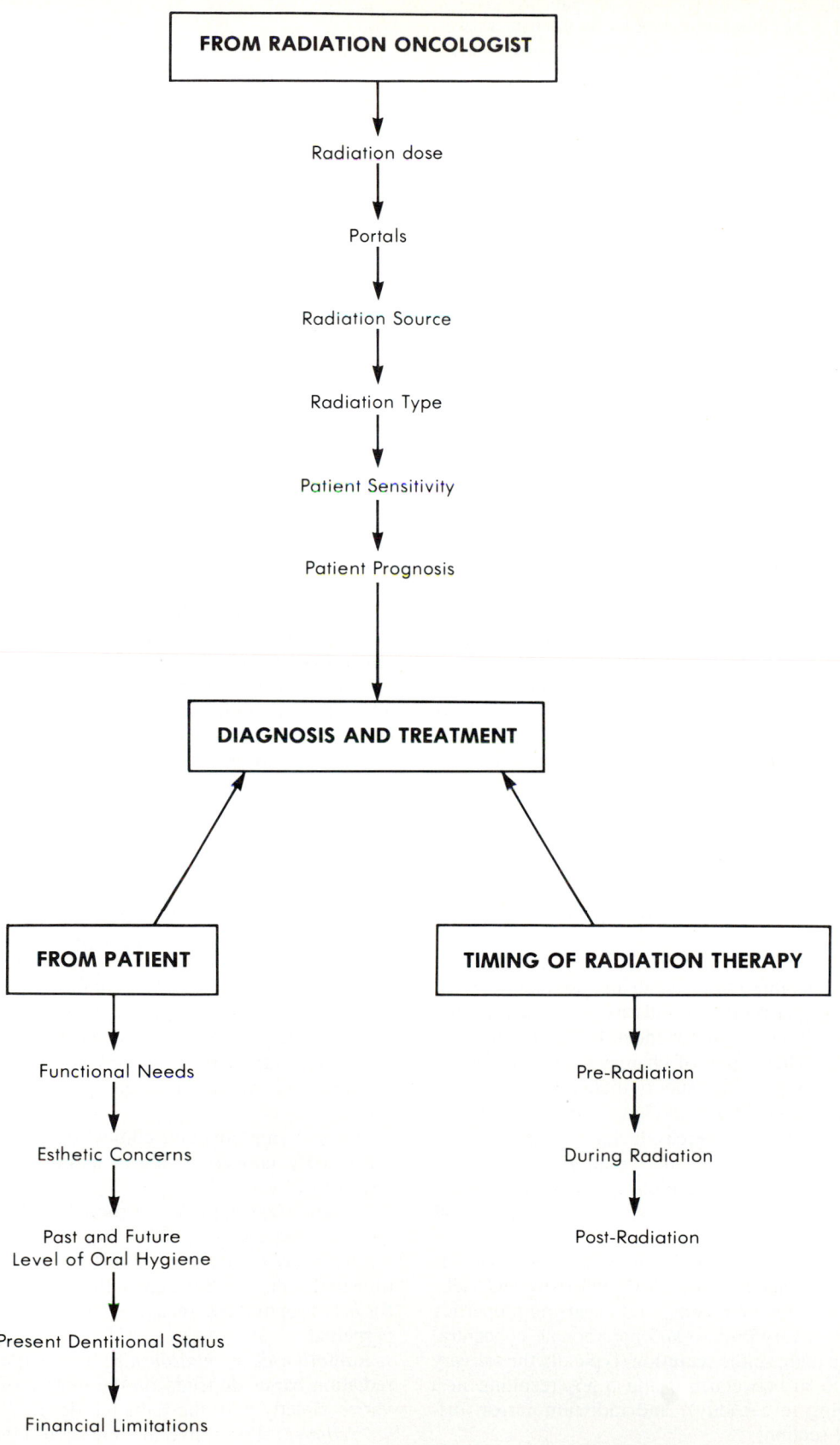

Fig. 4   Treatment plan for patients receiving radiation therapy.

or a soft-bristle brush for mechanical cleansing, along with a bland dentifrice.

5. Dietary adjustments such as requiring that patients ingest a bland, soft diet or recommending patients be fed with a nasogastric tube when an adequate oral diet cannot be maintained
6. Avoidance of over-the-counter mouthwashes, alcohol, and tobacco because of their irritative potential
7. Using the following medications for the treatment of secondary mucosal infections: antiviral medications such as acyclovir, or antifungal medications, such as nystatin, clotrimazole, and ketoconazole (See chemotherapy section for appropriate prescriptions)

Dysgeusia and glossodynia. In addition to the oral mucosa, radiation therapy also affects the tongue. Glossodynia is the result of glossitis and, like mucositis, is treated with topical anesthetics. Dysgeusia is the result of radiation damage to microvillae and outer taste cells on the tongue.

Signs and symptoms. Signs and symptoms include partial or complete loss of taste. With partial dysgeusia, bitter and acidic taste sensations are more radiation sensitive than salt and sweet sensations and therefore are affected first.

Onset. Symptoms are usually noticed within the first 2 weeks of treatment and frequently precede the symptoms of xerostomia and mucositis.

Duration. Some recovery is usually noted within 20 to 60 days following radiation therapy, but full recovery requires 60 to 120 days.

Reversibility. Recovery is usually to or approaching the preradiation therapy levels.

Radiation dose relationships. The degree of taste loss is directly proportional to the radiation dose. Initial symptoms can be seen at doses as small as 240 to 400 cGy, whereas radiation dosages in excess of 6000 cGy result in permanent taste loss.

Treatment. Palliative therapy can be provided in the form of zinc supplements. These dietary supplements have been shown to accelerate recovery, although they appear to be ineffective when used prophylactically. The usual dosage is 110 mg zinc sulfate with meals and at bedtime or 220 mg zinc sulfate twice a day.

SALIVARY CHANGES

Xerostomia. Xerostomia is the result of radiation-induced inflammation and degeneration of salivary gland acinar and ductal cells. The resulting salivary changes are both qualitative and quantitative, and the degree of change is virtually determined by the amount of parotid tissue irradiated. Serous glands tend to be more radiation sensitive and have better regenerative capacity than mucous glands, whereas ductal cells are the most radiation resistant. This sequence of radiation sensitivity is reflected clinically with saliva becoming more viscous initially (acinar cells) followed by a reduction in salivary volume (ductal cells).

Signs. Signs of xerostomia include diminished salivary volume that results in an increase in salivary viscosity and tackiness and a decrease in the lubricating and cleansing properties of saliva. Loss of salivary protein and bicarbonate concentrations that produce a more acidic secretion (typically the salivary pH drops from 7.0 to between 5.0 and 5.55, resulting in a diminished buffering in capacity), and radiation caries (discussed in the next section).

Symptoms. Symptoms of xerostomia include dryness, coughing, dysphonia, and dysphagia.

Onset. Symptoms are usually noticed within the first 2 weeks after radiation therapy.

Duration. The salivary changes are partially reversible. The degree of recovery is usually known within 6 to 12 months after radiation therapy.

Reversibility—radiation dose relationship. Signs and symptoms can be noted with a minimum radiation exposure of 1500 cGy, whereas irreversible changes require a 4000 to 6000 cGy dose.

Diagnosis. Diagnosis is determined by clinical signs and symptoms.

Treatment. Treatment is palliative and can include a combination of the following:

1. Alkaline rinses such as peroxide or bicarbonate, as described in the discussion of mucositis
2. Frequent sips of water, especially at night and during mastication (Patients often prefer this means of oral lubrication to the saliva substitutes, which are poorly tolerated.)
3. Saliva substitutes, which are usually a combination of glycerine, electrolytes, and fluoride (The agents commonly used include sodium carboxymethylcellulose and sorbitol. Saliva substitutes are intended to improve wetness and buffering capacity and to provide cariostatic support. The duration of effects is approximately 10 to 15 minutes, and the agents are prescribed on an as-needed basis.)
4. Saliva stimulants, which can include lemon drops, gum, or pilocarpine (Pilocarpine is prescribed in a 5 mg dose taken orally four times a day.)

ODONTOGENIC CHANGES

Radiation caries. Radiation caries is a rapid, diffuse demineralization, which is manifest as rampant cervical and cusp-tip decay. Cervical caries can amputate the crowns of teeth if left untreated. Fully mature teeth are not radiation sensitive; hence radiation caries is deemed the direct result of the aforementioned salivary changes. As such all teeth are affected, not just those within the radiation field.

Aside from the diminution in flow and the acidotic shift in pH, a reduction in salivary immunoproteins and electrolytes are part of the changes noted in salivary composition after radiation therapy. Together these changes result in a shift in the oral microflora to highly acidogenic and cariogenic microbes such as *Streptococcus mutans, Lactobacillus,* and *Actinomyces viscosis.* In addition to these microbial changes, patients' diets tend to favor nondetergent, high-carbohydrate foods. This dietary shift is an effort to placate the discomfort from xerostomia, mucositis, and dysgeusia, which further enhances the cariogenic microbial environment.

Signs and symptoms. Signs and symptoms are as stated above.

Onset. Symptoms and clinical evidence of radiation caries are usually noticed within 3 months of postradiation therapy.

Duration/reversibility. Although radiation caries are irreversible, they are preventable; hence prophylactic measures are the mainstay of therapy. Xerostomic patients remain susceptible to this disease throughout their lifetime; therefore the need for oral prophylactic measures and scrupulous oral hygiene is perpetual.

Radiation dose relationship. The patient's susceptibility to radiation caries depends on the degree of xerostomia, which varies directly with the radiation dose.

Treatment. Preventive therapy should include the following:

1. Emphasis on thorough and regular oral hygiene measures
2. Short oral hygiene recall appointments
3. Dietary counseling to minimize carbohydrate intake
4. Daily fluoride applications (Neutral preparations are preferred

to minimize tissue irritation. Stannous fluoride, 0.4%, or sodium fluoride, 1%, can be used in a carrier. The patient should place 5 to 10 drops in the carrier, hold the carrier in place for 5 minutes, and expectorate without rinsing. This treatment should be performed once a day, preferably at bedtime just after brushing.)

5. Chlorhexidine applications (Although chlorhexidine has not been tested on this patient population, the drug's anticaries and antimucositis activities would seem appropriate after radiation therapy.) (See chemotherapy section for possible dosage regimens.)

Developmental abnormalities. In the developing dentition, tooth number, tooth morphology, and condylar morphology can all be affected with radiation doses exceeding 500 cGy. These alterations can take the following forms:

1. Stunted condylar growth
2. Stunting or death of tooth buds
3. Altered crown or root morphology
4. Hypocalcification

FUNCTIONAL CHANGES
Nutritional impact. After radiation therapy, eating often becomes pleasureless because of the side effects of mucositis, xerostomia, dysgeusia, glossodynia, nausea, and vomiting.

Signs and symptoms. Signs and symptoms of radiation caries include anorexia, weight loss, dehydration, and poor nutrition (angular cheilitis, atrophic glossitis, and anemia), and a diet that favors a soft, bland, high-carbohydrate food selection at the expense of a more balanced menu.

Treatment. Treatment of radiation caries includes the following:

1. Dietary counseling and patient encouragement
2. Bland, balanced diet with vitamin and protein supplements
3. Creative menu preparations
4. Avoidance of cariogenic foods
5. Eating small, frequent meals
6. Palliative oral therapies such as topical anesthetics, alkaline rinses, analgesics, and saliva substitutes

Trismus. Fibrosis of the masticatory muscles or the temporomandibular joint can result in an insidious onset of trismus. The symptoms usually develop within 3 to 6 months after radiation therapy, and the treatment should be aimed at prevention of symptoms. Treatments include preradiation and postradiation home physiotherapy such as range-of-motion and isometric exercises.

ALVEOLAR CHANGES
Osteoradionecrosis. Osteoradionecrosis has been defined as an area of exposed bone in a field of radiation that is present for at least 3 months. The proposed pathophysiologic factors are as follows: Irradiation causes periarteritis and endarteritis, which lead to vessel wall thickening and loss of lumen size. As a consequence, the alveolar blood supply is compromised, resulting in the death of osteocytes and osteoblasts, which are replaced in the marrow by connective tissue and fat. The outcome is hypovascular, hypocellular, and hypoxic alveolar tissue with diminished repair and remodeling capabilities. In response to trauma this compromised tissue becomes infected, which can lead to progressive and extensive alveolar destruction.

The role that infecting microorganisms play in this process is controversial. The traditional perspective, expressed previously, places primary importance on the role of microbial infection in the development of osteoradionecrosis. Microorganisms associated with osteoradionecrosis include *Staphylococcus aureus* (most common), *Staphylococcus albus*, *Streptococcus hemolyticus*, *Streptococcus viridans*, *Pneumococcus*, *Pseudomonas*, and *Actinomyces* organisms, and *Escherichia coli*. However, recent data by Marx suggest that microorganisms are mere surface contaminants and that the underlying problem is not one of infection. Marx proposes that osteoradionecrosis represents the tissue's inability to keep up with the need for cellular turnover and collagen synthesis during healing. This reasoning likens the pathogenesis of osteoradionecrosis more to that of a diabetic ulcer than to that of osteomyelitis, as was traditionally thought.

Predictors of osteoradionecrosis. The following are predictors of osteoradionecrosis:

Radiation dose. Osteoradionecrosis is commonly seen in patients receiving total dosages ranging between 6000 to 6500 cGy and is infrequent in doses less than 6000 cGy.

Radiation field. Osteoradionecrosis is confined to the parameters of the radiation field and is most prevalent in the direct pathway of the radiation beam.

Dentition status. Significant controversy as to the role that dental disease plays in the development of osteoradionecrosis exists in the literature. A direct relationship cannot be confirmed at this time.

Type of radiation. Osteoradionecrosis is more likely with internal rather than external radiation because of the higher localized radiation dose delivered with an internal source.

Tumor location. The incidence of osteoradionecrosis increases as a tumor becomes more intimately associated with the alveolus. Tumors of the tongue and floor of the mouth are associated in this manner.

Tumor state. The incidence of osteoradionecrosis varies directly with the tumor stage except in the highest tumor staging, where patient survival time becomes a factor.

*Signs and symptoms.** Signs and symptoms of osteoradionecrosis include cellulitis, suppuration, fetid oral odor, oral cutaneous fistula, throbbing pain that is increased at night and with mastication, exposed bone, bony sequestrations, irregular radiographic radiolucencies, hemorrhage, and pathologic fracture.

Onset. Symptoms can be noticed within weeks or may take years to develop. However, the frequency of osteoradionecrosis is highest in the immediate postirradiation period and declines as the postirradiation period lengthens.

Incidence. The overall incidence of osteoradionecrosis is reported to be between 4% and 37.5% with a mean incidence of 10% to 15%. More than 90% of the cases occur in the mandible, which is due to a combination of effects. First, the greater bone density in the mandible allows a higher absorption of radiation dose and hence enhanced cell death. Second, mandibular preference is a manifestation of the poorer vascular supply in the mandible as compared with the maxilla.

Osteoradionecrosis also appears to be more common when radiation therapy is accompanied by radical neck dissection. This additional surgery involves sacrificing the external carotid artery whose branches supply the mandibular mucosa and periosteum, which further compromises mandibular blood supply. Finally, osteoradionecrosis is most commonly associated with postradiation trauma; however, spontaneous osteoradionecrosis has been reported in 5% to 39% of the patients examined in

---

*The signs and symptoms listed can be misleading because osteoradionecrosis is more commonly smoldering rather than virulent and acutely debilitating.

various studies and appears to be associated with high-radiation dosages.

Diagnosis. Diagnosis is based on clinical signs and symptoms, radiographs, and scintigraphy. Recent evidence suggests that the scintigraphic method of alveolar imaging may allow prediction or early diagnosis of osteoradionecrosis.

Treatment. Dentists must consider the following criteria to arrive at an appropriate individual treatment plan for osteoradionecrosis (see Fig. 4).

I. Prevention

The role of the general dentist in prevention is the cornerstone to the management of osteoradionecrosis.

A. The first determinant of care depends on information from the radiation oncologist cited previously, such as radiation dose, radiation field, expected oral complications, patient prognosis, and timing of radiation therapy. (Here the timing of radiation therapy refers to whether the patient is being treated before, during, or after irradiation.)

1. During the preradiation phase, the following measures are recommended.

a. Dentists should maintain an aggressive attitude concerning dental care to prevent the need for dental surgery after radiation therapy. This attitude is advised because postradiation extractions are associated with a higher incidence of osteoradionecrosis than are preradiation extractions.* Hence, all the teeth listed below, which usually have a poor prognosis, should be removed:

Impacted teeth
Unopposed teeth
Teeth with moderate to severe periodontitis
Teeth with extensive decay associated with pulpal impingement or those requiring extensive restorative efforts
Teeth with periapical lesions

When extracting teeth, the dentist should follow these procedures:

i. Extractions should be accompanied by radical alveolectomy and primary soft tissue closure. Here, sutures should not be placed too tightly to prevent pressure necrosis of the mucosa.

ii. Extractions should be accomplished 14 to 21 days before the beginning of radiation therapy to allow complete mucosal healing.

iii. Antibiotics may be used during this healing period. With the thinking on pathogenesis shifting away from infection and toward poor healing, there is less reason to support antibiotic therapy. Studies have questioned the validity of this practice.

b. There is no need for indiscriminate odontectomies. Although the sequelae of osteoradionecrosis can be devastating, its low overall incidence rate, coupled with the high rate of success after nonsurgical management, lends support to a more conservative approach to teeth with a good prognosis.

c. Prophylactic removal of exostosis and tori to eliminate the possibility of prosthetic impingement as a source of postradiation trauma should be considered.

d. Oral hygiene measures must be emphasized to the extent that the patient is competent and willing to engage in the rigorous and thorough measures needed to maintain their dentition following radiation therapy.

e. Psychologic preparation of patients to diminish fear and enhance motivation.

f. Schedule patients for short recall appointments to allow close follow-up monitoring throughout radiation therapy and thereafter.

2. Treating patients during or after radiation therapy requires a more conservative approach to the management of patients' dental problems. It is intended that the aforementioned aggressive attitude during preradiation therapy will lessen the need for extensive postradiation treatments. In contrast, during the postradiation period, an aggressive restorative therapy is stressed, with root canal therapy preferred to extractions. When necessary, extractions should be performed early in the postradiation period because of the higher incidence of osteoradionecrosis as the postradiation period lengthens. Recent evidence suggests that the residual healing deficit progressively worsens after irradiation treatment.

a. Alveoloplasty, low-tension primary closure, and possibly antibiotic therapy are advisable as with extraction in the preradiation patients.

b. Adjunctive preextraction and postextraction hyperbaric oxygen therapy must also be considered.

c. As with preirradiation patients, postirradiation patients should be counseled concerning their oral hygiene, nutrition, physical therapy, and psychologic expectations.

B. A second determinant of care is the information gained from the patient, such as the following:

1. The existing level of caries and periodontal disease
2. The patient's past oral hygiene motivation
3. The patient's past need and demand for dental therapy
4. The patient's present level of motivation and oral health awareness
5. The patient's functional and esthetic dental needs
6. The patient's financial capabilities

II. Treatment

A. Nonsurgical therapies

One approach to the treatment of osteoradionecrosis involves nonsurgical therapies comprised of irrigation, debridement, and analgesics in combination with 2 to 3 weeks of broad-spectrum antibiotics. Hyperbaric oxygen therapy can also be employed as an adjunct to stimulate healing. Hyperbaric oxygen increases tissue oxygenation and thereby enhances fibroblast mitosis, blood vessel budding, collagen synthesis, osteogenesis and osteoblastic activity, and leukocyte phagocytosis and may improve antibiotic actions and have some bactericidal and bacteriostatic properties. Typically patients are placed in a decompression chamber at 2 atmospheres for 2 hours each day. Each treatment is termed a "dive." Patients who are undergoing postradiation extractions and hyperbaric oxygen therapy commonly perform 20 dives before the extractions followed by 10 to 20 postextraction dives. Hyperbaric oxygen therapy is valuable in combination with the other aforementioned conservative measures but is of little assistance when used alone. In addition, cost ($300 per dive) and the poor availability of hyperbaric oxygen chambers have deterred widespread use of this therapeutic modality. After nonsurgical therapy, symptoms usually diminish within 1 to 2 weeks, with full healing in 50% to 75% of the patients within 1 year.

The success of nonsurgical therapy is inversely related to the radiation dose and the area of irradiated bone. In addition, nonsurgical therapy is less likely to be successful with internal radiation and postradiation extractions. Finally, there appears to be no relationship between the success of nonsurgical therapy and the timing of osteoradionecrosis.

B. Alveolar resection

A second mode mode of therapy for osteoradionecrosis is alveolar resection. This therapy is often combined with hyperbaric oxygen (as many as 50 dives) and is indicated in the following conditions:

1. Intractable pain

---

*There is conflicting evidence on the issue of preradiation versus postradiation extractions. There is growing evidence that the incidence of osteoradionecrosis is insensitive to the timing of extractions in relation to irradiation.

2. Recurrent severe infections
3. Pathologic fracture

BIBLIOGRAPHY

Aitasalo K and Ruotsalainen P: Effects of irradiation on mandibular scintigraphy, J Nucl Med 26:1263, 1985.

Baker DG: The radiobiological basis for tissue reactions in the oral cavity following therapeutic x-irradiation, Arch Otolaryngol 108:21, 1982.

Beumer III, J et al: Preradiation dental extractions and the incidence of bone necrosis, Head Neck Surg 5:514, 1983.

Beumer III, J et al: Osteoradionecrosis: predisposing factors and outcomes of therapy, Head Neck Surg 6:819, 1984.

Beumer III, J et al: Postradiation dental extractions: a review of the literature and a report of 72 episodes, Head Neck Surg 6:581, 1983.

Fishman SL: The patient with cancer, Dent Clin North Am 27:235, 1983.

Hariot JC et al: Systematic dental management in head and neck irradiation, Int J Rad Oncol Biol Phys 7:1025, 1981.

Larson DL et al: Major complications of radiotherapy in cancer of the oral cavity and oropharynx, Am J Surg 146:531, 1983.

Marciani RD and Ownby HE: Osteoradionecrosis of the jaws, J Oral Maxillofac Surg 44:218, 1986.

Marx RE: Osteoradionecrosis: a new concept of its pathophysiology, J Oral Maxillofac Surg 41:283, 1983.

Marx RE and Johnson RP: Studies in the radiobiology of osteoradionecrosis and thier clinical significance, Oral Surg Oral Med Oral Pathol 64: 379, 1987.

Rothwell RB: Prevention and treatment of the orofacial complications of radiotherapy, J Am Dent Assoc 114:316, 1987.

Dentist's role in the care of the terminally ill

Janet M. Kaye

The concept of "oral care" is an all inclusive one, embracing both therapy and solicitude. It can be defined as the diagnosis, prevention and treatment of oral disease and disability, with a concomitant expression of a conscious concern on the part of the therapist for the anxiety, pain and suffering of the patient, in question, and of his or her immediate family.

DUMMETT, 1971

Caring for terminally ill patients arouses anxiety in most people, and health care providers, including dentists, are no exception. The care of the dying arouses some of people's most pervasive fears: fear of extinction, helplessness, abandonment, disfigurement, and loss of self-esteem. Our attitudes toward the dying are a mixture of positive and negative emotions. It is our task to identify and assimilate all these feelings—not to deny them, but to recognize that it is human to have emotions. If we are to deal effectively with terminally ill patients, we need to deal first with our own feelings toward death. Just as each of us is unique, each approaches death in a different fashion. The most important point to keep in mind is that even when death is inevitable, the dental practitioner still may have much to offer.

In the past the dental profession showed little interest in terminally ill patients because dentistry was usually practiced on an ambulatory, relatively well population. Once death was imminent, dentists were inclined to transfer care of the terminally ill patients completely to the physician.

This has changed with the advent of holistic care and the concept of humanistic dentistry. Humanistic dentistry has been defined as concern for the total person who seeks dental treatment—not merely the teeth themselves, but the emotional and psychologic needs of that person.

Despite this new awareness in the literature, dental concerns for the dying patient remain grossly ignored. With the realization that proper dental care is an important component of general health care, dentists find themselves in a new role. They must provide comprehensive care to the terminally ill patient and often to family members, with whom they have had good rapport. Now when the patient and family are experiencing anxiety and fear, they look to all of their health-care providers including dentists for help. Dentists should not shy away from listening to the patient and family and offering whatever support is needed.

HELPING THE PATIENT

Different forms of help are extended to a person with a fatal disease at various stages of the disease. Initially help can be directed toward the fulfillment of a richer, more rewarding life. After this the patient may require help in decision making regarding care. When the prognosis is poor, the patient needs help in understanding and dealing with the prognosis and alternatives for treatment or lack of treatment without destroying all hope. Eventually, as the patient approaches the final stage, the health-care provider can help the individual to disengage from life and have a peaceful death.

Stages

In her landmark book *On Death and Dying*, Elisabeth Kübler-Ross organized her observations on the dying process as a series of stages through which a dying person goes:

1. Denial and isolation
2. Anger
3. Bargaining
4. Depression
5. Acceptance

This book was important in that it sensitized both the public and health-care providers to the needs of the dying. Dying was presented as a process to be understood rather than to be feared or ignored.

Unfortunately, many professionals have interpreted these five stages as fixed and universal. Kübler-Ross never meant to present the stages as rigid and invariable. Many patients do not move through all of these stages, and some seesaw back and forth. Rather than attempt to classify a patient, it is more important to observe the patient's physical and emotional condition. The dentist then is able to listen actively and respond in a manner that is relevant and meaningful to the patient at that time.

Problems of the terminally ill patient

Even in a dying patient, the mouth and its care assume great importance. The mouth remains one of the last sources of satisfaction with which the patient speaks and eats. It is also the vehicle through which the patient expresses love, fear, and anger to others. Consequently, proper oral health may be an important focus of the terminally ill patient.

The patient's physical appearance influences how he perceives himself and his social worth. For example, having her hair washed and set may be of great psychologic importance to a dying woman. If oral tissues and facial contours are affected by disease or neglect of care, psychologic and physiologic issues can arise and disturb patients' relationships with their families and their professional caregivers. The patient deserves to have these dental needs addressed.

There are other common sources of pain and discomfort for the dying patient that should not be ignored. Some of these are toothaches, soreness and pain of the tongue or mouth, mouth dryness, *Candida* and other oral infections, taste disturbances, mouth odor, and loss of taste perception. Many of

THE BILL OF RIGHTS FOR A DYING PERSON

1. The right to be treated as a living human being until death.
2. The right to maintain a sense of hopefulness, however changing it may be.
3. The right to be cared for by those who can maintain a sense of hopefulness, however changing that might be.
4. The right to express feelings and emotions about approaching death.
5. The right to participate in decisions concerning care.
6. The right to expect continuing medical and nursing attention even though cure goals must be changed to comfort goals.
7. The right not to die alone.
8. The right to be free from pain.
9. The right to have questions answered honestly.
10. The right not to be deceived.
11. The right to have help from and for the family in accepting death.
12. The right to die in peace and dignity.
13. The right to retain my individuality and not be judged for my decisions, which may be contrary to the beliefs of others.
14. The right to discuss and enlarge my religious and/or spiritual experiences regardless of what they may mean to others.
15. The right to expect that the sanctity of the human body will be respected after death.
16. The right to be cared for by caring, sensitive, knowledgable people, who will attempt to understand my needs, and who will be able to gain some personal satisfaction in helping me face my death.

Modified from Donovan M and Girton S: Cancer care nursing, ed 2, Norwalk, Conn, 1984, Appleton-Century-Crofts.

these symptoms can and should be alleviated by oral therapy in the dying just as they would be addressed in the healthy.

The "Bill of Rights for a Dying Person," (see box) should serve as a guide to all caregivers.

BIBLIOGRAPHY

Buckingham R: Dental care policies for treating the terminal cancer patient, Dent Hyg 55:23, 1981.

Donovan M and Girton S: Cancer care nursing, ed 2, Norwalk, Conn, 1984, Appleton-Century-Crofts.

Dummett C: Community dentistry's contribution to oral care of the aged and patients in terminal illness, J Am Coll Dent 38:152, 1971.

Kübler-Ross E: On death and dying, New York, 1969, Macmillan.

Kutscher A: The terminal patient: Oral care, New York, 1973, Foundation of Thanatology, distributed by Columbia University Press.

Pearson P: The dying patient with oral malignant disease, Otolaryngol Clin North Am 12:241, 1979.

CARDIOVASCULAR DISEASES

Edited by **Toby R. Engel**

85·INTRODUCTION TO CARDIOVASCULAR DISEASE

Toby R. Engel

Cardiologists deal with heart and vascular disease in terms of a physiologic division of symptoms and their management. They tend to be concerned with abnormal anatomy and physiology rather than with etiologic factors, pathogenesis, or biochemical derangements. The recent excitement about improving coronary perfusion by removing anatomic obstructions (with dissolution of clots or with balloon angioplasty) illustrates this focus.

Most patients with cardiovascular disease are lumped under just a few rubrics: hypertensive diseases, congenital diseases, valvular diseases, myocardial or pericardial diseases, and coronary and other arterial diseases. The cardinal symptoms of patients with cardiovascular disease (chest pain, dyspnea, edema, syncope) are common to a variety of these diseases. Pain is described in relation to coronary artery and aortic structure. Dyspnea and edema are dealt with as disorders of hemodynamic physiology tempered by the structural alterations of all the above diseases. Syncope and sudden death are discussed in terms of electrophysiologic mechanisms. Thromboemboli are described in relation to their anatomic distribution (pulmonary, peripheral, coronary). Even the special diseases involving younger patients are dealt with along anatomic or physiologic lines.

The physiologic abnormalities and approaches to therapy are similar for each disease. For example, vasodilation is beneficial in reducing peripheral vascular resistance in heart failure, as well as hypertension, certain forms of valvular disease, ischemic heart disease, and aortic dissection. The common denominator in managing all cardiovascular disorders is the expression of clinical difficulties and the measurement of therapeutic responses by simple physiologic measurements (for example, pulmonary capillary pressure or the intervals on the electrocardiogram).

86·CONGESTIVE HEART FAILURE

Joseph A. Franciosa *and* **W. Bruce Dunkman**

Congestive heart failure is a common outcome of many cardiovascular lesions and a major cause of physical disability. It should be regarded as a complex clinical syndrome rather than a distinct disease process, since its causes are multiple and its clinical expression variable. Nevertheless, congestive heart failure results from an interplay of pathogenetic mechanisms that are similar despite their development in response to diverse cardiovascular insults. Therefore a common clinical and pathophysiologic entity develops, which usually can be managed by similar interventions. The purpose of this chapter is to emphasize those common pathophysiologic features of congestive heart failure that facilitate understanding of its clinical presentations and from which a rational basis for its management can be derived.

DEFINITION. Congestive heart failure is a clinical syndrome that results from the inability of the heart to adequately perfuse peripheral tissues to enable them to meet their metabolic requirements. This can result from either inadequate systolic emptying or from impaired diastolic filling. Perfusion can be considered inadequate when it is absolutely reduced or when it is maintained at normal levels but is accomplished only under abnormal hemodynamic conditions that interfere with local tissue function. An example of the latter is acute hypertensive heart failure, in which pulmonary blood flow can be maintained at normal levels but is accomplished at an elevated pressure that can interfere with alveolar capillary gas exchange.

Congestive heart failure must be distinguished from other causes of inadequate tissue perfusion. These include shock of various noncardiac origins such as hypovolemia or sepsis and other states of vascular congestion such as cirrhosis and uremia. In these other conditions the clinical presentation can simulate heart failure, but a cardiovascular lesion is not present, ventricular emptying is not impaired, and the heart usually functions normally for the kind of loading conditions to which it is subjected.

ETIOLOGY. The lesions responsible for heart failure can directly involve the heart or can be located outside the heart in the vascular system but lead to impairment of cardiac function. Some common causes of congestive heart failure are outlined as follows:

I. Intracardiac
   A. Myocardial
      1. Acute myocarditis
         a. Toxic
         b. Infectious
            (1) Viral
            (2) Bacterial
            (3) Fungal
            (4) Parasitic
      2. Infiltrative diseases
         a. Amyloidosis
         b. Hemochromatosis
         c. Tumors
      3. Chronic inflammation
         a. Sarcoidosis
         b. Rheumatic fever
         c. Collagen-vascular diseases

401

4. Cardiomyopathies
   a. Congestive
     (1) Ischemic
     (2) Alcoholic
     (3) Postviral
     (4) Postpartum
     (5) Idiopathic
   b. Restrictive
   c. Hypertrophic
   d. Heredofamilial
 B. Endocardial
  1. Valvulopathies
   a. Rheumatic heart disease
   b. Infective endocarditis
   c. Degenerative valvular disease
  2. Collagen-vascular diseases
  3. Endocardial fibroelastosis
 C. Pericardial
  1. Inflammatory
   a. Acute
   b. Chronic
  2. Neoplastic
II. Extracardiac
 A. Systemic hypertension
 B. Pulmonary hypertension
  1. Parenchymal lung disease
  2. Pulmonary embolism
  3. Idiopathic
 C. High-output states
  1. Anemia
  2. Hyperthyroidism
  3. Beri-beri
  4. Alcoholic liver disease
  5. Arteriovenous fistula

Among the cardiac lesion sites, the *myocardium, endocardium,* and *pericardium* can be involved alone or in combination. The *myocardium* can be the site of inflammatory lesions such as myocarditis of toxic, viral, or bacterial origin. Infiltrative processes such as amyloidosis, sarcoidosis, and tumor, or chronic inflammatory lesions such as rheumatic carditis and rheumatoid arthritis or other collagen-vascular diseases can also involve the heart. Although these forms of myocarditis often are discovered to involve the heart when it is examined pathologically, they are relatively rare as causes of clinically manifest congestive heart failure, either because the disease entities are uncommon or because their cardiac involvement is not extensive.

By far the most common causes of myocardial disease are ischemic and idiopathic cardiomyopathy. Ischemic cardiomyopathy is due to severe coronary obstructive disease and may or may not be associated with typical ischemic events such as acute myocardial infarction or angina pectoris. Ischemia with electrocardiographic changes but no angina is called "silent ischemia." Pathologically, large coronary arteries are involved, and the lesions are indistinguishable from those observed in patients with other clinical presentations of ischemic heart disease. Although the existence of "small vessel coronary artery disease" has been postulated as a cause of ischemic cardiomyopathy, this has not been clearly demonstrated. Such "small vessel disease" has been seen in patients with diabetes or collagen-vascular diseases. Idiopathic cardiomyopathy is characterized by diffuse myocardial fibrosis with normal coronary arteries. It is seen in association with chronic alcoholism and following pregnancy and viral infections. Alcohol can produce direct cardiac depression, but the cardiomyopathy associated with excessive alcohol ingestion is not usually resolved by cessation of alcohol intake. Idiopathic cardiomyopathies can

involve the myocardium diffusely and lead to ventricular dilation and the typical clinical presentation of cardiovascular congestion, or they can lead to diffuse interstitial fibrosis resulting in stiffening of the myocardium with restriction of cardiac filling. Finally, the myocardium can be involved predominantly in specific areas leading to localized hypertrophy (hypertrophic cardiomyopathy). The idiopathic and hypertrophic cardiomyopathies are discussed in detail in Chapter 95.

Clinical congestive heart failure also can result from lesions of the *endocardium* or *heart valves*. These can be congenital or acquired, such as after rheumatic fever or bacterial endocarditis. These lesions are discussed in detail in Chapter 94. They lead to heart failure by causing a pressure overload on the ventricle (valvular obstruction) or a volume overload (valvular regurgitation or an abnormal communication between heart chambers).

The *pericardium* can be the site of inflammatory lesions from infection, myocardial infarction, pericardiotomy, or tumor infiltrates. These lesions usually do not lead to heart failure unless they cause pericardial fibrosis severe enough to produce adhesions or constriction great enough to restrict cardiac diastolic filling. Accumulation of fluid in the pericardial cavity as a result of any of these processes can limit cardiac diastolic filling and lead to pericardial tamponade, a low–cardiac output state requiring emergency treatment. Tamponade is seen most commonly with uremic or malignant pericarditis but can rarely occur with other types of pericarditis.

Cardiac dysfunction severe enough to lead to clinically overt heart failure can result from *extracardiac* lesions. The most important of these is systemic hypertension, which is the most common precursor of all forms of congestive heart failure. An explanation for this relationship is that elevated blood pressure increases resistance to left ventricular outflow and this chronic pressure overload leads to ventricular hypertrophy and dilation. Regression of left ventricular hypertrophy follows normalization of blood pressure with agents that inhibit the sympathetic nervous system. However, it does not follow equivalent blood pressure lowering with vasodilator drugs that reflexly increase sympathetic influences. Hypertension is also important as a cause of heart failure because it is a major risk factor for coronary artery disease.

In some cases of noncardiac lesions, increased venous return to the heart via abnormal arteriovenous communications can induce a congested state. Such volume overload from congenital or acquired arteriovenous fistulas is unusual, and large flow volumes are required before cardiac function is compromised.

Disease processes involving the *pulmonary vessels* or *lung parenchyma* can lead to congestive heart failure by raising pulmonary arterial pressure, thereby overloading the right ventricle and causing failure. Acute right ventricular failure can be caused by sudden increases in pulmonary pressure from pulmonary embolization or severe pneumonia. More commonly, the cause of pulmonary hypertension is chronic obstructive lung disease associated with severe structural changes of pulmonary vessels. Less frequently, pulmonary hypertension is primary and idiopathic (see Chapter 92). This form is most common in younger age-groups and has been thought in some cases to be the result of recurrent microembolization to the pulmonary arterial bed.

In "high-output" heart failure, cardiac output is at normal or above-normal levels. This occurs in anemia, hyperthyroidism, beri-beri, and alcoholic liver disease when cardiac output is inadequate to meet metabolic demands or its distribution is altered so that certain tissues are underperfused.

EPIDEMIOLOGY. Since heart failure results from a variety of cardiovascular lesions, its epidemiology reflects its multifactorial origin. Factors determining the incidence and severity of coronary artery disease, rheumatic fever, and hypertension have a great bearing on the prevalence of congestive heart failure in the population. These include age, sex, cigarette smoking, diet, serum cholesterol, blood glucose, body weight, family history, physical activity, and personality type.

It is estimated that heart failure affects more than 2 million individuals in the United States and was responsible for over 1,500,000 hospitalizations in 1982. In the Framingham study the annual rate of development of heart failure was 3.7 per 1000 for men and 2.5 per 1000 for women. The incidence rose with age, especially after 50 years of age. Hypertension was the most important precursor of congestive heart failure; 75% of patients with heart failure had a history of hypertension.

Hypertension significantly increases the risk of heart failure when it is associated with other heart disease, such as rheumatic or coronary artery disease. Other diseases commonly associated with heart failure include diabetes, cerebrovascular accident, chronic lung disease, and peripheral vascular disease.

NORMAL CARDIOVASCULAR FUNCTION

Myocardial ultrastructure. The light and electron microscopic structure of the myocardium is illustrated in Fig. 86-1. Individual myocardial cells abut on more than two neighboring cells, resulting from branching of myocardial fibers. Within the myocardial cell are multiple cross-banded, parallel myofibrils. The myofibrils are composed of numerous individual contractile elements called sarcomeres, which are connected in series. Investing the myofibrils is the sarcoplasmic reticulum, comprised of the sarcolemma, its inward tubular invaginations called the transverse tubules or T system, and similar tubules oriented lengthwise called the longitudinal system. These structures provide for the intracellular transport of electrolytes and metabolites required for cellular function.

Within the sarcomeres are two types of myofilaments, a set of thinner ones comprised principally of the protein *actin* and thicker ones comprised primarily of the protein *myosin*. Their spatial arrangement (Fig. 86-1) gives rise to light and dark bands. The actin and myosin filaments are believed to remain constant in length, with shortening of the sarcomere accomplished by the thin filaments being actively drawn deeper into the lattice of thick filaments during the contractile process (Fig. 86-2). This is achieved by serially making and breaking the linkages between actin and myosin in a process dependent on Ca^{++}, Mg^{++}, and high-energy adenosine triphosphate (ATP). The maximal contractile force that can be produced by the myocardium is determined by the overlap of actin and myosin filaments that allows the greatest number of force-generating bonds between them. This concept fits nicely with the known length-dependent property of skeletal and cardiac muscle (Frank-Starling principle) illustrated in Fig. 86-2. A variety of ultrastructural abnormalities of the myocardium have been described in hypertrophied and failing hearts, although simple alteration of sarcomere length and filament overlap does not appear to be responsible for heart failure. A number of biochemical abnormalities, including decreases in high-energy phosphates, actomyosin ATPase, and myocardial norepinephrine, have been observed and probably contribute to the impairment of myocardial cellular function.

Myocardial mechanics. Myocardial function can be described in terms of three fundamental parameters: *preload,* *afterload,* and *contractility.* These terms are most easily understood from the study of the isolated cat papillary muscle (Fig. 86-3). One end is attached to a fixed tension transducer, and the other is attached to a fulcrumed lever, whose position is determined by a stop at one end of the fulcrum and a tray, to which various weights can be added, at the other. The length of the muscle before contraction can be determined by the position of the stop, and the force against which the muscle contracts by the weight added to the tray; muscle contraction is initiated by applying an electrical stimulus.

When the weight in the tray is greater than the muscle can lift, an isometric contraction results. The force (tension) that the muscle develops under these circumstances is found to depend on its length. To a certain point of stretch the isometrically contracting muscle develops increasing force with increasing initial length. The weight of the tray and any added weights can also be used as a measure of stretch; thus stretch can be expressed in units of weight or mass as well as length (and in whole heart as pressure, which equals force/area). This length-dependent property of cardiac muscle is the Frank-Starling principle, and the mass (pressure) required to achieve any degree of stretch is termed the "preload." These relationships are depicted in Fig. 86-4 (force-length curve) and Fig. 86-5 (Frank-Starling curve). (In the intact heart, both end-diastolic volume and end-diastolic pressure have been used as measures of preload. The change in diastolic pressure associated with a given change in volume is termed "compliance." The lower curve in Fig. 86-4 and the dashed curve in Fig. 86-5 represent compliance.)

When the weight in the tray is restricted to values that allow the muscle to shorten, it is found that the initial velocity of shortening varies inversely with the weight the muscle is required to lift. The force against which the muscle shortens is termed the "afterload."

When both preload and afterload are varied, a maximal velocity (V_{max}) of shortening can be extrapolated as if a zero afterload were achieved. Similarly, as the preload and stretch are increased, there is a value beyond which further increases in preload do not result in the development of increased force of contraction. This is the maximal force a given muscle can develop and is termed P_o. Both V_{max} and P_o have been proposed as measures of the third fundamental property of muscle, "contractility." However, neither measurement is adequate to describe contractility clinically.

Work with the isolated cat papillary muscle appears to confirm the Frank-Starling law of the heart, which states that the force developed by the contracting heart is proportional to its initial length (preload). Changes in contractility are represented as shifts in both the force-length and force-velocity curves, upward in the case of increased contractility and downward in the case of decreased contractility (Fig. 86-5). The Frank-Starling principle fails to describe adequately changes in cardiac function that occur as a result of alterations in afterload. Furthermore, the intact heart operating at pressures in the physiologic range appears to function only on an ascending limb of its force-length relationship (that is, a descending limb of the Frank-Starling curve has not been demonstrated), and the force-length curves for different inotropic states (degrees of contractility) are nonparallel.

Afterload determines the degree of shortening of cardiac muscle, and afterload, as well as the other parameters determining myocardial performance, varies continuously during cardiac contraction. Thus the terms "instantaneous force," "instantaneous length," and "instantaneous shortening" (or "afterload") have been used. These terms serve to emphasize the dynamic nature of the circulatory system. The contracting heart is able to empty until it reaches a point on its maximal force-length curve (contractile state) that is determined by preload and afterload conditions.

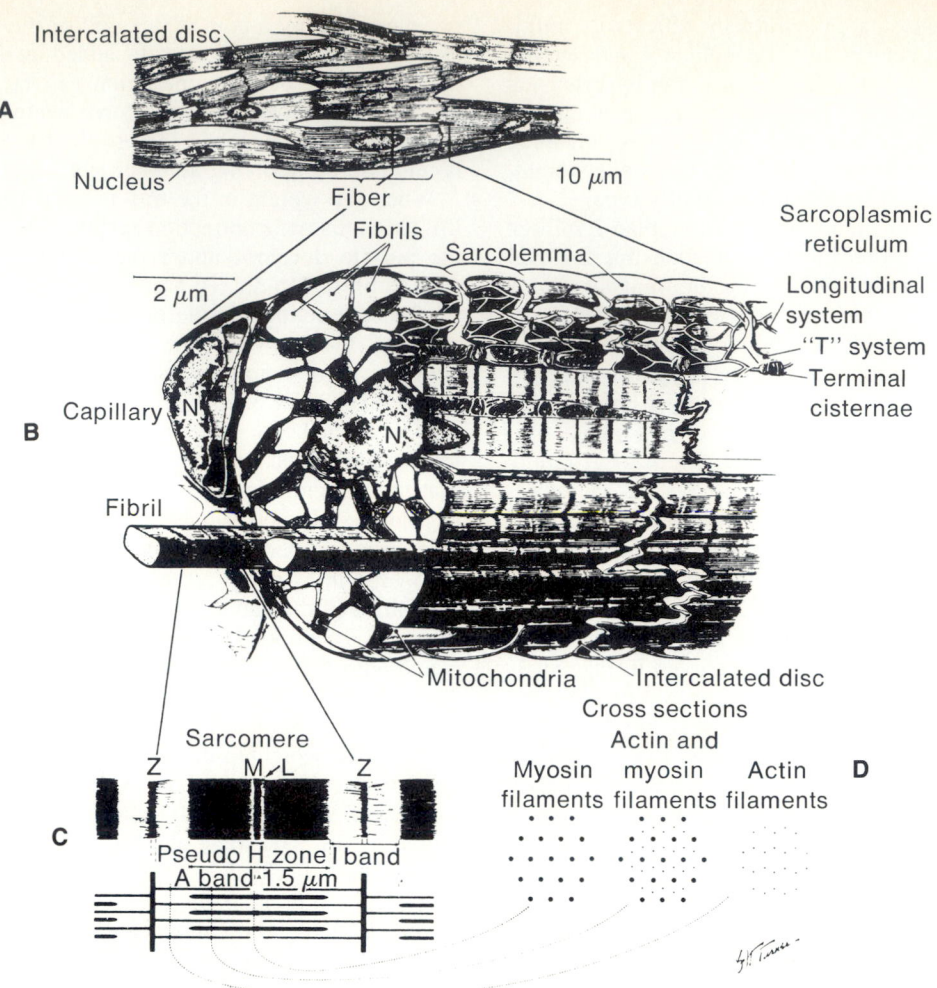

Fig. 86-1 Microscopic structure of heart muscle. **A,** Myocardium as seen under light microscope. Branching of fibers is evident, each fiber containing centrally located nucleus. Fibers or cells are connected by intercalated discs. **B,** Myocardial cell or fiber reconstructed from electron micrographs, showing arrangement of multiple parallel fibrils that compose cell and of serially connected sarcomeres that compose individual fibril (*N* = nucleus). Sarcotubular system that mediates activation, including sarcolemma and sarcoplasmic reticulum, is also shown. Intercalated disc in center of reconstruction serves to separate two cells. **C,** Individual sarcomere from myofibril, and below it, diagrammatic representation of arrangement of myofilaments that make up sarcomere. Thick filaments, approximately 1.5 μm in length, composed of myosin are localized to the A band, while thin filaments, 1 μm in length and composed primarily of actin, extend from the Z line through the I band into the A band, ending at the edges of the central H zone. The H zone is the central area of the A band where thin filaments are absent. Thick and thin filaments overlap only in the A band. **D,** Diagrammatic cross-section of sarcomere showing specific lattice arrangements of myofilaments. In center of sarcomere *(left)* only thick (myosin) filaments arranged in a hexagonal array are seen. In distal portions of A band *(center)* both thick and thin (actin) filaments are found, with each thick filament surrounded by six thin filaments. In I band *(right)* only thin filaments are present. (From Braunwald E, Ross J, Jr, and Sonnenblick EH: Mechanisms of contraction of the normal and failing heart, ed 2, Boston, 1976, Little, Brown & Co.)

Regulation of the circulation. The function of the heart is to provide peripheral tissues with sufficient blood to meet their metabolic requirements. The metabolic requirements of the tissues vary enormously from a basal state to one nearly 20-fold greater as reflected by total oxygen consumption. To account for this required variation, elaborate control mechanisms have evolved.

The mechanisms for regulation of the circulation (determination of the cardiac output and distribution of the cardiac output among the various tissues) can be grouped into two main categories, *neurogenic* and *endocrine*. A third category, *autoregulation,* involves local tissue factors and interplay of the neurogenic and endocrine mechanisms.

The *autonomic nervous system* plays an important role in the regulation of cardiac output. The balance of sympathetic and parasympathetic tone is the prime determinant of heart rate, the former accelerating it and the latter slowing it. Cardiac output is the product of stroke volume and heart rate. Control of heart rate is the principal acute determinant of cardiac output; stroke volume varies less in response to acute changes in physical activity or metabolic status. Changes in stroke volume do occur over time with physical training or in response to regurgitant valvular lesions or arteriovenous shunts. Control of heart rate by the autonomic nervous system is achieved via baroreceptors and other receptors in the blood vessels, heart, and lungs as mediated by various reflex arcs. The autonomic nervous system is critical in the control of regional and total systemic vascular resistance via vasoconstrictor and vasodi-

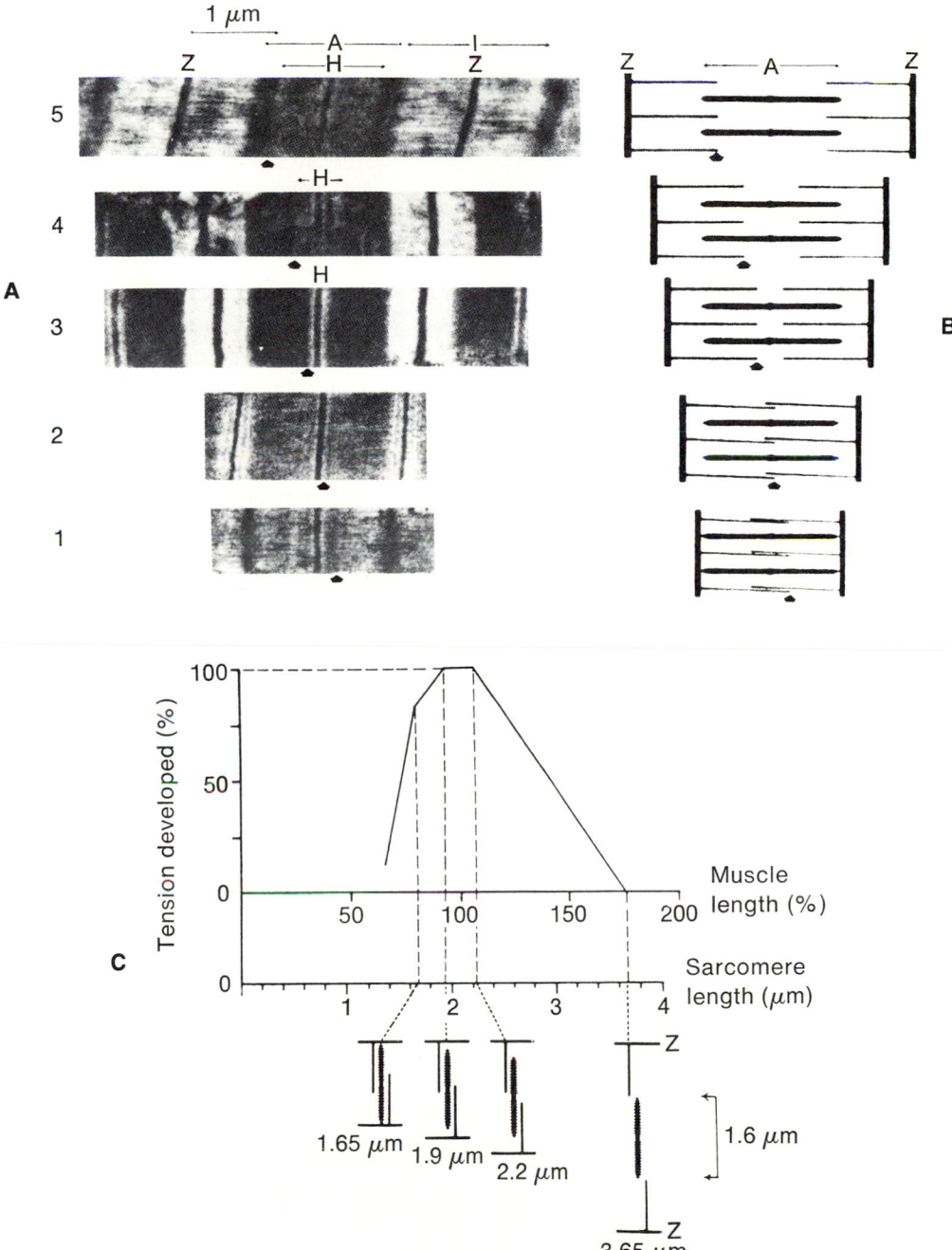

Fig. 86-2 Relationship between electron microscopic band patterns, sarcomere length, and tension development in skeletal muscle (frog sartorius). **A,** Band patterns as seen electron microscopically. **B,** Schematic representation of actin-myosin interaction during contraction of sarcomere. **C,** Maximal tension is developed when actin and myosin filaments are positioned to allow for development of greatest number of sites of interaction. Excessive overlap or separation results in decreased tension development. Similar relationship is probably present in cardiac muscle and may be in part the basis of the Frank-Starling principle. (**A** and **B** from Braunwald E, and others: Am. J. Cardiol 20:705, 1967. Used by permission of the American Heart Association, Inc. **C,** from Hanson J, and Lowy J: Br Med Bull 21:264, 1965.)

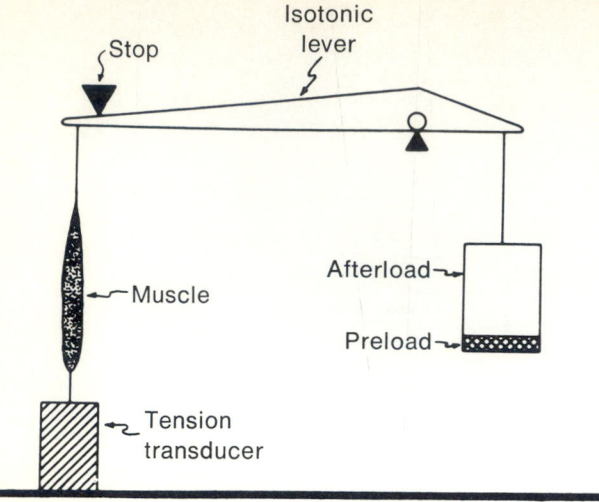

Fig. 86-3 Diagrammatic representation of isotonic lever system. Papillary muscle is stimulated by electrodes along its lateral aspect. Lower end of muscle is attached to extension from tension transducer, while upper free end is attached to end of lever system that is free to move. Fulcrum of lever system is shown at right. Small weight (preload) is placed on opposite end of lever and stretches muscle to length consistent with its resting length-tension relation. Stop is then fixed above tip of lever so that any added weight over and above preload will not be sensed by muscle until it attempts to contract. Additional loads (afterloads) can be added to preload. Total load equals sum of preload and afterloads. (From Braunwald E, Ross J, Jr, and Sonnenblick EH: Mechanisms of contraction of the normal and failing heart, ed 2, Boston, 1976, Little, Brown & Co.)

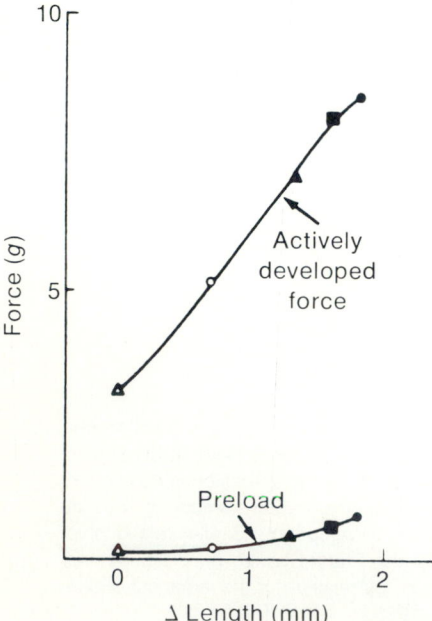

Fig. 86-4 Effects of varying initial muscle length on force-velocity relation of isolated cat papillary muscle. As initial length is increased by increasing preload *(lower line)*, actively developed force increases *(upper line)*, illustrating Frank-Starling principle. (Modified from Sonnenblick EH: Am J Physiol 207:1330, 1964.)

latory fibers that are regulated from the medullary vasomotor center, which in turn is influenced by the cerebral cortex, hypothalamus, and other neural centers.

Several important endocrine factors regulate the circulatory system. During activity or stress and in certain chronic conditions, the circulating catecholamines epinephrine and norepinephrine influence the heart rate, myocardial contractility, and peripheral vascular resistance. Angiotensin, a peptide produced from activation of angiotensinogen (produced in the liver) by renin (produced in the juxtaglomerular cells of the kidney), is the most potent pressor substance known and exerts its effect directly on arteriolar smooth muscle. Angiotensin, as well as potassium and adrenocorticotropic hormone (ACTH), also stimulates release of the mineralocorticoid aldosterone, which has an important sodium-retaining action, from the adrenal cortex. Antidiuretic hormone (ADH, vasopressin) is synthesized in the hypothalamus and is stored in and released from the posterior pituitary gland. It effects water conservation by the kidney and serves to regulate total body water and circulating blood volume. There is evidence that other humoral factors such as atrial natriuretic factor, bradykinin, and prostaglandins may also be important in vascular control.

The third major mechanism in the regulation of the circulation is autoregulation, which serves to enhance the blood supply to organs or muscle groups with augmented metabolic needs. Changes in vascular tone are mediated by local changes in pH, Po_2, Pco_2, $[K^+]$, $[Ca^{++}]$ and concentrations of metabolic products. Local tone regulates blood flow in response to varying metabolic needs. The autonomic nervous system and endocrine mechanisms also serve to increase blood flow to regions with increased metabolic demands.

Decreases in total blood volume with change in body posture, venous compression by skeletal muscle during exercise, and changes in intrathoracic and intrapericardial pressure can also have an important influence on cardiac output.

PATHOPHYSIOLOGY. In congestive heart failure of myocardial origin, decreased myocardial contractility is primary. There are changes in preload and afterload that are usually secondary but are of pathophysiologic and therapeutic importance.

Left ventricular failure. Clinically, the most common measure of myocardial contractility is the left ventricular ejection fraction (stroke volume ÷ end-diastolic volume), as determined angiographically or noninvasively by echocardiography or radionuclide blood pool scanning. If the primary defect in left-sided congestive heart failure is impaired contractility evidenced by decreased left ventricular ejection fraction, stroke volume decreases or left ventricular end-diastolic volume increases or both. It follows that generally there is a fall in cardiac output or a rise in left ventricular end-diastolic pressure. The latter tends to augment left ventricular contractility via the Frank-Starling mechanism and thereby to increase stroke volume, compensating for decreased contractility. When the decrease in myocardial contractility is mild or moderate, this compensatory increase in stroke volume can restore cardiac output to normal. However, the consequence of increased left ventricular end-diastolic pressure is increased left atrial pressure and therefore increased pulmonary venous and capillary pressures. These latter increased pressures constitute the hemodynamic criteria for left ventricular failure and are important in symptom production (for example, dyspnea) in so-called backward left-sided congestive heart failure. If left ventricular compliance is abnormally decreased while ejection fraction and volume of the left ventricle remains normal, cardiac output is maintained by elevation of left ventricular diastolic pressure.

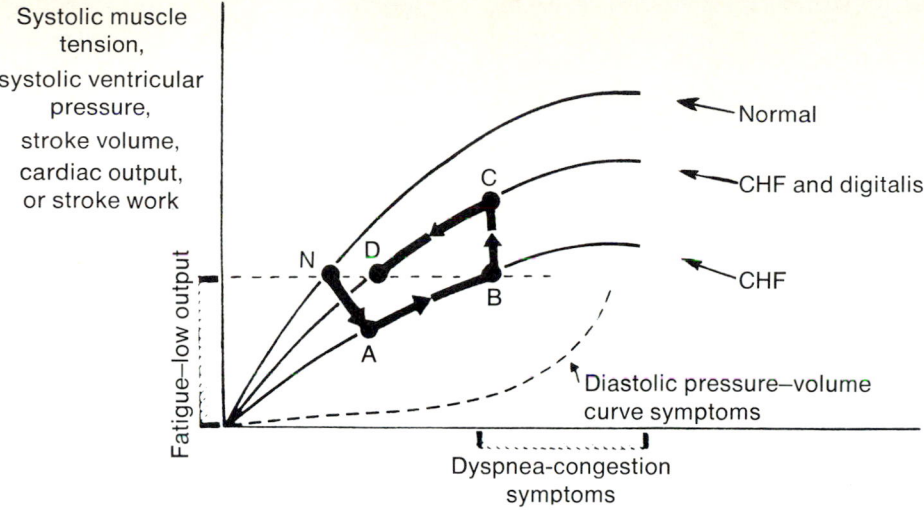

Fig. 86-5   Diagrammatic representation of Frank-Starling principle in congestive heart failure. Three curves represent length-tension or ventricular function curves in normal, congestive heart failure, and heart failure after treatment with digitalis. Points N through D (following the arrows) represent in sequence: depression of contractility, Frank-Starling compensation, increase in contractility with digitalis, and reduction in use of Frank-Starling compensation that digitalis allows. Of note is the fact that points N, B, and D all lie on same line in vertical axis and thus represent same stroke volume, but each is on a different end-diastolic pressure on horizontal axis. Levels at which symptoms of congestion, such as dyspnea, and symptoms of low cardiac output, such as fatigue, occur are represented by cross-hatched areas. Dashed curve represents diastolic pressure-volume curve relating end-diastolic pressure on ordinate to end-diastolic volume or muscle length on abscissa. (Modified from Spann J F, Mason D T, and Zelis R F: Mod. Concepts Cardiovasc Dis 39:79, 1970. Used by permission of the American Heart Association, Inc.)

With failure to maintain a normal cardiac output for the body's metabolic demands, relative peripheral perfusion falls. This results in impaired organ function and the symptoms of so-called forward left ventricular failure.

Depressed contractility does not always indicate clinical heart failure because reduced left ventricular ejection fraction can be present without any signs or symptoms of heart failure. Such asymptomatic cardiac depression can represent a stage of latent heart failure with adequacy of compensatory mechanisms. Conversely, clinically manifest heart failure can exist in association with normal left ventricular ejection fraction when diastolic dysfunction manifested by decreased compliance abnormally limits end-diastolic volume or valvular regurgitation increases stroke volume. Though left ventricular dysfunction is usually present in clinical heart failure, documentation of abnormal cardiac performance does not by itself establish the diagnosis of clinical congestive heart failure.

Right ventricular failure. The most common cause of right ventricular failure is left ventricular failure, although the findings in right ventricular failure are the same regardless of the cause. As indicated previously, the hallmarks of left ventricular myocardial failure are a decreased left ventricular ejection fraction and a rise in the left ventricular end-diastolic pressure, which is transmitted retrograde to the left atrium, pulmonary veins, and pulmonary capillaries. Since the right ventricle provides the active force for delivering blood to the left side of the circulation and the normal pulmonary circulation offers little resistance to forward flow, a rise in the pulmonary capillary pressure dictates a rise in right ventricular systolic pressure. To a degree, the right ventricle is capable of achieving this result without a rise in its filling pressure, but eventually the right ventricular end-diastolic pressure and therefore the mean right atrial pressure rise. These are the hemodynamic and clinical criteria for right ventricular failure.

Physiologic response to cardiac dysfunction. The same factors that regulate the systemic circulation in health have important roles in compensating for cardiac disease; failure of these compensatory mechanisms to return the circulatory system to normal results in symptom production and clinical congestive heart failure. An understanding of these compensatory mechanisms provides an understanding of the pathophysiology of congestive heart failure and its symptoms.

Heart rate. The compensatory response expressed most rapidly is increased heart rate. This may be evident first with modest exercise when increased muscle metabolism calls for increased blood flow (cardiac output). With greater myocardial impairment, tachycardia can be present at rest. Increases in heart rate are mediated by the autonomic nervous system and the endocrine mechanisms discussed previously.

Ventricular dilation and eccentric hypertrophy. Ventricular dilation is a major compensatory mechanism following myocardial injury or in volume overload lesions (regurgitant valvular lesions, atrial or ventricular septal defects, peripheral arteriovenous shunts). The volume of the ventricle increases with the cube of the radius, but thinning of the ventricular wall does not occur. The dilated ventricle may be able to maintain a normal stroke volume despite a decrease in ejection fraction. Ventricular dilation is accompanied by increased muscle mass, even if wall thickness remains normal. This is termed "eccentric hypertrophy."

Concentric hypertrophy. The left ventricular response to systemic hypertension, coarctation of the aorta, aortic valve stenosis, and other lesions, perhaps including ventricular dilation, is an increase in wall thickness ("concentric hypertrophy"). Concentrically hypertrophied myocardium has been demonstrated to have inherently decreased contractility. However, because of an increase in the number of contractile units, even though their individual contractility is less than normal, greater force can be developed by the concentrically hypertrophied myocardium than by normal myocardium, enabling the left ventricle to meet the demand imposed on it.

Thus maintenance of a normal stroke volume, despite decreased left ventricular ejection fraction, and maintenance of normal or higher than normal pressures, despite decreased contractility, are consequences of eccentric and concentric hypertrophy, respectively. Laplace's law indicates that wall stress is directly proportional to the pressure (P) in the chamber and its radius (r), and it is inversely proportional to the wall thickness (h) (wall stress = Pr/2h). Thus increased pressures and ventricular dilation result in increases in wall stress, but increased thickness of the wall tends to reduce the wall stress. A consideration of the compensatory mechanisms of heart rate, dilation, concentric and eccentric hypertrophy, and their interrelationships affecting wall stress is particularly important when myocardial oxygen delivery is limited as a result of obstructive coronary artery disease, since the four major determinants of myocardial oxygen demand are systolic wall stress, myocardial mass, heart rate, and contractile (inotropic) state.

Role of afterload in congestive heart failure. In recent years increased attention has been drawn to the role of afterload in the pathogenesis and treatment of congestive heart failure. Afterload, which is also termed "impedance" or "left ventricular outflow resistance," is the sum of all forces that oppose ejection of blood from the ventricle during systole. As indicated, this value varies with time during the process of ventricular emptying, but instantaneous variation is not easily quantitated. The two major determinants of afterload are the *compliance* of the large arteries that accept the ventricular ejectate and the *peripheral resistance* to blood flow (largely determined at the level of the small arteries and arterioles). These factors determine the systolic pressure rise in the left ventricle and systemic arteries for a given ventricular stroke volume. Other factors affecting the afterload are the viscosity of blood and the inertia of the static blood in the ventricle and proximal aorta, which must be overcome to initiate ventricular ejection.

The normal ventricle adjusts to changes in afterload and maintains a relatively constant stroke volume (homeometric autoregulation). When the ventricle fails, however, its output becomes inversely related to afterload. In congestive heart failure afterload has been found to be increased above normal. The responsible factors appear to be an increase in peripheral vascular resistance owing to enhanced sympathetic tone and an increase in circulating catecholamines and renin. Increased levels of atrial natriuretic factor, vasopressin, and prostaglandins may also play a role. In addition, the compliance of the large arteries is decreased owing either to age (arteriosclerosis) or to vascular smooth muscle congestion. The increased afterload tends to increase the work of the left ventricle at a time when its ability to perform work (inotropic state) is already decreased. In many instances the increased afterload appears to be more an adverse effect of myocardial failure than a beneficial compensatory mechanism; a vicious circle of increasing afterload resulting in further impairment of cardiac performance with resultant further increases in afterload is established.

Production of signs and symptoms in congestive heart failure. The severity of the clinical manifestations of congestive heart failure depends on the degree of myocardial impairment, the demands the individual's activities place on the heart, and the proportion of time spent in activity and at rest. With mild impairment of cardiac function, symptoms may be evident only with strenuous exertion or when the individual is very active for many hours each day. With more severe impairment of cardiac function, symptoms may appear at ordinary levels of activity and subside only slowly with rest. With severe impairment, the patient is symptomatic at rest or with minimal activity. In summary, patients are classified as asymptomatic (I), symptomatic with major exertion (II), symptomatic with mild exertion (III), or symptomatic at rest (IV). Functional capacity does not, however, correlate closely with resting measures of ventricular function, since patients with even marked depression of left ventricular ejection fraction can be asymptomatic.

Consequences of high ventricular filling pressures. The signs and symptoms of "backward" heart failure are the ones most commonly encountered. The cardinal clinical findings in congestive heart failure are *dyspnea* and *edema*. Inability of the failing ventricle to empty completely during systole or decreased compliance in diastole results in a rise in left ventricular end-diastolic pressure and a subsequent rise in left atrial, pulmonary venous, and pulmonary capillary pressures. How pulmonary venous hypertension leads to dyspnea is unclear, but it does not cause arterial hypoxemia or hypercapnia. Although reduced pulmonary compliance and increased work of breathing can result from pulmonary congestion, these usually produce typical changes in ventilation and blood gases that are usually absent when dyspnea is due to heart failure. There is evidence that passive elevation of pulmonary arterial pressures and total pulmonary resistance raise the afterload of the right ventricle, impeding its output and filling of the left ventricle, thereby limiting left ventricular output. Thus, dyspnea may actually represent an appropriate hyperventilatory response to inadequate systemic blood flow and lactate accumulation in underperfused tissues.

Dyspnea must be distinguished from *tachypnea*, an increased respiratory rate in response to metabolic needs that is not necessarily an appropriate hyperventilatory response to enhance gas exchange but is not perceived as shortness of breath by the patient.

When the elevated pulmonary capillary pressure exceeds the oncotic pressure, transudation of fluid into the alveoli, termed "pulmonary edema," occurs. The presence of fluid in alveoli is one cause of pulmonary rales heard on physical examination. The edema results in impaired gas exchange and increases the work of breathing beyond that imposed by pulmonary venous engorgement alone. Pulmonary edema can occur insidiously with the salt and water retention that develops in chronic congestive heart failure, or it can occur abruptly (*acute pulmonary edema*) following acute myocardial infarction, with acute aortic or mitral insufficiency, or without apparent cause.

Orthopnea is dyspnea when the patient is supine, alleviated by elevation of the trunk. Elevation of the thorax above the lower extremities decreases the hydrostatic pressure in the pulmonary capillaries and veins (especially in the upper lobes) and decreases venous return. Both factors contribute to a fall in pulmonary capillary and venous pressure that relieves the dyspnea. With mild orthopnea, sleeping on two or three pillows may provide relief. When orthopnea is more severe, the patient may be able to rest and sleep only bolt upright.

Another symptom of "backward" failure is *paroxysmal nocturnal dyspnea*. Patients with this symptom wake from sleep with shortness of breath that is relieved by sitting up or standing, especially before an open window. The pathophysiology of this symptom is in part similar to that of orthopnea, and sleeping with the thorax and head elevated may prevent it. However, it is possible that depression of the respiratory center during sleep results in hypoxia in the patient with already compromised gas exchange or that decreased adrenergic stimulation of the failing myocardium during sleep is pathophysiologically important.

The consequences of backward failure of the right ventricle are less life threatening than those of left ventricular failure. The sequences of pressure phenomena are identical, but elevation of the filling pressure of the right ventricle (right atrial pressure, jugular venous pressure, systemic venous pressure) does not interfere with as vital a process as respiratory gas exchange. The most common sign of right ventricular failure is *peripheral edema*, the result of chronic elevation of systemic venous pressure to a level that exceeds the oncotic pressure. When the patient spends considerable time in the upright position, edema is present at the ankle and pretibially. In the bedridden patient edema is commonly found in the dependent aspect of the trunk ("presacral" edema). Frequently when edema is present, the jugular venous pressure is elevated on physical examination. However, since the right-sided pressures may be elevated only with exertion, this finding may be absent during examination after a period of rest.

A second result of elevation of the systemic venous pressure is *hepatomegaly* and gastrointestinal venous congestion. Hepatic congestion results in parenchymal distention within a less distensible liver capsule, and epigastric or right upper quadrant discomfort is common. Manual compression of the abdomen causes a transient delivery of volume to the right atrium with concomitant elevation of the jugular venous pressure (hepatojugular reflux) visible by inspection. Care must be taken to distinguish this quite specific finding from venous distention produced by a Valsalva maneuver induced by vigorous palpation of the abdomen. Abdominal discomfort can also be due to edema of the gastrointestinal tract with disturbances of digestion and elimination. In severe right-sided heart failure, transudation of edema into the bowel lumen can result in protein-losing enteropathy. In advanced right heart failure ascites can be present.

Pleural effusion is a common finding in congestive heart failure. Since the pleural veins drain into both the pulmonary and systemic venous systems, pleural effusion usually signifies coexisting left and right heart failure. Occasionally pleural effusion can result from marked elevation of pressure in either venous system alone. Modest accumulation of fluid in the pericardium can also occur in heart failure, but pericardial effusions resulting from congestive heart failure are rarely large enough to cause tamponade. Cardiac tamponade can be considered a form of heart failure, but the cause is seldom myocardial. When tamponade is present, a pericardial origin should be sought.

Peripheral edema or accumulation of fluid in the pleural or peritoneal cavities tends to cause an increase in body weight. Anorexia of cardiac or other origin can cause loss of tissue mass concomitant with fluid retention so that no change in body weight occurs or the weight can actually decrease.

Consequences of reduced cardiac output. The "forward" signs and symptoms of heart failure are subtle and more difficult to evaluate than those caused by increased filling pressures. In part, this is because increased filling pressures and other compensatory mechanisms are able to sustain a normal resting cardiac output, as well as increases in the cardiac output sufficient to meet the demands imposed by modest to moderate physical activity.

Normal individuals can increase their cardiac output approximately fivefold with exercise and, by increasing peripheral tissue oxygen extraction, can increase oxygen consumption eightfold over resting levels. Trained athletes can raise their cardiac output sevenfold with exercise and their oxygen consumption nearly 20-fold. Neither normal individuals nor trained athletes attain much elevation of ventricular filling pressures to achieve these high levels of performance.

In contrast, the individual with congestive heart failure has a limited capacity to increase cardiac output and oxygen consumption and does so at the expense of elevated ventricular filling pressures, with the consequences previously detailed. Measurement of exercise capacity (work load), cardiac output, oxygen consumption, and the filling pressure required to achieve these maximal values assesses an individual's degree of impaired myocardial performance.

The signs and symptoms of reduced cardiac output in congestive heart failure are related to the changes in distribution of available cardiac output among the organ systems. Although skeletal muscle tends to receive its normal share of the cardiac output at rest, its demands cannot be met during exercise, and *easy fatigability* is a common symptom in congestive heart failure. Because of compensatory vasoconstriction to shift blood to more vital beds, the skin, splanchnic, and renal circulations are subject to the greatest reductions in blood flow when the cardiac output is reduced. Thus *pallor* of the skin and impaired temperature regulation accompany congestive heart failure. Reduced splanchnic circulation adds to the abdominal discomfort and impaired function caused by venous congestion and edema. Hepatic clearance of ADH and aldosterone is reduced.

Renal underperfusion results in reduced glomerular filtration, oliguria, and "prerenal" azotemia (usually without proportionate elevation of the serum creatinine level). Impaired sodium and water excretion contributes importantly to the development of edema. In addition, renal hypoperfusion induces release of renin that results in increased circulating angiotensin and, in turn, increased aldosterone release. Angiotensin contributes to vasoconstriction, and aldosterone further promotes sodium retention and accumulation of fluids.

Cerebral and coronary perfusion is decreased less than that of other organs in congestive heart failure. Perfusion of the hypothalamus is frequently reduced enough to result in the release of increased amounts of ADH. Reduction in cerebral blood flow can result in anxiety or difficulty in concentration and less commonly in confusion (especially if cerebrovascular disease coexists). Marked obtundation and coma rarely result from congestive heart failure. When the coronary arteries are free of atherosclerosis, there is not enough decrease in coronary perfusion in congestive failure to be of clinical importance. However, when the coronary circulation is limited by occlusive atherosclerotic disease, normal autoregulative processes may not be operative and the reduced coronary flow, in combination with the marked increase in myocardial oxygen consumption dictated by ventricular dilation, can cause an increase in angina pectoris or result in myocardial infarction.

LABORATORY FINDINGS. Of the routine laboratory tests, those most commonly affected by heart failure are renal and liver function tests and arterial blood gas studies. Renal function abnormalities result from kidney underperfusion and the effect of diuretic agents. Blood urea nitrogen is sensitive to decreases in renal blood flow and tends to rise earlier in congestive failure and to a greater degree than serum creatinine. Diuretic agents can also disproportionately raise blood urea nitrogen via direct renal action or by further decreasing renal blood flow. Serum electrolyte abnormalities occur commonly in heart failure. Hyponatremia can result from water retention or from excess urinary sodium loss in response to diuretics. Heart failure in patients with hyponatremia usually responds well to angiotensin-converting enzyme inhibitors. The serum sodium may be restored towards normal, although occasionally symptomatic hypotension results from these drugs. Hypokalemia occurs commonly as a manifestation of secondary aldosteronism or as a side effect of diuretics and responds to angiotensin-converting enzyme inhibitors. Hypochloremia can also result from diuretic therapy.

Liver function test findings are often abnormal in right-sided congestive heart failure because of hepatic venous congestion and hypoxia. Mild to moderate elevations of serum bilirubin, transaminases, and alkaline phosphatase are common. Occasionally these values reach such high levels that distinction from hepatitis is difficult. The prothrombin time is frequently prolonged and can be refractory to correction with vitamin K administration. Since alcoholic or other liver disease can be present in some patients with heart failure, distinction between primary and secondary liver disease is sometimes difficult.

With pulmonary congestion, oxygenation is impaired and arterial hypoxemia occurs. Hypercapnia can occur but only in the most severe cases. In chronic heart failure a low arterial oxygen tension is common, and arterial PCO_2 is often low owing to hyperventilation in an attempt to achieve adequate oxygenation. Arterial pH is often alkalotic as a result of both hyperventilation and diuretic-induced metabolic alkalosis. However, in severe low–cardiac output states, arterial pH can be at acidotic levels because of CO_2 retention and anaerobic metabolism.

The *electrocardiogram* can reflect the underlying cardiovascular pathologic condition but does not specifically diagnose congestive heart failure. Common features in heart failure are arrhythmias, left ventricular hypertrophy, conduction defects, and ST-T wave changes that can reflect underlying pathophysiology or the effects of digitalis and diuretics. A completely normal electrocardiogram can be seen occasionally.

The *chest roentgenogram* is a sensitive indicator of the presence of congestive heart failure. It is affected by the duration of heart failure and to some degree by its severity. Acute onset of left ventricular failure usually causes little if any change in heart size or contour, but in its earliest stages it produces pulmonary venous hypertension manifested as dilation and prominence of pulmonary veins. As the severity of pulmonary vascular congestion increases, vascular markings become more prominent, especially in the upper lobes. In the most severe cases transudation of fluid into the alveoli can occur and appears as infiltrates with an alveolar distribution. In chronic heart failure heart size is increased, with the cardiothoracic ratio usually exceeding 50%. Signs of long-standing pulmonary congestion are interstitial edema (Kerley's lines) and pleural effusion. Pericardial effusion can also contribute to increased heart size on roentgenogram. Lateral and oblique views of the heart may be necessary to demonstrate specific chamber enlargement. It should be recognized that neither acute nor chronic roentgenographic changes correlate closely with the hemodynamic findings or symptomatic status of patients.

Echocardiography is discussed in Chapter 89. In left-sided failure the echocardiogram frequently shows left ventricular dilation. Wall motion abnormalities, especially hypokinesis, can also be present. In restrictive and constrictive disease the chamber size can be normal, although valve motion patterns can reflect abnormal hemodynamics. The ability of two-dimensional echocardiography to assess ventricular function is good and can be enhanced by Doppler flow-velocity studies.

Cardiac catheterization is of particular value in diagnosing heart failure and in some instances in determining its cause. Hemodynamic findings consistent with heart failure include elevated ventricular filling pressures, decreased cardiac output, and decreased ejection fraction. Depressed contractility is usually evident on ventriculograms.

Right-sided heart catheterization can be performed safely at the patient's bedside using balloon-tipped flotation catheters, which can be equipped with thermistors for measurement of cardiac output by thermodilution. Since left ventricular pressures in diastole are transmitted back through the left atrium to the pulmonary vessels if the mitral valve is normal, pulmonary artery diastolic pressure or pulmonary capillary wedge pressure is virtually equal to left ventricular end-diastolic pressure. The right ventricular filling pressure can be estimated fairly accurately at the bedside by inspection of jugular venous pulsations. In chronic conditions, when the right and left ventricular filling pressures rise and fall together, physical examination alone may suffice to determine the appropriate therapeutic intervention. However, when right and left ventricular filling pressures are affected by disease processes that influence them independently, there may be little or no correspondence in values estimated at physical examination. Outstanding examples are cor pulmonale, in which pressures on the right side greatly exceed those on the left; myocardial infarction when abrupt elevation of the left-sided pressures has not yet been reflected on the right side of the circulation; and the respiratory distress syndrome when both right and left ventricular filling pressures can be elevated. In these situations simultaneous bedside determination of right- and left-sided filling pressures may be of great clinical value. For example, a pulmonary arterial diastolic pressure more than 5 mm Hg above pulmonary capillary wedge pressure suggests pulmonary hypertension from pulmonary parenchymal disease or pulmonary thromboembolic disease; in acute myocardial infarction a disproportionate elevation of right atrial pressure to levels as high as or higher than the pulmonary wedge pressure suggests right ventricular infarction.

DIAGNOSIS. The diagnosis of congestive heart failure is usually established from the history and physical findings. In addition to the common symptoms of dyspnea or easy fatigability, presenting features can include weight gain, anorexia, abdominal pain, and coughing with little or no sputum production. Because patients often modify their lifestyle to adapt to limitations imposed by the development of heart failure, they may appear asymptomatic. Meticulous interrogation may be required to uncover subtle symptoms or gradual changes in daily activities used to avoid symptoms. The presence of symptoms in association with a history suggesting a cardiac lesion, such as a murmur from rheumatic disease, angina pectoris, previous myocardial infarction, or hypertension, should lead to a suspicion of congestive heart failure. Physical findings can confirm the diagnosis. The most useful of these are elevation of the jugular venous pressure, a hepatojugular reflux, pulsus alternans, an S_3 gallop, pulmonary rales, peripheral edema, and Cheyne-Stokes respirations. Although the presence of these signs usually indicates heart failure, the signs are often absent. Diagnosis therefore frequently requires demonstration of objective evidence of cardiac dysfunction such as cardiac enlargement as shown by chest roentgenogram, abnormal cardiac size or motion as shown by echocardiography, or even abnormal ventricular function as shown by cardiac catheterization or radionuclide angiography. Finally, because of the poor correlation between these objective measurements and symptoms, or between subjective symptoms and measured exercise capacity, exercise testing may be needed to document the degree of functional limitation. Exercise testing has become an accepted technique in the diagnosis and management of heart failure. Specially modified protocols using low-level exertion are employed and under these conditions exercise testing is safe and reliable in patients with heart failure.

Congestive heart failure must be distinguished from other causes of dyspnea and fatigue. The most common noncardiac causes of shortness of breath are pulmonary disorders, identified by a history of pulmonary disease, abnormal pulmonary function tests, and abnormal blood gas studies. Sometimes the two disorders coexist, rendering their differentiation more difficult and occasionally requiring hemodynamic measurements to distinguish between heart failure and pulmonary disease as the cause of shortness of breath. Other causes of congested states simulating heart failure include renal failure, cirrhosis, and excess fluid administration. These are usually apparent from the clinical presentation and laboratory tests. However, pulmonary congestion resulting from excess fluid administration should prompt a careful search for the presence of previously unrecognized heart disease, since volume loading is usually well tolerated by patients with normal cardiovascular function. Finally, other causes of low cardiac output must be excluded. These include shock from sepsis, pulmonary embolism, hypoadrenalism, and hypovolemia (see Chapter 88).

COURSE AND PROGNOSIS. Although patients with congestive heart failure frequently have symptomatic improvement following the institution of therapy, the course is usually one of progressive deterioration. According to data collected in the Framingham study, the 5-year survival rate from the time of diagnosis of congestive heart failure is less than 50%. This ominous prognosis is as bad as or worse than that of all forms of cancer considered together. Patients with moderate to severe heart failure have a mortality as high as 50% to 60% within 12 to 24 months of the time of diagnosis.

The mode of death in congestive heart failure is commonly sudden and unexpected, whether the failure is due to ischemic heart disease or other forms of cardiomyopathy. It is difficult to predict the course on the basis of clinical findings. However, some hemodynamic measures of left ventricular function appear to be related to prognosis. Survival has been shown in some studies to be related to resting cardiac output. Probably the most powerful predictor of survival is the left ventricular ejection fraction. The prognosis is poor with ejection fractions below 20%, and 36-month survival is almost twice as great among patients with ejection fractions over 20%.

This ominous prognosis applies primarily to patients with chronic congestive heart failure of ischemic or idiopathic origin. In other cases congestive heart failure can be "cured." This is most likely when a specific cause such as myocarditis can be found and effectively treated. In patients with acute myocardial infarction, heart failure can be severe during the acute phase but transient and nonrecurrent. Patients with congestive heart failure resulting from valvular heart disease or ventricular aneurysm often improve following surgical therapy. This is more likely in patients whose ventricular function has remained sufficiently unimpaired by valvular disease. Improvement also occurs in cases of ventricular aneurysm when enough functioning myocardium is uninvolved by the aneurysm

that correction of the mechanical problem results in good residual function and thus symptomatic relief. The long-term prognosis is very good in such "cured" patients.

Patients with congestive heart failure are subject to other complications of their heart disease. *Arrhythmias* are frequent and range from relatively benign supraventricular to serious ventricular arrhythmias. These occur with ischemic heart disease but are also frequent in other forms of heart disease. The prevalence of arrhythmias appears to be greater in patients with more severe failure, and it is possible that the degree of hemodynamic abnormality, altered cardiac chamber size, and loading conditions are predisposing factors in some cases. *Embolic phenomena* are a common complication of congestive heart failure. Pulmonary embolism usually originates from the peripheral venous bed when there is stasis, particularly in patients with marked peripheral edema and right-sided heart failure. Systemic emboli to the cerebral, renal, and mesenteric beds originate from the left side of the heart (either atrium or ventricle) as a result of clot formation in these chambers. Atrial fibrillation, which is frequently present in patients with congestive failure, facilitates clot formation in the noncontracting atria.

In some patients with stable heart disease, symptoms develop acutely in response to arrhythmias, a new ischemic event, a change in medication, failure to take prescribed medication, or dietary indiscretion. Patients with heart failure are also subject to acute exacerbations of their disease for reasons that are not always apparent. When no apparent cause is found exacerbations commonly are attributed to dietary indiscretion or to noncompliance with medical regimens, but frequently these factors are not responsible for worsening the patient's clinical status. Excessive salt and fluid ingestion can unquestionably increase the severity of the symptoms of heart failure, but adjustment of diuretic dosage can usually compensate for minor increases in salt and water consumption. It is likely that acute exacerbations of congestive heart failure without apparent cause represent progression of the disease process. The vicious cycle of compensatory mechanisms leading to high peripheral resistance, increased afterload, and worsened left ventricular function may account for this steady course punctuated by acute episodes during which therapy must be readjusted.

MANAGEMENT. The major principles in the treatment of heart failure are outlined in Table 86-1. Certain general measures are recommended for the majority of patients with congestive heart failure. During periods of marked symptomatology patients are usually advised to rest and avoid undue exertion. Such a recommendation from the physician is rarely necessary because patients voluntarily curtail activities when their symptoms become more severe with exertion. The prescription of prolonged bed rest (for periods up to 6 months to 1 year) in acute myocarditis or idiopathic cardiomyopathy is no longer enforced in most cases, since it is difficult to achieve and can make patients susceptible to other complications, especially emboli. Diet is important, and obesity should be corrected to decrease the metabolic work load on the heart. In addition, patients are advised to curtail sodium intake, but this need not require great patient discomfort because excess sodium accumulation can be controlled by appropriate diuretic administration in all but the most severe cases.

Other factors that can aggravate or impose an increased load on cardiac performance should be controlled. Hypertension should be rigorously controlled by appropriate medications. Caution is advised in the prescription of antihypertensive drugs that can depress cardiac function; these include sympatholytic agents such as methyldopa, β-adrenergic blockers, certain cal-

Table 86-1   Treatment of congestive heart failure

	Acute heart failure	Chronic heart failure

General measures	Bed rest
	Strict sodium restriction
		Reduced activities
		Moderate sodium restriction
		Control associated disorders:
		   Hypertension
		   Obesity
		   Pulmonary disease
		   Arrhythmias
		Risk factor modification:
		   Smoking
		   Hyperlipidemia

Pharmacologic therapy	Oxygen Morphine Treatment of arrhythmias Correction of pH Diuretics (furosemide) Vasodilators (nitroprusside) Inotropic agents (sympathomimetics)	Inotropic agents (digitalis) Preload reduction (diuretics) Afterlaod reduction (vasodilators)
Other therapy	Mechanical circulatory assistance Surgery for specific lesions	Surgery for specific lesions Cardic transplantation

cium channel blockers, and reserpine. Other associated disorders such as pulmonary disease must be treated vigorously because they can have significant effects on the circulation by directly imposing a load on the right ventricle, thus limiting systemic oxygen delivery.

Drug treatment remains the cornerstone of therapy in clinically overt heart failure. The medications currently used fall into three categories: (1) inotropic agents that enhance contractility and thereby cardiac performance; (2) agents that reduce ventricular filling pressures and thereby decrease pulmonary and systemic venous congestion; and (3) impedance-reducing agents that decrease left ventricular outflow resistance, thereby allowing the failing ventricle to eject a greater portion of its diastolic volume and improve cardiac output.

Oral inotropic agents useful in congestive heart failure currently include only digitalis preparations, of which the most commonly used is digoxin. Although digitalis improves indices of myocardial contractility, several studies in recent years have demonstrated that the effects of digitalis are less than may be desired. Left ventricular filling pressure and cardiac output are not consistently improved by short- or long-term administration of digitalis. Because of the questionable hemodynamic efficacy and relatively high toxicity associated with digitalis administration, its routine use in the long-term management of congestive heart failure has recently been questioned. Some studies have shown that the agent can be withdrawn without deterioration in patients with chronic stable congestive heart failure, whereas others have indicated that withdrawal is associated with symptomatic deterioration. The use of digitalis (for example, digoxin in doses of 0.125 to 0.375 mg/day) is still recommended in chronic congestive heart failure. In contrast, acute digitalization for hemodynamic improvement does not appear warranted, since the effects of the agent are quite mild and more potent agents are available. The term "digitalization" merely means achievement of effective blood and tissue levels of digitalis, and because of the narrow therapeutic margin with this agent, it is no longer recommended that digoxin be rapidly given or that high doses be used in an attempt to achieve a greater inotropic effect. Daily maintenance doses result in digitalization over a period of days. Therapy may be guided by the use of blood levels, with values from 0.7 to 2 ng/ml

considered to be in the therapeutic range. Levels above 2 ng/ml are considered toxic. Higher doses should be avoided. However, the correlation between drug effect and digoxin blood levels is poor, and therapy is still best guided by clinical criteria. Other inotropic drugs are currently being developed, but none is now available for long-term oral administration.

The primary preload-reducing agents are diuretics, which decrease intravascular volume, thereby reducing ventricular filling pressures along with pulmonary and systemic venous congestion. Diuretics do not alter cardiac function because they simply shift ventricular performance along the same Frank-Starling curve. The reduction in preload is generally accompanied by no change or a slight fall in cardiac output. These agents should be used with caution in patients operating on a critical volume-dependent portion of the ventricular function curve (the more vertical portions on the left in Fig. 86-5), since a reduction in filling pressure can result in a substantial fall in cardiac output. Hypotension, azotemia, and other signs of low output can ensue. Furthermore, diuretic administration frequently results in electrolyte imbalance, including hyponatremia, hypokalemia, and metabolic alkalosis. Potassium supplementation is usually necessary with diuretic agents, especially when digitalis is used. The most commonly used diuretics are the potent loop diuretics furosemide (20 to 300 mg/day), ethacrynic acid (25 to 200 mg/day), and bumetanide (0.5 to 2 mg/day). Because these agents are short acting, they should usually be given at least twice a day in doses that prevent edema or weight gain. In some cases these agents alone produce an insufficient clinical response, but combining them with other diuretics such as thiazides, which act at a different site in the nephron, can lead synergistically to a marked increase in urinary sodium excretion. If hypokalemia becomes prominent, potassium-sparing diuretics such as spironolactone (25 to 150 mg/day) or triamterene (50 to 200 mg/day) may be beneficial.

The third class of agents used in heart failure are the vasodilators, which decrease resistance to left ventricular ejection. Of these, nitroprusside (0.5 to 8 μg/kg/min) is the agent of choice for parenteral use in acute left ventricular failure. Although many vasodilators produce sustained hemodynamic benefits, only those agents with venodilating ability have produced long-term improvement in symptoms and exercise capacity. Thus long-acting oral nitrates (isosorbide dinitrate [160 mg/day]) and angiotensin-converting enzyme inhibitors (captopril [75 to 150 mg/day], enalapril [5 to 20 mg/day], and lisinopril [10 to 40 mg/day]) have been the only effective vasodilators for chronic heart failure. Enalapril and nitrates in combination with hydralazine have been shown recently to be the first pharmacological interventions to reduce mortality in patients with chronic heart failure. The angiotensin-converting enzyme inhibitors are especially attractive because of their relatively specific action in interfering with a basic pathogenetic mechanism (that is, increased renin activity, which stimulates angiotensin production, thereby promoting vasoconstriction and secondary aldosteronism with sodium retention). Although vasodilators are currently used as adjuncts to conventional therapy with digitalis and diuretics in patients refractory to standard treatment, they are likely to be used earlier and in cases of milder heart failure in the future. They are also being tested as agents to prevent or delay the onset of clinical heart failure in patients with asymptomatic cardiac dysfunction.

Acute pulmonary edema is a medical emergency. The most outstanding abnormality in this condition is marked elevation of the pulmonary venous pressure leading to severe dyspnea. Cardiac output can be normal or occasionally even elevated. The immediate therapeutic goal is to reduce the high filling pressure. Initial therapy includes the administration of oxygen to improve oxygenation and morphine to interrupt disadvantageous cardiopulmonary reflexes and relieve anxiety. Diuretic agents are also useful. If a clinical response is not obtained in 20 to 30 minutes, the addition of impedance-reducing agents should be considered. The agent of choice in this instance is the potent vasodilator sodium nitroprusside. Decreasing impedance to left ventricular ejection allows an increase in cardiac output while simultaneously reducing left ventricular filling pressure. This desirable combination of effects has been consistently demonstrated in patients with acute pulmonary edema. In addition, the effects of nitroprusside can be finely titrated. In contradistinction, diuretics have delayed, limited, and inconsistent hemodynamic effects in acute pulmonary edema.

In patients with symptoms of low output (a shocklike state, oliguria, cerebral underperfusion, and cutaneous vasoconstriction), it may be necessary to add inotropic agents more potent than digitalis for short-term management. These patients usually are already receiving digitalis, and there is no evidence that giving additional digitalis is beneficial. The potent inotropic drugs available are the sympathomimetic agents isoproterenol, dopamine, dobutamine, and norepinephrine. These drugs enhance myocardial contractility and usually raise cardiac output. In high doses their peripheral vasoconstricting effect can limit the rise in cardiac output because of an associated increase in afterload. A useful approach therefore has been the combination of a vasodilating agent such as nitroprusside with a potent inotropic agent such as dopamine or dobutamine (see Chapter 88). This combination raises cardiac output more than either agent alone and is useful in severely low output states. A similar result can be achieved with amrinone, which has both vasodilator and positive inotropic effects. In patients with acute exacerbations of severe chronic congestive heart failure, it is usually necessary to continue these regimens for several days before instituting therapy with oral agents.

Many new treatments are currently being evaluated for use in heart failure. Milrinone is a new inotropic-vasodilator agent that improves hemodynamics, but its clinical efficacy is yet to be established. Xamoterol is a new partial β-agonist that combines positive inotropic action with antiadrenergic activity. The β-blocker metoprolol has had long-term efficacy in selected patients who tolerate its cardiac-depressing effects. Long-term β-blockade could be beneficial by attenuating the adverse effects of excessive sympathetic nervous activity. Some calcium channel blockers (nifedipine and diltiazem) are effective vasodilators, but are limited by their negative inotropic action (verapamil). In patients refractory to medical treatment, cardiac transplantation is now firmly established as an effective therapy. In some centers the results are better than for valvular surgery, and a greater than 80% 1-year survival rate can be anticipated. Cardiac transplantation is limited by the availability of suitable donor hearts.

Although the prognosis for congestive heart failure remains poor, the pathogenesis is becoming clearer. Factors adversely affecting prognosis include elevated ventricular filling pressures and circulating catecholamines, depressed cardiac output and left ventricular ejection fraction, and arrhythmias, all of which are amenable to intervention. Current emphasis is shifting to application of sensitive noninvasive diagnostic techniques for early recognition and therapeutic interventions to prevent or delay the onset of heart failure in patients with asymptomatic cardiac dysfunction. Other interventions are aimed at preventing or treating the cardiac lesions responsible for heart failure.

BIBLIOGRAPHY

Applefeld MM, editor: Contemporary issues in the management of chronic congestive heart failure, Am J Med 80(suppl 2B):28, 1986.

Cohn, JN (Symposium Chairman): New concepts in the mechanisms and treatment of congestive heart failure, Am J Cardiol 55 (2):1A, 1985.

Cohn JN and others: Effect of vasodilator therapy on mortality in chronic congestive heart failure, N Engl J Med 314:1547, 1986.

DelGreco F: The kidney in congestive heart failure, Mod Concepts Cardiovasc Dis 44:47, 1975.

Dodge HT and Baxley WA: Left ventricular volume and mass and their significance in heart disease, Am J Cardiol 23:528, 1969.

Franciosa JA: Exercise testing in chronic congestive heart failure, Am J Cardiol 53:1447, 1984.

Franciosa JA: Epidemiologic patterns, clinical evaluation, and long-term prognosis in chronic congestive heart failure, Am J Med 80(suppl 2B):14, 1986.

Franciosa JA, Baker BJ, and Seth L: Pulmonary versus systemic hemodynamics in determining exercise capacity of patients with chronic left ventricular failure, Am Heart J 110:807, 1985.

Francis GS: Neurohumoral mechanisms involved in congestive heart failure, Am J Cardiol 55:15A, 1985.

Kannel WB, Savage D, and Castelli WP: Cardiac failure in the Framingham study: twenty-year follow-up. In Braunwald E, editor: Congestive heart failure: current research and clinical applications, New York, 1982, Grune & Stratton.

Mason DT: Regulation of cardiac performance in clinical heart disease: interactions between contractile state, mechanical abnormalities and ventricular compensatory mechanisms, Am J Cardiol 32:437, 1973.

McCall D and O'Rourke RA: Congestive heart failure. II. Therapeutic options, old and new, Mod Concepts Cardiovasc Dis 54:61, 1985.

Smith WM: Epidemiology of congestive heart failure, Am J Cardiol 55:3A, 1985.

Sonnenblick EH and Strobeck JE: Derived indices of ventricular and myocardial function, N Engl J Med 296:978, 1977.

Weber KT and Janicki JS: The heart as a muscle-pump system and the concept of heart failure, Am Heart J 98:371, 1979.

87·SYSTEMIC HYPERTENSION

Robert L. Grissom

Hypertension is the principal reason for office visits to physicians, and of all diseases it results in the largest number of outpatient prescriptions. A national survey has shown that most American adults who have hypertension are aware of it and know that high blood pressure is a serious disease that cannot

Table 87-1 Classification of blood pressure in adults aged 18 years or older*

BP range, mm Hg	Category†
DBP	
<85	Normal BP
85-89	High-normal BP
90-104	Mild hypertension
105-114	Moderate hypertension
≥115	Severe hypertension
SBP, WHEN DBP <90 mm Hg	
<140	Normal BP
140-159	Borderline isolated systolic hypertension
≥160	Isolated systolic hypertension

From the Joint National Committee on Detection, Evaluation, and Treatment of High Blood Pressure: Arch Intern Med 148:1024, 1988.
*Classification based on the average of two or more readings on two or more occasions. BP, blood pressure; DPB, diastolic blood pressure; and SBP, systolic blood pressure.
†A classification of borderline isolated systolic hypertension (SBP, 140 to 159 mm Hg) or isolated systolic hypertension (SBP, ≥160 mm Hg) takes precedence over high-normal BP (DBP, 85 to 89 mm Hg) when both occur in the same person. High-normal BP (DBP, 85 to 89 mm Hg) takes precedence over a classification of normal BP (SBP, <140 mm Hg) when both occur in the same person.

Table 87-2 Classification of hypertension in the young*

Age group	≥95th percentile	≥99th percentile
NEWBORNS, d		
7 (SBP)	≥96	≥106
8-30 (SBP)	≥104	≥110
INFANTS (≤2 y)		
SBP	≥112	≥118
DBP	≥74	≥82
CHILDREN, y		
3-5		
SBP	≥116	≥124
DBP	≥76	≥84
6-9		
SBP	≥122	≥130
DBP	≥78	≥86
10-12		
SBP	≥126	≥134
DBP	≥82	≥90
13-15		
SBP	≥136	≥144
DBP	≥86	≥92
ADOLESCENTS (16-18 y)		
SBP	≥142	≥150
DBP	≥92	≥98

From the Joint National Committee on Detection, Evaluation, and Treatment of High Blood Pressure: Arch Intern Med 148:1033, 1988.
*SBP, systolic blood pressure; DBP, diastolic blood pressure. Classification based on report of Second Task Force on Blood Pressure Control in Children—1987. All values expressed as millimeters of mercury.

be cured but only controlled by continued treatment. Yet it is estimated that the disease is adequately controlled in fewer than half of the 58 million American adults who have it. Hypertension in the United States becomes more prevalent as people age. The rate for black Americans, especially males, far exceeds the rate for white Americans. The number of people under treatment has increased significantly over the past dozen or so years, since hypertension began receiving considerable publicity as a public health problem. In recent years morbidity and mortality from strokes have declined markedly, a fact attributed in large part to better management of hypertension. The incidence of coronary artery disease has diminished also, but how much of that reduction is attributable to hypertensive treatment is a matter of dispute. Since hypertension also contributes to heart failure and renal disease, they, too, may be expected to decline in frequency. Every health encounter, including dental visits, should be an occasion to consider measuring a patient's blood pressure. Knowledge of the disease and its treatment is important in managing oral and dental problems. Dentists have a unique opportunity to detect cases of high blood pressure, since semiannual dental visits are encouraged. Many men who otherwise are well may not see their physicians more often than every 3 to 5 years.

Blood pressure is remarkably well controlled by a series of reflexes and adjustments made throughout the day and night. The level stays within a fairly narrow range with almost all activities but varies normally so that it generally is lowest at night and highest in mid- to late morning. Anxiety, pain, exercise, and tenseness transiently raise the pressure, whereas relaxation, prolonged bed rest, and sleep lower it.

Some have questioned whether a dividing line exists between normal and high blood pressure. Sir George Pickering argued that there is no "bimodal distribution," that is, a separate and set number at which a person suddenly becomes hypertensive. Rather, he said, the model is a continuum; the higher the blood pressure, the more vascular damage occurs. Others hold to the concept of a distinct abnormal condition. The Department of Health and Human Services' Fourth Joint National Committee on Detection, Evaluation, and Treatment of High Blood Pressure (1988) and the American Heart Association arbitrarily set the dividing line for individuals over 18 years of age at 140/

90 mm Hg; the World Health Organization has chosen 160/95 for most adults as the point of which a diagnosis of hypertension ought to be made. At the same time, physicians and other health-care professionals are cautioned not to be overzealous in diagnosing hypertension when a single or occasional reading is elevated, since this may result from any of the several causes of transient hypertension.

The consensus report of the previously mentioned Fourth Joint National Committee set arbitrary limits for resting and seated arm blood pressure; these limits are given in Table 87-1.

Values in children may be considerably lower. The suggested upper limits of normal blood pressure in children by age category are given in Table 87-2.

Values in pregnancy, when the uterus and fetus produce a large arteriovenous shunt, tend to be lower than in nonpregnant women despite increased plasma renin activity.

MEASUREMENT OF BLOOD PRESSURE. It is important to measure the pressure accurately. Generally the first of three readings tends to be highest. In surveys a mean value of three determinations commonly is used, but in office practice two readings usually are taken and an average recorded.

The proper cuff size should be chosen to fit the arm well; thus a larger cuff diameter is used for a larger arm. A too small cuff on an obese or large, muscular arm falsely elevates the reading; a too large cuff on a small arm gives a falsely low reading.

The patient should be comfortably seated with the arm bared and approximately at heart level. The manometer pressure should be raised above the systolic level in the preliminary reading to find the systolic level by palpation of the radial or brachial pulse; this is to avoid being misled by an "auscultatory gap" with resulting overestimation of the diastolic pressure or underestimation of the systolic pressure with the usual auscultatory method.

The manometer pressure should be raised rapidly to avoid undue congestion of the arm and then reduced slowly for accurate reading of the systolic and diastolic levels. The latter is taken in adults at the point where the sounds disappear (Korotkoff fifth sound phase). In children and young adults the blood pressure sounds sometimes can be heard at zero pressure. In that case the practitioner also records where the sounds diminish in intensity (Korotkoff fourth sound phase). A similar technique is used in cases of aortic insufficiency when peripheral resistance is markedly lowered. On occasion arm blood pressure sounds may be weak and difficult to hear. In such cases it is useful to raise the arm to a vertical position over the head for several seconds to diminish the venous content of the arm veins. The pressure cuff then is pumped up over the systolic level, at which point the arm is brought back to a horizontal position. The sounds should be louder after this augmentation maneuver.

Hospitals, physicians' offices, and probably dentists' offices will find standard mercury manometer equipment and a stethoscope the most reliable and durable equipment to use. Spring-type manometers have proved serviceable but may be inaccurate if accidentally dropped. Calibration for accuracy, especially with nonmercury manometers, should be checked at least twice yearly. Newer electronic devices sometimes use heart sounds as endpoints, sometimes other pulsatile phenomena. They may simplify measurement by patients and also may be useful in surveys, but they can be expensive and sometimes inaccurate and fragile. For the individual patient, when comparison values over a long period may be most important, these devices can be useful for self-measurement; however, the standard for blood pressure measurement remains the mercury manometer.

DEFINITIONS AND PATHOGENESIS. "Primary hypertension" is a commonly used term. "Essential" or "idiopathic" hypertension is a synonymous term meaning that no cause other than genetics can be found. Indeed, heredity is important, although how the trait is transmitted is unknown. A discussion of the genetics of hypertension is beyond the scope of this chapter, but a study of families in Framingham, Massachusetts, showed some pertinent correlations.

The total peripheral arterial resistance in the systemic circulation is directly related to the pressure. Most resistance is in the arterioles, and because of the large flow to the kidneys (which receive approximately a quarter of the cardiac output), the renal afferent arterioles have a dominant influence on the pressure. In pulsatile flow Poiseuille's coefficient shows that blood pressure resistance increases inversely as the fourth power of the radius. This critical measurement is most evident in the arterioles because of their narrow diameter. Thus if the radius of an arteriole is reduced by half, resistance increases by a factor of 16 ($2 \times 2 \times 2 \times 2$).

Resistance is inversely related to blood flow, as expressed by the useful formula

$$R = \frac{P}{F}$$

Here R is total resistance, P is mean pressure, and F is systemic flow. For the systemic circulation as a whole, blood flow usually is considered to be cardiac output. Although cardiac output may be elevated in several conditions causing hypertension (thyrotoxicosis, acute glomerulonephritis, and other hyperdynamic states), in established primary hypertension cardiac output generally is normal. Thus the total mean pressure varies directly with the total resistance.

Total resistance cannot be measured directly. Resistance in the various parts of the body (including the arm) is not constant. For example, resistance in an exercising arm falls as the need for muscle flow increases. The *sum* of all resistance in the systemic circulation is called the total peripheral resistance (TPR). In fairly controlled resting conditions, as in an office, it remains relatively constant.

In addition to cardiac output and TPR, aortic impedance plays a role; this is the variable aortic expansion as the heart pumps a bolus of blood into the aorta with each beat. As the patient ages, impedance changes, because the aorta becomes more rigid and less elastic. This gives rise to a wider pulse pressure (the difference between systolic and diastolic pressures) so that readings as high as 160/75 mm Hg may be normal. Blood volume also is a factor, especially the diastolic blood volume. Blood volume, too, is altered in many situations. It diminishes in chronic illness or with prolonged bed rest. In acute blood volume reduction, as with hemorrhage, significant change in the blood pressure generally is a late rather than early response to blood volume changes.

Even under standard resting conditions blood pressure is not the same in all four extremities. It usually is similar in the two arms, but some varieties of congenital coarctation can make it higher in the right arm that in the left. Also, if one arm has partial atherosclerotic obstruction to the subclavian artery, the systolic pressure in that arm is correspondingly lower. The measured lower extremity pressure in the thigh, even in the recumbent position, is higher than upper extremity pressure because of the greater mass of underlying tissue and the phenomenon of reflected pressure waves. In practice only the systolic pressure in the leg is measured in the search for congenital coarctation, since the systolic reading alone suffices. More commonly, the practitioner simultaneously palpates the femoral and radial pulses for discrepancy in volume and timing. Normally the pulse wave should be felt simultaneously in each location; in the patient with coarctation, the "damped" femoral pulse arrives later than the radial pulse.

In the standing position systolic pressure tends to fall slightly and diastolic pressure to rise. If the diastolic rise while standing is more marked, it may signify elevated cathecholamine (norepinephrine) levels, as is sometimes found in young persons. However, the major change with standing is found in the elderly, especially those with reduced blood volume, in whom systolic pressure may fall 20 to 30 mm Hg or more on standing. In some individuals this fall may cause symptoms of light-headedness. The remedy for this may simply be more salt in the diet to expand the blood volume or less or no diuretic medication. Occasionally a salt-retaining hormone such as fludrocortisone is required.

Control of the pulmonary circuit pressure is fairly independent of the systemic pressure. In the absence of heart failure, pulmonary pressure remains approximately normal even when systemic pressure is very high. Measurement of pulmonary artery pressure requires cardiac catheterization.

Early primary hypertension

Hypertension is defined as chronic abnormal elevation of the resting systolic or diastolic pressure or both, and if persistent it carries a greater risk of complications. These complicating sequelae, rather than the elevated pressure itself, are the more serious consequences. The higher the pressure on a chronic basis, the greater the hazard. The major problems are coronary heart disease, heart failure, renal failure, stroke, and peripheral vascular disease. Because of this "target organ" damage, the diagnosis of hypertension carries serious implications for the patient and should not be made hastily. In one study more than 30% of patients with diastolic pressure higher than 95 mm Hg had normal pressure (that is, less than 90 mm Hg) on subsequent visits. For obvious reasons, in a dental office elevated pressure should be reported to the patient as a finding rather than as a diagnosis of hypertension.

For several years before chronic pressure elevation develops, transient rises may be observed in stressful circumstances such as during a dental visit. Such transient elevations often are called "labile hypertension." However, since all blood pressure levels fluctuate and therefore are labile, it seems better to label this phenomenon "transiently elevated pressure." In some instances of transiently elevated pressure, especially in young persons, cardiac output is increased. Some but not all such individuals later develop chronic hypertension. The stronger the family history of hypertension, the more likely the person with transiently elevated pressure will develop chronic hypertension.

Athletes with increased vagal tone and a slow heart rate may show transient systolic pressure elevation. Strong isometric maneuvers, as in weight lifting, transiently raise the pressure.

Symptoms may be few or nonexistent for many years. Unsteadiness, early morning headaches, nocturia, occasional blurred vision, and feelings of depression are described. Impotence is not infrequent. Often the first symptoms arise from side effects of treatment rather than from the hypertension itself. Since hypertension is a common cause of congestive heart failure, symptoms also may arise from that condition. Angina or transient ischemic attacks in the brain, reflecting coronary or cerebrovascular disease, may occur. If the blood pressure is only modestly elevated, organ damage may be delayed for many years or may never become significant. However, the pressure in both primary hypertension and secondary hypertension (as discussed later) may become progressively elevated and cause greater damage as it enters an accelerated or even malignant phase.

Accelerated hypertension

Also known as *severe* or *malignant hypertension,* accelerated hypertension arbitrarily is defined by diastolic pressures higher than 125 mm Hg plus evidence of target organ damage of the heart, eyes, central nervous system, or kidneys. If "choking" or edema of the optic disc is present, the term "malignant" is applied. This calls for urgent treatment, since it is associated with vascular fibrinoid necrosis, particularly of the renal arterioles, and portends early death.

Isolated systolic hypertension

Isolated systolic hypertension is seen with such metabolic abnormalities as thyrotoxicosis, but it is more commonly found in elderly individuals whose major vessels, including the aorta, have less elasticity. The aorta receives the pressure wave and the bolus of blood with less resilience, hence the systolic rise found in the brachial artery. In the past, this was thought to be a condition of aging that caused no damage; more recent studies have found an association with strokes and other hypertensive complications. Accordingly, gentle reduction now is recommended, with close attention to standing pressure to avoid sudden reductions in the cardiac output and cerebral blood flow. Somewhat related is *pseudohypertension,* in which quite rigid arm blood vessels are not easily compressible by the pressure cuff, with resultant Korotkoff's sounds at a falsely high level. A clue to pseudohypertension is a poorly compressible radial pulse that may be palpable even when the blood pressure cuff reading is high above the expected systolic level. In this unusual situation an intraarterial measurement will disclose the true level.

Secondary hypertension

Secondary hypertension should be considered, especially in younger individuals (that is, those under 40 years of age), in people with more severe hypertension, or in the patients for whom the pressure is difficult to control or in whom other clinical clues are present. These patients need more extensive evaluation, especially of the kidneys and adrenal glands. Formerly, an excretory urogram (intravenous pyelogram) was obtained regularly, but renal arteriography or digital subtraction angiography, looking especially for renal arterial stenosis, now is preferred. Plasma renin activity, aldosterone, and compounds secreted by pheochromocytomas are measured as well. Generally, high aldosterone activity suppresses plasma renin. Hormone secretions usually are measured both in urine and plasma.

For nearly 90 years the renal enzyme renin has puzzled investigators. It first was found that a crude extract of rabbit kidneys raised the pressure when injected into rabbits. In 1934 Goldblatt showed that a pressor substance was secreted into the plasma from an ischemic kidney. Subsequently this substance was isolated and called renin. It was found to act on a protein produced in the liver to yield angiotensin I. In turn angiotensin I is acted on by a plasma-converting enzyme to yield a powerful vasoconstrictor, angiotensin II, a protein that causes increased secretion of aldosterone.

Various causes of secondary hypertension can be corrected surgically; the one that occurs most frequently is renal arterial stenosis. Estimates of its prevalence range from less than 1% to 18% of patients with hypertension, but most would put the number at 3% or less. In adults under 40 years of age, the condition is most common in women, who are more apt to have renal arterial fibrous dysplasia. Over 50 years of age, when arteriosclerotic vascular occlusion of the renal arteries occurs more frequently, the condition may be superimposed on primary hypertension. In severe hypertension (diastolic blood pressure higher than 125 mm Hg), renal artery occlusive conditon is more common in whites than blacks. In one-sided renal arterial stenosis, catheter samples of effluent blood show an elevated plasma renin activity greater than 50% more from the renal veins of the ischemic kidney than from the opposite kidney veins or from the inferior vena cava below those renal veins. In one study of renovascular hypertension, 31% of lesions were bilateral. Operative repair has had varying success; balloon dilation has been successful at all ages and particularly in some older patients.

Several drugs used to manage hypertension affect plasma renin activity. Recently investigation has focused on the role of the kallikreins, various kinins, prostaglandins, endogenous digitalis-like factors, the atrial natriuretic factor, and a circulating substance in the serum of patients with primary hypertension that affects the level of cytosol calcium in platelets from nonhypertensive subjects. The interrelation of sodium, potassium, and calcium in patients with hypertension continues to intrigue workers in the field. It is clear that patients with hypercalcemia caused by hyperparathyroidism have a significantly greater likelihood of developing hypertension. It is expected that some patients now thought to have primary hypertension may be reclassified as having secondary hypertension as the cause of the hypertension becomes more firmly established.

A list of secondary hypertensive diseases is given in Table

Table 87-3   Chronic secondary hypertension

Cause	Mechanism
TYPES OF CHRONIC SECONDARY HYPERTENSION CURED OR HELPED BY SURGERY	
Renal artery obstruction ⎱ Renin-producing tumors ⎰	Excess stimulation of renin-angiotensin axis
Hypercalcemia caused by parathyroid tumor	Excess calcium
Adrenal cortical disease Cushing's syndrome Primary aldosteronism	Sodium retention, usually with suppression of plasma renin through feedback mechanisms
Adrenal medullary disease Phepchromocytoma	Excess secretion of catecholamines
Extraadrenal chromaffin tumors	Excess secretion of catecholamines
Coarctation of aorta	Increased resistance and stimulation of renin-angiotensin axis
Brain tumor	Cerebral regulatory factors
Atrioventricular fistula	Systolic hypertension through increased cardiac output
TYPES OF CHRONIC SECONDARY HYPERTENSION CURED OR HELPED BY MEDICATION	
Hypothyroidism and hyperthyroidism	Corrects metabolism
Pyelonephritis (especially with chronic renal failure)	Antibiotics clear infection
TYPES OF CHRONIC SECONDARY HYPERTENSION CURED OR HELPED BY REDUCTION OR ELIMINATION OF A SUBSTANCE	
Birth control medications, estrogen medications, licorice, sympathetic-stimulating drugs (nasal decongestants, diet pills) tyramine-containing foods (e.g., some cheeses in people taking monamine oxidase inhibitors)	Alteration of the renin-angiotensin-aldosterone axis
Alcohol	Pressor effect (may account for 10% of hypertension cases; recommended reduction to less than 2 oz/day)
TYPES OF CHRONIC SECONDARY HYPERTENSION FOR WHICH SURGICAL OR MEDICAL THERAPY CAN ONLY REDUCE ADVERSE EFFECTS	
Renal parenchymal disease, polycystic disease, connective tissue diseases (e.g., lupus), diabetic glomerulonephritis, renal hydronephrosis, acromegaly, carcinoid, quadriplegia, porphyria, lead poisoning, Paget's disease, aortic rigidity	Changes in renal function, renin-angiotensin, or cardiac and vascular function

87-3 indicating those that show marked improvement or cure with surgical or medical therapy directed at the cause.

Pregnancy-induced hypertension

Pregnancy-induced hypertension, formerly called pre-eclampsia, involves widespread vasospasm. It tends to occur in the first pregnancy, particularly in mothers under 20 years of age and in pregnancies complicated by diabetes or involving twins. The condition accelerates toward the end of the pregnancy. It often is associated with edema and albumin in the urine. Curiously, it tends to resolve after delivery. Uteroplacental hypoperfusion is thought to be a cause, with resulting renin-angiotensin and prostaglandin abnormalities. Prevention of the full syndrome is the routine strategy for treatment, but many antihypertensive drugs have been insufficiently tested for their effects on the unborn child. Methyldopa, hydralazine, and β-adrenergic blockers currently are the drugs of choice. It is important to distinguish pregnancy-induced hypertension from preexisting primary or secondary hypertension, which is worsened by the pregnancy.

DIAGNOSTIC APPROACH. The examiner should consider several questions when evaluating a patient with elevated pressure: Is the hypertension definitely established? Is the hypertension primary (that is, without demonstrable cause)? Has target organ damage occurred? Do any other conditions aggravate the potential target organ damage (for example, smoking or elevated cholesterol)? Will the patient respond positively to recommendations for treatment? The patient should understand that the pressure exceeds the normal range, that long-term treatment is necessary, that symptoms or lack of them do not indicate pressure levels, and that treatment is unlikely to result in a cure. However, with successful management, a normal life-style and excellent prognosis are expected.

Important elements of the patient's history include the degree and duration of the hypertension, the drugs used, and the patient's response. The patient should be asked about aggravating substances such as estrogens and nose drops and whether he has had any symptoms of target organ damage such as chest pain, headaches, or transient neurologic symptoms.

The more effective antihypertensive drugs now available lower the pressure in secondary types of hypertension but generally are less successful than in primary hypertension; this may be a clue to the careful physician. The physical examination gives other clues when hypercorticism exists, as with Cushing's syndrome. Routine palpation of femoral artery pulses will disclose a proximal obstruction from coarctation. Endocrine causes may be fairly obvious, as with hyperthyroidism and its concomitant hyperdynamic circulation and rapid pulse, or rather obscure, as in aldosteronism, in which persistent low blood potassium levels may be the first hint. High urinary aldosterone levels, calibrated against sodium-potassium excretion, and suppressed plasma renin activity assist the diagnosis.

During an examination the blood pressure should be measured in both arms and, in the older patient especially, compared with blood pressure level and pulse rate in the standing position. The general appearance may suggest thyroid dysfunction, acromegaly, or neurofibromatosis (which is associated with pheochromocytoma). Fundoscopic examination is the only means of seeing the arterioles, which tend to mimic changes in the kidneys. The ophthalmoscopic examination may give clues to arteriosclerotic changes, advanced diabetic lesions (hemorrhages and exudates), acute nephritis, or malignant hypertension with edema in a raised optic disc. The heart shows the effects of hypertension in the left atrium and ventricle. Evaluation of the apical impulse may show an outward thrust with hypertrophy, sometimes preceded by a palpable fourth sound that indicates decreased compliance of the left ventricle when the atrium contracts. Later, systolic murmurs may develop at both the apex and base. In severe hypertension, eventration of an aortic cusp may cause a diastolic regurgitant murmur. Since hypertension accelerates atherogenesis, clues may be found in the carotid or femoral arteries or the abdominal aorta with vascular bruits. Especially in middle-aged women, auscultation of the flanks may reveal a renal artery bruit, a clue to fibromuscular dysplastic lesions; in older adults, flank bruits may point to partial arteriosclerotic renal artery lesions. Either renal artery lesion potentially can be cured by surgery or palliated by angioplasty.

Because of the relatively chronic nature of hypertension and the cost-versus-benefit factor, extensive evaluation is not commonly done on first observation of patients with hypertension. In its 1988 report the Joint National Committee on Detection, Evaluation, and Treatment of High Blood Pressure recommended the following tests and procedures: hemoglobin and hematocrit, urinalysis (including microscopic evaluation), serum potassium, a measure of calcium, creatine, cholesterol, high density lipoprotein, triglycerides, glucose, and serum uric acid (blood urea nitrogen or creatinine), and a baseline electrocardiogram. An endocrine work up is not suggested unless conditions such as hyperthyroidism or Cushing's syndrome—causes of secondary hypertension—are suspected. With multichannel analysis the panel of tests often can be obtained economically. These tests are conducted to exclude the more common secondary causes, to provide a baseline for follow-up (as with serum potassium), and to seek other risk factors that may affect prognosis (for example, cholesterol and high-density lipoproteins). I have found creatinine clearance to be a useful way to assess kidney function annually or biennially. In the same 24-hour urine collection I measure sodium and potassium excretion to help the patient achieve the goal of limited sodium intake (75 to 90 mEq/day) and adequate potassium in the diet.

MANAGEMENT OF PRIMARY HYPERTENSION. It generally is agreed that drug administration has vastly improved prognosis and reduced target organ damage. Yet drug management is not the first consideration in treating mild or even moderate hypertension. Reduction of body weight in the obese patient, elimination of birth control tablets, increased exercise, and alleviation of stress may be all that are needed for some patients. Epidemiologic studies have shown a relationship between alcohol abuse and hypertension, a factor claimed to be significant for 10% of adults with hypertension. Daily consumption of more than 2 ounces of straight alcohol or its equivalent in beer or wine is associated with a rise in blood pressure to an abnormal level. Each of these factors must be sought and eliminated so far as possible in all patients, whether or not they are taking antihypertensive medication.

The ideal amount of salt ingestion has caused considerable debate. Animal studies have shown that some hypertensive rats may be salt-sensitive and others salt resistant. In humans, if salt restriction is to succeed by itself, severe restriction may be necessary. However, most commonly used antihypertensive medications other than diuretics cause some salt retention. Elderly patients appear to be more sensitive to sodium restriction than younger patients. When the family history strongly suggests a hereditary influence in hypertension, salt restriction may be useful even in normotensive offspring as a lifelong life-style of limited salt intake. My usual recommendation is 75 to 90 mEq sodium per day (about 5 g of sodium chloride). This requires no added salt in food preparation and avoidance of known salty foods such as potato chips and luncheon meats. If the patient is taking diuretics, limiting salt in this way helps avoid hypokalemia.

Since hypertension is one of several predisposing factors for premature coronary heart disease, it is important to look for other factors that may add to that risk, especially hyperlipidemia and cigarette smoking. Diabetes and physical inactivity likewise are important.

In 1980 the Joint National Committee on High Blood Pressure proposed a "step care" drug program that starts with a diuretic. In a high proportion of mild to moderate cases of hypertension, this alone may suffice. At least initially relatively few side effects occur. However, since hypertension is apt to be chronic over many years, some consequences of long-term diuretic use raise concern, including mild but persistent hypokalemia, an increase in plasma renin activity, and a slight tendency for increases in serum lipids, glucose, and uric acid. To counter these effects, smaller and smaller doses of diuretics have been recommended. Currently, 25 mg of hydrochlorothiazide daily or its equivalent with other diuretics is advocated. In patients with multiple-drug therapy, diuretics are useful to help prevent tolerance to adrenergic or vasodilating drugs, because the latter often lead to some sodium retention. Hyperuricemia and secondary gout are occasional problems causing a relative contraindication to their continued use. Most of the diuretics are related to sulfonamides and in rare cases may cause reactions in the mouth from allergic sensitivity. By far the major problem with their use has been undue loss of potassium. They are seldom used in pregnant patients because of concern about hypoperfusion of the placenta.

Longer-acting diuretics appear to cause more hypokalemia. Potassium-sparing agents may be given with the diuretic, such as amiloride, triamterene, or spironolactone, an aldosterone antagonist. Although commonly used, these drugs add to the cost of treatment. The need for potassium chloride supplement can be determined by testing potassium concentrations in the blood. Potassium-rich foods generally are favored over potassium medication. Elderly patients are especially prone to hypokalemia, so small daily amounts of a diuretic or an alternate-day regimen may be advisable.

Since the concept of step care was initiated, a variety of other drugs have become available that have been approved as the first step in place of diuretics or as monotherapy. These drugs, their side effects, and special considerations are listed in Table 87-4.

β-Adrenergic blockers, of which several compounds are now available in the United States, lower blood pressure to a degree similar to the diuretics. They may be useful in the patient with angina, a fast heart rate, or other conditions such as migraine for which some β-blockers have been approved. The various β-blockers appear to be about equally effective in controlling hypertension, although side effects may make one more acceptable than another.

Likewise sympatholytic drugs may be used as first step medication. These include the central nervous system α-adrenergic agonists (clonidine, α-methyldopa, guanabenz, guanfacine), the peripheral α-blocker prazosin, and the ganglionic blockers guanethidine and guanadrel.

Hydralazine is one of the older antihypertensive drugs still in use. At first it mainly was used alone and in larger doses than currently are given. Hence it also had more serious side effects. Its direct and indirect action lead to decreased peripheral vascular resistance. It has found its major use as part of a triple-drug program—diuretic plus β-blocker plus hydralazine—which seems to have minimized its side effects. It has been used extensively in pregnancy by both the oral and intravenous routes. Hydralazine and minoxidil, direct vasodilators, relax the smooth muscle in the peripheral vascular beds. Both drugs cause some tachycardia and increase plasma renin activity. Hydralazine has been a cause of a lupuslike syndrome, which fortunately can be reversed by discontinuing the drug. The major problem with minoxidil has been increased body hair growth (hypertrichosis), which is reported in 80% of patients. Fluid accumulation with this drug has made concomitant use of a diuretic necessary.

Prazosin, an α₁-adrenergic antagonist, reduces both preload and afterload through its relaxant effect on veins and arteries. It has proved a versatile drug, effective as monotherapy and

Table 87-4   Oral medications useful in hypertension

Drugs	Side effects and special considerations	Drugs	Side effects and special considerations
DIURETICS		**PERIPHERAL-ACTING ADRENERGIC INHIBITORS**	
Thiazides and related sulfonamides 13 in all, but hydrochlorothiazide most commonly used	Hypokalemia (increases digitalis toxicity, especially with long-acting thiazides), hyperuricemia (may precipitate acute gout), glucose intolerance, hypercholesterolemia, hypertriglyceridemia, sexual dysfunction; may be ineffective in renal failure	Guanadrel Guanethidine *Rauwolfia* alkaloids, including reserpine	Sexual dysfunction, nasal congestion, diarrhea, orthostatic hypertension Contraindicated in patients with a history of mental depression, nasal stuffiness
		α_1-Adrenergic blockers Prazosin Terazosin	"First dose" syncope, orthostatic hypotension, weakness, palpitations
Loop diuretics Furosemide Ethacrynic acid Bumetanide	Effective in chronic renal failure; may cause hypokalemia, hyperuricemia, and hyponatremia (especially in elderly patients)	**COMBINED α- and β-ADRENERGIC BLOCKERS**	
		Labetalol	Asthma, nausea, fatigue, dizziness, headache; avoid in cardiac failure, chronic obstructive pulmonary disease, sick sinus syndrome, heart block (greater than first degree); use with caution with diabetes
Potassium-sparing agents usually used in combination with diuretics	Slight danger of hyperkalemia in patients with renal failure		
Amiloride	Sexual dysfunction	**VASODILATORS**	
Spironolactone	Gynecomastia, mastodynia, sexual dysfunction	Hydralazine	Headache, tachycardia, fluid retention Positive antinuclear antibody test; lupus syndrome may occur (rare at recommended doses)
Triamterene	Rare nausea; rare blood dyserasia; rise in blood urea; low-salt syndrome	Minoxidil	Hypertrichosis
β-ADRENERGIC BLOCKERS		**ANGIOTENSIN-CONVERTING ENZYME INHIBITORS**	
Acebutolol Atenolol Metoprolol Nadolol Penbutolol Pindolol Propranolol Timolol	Bradycardia, fatigue, insomnia, bizarre dreams, sexual dysfunction, hypertriglyceridemia, decreased high-density lipoprotein cholesterol; avoid in asthma, chronic obstructive pulmonary disease, congestive failure, heart block (greater than first degree), and sick sinus syndrome; use cautiously with diabetes and peripheral vascular disease	Captopril Enalapril Lisinopril	Angioedema (enalopril), excessive hypotension, rash, neutropenia, especially with autoimmune-collagen disorders, proteinuria
		SLOW CHANNEL CALCIUM-ENTRY BLOCKING AGENTS	
CENTRAL-ACTING ADRENERGIC INHIBITORS		Verapamil Diltiazem Nifedipine Nitrendipine	Headache, hypotension, dizziness, nausea, flushing, edema, constipation; use with caution in patients with congestive failure or heart block
Clonidine Methyldopa Guanabenz Guanfacine	Drowsiness, dry mouth, fatigue, sexual dysfunction; rebound hypertension may occur on abrupt discontinuation; in rare cases depression, liver damage, positive direct Coombs' test with methyldopa		

From the Joint National Committee on Detection, Evaluation, and Treatment of High Blood Pressure: Arch Intern Med 148:1028, 1988.

in combination with other drugs. It also has been useful in cases involving coexistent heart failure. Postural hypotension has been a major side effect, especially when the drug is first given.

More recently the converting enzyme inhibitor captopril has been used two or three times a day as a first step drug. Enalapril, also a converting enzyme inhibitor, usually is given only once a day.

Slow channel calcium antagonists also have been applied in hypertension management. Successful results have been published with verapamil, diltiazem, and nifedipine. Patients most apt to benefit are blacks, obese individuals, and those with isolated systolic hypertension. Although many published reports testify to the usefulness of nifedipine and diltiazem, these drugs have not yet been approved by the Food and Drug Administration for use in hypertension. Verapamil recently was approved in a sustained action form for treatment of hypertension.

Several of these drugs may be used together, although generally only one in each grouping should be considered for concomitant use. Judicious combinations may decrease side effects. Some drugs affect a common end organ; for example, propranolol and verapamil slow conduction in the atrioven-

tricular node, so caution should be used when such combinations are prescribed, particularly in older age-groups. Some drugs for associated illness such as nonsteroidal antiinflammatory drugs (for example, indomethacin for arthritis) partially negate a diuretic effect. Tricyclic drugs given for mental illness may erase part or all of the benefit of guanethidine, clonidine, or methyldopa and even furosemide.

In more than 90% of patients hypertension can be controlled using one, two, or three drugs. Although the half-life of these agents vary considerably, in practice clinicians have found that almost all can be given once or twice a day, a feature that promotes compliance.

MANAGEMENT OF SECONDARY HYPERTENSION. These less common patients often respond to the same medications that control primary hypertension. As a class, however, they do less well, and failure to respond should alert the physician to the possibility of secondary hypertension. On the other hand, individuals with the most prevalent of the curable hypertensions, those caused by unilateral or bilateral renal arterial stenosis, may be unusually sensitive to captopril or enalapril. Indeed, this response has been proposed as a diagnostic test. In most secondary cases treatment depends somewhat on the cause. For example, in severe chronic renal failure, excessive blood volume often is critical and a dramatic reduction in pressure may follow dialysis with correction of fluid overload. Loop diuretics such as furosemide are used in place of thiazide diuretics when the blood creatinine level exceeds 2.5 mg/dl.

SPECIAL ASPECTS RELATED TO DENTISTRY. Improved blood pressure control has caused less concern that epinephrine in injectable dental anesthetics may cause an excessive rise in pressure. Orthostatic hypotension may be a problem, and operative procedures in the sitting position could pose a hazard. Aspirin now is commonly taken by patients with hypertension to decrease associated coronary or cerebral vascular thrombotic disease, and aspirin may cause bleeding problems. Many patients with hypertension develop systolic heart murmurs, in which case prophylaxis for endocarditis may be indicated.

Few antihypertensive medications affect the mouth. The α-agonists (methyldopa, clonidine, guanabenz, and guanfacine) may cause dryness of the mouth. For example, methyldopa has been associated with sore tongue, pigmentation, sialadenitis, and lip ulcers. Rare cases of oral reactions have been reported with almost all the drugs used in hypertension. Reserpine-type drugs may cause nasal stuffiness.

With anesthesia for general surgical conditions, good blood pressure control has been sought to avoid surgical complications. Omission of medication before surgery currently is not generally recommended, and the same guideline should apply to dental anesthesia. General anesthetics tend to cause vasodilation, and therefore the anesthetist should be informed of the medication being taken. Hypokalemia as a result of diuretics may be associated with arrhythmias. Some inhalant anesthetics (halothane, enflurane, and isoflurane) are similar in action to calcium slow channel antagonists. Finally, sudden witholding of an α-agonist such as clonidine may precipitate hypertension rebound.

In summary, the dentist frequently encounters hypertension as our population grows older, and he performs a real public service in measuring a patient's blood pressure. The dentist can discuss life-style with the patient, such as smoking and reducing anxiety, not only as it relates to the mouth but also as it affects the more general problems of hypertension and atherosclerosis. Additionally, drugs used in hypertension occasionally affect the mouth and dentition. Insofar as operative safety is concerned, the patient with an optimum blood pressure poses the least risk.

BIBLIOGRAPHY

Canadian Hypertension Society: Report of the consensus development conference on the management of mild hypertension in Canada, Toronto, 1984.
Cressman MD and Gifford RW: Hypertension and stroke, J Am Coll Cardiol 1(2):521, 1983.
Erne P and others: Correlation of platelet calcium with blood pressure: effect of antihypertensive therapy, N Engl J Med 310:1084, 1984.
Friedman GD, Klatsky AL, and Siegelaub AB: Alcohol, tobacco, and hypertension, Hypertension 4 (suppl) 111:143, 1982.
Joint National Committee on Detection, Evaluation, and Treatment of High Blood Pressure: The 1988 report of the Joint National Committee on Detection, Evaluation, and Treatment of High Blood Pressure, Arch Intern Med 148:1023, 1988.
Kaplan NM: Clinical hypertension, ed 4, Baltimore, 1986, Williams & Wilkins.
McAreavey D and others: Third drug trial: comparative study of antihypertensive agents added to treatment when blood pressure remains uncontrolled by a beta blocker plus thiazide diuretic, Br Med J 288:106, 1984.
Needleman P and Greenwald JE: Atriopeptin: a cardiac hormone intimately involved in fluid, electrolyte, and blood pressure homeostasis, N Engl J Med 314:828, 1986.
Prys-Roberts C: Anaesthesia and hypertension, Br J Anaesth 36:711, 1984.
Veterans Administration Cooperative Study Group on Antihypertensive Agents: Low dose captopril for the treatment of mild to moderate hypertension. Results of a 14-week trial, Arch Intern Med 144:1947, 1984.

88 · SHOCK

Carl V. Leier

Shock is an extreme state of circulatory failure in which inadequate perfusion of tissues by blood is the predominant pathophysiologic feature. Impaired tissue perfusion leads to general cellular dysfunction and cell death. The patient prototype, "a patient in shock," is a lethargic or somnolent individual with profound weakness (inability to stand) and cool, pale skin. The hands often are cold and moist ("clammy"). The pulse is weak (diminished amplitude) and rapid. Indirect (sphygmomanometer) blood pressure measurements are unobtainable or very low. Renal dysfunction with a reduced urine output develops early. If proper therapy is not initiated or if the therapeutic interventions fail, this circulatory collapse state deteriorates further and cell death occurs; the loss of tissue and cellular viability heralds a state of "irreversible shock" and death of the individual.

CLASSIFICATION. Extreme circulatory failure and shock can be caused by any or a combination of the three major mechanisms outlined below:

I. Reduction in intravascular volume (hypovolemic or cold shock)
   A. Loss of blood volume—hemorrhage
      1. External loss such as gastrointestinal bleeding, trauma
      2. Internal sequestration such as hemothorax, hemoperitoneum, fractures
   B. Loss of plasma volume
      1. Severe burns, exudative lesions
      2. Dehydration caused by vomiting, diarrhea, diabetic ketoacidosis, insensible water loss without replacement, adrenal insufficiency, diabetes insipidus
II. Increased vascular capacitance (warm shock)
   A. Drugs such as anesthetics and antihypertensive agents; overdosage of tranquilizers or sedatives
   B. Toxins and humoral substances such as endotoxins (gram-negative bacillary bacteremia), immune-mediated substances released during anaphylaxis
   C. Neurogenic disorders such as vasodepressor syncope ("faint"), orthostatic hypotension, acute spinal cord injury
III. Failure of the heart as a pump (congestive shock)
   A. Inadequate filling of cardiac chambers as in pericardial tamponade, tension pneumothorax
   B. Inadequate emptying of the ventricles as in myocardial infarction with failure, ruptured papillary muscle, dysrhythmias
   C. Combined inadequate filling and emptying, as from pulmonary embolus and intracardiac tumors

Shock caused by severe reduction in intravascualr volume generally is referred to as "hypovolemic shock" because of the low intravascular volume or "cold shock" because of the marked compensatory vasoconstriction with resultant cold extremities. The causes of this form of circulatory shock are related to either the excessive loss of blood or less commonly the excessive loss of plasma volume (rate of loss exceeding rate of replacement). The more common causes of acute and excessive blood loss are trauma with disruption of the wall of an artery or large vein or damage to a heavily vascularized structure such as the spleen, lung, liver, or kidney; gastrointestinal disorders such as peptic ulcer disease with erosion of the ulcer into an artery, ruptured esophageal varices in a patient with cirrhosis of the liver and portal hypertension, or hemorrhage from ulcerative colitis; defective mechanisms of blood clotting as seen in leukemia, hemophilia, and thrombocytopenia; and structural defects of the vascular system, exemplified by hereditary hemorrhagic telangiectasia with uncontrolled bleeding from the telangiectasia (nose, gastrointestinal, or lung), rupture of a saccular aneurysm of the aorta or artery, or dissecting aneurysm of the aorta. The more common causes of excessive loss of plasma volume include severe burns, pancreatitis, and peritonitis, with seepage of extracellular fluid (water, electrolytes, and proteins) from the burn or inflamed site. Situations that may lead to severe dehydration and hypovolemia include excessive vomiting or diarrhea, diabetic ketoacidosis (osmotic diuresis of water and electrolytes), inadequate intake of fluids, and untreated adrenal insufficiency, since lack of aldosterone effects a renal loss of water and electrolytes.

The severity of hypovolemic shock generally is related to the amount and rate of loss of the intravascular volume and the responsiveness of the individual's compensatory mechanisms to the sudden or excessive loss of volume. The acute loss of 25% or more of the intravascular volume is required to put a normal subject into circulatory shock; exsanguination in excess of this amount usually overwhelms the compensatory mechanisms and results in severe hypotension and inadequate tissue perfusion. Loss of the same volume over several days generally would not produce circulatory shock, because the compensatory mechanisms could maintain an adequate intravascular volume and perfusion pressure. The compensatory mechanisms of circulatory shock are discussed in the next section of this chapter.

An increase in total vascular capacitance without a change in intravascular volume produces hypotension and, if severe, circulatory shock. In contrast to the vasoconstricted cold extremities of hypovolemic shock, the extremities in this form of shock usually are warm as a result of generalized vasodilation; the term "warm shock" has been applied to this type of circulatory collapse. The excessive dilation of the vasculature may be caused by any of several factors: drugs—through a primary effect (such as that of antihypertensive drugs), an overdosage, or an idiosyncratic reaction; toxins such as endotoxin produced in certain bacterial infections and responsible for bacteremic or septic shock; humoral substances, exemplified by the immune-mediated substances released during an anaphylactic reaction to a drug such as penicillin or lidocaine, insect stings, or food allergies; and abnormalities in neurologic control of the vascular system such as spinal cord injury.

Shock resulting from failure of the heart as a pump may be referred to as "congestive shock" because an elevated venous pressure (systemic and/or pulmonary) is an accompanying feature. Failure of the heart's pumping mechanism may result from inadequate filling or emptying of the ventricles. The prototype for inadequate ventricular filling is pericardial tamponade, in which the pericardial space is filled by fluid or blood under high pressure, preventing adequate filling of the ventricular and atrial chambers by blood. The resultant stroke volume is small, and hypotension with poor tissue perfusion occurs. Failure of the heart to empty adequately or eject enough blood to maintain tissue perfusion generally is referred to as *cardiogenic shock*. The most common cause is myocardial infarction. Cardiogenic shock resulting from myocardial infarction has a mortality of greater than 60%. Acute valvular insufficiency such as that caused by rupture of a left ventricular papillary muscle may lead to shock on the basis of inadequate ejection of blood into the aorta; most of the blood is diverted into the left atrial chamber because of its lower resistance. Certain cardiac arrhythmias such as ventricular tachycardia or rapid supraventricular tachycardia often lead to inadequate

emptying of the ventricles. The ventricle in fibrillation or asystole does not eject any blood; if this condition is not corrected, the sudden onset of shock and death is imminent. A massive pulmonary embolus may lead to circulatory shock by preventing the emptying of the right ventricle and the filling of the left ventricle.

Although most causes of circulatory shock can be categorized into one of the three major types outlined previously, many shock states possess features of two or more types. Septic shock is accompanied by ventricular dysfunction (inadequate filling and/or emptying). Hypovolemic shock is largely a manifestation of poor venous return and diminished ventricular filling.

PHYSIOLOGIC ADAPTATIONS AND COMPENSATORY MECHANISMS. The reduction in arterial pressure and tissue perfusion initiates vital compensatory mechanisms. The major compensatory mechanisms are baroreceptor reflexes, release of endogenous vasoactive substances, and physiologic responses to increase and maintain an effective vascular volume.

Hypotension results in a decrease in the pressure that is sensed by the baroreceptors in the carotid sinuses and aortic arch; this effects a reduction in vagal tone and an increase in sympathetic tone. The enhanced sympathetic tone increases arteriolar and venous vasoconstriction, heart rate, and inotropy of the myocardium. These effects, in turn, increase and maintain perfusion pressure and blood flow to the brain and heart. The clinical manifestations of the increased sympathetic tone in hypovolemic shock are cool, moist extremities and tachycardia. In warm shock, such as sepsis, vasodilation occurs, and as a consequence the extremities may be normothermic or warm; however, the tachycardia from increased sympathetic tone persists. Patients with shock caused by dehydration states usually have cool, dry extremities and tachycardia.

The major endogenous vasoactive substances released during circulatory shock are the catecholamines, vasopressin, and angiotensin. The increased levels of the circulating catecholamines epinephrine and norepinephrine are part of the augmented sympathetic nervous system activity. Vasopressin, a potent vasoconstrictor, is released from the posterior pituitary gland in hypotensive states. Decreased renal perfusion stimulates the release of renin, which converts angiotensinogen to angiotensin. Angiotensin is a powerful vasoconstrictor and, interestingly, stimulates the brain thirst center. The endogenous release of these vasoactive substances contributes to reduction of vascular capacitance and redistribution of flow to the brain and myocardium. The role of the ubiquitous prostaglandins in shock states has not yet been defined.

The reabsorption of extravascular fluid and renal conservation of sodium chloride and water constitute a major compensatory mechanism serving to increase and maintain an adequate intravascular volume. These adaptations result in a decrease in hematocrit and plasma oncotic pressure in most forms of shock. Up to 1 L of extravascular fluid may be reabsorbed or autotransfused within the first hour of hypovolemic shock. Besides serving as a vasoconstrictor, angiotensin stimulates the release of aldosterone from the adrenal gland. Aldosterone, along with increased levels of adrenocorticosteroids and vasopressin (antidiuretic hormone), augments the renal reabsorption of sodium chloride and water.

CLINICAL MANIFESTATIONS. The spectrum of circulatory shock is very wide. The event can be transient and mild, as in vasodepressor syncope ("faint"),* or prolonged with a grave

---

*Not classified as a shock state by some investigators because of its transient, self-limited features.

prognosis, as in cardiogenic shock caused by a myocardial infarction.

Prolonged hypotension and poor tissue perfusion lead to general cellular dysfunction, which is manifest by varying degrees of organ failure. Although diminished renal perfusion provides certain compensatory mechanisms, prolonged and severe reduction in renal blood flow may lead to renal failure. Hepatic dysfunction and intestinal ileus with ischemia and infarction may occur in severe shock states. Circulatory shock can be accompanied by a progressive deterioration of pulmonary function resulting from accumulating secretions, atelectasis, pneumonia, ventilation-perfusion abnormalities, and interstitial-alveolar edema from alveolar damage (adult respiratory distress syndrome or "shock lung"). Abnormalities of the reticuloendothelial system combined with the accumulation of toxic products and vascular injury may complicate circulatory shock by eliciting diffuse intravascular coagulation, a condition characterized by diffuse hemorrhage and by thrombosis of the microvasculature. Failure of the compensatory mechanisms to maintain adequate cerebral blood flow manifests as lethargy, somnolence, coma, abnormal patterns of respiration (tachypnea, Cheyne-Stokes respiration, or apnea), and loss of central control of the entire nervous system. A reduction in coronary artery perfusion may produce myocardial ischemia and infarction, particularly in patients with underlying atherosclerotic coronary artery disease or myocardial hypertrophy. A *myocardial depressant factor* may be a contributory factor in certain forms of shock (for example, septic shock).

Untreated or intractable circulatory shock thus evolves into a vicious circle of deterioration. The cycle is perpetuated by the progressive development of the complications of shock just noted. Diffuse cell injury and cell death occur with the release of metabolic products (lactate, enzymes, and so forth). Systemically the metabolic products cause acidosis. Locally they disrupt the neural and humoral regulation of vascular smooth muscle, resulting in dilated, nonresponsive blood vessels (further worsening the shock state) and heralding the onset of irreversible shock. "Irreversible shock" is a term applied to terminal shock states incapable of responding favorably to treatment. Circulatory shock (untreated or intractable) is thus a syndrome involving multiple systems and evolves from extreme cardiovascular failure to failure of most of the body systems and death.

MANAGEMENT. The overall therapeutic approach should be concentrated in four major areas: prevention, treatment directed at the cause of the shock state, cardiovascular support, and management of complications.

Each member of the medical community has the responsibility to avoid and prevent events that may lead to circulatory shock. For example, inquiring about drug allergies before the administration of drugs is mandatory. A patient with easy bleeding and bruisability should be evaluated by a medical specialist before a dental or surgical procedure. Salicylates should not be administered to patients with a history of peptic ulcer disease. Bacterial infections should be treated properly and promptly, especially in immunocompromised patients, to prevent overwhelming bacteremia and sepsis.

The initial efforts in managing a patient in circulatory shock should be directed at providing cardiovascular support and determining the cause of the shock state; most often these activities are performed simultaneously. Except for congestive shock states, increasing intravascular volume is the most important part of therapy; infusion of saline and/or other volume expanders should be rapidly initiated, and large volumes (even 5 to 10 L) may be necessary to restore perfusion. To prevent complications of shock, this should be started while monitoring and diagnostic studies are being initiated. Cardiovascular monitoring should be performed in an intensive or coronary care unit and for most forms of shock should include continuous electrocardiography to determine heart rate and rhythm changes and indwelling catheters to measure central and peripheral blood pressures. The flow-directed triple-lumen pulmonary artery catheter (Swan-Ganz catheter) currently is the optimal hemodynamic monitoring device, because it provides direct-pressure recordings of the right atrium and pulmonary artery, indirect measurements of the left ventricular filling presure (via pulmonary arterial occlusive pressure), and cardiac output determinations, generally by a thermodilution technique. This catheter is particularly useful in the management of cardiogenic or congestive shock.

Urine flow of 30 ml or more per hour (which may require an indwelling urinary bladder catheter for measurement) indicates adequate renal perfusion. With diminished urine flow, a low urine sodium concentration (less than 20 mEq/L) indicates sodium reabsorption to conserve intravascular volume. However, the decreased urine flow causes the serum urea nitrogen to be elevated disproportionately (by more than 10 times) to serum creatinine. When diminished urine flow reflects acute renal tubular necrosis caused by shock, the urine sodium is high (more than 20 mEq/L), reflecting failure of reabsorption, and the serum urea nitrogen is elevated proportionately to creatinine (about 10 times that of creatinine). Gastrointestinal bleeding disproportionately elevates urea nitrogen.

Monitoring of the respiratory, metabolic, and hematologic status is accomplished by the intermittent determination of arterial blood gases, lactate concentrations, serum oncotic pressure, hematocrit, and blood clotting parameters. Intensive monitoring provides specific direction in therapeutics. For example, low central venous and left ventricular filling pressures indicate the need for administration of additional fluids. With a normal or high central venous pressure (higher than 8 mm Hg) and left ventricular filling pressure (a pulmonary wedge pressure higher than 14 mm Hg), inotropic agents are needed. Dopamine should be given in doses of 200 to 1000 μg/min to increase cardiac output and systemic blood pressure. This dose may dilate the renal and mesenteric arteries. It may be necessary to use higher doses such as 1500 to 3000 μg/min. These doses raise blood pressure further by causing peripheral vasoconstriction and are often administered with a vasodilator such as nitroprusside (16 to 200 μg/min).

The determination of the precise cause of shock permits direct intervention and reversal of the shock state. A history of a penicillin injection immediately before sudden clinical deterioration and shock strongly suggests an acute anaphylactic reaction; the expeditious administration of epinephrine, corticosteroids, and intravenous fluids usually prevents this form of shock from deteriorating into severe and irreversible shock. Hypovolemic shock in a patient with a history of peptic ulcer disease requires the placement of a nasogastric tube and analysis of gastric contents; if gastrointestinal bleeding is present, volume replacement with blood, saline, or volume expanders and control of the bleeding, possibly by surgery, are indicated. Besides fluid administration, septic shock is treated immediately with antibiotics directed at all suspected organisms until culture reports are available. Failure to detect and treat a remediable cause of shock often condemns the patient to irreversible shock regardless of how brilliant and aggressive the initial cardiovascular support may have been.

The primary thrust in the management of circulatory shock should be directed at prevention. However, once circulatory shock has developed, the patient's survival depends on aggressive and meticulous interaction of cardiovascular support, cardiovascular and systemic monitoring, and early detection and management of complicating problems.

BIBLIOGRAPHY

Abel FL and Kessler DP: Myocardial performance in hemorrhagic shock in dog and primate, Circ Res 32:492, 1973.

Cowley RA and Trump BF, editors: Pathophysiology of shock, anoxia and ischemia, Baltimore, 1982, Williams & Wilkins.

Kreis DJ Jr and Baue AE, editors: Clinical management of shock, Baltimore, 1984, University Park Press.

Lefer AM and Schumer W, editors: Molecular and cellular aspects of shock and trauma. In Progress in clinical and biological research, vol 3, New York, 1983, Alan R Liss.

Leier CV, Magorien RD, and Unverferth DV: Inotropic drugs in emergency management of cardiovascular disease. In Rund DA and Wolcott BW, editors: Connecticut, 1983, Appleton & Lange.

Selkurt EE: Current status of renal circulation and related nephron function in hemorrhage and experimental shock, Circ Shock 1:3, 1974.

Skjoldborg K, editor: Scanticon shock seminar, Amsterdam, 1978, Excerpta Medica.

Vatner SF: Effects of hemorrhage on regional blood flow distribution in dogs and primates, J Clin Invest 54:225, 1974.

Winslow EJ and others: Hemodynamic studies and results of therapy in 30 patients with bacteremic shock, Am J Med 54:421, 1973.

Zeifach BW and Fronek A: The interplay of central and peripheral factors in irreversible hemorrhagic shock, Prog Cardiovasc Dis 18:147, 1975.

89 · DIAGNOSTIC PROCEDURES IN CARDIOLOGY

David G. Meyers

The medical history and physical examination, which provide extensive information at low cost, remain the main sources of pertinent patient information. However, several specialized cardiac laboratory procedures have appreciably improved the care and understanding of cardiac diseases. Indeed, many important parameters of cardiac structure and function can be evaluated only by tests such as echocardiography and cardiac catheterization. Procedures such as cardiac catheterization have evolved from diagnostic tests into therapeutic procedures for coronary artery disease and myocardial infarction.

Electrocardiography

GENERAL PRINCIPLES. Myocardial contraction is induced by electrical depolarization. This electrical activity can be recorded graphically as an electrocardiogram (ECG). Myocardial cells have semipermeable membranes that allow development of ionic gradients, thereby producing electrical potential differences. By active transport via sodium-potassium adenosine triphosphatase (Na-K ATPase), the resting cell has an intracellular sodium concentration of about 10 mEq/L compared to 132 to 142 mEq/L in the extracellular fluid; the intracellular potassium concentration is approximately 150 mEq/L versus 3.5 to 5 mEq/L in extracellular fluid. This results in a -90 mV potential difference across the cell membrane. By either slow, spontaneous inward diffusion of sodium or by very rapid diffusion induced by electrical stimulation, myocardial cells depolarize to approximately $+20$ mV. This change in electrical polarity propagates from cell to cell. In the myocardium, depolarization causes muscle contraction by triggered inward calcium diffusion and release of stored intracellular calcium. The specialized pacemaker cells in the sinoatrial (SA) and atrioventricular (AV) nodes differ from other cells in that they use only calcium, not sodium, as the ionic trigger of depolarization.

Normally, depolarization begins in the SA node and spreads through the atria, causing atrial contraction (Fig. 89-1, A). The insulating effect of the atrioventricular ring prevents the electrical impulse from entering the ventricles by means other than through the AV node. From the AV node the depolarization wave is carried by the specialized conducting tissue of the His-Purkinje system, which consists of the common, or His, bundle, the right and left bundle branches, and the arborized Purkinje fibers that connect with the myocardial cells. The conducting system allows for both synchronous muscle contraction within cardiac chambers and proper coordination between the atria and ventricles.

The electrocardiograph detects electrical potential differences between electrodes placed on the chest and extremities. Since the electrodes are distant from the heart, only large potential differences, specifically those produced by atrial and ventricular muscle depolarization, are detected, whereas electrical impulses coursing through the His-Purkinje system are not detected. By convention when the electrical depolarization wave moves toward the monitoring electrode, the electrocardiograph inscribes an upward or positive deflection; when the impulse moves away from the electrode, the electrocardiograph inscribes a downward or negative deflection. The amount and direction of propagation of the electrical potential difference—the so-called electrical vector—is best measured by simultaneously monitoring several electrodes positioned on the extremities and chest. Constant motion of the graph paper at 25 mm/sec permits timing of the electrical events. The heart rate can easily be determined (Fig. 89-1, C). Voltage is measured on the verticle axis, where 1 mm = 0.1 mV. The more myocardial cells depolarizing at any given instant, the greater the potential difference and in turn the larger the vertical deflection (either positive or negative, depending on which direction the depolarization wave is traveling).

Each of the several deflections on the ECG correlates with an event in the cardiac cycle (Fig. 89-1, B). The first is the P wave, produced by depolarization of atrial muscle cells. After an interval this is followed by a series of positive and negative deflections called the QRS complex, which correlates with ventricular depolarization. The time from the beginning of the P wave until the beginning of the QRS complex approximates the time required for the depolarization wave to pass through the atria, the AV node, and the His-Purkinje system. The next deflection to occur in each cardiac cycle is the T wave, produced by repolarization of the ventricular muscle, when the resting membrane potential of -90 mV is reestablished through active exchange of sodium and potassium. The interval between the QRS complex and the T wave is called the ST segment.

ABNORMALITIES OF THE ELECTROCARDIOGRAM. Abnormalities of electrical impulse conduction are produced by damage to the AV node, the His bundle, or one of the bundle branches. AV nodal dysfunction may be caused by alterations in blood supply (myocardial infarction), digitalis, calcium blockers such as verapamil or β-adrenergic blocking agents such as propranolol. AV nodal block may be first-degree (1°), which is characterized by prolongation of the PR interval beyond its normal 200 milliseconds; Wenckebach-type second-degree (2°), which is characterized by a recurring sequence of progressive lengthening of the PR interval that culminates in a P wave not immediately followed by a QRS-T complex; or third-degree (3°), which is complete AV block, in which the atrial impulse is never conducted through the AV node and into the ventricles (Fig. 89-2).

When either bundle branch fails to conduct the impulse, the

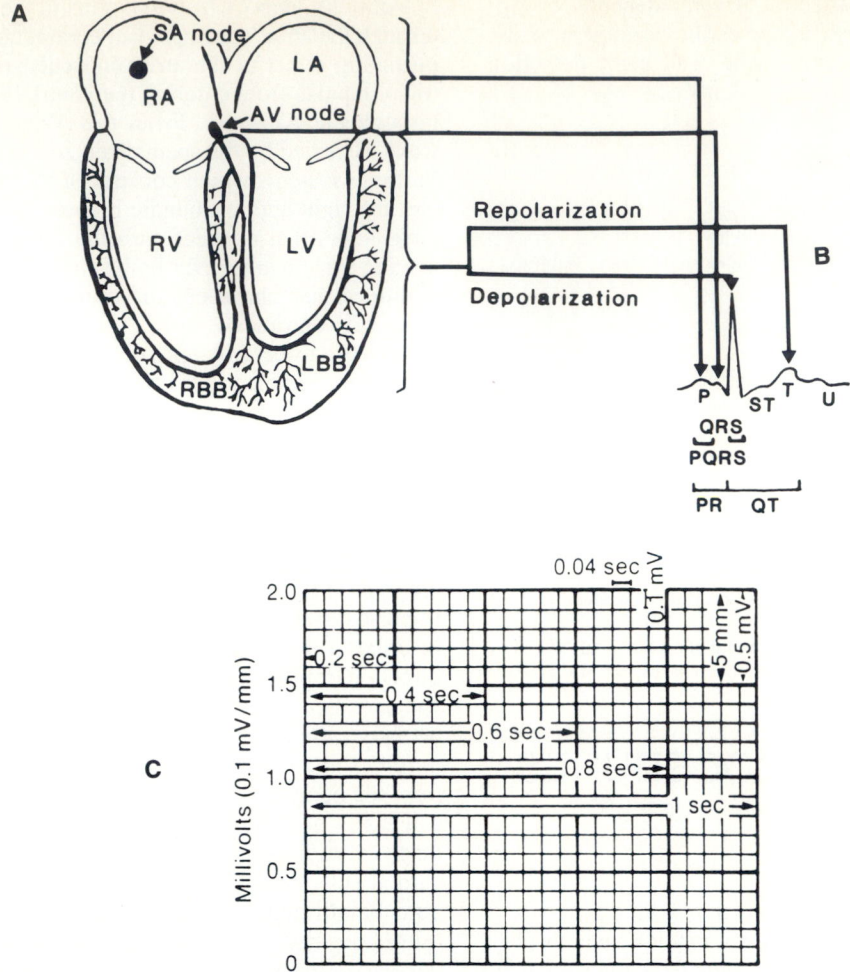

Fig. 89-1   A, Schematic representation of cardiac conduction system. Normally, impulse begins in sinoatrial node (SA), spreads through atria to reach atrioventricular node (AV), then courses through His bundle and, via right bundle branch (RBB) and left bundle branch (LBB), reaches myocytes. **B,** Schematic of electrical events of cardiac cycle, correlating P, QRS, and T deflections with electrical events such as ventricular depolarization. **C,** Ruler for measuring heart rate and QRS amplitude.

spread of the depolarization in the ventricle concerned cannot be entirely transmitted by the arborized conduction system. Instead conduction occurs directly from cell to cell. This produces delayed and asynchronous activation of ventricular muscle, manifest graphically by prolongation of the QRS duration beyond 120 milliseconds—the cardinal sign of bundle branch block. The delayed activation of the right ventricle produced by right bundle branch block is manifest by a rightward terminal QRS vector. This produces terminal R waves (positive deflection) in leads aVR and V_1, the electrocardiographic leads that monitor right ventricular activity (Fig. 89-2). By a similar mechanism left bundle branch block produces delayed left ventricular activation with terminal R waves in leads I, aVL, and V_6, the leads that monitor left ventricular activation.

Mobitz type II AV block is due to block either in the common bundle or as a simultaneous block in the left and right bundle branches. Mobitz type II heart block produces regular periodic failure of a P wave to conduct to the ventricles.

Complete heart block (or third-degree heart block) is caused by either bilateral bundle branch block, His bundle block, or AV nodal block. Ventricular depolarization occurs because a focus within the conduction system or ventricular muscle begins to spontaneously depolarize (an escape pacemaker). This results in AV dissociation (atrial and ventricular muscle acti-

vation occur independently instead of in the normal sequence of atrial conduction followed at a regular interval by ventricular contraction). AV dissociation may significantly reduce the heart's pumping efficiency.

Myocardial infarction produces two electrocardiographic patterns. One shows evolution of Q waves—negative (downward) deflections of more than 40 milliseconds' duration that occur at the beginning of the QRS complex in leads correlating with the affected area of the heart. For instance, Q waves in leads II, III, and aVF reflect inferior infarction, whereas Q waves in leads V_1, V_2, and V_3 reflect anteroseptal infarction. Q waves evolve over a number of hours to days. But in the first moments after the blood supply to the myocardium is compromised, the pattern shows tall (more than 10 mV) symmetrically peaked T waves, the so-called hyperacute T waves. These are followed by ST segment elevation (injury pattern) and progressive T wave inversion, changes that last several hours to many days. As the infarction evolves, Q waves appear, usually within 24 hours. While the ST-T changes usually resolve over several weeks, the Q waves most often are permanent. Thus Q waves mark the location of both recent and remote infarction.

The second pattern of myocardial infarction may not exhibit Q waves, merely ST segment depression and T wave inversion.

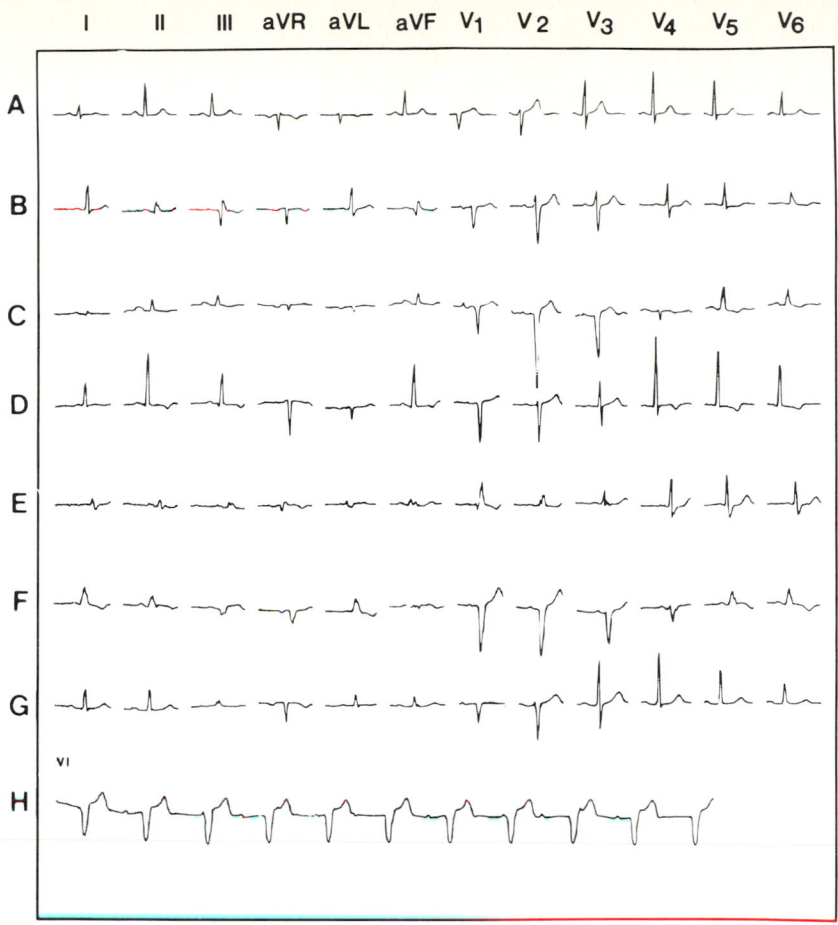

Fig. 89-2   Examples of several ECG patterns. *A,* Normal. *B,* Inferior myocardial infarction (Q waves in leads II, III, and AVF). *C,* Anteroseptal myocardial infarction (Q waves in leads V_1, V_2, V_3, and V_4) with ST segment elevation suggesting either acute injury or aneurysm. *D,* Left ventricular hypertrophy (LVH) manifest by S_{V2} + R_{V5} > 35 mv plus ST-T depression. *E,* Right bundle branch block (RBBB) demonstrated by QRS duration > 0.11 sec plus terminal wide S waves in leads I, AVL, and V_6 and wide terminal R waves in leads AVR and V_6. *F,* Left bundle branch block (LBBB) manifest as QRS duration > 0.11 sec; absence of initial "septal" Q waves in leads I, AVL, and V_6 plus wide R waves in same leads. *G,* First degree AV block (1°) with PR dissociation of P waves and QRS complexes. *H* Complete AV block with dissociation of P waves & QRS complexes. **H,** Complete AV blocks with dissociation of P waves and QRS complexes.

The evolution through peaked T waves and ST elevation does not occur in this setting.

Left ventricular hypertrophy exists when left ventricular muscle cells increase in size and volume in response to a stimulus such as hypertension. As the cells enlarge, they produce increased electrical potentials reflected in increased voltage (amplitude) of the QRS complex. The simplest electrocardiographic criterion of left ventricular hypertrophy is the sum of the S wave (negative deflection) voltage in lead V_1 or V_2 and the R wave (positive deflection) voltage in lead V_5 or V_6. When the sum is more than 3.5 mV (35 mm of vertical deflection), left ventricular hypertrophy is said to be present.

The electrocardiographic diagnosis of hypertrophy using these criteria has a significant rate of false positive and false negative tests. Diagnostic certainty is increased when the R-S sum appreciably exceeds 3.5 mV or when increased voltage is accompanied by depressed ST segments and inverted T waves, a left atrial abnormality, or markedly negative terminal P in V_1 and left axis deviation. Right ventricular hypertrophy is manifested by increased amplitude of the R wave in lead V_1 (Fig. 89-2). However, echocardiography (discussed later) is superior to electrocardiography in diagnosing hypertrophy.

EXERCISE ELECTROCARDIOGRAPHY. While wearing special electrodes, patients can be exercised at progressively increasing levels on a motorized treadmill or stationary bicycle. Exercise is increased until angina or exhaustion occurs or until a heart rate 80% of the maximum predicted for the patient's age is achieved. Ischemia is detected in about 70% of patients having hemodynamically significant coronary artery stenoses when horizontal or down-sloping ST segment depression of more than 1 mm when measured 80 milliseconds after the QRS complex is used to identify a positive test. This transient ST segment depression is believed to be caused by exercise-induced subendocardial ischemia. A negative test suggests the absence of significant coronary artery stenosis with about 80% certainty. Achieving 80% of maximum predicted heart rate without producing ST segment depression in a patient complaining of typical exertional angina pectoris does not exclude the diagnosis of angina, but it does suggest both a limited extent of coronary artery disease and a good prognosis. Although 1 mm of ST segment depression is a useful basis for interpreting an exercise test, other parameters (for example, ST segment depression of more than 2.0 mm) are highly predictive of severe coronary stenoses, multiple-vessel disease, or disease affecting the left main-stem artery. Diagnostic certainty and the probability of severe multiple-vessel disease increase when a given degree of ST change occurs at lower levels of exercise (for example, less than 6 minutes of progressive exercise), when it occurs at relatively low heart rates, or when the ST depression requires longer than 5 minutes to resolve with rest. Down-sloping ST depression is more important than horizontal changes, which in turn are more predictive than up-sloping ST segment depression. Normally systolic blood pressure increases with increasing levels of exercise, whereas a diastolic pressure decreases. A decline in systolic blood pressure during exercise suggests severe myocardial ischemia causing a decrease in cardiac output, an ominous finding.

In patients with atypical chest pain, ST segment depression of more than 1 mm increases the diagnostic probability that the pain is caused by myocardial ischemia but the finding is not specific. Exercise testing has been used to select angina patients for coronary angiography. A markedly positive test (ST segment depression of more than 2 mm or of 1 mm within 6 minutes) predicts both multiple-vessel disease and a high probability of ensuing cardiac events. Additionally, a complicated 1-year course is likely if ST segment depression, chest pain, and ventricular arrhythmias occur during a low level of exercise performed before discharge from the hosptial after myocardial infarction. In these settings coronary angiography usually is indicated. On the other hand, the screening of asymptomatic individuals by exercise testing is controversial because of its low specificity.

The efficacy of therapy for angina can be measured by exercise testing. However, exercise is contraindicated in patients with unstable angina and severe aortic stenosis. Because of resting ST segment alterations that confound interpretation, exercise testing without ancillary tests such as thallium scanning (discussed later) is not useful in patients with left bundle branch block or left ventricular hypertrophy or in those receiving digitalis.

AMBULATORY ELECTROCARDIOGRAPHY. Using tape-recording devices, the ECG can be continuously stored and later analyzed. This technique can identify serious arrhythmias and quantify isolated ectopic events (premature beats). Infrequent symptoms often make continuous ECG recordings impractical for diagnosis of their cause, but recorders that can be activated by the patient during symptoms and that store ECG data for a period starting before the moment of activation (retrograde memory) are available. Continuous out-of-hospital monitoring with radiotelemetry also is available. ST segment analysis of the tape recording can detect both symptomatic and asymptomatic myocardial ischemia, identified by transient ST segment depression. Focal coronary artery spasm is suggested by episodic ST segment elevation.

Echocardiography

Echocardiography uses pulsed sonic waves of 2 million to 3 million Hz (ultrasound). The piezoelectric crystal transducer transmits sound waves and then receives waves reflected from tissue density interfaces such as adjacent blood and muscle. Since the sound waves travel at a constant velocity, the time between transmitting and receiving the ultrasonic impulse is an indication of the distance between the transducer and the reflective tissue interface. By visualizing the moving heart, both cardiac structure and function can be assessed.

M-mode echocardiography is produced by a single stationary transducer emitting a discrete ultrasonic beam. When the reflected impulses received at the transducer are converted to a graphic format, the lines inscribed represent structural interfaces at varying depths from the transducer positioned on the chest. With the graph paper moving at a constant rate, both depth and time are portrayed (Fig. 89-3) and the motion of structures can be measured. By selectively directing the ultrasonic beam, different cardiac structures can be visualized graphically. This "ice pick" view permits only a limited examination of the heart, albeit in graphic format.

Two-dimensional (2-D) echocardiography rapidly moves the ultrasonic beam across an arc, thereby adding a second dimension and representing cardiac structures and motion in a real-time format that can be recorded on videotape. By virtue of the moving beam, a more inclusive examination of the heart is possible. Traditionally 2-D echocardiography visualizes the long axis, short axis, apical, and subxiphoid planes of the heart.

Whereas echocardiography uses ultrasound reflected from tissue interfaces lying perpendicular to the ultrasonic beam, Doppler ultrasonography uses impulses reflected from red blood cells moving parallel to the ultrasonic beam. Using the same principle that causes a train whistle to change pitch when the train moves toward or away from the listener, Doppler ultrasound measures the shift in frequency of the reflected ultrasound beam to determine the velocity and direction of the moving blood. Usually, Dopper ultrasound is transmitted in pulses. When coupled with a gating mechanism, this allows interrogation of flow at particular sites of interest such as downstream from the mitral valve. When flow velocity is very high (more than 6 m/sec), a continuous wave Doppler ultrasound more accurately determines blood flow velocity but with the loss of gating ability. Blood flow in the heart normally is laminar and nonturbulent. With laminar flow all adjacent red blood cells move with nearly equal velocity in the same direction, producing a uniform Doppler shift (Fig. 89-6). When cardiac valves become narrowed (stenotic) or allow leakage (regurgitation), the downstream blood flow becomes turbulent and blood cells move with many different velocities in many different directions. The nonuniform Doppler shift produced by turbulent flow is described as spectral broadening (Fig. 89-4). When flow velocities are color coded and incorporated in a moving 2-D echocardiographic image, a depiction of blood flow, as well as cardiac motion, is produced—so-called color flow Doppler duplex echocardiography.

EVALUATION OF CHAMBER SIZES AND WALL THICKNESS. Using both M-mode and 2-D echocardiography, the cardiac chambers and walls can be measured. The right ventricle is measured between the endocardial surfaces of the anterior wall and the right side of the interventricular septum at end-diastole. This dimension should be less than 2.6 cm, but it may be increased in pulmonary hypertension, right ventricular infarction, tricuspid or pulmonic valve insufficiency, or left-to-right shunting. A feature supporting right ventricular volume overload is paradoxical motion of the interventricular septum, whereby the septum moves anteriorly toward the right ventricle during systole instead of posteriorly toward the left ventricle. Left ventricular dilation is present when the end-diastolic dimension, measured from the endocardial surface of the left side of the interventricular septum to the endocardial surface of the posterior left ventricular wall, is more than 5.6 cm. Left ventricular dilation is a sign of heart failure, possibly from myocardial infarction, idiopathic dilated cardiomyopathy, aortic or mitral insufficiency, and right-to-left shunting. Left atrial size should roughly equal the short axis diameter of the aortic root or measure less than 4 cm. Left atrial enlargement generally is caused by mitral insufficiency or less often by mitral stenosis. The right atrium usually is not measured.

The walls of the left ventricle normally are of rather uniform

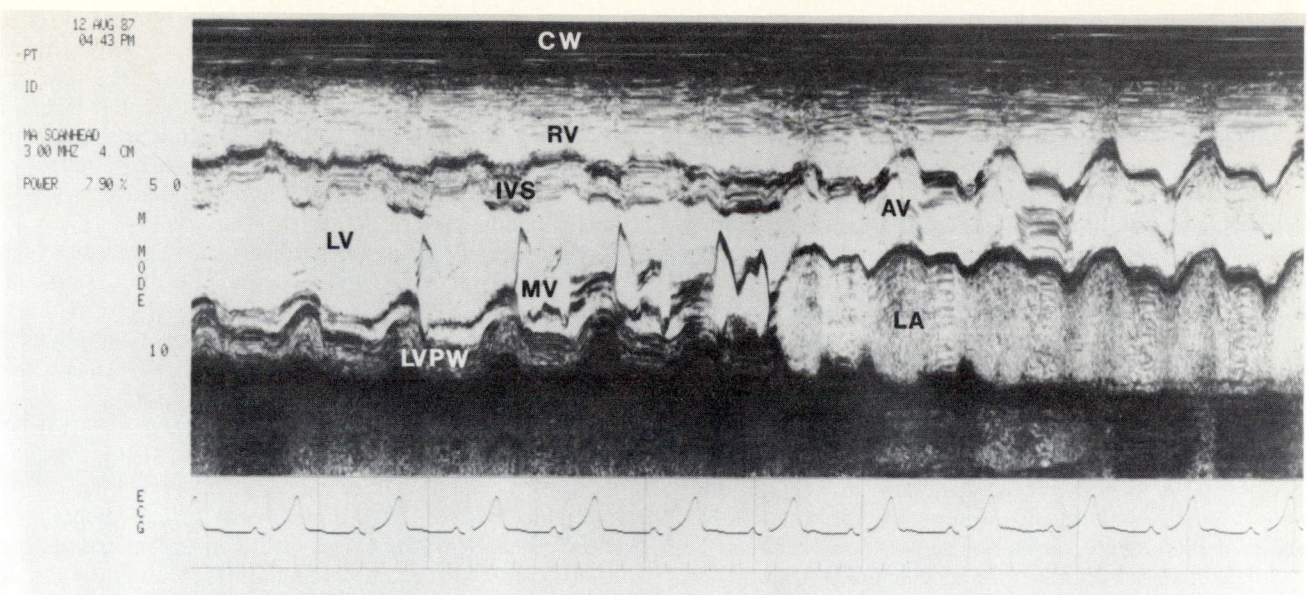

Fig. 89-3   M-mode echocardiographic scan from mid-left ventricle *(LV) (left)*, through mitral valve *(MV)*, to level of aortic valve *(AV)* and left atrium *(LA) (right)*. Note characteristic M-shaped diastolic motion of anterior mitral leaflet and parallelogram produced by opening of aortic valve. Interventricular septum *(IVS)* and left ventricular posterior wall *(LVPW)* both thicken and contract into left ventricular chamber during systole. Right ventricle *(RV)* and chest wall artifact *(CW)* are at top of tracing.

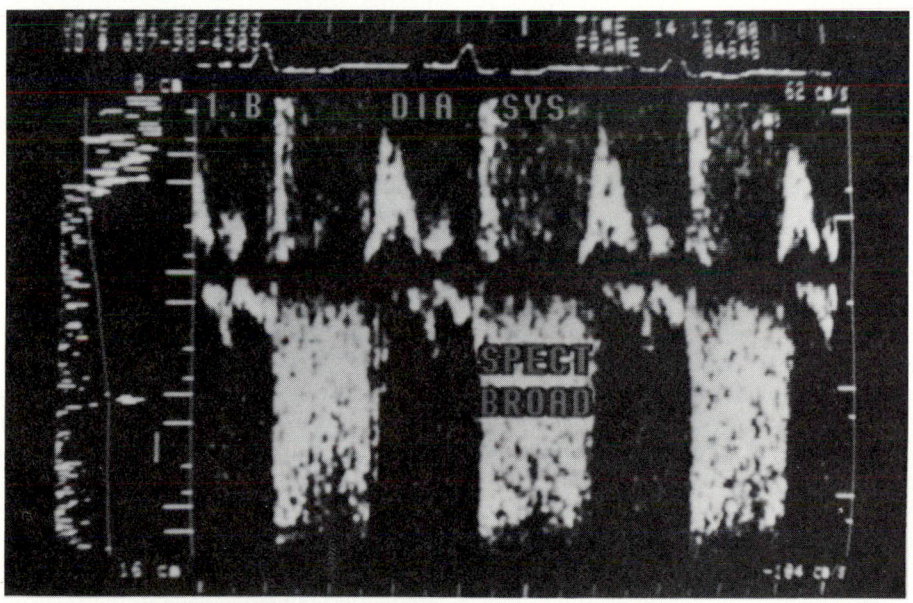

Fig. 89-4   Pulsed Doppler ultrasonogram with sampling taken at mitral valve, contrasting laminar flow during diastole (shown as discreet bright peaked line) with turbulent mitral regurgitation during systole, which graphically produces spectral broadening.

thickness. When measured in diastole, left ventricular wall thickness should be less than 1.1 cm. Concentric left ventricular hypertrophy produces uniform thickening of more than 1.1 cm. Focal or asymmetric thickening occurs in some forms of hypertrophic cardiomyopathy. Asymmetric septal hypertrophy is identified by a ratio greater than 1.3:1.0 of interventricular to posterior diastolic thickness. The ventricular walls may increase in thickness and in echodensity after infiltration of the myocardium with iron (hemochromatosis), protein (amyloidosis), or inflammatory cells (sarcoidosis). Conversely, the ventricular walls may become thinned and echodense after myocardial infarction.

EVALUATION OF LEFT VENTRICULAR FUNCTION. When the end-systolic short axis left ventricular internal dimension (LVIDs) is subtracted from the end-diastolic dimension (LVIDd) and the difference is then divided by the end-diastolic dimension, the result is left ventricular fractional shortening.

$$\text{Fractional shortening} = \frac{\text{LVIDd} - \text{LVIDs}}{\text{LVIDs}}$$

Fractional shortening (normal is 0.28 to 0.44) is a useful indicator of left ventricular systolic function and is proportional to the ejection fraction determined by nuclear or contrast ventriculography. When focal wall motion abnormalities such as a ventricular aneurysm or infarction-induced akinesis are present, fractional shortening no longer reliably represents left ventricular function. Other less widely used indicators of systolic function include systolic wall thickening, systolic excursion of individual left ventricular walls, and the mean rate of circumferential shortening.

Doppler ultrasonography also can be used to evaluate left ventricular function. In the simplest method peak transvalvular flow velocities are measured to estimate blood flow. If peak flow velocities are diminished, a low flow state such as forward heart failure may exist. However, underestimation of flow may occur, because Doppler flow velocity depends critically on the angle of beam incidence. For accurate measurement the ultrasound beam must be within 10 degrees of being parallel to the direction of blood flow. A more cumbersome technique depends on estimation of stroke volume calculated from the systolic flow curve obtained in the ascending aorta and the aortic cross-sectional area.

Echocardiography before and immediately after peak exercise can assess ventricular function by measuring the normal exercise-induced increase in fractional shortening. With ventricular dysfunction the fractional shortening may fail to increase or may even decrease during exercise. With significant coronary artery stenosis focal wall motion abnormalities absent at rest may be identified. Early results suggest that Doppler ultrasonography during exercise also might be useful.

EVALUATION OF CARDIAC VALVES. Valve structure and function can be evaluated by echocardiography. For the mitral valve, leaflet excursion and the maximum distance between the leaflets on M-mode studies provide a rough estimate of transmitral blood flow and orifice size. When the 2-D echocardiograph is directed through the leaflet tips in the cross-sectional (short axis) orientation, the area between the two leaflets accurately reflects mitral valve area, correlating with catheter-derived measurements ($r = 0.92$). But the valve area may be difficult to measure if the valve is heavily calcified, because the calcium is very echodense, reflects the echoes, and causes reverberation that diminishes clarity and resolution of the video display.

When the ultrasound beam is oriented parallel to the line of maximum flow, the peak velocity by Doppler estimates the transmitral gradient by the following formula: peak instantaneous pressure = 4 (peak velocity)^2. The mitral valve area also can be estimated by the pressure half-time formula, which refers to the time required to accomplish half of ventricular filling:

$$\text{Valve area (cm}^2\text{)} = \frac{\text{Pressure half-time (sec)}}{220}$$

Although the aortic valve cannot be visualized as well as the mitral valve, the degree of calcification can be assessed and the number of leaflets usually can be determined. Aortic stenosis produces thickening and calcification of the aortic valve leaflets. The leaflet edges fuse, thus decreasing the orifice through which blood may flow from the left ventricle to the aorta during systole. The severity of stenosis is difficult to determine accurately by echocardiography; Doppler ultrasonography is more precise. As described previously, the instantaneous peak gradient and the valve area by pressure half-time technique often can be determined when the valve cannot be visualized adequately. The sample volume of the gated pulsed Doppler transducer, when positioned in the left ventricular outflow track, can detect aortic insufficiency with a sensitivity unmatched by other techniques. Since no blood flow should occur just below the valve during diastole, the presence of turbulent regurgitant flow is easily detected as spectral broadening during diastole. The severity of aortic insufficiency cannot be measured precisely, but semiquantitative criteria have been applied.

Bacterial and fungal vegetations (from endocarditis) can appear on any valve. These are seen echocardiographically as thickening, deformation, and increased density of the valve leaflets. Since the best resolution of echocardiography is about 2 mm, many vegetations are not visualized. Thus a normal echocardiogram does not exclude endocarditis.

OTHER APPLICATIONS OF ECHOCARDIOGRAPHY. A left ventricular aneurysm is an area of scarring caused by a myocardial infarction that bulges or balloons outward during ventricular systole. Two-dimensional echocardiography permits delineation of the extent of the aneurysm and assessment of the other wall segments' functioning. Mural thrombi, which are not infrequent in a ventricular aneurysm, are seen well with 2-D echocardiography.

Echocardiography currently is the best technique for detecting pericardial effusion. Blood, purulent material, or serous fluid between two tissue densities (the viseral and parietal pericardia) appears as a dark non-echoreflective space between two echodense surfaces. The extent of pericardial fluid can be roughly quantified, assuming even distribution of fluid without loculation. Echocardiography is so sensitive it can detect a few cubic centimeters of normal pericardial fluid as a tiny, posterior echo-free space. However, echocardiography cannot discriminate between blood, purulent material, and serous fluid and thus does not replace pericardiocentesis for determining the cause of the effusion. Although the axial resolution of M-mode echocardiography is superior to 2-D echocardiography, the ability to visualize the distribution of pericardial fluid makes 2-D echocardiography the technique of choice.

Nuclear cardiology

NUCLEAR VENTRICULOGRAPHY. The γ-emitting isotope technetium 99m can be attached (tagged) to either red blood cells or albumin before injection intravenously. When the patient is positioned with the heart under a γ-camera, the cardiac blood pool (that blood in the ventricles and atria) can be approximated from the amount of γ-radiation measured. The radiation picture obtained can be gated by interfacing the γ-camera with the patient's ECG and a computerized data storage system. Gating involves accumulating and quantifying radiation counts at discrete periods during the cardiac cycle, for instance, in systole versus diastole (Fig. 89-5). A commonly used index of cardiac pump function is the ejection fraction (the percentage of blood pumped out of the heart with each beat). Ejection fraction by equilibrium nuclear ventriculography is calculated as

$$\frac{\text{Diastolic counts} - \text{Systolic counts}}{\text{Diastolic counts}} \times 100$$

A normal ejection fraction is 55% to 70%. Nuclear ventriculography also can examine the symmetry of ventricular systolic wall motion. Abnormal segments such as ventricular aneurysms can be visualized, although not with the clarity and resolution of 2-D echocardiography. If the leading edge of radiation is followed through the heart immediately on injection

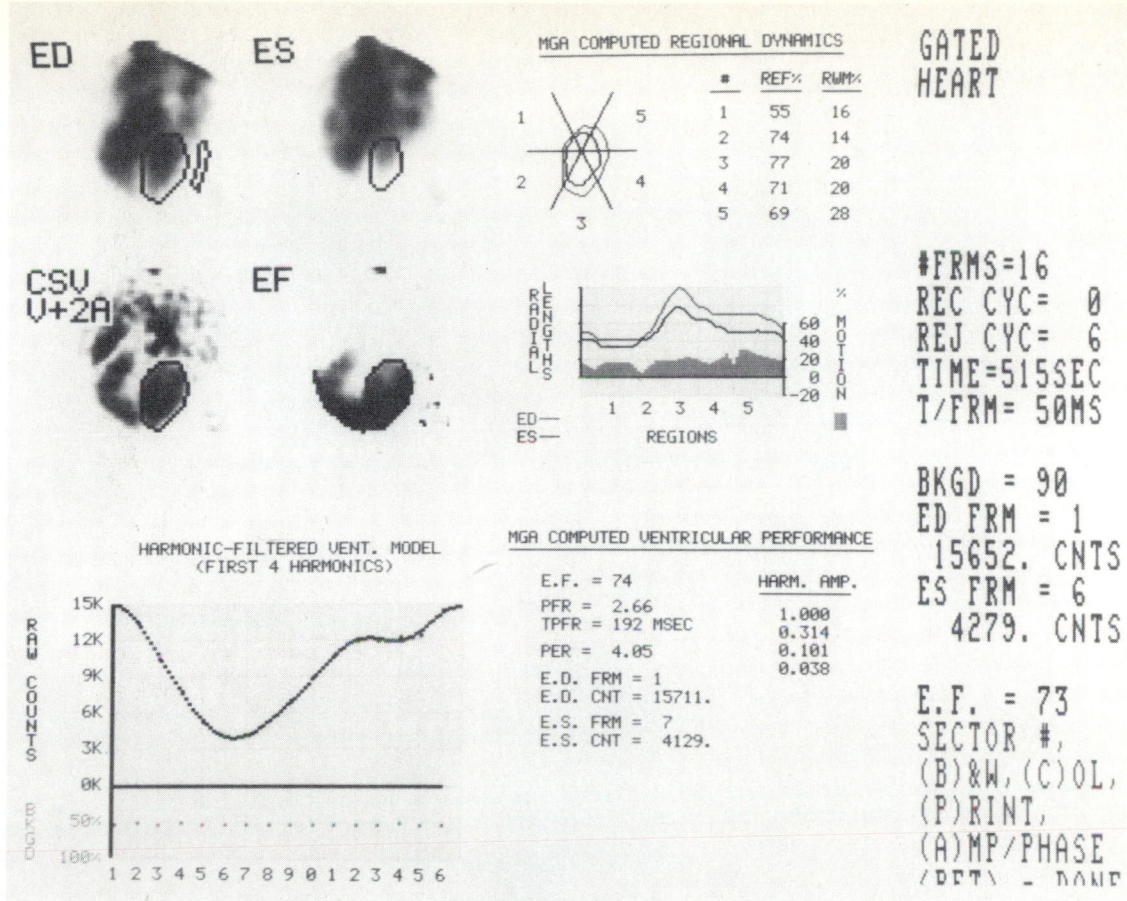

Fig. 89-5 Nuclear vertriculogram *(upper left quadrant)* and examples of analysis techniques. Ventriculogram is represented in end-diastole *(ED)* and systole *(ES)* as areas inscribed in dark lines. Overall scintillation counts over cardiac cycle are graphed in lower left quadrant. Upper right quadrant shows determination of regional wall motion in each of five radians. Lower right quadrant shows, as determined from diastolic-systolic/diastolic scintillation counts, ejection fraction of 59%.

of the radiolabeled carrier, right-to-left shunts can be identified. Using this *first-pass nuclear ventriculography* technique, a shunt is detected when the radiolabeled carrier appears prematurely in the left ventricle.

HOT SPOT SCANS. Technetium 99m is a calcium analog useful for detecting recent myocardial infarctions. Radiolabeling occurs because technetium 99m, like calcium, accumulates in dying myocardium, where it emits γ-radiation (a "hot spot"); in contrast, technetium 99m does not accumulate in normal myocardium. The amount of infarcted myocardium can be semiquantified by both the distribution (focal versus diffuse) and intensity of radiation. This technique is useful mainly when other more specific clinical indicators of myocardial infarction such as the ECG and cardiac enzymes are invalid. Hot spots persisting beyond 2 weeks reflect a poor prognosis.

COLD SPOT SCANS. Thallium 201 is a γ-emitting potassium analog that distributes within the myocardium parallel to the blood flow. Thallium 201 accumulates in myocardial cells that are well supplied with blood and metabolically active. When an artery becomes obstructed, blood flow ceases and the cells die (myocardial infarction). When thallium 201 is injected intravenously, the γ-scan shows homogeneous uptake of the isotope except in the infarct area (a "cold spot") (Fig. 89-6). Infarct-associated cold spots are permanent. Conversely, the cold spot produced by transient ischemia during exercise is

reversible and disappears in a few hours, as the ischemia resolves. Thus when thallium 201 is injected intravenously during peak exercise, any maldistribution of blood flow produced by a stenotic artery appears as an area of less intense γ-radiation (cold spot) compared to normal areas having a greater degree of uptake of thallium 201. After a few hours of rest the ischemia resolves and thallium 201 redistributes; that is, more isotope is taken up in previously ischemic cells while isotope exits the normal cells. A scan 4 to 5 hours after exercise-induced ischemia shows resolution of the cold spot. In summary, a transient cold spot indicates ischemia, whereas a permanent cold spot indicates infarction.

An exercise thallium 201 scan coupled with electrocardiography has two advantages over exercise electrocardiography alone: test sensitivity and specificity are improved, and the ischemic tissue is radiographically localized.

Cardiac catheterization

RIGHT-SIDED HEART CATHETERIZATION. Catheterization of the right side of the heart is accomplished by introducing a soft, flexible radiopaque plastic catheter into a large vein and, under fluoroscopic visualization, passing it through the right atrium and right ventricle into the pulmonary artery. Venous access may be obtained either via percutaneous puncture of the femoral, subclavian, or internal jugular veins or by dissection of the antecubital fossa with isolation of a brachial

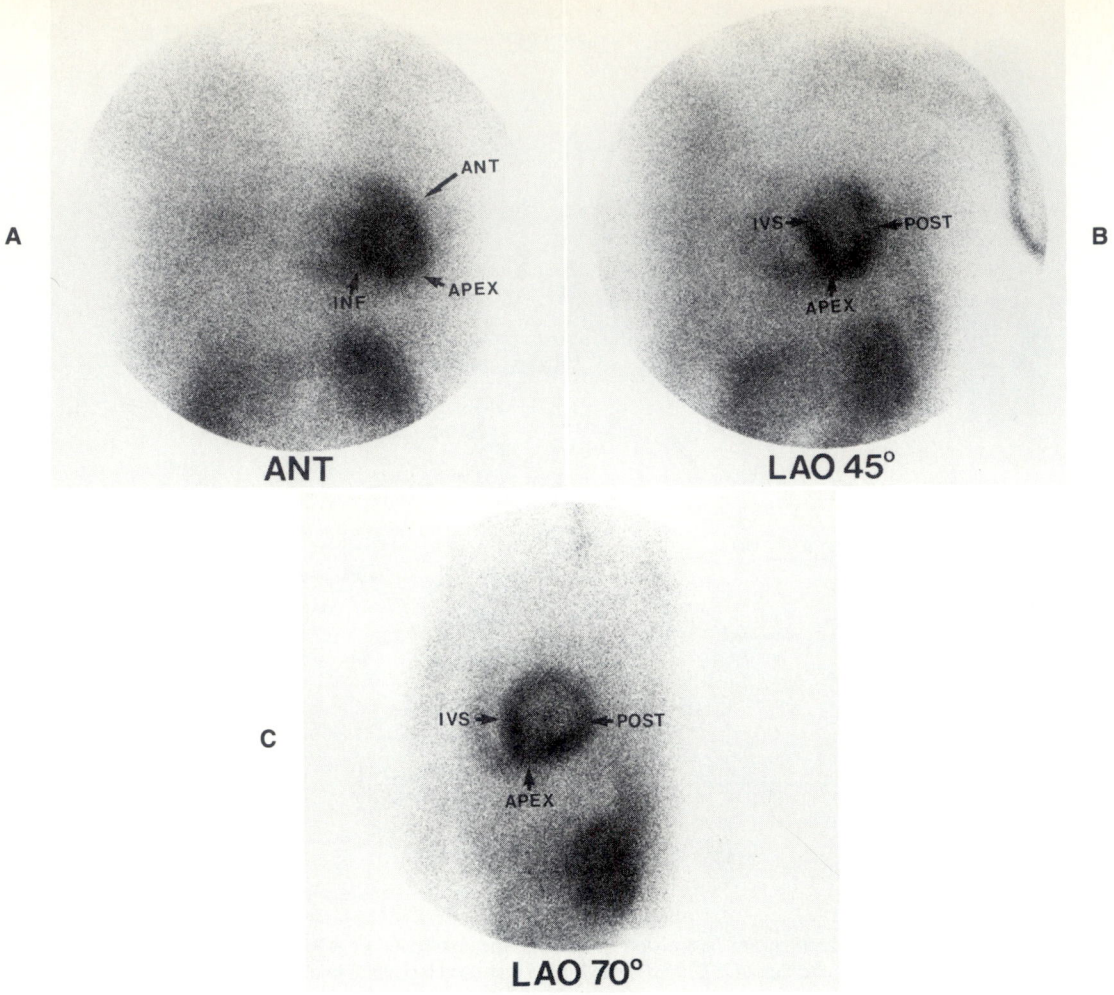

Fig. 89-6   Normal Thallium[201] cardiac scan in: **A,** Anterior; **B,** 45° left anterior oblique and; *C,* 70° left anterior oblique projections showing homogeneous distribution of isotope in anterior *(ant),* apical *(apex),* inferior *(inf),* posterior *(post),* septal *(IVS)* segments.

vein. The catheter devised by Swan and Ganz has a small air-filled balloon near its tip that, when inflated, allows it to be directed through the right heart by normal blood flow (Fig. 89-7). Often proper catheter positioning can be achieved without the use of fluoroscopy, an advantage in the intensive care unit. The pressure wave forms are characteristic of each chamber and identify the location of the catheter tip without the need for fluoroscopy (Fig. 89-8). When the distal balloon wedges in a pulmonary vessel of equal diameter, upstream (pulmonary artery) pressures no longer are recorded. Instead the distal lumen records the downstream pressure, called *pulmonary capillary wedge* (PCW) pressure, which reflects both left atrial and left ventricular diastolic pressures (when the mitral valve is open). These pressures reflect both the filling status of the left ventricle and the hydrostatic pressure responsible for transudation of fluid into the pulmonary interstitial and alveolar spaces.

LEFT-SIDED HEART CATHETERIZATION. The retrograde arterial approach via the femoral or brachial artery is the most widely employed technique of left heart catheterization and can be combined with left ventricular and coronary angiography. Measurement of aortic and left ventricular systolic pressure quantifies pressure gradients resulting from aortic stenosis. Measurement of left ventricular diastolic pressure estimates left ventricular filling and compliance. Simultaneous PCW pressure

and left ventricular diastolic pressure quantifies the transmitral valve pressure gradient in mitral stenosis.

ANALYSIS OF INTRACARDIAC PRESSURES. The normal atrial pressure tracing has a characteristic configuration comprising three positive waves: the "a" wave caused by atrial contraction, the "c" wave caused by atrioventricular valve closure, and the "v" wave caused by peak atrial filling near the end of ventricular systole. The x, x_1, and y waves represent the corresponding descent of the a, c, and v waves. Mean left atrial pressure normally exceeds that of the right atrium.

Modifications of atrial pressure pulse contour can be of diagnostic importance. In atrial fibrillation the "a" wave is absent. "A" waves are increased in ventricular hypertrophy because of reduced ventricular compliance and hypertrophied atria. These characteristics of the right atrial pulse often may be detected in the vena cava or jugular venous pulse, and those of the left atrial pressure pulse may be obtained from the PCW pressure tracing.

With atrioventricular valve regurgitation, blood enters the atrium both from its tributary veins and from the ventricle during ventricular systole, resulting in prominent v waves. In severe regurgitation through the atrioventricular valve, "ventricularization" of the atrial pressure pulse tends to occur; after ventricular relaxation the distended atrium empties rapidly, resulting in a steep y descent. However, patients with severe chronic regurgitation with enlarged compliant atria may have relatively normal pressures, whereas small, thick-walled (and less compliant) atria may have striking elevations of pressure with a smaller degree of regurgitation.

An early response to depressed myocardial contractility and to systolic ventricular overloading is ventricular dilation during diastole. Since elevated ventricular end-diastolic volume often is accompanied by elevated end-diastolic pressure, the latter may serve as an index of dysfunction in the absence of pericardial or endocardial disease. Elevated end-diastolic pressure in turn increases corresponding atrial and venous pressures, which ultimately are responsible for many symptoms of congestive heart failure.

Pulmonary artery pressure is abnormally low with severe obstruction to or diminution of right ventricular outflow and is elevated when there is left-sided heart disease and elevated diastolic pressures.

The contour of the pressure recorded in the central aorta and peripheral arteries is modified by aortic valve disease. With severe aortic stenosis the velocity of left ventricular ejection is diminished, the rise in central and peripheral arterial pressure is abnormally slow with a delayed peak, and the central aortic pressure tracing is characterized by prominent oscillations on the anacrotic (early or ascending) limb. Both the peak systolic pressure and dicrotic notch are delayed. In contrast, with hypertrophic cardiomyopathy (idiopathic hypertrophic subaortic stenosis), arterial pressure pulse rises more rapidly than normal since the left ventricle ejects a disproportionately large fraction of its stroke volume during early systole. In aortic regurgitation, the upstroke in both central and peripheral pulses is quite steep, the descending limb is collapsing, and the diastolic pressure is quite low in relation to peak systolic pressure. The dicrotic notch, signaling valve closure, is inconspicuous or absent in the peripheral pulse.

Cardiac output

Two methods, the Fick method and the indicator-dilution technique, are most often used to measure cardiac output (the quantity of blood pumped by the heart per unit of time). The Fick principle can be applied for the determination of blood flow to a variety of organs: total uptake or release of a substance by an organ is the product of organ blood flow and the difference in arterial and venous concentrations of the substance. The substance usually measured is oxygen content. The Fick principle may be used to measure pulmonary blood flow (total effective cardiac output in patients without circulatory shunts) by simultaneously determining oxygen uptake by the lungs and the difference in oxygen content between pulmonary arterial and venous blood. For example, if this difference is 4 ml/dl of blood, each 25 ml of blood must have acquired 1 ml of oxygen in lung transit. Thus if simultaneously determined oxy-

gen intake during 1 minute is 250 ml, this amount of oxygen must have been transported by 6250 ml (250 × 25) of blood during that 1 minute; this represents the cardiac output. In practice the value for pulmonary vein oxygen content generally is taken from the systemic arterial blood. Diffusion of oxygen across the pulmonary alveolocapillary membrane is assumed to be equal to oxygen uptake at the mouth and in the equilibrium state to oxygen consumption in peripheral tissues during the period of measurement. Since various tissues use different proportions of oxygen, it is essential to sample mixed venous blood to determine the overall arteriovenous oxygen difference in the body. Venous blood is well mixed in the pulmonary artery and usually in the right ventricle outflow tract. Total oxygen consumption must be determined with the patient in a stable or equilibrium state, that is ventilation and oxygen consumption must remain constant during the entire period of measurement.

The indicator-dilution method for measuring cardiac output is based on the principle that on injection of a known quantity of indicator into the circulation, its particles are dispersed so

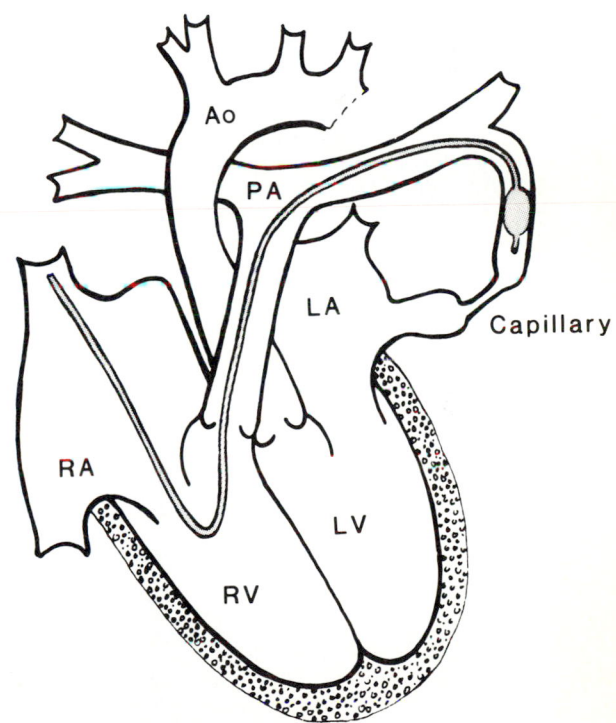

Fig. 89-7 Schematic of cardiac chambers showing passage of a balloon-directed catheter into the pulmonary capillary wedge position. *RA*, Right atrium; *RV*, right ventricle; *PA*, pulmonary artery; *LA*, left atrium; *LV*, left ventricle; and *Ao*, aorta.

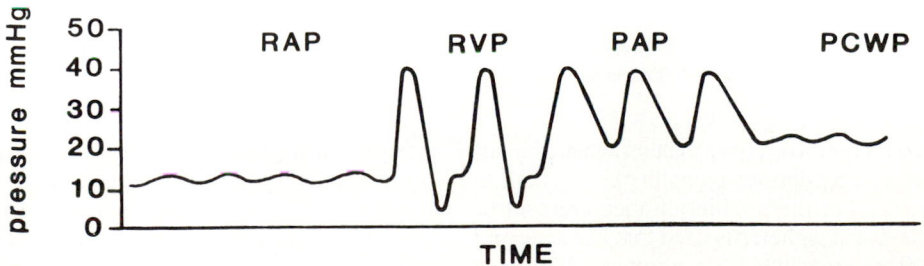

Fig. 89-8 Typical pressure wave contours produced by right atrium *(RAP)*, right ventricle *(RVP)*, pulmonary artery *(RAP)*, and pulmonary capillary wedge position *(PCWP)*.

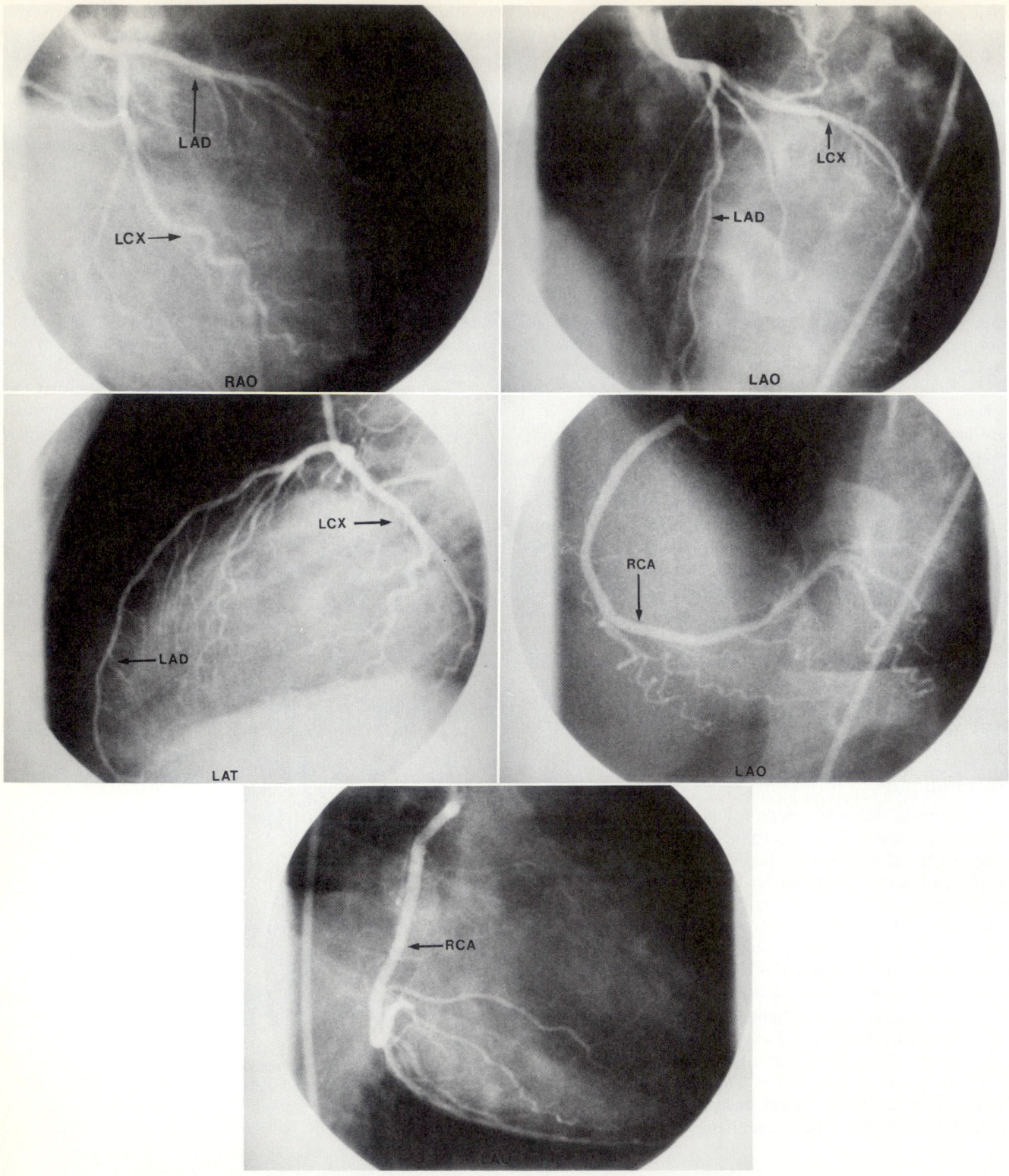

Fig. 89-9   Angiograms of normal left anterior descending *(LAD)*, left circumflex *(LCX)*, and right coronary artery *(RCA)* with their multiple branches in right anterior oblique *(RAO)*, cranially angulated left anterior oblique *(LAO)*, and lateral *(LAT)* projections.

that a smooth time-concentration curve results when the indicator is sampled at an appropriate point in the circulation beyond the injection site. For thermodilution measurement of cardiac output, a Swan-Ganz catheter is used that has a second lumen exiting 30 cm from the catheter tip, through which iced saline is injected. A thermister at the catheter tip positioned in the pulmonary artery continuously samples the change in blood temperature. Blood flow is inversely proportional to the change in temperature. When indocyanine green is used as the indicator, the dye is injected into the pulmonary artery or left ventricle and the change in dye concentration in peripheral arterial blood is determined by drawing blood through a densitometer or oximeter sensitive to changes in light transmission through whole blood. Calculation of the average concentration

NORMAL PRESSURE AND RESISTANCE VALUES

Right atrium	2-8 mm Hg
Right ventricle	15-30/2-8 mm Hg
Pulmonary artery	15-30/4-12 mm Hg
Pulmonary capillary wedge	2-12 mm Hg
Cardiac index	2.6-4.2 L/min/M²
Pulmonary vascular resistance	20-130 dyne-cm-sec⁻⁵
Systemic vascular resistance	700-1600 dyne-cm-sec⁻⁵

of indicator during inscription of the curve yields a measurement of the total volume of blood in which the indicator has been diluted during its passage from injection site to sampling site.

Since the adequacy of cardiac function can be related to the adequacy of oxygenation of peripheral tissues, the systemic arteriovenous oxygen difference is a simple and meaningful index. Regardless of the absolute level of cardiac output, an abnormally wide arteriovenous oxygen difference (more than 5.5 vol/dl with the patient at rest) signifies that the heart fails to deliver quantities of blood to peripheral tissues, thus causing peripheral oxygen extraction to be abnormally high.

Vascular resistance

Pulmonary vascular disease frequently accompanies disorders of the left side of the heart or pulmonary parenchyma, and determination of pulmonary vascular resistance is important. The pressure drop across the pulmonary vascular bed depends on the cross-sectional area of the pulmonary vessels and flow rate; resistance is calculated by dividing the mean pressure drop (mean pulmonary artery pressure minus mean left atrial or PCW pressure) by the cardiac output. Normally resistance offered by the pulmonary vascular bed is about one sixth that of the systemic vascular bed (see box). With pulmonary vascular disease the resistance to flow offered by the pulmonary vasculature is elevated and may even exceed systemic vascular resistance, causing severe right ventricular systolic pressure overload.

Systemic vascular resistance is obtained by dividing the mean arterial pressure minus the mean right atrial pressure by the cardiac output. Systemic vascular resistance is one determinant of left ventricular afterload. It is elevated by increased sympathetic tone in most individuals with hypertension or congestive heart failure and is reduced in states such as early sepsis, thyrotoxicosis, and arteriovenous shunts.

Valvular stenosis

The presence of significant obstruction to blood flow is demonstrable by a pressure gradient. The transvalvular pressure gradient is related to the square of flow rate (doubling of flow across the stenotic valve produces quadrupling of the pressure gradient). In other words, the valve orifice area is proportional to the rate of blood flow across the valve and inversely proportional to the square root of the pressure gradient. When valvular regurgitation coexists with stenosis, the flow rate across the valve is forward cardiac output plus the amount equal to regurgitant flow; thus if regurgitant flow is neglected in calculations, the orifice size is estimated incorrectly. And, unfortunately, there are no routine clinical techniques for precise measurement of regurgitant flow. In addition changes in heart rate modify the time during which blood flows across cardiac valves. Tachycardia shortens diastole relatively more

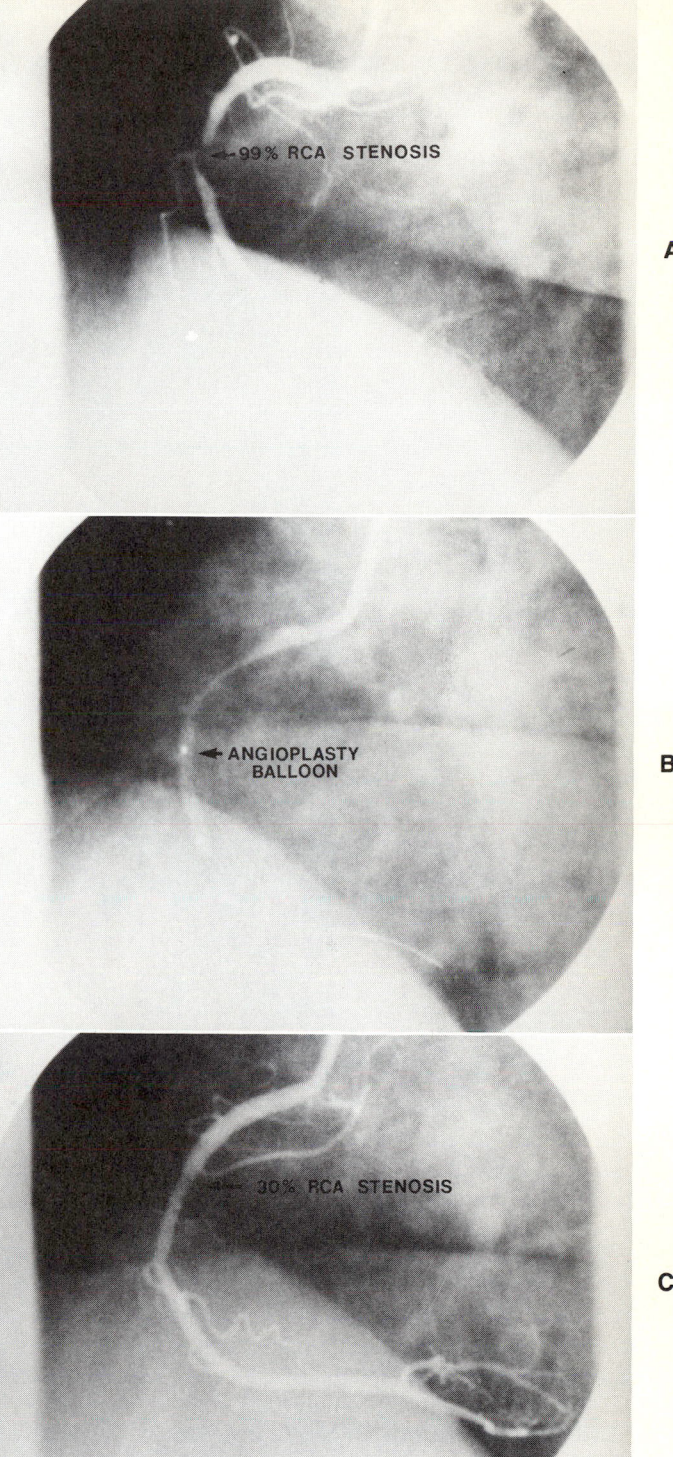

Fig. 89-10 Successful percutaneous transluminal coronary angioplasty (PTCA) of 99% right coronary artery stenosis (seen in LAO projection) results in residual 30% stenosis. **A**, PrePTCA. **B**, PTCA balloon inflated. **C**, PostPTCA.

than systole and thus augments the pressure gradient across stenotic atrioventricular valves.

Reduction of approximately 55% of the normal cross-sectional area of a heart valve must occur in the presence of normal blood flow before transvalvular pressure gradient develops. This implies that heart valves have a large functional

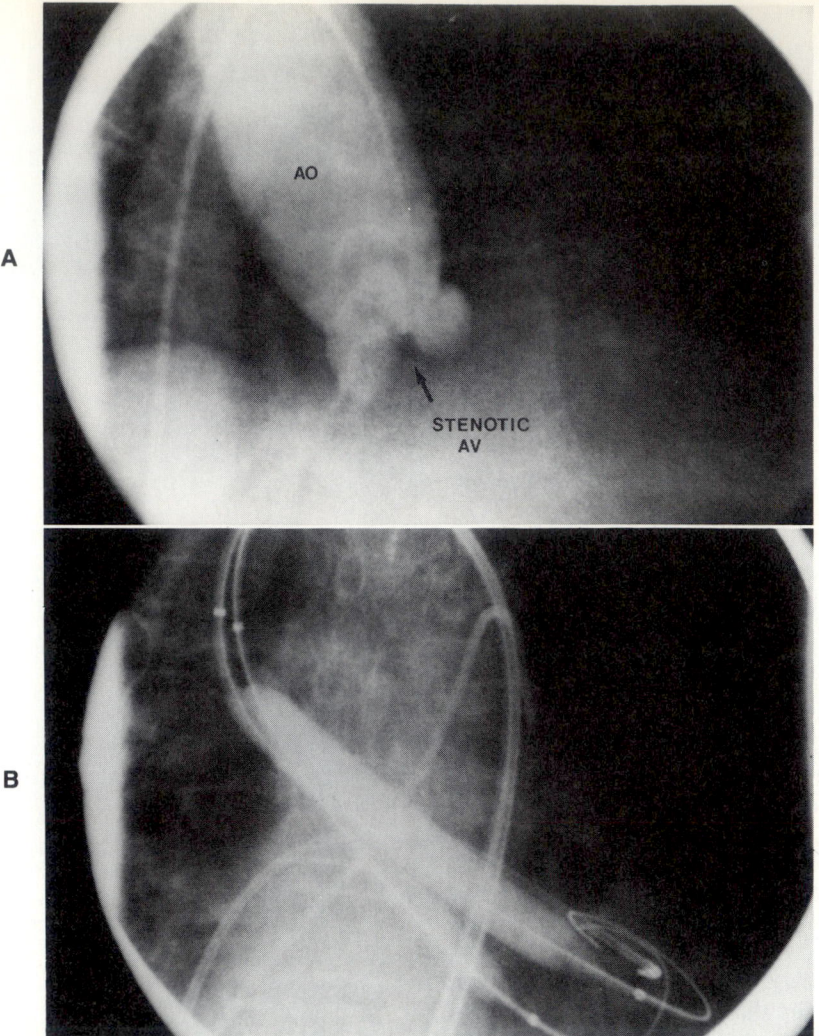

Fig. 89-11 **A,** Aortic *(Ao)* contrast injection showing stenotic aortic valve *(AV).* **B,** Inflation of two valvuloplasty balloon catheters positioned retrogradely across aortic valve.

reserve and that audible murmurs produced by turbulent flow across mildly stenotic valves are not necessarily accompanied by measurable pressure gradients. As stenosis increases in severity, however, a pressure gradient develops when cardiac output is elevated, as with exercise, anxiety, fever, anemia, or pregnancy. With more advanced stenosis, significant pressure gradients are recorded at rest. Finally, with very severe valvular obstruction, the cardiac output is reduced at rest and the transvalvular gradient thereby diminishes.

ENDOMYOCARDIAL BIOPSY. Because of the increasing use of cardiac transplantation and the need to histologically diagnose graft rejection, techniques have been developed for safely obtaining biopsy specimens of the heart. By percutaneous cannulation of either a large vein or artery, a semirigid bioptome catheter with small, closable cutting jaws on its tip is carefully advanced to the ventricle. Under fluoroscopic guidance, the tip is directed toward the interventricular septum, where a small amount of tissue (about 1 mm³) is extracted. Usually several samples are obtained for microscopic examiantion. Endomycardial biopsy also is useful for diagnosis of infiltrative processes and myocarditis, and because the bioptome is directed toward the interventricular septum, cardiac perforation is unusual. Thus risks and complications are similar to those of routine cardiac catheterization.

ANGIOGRAPHY. Radiopaque contrast agents can be injected at various sites during rapid-sequence roentgenography to produce either cine or stationary roentgenographic pictures. The gold standard test for pulmonary emboli is the pulmonary angiogram; a contrast agent is rapidly injected through a catheter in the main pulmonary artery or through a catheter positioned selectively in an individual lobar artery. Right atrial, right ventricular, and (by transatrial septal approach) left atrial angiograms are useful for evaluating congenital abnormalities. Left ventricular angiography not only detects and semiquantifies mitral regurgitation but also allows evaluation of ventricular wall motion. These abnormalities usually are classified as hypokinesis (diminished systolic motion), akinesis (absence of systolic motion), and dyskinesis (paradoxical systolic motion). The overall effect of segmental dysfunction can be quantified by calculating the ejection fraction (stroke volume divided by end-diastolic volume, where stroke volume equals end-diastolic volume minus end-systolic volume). The normal angiographic ejection fraction is 55% to 70%, and severe systolic dysfunction is considered to be present when the ejection fraction is less than 40%. Contrast injection within the proximal aorta allows semiquantification of aortic insufficiency. It also visualizes the aortic valve and root, necessary information for the surgeon before prostheses are selected for valve replacement.

Two techniques are used for coronary angiography. The Sones approach uses a single catheter to cannulate the right and left coronary ostia via the brachial artery. The Judkins approach uses preformed catheters for each of the coronary ostia with arterial access gained via percutaneous puncture of the femoral artery. In each case up to 10 ml of radiopaque contrast material is rapidly injected manually into the left main and right coronary artery. Rapid-sequence roentgenographic pictures produce a moving cineangiogram. Because the many branch vessels often overlap, several injections with pictures taken from several different angles are necessary. Coronary angiography only visualizes the arterial lumen (Fig. 89-9). If atherosclerosis, which is a subintimal process, is uniform and diffuse, the angiographer will not recognize the smooth diminution in luminal diameter. The hallmark of coronary atherosclerosis is the stenotic plaque. In these cases, discrete focal reduction in luminal diameter can be recognized. By adaptation of Poiseuille's law, a 70% reduction in luminal diameter is considered necessary to cause a significant impedance of blood flow and potential cause of ischemia. Underestimation of severity is inherent in coronary angiography, and apparent reductions in vessel diameter of between 50% and 70% are possibly hemodynamically significant. Yet coronary angiography, which gives anatomic and not physiologic information, cannot identify any one stenosis as the cause of clinical ischemia. Only physiologic tests such as exercise nuclear ventriculography, exercise echocardiography, and thallium cold spot scanning can define the physiologic significance of a stenosis. Yet in most cases the presence of stenosis greater than 70% is deemed adequate to explain symptoms and justify their treatment, as by coronary artery bypass grafting.

Despite yielding only anatomic information, coronary angiography currently is the definitive test for coronary arteriosclerosis, because it best delineates the extent of disease. Important facts necessary in making the choice between medical treatment, angioplasty (discussed below), and coronary artery bypass grafting include the number of stenosed coronary arteries, the location of these stenoses, and the condition and size of the distal portions of the arteries. The morbidity of coronary angiography is less than 1%, whereas the mortality is about 0.1%. The most common complications include bleeding and vascular damage at the arterial puncture site, emboli, ventricular arrhythmias, transient renal insufficiency, and allergic reactions to the contrast agent.

INTERVENTIONAL CATHETERIZATION. Cardiac catheterization is becoming an important part of the therapeutic armamentarium of coronary artery disease. Several years ago Gruentzig introduced the balloon angioplasty catheter for both peripheral and coronary artery stenosis (Fig. 89-10). Via a peripheral artery and through a large-diameter steering catheter, a small balloon-tipped catheter is advanced over a very fine, flexible guide wire through the arterial stenosis. When the balloon is within the stenotic segment, it is inflated to several atmospheres of pressure and held for 30 seconds to 3 minutes. This procedure is repeated until the stenosis is substantially reduced. In experienced hands the angioplasty catheter can compress and fissure the atherosclerotic plaque in 80% to 90% of attempts. Restenosis is noted after 1 year in about 30% of cases, but it responds to a second angioplasty. A catheter similar to but larger than the angioplasty catheter can effectively split stenotic cardiac valves without causing embolization or prohibitive valve insufficiency (Fig. 89-11). In initial trials this technique seemed most effective in the stiff, heavily calcified valves of elderly patients. If further experience proves suc-

cessful, balloon valvuloplasty will be widely used, because it can be accomplished at low risk and avoids the cost and complications of surgical valve replacement.

BIBLIOGRAPHY

Berger HJ and Zaret BL: Nuclear cardiology, N Engl J Med 305:799, 1981.
Ellestad MH: Stress testing: principles and practice, ed 3, Philadelphia, 1986, FA Davis Co.
Feigenbaum H: Echocardiography, ed 4, Philadelphia, 1986, Lea & Febiger.
Goldschlanger N: Use of the treadmill test in the diagnosis of coronary artery disease in patients with chest pain, Ann Intern Med 97:383, 1982.
Grossman W: Cardiac catheterization and angiography, ed 3, Philadelphia, 1985, Lea & Febiger.
Hatle L and Angelsen B: Doppler ultrasound in cardiology, ed 2, Philadelphia, 1985, Lea & Febiger.
Hess ML: Indications and results of endomyocardial biopsy, ACC Learning Center Highlights 2:6, 1985.
Marriott HJL: Practical electrocardiography, ed 8, Baltimore, 1986, Williams & Wilkins.
Pearlman AS, Scoblioko DR, and Saal AK: Assessment of valvular heart disease by Doppler echocardiography, Clin Cardiol 6:573, 1983.
Popp RL and others: Echocardiography: M-mode and two-dimensional methods, Ann Intern Med 93:844, 1980.
Rahimtoola SH: Catheter balloon valvuloplasty of aortic and mitral stenosis in adults, Circulation 75:895, 1987.
Reeder GS and Vlietstra RE: Coronary angioplasty: 1986, Mod Concepts Cardiovasc Dis 55:49, 1986.
Sharkey SW: Beyond the wedge: clinical physiology and the Swan-Ganz catheter, Am J Med 83:111, 1987.

90 · PULMONARY EMBOLISM

Steven G. Meister and **Toby R. Engel**

PATHOGENESIS. Thrombi and other solid objects that gain access to an arterial system are carried distally until they lodge in a branch and cause obstruction. This process is called embolization. Most emboli in the pulmonary arterial tree are thrombi formed in the larger systemic veins (usually in the legs and pelvis) that become detached from the vein wall, float into the right-sided heart chambers, and are expelled into the pulmonary artery. Embolization occurs most commonly to the lower lobes and more often to the right lung than the left.

Infected thrombi arise in veins that are draining areas of infection, particularly in the pelvis, and become septic emboli, resulting in abscesses when they lodge in the pulmonary tree. Less commonly the chambers or valves of the right side of the heart serve as a source of thrombi. Other substances such as fat, bone marrow, tumor fragments, air, vegetations from infected right-sided heart valves, and even foreign bodies such as shotgun pellets can embolize to the pulmonary circulation. However, in the following discussion the term "pulmonary embolism" refers to thrombotic material.

Emboli in the pulmonary arterial tree cause complete or partial obstruction of a branch. However, the pulmonary arterial circulation can absorb a remarkable amount of embolic material without an appreciable rise in overall resistance to blood flow. Approximately 50% of the pulmonary tree must be occluded for resistance to rise sufficiently to cause a measurable increase in pressure in the pulmonary artery.

Occasionally a large pulmonary embolus by itself can occlude a large portion of the pulmonary vasculature by "saddling" the bifurcation of the main pulmonary artery. More commonly symptomatic emboli are smaller but multiple, recurring several times over days and weeks. The effects of multiple emboli are additive and result in a rise in pulmonary arterial pressure when enough of the arterial tree has been occluded. In some patients emboli occur repeatedly and chronically over several weeks and months, creating chronic pulmonary hypertension, right ventricular hypertrophy, and eventual failure. This produces a clinical picture difficult to distinguish from chronic right-sided heart failure of other origins.

Another mechanism whereby pulmonary embolization results in pulmonary hypertension was suggested by infusion of small, fresh, experimentally produced thrombi into dogs, resulting in increased pulmonary vascular resistance and pressure. This effect was observed with emboli much too small to cause pulmonary hypertension from mechanical obstruction, suggesting that a vasoconstrictor substance was released from the thrombus itself. Increased resistance and pressure did not occur in animals pretreated with heparin.

The right ventricle is a thin-walled chamber designed for pumping blood at relatively low pressures. However, when abruptly called on to generate systolic pressures greater than about twice the normal pulmonary presure of 25 to 30 mm Hg, the right ventricle fails acutely. This in turn results in increased right atrial–systemic venous pressure and reduced cardiac output. On the other hand, a right ventricle that has undergone gradual hypertrophy because of pressure loading, as in mitral stenosis or chronic left-sided heart failure, frequently can sustain substantially higher pressures without failing.

Probably from the moment an embolis arrives in the pulmonary circulation, it is subject to thrombolytic mechanisms that work toward its gradual breakdown and eventual absorption. This process can proceed at variable rates and to different stages of completion. Serial angiographic studies in humans have emphasized this variability. In some patients massive pulmonary emboli have virtually disappeared in less than 2 weeks. In others, particularly the elderly, the clearing process is much slower and may never be completed.

Unlike most other tissues the pulmonary parenchyma has a dual blood supply consisting of the pulmonary arterial system and the bronchial arterial circulation arising from the aorta. This dual supply accounts for the infrequency of parenchymal infarction as a consequence of pulmonary embolization. Nevertheless, infarction and necrosis do occur, particularly with preexisting left ventricular failure. Necrosis produces a clinical picture similar to lobar or segmental pneumonitis. Infarctions ultimately are converted to relatively avascular scar tissue, causing a permanent loss of pulmonary vasculature.

The consequences of pulmonary embolization vary considerably, depending on whether the embolism is small or massive, whether emboli are single or multiple, whether pulmonary hypertension and right ventricular failure occur, and whether pulmonary infarction results. Therefore the clinical picture is extremely diverse and often confusing.

PREDISPOSING FACTORS. Acute pulmonary embolism seldom is an isolated entity. Its occurrence depends on a source of thrombotic material in either the large systemic veins or the right-sided heart chambers. These in turn seldom occur in the absence of an identifiable predisposing factor, recognition of which provides important clues to the diagnosis of the pulmonary embolism. Any factor that predisposes to phlebitis of the deep systemic veins predisposes to pulmonary embolism.

Among the most common factors in otherwise healthy individuals are orthopedic injuries, particularly of the lower extremities and pelvis. Leg casts, especially poorly fitting ones that compress the deep veins, often are associated with embolism. Hip fractures are an extremely common antecedent in the elderly. The extent of the orthopedic injury bears no relationship to the magnitude of the embolic syndrome that may be produced: a small cast on the lower leg may initiate a deep venous thrombosis that propagates proximally to the femoral or iliac veins and eventuates in a massive pulmonary embolism.

Major surgery of any type predisposes to deep venous thrombosis and pulmonary embolism so often that many surgeons advocate prophylactic anticoagulation with small doses of heparin before certain major procedures such as hip surgery.

Acute myocardial infarction, cardiogenic shock, and congestive heart failure also are predisposing factors, perhaps because reduction in cardiac output results in sluggish flow and consequent thrombus formation in the larger systemic veins. In congestive cardiomyopathies there is also mural thrombus formation, and thus emboli can arise from the right-sided heart chambers. Myocardial infarction involving the interventricular septum or the free walls of the right ventricle occasionally results in mural thrombosis and subsequent pulmonary embolization.

Pregnancy and oral contraceptives sometimes cause pulmonary embolism in healthy women. Compression of the inferior vena cava by the gravid uterus results in congestion and dilation of the veins of the pelvis and lower extremities, enhancing thrombus formation. The estrogenic component of contraceptives alters platelet adhesiveness and predisposes to thrombus formation.

Malignancies are another predisposing factor for venous thrombosis and pulmonary embolism. Recurrent *migratory* thrombophlebitis sometimes provides the first clue to the presence of a neoplasm. The mechanism whereby neoplasms induce venous thrombosis is not known.

CLINICAL MANIFESTATIONS. The most common symptom of acute pulmonary embolism is dyspnea at rest, typically of abrupt onset. Patients commonly complain of being unable to get enough air. Dyspnea at rest usually subsides after 1 to 2 hours but often is recurrent. Successive episodes often are noted to be of progressive severity and duration. The individual episodes probably correspond to successive embolic events. Subsidence of each episode may correspond to partial breakup and distal migration of the individual embolus. When dyspnea at rest has subsided, patients often describe persistence of dyspnea on slight exertion. Coughing of abrupt onset is also common.

A single massive embolus or many smaller emboli can result in pulmonary arterial obstruction sufficient to cause hypotension, light-headedness, or even syncope, but this is not common. Pain similar to that of acute myocardial infarction also is uncommon; when it occurs, it probably is a manifestation of sudden dilation of the pulmonary artery caused by hypertension.

With pulmonary infarction there is necrosis of a wedge-shaped segment of parenchyma that abuts on the pleura. Inflammation of visceral pleura overlying the infarct causes pain on deep inspiration, coughing, and sneezing. Hemoptysis is a consequence of the hemorrhagic nature of the infarct. Fever also may occur.

Some patients with chronic congestive heart failure complain only of a worsening of their congestive symptoms. Because of this it often is suggested that acute pulmonary embolism can cause acute pulmonary edema. The dyspnea associated with pulmonary embolism can be acute and severe and suggest pulmonary edema, but it is doubtful that the embolism actually causes pulmonary edema. Cardiac pulmonary edema results from increased pressure within the pulmonary capillary bed because of increased left atrial pressure, and pulmonary arterial obstruction tends to *lower* pulmonary capillary and left atrial pressures. Confusion may result because, as is subsequently detailed, pulmonary congestion resulting from left-sided heart failure causes false positive results in certain diagnostic tests for pulmonary embolism.

It is important to emphasize that many pulmonary emboli, particularly when small, cause no symptoms. They often are first discovered on the autopsy table. This is partly because physical findings of pulmonary embolism frequently are absent; emboli that cause neither right-sided heart failure nor pulmonary infarction seldom produce physical findings.

Acute right-sided heart failure causes elevated right ventricular diastolic pressure and consequently elevated right atrial and systemic venous pressure. The internal or external jugular veins become distended, with a pulsation at the time of right atrial contraction (timed with an S_4 gallop preceding the first heart sound). The pulmonic component of the second heart sound may be accentuated. The second sound may be widely split becuse of resistance to systolic ejection of the right ventricle, resulting in delayed closure of the pulmonic valve. Less commonly, a right ventricular S_3 gallop can be heard, which is loudest in the third and fourth intercostal space at the left sternal border and increases with inspiration. Occasionally a right ventricular lift is palpable at the lower left sternal border. A very unusual but well-documented finding in acute pulmonary embolism is pulsus paradoxus.

If infarction occurs, the findings are similar to bacterial pneumonia (rales, fever, signs of consolidation, pleural effusion, and/or friction rub).

The local findings of thrombosis of the deep veins of the legs or pelvis provide a clue to the presence of pulmonary embolism. However, deep venous thrombosis can be devoid of physical findings. In fact the loosely attached thrombi that are most likely to detach from the venous endothelium to become emboli also are the least likely to cause the complete venous obstruction and local inflammation responsible for the characteristic signs of thrombophlebitis. Furthermore, the responsible thrombus may well have embolized in its entirety to the lungs by the time the patient is evaluated for acute pulmonary embolism.

LABORATORY FINDINGS. The electrocardiogram (ECG) shows features of right ventricular overload only when pulmonary embolism is massive. The combination of an S wave in lead I, a Q wave in lead III, and an inverted T wave in lead III occurs with a right ventricular overload. Right precordial T inversion, abnormal rightward deviation of the QRS axis, and right bundle branch block are other signs. Increased right atrial pressure can be accompanied by enlargement of the P wave in leads II, III, and aV_F.

A variety of abnormalities are seen on the chest roentgenogram. Pulmonary infarction often is associated with an infiltrate, sometimes pyramidal in shape (with the apex pointing toward the hilum), corresponding to the segmental distribution of the occluded vessel. There may be elevation of the diaphragm on the affected side and horizontal streaks at the bases, representing thin, irregular bands of atelectasis.

In the absence of pulmonary infarction, underperfused areas may appear more radiolucent than adjacent normal areas. In the presence of massive pulmonary embolism, the nonembolized segments are overperfused and the resulting vascular engorgement may appear as an infiltrate. In the presence of

marked pulmonary hypertension, prominence of the main pulmonary arteries sometimes is notable.

It should be emphasized that these findings are inconstant and not specific. In fact a paucity of findings on the chest roentgenogram when the patient complains of severe dyspnea should suggest pulmonary embolism.

Arterial hypoxemia usually is present, regardless of whether there is right-sided heart failure or pulmonary infarction. It was noted in the early 1970s that the partial pressure of oxygen in the blood (PaO_2) was less than 80 mm Hg in most patients and less than 90 mm Hg in all patients with pulmonary embolism breathing room air. However, there have since been a number of cases of well-documented acute pulmonary embolism with PaO_2 in excess of 90 mm Hg. Thus normal PaO_2 does not completely exclude acute pulmonary embolism.

It also must be emphasized that an abnormally low PaO_2 is not specific and occurs in a number of conditions that may simulate the clinical picture of acute pulmonary embolus. Among these are congestive heart failure, chronic obstructive lung disease, viral and bacterial pneumonitis, and acute asthmatic attacks.

Other laboratory findings in pulmonary embolism may include decreased arterial $PaCO_2$, leukocytosis and elevated erythrocyte sedimentation rate, serum indirect bilirubin, serum lactic dehydrogenase, and fibrin-split products. However, these are not constant findings and therefore are of limited diagnostic value.

RADIONUCLIDE STUDIES AND PULMONARY ANGIOGRAPHY. Perfusion scanning of the lungs is a useful screening test for pulmonary embolism. Albumin is treated so that the molecules aggregate to a particle size that will not pass through the pulmonary capillaries and is labeled with a short-lived radioactive isotope of technetium. It is infused intravenously and passes to the pulmonary capillary bed, where the particles are trapped. Scintillation scanning of the thorax creates a series of images corresponding to the distribution of the labeled particles. When embolism is present, the particles are not distributed to lung segments supplied by obstructed arteries, creating filling defects on the scan (Fig. 90-1). The number of particles injected is too small to cause pulmonary vascular obstruction or hemodynamic consequences. (A rare exception is seen with advanced pulmonary vascular disease and extreme pulmonary hypertension, in which the injected particles may aggravate right ventricular failure and induce profound hypotension.)

Perfusion lung scanning is highly sensitive, and for practical purposes a normal scan excludes pulmonary embolism. Unfortunately, like the measurement of PaO_2, perfusion scanning is nonspecific and is abnormal in a variety of conditions, including some that have features resembling acute pulmonary embolism. In congestive heart failure reduced flow to the lower lobes often creates scan defects. Fluid in the lung fissures or at the bases also can cause false positive scans. In obstructive lung disease poorly ventilated segments have reduced perfusion on lung scan. Areas of pneumonitis also result in an abnormal scan.

Specificity can be improved by a variety of stragegies. Simple comparison of the lung scan to chest roentgenograms obtained at the same time is helpful in that scan defects corresponding to infiltrates and fluid collections should be disregarded. Determining whether the filling defects on scan correspond to the known segmental anatomy of the lungs is useful, since the pulmonary artery tree corresponds closely to segmental anatomy.

Combined ventilation-perfusion lung scanning contrasts the

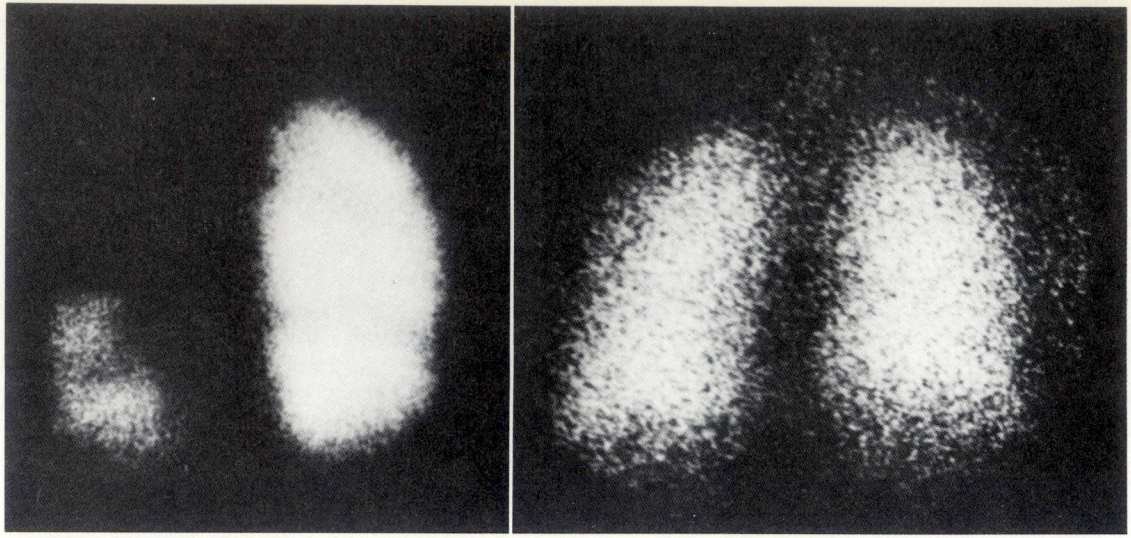

Fig. 90-1 Perfusion *(left)* and ventilation *(right)* scans in patient with massive pulmonary embolism involving lung. Note that one lung is nearly obliterated on perfusion scan and normally represented on ventilation scan.

images produced on standard perfusion scanning with those made following inhalation of radioactive xenon. Defects in the perfusion scan that are related to reflex underperfusion of poorly ventilated areas can be identified and disregarded (Fig. 90-1).

Pulmonary angiography is the most specific test for diagnosis of pulmonary embolism. It uses a radiopaque organic iodide-containing contrast meterial, which is introduced via a catheter passed through the right side of the heart into the main pulmonary artery or its subdivisions. The entire pulmonary arterial tree can be visualized clearly to the level of branches about 2 mm in diameter. Pulmonary embolism is demonstrated by an intravascular thrombus or an occluded ("cutoff") vessel (Fig. 90-2). A variety of normal anatomic features such as overlapping or branching vessels can resemble intravascular clots or cutoff vessels.

MANAGEMENT. The principal therapy for acute pulmonary embolus is anticoagulation. The rationale is prevention of additional thrombus formation at the site of origin to prevent further embolization while natural thrombolytic mechanisms digest the embolized clots. This is effective for most patients. It should be done initially in the hospital with heparin sulfate. Heparin therapy usually should be begun as soon as the diagnosis is strongly suspected while waiting for the diagnostic tests to be performed. Subcutaneous injection, intravenous bolus injection, and constant intravenous infusion are alternative approaches to heparinization. A single loading dose followed by a constant intravenous infusion is now widely used in hospitalized patients. Frequent monitoring of the partial thromboplastin time is used as a guide to dosage adjustment. Whichever is used, frequent monitoring of the partial thromboplastin time is useful to select the size and timing of subsequent doses and to avoid inadequate or excessive anticoagulation. A partial thromboplastin time one and one half to two and one half times longer than control values generally is considered optimal. When subcutaneous or intravenous bolus injecton is used, the partial thromboplastin time should be drawn 1 hour before the next scheduled dose, when it should be one and one half to two times control values. Constant intravenous infusion avoids the wide swings in partial thromboplastin times that occur when repeated boluses are used.

There is no evidence that anticoagulation with injected hep-

arin is any more or less effective than with oral warfarin (Coumadin). However, warfarin's effect (against hepatic synthesis of clotting proteins) is not seen for 48 hours. Thus "warfarinization" can be begun after heparinization has been achieved, and heparin should be continued until warfarin has prolonged the prothrombin time (PT) one and one half to two and one half times longer than control values.

Disadvantages of anticoagulation include bleeding at therapeutic levels in predisposed patients and in others when the therapeutic range is exceeded. Bleeding from heparinization is a common and serious in-hospital cause of drug-induced morbidity. Numerous common prescription and nonprescription drugs accentuate or diminish warfarin's action. Patients receiving long-term warfarin therapy should have PT checked *at least* once monthly. Three to 6 months of anticoagualtion generally is appropriate after embolization. Those with a predisposition to pulmonary embolism who have had documented emboli should be anticoagulated indefinitely.

Patients who cannot be anticoagulated or who have had recurrent pulmonary emboli while on *adequate* anticoagulation can have interruption of their inferior vena cava (IVC). Transverse compartmentalizaton of the IVC with a series of sutures or a specially designed clip permits continuing blood flow through the vessel without permitting passage of large thrombi. This procedure entails morbidity and potential mortality and should never be done without angiographic documentation of embolization. Alternatively, a sievelike device ("umbrella") can be implanted prevenously in the IVC via a specially designed catheter system. Recurrent embolism after IVC interruption has been reported; however, these recurrences generally have not been angiographically documented. Enlarged collateral vessels around the interruption were implicated, but these are less likely when plication or sieve implantation are used rather than ligation.

Acute submassive pulmonary emboli can result in asthmatic or shocklike states. This may result in part from release of vasoactive substances from platelets and other components of the emboli that cause bronchial and pulmonary arterial constriction. Initial therapy consists of heparin, oxygen, and agents such as dopamine to increase cardiac output.

In one extensive multiple-center trial the thrombolytic agents urokinase and streptokinase were found to induce faster clear-

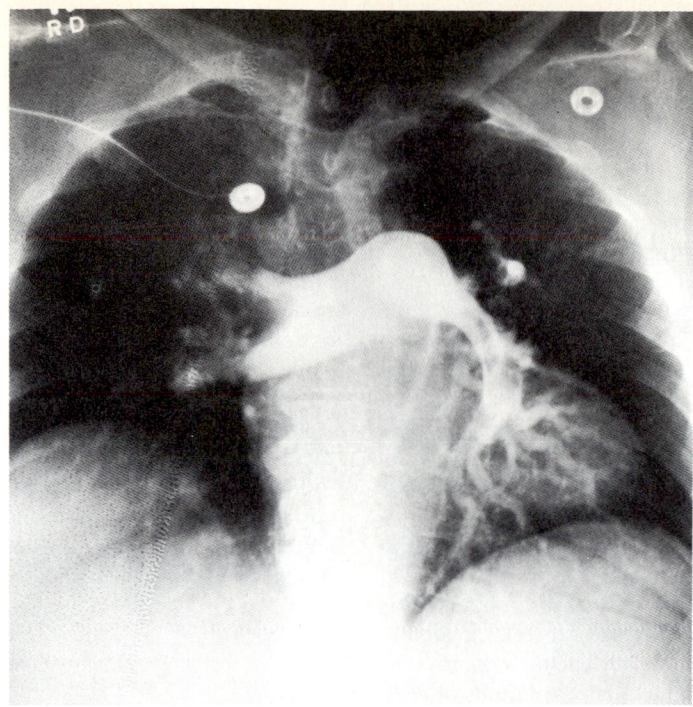

Fig. 90-2   Massive emboli to both lungs seen on pulmonary angiography. Major arteries to entire right lung and left upper lobe are occluded (cutoff). Left lower lobe artery contains several large, serpentine filling defects.

ing of emboli from the pulmonary vasculature than heparin alone. They are appropriate in patients in persistent circulatory shock from massive embolization. However, substantial morbidity and mortality from bleeding may result, and these agents should be used only when essential. An alternative approach in persistent shock is surgical embolectomy. However, most patients either become normotensive or die in the 1 or 2 hours required to prepare for open heart surgery.

Autopsy studies in the 1960s suggested that over 50% of patients dying in hospitals had pulmomary emboli. However, these studies used techniques that likely were oversensitive and overestimated the prevalence of clinically significant pulmonary emboli in these patients. The subsequent introduction of pulmonary perfusion scanning, which by itself frequently results in false positive diagnoses, greatly enhanced the tendency of clinicians to overdiagnose pulmonary embolism. The subsequent introduction of ventilation-perfusion scanning and more widespread utilization of pulmonary arteriography has markedly enhanced our ability to diagnose pulmonary embolism with great specificity is most instances. Since anticoagulation carries a definite risk of morbidity and mortality, the key to proper management of this disease is proper diagnosis. Thus, with infrequent exceptions, a firm diagnosis of pulmonary embolic disease should not be made without confirmation by ventilation-perfusion scanning or pulmonary arteriography. Although initiation of therapy with heparin is often appropriate before an accurate diagnosis can be established, continued or chronic anticoagulation and IVC interruption should not be done without definitive confirmation of the diagnosis.

BIBLIOGRAPHY

Bell WR and Simon TL: A comparative analysis of pulmonary perfusion scans with pulmonary angiograms (from a national cooperative study), Am Heart J 92:700, 1976.

Burdine JA and Wallace JM: Pulsus paradoxus and Kussmaul's sign in massive pulmonary embolism, Am J Cardiol 15:413, 1965.
Coon WW: Some recent developments in the pharamacology of heparin, J Clin Pharmacol 21:337, 1979.
Dalen JE and others: Resolution of acute pulmonary embolism in man, N Engl J Med 280:1194, 1969.
Dalen JE and others: Pulmonary embolism, pulmonary hemorrhage and pulmonary infarction, N Engl J Med 296:1431, 1977.
Gurewich V, Cohen ML, and Thomas DP: Humoral factors in massive pulmonary embolism: an experimental study, Am Heart J 76:784, 1968.
Gurewich V, Duncan PT, and Rabinov KR: Pulmonary embolism after ligation of the inferior vena cava, N Engl J Med 274:1350, 1966.
Hyland JW and others: Effect of selective embolization of various sized pulmonary arteries in dogs, Am J Physiol 204:619, 1963.
McIntyre KM and Sasahara AA: The hemodynamic response to pulmonary embolism in patients without prior cardiopulmonary disease, Am J Cardiol 28:288, 1971.
Poulose KP and others: Diagnosis of pulmonary embolism: a correlative study of the clinical, scan, and angiographic findings, Br Med J 3:67, 1970.
Robin ED: Overdiagnosis and overtreatment of pulmonary embolism: the emperor may have no clothes, Ann Intern Med 87:775, 1977.
Sagar S and others: Efficacy of low-dose heparin in prevention of extensive deep-vein thrombosis in patients undergoing total-hip replacement, Lancet 1:1151, 1976.
Szucs M Jr and others: Diagnostic sensitivity of laboratory findings in acute pulmonary embolism, Ann Intern Med 74:161, 1971.

91 · THROMBOPHLEBITIS

Steven G. Meister

PATHOPHYSIOLOGY. Thrombophlebitis is inflammation from thrombus formation within a vein. It is common and results from venous stasis, local injury to venous endothelium, or altered blood coagulability. Factors causing stasis of venous blood include congestive heart failure; myocardial infarction; prolonged bed rest; prolonged maintenance of the legs in a cramped position; pregnancy; tight, constricting casts or garments; and obesity. Damage to venous endothelium may result from physical trauma, intravenous lines and needles, infection, and vasculitis. A variety of systemic conditions, including carcinomatosis, the postoperative and postpartum states, polycythemia, and hyperviscosity syndrome, predispose to thrombophlebitis by altering blood coagulability. Thrombophlebitis at several sites, simultaneously or in rapid succession, is known as migratory thrombophlebitis. It suggests the presence of polycythemia or occult malignancy.

Thrombophlebitis occurs most commonly in the veins of the lower extremities and pelvis and may involve either the deep or the superficial veins. In the deep veins of the thighs and pelvis portions of the thrombi often break loose and are carried proximally to become pulmonary emboli. This rarely occurs with superficial phlebitis or phlebitis of the upper extremities. Deep vein thrombophlebitis also can damage the venous valves, causing them to become incompetent. This causes chronic venous stasis in the lower extremities and predisposes to recurrent phlebitis in the same veins.

CLINICAL MANIFESTATIONS. Superficial thrombophlebitis is an acute inflammation along the course of a superficial vein with redness, induration, and edema. Often the vein itself is visible or, more often, palpable and tender. Symptoms of deep vein thrombophlebitis range from none at all to severe pain. Most patients complain of nothing more than dull aching deep within the involved limb. Fever may be present.

Physical findings, when present, are related to venous inflammation or obstruction. Inflammation can give rise to a palpable, tender cord along the course of the vein. Obstruction produces distal swelling and congestion of the limb. The skin color is dusky, and the skin temperature is appreciably warmer than that of the uninvolved limb. The superficial veins distal to the obstruction also appear distended. Calf tenderness and Homans' sign, midcalf pain elicited by passive dorsiflexion of the foot, are present. Unfortunately, these findings are not always present. In fact those thrombi most loosely attached to the venous endothelium, and thus *least* likely to be associated with either inflammation or obstruction, are most likely to detach and become emboli. Accordingly, laboratory tests often are needed to establish a diagnosis of acute deep vein thrombophlebitis.

Damage to the venous valves from recurrent deep vein phlebitis results in chronic venous stasis with edema, pigmentation, and skin ulceration (postphlebitic syndrome).

LABORATORY FINDINGS. The most reliable test is injection of roentgenographic contrast medium into the veins of the feet. Serial roentgenograms are made as contrast material progresses through the deep venous system of the legs and pelvis. Thrombi appear as filling defects. This test is definitive; its drawbacks are that it is an invasive procedure involving moderate discomfort, slight risk, and considerable expense.

There are several noninvasive but less reliable alternative tests. Radioiodinated fibrinogen in taken up by an actively growing thrombus. Scintillation scanning reveals a "hot spot" over a thrombus. This is a highly sensitive technique for detecting even small thrombi distal to the midthigh, but it is less reliable for the more important proximal thrombi and is of little value in the pelvis. It is precisely these more proximal leg and pelvic thrombi that have been implicated in pulmonary embolism. Impedance phlebography measures minute fluctuations in electrical impedance of the legs that occur as a consequence of normal respiratory variations in blood volume. Both arterial and venous flow patterns are present and easily distinguishable. Absence of the normal venous fluctuations with inspiration is

found when deep veins are obstructed by thrombus. Doppler phlebography uses the phase shift of high-frequency sound waves reflected from moving blood cells to detect blood flow in large veins. It can detect absent flow when venous obstruction is present. Both phlebography tests show 80% to 90% sensitivity to obstructing thrombi in the iliac and femoral veins but are much less sensitive when a nonobstructing thrombus is present; this thrombus is less firmly attached and thus more likely to embolize.

MANAGEMENT AND PREVENTION. Superficial phlebitis is treated with analgesics, moist heat, elevation of the involved extremity, and bed rest. Deep vein phlebitis is treated in the same fashion, and anticoagulation is used as described in Chapter 90. Anticoagulation should be continued for 3 to 6 months. If thrombophlebitis is recurrent, long-term (even lifelong) treatment may be necessary.

Patients at risk for thrombophlebitis because of immobilization (for example, resulting from massive fractures, myocardial infarction, and major surgery) should be considered for prophylactic anticoagulation with heparin.

BIBLIOGRAPHY

Adar R and Salgman WE: Treatment of thrombosis of veins of the lower extremities, N Engl J Med 292:348, 1975.

Barber HM and others: A comparative study of dextran-70, warfarin and low-dose heparin for the prophylaxis of thrombo-embolism following total hip replacement, Postgrad Med J 53:130, 1977.

Dmochowski JR, Adams DF, and Couch NP: Impedance measurement in the diagnosis of deep venous thrombosis, Arch Surg 104:170, 1972.

Nicoliades AN and others: The origin of deep vein thromboses: a venographic study, Br J Radiol 44:653, 1971.

Provan JL and Thomson C: Natural history of thrombophlebitis and its relationship to pulmonary embolism, Can J Surg 16:284, 1973.

Rabinov K and Paulin S: Roentgen diagnosis of venous thrombosis in the leg, Arch Surg 104:134, 1972.

Steer ML and others: Limitations of impedance phlebography for diagnosis of venous thrombosis, Arch Surg 106:44, 1973.

Yao ST, Gourmos C, and Hobbs JT: Detection of proximal-vein thromboses by Doppler ultrasound flow-detection method, Lancet 1:1, 1972.

92 · PRIMARY PULMONARY HYPERTENSION

Nelson M. Wolf

Pulmonary hypertension, as defined by a pulmonary artery pressure of greater than 30/15 mm Hg, may be secondary to cardiac diseases. These include conditions that cause an increase in pulmonary venous pressure, such as left ventricular failure, mitral valve disease, and thrombus or myxoma of the left atrium. In addition, any condition that causes chronic hypoventilation such as chronic obstructive lung disease, neuromuscular disorders, or severe kyphoscoliosis also may result in pulmonary hypertension. Disorders that cause a reduction in the pulmonary vascular bed (including pulmonary emboli, arteritis, schistosomiasis, Eisenmenger's syndrome from congenital cardiac defects, and various interstitial parenchymal disorders such as interstitial fibrosis and interstitial granulomatosis) also may cause pulmonary hypertension.

The syndrome of *primary* pulmonary hypertension occurs with a frequency of about 0.2% to 0.17%. It is more common in individuals under 40 years of age, and females outnumber males 3:1. Although no cause has been determined, primary pulmonary hypertension has been associated with collagen vascular disease, Raynaud's syndrome, use of oral contraceptive agents, and the anorexic agent aminorex. Serum positive for

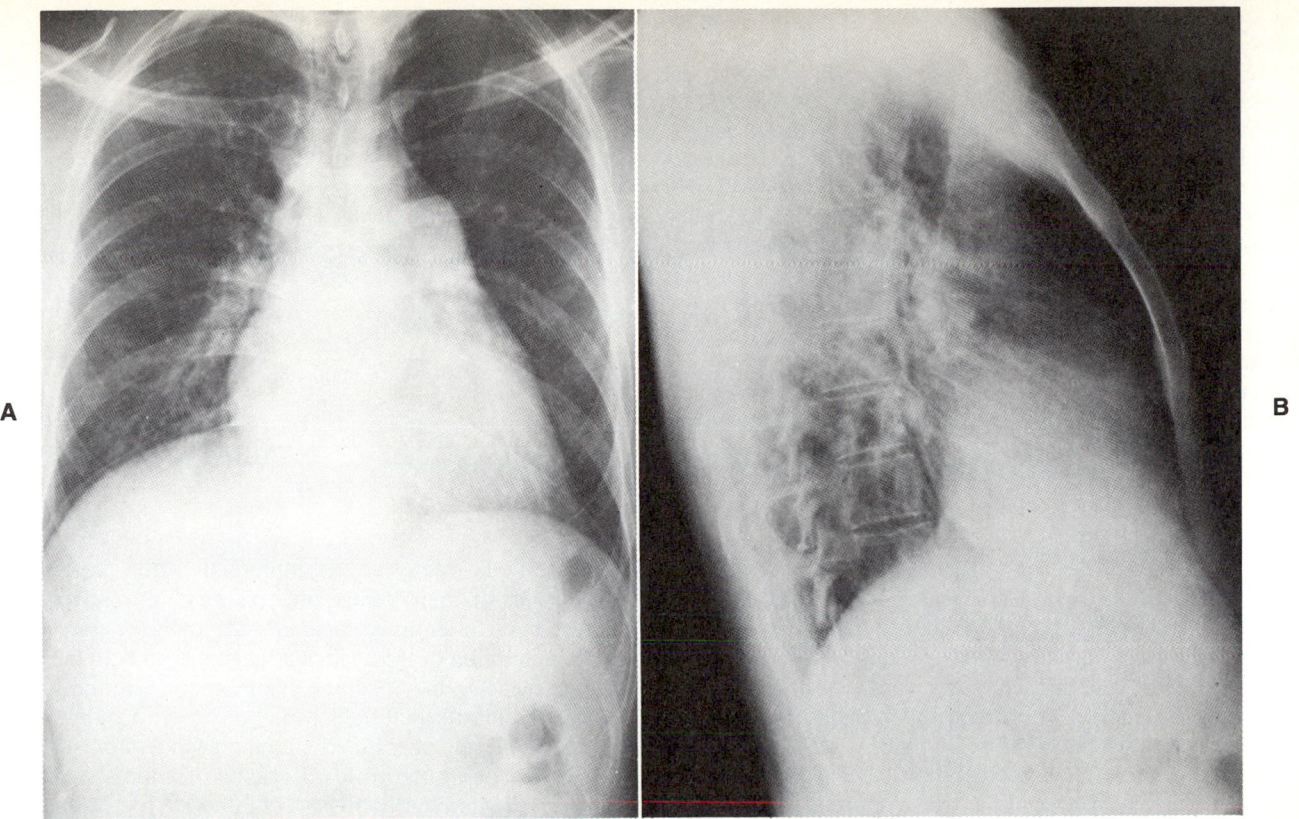

Fig. 92-1 **A,** Posteroanterior and **B,** lateral chest roentgenograms from 26-year-old male with primary pulmonary hypertension, showing cardiac enlargement, particularly of right ventricle, with prominence of main pulmonary arteries and attenuation of peripheral pulmonary arteries.

antinuclear antibodies has been described in 40% of patients with primary pulmonary hypertension.

PATHOLOGY. The histologic changes seen in the pulmonary arteries in primary pulmonary hypertension can be found in severe pulmonary hypertension of other origins. The changes are intimal proliferation, medial hypertrophy, plexiform lesions, fibrinoid necrosis, and arteritis. These pathologic changes involve primarily the pulmonary arterioles and small muscular pulmonary arteries. A grading system has been developed that correlates with altered hemodynamics. Grade 1 shows thickening of the medial and adventitial muscular coat. Grade 2 involves intimal cell proliferation in the smaller pulmonary arteries and arterioles. In grade 3 medial hypertrophy and progressive intimal proliferation occur. In grade 4 dilation of the pulmonary arteries occurs, and the plexiform lesion may be seen. In grade 5 chronic dilation occurs with medial and intimal fibrosis. At this point the intima may be acellular and essentially hyalinized. In grade 6 a necrotizing arteritis occurs. Beyond grade 4 the pulmonary hypertension is thought to be irreversible.

The pathogenesis of the disorder is not understood; however, two mechanisms have been proposed. One involves initial vasoconstriction of the smaller muscular pulmonary arteries and pulmonary arterioles. After prolonged vasoconstriction, the more advanced fixed lesions occur. The second mechanism proposed involves multiple small pulmonary emboli. At the advanced stage of disease the histology cannot be used to support one mechanism over the other.

CLINICAL MANIFESTATIONS. After an asymptomatic period of variable duration, the patient may experience several symptoms. As the pulmonary vascular bed is destroyed, cardiac output falls. Consequently, the heart is unable to increase its cardiac output with exertion. The patient may then suffer from exertional dyspnea, fatigue, effort syncope, or angina. Palpitations may occur as various arrhythmias occur. Eventually right-sided heart failure occurs; sudden death is a common outcome.

The physical findings are a reflection of right ventricular hypertrophy and pulmonary hypertension. The central venous pressure is elevated with prominent a waves (representing atrial contraction). As tricuspid regurgitation develops, this may be replaced by a regurgitant venous wave. The chest is clear to auscultation and percussion. Cardiac examination may reveal a left lower sternal lift; this is a reflection of the right ventricular dilation. The first heart sound usually is well preserved, and the second heart sound is characterized by an accentuated pulmonic valve component (P_2), which may be palpable. The second heart sound is closely split. An ejection sound, which reflects dilation of the main pulmonary artery, often is present. A fourth heart sound, originating from the right ventricle and varying with the respiratory cycle, often is heard. Cardiac murmurs, particularly those of tricuspid regurgitation or pulmonic valvular insufficiency resulting from pulmonary artery hypertension, may be audible in the later phases of the disease. If right-sided heart failure ensues, ascites and peripheral edema may be found. In addition, with tricuspid regurgitation, systolic pulsations of the liver may be palpated.

When the cardiac output becomes severely compromised, peripheral cyanosis may develop. In addition, with the elevation of the right atrial pressure, a foramen ovale may be opened and a small right-to-left shunt may occur, resulting in cyanosis.

The electrocardiogram reveals right axis deviation and right ventricular hypertrophy. The chest roentgenogram (Fig. 92-1) shows a prominent right ventricle, right atrium, and main pulmonary arteries. The smaller pulmonary arteries appear attenuated.

The echocardiogram shows an enlarged right ventricle and right atrium. The pulmonic valve motion is characterized by a relatively small a wave, as is noted with any cause of pulmonary hypertension. No evidence for left ventricular enlargement or mitral valvular abnormality is found. The septum may move in an abnormal fashion.

Pulmonary function studies show no appreciable abnormalities. The arterial blood gases reveal normal systemic saturation with some hypocapnia, indicative of hyperventilation.

Cardiac catheterization shows a markedly elevated pulmonary artery pressure with a normal wedge pressure. The calculated pulmonary vascular resistance is high, but no left-to-right shunt, mitral valvular disorder, or left ventricular dysfunction is found. Although the definitive diagnosis of primary pulmonary hypertension cannot be made before autopsy, a presumptive diagnosis can be made if the secondary causes are excluded.

The course of the disease varies; however, most patients average a life expectancy of 3 to 7 years once symptoms ensue. In rare cases a patient survives for longer than 10 years.

Patients with primary pulmonary hypertension tolerate pregnancy, anesthesia, sedation, surgery, cardiac catheterization, and angiography poorly, often with fatal results. Medications have been used to decrease the pulmonary vascular resistance with variable success. These medications have included oxygen therapy (particularly if hypoxia exists), isoproterenol, hydralazine, and diazoxide. However, systemic vasodilators may increase cardiac output, thereby increasing pulmonary hypertension and worsening symptoms. Since multiple pulmonary emboli cannot be excluded with certainty, anticoagulation has been used. Most recently certain calcium blockers have been used, with long-term reduction in the pulmonary hypertension and relief of symptoms. There is no evidence that any of these medicines prolong survival. Heart-lung transplantation has been performed successfully in desperate cases, with satisfactory results (better than 50% 1-year survival).

BIBLIOGRAPHY

Kleiger RE and others: Pulmonary hypertension in patients using oral contraceptives, Chest 69:143, 1976.

Rich R and others: Antinuclear antibodies in primary pulmonary hypertension, J Am Coll Cardiol 8:1307, 1986.

Rubin LJ and Peter RH: Oral hydralazine therapy for primary pulmonary hypertension, N Engl J Med 302:69, 1980.

Shettigar UR and others: Primary pulmonary hypertension, N Engl J Med 295:1414, 1976.

Wagenvoort CA and Wagenvoort N: Primary pulmonary hypertension: a pathologic study of the lung vessels in 156 clincially diagnosed cases, Circulation 42:1163, 1970.

Walcott G and others: Primary pulmonary hypertension, Am J Med 49:70, 1970.

Wang SWS and others: Diazoxide in treatment of primary pulmonary hypertension, Br Heart J 40:572, 1978.

Whittaker W and Heath D: Idiopathic pulmonary hypertension: etiology, pathogenesis, diagnosis and treatment, Prog Cardiovasc Dis 1:380, 1959.

93·CONGENITAL HEART DISEASE

Iain F.S. Black

Patients with congenital heart disease are referred to the internist, as adults, with increasing frequency and appear in

Table 93-1 Cardiac anomalies resulting from chromosomal abnormalities

Type	Frequency in live births	Common heart defects
Trisomy 21, Down's syndrome	1:800	Atrioventricular (AV) canal; ventricular septal defect; patent ductus arteriosus
Turner's syndrome	1:5500 females	Coarctation of the aorta
Trisomy 13	1:5000	Ventricular septal defect; patent ductus arteriosus; atrial septal defect; dextropositions
Trisomy 18	1:6000	Ventricular septal defect; patent ductus arteriosus

three settings. Many are asymptomatic after surgical cure or devolution of their defect; for example, a ventricular septal defect may be entirely repaired surgically or may disappear with maturation of the heart. Others are seen with the evolution of a defect that may become symptomatic after childbirth; for example, atrial septal defect may occur with right-sided heart failure in middle age. Finally, an increasing number of patients are experiencing the residual effects of anomalies that previously prevented survival past childhood; for example, those patients who have had surgical correction for transposition of the great vessels and no longer have shunts but may develop ventricular muscle dysfunction in adulthood. For these reasons the principles of pediatric cardiac physiology are directly related to the care of adults.

In 1952 when Dr. John Louis first closed an atrial septal defect using hypothermia and circulatory arrest under inflow occlusion, few people realized that this was to lead to the development of a highly sophisticated speciality for the care of children with congenital heart lesions. Yet despite all the advances that have been made, many children still die in infancy and others have problems for which a surgical solution is not yet available.

The incidence of congenital heart disease is 8:1000 live births. Some anomalies occur as part of chromosomal abnormalities (Table 93-1), and some occur in familial patterns unassociated with any currently detectable chromosomal abnormality. Most congenital heart lesions, however, occur without any known genetic mechanism. Problems occurring in familial patterns without known chromosomal abnormalities include hereditary familial cardiomyopathy, supravalvular aortic stenosis, glycogen storage disease, Holt-Oram syndrome (secundum atrial septal defect, hypoplastic thumb, accessory phalanx), and Laurence-Moon-Bardet-Biedl syndrome (mental retardation, retinitis pigmentosa, hypogonadism). In contrast, congenital heart disease resulting from a teratogenic agent clearly has an environmental cause. Thus there are many causes of congenital heart disease, and many lesions probably are acquired in utero as a result of interactions between genetic predisposition and subtle factors in the intrauterine environment.

Whereas most examples of congenital heart disease are isolated cases without familial pattern, if a child has congenital heart disease, this warrants some caution in counseling regarding subsequent pregnancy. The risk to a sibling is 2%, or about three times that of the general population.

HEMODYNAMICS OF CONGENITAL HEART DISEASE

All too often the approach to understanding congenital heart disease is to memorize the signs and symptoms of a long list of congenital heart lesions. A simple and more practical approach is to learn the fundamentals of blood flow and structural or vascular resistance as they apply to children with shunts or obstructive lesions. Before dealing with the structural abnormalities, it is necessary to review normal circulation as it applies to the fetus and the changes that occur after birth.

As the fetus grows, it is essential that the venous return to the right side of the heart be directed away from the lungs and through the patent ductus arteriosus to the mother's placenta. This is accomplished by vasoconstriction of the pulmonary arterioles, a mechanism that develops during the second trimester of pregnancy and persists until birth. The vasoconstriction is maintained by hypertrophy of the medial coat of the pulmonary arterioles in response to the low oxygen tension (19 to 22 mm Hg) of the blood returning to the right side of the heart.

Not all the venous blood returning to the heart enters the right ventricle. The inferior vena cava bloodstream, including the oxygenated blood returning from the placenta, is directed preferentially through a patent foramen ovale into the left atrium and left ventricle. By this method the coronary and cerebral circulations receive blood with a higher oxygen tension (25 to 28 mm Hg). Since a low oxygen tension is necessary to maintain the high pulmonary vascular resistance, the fetus uses a hemoglobin, called fetal hemoglobin, that allows the red blood cells to carry a larger quantity of oxygen for any given oxygen tension.

The placenta itself is an organ with a low vascular resistance, further encouraging the right ventricle to empty through the ductus arteriosus into the descending aorta. As a result the right ventricle functions as a systemic ventricle and maintains this role until birth.

At the time of birth the loss of the placenta establishes the normal systemic vascular resistance, which immediately reduces the right-to-left shunt across the ductus arteriosus. With the first breath the collapsed lungs expand and oxygen enters the alveoli. Sufficient oxygen diffuses across the wall of the alveoli to raise the oxygen tension in the tissues surrounding the arterioles so that the hypoxia is abolished. This causes the vasoconstriction to be relieved and the pulmonary vascular bed to open up. The rate of fall of the pulmonary vascular resistance is determined by the medial coat of the pulmonary arterioles, which, having been markedly hypertrophied, can retain a degree of vasoconstriction for some weeks after birth. Under normal circumstances the pulmonary vascular resistance drops rapidly at first and then more slowly until the normal baseline values are reached. This usually occurs in the first 2 to 4 weeks after birth but may be delayed in some children.

This capacity of the medial coat of the arterioles to retain a degree of vasoconstriction influences the clinical picture and progress of children born with systemic-to-pulmonary shunts. This is best illustrated by the child with a patent ductus arteriosus. It is usual for a patent ductus arteriosus to be closed functionally by 1 day of age and anatomically after approximately 15 days. If the ductus arteriosus remains open after birth, blood will flow through it from the circuit with the higher resistance to the circuit with the lower resistance. In the first hour or so after birth the higher pulmonary resistance still directs venous blood across the ductus arteriosus into the aorta, but as the pulmonary resistance falls further, the right-to-left shunt stops and is gradually replaced by one from the aorta into the pulmonary artery. As this shunt increases, excessive pulmonary flow occurs with volume overload of the heart and the clinical picture of congestive heart failure. Since the murmur of a patent ductus arteriosus is caused by the turbulence generated by the left-to-right shunt, if the pulmonary vascular resistance is slow to fall, it is possible for an infant to be discharged home on the third day of life with no abnormal cardiac findings, only to be seen 3 weeks later in the physician's office with an enlarged heart, congestive heart failure, and a loud, continuous murmur as a result of the large shunt. It often is difficult for parents to understand why, if the infant was born with this problem, the murmur was not heard during the hospital stay.

This delay in the appearance of signs and symptoms is common to all children with communications between the pulmonary and systemic circuits. The development of the typical clinical picture for each lesion depends on the degree and rate of fall of the pulmonary vascular resistance. If the pulmonary vascular resistance remains high at birth, little of the right ventricular output flows into the pulmonary vascular bed (being shunted instead from the pulmonary artery through the ductus arteriosus into the systemic circuit). This clinical picture is called "persistent fetal circulation," which aptly describes the mechanism involved. Should the high pulmonary vascular resistance persist, the infant will die as a result of hypoxia caused by inadequate pulmonary flow. Occasionally an infant is born in whom the pulmonary vascular resistance does not fall to normal levels. As a result some resistance to pulmonary flow remains that influences the clinical picture and prevents the development of cardiac failure by limiting the left-to-right shunt. Finally, in some cases the pulmonary resistance falls to normal after birth and then for reasons yet unexplained begins to rise again some months or years later. If the child has congestive heart failure, the gradual reduction in the left-to-right shunt as a result of the increasing pulmonary vascular resistance improves the clinical picture, which can be misleading if the increasing pulmonary vascular resistance is not appreciated.

The importance of the well-developed medial coat of the arterioles in maintaining vasoconstriction is well illustrated when considering premature infants born toward the end of the second trimester of pregnancy. If the ductus arteriosus remains open, it is essential that the pulmonary arterioles maintain adequate vasoconstriction to protect the lungs from a volume overload. However, since the medial coat of the pulmonary arterioles develops and matures during the last trimester of pregnancy, the premature infant has little muscle in the medial coat to maintain adequate vasoconstriction. It is for this reason that most premature infants with a large ductus arteriosus rapidly develop congestive heart failure and may be extremely difficult to manage medically.

These examples illustrate the important role of the pulmonary vascular bed in determining the clinical picture of children with intracardiac or extracardiac shunts. Although the size of the defect is important, the amount of blood flowing through the defect is in direct proportion to the vascular resistance of both pulmonary and systemic circuits.

THE PEDIATRIC ELECTROCARDIOGRAM

Whereas the pattern of an adult electrocardiogram (ECG) is one of left ventricular dominance, the ECG of the child has a pattern that depends on age. The systemic role of the right ventricle during fetal life requires that it be a hypertrophied

Table 93-2   Criteria for ECG diagnosis of hypertrophy

Type of hypertrophy	Key criteria	Less specific criteria
Right ventricular hypertrophy	R in V_1 > 20 mm > 29 mm (< 1 wk of age) S in V_6 > 20 mm (< 1 mo) > 10 mm (1-6 mo) > 5 mm (> 6 mo) Upright T in V_1, after 4 days	QR in V_1 or V_4 R R/S ratio in V_1 > 2 (> 6 mo) Right axis deviation
Left ventricular hypertrophy	S in V_1 > 25 mm R in V_6 > 20 mm (0-1 yr) > 25 mm (1-10 yr) > 30 mm (10-20 yr) Q in V_6 > 4 mm	R/S ratio in V_1 < 0.8 (< 1 yr) < 0.2 (1-5 yr) < 0.1 (> 5 yr)
Combined ventricular hypertrophy	Criteria for right and left ventricular hypertrophy Criteria for right ventricular hypertrophy plus R in V_6 > 15 mm or Q in V_6 > 3 mm Criteria for left ventricular hypertrophy plus R in V_1 > 15 mm	"Normal" ECG in presence of cardiomegaly

chamber; this explains why at birth there is a pattern of right ventricular dominance in the ECG. After birth, as the pulmonary vascular resistance falls, the right ventricle begins to lose its hypertrophy and develops the characteristics of a thinner-walled volume chamber. This development takes months to occur, and it may be a year or more before right ventricular dominance disappears from the ECG and the left ventricle assumes its dominant role. To one unfamiliar with the infant ECG, the prominent right ventricular forces often are incorrectly read as right ventricular hypertrophy.

The criteria listed in Table 93-2 exemplify the changing criteria used for the diagnosis of ventricular hypertrophy. The normal means frontal QRS axis also reflects changes during the newborn period, moving from 135 degrees to 75 degrees by 3 months. Further progression to the left is gradual after 3 months of age. Right atrial hypertrophy is diagnosed when tall, peaked P waves are present (2.5 mm if less than 1 year of age, 3 mm if older). Broad, notched, or prolonged P waves (0.1 second if more than 1 year of age) suggest left atrial enlargement.

PEDIATRIC ARRHYTHMIAS

Arrhythmias occurring in children are best classified as (1) tachycardias, (2) blocks, (3) extrasystolic rhythms, (4) preexcitation patterns, and (5) sinus node disorders. (See Chapter 97 for a more detailed discussion of these arrhythmias.)

Tachycardias

SUPRAVENTRICULAR TACHYCARDIA. The most common supraventricular tachycardia seen in children is that of the atrioventricular (AV) nodal reentrant type. The next most common is regular tachycardia from an ectopic focus in either atrium. Atrial flutter and fibrillation are relatively rare causes of supraventricular tachycardia.

Treatment is directed either to interrupting the reentrant cycle or suppressing the ectopic focus. In either case digitalis or verapamil is the drug of choice because they act to slow conduction through the AV node, thereby either abolishing the rhythm or slowing the ventricular response. Propranolol (Inderal) also is useful for prolonging AV conduction and suppressing ectopic foci. Quinidine is used to suppress ectopic foci.

VENTRICULAR TACHYCARDIA. Benign ventricular ectopy usually is seen as cycles of ventricular bigeminy or trigeminy. No treatment is indicated. Ventricular tachycardia most commonly is seen in the intensive care unit or cardiac intensive care unit. It is malignant, because it frequently produces a lower cardiac output, leading to cardiovascular collapse, and it may be a precursor to ventricular fibrillation. Initial treatment is lidocaine, first as a bolus and then as a continuous infusion. Procainamide and phenytoin are also effective in some cases.

Blocks

Acquired heart block may occur as an isolated finding of rheumatic carditis, myocarditis, or endocardial fibroelastosis. Most cases occur following surgical correction of lesions in which a ventricular septal defect is present. This is because the conducting system lies close to the margin of the defect and may be damaged by a suture as the patch is inserted. Complete congenital heart block is a rare lesion usually found as an isolated problem. Most of the children with this block are active and asymptomatic, but attacks caused by Stokes-Adams disease may occur and are most likely in children whose heart rates fall below 40 to 45 beats per minute. The occurrence of Stokes-Adams attacks is an indication for insertion of a pacemaker.

Preexcitation patterns: Wolff-Parkinson-White (WPW) syndrome

The incidence of WPW syndrome has been estimated to be about 0.1% in infants and children. The pattern results from an accessory conduction pathway that bypasses the AV node, causing early activation of a ventricle. This preexcitation produces a short PR interval and slurring of the upstroke of the QRS (called the δ wave).

The accessory pathway allows retrograde conduction from the ventricle to the atrium, which sustains an episode of tachycardia. The incidence of tachycardia in children with preexcitation patterns is not known but is thought to be about 50%. Digitalis is the drug of choice for management in children.

Sinus node disorders

Rhythms resulting from blocking the sinus impulse so that it does not enter the atrium, or sinus node dysfunction, are termed "sick sinus syndrome." Sinus arrest associated with Stokes-Adams attacks is an indication for a pacemaker.

It is becoming apparent that a number of the arrhythmias seen are complicated and require sophisticated diagnostic electrophysiologic study to unravel their origin. The techniques of investigation using His bundle catheters and atrial pacing are similar to those used in adults, with minor modifications to account for the pediatric age.

CHEST ROENTGENOGRAM IN CONGENITAL HEART DISEASE

Before the cardiac silhouette is interpreted, the roentgenogram should be evaluated for technique and any extracardiac findings. It is important that the patient be positioned properly with the two clavicles symmetric; this can be difficult in young children and infants and is a frequent cause of a technically poor film. Correct exposure is also important, since over- or underexposure leads to errors in interpretation of the pulmonary vasculature. The degree of inspiration also should be checked, with the crest of the diaphragm being no higher than the sixth anterior rib. Inadequate inspiration makes the heart appear enlarged and the pulmonary vasculature look increased.

Normal growth and individual variation from child to child require that initial roentgenographic evaluation of a heart include a minimum of the frontal, or posteroanterior (PA), and lateral views. Differences in chest configuration could result in errors of interpretation of cardiac size and shape if only a PA film is taken. Oblique views help visualize parts of the heart not readily observed on the standard PA and lateral views. The left anterior oblique view shows the relative size of the two ventricles and allows good visualization of the left bronchus (which becomes elevated in the early stages of left atrial enlargement). The right anterior oblique view also is useful for detecting minimal degrees of left atrial enlargement and gives indirect evidence of right ventricular size by demonstrating how much of the anterior border is in direct contact with the sternum.

In interpreting the chest roentgenogram it is important to understand the hemodynamics, especially with lesions in which there is enlargement of one or more parts of the heart because of volume overload. Enlargement can be localized to one chamber because of valvular insufficiency or involve a number of chambers and vessels as a result of the left-to-right shunt. The clinician often can deduce the hemodynamics involved by identifying which of the chambers are enlarged. For example, increased pulmonary flow with enlargement of both the left atrium and the left ventricle and dilation of the ascending aorta would be strongly indicative of a patent ductus arteriosus. However, if the increased pulmonary flow were associated with enlargement of the right atrium and right ventricle and the pulmonary artery, the roentgenographic findings would suggest an atrial septal defect (the left atrium would not be enlarged if it were able to empty efficiently across the atrial septal defect as well as through the mitral valve).

The chest roentgenogram is less helpful in the diagnosis of obstructive lesions. In children obstructive lesions rarely are associated with chamber enlargement unless there is associated cardiac failure. Only more subtle changes give a clue to the diagnosis. Dilation of the ascending aorta suggests aortic stenosis; a prominent pulmonary artery segment suggests pulmonary valve stenosis. If the apex of the left ventricle is displaced upward, one has to consider that right ventricular hypertrophy may be the cause. Some of these more subtle changes may be seen only in the oblique views.

The chest roentgenogram is particularly helpful in providing information regarding the pulmonary vascular bed. There is a definite correlation between the volume of blood shunted through the lungs and the size of the pulmonary arteries and veins. The size of any left-to-right shunt is usually expressed as a ratio of the pulmonary/systemic blood flow. In most lesions with a left-to-right shunt at ventricular or ductal level,

flow ratios in the range of 1.6:1 to 2:1 correlate with the roentgenographic pattern of a mild increase in vascular markings. Shunts at atrial level rarely show increased pulmonary vascular markings with a flow ratio less than 2:1. Any increase in pulmonary vascular markings requires the presence of a *significant* left-to-right shunt. Conversely, a chest roentgenogram with normal pulmonary vascular markings *does not exclude* lesions with a small left-to-right shunt.

CARDIAC CATHETERIZATION

Cardiac catheterization in infants and children requires a different set of skills and techniques from those used for adults. Most studies are done by percutaneous technique from the groin, since not only are the vessels larger than in the arm but approaching the heart from below facilitates passage of the catheter into the left side of the heart if there is a patent foramen ovale; this is useful in small infants when it is not desirable to enter an artery.

The risk to life is less than 1%, although figures as high as 3% or 4% have been quoted for the sick neonate undergoing a diagnostic study. Such risks are justified, since without definitive treatment survival cannot be expected. Excluding the newborn group, most cardiac catheterizations done in children are for:

1. Diagnosis when the clinical findings are confusing
2. Management when the decision is between the continuation of medical care or surgical intervention
3. Documentation of anatomy when surgery is being considered
4. Electrophysiologic evaluation of complex arrhythmias
5. Postoperative evaluation of reparative surgery
6. Therapeutic purposes such as the creation of an atrial septal defect with a specially designed balloon catheter in infants with transposition of the great arteries, tricuspid atresia, pulmonary atresia, and total anomalous pulmonary venous return (Balloon catheters are widely used to relieve pulmonary stenosis, aortic stenosis, and restenosis of coarctation of the aorta.)

The appearance of cyanosis suggests an unstable cardiac status and the need for early diagnostic intervention. Development of congestive heart failure is another indication for early catheterization unless the response to the introduction of digitalis therapy is prompt and satisfactory.

The measurement of pulmonary flow and the calculation of pulmonary vascular resistance are integral parts of a pediatric cardiac catheterization. The decision for medical or surgical management frequently depends on the ratio of the pulmonary/systemic flow and on the response of the pulmonary vascular bed to the left-to-right shunt. In the case of an asymptomatic child, the decision to recommend surgery is made on the basis of the natural history of the lesion.

Current research is concerned with refining techniques for treatment of congenital heart lesions using cardiac catheters. These techniques include closing atrial septal defects with an umbrella-like fixture that is introduced by the catheter and implanted in the atrial septum. A similar method employing a plug has been used for closing the defect in cases of patent ductus arteriosus. A catheter with a recessed knife at its tip has been developed to cut the atrial septum in children who have had a poor result following the standard balloon septostomy technique. Other types of catheters are now available for occlusion of shunts by embolization or occlusion of aortic collaterals.

NONINVASIVE STUDIES

The echocardiogram has become a very useful diagnostic tool for the evaluation of children with heart disease. The elucidation of cardiac anatomy made possible by echocardiography already has eliminated the need for cardiac catheterization in some children. It is expected that with time echocardiography will assume an even greater responsibility for primary diagnosis.

A major benefit of echocardiography is the addition of sufficient information regarding heart anatomy and function to reduce the necessity for several angiocardiographic injections during a cardiac catheterization. This reduces the duration of the study and the incidence of complications.

Echocardiography is being used more frequently as a tool for reevaluation. Repeated echocardiograms have been helpful in monitoring the response to cardiotoxic medications used for treating neoplastic lesions. Echocardiography also has assumed an increasing role in the evaluation of heart function in children with acquired heart disease, including sickle cell anemia, rheumatic heart disease, chronic renal disease, and systemic hypertension.

Exercise tests also are becoming an integral part of the diagnostic evaluation of children with cardiac disorders. The testing is done with either a treadmill or a bicycle ergometer following a strict protocol so that the performance of one child can be compared with others. Most studies report values for work, heart rate, blood pressure, and changes in the ECG at peak voluntary effort.

In children with specific heart lesions such as aortic stenosis, a reduction in work performance may be the first sign of a deteriorating cardiac status and an indication for surgery. Testing of a child after major open heart surgery evaluates the capacity to perform work and allows counseling as to how soon the child should return to active sports.

More interest probably will be shown in exercise testing in the next few years. Until recently the only hemodynamic data available were those obtained by cardiac catheterization in children under moderate to heavy sedation. There was no way of knowing how the same heart would perform if the child were active in an upright position. Data now being obtained from exercise testing give a new understanding of cardiac function and assist in identifying the child who needs surgical intervention.

SPECIFIC CONGENITAL HEART LESIONS

The malformations discussed in this chapter consist of all the major lesions and occur in over 80% of children with congenital heart disease. For information regarding the less common forms of congenital heart disease, the reader should refer to the bibliography. For convenience the lesions are separated according to the absence or presence of cyanosis. The acyanotic group is further subdivided into those with left-to-right shunts and those with obstructive lesions.

Acyanotic heart lesions with left-to-right shunts

In this group of lesions the connection between the systemic and pulmonary circulation may either be intracardiac or extracardiac. The left-to-right shunts not only cause murmurs but, if large enough, roentgenographic findings of cardiac enlargement, a prominent pulmonary artery, and increased vascular markings resulting from increased flow. The clinical findings of poor weight gain and congestive heart failure are present only if the shunt is large. The more common lesions are ostium secundum atrial septal defect, total and partial anomalous pulmonary venous return, endocardial cushion defects (ostium primum atrial septal defect or atrioventricular canal), ventricular septal defects, patent ductus arteriosus, and aorticopulmonary window and truncus arteriosus.

In all these the clinical picture depends on the magnitude of the left-to-right shunt, which in turn depends on the size of the defect and the level of the pulmonary vascular resistance. Small defects limit the amount of the left-to-right shunt and the increase in pulmonary flow. If the pulmonary vascular resistance is normal, a large septal defect will permit pulmonary flows to be as large as five times normal. In these larger defects the size of the left-to-right shunt also is controlled by the level of the pulmonary vascular resistance. An elevated pulmonary vascular resistance limits total pulmonary flow and reduces the size of the left-to-right shunt. The clinical picture is influenced accordingly.

The clinical picture of congenital heart disease in the premature infant is different from that of the term infant. The earlier the infant is born, the more immature is the pulmonary vascular bed, since the medial coat of the pulmonary arterioles does not develop its full vasoconstrictive capacity until close to term. If a premature infant is born with a shunt lesion, the pulmonary arterioles are ill-equipped to protect the vascular bed from a large blood volume. As a result the clinical picture is that of severe congestive heart failure developing in the first few days after birth.

OSTIUM SECUNDUM ATRIAL SEPTAL DEFECT. Ostium secundum atrial septal defect is the terminology given to an atrial septal defect located in the area of the fossa ovalis. The clinical picture is the direct result of the volume of blood shunting from the left atrium into the right atrium and overloading the right side of the heart. If the shunt is significant, the ECG will show right ventricular enlargement and the chest roentgenogram will show cardiac enlargement with increased pulmonary flow.

On auscultation there may be delayed closure of the pulmonic component of the second heart sound because of prolongation of the right ventricular ejection time. A systolic flow murmur is heard across the pulmonary valve and on occasion is soft enough to be mistaken for an innocent murmur. If the pulmonary-to-systemic flow ratio is 2.5:1 or greater, the volume of blood crossing the tricuspid valve generates a diastolic rumble heard best at the third and fourth left interspaces close to the sternum.

The clinical findings of atrial septal defect do not usually appear until at least 3 years of age. For the left-to-right shunt to develop, the right ventricle must lose its systemic characteristics, which are present at birth, and develop the role of a more distensible chamber that is required only to pump blood through the pulmonary circuit. As the right ventricle becomes more distensible, the left-to-right shunt at the atrial level increases. If the pulmonary/systemic flow ratio is 2:1 or greater, the average life expectancy is reduced and congestive heart failure or increased pulmonary vascular resistance is likely to develop after 30 years of age. A pulmonary/systemic flow ratio of 2:1 therefore is an indication for closure of the defect with cardiac bypass. In some centers, because of the low mortality associated with surgery, closure is considered with flow ratios as low as 1.5:1.

ANOMALOUS PULMONARY VENOUS RETURN. The basic malformation is failure of development of the common pulmonary veins from the left atrium. Although the pulmonary venous system can develop alternative drainage using other venous systems, the return to the heart still has to be via the superior vena cava or inferior vena cava or into the right atrium itself.

Survival requires an adequate atrial septal defect with sufficient flow into the left atrium and left ventricle to maintain systemic needs. The rapid fall in pulmonary vascular resistance after birth causes increased pulmonary flow with enlargement of the right side of the heart. The clinical findings are similar to those of atrial septal defect but more pronounced. If murmurs are present, they are flow murmurs and usually are not significant. If the atrial septal defect is of adequate size, many children respond well to digitalization and can be managed medically until corrective surgery with cardiac bypass is done electively at a later age. The clinical findings are different in children who have a degree of obstruction to their pulmonary veins. Even a moderate degree of obstruction significantly reduces pulmonary flow and the availability of oxygenated blood to the right side of the heart. This in turn reduces systemic saturation, with cyanosis resulting in some cases. Obstruction of the pulmonary veins is an unstable situation frequently requiring open heart surgery, with a high risk of mortality in the newborn period.

The clinical picture of partial anomalous pulmonary venous return depends on how many pulmonary veins are involved. If a small number are affected, the clinical picture is identical to that of the average secundum atrial septal defect, and the correct diagnosis can be established only at the time of cardiac catheterization. Management depends on the number of veins draining anomalously and their hemodynamic effects. A single anomalous pulmonary vein with a normal ECG pattern and chest roentgenogram and a documented small increase in pulmonary flow is compatible with a normal healthy life and does not require surgery.

ENDOCARDIAL CUSHION DEFECTS. In the development of the heart a crucial area is the site of the endocardial cushions, where the atrial and ventricular septum are in continuity and separate the mitral from the tricuspid valve. Abnormal development in this area causes a spectrum of lesions with various degrees of involvement of the atrial septum, ventricular septum, mitral valve, and tricuspid valve. The intracardiac communication is either that of an atrial septal defect, a ventricular septal defect, or a combination of both in which one of the septal defects dominates. The hemodynamic problem resulting from valvular involvement is that of insufficiency, which varies from minimal to severe.

Ostium primum atrial septal defect. This defect is low in the atrial septum and close to the mitral and tricuspid valves. Usually the mitral valve is deformed and often cleft, allowing a varying degree of mitral insufficiency. The clinical picture is that of an atrial septal defect, except the ECG has an axis of −60 degrees as a result of an abnormal pathway of the conducting system, a characteristic of endocardial cushion defects. In most cases the mitral insufficiency is mild and can be detected only by the presence of a systolic murmur at the apex.

Atrioventricular canal. In this disorder the upper portion of the ventricular septum and the lower portion of the atrial septum are absent. This single defect means that there is no septum to which the mitral and tricuspid valves can be attached for support. As a result the mitral and tricuspid valves are in continuity with each other (frequently appearing as one common valve either floating freely or attached to the lower rim of the ventricular portion of the defect). The clinical picture depends on the size of the defect between the two ventricles, the degree of incompetence of the mitral-tricuspid valve, and the level of the pulmonary vascular resistance. Frequently children with this defect are seen with a ventricular septal defect and severe congestive heart failure. The ECG, showing the characteristic axis of −60 degrees, suggests the diagnosis.

Initial management is medical with digitalization. The decision for surgery and its timing depend on the nature of the defects present and the status of the pulmonary vascular bed.

VENTRICULAR SEPTAL DEFECTS. Approximately 80% of ventricular septal defects are located in the membranous septum just below the aortic valve; 10% are in the posterior muscular septum behind the septal leaflet of the tricuspid valve, and the rest are situated low in the muscular part of the septum, where they may be multiple.

In defects with a pulmonary/systemic flow ratio of 2:1 or greater, the clinical picture is of cardiac enlargement with increased pulmonary flow. With the left-to-right shunt at ventricular level, the chest roentgenogram shows increased pulmonary flow with enlargement of the left atrium and left ventricle. Similarly the ECG shows left ventricular enlargement unless the shunt is sufficiently large to also increase the size of the right ventricle, in which case combined ventricular hypertrophy is seen on both ECG and chest roentgenogram.

The turbulence generated at the site of the defect causes a characteristic, harsh pansystolic murmur localized best at the third and fourth left interspaces close to the sternum. It may also be palpated as a thrill. If the pulmonary/systemic flow ratio is 2.5:1 or greater, a flow murmur is generated at the mitral valve and transmitted to the apex as a diastolic rumble.

Small ventricular septal defects (pulmonary/systemic flow ratios less than 2:1) are compatible with a full life. The only risk is of bacterial endocarditis (as high as 8% to 10% in adults). If the pulmonary/systemic flow ratio is greater than 2:1, there is a risk of increasing pulmonary vascular resistance or congestive heart failure in early adult life. In most centers if a child is progressing well but still has a pulmonary/systemic flow ratio greater than 2:1 at 4 or 5 years of age, the defect is closed with cardiac bypass. In infants with severe failure who fail to thrive or have repeated admissions to the hospital for pneumonia, surgery in the first year of life is indicated. The natural history of the lesion indicates that at least 50% of ventricular septal defects undergo a spontaneous reduction in size in the first few years of life; as many as 40% of those decreasing in size undergo spontaneous closure. For this reason conservative management for a 1-year-old child with a large shunt can be justified if the child has a low pulmonary vascular resistance, is making progress, and remains relatively free of serious infections. On the other hand, if the child has systemic pressure in the pulmonary artery with any findings to suggest possible risk for developing increased pulmonary vascular resistance, then surgical intervention would be justified. In some cases a repeat cardiac catheterization may be necessary to determine the correct plan of management.

"Eisenmenger's *complex*" refers to the development of increased pulmonary vascular resistance with cyanosis owing to right-to-left shunting across a ventricular septal defect (the term "Eisenmenger's *syndrome*" is used to describe cyanosis from any left-to-right communication that has resulted in abnormal pulmonary resistance and subsequent right-to-left reversal of the shunt).

PATENT DUCTUS ARTERIOSUS. The ductus that connects the pulmonary artery to the aorta usually closes within the first few hours of birth. If it does not, there is flow from the aorta into the pulmonary artery, which then returns normally to the left side of the heart and the aorta. As the pulmonary vascular resistance falls, the left-to-right shunt occurs in diastole as well as systole. The turbulence in both phases of the cycle generates a continuous machinery-like murmur best heard in the second left intercostal space close to the sternum. The murmur obscures the second heart sound. If the pulmonary/systemic flow ratio is greater than 2.5:1, the increased flow across the mitral valve causes a diastolic rumble heard at the apex. The development of the left-to-right shunt during diastole results in a widened pulse pressure detected as a strong bounding pulse.

Spontaneous closure of a patent ductus arteriosus can occur, particularly if it is associated with prematurity. If spontaneous closure does not occur, surgical ligation is recommended before 2 years of age regardless of the size of the shunt. The justification for closure in an asymptomatic child is the risk of bacterial endocarditis in later life, estimated to be as high as 13%, in comparison to the risk of surgery, which is 1% or less.

AORTICOPULMONARY WINDOW AND TRUNCUS ARTERIOSUS. The aorticopulmonary window is a rare lesion mentioned only because it can be seen with the clinical picture of a patent ductus arteriosus. The defect is a direct communication between the ascending aorta and the main pulmonary artery, with left-to-right shunt occurring during systole and diastole. The murmur is continuous, and the ECG and chest roentgenogram findings are similar to those of a patent ductus arteriosus. Diagnosis usually is made at cardiac catheterization, and open heart surgery is required for its closure.

Truncus arteriosus is another lesion that must be considered in the differential diagnosis of a patent ductus arteriosus. The intracardiac lesion is a ventricular septal defect with both ventricles emptying into one main arterial trunk arising from the base of the heart. There are varieties of truncus arteriosus, classified according to the method of blood supply to the lungs. The ECG is not diagnostic, showing only the biventricular enlargement of a large left-to-right shunt. The chest roentgenogram shows the same nonspecific findings. However, since some children with a truncus arteriosus have a right aortic arch, if this arch is seen on the chest roentgenogram or if the right pulmonary artery appears to branch higher than normal, the possibility of a truncus arteriosus should be considered. Palliative surgery consists of placing a constriction around the main pulmonary artery or both branches to reduce the flow into both lungs. More definitive surgery, which carries high risk, involves the use of cardiac bypass, at which time the ventricular septal defect is closed and the right ventricle is connected directly to the branches of the pulmonary artery by means of a conduit containing a valve. The left ventricle drains into the arterial trunk and supplies the systemic circuit.

Acyanotic heart disease with obstructive lesions

In discussing the obstructive lesions, it is necessary to separate infants from children older than 1 year of age. Both the clinical picture and the course of management are different. In both age-groups congenital mitral stenosis and congenital tricuspid stenosis are rare and are not discussed.

In children older than 1 year of age, the more common lesions are coarctation of the aorta, aortic stenosis, and pulmonary stenosis.

COARCTATION OF THE AORTA. In this lesion there is a localized constriction at or distal to the origin of the left subclavian artery from the aorta. The resulting narrowed pulse pressure distal to the obstruction causes weak or absent pulses in the lower limbs and occasionally in the left arm if the left subclavian artery is compromised by the constriction. There often is hypertension proximal to the coarctation. A systolic murmur usually is heard over the site of the coarctation in the back and transmitted to the left sternal border anteriorly. If the ascending aorta is dilated, there is an aortic ejection click that is best heard at the apex.

On chest roentgenogram the size of the heart usually is normal. Prominence of the left ventricle may be seen, as well as dilation of the ascending aorta. If the aortic knob and upper descending aorta are well visualized, the break in continuity

at the level of the coarctation may be identified. Left ventricular hypertrophy usually is seen on the ECG, although in some cases the finding is that of right ventricular hypertrophy. The reason for this ECG pattern in the absence of an associated right-sided heart lesion is not clear. The most commonly associated cardiac lesion is a bicuspid aortic valve that may occasionally cause aortic valve stenosis.

Turner's syndrome should be considered when a woman has coarctation of the aorta. Patients with Turner's syndrome have short stature, webbing of the neck, widely spaced nipples, a low hairline, and an increased carrying angle of the elbows.

AORTIC STENOSIS. Most lesions in aortic stenosis are valvular, although an occasional supravalvular or subvalvular obstruction is seen. Characteristically the aortic valve is thickened, deformed, and often bicuspid. In severe obstructions the left ventricle can generate systolic pressures greater than 200 mm Hg. Despite these high pressures the child may remain asymptomatic. Chest pain or angina is rare and occurs only if there is coronary insufficiency.

The turbulence generated across the obstruction causes a harsh crescendo-decrescendo murmur best heard in the first interspace close to the right sternal border and frequently associated with a thrill. If the ascending aorta is dilated, an apical ejection click is present. The second heart sound should remain split unless left ventricular emptying delays closure of the aortic valve to the point that it coincides with pulmonic valve closure, making the second heart sound appear single.

The chest roentgenogram may show dilation of the ascending aorta. The heart usually is of a normal size. The ECG may show left ventricular hypertrophy, but it may not reflect the severity of the aortic valve stenosis.

Surgery to relieve the obstruction is helpful, but the valve has an abnormal structure and may restenose or become calcified with time. In addition the deformed nature of the valve may result in aortic valve insufficiency after surgery. Most centers recommend surgery when the gradient across the valve is 50 mm Hg or greater, particularly if there are ST and T wave changes in the ECG. Other centers prefer to wait until the gradient is greater than 75 mm Hg, since the surgery is considered to be palliative and the results are not always satisfactory. With a badly deformed valve, replacement with a prosthetic valve may be the only option. Although the results from surgery are not optimal, the long-term prognosis without an operation is poor. Fibrosis of the myocardium with the development of left ventricular failure can be expected in adulthood. The risk of bacterial endocarditis and in severe cases sudden death also has to be considered.

PULMONARY STENOSIS. Pulmonary stenosis with an intact ventricular septum usually is valvular, although it may occur either proximal or distal to the valve. The proximal obstruction usually is at the infundibular level; occasionally it is a result of a muscle band high in the right ventricular cavity. Stenosis of the individual right and left pulmonary arteries is uncommon except following maternal rubella. The obstruction can be bilateral and severe. Regardless of the site of the obstruction, the hemodynamic result is an increase in right ventricular systolic pressure and work.

In valvular pulmonary stenosis the turbulence across the valve generates a harsh systolic murmur heard best at the second left interspace close to the sternum, usually associated with a thrill. In mild to moderate obstruction the pulmonary second heart sound is still split, with both components of normal intensity. An ejection click is heard at the upper left sternal border as a result of the dilation of the main pulmonary artery. The ECG shows right ventricular hypertrophy with right atrial enlargement if the obstruction is severe. The chest roentgenogram frequently is normal except for prominence of the main pulmonary artery because of its dilation.

Unlike aortic stenosis pulmonary valve stenosis rarely increases in severity. However, in moderate or severe stenosis, fibrosis of the myocardium develops with time, resulting in a gradual loss of right ventricular myocardial function. Congestive heart failure may be a late complication. In most centers a gradient of 50 to 75 mm Hg is considered justification for recommending surgery. As in aortic stenosis, even though the gradient may be abolished, the valve still is abnormal and antibiotic prophylaxis for bacterial endocarditis should be continued for life.

In the first year of life the obstruction to the pulmonary or aortic valve may be so severe that the ventricle dilates and fails. In the case of pulmonary stenosis, if there is a patent foramen ovale, a right-to-left shunt may occur, producing cyanosis. An enlarging right ventricle as a result of pulmonary stenosis is considered an emergency in the newborn period and an indication for immediate surgery.

Cyanotic heart lesions

Most heart lesions produce cyanosis because desaturated venous blood returning to the heart is pumped out into the systemic circuit without having been passed through the lungs for oxygenation. In tetralogy of Fallot, tricuspid atresia, and pulmonary atresia the obstruction to pulmonary flow results in a right-to-left shunt at the ventricular or atrial level. For cyanosis to be visible, at least 5 g/dl of desaturated hemoglobin must be present in the arterial blood. Infants with a mild degree of arterial desaturation may be pink at rest, becoming cyanotic only with crying as the right-to-left shunt increases. If the baby is anemic, cyanosis still may not be appreciated.

The cyanotic lesions discussed are tricuspid atresia, pulmonary atresia, tetralogy of Fallot, Ebstein's anomaly of the tricuspid valve, and transposition of the great arteries.

In the first three lesions there is diminished pulmonary flow as a result of obstruction of flow to the lungs. In the case of tricuspid atresia and pulmonary atresia, venous return to the right atrium cannot advance to the pulmonary artery and therefore crosses the atrial septum into the left atrium to become part of the left ventricular output. For an infant to survive, blood must enter the pulmonary circuit from the aorta through a patent ductus arteriosus. As long as the ductus maintains an adequate size, the child will survive. In tetralogy of Fallot, if there is pulmonary atresia, a patent ductus arteriosus is also necessary for survival. More commonly there is an obstructed but patent pulmonary valve that limits pulmonary flow and causes the remainder of the venous return to the right ventricle to cross the ventricular septal defect and enter the systemic circuit. The degree of cyanosis is proportional to the severity of the pulmonary valve obstruction.

TRICUSPID ATRESIA. Most commonly in this defect there is an atretic tricuspid valve with absence of both the right ventricle and the pulmonic valve. Hemodynamically there is a three-chambered heart, with the left ventricle maintaining not only systemic but pulmonary circulation through a patent ductus arteriosus. Since the usual pattern is for the patent ductus arteriosus to close in the hours or days after birth, the lesion constitutes one of the emergencies of the newborn period.

On examination the second heart sound is single because there is no pulmonary valve and if a murmur is present it is nonspecific. Occasionally a continuous murmur from the ductus arteriosus is heard. The chest roentgenogram shows a normal-sized heart with a small or absent pulmonary artery segment and evidence of decreased lung vascularity. The ECG characteristically shows absence of the right ventricular forces with left ventricular dominance and left axis deviation. Although 70% of cases of tricuspid atresia are associated with normally related great arteries, 30% do have transposition of the great arteries. Finally, tricuspid atresia may be associated with a ventricular septal defect, a small right ventricle, and a stenotic pulmonary outflow tract. Because of the ventricular septal defect, children with tricuspid atresia are not dependent for survival on a patent ductus arteriosus, but since many of them have small ventricular septal defects, pulmonary flow is limited and further compromised if the ventricular septal defect becomes smaller.

Even if there is an associated ventricular septal defect, the long-term prognosis is poor without surgery. In the absence of a right ventricle, surgery is palliative and usually consists of an anastomosis between the subclavian artery and the pulmonary artery (Blalock-Taussig operation) or a side-to-side anastomosis of the ascending aorta to the pulmonary artery (Waterston anastomosis). In recent years a more physiologic surgical procedure has been introduced called the Fontane procedure. This consists of connecting the right atrium directly to the pulmonary artery either with or without a conduit containing a porcine valve. If care is taken to select patients with low pulmonary artery pressures, the results are encouraging.

PULMONARY ATRESIA. This lesion differs from tricuspid atresia only in that the tricuspid valve is patent and associated with a right ventricular cavity that usually is small or hypoplastic. Hemodynamically the lesion is similar to that of tricuspid atresia, with the venous return shunting from right to left at atrial level. As in the case of tricuspid atresia, there is a single second heart sound and the systolic murmur, if present, is nonspecific. The chest roentgenogram is also similar to that of tricuspid atresia. The ECG has a vertical axis of approximately 90 degrees, and since there is a right ventricular cavity of varying size, right ventricular potentials are also seen. Since survival depends on patency of the ductus arteriosus, management in the newborn period is similar to that of tricuspid atresia.

TETRALOGY OF FALLOT. This lesion consists of a ventricular septal defect, pulmonary stenosis or atresia, and a systemic pressure in the right ventricle with a right-to-left shunt across the septal defect, as well as a 25% incidence of right aortic arch. The pulmonary stenosis is usually valvular or a combination of a valvular and infundibular obstruction. Occasionally pure infundibular stenosis is present.

As a result of the pulmonary obstruction, the pulmonary blood flow is reduced and often inadequate. The reduced venous return from the lungs, as well as the right-to-left shunt at the ventricular level, causes varying degrees of cyanosis and hypoxia. If cyanosis is not noted at birth, it usually appears in the first 6 months. The cyanosis becomes more noticeable, and as it increases in severity, dyspnea is common. Occasionally the infant or young child develops hypoxic episodes as a result of a sudden reduction in pulmonary blood flow. Irritability is followed by increased cyanosis and the sudden loss of consciousness. Although most of these episodes are brief, some may be prolonged and even cause death. One mechanism is thought to be a sudden constriction of the right ventricular outflow tract caused by muscle spasm. The treatment is to administer oxygen, morphine for sedation, and then a β-blocker such as propranolol (Inderal) if response to oxygen is poor.

The clinical findings are those of a single second heart sound (pulmonary valve closure not being heard) with a harsh systolic murmur at the upper left sternal border resulting from flow across the stenotic pulmonary valve. The chest roentgenogram shows a normal-sized heart with a small or absent pulmonary artery segment and decreased pulmonary flow. The ECG shows right ventricular hypertrophy.

The long-term prognosis without surgery is poor. With a severe pulmonary valve obstruction, the reduced pulmonary flow leads to fatigue, increasing cyanosis, polycythemia and its complications, and the risk of bacterial endocarditis. The appearance of hypoxic spells is an indication for early surgical intervention in the form of a palliative shunt in small infants. In infants older than 6 months of age, consideration is given to more definitive surgery, with closure of the ventricular septal defect and removal of the pulmonary obstruction. The decision to go ahead with a corrective procedure in the first year of life depends on the size of the pulmonary valve and right ventricular outflow tract. If these are of adequate size, corrective surgery is considered. If they are small or hypoplastic, most centers would consider doing a shunt, with corrective surgery being delayed until the child is older. A small right ventricular outflow tract with a hypoplastic pulmonary valve is not a contraindication to surgery, but if it is to handle a normal right ventricular output after closure of the ventricular septal defect, it has to be opened and enlarged with a patch. In such situations the pulmonary valve ring often is incompetent and the child may have severe pulmonary valve insufficiency after surgery.

Occasionally a child with a ventricular septal defect develops sufficient right ventricular outflow tract obstruction to cause both diminished pulmonary flow and a right-to-left shunt at the ventricular level. Hemodynamically the combination is behaving as a tetralogy of Fallot, but the anatomy, being that of a ventricular septal defect with infundibular pulmonic stenosis, is different and more favorable for successful corrective surgery. Occasionally the child is seen early with hypoxic spells that are not always recognized as such, since the child is acyanotic and has the clinical picture of a ventricular septal defect. If a child with a ventricular septal defect also had a right aortic arch, the likelihood of infundibular pulmonary stenosis developing is higher than in the child with a ventricular septal defect and a normal left arch.

EBSTEIN'S ANOMALY OF THE TRICUSPID VALVE. The tricuspid valve, instead of being in its usual position, is prolapsed into the right ventricle so that the ventricular cavity is greatly reduced in size. The septal and posterior cusps of the valve are grossly deformed and their attachment tends to separate the right ventricular cavity into two chambers, one at the apex and the other toward the outflow tract. Occasionally there may be a gradient between them. The hemodynamic effect of this anatomy is impairment of right ventricular function with a reduction in pulmonary flow. The right ventricular cardiac output is further compromised by insufficiency of the tricuspid valve. Because of an increase in right atrial pressure, there is frequently a right-to-left shunt at the atrial level with peripheral cyanosis (most noticeable in the early newborn period while the pulmonary vascular resistance is elevated). On auscultation there is frequently a triple rhythm, and a systolic murmur of tricuspid insufficiency usually is heard at the lower left sternal border. Occasionally a diastolic murmur as a result of tricuspid stenosis is present at the same area.

The chest roentgenogram shows a large heart caused primarily by right atrial enlargement. Right atrial enlargement also is a feature of the ECG, which often reveals characteristic conduction patterns of either a right bundle branch block or the Wolff-Parkinson-White syndrome (any supraventricular tachyrhythmia can occur).

In the asymptomatic child prognosis depends on the ability of the right ventricle to maintain an adequate cardiac output. Of those who survive infancy 80% die before 30 years of age. Tricuspid insufficiency is a cause of early right-sided congestive heart failure, and serious arrhythmias carry the risk of early death.

TRANSPOSITION OF THE GREAT ARTERIES. This lesion is unusual in that the intracardiac anatomy is normal; the only abnormality is the switching, or transposition, of the great arteries leaving the heart. As a result the venous return to the heart is pumped from the right ventricle into the aorta, and oxygenated blood returning from the lungs is directed from the left ventricle into the pulmonary artery. This situation—return of desaturated blood to the systemic circuit—is incompatible with life unless there are connections between the two circuits to permit mixing with reasonable oxygenation of the systemic blood. In fetal life adequate communication exists by means of a patent foramen ovale and a patent ductus arteriosus.

The clinical picture develops rapidly after birth as the patent ductus arteriosus begins to close. Cyanosis appears immediately or within a few hours of birth, and if the seriousness of the condition is not recognized quickly, there is rapid deterioration with early death. Management consists of correcting the inadequate mixing between the two circuits by creating an atrial septal defect to allow mixing at that level. Since the mortality is high when this is done by surgery in the newborn period, it is preferable to create one at the time of the cardiac catheterization using a special catheter. The catheter incorporates a balloon at its tip and is passed across the foramen ovale into the left atrium. The balloon is inflated and jerked back hard against the atrial septum. The tear that results is usually large enough to permit adequate mixing.

The diagnosis is difficult to make. On auscultation the second heart sound is normal, although there tends to be accentuation of the aortic component as a result of the anterior position of the aorta. Usually no murmurs are present, because the intracardiac anatomy is normal. Frequently the chest roentgenogram is read as normal, although features may be present that would provide a clue to the diagnosis. If no thymus is present, it may be noted that the mediastinum is narrow because the main pulmonary artery segment is lying more medial than usual. This gives the heart an "egg on a string" appearance, which is characteristic of a transposition of the great arteries.

If a successful balloon septostomy has been done, most infants do well for a number of months. At 6 months of age or older open heart surgery is performed to restore normal hemodynamics. The current surgical procedure is Mustard's operation, in which the atrial septum is removed and a piece of either the patient's pericardium or prosthetic material is inserted to direct the pulmonary venous return to the right ventricle and the systemic venous return to the left ventricle. The long-term prognosis for this operation is not yet known, but there is some concern about the ability of the right ventricle to continue to function efficiently as a systemic ventricle for the remainder of a patient's life. Another complication is the moderately high incidence of supraventricular arrhythmias after surgery.

The concern about the role of the right ventricle has reawakened interest in the surgical technique of repositioning the transposed great arteries over their appropriate ventricles. A major objection had been that the coronary arteries would remain with the pulmonary circuit, a contraindication to the operation. Newer surgical techniques have been developed to maintain continuity of the coronary arteries with the repositioned aorta. The best results with this operation are obtained when the left ventricular pressure is at or close to systemic levels, which is either in the first few days of life or in older children with associated lesions such as ventricular septal defect and a banding of the pulmonary artery.

When transposition of the great arteries is associated with a moderately large ventricular septal defect, the presenting clinical picture usually is that of a ventricular septal defect in congestive heart failure. There may be no cyanosis, although intermittent duskiness often is noted. In such patients closure of the ventricular septal defect would not be beneficial unless Mustard's operation was done at the same time. Apart from the congestive heart failure, a major concern of this combination of defects is that increased pulmonary vascular resistance can develop early in life. There also are partial forms of transposition of the great arteries with ventricular septal defects and other associated anomalies such as pulmonary stenosis. The reader should refer to one of the standard pediatric cardiology texts for details of these lesions.

MYOCARDIAL FAILURE IN CONGENITAL HEART DISEASE

Myocardial function can be impaired as a result of a viral infection, rheumatic fever, or a cardiomyopathy. If the ventricle cannot maintain a satisfactory cardiac output, passive congestion develops with the picture of congestive heart failure. More commonly in infants and children the myocardium is healthy but gradually fatigues as a result of having to cope with prolonged stress. In the presence of a left-to-right shunt the ventricle dilates, increasing the force of contraction by the stretching of each individual myocardial fiber (Starling's law). If the individual muscle fibers stretch to the point that they no longer contract efficiently and the end-diastolic pressure in the ventricle rises, passive congestion occurs and the picture of congestive heart failure becomes more apparent. Digitalis improves contractility and reduces the end-diastolic pressure. Because so many cases of congestive heart failure in children result from fatigue of normal myocardium, the response to digitalis usually is prompt and dramatic. Failure to show any real improvement after an adequate program of digitalization may be considered an indication for surgical intervention in an operable lesion.

SURGICAL MANAGEMENT OF CONGENITAL HEART DISEASE

If surgery is viewed as a method of improving cardiac function to allow a child to live a longer and more active life, the benefits and limitations are more easily understood. The term "corrective surgery" is misleading, since many of the major lesions may have mild residual defects after surgery. For example, the repair of a tetralogy of Fallot involves reconstruction of the right ventricular outflow tract, with the result that there is usually residual mild pulmonary valve insufficiency. The term "definitive surgery" is preferable to "corrective surgery."

Most of the surgery performed in the first 6 months of life is palliative in that it does not attempt to correct the causal lesion but compensates for it until such time as definitive repair is feasible. Examples are the Blalock-Taussig and Waterston shunts for infants with tetralogy of Fallot and the balloon septostomy done at the time of catheterization for transposition of the great arteries. A number of centers perform definitive repair

in this age-group but only in selected cases. Most surgeons prefer to delay surgery until after 6 months of age, when it is technically easier and the chances for survival are greater.

The aim of definitive surgery is to restore a flow pattern as close to normal as possible. In some lesions, such as ligation of a patent ductus arteriosus or closure of an atrial septal defect, the results are hemodynamically and structurally excellent. In other lesions, such as pulmonary stenosis, tetralogy of Fallot, atrioventricular canal, and aortic stenosis, valvular abnormalities remain even though satisfactory hemodynamic results have been obtained. The family must be told that despite the obvious immediate benefits, some uncertainty exists regarding the long-term prognosis.

In recent years one of the most important advances in the surgical management of congenital heart disease has been the development of the extracardiac conduit containing a valve. This is used to replace absent or hypoplastic valves and arteries and to reroute blood flow patterns in and around the heart. This conduit is being used for many lesions, including transposition of the great arteries with a ventricular septal defect and left ventricular outflow tract obstruction, pulmonary atresia, tetralogy of Fallot with a hypoplastic outflow tract, truncus arteriosus, tricuspid atresia, and single ventricle. Valved conduits also are being used between the left ventricle and the descending aorta in cases of severe aortic obstruction that is not suitable for direct repair. Although many children have benefited from the conduit surgery, it now appears that the heterograft pig valve may have a limited life span; some have developed fibrosis and have had to be replaced.

The availability of some form of surgery, including cardiac transplantation, for even the most complex lesions is prolonging the expected life span for most children with cardiac defects. Currently it is not possible to say what the long-term prognosis will be for most of them. Will the systemic right ventricle of a transposition of the great arteries function efficiently for the rest of a child's life? What is the long-term prognosis for the right ventricle of a child with tetralogy of Fallot in whom the pulmonary valve and right ventricular outflow tract needed to be patched? If complete right bundle branch block develops during the closure of a ventricular septal defect, will it cause problems in the future? Will the scar resulting from a ventriculotomy impair ventricular function at a later date? Will the long-term results of cardiac transplantation justify its increasing use? These questions and others will be answered in time.

BIBLIOGRAPHY

James FW: Exercise testing in children and young adults: an overview. In Wenger NK, editor: Cardiovascular clinics: exercise and the heart, Philadelphia, 1978, FA Davis Co.

Keith JD, Rowe RD, and Viad P: Heart disease in infancy and childhood, New York, 1967, MacMillan Publishing Co.

Krovetz LJ, Gessner IH, and Schiebler GL: Handbook of pediatric cardiology, New York, 1969, Harper & Row, Publishers, Inc.

Moller JH: Essentials of pediatric cardiology, Philadelphia, 1978, FA Davis Co.

Moss AJ and Adams FH: Heart disease in infants, children and adolescents, Baltimore, 1977, Williams & Wilkins.

Nadas AS and Fyler DC: Pediatric cardiology, Philadelphia, 1972, WB Saunders Co.

Perloff JK: The clinical recognition of congenital heart disease, Philadelphia, 1970, WB Saunders Co.

Rudolph AM: The changes in the circulation after birth, Circulation 41:343, 1970.

Taussig HB: Congenital malformations of the heart, Cambridge, 1960, Harvard University Press.

Vince DJ: Essentials of pediatric cardiology, Philadelphia, 1978, FA Davis Co.

Watson DG: Pediatric cardiology notes, Jackson, Miss, 1975, University of Mississippi Medical Center Publications.

Watson H: Paediatric cardiology, St Louis, 1968, The CV Mosby Co.

Wellens HJ, Lubbers WJ, and Losekoot TG: Preexcitation. In Roberts NK and Gelband H, editors: Cardiac arrhythmias in the neonate, infant and child, New York, 1977, Appleton & Lange.

94 · VALVULAR HEART DISEASE

Alexis B. Sokil *and* **Michael J. Barrett**

The causes of valvular heart disease have been changing over the last few decades. Rheumatic fever and its valvular sequelae are diagnosed less often, and they are being replaced by congenital valvular disease such as bicuspid aortic valve and by less well-defined disorders such as myxomatous degeneration of the mitral valve. Associated with these changes in the cause of valvular heart disease is the shifting age of the population being treated. For example, with aortic valve disease more and more patients over 60 years of age undergo successful valvular surgery. With mitral valve disease younger patients continue to predominate, especially because of mitral valve prolapse. Along with the changing causes and age-groups, newer techniques such as two-dimensional (2-D) echocardiography with Doppler ultrasonography enable the clinician to identify valve pathology and disturbed physiology at a much earlier stage in the patient's disease. It is hoped that such improvements in diagnostic and therapeutic armamentarium will result in optimal timing of valvular surgery and improve survival of patients with valvular heart disease. With all valvular heart disease antibiotic prophylaxis must be considered in association with dental procedures and other types of surgery (see discussion of "Infective endocarditis" in Chapter 40).

MITRAL REGURGITATION

The mitral valve consists of five components: the mitral anulus, mitral leaflets, chordae tendineae, papillary muscles, and ventricular myocardium supporting these muscles. All five components must work in synchrony for the mitral valve to remain competent.

Mitral regurgitation results when any one of these five elements is impaired; for example, when the mitral anulus becomes calcified, it loses its sphincterlike action and mild mitral regurgitation results. Rheumatic fever may cause thickening, scarring, and eventual calcification of the leaflets themselves. Commissures become adherent and the chordae shorten and retract the leaflets, thereby preventing adequate apposition of the mitral leaflets and resulting in mitral regurgitation. Another example is myxomatous degeneration of the leaflets, in which the leaflets increase markedly in size so that in systole they prolapse into the left atrium. Papillary muscles may become ischemic or infarcted and fibrotic, resulting in inadequate shortening during systole, which once again results in mitral regurgitation. Finally, the ventricular myocardium may offer inadequate support for the mitral apparatus. This can be a result of myocardial infarction or dilation of the left ventricular cavity, causing malposition of the papillary muscles.

CLINICAL MANIFESTATIONS. The most prominent symptom of mitral regurgitation is *dyspnea,* which may progress to orthopnea and paroxysmal nocturnal dyspnea. As mitral regurgitation increases, left atrial pressure rises. This pressure is transmitted into the pulmonary veins, eventually causing exudation of fluid into the capillaries of the lung. The larger the amount of mitral regurgitation, the higher the back pressure in the left atrium and pulmonary veins and the more severe the dyspnea. A second symptom is *fatigue,* which occurs fairly late in the course of the disease. This is caused by diminished cardiac output, because a large volume of blood is being regurgitated into the left atrium with each ventricular contraction. Decreased ventricular contractility, a late complication of this disease, also may contribute to diminished cardiac output.

Mild mitral regurgitation may remain asymptomatic for years. Age at the onset of symptomatology varies with the cause of mitral regurgitation. Rheumatic mitral regurgitation may follow an episode of rheumatic fever by 5 or 10 years and become evident in adolescence. Women experience rheumatic mitral regurgitation almost three times as often as men. In individuals over 40 years of age coronary artery disease often is responsible for mitral regurgitation because of either ischemic papillary muscles or ventricular dilation. Men and women are equally affected by this condition. On occasion a chorda tendineae ruptures spontaneously (seen in systemic hypertension or as a consequence of endocarditis) and causes symptoms soon thereafter.

Mitral regurgitation exerts its effect on the left ventricle by increasing the amount of blood required to be pumped to compensate for the regurgitation. When this regurgitant fraction is significant, the left ventricle enlarges, with the apex displaced beyond the midclavicular line. Typically an apical plateau-shaped holosystolic murmur radiating from the apex to the base of the heart or to the axilla is heard. Milder degrees of mitral regurgitation produce only a late systolic murmur, often crescendo in nature. Acute mitral regurgitation resulting from rupture of a chorda tendineae may be found as an early systolic murmur. With the advent of secondary pulmonary hypertension, P_2 (the sound of pulmonic valve closure) is increased and splitting of the second heart sound is slightly accentuated. A third heart sound (S_3 gallop) is present in all but the mildest cases. The gallop does not necessarily signify heart failure but may reflect early diastolic filling. Fourth heart sounds (S_4 gallop) are absent until late in the disease.

LABORATORY FINDINGS. The chest roentgenogram shows left ventricular enlargement and cardiomegaly over time. The left atrium also enlarges with time and may be seen as a "double density" under the left main-stem bronchus (see section on "Mitral stenosis" for roentgenographic findings). Late in the course of the disease the pulmonary arteries enlarge, as does the right ventricle. With acute mitral regurgitation there is a normal cardiac silhouette with pulmonary congestion.

The electrocardiogram (ECG) reveals sinus rhythm in the early stages. Left atrial enlargement is reflected by large negative P waves in V_1. With increasing left atrial dilation, atrial fibrillation is common. Left ventricular hypertrophy causes increased QRS voltage and repolarization abnormalities in the ST segments and the T waves.

Echocardiography (2-D combined with M-mode) reveals a dilated left ventricle and left atrium in cases of chronic mitral regurgitation; it can pinpoint the structural abnormality of the mitral apparatus responsible for the regurgitation, such as rheumatic disease, prolapse, a flail leaflet or vegetations from endocarditis. Mitral annular calcification can be readily detected. Overall and segmental wall motion can be assessed. Doppler echocardiography is accurate in detecting mitral regurgitation by identifying turbulent retrograde systolic flow within the left atrium. Mapping the extent of the turbulent jet with pulsed or color Doppler ultrasound can provide a good semiquantitative estimate of the severity of this lesion.

With the advent of Doppler echocardiography, cardiac catheterization no longer is necessary to document the presence and severity of mitral regurgitation, but catheterization can assess the hemodynamic burden and determine the presence and severity of any concomitant coronary artery disease. Before marked left atrial dilation, large atrial v waves reflecting the regurgitant blood are found. The severity of regurgitation into the left atrium is assessed by contrast injection into the left ventricle. As this disease progresses, left ventricular end-diastolic pressure rises when left ventricular contractility falters.

MANAGEMENT. Mild mitral regurgitation usually is asymptomatic and requires no specific therapy aside from prophylaxis against endocarditis. As the severity of mitral regurgitation increases or left ventricular contraction falters, dyspnea, orthopnea, paroxysmal nocturnal dyspnea, and fatigue appear. These symptoms call for dietary sodium restriction and/or diuretic therapy and digitalis (doses determined by symptomatic response and digoxin blood levels). Atrial fibrillation should be converted to sinus rhythm as long as the left atrium is not excessively dilated. Otherwise, the rate of the ventricular response to atrial fibrillation is controlled with the digitalis. Patients with dyspnea and fatigue often benefit from arterial vasodilators to reduce afterload, which in turn reduces the fraction of blood ejected by the ventricle that is regurgitated instead of entering the aorta.

When patients with mitral regurgitation become dyspneic with mild exertion despite medical therapy, the mitral valve should be replaced. Those whose left ventricular contractility is still normal improve significantly. The risks of surgery rise proportionately to decreased left ventricular function. Mitral valve replacement can be performed using either a prosthetic disk or ball valve or a porcine heterograft. The disk valves function well but require lifelong anticoagulation. Porcine heterografts are preferred in patients with bleeding disorders, because they do not require anticoagulation.

MITRAL VALVE PROLAPSE

Mitral valve prolapse is characterized by redundant mitral leaflets that bulge into the left atrium during systole. The clinical hallmarks of this disease are systolic clicks and a late systolic murmur.

Most cases are idiopathic, but a few are seen with Marfan's syndrome, atrial septal defect, congenital heart disease, or rheumatic valve disease. In some patients microscopic evidence of myxomatous degeneration of the enlarged mitral leaflets has been demonstrated. Prolapse may also occur secondary to bacterial endocarditis of the mitral valve.

CLINICAL MANIFESTATIONS. When isolated systolic clicks appear without a murmur, there often is no mitral regurgitation. The presence of a late systolic murmur indicates mitral regurgitation, usually of a mild degree. In early systole the valve is competent and no murmur is present. However, as the valve prolapses into the atrium, the leaflets separate and regurgitation results. Maneuvers that decrease ventricular volume such as standing enhance the prolapse and make the murmur occur earlier and last longer. Maneuvers that increase ventricular volume such as squatting move the click later in systole, and the murmur becomes shorter.

The prevalence of mitral valve prolapse is not known, but the disorder is common. Estimates vary from 0.3% to 15% and depend on the population studied and criteria used for diagnosis. Most patients are under 40 years of age, and women far outnumber men. Nonanginal chest pain is common and often causes the patient to seek medical attention. Arrhythmias such as atrial or ventricular premature beats and preexcitation syndromes are frequent. Sudden death has been reported but

is rare. In one report middle-aged patients with cerebral emboli showed a higher than expected incidence of mitral valve prolapse; the emboli could have emanated from the valve itself or from the left atrium.

Bony abnormalities of the thorax are common, including pectus excavatum, straight back syndrome, and mild thoracic scoliosis. Systolic clicks occur in mid- or late systole. The findings are notoriously variable, even when auscultation is done in the same position. Clicks may come and go, often making the diagnosis difficult.

LABORATORY FINDINGS. Inverted T waves may occur on the ECG especially in the inferior leads. Prolonged QT intervals are frequent and are associated with cardiac arrhythmias or sudden death.

The M-mode echocardiogram demonstrates late systolic displacement of one or both leaflets of the mitral valve. Holosystolic prolapse may be seen. With 2-D echocardiography, prolapse is diagnosed when any part of the leaflet is seen to protrude into the left atrium during systole. Associated mitral regurgitation can be detected by Doppler ultrasonography. Mild angiographic mitral regurgitation may be present during contrast left ventriculography, which shows the leaflets protruding beyond their closure line into the left atrium.

MANAGEMENT. Many physicians treat patients with mitral valve prolapse with antibiotics during dental and surgical procedures to prevent endocarditis, but such prophylaxis is controversial. Premature contractions usually are not treated. The degree of regurgitation (assessed by Doppler ultrasonography) determines the risk of arrhythmias or sudden death. Propranolol may be helpful in treating patients with chest pain, but there is no evidence that it is beneficial.

MITRAL STENOSIS

Rheumatic fever causes mitral stenosis. The acute episode usually occurs in childhood, but the consequences become evident 10 to 15 years later. Subclinical forms of the disease often occur, and almost half of the patients with rheumatic valvular involvement give no history of prior rheumatic fever.

The rheumatic process results in scarring and thickening of the leaflets, which narrows the valve orifice. In addition shortening and thickening of the chordae tendineae occur and may contribute to associated mitral regurgitation. As the disease progresses, left atrial size increases and thrombi may form as a result of stasis of blood in the left atrium.

CLINICAL MANIFESTATIONS. As the obstruction to flow from the left atrium to ventricle worsens, pressure in the left atrium increases and is transmitted to the pulmonary veins. The patient complains of dyspnea initially and orthopnea eventually. A late complication of mitral stenosis is pulmonary arterial hypertension caused by (1) the transmission of elevated left atrial pressure into the pulmonary veins and (2) a reactive increase in pulmonary arteriolar resistance that occurs as a secondary phenomenon. With the appearance of a dilated atrium, atrial fibrillation is common.

Following an acute episode of rheumatic fever in early childhood, symptoms become evident in adults in their thirties or forties. Women predominate over men almost 3:1. Patients first complain of dyspnea on exertion, which eventually progresses to dyspnea when lying flat (orthopnea) or paroxysmal nocturnal dyspnea. Symptoms may be heralded by the sudden onset of atrial fibrillation with a rapid ventricular response. Systemic emboli from the left atrium may be the first manifestation of mitral stenosis. With the onset of pulmonary hypertension, right ventricular failure with pedal edema, ascites, and hepatomegaly appears.

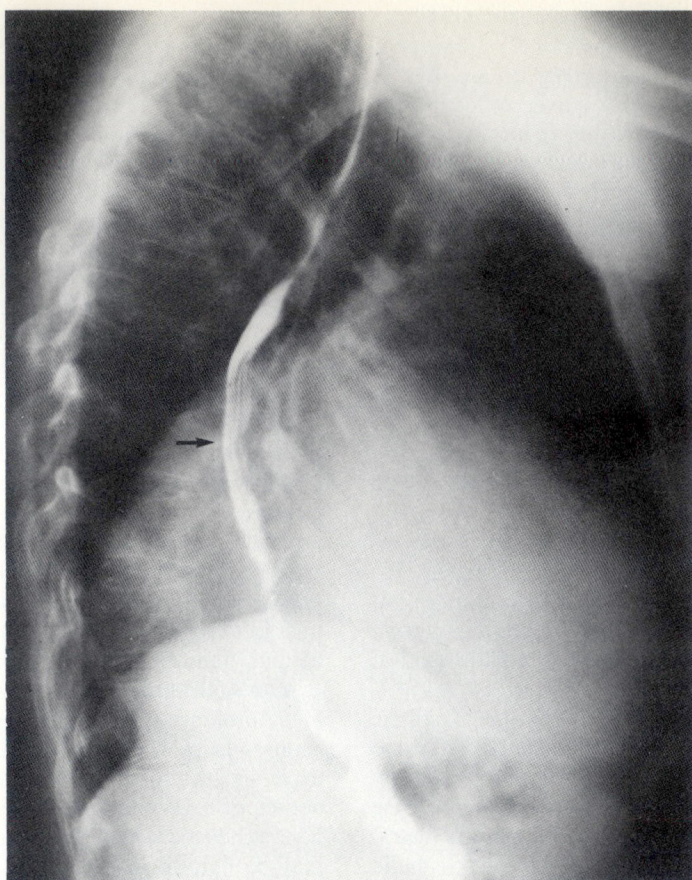

Fig. 94-1 Lateral chest roentgenogram with barium swallow demonstrating left atrial enlargement *(arrow)*. Left atrium enlarges posteriorly, displacing barium-filled esophagus.

The hallmarks of mitral stenosis can be overlooked on physical examination unless specifically sought. The first heart sound is increased and often is palpable at the left sternal border in all but severely calcified valves. Systole usually is quiescent except with associated mitral regurgitation. The second heart sound is split with accentuation of P_2 in cases of pulmonary hypertension. An opening snap of the mitral valve follows the P_2 by 0.06 to 0.11 second and inaugurates a low-frequency diastolic rumble. This opening snap may soften or even disappear if the valve becomes heavily calcified. The diastolic rumble is heard best with the bell of the stethoscope at the apex of the heart and with the patient in the left lateral decubitus position. In sinus rhythm there is a presystolic accentuation of the rumble timed with atrial contraction. As pulmonary hypertension appears, the right ventricular impulse becomes palpable at the left sternal edge.

LABORATORY FINDINGS. The chest roentgenogram reveals left atrial enlargement, manifest by a double density beneath an elevated left main-stem bronchus. Left atrial size is best demonstrated by a barium swallow in the lateral view (Fig. 94-1). Pulmonary venous congestion may be evident. With pulmonary hypertension pulmonary artery size is increased. A calcified mitral valve may be visible in the lateral chest roentgenogram or on fluoroscopy. Cardiomegaly is rare.

In the early stages of the disease the ECG reveals normal sinus rhythm and left atrial enlargement (manifest by a prominent negative P wave in V_1 and a wide notched P wave in II). As the disease progresses, right axis deviation becomes apparent. The combination of left atrial enlargement and right axis deviation suggests mitral stenosis.

An M-mode echocardiogram can establish the presence of mitral stenosis but cannot reliably quantify its severity. The 2-D echocardiogram can provide an estimate of the stenotic mitral valve area (Fig. 94-2). The obstruction to flow across the valve causes high diastolic flow velocities that are readily detectable by Doppler ultrasonography. A continuous-wave display of these velocities can be used not only to estimate the pressure gradient across the valve but also to derive an accurate, noninvasive measurement of the valve area. Cardiac catheterization further documents this pressure gradient between the left atrium and left ventricle in diastole; the mitral valve area is calculated by taking into account transvalvular blood flow (cardiac output), the pressure gradient, and diastolic filling time.

Atrial myxomas, which may produce the same symptoms as mitral stenosis, may be of right atrial or left atrial origin. The physical findings of atrial myxoma can precisely mimic those of mitral stenosis. Occasionally patients with left atrial myxoma have been followed for years with the mistaken diagnosis of mitral stenosis. Patients in later life are seen with myxoma, often after embolization; true metastases are not seen. At other times patients have unexplained signs of pulmonary hypertension, with syncope or with apparent culture-negative endocarditis. Atrial myxoma can be detected easily by echocardiography.

MANAGEMENT. The symptoms of mild to moderate mitral stenosis are principally those of pulmonary congestion and dyspnea. These usually respond to sodium restriction and/or a diuretic; only atrial fibrillation should be treated with digoxin. Propranolol can be used to control the ventricular rate if there

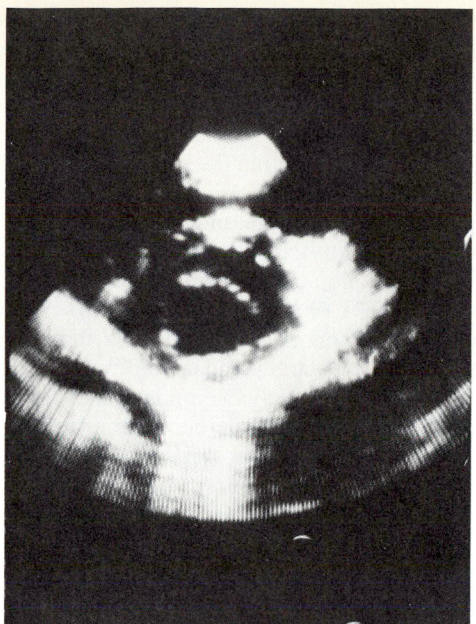
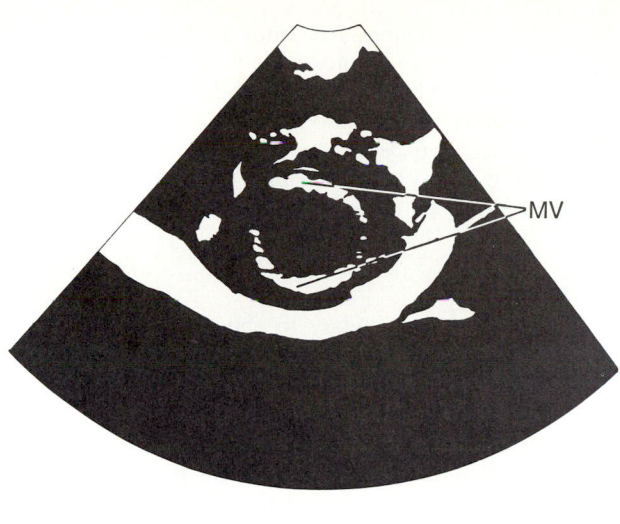

Fig. 94-2 On left is stop frame; on right is idealized drawing from 2-D echocardiogram demonstrating normal mitral valve, *MV,* in short axis view. Anterior leaflet forms top of this valve, and posterior leaflet forms bottom. Left ventricle appears as circle in this view.

is no regurgitation or diminished ventricular contractility from rheumatic carditis or pulmonary hypertension. Patients in atrial fibrillation should have electrical cardioversion to decrease the risk of emboli. Patients with atrial fibrillation should receive anticoagulation therapy with warfarin (Coumadin) to prevent systemic emboli unless a contraindication is present.

When patients become symptomatic with minimal exertion, they should undergo surgery. Some practitioners also consider recurrent emboli an indication for surgery. Patients with non-calcified valves and without associated regurgitation can have commissurotomy (leaflets directly separated), and this may relieve symptoms for many years. Severely distorted and calcified valves must be replaced with either a mechanical or tissue prosthesis. If chronic anticoagulation is contraindicated, a tissue prosthesis is preferred, but these degenerate and calcify with time and may be unsuitable for younger patients.

AORTIC STENOSIS

The most common cause of aortic stenosis today is congenital bicuspid valves (1% of the general population). Rheumatic disease also may result in stenosis of the aortic valve but is almost always accompanied by mitral disease as well.

CLINICAL MANIFESTATIONS. As the orifice of the aortic valve decreases, the pressure that the left ventricle must generate to eject a normal stroke volume increases. The diminished orifice size causes a pressure gradient across the valve. The turbulence of blood flow generates a murmur. To maintain flow across this narrowed valve, the left ventricle hypertrophies. As the severity increases, flow across the valve becomes fixed and the patient cannot increase cardiac output during exercise. The increased flow to the extremities with exertion causes a decrease in cerebral blood flow and results in dizziness or syncope. Despite severely increased intraventricular pressures, the left ventricle remains compensated as long as its size is normal. Later, myocardial contractility falls and the left ventricle dilates. Diastolic ventricular and left atrial pressures further increase. At this point dyspnea on mild exertion appears. Angina results from the increased oxygen requirements of the mas-

sively hypertrophied ventricle, even without coexistent coronary artery disease.

Aortic stenosis occurs in three times as many males as females. The murmur may be present for years before the onset of symptoms. However, from the time of the onset of dyspnea, angina, or syncope, survival is on the average only 5 years. Sudden death may occur when stenosis is severe.

The carotid pulse has a delayed rise with a small pulse volume. A systolic thrill may be felt in the second right intercostal space directly over the aorta. The left ventricular impulse is diffuse, and a palpable fourth heart sound is present. S_1 is normal and S_2 is soft or absent in severe aortic stenosis. The murmur is midsystolic, has a harsh character with a distinct late peaking, and radiates to the carotid arteries with a palpable thrill. With bicuspid valves an ejection sound is often present at the second right intercostal space.

LABORATORY FINDINGS. The chest roentgenogram shows a dilated aorta (poststenotic dilation), but at first the heart size is normal. Cardiomegaly is present later, as well as pulmonary congestion. A calcified aortic valve is often visible in the lateral chest roentgenogram. The ECG shows left ventricular hypertrophy.

The echocardiogram detects thickened aortic leaflets with decreased excursion. The pressure gradient across the valve reflects the severity of the stenosis and can be approximated using Doppler ultrasonography. Although this technique can provide a noninvasive assessment of stenosis, cardiac catheterization often is required. The gradient is determined not only by the severity of the stenosis but also by the flow across the valve (cardiac output). Both gradient and flow are measured at catheterization to calculate the effective valve area. As a rule, critical aortic stenosis is present when the pressure gradient across the valve is 50 mm Hg or higher, but the gradient is smaller with a reduced cardiac output across a critically narrowed valve.

MANAGEMENT. Patients with mild aortic stenosis are asymptomatic and require no therapy aside from prophylaxis against endocarditis. When angina, dyspnea, or syncope appear, cardiac catheterization should be done to assess the severity of the stenosis (as well as the coronary anatomy if there is angina). The treatment for severe aortic stenosis is valve replacement. A mechanical prosthesis requires lifelong anticoagulation. Other complications of prosthetic valves include endocarditis (antibiotic prophylaxis remains indicated), paravalvular leak, and systemic embolization despite anticoagulation. Porcine heterografts and pericardial xenografts do not require anticoagulation but may not withstand wear and tear over the years; these tend to be more suitable for elderly patients.

AORTIC REGURGITATION

Aortic regurgitation can be secondary to abnormal leaflet structure such as from endocarditis or rheumatic lesions. Calcific aortic stenosis often is associated with some regurgitation when the leaflets become rigid. Aortic regurgitation also may be caused by dilation of the aortic root so that the cusps do not approximate each other normally. Diseases of the aorta such as Marfan's syndrome or cystic medial necrosis, syphilis, ankylosing spondylitis, and dissection cause aortic regurgitation. Cardiac trauma can cause disruption of the leaflets or aortic ring.

CLINICAL MANIFESTATIONS. Blood ejected into the aorta in systole reenters the left ventricle in diastole. To compensate, the left ventricle must increase its stroke volume (by increasing end-diastolic pressure and volume and hence left ventricular size). Unlike mitral regurgitation, left atrial pressure is not elevated because the mitral valve prevents retrograde transmission of the elevated left ventricular pressure. The mitral valve may even close prematurely when diastolic aortic regurgitation quickly causes ventricular pressure to exceed atrial pressure, detracting from ventricular filling. With time the left ventricular enlargement becomes excessive and left ventricular diastolic pressure and hence left atrial pressure become elevated. Mitral regurgitation then can occur as a consequence of malposition of the papillary muscles. The elevated left atrial pressure results in dyspnea. Acute aortic regurgitation from bacterial endocarditis causes a rapid elevation in both left ventricular and left atrial pressures, with prominent symptoms of dyspnea.

Aortic regurgitation usually is well tolerated in its early stages. Exercise tolerance in particular is well maintained, since the vasodilation accompanying exercise serves to enhance forward stroke volume and thereby lessens regurgitation. Patients may become aware of the large stroke volume and note a forceful heartbeat or palpitations. Angina is not typical of aortic regurgitation (as compared to stenosis) and suggests coexistent coronary artery disease. Syncope can occur as a result of an arrhythmia.

The markedly increased stroke volume produces a wide pulse pressure. The carotid, brachial, and femoral artery pulses demonstrate a brisk upstroke with a rapid falloff (water-hammer pulse). In advanced cases the head bobs gently up and down and the nail beds alternately blanch and fill with each cardiac contraction. The left ventricular impulse is displaced beyond the midclavicular line. S_1 is soft. In cases of aortic root dilation an early systolic ejection sound may be heard in the second right intercostal space. S_2 splits normally, and its aortic component often is increased and may have a tambourlike quality. S_3 and S_4 gallops are common. The murmur of aortic regurgitation is a high-frequency, early diastolic blow often heard best at the third left intercostal space (Erb's point). The duration of the murmur varies with blood pressure and does not nec-

essarily reflect the severity of regurgitation. For instance, mild regurgitation may cause a brief murmur, but acute severe regurgitation also may result in only a very brief murmur that halts when the diastolic pressure equalizes in the aortic root and left ventricle. Most patients with aortic regurgitation have a systolic murmur reflecting the increased flow across the aortic valve. An apical diastolic Austin-Flint murmur caused by the regurgitant jet striking the anterior leaflet of the mitral valve mimics rheumatic mitral stenosis. However, there is no opening snap or presystolic accentuation of the murmur.

LABORATORY FINDINGS. The chest roentgenogram shows dilation of the ascending aortic root. With progressive disease the left ventricle enlarges and cardiomegaly results. Calcium may be seen in the aortic valve on lateral chest roentgenogram. Syphilis results in linear calcifications of the ascending aortic root.

The M-mode echocardiogram reveals the dilated left ventricle and dilated aortic root, as well as fluttering of the anterior leaflet of the mitral valve. In acute aortic regurgitation or in severe chronic regurgitation, premature closure of the mitral valve may be observed (the mitral valve is considered to close prematurely when its closure precedes the onset of the Q wave). Two-dimensional echocardiography may reveal vegetations on the leaflets or rheumatic involvement of these leaflets. The aortic valve may be seen to prolapse into the left ventricle in diastole.

Doppler echocardiography detects the regurgitant jet; high-velocity diastolic turbulent flow directed below the aortic valve into the left ventricular cavity is the characteristic Doppler finding in aortic regurgitation. The severity of the leak can be assessed by mapping the extent of the regurgitant flow. At cardiac catheterization an elevated left ventricular end-diastolic pressure indicates a significant hemodynamic burden imposed on the left ventricle; the severity of regurgitation is estimated from an aortogram.

MANAGEMENT. The first appearance of clear-cut pulmonary edema or other signs of left ventricular failure are an indication for surgical intervention. Patients who are allowed to persist for some time in left ventricular failure often have poor surgical results, since left ventricular contractility becomes irreversibly impaired. On the other hand, surgery is not recommended for only mild aortic regurgitation, because a mild lesion is well tolerated for several years. The usual indications for surgical intervention are increasing heart size on chest roentgenogram or clinical evidence of left ventricular failure. The long-term results of surgery often are good, although operative mortality is 10%.

TRICUSPID AND PULMONIC VALVE DISEASE

Tricuspid stenosis is rare as an isolated lesion. Usually it accompanies rheumatic involvement of other heart valves, but it is clinically significant in only 5% of such patients. Other causes of tricuspid stenosis include endocardial fibroelastosis, congenital malformations, and right atrial myxoma.

Tricuspid stenosis should be suspected in patients with multiple-valve disease who have severe venous congestion without marked pulmonary hypertension. On physical examination the jugular venous pressure is elevated and, in patients in sinus rhythm, there is a prominent jugular atrial a wave contraction. There is a characteristic slow fall in the jugular v wave caused by obstruction to right atrial emptying. On palpation of the precordium the right ventricle is not enlarged, although a diastolic thrill may be palpated over it. This diastolic rumble of tricuspid stenosis may not be heard unless specifically sought at the lower left sternal border. It resembles mitral stenosis but differs in that it becomes louder with inspiration.

The ECG reveals tall positive P waves in leads II and V_1 when sinus rhythm is present and later reveals atrial fibrillation. There usually is no evidence of right ventricular hypertrophy. Chest roentgenograms may show right atrial enlargement.

Surgical treatment usually is not indicated for mild tricuspid stenosis alone. However, if surgery is to be undertaken for other valvular lesions, the tricuspid valve first should be carefully evaluated, since tricuspid stenosis is sometimes recognized only when unexpected signs of venous congestion develop postoperatively.

Tricuspid regurgitation usually is caused by dilation of the right ventricle, which results from pulmonary hypertension. Tricuspid regurgitation also may result from traumatic injury, congenital defects such as Ebstein's anomaly, or bacterial endocarditis. Regurgitation is reflected by large v waves (regurgitant) in the jugular venous pulse. Systolic hepatic pulsations often are present, and there may be marked hepatomegaly, ascites, and peripheral edema. If pulmonary hypertension is present, a palpable pulmonary artery impulse may be felt in the second left intercostal space and an accentuated P_2 may be evident. With severe tricuspid regurgitation the right ventricle is enlarged and a systolic thrill is palpable at the lower left sternal border. The holosystolic murmur heard over the right ventricle increases with inspiration (Carvallo's sign).

The ECG reveals right ventricular hypertrophy and often atrial fibrillation. Chest roentgenograms show enlargement of the right atrium and ventricle.

Treatment of tricuspid regurgitation consists of sodium restriction, diuretics, and digitalis. If surgery is undertaken for associated mitral or aortic valve disease, functional tricuspid regurgitation improves as pulmonary hypertension is decreased. However, in organic lesions of the tricuspid valve, plication or a prosthetic valve is preferred.

Pulmonic regurgitation in adults is almost exclusively secondary to pulmonary hypertension or bacterial endocarditis. It is difficult to separate from aortic regurgitation. Pulmonic stenosis almost always is congenital, although subpulmonic stenosis may be seen in association with hypertrophic subaortic stenosis.

BIBLIOGRAPHY

Braunwald E and others: Aortic stenosis: physiologic, pathological and clinical concepts, Ann Intern Med 58:494, 1963.

Criley MJ and others: Prolapse of the mitral valve: clinical and cineangiographic findings, Br Heart J 28:488, 1966.

Frank S, Johnson A, and Ross J Jr: Natural history of valvular aortic stenosis, Br Heart J 35:41, 1975.

Goldschlager N and others: The natural history of aortic regurgitation: a clinical and hemodynamic study, Am J Med 54:577, 1973.

Gorlin R and Gorlin SG: Hydraulic formula for calculation of the area of stenotic mitral valve, other cardiac valves and central circulatory shunts, Am Heart J 41:1, 1951.

Jeresaty RM: Mitral valve prolapse click syndrome, Prog Cardiovasc Dis 15:623, 1973.

Kitchin A and Turner R: Diagnosis and treatment of tricuspid stenosis, Br Heart J 26:354, 1964.

Korn E, DeSanctis RW, and Sell S: Massive calcification of the mitral annulus: a clinico-pathological study of fourteen cases, N Engl J Med 267:900, 1962.

Nishimura RA and others: Doppler echocardiography: theory, instrumentation, technique, and application, Mayo Clin Proc 60:321, 1985.

Roberts WC: The structure of the aortic valve in clinically isolated aortic stenosis: an autopsy study of 162 patients over 15 years of age, Circulation 42:91, 1970.

Selzer A and Cohn KE: Natural history of mitral stenosis: a review, Circulation 41:878, 1972.

95·DISEASES OF THE HEART MUSCLE

Bruce M. McManus

Cardiomyopathies are diseases characterized by cardiac dysfunction in which the main abnormality lies in the working myocardium. Cardiomyopathies can be divided into two groups: primary (idiopathic) and secondary (Table 95-1). In defining the cardiomyopathies clinically, it is useful to recognize the varied spectrum of pathophysiology that they express. Both the primary and secondary categories have three possible functional states: (1) hypertrophic, hyperdynamic; (2) dilated, congestive; and (3) restrictive. To designate a cardiomyopathy as primary, acquired valvular, coronary, pericardial and aortic disease, and congenital cardiac defects must be excluded. Myocardial storage diseases and secondary endocardial diseases also must be sought and excluded as major causes of cardiac dysfunction. Although therapy at times may be similar for primary and secondary myocardial diseases, treatment often is distinctly different, and the specific diagnosis may carry a different prognosis.

The following discussion focuses on the physiologic subsets of idiopathic cardiomyopathy and subsequently on those cardiomyopathies with a known cause.

IDIOPATHIC CARDIOMYOPATHIES
Hypertrophic cardiomyopathy

DEFINITION. Hypertrophic cardiomyopathy has received much attention since it was first described as a distinct pathologic entity nearly 30 years ago. In this disorder the heart is hypertrophied and hyperdynamic. Systolic ejection generally is in the range of 70% to 80% of left ventricular end-diastolic volume, and "heart failure" results partly from difficulty in diastolic filling of the hypertrophied, poorly compliant, small cavity ventricle. Impaired relaxation and increased wall stress contribute to diminished rate and degree of diastolic filling. Because a midsystolic subaortic gradient frequently is present, hypertrophic cardiomyopathies are subdivided into those with obstruction and those without. It has never been clarified whether the gradient reflects a real obstruction to blood flow or whether the finding is an incidental one in a hyperdynamic heart that obliterates the left ventricle in systole. Since patients with gradients do no worse and possibly even better than patients without gradients and since the gradients tend to vary in the same patient, the subclassification by "obstruction" has become less meaningful in management.

PATHOGENESIS. Since hypertrophic cardiomyopathy only recently has been defined, it is not surprising that its pathogenesis is as yet unresolved. It has become apparent in recent years that the morphologic and clinical spectrum of hypertrophic cardiomyopathy is varied.

In some patients hypertrophic cardiomyopathy is a familial disorder associated with asymmetric hypertrophy of the ventricular septum (Fig. 95-1) and with abnormal myocardial histology highlighted by disarray of myocardial fibers and abnormal intramural coronary arteries. This form of hypertrophic cardiomyopathy was first described in 1958 by Donald Teare, who observed it at autopsy as the cause of sudden death in seven young adults. Teare noted that the cardiac structure was so abnormal, he believed it most likely was caused by some developmental anomaly or congenital lesion of the heart. Familial studies of this form of cardiomyopathy support the idea

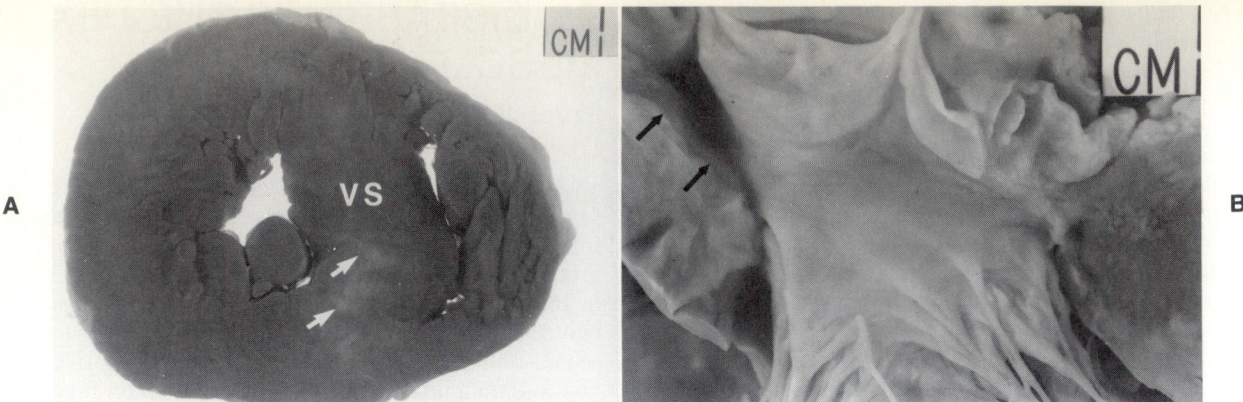

Fig. 95-1   Autopsy specimen from 17-year-old youth who died suddenly while playing basketball. **A,** Transverse section of left and right ventricles reveals preferential hypertrophy (thickening) of ventricular septum *(VS)* with scarring *(arrows)*. **B,** Anterior leaflet of mitral valve is thickened by fibrous tissue and associated with discrete endocardial fibrous plaque *(arrows)* just apical to aortic valve.

Table 95-1   Classification of cardiomyopathies

Functional type	Primary	Secondary
Hypertrophic, hyperdynamic	Idiopathic Familial Nonfamilial	Aortic stenosis, systemic hypertension, glycogen storage disease
Dilated, congestive	Idiopathic	Ischemic heart disease, scleroderma, sarcoidosis, hemochromatosis
Restrictive	Idiopathic endocardial fibroelastosis	Amyloidosis, secondary endocardial fibroelastosis, hemochromatosis

that hypertrophic cardiomyopathy may reflect an underlying genetic defect, ultimately manifest in abnormal cardiac structure and function. The muscle fiber disarray may reflect abnormal wall stress and tension created by the abnormality of cardiac shape or genetically determined functional abnormalities of left ventricular contraction (as might be seen with a derangement in the sympathetic nervous system). If present early enough in embryonic life, functional abnormalities could result in the congenital abnormality of heart structure. The precise interaction of structure and function in this condition remains unknown. However, this interplay may determine why the disease is manifest in some people very early in life and in others later.

Variants of hypertrophic cardiomyopathy of the "non-Teare type" exist. The heart functionally is abnormal, with hyperdynamic ejection, abnormal systolic anterior mitral valve motion, and unexplained hypertrophy (without asymmetric hypertrophy or myocardial fiber disarray). Thus hypertrophic cardiomyopathy may exist in two pathogenetically distinctive forms—familial (asymmetric) with autosomal dominant inheritance, and sporadic (symmetric). The relationship of the sporadic form to systemic hypertension remains unclear.

Secondary forms of functional symmetric hypertrophic cardiomyopathy may be difficult to distinguish from primary cardiomyopathy. Long-standing systemic hypertension and aortic stenosis can lead to this secondary condition. Even when the aortic valve is replaced, if the hypertrophy is advanced and the left ventricular cavity is normal to small in size, hypertrophic hemodynamics associated with rapid and almost complete systolic ejection and with cavity obliteration may occur.

Patients with normal hearts but hypercontractile states, such as may result from pressor administration, may develop a murmur and other features of hypertrophic cardiomyopathy. Thus in dealing with a patient with clinical features of hypertrophic cardiomyopathy, the practitioner must try to identify where those clinical features fall in the pathogenetic spectrum of the disorder. The interplay of left ventricular hypertrophy with abnormal diastolic function, subaortic obstruction, and ischemia is complex and provides for the myriad of clinical presentations.

CLINICAL MANIFESTATIONS. Patients with hypertrophic cardiomyopathy may be asymptomatic or may experience angina, syncope, congestive heart failure, ventricular arrhythmias, or sudden death. Thus hypertrophic cardiomyopathy may mimic the symptoms of both ischemic heart disease and aortic stenosis. On physical examination, however, rather than the delayed blunted pulse of aortic stenosis, the carotid pulse in hypertrophic cardiomyopathy has a brisk upstroke, a bifid peak, and a rapid decay. A loud, precordial holosystolic murmur usually is present. It is most prominent at the left lower sternal border and increases in intensity with the Valsalva maneuver. The electrocardiogram (ECG) may show nonspecific ST and T wave changes, left ventricular hypertrophy, and at times a Wolff-Parkinson-White conduction pattern. Deep septal Q waves sometimes are present in the precordial leads, leading to a "pseudoinfarct" pattern. The chest roentgenogram may be normal or may show cardiomegaly. M-mode and two dimensional echocardiography are especially useful in recognizing this disorder with visualization of increased left ventricular wall thickness and, in those patients with the familial form of hypertrophic cardiomyopathy, the asymmetric hypertrophy of the septum. Systolic anterior motion of the mitral valve is another useful echocardiographic sign of this condition, as is premature closure of the aortic valve. The left ventricular cavity usually is small, the left atrium may be enlarged, and the ejection fraction is increased. In patients with asymmetric hypertrophy of the septum, the septum usually exhibits poor excursion.

Arrhythmias are prevalent in some patients with hypertrophic cardiomyopathy. Malignant ventricular arrhythmias, including ventricular tachycardia and ventricular fibrillation, have been demonstrated in the familial form of this disorder and may account for sudden death in many patients with hypertrophic cardiomyopathy. Ventricular tachycardia appears to be related to the overall degree of cardiac hypertrophy. In patients with hypertrophic cardiomyopathy, especially with a family history of sudden death, 24-hour ambulatory monitoring is indicated. The finding of nonsustained ventricular tachycardia during ambulatory monitoring may portend later sudden death. Hypertrophic cardiomyopathy must be considered in the differential diagnosis of syncope and sudden death in a young patient. Supraventricular tachycardias, bradyrhythmias, accessory atrioventricular pathways, and complete heart block also may occur. Atrial fibrillation is especially poorly tolerated because of the hypertrophied ventricle and may lead to the development or worsening of heart failure or to systemic embolization.

DIAGNOSIS. The diagnosis of hypertrophic cardiomyopathy is based on the symptoms, physical examination, and laboratory evaluation, especially the echocardiogram. It is useful to determine whether the condition is the familial type with asymmetric hypertrophy, an idiopathic symmetric form, or the type secondary to long-standing systemic hypertension. Such a diagnostic distinction has prognostic implications. Studies of the familial form of this condition (when symptomatic) suggest a 4% annual mortality. For the nonfamilial or asymptomatic form of the condition, however, the prognosis is unknown. Implications for offspring and possible genetic counseling become important if the diagnosis is hypertrophic cardiomyopathy of the Teare type.

MANAGEMENT AND PROGNOSIS. Hypertrophic cardiomyopathy is treated if it is symptomatic. Since the 1960s propranolol and other β-adrenergic blocking agents have been the mainstay of therapy, and their presumed efficacy is based on their negative inotropic effect on myocardial contractility. Propranolol in doses of 160 to 640 mg/day usually is effective in reducing the angina. More recently, calcium antagonists such as verapamil have been used, but their vasodilating properties could result in worsening of the left ventricular cavity obstruction. Disopyramide and amiodarone may be particularly effective in treating the arrhythmias of hypertrophic cardiomyopathy. No definite evidence of efficacy in preventing sudden death can be attributed to any antiarrhythmic agent. Under most circumstances positive inotropic agents such as digitalis should be avoided, and diuretics must be used with caution, as volume depletion can lead to impaired left ventricular filling or intracavitary obstruction. Diuretics in conjunction with β-adrenergic blockers or verapamil may reduce pulmonary congestion. Prophylaxis with antibiotics before dental procedures is prudent, considering the increased risk of infective endocarditis.

For patients who have intractable symptoms despite medical therapy, surgical myotomy and myectomy of portions of the ventricular septum have been performed. Septal myectomy has proved successful in improving symptoms and in diminishing or abolishing the left ventricular outflow tract gradient in most patients, but it does not seem to prolong life. Since patients without outflow tract gradients appear to have the worst prognosis, this is not surprising. Mitral valve replacement has been performed for this condition, but its value is less widely accepted.

DILATED (CONGESTIVE) CARDIOMYOPATHY

DEFINITION. The second major form of idiopathic cardiomyopathy is dilated (congestive) cardiomyopathy, which is characterized by hypodynamic function, cardiac dilation and hypertrophy. As with hypertrophic cardiomyopathy, the cause is unknown. In dilated cardiomyopathy the heart is enlarged, with dilation out of proportion to hypertrophy (Fig. 95-2). Although the heart may weigh up to 1000 g (normal is less than 350 to 400 g), the actual wall thickness may be normal or even thin. Typically the heart acquires a globular shape, the myocardium looks normal grossly, and minor nonspecific

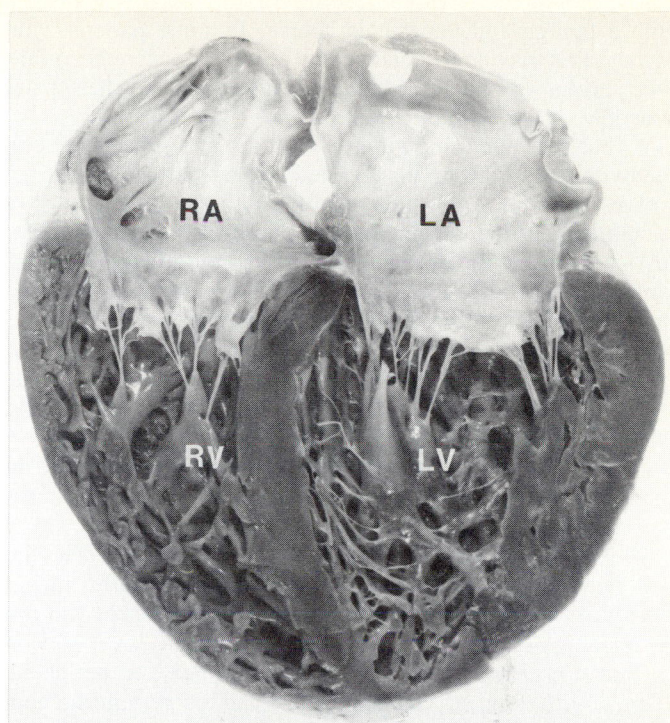

Fig. 95-2   Autopsy specimen from 35-year-old man (four-chamber echocardiographic cut). All four chambers are markedly dilated (dilated idiopathic cardiomyopathy). The atrioventricular valves are normal and no scars or mural thrombi are evident. *LA,* Left atrium; *LV,* left ventricle; *RA,* right atrium; *RV,* right ventricle.

changes, including cell hypertrophy and increased interstitial fibrosis, are present histologically. Mural thrombi frequently are present in all four cardiac chambers. The coronary arteries and cardiac valves are normal. Ultrastructural abnormalities present in biopsy specimens from patients with dilated cardiomyopathies are not specific.

PATHOGENESIS. Although the cause of idiopathic dilated cardiomyopathy has not been identified, it often is associated with potential etiologic factors, particularly alcohol and certain viral infections. For more than a century a link has been seen between alcohol and cardiomyopathy in humans and experimental animals, and the impact of alcohol often is attributed to a direct toxic effect on the myocardium. Indirect adverse effects of alcohol via nutritional deficiencies also have been suggested. Recently the acute and chronic toxic effects of alcohol on the myocardium have been studied. Although studies have shown temporary depression of myocardial contractility after acute alcohol ingestion and the accumulation of fatty acid ethyl esters in the myocardium, there is little direct evidence that alcohol per se has a direct and irreversible toxic effect on myocardial structure or function. In animals, prolonged exposure to high doses of alcohol has not produced cardiomyopathy. In humans indulging in chronic alcohol ingestion, the incidence of cardiomyopathy is unpredictable. Thus although alcohol is in some fashion linked to cardiomyopathy, a strict cause-and-effect relationship has not been established. Alcohol probably is a contributory factor but not a sole cause of this condition.

Viral infections may affect the heart and lead to a clinical picture of cardiomyopathy. Viruses that have been shown clinically to affect the heart include groups A and B coxsackieviruses, echoviruses, cytomegalovirus, and influenza viruses. When viral myocarditis occurs, it most often is asymptomatic with a benign and undetected course. In some patients viral myocarditis may be associated with acute congestive heart failure, serious rhythm or conduction disturbances, chest pain, syncope, and even sudden death.

A link between acute viral myocarditis and subsequent cardiomyopathy is strongly suggested but as with alcohol is not well established. The actual role of viral infections, clinical or subclinical, in the development of chronic congestive cardiomyopathy needs further definition before practitioners can contemplate the feasibility of preventive treatment with vaccines directed against the major cardiotoxic viruses.

Besides the two broad etiologic categories, other conditions on occasion may be linked in a direct or indirect fashion to the development of idiopathic dilated cardiomyopathy. These include the dilated cardiomyopathy of hypothyroidism and that occurring in the postpartum patient; to what extent viral infection or nutritional abnormalities might bear on the latter is not known.

CLINICAL MANIFESTATIONS AND DIAGNOSIS. The clinical picture of patients with dilated cardiomyopathy ranges from unexplained asymptomatic cardiac enlargement and minor electrocardiographic (ECG) abnormalities to severe biventricular congestive heart failure with dyspnea and peripheral edema, arrhythmias, and pulmonary and/or systemic embolism.

Chest pain is present in as many as 25% of patients and may lead to mistaken diagnosis of coronary heart disease. Physical examination reveals an enlarged heart with a right ventricular heave and an outwardly displaced but often poorly palpable apex beat. S₃ and S₄ gallops and murmurs of mitral regurgitation usually are present and at times of tricuspid regurgitation. Rales in the lungs, jugular venous distention, often with hepatomegaly, and peripheral edema may be present. At times patients have acute pulmonary edema or even cardiogenic shock.

The ECG almost always is abnormal, at the very least showing nonspecific ST and T wave changes. Pathologic Q waves are present in as many as 10% of patients. Conduction disturbances may occur, including bundle branch and complete heart blocks. Atrial arrhythmias, particularly chronic atrial fibrillation, may develop in the advanced stages of the disease; recurrent ventricular arrhythmias of all classes of severity may become a major source of morbidity and mortality. Left ventricular hypertrophy develops over time in some patients with congestive cardiomyopathy and may be a favorable sign for the patient's prognosis.

Noninvasive techniques have become especially useful in making the diagnosis of congestive cardiomyopathy. The echocardiogram may be useful in sorting out silent valvular or congenital abnormalities that sometimes mimic cardiomyopathy and also in detecting the characteristic dilated, diffusely hypodynamic ventricle and enlarged atria of cardiomyopathy. Nuclear myocardial scans using thallium 201 and gated cardiac blood pool scans help exclude ischemic heart disease. When the cause of the cardiomyopathy remains unclear and coronary disease has not been excluded, a cardiac catheterization may be necessary to define the coronary anatomy.

MANAGEMENT AND PROGNOSIS. Prognosis usually is poor in this condition. The disease tends to run a slowly progressive course with a 5-year mortality from the time of initial symptoms greater than 75%. Women with idiopathic dilated cardiomyopathy may have a somewhat better life expectancy than men. There is some evidence that patients who develop left ventricular hypertrophy (as detected by ECG) have a better prognosis, with survival for 10 to 20 years, whereas those without signs of hypertrophy (and possibly without the capa-

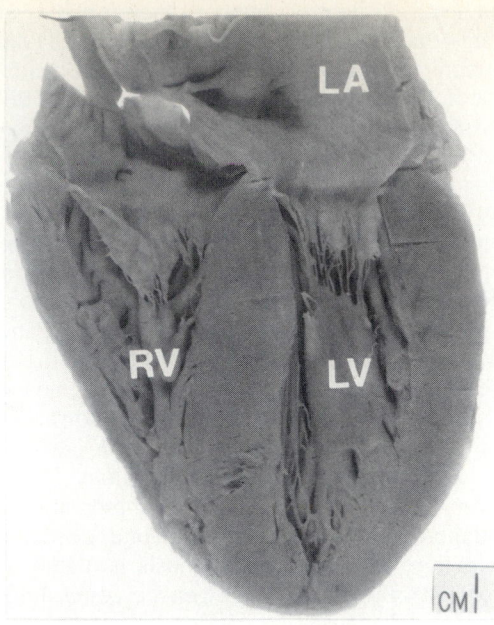

Fig. 95-3 Autopsy specimen from 47-year-old man (four-chamber echocardiographic cut). This man had cardiac amyloidosis causing restrictive hemodynamics. There is modest hypertrophy of left *(LV)* and right ventricular *(RV)* myocardium and minimal chamber dilation apart from left atrium *(LA)*.

bility of hypertrophy) have a more rapidly progressive downhill course, with survival for only months.

The treatment of cardiomyopathy is fundamentally treatment of symptoms. The congestive heart failure is treated with digitalis, diuretics, and vasodilator therapy, including hydralazine and nitrates (see Chapter 86). Arrhythmias are treated when they cause symptoms (see Chapter 97). Anticoagulants should be given routinely for antiembolic benefit.

RESTRICTIVE CARDIOMYOPATHIES

DEFINITION. The most infrequent of the idiopathic muscle diseases of the heart are the restrictive cardiomyopathies. The restrictive cardiomyopathies make up a heterogeneous group of diseases involving endocardium and/or myocardium, including Löffler's endocarditis, endomyocardial fibrosis, and endocardial fibroelastosis. These disorders have in common impaired left ventricular filling but near normal systolic function. Clinically and hemodynamically these cardiomyopathies mimic constrictive pericarditis. The restrictive hemodynamics may reflect diminished left ventricular compliance resulting from infiltration or scarring of myocardium or endocardium.

CLINICAL MANIFESTATIONS AND DIAGNOSIS. Patients with restrictive cardiomyopathy typically have symptoms of biventricular congestive failure with dyspnea and peripheral edema. They also may have atypical chest pain. On physical examination an early and prominent gallop usually is heard, and mitral insufficiency often is present, especially in those with endomyocardial fibrosis. The ECG shows abnormal ST-T wave changes and, in some patients, evidence of left ventricular hypertrophy. Atrial fibrillation may be present, and as would be expected in a condition associated with restricted diastolic filling, the onset of atrial fibrillation often is associated with abrupt and marked deterioration in clinical status. The chest roentgenogram may show cardiac enlargement, but in some patients cardiac size may be entirely normal despite the presence of heart failure.

The diagnosis of restrictive cardiomyopathy ultimately rests

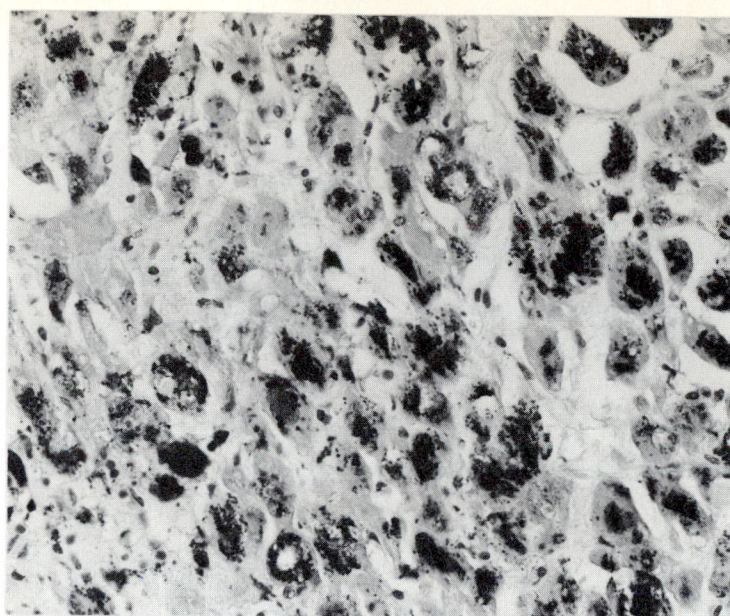

Fig. 95-4   Photomicrograph of myocardium of 23-year-old woman with transfusional hemosiderosis. Dark deposits in myocytes are iron. (Gomori's iron; magnification ×330).

on hemodynamic characterization of the entity. Since the causes of restrictive hemodynamics are so varied, treatable "secondary" causes of restrictive hemodynamics, especially constrictive pericarditis, must be considered. The echocardiogram is particularly useful in documenting the degree of normality in systolic function.

Morphologic features of endomyocardial fibrosis include a small cavity, thin-walled ventricle and a markedly thickened endomyocardium. Endocardial thickening typically is more prominent at the apex and in the body of both ventricles. The endocardial process may lead to diminished trabeculation and smoothness of the ventricular endocardium.

MANAGEMENT AND PROGNOSIS. The cause of primary restrictive cardiomyopathy is unknown. Hypereosinophilia caused by either parasitic infiltration or eosinophilic leukemia may play a role in some forms of this disease. No specific treatment exists for primary restrictive cardiomyopathy, and the course generally is one of relentless heart failure. In a few cases endocardial resection and valve replacement have been successful. Recent evidence suggests that a few patients with restrictive hemodynamics in whom no specific cause can be established may have a benign course with resolution of symptoms, but other patients will be plagued by arrhythmias.

SECONDARY CARDIOMYOPATHIES

Secondary cardiomyopathies constitute a mixed and often unusual assortment of diseases, including glycogen storage disease, hypertensive heart disease, aortic stenosis, supravalvular aortic stenosis and coarctation, sarcoidosis, scleroderma, ischemic heart disease, amyloidosis, hemochromatosis, metabolic or nutritional disorders, and toxic cardiomyopathies.

These secondary cardiomyopathies may behave functionally as a dilated congestive, hypertrophic, or restrictive cardiomyopathy and sometimes as a mixture of these functional states. Diagnosis of the many secondary cardiomyopathies depends first on recognition of the underlying disease process. This may be achieved by endomyocardial biopsy. Therapy includes treatment of the underlying disease and conventional treatment of the heart failure or arrhythmias as they are clinically manifested.

Secondary hypertrophic cardiomyopathies

One form of glycogen storage disease, Pompe's disease, is associated with cardiac dysfunction in early childhood that is clinically akin to hypertrophic cardiomyopathy. Cardiac catheterization may document a provokable left ventricular outflow tract gradient. The secondary hypertrophic state associated with long-standing systemic hypertension or valvular aortic stenosis, supraaortic stenosis and aortic coarctation, may be seen as hypertrophic cardiomyopathy, as already discussed, and represents a form of secondary myocardial disease.

Secondary congestive cardiomyopathies

Sarcoidosis may involve the heart by direct infiltration of myocardium with granulomas. The infiltrative lesions may be extensive enough to replace sizable portions of myocardium and lead to cardiac dilation, dysrhythmias, heart failure, and sudden death. As such the entity may mimic congestive cardiomyopathy.

Similarly, scleroderma may involve the heart and lead to extensive necrosis and fibrosis of all four cardiac chambers (possibly mediated by coronary microvascular abnormalities). Since sclerodermatous myocardial disease involves muscle injury and may lead to cardiac dilation with diffusely impaired function, it also may mimic an idiopathic dilated type of cardiomyopathy.

The most common of the secondary cardiomyopathies is that caused by ischemic heart disease. Recurrent myocardial damage as a result of multiple-vessel coronary occlusion may lead to a progressive remodeling of heart shape and size such that the heart becomes globular, diffusely dilated, and hypodynamic. In some patients with ischemic cardiomyopathy the clinical history may be quite vague and the myocardial infarctions clinically silent, so that it is not readily apparent that coronary disease is the cause; in these cases coronary angiography is necessary to identify the etiologic factor.

Secondary restrictive cardiomyopathies

Cardiac amyloidosis may lead to a secondary cardiomyopathy by virtue of diffuse infiltration of the myocardium by amyloid protein. Although cardiac amyloidosis often goes unrecognized in life, when the amyloid deposits around myocardial cells and in small vessels of the heart become extensive enough, abnormalities of cardiac function may become apparent. Cardiac amyloidosis may also present a clinical picture of restrictive cardiomyopathy (Fig. 95-3).

Hemochromatosis is another infiltrative disorder that may be seen as a cardiomyopathy of the restrictive or congestive form. Both amyloidosis and hemochromatosis (and iron-overload hemosiderosis) may be diagnosed by endomyocardial biopsy. Amyloidosis is characterized by interstitial and vascular amyloid deposits, whereas in hemochromatosis iron deposition occurs within cardiac myocytes (Fig. 95-4). Only hemochromatosis may be treated.

Secondary metabolic or nutritional cardiomyopathies

Another subgroup of secondary cardiomyopathies is the heterogeneous metabolic or nutritional category, caused by conditions such as hyperthyroidism, hypothyroidism, beriberi, chronic anemia, and selenium deficiency. Excess thyroid hormone is associated with increased cardiac output coinciding with an overall hypermetabolic state. Thyroid hormone causes enhanced myocardial contractility; it also decreases peripheral resistance. The high-output state of thyrotoxicosis has been cited as a cause of "high-output congestive heart failure." However, that thyroid hormone excess alone can then lead to chronic cardiomyopathy in an otherwise normal heart has not been established. Similarly, hypothyroidism may be associated with decreased cardiac output and depressed myocardial contractility, but the extent to which a chronic cardiomyopathy can be caused by this hormone deficiency also is unclear. Coronary artery disease in the hyperlipidemic hypothyroid state may contribute to myocardial injury and failure. Nevertheless, for these and other nutritional and metabolic "cardiomyopathies," judicious correction of the hormonal, vitamin, or other deficiency leads to correction of the myocardial abnormality.

Secondary toxic cardiomyopathy (anthracyclines)

Although recognized only for the past two decades, the causal relationship between doxorubicin administration and cardiomyopathy is firmly established. *Cardiotoxicity* is the major harmful side effect of this important chemotherapeutic agent. The toxicity may be asymptomatic and manifested only by nonspecific T wave changes, or it may evolve into a florid cardiomyopathy with rapidly progressive biventricular heart failure. Cardiotoxicity is almost always related to the total dosage of drug administered, and if that dosage is kept below 450 to 550 mg/m^2, the cardiomyopathy is unlikely to occur. Unlike many cardiomyopathies, doxorubicin cardiomyopathy is associated with distinctive morphologic abnormalities, including focal myocardial cell necrosis, vacuolar degeneration, and myofibrillar dropout. Moreover, these structural abnormalities, as detected by right ventricular biopsies, have been shown to correlate roughly with the functional abnormalities of myocardium.

BIBLIOGRAPHY

Abelmann WH: Classification and natural history of primary myocardial disease, Prog Cardiovasc Dis 27:73, 1984.
Benotti JR, Grossman W, and Cohn PF: Clinical profile of restrictive cardiomyopathy, Circulation 61:1206, 1980.
Braunwald E and others: In Idiopathic hypertrophic subaortic stenosis: a description of the disease based upon an analysis of 64 patients. In Idiopathic hypertrophic subaortic stenosis, American Heart Association Monographs, No. 10 (suppl. 4):1964.
Brock RC: Functional obstruction of the left ventricle (acquired aortic subvalvular stenosis), Guy's Hosp Rep 106:221, 1957.
Bulkley BH and others: Thallium 201 imaging and gated cardiac blood pool scans in patients with ischemic and idiopathic congestive cardiomyopathy: a clinical and pathologic study, Circulation 55:753, 1977.
Chatterjee K and Parmley WW: The role of vasodilator therapy in heart failure, Prog Cardiovasc Dis 19:301, 1977.
Maron BJ and others: Hypertrophic cardiomyopathy: interrelations of clinical manifestations, pathophysiology, and therapy. I, N Engl J Med 316:780, 1987.
Maron BJ and others: Hypertrophic cardiomyopathy: interrelations of clinical manifestations, pathophysiology, and therapy. II, N Engl J Med 316:844-852, 1987.
Roberts WC, Seigel RJ, McManus BM: Idiopathic dilated cardiomyopathy: analysis of 152 necropsy patients, Am J Cardiol 60:1340, 1987.
Silverman KJ, Hutchins GM, and Bulkley BH: Cardiac sarcoid: a clinicopathologic study of 84 unselected patients with systemic sarcoidosis, Circulation 58:1204, 1978.
Teare RD: Asymmetrical hypertrophy of the heart in young adults, Br Heart J 20:1, 1958.

96 · CORONARY HEART DISEASE

James B. Young, Craig M. Pratt and **Robert J. Luchi**

CORONARY ARTERY ANATOMY AND MYOCARDIAL PERFUSION

ANATOMY. The myocardium is perfused by two coronary arteries, the right and the left, arising respectively from the right and left sinuses of Valsalva (Fig. 96-1). It is not uncommon for the *right coronary artery* to arise from two ostia. When this occurs, the upper ostium gives rise to a vessel called the conus artery that supplies the right ventricular outflow tract. When a separate opening for the conus artery is not present, the first major branch from the right coronary artery supplies the right ventricular outflow tract. The major trunk of the right-coronary artery descends in the right atrioventricular groove. In this groove it curves around the acute margin of the heart after sending off one or more anterior right ventricular branches. In most patients the right coronary artery continues beyond the acute margin of the heart to extend to or past the crux of the heart, that point where the atrioventricular groove, together with with the interatrial and interventricular grooves, forms a cross. Extension of the right coronary artery to or beyond the crux of the heart is called right coronary artery dominance. As the right coronary artery courses in the posterior atrioventricular groove, it sends branches to the posterior right ventricle, to the interventricular septum, and to the inferior and posterior portions of the left ventricle. In most patients in whom the right coronary artery terminates at or near the acute margin of the heart, the inferior and posterior parts of the left ventricle are supplied by the circumflex artery.

The *left coronary artery* branches after a variable but usually short distance into the *anterior descending* and *circumflex coronary arteries*. The circumflex coronary artery proceeds along the groove between the left atrium and left ventricle, around the obtuse margin of the heart, where it gives off a large vessel called the obtuse marginal artery. The circumflex artery courses a variable distance in the left atrioventricular groove. When left coronary artery dominance is present, that is, when the circumflex artery reaches the crux of the heart, it is the circumflex artery that gives off branches to the inferior and posterior portions of the left ventricle. The left anterior descending

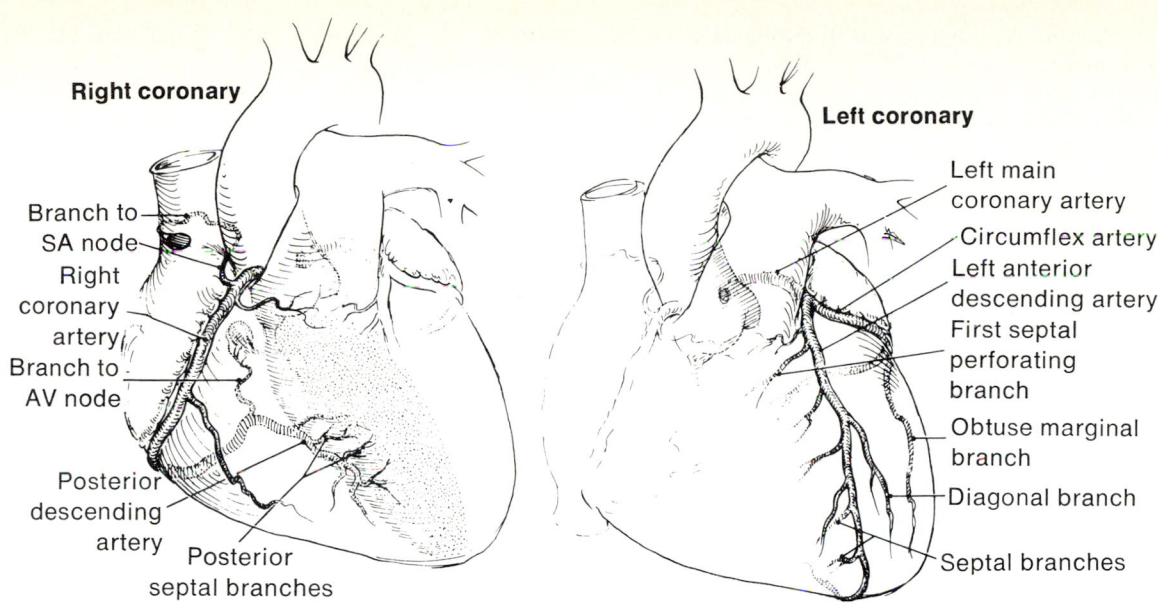

Right coronary

Branch to
SA node

Right
coronary
artery

Branch to
AV node

Posterior
descending
artery

Posterior
septal branches

Left coronary

Left main
coronary artery

Circumflex artery

Left anterior
descending artery

First septal
perforating
branch

Obtuse marginal
branch

Diagonal branch

Septal branches

Fig. 96-1   Typical coronary artery anatomy.

coronary artery nourishes a large part of the left ventricle as it descends in the anterior interventricular groove. It sends large perforating branches to the septum and several large diagonal branches that course over the anterior surface of the left ventricle. The anterior descending coronary artery reaches the apex, curves around it, and supplies a variable portion of the inferior wall of the left ventricle. The left coronary artery may trifurcate rather than bifurcate into circumflex and left anterior descending vessels. When a trifurcation exists, the third vessel is called the *ramus intermedius*. The ramus intermedius generally supplies an area of the lateral left ventricle.

The artery supplying the sinus node arises from the right coronary artery in 55% to 60% of individuals. In the remainder the sinus node artery is a branch of the left circumflex coronary artery. The artery to the atrioventricular node arises at the crux of the heart, from the right coronary artery in approximately 85% of individuals and from the left coronary artery in 15%. The blood supplied to the interventricular septum is provided predominantly from the left anterior descending coronary artery, although a small portion of the posterior and inferior septum is supplied from the right coronary artery. However, in patients in whom the left circumflex artery reaches the crux of the heart, the entire interventricular septum may receive its blood supply from the left coronary artery system.

Occlusions of the left anterior descending coronary artery may result in myocardial infarctions of the left ventricular anterior wall and the septum. Occlusions in the right coronary artery give rise to inferior and posterior wall infarctions of the left ventricle unless the right coronary artery does not reach the crux of the heart. The left circumflex artery supplies the lateral left ventricle; if fit extends to the crux of the heart or beyond, occlusions of the circumflex artery give rise to inferior and posterior wall myocardial infarctions.

Occlusions of the right coronary artery may result in infarctions of the right ventricle. Right ventricular infarction usually occurs in conjunction with inferior and posterior wall infarctions of the left ventricle that involve the interventricular septum. Only rarely does right ventricular infarction occur independently or left ventricular infarction.

Anatomically humans have only two coronary arteries. Nevertheless, it has become a clinical convention to describe coronary atherosclerosis as one-, two-, or three-vessel disease, the vessels being the *right coronary artery, left anterior descending coronary artery,* and *left circumflex coronary artery.*

The coronary venous system is more variable than the coronary arterial system. Veins generally follow the course of the major coronary arteries, but exceptions are common. The coronary veins draining the left ventricle ultimately empty into the coronary sinus, which lies posteriorly in the atrioventricular groove. The coronary sinus empties into the right atrium. Venous blood draining the right ventricle usually, but not always, also empties directly into the right atrium and right ventricle.

Either the right or the left coronary artery may congenitally be quite small and occasionally absent. The left coronary artery may arise from the pulmonary trunk. Severe symptoms of myocardial ischemia usually are present during infancy in these individuals. There may be a congenital coronary arteriovenous fistula (an abnormal communication between a coronary artery and vein), which, depending on its size, gives rise only to a localized continuous murmur or additionally to signs of ischemia or heart failure.

PHYSIOLOGY. The myocardium consists of cells dependent on oxygen for metabolism. They become injured or die when deprived of oxygen. As just described, the myocardium is supplied by a rich vascular network, although the endocardium is less well supplied than other regions of the myocardial wall. Coronary artery flow depends on the cardiac output and pressure gradient between the aorta and the right atrium, which receives the drainage from the coronary sinus, the major coronary venous channel. Blood flow to the myocardium occurs during both systole and diastole, but diastolic flow is greater because the compressing action of the contracting myocardium on intramyocardial blood vessels raises intramyocardial resistance during systole. Diastolic flow is related to the duration of diastole and therefore is limited during tachycardia when the proportion of the cardiac cycle spent in diastole is shortened.

Resistance along the coronary circuit includes (1) a basal viscous resistance defined as the resistance to flow offered by the fully dilated coronary vascular channels during the diastolic phase of the cycle; (2) an autoregulatory resistance determined by tonic contractions of the vascular smooth muscle of the coronary arterioles; and (3) the already mentioned resistance resulting from compression of vascular structures by the contracting myocardium. In the normal, intact, beating heart, overall coronary resistance is determined predominantly by the coronary arteriolar resistance. Resistance in the epicardial coronary arteries normally is small. Commonly, however, resistance in the epicardial coronary vessels is increased by coronary atherosclerosis, a resistance that is either fixed or slowly progressive. Coronary artery spasm produces a reversible and often severe increase in epicardial coronary artery resistance. Occasionally the left anterior descending coronary artery may tunnel through an area of the myocardium capable of active contraction. In this circumstance systolic contraction of the myocardium may sharply increase resistance and may curtail flow in the left anterior descending coronary artery to a clinically significant degree. Elevation of the diastolic pressure in the cavity of the left ventricle also may increase resistance to flow in the endocardial coronary vasculature by exerting a compressive effect on these vessels.

EPIDEMIOLOGY AND PREVENTION OF CORONARY HEART DISEASE

EPIDEMIOLOGY. The prevalence of coronary artery disease (CAD) varies greatly among different populations, and within these cohorts the incidence also varies with age, geographic location, and personal habits. It became clear in the 1930s and 1940s that to study the phenomenon of changing death rates in the world and specifically in the United States, long-range, population-based, prospective epidemiologic studies would be required. Subsequently, the Framingham Heart Study, the National Cooperative Pooling Project, the Tecumseh Study, the Western Collaborative Group Study, the Goteborg Study (Sweden), and the Ni-Hon-Sam Study (Japan) were initiated. To be sure, problems unique to long-term, pooled, epidemiologic studies were evident in these programs. However, they still provide the most accurate data base available to study the natural history of coronary heart disease. The most significant limitation of these surveys is applying conclusions from data gathered in the 1950s to current life-styles.

Important observations in these studies included an assessment of the CAD occurrence rate and discrimination of factors affecting and determining the incidence and natural history of the disease. The studies demonstrated a wide variation in CAD incidence according to individual habits and place of residence. By the 1950s it was clear that CAD was the leading cause of death in North American men and that this disease did not occur randomly. Important variables affecting incidence included age, race, sex, serum cholesterol level, hypertension, hyperglycemia, obesity, cigarette smoking, lack of exercise, high dietary fat intake, genetic factors, and psychosocial influences.

Overall incidence. The United States' crude monthly mortality for CAD in 1976 was 301 per 100,000. However, patterns of geographic variation are evident, with the highest age-adjusted death rate noted in the eastern United States (2310 per 100,000 along the Atlantic Coast and in the Southern Sunbelt, 711 per 100,000 in the Great Plains region, and 925 per 100,000 in the Western states). Variation in these rates also is noted among industrialized nations. The highest CAD age-adjusted death rate is found in Finland (2399 per 100,000) and the lowest in Japan (1285 per 100,000). Poorly kept epide-

miologic records in Asia, Africa, and Latin America prevent truly accurate comparison of these areas' CAD death rates with those of the recognized industrialized nations.

Sex. Men have a higher incidence of CAD than do women. In 1976 the male mortality from CAD was 5.2 times greater than the female mortality for the 35- to 44-year-old age-group and 2.3 times greater for those 65 to 74 years of age. These differences may be changing as trends and social practices evolve, such as the greater number of female smokers and the diminished emphasis on sexual distinction in the work force.

Time trends. CAD mortality increased throughout the 1960s for all age, sex, and race groups in the United States; however, a definite decline in mortality became apparent in the early 1970s, and it has continued through the 1980s. Some have attributed this decline to changes in life-style that altered CAD risk factors. Theoretically, an individual who modified such risk factors in his life-style would have reduced the likelihood of developing clinically significant CAD.

Age. The incidence of CAD increases with age. When CAD is present in younger individuals, it usually is associated with hyperlipidemia, hypertension, and a strong family history of CAD.

Lipids. It is useful to precisely characterize the various hyperlipoproteinemias because of their variable implications and treatment. CAD is more closely associated with hypercholesterolemia than with hypertriglyceridemia. Hyperlipidemia may be primary or secondary. The most frequent causes of secondary hyperlipidemia are diabetes, myxedema, alcoholism, cirrhosis, and nephrosis. The ratio of high- to low-density lipoproteins clearly is less in patients with CAD. High-density lipoprotein (HDL) is structurally distinct from the atherogenic lipids and participates in the removal of lipids from cells with subsequent delivery to the liver for metabolism. HDL levels can be increased with fat-controlled diets, exercise, and estrogen use.

Smoking. Smoking is clearly related to death from cardiovascular disease. Male smokers have a fivefold greater risk of cerebrovascular accident and a threefold greater risk of fatal myocardial infarction than do nonsmokers. Smoking causes adverse hemodynamic effects (tachycardia and hypertension) that are mediated by adrenergic amines. Nicotine probably is the factor responsible for inciting the adrenergic stimulation. Smoking also causes an increased blood glycerol level and lactate/pyruvate ratio. Carbon monoxide is detrimental, because it impairs left ventricular contractility.

Cigarette smoke also is harmful to nonsmokers when they are exposed to the noxious atmosphere created by smokers. Angina is induced at lower workloads in nonsmoking CAD patients exposed to cigarette smoke. It also has been shown that smoke inhalation impairs the diffusion of oxygen into the mitochondria.

Blood pressure. Both systolic and diastolic hypertension are related to the development of CAD, with systolic hypertension better correlated to the prevalence of CAD than either mean or diastolic blood pressure.

Establishing normal values for blood pressure is difficult, since both systolic and diastolic pressure have a continuous unimodal association with cardiovascular complications. Prudent points of intervention in any patient would be a systolic blood pressure of 160 mm Hg or greater or a diastolic pressure of 95 mm Hg or higher (see Chapter 87). These levels of hypertension should be treated aggressively, particularly in younger individuals. Despite the fact that systolic hypertension generally is better correlated with cardiovascular catastrophes, it would be unwise to dismiss isolated diastolic hypertension. Indeed, in younger men diastolic hypertension is a more potent risk factor for CAD. Likewise, isolated systolic hypertension should not be regarded as an inevitable concomitant finding of aging. Even in elderly age-groups, systolic hypertension carries significant implications for the development of CAD.

Diabetes and obesity. The risk of a cardiovascular event is doubled when diabetes mellitus is present. Obesity also may be a risk factor. The Framingham Study demonstrated an association between obesity and elevated low-density lipoprotein cholesterol. In addition to higher lipid levels, obese patients tend to have systolic hypertension and glucose intolerance.

Physical conditioning. Although reports demonstrate CAD in well-conditioned marathon runners, physical training does seem to be associated with a reduced risk of coronary disease.

Personality. A behavior pattern has been associated with CAD. The "coronary-prone" or "type A" personality describes individuals who have enhanced personality traits of aggressiveness, ambitiousness, and competitiveness, are chronically impatient, and have a passionate sense of time urgency. "Type A" behavior patterns have been associated with increased severity of CAD even when age, sex, blood pressure, smoking, and cholesterol level were comparable.

Coffee. It is controversial whether caffeine intake adversely affects the risk of developing CAD. The Boston Collaborative Drug Surveillance Program suggested a relationship between coffee consumption and acute coronary events in a retrospective study. However, the Framingham Study, a prospective study, failed to corroborate this observation. Also, in reports from the Evans County (Georgia) epidemiologic survey, coronary heart disease mortality was not associated with coffee consumption in several race and sex groups.

Oral contraceptives. It has been suggested that oral hormonal contraception is a CAD risk factor in younger women who smoke. The Lipid Research Clinic Program Prevalence Study demonstrated that patients under 45 years of age who were taking oral contraceptives had higher serum cholesterol and triglyceride levels. This study also reported that using oral contraception in the presence of other major cardiovascular disease risk factors increases the likelihood of death when a myocardial infarction does occur.

Ethanol consumption. Several recent studies have suggested that moderate alcohol consumption plays a *preventive* role in the development of CAD, although others have presented opposing data. The beneficial effects of alcohol may be related to its association with increased serum levels of high-density lipoproteins.

PREVENTION. To avert CAD, prevention and management of adverse risk factors before coronary atherosclerosis becomes clinically apparent seem important. Thus it appears wise to encourage cessation of smoking, control hypertension, modify hypercholesterolemia, and optimize weight and physical conditioning. Oral contraceptives should not be taken by women with other cardiovascular risk factors such as hypertension.

Reversibility of the atherosclerotic process by dietary manipulation has been demonstrated in animal studies. In humans it is difficult to assess the extent of atherosclerosis at the beginning of any study and maintain dietary compliance in human studies.

Recent evidence has substantiated the long-held belief that lowering lipid levels reduces cardiovascular mortality and morbidity. Results of large prospective epidemiologic studies such as the Lipid Research Clinic Program Study and the Helsinki Heart Study indicate that for each 1% reduction in total cholesterol, a 2% decrease in the incidence of coronary heart disease can be anticipated. Drugs such as cholestyramine and gemfibrozil have been used to lower cholesterol in these trials, but newer agents may be even more effective. A consensus conference of the National Institutes of Health has provided guidelines for identifying and managing adults with high blood cholesterol. Dietary modification and weight control should be the first steps in trying to lower even very high lipid levels. If drug treatment also is necessary, bile acid sequestrants (colestipol or cholestyramine) and nicotinic acid are the agents of first choice when triglycerides are not elevated. The new class of lipid-lowering agents, 3-hydroxy-3-methylglutaryl coenzyme A reductase inhibitors (such as lovastatin), are quite effective in reducing cholesterol levels, but their long-term safety and effects on coronary heart disease have not yet been completely defined.

It would seem that pharmacologic control of glucose intolerance would limit the development and progression of CAD. There is controversy, however, concerning the manner of control of hyperglycemia. The University Group Diabetes Program compared various oral hypoglycemic agents with insulin in ameliorating or retarding the vascular complications of diabetes. This study suggested that diabetic patients controlled with oral agents had a higher incidence of atherosclerotic complications. Therefore it would be prudent to control diabetes by modifying the diet and normalizing weight if possible. Failure to establish reasonable fasting and postprandial glucose levels with this protocol should prompt consideration of insulin administration.

ANGINA PECTORIS

DEFINITION. "Angina pectoris" literally means chest pain. The word "angina," derived from both Greek and Latin, is translated as a choking or strangling sensation. "Pectoris" means of the chest. Although many pathophysiologic events unrelated to the cardiovascular system may cause chest discomfort, convention has decreed that this term be used to refer to chest pains characteristic of ischemic heart disease. The mechanism for production of pain of this nature is always a discrepancy between myocardial oxygen demands and the ability of the coronary arteries to deliver this substrate. Angina pectoris therefore usually is caused by atherosclerotic heart disease.

Angina pectoris was first described by William Heberden in 1768. We report his description because of its accuracy and completeness, as well as its historical importance.

But there is a disorder of the breast marked with strong and peculiar symptoms, considerable for the kind of danger belonging to it, and not extremely rare, which deserves to be mentioned more at length. The seat of it, and sense of strangling, and anxiety with which it is attended, may make it not improperly be called angina pectoris.

They who are afflicted with it, are seized while they are walking, (more especially if it be up hill, and soon after eating) with a painful and most disagreeable sensation in the breast, which seems as if it would extinguish life, if it were to increase or continue; but the moment they stand still, all this uneasiness vanishes.

In all other respects, the patients are, at the beginning of this disorder, perfectly well, and in particular have no shortness of breath, from which it is totally different. The pain is sometimes situated in the upper part, sometimes in the middle, sometimes at the bottom of the os sterni, and often more included to the left than to the right side. It likewise very frequently extends from the breast to the middle of the left arm. Males are most liable to that disease, especially such as have passed their fiftieth year.

ETIOLOGY. Clinically, myocardial ischemia is most commonly associated with coronary atherosclerosis. Atheromas produce clinically significant reduction of coronary blood flow when the internal luminal area is reduced by 50% or more. Myocardial oxygen demands may be met while the patient is at rest, but during exercise, when myocardial oxygen requirements are raised by an increase in heart rate, myocardial contractility, and tension of the ventricular wall, myocardial demands for oxygen exceed the coronary arteries' capacity to deliver the requisite blood flow. This results in myocardial ischemia.

Myocardial ischemia also may result when there is a primary reduction of blood flow without an increase in myocardial oxygen demands. The most typical example of a primary reduction in blood flow is coronary artery spasm. Coronary artery spasm has been clearly demonstrated to be the major pathogenetic factor in *variant angina* (discussed later in the chapter), and there is evidence that it may be important in classic effort-induced angina, unstable angina, and myocardial infarction. Coronary artery spasm may be caused by mechanical, neural, or chemical factors. Reflex coronary artery spasm on exposure to cold has been demonstrated. Coronary artery spasm also has been documented in association with exercise. Coronary artery spasm appears to be more frequent when atherosclerotic heart disease is present. It is not known whether spasm can occur in a coronary artery completely free from atherosclerosis. A primary reduction in myocardial blood flow also may occur when the left anterior descending coronary artery is compressed during systole by an overlying band of myocardium.

Myocardial ischemia may result when blood pressure and cardiac output are severely reduced, as in shock, severe aortic stenosis, severe aortic insufficiency, sclerosis of the coronary ostia secondary to syphilitic aortitis, coronary arteritis, coronary embolization, and coronary thrombosis. Anemia and increased diffusion distances from capillary to myocardial cell, as in massive ventricular hypertrophy, worsen the myocardial oxygen deficits caused by any reduction in coronary blood flow. It is not uncommon for many of these factors to act in concert. Thus coronary thrombosis may completely occlude a vessel only partially occluded by atherosclerosis, coronary artery spasm may occur at a point where the vessel is partially obstructed by coronary atherosclerosis and complete the obstruction, or shock in conjunction with coronary atherosclerosis may produce myocardial ischemia more severe than that caused by either alone. Although myocardial ischemeia may occur in the absence of coronary atherosclerosis, it is much more common in association with it.

Silent myocardial ischemia recently has been recognized to have independent adverse prognostic implications. These patients, particularly those with diabetes or extensive coronary disease, have documented myocardial ischemia, sometimes without concomitant exertion and at normal heart rates, but they have no pain or other symptoms that might suggest an ischemic process clinically. It is currently unclear how silent ischemia should be managed.

PATHOPHYSIOLOGY. Resting myocardial oxygen consumption is approximately 100 ml of oxygen per 100 g of ventricular tissue per minute. Myocardial oxygen extraction averages 70% of the arterial oxygen content. The major determinants of oxygen consumption by the myocardium are the contractile state of the heart, the heart rate, and the tension generated in the myocardium. The tension generated is directly proportional to the pressure developed by the ventricle and the diameter of the ventricular cavity and inversely proportional to ventricular wall thickness. The extent of myocardial shortening, the energy required for activation of myocardial contraction, and "basal" cellular oxygen requirements are other determinants of myocardial oxygen consumption that are of little importance clinically. The so-called double product, that is, the product of the heart rate and the systolic blood pressure, serves as a useful bedside clinical index of myocardial oxygen consumption.

During periods of exercise and stress, myocardial oxygen demands increase. These demands are met primarily by coronary vasodilation, which increases coronary blood flow fourfold or fivefold. Some increase in myocardial oxygen extraction may occur, but only when myocardial oxygen demands are greatly increased. The stimulus to coronary vasodilation is unknown; however, metabolic products (such as adenosine), neural mechanisms, and prostaglandins probably are involved.

When an imbalance exists between myocardial oxygen demands and coronary blood flow, myocardial ischemia results. There is a rapid release of lactate, phosphate, and potassium from the ischemic myocardial cells. Creatine phosphate and ATP decline despite some shift to anaerobic metabolism. If the ischemia is severe or prolonged, anaerobic metabolism may fail to maintain cellular integrity and myocardial infarction results.

The consequences of myocardial ischemia include chest pain, reduced myocardial contractility and diastolic compliance, dyssynergic ventricular contraction, and ECG abnormalities, including ST segment elevation or depression, T wave inversion, and arrhythmias. Prolonged or severe myocardial ischemia may result in necrosis of myocardial cells, referred to as myocardial infarction.

Angina pectoris is produced when myocardial ischemia activates visceral efferent pain fibers. The biochemical events and nerve pathways involved are not completely understood. It is believed that the nerve impulses travel via unmyelinated sympathetic nerve fibers to the upper thoracic and lower cervical cord segments and from there to the thalamus and higher cortical centers. Activation of internuncial neurons in the lower thoracic and upper cervical segments may cause referral of pain to the arm, neck, jaw, and back.

CLINICAL MANIFESTATIONS. The patient's history is the key to the diagnosis of angina pectoris. The hallmark of effort-induced angina pectoris is a history of chest discomfort brought on by exercise or emotion and relieved by rest. Because the chest discomfort arises in a visceral organ, it often is difficult for the patient to characterize and clearly define its location. The discomfort commonly is described as a pain, heaviness, tightness, or squeezing sensation. The location of the discomfort usually is retrosternal, but it may occur in the epigastrium or in the precordial area. When the discomfort is located primarily in the epigastrium or precordial area, careful questioning often reveals that the retrosternal area is included. When severe, the discomfort commonly radiates to the jaw, neck, back, left shoulder, and/or inner aspect of the left arm down to the ring and little fingers of the left hand. Occasionally the patient may complain of discomfort only in the areas of referral, such as the jaw or left elbow. The duration of the discomfort varies, usually lasting between 5 and 10 minutes. Attacks lasting less than 5 minutes, however, are not uncommon; an attack persisting beyond 20 minutes suggests a form of unstable angina or myocardial infarction.

Because of the vague nature of the discomfort and the patient's difficulty in describing it precisely, the physician may be misled by the history. The most important characteristic of effort-induced angina pectoris is the relationship between chest discomfort and exertion and emotion and the relief of the chest discomfort by rest.

Severe discomfort may be associated with nausea, salivation, a feeling of generalized weakness, and light-headedness. The frequency and severity of the anginal discomfort may vary from day to day despite similar degrees of exertion. Usually the explanation for this variability can be found in the patient's emotional state (anxiety, for example, increases the metabolic demands of the heart) or in ambient weather conditions. Cold weather, particularly walking into a cold wind, brings on the discomfort sooner and increases its severity. On the other hand, when the amount of exercise and the patient's emotional state can be more or less controlled, as in the exercise laboratory, the amount of exercise that produces chest pain is reasonably constant from test to test.

Examination during an anginal attack may show an increased pulse rate and blood pressure. The patient may have pallor and increased facial sweating, and salivation may be increased. An S_4 gallop may be heard for the first time or may increase in intensity. If there is ischemia of a papillary muscle, a systolic apical murmur resulting from mitral insufficiency may be heard during angina and diminish in intensity or disappear when the attack has passed. Between anginal attacks examination may be normal or show changes of associated cardiac conditions such as hypertension or valvular heart disease.

A number of conditions can closely simulate the symptoms of angina pectoris. One of the more common is pain arising in the precordial chest wall. The nature of this chest pain is poorly understood. It may arise in muscle or in the costochondral or chondrosternal articulations (Tietze's syndrome). The chest wall often is tender to palpation. Pain originating in afferent nerves irritated by arthritis of the cervical and upper thoracic spine also may simulate angina pectoris. The discomfort of esophageal spasm or mucosal inflammation, the pain of peptic ulcer, and the pain of gallbladder disease, particularly chronic calculous cholecystitis, may mimic closely the discomfort of angina pectoris. The physician must consider these conditions in a patient whose symptoms are suggestive of angina. The patient's history and physical signs help discriminate between angina pectoris and these other conditions. However, the most helpful sign is the relationship of chest discomfort to exercise or emotion and its relief with rest or nitroglycerin in angina pectoris.

LABORATORY ASSESSMENT. The history and physical examination can be complemented by laboratory evaluation when indicated. Conditions such as anemia or thyrotoxicosis, which may exacerbate angina by increasing myocardial oxygen demands, should be excluded. Fasting and 2-hour postprandial blood sugar analyses should be performed to detect carbohydrate intolerance. Measurement of the patient's serum cholesterol and fasting serum triglycerides should be obtained. More sophisticated lipid analyses may be required to define various abnormal lipoprotein states.

DIAGNOSIS. The electrocardiogram (ECG) is an important tool in evaluating patients with angina pectoris. A normal resting ECG does not rule out angina pectoris. A resting ECG showing clear evidence of a previous myocardial infarction supports the clinical impression of angina pectoris. Other changes on the resting ECG such as left bundle branch block and nonspecific ST-T changes cannot be used as evidence to support a diagnosis of angina pectoris. Exercise electrocardiography (exercise stress testing) is important in the diagnosis of angina and in evaluating the response to therapy. The purpose of exercise stress testing is to document the ECG, blood pressure, and symptomatic response. Various exercise protocols are used, but all employ graded increases in exercise with constant ECG and blood pressure monitoring until the patient can exercise no further because of cardiovascular symptoms or fatigue. In a stress test exercise may be stopped at a predetermined heart rate, typically 85% of the maximum predicted on the basis of the patient's age.

One purpose of exercise stress testing is to correlate the patient's symptoms with certain cardiovascular changes suggesting myocardial ischemia. Another is to define the patient's exercise capacity. Although the test is relatively safe, occasionally ventricular tachycardia or ventricular fibrillation may be precipitated, and the physician must be prepared to handle these catastrophes. Exercise stress testing is contraindicated in the first several days after acute myocardial infarction and in patients with unstable angina pectoris with rest pain, severe significant tachycardia or bradycardia, advanced or untreated heart failure, aortic stenosis complicated by effort-induced syncope, and orthopedic or muscular disorders that prevent the patient from exercising adequately.

The normal response is one in which the patient has no episodes of chest discomfort and no horizontal or down-sloping ST segment depression of 1 mm or greater after reaching the target heart rate. A normal resting ECG simplifies interpretation of the changes occurring during exercise. A positive test is defined by chest discomfort and a horizontal or down-sloping ST segment depression of 1 mm or greater. Greater ST segment depression (for example, 3 to 4 mm) suggests greater degrees of ischemia, as does ST segment depression occurring early in the exercise protocol, failure of the systolic blood pressure to increase with exercise, or a drop in systolic blood pressure after it has risen. ST segment elevation may occur during exercise stress testing. Most often ST segment elevation appears to be caused by abnormal left ventricular patterns of contractions; occasionally it may be the result of exercise-induced coronary artery spasm.

If no symptoms of ECG changes occur but the patient cannot reach his assigned heart rate because of poor physical conditioning, the test cannot be used to rule out ischemia. Difficulties in interpretation arise when the resting ECG is abnormal, when the patient has chest discomfort without ST segment change, or when horizontal or down-sloping ST segment depression of 1 mm or greater occurs without chest discomfort.

The exercise stress test often is evaluated in terms of its ability to predict occlusive disease in the coronary arteries. Approximately 10% of patients who show a positive test as previously described will have normal coronary arteries or minimal atheromatous change. The reason for false positive tests is unknown; they tend to occur in younger individuals, particularly women. The sensitivity of exercise electrocardiography in predicting critical coronary atheromatous disease is in the range of 60% to 70% of patients with significant obstructive coronary artery disease. Increased specificity can be obtained by using additional endpoints, but sensitivity is reduced when this is done. Thus exercise stress testing alone is less useful than coronary angiography in predicting cardiovascular mortality or morbidity. The two tests used together are somewhat better than angiography alone in making predictions.

The accuracy of the exercise stress test in predicting critical coronary atheromatous disease can be considerably improved by combining the test with thallium perfusion scintigraphy or blood pool scanning. Thallium uptake by the myocardium is proportional to myocardial blood flow. Areas of ischemia developing during exercise appear as "cold" areas, that is, areas with reduced thallium uptake. When ischemia is relieved during rest following exercise, former "cold" areas show normal uptake of thallium. Exercise-induced wall motion abnormalities and reduction in ejection fraction are important indicators of ischemia demonstrable by blood pool scanning. The isotope commonly used in gated blood pool scanning is technetium 99 attached to red blood cells or serum albumin. Images of the blood pool in the right and left ventricles are prepared by computer processing of information derived from precordial counting. Changes in size and configuration of the blood pools can be analyzed separately during systole and diastole. Thus the geometry of ventricular contraction can be recorded, and an ejection fraction (the fraction of the end-diastolic volume ejected during systole) can be calculated.

Rest and exercise blood pool imaging can be compared with images at rest in terms of systolic function or ejection fraction and left ventricular wall motion. An inability to increase the ejection fraction with exercise or development of segmental left ventricular wall motion abnormalities suggests myocardial ischemia.

Coronary angiography determines the anatomy of the coronary circulation, the number and location of critical obstructive lesions, and the suitability of the coronary anatomy for coronary artery bypass grafting or balloon angioplasty. Also, coronary artery spasm can be elicited with infusion of ergonovine or by exposing the extremities to a noxiously cold environment.

Angiography is not indicated in all patients with angina pectoris. There is a definite although small risk of death, myocardial infarction, and cerebrovascular accident, and the procedure is expensive. The clearest indication for angiography is to determine coronary anatomy and pathology and the ventricular function of a patient with angina pectoris who requires coronary artery bypass surgery. The procedure also may be used to evaluate patients with valvular heart disease in whom both valvular surgery and coronary artery bypass surgery may be required. Another indication is evaluation of patients with atypical chest pain, particularly individuals such as airline pilots on whose cardiovascular health many lives depend. Coronary arteriography and ventriculography also provide the physician with important predictive information concerning patients who suffer from angina or have had a myocardial infarction.

The procedure is performed by inserting a catheter via the brachial artery (Sones' technique) or the femoral artery (Judkins' technique). A 75% reduction in the luminal cross-sectional area (50% luminal diameter reduction seen in two planes) is considered to be "critical" or "significant" obstruction of the coronary artery. It is likely, however, that cross-sectional luminal reductions of less than 75% may be important under stress or exercise when high coronary flow rates are required, and obviously, if vasospasm is superimposed upon a minimal fixed obstruction, an additional and critical decrement in blood flow could occur. The location and extent of intercoronary collateral vessels can be determined. Ventriculography shows areas of reduced and abnormal wall motion, as well as ventricular aneurysms. An ejection fraction also can be calculated.

Despite the availability and importance of these ancillary tests, the diagnosis of angina pectoris still is made mainly by the history.

COURSE. The prognosis of patients with angina pectoris is related both to the extent of critical obstructing coronary artery lesions and to ventricular function. Without intensive medical or surgical treatment, annual mortality is 2% for patients with single-vessel disease, 7% for patients with two-vessel disease, and 11% for patients with three-vessel disease. Critical obstruction of the left main coronary artery increases the annual

Table 96-1 Cardiovascular effects of antianginal drugs

| Effects | β-blockers | Nitrates | Calcium blockers | | |
			Nif	Verap	Dilt
Coronary resistance	↑ (?)	↓	↓ ↓	↓	↓
Systemic resistance	↑	↓	↓ ↓ ↓	↓ ↓	↓
Heart rate	↓	0	↑	↓ ↓	↓
Atrioventricular condition	↓	0	0	↓	↓
Contractility	↓	0	0	↓	↓

Nif, nifedipine; *Verap,* verapamil; *Dilt,* diltiazem; ↓, decrease; ↑, increase; *0,* unchanged

mortality to approximately 30%. These data do not take into account ventricular function. Patients with ejection fractions greater than 55% fare better than those with lesser ejection fractions in a continuum of increasing risk of any combination of coronary vessel involvement.

MANAGEMENT. Attention should be given to factors that may precipitate or worsen angina pectoris. Smoking must be stopped. Obesity, diabetes mellitus, and hypertension must be controlled. Disorders of cholesterol and triglyceride metabolism should be corrected on the presumption that this may retard the progression of atheromatous disease. Congestive heart failure, anemia, thyrotoxicosis, and tachyrhythmias should be treated, because they all increase myocardial oxygen consumption and worsen angina.

A controlled exercise program may benefit some patients with angina pectoris. The exercise prescription should be guided by the results of an exercise stress test. There is no convincing evidence that exercise prolongs life, retards atherosclerosis, or increases coronary collaterals. Some individuals do show increased serum HDLs, which are thought to have a protective effect against the development of atherosclerosis. However, the most important benefit from regular exercise is improved cardiovascular efficiency. Patients who exercise regularly can achieve a given level of total body oxygen consumption with less myocardial oxygen consumption because of a lower heart rate and blood pressure. Thus after training any given level of exercise can be sustained by a lower myocardial oxygen requirement.

The nitrates have been used for many years in treatment of and prophylaxis against anginal pain. The beneficial effects of nitrates are thought to be mediated by preload and afterload reduction (Table 96-1), by decreased myocardial wall stress and oxygen demand, and possibly by increased blood flow via coronary collateral vessels. Nitrates also relieve coronary artery spasm, should spasm be important in the genesis of the angina. Nitroglycerin (0.4 mg sublingually taken early in the course of an anginal episode) typically relieves the chest discomfort in 1 to 5 minutes. Sublingual nitroglycerin also may be used prophylactically before climbing stairs or hills—situations likely to precipitate anginal attacks. Longer-acting nitrates also are useful. Isosorbide dinitrate given sublingually in doses of 5 or 10 mg exerts a protective effect for a few hours; when 10 to 20 mg of isosorbide dinitrate is given by mouth, the protective effect may extend to 4 hours or longer. Nitroglycerin preparations applied to the skin are absorbed relatively slowly and may give protection for 6 hours or longer. There now are several routes that can be used to deliver nitrate preparations: oral sprays, mucosal pledgets, and skin patches designed for prolonged release of the drug, even up to 24 hours.

Side effects of nitrates include headache and hypotension. A tachyphylaxis to the vasodilation that underlies these effects

Table 96-2 Side effects of antianginal compounds

Side effect	β-blockers	Nitrates	Calcium blockers		
			Nif	Verap	Dilt
Headache	0	+ + +	+ + +	+	+
Dizziness	0	+ + +	+ +	+	+
Hypotension	+	+	+ +	+	+
Heart failure	+ + +	0	0	+ +	+
Bradycardia	+ +	0	0	+ +	+
Heart block	+ + +	0	0	+ +	+
Nausea	+	0	0	0	0
Constipation	0	0	0	+ + +	0
Bronchospasm	+ +	0	0	0	0

Nif, nifedipine; *Verap,* verapamil; *Dilt,* diltiazem; +, present; *0,* absent.

may occur with time. Nitroglycerin tablets lose their effectiveness after a number of months if not stored in tightly stoppered, colored glass vials.

The β-blocking drugs reduce heart rate, myocardial contractility, and blood pressure (Table 96-1), thereby reducing myocardial oxygen consumption and restoring the balance between myocardial blood flow and oxygen consumption. These agents therefore are particularly useful in controlling angina caused by exercise-related tachycardia. They also have a beneficial effect on rest angina. Propranolol is the prototypic β-blocking drug. Orally administered propranolol is metabolized by the liver soon after absorption (first-pass effect), but propranolol reduces hepatic blood flow and retards its own metabolism, resulting in a delayed achievement of a steady state after initiation of therapy. One of its metabolites, hydroxypropranolol, retains cardiovascular activity. The daily oral dosage usually is 80 to 320 mg in four divided doses. The drug should be given until the resting pulse rate is between 50 and 60 beats/min. This endpoint is more useful clinically than blood level determinations.

Side effects of β-blocking drugs in general include gastrointestinal upset, diarrhea, insomnia, disturbing dreams, and sometimes loss of sexual desire and performance (Table 96-2). Propranolol blocks both β₁-receptors (such as cardiac receptors) and β₂-receptors (such as pulmonary receptors), therefore it may produce bronchospasm in patients with asthma or chronic obstructive lung disease. It should not be taken by patients who have marked bronchospasm. Metoprolol, a relatively selective β₁-blocker, is preferred for these patients. Because both drugs decrease myocardial contractility, they may be contraindicated in congestive heart failure. They also are relatively contraindicated in patients with various forms of bradycardia.

Many additional β-blocking drugs now are available. These vary in their metabolism, and some are very long acting, permitting administration once a day.

Calcium channel blockers are the newest group of drugs available to treat angina pectoris. Collectively these drugs inhibit the flux of calcium across a variety of cell membranes. Among other effects this action inhibits smooth muscle contraction and reduces muscle tone in the vascular bed. This reduces cardiovascular afterload, increases coronary blood flow by vasodilation, and relieves coronary artery spasm.

Three calcium channel blockers currently are approved for clinical use: nifedipine, diltiazem, and verapamil. Diltiazem and verapamil differ from nifedipine in several ways. They slow the heart rate and atrioventricular (AV) nodal conduction, and they also may have a more negative inotropic effect than nifedipine. Diltiazem and verapamil should be used with cau-

tion in patients with bradycardia, heart block, or left ventricular dysfunction with heart failure.

Because calcium channel blockers can decrease blood pressure, they also have been used effectively as antihypertensive agents. Intravenous verapamil now is considered the drug of choice for terminating some forms of supraventricular tachycardia because of its effects on AV nodal conduction. As a group calcium channel blockers are most effective in treating angina pectoris caused by a combination of coronary vasospasm and fixed coronary artery obstruction.

Coronary artery bypass grafting. One direct way to increase myocardial blood flow is by coronary artery bypass surgery. The procedure entails removing a portion of the saphenous vein from the leg and anastomosing one end of it to the aorta and the other end to a suitable coronary artery distal to an obstructing lesion. Occasionally the internal mammary artery is used instead of a saphenous vein. When the internal mammary artery is used, only one anastomosis, to the distal coronary artery, can be done. A "suitable" coronary artery is one in which distal ramifications are free of disease and large enough to receive a graft and nourish a significant amount of myocardium. In appropriately selected patients, coronary artery bypass surgery can be performed with an operative mortality of less than 2% or 3%. The left ventricular ejection fraction should be equal to or greater than 30% to reduce risk. The major morbidity is myocardial infarction during surgery.

The major indication for coronary artery bypass surgery is disabling angina pectoris refractory to medical treatment. Approximately 60% of patients have complete relief of angina after surgery, and another 20% or 30% have major or partial relief. Exercise tolerance measured by exercise stress testing also improves in most patients. In patients with critical obstruction of the left main coronary artery, bypass surgery improves survival. It is uncertain whether coronary artery bypass surgery improves survival in other patients; some studies suggest improved survival in those with good ventricular function and triple-vessel disease, but other studies do not. When triple-vessel disease is present with left ventricular dysfunction (depressed ejection fraction), bypass surgery probably attenuates mortality. Asymptomatic patients with single- or double-vessel disease and no significant ischemia detected by radionuclide scintigraphic studies have a reasonably low morbidity and mortality (provided the left main and proximal left anterior descending coronary arteries are normal) and probably do not require surgery. Diffuse distal small coronary vessel disease, paticularly with extensive calcification or stenosis of the terminal segments, is not amenable to coronary bypass surgery. The operation is not indicated as treatment for congestive heart failure.

Recurrences of anginal pain 5 to 7 years after cure by coronary artery bypass surgery have been reported. Continued follow-up examinations, control of risk factors, and medical treatment when indicated are therefore important.

Percutaneous coronary dilation. A new alternative to surgical bypass of atherosclerotic stenoses is to crush the plaques outward via expansion of a balloon placed in the coronary artery by catheter techniques. This procedure may restore luminal patency with little risk. It can be done during the coronary angiography, obviating thoracotomy, but its use is limited to incomplete, noncalcific plaques easily reached by the catheter. Although this procedure has gained tremendous popularity recently, its use in patients with coronary artery disease is not well defined. Restenosis of the dilated artery is a frequent problem. Furthermore, triple-vessel angioplasty, although complex, can be performed, but its superiority to surgical intervention has not been demonstrated. Decisions to operate or to perform angioplasty on patients with ischemic heart disease should be made with a surgeon, since a failed angioplasty may require surgical intervention.

Unstable angina

Unstable angina pectoris is a syndrome intermediate in severity between classic effort-induced angina and myocardial infarction. The syndrome may be manifest as an abrupt increase in the number of anginal attacks daily, an increase in the severity of the attacks as reflected by nitrate consumption or the development of angina unassociated with exertion, or postprandial and nocturnal ischemic pain. The ECG in these patients frequently demonstrates ST and T wave abnormalities that indicate ischemia, but Q waves and enzymatic evidence of myocardial necrosis are absent.

Patients with unstable angina have on the average the same degree of coronary atheromatous changes as patients with effort-induced angina and those with myocardial infarction. It has been postulated that coronary spasm and platelet aggregation may play important roles in the pathogenesis of unstable angina pectoris, and it seems that thrombosis with spontaneous clot lysis may sometimes occur in this syndrome. Coronary artery spasm was found with significant frequency in one study.

Unstable angina is important, because it carries a much more ominous prognosis than does classic effort-induced angina. Patients judged to have unstable angina should be admitted to a coronary care unit. They require monitoring for arrhythmias and aggressive therapy. Acute myocardial infarction should be excluded by enzyme determinations, serial ECGs, and perhaps technetium pyrophosphate or thallium scintigraphy. Rapid control of the pain of myocardial ischemia is imperative. Long- and short-acting nitrates, calcium channel blockers, and β-blockers all can be used. Frequently combinations of these compounds are required. For example, the combination of nifedipine and propranolol has been demonstrated to work synergistically to ameliorate symptoms.

Pain refractory to drugs may respond to intraaortic balloon pumping. The balloon inflates in diastole, augmenting diastolic coronary blood flow. It deflates just before the next cardiac systole, thereby reducing afterload and hence myocardial oxygen demand.

In most patients the acute phase of unstable angina can be controlled by medication alone. Subsequent consideration of angioplasty or a coronary artery bypass procedure should be determined by the patient's frequency of rest and effort-induced angina after discharge from the hospital. In the few cases of unstable angina that cannot be controlled by medication alone, intraaortic balloon pumping, urgent coronary arteriography, and mechanical intervention (angioplasty or coronary artery bypass surgery) should be considered. However, results of a national prospective randomized trial of medical therapy alone versus surgical therapy plus medical therapy in unstable angina revealed no difference in mortality after 3 years. The incidence of myocardial infarction (comparing perioperative and postoperative infarction in the surgical group with nonoperative myocardial infarction in the medically treated group) was the same. However, pain relief was more complete in patients who underwent a coronary artery bypass procedure, and there was a 35% crossover rate from medical to surgical therapy, the largest portion of which occurred in the first 6 to 12 months.

Prinzmetal's variant angina

Prinzmetal described a variant form of angina pectoris in which the pain occurred only while the patient was at rest. The characteristic ECG change was ST segment elevation rather than ST segment depression, the latter being the hallmark of exercise-induced angina. Prinzmetal postulated that this form of angina was caused by coronary artery spasm, and this has been confirmed by coronary angiography performed during the course of variant angina. The course of variant angina depends on the nature of the underlying coronary artery pathology. In patients with little or no atheromatous change in the coronary arteries, coronary artery spasm and anginal pain tend to regress with time. This does not mean that Prinzmetal's variant angina is entirely a benign condition; severe hypotension, bradycardia, ventricular tachycardia, ventricular fibrillation, myocardial infarction, and death have occurred in patients with minimal or no atheromatous change but marked coronary artery spasm. In general, however, the prognosis of myocardial infarction and death is more likely in patients with coronary artery atheromatous disease.

Prinzmetal's variant angina is characterized by chest discomfort similar to that of effort-induced angina except that it occurs at rest. It often is cyclic in nature and may occur at the same time of day over a period of days or weeks. ECGs characteristically show ST segment elevation that regresses as the pain regresses. Various atrial and ventricular tachyrhythmias and bradycardias such as heart block may be seen. Because chest pain occurs at rest with ST segment elevation, myocardial infarction must be excluded in the differential diagnosis.

A rigid separation of Prinzmetal's variant angina from classic effort-induced angina has been challenged. Although spasm is the principal pathogenetic mechanism in variant angina, spasm also has been identified in patients with classic effort-induced angina. Furthermore, patients with Prinzmetal's angina may show either ST segment elevation or depression. Coronary artery spasm now is also known to contribute frequently to the pathogenesis of ischemia in many patients with coronary disease syndromes.

Prinzmetal's variant angina is treated with nitrates and calcium channel blockers. β-blockers are not used, because theoretically they could cause coronary vasoconstriction. Coronary artery bypass surgery should be reserved for patients with critical atheromatous narrowing who do not respond to pharmacologic therapy.

Angina with normal coronary arteries

Chest pain clinically indistinguishable from that of classic angina pectoris has been described in patients who have normal coronary arteries, even with no demonstrable spasm. Some of these patients have an easily identifiable cardiac abnormality that may or may not be related to their chest discomfort, such as hypertrophic cardiomyopathy, mitral valve prolapse syndrome, aortic stenois, and (less frequently) aortic insufficiency. The chest pain associated with mitral valve prolapse syndrome is not understood. In the other conditions, reduced ventricular compliance, increased left ventricular end-diastolic pressure, increased diffusing distances between the capillaries and the center of the hypertrophied myocardial cell, increased myocardial oxygen requirements, and interference with coronary flow because of valvular abnormalities are important in the pathogenesis of the oxygen supply/demand imbalance.

There remains a group of patients with angina pectoris, normal coronary arteries, and no identifiable associated cardiac lesion, among whom women predominate. Their ECGs may show ST segment depression with exercise. Not infrequently, altered carbohydrate metabolism and lipoprotein abnormalities are present. In an appreciable minority of patients, lactate production may be observed when the myocardium is stressed by either pacing or isoproterenol infusion, indicating a shift to anaerobic metabolism. The cause of this condition is unknown. Coronary artery spasm, disease of coronary vessels beyond the resolution of angiography, and an intrinsic disorder of the myocardial cell all have been proposed but with little supporting evidence. The symptomatic response to drugs is poor. Although the condition generally is benign, both myocardial infarction and sudden death have been reported.

ACUTE MYOCARDIAL INFARCTION

DEFINITION. Acute myocardial infarction (MI) results from cardiac muscle ischemia severe and extensive enough to create irreversible necrosis of myocardial cells. Generally MI is associated with obstructive coronary atherosclerosis and limitation of nutrient blood flow, producing anoxic, metabolic cellular death.

ETIOLOGY. Most MIs occur in patients with ischemic heart disease. Only 2% of all patients with MI and 16% of patients with MI younger than 35 years of age do not have atherosclerotic coronary artery disease. The small subset of infarction patients with normal coronary arteries tends not only to be young but to have few risk factors for coronary artery disease. In addition, they have none of the usual MI prodromes. Generally they have an acute hospital course no different from that of atherosclerotic patients with infarctions. Postinfarct problems (recurrent MI, heart failure, and sudden death) are, fortunately, less likely when coronary disease is absent, and these patients usually have no postinfarct angina.

The pathogenesis of MI in patients with no apparent coronary atherosclerosis might be attributed to coronary artery emboli, acute coronary thrombosis with subsequent recanalization, anomalous coronary anatomy, coronary arteriovenous fistulas, trauma, arteritis, or clinically undetected small vessel coronary artery disease. All of these conditions create an oxygen supply and demand disproportion that might predispose a patient to MI.

EPIDEMIOLOGY. Acute MI is an extraordinarily common hospital diagnosis. In the United States alone the diagnosis is made over 1.3 million times yearly. North American men have a 20% likelihood of having an MI or sudden death before they reach 65. Death rates following MI are, unfortunately, four times higher than in the normal population; half of these deaths are sudden.

PATHOGENESIS. Interrelated factors are responsible for the malignant alteration of the normal oxygen supply and demand equation that results in myocardial tissue death. Infarction results whether these changes are acute in situ thrombosis of nutrient vessels previously diseased with atherosclerosis, occlusive spasm of a normal coronary artery, or an embolic episode. Acute thrombosis may not always be the pathophysiologic event leading to myocardial necrosis, but thrombus is seen in at least 80% of patients undergoing coronary angiography during the infarction. The presence of these clots has focused recent therapeutic attention on thrombolysis during MI. Coronary occlusion has been demonstrated to occur in the absence of tissue necrosis if the collateral circulation is adequate to maintain normal cellular respiration. In addition, infarctions can occur in the absence of coronary occlusion.

Cellular ischemia acutely increases intracellular lactate concentration with the subsequent repression of enzymes in the glycolytic pathway. An increase in cellular acylcoenzyme A (acyl-CoA) occurs (particularly in the mitochondria) when acyl-CoA esters inhibit the effective exchange of adenosine diphosphate (ADP) and adenosine triphosphate (ATP) between the cytoplasm and the mitochondria. A decline in high-energy phosphate stores occurs, and this, in conjunction with the cellular acidosis and metabolite accumulation, contributes to the rapid development of irreversible ischemic injury that ultimately leads to severe left ventricular dysfunction and death in these individuals.

Grossly visible changes consisting of discoloration and edema occur in the left ventricle 6 to 8 hours after infarction. A serofibrinous exudate develops over the epicardium in transmural infarctions 48 hours later, and in 8 to 10 days the infarct thins when necrotic muscle is removed by inflammatory cells.

On an ultrastructural level, disruption of sarcomeres, condensation of myofibrillar material, margination of nucleolar chromatin, and granulation in the myocardium occur over a 24-hour period.

CLINICAL MANIFESTATIONS. Chest discomfort is the major complaint of patients with MI. The pain is thought to arise from the nerve endings in injured or ischemic myocardium rather than from necrotic muscle. This pain generally is the symptom that forces the patient to consult his physician. The discomfort usually is present at rest, varies in intensity, and lasts longer than 30 minutes. Often an eliciting event plays a role, such as exertional or emotional stress. The patient may characterize the discomfort in many ways. Frequently it is described not as a "painful" feeling but as a constricting, crushing, oppressing, compressing, squeezing, choking, burning, boring, or stabbing sensation. The discomfort usually is located retrosternally, with radiation of variable intensity and extent to the neck, jaws, teeth, arms, and back.

Other symptoms may include nausea and vomiting (more frequent in inferior wall MI than in anterior wall MI), diarrhea, weakness, dizziness, perspiration, intractable hiccups, and the symptoms of pulmonary edema (that is, severe dyspnea). At least 10% to 20% of MIs are diagnosed retrospectively (particularly in diabetic patients). MI may simulate other diseases such as acute pericarditis, pleurodynia, pulmonary embolism, aortic dissection, costochondritis, pancreatitis, gastritis, cholecystitis, and peptic ulcer disease.

Potentially confounding presentations in which MI must be considered include unexplained congestive heart failure, classic angina pectoris, atypical pain locations (persistent toothache), "bursitis," backache, sudden confusion, mania or psychosis, syncope, overwhelming weakness, acute indigestion, and unexplained peripheral arterial embolization.

Physical findings are trivial unless cardiogenic shock, pulmonary edema, or sustained arrhythmias are present. Usually the patient is anxious and restless, and there may be findings associated with hypertension, diabetes, or atherosclerosis.

Important signs (by no means specific for MI) include pericardial friction rub, the mitral regurgitation murmur of papillary muscle dysfunction, and gallop rhythms. Signs of abrupt left ventricular failure (pulmonary rales, jugular venous distention, orthopnea, and S_3 gallop) are important. The presence of an S_3 gallop in a patient with an acute MI is an ominous prognostic factor. Signs of shock also may be present (hypotension, oliguria, and peripheral cyanosis, in combination with cold, clammy, sweaty skin with an ashen-gray hue). Signs of central nervous system hypoperfusion (transient cerebral ischemic events, overt cerebrovascular accident, confusion) may predominate, particularly in the elderly.

It is important to know that hypotension does not necessarily mean shock in MI patients. Additional causes of low blood pressure in patients with MI include the bradycardia-hypotension syndrome associated with inferior wall myocardial infarction (Bezold-von Jarisch reflex), hypovolemia, occult mi-

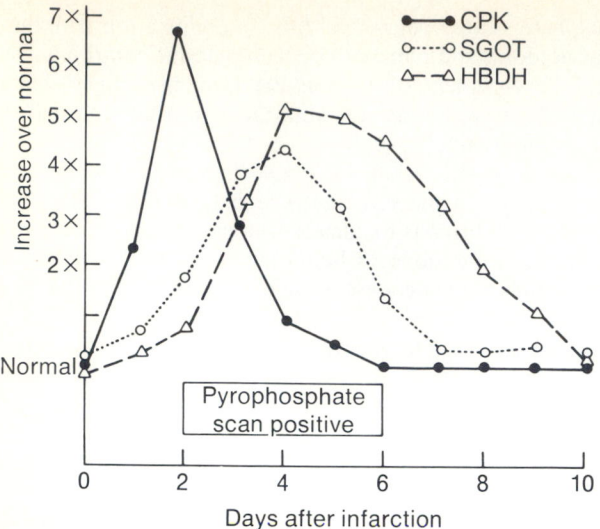

Fig. 96-2 Enzymatic elevation and technetium 99m pyrophosphate scan patterns in patients with acute myocardial infarction. *CPK,* creatine phosphokinase; *SGOT,* serum glutamicoxaloacetic transaminase; *HBDH,* hydroxybutyric dehydrogenase.

tral stenosis, pulmonary emboli, right ventricular infarction, and pericardial effusion.

Additional signs of MI include low-grade fever (most commonly after 24 to 48 hours) and Cheyne-Stokes respiration (secondary to central nervous system hypoperfusion, pulmonary edema, or opiate therapy).

The physical examination can provide prognostic information in the patient with acute MI. Patients with overt shock have a 60% to 80% mortality. The mere presence of bibasilar rales or an S_3 gallop suggests mortality of 10% to 15%. Morbidity and mortality after MI clearly relate to the presence of heart failure, which in turn depends on the size of the infarct. Because of this, considerable emphasis now is placed on early interventions that might decrease the amount of myocardial tissue ultimately necrosed.

LABORATORY FINDINGS. Certain enzymes liberated from necrotic myocardial cells are reasonably sensitive and specific indicators of MI. Indeed, the amount of enzyme liberation can grossly quantify the size of an infarction.

Creatine phosphokinase (CPK), isoenzymes, and isoforms may appear in serum almost immediately after the infarction (Fig. 96-2). Since CPK is liberated in significant amounts from injured brain, liver, thyroid, striated muscle, and smooth muscle cells, CPK elevation might mistakenly be attributed to cardiac muscle when in fact it is caused by hepatic, brain, or bowel infarction or more commonly by striated muscle trauma (most often resulting from intramuscular injection of irritating medication). A myocardial band (MB) of CPK can be detected by electrophoresis. If the CPK-MB exceeds 5% of the total CPK, myocardial cell damage can be assumed. The CPK level usually returns to normal within 4 to 6 days. Persistent elevation is an ominous sign, suggesting massive infarction or ongoing necrosis. Serum glutamic-oxaloacetic transaminase (SGOT) rises 6 to 12 hours after MI and returns to normal 5 to 7 days later. SGOT elevation also occurs in patients with liver disease, hepatic congestion, skeletal muscle disease, intramuscular injections, pulmonary emboli, shock, or pericarditis with epicardial involvement.

Lactic dehydrogenase (LDH) is the last enzyme to appear elevated in serum after MI, rising 48 hours after the event and

remaining elevated 7 to 9 days. LDH also is liberated in substantial quantities in hemolysis, megaloblastic anemia, leukemia, massive pulmonary emboli, shock, skeletal muscle disease, and myocarditis. Like CPK, LDH has an isoenzyme (hydroxybutyric dehydrogenase, HBDH) that is more specific for myocardial cell necrosis.

Additional abnormal laboratory findings in MI include leukocytosis, myoglobinuria, elevated erythrocyte sedimentation rate, and elevated hematocrit owing to hemoconcentration.

DIAGNOSIS. The diagnosis of acute MI is made by combined assessment of the history, physical examination, serum enzymes, ECG, and when available ancillary radionuclide imaging of the heart.

The ECG generally is abnormal in patients with an acute infarction. Indeed, for anterior MIs of reasonable size the ECG is positive in 95% of the cases. Not only is the ECG important for diagnosing MI, but it also helps determine extent of injury, the age and location of the infarction, and the presence of pericarditis or electrolyte disturbances. ECG monitorirng also is important for diagnosing rhythm disturbances.

The usual evolutionary pattern of ECG changes is early ST segment elevation with subsequent T wave inversion and Q wave formation. Q waves localize the region of myocardial necrosis. The usual evolution of ECG changes occurs over several weeks; persistent ST elevation beyond 6 weeks suggests the development of a ventricular aneurysm. Interestingly, 20% to 30% of ECGs normalize entirely after MI, making the retrospective diagnosis particularly difficult at times.

It is important to consider a right ventricular (RV) infarction in hypotensive patients with lateral or inferolateral MIs. Generally these patients have jugular venous distention, hypotension, and normal left ventricular filling pressures. The diagnosis must be made by right-sided heart catheterization. A first-pass radionuclide angiocardiogram with an abnormally low RV ejection fraction raises suspicion of an elevated RV filling (right atrial) pressure despite normal left ventricular (LV) filling (pulmonary capillary wedge) pressure. The treatment consists of intravascular expansion with saline, albumin, or crystalloid.

Radionuclide imaging may be useful in other respects. Technetium 99 pyrophosphate is taken up directly by acutely necrosed myocardial cells. This technique of myocardial imaging allows recognition, localization (of a "hot spot"), and estimation of the size of the infarction in most cases of transmural MI if the study is performed between 2 and 6 days after the acute infarction (pyrophosphate window in Fig. 96-2). In nontransmural MI a pattern of diffuse uptake may occur, which also can be present in non-MI situations.

Thallium 201 imaging, on the other hand, produces a "cold spot" in regions of diminished myocardial perfusion and therefore would be positive with MIs caused by acute coronary artery occlusion. This study theoretically should diagnose an MI at its earliest inception. However, the filling defect, or cold spot, would remain a persistent finding. Thus imaging with thallium after infarction cannot distinguish hypoperfusion resulting from an old scar from ischemic but viable myocardium. The greatest value of thallium 201 seems to be the imaging of cold spot regions with exercise-induced ischemia. (The perfusion scan is abnormal with exercise but normal at rest, suggesting adequate reperfusion.)

Radionuclide angiocardiography can yield serial estimates of left ventricular function by repeated determination of ejection fraction. A left-to-right shunt caused by acute ventricular septal defect (VSD) formation can be diagnosed. Marked mitral regurgitation also can be detected. This procedure thus can differentiate papillary muscle dysfunction or rupture from a

VSD. Radionuclide angiocardiography also may prove useful in differentiating true and false left ventricular aneurysms.

COURSE AND COMPLICATIONS. The actual mortality of acute MI is difficult to determine, because most patients who die don't reach the hospital alive. Some have estimated the prehospital mortality to be as high as 60%. Even patients surviving initial hospitalization have a subsequent high mortality, varying from 4% to 20% per year depending on the amount of left ventricular dyssynergy and number of diseased vessels.

Recently, definite MI has resulted in overall mortality of 10% to 15% and unstable angina in mortality of 1% to 5% while both groups were in the coronary care unit. Late hospital death accounted for 5% and 1%, respectively. Hypotension, heart failure, and ventricular arrhythmias are more common in MI patients than in those with unstable angina.

The following observations in the coronary care unit may be risk factors for death in patients with acute MI after discharge from the unit: the development of a new interventricular conduction defect, sinus tachycardia persisting more than 48 hours, ventricular fibrillation, atrial flutter or fibrillation, extensive anterior wall MI, left ventricular failure, and silent myocardial ischemia.

Hospital mortality depends on the extent of disease and the complications that occur. Arrhythmias are responsible for most deaths that occur on the first day. Ventricular fibrillation and tachycardia (which may lead to fibrillation) are the most common lethal arrhythmias. Trifascicular heart block also may occur early and is a poor prognostic sign. Shock or pulmonary edema usually occurs on the first or second day and carries a grave prognosis (60% to 80% and 20% to 50% mortality, respectively). Rupture of the intraventricular septum or papillary muscle may occur after several days and results in a loud systolic murmur and severe heart failure; rupture of the free ventricular wall may result in tamponade. A transient pericarditis (second or third day) from transmural infarction (seen in 15% with transmural MIs) and thromboembolic episodes (usually occurring after several days to weeks) carry a much less ominous prognosis.

Arterial emboli (cerebral, visceral, peripheral, coronary) may be caused by dislodgment of an acutely formed left ventricular mural thrombus. Phlebothrombosis, probably related to inactivity, occurs in as many as 10% of patients, and many have subsequent pulmonary emboli. Low doses of subcutaneously injected heparin have routinely been used in many hospitals to prevent this problem. Cerebral infarction from episodes of hypotension or tachyrhythmias may occur in patients with concomitant cerebrovascular and coronary artery disease. It is not uncommon to find an unsuspected MI in patients with cerebral infarction and vice versa. Acute renal failure may be secondary to either frank shock or transient hypotension.

Late complications (weeks to months) include formation of a ventricular aneurysm, delayed heart failure, postmyocardial infarction syndrome (Dressler's syndrome), and shoulder-hand syndrome.

Ventricular aneurysm often leads to heart failure, systemic embolism, or recurrent ventricular tachycardia. Patients often have a palpable double apical impulse, S_3 and S_4 gallops, and persistent elevation of ST segments on ECG. The chest roentgenogram may show a bulge on the heart border, and cineventriculography is diagnostic. If the aneurysm is causing symptoms not responsive to medical therapy, it can be resected.

Dressler's syndrome, thought to be an autoimmune reaction, consists of pericarditis, pleuritis, and pneumonitis. High titers of antimyocardial antibodies are present in the serum. If aspirin or nonsteroidal antiinflammatory agents do not give symptom-

Table 96-3 Intravenous versus intracoronary thrombolysis in acute myocardial infarction

	Intravenous	Intracoronary
Cardiac catheterization laboratory	Unnecessary	Mandatory
Cost	Minimal	High
Delay	15-30 min	1-3 hours
Applicability	All hospitals	Selected hospitals
Recanalization	35%-60%	50%-80%
Morbidity	Drug related	Procedure and drug related

atic relief, corticosteroids can be used. Anticoagulants should be avoided in patients with Dressler's syndrome, since life-threatening hemopericardium can result.

The shoulder-hand syndrome is a limitation of mobility in the shoulder and arm (usually on the left side) associated with pain. The treatment is physiotherapy.

MANAGEMENT. Admission to an intensive care unit has become standard practice when a patient's history and clinical findings suggest acute MI. The main benefit of the unit is continuous monitoring that allows early recognition of problematic arrythmias and complications of cardiac ischemia such as post-MI angina and heart failure. A cardiac care unit is a closely supervised area with well-trained individuals capable of recognizing and treating serious arrhythmias and initiating cardiopulmonary resuscitative efforts and defibrillation when appropriate. In addition, these units provide a place where pacemaker insertion and bedside hemodynamic monitoring with flow-directed pulmonary artery catheters can be accomplished.

Recently changes have been initiated in the approach to treating acute MI. Since progressive heart failure and sudden cardiac death constitute the two major mortality categories after MI, and since both are more likely to be seen in patients with large amounts of myocardium destroyed by the infarct, treatment has come to focus on interventions to decrease the size of the MI. To increase the blood supply to the periinfarct ischemic zone, thrombolytic agents could be given to patients arriving at the emergency room with less than 4 hours of chest pain and no contraindication to thrombolytic therapy (such contraindications include recent gastrointestinal bleeding, history of cerebrovascular accident, or clotting abnormalities). Clot lysis and reperfusion should be accomplished within 4 hours of the onset of symptoms to achieve consistent benefit.

Although intracoronary drug delivery may lyse more clots, the intravenous route has distinct advantages (see Table 96-3), since the most important consideration is delivery of thrombolytic agent as soon as possible after the infarct. Intravenous infusion of streptokinase recently has been demonstrated to reduce MI mortality in patients with anterior MI if given early after the onset of pain. Tissue-type plasminogen activator is one of the new thrombolytic agents developed using recombinant-DNA techniques. Theoretically, it is more fibrin specific and therefore safer to use with higher clot lysis rates. Whichever thrombolytic agent is chosen, care must be taken to avoid bleeding complications. Patients should not be treated with these compounds if there is a likelihood of hemorrhagic difficulty. Early administration after the infarction (within 3 to 4 hours) also must be reemphasized.

Despite successful early intervention with thrombolytic therapy, residual coronary stenosis generally is present in the infarct-related artery. Residual myocardium at risk and the potential for reocclusion and reinfarction may remain for such patients. Indeed, routine coronary angiography before discharge from the hospital in MI patients who had initially successful thrombolysis shows a high reocclusion rate, and frequently MI recurs within several months, with all the attendant risks of acute MI. Because of this, some patients who have had an infarction should undergo angioplasty after the infarct has been treated. Certainly it has been demonstrated that angioplasty can be performed safely and successfully following thrombolytic therapy. Indeed, some believe that angioplasty should be the treatment of choice in MI patients who seek help early. However, the disadvantage of this approach, as with intracoronary administration of thrombolytic agents, is the requirement of cardiac catheterization before achieving reperfusion (with all of the attendant delays) and the clinical importance of achieving reperfusion as soon as possible. Instead, after thrombolysis angioplasty or coronary artery bypass surgery can be considered on an elective basis. Assessment of the patient with noninvasive tests (limited treadmill exercise tests, nuclear scintigraphic studies, and arrhythmia detection devices) 7 to 10 days after the infarct can define the group at highest risk for reinfarction at a later date. Patients with residual ischemia should undergo coronary angiography, and if the coronary anatomy is reparable, they should undergo elective angioplasty or bypass surgery.

Adequate pain relief is important. Since pain is generated in the perinecrotic ischemic zone, its elimination suggests improvement of the oxygen supply and demand ratio in this region, which is at high risk for infarct extension. Morphine sulfate or meperidine may be given intravenously. Intramuscular injections should be avoided, especially when heart failure or shock is present, because of the variability of drug absorption in these states and the difficulty with interpretation of cardiac enzyme patterns. Nitrate administration (intravenous, sublingual, topical, or oral) also may be effective. This maneuver reduces left ventricular filling pressure and intramyocardial wall tension, thus decreasing myocardial oxygen demand and thereby eliminating ischemic chest pain. If pain following MI is particularly severe, prolonged, or intractable, intravenous administration of nitroprusside or nitroglycerin may relieve it. Intravenous nitrate administration also is useful for treating pulmonary congestion.

Sedation to relieve anxiety and continuous psychologic support usually are required. Low-flow oxygen administration should be considered in patients with hypoxia. The benefits of this maneuver in individuals with normal arterial P_{O_2} have not been clearly demonstrated, and it should be avoided if the patient finds it pleasant or uncomfortable.

A constipated patient straining at stool produces a Valsalva maneuver that increases peripheral vascular resistance, left ventricular wall stress, and myocardial oxygen demand, therefore potentially furthering ischemic injury. MI patients should receive stool softeners and appropriate laxatives, with permission to use a bedside commode as early as possible.

Early mobilization (after 2 to 5 days) of patients following infarction seems reasonable. The decision of when to mobilize an individual is rooted in common sense. However, early ambulation diminishes the likelihood of phlebothrombosis and restores patient self-confidence. With appropriate supervision, early ambulation and exercise after MI are safe.

Routine administration of anticoagulants to patients with acute MI remains controversial. There is no evidence to support the use of heparin or warfarin as primary interventional therapy during MI. These agents do seem to reduce morbidity and mortality associated with some thromboembolic complications,

including pulmonary embolism, systemic arterial embolism (sometimes the cause of stroke), left ventricular mural thrombosis, and deep venous thrombosis. Low-dose heparin (5000 units subcutaneously twice daily) can prevent some of these difficulties. Full-dose heparin administration frequently is given to MI patients after thrombolytic therapy to reduce the incidence of artery reocclusion, but these patients must be observed closely for hemorrhagic complications.

Agents that attenuate platelet aggregation (aspirin, dipyridamole, and sulfinpyrazone) also have been used mostly in patients after an infarct. Aspirin administered to patients with unstable angina has been demonstrated to reduce the occurrence of death and acute MI. Other agents have not produced such results. It should be emphasized that this therapy is not meant to replace conventional MI treatment. All antiplatelet agents have been evaluated to determine their efficacy in secondary prevention of recurrent MI and cardiac death after an infarction. Although use of these drugs seems to reduce the death rate from MI and the number of nonfatal infarctions, such a trend has not been supported by significant statistical evidence. Still, aspirin has been approved as a once-daily drug for MI patients.

Temporary transvenous pacemaker placement as prophylactic therapy to prevent sudden asystole or complete heart block and death should be considered in situations of complete heart block with slow idioventricular rhythm; atrioventricular dissociation with symptomatic, slow escape rhythm; symptomatic sinus bradycardia unresponsive to atropine; and new right bundle branch block with left anterior hemiblock, especially with first-degree or Mobitz type II second-degree heart block (see Chapter 97).

In the presence of an acute MI, specific arrhythmias that probably do not require pacing include asymptomatic Mobitz I (Wenckebach) second-degree heart block and asymptomatic junctional rhythm (atrioventricular dissociation) with an adequate ventricular rate. These arrhythmias are particularly common in inferior wall MIs. Indications for permanent pacing after infarction are controversial. Many would place a permanent pacemaker in individuals with complete heart block or unresolved Mobitz II block.

Since the physician must aggressively attempt to preserve as much myocardium from necrosis as possible, it is imperative that left ventricular hemodynamics be optimized. It is therefore important to accurately assess cardiac pump function in an individual with MI. Patients can be classified as to whether they have normal hemodynamics, hypovolemic hypotension, left ventricular systolic or diastolic dysfunction, or cardiogenic shock. Since the therapeutic requirements vary for these states, precise diagnosis is mandatory. Frequently this requires invasive hemodynamic monitoring with balloon-tipped, flow-directed, thermistor-equipped catheters passed percutaneously to the pulmonary artery. Invasive monitoring is required because of the frequent disparity between physical findings and actual hemodynamic measurements.

Guidelines for employing invasive hemodynamic monitoring include (1) hypotension unresponsive to simple measures (such as atropine administration in patients with bradycardia, or foot elevation); (2) persistent, unrelieved chest pain; (3) left ventricular failure manifested by dyspnea, rales, cardiomegaly, or chest roentgenographic findings of pulmonary vascular congestion; (4) refractory sinus tachycardia; (5) persistent or recurrent ventricular tachycardia; (6) unexplained or severe cyanosis, hypoxia, tachypnea, diaphoresis, or acidosis; and (7) clinical evidence of significant mitral regurgitation, ventricular septal defect, or pericardial effusion. Appropriate manipulation of preload and afterload can then be accomplished with fluids, vasodilators, and inotropic agents to optimize left ventricular function and preserve potentially salvageable ischemic myocardium.

There sometimes is a tendency to institute potent pharmacotherapeutic intervention in MI patients without measuring hemodynamic indices. For example, diuretics can cause a decline in ventricular filling pressure with subsequent hypotension if given to a patient with peripheral edema and a right ventricular infarction or to an individual with rales caused by pulmonary rather than myocardial pathology.

When shock or heart failure is present, adequate distal tissue perfusion must be ensured. In such cases measurement of hemodynamic parameters is essential. Sometimes low-output syndromes can be ameliorated by normalizing ventricular filling pressures with volume expansion. High systemic vascular resistance impairs efficient ventricular emptying, thereby lowering forward cardiac flow. Output can be increased in this setting if vasodilating drugs such as nitroprusside or nitroglycerin are used. These agents also can help lower pulmonary artery filling pressures and attenuate pulmonary edema. In hypotensive patients drugs that increase systemic resistance sometimes are required despite the side effects of decreased renal perfusion and increased oxygen demand. Phenylephrine and metaraminol are examples of agents that can achieve this effect, and they do sometimes restore appropriate arterial pressure, improving dynamics and effecting rises in cardiac output. Drugs such as dopamine, a primarily inotropic agent, may raise arterial pressure in hypotensive patients while avoiding problems with distal organ perfusion. Other drugs that exert a positive inotropic effect in the cardiovascular system include epinephrine and high doses of dopamine. Inotropic agents having a net vasodilatory effect on the periphery may actually cause a decline in systemic pressure. These include dobutamine and amrinone.

Percutaneously or surgically inserted, intraaortic balloon counter-pulsation devices can improve left ventricular hemodynamics in several ways. They augment diastolic aortic pressure and increase coronary perfusion, reduce left ventricular afterload and decrease myocardial oxygen requirements, lessen anaerobic metabolism, and diminish myocardial ischemia. Balloon counter-pulsation should be considered in the course of an MI in three circumstances: (1) hemodynamically unstable MI during cardiac catheterization (while searching for surgically correctable lesions); (2) cardiogenic shock unresponsive to medical management; and (3) persistent ischemic cardiac pain after maximal medical therapy.

Current problems encountered with balloon counter-pulsation include balloon dependence (difficulty in weaning the patient from the balloon) and peripheral vascular ischemia. Use of the balloon does not supplant surgery for correctable mechanical lesions; without such surgery the balloon does not improve overall mortality.

Other types of left ventricular assist devices also are now available but should be used only in desperate cases when other approaches have failed. These devices, as well as the total artificial heart, may implicate subsequent cardiac transplantation. Mechanical devices can be used to stabilize the patient while an appropriate donor heart is located. Appropriate patients usually are young, have massive MI and shock but no distal atherosclerosis, and have preserved vital organ function.

Surgical measures directed toward the heart in MI patients are indicated when a mechanical lesion such as ventricular septal defect or ruptured papillary muscle is present and clinical deterioration is occurring. In patients who have persistent ischemia after therapy, reoccluded coronary lesions after thrombolysis, or high-risk noninfarct-related coronary artery disease, bypass surgery can be considered before discharge from the hospital.

An important consideration with the MI patient is long-term drug therapy after discharge. What drugs should the patient take to prevent subsequent MI or premature mortality? β-Adrenergic blocking agents have been studied extensively in the MI patient with salutary results. The patients who benefit most from β-blocker therapy are those with recurrent or complicated MI, as long as overt congestive heart failure is not present. The timing of the institution of this therapy (whether short-term intravenous β-blocker therapy has an added benefit to long-term oral therapy started before discharge from the hospital) is not clear. Oral β-blocker therapy should be started sometime during the acute MI hospitalization and continued for at least 2 years. It is important to note that full β-blocking doses of a nonselective agent must be used to achieve the reduction in mortality seen in clinical trials. Long-term postinfarction therapy with other drugs such as nitrates or calcium channel blockers has not yet been demonstrated to affect mortality and morbidity. Diltiazem has been used prophylatically 24 to 36 hours after non-Q-wave MI, and angina and recurrent MI were less frequent at a 14-day endpoint.

SUDDEN DEATH

DEFINITION. A uniformly precise definition of sudden death is unavailable because of the wide-ranging interpretation of this phenomenon by epidemiologists, pathologists, clinicians, coroners, and the public. Three basic components seem interchangeable: (1) that a natural (atraumatic) process is present; (2) that the event was unexpected; and (3) that a short time frame surrounds the event. Thus the unanticipated occurrence of "sudden death" generally refers to an abrupt and unexpected change in continuity of a process (either health or disease) from the state immediately preceding death to the fatal episode itself.

The "suddenness" of the event has varied by definition but generally refers to death less than 6 hours after onset of symptoms when the death is observed, or death occurring within 24 hours of the time the subject is last seen and known to be well.

ETIOLOGY. Sudden death does not always denote cardiovascular pathology, but it is a very strong indicator of it and most often is associated with coronary artery disease (CAD). Indeed, heart disease can be inferred from the event of sudden death in 90% of the cases, with cardiovascular disease being present in virtually all cases in which death occurs less than 1 hour after symptoms appear. When confronted with an individual with clinical manifestations of sudden death, it becomes important to determine the most likely cause, since the type of emergency therapy required may be radically different depending on the mechanism. For example, a patient with sudden death owing to ventricular fibrillation is profoundly different from a patient with vasodepressor syncope ("vasovagal reaction" and common "faint"). Indeed, in sudden death an immediate decision is required as to whether the symptoms are caused by a self-terminating derangement, are the result of a cardiac condition, or are noncardiac in origin.

The most common noncardiac causes of sudden death originate in the central nervous system, although death ultimately results from an arrhythmia. Profound metabolic aberrations (sudden hypoxia, hypoglycemia, acidosis, hypercalcemia, and hyperkalemia) also may cause sudden death. Other important causes of sudden death not primarily cardiogenic include sepsis, anaphylaxis, electrical shock, and inadvertent drug toxicity

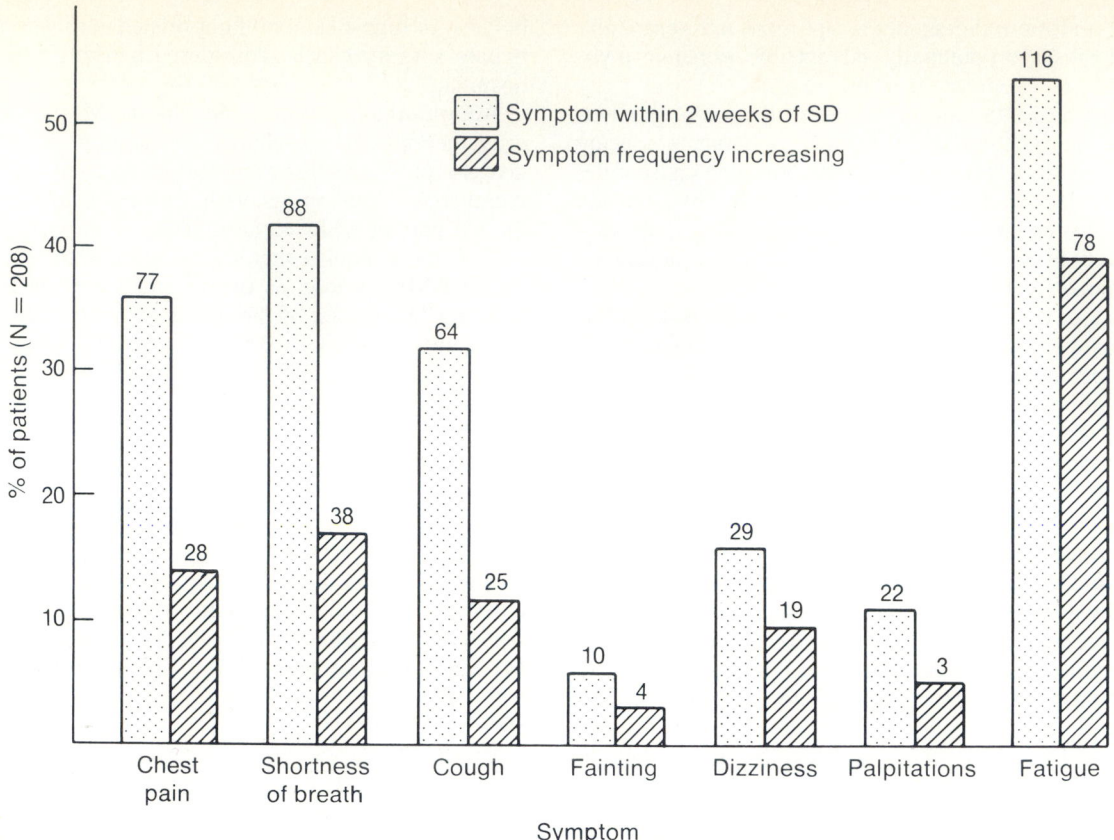

Fig. 96-3 Percentage of patients with atherosclerotic cardiovascular disease and sudden death, *SD,* who exhibited prodromes before their event. (Abstracted from Kuller L, Cooper M, and Perper J: Arch Intern Med 129:714, 1972.)

(as seen with tricyclic antidepressants, phenothiazines, diuretics, digitalis, quinidine, and procainamide).

Cardiovascular abnormalities precipitating sudden death can be divided into extracardiac problems (aortic dissection, cardiac tamponade, exsanguination, and hypovolemia) and intrinsic cardiac problems (by far the most significant of which are arrhythmias related to ischemic heart disease). Cardiac lesions other than CAD account for sudden death no more than 10% of the time. These lesions include mitral valve prolapse syndrome, bacterial endocarditis, obstructive cardiomyopathy, myocarditis, rheumatic heart disease, metastatic malignancies, congenital defects, and valvular abnormalities.

EPIDEMIOLOGY. The incidence of sudden death cannot be determined exactly. It appears, however, that 15% to 30% of all natural deaths should be categorized in this fashion. Sudden death seems to have a bimodal population distribution, with highest rates occurring at 1 to 6 months of age (sudden infant death syndrome seen in 3 of 1000 live-born infants) and 35 to 70 years. Males account for more deaths than females in all age-groups. Ninety percent of adults with sudden death occurring within 1 hour of the first symptoms have cardiovascular disease; 80% to 90% of this group have atherosclerotic cardiovascular disease. Significantly, 60% to 70% of atherosclerotic-related sudden death occurs out of the hospital, with 30% of patients with CAD having sudden death as their initial disease manifestation.

PATHOGENESIS. The final common pathway in sudden death is always an arrhythmia. Focal cardiac necrosis (acute or old MI) causes ventricular tachycardia and fibrillation.

One of the most important, potentially controllable associations with sudden death is the premature ventricular contrac-

tion (PVC). Several epidemiologic studies have shown that frequent PVCs indicate an increased risk for sudden death, presumably by inducing unstable ventricular arrhythmias such as ventricular tachycardia and fibrillation. The Framingham data demonstrated, however, that PVCs were a sudden death risk factor only when there was ECG evidence of atherosclerotic cardiovascular disease.

Three basic mechanisms could account for the development of ventricular arrhythmias following ischemic events: (1) unbalanced automaticity in multiple myocardial foci; (2) periinfarction or ischemic zone reentrant arrhythmias; and (3) depolarization afterpotentials. In the early period following myocardial necrosis, the important mechanism seems to be reentrant pathways created in the ventricular muscle as a result of slow conduction through ischemic or infarcted tissue. Later arrhythmias seem to arise in subendocardial Purkinje fibers, which develop spontaneous diastolic depolarization (and consequently slowed conduction), as well as prolonged action potential duration. A modifying element is parasympathetic/sympathetic imbalance, probably owing to modulating central nervous system factors.

In any event the ultimate consequence of the dysrhythmia (whether it be ventricular tachycardia, ventricular fibrillation, or asystole) is disruption of the cardiac pump function. Ineffectual pump output results in immediate tissue hypoperfusion with lactic acidosis and subsequent cellular death. Unless adequate tissue oxygenation can be maintained with effective cardiopulmonary resuscitation, cellular death with organism demise ensues. A vicious cycle persists as perpetuation of arrhythmias is encouraged by cellular acidosis and hypoxia.

CLINICAL MANIFESTATIONS. Sudden death may be truly

Table 96-4   Comparison between sudden death patients with MI and those without MI

	Sudden death with acute MI	Sudden death without MI
Prodromes	Yes	No
Duration of symptoms before sudden death	Minutes to hours	Seconds
Presence of PVCs	Yes	Yes (advanced grades)
Recurrence rate of sudden death	<5%	30%

unexpected, or it may follow a short period of prodromal warning. Prodromes are retrospectively recognized in 20% of cases. Fig. 96-3 demonstrates the incidence of different prodromal symptoms in a group of 208 patients with atherosclerosis and sudden death. These symptoms were ignored or minimized by most patients. Table 96-4 compares patients with sudden death and acute MIs to those without documented MIs. The patients with MIs have prodromes, with heralding symptoms present minutes to hours before the event. In addition, patients without associated acute MI are more likely to have recurrence of sudden death and usually have advanced forms of ventricular ectopia.

Fortunately, many individuals with sudden death can be saved. Cobb and others have reported on 400 patients who were resuscitated following sudden death owing to ventricular fibrillation. Of this group 35% had cardiopulmonary resuscitation (CPR) initiated by bystanders.

MANAGEMENT. Sudden death is potentially reversible. The prerequisites for reversibility are appropriate recognition of the event and immediate institution of basic life support measures. The value of CPR has been demonstrated in community-wide studies in which the 1-year survival rate of those successfully resuscitated was 70%.

CPR with effective maintenance of artificial ventilation and circulation must be instituted immediately. This should be followed by advanced life support measures that might include endotracheal intubation, cardiac monitoring for arrhythmias, defibrillation if indicated, maintenance of an intravenous infusion line, and pharmacotherapy to correct metabolic acidosis and aid in establishing an effective cardiac rhythm and circulation.

PREVENTION. Sudden death occurs mainly among patients with CAD. The identification of individuals at risk of sudden death is the subject of active investigation. Certain subsets of patients with recent MI who are predisposed to sudden death can be identified; for example, a patient with anterior infarction and bundle branch block would benefit from prolonged ECG monitoring to predict ventricular tachyrhythmias, as well as from evaluation for a pacemaker.

Rapid delivery of advanced CPR systems and wide-spectrum community training in CPR are also critical. Initiation of CPR by trained laymen lessens neurologic sequelae in survivors.

Identification of patients at risk for sudden death has been linked to complex forms of PVCs. A large survey demonstrated that the prevalence of ventricular ectopia was 0.6% on resting ECGs of 67,375 asymptomatic military men. Only 6 of 122,043 individuals clinically free from ischemic heart disease had complex ectopia such as multifocal PVCs or ventricular tachycardia. The mere presence of PVCs does not mean cardiovascular disease. Indeed, 24-hour ECG monitoring of asymptomatic medical student volunteers revealed that 50% had one or more PVCs (occasionally multiform). Also, the incidence of PVCs in any given population increases with age.

Several systems of PVC grading have been proposed to identify forms predicting sudden death. One fact is common to all grading methods: short bursts of ventricular tachycardia and PVC couplets increase the odds of an event. Also, multiple forms of PVCs carry an adverse prognostic index. Patients with advanced CAD and left ventricular dysfunction tend to have more complex PVC patterns.

Identification of those at risk for life-threatening arrhythmias using pacemaker stimulation techniques to induce arrhythmias and catheterization techniques for the selection of drug and surgical therapy is the subject of active and thus far fruitful investigation. The indicators for and measures of successful therapy soon may shift away from monitoring PVCs to inducing tachyrhythmias.

Available data demonstrate the effectiveness of prophylactic medical therapy in patients at risk for sudden death. It has been shown that titration of drug dose with blood levels can reduce sudden death from 30% to 10% in the subset of individuals who have once been resuscitated, although not all the monitored ventricular arrhythmias are abolished.

Finally, since many potentially fatal arrhythmias are linked to foci in the left ventricle and many of these foci are the borderline points of an aneurysm or scar, excision of these regions would seem beneficial. However, left ventricular aneurysmectomy alone has not always been effective in abolishing the dangerous arrhythmias. Endocardial and epicardial mapping techniques during induced ventricular tachycardia identify sites of tachycardia origination that can be surgically resected. Surgical therapy for recurrent ventricular tachycardia thus can be substantially improved by identification of the endocardial origin of the arrhythmia followed by appropriately guided surgical resection.

BIBLIOGRAPHY

Brodsky M and others: Arrhythmias documented by 24-hour continuous electrocardiographic monitoring in 50 male medical students without apparent heart disease, Am J Cardiol 39:390, 1977.

Calvert A, Lown B, and Gorlin R: Ventricular premature beats and anatomically defined coronary heart disease, Am J Cardiol 39:627, 1977.

Cobb LA and others: Resuscitation from out-of-hospital ventricular fibrillation: 4 years follow-up, Circulation 52(suppl):223, 1975.

Cohn PF: The role of noninvasive cardiac testing after an uncomplicated myocardial infarction, N Engl J Med 309:90, 1983.

DeWood MA, Spores J, and Notske RN: Medical and surgical management of myocardial infarction, Am J Cardiol 44:1356, 1979.

Ehrich DA and others: The hemodynamic response to intra-aortic balloon counterpulsation in patients with cardiogenic shock complicating acute myocardial infarction, Am Heart J 93:274, 1977.

Ellestad MH, Cooke BM Jr, and Greenbert PS: Stress testing: clinical applications and predictive capacity, Prog Cardiovasc Dis 21:431, 1979.

Eslami B and others: Acute myocardial infarction in the absence of coronary arterial obstruction, Ala J Med Sci 12:322, 1975.

Frick MH and others: Helsinki Heart Study: primary prevention trial with gemfibrozil in middle-aged men with dyslipidemia. Safety of treatment, changes in risk factors, and incidence of coronary heart disease, N Engl J Med 317:1237, 1987.

Frishman WH and Miller KP: Platelets and antiplatelet therapy in ischemic heart disease, Curr Probl Cardiol 11:1285, 1986.

Forrester JS and others: Medical therapy of acute myocardial infarction by application of hemodynamic subsets (in two parts), N Engl J Med 295:1356, 1404, 1976.

The GISSI Study Group: Effectiveness of intravenous thrombolytic treatment in acute myocardial infarction, Lancet 1:397, 1986.

The ISAM Study Group: A prospective trial of intravenous streptokinase in acute myocardial infarction (ISAM), N Engl J Med 314:1465, 1986.

Kannel WB and Feinleib H: Natural history of angina pectoris in the Framingham Study: prognosis and survival, Am J Cardiol 29:154, 1972.

Killip T III and Kimball JT: Treatment of myocardial infarction in a coronary care unit: a two-year experience with 250 patients, Am J Cardiol 20:457, 1967.

Krauss KR, Hutter AM Jr, and DeSanctis RW: Acute coronary insufficiency: course and follow-up, Arch Intern Med 129:808, 1972.

Kuller L, Cooper J, and Perper J: Epidemiology of sudden death, Arch Intern Med 129:714, 1972.

Lie KI and others: Lidocaine in the prevention of primary ventricular fibrillation: a double-blind randomized study in 212 consecutive patients, N Engl J Med 291:1324, 1974.

Lipid Research Clinics Program. The Lipid Research Clinics Coronary Primary Prevention Trial Results I. Reduction in incidence of coronary heart disease, JAMA 251:351, 1984.

Lipid Research Clinics Program. The Lipid Research Clinics Coronary Primary Prevention Trial Results II. The relationship of reduction in incidence of coronary heart disease to cholesterol lowering, JAMA 251:365, 1984.

McIntosh HD and Garcia JA: The first decade of aortocoronary bypass grafting, 1967-1977: a review, Circulation 57:405, 1978.

Pratt CM, Mahmariam JJ, and Young JB: Changing trends in the approach to acute myocardial infarction. In Taylor RW, editor: Critical care medicine, Philadelphia, 1988, JB Lippincott Co.

Revtyak GF and O'Rourke RA: Acute myocardial infarction: current concepts of pathophysiology and therapy, Baylor Cardiology Series 10:5, 1987.

Rifkind BM: Gemfibrozil, lipids and coronary risk, N Engl J Med 317:1279, 1987.

TIMI Study Group: Thrombolysis in myocardial infarction (TIMI) trial: phase I findings, N Engl J Med 312:932, 1985.

Topol EJ, Califf RM, and George BS: A randomized trial of immediate versus delayed elective angioplasty after intravenous tissue plasminogen activator in acute myocardial infarction, N Engl J Med 3:582, 1987.

Turi ZG and Braunwald E: The use of β blockers after myocardial infarction, N Engl J Med 314:1465, 1986.

Young JB and Roberts R: Medical options in chronic stable angina, Cardiovasc Med 10:21, 1985.

97·CARDIAC ARRHYTHMIAS

Jerry C. Luck *and* **Toby R. Engel**

A cardiac arrhythmia is a disturbance of rate, rhythm, or conduction, which may or may not be recognized by the patient. When the disturbance is apparent, the patient may complain of palpitations or dizziness. However, many arrhythmias go unrecognized by the patient and are detected only by special monitoring. Telemetry units with on-line electrocardiogram (ECG) monitoring and ambulatory tape-recorded monitoring facilitate detection and characterization. Some patients may complain of palpitations or dizziness but have only normal cardiac rate and rhythm recorded at the time. Ambulatory event-recorders have facilitated correlation of symptoms to an arrhythmia.

The significance of an episodic arrhythmia depends on its frequency, the type and severity of any underlying heart disease, and the form and rate of the arrhythmia. Quantification of arrhythmia depends on the degree of spontaneous variation. The frequency of ventricular premature complexes (VPCs) may vary daily by as much as 90%. An acute myocardial infarction (AMI) dramatically affects the frequency and type of arrhythmia by altering the substrate. Nearly 30% of AMI patients die before hospitalization, presumably from ventricular fibrillation. On hospitalization VPCs initially are ubiquitous. The danger of fibrillation lasts for 24 to 48 hours, but the risk then abates dramatically. Persistent frequent and complex VPCs in the months following AMI identify a high-risk group for sudden death in the year following AMI.

This discussion centers on the clinical relevance of arrhythmias, including those incidentally recorded. Proper classification of arrhythmias is important for selecting therapy. Mech-anisms are considered when they are relevant to therapy. Finally, controversial topics of therapeutic importance are discussed separately, including the indications for treating VPCs.

NORMAL CONDUCTION AND RHYTHM

The primary pacemaker is the sinus node, located at the high lateral right atrium. Blood flow is principally from an artery that arises from either the right or the circumflex coronary artery. Sympathetic fibers, more from the right stellate ganglion, and parasympathetic vagal fibers innervate the sinus node and surrounding atrium. A normal beat starts with conduction of the impulse from the node to the atrium (sinoatrial conduction).

The impulse spreads through the atrium (perhaps using special internodal tracts) into the atrioventricular (AV) node, which lies on the floor of the interatrial septum near the fibrous skeleton that supports the mitral and aortic valves. Blood flow to the AV node arises from the distal right coronary artery via an AV nodal branch in 90% of individuals. Both sympathetic left stellate fibers and parasympathetic vagal fibers richly innervate the AV node. The AV node modulates the conduction of impulses from the atrium to the common bundle and ventricles. The AV node thus acts as a gate, preventing too many atrial impulses from entering the ventricles (by a property called decremental conduction).

Infranodal conduction is first through the common bundle (His bundle), which traverses the fibrous body and muscular interventricular septum to trifurcate into a right bundle branch and anterior and posterior fascicles of the left bundle branch. The bundle branches ramify into a rapidly conducting network of Purkinje fibers. Branches of the left anterior descending coronary artery supply blood to the common bundle and much of the proximal bundle branches.

Electrocardiographic criteria for normal sinus rhythm are a P wave of sinus origin (normal axis, upright in lead II), a constant P morphology, a rate between 60 and 100 beats/min and a fairly constant P-P interval that varies at most by 0.16 seconds. The sinus rate is influenced by autonomic tone. For example, emotion, position, pain, fever, and drugs alter rate. Noncardiac illness may alter sinus rate, as does heart failure, which accelerates the rate to increase cardiac output. When the sinus node falters, a subsidiary pacemaker generally arises from the specialized conduction system. The atria, AV junction, and ventricle form a hierarchy of slower backup pacemakers.

Conduction defects can occur at any level. The most prevalent defects affect the sinus node, AV node, and the proximal infranodal structures. The ECG can diagnose conduction disturbances at these levels, but sinus node depolarization is not apparent on the ECG, and therefore sinoatrial conduction is not discernible. Profound slowing or absent P waves may indicate sinus dysfunction. A prolonged PR interval suggests an AV nodal defect. Bundle branch and fascicular blocks produce characteristic ECG patterns.

Arrhythmias may be classified as supraventricular or ventricular, and they are further subdivided according to rate. Normal sinus rates range between 60 and 100 beats/min. Tachycardia refers to rates greater than 100 beats/min, and bradycardia to rates less than 60 beats/min. Slower subsidiary pacemakers have different ranges of normal. For example, AV junctional subsidiary pacemakers have rates of 40 to 60 beats/min. Thus AV junctional tachycardia is a junctional rate greater than 60 beats/min, and AV junctional bradycardia is a junctional rate less than 40 beats/min.

TACHYCARDIAS
Supraventricular tachycardias

The commonly recognized supraventricular tachycardias are sinus, atrial, and paroxysmal supraventricular tachycardia (PSVT), atrial flutter, and atrial fibrillation (defined later). Only sinus tachycardia has physiologic causes; all others have pathologic causes. The QRS complexes usually are narrow.

Three mechanisms are invoked in abnormal tachycardia: automaticity, triggered automaticity, and reentry. Abnormal automaticity and triggered automaticity are forms of impulse formation, whereas reentry is a disorder of impulse conduction. Automaticity occurs when a cell exhibits repetitive spontaneous depolarization. A reduction in the maximum diastolic potential favors spontaneous discharge to the threshold voltage that causes the cell to fire. Triggered automaticity is diagnosed when a single cell demonstrates rapid firing initiated by a critically timed premature beat. This rapid firing must be initiated and is not a spontaneously occurring rhythm, but it is hard to diagnose clinically. Reentry is believed to be the most common cause of ectopy. During reentry the impulse travels in a circuit that leads back to its site of origin. Reentry requires at least two electrophysiologically disparate pathways that are connected distally—unidirectional block and an area of slow conduction. A critically timed premature complex can create unidirectional block in one pathway as a result of differences in refractory periods (or recovery). Slowed conduction in the remaining pathway allows for recovery in the blocked pathway, which permits retrograde conduction through the area of unidirectional block.

Sinus tachycardia

Sinus tachycardia generally ranges between 100 and 150 beats/min, and in adults the rate may exceed 150 beats/min in the presence of cardiovascular collapse, respiratory failure, or thyrotoxicosis. With maximal exercise the rate can increase to 180 to 200 beats/min. In children sinus rates can approach 230 beats/min. Sinus tachycardia frequently occurs because of emotion, fever, and anemia. Several drugs can accelerate sinus rate by direct action or by sympathomimetic or parasympatholytic action. Pulmonary causes are obstructive lung disease, embolism, asthma, and pneumonia. Any pathologic state that requires increased cardiac output should result in sinus tachycardia. In general, sinus tachycardia alone does not produce symptoms, and therapy is aimed at correcting the underlying cause.

Atrial tachycardia

Atrial tachycardia is a run of atrial complexes faster than sinus rhythm, with P waves that are not of sinus origin. Atrial tachycardias may be caused by reentry or enhanced automaticity and may be either regular or chaotic. Chaotic (multifocal) atrial tachycardia is diagnosed with P waves of at least three different forms in the same lead, irregular P-P intervals, and varying PR intervals. It commonly is mistaken for atrial fibrillation because of the irregular rhythm. Either may be seen in patients with decompensated chronic lung disease, severe heart disease (for example, dilated cardiomyopathy), and digitalis excess. Patients generally are elderly and often are severely ill, having associated electrolyte imbalance or septicemia. Digitalis excess frequently causes atrial tachycardia with AV block.

Paroxysmal supraventricular tachycardia

Paroxysmal supraventricular tachycardia (PSVT) applies to a group of regular tachycardias with rates between 150 and 250 beats/min. AV nodal reentrant tachycardia is the most common form and involves dual pathways within the node. A second common variety is based on reentry involving an accessory pathway (for example, Wolff-Parkinson-White syndrome). These account for nearly 90% of the regular PSVTs. Premature complexes are necessary to initiate the tachycardia. In the AV node, with two disparate pathways a critically timed atrial premature complex can create unidirectional block, conduct slowly down one pathway, and reenter retrogradely via the other to complete the circus movement. Premature ventricular complexes also can start reentry and initiate PSVT in individuals with an accessory pathway. In the latter instance the normal AV nodal pathway generally acts as the anterograde limb of the tachycardia, and the accessory pathway functions as the retrograde limb.

Wolff-Parkinson-White syndrome

Wolff-Parkinson-White (WPW) syndrome is associated with paroxysmal supraventricular tachyrhythmias. It has a characteristic ECG pattern (Fig. 97-1) with a short PR interval and a wide QRS complex with a slurred upstroke or δ-wave. Associated ST segment and T wave abnormalities also are present because of abnormal ventricular depolarization. The ECG of WPW syndrome can mimic myocardial infarction. The pattern and the PSVTs are explained by an accessory AV conduction pathway, present from birth, that provides an alternate route from the atria to the ventricles. This accessory connection has two properties different from the AV node, rapid conduction and recovery proportional to heart rate. The short PR ("preexcitation") thus is explained by the rapid AV conduction, and the QRS complex is a composite of two activation fronts, the anomalous ventricular activation at the site of insertion of the accessory pathway producing the δ-wave.

Since there are two AV connections, circus movements are possible, allowing for reentrant tachycardia, usually precipitated by an atrial premature complex taking the following pathway: atrium to AV node anterograde to the ventricle, and accessory pathway retrograde back to the atrium. These reentrant tachycardias often are much faster than is typical for PSVT of the AV node, frequently cause symptoms, and are more difficult to prevent with medication. Also, atrial fibrillation or flutter can occur, during which the gating mechanism of the AV node (decremental conduction) is circumvented and atrial impulses pass rapidly to the ventricles via the accessory pathway, producing extremely rapid ventricular rates and sometimes even ventricular fibrillation and sudden death. Sudden death usually is seen only after institution of digoxin or verapamil. Both agents frequently are used to treat reentrant PSVT but can facilitate AV conduction over the accessory pathway and are contraindicated in patients with WPW syndrome who have atrial fibrillation. However, these drugs are quite effective in patients with WPW syndrome who have reentrant PSVT but no atrial fibrillation. Digoxin can be used more safely in children with WPW syndrome, since atrial fibrillation and flutter are unusual in children.

Another preexcitation syndrome is Lown-Ganong-Levine syndrome, in which the ECG shows a short PR interval but a normally conducted QRS complex. In these cases rapid conduction occurs through or alongside the AV node, and reentrant tachycardia occurs as a result of the dual AV pathways. Less often an accessory pathway arises from either the AV node (nodoventricular) or the His bundle (fasciculoventricular) and inserts into the interventricular septum. This pathway comprises Mahaim fibers, which produce a normal PR interval but a wide QRS complex with a δ-wave.

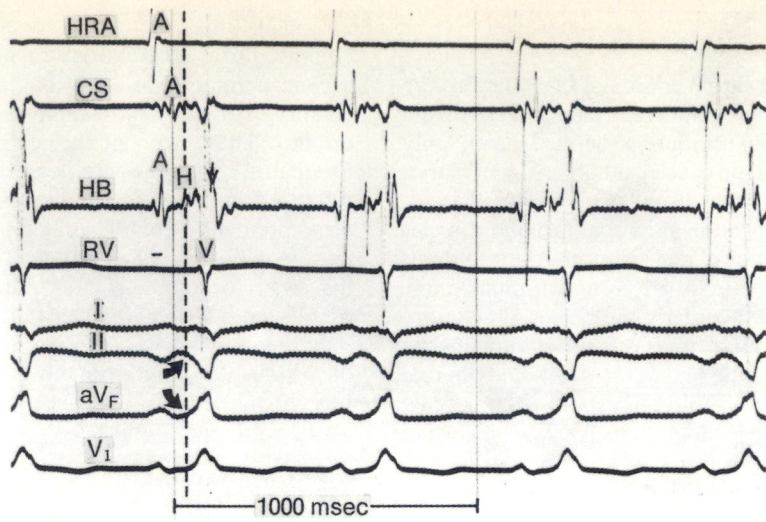

Fig. 97-1 Wolff-Parkinson-White (WPW) syndrome. Top four traces are intracardiac traces from high right atrium *(HRA)*, coronary sinus near left atrium *(CS)*, "His" bundle *(HB)*, and right ventricle *(RV)*. HB trace shows sequence of AV conduction from atrium to HB to ventricle. However, dotted line indicates ventricular activation (surface leads) simultaneous with activation of HB and is called "delta" wave. Presence of "delta" wave and simultaneous excitation of HB and ventricle (HV interval = 0) diagnose accessory pathway from atrium to ventricle.

The ECG is helpful in differentiating the anatomical site of the PSVT. In AV nodal reentrant tachycardia, the retrograde P wave commonly occurs simultaneously with or soon after the QRS complex. In patients with narrow QRS tachycardias involving an accessory pathway, the retrograde P always is recorded later, in the ST-T segment.

Atrial flutter

Classic (type 1) atrial flutter is characterized by an atrial rate of 250 to 350 beats/min and a 2:1 or 4:1 ventricular response. Occasionally, 1:1 AV conduction occurs, and this should suggest superimposed preexcitation (as in WPW syndrome) or drug therapy with parasympatholytics (quinidine). High degrees of AV block (greater than 4:1) in the absence of drug therapy suggest concomitant AV conduction disease. The ECG pattern of classic atrial flutter is a saw-toothed atrial pattern (best seen in leads II or V_1). Atrial flutter frequently is misdiagnosed as PSVT because the flutter waves are not obvious and the QRS response rate is 150 beats/min (Fig. 97-2). Atypical or impure type 2 flutter is characterized by faster atrial rates of 340 to 440 beats/min.

Atrial flutter may be chronic or paroxysmal. Chronic atrial flutter typically occurs with organic heart disease, especially rheumatic mitral valve disease. Paroxysmal atrial flutter may be seen in apparently healthy individuals, in those recovering from open heart surgery, and in patients with hyperthyroidism, WPW syndrome, pulmonary embolism, pericarditis, cardiomyopathy, diphtheria, chest trauma, alcohol excess, and sick sinus syndrome (discussed later). The paroxysmal form may degenerate into atrial fibrillation and frequently is seen in the transition from atrial fibrillation to sinus rhythm. Symptoms of atrial flutter depend on the ventricular response rate and the degree of underlying heart disease.

Atrial fibrillation

Atrial fibrillation is the most common tachyrhythmia. The ECG pattern for atrial fibrillation (Fig. 97-3) shows replacement of P waves by fibrillatory waves that are rapid, irregular oscillations (about 500/min), with an irregular ventricular response that is rapid (120 to 180 beats/min). When the ventricular response is very rapid (greater than 220 beats/min), WPW syndrome should be considered. Conversely, slow ventricular responses may be seen in the elderly, with AV nodal conduction slowed by drugs (β-blockers, digitalis, calcium channel blockers), or in underlying AV conduction disease (block). The QRS complex usually is narrow. However, a short R-R interval may impinge on refractoriness of only one bundle branch and cause aberrancy (a wide complex, discussed later).

Atrial fibrillation is seen most frequently in patients with organic heart disease. It is associated with rheumatic mitral valve disease, WPW syndrome, sick sinus syndrome, and congestive heart failure. It may occur in some patients with hyperthyroidism, excessive alcohol ingestion, and acute myocardial infarction. Atrial fibrillation is unusual in children without congenital heart disease. It may be chronic or paroxysmal, and patients with either type have an increased risk of embolic stroke. As with atrial flutter the severity of underlying heart disease and the ventricular response rate determine the hemodynamic status and symptoms of patients with atrial fibrillation. Treatment depends on the cause, the duration of the arrhythmia, and the patient's hemodynamic status.

Nonparoxysmal AV junctional tachycardia

Junctional pacemakers normally have rates of 40 to 60 beats/min. Nonparoxysmal AV junctional tachycardia (accelerated junctional rhythm) has a rate between 60 and 130 beats/min and almost always occurs in patients with heart disease. It may be seen with digitalis intoxication, acute inferior myocardial infarction, acute rheumatic fever, myocarditis, or open heart surgery. The rhythm is regular with a narrow QRS and absent, retrograde, or dissociated P waves. It seems to result from increased automaticity.

Ventricular tachycardia

Accelerated idioventricular rhythms (60 to 100 beats/min) probably reflect automatic foci. Since the ventricular rhythm

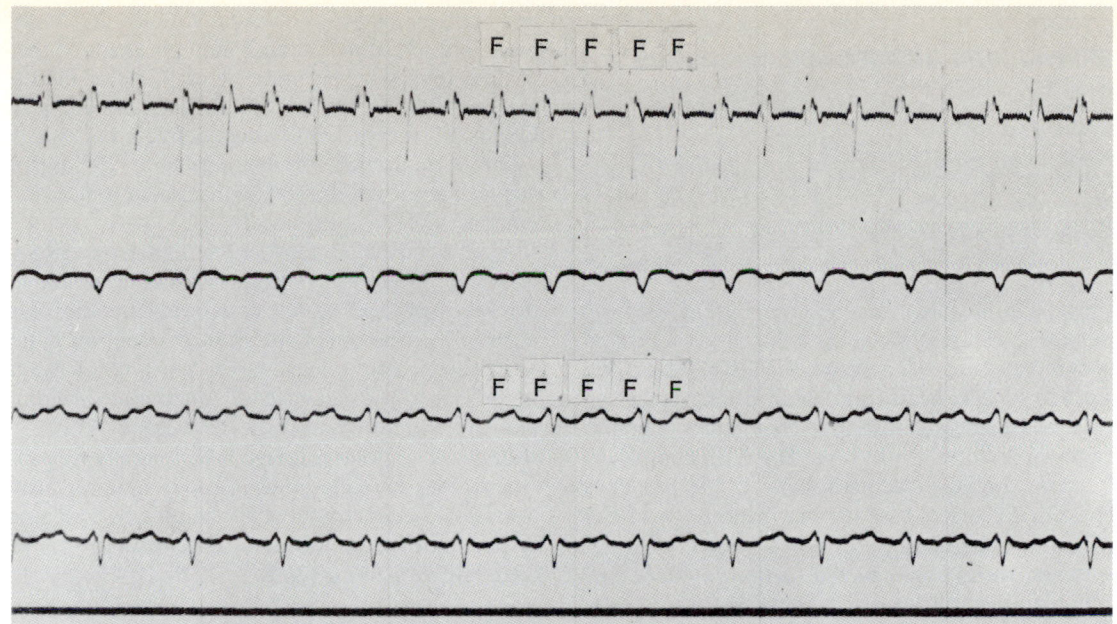

Fig. 97-2   Atrial flutter (250 bpm). Top trace is intracardiac atrial ECG and other three are surface leads. There are 1-second time lines. Regular atrial pattern is best seen in middle surface lead when aligned with atrial recording. There is 2:1 AV block. *F,* flutter waves.

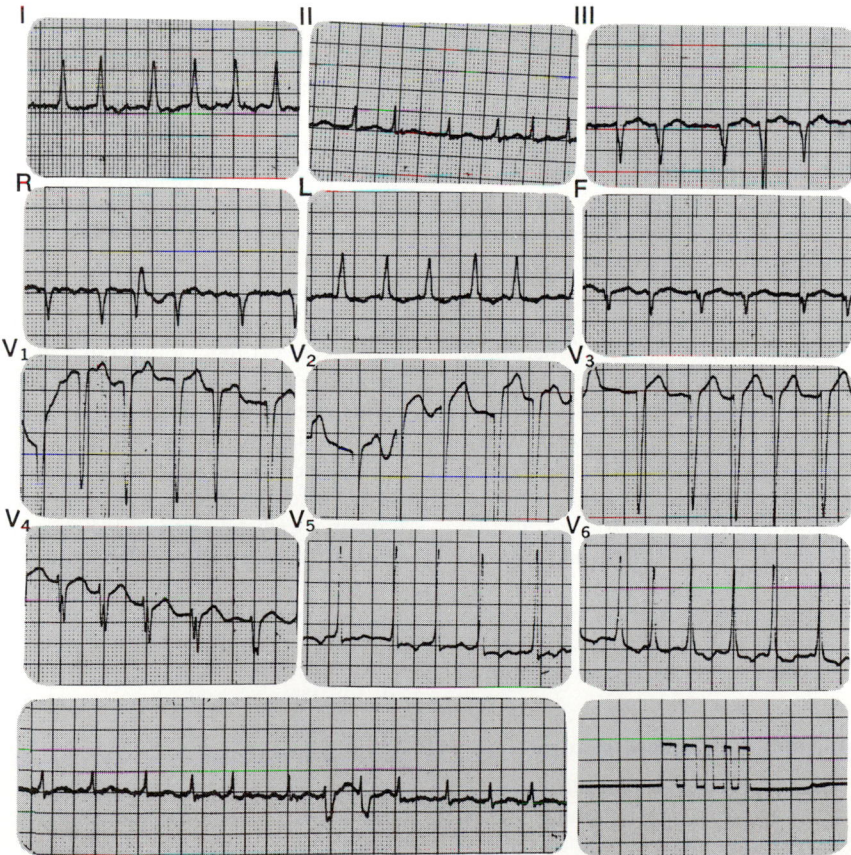

Fig. 97-3   Atrial fibrillation. Atrial activity is represented by irregular oscillations, and there is irregular rapid ventricular response. Some ventricular responses are aberrantly conducted, such as fourth beat in lead III, third beat in aV$_R$, and two beats in rhythm strip at bottom.

ETIOLOGIC FACTORS OF TORSADE DE POINTES

Congenital long QT: Jervell and Lange-Nielsen syndrome, Romano-Ward syndrome
Antiarrhythmic drugs: (classes 1 and 3)
Tranquilizers: (phenothiazines)
Severe bradycardia AV block
Nerve gas and organophosphate insecticides

---

and the sinus have similar rates there is competition resulting in fusion complexes. Ventricular tachycardia is a succession of ventricular complexes at rates faster than 100 beats/min (often reaching 120 to 240 beats/min) and usually based on reentry. It may be nonsustained, sustained for minutes to hours, or degenerate into ventricular fibrillation. The QRS complexes are wide and bizarre, because the ventricular origin produces an abnormal pattern of ventricular depolarization. The ECG diagnosis depends on recognizing atrial dissociation from the ventricles. Supraventricular captures and fusion complexes result from AV dissociation and further indicate that the focus is ventricular. Ventricular tachycardia usually occurs in the setting of organic heart disease, most commonly coronary heart disease, following recovery from myocardial infarction and frequently with ventricular aneurysm.

Incessant or frequently recurring ventricular tachycardia is rare but most often is seen when antiarrhythmic agents are being used. Bidirectional ventricular tachycardia (beats of alternating form or axis) suggests digitalis intoxication. Antiarrhythmic agents that prolong the QT interval can cause *torsade de pointes,* which is rapid paroxysms of ventricular tachycardia that appear to be revolving or turning on an axis. Any agent or condition that prolongs the QT interval potentially can produce this condition (see box).

Ventricular flutter and fibrillation

Ventricular flutter and fibrillation are not compatible with more than momentary survival, since they cause rapid hemodynamic deterioration. Ventricular flutter has rates of 250 to 350 beats/min and a sinusoidal QRS form. Ventricular fibrillation produces a chaotic pattern without discrete QRS potentials or periods of electrical quiescence.

The disease most frequently predisposing an individual to these lethal arrhythmias is coronary heart disease. Other forms of heart disease causing fibrillation or flutter are cardiomyopathy, rheumatic and degenerative valvular heart disease (particularly aortic stenosis), cardiac trauma, mitral valve prolapse, and the prolonged QT interval syndrome. Drug intoxication (digitalis, all class 1 antiarrhythmic drugs), cardiac surgery, and cardiac catheterization also can cause ventricular fibrillation. Finally, electrolyte imbalance, electrocution, and terminal noncardiac disease end in ventricular fibrillation. Flutter and fibrillation generally do not abate spontaneously. Rapid, direct current shock usually is necessary. The underlying cause is the primary factor determining whether electrical conversion will be effective.

Aberrant conduction versus ventricular ectopy

Wide QRS complexes and tachycardia can result from (1) a ventricular origin, (2) WPW syndrome, (3) bundle branch block, or (4) tachycardiac-related aberrancy. In the absence of AV dissociation and fusion complexes or sinus capture, the ECG diagnosis of ventricular tachycardia is uncertain. However, certain QRS morphologic features favor a ventricular origin: duration longer than 0.14 second, left axis deviation,

and certain patterns in leads V_1 and V_6. With right bundle branch block form, the morphologic features that suggest ventricular origin are an initial R in V_1 taller than the terminal R and a QS in V_6. In left bundle branch configurations, QR or QS in V_6 favors ventricular tachycardia. An irregular, very rapid (more than 220 beats/min) wide QRS tachycardia should suggest atrial fibrillation with conduction over an accessory pathway (WPW syndrome).

Supraventricular tachycardia has narrow QRS complexes unless there is WPW syndrome with anterograde conduction via the accessory pathways, underlying bundle branch block, or aberrancy. Aberrancy refers to conduction delay or block of supraventricular impulses over portions of the bundle branch system as a consequence of functional differences in bundle branch refractoriness. The QRS shows bundle branch block patterns of various degrees. Aberrancy is more likely to occur when the ventricular rate is rapid. During atrial fibrillation, aberrancy occurs frequently when a long R-R interval (causing dispersion of refractoriness) is followed by an abbreviated one (Ashman's phenomenon).

Treatment of tachycardias

Appropriate treatment of a tachycardia depends on an accurate diagnosis. Whenever possible a 12-lead ECG should be examined and interpreted in light of the clinical presentation. Narrow QRS tachycardia must be supraventricular in origin, but wide QRS tachycardia may be either ventricular or supraventricular. Vagal maneuvers (carotid massage, Valsalva maneuver, gagging) in a relatively stable patient may help diagnose or even terminate the tachycardia. Increased vagal tone slows conduction in the AV node, sometimes terminating supraventricular tachycardias that use the AV node as part of the reentrant circuit.

Supraventricular tachycardias are distressing but frequently well tolerated. However, for the patient with hypotension, pulmonary edema, or AMI, low-energy direct current (dc) cardioversion is the best therapy. A regular narrow QRS tachycardia (PSVT) in a stable patient may be treated with a rapid-acting agent such as verapamil (0.075 to 0.15 mg/kg intravenously over 2 minutes). However, verapamil given for ventricular tachycardia frequently is ineffective and produces hemodynamic decompensation. It is contraindicated in wide QRS tachycardias unless it is certain the origin is supraventricular. Atrial tachycardias, both regular and multifocal, frequently are secondary to an automatic focus, and class 1 antiarrhythmic agents often successfully suppress these foci. Multifocal atrial tachycardia also may respond to verapamil.

Sustained monomorphic ventricular tachycardia usually requires urgent cardioversion, but occasionally parenteral class 1 agents may be used. Electrophysiologic testing is recommended to determine appropriate therapy for prevention of a recurrence. The conventional class 1 antiarrhythmic agents are effective at preventing recurrence of ventricular tachycardia in a minority of patients. Amiodarone may be the most effective agent. However, it has a high frequency of intolerable side effects. Drug failures are managed with surgical excision of the focus (at high surgical risk) or by implantation of an automatic implantable cardioverter-defibrillator. Newer devices combine antitachycardia pacing with defibrillation. On the other hand, torsades de pointes frequently is caused by type 1 antiarrhythmic agents. In such cases discontinuing the offending agent usually suffices, but temporary pacing can suppress recurrences until the drug is metabolized.

The only therapy for ventricular fibrillation is immediate countershock.

BRADYCARDIAS AND HEART BLOCK

Symptomatic bradycardia results from sinus node dysfunction (sick sinus syndrome) or AV block. The consequences of bradycardia and heart block depend on the site and consequent rate of the escape pacemaker. Patients with very slow heart rates may have fatigue, dizziness, or frank syncope. Slow rates may aggravate heart failure. However, many bradycardic patients have few or no symptoms.

Sinus bradycardia refers to sinus rates less than 60 beats/min, but it often is asymptomatic until rates fall below 35 beats/min. Heart rate decreases with age, and it is not uncommon for the elderly to have sinus bradycardia. Well-trained athletes usually have sinus bradycardia. Periodic sinus bradycardia in an asymptomatic individual is not necessarily abnormal, and therapy is not indicated for bradycardia per se. Persistent or severe sinus bradycardia should alert the practitioner to the possibility of sinus node dysfunction, and patients with symptoms such as dizziness or syncope should be evaluated further.

Sinus node dysfunction

Severe sinus node dysfunction may show up as sinus arrest (a failure of automaticity) or sinoatrial block (a failure of conduction to the atrium). Since the sinus impulse is not appreciated on the surface ECG, first-degree (prolonged sinoatrial conduction internal) and third-degree (complete) sinoatrial block go unrecognized. Only second-degree sinoatrial block can be diagnosed by ECG, by the pattern of the P waves. Mobitz type 1 (Wenckebach) sinoatrial block is diagnosed by progressively shorter P-P intervals until a dropped P wave appears. Mobitz type 2 sinoatrial block is diagnosed by pauses that are multiples of the basic P-P interval. In contrast, sinus arrest shows a random pause that is not a multiple of the basic P-P interval (Fig. 97-4). Pauses as long as 2 or even 3 seconds sometimes are recorded in normal individuals (especially athletes or during sleep). Pauses longer than 3 seconds are abnormal, since subsidiary pacemakers should provide an escape before then.

Sinus node dysfunction may be a result of intrinsic disease, autonomic nervous system imbalance, or drug therapy. Associated atrial disease and tachyrhythmias frequently are present. About half of these patients also have recognizable AV conduction disease. Hypersensitive carotid sinus syndrome also causes sinus node dysfunction and is diagnosed when carotid stimulation produces pauses longer than 3 seconds (cardioinhibitory reflex). However, many older individuals with a hypersensitive carotid sinus reflex are asymptomatic.

Symptomatic sinus node dysfunction with dizziness, syncope, or fatigue is called *sick sinus syndrome,* a disorder that is more common in the elderly. The diagnosis is confirmed by ECG recordings of pauses during symptomatic periods, and it also should be considered if tachycardia-bradycardia episodes occur or if sinus arrest is present after dc shock of atrial fibrillation. Some patients have only persistent, severe, or inappropriate sinus bradycardia. If evidence of sinus node dysfunction (arrest, block, or tachycardia-bradycardia) is absent on monitoring, provocative testing can be employed to unmask sinus dysfunction, but these tests are insensitive. Carotid massage may produce sinus pauses or sinoatrial block. Exercise testing may show a blunted heart rate response. Many individuals fail to show the expected increase in heart rate after intravenous atropine. Finally, sinus node function can be evaluated using atrial overdrive pacing and the atrial extrastimulus technique. The postpacing interval (sinus node recovery time) is a measure of sinus automaticity. Abnormal recovery times are about 90% specific for sick sinus syndrome but only 75% sensitive. The sinoatrial conduction time can be estimated by programmed atrial extrastimulation, but it is prolonged in fewer than half of patients with sick sinus syndrome.

Pacing is not indicated for asymptomatic sinus bradycardia but only for patients who have symptoms while monitoring shows severe bradycardia or pauses. The symptomatic patient with mere sinus bradycardia should be evaluated and should receive a permanent pacemaker if prolonged sinus node recovery or sinoatrial conduction is recorded. Patients with tachycardia-bradycardia syndrome often are paced to ensure the safe use of antiarrhythmic therapy for suppressing the tachyrhythmias.

Some have advocated atrial or AV sequential pacing for patients with sick sinus syndrome. However, many with sick sinus syndrome eventually develop persistent atrial fibrillation. Also, half of patients with this disorder have associated AV conduction disease. Thus ventricular pacing often is appropriate, and rate-responsive pacing may be the optimal pacing modality.

AV block

AV block can occur at the level of the atrium, AV node, common (His) bundle or bundle branches. The surface ECG does not allow for the precise identification of the site of block, but recording of the His bundle electrogram identifies whether conduction abnormalities are above or below the common bundle.

AV block may be first-degree (prolonged PR interval), second-degree (intermittent AV block), or third-degree (complete AV block). The conduction interval through the node accounts for the major portion of the PR interval, and a prolonged PR interval suggests slow nodal conduction rather than delay below the His bundle.

Second-degree AV block is of two types. With Mobitz type 1 (Wenckebach) AV block, PR is progressively prolonged until a nonconducted P wave appears. The postpause PR interval is the shortest of all. The increments of PR prolongation are typically decremental, resulting in progressive R-R interval shortening. This Wenckebach periodicity is characteristic of defects in the AV node. In second-degree AV block, type 2, PR intervals are constant, with sudden failures in AV conduction. Type 2 block suggests infranodal disease.

In third-degree (complete) AV block, the atria and ventricles are controlled by separate pacemakers and the sinus impulse is never propagated to the ventricle. Complete AV block can be congenital or acquired. The defect can be at the level of the AV node, His bundle, or bundle branches (block at the atrial level is rare but may be seen in congenital heart block).

The conduction system below the His bundle is considered trifascicular. There is a right bundle branch and two divisions or fascicles of a left bundle branch. A characteristic ECG pattern is seen with block of each fascicle. Right bundle branch block shows a wide QRS (longer than 0.12 second), rSR', or QR in V_1, and deep S in I and V_6. Left bundle branch block is depicted by wide QRS longer than 0.12 second and a monophasic R wave in I, aVL and V_6. Left anterior fascicular block, the most frequent infranodal conduction abnormality, shows a frontal plane QRS axis less than -30 degrees, a small q in lead I and an r in lead III. The r in III and aVF may mask inferior myocardial infarction. Left posterior fascicular block produces right axis deviation greater than $+120$ degrees, a small q in lead III and a small r in lead I. Right axis deviation from lateral myocardial infarction or from right ventricular

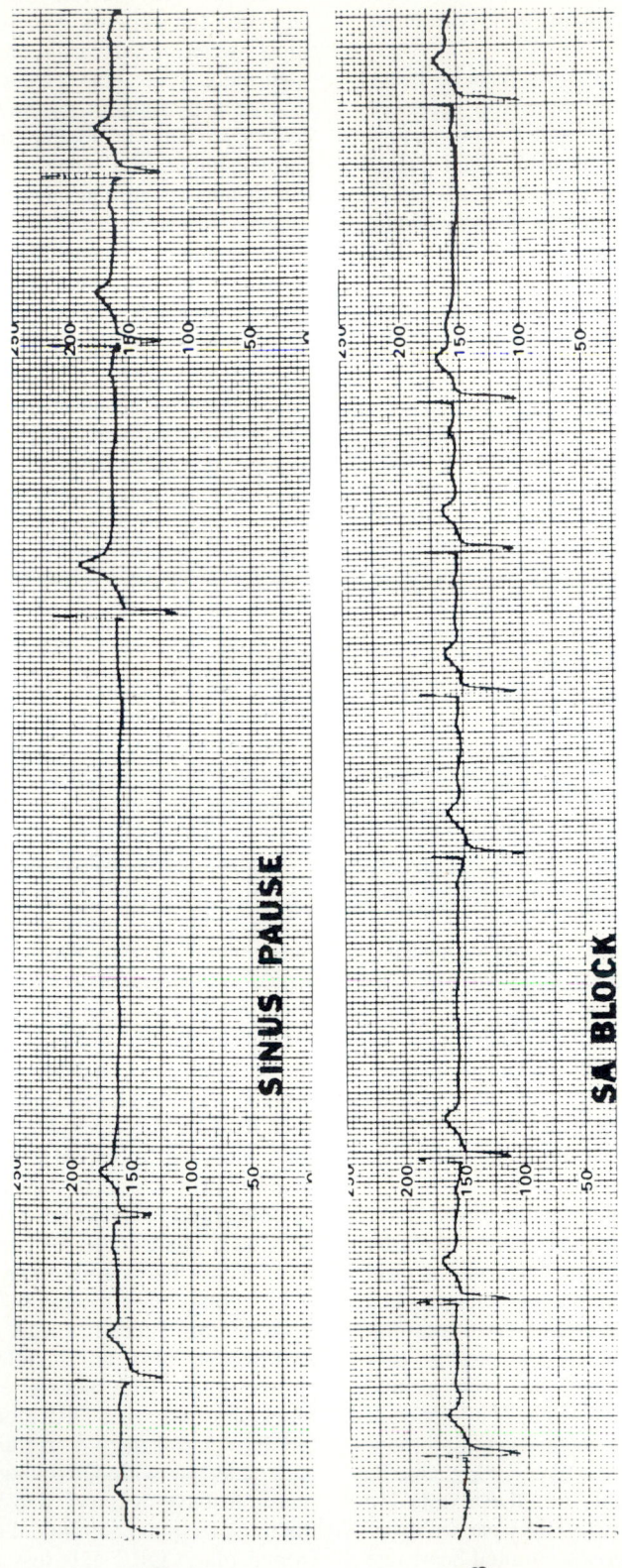

Fig. 97-4   **A,** Sinus pause or arrest. Pause is in excess of 4 seconds and is terminated by junctional escape beat. **B,** Sinoatrial block. Pauses are precisely twice basic sinus-cycle length.

hypertrophy caused by pulmonary or congenital heart disease must be excluded.

Interruption of conduction in a single fascicle causes right bundle branch or left fascicular block. Bifascicular block (block of two of the three infranodal fascicles) fortunately does not often progress to trifascicular or complete block in the absence of acute infarction. Patients with organic structural heart disease have a 5% incidence of progression, whereas patients with only primary conduction disease have a 1% incidence of progression to complete heart block. Management of patients with chronic AV conduction disease depends on the degree and site of blockage and the symptoms. First-degree AV block never requires pacing. Permanent pacemaker therapy is recommended for all symptomatic patients with intermittent (second-degree) or complete (third-degree) AV block. The asymptomatic patients with second- or third-degree AV block in the His bundle or below might warrant a permanent pacemaker. The asymptomatic patient with Mobitz type I (Wenckebach) AV block (implying that the defect is AV nodal, above the His bundle) can be followed without a pacemaker. Most children with congenital AV block are asymptomatic and do not require a pacemaker until symptoms develop. Asymptomatic patients with bifascicular block who are to undergo surgery do not need temporary pacemakers.

VENTRICULAR PREMATURE COMPLEXES (VPCs)

Normal individuals have some VPCs. In one study, half of healthy medical students had VPCs on a 24-hour tape-recorded monitor. Frequency was low, and complex forms were rare. VPCs increase with age and the severity of heart disease. When 811 men were monitored for 6 hours, 20% of the men 35 to 45 years of age had VPCs, whereas 80% of those over 65 years of age had VPCs. The presence of VPCs does not imply cardiac disease, but 90% of patients with coronary heart disease have VPCs. After myocardial infarction (MI), patients with more than 10 VPCs per hour have an increased risk of sudden death. Sudden death is clearly never a direct result of the VPCs. Rather, it results from ventricular fibrillation, whether with acute infarction or in the early months after infarction. For example, in acute infarction, frequent and complex VPCs do not necessarily precede ventricular fibrillation. Lidocaine prevents ventricular fibrillation in AMI but does not suppress many of the VPCs, that is, there is a dissociation between VPC suppression and prevention of ventricular fibrillation by lidocaine. Thus VPCs are markers of a risk of ventricular fibrillation but are inconsistent triggers of the event. In individuals who have no cardiac disease, VPCs are not associated with increased mortality.

After MI the risk of dying suddenly is greater, especially within the first 6 months. Patients with frequent and complex forms (multiformed, couplets, salvos of 3 or more), in the presence of moderate to severe left ventricular dysfunction, are at highest risk, but many patients with complex VPCs do not suffer sudden death. Only about 15% of infarction patients die in the year following discharge, but 33% to 50% have frequent and/or complex VPCs.

In the first 24 to 48 hours of AMI, prophylactic treatment with lidocaine reduces the incidence of ventricular fibrillation. However, after 48 to 72 hours the mechanism of ventricular arrhythmias (such as VPCs) is different. Drugs to prevent ventricular arrhythmias sometimes are selected on the basis of simple monitoring or by empiric use of antiarrhythmic agents. However, the drugs may worsen the arrhythmia or increase the risk of sudden death. Invasive electrophysiologic testing with tachycardia induction is recommended for identifying effective therapy to prevent ventricular tachycardia recurrence. Mere suppression of VPCs may not prevent ventricular tachycardia or ventricular fibrillation. Alternatively, antiarrhythmic therapy may prevent cardiac arrest without significantly reducing VPC frequency.

Patients with VPCs and structural heart disease other than coronary heart disease (such as dilated cardiomyopathy) have a somewhat increased risk of sudden death. On the other hand, asymptomatic patients with VPCs and without associated cardiac disease are not at increased risk of sudden death. Antiarrhythmic therapy is unwarranted.

AN OVERVIEW OF ANTIARRHYTHMIC AGENTS

Antiarrhythmic drugs are classified according to their electrophysiologic properties. Class 1 agents are local anesthetics that decrease conduction velocity by retarding the membrane sodium pump. The subgroups of class 1 agents (A, B, and C) are based on their speed of onset and offset. Group 1A includes the traditional agents quinidine, procainamide, and disopyramide. They slow conduction, widen QRS, and prolong refractory periods (prolong QT) at an intermediate rate. Drugs in these groups have a negative inotropic effect. They have an atropine-like property that may facilitate AV nodal conduction and can increase the ventricular response to atrial fibrillation or flutter. Quinidine causes hemolysis, thrombocytopenia, fever, diarrhea, and tinnitus. It increases the serum concentration of digoxin and digitoxin. Procainamide can cause fever, agranulocytosis, gastrointestinal disturbances, myalgias, and a lupuslike syndrome. Antinuclear antibodies form in nearly half of the patients, and arthritis develops in 20% of these. Most side effects of disopyramide are related to its atropine-like action (dry mouth, urinary retention, blurred vision, constipation, and exacerbation of glaucoma) and its exacerbation of heart failure.

Class 1B drugs include lidocaine, phenytoin, mexiletine, and tocainide. Mexiletine and tocainide are oral congeners of lidocaine. They may suppress VPCs but do not alter outcome after MI. This group shortens refractoriness and has little effect on conduction in normal myocardium. Thus the QRS duration and QT interval are not prolonged. Lidocaine in excess produces convulsions, mental confusion, and respiratory arrest. Orally administered phenytoin in excess produces ataxia and nystagmus. In rare cases it causes megaloblastic anemia, pseudolymphoma, or erythema multiforme. Mexiletine and tocainide frequently cause gastrointestinal disturbances and neurologic symptoms. Tocainide not infrequently causes agranulocytosis, and the complete blood count must be monitored. Lidocaine is the drug of choice for prophylaxis against ventricular fibrillation in the early phases of acute myocardial infarction. Phenytoin has been effective in reducing the incidence of sudden death in children with congenital heart disease (notably tetralogy) and frequent VPCs.

Class 1C includes flecainide, encainide, and propafenone. These agents dramatically affect conduction but not refractoriness. Thus AV conduction and the QRS duration routinely are prolonged, but otherwise the QT interval is not. These drugs can produce incessant ventricular tachycardia resistant to dc cardioversion. Flecainide frequently causes dizziness, blurred vision, and headache and can worsen congestive heart failure. Encainide also produces dizziness, diplopia, and paresthesia but does not worsen congestive heart failure.

Propranolol is the prototype class 2 β-adrenergic blocking drug. There are now a host of such drugs, including acebutolol, atenolol, esmolol (which is extremely short acting), metoprolol, sotalol, timolol, and nadolol. These drugs affect arrhyth-

Table 97-1 Generic pacemaker code (NASPE/BPEG)*

Position/ category	1 Chamber paced	2 Sensed	3 Mode of response	4 Programmable rate modulation	5 Antitachy function
Symbol†	O (none) V (ventricle) A (atrium) D (dual)	O V A D	O (none) I (inhibited) T (triggered) D (both)	O (none) P (simple-programmable) M (multiprogrammable) C (communicating [telemetry]) R (rate modulation)	O (none) P (pacing [antitachy]) S (shock) D (dual [P + S])

*NASPE/BPEG, North American Society of Pacing and Electrophysiology/British Pacing and Electrophysiology Group.
†*Examples:* **VVI,R:** ventricular paced, ventricular sensed, R-wave inhibited, rate modulation on; **DDD,C:** dual chamber pacing and sensing, atrial triggered and inhibited, ventricular inhibited, telemetry.

mias by altering the autonomic nervous system. They slow AV nodal conduction and are effective against supraventricular tachyrhythmias. These agents can cause bronchospasm and are contraindicated in asthma and moderately severe obstructive lung disease. They can mask the hypoglycemic effects of insulin overdose. Several (propranolol, metoprolol, timolol, atenolol) have been shown to reduce the incidence of sudden death following discharge from AMI, perhaps in part an antiarrhythmic effect.

Bretylium and amiodarone are class 3 drugs. Bretylium has both sympathomimetic and sympatholytic properties and increases the threshold for fibrillation. Initially it releases norepinephrine from postganglionic sympathetic nerves, increasing blood pressure transiently. Subsequently it blocks release and uptake of norepinephrine, causing orthostatic hypotension. It should be used for life-threatening ventricular arrhythmias refractory to lidocaine. Although classified in class 3, amiodarone has some group 1 effects. However, it markedly prolongs refractory periods out of proportion to its effect on conduction velocity. It may produce hypothyroidism or hyperthyroidism, pulmonary fibrosis, hepatitis, rashes, and microscopic corneal deposits. It presently is indicated only for documented life-threatening ventricular arrhythmias refractory to standard agents and when an electrophysiology laboratory is available.

Class 4 agents block calcium transport into cells. Verapamil and diltiazem have similar effects, principally on tissues that rely primarily on the calcium pump (the sinus and AV nodes). They suppress AV nodal reentrant tachycardia and control the ventricular response to atrial fibrillation and flutter. However, they may cause hypotension, bradycardia, or heart block.

Digoxin remains the mainstay for controlling the ventricular response to atrial fibrillation and for converting fibrillation and flutter to sinus rhythm. The combination of digoxin and diltiazem effectively controls the ventricular response rate in cases difficult to control with digoxin alone.

COUNTERSHOCK

Tachyrhythmias producing hemodynamic collapse, angina pectoris, or pulmonary edema require prompt countershock, which simultaneously depolarizes the entire myocardium, allowing for synchronous repolarization and resumption of sinus rhythm. The energy levels required depend on the type of arrhythmia. Organized tachycardias (PSVT, atrial flutter, ventricular tachycardia) generally respond to low energy levels (10 to 50 joules). Fibrillatory patterns usually require higher energy (100 to 300 joules). Multifocal atrial tachycardia and drug-induced tachyrhythmias resist cardioversion. Cardioversion synchronized to the QRS should be used for all tachycardias except ventricular fibrillation (which has no QRS). The shock is delivered in the safe period just after the peak of the QRS (a nonsynchronized shock may cause ventricular fibrillation when delivered on the T wave).

Digoxin often is discontinued before elective countershock of atrial flutter or fibrillation to avoid ventricular fibrillation, and anticoagulants are given to reduce the likelihood of thromboembolism on return to atrial systole. Generally, class 1 agents are started before cardioversion to maintain sinus rhythm after a successful cardioversion.

PACEMAKERS

Pacemakers were introduced to prevent syncope secondary to AV block. Symptomatic sick sinus syndrome also requires pacing. Pacemakers sometimes are used for termination of supraventricular tachycardia and occasionally for ventricular tachycardia. Automatic implantable cardioverter-defibrillators can be used to detect and shock recurrent ventricular tachycardia or fibrillation internally.

Pacemakers may be single or dual chamber (atrium and ventricle), inhibited or triggered multiprogrammable, and communicating. Three to five position codes are used to communicate information about a pulse generator, programmed mode, and the mode of response (Table 97-1). Originally pacemakers were single chamber units that paced the ventricle and sensed the ventricle in the demand mode (so called VVI mode). Currently, the most popular dual-chamber pacemaker is the DDD mode: both atrium and ventricle are paced, both are sensed, and both are triggered and inhibited. Rate-responsive pacemakers using physiologic sensors (for instance, skeletal muscle motion, temperature, stroke volume, and QT interval) now are available for VVI and soon will be available for DDD pacemakers.

Inadvertent pacemaker reprogramming may result from external electromagnetic noise. Many sources of interference exist in medical and dental settings and in daily life. Electrosurgery (such as cautery) and diathermal treatment are the main offenders. Broadcasting stations, electric pads, razors, or electric toothbrushes may cause interference. Electrotherapy is not contraindicated in patients with pacemakers, but ECG monitoring is mandatory to follow the patient's rhythm. During procedures using electrotherapy, pacemaker-dependent patients should have their units converted to an asynchronous mode by programming or simply by applying a magnet to the generator. Electrosurgery or cautery in the immediate field of the pacemaker may cause low-frequency currents to pass through the generator and lead to ventricular fibrillation. Damage to the generator can be avoided by not using the cautery within 4 to 6 inches of the generator. Should dc cardioversion be required, the paddles should be at least 6 inches from the pacemaker.

The automatic implantable cardioverter-defibrillator currently is used to terminate ventricular fibrillation and some tachycardias that cannot be prevented by drugs. Epicardial patch electrodes are used for defibrillation and either transvenous or epicardial leads are used for sensing. The current system identifies ventricular fibrillation or tachycardia and delivers a 25 to 30 joule shock. Once triggered, the device is committed to delivering a shock. The device can be activated (or deactivated) by a magnet externally placed over the generator. Future devices will also have demand pacing capabilities and sophisticated antitachycardia algorithms.

SUMMARY

The patient suspected of having a cardiac arrhythmia needs accurate characterization of the rhythm. Any disturbance recorded must be correlated with symptoms. The type and severity of underlying heart disease are important to management. Arrhythmia treatment requires recognition and removal of precipating causes and contributing factors. Antiarrhythmic agents frequently can worsen a cardiac arrhythmia. An ideal antiarrhythmic agent has not yet been developed, and sophisticated devices have become the preferred treatment for life-threatening arrhythmias.

BIBLIOGRAPHY

Barold SS, editor: Modern cardiac pacing, Mount Kisco, NY, 1985, Futura Publishing Co, Inc.

Beta Blocker Heart Attack Trial Research Group: A randomized trial of propranolol in patients with acute myocardial infarction. I. Mortality results. JAMA 247:1707, 1982.

Furman S, Hayes DL, and Holmes DR, editors: A practice of cardiac pacing, Mount Kisco, NY, 1986, Futura Publishing Co, Inc.

Horowitz LN and Morganroth J: Second generation antiarrhythmic agents: have we reached antiarrhythmic nirvana? J Am Coll Cardiol 9:459, 1987.

Horowitz LN and Zipes DP: A symposium: perspective on proarrhythmia, Am J Cardiol 59(11):1E, 1987.

Josephson ME and Kastor JA: Supraventricular tachycardia: mechanisms and management, Ann Intern Med 87:346, 1977.

Josephson ME and Wellens HJJ, editors: Tachycardias: mechanism, diagnosis and treatment, Philadelphia, 1984, Lea & Febiger.

Keefe DLD, Kates RE, and Harrison DC: New antiarrhythmic drugs: their place in therapy, Drugs 22:363, 1981.

Kennedy HL and others: Long-term follow-up of asymptomatic healthy subjects with frequent and complex ventricular ectopy, N Engl J Med 312:194, 1985.

Kostis JB and others: Premature ventricular complexes in the absence of identifiable heart disease, Circulation 63:1351, 1981.

Ludmer PL and Goldschlager N: Cardiac pacing in the 1980's, N Engl J Med 311:1671, 1984.

Pratt CM and others: Analysis of the spontaneous variability of ventricular arrhythmias: consecutive ambulatory electrocardiographic recordings of ventricular tachycardia, Am J Cardiol 56:67, 1985.

Surawitz B and Knoeble SB: Long qt: good, bad or indifferent? J Am Coll Cardiol 4:398, 1984.

Zipes DP and Rahimtoola SH, editors: State of the art consensus conference on electrophysiologic testing in the diagnosis and treatment of patients with cardiac arrhythmias, Circulation Supplement, Part 2, 75:(4), 1987.

98 • PERICARDITIS

Charles A. Bush *and* John M. Stang

The pericardium is a two-layered membranous structure surrounding the heart and great vessels. In its normal function the pericardium serves mainly as a protective structure, and the absence or surgical removal of the pericardium does not interfere with normal cardiac function. Like all other organic structures, the pericardium is subject to pathologic disorders resulting in various types of pericardial diseases. Unlike most valvular and congenital cardiac diseases, chronic pericardial disease does not require antibiotic prophylaxis for dental or surgical procedures to prevent endocarditis. Chronic pericardial disease does not contraindicate general anesthesia, but the disease must be accurately distinguished from myocardial ischemic problems.

ACUTE PERICARDITIS

DEFINITION. Acute pericarditis may be defined as active inflammatory disease of the pericardium that develops rapidly and is associated with the sudden onset of symptoms.

ETIOLOGY AND PATHOGENESIS. Acute pericarditis has a variety of causes. The common infectious causes include both viral and bacterial infections. The most common of the viral causes of acute pericarditis is coxsackievirus. Bacterial causes of acute pericarditis, although less common now with the availability of antibiotics, include suppurative bacterial infections of which pneumococcal, staphylococcal, and streptococcal infections are most prevalent. Prior surgical procedures and uremia are predisposing conditions to bacterial pericarditis. Tuberculosis as a cause of acute pericarditis is still common. Other infectious causes of acute pericarditis include fungal and parasitic infestations. Acute pericarditis is a frequent manifestation of connective tissue disease; common examples are systemic lupus erythematosus, rheumatoid arthritis, scleroderma, and mixed connective tissue disease. Acute pericarditis also may be a manifestation of an immunologic response or a hypersensitivity state. Causes for pericarditis in this subgroup include drug reactions, serum sickness, postmyocardial infarction syndrome, and postcardiotomy syndrome. The last two disorders apparently are immunologic responses to myocardial tissue damaged by infarction or surgery, resulting in pericardial inflammation. A variety of drugs, including procainamide and hydralazine, also cause acute pericarditis. Acute pericarditis frequently occurs with transmural myocardial infarction and is related to direct irritation of the pericardium by the infarcted myocardium. Acute pericarditis also may result from both penetrating and nonpenetrating wounds of the pericardium. Other causes are uremia, bacterial endocarditis, and acute rheumatic fever. However, the most common cause of acute pericarditis may be idiopathic or nonspecific pericarditis. This is usually a benign form of pericarditis for which no specific cause can be determined.

The pathogenesis of acute pericarditis depends on the underlying cause. Some type of infectious, immunologic, toxic, or mechanical insult to the pericardium appears necessary to start the process. The resultant pericarditis may be focal or diffuse. Focal pericarditis may be highly localized or spotty; diffuse pericarditis involves the entire pericardium. Acute pericarditis almost always involves at least the epicardial layer of the myocardium, and some of the manifestations of acute pericarditis are in fact related to myocardial involvement.

CLINICAL MANIFESTATIONS. The most common complaint of the patient with acute pericarditis is chest pain. The pain frequently is rather sudden in onset and persistent. It often is made worse by inspiration and lying supine; some relief may be obtained with sitting up and leaning forward. Dyspnea, or shortness of breath, is much less likely to occur with acute pericarditis. Fever is common in both infectious and noninfectious types of acute pericarditis. The pathognomonic physical finding of acute pericarditis is a pericardial friction rub. The pericardial friction rub frequently has three components that are synchronous with atrial systole, ventricular systole, and ventricular diastole. Occasionally the pericardial friction rub may be a two-component rub or a one-component rub. In the latter situation it may be difficult to distinguish a pericardial friction rub from a heart murmur.

It is important to point out that any or all of these findings may be absent with acute pericarditis.

LABORATORY FINDINGS. The specific laboratory findings of the underlying disease causing the acute pericarditis may suggest an examination for pericardial involvement. The white blood count may help indicate the presence of either viral or bacterial infection. Bacterial and viral cultures or viral titers of both acute and convalescent sera may be important in establishing the cause of acute pericarditis. The chest roentgenogram usually is not helpful in making a diagnosis of acute pericarditis, since the cardiac silhouette often is normal. The echocardiogram may be of benefit in identifying a small pericardial effusion. Occasionally a thickened pericardium also may be noted echocardiographically. The electrocardiogram (ECG) is the most useful laboratory study for the diagnosis of acute pericarditis. However, it is important to recognize that the abnormalities in the ECG are not necessarily specific for acute pericarditis, and frequently the ECG may be normal or show only nonspecific changes. In acute pericarditis affecting the pericardium diffusely, the ECG may demonstrate ST segment elevation or deep inverted T waves in all leads. In localized pericarditis the ST segment elevation and T wave inversion may be localized to specific leads. In the latter situation it is vitally important to exclude myocardial injury or infarction as a cause of these ECG changes. The patient with acute pericarditis does not develop Q waves, as does the patient with acute myocardial infarction. Another characteristic ECG change of acute pericarditis is depression of the PR segment. Atrial flutter or atrial fibrillation often is present.

DIAGNOSIS. The diagnosis of acute pericarditis is based on the history and physical findings and their correlation with laboratory studies, particularly the ECG. Acute pericarditis may be confused with acute myocardial infarction, dissecting aneurysm of the aorta, pleurisy, pneumonia, pneumothorax, and chest wall pain. It is important to recognize that acute pericarditis may coexist with all of these disease processes but may be particularly difficult to diagnose.

COURSE. Acute idiopathic and acute viral pericarditis are self-limited diseases that usually resolve gradually over days to weeks. Occasionally, acute pericarditis may be recurrent, and it is not unusual to have recurrent acute pericarditis on several occasions separated by several months. Acute pericarditis may become a chronic disease of the pericardium and may either result in chronic inflammation of the pericardium or evolve to chronic constrictive pericarditis. The course of acute pericarditis depends heavily on the underlying disease. If the underlying disease is progressive, the course of acute pericarditis probably will be chronic and progressive as well. Occasionally, acute pericarditis may be rapidly progressive, with either the rapid development of pericardial constriction or rapid fluid accumulation.

MANAGEMENT. The treatment of acute pericarditis necessitates a knowledge of the specific cause. Treatment of the underlying disease causing the acute pericarditis may be necessary to resolve pericarditis. Management of acute pericarditis in many situations involves supportive care and symptomatic treatment for pain relief. Antiinflammatory agents, including aspirin, indomethacin, and corticosteroids, may be of benefit. Occasionally pericardiectomy (surgical removal of the pericardium) is necessary for total relief of symptoms of pericarditis. This usually is necessary in the setting of chronic inflammatory disease or in recurrent acute pericarditis.

CONSTRICTIVE PERICARDITIS

DEFINITION. Constrictive pericarditis is a chronic disease of the pericardium, resulting from fibrosis and scarring of the pericardium, that interferes with atrial and ventricular diastolic filling of the heart.

ETIOLOGY. Constrictive pericarditis occurs most commonly as a sequela of inflammatory disease of the pericardium. It is most likely to occur secondary to bacterial infection, tuberculosis, radiation, or trauma. Constrictive pericarditis following open heart surgery is becoming increasingly common.

PATHOGENESIS. Chronic inflammation or irritation of the pericardium leads to increasing fibrosis. This eventually may result in scarring of the pericardium, adhesions of the pericardium to the epicardium, and ultimately dense calcification of the pericardium. This pathologic process results in loss of the normal pericardial viscoelastic properties, with formation of a rigid, nonelastic structure surrounding the heart. Depending on the degree of pericardial involvement and the intravascular volume, the physiology of constrictive pericarditis may be either occult or overt. Eventually the inability to fill the heart appropriately in diastole results in a diminution of cardiac output and an increase in venous pressure.

CLINICAL MANIFESTATIONS. The symptoms of a patient with constrictive pericarditis depend on the degree of pericardial involvement and the intravascular volume. Symptomatology may include vague nonspecific chest pain, dyspnea, and fatigue. In most severe cases the patient may have symptoms of right-sided heart failure, fluid retention, and markedly decreased cardiac output. The physical findings of the patient with constrictive pericarditis also depend on the intravascular volume. Frequently the patient demonstrates marked elevation of the jugular venous pressure, with prominent x and y collapses in the jugular venous pressure pulse. There usually is an inspiratory rise in the jugular venous pressure rather than the normal inspiratory fall. The liver frequently is enlarged, and significant peripheral edema may be present. The heart may be enlarged or normal in size. On examination the left ventricle generally is normal, and there are no signs of pulmonary congestion. On auscultation an early diastolic sound sometimes referred to as a pericardial knock is frequently heard.

LABORATORY FINDINGS. The ECG in constrictive pericarditis may be normal. Atrial fibrillation may be present, and the only other likely ECG abnormality is nonspecific ST-T wave changes. The chest roentgenogram and cardiac fluoroscopy can reveal a normal or enlarged cardiovascular silhouette. If pericardial calcification is present, it is a striking pathognomonic finding and appears as a dense, white shell around the heart (Fig. 98-1). The echocardiogram may demonstrate dense echoes of a thickened pericardium. Diagnosis of constrictive pericarditis is established best by cardiac catheterization. Classic findings of constrictive pericarditis at catheterization include characteristic pressure pulse configurations in both the right atrium and right ventricle. The right ventricular pressure pulse demonstrates a characteristic "dip and plateau." The most specific finding of constrictive pericarditis found at the time of catheterization is exact pressure equilibration in all cardiac chambers during ventricular diastole; specifically equilibration of the left ventricular diastolic pressure with left atrial pressure, with pulmonary artery diastolic pressure, with right ventricular diastolic pressure, and with right atrial pressure. This pressure equilibration results from the heart being limited in its filling by the extrinsic shell of the diseased pericardium rather than by the usual limiting factor of individual chamber stiffness. Thus filling the heart results in rapidly attaining a high diastolic

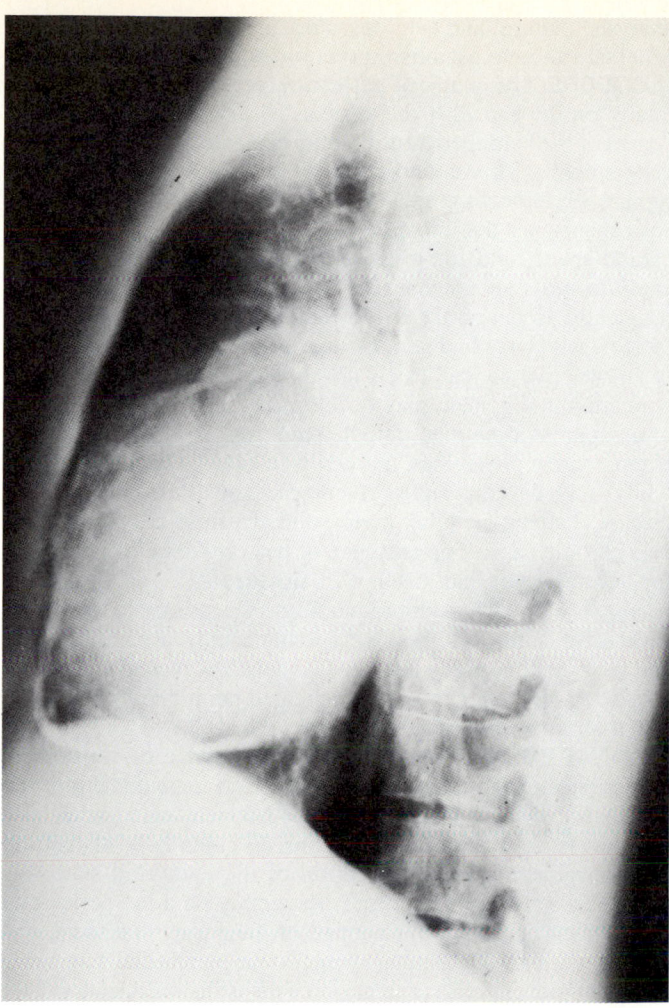

Fig. 98-1 Lateral chest roentgenogram of patient with constrictive pericarditis. Left atrium is enlarged because it is not enclosed within constricted pericardium. Roentgenogram shows a dense, white, calcified pericardium surrounding cardiac silhouette.

pressure that is transmitted equally through all chambers, much as putting air into a basketball results in a rapid rise in pressure within that chamber. When the pressure of filling equals the pressure within the chamber, flow stops and that pressure is maintained until contraction occurs.

DIAGNOSIS. The differential diagnosis of constrictive pericarditis includes valvular heart disease with congestive heart failure, congestive cardiomyopathy, restrictive myocardial disease, and cirrhosis. Each of these entities has subtle findings that enable the careful observer to differentiate constrictive pericarditis. However, in some cases restrictive myocardial disease may exactly mimic the findings of constrictive pericarditis, and the ultimate diagnosis may rest on a surgical and pathologic examination of the pericardium. It is important to realize that constrictive pericarditis may occur in association with other forms of heart disease. Diagnosis of constrictive pericarditis occurring coincidentally with other types of cardiac disease is difficult.

COURSE. Patients with occult constrictive pericardial disease may have a stable course or only a slowly progressive disease process. Many of these patients have a minor degree of disability from a disease that appears to be anatomically and physiologically stable. Patients with more overt constrictive pericarditis tend to have a progressive course. However, the

disease may have a particularly long course, and some patients with calcific constrictive pericarditis appear to be fairly stable with no major sequelae. The most common course of the patient with chronic constrictive pericarditis is one of progressive deterioration of cardiac output and progressive elevation of right-sided heart pressures with peripheral edema and hepatic congestion. The patient eventually may develop end-stage heart failure, with a markedly diminished cardiac output, or develop signs of cardiac cirrhosis with hepatic failure.

MANAGEMENT. Pericardiectomy is the treatment of choice for constrictive pericarditis if the patient is symptomatically disabled from that process. Likewise, pericardiectomy is recommended with signs of overt right-sided heart failure, hepatic congestion, or cardiac cirrhosis.

PREVENTION. Some clinicians believe that aggressive use of antiinflammatory agents early in the course of acute pericarditis prevents the later occurrence of constrictive pericarditis. The use of antibiotic therapy has reduced the incidence of constrictive pericarditis following bacterial pericarditis. Others think that concomitant corticosteroids prevent the development of constrictive pericarditis from tuberculous pericarditis.

EFFUSIVE PERICARDITIS

DEFINITION. When an abnormal amount of fluid accumulates in the pericardial space, this condition is known as effusive pericarditis. Fluid may develop in the pericardial space under little or no pressure, resulting in what is called a lax pericardial effusion. If fluid develops under pressure and there is cardiac compression, the resulting condition is pericardial tamponade.

ETIOLOGY. Inflammatory disease of the pericardium frequently is associated with pericardial effusion. With bacterial pericarditis the pericardial effusion may be pus. Fluid accumulation can occur in the pericardial space in connective tissue disorders and immunologic disorders; rheumatoid arthritis and systemic lupus erythematosus particularly may have significant pericardial effusions. A frequent cause of pericardial effusive disease is hypothyroidism. Bleeding into the pericardial space may result in a bloody pericardial effusion known as hemopericardium. This is likely to occur in relation to anticoagulant therapy, myocardial infarction, myocardial rupture following myocardial infarction, dissecting aneurysm of the aorta, and penetrating cardiac trauma. The patient with biventricular heart failure from any cause, including valvular heart disease, hypertensive heart disease, and ischemic heart disease, frequently has a pericardial effusion. Neoplastic disease metastatic to the pericardium is a common cause of large pericardial effusions. Metastatic adenocarcinoma of the lung is the most common primary source for pericardial metastatic disease.

PATHOGENESIS. Fluid accumulation in the pericardium may be related to either excessive production of pericardial fluid or inadequate drainage of the pericardial space. Excessive production of fluid is most likely to occur in inflammatory processes, connective tissue disorders, and metastatic neoplastic processes. Inadequate drainage of the pericardial space frequently results from alterations in lymphatic flow and may be the primary mechanism of fluid accumulation in patients with congestive heart failure. Blood accumulation in the pericardial space results almost exclusively from hemorrhage from a cardiac structure that lies within the pericardial space. The major determining factor as to whether a pericardial effusion is lax or under high pressure resulting in tamponade is the rate of fluid accumulation. The volume of pericardial effusion also plays a role in the intrapericardial pressure but probably is not as important as the rate of fluid accumulation. As little as 100 ml of pericardial effusion developing rapidly may result in a high pressure within the pericardial space, restricting cardiac filling and resulting in tamponade physiology. On the other hand, a pericardial effusion developing slowly over weeks or months may accumulate in excess of 1 L of pericardial fluid but may result in no elevation of intrapericardial pressure and therefore no cardiac compression.

CLINICAL MANIFESTATIONS. The patient with a *lax pericardial effusion* may be symptom free. If symptoms are present, they probably are only those of the underlying disease. The lax pericardial effusion frequently is diagnosed only by noting an abnormal cardiovascular silhouette on the chest roentgenogram. Some patients with a lax pericardial effusion may have vague, nondescript chest discomfort and some associated mild dyspnea or fatigue. The physical findings of a lax pericardial effusion may include an enlarged area of cardiac dullness on percussion, an apex impulse that is difficult or impossible to palpate, and diminished intensity of heart sounds. The patient with *pericardial tamponade* has symptoms of dyspnea, fatigue, and low cardiac output. Frequently the patient is acutely ill, demonstrating signs of marked respiratory distress and decreased tissue perfusion. Signs of a severely low cardiac output or shock may be present. Physical findings include hypotension with a narrowed pulse pressure. There is usually a dramatic inspiratory fall in systolic blood pressure (over that normally observed), sometimes associated with a completely absent palpable pulse during inspiration. This finding, with a decrease of more than 10 mm Hg, is known as a "paradoxical pulse"; this is in fact an exaggeration of the normal decrease in blood pressure with inspiration. The jugular venous pressure is markedly elevated. Tachycardia in the range of 100 to 160 beats/min is present.

LABORATORY FINDINGS. The laboratory diagnosis of a pericardial effusion is suggested by the chest roentgenogram, which demonstrates a markedly enlarged cardiac silhouette with a globular configuration. Cardiac fluoroscopy demonstrates diminished pulsation of the cardiac borders. The ECG is likely to demonstrate nonspecific ST and T wave changes. The most common ECG finding is one of diminished voltage in all leads. Alternating voltage (electrical alternans) of the QRS complex is a fairly specific finding for a large pericardial effusion. The echocardiogram is particularly helpful in establishing the presence of fluid in the pericardial space. Some estimate of the volume of fluid may be obtained by means of the echocardiogram. A nuclear cardiac scan also may demonstrate a large space between the inferior border of the heart and the liver, indicating a pericardial effusion. Right atrial angiography can demonstrate a discrepancy between the cardiac silhouette and the right atrial wall, which indicates the presence of pericardial fluid. Cardiac catheterization can delineate the physiology of the pericardial effusion.

DIAGNOSIS. The diagnosis of pericardial effusive disease is established by the echocardiographic or scan findings. Differential diagnosis of the enlarged globular cardiac silhouette must include congestive cardiomyopathy with primary myocardial disease and the rather rare entity of Ebstein's anomaly. Documentation of a significant pericardial effusion by echocardiogram and scan with normal-sized cardiac chambers helps to establish the diagnosis of pericardial effusion. It is important to recognize that a pericardial effusion can occur with other cardiovascular disorders and other underlying cardiac conditions, in which case there may be enlargement of the cardiac chambers. The etiologic diagnosis of a pericardial effusion is vital. This can be established by obtaining pericardial fluid for analysis, culture, and cytology. Pericardial biopsy may also be necessary to help establish the etiologic diagnosis.

COURSE. The course of pericardial effusive disease depends totally on the cause. If the pericardial effusion is bloody, the course of the hemopericardium may be acute and result in death very quickly. This is particularly true if the cause is cardiac rupture or dissecting aneurysm of the aorta. Occasionally a patient survives the immediate cause of bleeding into the pericardial space, and the process that resulted in the hemopericardium heals spontaneously. However, surgical intervention frequently is necessary to correct the underlying defect. In patients who have had hemopericardium, delayed development of constrictive pericarditis is not uncommon. The patient with pericardial tamponade may develop rapid deterioration related to a suppressed cardiac output, resulting in shock and death. If tamponade physiology gradually resolves, the patient eventually may develop signs of chronic constrictive pericardial disease. Patients with lax pericardial effusions may have them on a chronic basis. The presence of pericardial effusive disease for several years has been well documented and frequently results in little or no symptomatology. Occasionally such pericardial effusions may resolve spontaneously. Recurrent pericardial effusions are most common in neoplastic metastatic disease, with the recurrence of repeated tamponade physiology not at all uncommon.

MANAGEMENT. Treatment of pericardial effusive disease necessitates exact etiologic diagnosis, and management of the underlying disease is mandatory. Treatment of a pericardial effusion from hypothyroidism consists essentially of treating hypothyroidism. With resumption of the euthyroid state, the pericardial effusion disappears. Patients with a lax pericardial effusion may respond to drainage of the pericardial space and therapy with antiinflammatory agents or pericardial sclerosing agents to prevent reaccumulation of the effusion. Occasionally pericardiectomy is appropriate for management of a recurrent lax pericardial effusion. The management of acute pericardial tamponade is both medical and surgical. The immediate emergency therapy requires the rapid administration of large volumes of intravenous fluids to raise cardiac filling pressures and overcome the compressive effects of the pericardial fluid. Use of potent myocardial inotropic agents such as isoproterenol and dopamine also may be beneficial in aiding cardiac filling by increasing the contractility of the ventricle, thus assisting cardiac filling during the atrial x descent. A drainage procedure either by needle pericardiocentesis or by pericardial window technique ultimately is necessary to relieve cardiac compression and drain the pericardial space. The pericardial window technique involves a subxyphoid incision and placement of a drainage tube in the pericardial space. This procedure is not associated with many of the hazards of needle pericardiocentesis and is preferable for obtaining both fluid and tissue specimens for diagnostic studies.

OTHER LABORATORY TESTS AND PERICARDIAL DISEASES

The use of computed tomography scans and magnetic resonance imaging for diagnosis of pericardial disease should be limited to only those cases in which all other studies have failed to establish a diagnosis, as these tests are expensive and of limited usefulness.

The entity *effusive-constrictive pericarditis* is commonly associated with mediastinal irradiation. This form of pericardial disease has a thickened edematous pericardium with fluid in the pericardial space and is characterized by the hemodynamic findings of both pericardial constriction and pericardial effusion. This entity may respond to therapy with corticosteroids or antiinflammatory agents but most frequently necessitates pericardiectomy for symptomatic relief. *Mediastinal fibrosis* may involve all mediastinal structures, including the pericardium, and has findings not unlike those of constrictive pericarditis. Some *congenital defects* of the pericardium may be associated with near total or partial absence of the pericardium. Occasionally cardiac structures evaginate through partial pericardial defects, resulting in strangulation of some cardiac chambers. *Pericardial cysts* are not uncommon and frequently are benign; they may on occasion give rise to acute pericarditis. *Primary tumors* of the pericardium do occur but are rare.

BIBLIOGRAPHY

Agner RC and Gallis HA: Pericarditis: differential diagnostic considerations, Arch Intern Med 139:407, 1979.

Bush CA and others: Occult constrictive pericardial disease: diagnosis by rapid volume expansion and correction by pericardiectomy, Circulation 56:924, 1977.

Cohen MV and Greenberg MA: Constrictive pericarditis: early and late complication of cardiac surgery, Am J Cardiol 43:657, 1979.

Fowler NO: The electrocardiogram in pericarditis. Cardiovasc Clin 5:256, 1974.

Fowler NO and Holmes JC: Hemodynamic effects of isoproterenol and norepinephrine in acute cardiac tamponade, J Clin Invest 43:502, 1969.

Lorell B and others: Right ventricular infarction: clinical diagnosis and differentiation from cardiac tamponade and pericardial constriction, Am J Cardiol 43:465, 1978.

Reddy PS and others: Cardiac tamponade: hemodynamic observations in man, Circulation 58:265, 1979.

Robertson R and Arnold CR: Acute constrictive pericarditis, J Thorac Cardiovasc Surg 49:91, 1965.

Rubin RH and Moellering RC: Clinical, microbiologic and therapeutic aspects of purulent pericarditis, Am J Med 59:68, 1975.

Wood P: Chronic constrictive pericarditis, Am J Cardiol 7:48, 1961.

99 • DISEASES OF THE THORACIC AORTA

Lary A. Robinson

The aorta is the largest and most important blood vessel in the human body (Fig. 99-1). It originates from the left ventricle at the level of the anulus fibrosis, rises anteriorly and slightly to the right in the midmediastinum, courses transversely and posteriorly, and then descends via the left posterior chest through the diaphragm to the level of the lumbar vertebrae, where it divides into the common iliac arteries. In its course it gives off branches to the heart, brain, kidneys, gut, and extremities, carrying more blood than any other vascular channel. The thoracic aorta may be conveniently divided into the ascending, transverse (arch), and descending portions. Although the vessel is a continuum, many aortic diseases involve a specific anatomic section, and these arbitrary anatomic divisions may have important clinical implications in planning the surgical approach for a particular disorder.

ANATOMY OF THE AORTA
Ascending aorta

The heart, which is roughly the size of a clenched fist, is contiguous with the diaphragmatic pericardium as it rests tangentially in the midmediastinum. The ascending aorta begins at the level of the anulus fibrosis, the supporting structure for the aortic valve, which sits in the midmediastinum at the level of the third left costal cartilage, just behind the sternum. The lumen of the aorta is widest at its origin and tapers until it finally bifurcates into the iliac vessels. It rises from the heart vertically and slightly to the right for approximately 5 to 7 cm. The transition from the ascending aorta to the transverse aorta is marked by the branching off of the brachiocephalic artery. The ascending aorta is further distinguished from its remainder by pericardial envelopment, which is important to keep in mind in the diagnosis and treatment of ascending aortic dissections.

The bulbus aortae is the anatomic designation for the very slight dilation of the aorta at its origin just above the anulus of the aortic valve. The three cusps of the semilunar aortic valve divide this slightly dilated proximal aorta into three sinuses of Valsalva, designated the left, right, and posterior (noncoronary) sinuses. The ostium of the right coronary artery is located in the right sinus, and the left coronary ostium is found in the left sinus. The posterior sinus does not contain a coronary ostium; this fact is of some importance in planning an aortic valve replacement in a patient with an abnormally small aortic anulus, in whom the aortic root is widened by dividing through the noncoronary cusp and inserting a prosthetic patch and valve.

Arch of the aorta

The arch of the aorta may be thought of as beginning at the termination of the pericardial envelopment of the ascending aorta. Frequently referred to as the transverse arch, this portion of the aorta is protected by the upper sternum as it curves upward to the left and posteriorly at the level of the fourth vertebral body. The first major branch of the aortic arch is the brachiocephalic trunk (or innominate artery), which subsequently divides into the right subclavian and right common carotid vessels. Most commonly the left common carotid artery arises as a separate vascular branch of the arch 1 to 2 cm lateral to the origin of the brachiocephalic vessel. However, in a small percentage of individuals the left carotid artery arises from a common brachiocephalic trunk with the right carotid and right subclavian arteries. The left subclavian artery normally is the last branch of the aortic arch.

A patent ductus arteriosus, when present, arises from the lesser curvature of the thoracic aorta at the junction of the arch and the descending thoracic aorta just opposite the left subclavian artery, connecting the aorta with the left main pulmonary artery. This channel usually is obliterated shortly after birth and exists thereafter as the ligamentum arteriosum.

Within the concavity of the arch can be found the bifurcation of the main pulmonary artery and the left main bronchus. The left vagus nerve crosses the anterolateral portion of the arch, giving rise to the recurrent laryngeal nerve, which curves under the arch and ascends back into the neck, supplying the left vocal cord. All operative procedures involving the distal arch of the aorta, patent ductus arteriosus, or coarctation syndromes require careful surgical identification and preservation of the recurrent laryngeal nerve.

Descending aorta

The descending thoracic aorta occupies the left posterior mediastinum from the fourth to the twelfth thoracic vertebrae, moving gradually anteriorly as it descends from a position to the left of the vertebral column to one just in front of it at the level of the diaphragm. The branches of the descending thoracic aorta include the bronchial, esophageal, intercostal, pericardial, superior phrenic, and spinal arteries. In general any of these branches, with the exception of those supplying the spinal cord, may, if necessary, be ligated with impunity. The blood

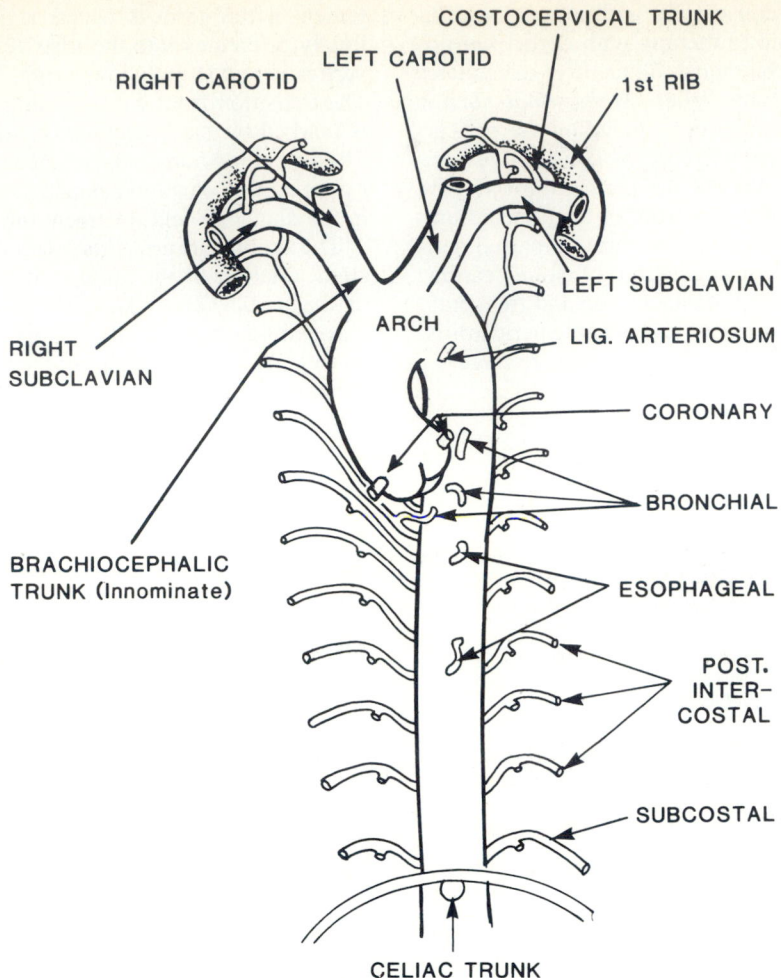

Fig. 99-1   Thoracic and aorta and its branches.

supply of the spinal cord is of particular concern to thoracic surgeons who perform procedures that require temporary cross-clamping with repair or grafting of sections of the thoracic aorta, since these actions may cause temporary or permanent spinal cord ischemia that may result in serious neurologic deficits such as paraplegia. The important branches of the descending thoracic aorta that supply the spinal cord seldom can be identified specifically during a surgical procedure. However, the principles of gentle handling of the aorta, minimal cross-clamping time, hypothermia, and use of cardiopulmonary bypass or heparinized shunts for maintaining spinal artery blood flow have been the keys to avoiding spinal cord ischemia.

CONGENITAL ANOMALIES OF THE THORACIC AORTA
Patent ductus arteriosus

Many patients with patent ductus arteriosus (see Chapter 93) appear to grow normally and are able to participate in normal activities. This often leads to the false assumption that the condition is compatible with normal longevity. However, it has been found that the subsequent life expectancy of patients with a patent ductus arteriosus who are alive at 17 years of age is approximately half that of the normal population.

Recently medical treatment aimed at nonoperative closure of patent ductus arteriosus, especially in premature and new-born infants, has been successful. Indomethacin, an inhibitor of prostaglandin E_1, causes closure of the patent ductus in a small percentage of infants, thus avoiding the need for thoracotomy and ligation. However, indomethacin itself has potential for renal or retinal toxicity when used in premature infants. In addition, indomethacin-induced closure of the ductus may be only temporary. If the ductus remains open despite drug treatment, and congestive heart failure or respiratory failure persist, surgical intervention is mandatory.

Surgical correction usually is recommended in young children with a persistent patent ductus arteriosus, even if no symptoms are present, since the long-term risks of pulmonary hypertension, endocarditis, or congestive heart failure are so appreciable. Operative risk is minimal.

Coarctation of the aorta

Coarctation (see Chapter 93) is congenital narrowing of the thoracic aorta, commonly occurring just distal to the left subclavian artery at the level of the patent ductus arteriosus or ligamentum arteriosum (Fig. 99-2). Less frequently the constriction is located proximal to the patent ductus arteriosus and then usually is associated with a major intracardiac defect, especially a ventricular septal defect. In its most severe form this variety represents interruption of the aortic arch. The more common so-called postductal coarctation is associated with a bicuspid aortic valve in 25% to 40% of cases, but other cardiac defects are uncommon. Most patients with this defect survive into adult life. Those who have hemodynamic difficulties in the neonatal or infant stages usually have associated intracar-

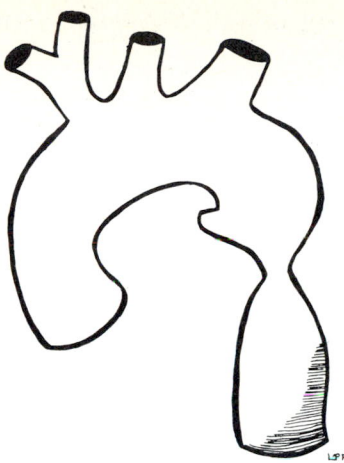

Fig. 99-2 Adult or postductal type of coarctation of thoracic aorta. (Illustration by Loretta P. Finnegan, M.D.)

diac anomalies. These infants with a so-called critical coarctation require prompt surgical repair to survive. Nevertheless, the operative risk in these cases is high.

In patients who survive beyond infancy, the physical and roentgenographic signs of persistent coarctation of the aorta are (1) upper extremity hypertension associated with lower extremity hypotension or absent pulses and (2) collateral arterial beds in the thoracic area. The internal mammary, intercostal, and subscapular vessels may become enlarged to three or four times normal size, are subject to dangerous aneurysm formation, and, in the case of the intercostal vessels, may produce notching of the ribs. Loud bruits may be heard over the posterolateral chest wall.

Most children are asymptomatic. The diagnosis usually results from the discovery of a bruit or upper extremity hypertension. When symptoms do exist, headache, dyspnea, general weakness, palpitations, and intermittent claudication may be present.

The diagnosis is established by comparing upper and lower extremity pulsations and blood pressures. It is essential to evaluate the blood pressure in both upper extremities, since variations may suggest involvement of the left subclavian artery in the coarctation. Systolic murmurs may be audible over the base of the heart or in the midback at the level of the sixth or seventh interspace. A diastolic murmur may represent flow through dilated intercostal arteries. Enlarged collateral chest wall vessels may produce palpable bruits over the chest wall. Evidence of left ventricular enlargement may be present and can be confirmed by an electrocardiogram (ECG). The definitive study is an aortogram, which demonstrates the site and severity of the coarctation and the most prominent collateral channels. If the physical examination or an echocardiogram suggest other associated abnormalities, complete cardiac catheterization is advisable.

Surgical therapy is indicated. Several studies have suggested that the life expectancy of an individual with untreated coarctation is approximately 30 to 40 years. Surgery between 7 and 14 years of age generally is recommended and allows the aorta to approach its adult size. The coarctated segment of aorta is excised. Usually an end-to-end anastomosis is possible. Occasionally it is necessary to insert a tubular Dacron graft. Because Dacron does not grow and because the incidence of recoarctation has been reported to be as high as 35%, especially if the patient is small at the time

of surgery, several alternate methods of handling coarctation of the aorta have been suggested. One is an aortic plastic technique, involving longitudinal opening of the coarctated segment with insertion of a diamond-shaped Dacron graft. However, long-term results have shown a high incidence of aneurysm formation with this method. Another method involves dividing the subclavian artery distally within the left side of the chest, opening it longitudinally in continuity with the coarctation, and folding it down as an onlay graft. The advantage of this so-called subclavian flap technique is, of course, that no prosthetic material is used and the coarctation is repaired with the patient's own tissue. This should allow normal growth of the segment. Follow-up studies have indicated excellent anatomic and hemodynamic results with this technique.

Vascular ring

A variety of congenital abnormalities of the aortic arch may form a vascular ring that constricts or obstructs the trachea or esophagus. Although most great vascular ring anomalies are asymptomatic, a few patients, usually infants, have stridor, frequent respiratory infections, wheezes, and even a "crowing" type of respiration. Occasionally the presenting complaint is difficulty swallowing or even aspiration pneumonia because of esophageal obstruction. The infant appears to get some relief by hyperextending the neck; respiratory obstruction may be accentuated by forcibly flexing the neck.

The congenital vascular ring that causes this sometimes fatal obstruction of the trachea and esophagus may arise from a double aortic arch, a right aortic arch with a ligamentum arteriosum completing a ring about the trachea, or an anomalous innominate, left common carotid, or subclavian artery. A barium swallow demonstrating the characteristic posterior compression of the esophagus, usually indicates the diagnosis. Rarely is arteriography necessary to demonstrate the anomaly. The condition is treated surgically, usually through the left chest, with division of the constricting ring or displacement of an aberrant vessel to provide more room for the trachea and esophagus.

THORACIC ANEURYSMS

An aneurysm of the thoracic aorta may be defined as a localized outpouching usually secondary to a weakness in the medial layer of the aorta. Aneurysms may occur on a congenital or an acquired basis and may be found anywhere in the thoracic aorta from the sinuses of Valsalva to the iliac bifurcation. The following are the known causes of thoracic aneurysms:

A. True aneurysms
1. Congenital—sinus of Valsalva
2. Arteriosclerotic
3. Cystic medial necrosis
4. Syphilitic
B. False aneurysms
1. Penetrating injury
2. Blunt injury
3. Iatrogenic—infected prosthetic graft or suture line

Dissection of the thoracic aorta secondary to intimal tear or trauma frequently has been associated with the term "aneurysm," hence the term "dissecting thoracic aneurysms." It must be understood that a dissecting hematoma within the wall of the aorta, either spontaneous or traumatic, is a different pathologic process from the formation of an aneurysm; this is discussed separately. Likewise, false aneurysms of the thoracic aorta represent organized hematomas secondary to tears in the thoracic aorta as a result of injury or surgery. These are called false aneurysms because their wall does not contain all three major layers of the aorta.

Aneurysms of the sinuses of Valsalva

Aneurysmal dilation of the sinuses of Valsalva may occur in association with Marfan's syndrome and in rare cases from syphilitic aortitis. False aneurysms of this area may occur secondary to bacterial endocarditis. However, the most commonly recognized aneurysms of the sinuses of Valsalva are congenital in origin and probably result from defective attachment of the aortic media to the fibrous base of the heart. The resulting localized weakness at the base of the aorta causes aneurysmal development and is most commonly found in the right coronary sinus, occasionally in the noncoronary sinus, and in rare cases in the left coronary sinus. The male to female occurrence ratio is 5:1.

Congenital aneurysms of the sinuses of Valsalva are extremely unusual except in Japan. Patients usually are asymptomatic until the fourth decade of life, when the aneurysm ruptures and forms a fistula protruding into a cardiac chamber (most frequently the right ventricle or right atrium but sometimes the pulmonary artery or pericardium). Unruptured aneurysms of the aortic sinuses also may produce clinical manifestations, including (1) obstruction of right ventricular outflow by a right coronary sinus aneurysm; (2) tricuspid regurgitation resulting from protrusion of an aneurysm of a noncoronary sinus into the right side of the heart in the area of the tricuspid valve; (3) heart block resulting from compression of the superior portion of the interventricular septum; (4) coronary insufficiency from compression of the left coronary artery; and (5) embolus.

Rupture of an aortic sinus aneurysm typically results in a left-to-right shunt into either the right ventricle or the right atrium. Fistulous communications with the left-sided cardiac chambers are distinctly rare. Although rupture of a sinus aneurysm may cause sudden death from congestive heart failure, most patients live approximately a year after fistula formation. Bacterial endocarditis within the sinus or the fistulous tract is the common cause of death after fistula formation. Sudden rupture of an aneurysm of the sinus of Valsalva into a cardiac chamber may produce severe chest pain, usually precordial in nature and occasionally simulating angina pectoris. Such a rupture may cause distortion of the aortic valve anulus with resultant aortic insufficiency.

Chest roentgenograms and ECGs usually are not diagnostic. The diagnosis can be established by cardiac catheterization and aortography. If rupture has not occurred, the aneurysm is visualized only as an outpouching of the sinus of Valsalva. If rupture has occurred, aortic root injection demonstrates flow of dye into the right atrium or ventricle. Chamber oxygen analysis also aids in locating the fistula.

A congenital aneurysm of the sinus of Valsalva is treated surgically. If the aneurysm is unruptured, it usually can be repaired through the aorta using cardiopulmonary bypass. Although the aneurysmal sinus occasionally can be repaired by local direct suture methods, it is not uncommon to require replacement of the ascending aorta with a woven Dacron graft. If the aneurysm has ruptured, it usually is repaired by a combined approach through the aorta and the chamber of intracardiac rupture. Replacement of the distorted and malfunctioning aortic valve with a prosthetic device also may be necessary. Mortality and morbidity associated with surgical correction of aneurysms of the sinus of Valsalva have steadily decreased, and all such aneurysms, with or without fistula formation and with or without symptoms, should be repaired surgically on discovery.

Aneurysms of the ascending aorta

Aneurysms that involve the entire ascending aorta from the valvular anulus to the branching off of the innominate artery usually are caused by cystic medial necrosis. Histologic examination of specimens obtained at surgery or autopsy generally shows thinning of the medial layer of the aortic wall with severe fragmentation or disappearance of the elastic fibers. As a result the ascending aorta becomes very thin and quite dilated. Associated distortion of the aortic valve may produce aortic regurgitation.

If the aortic valve is competent and not involved in the disease process, simple tubular graft replacement of the ascending aorta from a distance approximately 2 cm above the aortic valve to the level of the innominate vessels will suffice. Mild aortic regurgitation may be corrected in some instances by suture fixation of the commissural areas of the valve in such a way as to resuspend the leaflets and restore competence, thus avoiding aortic valve replacement. In cases in which aneurysms of the ascending aorta are associated with severe aortic insufficiency, replacement of the aortic valve and the ascending aorta with a commercially available valved conduit is the procedure of choice. This requires reimplantation of the coronary ostia into the side of the graft.

The advent of open heart surgery has resulted in several new problems in the ascending aorta and surgical methods for their correction. Aortic dissection or rupture at the site of cannulation for bypass surgery or placement of a proximal saphenous vein anastomosis has been reported. Dissection originating in the distal ascending aorta at the site of cannulation can be treated by removal of the cannula, temporary cessation of cardiopulmonary bypass, rapid cannulation of the femoral artery, and reinstitution of bypass in retrograde fashion. The cannulation site is then repaired.

Cracking or rupture of the aorta at the site of aortosaphenous anastomosis can be controlled by excision of that portion of the aorta, replacement with a Dacron patch, and subsequent anastomosis of the vein graft either to the Dacron patch or to other portions of the ascending aorta.

Aneurysms of the aortic arch

Before 1950 most reports indicated that aneurysms involving the arch of the aorta were nearly always syphilitic in origin and usually were extensions of aneurysms involving the ascending aorta. Now syphilis has nearly disappeared as a cause of major vascular disease, and arch aneurysms have become rare. Nearly all aneurysms of the transverse aortic arch reported today are arteriosclerotic in origin. An occasional posttraumatic false aneurysm has been reported in the arch.

A large aneurysm may produce symptoms by compressing branch arteries or adjacent structures, including the tracheobronchial tree, esophagus, pulmonary artery, and recurrent laryngeal nerve (producing hoarseness). Compression of the superior vena cava with resultant full-blown superior vena cava syndrome has been reported. Pain associated with rib or vertebral body erosion is not uncommon. Rupture of an arch aneurysm into the mediastinum, pleural space, esophagus, or tracheobronchial tree invariably results in immediate exsanguination.

The presence of aneurysms in the transverse arch may be suspected from simple roentgenograms, but aortography usually is required to define the true nature and extent of the lesion. Aneurysms of the transverse arch commonly involve the origins of the innominate, left carotid, and left subclavian arteries, and therefore surgical procedures designed to correct such aneurysms usually involve not only excision of the arch aneurysm but intraoperative preservation of areas supplied by the branches of the arch, particularly the brain.

Total prosthetic replacement of the aortic arch can be accomplished in a number of ways. Some perform resection and replacement of the ascending thoracic aorta using deep hypothermia, cardiopulmonary bypass, circulatory arrest, and myocardial cooling. Others have described an interesting method of approaching aneurysms of the aortic arch using surgically constructed bypass grafts and ultimately resecting the arch without the use of cardiopulmonary bypass. The surgical mortality (10% to 25%) and morbidity (especially stroke and renal failure) are considerable with aortic arch replacement by any method.

Aneurysms of the descending aorta

Most aneurysms of the descending thoracic aorta discovered today have an arteriosclerotic origin. The apparent increasing incidence of this disease may be related to the increased longevity of the population. These aneurysms usually are fusiform and arise just distal to the branching off of the left subclavian artery. Prior studies divided these aneurysms into fusiform and saccular types. However, most of these aneurysms have a common cause (arteriosclerosis), and they run the full spectrum from perfectly saccular to perfectly fusiform, all representing variations of the same disease process. Aneurysms may be reasonably well localized or extend the full length of the thoracic aorta and on into the abdominal area. They frequently are associated with aneurysms in other areas, most commonly the abdominal aorta in about 10% of patients. As would be expected, many patients with these aneurysms have associated cerebral and coronary vascular disease.

Although patients with descending thoracic aortic aneurysms can be asymptomatic, chest pain is frequent and usually caused by local erosion or compression. Pressure on the origin of the intercostal nerves or spine may produce extreme pain. Although these aneurysms have been reported to rupture into the tracheobronchial tree, esophagus, or pulmonary arterial tree, they most frequently rupture into the left pleural space, causing death by exsanguination. The suspicion of the presence of such aneurysms usually is provided by routine chest roentgenograms, although they may often be difficult to differentiate from other mediastinal masses. Aortography or computed chest tomography usually resolves the problem and is indicated when surgery is contemplated.

Effective surgical management involves the use of one of several techniques, including (1) cross-clamping of the aorta above and below the aneurysm with excision and rapid replacement with a prosthetic graft; (2) femoral cardiopulmonary bypass to protect the kidneys and spinal cord while the aorta is cross-clamped and the aneurysm is repaired; (3) left atrio-femoral bypass providing the same form of renal and spinal protection and ideally decompressing the left heart simultaneously, thereby reducing left ventricular work; and (4) internally heparin-coated shunts from the proximal aorta to the distal aorta or from the left ventricular apex to the femoral artery, allowing cross-clamping and repair of the aneurysm without heparinization or the use of bypass techniques.

When the period of aortic cross-clamp is kept to less than 30 to 40 minutes, the complication of paraplegia rarely occurs in aortic surgery. For longer periods use of a heparinized shunt or some type of bypass is advisable to lessen the potential for spinal cord ischemia with paraplegia or renal failure. Recent

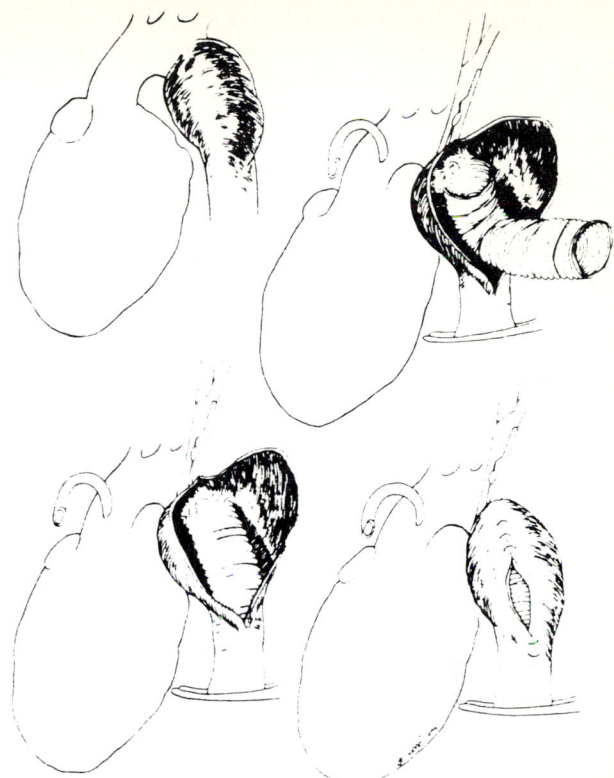

Fig. 99-3 Prosthetic grafting of aneurysm of descending aorta. In this case, heparin-coated shunt was inserted into ascending aorta and distal end of shunt was inserted into femoral artery (not shown). (From Lawrence GH, Hessel EA, Sauvage LR, Krause AH. J Thorac Cardiovasc Surg, 73:395, 1977.)

studies investigating the dreaded complication of paraplegia have suggested that additional measures such as systemic hypothermia (91° to 93° F [33° to 34° C]) and use of intravenous barbiturates may lessen the ischemic insult to the spinal cord. The surgery is illustrated in Fig. 99-3.

Much of the data concerning the natural history of aneurysms of the aorta are derived from patients with syphilis. Because syphilis has largely disappeared as a cause of vascular disease in this country, these older reports may no longer be applicable. In a more recent study in 1982 the 1-year survival of all patients with medically treated thoracic aneurysms was 58%; the 5-year survival was only 19% (however, rupture of the aneurysm accounted for just less than half of the deaths, cardiac disease being the leading cause of death). Significant risk factors for rupture include advanced age, an aneurysm greater than 6 cm in size, and hypertension. The surgical mortality for elective resection of an arteriosclerotic aneurysm is less than the risk of late rupture. The location of the aneurysm did not appear to influence the mortality, but the presence of symptoms clearly reduced survival. The development of symptoms usually indicates enlargement, often signaling prerupture expansion of the aneurysm. In general, the larger the aneurysm, the more likely the rupture, with recent symptomatic expansion often preceding this fatal event. After symptoms develop, the mean interval to rupture is only 2 years.

AORTIC DISSECTION

The unfortunate term "dissecting aneurysm" is attributed to Laennac. Although this term is well entrenched in the literature, it is incorrect and should be discarded. Aneurysm formation is not part of the pathogenesis of aortic dissection. The terms "aortic dissection" and "dissecting hematoma of the aorta" are more correct. A dissection occurs when an intimal tear develops, causing separation of the media by circulating blood to create a false lumen in the aorta.

Acute aortic dissection is the most common acute catastrophe involving the aorta, occurring in about 5 per million population per year and found in about 1 in 500 autopsies. Ruptured abdominal aneurysms occur at a rate of 3.6 per million population per year and ruptured thoracic aneurysms in only about 1 per million population per year.

Dissection of the thoracic aorta occurs most frequently in the 50- to 70-year age-group. The male to female incidence ratio is 2:1. It is unusual to see the lesion in patients under 40 years of age unless it is associated with full-blown Marfan's syndrome. Approximately 50% of cases of aortic dissection occurring in women under 40 years of age are associated with pregnancy. Dissection seems to be more common among blacks, possibly owing to the higher incidence of hypertension in that group.

PATHOGENESIS. There is no agreement concerning the cause of aortic dissection. Most agree that intimal tearing is the event that triggers dissection. The cause of the intimal tear is probably a combination of diseases within the aortic wall, including cystic medial necrosis, rupture of the vasa vasorum, and loss of elasticity, plus hemodynamic factors. Autopsy studies of patients who died from medial dissection have demonstrated clearly abnormal findings, including loss of elastic tissue, pooling of mucoid material, fibrosis, and apparent loss of cellular nuclei. The most common of these changes, cystic medial necrosis, has for decades been thought of as the primary pathologic lesion. However, it is clear that the media of normally aging aortas exhibit the same histopathologic features widely claimed to represent the specific medial defect underlying aortic dissection and that only quantitative differences exist between the pathology of aortic dissection and that of a normally aging aorta. The histologic features of the media, previously implicated as a specific underlying defect, appear to represent the morphologic substrata of a traumatizing and reparative process within the aortic wall consequent to hemodynamic forces. This process gradually may lead to dilation of the aorta. Hemodynamic tensions increase as the aneurysm enlarges. Local circumstances determine whether a dilated aorta ruptures or whether a dissection occurs.

The aorta in patients with Marfan's syndrome shows basically the same structural alterations. The underlying connective tissue disorder in these patients leads to complications at an earlier age.

In addition to the disease process or degenerative changes that must be present within the aortic wall for dissection to occur, the hemodynamic forces acting on the aortic wall also are of major importance. It has been shown experimentally that nonpulsatile flow at pressures up to 400 mm Hg produces no propagation of an aortic dissection. However, pulsatile pressure does cause propagation. Although an intimal tear is found in most aortic dissections at either surgery or autopsy, there is some controversy as to whether this tear is the primary initiating force in the creation of an aortic dissection or whether it is secondary to hemorrhage within the aortic wall as a result of rupture of the vasa vasorum.

CLINICAL MANIFESTATIONS. Extraordinarily severe chest pain is the most impressive chief complaint in nearly 90% of patients with aortic dissection. Patients usually report abrupt onset of the pain, which can be most severe in the anterior retrosternal area but may also be felt in or radiate to the intrascapular area, the epigastrium, or the back, often extending down into the legs. Arm pain is unusual. It is the simultaneous occurrence of the pain in several areas that helps to differentiate aortic dissection from acute myocardial infarction, although this distinction frequently is unclear; indeed, confusion with acute myocardial infarction is the most common diagnostic error made in patients with dissection. Pain may be minimal or absent in patients with spontaneous intimal lacerations, limited dissections, or even extensive classic dissections. It should be recognized that abrupt onset of neurologic symptoms may dull the patient's perception of pain and reduce or eliminate his ability to complain. The presence of neurologic signs in a patient with aortic dissection generally suggests involvement of the aortic arch and partial or complete occlusion of the innominate or left carotid arteries.

Most patients with thoracic aortic dissection appear acutely distressed and have measurable systolic and diastolic hypertension. Renal ischemia secondary to compromise of the renal artery flow by the dissecting channel may aggravate this hypertension. Low blood pressure is found almost exclusively with involvement of the ascending aorta, suggesting rupture into the pericardial sac and tamponade. Since the false channel created by the dissection can compromise the lumen of any branch of the aorta, evaluation of the pulse and blood pressure should be carried out in all four extremities. Occlusion of an arterial branch of the aorta produces definite loss or diminution of a pulse. The baseline pulse examination is especially important because of the possibility of subsequent propagation of the dissection, which is indicated by the loss of a pulse that originally was palpable.

The murmur of aortic regurgitation suggests retrograde dissection of the ascending thoracic aorta. This murmur is audible in approximately one third of all patients with aortic dissection but in less than 10% of those with a dissection distal to the left subclavian artery. Jugular venous distention may suggest cardiac tamponade but also can be caused by mediastinal hemorrhage and compression of the superior vena cava.

Any patient with a widened mediastinum on chest roentgenogram associated with free blood in the left pleural cavity as demonstrated by a limited thoracentesis should be considered to have a ruptured thoracic aorta until proved otherwise. In rare cases it may be necessary to carry out emergency surgery without performing angiography. However, the rapid availability of computed chest tomography almost always provides the surgeon some specific anatomic information for operative planning before surgery. The presence of a pericardial friction rub is ominous, usually indicating retrograde dissection into the pericardial cavity. However, there have been survivors, especially when the finding was noted immediately and surgery was undertaken without delay.

The presence of a new murmur of aortic insufficiency should suggest the possibility of the extension of the ascending dissection to involve the aortic anulus and valve. Severe aortic insufficiency also may appear at a later date in patients with healed ascending aortic dissections.

Neurologic complications of thoracic aortic dissection are of various types. One type represents altered states of consciousness in patients who have had profound episodes of hypotension and cerebral hypoperfusion. More focal neurologic disturbances occur when specific branches of the arch are compressed or totally occluded by the dissection. Ischemic paralysis of an extremity results from occlusion of the major vessel to that limb. It is more common in the lower extremities. Central nervous system symptoms including hemiplegia are secondary to carotid artery occlusion and are next in frequency. Paraplegia attributable to spinal cord ischemia occurs secondary to occlusion of intercostal or lumbar vessels. It is important to establish the patient's baseline neurologic status before undertaking surgical correction of the lesion, inasmuch as neurologic deficits as a result of the surgical procedure itself are not uncommon.

Retrograde aortic dissection resulting in coronary occlusion and myocardial infarction occurs in less than 5% of patients. It usually is a fatal event or at least precludes the possibility of major surgery. Two less commonly seen complications of aortic dissection are renal or splenic arterial occlusion and rupture of the dissection at the aortic root. The latter may produce complete heart block resulting from hematoma of the interatrial septum; left-to-right shunts created by rupture into the right atrium, right ventricle, or pulmonary artery; rupture into the left atrium resulting in a continuous murmur; obstruction of the pulmonary artery; or acute pericardial tamponade.

The following are common findings encountered in plain roentgenograms of patients with suspected or proven aortic dissection:

Mediastinal widening
Aortic root enlargement
Tracheal deviation
Depression of the left mainstem bronchus
An aortic shadow outside a calcified aortic knob
Left pleural effusion

It should be noted that a normal chest roentgenogram does not rule out the possibility of dissection. Possibly one third to half of patients initially may have a normal chest roentgenogram. Conversely, it should be remembered that a supine anteroposterior chest roentgenogram frequently suggests widening of the mediastinum when actually that is the normal roentgenographic appearance of the mediastinum in that position. Even when the clinical diagnosis of dissection seems well established, ECGs and enzyme determinations should be obtained to rule out the possibility of myocardial infarction.

CT of the chest recently has been used as the initial, noninvasive method of diagnosis of acute dissections. Nevertheless, contrast aortography remains indispensible for defining the site of the intimal tear, the extent of the false lumen, and the presence of aortic regurgitation—all necessary for surgical planning. DeBakey classified dissections on the basis of their origin and extent, offered in Fig. 99-4 because this classification is still often used. However, a more recent classification by Daily and associates based on therapeutic consideration is preferred: type A includes all dissections involving the ascending aorta regardless of the site of intimal tear; type B includes all dissections confined to the descending aorta distal to the left subclavian.

MANAGEMENT. The natural history of acute aortic dissection in patients managed before the introduction of modern pharmacologic and surgical treatment was poor. Of all patients with aortic dissection, 30% died within the first 24 hours, 50% within 48 hours, 70% by the end of 1 week, and 80% by the end of 2 weeks. The prognosis clearly was worse in patients with proximal (ascending aortic) tears and associated hypotension and was best in normotensive or hypertensive patients with distal (descending aortic) dissections.

All patients with any form of aortic dissection initially should be treated medically. A selection process then begins in an attempt to identify the patients most likely to benefit from surgical intervention.

The immediate goals of treatment are the reduction of pain, the control of systolic and diastolic blood pressure, and the decrease of tension in the aortic wall. Small intravenous doses

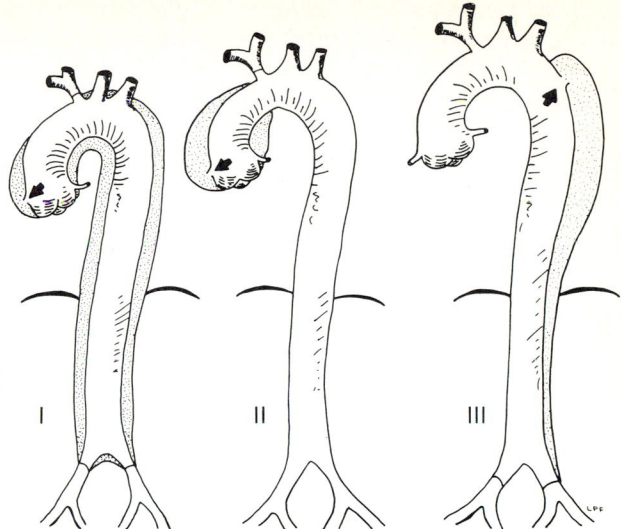

Fig. 99-4 DeBakey's classic categorization of dissection of thoracic aorta. In type *I*, dissection originates in *ascending* aorta *(arrow)* and extends throughout length of aorta. In type *II*, dissection originates in *ascending* aorta *(arrow)* but is limited to ascending aorta or proximal portion of arch. In type *III*, dissection originates in proximal *descending* thoracic aorta *(arrow)* and extends distally. (Illustration by Loretta P. Finnegan, M.D.)

of morphine sulfate reduce the patient's pain and allay anxiety. The intravenous administration of sodium nitroprusside usually results in a dramatic reduction of blood pressure with minimal side effects (see Chapter 87 for dosage); concomitant diuretic therapy (for example, furosemide) may be needed. Nitroprusside can result in transient increases in myocardial contractility that could conceivably contribute to extension of the dissection. Ventricular ejection velocity is lowered by small intravenous doses of propranolol (1 mg every 3 minutes to a total of 10 mg), thereby decreasing aortic wall tension. Patients who cannot tolerate sodium nitroprusside or whose blood pressure is not controlled with sodium nitroprusside in rare cases may require brief treatment with trimethaphan camphorsulfonate (Arfonad); however, tachyphylaxis develops rapidly with this drug.

As soon as the patient is stable, normotension has been achieved, and pain has been relieved, angiography can be accomplished. A percutaneous technique using the femoral approach is recommended. The purposes of the angiographic examination are (1) to confirm the diagnosis of aortic dissection, (2) to identify the site of origin (intimal tear) of the dissection, (3) to define the extent of the dissection, (4) to rule in or rule out involvement of the major branches of the aorta, and (5) to quantitate blood flow within the false lumen. Identifying the origin of the dissection is essential to proper planning of surgery. In an otherwise stable patient, surgery is relatively contraindicated if the intimal origin of the dissection cannot be identified.

Failure to opacify the false lumen roentgenographically, suggesting that the false lumen is clotted, indicates a more favorable prognosis for the patient. In one series long-term survival without surgery in patients without false lumen opacification was 89%, as compared at 43% of patients in whom the false channel could be filled with contrast media.

There is general agreement that surgery is the treatment of choice for proximal dissection (type A or DeBakey types I and II) involving the ascending aorta or the arch because progression of the hematoma in the direction of the aortic valve or branches of the aortic arch may have the devastating consequences of aortic insufficiency, pericardial tamponade, or neurologic compromise. It should be noted that a small group of patients with proximal dissection who refused surgery or in whom surgery was contraindicated because of age or associated medical illness were treated successfully with long-term medical therapy. As mentioned, some authorities believe that failure to identify the intimal tear within the proximal aorta is a relative contraindication to surgery in an otherwise stable patient.

Patients with a distal (type B or DeBakey type III) dissection initially should be treated medically as long as the dissection remains stable and uncomplicated. The slight advantage of medical therapy in this group, found in earlier studies, occurred at a time when the surgical mortality was similar to or greater than the medical mortality, particularly since patients with distal dissection tend to be somewhat older and have an increased incidence of associated atherosclerotic and cardiopulmonary disease. Recent advances in intraoperative and postoperative management have decreased the surgical mortality to as low as 11%. Because many patients with type B dissections require surgery in the chronic phase, often with complications leading to substantial operative risk, more centers are now advocating surgery in the acute phase after initial stabilization. However, surgical therapy is mandatory in patients with distal disease if there is evidence of rupture, impending rupture, pericardial tamponade, vital organ compromise, aortic insufficiency, or inability to control hypertension.

AORTIC TRANSECTION

Of all traumatic aortic injuries by far the most common is transection or acute rupture. High-speed vehicular travel has resulted in a marked increase in the frequency of this injury, with 15% of all automobile fatalities resulting from aortic rupture. Ninety percent of patients with aortic rupture die immediately at the scene. In the remainder, the adventitia or periaortic tissues contain the intravascular blood flow to create a false aneurysm. Early diagnosis is imperative, since the danger of free rupture into the pleural space and fatal exsanguination is a continuing danger.

The mechanism of injury usually is a rapid deceleration combined with compression, typically resulting in a circumferential tear. In more than 90% of cases the tear is located at the aortic isthmus just distal to the left subclavian artery; the remainder occur in the ascending aorta or in rare cases the aortic arch.

The clinical findings specifically related to aortic rupture may be minimal, especially in relation to the other major injuries usually found in these patients. The signs of a transection generally are caused by local compression by the false aneurysm and distal ischemia or perforation. These signs may include: back pain, hoarseness, pressure or pulse differences in the extremities, paraplegia, oliguria, systolic murmurs, hemoptysis, or Horner's syndrome.

The roentgenographic picture is the most suggestive, with a widened mediastinal shadow on the chest roentgenogram the most typical. Other findings on the chest roentgenogram may include pleural fluid or apical cap, abnormal aortic knob contour, downward displacement of the left main-stem bronchus, shift of the trachea or esophagus to the right, or left hemothorax without rib fracture. However, any patient with an acute deceleration injury with a widened mediastinum on chest roentgenogram should be assumed to have an aortic transection, and such patients urgently require an aortogram. Currently the use of computed chest tomography to determine the presence or *absence* of aortic rupture is controversial, but with refinements in instrumentation and interpretation, it may offer a reliable, less invasive diagnostic alternative.

The treatment of aortic transection is immediate surgical repair, often requiring a small prosthetic tubular graft to bridge the damaged area of the vessel. The results of surgery are excellent if aortic control is obtained before major hemorrhage.

AORTIC ARCH SYNDROME

The term "aortic arch syndrome" refers to a variety of acquired conditions that produce partial or total occlusion of one or all of the branches of the aortic arch. Although there are many known causes of aortic arch syndromes, in the United States over 90% of these lesions are secondary to atherosclerotic occlusive disease. Other causes to consider are trauma, neoplasm, syphilitic aortitis, Takayasu's arteritis or pulseless disease, and emboli. Also, many other diseases mimic aortic arch syndrome or produce brachiocephalic arterial obstruction. These include collagen vascular disease, thoracic outlet syndrome, and superior sulcus tumor.

When atherosclerosis is the cause of aortic arch syndrome, the left subclavian artery is the most commonly affected vessel, followed by the innominate and left common carotid arteries. In nearly half of the patients, several branches are involved.

CLINICAL MANIFESTATIONS. Although aortic arch syndrome is most common between 50 and 70 years of age, it is not rare in younger patients. Most patients show cerebral ischemia, which can be divided into four types: (1) a fixed neurologic deficit secondary to frank cerebrovascular accident, (2) transient ischemic attacks (TIAs), (3) reversible ischemic neurologic deficits somewhere between a cerebrovascular accident and a TIA, and (4) chronic deficits from hypoperfusion.

Physical examination should emphasize the evaluation of all peripheral pulses with particular attention to the carotid, temporal, brachial, and radial pulses. The detection of bruits along the course of any vessel demands additional evaluation by ultrasound. The definitive study is the angiogram. The aortic arch can be approached through either the brachial or the femoral artery, although most angiographers prefer the femoral approach.

Subclavian steal syndrome

Perhaps the best known of all the aortic arch syndromes is the subclavian steal syndrome. Ordinarily the pressure head is somewhat higher in the subclavian artery than in the basilar cerebral system, allowing antegrade flow in the vertebral vessel. However, with significant stenosis of the *proximal subclavian artery,* the pressure in the distal subclavian may fall below that of the basilar system, causing a reversal of flow in the vertebral artery system and subsequent diversion or "steal" of blood from the brain. Exercise of the involved upper extremity may increase flow beyond the subclavian lesion and pull even more blood from the cerebral circulation, which intensifies the cerebral symptoms associated with the flow reversal. The same syndrome has been described for the *innominate artery.* Significant stenosis at the base of this latter vessel can result in cerebral blood flow reversal. The possible greater danger is reversal of flow in the right carotid artery, as well as the right vertebral artery, intensifying the blood flow deficit in the brain.

In both steal syndromes surgical correction may be accomplished by attaching a Dacron bypass graft from the aorta to the involved vessel beyond the obstruction. However, the surgical procedures with far less risk for the patient include: (1) a prosthetic bypass graft from the left carotid artery to the left subclavian artery through a cervical incision or (2) an axillary artery to axillary bypass graft by the subcutaneous route. Both procedures are accomplished without entering the chest, thereby avoiding the morbidity and mortality of thoracotomy or median sternotomy needed for a bypass graft from the aorta, an especially important consideration in elderly patients, in whom the subclavian steal syndrome is so commonly found.

Takayasu's arteritis

Takayasu's arteritis or pulseless disease is an inflammatory panarteritis that may involve all the branches of the thoracic and the abdominal aorta. It has been reported worldwide but is rare in the United States. It is most commonly seen among young women of Oriental extraction.

Three major varieties of Takayasu's occlusive arteritis have been described, depending on the area of the vascular tree involved. In one variety, affecting approximately 50% of the patients, the aortic arch is the primary site of involvement. The second group, approximately one third of the patients, demonstrate involvement of all of the aorta. The third group, about 10% to 15% of the patients, have involvement of the distal thoracic aorta and abdominal aorta.

Most patients with Takayasu's arteritis or pulseless disease are under 40 years of age, and women predominate. Patients generally have systemic symptoms such as malaise, fever, anorexia, and weight loss. Many have cardiopulmonary complaints, including tachycardia, shortness of breath, and peripheral edema. The laboratory evaluation is not diagnostic, although many patients have anemia and leukocytosis.

Although the arteritis per se becomes inactive in many patients, the vascular obstructive lesions persist. If the inflammatory process continues unabated, early death owing to cardiac or cerebral complications is the rule. Corticosteroids have produced clinical remission in some patients. The value of anticoagulation therapy is unproved. Surgical correction may be indicated in the later fibrotic phase of the disease. However, because of the small size of the vessels involved, the revascularization effort is frequently less than ideal.

Syphilitic aortitis

Before the introduction of penicillin, syphilis was the most common cause of proximal aortitis and was responsible for most branch occlusions of the aortic arch. However, syphilitic aortitis is rare today. The diagnosis may be suggested if serologic tests for syphilis are positive and an angiogram confirms aortic arch involvement. Proper treatment consists of appropriate antibiotic therapy and prosthetic replacement grafts as indicated.

BIBLIOGRAPHY

Adams HD and VanGeertruyden HH: Neurologic complications of aortic surgery, Ann Surg 144:547, 1956.

Bergen JJ and Yao JST: Surgery of the aorta and its branches, New York, 1979, Grune & Stratton, Inc.

Bickerstaff LK and others: Thoracic aortic aneurysms: a population-based study, Surgery 92:1103, 1982.

Borrie J: Management of thoracic emergencies, New York, 1980, Appleton-Century-Crofts.

Ergin MA and others: Acute dissections of the aorta: current surgical treatment, Surg Clin North Am 65:721, 1985.

Hirst AE Jr, Johns VJ Jr, and Kime SW Jr: Dissecting aneurysm of the aorta: a review of 505 cases, Medicine 37:217, 1958.

Lam R, Robinson MJ, and Morales AR: Aortic dissection complicating aortocoronary saphenous vein bypass, Chest 68:729, 1976.

Nasu T: Pathology of pulseless disease: a systematic study and critical review of twenty-one autopsy cases reported in Japan, Angiology 14:255, 1963.

Reivich M and others: Reversal of blood flow through the vertebral artery and its effect on cerebral circulation, N Engl J Med 265:878, 1961.

Rob CG: The surgical treatment of occlusive disease of the extracranial cerebral arteries. In Dale WA, editor: Management of arterial occlusive disease, Chicago, 1971, Year Book Medical Publishers, Inc.

Robinson LA: Surgical intervention for acute cardiothoracic emergencies. In Ornato JP, editor: Cardiovascular emergencies, New York, 1986, Churchill Livingstone, Inc.

Ross RS and McKusick VA: Aortic arch syndromes, Arch Intern Med 92:701, 1953.

Schlatmann TJM and Becker AE: Histologic changes in the normal aging aorta: implications for dissecting aortic aneurysm, Am J Cardiol 39:13, 1977.

Schlatmann TJM and Becker AE: Pathogenesis of dissecting aneurysm of aorta, Am J Cardiol 39:21, 1977.

Stiles QR and others: Management of injuries of the thoracic and abdominal aorta, Am J Surg 150:132, 1985.

Taguchi K and others: Surgical correction of aneurysm of the sinus of Valsalva, Am J Cardiol 23:180, 1969.

Wheat MW Jr and others: Treatment of dissecting aneurysms of the aorta without surgery, J Thorac Cardiovasc Surg 50:364, 1965.

100 · DISEASES OF THE DISTAL AORTA AND BRANCHES OF THE AORTA

Marian F. McNamara

Mortality and morbidity from atherosclerotic arterial disease have reach epidemic levels in the United States. As the average age of the population increases, a further rise in atherosclerotic disease can be expected. Several risk factors, including hyperlipidemia, hypertension, cigarette smoking, and diabetes mellitus, are linked to the development of atherosclerotic plaque. Once symptoms are present, manipulation of these risk factors rarely results in palliation. Furthermore, early lesions commonly are asymptomatic, and the initial signs and symptoms are catastrophic events such as cerebrovascular accident, myocardial infarction, or severe limb ischemia resulting from arterial occlusion.

During the past three decades the natural history, pathophysiology, and response to therapy of arterial lesions in the aorta and its branches have been defined. Noninvasive diagnostic techniques and arteriography now allow objective quantification of arterial insufficiency and accurate localization of arterial lesions. Successful palliation is obtained in many patients by surgical treatment of segmental atherosclerotic lesions such as carotid stenosis, abdominal aortic aneurysms, and occlusive plaques in the aorta and limb vessels. The long-term success of these operations, however, depends on the progression of the atherosclerotic process, as well as the surgical techniques employed.

CEREBROVASCULAR DISEASE

Cerebrovascular accident (CVA, stroke) is the third leading cause of death in the United States, with an annual incidence of 1.7 per 1000 population. Morbidity results from paralysis, visual and sensory loss, and speech impairment. In 1951 Fisher drew attention to the importance of the *extracranial* arteries in CVA. Later the Joint Study of Extracranial Arterial Occlusion confirmed his initial opinion, demonstrating by arteriography that 75% of patients with CVA had lesions in surgically accessible sites.

PATHOPHYSIOLOGY. The most common sites of extracranial cerebrovascular disease are the common carotid artery at its bifurcation and the adjacent proximal internal carotid artery. Artherosclerotic plaques at these sites produce symptoms by ulceration with embolization and by stenosis. Ulcerated plaque is a focus for deposition of platelets and cholesterol debris. Embolization of this debris into the cerebral circulation results in transient ischemic attacks, amaurosis fugax, or CVA. Further deposition or growth of the plaque narrows the lumen of the artery. Stenosis of 50% or greater may result in decreased cerebral blood flow.

CLINICAL MANIFESTATIONS. Symptoms of cerebrovascular disease include completed CVA, transient ischemic attacks, and amaurosis fugax. Many lesions remain asymptomatic until CVA occurs. However, when transient deficits precede CVA, these events draw attention to the possibility of extracranial cerebrovascular disease and allow treatment before irreversible neurologic deficits arise. It is estimated that 30% of patients with transient ischemic attacks have a CVA within 5 years. By definition, transient ischemic attacks last less than 24 hours and resolve without residual neurologic deficit. These transient neurologic attacks may be related to the carotid system, vertebrobasilar system, or both. Unilateral motor or sensory loss, dysarthria, aphasia, and amaurosis fugax are indicators of disease in the carotid system. Dizziness, ataxia, vertigo, diplopia, and bilateral motor and sensory symptoms suggest lesions in the vertebrobasilar system. Occasionally bilateral carotid stenosis may cause vertebrobasilar symptoms by reducing total cerebral blood flow.

Physical examination of the patient with cerebrovascular disease should include palpation of the common carotid and upper extremity pulses. The internal carotid pulse is not palpable in the neck. Pulse evaluation may therefore be misleading, since the internal carotid artery frequently is occluded in the presence of a normal common carotid pulse. Bruits audible over the carotid bifurcation indicate stenosis. However, the absence of a bruit does not rule out hemodynamically significant stenosis, since bruits are absent in severe stenosis. In addition, many bruits heard in the neck radiate from the thorax or base of the neck and may be confused with intrinsic carotid bruits.

DIAGNOSTIC TESTS. Arteriography remains the definitive diagnostic test for cerebrovascular disease. Bilateral carotid injections are usually performed via the axillary or femoral route. An arch aortogram is desirable before selective catheterization of the cerebral vessels. If clinical findings suggest vertebrobasilar insufficiency, vertebral artery views are added. Despite improvement in arteriographic techniques, the complication rate for this study remains 1%.

Recently noninvasive tests have been introduced for the detection of atherosclerotic disease in the carotid artery. Many of these tests are based on monitoring the ophthalmic artery (the first branch of the internal carotid artery) as an indicator of internal carotid disease. Ocular pneumoplethysmography (OPG) allows accurate determination of ophthalmic artery pressure and significant carotid artery stenosis. This test usually is combined with analysis of a carotid bruit by carotid phonoangiography (CPA). Qualitative analysis of bruits by this method differentiates intrinsic carotid bruits from transmitted bruits. Systolic bruits are present with low-grade stenosis, and systolic-diastolic bruits are caused by high-grade obstruction. The combination of OPG and CPA correlates with angiographic findings in 90% of cases.

Ultrasound imaging provides anatomic information about the carotid bifurcation. However, calcified plaques may produce false positive results with this method. Duplex scanning combines real-time B-mode imaging and pulsed Doppler utrasound to overcome limitations inherent in each. It provides accurate anatomic information and characterizes the plaque. Plaques with homogeneous composition (fibrous plaques) can be differentiated from heterogeneous lesions (subplaque hemorrhage).

MANAGEMENT. The localized nature of atherosclerotic plaque at the carotid bifurcation makes this an ideal lesion for treatment by endarterectomy. Excision of the diseased intima restores luminal diameter and removes ulcerating plaques that may be a source of distal emboli. Indications for carotid endarterectomy include transient ischemic attacks, stable stroke, asymptomatic bruits, and in rare cases chronic cerebral ischemia. During the past 20 years, cerebral protective techniques including surgery under local anesthesia, electroencephalographic monitoring, use of an intraluminal shunt, and monitoring of carotid stump pressure and ophthalmic artery pressure have been suggested to further decrease operative mortality and morbidity. Operative mortality from carotid endarterectomy is now 1% to 2%, with neurologic deficits related to the operation in the range of 2% to 4%. The long-term patency of carotid arteries reconstructed by endarterectomy is high, and most patients undergoing surgery for transient ischemic episodes are asymptomatic in the postoperative period.

Patients with minimal neurologic deficit following CVA also are good candidates for carotid endarterectomy, since the incidence of recurrent CVA is great in this group.

The treatment of the asymptomatic bruit is controversial. It has been demonstrated that asymptomatic stenosis at the carotid bifurcation progresses in 60% of patients and that these patients have a 9% incidence of CVA without antecedent symptoms. A rational approach to the management of the patient with an asymptomatic bruit includes evaluation of its hemodynamic significance with noninvasive testing. In patients with hemodynamically significant lesions, arteriography and endarterectomy or close follow-up with testing at intervals is indicated to decrease the risk of CVA.

Direct reconstruction of arch branches by bypass from the ascending aorta is a safe, effective treatment. Exclusion of the diseased artery may be necessary if it has been a source of emboli. Extrathoracic bypass of atherosclerotic arch branches may be effectively achieved in high-risk patients, with a lessened morbidity.

Indications for vertebral reconstruction include vertebrobasilar symptoms with advanced lesions of a single or dominant vertebral artery. The risk of vertebral reconstruction is now known to be small in terms of death or neurologic deficit. Operative approach to vertebral stenosis initially was by endarterectomy of the origin of the vertebral artery or subclavian vertebral bypass. Proximal lesions now are treated by reimplanting the vertebral artery into the carotid artery, which is safer and more effective. More distal vertebral stenosis in the bony canal is managed by bypass to the distal vertebral at the C1 level.

ANEURYSMS

An aneurysm is a localized dilation of an artery caused by structural weakness in the wall. True aneurysms contain all anatomic layers present in the arterial wall: intima, media, and adventitia. In contrast, false aneurysms begin from a rupture of the arterial wall, surrounded by a fibrous sac or adventitia. Aneurysms are fusiform or saccular in configuration.

ETIOLOGY AND PATHOGENESIS. True aneurysms may be atherosclerotic, mycotic, or syphilitic. These processes weaken the media of the arterial wall and allow the artery to dilate.

Increased vessel diameter causes increased lateral wall tension as predicted by the law of Laplace. Increased lateral wall pressure causes further dilation, predisposing the thin vessel wall to rupture. Slow arterial flow through the dilated segment allows layered thrombus to be deposited along the wall. This thrombus does not protect against rupture and may give rise to emboli or complete thrombosis of the artery.

Atherosclerosis is the most common cause of true aneurysms in the United States. Over 95% of true aneurysms are located in the abdominal aorta below the renal arteries. Theories proposed to explain this segmental distribution include degeneration of elastic fibers from aging, turbulent flow, and anoxia caused by the occlusion of sparse vasa vasorum. Many patients with abdominal aortic aneurysms have generalized ectasia of the arterial tree or coexistent aneurysms in the popliteal, iliac, femoral, and renal arteries.

Mycotic aneurysms are rare. Infection of the arterial wall is caused by bacteremia, direct spread from adjacent structures such as osteomyelitis of the vertebral body, or contamination through an aortoduodenal fistula. Frequently an underlying atherosclerotic plaque or aneurysm is present. Infection results in destruction of the media and subsequent vessel dilation.

False aneurysms commonly are caused by trauma or disruption of vascular anastomoses. The trauma may be blunt or penetrating, acute or chronic. False aneurysms after vascular reconstruction result from disruption of the anastomosis. Degeneration of the arterial wall, fracture of suture material, infection, and degeneration of graft material are underlying causes.

EPIDEMIOLOGY. Atherosclerotic aneurysms are a disease of aging, diagnosed most frequently in the sixth, seventh, and eighth decades. A necropsy study of 4000 male veterans showed an increase in frequency of aortic aneurysms from 6% in the sixth decade to 14% in the ninth decade.

CLINICAL MANIFESTATIONS. Most abdominal aortic aneurysms are asymptomatic and are diagnosed at the time of physical examination or from roentgenograms of the abdomen or urinary tract. Symptoms are caused by compression, rupture, or embolization. Vague abdominal pain, back pain, or tenderness over the aneurysm may result from rapid enlargement, or it may be an early sign of rupture. Rupture produces blood in the retroperitoneal space, causing back pain and abdominal pain radiating into the groin. Shock and death follow the initial symptoms of rupture at a time interval that depends on the location and size of the rupture and the patients' cardiovascular stability. In rare cases abdominal aortic aneurysms are first manifested by emboli in the extremities. These emboli may be small, causing skin discoloration suggestive of petechial lesions, or large, causing major vessel occlusion. Thrombosis of the aneurysm mimicking aortic bifurcation embolus or acute aortic occlusion is rare.

DIAGNOSTIC TESTS. Plain roentgenograms reveal calcification in the aortic wall in 55% to 85% of abdominal aortic aneurysms (Fig. 100-1). However, the right wall of the aorta frequently overlies the vertebral column, obscuring calcification, and variation of the roentgenographic tube-to-patient distance can cause magnification of the lesion.

Ultrasound provides an accurate measurement of the aortic diameter to within several millimeters. This study can detect thrombus in the lumen of the aorta and can differentiate retroperitoneal lesions overlying the aorta from abdominal aortic aneurysms. However, it cannot give exact localization of the aneurysm in reference to the renal arteries or iliac vessels.

CT detects abdominal aortic aneurysms, assesses the diameter of the aorta, and differentiates residual lumen from

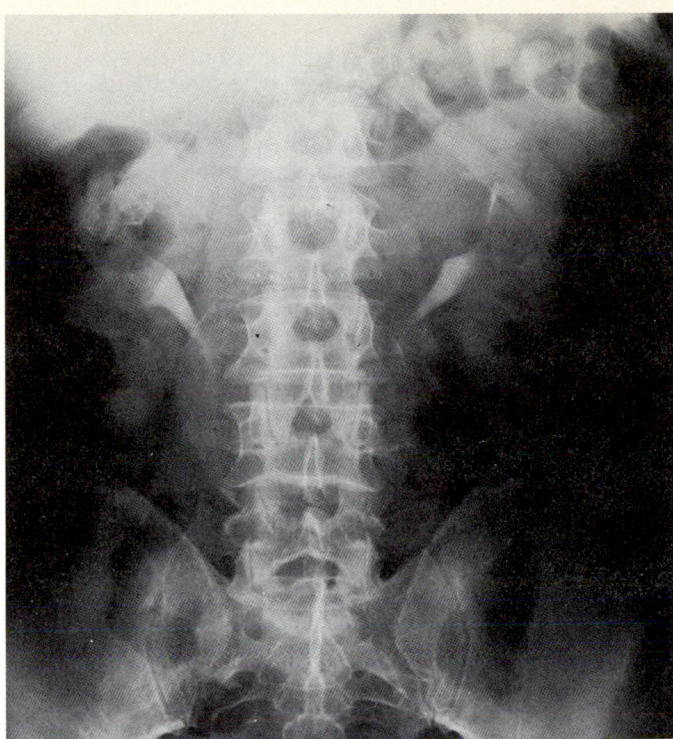

Fig. 100-1.   Roentgenogram of abdomen showing calcification in wall of 8.5-cm aortic aneurysm. There is dye in renal collecting system from a urogram.

overall diameter. Currently it is reserved for paralytic ileus in which ultrasound is ineffective and for detection of suspected retroperitoneal hematoma or infection.

Arteriography is a preoperative study. Since thrombus lining the aneurysm preserves normal luminal diameter in many patients, arteriography may not diagnose an abdominal aortic aneurysm. Current indications for preoperative arteriography include impaired renal function, renovascular hypertension, aneurysms extending above the renal arteries, renal anomalies such as horseshoe kidney, and the presence of lower extremity ischemia.

Elective aneurysm resection

Untreated aneurysms may rupture. Size is the factor correlating best with the risk of rupture; the 5-year risk of rupture of a 4 cm aneurysm is less than 15%, whereas it is over 75% for an 8 cm aneurysm. It generally is agreed that the risk of rupture for an aneurysm of 6 cm exceeds the risk of operative intervention.

Abdominal aortic aneurysms occur in patients with other manifestations of atherosclerosis, including coronary and cerebrovascular disease. In a series of 108 patients with abdominal aortic aneurysms, 43% had cardiac disease, 43% had hypertension, 19% had chronic obstructive pulmonary disease, and 19% had renal disease. Despite the coexistence of other disease processes, an aneurysm greater than 6 cm requires surgical intervention because of the risk of rupture. A survey of representative series published from 1959 through 1978 placed operative mortality in the range of none to 18%. Recent series report operative mortality ranging from 3% to 7%. Identifying unusual associated conditions, including multiple renal arteries, retroaortic renal veins, double vena cava, horseshoe kidney, and mycotic aneurysms, allows the most appropriate surgical management, further decreasing morbidity.

Complications of aortic aneurysm resection include renal failure, distal arterial insufficiency, colonic ischemia, infection of the prosthesis, and paraplegia. Proper fluid administration during and after aortic procedures is critical in preventing hypotension and subsequent renal complications. Early clamping of the iliac arteries and decreased manipulation of the aneurysm reduce distal arterial insufficiency from intraoperative embolization. Bowel ischemia rarely occurs in the absence of superior mesenteric artery stenosis. Evaluation of the colonic blood supply before abdominal closure allows intraoperative correction of this rare problem by reimplantation of the inferior mesenteric artery. Infection of the aortic prosthesis occurs during implantation or from bacteremia after insertion. To decrease the risk of graft infection, patients with aortic implants receive prophylactic antibiotics before and after surgery and during any subsequent procedure that could result in bacteremia. The likelihood of graft infection decreases as the pseudointimal covering develops. Spinal cord ischemia is a rare complication that occurs in patients with severe atherosclerosis and anomalous blood supply to the cord.

Ruptured abdominal aortic aneurysms

Abdominal aortic aneurysms most commonly rupture into the retroperitoneal space. This results in back pain and hypotension. The initial episode of hemorrhage generally causes transient symptoms followed by an asymptomatic period and then terminal cardiovascular collapse.

Despite improvements in surgical technique, the operative mortality associated with ruptured abdominal aortic aneurysms averages 50%. Factors that adversely influence survival are hypotension (systolic pressure less than 100 mm Hg), age, and severe blood loss. Symptomatic aneurysms require immediate surgery. Despite the high mortality of patients with ruptured abdominal aortic aneurysms, surgery is indicated even with marked hypotension, since the mortality of patients with unoperated ruptured aneurysms is 100%. Complications of resection of ruptured abdominal aneurysms include coagulopathy, bowel ischemia, renal failure, adult respiratory distress syndrome, arterial insufficiency of the extremities, and spinal cord ischemia. Myocardial infarction is a common cause of death despite successful resection. Mortality can be decreased by elective resection of aneurysms, thereby reducing the risk of rupture.

Popliteal artery aneurysms

Popliteal artery aneurysms are the most common extremity aneurysms, and atherosclerosis is the most common cause. Poststenotic turbulence produced by constriction at the adductor canal is thought to predispose patients to aneurysm formation at this level. Most patients with popliteal artery aneurysms are men in the 40- to 60-year age-group.

Aneurysms at other sites are common. Bilateral popliteal aneurysms were found in 59% of patients in one series. In contrast to abdominal aortic aneurysms that result in rupture, popliteal aneurysms produce symptoms of limb ischemia from thrombosis of the aneurysm or distal embolization. Large popliteal aneurysms may compress the adjacent popliteal vein and nerves.

A thrombosed aneurysm may be confused with an abscess, tumor, or Baker's cyst in the popliteal fossa. Likewise, a cyst overlying the popliteal artery may transmit its pulsation and be incorrectly diagnosed as a popliteal aneurysm. Ultrasound of the popliteal fossa allows differentiation between overlying structures and a widened popliteal artery. Most reported symptomatic popliteal aneurysms are 2.5 to 5 cm in diameter. However, isolated reports of larger lesions have appeared in the literature. Arteriography to evaluate the outflow tract is required in the preoperative evaluation of the patient with popliteal aneurysm. Emboli from the aneurysm commonly cause occlusive disease in vessels below the knee.

Treatment of popliteal aneurysm eliminates the risk of ischemic complications and restores adequate blood flow to the limb. Occasionally excision of the aneurysm with end-to-end anastomosis of the artery or interposition graft is possible. In most cases ligation of the aneurysm with vein bypass graft is the procedure of choice.

Elective treatment of patients with asymptomatic popliteal aneurysms has low morbidity and mortality. Asymptomatic lesions usually have an intact outflow tract, making reconstruction feasible. In contrast, popliteal aneurysms that are symptomatic as a result of embolization, rupture, or thrombosis often result in amputation. Long-term follow-up observation of these patients is required because of the frequent occurrence of other aneurysms, especially in the opposite popliteal artery and aorta.

ACUTE ARTERIAL INSUFFICIENCY

Acute arterial insufficiency is a sudden and marked decrease in arterial supply to an extremity. Sudden obstruction of a major artery not protected by adequate collateral circulation precipitates symptoms. The clinical manifestations are easily remembered by the mnemonic of five Ps: pain, paralysis, paresthesia, pallor, and pulselessness. Paralysis and paresthesia have important prognostic significance, since they result from ischemia of peripheral nerves and skeletal muscle. If paralysis or paresthesia is present, immediate intervention is required to save the limb.

The most common causes of acute arterial insufficiency are embolic and thrombotic occlusions. In young patients with known rheumatic heart disease, atrial fibrillation, or prosthetic valves, the diagnosis is straightforward. Patients in the atherosclerotic age range who have both significant cardiac disease and peripheral arterial disease present a diagnostic challenge. Less common causes of acute arterial insufficiency are dissecting aortic aneurysms with branch occlusion, intraarterial drug injection, and vasospasm induced by ergot abuse. Occasionally, extensive venous thrombosis may mimic acute arterial occlusion.

Emboli

The source of the embolus is the heart in 94% of cases. Mitral stenosis, atrial fibrillation, acute myocardial infarction, ventricular aneurysm, left atrial myxoma, bacterial endocarditis, and prosthetic heart valves are predisposing conditions. In a series of 338 patients with emboli, 231 had atrial fibrillation, 50 had acute myocardial infarction, and 7 had atherosclerotic plaques. The source of emboli in the remaining patients was undetermined.

Emboli lodge at branch points or areas of arterial tapering such as the adductor canal. Following impaction of the embolus, stagnant flow in the distal circulation allows distal clotting or formation of a tail thrombus. If collateral circulation is poorly developed, signs and symptoms of acute arterial insufficiency occur. Most emboli lodge in arteries supplying the lower extremities: 46% in the femoral arteries, 18% in the iliac arteries, and 11% in the popliteal tibial tree. Emboli in the upper extremities and the cerebral, renal, and mesenteric arteries are less frequent.

Clinical symptoms occur rapidly, including pain with decreased sensation and temperature of the limb. Examination of the pulses localizes the arterial occlusion. Neurologic evaluation determines the degree of ischemia. Decreased ability to differentiate light touch occurs before complete anesthesia. Paralysis and impaired motor function are late signs of severe arterial insufficiency. Loss of pliability of muscle mass indicates early tissue necrosis. Acidosis, hyperkalemia, and myoglobinuria result if treatment of acute arterial insufficiency is delayed, especially when large muscle masses are ischemic. Cardiac evaluation should exclude acute myocardial infarction, mural thrombosis, arrhythmia, and valvular disease. Abdominal examination is important at the time of initial evaluation, since there may be emboli in the mesenteric arteries. Abdominal distention or tenderness may indicate early bowel ischemia.

In patients in the atherosclerotic age-group, it is difficult to differentiate between embolic and thrombotic occlusion. Arteriography may be helpful in these patients to determine the cause and the extent of the operative procedure required.

MANAGEMENT. Operative removal of the embolus is indicated in all patients except those with terminal disease. During the initial 6 to 12 hours, emboli to the limb arteries can be removed with a minor surgical procedure using the Fogarty catheter. This restores arterial blood supply to the limb. Failure to remove emboli in the acute phase frequently results in amputation or major vascular reconstruction with higher morbidity and mortality.

Recently intraarterial infusion of urokinase or streptokinase has successfully restored perfusion in some patients if given early.

Anticoagulant therapy should be initiated as soon as a diagnosis of distal embolus is established. Anticoagulation before operative intervention prevents the propagation of distal thrombus and obstruction of collateral flow to the limb. Long-term anticoagulation is important to prevent recurrence. In one study of hospitalized patients, emboli recurred in 9% of those who had received anticoagulant therapy and in 31% of those who had not. Sympathectomy and vasodilating drugs are not indicated.

CHRONIC ARTERIAL DISEASES OF THE AORTA AND ITS BRANCHES

Atherosclerosis is the major cause of chronic arterial insufficiency. Less common causes include Buerger's disease (thromboangiitis obliterans), cystic disease of the popliteal artery, trauma, vasculitis, popliteal entrapment, and Takayasu's arteritis. Progressive narrowing of the arterial lumen by atherosclerotic plaque produces symptoms when peripheral demands exceed flow across the narrowed segment. Collateral vessels supplement arterial flow distal to the stenosed or occluded segment. However, arterial flow through collateral arteries is limited by their small size and high resistance.

Branch points, areas of posterior fixation, and areas of compression are preferentially involved in atherosclerosis because of turbulent flow at these points. The terminal aorta below the inferior mesenteric artery, the posterior wall of the common femoral artery, the superficial femoral artery at the level of the adductor hiatus, and the popliteal trifurcation are frequent sites of extensive atherosclerotic plaque. Segmental involvement is treated surgically by the bypass technique.

CLINICAL MANIFESTATIONS. Symptoms of chronic arterial insufficiency include claudication, rest pain, and skin lesions. Claudication is pain the the calf resulting from decreased arterial supply to the gastrocnemius muscle. The pain occurs with exercise because the impaired arterial system cannot meet the metabolic demands of the exercising muscle. Aortoiliac or superficial femoral occlusions may cause claudication. Similar exercise-induced pain in the hip or buttock results from iliac disease. Intermittent claudication varies in intensity and is not a sign of impending limb loss. In a study of 1440 patients with intermittent claudication, survival was 73% at 5 years and 38% at 10 years. Most deaths resulted from coronary or cerebrovascular disease. The amputation rate was 7.2% at 5 years and 12% at 10 years. Conservative treatment of claudication includes abstinence from nicotine, control of hyperlipidemia and hypertension, and exercise to develop collateral flow. Weight loss in the obese patient palliates symptoms by decreasing the work of exercise. Vasodilating drugs are of questionable benefit. Indications for surgical treatment depend on the degree of disability, site of occlusion, and the patient's medical status.

Rest pain, or pain in the distal portion of the foot and toes, indicates severe arterial insufficiency and impending tissue loss. This pain arises from ischemia of the skin and nerves of the foot. Symptoms initially occur at night because of loss of gravity-induced arterial inflow. Aggressive investigation and treatment by surgical reconstruction are indicated for limb salvage in this group of patients.

Ulcerations may occur spontaneously because of poor nutritional supply to the skin, but minor trauma is more commonly identified as the initiating event. Small traumatic lesions may progress to gangrene in a limb with arterial insufficiency. Signs of arterial insufficiency that precede ulceration or gangrene are atrophic nails and skin and hair loss.

DIAGNOSTIC TESTS. During the past 10 years development of techniques for noninvasive testing of arteries has introduced objectivity into the evaluation of occlusive disease. Doppler ultrasound (ankle blood pressure determinations and waveform analysis) and various plethysmographic techniques now are used to quantitate the degree of ischemia and define the level of hemodynamically significant arterial lesions. Blood pressure measurements obtained at the brachial, thigh, and ankle levels using the Doppler instrument as a sensor are the simplest of noninvasive testing methods. Blood pressure in the lower extremity should be equal to or greater than the brachial pressure in the absence of arterial obstructive lesions. Expression of the ankle pressure as a ratio over the brachial pressure may be used to quantitate ischemia. An index of 0.5 is compatible with claudication. An index of 0.3 indicates severe arterial insufficiency. Treadmill exercise testing is important to document the degree of disability from claudication and to differentiate neurogenic pain syndromes from arterial claudication.

Noninvasive testing has provided information on the natural history of arterial lesions. Pressure measurements have been used to predict the healing of traumatic ulcers of the foot, the success of revascularization procedures, and the level of amputation. Recently the measurement of penile arterial pressure has aided in the diagnosis of occlusion in patients whose impotence results from decreased arterial blood flow to the pelvis.

Although noninvasive testing gives the most accurate assessment of the effect of arterial occlusion on function of the extremity, arteriography provides a roadmap for the surgeon at the time of operation. Rapid sequence filming, advancements in catheter technique, and use of computer subtraction methods have provided clear visualization of the arterial tree. Films taken in multiple projections identify lesions in the iliac and femoral arteries previously undiagnosed by isolated anteroposterior projections. These advancements in arteriography allow optimal surgical treatment of arterial lesions by exact localization of the pathologic process. Arteriography is associated with low morbidity and mortality. The mortality of 0.5% results predominantly from hypersensitivity reactions to iodine contrast material. Serious complications, which have been reported in 0.3% to 2.3% of patients undergoing arteriography, include acute arterial occlusion caused by thrombus or subintimal dissection, hematoma, renal failure, and distal embolization.

Percutaneous transluminal angioplasty by balloon dilation with an intravascular catheter, performed after the lesions are identified through angiography or after the vessel is surgically exposed, effectively relieves stenosis by segmental atherosclerotic lesions in the aortoiliac, superficial femoral, and renal arteries. In some patients transluminal angioplasty is primary therapy, whereas in others it is used concurrently with distal reconstruction. Stenosis may recur, but patency for iliac lesions is 93.4% at 1 year, 82.2% at 2 years, and 79.4% at 3 years.

SPECIAL TREATMENT CONSIDERATIONS. Patients with severe arterial insufficiency frequently have occlusion at more than one level. Proximal aortoiliac lesions are corrected first, and this usually results in limb salvage. Bypass procedures to the posterior tibial, anterior tibial, or peroneal artery are now possible. Visualization of the leg vessels and plantar arch on arteriography is critical for the diagnosis of all lesions and may require delayed filming.

If the infrapopliteal arteries communicate with a patent plantar arch, patency rates are good. Limb salvage may result even in the presence of graft occlusion if the graft remains patent long enough to heal ischemic lesions. Sequential grafting from the popliteal to the distal tibial vessels has been suggested to improve outflow and patency rates.

The role of sympathectomy in the treatment of atherosclerotic occlusive disease is controversial, but direct arterial reconstruction, when possible, produces superior results. Sympathectomy is not indicated for claudication, since no increase in blood flow to the muscle results. Sympathectomy does increase blood flow to the skin to some extent and may be useful in healing small ischemic skin lesions. Complications include neuralgia and ejaculatory dysfunction or impotence in the male when bilateral sympathectomies at the first lumbar ganglion are performed.

Diabetic patients are at increased risk of lesions at all levels in the arterial tree. Classically lesions are most likely to occur in the infrapopliteal area. Patients with diabetes mellitus more often require amputation with peripheral arterial disease. This increased risk to the limb results from the preferential distal location of the arterial occlusion, presence of neuropathy, and decreased resistance to infection.

Noninvasive laboratory evaluation is used to localize lesions and distinguish pain caused by peripheral neuropathy from ischemic rest pain. Some diabetic patients have extensive calcification in the arterial wall that invalidates ankle pressure readings. Arteriography is associated with increased risk in patients with diabetic arterial disease. Dye excretion through a kidney with diabetic nephropathy is associated with an increased risk of acute tubular necrosis. Patients should be well hydrated before the evaluation.

Arterial reconstruction is possible in many patients with diabetic arterial disease. Segmental distribution of arterial occlusions and the state of the runoff vessels predict the success of the procedure, as in all patients with atherosclerotic disease. Sympathectomy should *not* be performed in patients with diabetic neuropathy that has resulted in autosympathectomy.

Leriche's syndrome (aortoiliac disease)

In 1940 Leriche described symptoms and signs of thrombotic obliteration of the aortic bifurcation in relatively young patients. These symptoms include (1) weariness of the lower extremities with exercise; (2) symmetric atrophy of both lower extremities without trophic skin or nail changes; (3) pallor of the legs and feet; and (4) inability to maintain an erection owing to decreased internal iliac arterial supply. Aortoiliac disease is progressive and may result in limb loss when sequential arterial occlusions develop. Because these patients are predominantly middle-aged (35 to 55 years of age), symptoms of claudication are more disabling than in the geriatric age-group. Operative intervention includes endarterectomy or bypass grafting. Today, aortofemoral bypass grafting is the preferred method of treatment in most hospitals. Mortality is in the range of 1% to 5%, with good 5- and 10-year patency rates. Complications include graft thrombosis, intraoperative embolization, false aneurysms at anastomosis, and graft infection. Retrograde ejaculation may result if dissection is performed at the aortic bifurcation.

Extraanatomic bypass (axillofemoral and femorofemoral grafts) are used for patients with aortoiliac involvement who cannot tolerate the aortoiliac or aortofemoral approach. Femorofemoral grafts are also employed as primary procedures for occlusive disease localized to one iliac artery. Five-year patency of 70% to 90% has been reported.

Superficial femoral occlusion

Occlusion of the superficial femoral artery is common in patients over 65 years of age. Symptoms are most severe at onset, and a small percentage of patients require immediate operative reconstruction because of severe arterial insufficiency. Most patients have a gradual improvement in exercise tolerance over a 6- to 12-month period. In this group mild residual claudication often does not require operative intervention. Patients with more severe claudication and poor collateral flow around the lesion are treated by femoropopliteal bypass. A saphenous vein of adequate luminal diameter is the prosthesis resulting in the best long-term patency. When a saphenous vein is not available, other materials such as expanded polytetrafluoroethylene are used. Complications include hematomas, thrombosis of the graft, saphenous nerve injury, edema of the lower extremity, and lymphocele. Patency rates are dependent on the status of the outflow system (runoff).

Buerger's disease (thromboangiitis obliterans)

In 1908 Buerger drew attention to a clinical syndrome caused by inflammation and occlusion of distal arteries by a specific pathologic process distinct from atherosclerosis. He named this syndrome thromboangiitis obliterans (TAO). Despite this precise description the terms "Buerger's disease" and "thromboangiitis obliterans" have been used by some to characterize distal arterial insufficiency and gangrene from any cause. Others have questioned the existence of the specific pathologic process originally described. These terms should be limited to the pathologic lesion characterized by transmural inflammation of distal arteries accompanied by thrombosis. Histologic evidence of inflammation in adjacent veins and nerves is common.

In contrast to atherosclerosis, Buerger's disease is a rare entity estimated to cause 1% of arterial insufficiency. The disease occurs most commonly in young men of Middle Eastern origin. The cause is unknown, although cigarette smoking has been closely linked to the onset and progression of the disease. Other etiologic factors that have been suggested include infection, genetic predisposition, trauma, and cold injury.

Clinical manifestations of Buerger's disease include rest pain, gangrene, claudication, Raynaud's phenomenon, thrombophlebitis, and hyperhidrosis. Arterial insufficiency caused by the disease usually has a sudden onset. Because of the distal location of the arterial occlusion, rest pain and gangrene are common initial symptoms. Calf or foot claudication is the first symptom in 20% of patients. Both upper and lower extremity involvement occurs in over 10% of the patients. A clinical diagnosis of Buerger's disease is usually made by identifying the following criteria: (1) upper and lower limb involvement, (2) distal site of lesion, (3) history of heavy cigarette smoking, (4) sparing of proximal arteries, and (5) phlebitis. Histologic examination of distal vessels is valuable in establishing the diagnosis and excluding atherosclerosis. Determination of the erythrocyte sedimentation rate, antinuclear antibodies, and rheumatoid factor is helpful in excluding other forms of vasculitis.

Treatment begins with prohibition of cigarette smoking. Smoking is the most important factor in predicting the progression of Buerger's disease. The distal site of arterial occlusion excludes arterial reconstruction in most patients. Rest pain and localized gangrene therefore are treated by sympathectomy and conservative amputation.

BIBLIOGRAPHY

Berguer RB: Selection of patients, choice of surgical technique, and results with vertebral artery reconstruction. In Berguer RB and Bauer RB, editors: Vertebrobasilar arterial occlusive disease. Medical and surgical management, New York, 1982, Raven Press.

Castanedo-Zuniga WE, editor: Transluminal angioplasty, New York, 1983, Thieme Medical Publishers, Inc.

Cranley JJ: Acute embolic occlusion of major arteries. In Bergen JJ and Yao JST, editors: Vascular surgical emergencies, Orlando, Florida, 1987, Grune & Stratton, Inc.

Crawford SE, Stowe CL, and Powers RW: Occlusion of the innominate, common carotid, and subclavian arteries: longterm results of surgical treatment, Surgery 94:781, 1983.

Hight DW, Tilney RL, and Couch NP: Changing clinical trends in patients with peripheral arterial emboli, Surgery 79:172, 1976.

Johnson JB and others: Natural history of asymptomatic carotid plaque, Arch Surg 120:1010, 1985.

Malone JM, Moore WS, and Goldstone J: The natural history of bilateral aortofemoral bypass grafts for ischemia of the lower extremities, Arch Surg 110:1300, 1975.

Porter JM, Taylor LM, and Baur GM: Nonatherosclerotic vascular disease. In Moore WS, editor: Vascular surgery—a comprehensive review, New York, 1983, Grune & Stratton, Inc.

Spence RV and others: Long-term results of transluminal angioplasty of the iliac and femoral arteries, Arch Surg 116:137, 1981.

Strandness DE: Echo-Doppler (duplex) ultrasonic scanning, J Vasc Surg 2:341, 1985.

Wakefield TW and others: Abdominal aortic aneurysm rupture: statistical analysis of factors affecting outcome of surgical treatment, Surgery 91:586, 1982.

DENTAL CORRELATIONS

Peter Quinn *and* **Louis F. Rose**

CONGESTIVE HEART FAILURE

Heart failure may be the outcome of virtually any aberrant cardiac process; therefore the syndrome must be considered a possibility in all patients of advanced age or indicative cardiac history. Following an evaluation designed to discover a history of specific cardiac lesions, individuals should be questioned about those symptoms classically associated with cardiac decompensation: fatigue, dyspnea on exertion, orthopnea, paroxysmal nocturnal dyspnea, and dependent edema. In patients known to have a history of previous cardiac failure, the answers to these same questions can provide important clues to the current state of compensation and the adequacy of therapy. Any change in such a patient's pattern of symptoms should prompt the dentist to postpone treatment and consult the individual's physician.

As has already been noted, the patient with early heart failure typically presents few signs when unstressed. The anxiety that many patients experience in the dental office can make a dental visit a substantial test of cardiac stamina, requiring the dentist's diligence in seeking out both frank and more subtle evidence of decompensation.

CLINICAL MANIFESTATIONS. Significant hypertension in a patient displaying symptoms of congestive heart failure is reason enough for immediate referral (see Chapter 87). Tachycardia, however, is not uncommon in dental surroundings and need not imply autonomic compensation for declining stroke volume. However, suspicions should be aroused when tachycardia is sustained or associated with other hard evidence of heart failure. An irregularity in the pulse may suggest arrhythmia as the basis of a patient's heart failure, but more often the disordered rhythm proves to be secondary to the underlying process actually producing the decompensation (such as valvular disease and cardiomyopathy). Since even short episodes of tachypnea are less common in the dental operatory than is tachycardia, respiratory rate may sometimes prove a more accurate barometer of cardiac reserve than heart rate. The reclining dental chair provides the practitioner with the means to observe any respiratory changes associated with recumbency (orthopnea).

Mucocutaneous color changes can accompany cardiac decompensation. Peripheral cyanosis (for example, as seen in the nail beds) results from exaggerated local extraction of oxygen from blood sluggishly pumped through reflexly constricted vessels. Chronic cyanosis in nail beds is manifested by "clubbing." When mucous membranes become blue (central cyanosis), a more serious condition occurs in which one may surmise the existence of significant intrapulmonary shunt. This latter situation is seen only when left ventricular filling pressures have risen high enough to produce pulmonary edema. This is the end result in left ventricular failure.

Patients suffering limited but chronic impairment of gas exchange may develop polycythemia in response to chronic hypoxia. Alone, absolute increases in hemoglobin level may be expected to produce a ruddiness in the complexion. However, when desaturation persists to the extent that 5 g/dl of hemoglobin remains reduced (the amount necessary for clinical cyanosis), the outcome is a curiously purple coloration of the skin. On occasion hypoxic stimulation of erythroid marrow elements is so pronounced that myeloid and megakaryocytic activity are depressed. When significant neutropenia is the result, particularly vigorous treatment of odontogenic infection is indicated. Oral purpuras may develop as a result of associated thrombocytopenia, but the dentist is obligated to exclude other causes of disordered primary hemostasis before settling on such a diagnosis.

Neck vein distention is important to evaluate but may be easily misinterpreted. Tight collars must be loosened and the patient's position taken into account before tenable conclusions may be drawn. For the dentist's purpose it is sufficient to observe the patient in the upright position, where the jugular veins may be considered as erect water manometers. Visible distention of these vessels occurs only when central venous pressure is sufficient to hold a column of blood above the level of the clavicles (approximately 12 cm H_2O). Such a pressure should be considered abnormal. Questionably abnormal observations may be tentatively corroborated by observation of peripheral veins. *In the absence of any peripheral obstruction to flow,* the veins on the dorsum of the hand should empty when elevated above the level of the heart. Continued distention of these vessels is further evidence of elevated central venous pressure. Other signs of right ventricular failure such as ascites and hepatomegaly may be present.

DENTAL MANAGEMENT. The practitioner first must assess the degree of failure and adequacy of treatment. Increasing dyspnea with less exertion, dyspnea at rest, several hospitalizations, and a constantly changing medical regimen are signs of progressive deterioration. Stable patients may undergo routine dental care if:

1. Appointments are kept short.
2. The supine position is avoided (this position allows peripheral blood to return to the central circulation and overwhelm the decompensated myocardium, resulting in orthopnea). A semirecumbent or erect position is mandatory.
3. Anxiety is controlled. (judicious use of mild sedatives can be helpful.)
4. Supplemental oxygen is provided.
5. The dentist is vigilant for iatrogenic problems in the patient who has had congestive heart failure, such as electrolyte disturbances from diuretics (for example, hypokalemia) and digitalis toxicity.

Acute dyspnea, anxiety, frothy productive cough, and cyanosis herald the onset of acute pulmonary edema. Should such signs occur in the dental office, the following list of actions is recommended:

1. Keep the patient erect.
2. Administer oxygen.
3. Administer meperidine hydrochloride (Demerol) (50 mg intramuscularly) or morphine sulfate (5-10 mg intramuscularly). (Be prepared to manage airway and support respirations.) This may help to reduce preload.
4. Apply tourniquets to the extremities to maintain blood pressure above venous pressures and below systolic arterial pressure. (This measure should be used only in extreme situations when the patient does not respond to the first three measures and hospital transportation is slow in coming.)
5. Arrange for transfer to a hospital, where definitive therapy with diuretics, nitroprusside, and more potent agents such as dopamine can be carried out.

Successful management of the hypertensive patient also depends on the adequacy of pain control. Both pain and its subsequent relief may produce exaggerated vasomotor responses. Thus it is best to provide adequate, long-lasting anesthesia so that the patient need not deal with either the stress or its precipitous removal. The long-expressed notion that pressors should not be used in the local anesthetic management of hypertensive patients has proved to be largely unfounded. It now is generally accepted that situations characterized by anesthesia of insufficient depth or longevity entail the release of endogenous catecholamines in amounts that far exceed those found in anesthetic preparations. This should not be interpreted to mean that these agents may be used with abandon but rather that the dentist should use the smallest quantity of medication consistent with the patient's comfort. Total epinephrine dosage should never exceed 0.2 mg in the healthy adult or 0.004 mg in the patient with cardiac disease (a 1:100,000 solution contains 0.018 mg of epinephrine). For the rare patient treated with the monoamine oxidase inhibitor, vasoconstrictor substances are contraindicated.

In those instances when dental manipulations are too involved to be performed effectively under local anesthesia, general anesthetics must, of course, be used. Because of the risks associated with these measures (and particularly the risk for

hypotension), it is not recommended that general anesthetics be used on an outpatient basis in patients with significant hypertensive cardiovascular disease. Medical consultation and hospitalization frequently are in the patient's best interest. For similar reasons, caution also must be exercised in the use of inhalation agents such as nitrous oxide for outpatient conscious sedation. Hypoxia may produce startling increases in arterial blood pressure, with calamitous results. Dentists should be familiar with the actions and side effects of the commonly used antihypertensive agents. Although less commonly employed today than in the past, reserpine preparations should evoke particular concern in the practitioner, being at times responsible for depression of affect, syncope, and profound hypotension. Because of the drug's mechanism of action (catecholamine depletion), hypotension is refractory to so-called indirect pressors (such as ephedrine) and should be treated with direct agents (such as norepinephrine or phenylephrine). Table 1 provides information on the side effects of the commonly used antihypertensive medicines.

SHOCK

True circulatory shock rarely occurs in the dental office. However, the dentist's indiscretion with surgical procedures or in prescribing drugs may make him or her culpable should the patient subsequently arrive at the hospital emergency ward in extremis. Only by eliciting a complete medical history can the practitioner hope to avoid those treatments likely to precipitate crisis in the compromised individual. Shock is classified by its origin:

Septic shock: infectious; secondary to a bacterial endotoxin that causes vasodilation; more common in gram-negative infections

Anaphylactic shock: cardiorespiratory collapse; caused by an IgE-mediated allergic response that releases chemical mediators from mast cells and basophils

Hypovolemic shock: inadequate cardiac function from volume depletion; results from bleeding, burns, renal disease, diuretics, and so on

Cardiogenic shock: decreased cardiac output after myocardial infarction ("pump failure")

Neurogenic shock (vasovagal): common fainting; relative hypovolemia from peripheral vasodilation and "pooling"

Septic and hypovolemic shock

Treatment modifications to prevent shock are few and easily implemented. When special risk of sepsis exists (for example, in a patient undergoing chemotherapy with steroids), aggressive management of dentoalveolar infection can do much to decrease the incidence of warm shock. The earliest evidence that infection no longer is localized and is spreading is indication enough for hospitalization of such individuals. Analgesic compounds containing aspirin must be prescribed with care so that the anticoagulated individual or ulcer patient is not threatened by serious hemorrhagic complications. Similarly, the patient with bleeding diathesis must command the use of unusual surgical precautions if a normally benign procedure is not to end in exsanguination.

Vasovagal syncope

The preceding comments concerning the rarity of shock in the dental office do not, of course, apply if one is to include vasovagal syncope within the definition of circulatory collapse. Syncope refers to an abrupt loss of consciousness, the causes of which are manifold. The common faint is a maladaptive cardiovascular response to stress, not infrequently associated

Table 1 Potential side effects and interactions of commonly used antihypertensive drugs

Antihypertensive drug	Side effects	Interactions
Thiazides	Gastrointensinal upset, weakness, photosensitivity, azotemia, hypokalemia, hyperglycemia	Enhance responsiveness to D-tubocurarine
β-blockers	Bradycardia, congestive heart failure, increased bronchial asthma, hallucinosis, Raynaud's phenomenon, weakness, depression	Epinephrine may produce bradycardia
Loop diuretics (furosemide)	Azotemia, hyperuricemia, hypokalemia, photosensitivity	Enhance D-tubocurarine
Potassium-sparing		
Spironolactone (Aldactone)	Hyperkalemia, gynecomastia, hirsutism	Aspirin may inhibit natriuresis
Triamterene	Hyperkalemia, diarrhea, nausea	
α-Methyldopa (Aldomet)	Orthostatic hypotension, drowsiness, depression, xerostomia, impotence, positive Coombs' test, gynecomastia	
Clonidine	Xerostomia, drowsiness, impotence, orthostatic hypotension, rebound hypertension with sudden cessation	
Reserpine	Drowsiness, sedation, weakness, nasal congestion, depression, bradycardia	Hypotension with general anesthesia
Hydralazine	Headache, tachycardia, palpitations, increased angina and congestive heart failure, "lupus" syndrome	
Guanethidine	Orthostatic hypotension	Alcohol increases orthostatic hypotension (hypotension with general anesthesia)
Prazosin	Orthostatic hypotension with syncope, dizziness, weakness, blurred vision, nausea, diarrhea, headache, palpitations	

with the sight of blood or hypodermic needles. A prodromal or presyncopal stage may include giddiness, confusion, visual disturbances, pallor, diaphoresis, or nausea and vomiting. If these symptoms are quickly addressed by placing the patient in a Trendelenburg position, loss of consciousness may be prevented. When such is not the case, true syncope follows, characterized by hypotension, bradycardia, and occasionally limited clonic activity. Treatment includes supination of the patient with elevation of the legs, airway protection, and administration of oxygen. Aromatic spirits of ammonia may be used to stimulate respiration, but only rarely are other forms of medical intervention required. When consciousness is not restored by these techniques and hypotension and bradycardia persist, slow intravenous administration of 0.5 to 1.0 mg atropine is indicated. The administration of atropine in doses of less than 0.5 mg is to be avoided, as this may produce idiosyncratic exacerbation of bradycardia.

Whenever fainting has occurred, the patient should be allowed to rest comfortably and encouraged to arise slowly. The patient with a history of atherosclerotic disease, who has responded to conservative treatment of syncope, should undergo at least cursory examination for evidence of end-organ damage. Whenever hypotension and bradycardia have been sustained enough to require the use of atropine, it is appropriate to arrange for examination of the patient by the physician. In either case the patient should be reappointed for dental treatment on a future date, before which time appropriate measures can be taken to deal with the anxiety that precipitated the syncope (for example, a plan for sedation).

Cardiogenic shock

For a discussion on cardiogenic shock refer to Chapter 96.

PULMONARY EMBOLISM

CLINICAL MANIFESTATIONS. Pulmonary embolism may occur in any setting, including the private dental office, although it is particularly common in the hospital, where patients are predisposed by both infirmity and incapacity.

It is good to remember that any of three conditions may predispose the patient to venous thrombosis: vascular stasis,

vessel wall disease, or disruption and hypercoagulability of blood. Statistically stasis is the most important of these conditions and is minimized by early postoperative ambulation or the use of support hose and daily leg exercise when extended bed rest is necessary. These measures are particularly important in patients with a history of phlebitic disease. The hospital dental practitioner should examine all patients at bed rest for signs of thrombophlebitis and should be alert to complaints of leg pain or swelling. Thrombophlebitis also is an important consideration in the differential diagnosis of postoperative fever, especially when such fever occurs several days after surgery and cannot be traced to wound infection or infection of the urinary tract. Although hypercoagulability of blood is an uncommon problem, the abrupt withdrawal of anticoagulants can produce rebound hypercoagulation on occasion.

DENTAL MANAGEMENT OF THE ANTICOAGULATED PATIENT

Coumarin. Coumarin preparations (for example, warfarin [Coumadin]) are the only agents currently used for outpatient anticoagulation. They exert their effect through the competitive inhibition of vitamin K, with subsequent depletion of those coagulation factors dependent on that substance for their synthesis (that is, factors II, VII, IX, and X). The half-life of these drugs requires that they be discontinued at least 2 days before the time at which normal coagulation studies might be desired. Only rarely, however, is the dentist's need for cessation of therapy compelling enough to justify the risk for thrombosis that accompanies such action. When contemplating procedures likely to cause bleeding, it is appropriate to ask that the physician make those dosage adjustments necessary to keep the prothrombin time between one and one half and two times the control. When this is accomplished, the hypoprothrombinemia is effectively countered with vigorous local hemostatic measures that, depending on the procedure performed, might include tension sutures over foam gelatin or the insertion of stents. Constant local pressure and soft diet frequently are beneficial.

Heparin. Anticoagulation is accomplished on an acute basis through the parenteral administration of heparin. Because effective hemostasis after extraction or mucogingival surgery is extremely difficult, only the most acute dental emergencies can be treated in the heparinized patient. When blood loss is anticipated, herparin must be discontinued for 4 to 6 hours before the procedure and should be reinstituted as soon as effective primary hemostatis has been observed.

• • •

When local hemostatic measures fail in the anticoagulated patient, pharmacologic manipulation becomes necessary. If the coumadinized patient can tolerate a wait of several hours, vitamin K administration will enhance his hemostatic ability. More urgent situations demand the transfusion of fresh-frozen plasma. When prompt reversal of heparin is in order, protamine sulfate is the drug of choice.

Rules useful in the treatment of the anticoagulated patient are as follows:

1. For treatments likely to cause bleeding (deep scaling, curettage, mucogingival surgery, or extraction), see that the coumadinized patient has a prothrombin time no greater than two times the control.
2. Use strict hemostatic surgical technique.
3. Employ vigorous local hemostatic measures, including primary closure when possible, foamed gelatin, soft tissue packs, and/or stents.
4. Remember that direct pressure is the most effective anti-hemorrhage measure, even in the anticoagulated patient.
5. Whenever possible use the Cavitron for gross scaling rather than curets, as the latter more commonly lacerates the gingiva and aggravates bleeding.
6. Acute dental conditions should not be prolonged; they should be given immediate attention.
7. Explain the nature of your treatment to the physician and enlist the physician's aid in management when medical intervention is required.

CONGENITAL HEART DISEASE

CLINICAL MANIFESTATIONS. Rarely does the dental patient with congenital heart disease betray his condition during the orofacial examination. Although it is the dentist's responsibility to be aware of those external physical characteristics that may suggest underlying cardiac abnormality, such as Down's facies or elfin facies, the dentist also must realize that the typical ambulatory patient with congenital cardiac impairment displays little physical evidence of such derangement. The blue mucosa and integument of central cyanosis so characteristic of right-to-left shunting lesions most often is observed in those too young and infirm to have come under the dentist's care. When some clinically detectable hypoxemia does persist on a chronic basis, a change in the depth of cyanosis should always be sought by the dentist as evidence of hypoxic decompensation. This may occur in patients who have previously undergone only palliative treatment or in an individual whose formerly marginal shunt has been increased by a second process (such as increasing pulmonary hypertension).

Anomalies of the dentition may bring children with cyanotic disease under the dentist's care, requiring each consultant to be aware of the frequent association between hypoplasia of the primary dentition and cyanotic heart disease. Delay in the formation of the permanent teeth also has been demonstrated in this group. Other reported oral findings such as furrowed tongue in tetralogy of Fallot and enlargement of maxillary incisor pulp chambers in coarctation of the aorta are too variable and nonspecific to be of great use in the clinical detection of disease.

Because the upper extremities are easily accessible to the dentist, they should always be examined for clubbing of the fingers.

DENTAL MANAGEMENT. Dentoalveolar infection is more common and potentially more devastating in individuals with congenital heart disease. In 1946 Kaner and others demonstrated that dentin is poorly calcified in those with congenital heart disease and that this may predispose such individuals to caries. Such vulnerability is particularly troublesome when it is coupled with the overindulgence of a parent concerned about the child's long-term prognosis. Indeed, studies have shown that oral hygiene and dietary habits are worse among individuals with congenital heart disease than among the general population.

As is true for individuals with endocardial disease of any variety, those marked by congenital cardiovascular anomaly are at increased risk of infective endocarditis, a risk that increases whenever surgical treatment of the disease requires the insertion of a prosthesis. Given the present recognition of the oral cavity as the most common origin of transient bacteremia, it is clear that the patient risks grave disease from both self-neglect and improper dental treatment. Optimal oral health is necessary to minimize the incidence of significant spontaneous *or* iatrogenic bacteremia. To further decrease risk in the treatment situation, antibiotic chemoprophylaxis usually is indicated. The reader is referred to the boxes on p. 509 concerning accepted antibiotic regimens and the relative risk of endocarditis in each of the disease states.

Systemic septic embolization, a form of so-called paradoxic embolization, is common among those with focal infection and congenital heart disease. Brain abscess is a dire consequence of such a process and should be suspected in any child with congenital heart disease who complains of headache. Because cultures of brain abscesses usually grow a mixed spectrum of anaerobic organisms and because the floral spectrum is so similar to that known to exist within the gingival crevice, oral infection and dental manipulations must be considered as important instigators of brain abscess in the child with congenital heart disease. Valachovic and Hargreaves believe pulpectomy to be contraindicated in the primary dentition of those with congenital heart disease, since root resorption can expose untreated accessory canals that might seed the blood with organisms. Citing a case of brain abscess traced to an endodontically treated primary tooth, they recommend extraction of any tooth with "clinical or radiographic evidence of apical or furcational periodontitis."

In summary, the treatment plan for those with congenital heart disease must include the following:

1. Medical consultation to learn the specific nature of the defect, specific past history, and risk of decompensation or arrhythmia.
2. Antibiotic prophylaxis for all dental procedures in an effort to avoid endocarditis and brain abscess.
3. Prompt and vigorous treatment of all oral infection, with extraction to be considered the preferred treatment for endodontically involved primary teeth.
4. A frank and open discussion with the parents and patient, detailing the importance of strict oral hygiene and regular dental care to both the oral and the general health of the patient.

VALVULAR HEART DISEASE

Damage to valves, causing stenosis or regurgitation, is a common cardiac problem. Ultimately it may present as congestive heart failure and/or arrythmia. The main concern of the dentist in these patients is the possibility of endocarditis.

During each patient evaluation a history of congenital or rheumatic heart disease must be sought, as well as a history

AMERICAN HEART ASSOCIATION—RECOMMENDED ANTIBIOTIC REGIMENS FOR ENDOCARDITIS PROPHYLAXIS*

FOR ADULTS UNDERGOING DENTAL OR RESPIRATORY TRACT PROCEDURES

Standard regimen

For dental procedures that cause gingival bleeding and oral surgery

Penicillin V, 2 g orally, 1 hour before, then 1 g 6 hours later. For patients unable to take oral medications, may substitute 2 million units of aqueous penicillin G intravenously or intramuscularly 30 to 60 minutes before a procedure and 1 million units 6 hours later

Pediatric doses: Dosage intervals are the same

Penicillin V, full adult dose if child weighs more than 60 lb; half the adult dose if child's weight is less than 60 lb

Aqueous penicillin G, 50,000 units/kg (25,000 units/kg as follow-up dose)

Special regimens

Parenteral regimen for use when maximal protection is desired, for example, for patients with prosthetic valves

Ampicillin, 1 to 2 g intramuscularly or intravenously, plus gentamicin, 1.5 mg/kg body weight intramuscularly or intravenously, 30 minutes before procedure, followed by 1 g of oral penicillin V 6 hours later. Alternatively, may repeat the parenteral regimen once 8 hours later

Oral regimen for patients allergic to penicillin

Erythromycin, 1 g orally 1 hour before, then 500 mg 6 hours later

Parenteral regimen for patients allergic to penicillin

Vancomycin, 1 g intravenously, slowly over 1 hour, starting 1 hour before; no repeat dose necessary

Pediatric doses: Dosage intervals are the same

Ampicillin, 50 mg/kg body weight per dose
Gentamicin, 2.0 mg//kg per dose
Erythromycin, 20 mg/kg for first dose, then 10 mg/kg
Vancomycin, 20 mg/kg per dose

*Adapted from Shulman ST and others: Prevention of bacterial endocarditis, Circulation 70: 1123A, 1984.

CATEGORIES OF RISK FOR SUBACUTE BACTERIAL ENDOCARDITIS

1. Greatly increased risk: regimen B
   a. Prosthetic valve
   b. Indwelling vascular catheter
2. Increased risk: regimen A or B
   a. Valvular heart disease
   b. Intracardiac shunts including patent ductus arteriosus, ventricular septal defect, and atrial septal defect of the primary type
   c. Hypertrophic cardiomyopathy (idiopathic hypertrophic subaortic stenosis, hypermetropic astigmatism)
   d. Hydrocephalus with ventricular-atrial shunt

3. Minimally increased risk: regimen A
   a. Mitral valve prolapse
   b. Transvenous cardiac pacemaker
   c. Artificial atrioventricular fistula for renal dialysis
   d. Synthetic arterial grafts
4. No increase in risk: no antibiotics
   a. Recent angiography or cardiac catheterization
   b. Uncomplicated atrial septal defect of secondary type
   c. Coronary artery surgery
   d. Shedding primary teeth

of heart murmur and rheumatic fever. When rheumatic fever is denied, it is wise to inquire specifically about childhood episodes of polyarthritis, "growing pains," chorea, or prolonged febrile infirmity. It is not uncommon for patients to be unaware that such illnesses may have been episodes of rheumatic fever.

Because so-called benign or functional cardiac murmurs are relatively common and require no modification of dental management, it is important that the practitioner make some effort to distinguish these from murmurs whose presence indicates organic disease. This often can be done with the help of the patient alone, since most people reporting a murmur will have been concerned enough about its significance to have queried their physicians. Whenever doubt remains, direct consultation with the physician is recommended. Also, since heart failure is the final common pathway in chronic heart disease, specific questions concerning this syndrome are appropriately included in the interrogation (for instance, dyspnea on exertion, paroxysmal nocturnal dyspnea, and orthopnea). Although such questions only occasionally lead to the discovery of new disease, they always provide valuable information concerning the

patient's cardiac reserve and his ability to meet the stress of treatment.

Hard physical findings within the dentist's realm are not the rule with valvular heart disease, but important information sometimes may be gleaned through careful evaluation of the vital signs and examination of the head, neck, and extremities. The physical findings herein described are variable and should not be considered pathognomonic of valvular disease. They may, however, prove important warning signs when discovered in those individuals with questionable history of rheumatic fever or murmur or known murmur previously assumed to be benign.

Systemic arterial blood pressure usually is normal in the ambulatory patient with mitral valve disease, but the patient with aortic insufficiency often shows systolic hypertension and a widened pulse pressure. In contrast, significant systolic hypertension is uncommon in the stenotic form of aortic valve disease.

Attention should be directed to the carotid pulse, where rate and regularity are noted. An irregular tachyrhythmia is likely atrial fibrillation, a rhythmic disturbance commonly associated with the dilated left atrium found in rheumatic mitral disease. Frequent extrasystole in a young woman may be the result of the ventricular automaticity seen in mitral valve prolapse.

Considering the pulse's character provides more data, a sharp, regular upstroke is common in mitral regurgitation (when normal sinus rhythm exists) and a slow, weak upstroke with delayed and sustained peak characteristic of aortic stenosis. Aortic insufficiency classically yields the bounding Corrigan or "water-hammer" pulse mentioned above, and this may have a double or bisferiens character (this latter quality also being seen in hypertrophic cardiomyopathy).

Tachypnea should never be ignored unless it is short-lived and obviously related to anxiety. When observed in a patient complaining of dyspnea, it should always prompt a search for other signs of decompensation. It is important to remember that some individuals with mitral disease are subject to chronic pulmonary transudation and are at increased risk for respiratory infection. Tachypnea may result from either the underlying problem or its sequelae. Similarly, the persistently febrile patient with known valvular disease may suffer if his fever is too quickly attributed to oral pathosis. Despite its relatively low incidence, infective endocarditis is responsible for morbidity and mortality sufficient in magnitude to justify a septic workup when fever has persisted for more than a week.

Just as symptoms of heart failure may be uncovered in the history, so must physical evidence of decompensation be sought during the examination. Jugular venous distention, ankle edema, and cyanosis are important signs that the dentist should not overlook (see Chapter 86).

Endocarditis

The dental patient with valvular heart disease faces three basic risks: heart failure, hemodynamically significant arrhythmia, and infective endocarditis.

Infection of the endocardius is a grave disorder, the incidence of which largely depends on the occurrence of transient bacteremia in those with existing valvular heart disease. Particularly distressing is the fact that these heart diseases may render their victims vulnerable to infection with endogenous organisms not ordinarily virulent in the human host.

Studies begun nearly five decades ago have shown the oral cavity to be the single most important area of regular bacterial ingress. Although the early works concerned themselves largely with postextraction bacteremia, more recent papers have established that virtually every dental procedure can seed organisms into the blood. In fact, simple mastication alone with no associated invasive tissue manipulation can produce bacteremia in many individuals. Logically the risk for such bacterial entry has been found to be related to the level of oral health, particularly of the periodontium.

Since the first work of Okell and Elliott in 1935, the significance of *Streptococcus viridans* bacteremia has been widely known. This group of organisms, whose ravages ordinarily are limited to the oral cavity, is one of the most common culprits in subacute bacterial endocarditis. Modern anaerobic culture techniques also have proved that anaerobes commonly found in the gingival sulcus are culpable in increasing numbers of cases.

DENTAL MANAGEMENT. The following are the most recent guidelines on prophylaxis from the American Heart Association. Coverage is indicated for all dental procedures likely to cause gingival bleeding (not simple adjustment of orthodontic appliances or shedding of deciduous teeth). These procedures include extractions, periodontal surgery, subgingival scaling and curettage, drainage of infectious tissue, and endodontic manipulation.

A list of cardiac conditions for which endocarditis prophylaxis is recommended follows:

Prosthetic heart valves
Most congenital cardiac malformations
Rheumatic and other acquired valvular defect
Idiopathic hypertrophic subaortic stenosis
Mitral valve prolapse *with* insufficiency
Previous history of bacterial endocarditis
Surgically created systemic-pulmonary shunts

A list of cardiac conditions for which endocarditis prophylaxis is NOT required follows:

Isolated secundum atrial septal defect
Secundum atrial septal defect corrected without a patch 6 or more months previously
Patent ductus arteriosus ligated and divided 6 or more months previously
Postoperatively after coronary bypass surgery
Cardiac catheterization and angiography

A commonly used list of disorders for which prophylaxis is believed to be required, and the relative risk for endocarditis in each, is given in the box on p. 509. Although the standards may be considered a near-consensus, they are empirically derived and hence subject to change.

It is important to note that despite the declining incidence of rheumatic fever, the dentist still can expect to encounter patients with a history of rheumatic heart disease who receive regular chemoprophylaxis against the recurrence of group A β-hemolytic *Streptococcus* infection and rheumatic fever (that is, monthly injections of benzathine or penicillin or daily oral doses). Such treatment should in no way be construed as adequate prophylaxis against subacute bacterial endocarditis. Because oral organisms resistant to the chronically administered medication are known to appear soon after the inception of such therapy, the dentist is advised to consult with the patient's physician to arrange for a substantial increase in the penicillin dose or for the substitution of another drug (usually erythromycin) during dental treatment.

As important as appropriate antibiotic prophylaxis is to the patient's continued health, it must be stated in summation that the dentist's efforts to foster optimal oral health are perhaps even more significant. As has been shown, dental manipulation is in no way essential to the genesis of bacteremia, and it must be assumed that frequent showers of organisms are the rule in individuals with neglected mouths. Perhaps the dentist performs the greatest service for this group when he or she succeeds in significantly modifying their oral hygiene behavior so that septic "suicide" can no longer be inadvertently accomplished.

BIBLIOGRAPHY

Batch AL and others: Bacteremia in patients undergoing oral procedures, Arch Int Med 1988:1084.

Benter IB and others: Comparative effects of local and systemic antibiotic therapy in the prevention of post-extraction bacteremia, J Am Dent Assoc 57:54, 1958.

Benter IB and Pressman RS: Antibiotic treatment of the gingival sulcus in prevention of postextraction bacteremia, J Oral Surg 14:20, 1956.

Burket LW and Burn CG: Bacteremia following dental extraction: demonstration of source of bacteria by means of a nonpathogen, J Dent Res 10:521, 1937.

Eisenbud L: Subacute bacterial endocarditis precipitated by non-surgical dental procedures, Oral Surg 15:624, 1962.

Feinstein AR and others: Prophylaxis of recurrent rheumatic fever, JAMA 206:565, 1968.

Hobson FG and Juel-Jensen BE: Teeth, *Streptococcus viridans*, and subacute bacterial endocarditis, Br Med J 2:1510, 1956.

McGowan DA and Tuohy O: Dental treatment of patients with valvular heart disease, Dent J, p 519, 1968.

Okell CC and Elliott SD: Bacteremia and oral sepsis with special reference to the etiology of subacute endocarditis, Lancet 2:869, 1935.

Shulman ST and others: Prevention of bacterial endocarditis, Circulation 70:1123 (A), 1984.

Spencer WH and others: Rheumatic fever, chemoprophylaxis, and penicillin-resistance gingival organisms, Ann Intern Med 73:683, 1970.

CARDIOMYOPATHY

CLINICAL MANIFESTATIONS. In general cardiomyopathy does not have clinical findings in the cervicofacial structures. Lipoidoses may reveal coarse facies, macrocephaly, or numerous angiomas.

DENTAL MANAGEMENT. Management is the same as that of heart failure and arrhythmia. The reader is referred to the appropriate sections for discussion of these topics.

CORONARY HEART DISEASE

CLINICAL MANIFESTATIONS. Pain is the most perplexing of the chief complaints; no other symptom is at once as demanding of solution and defiant of the doctor's analytic efforts. The discussion of the ischemic heart may provide the most appropriate framework within which to reiterate those clinical principles useful in the general interpretation of pain. Some of these principles may help to distinguish between like discomforts originating from systems as distinct and different as those devoted to circulatory and stomatognathic function.

The dentist should employ a standard protocol in the characterization of pain, in each instance seeking answers to the following questions:

Where is the pain located?
What kind of pain is it? Is it constant or intermittent, sharp or aching?
How long has it been present, and what was the nature of its onset?
Is there a pattern of referral?
Are there any initiating or exacerbating factors?
What, if anything, alleviates the pain?
Has the patient experienced similar pain in the past, and if so, how has this episode been different?
Are there any associated symptoms?

Although the location of a pain often is of great help in elucidating its nature, too great a reliance on this one characteristic has led many practitioners to unfortunate and inaccurate conclusions. A discomfort localized to the jaw with other characteristics atypical of gnathic affliction demands that related systems be evaluated. That 18% of all cardiac pain is localized solely in the teeth and jaws is ample evidence of the need for full evaluation in each case.

Admittedly, most who suffer with coronary artery disease are aware of the diagnosis before the dentist performs any evaluation. However, a knowledge of the character of pain is no less important when the history has revealed significant pathophysiology. Gauging a patient's ability to withstand stress must be largely based on the stability of the coronary occlusive process. This is most reliably determined by evaluating the ischemic pain pattern, and any change in the frequency or character of painful episodes necessitates postponement of dental treatment and cardiologic reevaluation.

DENTAL MANAGEMENT. Patients with angina whose pattern of pain is established and unchanging have low risk of angina in the dental office. For those who typically experience frequent bouts of angina after minor exertion, preoperative use of nitroglycerine is indicated. Although sedation also can be of great help in specific instances, it should, of course, be used judiciously. When the hypotension of deep sedation is superimposed on a critical coronary lesion, myocardial infarction may result. Indeed, the dentist must structure treatment to ensure the maintenance of that critical balance between myocardial oxygen demand and the ability of the coronary arteries to supply this substrate. Short morning appointments, adequate anesthesia, and sedation are among the measures that may help limit stress and therefore myocardial oxygen needs. Avoiding even small drug-related depressions in blood pressure protects the coronary perfusion that is so dependent on the maintenance of the gradient between diastolic arterial and left ventricular end-diastolic pressures.

The maximum allowable amount of epinephrine in the adult patient is 0.2 mg. In a patient with a history of cardiovascular disease, this is reduced to 0.04 mg, or one fifth of the adult dose. Remember that one carpule of local anesthesia with 1:1000,000 epinephrine contains 0.018 mg of epinephrine. Therefore two carpules is the maximum that could be used. The use of local hemostatic agents such as epinephrine-impregnated gingival cord cannot be condoned, since sizable doses of the drug may be absorbed through gingival vessels. Particular care should be exercised when epinephrine is administered to those receiving propranalol. The increased vagal tone resulting from epinephrine-related elevation of blood pressure normally has no bradycardic consequences, owing to the offsetting chronotropy of the drug. When this β-stimulatory effect is blocked by propranalol or other β-blockers, however, unopposed vagal stimulation can produce bradycardia and hypotension.

The dentist also may have an impact on the patient's well-being through ongoing concern for the control of atherosclerotic risk factors. Regular sphygmomanometric examinations are important in an effective antihypertensive program and may uncover changes in arterial impedance of critical significance to cardiac work load. Surprisingly, the detailing of oral damage attributable to tobacco use and dietary indiscretion may occasionally prove effective in modifying patient behavior.

When angina occurs during treatment the following steps should be taken:

1. Terminate the procedure.
2. Place the patient in a semisitting position.
3. Administer 100% oxygen.
4. Administer sublingual nitroglycerine, preferably the patient's own drug (0.32 or 0.4 mg are common doses); use the minimal dose needed for relief to avoid secondary hypotension.

Any pain that remains unrelieved after three doses of nitroglycerine given every 5 minutes, that lasts more than 15 to 20 minutes, or that is associated with diaphoresis, nausea, vomiting, syncope, or hypotension should prompt concern for myocardial infarction. The patient should continue oxygen, and 5 to 10 mg of morphine sulfate may be given intravenously for pain and anxiety. Vital signs must be closely monitored while arrangements are made for immediate transportation to a hospital.

Should cardiopulmonary arrest occur while aid is still forthcoming, it is the dentist's responsibility to make the diagnosis and institute treatment. The office staff should be trained in basic life support, and the dentist should be knowledgeable in advanced life support so that he or she may perform any advanced resuscitative measures that may be required (such as endotracheal intubation or central venous cannulation).

Following myocardial infarction elective dental treatment is contraindicated for a minimum of 6 months. After complete evolution of the myocardial scar, management depends on the clinical course, including postinfarction angina and arrhythmias. The physician should always be consulted to determine whether any specific contraindications to elective office therapy exist. If no problems are noted, the dentist may proceed with treatment, employing those principles used when caring for the patient with a cardiac condition. However, it is good to temper treatment, since the reinfarction rate remains disproportionately high for approximately 2 years in the postinfarction group.

ARRHYTHMIA

The dentist's detection of arrhythmia, whether through inquiry or examination, often justifies medical consultation before the initiation of therapy. Not every patient admitting to palpitation requires medical evaluation. Such an evaluation should be reserved for those who report frequent and distressing paroxysms; associated symptoms such as dizziness, angina, dyspnea, and syncope; or past history of significant heart disease.

CLINICAL MANIFESTATIONS. The dentist's examination occasionally may provide clues to the nature of the arrhythmia, but it should not be expected to substitute for communication with the physician. Regular waxing and waning of heart rate in concert with respiration is characteristic of sinus arrhythmia, a normal phenomenon in children and adults but a common harbinger of sinus node disease in the elderly. Irregular rhythms may have cyclical patterns, as in atrial or ventricular bigeminy, or may be characterized only by chaos (such as atrial fibrillation or multifocal atrial tachycardia).

Indeed, it generally is less crucial to identify an arrhythmia than to observe its circulatory impact. A short-lived paroxysm of supraventricular tachycardia that brings with it angina or syncope commands more of the dentist's concern than a chronic dysrhythmia lacking perfusion compromise. There are then but two major concerns in the evaluation of arrhythmia. The dentist must learn (1) the hemodynamic significance of the rhythm and (2) the propensity of that rhythm to degenerate into forms of even greater hemodynamic consequence. Both depend in large measure on the underlying process responsible for the observed alterations.

DENTAL MANAGEMENT. Before considering the dysrhythmias common to each of the major cardiopathologic processes, we should first describe those treatment principles essential to the management of any rhythmic disturbance occurring in the dental office. Cessation of therapy and the administration of oxygen are among those measures appropriate in all situations of new or sustained arrhythmia, as are an immediate hemodynamic evaluation and the summoning of medical help. An appraisal of the patient's mental alertness, blood pressure, heart rate, and skin temperature provides important clues to the adequacy of perfusion and does not depend on the presence of sophisticated monitoring equipment.

Hypotension demands the use of the Trendelenburg position but does not in itself justify pharmacologic intervention except when accompanied by persisting symptoms of end-organ oligemia (such as angina, confusion, or coma). In the setting of bradyarrhythmia, symptomatic hypotension is appropriately addressed with the intravenous administration of 0.5 to 1 mg atropine sulfate. Similarly, life-threatening hypotension with tachyrhythmia should be treated with vagal maneuvers. However, the risks of carotid massage require that the dentist use this technique only when it is truly necessary. The practitioner must be prepared to support the patient should syncope, cerebrovascular accident, or vagal arrest ensue.

Because medical treatment directed specifically at the arrhythmia often is impossible without electrocardiographic monitoring, definitive management usually must await the patient's transportation to the hospital. For those practitioners who possess the necessary skill and equipment, interventions beyond those already described may be appropriate. Fortunately, the supportive actions discussed usually suffice until medical help is available.

Patients with no underlying cardiac disease seldom suffer more than psychic disturbance from arrhythmia. Both atrial and ventricular ectopic beats are common in an otherwise healthy heart. In fact, it long has been held that stress and compulsive activity are the progenitors of much functional heart disease. The practitioner should employ those measures commonly used to reduce stress in the office, so that the patient does not come to expect the precipitation of symptoms with each dental visit.

Valvular heart disease commonly underlies arrhythmia; the atrial dysrhythmias of rheumatic mitral disorders are an example. When atrial fibrillation is chronic and ventricular rate is adequately controlled through digitalization, little need be done by the dentist save the implementation of standard endocarditis precautions. Should new atrial fibrillation develop in the dental office, the measures already described frequently provide the time required for transportation of the patient to an emergency facility.

The premature ventricular contractions of mitral valve prolapse are rarely of consequence, but paroxysms of supraventricular tachycardia may distress both dentist and patient alike. If the patient is unable to terminate his attack through accustomed vagal maneuvers, sedation and reassurance often prove effective. Most patients with supraventricular tachycardia do quite well and may be easily transported to a hospital if the rhythm persists.

Patients with cardiomyopathy are subject to a host of rhythmic disturbances, with atrial fibrillation, ventricular extrasystoles, and paroxysmal ventricular tachycardia being of particular note. The appearance of frequent multiformed premature ventricular contractions or bursts of ventricular tachycardia require treatment with intravenous lidocaine. Ventricular tachycardia with hypotension and obturation demands early asynchronous electric cardioversion.

Although premature ventricular contractions and ventricular tachycardia should also prompt the practitioner to suspect ischemic heart disease, the patient with coronary artery disease may occasionally suffer spontaneous ventricular fibrillation. Immediate 400 joule defibrillation helps avoid the intractable arrhythmias so common with the acidosis of prolonged circulatory arrest. Basic life-support measures are called for should defibrillation fail.

Although the dentist's role in the treatment of arrhythmic emergency may be a critical one, his or her part in the prevention of such catastrophies is of more far-reaching import. Combining knowledge of both the individual patient and the disease entities of concern, the dentist must modify the treatment plan in ways that accurately reflect the risks involved. Both impulsiveness and undue caution may precipitate a medical emergency. The young individual with functional disease or paroxysms of supraventricular arrhythmia should require little more than effective anxiety control. However, the elderly patient with ischemic disease is far more labile and may unexpectedly undergo cardiac arrest if ectopic warning signs are ignored.

Table 2 Commonly used antiarrhythmic agents

Agent	Side effects
Procainamide	Muscosal ulcers (secondary to agranulocytosis), lupuslike syndrome
Quinidine	Cinchonism, tinnitus, headache, nausea, vomiting, and visual disturbances
Disopyramide	Xerostomia, dry nose, dry eyes and throat, urinary hesitancy, and so on (anticholinergic)
Propranolol	Light-headedness, lassitude, bradycardia, heart failure, hypotension, ulcers (secondary to agranulocytosis), purpuras (thrombocytopenic and nonthrombocytopenic)

Inasmuch as any increase in sympathetic tone may contribute to the frequency of arrhythmia, it behooves the dentist to control the patient's anxiety. Because the group at greatest risk for serious arrhythmia largely comprises those with coronary artery disease or heart failure, the dentist coincidentally ensures against arrhythmic sequelae by attempting to prevent acute exacerbations of these underlying diseases.

Local anesthesia is preferred over general agents, since the hypoxia, hypercapnia, and sympathetic outbursts of induction may incite disordered rhythms. If general anesthesia is necessary in those at risk for ventricular arrhythmia, hospitalization and controlled ventilation anesthesia are indicated. The use of narcotics and local anesthetic agents during inhalation general anesthesia can help prevent the instigation of arrhythmias by peripheral stimuli. The fact that Halothane is known to sensitize the myocardium to catecholamines usually is reason enough to employ alternative agents. Balanced anesthesia using opiates, nitrous oxide, and high concentrations of oxygen is favored by many anesthesiologists for individuals at cardiac risk.

As is true in the treatment of any cardiac disease, the need to achieve adequate local anesthesia far outweighs the need to avoid vasoconstrictive agents such as epinephrine. The serial administration of short-lived anesthetics can do more to worsen an unstable cardiac rhythm than a single dose of anesthetic with epinephrine.

Pulp testors, motorized dental chairs, belt-driven handpieces, and cavitrons have all at one time been thought capable of producing pacemaker malfunction. Recent evidence suggests that electrosurgery units present the greatest risk to the paced heart. The demand type of pacemaker is the most common variety and the most sensitive to external electromagnetic sources. For these reasons it is appropriate for the dentist to confirm that all such office equipment is inoperative before the patient with the demand pacemaker arrives for an appointment.

A basic knowledge of antiarrhythmic pharmacology is essential to the competent treatment of these individuals. Mucosal ulceration may be the earliest evidence of agranulocytosis secondary to procainamide or propranolol toxicity. Xerostomia may be an anticholinergic consequence of disopyramide use. Since antiarrhythmic drugs in toxic amounts may precipitate arrhythmias, the dentist should heed signs of toxic syndromes such as cinchonism and lupuslike syndrome. Table 2 shows some side effects of the commonly used antiarrhythmic agents.

DISEASE OF THE AORTA AND ITS BRANCHES

Of the disorders discussed previously, cerebrovascular disease is of particular interest to the dentist. Involvements of other portions of the arterial tree have less dental significance, except when their therapy involves anticoagulation. This latter topic is considered in the chapter devoted to pulmonary embolism.

CLINICAL MANIFESTATIONS. All middle-aged and elderly patients should be queried about neurologic symptoms of vascular character. Those admitting to symptoms consistent with transient cerebral ischemia deserve medical referral. Needless to say, a history of completed stroke is always of note in that it identifies individuals whose cerebra may even yet be tenuously vascularized.

Beyond the carotid findings already mentioned, the head and neck examination usually reveals little in the patient with asymptomatic cerebrovascular disease. Opthalmoscopy may disclose asymmetric retinal deposition of cholesterol crystals in patients with unilateral carotid stenosis, but this is not an observation that the dentist would be expected to make. Thus in the elderly it is perhaps best to assume the existence of some cerebrovascular impairment, even when physical evidence is lacking.

Transient ischemia during the dental visit and fixed deficit from a previously completed stroke usually reveal themselves during the dentist's examination. Hemiparetic gait or aphasia may betray the history even as the dentist first greets a new patient. Evaluation of the cranial nerves is crucial to any examination, and the dentist should closely scrutinize the elderly for evidence of cranial nerve palsy. Jaw jerk and zygomatic reflexes may reveal subtle supranuclear fifth nerve involvement; a mild and barely discernible seventh nerve deficit may be the sole physical evidence of an old central nervous system insult. A careful search for infantile reflexes (such as sucking, snouting, and grasping) takes only a moment but can alert the practitioner to the presence of frontal lobe disease that may materially affect the dentist's treatment, especially in patients with associated apathy, impaired concentration, lability of affect, or inability to carry out planned tasks. Although these deficits most commonly are found in conjunction with idiopathic dementia, they also may result from ischemic deprivation of prefrontal areas.

The proposed relationship between oral erythrodiapedesis and cerebrovascular accident is noteworthy. It has been observed that the cytologic character of the oral washings may be related to the nature of a cerebrovascular accident. Large numbers of red cells commonly are found in the sediment of individuals with hemorrhagic intracerebral accidents. Subarachnoid bleeding and bland infarctions have low oral erythrodiapedesis, and the former are distinguished by the characteristic bloody or xanthochromic cerebrospinal fluid. These findings could prove useful in instances when a question as to the nature of the stroke creates difficulty in treatment planning (for example, whether to anticoagulate the patient).

Despite the fact that the atherosclerotic process is known to affect the facial vessels, it is uncommon for such involvement to be of measurable clinical import. The interpretation of studies designed to investigate the relationship between atherosclerosis and periodontal disease must await the development of reliable indices for rating the severity of these two processes. Fortunately, the collateralization of blood supply in the face all but prevents the occurrence of significant infarction of atheromatous origin. Although studies have shown atherosclerotic disease of the lingual arteries to be common, there are only a few reports of gangrene traceable to atheromas of these vessels.

DENTAL MANAGEMENT. Two major concerns arise in the dental management of those with cerebrovascular disease. The practitioner must (1) attempt to minimize the risk of additional neurologic insult during treatment and (2) contribute to the rehabilitation of the stroke victim.

Avoiding any substantial variation in cerebral blood flow is essential to the safety of these patients. Good hypertensive control limits the incidence of vasospastic or hemorrhagic infarction, and avoiding sedative-related hypotension can diminish the risk of bland stroke. For no other patient group are deliberate explanation and calm reassurance more important. The age-related and coincident increase in atherosclerosis and dementia should serve to remind us that the elderly individual often is poorly equipped to deal with the circulatory stress that confusion may provoke. Because disorientation commonly breeds paranoia, the dentist should spare no effort to keep an elderly patient informed. Sedatives may prove to be double-edged swords in these individuals, since small doses can increase disorientation and stress and larger doses may lead to hypnosis and cerebral oligemia. The practitioner should substitute experience and reassurance for sedative pharmaceuticals whenever possible.

Carotid sinus sensitivity among those with atherosclerotic cerebrovascular disease; occurs more often the dentist would do well to remember this when positioning and examining a patient. All three forms of carotid sinus syncope (vagal, depressor, and central) are potentially devastating for patients whose circulation is already compromised. Gentle palpation of the carotid pulses is essential to avoid such syncope and the inadvertent dislodgement and embolization of atheromatous material.

The individual who has sustained permanent cerebral injury presents several technical problems to the dentist, particularly concerning removable prosthetic procedures. The supportive tissues may undergo regressive change because of denture disuse around the time of the cerebrovascular accident. This is sometimes further complicated by the muscular flaccidity of the seventh nerve lesions. For these reasons denture relining and ultimate rebasing or refabrication usually are needed after a stroke. Other cranial nerve lesions may complicate the treatment process; fifth nerve disease with intraoral hypesthesia may lead to overextension of the denture bases, and ninth nerve palsy increases the chances of impression material aspiration. Frequent postinsertion adjustments and proper patient positioning for impressions are among the measures that may be taken to minimize these problems. Acrylic obliteration of the buccal vestibule on the affected side can be helpful to patients whose mimetic tonus is insufficient to keep the vestibule free of food debris. If and when such tonus returns, the added acrylic may be ground away.

Because stroke often brings dependency and depression to its victims, the dentist should do everything possible to help each patient remain orally self-sufficient. Designing partial dentures with extra clasps on the unaffected side simplifies their removal and eliminates a personal task for which the patient must otherwise enlist another's aid. Suction-mounted denture brushes also are helpful in the hemiplegic's hygiene efforts. Since the central goal is always the maintenance of oral health, however, the dentist must be prepared to encourage a patient to accept assistance, should that assistance prove essential to the success of the rehabilitative program (such as an apraxic individual who may remain unable to insert and remove a prosthesis).

Should a patient develop ischemic symptoms in the dental office, the practitioner must be prepared to support that individual until transportation to a hospital is available. The conscious patient requires oxygen and reassurance and should be allowed to rest comfortably in recumbency. If the patient loses consciousness, airway maintenance, including the removal of prostheses, becomes the cornerstone of treatment. In all instances the dentist should keep an accurate time record of the patient's level of consciousness, pupillary character, and vital signs. This information may prove invaluable to the medical team that assumes the care of the individual after transfer.

BIBLIOGRAPHY

Bradley JC: A radiological investigation into the age changes of the inferior dental artery, Br J Oral Surg 13:82, 1975.

Dreizen S and others: Human lingual atherosclerosis, Arch Oral Biol 19:813, 1974.

Reed C and Ingles MJ: Acute massive gangrene of the tongue, Br Med J 2:575, 1965.

Sakurai EH and Richardson JA: Vascular neck pain: a source of odontalgia, Oral Surg 25:553, 1968.

Selbey WG: Dental help for stroke patients, Br Dent J, p 409, 1977

Standards and guidelines for cardiopulmonary resuscitation and emergency cardiac care, JAMA 255:2905, 1986.

Stoica E and others: Oral at the onset of cerebrovascular accidents, Confin Neurol 33:277, 1971.

Zafran JN and Zayon GM: Prosthodontics and the stroke patient, J Am Dent Assoc 74:1250, 1967.

SECTION EIGHT

DISEASES OF THE KIDNEY AND DISTURBANCES IN ELECTROLYTE AND ACID-BASE METABOLISM

Edited by **Sandra P. Levison**

101 · INTRODUCTION

Sandra P. Levison

Patients with renal, electrolyte, or acid-base disorders may manifest any one of many symptoms or findings on physical or laboratory examination. These include hematuria, dysuria, oliguria, anuria, polyuria, hypertension, edema, stigmata of uremia, proteinuria, pyuria, crystalluria, azotemia, and alterations in the serum concentration of the sodium, potassium, hydrogen, bicarbonate, phosphate, calcium, or magnesium ions.

DETERMINING THE SITE OF INJURY

The signs, symptoms, and laboratory findings in various renal diseases may overlap considerably. Some patients may tolerate well the uremic symptoms of chronic renal failure, whereas similar decreases in renal function may cause severe illness in patients with acute renal failure. Hypertension usually is present in vascular or glomerular disease and variably present in tubular or interstitial disease. Edema may be a feature of tubular or glomerular disease, but it more commonly occurs early in glomerular disease characterized by the nephrotic syndrome or late in interstitial or glomerular disease when sodium excretion is decreased. The nephrotic syndrome rarely occurs with tubular, interstitial, or ureteral disease but is seen in glomerular disease or renal vein thrombosis.

Examining the urine sediment may help in determining the site of renal injury. A "bland" urine sediment with few findings can be seen with (1) vasculitis (such as periarteritis nodosa, hemolytic-uremic syndrome, and scleroderma); (2) renovascular disease (arterial thrombosis or embolus); (3) prerenal azotemia; and (4) postrenal azotemia. Crystalluria can be specific for the cause of renal injury. Uric acid crystals are seen in the urine of patients with tumor lysis syndrome. Calcium oxalate crystals are seen in ethylene glycol poisoning.

Gross hematuria may herald a tumor in the urinary tract, infection, or renal vascular disease, but it is very uncommon in tubulointerstitial disease. Microscopic hematuria is a nonspecific but potentially serious abnormality. Red blood cell (RBC) casts, however, suggest glomerular damage. White blood cells (WBCs) are a nonspecific inflammatory response seen in injury to the glomerulus, tubules, interstitium, or lower urinary tract.

HEMATURIA

Normally fewer than 1.5 million RBCs are excreted in the urine daily. When hematuria increases threefold, it can be detected microscopically. Fresh urine (15 ml collected by clean catch) is centrifuged for 5 minutes at 1500 rpm. After the supernatant is discarded, 0.25 to 0.5 ml of residual urine is used to resuspend the sediment. A drop of this suspension is examined using the high-dry objective ($\times 43$). An abnormal microscopic finding is more than 3 to 5 RBCs in each high-power field when many different fields are examined. Gross hematuria occurs when there is sufficient blood in the urine to make it obvious to the unassisted eye.

The presence of RBC casts or other casts that may accompany RBCs indicates that the kidney is the site of bleeding. Hypotonic urine may produce osmotic lysis of RBCs, and alkaline urine leads to the dissolution of casts. With gross hematuria, RBC casts are difficult to detect.

The dipstick test is used to detect hematuria. The test results may be negative when the number of RBCs is small and the cells are intact. Since the dipstick test also is positive for hemoglobin and myoglobin, conditions other than those associated with the hematuria should be considered when the test is positive and microscopic hematuria is absent. Myoglobinuria is associated with rhabdomyolysis, the most common causes of which are crushing or thermal injuries. The latter may follow prolonged exposure to extreme cold, heat stroke, or malignant hyperthermia caused by general anesthesia. Muscle injury also may follow vigorous exercise, particularly in unconditioned individuals, in alcoholic individuals, and in association with defects such as McArdle's syndrome.

Urine may falsely appear to contain blood in patients who have consumed considerable quantities of foods such as beets, berries, or substances containing red food dyes. A variety of drugs and their metabolites may cause a urine color resembling blood. Red-pink urine may follow the ingestion of phenacetin, sulfanilamide, quinine, phenytoin, methyldopa, doxorubicin, daunorubicin, the laxative phenolphthalein, and phenothiazines. Red-brown urine is seen following the administration of sulfanilamide, quinine, chloroquine, primaquine, metronidazole, phenytoin, the laxatives emodin and cascara, and phe-

515

nothiazines. Orange-red urine may be seen following the use of phenazopyridine, rifampin, and phenindione.

Hematuria requires thorough investigation to uncover the cause (see following outline). Hematuria usually does not require transfusion except after trauma and postoperatively.

Causes of hematuria

I. Urethral
  A. Foreign body
  B. Local trauma
II. Prostatic
  A. Benign hypertrophy
  B. Acute prostatitis
  C. Carcinoma
III. Bladder
  A. Infection
    1. Bacterial
    2. Viral
    3. Schistosomiasis
  B. Neoplasm
  C. Stones
  D. Foreign body
  E. Trauma
  F. Cyclophosphamide
IV. Ureteral
  A. Malignancy
  B. Stones
  C. Abdominal lesions causing ureteral inflammation
    1. Diverticulitis
    2. Appendicitis
    3. Salpingitis
    4. Gastrointestinal neoplasms
V. Renal
  A. Glomerulonephritis
    1. Not associated with systemic disease
      a. Poststreptococcal glomerulonephritis
      b. Acute nonstreptococcal glomerulonephritis
      c. Berger's disease (IgA nephropathy)
      d. Mesangiocapillary glomerulonephritis
      e. Rapidly progressive glomerulonephritis
      f. Chronic glomerulonephritis
    2. Associated with systemic disease
      a. Lupus erythematosus
      b. Polyarteritis nodosa
      c. Scleroderma
      d. Wegener's granulomatosis
      e. Vasculitis
      f. Goodpasture's syndrome
      g. Thrombotic thrombocytopenic purpura
      h. Preeclampsia, "toxemia" of pregnancy
      i. Hemolytic-uremic syndrome
      j. Infective endocarditis
  B. Infections
    1. Pyelonephritis
    2. Papillary necrosis
    3. Tuberculosis
  C. Neoplasms
  D. Hereditary diseases
    1. Adult polycystic kidney disease
    2. Alport's syndrome
    3. Hemoglobinopathies
      a. Sickle cell anemia
      b. Sickle cell trait
      c. Sickle thalassemia
      d. Sickle cell hemoglobin C
      e. Homozygous hemoglobin C
      f. Homozygous hemoglobin D
    4. Osler-Weber-Rendu disease
  E. Trauma
  F. Malignant hypertension
  G. Acute tubular necrosis
  H. Renal infarct
  I. Renal vein thrombosis
  J. Coagulation defects—hereditary, acquired, or associated with blood dyscrasias

PROTEINURIA

The normal urinary protein excretion is less than 150 mg each day. Proteins with molecular weights of less than 10,000 are filtered by the glomerulus and reabsorbed by the tubules. As molecular weight increases, filtered protein progressively decreases. Most proteins with molecular weights greater than 50,000 are not filtered. In glomerular disease increased amounts of protein appear in the urine, at times reaching as much as 25 g per day. Normally, fixed negative-charged components of the glomerular capillary wall restrict (via electrostatic hindrance) circulating albumin. With glomerular injury, the loss of negative charges in the membrane no longer repel albumin. When the proteinuria is "selective," the proteins are of a molecular weight slightly greater than 50,000 with almost undetectable amounts of high-molecular-weight proteins. Selective proteinuria usually is associated with a more favorable prognosis than unselective proteinuria. Large amounts of proteins with high molecular weights appear in the urine of patients with unselective proteinuria. Tubular proteinuria is characterized by incomplete tubular reabsorption of normally filtered proteins, with 1 to 4 g of protein excreted each day.

In patients with increased proteinuria whose protein excretion does not exceed 1 g each day, the problem is distinguishing insignificant proteinuria from that associated with organic disease. With *febrile illnesses* as much as 500 mg to 1 g of protein a day may be excreted. Febrile proteinuria ceases within days of defervescence. Up to 1 g of protein a day may be excreted by an unconditioned person after *strenuous exercise*. Hypertension, edema, azotemia, and abnormal urinary sediment are absent, and the proteinuria disappears within a few days of the exercise. *Orthostatic proteinuria* occurs when the individual is in the lordotic posture, and it disappears with recumbency. It usually is seen in young adults or children with no other associated symptoms. *Nephrotic proteinura* occurs when more than 3.5 g of protein is excreted per day. When renal insufficiency or renal failure develops in a patient with nephrotic syndrome, the total amount of protein excreted may appear to dimish.

The presence of increased urinary protein may be determined by several means. The dipstick is a convenient, simple method that is not specific for albumin nor accurate quantitatively. If the specimen is not dilute (the first morning specimen is optimal), a negative result of a dipstick test precludes albuminuria. It does not rule out the presence of other proteins such as Bence Jones proteins. Because strongly alkaline urine may give false positive results, dipstick-positive urine should be confirmed by measuring protein excretion in several urine samples before an evaluation for renal disease is undertaken. Accurate measurement of urinary protein excretion involves the collection of a 24-hour urine specimen and the precipitation of the protein by trichloroacetic acid and then measurement of the protein by biuret reaction. The completeness of collection should be determined by measuring the urinary creatinine excretion. False positive results have been reported with roentgenographic contrast media, chlorpromazine, and tolbutamide metabolites; following high doses of sulfonamides and various penicillins; and occasionally when the urine is extremely alkaline. Paper electrophoresis of the urine proteins separates the proteins according to charge and it helps detect the type of protein present. It distinguishes Bence Jones protein, albumin, and the various immunoglobulins. Separation techniques based on molecular weight also are available.

In the absence of clinical proteinuria, as measured by standard laboratory methods, elevated albumin excretion can be detected by radioimmunoassay or chemicoimmunoassay. Studies have documented that this *microalbuminuria* is important in predicting the development of renal disease, particularly in patients with diabetes.

To avoid the problems associated with the inaccuracies of 24-hour urine collections, a ratio of urine protein to creatinine can be determined from a urine aliquot. Ratios above 3 are associated with proteinuria greater than 3 g/day, whereas a ratio less than 0.2 is associated with less than 200 mg/day of protein. Ratios from first-voided urine collections cause inaccuracies.

PYURIA

Pyuria has been defined as the urinary excretion of more than 3 million WBCs each day. Normal urine has fewer than 5 WBCs in each high-power field. The most common cause of pyuria is the contamination of normal urine by improper collection techniques. Pyuria rarely is an isolated presenting symptom. Bacterial infection of the urinary tract (urethritis, cystitis, pyelonephritis, and prostatitis) is the most common pathologic cause of pyuria. Pyuria also is seen in the following circumstances: (1) granulomatous infections of the urinary tract (for example, tuberculosis); (2) neoplasms of the urinary tract; (3) foreign bodies in the urinary tract (stones or exogenously derived foreign bodies); (4) in association with inflammatory diseases in organs contiguous to the urinary tract (diverticulitis, appendicitis, colitis, ileitis, and pelvic inflammatory disease); (5) as a result of the ingestion of large quantities of phenacetin with the production of chronic interstitial nephritis (see Chapter 107); (6) as a result of the acute interstitial nephritis produced by penicillin analogs and furosemide (see Chapter 145); and (7) in association with other systemic events such as fever, congestive heart failure, and exercise.

Eosinophiluria is associated with interstitial nephritis, particularly allergic interstitial nephritis associated with nonsteroidal analgesics, allopurinol, and antibiotics. It also can be seen in patients with chronic urinary tract infection.

Examination of a centrifuged clean-catch midstream urine specimen, rather than a random urine, is more reliable in determining urine eosinophils. Hansel's and Pilot's stains are more sensitive than Wright's stain, because a urine pH less than 7 inhibits the ability of Wright's stain to detect urine eosinophils. Acute interstitial nephritis documented by renal biopsy may be associated with urine eosinophiluria in only 53% of cases and in some cases in the absence of peripheral eosinophilia. Some patients may have eosinophilia without eosinophiluria or eosinophiluria with pyuria.

102 · STRUCTURE AND FUNCTION OF THE KIDNEY

Pedro C. Fernandez

Each human kidney is composed of approximately 1 million anatomic and functional units called nephrons. Each nephron includes a glomerulus, which is continuous with a tubule. The glomerulus consists of a tuft of interconnected capillary vessels that branch off the afferent glomerular arteriole and reunite in an efferent glomerular arteriole. The glomerular capillary wall comprises three layers: the fenestrated capillary endothelium, the basement membrane, and the epithelial cells (podocytes). The podocytes exhibit a large number of cytoplasmic extensions (foot processes) that interdigitate with each other, leaving only a narrow slit between them. The glomerular capillary tuft is contained inside a balloonlike structure, Bowman's capsule, that opens into and is continuous with the proximal tubule. The glomerulus is the filtering component of the nephron. Approximately 180 L of plasma are filtered daily by the glomerulus and subsequently markedly reduced in volume and modified in composition during passage along the tubule.

The tubule is divided into several segments: the proximal tubule, the hairpinlike Henle's loop, the distal tubule, and the collecting duct. The last segment collects urine from several terminal distal tubules and opens directly into the renal papillae. The tubule is lined by a single layer of cuboid epithelial cells resting on a basement membrane. Marked morphologic differences exist among the epithelial cells lining the diverse tubular segments. From a functional point of view the proximal tubule's characteristics are quite different from those in the other nephron segments. The proximal tubule reabsorbs approximately 70% of the glomerular filtrate, but only minor or no changes in filtrate composition take place in this nephron segment. It thus can be functionally classified as a high-capacity, low-gradient system. As the filtrate moves distally along the nephron, the amount of filtrate reabsorbed by the remaining tubular segments decreases progressively. However, simultaneously, the tubule's ability to create and maintain steep ionic concentration differences between the tubular urine and the blood increases greatly (low-capacity, high-gradient system). Teleologically, the kidney's anatomic distribution of epithelia with different transport characteristics favors the formation of urine that may differ markedly in composition from the plasma.

The human kidney has two main populations of nephrons, with some variations between the two types. The cortical nephrons, located in the outer cortex, have short Henle's loops and are more numerous than the juxtamedullary nephrons. The latter nephrons are more deeply situated near the corticomedullary boundary and have long loops with well-developed descending and ascending limbs. There seems to be a direct relationship between maximal urine-concentrating ability and the relative length of the Henle's loop.

RENAL BLOOD FLOW AND GLOMERULAR FILTRATION

Normally the renal blood flow is approximately 25% of the cardiac output. The corresponding renal plasma flow is 600 ml/min, of which 120 ml/min is filtered at the glomerulus. The relationship between the glomerular filtration rate and the renal plasma flow is described by the filtration fraction, which is the ratio of the glomerular filtration rate to the plasma flow rate and which normally averages 20%.

It is characteristic of the renal circulation that both the renal blood flow and the glomerular filtration rate tend to remain quite constant in the face of changes in mean arterial pressure ranging from 80 to 180 mm Hg. This circulatory autoregulation mainly is a result of changes in the renal vascular resistance at the level of the afferent glomerular arterioles. The mechanisms of circulatory autoregulation are intrinsic to the kidney, and they may be modified by neurogenic and humoral factors (catecholamines, angiotensin, and prostaglandins). The bulk of the renal blood flow (90%) is distributed to the cortical area of the kidneys. Within the cortex itself, the outer part seems to have a larger blood flow than those areas closer to the renal medulla.

Glomerular filtration is a physical process determined by the interplay between the forces favoring filtration (glomerular capillary hydraulic pressure) and those opposing it (glomerular capillary oncotic pressure and hydraulic pressure in Bowman's capsule). The mean net filtration (that is, the difference between the capillary hydraulic pressure and both the hydraulic pressure in Bowman's capsule and the glomerular capillary oncotic pressure) is probably less than 10 mm Hg. Given the magnitude of glomerular filtration (180 L/day in adults), the low mean net ultrafiltration pressure suggests a high hydraulic conductivity of the glomerular capillary wall. This may be related in part to the large surface area displayed by the glomerular capillary bed.

The glomerular filtrate is a virtually protein-free ultrafiltrate of the plasma. Apart from the restriction to the passage of macromolecules, which is purely dependent on the pore size of the glomerular capillary wall, electrical charge also is an important factor in limiting the filtration of plasma proteins. Fixed negative charges that are present in the glomerular capillary wall significantly restrict the passage of negatively charged plasma proteins. In pathologic states proteinuria is at least partly caused by a decrease in the normal electronegativity of the glomerular capillary wall.

As a consequence of the formation of a protein-free ultrafiltrate, the plasma protein concentration and consequently the plasma oncotic pressure increase at the efferent end of the glomerular capillary bed. Since the blood supply to the proximal tubule is derived from the efferent arteriole, the oncotic pressure at the level of the peritubular capillaries normally is higher than that of the systemic blood. This high oncotic pressure represents a driving force for the net reabsorption of salt and water by the proximal tubule. Changes in the filtration fraction may thus influence proximal tubular reabsorption through concomitant changes in the oncotic pressure of peritubular capillaries.

RENAL HANDLING OF SODIUM AND WATER

Within a narrow range of variation, renal regulation and maintenance of the osmolality and volume of the extracellular fluid are accomplished through changes in urinary excretion of water and sodium, respectively.

The osmolality of the extracellular fluid normally is maintained between 280 and 290 mOsm/kg water, despite highly variable fluid intakes, the continuous addition of solute to the body by the diet and its metabolic products, and the continued loss of hypotonic fluids through the skin and respiration. The kidney can excrete a urine ranging in osmolality from one sixth to four times the plasma osmolality. Thus, the osmolality of the intake (taking into account extrarenal water losses) is closely matched by the osmolality of the urine, and a constant extracellular fluid osmolality is maintained. A feedback control system normally links the extracellular fluid osmolality to the renal concentrating and diluting mechanisms. This is the osmoreceptor–antidiuretic hormone secretory apparatus, located in the hypothalamus and posterior pituitary. The kidney needs antidiuretic hormone (ADH), which is released in response to increases in plasma osmolality, to produce a concentrated urine. In the absence of circulating ADH (decreased plasma osmolality), the renal concentrating mechanisms are interrupted, and a dilute urine is excreted.

The intrarenal mechanisms of urine concentration and dilution are located in the tubular segments distal to the proximal tubule. Isotonic fluid escaping reabsorption by the proximal tubule is rendered hypotonic as it emerges at the end of the ascending limb of Henle's loop. This results from the ability of the thick ascending limb to reabsorb sodium, potassium, and chloride without water ($Na^+ - K^+ - Cl^-$ cotransport system). The reabsorbed salts render the medullary interstitium hypertonic to the plasma. The countercurrent disposition of both limbs of Henle's loop accounts for the increase in tonicity observed in the innermost region of the renal medulla (countercurrent multiplication). In addition the hairpinlike medullary blood vessels act as a countercurrent exchanger, which prevents dissipation of the medullary hypertonicity. The process just described is instrumental in both urine concentration and urine dilution. In the absence of ADH the tubular segments beyond the loop are for the most part impermeable to water, and as they continue to reabsorb sodium chloride, a maximally dilute urine is produced. In the presence of ADH the water permeability of those most distal nephron segments is markedly increased, allowing osmotic equilibration, through water reabsorption, to take place between the tubular fluid and the surrounding interstitium. A maximally concentrated urine thus is produced as the tubular urine osmotically equilibrates with the maximally hypertonic medullary interstitium at the level of the terminal collecting duct.

Sodium is actively extruded from all cells in the body and is distributed primarily in the extracellular fluid, where sodium salts account for more than 95% of the osmolality of that fluid. Changes in sodium excretion by the kidneys are accompanied by parallel changes in renal excretion of water, as dictated by the ADH-renal mechanisms that control extracellular fluid osmolality discussed earlier. Therefore changes in the body content of sodium result in parallel changes in the volume of the extracellular fluid. The renal regulation of extracellular fluid volume is accomplished through the control of urinary sodium excretion. Normally a neutral sodium balance is maintained, in which the urinary output of sodium equals the intake minus the extrarenal losses of sodium. If the volume of extracellular fluid increases or decreases, appropriate changes in the urinary excretion of sodium rapidly take place to restore the altered volume of that fluid compartment. The feedback control system, which monitors changes in extracellular fluid volume and secondarily dictates the pattern of urinary sodium excretion, consists of an afferent volume-sensing limb and an efferent or effector limb that modulates the rate of urinary sodium excretion. Volume sensors exist on both the venous and arterial sides of the circulation; atrial volume receptors are the most important of those present on the venous side of the circulation. The arterial volume sensors include not only the carotid and aortic baroreceptors but also intrarenal receptors at the level of the juxtaglomerular apparatus.

The efferent limb controlling sodium homeostasis (and consequently extracellular fluid volume homeostasis) comprises the kidney and extrarenal and intrarenal neurohumoral factors able to influence the renal handling of sodium. About 22,000 mEq of sodium are filtered each day. Normally two thirds of the filtered sodium load is reabsorbed isotonically in the proximal tubule, 20% to 25% is reabsorbed by the ascending limb of Henle's loop, and the remaining 10% to 15% is reabsorbed in the distal tubule and collecting duct. The amount of sodium excreted in the final urine represents approximately 1% of the filtered sodium load. Although alterations in the filtered load of sodium mediated through changes in glomerular filtration rate are accompanied by parallel changes in urinary sodium excretion, sodium balance often is accomplished without any noticeable change in glomerular filtration rate, through proper adjustments in the rate of tubular sodium reabsorption. Proximal tubular sodium reabsorption is greatly influenced by peritubular physical factors such as colloid-osmotic and hydrostatic pressures, whereas at the level of the cortical collecting tubule sodium reabsorption depends at least partly on the levels of aldosterone. Although other substances such as angiotensin II, neuroamines, prostaglandins, and kinin have been shown experimentally to influence sodium reabsorption in different nephron segments, their role in the day-to-day maintenance of extracellular fluid volume homeostasis remains unclear, as it does under pathologic conditions.

More recently considerable attention has been focused on a circulating 28-aminoacid peptide, synthesized and stored by atrial muscle cells as a 126-aminoacid precursor. This peptide, called atrial natriuretic factor (ANF), is released from the atria in the circulation in response to an increase in atrial stretch or wall tension, such as occurs with expansion of extracellular fluid volume. Apart from being a potent vasodilator, ANF produces a dramatic increase in renal salt and water excretion. The mechanism of the ANF-induced natriuresis remains somewhat controversial; although a hemodynamically mediated increase in glomerular filtration rate is a major determinant of the natriuresis, the process seems to be mediated, at least in part, through ANF-induced inhibition of sodium reabsorption at the level of the medullary collecting duct.

Changes in sodium reabsorption in response to changes in the extracellular fluid volume occur in different nephron segments and through different mechanisms. The interactions between those several sites and mechanisms has not been clearly elucidated, but there is reason to believe that sodium homeostasis is maintained despite malfunction or failure of any individual control system by adjustments in other branches of the efferent limb. In other words, volume homeostasis is too important to be potentially compromised by a single control system, thus it is controlled by several interacting, fail-safe physiologic devices.

ROLE OF THE KIDNEY IN ACID-BASE HOMEOSTASIS

Despite wide variations in the dietary intake of acid or alkali, fecal loss of alkali, and metabolic production of nonvolatile acids, the pH of the blood normally is maintained between 7.36 and 7.44, mainly as a result of precise renal regulation of the plasma bicarbonate concentration. At the normal plasma bicarbonate concentraction of 24 mEq/L, approximately 4000 mEq of bicarbonate are filtered at the glomerulus each day. This amount greatly exceeds the body stores of bicarbonate, and from a quantitative point of view the main role of the kidney in acid-base homeostasis is reabsorption of the filtered bicarbonate. This reabsorption is practically complete at normal plasma bicarbonate concentrations. The proximal tubule accounts for 80% to 90% of that bicarbonate reabsorption, the remainder being reabsorbed beyond the proximal convolutions. Bicarbonate reabsorption is mediated through H^+ secretion by a Na^+/H^+ exchanger present at the apical cell membranes. Different carbonic anhydrase isoenzymes play a major role in the process of proximal bicarbonate reabsorption by preventing luminal accumulation of carbonic acid (brush border carbonic anhydrase) and by providing an adequate amount of H^+ for Na^+/H^+ exchange (cytosolic carbonic anhydrase).

The rate of proximal tubular bicarbonate reabsorption can be changed markedly by physiologic and pathologic regulatory factors. In general, proximal tubular bicarbonate reabsorption parallels glomerular filtration rate, so that increases in glomerular filtration rate produce near-proportional increases in bicarbonate reabsorption and do not result in urinary loss of large amounts of bicarbonate. However, at higher than normal plasma bicarbonate concentrations, reductions in glomerular filtration rate may not be accompanied by proportional decreases in proximal bicarbonate reabsorption. This often results in an inability to correct the elevated plasma bicarbonate concentration by allowing the urinary excretion of large amounts of bicarbonate. Independently of changes in the filtered load of bicarbonate, other factors also influence the bicarbonate reabsorptive capacity of the proximal tubule. Thus the capacity varies directly with the arterial P_{CO_2}, whereas it changes reciprocally with the effective volume of the extracellular fluid. Chloride deficiency seems to impair the kidney's ability to excrete a bicarbonate load, but this phenomenon may result from impairment of the Cl^- absorption/HCO_3^- secretion exchange mechanism present in the collecting tubules rather than from an alteration in proximal bicarbonate handling.

The metabolism of different foods produces 50 to 100 mEq of H^+ per day in the form of sulfuric, phosphoric, and several strong organic acids. These nonvolatile acids are buffered instantaneously by intracellular and extracellular buffers, including bicarbonate, which is titrated to water and carbon dioxide, the latter being eliminated by the lungs. Although these buffering systems provide an immediate defense against wide pH fluctuations, ultimately exhaustion of body buffers and overwhelming acidosis would occur if the kidneys were unable to excrete in the urine an amount of H^+ equivalent to that provided by the nonvolatile acids. Since only a negligible amount of free H^+ exists at even the lowest urine pH (4.5 to 5.2), most of the H^+ excreted in the urine is bound to buffers. About one third of the daily H^+ load is excreted bound to organic anions (phosphate and creatinine); the amount of H^+ excreted in this form (titratable acid) is equivalent to the amount of base required to titrate the urine to the pH of the blood. The remainder of the H^+ is excreted in the urine as NH_4^+, produced from the titration of NH_3 by secreted H^+; NH_3 is derived from glutamine by the renal tubular cells. In acidosis NH_3 production may increase 10-fold, thus allowing the excretion of increasingly large acid loads. It should be emphasized that H^+ excretion as titratable acid and NH^+ is highly dependent of the acidification of the urine to a pH considerably lower than that of the blood; that is, the tubular epithelium normally can create and maintain large H^+ concentration gradients between blood and urine.

The excretion of 1 mEq of H^+ in the urine either as titratable acid or NH^+ entails the generation and addition of 1 mEq of bicarbonate to the blood. Equimolar reconstitution of body buffers that had been titrated by metabolic nonvolatile acids thus is accomplished, and day-to-day acid-base balance is maintained.

RENAL HANDLING OF POTASSIUM

Of the 3500 to 4000 mEq of potassium present in the normal adult, less than 100 mEq are distributed in the extracellular fluid; potassium is the main intracellular cation. However, the concentration of potassium in the extracellular fluid is closely maintained between 3.5 and 5.5 mEq/L. Fluctuations outside this range may have deleterious effects on the function of excitable tissues, since the ratio of intracellular potassium concentration to extracellular potassium concentration is the main determinant of the cell membrane resting potential.

An average diet provides 50 to 100 mEq of potassium daily. Normally 90% of the ingested potassium is excreted in the urine. Although the kidneys are responsible for the day-to-day maintenance of potassium balance, the immediate disposition of an acute potassium load is largely effected via transfer of potassium into liver and muscle cells. This cellular uptake of potassium, which is highly effective in preventing the development of potentially dangerous hyperkalemia, is stimulated by insulin, β-adrenergic agonists, and aldosterone, whereas α-adrenergic agonists and glucagon have an inhibitory effect. The cell stores of potassium also minimize the degree of hypokalemia present in conditions of negative potassium balance, but little is known about the physiologic control mechanisms in this situation.

Marked fluctuations in potassium intake are followed by concomitant isodirectional changes in urinary potassium excretion, which ensure a practically constant body potassium content and serum potassium concentration. The extremely sensitive response of the adrenal cortex to minimal changes in serum potassium concentration with changes in aldosterone secretion seems to play a crucial role in the so-called renal potassium adaptation.

The renal handling of potassium is rather complex, as different tubular segments exhibit either net reabsorption or net secretion of potassium. Overall the proximal tubule, loop of Henle, and early distal tubule combined effect net removal of almost all the filtered potassium from the tubular fluid. Thus the amount of potassium excreted in the final urine mainly is determined by the net potassium secretory rate of the late distal tubules and cortical collecting ducts. Minimal potassium reabsorption seems to occur at the medullary collecting ducts.

The mechanisms underlying distal nephron tubular potassium secretion represent the interplay between chemical concentration gradients and electrical potential differences existing across the different cell membrane barriers of the distal tubular epithelium, coupled to active transport steps present at some of those barriers. Active cellular potassium uptake occurs at the basolateral cell membranes, whereas the maintenance of high intracellular potassium levels, together with the luminal electrical negativity, allow potassium secretion into the lumen to proceed passively down the electrochemical gradient for the ion. However, the rate of potassium secretion may exceed that expected on the basis of the existing electrochemical gradients, indicating the likely existence of an active secretory process. In addition active potassium absorption also occurs at the apical cell membranes, and it accounts for the net distal tubular absorption of potassium observed under conditions of potassium deprivation. The different cell types present in those most distal tubular segments may account for the apparent multiplicity of those potassium transport processes.

Several factors exert a major influence on the net rates of distal tubular potassium secretion. The most important are:

1. Aldosterone, which increases potassium secretion by increasing peritubular cell potassium uptake and/or facilitating potassium secretion across the apical cell membranes.
2. The rate of delivery of fluid and sodium to the potassium secretory sites, potassium secretion increasing with increasing delivery rates. Delivery of sodium with anions other than chloride further facilitates potassium secretion.
3. The cellular stores of potassium which at the level of the renal tubular cells depend not only on the total body potassium stores but also on the individual's acid-base status.

BIBLIOGRAPHY

Brenner BM and Rector FC Jr, editors: The kidney, ed 3, Philadelphia, 1986, WB Saunders Co.

Brenner BM and Stein JH, editors: Body fluid homeostasis. Contemporary issues in nephrology, vol 16, New York, 1987, Churchill Livingstone, Inc.

Cogan MG and Alpern RJ: Regulation of proximal bicarbonate reabsorption, Am J Physiol 247:F387, 1984.

Stanton B and Giebisch G: Mechanism of urinary potassium excretion, Miner Electrolyte Metab 5:100, 1981.

103 · DISTURBANCES IN FLUID, ELECTROLYTE, AND ACID-BASE METABOLISM

HUGH J. CARROLL *and* **MAN S. OH**

SODIUM AND WATER METABOLISM

To preserve the proper biochemical milieu, normal ionic strength must be maintained. The osmolality of cellular and extracellular fluid is about 280 mOsm/L. The osmolality of the body fluids is maintained within a narrow range through the combined action of the thirst mechanism and antidiuretic hormone (ADH). When an individual is dehydrated, the serum sodium concentration and total body fluid osmolality rise. This simultaneously stimulates the thirst mechanism and release of ADH from the posterior pituitary gland. With overhydration the serum osmolality and sodium concentration are low and ADH is suppressed. This allows the kidney to excrete dilute urine, and osmolality returns to normal. Hyponatremia and hypernatremia are observed clinically when an abnormality occurs in these control mechanisms.

HYPONATREMIA

Hyponatremia is defined as a reduction in sodium concentration in serum (extracellular) water. In *pseudohyponatremia*, which can be caused by hyperlipidemia or hyperproteinemia, sodium concentration is low in serum but the concentration in serum water is normal. Characteristically, effective osmolality is normal in pseudohyponatremia. However, normal effective osmolality with hyponatremia does not prove pseudohyponatremia; by chance, effective osmolality might be normal by accumulation of a solute other than sodium salts. Some authors extend the term "pseudohyponatremia" to hyponatremia caused by hyperglycemia or mannitol accumulation, perhaps on the basis that, in contrast to the low effective osmolality observed in the usual types of hyponatremia, the effective osmolality is increased in hyponatremia caused by glucose or mannitol accumulation. Such use of the term is unacceptable, however, just as the term "pseudonormonatremia" would be unacceptable for normal sodium in the presence of hyperglycemia.

PATHOGENESIS. The extracellular Na^+ concentration can be reduced by four mechanisms: (1) retention of water, (2) loss of sodium, (3) shift of sodium into the cell, and (4) shift of water from the cell to the extracellular fluid.

Primary water retention may occur either because of a greatly increased water intake, as in psychogenic polydipsia, or because of reduced water excretion. Reduced water excretion may be caused by renal failure, increased levels of ADH, or reduced urine flow through the distal nephron, as in conditions with a low effective arterial volume.

MECHANISMS FOR MAINTENANCE OF HYPONATREMIA

I. Excessive intake of water
II. Impaired renal excretion of water
   A. Severe renal dysfunction
   B. Increased release of ADH: appropriate or inappropriate
   C. Increased renal tubular responsiveness to ADH
   D. Decreased urine flow in the collecting duct

Reduced urine flow results from reduced glomerular filtration and enhanced reabsorption of water and sodium in the proximal nephron. Increased ADH activity may be caused by the low effective arterial volume in states in which edema develops, such as congestive heart failure, the nephrotic syndrome, and ascites, or in the syndrome of inappropriate ADH secretion

(SIADH). In SIADH the hormone is released from a tumor or from the posterior pituitary gland in response to various stimuli, including emetic stimulus, hypoxia, hypercapnia, hypoglycemia, physical and psychologic stress such as that caused by surgery, drugs such as β-adrenergic agonists and cyclophosphamide (Cytoxan), pulmonary diseases, and intracranial lesions. Other causes of SIADH include the following:

I. Tumors
   A. Cancer of the lung, pancreas, duodenum, ureter, bladder, or prostate
   B. Lymphoma, thymoma, mesothelioma, Ewing's sarcoma
II. Intrathoracic causes: virtually any pulmonary lesion
   A. Bacterial and viral pneumonia
   B. Lung abscess
   C. Asthma
   D. Pneumothorax
   E. Tuberculosis
   F. Aspergillosis
   G. Positive-pressure breathing
   H. Cystic fibrosis
III. Central nervous system abnormalities: virtually any brain lesion
   A. Encephalitis and meningitis
   B. Head trauma
   C. Cerebrovascular accidents
   D. Acute intermittent porphyria
   E. Brain tumors and abscesses
   F. Subdural hematoma
   G. Guillain-Barré syndrome
IV. Drugs: pathogenetic mechanism is unclear and poorly documented in most instances
   A. ADH analogs and oxytocin
   B. Drugs that increase ADH release directly or through emetic stimulus
      1. Sulfonylureas (?): chlorpropamide, tolbutamide
      2. Antimetabolites: vincristine, vinblastine, cyclophosphamide (?)
      3. Clofibrate (Atromid)
      4. Bromocriptine (Parlodel)
      5. Tricyclic antidepressants and related drugs: amitryptline (Elavil), protryptiline (Vivactil), desipramine (Norpramin)
      6. Narcotics: morphine, demerol
      7. Phenothiazines and related drugs: thioridazine (Mellaril), trifluoperazine (Stelazine), fluphenazine (Prolixin), thiothixene (Navane), haloperidol (Haldol)
      8. Cistplatin (Platinol)
   C. Drugs that enhance ADH effect on the kidney
      1. Chlorpropamide, tolbutamide
      2. Diuretics, especially thiazides
      3. Acetaminophen (Tylenol)
      4. Nonsteroidal antiinflammatory drugs: indomethacin (Indocin)
      5. Carbamazepine (Tegretol)
V. Surgical and emotional stress: emetic (?)
VI. Idiopathic

Hyponatremia may be primarily a result of sodium loss caused by sweating, diarrhea, vomiting, diuretic therapy, adrenal insufficiency, or certain types of renal disease. It may be caused in part by the shift of sodium into the cell in exchange for cell potassium in potassium-depleted states. Mild asymptomatic hyponatremia is observed in patients with chronic, debilitating disease and is referred to as the reset osmostat syndrome. This is a subtype of SIADH in which serum sodium concentration is regulated at a lower than normal level.

DIAGNOSIS AND MANAGEMENT. The patient with hypoosmolality and hyponatremia can be assigned to one of three categories, depending on the extracellular fluid (ECF) volume. That volume, estimated by physical examination of the patient, is low, expanded, or normal. When the ECF volume is low or expanded (edematous patients), urinary sodium usually is less than 20 mEq/L. The exception to this rule is hyponatremia caused by diuretic therapy or primary renal salt wasting such as occurs in Addison's disease. The mechanism of hyponatremia in patients with diminished ECF volume is volume-related stimulation of release of ADH and reduction in collecting duct urine flow as a result of enhanced proximal reabsorption. Patients with hyponatremia and diminished ECF volume are treated by administering isotonic sodium chloride. The kidney excretes whatever water is not needed and retains the salt. Patients with edema have an expanded extracellular space and increased total body sodium but a low effective arterial volume. The low effective arterial volume impairs urinary dilution by stimulating release of ADH and by reducing the urine flow at the collecting duct. The patients should be treated with the careful use of diuretics combined with inhibition of excessive water intake.

Hyponatremic patients with an apparently normal ECF volume usually have SIADH. Hyponatremia in SIADH is caused primarily by retention of water, but expanded effective arterial volume resulting from water retention tends to cause renal sodium wasting. However, it must be noted that physical examination is notoriously unreliable in determining the status of effective arterial volume. Patients with SIADH with expanded effective arterial volume often have a chronic debilitating disease and therefore may appear dehydrated. In these patients laboratory data such as urinary sodium, blood urea nitrogen, serum creatinine, and serum uric acid, generally are much more reliable than the physical examination. Patients with SIADH can be treated by water restriction with liberal salt intake. When the excess body water has been lost and the effective arterial volume is restored to a normal level, the renal salt wasting tendency stops.

At times hyponatremia must be treated with hypertonic saline, and the desirable rate of rise in serum Na is a matter of some debate. In our view, in hyperacute hyponatremia (development within 12 hours), the rate of correction may be as fast as 5 mEq/L/hr, and fuosemide may be given concomitantly with salt solutions to promote water excretion. For acute hyponatremia (less than 48 hours), the rate may be as high as 2 mEq/L/hr, but for chronic hyponatremia the rate should not exceed 0.5 mEq/L/hr. It is never necessary to raise the serum Na rapidly to normal. Rapid correction of hyponatremia should be reserved only for those patients with acute symptomatic hyponatremia to avoid central pontine myelinolysis, a demyelinating disease of the central pons that may occur when hyponatremia, especially chronic hyponatremia, is corrected too rapidly (at a rate greater than 0.5 mEq/L/hr).

HYPERNATREMIA

PATHOGENESIS. Hypernatremia usually is caused by excessive water loss (see box). It also can be caused by the addition of salt to the body along with or without loss of water. An example of the latter is the entry of hypertonic salt into the maternal circulation during an abortion procedure, drowning in the sea, and the use of hypertonic sodium bicarbonate during cardiac resuscitation.

Chronic hypernatremia in a conscious individual occurs only if the thirst mechanism is defective, since hyperosmolality provokes severe thirst and water drinking corrects hypernatremia. In essential hypernatremia defective osmoreceptor function prevents release of ADH and thirst perception in reponse to

---

CAUSES OF EXCESSIVE WATER LOSS

I. Renal water loss
  A. Diabetes insipidus
    1. Hypothalamic or pituitary (central) diabetes insipidus
      a. Primary and metastatic brain tumors
      b. Granulomas: sarcoidosis and tuberculosis
      c. Surgery or trauma
      d. Infection: meningitis and encephalitis
      e. Idiopathic
      f. Essential hypernatremia: defective osmoreceptor regulation for thirst and ADH

    2. Nephrogenic diabetes insipidus
      a. Congenital
      b. Acquired: drug-induced (lithium, demeclocycline, methoxyflurane) or various renal diseases (sickle cell disease, amyloidosis, obstructive uropathy, interstitial nephritis and so forth
  B. Osmotic diuresis: glucose, urea, or mannitol
II. Extrarenal water loss
  A. Cutaneous: sweating or burns
  B. Pulmonary: hyperventilation with fever
  C. Gastrointestinal: osmotic diarrhea or loss of gastric juice

---

hyperosmolality. Because ADH production mechanisms are intact in this condition, with sufficient dehydration ADH can be released through the baroreceptor mechanism and the urine becomes normally concentrated. In patients who are confused, comatose, physically unable to drink, or without access to water, hypernatremia also may occur without defective thirst.

DIAGNOSIS. Examination of the urine osmolality can help determine the cause of hypernatremia. If the urine osmolality is greater than 800 mOsm/L, the patient is simply water depleted and his kidneys are responding normally. If the dehydrated patient with severe hypernatremia is unable to raise the urine osmolality even to the level of the plasma osmolality, he is suffering from severe central diabetes insipidus or severe nephrogenic diabetes insipidus (inability to respond to ADH). If the urine osmolality is greater than plasma osmolality and less than 800 mOsm/L, the patient has severe osmotic diuresis, mild nephrogenic diabetes insipidus, or moderately severe central diabetes insipidus. Osmotic diuresis is obvious when the patient is excreting large amounts of solute. Central diabetes insipidus can be distinguished from nephrogenic diabetes insipidus; patients with the latter do not respond to the infusion of ADH with a significant increase in urine osmolality, whereas patients who lack ADH show a marked rise in urine osmolality when ADH is administered.

MANAGEMENT. Hypernatremia is treated by administering water in the form of isotonic or hypotonic glucose solution. The quantity of water required to treat a given degree of hypernatremia in a patient with water loss alone can be estimated from the following formula:

$$\text{Water requirement} = \text{TBW} \times \left(\frac{\text{Actual serum Na}}{\text{Desired serum Na}} - 1 \right)$$
$$= \text{TBW} \times \frac{\Delta \text{ Na}}{\text{Desired serum Na}}$$

where TBW is total body water and Δ Na the difference between actual and desired Na. For patients whose hypernatremia is also caused in part by salt accumulation, it may become necessary to use diuretics such as furosemide if urinary excretion of the extra salt does not promptly follow the administration of water. When hypernatremia complicates renal failure, the excess salt can be removed by dialysis.

VOLUME DEPLETION STATES
Effective osmolality and tonicity

The terms "effective osmolality" and "tonicity" both refer to the solute concentration that determines osmotic water movement across the cell membrane. Thus if the body fluid is hypertonic or effective osmolality is increased, water is pulled from the cell; if the body fluid is hypotonic or effective osmolality is decreased, water enters the cell. In contrast, if the body fluid osmolality is increased by substances that can enter the cell freely (for example, urea or alcohol), the effective osmolality remains normal, as does tonicity. An increase in extracellular osmolality caused by hypernatremia, glucose, or mannitol causes a shift of water from the cell, since sodium, glucose, and mannitol are virtually or completely restricted to the ECF; thus effective osmolality is increased.

Hypernatremia is always associated with increased effective osmolality, but hyponatremia is not always associated with decreased effective osmolality. Hyponatremia caused by hyperglycemia or mannitol is associated with increased effective osmolality. The total serum osmolality can be measured by an osmometer or can be estimated by using the following equation:

Serum osmolality (mOsm/L) = Sodium (mEq/L) × 2 +
$$\frac{\text{Glucose (mg/dl)}}{18} + \frac{\text{BUN (mg/dl)}}{2.8} - 10$$

However, because the osmometer does not distinguish between the solutes that can diffuse into the cell freely and those that cannot, the effective osmolality can only be estimated:

Effective osmolality =
  Serum osmolality − Osmolalities of freely diffusible solutes

Routes of fluid loss

About 200 to 300 ml of pure water is lost daily via the lungs. This volume increases with fever and hyperventilation. About 0.3 ml/calorie of pure water is lost through the skin in the absence of sweat. This amount is increased with fever and sweating; sweat contains about 50 mEq/L of sodium and 5 mEq/L of potassium. In the absence of fever or hyperventilation, the water loss by ventilation is almost exactly identical to the water production by metabolism. Therefore only the water loss through the skin needs to be considered in estimating insensible water loss.

The renal excretion of water and salt varies with intake, but the minimum water loss without renal failure is about 500 ml/day. An abnormal fluid loss through the kidney can occur with diuretic therapy, osmotic diuresis, metabolic acidosis, aldosterone deficiency, salt-losing renal disease, and the diuretic phase of acute tubular necrosis. Normally about 100 ml of water and 7 to 10 mEq of potassium are lost daily in the stool. An abnormal fluid loss can occur with vomiting or gastric lavage, diarrhea, drainage through a fistula, or enterostomy. When there is evidence of volume depletion without an obvious loss, fluid may be sequestered in the intestinal lumen because of mechanical obstruction or adynamic ileus, in the pleural cavity and peritoneal cavity, in the skin with burns, or in the extremities with thrombophlebitis.

Types of dehydration

Dehydration can be divided into three types—isotonic, hypertonic, and hypotonic—depending on the effective osmolality (tonicity) of the ECF.

ISOTONIC DEHYDRATION. Isotonic fluid loss may occur through the kidney or the gastrointestinal tract or directly from the ECF by drainage of pleural effusions, ascites, and so forth. Since water moves across cell membranes only in response to a change in the effective osmolality of the ECF, the intracellular volume remains normal and the fluid loss is only from the ECF space. The treatment consists of isotonic salt solution in the amount of the estimated ECF deficit.

HYPERTONIC DEHYDRATION. The primary aberration in hypertonic dehydration is loss of water because of either inadequate water intake or excessive water loss. Inadequacy or cessation of water intake may be caused by a defective thirst mechanism, as occurs with central nervous system lesions; impaired consciousness; lack of access to water because the patient is neglected, restrained, or paralyzed; or inability to drink water because of continuous vomiting or esophageal or pharyngeal tumors. Excessive water loss results from osmotic diuresis, diabetes insipidus, or sweating.

Dehydration caused by reduced water intake usually is slower to develop than that caused by abnormal water loss. Even when excessive water loss is the cause of hypertonic volume depletion, one of the conditions necessary for the limitation of water intake must be present to maintain hypertonicity. Otherwise, the stimulation of thirst by increased osmolality leads to increased water drinking and the correction of hypernatremia.

In hypertonic dehydration the salt content of the body may be normal, increased, or decreased. It is decreased if salt loss accompanied the water loss, as in osmotic diuresis or vomiting, but the salt loss is less than the water loss to maintain hypertonicity. In pure desiccation the salt content is normal, because the renal excretion of salt promptly stops as dehydration develops. If salt is administered to or ingested by a water-deficient person, it is largely retained because of volume depletion and the salt content of the body increases. In this case hypernatremia is the result not only of water loss but also of sodium retention. In pure water loss without a gain or loss of salt, the serum sodium concentration may be used as a fairly accurate index of the degree of desiccation. The estimated water deficit can be replaced with 2.5% or 5% glucose solution. (See p. 522 for calculation of water deficit.)

If salt retention is a cause of the hypernatremia, administering the total amount of water loss calculated on the basis of altered serum sodium leads to an overexpansion of the ECF volume. If the kidney is functioning normally, the excess salt and water are excreted. If renal function is impaired, the correction of hypernatremia in patients with sodium excess may require removal of sodium from the body by diuretics or dialysis in addition to administration of water.

HYPOTONIC DEHYDRATION. If renal function is adequate, a loss of salt alone does not occur because the resultant hyponatremia suppresses ADH and the kidney excretes water. More commonly both water and salt are lost, but salt loss exceeds water loss. Patients with hypotonic dehydration may present more evidence of compromised circulation for a given degree of fluid loss than patients with isotonic or hypertonic dehydration, because acute hypotonicity itself may significantly diminish vascular tone and cardiac output. In addition the reduction in the ECF for a given amount of total body water loss is greater in hypotonic dehydration than in other types, because water is lost from the body as well as into the cells.

Hypotonic dehydration may be treated by administering hypertonic saline to restore the serum sodium concentration to normal and adding normal saline to complete the restoration of the ECF volume. The amount of sodium necessary to normalize serum sodium is calculated as:

$$140 - \text{Serum sodium (mEq/L)} \times \text{Total body water (L)}$$

The total body water is used instead of the ECF volume for this calculation because an increase in extracellular sodium and hence osmolality would cause a shift of water from the cell. As indicated earlier, because of the danger of central pontine myelinolysis, the use of hypertonic saline is indicated only if the patient is suffering from acute symptoms of hyponatremia. Hypotonic dehydration commonly is treated by administering isotonic saline, with the rationale that with expansion of the ECF volume ADH will be suppressed and free water will be excreted to restore the serum sodium concentration to normal. However, a rapid increase in serum sodium still can occur with administration of normal saline, especially when a large amount of saline is administered with potassium supplement (uptake of potassium into the cell is accompanied by exit of sodium from the cell) to a patient who is only mildly volume depleted. The appraisal of volume depletion on clinical grounds often is inaccurate, and a chronically debilitated patient with hyponatremia and mild volume depletion may appear severely volume depleted. For these reasons the use of half-normal saline alternating with normal saline might be more prudent when the volume status is uncertain.

EDEMA

An inappropriate collection of interstitial fluid may be caused by a rise in capillary hydrostatic pressure, low plasma oncotic pressure (hypoalbuminemia), increase in capillary permeability (often idiopathic), or obstructed lymphatics. In most instances of generalized edema a reduced effective arterial volume causes renal salt and water retention. The treatment of edema involves restricting salt intake and, if renal function is adequate, using diuretics. Various diuretics work at different parts of the nephron. The diuretics that operate in the proximal tubule include acetazolamide (Diamox) and osmotic diuretics. The diuretics that operate in the ascending limb of Henle's loop include furosemide (Lasix), ethacrynic acid (Edecrin), and bumetanide (Bumex). The thiazide-like group diuretics (hydrochlorothiazide, chlorthalidone, and metolazone) operate in the early distal tubule. These diuretics have different degrees of potency and duration of action; metolazone is the most potent of the thiazide and thiazide-like diuretics. Diuretics in general cause potassium depletion. The diuretics that act in the collecting duct cause potassium retention; these include spironolactone (Aldactone), triamterene (Dyrenium), and amiloride (Midamor). Combinations of diuretics can be used for their synergistic effect or to allow the side effects of one (such as potassium loss) to offset the side effects of the other (such as potassium retention).

POTASSIUM METABOLISM

Most of the potassium in the body is contained in the cells, where the concentration is about 150 mEq/L of cell water; the plasma potassium concentration normally is 4 to 5 mEq/L. Clinical problems in potassium metabolism are caused by hypokalemia, a result of potassium loss or of a shift of potassium into the cells, or by hyperkalemia, in which potassium is retained in excess or shifted from the cells to the ECF. The mechanism of urinary potassium excretion involves secretion of potassium into the urine in the distal tubule and the collecting duct. Several factors modify the rate of potassium secretion.

HYPOKALEMIA

PATHOGENESIS. Hypokalemia is defined as a reduction in the extracellular potassium concentration. Potassium may be lost through the kidney or by extrarenal routes, the most important of which is the gastrointestinal tract. Gastrointestinal losses may be caused by diarrhea, laxative abuse, villous adenomas of the rectum, vomiting, or surgical drainage of the gastrointestinal tract. A shift of potassium into the cells can be caused by metabolic or respiratory alkalosis, ingestion of soluble barium salts, glucose and insulin infusion, β_2-adrenergic agonists (for example, salbutamol), and hypokalemic periodic paralysis.

Excessive renal potassium loss may occur with (1) increased aldosterone production, as in primary or secondary hyperaldosteronism (loss may not occur in these conditions if delivery of sodium to the distal nephron is reduced); (2) excessive production of deoxycorticosterone (as in adrenal cancer, ectopic adrenocorticotropic hormone (ACTH)–secreting tumor, 11- or 17-hydroxylase deficiency); (3) excessive ingestion of mineralocorticoid-like substances such as licorice or of exogenous mineralocorticoids; (4) excessive delivery of sodium to the distal nephron with normal or increased plasma concentrations of aldosterone, as in diuretic therapy, metabolic acidosis, or Bartter's syndrome; (5) increased delivery of poorly reabsorbable anions such as bicarbonate, sulfate, penicillin, or ketone anions to the distal nephron; or (6) unclear mechanisms such as magnesium deficiency, leukemia, or Liddle's syndrome.

PATHOGENETIC MECHANISMS OF HYPOKALEMIA

  I. Decreased intake
 II. Intracellular shift
     A. Glucose and insulin
     B. Alkalosis
     C. β_2-Agonists
     D. Hypokalemic periodic paralysis
III. Renal loss
     A. Hypermineralocorticoidism; primary and secondary hyperaldosteronism, exogenous mineralocorticoids
     B. Increased delivery of poorly reabsorbable anions to the collecting duct
     C. Increased delivery of sodium to the collecting duct; diuretics
     D. Unknown mechanisms; Liddle's syndrome, magnesium deficiency, acute leukemia

It can be concluded that the kidney is the route of potassium loss if the daily potassium excretion in the urine exceeds 40 mEq while the patient has a low serum potassium concentration. If a hypokalemic patient excretes less than 20 mEq of potassium in the urine daily, the route of potassium loss is extrarenal. It often is useful to measure the plasma renin activity and the plasma aldosterone concentration for the differential diagnosis of hypokalemia caused by renal potassium loss. Some of the important patterns are:

1. Low plasma renin activity with high aldosterone concentration—primary hyperaldosteronism caused by adrenal adenoma or bilateral adrenal hyperplasia
2. Increased plasma renin activity and increased aldosterone concentration—"secondary hyperaldosteronism" such as malignant hypertension, renal artery stenosis, Bartter's syndrome, and diuretic therapy
3. Decreased plasma renin activity and decreased aldosterone concentration—increased mineralocorticoid concentration other than that of aldosterone; ingestion of licorice; exaggerated salt reabsorption without excess mineralocorticoid (Liddle's syndrome)

CLINICAL MANIFESTATIONS. The important consequences of hypokalemia affect the neuromuscular system. The involvement of skeletal muscle is manifested by muscle weakness or paralysis. The involvement of visceral muscle may be represented by adynamic ileus. The effects on the heart include various types of heart block and arrhythmias.

MANAGEMENT. The treatment of hypokalemia involves correcting the underlying cause when possible, administering potassium by the oral or intravenous route, and, when it is required and feasible, reducing urinary potassium loss. The last requirement often can be met by using potassium-sparing diuretics such as amiloride and by reducing sodium intake.

HYPERKALEMIA

PATHOGENESIS. Hyperkalemia is defined as an increase in the extracellular potassium concentration. True hyperkalemia must be distinguished from pseudohyperkalemia, which is an elevated concentration of potassium only in vitro or in the local blood vessel from which blood is being drawn. Pseudohyperkalemia may be caused by the release of potassium during blood clotting in vitro from platelets or from leukocytes in thrombocytosis or severe leukocytosis. Plasma concentration is not elevated. In vitro hemolysis, using tourniquet with fist exercise or using tubes containing fluoride or potassium-ethylenediaminetetraacetic acid (EDTA), also may lead to in vitro "hyperkalemia." Hyperkalemia can be caused by reduced renal excretion, a shift of potassium from the cell to the ECF and by increased potassium intake. Increased potassium intake can be only a contributing factor, and only if renal excretion also is impaired. Potassium may be caused to shift out the cell by acute acidosis (primarily inorganic metabolic acidosis), rhabdomyolysis, hemolysis, increased catabolism, hyperosmolar states, β_2-blockers, and hyperkalemic periodic paralysis.

Causes of reduced renal potassium excretion

  I. Aldosterone deficiency
     A. Generalized adrenocortical insufficiency
        1. Addison's disease
        2. Enzyme defects
     B. Selective deficiency of aldosterone
        1. Chronic heparin therapy
        2. Hyporeninemic hypoaldosteronism
        3. Enzyme defects in the zona glomerulosa
 II. Tubular unresponsiveness to aldosterone (pseudohypoaldosteronism)
     A. Congenital
     B. Acquired; salt-losing nephropathy, potassium-sparing diuretics
III. Reduced delivery of sodium to the distal nephron; marked reduction in effective arterial volume such as hepatorenal syndrome, severe heart failure
IV. Advanced renal failure

DIAGNOSIS OF RENAL CAUSES OF HYPERKALEMIA. When it has been established that hyperkalemia results from deficient excretion of potassium by the kidney, the pattern of plasma renin activity (PRA) and plasma aldosterone concentration may be useful in establishing the cause:

1. High PRA and low plasma aldosterone concentration—selective aldosterone deficiency caused by adrenal disease, Addison's disease; chronic heparin therapy (heparin interferes with aldosterone synthesis)
2. High PRA and high aldosterone concentration—reduced delivery of sodium to the distal nephron; tubular unresponsiveness to aldosterone; potassium-sparing diuretics
3. Low PRA and low aldosterone concentration—hyporeninemic hypoaldosteronism

CLINICAL MANIFESTATIONS. Isolated in vitro hyperkalemia is clinically unimportant. True hyperkalemia causes changes in myocardial excitability ranging from electrocardiographic abnormalities consisting of tall T waves and decreased P waves to eventual atrial asystole, intraventricular block, and ultimately ventricular standstill. Neuromuscular symptoms occur only with severe hyperkalemia.

MANAGEMENT. Hyperkalemia is treated by combinations of three basic modalities:

I. Reduction in body potassium
   A. Reduced potassium intake
   B. Increased intestinal loss by use of sodium-potassium exchange resin; sodium polystyrene sulfonate (Kayexalate)
   C. Increased renal potassium excretion by increased sodium intake, diuretics, and mineralocorticoid therapy, e.g., fludrocortisone acetate (Florinef)
   D. Peritoneal dialysis or hemodialysis
II. Shift of potassium into the cell
   A. Administration of alkali
   B. Intravenous insulin and glucose
   C. Administration of β_2-agonists (salbutamol)
III. Antagonism of potassium in the heart
   A. Intravenous administration of calcium salts
   B. Administration of hypertonic sodium salts, usually as bicarbonate

ACID-BASE BALANCE

The concentration of hydrogen ion (H^+) in the body fluid must be maintained within a very narrow range for cellular biochemical reactions to perform properly. The H^+ concentration of body fluids is about 40 nEq/L. Current convention expresses this concentration as the pH, which is the negative logarithm of the H^+ concentration. The normal blood pH is about 7.4. The body is constantly threatened by addition of acids or alkali. To prevent gross deviation from the normal pH, the body is equipped with a set of buffering mechanisms that prevent an excessive rise or fall in the H^+ concentration. These buffers include the bicarbonate-carbonic acid system, which is the predominant buffering system of the ECF, and a variety of intracellular buffers, most important of which are the bone buffers. The bicarbonate-carbonic acid system is not only the most important buffer system of the body, it also is one that is readily available for study in the form of the arterial blood gases. Since the bicarbonate-carbonic acid buffer system is in equilibrium with other buffers, evaluation of the arterial blood gases gives a clue to the state of the other buffers in the body. Bicarbonate is produced by the kidney, and primary disturbances in bicarbonate concentration cause metabolic disturbances in acid-base regulation. Carbonic acid is produced by the reaction of CO_2 with water, and inappropriate retention or loss of CO_2 causes respiratory disturbances in acid-base regulation. There are four types of primary acid-base disturbances:

1. Metabolic acidosis, a primary decrease in bicarbonate
2. Metabolic alkalosis, a primary increase in bicarbonate
3. Respiratory acidosis, a primary increase in P_{CO_2}
4. Respiratory alkalosis, a primary decrease in P_{CO_2}

Metabolic acidosis

Each day the body produces about 70 mEq of acid from the metabolism of foods. This acid is buffered by the various body buffers and their anions are subsequently excreted by the kidney. In an attempt to maintain normal acid-base balance, the kidney excretes the same amount of acid, in the form of ammonium and titratable acids, and thereby generates bicarbonate.

PATHOGENESIS. Metabolic acidosis may be caused by one of two general mechanisms: extrarenal acidosis and renal acidosis. In extrarenal acidosis the serum bicarbonate concentration falls because acid production or ingestion is so great it exceeds the renal excretory ability. Examples of extrarenal acidosis include the generation of organic acids in diabetic ketoacidosis and D- and L-lactic acidoses, the intestinal loss of bicarbonate, and ingestion of acid, toxins, or precursors of acid. Renal acidosis occurs because the kidney is unable to excrete the normal amount of metabolic acid needed to regenerate the bicarbonate titrated by the normal production of endogenous acids. Impaired renal acid excretion may be caused by specific tubular defects, as in renal tubular acidosis, or by a reduction in the number of functioning nephrons as a result of renal disease, as in uremic acidosis.

Classification of metabolic acidosis

I. Renal acidosis
   A. Renal tubular acidosis (RTA): type I (classic distal RTA), type II (proximal RTA), and type IV (RTA caused by aldosterone deficiency or resistance)
   B. Uremic acidosis
II. Extrarenal acidosis
   A. Loss of bicarbonate in the stool
   B. Excessive organic acid production: ketoacids, d- and l-lactic acids
   C. Ingestion of exogenous acid or acid precursors
   D. Toxins; salicylate, methanol, ethylene glycol

COMPENSATORY MECHANISMS. The mechanisms the body uses to protect itself from the effects of metabolic acidosis and to restore itself to normal may be summarized as follows:

1. Buffering by bicarbonate and cellular and bone buffers.
2. Respiratory compensation in which the low blood pH stimulates ventilation. The P_{CO_2} appropriate for a given fall in bicarbonate can be calculated by the following equation:

$$\Delta P_{CO_2} = \Delta HCO_3^- \times 1.2 \pm 2$$

   For example, a patient whose serum bicarbonate level fell from 24 to 12 mEq/L ($HCO_3^- = 12$ mEq/L) should respond with a decrease in arterial P_{CO_2} by $12 \times 1.2 = 14.4$ mm Hg.
3. Excretion of acid by the kidney with simultaneous regeneration of bicarbonate. Phosphate and ammonia serve as major urinary buffers for the process.
4. Conversion of organic anions (lactate and ketone anions) to bicarbonate.

MANAGEMENT. Most patients with diabetes who have ketoacidosis have prompt reversal of the acidotic state following administration of insulin; the metabolism of ketone anions produces bicarbonate, and the kidney generates additional bicarbonate. L-lactic acidosis can be reversed only if the cause is corrected, but intravenous bicarbonate may be used to ameliorate acidosis while the basic problem is being managed. The effect of an experimental drug, dichloroacetate, is quite promising for treatment of lactic acidosis. D-lactic acidosis, which results from colonic overproduction of D-lactic acid in patients with short-bowel syndrome, can be treated with oral antibiotics.

Severe acidosis requires administration of bicarbonate to restore the pH to approximately 7.2, particularly in older individuals or those with compromised myocardial reserve, although some have argued against using alkali in the management of lactic acidosis. A good initial dosage is 1 mEq of bicarbonate per pound of body weight. This dosage can be repeated on the basis of arterial blood gas studies.

Patients with renal acidosis have no bicarbonate precursors circulating in the blood, and their kidneys are unable to regenerate sufficient bicarbonate to reverse the acidosis. Such patients must be treated by the administration of bicarbonate or by a bicarbonate precursor such as sodium citrate (Shohl's solution).

METABOLIC ALKALOSIS

PATHOGENESIS. Two pathogenetic mechanisms are required to maintain a high serum bicarbonate concentration: a mechanism to establish the high serum bicarbonate and a mechanism to prevent the excretion of bicarbonate in the urine by raising the renal threshold for bicarbonate.

Mechanisms for metabolic alkalosis

I. Mechanisms that produce a high serum bicarbonate concentration
  A. Gastrointestinal or renal H^+ loss
  B. Intracellular shift of H^+ in potassium depletion states
  C. Ingestion of alkali or precursors of alkali
  D. Conversion of organic anions to bicarbonate
  E. Loss of extracellular volume without loss of bicarbonate (contraction alkalosis)
II. Mechanisms that increase the renal threshold for bicarbonate excretion
  A. Low effective arterial volume
  B. Potassium depletion
  C. Hypercalcemia; hyperphosphatemia; hypoparathyroidism
  D. Chloride depletion (associated with volume depletion)
  E. Renal failure

CLINICAL MANIFESTATIONS. The major clinical categories of metabolic alkalosis are those with reduced effective arterial volume and those with expanded effective arterial volume. The disorders associated with low effective arterial volume are described as "chloride responsive" and are characterized by low urine chloride concentrations (less than 10 mEq/L). Exceptions to the rule of low urine chloride are Bartter's syndrome and diuretic therapy. When metabolic alkalosis is accompanied by reduction in effective arterial volume caused by edema-forming states, administering sodium chloride does not cause renal excretion of bicarbonate. The disorders associated with increased effective arterial volume are called "chloride resistant" metabolic alkalosis and are characterized by normal urinary chloride concentrations.

Categories of metabolic alkalosis

I. Metabolic alkalosis with reduced effective arterial volume (chloride-responsive alkalosis)
  A. Gastrointestinal H^+ loss caused by vomiting, gastric suction, congenital chloridorrhea (rare)
  B. Renal H^+ loss: diuretic abuse
II. Metabolic alkalosis with normal or increased effective arterial volume (chloride-resistant alkalosis)
  A. Primary aldosteronism, renin-secreting tumor, renal artery stenosis
  B. Cushing's syndrome (pituitary-adrenal and ectopic ACTH)
  C. Liddle's syndrome (resembles mineralocorticoid hyperresponsiveness)
  D. Excess licorice or carbenoxolone (resembles mineralocorticoid effect)
  E. Milk-alkali syndrome
  F. Potassium depletion

COMPENSATORY MECHANISMS. The body compensates for metabolic alkalosis in three ways: (1) tissue buffering by intracellular and bone buffers; (2) renal loss of bicarbonate when the cause is extrarenal; and (3) respiratory compensation. Hypoventilation with an increase in carbon dioxide can help ameliorate the rise in pH caused by increase in bicarbonate. However, this is the least satisfactory of all acid-base compensatory mechanisms, because it is limited by hypoxemia, an inevitable consequence of hypoventilation. It once was thought that the compensatory rise in PCO_2 rarely exceeded 60 mm Hg, regardless of the rise in bicarbonate, except in azotemic patients, but it now appears that respiratory compensation is proportional to the elevation of serum bicarbonate at any level of serum bicarbonate. The following equation predicts the normal compensation of metabolic alkalosis:

$$\Delta PCO_2 = \Delta HCO_3^- \times 0.7 \pm 5$$

MANAGEMENT. If possible, attempts should be made to remove factors that raise the serum bicarbonate concentration or that prevent renal bicarbonate excretion. In volume-depleted states administering chloride accomplishes this, and in potassium-depleted states correcting potassium depletion reverses alkalosis. Alternatively, direct titration of bicarbonate can be provided with ammonium chloride, hydrochloric acid of various normality, and lysine or arginine hydrochloride. Enhancing renal excretion of bicarbonate by administering acetazolamide may be effective when heart failure also is involved. Hemodialysis is useful in metabolic alkalosis with severe renal failure.

RESPIRATORY ACIDOSIS

PATHOGENESIS. Since carbon dioxide can be readily expelled by the body through ventilation, elevated levels of carbon dioxide in the body are traceable to disturbances of ventilation rather than to overproduction of carbon dioxide. Hypoventilation may be caused by a variety of mechanisms that involve the lung itself, the thoracic cage, the respiratory muscles and nerves, and the respiratory center in the brain (see the following list).

Causes of respiratory acidosis

1. Suppression of the respiratory center by central nervous system disease or pharmacologic agents; severe obesity (pickwickian syndrome)
2. Neuromuscular disorder—Guillain-Barré syndrome, myasthenia gravis, severe potassium depletion
3. Airway obstruction—aspiration, laryngeal edema, bronchospasm
4. Acute lung disease—pneumonia, massive embolism, pulmonary edema
5. Chronic lung disease—emphysema, bronchitis, interstitial lung disease
6. Alveolar hypoventilation—primary or caused by obesity
7. Thoracic cage disorder, trauma, kyphoscoliosis, flail chest, pneumothorax, severe obesity

COMPENSATORY MECHANISMS. Compensation for respiratory acidosis is accomplished through the generation and retention of bicarbonate. Bicarbonate is produced by two mechanisms: tissue buffering, which is rapid but increases the serum bicarbonate by at most 3 to 4 mEq/L, and renal excretion of H^+ with simultaneous generation of bicarbonate. This renal process requires 3 to 5 days to achieve its maximal effect; the increase in bicarbonate appropriate for a given rise in P_{CO_2} is calculated by the following equation:

$$\Delta HCO_3^- = \Delta P_{CO_2} \times 0.4 \pm 3$$

MANAGEMENT. Obvious causes of hypoventilation such as obstruction of the airway must be removed, and mechanical ventilation should be applied as necessary. In patients with pulmonary failure, efforts must be made to reestablish adequate ventilation so that oxygen can be administered at an appropriate rate. Care must be taken to avoid carbon dioxide narcosis in patients with protracted hypercapnia; P_{O_2} should be kept between 50 and 60 mm Hg. Dehydration and infection must be treated appropriately. Potassium and chloride deficits, if present, must be restored. The arterial pH must be monitored to avoid posthypercapnic alkalosis. When ventilation is restored and carbon dioxide levels decline, the alkaline pH allows renal excretion of bicarbonate and restoration of serum bicarbonate to a normal level. The factors that may prevent excretion of bicarbonate have been listed previously (see p. 526). In posthypercapnic states the most common reasons for persistent alkalosis are low effective arterial volume and potassium deficiency.

RESPIRATORY ALKALOSIS

PATHOGENESIS. Respiratory alkalosis is caused by excessive loss of carbon dioxide as a result of hyperventilation (see the following list).

Causes of respiratory alkalosis
1. Hypoxia from high altitude or lung disease
2. Drugs and toxins such as salicylate, progesterone, and epinephrine
3. Central nervous system disorders such as meningitis, brain tumor, cerebrovascular accident, or trauma
4. Psychogenic hyperventilation
5. Reflex stimulation caused by pneumothorax, pulmonary congestion, pulmonary emboli, or pneumonia
6. Sudden recovery from metabolic acidosis
7. Miscellaneous causes such as hepatic failure, gram-negative sepsis, or assisted ventilation

COMPENSATORY MECHANISMS. Compensation of respiratory alkalosis is accomplished by reducing the serum bicarbonate concentration. The bicarbonate concentration falls 3 to 4 mEq/L because of tissue buffering, which is completed within seconds. Renal compensation requires 2 to 3 days for maximal effect and consists of excretion of bicarbonate and reduced net acid excretion. Generation of lactic acid is increased in acute respiratory alkalosis. The appropriate degree of compensation is calculated by the following equation:

$$\Delta HCO_3^- = \Delta P_{CO_2} \times 0.5 \pm 2.5$$

The excellent compensation predicted by this equation often results in blood pH returning to normal.

MANAGEMENT. Treating respiratory alkalosis is difficult. Whenever possible the underlying disorder should be corrected. For hyperventilation caused by anxiety, rebreathing of carbon dioxide into a bag may help. Sedation with agents that suppress the respiratory center such as chlordiazepoxide (Librium) and phenobarbital sometimes may be indicated. In extreme cases pharmacologic paralysis and mechanical ventilation must be used.

Disorder	pH	HCO₃⁻	P_CO₂
Metabolic acidosis	↓	↓ 1°	↓ 2°
Respiratory acidosis	↓	↑ 2°	↑ 1°
Metabolic alkalosis	↑	↑ 1°	↑ 2°
Respiratory alkalosis	↑	↓ 2°	↓ 1°

Fig. 103-1 Primary and secondary events in acid-base disturbances. (From Carroll HJ and Oh MS: Water, electrolyte and acid-base metabolism, Philadelphia, 1989, JB Lippincott Co.)

MIXED ACID-BASE DISORDERS

The arterial blood gases serve to confirm the diagnostic impression of an acid-base disturbance, to determine the severity of a disturbance, and to permit an assessment of the appropriateness of the degree of compensation for the primary acid-base disturbance. Fig. 103-1 shows the primary and compensatory changes noted in uncomplicated acid-base disturbance. For each of the disorders in this scheme the formulas used to determine the appropriate compensation were supplied earlier. If the patient seems to be undercompensated or overcompensated, he may have an additional, unrelated primary acid-base disturbance. There are five types of mixed acid-base disorders that consist of pairs of primary disorders.

1. Respiratory acidosis with metabolic acidosis
2. Respiratory acidosis with metabolic alkalosis
3. Respiratory alkalosis with metabolic alkalosis
4. Respiratory alkalosis with metabolic acidosis
5. Metabolic acidosis with metabolic alkalosis

BIBLIOGRAPHY
Adrogue HJ and Madias NE: Changes in plasma potassium concentration during acute acid-base disturbances, Am J Med 71:456, 1981.

Anderson B: Regulation of water intake, Physiol Rev 58:582, 1978.

Arieff AI: Principles of parenteral therapy. In Maxwell MH and Kleeman CR, editors: Clinical disorders of fluid and electrolyte metabolism, ed 2, New York, 1972, McGraw-Hill, Inc.

Arieff AL and Carroll HJ: Non-ketotic hyperosmolar coma with hyperglycemia, Medicine (Baltimore) 51:73, 1972.

Blumberg A and others: Effect of various therapeutic approaches on plasma potassium and major regulating factors in terminal renal failure, Am J Med 85:507, 1988.

Carroll HJ and Oh MS: Water, electrolyte, and acid-base metabolism, Philadelphia, 1978, JB Lippincott Co.

Darrow DC: A guide to learning fluid therapy, Springfield Ill, 1959, Charles C Thomas.

Dubois GD and Arieff AL: Symptomatic hyponatremia: the case for rapid correction. In Narins R, editor: Controversies in nephrology and hypertension, New York, 1984, Churchill Livingstone, Inc.

Halperin ML and others: Interpretation of the serum potassium concentration in metabolic acidosis, Clin Invest Med 2:55, 1979.

Jacobson HR and Seldin DW: On the generation, maintenance, and correction of metabolic alkalosis, Am J Physiol 245:F425, 1983.

Kinney JM and Moore FD: Surgical metabolism in metabolism of body fluids. In Bland JH, editor: Clinical metabolism of body water and electrolytes, Philadelphia, 1963, WB Saunders Co.

Kurtzman NA: Acquired distal renal tubular acidosis, Kidney Int 24:807, 1983.

Laureno R and Karp B: Pontine and extrapontine myelinolysis following rapid correction of hyponatremia, Lancet I:1439, 1988.

Narins RG and Cohen JJ: Bicarbonate therapy for organic acidosis: the case for its continued use, Ann Intern Med 106:615, 1987.

Norenberg MD: The case for a more conservative approach. In Narins R, editor: Controversies in nephrology and hypertension, New York, 1984, Churchill Livingstone, Inc.

Oh MS and Carroll HJ: The anion gap, N Engl J Med 297:814, 1977.

Oh MS, Uribarri J, and Carroll HJ: Electrolyte case vignette: a case of unusual organic acidosis Am J Kidney Dis 11:80, 1988.

Oh MS and others: D-lactic acidosis in a man with short bowel syndrome, N Engl J Med 301:249, 1979.

Orwall ES: The milk-alkali syndrome. The current concept, Ann Intern Med 97:242, 1982.

Oster JR and others: Plasma potassium response to metabolic acidosis induced by mineral and non-mineral acids, Miner Electrolyte Metab 4:28, 1980.

Phelps K and others: The pathophysiology of the syndrome of hyporeninemic hypoaldosteronism, Metabolism 29:186, 1980.

Ponce SP and others: Drug-induced hyperkalemia, Medicine 64:357, 1985.

Relman AS, Lennon EJ and Lemann J Jr: Endogenous production of fixed acid and a measurement of net acid balance in normal subjects, J Clin Invest 40:1621, 1961.

Robertson GL: Abnormalities of thirst regulation, Kidney Int 25:460, 1984.

Robertson GL and Berl T: Water metabolism. In Brenner BM and Rector FC, editors: The kidney, Philadelphia, 1986, WB Saunders Co.

Rose BD: New approach to disturbances in the plasma sodium concentration, Am J Med 81:1033, 1986.

Simpson DP: Control of hydrogen ion homeostasis and renal acidosis, Medicine (Baltimore) 50:503, 1971.

Sterns, RH, Riggs JE, and Schochet SS Jr: Osmotic demyelination syndrome following correction of hyponatremia, N Engl J Med 314:1535, 1986.

Uribarri J, Oh MS, and Carroll HJ: Salt-losing nephropathy, Am J Nephrol 3:193, 1983.

Williams ME, Rosa RM, and Epstein FH: Hyperkalemia, Adv Intern Med 31:265, 91, 1986.

Zerbe RL and Robertson GL: Osmoregulation of thirst and vasopressin secretion in human subjects: effect of various solutes, Am J Physiol 224:F607, 1983.

104 · INVESTIGATION OF RENAL FUNCTION AND STRUCTURE

PEDRO C. FERNANDEZ

CLINICAL ASSESSMENT OF RENAL FUNCTION
Clearance measurements

The urinary excretion of any substance can be expressed in terms of its plasma clearance, which is equal to the urine/plasma concentration ratio for that substance times the urine volume ($C = U/P \times V$). The clearance of substances that are freely ultrafiltrable and not subjected to either tubular reabsorption or secretion equals the glomerular filtration rate (GFR). If a substance were completely extracted from the plasma and excreted in the urine in each single pass through the kidneys, its clearance would equal the renal plasma flow. Substances that undergo net tubular reabsorption have clearances lower than the GFR. When the clearance of a substance exceeds its GFR, that substance is subjected to net tubular secretion by the kidney.

The overall renal excretory function is best assessed clinically by determining the GFR. Determining the clearance of inulin or polyfructosan is the most reliable method of measuring the GFR. However, since these clearance determinations are cumbersome to perform, measuring the clearance of endogenous creatinine can be substituted in most clinical situations. Practically all the creatinine excreted in the urine is formed in the muscles at a relatively constant rate for a given individual. In humans, creatinine not only is filtered at the glomerulus but also undergoes tubular secretion. The latter probably accounts for a larger fraction of the urinary creatinine when renal function is decreased. Thus in normal individuals the creatinine and inulin clearances are almost equal, but when the GFR is decreased, the creatinine clearance exceeds the inulin clearance. Despite these reservations the creatinine clearance is a

useful parameter for determining the progression of renal disease. For clinical purposes the creatinine clearance is best determined using a 24-hour urine collection, which reduces the error caused by inaccurate timing and defective emptying of the bladder. The creatinine concentration in the plasma should be determined in the morning of the urine collection period. Although various analytic methods may be used to measure the urine creatinine, the method used to determine plasma creatinine should measure the true creatinine and not the so-called noncreatinine chromogens. Automated laboratory methods provide an adequate measurement of the plasma creatinine concentration. The determination of the creatinine clearance is valid only if the patient's renal function is in a steady state, that is, not changing while the clearance is being determined. Creatinine clearance normally averages 120 ± 20 ml/min in men and 110 ± 15 ml/min in women.

The GFR may be estimated from the plasma creatinine concentration. This is based on the fact that, if creatinine production remains constant, the plasma creatinine concentration varies with changes in the GFR. The inverse relationship between the plasma creatinine concentration and the GFR is given by a rectangular hyperbola, so that a doubling of the plasma creatinine concentration would mean that the GFR has been halved. Although this relationship is grossly correct, it should be mentioned that normal plasma creatinine concentrations range from 0.7 to 1.4 mg/dl, depending mainly on the body muscle mass. Consequently, the plasma creatinine concentration changes reliably reflect changes in the GFR only when the plasma creatinine concentration and creatinine clearance were previously known. In advanced renal failure this relationship does not hold true because of the decreased creatinine production and the increased contribution of tubular secretion to the urinary excretion of creatinine.

An inverse relationship also exists between the blood urea nitrogen (BUN) concentration and the GFR. Although the BUN increases with deteriorating renal function, this parameter is a less reliable indicator of renal function than the plasma creatinine concentration, mainly because urea production varies and is markedly influenced by factors such as protein intake and degree of protein catabolism.

Determining renal blood flow is rarely done for clinical purposes. The renal clearance of paraaminohippurate (PAH), a substance that in humans has a 90% index of extraction in a single pass through the kidney, closely approaches the value of the renal plasma flow. However, the adequacy of the blood supply to the kidney more often is clinically assessed by means of radioisotope studies, as discussed later in this chapter.

Measurements of renal concentrating ability

Although a diseased kidney loses the ability to maximally concentrate the urine, direct investigation of the renal concentrating ability is indicated mainly in the diagnosis of nonglucosuric polyuria. The test requires complete fluid deprivation for 12 hours or until the patient's body weight is reduced by 3% to 5%, whichever comes first. A patient with marked polyuria should be carefully observed to prevent the development of severe intravascular volume depletion. The patient empties the bladder at the end of the fluid deprivation period, and the osmolality of the urine voided in the next half hour is determined. Five units of aqueous vasopressin are then injected subcutaneously, and the osmolality of the subsequent urine sample is determined. Normal individuals excrete a urine with an osmolality of at least 800 mOsm/kg water following 12 hours of fluid deprivation. Moreover, the osmolality of their urine is not increased further by the exogenous administration of vasopressin.

Urinalysis

The urinalysis is the simplest, most economical, and most reliable screening test for detecting renal disease. It should be performed on a freshly voided, midstream, clean-catch urine specimen. Samples collected in the morning after an overnight fast allow estimation of the kidney's concentrating ability. A specific gravity greater than 1.02 in the absence of glucosuria is a strong argument against the presence of significant renal failure.

The urine should be tested routinely for the presence of protein, sugar, and blood. The widely available dipsticks impregnated with several reagents provide a simple, reliable method for qualitative chemical testing of urine samples.

The bromphenol-impregnated protein indicator reacts more strongly in the presence of albumin than of globulins and does not detect Bence Jones protein. False positive results may be seen with very alkaline urines. The detection of persistent proteinuria by routine urinalysis should be followed by its quantification on a 24-hour urine sample, by means of the sulfosalicylic acid, biuret, or Kjeldahl methods. The amount and type of proteins being excreted also may be determined by electrophoretic and immunologic techniques.

Glucose, but not other sugars, is specifically detected by the glucose oxidase–impregnated dipstick. The orthotolidine reagent of the dipstick detects both heme pigments and myoglobin; the urinary sediment should be examined microscopically to confirm the presence of red blood cells in patients with hematuria.

The pH indicator of the dipstick is of little clinical value, although a highly alkaline urine (pH of 8 or higher) suggests a urinary tract infection caused by urea-splitting organisms, usually *Proteus* organisms.

Careful microscopic examination of the urinary sediment is an essential part of the urinalysis. Ten to 15 ml of urine should be centrifuged, the supernatant decanted, and the sediment resuspended in 0.5 ml of urine. A thin film of the sediment, as obtained by depositing a coverslide over a droplet of the sediment, should then be examined with a subdued light under the low-power objective ($\times 10$) and the high-dry-power objective ($\times 40$), screening 15 to 20 different fields. Attention should be paid to the presence and type of cells, urinary casts, and crystals. Cell and cast quantification is expressed as the number of formed elements per high-dry-power field.

The normal urinary sediment contains one or no red blood cells and not more than three to five white blood cells in each high-power field in men and three or fewer red blood cells and six to eight white blood cells in women. Although hyaline casts may be seen in small numbers in normal individuals, other types of casts (granular, waxy, red cell, white cell, and renal tubular cell casts) are abnormal. Since urinary casts are formed exclusively inside the renal tubules, the presence of cellular casts suggests a pathologic condition in the kidney itself rather than or in addition to disease elsewhere in the urinary tract. The presence of red blood cell casts in patients with hematuria is strong evidence for glomerulitis. Other types of casts, specifically granular casts, are not useful for localizing disease.

With 3+ or 4+ proteinuria the sediment should be examined under polarized light for double-refractile bodies ("Maltese crosses"), which may be free in the sediment, encased in casts (fatty casts), or inside degenerated renal tubular cells (oval fat bodies). These double-refractile bodies are fat globules seen most often in patients with the nephrotic syndrome.

Assessment of proteinuria

Normal individuals excrete less than 150 mg of protein in the urine in each 24 hours. The most abundant protein in normal urine is the Tamm-Horsfall protein or uromucoid, a glycoprotein not present in the plasma. This protein is secreted by the distal nephron segments and tends to precipitate inside the tubules in pathologic states. It is the main constituent of the matrix of urinary casts. Most of the other urinary proteins, including albumin and various globulins, are normal plasma proteins. Some urinary proteins are derived from prostatic and urethral secretions or are enzymes released from renal tubular cells.

Pathologic proteinuria usually is persistent and may range in severity from less than 500 mg protein to more than 30 mg in each 24 hours. Animal experiments indicate that the normal glomerular filtrate contains less than 30 mg protein/L urine, mainly albumin. Since this protein does not appear in the excreted urine, most of it must be reabsorbed by the tubules. Tubular reabsorption of protein occurs at least in part by a process of endocytosis and seems to be a saturable process.

Three main mechanisms account for the development of pathologic proteinuria:

1. *The presence in the plasma of abnormal proteins, which can easily cross the glomerular wall owing to their low molecular weight* (less than 40,000). This type of proteinuria is exemplified by the urinary excretion of light chains of immunoglobulins (Bence Jones protein) in patients with multiple myeloma and sometimes in those with amyloidosis.
2. *Abnormal tubular reabsorption of normally filtered plasma proteins, seen mainly in the tubulointerstitial type of renal disease.* This "tubular" proteinuria usually is mild (less than 1.5 g/day), and most of the proteins appearing in the urine are low-molecular-weight globulins, especially β_2-microglobulin.
3. *Abnormal permeability of the glomerular capillary wall to normal plasma protein constituents, mainly albumin.* This is the most common cause of pathologic proteinuria. The proteinuria of glomerular disease may be of any degree of severity. Practically all patients with urinary protein in excess of 3 g/day ("nephrotic range" proteinuria) have some form of glomerular disease, as do most patients with 24-hour urinary protein ranging from 1.5 to 3 g.

Mild abnormal proteinuria (usually less than 1.5 g protein/24 hours) occasionally is seen in the absence of renal disease, such as in patients with congestive heart failure, in febrile illnesses, following heavy exercise, and in so-called orthostatic proteinuria. This last condition is characterized by the presence of proteinuria when the patient is erect, but not when he is recumbent. It most commonly is seen in young adults, and if associated with normal renal function and the absence of abnormalities in the urinary sediment, it has an excellent prognosis, often disappearing spontaneously.

Recent evidence about insulin-dependent diabetes suggests that the presence of abnormal but subclinical quantities of albumin, *microalbuminuria*, predicts the future development of diabetic nephropathy.

ROENTGENOGRAPHIC AND ULTRASONOGRAPHIC EXAMINATION OF THE KIDNEYS

Roentgenographic examination of the kidneys provides the physician with detailed anatomic information about the kidneys and the collecting system. Plain roentgenography of the abdomen may yield valuable information about the size and contour of the kidneys and the presence of opacities (renal calcifications or calculi) in the region of the kidney or the collecting system. This noninvasive examination is the preliminary step to the more accurate renal roentgenographic examinations in which radiopaque contrast material is administered to the patient. Triiodinated sodium or meglumine diatrizoate, iothalamate, and metrizoate are radiopaque contrast agents excreted only by glomerular filtration and concentrated in the urine by the tubular reabsorption of salt and water. The contrast agent is injected into a peripheral vein, and the renal concentration and excretion of the agent then are followed by means of an intravenous pyelogram or excretory urogram. Another technique is to insert a thin catheter percutaneously into a large peripheral artery or vein (usually the femoral vessels at the groin) and subsequently to move it into the renal arteries or veins. This allows direct injection of the radiopaque dye into the renal arteries (renal arteriography) or veins (renal venography) to assess the renal vasculature in detail. In certain cases the contrast material is injected directly into the collecting system. This may be done in two ways: (1) via a catheter passed percutaneously into the renal pelvis (antegrade pyelography) or (2) through a catheter inserted during cystoscopy into the ureter via the ureteral bladder orifices (retrograde pyelography).

Administration of iodinated roentgenographic contrast material may be followed by allergic reactions ranging in severity from an urticarial rash to bronchospasm and anaphylactic shock. Unless studies requiring administration of these dyes are absolutely necessary, they should not be performed in individuals with a history of allergy to contrast agents. If they are necessary, the patient must be pretreated with corticosteroids under expert guidance and an emergency resuscitation team must be available at the time of the procedure.

Acute renal failure following the intravascular injection of roentgenographic contrast agents has been reported relatively frequently in recent years. Predisposing factors to the development of acute renal failure are (1) preexisting renal insufficiency (serum creatinine concentration greater than 2 mg/dl); (2) diabetes mellitus, especially if long standing and associated with renal insufficiency; (3) multiple myeloma; (4) dehydration, which probably increases the inherent risk in otherwise predisposed patients, particularly those with multiple myeloma; and (5) advanced age, hypertension, and hyperuricemia, which are thought to constitute additional risk factors. Although the condition usually is transient and full recovery is the rule, diabetic patients with severe renal insufficiency (serum creatinine concentration greater than 5 mg/dl) may not regain renal function.

Intravenous urography

In intravenous urography intravenous administration of a bolus of a radiopaque contrast agent normally is followed by progressive opacification of the renal parenchyma within the first minute of the injection (the nephrogram). This is followed in the next 1 to 3 minutes by successive opacification of the calices, renal pelvis, and ureters (urogram). The dye normally disappears between 30 and 60 minutes after the injection.

Visualization of the renal parenchyma and perirenal structures is improved by tomographic sections, which eliminate overlying bowel gas from the renal image. Nephrotomography combined with continuous intravenous infusion of contrast material is particularly valuable in evaluating renal masses. Detailed visualization of the collecting system is facilitated by

external compression of the distal ureters by means of a pneumatic device applied over the lower abdominal wall. This prevents the rapid flow of contrast material into the bladder.

Intravenous urography remains the best initial study in roentgenographic evaluation of renal disease. The nephrogram shows the size and contour of the kidneys. Visualization of renal masses is best accomplished by nephrotomography. If the mass is cystic, a thin, regular wall suggests a benign cyst. The nephrogram also may provide useful functional information. In chronic renal failure the nephrogram is delayed and faint, whereas acute renal failure may present a rapidly appearing and abnormally persistent nephrogram. In urinary tract obstruction the nephrogram appears late and increases progressively in intensity.

The urogram makes it possible to study the anatomy of the collecting system. Distortion of the calices may be caused by renal mass lesions or by previous inflammatory disease of the kidneys. The calices and renal pelvis are dilated in urinary tract obstruction. Ulcerations and excavations of the renal papillae may be seen in renal tuberculosis and papillary necrosis. Stones or primary tumors of the collecting system appear as filling defects on the urogram. The urogram also provides diagnostically valuable functional information. In hypertension caused by stenosis of one renal artery, the urogram is delayed in the affected side in films taken at 1 or 2 minutes (rapid-sequence intravenous urogram). The urogram also is delayed in obstruction, and films taken at 6, 12, and 24 hours may show a dilated collecting system.

Retrograde pyelography

Retrograde pyelography is indicated mainly in two clinical situations. With renal failure the patient's history and other diagnostic procedures (ultrasonography, intravenous urography, radionuclide scanning) may lead the physician to suspect that urinary tract obstruction is the cause. In these cases the procedure usually is done on one side only (preferably the one on which the kidney is larger), since bilateral obstruction is implied when obstruction is the cause of renal failure. If obstruction is found and the catheter can be passed beyond the point of obstruction, it may be left in place to ensure urine drainage until a more definitive procedure is performed. Retrograde pyelography also is useful in the differential diagnosis of unexplained unilateral hematuria or filling defects in the collecting system that have not been sufficiently visualized with the intravenous urogram.

The main complication of retrograde pyelography is introduction of infection. For this reason, as well as the frequent need for general or spinal anesthesia with retrograde pyelography, antegrade pyelography is favored in the diagnosis and immediate management of urinary tract obstruction.

Antegrade pyelography

The major indication for diagnostic antegrade pyelography is suspected obstruction, as just discussed. In addition the antegrade insertion of draining catheters may be the temporary procedure of choice to relieve confirmed urinary tract obstruction. This is chiefly because antegrade pyelography is a more sterile procedure than retrograde pyelography and it is performed with local anesthesia.

Renal angiography

The main renal arteries can be visualized by injecting the contrast material into the aorta (aortography). Digital subtraction angiography is a new technique for visualizing the renal vasculature following intravenous injection of contrast material. However, detailed visualization of the intrarenal vasculature requires direct injection of the dye into the main renal artery or one of its branches (selective renal arteriography). The renal veins are faintly visible on the arteriogram within a few seconds of the injection. For more precise definition the contrast agent must be injected directly into the renal veins (renal venography).

The main indications for renal arteriography are (1) for evaluation of renal masses that have not been clearly defined by other examinations, (2) for confirmation of the diagnosis of hypertension associated with stenosis of the renal arteries, (3) in cases of renal trauma and posttransplant renal failure, and (4) therapeutically for the obliteration, by means of local embolization, of the vascular supply to tumors, arteriovenous fistulas, and lacerated blood vessels.

Renal venography is performed to determine if renal cell carcinoma has spread beyond the parenchyma into the renal veins. The procedure also is needed to confirm renal vein thrombosis, which may complicate the nephrotic syndrome. Finally, renal vein catheterization often is performed to obtain blood samples in cases of hypertension associated with renal artery stenosis. Renal vein renin concentration ratios of 1.5 or greater between the affected and the unaffected sides are the best criterion for surgical treatment of the hypertension.

Computed tomography

Computed tomographic (CT) scanning provides high-resolution transverse images of the kidneys, adrenal glands, and perirenal areas. The investigation is noninvasive and safe, except for the potential hazard of complications induced by iodinated contrast material, which generally is used in renal computed tomography.

CT is indicated in the further evaluation of mass lesions identified by intravenous urography or renal ultrasonography. The CT scan allows differentiation between cystic and solid lesions. The benign or malignant nature of arteriographically avascular masses can at times be ascertained by CT. The technique also is valuable in assessing the regional spread of proven renal malignancies. In addition it is useful in evaluating suspected cases of hydronephrosis, adrenal tumors, and other perirenal and retroperitoneal disease processes.

Renal ultrasonography

Ultrasonic waves from 1 to 10 MHz in frequency travel at a characteristic uniform velocity through a homogeneous medium, but they become refracted or reflected at the interface of two media with different acoustic properties. The combination of this basic principle with amplification and computer analysis of the reflected ultrasound beam ("echo"), as exemplified by gray-scale ultrasonography, allows demonstration of the contour, size, and morphologic details of the renal parenchyma.

Longitudinal and transverse ultrasonographic sections of the kidney usually are obtained. The normal renal cortex is echogenic, whereas the renal medulla and intrarenal collecting system are relatively echo free. Fluid-filled areas such as renal cysts or a dilated collecting system appear as sonolucent areas with occasional internal echoes owing to tissue debris from infection or tumor necrosis. Solid masses within the kidney may produce increased echoes, but they frequently are difficult to differentiate from normal parenchyma.

Renal ultrasonography is a benign, noninvasive procedure that is rapidly gaining popularity as the screening test for the study of the renal anatomy. In this respect it is particularly useful when there are absolute or relative contraindications to the intravenous urogram. Moreover, renal ultrasonography is mandatory in evaluating renal masses. With lesions 1.5 cm in diameter or greater, ultrasonography allows differentiation between solid masses (usually tumors) and fluid-filled structures. In the latter a smooth and sharply defined wall and the absence of internal echoes are highly characteristic of a benign cyst. If ultrasonographic findings are equivocal, the cystic lesion may be punctured under ultrasonographic guidance and the fluid processed for cytologic and chemical analysis.

Ultrasonography also is useful in detecting urinary tract obstruction and the diagnosis of polycystic kidney disease. Performing a percutaneous renal biopsy or antegrade pyelography is greatly facilitated by determining the exact location of the kidney with ultrasonography.

Radioisotope imaging

A large number of radiopharmaceuticals that are excreted by the kidney currently are available. The renal handling of different radiopharmaceuticals varies. Among the most commonly used agents are (1) technetium-labeled diethylenetriamine pentaacetic acid (Tc 99m DTPA), which is excreted almost exclusively by glomerular filtration; (2) radioactive iodine—labeled orthoiodohippuric acid (Hippuran I 131), which is excreted primarily by tubular secretion; (3) technetium-labeled dimercaptosuccinic acid (Tc 99m DMSA), which is bound by cortical tubular cells; and (4) technetium-labeled glucoheptonate (Tc 99m GHA), which combines the properties of DTPA and DMSA.

Current gamma camera external scanning techniques can produce roentgenographic images of the kidneys and collecting system (renal scan). In addition curves plotting the accumulation of the radioactive compound in the renal areas versus time can be constructed (isotopic renogram). Finally, since early accumulation of radioactive tracers in the kidneys depends mainly on the blood supply, the magnitude of the renal blood flow can be estimated by isotopic techniques. The choice of agent depends on the problem to be investigated; consequently the physician performing the test should be given the pertinent clinical information.

The imaging procedure is safe, since the radiation exposure risk of isotopic studies generally is less than that of standard urography. Its indications are quite broad and include (1) screening evaluation of patients suspected of having hypertension caused by renal artery stenosis; (2) evaluation of solid renal masses to distinguish between tumor and pseudotumor; (3) diagnostic evaluation of patients with acute and chronic renal failure, particularly to assess renal blood supply and the presence or absence of obstruction; (4) postoperative follow-up monitoring of renal function in renal transplant recipients.

RENAL BIOPSY

Although renal biopsy specimens may be obtained surgically, percutaneous renal biopsy usually is the procedure of choice in the morphologic evaluation of medical ailments of the kidney. The procedure is relatively simple and safe in experienced hands. The lower pole of the right kidney usually is chosen, its exact position being determined roentgenographically or by renal ultrasonography. With the patient under local anesthesia, the kidney first is located by means of a thin-bore spinal needle, and subsequently renal tissue is obtained using the Franklin modification of the Vim-Silverman biopsy needle or with a specially designed disposable needle (Travenol needle). Complete bed rest is prescribed, and the patient is carefully observed for the following 24 hours. The obtained tissue should be processed for light microscopy (and stained with hematoxylin-eosin, periodic acid–Schiff [PAS], PAS–silver methenamine, Masson trichrome, and if indicated other special stains), electron microscopy, and immunofluorescence studies. Light microscopy sections should not exceed 3 μm in thickness. For a biopsy specimen to be diagnostically adequate, it should contain at least 5 to 10 glomeruli.

The absolute or relative contraindications to percutaneous renal biopsy are patient uncooperativeness, the presence of a single kidney, bleeding and/or coagulation abnormalities, uncontrolled hypertension, and small, contracted kidneys. In the case of active or suspected renal infection or neoplasm, needle biopsy should not be performed, owing to the risk of dissemination.

Renal biopsy is particularly useful in the diagnosis of glomerular diseases, which currently are classified mainly on the basis of clinicopathologic correlations. Thus biopsies commonly are performed in patients with the nephrotic syndrome, acute nephritic syndrome, and persistent urinary abnormalities to diagnose the underlying disease, establish a prognosis, and select therapy. Renal biopsy also is frequently indicated to determine the degree and type of renal involvement in certain systemic diseases. Acute renal failure of obscure cause or protracted course is another indication for renal biopsy.

The immediate complications of percutaneous renal biopsy are laceration of the kidney or other intraabdominal organs and severe bleeding. Infection is uncommon. Formation of an arteriovenous fistula, manifested by hematuria and/or severe hypertension, is a rare late complication.

BIBLIOGRAPHY

Heinemann HO, Maack TM, and Sherman RL: Combined clinical and basic science seminar: proteinuria, Am J Med 56:71, 1974.

Kassirer JP and Gennari JF: Laboratory evaluation of renal function. In Earley LE and Gottschalk CW, editors: Strauss and Welt's diseases of the kidney, ed 3, Boston, 1979, Little, Brown & Co.

Muehrcke RC and Pirani CL: Renal biopsy: an adjunct in the study of kidney disease. In Black D, editor: Renal disease, ed 3, Oxford, England, 1972, Blackwell Scientific Publications, Inc.

Morrison RBI: Urinanalysis and assessment of renal function. In Black D, editor: Renal disease, ed 3, Oxford, England, 1972, Blackwell Scientific Publications, Inc.

Rosenfield AT, Glickman MG, and Hodson J: Diagnostic imaging in renal disease, New York, 1979, Appleton-Lange.

105·PRIMARY GLOMERULAR DISEASE

Pasha Agarwal *and* **Brajesh Agarwal**

Glomerular disease includes all renal conditions in which structural and functional abnormalities of the glomeruli are the primary features. The kidneys may be affected in multiple-system diseases of known cause, but in most cases of glomerulonephritis the cause is unknown. Basically, two immunologic mechanisms have been implicated in the pathogenesis of glomerulonephritis. Anti–glomerular basement membrane antibodies play a role in a few cases, but the more common pathogenetic mechanism involves the deposition of circulating antigen-antibody complexes in the glomeruli, which initiates an inflammatory reaction leading to glomerular damage. Recent studies suggest that free circulating antibodies may react with antigens already present in the glomerulus, resulting in situ immune-complex formation. Activation of the complement system plays a major role in the resultant inflammatory process.

The glomerular diseases may be clinically manifested in three different forms: asymptomatic urinary abnormalities, nephritic syndrome, or nephrotic syndrome.

ASYMPTOMATIC URINARY ABNORMALITIES

Asymptomatic proteinuria or hematuria may be associated with a benign course; mild to moderate proteinuria is present, sometimes only with lordotic posture. Gross or microscopic hematuria may be persistent or recurrent. Dysmorphic red blood cells are the hallmark of glomerular hematuria. Hypoproteinuria, hypertension, edema, and renal failure are absent.

NEPHRITIC SYNDROME

Nephritic syndrome is characterized by evidence of inflammation of the glomeruli and is manifest by the abrupt onset of macroscopic or microscopic hematuria, erythrocyte casts, and proteinuria. Usually nephritic syndrome is associated with edema and circulatory congestion, hypertension, and some degree of renal failure, and occasionally it is seen with oliguria. The course may be acute, subacute, or chronic. Most patients with acute glomerulonephritis have a short clinical course and recover spontaneously. Subacute or rapidly progressive glomerulonephritis is more insidious in onset and progressive in course. Patients usually are markedly oliguric, and severe renal failure rapidly develops. In patients with chronic glomerulonephritis caused by various inherited and acquired glomerular diseases, progressive renal functional impairment gradually develops, accompanied by varying degrees of proteinuria, hematuria, and hypertension.

Acute poststreptococcal glomerulonephritis

Acute poststreptococcal glomerulonephritis is a prototype of acute nephritic syndrome that can be seen in a variety of conditions including some nonstreptococcal infections (pneumococcal pneumonia, bacterial endocarditis, infected ventriculoatrial shunt, sepsis, leptospirosis, infectious hepatitis, infectious mononucleosis, coxsackievirus type B infection, mumps, varicella, echovirus infection, toxoplasmosis, malaria), collagen-vascular disorders, other systemic diseases, and some primary glomerular diseases (membranoproliferative glomerulonephritis, benign focal glomerulonephritis, and IgA nephropathy).

Only a few strains of group A β-hemolytic streptococci are nephritogenic. These strains are typed according to the M protein antigen present on the cell wall of the organism. The strains most frequently associated with nephritis include 1, 2, 4, 12, 18, 25, 49 (Red Lake), 55, 57, and 60. Poststreptococcal glomerulonephritis is an immune-complex disease, but the nature of the antigen is not well defined. However, it appears to be derived from the streptococcal organism.

PATHOLOGY. Acute poststreptococcal glomerulonephritis is characterized histologically by diffuse cellular proliferation involving all glomeruli. There is an increase in endothelial and mesangial cells, along with an infiltration of neutrophils. The capillary lumen may be narrowed and sometimes obliterated. Severe cases may show necrotizing changes, extravasation of debris, fibrin, neutrophils in Bowman's space, and formation of crescents because of proliferation of epithelial cells of Bowman's capsule. The tubules may be dilated and filled with red blood cells and casts. Edema and infiltration of inflammatory cells in the interstitium also may be noted. In the healing phase sclerotic changes in the glomeruli may occur. In some series a persistent increase in the cellularity in the mesangial stalk region has been described. This is a nonspecific finding and can occur in patients without a history of acute infection. Electron microscopy characteristically shows scattered subepithelial deposits of electron-dense material in the form of humps. Immunofluorescence reveals diffuse granular deposits of IgG, complement (C3), properdin, and fibrinogen.

CLINICAL MANIFESTATIONS. Poststreptococcal glomerulonephritis occurs in all age-groups but most commonly in children. The peak incidence is between 3 and 7 years of age, and the disease is more frequent in males. Characteristically there is a latent period of a few days between the onset of acute streptococcal infection (in the throat or skin) and clinical findings suggestive of acute glomerulonephritis. The clinical features in the elderly may be very atypical.

The onset may be heralded by vague constitutional symptoms. Usually the patient has a history of gross hematuria. Sometimes the urine is described as smoky or cola colored. Hematuria may be microscopic, and the disease may remain undetected if urinalysis is not performed carefully. Oliguria and anuria are uncommon and, when present, indicate a poor prognosis. Dull, aching pain in the abdomen or loins also may be present. In most symptomatic patients some degree of edema develops, most prominently in the face and eyelids in the morning. Later in the disease course dependent edema and anasarca may develop. The patient also may have mild to moderate hypertension, circulatory congestion, and in some cases pulmonary edema caused by volume expansion. During the acute phase one possible complication is severe hypertension resulting in hypertensive encephalopathy. In most cases in adults the course is that of slow healing with clinical improvement and return of the blood pressure to normal. Abnormal urinary findings such as mild proteinuria and microscopic hematuria may persist as long as 2 years after clinical resolution with a normal glomerular filtration rate. In the acute stage up to 5% of patients die of complications despite dialysis. A rapidly progressive decline in renal function leading to end-stage renal failure within a few weeks occurs in a few patients. In most of these cases extensive crescent formation is seen in renal biopsy specimens. Chronic glomerulonephritis also can develop occasionally after apparent clinical healing of acute poststreptococcal glomerulonephritis.

LABORATORY FINDINGS. Urinalysis is the most important test in diagnosing glomerulonephritis. The urine appears red or brownish, and red blood cells and some degree of proteinuria are almost always present. Red blood cell casts commonly are seen. Occasionally leukocytes, other casts, or proteinuria in the nephrotic range may be found.

The glomerular filtration rate varies from normal in asymptomatic patients to markedly decreased in symptomatic patients. The renal plasma flow and tubular functions are less affected, and the filtration fraction is decreased. The urine-concentrating ability is preserved until advanced renal failure supervenes. Some degree of normocytic normochromic anemia and hypoalbuminemia resulting from excessive fluid retention may be present. Intrinsic myocardial function remains normal, and pulmonary congestion with or without cardiac enlargement reflects an expanded vascular volume caused by sodium retention. The throat culture may be positive for group A β-hemolytic streptococci during the acute phase when the pharynx is isthe site of infection. Measurements of changing antibody titers to streptococcal antigens (antistreptolysin O [ASO], antihyaluronidase, anti-NADase, or streptozyme) help confirm the diagnosis. There seems to be no correlation between the degree of titer increase and the severity of disease. Titers may remain elevated for 6 months. Both the classic and alternate pathways of the complement system are activated in poststreptococcal nephritis. The total serum hemolytic complement (CH_{50}) and C3 components are decreased during the first 3 to 8 weeks.

MANAGEMENT. Streptococcal infection should be treated with antimicrobial drugs. Whether antibiotic treatment prevents the development of acute glomerulonephritis in patients who are already infected with nephritogenic streptococci is controversial. Once glomerulonephritis develops, no treatment modality changes the clinical course. There is no evidence that steroids, cytotoxic agents, or anticoagulants are of benefit, and their use is not recommended. Complications such as circulatory congestion, hypertension, and metabolic abnormalities should be prevented or treated promptly with appropriate diet, fluid and sodium restriction, diuretics, antihypertensives, and dialysis as indicated.

Rapidly progressive glomerulonephritis

Rapidly progressive glomerulonephritis is a clinicopathologic syndrome characterized by rapid deterioration of renal function leading quickly to uremia and by proliferation of extracapillary cells of Bowman's capsule (crescents). The cause may be unknown (idiopathic), or the disorder may be associated with other diseases, for example, poststreptococcal glomerulonephritis, hypersensitivity angiitis, Goodpasture's syndrome, Wegener's granulomatosis, systemic lupus erythematosus, Schönlein-Henoch purpura, hemolytic-uremic syndrome, thrombotic thrombocytopenic purpura, mixed cryoglobulinemia, and membranoproliferative glomerulonephritis.

PATHOGENESIS AND PATHOLOGY. The most striking findings are the proliferation of extracapillary cells and the formation of crescents in more than 60% of the glomeruli. Necrosis, neutrophilic infiltration, and fibrin deposition are present to a variable degree. Gross examination reveals a large, pale kidney with petechiae on the surface. The pathogenesis of idiopathic, rapidly proliferative glomerulonephritis may be (1) *anti–glomerular basement membrane* (anti-GBM) *disease,* in which linear deposits of immunoglobulins in an uninterrupted continuous pattern along the glomerular basement membrane and circulating anti-GBM antibodies are found in the serum; (2) *immune-complex disease,* in which immunoglobulin and complement are deposited in a granular pattern along the glomerular capillaries or in the mesangium; or (3) *nonimmune disease,* in which no deposits of immunoglobulins or complement are seen.

CLINICAL MANIFESTATIONS. The onset may be abrupt or insidious. A patient may have nonspecific constitutional complaints. At the time of the initial examination, oliguria or anuria commonly is present. Proteinuria, hematuria, and red blood cell casts, indicating glomerular damage, are almost always found. The blood urea nitrogen and creatinine values are elevated. Hypertension and edema sometimes may be present. In many cases no predisposing cause is obvious.

MANAGEMENT. In 90% of patients with rapidly progressive glomerulonephritis, end-stage renal failure develops within a short time. No treatment has been proved to be consistently effective. Steroids, immunosuppressive drugs, anticoagulants, and antiplatelet drugs alone and in various combinations have been tried. Recently large doses of steroids (prednisone, 30 mg/kg) given intravenously as a pulse therapy in varying regimens have been shown to be beneficial in more than 70% of cases of rapidly progressive glomerulonephritis not induced by anti-GBM antibodies. Plasmapheresis to reduce the circulating levels of anti-GBM antibodies, in combination with steroids and immunosuppressive drugs, has been found effective in reducing mortality and long-term morbidity. Even though recurrence of glomerulonephritis induced by anti-GBM antibodies is common in transplanted kidneys, patients do well for extended periods. Therefore transplantation of the kidney is not contraindicated.

Goodpasture's syndrome

The syndrome of pulmonary hemorrhage associated with glomerulonephritis is called Goodpasture's syndrome. This clinical picture is nonspecific and can be seen in other diseases (Wegener's granulomatosis, systemic lupus erythematosus, mixed cryoglobulinemia, and necrotizing vasculitis).

Renal biopsy reveals focal glomerulonephritis early in the disease, but with progression of lesions, crescent formation is seen in most of the glomeruli. Linear deposits of immunoglobulin along the glomerular basement membrane characteristically are found on immunofluorescence studies.

Goodpasture's syndrome usually is seen in young men. Associations with influenza and with exposure to volatile hydrocarbons have been reported in a few cases. Hemoptysis usually precedes the apparent onset of glomerulonephritis. Iron deficiency anemia develops, and the sputum contains hemosiderin-laden macrophages. Urinalysis reveals erythrocytes, casts, and proteinuria. Renal failure develops rapidly. Anti-GBM antibodies are present in the circulation. The most common course is that of waxing and waning pulmonary hemorrhages and development of progressive, often irreversible, renal failure. The treatment is similar to that of rapidly progressive glomerulonephritis (discussed in the preceding section). Bilateral nephrectomy and maintenance dialysis have been recommended to prevent possibly fatal pulmonary hemorrhage. Success with plasmapheresis appears to make this obsolete.

Focal glomerulonephritis

Focal glomerulonephritis includes several conditions in which some of the glomeruli are affected whereas others remain normal. Various syndromes in which focal glomerulonephritis is seen are recurrent or persistent hematuria, benign hematuria with focal glomerulonephritis, IgA nephropathy (Berger's disease), and hereditary nephritis. This lesion also occurs in some systemic diseases such as subacute bacterial endocarditis, Schönlein-Henoch purpura, systemic lupus erythematosus, and hypersensitivity angiitis.

The clinical features of the various syndromes of undetermined cause are similar, and they may have the same pathogenesis. Patients usually have recurrent or persistent hematuria and mild proteinuria. Hypertension, the nephrotic syndrome, and renal failure are uncommon, and the prognosis generally is good.

MESANGIAL PROLIFERATIVE GLOMERULONEPHRITIS. Renal biopsy in this subgroup shows proliferation of mesangial cells and an increase in mesangial matrix. Hematuria, along with proteinuria and nephrotic syndrome, are common clinical presentations. Besides individuals with an idiopathic type of the disease, some patients with resolving poststreptococcal glomerulonephritis, systemic lupus erythematosus, Schönlein-Henoch purpura, and other disorders may have similar histologic changes. The prognosis is good for those in the idiopathic group. Only patients with symptomatic nephrotic syndrome require therapy with prednisone. Cyclophosphamide can be used in patients resistant to prednisone. Very few patients develop advanced renal failure.

IgA NEPHROPATHY (BERGER'S DISEASE). The most clearly defined syndrome associated with focal nephritis is IgA nephropathy, or Berger's disease, which is characterized by deposits of IgA in the mesangial area of the glomeruli. IgG

and complement also are present but stain less intensely on immunofluorescence. Light microscopy shows a variable histologic picture, but segmental or diffuse proliferative changes may be seen. IgA nephropathy also is seen in association with gluten enteropathy, dermatitis herpetiformis, Crohn's disease, mucin-secreting adenocarcinoma, and cirrhosis.

Idiopathic disease is more common in boys and young men. Most patients have either episodes of gross hematuria, frequently preceded by an acute respiratory illness, or persistent microscopic hematuria. Heavy proteinuria occasionally has been noted, and renal failure may develop in as many as 20% of the cases. The response to corticosteroid treatment varies. IgA nephropathy commonly recurs in patients requiring renal transplantation.

Hereditary nephritis (Alport's syndrome)

Hereditary nephritis, or Alport's syndrome, consists of nephritis and nerve deafness. The mode of inheritance seems to be autosomally dominant with variable penetrance. Males are more severely affected, and the disease more often is transmitted through an afflicted female.

Histologic findings of mixed glomerular and tubulointerstitial diseases usually are present. The glomeruli may show segmental hypercellularity, sclerosis, and at times crescent formation. Foam cells in the interstitium and tubular dilation and atrophy commonly are found. The electron microscopic finding of longitudinal splitting and lamellation of the glomerular capillary basement membrane ("basket-weave pattern") is characteristic of hereditary nephritis.

The disease may be clinically latent for years, although laboratory abnormalities are present. A defect in hearing, which may be unilateral nerve deafness, is present in one third of the patients. Ocular abnormalities such as cataracts, keratoconus, myopia, and nystagmus also may be present in some cases.

Hematuria is the most common renal manifestation of the disease. Proteinuria is mild or absent in the early stages, but in the advanced stage heavy proteinuria may be present. Renal failure, often accompanied by hypertension, develops in the late second or third decade of life. The patients are treated with dialysis or transplantation or both.

NEPHROTIC SYNDROME

Nephrotic syndrome is characterized by heavy proteinuria (more than 3.5 g protein/1.73 m² body surface area/day) and usually is associated with hypoalbuminemia, hyperlipidemia, and edema. Lipiduria is a constant finding and can be demonstrated by light microscopy as oval fat bodies and fatty casts or as "Maltese crosses" under polarizing light. Abnormal tubular functions such as aminoaciduria and glycosuria also are noted in some patients. The following outline includes some of the conditions associated with nephrotic syndrome:

Causes and conditions associated with nephrotic syndrome

I. Primary glomerular diseases (idiopathic)
    A. Lipoid nephrosis
    B. Membranous nephropathy
    C. Membranoproliferative glomerulonephritis
    D. Proliferative glomerulonephritis
    E. Focal glomerular sclerosis
II. Allergens
    A. Bee sting
    B. Pollen
    C. Poison oak
    D. Poison ivy
    E. Insect repellent
III. Drugs

   A. Penicillamine
   B. Bismuth
   C. Gold
   D. Probenecid
   E. Trimethadione
   F. Captopril
   G. Heroin
   H. Nonsteroidal antiinflammatory drugs
 IV. Collagen-vascular diseases
   A. Systemic lupus erythematosus
   B. Polyarteritis nodosa
  V. Metabolic diseases
   A. Diabetes mellitus
   B. Amyloidosis
   C. Multiple myeloma
 VI. Infectious diseases
   A. Quartan malaria (*Plasmodium malariae*)
   B. Bacterial endocarditis
   C. Schistosomiasis
   D. Secondary syphilis
VII. Neoplastic diseases
   A. Bronchogenic carcinoma
   B. Hodgkin's disease
   C. Colonic carcinoma
VIII. Vascular diseases
   A. Constrictive pericarditis
   B. Renal vein thrombosis
   C. Inferior vena cava obstruction
 IX. Congenital nephrotic syndrome
  X. Heredofamilial nephrotic syndrome
 XI. Pregnancy

More than 70% of cases of nephrotic syndrome in Western countries are related to primary glomerular diseases. In the remaining cases the most common causes of nephrotic syndrome are diabetes, amyloidosis, multiple myeloma, and collagen-vascular diseases. The clinical course, prognosis, and response to treatment in patients with nephrotic syndrome correlate with the underlying disease.

PATHOGENESIS OF PROTEINURIA AND EDEMA. Increased glomerular basement membrane permeability caused by an immunologic, inflammatory, or metabolic abnormality results in proteinuria. Usually proteins of low molecular weight, such as albumin and α-globulin, are excreted in excessive amounts, whereas the higher-molecular-weight proteins are retained in the blood. When albumin synthesis cannot keep pace with excretion and the catabolic process, hypoalbuminemia develops. The plasma oncotic pressure falls, and in accordance with Starling's law, fluid shifts to the interstitial space from the intravascular compartment. A decrease in intravascular volume reduces the effective renal blood flow, decreases the glomerular filtration rate, and stimulates production of aldosterone (secondary to renin-angiotensin) and antidiuretic hormone. All these hemodynamic and endocrine changes cause excessive retention of sodium and water and edema formation.

CLINICAL MANIFESTATIONS. Except for cases in which heavy proteinuria is detected during routine urinalysis, most patients with nephrotic syndrome initially show edema in the lower extremities, followed by anasarca. Later, fluid accumulates in the serosal (peritoneal, pleural, and pericardial) cavities.

When the protein loss is massive, patients may show manifestations of malnutrition. Transverse white bands appear on the nails as the result of hypoalbuminemia. Unless accompanied by severe renal failure, anemia is uncommon. However, the patient appears pale. Hypertension develops in some patients. The incidence of myocardial infarction, atherosclerotic heart disease, renal vein thrombosis, and other thromboembolic complications is high. A transient deterioration of renal function, as evidenced by elevation of blood urea nitrogen and creatinine values and orthostatic hypotension, may occur as a result of overtreatment with diuretics and strict sodium restriction. These patients also are more susceptible to bacterial infections.

LABORATORY FINDINGS. Examination of the urine shows heavy proteinuria and lipiduria. In the blood the typical findings are hypoalbuminemia and hyperlipidemia. The pathogenesis of hyperlipidemia is unclear but may be related to increased synthesis of lipoproteins. Characteristically, patients with nephrotic syndrome also have decreased α_1-globulin levels and increased α_2- and β-globulin levels. Increased concentrations of fibrinogen, fibrinolytic inhibitors, and factors V, VII, VIII, and X have been observed. The serum T_4 level may be low, but the patients are clinically euthyroid. Hypomagnesemia also has been reported.

MANAGEMENT. All attempts should be made to diagnose the cause of nephrotic syndrome, and therapy should be guided accordingly (see the following and Chapter 106). A diet rich in protein (2 to 3 g protein/kg body weight/day) is recommended, since edema is a direct consequence of hypoalbuminemia. Supplementary vitamins also are suggested because vitamins may be lost with the proteinuria. Salt intake should be somewhat restricted, but with the availability of modern diuretics severe restriction is not necessary. Mild edema does not necessitate diuretic therapy, but patients with marked fluid retention are treated with the thiazide group of diuretics, and in resistant cases loop diuretics may be used. Because some bacterial infections in these patients may be caused by a loss of immunoglobulins in the urine, appropriate antibiotics should be started promptly to prevent overwhelming infection. The beneficial effects of pneumococcal polysaccharide vaccination in patients with nephrotic syndrome are being investigated. Attempts to decrease massive proteinuria with iatrogenic embolization through the renal arteries, surgical nephrectomy, and administration of indomethacin should be discouraged, because they may be harmful.

Primary glomerular diseases resulting in the nephrotic syndrome

LIPOID NEPHROSIS. Lipoid nephrosis, also called minimal lesion disease or nil disease, is characterized by the absence of significant glomerular abnormalities on light microscopy. Glomerular abnormalities can be seen only with the electron microscope. Fusion of the foot processes of the epithelial cells is consistently present. The basement membrane itself shows no abnormality. No immunologic abnormality in the blood or renal tissue has been demonstrated. The cause is unknown, but some patients have a history of exposure to an allergen. There is an increased incidence of this lesion in patients with Hodgkin's disease.

In the age-group of 1 to 5 years 95% of patients with nephrotic syndrome have lipoid nephrosis, whereas only 20% of nephrotic adults have it. The disease is characterized by an insidious onset of edema. The renal function remains stable for several years. Persistent hematuria and hypertension are absent. The prognosis is good; spontaneous remission occurs in 60% of the cases, and 90% show remission with corticosteroids. Initially prednisone (1 mg/kg body weight/day) is recommended. The daily dosage is reduced to 15 to 20 mg after remission occurs. The complications associated with steroids may be minimized by alternate-day prednisone therapy. Cyclophosphamide is used for patients with frequent relapses or those requiring high doses of prednisone.

MEMBRANOUS NEPHROPATHY. Membranous nephropathy is characterized by diffuse thickening of the basement membrane of the glomerular capillary walls without cellular proliferation. Early in the disease the basement membrane may not show much change on routine light microscopy. However, spikelike projections of the epithelial surface of the basement membrane may be demonstrated with silver methenamine staining, and electron microscopy reveals subepithelial deposits of electron-dense material. In the advanced stages diffuse thickening of the basement membrane becomes apparent on light microscopy. Immunofluorescence studies reveal deposits of immune complexes containing IgG and complement in a granular pattern in capillary walls. These morphologic lesions also have been seen in patients with systemic lupus erythematosus, carcinoma, sarcoidosis, renal vein thrombosis, diabetes mellitus, hepatitis B antigenemia, secondary syphilis, and schistosomiasis. Certain toxic drugs such as mercury (organic and inorganic), gold, penicillamine, and trimethadione also can cause nephrotic syndrome with similar histologic findings. However, in idiopathic membranous nephropathy no specific antigen has been demonstrated.

Idiopathic membranous nephropathy is a disease of adults and is rare in children. It is insidious at onset, and the clinical course varies. About 20% to 25% of the patients show spontaneous remission. Of the remaining patients some have rapid deterioration of renal function, leading to end-stage renal disease within 3 to 5 years. In others the course is indolent, and renal function declines slowly. Hypertension may be present, and in some cases microscopic hematuria also has been noted. Interestingly, renal vein thrombosis frequently occurs in these patients and seems to be the result rather than the cause of the disease.

Steroid therapy has been tried, but no consistent beneficial effect has been seen. In a recent study initiating steroid treatment early prevented a decrease in glomerular filtration in patients with membranous nephropathy and a normal glomerular filtration rate. Alkylating agents are not effective.

MEMBRANOPROLIFERATIVE GLOMERULONEPHRITIS. At least two and perhaps three subgroups make up the disorder called membranoproliferative glomerulonephritis or mesangiocapillary glomerulonephritis. The glomeruli usually are enlarged, and marked accentuation of the lobular pattern usually is visible. The characteristic findings are hypercellularity of the mesangial or centrilobular area with subendothelial extension of mesangial cells and matrix into the periphery of capillary walls, giving an appearance of duplicated basement membranes. In type I, a close relationship is found between membranoproliferative glomerulonephritis and classic lobular glomerulonephritis. Finely granular subendothelial and mesangial deposits commonly are demonstrable on electron microscopy. Immunofluorescence staining shows C3 and IgG along capillary walls. Complement is activated through the classic pathway. Type II shows dense intramembranous deposits giving an appearance of ribbonlike thickening of the basement membrane. On immunofluorescence these deposits stain only for complement. This disease usually occurs in adolescents or young adults. Onset of hematuria associated with proteinuria may be acute, but more commonly the onset is insidious. The disease also may be manifested by asymptomatic proteinuria and mild or no edema. In many cases hypertension develops. Partial lipodystrophy in women sometimes is associated with the type II lesion. The characteristic feature of this disease is persistent hypocomplementemia, which is more commonly seen with the type II lesion. The serum of these patients

contains a factor (C3 NeF) that can activate the alternate pathway of complement at the C3 step. Complement factors preceding C3 in the complement activation cascade may be normal while the level of C3 is low. The disease has a high incidence of recurrence in transplanted kidneys. Corticosteroid and antiplatelet agents seem to have a beneficial effect in type I cases.

PROLIFERATIVE GLOMERULONEPHRITIS. Proliferative glomerulonephritis is a heterogeneous group of diseases causing nephrotic syndrome. There is a definite increase in glomerular cellularity. The classic picture is seen in poststreptococcal acute glomerulonephritis (described previously). In some of these patients nephrotic syndrome follows an acute attack of glomerulonephritis. Generally the prognosis is good, and renal function returns to normal. Remission of nephrotic syndrome can occur as long as 12 to 18 months after onset. Proliferative glomerulonephritis with marked glomerular damage usually is associated with a poor prognosis. A good prognosis has been documented in patients with mild mesangial proliferative glomerulonephritis. These patients also show improvement with steroid treatment.

FOCAL GLOMERULOSCLEROSIS. The characteristic lesion in focal glomerulosclerosis is segmental sclerosis and hyalinization of some glomeruli, especially those in the deeper cortex. Usually only part of the capillary tuft is involved, but occasionally the affected glomeruli may be totally hyalinized. The capillary lumina are obliterated, and the involved capillary tuft shows adhesion to the adjacent Bowman's capsule. Tubular atrophy and interstitial fibrosis often are present. Electron microscopic examination may reveal various combinations of paramesangial, subendothelial, and intramembranous electron-dense deposits. No specific findings are consistently reported on immunofluorescence. The presence of fibrin or fibrinogen has been described in one third of the cases. Focal and segmental hyalinosis is not a specific disease entity. Similar histopathologic changes are seen in Alport's syndrome, hypertension, reflux nephropathy, analgesic abuse nephropathy, heroin abuse nephropathy, and persistent idiopathic proteinuria. However, when seen in nephrotic patients, hyalinosis is a significant finding. Focal and segmental hyalinosis should not be confused with focal and segmental glomerulonephritis in which proliferation of the cells and not hyalinization of the capillary tuft is the diagnostic finding.

Focal glomerulosclerosis most commonly affects children, but this lesion is also seen in adults and now is one of the most frequently observed lesions in biopsy specimens of adults. Onset is insidious. The disease is characterized by edema and heavy proteinuria. Microscopic hematuria is common. Hypertension and decreased renal function may be found when focal glomerulosclerosis is detected. In drug addicts with nephrotic syndrome focal glomerulosclerosis usually is the main histologic finding.

The prognosis is poor, and renal function deteriorates rapidly. Patients with total hyalinization of the glomeruli have a better prognosis than those with segmental sclerosis. The response to corticosteroids is better in children than in adults.

CHRONIC GLOMERULONEPHRITIS. Chronic glomerulonephritis is the final outcome of several different types of renal disease. Histologically, the most striking feature is hyalinization of most of the glomeruli. Undamaged glomeruli show a proliferation of cells. The capillary walls usually are thickened. In moderate chronic proliferative glomerulonephritis, tubular atrophy and interstitial scarring may not be extensive. There often is no history of renal disease, infection, or any systemic disease. Frequently the disease is manifested by the nephrotic syndrome and symptoms and signs of renal failure. The prognosis and response to treatment are poor.

BIBLIOGRAPHY

Bacani RA and others: Rapidly progressive (nonstreptococcal) glomerulonephritis, Ann Intern Med 69:463, 1968.

Baldwin DS and Schacht RG: Late sequelae of poststreptococcal glomerulonephritis, Annu Rev Med 27:49, 1976.

Cameron JS and others: The nephrotic syndrome in adults with "minimal change" glomerular lesion, Q J Med 43:461, 1974.

Coggins CH: An interhospital study of the adult idiopathic nephrotic syndrome and its response to treatment, Kidney Int 8:408, 1975.

Donado JV Jr and others: Idiopathic membranoproliferative (mesangiocapillary) glomerulonephritis: a clinicopathologic study, Mayo Clin Proc 54:141, 1979.

Glassock RJ: Clinical aspects of acute, rapidly progressive and chronic glomerulonephritis. In Earley LE and Gottschalk CW, editors: Strauss and Welt's diseases of the kidney, ed 3, Boston, 1979, Little, Brown & Co.

Gluck MC and others: Membranous glomerulonephritis: evolution of clinical and pathologic features, Ann Intern Med 78:1, 1973.

Gutman RA and others: The immune complex glomerulonephritis of bacterial endocarditis, Medicine 51:1, 1972.

Habib R: Focal glomerular sclerosis (editorial), Kidney Int 4:355, 1973.

Hayslett JP and others: Clinicopathological correlations in the nephrotic syndrome due to primary renal disease, Medicine 52:93, 1973.

McKenzie PE and others: Plasmapheresis in glomerulonephritis, Clin Nephrol 12:97, 1979.

Merrill JP: Glomerulonephritis, N Engl J Med 290:257, 1974.

Nissenson AR and others: Poststreptococcal acute glomerulonephritis: fact and controversy, Ann Intern Med 91:76, 1979.

Pierides AM and others: Idiopathic membranous nephropathy, Q J Med 182:163, 1977.

Sherman RL, Churg J, and Yudis M: Hereditary nephritis with a characteristic renal lesion, Am J Med 56:44, 1974.

Wilson CB and Dixon FJ: Antiglomerular basement membrane antibody induced glomerulonephritis, Kidney Int 3:74, 1973.

Wilson CB and Dixon FJ: Immunopathology and glomerulonephritis, Annu Rev Med 25:83, 1974.

Zimmerman SW and Burkholder PM: Immunoglobulin A nephropathy, Arch Intern Med 135:1217, 1974.

106 · RENAL LESIONS IN SYSTEMIC DISEASE

Brajesh Agarwal and **Pasha Agarwal**

COLLAGEN-VASCULAR DISEASES
Systemic lupus erythematosus

(See Chapter 16.)

Renal involvement is seen clinically in two thirds of the cases of systemic lupus erythematosus. In many patients the kidney is the initial organ involved. Although lupus nephritis commonly is accompanied by other systemic findings, it may be the sole manifestation during the entire course of the disease.

PATHOLOGY. Although the pathologic changes are present primarily in the glomeruli, occasionally only interstitial nephritis is present. Renal involvement may occur in the absence of abnormalities in urinalysis or renal function. Active disease is associated with glomerular hypercellularity, fibrinoid necrosis, cellular crescents, hyaline thrombi, and vasculitis. Chronic changes include tubular atrophy, fibrous crescents, interstitial fibrosis, and glomerular sclerosis. Prognosis and therapy are determined by the presence of these active or chronic lesions.

Regardless of clinical manifestations, most patients with lupus have deposits with complement and immunoglobulins. The World Health Organization (WHO) system frequently is used to classify renal biopsy specimens in patients with lupus. The five WHO classes are class I, a totally normal biopsy; class II, minimal lesions with some increase in mesangial structure; class III, focal and segmental proliferative glomerulonephritis; class IV, diffuse proliferative glomerulonephritis; and class V, membranous glomerulonephritis. Typical "wire looping" (a rigid-appearing eosinophilic glomerular capillary wall) is seen in association with proliferative lesions. Focal, segmental, or global sclerosis may be seen with classes IV or V. Interstitial nephritis also may be seen in classes II through V. Complexes initially are deposited in the mesangium and later extend to the subendothelial areas of the glomerular capillary walls. In the membranous form, immune complexes are deposited in the subepithelial aspect of the basement membrane. The clinical course of the disease seems to correlate with the histologic findings and with the amount and site of immune-complex deposition.

CLINICAL MANIFESTATIONS. The clinical presentation and course of the disease vary from mild asymptomatic urinary abnormalities to nephritic syndrome and rapidly progressive glomerulonephritis. Nephrotic syndrome or renal failure rarely develops in patients with minimal histologic changes, therefore these patients have a better prognosis. Patients with diffuse proliferative changes and subendothelial deposits have a worse prognosis. They usually have proteinuria and hematuria, and renal failure develops rapidly. Patients with membranous lupus nephritis often show the clinical symptoms of nephrotic syndrome. Renal function deteriorates slowly. Various immunologic abnormalities such as a low serum complement concentration and the presence of antinuclear antibodies, anti-DNA antibodies, circulating immune complexes, cryoglobulins, and rheumatoid factors can be detected in the serum.

MANAGEMENT. Treatment regimens for lupus nephritis vary, and results are controversial. Extrarenal manifestations of the disease must be considered in planning reasonable treatment. Since renal histology cannot be accurately correlated with urinary sediment and protein excretion and serologic abnormalities, a renal biopsy often is performed.

Patients with minimal histologic lesions can be treated with small oral doses of steroids (prednisone, 0.5 mg/kg/day). The serious morbidity and increased mortality associated with high doses of prednisone or cytotoxic drugs must be weighed against the inherent risk of the lesion. If there is no improvement or if toxicity develops, the steroid dosage should be tapered. The patient should be observed for signs of progression of the lesion to the diffuse form.

Suggestions for managing membranous lupus nephritis with nephrotic syndrome vary from no therapy to a 6-week trial of prednisone (1 mg/kg/day), followed by a lower dose or alternate-day therapy if remission is induced.

There is uniform agreement that diffuse proliferative glomerular lesions with proteinuria or azotemia should be treated aggressively, but therapeutic approaches vary. Regimens consisting of oral cyclophosphamide (2 to 2.5 mg/kg/day) and high doses of prednisone (1 mg/kg/day) alone or in combination have been advocated. Short-term intravenous steroid regimens (methylprednisolone, 1 g/day for 3 days) followed by low-dose steroids also are used. Pulse cyclophosphamide therapy in dosages up to 1 g/m² intravenously every 3 months with low-dose prednisone was found to be most effective and least toxic in one study. Chronic fibrotic renal damage recently was shown to be prevented by combinations of prednisone with azathioprine plus cyclophosphamide, or prednisone with intermittent intravenous cyclophosphamide. Plasmapheresis does not change the survival rate for lupus nephritis patients.

Scleroderma

(See Chapter 17.)

PATHOLOGY. Renal involvement in scleroderma (progressive systemic sclerosis) is not uncommon and adversely affects the prognosis. Pathologic changes such as concentric intimal proliferation and deposition of mucoid material are seen mainly in the arcuate and interlobular arteries. The vessel lumen may be partly or totally occluded. The arterioles show fibrinoid necrosis, and the glomeruli often are ischemic. Patchy bilateral renal cortical necrosis is found in patients with oliguric renal failure. Immunofluorescence studies show fibrinogen in the damaged vessels and glomeruli.

CLINICAL MANIFESTATIONS. Mild proteinuria, often intermittent, is the most common renal manifestation. Patients may have an abrupt onset of malignant hypertension, and renal failure rapidly develops. Some patients have normotensive oliguric renal failure. Azotemia with or without hypertension indicates a poor prognosis.

MANAGEMENT. No definite improvement in scleroderma has been seen with any specific therapy. Patients with hypertension and renal failure should be treated vigorously with antihypertensive medications and dialysis. With the use of antirenin drugs (propranolol and captopril) and vasodilators (minoxidil) in patients with severe hypertension, improvement in renal function has been documented. Bilateral nephrectomy and maintenance dialysis are recommended for patients with uncontrolled hypertension and irreversible renal failure. Transplantation has been performed successfully in a few patients.

Polyarteritis nodosa

(See Chapter 20.)

PATHOLOGY. Renal pathologic changes are very common in polyarteritis nodosa. Arteritis and obliteration of the vessel lumen with aneurysm formation may occur. In the classic form of polyarteritis, the medium-sized vessels are involved and renal cortical infarcts are common. Amphetamine abuse and chronic viral hepatitis may be associated with this lesion. Small vessels are diseased in the microscopic form of *hypersensitivity angiitis*. Diffuse or focal glomerulitis may be seen, with fibrinoid necrosis and microthrombus formation in glomerular capillaries. Crescent formation may occur, especially when small vessels are involved. Interstitial infiltrates of inflammatory cells and tubular atrophy may be present.

CLINICAL MANIFESTATIONS. Renal manifestations of polyarteritis usually are seen in association with symptoms and signs of other systemic involvement. The patients may have gross hematuria, and the clinical picture may resemble that of acute glomerulonephritis. There is a urine sediment containing erythrocytes, erythrocytic casts, fat cells, fatty casts, broad casts, granular casts, and waxy casts; this is referred to as a "telescoped" sediment. Hypertension and rapid deterioration of renal function are common.

MANAGEMENT. In most cases renal lesions contribute in some way to the patient's death. High doses of corticosteroids (prednisone, 1 mg/kg/day) are recommended. Azathioprine or cyclophosphamide is used in severe systemic necrotizing vasculitis, along with corticosteroid treatment.

Wegener's granulomatosis

(See Chapter 22.)

Wegener's granulomatosis is characterized by a necrotizing granulomatous vasculitis that may involve the nasopharynx, paranasal sinuses, lungs, ears, eye, heart, nervous system, skin, and joints. In the generalized form renal involvement is common and can be fatal.

PATHOLOGY. The classic renal lesion is a focal and segmental glomerulonephritis with proliferative changes and fibrinoid necrosis. In severe cases diffuse changes and crescent formation occur. In some cases localized subepithelial deposits of dense material are seen on electron microscopy. Immunofluorescence studies show staining for IgG and complement along the basement membrane.

CLINICAL MANIFESTATIONS. The presentation and urinary findings (proteinuria, erythrocytes, and erythrocyte casts) are typical of acute glomerulonephritis. Sinusitis, hemoptysis, and pulmonary infiltrates often are present. Renal function can deteriorate rapidly.

MANAGEMENT. Early diagnosis, frequently by biopsy, is important because Wegener's granulomatosis is a fatal disease if not treated promptly. Long-lasting remissions have been induced with cyclophosphamide (1 to 2 mg/kg/day).

Schönlein-Henoch purpura

(See Chapter 21.)

With Schönlein-Henoch purpura (anaphylactoid purpura), renal damage is more common in children than in adults. Other manifestations of this syndrome (arthritis, rash, and gastrointestinal hemorrhage) also are present in most cases.

PATHOLOGY. Focal and segmental proliferation occurs with fibrinoid necrosis of the glomerular capillary tuft and intracapillary deposition of fibrin. In severe cases crescent formation may occur. Immunofluorescence studies commonly show granular staining of the mesangium for fibrinogen, IgA, IgG, and C3, suggesting that the pathogenesis of renal damage is associated with deposition of immune complexes in the glomeruli. Serum complement and immunoglobulin levels usually are normal, however.

CLINICAL MANIFESTATIONS. Patients may remain asymptomatic or have hematuria, proteinuria, or renal failure. The clinical course usually is benign with spontaneous remission. However, in some patients with crescentic glomerular changes, advanced renal failure necessitating dialysis may develop.

MANAGEMENT. Besides symptomatic treatment, corticosteroids may be given to treat the extrarenal manifestations of Schönlein-Henoch purpura (see Chapter 21). In patients with progressive renal failure a trial of azathioprine or mercaptopurine may be used.

Hemolytic-uremic syndrome and thrombotic thrombocytopenic purpura

The hemolytic-uremic syndrome occurs most frequently in children, whereas thrombotic thrombocytopenic purpura is more common in adults. Both disorders are characterized by microangiopathic hemolytic anemia and thrombocytopenia. Platelet thrombi are seen in small arteries and capillaries throughout the body. In thrombotic thrombocytopenic purpura, pulmonary and cerebral manifestations may be significant and more marked than the renal involvement. In the hemolytic-uremic syndrome, disseminated intravascular coagulation occurs and renal involvement is severe. Local deposition of fibrin and platelets in the subendothelial space may result in focal or generalized renal cortical necrosis. The syndrome is characterized by oliguria or anuria, proteinuria, hematuria, and impaired renal function. The prognosis is poor, and the patients usually die of renal failure. The response to treatment with steroids and immunosuppressive drugs is inconsistent. Recently good results have been reported with exchange transfusion and plasmapheresis. Prompt diagnosis and early treatment improve the prognosis. Use of several antiplatelet drugs and vincristine also is recommended.

METABOLIC AND OTHER SYSTEMIC DISEASES
Diabetes mellitus

PATHOLOGY. The common renal lesions in diabetes mellitus are diffuse and nodular intracapillary glomerulosclerosis. Vascular lesions in the form of arteriosclerosis involving vessels of all sizes and hyaline thickening of arterioles, especially the efferent aterioles, are frequent findings. Interstitial fibrosis, glycogen deposition in renal tubules, pyelonephritis, and papillary necrosis also are seen.

CLINICAL MANIFESTATIONS. Microalbuminuria usually is the first manifestation of diabetic nephropathy. This occurs in the face of a normal filtration rate. Clinically evident renal disease (decreased filtration rate, proteinuria, and nephrotic syndrome) appears after 15 to 20 years of diabetes. Initially the kidney size and glomerular filtration rate may be above normal. It is the hyperfiltration that is thought to produce renal damage. As the disease progresses, hypertension and edema develop and the glomerular filtration rate drops. Hematuria is uncommon. In most cases other evidence of diabetic microangiopathy, particularly diabetic retinopathy, also is present.

Patients with acute papillary necrosis and pyelonephritis may have chills, fever, flank pain, oliguria or anuria, and rapid deterioration of renal function. Acute renal failure also may develop in diabetic patients following use of radiopaque contrast media.

MANAGEMENT. Diabetic nephropathy may be delayed by early euglycemia and maintenance of normal blood pressure in insulin-dependent patients. Experimental trials using angiotensin-converting enzyme inhibitors to prevent intraglomerular hyperfiltration are in progress. Diabetic patients maintained with hemodialysis have a poorer prognosis than hemodialysis patients who are not diabetic. The former frequently have problems with vascular access and have higher morbidity and mortality because of vascular complications. Blindness and loss of extremities commonly occur. Encouraging results with renal transplantation, especially if performed at an early stage, have been demonstrated in some centers. Long-term peritoneal dialysis may be the therapy of choice, particularly if vascular access is a problem.

Renal amyloidosis

(See Chapter 76.)

Accumulation of amyloid in the kidney occurs frequently in primary or secondary amyloidosis. This is most marked in the glomeruli but also may occur in the peritubular basement membrane, interstitium, and blood vessels. Characteristic amyloid fibrils can be seen by electron microscopy, or affected tissues can be stained with Congo red to demonstrate green birefringence under polarized light.

Proteinuria is the main manifestation of renal amyloidosis. Clinically, the patient may have nephrotic syndrome or renal insufficiency. Renal tubular disorders such as Fanconi's syndrome or distal renal tubular acidosis also may be present and may be associated with Bence Jones proteinuria. Hypertension, although uncommon, may occur. The kidney size may remain normal despite advanced renal failure. Death from renal causes is not uncommon. There is no effective therapy directed specifically at preventing or reducing amyloidosis. Cases associated with multiple myeloma show remission with alkylating agents, and those following chronic infection may resolve with cure of the infection. Inhibition of amyloid deposits is seen with colchicine therapy. Patients with advanced renal failure are treated with dialysis or transplantation or both. However, the disease commonly recurs in transplanted kidneys.

Multiple myeloma

(See Chapter 76.)

The kidneys frequently are affected in multiple myeloma. Many factors may contribute to renal injury, including hyperuricemia, hypercalcemia, plasma hyperviscosity, interstitial infiltration of plasma cells, pyelonephritis, urinary tract obstruction, and amyloidosis. Renal insufficiency progresses slowly over several months. Bence Jones proteins (light chains) may have a direct toxic effect on the renal tubules and may result in tubular atrophy and dysfunction. Large eosinophilic casts commonly are seen in tubular lumina. Glomerular changes are minimal. Isolated tubular defects without a reduction of glomerular filtration, such as Fanconi's syndrome, distal renal tubular acidosis, and urine-concentrating defects, are seen in association with excretion of light chains. Dehydration, use of roentgenographic contrast materials or nephrotoxic antibiotics, and hypercalcemia are some of the factors that may precipitate acute renal failure in patients with myeloma who have not previously had renal impairment. Light-chain nephropathy manifesting with heavy proteinuria and renal insufficiency is a distinct disorder and may occur in the absence of overt multiple myeloma. Light chains are deposited not only in the kidney but also in other tissues, such as the heart, liver, spleen, nerves, and gastrointestinal tract.

Symptomatic treatment (correction of volume depletion, hypercalcemia, and hyperuricemia) and avoiding the use of nephrotoxic antibiotics and roentgenographic contrast materials are recommended. Improved renal function has been noted when alkylating agents are used. Acute renal failure is treated with forced alkaline diuresis, dialysis, and chemotherapy. In patients with acute renal failure associated with an increased excretion of urinary light chains, plasmapheresis has been successful in restoring renal function. Patients with end-stage renal failure and multiple myeloma can be considered for dialysis and transplantation.

Waldenström's macroglobulinemia

(See Chapter 76.)

In contrast to multiple myeloma, in which glomerular disease is rare, Waldenström's macroglobulinemia may be manifested by large eosinophilic thrombi, nonspecific glomerulitis, or deposition of amyloid material in the glomeruli. Immunofluorescence studies and electron microscopic examination show intraluminal deposits of IgM between the endothelium and the inner aspect of the glomerular basement membrane. The tubules rarely are affected, but the interstitium may have infiltrates of lymphoid cells. Proteinuria is the most common clinical finding and may be nonselective or may have only light chains. Therapy includes the use of alkylating agents and plasmapheresis.

Essential cryoglobulinemia

Essential mixed cryoglobulinemia, usually of an IgG-IgM combination, may result in renal damage. There is glomerular proliferation with deposition of IgG and IgM. In some cases only one immunoglobulin is present. Occasionally crescent and intracapillary thrombi form. The clinical picture is that of acute glomerulonephritis, at times leading to acute renal failure. In some cases both renal lesions and symptoms disappear completely when the exacerbating condition is alleviated. In others renal failure may persist. In almost all cases renal lesions are associated with purpura. Extrarenal manifestations of mixed essential cryoglobulinemia include arthralgia, Raynaud's syndrome, extrarenal necrotizing angiitis, and peripheral neuropathy. Plasmapheresis is recommended in rapidly progressive renal failure. Adrenal corticosteroids and immunosuppressive drugs have not been found to be very effective.

Sickle cell disease

(See Chapter 67.)

Although a variety of functional abnormalities are noted in patients with sickle cell disease or uncomplicated sickle cell trait, morphologic defects are seen mainly in sickle cell disease.

PATHOLOGY. The kidneys show enlarged glomeruli with engorged capillaries filled with sickled red blood cells. In a few cases thickening of glomerular basement membrane, membranoproliferative glomerulonephritis, and segmental glomerular sclerosis also have been described. Patchy interstitial fibrosis, especially in the medulla, and papillary necrosis are common.

CLINICAL MANIFESTATIONS. Microscopic hematuria is the most common renal manifestation of both sickle cell disease and sickle cell trait. Recurrent bouts or a single episode of gross hematuria may occur, leading to severe anemia. Some patients have nephrotic syndrome. Papillary necrosis, seen in sickle cell disease, usually is insidious. Advanced renal failure is uncommon. Early in the disease the glomerular filtration rate may be supernormal. Maximal urine-concentrating ability is defective in the disease and the trait. Initially this defect can be reversed by transfusion of normal hemoglobin A, but eventually it is irreversible. The pathogenesis of the defect seems to be related to the loss of normal medullary and papillary architecture and to changes in the pattern of vasa recta caused by sickling of the cells. Impaired renal acidification of the urine and potassium excretion also have been described.

MANAGEMENT. Treatment of patients with massive hematuria has been frustrating, and no consistently successful regimen is available. A combined regimen of intravenous mannitol to promote osmotic diuresis, potent loop diuretics (furosemide or ethacrynic acid), and sodium bicarbonate to alkalinize the urine, along with infusion of hypotonic fluid, is recommended but often unsuccessful. ϵ-Aminocaproic acid has been found to be effective. In some patients the massive hematuria is caused by the association of von Willebrand's disease and sickle hemoglobin. Such patients respond to factor VIII infusion. Nephrectomy should be discouraged. Hemodialysis and transplantation have been used for terminal renal failure.

Sarcoidosis

(See Chapter 24.)

The kidneys frequently are affected in diffuse sarcoidosis. Although sarcoid granuloma formation is common, it rarely leads to severe renal failure. Impairment of renal function is correlated with the associated hypercalcemia, nephrocalcinosis, and hyperuricemia, and the therapy is directed specifically at those problems. Glomerular changes in the form of membranous glomerulopathy, focal glomerulosclerosis, and proliferative glomerulonephritis also have been reported. Patients with glomerular changes may have the nephrotic syndrome; otherwise, proteinuria usually is mild. Besides symptomatic treatment, corticosteroids are recommended.

Sjögren's syndrome

In Sjögren's syndrome chronic infiltration of lymphocytes and plasma cells in the renal interstitium results in severe tubular dysfunction. Distal renal tubular acidosis is seen with low serum bicarbonate concentration and hypokalemia; nephrogenic diabetes insipidus with polyuria and impaired renal concentrating ability; and chronic interstitial nephritis with azotemia. Vasculitis and glomerular lesions also are commonly seen. Symptomatic treatment includes replacing fluids, bicarbonate, and potassium. Corticosteroids are used in severe renal disease.

Glomerulonephritis associated with bacterial endocarditis and ventriculoatrial shunt infection

Glomerulonephritis may develop in patients with bacterial endocarditis and ventriculoatrial shunt infection. Usually this follows chronic indolent infection with organisms such as streptococci or *Staphylococcus albus*. However, development of the acute nephritic syndrome also has been seen in association with fulminant infections such as those caused by *Staphylococcus aureus*.

Kidney biopsy specimens show focal or diffuse proliferative changes in the glomeruli. In severe cases proliferation of epithelial cells (crescents) also can be seen. The development of the renal lesion appears to be related to the deposition of immune complexes rather than to bacterial embolization, since granular deposits of IgG and complement can be detected in the peripheral capillaries. Electron microscopy shows electron-dense material in the basement membrane in the subendothelial area of the capillary loops. During the acute phase rheumatoid factor, circulating immune complexes, and cryoglobulins can be detected in the serum, and serum levels of C1q, C3, and C4 are diminished. The symptoms and clinical course vary from asymptomatic hematuria and proteinuria to oliguria and advanced renal failure. The prognosis is good if the infection is promptly and successfully treated. In some patients, renal insufficiency and/or renal failure may complicate endocarditis as a result of the antibiotic therapy, which usually is prolonged. Nephrotoxic and allergic interstitial disease may be seen.

Renal disease in acquired immunodeficiency syndrome

Acute renal failure, proteinuria, and nephrotic syndrome are seen in patients with acquired immunodeficiency syndrome (AIDS). The renal lesion may be related to the disease itself, infection, various complications, or drug therapy. In one series 43% of patients had proteinuria of more than 0.5 g/day. On autopsy various glomerular lesions are found, including minimal, focal, and diffuse mesangial hyperplasia. However, the most common pathologic characteristic described is focal and segmental glomerular sclerosis. These lesions seem to be more prevalent in intravenous drug abusers than in homosexuals or other high-risk AIDS patients. In these patients the glomerular filtration rate falls rapidly, and asymptomatic proteinuria does not have any correlation with glomerular injury. Symptomatic treatment is recommended. Most patients do not survive long enough to require maintenance hemodialysis. However, dialysis therapy is not withheld from AIDS patients. Management of patients with renal failure and AIDS-related complex is individualized.

BIBLIOGRAPHY

Alleyne SAO and others: The kidney in sickle cell anemia, Kidney Int 7:371, 1975.

Aster RH: Thrombotic thrombocytopenic purpura: new clues to the etiology of an enigmatic disease, N Engl J Med 297:1400, 1977.

Baldwin DS and others: Lupus nephritis: clinical course as related to morphologic forms and their transitions, Am J Med 62:12, 1977.

Balow JE and others: Lupus nephritis, Ann Intern Med 106:79, 1987.

Berlyne GM and others: Dialysis in AIDS patients, Nephron 44:265, 1986.

Brouet J-C and others: Biologic and clinical significance of cryoglobulins: a report of 86 cases, Am J Med 57:775, 1974.

Cannon PJ: Medical management of renal scleroderma, N Engl J Med 299:886, 1978.

DeFronzo RA and others: Renal function in patients with multiple myeloma, Medicine 57:151, 1978.

Falls WF and others: Nonhypercalcemic sarcoid nephropathy, Arch Intern Med 130:285, 1972.

Fauci AS, Haynes BF, and Katz P: The spectrum of vasculitis: clinical, pathologic, immunologic, and therapeutic considerations, Ann Intern Med 89:660, 1978.

Gundersen HJ and others: Early and late changes in the diabetic kidney, Adv Nephrol 8:43, 1979.

Hecht B and others: Prognostic indices in lupus nephritis, Medicine 55:163, 1976.

Jacobs C and others: Treatment of end-stage renal failure in the insulin-dependent diabetic patient, Adv Nephrol 8:101, 1979.

Kaplan BS and Drummond KN: The hemolytic-uremic syndrome is a syndrome (editorial), N Engl J Med 298:964, 1978.

Kyle RA and Bayrd ED: Amyloidosis: a review of 236 cases, Medicine 54:29, 1975.

McCoy RC and Tisher CC: Glomerulonephritis associated with sarcoidosis, Am J Pathol 68:339, 1972.

Morel-Maroger L and Verroust P: Glomerular lesions in dysproteinemias, Kidney Int 5:249, 1974.

Pardo V and others: Glomerular lesions in acquired immunodeficiency syndrome, Ann Intern Med 101:429, 1984.

Rao TKS and others: Associated focal and segmental glomerulosclerosis in the acquired immunodeficiency syndrome, N Engl J Med 310:669, 1984.

Sebastian A and others: Renal amyloidosis, nephrotic syndrome, and impaired renal tubular absorption of bicarbonate, Ann Intern Med 69:541, 1968.

Wolff SM and others: Wegener's granulomatosis, Ann Intern Med 81:513, 1974.

Zlotnick A and Rosenmann E: Renal pathologic findings associated with monoclonal gammopathies, Arch Intern Med 135:40, 1975.

107 · INTERSTITIAL NEPHRITIS

Paul J. Kovnat

DEFINITION AND ETIOLOGY. "Interstitial nephritis" refers to a group of renal disorders characterized by functional and morphologic alterations in the renal tubules and interstitium. In this category of nephropathies the tubular and interstitial findings are increased out of proportion to the glomerular changes. Other terms for this disorder include "tubulointerstitial disorder," "interstitial nephropathy," "interstitial renal inflammation," and "tubulointerstitial disease." Many of the renal findings are nonspecific responses to noxious substances and systemic disease. In some instances specific tubular defects are present.

Until a few years ago chronic interstitial nephritis was known as chronic pyelonephritis and was thought to be caused by infection. Studies of patients with urinary tract infections, however, have led to the generally held view that urinary infections rarely if ever cause significant renal damage in adults in the absence of underlying kidney disease or urinary tract obstruc-

tion. Furthermore, most patients with interstitial nephritis and infection have the infection as a complication of their underlying disease rather than as the primary process. The infection may be the factor that causes symptoms and therefore triggers the investigation and identification of interstitial nephritis. It is estimated that most cases of chronic interstitial nephritis are preventable. Withdrawal of the inciting agent, with or without the addition of corticosteroid treatment of an acute immunologically mediated disorder, may stabilize or even reverse renal defects.

Causes of interstitial nephritis

I. Obstruction of urinary collecting system
II. Physical factors and environment
    A. Radiation nephritis
    B. Balkan nephritis—limited to Danube Valley (obscure environmental cause)
III. Metabolic causes
    A. Hypercalcemia or hypercalciuria
    B. Hypokalemia
    C. Hyperuricemia or hyperuricosuria
    D. Oxalosis or hyperoxaluria
IV. Hereditary causes
    A. Medullary cystic disease (nephronophthisis)
    B. Sponge kidney
V. Vascular causes
    A. Sickle cell disease
    B. Atheroembolic disease
    C. Nephrosclerosis
VI. Infiltrative causes
    A. Lymphoma
    B. Leukemia
    C. Myeloma
    D. Amyloidosis
VII. Immunologic and granulomatous causes
    A. Transplant rejection
    B. Systemic lupus erythematosus
    C. Sarcoidosis
    D. Sjögren's syndrome
VIII. Hypersensitivity
    A. Antibiotics
        1. Penicillins (especially methicillin)
        2. Sulfonamides
        3. Rifampin
    B. Nonsteroidal antiinflammatory agents
    C. Anticonvulsants
    D. Diuretics
    E. Cimetidine, allopurinol
IX. Toxicity
    A. Heavy metals
        1. Cadmium
        2. Copper
        3. Uranium
        4. Lead
    B. Analgesic abuse
    C. Aminoglycosides (gentamicin and tobramycin)
    D. Cyclosporine A
    E. Cis-platinum, methyl CCNU
X. Infection
    A. Tuberculosis
    B. Fungus
    C. Bacterial pyelonephritis (?)
XI. No known cause

PATHOLOGY. Interstitial nephritis is characterized by cellular infiltration, edema, and fibrosis of the potential space between nephrons, tubular dilation, and tubular cell atrophy. If edema and infiltration with polymorphonuclear cells are the major findings, the descriptive term "acute interstitial nephritis" is preferred. If tubular atrophy and fibrosis are the major findings, the disease is called "chronic interstitial nephritis." When eosinophils predominate in the interstitium, "allergic interstitial nephritis" is the preferred term. In immunologically mediated acute tubulointerstitial nephritis, the mechanisms include antitubular basement membrane antibodies, deposits of complexes around tubules, and direct T-cell-mediated damage. Papillary necrosis may occur, with sloughing of the renal papillae. Fibrosis around Bowman's capsule with secondary glomerular changes may be an attendant finding. In the patient with end-stage renal disease, the histologic findings of chronic interstitial nephritis may be similar to those of the end-stage kidney of chronic glomerular disease.

CLINICAL MANIFESTATIONS. Interstitial nephritis may come to the attention of the physician in one of several ways:

1. Patients may have known systemic disease or known exposure to a toxin, and investigation may show the findings of interstitial nephritis.
2. Patients may have urinary tract infections, and investigation may show evidence of underlying chronic interstitial nephritis as the predisposing factor.
3. Acute flank pain with fever and hematuria may signal papillary necrosis or urinary calculi as the first sign of interstitial nephritis.
4. After seeking treatment for other problems, patients may be found to have abnormal urinary findings, azotemia, or stigmata of chronic interstitial nephritis.
5. Patients may complain of polyuria or nocturia because of early loss of urine-concentrating ability.
6. Evidence for chronic interstitial nephritis may be found during investigation of family members or associates of patients with hereditary or environmental causes of kidney disease.
7. Patients may develop acute onset of fever, rash, eosinophilia, hematuria, eosinophiliuria, and mild proteinuria, developing 10 to 20 days after initiating drug therapy.
8. Unexplained acute renal failure, either oliguric or nonoliguric, may be the initial problem.

Interstitial nephritis should be considered in a patient with renal disease (elevated blood urea nitrogen and creatinine levels or abnormal findings on urinalysis) in whom characteristics of primary glomerular disease are absent. Because of its potential reversibility, interstitial nephritis must be differentiated from glomerulonephritis (Table 107-1). Tubular dysfunction may be seen as a specific defect such as salt wasting, loss of urine-concentrating ability (polyuria), or tubular acidosis.

Although tubular and interstitial abnormalities predominate, secondary changes occur in the microcirculation and glomeruli, with a resultant decline in the glomerular filtration rate.

DIAGNOSIS. Evaluation of a patient with interstitial nephritis should include a historical review for (1) exposure to radiation or heavy metal such as lead or cadmium; (2) symptoms of partial urinary obstruction or of gross hematuria, suggestive of stone disease or papillary necrosis; (3) family history of renal disease or sickle cell disease; (4) therapy with drugs such as penicillins, sulfonamides, nonsteroidal antiinflammatory drugs, rifampin, anticonvulsants, aminoglycosides, or methoxyflurane anesthetics; (5) chronic diarrheal states; or (6) analgesic abuse.

The physical examination and laboratory screening of patients with interstitial nephritis should search for evidence of systemic disease; elevated urine or serum levels of calcium, uric acid, or oxalate; hypokalemia; bacteriuria; or eosinophiliuria. Intravenous urography may be helpful in papillary necrosis or sponge kidney, but results often are not specific. Renal

Table 107-1   Comparison of glomerulonephritis and interstitial nephritis

Factor	Glomerulonephritis	Interstitial nephritis
Urinary sediment	Many cells and casts	Eosinophils, few cells and casts
Sodium excretion	Normal until late	Sodium wasting common
Hyperkalemia	Mild until oliguria	May occur early
Proteinuria	>3 g/day	<1 g/day
Type of protein	Primarily albumin	Nonselective with β-microglobulins and lysozyme
Hypertension	Usual	<50% of cases and usually mild
Acidosis	Normochloremic with increased anion gap	Hyperchloremic
Uric acid level	Mildly elevated	Frequently markedly elevated
Anemia	Moderate until renal failure	Disproportionately severe for degree of renal failure
Kidney biopsy	Often diagnostic	Usually nonspecific
Urine volume	Unremarkable	Frequently increased with poor concentrating ability

biopsy usually is not diagnostic, but eosinophils may suggest acute interstitial nephritis.

MANAGEMENT. The cornerstone of therapy is identification and removal or reversal of the underlying cause. A short course of corticosteroid therapy is indicated in some patients with allergic interstitial nephritis. Complicating factors such as infection, obstruction, volume depletion, congestive heart failure, hypertension, electrolyte disturbances, and administration of nephrotoxins must be prevented or if present appropriately treated. Hemodialysis, peritoneal dialysis, and transplantation may be used for patients with interstitial nephritis in whom renal failure develops despite therapy.

HYPEROXALURIA

Excessive urinary excretion of oxalic acid is caused by excessive production or excessive colonic absorption of oxalic acid. The hyperoxaluria leads to calcium oxalate nephrolithiasis or interstitial nephritis or both.

Causes of hyperoxaluria include (1) primary hyperoxaluria, an autosomal recessive disorder of glyoxalate metabolism; (2) toxicity from drinking antifreeze (ethylene glycol); (3) methoxyflurane-induced anesthesia; and (4) (more recently described) steatorrhea.

Steatorrhea commonly develops in people with chronic inflammatory bowel disease or jejunoileal bypass. In the presence of steatorrhea the calcium in the small-bowel lumen, which normally combines with oxalate to make a nonabsorbable compound, is bound by unabsorbed fatty acids. This leaves oxalate as sodium oxalate, rather than as insoluble calcium oxalate, making it abnormally available for absorption. The treatment is aimed at reversing the steatorrhea.

ANALGESIC ABUSE NEPHROPATHY

Analgesic abuse nephropathy, or analgesic nephropathy, is a form of interstitial nephritis usually characterized by papillary necrosis, which is attributable to excessive consumption of analgesics (for example, over 1 kg of phenacetin—six tablets a day for 3 years). This disorder originally was called "phenacetin nephropathy," but in recent years as many as one third of patients with analgesic nephropathy have had no history of significant phenacetin intake. Usually patients have consumed a mixture of analgesics, especially aspirin, phenacetin, and caffeine.

Many analgesic and nonsteroidal antiinflammatory agents, including phenylbutazone, mefenamic acid (Ponstel), indomethacin (Indocin), sulindac (Clinoril), and propoxyphene (Darvon), have produced papillary necrosis in laboratory animals. More recently clinical reports have implicated these and other nonsteroidal antiinflammatory agents as causes for nephropathy.

Analgesics and their metabolites are concentrated in the medulla of the kidney, where they inhibit local prostaglandin synthesis, which in turn reduces medullary blood flow. Papillary ischemia, fibrosis, and necrosis result. Salicylate, by uncoupling oxidative phosphorylation and thus inhibiting normal repair of the damaged renal medulla, further contributes to this process.

Analgesic abuse nephropathy may be manifested by symptoms of papillary necrosis such as flank pain, colic, and hematuria. However, patients also may have symptoms of chronic interstitial nephritis, such as nocturia, anemia, salt wasting, and metabolic acidosis, as well as evidence of chronic renal failure. Patients usually have a history of headaches and backaches and may have gastrointestinal symptoms of analgesic excess, such as gastritis or gastrointestinal bleeding. Some patients may not report analgesic use because of embarrassment or failure to recognize the importance of mentioning these nonprescription drugs.

Discontinuing use of all analgesics is an essential objective in the care of patients with analgesic abuse nephropathy. The prognosis is good if renal failure is not severe and marked proteinuria has not developed. Even patients with elevated serum creatinine concentrations may display some improvement. Recent evidence suggests an increased risk for development of transitional cell carcinoma of the bladder in patients with a history of analgesic abuse nephropathy.

Nonsteroidal antiinflammatory drugs (NSAIDs) and the kidney

Nonsteroidal antiinflammatory drugs (NSAIDs) are important therapeutic agents widely used for rheumatologic disorders. They include:

Aspirin
Fenoprofen (Nalfon)
Ibuprofen (Motrin)
Indomethacin (Indocin)
Meclofenamate (Meclomen)
Mefenamic acid (Ponstel)
Naproxen (Naprosyn)
Phenylbutazone (Butazolidin)
Piroxicam (Feldene)
Sulindac (Clinoril)
Tolmetin (Tolectin)
Zomepirac (Zomax)

The antiinflammatory properties of these agents are the result of their common ability to inhibit cyclooxygenase, a major enzyme in the biosynthesis of prostaglandins. The prostaglandins, unsaturated fatty acids, are synthesized immediately before release from arachidonic acid, derived from the phospholipid pool of cell membranes. The prostaglandins participate in many of the aspects of renal physiology, including autoregulation of renal blood flow and glomerular filtration, modu-

lation of renin release, and tubular ion and water transport. Diminished prostaglandin production appears to be the initiating factor in the pathophysiology of most forms of NSAID-associated renal dysfunction.

NSAIDs have little effect on the glomerular filtration rate and renal hemodynamics in normal individuals. However, in situations associated with effective volume contraction, prostaglandins are important in modulating renal function; and NSAIDs have an important effect by blocking prostaglandin production. The conditions associated with volume contraction in which these drugs affect glomerular filtration include reduced cardiac output, hypotension, cirrhosis, nephrotic syndrome, congestive heart failure, volume depletion, diuretics, and anesthesia. Volume contraction leads to activation of pressors, including the adrenergic and renin-angiotensin systems. The renal vasoconstrictive influences of norepinephrine and angiotensin usually are balanced by their stimulation of vasodilatory renal prostaglandins. Renal blood flow and glomerular filtration thus are maintained. When prostaglandin-mediated counterregulatory mechanisms are suppressed by drugs that inhibit cyclooxygenase, renal hemodynamics is impaired.

Any clinical situation in which elevated circulating levels of angiotension and catacholamines exist must be considered a high-risk setting for the development of NSAID-induced renal failure. In chronic renal diseases renal prostaglandins may enhance renal blood flow in surviving nephrons. Blocking prostaglandins with NSAIDs could cause a further fall in renal blood flow and the glomerular filtration rate.

Nephrotic syndrome may develop in patients using NSAIDs. This has been associated with biopsy findings of minimal change and interstitial inflammation. T-cell activation has been proposed as the underlying mechanism.

By blocking prostaglandins NSAIDs increase the tubular cellular response to antidiuretic hormone and decrease renal medullary blood flow. These effects maximize antidiuresis and can lead to water retention and hyponatremia.

Sodium retention is the most common side effect of NSAID therapy. They cause salt retention and edema in susceptible patients both by decreasing the glomerular filtration rate and by directly increasing tubular transport of sodium chloride. NSAIDs lead to sodium retention and increase the vasoconstrictive responses to pressor hormones, blunting the action of diuretics and β-blockers. Thus they may aggravate hypertension in some patients. Hyperkalemia may result in patients with mild renal failure who receive NSAIDs because prostaglandin blockage induces a hyporeninemic hypoaldosterone state.

Sulindac may offer advantages over other NSAIDs by relative sparing of renal prostaglandin activity. Sulindac is a prodrug that must be reduced to the active form in the liver. Oxidases in the kidney can oxidize the reduced form to the inactive prodrug, thereby preventing cyclooxygenase inhibition in the kidney. Whether Sulindac will be substantially safer clinically than other NSAIDs has yet to be demonstrated.

BIBLIOGRAPHY

Brenner BM and others: Tubulo-nephritis nephropathies. In Brenner BM, editor: Clinical nephrology, Philadelphia, 1987, WB Saunders Co.

Clive DM and Stoff JS: Renal syndromes associated with nonsteroidal antiinflammatory drugs, N Engl J Med 310:563, 1984.

Cotran R and others: Tubulo-interstitial disease. In Brenner B and Rector F, editors: The kidney, Philadelphia, 1986, WB Saunders Co.

Dunn MJ: Nonsteroidal anti-inflammatory drugs and renal function, Annu Rev Med 35:411, 1984.

108 · OTHER RENAL DISEASES

Steven J. Peitzman

NEPHROGENIC DIABETES INSIPIDUS

Polyuria occasionally results from a tubular inability to generate concentrated urine, even in the presence of antidiuretic hormone (ADH). The polyuria usually is less abundant than that seen in classic central diabetes insipidus, which is characterized by a lack of ADH. An otherwise healthy and alert person with nephrogenic diabetes insipidus therefore usually has little difficulty ingesting enough water to replace the amount voided. On the other hand, impaired access to water for any reason favors dehydration and hypernatremia. A rare congenital nephrogenic diabetes insipidus occurs, but most cases reflect toxic, ischemic, or mechanical damage to the distal tubule and collecting duct. Drugs capable of inducing this disorder include lithium, demeclocycline, and methoxyflurane. They probably interfere with the activation by ADH of adenyl cyclase–mediated cyclic adenosine monophosphate (AMP) and its effects on increasing the water permeability of the collecting duct. The polyuria caused by methoxyflurane appears to be attributable to a toxic effect of the fluoride ion released metabolically; fortunately, it rarely persists beyond several days. Other causes of nephrogenic diabetes insipidus include hypokalemia, hypercalcemia, obstructive nephropathy, sickle cell trait or disease, pyelonephritis, medullary cystic disease, Sjögren's syndrome, and amyloidosis.

The definitive diagnosis is established when the concentrating defect fails to respond to exogenous ADH (5 mU/min of aqueous vasopressin given intravenously slowly for 1 hour or 5 units vasopressin tannate in oil given intramuscularly).

HYPERCALCEMIC NEPHROPATHY

"Hypercalcemic nephropathy" is a regrettably indistinct term that comprises several adverse effects of calcium on the kidney. Acute renal failure is said to occasionally follow a rapid and severe rise of the plasma calcium level; the association has been documented most commonly in the hypercalcemia of multiple myeloma. Chronic hypercalcemia of any cause (see Chapter 193) more predictably leads to several phenomena. It may blunt concentrating ability and, much like hypokalemia, may bring on reversible nephrogenic diabetes insipidus. Some evidence supports hypercalcemia as a cause of moderate hypertension, which may vanish on correction of the calcium elevation. Whether this effect is mediated by a renal disturbance is uncertain.

Nephrocalcinosis is the roentgenographic or pathologic finding of diffuse calcium deposition, which usually is most intense in the renal interstitium. Although it may be wholly asymptomatic, nephrocalcinosis (at least when caused by primary hyperparathyroidism) may correlate with a gradual reduction in the glomerular filtration rate (GFR). If associated with hypercalciuria, hypercalcemia predisposes the patient to renal calculi. The treatment of any renal disorder resulting from hypercalcemia obviously would include attention to the underlying cause and specific measures to lower the plasma calcium content (see Chapter 193).

URIC ACID NEPHROPATHY

Throughout the later nineteenth century and most of the twentieth, physicians concerned with renal disease confidently held gout to be a common source of renal failure with chronic interstitial nephritis. Recently, however, this understanding has undergone a remarkable revision. Careful and prolonged prospective studies of patients with gout indicate that gout itself rarely induces renal failure. Hence the relationship between the histologic picture (interstitial sodium urate deposits with surrounding inflammation) and the clinical event (decrease in the GFR) now seems uncertain. Some individuals with gout undeniably suffer renal insufficiency but usually as a consequence of other disorders known often to accompany gout, such as uric acid stones with infection or obstruction, hypertension, and renal atherosclerotic vascular disease. One relatively distinct entity, lead poisoning, also produces the association of gout and renal failure. Chronic plumbism causes interstitial nephritis, hypertension, and at least under some circumstances hyperuricemia and saturnine gout. This confluence of findings occurs in some parts of the United States in those who drink "moonshine" alcohol, which often is distilled in improvised devices rich in lead.

Although gouty nephropathy has declined as an important disease concept—either in actuality or in the eyes of physicians—a new and important recognition of *acute* uric acid nephropathy has emerged. In this acute form a massive bulk of uric acid suddenly appears, is filtered or secreted into the tubular lumina, and precipitates. The crystalline material forms an effective intrarenal obstruction to urinary flow; the patient clinically seems to have oliguric acute renal failure. Most patients reported to have this complication had been recently treated with chemotherapeutic agents for leukemia or lymphoma. With the lysis of a large number of abnormal cells, abundant nuclear purines become available for metabolism to their end product, uric acid. Administering allopurinol reduces conversion of purines to uric acid and may be used to prevent renal failure in this setting. In rare cases acute intrarenal uric acid obstruction also occurs following the use of uricosuric drugs.

RENAL TUBULAR ACIDOSIS

In a sense all renal acidosis is tubular; the kidneys excrete the body's metabolic acid load by tubular secretion, not by filtration of hydrogen ion, which exists free in plasma only in negligible amounts. In addition the tubules, especially the proximal tubules, reabsorb from the luminal fluid all of the filtered bicarbonate. Retention of this bicarbonate, along with distal generation of new bicarbonate equivalent to metabolic acid generation, maintains normal systemic pH and buffering capacity. The term "renal tubular acidosis" (RTA), however, conventionally is reserved to describe certain diseases marked not by an overall loss of renal function (filtration and tubular transport) but by a dominant decline in tubular capacity to excrete acid.

The patient with *proximal* (type 2) RTA has only partial ability to proximally reabsorb bicarbonate from luminal filtrate. A stable metabolic acidosis occurs, and administered sodium bicarbonate largely is excreted through the urine without raising the plasma bicarbonate concentration to normal or completely correcting the acidosis. Although distal acidification (ability to secrete hydrogen ion) is normal in proximal RTA, the large quantities of sodium bicarbonate unclaimed by the proximal tubule exceed the bicarbonate-reclaiming ability of the distal tubule, resulting in bicarbonaturia. But with severe acidosis, bicarbonaturia stops and the urinary pH falls to normal, since with lowered plasma bicarbonate concentration the small filtered load of bicarbonate can be reabsorbed by the impaired proximal tubule, and distal bicarbonate delivery is not sufficient to prevent maximal lowering of pH.

Proximal RTA occasionally appears as an isolated defect,

but more often it is associated with other proximal defects *(Fanconi's syndrome),* as in cystinosis, Wilson's disease, hereditary fructose intolerance, multiple myeloma, medullary cystic disease, and acute lead nephropathy.

The underlying disorder associated with proximal RTA should be treated. If this is not feasible, large quantities of sodium bicarbonate (5 to 10 mEq/kg/day) are necessary to correct the acidosis. Potassium supplementation in increasing quantities is required with bicarbonate therapy.

Patients with the more common *distal* (type 1) RTA can reabsorb all filtered bicarbonate proximally but are unable to maximally acidify distal tubular fluid. The quantitative excretion of acid as fully saturated buffer requires a low luminal pH. The defects causing the inability to lower urinary pH are not fully known. It is postulated that some patients have "weak" hydrogen ion secretory pumps that cannot generate a gradient of protons. Failure to acheive this gradient results in a submaximal lowering of urinary pH. Other patients may have a defect in distal tubular permeability, which allows a "backflow" of hydrogen ions; this backflow prevents full maintenance of the hydrogen ion gradient. Like patients with proximal RTA, those with the distal form show hyperchloremic metabolic acidosis, which may be associated with hypokalemia. The hypokalemia sometimes is severe and can cause distresing muscle weakness, which is a symptom that may call attention to the disease. Part of the daily metabolic acid load that is not excreted is buffered by the skeleton; bone pain, osteomalacia, and rickets (in children) may result. The consequent dissolution of bone releases excess calcium into the plasma and hence into the urine. The hypercalciuria, a relatively high urinary pH, and decreased citrate excretion (a consequence of acidemia) contribute to the high incidence of calcium renal stones and renal parenchymal calcification (nephrocalcinosis) seen in distal RTA.

Distal RTA may be an independent disorder, or it may accompany other diseases, as shown in the following outline:

Disorders associated with distal RTA

I. Primary distal RTA
   A. Infantile
   B. Adult sporadic
   C. Genetic defect in carbonic anhydrase
II. Nephrocalcinosis (for example, primary hyperparathyroidism, hypervitaminosis D)
III. Hypergammaglobulinemic states (for example, Sjögren's syndrome, lupus erythematosus)
IV. Cirrhosis
V. Renal transplantation rejection
VI. Drugs and toxins
   A. Amphotericin B
   B. Toluene
   C. Spironolactone
   D. Amiloride
VII. Medullary sponge kidney
VIII. Obstructive nephropathy (discussed later)

The diagnosis of distal RTA is confirmed by demonstrating that the urine pH does not drop below 5.4 during spontaneously present acidemia or after infusing ammonium chloride (0.1 g/kg body weight).

When an underlying cause of distal RTA cannot be identified or cannot be specifically corrected, the acidosis should be treated with alkali replacement. Usually only modest quantities of sodium bicarbonate (1 to 3 mEq/kg/day) are required, and with this supplementation renal potassium loss may stop. Children require more bicarbonate to ensure growth.

"TYPE 4 RTA" AND HYPORENINEMIC HYPOALDOSTERONISM

Nephrologists recently have recognized a heterogeneous group of patients with moderately impaired or normal glomerular filtration rate, hyperkalemia, and hyperchloremic metabolic acidosis. This hyperkalemic distal renal tubular acidosis (sometimes termed "type 4") now seems more common than the classic forms discussed above. It clearly represents more than one mechanism.

Some patients have what has been called a *voltage-dependent* defect: their kidneys lack the ability to generate the usually present negative intraluminal voltage in the collecting duct. The underlying basis may be some abnormality in salt transport in or delivery of salt to this nephron segment (preferential active reabsorption of sodium in slight excess of chloride produces the negative intraluminal charge in the collecting duct). The diminished tubular negative charge is insufficient to attract adequate amounts of potassium and hydrogen ions into the luminal fluid, and their net excretion is impaired. Hyperchloremic acidosis and hyperkalemia result. The hyperkalemia may then worsen the acidosis, since excess cellular potassium hinders renal ammoniagenesis. This form of RTA has been described in the following situations: chronic urinary tract obstruction, chronic renal transplantation rejection, lupus nephritis, sickle cell nephropathy, and diabetes mellitus. Often the hyperkalemia is more dramatic than the acidosis.

Overlapping this syndrome is the disorder *hyporeninemic hypoaldosteronism.* Some patients with diabetic nephropathy and others with interstitial nephritis display hyperkalemia and hyperchloremic acidosis out of proportion to their overall loss of nephron function. In this disorder the renin-producing cells fail to generate renin and to trigger the renin-angiotensin-aldosterone pathway. Aldosterone is needed for maximal distal potassium secretion and probably also directly aids hydrogen ion secretion; the hyperkalemia also impairs ammoniagenesis and therefore acid excretion.

Defining the mechanisms that can cause hyperkalemic RTA may be important. Some patients require treatment with mineralocorticoid (to replace the absent aldosterone); others do not respond to this measure but might to a diuretic that can increase distal salt delivery.

BIBLIOGRAPHY

Berger L and Yu T: Renal function in gout, Am J Med 59:605, 1975.

Cox M and others: Disorders of thirst and renal water excretion. In Arieff AI and DeFronzo RA, editors: Fluid, electrolyte and acid-base disorders, vol 1, New York, 1985, Churchill Livingstone Inc.

DeFronzo RA: Hyperkalemia and hyporeninemic hypoaldosteronism, Kidney Int 17:118, 1980.

DeFronzo RA and others: Acute renal failure in multiple myeloma, Medicine 54:209, 1975.

Heptinstall RH: Pathology of the kidney, ed 2, vol 2, Boston, 1974, Little, Brown & Co.

Kokko JP: Primary acquired hypoaldosteronism, Kidney Int 27:690, 1985.

Kurtzman NA: Acquired distal renal tubular acidosis, Kidney Int 24:807, 1983.

Massry S: Effects of electrolyte disorders on the kidney. In Earley LE and Gottschalk CW, editors: Strauss and Welt's diseases of the kidney, ed 3, Boston, 1979, Little, Brown & Co.

Narins RG and others: Metabolic acid-base disorders: pathophysiology, classification, and treatment. In Arieff AI and DeFronzo RA, editors: Fluid, electrolyte and acid-base disorders, vol 1, New York, 1985, Churchill Livingstone, Inc.

Robinson RR and Yarger WE: Acute uric acid nephropathy, Arch Intern Med 137:839, 1977.

Schambelan M, Sebastian A, and Biglieri EG: Prevalence, pathogenesis, and functional significance of aldosterone deficiency in hyperkalemic patients with chronic renal insufficiency, Kidney Int 17:89, 1980.

109 · TOXIC NEPHROPATHY

Louis J. Riley, Jr., Christine P. Bastl, and
Robert G. Narins*

Acute tubular necrosis (ATN) develops most often in the settings of hypotension and sepsis and with potentially nephropathic drugs and toxins. An ever-lengthening list of common medications and poisons capable of injuring the kidneys has greatly increased the incidence of toxic nephropathy.

PATHOGENESIS

Several intrinsic properties of the kidneys sensitize them to drug- and toxin-induced damage. Although the kidneys make up less than 1% of body weight, they receive 25% of the cardiac output, thereby greatly enhancing their exposure to circulating toxins. Nephrotoxins are concentrated in tubular fluid by the reabsorption of more than 98% of toxin-free glomerular filtrate and by their direct secretion into the lumen. Some toxins are reabsorbed from the glomerular filtrate and accumulate within tubular cells, thereby directly compromising renal epithelium. Additionally, active enzyme systems in the kidney can activate drugs into reactive toxins. Thus the kidneys' unique functional and anatomic properties render them susceptible to toxic damage from various agents at blood concentrations not injurious to other organs.

Toxic nephropathy may be mediated by various processes, including immunologic mechanisms, direct epithelial damage, or obstruction.

Necrotizing vasculitis, polyarteritis, the nephrotic syndrome, and acute glomerulonephritis all may be caused by drug-induced *hypersensitivity* reactions. The administered agent, a metabolic product, or an associated contaminant may act as the antigen in sensitized individuals, evoking an antibody response and acute serum sickness. When immune complexes are deposited in the kidney, acute vasculitis or a variety of glomerular and tubular nephritides may result. The enormous endothelial surface provided by the renal blood vessels ensures a fertile ground for the development of allergic vasculitis. The potential for immune complex formation is present with almost any exogenously derived material such as foreign sera, toxoids, or drugs. Common offending drugs include the penicillins and sulfonamides. The hypersensitivity reactions usually give evidence of diffuse systemic involvement, manifested by some combination of fever, urticaria, arthralgias, and arthritis.

Toxins also may produce a chronic glomerulonephritis with the nephrotic syndrome or slowly progressive renal insufficiency or both. Depositon of antigen-antibody complexes mediates this lesion. The membranous nephritis associated with gold or penicillamine is a clear example of toxin-induced, chronic glomerulonephritis (see the discussion of "Glomerulopathies" later in this chapter). Evidence suggests that these drugs complex with tissue proteins, forming an antigen to which antibodies are produced. The deposited complex evokes an inflammatory reaction in the glomerulus.

Tubular and interstitial damage also may occur through immunologic mechanisms. Acute interstitial nephritis is a well-recognized reaction to therapy with the penicillins, especially methicillin. Patients usually have fever, eosinophilia, eosinophiluria, and rash, suggesting that their nephritis has an allergic basis. The penicilloyl haptenic group complexes with the tubular basement membrane, forming an antigen that incites an antibody response. Other drugs that may cause immune complex–mediated interstitial nephritis are rifampin, sulfonamides, furosemide, cephalothin, phenindione, and allopurinol.

Nephrotoxins also produce acute renal failure by direct damage to proximal renal tubular cells. ATN probably is the most common clinically recognized syndrome produced by nephrotoxins; however, the pathophysiologic events producing cell death remain unclear. The agents most commonly associated with ATN are listed in Table 109-1. Toxic epithelial cell damage may occur with minimal or no impairment of glomerular function. A diffuse defect of proximal tubular transport, *Fanconi's syndrome,* is caused by a variety of drugs and toxins. Outdated tetracyclines caused this syndrome in the past, but it also has resulted from exposure to heavy metals such as lead and mercury. Although gentamicin commonly caused acute renal failure, it also can cause renal tubular wasting of magnesium and potassium. Distal renal tubular acidosis is caused when amphotericin B disrupts luminal membrane integrity, thereby allowing secreted protons to diffuse back to blood. Hypokalemic renal alkalosis may result from the ability of high doses of penicillin, ticarcillin, or carbenicillin to cause distal tubular potassium and hydrogen ion wasting. Impaired distal tubular potassium secretion has been found with indomethacin and propranolol. Nephrogenic diabetes insipidus resulting from blockade of the tubular effects of antidiuretic hormone (ADH) is caused by lithium and demeclocycline.

Various agents also can produce acute uremia by obstructing urine flow. Ureteral obstruction may be caused by retroperitoneal fibrosis related to methysergide use. Most obstructive uropathies related to toxins are intrarenal in nature. The obstruction may be caused by crystallization and precipitation of the agent within the renal tubule, as occurs with large doses of methotrexate. Obstruction also may occur as a result of drug-induced generation of relatively insoluble substances such as uric acid, as seen with cancer chemotherapy. The acute renal failure associated with roentgenographic contrast material is thought to be at least partially caused by tubular obstruction. Although not well defined, the obstructing agent may be the contrast dye, uric acid, Tamm-Horsfall proteins, or a combination of these three. Endogenously released substances that cause obstructive uropathy by precipitation in distal tubules include myeloma proteins, myoglobin, and hemoglobin.

Chronic renal failure caused by chronic tubulointerstitial nephritis most commonly is seen with the combination analgesic drugs containing aspirin and phenacetin or acetaminophen. The cumulative consumption of large quantities of these drugs and their concentration in the papilla and medulla produces oxidative tissue damage.

The remainder of this chapter deals with a general review of the drug and toxin-induced glomerular, tubular, interstitial, renal vascular, and obstructive syndromes; this review in turn is followed by a more detailed outline of the effects of specific disorders caused by selected drugs and toxins.

CLINICAL SYNDROMES ASSOCIATED WITH NEPHROTOXICITY

The clinical presentations of the toxic nephropathies are dictated largely by which renal structures are involved (Table 109-1). Certain toxic nephropathies lead to renal failure that may evolve over a period of days or more insidiously progress over many months. Differentiating toxin-induced renal failure into

---

*Material in this chapter based in part on the first edition, written by T.K.S. Rao.

Table 109-1 Localization of the toxic nephropathies

Anatomic site	Urinary sediment	Proteinuria	Hypertension	Miscellaneous	Commonly associated drugs and toxins
Glomeruli	Red blood cells (RBCs); lipid; oval fat bodies; casts: RBC, pigmented, white blood cell (WBC)	2-4+	Unusual in rapidly progressive glomerulonephritis, common in other forms of acute glomerulonephritis	Look for signs of nephrotic syndrome	Pencillamine, gold, sulfonamides, penicillin, heroin, antiepileptics, nonsteroidal antiinflammatory drugs, mercury, probenecid, rifampin, captopril, tiopronin, aprotinin
Tubules (ATN)	Renal tubular epithelial cells (RTEs); casts: RTE, finely granular, coarsely granular, pigmented	1-2+	Variable	Sepsis, hypotension, renal tubular acidosis, diabetes insipidus, Fanconi's syndrome	Aminoglycosides, cephalosporins, lead (acute), glycols, hydrocarbons, roentgenographic dyes, lithium, methoxyflurane, amphotericin B, trichlorethylene, cisplatin, methotrexate, demeclocycline, cyclosporin, streptozotocin, azacytidine
Interstitium	RTEs, WBCs, eosinophiluria, RBCs; casts: RTE, WBC, RBC (rare)	1-2+	Variable	Fever, rash, eosinophilia, drug allergy	Penicillin homologues, thiazides, furosemide, cimetidine, phenacetin, anesthetics, lithium (?), phenytoin, rifampin
Blood vessels	RBCs are scant if preglomerular; RBCs with RBC casts if glomerular	2-4+	Variable but may be severe	Signs of multiple-system disease, drug allergy, hepatitis-associated antigen positive, renal aneurysms	Suflonamides, amphetamines, penicillin homologues, allopurinol, potassium iodide, cyclosporin
Ureter	Bland sediment	0-1+	Reversible hypertension with unilateral or bilateral hydronephrosis	Insidious renal failure, back pain in migrainous patients	Methysergide, ergots (rarely), methicillin
Bladder	RBCs	0-1+	Unassociated		Cyclophosphamide, semisynthetic penicillins

acute and chronic forms carries important diagnositc and therapeutic implications.

Acute renal failure

Rapidly occurring renal insufficiency may be caused by acute injury to any of the aforementioned anatomic areas. A carefully taken history, physical examination, and laboratory evaluation permit rapid differentiation of acute intrinsic renal insufficiency into discrete glomerular, tubular, interstitial, vascular, and obstructive syndromes (Table 109-1). Drug- or toxin-induced ATN may occur as oliguric (less than 400 ml of urine excreted daily) or nonoliguric renal failure.

Chronic renal failure

Several drugs and toxins can slowly destroy the kidneys, leading to the insidious onset of progressive renal failure. Prolonged exposure to certain analgesic compounds and heavy metals is the most common cause of this form of toxic nephropathy. In advanced cases the presence of small, shrunken kidneys, chronic anemia, or osteopenia allows these disorders to be differentiated from the acute syndromes of acute renal failure.

Glomerulopathies

Acute glomerulonephritis may develop as part of a systemic hypersensitivity reaction to drugs such as penicillin or sulfonamides (Table 109-1). The patients show deteriorating renal function, hypertension, proteinuria, and edema. Red blood cells (RBCs) and white blood cells (WBCs), both free and trapped within casts, are found in the urinary sediment, reflecting the acute glomerular inflammation. Deposition of immune complexes within the glomerulus or the presence of glomerular microvasculitis results in an aggressive proliferation of mesangial, endothelial, and occasionally epithelial cells. An

influx of WBCs and their penetration, along with RBCs, of the disrupted glomerular barrier account for the sedimentary changes observed.

Other nephrotoxins, also acting through immune mechanisms, produce a somewhat less dramatic and more indolent glomerulopathy characterized by varying degrees of proteinuria. Such patients often show a recent onset of edema or the serendipitous finding of albuminuria on routine urinalysis. Gold, penicillamine, and nonsteroidal antiinflammatory agents are only a few of the drugs capable of this more selective alteration of glomerular permeability. A renal biopsy usually reveals either minimal changes or thickening of the basement membrane and capillary wall. Portions of some glomeruli may reveal mild proliferative changes. These "bland" glomerular alterations usually are mirrored by an equally bland urinary sediment. Occasional RBCs, finely granular and hyalin casts, and oval fat bodies are typically found in the urine.

Tubular disorders

A variety of drugs and toxins (Table 109-1) may impair proximal or distal tubular function and thereby cause dramatic clinical syndromes. Agents damaging the proximal tubule may appear as isolated defects in the transport of phosphorus, glucose, uric acid, amino acids, or bicarbonate. Fanconi's syndrome is characterized by impaired transport of several of these substances normally processed by the proximal nephron. Bone pain, osteomalacia, and fractures reflect the phosphaturia, whereas muscle weakness, paresthesias, and cardiac arrhythmias are the consequences of bicarbonate and potassium wasting. Blood chemistries reveal hypobicarbonatemia and hyperchloremia, reflecting the presence of bicarbonaturia. Certain heavy metals, hydrocarbons, and antibiotics have been shown to cause these syndromes.

Several drugs and toxins may impair the distal nephron's

ability to reabsorb sodium, to secrete potassium and protons properly, and to process water effectively. Ingesting amphotericin B or lithium or sniffing glue (trichloroethylene) impairs distal hydrogen ion secretion and urinary acidification, thereby initiating a series of events that lead to potassium and calcium wasting. Lithium and demeclocycline inhibit the hydroosmotic effect of ADH and thereby cause polyuria and nephrogenic diabetes insipidus. Tubular reabsorptive defects are induced by some drugs as part of a more diffuse picture of renal damage. Magnesium wasting, for example, may complicate the acute renal failure occurring with gentamicin or cisplatin nephrotoxicity.

Interstitial disorders

The list of drugs causing acute diffuse interstitial nephritis is growing rapidly (Table 109-1). The clinical picture usually includes some manifestation of hypersensitivity such as fever, rash, or peripheral or urinary eosinophilia. WBCs, including eosinophils, renal epithelial cells, and finely and coarsely granular and cellular casts, characterize the urinary sediment. Salt wasting and potassium retention may be seen in some patients. The rising blood urea nitrogen and creatinine levels may be associated with oliguria or nonoliguria. A biopsy of these swollen, edematous kidneys reveals diffuse round cell infiltration often accompanied by eosinophils, whereas the glomeruli and tubules usually are well preserved.

Penicillins (especially methicillin), thiazides, furosemide, phenytoin, and many other drugs have been incriminated as causing this form of reversible renal failure.

Vascular disorders

Large- and small-vessel vasculitides can be caused by various drugs. The intravenous use of amphetamines may cause a polyarteritis nodosa–like syndrome that commonly attacks the kidney. Inflammation of medium-sized to small renal cortical arteries leads to the formation of vascular aneurysms that occasionally rupture. Progressive azotemia, hypertension, and a bland urinary sediment occur in many patients. The microvasculitides are characterized by proliferative glomerulitis (see previous discussion of "Glomerulopathies").

Obstruction

Methysergide (Sansert) therapy may lead to progressive retroperitoneal fibrosis with entrapment of one or both ureters, causing the insidious onset of progressive renal failure. Hypersensitivity reactions to drugs such as methicillin occasionally may lead to obstructive ureteral urticaria. Crystalluria, as occurs with hyperuricosuria and oxaluria, may cause intrarenal obstruction.

SPECIFIC NEPHROTOXINS

Specific toxins causing nephropathies are listed in Table 109-2.

Heavy metals

(See Chapter 138).

Inorganic *mercurial salts* avidly bind to sulfhydryl groups on key cellular proteins. Poisoning, industrial exposure, or more rarely mercurial diuretic therapy may result in ATN or nephrotic syndrome. The clinical picture is characterized by a metallic taste, various signs and symptoms in the upper and lower gastrointestinal tract, and shock. The therapy includes an emetic, gastric lavage with charcoal, and the intravenous use of the chelating agent dimercaprol (BAL) in doses of 3

Table 109-2 Specific nephrotoxins

Group	Agents
Heavy metals	
Common	Mercury, gold, lead, cadmium, cisplatin, beryllium
Rare	Bismuth, arsenic, copper, silver, thallium, uranium
Antibiotics	
Aminoglycosides	Streptomycin, neomycin, gentamicin, kanamycin, tobramycin
Cephalosporins	Cephaloridine, cephalothin
Sulfonamides	Sulfathiazole, sulfadiazine, sulfapyridine, sulfamethoxazole
Penicillins	Penicillin G, methicillin, ampicillin
Antituberculous drugs	Rifampin, aminosalicylate sodium, capreomycin
Others	Tetracyclines, amphotericin B, bacitracin, polymyxin, colistin
Analgesics and nonsteroidal antiinflammatory drugs	Phenacetin, aspirin, phenylbutazone, indomethacin, fenoprofen, naproxen, ibuprofen
Hydrocarbons and glycols	Carbon tetrachloride, trichloroethylene, tetrachloroethylene, ethylene glycol
Anesthetics	Methoxyflurane, enflurane, fluroxene
Diuretics	Thiazides, furosemide, triamterene
Pigments	Hemoglobin, myoglobin
Antiepileptics	Trimethadione, paramethadione, phenytoin
Antineoplastics	Cisplatin, semustine, mithramycin, mitomycin-C, 5-azacytidine, streptozotocin
Miscellaneous	Lithium, vitamin D, heroin, probenecid

mg/kg every 4 hours. If renal failure is present, hemodialysis must be initiated to remove the dimercaprol-mercury complex.

Gold salts as therapy for rheumatoid arthritis may cause membranous nephropathy with nephrotic syndrome. Although glomerular deposition of gold-induced immune complexes is the putative cause, there is no unequivocal proof for this mechanism. Neither the cumulative dose nor the serum or urinary gold levels are well correlated with the proteinuria that occurs in a small number of treated patients. Dermatitis and bone marrow depression may be associated findings. The proteinuria remits within weeks of discontinuing therapy. Steroids have not been proved beneficial in proteinuria, and they should not be used.

Acute *lead* intoxication, as seen with pica syndrome or the inhalation of tetraethyl lead fumes, causes reversible acute renal failure with proximal tubular damage and Fanconi's syndrome. Chronic exposure causes interstitial nephritis and irreversible chronic renal failure.

Acute lead syndrome occurs primarily in children 1 to 5 years of age who have repeatedly swallowed chips of lead-based paint. Industrial exposure, as with lead storage batteries or leaded gasoline products, causes intoxication in adults. Phosphaturia, glycosuria, aminoaciduria, and less often uricosuria, and bicarbonate wasting are part of the acute renal failure caused by a brief, high-dose lead exposure. Motor neuropathy, abdominal colic, and anemia with basophilic stippling of RBCs often are associated signs. Varying degrees of epithelial cell damage and acid-fast intranuclear inclusions in normal or damaged proximal tubular cells characterize this disorder.

Sustained exposure to lead insidiously leads to chronic renal failure resulting from interstitial nephritis. Industrial exposure or protracted use of illicit ("moonshine") alcohol produced in leaded stills causes most cases in adults. Gout occurs in more than 50% of patients and is a strong clue to the presence of chronic lead nephropathy. Extrarenal signs of lead toxicity are not usually found in the chronic syndrome. Interstitial scarring, round cell infiltration, and an occasional intranuclear inclusion are histologic findings.

The chelation of lead with parenteral ethylenediaminetetraacetic acid (EDTA) is effective treatment for acute renal and extrarenal manifestations of toxicity. Chronic lead nephropathy is best treated by simply avoiding further exposure. Chelation therapy has not been proved beneficial for this irreversible renal disease.

Acute *cadmium* toxicity may lead to the abrupt onset of reversible renal failure but more frequently causes Fanconi's syndrome. The proximal reclamation of low-molecular-weight (15,000 to 40,000 daltons) proteins normally filtered, reabsorbed, and metabolized in the early nephron is impaired, causing lysozymuria and light-chain proteinuria. Toxic exposure occurs primarily in the alkaline storage battery and metallurgic industries. Bone disease and acidosis resulting from renal tubular damage are the major clinical manifestations. Advanced renal failure has not been well documented, and therapy is limited to avoiding futher exposure.

Beryllium may cause a chronic granulomatous interstitial kidney and lung disease when it is inhaled in the manufacture of fluorescent lights. Hyperuricemia and small urinary calculi containing beryllium or calcium oxalate may occur, but the major clinical manifestation is chronic pulmonary disease.

Silver is a rare cause of ATN that occus in film developers.

Both *copper* and *ferrous sulfate* intoxication have resulted in acute renal failure, although part of the renal damage may be explained by shock and, in the case of copper, the development of hemolysis and sulfhemoglobinemia.

Antimony therapy for kalaazar and *cisplatin* therapy for various genitourinary tract malignancies have resulted in acute renal failure. Cisplatin causes acute interstitial nephritis characterized by magnesuria, hypomagnesemia, and tetany. Chronic renal insufficiency may ensue.

Thallium, used in rat poison and ectoparasiticide, has been reported to cause renal proteinuria.

Arsenic intoxication, in addition to causing well-recognized neurologic and gastointestinal symptoms, may also cause ATN. The exposure may be intentional or may occur accidentally with certain fertilizers, agricultural sprays, or arsine gas (used in the petroleum industry).

Roentgenographic dyes

Absorbed or parenteral iodinated contrast dyes cause ATN in some patients. The risk of nephrotoxicity appears to be greatest in patients with dehydration, azotemia, or diabetes mellitus and in the elderly. The pathogenesis of dye-induced renal failure is uncertain. Dehydration, dye-induced uricosuria, precipitation of Tamm-Horsfall or light-chain proteins, direct cellular toxicity, reduction in renal blood flow, and idiosyncratic reactions are possible but unproven mechanisms.

Cholecystographic, angiographic, and pyelographic dyes all have injured the kidney. No clear relationship exists between the total dose of dye and development of nephrotoxicity. Renal failure usually occurs within 24 to 72 hours of exposure to dye. Acute renal failure typically is mild and nonoliguric with peak serum creatinine levels of 5 to 6 mg/dl. Most patients show improved renal function within 5 to 7 days. Dialysis usually is not required, and severe hyperkalemia is unusual. Azotemic diabetic patients whose preexposure serum creatinine concentration exceeds 5 mg/dl tend to have more severe and

often permanent renal failure. Appropriate substitution of ultrasonography and avoiding dehydration may limit this complication. Newer nonionic dyes may be less nephrotoxic.

Antibiotics

All *aminoglycosides* are potential nephrotoxins, but the more widespread use of gentamicin and tobramycin makes them by far the most common offenders. Restricting the poorly absorbable neomycin to oral and topical therapy and further purification of streptomycin have markedly limited their renal toxicity. As with gentamicin and tobramycin, kanamycin causes ATN, but its use has greatly diminished over the years.

The pathogenesis of aminoglycoside-induced ATN is imperfectly understood, although decreased glomerular permeability and lysosomal and mitochondrial damage of proximal tubular epithelium have been demonstrated experimentally. Factors predisposing patients to aminoglycoside-induced ATN include excessive dosage, advanced age, dehydration, low salt intake, hypokalemia, and concomitant exposure to furosemide, cephalosporins, or methoxyflurane.

Although exceptions are common, aminoglycoside-induced renal failure is typically mild and nonoliguric with serum creatinine concentrations frequently peaking at 6 to 10 mg/dl before returning to baseline levels. Magnesium and potassium wasting may accompany the disorder. The concomitance of this otherwise mild renal failure with sepsis and other medical and surgical disorders makes the prognosis for survival guarded.

Cephaloridine unequivocally causes a dose-dependent acute renal failure. High doses of other *cephalosporins,* especially when associated with the same factors that sensitize patients to aminoglycoside nephrotoxicity, also may cause acute renal failure.

Sulfonamide antibiotics may cause acute renal failure by such mechanisms as precipitation in and obstruction of renal tubules and induction of hypersensitivity vasculitis or acute interstitial nephritis. Newer sulfonamides are far more soluble than older preparations, making drug precipitation and intrarenal obstruction extremely rare. Nevertheless, with dehydration, high dosage still can lead to sulfonamide crystalluria and obstruction. Vasculitis and interstitial nephritis usually are associated with fever, rash, and eosinophilia. Trimethoprim-sulfamethoxazole is mildly nephrotoxic but also may cause a functional decrease in the creatinine clearance by impairing the renal tubular secretion of creatinine, with true glomerular filtration being unimpaired.

Amphotericin B commonly causes a dose-dependent, nonoliguric ATN that frequently is associated with hypercalciuria, hypokalemia, and a distal renal tubular acidosis. Avoiding excessive dosage and maintaining brisk urine flows may limit toxicity.

The severe nephrotoxicity of *bacitracin, polymyxin,* and *colistin* limits their use mainly to topical therapy. *Capreomycin* and *rifampin,* antituberculous drugs, may cause acute renal failure. Rifampin nephrotoxicity, which often is associated with light-chain proteinuria, develops most commonly when patients resume therapy following discontinuance. Extrarenal metabolic effects of *tetracyclines* cause azotemia by impairing the anabolism of protein. Changes in the preservatives used in the manufacture of tetracyclines have eliminated drug-induced Fanconi's syndrome. Demethylchlortetracycline causes a dose-dependent nephrogenic diabetes insipidus that may lead to hypernatremia and azotemia.

Acute interstitial nephritis may be caused by the *penicillins,* especially methicillin, less commonly ampicillin, and least commonly penicillin G. Hypersensitivity-induced vasculitis is a reported but infrequent complication of these drugs.

Analgesics, nonsteroidal antiinflammatory agents, and drug abuse

The cumulative ingestion of 2 to 7 kg of *phenacetin*, usually in association with aspirin, causes chronic renal failure as a result of interstitial nephritis. Papillary necrosis and an increased incidence of transitional cell carcinoma have been noted. Acetyl-*p*-aminophenol, phenacetin's major metabolite, concentrates in the renal medulla, causing oxidative tissue damage. Discontinuing the drug often halts progressive azotemia and may result in improvement.

Methysergide, used to treat migraine headaches, not uncommonly causes retroperitoneal fibrosis. The resulting hydronephrosis may lead to insidious renal failure.

Nonsteroidal antiinflammatory drugs (NSAIDs) such as indomethacin, fenoprofen, naproxen, and ibuprofen, have been associated with reversible lipoid nephrosis and acute interstitial nephritis. Renal prostaglandins, the synthesis of which is inhibitied by NSAIDs, are regulators of renin secretion. The hyperkalemia sometimes associated with NSAIDs is caused by induced hyporeninemic hypoaldosteronism. Loss of the vasodilating prostaglandins may severely compromise renal blood flow and lead to acute renal failure in patients with preexisting dehydration, nephrotic syndrome, liver disease, or congestive heart failure or in those undergoing surgery. Patients with systemic lupus erythematosus appear particularly sensitive to the inhibitory effects of NSAIDs on the glomerular filtration rate and renal blood flow.

Heroin abuse causes nephrotic syndrome and renal failure by mechanisms that are unclear. Focal glomerular sclerosis is the most commonly associated lesion. Intravenously administered *amphetamines* are known to induce a polyarteritis nodosa–like syndrome with renal insufficiency and aneurysms of intrarenal vessels.

Hydrocarbons and glycols

Inhaling or ingesting *carbon tetrachloride,* a household cleanser, industrial solvent, and fire extinguisher, leads to severe hepatitis and oliguric renal failure. *Tetrachloroethylene,* a dry-cleaning and degreasing agent, causes a similar syndrome. Sniffing spot remover or glue containing *trichloroethylene* also leads to liver and renal failure. Fanconi's syndrome and distal renal tubular acidosis often are associated findings.

Ethylene glycol (antifreeze) is metabolized to oxalic and glycolic acids and impairs central nervous system activity, leading to renal and cardiopulmonary failure. An elevated anion gap metabolic acidosis caused by glycolic acid accumulation and calcium oxalate crystalluria are typical findings. The therapy entails using hemodialysis and parenteral ethanol to block metabolic conversion of ethylene glycol to its more toxic metabolites.

Pigments

Transfusion reactions or drug-induced hemolysis may produce increased hemoglobin, which may lead to acute renal failure. Alcohol, hypokalemia, hypophosphatemia, trauma, coma, and viral infections can induce rhabdomyolysis resulting in acute renal failure. Obstructing pigment casts or direct epithelial or glomerular damage may cause the nephrotoxicity. Both hemoglobin and myoglobin contain iron and may cause increased superoxide production. The oxygen free radicals are believed to be toxic. The early use of sodium bicarbonate and furosemide or mannitol diuresis may prevent renal failure in these cases of pigment nephropathy.

Antineoplastic agents

A number of antineoplastic agents are potentially nephrotoxic. *Methotrexate,* which inhibits folate synthesis, is excreted primarily by the kidney and in high doses frequently causes renal damage. Intratubular precipitation followed by obstruction is the most widely accepted mechanism of the agent's nephrotoxicity. Precipitation is favored by concentrated, acidic urine, making forced alkaline diuresis a reasonable prophylaxis. Methotrexate also is cytotoxic and may cause direct tubular damage. Leucovorin rescue may counteract methotrexate cytotoxicity even in patients with established acute methotrexate nephropathy.

Semustine, a nitrosourea compound, characteristically causes dose-related nephrotoxicity. Cumulative doses exceeding 1400 mg/m^2 cause slowly progressive and often irreversible renal failure in 25% of patients. Although the mechanism of nephrotoxicity remains obscure, pathologic findings reveal tubular atrophy, interstitial fibrosis, and glomerulosclerosis.

Streptozotocin, the most nephrotoxic of the nitrosourea compounds, also causes dose-related, cumulative renal damage. Mild proteinuria heralds later-appearing generalized proximal tubular dysfunction, that is, Fanconi's syndrome. Oligoanuria also has been reported. Monitoring for proteinuria and careful dose scheduling may prevent nephrotoxicity. Streptozotocin should be discontinued at the first evidence of proteinuria or tubular toxicity. Therapy may be carefully reinstituted upon resolution of nephrotoxic signs.

Mithramycin, a cytotoxic antibiotic, commonly is used to treat malignancy-associated hypercalcemia. Nephrotoxicity is cumulative and potentially irreversible, The mechanism of nephrotoxicity is unknown, but the pathologic changes include tubular degeneration, atrophy and necrosis.

Mitomycin, an alkylating agent, causes an idiosyncratic syndrome characterized by microangiopathic hemolytic anemia, thrombocytopenia, hypertension, and renal failure, a variant of the hemolytic-uremic syndrome. Fibrin thrombi deposit in glomeruli and small arteries, causing arteriolar hyperplasia and glomerular necrosis. Therapy with steroids and plasmapheresis has not been uniformly successful.

5-Azacytidine, a pyrimidine analog, causes azotemia with proximal and distal renal tubular dysfunction. Concentrating and acidifying defects, salt wasting, and Fanconi's syndrome all may appear as manifestations of 5-azacytidine nephrotoxicity.

Cisplatin's antitumor activity is similar to that of alkylating agents. Cytotoxic nephrotoxicity is likely, since renal concentrations are high and platinum is actively secreted by proximal tubular epithelium. Dose-related, cumulative effects include proximal and distal tubular necrosis, interstitial edema, and lymphocytic infiltration. Glomeruli remain uninvolved. Hypomagnesemia, the most common biochemical effect of cisplatin, results from magnesuria and often causes resistant hypokalemia and hypocalcemia. Forced diuresis with saline and loop diuretics or mannitol is effective prophylaxis for cisplatin nephrotoxicity.

Uric acid nephropathy may occur secondary to use of these agents. Intrarenal obstruction caused by increased uric acid production and excretion may occur in myeloproliferative disorders such as acute lymphocytic leukemia, chronic myelogenous leukemia, Hodgkin's disease, and reticulum cell sarcoma during treatment with chemotheapy or radiation of very responsive tumors. In these circumstances uric acid precipitates in the lumen of the nephron, producing acute hyperuricemic nephropathy with oliguanuria. Prevention includes inhibiting uric acid production with allopurinol for 2 to 3 days before tumor lysis and increasing urine flow with hydration while alkalinizing the urine (pH≥7) with sodium bicarbonate or acetazolamide. Once renal failure occurs, the size of the uric acid pool can be decreased by hemodialysis and allopurinol.

Miscellaneous toxins

Metabolism of the general anesthetic *methoxyflurane* (Penthrane) forms oxalic acid and releases fluoride. Nephrogenic diabetes insipidus and acute renal failure develop in some patients. Interstitial fibrosis and calcium oxalate crystallization are the hallmarks of this disorder. Other related anesthetics, *fluroxene* (Fluoromar) and *enflurane* (Ethrane), also have caused acute renal failure.

Lithium salts, used in treating certain psychiatric conditions, may cause a dose-dependent, slowly reversible nephrogenic diabetes insipidus. Lithium has been associated with chronic interstitial nephritis, but the causality has not been firmly established.

Hypersensitivity reactions to *thiazides, furosemide,* and the anticoagulant *phenindione* all have been reported to cause acute renal failure. Biopsy has shown acute interstitial nephritis.

Penicillamine, used in treating cystinuria, Wilson's disease, and a variety of collagen-vascular disorders, causes an immune-complex, membranous glomerulonephritis and nephrotic syndrome. Continued use of the drug may lead to rapidly progressive, crescentic glomerulonephritis. The membranous lesion usually is reversible with discontinuance of therapy.

Cyclosporine, a immunosuppressive agent with selectivity for T-cell–related immune responses, effectively treats transplantation rejection and certain autoimmune diseases. Nephrotoxicity with azotemia, hyperkalemic type 4 renal tubular acidosis, and hypertension, is the agent's key drawback. Nephrotoxicity may occur acutely, subacutely, or chronically. Cyclosporine causes hemodynamic changes and tubular dysfunction. Vasoconstrictive reduction in the renal blood flow and glomerular filtration rate raises the serum creatinine concentration, whereas the tubulotoxicity effects a hyperkalemic. hyperchloremic metabolic acidosis. Nephrotoxicity is dose related. Individualized drug regimens that maintain blood cyclosporine levels in an acceptable range or reducing the duration of therapy can minimize the potential for nephrotoxicity.

BIBLIOGRAPHY

Agarwal BN, Cabebe FG, and Hoffman BI: Diphenylhydantoin-induced acute renal failure, Nephron 18:249, 1977.
Appel GB and Neu HC: The nephrotoxicity of antimicrobial agents (in three parts), N Engl J Med 296:663, 722, 784, 1977.
Bastl CP, Rudnick MR, and Narins RG: Diagnostic approaches to acute renal failure. In Brenner BM and Stein JH, editors: Contemporary issues in nephrology, vol 6, New York, 1980, Churchill Livingstone, Inc.
Bennett WM: Basic mechanisms and pathophysiology of cyclosporine nephrotoxicity, Transplan Proc 17(suppl 1):297, 1985.
Border WA and others: Antitubular basement-membrane antibodies in methicillin associated interstitial nephritis, N Engl J Med 291: 381, 1974.
Byrd L and Sherman RL: Radiocontrast-induced acute renal failure: a clinical and pathological review, Medicine 58:270, 1979.
Carling PC and others: Nephrotoxicity associated with cephalothin administration, Arch Intern Med 135:797, 1975.
Citron BP and others: Necrotizing angiitis with drug abuse, N Engl J Med 283:1003, 1970.
Cogan MC and Arieff AI: Sodium wasting, acidosis and hyperkalemia induced by methicillin interstitial nephritis, Am J Med 64:500, 1978.
Gault MH and others: Syndrome associated with the abuse of analgesics, Ann Inter Med 68:906, 1968.
Graham JR and others: Fibrotic disorders associated with methysergide therapy for headache, N Engl J Med 274:359, 1966.

Hestbech J and others: Chronic renal lesions following long-term treatment with lithium, Kidney Int 12:205, 1977.
Humes HD and Weinberg JM: Toxic nephropathies. In Brenner BM and Rector FC Jr, editors: The kidney, ed 3, Philadelphia, 1986, WB Saunders Co.
Johansson S and Wahlqvist L: Tumors of urinary bladder and ureter associated with abuse of phenacetin-containing analgesics, Acta Pathol Microbiol Scand 85:768, 1977.
McCurdy DK, Frederic M, and Elkinton JR: Renal tubular acidosis due to amphotericin B, N Engl J Med 278:124, 1968.
Rao TK, Nicastri AD, and Friedman EA: Natural history of heroin associated nephropathy, N Engl J Med 290:19, 1974.
Schilsky RL and Anderson T: Hypomagnesemia and renal magnesium wasting in patients receiving cisplatin, Ann Intern Med 90:929, 1979.
Singer J and Rotenberg D: Demeclocycline-induced nephrogenic diabetes insipidus, in vivo and in vitro studies, Ann Intern Med 79:679, 1973.

110·ACUTE RENAL FAILURE

Robert E. Gerhardt *and* **Charles J. Wolf***

DEFINITION. Acute renal failure (ARF) may be defined as an abrupt reduction in glomerular and renal tubular function resulting in azotemia. Oliguria (daily urine output less than 400 ml) and anuria (daily urine output less than 50 ml) with azotemia long have been considered hallmarks of this syndrome, yet a nonoliguric form is commonly encountered in clinical practice. ARF may be dramatic, at times a life-threatening syndrome, or alternatively subtle in severity and gradual in onset. Reduced renal function from any cause is associated with retention of blood urea nitrogen (BUN), creatinine, phosphorus, uric acid, and several other substances not usually measured in clinical practice. During ARF the serum creatinine concentration usually increases by 1 to 2 mg/dl/day and the BUN level by 10 to 20 mg/dl/day. In diseases associated with hypercatabolism, such as following trauma or rhabdomyolysis, the increase in BUN and creatinine levels may be three to five times this rate. The major emphasis in this chapter is on the variety of ARF known as acute tubular necrosis (ATN). Synonyms for ATN include "shock kidney," "lower nephron nephrosis," "nephrotoxic nephropathy," and "vasomotor nephropathy."

ETIOLOGY AND PATHOGENESIS. In a recent review of 2200 cases of ARF collected from around the world, 43% were related to surgery, 26% occurred in a medical setting, 13% were related to complications of pregnancy, 9% were related to trauma, and 9% were a result of nephrotoxins. A rational approach to the patient with ARF requires differentiating the causes of azotemia into prerenal, renal, and postrenal, as shown in Fig. 110-1. Examining the urine, along with the history and physical examination, can help suggest the cause of the renal failure. Scant findings in the urine is a feature compatible with prerenal azotemia, obstruction, renal vascular disease, or vasculitis. Red blood cells and red blood cell casts are seen with glomerulonephritis or interstitial nephritis. Granular casts are seen in ATN. Crystalluria suggests uric acid nephropathy or calcium oxalate production as in ethylene glycol ingestion. Eosinophiles are seen in acute interstitial nephritis. White blood cells or white blood cell casts are present in pyelonephritis and acute interstitial nephritis.

Prerenal failure

Decreased renal perfusion, resulting from lowered effective arterial volume from any cause, can lead to decreased renal

---

*Material in this chapter based in part on the first edition, written by T.K.S. Rao.

I. **Prerenal**
  A. **Gastrointestinal losses** (vomiting, diarrhea, nasogastric suction, colostomy, ileus)
  B. **Excessive sweating**
  C. **Hemorrhage**
  D. **Burns with sequestration of fluids**
  E. **Renal losses** (diuretics, renal salt wasting)
  F. **Cardiovascular failure**
    1. Congestive heart failure
    2. Myocardial infarction with shock
    3. Cardiac tamponade
  G. **Hepatic failure**
    1. Cirrhosis with ascites
    2. Hepatorenal syndrome

III. **Postrenal**
  A. **Bilateral ureteric obstruction or ureteric obstruction in a solitary kidney**
    1. Retroperitoneal fibrosis
    2. Tumor
    3. Stones
    4. Surgical ligation
    5. Papillary necrosis
  B. **Bladder obstruction** (prostatic hypertrophy, stones, neurogenic)
  C. **Disruption of bladder** (with intraperitoneal extravasation of urine)
  D. **Urethral obstruction** (stones, strictures)

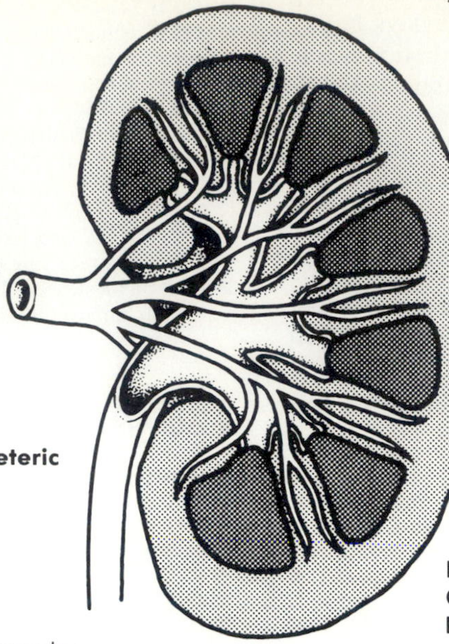

II. **Intrinsic Renal**
  A. **Acute tubular necrosis** (vasomotor nephropathy)
    1. Hypovolemia
    2. Septic shock
    3. Drug-induced (aminoglycosides, amphotericin B)
    4. Roentgenographic contrast media
    5. Anesthetics (methoxyflurane)
    6. Nephrotoxins (environmental and industrial)
      a. Carbon tetrachloride
      b. Methyl alcohol
      c. Heavy metals (bismuth, lead, uranium, inorganic mercurials)
    7. Posttraumatic and postoperative
    8. Rhabdomyolysis with myogloburinuria (trauma, fever, heat stroke, severe viral infections)
    9. Hemolysis with homoglobinuria
    10. Obstetric (septic abortion, uterine hemorrhage)
  B. **Bilateral cortical necrosis**
  C. **Glomerulonephritis, severe acute form**
  D. **Vasculitis**
    1. Polyarteritis
    2. Wegener's granulomatosis
  E. **Malignant hypertension**
  F. **Accelerated scleroderma**
  G. **Allergic interstitial nephritis** (antibiotics, anticonvulsants)
  H. **Miscellaneous** - hypercalcemia, hyperuricemia, multiple myeloma, homograft rejection)

Fig. 110-1 Causes of acute renal failure.

function. Some causes of decreased effective arterial volume include excessive blood loss from hemorrhage, sequestration of fluids following severe burns, intestinal obstruction, or cardiac failure. The common pathophysiologic factor in these states is reduced renal blood flow without intrinsic injury to glomeruli and tubules. The renal response to hypovolemia is an attempt to maintain the extracellular fluid volume by retaining salt and water. Initially this is associated with excretion of concentrated urine. Prompt restoration of vascular volume and improvement in cardiac function result in increased urine output and correction of azotemia.

Intrinsic renal failure

Of the various causes of intrinsic renal failure listed in Fig. 110-1, this chapter is limited mainly to discussion of acute tubular necrosis syndrome. This term is a misnomer, however, because renal tubular necrosis is not always present, and little correlation exists between histologic lesions in the kidney and the severity of renal failure (that is, histologic findings may be normal despite uremia). Renal ischemia and nephrotoxic agents are the two major factors involved in the pathogenesis of ATN. In both, significant intrarenal hemodynamic alterations account for the development of renal failure.

Renal ischemia

Although hypotension itself rarely leads to ATN, hypotension in the presence of trauma, sepsis, surgery, or other coexisting insults frequently results in this syndrome. Because of a lack of good animal models of ATN and since patients, for unknown reasons, vary in their susceptibility to the disorder, the exact relationship of coexisting conditions and ischemia in

the development of ATN is not always clear. In clinical situations a specific insult causing ATN cannot be ascribed in 30% to 40% of cases. Factors such as excess renin-angiotensin production, intrarenal vascular coagulopathy, or other unknown mechanisms contributing to ATN in ischemia are poorly understood and at present not generally amenable to therapy.

Although the kidney is provided with an excellent supply of blood and oxygen, the medulla, particularly the thick ascending limb (TAL), with its high metabolic activity and oxygen consumption, is susceptible to hypoxia. It is now thought that renal underperfusion caused by hypovolemia or by agents that cause oxygen free-radical (superoxide) production causes tubular injury. Currently efforts to preserve renal perfusion (for example with mannitol) preoperatively or to restore perfusion in shock and sepsis are undertaken in an attempt to reduce renal ischemia in these situations.

Nephrotoxins

Industrial chemicals (carbon tetrachloride and ethylene glycol), heavy metals (mercury and lead), nephrotoxic drugs (aminoglycoside antibiotics), anesthetic agents, and roentgenographic contrast media (intravenous pyelography, oral cholecystography, and angiography dyes) are some of the commonly encountered agents implicated in the production of ATN in humans. Careful monitoring of blood levels of nephrotoxic drugs and careful use of roentgenographic contrast agents has decreased ATN from these causes. Significant risk factors in the use of contrast agents include diabetes mellitus, old age, preexisting volume depletion, elevated baseline serum creatinine, and multiple myeloma. The release of large amounts of hemoglobin (intravascular hemolysis) or myoglobin (in rhabdomyolysis) into the circulation in patients who are dehydrated and acidotic also may result in ATN. These agents probably produce renal tubular injury by a direct toxic mechanism. Hemoglobin and myoglobin contain iron and accelerate formation of free radicals.

In both ischemic and nephrotoxic ATN, once the initiating events produce an acute reduction in renal function, many factors may be responsible for maintaining renal failure, including persistent profound renal vasoconstriction, renal tubular obstruction by inspissated debris, and back leakage of tubular fluid through disruptions in the tubular wall.

Postrenal failure

In the postrenal group of disorders renal failure is caused by obstruction of urine flow in various segments of the urinary tract. The need for prompt diagnosis and relief of obstruction cannot be overemphasized, since this reversible cause of ARF can progress to permanent renal damage if left undetected.

CLINICAL MANIFESTATIONS

Oliguric phase. In most patients with ATN the endogenous creatinine clearance falls to 1 ml/min or less. Within a day of the precipitating event, oliguria with azotemia usually is seen, but at times it may be delayed for 1 or 2 weeks. The average duration of oliguria is 7 to 14 days, but it may abate in a few hours or persist for several weeks. The daily urine output averages 200 to 300 ml, and anuria is rare. In the nonoliguric form of ATN, the glomerular filtraton rate (GFR) still is markedly reduced, but the creatinine clearance is not less than 3 to 5 ml/min and the daily urine output generally is more than 500 ml. Regardless of urine volume, the concentration of BUN, creatinine, uric acid, phosphorus, and the other products of nitrogen metabolism progressively increases. Retention of 50 to 100 mEq of fixed acids daily results in metabolic acidosis, which is reflected biochemically as a decrease in plasma bicarbonate concentration and a reduction in arterial pH. Hyperkalemia generally develops, its severity depending on potassium intake, release of potassium from the tissues, and systemic pH. Hyperkalemia generally is the most dangerous consequence of ATN and the most common cause of mortality; it should always be watched for and treated. The effects of hyperkalemia on the electrocardiogram (ECG) include (in sequence) tall, peaked T waves in the precordial leads, prolongation of the P-R interval, complete heart block, absent P waves, prolongation of the QRS complexes, ventricular fibrillation, and cardiac arrest. The electrophysiologic effects of hyperkalemia on the myocardium are potentiated by other electrolyte disturbances such as hyponatremia and hypocalcemia.

Salt and water retention, with the development of peripheral edema and pulmonary congestion, is a frequent complication of ATN. With persistent renal failure uremic syndrome develops, including many abnormalities. Neurologic manifestations may include stupor, mental confusion, axterixis, convulsion, and coma. Gastrointestinal bleeding resulting from uremic gastritis or colitis may at times be severe enough to require blood transfusion. Anemia, platelet dysfunction, hypocalcemia, poor wound healing, and an increased tendency to develop infections are some of the other findings that may be present. Pericardial effusion and tamponade may occur in rare cases.

Diuretic phase. After 1 to 2 weeks of oliguria, if recovery is to occur, urine output increases progressively, generally 2 to 3 L a day but at times exceeding 5 to 10 L daily. The onset of diuresis signals the beginning of recovery from ATN. Since diuresis precedes the decline in BUN and creatinine levels by a few days, uremic symptoms may progress, requiring dialysis.

Table 110-1 Differential characteristics of prerenal azotemia and acute renal failure

Laboratory study	Prerenal azotemia	ARF
BUN/serum creatinine concentrations	>10:1	10:1
Urine/plasma osmolality	>1.4:1	1
Urinary sodium concentration	<20 mEq/L	>20 mEq/L
Fractional excretion of sodium*	<1	>4
Urine output	500-600 ml/day	<400 ml/day
Urine sediment	None	Renal failure, broad granular casts

$$*\text{Fractional excretion of sodium} = \frac{\text{Urine Na}^+ \times \text{Plasma creatinine}}{\text{Urine creatinine} \times \text{Plasma Na}^+} \times 100$$

The magnitude of the diuresis depends on three factors: the degree to which urea and other endogenous solutes accumulate during oliguria, the degree of extracellular volume expansion caused by salt and water retention, and the rate of recovery of tubular reabsorptive capacity. Significant fluid and electrolyte losses occasionally occur because of the recovering tubules' inability to concentrate the urine. Following the onset of diuresis, the GFR improves gradually, as reflected by a fall in BUN and creatinine levels. Normal values usually are achieved in 2 to 3 weeks. Recovery of renal function following more than 3 weeks of oliguria is uncommon but does occur. Infection is the major complication during the diuretic phase, the most common being urinary tract infection from indwelling bladder catheters and septicemia from intravenous infusions or operative trauma sites.

Recovery phase. During the recovery phase renal function continues to improve and achieves a level compatible with normal life. After a few months testing may reveal a minor reduction in the GFR and a diminution in the kidneys' ability to concentrate and acidify the urine. These functional derangements are of no practical clinical significance except when ARF is superimposed on chronic renal failure. In rare cases patients with ATN fail to recover, and irreversible renal failure requiring maintenance hemodialysis develops.

DIAGNOSIS. The approach to the patient with acute onset of oliguria and azotemia should be as follows:

Tests for prerenal azotemia. A careful history is taken and a physical examination is performed to uncover underlying predisposing factors such as evidence of a toxin, volume depletion, or cardiac failure. Laboratory studies (Table 110-1) also can help distinguish prerenal azotemia from ARF. In prerenal azotemia, oliguria is associated with a concentrated urine (specific gravity greater than or equal to 1.02), a urine/plasma osmolality ratio greater than 1.4:1, a low urinary sodium concentration (less than 20 mEq/L), and a fractional sodium excretion of less than 1. The BUN/creatinine ratio is abnormally increased (greater than 10:1), because urea clearance is more sensitive to urine flow than creatinine clearance. By contrast, in the oliguric patient with ARF the urine is isosmolar to blood, the urine sodium concentration and fractional excretion of sodium are high, and BUN and creatinine levels rise proportionately. If the diagnosis of prerenal azotemia is made, rapid and appropriate expansion of the plasma volume should be initiated with saline, albumin, plasmanate, or blood while the patient's cardiovascular status is monitored by auscultation of the lungs for rales and central venous or pulmonary wedge pressure measurements. Patients with prerenal azotemia resulting from hypovolemia generally respond to expansion of their intravascular volume. The heart rate falls, blood pressure rises, and urine output increases. A satisfactory response consists of an increase in urine volume to more than 50 ml/hr.

Tests for urinary tract obstruction. The extent of the search for obstruction varies and depends on the clinical situation. Prostate hypertrophy, causing outlet obstruction, is common and can be determined after rectal examination and measurement of the residual urine volume by percussion of the bladder, bladder sonography, or bladder catheterization. Plain films of the abdomen can detect radiopaque calculi. A renal sonogram is noninvasive and should always be obtained in ARF to confirm the presence of two kidneys, to rule out dilation of the collecting system, and to evaluate bladder function. CT scans of the abdomen without contrast media can be obtained to uncover extrinsic mass lesions that may be compressing the ureters. If ureteral obstruction is likely, retrograde ureteral catheterization is performed. The risks of this procedure are infection and edema of the ureter, or in rare cases perforation of the uterer or renal pelvis. More recently most hospitals are equipped to perform percutaneous antegrade nephrostomy using ultrasound guidance. This is especially useful in patients with intrinsic obstruction of the ureters, when retrograde catheterization is technically impossible.

Other intrinsic renal diseases. Since ARF can be caused by systemic diseases, as well as by bilateral primary renal diseases other than ATN, a careful search must be made for other causes via the history, physical examination, and laboratory tests. Allergic interstitial nephritis from commonly used drugs (for instance, penicillins and derivatives; sulfa drugs and derivatives, including most diuretics; nonsteroidal antiinflammatory agents; and phenytoin) may *exactly* mimic ATN in presentation and time course. Fever, skin rash, eosinophiles in the urine, and high peripheral eosinophil count, when present, suggest allergic interstitial nephritis as the cause of ARF.

MANAGEMENT
Oliguric phase. ATN usually follows its own self-limited course, and currently no specific therapy can hasten the recovery of renal function. Consequently the treatment is aimed at careful management of the primary problem, be it medical, surgical, traumatic, or obstetric, while avoiding additional nephrotoxic injury and minimizing the complications of uremia.

The principles of management during the oliguric phase of ATN consist of restricting sodium, fluids, and potassium; maintaining nutrition; and instituting early dialysis before the development of complications.

Fluids and nutrition. The daily sodium and fluid intake in oliguric patients should be restricted to an amount equal to the sum of urinary output and extrarenal losses (from insensible losses, nasogastric suction, colostomy drainage, and diarrhea). The fluid balance is determined by weighing the patient daily and accurately recording all intake and output volumes, as well as by measuring electrolyte excretion. Nutrition must be maintained by prescribing an adequate diet. If the patient is unable to tolerate oral feeding, aseptic hyperalimentation techniques must be instituted to provide adequate caloric intake. Further evaluation is required before the routine uses of hyperalimentation in uncomplicated ATN can be recommended. Appropriate fluid and nutritional intake is associated with no weight gain (for example, from edema fluid). Because of the catabolism attendant with the illness, lean body mass is lost and nonedematous patients lose 1 to 2 lbs/day.

Multivitamins are prescribed to prevent a vitamin deficiency. If significant metabolic acidosis (pH less than 7.3) is present, sodium bicarbonate should be administered (see Chapter 103). Using sodium bicarbonate in oliguric patients is limited by the high sodium content of each ampule (which has equal quantities of sodium and bicarbonate). Severe acidosis, especially in the face of volume overload, requires intervention with dialysis. Other measures include using antacids containing aluminum or calcium to prevent absorption of phosphate from the gut and avoiding products containing magnesium; both phosphate and magnesium are retained in renal failure.

If significant pulmonary congestion develops despite the preceding measures, dialysis should be instituted as early as possible. During dialysis excess fluid can be removed by ultrafiltration. In an emergency situation, if dialysis or ultrafiltration cannot be instituted immediately, phlebotomy with the removal of 250 to 500 ml of blood (if the hematocrit level is greater than 30%) may be indicated to treat severe fluid overload.

Hyperkalemia. The myocardial effects of hyperkalemia can provoke the most lethal complications of ATN. Efforts to prevent hyperkalemia include avoiding potassium supplements, potassium-rich foods, and potassium-sparing diuretics (spironolactone and triamterene). Since hyponatremia and acidosis accompany renal failure and aggravate myocardial sensitivity to potassium, it is difficult to label any specific potassium concentration as safe. During the oliguric phase of ATN, frequent determinations of sodium, potassium, and bicarbonate concentrations and ECG monitoring are essential to detect hyperkalemia early. Despite severe potassium restriction, hyperkalemia commonly occurs in the course of ATN, particularly in catabolic patients.

Treatment of hyperkalemia depends on the speed of correction required. With arrhythmias or ECG changes of hyperkalemia, intravenous calcium gluconate can be given in patients not receiving digitalis. Calcium acts almost immediately to stabilize the myocardial cell membranes and block the effects of hyperkalemia.

Potassium also may be driven into cells by using glucose (with or without insulin) or sodium bicarbonate. Glucose and bicarbonate are slower to act than calcium, taking 15 to 30 minutes for effect, but they last up to 60 to 90 minutes. However, none of the above methods remove potassium from the body.

Potassium can be removed from the body by using a sodium-potassium exchange resin such as sodium polystyrene sulfonate (Kayexalate) or by dialysis. Resins may be given orally or by retention enema and are more effective than peritoneal dialysis. However, sodium is retained by the body in exchange for potassium and may result in volume overload. Hemodialysis is the quickest and most effective way to eliminate potassium from the body; hyperkalemia frequently is the precipitating factor for initiating dialysis in ARF.

Infection. Every attempt should be made to prevent sepsis from developing in patients with ATN, including avoiding indwelling bladder catheters, proper surgical management of trauma, adequate pulmonary toilet, and antiseptic care of infusion sites. Infection must be recognized early, because the response may be blunted with uremia. If infection does develop, a careful search for the source and identification of the organism and its antibiotic sensitivity should be undertaken. Aggressive therapy should be initiated promptly to prevent overwhelming sepsis. When nephrotoxic antibiotics (aminoglycosides) are needed, the dosage should be modified after the first dose, according to the residual renal function and dialyzability of the drug. As soon as the organism is identified and sensitivities are available, regimens can be established that avoid nephrotoxic antibiotics whenever possible.

Dialysis. When conservative measures fail to maintain an optimal clinical status, dialysis therapy should be instituted. Indications for dialysis include hyperkalemia, acidosis, fluid overload, uremia-induced nausea and vomiting, septicemia, bleeding diathesis or pericarditis resulting from uremia, asterixis, and uremic coma. Early dialysis currently is recommended to avoid these serious complications. Both peritoneal dialysis and hemodialysis are acceptable modes of treatment in ATN; the mode selected depends on the patient's clinical state and the hospital's resources. Generally patients are hemodialyzed every other day, but if the clinical status deteriorates or a hypercatabolic state exists, daily dialysis may be needed.

Diuretic phase. During the diuretic phase the goal of management is to maintain a normal fluid balance. At this time most patients excrete the excess fluid retained during the oliguric phase. Occasionally, however, dehydration may occur because of excessive diuresis resulting from tubular injury, and provisions should be made to replace fluid and electrolytes to maintain a normal vascular volume. Body weight, urinary output, tissue turgor, the presence or absence of edema, and serum and urinary electrolyte levels serve as guides to proper replacement therapy. Infection and uremic complications are still a problem during the diuretic phase, and the principles previously outlined should be followed. Hyperkalemia is rare during diuresis.

PROGNOSIS. Death in ATN usually is a result of the underlying disease. The highest mortality occurs when renal failure is precipitated by trauma, surgery, or infection. Reported fatality in such patients ranges from 50% to 75% and largely is attributable to respiratory insufficiency, sepsis, and gastrointestinal bleeding. The mortality in obstetric-related or nephrotoxin-induced ATN generally is less than 10%. The prognosis is good for patients who recover from ARF, because the residual renal damage is minimal.

BIBLIOGRAPHY

Anderson RJ and others: Nonoliguric acute renal failure, N Engl J Med 296:1134, 1977.

Brezis M, Rosen S, and Epstein FH: Acute renal failure. In Brenner BM and Rector FC Jr, editors: The kidney, ed 3, Philadelphia, 1986, WB Saunders Co.

Brezis M and others: Renal ischemia: a new perspective, Kidney Int 26:375, 1984.

Knochel JP: Complications of total parenteral nutrition, Kidney Int 27:489, 1985.

Levinsky NG: Pathophysiology of acute renal failure, N Engl J Med 296:1453, 1977.

Linton AL and others: Acute interstitial nephritis due to drugs, Ann Intern Med 93:735, 1980.

111·CHRONIC RENAL FAILURE

Raphael Cohen *and* Michael Rudnick

DEFINITION AND ETIOLOGY. Chronic renal disease implies structural renal damage that limits or reduces the glomerular filtration capacity of the kidneys. The damage usually is irreversible and, more ominously, structural and functional impairment is slowly progressive. Throughout the period of deterioration, covering a wide spectrum of deranged renal function, adaptive mechanisms by both the kidneys and the patient as a whole allow for states of compensated homeostasis. Thus for prolonged periods chronic renal failure (CRF) at any point is a steady-state condition without demonstrable fluctuation in renal function or day-to-day changes in body composition.

Ultimately, with advanced disease and severe impairment of glomerular filtration and other renal functions, compensatory mechanisms either break down or themselves lead to secondary maladaptive consequences, resulting in a deranged internal milieu and multiple-system dysfunction, collectively known as uremia.

The reported incidence of CRF depends on the cut-off level of renal function used to define that state. Thus chronic renal disease generally is much more prevalent than, say, end-stage CRF, which necessitates renal replacement therapy. In the United States in 1985, almost 30,000 new patients with CRF began dialysis, for an annual incidence of 0.01% of end-stage renal disease (ESRD) in this country. Such statistics vary from country to country and even vary nationally in different geographic, demographic, and ethnic subgroups, depending on the prevalence of diseases that cause chronic renal injury. As outlined in preceding and succeeding chapters, the list of diseases causing CRF is diverse and includes: chronic immunologic glomerulopathies (either intrinsic to the kidney or secondary to systemic illnesses), hypertensive nephrosclerosis, chronic tubulointerstitial diseases (for example, those secondary to infection, urologic or obstructive diseases, or toxic nephropathies such as analgesic abuse), metabolic diseases such as diabetes mellitus, and congenital and hereditary renal conditions such as polycystic kidney disease (PCKD). In the United States the leading cause of ESRD usually is quoted to be chronic glomerulonephritis (30% to 40%), with diabetes, PCKD, and nephrosclerosis each contributing 5% to 10%. However, diabetes mellitus is moving up in frequency. In the black population in the United States, in whom hypertension is a greater public health problem, nephrosclerosis as a cause of CRF undoubtedly is more frequent. In other locales, other unique diseases predominate; for example, in Australia, analgesic nephropathy has been a leading cause of CRF. The cause of CRF remains unknown in many patients who are seen late in their course, because in the end-stage phase the clinical and structural manifestations of renal scarring tend to merge toward a single entity.

COURSE (Fig. 111-1). As mentioned previously, the course of CRF is a slow evolution of steady-state conditions characterized by a continuum of functional impairment and offsetting adaptations in the patient. Early on, the anatomic damage in the kidney may not be readily apparent from a functional standpoint, with a relatively well-preserved overall glomerular filtration rate (GFR) of 70% to 100% and normal serum creatinine. The damage can be discerned only by noting an abnormal urinalysis or by ascertaining a diminished reserve of renal function (for example, diminished maximal concentrating ability in the face of water deprivation or limited ability to further augment GFR in response to physiologic challenges such as pregnancy or protein loading). Later, as damage continues and the GFR falls to 30% to 50% of normal, more easily noticed elevations in nitrogenous wastes become apparent. Hypertension may be an early concomitant of renal injury, or it may ensue along with other manifestations of volume overload as renal function falls further to ranges of 10% to 25%. At this point the steady-state condition also is characterized by worsening anemia, metabolic acidosis, and hyperphosphatemia. When the GFR falls to less than 5% to 10% of normal, the patient usually develops a symptom complex encompassing dysfunction of several organ systems and generalized metabolic disturbance, a syndrome referred to as uremia. At this extreme of renal failure, a steady-state condition cannot be maintained and the uremic syndrome becomes manifest. No matter how the kidney is injured initially, the uremic endpoint clinically

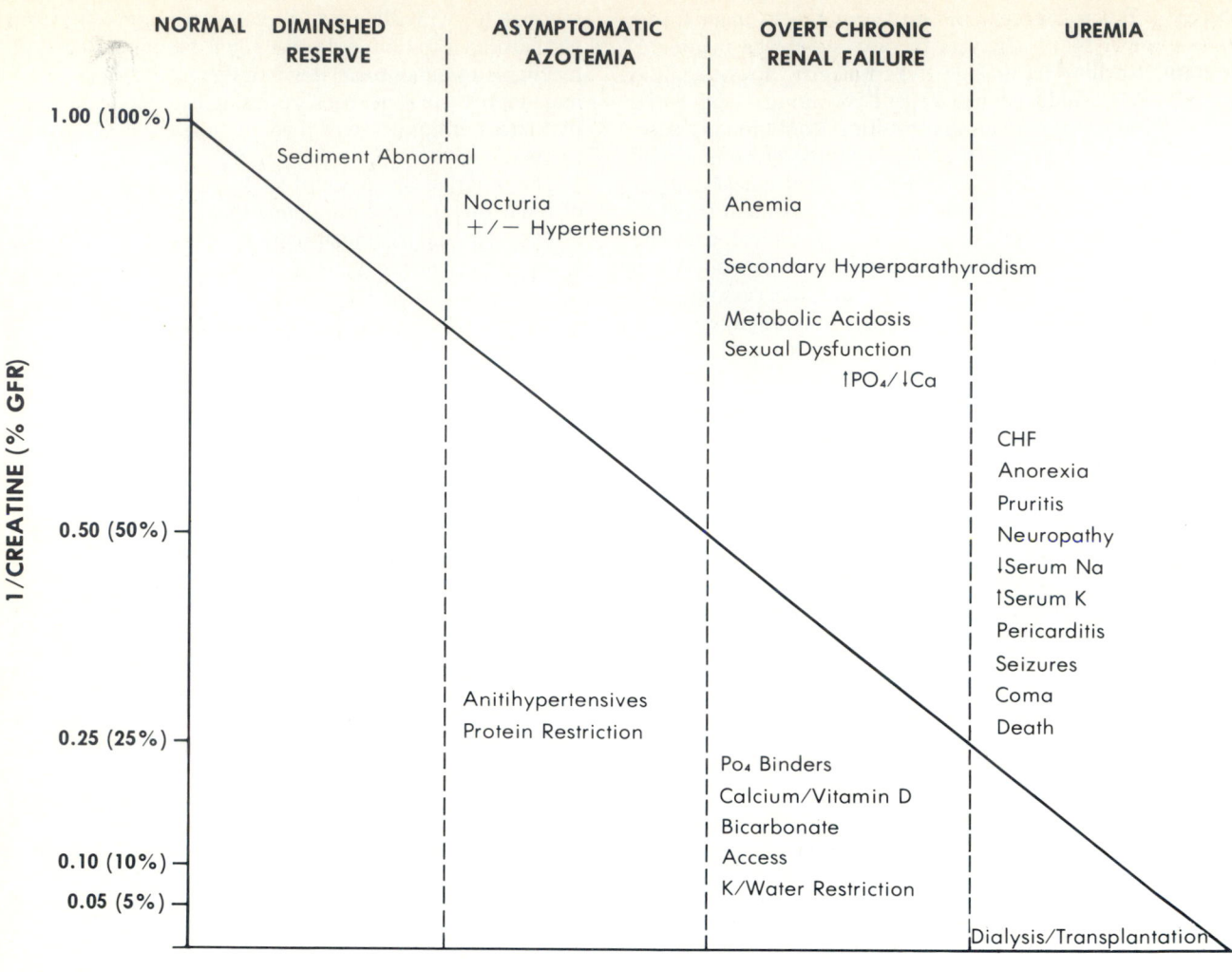

Fig. 111-1   Schema of course of chronic renal failure.

looks the same and the end-stage kidney usually is shrunken with a histologic appearance of hyalinized or sclerotic glomeruli, with a reduced number of dilated tubules separated by interstitial scar tissue.

The rate at which renal function deteriorates and the patient evolves through the four overlapping clinical stages—diminished renal reserve, asymptomatic azotemia, overt CRF, and uremia—varies considerably, depending on the different underlying disease processes. Moreover, different individuals with the same diagnosis may have dramatically different courses. However, it has been observed that in a given patient, the rate of decline usually is predictable. (For many there is a linear fall-off in GFR with time. Since the nitrogenous waste creatinine is excreted predominantly by glomerular filtration, the endogenous creatinine clearance [expressed as the amount of creatinine excreted in the urine per unit time divided by the serum creatinine] approximates the GFR. In steady states an individual's excretion of creatinine per unit time should be relatively constant; hence the estimated GFR should be proportional to 1/serum creatinine. Thus over the course of CRF in a given patient, a linear down slope of 1/creatinine versus time frequently can be plotted. In other patients a plot of log creatinine versus time gives a better linear correlation.)

Although many of the original insults to the kidney from disease processes may be long-term problems and may contribute to the progressive loss of renal function over protracted periods, in other situations the injurious process or toxic exposure can be attenuated or removed. Nevertheless, it has become perplexingly obvious that once a certain undefined critical renal mass has been damaged, frequently the remaining mass and function inexorably decline, even if the original insult is eliminated. In attempts to explain this progression, other factors have been explored. Little evidence supports the hypothesis that early structural damage in the kidney releases tissue components that then trigger a secondary and ongoing autoimmune injury to the kidney. The observed tissue deposition of calcium-phosphate salts in CRF has been suggested as another ongoing physical injury to the sick kidney. Uncontrolled hypertension has been documented in human and animal studies to affect dramatically the rate of progression of a variety of renal diseases. Interestingly, high protein intake accelerates the structural and functional deterioration in a variety of animal models of renal failure, whereas reduction of protein intake can retard this progression. Recent studies of modulation of protein intake in human renal failure also suggest the important role of protein as a factor modulating the course of chronic renal disease. The mechanisms underlying the modifying effects of protein intake and hypertension have not been completely unraveled but may be linked to alterations in intrarenal hemodynamics. Laboratory investigation over the past decade has demonstrated that with renal injury or ablation, surviving nephrons undergo structural and functional hypertrophy, which underlies some of the homeostatic adaptations of the kidney as a whole in CRF. These adaptations include relative vasodilation in the microcirculation of functioning glomeruli, allowing for greater intraglomerular perfusion pressures that can augment the remnant nephrons' GFR. Teleologically, this compensates for the loss of filtration from drop out of other units or loss of filtering surface in diseased glomeruli and thus helps in the short term to preserve overall GFR. However, in the long run the resultant "barotrauma" of heightened intracapillary pressure in glomeruli may extend glomerular damage, and experimental reduction of intraglomerular capillary pressures has slowed the progression of renal disease in animal models of renal failure. These reductions have been accomplished precisely through modulation of such factors as systemic hypertension and protein intake. The implication that seems to be emerging from the experimental and clinical observations is that renal failure can progress independently of the initiating insults. Chronic renal injury then is a snowballing phenomenon, with compensating adaptive mechanisms that are increasingly recruited, but which ultimately extend renal damage and prove maladaptive.

PATHOPHYSIOLOGY AND PATHOGENESIS. As noted previously, during the course of CRF the normal body internal milieu is progressively deranged, leading ultimately to alteration of cellular and organ functions. The departure from normal homeostasis and body composition occurs gradually in the continuum from asymptomatic renal disease to uremia and is characterized by retention of nitrogenous wastes, renal biosynthetic and biodegradative failure, and alterations in fluid and electrolyte handling.

Nitrogenous wastes. The term "uremia" stresses the view that retained nitrogenous waste compounds generated from dietary and endogenous protein catabolism, which normally are eliminated in the urine, are the "toxins" accounting for the uremic syndrome. Clearly their accumulation precedes the multiple-system breakdown of uremia, and reducing the body pools of nitrogenous waste with dietary therapy or dialysis attenuates the symptoms of uremia. The list of compounds that have been incriminated as uremic toxins is long and includes: urea, guanidinium compounds, aromatic compounds, aliphatic amines, peptides, and "middle molecules." Routinely the only compounds measured clinically are the blood urea nitrogen (BUN) and the creatinine. The rate of accumulation of the various substances varies with different rates of production and excretion, the latter fluctuating with both variable renal and nonrenal clearances.

Urea is quantitatively the most abundant of the products of protein degradation, accounting for 85% of the excreted urinary nitrogen, and historically was incriminated as the first toxin. Except at very high concentrations that have been produced in experimental situations, urea produces only subtle symptoms of headache and malaise, and in patients uremic symptoms have been relieved without changing the BUN level. In addition, the BUN is a relatively poor marker of endogenous GFR, because its clearance is also modified by variable reabsorption by the kidney after its filtration and because of the highly variable production rate relating to protein intake, gastrointestinal blood loss, and catabolic stresses. The production rate of creatinine, which is the by-product of the pool of muscle creatine, is more constant, because muscle mass changes only gradually. Its frequent use as the endogenous marker of GFR suffers mainly from changes in nonrenal elimination with time

and variable tubular secretion by the kidney. Moreover, there is no overt evidence that creatinine itself is a toxic compound. The role of elevated levels of uric acid in CRF has been denigrated by the consensus that uric acid alone does not seem to be nephrotoxic. Experimental evidence is stronger that guanidine and its metabolic derivatives are more important uremic toxins and that these compounds have been linked to some of the neurologic, gastrointestinal, and hematologic disturbances noted in uremic patients. Similarly, the experimental toxicology of various polyamines that are aliphatic, cationic nitrogenous molecules such as spermine and spermidine, with their specific effects on cell membrane transport functions, seems to mimic some of the clinical and biochemical characteristics of uremia.

Much of the hunt for the elusive uremic toxins in the past decade has focused on "middle molecules," apparent peptides with molecular weights ranging from 300 to 2000. Their in vitro toxicity and the purported different impacts on uremia of dialytic techniques with different middle molecule clearance, have lent credence to their significance as uremic toxins. However, they remain poorly purified and characterized biochemically, and as with the host of other purported uremic toxins have not definitively satisfied "Koch's postulates" as the "pathogens" in CRF.

Biosynthetic and degradative failure. Beyond its excretory role, the kidney is an important endocrine organ, being the major physiologic source of erythropoietin and 1,25 dihydroxy-vitamin D. Erythropoietin is the prime humoral stimulator of erythropoiesis in the bone marrow, and the progressive anemia of CRF is related to the relative lack of erythropoietin in the setting of progressive loss of renal mass. 1,25 Dihydroxyvitamin D is the renal hydroxylation product of the hepatic precursor 25 hydroxyvitamin D and is intimately involved in calcium homeostasis. The absolute deficiency of this hormone in CRF is one cause of the altered calcium balance. Biosynthetic deficiency as renal disease progresses also is reflected in other areas such as acid-base balance, in which diminished renal production of ammonia, the major urinary buffer, ultimately limits net acid excretion and in carbohydrate metabolism, in which the lack of renal contribution to gluconeogenesis can contribute to the increased susceptibility of CRF patients to hypoglycemia in the setting of prolonged fasting.

Aside from the renal clearance of relatively small solutes, the kidneys bind and metabolize a variety of peptides, including hormones such as insulin, prolactin, and growth hormone, and in CRF altered levels of these compounds may be involved in the endocrinologic and metabolic derangements that develop. Exogenous compounds (drugs) as well may have altered pharmacokinetics not only in the face of diminished GFR but also as a result of altered tubular secretion, metabolism, and protein binding.

Alterations in fluid and electrolyte handling. The critical role of the kidneys in regulating the excretion of water and electrolytes is maintained in the face of progressive renal damage. However, the physiologic strategies differ from those of normal kidneys, and the range over which external balance can be maintained is inexorably narrowed until the excretory function no longer can keep pace with even the basal body needs. Moreover, some of the mechanisms employed to allow the kidney to maintain steady-state conditions may prove deleterious in other respects, further paving the road to uremia.

Water. The kidneys normally can defend against the dilution of the solute content of body fluids by excreting up to 30 L/day of very dilute urine and can maintain water balance in the face of relative water deprivation by excreting the daily solute load in a highly concentrated urine. One of the earliest functional defects with structural renal disease is impairment of the urinary concentrating mechanism, accounting for patients' complaints of polyuria and nocturia. This defect also makes patients with renal failure susceptible to dehydration and hypernatremia if they lose access to fluids, as with overzealous fluid restriction in the hospital. Later in the progression of their disease, renal patients lose the ability to maximally dilute the urine, and the ability to excrete water loads and defend against hyponatremia falls off progressively with loss of GFR. The urine tends to be isosthenuric. Estimating a daily solute excretion rate of 600 mOsm, urinary output becomes locked in at around 2 L/day.

Salt. The kidneys help maintain relative constancy of the size of the extracellular fluid (ECF) compartment by regulating the external balance of sodium chloride, the major determinant of the ECF volume. To maintain salt balance over a wide range of salt intake, the renal excretion of sodium chloride also must vary despite relative constancy of the amount of sodium chloride filtered. Thus depending on intake the fraction of filtered sodium that is excreted can vary from less than 0.1% to more than 20% (less than 20 mEq/day to 400 mEq/day). As GFR gradually declines in the course of CRF, the patient's fractional excretion of sodium must progressively increase to stay in balance at constant sodium intake. The mechanisms allowing for higher fractional excretion of sodium at a given intake and a given ECF size are not completely understood, but they may involve humoral mechanisms that not only influence renal sodium excretion but that ultimately also alter sodium handling across cell membranes of other tissues. The resultant maladaptive transcellular cation distributions are thought to play a pathologic role in neuromuscular and vascular dysfunction of uremia. Moreover, in the steady-state condition of CRF, the kidneys' ability to rapidly augment or reduce the excretion of sodium in response to sudden increases or decreases in salt intake is dramatically slowed. Thus patients are more susceptible to salt and volume overload with sudden increases in the salt intake, but they also are subject to salt depletion and volume contraction when dietary sodium is suddenly diminished. In advanced renal failure, fractional excretion of sodium ultimately can't keep pace with even normal intake, and to prevent complications of ECF expansion such as hypertension, congestive heart failure (CHF), or severe edema, dietary sodium must be restricted and potent loop diuretics prescribed to try to further augment fractional excretion. Some chronic renal diseases, especially those causing early and severe medullary structural damage, are characterized for most of their course by a distinct inability to conserve sodium, and in these salt-wasting patients particular care must be taken to avoid salt depletion and volume contraction, which can lower blood pressure and renal blood flow and further impair glomerular filtration.

Potassium. Renal excretion of potassium, again the major control point for external potassium homeostasis, depends not so much on glomerular filtration and the degree of tubular reabsorption of filtered potassium as on secretion in distal portions of the nephron. Distal potassium secretion primarily depends on adequate urinary flow and sodium delivery to these sites. Thus external potassium balance usually is rather well defended until the very late stages of CRF, when markedly diminishing urinary output limits excretion. Once again, however, throughout their course the patient's ability to excrete acute loads of potassium intake is limited. Moreover, the patient is very susceptible to developing hyperkalemia when urinary flow is suddenly diminished in the face of volume depletion or hypotension. Similarly, the patient may be very sensitive

to drugs that can interfere with mechanisms of distal potassium secretion. Nonsteroidal antiinflammatory drugs and converting enzyme inhibitors can interrupt adequate aldosterone generation, whereas "potassium-sparing" diuretics such as spironolactone and amiloride are dangerous because they directly affect distal tubular potassium secretion. Some patients with chronic tubulointerstitial renal disease, especially those with diabetes, may develop problems with hyperkalemia much earlier in the course of their renal disease. They appear to have either a relative lack of aldosterone or distal tubular unresponsiveness to mineralocorticoid, which prevents adequate distal tubular secretion of potassium even with preserved distal urine flow. All these potential and inevitable problems in maintaining external potassium balance in CRF are exacerbated by derangements of internal potassium homeostasis. Altered cell membrane $Na^+ - K^+$ ATPase activity does not allow for the normal active cellular uptake of potassium and extrusion of sodium, and this maldistribution of extracellular/intracellular potassium may be accentuated by acidemia, insulin deficiency (diabetes), lack of aldosterone, and drugs such as β-blocking agents (which interfere with catecholamine-mediated cellular potassium uptake). In fact, total body potassium is depleted in many CRF patients in the face of anorexia and poor oral intake. The combination of extracellular hyperkalemia and intracellular potassium depletion alters transmembrane electrical potentials and basic cell physiology. Clinically, this manifests most noticeably as neuromuscular dysfunction, contributing to symptoms of muscle weakness, gastrointestinal dysfunction, and most ominously to cardiac arrhythmias.

Acid-base balance. Normal metabolism generates volatile acids (excreted as CO_2 via the lungs) and nonvolatile acids, both organic and inorganic, which are handled by the kidneys. The anions of these fixed acids are filtered (and to a certain extent secreted) and excreted in the urine while the distal parts of the nephrons secrete hydrogen ions into the urine, where they are buffered and carried out in the form of ammonium and titrated phosphates. The process of distal hydrogen ion secretion generates bicarbonate back into the circulation to replenish the base that was consumed by the initial acid production. In basal states these functions balance the production and excretion of 50 to 100 mEq/day of acid and can be stimulated to excrete several hundred milliequivalents per day by increasing ammonia buffer production in the urine and the rate of distal proton secretion. An important feature is that renal proximal tubules reabsorb the filtered load of bicarbonate to prevent base depletion, handling quantitatively a much heavier acid-base traffic of about 4500 mEq/day. In most renal diseases the remaining functional distal tubular proton secretion can continue to generate a highly acid urine (pH less than 5.5), but the absolute acid elimination is limited by the overall deficiency in net ammonia production. The adaptive increases in urinary acidification and ammonia production by individually functioning nephrons usually offset the intrinsic defects so that metabolic acidosis with a fall in serum bicarbonate is not usually apparent until GFR is less than 30% to 40% of normal. Increases in net acid production (for example, with diarrhea, when bicarbonate is lost from the body and must be regenerated by increased distal acid excretion), however, may unmask the tendency toward metabolic acidosis. As with potassium handling, diseases that early on impair distal tubular function may result in an earlier expression of metabolic acidosis. There also is some controversy as to whether proximal tubular bicarbonate reabsorption is defective, which would result in further base deficit. The accumulation of the anions of the fixed acids caused by reduced elimination by glomerular filtration tends to become noticeable as the GFR falls below 30% of normal, resulting in a rise in the serum level of these unmeasured anions. Thus as renal function deteriorates, there is a discordant failure of excretion of anions of fixed acid and distal tubular proton elimination, resulting in variable combinations of nonanion-gap (hyperchloremic) and high anion-gap metabolic acidosis. Interestingly, despite continued positive acid balance in CRF, it is unusual to see the serum bicarbonate fall much below 12 to 14 mEq/L, implying the recruitment of body buffer stores to prevent further titration of bicarbonate. Bone dissolution has been hypothesized as the reservoir for this base, an adaptation with conceivably adverse effects on skeletal physiology and structure. Aside from the deleterious effects on bone, the acidemia of CRF presumably alters intracellular pH of other tissues and ultimately plays a role in organ dysfunction of uremia.

Divalent ions. Renal function is central to the physiology of calcium, magnesium, and phosphate, all most abundant in the bone, where they make up the major mineral backbone of the skeleton. The small amount of extraskeletal phosphate is found predominantly inside cells, where it is a major intracellular anion and a substrate for high-energy phosphate intermediates of metabolism and phosphorylated proteins. The external balance of phosphate in the body is maintained by matching its renal excretion (by filtration and variable reabsorption along the nephron) to dietary intake. In renal failure, as filtration of phosphate progressively falls, a normal overall rate of excretion is maintained by suppression of tubular reabsorption, mediated by a feedback loop involving parathyroid hormone (PTH). Any slight rise in serum phosphate concentration tends to lower, through physical interaction, serum ionized calcium, which is a potent stimulus for PTH secretion. The augmented PTH effect on remaining kidney function blunts renal phosphate reabsorption, allowing for greater fractional excretion of phosphate. Ultimately, when GFR falls below 20% to 30% of normal, the augmented PTH effect cannot maintain enough phosphate elimination and frank hyperphosphatemia with the attendant depression of ionized calcium becomes apparent. Thus parathyroid overactivity is a hallmark of CRF, but this adaptation to maintain extracellular calcium and phosphate in physiologic range may have a far-reaching impact on bone and possibly other functions. The hyperparathyroid milieu in CRF has been suggested to contribute to altered nerve conduction, red blood cell membrane instability, diminished insulin release, altered platelet function, hypertension, myocardial dysfunction, peripheral myopathy, and soft tissue calcium deposition. Thus the body's attempt to maintain physiologic calcium concentration through secondary hyperparathyroidism is a "trade-off" against a host of other possible problems.

The development of hypocalcemia is abetted by inadequate gastrointestinal calcium absorption resulting from the deficiency of 1,25 dihydroxyvitamin D, the most potent vitamin D metabolite for bone mineralization and gastrointestinal calcium absorption. As previously noted, as renal mass is lost to the scarring of CRF, the metabolic capacity of 1-hydroxylation of the 25 hydroxyvitamin D is lost. High circulating levels of PTH help to stimulate the remnant hydroxylase activity in the kidney, whereas hyperphosphatemia late in renal failure blunts the hydroxylase activity. The absolute deficiency of 1,25 dihydroxyvitamin D in CRF not only contributes to hypocalcemia by reducing gut calcium absorption, it also may blunt the calcemic response of bone to PTH. On the other hand, there is evidence that low 1,25 dihydroxyvitamin D levels may decrease the sensitivity of parathyroid glands to calcium, further exacerbating the hyperparathyroidism of CRF. This crucial vitamin D metabolite also may have important effects directly on muscle, and its lack may contribute to uremic myopathy.

Magnesium absorption from the gut is less dependent on vitamin D, but its overall balance does depend on renal excretion. Thus hypermagnesemia can occur in CRF, especially if magnesium-containing antacids or laxatives are ingested frequently. With severe hypermagnesemia, dangerous neuromuscular depression and cardiac arrhythmias can occur.

The pathophysiology of uremia thus should be viewed not only as a result of the accumulation of nitrogenous wastes but also as the consequence of adaptive physiologic trade-offs that the body makes to try to maintain a constant environment. Ultimately, electrolyte homeostasis does break down with further changes in body fluid composition. Not only does the ECF expand with salt retention, impairment of critical membrane functions allows for changes in the intracellular fluid compartment and alterations of neuromuscular activity. Although the intracellular fluid compartment may be expanded along with total body water, total body potassium, along with actual lean body mass and nitrogen stores, are diminished. Energy utilization becomes inefficient in uremia, and basal body temperature may be low. Basic nitrogen, carbohydrate, and fat metabolism may be altered, and a state akin to protein malnutrition may exist. With these changes in extracellular and intracellular composition and impaired membrane and cellular metabolic activities, the multiple-system dysfunction of uremia inevitably manifests clinically.

CLINICAL MANIFESTATIONS OF UREMIC SYNDROME. Whereas clinically silent renal damage and later overt azotemia may leave the CRF patient asymptomatic for years, when GFR falls below 5 to 10 ml/min, symptoms develop. The patient's complaints are not pathognomonic for renal failure. Uremic syndrome, then, is a constellation of signs and symptoms in the patient with advanced renal failure highlighted by generalized malaise and fatigue. These signs and symptoms are described below in an organ system approach.

Integumentary system. The sallow appearance of uremic patients is likely a result of pallor from the underlying anemia and deposition of accumulated poorly defined pigments. The skin is dry, and there may be ecchymoses resulting from bleeding tendencies. Excoriations underscore the patient's complaints of intense pruritus, which has questionably been attributed to calcium and phosphate deposition in the skin and high circulating PTH levels. In advanced uremia a white, powdery uremic "frost" may evaporate on the skin surface with a fishy ammoniacal odor. The patient frequently complains of brittle nails, and oncholysis may be prominent.

Cardiovascular system. Hypertension develops during the course of CRF in 90% of patients. Ultimately it can be related to overt sodium overload and ECF expansion, but even before this stage inappropriate renin-angiotensin homeostasis and altered volume/vascular tone relationships play a role. The hypertension of CRF undoubtedly contributes to other problems, including the development of cardiomyopathy, accelerated atherogenesis, and the progression of the renal failure itself.

Pericarditis may occur in the uremic patient as a late manifestation. In the predialytic era, this heralded imminent mortality. Commonly the pericarditis appears as pleuritic chest pain with a friction rub and fever on examination, often with a leukocytosis and compatible electrocardiogram (ECG) changes on laboratory investigation. A chest roentgenogram shows cardiac enlargement, and an echocardiogram reveals a pericardial effusion. Routine use of ultrasound, moreover, frequently reveals pericardial effusions in CRF patients without symptoms of pericarditis. In rare cases the patient develops cardiac tamponade as a result of the build-up of pericardial fluid or sudden hemorrhage into the effusion.

Uremia is a state of accelerated atherogenesis, although it is hard to separate individual etiologic factors such as hypertension and hyperlipidemia. Cardiovascular complications remain a major source of mortality in the CRF population. In rare cases the CRF patient (more commonly late in the course while already on dialysis) develops digital ulcerations and infarctions (calciphylaxis) related to severe small vessel arteriosclerosis and calcification, thought to be abetted by the state of hyperparathyroidism.

Pulmonary system. Pleurisy, with its associated chest pain, fever, pleural rub, and effusion, may be another representation of the generalized serositis that occurs in uremia. It is manifested less frequently and often concurrently with pericarditis. "Uremic lung," a butterfly-shaped pulmonary infiltrate on chest roentgenogram associated with dyspnea and hypoxemia, is another controversial entity in terms of its uniqueness in the uremic milieu. It may simply be a manifestation of congestive heart failure in the uremic patient with fluid overload and left ventricular dysfunction. However, there may be a leaky capillary syndrome in uremia. Pulmonary calcification, another soft tissue consequence of altered calcium/phosphate homeostasis, may occasionally be seen on chest roentgenogram in CRF patients or may show up more impressively on technetium bone scanning. These deposits may be asymptomatic or may result in impaired oxygen exchange and restrictive pulmonary function.

Gastrointestinal system. Anorexia and nausea become progressively more frequent complaints as a patient becomes uremic. Frequently morning nausea is most prominent, and the patient notes a specific aversion to meat. There is an increased incidence of gastrointestinal bleeding in CRF patients, and the frequent finding of gastritis, duodenitis, and even colitis may reflect generalized mucosal damage in uremia. The incidence of frank peptic ulceration is not clearly increased nor is there augmented gastric acid production in CRF, although circulating gastrin levels are high. The recently noted increased incidence of gastrointestinal angiodysplasias in CRF patients likely contributes to their gastrointestinal blood loss. Liver disease is not a specific consequence of CRF, although the liver may be involved by diseases affecting the kidney (for example, polycystic kidney disease) or may be injured by drugs or transfusions used in treating the renal condition and the complications of CRF. The frequently elevated serum amylase and lipase levels in CRF patients are of unclear clinical significance.

Hematologic system. Once the GFR is less than 40% to 50% normal, a normocytic normochromic anemia predictably develops, the severity of which progressively parallels the course of the renal decline. A nadir hemoglobin as low as 6 to 7 gm/dl usually is reached in ESRD. A blood smear may show corrugated erythrocytes (burr cells). Typically, iron stores are normal on bone marrow biopsy, as reflected by normal to high serum ferritin levels, with variable iron levels and low transferin concentrations, as in other chronic disease states. The reticulocyte count is inappropriately low, and the bone marrow appearance is nonspecific, usually normocellular or occasionally hypocellular. The major etiologic factor in this hypoproliferative anemia is the relative lack of erythropoietin in the face of destruction of its source of production by renal tissue, and anephric patients tend to have the most severe anemia. Erythropoietin is not completely absent, however, and other clinical and in vitro evidence suggests that a variety of purported marrow toxins in the uremic environment also blunt the erythropoietic response of the marrow. (Nevertheless, ex-

ogenous erythropoietin can completely reverse the anemia.) Exacerbating the situation is the shortened red blood cell life span in uremia, attributed to extracorpuscular toxic factors that increase the fragility of erythrocytes and impair their ability to withstand oxidative stresses. The ongoing mild extravascular hemolysis may be exacerbated by drugs with a high oxidative potential, microangiopathy of malignant hypertension, development of hypersplenism, hypophosphatemia from overaggressive medical therapy, and accidental physical stresses imposed by faulty dialysis, a treatment that usually ameliorates the anemia to a mild degree. Superimposed on these problems may be the development of iron deficiency in the face of gastrointestinal bleeding or nutritional or dialysis-related folate deficiency. Some CRF patients, in particular those with PCKD, maintain fairly normal hematocrits as their disease progresses, likely related to higher erythropoietin production from their kidneys. The frank polycythemia that occasionally develops with CRF also has been linked to the recently recognized polycystic degeneration of end-stage kidneys.

Although the peripheral white blood count and marrow production are normal in CRF, in vitro demonstrations of chemotactic and phagocytic defects in granulocytes in the uremic environment are implicated in the increased susceptibility to and mortality from infections in patients with renal failure. The altered granulocyte function occurs despite relatively normal complement and immunoglobulin levels, although specific humoral antibody production may be blunted in uremia, as evidenced by subnormal response to vaccines. This alteration in B-lymphocyte function may be more a reflection of altered T-lymphocyte responsiveness, as suggested by the lymphopenia in CRF, the frequency of anergy, and impaired in vitro mitogen responsiveness of T cells.

Despite relatively normal clotting factor concentrations and normal prothrombin time, partial thromboplastin time, and platelet counts, hemostasis is impaired in late CRF as a result of platelet dysfunction. The decreased in vitro adhesivensss and aggregability in response to adenosine diphosphate (ADP) and the decreased release of platelet factor 3 are reflected in vivo by prolonged bleeding times. Certain nitrogenous compounds have shown in vitro platelet toxicity, and the roles of altered prostaglandin-thromboxane production, abnormal factor 8 component biochemistry, and elevated levels of PTH in relation to the platelet dsyfunction and bleeding diathesis have yet to be fully defined.

Renal osteodystrophy. Renal osteodystrophy classically refers to the spectrum of bone disease that occurs in CRF patients both before and after starting dialysis. Bone biopsy with dynamic tetracycline labeling demonstrates an overlapping range of abnormalities in up to 90% of patients. The spectrum encompasses osteitis fibrosa (OF), characterized by increased osteoclastic bone reabsorption and marrow fibrosis associated with normal mineralization; osteomalacia (OM), characterized by increased osteoid, impaired mineralization, decreased osteoclastic activity, and absent marrow fibrosis; and aplastic or adynamic bone, characterized by generalized decrease in cellular activity in bone without excess osteoid or marrow fibrosis. Most commonly a mixture of OF and OM is seen, usually with a predominance of OF. Superimposed on the morphologic abnormalities may be increased or decreased bone mass, resulting roentgenographically in osteosclerosis or osteopenia, respectively. Etiologically, the abnormal mineral metabolism and hormonal responses outlined above are felt to be most influential, and the potential impact of chronic acidosis on bone physiology also is alluded to. Ironically, over the last decade evidence has mounted indicating that the zealous use of aluminum hydroxide as an enteral phosphate binder to prevent hyperphosphatemia and the ensuing secondary hyperparathyroidism can itself result in the toxic accumulation of aluminum in bone, generating a debilitating form of osteomalacia. The clinical correlates of these different pathologic manifestations of metabolic bone disease in CRF usually are not sufficiently diagnostic or specific to differentiate the various histologic and pathophysiologic processes. Biochemical abnormalities are seen in more than 70% of patients. Serum calcium usually is low but may be frankly elevated in severe OF or in patients with aluminum OM or those overtreated with vitamin D supplements. Alkaline phosphatase tends to be higher in those patients with OF, as do aminoterminal PTH levels, but significant overlap occurs. Screening serum aluminum levels, which generally are high in CRF, does not differentiate patients with aluminum bone toxicity. Rather, mobilization tests with chelating agents may unmask the patients with aluminum toxicity. Bone histology and special staining most reliably sort out the underlying pathology and the extent of the osseous aluminum accumulation. Depending on how diligently it is sought, roentgenographic evidence of the underlying metabolic diseases can be delineated in more than 50% of late-stage patients. The subperiosteal reabsorption of cortical bone seen in fingers, clavicles, and the lamina dura of the mandible and "brown tumors" are suggestive but not diagnostic of OF. The "rugger-jersey" spine reflecting the cortical sclerosis of the vertebral bodies is a characteristic finding in CRF patients.

Overt symptoms of the bone disease such as pain and fractures may manifest in a few patients. Hypercalcemic complications may develop in severely hyperparathyroid, aluminum toxic, or vitamin D–overdosed patients. Other patients may be plagued by problems frequently included under the rubric of renal osteodystrophy. Pruritus, severe vascular calcification with digital necrosis (calciphylaxis), proximal myopathies, metastatic calcification in periarticular locations and joints with chondrocalcinosis, and possibly metastatic calcification in visceral tissues such as myocardium, lung, and the kidney itself have been linked to the abnormal humoral and mineral milieu of CRF. Excess PTH may play a role in the neurotoxicity and anemia of CRF, whereas CNS aluminum accumulation can cause a progressive fatal dementing illness in CRF patients. Thus slowly progressive renal osteodystrophy has a far-ranging impact in uremia. Other rheumatologic problems also may occur more frequently in CRF patients, such as pseudogout from calcium pyrophosphate crystal deposition, synovitis attributed to hydroxyapatite or calcium oxalate crystals, and carpal tunnel syndrome caused by amyloid deposition composed of β_2-microglobulin. However, the incidence of gout does not seem increased despite an almost universal development of hyperuricemia as renal function deteriorates.

Neurologic system. Systemic diseases that lead to CRF also may damage the central and peripheral nervous systems. Thus early on a patient may suffer from the autonomic neuropathy of amyloid, the symmetric polyneuropathy of diabetes, or vasculitic mononeuropathies and cerebritis. Typically, however, all patients with CRF develop central and peripheral neurologic signs and symptoms as they become uremic. The peripheral neuropathy manifests most commonly as a symmetric sensory stocking-glove polyneuropathy similar to that in diabetes. Early on nerve conduction tests may detect slowing, and later, in untreated patients, frank motor weakness may develop, leading to footdrop and wristdrop. Characteristically, however, patients complain of cramps, "burning feet," or "restless legs." Subtle central nervous dysfunction may manifest as restlessness, irritability, and changes in sleep pattern, and the electroencephalogram (EEG) may show slowing changes compatible with metabolic encephalopathy. Cognitive function becomes impaired, with forgetfulness and inability to perform mental tasks. Ultimately confusion, disorientation, and lethary develop, along with asterixis and myoclonus. Encephalopathy progresses in the end-stage to stupor, coma, and/or seizures. As for other manifestations of CRF, the search for the uremic neurotoxin continues, with considerable attention given to the possibility of false neurotransmitters, middle molecules, and effects of excess PTH.

Endocrine-metabolic system. CRF is a state of carbohydrate intolerance with peripheral insulin resistance resulting from impaired insulin binding to target tissues, as well as postreceptor defects. Although similar to that in patients with type II diabetes, the glucose intolerance is not as severe and hypoglycemic therapy rarely is indicated. Somewhat paradoxically, patients with insulin-dependent diabetes with progressive renal failure frequently note a diminished need for exogenous insulin, likely related to decreased intake and the prolonged biologic half-life of both exogenous and endogenous insulin, which is metabolized by the kidneys. In diabetic patients, hemoglobin AIc monitoring can be misleading, because in azotemia carbamylated hemoglobin can interfere with the electrophoresis. In addition to altered carbohydrate homeostasis, uremic patients characteristically demonstrate hypertriglyceridemia with elevated levels of very-low-density lipoprotein, attributed to diminished peripheral lipoprotein lipase activity. Finally, although the intracellular mechanisms have not been elucidated, protein metabolism in uremia is altered and abnormal extracellular amino acid patterns are seen. Some investigators have likened uremia to a state of functional malnutrition.

Some of the clinical features of uremia suggest a diagnosis of hypothyroidism. In fact, there is an increased incidence of goiter in CRF patients, and total thyroxine and especially triiodothyronine values may be low. The relatively normal free T_4 and thyroid-stimulating hormone levels, along with high reverse T_3 levels and low free T_3 levels, are more consistent with the "sick euthyroidism" seen in other chronic illnesses.

Most bothersome to uremic patients is the almost inevitable sexual dysfunction that occurs. Men complain of diminished libido and erectile impotence and frequently are found to have testicular atrophy with altered histology, low testosterone levels, and oligospermia or azoospermia. Some develop gynecomastia. Although primary gonadal failure is implied, hypothalamic-pituitary dysfunction also is suggested by high but still inappropriate gonadotropin levels. While the psychologic factors of chronic illness and the physical effects of vascular disease, neuropathy, and medications no doubt play a role, the uremic male's sexual dysfunction has been linked alternatively to zinc deficiency and hyperprolactinemia. Thus supplemental zinc therapy in some and bromocriptine use in others have been reported to improve sexual function in impotent uremic men. Similar abnormalities may contribute to the complicated web of deranged reproductive endocrinology in azotemic women, who commonly become infertile with or without oligomenorrhea or amenorrhea. These women manifest a combination of ovarian failure with low normal estrogen and progesterone production and altered central hypothalamic-pituitary function, with disproportionate changes in leutinizing hormone (LH) and folicle-stimulating hormone levels, along with impaired feedback control by estrogen on LH secretion. Although it is rare for a woman with advanced CRF to conceive, contraception must be considered for those still menstruating, although both IUDs and hormonal manipulation are less than desirable in hypertensive patients prone to infection. Although anovulatory cycles and menstrual irregularity appear late in renal disease, even in asymptomatic stages of chronic renal disease, with a GFR less than 30% normal, it is unusual for pregnant women to carry a gestation successfully, with extremely high rates of fetal wastage and maternal complications. Patients with GFR between 30% to 60% of normal (creatinine 1.5 to 2.5 mg/dl) may have a successful pregnancy, but up to a third of mothers suffer deterioration of renal function and worsening of their hypertension. Women with chronic renal disease but with preserved GFR (creatinine less than 1.5 mg/dl) who are managed in high-risk clinics under meticulous obstetric and medical supervision with highly controlled blood pressure have excellent gestational results, but with increased incidences of prematurity in the infants and frequent transient worsening of their proteinuria, along with an increased risk of toxemia of pregnancy.

Approach to the patient with CRF

Diagnosis. When confronted with newly discovered symptomatic or asymptomatic azotemia in a patient, the practitioner must differentiate between acute and chronic renal failure. Observation over several days establishes whether a patient is in a steady-state condition consistent with chronic disease, whereas oliguria with progressive derangement of fluid and electrolyte balance and rising creatinine levels denote acute renal failure. Detective work may uncover crucial historical information documenting evidence of previous renal disease. With advanced CRF it is suspicious not to find the patient anemic with at least biochemical if not roentgenographic evidence of renal osteodystrophy. Small kidney size also is suggestive of chronic renal scarring. Even with chronic disease, a diligent search for exacerbating factors that could cause further acute reversible deterioration in renal function should be made. In this sense it is useful to follow the 1/creatinine-versus-time curve to detect unexpected deviations from the extrapolated linear relationship that might signal a new acute insult superimposed on the chronic process. Thus the history and physical examination should be aimed at screening for evidence of "prerenal failure" secondary to volume depletion or diminished cardiac output, "postrenal failure" from urinary obstruction, and toxic effects of drugs leading to acute tubular necrosis (ATN) or parenchymal hypersensitivity reactions.

A thorough history and physical examination also may elucidate the nature of the underlying chronic renal disease. The practitioner should focus on evidence for systemic illness (such as diabetes, vasculitis, or connective tissue disorders), vascular disease (that is, hypertension), urologic disease, family history of renal disease, and chronic drug or toxin exposure (for example, lead or analgesics). The urinalysis may point to a primary glomerulopathy or tubulointerstitial process. Routine laboratory tests should assess the degree of anemia, the concentration of extracellular electrolytes, and acid-base status, and derangement in calcium/phosphate metabolism, as well as screen for the presence of any associated liver disease or gammopathies. Further blood tests usually are dictated by the physical examination and historical findings. Roentgenographic flat plates of the abdomen may detect stones or nephrocalcinosis, and ultrasound can rule out obstruction and assess kidney size. Contrast studies, such as an intravenous pyelogram, can delineate calyceal deformity and parenchymal scarring of chronic pyelonephritis and the papillary necrosis seen in diabetics and

sickle cell patients, but frequently it can add little to the clinical information and should not be routinely undertaken, especially because of the greater likelihood of inducing contrast ATN in patients with underlying renal dysfunction. Arteriography rarely is helpful except when there is a strong suspicion of underlying renovascular occlusive disease compromising renal function, and it is fraught with potential nephrotoxic complications. Outside of academic investigation, renal biopsy in the setting of CRF has a limited role, especially if its aim is to potentially alter patient management. By definition, chronic renal disease implies a scarring process and usually can't be undone. Also, in advanced cases the disruption of normal kidney architecture takes on a similar appearance and biopsy may not give specific answers. Biopsy may be indicated to differentiate acute from chronic processes or to sort out the cause of a more rapid deterioration than anticipated in the course of a CRF patient. In addition, defining the nature of the underlying chronic disease process may have prognostic significance for patients, since some diseases progress more rapidly and inexorably than others and an early insight into the course of the illness may help a patient with future plans. Finally, an exact histologic diagnosis may be important in some disorders that are hereditary or that have a high propensity for recurrence after transplantation.

PREVENTING PROGRESSION. Specific measures aimed at the underlying pathologic condition may arrest progression of the renal disease. These measures may include relieving obstruction, treating hypercalcemia, correcting critical renovascular stenoses, and eradicating paraproteins in lymphoid neoplasias. Early and sustained glycemic control in patients with diabetes has been hypothesized but not proved, to prevent subsequent development of diabetic nephropathy. The role of immunosuppressive therapy and plasmapheresis to treat immunologic renal disease is discussed in other chapters.

In all situations vigilance must be maintained against superimposed volume depletion, obstruction, and toxic effects of new medications. In particular, nonsteroidal antiinflammatory drugs and nephrotoxic antibiotics must be used with great caution. Many other commonly used drugs that depend on renal excretion also accumulate if used in standard dosages, and the dose must be adjusted at different stages of CRF to avoid nonrenal toxicity. Urinary tract infections should be treated, and instrumentation (for example, use of a Foley catheter) should be avoided to prevent bacterial colonization.

Clinical application of the exciting empiric observations of the effects of protein restriction and blood pressure control on subsequent renal function deterioration will potentially alter the conservative management stance taken with patients with chronically progressing renal disease. Thus the consensus is developing that the commonly encountered hypertension of renal disease should be treated aggressively. Classically, a "stepped care" approach to antihypertensive therapy in CRF has been used, with salt restriction and diuretic therapy as the first step. Usually more potent loop diuretics are necessary once GFR is less than 50%, although synergy with thiazides such as metolazone may be needed in late renal failure with severe salt retention. The use of "central acting" agents such as α-methyldopa, clonidine, and guanabenz can be used, as in nonazotemic patients with the same modest potency and frequency of side effects. β-Blockade can be undertaken with the knowledge that the newer, longer-acting β-blocking drugs depend on renal excretion, and that maximal doses must be adjusted for renal dysfunction. Similarly, nonselective β-blocking drugs can impair extrarenal potassium uptake and contribute to hyperkalemia in patients with advanced renal failure. Vasodilator therapy, especially with the potent agent minoxidil, sometimes is required as well but may exacerbate salt retention.

Calcium channel blocking drugs offer another attractive therapeutic tool, theoretically without the adverse effects on renal blood flow and GFR associated with other agents. Finally, converting enzyme inhibition is effective and is being explored for its potentially unique intrarenal hemodynamic effects that may allow for greater reduction of intraglomerular hydrostatic pressure and a more dramatic retardation of snowballing glomerulosclerosis. Converting enzyme inhibition may become the preferred antihypertensive for CRF patients, so long as it is used cautiously so as not to exacerbate underlying tendencies toward hyperkalemia and is not used injudiciously in patients with bilateral renovascular disease.

Just as aggressive antihypertensive therapy should be initiated early, growing evidence indicates that protein restriction early in the course of progressive renal disease may attenuate the perpetuating damage from glomerular hyperfiltration. Although large-scale prospective studies are being conducted to determine how early and to what extent protein restriction may alter the course of renal failure, a conservative recommendation of limiting protein intake to 0.6 gm/kg of body weight/day can be made without impairing nutrition. Lower protein diets may be feasible but may need supplementation with essential amino acid or amino acid ketoanalogs.

TREATING SPECIFIC COMPLICATIONS. Manifestations of salt overload such as hypertension, congestive heart failure, and severe edema should be managed with dietary salt restriction and potent diuretics, usually on a twice daily schedule. Although there is still controversy over the detrimental effects of mild acidosis of CRF, most nephrologists initiate supplemental sodium bicarbonate therapy (40 to 80 mEq/day) to maintain serum bicarbonate at around 20, realizing that the added sodium load may exacerbate problems related to ECF expansion.

Dietary phosphate restriction has been pushed to try to break the triggering effect of mild hyperphosphatemia on the secondary hyperparathyroidism of renal osteodystrophy, but it is difficult to obtain diets of less than 800 mg/day without also severely limiting calcium intake. Thus over the past decade progressively earlier and more aggressive use of aluminum hydroxide phosphate–binding medications was initiated to prevent a maladaptive hyperparathyroid response. The recommendations now are tempered by the recognition of aluminum toxicity in CRF. New enteral phosphate binders are being researched, and a flurry of recent interest has centered on the use of calcium salts themselves in high doses to lower the gastrointestinal uptake of phosphate. Thus once GFR is less than 25% to 30% normal, a combination of aluminum hydroxide and calcium salts should be taken postprandially to keep serum phosphate within normal range, being careful to avoid hypophosphatemia. If serum calcium remains low with well-controlled phosphate levels, supplemental calcium should be added and the use of synthetic vitamin D metabolites, in particular 1,25 dihydroxyvitamin D, should be slowly and progressively increased to maintain serum calcium within normal limits. Again, hypercalcemia and worsening hyperphosphatemia should be screened for when using vitamin D therapy. After many years of CRF, usually when a patient is already on dialysis, severe manifestations of renal osteodystrophy related to unremitting hyperparathyroidism can be ameliorated by total parathyroidectomy with partial autotransplantation of parathyroid tissue into the subcutaneous tissue of the forearm.

In treating the progressive anemia of CRF possibilities of superimposed iron deficiency and nutritional deficiencies of folate or vitamin B_{12} should be eliminated. Hemolysis in the setting of oxidative stresses from drugs should be avoided. Excessive phlebotomy from the temptation to overzealously monitor abnormal but relatively stable blood studies must be eliminated. Androgen and synthetic androgen analogs, which are used in advanced stages of CRF, have been found to ameliorate the anemia in many patients. They do not appear effective in patients who have been nephrectomized, and their mode of interaction with circulating erythropoietin on the bone marrow is not understood. On the horizon is the use of synthetic erythropoietin to modulate the hemoglobin level in patients with CRF and other chronic anemias. Although the symptoms of chronic anemia may be hard to distinguish from the other manifestations of uremia, patients usually tolerate hemoglobin levels in the range of 6 to 8 gm/dl. Transfusional therapy, with the attendant risks of infection transmission and iron overload, should be resorted to only for disabling angina, congestive heart failure, or other clear-cut symptoms of the anemia. For uremic patients with prolonged bleeding times caused by qualitative platelet dysfunction, infusions of a synthetic vasopressin analog (DdAVP), cryoprecipitate, or conjugated estrogens have been found to reverse the coagulopathy over the short term and may be necessary with poorly controlled active bleeding or prophylactically with major surgery.

DIETARY THERAPY. Dietary salt restriction may become necessary to treat hypertension or congestive heart failure in CRF patients. However, it should not be implemented routinely, since some patients may be frank salt wasters, whereas all patients will have difficulty adjusting to very low salt intake and thus may become volume depleted if inappropriately placed on low sodium intake. Similarly, until end-stage most patients will have an obligate water requirement excreting isosthenuric urine. Thus unless the patient is hyponatremic, fluid restriction should not be enforced, although water loads of more than about 3 L/day can cause hypotonicity in patients with advanced disease. Unless patients have superimposed hypoaldosteronism, tight potassium restriction under 60 to 80 mEq/day need not be practiced until they become oliguric. Diets with phosphate of 700 to 800 mg/day should be outlined to patients by the time the GFR is about one-third normal. Protein restriction of 0.6 gm/kg/day, instituted early on, may slow progression of azotemia, whereas late in the course even more stringent protein restriction over the short-term will diminish the generation of nitrogenous wastes and lessen uremic symptoms. High caloric intake of 30 to 40 kcal/kg should be maintained throughout the course to minimize the catabolic tendency of uremic patients. With adequate nutritional intake, routine vitamin supplementation other than vitamin D metabolites usually is not needed until patients begin dialysis therapy. High-dose vitamin administration, in fact, may be deleterious with potential for vitamin A toxicity and vitamin C–exacerbated oxalosis. Similarly, overzealous iron therapy with ineffective iron utilization can hasten the development of secondary hemosiderosis.

DENTAL IMPLICATIONS IN CRF. The oral cavity may be involved by systemic diseases that also lead to CRF, but aside from the oral manifestations of renal osteodystrophy mentioned above, few oral pathologic features are related specifically to CRF. Increased incidence of stomatitis may reflect the underlying susceptibility of gastrointestinal mucosa in general in uremia. The questionably increased incidence of parotitis may be related to episodic dehydration, but there is little data on salivary gland function and oral microbiology in CRF. Dental management of these patients requires awareness of the systemic complications of CRF, which have been discussed previously. Direct contact between nephrologist and dentist can alert the dentist to relevant problems in the patient and facilitate the development of the overall dental treatment plan.

In patients on hemodialysis, dental work optimally is scheduled on the day following dialysis treatment, at the peak of patient well-being and electrolyte balance and when the anticoagulent effect of the transient heparinization of dialysis has been reversed. For oral surgical procedures and extensive periodontal surgery, a bleeding time along with the other routine coagulation screening tests should be obtained, and if significantly prolonged, postoperative bleeding problems should be anticipated with back-up availability of DdAVP or cryoprecipitate for infusion if needed. For patients on hemodialysis or peritoneal dialysis, antibiotic prophylaxis similar to that used for rheumatic fever and endocarditis prophylaxis should be employed to prevent the anachoretic infection of the dialysis access. Preoperative consultation with the nephrologist may allow for parenteral administration of the antibiotics at the time of dialysis before surgery. Information about the patient's hepatitis status is readily available from the nephrologist so that appropriate measures can be taken to avoid transmission of the disease. Altered drug pharmacokinetics in CRF requires careful review of antibiotic regimens (see Table 111-1), as well as those for analgesia and anesthesia. Standard dosages of oral penicillins commonly used for odontogenic infections are well tolerated by CRF patients, but parenteral high-dose penicillin therapy requires dose adjustment. Clindamycin and erythromycin, which are hepatically metabolized, are also used in unchanged dosages, whereas tetracycline should be avoided because of its catabolic effect. Most later-generation cephalosporin and penicillin derivatives, along with all aminoglycosides, need to be dose adjusted for the degree of renal impairment and dialytic therapy.

Among analgesics aspirin exacerbates the qualitative platelet dysfunction in advanced renal failure. Popular nonsteroidal antiinflammatory agents should be avoided in azotemic patients because of their tendency to acutely worsen GFR. This is not a consideration in patients already on dialysis, although the gastrointestinal toxicity of such agents in these patients must be feared. Most narcotics can be used without dose alteration. However, increased sensitivity to morphine from altered drug binding or accumulation of metabolites and central nervous system side effects from high-dose meperidine dictate that these agents should be used with caution in patients with advanced renal insufficiency. Since most local anesthetics are predominantly metabolized to less active forms before renal excretion, only modest dose reductions of these agents need be employed in CRF patients. In addition, there is no contraindication to the use of local vasoconstrictors. Similarly, short courses of sedative drugs such as diazepam do not require dose adjustment. The use of intravenous and inhalation anesthetic agents should be modified according to the usual anemic and hypertensive state of these patients. Regimens using short-acting barbiturates such as methohexital and narcotics such as fentanyl, along with nitrous oxide-oxygen, usually are well tolerated. Among neuromuscular agents pancuronium and gallamine should be avoided, and succinylcholine can exacerbate hyperkalemia.

Planning therapy for end-stage renal disease

Recognizing the progressive nature of chronic renal disease and the limitations of conservative therapy, patients must be seen regularly, the frequency of follow-up depending on the rate of progression and the patient's clinical stability. Evaluations should include assessment of volume status, blood pressure control, compliance with drug and dietary regimens, metabolic and electrolyte status, and an estimate of the GFR by obtaining BUN and creatinine values. Urinalysis should screen for infection or signs of superimposed renal injury and inflammation. The degree of anemia should be checked, and in later stages symptoms and signs of developing uremia should be sought—including development of pruritus, appetite changes, mental status alterations, asterixis, and pericardial friction rub. Management of the patient with progressive disease also should incorporate ongoing education of the patient and family about the nature of the disease and the long-term medical and social implications of end-stage renal disease (ESRD). Generally, the tempo of the disease progression as assessed by the 1/creatinine versus time plot allows a rough extrapolation as to when the patient will become uremic (GFR less than 5% to 10% normal) and be in need of renal replacement therapy beyond the conservative regimen outlined above. Well before this stage is reached, the options of various forms of dialysis and transplantation should have been reviewed and explored with the

Table 111-1   Guidelines for antibiotic therapy in dental treatment of patients with renal disease

| Drug | Normal dose regimen | Adjusted dosage for percentage of normal GFR | | | Extra dose postdialysis |
		>50%	10%-50%	<50%	
Amoxicillin	250-500 mg q8h	—*	½†	½	Yes
Ampicillin	500 mg-2 g q6h	—	½	½	Yes
Penicillin G	600,000-3 million units q6h	—	½	½	Yes
Penicillin VK	500 mg q6h	—	—	—	No
Oxacillin	1-2 g q4h	Limit to 6 g/day	Limit to 6 g/day	Limit to 6 g/day	No
Dicloxacillin	500 mg q6h	—	—	—	No
Clindamycin	300-600 mg q6h	—	—	—	No
Erythromycin	500 mg-1 g q6h	—	—	—	No
Tetracycline	500 mg q6h	½	Avoid	Avoid	Avoid
Gentamicin‡	Load 1.7 mg/kg, then 1 mg/kg q8h	½	¼	⅛	Yes
Cephalexin	500 mg q6h	—	½	½	Yes
Cephalothin	500 mg-2 g q6h	—	½	¼	Yes
Cefazolin	½ g q8h	—	½	¼	Yes

Modified with permission from: Bennett WM and others: Drug therapy in renal failure, Ann Intern Med 93:61, 1980.

*Dashes indicate no change in dosage.

†Fraction of normal dose.

‡Use of dosages derived from nomograms is recommended, and serum levels should be monitored.

patient and family, and if possible visits to dialysis units to meet with patients on both peritoneal and hemodialysis should be arranged. With a more clear-cut understanding of available therapeutic modalities, the patient and the physician can formulate well ahead of time a plan of action to deal with ESRD. A team approach incorporating input from social worker, dietitian, physician, and nurses, along with the patient and his family, should be stressed. Planning should include the timing of creation of either angioaccess for hemodialysis or placement of an indwelling catheter for peritoneal dialysis. The forearm vasculature of CRF patients should be zealously guarded from trauma such as venipuncture to ensure better results of later fistula creation. Although most ESRD patients need dialytic therapy as symptoms develop, early evaluation for suitability for future transplantation also should be undertaken and discussions with and screening of potential family donors can be instituted before dialysis is begun.

Prognosis and future developments

Twenty-five years ago, in the predialytic and pretransplant era, presentation with advanced uremic findings of seizures, coma, or pericarditis heralded a very short survival. Renal replacement therapy initiated well before the development of such flagrant signs of uremia allows for correction of volume overload and electrolyte and acid-base imbalances. Anorexia improves, the encephalopathy clears, and sensory neuropathic symptoms usually abate. Anemia improves only mildly, whereas platelet dysfunction also frequently persists. A need for phosphate restriction and binders, along with calcium and vitamin D supplementation continues. Patients frequently remain anergic and unless they receive a transplantation, continue to be impotent or sterile. Thus dialysis certainly does not restore health to normal, but in many instances allows for enough recuperation and rehabilitation for a patient to resume a semblance of normal activity.

The high incidence of infection and cardiovascular complications continues to be the major source of morbidity and mortality for ESRD patients, but the overall prognosis and longevity with dialysis depends strongly on the patient's age and the presence of absence of underlying end-organ diseases or systemic illness such as diabetes mellitus. Thus the meaning of average annual mortality figures of 10% in the dialysis population becomes less relevant to the individual patient.

The prognosis of CRF patients in the future depends to a large extent on improvements in medical care in general and technical breakthroughs in the field of dialysis and transplantation. However, work at the exciting frontiers in the understanding of the pathophysiology of renal disease and its mechanism of progression, along with the causes and control of major public health menaces such as diabetes mellitus and hypertension, promises significant future changes in CRF.

BIBLIOGRAPHY

Bennett WM and others: Drug therapy in renal failure: dosing guidelines in adults (in two parts), Ann Intern Med 93:61, 286, 1980.
Brenner BM and others: Dietary protein intake and the progressive nature of kidney disease: the role of hemodynamically mediated glomerular injury in the pathogenesis of progressive glomerular sclerosis in aging, renal ablation, and intrinsic renal disease, N Engl J Med 307:652, 1982.
Bricker NS and others: Magnification phenomenon in chronic renal disease, N Engl J Med 299:1287, 1978.
Eknoyan G and Knochel JP: Systemic consequencs of renal failure, New York, 1984, Grune & Stratton, Inc.
Eschbach J and Adamson JW: Anemia of ESRD, Kidney Int 28:1, 1985.
Harris RC and others: Pathophysiology of renal disease. In Brenner BM and Rector FC Jr, editors: The kidney, ed 3, Philadelphia, 1986, WB Saunders Co.
Knochel JP: The pathophysiology of uremia, Hosp Practice 16:65, 1981.
Mitch WF: The infuence of the diet on the progression of renal insufficiency, Annu Rev Med 35:249, 1984.
Morrison G and Murray TC: Electrolyte acid-base and fluid homeostasis in chronic renal failure, Med Clin Noth Am 65:429, 1981.
Raskin NH and Fishman RA: Neurologic disorders in renal failure, N Engl J Med 294(3):143, 204, 1976.

112 · TREATMENT OF IRREVERSIBLE RENAL FAILURE BY DIALYSIS

Lois Anne Katz

Patients with uremia caused by acute or chronic renal failure are treated with peritoneal dialysis or hemodialysis. These techniques also may be used to remove poisons or to correct severe fluid or electrolyte abnormalities. During dialysis, solutes diffuse down a concentration gradient and across a semipermeable membrane that separates blood from a balanced salt solution (dialysate). This protein-free solution approximates the composition of normal plasma water, although the sodium concentration usually is slightly lower than the normal physiologic level and the potassium concentration varies depending on the patient's serum potassium level. The dialysate does not contain those substances (urea, creatinine, and uric acid) that are to be removed from the patient but does have relatively high concentrations of buffer (usually acetate, lactate, or bicarbonate) and calcium so that these solutes can diffuse into the patient's plasma. Metabolism of the acetate to bicarbonate corrects acidosis. How quickly solutes are removed from the blood depends on their size, the area and permeability of the membrane, blood flow, and dialysate flow.

PERITONEAL DIALYSIS

In peritoneal dialysis a plastic catheter is inserted percutaneously into the abdominal cavity and dialysate is infused. The peritoneum, which has a functional surface area of about 1 m^2, acts as the semipermeable membrane. It is permeable to small- and middle-molecular-weight (500 to 6000 daltons) solutes; some proteins also cross this membrane. In adults 1 to 2 L of sterile dialysate warmed to body temperature is infused rapidly, allowed to remain in the abdomen for a variable period (up to 30 minutes), and then drained by gravity. Each complete exchange takes 30 to 60 minutes. Small amounts of heparin may be added to the dialysate to maintain catheter patency. Fluid removal depends on the osmolality of the dialysate, which is determined by its glucose concentration. Commercially available dialysate containing 1.5 g/dl dextrose is slightly hypertonic to plasma and leads to some water loss. To remove more fluid from overhydrated patients, solutions containing 2.5 or 4.25 g/dl of dextrose are available. In acute dialysis, exchanges are continued for 36 to 48 hours or until the desired correction of plasma abnormalities is obtained.

Because peritoneal dialysis is a relatively simple technique requiring no complicated equipment, it is widely available. There are few contraindications, although it may be difficult to perform in a patient with previous abdominal surgery and adhesions. Technical problems include abdominal discomfort or pain, intraabdominal bleeding, inadequate drainage, and leakage around the catheter site. When 4.25% dextrose solutions are used, hyperglycemia may develop, especially in diabetic patients. Removal of too much water may result in hypernatremia. Perforation of a viscus (such as the colon or bladder) or blood vessel may complicate catheter placement. The most common problem is peritonitis, subclinical (cloudy fluid and positive cultures) or clinical (with fever and abdominal pain). Intraperitoneal and systemic antibiotics are used to treat peritonitis when it occurs.

Chronic peritoneal dialysis may be used in the treatment of end-stage renal failure. A permanent Silastic catheter with Dacron cuffs is inserted surgically. Patients are dialyzed intermittently for 8 to 12 hours three or four times a week in a hospital unit or at home or continuously using a technique known as continuous ambulatory peritoneal dialysis (CAPD) or continuous cycling peritoneal dialysis (CCPD). Patients undergoing CAPD use dialysate in plastic bags that are connected by tubing to the permanent catheter. After the dialysate is instilled into the abdomen, the empty bag is rolled up and worn for several hours. Then the bag is unrolled, used to drain the dialysate, and discarded. Bagless methods of CAPD also are available; the patient discards the empty bag after infusing the dialysate. Four or five exchanges are done daily. Patients receiving CAPD are independent and ambulatory even while being dialyzed. Because the dialysis is continuous, they have fewer dietary and fluid restrictions than those receiving intermittent dialysis, and their blood pressure usually is normal without medications. Since protein losses are significant with CAPD, high-protein diets are prescribed. The main disadvantage of CAPD is frequent peritonitis, which usually responds to antibiotics but sometimes requires removal of the catheter. Patients who adhere strictly to the required aseptic techniques may develop peritonitis as infrequently as once every 12 to 18 months.

HEMODIALYSIS

When hemodialysis is performed, dialysate and anticoagulated blood flow on opposite sides of a synthetic semipermeable membrane contained in a disposable dialyzer or artificial kidney. Types of dialyzers include hollow-fiber and plate dialyzers; most have membranes made of cuprophan or polyacrylonitrile with surface areas of 1 to 2.5 m². Dialyzers may be used once or reused up to 10 to 20 times. Most patients with no residual kidney function are dialyzed for 4 hours three times a week.

Vascular access is necessary. Surgically constructed internal arteriovenous (AV) fistulas are commonly used; in patients whose own vessels are poor, synthetic vascular prostheses may be used to create a fistula. Once the veins near the fistula dilate, one or two needles can be inserted to provide flow of blood to and from the dialyzer. An alternative method of access is the cannulation of vessels to form an external AV shunt. Shunts obviate the need for venipunctures but are easily infected or thrombosed. Catheters can be inserted into the femoral or subclavian veins for blood access; this method is usually reserved for acute dialyses. Blood flows of 200 to 300 ml/min are used.

Dialysate, prepared from specially treated water, is mixed, heated, monitored, and pumped at flow rates of about 500 ml/min to the dialysate compartment of the artificial kidney. Urea and creatinine are easily cleared; the removal of toxins of middle molecular weight depends on the dialyzer size and the length of treatment. Hydrostatic pressure across the membrane, not dialysate osmolality, determines fluid removal or ultrafiltration. Positive pressure on the blood side and negative pressure created in the dialysate compartment result in a transmembrane pressure gradient that is adjusted to remove an appropriate amount of fluid.

To prevent blood from clotting when it is exposed to the tubing or membrane, heparin is infused systemically. In patients who are actively bleeding or likely to bleed, several techniques are available. It is possible to use citrate instead of heparin for anticoagulation. Low doses of heparin or regional heparinization (heparin infused into blood going to the dialyzer and protamine infused into blood returning to the patient) also may be used. Unfortunately, bleeding may occur despite this treatment. In some circumstances high blood flow can obviate the need for heparin. However, significant bleeding, hypotension, or cardiovascular instability are contraindications to hemodialysis.

The technical complications of hemodialysis include blood leaks, air emboli, and hemolysis caused by contaminated or improperly prepared dialysate. Hypotension, bleeding, muscle cramps, cardiac arrhythmias, fever, infection, pruritus, and disequilibrium (headaches, nausea and vomiting, and seizures) may occur during dialysis.

Patients undergoing hemodialysis may be infected by the hepatitis virus, and many become chronic carriers, with the virus found in blood, saliva, and other body secretions. Most dialysis units routinely test for hepatitis B surface antigen (HBsAg) and isolate patients who are carriers. More recently, dialysis patients have been infected with non-A, non-B hepatitis. Patients who are HIV-positive are similarly isolated.

Because of the risk of septicemia and endocarditis in patients with AV fistulas, such patients should probably receive prophylactic antibiotics for dental or surgical procedures. Well-dialyzed patients have normal coagulation profiles between dialyses; however, patients with AV shunts are anticoagulated with warfarin (Coumadin). Patients receiving dialysis often have occult or overt gastrointestinal bleeding resulting from duodenal ulcer disease or gastritis; therefore, for routine analgesia acetaminophen is prescribed instead of aspirin. Drugs containing magnesium should not be given. Many other drugs such as antibiotics, which are normally excreted by the kidneys, must be given in reduced dosage to dialyzed patients.

Patients receiving dialysis must follow certain dietary limitations; protein, salt, and potassium are moderately restricted, and fluid intake is severely reduced to avoid excessive weight gain between treatments.

Hemodialysis may be done in a hospital, in a satellite clinic, or at home. Most patients feel well following dialysis; their urea and creatinine levels are significantly lowered, and their fluid and electrolyte metabolism is normalized. Dialysis substitutes for the excretory functions of the kidney but not for its endocrine functions.

Dialysis treatments usually are begun when a patient's creatinine clearance is less than or equal to 5 ml/min or when uremic signs or symptoms supervene. Advanced age and systemic illnesses no longer are contraindications to maintenance dialysis. Currently, most patients are hemodialyzed, although children and elderly and diabetic patients may do better with peritoneal dialysis. Peritoneal dialysis does not require vascular access or anticoagulation; because it is less efficient than hemodialysis, changes occur slowly, and hypotension and disequilibrium are seen less frequently. For these reasons peritoneal dialysis may be the preferred mode of therapy in patients who have small or fragile veins, bleeding, severe angina, or neurologic problems likely to be complicated by disequilibrium.

NEW DEVELOPMENTS

Several new developments in the treatment of uremia include hemoperfusion, hemofiltration (convectional dialysis technique in which clearance of large and small molecules is equal), sequential dialysis (ultrafiltration without dialysis followed by dialysis without fluid removal), and oral sorbents. Work is under way to construct a wearable, continuously working hemodialyzer. More efficient dialyzers and new types of membranes, including some that are more biocompatible, are now available. A new technique of rapid or high flux hemodialysis uses higher blood and dialysate flows, bicarbonate as the buffer, and controlled ultrafiltration. Although treatments may be shortened to 2 to 2½ hours with rapid dialysis, long-term adequacy of this therapy is still being assessed.

COMPLICATIONS

Even if patients tolerate the dialysis treatments without serious problems, patients undergoing hemodialysis or peritoneal dialysis are subject to numerous long-term complications. Many dialyzed patients have hypertension, usually related to volume overload but occasionally renin dependent. Hypertension and lipid abnormalities may predispose patients to accelerated atherosclerosis. There is a high incidence of fatal and nonfatal cardiovascular complications, especially atherosclerotic heart disease.

Most patients have chronic anemia, which may be treated with iron, androgens, or synthetic erythropoietin. Neurologic abnormalities include peripheral neuropathy, autonomic neuropathy (which may be manifested as orthostatic hypotension), and dialysis encephalopathy, a progressive dementia related to accumulation of aluminum in the brain. Another problem is disordered calcium-phosphorus metabolism leading to secondary hyperparathyroidism and bone lesions known as renal osteodystrophy. High serum phosphorus concentrations, hypocalcemia caused by decreased production of the active metabolite of vitamin D (an endocrine function of the kidney not corrected by dialysis), and acidosis contribute to the hyperparathyroidism. An early sign may be loss of the lamina dura of the teeth. The use of phosphate-binding antacids, active vitamin D metabolites, dialysate with a high calcium content, and calcium supplements may prevent the development of parathyroid hyperplasia. Some patients develop bone disease from aluminum deposition. The usual source of the aluminum is ingestion of aluminum hydroxide or carbonate for phosphate binding. Dialyzed patients are susceptible to all kinds of infections; pneumonias, tuberculosis, and skin infections commonly occur. Most dialysis-related deaths are a result of cardiovascular disease or infection. Mortality is highest in the first year of treatment; the overall mortality is about 8% to 15% a year. Despite the medical and psychosocial problems associated with the treatment of uremia, dialysis does restore many individuals to happy and productive lives.

BIBLIOGRAPHY

Alfrey AC: Dialysis encephalopathy, Kidney Int (suppl 18) 29:S53, 1986.
Bennett WM and others: Drug prescribing in renal failure: dosing guidelines for adults, Am J Kidney Dis 3:155, 1983.
Coburn JW and Slatopolsky E: Vitamin D, parathyroid hormone, and renal osteodystrophy. In Brenner BM and Rector FC Jr, editors: The kidney, ed 3, Philadelphia, 1986, WB Saunders Co.
Friedman Eli A: Critical appraisal of continuous ambulatory peritoneal dialysis, Annu Rev Med 35:233, 1984.
Manis T and Friedman EA: Dialytic therapy for irreversible uremia (in two parts), N Engl J Med 301:1260, 1979.
Merrill JP: Dialysis versus transplantation in the treatment of end-stage renal disease, Annu Rev Med 29:343, 1978.
Popovich RP and others: Continuous ambulatory peritoneal dialysis, Ann Intern Med 88:449, 1978.
Quarles LD: The renal osteodystrophies therapeutic principles, The Kidney 18:11, 1985.
Reed WE Jr and Sabatini S: The use of drugs in renal failure, Semin Nephrol 6:259, 1986.
Sherrard DJ: Aluminum and renal osteodystrophy, Semin Nephrol (suppl 1) 6:5, 1986.

113·RENAL TRANSPLANTATION

Robert A. Grossman

Dialysis and renal transplantation must be considered complementary forms of therapy for chronic renal failure. Although dialysis can exist without transplantation, the reverse is not true. The advantages of transplantation over dialysis include a more nearly normal life-style, an improved sense of well-being, better rehabilitation, the chance for reproduction, and perhaps a longer life span. The widespread use of cyclosporine as the major immunosuppressive drug, starting in 1983, has caused a modest revolution in renal transplantation. Its use has dramatically increased success rates of cadaveric transplantation, reduced mortality, and shortened the hospital stay, making renal transplantation more desirable. However, transplantation should be considered a form of therapy for renal disease, not a cure. In 1985 about 7700 renal transplantations were performed at 170 transplantation centers in the United States.

PATIENT SELECTION AND PREPARATION

The indications of renal transplantation have become so broad that it is simpler to list the contraindications: extremes of age, metastatic cancer, active infection, and destructive psychosis. Severe vascular disease affecting the heart, extremities, or brain or severe chronic lung disease dramatically increase the risk of surgery and immunosuppression and may prohibit renal transplantation. Diseases such as diabetes mellitus, systemic lupus erythematosus, Wegener's granulomatosis, scleroderma, and amyloidosis are no longer contraindications for renal transplantation.

The patient should be in optimal condition at the time of transplantation surgery. Hypertension and diabetes should be controlled, coronary artery disease should be stable, and gastrointestinal disease such as peptic ulcers, gastritis or diverticulitis should be in remission. Active infection must be cured, and potential infectious sources must be eliminated before transplantation and immunosuppression can proceed. The most common potential source of infection is the urinary tract. Infected hydronephrotic, calcareous, or pyelonephritic kidneys must be removed. The urinary bladder must function normally; if not, it must be repaired or a bowel conduit created before transplantation.

Bilateral nephrectomy is performed for chronic renal infection; with the advent of more potent antihypertensive drugs, bilateral nephrectomy is performed only rarely for hypertension. Splenectomy is almost never performed before transplantation; unlike older drugs, cyclosporine is not a bone marrow suppressant, so the level of the white blood cell and platelet counts are not of great concern so long as they are adequate.

In the period from 1975 to 1985 a substantial body of evidence developed suggesting that transplantation recipients who had received blood transfusions had a greater success rate than those who had never been transfused. The mechanism for the increase in transplantation success following transfusion was never firmly established; however, it was necessary to have white cells and platelets or their fragments in the blood preparation to attain the increase in graft success. Because of the increment in graft success, many centers required that all recipients of kidney transplants receive blood transfusions before transplantation. As a corollary of this, many centers were using "donor-specific transfusions." Blood from a mismatched living donor was purposely administered to the potential donor before transplantation. A minority of the recipients would form human leukocyte antigen (HLA) antibodies against the donor so that the donor could not be used. Most patients who received transfusions from the donor would then tolerate the graft with a dramatic improvement in graft success. Since the advent of cyclosporine this transfusion effect has inexplicably waned, and many centers are discontinuing their mandatory transfusion policy.

Histocompatibility determination

An absolute prerequisite for renal transplantation is ABO (red blood cell) compatibility, not necessarily identity, between recipient and donor. Rh factor, positive or negative, is not relevant in renal transplantation, since Rh is expressed only on red blood cells; ABO antigens are found on all cells of the body.

The HLA system, part of the major histocompatibility complex (MHC), is found on the short arm of chromosome 6. Many loci have been described as a part of the MHC, but only four are relevant in clinical transplantation. These are the HLA-A, HLA-B, HLA-D, and HLA-DR loci. The A and B loci were the earliest described antigens. They may be determined serologically in a few hours and are class I antigens. The D locus is a class II antigen and can be determined only by performing a mixed lymphocyte reaction, a complicated test that takes several days. Since the "shelf life" of a cadaver kidney is only about 48 hours, it is impossible to determine D loci in the donor before transplantation. In the past decade it has become possible to determine the D-related (DR) class II antigens serologically on the surface of B lymphocytes. The body's immune system recognizes differences at class II loci and mounts an immunologic attack against class I antigens. Each of the antigens is present in duplicate, since an individual has two number 6 chromosomes, one from each parent. Parents match children for one number 6 chromosome, a one haplotype (chromosome) match. Siblings may match for two haplotypes, one haplotype, or no (zero) haplotypes. In family studies it is possible to show a decrement in graft success going from a two haplotype match to a one haplotype match to a zero haplotype match. In cadaveric transplantation the relationship between HLA matching and graft success is cloudy. Since the advent of cyclosporine therapy, the usefulness of HLA matching is being called into question. A "perfect" match cadaveric kidney has a success rate a few percentage points higher than average. However, the chance of finding this perfect match varies between one in several hundred and one in several tens of thousands, depending on the frequency distribution in the population of the recipient's HLA type. Conversely, a cadaveric graft that matches for no antigens probably will have a success rate a few percentage points worse than average. It appears that the success rate for all matches between the perfect match and a zero antigen match are about the same.

The HLA system also is important for defining sensitization before transplantation. In some individuals exposure to foreign tissue through pregnancies, blood transfusions, or before transplantation results in the formation of antibodies against HLA loci. All transplantation centers determine the presence of preformed HLA antibodies by screening the recipient's serum against a panel of cells that represent all known HLA types. By this means the identity and level of preformed antibodies may be determined. In addition, a "direct cross-match" is performed immediately before each transplantation. With this technique recipient serum is mixed with donor lymphocytes in the presence of complement. After adequate incubation, the specimen is examined for lymphocyte killing using phase contrast microscopy. Killing above a predetermined level strongly suggest the presence of preformed antibodies in the recipient

directed against antigens found in the donor, a positive cross-match. If transplantation were to proceed in the face of the positive cross-match, there is a >90% chance that hyperacute rejection will occur.

Cadaver donors

Although a kidney from a family member with one or two matching haplotypes has a better chance of success than does a kidney from a cadaveric donor, the trend in the United States and around the world is toward cadaveric rather than family donors. The reasons include the increasing age of recipients with fewer donors available, as well as ethical questions about the use of living donors.

Cadaver donor procurement. Currently there is a dramatic shortage of cadaver donors for kidneys, as well as other organs. The waiting time for a cadaver kidney can vary from a few months to 2 or more years depending on the recipient's blood type and the presence of preformed HLA antibodies. Although blood type "O" is the most common type, there is a greater shortage of "O" kidneys than any other. The reason for this anomaly is not clear. Surveys have suggested that, if all potential organs were harvested, there would be an adequate supply of kidneys. However, the harvest rate is probably only 20% to 25% of available organs. This low rate is due to both physician and public ignorance of the desperate need for cadaver organs. Several states have recently mandated that all persons dying in hospitals in that state must be *considered* for organ donation; of course, they must be medically suitable and the family must consent. The Uniform Anatomic Gift Act that has been enacted by most states has not dramatically increased the supply of organs; even if the deceased patient had carried a donor card, the body is still considered the property of the next of kin and consent is always obtained before donation.

Any patient under 60 years of age with actual or impending brain death and normal kidney fucntion should be considered as a kidney donor. The presence of malignancy (except for nonmetastasizing cerebral tumors), infection, renal disease, long-standing diabetes, or moderate to severe hypertension makes a potential donor unacceptable. Most donors who meet medical criteria for brain death have suffered severe head trauma or spontaneous cerebral hemorrhage.

Organ preservation

Unlike the liver, heart, and pancreas, which must be implanted in the recipient within 6 hours, the kidney can be stored for up to 48 hours and occasionally longer with acceptable success rates. There are two methods of cadaver kidney preservation. Once removed, the kidney can be flushed with a hyperosmolar solution such as Collins' solution and stored in iced slush. Alternatively, the kidney may be placed on a pulsatile perfusion apparatus, where it is continually perfused with oxygenated plasma or albumin solutions at 40° F (4° C). Pulsatile perfusion is more expensive than simple cold storage with no proven increase in success; for this reason most kidney transplantation centers in the United States have abandoned pulsatile perfusion. Although kidneys can be preserved for up to 48 hours or longer, with the use of cyclosporine, there is evidence that transplanting the organ in less than 24 hours may improve success rates.

SURGICAL PROCEDURE

Cadaveric and living donor kidney transplantations are performed with identical surgical techniques. The kidney is placed in a heterotopic position retroperitoneally in either iliac fossa. An arterial anastamosis is created with the recipient's external iliac artery in an end-to-side fashion. Alternatively, the artery of the kidney can be attached in an end-to-end fashion with the recipient's internal iliac (hypogastric) artery. The renal vein is attached end-to-side to the recipient's external iliac vein. The donor ureter usually is tunneled into the bladder in a nonrefluxing manner (ureteroneocystostomy).

IMMUNOSUPPRESSIVE THERAPY

Since 1983 the major immunosuppressive drug in all solid organ transplantations has been cyclosporine. This drug, which is of fungal origin, is a novel cyclic polypeptide containing 11 amino acids. Its proposed mechanism of action differs from any other immunosuppressive agent presently available; it appears to block the formation and release of interleukin 2 and thus prevents amplification of the T-cell response to a foreign antigen. Unlike most other immunosuppressive drugs, it does not interfere with bone marrow function; hence leukopenia and thrombocytopenia are not problems in its use. In most centers in the United States cyclosporine is used in combination with low doses of glucocorticoids, usually prednisone. The introduction of cyclosporine has increased the success of cadaveric renal transplantation 20% to 25% over that obtained with azathioprine and steroids. In addition, mortality has fallen, the incidence of rejection is lower, the hospital stay has been shortened, and rehospitalization rates have been reduced. Cyclosporine is used in most institutions for all renal transplantations with the exception of the two-haplotype-matched (identical) family donor, in which cases the success rate at 1 year already exceeds 95%.

Cyclosporine does cause some problems, however. It is nephrotoxic with acute reversible decrements in renal function when dose levels are too high, and it may cause possible long-term renal fibrosis even when the dosage is therapeutic. Drug absorption from the gastrointestinal tract is poor and differs from individual to individual; it also differs in the same individual over time. For this reason levels in the blood must be monitored carefully by radioimmunoassay or high-performance liquid chromatography. Dosage requirements usually stabilize over several weeks to a few months. Other problems with cyclosporine use incude hirsutism, gingival hyperplasia, tremors, and hepatic dysfunction. All these side effects can be ameliorated by careful attention to drug levels in the blood. The final problem with cyclosporine is its cost; for the average patient the drug costs about $5000 a year. In 1986 federal legislation provided for reimbursement for the cost of the drug for 1 year. Beyond this point there are a few patients for whom funding for cyclosporine cannot be found, and they must be switched to azathioprine because it is much less expensive. Fortunately, by 1 year after transplantation about 90% of patients taking cyclosporine can be changed to azathioprine with relative impunity.

Prednisone is used in addition to cyclosporine in almost all programs. In most institutions the patient is discharged 2 weeks after the transplantation on a regimen of 20 to 30 mg/day of prednisone. If rejection does not develop, the dose is tapered to 10 mg/day or 20 mg on alternate days by 3 months after surgery.

Some centers use a combination of prednisone, cyclosporine, and azathioprine as initial therapy for renal transplantation. The cyclosporine and azathioprine are each used in lower doses than would be prescribed if they were administered alone with prednisone. There are two reasons for this type of therapy: (1) cyclosporine at full dosage increases the duration of acute tubular necrosis; the lower dose ameliorates but does not remove this problem; and (2) cyclosporine and azathioprine inhibit the immune system at different points; there is some evidence that more effective immunosuppression may be attained with a combination of the two drugs.

Some centers do not use cyclosporine at all in the first few days after transplantation. A combination of prednisone, azathioprine, and either heterologous antilymphocyte serum or monoclonal antibody directed against T cells is administered for the first 5 to 14 days after transplantation. When the graft is functioning well, cyclosporine is added and the azathioprine and antilymphocyte serum or monoclonal antibody is stopped. By using this drug therapy the interference of cyclosporine with primary graft function is eliminated.

COMPLICATIONS
Rejection reactions

Rejection can be divided into three types: hyperacute, acute, and chronic.

Hyperacute rejection occurs when the recipient has preformed circulating antibodies directed against the HLA loci of the donor kidney. It takes place within minutes to hours of the opening of the arterial anastomosis and always results in loss of the graft. The preformed antibodies react with antigens on the vascular endothelium of the graft; activation of the complement, clotting, and kinin cascades occurs with thrombosis of the involved vessels. Hyperacute rejection usually can be prevented by careful pretransplantation cross-matching of the donor and recipient. However, a rare patient having levels of cytotoxic antibodies too low to be detected by cross-matching techniques suffers a hyperacute rejection. Hyperacute rejection usually is recognized during surgery; the kidney never "pinks up" but remains soft and blue even though the arterial anastomosis is clearly patent.

Acute rejection usually occurs between 1 and 12 weeks after transplantation. It usually is recognized by a decrement in graft function. In the cyclosporine era the previously important signs of acute rejection—fever, graft tenderness, weight gain, and a decrease in urine output—often are absent. Since cyclosporine itself may cause a decrement in graft function, it often is necessary to distinguish between acute rejection and cyclosporine nephrotoxicity. This is accomplished by biopsy of the graft (a bedside procedure). There is no other specific test to determine the presence of rejection. Acute rejection is characterized histologically by the presence of edema and an interstitial round cell infiltrate in the graft. Cyclosporine nephrotoxicity is defined by a decrement in graft function *without* the histologic findings of rejection. Although cyclosporine levels are helpful in defining nephrotoxicity, toxicity can occur in the presence of "normal" levels and rejection can be present with "toxic" levels; thus the importance of the biopsy. If rejection is present, it can be treated in one of several ways. The dose of steroids can be increased either as oral prednisone or with the use of "pulse" methylprednisolone (250 to 1000 mg/day intravenously for 3 to 5 days). Alternatively, acute rejection can be treated with heterologous antilymphocyte or antithymocyte serum or with monoclonal antibodies directed against T cells.

Chronic rejection is an insidious process causing a gradual loss of graft function over months to years. It is characterized pathologically by obliteration of small vessels by endothelial proliferation with interstitial fibrosis. There currently is debate over whether part of what is now called chronic rejection may in reality be chronic cyclosporine nephrotoxicity; histologically, the two conditions are identical. There is no effective treatment for chronic rejection. Increased levels of immunosuppression increase morbidity and mortality without decreasing the rate of graft loss.

Primary graft nonfunction

Virtually all grafts from living donors and about two thirds of those from cadaver donors function immediately. Most kidneys that do not function promptly after surgery have acute tubular necrosis (ATN), for which the treatment is watchful waiting. Although the presence of ATN should not decrease eventual graft success, most large series now show a 10% to 15% decrement in 1-year graft survival in patients in whom ATN has occurred. This observation may have two causes. First, as noted earlier, the use of cyclosporine can dramatically increase the recovery time from ATN and in a few cases may prohibit recovery entirely. Second, with the absence of graft function, the use of cyclosporine may entirely mask other signs and symptoms of acute rejection, allowing rejection to be missed entirely. Other conditions causing immediate graft nonfunction are venous or arterial thrombosis and ureteral obstruction. The diagnosis of these conditions usually can be made easily by a combination of radionuclide and Doppler ultrasonic scanning and the judicious use of arteriography.

Infection

Infection is a major complication and cause of death in kidney transplantation. Infections range from simple cystitis in 40% to 50% of recipients to life-threatening pulmonary and systemic infections. Since the advent of cyclosporine therapy, opportunistic infections have become less common; yet infections with *Pneumocystis* organisms, cytomegalovirus, herpes simplex and zoster, and *Cryptococcus* organisms still occur. If suspected, evaluation must be rapid and complete, since overwhelming infection can occur in a short period of time in the immunosuppressed host.

Hypertension

Hypertension occurs in most patients receiving kidney transplantation; its incidence actually has increased since the introduction of cyclosporine. This may be the result of renal vasoconstriction induced by the drug, although the mechanism of cyclosporine-induced hypertension has not been fully elucidated. In general, treatment of the hypertension does not differ substantially from that in the general population. However, there is a 5% to 10% incidence of transplant renal artery stenosis in the first few months following surgery; this condition often is amenable to treatment by balloon angioplasty.

Recurrent disease

The incidence of recurrence of the original kidney disease in the transplanted organ is remarkably small, perhaps because of immunosuppressive therapy. Focal segmental glomerulosclerosis, membranoproliferative glomerulonephritis, anti–glomerular basement membrane nephritis (Goodpasture's syndrome), and IgA nephropathy (Berger's disease) all have been reported to recur in a small number of patients.

Malignancy

In the United States there is a 6% incidence of malignancy in the few years following renal transplantation. About three fourths of these are cancers on the skin, lips, and uterine cervix that are amenable to surgical excision. Of the remaining 25% the most are lymphoproliferative disorders of the brain or gut that are histologically indistinguishable from diffuse histiocytic lymphomas; however, these "lymphomas"; usually are polyclonal in origin, whereas true lymphomas are monoclonal. When they occur in the gastrointestinal tract, these "lymphomas" usually can be treated by a combination of surgical re-

Table 113-1   Graft and patient survival following renal transplantation

Kidney source	1-year survival (%) Graft	1-year survival (%) Patient	10-year survival (%) Graft	10-year survival (%) Patient
HLA-identical sibling (four-antigen match)	> 95	> 99	80-85	90-95
One haplotype (two-antigen match)	90	97	60-65	80-85
Cadaver	80	95	50*	?†

*Projected from 3- to 5-year data with cyclosporine where a linear 3% yearly loss of kidneys occurs.
†There are no long-term data for patient survival with cyclosporine therapy.

section and decrease or cessation of immunosuppression; those of the central nervous system usually are fatal.

Other complications

Urinary leakage, obstruction, or fistula formation may occur because of ureteral ischemia or errors in surgical technique. Lymphocele formation occurs in 2% to 3% of patients when lymph collects between the kidney and the intact peritoneal membrane. This collection may compress the ureter, causing obstruction to urine flow. Any of the recognized complications of steroid therapy may occur, including diabetes, aseptic necrosis of bone, peptic ulcer disease, and posterior subcapsular cataracts.

OUTCOME

The results of renal transplantation may be expressed in two ways, graft survival and patient survival (Table 113-1). The best results for both patient and graft survival occur with transplantation from a living related kidney donor; with this type of transplantation patient survival exceeds that for dialysis therapy. With cadaveric transplantation, no statement can be made about patient survival compared with dialysis; however, with the dramatic fall in patient mortality seen since the introduction of cyclosporine, it is possible that patient survival with cadaveric transplantation will exceed that of dialysis in the future.

BIBLIOGRAPHY

Bennett WM and Norman DJ: Action and toxicity of cyclosporine, Annu Rev Med 37:215, 1986.
Carpenter CB and Milford EL: Renal transplantation: immunobiology. In Brenner BM and Rector FC Jr, editors: The kidney, ed 3, Philadelphia, 1986, WB Saunders Co.
Opelz G: Improved kidney graft survival in non-transfused recipients, Transplant Proc 19:149, 1987.
Strom TB and Tilney NL: Renal transplantation: clinical aspects. In Brenner BM and Rector FC, Jr, editors: The kidney, ed 3, Philadelphia, 1986, WB Saunders Co.
Tolle SW and others: Responsibilities of primary physicians in organ donation, Ann Intern Med 106:740, 1987.

114 • NEPHROLITHIASIS

Mary Catherine Stom *and* **Elizabeth D. Labovity**

Kidney stones predominate in industrialized areas, whereas bladder stones are more common in underdeveloped and nonurban areas. Kidney stones occur in 1% to 5% of the U.S. population. If infectious stones are eliminated, men have four times as many stones as do women. The prevalence is higher in whites than in blacks and in white-collar workers than in laborers. The peak incidence of initial stone formation is in the third decade of life. Most patients average more than 3.5 stones in their lifetime, with 50% of patients having a second stone within 5 years and 60% within 9 years. There appear to be "stone belts"; in the southeastern United States, stones are more common than other regions.

Calcium stones predominate. Of all analyzed stones, calcium oxalate and calcium phosphate account for more than 80%, struvite for 10% to 15%, uric acid for 5% to 10%, and cystine for 1% to 3%.

The presentation of kidney stones ranges from asymptomatic hematuria and minimal proteinuria to dysuria, colic, costo-vertebral angle tenderness, and the passing of clots, sludge, or stones. The initial syndrome may result from the complications of stones, including obstruction, renal failure, infection, and hematuria.

Normal urine is commonly supersaturated with calcium, ox-alate, and phosphate. Stone formation, however, is multifac-torial and is affected by the saturation and solubility of salts, promoters and inhibitors of crystal growth and aggregation, and local physical factors (obstruction, infection, and urine pH). The crystal nidus may be homogeneous or heterogeneous. Crystals of similar lattice size may grow on one another; thus calcium oxalate, calcium phosphate, and monosodium urate crystals, all of similar dimensions, augment the precipitation of one another. The existence of inhibitors has been known for more than 20 years. The main inhibitors in vivo seem to be inorganic phosphate, citrate, and magnesium; however, in vitro studies have identified other inhibitors such as urine, zinc, polyelectrolytes, and proteins. Inhibitors delay nidus forma-tion, growth, and aggregation. One theory of the mechanism of inhibition is based on the fact that less than 1% of the crystal surface need be bound by an inhibitor to prevent crystal growth. It is not known if patients with stones overall have less inhib-itors.

The physical chemistry involved in stone formation has clinical and therapeutic relevance. The therapy should be di-rected at increasing solubility, decreasing saturation, increasing inhibitors, and impairing crystal nidus formation. Therapeutic maneuvers include hydration, drugs, and alteration in the urine pH.

CALCIUM STONES

Nephrocalcinosis, in distinction to kidney stones, is the de-position of calcium within *renal* tissue. It may be demonstrable roentgenographically or histologically. Hypercalciuria and/or hypercalcemic states, infection, and renal degenerative changes predispose patients to nephrocalcinosis. Nephrocalcinosis is an asymptomatic phenomenon and may or may not be associated with calcium stones. The following disccusion is limited to kidney stones.

Although there are two types of calcium stones (oxalate and phosphate), there are diverse metabolic causes that must be delineated to devise appropriate therapy. In one study that eval-uated 460 consecutive calcium stone–forming patients, it was found that 80% had known causes of stone disease (Table 114-1).

It has been long recognized that stone formation may be a consequence of inadequate inhibitors of crystal growth. The well-defined inhibitors—citrate, magnesium, and pyrophos-phate—are important deterrents against calcium phosphate crystalization. However, most calcium stones are of oxalate salt and not phosphate. Thus studies that have demonstrated an abnormal glycoprotein inhibitor (nephrocalcin) of calcium

Table 114-1 Metabolic and clinical disorders in 460 consecutive calcium stone formers

Disorder	No. of patients	%
Idiopathic hypercalciuria	95	20.7
Marginal hypercalciuria*	53	11.5
Hyperuricosuria†	67	14.6
Hypercalciuria and hyperuricosuria‡	54	11.7
Hyperuricemia	26	5.7
Primary hyperparathyroidism	24	5.2
Renal tubular acidosis§	17	3.7
Inflammatory bowel disease‖	21	4.6
Medullary sponge kidney	7	1.5
Sarcoidosis	3	0.7
No disorder found	93	20.2
TOTAL	460	

Reproduced with permission from Coe FL: Nephrolithiasis–pathogenesis and treatment. Copyright © 1978 by Year Book Medical Publishers, Inc, Chicago.
*Urine calcium > 140 mg/g creatinine.
†Urine uric acid above 800 mg (men) and 750 mg (women) in at least one of two 24-hour urine collections.
‡Marginal hypercalciuria not included.
§Distal hereditary form.
‖Regional enteritis, ulcerative colitis, granulomatous ileocolitis.

oxalate crystal growth in the urine and stone organic matrix of patients with stones perhaps will allow practitioners to mark predisposed patients and provide the normal inhibitor for cal-cium oxalate nephrolithiasis.

Hypercalciuria

The most widely accepted normal levels of daily calcium excretion are 250 mg for women and 300 mg for men, or 4 mg/kg body weight. These values are based on studies showing that 95% of non-stone-forming patients excreted less than 250 to 300 mg of calcium a day and that more than 30% of stone-forming patients excreted more than this. Marginal hypercal-ciuria is defined as excretion of more than 150 mg calcium/1 g creatinine/day.

If hypercalciuria occurs with hypercalcemia, the approach to the patient is directed toward diagnosis of the hypercalcemia; for example, hyperparathyroidism, tumor, Paget's disease of bone, vitamin D excess, sarcoidosis, immobilization, milk-alkali syndrome, hyperthyroidism, adrenocortical insuffi-ciency, infantile hypercalcemia, renal transplantation, and the recovery phase of acute renal failure. If the patient is nor-mocalcemic, several causes of hypercalciuria must be excluded; for example, hyperparathyroidism, renal tubular acidosis, sar-coidosis, Cushing's disease, hyperthyroidism, Paget's disease, immobilization, medullary sponge kidney, and drugs such as vitamins A and D, furosemide, ethacrynic acid, and perhaps spironolactone. Therapy for the hypercalciuria is then directed at the underlying cause.

Hyperparathyroidism is the most common cause of hyper-calcemic hypercalciuric stone formation. An inappropriately high serum parathyroid hormone (PTH) level is the prime in-dicator of the diagnosis. Hypercalcemia of neoplasm is com-mon, but stones are rare. Sarcoid patients have normal or high serum calcium concentrations, low serum PTH levels, and hy-percalciuria from both increased levels of and increased gut sensitivity to hydroxylated vitamin D_3, or 1,25-dihydroxy-cholecalciferol (1,25[OH]$_2$D$_3$). In sarcoidosis the hypercalci-uria is reversed in 5 to 14 days with 15 mg of prednisone daily.

Distal renal tubular acidosis is a disease associated with metabolic acidosis caused by renal inability to secrete H^+ and acidify the urine to a pH less than 5.8 (see Chapter 144). It is a cause of normocalcemic, hypercalciuric stone formation. Patients with this disease have hypercalciuria, phosphaturia, and lowered urinary citrate levels. The hypercalciuria, phosphaturia, alkaline urine (a result of the basic metabolic defect), and low urine levels of citrate (a necessary inhibitor), are associated with the common occurrence of calcium phosphate stones. Specific therapy for the hypercalciuria is directed toward resolution of the acidosis with 0.5 to 2 mEq base/kg body weight/day in four equally divided doses.

In medullary sponge kidney 50% of patients have calcareous deposits in the cysts and 40% have hypercalciuria (see Chapter 152). Hypercalciuria should be treated.

Idiopathic hypercalciuria is the syndrome of normocalcemia, recurrent calcium stones, and hypercalciuria of undetermined cause. Controversy exists concerning the definition and pathogenesis of idiopathic hypercalciuria. Two pathogenetic mechanisms—renal hypercalciuria and absorptive hypercalciuria—have been described. In renal hypercalciuria the primary defect is an impairment of renal tubular calcium reabsorption, perhaps as a result of renal phosphate leak and phosphate depletion. Regardless of the cause, the calcium loss stimulates PTH release and further phosphate depletion, both of which lead to increased $1,25(OH)_2D_3$ formation. This enhances the intestinal absorption of calcium.

Absorptive hypercalciuria has as its primary defect an increased intestinal absorption of calcium. This presents an increased calcium load to the kidney, suppresses PTH, and results in hypercalciuria. One third to one half of these patients have elevated levels of $1,25(OH)_2D_3$. Some suggest that the primary defect is again renal tubular phosphate wasting, with phosphate depletion stimulating formation of the active vitamin D. It is believed that phosphate depletion and $1,25(OH)_2D_3$ decrease PTH release.

In both renal and absorptive hypercalciuria the urine calcium, $1,25(OH)_2D_3$, and intestinal calcium absorption is high and serum phosphate concentrations are normal or low. The higher PTH concentration in renal hypercalciuria helps distinguish the two conditions. In renal hypercalciuria a high urinary calcium level persists after both a low-calcium diet (400 mg/day for 5 to 7 days) and a high-calcium diet (1000 mg/day for 5 to 7 days), whereas in absorptive hypercalciuria increased urine calcium results only after the high-calcium diet. In addition, after overnight fasting a 2-hour urine sample shows a calcium/creatinine excretion ratio of less than 0.11 in absorptive hypercalciuria and greater than 0.12 in renal hypercalciuria.

Therapy is directed toward lessening the urine calcium concentration, increasing urine inhibitor concentration, or both. Thiazide diuretics accomplish this (1) by stimulating calcium resorption via PTH, (2) by producing volume depletion, which increases proximal tubular calcium resorption, and (3) perhaps by potentiating the action of PTH by inhibiting the degradation of renal cyclic AMP. Impairment of the effectiveness of thiazides may be a result of volume repletion and hypoparathyroidism. Decreased stone formation is found in as many as 90% of treated patients. Suggested mechanisms for this include hypocalciuria, increased urine volume, reduced oxalate excretion, or increased urine phosphate and magnesium. In some patients treated with thiazides there may be a slight rise in the total serum calcium concentration. The serum PTH level should not rise and in fact may decrease if the renal calcium "leak" of renal hypercalciuria is resolved with thiazides. If the serum calcium concentration remains at 11 mg/dl for more than 4 to 6 weeks, despite discontinuing the thiazides, other causes of

hypercalcemia, especially hyperparathyroidism, should be pursued. Agents that bind calcium in the intestinal tract are also used in the therapy for idiopathic hypercalciuria. Orthophosphates (1.5 to 2 g/day in divided doses) decreased stone activity in 90% of study patients. Stone prevention may result from decreased gastrointestinal calcium absorption, increased urine phosphate levels, or decreased urine calcium levels. Neutral phosphate preparations are preferable to acid preparations because acidosis decreases renal calcium resorption. Diarrhea, the most common side effect, may be obviated by prescribing the phosphates for postprandial use. An increased urine oxalate level may occur, which in theory may increase calcium oxalate stone formation. Phosphates should be avoided in patients with renal failure or phosphate stones (for example, patients with renal tubular acidosis and those with struvite stones). Cellulose phosphate is a nonabsorbable cation-binding resin that binds calcium and magnesium in the intestine, thus decreasing absorption. A negative calcium-magnesium balance may ensue. For these reasons the drug should be reserved for patients with absorptive hypercalciuria who do not respond to other therapies.

Citrate or trace metal citrate ion complexes are inhibitors of both calcium phosphate and oxalate crystal growth. Furthermore, citrate reduces the urine saturation by complexing with calcium. Potassium citrate may increase renal calcium absorption (as opposed to sodium citrate, which would enhance urine calcium as a result of the linked natriuresis-calciuresis). Finally, hypocitraturia is the only metabolic risk factor for many patients with stones. Patients with hypercalciuria and hyper-uricosuric calcium stones who are resistant to therapy have been found to have a thiazide-induced hypocitraturia. Both of these groups of patients have been successfully treated with potassium citrate and thiazide and/or allopurinol.

Potassium citrate then is indicated as therapy for patients with calcium stones with distal renal tubular acidosis (RTA; hypocitraturia), diarrhea, thiazide and/or allopurinol unresponsiveness, hyperoxaluria, and renal failure.

Hyperuricosuric, calcium oxalate nephrolithiasis

Both hyperuricosuria (urinary uric acid excretion greater than 750 mg/day in females and greater than 800 mg/day in males) and hyperuricemia have been recognized as risk factors for calcium stones. With allopurinol treatment, stone formation is reduced to 6% of predicted cases. These patients have a different clinical syndrome than other stone-forming patients; the onset is later, the formation rates are higher, the interval times are shorter, and surgical manipulation is more common.

Hyperoxaluria

Hyperoxaluria (oxalate excreted in urine greater than 40 mg/day) results from increased intestinal absorption or overproduction of oxalate. Increased absorption occurs with overingestion (rare), small bowel bypass surgery (because of fatty acid malabsorption), and ingestion of cellulose phosphate. Fatty acids and cellulose phosphate bind intestinal calcium, leaving oxalate free to be absorbed. The overproduction of oxalate may be primary (hereditary) or secondary. Ascorbic acid, ethylene glycol, and methoxyflurane are converted to substrate for oxalate formation, causing hyperoxaluria. Cholestyramine, a low-fat diet, calcium tablets, and oxalate restriction should be therapeutic in hyperabsorption states. Pyridoxine may be used in overproduction states. Citrate inhibits oxalate crystal growth.

Idiopathic calcium stones

In patients with idiopathic calcium stones, treatment with low-calcium diets and hydration produces modest success. Thiazides, allopurinol, orthophosphates, and potassium citrate have caused decreased stone activity in some studies.

STRUVITE STONES

Struvite stones are associated with infection. Urease-forming bacteria (most often *Proteus* organisms) form an alkaline urine, resulting in magnesium–ammonium phosphate (struvite) stones. This begins a vicious circle, since the stone harbors the infection, which in turn increases growth of the stone. Struvite stones can grow rapidly in this infectious environment and are often staghorn calculi when the patients (usually young women, elderly men, and patients with indwelling Foley catheters and ileostomies) are discovered. The diagnosis involves metabolic evaluation (any stone may have been the nidus), definition of the bacteria, and roentgenographic evaluation for an anatomic defect. The therapy is then directed at eradication or long-term suppression of the infection, surgical removal of all stones, repair of the anatomy, and treatment of any metabolic disorder. Because recurrence after surgical removal is high, lithotripsy (percutaneous or extracorporeal) may be the preferred manner of stone removal. Urease inhibitors recently have been found effective in patients refractory to treatment. However, the high prevalence of adverse effects and the unknown chronic toxicity should limit their use to patients who cannot receive surgical or lithotripsy procedures or patients during the immediate postoperative period.

URIC ACID STONES

Uric acid stones account for 10% of all cases of renal stones in the United States, but this varies in other parts of the world. Pure uric acid stones are radiolucent, but often calcium oxalate or phosphate crystals are part of the stone, which then is radiopaque.

Hyperuricosuria may result from hyperuricemia or an abnormality in renal proximal tubular transport. Because of the low pK of uric acid (5.75), it is almost completely dissociated at blood pH into its ionized soluble form, monosodium urate. In the tubules, as the pH falls, ionized urate is transformed into free undissociated uric acid, whose solubility is much less. The precipitation of uric acid crystals depends on the quantity excreted and a urinary pH of less than 6. Decreased ammonia excretion rates in patients with uric acid stones, leading to increased urinary acidity, may be important in the pathogenesis. Other clinical techniques and syndromes (ileostomies, diarrhea, and volume depletion states) that dispose patients to aciduria may be manifested by normal serum uric acid levels but uric acid stones as well.

Uric acid stone formation is correlated with hyperuricemia and hyperuricosura. The disorders of uric acid overproduction include gout, myeloproliferative diseases, Lesch-Nyhan syndrome and other enzyme deficiency states, and glycogen storage diseases. The therapy is directed at alkalinizing urine (pH 6 to 7), increasing urine volume (3 L/day), and decreasing serum and urine uric acid levels (as with allopurinol). Potassium citrate is useful because it alkalinizes urine and reduces urinary calcium excretion.

CYSTINE STONES

Cystine stones, a familial disease, occur in males and females with equal frequency and at any age. They are moderately radiopaque because of their sulfur bonds. Of stones passed by cystinuric patients, 50% are pure, 40% are mixed, and alomst 10% have no cystine; thus stone analysis alone is insufficient, and the diagnosis is based on the urinary excretion of cystine. Hexagonal flat crystals on urinalysis are strong evidence. The excretion of increased amounts of cystine is determined with the nitroprusside screening test of the urine, which detects greater than 75 mg cystine/1000 mg creatinine. False positive results occur in patients with cystinosis, homocystinuria, or acetonuria. The normal excretion of cystine is less than or equal to 30 mg/day. Decreased solubility occurs in an acid pH. The therapy includes hydration, urinary alkalinization (pH greater than 7), and possibly penicillamine, which complexes with and solubilizes cystine. Penicillamine side effects may be significant.

MANAGEMENT OF ACUTE UROLITHIASIS

The initial therapy for acute symptomatic urolithiasis involves administering adequate analgesics and ensuring a fluid intake of more than 3 L/day. Infection should be treated, and if gram-negative bacillary bacteremia with shock occurs, emergency intervention may be required to remove an obstructing stone. This may be open surgery or lithotripsy, either percutaneous (PL) or extracorporeal shock wave (ESWL). In PL, ultrasound and electrohydraulic sources of energy fragment and remove stones from the urinary tract. In ESWL, spark-induced shock waves propagate through water and focus on the kidney stone of the patient, who is placed strategically in a tank of water. Currently, both of these procedures are used for symptomatic and asymptomatic stones, staghorn stones, and ureteral lithiasis, as well as renal stones.

Calculus chemolysis recently has been undertaken to lyse renal stones via a nephrostomy tube. However, this therapy may cause systemic toxicity or renal damage.

Eradication of bacteriuria or long-term suppression or metabolic intervention may help prevent the formation of new stones or the propagation of stones already present.

BIBLIOGRAPHY

Broadus AE and Thier S: Metabolic basis of renal-stone disease, N Engl J Med 300:839, 1979.

Coe FL, editor: Nephrolithiasis—pathogenesis and treatment, Chicago, 1978, Year Book Medical Publishers, Inc.

Drach GW and others: Report of the United States cooperative study of extracorporeal shock wave lithotripsy, Urol 135:1127, 1986.

Hosking DH and others: Urinary citrate excretion in normal persons and patients with idiopathic calcium urolithiasis, J Lab Clin Med 106:682, 1985.

Labovitz ED: Hyperuricemia and the kidney. In Jepson JH, editor: Hematologic problems in renal disease, Reading, Mass, 1979, Addison-Wesley Publishing Co, Inc.

Lang EK: Percutaneous nephrostolithotomy and lithotripsy: a multi-institutional survey of complications, Radiology 162:25, 1987.

Mulley AG Jr: Shock-wave lithotripsy. Assessing a slam-bang technology, N Engl J Med 314:845, 1986 (editorial).

Nakagawa Y and others: Isolation from human calcium oxalate renal stones of nephrocalcin, a glycoprotein inhibitor of calcium oxalate crystal growth, J Clin Invest 79:1782, 1987.

Pak CY, editor: Symposium on urolithiasis, Kidney Int 13:341, 1978.

Pak CY: Physiological basis for absorptive and renal hypercalciurias, Am J Physiol 237:415, 1979.

Pak CYC, Sakhaee K, and Fuller C: Successful management of uric acid nephrolithiasis with potassium citrate, Kidney Int 30:422, 1986.

Pak CYC and others: Correction of hypocitraturia and prevention of stone formation by combined thiazide and potassium citrate therapy in thiazide-unresponsive hypercalciuric nephrolithiasis, Am J Med 79:284, 1985.

Williams JJ, Rodman JS, and Peterson CM: A randomized double-blind study of acetohydroxamic acid in struvite nephrolithiasis, N Engl J Med 311:760, 1974.

115·MALFORMATIONS OF THE URINARY TRACT

Linda B. Hiner

RENAL ANOMALIES
Renal agenesis

Bilateral renal agenesis occurs in about 1 in 4000 births and is incompatible with life. The absence of intrauterine micturition leads to oligohydramnios with ensuing lung hypoplasia, facial dysmorphism (Potter's facies), and limb anomalies. Severe pulmonary hypoplasia commonly leads to death within hours.

Unilateral renal agenesis is sporadic, occurring in about 1 in 1000 births. It is commonly associated with ipsilateral agenesis of the ureter and bladder hemitrigone or adrenal gland and is occasionally associated with abnormalities of the genital tract such as absence of a gonad or a uterine horn. The solitary kidney is large from birth; it may be more susceptible to infection, stone formation, and tumor.

Renal hypoplasia

The term "hypoplasia" describes a kidney the histology of which is normal but in which total size or number of ureteral divisions is reduced. Unilateral renal hypoplasia occurs in about 1 in 500 live births. Since small renal size may result from abnormal renal growth in utero or after birth, a diagnosis of true renal hypoplasia requires histologic evaluation. Because these kidneys are prone to develop infection, stones, and vascular disease, the diagnosis usually is discovered incidentally during evaluation for one of these complications.

The Ask-Upmark kidney is a form of segmental renal hypoplasia or perhaps atrophy characterized by bands of aglomerular or hypoglomerular tissue that cut deep clefts into the cortex and medulla of the involved kidney. The cause of the malformation in some cases is scarring from infection associated with vesicoureteral reflux. It may be associated with severe childhood hypertension, which usually is corrected by nephrectomy or segmental nephrectomy.

Oligomeganephronia is a nonfamilial form of bilateral renal hypoplasia associated with a reduced number of calyceal divisions. Nephrons are increased both in length and in volume. Affected individuals generally are children who tend to "outgrow" their fixed, limited renal function within the first decade of life. They may have associated progressive glomerulosclerosis and interstitial fibrosis. These children are good candidates for renal transplantation.

True bilateral renal hypoplasia is unusual. Both kidneys appear as miniatures with a normal number of calyceal divisions. This defect may occur with other congenital abnormalities, especially those of the central nervous system. The outlook for infants with renal hypoplasia may not be so grim as in the past, since techniques for infant dialysis and transplantation are improving.

Renal dysplasia

Gross disorganization of tissue differentiation results in dysplasia of the kidney. Dysplastic kidneys may also be hypoplastic, but the term "hypoplasia" is reserved for kidneys with normal tissue differentiation. The disorganized renal tissue may contain areas of squamous epithelium, fibrous tissue, bone, or cartilage. Renal cysts are common.

Renal dysplasia usually is sporadic. There may be concurrence within families for the functionally or mechanically obstructive lesions that lead to renal dysplasia. It generally is believed that abnormal differentiation results from in utero obstruction to urine flow. Such obstruction may be of varying degrees and result from such causes as ureteral atresia, obstruction to bladder emptying, or obstruction at the ureteropelvic junction.

Multicystic kidneys caused by *bilateral* ureteral atresia are large, grossly cystic, and have a completely disorganized structure. This condition is not compatible with life. Affected children are oliguric in utero and have oligohydramnios, Potter's facies, and pulmonary hypoplasia.

Unilateral multicystic renal dysplasia is associated with severe in utero urinary obstruction on the involved side and usually appears as an abdominal mass in the newborn. The treatment is nephrectomy, usually in the first 2 years of life. The remaining kidney may not be entirely normal, and there may be associated bladder or ureteral abnormalities. The prognosis, however, usually is good.

Anomalies of renal position

Abnormal ureteral and renal migration or renal rotation during embryogenesis may lead to such anomalies as horsehoe kidney or ectopic kidneys. There may be areas of dysplasia within such abnormally placed kidneys. Susceptibility to infection and stone formation is increased, and the incidence of progressive interstitial fibrosis with loss of renal function may be increased.

Ureteral anomalies

A complete duplication of the collecting system, or "double kidney," refers to a double pelvis within the substance of one kidney. There may be a single terminal ureter or completely duplicated ureters that reach the bladder independently. True supernumerary kidneys are rare. The ureter from the upper pole of the kidney often opens ectopically into the bladder and is associated with vesicoureteral reflux. The upper pole ureter also may open ectopically into the urethra, the vagina, or the rectum.

Although a variety of anomalies of the bladder and ureter are described, often with associated abnormal renal morphogenesis, clinically the most significant are those leading to vesicoureteral reflux. Reflux of bladder urine into the ureter results from incompetent flap-valve function of the bladder wall and the intramural ureter.

Anatomic situations associated with vesicoureteral reflux include a shortened intramural ureteral tunnel, a large-diameter intramural ureter, abnormal placement of the ureteral orifice with associated loss of normal detrusor function, and decreased pliability of the bladder wall.

Urine that has refluxed into the ureter and kidney serves as a reservoir and increases the risk of urinary infection (see discussion of "Urinary tract infection and perinephric abscess" in Chapter 40). There may be mechanical damage to the kidney, especially if an associated obstruction is present. Although it is commonly thought that refluxed urine exposes the upper tract to bacteria, p-fimbriated *Escherichia coli* may ascend the ureters in the absence of vesicoureteral reflux. Severely involved individuals with massive hydroureteronephrosis often have dysplastic kidneys, the function of which cannot be much improved by ureteral reimplantation.

Although vesicoureteral reflux is uncommon in adults with urinary tract infection, it is found in 30% or more of young girls whose urinary tracts are evaluated after cystitis or pyelonephritis. Such reflux is more common in girls than boys and in whites than blacks.

Reflux can be evaluated by its appearance during contrast voiding cystourethrogram. The International Classification's fine grades of vesicoureteral reflux are as follow:

I. Ureter only
II. Ureter, pelvis, calyces; no dilation; normal fornices
III. As in Grade II, but mild dilation of and/or tortuosity of the ureter; mild dilation of the pelvis; minimal blunting of fornices
IV. Moderate dilation of the ureter, pelvis, calyces; angles of fornices blunted; papillary impression present
V. Gross dilation of ureter, pelvis, calyces; fornices blunted or lost and no papillary impressions in most calyces

Since the roentgenographic grade of reflux correlates with spontaneous cessation of reflux, cystoscopy for assessment of the ureteral orifice is no longer routinely performed and has little prognostic significance. The tendency to cease refluxing falls with increasing grade and is minimal for grades IV and V. Cessation of reflux in grade III ureters is being assessed as a part of a collaborative study of conservative versus surgical treatment of vesicoureteral reflux. Maintenance of an infection-free urine prevents or markedly reduces scar formation during the period of growth leading to cessation of reflux. Prevention of scars is important, since 20% of children with bilateral renal scars become hypertensive.

Reflux may produce progressive renal disease associated with hypertension, proteinuria, glomerulosclerosis, and interstitial fibrosis. Ureteral reimplantation after the development of proteinuria and hypertension may not stop loss of renal function.

BLADDER ANOMALIES

Congenital bladder anomalies are rare. The more severe ones require urinary diversion in childhood. Agenesis of the bladder, hypoplasia, duplications, and diverticulae have been described. Failure of closure involving the rectum (cloacal extrophy) can occur. Children with sacral agenesis or meningomyelocele may have accompanying neurogenic bladder.

URETHRAL ANOMALIES

Minor urethral anomalies include urethral stenosis, which may require surgical correction to prevent urinary obstruction or infection. Hypospadius (presence of a proximal ventral meatus) is the most common urethral abnormality in males and often requires surgical correction. Epispadius (abnormal dorsal opening of the urethra) occurs in both sexes and is either entirely asymptomatic or produces incontinence. Two other rare anomalies are megalourethra, which is associated with lack of development of the erectile bodies of the penis, and urethral diverticula.

BIBLIOGRAPHY

Bernstein J: Congenital malformations of the kidney. In Early LE and Gottschalk CW, editors: Strauss and Welt's diseases of the Kidney, ed 3, Boston, 1979, Little Brown & Co.
Bellinger MF: The management of vesicoureteral reflux, Urol Clin North 12:23, 1985.
Duckett JW: Vesicoureteral reflux: a "conservative" analysis, Am J Kidney Dis 3:139, 1983.
Shindo S, Bernstein J, and Arant, BS Jr: Evolution of renal segmental atrophy (Ask-Upmark kidney) in children with vesicoureteric reflux: radiographic and morphologic studies, J Pediatr 102:947, 1983.
So SKS and others: Growth and development in infants after renal transplantation, J Pediatr 110:343, 1987.
Stickler GB and others: Primary interstitial nephritis with reflux: a cause of hypertension, Am J Dis Child 122:144, 1971.

Torres VE and others: The progression of vesicoureteral reflux nephropathy, Ann Intern Med 92:776, 1980.

116·RENAL CYSTS AND CYSTIC DISEASES OF THE KIDNEY

Linda B. Hiner

Renal cysts are present in about half of individuals over 50 years of age. These cysts may be "simple" or may occur in association with other renal problems. They may arise from the renal parenchymal epithelium, renal capsule, or within the peripelvic renal lymphatics. Renal cysts have been described in congenital syndromes associated with multiple dysmorphic features and in dysplastic or congenitally obstructed kidneys. Renal cysts may be the primary manifestation of hereditary kidney disease in both adults and children. They also may develop in renal tumors.

SIMPLE CYSTS

Half of all individuals over 50 years of age have one or more simple renal cysts. Since these cysts are uncommon in children, they appear to be acquired lesions. Unless they are very large, renal cysts are asymptomatic and are discovered fortuitously during abdominal imaging studies performed for other purposes. If cysts rupture, hemorrhage, or become infected, they may cause pain and hematuria. Hemorrhage is unusual in simple renal cysts.

Simple cysts may vary from a few milliliters to more than a liter in volume. Very large cysts may be palpable through the abdominal wall. Their walls are translucent and parchmentlike. The fluid within them usually is straw colored and resembles an ultrafiltrate of plasma. The lining cells are flattened epithelium with occasional papillary projections. The cyst capsule contains some collagen, some mononuclear cells, and occasionally focal deposits of calcium or hemosiderin. The appearance of calcium in a cyst or bleeding into a cyst suggests possible nephrocarcinoma.

Renal cortical cysts may be solitary or multiple, unilateral or bilateral. Available imaging modalities can confirm the likelihood of a simple cyst 95% of the time.

AUTOSOMAL DOMINANT POLYCYSTIC KIDNEY DISEASE

Autosomal dominant polycystic kidney disease (ADPKD) accounts for about 8% of all of the dialysis and renal transplantation patients in the United States. The gene for ADPKD has been localized to the short arm of chromosome 16 and is closely linked to the α-globin genes (3' HVR). Penetrance is high if individuals are followed into their seventies and eighties. Although adult polycystic disease tends to become clinically apparent within the third to sixth decades, it has been described in newborns. Since polycystic disease usually is not clinically apparent until after an individual is well into reproductive age, some individuals at risk may request an imaging evaluation for this disorder for purposes of genetic counseling. Most who are destined to express polycystic disease can be identified in their twenties. However, negative evaluation does not always mean that the individual is unaffected, and a family study, including DNA markers for chromosome 16, can be a more reliable means of predicting the presence of the disorder. The cause of ADPKD is unknown. A similar entity may be induced chemically in genetically predisposed mice. When raised in a germ-free environment, these mice do not manifest the disease.

In humans with ADPKD the kidneys may be huge. The cysts are distributed throughout the renal parenchyma and may vary in diameter from a few millimeters to several centimeters. The cysts are derived from tubular segments, and analysis of their contents may indicate their tubular sites of origin. Most cysts are lined with a single layer of cuboidal or columnar epithelium. They may be continuous with the glomerular tuft. There is interstitial fibrosis of varying amounts but no dysplasia.

Electron microscopy reveals splitting and lamination of the basement membrane of the renal tubules. There are no immune complexes. Cysts may be found in organs other than the kidneys including the liver (one third of ADPKD patients) spleen, lung, ovary, endometrium, epididymis, and seminal vesicles.

Abdominal pain (30%) and hypertension (21%) are the most common initial symptoms. During their course more than 60% of patients experience acute abdominal pain associated with their disease. Urinary infection, cyst hemorrhage or rupture, and nephrolithiasis often are associated with painful episodes. Seventy-five percent of women and nearly 25% of men may develop symptomatic urinary infection. As many as 30% of patients may develop renal stones. Hypertension eventually occurs in more than 60% of the patients. Aneurysms of cerebral arteries occur and may cause hemorrhage.

Gross hematuria occurs in more than 40% of patients, and hematuria occurs in more than 60%. Proteinuria occurs in nearly 70% of patients but usually not in large quantities. Qualitatively larger amounts appear in those with well-preserved renal function whose specimens are concentrated.

Hematocrit levels in these patients usually are similar to those of patients with other renal diseases and comparable degrees of renal function. An occasional patient may demonstrate the erythrocytosis that has been described in association with renal cysts. This is felt to be the result of increased production of erythropoietin.

The rate of deterioration of renal function can be estimated for each patient by assessing the rate of decline of the reciprocal of the serum creatinine (when the reciprocal is 0.6 or less). The rate of decline is established by use of at least three serum creatinine levels within 1 year. Functional deterioration varies among patients; it may take as long as 30 years or may progress as fast as about 7% per year.

Therapy involves control of hypertension and urinary tract infection, maintenance of acid-base and electrolyte equilibrium, and prevention and treatment of renal osteodystrophy. Potent diuretics may increase cyst size. These patients are excellent candidates for renal transplantation and dialysis.

INFANTILE POLYCYSTIC DISEASE OF THE KIDNEY

Infantile polycystic disease is an autosomal recessive disorder that is always associated with variable amounts of hepatic fibrosis and intercommunicating bile duct ectasia. The clinical expression varies. In some children the renal expression is so severe that there is oligohydramnios from oliguria in utero and renal failure, Potter's facies, and pulmonary hypoplasia from birth. Others may develop severe renal insufficiency later in infancy or childhood. In some the renal involvement is less severe, but portal hypertension with gastrointestinal bleeding may occur before significant renal failure ensues.

Large flank masses may be palpable at birth. If not discovered in the newborn, this disorder usually is diagnosed later in infancy. Hepatomegaly occurs in infancy or early childhood. Renal infection, stone formation, and hemorrhage are not characteristic of this disorder.

Affected kidneys are large, spongy-looking organs with dilated cortical collecting ducts seen as radial stripes on the renal surface. The numbers of nephrons and degree of ductular branching are normal. Progressive cyst formation does not occur, and relative renal size may diminish with somatic growth. Glomerular obsolescence, interstitial fibrosis, and tubular atrophy may be present. Extrarenal cysts occur less commonly than in adult polycystic disease, and cerebral aneurysm formation is rare.

Sonographic and urographic findings consistent with infantile polycystic disease differentiate it from cystic dysplasias of the kidneys. Older infants and children with end-stage renal disease caused by this disorder are good candidates for dialysis and transplantation. Advances in dialysis and transplantation techniques may improve the chances for a near-normal childhood for severely affected infants as well.

MEDULLARY CYSTIC RENAL DISEASE COMPLEX

Three renal disorders with different ages of onset, associated extrarenal findings, and modes of inheritance makeup this group of clinical entities. The renal functional changes and renal biopsy findings are similar. All are characterized histologically by cysts at the corticomedullary junction, glomerular sclerosis, interstitial fibrosis, and tubular dilation with deposition of periodic acid-Schiff (PAS)–positive material along the tubules. Hyposthenuria is the rule, and polyuria is the first manifestation. Salt wasting occurs and may lead to symptomatic volume contraction. In some forms of the disorder anemia occurs early and is disporportionate to the degree of renal insufficiency.

Juvenile medullary nephronophthisis and *renal-retinal dysplasia* are autosomal recessive disorders. Clinical onset occurs in the first decade of life and end-stage renal failure usually occurs by the end of that decade or in the teens. Some families have members who maintain adequate renal function longer. Anemia, growth failure, and renal osteodystrophy may be severe in these children. Hypertension is rare until end-stage renal disease supervenes. Those children with retinal degeneration may have associated cerebral dysfunction, deafness, and hepatic fibrosis. Some have iminoglycinuria.

Medullary cystic disease is inherited in an autosomal dominant pattern. Its onset usually is later, often in the second decade of life. Its clinical expression and histologic findings are nearly identical to those of nephronophthisis.

The diagnosis of these disorders usually is suspected by the clinical presentation, family history, and associated findings, including retinal changes. Renal biopsy demonstration of the typical histologic features confirms the diagnosis. These patients are excellent candidates for dialysis and renal transplantation.

MEDULLARY SPONGE KIDNEY

Medullary sponge kidney is a condition in which there is cystic dilation of the terminal collecting ducts. This dilation may be present at birth. It may remain asymptomatic throughout the life of an individual, being discovered fortuitously during excretory urography done for other reasons. Other patients may have urinary infection, nephrolithiasis, or hypercalciuria. Adequate therapy of these complications, when they occur, may preserve renal function.

BIBLIOGRAPHY

Anand SK and others: Cystic diseases of the kidney in children, Adv Pediatr 31:371, 1984.

Delaney VB and others: Autosomal dominant polycystic kidney disease: presentation, complications, and prognosis, Am J Kidney Dis 5:104, 1985.

Grantham JJ: Polycystic renal disease. In Early LE and Gottschalk CW, editors: Strauss and Welt's diseases of the kidney, ed 3, Boston, 1979, Little, Brown, & Co.

Lieberman E and others: Infantile polycystic disease of the kidneys and liver: clinical, pathological and radiological correlations and comparison with congenital hepatic fibrosis, Medicine 50:277, 1971.

Milutinovic J and others: Autosomal dominant polycystic kidney disease: symptoms and clinical findings, Q J Med 212:511, 1984.

Romero R and others: The diagnosis of congenital renal anomalies with ultrasound. II. Infantile polycystic kidney disease. Am J Obstet Gynecol 150:259, 1984.

Werder AA, Cuppage FE, and Nielson AH: Naturally occurring polycystic renal disease in CFW, mice, Kidney Int 8:464, 1975.

117·OBSTRUCTIVE NEPHROPATHY

Jose de la Rosa *and* **Sandra P. Levison**

Obstructive nephropathy occurs in a wide variety of clinical circumstances. It is important to identify obstruction early, since irreversible loss of functional nephron mass is related to the duration of obstruction.

DEFINITIONS. Although "obstructive nephropathy," "obstructive uropathy," and "hydronephrosis" are terms used interchangeably to describe obstruction of the urinary collecting system, there are subtle differences in each term. Obstructive nephropathy refers to the renal disease that occurs as a result of impedance to urine flow. Obstructive uropathy is the term used to described the structural changes in the urinary tract caused by obstruction of urine flow. Hydronephrosis is the distention of the renal pelvis and calices as a result of the back pressure that occurs because of obstruction of the ureter.

It is important to remember that dilation of the collecting system does not necessarily mean obstruction. There are other nonobstructing causes of dilation such as reflux nephropathy and primary megaureter.

INCIDENCE. Obstructive uropathy is most common in children because of the increased incidence of congenital abnormalities in this age-group. It is equally prevalent in males and females. At 15 years of age the occurrence of obstruction begins to decline until it reaches its lowest incidence at middle-age. The incidence begins to rise again in males at 60 years of age as a result of prostate disease.

CAUSES OF URINARY TRACT OBSTRUCTION. Obstructive uropathy can result from functional defects or from intrinsic or extrinsic mechanical blockage of urine anywhere along the genitourinary tract. A list of common functional and mechanical causes of urinary tract obstruction follows:

Common causes of functional urinary tract obstruction

I. Ureter
   A. Ureteropelvic dysfunction
   B. Ureterovesical dysfunction
   C. Adynamic ureteral segment
   D. Spinal cord trauma
   E. Cerebrovascular disease
   F. Drugs
II. Urinary bladder
   A. Congenital
      1. Myelodysplasia
      2. Spinal cord defect
   B. Acquired
      1. Tabes dorsalis
      2. Diabetes mellitus
      3. Multiple sclerosis
      4. Parkinson's disease
      5. Anticholinergic drugs

Common causes of mechanical urinary tract obstruction

I. Congenital
   A. Ureter
      1. Ureteropelvic junction narrowing or obstruction
      2. Ureterovesical junction narrowing or obstruction
      3. Ureterocele
      4. Retrocaval ureter
   B. Bladder
      1. Bladder neck obstruction
      2. Ureterocele
   C. Urethra
      1. Posterior urethral valve
      2. Meatal stenosis
      3. Phimosis
II. Aquired intrinsic defects
   A. Ureter
      1. Calculi
      2. Inflammation
      3. Sloughed papillae
      4. Blood clots
      5. Uric acid crystals
   B. Bladder
      1. Benign prostatic hypertrophy
      2. Cancer of prostate
      3. Cancer of bladder
      4. Calculi
      5. Diabetic neuropathy
      6. Spinal cord disease
   C. Urethra
      1. Stricture
      2. Tumor
      3. Calculi
      4. Trauma
      5. Phimosis
III. Acquired extrinsic defects
   A. Ureter
      1. Pregnant uterus
      2. Retroperitoneal fibrosis
      3. Aortic aneurysm
      4. Radiation
      5. Carcinoma of the uterus, prostate, bladder, colon, rectum
      6. Retroperitoneal lymphoma
      7. Iatrogenic (surgical)
   B. Bladder
      1. Carcinoma of cervix
      2. Endometriosis
   C. Urethra
      1. Trauma

Obstruction can be unilateral or bilateral, partial or complete, acute or chronic and can cause temporary or permanent damage to the kidney.

In congenital functional defect of the collecting system, the most commonly involved site is the ureteropelvic junction. The left kidney usually is affected. This defect is attributed to the presence of more longitudinal rather than circular muscles in this area.

Among the intrarenal causes of obstructive uropathy two frequently encountered conditions that clinicians overlook are uric acid nephropathy and multiple myeloma. Uric acid crystals can be deposited in the tubular lumen as a complication of administering alkylating agents to patients who have hematological malignancies or malignancies with a very high cellular turnover. Uric acid is released when the cells lyse and the hyperuricemia and hyperuricosuria result in precipitation of uric acid stones. In multiple myeloma light-chain or Bence Jones proteins are deposited in the tubules.

Urinary calculi are the most common causes of extrarenal obstruction, with calcium oxalate stone as the most common form. The genitourinary tract has four normal anatomic narrowings. These points of narrowing include the ureteropelvic junction, ureterovesical junction, bladder neck, and the urethral meatus. The stone is liable to lodge in these areas of physiologic narrowing. Calculi are three times more prevalent among males, and the peak incidence occurs in the second and third decades of life.

Pregnancy is the most common cause of obstructive uropathy in females. The right ureter is more commonly affected than the left. The obstruction is thought to be the result of the presence of the enlarged uterus and elevated serum progesterone level that occur during pregnancy. Progesterone has been shown to decrease the peristaltic movement of the ureters.

Abdominal aneurysm is the most common form of vascular abnormality, causing obstruction to the collecting system. Ten percent of patients with this abnormality can develop urologic complications.

Benign prostatic hypertrophy is the most common condition causing obstruction to urine flow from the bladder, although inflammatory diseases and cancer of the prostate also are common.

PATHOPHYSIOLOGY. With obstruction urine distends the ureters and renal pelvis and flows back to the renal tubules. Based on experimental observations the flow of urine in the unobstructed ureter is facilitated by both longitudinal and circular muscle forces. The initial motion of the ureter during the propulsion of urine is an upward motion. This upward motion stimulates the proximal circular muscles to coaptate. This coaptation gives rise to the formation of a bolus of urine. This is then followed by contraction of the longitudinal muscles with a consequent propagation of the bolus of urine down the ureter. With obstruction, proximal coaptation does not occur and the pressure generated by ureteral wall tension is transmitted directly to the renal parenchyma. The resulting increase in the intratubular pressure is felt to contribute to the functional and morphologic abnormalities that occur with obstruction. In far advanced cases of obstruction the kidney is transformed into a thin-walled cystic structure.

In the acute phase of bilateral ureteral obstruction, the renal blood flow increases initially. This initial increase is felt to be caused by the augmented production of vasodilatory prostaglandins (PGE_2 and prostacyclin) by the obstructed kidney. Although renal blood flow increases, there is a concomitant decrease in glomerular filtration rate and medullary blood flow. In the chronic stage of obstruction renal blood flow progressively decreases because of an increase in the production of the vasoconstrictor prostaglandin, thromboxane A_2, and a further decrement in glomerular filtration rate ensues. There is also an increase in production of renin-angiotensin.

Alterations in renal tubular function occur with obstruction, with impaired ability to concentrate urine being the most commonly observed defect. Experimental observations in animals with obstruction suggest that nephrogenic diabetes insipidus develops because of a decrease in the tubular generation of cyclic adenosine monophosphate (AMP) in response to endogenous and exogenous vasopressin.

There is also defective urinary acidification in both unilateral and bilateral obstruction. When patients with obstruction are given an ammonium chloride–loading test, they cannot lower their urinary pH below 5. They develop a hyperchloremic, hyperkalemic metabolic acidosis caused by either a renal secretory defect or selective hypoaldosteronism.

Persistent obstruction for more than 3 to 4 months results in irreversible renal damage.

With relief of obstruction of a solitary kidney or bilateral obstruction patients may exhibit a postobstructive diuresis. This is caused by the defect in concentrating ability that occurs with obstruction, increase solute load per nephron secondary to the accumulation of urea and sodium when the patient is obstructed, and the presence of increased atrial natriuretic factors.

CLINICAL MANIFESTATIONS OF OBSTRUCTION. In patients who develop uremia with no apparent past history of renal disease or with relatively normal urinary sediments, obstructive uropathy should be considered. Obstruction also should be sought in patients with a history of stable renal disease who develop an abrupt decline in renal function that is otherwise unexplained.

In patients with recurrent urinary tract infection with no apparent cause, obstruction should be suspected and a detailed evaluation of the collecting system for structural abnormalities should be undertaken.

Complete bilateral obstruction or complete unilateral obstruction with only one functioning kidney usually results in anuria. If the obstruction is partial, polyuria may become a prominent symptom. A characteristic finding of intermittent obstruction is the occurrence of alternating oliguria and polyuria. This is especially seen in elderly individuals. Significant urinary obstruction can occur with normal urine output.

Pain in the affected kidney is one of the hallmarks of acute obstruction, but obstruction may be painless. In long-standing obstruction the kidney size also may increase.

Polycythemia has been reported in some cases of obstructive nephropathy. Animal studies suggest that there is augmented production of erythropoietin by the obstructed kidney.

In complete bilateral obstruction hypertension can develop as a result of a volume-related mechanism produced by sodium and water retention. In unilateral obstruction hypertension also may develop because of increased production of renin by the obstructed kidney.

When there is a strong clinical suspicion of obstruction, a thorough history directed toward symptoms of urinary tract infection, dysuria, hematuria, frequency, or terminal dribbling should be sought. The physical examination should be directed to the presence of flank or abdominal mass, suprapubic mass, or a rectal mass. A thorough gynecologic evaluation is required.

DIAGNOSTIC STUDIES. A urinalysis should be performed on a freshly collected urine sample. If hematuria is present, calculus, sloughed pappila, or a tumor should be suspected. When the urine contains bacteria with coexisting white blood cell casts, it may indicate coexisting pyelonephritis. The urine should be strained for tissue papillae or stones. Urine should be examined thoroughly for crystals, as these may indicate the type of stone causing the obstruction. Other laboratory studies should include measurement of blood urea nitrogen and serum creatinine aside from the usual hematologic studies.

In the early 1960s, Swartz and associates produced evidence showing that an intravenous pyelogram was an invaluable and practical way of diagnosing obstruction. This technique came under scrutiny in the 1970s because of published reports of dye-induced renal failure. In the late 1970s modern ultrasonography and computed axial tomography came into vogue as noninvasive methods for identifying obstruction and renal size. None of these studies are infallible, and false negative studies may be seen early in the course of obstruction. Hydronephrosis

---

CHOICE OF IMAGING TECHNIQUES TO DETERMINE OBSTRUCTIVE UROPATHY	
FLANK PAIN WITHOUT IMPAIRED RENAL FUNCTION	**FLANK PAIN WITH IMPAIRED RENAL FUNCTION**
1. Plain film of the abdomen (shows the size, contour of the kidney and presence of radiopaque stones)	1. Ulrasonography
2. Intravenous pyelogram (allows the clinician to estimate the degree of obstruction and assists in ascertaining if pain is caused by radiolucent stones.	2. Computed tomography without dye
	3. Radionucleid scan
	4. Retrograde or antegrade pyelography

may take 24 to 48 hours to develop or may be absent when the filtration rate is very low or when dehydration is significant.

MANAGEMENT OF URINARY TRACT OBSTRUCTION. Obstruction should be diagnosed and relieved promptly so as to avoid metabolic and structural sequelae. High-grade or total bilateral obstruction requires surgical or instrumental intervention as soon as possible. In partial unilateral obstruction especially that caused by stones, immediate intervention is not necessary but attention should be given in the evaluation of renal function. The obstruction should be relieved. If infection is present along with obstruction, antibiotic therapy is needed along with correction of the obstruction. When a postobstructive diuresis follows relief of obstruction, therapy includes careful and adequate fluid replacement based on measurements of urine output, daily weight, and determination of ideal body weight.

BIBLIOGRAPHY

Diagnosing obstruction in renal failure, Lancet 8407:848, 1984.

Saulo Klahr: Pathophysiology of obstructive nephropathy, Kidney Int 25:914, 1983.

Sherman RL and Schneider M: Obstructive uropathy as seen by the internist: the role of ultrasound and CT scanning, DM 12:1, 1984.

Shlueter W and Batlle D: Chronic obstructive nephropathy, Sem Nephrol 8:17, 1988.

118 · NEOPLASMS OF THE URINARY TRACT

Linda B. Hiner and **Lester Karafin**

RENAL ADENOCARCINOMA

PATHOLOGY. The most prevalent malignant renal neoplasm among adults is renal adenocarcinoma. It is more common in men than women and occurs only rarely in children. There are three major cell types of renal adenocarcinoma: clear cells that resemble renal tubular epithelial cells, granular eosinophilic cells, and spindle cells. These cells can form tubular structures, acini, or papillae, as well as cystic or solid masses.

Patient outcome is related to several factors including extension into the immediate perirenal tissues, renal vein, inferior vena cava, regional lymphs nodes, and contiguous structures. It is also affected by the presence of distant metastases. The staging classification of the American Joint Committee of Cancer, a TNM (tumor, lymph node, metastasis) format, addresses these prognostic factors. The tumor is assigned designations based on size, local extension, vein involvement, and invasion of contiguous structures.

T_0	No tumor
T_1	Small tumor, little renal distortion
T_2	Large tumor, renal distortion
T_{3a}	Perinephric tissue extension
T_{3b}	Renal vein involvement
T_{3c}	Renal vein and subdiaphragmatic IVC
T_4	Adjacent structures involved

Lymph node involvement is categorized by number and degree of fixation.

N_0	No nodes involved
N_1	Single node on same side
N_2	Multiple regional nodes
N_3	Fixed regional nodes

The occurrence of distant metastases, primarily to lung, bone, and liver, is designated by adding the stage assignment M_1. Tumor size at the time of diagnosis is not an isolated sign. Small tumors can metastasize widely. The degree of cellular anaplasia can be more closely related to tumor extension than size alone.

$T_{1-2}N_0$ patients have a 5-year survival rate of between 60% and 82%, which drops to 45% if Gerota's fascia is invaded (T_{3a}). Few T_4 patients live 5 years. Lymph node involvement correlates with 5-year survival rate of only 0% to 30%. The presence of distant metastases limits survival statistics markedly; only 5% to 20% of patients with distant metastases are living at the end of 1 year. More than 25% of patients may have distant metastases at the time of diagnosis.

CLINICAL MANIFESTATIONS. Renal adenocarcinomas are among the "great imitators" of medicine. Painless hematuria is the most common initial symptom (60%). Other signs and symptoms at the time of diagnosis are related to tumor extension, compounds produced by tumor cells and released into the circulation, or the individual's immune response to the tumor. Such signs and symptoms include fever from tumor-produced pyrogens; elevated erythrocyte sedimentation rate, anemia, and amyloidosis; or neuropathy from immune responses. Involvement of the inferior vena cava can lead to leg edema or varicocele formation.

A variety of endocrinopathies can result from tumor cell production of hormonelike substances. Polycythemia can occur from an erythropoietin-like substance. A syndrome resembling Cushing's disease can occur from production of adrenocorticotropic hormone–like peptides, or masculinization from excessive production of gonadotropin-like proteins. Hypercalcemia can occur from production of a parathyroid hormone–like substance or from bone metastases. Hypercalcemia can also occur from prostaglandin-induced bone resorption. When this occurs, the hypercalcemia may respond to therapy with prostaglandin inhibitors like indomethacin.

These endocrinopathies are most likely to occur when the primary tumor is of an undifferentiated cell type. Hematuria may not coexist with the constitutional symptoms.

Hepatic dysfunction with hepatocellular degeneration and portal triaditis can occur independently from metastases in the liver or local invasion. When this occurs, it may regress when the primary tumor is removed.

DIAGNOSIS. Renal adenocarcinomas are often discovered

during abdominal imaging studies, such as computed tomography (CT), ultrasound, or even intravenous pyelography (IVP) performed for unrelated reasons or during evaluation for painless hematuria. A variety of imaging modalities are available to assist in the assessment of renal masses and to evaluate the extent of local or distant tumor spread.

Ultrasound-guided cyst puncture to obtain fluid for cytologic examination and enzyme determination can be used to differentiate simple cysts from cystic renal adenocarcinoma. Abdominal CT can provide staging information and localization of the tumor by showing the extent of local spread, spread to contiguous structures, and nodal involvement. Nodes can be enlarged from inflammatory response to the tumor as well as from tumor spread. CT can demonstrate renal vein or caval involvement, but these are probably better assessed by venography. Magnetic resonance imaging (MRI) may turn out to be superior to venography for assessing venous involvement. Arteriography is rarely used except to assess vasculature before partial nephrectomy.

MANAGEMENT. Radical nephrectomy, removal of Gerota's fascia and its contents, perhaps with limited node dissection, offers the best chance for survival for patients with stage $T_{1-2}N_0M_0$ renal carcinoma. Any statistical advantage of preoperative angioinfarction of the involved kidney is not proven. Radiation therapy, either preoperatively or postoperatively, does not increase survival for these patients even if they prove to have limited lymph node involvement.

Chemotherapy, hormonal therapy, and immunotherapy do not seem to prolong survival when regional nodes are involved or distant metastases are present. In the presence of metastatic disease, nephrectomy or tumor debulking are indicated primarily for control of pain or bleeding, severe endocrinopathy, or in the presence of a solitary distant metastasis that can be excised or irradiated. Hormonal therapy with progestational agents can have a palliative effect in some patients with metastatic disease.

WILMS' TUMOR (NEPHROBLASTOMA)

Wilms' tumor, also called nephroblastoma or embryonal carcinosarcoma, is the second most common retroperitoneal malignant neoplasm of childhood. It accounts for 22% of all childhood abdominal masses and 10% of all childhood malignant tumors. This tumor most often appears in patients under 8 years of age and is rarely seen in adults and adolescents. The mean age at diagnosis is 3 years. There is no race or sex predilection for this tumor. There is an increased incidence in individuals with spontaneous aniridia, hemihypertrophy of the face or extremities, urogenital anomalies, and certain chromosomal abnormalities; and there are reports of its occurrence in several members of the same family.

PATHOLOGY. Wilms' tumors contain epithelial, blastemal, and stromal elements that can demonstrate variable degrees of differentiation. The outcome for patients with this tumor can be related to tumor structure, the child's age, lymph node involvement, and tumor weight.

The National Wilms' Tumor Study (NWTS) divided patients into five categories based on the extent of the tumor's spread and the success of the surgical resection. These groups were as follows:

STAGE I: Tumor is limited to the kidney; resection is complete.
STAGE II: Local spread is evident into paraaortic nodes or into blood vessels outside the kidney; no residual tumor remains beyond the resection.
STAGE III: Residual tumor remains within the abdomen because of intraoperative tumor rupture, peritoneal implants, node involvement

beyond abdominal paraaortic nodes, or inability to resect the tumor completely.
STAGE IV: Hematogenous metastases are present at initial diagnosis.
STAGE V: Bilateral renal involvement is present.

The stages have been somewhat revised for the third phase of the NWTS (presently ongoing).

The NWTS has shown that the degree of epithelial differentiation is not of prognostic significance. There are, however, a minority of Wilms' tumors whose histology is considered unfavorable. These tumors are divided into groups called anaplastic and sarcomatous. There are well-defined histologic criteria for inclusion in each group, and together they account for about 10% of Wilms' tumors.

CLINICAL MANIFESTATIONS. Wilms' tumor is usually discovered because a child's mother notes abdominal swelling or an abdominal mass (83%) in the child. The child may complain of abdominal pain (37%) or have hematuria (21%). Hypertension is a variable finding. Patients may initially show signs of tumor spread such as hepatomegaly, ascites, or venous engorgement from involvement of the inferior vena cava. They may show signs of tumor rupture such as acute abdominal emergency with anemia.

DIAGNOSIS. The evaluation of the child with an abdominal mass should be designed to efficiently and quickly establish the location and the nature of the mass. The initial laboratory evaluation should include a complete blood count, blood urea, nitrogen and creatinine level determinations, liver function tests, and urinalysis. Imaging studies should establish the presence of an intrarenal mass, the status of the contralateral kidney, the presence or absence of involvement of the inferior vena cava, or of pulmonary metastases. Evaluation for the presence of bone metastases is reserved for those tumors whose structure is of the unfavorable sarcomatous pattern. The imaging modalities to be employed should be selected only after discussion with the consulting pediatric radiologist, since the choice is dependent on both the availability of equipment and the experience of the radiologist. The choices may change rapidly as information is gained about the application of newer imaging techniques, such as MRI, to pediatric patients.

MANAGEMENT. Treatment modalities include surgical removal, chemotherapy, and postoperative irradiation. Stage I (favorable histology) tumors require only chemotherapy with vincristine sulfate and actinomycin D. Preliminary data from the third NWTS suggest that irradiation may prove unnecessary for stage II tumors, and that less irradiation than previously used can be effective for stage III tumors. Pulmonary metastases are treated with whole lung irradiation and combination chemotherapy.

Wilms' tumor usually occurs in children. Patients may have complications, primarily from radiation therapy, that only become apparent later in childhood or adulthood. Complications have included scoliosis of the spine, vascular abnormalities, and secondary tumors (1% annual incidence). Newer study protocols demonstrating the need for less irradiation will help to reduce these consequences in the future.

UROTHELIAL TUMORS OF THE KIDNEY

Tumors of the renal pelvis and ureters are uncommon. Transitional cell tumors of both the upper and lower urinary tract are associated with certain industrial exposures. More men than women have transitional cell tumors, which may reflect greater exposure to potential carcinogens. In the United States and Australia cigarette smoking has been linked to the development of these tumors.

Two groups of individuals have an increased incidence of urothelial tumor of the renal pelvis without an associated increased risk of bladder tumor; the first are those with so-called Balkan nephropathy, and the second are those with interstitial nephritis caused by the chronic use of analgesics containing aspirin and either phenacetin or acetaminophen. In both of these groups of patients, the usual male preponderance is lacking.

PATHOLOGY. Transitional cell carcinomas constitute 85% to 90% of the tumors. Tumors are graded by the degree of cellular differentiation and assigned stages by their degree of infiltration and spread. They can occur as carcinomas in situ or invade locally. They metastasize usually to lung, bone, liver, and brain. They tend to spread locally first into Gerota's fascia or into the renal parenchyma, then to the regional lymph nodes and adjacent organs. The high incidence of simultaneously occurring or recurring tumors lower in the ureters or bladder on the same side suggests that cells shed from the tumor can implant lower in the urinary tract. There may be a generalized abnormality of the uroepithelium in these patients, leading to the presence of multiple tumors and to apparent recurrences. In patients with multiple primary tumors, classification is by the worst stage and grade.

CLINICAL MANIFESTATIONS. Urothelial tumor of the renal pelvis and ureter can have an insidious onset. The muscular wall of these structures is thin and the tumor can extend quite easily. About 75% of the patients have hematuria, either gross or microscopic, at the time of diagnosis. Only about 26% complain of pain. There is rarely a palpable mass. Patients can have associated bladder tumors and symptoms of bladder irritability.

DIAGNOSIS. The tools that are available for the diagnosis and evaluation of the patient who may have a urothelial tumor of the upper urinary tract include intravenous urography, cystoscopy with retrograde pyelography, and cytologic study of urine or ureteral washings obtained with or without brush biopsy. Operative nephroscopy can be used in some cases. A lucent defect in the renal pelvis or upper ureter seen on excretory urography can be caused by a blood clot, radiolucent stone, pyelitis cystica, an area of leukoplakia with squamous metaplasia, or even a vascular impression. Ultrasound and CT have been used to assist in differentiating among these causes. Examination of the bladder and the contralateral kidney is imperative. Chest radiographs, bone and liver scans, and liver function tests can be used to determine the presence of distant metastases.

MANAGEMENT. Classically the treatment has been nephroureterectomy with removal of a cuff of bladder adjacent to the site of ureteral entry. When the tumor is bilateral or of an apparently low grade and stage, segmental nephrectomy or segmental ureterectomy have been used. Segmental ureterectomy for ureteral tumors has been more successful than that for tumors of the renal pelvis. Segmental nephrectomy has been tried for patients with solitary kidneys. Operative nephroscopy at the time of segmental nephrectomy determines if the remainder of the kidney appears free from tumor. Neither radiation nor chemotherapy has been a consistently helpful. New multiple drug regimens using methotrexate, vinblastine sulfate, adriamycin, and cisplatin are being assessed and can prove helpful.

The outcome of management seems related more to the grade and extent of tumor spread than to the procedure performed. Over 50% of the patients already have or will have a urothelial tumor in the bladder (48%) or contralateral kidney (1% to 2%) within 2 years.

BLADDER NEOPLASMS

Carcinoma of the bladder is the second most prevalent genitourinary tract tumor (carcinoma of the prostate is the leading cause of death from genitourinary tract malignancy). Although it can occur at any age, it occurs most often in middle age and beyond. Predisposing factors include exposure to many of the same environmental agents as are associated with urothelial carcinomas of the renal pelvis and ureter, including cigarette smoking.

Transitional cell carcinomas comprise 90% of all bladder tumors. They are usually papillary (70%), but can be sessile. They can be superficial or invasive. Like urothelial tumors of the upper tract, they are graded by degree of cellular anaplasia and staged by extent of tumor invasion and spread. The occurrence of carcinoma in situ together with visible lesions carries a more ominous prognosis.

Hematuria is the initial sign in 75% of patients. Symptoms of bladder irritability such as dysuria, frequency, and urgency occur in some patients with carcinoma in situ and in as many as 30% of patients with invasive disease. Flank pain from ureteral obstruction and pelvic pain from tumor extension can also be initial symptoms in individuals with invasive bladder tumors.

Therapeutic modalities are based on whether the tumors are superficial or invasive. Superficial tumors are often multiple and recurrent. For single or small numbers of superficial papillary lesions therapy includes cytoscopy and transurethral resection with biopsy of specified areas of apparently uninvolved bladder. Regular reassessment for possible recurrences is mandatory.

When superficial tumors are multiple or recurrent, resection plus intravesical instillation of chemotherapeutic agents can be useful. Triethylenethiophosphoramide (Thiotepa), adriamycin, and mitomycin C have all been used. Immunotherapy with Bacille bilié de Calmette-Guérin (BCG), laser therapy, and phototherapy following cell sensitization with heme derivatives have also been used. Cystectomy is rarely indicated for superficial lesions unless there are multiple recurrences after topical chemotherapy.

Radical surgery remains the major treatment modality for invasive bladder carcinoma. The roles of radiotherapy and combination chemotherapy are controversial. New multidrug regimens including methotrexate, vinblastine sulfate, adriamycin, and cisplatin may prove helpful for patients with metastatic disease.

PROSTATIC CARCINOMA

The prevalence of carcinoma of the prostate is second only to that of cancer of the lung in men. Its incidence is rising and is now nearly 70 to every 100,000 men. This tumor occurs primarily in men over fifty years of age, and the high incidence of deaths from other disease processes that occur in this age-group makes survival statistics difficult to interpret. Prostatic carcinoma seems to be more common and perhaps more aggressive in blacks.

PATHOLOGY. Adenocarcinoma accounts for 95% of these tumors, which are felt to originate in peripheral parts of the gland. Tumors are graded by degree of cellular anaplasia and disruption of glandular structure. Even when very small areas are of poorly differentiated cell type, the prognosis is worse. Prostatic tumors spread medially and later penetrate the capsule extending locally to sites including the seminal vesicles, bladder, urethra, and pelvic walls. Lymphatic spread is first to hypogastric and obturator nodes, then to presacral paraaortic chains. Metastases to bone involve the axial and appendicular skeleton, primarily pelvis, lumbar spine, femur, then thoracic spine and ribs. Parenchymal metastases occur in lung, liver, and adrenal glands.

CLINICAL MANIFESTATIONS. Localized symptoms are usually bladder outlet obstruction or bladder irritation. Unless leg edema occurs, lymph node extension is usually asymptomatic. Pain from skeletal metastases can closely mimic symptoms from degenerative arthritis, leading to a delay in diagnosis.

DIAGNOSIS. The diagnosis is suspected on the basis of the digital examination and confirmed by needle core or aspiration biopsy. The extent of local spread is assessed by digital bimanual examination, CT, and pelvic ultrasound examination. The role of MRI is yet to be established. The presence of spread to lymph nodes in the pelvis is better established with staging lymphadenectomy than with lymphangiogram, which has as high as a 40% false negative rate when only hypogastric and obturator nodes are involved. When nodes are seen using CT, the spread is usually extensive. Bone scans are more sensitive than skeletal radiographs to assess the presence of bone metastases. Clear elevations of serum acid phosphatase almost always herald the future occurrence of bone lesions, even when they are not demonstrable at first assessment.

MANAGEMENT. Surgery is the primary therapy for individuals with localized tumors whose overall health allows it. Radiation therapy may not offer additional benefits to survival if initial staging was correct. Its use can be curative as primary therapy in a reduced percentage of patients. Once the tumor has spread, hormonal therapy is used. Such therapy includes treatment with estrogen or removal of androgens. The latter can be accomplished by orchiectomy, the use of medications to block androgen receptors, and suppression of androgen synthesis.

BIBLIOGRAPHY

Adenocarcinoma of the kidney

Beahrs OH and Myers MH, editors: American Joint Committee on Cancer: manual for staging of cancer, ed 2, Philadelphia, 1983, JB Lippincott.
de Kernion JB: Management of renal adenocarcinoma. In de Kernion, JB and Paulson, DF, editors: Genitourinary cancer management, Philadelphia, 1987, Lea and Febiger.
Siminovitch JM, Montie JE, and Straffon RA: Prognostic indicators in renal adenocarcinoma, J Urol 130:20, 1983.

Wilm's tumor

Beckwith JB: Wilm's tumor and other renal tumors of childhood: an update, J Urol 136:320, 1986.
Green DM: The diagnosis and management of Wilm's tumor, Pediatr Clin North Am 32:735, 1985.
Merten DF and Kirks DR: Diagnostic imaging of pediatric abdominal masses, Pediatr Clin North Am 32:1397, 1985.

Urothelial tumors of the kidney

McDonald MW and Zincke H: Urothelial tumors of the upper urinary tract. In deKernion, JB and Paulson, DF, editors: Genitourinary cancer management, Philadelphia, 1987, Lea and Febiger.

Bladder tumors

Maldazys JD: Management of superficial bladder tumors and carcinoma in situ. In de Kernion, JB and Paulson, DF, editors: Genitourinary cancer management, Philadelphia, 1987, Lea and Febiger.
Olsson CA: Management of invasive carcinoma of the bladder. In de Kernion, JB and Paulson, DF, editors: Genitourinary cancer management, Philadelphia, 1987, Lea and Febiger.

Tumors of the prostate

Paulson DF: Management of prostatic malignancy. In de Kernion, JB and Paulson, DF, editors: Genitourinary cancer management, Philadelphia, 1987, Lea and Febiger.

119·VASCULAR DISORDERS OF THE KIDNEY

Stuart M. Homer

RENAL ARTERY STENOSIS

Renal artery stenosis is an important cause of secondary hypertension. Estimates of its incidence range from 1% to 4% of the hypertensive population. Its incidence is substantially higher in patients with malignant hypertension (approaching 30%). Recent attention has been directed toward the role of this disorder in producing progressive renal insufficiency and chronic renal failure. Initial signs of the disease are most commonly hypertension or hypertension and azotemia.

Atherosclerotic disease of the renal artery and aorta and fibromuscular dysplasias represent the pathologic factors underlying over 95% of cases. A number of diagnostic screening tests exist to detect this condition, including hypertensive intravenous pyelography (IVP), radionuclide renal scanning, peripheral vein renin levels and digital subtraction angiography; however, none of these have proved entirely ideal. The standard test remains renal arteriography.

The discovery of an anatomic lesion of the renal artery does not prove its physiologic or clinical significance. A number of clinical and biochemical parameters have been applied to improve patient selection for surgical (renal revascularization or nephrectomy) or radiologic (percutaneous transluminal renal angioplasty [PTRA]) intervention. The importance of this disorder is its potential reversibility. The key to its management is the recognition of the setting in which it occurs and an aggressive diagnostic approach.

ETIOLOGY. Atherosclerosis is the cause of renal artery stenosis in approximately 65% of cases. The process involves the proximal one third of the renal artery and is usually part of a generalized atherosclerotic process. Lesions affecting the aorta can involve the ostia of the renal arteries with the same physiologic consequences as other lesions. As with atherosclerotic disease in general, renal arterial disease occurs more commonly in men over 50 years of age. This disease also tends to progress. One study found that over a 52 month interval, 44% of lesions worsened, some to complete occlusion. In general, the more severe the stenosis, the more likely it will worsen.

Fibromuscular dysplasia is the other disorder commonly producing renal artery stenosis. This is a dysplastic process involving medium-sized arteries throughout the body, although the clinically important lesions seem confined to the renal arteries. The disorder is classified into intimal, medial, and periadventitial groups, depending on the portion of the vessel wall involved. Ninety-seven percent of cases involve the vessel media. These have been further subdivided into (in descending order of frequency) medial fibroplasia, perimedial fibroplasia, medial hyperplasia, and medial dissection. Radiologically, the stenosis can appear focal, multifocal, or tubular, but most classically it appears as a series of dilatations and stenoses resembling a "string of beads." It involves the distal two thirds of the renal artery or its branches. Fibromuscular lesions usually do not progress to complete occlusion. The disorder occurs in people between 20 and 40 years of age and is much more common in women than men. The disorder is rarely seen in blacks.

There are a number of uncommon causes of renal artery stenosis. Stenosis of the artery to a transplanted kidney occurs not infrequently and can be related to surgical technique or rejection phenomena. Arteritis of a variety of causes including Takayasu's disease can involve the renal arteries. Neurofibromatosis has also produced stenosis of the renal arteries. Renal artery embolism or thrombosis or extrinsic compression of the renal artery by a mass or tumor have all been reported to produce renal artery stenosis.

PATHOPHYSIOLOGY. In 1934 Goldblatt demonstrated that sustained hypertension could be produced in experimental animals by constricting one renal artery while leaving the kidneys intact (two kidney–one clip model). Hypertension could also be produced by unilateral renal artery constriction and removal of the contralateral kidney (one kidney–one clip model). Human disease more closely resembles the two kidney–one clip model, although the one kidney–one clip model has relevance for patients with one functioning kidney and stenosis of that artery (as can occur following renal transplantation).

The pathophysiologic process can be divided into an initiation phase responsible for the production of hypertension and a chronic phase responsible for its maintenance. The initiation phase occurs promptly following the induction of renal ischemia and is due to renin release from the ischemic kidney. Renin release leads to the generation of angiotensin II, which via its potent vasoconstrictor activity results in elevation of blood pressure. This blood pressure rise can be blocked with the use of angiotensin II antagonists or inhibitors of angiotensin II–converting enzyme.

The chronic phase appears, in part, to be renin-mediated, but is also a consequence of volume expansion caused by sodium retention mediated via a variety of mechanisms (increased aldosterone levels, intrarenal mechanisms, and increased renal sympathetic activity) and via microvascular injury to the contralateral kidney resulting from systemic hypertension.

The implication of these experimental observations is that early intervention to correct the stenosis or block angiotensin II generation or effect restores blood pressure to normal. However, late intervention is not always effective. These observations in experimental disease have been borne out in clinical practice.

DIAGNOSIS AND LABORATORY FINDINGS. The diagnosis of renovascular disease should be considered in the following circumstances: onset of hypertension late in life (after 50 years of age) especially when there is other evidence of atherosclerotic diseases, renal insufficiency, or both; hypertension that is suddenly more difficult to control; accelerated or malignant hypertension, especially with grades III or IV retinopathy in nonblacks; the development of renal insufficiency following the attainment of normotension by the use of antihypertensive therapies, in particular, following the use of angiotensin II–converting enzyme inhibitors; severe hypertension in patients under 30 years of age, especially in white women; the presence of an abdominal or flank bruit in a hypertensive individual; significant hypokalemia either initially or following the use of standard doses of diuretics (suggesting a hyperaldosteronemic state).

There are a number of laboratory and radiologic studies designed to assist in the diagnosis of renal artery stenosis. Ideally these tests would not only identify those patients with anatomic lesions of the renal artery, but suggest which lesions are of physiologic significance. Unfortunately, none of the screening studies are ideal. Rapid sequence IVP has been the classic screening study for renovascular hypertension. When positive by the classic criteria of asymmetric kidney size, increased pyelographic density of the affected kidney, and de-

layed appearance of contrast in the collecting system, the test is reasonably specific in indicating the presence of disease (85% to 90%). However, a normal study can have from 17% to 38% false negative rate for unilateral disease and an even higher rate (greater than 50%) for bilateral disease. Radionuclide scanning is probably less sensitive than the IVP; estimates of vascular perfusion and flow tend to reflect the prevailing level of renal function. Digital subtraction angiography (DSA) allows visualization of the renal arteries with an intravenous injection of contrast. Current limitations of the technique include the requirement for relatively large doses of intravenous contrast material, difficulty in visualizing branches of the renal arteries and in obtaining oblique views, and a 7% incidence of technically uninterpretable studies (such as patient movement, bowel gas). If these technical difficulties can be overcome, DSA will become the screening study of choice.

Random peripheral vein renin determinations have not proved useful in screening for renal arterial disease. Renin profiling, which combines peripheral vein renin determination with a 24-hour urinary sodium excretion measurement, has been espoused by some investigators, but has not been widely accepted. Blood pressure response to converting enzyme inhibition or angiotensin II antagonists reflect the prevailing levels of circulating angiotensin II; however, it does not accurately predict the presence of renal artery stenosis.

Selective renal arteriography with oblique and magnification views remains the standard diagnostic procedure for anatomic renal artery stenosis. The risks of the study, which include hematoma, contrast-induced acute renal failure, and vascular trauma, approach 1% to 2% morbidity in large series. Intraarterial DSA allows the administration of small contrast loads that decrease the risk of contrast nephropathy yet usually produce good visualization of the renal arteries.

Efforts have been made to ascertain the physiologic significance of the anatomic lesion before attempts at surgical correction. Angiographic criteria such as degree of stenosis, poststenotic dilation, or presence of collaterals have not been good predictors of surgical success. The duration of hypertension has been a useful predictor of outcome; patients with hypertension of shorter duration (less than 5 years) generally respond more favorably.

Determining the concentration of renin in the renal venous effluent of both kidneys has been used as a predictor of outcome for 25 years. When the ratio of the renin concentration of the affected kidney to that of the contralateral kidney is 1.5:1 or greater (indicating increased secretion from the affected kidney with suppression of renin release from the contralateral kidney), there is a high likelihood of success from surgical intervention. However, a negative study does not exclude the possibility of a beneficial result. To optimize interpretation of test results, antirenin therapy (β-blocking agents) should be discontinued several days before sampling. Maneuvers to augment renin secretion, such as sodium restriction and, more recently, captopril administration, have also been applied to enhance the test's sensitivity.

MANAGEMENT. Therapy can be either medical or interventional. The intervention can be either removal of the ischemic kidney or an attempt to restore normal blood flow to the organ. Normal flow can be restored via a surgical bypass procedure or via dilatation of the stenotic vessel by percutaneous transluminal renal angioplasty (PTRA).

Medical therapy consists of administration of antihypertensive agents that control blood pressure. With the modern therapeutic armamentarium, including the use of β-blocking agents capable of inhibiting renin release, converting enzyme inhibitors, and potent vasodilators, it is rare that blood pressure levels cannot be restored to normal. The risks of medical management include adverse drug effects, noncompliance with therapy, and the possibility that renal artery stenosis (particularly atherosclerotic disease) will progress and result in diminished functioning renal mass. In general, medical therapy is reserved for those for whom interventional therapy is felt to present an excessive risk.

Surgical therapy usually consists of efforts to revascularize the ischemic kidney, most commonly with the use of aorticorenal saphenous vein bypass graft. A major advance in surgical therapy has been the recognition that patients with atherosclerotic disease of the renal arteries may have clinically significant disease of the coronary and carotid vessels as well. Therefore before undergoing renal revascularization, evaluation and surgical therapy, if necessary, is directed at these other critical vascular systems. Simple nephrectomy is carried out if revascularization is technically impossible or if the involved kidney is making a negligible contribution to renal function, which appears unlikely to improve following restoration of blood flow. Small kidneys (less than 8 cm) are unlikely to benefit from revascularization. Approximately 95% of patients with unilateral fibromuscular disease and 90% of those with unilateral atherosclerotic disease are benefited by the procedure. Surgical mortality is quite low in patients with fibromuscular disease (less than 1%) but is significantly higher in those with atherosclerotic lesions.

PTRA, first introduced by Gruntzig in 1974, is performed by an interventional radiologist. The procedure has a high rate of technical success in fibromuscular disease (90%), with 90% of those experiencing long-term benefit. In unilateral atherosclerotic disease both the technical success rate (70% to 90%) and benefit rate (80%) are lower. In bilateral atherosclerotic disease the success rate is lower still (50%). However, repeated dilation can be performed without additional risk. The risks of the procedure include those of radiocontrast and of the catheter, including thrombotic arterial occlusion, cholesterol emboli, intimal dissection, and even rupture of the renal artery. Although the incidence of morbid events requiring surgical intervention is quite low (about 1% to 2% in experienced centers), patients undergoing the procedure should be considered candidates for surgery, and a qualified vascular surgical team should be available for immediate intervention.

PROGNOSIS. Outcome can be measured as overall mortality, control of hypertension, and preservation of renal function. By all these criteria, interventional therapy is better. Therefore it behooves the clinician to be alert to the diagnosis and pursue it appropriately.

RENAL VEIN THROMBOSIS

Renal vein thrombosis (RVT) occurs both as an acute syndrome characterized by renal failure, flank pain, and hematuria, and a more insidious process complicating preexisting renal disease with worsening of proteinuria, edema, and pulmonary embolism. The former syndrome occurs in infancy; the latter, in the adult with nephrotic syndrome. This discussion focuses primarily on the second syndrome.

ETIOLOGY. As with other causes of venous thrombosis, local stasis of blood flow, hemoconcentration, and defects in the coagulation system contribute to the development of renal vein thrombosis. Profound diarrhea illness and sepsis in infants produces dehydration, hemoconcentration, and possibly disseminated intravascular coagulation resulting in thrombosis. Obstruction of the renal veins can produce thrombosis and be either extrinsic, secondary to paraaortic adenopathy, tumor, or trauma, or intrinsic, with extension of renal carcinoma into the renal vein. Thrombosis also occurs with systemic hypercoagulable states, such as with certain carcinomas, pregnancy, or oral contraceptive use and in the nephrotic syndrome. Older reports of renal vein thrombosis in association with constrictive pericarditis, congestive heart failure, or massive obesity did not exclude intrinsic glomerular pathology as the proximate cause of the thrombosis and should not be included in modern listings of associated conditions.

PATHOPHYSIOLOGY. In infants and children with sepsis and diarrhea or dehydration from other causes, hemoconcentration, volume depletion, and possibly disseminated intravascular coagulation (DIC) appear to be the predominant pathophysiologic factors in the genesis of renal vein thrombosis.

In the adult, current thought suggests that renal vein thrombosis most commonly is a consequence of a primary renal disease producing the nephrotic snydrome. It had previously been held that elevated renal venous pressure associated with renal vein thrombosis would in itself produce the nephrotic syndrome. This concept has had to be abandoned because, in most species, experiments to produce nephrotic syndrome following thrombosis or ligation of the renal veins have failed. In humans renal vein and inferior vena cava thrombosis have both been reported without nephrotic range proteinuria. Conversely, relief of venous hypertension in patients with constrictive pericarditis or after anticoagulation or thrombolytic therapy for renal vein thrombosis does not result in resolution of the nephrotic syndrome, either clinically or histologically.

Rather, it is the nephrotic syndrome itself that induces a systemic hypercoagulable state. The exact mechanism for this is uncertain, but it appears to be related to loss of clot-inhibiting factors into the urine. Low levels of anti–thrombin III have been reported in patients with nephrotic syndrome and renal vein thrombosis. Investigations are currently in progress to evaluate the role of plasma protein C, an important endogenous anticoagulant.

Membranous glomerulopathy occurs in association with RVT with a disproportionately high incidence, whereas it is proportionately less common in minimal change disease. The reason for these associations is not known.

DIAGNOSIS AND LABORATORY FINDINGS. Acute renal vein thrombosis in the infant can lead to complete or partial renal thrombosis and infarction with flank pain, fever, leukocytosis and hematuria, and a flank mass. If both kidneys are involved, oliguria and renal failure ensue.

In the adult, renal vein thrombosis is more insidious and usually accompanies preexisting nephrotic syndrome. It can be completely asymptomatic, without local or systemic consequence. Possible renal effects include worsening of proteinuria, modest impairment of glomerular filtration, and a variety of tubular defects that can mimic a Fanconi's syndrome, such as hyperchloremic acidosis, phosphaturia, glycosuria, and aminoaciduria. It is not certain whether these abnormalities reflect the effect of renal vein thrombosis or the primary renal disorder.

Pulmonary embolism and venous obstruction of the inferior vena cava with worsening edema can be initial manifestations of RVT. Hypertension has also been reported in association with unilateral renal vein thrombosis.

The diagnosis is made radiographically. An IVP can be suggestive if the disease is unilateral and the classic findings of an enlarged kidney with poor concentration of dye and notching of the ureters indicating the presence of collateral vessels is seen. However, renal venography via a percutaneous femoral approach is the current method of choice. High blood flow rates from the renal veins can make interpretation difficult, and there is a risk of dislodging a clot and producing a pulmonary embolism. Alternative diagnostic methods, including CT scan, ultrasound, Doppler and nuclear magnetic resonance imaging, are under investigation.

Renal biopsy may show an increased number of leukocytes marginated in glomerular capillaries and increased interstitial edema. A biopsy should not be performed to make the diagnosis. Whether patients with membranous glomerulopathy should undergo routine renal venography before the development of symptoms or signs of RVT is still unclear. Since the true frequency of the disorder in this population is unknown, most clinicians await the development of a specific indication to pursue the diagnosis.

MANAGEMENT. The current treatment for RVT is systemic anticoagulation with heparin and then warfarin. Streptokinase and tissue plasminogen activator have also been used, but data on whether they are better than conventional therapy are lacking. Long-term anticoagulation can result in the resolution of the thrombosis and a decrease in the risk of pulmonary embolism. Proteinuria or renal function may be improved as well. The duration of anticoagulant therapy is unclear, but the thrombotic diathesis persists as long as the patient remains nephrotic. Some clinicians continue treatment for an arbitrary 3 to 6 months; others continue anticoagulation until the nephrotic syndrome resolves or uremia develops. There is no established role for surgery in this disease.

BIBLIOGRAPHY

Harrington J and Kassirer S: Renal vein thrombosis, Annu Rev Med 33:255, 1982.

Lach F, Papper S, and Massry S: Critical spectrum of renal vein thrombosis, acute and chronic, Am J Med 69:819, 1980.

Madias N: Renovascular hypertension, AKS Nephrol Let 3:27, 1986.

Schreiber MJ, Pohl MA, and Novick AC: Natural history of atherosclerotic and fibros renal artery disorders, Neurol Clin North Am 11:383, 1984.

Ying C and others: Renal revascularization in azotemic, hypertensive patients resistant to therapy, N Eng J Med 311:1070, 1984.

120 · RENAL DISEASE IN PREGNANCY

Stuart M. Homer

Renal function and structure are affected significantly by pregnancy. This section reviews the changes in renal function associated with pregnancy and the interaction of a variety of disorders of the kidney with the pregnant state. Specific attention is focused on the effect of this interaction on fetal outcome (mortality) and maternal outcome (hypertension and renal functional impairment).

Anatomically, pregnancy results in a modest increase in renal size (approximately 1 cm). This is due to vascular engorgement and an increase in interstitial fluid occurring as a consequence of increases in renal blood flow and a generalized increase in interstitial fluid throughout the body. A more prominent and more important change is the general dilation of the collecting system (which includes the renal pelvis and ureters) to the level of the pelvic brim, which results in the slowing of peristalsis and urine flow. This change occurs in the first trimester and persists to term. It most likely is due to the hormonal milieu of the pregnant state, although uterine obstruction of urine flow may be a factor, particularly near term. The ureteral dilation and slowed urine transit rates enhance the likelihood of pyelo-

nephritis when bladder infection is present. The dilation can persist for up to 12 weeks post partum.

Renal blood flow increases early in pregnancy, reaching flow rates 50% to 80% above nongravid values (800 ml/min) in the first and second trimesters and declining modestly near term (700 ml/min). This occurs as a consequence of the overall increase in cardiac output and a specific fall in renal vascular resistance. Glomerular filtration rate (GFR) also increases very early in pregnancy to values 50% over the pregravid state. This increase is maintained to term, implying an increase in filtration fraction in the third trimester. The increase in GFR largely reflects the increase in renal plasma flow, and to a lesser extent the hypoalbuminemia of pregnancy. Reflecting the changes in GFR, normal values for blood urea nitrogen (BUN) and creatinine are lower in pregnancy, averaging 8.7 mg/dl and 0.46 mg/dl respectively. A BUN value greater than 13 or a creatinine value over 0.8 mg% is abnormal and should prompt a vigorous search for a superimposed or underlying renal disease.

A number of alterations in tubular function are noteworthy. Uric acid clearance doubles during pregnancy, resulting in serum urate levels in the 2.5 to 4.0 mg/dl range. An elevation in serum uric acid is a sensitive indicator of the development of preeclampsia or the presence of preexisting renal disease. Glucosuria occurs in most normal pregnancies, largely because the tubules cannot reabsorb the increased filtered load produced by the increased GFR. The glucosuria is not related to blood glucose levels and resolves by 1 week post partum. Aminoaciduria can occur as well but appears restricted to certain amino acids, specifically, histidine, glycine, threonine, serine, and alanine. Amino acid losses can approach 2 g daily. The mechanisms for this have not been well defined.

Protein excretion also increases in pregnancy, reaching 300 mg/24 hours. Potential mechanisms for this include the increase in GFR, increased renal venous pressure caused by compression of the renal veins by the gravid uterus, and the lordotic posture assumed in late pregnancy. This degree of proteinuria can be detected by dipstick; therefore a 24-hour urine protein test must be carried out before determining whether the degree of proteinuria is a pathologic characteristic.

Normal pregnancy is characterized by a chronic respiratory alkalosis secondary to a progesterone-stimulated increase in the respiratory drive. Pco_2 falls to 31 torr, and plasma bicarbonate levels fall to 18 to 22 mEq/L. As a consequence of the renal adjustment to hypocapnia, the pH rises modestly to 7.44.

There is a fall in plasma osmolality of 8 to 10 mOsm/kg and a fall in serum sodium concentration of 4 to 5 mEq/L early in pregnancy. This appears to be a consequence of a "reset" osmostat with alterations in the threshold for thirst and antidiuretic hormone (ADH) secretion. There is also a mild water-excreting defect in pregnancy; that is, as compared to the nonpregnant state, pregnancy impairs the ability to excrete a water load. However, maximum urinary diluting ability is normal. Urinary concentrating ability is normal as well.

The pregnant woman is volume expanded, retaining 7 L of fluid near term. This fluid is shared between the fetus and uteroplacental bed, and the maternal tissues and circulation. There is expansion of both maternal plasma volume and interstitial fluid volume. Nonetheless, renal sodium handling is probably normal, at least as measured in acute studies of salt loading and deprivation.

Blood pressure decreases in pregnancy during the first trimester, remains low during the second trimester, and tends to rise toward pregravid levels near term. The decrement can average about 10 mm/Hg and is due to a decrease in overall peripheral vascular resistance (PVR). The drop in PVR is related both to the uteroplacental circulation, which acts as an arteriovenous fistula, and to the effects of pregnancy-related hormones and prostaglandins on vascular smooth muscle. A diastolic blood pressure greater than 85 mm/Hg in the third trimester or greater than 75 mm/Hg in the first or second trimester is considered excessive and should prompt a search for preexisting hypertension or renal disease or the superimposition of preeclampsia.

PREEXISTING RENAL DISEASES IN PREGNANCY

Renal disease can antedate pregnancy, occur as a consequence of pregnancy, or be a part of a systemic process affecting both the pregnancy and the kidney. Renal disease has an impact on the outcome of pregnancy, both fetal and maternal. In addition, pregnancy itself can have an important impact on the future course of renal disease.

There is a substantial body of literature, much of it controversial, that examines the interaction of preexisting renal disease and pregnancy. In general, if renal function is well preserved (creatinine level 1.4 mg/dl or below) at the start of pregnancy and blood pressure is normal or easily controlled, the outlook for the pregnancy and for future maternal renal function is good. The converse is also true. Hypertension and more severe renal impairment result in a higher incidence of fetal prematurity and mortality and can accelerate maternal renal failure. Renal insufficiency (serum creatinine level over 2.0 mg/dl) is associated with impaired fertility. However, this association is not invariable; there are scattered case reports of dialysis patients carrying a pregnancy successfully to term.

For most glomerular diseases, the above formulation applies. The course of IgA nephropathy, focal sclerosis, and membranoproliferative glomerulonephritis in pregnancy and postpartum have been a subject of controversy caused by variations in data from different centers. Systemic diseases such as polyarteritis nodosa and scleroderma have a notoriously bad outcome in pregnancy, characterized by the development of malignant range hypertension and azotemia. The course of systemic lupus erythematosis (SLE) remains controversial. In general, if the disease has been in remission for a period of time before conception the outlook is good, whereas a high index of disease activity augurs a difficult course. Exacerbations of SLE postpartum have been well described. Diabetic nephropathy is commonly associated with worsening of hypertension and nephrotic syndrome, but these abnormalities usually return towards baseline post partum.

In patients with preexisting proteinuria, protein excretion always increases during pregnancy, sometimes reaching the nephrotic range. In general, hypoalbuminemia is well tolerated by mother and fetus. Severe hypoalbuminemia can lead to small-for-dates babies and aggravate maternal fluid retention. Minimal change disease, when it exacerbates during pregnancy, can be treated with corticosteriods if a significant clinical indication is present.

Polycystic kidney disease in the childbearing years is usually well tolerated. Reflux nephropathy is thought by most not to adversely influence pregnancy except when hypertension or renal insufficiency are present.

Renal transplant recipients of childbearing age can conceive and bear children. In general, the prognosis for mother and fetus correlates with renal function and blood pressure control. Immunosuppressive medication is *not* discontinued. The course of these patients is fraught with potential complications and requires the close cooperation of specialists.

DE NOVO RENAL DISEASE IN PREGNANCY

Renal disease can arise de novo during pregnancy. Pyelonephritis occurs with increased frequency as a consequence of the dilation and stasis present in the upper tracts. There appears to be no increased frequency of bladder infection, however.

Acute renal failure (ARF) can occur during pregnancy; when it does, there is a higher incidence of renal cortical necrosis than in other settings. Previously, the most common cause of ARF in pregnancy was septic abortion. This complication has largely disappeared in this country since the liberalization of laws restricting access to abortions. There remains a significant incidence of ARF associated with toxemic disorders and obstetric catastrophes such as abruptio placentae.

Two rare disorders unique to pregnancy result in acute renal failure. Acute fatty liver of pregnancy results in liver failure, jaundice, and in 60% of cases oliguria and acute renal failure. Its pathogenesis is obscure. Idiopathic postpartum acute renal failure can mimic clinically and pathologically acute hemolytic-uremic syndrome. The disease occurs up to 2 months post partum and is characterized by oliguria, microangiopathic hemolytic anemia, thrombocytopenia, and, often, neurologic signs such as seizures and fluctuations in the level of consciousness. For those who survive the acute disease, chronic renal failure is the usual sequela.

HYPERTENSIVE DISORDERS OF PREGNANCY

The hypertensive disorders of pregnancy are divided into four categories as provided by the American College of Obstetrics and Gynecology: Preeclampsia and eclampsia, chronic hypertension, chronic hypertension with superimposed preeclampsia, and late or transient hypertension.

Preeclampsia occurs in 10% to 20% of primagravidas and between 5% to 7% of all pregnancies. It occurs more commonly in diabetics, in those with preexisting hypertension or renal disease, in the very young (less than 17 years old), in the relatively older pregnant woman (greater than 35 years), and in those with a previous episode of preeclampsia. The syndrome is characterized by the development of hypertension, edema, and proteinuria; there is often evidence for disseminated intravascular coagulation. It occurs after the twentieth week of gestation and can progress in a rapid and dramatic manner. When convulsions occur, the disorder is called eclampsia. Symptoms of headache, abdominal pain, and apprehension can presage the development of frank eclampsia. Rapid weight gain, rise in blood pressure, and hyperreflexia are characteristic physical findings. Laboratory evidence of preeclampsia includes hyperuricemia, a rise in BUN and creatinine values above those normal for pregnancy, proteinuria (occasionally, nephrotic syndrome), and sometimes thrombocytopenia and elevation of fibrin split products. Oliguria and renal failure can occur. Renal pathology reveals the classic lesion of glomerular endotheliosis. The glomerulus is swollen and bloodless; glomerular endothelial cells are swollen and contain numerous vacuoles. Also observed, but of lesser importance, is the appearance in some specimens of histologic evidence of disseminated intravascular coagulate (DIC), including subendothelial fibrin deposits. Renal biopsy is performed only rarely in pregnancy because of the higher incidence of bleeding complications in this setting and because of this it is usually not an acceptable diagnostic tool.

The pathogenesis of preeclampsia is not known. Normally pregnant women are relatively resistant to blood pressure elevations caused by infusions of angiotensin II. In preeclampsia, this insensitivity is lost, even before the clinical manifestations of the disease appear. In addition, plasma volume is diminished and central venous pressure is low despite the presence of edema, again suggesting increased vasoconstriction as the source of elevated blood pressure. Despite the observation of intravascular volume depletion, efforts to treat preeclampsia with volume expansion must still be considered experimental and quite risky. Various pathogenetic hypotheses have been advanced, including uteroplacental insufficiency, inadequate production of vasodilatory prostaglandins, and abnormal placental development.

Management is directed toward confirming the diagnosis and delivering the fetus at an opportune moment. Most authorities consider even the clinical suspicion of preeclampsia as an indication for hospitalization and observation. Patients with elevated blood pressure are treated with bedrest in the left lateral decubitus position. Diuretics are avoided; sometimes α-methyldopa, hydralazine, or both are given for moderate blood pressure elevations. Magnesium sulfate is administered parenterally for neuromuscular irritability, for hyperreflexia, or as seizure prophylaxis. The treatment of choice is the delivery of the fetus. In the absence of obvious signs of clinical improvement with conservative therapy, steps should be taken to deliver the fetus promptly. Failure to do so can increase maternal morbidity or mortality and does not help the fetus, for whom the uterus has become a hostile environment.

Maternal mortality from frank eclampsia ranges from 2% to 5%, and fetal mortality is increased. Blood pressure usually returns to normal within 2 weeks after delivery. Data do not support a role for preeclampsia in producing subsequent hypertension or chronic renal disease in the mother.

CHRONIC HYPERTENSION

Women with chronic hypertension can and do become pregnant. Diagnostic confusion can occur when the pregnant patient has hypertension for the first time in the third trimester. Blood pressure may have been normal in the first and second trimesters because of the pregnancy-induced drop in systemic vascular resistance and may simply be returning to baseline values at term. Careful evaluation is required to exclude preeclampsia in these individuals.

Much controversy exists regarding management of hypertension in pregnancy. Most practitioners would not institute drug therapy for mild blood pressure elevations. When drug therapy is required, hydralazine and methyldopa are the best studied and are proven safe. Diuretics are generally avoided, although they are sometimes continued if the patient had received them before pregnancy. β-blockers are probably safe, although some data suggest they may be associated with fetal bradycardia, hypoglycemia, intrauterine growth retardation, and intrapartum fetal loss. Angiotensin-converting enzyme inhibitors must be avoided; animal studies have demonstrated a high frequency of intrauterine death. The clinical safety of calcium channel blockers in pregnancy is unknown.

In general, with control of blood pressure and avoidance of preeclampsia, the outlook for mother and fetus in chronic hypertension is good. This is true even for secondary forms of hypertension, including hyperaldosteronism or renal artery stenosis. The exception to this is pheochromocytoma, which, when undiagnosed, can lead to substantial maternal and fetal mortality.

SUMMARY

Many types of preexisting renal disease pose only a modest increase in risk of progressive renal disease to the mother.

Certain types of renal pathology are more problematic, such as systemic lupus, IgA nephropathy, and membranoproliferative glomerulonephritis. Scleroderma and polyarteritis nodosa should be considered contraindications to pregnancy. Patients with active lupus should not become pregnant until the disease is quiescent.

Chronic hypertension is usually well tolerated in pregnancy. Care must be taken to watch for the possible superimposition of preeclampsia. Preeclampsia itself must be diagnosed promptly and managed aggressively.

BIBLIOGRAPHY

Burrow GN and Ferris TF: Medical complications during pregnancy, ed 3, Philadelphia, 1988, WB Saunders Co.

Fink L and others: Systemic lupus erythematosis in pregnancy, Ann Intern Med 94:667, 1987.

Hou S, Grossman M, and Madias N: Pregnancy in women with renal disease and moderate renal insufficiency, Am J Med 78:185, 1985.

Jungers P: Chronic kidney disorders in pregnancy, Adv Nephrol 15:103, 1986.

Lindheimer N and Katz A: The kidney in pregnancy. In Brenner B and Rector F, editors: The kidney, ed 3, Philadelphia, 1986, WB Saunders Co.

Dental correlations

Burton H. Goldstein

Patients with renal disease generally have clinical manifestations related to the functional status of their kidneys regardless of the cause of their disease. Their problems and concomitant dental treatment are frequently associated with the various drugs and life-saving treatment modalities such as dialysis and transplantation.

ORAL MANIFESTATIONS. Oral lesions related to renal disease are generally nonspecific. However, many of the metabolic and physiologic body alterations that accompany renal disease have oral manifestations. Clinicians should be aware that some of the signs and symptoms manifested in the oral cavity can suggest the presence of renal disease, especially in the more advanced stages. Since laboratory techniques have become more reliable and sophisticated, renal and electrolyte disorders are frequently discovered before the patient is symptomatic.

Elevation of blood urea nitrogen in renal failure results in a high concentration of urea in the saliva; a breakdown product, ammonia, results. The increased concentrations of ammonia result in some distinguishing oral manifestations. Dysgeusia, often described as a salty or metallic bad taste and frequently perceived as halitosis, is a common occurrence. Uremic stomatitis can occur in severe untreated renal failure. This is most often noted in patients with a blood urea level exceeding 30 mmole/L. Baries' classification of uremic stomatitis consists of two types. *Type I, erythemopulaceous,* initially manifests a red thickening of the buccal mucosa, which later includes a gray, thick, pasty, gluey exudate and pseudomembrane covering the gingiva, fauces, and oral mucosa. When the pseudomembrane is removed with a tongue blade, a swollen, dry, red but not ulcerated mucosa is found. Associated manifestations for type I include fetor oris, dry burning sensation, excessive saliva, and perversion of taste. *Type II, ulcerative form,* is similar to type I but includes loss of integrity of the mucosa with frank ulceration. The ulcers can be superficial or deep and frequently involve the gingiva. Purpura can also be seen on the mucosa as a result of factor III deficiency. Bone marrow depression results in anemia. Excessive salivation is again noted. Parotid and submandibular gland swelling may be seen in patients with chronic renal failure without accompanying uremic stomatitis.

The cause of uremic stomatitis is partially related to the high salivary urea level with consequent breakdown into ammonia and to the presence of other harmful metabolites, which are not being executed by the kidneys. Histologic uremic stomatitis appears as an intense polymorphonuclear inflammation and extensive necrosis of mucosa; the friable mucosa is highly susceptible to secondary infection. The most common bacteria involved are Vincent's organisms, fusobacterium. As in the treatment of acute necrotizing ulcerative gingivitis (ANUG), local debridement and systemic antibiotics (for example, penicillin or erythromycin) are useful therapy.

Patients with uremic stomatitis are severely ill, and the oral lesions can take 2 to 3 weeks to resolve after the onset of dialysis. During this period dental management is generally palliative (for example, hydrogen peroxide, mouth rinses, or topical anesthetics).

Bleeding disorders are associated with uremia and have nonspecific oral manifestations such as ecchymoses, petechiae, and spontaneous gingival bleeding. The same bleeding disorders also contribute to the crusting seen in uremic stomatitis. The mechanisms of these hemostatic defects are complex, and although thrombocytopenia can occur in many uremic patients, the major cause of the clinical bleeding problem is considered to be platelet dysfunction. This abnormality is caused by a dialyzable substance, and the control of the bleeding and associated oral manifestations is related to systemic improvement by dialysis.

Chronic renal failure is frequently accompanied by anemia. The anemia can be severe, with hemoglobin levels of 5 g/dl or less. Oral mucosal and gingival pallor can be present in such situations. This anemia is often well tolerated by the patient and does not usually respond to treatment of renal failure. If other factors compound the anemia of chronic renal failure, such as pernicious anemia, a glossitis may be seen.

Several other factors also cause oral signs in uremic patients. Hyperuricemia secondary to renal failure can cause deposition of urate crystals in the temporomandibular joint or oral soft tissues. Edema, secondary to decrease in osmotic pressure from loss of plasma protein (as in nephrotic syndrome), manifests itself orally in the tissues of low resistance. Therefore the uvula is apt to show signs of congestion with edema. Passive venous congestion secondary to cardiac insufficiency may be evident by swelling on the base and lower surface of the tongue.

Neuropathy occurring with severe renal failure can be manifested as dysesthesia of the lingual nerve. The patient may complain of tingling or numbness of the tongue.

Severe orofacial and odontogenic infections sometimes associated with unusual oral flora can also occur in the debilitated or immunosuppressed renal failure patient. In a series of immunosuppressed and control patients dental infection occurred as frequently as pneumonia or urinary tract infections in the transplant patients. Patients who developed acute alveolar abscesses tended to be immunosuppressed for more than 5 years and had lymphocyte counts less than 400 ml³. The importance of good dental health before transplantation and maintenance of dental health was emphasized, although none of the patients in the study died as a result of dental infection–related sepsis. (See "Dental management".)

The most commonly seen changes on dental radiographs of patients with chronic renal failure are altered trabeculation, altered radiodensity, subperiosteal cortical bone resorption, and partial loss of the lamina dura. Periapical and panoramic radiography can reveal both osteoporotic and osteosclerotic appearances, often termed "chalky," "ground glass," or "granular" because of the delicate, finely meshed trabecular pattern.

The much discussed loss of lamina dura associated with chronic renal failure, although present in some patients, should not be considered diagnostic or specific for renal disease, since it can occur in localized inflammatory disorders as well as in many systemic diseases. The associated "triad" of loss of lamina dura, altered trabecular pattern, and density changes is suggestive or renal osteodystrophy. Temporomandibular joint involvement has been documented to include decreased bone density; subcortical cysts of the condyle; irregularity of the condyle, glenoid fossa, or both; and in the most severe cases, complete resorption of the condylar head and process with resultant acquired dentofacial deformity.

If the process of renal osteodystrophy begins at an early age, during the development of the teeth, the teeth can appear highly calcified, because teeth are depositories of calcium but do not release calcium. Cystic lesions of the jaws (osteoclastomas) may also be evident. These giant cell lesions can cause a thinning of the cortex and can be palpable as surface swellings. Such lesions may be seen in the calvarium, mandible, and maxilla as well as the long bones, pelvis, and phalanges.

The oral manifestations of hyperparathyroidism secondary to renal failure during childhood are important since they affect growth and development of the dentoalveolar complex. Young patients, especially those undergoing dialysis, must be provided with sufficient calcium for proper development of teeth. These patients generally have a low caries incidence, although excessive calculus deposits are detected on the teeth secondary to an increased calcium-phosphate solubility product.

Vitamin D–resistant rickets caused by renal tubular defects cause unique oral manifestations involving the structure of the tooth. Such defects cause the formation of globular dentin with clefts and defects in the dentinal tubules. Pulp horns become elongated and extend to the dentinoenamel junction. The abnormality in dentin formation is a direct cause for frequent bacterial invasion of the pulp without evidence of tubular destruction of the dentin normally seen in the cariously involved tooth. Periapical involvement is seen without apparent tooth involvement. Dental radiographs reveal the presence of lamina dura and an abnormal alveolar bone pattern.

Dental alterations observed in patients with renal disease include both intrinsic staining from previous tetracycline administration and extrinsic staining from iron medications. Enamel hypoplasia, retarded growth, and tooth eruption can be seen, and an increased tendency toward heavy dental calculus formation has been reported.

Malignant renal tumors can metastasize to the jaws, the oral structures, or both. Renal cell carcinoma has been reported to represent 15% of the primary cancers with jaw metastases. The mandible was more frequently involved than the maxilla. These tumors can be accompanied by soft tissue swelling and mobility of the teeth in the area of the lesion. Such rare lesions can be suspected if an extraction socket fails to heal. Direct soft tissue involvement is also rare, in which case the carcinoma can be found in the gingiva, lips, tongue, or salivary glands. The lesions have been described as red-brown in appearance, friable, and cystlike.

Orofacial abnormalities are seen in a number of syndromes that involve renal abnormalities. Patients with chromosomal syndromes, especially trisomy 18 or Turner (XO) syndrome, can have associated renal anomalies, including horseshoe kidney. Cleft palate patients have a higher incidence of renal anomalies than the general population and warrant investigation. Any family history of an infant death related to renal disease should be investigated for the possible presence of renal agenesis or renal dysplasia, which can be associated with Potter syndrome (oligohydramnios syndrome) and bilateral renal agenesis, also associated with micrognathia, cleft lip, and cleft palate. Patients with Reiter's syndrome may have oral lesions; occasionally their involvement of the urinary tract includes nephritis. Multiple oral fibromas are seen in tuberous sclerosis (Bourneville-Pringle syndrome), and 40% of these patients have renal hamartomas. Oral and facial angiokeratomas (multiple red-purple pinpoint lesions especially on the lips) are seen in Fabry's syndrome (angiokeratoma corporis diffusum). These patients suffer progressive renal failure from the accumulation of a glycosphingolipid. Further specific discussion of these and the many other syndromes that can be associated with both oral and renal involvement is available.

DENTAL MANAGEMENT. Dental treatment for patients with end-stage renal disease and transplants is recognized as an essential health service. Dental management is complicated because of the oral disease and the medical problems seen in this population. These patients survive under narrowly controlled conditions of intake and activity as well as under great physiologic and psychologic stress with medications, diet, invasive treatments, limited life-style, and dependency on others. Dental treatment, even minor dental procedures, can present major problems and should be considered particularly stressful when superimposed on such situations.

Hemodialysis is by far the most prevalent therapy for end-stage renal disease. In a survey of 100 hemodialysis patients, more than 60% were in need of dental treatment and 88% had natural teeth present in one or both arches. All renal dialysis patients should be informed of the importance of oral health in preventing complications caused by infection or dietary difficulties. Comprehensive oral evaluation and dental treatment are part of the basic health care of the end-stage renal disease patient. Many hospitals provide dental services, although most medically controlled renal failure patients can be safely and adequately treated in the private dental office.

A healthy dentition and oral cavity should be considered a basic precondition to renal transplantation. The consequences of oral infection can be life-threatening in the immunosuppressed patient. Dental management of the transplant patient is complicated by the potent medications often used to prevent or treat graft rejection. In 21 patients with fever of unknown origin after renal transplantation, 16 had oral pathology including infected nonvital teeth, impacted teeth with the possibility of oral communication, advanced periodontitis with furcation involvement and pockets over 5 mm in depth, and osteomyelitis. Six of these patients' fevers resolved within 12 hours of dental treatment.

The following considerations are important when evaluating and treating the dental patient with renal disease.

Timing. The best time for dental treatment is the day after dialysis. This will avoid bleeding problems related to systemic anticoagulation as well as provide an optimal metabolic condition for the patient. Individual dental or medical considerations can be coordinated with regional anticoagulation techniques, in-hospital dental treatment, and other treatment modifications as suited to individual patient needs.

Asepsis. All patients with end-stage renal disease, including renal transplant recipients, are potential carriers of hepatitis B. Laboratory testing to determine hepatitis B surface antigen (HBsAg) should be routinely obtained for these patients before dental treatment and updated frequently. HBsAg-negative or HBsAb-positive patients can be treated routinely, and HBsAg-positive patients should be treated with currently recommended procedures to minimize the potential transmission of hepatitis B. The presence of hepatitis B antigen does not contraindicate

dental office treatment but rather indicates the need for special care and meticulous techniques. In view of the universal precautions to protect against AIDS, these tests are now virturally mandatory.

Hematologic and physiologic status. The multiple hematologic abnormalities that accompany renal disease and the treatment of renal failure must be considered for each patient as potential modifying factors for dental treatment. Clinical and laboratory evaluation for anemia, bleeding disorders, and white cell abnormalities may be indicated, depending on the status of renal disease or therapeutic modality and the type of dental treatment anticipated. Fluid and electrolyte balance can also be subject to wide ranges of alterations in patients undergoing dialysis and with varying stages of renal failure. Evaluation and stabilization of these alterations should be accomplished before dental treatment.

Maintenance of the vascular access device of the hemodialysis patient is important. The location of the shunt or fistula should be noted and care taken to avoid venipuncture, blood pressure cuff compression, or any trauma to the area. Dental procedures should be delayed for at least 2 weeks after placement or revision of a vascular access and should be avoided during periods of infection or thrombosis of the access.

Patients on continuous ambulatory peritoneal dialysis (CAPD) should be treated similarly to hemodialysis patients. CAPD patients are often more physiologically normal than hemodialysis patients and are not systematically anticoagulated. Dental procedures should be delayed for the first 30 days following placement of the indwelling peritoneal catheter to allow a proper seal to form and should be avoided during any periods of peritoneal or catheter-related complications.

Immunosuppression and corticosteroid medications. Many renal transplant patients are on a regimen of antiinflammatory and immunosuppressive medications. These medications can mask the early signs and symptoms of infection and inflammation, making timely diagnosis difficult and producing a tendency toward more severe problems when first recognized. The prophylactic use of antibiotics for dental treatment must be considered for each patient and each procedure. At present, there is no documented evidence of the efficacy of antimicrobial prophylaxis in the renal transplant patient; however, many dentists and physicians think the benefits of potential protection far outweigh the risks of potential infection. The nature of each dental procedure as well as the individual patient's physical and psychologic status must also be considered. Chronic systemic steroid administration suppresses the patient's ability to respond to stress by causing adrenal atrophy. Supplemental steroids should be considered before stressful dental procedures.

Medications and drug therapy for dental purposes. The practitioner prescribing or administering medications to patients with compromised renal function must be familiar with the metabolism and excretion of each of the agents involved and the functional status of the individual patient's kidneys. To provide safe yet effective drug therapy, modification of the usual dosage regimen may be necessary. For drug administration for dental purposes, two dosage categories are sufficient, both distinguished by amounts of kidney function: patients with mild to moderate renal failure or renal insufficiency and patients with severe renal failure or who are functionally anephric. Guidelines are presented in tabular form and discussed according to therapeutic use. (See Table 1.)

Local anesthesia. Renal failure, renal dialysis, renal transplantation, and other medically controlled conditions related to end-stage renal disease, such as hypertension, do not con-

Table 1 Guidelines for drug therapy in dental treatment of patients with renal disease

Drug	Normal dosage regimen	Dosage adjustment in	
		Renal insufficiency	Anephric patient
ANALGESICS			
Acetaminophen	q3-4h	Unchanged	Avoid
ASA	q3-4h	q4-6h	q8-12h
Phenacetin	q3-4h	Avoid	Avoid
Codeine	q4h	Unchanged	Unchanged
Meperidine	q4h	Unchanged	Unchanged
Morphine	q4h	Unchanged	Unchanged
Pentazocine	q4-6h	Unchanged	Unchanged
SEDATIVES			
Diazepam	q8h	Unchanged	Unchanged
ANTIMICROBIAL AGENTS			
Clindamycin	q6h	Unchanged	Unchanged
Erythromycin	q6h	Unchanged	Unchanged
Tetracycline	q6h	Avoid	Avoid
Doxycylcine	q24h	Unchanged	Unchanged
Penicillin G	q8h	Unchanged	q12-16h*
Penicillin V	q8h	Unchanged	q12-16h*
Amoxillin	q8h	q8-12h	q12-16h
Ampicillin	q6h	q8h	q12h
Cloxicillin	q6h	Unchanged	Unchanged
Dicloxicillin	q6h	Unchanged	Unchanged
Oxacillin	q6h	Unchanged	Unchanged
Methicillin	q6h	Unchanged	Unchanged

These guidelines are suggested estimates aimed at providing optimal therapeutic effects with minimal side effects. Individual patient variation in serum levels can be significant, and this table in no way implies that these regimens are "safe" or rigid requirements. Modified and adapted from Bennett, Singer, and Coggins: JAMA 230:1544, 1974; Heard, Staples, and Czerwinski: J Am Dent Assoc 96:792, 1978; Kelly and others: Oral Surg 50:372, 1980.
*The potassium salt has 1.7 mEg K^+ per 1 million units.

traindicate the use of local anesthetics or vasoconstrictors in dentistry. Provision of adequate pain relief for dental procedures sometimes necessitates the use of vasoconstrictor-containing local anesthetic solutions. The kidney is the main excretory organ for all the local anesthetics commonly used in dentistry and their metabolites. The amide-type local anesthetic agents are excreted approximately 15% or less unchanged, and the ester-type agents are excreted unchanged in even smaller amounts. Significant impairment of renal function can therefore result in increased blood levels of the local anesthetic or its metabolites (which are generally less toxic than the parent compounds), which can cause adverse systemic effects. The use of cocaine is specifically contraindicated since it is excreted entirely unchanged in the urine. On the basis of clinical experience, it is recommended that the slow administration of not more than 25% of the maximum total recommended dosage for the "normal" patient is a practical and safe guideline for local anesthetic injections for dental purposes in the medically controlled patient with absent renal function and not more than 50% of the maximum "normal dose" in the patient with renal insufficiency. Specific information regarding a safe local anesthetic dosage in the patient with end-stage renal disease is not available.

Inhalation sedation. The administration of nitrous oxide and oxygen to produce conscious sedation and analgesia should be carefully performed in the patient with impaired renal function. The degree of anemia and oxygen-carrying capacity of the blood must be considered. However, it appears to be clinically safe and well tolerated to administer up to 50% nitrous oxide and 50% oxygen to the monitored and medically controlled

patient with end-stage renal disease. A knowledge of the patient's hemoglobin level and serum potassium is helpful before the use of inhalation sedation agents.

Parenteral sedation. Anxiety control in dentistry sometimes requires the use of sedative drugs. In patients with end-stage renal disease, diazepam is the safest and most commonly used agent. Whether given orally, intramuscularly, or intravenously, careful administration and especially titration of the intravenous dose should be employed. Diazepam is removed by hemodialysis, and modification of the dosage for single episodic sedative purposes is usually unnecessary. Diazepam and its metabolite oxazepam can linger. All sedated patients should be monitored closely after the procedure and should have someone accompany them home when discharged.

General anesthesia. The administration of general anesthesia to the patient with impaired renal function should be performed by a specialist with knowledge, training, and ability to manage the complex potential problems associated with an anemic hypertensive and metabolically unstable patient. Efficient use of general anesthetic time to accomplish maximal services should be considered and hospitalization is indicated. The clinician should know that inhalation or parenteral sedation is on a continuum with general anesthesia. Therefore the dentist should be able to manage and support the unconscious patient if the administration of any of these agents is considered.

Analgesics. Doses of the nonnarcotic analgesics commonly used in dentistry must be modified for patients with renal failure (Table 1). Both aspirin and acetaminophen are removed by hemodialysis. The use of acetaminophen should be avoided in severe renal failure because of nephrotoxic side effects. Doses of the narcotic analgesics are usually not modified, since they are detoxified primarily by the liver.

Antibiotics. Penicillin is the drug of choice for the treatment of most oral and odontogenic infections. It can be prescribed in usual doses (less than 3 million units/day) for periods up to 5 days. However, high-dose or long-term therapy requires regimen modification, with special caution in using the potassium salt of penicillin G or penicillin V (Table 1). Amoxicillin, ampicillin, and carbenicillin are removed by hemodialysis, whereas the other commonly used penicillins are not. Tetracyclines are usually avoided with renal functional impairment because of their catabolic effects, but if they must be prescribed doxycycline is recommended for uremic patients. Erythromycin and clindamycin can be given in usual doses.

Antibiotic prophylaxis for the patient with renal disease should be considered based on individual patient dictates. Many authors recommend the American Heart Association antibiotic prophylaxis regimen for patients on hemodialysis because of the increased risk of endocarditis as well as to protect the dialysis fistula.

SUMMARY

Guidelines for dental treatment of the patient with renal disease follow:

Renal failure and dialysis patient

1. Consult with the treating physician; consider the patient's clinical status, medications, timing of dialysis and dental treatment, and laboratory data at the time of the dental procedure (coagulation, clotting, electrolytes, and blood chemistry)
2. Use antibiotic prophylaxis if indicated
3. Calculate the appropriate dosage of local anesthetics, therapeutic antibiotics, and analgesics
4. Establish or continue preventive dental care

Renal transplant patient

1. Pretransplant oral health established
2. Consult with treating physician; consider the patient's clinical status, medications, and laboratory data at the time of the dental procedure (hematology and blood chemistry)
3. Use antibiotic and corticosteroid prophylaxis if indicated
4. Administer therapeutic antibiotics if indicated
5. Eliminate odontogenic infection rapidly
6. Establish or continue preventive dental care

BIBLIOGRAPHY

Alexander RE: Hepatitis risk: a clinical perspective, J Am Dent Assoc 101:182, 1981.

Bennett WM and others: Drug prescribing in renal failure: dosing guidelines for adults, Am J Kidney Dis 3(3):155, 1983.

Cappellini G and others: Temporomandilbular joint changes in renal osteodystrophy, Radiol Clin 47:330, 1978.

The choice of antimicrobial drugs, Med Letter 549(22):9, 1980.

Chow M and Peterson D: Dental management for children with chronic renal failure undergoing hemodialysis therapy, Oral Surg 48(1):34, 1979.

Clausen F and Poulsen H: Metastatic carcinoma to the jaws, Acta Pathol Microbiol Scand 57:361, 1963.

Comore B, Collins L, and Crane M: Internal medicine in dental practice, Philadelphia, 1943, Lea & Febiger.

Covino BG and Vassallo HG: Local anesthetics: mechanisms of action and clinical use: the scientific basis of clinical anesthesia series, New York, 1976, Grune & Stratton, Inc.

Eigner TL, Jastak JT, and Bennett WM: Achieving oral health in patients with renal failure and renal transplants, JADA 113:612, 1986.

Epstein SR, Mandel I, and Scopp IW: Salivary composition and calculus formation in patients undergoing hemodialysis, J Periodontol 51:336, 1980.

Fletcher P, Scopp I, and Hersh R: Oral manifestations of secondary hyperparathyroidism related to long term hemodialysis, Oral Surg 43(2):1218, 1977.

Gorlin RJ, Pindborg JJ, and Cohen MM Jr: Syndromes of the head and neck, ed 2, New York, 1976, McGraw-Hill Book Co.

Greenberg M and Cohen G: Oral infection in immunosuppressed renal transplant patients, Oral Surg 43(6):874, 1977.

Guttman RD: Renal transplantation, N Engl J Med 301:975, 1979.

Heard E Jr, Staples AF, and Czerwinski AW: The dental patient with renal disease: precautions and guidelines, J Am Dent Assoc 96:792, 1978.

Hovinga J, Roudovoets AP, and Gaillard J: Some findings in patients uraemic stomatitis, Dent Health 17:15, 1978.

Kelly WH and others: Radiographic changes of the jawbones in end stage renal disease, Oral Surg 50:372, 1980.

Krekeler G, Wilms H, and Akuamoa-Boateng E: Inflammatory pathology in the dental system in renal transplantation, Int J Oral Surg 9:383, 1980.

Payne W and others: Reconstruction of the temporomandibular joints in a patient with renal osteodystrophy, J Oral Surg 35:394, 1977.

Potter JL and Wilson NHF: A dental survey of renal dialysis patients, Public Health, 93:153, 1979.

Shafer W, Hine H, and Levy B: Oral pathology, Philadelphia, 1974, WB Saunders Co.

Sowell SB: Dental care for patients with renal failure and renal transplants, J Am Dent Assoc 104:171, 1982.

Spolnick KJ and others: Dental radiographic manifestations of end-stage renal disease, Dent Rad Photog 54:21, 1981.

Thoma KH: Oral Pathology, St Louis, 1950, The CV Mosby Co.

Van Scoy RE and Wilson WR: Antimicrobial agents in patients with renal insufficiency, Mayo Clin Proc 52:704, 1977.

Westbrook SD: Dental management of patients receiving hemodialysis and kidney transplants, J Am Dent Assoc 96:464, 1978.

Wintrobe MM and others: Clinical hematology, ed 7, Philadelphia, 1974, Lea & Febiger.

SECTION NINE

RESPIRATORY DISEASES

Edited by **William L. Morrissey**

121 · INTRODUCTION TO THE RESPIRATORY SYSTEM

Sanford Levine, Samuel T. Kuna *and*
David J. Henson

DEFINITIONS

"Respiration" can be defined as the processes that effect gas exchange between an organism and its environment. The term "respiratory system" describes the organs and tissues involved in respiration: the nose, mouth, oropharynx, extrapulmonary airways, thoracic cage, respiratory muscles, pleura, lungs, nerves, spinal cord, brain, and cardiovascular system. In this chapter we have restricted discussion of pathologic conditions of the respiratory system to the extrapulmonary and intrapulmonary airways, lungs, pleura, chest wall, and muscles of respiration.

OVERVIEW OF RESPIRATION

The major function of the lung is to add oxygen to and remove carbon dioxide from venous blood. This task is accomplished through two different conducting systems: a gas-conducting system and a blood-conducting system. The gas-conducting system terminates in blind pouches, or alveoli; the major function of this system is to maintain gas tensions in these alveoli in the direction of ambient gas. The blood-conducting system transports venous blood to alveolar walls; the blood is contained in these walls in thin-walled exchange vessels, or pulmonary capillaries. The surface area of the pulmonary capillary-alveolar interface constitutes the major area of gas exchange. In adults the surface area of this interface is about 70 m², or approximately 40 times the surface area of the body. To further facilitate gas transfer between alveoli and pulmonary capillary blood, the membrane separating these structures is only 1 or 2 μm thick.

The gas-conducting system begins at the two nasal passages (sometimes a third passage, the mouth, also is used), which subsequently merge into one tube, the trachea. The trachea subdivides into two main branches, the left and right main-stem bronchi. Each main-stem bronchus passes to its corresponding lung (for example, the left main-stem bronchus to the left lung) and then has 20 to 23 further subdivisions (or bifurcations). These subdivisions have about 1 million terminal conducting tubes, and the 300 million alveoli (the number in the two lungs of adults) arise from these terminal conducting tubes. The diameters of the alveoli range from 75 to 300 μm.

During quiet breathing the diaphragm is the principal muscle of inspiration, and it accounts for the movement of more than two thirds of the air that enters the lung. When the diaphragm contracts, its domes descend and the chest expands longitudinally. At the same time, because of the vertically oriented attachment of the diaphragm to the costal margins, contractions elevate the lower ribs.

Contraction of the intercostal muscles (external intercostal and parasternal intercartilaginous muscles) also raises the ribs during inspiration. As the ribs are elevated, the anteroposterior and transverse dimensions of the thorax enlarge as a result of the movement of the ribs around the axes of their necks. Upward displacement of the upper ribs increases the anteroposterior dimension, whereas elevation of the lower ribs increases the transverse dimension of the chest.

Besides the diaphragm and intercostal muscles, other inspiratory muscles may play a role in enlarging the thorax in certain circumstances. The scalene muscles make their major contribution during high levels of ventilation, when the upper parts of the thorax must be enlarged. These muscles arise from the transverse processes of the lower five cervical vertebrae and insert into the upper aspect of the first and second ribs. Contraction of these muscles elevates and fixes the uppermost part of the rib cage.

Another accessory muscle, the sternocleidomastoid, normally becomes active only at high levels of ventilation. Contraction of the sternocleidomastoid muscle frequently is apparent during severe asthmatic or bronchitic episodes. The sternocleidomastoid muscle elevates the sternum and slightly enlarges the anteroposterior and longitudinal dimensions of the chest.

In contrast to inspiration, expiration during quiet breathing occurs passively as a result of lung recoil. However, expiration does become active at higher levels of ventilation and when movement of air out of the lungs is impeded. The muscles involved in active expiration include the internal intercostal muscles and the transversus and rectus abdominis muscles, which compress the abdominal contents, depress the lower ribs, and pull down the anterior part of the lower chest.

TOTAL VENTILATION VERSUS ALVEOLAR VENTILATION

Total ventilation is the volume of air entering or leaving the respiratory system during each breath (tidal volume) or each minute (minute ventilation or minute volume).

Alveolar ventilation is the volume of gas entering the alveoli during each breath or each minute. This gas entering the alveoli arises from two sources. In early inspiration the alveoli are filled with gas remaining in the conducting airways after the last expiration, whereas during the latter portion of inspiration freshly inspired gas enters the alveoli. Alveolar ventilation is always less than total ventilation; the difference between the two depends on the anatomic dead space (the internal volume of the conducting airways), tidal volume, and respiratory frequency.

ALVEOLAR VENTILATION AND ARTERIAL CARBON DIOXIDE TENSION

The following relationship exists between alveolar ventilation, arterial carbon dioxide tension (Pa_{CO_2}), and CO_2 production:

$$Pa_{CO_2} \propto \frac{CO_2 \text{ production}}{\text{Alveolar ventilation}}$$

This indicates that Pa_{CO_2} represents a quantitative statement of the ratio between tissue CO_2 production and alveolar ventilation. Strictly speaking,

$$Pa_{CO_2} \text{ in mm Hg} = \frac{CO_2 \text{ production} \times 0.863}{\text{Alveolar ventilation}}$$

when CO_2 production is stated in milliliters per minute at standard temperature and pressure of dry gas (STPD), and alveolar ventilation is stated in milliliters of gas per minute at body temperature and pressure saturated with water vapor (BTPS). In normal humans at sea level, a Pa_{CO_2} of 36 to 42 mm Hg represents an appropriate value. The terms "hypoventilation" and "hyperventilation" describe abnormal relationships between alveolar ventilation and tissue CO_2 production. Hypoventilation is characterized by an increase in Pa_{CO_2} (that is, greater than 42 mm Hg); this disorder indicates a decrease in alveolar ventilation per unit of CO_2 production. In contrast, hyperventilation is characterized by a decrease in Pa_{CO_2} (that is, less than 36 mm Hg); this latter disorder exhibits an increase in alveolar ventilation per unit of CO_2 production.

Some clinicians erroneously use Pa_{CO_2} as a quantitative measure of alveolar ventilation, believing that a constant Pa_{CO_2} implies no change in alveolar ventilation. This generalization is true only for circumstances in which tissue CO_2 production remains constant. However, during moderate muscular exercise, an unchanged Pa_{CO_2} accompanies twofold to sixfold increases in both alveolar ventilation and tissue CO_2 production.

COMPOSITION OF ALVEOLAR GAS AND ARTERIAL OXYGEN TENSION

Alveolar gas can be thought of as a compartment of gas lying between atmospheric air and alveolar capillary blood. O_2 is continuously removed from the alveolar gas and CO_2 continuously added to it by blood flowing through alveolar capillaries. Alveolar gas tensions (Pa_{O_2}, Pa_{CO_2}) exhibit three important phenomena: (1) in each alveolus the gas tensions vary throughout every breath; P_{O_2} is highest and P_{CO_2} is lowest at end-inspiration; (2) in the same alveolus gas tensions vary from breath to breath; and (3) gas tensions differ considerably between different alveoli.

Despite these statements about the heterogeneity of alveolar gas, calculating the *mean* Pa_{O_2} is useful. Even in normal subjects, mean Pa_{O_2} is always greater than Pa_{O_2}. The difference between alveolar and arterial P_{O_2} is termed the "alveolar-arterial P_{O_2} difference," or $P(A-a)_{O_2}$; it is a measure of the lung's efficiency in transferring O_2 between the alveolus and blood. In normal young subjects breathing room air, the $P(A-a)_{O_2}$ usually is less than 12 mm Hg, whereas in patients with lung disease this difference is greater than 15 mm Hg. When patients with lung disease hyperventilate, their Pa_{O_2} is sometimes raised to normal values; however, their $P(A-a)_{O_2}$ remains abnormally high (greater than 15 mm Hg).

Calculation of mean Pa_{O_2}

An approximate clinical method of calculating mean Pa_{O_2} is as follows:

$$Pa_{O_2} = P_{I_{O_2}} - \frac{Pa_{CO_2}}{R}$$

where

Pa_{O_2} = Mean alveolar P_{O_2}
$P_{I_{O_2}}$ = Moist inspired P_{O_2}, that is $F_{I_{O_2}} \times$ (barometric pressure − water vapor pressure)
Pa_{CO_2} = Mean arterial P_{CO_2}
R = Respiratory exchange ratio, that is, milliliters of CO_2 excreted / milliliters of O_2 taken up
$F_{I_{O_2}}$ = Fractional concentration of O_2 in inspired gas

For normal humans in steady-state conditions at sea level, the $P_{I_{O_2}}$ of moist inspired air (that is, tracheal gas) is approximately 150 mm Hg, Pa_{CO_2} approximates 40 mm Hg, and R varies between 1.0 and 0.7. For an R of 1.0, $Pa_{O_2} = 110$ mm Hg, whereas an R of 0.7 results in a Pa_{O_2} of 93 mm Hg. For clinical purposes, an R of 0.8 usually is assumed.

PULMONARY PERFUSION

The lung has a dual blood supply: the pulmonary circulation and bronchial circulation. Bronchial arteries arise from the thoracic aorta and hence have systemic pressures. They perfuse the tracheobronchial tree and anastomose with the pulmonary circulation. Most major episodes of hemoptysis are caused by abnormalities in the tracheobronchial tree.

Some of the blood in the bronchial circulation does not come into contact with the alveoli and is desaturated when it enters the left atrium. Blood from the bronchial circulation and the thebesian veins of the left ventricle accounts for the normal right-to-left anatomic shunt that is about 6% of the resting cardiac output.

The pulmonary circulation arises from the right ventricle. It is a low-pressure system. The normal pulmonary artery pressure (PAP) is 20/10 mm Hg with a mean of 14 mm Hg. Although the pulmonary circulation has almost the same blood flow as the systemic circulation, the pressures are lower in the former because of the low pulmonary vascular resistance (PVR). The normal PVR is less than 1 mm Hg/L/sec and is less than 10% of systemic vascular resistance. With increases in pulmonary blood flow, as during exercise, PVR decreases and mean PAP increases only slightly. This decrease in PVR results from an increase in the total cross-sectional area of the vascular bed from distention of vessels that already contain circulating blood and recruitment of previously collapsed vessels. The ability of the pulmonary circulation to adapt to changes in blood flow is dramatically demonstrated after a pneumonectomy. Despite doubling of blood flow to the remaining normal lung, PAP remains normal. More than 50% of the pulmonary vascular tree must be obliterated for this condition to be the sole cause of increased PAP. Other factors that can increase PAP are (1) increased left atrial pressure, (2) alveolar hypoxia, (3) acidemia, and (4) humoral substances such as histamine, catecholamines, and prostaglandins. Release of these humoral substances is the proposed mechanism for the rise in PAP after major pulmonary emboli that occlude less than 50% of the pulmonary vascular bed.

RELATIONSHIP BETWEEN ALVEOLAR VENTILATION AND PULMONARY CAPILLARY BLOOD FLOW
Distribution of pulmonary capillary blood flow

Gravity plays a major role in the distribution of pulmonary capillary blood flow. In the upright human lung, capillary blood flow decreases almost linearly from bottom to top. When the subject lies supine, the apical zone blood flow increases significantly and the blood flow distribution from apex to base becomes fairly uniform. However, in this posture, blood flow in the posterior (dependent) regions of the lung exceeds flow in the anterior parts. Measurements on human subjects suspended upside down show tht apical blood flow exceeds basal blood flow in this position.

The role of gravity in accounting for the vertical distribution of pulmonary capillary blood flow in upright humans can be explained by hydrostatic pressure differences in the pulmonary blood vessels. Viewing the pulmonary arterial system as a continuous column of blood, the difference in pressure between the top and bottom of a vertically suspended lung 30 cm high is about 30 cm of water, or 23 mm Hg. This is a large pressure difference for the low-pressure pulmonary circulation (normal pressure equals 20/10), and its effects account for the distribution of pulmonary capillary blood flow in the upright position.

Distribution of alveolar ventilation

The alveoli are not uniformly ventilated in human lungs. Some alveoli are hyperventilated, whereas others are hypoventilated. The presence of nonuniform alveolar ventilation can be demonstrated by many tests such as nitrogen washout, closing volume, and radionuclide techniques.

Matching of alveolar ventilation and pulmonary capillary blood flow

For the entire respiratory system, the matching of alveolar ventilation to pulmonary capillary blood flow usually is quantitated by the ventilation-perfusion ratio ($\dot{V}A/\dot{Q}c$). In healthy humans under basal conditions (that is, 4 L/min of alveolar ventilation and 5 L/min of pulmonary blood flow), the $\dot{V}A/\dot{Q}c$ for the entire respiratory system is 0.8.

Just as there is a $\dot{V}A/\dot{Q}c$ ratio for the entire respiratory system, each of the 300 million alveoli in the two lungs has its own $\dot{V}A/\dot{Q}c$ ratio. The $\dot{V}A/\dot{Q}c$ of each alveolus is determined by the ratio of ventilation to blood flow for that alveolus. Fig. 121-1 presents a schematic diagram of three representative alveoli. Alveolus B has a normal $\dot{V}A/\dot{Q}c$ ratio, approximately 0.8. In Fig. 121-1 this alveolus has a Po_2 of 100 mm Hg and a Pco_2 of 40 mm Hg. Alveolus A is distal to an obstructed bronchus; since this alveolus is not ventilated, it has a $\dot{V}A/\dot{Q}c$ ratio of 0. The gas tensions in this alveolus are in equilibrium with mixed venous blood; the Po_2 is 40 mm Hg and the Pco_2 is 45 mm Hg. Perfusion has been eliminated in alveolus C; since this alveolus is not perfused, its $\dot{V}A/\dot{Q}c$ ratio is infinite. The gas tensions in this alveolus are identical to those in moist ambient gas; the Po_2 is 150 mm Hg, and the Pco_2 is 0 mm Hg. Even normal individuals may have a few alveoli with a ratio of 0 or infinity, but most are close to four fifths, or 0.8. Patients with pulmonary disease have more alveoli with a ratio of 0 or infinity and many more that deviate significantly from 0.8.

Effects of $\dot{V}A/\dot{Q}c$ abnormalities on $Paco_2$

Fig. 121-2, A, indicates that over the physiologic range, a linear relationship exists in blood between Pco_2 and CO_2

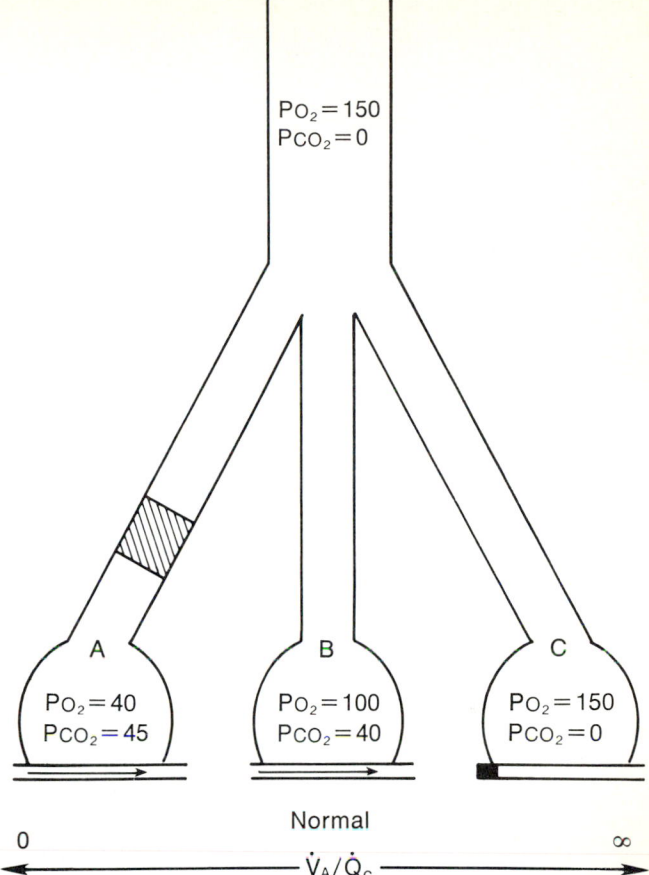

Fig. 121-1   Relationships of alveolar ventilation to pulmonary capillary blood flow (VA/QC).

content. Alveoli with infinite $\dot{V}A/\dot{Q}c$ ratios have no blood flow and therefore play no role in determining $Paco_2$. However, alveoli with high $\dot{V}A/\dot{Q}c$ ratios are extremely effective. Alveoli with high $\dot{V}A/\dot{Q}c$ ratios can compensate for alveoli with low $\dot{V}A/\dot{Q}c$ ratios with respect to pulmonary CO_2 elimination and thereby maintain a normal $Paco_2$.

Effects of ventilation-perfusion abnormalities on Pao_2

Alveoli with low $\dot{V}A/\dot{Q}c$ ratios cause arterial hypoxemia regardless of the presence of alveoli with high $\dot{V}A/\dot{Q}c$ ratios. Fig. 121-2, B, shows the oxyhemoglobin dissociation curve. Because of the nonlinear shape of this curve, the decrement in arterial blood O_2 content caused by alveoli with low Po_2 cannot be compensated for by alveoli with relatively high Po_2, and arterial hypoxemia results.

ROLE OF DIFFUSION IN ALVEOLAR-CAPILLARY GAS TRANSFER

Diffusion is the process by which gas transfer occurs between the alveolus and the capillary; it is determined by the following variables: surface area of the alveolar-capillary membrane, thickness of the alveolar-capillary membrane, and difference in partial pressure between the two sides of the membrane (that is, the alveolar-capillary gradient). Decreases in tissue surface area of the alveolar-capillary membrane, increases in thickness of this membrane, and decreases in the alveolar-capillary gradient all decrease the rate of gas transfer between the alveolus and pulmonary capillary. This rate of gas transfer also is pro-

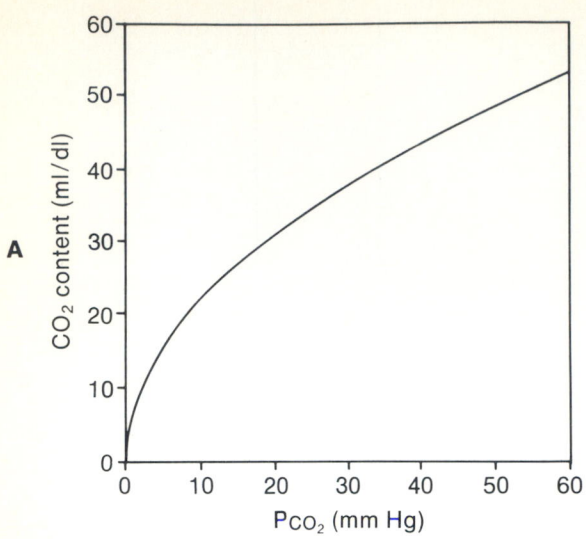

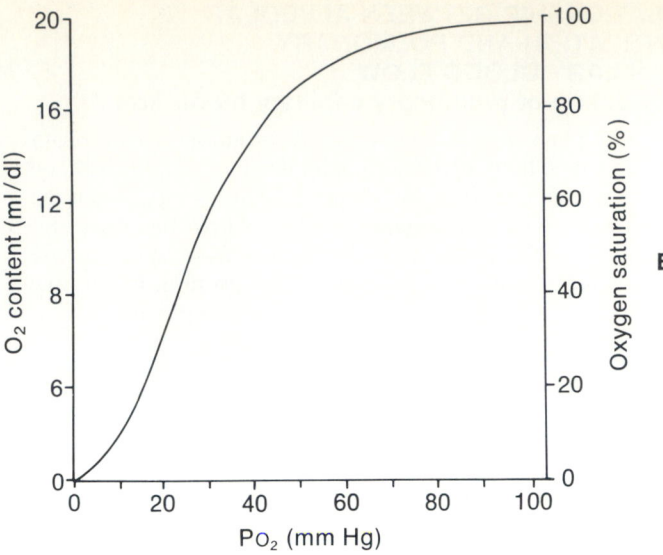

Fig. 121-2   Relationship between gas contents and partial pressure. **A,** Relationship between P_{CO_2} (abscissa) and CO_2 content (ordinate). **B,** Relationship between P_{O_2} (abscissa) and O_2 content and percent of saturation (ordinate). O_2 content data assume 15 g hemoglobin/dl blood.

portional to a diffusion constant that depends on the properties of the tissue and the particular gas.

Under resting conditions the red blood cell (RBC) spends about 0.75 second in its passage through the pulmonary capillary. The P_{O_2} in an RBC entering the pulmonary capillary is about 40 mm Hg. Since the alveolar P_{O_2} is 100 mm Hg, this large pressure difference causes the P_{O_2} in the RBC to rise rapidly; RBC P_{O_2} very nearly reaches P_{AO_2} by the time the RBC is one third of its way along the capillary. Under normal circumstances there is no measurable P_{O_2} difference between alveolar gas and end-capillary pulmonary blood; therefore diffusion is not a rate-limiting factor in alveolar-capillary O_2 exchange in resting humans.

During severe exercise the time spent by the RBC in the pulmonary capillary may diminish to 0.25 second. Therefore the time available for oxygenation is less, but in normal subjects breathing ambient air there is still no alveolar–end pulmonary capillary P_{O_2} gradient. However, if the alveolar-capillary membrane is abnormal, O_2 is transferred across the alveolar-capillary membrane at a slower rate and the end-capillary RBC P_{O_2} may be less than the P_{AO_2}. In this case diffusion constitutes a rate-limiting process in oxygenating pulmonary capillary blood.

Another method of demonstrating diffusion limitation of O_2 transfer is to reduce P_{AO_2} (for example, to 50 mm Hg). In this case the P_{O_2} of RBCs entering the pulmonary capillaries may be only about 20 mm Hg; however, the alveolar-capillary O_2 gradient has been reduced from a normal of 60 mm Hg to 30 mm Hg. Therefore transfer of O_2 occurs at a slower rate. In the normal individual an alveolar–end capillary P_{O_2} gradient may not occur under these circumstances; however, in cases in which the alveolar-capillary membrane is abnormal, end-capillary P_{O_2} is less than P_{AO_2}. Thus once again in the abnormal lung, diffusion constitutes a rate-limiting process in oxygenating pulmonary capillary blood.

The role of diffusion as a rate-limiting factor in the oxygenation of pulmonary capillary blood in normal subjects remains controversial. However, some authorities believe that exhausting exercise at high altitudes (that is, hypoxic conditions) constitutes a situation in which diffusion impairment of

O_2 transfer can be demonstrated in normal humans. Therefore it follows that an individual with an abnormal blood gas barrier probably would show diffusion impairment of oxygenation in the laboratory while breathing hypoxic gas mixtures during exercise.

Measurements of diffusing capacity

Carbon monoxide (CO) generally is used in diffusion capacity measurements, because it provides certain technical advantages; in addition, this gas is transported and absorbed in the same manner as O_2. The CO diffusing capacity (D_{LCO}) is equal to CO uptake per minute divided by the mean pressure gradient for CO between alveolar gas (P_{ACO}) and pulmonary capillary blood.

Clinical relevance of D_{LCO}

The main clinical problem with D_{LCO} is that it is not a specific test of abnormality of the alveolar-capillary membrane; for example, a patient who has undergone a pneumonectomy with no obvious pathologic condition in the remaining lung has a significant decrease in D_{LCO}. After many years of using this test, most experts now agree that D_{LCO} is affected by the following variables: lung volume, pulmonary capillary blood volume, blood hemoglobin concentration, and $\dot{V}_A/\dot{Q}_C$ mismatch. Decreases in lung volumes, pulmonary capillary blood volume, and hemoglobin concentration all decrease D_{LCO}; increases in $\dot{V}_A/\dot{Q}_C$ mismatch also decrease D_{LCO}. Because so many pathologic processes other than diffusion can decrease D_{LCO}, the British literature uses the less specific term "CO transfer factor" rather than "diffusing capacity."

The precise relationship between decreases in D_{LCO} and resting arterial hypoxemia remains somewhat controversial. However, most authorities believe that patients with interstitial lung disease without obvious $\dot{V}_A/\dot{Q}_C$ abnormalities can show decreases in D_{LCO} in the absence of resting arterial hypoxemia.

CONTROL OF VENTILATION

The respiratory center in the medulla oblongata regulates the neural drive to the muscles of ventilation; the output from this center is modulated by multiple inputs. Afferents from the

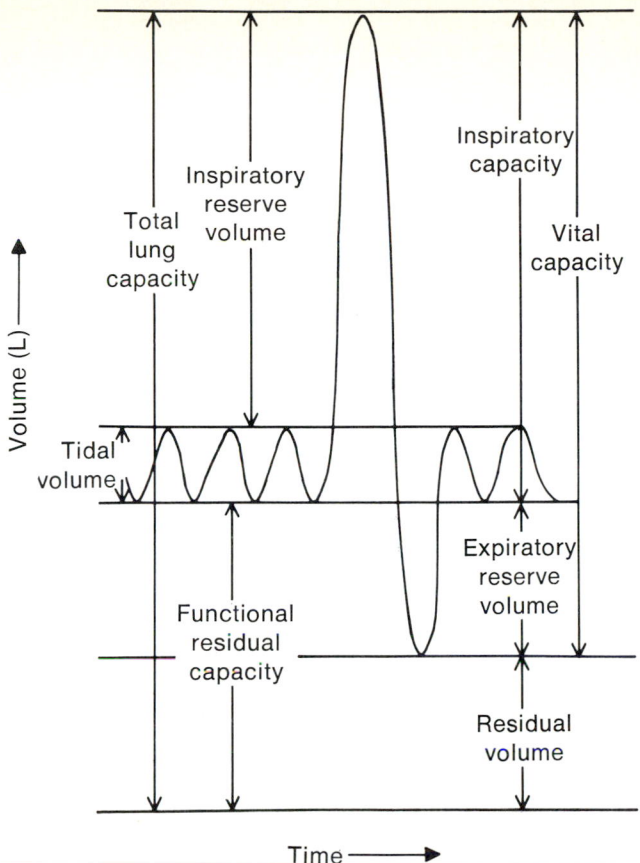

Fig. 121-3   Lung volumes and capacities.

the lungs, which become very stiff at high lung volumes). Loss of lung recoil in conditions such as emphysema allows the inspiratory muscles to shorten further, resulting in increased TLC.

Vital capacity (VC) is defined as the amount of gas that a person can exhale from TLC. The VC is always decreased in restrictive ventilatory disorders (such as pulmonary fibrosis), and it may or may not be decreased in obstructive pulmonary disease.

Residual volume (RV) is the amount of gas remaining in the lung at the end of a maximal expiration. In young individuals the RV is determined by the point at which the inward pressure developed by the expiratory muscles and the lung is equal and opposite to the outward recoil of the chest wall. (Actually at RV the inward recoil pressure of the lung is quite small; on the other hand, the outward recoil of the chest wall is large.) In older individuals the RV is governed mainly by factors that regulate the caliber and patency of peripheral airways; thus even though the expiratory muscles are capable of greater thoracic compression, further exhalation of gas is prevented by airway closure.

Lung volumes and capacities vary among healthy individuals according to their age, sex, and physical characteristics (especially height). Because body build varies slightly from one ethnic group to another, it is important to have normal data that pertain to the population being studied. Measured lung volumes and capacities are usually expressed as both the observed value and the percentage of the predicted value for a normal subject of the same age, sex, and height:

$$\text{Percent predicted} = \frac{\text{Observed value}}{\text{Predicted value}} \times 100$$

Measured values for lung volumes and capacities should not be considered abnormal unless they are clearly outside the range of values likely to be found in normal individuals (100% ± 20% for VC, TLC, and RV).

Measurement of the forced expiratory vital capacity

Measurement of the forced expiratory vital capacity (FVC) is probably the most commonly used test of pulmonary performance. In this test the subject (wearing noseclips) inspires maximally to TLC and then forcefully expires into a spirometer until RV is reached. The most commonly used spirometer, the water-filled spirometer, presents a record of volume on the ordinate versus time on the abscissa. Fig. 121-4,A, presents a representative volume-time record of an FVC of a normal subject. In normal individuals the FVC equals the VC from a slow or nonexpulsive maneuver. However, in patients with obstructive airways disease, vigorous expiration may cause airways to narrow or close so that the FVC may be less than the slow VC.

Additional information about airway function can be obtained from the forced expiratory volume in 1 second ($FEV_{1.0}$), the forced expiratory volume in 3 seconds ($FEV_{3.0}$), and the flow rate between 25% and 75% of the VC (FEF_{25-75}). The volume-time plot in Fig. 121-4, A, shows all of these measurements. In normal individuals the ratio between $FEV_{1.0}$ and FVC ($FEV_{1.0}/FVC$) is greater than 75%, and the ratio between $FEV_{3.0}$ and FVC ($FEV_{3.0}/FVC$) is greater than 97%. In patients with obstructive pulmonary disorders, $FEV_{1.0}/FVC$ is less than 75%, $FEV_{3.0}/FVC$ is less thn 97%, and FEF_{25-75} is appreciably less than the predicted normal measurement.

Other types of spirometers (such as a rolling seal) present a recording of flow on the ordinate versus volume on the abscissa;

cerebral cortex can bring ventilation under conscious control. Other afferents relay information about the effectiveness of gas exchange by monitoring the tensions of O_2 and CO_2 is arterial blood. The input from these chemoreceptors is referred to as the chemical drive to ventilation. The Po_2 of arterial blood is monitored by the carotid and aortic bodies. This information is transmitted to the brain via the glossopharyngeal and vagus nerves. Removal of the carotid bodies in humans ablates the ventilatory response to arterial hypoxia. However, although both the carotid and aortic bodies respond to increases in arterial Pco_2, removal of these structures does not ablate the ventilatory response to hypercapnia; the reason for this is that an important CO_2 or H^+ receptor is located on the surface of the medulla oblongata.

Receptors in the trachea and lungs transmit information about the mechanical state of the lung to the respiratory center via the vagus nerves and spinal cord. Receptors innervated by the vagus nerves include irritant receptors, stretch receptors, and J receptors; inputs from these receptors constitute the mechanical drive to ventilation. Without an increased chemical drive to ventilation, an increased mechanical drive may explain the tachypnea seen in lung disorders such as pulmonary edema and asthma.

EVALUATION OF PULMONARY PERFORMANCE
Measurement of lung volumes and capacities

Fig. 121-3 presents a schematic diagram of the lung volumes and capacities. When the lungs are fully expanded, the amount of gas they contain is called the total lung capacity (TLC). TLC is determined by the point at which the pressure developed by the inspiratory muscles is equal and opposite to the combined recoil pressures of the lungs and chest wall (principally

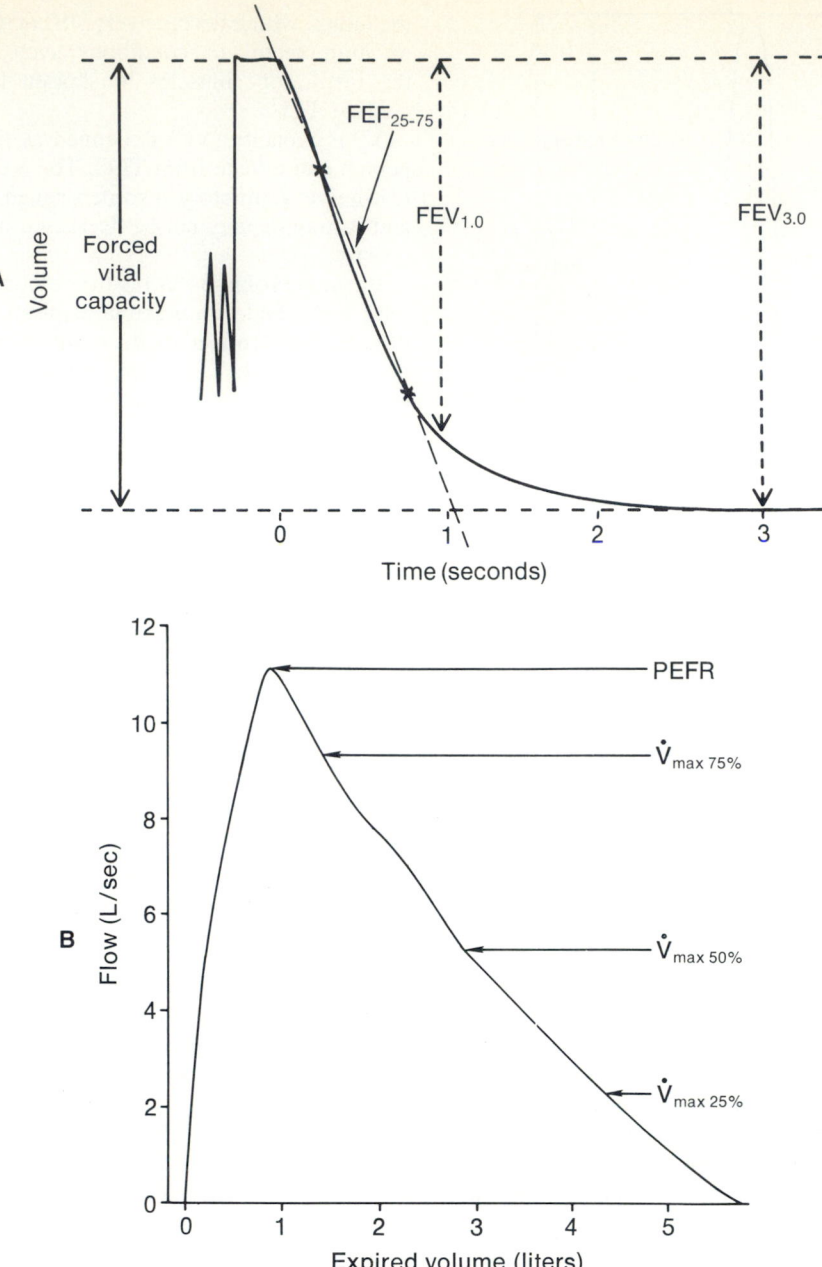

Fig. 121-4   Forced expiratory vital capacities. **A,** Volume-time representation, FEF_{22-75} mean flow rate between 25% and 75% of vital capacity; $FEV_{1.0}$ forced expired volume in 1 second; $FEV_{3.0}$ forced expired volume in 3 seconds. **B,** Flow-volume representation of forced expiratory vital capacity. *PEFR,* peak expiratory flow rate; other markings on flow-volume loop indicate maximal flow *rates* at 75% of FVC($V_{max75\%}$). 50% of FVC ($V_{max50\%}$). and 25% of FVC ($V_{max25\%}$).

Fig. 121-4, *B,* presents a representative flow-volume record of an FVC of a normal subject. The markings on this diagram indicate peak expiratory flow rate (PEFR) and maximal flow rates at 75% of FVC ($\dot{V}_{max\ 75\%}$), 50% of FVC ($\dot{V}_{max\ 50\%}$), and 25% of FVC ($\dot{V}_{max\ 25\%}$). From the flow-volume loop, all of the maximal flow rates at any fraction of the VC can be determined and reported as percentages of the predicted values for an individual of the same age, sex, and body size.

The early portion of the maximal expiratory flow-volume curve, which includes peak flow and probably $\dot{V}_{max\ 75\%}$, is determined largely by the effort exerted by the subject and is called the effort-dependent segment. Below 75% of the VC, increasingly expiratory effort fails to augment the velocity of

airflow; therefore this latter portion is called the effort-independent segment. Effort independence of expiratory flow (at intermediate and low lung volumes) is explained by a combination of circumstances through which increasing expiratory effort narrows airways by the phenomenon of dynamic compression and increases airway resistance by the amount necessary to offset the effect of the increased driving pressure.

Measurement of functional residual capacity

Functional residual capacity (FRC) is the volume of gas remaining in the lungs at the end of a normal expiration. Currently two techniques are used to measure FRC: inert gas dilution and body plethysmography.

The closed-circuit helium dilution method is the most commonly employed inert gas dilution method. In this method a spirometer is initially filled with a mixture of approximately 10% helium in air. Starting precisely at FRC, the patient begins to breathe from the closed spirometer system. The spirometer contains a CO_2 scrubber to absorb all the CO_2 produced by the patient. This scrubbing of CO_2 would decrease the total volume of gas in the spirometer; however, O_2 is added by the operator to maintain a constant volume. As the helium in the spirometer mixes with the gas in the patient's lungs, the concentration of helium continuously falls until a constant level is achieved. Since helium does not cross the alveolar-capillary membrane, the total volume of helium in the patient's lungs plus the spirometer system does not change during the rebreathing period. Therefore the initial concentration of helium multiplied by the initial volume of the spirometer system must equal the final concentration of helium multiplied by the total volume of the spirometer-patient system at the end of the test (that is, the sum of the patient's FRC and the final volume of gas in the spirometer system). The patient's FRC can be easily computed from the relationship previously noted. However, FRC measurements by all of the inert gas dilution techniques measure only the volume of gas that freely communicates with the airways during the breathing maneuver; dilution techniques do not detect gas trapped beyond closed (or narrowed) airways and in poorly communicating regions such as those with bullae.

Body plethysmography involves placing the patient in the plethysmograph, a large, airtight box resembling a telephone booth. The patient initially breathes through a mouthpiece, which is then occluded by a shutter at the end of a normal expiration (that is, FRC). The individual then pants against the occluded mouthpiece. During panting, with its associated thoracic volume changes, pressure is measured at the mouth and in the plethysmograph; changes in the plethysmograph pressure reflect changes in thoracic volume. From application of Boyle's law, which states that the pressure times the volume of a gas is constant if the temperature remains the same, the volume of gas in the thorax can be calculated. The body plethysmograph measures all of the gas present during breathing, including that in freely communicating airspaces and any that may be trapped behind poorly communicating airways (as in bullous emphysema) or in closed spaces (as in pneumothorax).

At FRC the inward recoil pressure of the lungs is equal but opposite to the outward recoil pressure of the chest wall. Therefore the FRC is reduced by conditions characterized by an increased recoil pressure of the lungs (such as pulmonary fibrosis); similarly, the FRC is increased in conditions characterized by a decreased recoil pressure of the lungs (such as emphysema).

Exercise testing

Muscle O_2 consumption and CO_2 production increase greatly during exercise. Coincident with these alterations in muscle metabolism, mixed venous blood shows decreases in P_{O_2} and increases in P_{CO_2}. In addition, the time that a given volume of blood spends in the pulmonary capillary decreases significantly. Nonetheless, the normal respiratory system maintains Pa_{O_2} at resting levels and Pa_{CO_2} at or below resting levels. Exercise-induced hypoxemia is commonly the first abnormality noted in early interstitial lung disease; this abnormality is a good indicator for evaluating therapy in interstitial lung disease. Many patients with obstructive lung disease also manifest exercise-induced arterial hypoxemia. Last, in all types of lung disease, exercise testing provides the physician with objective measurements of work tolerance (such as maximal O_2 con-

sumption); these measurements should enable the physician to provide better occupational guidance to the patient.

Airway resistance

The driving pressure producing airflow along the tracheobronchial tree is the difference between alveolar pressure and pressure at the airway opening. Airway resistance (R_{aw}) is defined as the quotient of driving pressure divided by the rate of airflow. Resistance to airflow is affected chiefly by the caliber of the airways. R_{aw} is measured in a plethysmograph similar to that used for determining FRC.

The diameter of individual members of each successive generation of airways decreases from the trachea to the peripheral airways. However, the total cross-sectional area of the tracheobronchial tree progressively increases from the trachea to the peripheral airways. These anatomic observations indicate that most of the resistance of the human tracheobronchial tree resides in large airways; direct measurements reveal that about 80% of total R_{aw} originates in airways more than 2 mm in diameter. A corollary of this observation is that decreases can occur in the caliber of the small peripheral airways (that is, less than 2 mm), without having much effect on total R_{aw}. Therefore small peripheral airways sometimes are referred to as the lung's "quiet zone."

Changes in the cross-sectional area of the airways can be effected by the following mechanisms: (1) changes in lung volume, (2) diseases of the lung parenchyma, and (3) diseases of the airways. First, the caliber of individual airways progressively increases as the subject approaches TLC; conversely, airway caliber decreases as the subject approaches RV. The reason underlying this association between airway caliber and lung volume is that lung parenchyma normally serves as radial supports to maintain the patency of airways; at high lung volumes these tethers are taut, increasing the elastic recoil of the lung and maintaining the airways in a fully patent state. However, at low lung volumes the tethers are lax, decreasing the elastic recoil of the lung and allowing the airways to be partially collapsed. In diseases such as emphysema the airways are not maintained in a fully patent state because of a decrease in elastic recoil of the lung at any given lung volume. Airway narrowing also can result from bronchospasm, edema of the mucosal lining, and secretions within the lumen.

CATEGORIZATION OF LUNG DISEASE

Lung diseases that cause abnormalities of ventilation usually are divided into two categories: restrictive and obstructive ventilatory disorders. It has been pointed out that this classification is somewhat unsatisfactory, since it ignores the fact that disturbances of the distribution of ventilation are the earliest and probably the most common abnormality of ventilation. Moreover, abnormalities in the distribution of ventilation can occur in the absence of manifestations of either obstructive or restrictive disorders. Table 121-1 presents characteristic changes in both lung volumes and flow rates in patients with restrictive and obstructive ventilatory disorders.

Restrictive ventilatory disorders

Restrictive ventilatory disorders are characterized by reductions in lung volumes. The hallmark of restriction is a decreased VC and TLC. A decrease in VC also sometimes occurs in obstructive ventilatory disorders; therefore if only the VC is measured, the presence of airway obstruction must be ruled out by the ratios $FEV_{1.0}/FVC$ and $FEV_{3.0}/FVC$.

Restrictive ventilatory disorders (kyphoscoliosis) can develop in conditions that (1) stiffen the chest wall or weaken

Table 121-1   Characteristic changes in lung capacities, volumes, and forced expiratory spirograms in patients with restrictive and obstructive ventilatory disorders

Test	Restrictive	Obstructive
FVC	Decreased	Decreased or normal
RV	Decreased	Increased
TLC	Decreased	Normal or increased
RV/TLC	Normal or increased	Significantly increased
$FEV_{1.0}/FVC$	Normal or increased	Decreased
$FEV_{3.0}/FVC$	Normal or increased	Decreased
FEF_{25-75}	Normal or decreased	Decreased

the respiratory muscles (myasthenia gravis), (2) cause infiltrates in the lung parenchyma or airspaces (diffuse interstitial fibrosis and pulmonary edema), (3) involve the pleura (pleural thickening), (4) occupy space within the thorax (tumors, effusions, and cardiac enlargement), and (5) occur after lung resection.

Obstructive ventilatory disorders

Obstructive ventilatory disorders are characterized by abnormalities in the FVC; an $FEV_{1.0}/FVC$ ratio less than 75% is a widely used criterion for diagnosis of these disorders. However, maximal flow-volume relationships (particularly flow rates obtained at low lung volumes) are being increasingly used in the diagnosis of obstructive pulmonary disorders, and these relationships appear to be more sensitive for the early diagnosis of peripheral airway obstruction.

Obstructive ventilatory disorders are found in patients with asthma, bronchitis, emphysema, advanced bronchiectasis, and other diseases that cause narrowing of the tracheobronchial system. When the term "obstructive disorders" originally was coined, it was not possible to differentiate among these various entities; therefore they were lumped together in the nonspecific category of chronic obstructive pulmonary disease (COPD). However, specialized tests now can sort out these various diseases even when they coexist.

INITIAL EVALUATION OF ARTERIAL BLOOD GAS MEASUREMENTS

Blood gas measurements are subject to technical error, therefore the physician must determine whether a given set of blood gas values is theoretically possible for the FIO_2 being delivered to the patient. As an example of this principle, we analyze the measurements of PaO_2 and $PaCO_2$ in a patient with severe COPD who was spontaneously breathing room air: in a measured blood sample PaO_2 equals 80 mm Hg and $PaCO_2$ equals 65 mm Hg. Assuming a respiratory exchange ratio (R) of 0.8 and substituting in the simplified alveolar air equation:

$$PAO_2 = 150 - \frac{65}{0.8} = 69 \text{ mm Hg}$$

The $P(A\text{-}a)O_2$ is determined as follows:

$$P(A - a)O_2 = 69 - 80 = -11 \text{ mm Hg}$$

Since the $P(A\text{-}a)O_2$ can never be negative, it is assumed that an error exists in the reported blood gas measurements. Although clinicians often blame the laboratory for such errors in blood gas determinations, faulty technique in drawing arterial blood gas specimens (such as allowing room air into the syringe) may be responsible for these erroneous measurements.

ARTERIAL HYPERCAPNIA

In determing a therapeutic approach to the patient with arterial hypercapnia, the physician first must determine if the arterial hypercapnia is acute or chronic and what deleterious effects (if any) it is causing.

Acute versus chronic arterial hypercapnia

Acute increases in $PaCO_2$ cause significant decreases in arterial pH levels. On the other hand, in response to chronic increases in $PaCO_2$, renal mechanisms increase the blood bicarbonate concentration; therefore chronic hypercapnia is accompanied by only a small decrease (if any) in arterial pH levels. Another excellent clue is provided by the patient's past record; did the patient have arterial hypercapnia when last discharged from the hospital or seen as an outpatient at the physician's office?

Patients with COPD commonly have acute hypercapnia superimposed on chronic hypercapnia. In these situations the patient's history, previous records, and nomograms (graphs showing the relationship between arterial pH levels and $PaCO_2$ for both acute and chronic hypercapnia) allow the physican to estimate the magnitude of the acute increase in $PaCO_2$.

Physical signs of hypercapnia

The clinical signs of hypercapnia are nonspecific, and these effects are often difficult to distinguish from those of hypoxemia in ventilatory failure. Minor degrees of hypercapnia usually produce an increase in systemic blood pressure, drowsiness, irritability, and headache. Significant elevations of $PaCO_2$ result in muscle twitching and a further deterioration of mental function that can progress to coma. However, the cerebral effects of hypercapnia depend to a large extent on the acuteness of the change, so that in some instances a patient with chronic CO_2 retention at a level of 80 mm Hg may be fully conscious, whereas another patient with acute elevation of $PaCO_2$ to 80 mm Hg may be stuporous.

Therapy for acute symptomatic hypercapnia

If acute hypercapnia and coma are caused by a drug overdose, specific pharmacologic antagonists to the offending drug should be administered immediately if available. If the acute hypercapnia and associated coma are not caused by a drug overdose, the patient should be intubated and receive mechanical ventilation.

Relationship of arterial hypercapnia to lung disease

Patients with restrictive ventilatory disorders rarely manifest arterial hypercapnia throughout the course of the disease. However, hypercapnia sometimes develops in these patients as a terminal event.

In contrast, hypercapnia commonly develops in patients with COPD. The development of arterial hypercapnia is poorly correlated with most tests of pulmonary function. However, in patients with COPD hypercapnia rarely develops until the $FEV_{1.0}$ decreases to below 1.25 L. If arterial hypercapnia develops in a patient with COPD and an $FEV_{1.0}$ greater than 1.25 L, he should be evaluated for the following clinical entities: (1) administration of drugs capable of depressing ventilation, (2) metabolic alkalosis, or (3) a disorder of respiratory regulation.

ARTERIAL HYPOXEMIA

Five physiologic mechanisms are known to cause arterial hypoxemia: (1) inspiring air (or a gas mixture) with a low

PO_2, (2) hypoventilation, (3) decreased diffusion, (4) ventilation-perfusion mismatching, and (5) right-to-left shunting of blood.

Inspiring air (or a gas mixture) with a low PO_2

At sea level individuals trapped in a fire inspire air with a low PO_2, since the ambient PO_2 has been reduced by the consumption of O_2. Obviously, the therapy for this condition is to remove the individual from the environment of the fire.

The most common cause of arterial hypoxemia is a sojourn at a high altitude. The decreased barometric pressure at high altitudes quantitatively accounts for the hypoxemia seen in mountain dwellers; in these individuals the $P(A-a)O_2$ is normal. The magnitude of altitude-induced hypoxemia can be quite severe. For example, normal individuals living at 3050 m above sea level exhibit an arterial PO_2 of 53 mm Hg. In most of the United States, altitude-induced hypoxemia is of little practical importance. However, in Denver (altitude 1560 m) the normal PaO_2 is approximately 70 mm Hg. Therefore patients with lung disease may require supplemental O_2 earlier in the course of their disease when living at high altitudes.

Alveolar hypoventilation

Alveolar hypoventilation is manifested by an increase in both arterial and alveolar PCO_2. Since the sum of the partial pressures of the alveolar gases must equal barometric pressure, increases in $PACO_2$ must be accompanied by decreases in PAO_2, because the alveolar pressures of nitrogen and water vapor remain virtually constant. At sea level "pure alveolar hypoventilation" is the only disease causing arterial hypoxemia with a normal $P(A-a)O_2$.

Since the $P(A-a)O_2$ is normal in pure alveolar hypoventilation, this entity cannot result from intrinsic lung disease in itself. Rather, pure alveolar hypoventilation usually is caused by depression of the central nervous system resulting from anesthetic agents or sedatives. It also can be a result of neuromuscular disease such as myasthenia gravis or Guillain-Barré syndrome.

The principal point in the management of pure alveolar hypoventilation is the realization that the patient is rarely if ever in a steady state; he will continue to hypoventilate, and $PaCO_2$ will continue to increase progressively. Therefore this medical emergency must be treated promptly. A patient suffering from a drug overdose should be given a specific antidote for the offending agent (such as naloxone for opiate intoxication). If the patient does not show a notable improvement following the administration of the pharmacologic antagonist or if no history of drug ingestion is obtained, the patient must be intubated and undergo mechanical ventilation.

Diffusion

Diffusion abnormality in the absence of ventilation-perfusion mismatch does not cause resting arterial hypoxemia.

Ventilation-perfusion mismatch

The most common cause of arterial hypoxemia at sea level is $\dot{V}A/\dot{Q}c$ mismatch, and this mechanism accounts for the hypoxemia of both obstructive and restrictive ventilatory disorders. The fact that alveoli with low $\dot{V}A/\dot{Q}c$ ratios can result in hypoxemia has been previously noted.

The patient with acute hypoxemia caused largely by $\dot{V}A/\dot{Q}c$ mismatch, who also manifests severe signs of acute hypercapnia (such as coma and depressed breathing), should be intubated and undergo mechanical ventilation.

If acute hypoxemia resulting from $\dot{V}A/\dot{Q}c$ mismatch is associated with hypercapnia in the absence of clinical manifestations of hypercapnia, controlled O_2 therapy (that is, small increases in FIO_2) is begun. The goal of this therapy is to raise the PaO_2 to approximately 60 mm Hg; the oxyhemoglobin dissociation curve indicates that the arterial O_2 saturation is approximately 90% at this point.

If the PaO_2 is raised above 60 mm Hg (or even in some patients to 60 mm Hg), the hypoxemia-induced chemical drive to ventilation is eliminated, and the patient may hypoventilate further. If after the administration of O_2 therapy the patient shows severe clinical manifestations of acute hypercapnia, he should be intubated and receive mechanical ventilation.

Right-to-left shunt

A right-to-left shunt is characterized by the failure of some mixed venous blood to come into contact with ventilated alveoli; rather, this fraction of mixed venous blood passes directly into the left side of the heart. The thebesian and bronchial veins account for the normal anatomic right-to-left shunt. Many types of congenital heart disease are characterized by pathologic right-to-left shunts (such as tetralogy of Fallot, tricuspid atresia, and pulmonary atresia). Other types of congenital heart disease initially appear as a left-to-right shunt and then develop pulmonary hypertension. Once pulmonary hypertension has become established, these conditions become transformed into right-to-left shunts; examples of this type of condition include atrial septal defect, ventricular septal defect, and patent ductus arteriosus. Pulmonary arteriovenous fistulas and blood flow to a collapsed lung are examples of intrapulmonary right-to-left shunts.

Arterial hypoxemia from a right-to-left shunt can be distinguished from that caused by $\dot{V}A/\dot{Q}c$ mismatch by having the patient inspire 100% O_2. The breathing of 100% O_2 flushes nitrogen out of the lungs and creates a high gradient for O_2 across the alveolar-capillary membrane; this gradient is sufficiently large to fully oxygenate even pulmonary capillary blood passing through low $\dot{V}A/\dot{Q}c$ regions. Thus when arterial hypoxemia is caused by a ventilation-perfusion imbalance, the $P(A-a)O_2$ difference becomes normal (about 80 mm Hg) when the patient is breathing 100% O_2. In contrast, in a right-to-left shunt the shunted desaturated blood never comes in contact with the O_2-enriched alveoli, and the $P(A-a)O_2$ difference remains elevated.

The presence of a major right-to-left shunt in such a common pulmonary disease as adult respiratory distress syndrome (ARDS) has important implications. As noted, breathing 100% O_2 does not appreciably correct the arterial hypoxemia. On the other hand, inspiration of 100% O_2 for a prolonged time results in pulmonary O_2 toxicity (whether arterial hypoxemia is present or not). Therefore when faced with hypoxemia resulting from a right-to-left shunt caused by ARDS, the physician must resort to such therapeutic modalities as positive end-expiratory pressure (PEEP).

BIBLIOGRAPHY

Bates DV, Macklem PT, and Christie RV: Respiratory function in disease: an introduction to the integrated study of the lung, ed 2, Philadelphia, 1971, WB Saunders Co.

Campbell EJM, Agostoni E, and Davis JN: The respiratory muscles: mechanics and neural control, ed 2, Philadelphia, 1970, WB Saunders Co.

Comroe JH Jr: Physiology of respiration: an introductory text, ed 2, Chicago, 1974, Year Book Medical Publishers, Inc.

Comroe JH Jr and others: The lung: clinical physiology and pulmonary function tests, ed 2, Chicago, 1962, Year Book Medical Publishers, Inc.

Fenn WO and Rahn H, editors: Handbook of physiology: respiration, vols 1 and 2, Washington, DC, 1965, American Physiological Society.

Fishman AP: Pulmonary diseases and disorders, New York, 1980, McGraw-Hill Book Co.

Jones NL and others: Clinical exercise testing, Philadelphia, 1975, WB Saunders Co.

Murray JF: The normal lung: the basis for diagnosis and treatment of pulmonary disease, Philadelphia, 1976, WB Saunders Co.

Nunn JF: Applied pulmonary physiology, London, 1977, Butterworth & Co, Ltd.

West JB: Respiratory physiology: the essentials, ed 2, Baltimore, 1979, Williams & Wilkins.

122·RESPIRATORY DIAGNOSTIC PROCEDURES

Samuel T. Kuna, Sharon Levy, *and* **Sanford Levine**

Despite their wide diversity, respiratory diseases and disorders have common patterns of clinical presentation. Determining the specific etiologic factors of a particular respiratory symptom usually requires one or more diagnostic procedures. These diagnostic techniques range from a specialized physical examination of the respiratory system to complex invasive procedures that may produce morbidity (and in rare cases mortality). Deciding the course of the diagnostic evaluation depends not only on the balance between diagnostic yield and risk of injury but also on the severity and progression of the disease state, as determined by medical history and physical examination. An acutely dyspneic patient requires a rapid diagnostic evaluation. In such an emergent situation, higher-risk invasive procedures may be justified earlier in the evaluation to establish the diagnosis quickly and initiate therapy.

This chapter presents the following respiratory diagnostic techniques: specialized physical examination, chest roentgenographic examination, sputum examination, radionuclide scans, ultrasonography, thoracentesis, bronchoscopy, percutaneous needle aspiration, open lung biopsy, mediastinoscopy and mediastinotomy, pulmonary angiography, and polysomnography. Arterial blood gas studies and other tests of pulmonary performance are discussed in Chapter 121.

SPECIALIZED ASPECTS OF THE PHYSICAL EXAMINATION OF THE RESPIRATORY SYSTEM
Examination of nonthoracic areas

CYANOSIS. The physician should note the color of the nailbeds and lips. A bluish discoloration of these areas is termed cyanosis. Hypoxemia is associated with cyanosis when the concentration of reduced hemoglobin in mucosal and/or cutaneous capillaries reaches 5 g/dl of blood. The distribution of cyanosis frequently provides a clue to the cause. Patients with respiratory-related cyanosis exhibit both peripheral (nailbed) and central (perioral) discoloration. In contrast, generalized systemic arteriolar vasoconstriction, as occurs in low cardiac output states, is associated with peripheral but not central cyanosis.

A peculiar distribution of cyanosis is observed in patients with patent ductus arteriosus associated with pulmonary hypertension and a predominant right-to-left shunt; in this complicated condition a pink right upper extremity is accompanied by cyanosis of the left upper and both lower extremities. Patients with cardiovascular lesions may show various patterns of cyanosis; these patterns strongly suggest that arterial hypoxemia caused by intrinsic lung disease cannot account for the observed cyanosis.

The relationship between an abnormal red blood cell count, such as in anemia and polycythemia, and cyanosis is important. Patients with severe anemia (hemoglobin concentration less than 5 g/dl of blood) never exhibit cyanosis, regardless of the severity of the arterial hypoxemia. Conversely, patients with significant degrees of polycythemia may manifest cyanosis coincident with moderate arterial hypoxemia.

Occasionally, significant "global" cyanosis is observed in patients whose measured arterial O_2 tension (PaO_2) is perfectly normal (100 mm Hg). This combination of findings suggests that the blood of the patient contains an abnormal hemoglobin such as methemoglobin or sulfhemoglobin. The physician can confirm this by drawing another blood specimen from the patient (venous blood is adequate) and demonstrating that the blood fails to become red when it is aerated in a syringe with room air or a hyperoxic gas mixture. Although exact definition of the abnormal hemoglobin must await specialized hematologic tests, this simple test allows the astute physician to conclude that the perceived cyanosis is unrelated to arterial hypoxemia.

CLUBBING. "Clubbing" is the term used to refer to changes in the distal segment of a digit that result from an increase in soft tissue. This selective increase in soft tissue is accompanied by sponginess at the nail base, widening of the angle formed at the junction of the nail base and periungual skin, and increased curvature of the nails in both the coronal and longitudinal planes.

Clubbing can be divided into two categories, hereditary and acquired. Hereditary clubbing involves all digits, is present throughout life, and occurs in individuals with a strong family history. Hereditary clubbing is the commonest form of clubbing and is particularly prevalent in black populations.

In contrast, acquired clubbing may affect only some digits, and it occurs in patients with pulmonary and nonpulmonary diseases. Pulmonary diseases generally associated with clubbing include primary or metastatic carcinoma of the lung and diseases of chronic pulmonary suppuration, including bronchiectasis, empyema, and lung abscess. It also can be associated with pulmonary fibrosis and cystic fibrosis. Clubbing is an unusual finding in chronic obstructive pulmonary disease (COPD) in the absence of chronic infection, and it also is unusual in tuberculosis unless significant pulmonary fibrosis or empyema is present.

As mentioned earlier, clubbing is not a specific sign of pulmonary disease; it also can be associated with hepatic cirrhosis, regional enteritis, ulcerative colitis, subacute bacterial endocarditis, and congenital cyanotic heart disease.

HYPERTROPHIC PULMONARY OSTEOARTHROPATHY. Some patients with acquired clubbing associated with lung cancer also exhibit hypertrophic pulmonary osteoarthropathy (HPO). HPO is the occurrence of subperiosteal new bone formation in the distal portions of the long bones of the extremities. This is an extremely painful condition, and its precise etiologic factors remain unknown. However, the pain of HPO often is dramatically relieved by indomethacin or by removal of the tumor.

Examination of the thorax

Examination of the thorax includes inspection, palpation, percussion, and auscultation.

INSPECTION. The rate and pattern of breathing are easily appreciated and serve as important indices of respiratory function. An abnormality in respiratory rate or pattern raises the immediate concern of inadequate exchange of oxygen and carbon dioxide across the lung. This possibility must be evaluated quickly with an arterial blood gas analysis. In acutely dyspneic patients, a respiratory rate greater than 40 breaths/min is non-sustainable and, barring prompt therapeutic intervention, inevitably leads to fatigue of the inspiratory muscles and cardio-respiratory collapse.

Most if not all severely dyspneic patients switch from nasal to mouth breathing. The nasal passages account for about half of the total resistance of the respiratory airways. Although the exact stimulus for this switch in breathing route is unknown, the initiation of mouth breathing decreases the work of breathing. During mouth breathing many patients with severe obstructive pulmonary disease exhale through pursed lips. Pursed lip breathing (PLB) relieves dyspnea both at rest and during exercise. PLB presumably maintains the patency of bronchi during expiration. Two possible mechanisms account for the subjective benefit elicited by PLB: (1) a change in the length-tension relationship of the respiratory muscles, or (2) relief from any discomfort associated with the narrowing or collapse of bronchi during forced exhalation.

A diminished or asymmetric thoracic excursion as the individual breathes with moderately large tidal volumes frequently is the first clue to an underlying abnormality of the respiratory apparatus. Skeletal abnormalities such as an abnormal curvature of the spine or abnormal orientation between ribs and sternum may be the cause of respiratory symptoms. In asthenic patients with COPD, the clinician often can appreciate a barrel-shaped configuration of the chest wall secondary to air trapping and decreased lung elastic recoil. Patients with obstructive pulmonary disease and dyspnea invariably use the accessory muscles of respiration such as the anterior scalenes and sternocleidomastoids. The phasic inspiratory contractions of these muscles are best appreciated by palpation rather than by inspection. The presence of intercostal retractions in patients with asthma and COPD indicate severe respiratory dysfunction.

PALPATION. Palpation should include a meticulous search for axillary and supraclavicular lymph nodes. The trachea is palpated in the suprasternal notch to check for mediastinal shifts.

Palpation also is used to perceive vocal fremitus. To produce fremitus the patient should slowly repeat some phrase such as "ninety-nine" loudly and in as low a pitch as possible; the physician should be able to palpate vibrations induced by these sounds over all areas of the chest wall covering the lung. Fremitus normally is decreased or absent if the patient's voice is not sufficiently forceful and resonant. It also is diminished by a thick layer of fat in the thoracic wall and especially by large breasts.

Fremitus is pathologically increased whenever the ratio of lung tissue or solid matter to air in a particular lung region is increased, provided that the bronchus to that area is patent. An example is the increased fremitus palpable over a pneumonic infiltrate with a patent bronchus. However, fremitus is decreased or absent if the bronchus supplying that region is occluded, thereby preventing the transmission of sound down the tracheobronchial tree. Examples of the latter type of pathologic entities include extrinsic compression, endobronchial tumor, foreign body, or retained secretions.

Air in the pleural cavity (pneumothorax) or any type of pleural effusion separates the lung from the chest wall and blocks the transmission of vibrations from the lung to the chest wall; in these situations fremitus is diminished or absent.

PERCUSSION. The percussion note over the thorax is de-termined by the ratio of air to solid tissue. A relative increase in the amount of air gives a more booming note; a relative decrease results in a duller or flatter sound. The term "resonant" describes the percussion note over healthy lung tissue.

Dullness represents the composite sound produced by resonance from the lung, plus a more pronounced element from solid, airless tissue. It normally is present over the heart, mediastinum, upper portion of the liver, and spleen—organs that are solid but also adjacent to the air-containing lung.

The finding of dullness over normally resonant areas of the chest indicates a pathologic change in the underlying tissues. Among the abnormal conditions causing dullness are pleural effusion, atelectasis, pneumonia, and fibrothorax.

AUSCULTATION. Auscultation of the respiratory system can be subdivided into breath sounds at the mouth and breath sounds transmitted to the chest wall; a stethoscope is required only for the latter category.

Breath sounds at the mouth. The breath sounds of healthy, awake individuals are inaudible at a distance of a few centimeters from the mouth unless the patient is panting, gasping, or sighing. In contrast, the resting ventilation of many patients with obstructive airways disease is accompanied by noise that can be heard across the room. In chronic bronchitis and asthma the intensity of the *inspiratory* noise correlates well with the forced expiratory volume in 1 second ($FEV_{1.0}$), peak expiratory flow rate, and other indices of obstruction to airflow. However, in emphysema the sound of inspiration at the mouth is faint, even in the presence of severe airflow obstruction. Therefore the amplitude of the inspiratory sound constitutes one criterion for distinguishing emphysema from chronic bronchitis and asthma.

Breath sounds transmitted to the chest wall. Breath sounds vary according to the location of the stethoscope. The breath sounds heard over the trachea have a short inspiratory phase and a long expiratory phase; these breath sounds remain audible to the end of expiration. They have been called bronchial breath sounds. Normal breath sounds heard over the chest (formerly termed "vesicular" breath sounds) have a long inspiratory phase and a short expiratory phase, becoming inaudible throughout the major portion of expiratory airflow. Normal breath sounds over the chest are believed to originate in the upper airway, trachea, and proximal segments of the bronchial tree. The aerated lung and chest wall act as a low-pass filter that attenuates this sound. Fluid or air in the pleural space establishes a complete acoustic barrier. Consolidated lung tissue transmits breath sounds almost without attenuation. The breath sounds over such areas of consolidation are similar to those over the trachea. Increased transmission of voice also occurs over areas of lung consolidation. This clinical sign is termed "bronchophony" or "whispered pectoriloquy."

Adventitious lung sounds include crackles and wheezes. Crackles are discontinuous popping sounds that are believed to be caused by the reequilibration of pressure with sudden reinflation of collapsed alveoli and peripheral airways. Crackles can occur during inspiration and expiration. They can be scanty or profuse, loud or faint, and high pitched or low pitched. Crackles are a characteristic physical finding in pneumonia, pulmonary edema, atelectasis, and interstitial diseases.

Wheezes are continuous musical sounds. They are believed to be generated by the oscillation of the walls of airways between the closed and barely open positions. Wheezing can be elicited in normal individuals during the dynamic airway compression of a maximal forced expiration. Nonetheless, wheezing should be thought of as a clinical sign of potentially reversible airway obstruction. Wheezing may consist of constant musical notes that start and stop at different times during inspiration and expiration. Such a pattern is characteristic of asthma. Alternatively, wheezes can be variable musical sounds occurring throughout expiration. These wheezes occur in many chronic pulmonary diseases.

CHEST ROENTGENOGRAPHIC EXAMINATION
Posteroanterior and lateral chest views

The chest roentgenographic examination is an invaluable diagnostic tool in the evaluation of diseases of the thorax. Although different pulmonary diseases may have similar clinical presentations, they often can be distinguished on the basis of their characteristic roentgenographic appearance in conjunction with the history and physical examination. These patterns of presentation frequently determine the diagnostic and therapeutic approach to a particular clinical problem. The importance of past films cannot be overemphasized. An abnormality that is roentgenographically stable over a 2-year period rarely warrants further evaluation. Conversely, a changing roentgenographic appearance identifies an active process that requires further investigation. In the workup of any pulmonary disorder, every effort should be made to obtain results of previous studies.

The standard posteroanterior and lateral views reveal whether a disorder is intraparenchymal, extraparenchymal, or both. If the abnormality is not apparent on both of these films, oblique views can help make this distinction. An intraparenchymal infiltrate may be alveolar or interstitial. An alveolar infiltrate is fluffy and irregular. Confluent alveolar infiltrates obliterate the borders of adjacent thoracic structures such as the diaphragm, heart, or mediastinum; this loss of margins is called the "silhouette sign."

Airways surrounded by fluid-filled alveoli produce air bronchograms. Common respiratory disorders that produce an alveolar pattern include pneumonias and pulmonary edema. The location of the infiltrate helps establish a differential diagnosis. For example, whereas a bilateral perihilar alveolar infiltrate is typical for pulmonary edema, a unilateral alveolar infiltrate is much more likely to result from an infectious process.

An interstitial infiltrate is more discrete and sharp. Air bronchograms are not characteristic. Interstitial patterns can be micronodular, reticular, or linear. The type of interstitial pattern, as well as its location, can help determine its cause. For example, a micronodular pattern with predominance in the apices would be a typical roentgenographic presentation for sarcoidosis. A micronodular interstitial infiltrate uniformly distributed throughout the lung fields would be a representative presentation for miliary tuberculosis.

Usually the roentgenographic examination gives the first indication of a solitary pulmonary nodule. This often initiates an extensive diagnostic evaluation. Of the many possible causes of a solitary pulmonary nodule, bronchogenic carcinoma, tuberculosis, and fungal infections are among the most common. The roentgenographic appearance of the nodule may help determine its cause. The presence of "popcorn calcifications" on tomography is suggestive of a hamartoma. In general, well-circumscribed lesions are more likely to be benign. As previously noted, past films are important to determine if the nodule is changing in size or is roentgenographically stable. Pneumonitis also can manifest as a nodule. If previous films are not available, it is important to document that the lesion is not evanescent by repeating the roentgenographic examination after an interval of at least 1 week.

An opacification in the lung may represent atelectasis. Obstruction of airways leads to resorption of air distally and collapse of these lung units. When involving peripheral airways, this collapse can appear as discoid or platelike opacities. Atelectasis is particularly common after upper abdominal surgery and is manifested clinically by fever. Obstruction of a central bronchus can result in the collapse of a lobe or even an entire lung. Collapse of each individual lobe has a characteristic roentgenographic appearance. The central obstructing lesion usually is the result of a mucous plug, endobronchial tumor, or foreign body.

The film also can show areas of decreased density in the lung. Localized hyperlucent airspaces may represent bullae, blebs, or cysts. Bullae are airspaces within the lung that occur in association with emphysema. Blebs are collections of air adjoining the visceral pleura, usually in the apices. Cysts are airspaces that have an epithelial lining. Some are congenital malformations of the bronchial tree; others result from persistent postinfectious cavities that reepithelialize. Hyperlucent areas also can be caused by a decrease in vascular perfusion, for example, from pulmonary embolus. Diffuse hyperlucency is typical in emphysema, a disease of lung destruction. In contrast, a unilateral hyperlucent lung suggests the following possibilities: (1) a technical error resulting when one side of the chest is not flush with the film cassette, (2) a difference in soft tissue mass overlying each hemithorax, for example, after mastectomy, (3) a unilateral pleural effusion in a film taken with the patient in a supine position, (4) decreased perfusion to one lung caused by postinfection ventilation abnormalities (Swyer-James or Macleod's syndrome), and (5) pneumothorax.

The film may reveal an extrapulmonary abnormality involving the heart, mediastinum, and pleura. Pleural disease frequently escapes detection during physical examination. The most common pleural abnormality is a pleural effusion. Accumulation of fluid between the visceral and parietal pleura appears in the dependent portion of the thorax and initially causes blunting of the costophrenic angle. Blunting on the erect posteroanterior film occurs only after the accumulation of 300 to 500 ml of fluid.

Special views

Small pleural effusions can be seen on the lateral projection, but a lateral decubitus view is the most sensitive roentgenographic technique to document pleural fluid. The lateral decubitus view also differentiates blunting caused by pleural fluid from other causes of blunting such as pleural fibrosis. A subpulmonic effusion, which follows the contour of the diaphragm on an upright film with relative preservation of the costophrenic angles, also layers out on the decubitus view. A loculated pleural effusion, however, does not change position but can be diagnosed as fluid with ultrasonography (see "Ultrasonography").

In the standard posteroanterior view of the chest, parenchymal abnormalities in the lung apex may be obscured by the overlying clavicles and first rib. In an apical lordotic view these structures are no longer superimposed, enabling better interpretation of the apical infiltrate.

Abnormalities in other areas of the film that are difficult to interpret can be better defined by oblique views and tomography (that is, roentgenographic slices of lung tissue). Currently lung tomograms are indicated to (1) confirm the presence of cavitation that is only suggested on standard films, (2) detect calcification in a solitary pulmonary nodule, (3) distinguish hilar adenopathy and abnormal mediastinal masses, and (4) demonstrate the presence of fungus balls or mycetomas in cavities. Additionally, whole lung tomograms may reveal evidence of multiple pulmonary metastases. Tomograms also give a good outline of the trachea and bronchi and are useful in evaluating a possible central obstructing lesion.

Although more expensive than conventional roentgenograms, computed tomography (CT) has assumed an important role in the roentgenographic evaluation of the thorax. Computed tomography is useful in (1) detecting small parenchymal nodules, (2) identifying pleural disease, (3) distinguishing tissue masses from vascular structures, and (4) evaluating hilar and mediastinal lymph node enlargement. Although CT scans are exquisitely sensitive for identifying lymph node enlargement of greater than 2 cm, histologic examination of these nodes may reveal an inflammatory process rather than neoplastic disease. Besides CT scanning, the newer technique of nuclear magnetic resonance imaging may have important applications in pulmonary medicine, but its role in thoracic imaging is still being evaluated.

SPUTUM EXAMINATION

Sputum from the tracheobronchial tree can contain many different types of cells, including ciliated epithelial cells, polymorphonuclear leukocytes, and alveolar macrophages. Grossly, sputum may appear mucoid or purulent. Purulent sputum usually indicates the presence of either an infectious or an allergic disorder. Purulent sputum with a foul odor suggests an infection caused by anaerobic organisms. Sputum from bronchiectasis forms three distinct layers when collected and allowed to stand. Pink, frothy sputum suggests pulmonary edema. However, none of these findings are diagnostic.

Microscopic examination of freely expectorated or induced sputum can yield important information. A useful routine is to examine a wet mount of the sputum specimen before staining it. A drop of sputum is spread under a coverslip and screened for the presence of squamous cells and alveolar macrophages. The presence of many squamous cells indicates that the specimen must have originated above the level of the larynx. In contrast, the presence of alveolar macrophages indicates that the specimen originated from the tracheobronchial tree and is an appropriate sample for staining. The number of eosinophils on the wet mount can also be determined and could suggest an allergic disorder responsive to steroids. After the coverslip is removed, the slide dries and is stained for bacteria or acid-fast mycobacteria. The presence of many leukocytes, as well as bacteria, on a sputum Gram stain is indicative of infection. Appropriate antibiotic coverage is determined by the morphologic structure of the organisms and the appearance of the roentgenographic film. A sputum culture is used to help verify this therapeutic decision.

Cytologic examination of the sputum is useful in diagnosing neoplasms located in endobronchial sites. The diagnostic yield of this procedure increases with up to five separate sputum collections. Since sputum is also composed of extrapulmonary secretions, malignant cells on sputum cytologic examination may originate from the extrathoracic airway or an esophageal tumor.

RADIONUCLIDE SCANS
Perfusion scan

One type of radionuclide scan assesses the distribution of perfusion in the lungs. The perfusion scan is performed by intravenous injection of technetium Tc 99m human albumin microspheres. These particles have a diameter larger than that of the capillary lumen and are retained in the pulmonary capillary bed. This microembolization is transient and of no clinical consequence. The distribution of pulmonary blood flow is determined by quantifying the relative distribution of the radioactive-labeled albumin with scintillation scanning over the thorax.

Ventilation scan

Another type of radionuclide scan assesses the distribution of ventilation in the lungs. The ventilation scan is performed by having the patient breathe a radioactive gas, usually xenon 133, from a spirometer. Scintillation scanning that monitors the distribution of xenon is used as a marker for the distribution of ventilation. The distribution of ventilation is evaluated under the following circumstances: (1) initially, on inspiration to total lung capacity (TLC), (2) during equilibration of the labeled xenon in the lungs with normal tidal breathing (wash-in), and (3) during elimination of the labeled xenon from the lungs when breathing room air (washout). Areas of decreased ventilation are characterized by delayed appearance of the radionuclide during wash-in and prolonged retention of the radionuclide on washout.

Use of radionuclide scans in the diagnosis of pulmonary emboli

In most institutions perfusion scans are routinely used in the diagnostic workup for pulmonary emboli. Embolic occlusion of branches of the pulmonary arterial tree results in segmental areas of decreased or absent perfusion. Therefore an entirely normal perfusion scan constitutes strong evidence against the diagnosis of pulmonary emboli.

An abnormal perfusion scan, however, requires careful interpretation. The finding of multiple segmental areas with a ventilation-perfusion mismatch (that is, presence of ventilation but absence of perfusion) is consistent with the diagnosis of pulmonary thromboembolism. However, a matched decrease in both ventilation and perfusion may be secondary to other pulmonary parenchymal disorders. Any alveolar filling process, such as a pneumonia, decreases ventilation to the involved area of the lung, which in turn elicits a secondary decrease in perfusion to the same area. Therefore it is important to correlate the results of the perfusion scan with a concurrent chest roentgenographic examination.

In patients with obstructive pulmonary disease, regions characterized by low $\dot{V}A/\dot{Q}c$ ratios may show up as areas of decreased perfusion on the perfusion scan. However, a ventilation scan can demonstrate that the perfusion defects are occurring in areas of low $\dot{V}A/\dot{Q}c$ ratios.

Use of perfusion lung scans in the preoperative assessment of patients undergoing lung resection

Perfusion lung scans are used in the preoperative assessment of patients with marginal respiratory reserve who are scheduled for lung resection. If the area of the lung to be removed has poor perfusion, resection probably will not significantly impair respiratory function. In evaluating a patient for pneumonectomy, the perfusion lung scan can quantify the percentage of pulmonary blood flow to each lung. On this basis it is possible to estimate from routine tests of pulmonary performance (see Chapter 157) the pulmonary function that remains following removal of the involved lung and to predict whether the patient can tolerate a pneumonectomy.

ULTRASONOGRAPHY

Ultrasonography often helps determine the presence and location of fluid in the pleural space. When the high-frequency sound waves are directed into the normal thoracic cavity, the sound is almost completely reflected by the air-containing lung at the surface. However, when pleural fluid is present, an echo-free space is demonstrated between the chest wall and the aerated lung. The fluid transmits the sound so that echoes are produced only when the sound waves are reflected from the underlying lung.

THORACENTESIS

Thoracentesis is performed for both diagnostic and therapeutic purposes. The diagnostic indication is to elucidate the cause of the pleural effusion, whereas the therapeutic indication is symptomatic relief from dyspnea.

Methodology and complications

To perform a thoracentesis in a free-flowing effusion, the best site for introduction of the needle in a sitting subject is the posterior eighth intercostal space at the midscapular line. A helpful landmark is the scapular tip that overlies the seventh rib when the arms are flush with the body. A loculated pleural effusion should be localized by ultrasonography before a decision is made concerning the site for introducing the needle.

The complications of thoracentesis include pneumothorax, hemothorax, reexpansion pulmonary edema, and in rare cases air embolism. Leakage of air into the pleural space through the thoracentesis needle is the most common cause of pneumothorax associated with thoracentesis. However, in a few instances pneumothorax follows laceration of the visceral pleura; the leak usually seals itself quickly. If the pneumothorax is large or causes dyspnea, aspiration of the air or even placement of a chest tube is indicated. Hemothorax usually follows trauma to an intercostal vessel.

Reexpansion pulmonary edema is believed to result from increasingly subatmospheric intrathoracic pressure following removal of a large amount of fluid. The balance of forces across the alveolar-capillary membrane, described in Starling's law, is disrupted, resulting in transudation of fluid into the alveoli. The incidence of this complication can be decreased by limiting fluid aspiration during each thoracentesis to 1 L or less.

In rare instances laceration of lung tissue by the thoracentesis needle allows air from alveoli to enter adjacent pulmonary veins, producing air embolism. When this complication is suspected, the patient is placed on his left side with the head lower than the trunk to trap gas in the right atrium, thereby minimizing pulmonary and systemic air embolism.

Pleural fluid analysis

If pus is aspirated from the pleural space or organisms are present on stains of the pleural fluid, an infection is the cause of the pleural effusion and should be treated appropriately. Even if there is no initial evidence to suggest bacterial infection, a specimen of fluid is still sent for culture. In addition, chemical studies of the fluid are made to determine whether it is a transudate or an exudate. Table 122-1 presents simple chemical criteria for distinguishing between transudative and exudative pleural effusions.

The cellular profile of pleural fluid may provide some suggestions regarding cause. Bloody pleural effusions with red blood cell counts higher than 100,000/ml result most commonly from trauma, malignancy, and pulmonary thromboembolism. A lymphocytic pleural effusion with greater than

Table 122-1 Criteria for distinguishing pleural transudates from exudates

	Transudate	Exudate
General criteria		
Pleural fluid specific gravity	<1.016	>1.016
Pleural fluid total protein	<3 g/dl	>3 g/dl
Criteria of Light, et al		
$\frac{\text{Pleural fluid total protein}}{\text{Serum total protein}}$	<0.5	
Lactic dehydrogenase (LDH)	<200 units	
$\frac{\text{Pleural fluid LDH}}{\text{Serum LDH}}$	<0.6	

*Diagnosis of transudative effusion requires that all three criteria be fulfilled.

50% lymphocytes suggests a tuberculous or malignant origin. Eosinophilia in pleural fluid is a nonspecific finding.

Transudative effusions

Pleural fluid formed through normal capillary membranes is termed a transudate; transudates contain little protein or other large molecules (Table 122-1). Transudates occur when normal relationships between capillary hydrostatic pressure and colloid osmotic pressure are disturbed so that fluid formation within the pleural space exceeds its resorption. The following physiologic disturbances favor the accumulation of a transudate in the pleural space: increases in systemic capillary pressure, increases in pulmonary capillary pressure, and decreases in the colloid osmotic pressure of plasma. Common causes of transudates are left ventricular failure, nephrotic syndrome, and cirrhosis with ascites. Pleural effusions associated with ascites usually are caused by hypoalbuminemia and by transdiaphragmatic passage of peritoneal fluid (via lymphatics) into the pleural space. The finding of a transudative pleural effusion in the appropriate clinical setting should focus attention on treating the underlying clinical disorder.

Exudative effusions

Pleural fluid formed through abnormally permeable capillary membranes is termed an exudate; exudates contain higher concentrations of protein than transudates (Table 122-1). The altered membrane permeability is usually produced by inflammatory changes in the pleura caused by infection, pulmonary infarction, or neoplasm. Given its many possible causes, an exudative pleural effusion usually requires further diagnostic studies as dictated by the clinical setting. However, portions of the fluid are routinely submitted to cytopathology to rule out the presence of malignant cells exfoliated from pleural surfaces. The pleural fluid amylase concentration is elevated when the effusion is caused by pancreatitis or esophageal rupture. The complement concentration is decreased in pleural fluid resulting from systemic lupus erythematosus. The rheumatoid factor level is elevated and the glucose concentration is characteristically less than 10 mg/dl in pleural fluid associated with rheumatoid arthritis.

Frequently, after empyema is ruled out, the chemical profile of the exudative fluid does not establish its cause. It then becomes important to exclude two diagnoses: tuberculous pleural effusion and malignant pleural effusion. For this purpose another thoracentesis is performed in conjunction with biopsies of the parietal pleura. Several biopsies are submitted for histopathologic examination to look for malignant cells or granulomas. Another biopsy is sent for mycobacterial culture. The addition of this low-risk procedure greatly increases the diagnostic yield of the thoracentesis. Repeating the pleural biopsies and thoracentesis, if the first attempt does not establish the diagnosis, also increases the likelihood of identifying a tuberculous or malignant pleural effusion. Continued failure to establish a diagnosis may necessitate an open pleural biopsy.

BRONCHOSCOPY

The fiberoptic bronchoscope is an invaluable diagnostic tool in the evaluation of pulmonary diseases, providing diagnoses that previously could be made only by thoracotomy. Bronchoscopy is a low-risk procedure. In one large series the mortality was 0.01% and the morbidity 0.08%. With direct vision for guidance, the flexible bronchoscope can reach the first generations of subsegmental bronchi. More distally the airways become too narrow to allow further passage of the bronchoscope. When an abnormality is identified using direct vision, endobronchial biopsies and brushings are performed. Many abnormalities, however, are more peripheral in location and are beyond the field of bronchoscopic vision. In these situations forceps and brushes are advanced through the bronchoscope and guided into the lesion with the aid of fluoroscopy. A biopsy from the lung periphery should include alveoli, as well as bronchiolar tissue, and is called a transbronchial biopsy. Additionally, a needle catheter can be inserted through the tracheal wall at the level of the main carina and into subcarinal nodes to search for local metastatic involvement from a bronchogenic carcinoma. Thus regardless of location specimens can be obtained directly from the abnormal area and sent for culture, as well as cytologic and histologic examination.

Bronchoscopy is of particular value in the evaluation of hemoptysis, atelectasis, and mass or cavitary lesions found on roentgenographic examination. It is also useful in determining the cause of diffuse interstitial patterns found on roentgenographic examination. With transbronchial biopsy the diagnostic yield in sarcoidosis is said to be greater than 80%. Bronchoscopy is generally of limited use in establishing the infectious cause of bacterial pneumonias, but the use of sterile catheter-sheathed brushes helps reduce the likelihood of contamination from upper airway secretions. This newer technique, along with quantitative cultures, may increase the usefulness of bronchoscopy in diagnosing the cause of pneumonias.

Bronchoalveolar lavage is a very useful technique for diagnosing pulmonary infection by unusual pathogens such as *Pneumocystis carinii* and cytomegalovirus in the immunocompromised host. The tip of the bronchoscope is wedged into a segmental or subsegmental bronchus, and 40 ml aliquots of normal saline are instilled into the lung and immediately suctioned out. From 60% to 80% of the fluid is recovered, containing cells from the bronchial tree and alveoli. Recent work has attempted to determine if a particular cellular profile in the bronchoalveolar fluid can be used to diagnose specific disease states or aid therapeutic management. This application of bronchoalveolar lavage remains experimental.

Because of its versatility the flexible bronchoscope has virtually replaced the rigid bronchoscope. However, the rigid bronchoscope is still preferable to obtain large endobronchial biopsy specimens, to remove foreign bodies, to evaluate tracheal lesions, and to allow bronchoscopy in the presence of profuse bleeding.

PERCUTANEOUS NEEDLE ASPIRATION

Percutaneous needle aspirations are playing an increasingly important role in the diagnostic evaluation of nodules and masses in the chest. Use of a narrow-gauge needle has decreased the incidence of bleeding and pneumothorax. Needle guidance with biplane fluoroscopy or computed tomography greatly increases the diagnostic yield and is the procedure of choice for peripheral lung lesions.

Percutaneous needle aspiration provides a cytologic, rather than a histologic, diagnosis. Although percutaneous needle aspiration also is used for the diagnosis of pulmonary infections, the risk of complications in these particular patients, especially the immunocompromised host, appears to be greater than that with bronchoscopy.

OPEN LUNG BIOPSY

Failure to establish the cause of a parenchymal abnormality with any of these techniques may lead to an open lung biopsy. This surgical procedure requires general anesthesia. Open lung biopsy provides a larger specimen of lung tissue, permitting an analysis of lung architecture. This is of particular importance in reaching a diagnosis in the diffuse nonnodular interstitial infiltrates. Open lung biopsy is also useful in diagnosing opportunistic pulmonary infections in the immunocompromised host.

MEDIASTINOSCOPY AND MEDIASTINOTOMY

Mediastinoscopy is an operative procedure performed by blunt dissection along the thoracic trachea and paratracheal structures through a transverse incision across the suprasternal notch. Lymph nodes visualized through a mediastinoscope can be biopsied. It is technically difficult to reach left-sided structures by this approach. The left side of the mediastinum can be evaluated by mediastinotomy, dissecting down into the mediastinum through a transverse incision over the second left anterior costal cartilage. These procedures are used to stage a bronchogenic carcinoma for local spread to hilar and paratracheal nodes. There are few false negative results, and the mortality should be no greater than that from general anesthesia. Finding carcinomatous mediastinal lymph nodes usually obviates the need for thoracotomy. In addition, when the roentgenographic examination shows lymphadenopathy consistent with such diagnoses as sarcoidosis, Hodgkin's disease, and tuberculosis, mediastinoscopy or mediastinotomy can be used to obtain lymph node tissue for pathologic examination. The superior vena cava syndrome and prior mediastinoscopy are considered to be contraindications to mediastinoscopy.

PULMONARY ANGIOGRAPHY

Pulmonary angiography provides a visualization of the pulmonary vascular tree. This invasive procedure is the most sensitive technique available for diagnosing pulmonary thromboembolism. It is indicated (1) when findings on the lung scan are equivocal; (2) in the presence of an underlying pulmonary disease such as emphysema, which would make the interpretation of the lung scans difficult; (3) for firmly establishing the diagnosis of pulmonary thromboembolism in a patient who is at high risk of complications from anticoagulant therapy; and (4) in cases of life-threatening pulmonary embolism before starting thrombolytic therapy. Complications of pulmonary angiography include arrhythmias, hematoma formation, vasovagal reactions, and acute right ventricular failure in patients with severe pulmonary hypertension.

Angiography of the bronchial circulation, although not of diagnostic usefulness, is currently performed in some medical centers in the treatment of significant hemoptysis. Angiography is used to guide therapeutic embolization of the bronchial circulation in an effort to stop bleeding from the tracheobronchial tree. Angiography also identifies whether a spinal artery arises from the bronchial artery, which is a contraindication to embolization.

POLYSOMNOGRAPHY

The growing recognition that some patients have severe respiratory abnormalities during sleep has led to a steady increase in diagnostic sleep evaluations. The following parameters are usually monitored: (1) electroencephalogram, (2) oxygen saturation by ear oximeter, (3) rib cage and abdominal motion by impedance plethysmography, and (4) airflow at the nose and mouth by thermistors or CO_2 sensors. Subjects with obstructive sleep apnea develop several intermittent episodes of airway closure during sleep, as detected by an absence of airflow at the nose and mouth despite continuing respiratory efforts. This upper airway closure sometimes can be successfully prevented by application of positive airway pressure during sleep through a nose mask. Some patients with chronic obstructive pulmonary disease develop severe arterial oxygen desaturation during sleep, which may be caused by a decrease in neural activation of accessory and external intercostal muscles, worsening $\dot{V}A/\dot{Q}c$ mismatch, or both. This nocturnal oxygen desaturation can be reversed with supplemental oxygen.

BIBLIOGRAPHY

Anderson HA and Faber LP: Diagnostic and therapeutic applications of the bronchoscope, Chest (suppl) 73:685, 1978.
Bordow RA and Moser RM: Manual of clinical problems in pulmonary medicine, Boston, 1985, Little, Brown & Co.
Epstein RL: Constituents of sputum: a simple method, Ann Intern Med 77:259, 1972.
Fishman AP: Pulmonary diseases and disorders, New York, 1980, McGraw-Hill Book Co.
Forgacs P: The functional basis of pulmonary sounds, Chest 73:399, 1978.
Fraser RG and Pare JAP: Diagnosis of diseases of the chest, Philadelphia, 1978, WB Saunders Co.
George RB, Light RW, and Matthay RA: Chest medicine, New York, 1983, Churchill Livingstone, Inc.
Light RW and others: Pleural effusions: the diagnostic separation of transudates and exudates, Ann Intern Med 77:507, 1972.
Sackner MA: Diagnostic techniques in pulmonary disease. Parts I and II, New York, 1980, Marcel Dekker, Inc.

123·CHRONIC BRONCHITIS AND EMPHYSEMA

Paul D. Siegel and **Frank Barch**

Chronic obstructive pulmonary disease (COPD) may be the consequence either of primary airway disease, typified by chronic bronchitis, or of parenchymal disease, represented by emphysema. These two diseases have many overlapping characteristics such as a reduction in expiratory flow rates and a relationship to smoking. These similarities allow them to be considered jointly. In addition, the two diseases frequently coexist, and it is often impossible to separate the various facets of each disease as they occur in a particular patient. If a patient has significant chronic bronchitis with obstruction that is resistant to bronchodilators, associated emphysema is a likely pathologic finding. In addition, the patient with predominantly emphysematous lung disease may exhibit features of chronic bronchitis.

Airway obstruction usually is defined in terms of a diminished flow of air during forced expiration, and a variety of tests have evolved to measure this. The volume of air exhaled in the first second of forced expiration ($FEV_{1.0}$) is one of the most commonly used measures; predictive equations based on sex, height, and age have been devised. Values less than 75% of the patient's predicted $FEV_{1.0}$ levels are likely to be abnormal, values less than 65% of those predicted strongly suggest abnormality, and values less than 1 L for the $FEV_{1.0}$ indicate severe disease and often are associated with CO_2 retention.

The airway obstruction found in COPD can be compared to flow obstruction in a water pipe. If deposits on the pipe wall reduce the size of the lumen or if the walls have been squeezed together in some areas, the resistance to flow increases, turbulence may develop and further increase resistance, and transport of fluid through the pipe takes longer. Although this conception describes an airway partially occluded by mucus or narrowed by bronchospasm in chronic bronchitis, it does not explain the airway obstruction that occurs in emphysema. In this form of COPD the forces that must be overcome to exhale during a forced expiratory effort must be considered. Chest wall and lung inertia and tissue viscous resistance are minimal, and therefore airway resistance is the major component. Airway pressure must be greater than atmospheric pressure to allow flow to occur. This pressure is produced by a combination of pressures generated by the expiratory muscles of the chest cage and by the elastic recoil of the lung itself. The bronchioles lack cartilage and are surrounded by lung tissue that is under compressive force generated by the chest wall during expiration. The driving pressure for flow through the bronchioles is equal to the static recoil pressure of the lung plus the pressure generated by the expiratory muscles of the chest wall. Along the airway from alveolus to mouth, the pressure decreases as a consequence of flow resistance. At some point (the equal pressure point) this pressure within the lumen equals the pressure in the surrounding lung. Because the pressure closer to the mouth along this airway is less than the surrounding lung pressure, "dynamic compression" of the airway tends to occur. However, at this point in the normal lung the bronchioles are rigid enough to prevent collapse.

If lung elastic recoil is diminished, as in emphysema, the alveolar driving pressure and the retractile force of the lung, acting to increase airway pressure and keep the bronchiole lumen patent, are diminished. The point of dynamic compression then occurs more distally in less rigid bronchioles, decreasing expiratory flow. If a stronger expiratory effort is applied, driving pressure is increased, along with dynamic compression, and the flow changes very little.

CHRONIC BRONCHITIS

DEFINITION. Chronic bronchitis is a pulmonary response to chronic irritant exposure. It is defined as the presence of a productive cough on most days for at least 3 months of at least 2 consecutive years. Some patients with chronic bronchitis manifest a reduction in forced expiratory flow rates, wheezing, shortness of breath, or dyspnea on exertion. Patients with "simple" chronic bronchitis have been said to lack evidence of airway obstruction, but sensitive tests of small airway function show abnormal lung function in many of these patients. Although some patients with chronic bronchitis only produce excessive mucus, which is easily cleared and does not significantly obstruct the airways, for this discussion the term "chronic bronchitis" implies significant associated airway obstruction.

EPIDEMIOLOGY. COPD is a major cause of chronic disability in the United States. Valid statistics concerning COPD are difficult to accumulate. Much disease probably goes undiagnosed, and data collected from sources such as death certificates underrepresent its prevalence. An associated disease such as pneumonia or lung cancer is commonly the terminal event for patients with COPD.

Epidemiologic studies using questionnaires suggest that 10% to 25% of the adult American population have chronic bronchitis; however, the National Health Survey in 1970 reported a more conservative prevalence rate of 29.5:1000 adults. According to the Social Security Administration, COPD ranks second only to coronary artery disease as a cause of disability. A male to female ratio of 9:1 has been reported, but this number may be changing to reflect the increasing incidence of smoking among women. More recent data suggest a 7:1 ratio.

ETIOLOGY. Chronic airway irritation from cigarette smoking is the primary cause of chronic bronchitis and emphysema. Nonsmoking Seventh-Day Adventists show reduced mortality from COPD, suggesting that smoking is important in its development. For example, the data from the Tecumseh study suggest that a 45-year-old male nonsmoker with a normal expiratory airflow has a 1 in 200 chance of developing obstructive airway disease in the next 15 years. If the same man has maximal airflow of 80% of predicted and smokes 40 cigarettes per day, his risk is 1 in 5 or 6. If he stops smoking, his risk declines to 1 in 15.

Air pollution can play a significant role in COPD, especially in smokers, since the mortality from COPD correlates with worsening of air quality. Chronic bronchitis is twice as common in London as in rural England. In normal children ventilatory function after exercise is impaired by air pollutants. Exposure to a dusty atmosphere is associated with chronic bronchitis, including evidence of airflow obstruction. Hereditary factors also play a role in COPD, as demonstrated in *Kartagener's syndrome,* which consists of chronic bronchitis with bronchiectasis, sinusitis, and situs inversus.

Impaired airway clearance related to alterations in the phagocytic activity of macrophages and polymorphonuclear leukocytes in COPD allows deposited bacteria to proliferate for prolonged periods before removal; however, a causative role of infection in COPD is not clear. During acute exacerbations of COPD, with changes in sputum and other pertinent findings, antibiotics can decrease the duration of morbidity and effect more rapid recovery of decreased peak expiratory flow rates. Although the use of these drugs prophylactically seems to decrease the duration of exacerbations, the total number of episodes does not change, implying that viral infections may initiate or exacerbate symptoms and that bacteria contribute to the persistence of the worsened symptomatology.

Diplococcus pneumoniae and *Haemophilus influenzae* are commonly cultured from the sputum of patients with chronic bronchitis; *Mycoplasma* organisms and L-forms also have been implicated in exacerbations, but their ubiquity in bronchitic patients and the lack of host-antibody response to their presence make assessment of their role difficult. Recurrent exacerbations seem to be related to the gradual progressive decline in pulmonary function exhibited by patients with chronic bronchitis.

PATHOGENESIS AND PATHOLOGY. Chronic bronchitis is a clinical diagnosis with variable pathologic findings. Characteristic findings include hypertrophy of mucous glands and hyperplasia of goblet cells. The Reid index is an attempt to quantify these; it is defined as the ratio of mucous gland depth to bronchial wall thickness, with the upper limit of normal being 0.4. A correlation between the Reid index and the volume of sputum produced exists; however, this correlation is a bell-shaped curve skewed toward patients with chronic bronchitis

rather than a bimodal distribution of both normal individuals and bronchitic patients. An associated inflammatory infiltrate frequently is found in and around the bronchial walls but is of highly variable severity. There also may be associated mucous plugging or even obliteration of smaller airways.

Airway irritants, especially cigarette smoke, impair pulmonary defense mechanisms, decrease ciliary activity, interfere with normal scavenger cell activity, cause bronchospasm, increase scavenger cell populations, and increase mucus viscosity and volume. Mucus stasis and impaired phagocytic cell function promote colonization of the airways by bacteria. Retained secretions plus inflammation may accouont for the reduction in small airway function.

CLINICAL MANIFESTATIONS. COPD is usually a combination of chronic bronchitis and emphysema. In most cases a chronic productive cough that was insidious in onset has been present for many years. The patient may even deny having this symptom initially and later admit to having a "smoker's cough." Episodes of tracheobronchitis with mucopurulent secretions occur later. These episodes tend to resolve spontaneously, although slowly.

Accounts of repeated "colds" characterized by cough and sputum production and lasting for a protracted period can commonly be elicted. Dyspnea on exertion, wheezes, rhonchi, and diminished expiratory flow rates are found. Posttussive wheezing and cough provoked by forced expiratory effort underscore the irritable airways found in chronic bronchitis with associated obstructive airways disease.

The patient with chronic bronchitis may have less dyspnea than the patient with relatively pure emphysema who demonstrates comparable ventilatory insufficiency, but hypoxemia and CO_2 retention usually are more severe in bronchitis. Hypoxemia and hypercarbia induce pulmonary vasospasm, which can lead to right-sided heart strain and eventual right ventricular failure. The disorder occasionally may be erroneously diagnosed as biventricular heart failure, since the patient complains of orthopnea (caused by worsening ventilation-perfusion matching when the patient is supine), paroxysmal nocturnal dyspnea (from retained pulmonary secretions), dyspnea on exertion, shortness of breath even at rest, and dependent edema. Lethargy and somnolence also may be present.

The physical examination may demonstrate wheezing (as in cardiac asthma), rhonchi, and rales. In addition, the patient may show signs of right ventricular failure with neck vein distention, hepatojugular reflux, and bipedal edema. If the absence of a left ventricular gallop is not appreciated, the presence of a right ventricular gallop, an increased P_2, and a right ventricular heave may lead to an erroneous diagnosis of biventricular heart failure.

Differentiating chronic bronchitis with cor pulmonale from biventricular failure sometimes requires an exhaustive history and a careful physical examination. The physical examination of patients with chronic bronchitis should reveal evidence of airway obstruction with a decrease in forced expiratory flow rates. A simple test showing fair correlation with spirometric testing results requires the patient to make a forced expiratory effort from full inspiration with his mouth wide open while the physician listens over the trachea with a stethoscope. If air movement can still be heard after 4 seconds of expiration, significant airway obstruction is suggested. Hyperinflation, decreased respiratory excursion, use of the accessory muscles of respiration, and depression of the diaphragmatic position are less marked than in advanced emphysema.

Digital clubbing is rare in chronic obstructive bronchitis and should raise the suspicion of complicating bronchiectasis or lung tumor. Cyanosis may be noted but is an unreliable sign of arterial hypoxemia.

LABORATORY FINDINGS. Although chest roentgenography cannot establish the diagnosis of chronic bronchitis, it plays an important role in the evaluation of chronic cough by helping to rule out other causes of the symptom such as neoplasia, inflammatory lesions, and left ventricular failure. The chest roentgenogram is abnormal in up to 80% of patients with chronic bronchitis, with common findings including hyperinflation (best detected by finding a flattened diaphragm on the lateral film), ring shadows and parallel lines (representing thickened bronchial walls), and increased peripheral markings.

The electrocardiogram (ECG) is frequently abnormal in COPD. Atrial and ventricular arrhythmias are common in the presence of pulmonary hypertension, hypoxia, or respiratory acidosis. About half of hospitalized patients demonstrate arrhythmias, with atrial tachycardia and multifocal atrial tachycardia (MAT) being the most common. MAT incidence also is correlated with the use of theophylline compounds, and the disorder recently has been found to respond reasonably well to treatment with certain calcium channel blocking drugs. With 72-hour monitoring the incidence of arrhythmias approaches 90%, often occurring with severe hypoxemia, which may be found in patients with chronic bronchitis during rapid eye movement (REM) sleep.

Unfortunately, improvement in the patient's arterial blood gases correlates poorly with resolution of the arrhythmia. Other ECG abnormalities generally reflect pulmonary hypertension: tall, peaked P waves, a shift to the right of the P wave axis, and evidence of right ventricular hypertrophy. In the absence of conduction defects, an S_1-Q_3 pattern, an S_1-S_2-S_3 pattern, an R/S ratio in V_6 less than $1:1$, and a right axis deviation greater than 110 degrees are most suggestive of right ventricular hypertrophy. Combinations of these findings increase the accuracy of the diagnosis of right ventricular hypertrophy.

In patients with COPD the leukocyte count usually is normal unless a bacterial infection has supervened. Hematocrit values and hemoglobin levels may be elevated, reflecting secondary polycythemia resulting from hypoxemia, "stress," or diuretic therapy. These changes may be obscured by the increased plasma volume of right ventricular failure.

Sputum examination in the patient with chronic bronchitis usually is of minimal help, since leukocytes often are found in the patient's sputum regardless of the clinical status; colonization of the lower respiratory tract with a variety of organisms is the common finding. Nevertheless, gross and microscopic sputum examination should be performed, since the finding of pus or the predominance of a single organism may influence therapy.

Early in the course of chronic bronchitis, routine pulmonary function tests often reveal normal findings. In contrast, the more sensitive tests, which reflect small airway function such as frequency dependence of compliance, closing volume, maximal midexpiratory flow rate, and change in flow rates at lower lung volumes when the patient breathes helium-oxygen mixtures instead of air (volume of isoflow), often are abnormal. These tests are not in general clinical use because of their poor standardization, technical difficulty, and expense. Furthermore, they often are abnormal in young, healthy smokers. As the obstructive defect worsens, there is evidence of a decrease in maximal expiratory flow rates, such as the $FEV_{1.0}$ and peak expiratory flow, as well as a decrement in

the maximal voluntary ventilation. Such flow reduction may or may not respond to bronchodilators. The residual volume may be elevated with a relatively unchanged total lung capacity. The diffusing capacity frequently is unimpaired, although this test can be affected by a severe ventilation-perfusion mismatch.

Compliance measurements occasionally are used in the evaluation of COPD, although they tend to be time consuming and uncomfortable for the patient. Compliance is a means of expressing the volume-pressure relationship of the lung and thorax. The tidal volume generated by a measured change in transpulmonary pressure is divided by that pressure change. Static compliance is calculated at a time when air flow has ceased, whereas dynamic compliance is measured during an uninterrupted respiratory cycle. Static compliance is normal or reduced in bronchitis, clearly distinguishing it from emphysema, in which the static compliance is increased. Dynamic compliance, however, is diminished in both diseases and decreases more with increasing respiratory frequency (frequency dependence of compliance).

MANAGEMENT. Avoidance of bronchoirritants, especially cigarettes, should be the mainstay of patient management, especially during exacerbations of respiratory symptoms. Smoking contributes to bronchospasm, mucus production, and decreased ciliary motion and raises the carboxyhemoglobin levels.

Therapy also should be directed toward relieving airway obstruction, reducing cough and sputum production, treating infections, preventing complications, and managing acute respiratory insufficiency. Airway obstruction usually has been managed with oral bronchodilators, specifically theophylline or other xanthines. The pharmacology of these drugs is complex. Metabolism is diminished in severe COPD, congestive heart failure, liver disease, old age, and with the use of some histamine (H_2) antagonist drugs and is increased by cigarette smoking and the ingesting of barbiturates. Nausea and anorexia are the early warning signs of excessive theophylline dosage. Although serious toxic reactions (coma, seizures, shock, or respiratory arrest) may occur without warning when theophylline dosage is excessive, these serious reactions are rare. The emetic quality of theophylline is believed to be mediated through the central nervous system; thus preparations designed to minimize gastric exposure to theophylline have been disappointing. The usual initial dose is about 100 to 200 mg of theophylline four times daily. Extended-release preparations appear to offer some advantages.

Adrenergic agonists, especially selective β_2-agents, are of potential benefit not only for their bronchodilator activity but also for their ability to speed up mucous transport. Recently the trend has been toward greater use of aerosolized β_2-adrenergic agonists rather than the ingested forms of these drugs. These aerosols can be delivered by intermittent positive-pressure breathing (IPPB) machines, but they are more commonly delivered by hand-held nebulizers or by propellant-driven metered-dose inhalers. If O_2 is used to power the IPPB machine, the resulting high inspired O_2 concentration can aggravate CO_2 retention in the O_2 sensitive, severely compromised patient with COPD. Physical therapy involving the chest and postural drainage may help to loosen and raise thick, viscous secretions, especially with decreased cough or severe debility.

Oral expectorants have less than convincing benefit. Atropine-like agents, including antihistamines, have been thought to be contraindicated because of their adverse effect on sputum viscosity, but recent work using inhaled anticholingergic agents to treat bronchospasm has shown enough promise that these agents are now available in metered-dose inhaler form.

The role of corticosteroids is not clearly defined. Methylprednisolone has been shown to improve $FEV_{1.0}$ when used with bronchodilators in hospitalized patients with chronic bronchitis. Some stable outpatients may demonstrate an improvement in expiratory flow rates with steroids (such as prednisone, 5 to 10 mg/day) administered in association with their usual bronchodilators. Long-term metabolic side effects may seriously impair the usefulness of steroids in this group of chronically ill patients.

Antibiotics have been widely used to treat exacerbations of symptoms. Ampicillin, tetracycline, erythromycin, and trimethoprim-sulfonamide combinations have been shown to be effective in decreasing morbidity. A common indication for therapy is a change in sputum consistency, amount, or color associated with a worsening of dyspnea. A sputum Gram stain usually confirms an increased number of leukocytes. Frequent exacerbations may be managed with prophylactic antibiotics. Regimens have included daily therapy during the winter, 4 days a week during the winter, or a 5- to 7-day course at the first sign of exacerbation. Unfortunately, although such prophylactic therapy has reduced the severity and duration of exacerbations, their frequency generally has been unaffected.

The use of O_2 therapy for 12 to 16 hours daily has been evaluated and is effective in decreasing cor pulmonale, pulmonary hypertension, secondary polycythemia, nocturnal hypoxemia, and associated arrhythmias. O_2 therapy may be warranted when a patient demonstrates severe hypoxemia on mild exercise or when O_2 improves exercise tolerance. Cough suppressants, sedatives, and hypnotic agents pose a serious threat to patients with severe chronic bronchitis. Patients with hypercapnia are particularly susceptible to respiratory depression. The suppression of cough may lead to retention of pulmonary secretions with resultant worsening of hypoxia and hypercapnia; this in turn causes central nervous system depression.

Cor pulmonale. Except for reducing pulmonary hypertension, little can be done to treat cor pulmonale. If polycythemia is significant, a decrease in resistance to blood flow may occur with a decrease in the hematocrit. This is best accomplished by reducing hypoxia with supplemental O_2; however, phlebotomy is occasionally indicated. Diuretics may control peripheral edema but further compromise cardiac output and contribute to electrolyte abnormalities. Abnormalities of left ventricular function in patients with cor pulmonale usually are minor. Digoxin has been used to improve right ventricular function but usually is without significant benefit, and these patients may be particularly susceptible to drug-induced side effects.

EMPHYSEMA

DEFINITION. Emphysema is an abnormal morphologic finding consisting of alveolar enlargement with destruction of alveolar walls. It usually is subdivided into centrilobular, panlobular, and localized forms. Centrilobular emphysema commonly is ascribed to chronic bronchitis and is associated with disease of the conducting airways. Panlobular emphysema is a parenchymal abnormality, typically represented by the patient with α-1-antitrypsin deficiency.

EPIDEMIOLOGY. Emphysema has been estimated by the National Health Survey to have a prevalence of 9.8:1000 adults, or about one third that of chronic bronchitis. In the patients surveyed, activity limitation from emphysema was present in about 35%, whereas such limitation affected only 5% of the bronchitis group. Although much attention has been given to patients deficient in α-1-antitrypsin because of implications regarding pathogenesis, this autosomal recessive gene appears in its homozygous form in only about 0.1% of the U.S. population.

PATHOGENESIS AND PATHOLOGY. A clear distinction between centrilobular and panlobular emphysema frequently cannot be made. Such differentiation clinically is of little consequence. The hypotheses of pathogenesis receiving the greatest attention at present are those involving lung damage from proteolytic enzymes in the presence of abnormal controlling factors. This reasoning grew out of the discovery that some nonsmoking patients with pure emphysema of early onset lacked certain serum proteins originally termed α-1-antitrypsin but more accurately described as α-1-antiproteases. Various degradative enzymes inhibited by these proteins have been shown to cause emphysema when administered to experimental animals. The effect of smoking on the balance between proteolytic enzymes and inhibitor proteins is under investigation.

ETIOLOGY. Genetic predisposition is more clearly present in emphysema than in chronic bronchitis. The homozygous antitrypsin-deficient patient is rare and very susceptible to panlobular emphysema. The heterozygous antitrypsin-deficient patient may be at increased risk for COPD, especially if subjected to stress such as cigarette smoke. Cigarette smoking remains the greatest risk factor for the development of emphysema, although air pollution and infection may contribute by provoking chronic bronchitis.

CLINICAL MANIFESTATIONS. In relatively pure emphysema there is a gradual onset of dyspnea on exertion without a productive cough. Over the ensuing years shortness of breath at rest, fatigue, and weight loss develop. The physical examination demonstrates the findings of the classic "pink puffer"; a thin and sometimes wasted acyanotic patient with a hyperinflated (barrel) chest and low-lying diaphragms. There is increased use of the accessory muscles of respiration. The chest wall appears to move more vertically and on inspiration lacks the normal increase in the anteroposterior diameter and widening of the intercostal spaces. Intercostal and supraclavicular retractions may be noted. The lungs are hyperresonant to percussion with diminished breath sounds. Dry, crackling rales occasionally are heard.

The cardiac examination frequently is difficult because of the air-filled lung interposed between chest wall and heart. The heart frequently assumes a rather vertical position behind the sternum. The apical impulse and cardiac sounds may be best noted in the subxyphoid area. A loud pulmonary closure sound suggests pulmonary hypertension, and a right-sided gallop indicates right ventricular failure.

Abdominal examination may demonstrate a palpable liver edge; however, percussion of the superior border usually reveals a low-lying rather than an enlarged liver. Clubbing of the extremities is not present unless a complicating disease such as lung cancer has developed.

LABORATORY FINDINGS. Moderate or advanced emphysema often can be diagnosed from a routine chest roentgenogram, although a normal chest film does not exclude significant disease. The roentgenographic findings reflect two major physiologic changes: lung hyperinflation and damage to lung parenchyma. The more reliable signs of hyperinflation are an increased retrosternal airspace and flat or scalloped diaphragms. Less specific findings are low-lying diaphragms, hyperlucency of the lung fields, increased intercostal spaces, and an increased anteroposterior diameter (Fig. 123-1). Vascular changes include prominent hila with diminished peripheral ves-

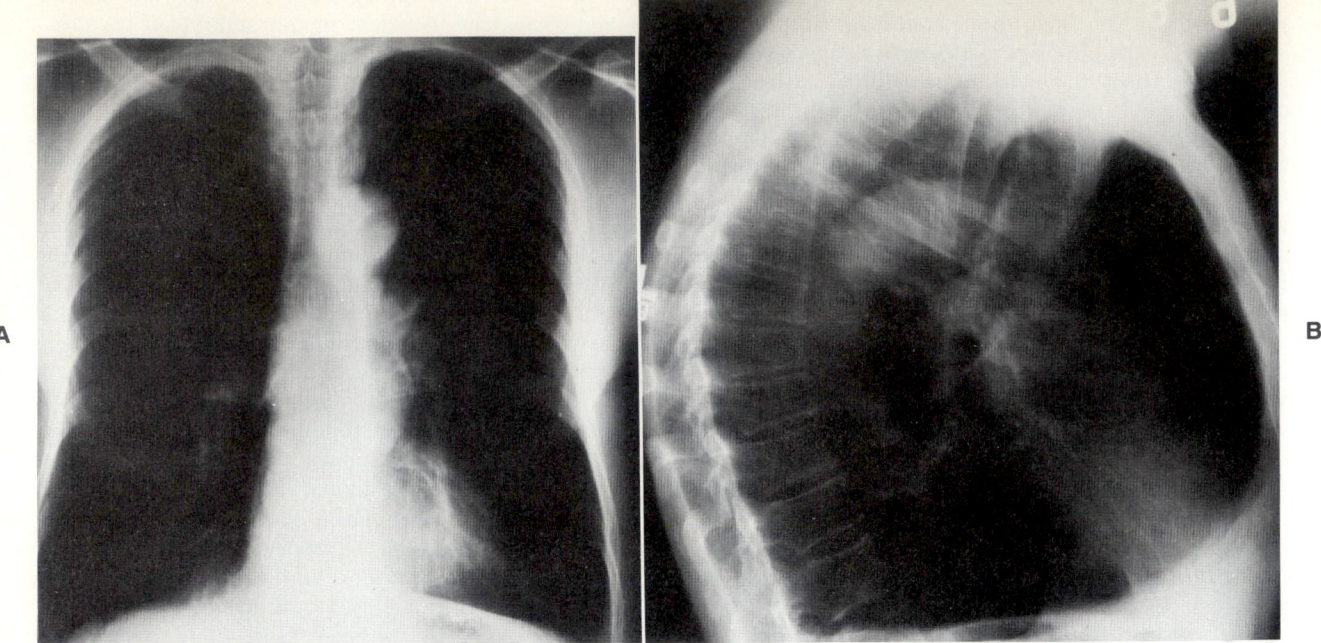

Fig. 123-1 **A,** Posteroanterior and, **B,** lateral chest roentgenograms of 67-year-old man with emphysema. Note increased retrosternal air space, flat diaphragms, and increased anteroposterior diameter. (Courtesy of George Popky, MD.)

sels and a "pruned" appearance (loss of visible distal divisions) of the vascular tree. The cardiac silhouette may appear narrow with a vertical axis. Irregular patches of lucency suggest emphysema. The diagnosis of a bulla is usually reserved for a radiolucent area clearly surrounded by a visible ring of lung tissue.

The ECG changes in emphysema are comparable to those in chronic bronchitis but tend to occur later in the disease process. Diffuse low voltage may also be seen.

Infectious airway disease is not a typical feature of pure emphysema; when it occurs, it usually is associated with tracheobronchitis or pneumonia. Sputum usually is minimal in the patient with stable emphysema, and hematologic abnormalities are likewise absent. A serum protein electrophoresis may show near absence of the α-1 region in the α-1-antitrypsin–deficient homozygote. A normal α-1 region on serum protein electrophoresis does not rule out the heterozygous state or an abnormal α-1-antiprotease. Further studies are indicated if a low α-1 level is noted.

Tests for airway obstruction show similar results in both chronic bronchitis and emphysema with the exception of the static lung compliance, which is increased in emphysema, and the diffusion capacity, which is generally more severely impaired in emphysema. Pure emphysema demonstrates bronchodilator-resistant airway obstruction, but so may chronic bronchitis. Flow rates in emphysema may show a disproportionate reduction in comparison with lung volumes, which may be increased. Arterial O_2 levels are commonly depressed, but CO_2 retention is less common and occurs later in the course of emphysema.

MANAGEMENT. Currently little can be done for the patient with pure emphysema. However, for those with α-1-antitrypsin deficiency, infusions of an α-1-antitrypsin preparation twice weekly over a 6-month period have been shown to reverse the biochemical abnormalities in serum and lung fluid but not to improve lung function. Avoidance of smoking, of carbon mon-

oxide exposure, and of the stress of other illnesses is important. When hypoxia-related polycythemia, central nervous system dysfunction, or pulmonary hypertension occurs, O_2 therapy may be of help. Cor pulmonale, however, is not usually the result of pulmonary vasospasm but often reflects the decreased pulmonary vascular bed. O_2 usually fails to significantly improve the cor pulmonale associated with emphysema.

The decision to intubate and artificially ventilate a patient with emphysema-related ventilatory failure is always difficult. This reflects the recognition that the respiratory failure resulting from emphysema, in the absence of acute correctable complications such as pneumonia, is not associated with a reversible condition, and artificially ventilated patients with emphysema may be dependent on the ventilator for the remainder of their lives.

BIBLIOGRAPHY

Anthonisen NR and others: Antibiotic therapy in exacerbations of COPD, Ann Intern Med 106:196, 1987.

Ayers S: Cigarette smoking and lung diseases, Basics of Respiratory Disease, vol 3, no 5, 1975.

Boushay H and others: Bronchial hyper-reactivity, Am Rev Respir Dis 121:389, 1980.

Brashear R and Rhodes M: Chronic obstructive lung disease, clinical treatment and management, St. Louis, 1978, The CV Mosby Co.

Burrows B and Earle R: Course and prognosis of chronic obstructive lung disease, N Engl J Med 280:397, 1969.

Fishman A: Chronic cor pulmonale, Am Rev Respir Dis 114:775, 1976.

Fletcher C and Peto R: The natural history of chronic airflow obstruction, Br Med J 1:1645, 1977.

Goldsmith J: Health effects of air pollution, Basics of Respiratory Disease, vol 4, no 2, 1975.

Gump D and others: Role of infection in chronic bronchitis, Am Rev Respir Dis 113:465, 1976.

Higgins MW and others: An index of risk for obstructive airway disease, Am Rev Respir Dis 125:144, 1982.

Hogg J and others: Site and nature of airway obstruction in chronic obstructive lung disease, N Engl J Med 278:1355, 1968.

Hugh-Jones P and Whimster W: The etiology and management of disabling emphysema, Am Rev Respir Dis 117:337, 1978.

Jeanne J: The clinical pharmacology of bronchodilators, Basics of Respiratory Disease, vol 6, no 1, 1977.

Kueppers F and Black L: Alpha-1-antitrypsin and its deficiency, Am Rev Respir Dis 110:176, 1974.

Lertzman M and Cherniack R: Rehabilitation of patients with chronic obstructive pulmonary disease, Am Rev Respir Dis 114:1145, 1976.

Macklem P: Disease in small airways, Basics of Respiratory Disease, vol 4, no 5, 1976.

Rodman T and Sterling F: Pulmonary emphysema and related lung disease, St. Louis, 1969, The CV Mosby Co.

Thurlbeck W: Chronic obstructive lung disease—a comparison between clinical, roentgenologic, functional and morphologic criteria in chronic bronchitis, emphysema, asthma and bronchiectasis, Medicine 49:81, 1970.

Thurlbeck W: Chronic bronchitis and emphysema—the pathophysiology of chronic obstructive lung disease, Basics of Respiratory Disease, vol 3, no 1, 1974.

US Department of Health and Human Services: Smoking and health, a report of the Surgeon General, Pub No 79-50066, Washington DC, 1979, US Government Printing Office.

Wewers MD and others: Replacement therapy for α-1-antitrypsin deficiency associated with emphysema, N Engl J Med 316:1050, 1987.

124 • PULMONARY HYPERTENSION AND COR PULMONALE

William L. Morrissey

When the right ventricle faces increased pressures in the pulmonary vascular system, right ventricular enlargement and dilation ensue. These changes of right ventricular overload are manifested clinically by the signs and symptoms of right-sided heart failure, including right ventricular prominence, right ventricular gallop rhythm, jugular venous distention, and peripheral edema. The electrocardiogram shows evidence of right atrial hypertrophy (peaked P waves, or P pulmonale) and right ventricular strain.

Most commonly the increased pulmonary vascular pressures merely reflect the elevated left-sided heart pressures caused by left ventricular failure or mitral valve disease. However, pulmonary hypertension may develop in spite of normal left-sided pressures. The resultant right ventricular failure is then termed "cor pulmonale," or heart disease resulting from lung disease. This form of pulmonary hypertension is the result of either pulmonary parenchymal disease or airways hypoxia, or it may be primary, as in primary pulmonary hypertension.

Pulmonary parenchymal disease may involve loss of alveoli with concurrent loss of associated capillaries, as in emphysema, or isolated loss of the capillary bed, as in pulmonary vasculitis resulting from collagen vascular disease or illicit intravenous drug use. Other causes of a diminished vascular bed include recurrent pulmonary emboli, primary pulmonary hypertension, and pulmonary venoocclusive disease. Primary pulmonary hypertension is a disease of unknown cause occurring predominantly in young women and confirmed histologically by finding pulmonary arterial hypertrophy and hyperplasia. Pulmonary venoocclusive disease begins with fibrous narrowing of pulmonary venules and progresses to occlusion and subsequent pulmonary arterial changes. Therapy for pulmonary vascular diseases is generally unsatisfactory, although prevention of pulmonary emboli is a worthwhile goal.

Hypoxia, usually caused by chronic obstructive pulmonary disease, results in pulmonary hypertension by inducing vasoconstriction. This apparently inappropriate reaction to hypoxia is the unfortunate extension of the body's normal and appropriate attempt to divert blood away from areas in which it is being poorly oxygenated. The therapy is directed at the underlying lung disease, but relief of hypoxia is crucial to improvement. The administration of supplemental oxygen to raise the arterial oxygen level to 50 to 60 mm Hg usually is required. Diuretic therapy may improve peripheral edema, but digitalis is not particularly helpful.

BIBLIOGRAPHY

Fishman AP: Chronic cor pulmonale: state of the art, Am Rev Respir Dis 114:775, 1976.

125 • BRONCHIECTASIS

Paul D. Siegel and **Frank Barch**

DEFINITION. Bronchiectasis is a morphologic change consisting of persistent abnormal dilation of bronchi. It may occur diffusely throughout the tracheobronchial tree, usually in a patchy distribution, or it may be localized to a segment or lobe. It may be associated with recurrent cough, fever, pneumonia, sporadic hemoptysis, or frequently if not always, copious purulent continuous sputum production; or it may be of no clinical importance and unaccompanied by symptoms.

ETIOLOGY AND EPIDEMIOLOGY. Bronchiectasis has a number of causes and predisposing factors. It also can occur without any discernible cause, in which case it often is presumed to have followed an unrecognized bronchopulmonary infection.

Bronchiectasis is associated with several congenital anomalies. Pulmonary sequestration is a localized abnormality usually accompanied by bronchiectasis. Yellow nail syndrome is a condition in which bronchiectasis coexists with lymphedema and yellow nails. Bronchiectasis is a common complication of cystic fibrosis (mucoviscidosis).

The association of bronchiectasis, sinusitis, and situs inversus has been referred to as Kartagener's syndrome or triad. Bronchiectasis occurs in 15% to 25% of patients with situs inversus, strongly suggesting a congenital origin. In Kartagener's syndrome structural abnormalities of the bronchial cilia have been described, with subsequent impaired motility of the cilia. This hinders mucus clearance and sets up nidus for recurrent infection. Spermatozoa of these patients also are immotile and have the same microtubular deficiency.

Bronchiectasis commonly occurs as a complication of congenital or acquired disorders of humoral immunity. A defect in humoral immunity renders a patient susceptible to pyogenic bacterial infections. Recurrent pneumonia with *Streptococcus pneumoniae* is common, and *Streptococcus pyogenes, Pseudomonas aeruginosa,* and *Haemophilus influenzae* also are commonly found pathogens. Presumably, bronchiectasis is the result of repeated injury to the tracheobronchial tree as a consequence of infection with these organisms.

Bronchiectasis may occur following childhood pneumonia, especially that subsequent to measles or pertussis. Bronchial obstruction by a tumor, foreign body, or stenosis also is commonly followed by bronchiectasis. Tuberculosis may be associated with bronchiectasis that persists after the organism is eradicated. A localized, proximal form of bronchiectasis can be seen in asthmatic patients whose bronchi are colonized by *Aspergillus* species.

Exposure to the oxides of sulfur or nitrogen most commonly results in obliterative bronchiolitis as a late sequela, but occasionally bronchiectasis may occur. This was seen more often in the past after exposure to mustard gas.

PATHOLOGY AND PATHOPHYSIOLOGY. Bronchiectasis can be divided into a cylindric type, a saccular form, and an intermediate irregular ectasia known as varicose. Cylindric bronchiectasis may occur following pneumonia and is reversible, whereas saccular bronchiectasis usually is considered irreversible.

In addition to luminal dilation, substantial inflammatory changes occur in the bronchial walls. All layers of the wall may be infiltrated with inflammatory cells, and smaller branches may be plugged by mucus or fibrous tissue. Large anastomotic channels develop between the bronchial and pulmonary circulations, with an increase in bronchial artery blood flow. These changes result in a ventilatory pattern resembling that of chronic bronchitis. The vital capacity is decreased, with more severe decreases found in the expiratory flow rates. The maximal voluntary ventilation is decreased, and the ratio of residual volume to total lung capacity is increased. The venous admixture is increased because of abnormal ventilation-perfusion ratios and a decrease in diffusing capacity.

CLINICAL MANIFESTATIONS. Although patients with bronchiectasis may be asymptomatic, the symptoms are characteristically those of recurrent bronchopulmonary infections. Cough, producing copious three-layered sputum containing pus on the bottom, saliva in the center, and mucus on the top, is a classic symptom. This type of presentation currently is less common because of widespread antibiotic therapy. Recurrent fevers frequently are present, and chronic fatigue is common. Hemoptysis is not uncommon and may be massive. Hemoptysis may be the initial symptom in cases of upper lobe bronchiectasis, since excessive sputum production is uncommon. These cases often are referred to as dry bronchiectasis or bronchiectasis sicca. The most characteristic finding in bronchiectasis is the detection of crackles over the affected lung lobe or segment. These may be accompanied by wheezes and usually persist even when the patient is asymptomatic. Clubbing of the fingers also is a common occurrence in bronchiectasis.

LABORATORY FINDINGS. Routine chest roentgenograms rarely are normal in bronchiectasis but seldom can establish the diagnosis. Bronchography, in which a radiopaque contrast medium is instilled into the tracheobronchial tree, provides a morphologic diagnosis of bronchiectasis and also delineates the extent of involvement. Patients with impaired pulmonary function should be evaluated with caution, since bilateral bronchography produces a temporary 30% to 50% decrease in lung function. Care must be taken not to diagnose irreversible bronchiectasis when cylindric changes are found in a lobe or segment for up to 4 months following an episode of pneumonia; these changes may be reversible.

DIAGNOSIS. The diagnosis of bronchiectasis is based on the clinical history and the findings of persistent crackles and wheezes during the physical examination. If clubbing of the fingers is present, this diagnosis is even more likely. Asthma often is confused with bronchiectasis, but in asthma the physical examination should not reveal persistent crackles and the airway obstruction should be largely reversible.

Computed tomographic (CT) scan of the chest is a sensitive method for diagnosing bronchiectasis. In patients with cylindrical or varicose brochiectasis, the normally invisible intraparenchymal bronchi are thickwalled and dilated. In patients with cystic bronchiectasis the characteristic CT findings are thick-walled cystic spaces that are either grouped together in a cluster or strung together in a linear fashion.

Fluid levels in cysts are readily seen on CT scans. Bronchography, formerly the definitive method for establishing the diagnosis has rarely been needed since the advent of chest CT scanning.

COURSE AND PROGNOSIS. The course and prognosis of bronchiectasis depend largely on the extent and severity of the disorder. Bronchiectasis localized to a lobe or segment often causes little or no difficulty and is amenable to surgical correction. Generalized bronchiectasis with recurrent infections and sepsis formerly resulted in death within several years after the diagnosis. The introduction of antibiotics has enabled most patients to live more than 15 years after the diagnosis is first established. Those with cystic fibrosis or immunologic deficiencies continue to have a much poorer prognosis. Pulmonary function tends to decline rather slowly, so that respiratory insufficiency and cor pulmonale develop rather late in the course of the disease, if at all.

MANAGEMENT. The mainstay of medical therapy for bronchiectasis is the maintenance of a clear airway, which prevents pooling of secretions and subsequent infection. This can be accomplished by postural drainage, in which the bronchi draining the involved segments or lobes are placed in a dependent position for 10 to 20 minutes at least twice daily. Chest percussion or vibration over the involved area may further facilitate drainage. If nebulized acetylcysteine is used to loosen viscid secretions, it should be combined with a bronchodilator aerosol. The use of bronchodilator and decongestant aerosols before postural drainage may make the latter more productive. Oral antibiotics usually are reserved for the treatment of exacerbations of bronchopulmonary infection. Selected patients with persistently purulent sputum or frequently recurring attacks of bronchopulmonary infection have been reported to benefit from the intermittent administration of tetracycline or ampicillin. Acute infections should be treated with an appropriate antibiotic chosen on the basis of a sputum Gram stain and culture results.

Ampicillin or tetracycline usually is effective except in cystic fibrosis, in which the frequent occurrence of staphylococcal and *Pseudomonas* infections often requires use of a penicillin, an aminoglycoside, or a third-generation cephalosporin (ceftazidime) respectively.

Hemoptysis usually is managed adequately with rest, cough suppressants, and treatment of infection. Blood replacement rarely is necessary. Emergency resection of a segment or lobe to stop life-threatening bleeding is even less commonly needed. Elective surgical resection is reserved for cases in which the disease is localized to a segment or lobe. In these individuals failure to control recurrent infection, hemoptysis, or chronic debilitating cough might be considered an indication for surgery. Before any surgery, bronchography should be performed to outline the extent of the disease. Pulmonary function studies are useful to indicate the patient's ability to tolerate the surgery.

PREVENTION. Prevention of bronchiectasis requires an understanding of the role of bronchial obstruction and infection. Aspirated foreign bodies should be promptly removed, and the prevention or prompt reexpansion of postoperative atelectasis also is important. Vigorous treatment of bronchopneumonia is mandatory, and slowly resolving pneumonias must be followed to full resolution. If this does not occur spontaneously within an appropriate time (generally 6 weeks), measures such as bronchoscopy, physiotherapy, and respiratory therapy should be taken to encourage resolution. If there is no response to initial therapy or if there is evidence of an obstructing lesion, bronchoscopy should be considered much sooner. Prompt treatment of primary tuberculosis may prevent bronchial compression and atelectasis with the subsequent development of bronchiectasis.

BIBLIOGRAPHY

Barker AF and Bardana EJ, Jr.: Bronchiectasis: state of the art, Am Rev Resp Dis 137(4):969, 1988.

Guenter CA and Welch MA: Pulmonary medicine, Philadelphia, 1978, JB Lippincott Co.

Naidich DP and others: Computed tomography of bronchiectasis, J Comput Assist Tomogr 6:437, 1982.

Rosenberg M and others: Clinical immunologic criteria for the diagnosis of allergic bronchopulmonary aspergillosis, Ann Intern Med 86:405, 1977.

Sturgess JM and others: Cilia with defective radial spokes, N Engl J Med 300:53, 1979.

126·LUNG ABSCESS

Donald Kaye

ETIOLOGY AND PATHOGENESIS. Lung abscess occurs when lung parenchyma in an area of infection undergoes necrosis. Many of these areas communicate with bronchi and therefore undergo cavitation with formation of an air-fluid level. Cavitation may occur as a part of acute bacterial pneumonia; it is common in staphylococcal, *Klebsiella, Pseudomonas,* and other pneumonias, except for those caused by pneumococci and by *Mycoplasma pneumoniae* and *Haemophilus influenzae*. However, the term "lung abscess" often is reserved to describe a more chronic process in which the most common cause is a combination of anaerobic and microaerophilic bacteria, often in association with aerobes.

The most common pathogenetic mechanism of lung abscess is identical with that of mixed flora pneumonia—aspiration of the contents of the mouth. The material aspirated plugs off a bronchus or bronchiole, providing an anaerobic environment and allowing the anaerobic bacteria that are always present to grow. An acute aspiration or necrotizing mixed flora pneumonia that is cavitary may result, or a lung abscess may be discovered after days or weeks of fever.

Aspiration most often occurs during an episode of unconsciousness (for example, from alcohol, drug overdose, head trauma, anesthesia, seizure, or coma from any cause), in association with neuromuscular disease of the oropharynx or esophagus, or following operative procedures in the mouth. The patient's oral hygiene often is poor, and a gag reflex may be absent.

Lung abscess also tends to occur beyond obstructive disease of the bronchus such as beyond a tumor. Lung abscess in an edentulous person who has few anaerobes in the mouth suggests tumor. Bronchiectasis is another predisposing factor. Lung abscess occasionally results from secondary infection of a bronchogenic cyst, uninfected cavity or bulla, or from infection of a bland infarct. Lung abscess may also occur from a subdiaphragmatic process extending to the lung, such as amebic abscess of the liver causing right lower lobe infection.

Solitary or multiple lung abscesses may occur as the result of metastasis from suppurative pelvic or jugular thrombophlebitis, usually caused by anaerobes; from right-sided endocarditis, usually caused by *Staphylococcus aureus* (particularly in intravenous drug abusers); and occasionally from bacteremia from other sites.

CLINICAL MANIFESTATIONS. The patient with aspiration pneumonia has an acute onset of fever and cough productive of purulent sputum with or without blood. Pleuritic chest pain may be present if empyema develops. The physical examination reveals evidence of dullness to percussion and rales.

Patients with lung abscess often give a history of fever, anorexia, weight loss, malaise, and cough for days, weeks, or even months, with or without an initial acute onset. The sputum is commonly blood tinged and in most patients has a foul odor. Physical examination of the chest may reveal dullness, am-

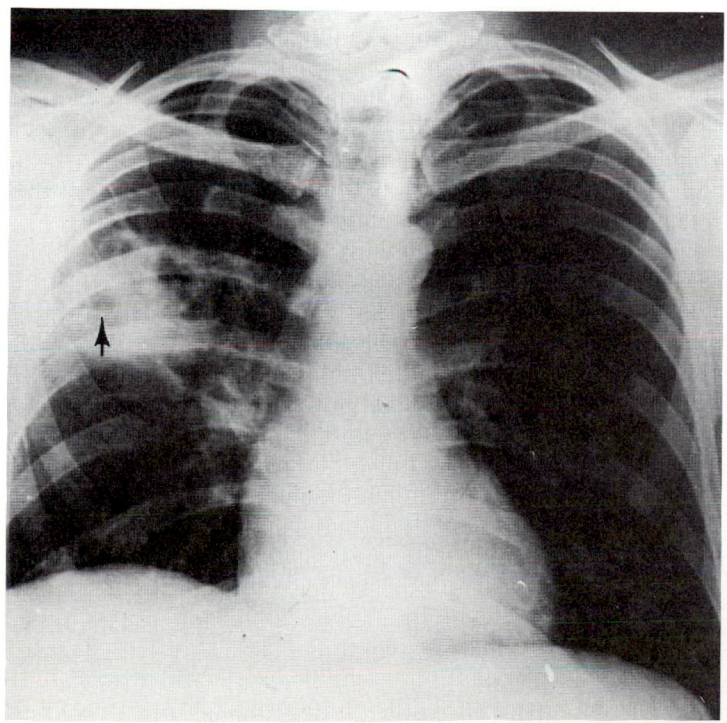

Fig. 126-1 Lung abscess demonstrating air-fluid level *(arrow).*

phoric breathing, and rales but often is negative. Clubbing of the fingers may occur.

LABORATORY FINDINGS. The microscopic examination of sputum in both aspiration pneumonia and anaerobic organism lung abscess reveals many polymorphonuclear leukocytes and a mixed flora of gram-positive cocci in chains, mixed gram-negative bacilli, gram-negative cocci, and/or gram-positive bacilli. Cultures usually reveal "normal flora." In fact, sputum cultures are of no value, because the organisms that cause lung abscess are present in the mouth in huge numbers. The diagnosis usually is apparent clinically and from the roentgenographic examination. Although percutaneous transtracheal aspiration is not usually indicated clinically, proper culturing of the aspirate reveals a mixed flora of anaerobes with or without aerobes. The organisms most commonly isolated are *Fusobacterium*, *Peptostreptococcus*, and *Peptococcus* organisms, microaerophilic streptococci, and *Bacteroides melaninogenicus*.

Chest roentgenography reveals the infiltrate of pneumonia, often with multiple cavities in aspiration pneumonia. A lung abscess usually shows a well-defined cavity surrounded by a rim of infiltrate. Air-fluid levels are common and strongly suggest abscess rather than tuberculosis (Fig. 126-1). The infiltrate usually is in the midlung fields, since most patients aspirate while lying on their backs or sides and aspirate into the dependent areas of the lungs, most commonly the posterior segment of the right upper lobe, the posteroapical segment of the left upper lobe, or the superior segments of the lower lobes.

If empyema occurs, the roentgenographic examination reveals pleural effusion, and an aspirate yields pus containing one or more of the etiologic agents. The fluid may have a foul odor. Blood cultures are positive in patients with metastatic lung abscesses. Cavitating carcinoma, tuberculosis, fungal infection, and Wegener's granulomatosis may simulate lung abscess.

MANAGEMENT. In contrast to abscesses elsewhere, surgical drainage is rarely indicated in lung abscess. Postural drainage is important, and drainage usually occurs through the bronchi provided they are unobstructed. In the presence of apparent obstruction, such as with atelectasis, bronchoscopy should be performed promptly to determine the patency of the airways.

The primary approach to the treatment of mixed flora lung abscess and aspiration pneumonia is antibiotic therapy directed toward the mouth flora (mainly anaerobic microorganisms) that cause most of these infections. Many of the anaerobes isolated from the mouth are sensitive to penicillin G, ampicillin, cephalothin, cefazolin, and cephalexin, and these agents have been used successfully. However, *B. melaninogenicus* (which is commonly isolated in lung abscesses and aspiration pneumonias) and *B. fragilis* (which is isolated in 10% to 15% of cases) often produce β-lactamase. For this reason preferred regimens are clindamycin (600 mg parenterally every 8 hours), ampicillin-sulbactam (3 g intravenously every 6 hours), cefoxitin (2 g intravenously every 4 hours), penicillin G plus metronidazole (20 million units penicillin each day plus 500 mg metronidazole intravenously every 6 hours) or ticarcillin-clavulanic acid (3 g intravenously every 4 hours). After response, oral clindamycin or amoxicillin-clavulanic acid can be used.

Aspiration pneumonia usually requires 2 weeks of therapy. There is no established duration of therapy required to prevent relapse after the treatment of anaerobic organism lung abscess. Although some lung abscesses have been cured with 2 or 3 weeks of therapy, those acquired by the bacteremic route usually require 4 to 6 weeks of therapy, and some acquired following aspiration may require 6 or even more weeks of therapy.

The lung abscesses that occur as a result of infection by a single organism such as *S. aureus* or *Klebsiella* are treated with antimicrobial agents directed specifically at the causative organism, for example, nafcillin for *S. aureus* infections.

Empyema should be drained. Abscesses at distant sites, such as a pelvic abscess in a patient with metastatic lung abscesses, should also be drained. Heparin therapy and vein ligation may be required in patients with septic phlebitis who continue to have pulmonary emboli.

PROGNOSIS. The prognosis in appropriately treated aspiration pneumonia depends partially on the underlying disease, but the overall mortality is about 20%. With multiple cavities the course is more severe. Anaerobic organism lung abscess has a mortality of about 10%. Pneumonias caused by *S. aureus*, *Klebsiella* organisms, and other gram-negative bacilli have a mortality of 25% or higher even with appropriate therapy.

BIBLIOGRAPHY

Bartlett JG and Finegold SM: Anaerobic pleuropulmonary infections, Medicine 51:413, 1972.
Bartlett JG and others: Bacteriology and treatment of primary lung abscess, Am Rev Respir Dis 109:510, 1974.
Levison ME and others: Clindamycin compared with penicillin for the treatment of anaerobic lung abscess, Ann Int Med 98:466, 1983.

127·CYSTIC FIBROSIS

Paul D. Siegel *and* **Frank Barch**

Cystic fibrosis is transmitted as a simple autosomal recessive trait. It is one of the most commonly inherited disorders of the white population of the United States, occurring in about 1 in 2000 live births. About 5% of the white population of the United States are heterozygous carriers. The basic abnormality appears to be an elevation of viscosity of the mucous secretions of the body. In the pancreas this results in the obstruction of secretory ducts, with subsequent exocrine insufficiency and malabsorption. In the bronchi extensive plugging occurs with obstruction, infection, and consequent destruction of bronchial walls. The inadequate clearance of secretions and resultant bronchiectasis commonly involve the upper lobes, whereas the usual idiopathic bronchiectasis preferentially affects the lower lobes.

The secretory abnormality that provides confirmation of the diagnosis of cystic fibrosis is elevation of the concentration in sweat of both sodium and chloride to greater than 60 mEq/L provided the standard pilocarpine iontophoresis method is used.

Complications include pneumothorax, massive hemoptysis, and cor pulmonale, as well as hypertrophic pulmonary osteoarthropathy and inappropriate secretion of antidiuretic hormone. Infection with *Staphylococcus aureus* and especially *Pseudomonas aeruginosa* is common, and death before 20 years of age formerly was the rule. Recently, however, with aggressive respiratory and physical therapy and more appropriate antibiotic treatment, including the use of aerosolized antipseudomonal antibiotics, more than 30% of patients with cystic fibrosis survive past the age of 18.

BIBLIOGRAPHY

Davis PB and diSant'Agnese PA: Diagnosis and treatment of cystic fibrosis: an update, Chest 85:802, 1984.

Stern RC and others: The course of cystic fibrosis in 95 patients, J Pediatr 89:406, 1976.

Tomashefski JF, Christoforidis AJ, and Abdullah AK: Cystic fibrosis in young adults, Chest 57:28, 1970.

128·BULLOUS EMPHYSEMA AND LUNG CYSTS

Paul D. Siegel and **Frank Barch**

BULLOUS EMPHYSEMA

DEFINITION. A bulla is an emphysematous space exceeding 1 cm in diameter. In contrast, blebs are collections of air within the visceral pleura, and cysts are airspaces lined completely by epithelium. Bullous emphysema is said to exist when one or more bullae are present.

ETIOLOGY AND PATHOGENESIS. Bullae can be associated with chronic bronchitis or panacinar (panlobular) emphysema. They also complicate the late stages of both pneumoconiosis and pulmonary sarcoidosis. In addition, bullae can appear without accompanying disease of the airways or interstitium. This latter type comprises true bullous disease of the lung or bullous emphysema, whereas the others are more properly referred to as emphysema with bullae, sarcoidosis with bullae, and so on.

Bullae are formed by the same processes responsible for emphysema, including atrophy and overinflation and destruction of lung tissue. Progressive trapping of air causes bullae to enlarge and in some cases to eventually reach remarkable size.

CLINICAL MANIFESTATIONS. Bullae that occur in a relatively normal lung usually are detected at the time of routine chest roentgenography as areas of hyperlucency bordered by curvilinear densities. Occasionally they may become large enough to interfere with the function of the remaining normal lung and then can cause shortness of breath. A sudden enlargement of a bulla or the development of spontaneous pneumothorax from rupture of a bulla can result in acute dyspnea or severe pleuritic chest pain. Bullae may become infected, leading to cough, fever, chills, and sputum production. The physical findings are those of decreased or absent breath sounds with a hyperresonant percussion note over the bulla, in addition to the signs of any underlying lung disease.

LABORATORY FINDINGS. The roentgenographic findings consist of areas of increased radiolucency that are sharply defined and bordered, at least to some extent, by fine opaque lines representing fused connective tissue septa. Perfusion lung scans show an absence of perfusion in the bullae. However, ventilation scans may show normal, diminished, or absent ventilation depending on the patency of the bronchus leading to the bulla.

The results of pulmonary function studies in patients with bullae and normal intervening lungs are normal except for an increase in functional residual capacity when measured by body plethysmography. If the bullae communicate very poorly with the airway, this increase may not be reflected in the functional residual capacity measured by dilutional techniques.

In patients with underlying emphysema or chronic bronchitis, the pulmonary function studies are abnormal and consistent with the severity of the underlying disease.

MANAGEMENT. Bullae in an asymptomatic patient with normal lung function require no therapy other than cessation of smoking and periodic evaluation for enlargement of the bullae.

Infected bullae should be treated with appropriate antibiotics as determined by a sputum smear and culture. The major decision to be made in the management of bullae is whether surgical removal or obliteration of the bullae should be performed. Each case must be considered on an individual basis, but generally the indications for surgery include dyspnea, recurrent pneumothorax, infection, and hemoptysis. The best results from surgery are obtained in patients with giant bullae (especially if confined largely to one lung), with evidence of atelectasis of adjacent tissue, with lesser degrees of chronic obstructive pulmonary disease, and in whom simple plication or excision of bullae rather than lobectomy is possible.

LUNG CYSTS

DEFINITION. A lung cyst is defined as an abnormal space lined with bronchial epithelium. This space may be either fluid- or air-filled.

BRONCHOGENIC CYSTS. Bronchogenic cysts are rare developmental abnormalities resulting from abnormal budding of the developing foregut; they may lie within either the mediastinum or the lung. They are usually first discovered in the patient's third decade of life as an incidental finding on the chest roentgenogram. Pathologically a cyst usually is thin walled and lined with either ciliated or nonciliated epithelium. If it is centrally located, it may contain mucous glands, cartilage, muscle tissue, and elastic fibers. Central cysts are usually solitary and do not communicate with the major bronchi. In contrast, peripheral cysts, usually located within the parenchyma, are more often multiple and may retain communication with normal bronchi. The presence of ciliated or nonciliated respiratory epithelium is noted in the absence of infection; however, infection may destroy the epithelium. Mucous glands and cartilage are usually absent in peripheral bronchogenic cysts; muscle is nearly always absent, whereas elastic fibers are more common. Calcium deposits in either central or peripheral bronchogenic cysts are rare.

ACQUIRED CYSTS. Acquired lung cysts are more common than the congenital variety. The term implies that the abnormal space is air filled. The terms "bulla," "bleb," and "cyst" are somewhat variable, in part reflecting the fact that pathologic examination is often necessary to distinguish among them. A postinfection cavity is one of the most common precursors of such cysts.

CLINICAL MANIFESTATIONS. Most cysts are asymptomatic. If a cyst is intrapulmonary, hemoptysis is the most common symptom. Although pneumothorax is rare, air embolism has been noted following decompression in tunnel workers with pulmonary bronchogenic cysts. In contrast, mediastinal cysts give rise to symptoms produced by local pressure, especially when present in confined areas such as near the carina. Cough, dyspnea on exertion, stridor, and dysphagia may also be reported.

Roentgenographic discovery of these lesions unfortunately does not often allow a definitive diagnosis. The cysts are usually sharply marginated, round, dense tissue masses that are commonly stable in size but may occasionally change. Intrapulmonary cysts favor the lower lobes of both lungs.

Mediastinal cysts often occur as sharply defined masses below the carina. Esophageal displacement or tracheobronchial compression may be reported. Infection eventually occurs in a high proportion of patients with lung cysts. In the presence of infection it may be difficult to differentiate, even pathologically, between a bronchogenic cyst and an acquired lung cyst resulting from an abscess that has already healed. A definitive diagnosis may require thoracotomy. If symptoms occur, surgical resection may be necessary.

BIBLIOGRAPHY

Fraser R and Paré J: Diagnosis of diseases of the chest, vol 1, Philadelphia, 1977, WB Saunders Co.

Landing B: Congenital malformations and genetic disorders of the respiratory tract, Am Rev Respir Dis 120:151, 1979.

Murphy DMF and Fishman AP: Bullous emphysema. In Fishman AP, editor: Pulmonary diseases and disorders, New York, 1980, McGraw-Hill Book Co.

Poe RH and others: Perfusion-ventilation scintiphotography in bullous disease of the lung, Am Rev Respir Dis 107:946, 1973.

Wesley JR, Macleod WM, and Mullard KS: Evaluation and surgery of bullous emphysema, J Thorac Cardiovasc Surg 63:945, 1972.

129 · ATELECTASIS

Paul D. Siegel *and* **Frank Barch**

DEFINITION. Atelectasis is the collapse of lung tissue that has been previously expanded. Since the alveoli in the affected portion of the lung are no longer filled with air, blood flowing past this area is not oxygenated and the area functions as a venoarterial or right-to-left shunt.

ETIOLOGY. Any lesion obstructing a bronchus to a lung, lobe, or bronchopulmonary segment can cause atelectasis of that portion of lung. These lesions can include foreign bodies, such as dental bridges or portions of teeth, aspirated mucus or food, and endobronchial tumors. Extrabronchial compression by lymph nodes or tumors may be of sufficient magnitude to cause bronchial obstruction. Broncholiths caused by the erosion of calcified lymph nodes into a bronchus can also cause bronchial obstruction.

Atelectasis may develop without bronchial obstruction following radiotherapy. Small areas of collapse, termed "microatelectasis," may develop whenever respiration is impaired and pulmonary surfactant is diminished, as in the postanesthetic state or in the adult respiratory distress syndrome. Linear or platelike atelectasis also may develop as a result of pulmonary infarction, pleural effusion, or other conditions that restrict or limit chest wall or diaphragm motion. These include obesity, ascites, pleuritic pain, paralytic or obstructive ileus, and subdiaphragmatic masses or abscesses. Basilar atelectasis may develop in the postoperative period, especially after upper abdominal or thoracic surgery.

PATHOGENESIS. When a bronchus is occluded, the air distal to the obstruction is absorbed into the blood. This occurs because the sum of the partial pressures of the gases in venous blood is less than that in alveolar air, since the fall in P_{O_2} in tissue greatly exceeds the rise in P_{CO_2} in the same tissue. If room air is being breathed, the area distal to an obstruction will collapse in several hours. If O_2 is being breathed, the pressure gradient is greater and collapse may occur in a few minutes. With occlusion of a smaller bronchus, collapse may be prevented by openings in the alveolar wall that allow passage of air from one lobule to another. However, it is known that collapse can occur even under these circumstances, probably because of blockage of the collateral channels or local loss of surfactant.

A sharp reduction in vital capacity occurs following upper abdominal and thoracic surgery. Small areas of atelectasis subsequently develop, presumably because of impaired expansion of the lung or because of deactivation of surfactant. As the vital capacity becomes smaller, more alveolar units approach their closing volume and thus become atelectatic, requiring

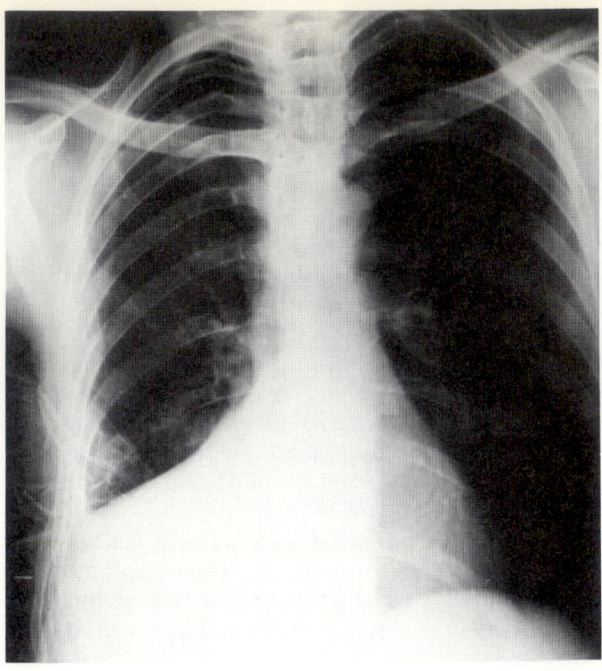

Fig. 129-1   Right lower lobe atelectasis with obliteration of shadow of diaphragm. There is no bronchogram. (Courtesy of George Popky, MD.)

greater than normal pressures to reexpand. In many critically ill patients, persistent collapse of lung tissue results from retained secretions in the airway, impaired regional ventilation, and altered compliance of lung tissue.

CLINICAL MANIFESTATIONS. If a main bronchus to the right or left lung is occluded, respiratory distress with tachypnea, tachycardia, and fever (probably from pneumonia) can follow. Arterial O_2 saturation drops initially, and cyanosis may become evident. If atelectasis involves only one lobe or part of a lobe, the only symptoms may be fever or dyspnea. Tachypnea and tachycardia may also occur but may be less pronounced.

LABORATORY FINDINGS. The findings on physical examination depend on the location and extent of the atelectasis. Uninflated portions of the lung generally show dullness to percussion, decreased or absent breath sounds, and sometimes rales and egophony. With a major loss of volume there is a shift of the trachea and mediastinum toward the involved side or an elevation of the diaphragm. The only significant laboratory findings are usually the abnormalities in arterial blood gases. The Pa_{O_2} is decreased as a result of the shunt effect from blood perfusing the unventilated lung. The Pa_{CO_2} may drop significantly as the result of the compensatory hyperventilation of the remaining lung. The white blood cell count often is elevated.

DIAGNOSIS. The diagnosis is suspected by recognizing the patient at risk and heeding the clinical findings described previously. For major areas of atelectasis the chest film is the most important diagnostic tool, showing collapsed lobes and abnormal locations of interlobar fissures (Fig. 129-1).

Air bronchograms produced by the contrast between endobronchial gas and collapsed tissue on the chest roentgenogram may have therapeutic significance, since they correlate with patency of major airways. In atelectasis caused by proximal airway obstruction, usually there is no air remaining in the bronchus, and an air bronchogram is not found; this suggests that bronchoscopy may be helpful in relieving the obstruction.

COURSE, MANAGEMENT, AND PREVENTION. If untreated, atelectasis, particularly if caused by an obstructed bronchus, can lead to secondary infection and bacterial pneumonia. The secretions retained in the obstructed or unventilated portion of the lung serve as a medium for bacterial growth and eventual pneumonia. If the bronchus to the atelectatic area is obstructed, infection is likely to be caused by anaerobic or other bacteria and to result in lung abscess. Whether pneumonia develops or not, atelectasis can progress to eventual fibrosis and permanent volume loss if the affected pulmonary tissue is not reexpanded. As with almost any pathologic process, prevention is preferable to treatment.

Since atelectasis is a rather common complication of upper abdominal and chest surgery, this situation has been intensely studied. Although there remains considerable controversy as to the best technique, the major factor in the prevention of postoperative atelectasis appears to be periodic expansion of the lungs with large volumes of air. Formerly intermittent positive-pressure breathing (IPPB) therapy was used to achieve this result, but more recently incentive spirometry and other techniques have been used. Currently it would appear that none of these methods offers any advantages over the others in most cases.

The patient's own bronchoalveolar clearing mechanisms also should be used. This requires training in cough techniques, encouragement to cough, early postoperative mobility, and avoidance of suppression of the cough reflex with sedation or pain medication. Chest percussion to loosen secretions and adequate airway hydration to prevent excessive drying and inspissation of mucus also are important in preventing atelectasis. Once atelectasis has occurred, the treatment depends to some extent on the cause. If there is proximal airway obstruction by a foreign body, this should be promptly removed by rigid bronchoscopy. If there is no proximal obstruction or obstruction only by mucus plugs, vigorous respiratory therapy, including airway humidification, aerosolized bronchodilators, mucolytic agents, chest percussion, and postural drainage techniques, should be employed. If these measures are unsuccessful, fiberoptic bronchoscopy is recommended for aspiration of mucus plugs and saline lavage of occluded areas. In addition, bronchodilators, decongestants, and mucolytic agents may be instilled locally to aid in the removal of mucus plugs.

MIDDLE LOBE SYNDROME

Middle lobe syndrome is atelectasis of the right middle lobe, with the cause generally attributed to compression of the lobe's orifice by enlarged peribronchial nodes. Recently, however, this concept of cause has been challenged, since numerous cases have been reported in which no bronchial obstruction could be documented by bronchoscopy and bronchography. The right middle lobe has been singled out for special consideration because chronic atelectasis, with no readily discernible cause, appears to occur most commonly in this lobe. Theories advanced for the predilection of this lobe to volume loss now include (1) the prominent collection of lymph nodes surrounding the right middle lobe bronchus, (2) the drainage of much of the right lung and some of the left lung into these nodes, (3) the acute angulation of the right middle lobe bronchus, (4) the relatively narrow caliber of the right middle lobe bronchus compared to other bronchi subserving similar lung volumes, (5) the relatively long length and easy compressibility of the right middle lobe bronchus, and (6) the relatively poor collateral ventilation of the right middle lobe, attributed to the greater ratio of pleural surface to nonpleural surface of this lobe when compared to other lobes.

The symptoms of right middle lobe syndrome vary and include a history suggestive of bronchial asthma or episodes of recurrent respiratory infections. Chronic cough, fever, anterior chest pain, and hemoptysis also may be complaints.

The roentgenographic findings are those of volume loss in the right middle lobe. This may be difficult to detect unless a lateral film of the chest is carefully scrutinized. When right middle lobe atelectasis is discovered, bronchoscopy and possible bronchography are required to evaluate the lesion, since in the adult population about 40% of such lesions are caused by malignant tumors. Treatment of the right middle lobe syndrome is the same as that for any other lobar atelectasis, except that the tendency toward chronicity may necessitate long-term respiratory therapy on an outpatient basis. Because of the chronicity and recurrent nature of right middle lobe atelectasis, surgical removal of the lobe is required more frequently than in other forms or areas of atelectasis, but this is still rarely necessary.

BIBLIOGRAPHY

Culiner MM: The right middle lobe syndrome, a non-obstructive complex, Dis Chest 50:57, 1966.

Fraser RG and Paré JA: Diagnosis of diseases of the chest, Philadelphia, 1977, WB Saunders Co.

Inner CR and others: Collateral ventilation and the middle lobe syndrome, Am Rev Respir Dis 118:305, 1978.

Iverson L and others: A comparative study of IPPB, the incentive spirometer and blow bottles: the prevention of atelectasis following cardiac surgery, Ann Thorac Surg 24:197, 1978.

Latimer RG and others: Pulmonary complications after upper abdominal surgery by pre-operative and post-operative computerized spirometer and blood gas analysis, Am J Surg 122:622, 1971.

Mahajan VK, Catron PW, and Huber GL: The value of fiberoptic bronchoscopy in the management of pulmonary collapse, Chest 73:817, 1978.

Marini JJ, Pierson DJ, and Hudson LD: Acute lobar atelectasis: a prospective comparison of fiberoptic bronchoscopy and respiratory therapy, Am Rev Respir Dis 119:971, 1979.

Schlenker JD and Hubay CA: The pathogenesis of post-operative atelectasis, Arch Surg 107:846, 1973.

130 · ASTHMA

Lee W. Greenspon

DEFINITION. Asthma is a disease process in which airway smooth muscle shows an increased responsiveness to a variety of nonspecific stimuli, which can result in widespread narrowing of the airways and obstruction to airflow. Airflow obstruction is reversible, either spontaneously or through therapy. Clinically, asthma is characterized by paroxysms of dyspnea, coughing, and wheezing. Exacerbations may be short-lived or prolonged and often are interspersed with periods of complete clinical recovery. However, the spectrum and severity of the disease varies greatly between patients, with some chronically symptomatic despite therapy and others only occasionally symptomatic after viral upper respiratory tract infections.

PREVALENCE AND NATURAL HISTORY. It is now estimated that 4% of the adult population and as many as 10% of children have this disorder. Asthma occurs at all ages, but about 50% of cases develop before 10 years of age and another 30% by 40 years of age. There is a significant male to female preponderance only in childhood onset disease. Most asthmatic children have complete remission of their disease, but remission is less likely if the asthma is severe in childhood or if it is accompanied by infantile eczema or chronic sinusitis. Adult-onset asthma is less likely to go into remission. Death from asthma is relatively rare, with fewer than 2% of these patients dying of the disease.

PATHOGENESIS. Experimental models now suggest that airway hyperresponsiveness relates to the development of airway inflammation. Several factors can induce or exacerbate the asthmatic condition, including exposure to allergens, environmental toxins, occupational factors, and respiratory infections.

ETIOLOGIC FACTORS

Allergens. Allergic asthma depends on sensitized IgE antibody, which is bound to mast cells. Mast cells line the tracheobronchial tree and are proinflammatory. Binding of allergens to bound antibodies induces an immediate hypersensitivity reaction, with release of preformed chemical mediators of anaphylaxis such as histamine and generation of other potent mediators such as leukotrienes (slow-reacting substance of anaphylaxis) and prostaglandins (PGG_2, $PGF_{2\alpha}$, PGD_2). The result is an intense inflammatory reaction with smooth muscle constriction, vascular congestion, and edema formation. Chemotactic factors for neutrophils (NCF-A) and eosinophils (ECF) bring these cells to the site of the reaction hours later and are responsible for the late-phase allergic response. Allergen inhalation in the laboratory may induce airway hyperresponsiveness that lasts for up to 2 weeks.

A significant proportion of childhood-onset asthma occurs in individuals who are also allergic. For example, in a group in which the age of onset was 15 to 29 years, 83% were felt to have an allergic or extrinsic component. Adult-onset asthma is less likely to be associated with allergies.

Environmental toxins. Ozone is the major oxidant generated in photochemical smog. Healthy volunteers exposed to 0.6 ppm of ozone for 2 hours demonstrate airway hyperresponsiveness that may last for up to 1 week after exposure. In the animal model development of airway hyperresponsiveness depends on neutrophil influx into the airway wall, indicating a local inflammatory response. Other oxidants such as sulphur dioxide (5 ppm) and nitrogen dioxide (1 ppm) also induce hyperresponsiveness. Whether chronic low-level exposure can induce asthma has not been established; however, levels of sulphur dioxide as low as 0.1 ppm can induce bronchospasm in exercising asthmatic individuals.

Occupational agents. Many kinds of occupational exposure are associated with inducing the asthmatic condition. Often these associations are used to describe the type of asthma; for example, baker's asthma, western red cedar asthma, and meat wrappers asthma. Among the most common agents is toluene diisocyante (TDI), which is used in the plastics and insulation industries. Approximately 15% of workers exposed may develop asthma. Unfortunately, only 50% of sensitized workers who leave the workplace go into remission even after 2 years.

With occupational exposure there is a characteristic cyclic history. The patient is well in the morning, but symptoms may develop by the end of the shift and progress after leaving the work site. Workers usually are free of symptoms on weekends and on holidays.

Infections. A viral upper respiratory tract infection is the most common stimulus that exacerbates asthma and perhaps induces the condition. For example, it has been shown that approximately 30% of children infected with respiratory syncytial virus (RSV) in the respiratory tract develop a prolonged wheezy syndrome typical of asthma. The most important viruses producing this syndrome have been found to be rhinoviruses (common cold agents), influenza virus, and RSV. Pneumonia caused by *mycoplasma* organisms also has been associated with the precipitation of attacks, but bacterial infection has not been implicated. The mechanism by which viruses induce asthma is unknown but probably relates to a local inflammatory response in the airway mucosa. Recent studies have shown virus-specific IgE antibody and histamine in nasal secretions of children with acute respiratory illnesses, suggesting an acquired immediate hypersensitivity to viral antigens.

Modifiers. Many factors may worsen the asthmatic condition in individuals with preexisting disease. Exercise triggers bronchospasm in most asthmatic individuals if the exercise is at a high enough level to cause significant drying and heat loss from the airway. The colder and drier the ambient air and the higher the minute ventilation, the more intense the bronchoconstriction. Hyperventilation of cold, dry air by a stationary subject produces the same response, indicating that exercise itself is not the stimulus. Emotional factors interact with the asthmatic condition and may worsen the disease process but usually are not the sole cause responsible for an acute exacerbation. The central nervous system also can control or modulate airway tone through control of parasympathetic vagal nerve efferent activity.

PATHOLOGIC CHANGES AND CLINICAL MANIFESTATIONS. In patients dying of asthma, the pathology is distinctive. The lungs are overinflated, and there are numerous gelatinous plugs of mucus throughout the tracheobronchial tree down to the terminal bronchioles. Histologic examination shows eosinophilic infiltration of airway mucosa, denudation of surface epithelium, hypertrophy of airway smooth muscle, and thickened basement membranes. These changes, even in milder form, explain the obstruction to airflow and the complaints of cough, wheezing, and shortness of breath. In fact, early mild disease may be manifested with only one of these complaints, such as persistent cough.

Physical examination of the asthmatic individual during an acute exacerbation often reveals tachypnea, tachycardia, and an inability to lie flat comfortably. Use of accessory muscles of respiration (sternocleidomastoids) and an exaggerated decrease in systolic blood pressure on inspiration (pulses paradoxus) indicate severe airway obstruction. This often is accompanied by hyperinflation of the chest. The intensity of wheezing does not correlate with the severity of disease. Since severity may be difficult to determine by physical examination alone, various laboratory tests should be employed to evaluate objectively the degree of airflow obstruction and the response to therapy (see "Laboratory findings").

Certain variant forms of asthma require special consideration. Approximately 10% of individuals with asthma demonstrate aspirin hypersensitivity. The problem usually begins with perennial rhinitis that is followed by rhinosinusitis with nasal polyps. On exposure to very small amounts of aspirin, severe episodes of airway obstruction with nasal congestion may develop. There is cross-reactivity with other nonsteroidal compounds such as indomethacin, as well as with tartrazine and other yellow dyes. The mechanism of this reaction remains unknown.

Allergic bronchopulmonary aspergillosis is an immune hypersensitivity to antigens of the fungus *Aspergillus*. This fungus may colonize the airways of patients with asthma and the individuals may develop a reaction characterized by expectoration of brown plugs of sputum; pulmonary infiltrates; elevated serum IgE levels; and blood and tissue eosinophilia. It is important to recognize this syndrome, because untreated patients may develop central bronchiectasis and pulmonary fibrosis. Corticosteroid therapy often is effective.

LABORATORY FINDINGS. Asthma is characterized by reversible airflow obstruction. During active episodes spirometry is always abnormal and demonstrates decreased airflow at all lung volumes. In patients who come to the emergency room for therapy, the volume of air exhaled in the first second of forced expiration ($FEV_{1.0}$) commonly is reduced to approximately 30% of the predicted value, with a ratio of $FEV_{1.0}$ to forced expiratory vital capacity (FVC) of less than 50%. Simpler measurements of airflow such as peak expiratory flow rate (PEFR) may also be reduced to 30% of predicted value, or about 100 L/min. In gauging the severity and management of asthma, it is important to have documented, objective improvement in airflow (an increase in $FEV_{1.0}$ by at least 30%) 1 hour after aggressive bronchodilator therapy. Patients that fail to respond to this degree should be hospitalized and treated with frequent bronchodilator aerosol therapy and corticosteroids.

The chest roentgenogram is nonspecific, demonstrating hyperinflation in only 30% of cases. A chest roentgenogram is warranted only if pneumonia is a consideration. Sputum and blood eosinophilia is common but nonspecific. Analysis of arterial blood gases is an important determination in severe cases. Hypoxemia (decreased PaO_2) is a universal finding duirng acute attacks. Most asthmatic individuals also have hypocapnia (decreased $PaCO_2$) and respiratory alkalosis. A normal carbon dioxide tension during an acute attack tends to be associated with severe obstruction accompanied by respiratory muscle fatigue, and it should be viewed as a sign of impending respiratory failure.

THERAPY. Patient education about the nature of airway hyperresponsiveness and the factors that may induce bronchospasm is critically important in the management of asthma. Eliminating causative agents may be the most successful form of therapy. Specific drug therapy is reviewed briefly.

Adrenergic agents. Catecholamines (epinephrine, isoproterenol, and isoetharine), resorcinols (metaproterenol and terbutaline), and saligenins (salbutamol) all are used in clinical practice. The resorcinols and saligenins have greater clinical efficacy in that they can be administered by the intravenous, oral, or inhaled route. In addition, they have β_2-adrenergic selectivity with many fewer direct cardiac effects. Epinephrine by the subcutaneous route still is commonly used in the emergency situation. The usual adult dose is 0.3 ml of a 1:1000 solution administered subcutaneously. Because of significant cardiac and α-adrenergic effects, this drug is not recommended in asthmatic individuals over 40 years of age. The preferred method of delivery of adrenergic agents is by inhalation. Most of these preparations are packaged in pocket-sized metered-dose inhalers or as a solution that can be nebulized in a hand-held device. The side effects of these agents include tremor, tachycardia, and nervousness.

Methylxanthines. Theophyllines act as bronchodilators. These drugs are less potent than the adrenergic agents and have a narrower therapeutic to toxic ratio. The mechanism responsible for the bronchodilator effect is unknown. It formerly was thought that these drugs increased cyclic adenosine monophosphate (AMP) by inhibition of phosphodiesterase. However, recent evidence no longer supports this concept. The therapeutic serum concentration of theophylline is between 10 and 20 μg/ml. For initiation of intravenous therapy with aminophylline, the recommended loading dose is 5 to 6 mg/kg given over 30 minutes and then a constant infusion of 0.5 mg/kg/hr. Theophylline metabolism and clearance vary widely from patient to patient. Theophylline is primarily metabolized in the liver. Therefore acute and chronic hepatic dysfunction or passive congestion of the liver (as in heart failure) dramatically decreases clearance rates. Clearance is increased in children and smokers and falls with concurrent use of cimetidine or erythromycin. The most common side effects of theophylline

toxicity are tremulousness, nervousness, nausea, vomiting, and tachycardia. Plasma levels of 40 μg/ml increase the risk of seizures and potentially lethal cardiac arrythmias.

Glucocorticoids. Glucocorticoids, which are potent airway antiinflammatory agents, are essential in the management of severe airway disease. In any acute asthmatic exacerbation that is worsening despite optimal bronchodilator therapy, steroids may be helpful in abating the attack. The exact dosages and duration of therapy are controversial. For the asthmatic patient with severe disease who requires hospitalization, most practitioners would agree to use intravenous corticosteroids in moderate to high doses (for example, 60 mg of solumedrol every 6 hours). For outpatient exacerbations, corticosteroids may be given orally for short courses of 1 to 2 weeks. Occasionally, particularly in the adult asthmatic patient, a maintenance regimen of corticosteroids is required. To avoid the systemic side effects of high-dose oral steroids, an attempt should first be made to use inhaled steroids such as beclomethasone. Inhaled steroids exert their action locally and undergo little systemic absorption, so inhibition of the pituitary-adrenal axis is minimal. An occasional asthmatic individual may also be maintained on alternate-day oral corticosteroid therapy.

Cromolyn sodium. The mechanism of action of cromolyn sodium is still poorly understood. It appears to stabilize the mast cell and thereby prevent release of various mediators that result in bronchospasm, especially those induced by allergens. However, cromolyn also inhibits bronchoconstriction induced by cold air, exercise, and sulphur dioxide. Cromolyn has a greater role as a prophylactic agent and may inhibit transient spells of bronchospasm. Because it has no role as a direct bronchodilator, cromolyn may be useful between attacks and can be used in combination with other agents to control symptoms and perhaps to decrease corticosteroid requirements. Currently it is available for inhalation as a powder, in solution, and as a metered-dose inhaler.

Anticholinergic agents. Atropine and ipratropium bromide (Atrovent) are available in the United States as anticholinergic bronchodilators. Since the major innervation of airway smooth muscle is by vagal parasympathetic nerves, these agents cause relaxation of bronchial smooth muscle and inhibit reflex bronchoconstriction. Generally, these agents have no greater effect in individuals with asthma than do standard β-adrenergic bronchodilators. However, in a particular patient there occasionally is a much greater response to an anticholinergic agent than to a β-adrenergic agent. The newer anticholinergic agent ipratropium bromide has little systemic absorption when delivered by the inhalation route and has a wide margin of safety.

STATUS ASTHMATICUS. Status asthmaticus refers to the acute and severe asthma exacerbation that does not respond to aggressive medical therapy. Severe asthma is a life-threatening condition. The pathologic description of individuals who die of this disease indicates that airway inflammation and mucous impaction of the airway are more important determinants than bronchoconstriction. These changes may take days to weeks to correct, and these severe cases need attention in an intensive care unit. Good hydration, oxygen therapy, and occasionally assisted mechanical ventilation is necessary.

BIBLIOGRAPHY

Bailey WC: Asthma, Clin Chest Med 5:4, 1984.
Epstein SW and Middleton EW: Advances in assessment and therapy of asthma, Chest (suppl)82:1, 1982.
Fanta CH, Rossing TH, and McFadden ER: Emergency room treatment of asthma, Am J Med 72:416, 1982.
McFadden ER: Pathogenesis of asthma, J Allergy Clin Immunol 73:413, 1984.

131·RESPIRATORY FAILURE

Sandeep Dhand and **Marda E. Donner**

Respiratory failure implies a severe derangement of the gas exchange function of the lungs. Normal pulmonary physiologic mechanisms (see also Capter 157) are described here initially; a discussion of repiratory failure follows.

OXYGEN TRANSPORT

O_2 transport to tissues depends on O_2 content and cardiac output. The former is a function of hemoglobin (Hb), O_2 saturation of Hb (SaO_2), and arterial O_2 tension (PaO_2), as shown in the equation:

$$O_2 \text{ content} = O_2 \text{ carried by Hb} + O_2 \text{ dissolved in plasma}$$
$$= (1.34 \times \text{g Hb} \times SaO_2) + (0.003 \times PaO_2)$$

For a normal Hb concentration (15 g/dl), PaO_2 (100 mm Hg), and SaO_2 (100%) the value of O_2 content carried by Hb is 20.1 volume percent. The Hb is the major determinant of the total amount of O_2 carried by blood under normal conditions.

The normal oxyhemoglobin dissociation curve is shown in Fig. 131-1. Usually a PO_2 of 55 to 60 mm Hg is associated with acceptable saturation of the hemoglobin and O_2 delivery to tissues. A shift of the curve to the right or left indicates a change in the Hb affinity for O_2 and is measured as the PaO_2 at which 50% of the Hb is saturated with O_2. A shift of the curve to the right occurs with acidemia, high $PaCO_2$, high temperature, and increased red blood cell 2,3-diphosphoglycerate (2,3-DPG); it results in reduced O_2 content but aids in the transfer of O_2 from blood to tissue.

The Fick equation ($\dot{V}O_2 = \dot{Q}[CaO_2 - C\bar{v}O_2]$), in which $\dot{V}O_2$ is O_2 consumption, $\dot{Q}$ equals cardiac output, CaO_2 is arterial O_2 content, and $C\bar{v}O_2$ equals mixed venous O_2 content, indicates that if $\dot{V}O_2$ is constant, cardiac output is inversely related to the arterial to venous O_2 content difference ($C[a-\bar{v}]O_2$). A reduction in $C\bar{v}O_2$ or increase in $C(a-\bar{v})O_2$ signifies decreased cardiac output. The $C\bar{v}O_2$ can be measured in pulmonary arterial blood via a Swan-Ganz catheter, or cardiac output can be estimated directly by a thermodilution technique.

Thus even with a normal PaO_2, O_2 delivery may be inadequate if cardiac output is reduced or hemoglobin is low or inefficient for O_2 transport.

CARBON DIOXIDE TRANSPORT

Carbon dioxide elimination differs in several important aspects from oxygen delivery. CO_2 is present mainly as dissolved gas in blood and tissues, and the body has a major buffering system for CO_2 that aids in maintaining CO_2 homeostasis.

The Henderson-Hasselbalch equation indicates the relationship of pH, HCO_3^- and PCO_2

$$pH = pK' + \log \frac{[HCO_3^-]}{0.03 \times PCO_2}$$

where pK is the dissociation constant in plasma at 98.6° F (37° C). In the normal situation this equation becomes

$$7.4 = 6.1 + \log \frac{(24)}{0.03 \times 40}$$

In chronic respiratory acidosis the elevation in the $PaCO_2$ is chronic, thus allowing time for the renal compensatory response, which results in an increase in HCO_3^-. Hence the fall

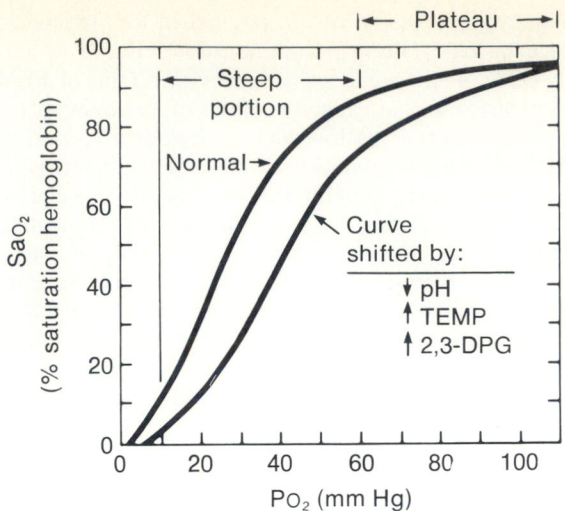

Fig. 131-1   Normal oxyhemoglobin dissociation curve, with pH 7.4 and temperature 98.6° F (37° C). Shifted curve depicts rightward shift caused by decrease in pH, increase in temperature, and increase in red blood cell 2,3-diphosphoglycerate.

in pH is not significant. In acute respiratory acidosis, however, an acute increase in $PaCO_2$ results in a significant drop in pH because of the lack of time for a compensatory rise in HCO_3^-.

HYPOXEMIA AND ITS MECHANISMS

Hypoxemia indicates a reduced level of oxygen in the blood (low PaO_2). The four basic mechanisms of hypoxemia are ventilation-perfusion ($\dot{V}A/\dot{Q}c$) mismatch, right-to-left shunting of blood (venous admixture), diffusion defects, and alveolar hypoventilation. Of these, $\dot{V}A/\dot{Q}c$ mismatch is the most common.

The alveolar-arterial (A-a) oxygen gradient is the difference between the PO_2 in alveolar air and that in arterial blood; it normally is less than 12 mm Hg in an individual breathing room air. This difference is related to some normal intrapulmonary right-to-left shunting of blood and some $\dot{V}A/\dot{Q}c$ mismatch. $P(A-a)O_2$ is increased with most causes of hypoxemia except pure alveolar hypoventilation.

Normal values of arterial blood gases measured during room air breathing are 80 to 90 mm Hg PaO_2 (decreasing with increasing age), 36 to 42 mm Hg $PaCO_2$, 7.38 to 7.42 pH, and 95% to 100% SaO_2. The mixed venous O_2 ($P\bar{v}O_2$) normally is about 40 mm Hg. A reduction in PaO_2 below 50 mm Hg with or without an elevation of the $PaCO_2$ above 50 mm Hg indicates respiratory failure.

CLASSIFICATION OF RESPIRATORY FAILURE

Respiratory failure may be acute or chronic and hypoxemic alone or hypoxemic and hypercarbic. Acute respiratory failure is characterized by a rapid change in the PaO_2 or $PaCO_2$, either in individuals with previously normal lungs or in those with underlying chronic respiratory failure. It is a medical emergency. Chronic respiratory failure is suggested by the presence of an elevated HCO_3^- caused by renal compensation for a chronically elevated PCO_2. The causes of respiratory failure follow:

I. Failure to oxygenate arterial blood (hypoxemic respiratory failure)
  A. Adult respiratory distress syndrome (ARDS)
  B. Cardiac pulmonary edema
  C. Neurogenic pulmonary edema
  D. Pneumonia
  E. Atelectasis

F. Other causes of $\dot{V}/\dot{Q}$ mismatch or shunt (pulmonary embolus, interstitial lung disease)
II. Failure of CO_2 excretion (hypoxic and hypercarbic respiratory failure)
   A. Chronic obstructive pulmonary disease (COPD)
   B. Severe bronchial asthma
III. Failure with normal lungs (predominantly hypercarbic respiratory failure)
   A. Brain: sedative overdose, central and obstructive sleep apneas, primary alveolar hypoventilation
   B. Spinal cord and chest wall (chest bellows): obesity hypoventilation syndrome, kyphoscoliosis, thoracoplasty, flail chest, cervical cord injury, other neuromuscular diseases
   C. Upper airways: severe laryngospasm, foreign body, tumor, stenosis

HYPOXEMIC RESPIRATORY FAILURE

ARDS is one of the most common causes of acute hypoxemic respiratory failure. Other synonyms for this disorder are shock lung and Da Nang lung. The causes of ARDS include gram-negative sepsis, major trauma, multiple transfusions, gastric aspiration, pancreatitis, drug reaction or overdose, hypotension, fat emboli, and viral pneumonia.

The patient usually has no underlying cardiac or pulmonary disease. Symptoms and signs develop after a latent period of up to 48 hours following an insult. The earliest features are tachypnea and apprehension. These gradually worsen and eventually are accompanied by grunting respirations and use of the accessory muscles of respiration. Rales and rhonchi may be audible during auscultation of the chest. Hypoxemia minimally responsive to oxygen therapy (indicating intrapulmonary right-to-left shunting of blood) is evident. The chest roentgenogram shows bilateral patchy, fluffy infiltrates that gradually progress to a "lung white-out." Air bronchograms are commonly prominent.

ARDS is characterized by an increase in extravascular lung water, which may result from a number of mechanisms, as predicted by Starling's law. The permeability of the alveolar-capillary membrane is increased in ARDS with a resultant fluid flux from vessels to extravascular lung tissues. This increase may be related to direct damage, as from aspiration of gastric contents with a low pH, or to release of proteolytic enzymes and complement activation, particularly in pancreatitis and sepsis. Low protein osmotic pressure and increased hydrostatic pressure may play a small role in some cases of ARDS. The pulmonary capillary wedge pressure (PCWP), as measured by a Swan-Ganz catheter, is a reflection of left ventricular filling pressures and therefore cardiac function and is normal in ARDS, thus differentiating it from cardiogenic pulmonary edema.

In ARDS, lung mechanics, lung volumes, and gas exchange are altered. The lung compliance is decreased as a result of increased lung water and decreased surfactant. The functional residual capacity (FRC) is consistently reduced as a result of atelectasis and reduced compliance. Hypoxemia is present, as indicated by widening of the $P(A\text{-}a)O_2$. An intrapulmonary right-to-left shunt is suggested by the lack of response of the hypoxemia to inhalation of 100% O_2. This shunt occurs when lung units become filled with edema fluid and are not ventilated. Perfusion continues so that the $\dot{V}A/\dot{Q}c$ ratio in these involved lung units approaches zero. Hypercarbia in patients with ARDS is a late and ominous sign. The diagnosis of ARDS is made by finding appropriate clinical circumstances, diffuse alveolar shadows on the chest roentgenogram with a normal heart size (Fig. 131-2), hypoxemia resistant to

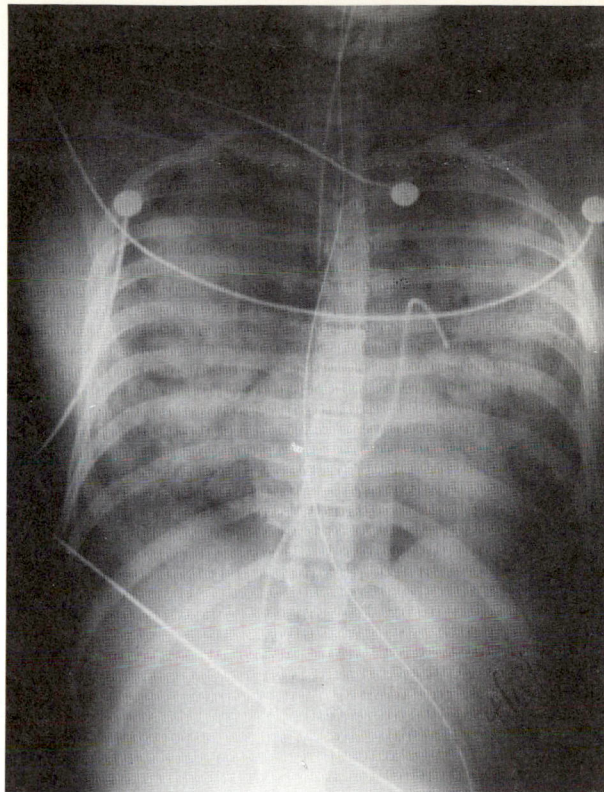

Fig. 131-2 Acute respiratory distress syndrome in 17-year-old girl with overwhelming bacteremia. There are bilateral alveolar infiltrates with normal heart size.

O_2 therapy, decreased lung compliance and FRC, and normal PCWP.

MANAGEMENT. The aim of treatment in ARDS is to maintain adequate O_2 transport and thus good tissue oxygenation. Swan-Ganz catheters help in the measurement of $P\bar{v}O_2$, cardiac output, and PCWP. The PCWP is a better indicator of left ventricular function and overall fluid status than is the central venous pressure.

Adequate oxygenation in patients with ARDS can be obtained by proper fluid management guided by the PCWP (keeping it between 10 and 12 mm Hg to reduce the lung water), diuretics as necessary, supplemental high concentrations of oxygen, and early mechanical ventilation. The value of positive end-expiratory pressure (PEEP) in ARDS has been well documented. Recruiting collapsed alveoli and hence increasing FRC reduces the areas of low $\dot{V}A/\dot{Q}c$ or shunt. This increases the PaO_2 obtained with a given inspired O_2 concentration (FIO_2) and helps prevent O_2 toxicity by allowing reduction of the FIO_2.

The hazards of PEEP include barotrauma and hemodynamic impairment. The former consists of subcutaneous emphysema, pneumothorax, and pneumomediastinum. The hemodynamic consequences of PEEP mainly involve a reduction in cardiac output, which is in part caused by decreased venous return and by decreased left ventricular compliance. As demonstrated earlier by the Fick equation, a decrease in cardiac output may offset any advantage gained by an increase in PaO_2, since systemic O_2 transport depends on both of these factors. The $P\bar{v}O_2$, cardiac output, and effective compliance can all be used as guides for the level of PEEP that leads to the most favorable combination of PaO_2 and cardiac output. Ideally, the PaO_2 is kept between 60 and 80 mm Hg, the $P\bar{v}O_2$ above 30 mm Hg,

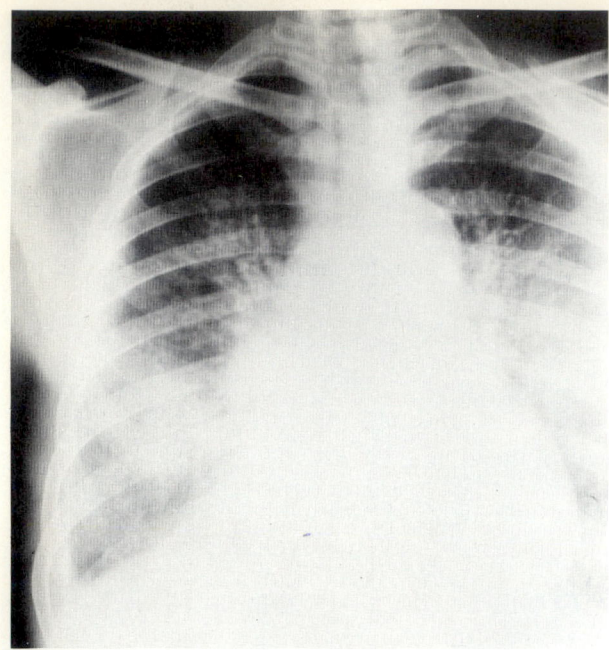

Fig. 131-3   Heart failure in 42-year-old man demonstrating enlarged heart with marked venous congestion and pulmonary edema. (Courtesy of George Popky, MD.)

the FIO_2 at 0.5 or lower, and the PCWP between 10 and 12 mm Hg.

The use of corticosteroids in ARDS is controversial and probably not indicated in most settings. Adequate nutritional support is essential. The prognosis is poor, with mortality ranging from 20% to 50% in fully developed ARDS. Death usually is related to systemic complications such as infection, renal failure, gastrointestinal bleeding, or cardiac failure rather than the pulmonary dysfunction.

PULMONARY EDEMA

Cardiac pulmonary edema is characterized by increased lung water, bilateral infiltrates, cardiomegaly, and increased PCWP, as measured by means of the Swan-Ganz catheter (Fig. 131-3). In accordance with Starling's law, the increase in pulmonary capillary hydrostatic pressure related to left ventricular failure or mitral stenosis leads to increased fluid flux into the lung interstitium and then into the alveoli.

Patients with pulmonary edema have tachypnea, cardiac enlargement, and an S_3 gallop. They usually have an underlying cardiac condition and respond quickly to diuretics, digitalis, and fluid restriction. Hypoxemia and respiratory alkalosis are common in the early phases, but with severe pulmonary edema, respiratory acidosis supervenes and assisted ventilation may be necessary. Usually, however, supplemental O_2 administered by nasal prongs or a mask is sufficient.

Neurogenic pulmonary edema (usually following head injury) also is related in part to elevated hydrostatic pressure. The mechanism is thought to be hypothalamic stimulation leading to pulmonary venoconstriction and shifting of blood from the systemic to the pulmonary circulation. Adrenergic blocking agents may be helpful in this form of edema.

CHRONIC OBSTRUCTIVE PULMONARY DISEASE AND ASTHMA

Most patients with COPD who have respiratory failure also have severe chronic bronchitis (giving the characteristic "blue bloater" appearance). Severe bronchial asthma (status asthmaticus) and cystic fibrosis are less common causes of respiratory failure. Patients with these disorders usually have a long history of disease. The chronic bronchitis group may have chronic well-compensated respiratory failure, and acute respiratory failure may be superimposed on chronically abnormal blood gas levels. One third of cases of acute respiratory failure in intensive care units are caused by acute exacerbations of COPD.

The mechanisms of airway obstruction in patients with COPD or asthma are intraluminal obstructions (mucus plugs), intramural narrowing (edema and smooth muscle contraction), and loss of extramural support (decreased elasticity in emphysema). Airway obstruction leads to nonhomogeneous distribution of ventilation and hence to areas with abnormal $\dot{V}A/\dot{Q}c$ ratios. Low $\dot{V}A/\dot{Q}c$ ratios lead to hypoxemia and high $\dot{V}A/\dot{Q}c$ ratios result in increased alveolar dead space and ultimately hypercapnia. Increased work of breathing caused by the abnormal airway resistance also may worsen gas exchange abnormalities. Recent work has demonstrated the significance of respiratory muscle fatigue in the pathogenesis of respiratory failure.

Acute respiratory failure complicating chronic respiratory failure is characterized by sudden worsening in the blood gases from their baseline abnormalities and may be precipitated by infection, bronchospasm, congestive heart failure, sedatives, or high concentrations of O_2.

The clinical manifestations of the acute phase are those of hypoxemia and hypercapnia. The former results in confusion, restlessness, tachycardia, supraventricular tachyrhythmias, and peripheral vasoconstriction, whereas hypercapnia leads to headache, drowsiness, coma, papilledema, hypertension, and tachycardia. Semicoma or coma generally is observed only when the $PaCO_2$ exceeds 75 mm Hg or the PaO_2 is less than 35 mm Hg. The patient with chronic respiratory failure has similar symptoms of hypoxemia, but the increased $PaCO_2$ is well compensated for and the symptoms of CO_2 narcosis are less prominent. Features of chronic hypoxemia are evident in the form of pulmonary hypertension, cor pulmonale, and polycythemia.

MANAGEMENT. Since hypoxemia provides a more immediate danger to life than hypercapnia, correction of the low PO_2 is of utmost importance. The goal is to increase the PaO_2 to 50 to 60 mm Hg, that is, above the steep portion of the oxyhemoglobin dissociation curve. Patients with COPD and acute respiratory failure are very O_2 sensitive. Since their ventilatory drive depends on hypoxemia, removing this hypoxic stimulus with excessive O_2 may cause them to hypoventilate and retain CO_2. Controlling O_2 at a fixed FIO_2 is very important in these patients. Venturi masks or nasal prongs administering O_2 at 1 to 2 L/min can be used. Nasal prongs allow for better patient comfort and expectoration, which should be encouraged. Arterial blood gas measurements must be repeated at frequent intervals to ensure a safe PaO_2 and to avoid significant CO_2 retention. However, the fear of CO_2 retention should not be a contraindication to O_2 therapy, since hypoxemia poses a more immediate threat to life.

Bronchodilators help by reducing the airway narrowing and thus improving the $\dot{V}A/\dot{Q}c$ abnormality and the work of breathing. The drugs available include theophyllines (intravenous and oral), adrenergic agonists (oral, inhaled, and subcutaneous), and anticholinergics. Theophyllines also reduce diaphragmatic muscle fatigue. Intravenous aminophylline can be used during acute respiratory failure related to

COPD or asthma. In patients not previously receiving theophylline preparations, a loading dose of 6 mg/kg body weight is given over 20 minutes followed by a maintenance infusion of 0.3 to 0.9 mg/kg/hr to achieve a therapeutic blood level (10 to 20 μg/ml). Patients over 50 years of age or those with associated congestive heart failure or liver disease require reduction in the maintenance dose. In the obese patient total body weight is used in calculating the loading dose, but lean body weight is used for the maintenance dose. If theophylline has been given in the preceding 12 hours, only half the usual loading dose is given until after the theophylline level is available. Inhaled brochodilators can be delivered by compressor-powered nebulizer or by freon-propelled metered-dose inhaler.

Antibiotics such as tetracycline or ampicillin may be indicated, especially if the sputum is purulent and the Gram stain reveals pus cells. The most common organisms found are *Streptoccoccus pneumoniae* and *Haemophilus influenzae*. Pneumonia, if present, must be aggressively treated, because it may be the precipitating cause of the respiratory failure. Viral infections also are important in exacerbations.

Corticosteroids have been used extensively in this setting, and they help by reducing inflammation and by sensitizing adrenergic receptor sites to adrenergic agonists. Significant wheezing, unresponsiveness to bronchodilators, and sputum or blood eosinophilia are considered by some to be indications for using steroids.

Approximately 15% to 25% of patients with COPD who are experiencing acute respiratory failure require therapy with an artificial airway and mechanical ventilation. Indications for this therapy include apnea, marked respiratory acidosis with a pH of less than 7.2, and an associated metabolic acidosis related to hypotension or hypoxemia. It is important to lower the $PaCO_2$ slowly, because acute CO_2 reduction in the presence of bicarbonate retention can lead to severe alkalemia and possibly seizures or arrhythmias.

In patients with acute respiratory failure, cor pulmonale, and right ventricular failure, the use of digitalis is controversial and may be associated with an increased incidence of arrhythmias. Respiratory stimulants have no proven benefit.

Roughly 70% of patients with COPD survive a given episode of acute respiratory failure. However, the long-term prognosis is poor, with 1-year survival rates of 50% and 2-year survival rates of 30% reported following episodes of acute respiratory failure in COPD patients.

RESPIRATORY FAILURE WITH NORMAL LUNGS

Chemoreceptors and neuroreceptors send signals to the respiratory centers in the brainstem. Chemoreceptors in the carotid and aortic bodies are sensitive to changes in the O_2 level in the blood, and chemoreceptors in the brainstem respond to changes in the hydrogen ion level. A reduction in blood O_2 tension or an elevation of hydrogen ion content is detected by these chemoreceptors and results in increased levels of ventilation.

Neuroreceptors in the lung include stretch, irritant, and juxtapulmonary capillary receptors. Neuroreceptors detect changes in the mechanical status of the lung and send impulses to the medullary brain centers.

Abnormal respiratory control

Alveolar hypoventilation is most commonly caused by changes in the lung parenchyma or airways, but it also can occur in patients with normal lungs. Abnormal respiratory mechanics can develop with severe obesity, one of the sleep apnea syndromes, or with primary alveolar hypoventilation. A number of disease entities fall into this category of respiratory failure with normal lungs (see outline p. 622).

Hypoventilation related to sedative overdose is manifested as coma, with the patient having slow, shallow respirations. At times ventilation may have to be immediately supported mechanically without waiting for results on arterial blood gases.

The sleep apnea syndromes (central and obstructive) were described only recently. Central sleep apnea is the occurrence of frequent episodes of cessation of respiration caused by failure of the normal neurologic impulses to reach the respiratory muscles. These episodes must occur during non–rapid eye movement sleep, must last longer than 10 seconds, and must recur more than 30 times in a night to be considered significant. Obstructive sleep apnea differs from the central type only in that neurologic impulses and respiratory muscle activity persist throughout the apneic episode, with transient upper airway obstruction temporarily interrupting airflow. Chronic disease is characterized by cyanosis, somnolence, polycythemia, pulmonary hypertension, and cor pulmonale. Most of the clincial abnormalities can be explained on the basis of chronic hypoxemia and hypercapnia. Snoring is an obvious finding in obstructive sleep apnea, particularly when it is associated with obesity. Sedation or a lower respiratory tract infection exacerbates the gas exchange abnormality and can lead to acute respiratory failure. Treatment involves measures to decrease the obstruction such as weight loss, nasal continuous positive airway pressure (CPAP) (which appears to use CPAP as a splint to keep the oropharynx patent), or tracheostomy. In some cases a respiratory stimulant such as progesterone or protryptyline is useful. Oxygen administration may lessen the degree of hypoxia but does not correct the obstruction.

Alveolar hypoventilation resulting from defective brainstem regulation (primary alveolar hypoventilation) is uncommon but not rare. Some cases are associated with neurologic disorders such as encephalitis, whereas others are not associated with central nervous system disease other than the loss of respiratory control. In this disorder the respiratory centers do not respond to CO_2 or acid stimuli and depend on hypoxic drive to maintain respiration. The suppression of hypoxic drive by the use of excessive O_2 or the administration of sedative or tranquilizing drugs results in CO_2 narcosis. Such patients can ventilate voluntarily to normal levels.

Treatment is directed at maintaining safe but not excessive levels of oxygenation. Assisted ventilation with mechanical devices, rocking beds, and electrophrenic pacemakers may be required, particularly at night.

Chest bellows disease

Chest bellows disease can be divided into mechanical and neuromuscular categories. The former category includes obesity hypoventilation syndrome, kyphoscoliosis, and thoracoplasty; the latter category encompasses amyotrophic lateral sclerosis, poliomyelitis, myasthenia gravis, multiple sclerosis, spinal cord injury, and Guillain-Barré syndrome. Respiratory failure is fairly common and progresses slowly with these diseases.

In chest bellows disease lung function is impaired because of reduced ability to cough, leading to retained secretions, infections, and atelectasis. These can result in a severe degree of V_A/Q_C mismatch. Vital capacity (VC) is progressively reduced, and its measurement is a better prognostic indicator than are arterial blood gases. A VC greater than 1 L, exceeding three times the tidal volume, or above 10 to 15 ml/kg body weight usually is adequate. Any reduction below these levels leads to significant hypoventilation, $\dot{V}_A/\dot{Q}c$ abnormalities, and respiratory failure. The chest wall compliance in this group of diseases is low, and the work of breathing is high. This coupled with the reduction in FRC below the level of closing capacity causes further impairment of gas exchange. With increasingly severe disease patients cannot maintain the high level of respiratory work required, and alveolar hypoventilation ensues. Lower respiratory infections, sedatives, or underlying obstructive lung disease may precipitate acute respiratory failure.

Although many obese patients maintain normal levels of oxygen tension and alveolar ventilation, some have hypoxemia, whereas others have both hypoxemia and hypoventilation. Obesity hypoventilation syndrome is characterized by alveolar hypoventilation with Pa_{CO_2} elevation, hypersomnia, cyanosis, and polycythemia; cor pulmonale is common (such patients have been called "pickwickian" because of their resemblance to a character in Charles Dickens' *Pickwick Papers*). Inspiratory capacity, tidal volume, and total lung capacity are preserved, but the FRC and expiratory reserve volume are reduced. Hypoxemia can be an early development because of inadequate ventilation to perfused units at the bases of the lungs.

The cause of this syndrome is not yet completely understood, but some factors appear related if not causative. The work of breathing is increased, and the chest wall compliance is reduced in obese patients with this syndrome, but both remain at normal levels in obese patients who do not have the syndrome. In addition, decreased responsiveness of the respiratory center to CO_2 has been demonstrated. Intermittent obstruction of the upper airways, such as at the glottis, is another feature of this disorder. Treatment of this syndrome includes drastic weight reduction, which is sometimes successful in reversing the syndrome. Relief of nocturnal airway obstruction and correction of hypoxemia also are important in management. Correction of acid-base status, appropriate use of diuretics, and pharmacologic agents such as theophylline and medroxyprogesterone to stimulate ventilation are useful in some patients.

In kyphoscoliosis the angle of scoliosis determines the degree of functional impairment. The risk of respiratory failure increases with an angle of scoliosis exceeding 70 degrees, and at more than 120 degrees alveolar hypoventilation commonly results. In patients with scoliosis or thoracoplasty the use of periodic hyperinflation with an intermittent positive-pressure breathing (IPPB) device or an incentive spirometer has been shown to improve lung compliance and hypoxemia for several hours. Chronic hypoxemia also should be treated with controlled O_2 therapy. The use of orthopedic procedures for correcting kyphoscoliosis and thereby attempting to prevent progression of ventilatory impairment shows little long-term benefit.

Hypercapnia is rare in flail chest, and hypoxemia occurring in this condition is related to lung contusion, which causes decreased FRC and $\dot{V}_A/\dot{Q}c$ mismatching.

Patients with injury to the cervical spinal cord cephalad to the third cervical vertebrae have no diaphragmatic function; with injury at the third to fifth cervical vertebrae diaphragmatic function is partially lost. Either situation can result in the neuromuscular type of respiratory failure. Guillain-Barré syndrome at times may develop rapidly and be accompanied by respiratory failure. Patients with myasthenia gravis may have intermittent episodes of respiratory failure.

Respiratory infections must be treated vigorously. Tracheostomy should be considered in obstructive sleep apnea or in obesity hypoventilation syndrome and diaphragmatic pacing in cervical cord paralysis.

If these measures do not suffice and chronic respiratory failure persists, modalities such as a negative-pressure body respirator, a rocking bed, or frog breathing (a glossopharyngeal maneuver that forces air into lungs) can be used.

Assisted mechanical ventilation may be necessary during respiratory infections in a patient with kyphoscoliosis, during the acute phase of cervical cord injury, in obesity hypoventilation syndrome with severe congestive heart failure, or during periods of marked neuromuscular weakness in Guillain-Barré syndrome or myasthenia gravis.

Upper airway obstruction

Upper airway obstruction frequently is overlooked in the initial evaluation of dyspnea and wheezing.

Obstruction of the trachea may occur precipitously, as in the "cafe coronary" with foreign body obstruction. The individual is in acute respiratory distress but unable to speak, since the obstruction prevents airflow. Wheezing is not heard. Therapy consists of attempts to relieve the obstruction by abdominal thrusts (Heimlich maneuver), back pounding, or, as a last resort, manual removal with the fingers. Failure to relieve the obstruction results in death. Less than complete obstruction can be identified by noisy respiration, and this situation is best handled by transferring the victim to an emergency care facility. More aggressive intervention may only convert partial obstruction into complete obstruction.

Tracheal obstruction also can result from tracheal or vocal cord tumor and from stenosis caused by previous tracheal intubation or injury, in which case signs and symptoms develop insidiously. Although inspiratory stridor usually is obvious when listened for over the trachea, the condition often is initially diagnosed as asthma. Occasionally these patients are even admitted to an intensive care unit for treatment of status asthmaticus before the correct diagnosis is made. The findings, besides inspiratory stridor, may be limited to an abnormal laryngoscopic or bronchoscopic examination. Flow-volume loops may be extremely useful in diagnosing occult forms of upper airway obstruction. Therapy includes maintenance of the upper airway by careful intubations or tracheostomy. The definitive therapy usually is surgical. More recently lasers have been used in this setting.

Respiratory failure related to upper airway obstruction responds rapidly to removal of the obstruction or to tracheostomy. Prolonged ventilatory support and oxygen therapy are rarely indicated.

BIBLIOGRAPHY

Briston G: Respiratory emergencies: acute asthma, Sem. Resp. Med. 1:16, 1980.

Libby DM and others: Acute respiratory failure in kyphoscoliosis, Am J Med 73:532, 1982.

Maunder RJ, Hudson LD, et al: Prediction of ARDS by Clinical Risk Factors. Am. Rev. Resp. Dis. 131:A137, 1987.

Murray JF: Mechanisms of acute respiratory failure, Am Rev Respir Dis 165:1071, 1977.

Rosen RL: Acute respiratory failure and chronic obstructive lung disease, Med Clin North Am 70:895, 1986.

Roussos C: Function and fatigue of respiratory muscles, Chest (suppl) 88:2/ 124S, 1985.

Staub NL: Pulmonary edema, Physiol Rev 54:678, 1974.

Strohl KP and others: Physiologic basis of therapy of sleep apnea. State of the art, Am Rev Respir Dis 134:791, 1986.

132·DIFFUSE LUNG DISEASES

Morton Rubenstein

PULMONARY FIBROSIS
Idiopathic pulmonary fibrosis

Idiopathic pulmonary fibrosis (IPF) typifies many of the clinical, roentgenographic, and physiologic features of the interstitial lung diseases. It is characterized by dyspnea, interstitial infiltrates on the chest roentgenogram, inflammation and fibrosis of the alveolar walls, and a relatively poor response to therapy. After known causes are excluded, IPF accounts for about 40% to 60% of interstitial disease. It commonly occurs in the fourth and fifth decades of life, but there is no clear-cut sexual, racial, or geographic predilection.

ETIOLOGY AND PATHOLOGY. Although no single pathogenetic mechanism has been described that accounts for all features of IPF, some evidence suggests participation of the immune system, perhaps in response to alveolar injury. Autoantibodies such as rheumatoid factor and antinuclear antibody, circulating immune complexes, alveolar deposition of IgG and complement, increased amounts of immunoglobulins and inflammatory cells in lavage fluid, and the occasional improvement following treatment with steroids or immunosuppressive agents support the concept of an immune mechanism.

The histologic features of IPF vary. In some cases hyperplasia of type II alveolar cells and the presence of large numbers of mononuclear cells (predominantly macrophages) lying within the alveoli are prominent findings; this condition has been termed "desquamative interstitial pneumonitis" (DIP). Despite the presence of alveolar wall inflammation in DIP, collagen deposition is minimal. In the forms of IPF termed "usual interstitial pneumonitis" (UIP), alveolar walls are thickened by chronic inflammatory cells and fibrous tissue. As fibrous tissue replaces alveolar walls, the inflammatory changes subside. Mural fibrosis is marked by a distortion of alveolar architecture, and the alveoli coalesce into cysts or blebs to produce the roentgenographic picture called *honeycombing* that commonly is most pronounced at the lung bases. With advanced disease changes of pulmonary hypertension occur, characterized by medial hypertrophy and luminal narrowing in pulmonary arterioles. Although DIP, UIP, and mural fibrosis once were believed to be distinct entities, they have been found to coexist in different areas of the same lung and probably represent stages of IPF.

The pathogenesis of IPF is incompletely understood. Lung B cells, although present in normal proportion to other inflammatory cells, are increased in absolute number. IgG levels are higher as well. Presumably the immune complexes found in the lower respiratory tracts of IPF patients are derived from the immunoglobulins produced by B cells. Since the number of B cells and the levels of IgG in blood are normal or minimally increased, the immune reaction appears to be localized to the lung. The antigen that triggers this immune reaction is not known; although symptoms of viral infection have been noted to precede some cases of IPF, no clear association between viral disease and IPF has been established.

It appears that alveolitis develops early in the disease process, initially with intense inflammation and only mild derangement of alveolar walls but later with less inflammation and more pronounced mural fibrosis. Bronchoalveolar lavage studies demonstrate increases in total numbers of inflammatory cells; macrophages and neutrophils are most prominent in perpetuating the alveolitis, although lesser numbers of other cells (eosinophils, lymphocytes) are involved. Immune complexes may stimulate macrophages to produce chemotactic factors for neutrophils; both neutrophils and macrophages may have cytotoxic effects on normal alveolar cells. Additionally, macrophages release factors (fibronectin, alveolar macrophage–derived growth factor) that promote fibroblast replication and activity, in turn leading to increased collagen synthesis and development of interstitial fibrosis.

CLINICAL MANIFESTATIONS. The cardinal symptom of IPF is dyspnea, which often develops insidiously. A dry cough usually is present. On auscultation, bilateral basilar crackling rales may be heard with inspiration. As the disease advances, tachypnea, tachycardia, and cyanosis may develop. When pulmonary hypertension develops, jugular venous distention, a right ventricular "tap," pulmonic flow murmur, S_3 and S_4 heart sounds, hepatomegaly, and peripheral edema may be found. Digital clubbing is common in advanced cases. IPF and the collagen-vascular diseases may have certain features in common, including digital vasculitis, Raynaud's phenomenon, arthralgias, and discoid lupus erythematosus.

DIAGNOSIS. The chest roentgenogram typically shows bilateral reticular or reticulonodular densities, predominantly in the lower lung zones, and loss of volume (Fig. 132-1). In advanced cases, "honeycomb" changes and evidence of pulmonary hypertension develop. Small cystic spaces occasionally may rupture, resulting in pneumothorax.

Routine laboratory studies usually contribute little additional diagnostic information. An elevated sedimentation rate often is found. The presence of rheumatoid factor, antinuclear antibody, Coombs'-positive hemolytic anemia, and idiopathic thrombocytopenic purpura has been reported. Pulmonary function tests typically reveal arterial hypoxemia and a decrease in lung volumes and diffusing capacity. Early in the course of the disease the chest roentgenogram, resting arterial blood gas values, and pulmonary function tests may be normal, but an exercise study usually reveals evidence of impaired oxygenation.

Although the diagnosis of IPF requires the exclusion of known causes of interstitial pneumonitis, the clinical picture usually suggests the diagnosis. Because a number of other disorders closely resemble IPF, because the course, prognosis, and therapy of some of these disorders may differ from those of IPF, and because the course of IPF often is defined by the histologic features, a lung biopsy usually is required. In some centers transbronchial biopsy is performed initially. Because a relatively small amount of tissue is obtained, however, this procedure tends to yield diagnostic information in cases of sarcoidosis or malignancy but often gives insufficient or even misleading information in IPF and other diffuse lung diseases. Thus open biopsy may still be required if transbronchial biopsy does not provide an adequate diagnostic picture.

MANAGEMENT AND PROGNOSIS. Corticosteroids are the mainstay of therapy, which usually is begun following diagnosis, since IPF is a progressive disorder that rarely exhibits spontaneous remission. These drugs presumably decrease inflammation and subsequent fibrosis, so that those patients with biopsy evidence of active alveolitis and relatively little fibrosis are more likely to respond favorably to therapy. The paucity of controlled trials of corticosteroid therapy makes it difficult to judge the effect of corticosteroids on the course and outcome of IPF. Retrospective studies suggest that about 40% to 50% of patients show improvement of dyspnea, about 15% to 20% show objective response on pulmonary function testing or chest roentgenography, and those responding to initial therapy survive longer.

The optimal method for evaluating patient progress has not

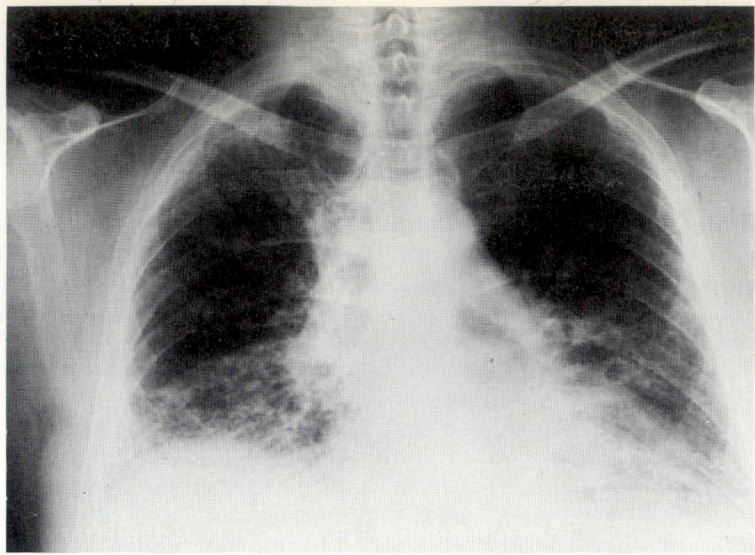

Fig. 132-1 Idiopathic pulmonary fibrosis (IPF) in 39-year-old man. There is bilateral interstitial infiltration, most pronounced at bases and obliterating diaphragms and cardiac borders.

been established. Symptoms, physical findings, and chest roentgenograms are not adequate. Lung volumes, diffusing capacity, and Po_2 (at rest and especially with exercise) are more sensitive parameters. Corticosteroid therapy usually is initiated with prednisone at a dosage of 1 mg/kg/day. After reevaluation following an adequate duration of therapy (typically 6 to 12 weeks), prednisone is tapered and discontinued in nonresponders and very slowly decreased in those who demonstrate objective evidence of improvement (by pulmonary function testing and chest roentgenography) to the lowest dose required to maintain remission as judged by follow-up testing. Those who fail to respond to corticosteroids or who subsequently develop progressive disease may be administered immunosuppressive drugs such as azathioprine or cyclophosphamide.

Measurement of circulating immune complexes, bronchoalveolar lavage (by fiberoptic bronchoscopy), and gallium citrate lung scanning have been used in recent years to study patients with IPF. Although these techniques have yielded useful research data, they have not been completely successful in accurately identifying those patients with the more cellular or inflammatory changes on lung biopsy, and their results do not reliably predict steroid responsiveness in IPF. They also tend to be costly. For these reasons routine use in patient care does not appear warranted, although it may help in clinical decision making in selected cases.

Patients with IPF are susceptible to chest infection and may need antibiotics and chest physical therapy. Supplemental oxygen may improve cor pulmonale and right-sided heart failure, decrease elevated red blood cell mass, and improve exercise tolerance. Nutritional supplementation also may be useful.

The course and prognosis of IPF vary. A fulminant course leading to death within 1 year, called the Hamman-Rich syndrome, is unusual; mean survival in IPF is about 3 to 6 years. About 20% of patients show little progression of lung disease and have prolonged survival. The duration of survival seems to correlate with the severity of functional impairment at the time of recognition; the appearance of the chest roentgenogram correlates poorly with survival. The most common cause of death is respiratory failure, often accompanied by pulmonary infection.

Lymphocytic interstitial pneumonitis

Lymphocytic interstitial pneumonitis (LIP) is characterized by a histologic pattern of pulmonary interstitial infiltration with a uniform population of lymphocytes. The mode of onset, physical findings, appearance of the chest roentgenogram, and pulmonary function data are indistinguishable from those of IPF, except that digital clubbing is relatively uncommon, chest infection is possibly more common, and the pattern of infiltration on the chest film may be more coarsely nodular. Patients also may have dysproteinemias, defects in delayed hypersensitivity, and other immune phenomena. Lymphocytic infiltrates may involve the salivary glands, thyroid, kidney, and liver. Patients may have Sjögren's syndrome, Hashimoto's thyroiditis, renal tubular acidosis, or chronic active hepatitis.

The clinical course of LIP varies, although only a limited number of cases have been observed. Respiratory failure does not appear to be a common cause of death. The disorder has been treated with corticosteroids and immunosuppressive agents, but response has been infrequent.

Systemic lupus erythematosus

(See Chapter 16.)

The pulmonary manifestations of systemic lupus erythematosus (SLE) may take the form of pleural disease, atelectasis, acute pneumonitis, and chronic interstitial disease. Pleural pain is a frequent symptom, and pleural effusion often is present. Transient atelectasis, commonly consisting of linear or patchy involvement of the lung bases, often is found. Acute lupus pneumonitis is relatively uncommon; it is characterized by fever, dyspnea, cough, and patchy infiltrates. Since patients with SLE are susceptible to infectious pneumonitis because of their underlying disease and treatment with corticosteroids or immunosuppressive agents, a diagnosis of acute lupus pneumonitis should be considered only after infection has been carefully excluded.

The chronic interstitial abnormalities seen in SLE include an interstitial pneumonitis and fibrosis, a lymphocytic interstitial reaction, hemosiderosis, and a small-vessel vasculitis. Clinically apparent interstitial disease, most commonly fibrosis, occurs in about 10% of SLE cases.

Scleroderma (progressive systemic sclerosis)

(See Chapter 17.)

Scleroderma or progressive systemic sclerosis (PSS) is the collagen-vascular disease most frequently associated with interstitial disease. Dyspnea develops in approximately 40% of patients with PSS, and a similar percentage have evidence of increased interstitial density or chest roentgenograms. At autopsy as many as 90% of patients have evidence of lung involvement that commonly resembles IPF, but occasionally a hypersensitivity angiitis picture is found. Pleural disease also is seen on occasion, usually in the form of pleural thickening.

The interstitial fibrosis seen in PSS seems to progress more rapidly than that associated with the other collagen-vascular diseases, yet less rapidly than with IPF. The 5-year survival in patients with PSS-related intersitital fibrosis is about 50%, and death from PSS is more commonly related to renal or cardiac failure.

The high incidence of disorders of esophageal motility and swallowing associated with PSS may lead to aspiration and recurrent pulmonary inflammation, infection, and scarring. PSS also has been reported to be associated with an increased incidence of bronchoalveolar cell carcinoma.

Rheumatoid arthritis

(See Chapter 10.)

Interstitial fibrosis of the IPF type is the most common pulmonary manifestation of rheumatoid arthritis (RA). It usually is milder and less progressive than IPF, and death resulting from respiratory failure is uncommon. Interstitial fibrosis is more common in males. There is no clear-cut correlation of fibrosis with the duration and extent of articular disease nor with the titer of rheumatoid factor. Pulmonary function abnormalities are present in about 40% of patients with RA, but only half of these have detectable abnormalities on chest roentgenograms.

The diagnosis is based on the presence of clinical features of RA in a patient with concomitant interstitial fibrosis. The diagnosis is complicated by the facts that about 20% of IPF patients may have either arthralgias or a positive test for rheumatoid factor and that in RA interstitial disease can occasionally precede the development of joint symptoms.

Other pulmonary manifestations of RA include pleural disease, pulmonary nodules, and pulmonary vasculitis. Pleural effusion is more common in males, is associated with high titers of rheumatoid factor and with extraarticular disease, tends to follow the development of joint symptoms, and is seldom massive. The fluid is an exudate that commonly has a markedly reduced glucose content (often less than 20 mg/dl). Lung nodules may be single or multiple, solid or cavitary, and variable in size. They usually occur in patients who also have subcutaneous nodules that are identical histologically to the pulmonary lesions. The treatment of nodules is unnecessary unless hemoptysis or rupture into the pleural space occurs. In Caplan's syndrome pulmonary nodules form in patients with coexisting RA and pneumoconiosis.

Polymyositis-dermatomyositis

(See Chapter 19.)

Pulmonary fibrosis resembling IPF is an uncommon complication of polymyositis, occurring in about 5% to 10% of patients. Bronchogenic carcinoma may be associated with adult polymyositis.

Mixed connective tissue disease (overlap syndrome)

(See Chapter 17.)

In mixed connective tissue disease, also called the overlap syndrome, the features of two or more of the collagen-vascular diseases coexist. In a substantial number of patients with overlap syndrome, pulmonary abnormalities develop that are similar in histopathology to IPF.

Sjögren's syndrome

(See Chapter 10.)

Interstitial pulmonary disease occurs in about 3% of patients with this chronic inflammatory disorder. An IPF-like alveolitis may occur, or LIP-like infiltrates may develop. The latter may follow a benign course and cause minimal dysfunction, but occasionally they may progress rapidly to end-stage fibrosis. Malignant lymphoma is a reported complication of the LIP of Sjögren's syndrome.

These patients also develop nonparenchymal abnormalities. Pleuritis with or without effusion may occur. Desiccation of the tracheobronchial tree (related to lymphocytic infiltration and destruction of mucous glands) may lead to inspissated secretions and respiratory infection.

Ankylosing spondylitis

(See Chapter 12.)

Patients with ankylosing spondylitis occasionally have upper lobe fibrosis. This usually is bilateral and on a chest roentgenogram may resemble tuberculosis. In its early stages the fibrosis may appear as linear fibrotic stranding, later becoming coarser to form large, dense infiltrates. Cavitation is common and may be the site of mycetoma formation. As fibrosis advances, lung distortion and bronchiectasis can lead to the development of cough, sputum production, and recurrent chest infection.

INTERSTITIAL DISEASES OF UNKNOWN CAUSE
Sarcoidosis

(See Chapter 24.)

Sarcoidosis is a systemic granulomatous disease of unknown cause. It most often affects young adults and is commonly manifested by bilateral hilar adenopathy, lung infiltrates, ocular disease, or cutaneous lesions. Other commonly occurring features include abnormalities of the immune system and hypercalciuria, occasionally associated with hypercalcemia. The diagnosis is based on clinical and roentgenographic evidence coupled with histologic evidence of noncaseating epithelioid-cell granulomas.

EPIDEMIOLOGY. The worldwide distribution and prevalence of sarcoidosis have proved difficult to determine because of variability in both diagnostic criteria and availability of diagnostic modalities. In the United States the disease occurs over a wide age range, but the highest incidence is in young adults. There is a slight female preponderance. American blacks are affected about 10 times more frequently than whites. About 50% have respiratory symptoms, about 25% have systemic symptoms such as fever, anorexia, and weight loss, less than 10% manifest symptoms of localized extrathoracic disease, and 20% are asymptomatic and are discovered by chest roentgenography.

CLINICAL MANIFESTATIONS. Pulmonary involvement is the leading cause of disability and death in sarcoidosis, and about one third of the patients with this disorder have dyspnea at some time. Even in patients with only hilar adenopathy and roentgenographically clear lung parenchyma, abnormalities may be present on pulmonary function testing, and granulomas may be demonstrated by lung biopsy. Cough develops in about one third of patients and may be due to endobronchial granulomas. If parenchymal fibrosis and secondary bronchiectasis occur, purulent secretions and chronic pulmonary infection can develop. Chest pain occurs in less than 20% of cases and hemoptysis in less than 5%.

The physical examination may reveal no abnormality referable to the lungs. With advanced disease there may be tachypnea, harsh breath sounds, or bibasilar inspiratory crackles. Wheezes suggest the presence of endobronchial disease. Diminished breath sounds may signify the development of bullae or compensatory emphysema as pulmonary fibrosis occurs. Pleural effusion develops in only a small percentage of cases, generally as a small, unilateral, asymptomatic exudate. The fluid contains predominantly lymphocytes, and the pleural biopsy may reveal noncaseating granulomas. End-stage pulmonary fibrosis, which occurs in less than 5% of cases, resembles end-stage fibrotic lung disease of other causes.

A host of extrathoracic manifestations are known to occur. Palpable adenopathy usually is nontender. Splenomegaly, which occurs in 10% to 20% of cases, rarely leads to clinical complications. Erythema nodosum, a nonspecific cutaneous vasculitis of the lower extremities, occurs in less than 5% of patients. Erythema nodosum and bilateral hilar adenopathy (*Löfgren's syndrome*) portend a favorable outcome.

Skin lesions, which are seen in 30% of cases, often consist of small papules that on biopsy reveal typical granulomas. *Lupus pernio* is a severe destructive cutaneous infiltration occurring over the nose, cheeks, lips, and ears.

Ocular involvement (in 20% of cases) is most commonly manifested as acute anterior uveitis. Chronic uveitis, glaucoma, corneal and lenticular opacities, retinitis, papillitis, and blindness may occur. The association of uveitis with granulomatous involvement of the salivary glands has been designated *Heerfordt's syndrome*. Central nervous system involvement (in 5% of cases) may take the form of cranial nerve palsies, basilar meningitis, or intracerebral granulomatous disease.

Granulomatous disease of the myocardium is found at autopsy in 20% of patients. Clinical disease occurs less often and is most commonly manifested by conduction disturbances, ventricular arrhythmias, or left ventricular failure. In end-stage lung disease there may be cor pulmonale. Although percutaneous biopsy shows granulomatous disease of the liver in 50% to 80% of the patients, hepatomegaly occurs in only 10% to 20% and clinically significant liver disease is rare. Less than 5% of patients have detectable renal involvement, with nephrocalcinosis and nephrolithiasis being most frequent.

Almost all patients with sarcoidosis have decreased plasma levels of parathyroid hormone, 10% to 30% have hypercalciuria, and 2% to 3% have hypercalcemia. Increased absorption of calcium from the gastrointestinal tract, suggesting a heightened sensitivity to vitamin D, seems to underlie the abnormalities of calcium metabolism. Musculoskeletal complaints may include transient polyarthralgias and polyarthritis, usually involving the knees and ankles. Muscle biopsy (especially of the gastrocnemius muscle) may demonstrate granuloma formation, but overt myopathy is rare.

LABORATORY FINDINGS AND DIAGNOSIS. A variety of largely nonspecific laboratory findings have been associated with sarcoidosis. Hematologic studies may demonstrate mild anemia or lymphocytopenia. Thrombocytopenia, hemolytic anemia, eosinophilia, and pancytopenia resulting from hypersplenism are rare. Urinalysis may demonstrate an impaired

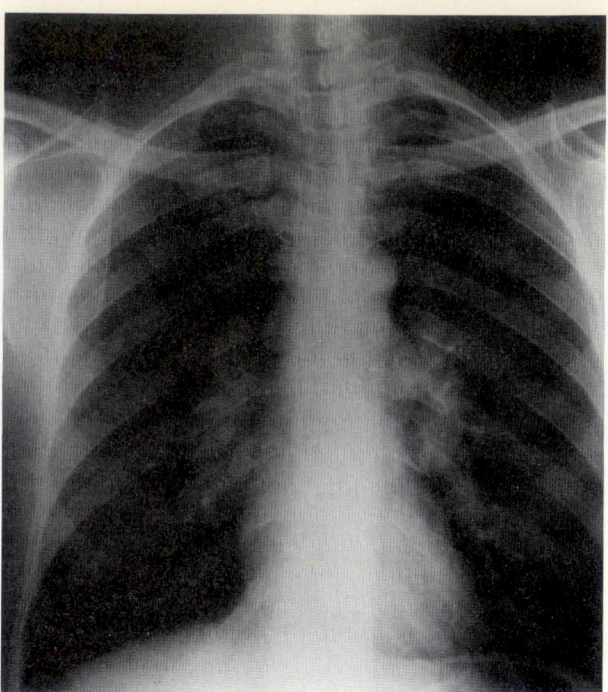

Fig. 132-2 Bilateral hilar adenopathy in patient with sarcoidosis. No parenchymal involvement can be seen (stage I). (Courtesy of George Popky, MD.)

concentrating ability owing to diabetes insipidus (from pituitary involvement) or to hypercalcemic nephropathy. Elevated levels of hepatic enzymes may also be found.

There has been interest in angiotensin-converting enzyme (ACE) as a serologic marker of this disease. This enzyme catalyzes the conversion of angiotensin I to the vasoconstrictor angiotensin II and the conversion of the vasodilator bradykinin to inactive metabolites. Most ACE is found on the luminal surface of vascular endothelium and on the brush border of cells lining the proximal convoluted tubules of the kidney. However, the source of elevated ACE in sarcoid is probably the epithelioid cells of sarcoid granulomas. Although ACE elevations once were felt to be a sensitive and specific serum marker for sarcoidosis, subsequent studies have disclosed that a large number of conditions other than sarcoidosis may be associated with increased serum ACE, including histoplasmosis, hyperthyroidism, chronic renal failure, alcoholic liver disease, primary biliary cirrhosis, silicosis, diabetes mellitus, and others. Although elevated ACE levels tend to fall in patients who remit either spontaneously or with corticosteroid therapy, ACE levels may vary in a nonspecific way and may fail to correlate with disease activity, so that routine ACE measurements cannot be used reliably to follow a patient's progress.

Often the chest roentgenogram provides the initial clue to the correct diagnosis. The roentgenographic findings have been divided into four categories:

1. *Stage O.* Patients in this category (10%) have a normal chest roentgenogram.
2. *Stage I.* In these patients (50%) bilateral hilar adenopathy is present, but the parenchyma is clear. The enlarged lymph nodes are smooth and lobulated. A clear space is usually present between the nodes and the remainder of the hilus (Fig. 132-2). Right paratracheal adenopathy is present in about half.
3. *Stage II.* These patients (25% to 30%) have parenchymal infiltrates in addition to bilateral hilar adenopathy. The pattern

usually is nonspecific and can be quite variable with diffuse small nodules, linear densities, reticulonodular changes, larger confluent shadows, and/or atelectasis.

4. *Stage III*. These patients (10% to 15%) have infiltrates without evidence of hilar adenopathy. Linear fibrotic strands, cystic changes, and bullous disease may occur.

Other roentgenographic changes include nephrolithiasis and lytic bone lesions of the phalanges. The latter are most likely to be found when there are pain and swelling in the overlying soft tissues.

Pulmonary function tests are generally more sensitive than the chest roentgenogram in detecting parenchymal lung involvement. Serial measurements of pulmonary function serve as important guides to therapy, but the initial severity of impairment is not an accurate predictor of the future clinical course. The diffusing capacity is perhaps the most useful test with which to follow the patient with sarcoidosis, and it is diminished in more than half of patients with stage I disease.

In more advanced parenchymal disease the lung volumes and diffusing capacity are diminished in a manner typical of restrictive disease. There may be arterial hypoxemia, and exercise testing may reveal significant exertional limitation and oxyhemoglobin desaturation. Airway obstruction may be caused by endobronchial or peribronchial involvement or by airway distortion owing to parenchymal fibrosis.

Sarcoidosis is associated with a variety of abnormal findings related to the immune system. However, it has proved difficult either to identify a causative antigen or to fit the known immunologic abnormalities into a clearly defined pathogenetic mechanism. Among the features that suggest involvement of the immune system are polyarthralgias, erythema nodosum, and evidence of depressed cellular immunity (such as lymphopenia, decreased numbers of circulating T cells, impaired T-cell proliferative response to mitogens, and cutaneous anergy to skin test antigens and synthetic skin sensitizers). In patients with inactive or resolved disease many of the abnormalities disappear. The defect in cellular immunity is relatively mild, and sarcoidosis is not associated with an increased incidence of opportunistic infection. Cells obtained by lung lavage from patients with sarcoidosis reveal an increased number of activated T lymphocytes, a finding that seems to support the belief that the lung is the site of an immune response in the form of a T-cell alveolitis.

Since there are no pathognomonic features, the diagnosis must be based on a compatible clinical picture, biopsy evidence of noncaseating granulomas, and exclusion of other granulomatous disorders. The biopsy procedures that most often yield noncaseating granulomas are mediastinoscopy, open lung biopsy, and multiple transbronchial biopsies. These are positive in over 90% of patients with roentgenographic evidence of disease. Percutaneous liver biopsy has a high yield (60% to 90% positive), but hepatic noncaseating granulomas may be seen in a variety of other illnesses. Skin lesions and palpably enlarged lymph nodes may yield granulomas. Other sites used to obtain material for histologic study include the lacrimal glands, major salivary glands, labial salivary glands, and gastrocnemius muscle.

MANAGEMENT. Corticosteroids (initially 1 mg/kg/day of prednisone, which is then tapered) appear to diminish the granulomatous inflammation, but whether the final degree of fibrosis is modified is unknown. As a rule, patients with minimal or no pulmonary function impairment are not treated. Patients with symptomatic lung disease, marked function changes, or evidence of progressive lung disease on serial chest roentgenograms and pulmonary function tests generally receive therapy. Treatment also is indicated for disfiguring skin lesions, myocardial or central nervous system disease, severe constitutional symptoms, and ocular disease. Mild anterior uveitis may be controlled with topical therapy, but this should be carried out under the supervision of an ophthalmologist. Hypercalcemia also responds to corticosteroid therapy, which may minimize or prevent nephropathy. In patients whose lung disease progresses to fibrosis and bronchiectasis, bronchial infection may occur and require antibiotic therapy. Massive hemoptysis may require surgical resection of the source of bleeding. Mycetoma formation generally is asymptomatic, but surgery may be needed if hemoptysis results.

Significant pulmonary uptake on gallium scan and bronchoalveolar lavage fluid lymphocytosis tend to correlate with the presence of active alveolitis and tend to fall with spontaneous or corticosteroid-induced remission. These studies are not specific for sarcoid, are somewhat expensive, and are not as accurate in predicting the presence of alveolitis or the likelihood of corticosteroid response as would be desired. Thus their role in routine management is not fully established.

PROGNOSIS. The prognosis varies. The mortality from sarcoidosis is less than 5%. The causes of death most commonly include respiratory insufficiency, massive hemoptysis, and severe disease of the heart, brain, kidneys, or liver. Of patients with stage I disease, 75% achieve remission within 2 years of diagnosis and 25% develop pulmonary infiltrates. Of those with infiltrates at the time of diagnosis, 50% are improved within 2 years; in the rest the infiltrates either do not change or worsen. Roughly 10% of all sarcoid patients show roentgenographic evidence of fibrosis. Chronic uveitis, skin lesions, bone cysts, and upper respiratory granulomas are said to portend the development of major pulmonary impairment.

Histiocytosis X

(See Chapter 19.)

Histiocytosis X refers to three rare diseases: eosinophilic granuloma, Hand-Schüller-Christian disease, and Letterer-Siwe disease. However, about half the patients do not fit unequivocally into any one of these three disease categories. The common histologic feature is an infiltration containing large, irregularly shaped histiocytes with pale, eosinophilic, "foamy" cytoplasm.

Eosinophilic granuloma is the form most often associated with pulmonary disease in adults. In about 25% of cases the disorder is generalized, but in most adults the disease is confined to the lungs. Eosinophilic granuloma may be detected in an asymptomatic patient on routine chest roentgenogram or may present with dyspnea and cough. Spontaneous pneumothorax may occur. The disease may have systemic manifestations such as fever, weakness, and cachexia. Early in the disease the chest roentgenogram reveals a widespread symmetric interstitial infiltrate, usually distributed uniformly from base to apex but occasionally more prominent in the upper lobes. The diagnosis of lung disease caused by eosinophilic granuloma usually requires open biopsy. Typically there are poorly demarcated areas of alveolitis dominated by mononuclear phagocytes (histiocytes). Ultrastructural studies have shown these cells to be a mixture of pigment-laden macrophages and histiocytosis X cells. The latter resemble the Langerhans' cells seen in normal skin and, like Langerhans' cells, may contain the surface antigen OKT6. Thus immunocytochemical staining for this marker may aid in diagnosis. Electron microscopy of histiocytosis X cells demonstrates characteristic rodlike intracellular inclusions (X bodies). These cells may also be recovered and identified in bronchoalveolar lavage fluid.

The course and prognosis of eosinophilic granuloma vary, ranging from a single stable bone lesion to a multiple-system progressive disease with a rapidly fatal course. Similarly, lung involvement may be functionally mild or may evolve into a progressive fibrotic process resulting in extensive cystic change and respiratory insufficiency. Most adult cases that are confined largely to the lungs have a benign course. The disease has been treated with steroids, but although apparent benefit occasionally has been noted, the rarity of eosinophilic granuloma and the variability of its natural history have made it difficult to assess the usefulness of this therapy.

Hand-Schüller-Christian disease, occurring most often in childhood, is a widespread disease whose manifestations include skin lesions, bone lesions, otitis media, mastoiditis, adenopathy, splenic enlargement, and interstitial lung disease. Exophthalmos, diabetes insipidus, and bony lesions of the skull are a characteristic triad. The course is variable. Recovery may occur, although occasionally with persistence of the diabetes insipidus.

Letterer-Siwe disease affects children under 3 years of age and is regarded as a lymphomatous proliferation of histiocytes. The manifestations include adenopathy, hepatosplenomegaly, skin and bone lesions, and marrow involvement with pancytopenia, bleeding, and infection. The illness usually is rapidly fatal.

Amyloid

(See Chapter 16.)

Amyloid may involve the lung parenchyma as one or more nodular deposits (usually asymptomatic) or in the form of widespread interstitial infiltrates. The latter picture usually accompanies generalized amyloidosis and may produce significant lung restriction. Tracheobronchial amyloid deposits occasionally produce signs and symptoms of localized obstruction.

PULMONARY VASCULITIDES
Polyarteritis nodosa and related vasculitides

(See Chapter 20.)

At one time medical textbooks described asthma, eosinophilia, and pulmonary infiltrates as manifestations of polyarteritis nodosa. However, it is now recognized that polyarteritis nodosa is largely a necrotizing disorder of medium-sized muscular arteries that is unlikely to affect pulmonary vessels and rarely is associated with lung disease. Patients with the constellation of wheezing, fever, eosinophilia, and vasculitis are more likely to have *Churg-Strauss syndrome,* a disorder essentially confined to asthmatic individuals and most commonly involving the lung (diffuse alveolitis with granulomas and fibrosis), skin, gastrointestinal tract, and peripheral nerves (Fig. 132-3).

Hypersensitivity (allergic) angiitis is a systemic small-vessel vasculitis that may be associated with both alveolitis and interstitial fibrosis. About half the cases are of unknown cause; drugs or infection appear to precipitate some cases. The disorder is thought to result from the deposition of immune complexes in the walls of small blood vessels, activation of complement, and subsequent inflammation.

Some patients with necrotizing vasculitis cannot be easily classified as having one of the well-defined vasculitides such

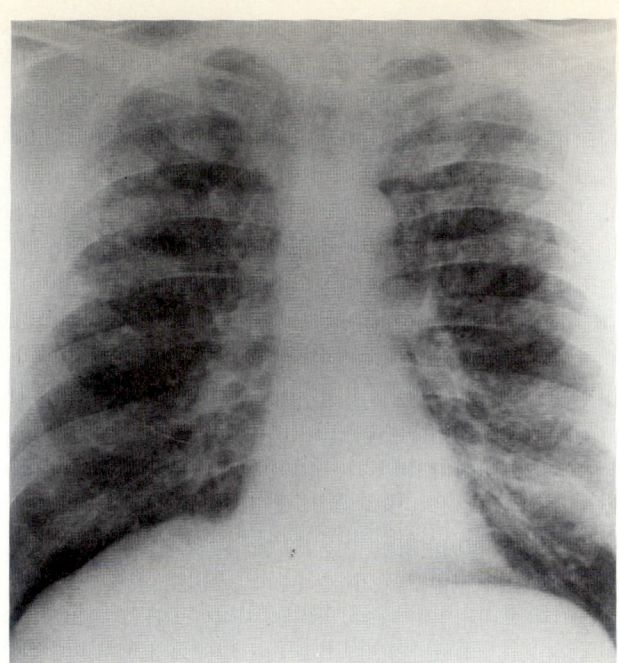

Fig. 132-3   Diffuse pulmonary disease (Churg-Strauss syndrome). (Courtesy of George Popky, MD.)

as polyarteritis nodosa, Churg-Strauss syndrome, or hypersensitivity angiitis. The term "overlap vasculitis" has been used to describe such patients, who often have pulmonary involvement characterized by interstitial fibrosis and necrotizing vasculitis.

Wegener's granulomatosis

(See Chapter 22.)

Wegener's granulomatosis is a multisystem disorder characterized by necrotizing vasculitis of the upper and lower respiratory tract, glomerulonephritis, and disseminated vasculitis involving small vessels. Respiratory tract involvement usually is clinically evident, whereas the renal disease may be subclinical. A renal biopsy may show focal glomerulonephritis. Upper respiratory tract involvement may include paranasal sinusitis, otitis media, scleroiritis, and nasopharyngeal ulceration. With nasal involvement there may be bacterial infection, septal perforation, and saddle nose deformity. Involvement of the lung may take the form of transient infiltrates associated with few or no symptoms. Commonly, however, there are nodular lesions that may cavitate and may be associated with fever, cough, chest pain, or hemoptysis. Pleural effusion and adenopathy are uncommon.

The major recent therapeutic advance in this once rapidly fatal disorder was the discovery that cyclophosphamide induces long-term remission in most patients.

DIFFUSE HEMORRHAGIC LUNG DISEASE AND PULMONARY HEMOSIDEROSIS

Among the disorders associated with lung hemorrhage or the widespread deposition of iron in lung tissue are mitral stenosis, long-standing left ventricular failure, repeated blood transfusions or excessive administration of parenteral iron preparations, Goodpasture's syndrome (lung hemorrhage with nephritis), and idiopathic pulmonary hemosiderosis. In all these entities the parenchymal iron deposition may lead to pulmonary fibrosis and restriction.

Goodpasture's syndrome

Goodpasture's syndrome is an immune-complex disease manifested by interstitial and intraalveolar hemorrhage (with or without gross hemoptysis), iron deficiency anemia, and acute glomerulonephritis. It is a disease of young adults (usual age range 16 to 30 years), with more than 75% of the cases occurring in males. About 20% of the cases follow viral respiratory illnesses.

The pathogenesis is believed to be related to the antigenic similarity of alveolar and glomerular basement membranes. Injury to one of these membranes may result in the alteration, release, or "unmasking" of membrane antigen that triggers the production of anti–basement membrane antibody. This antibody attaches to the alveolar and glomerular basement membrane, binds complement, and causes a cytotoxic reaction that damages the involved structures. In the lung there is bleeding from the damaged pulmonary capillaries into the interstitial spaces and alveoli.

Hemosiderin remains in the lung parenchyma as a result of the breakdown of blood; this eventually leads to fibrosis and may contribute to iron deficiency anemia (because iron from the lung hemorrhage apparently remains sequestered in the lung, unavailable for hemoglobin synthesis). The finding of linear deposits of IgG along the glomerular basement membrane with immunofluorescent staining, the presence of acute glomerulonephritis on kidney biopsy, the demonstration of bound immunoglobulin and complement in the lung, and the nearly universal presence of circulating anti–glomerular basement membrane antibody (anti-GBM) are characteristic of this disorder.

Hemoptysis often is the initial symptom. Although massive hemorrhage may occur, repeated small hemorrhages resulting in pulmonary fibrosis are more common. Macrophages take up the breakdown products of blood in the lung parenchyma, and hemosiderin-laden macrophages may be recovered in the sputum or on bronchoscopy, which is usually otherwise normal. Other manifestations include rales and rhonchi as the result of lung hemorrhage and pallor as the result of anemia. Systemic symptoms such as weight loss, malaise, and exertional dyspnea also may occur. The chest roentgenogram may show patchy densities that vary in appearance from day to day, reflecting the recurrence or resolution of hemorrhage. Eventually an interstitial pattern develops, and there may be fibrosis that appears indistinguishable from fibrosis caused by other diffuse parenchymal diseases.

Progressive renal disease causes the appearance of albuminuria, microscopic hematuria, and cellular and granular casts. Uremia may develop rapidly and was formerly the most common cause of death. Because this complication has been postponed in some cases by dialysis and renal transplantation (glomerulonephritis also may develop in the transplanted kidney), death now more often results from lung hemorrhage and respiratory insufficiency. Bilateral nephrectomy may lead to a cessation of lung hemorrhage, presumably by removing the source of antigen. Steroids, immunosuppressive agents, and plasmapheresis (to remove circulating anti-GBM) may lead to sustained remissions. It may prove useful to follow such patients with serial measurements of the diffusing capacity, since a sudden increase in diffusing capacity, presumed to result from carbon monoxide uptake by the red blood cells in areas of lung hemorrhage, may serve as an indication for repeated plasmapheresis.

Idiopathic pulmonary hemosiderosis

Idiopathic pulmonary hemosiderosis most often affects children and is rare in individuals over 20 years of age. The sex distribution in affected children is about equal, although males seem to be more commonly affected in the young adult age-group. The clinical and roentgenographic manifestations are indistinguishable from those of Goodpasture's syndrome, except for the absence of renal involvement. The histologic findings in the lung also are identical, except that in idiopathic pulmonary hemosiderosis, anti-IgG antibody is not demonstrated by immunofluorescent staining.

The diagnosis is based on the clinical picture of hemoptysis, iron deficiency anemia, chest roentgenogram abnormalities (as previously described for Goodpasture's syndrome), the finding of hemosiderin-laden macrophages in the sputum, and the absence of both renal involvement and anti-GBM. The disorder is usually fatal with a course of several weeks to several years. Death may result from large hemorrhages with hypoxemia or from recurrent smaller hemorrhages leading to the development of interstitial fibrosis and cor pulmonale.

EOSINOPHILIC DISEASES
Pulmonary infiltrates with eosinophilia (PIE syndrome)

PIE syndrome (infiltrative lung disease with blood eosinophilia) may follow either a brief, self-limited course or a more severe and protracted one. Cases occur that are not easily classified as one of the two major idiopathic varieties of PIE syndrome, Löffler's syndrome and chronic eosinophilic pneumonia. In addition, a large number of disorders (principally neoplasms, infections, and drug-induced disease) have been recognized that may also cause eosinophilia and pulmonary infiltrates. The following outline lists the subtypes of PIE syndrome:

Classification of PIE syndrome

I. Löffler's syndrome
II. Chronic eosinophilic pneumonia
III. Known causes
    A. Tumor
        1. Leukemia, lymphoma (especially Hodgkin's disease)
        2. Metastatic carcinoma
        3. Bronchogenic carcinoma
    B. Parasitic disease
        1. Infection with *Ascaris, Stronglyoides,* and *Ancylostoma* species and others
        2. Visceral larva migrans (*Toxocara canis*)
        3. Tropical eosinophilia (microfilaria)
    C. Other infections, especially viral pneumonitis
    D. Sarcoidosis
    E. Drug reactions such as those caused by nitrofurantoin, para-aminosalicylic acid, penicillin, sulfonamides, chlorpropamide, isoniazid, aspirin, methotrexate, disodium cromoglycate
    F. Bronchopulmonary aspergillosis
    G. Vasculitis such as Churg-Strauss syndrome

LÖFFLER'S SYNDROME. Löffler's syndrome is a self-limited disorder that usually runs its course in several weeks. There are transient migratory infiltrates and blood eosinophilia. Patients may be asymptomatic or may manifest symptoms such as cough, fever, headache, and malaise. Wheezing may be present. The histologic picture is not well defined; patients have such mild symptoms and the illness is of such short duration that a lung biopsy is usually not performed.

CHRONIC EOSINOPHILIC PNEUMONIA. Chronic eosinophilic pneumonia is clinically a more severe disorder than Löffler's syndrome. It is characterized by cough, dyspnea, and occasionally hemoptysis. There may be systemic symptoms such as weight loss, fever, chills, and diaphoresis. The blood eosinophil count is normal in one third of the patients. The chest roentgenogram characteristically shows peripherally located infiltrates that spare the perihilar areas. A biopsy shows increased numbers of eosinophils in the tissues. The disorder may persist for months or years, but both the symptoms and roentgenographic densities clear rapidly with corticosteroid therapy.

FAMILIAL DISEASES
Gaucher's disease

(See Chapter 195.)

Gaucher's disease, a lipid storage disease caused by a deficiency of the enzyme glucocerebrosidase, is associated with the accumulation of lipid material in reticuloendothelial cells. The resulting *Gaucher's cells* may infiltrate a number of organs. Involvement of the pulmonary interstitium and pulmonary fibrosis may occur.

Niemann-Pick disease

(See Chapter 195.)

Niemann-Pick disease, another lipid storage disease, is caused by a deficiency of the enzyme sphingomyelinase. It is associated with the accumulation of sphingomyelin in histiocytes, giving them a foamy appearance. These foam cells, in addition to infiltrating the liver, spleen, lymph nodes, and central nervous system, may cause interstitial pulmonary disease.

Familial interstitial pneumonitis

An interstitial pneumonitis indistinguishable from idiopathic pulmonary fibrosis may occur on a familial basis. The mechanism of inheritance has not been clarified but may be autosomal dominant with incomplete penetrance.

Neurofibromatosis

(See Chapter 156.)

Neurofibromatosis, also known as von Recklinghausen's disease, is an autosomal dominant disorder characterized by neurofibromas in the skin and peripheral and central nervous system and by cutaneous café au lait spots. About 10% to 20% of the cases in adults are associated with interstitial fibrosis that is histologically indistinguishable from the idiopathic variety.

Tuberous sclerosis

(See Chapter 156.)

Tuberous sclerosis is a rare disorder characterized by mental deficiency, seizures, adenoma sebaceum, and hamartomatous involvement of multiple organs. Intersitital pulmonary fibrosis occurs in about 10% to 20% of the cases.

DRUG-INDUCED DISEASE

The wide variety of drugs in clinical use today and the large quantities administered have significantly increased the risk of adverse drug reactions. The problem is heightened by the frequent use of multiple-drug therapy, which increases the opportunities for adverse drug interactions, by the ready availability and widespread use of nonprescription drugs, and by the surreptitious use of narcotic and mood-altering drugs. The lung parenchyma may be affected by drugs through a variety of mechanisms. Common types of drug-induced disease and some of the agents that cause them are listed in the following outline:

Common agents causing drug-induced lung disease

I. Acute pulmonary infiltrates
   Amitriptyline
   Azathioprine
   Chlorpropamide
   Imipramine
   Isoniazid
   Mephenesin
   Methotrexate
   Nitrofurantoin
   Paraaminosalicylic acid
   Penicillamine
   Penicillin
   Procarbazine
   Sulfonamides
II. Chronic interstitial fibrosis
   Amiodarone
   BCNU
   β-blocking drugs (practolol, propranolol, pindolol)
   Bleomycin
   Busulfan
   Cyclophosphamide
   Gold salts
   Hexamethonium
   Mecamylamine
   Melphalan
   Methotrexate
   Nitrofurantoin
   Oxygen
   Penicillamine
   Tocainide
III. Increased permeability of alveolar-capillary membrane
   Chlordiazepoxide
   Ethchlorvynol
   Heroin
   Methadone
   Propoxyphene
   Salicylates
   Thiazides
IV. SLE syndrome
   Acebutolol
   Allopurinol
   Hydralazine
   Isoniazid
   Mephenytoin
   Methyldopa
   Methylthiouracil
   Phenytoin
   Procainamide
   Propylthiouracil
   Reserpine

RADIATION PNEUMONITIS AND FIBROSIS

(See Chapter 138.)

Radiation damage to the lung results most commonly from the therapeutic use of radiation in a variable percentage of patients treated for malignancies of the breast, mediastinal structures, and lung. Such damage usually is divided into an early stage (radiation pneumonitis) and a late reaction (radiation fibrosis). Although radiation pneumonitis occasionally may resolve completely and without sequelae, it more often is followed by at least some degree of fibrosis.

Radiation pneumonitis develops insidiously, usually 2 to 6 months after radiation therapy but occasionally as early as 4 weeks. Earlier reactions are associated with more severe damage. The degree of lung involvement is related to the volume of lung irradiated, the total dose of radiation and its rate of delivery, the concomitant use of chemotherapeutic agents, the withdrawal of steroid therapy during or after radiation therapy, and the administration of radiation to an area previously irradiated. Radiation damage is likely to be tolerated poorly by individuals with previously impaired pulmonary function.

An early symptom of radiation pneumonitis is cough, usually hacking and nonproductive (although scant amounts of pink-tinged sputum may be produced). The major symptom of radiation pneumonitis is dyspnea, present only on exertion in most cases but progressing to severe respiratory distress at rest in some. Fever and other constitutional symptoms may accompany severe cases as well. There may be rales, signs of consolidation, a pleural friction rub, and skin changes overlying the port of radiation.

Histologic findings include engorged and thrombosed pulmonary capillaries, hyperplasia and desquamation of alveolar lining cells, hyaline membranes, and edema and mononuclear cell infiltrates of the interstitial space. Roentgenographic changes initially consist of diffuse haziness in the area of involvement, and the normal lung markings become indistinct. As the process progresses, alveolar infiltrates may develop, and in advanced cases consolidation accompanied by air bronchograms may be seen. Pleural and pericardial effusions may develop, and the mediastinum may become widened and blurred. Lung cavitation is unusual; its occurrence should suggest the development of either infection or necrosis of the underlying tumor. Classically, the roentgenographic density has relatively sharp margins that correspond to those of the radiation port, but diffuse and poorly marginated pneumonitis also may occur. Corticosteroid therapy may be of benefit, but data concerning efficacy in controlled trials are lacking.

Radiation fibrosis, which in some degree usually follows symptomatic radiation pneumonitis by 6 months or more, occasionally may result in severe dyspnea and even chronic respiratory failure. With unilateral irradiation there may be volume loss with a shift of the mediastinal structures toward the affected side. The involved area becomes progressively contracted, the diaphragms may become tented, and pleural thickening may develop. Finally a densely fibrotic and contracted portion of lung may be left, and bronchiectatic changes may develop in the area. There is no known effective therapy for the fibrotic stage.

BIBLIOGRAPHY

Baum GL, editor: Textbook of pulmonary diseases, ed 2, Boston, 1974, Little, Brown & Co.

Carrington CB, Addington WW, and Goff AM: Chronic eosinophilic pneumonia, N Engl J Med 289:787, 1969.

Carrington CB and others: Natural history and treated course of usual and desquamative interstitial pneumonia, N Engl J Med 298:801, 1978.

Colp C: Sarcoidosis: course and treatment, Med Clin North Am 61:1267, 1977.

Daniele RP, Dauber JH, and Rossman MD: Immunologic abnormalities in sarcoidosis, Ann Intern Med 92:406, 1980.

Davis WB and Crystal RG: Chronic interstitial lung disease. In Simmons DH, editor: Current pulmonology, vol 5, New York, 1984, John Wiley & Sons.

Dreisin RB and others: Circulating immune complexes in the idiopathic interstitial pneumonias, N Engl J Med 298:353, 1978.

Fulmer JD and Crystal RG: Interstitial lung disease. In Simmons DH, editor: Current pulmonology, Boston, 1979, Houghton Mifflin Co.

Hinshaw HD and Murray JF: Diseases of the chest, ed 4, Philadelphia, 1980, WB Saunders Co.

James DG, editor: Sarcoidosis of the respiratory system, Semin Respir Med 8(1), 1986.

Liebow AA and Carrington CB: The eosinophilic pneumonias, Medicine 48:251, 1969.

Mitchell DN and Scadding JG: Sarcoidosis, Am Rev Respir Dis 110:774, 1974.

Morrissey WL and others: Chronic eosinophilic pneumonia, Respiration 32:453, 1975.

Schwartz MI: Idiopathic interstitial lung disease, Semin Respir Med 1:47, 1979.

Sostman HD, Matthay RA, and Putman CE: Cytotoxic drug–induced lung disease, Am J Med 62:608, 1977.

Strimlan CV and others: Lymphocytic interstitial pneumonitis, Ann Intern Med 88:616, 1978.

Turner-Warwick M, editor: Interstitial lung disease, Semin Respir Med 6(1), 1984.

Weinberger SE and others: Bronchoalveolar lavage in interstitial lung disease, Ann Intern Med 89:459, 1978.

Winterbauer RH and Hammar SP: Sarcoidosis and idiopathic pulmonary fibrosis: a review of recent events. In Simmons DH, editor: Current pulmonology, vol 7, Chicago, 1986, Year Book Medical Publishers, Inc.

Zeck RT and Cugell DS: Diffuse infiltrative lung diseases, Med Clin North Am 61:1251, 1977.

133·OCCUPATIONAL AND ENVIRONMENTAL LUNG DISEASE

David M.F. Murphy

The importance of occupation as a cause of disease has been recognized for centuries. Whenever an occupational lung disease is suspected, it is essential to take a detailed history, as the patient often does not realize the potential significance of a particular occupation. With recent advances in technology, a previously unrecognized condition may be brought to light, and careful documentation of any exposure to dusts, fumes, gases, or chemicals is important. Such exposures may occur not only at work but also in the home or during recreational activity. Exposure may be occupational, paraoccupational, household, or environmental. Paraoccupational exposure occurs when a worker who does not directly handle a noxious material is exposed by associating with a worker who does.

The diagnosis of an occupational lung disease is based on two factors: an occupational history that is pertinent to the condition and a chest roentgenogram that reveals a characteristic pattern compatible with the condition. Functional impairment may be assessed by pulmonary function tests, and occasionally an open lung biopsy must be performed to make the diagnosis. It is important to be precise about definition. A *disease* is defined as the failure of an organism's adaptive mechanisms to counteract adequately the stimuli or stresses to which it is subject, resulting in a disturbance in function or structure of any part, organ, or system of the body. A *disorder* is defined as a disturbance or derangement of regular normal physical health or function.

Occupational lung diseases can be divided into two broad groups: those caused by exposure to organic agents, and those caused by exposure to inorganic agents. Inorganic dusts have caused lung disease for centuries. As metal mining was associated with the progress of civilization, so exposure to silica occurred with both its procurement and refinement. Coal dust and more recently asbestos dust became important causes of lung disease as these agents acquired technologic importance. Inorganic dusts also may be associated with industrial bronchitis and pulmonary neoplasms, but they mainly are associated with the development of pneumoconiosis. Pneumoconiosis is defined as the accumulation of dust in the lungs and the lung tissue's reaction to its presence.

In certain susceptible individuals organic dusts may give rise to occupational asthma, hypersensitivity pneumonitis, or bronchitis. When inhaled as vapors, chemicals may cause acute upper airway injury or acute pulmonary edema, and late sequelae may include adult respiratory distress syndrome (ARDS) and bronchiolitis obliterans.

The medical consequences of inhaling a particular agent depend on the type of agent and the individual's susceptibility. For a dust particle to penetrate to the gas-exchanging part of the lung (that is, beyond the terminal bronchioles), it must be small enough to bypass the filtering mechanism of the upper airways and the nose. In general, only particles measuring less than 7 μm in diameter can reach beyond the distal airways. Particles of this size make up the "respirable fraction." Inertial impaction, sedimentation, and diffusion result in deposition of particles on the walls of the airways; scavenging macrophages remove the particles and transport them to the lymphatic system. As inorganic dust particles tend to accumulate around the respiratory bronchioles, this site usually manifests the first histologic evidence of disease. Organic dusts, on the other hand, produce immunologic reactions at the alveolar level in susceptible individuals, leading to the formation of granulomas in hypersensitivity pneumonitis or, as in the case of occupational asthma, bronchiolar smooth muscle hypertrophy.

ASBESTOS-RELATED CONDITIONS

Asbestos is a naturally occurring fibrous silicate that has two main types of fiber: curly fibers, or the serpentine form, and needlelike fibers, or the amphibole form. Of the serpentine form, white asbestos, or chrysolite, is mined mainly in Canada and the Soviet Union. The amphibole group includes blue asbestos, or crocidolite, found especially in South Africa; amosite, or brown asbestos, from the Transvaal in South Africa; and anthophyllite, a white form found in Finland. Tremolite and actinolite are less common forms of asbestos. Most of the asbestos currently used in the United States is chrysolite.

Asbestos is remarkably resistant to heat and chemical destruction, a property that reflects the chemical structure of the fibrous silicates, which contain silicon and oxygen with varied concentrations of iron, calcium, sodium, and magnesium. As a result asbestos is used especially for insulation and fireproofing. During World War II and later, large numbers of ships were insulated by spraying the inside of the holds with asbestos. Many of these vessels are now being refitted, and the insulation removed creates a risk of exposure. A similar hazard exists when dry lagging (covering) of pipes and electrical lines is removed. Asbestos also is used as grouting material in furnaces, in cement products, tiles, gutters, roofing material, and brake linings and in the paper, paint, and plastics manufacturing industries. Paraoccupational exposure to asbestos is not uncommon in the shipyard industry, and environmental exposure may occur in residents living near asbestos dumps, mines, or mills. Household exposure may result from exposure of other family members to a worker's dusty overalls or from home improvement projects involving installation of insulation. The lung conditions associated with asbestos exposure include pleural plaques, diffuse pleural thickening, pleural effusion, asbestosis, diffuse malignant mesothelioma of the pleura, and bronchogenic carcinoma.

Pleural plaques

Bilateral pleural plaques usually are regarded as evidence of asbestos exposure. They may occur over the diaphragm or on the parietal surface of the costal pleura and may be hyaline or calcified. When uncalcified they appear as protuberant densities along the walls of the chest, commonly in the middle or lower zones. When calcified they often are visible as thin, linear calcifications over the surface of the diaphragm or along the costal margins. Oblique views often are useful in detecting pleural plaques. When the plaque is unilateral, it should be considered as caused by asbestos exposure only when other causes such as previous pleurisy or tuberculosis have been excluded and when a history of exposure to asbestos has been obtained. Currently there is no evidence that plaques precede the development of diffuse malignant mesothelioma of the pleura; however, there is some evidence that the presence of pleural plaques doubles the risk of developing bronchogenic carcinoma. Their presence also may indicate increased risk of developing laryngeal carcinoma. Although pleural plaques are remarkably good markers for asbestos exposure, autopsy studies reveal that only about 25% of plaques are detected by roentgenography. The lung asbestos body count is not always elevated in patients who have pleural plaques, and asbestos bodies are not usually found in pleural plaques, although uncoated asbestos fibers can be detected.

Diffuse pleural thickening

Bilateral diffuse pleural thickening may be associated with asbestos exposure. This thickening may be minimal or extensive. With the more severe forms the costrophrenic angles are obliterated and there is significant restriction, constituting a form of fibrothorax.

Pleural effusion

An exudative pleural effusion is the most common lung condition associated with asbestos exposure in the earlier years of exposure. This diagnosis is made only after exclusion of other causes of pleural effusion. Asbestos-related pleural effusions often are blood tinged and recurrent.

Asbestosis

Asbestosis is defined as fibrosis of the lungs caused by inhaled asbestos dust. Up to a certain level, the greater the amount of asbestos dust inhaled, the greater the fibrosis that results, but progression from moderate to severe fibrosis seems to be related to other factors. Progressive fibrosis is associated with a progressive decrease in total lymphocyte count. Antinuclear antibodies occur more commonly in exposed individuals in whom clinical disease develops than in those in whom it does not.

Fibrosis develops first in subpleural areas and then extends deeper into the lobe. Lower lobes tend to be affected first, with the disease then spreading to middle and upper lobes. Honeycomb cysts and emphysema may be seen later. Lesions similar to the massive fibrosis of complicated coal workers' pneumoconiosis are very uncommon. The earliest stage identified microscopically is a peribronchiolar fibrosis with subsequent fibrosis of alveolar walls. Ferruginous bodies or uncoated asbestos fibers also may be seen. The initial symptom usually is inappropriate breathlessness following exertion. Nonproductive cough and chest pain also occur. Later, cellophane-like late inspiratory crackles are audible on auscultation at the lung bases. Clubbing of the fingers occurs in some cases. Irregular or round opacities are seen roentgenographically, particularly in the lower zones. A ground-glass appearance also may occur, and cystic changes or "honeycomb lung" may be seen in the late stages of the disease. When a mixed dust exposure occurs (for example, with silica), the opacities tend to be more rounded.

Usually asbestosis results in a restrictive pattern of functional impairment with a reduction in the vital capacity (VC) and total lung capacity (TLC). The diffusing capacity frequently is decreased, and arterial oxygen desaturation may be demonstrated on exercise. About 20% of cases demonstrate an obstructive pattern with reduction in the ratio of the 1-second forced expired volume ($FEV_{1.0}$) to the forced vital capacity (FVC), and a further 20% reveal a mixed obstructive and restrictive pattern. The diagnosis is definitely established when an appropriate exposure history is obtained in association with the roentgenographic changes of parenchymal disease, lung function impairment, and appropriate clinical findings. There is no evidence that removal from the source of exposure affects the outcome of the disease.

Treatment of infections may be important, since it has been suggested that nonspecific inflammation may contribute to progression of the fibrosis. Corticosteroid therapy is not advocated. Supplemental oxygen may provide some symptomatic relief of dyspnea.

Malignant mesothelioma

There is a clear association between pleural or peritoneal mesothelioma and inhalation of crocidolite asbestos. The tumor is not related to the amount of inhaled asbestos fiber, and there is a latent period of about 40 years from exposure to development of the tumor. Some cases of mesothelioma have been reported in association with other types of asbestos.

A definite diagnosis can be made only by histologic examination of the tumor tissue. Since these tumors contain a variety of cell types and arrangements, diagnosis often is difficult. If a mesothelioma is suspected, tissue should be obtained by open pleural biopsy rather than by needle biopsy, since the latter usually provides an insufficient specimen and the tumor may grow down the needle track. Cytologic examination of the pleural fluid usually is unhelpful.

Roentgenographic findings include pleural effusion (which may hide the lobulated pleural mass), hydropneumothorax, chest wall masses, and satellite lung lesions. Although various types of treatment have been tried, including surgical resection, chemotherapy, and radiation therapy, there is no curative therapy. The average survival time is about 6 months from the onset of symptoms. Surgery, which was the most effective treatment in the past, does not affect the median survival rate. Instillation of radioactive colloidal gold into the pleura occasionally has prolonged survival. Removal of pleural fluid to relieve breathlessness helps provide symptomatic relief.

Bronchogenic carcinoma

It has been clearly established that significant exposure to asbestos is associated with an increased risk for the development of lung cancer. About 20% of men with asbestosis die of lung cancer. When asbestos exposure is combined with cigarette smoking, the risk is multiplied; a heavily exposed smoker has 90 times as great a risk of developing lung cancer as a nonexposed nonsmoker. Most are adenocarcinomas of the squamous cell type, whereas oat cell carcinomas are uncommon. Other cancers shown to be associated with asbestos exposure include carcinoma of the larynx and gastrointestinal carcinomas.

COAL WORKER'S PNEUMOCONIOSIS

ETIOLOGY AND EPIDEMIOLOGY. Coal worker's pneumoconiosis (CWP) results from the prolonged inhalation of coal dust of respirable size. In most cases at least 10 years' exposure is required before roentgenographic disease is evident. The condition is defined as the accumulation of coal dust in the lungs and the reaction of tissue to its presence. The disease takes two forms, simple and complicated. Although originally believed to have little effect on life expectancy, CWP was recognized in the 1930s as an important cause of excessive mortality in the coal miners of southern Wales.

Most coal mined in the United States is bituminous coal; however, small amounts of anthracite coal are still mined in eastern Pennsylvania. There are about 120,000 underground coal miners in the United States. The overall prevalence of simple CWP in the exposed population of the United States is about 10%, whereas the prevalence of the complicated form is about 0.4%. In coal miners exposed to high concentrations of silica dust such as occurs in roof bolting, silicosis may develop in addition to CWP. Strip mining is not associated with CWP.

Coal dust of respirable size accumulates in the lungs. It first is deposited in the alveoli and ingested by alveolar macrophages, which migrate to the region of the respiratory bronchiole. Coal dust is not toxic to the macrophages if it does not contain free silica. Accumulation of coal dust around the respiratory bronchiole produces a pathologically distinct lesion, the *coal macule*. Besides the coal dust, a few fibers of reticulin also are laid down. In some cases atrophy of the smooth muscle of the respiratory bronchiole, along with traction on the wall of the bronchiole by the muscle, leads to *focal emphysema*. Collections of coal dust also may be found in the hilar lymph nodes and in the lymphatics leading to the nodes.

Complicated CWP, or progressive massive fibrosis (PMF), usually develops with advanced simple CWP. The precise factors responsible for development of the complicated form remain a mystery, but the condition is characterized by the development of unilateral or bilateral black fibrotic masses larger than 1 cm in diameter in the upper lobes of the lungs. This results in upward retraction of the hila, and bullous emphysema also may develop. The fibrotic masses tend to increase progressively in size, resulting in distortion of the airways and destruction of the pulmonary vasculature. The condition may be complicated by pulmonary tuberculosis, but this occurs less commonly than in silicosis. The massive lesions may cavitate because of ischemic central necrosis or coincident mycobacterial infection.

CLINICAL MANIFESTATIONS AND LABORATORY FINDINGS. Simple CWP has few symptoms and signs. Chronic cough and sputum production are most likely to result from coincident chronic bronchitis caused by cigarette smoking. PMF is associated with shortness of breath and a local decrease in tone of the percussion note. If cor pulmonale develops, signs of right-sided heart failure are present. Clubbing of the fingers is not seen in CWP or silicosis.

Simple CWP appears roentgenographically as uniform nodules, usually more profuse in the upper lung zones and varying in size from 1.5 to 10 mm. Bilateral masses can cause an "angel's wings" appearance in complicated CWP. Since this appearance is also associated with simple CWP, which usually is obvious roentgenographically, these large masses usually are not confused with carcinoma of the lung or pulmonary tuberculosis. Simple CWP is not associated with clinically significant decreases in ventilatory capacity. Complicated CWP, on the other hand, may be associated with airflow obstruction. The large masses may cause a reduction in lung volume, and the diffusing capacity is decreased in proportion to this reduction. Exercise often is accompanied by a reduction in arterial oxygen tension.

MANAGEMENT AND PREVENTION. Prevention is the only effective measure. The reduction of dust levels in the coal mines eventually will reduce the prevalence of the disease. Symptomatic management as described in the discussion of silicosis may be of value in some cases.

SILICOSIS

ETIOLOGY AND EPIDEMIOLOGY. Silicosis is a common occupational lung disease in the United States. It is defined as a fibrotic lung disease resulting from the inhalation of dust containing silicon dioxide, or silica. More than 1 million workers in the United States are believed to be exposed to free silica. Industries associated with a silica hazard include metal mining, coal mining, Foundry work, and stone, clay, and glass production. Sandblasting of stone and metal is particularly hazardous.

Simple silicosis is rarely seen in workers with less than 20 years' exposure to free silica, but an accelerated form of silicosis that occurs after 10 to 15 months of exposure has been described in sandblasters.

PATHOGENESIS. When deposited in the alveoli, silica particles are ingested by alveolar macrophages and enclosed within their phagosomes. A reaction between the phagosomal wall and the inhaled silica particle subsequently takes place, leading to the release of phagosomal proteolytic enzymes within the macrophage. This results in destruction of the macrophage and ultimately in release of the silica particle. The released silica particle is then ingested by another macrophage, and the process repeats itself. Destruction of the macrophage also leads to release of at least two factors: a chemotactic factor for other macrophages and a factor involved in the production of collagen. The continual formation of fibrous tissue leads to the production of the characteristic "silicotic nodule," which has a whorled appearance caused by concentric layers of connective tissue. Silicotic nodules usually are seen adjacent to respiratory bronchioles or pulmonary arterioles. For reasons currently unclear, large numbers of nodules tend to conglomerate in the upper lobes with increased fibrosis. This more advanced stage of the disease is known as "conglomerate silicosis."

Silicosis sometimes is associated with infection with *Mycobacterium tuberculosis*. In these cases the pathologic findings of pulmonary tuberculosis also may be found in the lungs. Cavitation of the conglomerate masses may result from either ischemia or tuberculous infection. An abnormal immunologic reaction also may be important in the pathogenesis of silicosis, since there is an increased prevalence of autoimmune disease in patients with this disorder.

CLINICAL MANIFESTATIONS. Silicosis can be classified into three main types: simple, conglomerate, and acute. The simple type is characterized by few symptoms other than shortness of breath and cough, which occur only in its later stages. Conglomerate silicosis is associated with more severe dyspnea, paroxysmal coughing, and, in the later stages of the disease, tachypnea and use of the accessory muscles of respiration. Acute silicosis is associated with rapidly progressive dyspnea, cough, and a fulminant course.

The physical signs include some degree of dullness to percussion over areas of conglomeration, which usually are located in one or both upper lobes. Bullous emphysema often complicates conglomerate silicosis and may mask this decreased resonance. Distortion of the airways by the large masses can cause signs of airflow obstruction. Pulmonary hypertension may develop as a result of hypoxemia and reduction in the pulmonary vascular bed and lead to cor pulmonale and ultimately death.

LABORATORY FINDINGS. The simple form of silicosis is characterized on the chest roentgenogram by multiple small

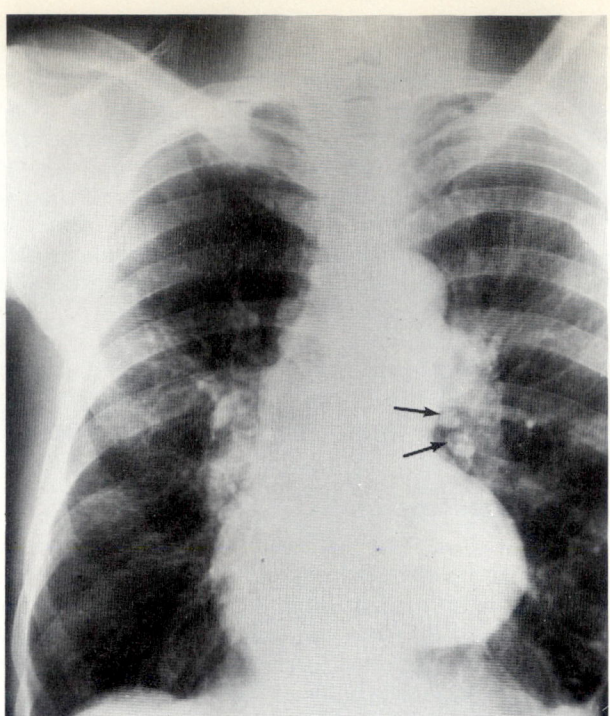

Fig. 133-1 Silicosis showing "eggshell" calcifications of hilar lymph nodes *(arrows)*. There is mild fibrosis in midlung regions. (Courtesy of George Popky, MD.)

nodules, predominantly in the upper lobes. These nodules usually are fairly uniform in size and vary from 1.5 to 10 mm in diameter. They occasionally calcify. More commonly, calcification of hilar lymph node capsules gives rise to "eggshell" calcification (Fig. 133-1).

Conglomerate silicosis is characterized roentgenographically by fibrotic masses greater than 1 cm in diameter that develop in the upper lobes in patients with simple silicosis. These masses migrate toward the hilum, causing it to retract upward. A peripheral zone of bullous emphysema often develops beyond the mass, and bullae also may develop at the lung bases. It usually is impossible to distinguish the presence of concomitant tuberculosis using roentgenography alone.

Acute silicosis occasionally is seen in workers exposed to high levels of respirable free silica over relatively short periods. Roentgenograms of the chest show a bilateral alveolar filling pattern spreading out from the hila.

Simple silicosis has little effect on lung function, whereas conglomerate disease may give rise to an obstructive and/or restrictive pattern accompanied by a reduction in diffusing capacity.

PREVENTION AND MANAGEMENT. Prevention is the best course. If a dust hazard is recognized, the concentration of silica dust must be maintained below levels believed to be associated with an acceptable incidence of disease. Because simple silicosis may progress, workers with the disease should avoid further exposure to free silica. Patients with conglomerate silicosis may require supplemental oxygen, cardiac glycosides, and antibiotics to counter respiratory infections. Concomitant tuberculosis should be treated with appropriate chemotherapeutic agents. A positive skin test for tuberculosis (in the absence of active tuberculosis) is an indication for prophylactic chemotherapy with agents such as isoniazid (300 mg/day for 1 year). The polymer poly-2-vinyl pyridine-N-oxide

(PVNO) has been shown to protect animals from the effects of inhaled silica and may prove to be of value in the future.

DENTAL TECHNICIAN'S PNEUMOCONIOSIS

Dental technicians can develop pneumoconiosis. In the course of their job they often are exposed to a variety of dusts, including silica, asbestos, and silicon carbide and also to metallic alloys containing cobalt, chromium, molybdenum, beryllium, and nickel. Many of these technicians are relatively young, with an average age of about 30 years, with exposures to dust of only about 12 years. It is not certain what causes dental technician's pneumoconiosis, but materials from abrasives have been suspected. Recent reports of mineralogic analysis of dust suggest that particles originating from vitallium prostheses may be important. Investigations in Europe have indicated that about 50% of dental technicians report respiratory symptoms and one third have chest roentgenographic abnormalities. These are reticulonodular in nature and have an upper zone distribution. Pulmonary function abnormalities include reduced lung volumes, decreased diffusing capacity, and hypoxemia at rest and with exercise.

OCCUPATIONAL ASTHMA

Occupational asthma may be defined as asthma that develops after a variable period of symptomless exposure to a sensitizing agent at work. It usually is necessary first to make a diagnosis of asthma and then to demonstrate its relationship to the patient's occupation. The prevalence of occupational asthma is estimated at about 2% of all cases of asthma. Since it is estimated that 4% to 8% of the United States' population suffer from some form of asthma, this means that anywhere from 160,000 to 320,000 people may have occupational asthma. Of course the incidence varies from industry to industry. For example, up to 35% of animal handlers and certain workers in the cotton industry may be affected, whereas the incidence of occupational asthma in western red cedar mills or with exposure to toluene diisocyanates (TDI) is about 5%.

Four mechanisms are believed to be important in the pathogenesis of occupational asthma. (See outline below.) These comprise reflex, inflammatory, pharmacologic, and allergic mechanisms.

Mechanisms of occupational asthma

Reflex (SO_2, NH_3, inert particles)
Inflammatory (H_2S, NH_3)
Pharmacologic (cotton, tropolones, TDI, organophosphates, western red cedar extracts)
Allergic
  High-molecular-weight agents: enzymes, animal dander, insects, grain, flour
  Low-molecular-weight agents: anhydrides, TDI, metals, salts, colophony

Asthma may be activated through nonspecific reflex mechanisms when receptors are stimulated by irritant gases or fumes. The irritant receptors activate a vagal-mediated reflex that produces bronchoconstriction. Inflammatory mechanisms may operate after exposure to gases or fumes, resulting in damage to the surface epithelium of the airways. With the inflammation there is an associated reduction in the stimulus threshold of the irritant receptors. Nonspecific stimuli may then induce bronchoconstriction. A variety of pharmacologic mechanisms also have been proposed, including direct release of lung tissue histamine and β-adrenergic blockade.

Allergic mechanisms are the best described and include the development of specific IgE against the occupational agent.

Table 133-1 Classification of agents causing occupational asthma

Groups	Example
Animal origin	Dander, molds, bacteria, insects, fish, mites
Vegetable origin	Cotton, flax, hemp, beans, woods, flour, grain, jute, enzymes, seeds, tea, tobacco, gum
Chemical origin	
Inorganic	Sulfur dioxide, chlorine, nitrogen dioxide, ammonia, platinum, nickel, chromium, aluminum
Organic	Diisocyanates, polyvinyl citronide, organophosphates, dyes, anhydrides, formaldehyde, fluxes, antibiotics

Lower-molecular-weight compounds may act as haptens after combining with human serum protein. Specific IgE may then be produced against the hapten. Allergens combine with specific IgE on the surface of the mast cell, resulting in an immediate or delayed release of chemical mediators that in turn produce immediate or delayed bronchoconstriction.

Certain predisposing factors are important in the development of occupational asthma, including atopy, nonspecific bronchial hyperreactivity and the duration of exposure. More than 200 agents have been identified as potential cases of occupational asthma. These are classified in Table 133-1. Some of the better-described types of occupational asthma follow exposure to grain dust, flour, animal dander, insects, western red cedar wood, enzymes, isocyanates, organophosphates, drugs, cotton, metal salts, soldering fluxes, beans, and formaldehyde.

Patients may manifest symptoms of breathlessness, cough, wheezing, or chest tightness upon exposure to a particular agent. In these circumstances the worker often recognizes the relationship between the exposure and the symptoms. However, the relationship is less obvious when symptoms occur after work or in the early hours of the morning. In addition wheezing is not always a presenting symptom, and cough perhaps associated with rhinitis may be dismissed as bronchitis. Disappearance of symptoms on the weekend or during vacation with recurrence upon return to work is important evidence suggesting an occupational relationship. When tracing an occupational history, knowledge of the more common causes of occupational asthma is valuable.

Physical examination may reveal the signs of asthma or may be normal. Pulmonary function tests may be normal or may show an obstructive pattern. Skin tests and specific IgE testing may provide additional diagnostic evidence, but the most valuable information is obtained from challenge tests with the specific occupational agent. Such testing includes exposure to a innocuous control material. The test should simulate the occupational exposure as closely as possible. Monitoring should be carried out by experienced personnel in a hospital setting. Such challenge testing has shown immediate, delayed, dual, and recurrent patterns of reduction in lung function.

Treatment of occupational asthma is similar to the treatment of other forms of asthma. Disodium chromoglycate may be useful in preventing attacks, as it has been shown to inhibit the immediate and delayed reactions produced by challenge. Steroids inhibit only the delayed reaction. Avoiding the offending agent or substituting materials may be necessary to control the condition. Identifying susceptible workers by routine monitoring of symptoms, pulmonary function tests, or skin tests also may be helpful in preventing the development of this disorder.

Table 133-2 Inhaled gases and vapors commonly involved in direct respiratory tract injury

Substance	Source
Ammonia	Fertilizer production
	Commerical refrigerant
Cadmium	Heating or smelting of ores and metals
	Welding
Chlorine	Manufacture of alkalies and bleaches
	Water purification
Nitrogen oxides	Silage (silo filler's disease)
	Arc welding in enclosed spaces
	Burning of nitrogen-containing substances
	Manufacturing processes
Ozone	Inside high-altitude, high performance aircraft
	Photochemical smog
	Arc welding
Sulfur dioxide	Multiple industrial processes (especially manufacturing of paper and chemicals)
	Smog

Byssinosis

Byssinosis usually is included under occupational asthma and may occur among cotton, flax, or soft hemp workers. In the cotton industry the prevalence is highest in cardroom workers and spinners. Washing and steaming of cotton may reduce the incidence of the disease, as the active agent is water soluble. A pharmacologic mechanism has been felt to be responsible for this condition, since histamine is liberated directly from lung tissue by extracts made from the bracht of the cotton boll. Recent studies have suggested that endotoxins from gram-negative bacteria that contaminate cotton dust also may be important.

The disease is characterized by chest tightness, which develops usually only on the afternoon of the first workday. As the condition progresses, symptoms occur on more than one day and eventually the disease may become chronic, with persistent symptoms and permanent reduction in ventilatory capacity. Smoking is felt to be an important predisposing factor.

Inhaled gases and vapors

A number of gases and fumes can damage the lungs. Exposure to these agents often occurs as a result of industrial accidents. Table 133-2 lists some of the more common gases, along with their sources. Depending on the nature of the gas a variety of effects can occur, ranging from acute asphyxia to long-term sequelae such as bronchiolitis obliterans. How the lungs are affected depends on the type of gas and its concentration, solubility, and irritant potential. Gases such as carbon monoxide, carbon dioxide, nitrogen, methane, cyanide, and hydrogen sulphide can cause asphyxiation.

The more irritating and soluble the gas, the more likely is the exposed individual to experience immediate unpleasant symptoms such as burning of the eyes, nasal lacrymation, facial burns, or mucosal edema, which may result in upper airway obstruction. Gases such as anhydrous ammonia and hydrochloric acid can cause these effects. These markedly irritating fumes force the exposed worker to obtain relief by urgently seeking escape from the contaminated area. Survival from acute injury carries a good prognosis, although some patients suffer acute pulmonary edema, and bronchiolitis obliterans occasionally has been reported as a late sequelae.

A large number of inorganic and organic agents have been reported to cause acute tracheobronchitis, pneumonitis, or frank pulmonary edema. These include chlorine, cadmium, cobalt, hydrogen fluoride (also sulphide and selenide) mercury,

nitrogen dioxide, ozone, sulphur dioxide, and zinc chloride. The organic compounds include acetaldehyde, acrolein, nickel carbonyl, and phosgene. The usual symptoms after exposure are dyspnea and cough, with noncardiogenic pulmonary edema identified roentgenographically. Pathologically, the picutre is that of diffuse alveolar damage with an initial exudative phase followed by a proliferative phase. The exudative phase is characterized by interseptal and intraalveolar edema followed by the development of hyaline membranes.

Electron microscopy reveals sloughing of alveolar lining cells and denudation of the alveolar basement membrane. After about a week an interstitial inflammation consisting of lymphocytes, plasma cells, and histiocytes becomes prominent. The reparative process is characterized by proliferation of alveolar lining cells, which have been shown to be type II pneumocytes. Later, organization occurs with the development of loose fibroblastic proliferation and a focal intraalveolar fibrosis. Bronchiolitis obliterans occurs in the late stages in a few cases. In addition, exposure to cadmium can produce emphysema.

A third pattern of disease occurs with minimally irritating gases such as nitrogen dioxide and nickel carbonyl. *Silo fillers' disease* is an example. In this condition farm workers may be exposed to nitrogen dioxide if they enter a silo where silage has been freshly prepared (usually in the first week after filling). The nitrogen dioxide probably comes from a chemical reaction whereby the nitrates in soil treated with nitrogen-rich fertilizers are oxidized. Initial symptoms of cough, dyspnea, and weakness rapidly resolve, but after 48 hours fever, chills, myalgia, dyspnea, and hypoxemia can occur. Rales become audible, and the chest roentgenogram shows noncardiogenic pulmonary edema, sometimes with a nodular component. Although spontaneous resolution often follows, death may occur in either the first or second stages. Treatment with steroids, supplemental oxygen, and mechanical ventilation may be necessary. The pathologic findings are those of an interstitial lymphocytic infiltrate and bronchiolitis obliterans. Pulmonary function abnormalities may persist for up to 3 years.

Hypersensitivity pneumonitis

The hypersensitivity pneumonitis conditions are defined as a group of pulmonary disorders in which inhalation of organic dust results in hypersensitivity reactions at the alveolar level usually associated with the production of serum precipitins. Many of these disorders are occupationally related. Table 133-3 lists the more common conditions.

In most cases hypersensitivity pneumonitis results from the inhalation of organic dust containing proteinaceous material that acts as an allergen. Although precipitating antibodies against the allergens have been detected in exposed workers, not all subjects with precipitating antibodies develop disease. It is not known why the disease, which occurs in both acute and chronic forms, develops only in some workers. Many of the allergens identified have been bacterial or fungal spores. These spores are less than 5 μm in diameter and so can penetrate to the alveolar level. Spores from thermophilic bacteria particularly have been associated with the condition. These bacteria grow in the high temperatures generated in moldy hay, bagasse, or mushroom compost. It is believed that large numbers of spores are liberated when moldy hay is turned, and in exposed workers up to 750,000 spores can be deposited in the lung each minute.

In affected individuals a cellular reaction occurs at the alveolar level. In the early stages this consists of infiltration of the alveolar walls with lymphocytes, plasma cells, and foamy histiocytes. Alveolar macrophages are found in the alveolar

Table 133-3 Common types of hypersensitivity pneumonitis

Clinical condition	Source of offending agent	Agent
Farmer's lung	Moldy hay	*Micropolyspora faeni*
		Thermoactinomyces vulgaris
Bagassosis	Moldy bagasse	*Thermoactinomyces vulgaris*
Mushroom worker's lung	Mushroom compost	*Micropolyspora faeni*
		Thermoactinomyces vulgaris
Suberosis	Cork dust	Cork dust
Maple bark disease	Maple bark	*Cryptostroma corticale*
Sequoiosis	Redwood sawdust	*Aureobasidium pullulans*
Wood pulp worker's disease	Wood pulp	*Alternaria* spp
Malt worker's lung	Moldy barley	*Aspergillus clavatus*
Wheat weevil disease	Wheat flour	*Sitophilus granarius*
		Aspergillus fumigatus
Furrier's lung	Animal hairs	None shown
Coffee worker's lung	Coffee beans	Coffee bean dust
Paprika splitter's lung	Paprika	*Mucor stolonifer*
Cheese washer's lung	Moldy cheese	*Penicillium caseii*
Bird fancier's lung (pigeon breeder's lung)	Pigeon, parrot, and other bird droppings	Serum and droppings
Pituitary snuff taker's lung	Bovine and porcine pituitary snuff	Pituitary antigens
Turkey raiser's disease	Turkey protein	Turkey serum
Chicken raiser's disease	Chicken protein	Chicken feathers, serum, and droppings

spaces. Loosely formed granulomas are an important histologic characteristic of this disorder. In some cases bronchiolitis obliterans also occurs. In the late stages irreversible interstitial fibrosis and honeycombing are the predominant findings.

It has been suggested that the immunologic mechanism involved in initiating the cellular reaction is a hypersensitivity response. It is characterized by the onset of systemic symptoms, including fever, malaise, or myalgia 4 to 6 hours after exposure to the organic dust, associated with rales on auscultation of the chest and a mixed reticular-nodular pattern on the chest roentgenogram. Lung function tests reveal a restrictive pattern with an associated defect in gas transfer. Precipitating antibodies of the IgG class may be demonstrated against the allergen. Bronchial inhalation challenge with the appropriate allergen is valuable in establishing the diagnosis.

Treatment involves avoiding the allergen, which may entail a change of occupation. Acute hypersensitivity pneumonitis may be rapidly fatal and should be treated with steroids, supplemental oxygen, and mechanical ventilation if respiratory failure ensues.

Smoke inhalation and burn injury

Smoke inhalation can cause pulmonary injury by thermal, chemical, or hypoxic means. When hot gases or particulates are inhaled, mucosal edema occurs in the nasopharynx, pharynx, and upper airway, leading to acute upper airway obstruction. Because a large number of materials are used in home construction, combustion produces a variety of toxic substances, including hydrochloric acid, acrolein, phosgene, cyanide, nitrites, and aldehydes. These can cause chemical injury resulting in mucosal edema, peribronchial edema, bronchoconstriction, or bronchorrhea. Hypoxemia results from asphyxia, upper airway obstruction, or carbon monoxide poisoning.

Carbon monoxide combines readily with hemoglobin, displacing oxygen and forming carboxyhemoglobin. As a result the oxygen available to the tissues is markedly reduced. Small concentrations of carbon monoxide have disproportionately adverse effects on the oxygen-carrying capacity of hemoglobin. In addition the oxygen dissociation curve's shift to the left reduces the amount of oxygen released to the tissues. The combination of these effects leads to severe tissue hypoxemia

in the presence of normal arterial oxygen tension. Headaches and nausea occur at lower levels of carboxyhemoglobin, but as the levels increases, dizziness, ataxia, behavioral changes, and visual impairment develop. When levels of carboxyhemoglobin are in the range of 50%, convulsions, coma, and death may result. Patients who have suffered smoke inhalation or burns often have dyspnea, cyanosis, wheezing, hoarseness, or stridor. Signs of upper and lower airway obstruction should be sought. Evaluation may require transnasal fiberoptic bronchoscopy, and if life-threatening upper airway obstruction is present, immediate endotracheal intubation or tracheostomy may be required.

Bronchospasm may respond to bronchodilators, but corticosteroids may be required if bronchospasm is intractable. Administering supplemental oxygen relieves hypoxemia and increases the dissociation of carbon monoxide from hemoglobin. Hyperbaric oxygen therapy has been used successfully for patients with severe carbon monoxide intoxication, but endotracheal intubation or tracheostomy with mechanical ventilation may be required to treat hypoxemic respiratory failure. A few patients develop ARDS after a symptom-free interval following the event, and a third group develops pneumonia weeks after the initial injury. Up to one fourth of patients who suffer significant burns develop pulmonary complications.

Oxygen toxicity

Although humans need oxygen to exist, human tolerance for this gas is limited. In a classic example of too much of a good thing, exposure to greater than normal partial pressures of O_2 can result in lung injury. This generally occurs because of therapeutic intervention during disease states causing hypoxia, but divers, aviators, and workers in hyperbaric chambers also may be exposed to increased pressures of O_2, and it is the pressure of inspired O_2 rather than the concentration that appears to be the major determinant of toxicity.

Some studies have shown impairment of mucociliary transport mechanisms and alveolar macrophage activity at relatively low levels of O_2 supplementation, but at normal atmospheric pressure up to 40% O_2 is considered safe. Most practitioners agree that concentrations greater than 60% generally are toxic, but there is disagreement about the safety of intermediate concentrations. However, the consensus is that (1) O_2 supplementation is indicated only for the treatment of hypoxia, (2) other means of improving oxygenation should also be used, (3) the minimal concentration necessary to relieve hypoxia should be employed, and (4) O_2 supplementation should be decreased and discontinued as soon as feasible.

The initial manifestations of O_2 toxicity are increasing discomfort on inspiration and dry cough. Lung volumes are reduced, and diffusion is impaired. Arterial O_2 pressures begin to fall as the alveolar-arterial O_2 difference increases. If hypoxia is present, O_2 supplementation may have to be further increased, even though this can exacerbate the degree of toxicity. Pathologically, interstitial edema, cellular infiltration, patchy atelectasis, and hemorrhagic pneumonitis develop. Often the pathologic picture is complicated by the presence of the initial disease entity that necessitated O_2 supplementation. Therapy other than that directed at the underlying disease process and other than continued efforts to decrease the pressures of O_2 being used has been unsatisfactory.

BIBLIOGRAPHY

Bailey WC and others: Silico-mycobacterial disease in sandblasters, Am Rev Respir Dis 110:115, 1974.

Becklake MR: Asbestos related diseases of the lung and other organs: their epidemiology and implications for clinical practice, Am Rev Respir Dis 114:187, 1976.

Criteria document—recommendations for an occupational exposure standard for crystalline silica, US Department of Health, Education and Welfare, Washington, DC, 1974, US Government Printing Office.

Devuyst P and others: Dental technicians pneumoconiosis: a report of two cases, Am Rev Respir Dis 133:312, 1986.

Elmes PC and Simpson MJC: The clinical aspects of mesothelioma, Q J Med 45:427, 1976.

Jacobson G and Lanihart WS: ILO/UC 1971 international classification of radiographs of the pneumoconioses, Med Radiogr Photogr 48:67, 1972.

Legha SS and Muggic FM: Therapeutic approaches in malignant mesothelioma, Cancer Treat Rev 4:13, 1977.

Morgan WKC: Byssinosis and related conditions. In Morgan WKC and Seaton A, editors: Occupational lung diseases, Philadelphia, 1975, WB Saunders Co.

Morgan WKC and Lapp NL: Respiratory disease in coal miners, Am Rev Respir Dis 113:531, 1976.

Schlueter DP: Response of the lung to inhaled antigens, Am J Med 57:476, 1974.

Slavin RG: Asthma in adults. III. Occupational asthma, Hosp Practice 13:133, 1978.

Wagner JC, Sleggs CA, and Marchand P: Diffuse pleural mesothelioma and asbestos exposure in the north-west Cape Province, Br J Ind Med 17:260, 1960.

Weil H and Ziskind MM: Occupational pulmonary diseases. In Fishman AP, editor: Pulmonary diseases and disorders, New York, 1980, McGraw-Hill, Inc.

134 • DISEASES OF THE PLEURA

William L. Morrissey*

The pleura, which is composed of connective tissue, is the very thin covering or lining of the lung. It contains lymphatics, blood vessels, smooth muscle fibers, and pain fibers.

The parietal pleura lines the inner surface of the chest wall and becomes the visceral pleura at the hilum; thus pleura encases the entire lung. It creates a saclike structure, the pleural cavity, that has no air within it but does contain a thin layer of fluid that serves to decrease the friction between the two layers of pleura. This lymph fluid within the pleural space is

*Material in this chapter is based in part on the first edition, written by Maurice Sones.

not static but is slowly being formed and removed. The presence of this fluid can be demonstrated by roentgenographic techniques in 10% of normal individuals and up to 40% of postpartum women. The turnover of pleural fluid may amount to several milliliters daily. The generally accepted physiologic mechanisms by which this fluid enters and leaves the pleural space depend on several pressures. The parietal capillary hydrostatic pressure (30 cm water) plus the negative pleural space pressure (5 cm water) plus the pleural fluid osmotic pressure (6 cm water) totals 41 cm of water pressure. The colloid osmotic pressure of the blood within the capillaries is 32 cm of water. The resulting difference of 9 cm of water pressure produces a flow of fluid from the parietal pleura into the pleural space. In the visceral pleura, however, the capillary hydrostatic pressure is only 11 cm of water as opposed to 30 cm in the parietal pleura. This reduced pressure allows a constant movement of fluid from the pleural space into the visceral pleura, that is, from the area of higher pressure to one of lower pressure. More recent studies suggest that lymphatics may provide the major exit route of pleural liquid. Interruption of this process can interfere with normal fluid transport or result in increased friction between pleural layers.

PLEURITIS

Pleuritis is an inflammation of the pleura. Most commonly it is caused by tuberculosis, bacterial pneumonia, lung abscess, malignancy, or pulmonary embolism. One type of tumor affecting the pleura is mesothelioma, usually related to asbestos exposure. By interfering with the normal fluid transport, all of these conditions result in increased friction between the layers of pleura.

The most prominent symptom associated with pleurisy is pain, which usually is sharp and lancinating and is accentuated by inspiration. Cough is common and aggravates the pain. The most severe pleuritic-like pain is noted in Bornholm disease, frequently called the "devil's grip" (it is more likely a result of involvement of the intercostal muscle or nerve than of the pleura and is caused by coxsackievirus, type B.) Other symptoms may be present that usually are related to the underlying disease process. The cardinal physical finding is a pleural friction rub, which may be absent if marked splinting of the affected side occurs. Chest wall tenderness may be present. Breathing can become very distressing and consequently can be quite shallow. Fever also may be present, especially with infections. An insidious onset of pleuritis with gradual deterioration of health in patients over 40 years of age suggests malignancy.

Laboratory studies should be directed at the suspected underlying cause. Chest roentgenograms generally reveal poor expansion and/or the presence of underlying parenchymal disease or pleural fluid. An examination of pleural effusion, if present, is critical (see following discussion of "Pleural effusion"). The progression of pleuritis can result in the formation of a pleural effusion either by increasing fluid production or by inhibiting its uptake. The therapy is symptomatic once the underlying cause has been identified and removed.

PLEURAL EFFUSION

The systematic approach to abnormal fluid accumulation in the pleural space, or pleural effusion, begins with a complete history and physical examination, followed by appropriate chest roentgenograms that include posteroanterior and lateral decubitus views. Computed tomography (CT) scans and ultrasound examinations may aid in localizing fluid, but they usually are not helpful in determining etiologic factors. Skin tests for tuberculosis, as well as examination of the pleural fluid for bacteria, tubercle bacilli, fungi, malignant cells, and *Entamoeba histolytica,* may be useful. When the cause of the effusion is unclear, examining the pleura itself by needle biopsy often can be revealing. Lymph node biopsy, mediastinoscopy, sputum examination, open pleural biopsy, and exploratory thoracotomy are other techniques that may have to be considered when evaluating pleural effusions.

An area of dullness to percussion found posteriorly above the diaphragm, which becomes resonant when the patient bends forward, suggests the presence of shifting or mobile pleural fluid. Breath sounds are absent in the area. Clubbing of the fingers can be seen with effusions caused by chronic infections such as bronchiectasis or empyema and also with malignancies. The chest roentgenogram shows a homogeneously increased density above the diaphragm and adjacent to the chest wall. A decubitus view allows detection of lesser amounts of fluid.

Any of a number of diseases may cause pleural effusion (see list, p. 640). It may be a prominent finding in patients with congestive heart failure, tuberculosis, pneumonia, and pulmonary embolism. Rheumatoid arthritis also may result in a pleural effusion. Pleural effusion may occur with pelvic tumors in females (Meigs' syndrome). Nephrotic syndrome may be associated with pleural effusions, as well as with marked peripheral edema and ascites.

Pleural effusions also have been reported in pancreatitis, chylothorax resulting from traumatic or surgical injury to the thoracic duct, ankylosing spondylitis, cirrhosis of the liver with ascites, amebiasis, sarcoidosis, disseminated lupus erythematosus, insertion of central venous cannulas, and uremia. There is about a 50% incidence of small pleural effusions after abdominal surgery.

Pleural effusions can be divided into transudates and exudates. A transudate is a filtrate of plasma containing small amounts of protein that has passed through a membrane as a result of an alteration in the mechanics of fluid homeostasis. An exudate is the result of the passage of fluid, protein, and white blood cells through vessel walls that have been made permeable because of localized disease and interference with lymphatic drainage. Transudates occur in congestive heart failure, cirrhosis, and nephrotic syndrome, whereas exudates are found with pneumonia, tuberculosis, malignancy, and pulmonary embolism.

Transudates usually are clear with a specific gravity of 1.015 or less, a protein content of less than 3 g/dl, and a lactic acid dehydrogenase (LDH) concentration of less than 200 units. The ratio of pleural fluid to serum protein generally is less than 0.5 and that for pleural fluid to serum LDH less than 0.6.

With exudates these parameters are increased: protein content is greater than 3 g/dl; the pleural fluid to serum protein ratio is more than 0.5, and the pleural fluid to serum LDH ratio greater than 0.6.

Milky fluid (chylothorax) most often is seen following trauma or with disease involving the thoracic duct. In this case pleural fluid triglycerides often exceed 110 mg/dl. Long-standing effusions containing excessive amounts of cholesterol and exhibiting a satinlike sheen are called pseudochylous effusions.

A pH less than 6 (particularly if accompanied by an elevated amylase) suggests gastric contents from esophageal rupture, and a pH between 6 and 7 implies empyema. Samples for pH determination must be collected anaerobically.

If the pleural fluid is bloody or turbid, with the red cell count exceeding 100,000/mm³, malignancy is found in more than 50% of cases. Bloody fluid also may be found in trauma or pulmonary embolism and in rare cases in congestive heart failure, infections, and cirrhosis of the liver.

A white blood cell count of more than 1000/mm³ in the absence of red cells suggests that the fluid is related to inflammation such as bacterial or tuberculous infection. If at least 50% of the white blood cells are polymorphonuclear, bacterial infection usually is the cause of the effusion. A preponderance of lymphocytes is seen in effusions caused by tuberculosis. Neoplasm or sarcoidosis occasionally may also cause pleural fluid lymphocytosis. Congestive heart failure rarely results in pleural white cell counts higher than 1000/mm³.

Eosinophil counts of 10% to 50% can be seen in Löffler's syndrome, polyarteritis nodosa, tropical eosinophilia, and Hodgkin's disease. When blood eosinophilia coexists, hypersensitivity reactions are suggested. Pleural fluid eosinophilia in the absence of blood eosinophilia often is of occult origin but has been related to pulmonary infection, trauma, malignant tumor, pulmonary infarction, or cirrhosis of the liver with ascites. Mesothelial cells may or may not be present, but more than 5% mesothelial cells virtually rules out tuberculous pleurisy.

Glucose should be measured during the fasting state, and if it exceeds 85 mg/dl in pleural fluid, the fluid is probably not caused by infection in the pleural space. In the absence of acute bacterial infection, levels of glucose less than 60 mg/dl suggest tuberculosis or malignancy, and a glucose concentration under 30 mg/dl most commonly is seen in patients with rheumatoid arthritis.

When abdominal pain accompanies pleural effusion, pancreatitis should be suspected, and in that case the pleural fluid amylase level will be higher than the serum amylase concentration. Pleural fluid that is gelatinous and bloody and contains elevated levels of hyaluronic acid suggests an underlying malignant mesothelioma.

In pleural effusions caused by malignancy there is a 50% chance of finding tumor cells by cytologic examination of a single specimen. If three or more specimens are obtained and a pleural biopsy is performed, up to 90% of malignant effusions can be correctly diagnosed.

Cultures of pleural fluid often are positive in empyema but are not diagnostically helpful in the patient with pneumonia and a sterile sympathetic effusion. If the fluid is foul smelling, anaerobes are the cause, but they may be difficult to isolate. Turberculosis can be diagnosed by direct smear and culture in less than 30% of cases, possibly because pleural effusions resulting from tuberculosis often are caused by a hypersensitivity reaction to the tubercle bacillus, and thus few bacilli may be present. If possible, large amounts of fluid should be examined to improve the chances of obtaining a positive culture.

Biopsy techniques may be important in evaluating pleural effusions. A pleural biopsy should be performed in the case of an exudative effusion if the diagnosis has not been made by other means. Complications are uncommon but include pneumothorax and bleeding. Implantation of carcinoma in the needle tract also is reported in rare cases. The contraindications to pleural biopsy are an uncooperative patient, severe coagulation defects, and limited respiratory reserve. A tissue diagnosis can be made in 75% of cases of tuberculous fluid accumulation and in more than 50% of cases of effusion caused by malignancy or rheumatoid disease. Biopsy of the internal mammary nodes via the second intercostal space gives positive findings in up to 50% of cases of effusions resulting from tuberculosis or malignancy. The diagnosis can be established by thoracoscopy or pleuroscopy (procedures that allow direct visualization of the pleura) in about 90% of cases caused by tuberculosis or malignancy. Open pleural biopsy as a diagnostic procedure should be considered only when other procedures have failed.

Pleural effusions have numerous causes, which are given in the following list:

Causes of pleural effusion

Common
Malignancy
Congestive heart failure
Peritoneal dialysis
Pulmonary infarction
Infection (bacterial, fungal, parasitic, tuberculous, viral)
Pancreatitis
Cirrhosis with ascites
Collagen diseases
Renal diseases (nephrotic syndrome)
Subphrenic abscess
Trauma to lung, mediastinum, or spine
Postmyocardial infarction (Dressler's syndrome)
Postcardiac injury
Idiopathic

Rare
Amiodarone
Amebiasis
Benign asbestos pleurisy
Catamenial pneumothorax
Central venous cannula insertion
Coagulation defects
Drug-induced lupus pleuritis
Emphysema
Hepatitis B infection
Hydrocarbon ingestion
Hypoproteinemia
Iatrogenic (surgery, instillation of drugs)
Infectious mononucleosis
Löffler's syndrome
Malignant mesothelioma
Familial Mediterranean fever
Meig's syndrome
Methysergide therapy
Myxedema
Niemann-Pick disease
Nitrofurantoin
Pneumoconioses
Obstructed superior vena cava or azygos vein
Radiation therapy
Respiratory distress syndrome
Ruptured aneurysm
Ruptured dermoid cyst
Ruptured esophagus
Sarcoidosis
Spontaneous chylothorax
Trapped lung syndrome
Waldenström's macroglobulinemia
Wegener's granulomatosis
Whipple's disease
Yellow nail syndrome

The most common causes of pleural effusions are cancer, congestive heart failure, infection, and pulmonary embolism. If there is evidence of congestive heart failure, the fluid should resolve with drug treatment and nothing more need be done. If it does not resolve, however, or if there is no evidence of congestive heart failure, thoracentesis should be performed. A protein measurement, cell count and differential, and cytologic examinations should be ordered routinely.

If the primary diagnosis being considered is cancer or lymphoma, depending on the characteristics of the pleural fluid, only protein measurement and cytologic studies ordinarily need be obtained. If the effusion is chylous in nature, a determination of fat content (triglyceride and cholesterol) also is in order. If the fluid is purulent, routine culture and Gram stain should be added. However, other studies that have a high correlation with the specific diagnosis being considered should be included, such as the glucose concentration in rheumatoid disease, the amylase level in pancreatitis, and appropriate stains and cultures in tuberculosis and fungal infections. If the diagnosis still has not been established, pleural biopsy and other studies are indicated. This approach to the diagnosis of pleural effusion is more reasonable and economical than ordering all studies at the initial examination without taking the time to evaluate and proceed in an orderly fashion.

Therapy depends on the underlying cause and nature of the fluid, but repeated thoracentesis or instillation of sclerosing agents such as tetracycline may be necessary for recurring effusions.

PNEUMOTHORAX

Spontaneous pneumothorax most commonly occurs in young men when a bleb ruptures, allowing air to escape into the pleural space, and results in partial or total collapse of a lung. Occasionally the tension within the chest may increase from the trapping of more air, which results in the collapse of a large part of the lung with a shift of the heart and mediastinum to the opposite side; this is called a tension pneumothorax, an extremely dangerous situation, because it compromises the opposite lung. The patient initially may note pain, which is followed by increasing dyspnea. Inadequate blood supply to the lungs and heart may result in a pale, sweaty, dyspneic patient.

Physical examination reveals hyperresonance with absent breath sounds over the pneumothorax. The chest roentgenogram exhibits an area of hyperlucency with an absence of lung markings. The collapsed lung may be evident as an area of increased density. With tension pneumothorax the diaphragm is pushed down, and mediastinal structures are displaced to the contralateral side.

Chronic obstructive pulmonary disease, pneumonia and other infections, malignancies, the pneumoconioses, and sarcoidosis are other conditions in which spontaneous pneumothorax may occur. If done incorrectly, cannulation of a subclavian vein also may result in this complication. Pneumothorax is a common finding in infants with respiratory distress syndrome, the incidence varying with severity of the syndrome, intensity of respiratory assistance, and use of continuous positive airway pressure (CPAP) or positive end-expiratory pressure (PEEP).

Recurring spontaneous pneumothorax may be associated with menses. This entity, catamenial pneumothorax, is found predominantly on the right side and usually is associated with endometriosis. The management of patients who have received respiratory therapy also is occasionally complicated by subcutaneous emphysema, pneumomediastinum, and pneumothorax.

Pneumothorax can be relieved by inserting a large-bore needle or catheter under a water seal to permit the air to escape, thus allowing the lung to reexpand and relieving the dyspnea and pain. In the case of a tension pneumothorax a medical emergency exists until the air is released. A conservative approach should be used in clamping or removing a tube thoracostomy. Before removal there should be no air leak and full lung expansion. Removal should be preceded by a trial of tube clamping for 24 to 48 hours with no recurrence of the pneumothorax.

The rent in the lung frequently closes over, and the lung completely reexpands; however, recurrence is common. Pleurodesis often can be accomplished with talc or tetracycline instillation; if this does not correct the situation or if three or more episodes occur, surgical intervention usually is necessary.

PLEURAL TUMORS

Primary pleural tumors are of two varieties: a localized fibrous mesothelioma that often is pedunculated, benign, and treated by localized excision, and a highly malignant, diffuse mesothelioma related to asbestos exposure in up to 40% of cases (see Chapter 133).

The benign mesotheliomas may be associated with hypoglycemia and rheumatoid-like symptoms, both of which are cured with removal of the tumor. The chest roentgenogram, often the first evidence of abnormality, reveals a localized, encapsulated lesion, commonly along pleural planes. The therapy is surgical removal, and the prognosis is good.

Malignant mesothelioma often is characterized chiefly by the signs and symptoms of a pleural effusion. It may be manifested by pleuritic pain, dull, aching chest pain, or shortness of breath. Chest roentgenograms reveal a pattern similar to that of a rapidly progressing pleural effusion. Instillation of tetracycline, quinacrine, or radioactive phosphorus may obliterate the pleural space and temporarily prevent the further formation of fluid, but the treatment of malignant mesothelioma often is unsatisfactory. A patient occasionally partially responds to total pleurectomy, chemotherapy with variety of drugs, radiation therapy, or a combination of these. The overall outlook is generally grave, with most patients dying within the year following diagnosis.

Metastatic tumors arising from the lung, breast, pancreas, ovary, and colon may involve the pleura. Thymoma and lymphoma also can spread to the pleura. Therapy includes local irradiation for pain relief and management appropriate for the primary lesion.

BIBLIOGRAPHY

Arai H and others: Significance of the quantification and demonstration of hyaluronic acid in tissue specimens for the diagnosis of pleural mesothelioma, Am Rev Respir Dis 120:529, 1979.

Ayvazian L: Diagnostic aspects of pleural effusion, Bull NY Acad Med 53:532, 1977.

Barrocar A: Catamenial PNX: case report and review of the literature, Am Surg 45:340, 1979.

Ellis K and Wolff M: Mesotheliomas and secondary tumors of the pleura, Semin Roentgenol 12:303, 1977.

Felson B, editor: Causes of pleural fluid, Semin Roentgenol 12:327, 1977.

Herman MA: Recurring spontaneous pneumothorax associated with menses, South Med J 69:488, 1976.

Light RW and George RB: Incidence of pleural effusion after abdominal surgery, Chest 69:621, 1976.

Ogata ES and others: Pneumothorax in the respiratory distress syndrome: incidence and effect on vital signs, blood gases and pH, Pediatrics 58:177, 1976.

Sahebjami H and Loudon RG: Pleural effusion: pathophysiology and clinical features, Semin Roentgenol 12:269, 1977.

Sahn SA, editor: Diseases of the pleura, Semin Respir Med 9(1):1 1987.

Storey DD, Dines DE, and Coles DT: Pleural effusion, a diagnostic dilemma, JAMA 236, 2183, 1976.

Zimmerman JE, Dunbar BS, and Klingenmaier CH: Management of subcutaneous emphysema, pneumomediastinum and pneumothorax during respirator therapy, Crit Care Med 3:69, 1975.

135 · DISEASES OF THE MEDIASTINUM, DIAPHRAGM, AND CHEST WALL

Stanley L. Altschuler

MEDIASTINAL DISEASE

The mediastinum is located in the midthorax and separates the two pleural cavities. From the thoracic inlet to the diaphragm the mediastinum is divided into three major compartments: anterior, middle, and posterior. The anterior mediastinum is situated in front of the heart and contains the thymus gland, the anterior mediastinal lymph nodes, and the internal mammary arteries and veins. The middle mediastinal compartment contains the pericardium and heart, the great vessels, the phrenic and part of the vagus nerves, the trachea and main bronchi, and lymph nodes. The posterior mediastinum contains the descending thoracic aorta, esophagus, thoracic duct, azygos and hemiazygos veins, the sympathetic nerves and portions of the vagus nerve, and posterior mediastinal lymph nodes. Diseases of the mediastinum are predominantly infectious, tumor related, or the result of abnormalities of the contained structures. Chest roentgenograms often are crucial in diagnosing diseases of the mediastinum, and the use of computed tomography of the chest has significantly enhanced the diagnoses of these diseases.

Mediastinitis

Acute infections of the mediastinum usually result from esophageal perforation. The esophagus may be perforated from carcinoma, from an impacted foreign body, as a complication of esophagoscopy, or spontaneously after vomiting. Infection from adjacent tissues also can spread into the mediastinum. The clinical manifestations of mediastinitis include severe retrosternal pain associated with chills and high fever. Subcutaneous emphysema may be present in the soft tissues of the neck. The diagnosis is suggested by the clinical presentation and substantiated by roentgenographic findings, including widening of the mediastinum, the presence of air in the mediastinum or soft tissues of the neck, and the presence of pneumothorax or hydropneumothorax. Untreated mediastinitis can result in abscess formation, with perforation of the abscess into the pleural cavity, esophagus, or bronchus. Treatment involves the use of appropriate antibiotics, maintenance of fluid balance, and identification and treatment of the originating insult.

Chronic mediastinitis usually develops slowly and asymptomatically. The diagnosis often is first suspected on the basis of a routine chest roentgenogram or occasionally because of symptoms related to pressure on one of the mediastinal structures. Chronic mediastinitis can be granulomatous or sclerosing.

The cause of granulomatous mediastinitis is seldom established, but histoplasmosis or tuberculosis sometimes is implicated. Sarcoidosis, silicosis, and other fungal infections can also be responsible. Most patients are asymptomatic, but obstruction of the superior vena cava and the esophagus may be the initial manifestation. *Superior vena caval syndrome* is characterized by puffiness of the face and neck, cyanosis, headaches, epistaxis, and light-headedness.

The cause of sclerosing mediastinitis is only rarely established; it is sometimes associated with retroperitoneal fibrosis or other sclerosing conditions, leading to the concept of a multifocal fibrosclerosis. This association has been reported in cases of systemic lupus erythematosus, rheumatoid disease, and during treatment with methysergide maleate. The diagnosis is suspected by finding a widening of the upper half of the mediastinum on chest roentgenogram, but a biopsy is required for confirmation. Clinical manifestations include superior vena caval obstruction and obstruction of the tracheobronchial tree and esophagus. Treatment is directed at correcting the underlying cause and relieving obstruction.

Pneumomediastinum

The presence of gas in the mediastinum, or pneumomediastinum, is relatively rare. It usually occurs spontaneously but may result from trauma or follow rupture of the esophagus or tracheobronchial tree during endoscopy. Spontaneous pneumomediastinum usually results from severe coughing or vomiting, deep inspiratory efforts, or Valsalva's maneuver and may occur in the mother during the time of delivery, particularly when labor is prolonged. Gas accumulates in the mediastinum and hilar areas and also can result in pneumothorax. These findings are evident on the chest roentgenogram as abnormal hyperlucent areas. The air usually passes into the neck, resulting in gas in the tissues or subcutaneous emphysema. If the gas is unable to leave the mediastinal compartment, pressure may develop, causing compression of vascular or respiratory structures. Air also may enter the mediastinum as a result of dental extractions or following trauma to the neck.

The clinical manifestations include the sudden onset of retrosternal pain radiating to the shoulders and arms. Swallowing and respiratory efforts may increase the pain, and dyspnea may be severe. Subcutaneous emphysema is sometimes noted in the neck or over the thoracic wall. Pneumomediastinum usually resolves spontaneously or after correction of the underlying cause. Chest tube drainage of air for reexpansion of the lung may be required if a pneumothorax also develops.

Anterior mediastinal masses

Thymomas, germinal tumors, thyroid lesions, and lipomas constitute most abnormal masses in the anterior mediastinum.

Thymomas are the most commonly occurring neoplasms in the anterior mediastinum and may be benign or malignant. Thymomas are often associated with myasthenia gravis, and most of the symptoms related to thymomas are the result of this condition.

Germinal tumors include dermoid cysts, teratomas, seminomas, choriocarcinomas, and embryonal carcinomas. These tumors arise from primitive germ cell nests and are present from birth although they are manifested only later in life. Dermoid cysts contain only epidermis and its appendages, whereas teratomas contain all three embryonic derivatives. Most of these lesions are benign and asymptomatic and are discovered on routine chest roentgenograms. Thoracic seminomas are histologically similar to testicular seminomas and ovarian tumors. Most choriocarcinomas of the mediastinum occur in males; they grow rapidly and produce symptoms such as dyspnea, hemoptysis, Horner's syndrome, and gynecomastia. The possibility of metastasis from the testes must be eliminated in both seminoma and choriocarcinoma.

Thyroid goiters are usually asymptomatic and also are discovered on routine chest roentgenograms. Clinical manifestations include respiratory distress caused by tracheal compression, as well as stridor and hoarseness resulting from involvement of the recurrent laryngeal nerve. Usually an enlarged gland can be palpated in the neck region when a thyroid-related mediastinal mass is present.

Lipomas can occur in any of the mediastinal compartments but usually are found anteriorly. They often are visualized on chest roentgenograms and appear to have a density lower than surrounding tissues. Occasionally fatty deposition in the anterior mediastinum can be the result of corticosteroid administration. Fibromas, hemangiomas, and lymphangiomas are other mesenchymal tumors that may rarely appear in the anterior mediastinum.

Middle mediastinal masses

Lymph node enlargement in Hodgkin's disease and non-Hodgkin's lymphoma usually occurs in the middle mediastinum. Metastasis from cancer in the lungs, gastrointestinal tract, prostate, or kidneys can also result in lymph node enlargement; other causes include tuberculosis, histoplasmosis, and sarcoidosis.

Bronchogenic cysts are congenital abnormalities usually located near the carina. They often have a cavitary appearance on chest roentgenograms. These cysts are mostly asymptomatic but occasionally cause tracheal compression. Pericardial cysts usually are located in the cardiophrenic angles and remain asymptomatic but sometimes cause dyspnea.

Dilations or aneurysms of major vessels in the mediastinum also can occur as mediastinal masses. Dilation of the main pulmonary artery usually is the result of pulmonary hypertension or a left-to-right shunt. Aortic aneurysms may result from arteriosclerosis, syphilis, trauma, dissection, stenosis, or infection. Patients with aortic aneurysms commonly are asymptomatic, but symptoms related to compression of the superior vena cava, recurrent laryngeal nerve, or tracheobronchial tree may develop. Dissecting aneurysms usually result in severe retrosternal pain radiating to the back.

Posterior mediastinal masses

Neurogenic neoplasms can arise from nerve sheaths, nerve cells, or all nerve elements and usually occur in the posterior mediastinum. Nerve sheath tumors are usually benign, whereas tumors arising from other nerve elements are often malignant. Mediastinal neurofibromas and neurilemomas arise from peripheral nerves. Sympathetic ganglia may give rise to neuroblastomas and pheochromocytomas. Chemodectomas arise from paraganglionic cells.

Esophageal lesions, including neoplasm, diverticulum, hiatus hernia, and megaesophagus, are located in the posterior mediastinum. Esophageal neoplasms frequently are malignant, although benign lesions also occur. Esophageal diverticula are of three types and can be differentiated on the chest roentgenogram on the basis of location. Zenker's diverticula are located in the pharyngeal region. Traction diverticula are commonly the result of granulomatous processes such as histoplasmosis or tuberculosis and are located in the middle portion of the esophagus. Pulsion diverticula are located in the lower esophagus and are the result of mucosal outpouchings. Dilation of the esophagus may be caused by scleroderma, carcinoma, achalasia, or gastric regurgitation.

All of the various mediastinal masses can appear as localized lesions on chest roentgenograms. Surgical exploration often is required for both diagnosis and therapy.

DIAPHRAGMATIC DISEASE

The diaphragm is a musculotendinous structure that separates the thoracic and abdominal cavities. Muscle fibers arise from the thoracic ribs, lumbar vertebrae, and the xiphoid process and insert into a central tendon. Contraction of the muscles results in a downward movement of the diaphragm and expansion of the thoracic cage. In the normal individual diaphragmatic contraction is responsible for most of the air that is inspired during ventilation. Diaphragmatic excursion can be measured by roentgenographic techniques as well as by physical examination and is usually approximately 3.5 cm.

Abnormalities of motion

Although paralysis of the diaphragm may have any of several causes, the most common is phrenic nerve invasion by carcinoma. Other causes of diaphragmatic paralysis include disc degeneration in the cervical area, abnormalities of nerve roots from the third to the fifth cervical vertebrae, and viral neuritis. Other disorders of diaphragmatic motion include tonic contractions, diaphragmatic flutter, and persistent hiccups. Pain and dyspnea may result from these abnormal contractions. Elevation of a hemidiaphragm, abnormal motion during respiration, mediastinal swing during respiration, or paradoxic motion with sniffing can be demonstrated fluoroscopically in patients with abnormal diaphragmatic activity. The therapy is directed at the underlying cause.

Eventration

Eventration is a congenital anomaly with abnormal muscular development of a hemidiaphragm. A portion of the diaphragm consists of a thin, membranous sheath rather than the normal muscle fibers. The abnormality usually is found on a routine roentgenographic study, and the diagnosis can be confirmed if necessary by the induction of a pneumoperitoneum. This abnormality usually is asymptomatic but occasionally results in respiratory or cardiac distress. Generally no therapy is required.

Herniation

Herniation of abdominal contents into the thoracic cavity can occur as a result of trauma or disruption through congenitally weak areas of the diaphragm. Herniation through the esophageal hiatus (hiatus hernia) is the common form of diaphragmatic hernia. Most patients with esophageal hiatus hernia are asymptomatic; however, retrosternal pain, particularly when the patient lies flat, is the most frequent clinical manifestation. On occasion the entire stomach may herniate through the esophageal hiatus and become incarcerated or strangulated. Hiatus hernia may result in the air-fluid level in the stomach being seen behind the heart on a chest roentgenogram. Treatment includes avoiding recumbent positions and using antacids.

Herniation through the posterior hiatus, or the foramen of Bochdalek, occurs in infants but rarely in adults. Herniation through the anteriorly situated Morgagni's foramen is also rare. These two unusual forms of hiatus hernia are relatively asymptomatic in adults.

Miscellaneous conditions

Other abnormalities of the diaphragm include intradiaphragmatic cysts, known as extralobar sequestration, and tumors of the diaphragm. Extralobar sequestration of lung tissue results when a lung bud develops within the diaphragm during embryonic development. The sequestered lung is aerated via the tracheobronchial tree. Blood is supplied by the abdominal aorta, and drainage occurs via systemic veins. Tumors of the diaphragm can be benign or malignant, but both types are quite rare. The diagnosis is suspected when an abnormal diaphragmatic mass is noted on the chest roentgenogram, but a definitive diagnosis often requires open biopsy. The therapy depends on the tumor type, but surgical removal at the time of diagnostic thoracotomy is the common procedure.

CHEST WALL DISEASE
Rib lesions

Accessory ribs arising from the seventh cervical vertebra are known as cervical ribs and often are asymptomatic; they are roentgenographically evident as simply a smaller set of ribs. These accessory ribs can compress subclavian vessels or the brachial plexus. The symptoms include arm pain, reduction of the peripheral pulse, and weakness of the upper extremities. If the symptoms are disabling, surgical removal of the cervical rib is required.

Notching of the ribs seen on the chest roentgenogram most commonly is caused by the dilation of intercostal arteries, which usually results from coarctation of the aorta. Rib notching may be associated with various other congenital cardiovascular defects.

Costochondral osteochondritis, or Tietze's syndrome, involves inflammation of the costochondral or costosternal joints. The disorder usually occurs in patients 20 to 40 years of age and is a self-limited disease characterized by anterior chest wall pain. Acute myocardial infarction may have to be ruled out in patients with this syndrome. In addition to chest pain with movement and respiratory effort, there is localized tenderness over the costosternal junction or cartilaginous aspect of the anterior rib cage. Roentgenographic studies are unrewarding. This condition is treated with aspirin or other antiinflammatory agents.

Neoplasms of the rib cage are almost always metastatic, with the primary source usually the lung or breast. Multiple myeloma and Hodgkin's disease less commonly involve the rib cage. Paget's disease also may be observed on roentgenographic examination of the ribs.

Sternal abnormalities

Pectus excavatum, or "funnel chest," is a depression of the sternum with the ribs protruding anteriorly. It often is associated with connective tissue disorders such as Marfan's syndrome or with multiple congenital defects. Most patients with pectus excavatum have normal pulmonary function studies and little or no respiratory disability. Surgery is required to correct the defects, but it is only rarely indicated and usually performed primarily for cosmetic purposes.

Pectus carinatum, or "pigeon breast," is a deformity in which the sternum protrudes anteriorly more than normal. This disorder frequently is associated with atrial or ventricular septal defects of the heart and occasionally associated with severe asthma of early childhood. Surgical correction is rarely if ever indicated.

Thoracic spinal abnormalities

Kyphosis is an abnormal posterior curvature of the thoracic spine, and *scoliosis* is an abnormal lateral curvature. Kyphoscoliosis can be classified as congenital, paralytic, or idiopathic. Congenital kyphoscoliosis may be associated with neurofibromatosis, Marfan's syndrome, or other hereditary disorders. Poliomyelitis is the most common cause of paralytic kyphoscoliosis. The cause of kyphoscoliosis may remain unknown, and in this case there is a female predominance.

Kyphoscoliosis can alter the mechanical properties of the respiratory system. Chest wall compliance is reduced, and the work of breathing is increased. Lung volumes, including tidal volumes, are smaller than normal. Eventually alveolar hypoventilation ensues, and complications associated with respiratory failure develop. These include pulmonary artery hypertension and right-sided heart failure, hypoxemia and hypercapnia, acid-base disturbances, and recurrent respiratory infections.

Corrective surgery and orthopedic devices may be helpful in the adolescent patient with kyphoscoliosis. Straightening of the curvature followed by fixation of the spine results in increased lung volumes and diminished mechanical abnormalities of the thoracic cage. Treatment of kyphoscoliosis in the advanced stage is directed at correction of hypoxemia and heart failure, as well as prevention of respiratory infections. Assisted ventilation by means of positive-pressure machines, negative-pressure devices such as cuirass respirators, or rocking beds can improve alveolar ventilation. Surgery usually is not recommended for advanced disease.

Ankylosing spondylitis

(See Chapter 12.)

Ankylosing spondylitis is a rheumatologic condition in which bony ankylosis of zygapophyseal joints and ossification of paravertebral structures result in fixation of the chest cage in inspiration. The male to female ratio is approximately 8:1. The association of ankylosing spondylitis with the histocompatibility antigen HLA-B27 supports a genetic relationship.

Low back pain and stiffness, sometimes associated with fever, fatigue, and weight loss, herald the onset of ankylosing spondylitis. Symptoms progress cephalad, eventually involving the thorax. Respiratory mechanics are altered, and alveolar hypoventilation with carbon dioxide retention develops. Pulmonary function testing reveals an increased residual volume and reduced vital capacity without evidence for airway obstruction.

Some patients with ankylosing spondylitis also develop pulmonary interstitial fibrosis. Other extraarticular manifestations include iridocyclitis, aortic insufficiency, and cardiac conduction abnormalities. The diagnosis is confirmed by the classic roentgenographic features, which include a "bamboo spine."

Treatment comprises exercise, physical therapy, and suppression of pain and inflammation. Indomethacin and phenylbutazone are the most effective antiinflammatory agents, but an initial trial of salicylates is recommended.

BIBLIOGRAPHY

Bergofsky EH: Respiratory failure in disorders of the thoracic cage, Am Rev Respir Dis 119:643, 1979.

Caillet R: Scoliosis diagnosis and management, Philadelphia, 1975, FA Davis Co.

Dines DE and others: Mediastinal granuloma and fibrosing mediastinitis, Chest 75:320, 1979.

Gacad G and Hamosh P: The lung in ankylosing spondylitis, Am Rev Respir Dis 107:286, 1973.

Gale A and others: Neurogenic tumors of the mediastinum, Ann Thorac Surg 17:434, 1974.

Gibson GJ and others: Pulmonary mechanics in patients with respiratory muscle weakness, Am Rev Respir Dis 115:389, 1977.

Heitzman ER: Computed tomography of the thorax: current perspectives, AJR 136:2, 1981.

McCredie M, Lovejoy FW, and Kaltreider NL: Pulmonary function in diaphragmatic paralysis, Thorax 17:213, 1962.

Proceedings of the International Symposium on the Diaphragm, Am Rev Respir Dis 119:1, 1979.

Salyer D, Salyer W, and Eggleston J: Benign developmental cysts of the mediastinum, Arch Pathol Lab Med 101:136, 1977.

136 · PRIMARY MALIGNANCIES OF THE LUNG

William Weiss

Pulmonary tumors may be benign or malignant. They have been classified by the World Health Organization into 13 types, with the distribution varying somewhat with geographic location and population subgroup. Almost 50% of the cases occurring in the general U.S. male population are squamous cell carcinomas, 15% to 20% are small cell carcinomas, 15% to 20% are adenocarcinomas, 10% are large cell carcinomas, and the remainder includes mixtures of squamous cell carcinoma and adenocarcinoma, carcinoids, bronchial gland tumors, and a few rarer types. In females squamous cell and small cell carcinomas are less common, and adenocarcinomas account for a larger proportion of the cases.

ETIOLOGY AND EPIDEMIOLOGY. Lung cancer is a disease of increasing importance, not only because of its frequency but also because current knowledge about its chain of causation makes prevention a possibility. Primary lung cancer has increased strikingly in incidence during this century, from a rare disease to the most common cause of cancer mortality in both men and women. More than 140,000 deaths result from lung cancer each year in the United States. It is almost entirely a disease of people 45 years of age or older, with an age-specific peak in the seventh decade of life. The drop in incidence after the seventh decade occurs primarily because of a cohort effect, that is, the oldest people today were born into cohorts whose lifelong risks of lung cancer were lower than those of later birth cohorts, probably as a result of lower exposure to carcinogens. Individual birth cohorts show a steadily increasing risk with increasing age. In recent years the risks have become higher in blacks than in whites. The reason for this is unclear. Recently the increase of the rates among men has slowed somewhat and even declined in white males, but the rates among women have increased exponentially. As a result, the male to female ratio has been falling from about 7:1 two decades ago to about 2:1 currently.

The explanation for these age, sex, and temporal characteristics lies in a strong association between the incidence of lung cancer and the prevalence of cigarette smoking in a given population, allowing for a lag of 20 to 40 years. The judgment that this association is one of cause and effect is based on a great deal of corroborated evidence that includes the following: (1) the incidence is negligible in people who have never smoked; (2) there is a stong dose-response relationship between the number of cigarettes smoked daily and the incidence of the disease; (3) this relationship holds for all histologic types of lung cancer, although it is not as strong for adenocarcinoma as for the other major types; (4) the association is consistent with what is known about lung cancer, such as its predilection for men, who in the past have been smokers more commonly than have women; (5) the incidence decreases among people who stop smoking until at 20 years after cessation it reaches a level almost as low as the incidence in nonsmokers; and (6) lung cancer has been produced in animals exposed to cigarette smoke.

The relationship of lung cancer to cigar and pipe smoke is much weaker, probably because most smokers of these forms of tobacco inhale relatively little smoke. At present smoking can account for 95% to 99% of lung cancer in men and 70% in women. Since women contribute only about 33% of the cases, it can be calculated that smoking can account for more than 86% of all cases. Therefore smoking must be taken into account when evaluating other causes of this disease.

A small proportion of lung cancer cases is caused by occupational exposure such as to asbestos, ionizing irradiation, coke oven fumes, arsenic, nickel, chromates, chloromethyl ethers, and mustard gas. When it has been studied, the interaction of these agents with cigarette smoke varies. It is more than additive in asbestos workers and uranium miners but one of antagonism in chloromethyl ether workers.

It is not clear whether ambient air pollution plays any significant role in causing lung cancer. The association is weak, inconsistent, and possibly spurious when positive because people in lower socioeconomic levels tend to live in more polluted areas and also are more commonly smokers than those in higher socioeconomic levels.

Lung cancer does not develop in everyone exposed to a pulmonary carcinogen. The lifetime risk of a heavy cigarette smoker is probably about 15%. Host factors must also be important in determining susceptibility, but much of the explanation for lung cancer not developing in most smokers lies with the induction-latent period, which may range from 30 to 60 years; thus competing causes of death remove many people from risk before the malignant process reaches clinical proportions.

The histologic type is important when considering etiologic factors. Recent data show that small cell carcinomas commonly are found in uranium miners and chloromethyl ether workers.

PATHOGENESIS. The evolution of changes in the bronchial epithelium in relation to the most common carcinogenic exposure, cigarette smoke, has been carefully studied. There is a loss of epithelial cilia, an increase in the number of cell rows, and the development of squamous metaplasia and cellular atypia. These abnormalities show a dose-response relationship to cigarette consumption and are less common in pipe and cigar smokers, presumably because they inhale less smoke. Eventually foci of carcinoma in situ develop in several areas, and sooner or later one or more of these become invasive. This observation accounts for the 10% of patients who have multiple cancers. People who stop smoking show regression of the epithelial abnormalities.

Lung cancer is predominantly a tumor of the medium-sized and small bronchi; thus it most often originates as a peripheral lesion. Tumors occur most commonly in the upper lobes. The lobar distribution is consistent with the pattern of particulate deposition in hollow casts of the human bronchial tree. Cancers that develop in the larger bronchi tend to produce enlargement of the hilar structures and bronchial obstruction. If the obstruction is partial, it may cause localized obstructive emphysema through a check-valve mechanism, but more commonly it progresses to produce atelectasis, distal pneumonitis, or suppuration. Occasionally the tumor itself cavitates and may be mistaken for an abscess. Sometimes there is direct invasion of surrounding organs. Characteristically lung cancer metastasizes early to regional nodes, mediastinal nodes, the liver, bone, adrenal glands, and the brain and less often to many other organs.

CLINICAL MANIFESTATIONS. The symptoms and signs of lung cancer are related to the primary tumor, extension to neighboring structures, metastases, and systemic effects. Some patients are asymptomatic at the time the tumor is detected, usually by routine chest roentgenograms, but most have clinical manifestations.

Symptoms related to the primary lesion most commonly include dyspnea and a chronic cough productive of small

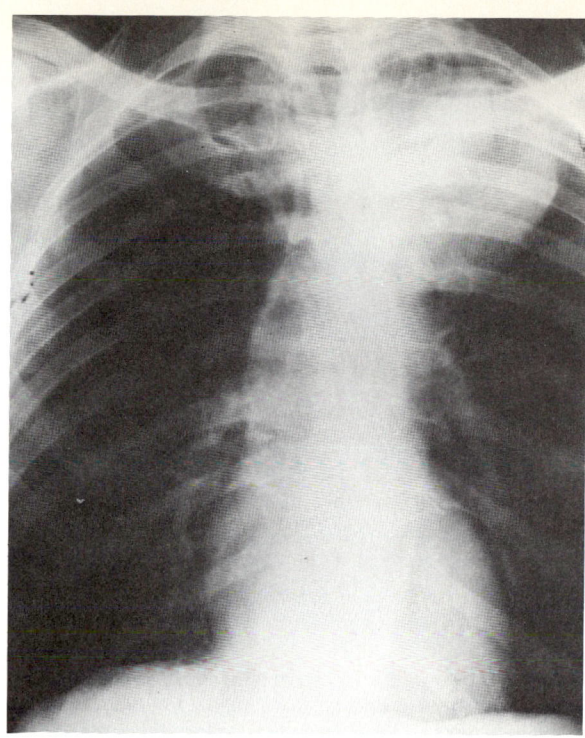

Fig. 136-1   Bronchogenic carcinoma at apex of left lung and invading brachial plexus (Pancoast's tumor). (Courtesy of George Popky, MD)

amounts of nonpurulent sputum. However, since most patients with this disease are cigarette smokers, chronic bronchitis and emphysema are common and often account for the cough and dyspnea. Less common symptoms include hemoptysis, usually limited to blood-streaked sputum, and in rare cases unilateral wheezing caused by partial obstruction of a major bronchus by the neoplasm. Distal infection may produce manifestations of pneumonia or suppuration, including chills, fever, and purulent sputum. Obstruction can also lead to signs of atelectasis of a lobe or an entire lung. When the tumor extends beyond the lung, many other symptoms and signs may develop. Pleural extension causes pleuritic pain and pleural effusion. Chest wall involvement often produces chest pain of a dull, boring, and persistent nature. Extension to the esophagus may cause dysphagia. Involvement of the recurrent laryngeal nerve paralyzes a vocal cord with resultant hoarseness. Superior vena caval obstruction is followed by edema of the face, neck, and upper extremities and dilated veins in these areas, sometimes with headache, dizziness, and vertigo (*superior vena caval syndrome*). Invasion of the brachial plexus by a neoplasm at the apex of the lung causes pain along the nerve distribution, muscle weakness, sensory disturbances of the upper extremity, and other abnormalities caused by neural involvement such as *Pancoast's syndrome* (Fig. 136-1.)

Distant metastases may produce visible or palpable superficial tumors, bone pain, headache, and paralyses or other neurologic manifestations. Lymph node enlargement, especially in the neck, is common. Hepatic involvement may cause epigastric distress and jaundice.

Systemic effects include anorexia, weight loss, fatigue, and weakness. In a small percentage of patients endocrine syndromes develop because of the secretion of hormonelike substances by the tumor; these syndromes include the syndrome of inappropriate antidiuretic hormone secretion (SIADH), Cushing's syndrome, gynecomastia, and hypercalcemia (see

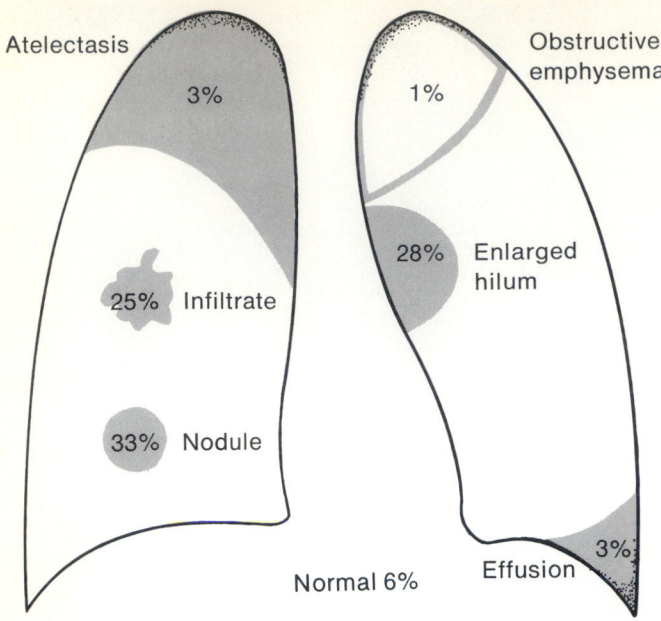

Atelectasis   3%

Obstructive emphysema   1%

28% Enlarged hilum

25% Infiltrate

33% Nodule

3%

Normal 6%   Effusion

Fig. 136-2   Early roentgenographic appearance of lung cancer found as result of semiannual chest x-ray screening of older men in Philadelphia Pulmonary Neoplasm Research Project (From Weiss W: J Respir Dis 1[3]:41, 1980.)

Chapter 192). Hypertrophic pulmonary osteoarthropathy, usually of the long bones, may cause pain, limitation of motion, and tenderness and is often associated with clubbing of the digits. Clubbing also often occurs alone. These manifestations tend to disappear after successful complete resection of the tumor.

Some neurologic and neuromuscular syndromes not caused by metastases may occur, such as cerebellar degeneration, neuropathy, and myopathy. These usually do not regress after resection of the tumor. Thrombophlebitis is fairly common, and nonbacterial thrombotic endocarditis with embolic phenomena may develop.

LABORATORY FINDINGS. Useful laboratory studies in lung cancer are limited mainly to the chest roentgenogram and cytologic examination of the sputum. Other laboratory studies depend on the clinical evidence of disease beyond the lung or of systemic syndromes. A chest roentgenogram should be obtained when pulmonary disease is suspected. Its use as a periodic screening device has been disappointing in improving the cure rate, because metastases usually have occurred by the time a tumor is large enough to be seen on the chest roentgenogram. Most lung cancers can be seen on a posteroanterior roentgenogram, but other views and types of examination may be useful. Early in the course of the disease most cancers are manifested as peripheral lesions; of these approximately half are round nodules or masses and half are ill-defined nonhomogeneous infiltrates that are sometimes mistaken for inflammatory disease (Fig. 136-2). Most of the remaining cancers, especially small cell carcinomas, arise in the central bronchi and are manifested as enlarged hilar shadows or mediastinal widening. Occasionally a pleural effusion or localized obstructive emphysema may be the first sign. In rare cases, but particularly when the tumor is entirely endobronchial, the chest roentgenogram may be normal.

With time atelectasis and pleural effusion become more commonly noted on the roentgenogram. These are most frequently found when the diagnosis is made after serious symptoms have led the patient to seek medical care. Lung cancers sometimes develop gross necrosis and excavate, producing cavities whose walls are characteristically irregular and nodular; these are usually best demonstrated by tomographic techniques.

Cytologic examinations of sputum are simple to perform, but good, deep cough specimens are essential in these studies and at least three should be examined. The inhalation of hypertonic saline vapor may be used to induce sputum. Cytologic studies of sputum occasionally show the presence of tumor cells even though the chest roentgenogram is normal. The diagnosis can often be confirmed by this method, but frequently it is not possible to determine the histologic type of cancer. A tissue specimen is preferred for this purpose.

DIAGNOSIS. The steps in making a diagnosis of lung cancer, in order of increasing complexity, cost, and hazard, are as follows: history, physical examination, chest roentgenogram, cytologic examination of sputum, bronchoscopy with cytologic examination of secretions and brushings, biopsy of easily accessible lesions, mediastinoscopy, and thoracotomy. A diagnosis can be only presumptive until cytologic or histologic evidence is obtained. Such evidence is highly desirable, because although surgery is the treatment of choice for other types, it is essentially worthless for small cell carcinoma.

Bronchoscopy is a minor, essentially risk-free procedure and, since the advent of the fiberoptic instrument a decade ago, offers little discomfort. Its efficacy in confirming the diagnosis is high as a result of cytologic examination of bronchial secretions and brush specimens and transbronchial biopsy. With these techniques it is possible to establish the presence of lung cancer in 80% to 90% of cases. In addition bronchoscopy can help determine the extent of the disease within the lung.

Biopsy of these lesions may be accomplished in other ways. In cases of peripheral lesions in the lung that cannot be reached with the bronchoscope, a needle biopsy under fluoroscopic control sometimes can provide a diagnostic specimen. If the cancer is large and adjacent to the chest wall, this technique offers no particular difficulty, but if it is small and deep in the lung, the procedure should be performed by an experienced physician with the recognition that pneumothorax and hemoptysis may result. Some metastases are readily sampled by biopsy, and thus the diagnosis may be easily made.

In a small percentage of cases an important step in establishing a diagnosis is mediastinoscopy. This is a minor procedure taking only half an hour. It can be performed with the patient under local anesthesia; the associated morbidity is about 1.5%, and the mortality is negligible. The procedure consists of making a small incision in the suprasternal notch, entering the superior mediastinum anterior to the trachea, and employing blunt dissection and an instrument similar to a laryngoscope. A biopsy of a lymph node may be made through the mediastinoscope. Mediastinoscopy can also be used in the staging of lung cancer.

Thoracotomy, the ultimate step in the diagnostic evaluation, is seldom necessary today. It should not be undertaken lightly, because the type of patient (aged and often with cardiac problems or chronic obstructive lung disease) who has lung cancer has a significant operative mortality of 2% to 10%, depending on how carefully patients are selected for surgery.

COURSE. Much of the natural history of lung cancer has been learned piecemeal and some from prospective periodic screening studies. Although many pieces of the puzzle are still

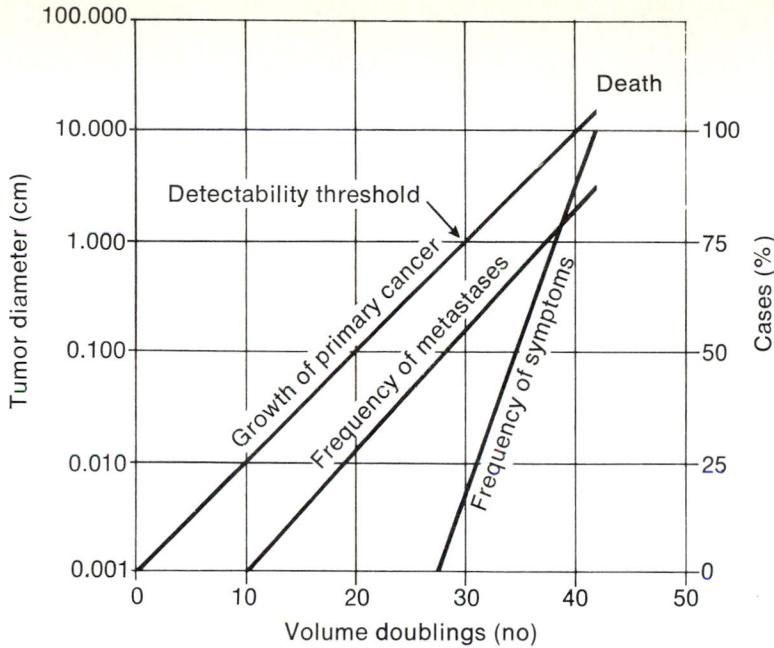

Fig. 136-3   Diagram of hypothetical natural history of lung cancer (see text for explanation). (From Weiss W: J Respir Dis 1:41, 1980.)

missing, a fairly clear picture is emerging, as diagrammed in Fig. 136-3.

The growth rate of cancer cells probably is close to exponential, since one cell divides to form two, two make four, and so on. This growth rate can be seen as a straight line by plotting the number of volume doublings on an arithmetic scale along the horizontal axis and the tumor size or diameter (which in a sphere bears a constant relationship to the volume or number of cells) on a logarithmic scale along the vertical axis. To simplify calculations, this model assumes that the average diameter of a cancer cell is 0.001 cm (10 μm); changing the cellular diameter would make little difference in the details.

A tumor diameter of 1 cm is at the threshold of detectability by chest roentgenogram, and some tumors are missed even at diameters of 2 or 3 cm. About 30 doublings are required for the tumor to reach a diameter of 1 cm, and symptoms rarely appear before this point. However, by 40 doublings the tumor reaches a diameter of 10 cm, at which point only a few patients survive. Metastases probably begin very early, arbitrarily designated in Fig. 136-3 at the tenth doubling. They are discernible in 85% of patients by the fortieth doubling. This model suggests that the diagnosis of lung cancer usually is made in the last quarter of a tumor's life cycle. Early diagnosis, allowing time for cure by resection, is possible only in the few patients whose cancers spread very late or not at all. This happens sometimes in squamous cell carcinoma but seldom in small cell carcinoma or adenocarcinoma. It is difficult to relate the number of volume doublings to units of time because doubling time varies in individual tumors by an order of magnitude.

MANAGEMENT. The treatment of choice for lung cancer is resection whenever feasible, except in patients with small cell carcinoma, which almost always has metastasized by the time of diagnosis and thus rarely is amenable to removal. The decision for resection depends on the stage of the disease and the patient's ability to tolerate major chest surgery.

A lung cancer may be staged after clinical evaluation, which includes all the steps taken to arrive at a diagnosis except thoracotomy. An elaborate classification of the extent of disease has been devised, but the final criteria for the decision against surgical treatment include: (1) the presence of distant metastases, (2) evidence of spread beyond the confines of the lung, or (3) a distance of less than 2 cm from the neoplasm to the carina of the trachea. If there is no evidence of such involvement by history, physical examination, chest roentgenogram, or bronchoscopy, the logical next step is mediastinoscopy. In preoperative evaluation the results of this simple procedure distinguish the resectable from the unresectable cases with considerable accuracy. Even small peripheral cancers may involve mediastinal nodes in up to 30% of the cases. Such an extension is considered a contraindication to surgery by most physicians. The low morbidity and negligible mortality of mediastinoscopy make it an excellent method for avoiding the hazards of thoracotomy.

There is some question as to how far the search for distant metastases should go if the clinical evaluation up to and including mediastinoscopy shows no evidence of spread. Liver and brain scans are warranted only if chemical tests of liver function show abnormalities or there are abnormal neurologic manifestations. In the absence of such abnormalities, scans seldom add information and are sometimes falsely positive. Roentgenographic bone surveys and scans in asymptomatic patients similarly are unjustified. Gallium citrate Ga 67 scans currently are under investigation.

Since lung cancer is a disease of middle to old age, the patients often have other health problems, some of which make chest surgery unfeasible. Most common among these problems are cardiac disease and chronic obstructive pulmonary disease. A patient with severe coronary disease or any other condition that suggests survival of less than 1 year is not generally considered a candidate for resectional surgery.

Because lung cancer patients usually are smokers, chronic bronchitis and emphysema are common complications that require an evaluation of pulmonary function. In some cases the clinical assessment suffices to determine the very good and the very bad risk cases. For cases between these extremes, pulmonary function tests should be performed. Unfortunately, there are no hard and fast rules or reliable critical values that allow more than a reasonable estimation of who is at low risk for surgery. It is also unfortunate that surgery may make the patient a respiratory cripple even though it cures his cancer. The judgment of operability is further complicated by the question of how much of the patient's dysfunction is caused by the cancer and how much is the result of other pulmonary diseases.

Given 100 patients, with a conservative approach to surgery, a clinical evaluation, including bronchoscopy, is likely to eliminate 75 cases as surgical candidates; mediastinoscopy may remove another 10, so that only 15 are candidates for thoracotomy. Of these only 13 are likely to have a completely resectable lesion. If the approach is more radical, a larger proportion of patients will undergo surgery, but the result will be essentially the same, with only a 11% to 13% 5-year survival rate overall.

Rarely does any other form of treatment have a significant curative impact. Radiotherapy often shrinks the primary tumor and may even kill all the malignant cells in it, but the distant metastases are unaffected. It may, however, provide palliation for superior vena caval syndrome, brain metastases, and bone pain. Early results of trials with multiple-drug regimens in patients with small cell carcinoma suggest some prolongation of life. Since this type of cancer is almost never detected before metastases occur, radiotherapy and chemotherapy are the treatments of choice. These therapies also may be of some value in patients unsuitable for surgery for other reasons.

PREVENTION. Because of the overall poor results in the management of lung cancer, prevention deserves more attention. Campaigns against cigarette smoking and exposure to carcinogens in the workplace are important. It is likely that the elimination of tobacco and industrial carcinogens would result in the almost complete disappearance of this dread disease and return its incidence to the rarity it had early in this century— a far cry from the approximately 140,000 deaths it now causes annually in the United States.

BIBLIOGRAPHY

Archer VE, Gillam JD, and Wagoner JK: Respiratory disease mortality among uranium miners, Ann NY Acad Sci 271:280, 1976.

Ashbaugh DG: Mediastinoscopy, Arch Surg 100:568, 1970.

Auerbach O and others: Changes in bronchial epithelium in relation to sex, age, residence, smoking, and pneumonia, N Engl J Med 267:111, 1962.

Benfield JR and others: Current and future concepts of lung cancer (UCLA Conference), Ann Intern Med 83:93, 1975.

Doll R and Peto R: Mortality in relation to smoking: 20 years' observations on male British doctors, Br Med J 2:1525, 1976.

Fox W and Scadding JG: Medical Research Council comparative trial of surgery and radiotherapy for primary treatment of small-celled or oat-celled carcinoma of bronchus, Lancet 2:63, 1973.

Geddes DM: The natural history of lung cancer: a review based on rates of tumor growth, Br J Dis Chest 73:1, 1979.

Hammond EC, Selikoff IJ, and Seidman H: Asbestos exposure, cigarette smoking, and death rates, Ann NY Acad Sci 330:473, 1979.

Tisi GM: Preoperative evaluation of pulmonary function, Am Rev Respir Dis 119:293, 1979.

Weiss W: Lung cancer due to chemicals, Comp Ther 5:18, 1979.

Weiss W: The Philadelphia Pulmonary Neoplasm Research Project, Appl Radiol 8:50, 138, 1979.

Weiss W: Lung cancer: diagnosis and preoperative evaluation, J Respir Dis 1:41, 1980.

Weiss W and others: Risk of lung cancer according to histologic type and cigarette dosage, JAMA 222:799, 1972.

137·TUMORS OF THE LUNG OTHER THAN BRONCHOGENIC CARCINOMA

William L. Morrissey

Although primary malignant lung tumors constitute the most common and most serious form of pulmonary tumors, other lung tumors are not uncommon. Included in the latter category are bronchial adenomas, lymphomas, fibromas, chondromas, papillomas, lipomas, hamartomas, and metastatic tumors. Benign neoplasms constitute less than 10% of primary pulmonary neoplasms.

BRONCHIAL ADENOMA

Bronchial adenoma accounts for somewhat less than 5% of all tumors of the lung but may represent 50% of benign lesions. There is now a tendency to classify it as malignant because of its aggressive local invasion and rare distant metastases. Bronchial adenoma originates from cells in the bronchial wall, usually in proximal airways. It generally is only locally invasive and histologically is either of the carcinoid or cylindromatous (cystadenoma) type; 90% are carcinoid. Bronchial adenoma is associated with hemoptysis or the sequelae of obstruction such as pneumonia in patients over 30 years of age. In rare cases the carcinoid form may produce the carcinoid syndrome with wheezing, episodic flushing, cyanosis, diarrhea, right-sided valvular heart disease, increased serum levels of 5-hydroxytryptamine (serotonin), and increased urine levels of 5-hydroxyindoleacetic acid (5-HIAA). This syndrome also may occur with carcinoid tumors of the intestinal tract, invariably after hepatic metastasis, and with oat cell or undifferentiated bronchogenic carcinoma.

The carcinoid syndrome is treated symptomatically if local resection for the adenoma is not curative. Although endoscopic removal has been attempted in the past, this has proved unsatisfactory and should be reserved for patients unable to tolerate thoracotomy. The prognosis for long-term survival is good, although extensive local spread or (in rare cases) distant metastasis may be fatal.

LYMPHOMA AND LYMPHOPROLIFERATIVE DISORDERS

Primary pulmonary lymphoma without extrathoracic or mediastinal involvement is rare, but lymphomatous involvement of the lung, including both parenchymal and pleural manifestations, may occur in up to 40% of patients with disseminated lymphoma. Hilar adenopathy, nodular or infiltrative parenchymal lesions, and, less commonly, pleural effusions may all occur. The symptoms include dyspnea, pain, cough, localized wheezing, hemoptysis, and systemic manifestations.

Other lymphoproliferative disorders affecting the lungs include lymphocytic interstitial pneumonia, Sjögren's syndrome, pseudolymphoma, Waldenström's macroglobulinemia, leukemia, amyloidosis, and multiple myeloma.

BENIGN TUMORS

Benign endobronchial tumors include fibroma, chondroma, papilloma, and lipoma, with the first two accounting for 80% of these lesions. They are usually manifested by obstructive related symptoms, may be confused with bronchial adenoma, and require local or endoscopic removal.

Hamartomas are benign but disorganized collections of nor-

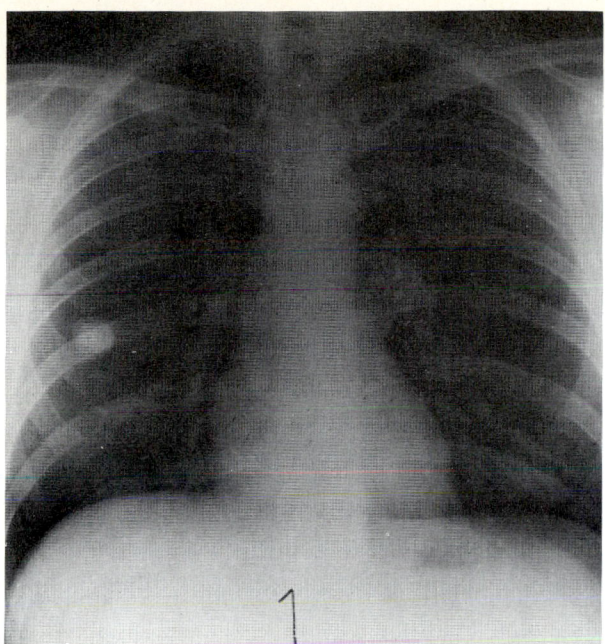

Fig. 137-1   Hamartoma manifest as solitary pulmonary nodule containing calcium. (Courtesy of George Popky, MD.)

mal tissue. In the lung they usually contain primarily muscle, collagen, or cartilage. Most are discovered in asymptomatic individuals in whom the chest roentgenogram was obtained for other reasons. The lesion usually is round, less than 5 cm in diameter, and may be flecked with calcium (popcorn calcification) (Fig. 137-1). Resection may be necessary to confirm the diagnosis and to rule out malignancy.

METASTATIC TUMORS

Metastatic tumors may involve the lung in several ways. Multiple nodular densities, particularly from kidney, breast, thyroid, or testicular primary sites, may be seen on the chest roentgenogram. Diffuse spread of tumor cells throughout the lung (lymphangitic carcinomatosis) results in rapidly progressive pulmonary disease terminating in respiratory failure; the most common primary sites for this type of tumor spread include the stomach, colon, bronchus, larynx, breast, prostate, and pancreas. Progressively severe dyspnea is common, but pleuritic chest pain, cyanosis, tachypnea, shallow respirations, and signs and symptoms of cor pulmonale may develop. The chest roentgenogram usually shows bilateral diffuse linear shadows or fine nodular shadows. Less commonly, hilar enlargement or a parenchymal mass lesion also may be seen. The syndrome may be difficult to distinguish from other causes of diffuse lung disease without resorting to lung biopsy. In patients receiving chemotherapy or irradiation of the thorax, tumor spread may have to be differentiated from radiation-induced or drug-induced changes as well as from opportunistic infections, such as those caused by *Pneumocystis carinii*. The therapy available is generally unsatisfactory, although steroids may provide some symptomatic relief.

SOLITARY PULMONARY NODULE

The solitary pulmonary nodule discovered on routine roentgenographic examination of the chest in the asymptomatic individual may have one of many origins. Because of this, it represents a difficult diagnostic and therapeutic problem.

Referred to as a coin lesion, this nodule appears as a rounded abnormal shadow on the chest roentgenogram. It is well circumscribed, round or oval, surrounded by normal lung, smooth bordered, homogeneous, noncavitated, and with no associated satellite lesions. Overall it appears that about 5% are malignant, although some surgical series report up to a 50% rate of malignancy. The risk of malignancy is increased in males, smokers, and those over 40 years of age. The differential diagnosis includes granulomas (the most common benign cause), hamartomas, and other benign lung tumors. Pulmonary infarcts and interlobar effusions (vanishing tumor) are other possibilities. Additional causes include primary lung malignancies and metastatic lesions. If metastatic, the primary site is most often the kidney, colon, or nasopharyngeal area.

Although age, smoking history, previous granulomatous infections, and positive skin and serologic tests for fungi or tuberculosis may be helpful, they rarely allow a definitive diagnosis. The availability of previous chest roentgenograms may diminish the need for further evaluation, since the doubling time for carcinomatous lesions varies from about 6 weeks to 18 months. More rapid growth suggests an inflammatory process, whereas roentgenographic stability longer than 2 years makes malignancy unlikely. The presence of laminated or stippled calcification also suggests a benign lesion. The introduction of computed tomography has been reported to increase the ability to detect calcium.

Bronchoscopy or percutaneous transthoracic needle biopsy sometimes can establish the diagnosis, but generally thoracotomy is required. Extensive workup for a primary tumor elsewhere before thoracotomy is unwarranted unless there are specific symptoms or laboratory abnormalities referable to another organ system. Mediastinoscopy is rarely helpful in the diagnosis.

Resection has therapeutic as well as diagnostic value. Surgical removal of a primary lung tumor occurring as a solitary nodule may result in a 50% 5-year survival rate. Resection of a solitary metastasis from a known primary tumor may be indicated if the primary tumor has been completely eradicated and there are no other known metastases; the best results have been obtained in cases of sarcoma and colonic cancer.

BIBLIOGRAPHY

Filly R, Blank N, and Castellins RA: Radiologic distribution of intrathoracic disease in previously untreated patients with Hodgkin's disease and non-Hodgkin's lymphoma, Radiology 120:277, 1976.

Goodwin JD: Carcinoid tumors: an analysis of 2837 cases, Cancer 36:560, 1975.

Heitzman ER, Markarian B, and DeLise CT: Lymphoproliferative disorders of the thorax, Semin Roentgenol 10:73, 1975.

Lillington GA: The solitary pulmonary nodule—1974, Am Rev Respir Dis 110:699, 1974.

Okike N, Bernatz PE and Woolner LB: Carcinoid tumors of the lung Ann Thorac Surg 22:270, 1976.

Yang S, and Lin C: Lymphangitic carcinomatosis of the lungs, Chest 62:179, 1972.

Dental correlations

Peter D. Quinn

Statistically, the most common respiratory diseases of impact in the outpatient setting are bronchitis, emphysema, and asthma. The first two are discussed together under chronic obstructive pulmonary disease (COPD). Considering bronchitis and emphysema together is a somewhat arbitrary coupling, made because these diseases rarely exist singly in pure form. Especially in the patient with long-standing disease, both bronchitis and emphysema are more than likely present. These two are dealt with separately from asthma to point out an important difference: COPD is largely irreversible. The damage to the tracheobronchial tree and alveolar walls is demonstrable. Although some of the edema, inflammation, and sputum production decreases with cessation of smoking in chronic bronchitis, the underlying pathology tends to continue. The destruction and dilation of terminal alveoli in emphysema is truly irreversible. Asthma, on the other hand, is acute and episodic with no inherent tissue damage. It is more of an abnormal and excessive responsiveness of the tracheobronchial tree.

CHRONIC BRONCHITIS

It must be remembered that chronic bronchitis is a clinical diagnosis made by documenting a chronic cough and sputum production for at least 3 months for two consecutive years. Smoking is the leading cause of COPD, but in a patient without risk factors (that is, tobacco use, environmental pollutants, and chronic viral or bacterial infection), α-antitrypsin deficiency should be ruled out. Formerly these patients were referred to as "blue bloaters" because most were obese with some evidence of cyanosis. These patients give a history of frequent, protracted "colds," which actually are exacerbations of the underlying disease process brought on by infections (viral, bacterial, or atypical). The slowly progressive course of the disease is punctuated by these episodic infections. In the later stages of bronchitis the Po_2 can be decreased (less than 70 torr) and the Pco_2 is elevated. The hypoxia can cause secondary cor pulmonale and polycythemia.

MANAGEMENT. The dentist can assess the degree of impairment caused by bronchitis by reviewing symptoms and therapy. The degree of dyspnea is paramount. Dyspnea only with marked exertion portends a better prognosis than dyspnea at rest or with mild exertion. Therapy includes the following:

1. Cessation of smoking and avoidance of other respiratory irritants
2. Adequate fluid intake to decrease the viscosity of secretions (increased humidity also can be helpful)
3. Bronchodilators: theophylline or other zanthines, which can be tested for efficacy by measuring forced expiratory volume before and after administration
4. Adrenergic agents: β_2 selective agents such as terbutaline cause bronchodilation while avoiding β_1 cardiac effects; some of these drugs can be administered with inhalants
5. Corticosteroids: beneficial in certain cases but usually avoided because of long-term side effects
6. Antibiotics: appropriate antibiotics, guided by cultures and sensitivity of a sputum specimen, for upper respiratory tract infections
7. Oxygen therapy: indicated only when severe hypoxemia is present or when O_2 is shown to improve exercise tolerance

EMPHYSEMA

In contrast to bronchitis, emphysema is a pathologic diagnosis, made by demonstrating destruction of lung parenchyma and loss of elasticity of the alveoli. The result is a marked decrease in forced expiratory volume with overinflation of the lungs. Clinically, these patients have dyspnea with increased anteroposterior chest diameter ("barrel chest"), decreased breath sounds, and hyperresonant lung fields. These patients have been referred to as "pink puffers," because unlike bronchitis patients they are more asthenic, less edematous, and not cyanotic. Expiration is sometimes associated with "pursed lips" in an attempt to stop collapse of alveoli on end-expiration. In smokers, bronchitis usually precedes emphysema, whereas a "pure" form of emphysema without bronchitis can be associated with α-antitrypsin deficiency. The clinical course of emphysema is more relentless and less responsive to treatment than that of bronchitis.

MANAGEMENT. Therapy is limited for the irreversible lung damage in emphysema. Some of the measures mentioned for bronchitis (that is, bronchodilators, corticosteroids, antibiotics, and physical therapy) at times can be helpful. Oxygen therapy often is warranted in severe disease but should be used with caution. O_2 therapy is designed to increase oxygenation without suppressing the drive to breath. Because of chronic CO_2 retention, patients with emphysema become less sensitive to hypercapnia (increased CO_2). They can develop a respiratory drive stimulated only by hypoxia. Increasing their O_2 could potentially cause hypoventilation by removing the respiratory stimulus.

Dental management of patients with COPD

1. Assess the degree of disease. Dyspnea at rest or with mild exertion calls for special caution.
2. Look for signs of cardiac disease secondary to COPD. Atrial and ventricular arrythmias are common with pulmonary hypertension, hypoxia, or respiratory acidosis. Vasoconstrictors are contraindicated.
3. Avoid long appointments or complicated, stressful procedures.
4. Defer nonemergency care during exacerbations such as upper respiratory tract infections.
5. Avoid using sedatives or narcotics. They can depress the respiratory drive and cause increased hypoxia and carbon dioxide retention.
6. When enough alveolar septae are destroyed in emphysema, spaces greater than 1 cm can form. They are called "bulla" and can spontaneously rupture, causing pneumothorax. Positive pressure ventilation also can lead to rupture. Therefore general anesthesia should be avoided or undertaken with extreme care and after consultation.
7. Avoid vasoconstrictors in patients on bronchodilator therapy. The combination could cause cardiac arrythmia.
8. For patients on corticosteriod therapy, use prophylaxis for adrenal suppression when indicated.
9. Use oxygen with care. In patients with chronic CO_2 retention, O_2 can cause respiratory depression.
10. In general, maintain patients in an upright position. The supine position increases the work of breathing and can precipitate pulmonary edema.

ASTHMA

Of the statistically common respiratory ailments, asthma is potentially the most problematic in dental practice. It is a hypersensitivity of the airway to certain stimuli. It can be acute and life threatening. Since 2% to 3% of the population has this disease, a thorough understanding of its pathophysiology and treatment is vital. Historically, the disease has been divided into two categories.

Extrinsic asthma	Intrinsic asthma
Age	
Begins before age 35; usually stops before adulthood	Usually affects adults after age 35
Etiology	
Exposure to specific allergen (for example, foods, animal hair, and so forth)	Nonallergic factors (for example, respiratory tract infection, emotional stress, cold, exercise, and irritants such as smoke)
IgE levels	
High	Normal
Skin testing	
Positive for specific allergens	Usually negative

As in COPD, patients can exhibit some aspects of both

asthma processes. Another subgroup comprises patients with the triad of nasal polyps, seasonal rhinitis, and aspirin-induced bronchospasm. All prostaglandin inhibitors can be implicated, and the nonsteroidal antiinflammatory drugs should be avoided as well.

The most important distinction between asthma and COPD is the reversibility of the asthmatic attack. With proper evaluation and management attacks can be largely avoided, but if they occur, proper management can be lifesaving. The most severe form of bronchospasm, which is unresponsive to usual therapy, is status epilepticus. Death can occur from respiratory acidosis, hypoxia, and hypercapnia.

It should be apparent that the dentist's most important task is identifying and avoiding precipitating factors. A patient who gives a history of wheezing only after an hour of vigorous exercise certainly is easier to manage than an extremely anxious patient who reports severe asthmatic attacks triggered by emotional stress. For many individuals surroundings can cause considerable anxiety. Psychologic management techniques and possibly an anxiolytic drug may be indicated. The dentist can assess the severity of the disease by listening to the patient. A patient who has been in the emergency room several times in the previous 6 months for an epinephrine injection to "break an attack" warrants more caution than the patient who reports childhood wheezing that he "grew out of." The patient's current status can be assessed by evaluating the level of treatment. Since prevention is the main goal of therapy, many patients receive long-term medication therapy.

MANAGEMENT. Management includes:

1. Theophyllines. These are the mainstay of long-term therapy. Maintaining a proper blood level depends on compliance. Often when patients stop taking their medication the decrease in circulating serum concentrations can precipitate an attack. The drugs also are used in conjunction with other medications to treat an acute attack.
2. Sympathomimetic agents. Epinephrine is still used to treat an acute attack unresponsive to aerosol bronchodilators, but there has been considerable refinement in other β-agonist drugs. Since epinephrine has both β_1 and β_2 effects, significant undesirable cardiac (β_1) effects sometimes can occur. These include tachycardia and other arrythmias, increase in cardiac contraction with resultant ischemia, and possibly angina. The newer agents are specific for β_2 (bronchodilator) effects. They include terbutaline, metaproterenol, and albuterol. There are oral forms for prophylactic dosage and aerosols for direct delivery to the tracheobronchial tree.
3. Corticosteroids. These can be used for acute or chronic management. Obviously they are avoided because of the numerous deleterious side effects, including adrenal suppression, risk of infection, osteoporosis, diabetes, and purpura. A patient who requires chronic steroid therapy to control symptoms runs a greater risk of experiencing problems during dental therapy. Recently, delivery of steroids such as beclomethasone by aerosol has proved successful in obtaining beneficial local effects while avoiding systemic side effects.

Asthma is a disease with a wide spectrum of manifestations. When treating such patients, the dentist must observe the following protocols:

1. Assess the severity of the disease. Ask about multiple hospitalizations, frequent visits to the emergency room, and the degree to which the disease affects normal functioning. Look at current therapy to assess the refractoriness of the disease. Make sure current medications are being taken, and consult with the physician.
2. Identify what precipitates an attack. If those precipitants exist in the treatment scenario (for example, stress or certain medications), take appropriate steps to control them. For example, an anxious patient who exhibits symptoms under pressure should be sedated. Long appointments should be avoided.

3. Prophylactically, some patients benefit from using their own bronchodilators before treatment. This may have real protective effects by blocking an attack and a definite psychologic effect by introducing an element of control over possible exacerbations.
4. Avoid certain drugs such as epinephrine in the local anesthesia. It can have a negative cumulative effect in combination with other sympathomimetic agents.
5. Be aware of indicated precautions for adrenal suppression in the patient on corticosteroid therapy.

BRONCHIECTASIS

This disorder is characterized by permanently dilated bronchi. It can be caused by congenital malformation or necrotizing pneumonia. In some cases the bronchopulmonary infection is unrecognized. It can have a patchy distribution or be panlobar. Classically, it is manifest by cough; voluminous sputum production ("three-layered" sputum with pus on the bottom, saliva in the center, and mucus on top); hemoptysis; chronic fatigue; and recurrent fevers.

Therapy consists of chest physical therapy with aerosols to keep the airways clear and antibiotics when indicated. The dental patient with bronchiectasis should be treated similarly to COPD patients, with special emphasis on avoiding aspiration from dental aerosols.

CYSTIC FIBROSIS

PATHOPHYSIOLOGY AND MANIFESTATIONS. This is a generalized disorder of exocrine gland secretion. The clinical picture of pulmonary complications caused by retained secretions and airway plugging leads to bronchiectasis with recurrent bronchopneumonia. Other glandular malfunction such as pancreatic insufficiency also is present. The presence of high concentrations of sodium and chloride in sweat is diagnostic. Death from bronchopulmonary infection used to be common, but aggressive physical therapy with hydration, postural drainage, and proper antibiotic therapy has lead to increased survival rates.

MANAGEMENT. The dentist must avoid exacerbating the underlying disease in the patient with cystic fibrosis. High flow rates of unhumidified gases such as oxygen or nitrous oxide can dry out respiratory secretions that already have increased viscosity. This can lead to further plugging and infection. Rubber dams should be used to decrease the possibility of aspiration from dental handpiece aerosols. Long appointments that interfere with the schedule of respiratory physical therapy should be avoided, and routine dental care should be scheduled only when there is no evidence of current exacerbation of the underlying disease. Sedatives should be avoided, and consultation is indicated, especially when oral infection is present, to review the patient's history of antibiotic use.

DIFFUSE LUNG DISEASE

A number of disorders ultimately compromise gas exchange, including the following:

Pulmonary fibrosis
Systemic lupus erythematosus
Scleroderma
Rheumatoid arthritis
Connective tissue disorders
Sarcoidosis
Amyloidosis
Histiocytosis X
Pulmonary vasculitides
Radiation pneumonitis
Occupational lung diseases

Symptoms can include dyspnea, cough, cyanosis, digital clubbing, pulmonary hypertension, and asthma. The degree of dyspnea is the best guideline to the degree of underlying disease. Early-stage disease with minimal shunting should not present severe difficulties with dental care, but when dyspnea is severe and hypoxia and hypercapnia are present, management as outlined for the COPD patient is warranted after consultation.

SECTION TEN

ENVIRONMENTAL INJURIES

Edited by **Donald Kaye**

138 · CHEMICAL AND ENVIRONMENTAL INJURIES

Nancy E. Bennet*

RADIATION INJURY

DEFINITION. Common types of ionizing radiation are non-penetrating (α- and β-rays) and penetrating (γ-rays and x-rays). α-Rays comprise two protons and two neutrons; they are positively charged and are converted to helium atoms by the acquisition of two electrons. β-Rays are electrons ejected from the nucleus of an atom undergoing radioactive decay. γ-Rays have great penetrating power and are electromagnetic radiation emitted by the nucleus of a radioactive substance. X-rays are similar waves of even shorter wavelength and greater penetrating power; they are produced by the bombardment of a substance by a stream of electrons at very high velocity, as in a vacuum tube.

Several terms and concepts are required to understand the expressions of amounts of radiation. The *roentgen* (R) is a measure of the amount of radiation passing through air. However, for medical use and for damage to tissue to occur, the radiation must be absorbed by tissue and not just pass through air. The *rad* is a unit defined as the amount of radiation energy equal to the absorption of 100 ergs of energy per gram of material. The type and thickness of tissue absorbing the rad are important; the greatest absorption is by the deeper tissues. The length of time of radiation absorption is also important; the greater the time, the less tissue damage resulting from the exposure. This is of great use in radiation oncology because a tumoricidal dose can be given with less damage to normal tissues.

PATHOPHYSIOLOGY. At the molecular level the penetrating radiation starts a cascade reaction that culminates in cellular death or injury. First, penetrating particles or waves react with nuclei or intracellular atoms to produce ion pairs; these then react with water molecules to produce the toxic products H_2O_2 and HO_2. Finally, these products react with essential intracellular regulators such as deoxyribonucleic acid (DNA) and enzymes, leading to altered function or death of the irradiated cells. At the cellular level the type of damage done depends on the dosage factors mentioned previously. Very low doses may produce chromosomal mutations such as breaks or dele-

*Material in this chapter is based in part on the first edition, written by Geoffrey Lefferts and David T. Lush.

tions; somewhat higher doses can cause a transient abnormal chromosomal function such as slowed mitosis. A few hundred rad can cause permanent cessation of mitotic activity without altering the other cell functions. Higher doses directly kill cells by preventing normal metabolic functions.

At the tissue level, rapidly reproducing areas are affected earlier and by lower radiation dosages; for instance, bone marrow and skin are affected by much smaller doses than are needed to affect bone, muscle, or the central nervous system (CNS), which are slowly proliferating or nonproliferating tissues.

There is considerable debate concerning the amount of radiation needed to produce an effect on cell components, especially DNA. One school of thought advocates a "threshold effect," with no damage of any kind occurring until a variable and unknown threshold dosage level is reached and with a linear relationship between dosage and damage above this threshold. The other school believes that current evidence suggests there is no safe lower limit and that the linear dose-damage relationship starts at dose 0 and increases from there; this group argues that the time from exposure to noticeable effect can be so long for some minor chromosomal aberrations that the ultimate damage is easy to overlook.

CLINICAL MANIFESTATIONS. As can be seen in Table 138-1, the part of the body affected by a particular amount of radiation is hard to predict. Most exposures are accidental, and thus specific details on dose or distribution are unknown; only by observation of the clinical course can a retrospective conclusion be reached. The side effects of radiation are commonly divided into acute and delayed effects. Diffuse or local exposure is another useful way to categorize the syndromes.

Acute diffuse exposure results in three syndromes. One is the cerebral syndrome, a usually fatal result of massive exposure. The course is progressive loss of consciousness followed by irreversible cardiovascular collapse, developing over 1 to 2 days. The second is the hematopoietic syndrome. This has many variations, as noted in Table 138-1, depending on which bone marrow cell line is the most affected. In terms of rapidly fatal effect, the loss of neutrophils is most threatening, since fatal bacterial infection commonly occurs rapidly after cell counts fall to less than a few hundred cells per cubic millimeter. The third syndrome, the gastrointestinal syndrome, results when radiation damage prevents the normal rapid turnover of gastrointestinal epithelial cells. This leads to the rapid loss of fluid and electrolytes and to severe dehydration. Regeneration can occur if the patient receives supportive therapy through the first few weeks.

Acute local exposure can cause severe damage to the skin

657

Table 138-1   Effects of radiation on body systems

Organ or effect	Time to onset	Time to maximal effect	Total time from first dose to recovery	Dose requirement to cause injury (rad)	Major consequences
Cerebral syndrome	Few hours	1-2 days	Usually fatal	3000	Irreversible coma and cardiovascular collapse
Hematologic syndrome					
Granulocyte depletion	1-2 weeks	4 weeks	6-8 weeks	200-400	Bacterial infection
Lymphocyte depletion	Few hours	1-2 days	4-8 weeks	200-400	Nonbacterial infection (virus, tuberculosis)
Platelet depletion	1-2 weeks	4 weeks	6-8 weeks	200-400	Bleeding
Gastrointestinal syndrome	3-4 days	6-7 days	2 weeks	600-2000	Fluid and electrolyte loss from mucosal sloughing
Skin lesions					
First-degree burn	Few hours	2-3 weeks	6-8 weeks	200	
Second- or third-degree burn	Few days	1-2 weeks	8-12 weeks	1000	May need skin grafts
Hair loss		3 weeks	3-4 months	300	Permanent if greater than 700-800 rad
Sterility	—	Few days to few weeks	—	600-700	Permanent infertility
Hypothyroidism	—	Several years	—	Variable	Myxedema
Cataract	—	Several years	—	300-600	Visual loss
Leukemia	—	5-7 years	—	Unknown	Fatal
Solid tumors (thyroid, bone, breast, lung)	—	Many years	—	Unknown	Usually fatal, except thyroid tumors

and its appendages (hair) even if no internal organs or systems are damaged. Depending on the dosage and duration of exposure, changes may range from mild redness and itching, resembling a sunburn, to painful, full-thickness necrosis. Hair loss can occur with doses that do not cause much obvious skin damage; it may or may not be permanent, depending on dosage and duration of exposure.

Delayed effects are arbitrarily defined as those that take years to become noticeable. Sterility, hypothyroidism, lenticular cataracts, and neoplasia are the most common late effects. Leukemias are the most publicized cancers associated with irradiation, but various solid tumors such as those of the thyroid, bone, lung, and breast are also noteworthy.

MANAGEMENT. For treatment of the acute cerebral syndrome only supportive measures are available, such as intravenous fluids, respiratory support, and anticonvulsant therapy. For the more common hematologic syndrome the object is to support the patient through the stage of absence of the various cell lines until recovery can occur. If bacterial infection can be prevented or successfully treated until granulopoiesis is reestablished, the patient should recover. In severe cases, as occurred in the Chernobyl nuclear accident in the Soviet Union, bone marrow transplantation has been used with moderate success. The prevention of infection is important; instrumentation and invasive procedures should be avoided if possible, and reverse isolation can be used, depending on the individual situation and severity. The gastrointestinal syndrome, as mentioned previously, is best managed by vigorous support with fluids and electrolytes. Intravenous hyperalimentation is useful because this syndrome is theoretically reversible.

Local injury to skin and appendages is managed in much the same way as a burn. Mild lesions need no specific treatment, whereas third-degree, full-thickness lesions may require debridement and grafting. Permanent hyperpigmentation may result from even mild lesions. Neither prophylactic nor therapeutic treatment is available for hair loss.

Treatment of the delayed effects is the same as when these conditions arise for any other reason and is beyond the scope of this chapter. These conditions may appear many years after the exposure; periodic examination for them is important so that they can be diagnosed in the earliest and most treatable stage.

Dental radiation dosage

Robert Beiderman

Dental radiation doses are generally well below those delivered by medical practitioners. Nevertheless, low, repeated x-radiation doses delivered to limited body sites over a period of days, weeks, or years should be considered. In 1959 the National Council on Radiation Protection and Measurement (NCRP) established that available evidence was insufficient to establish the dose-response relationship at low doses. They proposed that the direct proportional relationship be assumed to exist until proved otherwise. In effect this statement requires that dentists realize that *any* exposure to themselves or their patients may carry potential somatic or genetic effect. On June 29, 1981, before the National Center for Health Care Technology Assessment Forum: Dental Radiology, Dr. Lauriston S. Taylor, Honorary President of the NCRP, made the following comments:

1. The public tends to believe that it is at much greater risk of harm from radiation than actually exists.
2. The doses of radiation normally used in dental radiology are so low as to pose little if any risk. Nevertheless, because any exposure to radiation might possibly cause harm, x-rays should be used only when the patient is expected to benefit.

Total oral radiation doses to the head and neck for a complete mouth series range from 4 to 6 rad. Although this seems small, it is possible for the eye lenses and the thyroid gland to receive a total dose of somewhat less than 2 rad. It is not known whether this amount is significant, especially if dental needs dictate repeating this dose serially for several years. For this reason, use of thyroid shields may be indicated.

Genetic doses from head and neck irradiation are extremely small. About 1/10,000 rad reaches the unshielded reproductive cells for each rad of head and neck exposure. Again, the dose is low but may be significant, and body shielding of dental patients is recommended.

Elective oral radiologic treatment is generally delayed until the last two trimesters of pregnancy. The reason for this is usually patient apprehension or physician recommendation to pregnant patients. According to available indications, a pregnant patient who is properly shielded could receive dental x-ray doses at any time. However, exposure of first-trimester pregnant women is usually confined to emergency dental situations. These patients, of course, should be shielded.

The specific effects of dental radiation doses are not known. The effects of usually larger medical doses cannot be extrapolated in direct proportion. Dentists should obtain a clinical history and perform clinical examinations of patients to minimize patient exposure yet maximize necessary diagnostic information. The practitioner should consider dose rate, age, sex, individual variations, and relative tissue radiosensitivity variations before prescribing oral radiographs.

ELECTRICAL INJURY

EPIDEMIOLOGY. Electrical injuries, which cause approximately 1200 deaths per year, are caused by lightning injuries (20%) and by technical electrical injuries (80%). The clinical features of these two types of injuries vary dramatically, and only technical electrical injuries are discussed here in greater detail.

PATHOPHYSIOLOGY. Technical electrical injuries usually involve prolonged exposure to alternating current (AC). Two major problems result: cardiorespiratory arrest, for which immediate resuscitation is needed, and localized "crush" injury caused by massive thermal damage to muscle and vascular tissue. Tissue damage is more severe with AC than with direct current because the former causes tetanic muscle contractions that keep the victim from releasing contact with the source. Location of the entrance and exit points of the current is important, since a short path may cause less damage than a path through the length of the body. The amount of current passing through the body is also crucial: the flow of current is directly proportional to the difference in voltage between its source and destination and inversely proportional to the electrical resistance between these points (Ohm's law).

CLINICAL MANIFESTATIONS. The severity, nature, and time course of clinical signs of electrical injury can vary widely. The most severe symptoms are caused by apnea and cardiac standstill: these are fatal unless resuscitation is begun within 2 to 4 minutes. Fractures, especially of the spine or proximal long bones owing to tetanic contracture of axial or proximal muscles, require early diagnosis and immobilization. Musculoskeletal injuries involving ischemic and coagulation necrosis are common, and amputation may be required. Renal damage occurs in 6% to 22% of cases and is usually caused by myoglobin deposition. This can lead to oliguria, hyperkalemia, and metabolic acidosis in severe cases. Neurologic injuries, ranging from mild confusion to spinal cord injury to coma, are also common. Gastrointestinal and pulmonary injuries can be of significance, and late complications such as sepsis are often seen.

MANAGEMENT. The first priority in treatment is the safe removal of the victim from contact with the source of current. Either the current should be turned off, if possible rapidly, or the victim should be pulled away; if the source cannot be turned off, the rescuer must use a nonconductive (wood, leather, or rubber) shield or guard when touching the victim to avoid becoming part of the electrical circuit. After this, if the victim is not breathing or has no pulse, cardiopulmonary resuscitation must be started at once and continued until breathing or circulation has returned or until an hour has passed with no response, indicating that response is unlikely.

Treatment in the next few hours centers on wound care, fracture diagnosis and management, and fluid and electrolyte therapy. Careful physical and roentgenographic examination of deformed or tender bony areas is important. The vertebrae are especially susceptible to fracture. The wound management is standard, with debridement, irrigation, and review of tetanus immunization status most important. Fluid management can be crucial because a large portion of plasma volume can escape into the muscle compartments. Close monitoring of the pulse rate, blood pressure, urine volume and specific gravity, and serum electrolyte levels is necessary. Intravenous fluids are needed if any of these parameters indicate the presence of hypovolemia.

After the initial stabilization steps, taken during the first few hours of hospital care, several more definitive steps are needed over the next several days:

1. Devitalized tissue, usually skin or muscle, may require removal and eventual grafting. If the current has caused the death of an area of muscle, it must be surgically removed to prevent infection and sloughing.
2. Late vascular damage in the form of thrombosis or hemorrhage may occur at sites distant from the entrance or exit wounds, and close observation for several days is needed to detect and treat these problems. Bowel, extremity, or renal tissue and arterial or venous vessels may be involved.
3. Renal sequelae related to large tissue injury may occur; myoglobin released from damaged muscle may precipitate in the renal tubules and cause acute renal failure. This is manifest as oliguria, rising blood urea nitrogen (BUN) and creatinine concentrations, and a positive result of a urine test for myoglobin. Standard treatment for acute renal failure is needed. Recovery may take several weeks, and the mortality rate is high (25% to 50%).
4. The incidence of gastritis and stress gastric ulcers is high in patients with severe injuries of any type, and electrical injury is no exception. Monitoring of hematocrit and stool for occult blood loss is important. Prophylaxis with frequent (every 2 to 3 hours) administration of antacid, H_2 blockers, or both is indicated.
5. Neurologic sequelae may result from damage to the peripheral nerves, spinal cord, or brain; discovery of this may be delayed by the other complications and may take several weeks. The nature of the deficit depends on the particular nerve or cord level involved; the treatment is supportive and rehabilitative, and no preventive measures are known.

POISONINGS
Heavy Metal Toxicity

Heavy metal poisoning is noteworthy for two reasons. First, these diseases are common enough, although not an everyday occurrence, to warrant a basic knowledge of them by all practitioners. Second, most are treatable if the diagnosis is made early enough.

Lead Poisoning

ETIOLOGY. Lead enters the body through ingestion and inhalation. Ingestion occurs commonly from eating paint made with various lead compounds. The usual victims are children who are less than 5 years of age and live in older housing that has not been repainted for years, since paints made in recent years contain little or no lead. Lead ingestion also occurs in minor epidemic form among users of homemade whiskey distilled in auto radiators containing lead. Inhalation usually occurs in an industrial setting, especially in the production of leaded gasoline and in the production or the burning for reuse of storage batteries. Metal workers and jewelers are also at risk.

Once lead is ingested, about 10% is absorbed from the gastrointestinal tract, transported to the liver, released into the circulation, and deposited in bone marrow and red cell precursors and in bone. The lead stored in bone is inert and does not contribute to the toxic effect unless mobilized. Lead is cleared rapidly from the blood by these storage sites. Inhaled lead is absorbed directly into the blood through the respiratory mucosa.

CLINICAL MANIFESTATIONS. The signs of lead poisoning usually develop slowly because prolonged exposure is needed for enough lead to accumulate to cause symptoms and signs. A high index of suspicion is needed because the early symptoms are vague and may be intermittent.

The most common symptoms occur in three main sites: the gastrointestinal tract, peripheral nerves, and CNS. Bouts of severe gastrointestinal pain occur in varying locations with or without nausea and vomiting. An examination while pain is present does not show abdominal tenderness or other signs of intraperitoneal inflammation. The cause of the pain is spasm of the bowel wall musculature. Fever and leukocytosis do not occur. Results of liver function tests may be abnormal, however.

Peripheral neuropathy is the second symptom complex; weakness without sensory loss is the key finding. The upper extremities are affected more severely than the lower. Recovery after treatment is common if the condition has not resulted in severe atrophy by the time of diagnosis.

CNS symptoms are also common. Extensive neuropsychiatric testing has frequently detected memory and cognitive defects not apparent to the casual observer. Frank encephalopathy occurs primarily in children. It can progress rapidly to seizures, stupor, and coma if untreated.

In patients with poor oral hygiene, lead sulfide may be deposited in a black line (lead line) along the gingival margin of the teeth.

Recent reports have documented that anemia occurs in less than one third of cases of chronic lead exposure. The "classic" findings of microcytosis and basophilic stippling also are only occasionally present. Interestingly, when severe anemia has been present, it has often been found to involve significant hemolysis.

Lead levels in whole blood, when measured correctly, are the most useful diagnostic tests for lead exposure. Levels greater than 40 μg/dl indicate significant exposure. A newer assay in whole blood, protoporphyrin level, has also been found useful in assessing occupational exposure in humans.

Although urine tests for lead exposure have been used less frequently in recent years, measurements of 24-hour lead excretion after injection of calcium ethylenediaminetetraacetic acid (EDTA) chelation challenge test correlate well with total body lead stores and are a useful confirmatory test.

MANAGEMENT. The permanent elimination of the source of lead is essential. Encephalopathy requires emergency treatment by lowering the intracranial pressure with osmotic agents or steroids. Next, calcium EDTA is used as a chelating agent, followed by penicillamine.

Mercury poisoning

Mercury can cause three different syndromes—acute inorganic poisoning, chronic inorganic poisoning, and organic mercurial toxicity—that can result from the ingestion of mercuric chloride. This industrial corrosive extensively damages any gastrointestinal mucosa with which it has contact; after absorption it denatures enzymes by combining with their sulfhydryl groups, especially in the renal tubular cells where the substance is concentrated for potential excretion. Severe diffuse enteritis and uremia result. There is an early need for massive replacement of the fluid loss of enteritis and a later need for fluid restriction and a program for the treatment of renal failure. The prognosis is poor.

Chronic intoxication is usually the result of industrial exposure. Photoengraving, the manufacture of scientific and electrical instruments, scientific research laboratories, mining, and the production of industrial and marine paints are all enterprises using large amounts of mercury, and workers in these industries can have long-term contact with the substance. The symptoms and signs are diffuse and can appear unrelated if they wax and wane over months or even years. Painful bleeding gums, often with a blue, metallic-appearing line along the margin, loosening of teeth, and a generally painful stomatitis are common. Neuropsychiatric manifestations of facial or distal extremity tremors, irritability, and bizarre behavior or frank psychosis constitute a second large group of symptoms. The nephrotic syndrome with its massive proteinuria may appear early or late in the course. Treatment with dimercaprol (BAL) and penicillamine as a chelating agent is effective if used early in the therapy, but residual damage is not unusual.

The organic mercurials' ethyl and methyl compounds seem to concentrate in the nervous system, causing ataxia, peripheral neuropathy, loss of vision, and a dementia or retardation syndrome. As with the chronic inorganic syndrome, when high levels have been present in tissue for a prolonged period, treatment with chelating agents is seldom helpful.

Poisoning with arsenic and thallium

Arsenic is a main ingredient of many insecticides and pesticides used in homes and commercial agriculture. Poisoning usually occurs by accidental or intentional ingestion of one of these products; in rare cases agricultural workers have enough exposure to cause symptoms.

In just a few hours, acute arsenic poisoning can cause death from cardiovascular collapse and shock, after a period of severe vomiting, diarrhea, and abdominal pain. Chronic poisoning depends on the frequency and amount of exposure. Since several weeks are required for the excretion of just one dose, very small doses at even weekly intervals can gradually accumulate to cause a problem. Arsenic is stored in nervous tissue, liver, and keratin-containing tissue such as hair and nails. Neurologic signs of severe mixed peripheral neuropathy, headache, depressive symptoms, fatigue, and even convulsions are common. Skin signs, especially hyperpigmentation, hyperkeratosis, scaly dry rash, and transverse white lines in the fingernails are also important.

The diagnosis is confirmed by the analysis of urine, hair, or nails for arsenic. Since arsenic exists in low levels in food and water, some arsenic is normally present in the body. A urine excretion greater than 0.2 mg/L or hair levels greater than 0.1 mg/100 g of hair strongly indicate arsenic poisoning. The treatment is removal of the source of toxicity, plus BAL for the acute syndrome; BAL is not very effective for chronic poisoning.

Although the use of thallium in household products was banned by the U.S. government in 1965, it is still found in leftover insecticides and pesticides. Accumulation in nervous tissue and hair loss dominate the clinical picture of thallium poisoning. The treatment is purely supportive because the chelating agents do not much effect on thallium.

Carbon monoxide poisoning

Carbon monoxide (CO) is an odorless gas produced by the combustion of almost any carbon-containing material except natural gas. It is dangerous because its affinity for hemoglobin is over 200 times as great as oxygen's; thus it displaces oxygen and causes tissue hypoxia. A tiny amount of CO, enough to cause about 0.5% of hemoglobin to be carboxyhemoglobin (COHb), is produced endogenously as part of normal metabolism. Although automobile exhaust and poorly ventilated gas and coal stoves are well-known sources of CO, less well-publicized is a much more common source, the cigarette. Long-term smokers can have up to 10% COHb, which is more than 10 times the amount normally produced endogenously. More than 3000 deaths occur each year from accidental or suicidal exposure to high concentrations of CO.

The symptoms usually do not develop until the COHb level exceeds 20%, at which point headache, lightheadedness, nausea, or confusion may appear. As the blood concentration rises above 40%, changes in the level of consciousness start to occur, culminating in seizures or coma and eventual death as levels exceed 60%. In people with previously existing ischemic heart disease or chronic pulmonary disease, the symptoms occur at lower levels of COHb. The diagnosis is confirmed by a low level of measured (not calculated) oxygen saturation or by a high level of COHb. Arterial oxygen tension remains normal despite significant tissue hypoxemia because overall plasma content of oxygen remains unchanged.

Treatment of CO poisoning requires removal from the causative environment, followed by effective ventilation with high O_2 tension. Administration of 100% O_2, by artificial ventilation if necessary, helps displace the CO from hemoglobin sites and increases the O_2 delivered to hypoxic tissues by increasing dissolved O_2. Decreasing O_2 demand by strict rest, lowering any elevated temperature, and keeping the hematocrit normal by transfusion if needed are also useful steps. Hyperbaric O_2 should be used when COHb levels exceed 20% or when significant symptoms are present. Recovery is slow in serious cases; improvement in neurologic signs may continue for many days or weeks after the initial presentation.

Other common poisons

In addition to the heavy metals and CO, a number of other substances can cause acute poisoning. Those commonly found in the home are discussed here.

ACIDS, ALKALIES, AND BLEACHES. Lye (sodium hydroxide), washing soda (sodium carbonate), and other strong alkalies and acids are commonly used as cleansing agents and drain solvents. Ingestion of these substances causes severe and almost immediate irritant burns of all mucosal surfaces contacted; the esophagus and stomach may be perforated from the lesion. Death usually results from peritonitis or mediastinitis caused by perforation. The initial treatment is dilution of the poison with large amounts of water or milk. Vomiting should not be induced, since it increases the risk of perforation. Beyond this, the treatment is that of shock or intestinal perforation.

INSECTICIDES. Chlorinated insecticides such as DDT are seen much less often since they were banned by the U.S. government. However, they are still present in many households and can cause diffuse central nervous system and muscle hyperexcitability if ingested in large amounts. The treatment

is induced emesis followed by supportive measures for seizures and ventilatory failure.

Cholinesterase inhibition–type insecticides are quite common; they can be inhaled, ingested, or absorbed through the skin. They produce damage by allowing acetylcholine to accumulate at the nerve endings and cause diffuse autonomic and CNS effects. Central depression occurs, leading to coma; peripheral muscle weakness or fasciculation, vomiting or diarrhea, blurred vision, excess salivation, and sweating also occur. The combination of signs makes the diagnosis likely. The treatment is induced emesis to remove the poison, followed by atropine injections to block the central and parasympathetic acetylcholine effects.

Fluorinated insecticides are also common. Their damage is caused by enzyme inhibition, which blocks cellular chemical reactions. Fluoride can also precipitate with calcium and thus deplete serum calcium, leading to neuromuscular hyperirritability. Ingestion is treated by the administration of oral calcium to precipitate the fluoride before it is absorbed. This is followed by general supportive measures.

PETROLEUM PRODUCTS. The accidental or intentional ingestion of gasoline or kerosene can lead to aspiration of the material into the lungs, where pulmonary edema and chemical pneumonitis may result. Induced emesis and gastric lavage are not indicated as emergency measures unless a cuffed endotracheal tube is in place to reduce the danger of aspiration of these products. Otherwise, the treatment is symptomatic.

NEAR-DROWNING

Near-drowning is the occurrence, after immersion in water, of symptoms sufficient to bring the victim to medical attention. The incidence is unknown, but its importance can be inferred from the fact that more than 7000 people drown each year in the United States. Most drownings and near-drownings are accidental, occur in the summer, involve young people, and take place during a water sport activity such as boating, swimming, or fishing.

DIAGNOSIS. The diagnosis is usually obvious from the circumstances; the victim rarely comes to medical attention unless the accident or episode is witnessed and the observers become rescuers. As much information as possible should be obtained from these observers. Details of where and how the victim was found, names of other witnesses, circumstances of any possible trauma, and the victim's initial condition are likely to be useful in evaluating the patient for complications and in dealing with any legal aftermath of the event.

PATHOPHYSIOLOGY. Hypoxia is the cause of death in most cases. It can occur in either of two ways. More commonly the submerged victim holds his breath and struggles to reach the surface; if unable to do so after an individually variable period, he takes gasps of water instead of air into his lungs. While he is holding his breath, blood oxygen and remaining alveolar oxygen are used up and carbon dioxide accumulates. The resulting hypoxia is fatal if some air does not enter the lungs within at least 4 minutes. Less commonly the victim does not aspirate water into his lungs because of an unconscious reflex laryngospasm; if the airflow is restarted within the 3- or 4-minute period necessary for brain death from hypoxia, recovery may be complete.

If water has entered the lungs and then airflow is reestablished, the prognosis depends on how much lung tissue has been filled with water and whether the water is salt water or fresh water. Salt water generally has a worse prognosis. The very high sodium and chloride content of seawater causes vascular water to enter the alveoli in an attempt to dilute the ion concentration; this worsens the picture because more fluid is drawn into the lungs, and a borderline situation may become fatal. Fresh water has the opposite effect; it is hypotonic and is drawn out of the alveoli into the plasma for osmotic reasons. However, the alveolar membrane has been damaged and atelectasis or collapse of the alveoli may result, with no subsequent improvement in oxygenation of blood because a water-filled alveolus is replaced by a collapsed one. If enough fresh water enters the circulation, hemodilution leading to hemolysis and hyponatremia can result, further decreasing the oxygen-carrying capacity of the blood. However, these fluid and electrolyte shifts and abnormalities are fatal in only a small minority of late deaths; hypoxemia resulting from aspiration or laryngospasm is the dominant factor.

CLINICAL MANIFESTATIONS. The initial condition of the victim can range from death to normal wakefulness, depending on the length of time of submersion and the amount of water aspirated. Generally the neurologic state is at its worst point initially, with recovery depending on how much brain damage has occurred before rescue. Recovery may take several days or even weeks; older people have longer recovery periods. In the pulmonary system, signs of alveolar consolidation (dullness to percussion and bronchial breath sounds) are found in areas of aspiration. Areas of atelectasis showing dullness to percussion and decreased breath sounds may also be present. Unlike the neurologic picture, the respiratory signs may worsen during the first few days as fluid shifts occur.

A number of complications may occur. Gastric distention from aspiration or reflex phenomena, pneumonia, pulmonary edema, or acute renal failure can occur in severe cases.

Associated injuries must be sought aggressively. It cannot be assumed that all the patient's problems are due to immersion. There may be fractures, drug overdose, intracranial bleeding, and soft tissue injuries resulting from trauma. The victim may have fallen during the accident causing the drowning; the possibility of a suicide attempt must also be kept in mind.

MANAGEMENT. The most important part of treatment is first aid at the discovery site. Standard cardiopulmonary resuscitation must be started immediately after the discovery of a nonbreathing or pulseless victim. Any delay can be fatal, since the brain can tolerate only a few minutes of hypoxia and the victim has already been immersed for an unknown period. Resuscitation should be continued until spontaneous breathing returns or until the victim can be taken to a hospital. Oxygen administration should be started as soon as possible.

Even if a near-drowning victim appears fully recovered, overnight hospital observation for complications is recommended. Several studies should be performed immediately in all cases: chest roentgenography, serum electrolyte determination, arterial blood gas study, complete blood cell count, and renal function determination. If oxygenation is abnormal, oxygen therapy should be given. Endotracheal intubation may be needed if the defect is severe, although nasal administration of oxygen may suffice if the aspiration or atelectasis has been minor. For an unconscious victim, full supportive measures with intravenous fluids, careful neurologic observation, and respiratory support (if needed) are used. The recovery period may be prolonged, and a poor prognosis cannot be assigned early in the course. Any previously existing diseases and any traumatic injuries should be vigorously treated with standard measures for the conditions found.

ABNORMALITIES OF TEMPERATURE REGULATION

Body temperature is closely controlled by neural, vascular, and metabolic mechanisms that permit only a few degrees of variation despite wide fluctuation in ambient temperature. The temperature of circulating blood is sensed by regulatory cells in the hypothalamus, which initiates compensatory changes if the blood is too warm or too cool. The range of normal is 96° F (35.8° C) to 99° F (37.2° C); a diurnal rhythm occurs with the lowest values in the early morning and a peak of 1° to 2° F higher in the early evening.

Excess body heat is lost through four different mechanisms. Conduction is direct transfer by contact from one surface to another and is a minor consideration, except during water immersion, in humans. Convection is transfer from the body surface to the ambient air; wind accelerates this considerably. Radiation is transfer of heat energy by nonparticulate means; this can be responsible for the loss of half the body's heat production at temperatures near freezing. Evaporation of water cools the body surface and is the main object of sweating. Heat is produced by metabolic reactions in body tissues, the largest component of which is muscle tissue. Shivering, a reflex response to cool circulating blood, increases heat production in muscle tissue. The main regulating device of these mechanisms of heat production or loss is blood flow to skin vessels, which contract or dilate depending on the need to conserve or lose heat; the amount of sweat produced can also vary because sweat glands of the skin respond to sympathetic nerve stimulation.

Heat syndromes

Two major mechanisms cause heat syndromes. The first is prolonged sweating without adequate replacement of water and sodium chloride; the second is cessation of sweating and failure of the evaporation mechanism of heat loss. Heat cramps, heat syncope, and heat exhaustion are related to the first mechanism, and heat stroke is caused by the second. Heat stroke is the most serious of these syndromes and has a mortality of up to 70% in some series.

HEAT CRAMPS. Heat cramps are painful spasms of the voluntary muscles, usually after sudden or strenuous use of the involved muscle during hot weather and after excess sweating. The replacement of sodium chloride and water is therapeutic, and the use of sodium chloride tablets before such activity may be prophylactic.

HEAT SYNCOPE. Heat syncope occurs when a person working in a hot, humid environment becomes lightheaded or weak and then faints without other discoverable cause. Cutaneous vasodilation, loss of circulating volume resulting from excess sweating with inadequate water intake, lack of salt replacement, and lack of acclimatization to the hot surroundings contribute to the event. The physical findings are tachycardia, hypotension, and cool sweaty skin. The treatment is usually quick and easy and consists of rest, a supine position, and replacement of water and salt.

HEAT EXHAUSTION. Heat exhaustion is a general term used to describe a more prolonged and generalized syndrome than either heat cramps or syncope, although both are usually part of the picture. Prolonged sweating for several days leads to a symptom complex of weakness, nausea, unsteadiness, thirst, loss of concentration, muscle cramps, and eventual collapse or delirium. Again, the cause is thought to be prolonged underreplacement of salt and water. Treatment is replacement of salt and water by the oral or intravenous route, whichever is needed to replace 6 to 8 L of fluid each day. This syndrome is common and can occur with little physical work in people with chronic diseases such as heart failure or arteriosclerosis or those in the geriatric age group. Nursing home patients are especially susceptible during prolonged periods of high heat and humidity.

HEAT STROKE. Heat stroke, or heat pyrexia, results from the cessation of sweating despite a high ambient temperature and humidity. The exact cause is unknown. As with heat syncope, the incidence is higher in older people and those with chronic circulatory ailments. Symptoms similar to those of heat exhaustion may or may not precede the onset. Cessation of sweating and a rapid rise in body temperature to 105° or 106° F (41.1° C) signal the onset. The skin is hot and dry, and the patient is tachycardic and disoriented or delirious. Complications can follow quickly if the treatment is not immediate; shock, coagulopathy with diffuse bleeding, heart failure, or renal failure can occur within 1 to 2 days. Treatment consists of evaporative cooling—keeping the patient wet with frequent applications of warm water and providing maximal dry air circulation with fans. This method has been found safer and more efficient than the ice water bath technique. If the high temperature is not reduced, it will permanently damage intracellular enzymes in neural, renal, and other tissues. Once the temperature falls to about 101° F (38.3° C), cooling can be stopped and general supportive measures should be continued. The intravenous administration of fluids and electrolytes is guided by laboratory measurements and hemodynamic parameters.

Hypothermia

Hypothermia occurs when heat loss exceeds heat production for long periods, or during a short period of immersion in cold water. The numerical definition is a central (rectal or esophageal) temperature less than 95° F (35° C). Since standard medical thermometers are not calibrated lower than this level, incubator thermometers or other wider-range instruments must be used to confirm the diagnosis.

The physiologic effects of hypothermia are numerous. Neurologic abnormalities include confusion and, later, coma. Cardiac irritability is pronounced and is the most common cause of death (arrhythmias can occur during rewarming as well). Myocardial contractility is also depressed. Hypovolemia is invariably present because of renal dysfunction and marked "third spacing" of the vascular volume into the body's interstitial compartment. To complicate matters, numerous acid-base derangements take place during hypothermia, and the patient undergoes pulmonary changes, initially hyperventilation and then hypoventilation as temperature falls to less than 31° C.

Hypothermia can be caused by many metabolic diseases (hypothyroidism, hypoglycemia, hypopituitarism, malnutrition, and Wernicke's encephalopathy). In addition, drug use (for instance, alcohol, barbiturates, phenothiazines, and general anesthetics) and numerous other disorders (sepsis, stroke, head trauma, burns, and erythroderma) can be involved. Renal failure and hepatic failure can also cause a mild decrease in core temperature. Environmental exposure is the most common cause of severe hypothermia. Persons at greatest risk for hypothermia are elderly, alcoholic, malnourished, or otherwise socially deprived.

Unfortunately, the presence of hypothermia is easy to overlook because its initial clinical manifestations are often numerous and nonspecific. The *sine qua non* for the diagnosis, of course, is a core temperature reading of less than 35° C. Hypothermic patients are frequently stuporous or comatose and bradycardic. Hypotension, body stiffness, and shallow respiration are also common. The most common electrocardiographic manifestations are bradycardia, atrial fibrillation, ventricular arrythmias, and the classic Osborne wave at the end of the QRS complex. It is important that death not be declared prematurely in a potentially hypothermic patient.

Prehospital management of a hypothermic patient should include passive rewarming (insulation of the patient from the environment with unwarmed blankets) and administration of heated and humidified oxygen if available. Cardiopulmonary resuscitation should be employed only for ventricular fibrillation, pulseless ventricular tachycardia, and true asystole. Volume expansion is indicated if feasible. Active or passive stimulation of the patient should be minimized because they have been reported to induce ventricular fibrillation in some cases.

Hospital management consists of the usual supportive measures for a critically ill patient, along with a search for significant associated illness, aggressive fluid resuscitation, and rewarming techniques, preferably peritoneal dialysis. The use of active external rewarming (use of warm blankets, water immersion, and so on) has been controversial, and several reports have documented an increased mortality associated with its use.

Despite the severity of illness of many patients with hypothermia, almost all of its manifestations are fully reversible. Overall mortality for this condition is approximately 38%.

BIBLIOGRAPHY

Callahan M: Heat illness. In Rosen, P, et al, editors: Emergency medicine: concepts and clinical practice, ed 2, St Louis, 1987, The CV Mosby Co.

Chisolm JJ Jr: Poisoning due to heavy metals, Pediatr Clin North Am 17:591, 1970.

Cullen M and others: Adult inorganic lead intoxication, Medicine 62:221, 1983.

Dalrymple GV and others: Medical radiation biology, Philadelphia, 1973, WB Saunders Co.

Epstein F and Eilers M: Carbon monoxide poisoning. In Rosen, P, et al, editors: Emergency medicine, concepts and clinical practice, ed 2, St Louis, 1987, The CV Mosby Co.

Ferguson J et al: Accidental hypothermia. Emerg Med Clin North Am 1:619, 1983.

Jablon S and Kato H: Studies of the mortality of A-bomb survivors. V. Radiation dose and mortality, 1950-1970, Radiat Res 50:649, 1972.

Joselow MM, Louria DB, and Browder A: Mercurialism: environmental and occupational aspects, Ann Intern Med 76:119, 1972.

Kizer KW: Resuscitation of submersion casualties, Emerg Med Clin North Am 1:643, 1983.

Kunkle RF: Electrical injuries. In Rosen, P, et al, editors: Emergency medicine: concepts and clinical practice, ed 2, St Louis, 1987, The CV Mosby Co.

Modell JH: Biology of drowning, Annu Rev Med 29:1, 1978.

Reuler JB: Hypothermia: pathophysiology, clinical settings and management, Ann Intern Med 89:519, 1978.

Rouse RG and Dimick AR: The treatment of electrical injury compared to burn injury: a review of pathophysiology and comparison of treatment protocols, J Trauma 18:43, 1978.

Stannard JN: Toxicology of radionuclides, Annu Rev Pharmacol 13:325, 1973.

NEUROLOGIC DISEASES

Edited by **Rosalie A. Burns**

139 · INTRODUCTION TO NEUROLOGY

Rosalie A. Burns

The subject of neurology deals with diseases of the brain, spinal cord, nerve roots, peripheral nerves, neuromuscular junctions, and muscles. These are often referred to using the Greek or Latin derivative as encephalopathies, myelopathies, radiculopathies, neuropathies, myoneural junction disturbances, and myopathies. Encephalopathies can be further broken down into encephalopathies mainly affecting gray matter, or polioencephalopathies, and encephalopathies affecting white matter, or leukoencephalopathies. For the most part, neurologic disorders are destructive, with symptoms reflecting loss of function or deficits. Irritative phenomena occur with lesions in the cerebral cortex, however, resulting in seizure activity. Neurologic disorders may be focal, as in a cerebral infarction or hemorrhage; may be diffuse, as in a metabolic encephalopathy; or may follow an anatomic pattern in which specific combinations of anatomic pathways or systems are affected, as in motor neuron disease or combined system disease (so-called system disorders).

Whereas the neurologic examination points to lesion localization, the case history suggests the cause and the differential diagnosis. To be effective, the case history must indicate the nature of the problem, the type of onset, and whether progression or improvement has occurred. Specific information of importance in a neurologic history includes detail regarding headaches, vertigo, hearing loss, disturbed vision, speech disturbance, dysphagia, sensory or motor disturbance, seizures, syncope, sphincter disturbances, sexual dysfunction, and disorders of cerebration. The patient's medical history may disclose underlying relevant medical illnesses such as pernicious anemia in combined system disease or a previous myocardial infarction in an embolic cerebrovascular accident. A previous head injury may be the cause of a seizure disorder, or meningitis may be the cause of eventual normal pressure hydrocephalus. The patient's educational history is important as background for evaluating dementia. The family history is relevant, for example, in diagnosing many degenerative disorders. An occupational history and a history of exposure to toxins and the use of medications, drugs, or alcohol are also important for diagnosing a variety of central and peripheral disorders. The emotional impact of neurologic disorders must always be assessed.

Because the deficits discovered during the neurologic examination correlate with the localization of lesions, a basic knowledge of neuroanatomy is a prerequisite for analyzing a neurologic problem. Any case analysis should begin with anatomic localization. The cerebral hemispheres can be visualized well using either computed tomography (Fig. 139-1) or magnetic resonance imaging. In appropriate horizontal sections, for example, it is possible to see the frontal, parietal, temporal, and occipital lobes, the cortical sulci, the sylvian fissures, the basal ganglia, the ventricular system with the lateral and third ventricles, the fourth ventricle, the cerebellum, and the brainstem.

NEUROLOGIC LESIONS
Lesions of the frontal lobe

Lesions of the frontal lobe affecting the motor cortex result in a contralateral hemiplegia or paresis affecting fine and skilled movements to a greater extent than gross movements. Weakness is classified as paresis when the paralysis is partial and as plegia when the paralysis is complete. The paralysis may be initially flaccid (hypotonic), but ultimately spasticity develops (an increased tone of the limbs, noted maximally during initial passive movement). Spasticity is generally greater in the adductors and flexors of the arm and the extensors of the leg. Associated with this tone change are increased deep tendon reflexes, pathologic reflexes such as the Babinski sign, and absent superficial abdominal reflexes. Whereas the lower face and the limbs are affected by unilateral corticobulbar and corticospinal tract involvement, various midline structures are uninvolved because their innervation derives from both cerebral hemispheres (upper face, pharynx, larynx, neck muscles, diaphragm, and trunk). There may be minor degrees of motor deficit such as a minimal flattening of the nasolabial fold, decreased arm swing during walking, a slight downward drift of an outstretched arm, or an eversion of the leg while the patient is reclining. The frontal eye field, which lies anterior to the motor cortex, is thought to be the source of a saccadic (rapid voluntary) polysynaptic eye movement pathway (frontomesencephalic) from the cerebral hemisphere to the opposite pontine paramedian reticular formation (PPRF). Patients with lesions in this cerebral region tend to look toward the side of the lesion. This is commonly transient and can be overcome by using ice-water labyrinthine stimulation or the doll's head reflex. Seizure discharges in this region cause the head and eyes to turn toward the opposite side.

Focal lesions affecting the dominant frontal lobe are likely to cause an expressive language disturbance known as nonfluent aphasia, or Broca's aphasia, and may cause some forms of apraxia. Apraxia, the inability to perform a motor act when

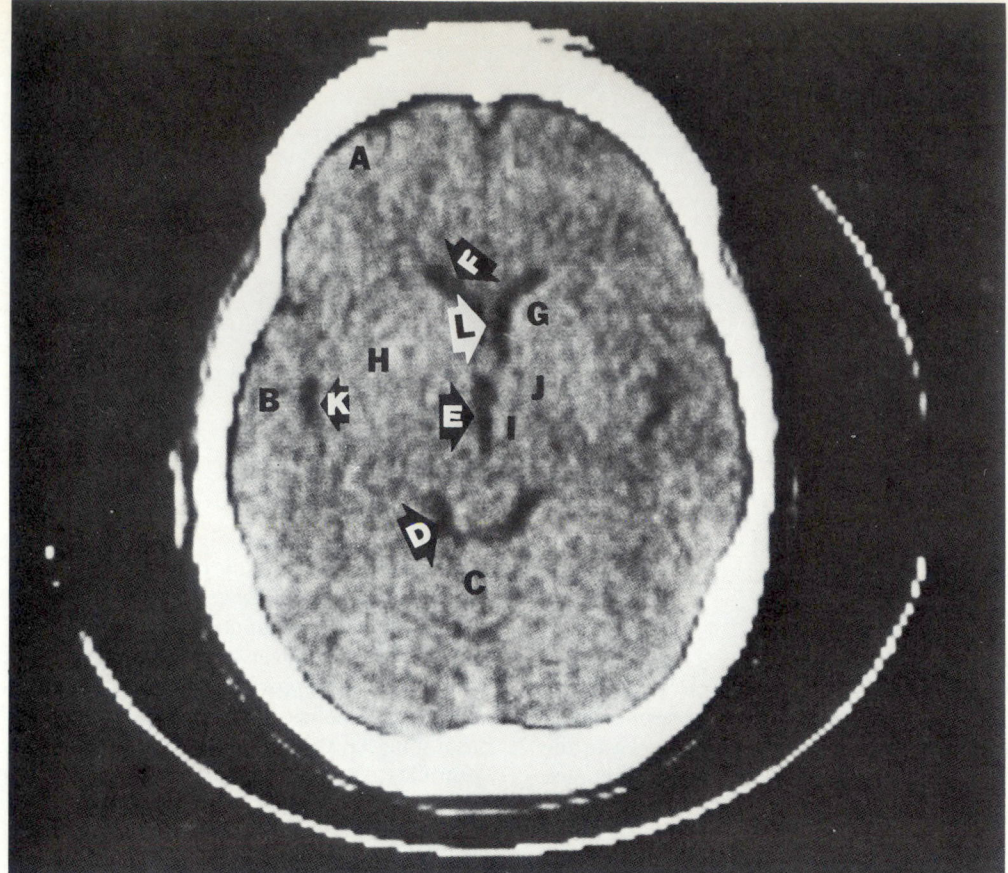

Fig. 139-1   Anatomic designations of computed tomogram. *A,* frontal lobe; *B,* temporal lobe; *C,* superior vermis of cerebellum; *D,* quadrigeminal cistern; *E,* third ventricle; *F,* frontal horn of lateral ventricle; *G,* caudate nucleus; *H,* lenticular nucleus; *I,* thalamus; *J,* internal capsule; *K,* sylvian cistern; *L,* septum pellucidum.

the necessary motor, sensory, and cerebellar skills are intact, occurs with disconnection lesions of white matter pathways coursing between the dominant parietal and frontal areas, the corpus callosum, and the nondominant frontal area. An example of apraxia is the inability of a patient to mimic eating on command, although the patient understands the command and has no difficulty handling his own meals (see Chapter 142). A patient who has difficulty in walking and who walks with small steps, a narrow base, shuffling, and the feet seemingly stuck to the floor is said to suffer from apraxia of gait. It has been attributed to bilateral frontal lobe disease.

A variety of pathologic reflexes known as primitive reflexes or frontal release signs are common with frontal lobe lesions and resemble the reflexes seen in an infant. These include the suck, snout, root, and grasp reflexes. The suck reflex is a pouting movement in response to tactile stimulation of the lips; the snout reflex is a pursing of the mouth in response to pressure on the upper lip; the root reflex involves a movement of the angle of the mouth toward a stimulus on the corner of the lips or cheek; and the grasp reflex involves a flexion of the patient's fingers over the examiner's fingers with moving palmar stimulation. Paratonia, or gegenhalten, is also seen with frontal lobe lesions; it is a seeming inability of the limbs to relax for testing of passive movements.

Lesions of the parietal lobe

Manifestations of parietal lobe lesions may include cortical sensory loss, agnosias, apraxia, seizures, visual field defects, and disruption of optokinetic nystagmus.

Cortical sensory loss resulting from the involvement of the postcentral gyrus may include deficits in pain, touch, and temperature. This loss is generally considered to affect discriminative sensations, so deficits may involve position sense, touch localization (atopognosia), two-point discrimination, the ability to identify an object by modalities such as texture, size, and weight (astereognosis), the identification of numbers outlined on the palm (agraphesthesia), and the appreciation of double simultaneous stimuli (extinction). Vibration sense is thought by many to be a thalamic function.

The term "agnosia" is used when the patient has impaired recognition or awareness of something through otherwise intact sensory modalities such as visual, auditory, or tactile (see Chapter 142). Some patients with lesions of the nondominant parietal lobe may be unaware of their deficit or illness (anosognosia). They may have a disorder of awareness of space and of body schema resulting in unilateral neglect (amorphosynthesis). They may also have constructional apraxia, which is a difficulty with drawing and copying.

Patients with lesions of the dominant parietal lobe may have difficulty carrying out acts because of apraxia. They may have Gerstmann's syndrome, in which they cannot distinguish right from left (right-left disorientation), have difficulty doing simple mathematical problems (acalculia), are unable to identify or name body parts, particularly digits (finger agnosia), and are unable to write spontaneously (agraphia).

Aphasia and alexia may also occur with lesions of the dominant parietal lobe. The aphasia is fluent in the sense that speech production may approach the normal in the number of words used and in rhythm, but language content is abnormal. The abnormality consists of substituting incorrect words or phrases (paraphasias) for the intended ones. When fluent aphasia is due to a lesion of the arcuate fasciculus in the subcortical parietal lobe, comprehension of the spoken word is normal, but an examiner's words cannot be repeated correctly (conduction aphasia). Parietal alexia is accompanied by agraphia, is present in the absence of significant aphasia, and is found in lesions of the dominant angular gyrus.

Seizure disorders manifested by sensory phenomena may occur with irritative lesions of the parietal lobe. Lesions involving the parietal optic radiations produce inferior quadrantanopsias. Optokinetic nystagmus (OKN) is a normal phenomenon that may be disrupted with parietal lobe disease. A series of stripes or bars moved across the patient's field of vision produces OKN. This visually induced nystagmus consists of two phases, a slow (pursuit) phase in the direction of the moving objects and a fast (saccadic) phase in the opposite direction. Although the precise pathways have defied elucidation and abnormalities are not dependent on visual field defects, two clinicoanatomic correlations deserve mention. First, because vision is a prerequisite, OKN is absent if the patient is blind (for example, cortical blindness) but is present if the patient is feigning blindness (that is, functional blindness). Thus the presence of OKN proves that there must be *some* residual vision. Second, if the moving objects are directed toward a damaged parietal lobe, OKN may be abnormal in rate, rhythm, or amplitude. Thus unilateral disruption of OKN is a clinical sign of parietal lobe damage.

Lesions of the temporal lobe

Manifestations of temporal lobe lesions include Wernicke's aphasia, complex partial (psychomotor) seizures, and memory disorders (see Chapters 142 and 145). Cortical deafness is uncommon; it requires bilateral lesions of the primary auditory cortex located in the superior temporal gyri. Involvement of the temporal optic radiations may produce superior quadrantanopsias. The anterior 5 cm of one temporal lobe can be removed without causing a significant deficit.

Lesions of the occipital lobe

Manifestations of occipital lobe lesions involve mainly disorders related to vision. There may be homonymous hemianopsias caused by involvement of the geniculocalcarine system. Central vision, or macular vision, is often preserved; this is called "macular sparing." Homonymous scotomas in the macular or paramacular visual fields may occur. Cortical blindness with preservation of pupillary light reflexes may develop with bilateral occipital lobe infarction (see Chapter 152). Occipital lobe seizures are manifested by the patient perceiving abstract forms and colors. A polysynaptic occipitomesencephalic pathway is involved with horizontal slow pursuit or following movements of the eyes.

Lesions of basal ganglia

Evaluating lesions of the basal ganglia (extrapyramidal lesions) involves assessing muscular tone, looking for rigidity (increased resistance throughout a range of passive movement), and observing for abnormal involuntary movements such as chorea, athetosis, hemiballismus, or dystonia (see Chapter 150).

Lesions of corticospinal pathways

Lesions of the corticospinal pathways anywhere in their course produce the upper motor neuron signs of increased deep tendon reflexes, spasticity, and weakness. A unilateral corticospinal lesion at the level of the internal capsule results in hemiparesis or hemiplegia.

Lesions of the thalamus

Lesions of the thalamus may produce nondiscriminative sensory deficits (for example, with pain, touch, temperature, and vibration) resulting from involvement of the ventral posterior nucleus. Thalamic pain may develop (see Chapter 152). Lesions of the dorsal medial nucleus of the thalamus have been associated with the amnestic syndrome (Korsakoff's psychosis) in Wernicke's disease (see Chapter 154).

Lesions of the cerebellum

Lesions of the cerebellum in general may affect equilibrium (involvement of midline cerebellum or vermis) or limb coordination (involvement of cerebellar hemispheres). Patients with midline cerebellar lesions have gait ataxia and truncal ataxia. The gait is often described as wide based. These patients perform tandem gait poorly and may be unable to stand with their feet together and eyes open. With lesions of the cerebellar hemispheres, patients display dysmetria and intention tremor on a variety of coordination tests such as the finger-to-nose and heel-to-shin maneuvers and the performance of rapid, rhythmic, alternating movements. Diffuse cerebellar lesions may produce an intermittent explosiveness of speech known as "scanning." Patients may have hypotonia on passive movement and may be unable to check movement, resulting in a rebound phenomenon when resistance to muscle contraction is suddenly removed.

Lesions of the brainstem

Lesions of the brainstem produce cranial nerve, motor, sensory, and cerebellar system deficits. Involvement of the reticular system results in a loss of consciousness. A review of the vascular disorders of the brainstem (see Chapter 152) gives an overview of the anatomy of this region. The cranial nerve deficits are ipsilateral to the site of the lesion, and the sensory and motor deficits are usually contralateral. A major portion of the brainstem can be assessed by evaluating pupillary responses to light, voluntary extraocular movements, and reflex extraocular movements such as the oculocephalic or doll's head (or eye) reflex and the oculovestibular or caloric response (see Chapter 140). Ophthalmoplegias may be internal (pupillary paralysis) or external, involving eye movements. Involvement of the extraocular muscles supplied by the third, fourth, and sixth cranial nuclei or their nerves (nuclear or infranuclear) results in dysconjugate gaze (unequal limitation of eye movement) and diplopia. Internuclear ophthalmoplegia or the syndrome of the medial longitudinal fasciculus is a supranuclear dysconjugate gaze abnormality (see discussion of multiple sclerosis in Chapter 148). The paralysis of horizontal conjugate gaze that occurs with lesions of the pontine gaze center (PPRF) is usually persistent and involves both saccadic and pursuit movements. It is not overcome by ice-water labyrinthine stimulation.

Nystagmus is an oscillation of the eyes that occurs with brainstem disease. It also may be normally induced, as in OKN, may be congenital (pendular), may be associated with a severe reduction in visual acuity, may be related to ingesting drugs such as phenytoin, may reflect labyrinthine disease, or may result from a supranuclear gaze paresis (to the side of the paresis). The oscillatory eye movements in nystagmus may be pendular (of equal amplitude in both directions) or have a jerklike quality with slow and fast components. Jerk nystagmus is usually named by the direction of the more easily visualized fast component (for example, horizontal to the right); it occurs in brainstem disease and may be horizontal, rotatory, or vertical. Conjugate horizontal nystagmus on lateral gaze may be gaze evoked ipsilaterally as a result of either a conjugate gaze paresis or a cerebellar pathway involvement with a pontine lesion. It may also be caused by involvement of the vestibular nuclei, occurring either in the primary position or as a gaze-evoked nystagmus to the side opposite the lesion. Rotatory nystagmus suggests involvement of the vestibular nuclei. Vertical nystagmus always indicates brainstem disease if drug intoxication is excluded. Upbeat nystagmus can be more specifically localized to the medullary area when it is present in the primary position but increases in intensity on downward gaze. A large-amplitude upbeat nystagmus in the primary position that increases during upward gaze suggests a lesion in the anterior vermis of the cerebellum. Downbeat vertical nystagmus suggests a medullary lesion, commonly associated with Arnold-Chiari malformations or other abnormalities of the craniovertebral junction. A horizontal nystagmus in the primary position that changes direction periodically is known as periodic alternating nystagmus and requires careful observation to be noted. It suggests a lesion in the caudal medullary region. Seesaw nystagmus (one eye up and one down) suggests a diencephalic lesion. Retraction nystagmus and convergence nystagmus are associated with paralysis of upward gaze (Parinaud's syndrome) and suggest a pretectal lesion.

Although evaluating the trigeminal nerve assesses pontine function, lesions of the spinal tract of the trigeminal nerve, which descends as low as the upper cervical cord, may decrease peripheral facial pain sensation. Whereas involvement of supranuclear or corticobulbar fibers to the seventh cranial nerve nucleus results only in weakness of the contralateral lower face, a lesion of the seventh nerve nucleus in the pons or in the nerve itself involves both the upper and the lower halves of the face on the same side. A peripheral seventh cranial nerve palsy may decrease lacrimation and possibly salivation and taste on the same side and may produce hyperacusis by involving, respectively, branches to the greater superficial petrosal nerve, the chorda tympani, and the nerve to the stapedius muscle.

Nerve deafness and vestibular disturbances are discussed in Chapter 147. Bulbar palsy, with the patient having difficulty in speaking and swallowing (dysarthria and dysphagia), occurs with lesions involving the ninth, tenth, and twelfth cranial nuclei or cranial nerves. With twelfth cranial nerve lesions, atrophy and fasciculations of the tongue are present, with deviation of the protruded tongue toward the side of the lesion.

Lesions of the spinal cord

Lesions of the spinal cord may be localized at a transverse level or may be diffuse. Localized lesions at a transverse level involve segmental structures such as the secondary sensory neurons for pain and temperature that cross in the anterior commissure and long tract functions below the level of the lesion. Unilateral long tract lesions produce ipsilateral proprioceptive loss when in the posterior columns, contralateral pain and temperature sensation deficits when in the lateral spinothalamic tracts, and ipsilateral motor dysfunction when in the corticospinal pathways. In unilateral localized lesions of the spinal cord the perception of touch is commonly spared, as compared to the perception of pain (dissociated sensory loss). This occurs because touch sensation traverses the anterior spinothalamic tracts and posterior columns bilaterally, providing alternate pathways, whereas pain sensation only traverses the opposite lateral spinothalamic tract. Involvement of corticospinal tracts results in weakness below the level of the lesion with increased deep tendon reflexes and increased tone (in acute spinal shock, flaccidity and decreased deep tendon reflexes are noted). The Babinski sign may be present, and incontinence may occur. Preservation of sacral sensation, or "sacral sparing," may occur with intramedullary mass lesions. Pain is commonly associated with extramedullary mass lesions. Localized spinal cord disorders may include transverse myelitis as from multiple sclerosis, intramedullary syrinx or tumor, or extramedullary compression by mass lesions. Other lesions of the spinal cord may involve combinations of particular tracts or systems, as in the posterior column and corticospinal tract involvement of combined system disease.

Diffuse involvement of anterior horn cells, as in amyotrophic lateral sclerosis, results in widespread atrophy, weakness, fasciculations (contraction of muscle fibers of a single motor unit), and a decrease in deep tendon reflexes.

Lesions of nerve roots, peripheral nerves, neuromuscular junction, and muscle

Lesions of nerve roots and peripheral nerves result in atrophy, weakness, fasciculations, a decrease in deep tendon reflexes, and sensory deficit, all appropriate to their myotomal or dermatomal origin. Deep tendon reflexes are mediated by specific spinal cord segmental levels as follows: biceps—fifth and sixth cervical; radial—fifth and sixth cervical; triceps—sixth, seventh, and eighth cervical; patellar—third and fourth lumbar; and Achilles—first sacral.

Lesions of the neuromuscular junction, such as myasthenia gravis, are characterized by a weakness of muscle that varies with activity. The muscle mass is usually retained, and deep tendon reflexes may be decreased during muscle fatigue.

In muscle disease, weakness is often proximally distributed. Deep tendon reflexes are lost only with significant muscle atrophy, which may occur with time (see Chapter 155).

DIAGNOSTIC TESTS

To correctly use the variety of diagnostic tests available for neurologic disorders, it is essential to base the study selection on a careful assessment of the history and physical examination. Details regarding diagnostic tools are specifically discussed in appropriate sections of this book. Some generalizations are mentioned here regarding selected procedures.

Computed tomography (CT) is a roentgenographic technique using computer analysis of digitized, fine-beam roentgen ray transmission data. It produces a cross-sectional anatomic image with extremely high tissue density discrimination, detecting destructive, hemorrhagic, neoplastic, atrophic, and demyelinative brain lesions. There are pitfalls in using CT scanning of the head. Studies both with and without contrast medium should be obtained when the patient does not have an allergy to iodinated material. This increases the likelihood of demonstrating one of the many lesions associated with a breakdown in the blood-brain barrier. Some subdural hematomas may be difficult to define because they may be isodense with the surrounding brain and may be bilateral without a shift of intracranial structures. Arteriovenous malformations and aneurysms may not be demonstrated by a CT scan. Current scanners do not always define brainstem infarction. However, because of its high density discrimination the CT scan may detect faint calcification and small hemorrhages and may distinguish intracerebral brain abscesses, tumors, and infarctions. Using echoencephalography for determining a shift of the mid-

---

FACTORS AFFECTING SIGNAL INTENSITY ON MRI

	Hypointensity	Hyperintensity

T_1 WEIGHTED IMAGE	Long T_1 relaxation time
	  Cerebrospinal fluid
	  Most brain lesions
	Rapidly moving protons
	  Pulsatile Cerebrospinal fluid
	  Rapid blood flow
	Decreased proton density
	  Bone, dura
	  Calcified lesions
		Short T_1 relaxation time
		  Fat
		  Paramagnetic effect
		  Subacute blood clots
		  Paramagnetic agents (gadolinium-DPTA)

T_2 WEIGHTED IMAGE	Short T_2 relaxation time
	Rapidly moving protons
	  Pulsatile Cerebrospinal fluid
	  Rapid blood flow
	Intracellular paramagnetic effect (acute or chronic
	  blood products)
	Decreased proton density
	  Bone, dura
	  Calcified lesions
		Long T_2 relaxation time
		  Nonpulsatile cerebrospinal fluid
		  Most brain lesions
		  Cysts, abscess cavities
		  Subacute blood clot

---

line structures is rarely warranted when a CT scan can be obtained.

The skull roentgenogram remains useful in detecting skull fractures and abnormalities in the region of the sella turcica and at the base of the skull, as in foraminal erosions. The isotope brain scan rarely is used today.

Magnetic resonance imaging (MRI) results in clear brain and spinal cord images, which are obtainable in any plane without the use of ionizing radiation. The image is created by stimulating spinning protons in a magnetic field with radiofrequency waves, which causes them to absorb energy and change their orientation. During the dissipation of the excess energy, or "relaxation," the protons reorient at different rates depending on the size of their associated molecules and other factors. The signal intensities within the images differ with the proton density and the relaxation times of the tissues, known as T_1 and T_2 (see box above). T_1 is a time constant that represents the restoration of the longitudinal magnetization. T_2 is a time constant associated with transverse relaxation. The detection of either T_1 or T_2 tissue properties varies with the different imaging sequences. Pathologic conditions alter the relaxation times. Paramagnetic ions such as gadolinium-DPTA enhance lesions by affecting relaxation times and are used like injectable radiographic contrast agents, which increase the sensitivity and specificity of MRI.

Cerebral angiography, accomplished most often today by catheterization via the femoral artery, is performed to diagnose lesions when they are not outlined by other techniques and when management will be influenced by the findings. An example of a lesion that warrants cerebral angiography to disclose it is an arteriovenous malformation or aneurysm that might be shown to be surgically accessible. Another purpose of cerebral angiography is to visualize stenosed or occluded extracranial or intracranial cerebral vessels, with the goal of endarterectomy.

Computed digital angiography and dynamic CT scanning are techniques using the rapid injection of an intravenous bolus of contrast media. At times, they may replace some arterial vascular studies.

Pneumoencephalography has been entirely replaced by CT scanning and MRI. Introducing air into the subarachnoid space

and the ventricular system is no longer necessary to outline the anatomic structures.

Positron emission tomography (PET) is a research technique using appropriately labeled, positron-emitting isotopes, which can be imaged in a manner similar to roentgenographic CT scanning, to study metabolism and physiologic alterations in the brain.

Spine films are important in demonstrating subluxations, dislocations, compression fractures, erosions, and intervertebral disc space abnormalities. MRI is an excellent modality for the demonstration of extramedullary and some intramedullary spinal cord lesions. Myelography, the introduction of water-soluble, or occasionally nonsoluble (iophendylate [Pantopaque]), contrast agents into the spinal subarachnoid space, is still used for diagnosing many spinal canal disorders for which surgery or radiotherapy would be advised. This includes intramedullary mass lesions and extramedullary mass lesions of the spinal cord, foramen magnum, and cauda equina such as tumors, syrinxes, and arteriovenous malformations. Spinal CT scanning, with and without the water-soluble contrast agents and with the appropriate equipment, can demonstrate extramedullary spinal lesions and some intramedullary spinal cord lesions. Spinal CT scanning may sharply delineate lumbar disc protrusions. With the use of intrathecal water-soluble contrast media, many intradural lesions can be better defined than they are with routine myelography.

Spinal angiography is important in diagnosing spinal arteriovenous malformations, but because of the danger of spinal cord injury it should be reserved for patients in whom the index of suspicion is very high and for whom surgery is justified.

Lumbar puncture, with the assessment of intracranial pressure and the evaluation of cerebrospinal fluid for cells, protein, sugar, serology, and organisms, is essential in the diagnosis and differentiation of meningitis and encephalitis. Lumbar puncture remains important in the diagnosis of subarachnoid hemorrhage if blood in the subarachnoid space is not defined on a CT scan. Although lumbar puncture presents the real danger of cerebral herniation when increased intracranial pressure is present, it is not contraindicated and must be performed if a CT scan fails to define a mass and a central nervous system infection remains possible. In such a situation, lumbar puncture can differentiate pseudotumor cerebri from meningitis. Patterns of altered cerebrospinal fluid are described under specific disorders in this text.

Audiograms, caloric testing, and electronystagmography are discussed in Chapter 147.

Noninvasive extracranial vascular diagnostic tests are discussed in Chapter 100.

Electromyography (EMG) may be used to differentiate nerve and muscle disease and to evaluate neuromuscular disorders. Measurement of nerve conduction velocity is particularly helpful in detecting the demyelinative neuropathies and compression peripheral neuropathies. Details regarding these procedures and muscle biopsy are discussed in Chapter 155.

Electroencephalography, recording the electrical activity of the most superficial layers of the cerebral cortex, is important in the diagnosis of seizure disorders, metabolic encephalopathies, dementia, focal versus diffuse pathologic conditions, and cerebral death. The normal background activity consists of α-waves at 8 to 12 Hz, most prominent posteriorly, and low-voltage fast β-waves at 13 to 30 Hz anteriorly. Significant degrees of slower activity, such as δ-waves at 0.5 to 3 Hz and θ-waves at 4 to 7 Hz, either diffusely or focally distributed, can be correlated with destructive lesions. Metabolic encephalopathies should be associated with diffuse slow-wave activity. Destructive focal lesions, such as tumor or infarction, may cause focal slow-wave activity. Cerebral dysrhythmias are associated with seizure disorders (see Chapter 145). Provocative techniques that may be used to bring out seizure activity include sleep tracings, photic stimulation, hyperventilation, and in special instances pentylenetetrazol (Metrazol) activation. Special sleep tracings may be useful in diagnosing sleep disorders such as narcolepsy and sleep apnea.

Within the last decade the scope and usefulness of electrophysiologic methods employed in neurologic diagnosis have expanded. Although standard electroencephalography (EEG) and EMG techniques are still the main methods, using a minicomputer with them has increased their usefulness. By using computer averaging, the evoked potentials for a series of visual, auditory, or somatosensory stimuli can be calculated and compared to normal levels for stimulus latency, interwave latency, and amplitude. The visual evoked response (VER) is useful in diagnosing dysfunction in the optic nerve and optic chiasm, as occurs with multiple sclerosis and chiasmatic tumors. The brainstem auditory evoked response (BAER) can localize dysfunction in the auditory system from the cochlea to the medial geniculate body. Lesions that impair the auditory pathways include multiple sclerosis, tumors, and vascular disease. The somatosensory evoked response (SER) is useful in defining peripheral nerve plexus dysfunction and spinal cord dysfunction. These clinical neurophysiologic techniques often show abnormalities earlier than other studies.

BIBLIOGRAPHY

Baker AB and Baker LH, editors: Clinical neurology, New York, 1980, Harper & Row Publishers, Inc.

Critchley M, O'Leary JL, and Jennett B, editors: Scientific foundations of neurology, Philadelphia, 1972, FA Davis Co.

Haymaker W: Bing's local diagnosis in neurological diseases, St Louis, 1969, The CV Mosby Co.

140·ALTERATIONS IN CONSCIOUSNESS

Richard N. Harner*

The behavior of the human central nervous system alternates between wakefulness and sleep in periods closely tied to circadian rhythms. During wakefulness, objective interaction with the environment is always accompanied by the awareness of private brain events, called thoughts, intimately related to behavior and occurring in an uninterrupted stream called *mentation*.

Introspectively we can distinguish two components of human mentation. *Cognition* produces a coherent view of the internal and external environment by identifying, analyzing, classifying, and storing data collected by the senses. *Affect,* or *emotion*, identifies primal sensations that occur spontaneously or by learned association with cognitive functions. Awake behavior is then the result of the integration of cognitive patterns of response, learned and perfected through experience (learned behavior), and built-in patterns of emotional nature (instinctive behavior).

Anatomically and physiologically, at least three parts of the brain are involved in producing awake behavior. The first is phylogenetically ancient and is located in the reticular core of the upper brainstem and diencephalic region. It activates and coordinates the most general patterns of reactivity to the environment, giving a person the appearance of alertness and vigilance. When these structures are destroyed or when their physiology is disturbed, waking behavior decreases or ceases completely, resulting in the pathologic states of stupor or coma.

The second anatomic subdivision consists of phylogenetically recent structures, such as the cortical mantle and its connections, that have developed in parallel with the increasing variety of complex cognitive aspects of vertebrate behavior. The development of these structures in the human is the anatomic feature that most distinctively separates us from other animals, allowing us to be in contact with a large and complex environment and simultaneously draw the detailed distinctions between the environment and ourselves that we call self-awareness. Damage to the neocortex or its connections results in pathologic states characterized by a decrease in the capacity to analyze data and a decrease in the versatility of responses to the environment (learned behavior). Localized damage may result in isolated deficits of cognition in one sensory modality (agnosia) or in the impairment of language (aphasia), memory (amnesia), or motility (apraxia). Diffuse damage may result in a general impoverishment of all cognitive functions and learned behavior, called dementia. Widespread, severe loss of neocortical function results in impaired consciousness.

The third part is the anatomic substrate of emotional, or instinctive, behavior. It is located in the phylogenetically ancient part of the brain called the limbic lobe and mediates some patterns of behavior that determine the survival of the individual or the species, such as mating, aggression, fear, and affection. Damage to the limbic system or interference with its physiology results in distortions of perception, behavior, and consciousness.

---

*Material in this chapter is based in part on the first edition, written by Leopold Canales.

Table 140-1   Classification of stupor and coma

Level of consciousness	Response to stimulation*		Comments
	Verbal	Painful	
Awake	+++	+++	Alert and fully oriented
Sleep	++	+++	Returns to alertness and orientation when stimulated
Delirium	++	+++	Confused, disoriented, agitated, combative; hallucinations may occur
Obtundation	+	++	Remains drowsy, confused, and disoriented when awakened; wakefulness maintained only by continuous stimulation
Light stupor	−	++	Withdraws quickly and forcefully from moderately intense pain, localizing the stimulus
Deep stupor	−	+	Responds only to a strong stimulus but is unable to localize it; decerebration or other stereotyped responses may be present
Coma	−	−	Although unresponsive to stimulation, vital signs may be stable without assistance; some brainstem and spinal cord reflexes may still be present; EEG shows electrical activity
Cerebral death	−	−	Vital signs artificially maintained; no reflexes; electrical silence on EEG

+, Responds to a strong stimulus; ++, responds to a mild stimulus; +++, responds normally; −, no response to stimulus.

STUPOR AND COMA

In clinical neurology the term "consciousness" has been used to imply not only the appearance of wakefulness but also the presence of some form of mental function. The general reactivity of the nervous system to stimuli that we call wakefulness or alertness depends on the interaction of the reticular activating system located in the upper brainstem and diencephalic region with the cerebral hemispheres. Structural or metabolic damage to these structures produces states of decreased alertness or unconsciousness that range from drowsiness to stupor to the complete unresponsiveness of coma (Table 140-1).

A practical way to classify the level of consciousness of a patient is to observe responses to verbal and painful stimulation. A normal person during wakefulness responds readily and appropriately to verbal and painful stimuli. At the end of a period of wakefulness, which for most people is around 16 hours, or in the presence of a nonstimulating environment, the nervous system drifts into sleep, but when aroused it rapidly regains an alert and fully oriented mental state.

The earliest stages of a pathologic decrease in consciousness that are clearly distinguishable are *delirium* and *obtundation*. In delirium the impairment of consciousness is not severe enough to completely abolish voluntary behavior but impairs

mentation sufficiently to produce confusion, disorientation, distortions of perception, dysphoria, and psychomotor agitation. This is seen commonly in metabolic encephalopathies and transiently in patients who are going slowly into coma or recovering from coma. In obtundation the impairment of consciousness has progressed to what looks like deep sleep, but when aroused the patient is unable to regain a normal state of alertness, remains confused and disoriented, and can be kept awake only through constant stimulation.

In the further deteriorated state of consciousness called *stupor*, the patient no longer responds to verbal stimuli but still responds to pain. In lighter states of stupor the response to pain is quick and well coordinated, sometimes including verbal manifestations of anger and defensive movements. When a deeper state of stupor is present, a stronger stimulus is needed to elicit a response; at this point the patient is unable to localize the stimulus and the response is slower and usually stereotyped. In the deeper state of unconsciousness called *coma*, the patient no longer responds to painful stimuli but may be able to manifest some brainstem and spinal cord reflexes. This is often seen in severe barbiturate intoxication, anoxic encephalopathy, and transiently in postictal states.

Unfortunately, no unanimity in the medical literature exists concerning the nomenclature used to define different states of unconsciousness. Some authors call any degree of unresponsiveness stupor or use terms such as "semicoma" or "semistupor" without precisely describing the degree of patient responsiveness. Because of this lack of agreement, the physician should always add a description of the behavior of the patient and the type of stimulus employed to clarify the meaning of the terms.

Some states of consciousness exist in which the degree of interaction between a patient and the environment is greatly reduced, giving the appearance of unresponsiveness. However, on closer inspection evidence of preserved alertness or at least some degree of mental function sometimes exists.

The *locked-in syndrome*, or de-efferented state, is a condition in which a lesion in the ventral portion of the brainstem severely damages the corticospinal and corticobulbar tracts, producing extensive paralysis and in some cases sparing only vertical eye movements. Some patients with this condition have learned to translate their remaining eye movements into Morse code and thus reveal an intact mind.

The *apallic state* refers to the state of severely decreased responsiveness resulting from extensive bilateral lesions in the cerebral hemispheres. The combination of cortical lesions and deeper white matter and gray matter lesions produced by trauma, prolonged anoxia, hypoglycemia, carbon monoxide exposure, or the end state of a degenerative disease damages motor, cognitive, and affective mechanisms.

Akinetic mutism is a state in which patients give the appearance of vigilance by following objects with their eyes and occasionally chewing and swallowing food but remaining otherwise relatively immobile and mute. This condition, also called coma vigil, has been associated with a variety of deep brain lesions, such as communicating hydrocephalus, septal and hypothalamic lesions, lesions near the third ventricle, and paramedian infarctions in the mesencephalic region.

Catatonic stupor is seen most commonly in young people affected by catatonic schizophrenia. The patient lies with eyes open or tightly closed, resisting passive eye opening. Patients have no spontaneous movements, but optokinetic stimulation and caloric testing produce nystagmus. Sometimes the phenomenon of catalepsy is found in which passive postures of the limbs are maintained for a prolonged time. This state of unresponsiveness may be interrupted by catatonic excitement in which the patient is wildly agitated and combative. The electroencephalogram (EEG) during catatonic stupor usually shows fast low-voltage activity instead of the slow frequencies found in unconscious patients.

Although in *hysterical unresponsiveness* the patient may appear to have no response to verbal and painful stimuli, neurologic examination reveals normal pupillary reflexes, nystagmus in response to caloric stimulation, and an EEG pattern indicating an awake state.

PATHOPHYSIOLOGY OF UNCONSCIOUSNESS

Early pathologic accounts of patients with encephalitis suggested that lesions in the tegmental region of the upper midbrain were responsible for the decrease in consciousness. The classic animal experiments of Bremer in 1935 demonstrated that transections through the lower part of the brainstem (encephale isolé) show the behavior and EEG characteristics of cycles of wakefulness and sleep, whereas transections through the upper midbrain (cerveau isolé) put the animal into a state resembling perpetual sleep. The initial interpretation of these experiments, which followed pavlovian doctrines, suggested that sensory inflow was responsible for maintaining wakefulness.

In 1949 Magoun and Moruzzi discovered the ascending reticular activating system (ARAS). This system, within the reticular formation of the brainstem and diencephalon, produced awakening of the animal with electrical stimulation. Destruction of the ARAS produced the behavior and EEG patterns of coma that were irreversible to stimulation via intact sensory pathways. Further experience with pathologic specimens and experimental preparations indicates that, to produce unconsciousness, lesions in the brainstem reticular formation must be bilateral and rostral to the lower third of the pons. Patients with pontine lesions that cause unconsciousness may show awake EEG patterns.

Lesions of the cerebral hemispheres also can produce a decrease in consciousness, but whereas in the brainstem a discrete well-localized lesion can devastate wakefulness, hemispheric lesions must be bilateral and extensive to do so.

INITIAL EXAMINATION OF THE PATIENT IN COMA

The metabolism of the brain is critically dependent on blood flow, oxygenation, glucose, and thiamine. Whatever the cause of coma, outcome depends on the physician's ability to establish adequate airway, breathing, and circulation (ABC). After three tubes of blood are drawn, glucose (25 g) and thiamine (100 mg) are administered quickly while the clinical assessment proceeds.

A *general physical examination* should precede the neurologic evaluation. Evidence of trauma should be sought by palpating the scalp carefully and looking for an accumulation of blood in the subcutaneous orbital and mastoid regions and behind the tympanic membranes. Blood in these locations or leakage of cerebrospinal fluid (CSF) through the nose or ear canal is evidence of a basilar skull fracture. Obvious signs of head trauma should alert the physician to the possibility of an accompanying cervical spine injury, and passive neck movements should be avoided until cervical roentgenograms are taken. Inspection of the mouth may show evidence of tongue biting and hypertrophic gums (a side effect of the anticonvulsant phenytoin) that point to seizures as the cause of the loss of consciousness. The general physical examination also may show evidence of bleeding diathesis, cirrhosis, respiratory dis-

ease, or other systemic illness that could be the primary cause of or a contributing factor to the loss of consciousness.

The *neurologic examination* of an unconscious patient is a challenge. Since the patient is unable to cooperate, the examination is directed toward establishing the degree of responsiveness to specific stimuli ("level of consciousness") and the anatomic localization of the lesion.

The parameters that are most informative in unconscious patients are the ocular fundi, pupillary reflexes, spontaneous and reflex motor behavior, spontaneous and reflex eye movements, and respiration.

OCULAR FUNDI. Careful observation of the ocular fundi without using mydriatics that interfere with pupillary reflexes may produce information about chronic arterial hypertension, diabetes, subhyaloid hemorrhages (the result of sudden severe intracranial hypertension, as in subarachnoid hemorrhage), and the presence or absence of papilledema.

PUPILLARY REFLEXES. Pupillary reflexes depend on the function of centers situated in the diencephalon and the brainstem. Horner's syndrome (ptosis, miosis, and anhidrosis) is caused by damage to the sympathetic fibers that descend from the hypothalamus through the brainstem and the cervical spinal cord toward the second neuron in the upper thoracic region and then return to the cranium to dilate the pupil via peripheral sympathetic nerves accompanying the carotid artery. Any lesion along this circuitous route could produce Horner's syndrome, but in the presence of stupor or coma a diencephalic lesion or a brainstem lesion is likely. Pupils that are midposition in range and unreactive to light suggest a midbrain lesion in the tectal or pretectal region, but the additional presence of bilateral external oculomotor paralysis points to a more tegmental location involving third nerve nuclei or fibers. Bilateral pinpoint pupils indicate a pontine lesion. The light reflex is still present, although a magnifying lens may be required to observe it.

A unilaterally dilated pupil suggests peripheral compression of the third nerve. The pupillary fibers are located in the periphery of the nerve and are the first to be affected in the process of transtentorial herniation when the uncus of the temporal lobe presses on the nerve, stretching its fibers.

Systemic metabolic processes leading to unconsciousness do not affect pupillary reflexes except for intoxication with atropine-like drugs, glutethimide, and opiates. Atropine-like drugs produce fully dilated, unresponsive pupils in addition to dry skin, dry mucous membranes, and hyperthermia. Glutethimide is a hypnotic; an overdose produces midposition pupils or moderately dilated pupils. Opiates such as heroin or morphine constrict the pupils to pinpoint size but preserve the light reflex.

SPONTANEOUS AND REFLEX MOTOR BEHAVIOR. In cases in which unconsciousness progresses from obtundation into coma, a concomitant deterioration of spontaneous and reflex motor behavior occurs. In obtundation it is common to see the patient spontaneously changing posture in bed, drawing up the bed sheets, and trying to pull out intravenous needles and indwelling catheters. When painful stimuli are used, the patient accurately localizes the stimulus and fights forcefully, sometimes accompanying the response with vocalization and grimacing. Asymmetry of spontaneous movement, confirmed by a similar pattern of response to pain, may indicate a hemiparesis or monoparesis. A variety of painful stimuli are used by clinicians to reach a diagnosis. Some are ineffective, damaging, or degrading. Bilateral upward *pressure on the styloid processes* with the examiner's thumbs placed just behind the mandible is best. In stupor or light coma this produces a bilateral facial grimace that allows evaluation of facial weakness, as well as symmetric stimuli for evaluation of eye opening, voluntary movement, and posture. As unconsciousness deepens, the resting posture becomes less natural and spontaneous movements no longer occur. Motor asymmetries become less apparent as the response to pain becomes less elaborate and forceful; they may be replaced by stereotyped responses having specific anatomic or pathologic connotations. These responses include the following:

1. *Decorticate posture*. The arms and wrists are flexed, and the legs are extended with internal rotation and plantar flexion. This posture is seen in cases of extensive hemispheric lesions involving the corticospinal pathways.
2. *Decerebrate posture*. In this posture the arms are extended and pronated and the legs are extended with plantar flexion (sometimes accompanied by trismus and opisthotonos) spontaneously or as a response to pain. A lesion between the red nuclei and the vestibular nuclei of the brainstem is implicated.

External rotation of one leg may be caused by hip fracture, leg weakness, or hemiparesis. *Focal seizures* may be manifested by minor deviation of gaze, usually with a clonic quality, head rotation, or twitching of the face or fingers. Generalized *myoclonic contractions* are commonly seen in uremia or anoxia. Coarse and irregular tremor and *asterixis* are often seen in metabolic encephalopathies, especially hepatic ones.

SPONTANEOUS AND REFLEX EYE MOVEMENTS. Unconscious patients in whom the centers that mediate eye movements are intact commonly have a slightly divergent, straightforward gaze and slow, horizontal conjugate movements (roving eye movements). In these patients, turning the head briskly from side to side elicits conjugate eye movements directed opposite to the head rotation. This is the oculocephalic, or doll's eye reflex, which is absent in the normal alert individual. Stimulation of the semicircular canals by irrigating the external ear canal with 50 ml of ice water (caloric stimulation) produces tonic eye deviation toward the stimulated side. In a normal individual this type of stimulation causes nystagmus with the rapid component away from the stimulated side.

Full horizontal excursion of the eyes to both sides is possible only when the nuclei and the internuclear connections between the third and the sixth nerves are preserved. Because these structures are located in the tegmentum of the pons and the midbrain, the presence of horizontal eye movements suggests that the immediately adjacent reticular activating system is also intact and that the cause of unconsciousness is not a structural brainstem lesion.

Unilateral lesions in the pontine gaze center (region of the abducens nucleus) produce a paralysis of ipsilateral conjugate gaze and a contralateral conjugate deviation of the eyes. Caloric stimulation fails to move the eyes beyond the midline.

The pathway connecting the pontine gaze center to the midbrain oculomotor nuclei is called the medial longitudinal fasciculus (MLF). When its fibers are damaged, the ipsilateral medial rectus muscle fails to contract when required for voluntary or reflex conjugate horizontal gaze. This is called internuclear ophthalmoplegia and can be demonstrated by oculocephalic or caloric testing in the unconscious patient. Paresis of vertical gaze as indicated by loss of doll's eye reflex to neck flexion or bilateral ice-water (caloric) stimulation indicates midbrain involvement. Observations of spontaneous eye movements in comas caused by a brainstem lesion may reveal both conjugate and dysconjugate activity, ocular bobbing, and ocular myoclonus.

Skew deviation of the eyes (one up or down) is an indication of brainstem lesions. Forced downward and inward deviation of the eyes (looking at the tip of the nose) has been described in cases of thalamic hemorrhage and is usually accompanied by nonreactive pinpoint pupils.

RESPIRATION. The abnormal respiratory patterns most commonly identified in unconscious patients are Cheyne-Stokes respiration, central neurogenic hyperventilation, and apneustic and ataxic breathing.

Cheyne-Stokes respiration is the respiratory rhythm that alternates between periods of hyperpnea (increased rate and depth of ventilation) and apnea (absence of respiratory movements). After the apnea the hyperpnea starts in a crescendo fashion until a peak is reached, after which a decrescendo period starts, ending in apnea again. It is commonly caused by deep, bilateral hemispheric lesions, either structural or metabolic.

Central neurogenic hyperventilation is a transient pattern of rapid, regular respiration described with tegmental lesions of the upper brainstem but probably pulmonary in origin.

Apneustic breathing is the result of a lesion in the pontine respiratory center. The inspiratory and expiratory phases of the respiratory cycle are separated by pauses of 2 to 3 seconds.

Ataxic respiration is a disorganized pattern of inspiratory and expiratory movements seen in association with lesions of the medullary respiratory center.

From these descriptions it can be concluded that if the pattern of the respiratory cycle is disturbed, there is a lesion in the ponto-medullary respiratory center. Lesions above this level affect only the respiratory rate and amplitude.

LESIONS PRODUCING UNCONSCIOUSNESS

Lesions producing unconsciousness can be divided into three groups: supratentorial mass lesions, infratentorial lesions, and diffuse encephalopathies.

Supratentorial mass lesions

The intracranial cavity is divided into two compartments by a portion of the dura called the tentorium cerebelli. The supratentorial compartment harbors the cerebral hemispheres and the diencephalon, whereas the infratentorial compartment or posterior fossa contains the cerebellum and the brainstem. The anterior attachment of the tentorium is to the edges of the petrous bone and the clinoid processes of the sella turcica. Between the clinoid attachments the edge of the tentorium recedes to form an opening called the incisura, through which the midbrain, the CSF contained in the mesencephalic subarachnoid cisterns, and the posterior cerebral arteries enter the supratentorial space. This incisura is the only connection between the supratentorial and infratentorial compartments.

Because of the nondistensible properties of the adult skull, an expanding mass in the supratentorial space produces progressive displacement of brain parenchyma and increased intracranial pressure that eventually pushes the tissues through the only possible exit, the incisura. The passage of the supratentorial structures through the incisura is called *transtentorial herniation* and causes a number of clinical signs that can be grouped into two syndromes: central and uncal herniations.

Central transtentorial herniation occurs when the displacement of tissues is symmetric and the resultant vector of forces converges in the midline to push the diencephalon down through the incisura. Acute hydrocephalus and vertex, frontal, or occipital mass lesions are the most common causes of central transtentorial herniation. The impairment of diencephalic function and the downward displacement of the brainstem initially produce obtundation or light stupor accompanied by Cheyne-Stokes respirations and small pupils. Roving eye movements may be present, and the eyes move conjugately toward the side of caloric stimulation, implicating the structural integrity of the brainstem. Preexisting hemiparesis may worsen, whereas paratonia (active resistance to passive movements) develops bilaterally, accompanied by bilateral Babinski's sign and decorticate posture. As the herniation progresses, signs of hypothalamic distress (diabetes insipidus, hyperthermia, or hypothermia) may occur, and signs of midbrain involvement begin to characterize the clinical picture. Cheyne-Stokes respiration is replaced by central hyperventilation, the pupils enlarge to midpoint, caloric testing produces dysconjugate movements, and decorticate posture is replaced by spontaneous, or pain-elicited, decerebrate rigidity.

Further progression shows signs of lower brainstem involvement with the development of generalized flaccidity and an absent response to caloric stimulation. At this point the combination of pressure and downward displacement of the brainstem produces ischemia and herniation of the medulla and the cerebellar tonsils through the foramen magnum, resulting in respiratory depression and hypotension. Respiratory arrest and dilated pupils signal the end of the process. If vital signs are artificially maintained with ventilators and pressor agents, the intracranial pressure may continue to rise, becoming equal to the arterial systolic pressure, at which point no brain perfusion is possible.

The inferior surface of the temporal lobe rests on the tentorium, and the most medial portion, the uncus, slightly overhangs the edge. Expanding temporal or parietal lesions produce a medial displacement of the hemisphere, which, in addition to the increased intracranial pressure pushes the ipsilateral uncus through the incisura. This is called uncal herniation. The third cranial nerve runs parallel to the incisural edge in such a way that the herniated uncus descends on the nerve, stretching its fibers and producing ipsilateral pupillary dilatation.

At this point consciousness may be normal or impaired, depending on how much the supratentorial displacement of the tissues is affecting the diencephalic region. Further herniation of the uncus compresses the midbrain against the opposite edge of the tentorium. Signs of progressive deterioration of brainstem function include further depression of consciousness, abnormal respiratory pattern, sluggish or absent caloric response, decerebrate posture, dilation of the pupil opposite the one originally dilated, and hemiparesis ipsilateral to the mass lesion. Such hemiparesis is explained as the result of the pressure of the cerebral peduncle contralateral to the herniating temporal lobe against the tentorial edge (Kernohan's notch). The time between the initial pupillary dilatation and the signs of midbrain distress can be quite short if the expanding lesion is rapidly enlarging (for example, in epidural hematoma). After this point the clinical picture is identical to central transtentorial herniation. Postmortem specimens from patients who have sustained prolonged herniation have shown that the compression and displacement of the brainstem result in tegmental hemorrhagic lesions caused by compression of venous drainage through the incisura.

Infratentorial lesions

Two types of posterior fossa lesion (infratentorial lesions) cause unconsciousness: destructive lesions that directly destroy the reticular activating system in the brainstem tegmentum and expanding lesions that compress the brainstem or CSF pathways.

In destructive lesions a rapid loss of consciousness occurs

Table 140-2 Metabolic causes of unconsciousness

General causes	Specific manifestations and drugs
Lack of energy substrate	Anoxia, hypoglycemia, decreased brain blood flow, deficient thiamine and niacin
Endogenous causes	
Organ system failure	Liver, kidney, lung, endocrine system
Fluid and electrolyte imbalance	Dehydration/water intoxication, hyponatremia/hypernatremia, hypomagnesemia/hypermagnesemia, hypocalcemia/hypercalcemia, acidosis/alkalosis
Toxic products or direct effect of infection	Sepsis, meningitis
Disturbance of temperature regulation	Hypothermia/hyperthermia
Exogenous causes	Sedative drugs, ethanol, anticholinergics, opiates, heavy metals, cyanide, methyl alcohol, ethylene glycol, organic phosphates

simultaneously with signs of midbrain or pontine dysfunction. Brainstem infarction caused by basilar artery thrombosis and pontine hemorrhage are the most common pathologic conditions destroying the brainstem tegmentum.

Expansive lesions, or mass lesions, produce a disturbance of consciousness either by directly compressing the brainstem or by blocking CSF flow through the fourth ventricle and thereby producing acute hydrocephalus. Cerebellar hemorrhage, infarction, tumor, and abscess account for the majority of these cases.

Diffuse encephalopathies

Diffuse disturbances of neuronal function occur when the substrates required for neuronal energy metabolism are in short supply, when the internal environment of the cell is disturbed by external agents such as drugs or environmental poisons, or as a complication of the failure of another organ system such as the renal, hepatic, endocrine, cardiovascular, or respiratory system.

Metabolic encephalopathy is the most common cause of decreased consciousness and accounts in any large hospital for more than half of the patients with coma of unknown origin. The metabolic causes of unconsciousness are listed in Table 140-2.

When the metabolic impairment is mild, the onset of symptoms can be insidious and nonspecific. Subtle changes in mentation such as decreased attention span, mild drowsiness, dullness of affect, and decreased motor coordination precede for variable periods of time the more overt pathologic picture of an advanced metabolic impairment. As neuronal dysfunction progresses, confusion, disorientation, and perceptual distortions such as illusions, delusions, or hallucinations, accompanied by combativeness and agitation, may dominate the clinical picture for a prolonged time or may be a short prelude to a more severe impairment of consciousness.

Motor phenomena such as tremor, asterixis, myoclonus, or seizures are usually seen during the course of the disease. The level of consciousness often fluctuates, so a patient who is at one moment confused and agitated may quiet down to a stuporous state for a variable period and then return spontaneously to psychomotor agitation.

Metabolic encephalopathy is generally characterized by impairment of consciousness without signs of focal neurologic deficit. Nevertheless, exceptions exist. Focal signs suggestive of a structural lesion such as hemiparesis, aphasia, and focal seizures may occur in hypoglycemia. Hemiparesis, gaze palsies, and bilateral Babinski's sign may be present transiently in hepatic failure. Signs of meningeal irritation, with CSF pleocytosis and focal seizures, can be seen in uremic encephalopathy. The opposite situation, in which focal or multifocal pathologic conditions behave clinically as diffuse brain disorders, is also important to remember in the differential diagnosis. Chronic subdural hematoma, frontal and temporal lobe tumors, fat embolism, systemic lupus erythematosus, cerebral malaria, and thrombotic thrombocytopenic purpura are examples of such a situation.

Elderly demented patients seem to be more susceptible to metabolic encephalopathies and take longer to recover from them than younger patients with healthy brains. In this respect the prolonged use of drugs, especially sedatives and analgesics, is of particular concern because it is one of the most common causes of such problems in these patients.

Epilepsy is a common cause of stupor and coma, particularly in the postictal state, in which severe impairment of consciousness may occur and last for many hours. Intoxication with antiepileptic drugs, accidental or volitional, may be seen. Pseudoseizures may result in prolonged apparent unresponsiveness. *Ictal coma* is recognized increasingly as a cause of impaired consciousness. Persistent focal or multifocal seizure activity may impair consciousness in patients with cerebral infarction, hemorrhage, or tumor. Patients with primary generalized epilepsy may develop *spike-wave stupor* in childhood or even in later life.

LABORATORY DATA IN THE DIAGNOSIS OF UNCONSCIOUSNESS

The basic battery of tests supplementing the clinical analysis of the history and physical examination consists of computed tomography (CT scans), EEG, and serum chemistry tests. The CT scan produces information about structural lesions in the supratentorial and infratentorial spaces and is the ideal test for diagnosing tumors, hematomas, hydrocephalus, cerebrovascular accidents, and brain swelling. Intrinsic brainstem lesions are still difficult to visualize with current techniques.

The EEG tests neuronal physiology and is therefore important in the diagnosis and follow-up of metabolic encephalopathies and toxic encephalopathy and in the diagnosis of ictal stupor. Serum chemistry tests should cover the spectrum of biochemical abnormalities that may result from an organ system failure or fluid and electrolyte imbalance capable of impairing brain function.

CSF examination is important when the differential diagnosis includes a central nervous system infection or a subarachnoid hemorrhage. Screening serum and urine for toxic agents becomes necessary when the cause of coma is not obvious.

Skull roentgenograms, isotope brain scans, or cerebral angiograms may become important in the diagnosis of coma if a CT scan is not available. Skull roentgenograms should be obtained in every case of craniofacial trauma.

BIBLIOGRAPHY

Fisher CM: The neurological examination of the comatose patient, Acta Neurol Scand 45(suppl 36):1, 1969.

Harner R and Naquet R, editors: Altered states of consciousness, coma, and cerebral death, Vol 12. In Remond A, editor: Handbook of electroencephalography, Amsterdam, 1975, Elsevier.

Plum F and Posner J: The diagnosis of stupor and coma, ed 3, Philadelphia, 1982, FA Davis Co.

Ropper AH: Coma and acutely raised intracranial pressure. In Asbury AK,

McKhann G, and McDonald I, editors: Diseases of the nervous system, Philadelphia, 1986, WB Saunders Co.

141·SLEEP DISORDERS
June M. Fry

The clinical application of acquired scientific information regarding sleep physiology and biologic rhythm functions has led to the formulation of a diagnostic classification of sleep and arousal disorders and new diagnostic tests and treatments for these disorders. The diagnostic classification includes four major divisions: disorders of initiating and maintaining sleep (insomnias); disorders of excessive somnolence; disorders of the sleep-wake schedule; and dysfunctions associated with sleep, sleep stages, or partial arousals (parasomnias).

Clinical polysomnography provides objective measurements of physiologic and pathologic changes during sleep. These continuous polygraphic recordings of edetroencephalography (EEG), surface electromyography (EMG) of mentalis muscles for detection of muscle activity loss during REM sleep, and anterior tibialis muscles for detection of leg movements, electrooculography (EOG) for detection of eye movements, electrocardiogram (ECG), respiration (airflow at nares and mouth), respiratory effort, and oxygen saturation by oximetry are now routinely used in sleep disorders centers.

Wakefulness and sleep states are characterized by typical patterns on EEG, EOG, and chin EMG. Sleep is an active, complex state with two phases: non–rapid eye movement (non-REM) sleep and rapid eye movement (REM) sleep. Non-REM sleep is composed of four stages of progressive slowing of the EEG with low-voltage, mixed-frequency activity in stage 1, moderately low-voltage background EEG with sleep spindles (0.5- to 2-second bursts of 12 to 14 Hz activity) and K complexes (brief high-voltage biphasic discharges) in stage 2, and high-amplitude slower-frequency activity in stages 3 and 4, also called delta sleep. REM sleep consists of low-voltage, mixed-frequency EEG, intermittent sawtooth waves (3 to 5 Hz triangular waveforms), bursts of rapid, conjugate eye movements, suppressed or absent chin EMG caused by an active inhibition of muscle activity, and intermittent irregular bursts of muscle discharges. During REM sleep heart and respiration rates are increased and irregular, and vivid dreaming and penile tumescence occur.

Transient insomnia lasts less than 3 weeks and is usually situational, caused by emotions such as excitement, sorrow, or anxiety. Hypnotic drugs may be an effective treatment but should be prescribed for less than 2 weeks, and the patient should be warned that sleep disruption and anxiety may recur when the drug is discontinued. Benzodiazepines are the drugs of choice, and no other hypnotics should be prescribed with them.

When insomnia continues for more than 3 weeks, it is termed persistent insomnia, and there are many causes. The specific cause (for example, psychiatric disorder, pain, gastroesophageal reflux, hypnotic drug use, or alcohol abuse) must be determined and treated.

Persistent psychophysiologic insomnia often follows situational insomnia and results from somatized anxiety manifested as restlessness, apprehension, ruminative thoughts, and hypervigilance, all of which interfere with sleep and lead to negative conditioning. The most effective treatment is behavioral therapy including relaxation therapy, stimulus control, and sleep hygiene.

Nocturnal myoclonus (periodic leg movements in sleep) is often associated with insomnia but may also lead to fatigue and daytime sleepiness. Stereotypic contractions of lower leg muscles occur in rhythmic series during sleep and often cause brief arousals. Clonazepam (0.5 to 2 mg orally at bedtime) is the most commonly used treatment. Before drug treatment is begun, deficiencies of folic acid and iron should be sought and treated if present.

All patients with excessive daytime sleepiness require diagnostic evaluation. The two most common disorders of excessive somnolence are obstructive sleep apnea and narcolepsy.

Patients with obstructive sleep apnea are typically obese, middle-aged and older men who snore loudly and have breathing pauses followed by loud, snorting snores and arousals during sleep. Apnea episodes may occur hundreds of times during nocturnal sleep and are usually caused by obstruction in the oropharynx or hypopharynx. Obstructive sleep apnea is rare in women except after menopause or in the presence of structural abnormalities such as micrognathia or enlarged tonsils and morbid obesity. In severe cases of obstructive sleep apnea, in addition to chronic daytime drowsiness, essential hypertension and cardiac arrhythmias may develop.

The most common nonsurgical treatment for sleep apnea is nasal continuous positive airway pressure (CPAP), which is administered by delivering air from a blower controlled by a pressure valve to a nasal mask via tubing. The treatment is first tried during polysomnography so that the pressure required for the alleviation of airway obstruction during sleep can be determined. If the treatment is successful and well tolerated, a commercially available nasal CPAP unit is prescribed for home use. A tongue-retaining device and an orthodontic appliance worn during sleep may benefit select patients. In most cases weight loss is the ideal treatment. In some cases, especially in children and young adults, excision of enlarged tonsils and adenoids results in cure. The surgical procedure, uvulopalatopharyngoplasty, is inconsistently beneficial, and selection criteria are not well established. Tracheostomy is always successful by providing an airway below the obstruction. Central sleep apnea characterized by intermittent loss of respiratory effort also occurs but is uncommon. It presumably is caused by central nervous system dysfunction but specific lesions are rarely identified.

Narcolepsy is a specific neurologic disorder characterized by excessive daytime sleepiness causing obligatory naps that are often refreshing. Approximately 80% to 90% of narcoleptic patients develop cataplexy, which consists of brief episodes of paralysis or weakness precipitated by strong emotions such as laughter, anger, and surprise. Other symptoms may include hypnagogic hallucinations, vivid dreamlike images that occur during sleep onset or upon waking, and sleep paralysis, a global paralysis of voluntary muscles that also occurs at sleep onset or upon waking. These auxiliary symptoms are thought to be dissociated REM sleep phenomena. Narcolepsy is a genetic disorder that usually begins during the second decade of life. It is incurable but is treated with medications aimed at the relief of symptoms. Many patients benefit from regularly scheduled deliberate brief naps, but most patients also require stimulants, which include pemoline (18.75 to 112.5 mg/day), methylphenidate (5 to 60 mg/day), or dextroamphetamine (5 to 60 mg/day). Incomplete control of symptoms, side effects, and tolerance may occur with these drugs. If cataplexy is frequent or disabling imipramine (25 to 100 mg/day), or protriptyline (15 to 40 mg/day) usually provides effective treatment.

The differential diagnosis of excessive daytime sleepiness includes many other conditions and disorders. These include chronic sleep deprivation, use of drugs and alcohol, idiopathic CNS hypersomnolence, and the Klein-Levin syndrome. Klein-Levin syndrome is a rare disorder characterized by recurrent episodes of excessive sleepiness lasting 1 day to 4 weeks and is accompanied by abnormal behavior including increased appetite and sexual disinhibition and mental disturbances.

BIBLIOGRAPHY

Coleman R, Pollak CP, and Weitzman ED: Periodic movements in sleep (nocturnal myoclonus): relation to sleep disorders, Ann Neurol 8:416, 1980.

Fujita S et al: Surgical correction of anatomic abnormalities in obstructive sleep apnea syndrome: uvulopalatopharyngoplasty, Otolaryngol Head Neck Surg 89:923, 1981.

Guilleminault C, editor: Sleeping and waking disorders: indications and techniques, Menlo Park, Calif, 1981, Addison-Wesley.

Guilleminault C, editor: Narcolepsy, Sleep 9:99, 1986.

Guilleminault C and Lugaresi E, editors: Sleep wake disorders: natural history, epidemiology, and long-term evolution, New York, 1983, Raven Press.

Hauri P, editor: The sleep disorders. In Current concepts, Kalamazoo, Mich., 1982, Upjohn Co.

National Institute of Mental Health Consensus Development Conference: Drugs and insomnia: the use of medication to promote sleep, JAMA 251:2410, 1984.

Roffwarg HP: Diagnostic classification of sleep and arousal disorders, Sleep 2:1, 1979.

Roffwarg H and Erman M: Evaluation and diagnosis of the sleep disorders: implications for psychiatry and other clinical specialities, Psychiatr Update 4:294, 1985.

Sullivan CE et al: Reversal of obstructive sleep apnea by continuous positive airway pressure applied through the nares, Lancet 1:862, 1981.

Thawley SE, editor: Symposium on sleep apnea disorders, Med Clin North Am 69:6, 1985.

Weitzman ED et al: Biological rhythms in man: relationship of sleep-wake cycle, cortisol, growth hormone and temperature during temporal isolation. In Martin JB, Reichlin S, and Bick K, editors: Neurosecretion and brain peptides, New York, 1981, Raven Press.

Weitzman ED: Sleep and aging. In Katzman R and Terry R, editors: Neurology of aging, Philadelphia, 1983, FA Davis Co.

142·DISORDERS OF COGNITION

Neil M. Sussman*

The study of cognitive disorders has been historically based on clinical descriptions of abnormal behavior associated with brain lesions. Terminology is based on these behavioral defects. When the predominant feature is a failure to identify or recognize a stimulus and sensation is intact, the syndrome is called *agnosia*. When there is a failure to execute a response (in the absence of paralysis), it is called *apraxia*. Disorders of language production and comprehension are called *aphasias*, and disorders of memory are known as *amnesias*.

Much literature has accumulated over the years and has produced conflict and controversy in the classification, anatomic correlation, and inferred pathophysiology of many cognitive dysfunctions. At the core of the problem is our ignorance of the pertinent normal anatomic structures and physiologic mechanisms involved. Without such knowledge the various definitions, classifications, and anatomic inferences based on diseased structures are often incomplete and inaccurate. The problem is compounded because human behavior is complex, and when disease occurs, the normal pathways that remain

---

*Material in this chapter is based in part on the first edition, written by Leopold Canales.

INFORMATION PROCESSING OPERATIONS

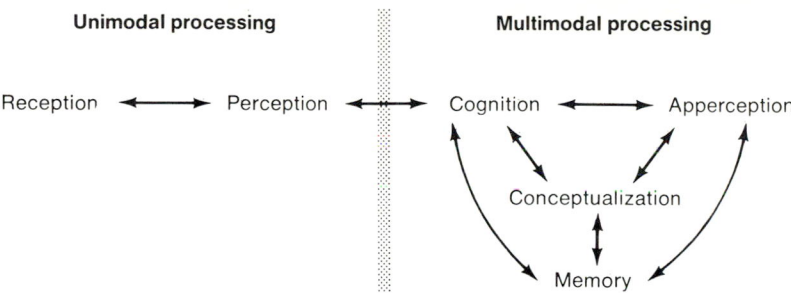

Fig. 142-1   Model for information processing. Each sensory modality undergoes some degree of unimodal processing before entering the pool of multimodal information, which is integrated by special areas of the association cortex.

produce syndromes that can conform to almost any classification.

To understand the function of the nervous system, one must realize that it is clearly concerned with processing information. Anatomically, the great development of the cortex of the cerebral hemispheres is the most striking phylogenetic feature differentiating the human brain from the brains of other mammals. This development is based primarily on the increase in the area occupied by the association cortex and its connections. The human brain therefore possesses additional machinery that enables it to process information quantitatively and qualitatively better than any other comparable nervous system. We can also assume that damage to the hemispheres would result in syndromes that in one way or another would result in failure of information processing.

To use information processing as a conceptual tool requires a correlation between our knowledge of anatomy and physiology and a general model of human information processing. This correlation is unavoidably tentative because of the need to generalize about complex mechanisms that at present cannot be defined more precisely and because of our modest knowledge of the anatomy and physiology of the different sensory channels. In recent years knowledge about information processing by the visual cortex has become available, and indications that the same type of processing occurs in other sensory modalities exist.

The basic premise of the model can be summarized as follows: each sensory modality undergoes some degree of processing before entering the pool of multimodal information; this pool is integrated in different ways by special areas of the association cortex, leading to unique forms of behavior (Fig. 142-1).

INFORMATION PROCESSING AND FOCAL HEMISPHERIC LESIONS

Different types of environmental energy are constantly stimulating our peripheral receptors. The transduction of energy taking place at the receptor area (for example, in the retina and cochlea) generates a signal that contains all the information of that modality at a given moment. This operation, called *reception*, constitutes the first step of the information processing model. Lesions at this point produce unimodal and primary deficits. The lesion affects only one sensory modality, destroying raw information (for example, a complete lesion destroys all information for sight or sound, producing blindness or deafness).

From the receptor area the information is transported to the primary receptive cortex of each modality via those thalamic nuclei that are also modality specific. This anatomic arrangement is common to most sensory channels. (The sense of smell does not pass through the thalamus.) Once the information reaches the primary receptive cortex, it travels to the immediately adjacent cortical regions, called the association cortex. In the primary and association cortices the raw information begins to be analyzed and organized into familiar patterns. This constitutes the second operation of sensory processing, called *perception*. Lesions limited to these cortical regions are uncommon. The few cases reported have been caused by carbon monoxide poisoning, anoxia, and rarely infarctions. An example is visual agnosia in which, in the presence of good visual acuity and intact visual fields, the patient is unable to identify or copy objects.

In the association cortex the information travels via subcortical fibers to the nonspecific thalamic nuclei, to other association cortical regions and limbic structures ipsilaterally, and via commissural fibers to the homotopic cortex in the contralateral hemisphere. In the association cortex and its connections the unimodal information coming from the primary receptive cortices is integrated and further elaborated into multimodal levels. In this process, called *gnosis* or *cognition*, perceptions are identified and classified on the basis of past experience (recognition) or by association with other sensory modalities (cross-modality reference). Hallucinations are disorders of perception in which thought is distorted and perceived by the patient as being real.

Discrete lesions of the association cortex or its connecting fibers result in disconnection syndromes. Many types of agnosias and apraxias are easily explained by this mechanism. Alexia (inability to read) without agraphia (inability to write) and with color anomia results from a combined lesion of the left occipital cortex and the splenium of the corpus callosum. Surgical section of the corpus callosum results in an "aphasic right hemisphere" (alexia and anomia in the left visual field and apraxia and tactile anomia in the left hand). In visual association agnosia the patient can copy drawings without difficulty but is unable to identify them. In visual object agnosia the patient has an inability to name objects that can be described in detail and can be named when touched. Both visual association agnosia and visual object agnosia suggest a disconnection between the visual and language centers.

Based on visual and somesthetic information, the parietal cortex can abstract the *concepts* of self-image (somatognosia) and external space. Arithmetic calculation, the sensing of volume and shape (stereognosis), the sensing of weight (barognosis), and the ability to read and write are also made possible by the capacity of the parietal cortex to codify, abstract, and integrate information into concepts.

Lesions of the parietal cortex produce syndromes that represent the conceptual loss of self-image, external space, and their relationship. Neglect of the contralateral space or of the limbs, spatial disorientation, right versus left confusion, dressing apraxias, constructional apraxias, and astereognosis are the predominant features of right-sided lesions. Alexia, agraphia, acalculia, and finger agnosia are seen with left-sided lesions.

The language-processing cortex is located at the convergence of the temporal, parietal, and frontal regions and is in the left hemisphere in almost all right-handed people and the large majority of left-handed people. This area of the association cortex with its connections can encode cognitive and affective information into a system of symbols called verbal language and can also produce the reverse process of decoding verbal language into cognition and emotion. This process of codifying information provides the brain with an extraordinary capacity to receive, extract, store, and transmit vast amounts of information that would be otherwise inaccessible. The operations possible with the use of this code (including abstraction, association, synthesis, induction, and deduction) result in what is called the *verbal conceptual* level of information processing. It occupies the major portion of mentation and has become the most important mental instrument to interpret the environment.

Damage to the language-processing cortex results in syndromes called aphasias. If the lesion affects the posterior aspect of this area (Wernicke's area), the patient's difficulty is primarily with the decoding process (an inability to understand spoken and written language). Patients have a marked increase in verbal output, and the language used is often filled with errors. Lesions in the anterior aspect of the language-processing area, toward the posterior and inferior portions of the frontal lobe, result in difficulty or inability to encode language (Broca's aphasia) with difficulty in verbal expression. Patients have a marked reduction in verbal output with poor use of connecting words such as adjectives and prepositions. Subcortical lesions that connect Broca's area in the frontal lobe and Wernicke's area in the posterior temporal lobe can produce difficulties in repeating phrases on command even when the patient comprehends well and produces language fluently. This is called conduction aphasia.

Another special area of multimodal convergence is the prefrontal cortex. It is extensively connected with the rest of the cerebral cortex and the limbic system, which suggests that its function deals with the interface between cognition and emotion. In general the prefrontal cortex seems concerned with integrating cognitive information and emotional needs, resulting in forms of behavior that produce the most adequate emotional response to a given environmental situation. From the clinical description of patients with bilateral prefrontal lesions, it seems clear that these patients suffer changes in their emotional reactions. The terms "witzelsucht" and "moria" have been used to describe the facetiousness and silly joking these patients often display. Changes in goal-oriented behavior are commonly prominent and are manifested as a lack of insight and foresight, a loss of the sense of what is socially appropriate, and a loss of ethical and esthetic values.

The next operation in information processing is *apperception*. This involves the choice of material brought from cognition and emotion into the stream of thought (mentation). Apperception also determines what information is incorporated as memories. Its anatomic and physiologic substrates represent the collective effort of cortical and limbic structures, as well

as diencephalic mechanisms that deal with arousal and attention. Damage to any of these structures impairs mentation.

The last operation in information processing is *memory*, which is the ability to store and retrieve information. Memory is one of the most important features of human information processing. It is the basis of learned behavior because without it the nervous system would depend entirely on a limited repertory of built-in responses (reflex behavior).

The anatomic structures that have so far been implicated in memory function are located mainly in the limbic system, suggesting a link between emotions and memory. Assuming a nervous system model in which emotions are a primary impulse for action, the learning process is directed at retaining data that produce emotional experiences intense enough to induce a motor response (pursuit or avoidance depending on the nature of the emotional experience). The learning process is demonstrated when the stereotyped response to the same stimulus under the same circumstances is repeated. This is even more clearly demonstrated when the response is to only a portion of the original stimulus. Our conscious experience using memory processes clearly shows the utility of such a model. Data related to intense emotional situations enter our memory without difficulty and are not only easy to remember but often impossible to forget, whereas daily events with a minimum of emotional association escape our memory completely or are retained for only short periods. The purposeful use of memory, unrelated to emotional experience, requires laborious recruitment of attention, tedious repetition, and periodic rehearsal to prevent decay. Lesions of the hippocampi, fornices, mammillary bodies, and dorsomedial nuclei of the thalamus have been associated in different degrees with amnestic syndromes. The most consistent evidence so far concerns lesions of the hippocampus; its bilateral excision, called Korsakoff's syndrome, produces the most severe and discrete amnestic syndrome sparing all other cognitive functions.

Memory can be clinically categorized and selectively affected in the following ways.

Immediate memory, or *instant recall,* is the ability to retain data long enough to maintain a coherent thread of thought, to execute sequential tasks, or to perform mental calculation and digit span (repeating a series of digits after hearing them). Even in some patients with bilateral hippocampal lesions (Korsakoff's syndrome), immediate memory can be maintained for a few minutes if there is no distraction. Immediate memory is impaired in processes that decrease the attention span, such as metabolic encephalopathies and dementia; in normal individuals a decrease in concentration can occur from distractibility, excessive fatigue, or tiredness.

Short-term memory is the ability to retain and retrieve data for more than a few minutes. Its loss represents the amnestic syndrome and can be produced by bilateral hippocampal lesions caused most commonly by thiamine deficiency or head trauma. Old memories and skills are retained, but new learning is impossible (anterograde amnesia). Transient forms of short-term memory deficits have been described in cases of temporal lobe epilepsy or idiopathic transient global amnesia. Patients with the latter usually have difficulty recalling recent events before the attack (retrograde amnesia) in addition to having the memory defect during the attack. A unilateral hippocampal lesion on the left side may impair verbal recent memory, whereas a hippocampal lesion on the right side may impair nonverbal recent memory.

Long-term memory is the ability to retain and retrieve data extending from events of a few months back to events of childhood. It is affected in retrograde amnesia most commonly seen in cases of severe head injury. The defect rarely persists beyond a few months and tends to lessen with time.

In summary, focal lesions to the hemispheres produce clinical syndromes through the following defects of information processing:

1. Deterioration of the signal through damage to the thalamocortical projections, producing deficits in primary sensation such as visual field defects or hypesthesia
2. Perceptual disorders resulting from failure to complete the processing of unimodal information because of damage to the cortical extraction mechanisms
3. Disconnection syndromes resulting from failure of cross-modality referencing and multimodal processing because of lesions affecting connecting fibers (commissural or subcortical) from their neurons of origin
4. Inability to integrate multimodal information to a conceptual level because of damage to the special areas of multimodal convergence such as the parietal, language-processing, and prefrontal cortices
5. Inability to store or retrieve information because of damage to limbic structures or certain thalamic nuclei

These syndromes are seldom found in pure form because hemispheric lesions rarely remain limited to the cortex or to discrete connecting fibers. The most common syndrome is a mixture of these mechanisms, the result depending on the type and location of the lesion.

INFORMATION PROCESSING DEFECT AND DIFFUSE HEMISPHERIC PATHOLOGY (DEMENTIA)

DEFINITION AND DIAGNOSIS. The impairment of all cognitive functions and learned behavior is called dementia. It can be caused by diffuse damage to the cortex or its connections or by one or several focal lesions large enough that the resulting cognitive loss severely impairs general behavior and cannot be compensated for by the remaining healthy tissue. Dementia is a common and nonspecific clinical syndrome that can result from any of the pathologic processes known to affect the central nervous system.

It is estimated that dementia is severe enough in about 5% of the population older than 65 years of age to render them unable to perform the activities of daily living. It is the most common reason for needing nursing home care. Dementia is expected to increase in prevalence as the older segment of the population increases. For many years the classification of dementia has included a division between senile and presenile types. This is an arbitrary distinction because no specific clinical or pathologic characteristics exist to differentiate dementias starting before or after 65 years of age.

Because many different causes of dementia exist, there may be variations in the chronology of the evolution and in the neurologic signs accompanying the cognitive impairment. Clinically, generalized cognitive and behavioral deterioration is manifest in the neurologic examination as an impairment of data processing (a decrease in memory, abstraction, and attention span) and as an inappropriate response to the environment (impaired judgment and affect). The physician first notices whether the patient is groomed properly. Patients with dementia often show a decline in social skills and hence wear clothing that is dirty or not color coordinated. The physician then tests several parameters while taking the history. Patients' abilities to maintain a coherent thread of thought, their attention spans, and the information content of their language give the physician a general idea of their intellectual capacities. Direct mental testing of every parameter should be performed in progressive degrees of complexity. It is always important to test attention

span and language function first because they are the main factors limiting the degree of complexity possible in the rest of the neurologic examination. The physician should test patients' attention using a series of numbers repeated forward and backward in escalating degrees of difficulty (normal is seven numbers forward and five backwards). Subtracting serial sevens from 100 is another good test. Memory can be tested by asking patients to repeat three items 5 minutes after they hear them or to retell immediately a simple but detailed story. Abstraction is tested by asking patients to perform the similarities test that is described as follows. The physician asks "What are the similarities between an apple and an orange?" Answer: "They are both fruits." This may be used also as an example. Then ask patients the similarities between bus and boat, dog and lion, and eye and ear. Patients who are college graduates can be asked the similarities between praise and punishment. The normal respondent gives similarities. In dementia, patients often give differences. The remainder of the neurologic examination may show severe deficits of cortical function involving visuospatial tasks, body scheme, apraxias, and agnosias of different kinds.

Cognitive motor testing is of great interest because the findings point to a process of disintegration of function that reverses ontogenetic development. Infants react to the environment reflexly. Stimulating the lips or circumoral region causes the infant to pursue the stimulus and begin sucking. Stimulating the palmar surfaces of the hands and feet causes grasping. Dorsiflexion of the foot elicits a stepping reaction, and stroking the thenar eminence produces the contraction of the mentalis muscle (palmar mental response). In infancy, myelination of the hemispheres has not yet taken place, and therefore the command of motor behavior occurs mainly at the diencephalic, limbic, and brainstem levels. With the progressive maturation of the nervous system, learned behavior replaces reflex behavior, culminating years later in mature individuals who have an immense repertory of responses at their disposal. This process of learning is preceded by the progressive myelination of the hemispheres that become incorporated in processing information and commanding motor behavior (cortication).

In a degenerative process such as Alzheimer's disease, which is characterized by progressive cortical neuronal loss, the cerebral hemispheres begin to lose their role in behavior (decortication), sending the command back to the diencephalic and brainstem reflex levels. The reappearance of infantile reflexes and findings of motor impersistence, perseveration, and generalized hyperreflexia are classic in advanced dementia. In the end stage of motor deterioration the patient returns to the fetal position (pelvicrural contraction).

Alzheimer's disease

Alzheimer's disease, characterized pathologically by neuronal loss, senile plaques, and neurofibrillary tangles, affects primarily the association cortex and hippocampus and in some series accounts for up to 55% of cases of dementia. The early manifestations of Alzheimer's disease can be insidious and more obvious to relatives and co-workers than to the physician examining the patient for the first time or to the patient himself. The account by an observant relative, familiar with the patient's emotional and intellectual characteristics, points to a subtle but progressive personality change. Negative personality traits, which in an unaffected person are kept in bounds because of good judgment, begin to express themselves more overtly at the same time that positive aspects of the personality begin to diminish. Suspiciousness may turn into paranoia, assertiveness into belligerence, and tenaciousness into stubbornness as intellectual drive, sense of humor, and subtlety of observation begin to deteriorate. At this point the patient may be aware of an inability to interact with the environment as effectively as before. Consequently in as many as 25% of these patients a mild reactive depression develops.

As the disease progresses, the abnormalities of behavior become more obvious. Relatives become increasingly aware of the patient's unreliability in handling money, conveying messages, and making decisions. Accidents resulting from carelessness begin to occur at home or at work, and the patient's social life and outside interests are greatly reduced or become nonexistent. Disorientation in space progresses, so the patient is easily lost when away from home, and the conversation is reduced to clichés and formula courtesies. At this point the diagnosis of dementia is obvious. The neurologic examination shows signs of dysfunction in the mental status examination, as well as the presence of infantile reflexes.

A more advanced state of Alzheimer's disease renders the patient unable to perform activities of daily living. The patient must be dressed, bathed, and fed. Sphincter control disappears, and apathy and mutism ensue. The patient may spend the whole day sitting in a chair staring at the walls, and motor behavior is reduced to occasional clumsy attempts to stand up.

Other causes of dementia

Among other disorders that cause dementia are mass lesions, such as tumors or chronic subdural hematomas, the spongiform encephalopathies, such as Creutzfeldt-Jakob disease, Pick's disease, Huntington's chorea, parkinsonism (see Chapter 150), multiple sclerosis (see Chapter 147), progressive multifocal leukoencephalopathy, progressive supranuclear palsy, Hallervorden-Spatz disease, normal pressure hydrocephalus, vitamin B_{12} deficiency, dementia paralytica caused by syphilis or other chronic central nervous system infections (see Chapter 51), subacute sclerosing panencephalitis (see Chapter 151), and a variety of storage diseases and leukodystrophies in childhood (see Chapters 148 and 195). Vascular disease may cause dementia when multifocal infarctions or lacunae are present.

A variety of toxic and metabolic derangements, such as those induced by drug ingestion, hypothyroidism, and hypercalcemia, may result in impaired mentation. These disorders are not classified as dementia, since they are reversible.

Creutzfeldt-Jakob disease

Although the spongiform encephalopathy Creutzfeldt-Jakob disease accounts for a small number of cases of dementia, it has become the subject of much attention since its infectious origin as a slow virus disorder was demonstrated in 1969. It is characterized by dementia, myoclonic jerks, rigidity, cerebellar incoordination, and occasionally motor neuron disease. The course of the illness is relatively rapid. The average duration is 15 months, although some patients have survived for as much as 6 years. It is characterized by diffuse neuronal loss in the cortex, basal ganglia, and cerebellum. The treatment is symptomatic. Because of the possibility of contagion, caution is advised in handling tissues and cerebrospinal fluid (CSF) from both patients and contaminated instruments.

AIDS-related dementia

Human immunodeficiency virus (HIV) produces the disease acquired immunodeficiency syndrome (AIDS) and its related disorders such as the lymphadenopathy syndrome and AIDS-related complex (ARC). These syndromes are associated with disorders of cognition and can produce dementia. Patients with AIDS are susceptible to direct HIV involvement of the central nervous system, as well as by a variety of other viral syndromes, invasive organisms, and neoplasms including herpes simplex encephalitis, progressive multifocal leukoencephalopathy, subacute encephalitis, toxoplasmosis, cryptococcosis, candidiasis, mycobacterial infection, *Treponema pallidum* infection, primary central nervous system (CNS) lymphoma, systemic lymphoma with CNS involvement, and metastatic Kaposi's sarcoma. Patients may be infected by several organisms and neoplasms at the same time.

Pick's disease

Pick's disease is a rare cause of dementia. Its course is progressive and lasts from 2 to 15 years. Pathologically, atrophy of the frontal and temporal cortices is prominent. The parietal cortex is less involved, and the occipital lobes are usually spared. Pick's disease is clinically indistinguishable from Alzheimer's disease. The treatment is symptomatic.

Huntington's chorea

Huntington's chorea is a degenerative hereditary disorder characterized by rapid, sudden involuntary movements and progressive dementia. Symptoms begin around the fourth decade of life, although there is a range from 15 to 65 years of age. Rarely, it may be seen in childhood. Sporadic cases have been found, but its transmission is almost exclusively in a dominant hereditary pattern. Pathologically there is atrophy of the caudate nucleus and the cerebral cortex. Less prominent degenerative changes are also found in other subcortical gray structures. No specific treatment for this condition exists, but choreic movements are lessened by using reserpine, phenothiazines, or haloperidol.

Progressive supranuclear palsy

Progressive supranuclear palsy is a degenerative disorder that begins late in life and is characterized clinically by supranuclear ophthalmoplegia, pseudobulbar palsy, and axial dystonia. Mild dementia may also be present. L-Dopa may produce some improvement in the motor disability.

Hallervorden-Spatz disease

Hallervorden-Spatz disease is a recessively inherited disorder characterized by deposits of iron in the basal ganglia. It produces neuronal degeneration affecting primarily the red nucleus, globus pallidus, and substantia nigra. Rigidity, dystonia, choreoathetosis, spasticity, and progressive dementia are all present. Onset is in late childhood; treatment is symptomatic.

Normal pressure hydrocephalus

Normal pressure hydrocephalus (NPH) is a rare but treatable cause of dementia. Known causes include brain tumor, head trauma, subarachnoid hemorrhage, and meningitis, but in most cases the cause is uknown. Progressive dementia, urinary incontinence, and gait disturbance accompany the dilation of the ventricles, which probably results from the impairment of CSF flow through the subarachnoid space. The slowly progressive dilation of the ventricles accounts for the CSF pressure being maintained within normal limits. The most important diagnostic test is the computed tomographic (CT) scan, which shows severe dilation of the entire ventricular system in the absence of cortical atrophy. Another important test is isotope cisternography, which studies the flow of radioactive-labeled substances in the subarachnoid space. In cases of NPH the radioactive material injected into the lumbar sac enters the ventricular system instead of flowing toward the cerebral convexities and concentrating along the sagittal sinus. Isotope retention in the ventricular system for more than 48 hours has been associated with a good prognosis for improvement with CSF shunting procedures.

MANAGEMENT. Because of the large number of diseases included in the differential diagnosis of dementia, it is considered practical to direct clinical efforts to detecting the treatable causes of dementia and impaired mentation. Chronic central nervous system infections (syphilis and fungi), mass lesions (tumors and chronic subdural hematoma), chronic intoxication (sedatives and heavy metals), deficiency states (pellagra and vitamin B_{12} deficiency), hormonal dysfunction (of thyroid, parathyroid, and adrenal glands), and NPH should be investigated before assuming that an untreatable degenerative disorder is the cause.

LABORATORY FINDINGS. A CT scan of the head is imperative in the diagnosis of dementia. Hydrocephalus, brain atrophy, and mass lesions are easily demonstrated with this test. A lumbar puncture is essential to rule out infection, and serum chemistry tests, including drug and heavy metal screening, can detect the other possible causes. Magnetic resonance imaging (MRI) is a new diagnostic tool for the evaluation of structural lesions. MRI may supplant CT scans as the imaging test of choice.

Depression in the elderly can produce manifestations of behavior that resemble dementia. In most cases the patient has a history of psychiatric care, and in some patients crying spells, sadness, and self-deprecatory statements may betray the underlying depression. In cases in which the diagnosis remains in doubt, a therapeutic trial with antidepressants is warranted.

BIBLIOGRAPHY

Benson DF: Aphasia, alexia and agraphia, New York, 1979, Churchill Livingstone.

Filskov SB and Boll TJ: Handbook of clinical neuropsychology, New York, 1981, John Wiley & Sons.

Mcsulam MM: Principles of behavioral neurology, 1985, Philadelphia, FA Davis Co.

Heilman KM and Satz P: Neuropsychology of human emotion, 1983, New York, the Guilford Press.

143 · CENTRAL NERVOUS SYSTEM INTOXICATIONS

Paul L. Schraeder

The clinical practitioner is often confronted with patients having varying degrees of central nervous system (CNS) intoxication, ranging from mild isolated exposure to intoxicants to full-blown chronic drug abuse. Persons of all ages and social and educational levels are affected. The patient may also be taking more than one type of drug with combined toxicity, producing a more complicated problem such as when the toxicity of alcohol is enhanced with use of a sedative drug of the barbiturate or benzodiazepine group. Although self-inflicted CNS intoxications are common, all too often the patient's problems are a result of the physician's overreliance on the prescription pad as a substitute for empathic listening.

CNS DEPRESSANTS

The most commonly encountered CNS depressant is ethyl alcohol, although lay people widely believe that it is a CNS stimulant. Up to 7% of the adult population of the United States is estimated to have major alcohol-related problems. Symptoms of alcohol intoxication result in about 50% of those persons who achieve a blood alcohol level of 50 mg/dl or greater,

although habitual imbibers have few signs of intoxication at this blood level. (A blood alcohol level above 400 mg/dl produces stupor or coma.) The widespread potential for alcohol abuse can be appreciated when one realizes that two thirds of the adult population in the United States use alcohol at least intermittently and that an increasingly higher percentage of alcoholics are in their teens. The common symptoms of adult alcohol intoxication are well known and include dysarthria, ataxia, and changes in behavior. With increasing blood alcohol levels, the generalized CNS depressant effect becomes increasingly manifested by impaired sensory, motor, and judgmental functions.

An uncommon but dramatic manifestation of alcohol ingestion is pathologic alcoholic intoxication. This violent and at times self-destructive state can be associated with hallucinations or delusional thinking and may be more likely to occur in persons with underlying psychopathologic conditions. In a susceptible person pathologic intoxication may result from ingesting a relatively modest amount of alcohol.

The withdrawal states that occur as the depressant effect of alcohol wears off are a major problem encountered among alcohol abusers. The most benign set of symptoms is the self-limited, morning-after hangover that includes irritability, malaise, slight tremulousness, and headache. If the person has been drinking heavily for several days or longer, a more severe state of tremulousness may occur. The patient has tremors that are often quite severe, with mental irritability, mild disorientation, insomnia, and autonomic symptoms including tachycardia, nausea, and vomiting. The symptoms usually subside after a few days but can take as long as 2 weeks to disappear.

Withdrawal seizures or "rum fits" occur 6 to 48 hours after the patient has had the last drink. One or more seizures can occur and are usually generalized; if any focal component is present, cerebral pathologic conditions are highly suspect. Anticonvulsants should not be used to treat these seizures. Alcoholics are unreliable, take anticonvulsants irregularly, and commonly withdraw from alcohol and anticonvulsants simultaneously when treated with anticonvulsants, almost guaranteeing severe withdrawal seizures. It should be remembered, however, that alcohol withdrawal, even of a minimal degree, can aggravate an independent seizure disorder. A thoughtfully obtained, nonjudgmental medical history should easily clarify which patients also have seizures occurring independently of the withdrawal state. This important information can usually be obtained by asking the patient or the friends and family whether the patient has ever had seizures while abstaining from alcohol for extended periods. Likewise, a history of childhood seizures is suggestive of an independent seizure disorder. To make a diagnosis of alcohol withdrawal seizure alone, it must be determined that the seizures occur only when the patient is withdrawing. Status epilepticus (continuous seizure activity) or two or more seizures occurring without a return of consciousness should be treated in the manner discussed in Chapter 145.

Delerium tremens, or the "DTs," is the most severe form of alcohol withdrawal. Delirium tremens may be mild or severe, with onset 1 to 4 days after the beginning of abstinence. Although not the usual case, this state may be preceded by one or more seizures. In the milder syndrome the patient is diaphoretic, confused, tremulous, fearful, and often has hallucinations. In the majority of cases the symptoms are more severe, manifested by frighteningly vivid auditory and visual hallucinations with prominent autonomic overactivity (including diaphoresis, tremulousness, and tachycardia). Without treatment the mortality is usually 5% to 15% but has been reported as high as 50%. A rare but dramatic withdrawal syndrome is alcoholic hallucinosis, in which auditory hallucinations are the major symptom, without tremulousness or clouding of consciousness. Repeated bouts of this syndrome may indicate an underlying schizophrenic state.

The treatment of the alcohol withdrawal state starts with the presumption that underlying intracranial disease is present. Cerebral trauma often precedes or accompanies the withdrawal state, and a subdural hematoma should be suspected. Likewise, CNS infection should be considered in the debilitated chronic alcoholic patient who has fever with confusion or seizures. The initial evaluation should include a computed tomographic (CT) scan. A lumbar puncture is indicated if symptoms of meningitis such as unexplained fever or nuchal stiffness exist. The parenteral administration of fluids is important but must include vitamins, especially thiamine, from the beginning, particularly if glucose solutions are given initially. The specific drug treatment of alcohol withdrawal is often the subject of heated discussion among knowledgeable professionals, but as a general rule drugs cross-tolerant (that is, producing a similar clinical response) with alcohol are best; these include benzodiazepines and paraldehyde. Phenothiazines should not be used in treating withdrawal because they are not cross-tolerant with alcohol and can aggravate a seizure diathesis. Barbiturates may cause excessive sedation and respiratory depression. Many drug regimens are used, but several studies have shown that modern drugs have minimal or no advantage over paraldehyde, which may be given in doses of 7.5 to 10 ml, either orally or as oil retention enemas every 4 hours. Parenteral administration of this drug should be avoided, since it is potentially hazardous. Sterile abscesses can result from an intramuscular injection, and the presence in old vials of the breakdown product acetaldehyde, a metabolic poison, makes intravenous injection risky. In severe delirium tremens the successful treatment of withdrawal symptoms requires parenteral doses of chlordiazepoxide with up to 400 or 500 mg being administered during the course of treatment. The benzodiazepines are also effective treatments. The most important aspect of drug treatment, however, is to choose a drug that works and learn to use it safely and effectively.

The outpatient management of patients with suspected delirium tremens is discouraged because there is no way of determining the prognosis based on a cursory evaluation of early symptoms. Likewise the physician should keep in mind that delirium tremens develops in one third of patients with withdrawal seizures, and these patients should be observed for at least 72 hours. Status epilepticus should be treated in the manner discussed in Chapter 145.

Because *methyl alcohol* is found occasionally in illegally produced alcoholic beverages, methyl alcohol poisoning deserves mention. This compound is oxidized to formic acid and formaldehyde, which produce delayed toxic manifestations. Severe acidosis and blindness caused by retinal ganglion cell damage may result. The treatment consists primarily of giving bicarbonate intravenously, with hemodialysis reserved for severe poisoning.

Intoxication with depressant drugs other than ethanol is a major problem, in part brought on by the public expectation that medication can cure all human ills, whether physical or emotional. Barbiturates are ubiquitous and consequently are responsible for a major proportion of intoxications. Acute intoxication with the shorter-acting barbiturates is more hazardous; the patient rapidly becomes comatose with relatively low blood levels (as low as 10 μg/ml). Long-standing drugs such as phenobarbital require higher blood levels (60 μg/ml) to produce coma, and consequently they take more time to achieve the same degree of CNS depression than with the shorter-acting barbiturates. The varying signs of acute barbiturate intoxication are similar to alcohol intoxication, ranging from minimal mental dysfunction, dysarthria, ataxia, and nystagmus to more severe depression and apnea. In the early differential diagnosis of drug intoxication, serum blood levels are important. Likewise, the electroencephalogram (EEG) is sometimes useful as a diagnostic tool because mild degrees of intoxication result in prominent fast (greater than 13 Hz) beta activity, whereas more severe degrees of intoxication result in slower (1 to 3 Hz) delta activity intermixed with the beta rhythm. Bilateral burst suppression patterns, that is, periodic complexes (repetitive waveforms) mixed with the absence of EEG waves, are often present on the EEG in severely intoxicated persons.

The treatment of acute barbiturate intoxication consists of maintaining respiration, using endotracheal intubation and artificial respiratory support if needed. Diuresis aided by alkalinization of the urine is the major means of ridding the body of barbiturates. Although hemodialysis is also effective, it is usually reserved for patients who have renal failure.

In persons withdrawing from chronic barbiturate abuse, prominent symptoms include tremulousness, insomnia, seizures, and a hallucinatory delirium similar to that in alcohol withdrawal. To suppress the symptoms, pentobarbital substitution is often used in doses to cause mild intoxication. Usually, 200 to 400 mg every 6 hours is sufficient to achieve stabilization; 1 to 2 days thereafter the pentobarbital is gradually withdrawn at a rate of 100 mg daily. Temporary increases in dosage may be needed to suppress symptoms during withdrawal.

Other depressants besides barbiturates are often the cause of CNS intoxication. Although once commonly used, bromides are now infrequently prescribed. Nonetheless, occasional intoxication cases appear. Chronic bromism can be manifest as confusion, memory problems, delirium, and, in severe cases, coma. Skin lesions, conjunctivitis, and gastritis are common. Blood bromide levels above 75 mg/dl are in the toxic range. A high sodium intake and diuretic treatment cause bromide excretion diuresis; hemodialysis is effective in severe cases of intoxication.

Benzodiazepines, including chlordiazepoxide, diazepam, and flurazepam, are among the most commonly abused CNS depressants. The symptoms of intoxication are nonspecific and include gait ataxia, drowsiness, slurred speech, and confusion. Other types of nonbenzodiazepine depressant drugs, including glutethimide and methaqualone, have similar clinical properties. Chronic abuse of most of the depressant drugs can result in the same symptoms of withdrawal as described with alcohol and the barbiturates; these symptoms require the same type of treatment. As in the withdrawal from alcohol, phenytoin is of little use in preventing the seizures that are often the early part of the abstinence syndrome. Phenothiazines should be avoided in any form of abstinence syndrome.

CNS STIMULANTS

The most commonly used CNS stimulant is caffeine. The average cup of coffee or tea contains 80 to 150 mg of the drug, and a 12-oz bottle of cola contains 35 to 50 mg. Caffeine counteracts fatigue and promotes wakefulness while producing clearer thinking and a better appreciation of sensory stimuli. Overdosage leads to insomnia, diuresis, tachycardia, and cardiac arrhythmias.

Amphetamines are commonly abused drugs. Although their mechanism of action is unclear, it appears that they may cause the release of norepinephrine from the brain. The CNS effects include stimulated alertness, diminished appetite, mood elevation, and increased motor and speech activity. Prolonged use results in a debt of wakefulness that must be paid off by a significant degree of fatigue and depression. The acute CNS toxic effects of amphetamines are exaggerations of the therapeutic effects and include arrhythmia, irritability, insomnia, and weakness. Confusion, anxiety, delirium, and even suicidal or homicidal tendencies can occur, particularly in persons predisposed to mental illness. The treatment of acute intoxication includes increasing urinary secretion by acidifying the urine with ammonium chloride in conjunction with chlorpromazine and antihypertensives. Chronic amphetamine intoxication results in many of the same symptoms found in acute intoxication. Profound weight loss and a paranoid psychosis, however, are also usually present. The intravenous use of amphetamines is associated with the occurrence of autoimmune vasculitis and endocarditis.

Methylphenidate is structurally related to the amphetamines, having similar therapeutic and toxic properties. As with the amphetamines, the only valid clinical indications for its use are for the childhood hyperactivity syndrome and narcolepsy.

OTHER COMMONLY ABUSED DRUGS

The opiates and other analgesic drugs, cocaine, and various illegal compounds constitute other commonly abused drugs that have a profound socioeconomic impact. Both compulsive drug use and physical dependence are widespread problems with which all groups of medical practitioners must deal. It is important that all prescriptions for potentially addicting drugs be written only after the physician thinks carefully about the specific needs of the patient. Opium derivatives must be used only when no other category of drug provides relief. A balance must be maintained between the need to relieve unnecessary suffering and the concern for prescribing a potentially addicting drug (for example, for a patient with a terminal malignancy).

The most common cause of illegally obtained drug-related deaths in the United States is acute opiate intoxication (for example, from heroin, morphine, or meperidine). The symptoms of opiate intoxication include respiratory depression, pinpoint pupils, hypothermia, hypotension, and bradycardia. Death results from acute respiratory failure. Pulmonary edema is commonly seen. A patient with the combination of coma, pinpoint pupils, and depressed respirations should prompt suspicion of acute opiate intoxication; another important and apparent clue is needle marks on the arm.

If the drug is taken orally, the treatment starts with gastric intubation and aspiration, since opiates cause gastric retention. Because of the high risk of respiratory arrest, an endotracheal tube is needed along with respiratory support. The opiate antagonist naloxone (Narcan) should be given in a dose of 0.5 to 0.7 mg intravenously to improve spontaneous respirations. Subsequent intramuscular doses can be used as needed to maintain the response. Since many persons suffering from acute opiate intoxication are also habitual users of opiates, the patient must be observed for the precipitation of acute withdrawal symptoms.

Opiate addiction is a major public health problem. Various studies estimate that more than 500,000 heroin addicts live in the United States, with two thirds of these having used opiates before 21 years of age. With repeated use increasingly larger doses are needed to produce the desired euphoria, so in many cases massive doses are eventually tolerated. The severity of the abstinence symptoms is proportional to the daily dosage of the drug and the length of time the patient has been addicted.

The abstinence symptoms are both purposive, that is, related to the environment and oriented toward obtaining more drugs, and nonpurposive, which includes uncontrolled symptoms and signs such as mydriasis, muscle twitching, gooseflesh, extreme restlessness, vomiting, diarrhea, and alternating feelings of hot and cold. The symptoms start at 8 to 16 hours after the last dose, peak at 2 to 3 days, and are usually gone within 1 to 1½ weeks. Although complete abstinence as a treatment is usually not life threatening as long as a sufficient fluid and electrolyte balance is maintained, modern withdrawal management includes an initial dose of methadone of 15 to 20 mg orally. Further maintenance doses are given at a ratio of 1 mg methadone for 4 mg of morphine, 2 mg of heroin, or 20 mg of meperidine, followed by a reduction of 20% of the total dose each day. After 10 days the withdrawal is usually complete. Preventing further addiction at this time involves using daily methadone doses that block the euphoria of intravenously injected heroin. Neurologic complications of opiate addiction include transverse myelopathy, various types of neuropathies, acute myopathies, and CNS infections (meningitis and abscess). Some of these complications may be the result of contaminating agents mixed with the opiates.

After many years of being a relatively minor source of drug abuse, cocaine again is becoming much more widely used. The drug produces a euphoria often indistinguishable from that caused by amphetamines. With high doses, increased CNS irritability, including seizures, appears. High body temperatures are a common symptom of cocaine intoxication, and signs of increased sympathetic activity are evident. Thus the symptoms of cocaine intoxication include restlessness, tachycardia, fever, mydriasis, delirium, convulsions, and finally respiratory arrest. The treatment involves intravenous administration of sedatives such as barbiturates or benzodiazepines.

Chronic cocaine abuse, especially with the freebase form ("crack"), is also associated with cerebral hemorrhages or infarctions as a complication of drug-related CNS vasculitis.

Although a wide variety of other drugs have varying degrees of popularity with drug users, cannabis (marijuana) and lysergic acid diethylamide (LSD or "acid") are the best known. The active agent in cannabis is tetrahydrocannabinol. The desired effect is a feeling of euphoria, relaxation, and sleepiness. A sense of unreality about self is also reported, along with more vivid sensory perceptions and altered time perception. High doses produce a toxic psychosis. The so-called hard drug effect of hallucinogenic agents such as LSD is typically described as a feeling of being a passive spectator to one's own experiences, which also acquire a unique meaning to that person. Visual illusions and hallucinations are common, and complex sensory and affective interactions frequently occur. Auditory hallucinations, however, are rare. A common adverse reaction is the so-called bad trip or panic response. Flashbacks, or recurrences of drug effects previously experienced, are common. The treatment for these phenomena is sedation, using agents such as diazepam, and talking down the patient. Habitual use of LSD can result in a permanent psychosis.

Phencyclidine (PCP, or "angel dust") has become a major illegal drug. It is used as a veterinary anesthetic and is related to the commonly used human anesthetic ketamine. Its psychotomimetic effects preclude its legal use in humans. Phencyclidine can be taken orally or smoked. The symptoms and signs of phencyclidine intoxication include nystagmus, hypertension, tachycardia, flushing, sweating, ataxia, and CNS depression. Abnormal meiosis is a variable finding. Patients exhibit a dramatic variation between hyperactivity resembling mania and hypoactivity resembling catatonia. Complex bizarre behavior is also commonly seen. Laryngeal stridor, seizures, and renal failure may occur with overdosage. In contrast to LSD, hallucinations are uncommon. Phencyclidine intoxication must be suspected in any young person with an acute psychosis and hypertension. The treatment includes gastric lavage and increasing urinary excretion by acidifying the urine with ascorbic acid or ammonium chloride. Treatment with phenothiazines tends to lower the blood pressure too precipitously, but diazepam or haloperidol therapy may be useful. In mild intoxication a dark, quiet environment is sufficient treatment. As with any illegal drug use, patients often take mixtures of several drugs, making a diagnosis of any particular drug as the cause of the patient's symptoms a difficult task.

NEUROLOGIC EFFECTS OF COMMONLY PRESCRIBED DRUGS

This section describes the various CNS and peripheral nervous system complications that may be seen with drugs in the phenothiazine, antidepressant, antibiotic, antituberculous, steroid, and antimetabolite groups.

Phenothiazines are indicated for various psychoses, but they are commonly and inappropriately used in treating less severe symptoms such as anxiety. The major neurologic side effects are extrapyramidal. Typical symptoms of parkinsonism may be seen, including rigidity, tremor, masked facies, and bradykinesia. Various types of extrapyramidal symptoms and dyskinetic symptoms are common in sensitive persons after only one dose of a phenothiazine, but they usually respond quickly to intravenous administration of 25 to 50 mg of diphenhydramine (Benadryl). Unfortunately, the most chronic movement disorder, tardive dyskinesia (continuous facial, lip, and chewing movements as a result of long-term phenothiazine use), is not responsive to therapy. It must also be remembered that phenothiazines tend to lower the seizure threshold. Anticholinergic drugs diminish the parkinsonian symptoms but may increase the tardive dyskinesia.

The antidepressant drugs most commonly used are in the tricyclic group (for example, imipramine, amitriptyline, and desipramine). The neurologic side effects of these drugs are of a wide variety. A fine tremor is common in 1 out of 10 patients. As with phenothiazines, elements of parkinsonian symptoms can also be found. Likewise, generalized major motor seizures have been reported to follow high doses of these drugs. In severe poisoning, hyperpyrexia, elevated blood pressure, choreoathetosis, delirium, and seizures can occur. The treatment for overdosage is intravenous physostigmine to reverse these CNS anticholinergic symptoms. Propranolol and lidocaine may be needed to control cardiac arrhythmias.

Another commonly used drug is lithium carbonate, which is important in treating manic depressive illness. At therapeutic levels of 0.9 to 1.4 mEq/L neurologic symptoms such as ataxia, slurred speech, and fine tremor appear. Higher levels result in more severe manifestations such as impairment of consciousness or even coma, severe tremor, hyperreflexia, fasciculations, and convulsions. The treatment involves diuresis, intravenous administration of sodium bicarbonate, and in severe cases dialysis.

The atropine group of drugs can produce delirium, as can any agent with major anticholinergic effects (for example, phenothiazines, antidepressants, and antiparkinsonian agents). With increasing dosages they can also produce memory loss and visual hallucinations. Older patients seem more susceptible to these symptoms, and for such patients any of these drugs

should be used cautiously. Physostigmine is used to treat anticholinergic overdose.

Peripheral polyneuropathies can be caused by many different drugs. In the past, before the concurrent use of pyridoxine (vitamin B_6), using isoniazid to treat tuberculosis commonly resulted in the appearance of a neuropathy after several months. This neuropathy was thought to result from interference with the production of pyridoxal phosphate. Nitrofurantoin, a drug commonly used to treat urinary tract infections, also can produce peripheral neuropathy after several weeks of use. In both instances the earliest symptoms are paresthesias of the feet, followed by an increasing diffuse sensory loss, primarily in the lower extremities, along with increasing weakness and loss of deep tendon reflexes. Other common drug-related polyneuropathies are produced by disulfiram and vincristine.

Corticosteroids are implicated as the cause of several types of neurologic symptoms. Pseudotumor cerebri (increased intracranial pressure not caused by structural disease) is an uncommon but well-established reaction to withdrawal from these compounds. A myopathy, with the usual emphasis on proximal limb weakness, can be seen in patients undergoing long-term, high-dose corticosteroid therapy. Even with withdrawal, this weakness resulting from muscle dysfunction may persist. In addition, these compounds commonly produce psychiatric symptoms such as depression or psychosis of a schizophrenic type.

BIBLIOGRAPHY

Adams RD and Victor M: Principles of neurology, ed 3, New York, 1985, McGraw-Hill Inc.

Gilman AE and others: The pharmacological basis of therapeutics, ed 7, New York, 1985, MacMillan Inc.

Kaye BR and Fainstat M: Cerebral vasculitis associated with cocaine abuse, JAMA 258:2104, 1987.

Kissin B, Lowinson JH, and Millman RB, editors: Recent developments in chemotherapy of narcotic addiction, Ann NY Acad Sci 311:1, 1978.

Rowland LP, editor: Merritt's textbook of neurology, Philadelphia, 1984, Lea & Febiger.

144 · SYNCOPE

Paul L. Schraeder

Syncope, or fainting, refers to an impairment of consciousness with an associated loss of postural tone. Although syncope is one of the most common symptoms encountered by the physician, patients often considerably confuse terms when attempting to describe their symptoms. Patients often describe dizziness, light-headedness, unsteadiness, and other ill-defined feelings of weakness as fainting spells. One of the common yet difficult differentiations to make is between fainting and seizures. In making this differentiation, no series of laboratory tests is as important as a carefully taken history. Because the patient may poorly recall what happened, the sequence of events as related by friends or family usually is important in helping the physician determine the cause of the patient's symptoms.

Syncope of whatever cause usually is preceded by symptoms of varying duration. Commonly, feelings of light-headedness are accompanied by sweating, pallor, nausea, impaired vision, and an inability to think. The patient with a seizure often receives no warning, or if there is a warning or an aura, the symptoms are more specific and stereotyped before each event. The patient with syncope often complains of palpitations before losing consciousness. Likewise, at the time of the event the patient may have an occasional convulsive jerk. These so-called syncopal seizures should not be confused with a seizure disorder. Usually as the patient lies down the symptoms abate rapidly because of an improvement of blood flow to the brain. In contrast to the patient with a seizure who is often confused for varying periods after regaining consciousness, the patient with syncope rapidly resumes a fully alert state with no hint of confusion, lethargy, or headache.

The causes of fainting are divided into two broad categories. The cardiovascular category includes events that cause diffusely impaired cerebral blood flow because of changes in vascular resistance or a drop in cardiac output. The metabolic category encompasses causes such as hypoglycemia and hypoxia. The following are the most common etiologic factors in each category.

In the cardiovascular category the most common cause of fainting is vasovagal syncope, which usually occurs in healthy persons. Almost every physician can recall classmates who fainted when first confronted with venipuncture, illustrating that sudden, severe, emotional stress or pain can cause peripheral vasodilatation with a resulting drop in brain perfusion. Likewise, most people at one time or another have felt close to fainting in closed, hot, unventilated quarters. The patient with vasovagal syncope often is pale, sweaty, nauseated, and mildly short of breath before losing consciousness. Because of excessive vagal stimulation, the cardiac rate does not increase in compensation for the drop in blood pressure. Placing the patient in a recumbent position usually restores consciousness with no sequelae. A behavioral approach to treatment, desensitizing the patient to stressful circumstances, may be helpful in preventing such events in some patients.

Micturition syncope is probably also related to excessive vagal reflex activity, occurring in males emptying an overfull bladder. This nonpathologic state, often unwitnessed, is commonly confused with a nocturnal seizure. The patient, however, may be able to relate a sequence of symptoms that are compatible with a rapidly progressive onset of faintness and with a rapid return of alertness after lying on the floor. In these circumstances head injury and some urinary incontinence may give the erroneous impression of a seizure.

Some patients have episodes of decreased cerebral perfusion because of postural hypotension. Often such persons are taking diuretics or antihypertensive medications and typically experience the rapid progression of symptoms associated with syncope when standing up quickly from a recumbent position. Also susceptible to postural hypotension are persons taking phenothiazine drugs or L-dopa. Diabetic patients commonly have an autonomic component as part of a peripheral polyneuropathy, with vasomotor instability on arising. It should be kept in mind, however, that many otherwise normal persons may suffer syncope if they arise too quickly from a prolonged state of recumbency. The diagnosis of postural hypotension usually can be suspected from the patient's history. The diagnosis is confirmed by having the patient lie supine for several minutes, taking a baseline blood pressure reading, and then having the patient stand up suddenly; the blood pressure determination is repeated several times. Any more than a minor transient drop in blood pressure is considered suspect, especially if the patient complains of appropriate symptoms in conjunction with a significant drop in pressure. The treatment consists of readjusting dosages of any offending medication, advising the patient to arise from a recumbent position gradually, and recommending that the patient wear supportive hose. In nonhypertensive patients, extra salt in the diet may raise intravascular volume.

Cardiac syncope most commonly results from an arrhythmia. Whether it is a form of bradycardia or tachycardia, the net result is impaired cerebral circulation. The best-known cause of cardiogenic syncope is Stokes-Adams syndrome resulting from a cardiac conduction block. In these patients ventricular standstill may last for several seconds with a rapid onset of unconsciousness. Often there are a few clonic jerks, which should not be confused with seizures. The episodes of syncope can occur several times daily and are unrelated to posture. It is important to obtain continuous 24-hour electrocardiographic monitoring for patients suspected of having Stokes-Adams syndrome.

Carotid sinus syncope is the result of an exaggerated normal response to stimulation, although in some instances no history suggestive of a sensitivity to carotid sinus stimulation can be obtained. In susceptible persons a minor stimulus such as shaving over the sinus and tilting back or turning the head can result in an attack with a sudden loss of consciousness, falling, and some clonic motor activity. The unconsciousness lasts no more than a few minutes, with a complete return of alertness when consciousness returns. Three mechanisms are used to explain the syncope: the vagal type of response, resulting in cardiac slowing of varying degrees; the depressor type of response, resulting in a fall of arterial pressure without a change in heart rate; and the central type of response, with an impairment of cerebral perfusion caused by carotid artery stenosis. The treatment is preventive with efforts to remove offending stimuli such as tight collars. Atropine may occasionally be needed to prevent bradycardia, whereas sympathomimetic drugs such as ephedrine may be useful for persons susceptible to hypotensive episodes. Neither cardiac pacemakers nor carotid sinus denervation is usually needed, but they may produce dramatic results in severely affected persons. Finally it should be kept in mind that frequently a carotid artery arteriosclerotic plaque may predispose a patient to hypersensitivity; in such instances too much pressure on the sinus may actually impair the blood supply to the brain.

Hypoglycemia is a common noncardiovascular cause of syncope or near-syncope. Usually, reactive hypoglycemia occurs 2 to 4 or more hours after eating a high-carbohydrate meal. The history is of a gradual onset of sweating, tremor, confusion, and often an urge to eat. Coma and seizures occur only when blood sugar levels are below 20 mg/dl. In such severe cases islet-cell pancreatic tumors, endocrinopathies of the pituitary-adrenal axis, or excessive doses of exogenous insulin in diabetic patients should be considered as possible causes. The diagnosis, as always, hinges on a good history, especially in the patient with reactive hypoglycemia. The relationship of the syncope to meals is the most important point to seek, and the diagnosis can be confirmed with a glucose tolerance test. Treatment focuses on preventing unusual glucose loads.

Hyperventilation syndrome can cause a faint feeling but uncommonly results in a complete loss of consciousness. Along with the causative anxiety, the patient complains of having a pounding in the chest. Patients may admit feeling short of breath when asked, but many times patients are unaware of any such feeling even when the question is emphasized. Associated symptoms include paresthesias of the fingers and the perioral area. Hyperventilation results in hypocapnia with concomitant cerebral vasoconstriction and decreased cerebral blood flow. Transient systemic alkalosis may contribute to protein binding of calcium, with resultant peripheral nerve symptoms in the form of paresthesias and muscle spasms. The treatment consists of telling the patient to breathe into a paper bag or voluntarily inhibiting the respiratory rate to elevate the carbon dioxide pressure rapidly. Explaining the cause and mechanism of these often frightening symptoms to the patient usually is sufficient to provide relief. In cases of severe recurrent anxiety and hyperventilation, however, psychotherapy is recommended.

BIBLIOGRAPHY

Adams RP and Victor M: Principles of neurology, New York, 1985, McGraw-Hill Inc.

145·EPILEPSY (SEIZURE DISORDERS)

Paul L. Schraeder

DEFINITION. A seizure is an uncontrolled paroxysmal discharge of the central nervous system that interferes with normal function; "epilepsy" is a term used to denote the repeated occurence of any of the various forms of seizures. A prodrome refers to the mood or behavior change that often precedes a seizure by hours or even days. An aura is the localized symptom that may be the first part of a seizure originating from a localized region of the cerebral cortex, but often it can occur alone. Neither seizure nor epilepsy defines a disease state but rather is only a symptom of some underlying disease of the brain, whether structural, biochemical, or genetic. In many patients, if not the majority, a concise mechanism cannot be defined. This uncertainty and lack of understanding contribute to the difficulty in management of these patients and to the negative attitudes toward epileptic persons that are frequently encountered.

Despite the relative ease of defining prodrome and aura on paper, it should be remembered that patients often cannot clearly describe what they experience. A reliable patient may only be able to say, "I just knew that I was going to have a seizure." Likewise, the amnesia commonly associated with the seizure often precludes an accurate description of the prelude of the seizure. Auras may be considered as minor, recurrent symptoms that stand alone, making them psychologically debilitating occurrences, since the patient can never be certain when the aura will proceed to a severe seizure. The aura acts as a pointer, indicating from which part of the brain the seizure originated.

CLASSIFICATION AND PATHOPHYSIOLOGY. The classification of epileptic seizures is of much more than academic importance. For many years the description of seizure types was limited to focal motor (jacksonian), psychomotor (temporal lobe), grand mal, and petit mal. As knowledge of the electroencephalographic (EEG) and clinical manifestations accumulated, it became evident that many observed phenomena did not fit into these categories. Seizures originating in the temporal lobe also can be so subtle that they escape recognition as a seizure by all but the most experienced observer. In the 1960s the International League Against Epilepsy made a major effort to formulate a more rational and useful classification, based on both clinical and EEG observation of seizures of all types. This international classification of epileptic seizures was recently revised.

Before describing this classification further, it is important to consider the possible pathophysiologic nature of epilepsy, keeping in mind that the actual mechanisms of seizures are still unknown. Seizures may be focal or generalized or both. If a population of cortical neurons loses inhibitory control, it can

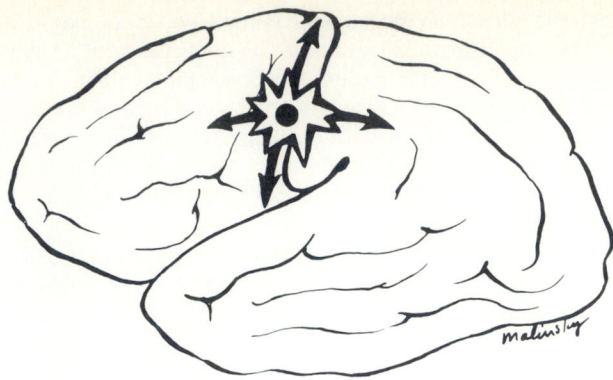

Fig. 145-1 Focal seizure involves spread of discharge over limited area of cerebral cortex.

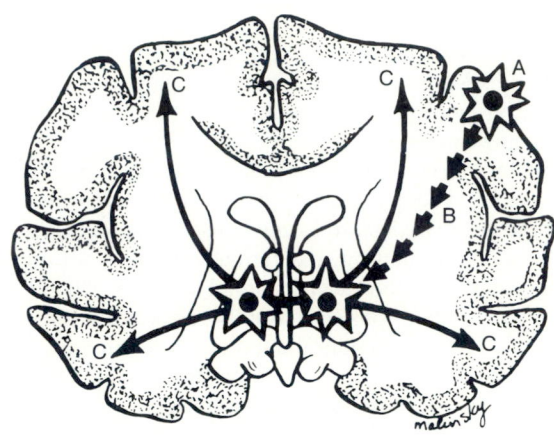

Fig. 145-2 *A,* cortical focus of epileptogenic discharge. *B,* spread of discharge to thalamus and reticular activating formation. *C,* secondary spread to both hemispheres, causing generalized seizure. *C,* without *A* and *B,* occurs in idiopathic epilepsy.

start firing in a synchronized fashion. One of the results can be a localized seizure that involves only the cortex contiguous to the focus. At most this activity involves one hemisphere (Fig. 145-1). If this focal seizure activity involves the reticular activating formation and the diencephalic structures, however, a secondarily generalized seizure can occur with a loss of consciousness. Although the mechanism is not entirely understood, these deep midline structures are thought to play an important primary role in causing primarily generalized (idiopathic) seizures (Fig. 145-2). The International Classification of Epileptic Seizures (see the box on p. 687) is a categorization of seizures that can be easily understood, keeping in mind the concepts just described.

Partial seizures. Partial seizures are so named because they originate from a localized area of the brain and usually do not involve the whole brain as do generalized seizures. In a partial seizure with elemental symptoms, whether they are focal motor, sensory, or autonomic, the patient remains conscious. When elemental or simple partial seizures are of the focal motor type, they usually originate in the contralateral precentral gyrus, with the first symptoms occurring in the body part controlled by that brain region (for example, the hand or face). This motor activity can spread (as seen in the classic jacksonian seizures) to involve the whole limb and often the entire half of the body. Continuous, well-localized, clonic seizure activity usually occurring in the face or hand is known as epilepsia partialis continua. Elemental sensory seizures are uncommon,

THE INTERNATIONAL CLASSIFICATION OF EPILEPTIC SEIZURES

I. Partial (focal, local) seizures
   A. Simple partial seizures (consciousness not impaired)
      1. With motor symptoms
      2. With somatosensory or special sensory symptoms
      3. With autonomic symptoms
      4. With psychic symptoms
   B. Complex partial seizures (with impairment of consciousness)
      1. Beginning as simple partial seizures and progressing to impairment of consciousness
         a. With no other features
         b. With features as in I.A.1–I.A.4
         c. With automatisms
      2. With impairment of consciousness at onset
         a. With no other features
         b. With features as in I.A.1–I.A.4
         c. With automatisms
   C. Partial seizures evolving to secondarily generalized seizures
      1. Simple partial seizures evolving to generalized seizures
      2. Complex partial seizures evolving to generalized seizures
      3. Simple partial seizures evolving to complex partial seizures to generalized seizures
II. Generalized seizures (convulsive or nonconvulsive)
   A. Absence seizures
      1. Absence seizures
      2. Atypical absence seizures
   B. Myoclonic seizures
   C. Clonic seizures
   D. Tonic seizures
   E. Tonic–clonic seizures
   F. Atonic seizures (astatic seizures)
III. Unclassified epileptic seizures—includes all seizures that cannot be classified because of inadequate or incomplete data and some that defy classification in hitherto described categories. This includes some neonatal seizures, e.g., rhythmic eye movements, chewing, and swimming movements.

originate from the postcentral gyrus, and are manifested by various degrees of paresthesias or numbness. Simple focal seizures commonly have mixed motor and sensory symptoms. So-called psychic symptoms may include recurrent feelings of dissociation from one's body or surroundings and sudden overwhelming affective symptoms such as fear.

Partial seizures with complex symptoms (also known as psychomotor seizures or temporal lobe seizures), in contrast to partial seizures with elemental symptoms, are often associated with an impairment of consciousness. Indeed, as seen in the classification, an impairment of consciousness may be the only manifestation and may be difficult to differentiate from the petit mal absence described in the following section. The older age of onset, the presence of an aura, and varying periods of postictal confusion are three of the main differentiating features in the partial seizure. Commonly occurring auras, simple partial seizures, include a visceral rising sensation from the epigastrium to the throat, olfactory sensations, and overwhelming feelings of familiarity (déjà vu). The most common observable manifestation of complex partial epilepsy is the ictal automatism. These uncontrolled motor activities are stereotyped and include lip smacking, chewing movements, fumbling movements of the fingers, inappropriate verbalizations, and even complex acts. These seizures can also consist of impairment or distortions of perceptions, including complex delusions and hallucinations. In many cases varying combinations of symptoms occur at different times. Purposeful, directed, violent behavior is not an epileptic phenomenon; however, often the patient reacts defensively if efforts are made at restraint during complex partial seizures or periods of postictal confusion.

Generalized seizures. Generalized seizures without onset from a focal cortical discharge are usually either absences (petit mal) or tonic-clonic (grand mal). Since there is no focal component, prodromes, auras, and focal motor or sensory symptoms are not expected. No brain disease is diagnosable, and the seizures are thought to be the result of a diathesis involving corticoreticular interaction. Except in the case of psychogenic pseudoseizures, the diagnosis of tonic-clonic activity is obvious. Petit mal absences, however, often have subtle manifestations. The onset of absence seizures is usually between 4 and 10 years of age, with the frequency of episodes tending to wane after puberty. Children with this disorder are often diagnosed as having behavior or learning problems, when in reality their functioning may be altered by repetitive periods of impairment of consciousness occurring each day. In recent years automatisms have been observed as part of petit mal seizures, making differentiation from complex partial seizures difficult without the use of the EEG. It should also be remembered that generalized tonic-clonic seizures develop at puberty in as many as 50% of persons with a petit mal seizure disorder.

Generalized seizures also can be the result of the secondary generalization of focal cortical discharges and clinically are often difficult to differentiate from primarily generalized tonic-clonic seizures. Tonic-clonic seizures resulting from a focus of cortical irritability tend to have an onset after adolescence. The older the patient when the first seizure occurs, the more probable that it results from a cortical pathologic condition. In secondarily generalized tonic-clonic seizures an aura may occur or the patient may also have a focal (simple partial or complex partial) seizure just before the tonic-clonic activity. One of the most common clinical problems in neurology is making the differentiation between primarily and secondarily generalized tonic-clonic seizures.

Finally, generalized seizures such as infantile spasms (massive myoclonic seizures), clonic seizures, tonic seizures, and atonic seizures (sudden loss of muscle tone with falling) require brief mention. These seizure types are usually found in childhood and are often associated with the presence of various types of perinatal, metabolic, and genetic brain disease. The prognosis for normal development in these young patients is, unfortunately, often poor, and the treatment is less successful than with other seizure types.

ETIOLOGY

Genetic factors. In general, epilepsy is not a predictable, inherited entity except in rare autosomal dominant diseases such as tuberous sclerosis, Sturge-Weber syndrome, and neurofibromatosis. For the more common types of primarily generalized seizures, the patterns of inheritance are not fully understood. The only well-defined inherited pattern is that of the classic 2.5 to 3/sec spike-and-wave pattern on the EEG. More than 40% of siblings of patients with petit mal seizures have this EEG trait, yet less than 8% of siblings have seizures. The EEG trait has its highest prevalence before 15 years of age, then diminishes rapidly; it is a marker of a dominantly inherited seizure diathesis with incomplete penetrance of the trait. In a broader population of epileptic patients with diverse seizure types, 3.2% of near relatives also have epilepsy. This incidence increases to 7.6% of relatives of infants with seizures. If the seizure onset is after 30 years of age, the incidence in relatives is much lower, less than 2%. Although inheritance is thought to be a major risk factor in the development of seizures, environmental risk factors play a significant role. For example, certain circumstances such as head trauma, brain tumor, and stroke are known to result in the development of seizures. Persons with a family history of epilepsy are in a higher risk category of developng epilepsy as a result of such environmental risk factors than are persons without such a family history.

Acquired factors. Although many disorders of brain structure and metabolism cause seizures, the following are the most common etiologic factors. Head injury is one of the major causes of epilepsy and is the most commonly acquired cause of seizure in the young adult. The more severe the head trauma, the greater the chance of seizures, with the risk approaching 50% in persons with open head injuries. More than 90% of seizures resulting from head trauma occur within 2 years. Paradoxically, if seizures occur within 1 week after head trauma, the risk of subsequent seizures developing is small. In persons whose onset of seizures occurs after age 21 and who have no known history of trauma or alcohol abuse, the next most likely cause is a tumor, with a probability of 10%. After age 50 the chance of a tumor as a cause of adult-onset seizures approaches 15%; if the seizure is focal, the risk of neoplasm is even greater. Cerebrovascular disease, nonetheless, is the most common cause of seizure onset after age 50, with more than 7% of persons with brain infarction ultimately having seizures. The risk is higher if hemorrhage is present. As in the case of head trauma, the patients whose seizures develop early in the postinfarction period have less risk of subsequent seizures than those with later (after 2 weeks) onset of seizures.

Alcohol withdrawal seizures are common in urban emergency rooms and are usually generalized without focal features. These seizures typically occur 7 to 48 hours after the cessation of drinking. Unfortunately, it is often difficult to differentiate so-called rum fits from an underlying seizure disorder that is precipitated by alcohol withdrawal. If focal seizures occur during withdrawal states, other causes must be considered, including subdural hematoma and brain contusion.

As a generalization, an adult onset of seizures implies serious structural disorders until proved otherwise. The physician must avoid the pitfall of categorizing the cause of a seizure (for example, alcohol withdrawal) on the basis of a superficial evaluation and must remember that a seizure is a symptom, not a diagnosis.

CLINICAL EVALUATION AND MANIFESTATIONS

History. A thorough history is the most important factor in establishing the probable nature of the patient's problem. Every effort must be made to obtain information from observers and family members, as well as from the patient. Specific points that must be covered include the presence of a prodrome or an aura, whether the seizure onset was focal, a clear description of the seizure, and the number and length of seizures. The physician should also inquire about acute precipitating causes such as noncompliance with anticonvulsant medication, drug use, alcohol or drug withdrawal, and the relation of the seizure to menses. The previous seizure history (that is, types and frequency of seizures), anticonvulsant medication used, and family history are important. Additional information concerning specific medical and neurologic causes of seizures should include inquiries about head trauma, headaches, fever, focal neurologic symptoms, visual symptoms, personality change, previous neurologic disorders (for example, encephalitis or stroke), diabetes, heart disease, renal disease, liver disease, and hypertension.

Examination. The general physical examination should include some emphasis on observation. For example, tremulousness might indicate alcohol withdrawal or other drug withdrawal, fetid breath might indicate metabolic derangement (for example, hepatic failure), cyanosis might indicate hypoxia, and skin lesions such as café au lait spots or adenoma sebaceum (collections of raised lesions resembling pimples, primarily around the nasolabial fold on the face) could indicate neurofibromatosis or tuberous sclerosis, respectively, as probable causes of the seizure. Evidence of trauma such as scalp ecchymosis or other injuries to the head should be sought. The tympanic membranes should be examined to search for evidence of blood in the middle ear, as is seen in basilar skull fracture. A cardiovascular examination should be performed, since cardiac arrhythmias may result in cerebral emboli accompanied by seizures.

In examining the patient neurologically, one should note the state of consciousness, for subsequent comparison, to see if the patient is becoming less or more alert. If the patient is having a seizure while being examined, the seizure should be described and its duration noted. Any focal signs during the seizure (for example, focal motor activity or tonic deviation of the eyes) should be noted, as should any focal signs postictally (for example, transient focal paralysis). The presence of nuchal rigidity raises the question of a subarachnoid hemorrhage or a CNS infection. The extraocular movements should be evaluated, and if the patient is unresponsive, the oculocephalic or doll's eye reflex should be observed. Pupillary responses are important to note because asymmetries could be the result of early brain herniation with pressure on the third nerve. The funduscopic examination is necessary, with emphasis on looking for signs of elevated intracranial pressure such as loss of venous pulsation, early disc elevation, or hemorrhage. Patients should be examined for any focal motor weakness, but if they are unconscious, the examiner may have to depend on looking for asymmetries of withdrawal to painful stimuli or for any differences in muscle tone. A unilateral Babinski's sign is important in localization, as in an asymmetry of the deep tendon reflexes. Testing cerebellar function usually includes evaluating the patient's equilibrium or gait, as well as evaluating coordination by finger-to-nose movements and the performance of rapid alternating hand movements; however, in a confused or stuporous patient it is often impossible to perform this aspect of the examination. The same is true for the sensory examination, which, if it is performed adequately, requires the patient's full alertness and cooperation. In a postictal patient the response to superficial pain or deep pain may often be the only sensory information available to the examiner.

In short, the examination of the patient with a recent or ongoing seizure should focus on observations of possible acute causes, such as trauma, CNS hemorrhage, metabolic disease, infection, or cardiovascular disorder. Emphasis during the neurologic examination should be directed toward seeking evidence of deterioration of the state of consciousness and any focal signs indicating recent localized brain disease (for example, a subdural hematoma with early brainstem herniation) or long-standing localized brain disease (for example, an old perinatal injury).

Diagnostic procedures. The diagnostic procedures used to evaluate an initial seizure in an adult in the acute phase should, at a minimum, include a complete blood count, urinalysis, and tests for blood glucose, serum calcium, phosphorus, electrolytes, blood urea nitrogen, blood alcohol level, and urine screening for various drugs. If evidence of trauma, focal signs on neurologic examination, or of increased intracranial pressure exists, a computed tomographic (CT) scan should be obtained immediately to look for the structural causes of seizures that might warrant early treatment. A lumbar puncture should not be performed routinely unless there is a strong suspicion of a CNS infection or a subarachnoid hemorrhage; lumbar puncture is contraindicated in patients who have signs of increased intracranial pressure (for example, papilledema, third nerve palsy, or a space-occupying mass on a CT scan). It is prudent to obtain a CT scan before doing an emergency lumbar puncture. When performing a lumbar puncture, the physician should use a small (20-gauge) needle and examine the cerebrospinal fluid immediately. In young children who have a febrile seizure, a lumbar puncture is absolutely necessary to rule out a CNS infection, provided no evidence of increased intracranial pressure exists.

CT scanning is revolutionary in allowing definitive evaluation for most structural causes of seizures, and the newer technique of magnetic resonance imaging (MRI) appears to provide even greater diagnostic information, Either CT scanning or MRI is required for the study of all adults with the recent onset of seizures and of persons with a change in established seizure patterns. Cerebral angiography has remained useful, particularly in looking for various types of vascular abnormalities such as arteriovenous malformations.

The EEG is important in evaluating persons with seizures. An epileptogenic discharge on an EEG often clarifies an otherwise equivocal seizure history. Although as many as 50% or more of persons with epilepsy eventually have abnormal discharges on the EEG, a negative EEG does not exclude epilepsy. The probability of finding a positive EEG is a function of the severity of the seizure disorder, the number and duration of EEGs, and the use of procedures that activate epileptogenic activity, such as sleep, photic stimulation, and hyperventilation. Photic stimulation and hyperventilation are useful in certain patients with petit mal seizures, whereas sleep and hyperventilation are useful in complex partial seizures. Sleep is a benign activating procedure that, when used in combination with noninvasive nasopharyngeal electrodes, increases the yield of epileptogenic activity by 25% or more during a routine awake study. Closed circuit television monitored EEG and 24-hour ambulatory EEG also provide additional information about the clinical seizures and the fre-

quency of ictal activity. It should be remembered that the differentiation between petit mal absences or automatisms and complex partial absences or automatisms may hinge on finding classic 3/sec bilateral symmetric spike-and-wave discharges as opposed to temporal lobe discharges. This differentiation is important because the therapeutic antiepileptic drugs for these two seizure types are quite different. Nonetheless, despite all our sophisticated technology, the most useful diagnostic procedure is a thorough history, a careful neurologic examination, and consistent and careful follow-up monitoring of the patient.

MANAGEMENT. The immediate treatment of the patient with a seizure is less involved than the long-term management of the epileptic patient. A soft object should be placed under the head of patients having seizures to prevent them from hurting themselves. Positioning patients on their sides with the head extended also minimizes the danger of aspiration; it is not necessary to use the traditional padded tongue blade. Intravenous medication is not needed for the patient with a single, short, self-limited seizure. In prescribing long-term maintenance anticonvulsant drugs, every physician should adhere to the following basic principles:

1. Use the correct drug for the type of seizure.
2. Use one drug until enough is given to achieve seizure control or until appearance of toxic effect.
3. Monitor blood drug levels in patients with poor seizure control or with signs of toxicity.
4. If the first drug inadequately controls seizures at therapeutic levels, add a second drug to achieve therapeutic levels, discontinuing the first drug gradually only if the second is effective in controlling the seizures.
5. Because status epilepticus may ensue, do not abruptly withdraw any drug.

Table 145-1 lists some of the major anticonvulsants used for the common types of seizures, along with the usual dosage schedule and the therapeutic blood levels.

Phenytoin can be given safely to adults at an initial oral loading dose of 900 to 1000 mg, which achieves therapeutic blood levels rapidly. Intravenous use of this drug is reserved only for status epilepticus, and intramuscular use is never recommended because of the marked unpredictability of absorption by this route of administration. Within 12 hours of the loading dose, the patient should receive another 300 to 400 mg to maintain the therapeutic blood level. Thereafter, many patients can take phenytoin once every 24 hours to maintain seizure control, but in some individuals who are rapid metabolizers the anticonvulsant half-life may be sufficiently short (for example, 12 hours) to require divided dosage.

Phenobarbital is a long-respected and effective drug that is forgiving of occasional missed doses because of its long half-life. It can be administered routinely as a single oral daily dose. In using primidone, carbamazepine, and ethosuximide, divided doses are needed to achieve a relatively stable therapeutic level of anticonvulsant medication. No matter which drug is used, however, unless a consistent therapeutic blood level is maintained, effective seizure control is unlikely. Nonetheless, if the patient is seizure free with less-than-therapeutic levels in the blood, raising the dosage is usually not helpful. In contrast, if a patient necessarily maintains higher-than-therapeutic serum levels of medication to achieve seizure control yet shows no signs of toxicity, dosage should not be diminished. In summary, the physician should treat the patient, not the levels, and should rely on levels only when poor seizure control or drug toxicity is present.

Table 145-1 Commonly used initial antiepileptic agents

Seizure type	Drugs	Usual adult dose	Therapeutic level	Common side effects	Monitoring
Generalized (primarily tonic-clonic or grand mal and secondarily generalized), simple partial, and complex partial seizures	Phenobarbital	90-180 mg/day	20-40 μg/ml	Dose related—nystagmus, ataxia, drowsiness Idiosyncratic—megaloblastic anemia, rash, paradoxical hyperkinesis	Annual complete blood count (CBC)
	Phenytoin (Dilantin)	300-400 mg/day	10-20 μg/ml	Dose related—nystagmus, ataxia, lethargy, diplopia Idiosyncratic—rash, adenopathy of pseudolymphoma, lupus erythematosus, blood dyscrasias Other—gum hyperplasia, hypertrichosis, hyperglycemia, hypocalcemia, megaloblastic anemia	Annual CBC
	Primidone (Mysoline)	750-1500 mg/day	8-12 μg/ml	Essentially similar to phenobarbital	Annual CBC
	Carbamazepine (Tegretol)	900-2000 mg/day	8-12 μg/ml	Dose related—ataxia, nystagmus, dizziness, diplopia Idiosyncratic—agranulocytosis and thrombocytopenia, rash, hepatic dysfunction	CBC with platelet count, urinalysis, liver function studies monthly for 3 months, then quarterly
Primarily generalized absences (petit mal)	Ethosuximide (Zarontin)	Up to 2 g/day	40-80 μg/ml	Dose related—nausea, vomiting, fatigue, vertigo, lethargy Idiosyncratic—rash, leukopenia, lupus erythematosus	CBC every 3 months for 1 year, then annually
	Valproic acid (Depakane)*	Up to 4 g/day	50-120 μg/ml	Dose related—GI upset, elevated liver enzymes, tremor, hyperammonemia, nausea Idiosyncratic—liver failure, fetal neural tube defects, pancreatitis, weight gain, alopecia	CBC, platelet count, and liver function studies monthly for 3 months, then quarterly

*Also effective in treating primarily generalized tonic-clonic seizures and myoclonic seizures.

Drug interactions should be kept in mind. For example, valproic acid inhibits phenobarbital metabolism and results in an elevation of the phenobarbital blood level. Likewise, valproic acid lowers total serum phenytoin levels yet increases the amount of active unbound phenytoin. Isoniazid is metabolized by the same pathways as phenytoin; thus when it is used in combination with standard doses of phenytoin, toxic levels of phenytoin often result.

Several other important points are relative to an adequate therapeutic approach in managing the patient who has a seizure disorder. Consideration must be given to dietary and personal habits, other drug use, and emotional factors, since these may significantly influence the patient's seizure control. For example, an unusually high intake of caffeine in the form of coffee, tea, or cola drinks may impair seizure control. Likewise, some persons with a seizure disorder may find that seizures occur after they consume even moderate amounts of alcohol. Insufficient rest is another factor that increases seizure frequency, and every patient with a seizure disorder should have regular sleeping habits. Some college students with a seizure disorder have seizures after staying up all night studying for an examination. Many times patients receive medications from more than one physician, so inadvertent incompatibilities may occur. Some persons with seizure disorders are subject to increased frequency of seizure as a result of taking antihistamines, phenothiazines, and tricyclic antidepressants. The local anesthetic lodocaine (Xylocaine) also can induce seizures in susceptible persons, although this is an uncommon occurrence. Finally, the importance of emotional factors in increased seizure frequency should be mentioned. Emotional stresses of various types may precipitate seizures, but often this factor remains unknown unless the patient is asked about any adverse circumstances that may be occurring at home or at work.

The treatment of the patient who has a history of alcohol or drug withdrawal seizures is follow-up monitoring, abstinence, and multivitamin therapy. If the patient had a recent seizure that is thought to be the result of withdrawal, however, that person has a 30% risk of fulminating delirium tremens. Consequently, despite the reluctance of many physicians to deal with alcoholic patients, it is important that all patients with so-called rum fits be admitted for at least 48 to 72 hours of observation, since the withdrawal seizure can precede the full abstinence syndrome by that much time. The specific therapy for the withdrawal or abstinence state is discussed in Chapter 180. Except for the rare patient who has status epilepticus, the use of anticonvulsants is not indicated. One of the consequences of prescribing antiepileptic medication for a known alcoholic patient without specific indication is introducing the opportunity for subsequent withdrawal from both alcohol and the antiepileptic agent. Unfortunately, some alcoholic patients also have an independent seizure disorder, often the result of the many head traumas they have sustained. The history may be difficult to obtain, and patients may be noncompliant; they may need long-term anticonvulsant therapy and often present therapeutic dilemmas that can be resolved only if they resolve their drinking problems.

STATUS EPILEPTICUS

Pathogenesis. Status epilepticus is defined as two or more seizures occurring without the patient regaining alertness, or a state of continuous seizure activity. This clinical state may be most dramatically manifested by tonic-clonic seizure activity but is also demonstrated by continuous focal motor seizures without an impairment of consciousness. In addition, petit mal status epilepticus and psychomotor status epilepticus (although usually not recognized as seizure activity) are manifest by a confusional state or inappropriate behavior. The greatest risk of complications such as anoxia or aspiration pneumonia occurs as a result of generalized grand mal or tonic-clonic status epilepticus. The risk of cardiac arrhythmias also increases. Common causes of status epilepticus include abrupt anticonvulsant withdrawal, various metabolic derangements such as electrolyte imbalance, hypoglycemia, renal failure, or hypoxic encephalopathy, CNS infections, and hemorrhage. Blood samples for a complete blood count and for deteramination of levels of calcium, phosphorus, magnesium, blood urea nitrogen, glucose, and electrolytes should be drawn. Arterial blood gas values should also be obtained if circumstances permit.

Management. The most important early steps in treating status epilepticus are establishing an airway, providing oxygen, properly positioning the patient on his side with the head slightly extended and cushioned, and administering drugs intravenously. A discussion of the drug therapy for status epilepticus among a group of neurologists usually results in as many opinions on the correct approach as there are members of the group. The fundamental principle, however, is to give enough medication intravenously to stop the seizure. More important than discussing which drug is best is the principle of having a plan before being faced with the emergency. The following plan is one approach to treating status epilepticus:

1. Initially, after drawing blood glucose, give 50% dextrose with 100 mg of thiamine intravenously.
2. If this is unsuccessful, give diazepam (Valium) intravenously at a rate of 2.5 mg/min until the seizure stops or to a maximum of 20 to 30 mg. The diazepam is infused through a separate vein or through intravenous tubing containing a 0.9% saline solution (diazepam and phenytoin are poorly soluble in glucose solution).
3. Next, 18 mg of phenytoin/kg body weight should be given to an adult at a rate no faster than 50 mg/min intravenously, through a separate vein or through intravenous tubing containing saline. An ECG monitor should be used. Phenytoin should be given as soon as the diazepam stops the seizure because of the short time (15 to 20 minutes) that intravenous diazepam is effective. In elderly or severely ill patients the infusion rate of phenytoin should not exceed 25 mg/min.

In the uncommon event that this dosage schedule does not work, phenobarbital should be given. The concurrent use of diazepam and phenobarbital intravenously may produce severe respiratory depression. If the patient is adequately intubated and has adequate respiratory assitance, however, 200 to 400 mg doses of phenobarbital can be given intravenously to a total dose of 15 mg/kg if the seizures continue unabated. As an alternative 5 to 10 ml of paraldehyde as an oil retention enema may be tried. If all else fails, general anesthesia is needed.

BIBLIOGRAPHY

Adams RD and Victor M: Principles of neurology, ed 3, New York, 1985, McGraw-Hill Inc.

Brown TR and Feldman RG, editors: Epilepsy: diagnosis and management, Boston, 1983, Little, Brown & Co Inc.

Gilman AE and others, editors: The pharmacological basis of therapeutics, ed 7, New York, 1985, MacMillan Publishing Co.

Porter RJ: Epilepsy: 100 elementary principles, London, 1984, WB Saunders Co.

Woodbury DM, Penry JK, and Pippender CE: Antiepileptic drugs, New York, 1982, Raven Press.

146 · HEADACHE AND FACIAL PAIN

Roy A. Jackel*

Headache is an exceedingly common symptom. Fortunately, most causes of head pain are benign and self-limited. In understanding the pathophysiology of head and face pain, it is important to realize that the brain parenchyma itself is insensitive to pain. Additional structures that are insensitive to pain include the ependymal lining of the ventricles, the choroid plexuses, the pia arachnoid membrane, parts of the dura mater, and the skull itself. The intracranial pain-sensitive structures include the venous sinuses and their tributaries, parts of the dura at the base, the dural arteries, and the arteries at the base of the brain. Extracranial structures sensitive to pain include the skin, scalp, fascia, muscles, arteries, and mucosa. The fifth cranial nerve contains the pain fibers above the tentorium cerebelli, with pain referred to the frontal and temporal areas as far back as a line drawn coronally above the ears. Below the tentorium cerebelli, pain is mediated by the ninth and tenth cranial nerves and the first two or three cervical nerve roots, with pain usually located in the occipital areas or in the upper cervical areas.

As indicated anatomically, headaches may arise from intracranial and extracranial locations and may be classified this way clinically. Trigeminal neuralgia and other more atypical facial pain syndromes also must be considered in the differential diagnosis of head and face pain.

Diamond and Dalessio have classified headaches into three main categories: vascular headaches, muscle contraction headaches, and traction and inflammatory headaches. Vascular headache includes migraine, cluster, hypertensive, and toxic-vascular headache. Muscle contraction headaches include those related to muscle strain, anxiety, depression, or cervical osteoarthritis. The category of traction and inflammatory headache refers to headache caused by intracranial mass lesions, such as tumors and cerebral hemorrhages, diseases of the eyes, throat, and teeth, arteritis, cranial neuralgias, and temporomandibular joint (TMJ) disease. Overlap occurs between these categories, and these classifications do not necessarily suggest etiologic mechanisms.

VASCULAR HEADACHE

Extracranial causes of headache most commonly include vascular and muscle contraction mechanisms. In vascular headache, pain is caused by extracranial vasodilation involving branches of the external carotid artery.

Migraine

Migraine, a major category of vascular headache, is characterized by recurrent unilateral throbbing headache often associated with autonomic symptoms. It is often familial and has some predilection for young women. A positive history of migraine headache can be obtained in 50% to 60% of the parents and as many as 27% of the siblings of migraine sufferers. The onset of migraine headache is before 40 years of age in 90% of patients. An onset after the age of 40 raises the likelihood of another diagnosis. The majority of migraine sufferers younger than 10 years of age are boys. In classic mi-

---

*Material in this chapter is based in part on the first edition, written by Vasant Dhopesh.

graine, which occurs in the minority of cases, an aura or prodrome occurs, consisting most often of visual phenomena in
which scintillating scotomata appear in half of the visual field.
Researchers think this is caused by an ischemia of the occipital
cortex resulting from vasoconstriction of the cerebral arteries.
Prodromes may consist of other sensory, motor, mood, behavioral, or perceptual disturbances. A prodrome can precede
the headache by hours to days. Prodromes are associated with
a cortical hypoperfusion, which may be localized or may move
slowly across the cortex as in a well-known cerebral electrical
phenomenon, "the spreading depression of Leão." Severe
throbbing unilateral headache follows most commonly in the
temporal and frontal regions but also in the retroorbital, parietal, or occipital areas. Almost always anorexia and nausea
are present. Other regularly accompanying features are photophobia and sonophobia, and most patients prefer to lie down
in a dark quiet room. Variations include common migraine,
the most common variety of vascular headache, in which the
aura is absent, and rare varieties of complicated migraine, such
as hemiplegic and ophthalmoplegic types, in which transient
neurologic signs and symptoms occur. The neurologic deficit
may occur without a headache and is then known as a migraine
equivalent. This entity tends to occur after 40 years of age and
must be differentiated from transient cerebral ischemia.

Many factors are known to precipitate a migraine attack.
Some say that migraine sufferers are perfectionists and at times
have a compulsive personality structure. Any undue stress or
fatigue may provoke a headache. In dietary migraine, certain
tyramine-rich foods (aged cheese, chicken liver, broad beans,
and certain red wines) bring on an attack. Migraine is associated
with hormonal changes, although the exact relationship is unknown. Migraine may be associated with menstruation and
often disappears during pregnancy. Oral contraceptives increase the frequency and severity of migraine attacks.

The exact pathogenesis of migraine is unclear. The humoral-
vascular theory proposes that circulating vasoactive amines
produce the prodromes through an intracranial vasoconstrictive
phase and that the headaches are the consequence of subsequent
extracranial vasodilation. A neurogenic hypothesis suggests
that vasoconstriction and vasodilation are secondary to a primary neurologic trigger involving intrinsic monoamine pathways in the brain. Another theory considers that the primary
abnormality may involve the release of serotonin from platelets. Recent studies have shown that serotonin levels rise during
the prodromal phase and drop during the headache phase and
that the urinary excretion of 5-hydroxyindoleacetic acid (5-
HIAA), a metabolite of serotonin, is increased during the attack. Platelet aggregability, which increases just before a migraine episode, is presumably responsible for the release of
serotonin. Migraine is not thought to be an allergic phenomenon.

The treatment of migraine can be divided into two parts,
symptomatic and prophylactic. The therapy for an acute attack
consists of vasoconstrictor agents such as the ergot aklaloids.
The most commonly used drug is 1 to 2 mg ergotamine tartrate
every half hour, given orally, sublingually, by inhalant, or
rectally until the patient is relieved. No more than 6 mg/day
or 10 mg/week should be administered. Various commercial
preparations of ergotamine tartrate combined with antiemetic,
anticholinergic, or sedative agents are available. For migraine
status, in which headache persists for days to weeks, dihy-
droergotamine may be intravenously administered. Treatment
with ergotamines should begin early in the course of the headache. Caution should be used in patients who have complicated
migraine and in whom further vasoconstriction is not desirable.

Toxic doses may cause intense vasoconstriction and gangrene
in the limbs and rarely in the tongue. The prophylactic treatment consists of avoiding known precipitating factors such as
foods containing high levels of tyramine. Prophylactic medications may be administered to patients whose headaches are
frequent enough to interfere with their ability to function or in
whom vasoconstrictors are contraindicated. β-Adrenergic
blockers, particularly propranolol, are the drugs of choice for
prophylaxis in selected patients. The propranolol dosage is 20
to 60 mg four times a day. A long-acting form of propranolol
can be given once a day. Methysergide, a lysergic acid derivative, is effectively prophylactically. Resembling serotonin in
its structure, methysergide is thought to be a competitive serotonin inhibitor that simulates the vasoconstrictor-potentiating
effects of serotinin on catecholamines. The dosage is 2 mg
three times daily. Retroperitoneal fibrosis is a serious side effect. Other prophylactic agents include amitriptyline, cyproheptadine, naproxen, calcium-channel blockers, and the anticonvulsant agents phenytoin and carbamazepine. Electromyographic or thermal biofeedback may be useful.

Many other conditions are known to produce vascular headache, including febrile states, bacteremia, carbon monoxide
inhalation, nitrite ingestion, hypoxia, the postictal state following seizures, and caffeine withdrawal. Because the knowledge of these conditons is obtained readily by eliciting a thorough history, the diganosis is relatively straightforward, and
an elaborate differential diagnosis is unnecessary. The treatment is directed toward the primary offending agent.

Cluster headache

Cluster headaches (Horton's, or histamine, headache) are
unilateral and vascular and belong to the migraine family; however, the characteristic features are distinct enough to classify
them as a separate entity. Cluster headache can mimic face
pain. It is more common in males and usually occurs in the
third and fourth decades of life. The outstanding clinical feature
is the periodicity of the headache, occurring in small groups
or clusters separated by brief intervals (chronic, nonremitting
forms, however, have been described). The pain is commonly
nocturnal, recurring at the same time, and is usually located
in and behind the eyeball, temple, and forehead. It is throbbing,
stabbing, or burning and so severe that patients cannot sit still
and may walk around in the hope of getting some relief. There
is no prodrome or appreciable nausea. Other autonomic symptoms, however, such as eye tearing and nasal congestion on
the same side, are prominent. A Horner's syndrome manifested
by partial lid ptosis and pupillary miosis may be seen, and this
occasionally can be permanent. The recurrent brief attacks of
headache most commonly last 30 to 45 minutes but may continue for hours. They recur for weeks, then abruptly disappear
for months or years, only to recur again in another cluster.
Cluster headaches must be differentiated from atypical facial
neuralgia and may mimic Raeder's syndrome, both of which
are discussed later in this section. The exact mechanism of the
production of cluster headache is unknown, although increased
histamine with resultant vasodilation, hypothalamic dysfunction, and sphenopalatine ganglion hypersensitivity have been
incriminated. Although cluster headaches are vascular, the response to ergot preparations is less than in migraine, and other
approaches have been tried. Prednisone (40 mg/day for 5 days
and then tapered during 3 weeks) has been used to abort attacks.
Lithium in doses up to 900 mg/day, with monitoring of serum
levels, is useful as a prophylactic agent. Antiserotinergic agents
such as cyproheptadine (4 mg four times a day) and methysergide (2 mg three times a day) are successful as prophylactic

agents, although methysergide has a potential risk. Other treatments have included 100% oxygen inhalation, somatostatin administered intravenously, and cocaine or lidocaine administered intranasally. Prednisone and lithium are particularly useful in chronic cluster headache. Medication should be limited to the length of the cycle and restarted with the occurrence of the next cycle. Since alcohol is a common precipitating factor, it should be avoided.

An unusual variant of the cluster headache, chronic paroxysmal hemicrania, has been recognized in women. These brief headaches occur repeatedly throughout the day and respond dramatically to indomethacin in doses of between 25 to 50 mg three times a day.

Hypertensive headache

Hypertensive headache occurs in about 10% to 15% of hypertensive patients. These headaches are more common after awakening, predominantly occipital, and throbbing in type. They are thought to have both vascular and muscle contraction components and may be relieved with effective antihypertensive treatment.

Toxic vascular headache

Many factors, including febrile states, bacteremia, carbon monoxide inhalation, nitrite ingestion, hypoxia, postictal states after seizures, caffeine withdrawal, and "hangover" reactions, produce vascular headaches. Physicians know about these factors if they take a thorough history. The treatment is directed toward the primary offending agent.

MUSCLE CONTRACTION (TENSION) HEADACHE

Muscle contraction headache, also known as tension headache, is the most common type of head pain encountered clinically. Most series report a preponderance of this condition in women and a higher incidence in adults between 20 to 40 years of age, but symptoms may persist in later years. The headache pain characteristically is slow in onset and develops into a steady ache of mild to severe intensity, increasing as the day progresses. It may be confined to the frontal, temporal, or occipital regions or be diffuse, and although most often bilateral, it may have a unilateral component. Some patients describe it as a tightness, pressure, or bandlike sensation around the head. Other associated symptoms such as nausea, vomiting, and photophobia are absent unless the headaches are severe or a vascular component is present. Some patients report a continuum between muscle contraction headache and migraine because of their frequent coexistence and the presence of overlapping symptoms. Muscle contraction headache may also be caused by local diseases of the spine, eyes, teeth, or paranasal sinuses.

The role of emotional factors such as anxiety, repressed hostility, and unresolved dependency in the causation of muscle contraction headache is well established. The observation that many patients with muscle contraction headache are depressed and have other somatic complaints such as anorexia and insomnia has led some authorities to believe that the headache is a symptom of depression.

The pathophysiology of muscle contraction headache is not clear. It is known that muscle fatigue and pain can be induced by volitional or sustained contraction of muscles. Some researchers have suggested, however, that muscle contraction is a product, rather than a cause, of the headache. The chemical microenvironment plays an important role and includes changes in substances such as bradykinin, lactic acid, serotonin, and prostaglandins.

The aim of treatment is to reduce both muscle and emotional tension. Mild headaches respond to simple analgesics, such as aspirin, or nonsteroidal antiinflammatory agents, such as 400 to 800 mg of ibuprofen three to four times per day. Massage, heat, physical therapy, and exercise are important adjunct treatments. Anxiolytic agents such as diazepam, combination medications such as those containing mild analgesics with butalbital, and amitriptyline (50 to 150 mg/day) are of considerable value, especially in depressed patients. In severe and more resistant cases psychotherapeutic interventions may be necessary. Various other modalities such as biofeedback, hypnosis, and acupuncture are being used to treat resistant cases.

Posttraumatic syndrome

Posttraumatic, or postconcussion, syndrome with headache may develop as a sequela to head injury along with other symptoms such as dizziness, light-headedness, and lack of concentration. Researchers think that these headaches are caused by muscle contraction, vascular dilation, or direct injury to the scalp. They are notoriously resistant to any form of treatment but eventually subside. They should be differentiated from headaches caused by subdural hematoma.

TRACTION AND INFLAMMATORY HEADACHE
Traction headache

The brain is not sensitive to pain but is surrounded, especially at the base, by pain-sensitive structures (arteries, veins, and cranial nerves) that produce referred head pain when stretched or displaced by a mass lesion. Although a mass lesion classically suggests a tumor, other conditions such as an abscess, hematoma, or brain edema can produce headache through a similar traction mechanism. These traction headaches are often deep and dull, with a steady ache that is usually worse in the morning and is aggravated by the coughing and straining that result in transiently increased intracranial pressure. The location of the pain may serve as a rough guide to the location of the mass, corresponding in position in 70% to 80% of the cases in the absence of diffusely raised intracranial pressure. For example, in posterior fossa tumors, the headache is almost always occipital. Focal neurologic signs suggestive of a structural lesion may be found, and papilledema, when present, supports the impression of increased intracranial pressure caused by a mass lesion.

Appropriate laboratory tests pinpoint the location and nature of the mass. Computed tomographic (CT) scanning and magnetic resonance imaging (MRI) have essentially eliminated the need for more complex roentgenographic procedures. Electroencephalography and cerebral angiography may be useful. The therapy usually consists of surgically removing the mass. In specific instances radiation therapy, steroids, or antibiotics may be advisable.

Lumbar puncture headache

Lumbar puncture headache also is classified as traction headache because the mechanism is presumed to be a leakage of cerebrospinal fluid (CSF) after puncture of the dural sac, with a subsequent minimal displacement of pain-sensitive structures. These headaches are occipital or frontal, are precipitated or worsened by assuming an erect posture, and are relieved by recumbency. Simple analgesics and bed rest usually bring relief. Rarely, in incapacitating cases, intravenous fluids and small doses of codeine may be necessary for 24 hours.

Headache in pseudotumor cerebri

Pseudotumor cerebri, also called benign intracranial hypertension, is a syndrome that occurs mainly in young, obese women. The patient has diffuse headaches caused by increased intracranial pressure that may be associated with blurred vision or visual obscurations. On examination the main sign elicited is papilledema. Sixth nerve palsies and an enlarged blind spot may occur. The CSF is normal except for increased pressure. The pathogenesis of this increased pressure is unknown, but various factors have been associated with it, such as venous sinus thrombosis, vitamin A excess, pregnancy, and taking birth control pills. As the name implies, the prognosis is usually good. Treatment to relieve the headache and to preserve vision consists of elimination of any known instigating factors, weight loss, repeated lumbar punctures, and occasionally diuretics (acetazolamide) and steroids. If patients do not respond medically, lumboperiotonal shunts may be considered.

Headache in subarachnoid hemorrhage

Subarachnoid hemorrhage may be caused by the rupture of a cerebral artery aneurysm with the onset of sudden severe and generalized headache. Patients may or may not lose consciousness and may or may not have focal neurologic signs. As a result of chemical meningitis caused by the presence of blood, nuchal rigidity frequently develops. The diagnosis can be based on the demonstration of blood on a noncontrast CT scan or by a spinal tap that reveals red blood cells and xanthochromia of the supernatant fluid. If an aneurysm is suspected, angiography is indicated to confirm its presence and suitability for surgical treatment.

Headache in meningitis

Headaches that occur with various forms of meningitis have a variable onset, are severe, and are aggravated by any movement of the head. Patients with these headaches are febrile and have signs of meningeal irritation. Researchers think that the pain is caused by a chemical irritation of the nerve endings in the meninges. A spinal tap with careful CSF examination is essential to establish the diagnosis and determine proper treatment.

Headache in temporal arteritis

Temporal arteritis is also called cranial arteritis and giant cell arteritis. A biopsy of the superficial temporal artery and other cranial and noncranial arteries may reveal the presence of giant cells and perivascular inflammatory exudate. Extracranial and intracranial arteries, especially the ophthalmic arteries, may be involved. Termporal arteritis is included in the group of so-called collagen-vascular diseases because the pathogenesis of this condition is thought to be caused by an autoimmune mechanism. It typically affects patients older than 60 years of age. The headache is commonly located in the temporal area and may be accompanied by vision loss caused by ophthalmic artery involvement. Temporal arteries may be seen as enlarged, tortuous vessels or may be felt as firm, tender cords on palpation. The most useful laboratory test is determination of the erythrocyte sedimentation rate (ESR), which usually is markedly elevated. The diagnosis may be confirmed by a temporal artery biopsy, which may reveal the presence of giant cells and perivascular inflammatory exudate, although occasionally biopsies may be normal. The condition dramatically responds to corticosteroids such as orally administered prednisone in a dosage of 60 mg/day, which should be instituted early to prevent visual loss. The prednisone should be tapered to 40 mg/day after 1 week, and after 4 to 6 weeks it should be reduced further to a maintenance dosage of 5 to 10 mg/day, which should be continued for about 2 years. The ESR should be used as a guide to management.

Headache from sinus or eye disease

Headache in sinusitis results from an inflammation of the ostia and the turbinates. The pain is characteristically dull and aching and is present in the morning with improvement as the day progresses. Tenderness may be present over the affected sinus. Pain in frontal sinusitis is felt over the forehead, in ethmoid sinusitis between the orbits, and in maxillary sinusitis over the cheek and upper jaw. The treatment consists of decongestants, antibiotics, and surgical drainage if a fluid level is present on roentgenograms of the sinuses. Errors of refraction, glaucoma, or inflammatory conditions of the eye produce headache, with pain usually localized to the eye. Careful ophthalmologic evaluation can determine pathologic conditions of the eye.

TRIGEMINAL NEURALGIA

Trigeminal neuralgia (tic doulourex) is characterized by brief paroxysmal attacks of severe pain in the distribution of one of the three divisions of the trigeminal nerve. The pain is so excruciating that it often causes the patient to wince with obvious facial contraction; hence the name tic douloureux. Similar paroxysmal attacks of pain in the throat are known as glossopharyngeal neuralgia.

The pathogenesis of trigeminal neuralgia is unknown but may involve failure of segmental inhibition secondary to trigeminal nerve damage. Compression of the root entry zone of the trigeminal nerve by a tortuous branch of the basilar artery has been shown to be responsible for a number of cases of trigeminal neuralgia. This syndrome also can occur in cases of multiple sclerosis, gasserian ganglion or cerebellopontine angle tumor, or brainstem infarction. Differentiation can be made because trigeminal neuralgia should not be accompanied by neurologic deficit.

The idiopathic form of this disorder occurs in midlife or late life and is slightly more common in females. The second and third divisions of the fifth nerve are most commonly involved. The pain is described variously as "like lightning jabs" or "electrical shocks" and lasts only a few seconds. The attacks are recurrent for weeks or months, although there may be spontaneous remissions. Frequently there are tender areas or trigger zones, and any mechanical activity such as smiling, talking, chewing, or touching the face sets off an attack. A neurologic deficit in the distribution of the fifth cranial nerve demands an urgent search for structural causes. The diagnosis is based on the characteristic history. Differentiation from atypical facial neuralgia is discussed later in this chapter.

Because it is believed that the pain of trigeminal neuralgia is caused by the temporal summation of afferent impulses in the spinal nucleus of the fifth cranial nerve, anticonvulsants have been tried; these agents have been found effective. The drug of choice is carbamazepine (Tegretol) in doses of 400 to 1200 mg/day, starting with small doses to prevent side effects. Rarely, severe bone marrow depression can occur as an idiosyncratic reaction; therefore periodic blood counts are advisable. Another anticonvulsant, phenytoin (Dilantin), in doses of 300 to 600 mg/day also has been useful. Other medical therapy includes chlorphenesin (800 to 2400 mg/day) or baclofen (30 to 80 mg/day). If medical treatment fails and renders the patient incapacitated, surgery may be undertaken. A number of procedures are available, each with their own advantages and disadvantages. The choice of the procedure should depend in part on the patient's age and medical situation. Radiofrequency rhizotomy of the trigeminal root, glycerol injection of Meckel's cave (trigeminal cistern), or local ablation of the peripheral trigeminal nerve affected are destuctive procedures to the nerve itself, often resulting in a neurologic deficit such as facial sensory loss or masseter muscle weakness. Microvascular decompression developed by Jannetta interposes a prosthetic implant between a vessel (often the superior cerebellar artery) and the root entry zone of the trigeminal nerve. This procedure requires a major craniotomy with possible surgical complications as well as a longer hospital stay.

ATYPICAL FACIAL NEURALGIA

There are as many syndromes as there are structures of the head and face that are characterized by forms of atypical facial neuralgia, or "lower half headache." Sluder's sphenopalatine ganglion neuralgia and Vail's vidian neuralgia are included in this category, and the profusion of eponyms compounds the confusion. It is often impossible to pinpoint the exact source of the pathologic condition. Frequently this condition is diagnosed as trigeminal neuralgia. They are differentiated from those with trigeminal neuralgia, however, by the absence of trigger zones, by the occurrence in a younger age group, and by the character of the pain, which may be dull, throbbing, boring, and either constant or episodic. Some autonomic symptoms such as eye tearing, nasal congestion, and nausea may be present. The pain is located at the base of the nose or in the orbit, upper cheek, jaws, and teeth and may radiate to the temple or forehead. Sluder believed that the cause was in the sphenopalatine ganglion and termed the disorder "sphenopalatine ganglion neuralgia." Vail ascribed the same condition to an irritation of the vidian nerve caused by sphenoid sinusitis and coined the term "vidian neuraliga." Destroying either the sphenopalatine ganglion or the vidian nerve does not abolish the pain in all cases. It is therefore believed that atypical facial neuralgia is caused by multiple factors, including vascular phenomena. It may resemble vascular headache of the migraine type, especially cluster headache, from which it may be difficult for the physician to differentiate. Unfortunately, the therapeutic response to various treatments, including ergot alkaloids, is poor.

Raeder described patients with orbital pain and supraorbital pain associated with oculosympathetic paralysis. Raeder's syndrome is also referred to as paratrigeminal neuralgia, since a lesion in the paratrigeminal location could involve the ophthalmic division of the trigeminal nerve and the oculosympathetic fibers traveling with the internal carotid artery. Most often no definitive cause is found. Men are affected more commonly than women. Researchers believe that the oculosympathetic paralysis is caused by pressure from dilation of the internal carotid artery in the cavernous sinus. The resultant partial Horner's syndrome is manifested as miosis and partial ptosis. Usually there is normal facial sweating or loss of sweating only in a localized supraorbital area, since the lesion involves sympathetic fibers along the internal carotid artery and sudomotor fibers to the face travel along the branches of the external carotid artery. If studies exclude a parasellar lesion, the treatment of Raeder's syndrome is the same as that for cluster headache, which many physicians believe is synonymous with Raeder's syndrome.

"Atypical facial pain" is a term that is used when pain does not have characteristics of any of the conditions described previously. The pain usually persists for months or years and in some cases attains the status of a delusion. It is presumed psychogenic and therefore may be resistant to any kind of therapy.

CAROTIDYNIA

Carotidynia is pain that occurs on one side of the neck in the area of the bifurcation of the common carotid artery. It may radiate to the face, jaw, and temple and characteristically occurs in young or middle-aged adults. Swelling and tenderness in the carotid artery at the carotid sinus may be present. Similarities to migraine headache have been noted, and carotidynia may respond to similar medications. Otherwise the treatment is symptomatic.

Temporomandibular joint pain dysfunction syndrome (myofascial pain dysfunction syndrome)

The TMJ pain dysfunction syndrome involves a dull and aching pain that is localized to the area of the jaw, neck, ear, and temple. The pain is usually unilateral and may be continuous for prolonged periods. There may be tenderness and spasm of the muscles of mastication with limitation of jaw motion. Although the etiologic factors are not always completely understood, TMJ pain may be caused by muscle spasm, as in the myofascial pain dysfunction (MPD) syndrome), or by articular disorders. The muscle spasm may be caused by psychologic factors, or it may be precipitated by an overcontraction secondary to malocclusion. Articular disorders may be studied with MRI, which may show displacement of the joint meniscus. Treatment should be directed toward relief of the muscle spasm with heat, massage, salicylates, and muscle relaxants. Dental splints may be helpful.

● ● ●

From the foregoing discussion, it is clear that for a patient with the complaint of headache or face pain, a detailed history is essential. The physician should ask pertinent questions about onset, location, quality, intensity, relationship to the time of day, inciting events, and associated symptoms. Although in the majority of instances pain involving the head and face falls into well-defined syndromes, it may be difficult to determine whether the pain results from diseased teeth, TMJ disease, a sinus disorder, vascular headache, or neuralgia. In such cases a multidisciplinary evaluation is required so that patients are spared unnecessary treatments such as extraction of teeth. Conversely, patients with dental dysfunction or TMJ disease should not be subjected to neurosurgery or other inappropriate procedures.

BIBLIOGRAPHY

Ad Hoc Committee on Classification of Headache: Classification of headache, JAMA 179:127, 1962.
Blau JN: Migraine pathogenesis: the neural hypothesis reexamined, J Neurol Neurosurg Psychiatry 47:437, 1984.
Dalessio DEJ: Wolff's headache and other head pain, ed 5, New York, 1987, Oxford University Press.
Diamond S and Dalessio DJ: The practicing physician's approach to headache, ed 4, Baltimore, 1986, Williams & Wilkins.
Featherstone HJ: Migraine and muscle contraction headaches, Headache 25:194, 1985.
Fisher CN: Late-life migraine accompaniments as a cause of unexplained transient ischemic attacks, Can J Neurol Sci 7:9, 1980.
Hanington E: The platelet and migraine, Headache 26:411, 1986.
Packard RC, editor: Headache. In Neurologic clinics. 1, No. 2, Philadelphia, 1983, WB Saunders Co.
Raskin NH and Appenzeller O: Headache, Philadelphia, 1980, WB Saunders Co.
Reik L: Unnecessary dental treatment of headache patients for temporomandibular joint disorders, Headache 25:246, 1985.
Reik L and Hale M: The temporomandibular joint pain-dysfunction syndrome: a frequent cause of headache, Headache 21:151, 1981.

147·DIZZINESS, VERTIGO, AND HEARING LOSS

Joseph U. Toglia

DIZZINESS

"Dizziness," a nonspecific descriptive term that is often used to refer to a sensation of disequilibrium, may be ophthalmogenic (as when a patient wears glasses with the wrong refractive correction or has cataracts) or somatosensory (as when a patient has lost proprioceptive sensation in conditions such as peripheral neuropathy or cervical spondylosis). Odontogenic dizziness is associated with abnormal dental occlusion and temporomandibular joint (TMJ) dysfunction, in which disorders and symptoms such as tinnitus, hearing loss, facial pain, and nausea also are reported (see the discussion of dental correlations in this chapter). Dizziness may also result from hyperventilation. The overbreathing and resultant hypocapnia produce cerebral vasoconstriction and a diminished cerebral blood flow. A patient with the hyperventilation syndrome also complains of paresthesia of the extremities and lips. Nystagmus is absent, and caloric test results are normal. If more than one of these situations occur, as with various combinations of ophthalmogenic, somatosensory, and odontogenic types, dizziness may become incapacitating. Such combinations often occur in elderly patients with multisystem disorders, such as diabetes mellitus, cataract, and cervical spondylosis.

VERTIGO

The term "vertigo" implies a sensation of rotation in space of either the patient or the environment, caused by altered physiology of the labyrinth or the central vestibular pathways of the ear. Vertigo may be physiologic, as experienced after sudden rotatory acceleration or deceleration (Bárány's test), or pathologic, as experienced with disorders of the labyrinth or with lesions of the central vestibular pathways.

The differential diagnosis between peripheral or otogenic vertigo and central or neurogenic vertigo is based on clinical observations and a laboratory evaluation.

CLINICAL MANIFESTATIONS. Otogenic vertigo is usually influenced by position and movement of the head in space. The duration varies from hours to several days. The patient loses his balance and has a tendency to fall to one side. Autonomic symptoms such as sweating, pallor, nausea, and vomiting occur almost constantly. Tinnitus and hearing loss are often noted. A jerky, horizontal-rotatory, unidirectional nystagmus is associated with the vertigo and is seen better when visual fixation is abolished. Other neurologic signs and symptoms are characteristically absent. Otogenic, or benign, vertigo can be elicited when the seated patient is suddenly placed in a supine position with the head hanging off the examining table (the Hallpike maneuver). In this position, and usually when the pathologic vestibular apparatus is undermost, a rotatory nystagmus develops. If the head position is turned, this nystagmus remains direction fixed, but it reverses direction when the patient returns to the sitting position. The nystagmus appears after 3 to 5 seconds of latency and lasts for 10 to 15 seconds. Neither the nystagmus nor the vertigo recurs if several positional tests are performed consecutively.

Neurogenic central, or nonbenign, vertigo is not influenced by the position of the head in space but in some cases may be influenced by rotating and extending the neck. Autonomic symptoms are usually absent except in cases of acute vascular lesions of the medulla or cerebellum. Audiologic symptoms are usually absent except in cases of acoustic neurinoma or other lesions in the cerebellopontine angle. Signs of cerebellar dysfunction are often present. These include ataxia of the extremities, dysarthria, tremor, and falling. Signs of cranial nerve dysfunction are frequent. At no time should vertigo be attributed to end-organ disease if the examination shows paralysis of any but the seventh and eighth cranial nerves, which may be disrupted in patients with either neurologic or otologic disease. The most common cranial nerve deficits include facial paresthesia, dysphonia, dysphagia, and paralysis of the tongue, palate, larynx, and sternocleidomastoid muscles. Nystagmus is the most important neurologic sign. Central nystagmus may be vertical, purely rotatory, multidirectional, monocular, pendular, retractory, convergent, see-saw, or alternating and is usually not inhibited by visual fixation.

A direction-changing positional nystagmus, elicited in the Hallpike maneuver, suggests central nervous system disease. The nystagmus has no latency period, no specific directionality, and no fatigability. It remains unchanged as long as the critical head position is maintained. When the head position is reversed, a similar nystagmus develops in the opposite direction.

LABORATORY DIAGNOSIS. The most specific tests for evaluation of vertigo are those that check labyrinthine function by means of caloric and rotatory stimulations. The rotatory tests are performed by rotating the patient in a rotatory chair and measuring the nystagmus induced by acceleration and deceleration. The caloric tests are performed by irrigating the ear canal alternately with cold and warm water while the patient's head is positioned in the midsagittal plane so that a line between the external ear orifice and the lateral canthus of the eye is perpendicular to the floor. About 30 seconds after the irrigation stops, the patient's eyes develop a jerky, horizontal-rotatory nystagmus, with the fast phase beating away from the ear irrigated by cold water or toward the ear irrigated by warm water. The nystagmus lasts about 1 minute, and nausea and other autonomic symptoms may develop. The caloric tests show abnormalities in both peripheral and central vestibular dysfunction. The caloric responses are best evaluated with relation to latency, duration, amplitude, and frequency using electronystagmography (ENG). This technique is based on the existence of a corneoretinal electrical potential, and it allows the recording of eye movement direction, as well as amplitude, frequency, and speed. The recorded movements may be physiologic or pathologic. ENG is particularly useful when the patient complains of vertigo and both the otologic and neurologic examinations are normal. The ENG may be performed either in the dark or with the patient's eyes closed. The presence of nystagmus under these circumstances can be of paramount importance in establishing objective evidence of organicity.

Additional tests of value in specific instances include audiograms, brainstem auditory evoked potentials (see discussion of "Hearing loss" in this chapter), skull and mastoid roentgenograms, complex motion tomography of the temporal bone, computed tomography of the brain, high-resolution computed tomographic (CT) scans of the inner ear, CT cisternography with air or metrizamide, Pantopaque encephalography, magnetic resonance imaging (MRI), cervical spine roentgenograms, cerebrospinal fluid (CSF) examination, and occasionally cerebral angiography. The selection of these additional tests depends on the clinical history and the physical examination.

Diseases causing vertigo

DISEASES OF THE LABYRINTH. The function of the labyrinth may be disrupted by a variety of pathologic processes, including infectious labyrinthitis, drugs (gentamicin, strepto-mycin, kanamycin, and neomycin), metabolic disorders (diabetes, dysproteinemia, and uremia), vascular diseases, and head trauma. The most common diseases of the labyrinth are acute labyrinthitis, traumatic labyrinthopathy, Ménière's syndrome, and benign positional vertigo.

Acute labyrinthitis usually occurs with chronic middle ear infection, especially associated with cholesteatoma. Vertigo, ataxia, nausea, and vomiting are always present, and hearing loss may occur. Nystagmus beats to the opposite side, and the caloric responses are diminished on the side of the pathologic condition. Usually there is no fever. Bacterial labyrinthitis or suppurative labyrinthitis, in which there are abnormalities in hearing, should be distinguished from a viral form or from vestibular neuronitis, in which cochlear signs and symptoms are conspicuously absent. The prognosis in labyrinthitis is usually benign, and recovery takes place within several days to a few weeks. Occasionally bacterial infection spreads to the central nervous system, produces a middle ear cholesteatoma, or causes a fistula of the labyrinth. The therapy is with antibiotics, myringotomy, symptomatic medication, or all three for vertigo and nausea. Mastoidectomy is indicated in cases of chronic osteitis and fistula of the labyrinth.

Ménière's syndrome usually is attributed to hydrops of the membranous labyrinth caused by a defective reabsorption of the endolymph. Its cause is unknown, although it is associated with allergies, metabolic and endocrine disturbances, and dysfunction of the autonomic nervous system.

Symptoms and signs include a fluctuating fullness and hearing loss in one ear associated with episodes of vertigo, tinnitus, unsteadiness, nausea, and vomiting. Most symptoms abate within several hours. These attacks occur periodically and at varying intervals. Nystagmus is active during the acute attack and may persist for weeks after the vertigo has subsided. Caloric test results are always abnormal. Audiologic tests show specific abnormalities (see discussion of "Hearing loss" in this chapter).

The attacks become less frequent after several years, but the hearing loss gets progressively worse. In about 10% of these patients the other ear also eventually becomes involved. When possible, therapy should be addressed to a specific cause. Nevertheless, medications such as antihistaminics are needed for acute symptoms. A variety of regimens, including diuretics, anticonvulsants, and desensitization, are used prophylactically. When medical therapy has failed and the attacks continue to be incapacitating, and particularly if the hearing loss is already severe, various surgical procedures should be considered. These include labyrinthotomy, labyrinthectomy, and vestibular nerve section.

In benign positional vertigo, short periods occur during which vertigo is noted only on change of position. There may or may not be evidence of vestibular dysfunction of the benign type. The condition is self-limited, and no specific therapy is indicated.

DISEASES OF THE CENTRAL NERVOUS SYSTEM. Vertigo occurs in many diseases of the central nervous system (CNS), including intracranial infections (cerebellar or temporal lobe abscess), vascular disease (vertebrobasilar artery insufficiency, brainstem and cerebellar infarction, and cerebellar hemorrhage), multiple sclerosis, migraine, epilepsy, encephalitis, CNS trauma, degenerative diseases, and CNS neoplasms. Only a few of these conditions are discussed here in detail.

Vascular diseases. *Vertebrobasilar artery insufficiency.* Patients with vertebrobasilar artery insufficiency have transient neurologic symptoms and deficits that may result from com-

binations of intrinsic vascular disease and from mechanical causes of decreased perfusion pressure. A common example of the latter is obstruction of the vertebral arteries by arthritic osteophytes.

Patients with vertebrobasilar artery insufficiency may experience vertigo, transitory visual disturbances, syncope dysarthria, drop attacks, or numbness. If vertigo is caused by ischemia of the labyrinth, the patient most often complains of tinnitus and hearing difficulty. The symptoms may be induced by postural changes of the neck, by sudden arising from a sitting or supine position, or by exercise of the upper extremities (subclavian steal syndrome). Special tests include cervical spine roentgenograms, ENG, and in some cases angiography.

Infarctions and hemorrhages. Infarctions and hemorrhages cause vertigo when they are localized in the posterolateral area of the medulla or in the cerebellum.

The symptoms include many of those seen in cases of vertebrobasilar artery insufficiency, but the deficits are not transient. They often can be grouped in specific syndromes according to the anatomic blood supply (for example, Wallenberg's syndrome). ENG and brainstem auditory evoked potentials are particularly useful tests for diagnosing brainstem lesions.

The prognosis varies with the severity of the vascular disease and the localization of the lesion in the brainstem.

Multiple sclerosis. Although vertigo is a common complaint of patients with multiple sclerosis, the latter disorder begins with vertigo in only about 5% of the cases.

Paroxysmal vertigo with or without autonomic symptoms or loss of balance may suggest multiple sclerosis in a young patient, particularly if it is associated with other oculomotor abnormalities or with visual abnormalities. Vertigo in this instance is seldom associated with tinnitus or loss of hearing. Nystagmus occurs in 70% of cases and in a variety of forms, especially monocular and vertical. ENG may demonstrate abnormalities of eye movement that are not evident on direct visual inspection. Vertibular test results are almost always abnormal. Visual, auditory, and somatosensory evoked potentials are frequently abnormal. The diagnosis depends on the course of the illness and the elevation of CSF γ-globulins. The prognosis and therapy are discussed further in Chapter 148.

Epilepsy. An epileptogenic lesion in the temporal lobe may cause vertiginous seizures, in which case the vertigo usually occurs as the aura of a generalized attack. It is frequently associated with an epigastric sensation but not with hearing loss or nystagmus. The diagnosis is established by electroencephalography (EEG). Vertiginous epilepsy must not be confused with vestibulogenic epilepsy in which seizures are induced by stimulation of the labyrinth.

Migraine. Paroxysmal vertigo may occur in place of a migraine attack (migraine equivalent) or as one of the multiple manifestations of basilar artery migraine. Vertigo typical of Ménière's syndrome may replace the attacks of migraine in later life. At times, attacks of migraine and Ménière's syndrome may occur independently in the same patient.

Head trauma is a common cause of labyrinth dysfunction, or traumatic labyrinthopathy. The trauma may cause extravasation of blood into the labyrinth, producing permanent damage, or may result only in a transient loss of labyrinthine function (labyrinthine concussion). An acute flexion-extension injury of the neck also causes labyrinthine dysfunction, through concussion of the labyrinth, through ischemia in the distribution of branches of the vertebral artery, or through disruption of proprioceptive cervical impulses. Vertigo occurs in the immediate posttraumatic period. Several days later the vertigo is usually present only after the assumption of certain postures, and the patient may complain only of postural disequilibrium. Nystagmus and abnormal results of caloric tests recorded by ENG occur in about 40% of these patients. The degree of tinnitus and hearing loss varies according to the severity and type of head trauma and is particularly severe with fractures of the petrous bone.

The prognosis varies according to the severity of the trauma. Even minor injuries may cause protracted symptoms, especially when a medicolegal settlement is pending or if the patient has a psychiatric disorder. The therapy is symptomatic. These patients often require mild tranquilizers and psychotherapy.

Tumors. Vertigo may occur in patients with CNS tumors, particularly when the tumor is located in the posterior fossa. It also may occur with tumors in the anterior cranial fossa, particularly the temporal lobe, but the incidence is low. Posterior fossa tumors causing vertigo are found in the cerebellum, brainstem, fourth ventricle, and cerebellopontine angle (CPA). Their location is clinically identifiable by a variety of neurologic symptoms and signs and by ancillary tests such as CT scan and MRI.

CPA tumors include acoustic neurinomas (ANs), which represent 70% to 80% of CPA tumors, and meningiomas. The initial symptoms of AN are tinnitus and hearing loss. Vertigo occurs as the initial symptom in a small percentage of cases, but once the tumor has expanded, the incidence of dizziness and vertigo increases to as much as 58%. Spontaneous nystagmus occurs in the majority of cases. Other cranial nerve palsies include those of the trigeminal and abducens and the fourth, seventh, tenth, and eleventh cranial nerves. Other neurologic signs include cerebellar ataxia and signs of increased intracranial pressure. The diagnosis of AN is based on ancillary studies, starting with audiologic and vestibular tests. Audiograms reveal sensory neural hearing loss, poor speech discrimination, tone decay, and poor stapedium reflex in the vast majority of the patients. Loss of vestibular function with the caloric test is found in 85% to 90% of cases. Additional useful tests include brainstem auditory evoked responses, ENG, complex motion tomography of the temporal bone of the posterior fossa, high-resolution CT scans of the inner ear, CT cisternography with air or metrizamide, isophendylate encephalography, and MRI. The spinal fluid protein level is elevated in a large percentage of cases. The surgical prognosis is good, especially in cases that are diagnosed early.

Meningioma is the second most common tumor in the CPA. Paralysis of the fifth, seventh, and eighth cranial nerves occurs in the majority of cases, as with AN, but paralysis of the other cranial nerves occurs more often than in AN. Papilledema, ataxia, cerebellar signs, and nystagmus also occur in the majority of cases. Vestibular hyporeflexia and hearing loss are less frequent than in AN.

TRAUMA. Head trauma may cause vertigo by more than one mechanism. It may damage the vestibular nerve through fracture of the petrous portion of the temporal bone, or it may produce an epileptogenic focus in the cerebral cortex. Vertigo may also occur as a symptom of concussion or with flexion-extension injuries of the neck. When vertigo is induced by temporal bone fracture, the clinical findings may include otorrhagia hemotympanum, CSF otorrhea, laceration of the tympanic membrane, ecchymosis of the mastoid region, and vestibular and auditory abnormalities. The incidence of dizziness and vertigo in patients with fracture of the temporal bone is reported to range from 75% to 93% compared with vertigo in only 56% of patients with skull fracture in other location.

HEARING LOSS

The human ear detects tones ranging in frequency between 16 Hz and 16,000 Hz. The greater the frequency, the higher the pitch. Persons who clearly detect frequencies between 500 and 2000 Hz can hear adequately but may not appreciate the many qualities of sound. The loudness of sound depends on the amplitude of the sound wave. The greater the amplitude, the louder the sound.

Normal hearing levels are defined by an international standard. The intensity of sound is defined in decibels (db), with 0 being barely audible. A patient's hearing level is the difference in decibels between the faintest pure tone that can be heard and the normal reference level given by the standard. Normal conversation has a level of about 60 db. Mild hearing loss often starts at 4000 Hz and is rather common after 65 years of age, but it is noted also among younger people, especially those exposed continually to intense noise. A hearing loss of 15 db at the frequencies of 500, 1000, or 2000 Hz is considered a minor impairment, and a loss of 80 db at the same frequencies may be considered deafness, at least in a social context. Hearing loss may be caused by diseases of the middle ear (conductive hearing loss), the cochlea and cochlear nerve (sensorineural hearing loss), and the central auditory pathways (central hearing loss).

Hearing loss may be evaluated as a screening procedure (Weber's and Rinne tests) with a tuning fork at either 256 or 512 Hz or more thoroughly in special environments with audiometry. In Weber's test the tuning fork is struck and placed on the forehead. If hearing is equal in both ears, the patient does not lateralize the vibratory sound to either ear. If the sound is lateralized to the right ear, for example, this means either that the left ear has sensorineural hearing loss or that the right ear has conductive hearing loss. In the Rinne test the tuning fork is struck and placed alternately near the ear and against the homolateral mastoid bone. If the hearing is normal, the sound is heard about twice as long by air conduction as by bone conduction. If bone conduction is equal to or greater than air conduction, the hearing loss is conductive and not sensorineural.

Conventional pure tone audiometric testing reveals the patient's level and configuration of hearing loss by both air and bone conduction. Speech audiometry tests measure the patient's threshold for speech and the ability to discriminate its finer qualities. Special auditory tests (impedance audiometry, Békésy audiometry, and loudness balance and tone decay tests) are useful clinically in differentiating conductive hearing disorders, cochlear and retrocochlear lesions, and pathologic conditions of the CNS.

The three basic types of hearing loss are conductive, sensorineural, and central.

Conductive hearing loss

Conductive hearing loss is caused by pathologic conditions of the external or middle ear; common causes are otitis media and otosclerosis. Otitis media may be infectious (suppurative) or noninfectious (serous). Suppurative otitis may spread to the inner ear, mastoid, and CNS. Chronic otitis may produce a cholesteatoma; this tumor may invade the inner ear, resulting in mixed conductive and sensorineural hearing loss. In otosclerosis, which is commonly familial, there is decreased mobility of the middle ear ossicles, the hearing loss begins in late adolescence, and the deficit is conductive. Audiometric tests in middle ear disease reveal an essentially normal level of hearing of pure tones by bone conduction and a substantial loss of air conduction.

Sensorineural hearing loss

Sensorineural hearing loss, typical of Ménière's disease and acoustic neurinoma, is caused by lesions of the cochlea or the cochlear nerve. Patients note difficulty in understanding conversation in a noisy place and cannot tolerate loud speech.

In sensoineural hearing loss, air conduction is greater than bone conduction on the Rinne test, although both are diminished; on Weber's test the sound is lateralized to the normal ear. Audiometric tests reveal that pure tone air and bone conduction thresholds are both impaired, mostly in the higher frequencies. The presence of recruitment (a disproportionate increase in loudness perceived relative to intensity delivered) suggests a lesion of the cochlea, as in Ménière's disease, and early impairment of speech discrimination suggests a nerve lesion, as in a tumor of the eighth cranial nerve (acoustic neurinoma).

In Ménière's disease the hearing loss is almost always unilateral and of moderate degree for all frequencies, and hearing sensitivity fluctuates in the early stage of the disease. Tinnitus and vertigo are the other two complaints in this syndrome.

In the past, acoustic neurinoma was rarely seen until the involved ear was essentially deaf. However, thanks to current specific neuroimaging tests, the tumor may be diagnosed when the hearing loss is as little as 15 db. Tinnitus is the earliest symptom, and vertigo is either absent or seen in the later stage of the disease (see the discussion of Vertigo, diseases of the CNS in this chapter). Brainstem auditory evoked potential testing is an excellent method for localizing the site of the lesion.

Sudden hearing loss may be caused by acute ischemia in the distribution of the internal auditory and anterior inferior cerebellar arteries, which supply the labyrinth and brainstem cochlear nuclei. Other causes of sensorineural hearing loss include trauma, presbycusis, and ototoxicity.

Central hearing loss

Central hearing loss is caused by pathologic conditions of the central auditory pathways (cochlear and dorsal olivary nuclei, inferior colliculi, medial geniculate bodies, and temporal lobe cortex). This is rather uncommon, although it may be seen in multiple scherosis, encephalitis, and brainstem infarction. The hearing loss is evident most often against a background of multiple sensory stimuli.

Audiometry tests reveal normal pure tone audiometry and conventional speech audiometry. Localization audiometry and brainstem auditory evoked potentials are the most useful tests for diagnosing central hearing loss.

The technique of brainstem auditory evoked potentials is relatively simple: the responses to auditory stimuli are averaged in an evoked response recording device via scalp electrodes. A normal response is characterized by a series of seven electrical potentials that are generated in the auditory nerve, the cochlear nuclei, and the interconnecting pathways. Lesions of the central auditory pathways alter the latencies and amplitude of these evoked responses.

BIBLIOGRAPHY

Nylen CO: Positional nystagmus, J Laryngol Otol 64:295, 1950.
Paparella MM and Shumrick DA, editors: Otolaryngology, Philadelphia, 1973, WB Saunders Co.
Toglia JU: Labyrinth versus central nystagmus: electronystagmographic observation, Dis Nerv System 40:110, 1971.
Toglia JU: Dizziness in the elderly. In Fields WS, editor: Neurological and sensory disorders in the elderly, Houston neurological symposium, Houston, 1975, University of Texas Press.
Toglia J: Electronystagmography: technical aspects, Springfield, Ill, 1976, Charles C Thomas, Publisher.
Toglia JU, Thomas D, and Kuritzky A: Common migraine and vestibular function, Ann Otol Rhinol Laryngol 90:267, 1981.

148·DEMYELINATING, DEGENERATIVE, AND HEREDOFAMILIAL DISEASES OF THE CENTRAL NERVOUS SYSTEM

Wallace W. Tourtellotte and **Michael J. Walsh**

DISEASES OF WHITE MATTER

Diseases of white matter constitute a heterogeneous group of disorders, with damage confined predominantly to the white matter, loss of the oligodendrocytes and their myelin sheaths, and relative sparing of the neurons and the axons. It is useful to divide these disorders into *demyelinating* and *dysmyelinating* types. Demyelinating refers to disorders in which myelin is apparently formed normally but because of various insults is broken down; dysmyelinating refers to disorders in which it is presumed that the myelin membrane is abnormal qualitatively or quantitatively at the time of formation. Most demyelinating disorders are of unknown origin, but some are thought to be virally and immunologically mediated, whereas dysmyelinating disorders are caused by known or presumed genetically determined disturbances of myelin formation and breakdown. These two categories of white matter disease differ epidemiologically, clinically, and prognostically. Multiple sclerosis and its varients are the prototypes of the demyelinating diseases, and metachromatic leukodystrophy and its relatives are the best characterized of the dysmyelinating diseases. Also included with the dysmyelinating diseases are adrenoleukodystrophy, globoid cell leukodystrophy, sudanophilic leukodystrophy, spongy sclerosis, fibrinoid leukodystrophy, and some of the aminoacidurias (phenylketonuria) and lipidoses. Phenylketonuria is potentially treatable if the diagnosis is made at birth, but no therapy is yet available for the other disorders. The metabolic disturbance that is presumed to underlie most of these disorders is known in only a few instances, and diagnosis is sometimes impossible during life. The advent of computed tomography (CT) and magnetic resonance imaging (MRI) of the brain has made possible a noninvasive differentiation of gray matter from white matter, which reveals changes in white matter that may be helpful in the differential diagnosis. These noninvasive tests may also confirm the presence of bilateral disease when the patient has focal symptoms suggesting a mass lesion. Enhancement of the lesion by injection of contrast media may be demonstrable when considerable inflammation and disruption of the blood-brain barrier is present.

Demyelinating diseases

MULTIPLE SCLEROSIS. Multiple sclerosis (MS) is the most common of the human demyelinating diseases. The disease has been known as a clinical and pathologic entity for the past century, but its cause is still not established and no known therapy reverses the demyelination or prevents the progression of this disease. There is no diagnostic test for MS, although a constellation of clinical and laboratory findings is suggestive when a restricted number of other disorders are excluded. The disease derives its name from the autopsy picture of the brain, where grossly apparent and microscopic plaques are scattered throughout the white matter of the central nervous system (CNS). The clinical picture also reflects the presence of multiple disseminated lesions of the brain. Another remarkable feature of this disease is the tendency for serious symptoms such as blindness and hemiplegia to remit. These aspects—dissemination over time and evidence of multiple lesions in the CNS—are prerequisites for a clinical diagnosis of MS. Not all patients, however, meet the stringent clinical criteria for diagnosis, and laboratory investigations may be equivocal. In these instances the physician may have to perform exhaustive studies to exclude other diseases and may have to postpone making a definitive diagnosis. However, it is usually possible to make the diagnosis with assurance, and recently developed techniques for noninvasive investigation of the CNS, especially MRI, sometimes provide strong support for the clinical diagnosis.

Etiology. No single hypothesis with experimental validation has emerged that explains adequately all the features of MS. Morphologic, genetic, virologic, epidemiologic, immunologic, and clinical peculiarities abound in this disease more than any other disorder of the CNS. Because MS affects so many young people and seems potentially treatable if the inciting events and the factors that induce its exacerbation and progression are identified, an enormous research effort has been under way for almost a century to establish the cause and therapy for this disorder. The following are the most reliable observations on which an etiologic hypothesis might be established.

Morphology. The lesions of MS, particularly perivascular lymphocyte cuffing and periplaque and white matter infiltration by plasma cells and lymphocytes, are characteristic of lesions seen in viral and postvaccinal disorders of the CNS, leading some to consider a viral cause. The morphologic conditions are also reminiscent of those in experimental allergic encephalomyelitis, a disorder induced by immunization with brain homogenate combined with adjuvant.

Genetic aspects. An individual who has an identical (monozygotic) twin affected with MS has a 26% risk of the disease. The risk of a nonidentical (dizygotic) twin is 2%, the same as it is for nontwin siblings. Accordingly twin studies show a major genetic component in susceptibility to MS.

Immunogenetic data that tend to implicate certain histocompatibility antigens in the genesis of MS have accumulated during the past few years. It appears that certain human lymphocyte antigens (HLAs) are significantly overrepresented in patients with MS (HLA-A3, HLA-B7, and HLA-DR2).

Virology. Patients with MS tend to have higher titers of antibody in both serum and cerebrospinal fluid (CSF) to a large number of viruses, most notably measles, rubella, mumps, parainfluenza, Epstein-Barr virus, herpes simplex type 1 and 2 virus, and HTLV-1 (although the latter is controversial). The observed differences, although significant, are relatively small in most studies, generally on the order of a twofold or smaller titer elevation. Morphologic studies using electron microscopy sometimes demonstrate filamentous structures resembling paramyxovirus nucleocapsid in mononuclear cell nuclei in MS brain lesions, but no immunologic evidence points to this material as being a virus. Efforts to culture virus from the brain have been unsuccessful except in a few instances. Clustering of MS in families and communities may suggest a common agent such as virus, but other environmental and genetic hypotheses are also plausible • explanations.

Epidemiology. Numerous studies have confirmed the well-known association between disease prevalence and distance from the equator. Geographically, MS is most common in western Europe, southern Canada, southern Australia, and New Zealand. Clusters of the disease have occurred in such places as the Faroe Islands. Although these islands had not experienced a high incidence of MS, there was a virtual epidemic of disease attributed to the presence of British forces on the islands during World War II. The epidemiologic studies in the Faroe Islands seem compatible with a transmissable viral infection of the CNS introduced at that time. Other studies evaluated the impact of migrations of populations on the prevalence of MS. It appears that individuals who move from areas of higher prevalence to areas of lower prevalence after 15 years of age retain the risk of MS of their previous environment. Those who move before 15 years of age acquire the risk prevalence of their new environment. Various hypotheses may account for these differences. Children from areas of high prevalence may have an infection in the early years of life that predisposes them to subsequently having MS. Alternatively, infection may be common in areas of low risk for MS and may provide protection later against the disease. Virus infection may also affect age groups differently. For example, when poliomyelitis occurs at an early age, it may be asymptomatic, whereas in later life it tends to produce paralytic disease. Lifelong immunity occurs in both instances. Epidemiologic investigations have also raised the question of a dietary factor (deficiency of unsaturated fats) being associated with the increased incidence of MS in certain regions of the world.

Immunologic aspects. The CSF shows abnormalities in 90% of patients with MS, most notably increased intra–blood brain barrier IgG synthesis (rate by formula and unique CSF IgG oligoclonal bands by isoelectric focusing and immunofixation). Evidence exists that the majority of IgG is synthesized in situ within the CNS independent of the systemic immune system. It has long been speculated that this immunoglobulin is directed against MS antigen(s), but studies to determine the specificity of this IgG have been inconclusive.

It seems that suppressor lymphocyte function is altered in MS and that acute deteriorations in this disease are accompanied or perhaps preceded by defective immunoregulation that allows unimpeded damage to oligodendrocytes and the myelin membrane. Remission, however, is accompanied by a rebound elevation in suppressor function. Whether the suppressor abnormality is of pathogenetic significance or is merely a secondary manifestation of a more complex immune perturbation is unknown.

In summary, both virally and immunologically mediated injury may give rise to human demyelination with features identical to those seen in MS. Genetic factors play a role in MS, but there is no haplotype or genetic characteristic yet known that is obligatory for disease expression. Some evidence exists that a disturbance of fatty acid and prostaglandin metabolism may play some part in the disease's pathogenesis. Such a disturbance may render myelin more susceptible to an immune attack and permit injury to the oligodendrocytes and the myelin membranes by cytotoxic cells and serum factors that gain access to them. It is also possible that MS is not one disorder but a consequence of various insults to the CNS acting alone or in unison, in the same way that pneumonia has many causes.

Neuropathology. The external surface of the brain is normal. Sometimes the brain weight is diminished and the ventricles are enlarged. Staining of the myelin sheath in sections of the cerebral hemispheres, brainstem, cerebellum, and spinal cord may reveal multifocal discrete plaques of demyelination. In the cerebral hemispheres there is a predilection for plaques to be present in the periventricular areas, particularly around the third and fourth ventricles. The optic nerves are often shrunken because of demyelination. A mild lymphocytic meningitis may accompany the parenchymal changes, predominantly a perivenulitis that is most apparent in the deep sulcal recesses. Although MS is primarily a disorder of myelin, some axonal damage may occur, and gliosis develops with time. The peripheral nerves are not involved.

Pathophysiology. Demyelination leads to four important central disturbances that are relevant to the clinical appearance of MS: decreased nerve conduction velocity, differential rate of transmission of impulses resulting from slowing in the fibers of particular nerves or tracts, frequency-related conduction block, and complete failure of impulse transmission.

Minor fluctuations in temperature may produce major changes in the severity of signs and symptoms of MS. Increases of 0.2° F may produce decreased visual acuity, additional weakness, and pathologic reflexes. The disease's tendency to be aggravated by increasing temperature is the basis for the hot bath test still used diagnostically by some physicians. It has also been observed that hyperventilation may produce transitory amelioration of some manifestations such as scotomas; sodium bicarbonate infusions may have similar effects. This is believed to result from an effect on ionized calcium, since hypocalcemia increases the excitability of damaged fibers and may facilitate conduction in demyelinated nerves and tracts.

Clinical manifestations. The clinical manifestations of MS reflect the effect of the widespread and multifocal demyelination of the CNS both in place and time (that is, multiple sites and episodes). The disease process tends to affect some systems preferentially, so certain manifestations commonly occur whereas other signs and symptoms occur only rarely. Furthermore, not all lesions of the CNS are manifest clinically, and the lesions at autopsy may be extensive although the known manifestations in life were trivial. As electrophysiologic and roentgenographic techniques continue to develop, it is likely that more clinically inapparent lesions will be identified; for example, evoked potential recordings of the brainstem and visual system are often abnormal even though clinical testing shows no abnormality.

The cardinal manifestations of MS are caused by injury to the visual, motor, and sensory fiber systems and are easily categorized.

Visual manifestations are of great importance because 60% or more of patients have significant temporary or permanent visual complaints. Moreover, some eye signs elicited by the physician, causing little or no symptoms, are extremely helpful in supporting a diagnosis in difficult cases. The interrogation of the patient is important in establishing evidence of disease dissemination with time. Some patients initially deny all visual complaints, but when queried repeatedly and by different examiners, they may recall long-forgotten episodes of temporary visual disturbances.

Optic neuritis is the most serious of the visual manifestations. It may be the first symptom of MS, preceding other manifestations by many years, or may appear at the onset or at any time during the course of the disease. It may be unilateral or bilateral and the eyes may be affected together or separately. Patients may complain of the sensation of having a patch or a fog over one eye, or they may complain of visual blurring. When a central scotoma is the main feature, the patient may appreciate that the peripheral field of vision is unaffected. Paracentral scotomas, quadrantanopsia, altitudinal field defects, and less commonly homonymous field defects may occur. Optic neuritis is usually subacute at onset with gradual and maximal visual impairment developing for several days; this is in contrast to ischemic optic neuropathy, in which visual loss is usually acute and total. Sudden visual loss, however, does

occur. Frontal headache or pain on moving or touching the eye is common, as is photophobia. Visual acuity in most patients falls to 20/100 or worse. Gradual recovery occurs for 2 to 4 weeks in most patients, but many are left with subjective residua of the primary attack. Some notice that colors appear desaturated, and defects in color perception may be elicited. Vision may be transiently reduced with vigorous exercise or increased temperature (Uhthoff's symptom).

During the episode of optic neuritis, disc edema resembling papilledema may occur; however, in papilledema the visual acuity is normal. The edema is now considered to be caused by a disturbance of axoplasm flow at the optic nerve head. The term "retrobulbar neuritis" is used when funduscopy is normal. An important physical sign to look for in every patient is an afferent pupillary defect (Marcus Gunn's pupillary sign, or the swinging flashlight sign). This test is positive in most patients who have had unilateral optic neuritis and also may be elicited in patients in whom there is no clear history to suggest previous eye disease. To elicit this sign, the physician shines the light in each eye separately. When the light is swiftly shifted from the normal to the affected eye, the pupil dilates rather than constricts in response to direct light stimulation. The optic disc becomes pale in patients with previous optic neuritis, chiefly temporally at first. Optic pallor, however, is not a useful sign because it depends on a subjective evaluation. A more reliable assessment is possible by counting the small vessels intervening on the disc between the major grouping of superior and inferior retinal vessels; normally there are six to eight small vessels, but in optic neuritis there may be only two to four.

MS eventually develops in 40% or more of all patients with optic neuritis. Predictive tests, however, are of no value at this time in attempting to predict which patients will have multifocal demyelinating disease.

Another category of visual system abnormality reflects disease of the oculomotor system. Whereas palsies of individual muscles and nerves occur infrequently, internuclear ophthalmoplegia is a common sign and should be carefully sought. The cardinal manifestations of internuclear ophthalmoplegia are unilateral nystagmus in the abducting eye and contralateral impaired adduction. The signs are indicative of a lesion of the medial longitudinal fasciculus on the side contralateral to the nystagmus.

Motor manifestations are common and occur in almost all patients at some stage of the illness; they are responsible for most of the chronic disability seen in MS. Excessive fatigue may herald disease onset and may be prominent at a time when there is no easily identifiable objective motor finding. A sense of stiffness or heaviness, especially in the lower extremities, is a common patient complaint. Dragging of an extremity or stumbling may occur. Involvement of the upper extremities is usually preceded by or is simultaneous with involvement of the lower extremities. Unilateral upper extremity monoparesis is manifested by "the useless hand," a clumsiness or diminished facility for tasks requiring skilled motor function, such as handwriting or typing. A feature of the motor signs and symptoms is their tendency to fluctuate from day to day or hour to hour at disease onset. This is especially true for signs such as the Babinski sign, which may alternate from flexor to extensor with repeated testing. Exercise or an increase in body temperature may render an equivocal plantar response plainly extensor. The important accompaniments of motor involvement are increased tone, spasticity, increased reflexes, and alteration in cutaneous reflexes. The Babinski sign is found in most patients with established disease, and clonus at the ankle and knee is elicited. The superficial abdominal and cremasteric reflexes are altered and lost, but abdominal reflexes are often difficult to assess when the patient is obese or has abdominal scarring. A downward drift of the outstretched arms is a useful indication of disease. The motor disability may remit or progress to paraparesis or paraplegia, sometimes with equal severity in the upper extremities. Cerebellar signs commonly accompany the corticospinal disturbance, but not invariably. At times chronic spastic paraparesis, as either a stable or a slowly progressive deficit, is the only manifestation, and the diagnosis is then difficult to make because the criteria of the dissemination of the disease in place and time cannot be confirmed.

The prominence of cerebellar abnormalities has been known since the time of Charcot, and the triad of scanning speech, nystagmus, and intention tremor is sometimes known by this name. Along with corticospinal tract involvement, this is the most disabling of the major manifestations of MS. Incoordination, disequilibrium, falling, and stumbling are distressing. Skilled use of the hands for writing and work may be impossible. Sometimes only mild tremor is present; this is predominantly a proximal tremor and is accentuated greatly with the initiation and persistence of movement. The tremor may be predominantly truncal, in which case the patient has difficulty with gait and has titubation of the head. Marked dysarthria may make speech unintelligible. The tremor may be so manifest and powerful that the patient's bed or wheelchair may shake in synchrony.

Sensory manifestations are common, and patient complaints related to sensory disturbance may greatly exceed what might be demonstrable on physical examination. Paresthesias are the most common complaint, but the patient may describe a complex pattern of sensory alteration. The impairment may be so great that the patient is unaware of the position of a limb in space and needs to visually identify its location. Patients complain of both lower extremities feeling dead, heavy, or like wood. They may note sensations like a constricting bandage, for example, around all or part of the circumference of the abdomen. Disturbance of temperature, with an entire limb or the lower half of the body unable to appreciate the degree of heat or cold, such as while swimming or bathing, is a feature in some cases. Lhermitte's sign refers to a sensation of electricity or shock that may extend down the arms and back in association with sudden neck flexion. Although this is described by some patients with MS, it also occurs after trauma and with cervical spondylosis or cord tumor. Testing of sensory function usually discloses that the most prominent disturbance is in posterior column modalities, including vibration sense and position sense.

Bladder complaints are found in most instances of established disease. Urgency, precipitancy, poor urinary stream, frequency of urination, and urinary incontinence are found in various degrees. It is common for the examiner to be able to identify some disturbance of corticospinal disease when urinary complaints are prominent. Abnormalities in the bladder muscle (detrusor) reflex function in MS arise from either an interruption of the corticoregulatory tracts or a demyelination in the conus medullaris; the former leads to detrusor hyperreflexia and the latter to detrusor areflexia. Almost all patients have abnormalities, hyperreflexia being twice as common as hyporeflexia. Diminished facility and frequency of penile erection and actual impotence may result from the disease in some cases. Psychologic factors may be at fault and should be assessed fully in any evaluation. Cystometrography and anal sphincter electromyography are useful to categorize the urinary and sexual complaints.

Other manifestations such as aphasia and myoclonus occur uncommonly. Some authors report an increased frequency of epilepsy. Cranial nerve palsies are rare; facial palsy is usually of the central type but peripheral seventh nerve palsy can occur. It is rare for the acoustic division of the eighth nerve to be affected, but vestibular symptoms occur occasionally and a severe episode with vertigo, nausea, and vomiting may herald the onset of MS. An important paroxysmal syndrome seen in 2% to 5% of patients is trigeminal neuralgia. Other painful syndromes include glossopharyngeal neuralgia, atypical facial pain, and shooting pains similar to the pain of tabes dorsalis. Some patients have facial myokymia, a movement disorder affecting the facial muscles and manifested as undulant, poorly synchronized movements that may occur bilaterally or unilaterally. Paroxysmal syndromes, including tonic spasms, facial myokymia, and trigeminal neuralgia, may arise from cross-communication between nude axons. Intellectual impairment is not a prominent feature of MS but may result from the cumulative effects of long-standing disease and extensive demyelination.

Diagnosis. Because multiple lesions in the CNS are expected in MS, any patient with neurologic signs pointing to a single lesion should be investigated for a localized disorder such as a spinal cord or foramen magnum tumor, a cervical disc, or a spinal malformation. In spinal cord or foramen magnum tumors, cervical discs, or spinal malformations pain may occur, and the course is more likely to be one of progression rather than of remission and exacerbation. Spinocerebellar degenerations have characteristic patterns of inheritance and involve particular pathways in the CNS. Subacute combined degeneration gives signs characteristic of symmetric involvement of posterior and lateral columns of the spinal cord, generally in a patient with a low serum vitamin B_{12} level. Syringomyelia commonly includes a segmental sensory involvement not typical of MS. Collagen disorders, particularly lupus erythematosus, may mimic MS, since vasculitis can cause multifocal CNS disease. A diagnosis of hysteria is sometimes considered early in MS, when neurologic signs may be transient or not prominent. Such a psychiatric diagnosis should be suggested by a history of psychiatric disturbances and not by the absence of neurologic signs. Multiple sclerosis generally does not produce signs of peripheral neuropathy or anterior horn cell disturbance, and its onset is uncommon beyond 50 years of age.

Laboratory findings. No definitive laboratory tests exist for MS. The physician should perform a CSF analysis for every patient suspected of having this disorder. This analysis should include a cell count with differential count, estimation of total protein and IgG concentration, and electrophoresis to check for the presence of oligoclonal IgG bands. The CSF leukocyte count is greater than five cells (lymphocytes)/mm³ in about 30% of cases. A count that exceeds 50 cells/mm³ or the presence of polymorphonuclear leukocytes should cast doubt on the diagnosis or suggest a complication. The total protein level in the CSF is usually normal. A protein value greater than 100 mg/dl warrants a reevaluation of the diagnosis. Intra–blood brain barrier IgG synthesis is demonstrated in almost all patients with the diagnosis of clinical definite multiple sclerosis. This profile may be mimicked in part by neurosyphilis, subacute sclerosing panencephalitis, and certain other diseases, including chronic infections. The serum IgG concentration should be normal in MS. In addition, myelin basic protein can be measured in the CSF by radioimmunoassay and may be increased in the CSF during an acute exacerbation, reflecting the myelin breakdown process. Concentrations of measles antibodies and other common viral antibodies are increased, more in CSF than in blood.

MRI of the brain and spinal cord may show areas of high attentuation (T_2 weighted images), especially surrounding the ventricles. Ventricular enlargement and cerebral atrophy are seen with longstanding disease. A large plaque of demyelination may be difficult to differentiate from a tumor if no other lesions are demonstrable.

Electrophysiologic studies of sensory function have been useful in evaluting the patient with suspected MS. This has involved using auditory, visual, and somatosensory evoked potentials. The visual evoked response is abnormal in acute optic neuritis. Delayed latency of the response, an altered waveform, and an altered amplitude of the response occur. The amplitude of the response recovers with improving visual acuity, but the delayed latency, once established, persists indefinitely. Visual evoked responses are impaired in more than 85% of patients with clinical definite MS regardless of the findings on ophthalmologic examination. Similarly, spinal cord, subcortical, and rolandic somatosensory responses may show abnormalities in MS, and brainstem evoked responses are often abnormal. These recordings may be made before, during, and after artificially raising the body temperature and may yield additional information on disease dissemination. Thus a combination of electrophysiologic recordings can facilitate assessing the major fiber tracts in the CNS for clinically inapparent disease, can provide evidence for disease dissemination in the presence of isolated signs and symptoms, and may be useful in following the course of the illness and the response to various putative therapies.

Course. Remissions, which may be complete or partial, are common, particularly in cases beginning in young adult life. The course is more likely to be progressive, without remissions occurring, in cases of MS beginning at a later age. The mechanism of relapse and remission has long been a perplexing problem in MS. Pathologic studies suggest that remyelination may take place; however, this is usually limited in extent and may not contribute much to restoring lost function. An alternative mechanism of recovery involves structural and cytochemical alterations in the internodal axon that permit a continuous conduction of impulses along the nerve fiber. This may involve the development of new sodium channels along the entire axon. Recovery from some acute deficits may simply result from resolution of the edema that is known to accompany acute lesions. Corticosteroids or adrenocorticotropic hormone (ACTH) may be of some benefit in accelerating this resolution.

Remissions tend to become less complete with time. Despite varying degrees of disability, longevity is better than generally believed; more than 70% of patients with MS are alive 25 years after its onset.

Management. The treatment of MS is symptomatic and is aimed at alleviating the neurologic and psychologic consequences of demyelination and its complications. The uncertainty of diagnosis in some instances and the tendency of the disease to go into remission and then to relapse have made quantifying responses to various interventions difficult.

Incoordination, spasticity, and bladder difficulties constitute the three symptoms that are most disabling for patients with MS. At this time no drug is reliably helpful for tremor and incoordination. Propranolol in low doses (40 to 240 mg/day) is sometimes helpful for short periods in reducing the intensity of the tremor. When tremors are severe and disabling for long periods, contralateral thalamotomy may give relief for some years. Spasticity and flexor spasm can be both painful and disabling. Baclofen (Lioresal) has proved a significant development in the symptomatic management of such patients. The dosage is 5 mg three times a day, increasing until an optimal effect is achieved (usually 15 to 25 mg three times a day). Diazepam may be useful in moderating the intensity of spasticity, but the required doses often lead to sedation.

In bladder disorders, anticholinergic agents such as propantheline and oxybutynin reduce detrusor reflex activity and diminish urgency and precipitancy in some cases. Baclofen is also helpful. Bethanechol may help patients with decreased detrusor reflex contraction and bladder tone. Various surgical procedures have been devised, such as intermittent urinary catheterization, which prevents excessive bladder distention. When neurologic impotence is present, a penile prosthesis may be inserted. Dorsal column stimulation has not been useful in treating any of these complications of MS.

Every attempt should be made to maintain patient mobility and to prevent deformities and contractures. Because premature fatigue may be an overwhelming symptom in MS, physiotherapy should be modified in accordance with the stamina of the patient. Hydrotherapy is of great value to patients with MS because buoyancy permits more vigorous and precise movement and dissipates the heat that so frequently aggravates MS symptoms.

Corticosteroids and ACTH do not appear to alter the progression of neurologic injury or to reverse preexisting injury to the CNS. Clearly there are potentially serious complications from their use for long periods in immobilized patients with bladder dysfunction and increased liability to infection and osteoporosis. Corticosteroids and ACTH should be reserved for instances of acute neurologic deterioration, such as optic neuritis with severe visual impairment, bilateral optic neuritis, acute transverse myelitis, and the uncommon instances when the lesion ascends with quadriparesis and bulbar paresis. In these situations, adrenocorticotropic hormone (ACTH) or prednisone (40 to 60 mg/day) is used for 8 to 10 days. Nonspecific immunosuppressive therapy (for example, azathioprine and cyclophosphamide) should be considered highly experimental in treating MS.

ACUTE DISSEMINATED ENCEPHALOMYELITIS AND ACUTE NECROTIZING ENCEPHALOMYELITIS. Acute disseminated encephalomyelitis (ADE) and acute necrotizing encephalomyelitis (ANE) constitute a spectrum of pathologic injury to the CNS characterized chiefly by a white matter injury, often with a predilection for the white matter of the cerebrum, brainstem, and spinal cord. The peripheral nervous system may also be affected. The relationship of ADE to ANE is controversial, but present evidence suggests that both are responses to an immune-mediated injury to the CNS. In both disorders perivenous inflammation with myelinoclasis is common, but the destruction of white matter may be more extensive in ANE.

ADE is most common in childhood but also occurs in adult life. A history of preceding viral infection may be obtained, or both may occur concurrently. Sometimes the disorder is consequent to immunization, in which case the term "postvaccinal encephalomyelitis" is appropriate. Postvaccinal encephalomyelitis has been seen after rabies and smallpox vaccination. The clinical picture in ADE is characterized by the acute onset of headache, high fever, stiff neck, and alteration in mental status with delirium and obtundation. Seizures may occur. Focal signs depend on the predominant site of injury. In cases of predominant spinal cord injury, areflexic flaccid paraplegia or quadriplegia with sensory disturbance and sphincter failure may occur as a manifestation of transverse myelitis. Guillain-Barré syndrome with neuropathic features may be the major manifestation. A brainstem syndrome may predominate, in which nystagmus, ophthalmoplegia, facial paresis, and various motor and sensory findings are combined. The CSF demonstrates pleocytosis with increased protein concentration but is occasionally normal.

ANE may be similar clinically to ADE but is more fulminating and more frequently characterized by focal symptoms and signs. The disease tends to occur in children and young adults and often is preceded by an upper respiratory tract infection.

Both disorders may be fatal in hours or days, but patients with ADE commonly recover partially or fully. In occasional instances both disorders may recur after full recovery, sometimes in association with some new antigenic stimulus such as drug ingestion or vaccination. Most clinicians believe that corticosteroids or ACTH are useful if given in time.

CENTRAL PONTINE MYELINOLYSIS. Central pontine myelinolysis (CPM) is a unique disease of the brainstem characterized by demyelination, affecting chiefly the basis pontis but sometimes extending into the pontine tegmentum or more diffusely throughout the CNS. Despite demyelination and loss of oligodendrocytes, the neurons and their axons are usually normal. Mild perivenular inflammatory cuffing is seen in early cases. Microcavitation may occur, as may fibrillary gliosis with older lesions. The disorder is diagnosed in both sexes and is described as occurring in childhood and in adulthood. Most cases are seen in alcoholic patients suffering from malnutrition, but the disorder also occurs in association with malignancy, cachectic states associated with severe medical illness, and cytotoxic chemotherapy. In almost all instances there is severe metabolic disturbance with hyponatremia. The clinical picture is characterized by obtundation and mental status abnormality with disorientation. Tremulousness, ataxia, and hallucinations may be present, especially in alcoholic patients. The latter stages of disease are accompanied by bilateral corticospinal and corticobulbar signs, chiefly extensor plantar responses, spasticity, and posturing of the extremities. Bilateral facial paresis and pseudobulbar or bulbar palsy may be seen. A locked-in syndrome (see Chapter 189) may occur. More extensive demyelination may lead to pupillary abnormalities and abnormalities of eye movements. The disorder should be suspected in appropriate clinical settings when patients manifest bilateral neurologic signs and evidence of brainstem dysfunction without obvious explanation. The presence of hyponatremia and recent massive volume replacement (that is, fluid infusions) should increase suspicion of the diagnosis. CT with careful delineation of the brainstem may show a low-density zone, lucency, or evidence of cavitation in the ventral pons when the lesion is large; MRI (T_2 weighted mode) appears even more sensitive in detecting the demyelinating lesion. The disorder is usually fatal, but the lesion is sometimes seen in autopsies of patients who died from other causes, and recovery has occurred in patients with evidence of severe pontine dysfunction. Treatment measures should be designed to combat or prevent cerebral edema. Electrolyte disturbances should be corrected without aggravating the preexisting hyponatremia commonly associated with CPM. Hypertonic saline and diuresis may be required. When inappropriate antidiuretic hormone (ADH) secretion is present, the usual measures to treat this disorder should be instituted, including fluid restriction and drugs when necessary. The cause of CPM is unknown, but factors suggested as important in its pathogenesis include malnutrition, electrolyte disturbance (hyponatremia), transient hypotension, cerebral edema, and vulnerability of the basis pontis to vascular damage.

MARCHIAFAVA-BIGNAMI DISEASE. Marchiafava Bignami disease is a rare demyelinating disorder that symmetrically affects the corpus callosum and at times the anterior and posterior commissure, the cerebellar peduncles, and the cerebral association bundles. Originally described in wine-drinking Italian men, this disease is now known to occur in individuals of varying nationalities. It does occur predominantly in middle-aged or elderly men, and is usually, although not exclusively, associated with alcoholism. Although malnutriton and alcohol have been implicated, the cause of this disease is not well understood. The clinical picture is nonspecific and poorly defined because of the rarity of the disease and its overlap with other complications of alcoholism. Dementia, aberrant behavior, apraxia, aphasia, dysarthria, hemiparesis, incontinence, seizures, stupor, and coma have all been described as features. Remissions are thought to occur, although the disease is said to have a progressive course leading to death in 3 to 6 years. Other causes of dementia should be considered in the differential diagnosis. No specific treatment exists.

LEUKOENCEPHALOPATHY WITH NEOPLASIA. Neoplasia may be accompanied by various neurologic syndromes reflecting white matter damage. These include progressive multifocal leukoencephalopathy (see Chapter 188) and central pontine myelinolysis. Disseminated necrotizing encephalomyelopathy is a white matter disorder associated with the treatment of neoplasia, most often occurring in children receiving the combination of intrathecal methotrexate with craniospinal irradiation for leukemia and sarcoma. In occasional instances similar clinical and pathologic findings have followed intravenous administration of methotrexate in high doses without craniospinal irradiation. The clinical picture is variable. Patients may be asymptomatic or show minor deficits in the face of evidence of white matter loss on CT or MRI. In the severe disorder behavioral and personality change may occur early, followed by motor manifestations with spasticity and paresis. Intellectual decline, memory impairment, language disturbance, and seizures can occur. The diagnosis is suspected when evidence of widespread and progressive injury to the brain exists. Infection by opportunistic organisms must be excluded. CT or MRI may show focal or diffuse white matter injury. Pathologically, multifocal patchy coagulative necrosis of the white matter or diffuse symmetric demyelination is seen. Axonal swelling is a constant and early feature, as are demyelination and areas of gliosis. No treatment exists for this disorder.

Dysmyelinating diseases

METACHROMATIC LEUKODYSTROPHY. Metachromatic leukodystrophy is the most common of the leukodystrophies. The disease is inherited as an autosomal recessive trait; late infantile, juvenile, and adult forms occur. In the late infantile form development seems normal until the end of the first year of life. At this time incoordination and gait disturbance appear. The patient has flaccid paraparesis or quadriparesis with absent or diminished reflexes. Rarely, spastic diplegia without increased stretch reflexes occurs. Speech deteriorates because of dysarthria and dysphasia. Optic atrophy may be seen. Eventually the patient has quadriplegia with decorticate or decerebrate posturing. Dysphagia caused by bulbar and pseudobulbar palsy occurs. Dementia ensues, and the patient usually dies 2 to 4 years after the onset of symptoms.

The progression of the juvenile form is similar to the infantile variety, except deterioration is not as rapid.

The adult form of metachromatic leukodystrophy may be difficult to diagnose because for many years the patient may appear to suffer from a functional disorder. Later, seizures, movement disorders with extrapyramidal signs, and intellectual impairment confirm the organic nature of the disease.

In this disease galactosyl ceramide esterified with sulfuric acid accumulates in nervous tissue, the kidney, and the biliary system. The defect in this disease results from a lack of arylsulfatase A, which hydrolyzes the sulfuric acid ester from galactose. Patients excrete large quantities of this material, and it also accumulates in the nervous tissue. The material is stained with the dye cresyl violet, and the orange-brown color produced is known as metachromasia.

Pathologically, white matter is involved extensively, usually symmetrically. The ventricles may be enlarged because of shrinkage of the white matter. Myelin is principally affected, but axons and neurons also undergo degeneration. Macrophages filled with debris are evident in areas of myelin breakdown. Nerve cells are ballooned and swollen, containing cerebroside sulfatide. Metachromatic material is seen also in oligodendrocytes, some neurons, and Schwann cells.

The diagnosis is made by measuring urinary arylsulfatase A activity or by demonstrating metachromatic material in tissue from the kidney or peripheral nerve. The diagnosis of the heterozygote state can be made by assaying enzyme levels in cultured fibroblasts. The CSF almost always shows an increase in total protein. CT scans may show decreased density surrounding the lateral ventricles, which is consistent with a diffuse demyelinating process, whereas MRI in the T_2-weighted mode shows hyperintensity surrounding the lateral ventricles. Nerve conduction velocities are slowed, and a sural nerve biopsy stained with acidified cresyl violet may show the metachromatic staining of stored sulfatide. Prenatal diagnosis is possible by amniocentesis.

ADRENOLEUKODYSTROPHY. The typical age at onset of adrenoleukodystrophy is between 5 and 10 years. The initial symptoms are behavior disturbance and intellectual failure. Visual loss (cortical) and motor deficits occur, and seizures may develop later. Unilateral symptoms may initially predominate. In children signs of adrenal insufficiency are not prominent, although their skin may show a bronze pigmentation. When familial, the disease shows an X-linked recessive pattern of inheritance. An enzyme defect is presumed in this disorder, but its nature is unknown. A brain biopsy shows the key feature of demyelination. Subcortical arcuate fibers are usually not involved. On light microscopy adrenoleukodystrophy may look identical to multiple sclerosis. An ultrastructural study may reveal characteristic trilaminar cytoplasmic inclusions within the macrophages. Similar changes are found in the peripheral tissues, and a biopsy of one of these peripheral sites may allow a diagnosis to be made in life. CT scanning is useful in excluding tumor and shows extensive, usually symmetric, low-density lesions in the white matter. MRI may be even more sensitive and discriminative. Some lesions may be enhanced with injection of contrast media. ACTH stimulation reveals an impaired adrenal reserve. The CSF total protein is often increased. Many cases of adrenoleukodystrophy were described in the past under the eponym "Schilder's disease."

GLOBOID CELL LEUKODYSTROPHY (KRABBE'S DISEASE). Globoid cell leukodystrophy, or Krabbe's disease, is a rare dysmyelinating disease in which symptoms begin within the first 3 to 6 months of life with irritability, stiffness of the extremities, and febrile episodes. The infant becomes sensitive to external stimulation and cries constantly for no apparent reason. Progressive intellectual deterioration, decorticate posturing, and death within months to several years ensue. The disorder is associated with a deficiency of a β-galactosidase (cerebrosidase) and is transmitted as an autosomal recessive trait. Extensive demyelination of the brain and spinal cord occurs. The gray matter is usually spared. Large multinucleated globoid cells with abundant cytoplasm and containing para-aminosalicylic acid (PAS) positive staining material are found in the CNS. Peripheral nerve involvement is present. The urine sediment shows galactosyl ceramide. Reduced levels of β-galactosidase (cerebrosidase) are found in leukocytes and fibroblasts. Nerve conduction velocities are slowed. A CT scan and MRI may show the white matter loss. The CSF protein is increased. Prenatal diagnosis is possible by amniocentesis.

SUDANOPHILIC LEUKODYSTROPHY (PELIZAEUS-MERZBACHER DISEASE). Sudanophilic leukodystrophy, or Pelizaeus-Merzbacher disease, is a rare dysmyelinating disorder affecting principally the white matter. It is most commonly a sex-linked recessive disorder. The clinical picture is variable; it may begin in the first few months of life or later in childhood. The earliest and most characteristic signs are pendular and rotary nystagmus, chaotic eye movement, and intermittent shaking movements of the arms and the head. The disease may progress slowly for many decades. In cases occurring later in life, spasticity, dysarthria, ataxia, and choreoathetosis occur. In all cases intellectual deterioration occurs and seizures are common. Optic atrophy and blindness eventually appear. The characteristic pathologic condition is a symmetric, diffuse hypomyelination with areas of gliosis interspersed with islands of normal myelination. The white matter disturbance, interpreted as an arrest of myelination, is most prominent in the cerebrum and cerebellum. The subcortical U fibers and the axons are spared. Diagnostic tests and treatment are not available for this disease.

SPONGY DEGENERATION OF THE WHITE MATTER (CANAVAN'S DISEASE). Spongy degeneration of the white matter, or Canavan's disease, is an autosomal recessive disorder usually classified with the dysmyelinating disease. More than 30% of reported cases have occurred in Ashkenazi Jews (of eastern European descent), but cases have been reported in all races. Most cases begin in infancy with hypotonia of the head and neck noticeable at 3 to 4 months of age. Megalencephaly and psychomotor retardation are apparent by 6 months of age. Decerebrate and decorticate posturing in response to sensory stimuli is superimposed on generalized hypotonia. Myoclonic seizures and choreoathetosis are added to the evolving clinical picture. Autonomic crises (for example, blood pressure fluctuations and diaphoresis) may occur. Optic atrophy, nystagmus, and rolling eye movements are noted. Most patients die in the first 2 years of the disease. The first signs of Canavan's disease may be noted later in the first decade, in which case a cerebellar syndrome with optic atrophy, spasticity, and intellectual deterioration occurs, but megalencephaly is usually not present. Pathologically, the brain is enlarged. There is little stainable myelin, along with marked vacuolation of the myelin sheaths and secondary degeneration of the myelin membrane. The water content of the brain is increased, and both edema and a spongy state have been described on microscopic examination. There is a generalized enlargement of the protoplasmic astrocytes, which contain bizarre and enormously elongated mitochondria with a crystalline substructure. Alzheimer's type 2 cells are also present in great numbers. Diagnostic tests and therapy are not available for this disorder.

FIBRINOID LEUKODYSTROPHY (ALEXANDER'S DIS-

EASE). Fibrinoid leukodystrophy, or Alexander's disease, is the rarest of the hereditary disorders of myelin. Its mode of transmission is unknown, but the disease affects males much more frequently than females. Neurologic deterioration with a rapidly enlarging head begins early in infancy. The head enlargement usually results from megalencephaly, but hydrocephalus may occur. Seizures and spasticity are characteristic symptoms. If hydrocephalus results from stenosis of the aqueduct of Sylvius, there may be a temporary response to shunting. Most affected children die before 5 years of age. At autopsy the brain is heavier and larger than normal. There is a pronounced lack of myelin staining of the cerebral and cerebellar white matter. Multiple hypertrophic astrocytes with eosinophilic inclusions within their cytoplasm are seen; these inclusions are known as Rosenthal fibers and are thought to represent glial degradation products. The axis cylinders are preserved. No inflammatory cells are present. No degenerating sudanophilic material exists to indicate myelin breakdown. There is no diagnostic test for this disease, and its cause is unknown.

Other dysmyelinating diseases. Other dysmyelinating diseases include phenylketonuria, an autosomal recessive disorder classified in the aminoacidopathies, and the lipidoses (for example, Tay-Sachs disease) (see Chapter 102).

DEGENERATIVE DISORDERS
Motor neuron disease

The term "motor neuron disease" refers to a group of disorders characterized pathologically by injury and a loss of motor neurons in the cerebral cortex, brainstem, and spinal cord and clinically by muscular atrophy, spasticity, and weakness. Significant sensory symptoms are absent in all instances. The nomenclature established for these diseases is reasonably descriptive of the clinical and pathologic findings. Amyotrophic lateral sclerosis (ALS) refers to cases in which upper motor neuron findings are prominent, in addition to atrophy and fasciculations as manifestations of lower motor neuron involvement. Involvement of the bulbar muscles usually occurs at some point during the course of the disease. Progressive bulbar palsy is a variant of ALS; its chief features are paresis and wasting of muscles innervated by the lower cranial nerves, and it is characterized clinically by dysphonia, dysphagia, dysarthria, and difficulty with respiration and clearing of secretions. Progressive muscular atrophy is characterized by findings chiefly reflecting an injury to anterior horn cells. It is not a single entity and includes a number of disorders with differences in age of onset, severity, genetics, and prognosis, such as Werdnig-Hoffman syndrome of infancy and Kugelberg-Welander disease of late childhood or early adulthood. The neuronal form of Charcot-Marie-Tooth disease may be included in this category.

AMYOTROPHIC LATERAL SCLEROSIS. ALS is the most common variant of motor neuron disease, with an estimated prevalence of 2 to 7:100,000 persons in the United States. A clustering of cases occurs in the western Pacific region, where the disease is perhaps 50 times more common than in other regions. The mean age of onset is between 50 and 60 years of age, but the disease also may occur in the very aged. ALS has a slight male preponderance, and familial cases occasionally occur.

Etiology. The cause of ALS is not established. The clustering of cases found in the western Pacific, especially in Guam, and the occasional occurrence of an ALS syndrome many years after a poliovirus infection have raised the question of the disease being a slow virus infection. Efforts to transmit this disease have not been successful, virologic studies have not disclosed any disease-specific abnormality, and the majority of ultrastructural studies for virus material have been negative or inconclusive. Immunologic factors involved in its pathogenesis are suggested by the finding of immune complex deposition in the glomeruli of some patients with ALS and the cytotoxicity of ALS serum to anterior horn cells in tissue culture. Histocompatibility typing in some studies has shown a preponderance of some HLA types.

Pathology. In the cerebrum, atrophy of the cortex, particularly of the precentral gyrus, may be grossly apparent. Microscopic changes are confined to the upper motor neurons and to the lower motor neurons and their tracts. The Betz cells of the motor cortex are reduced in number and size. There is loss of the motor neurons of the brainstem except for those subserving the extraocular muscles. In the spinal cord a loss of large motor neurons is found and corticospinal tract degeneration is noted. In the Guamanian form neurofibrillary degeneration is prominent. In some familial cases of ALS, degeneration of the posterior columns and spinocerebellar tracts occurs, linking this subtype to other degenerations of the nervous system.

Clinical manifestations. Signs of anterior horn cell disease may predominate initially, or the patient may have pyramidal tract signs alone. Eventually, combinations of findings develop in which, despite atrophy and fasciculations of anterior horn cell disease, reflexes may be increased pathologically and there may be reflex spread. The principal symptom is weakness that begins in the upper extremities and is often unilateral at onset. Atrophy, cramps, and fasciculations develop. The weakness and wasting often are first apparent in the small muscles of the hand and result in loss of dexterity for fine hand movements and in clumsiness. In a minority of patients the weakness and atrophy are first apparent proximally in the sholder girdle muscles. At a time when the hands and upper extremity muscles have been greatly damaged by disease, the lower extremities may be unimpaired, although examination may disclose fasciculations and brisk reflexes. Conversely, spastic paraparesis may occur. Unilateral involvement may be present for a long time, sometimes masquerading as a localized lesion. In such cases, however, careful examination for fasciculations throughout the body, using reflected light and muscle percussion, commonly discloses multifocal twitching. Sometimes the first evidence of ALS is in the lower extremity, manifested by footdrop and mimicking a mononeuropathy of the peroneal nerve for some time. The time of onset and rate of progression of bulbar palsy are variable; the first signs usually include fasciculations and atrophy of the tongue. The patient complains of dysphagia, and dysphonia and dysarthria appear. Significant sensory findings do not occur; if present, they are caused by some complicating process such as metabolic disease, entrapment neuropathy, radiculopathy, or spondylosis. Sphincter involvement does not usually occur except in the later stages of the illness.

Differential diagnosis. The neurologic examination usually is adequate to establish the differential diagnosis. Nevertheless, some conditions may mimic ALS. Foremost among these disorders are spinal cord disease such as cervical spondylosis with myelopathy and radiculopathy. Tumors of the spinocranial junction, especially foramen magnum meningiomas, may be missed if this region is not carefully examined by MRI or CT myelography. Demyelinating disease must be considered when the patient is young and complains of such symptoms as a useless hand. Syringomyelia may be considered when there are atrophy in the arms and spasticity in the legs, but prominent and characteristic sensory signs establish the diagnosis of syringomyelia.

Laboratory findings. No specific laboratory abnormality occurs in ALS. Creatine phosphokinase may be elevated to twice its normal values. Circulating immune complexes may be found, but the antigen has not been identified. The CSF may show a mild elevation of total protein with a normal intra-blood brain barrier IgG synthesis and a normal cell count. The MRI or CT myelography may be normal or may show a shrunken spinal cord. Both CT scanning and MRI of the brain are normal or show cerebral atrophy. The electromyogram may show remarkable abnormalities and is useful in confirming a diffuse process in patients who have monoparetic or unilateral forms of disease; it typically shows widespread fibrillations associated with giant polyphasic potentials and fasciculations. Motor and sensory nerve conduction velocities are typically normal. A muscle biopsy usually shows the abnormalities and changes of denervation.

Course. The course of ALS is usually unremittingly progressive. Patients survive for 3 to 5 years or less, although the survival rate may range from 1 to 10 years. Variations in the initial symptoms and in the course of ALS occur, and since the prognosis depends to a large extent on the degree of the involvement of the bulbar musculature, the early development of bulbar paralysis is associated with a shorter course compared to that found with its late onset. One familial variant of ALS is characterized by an illness of long duration.

Management. No specific treatment for ALS is known. Immunosuppressive therapy is not useful. Patients should maintain their mobility, and their morale may be helped by an active hydrotherapy exercise program. When spasticity and clonus are painful or cause gait difficulty, either diazepam (5 mg three times a day) or baclofen (5 mg three times a day, increasing to its optimal effect, usually 15 to 25 mg three times a day) may be used. Drug therapy may help to reduce secretions in bulbar paresis, and a cricopharyngeal myotomy may alleviate dysphagia.

PROGRESSIVE SPINAL MUSCULAR ATROPHIES

Werdnig-Hoffman disease (infantile muscular atrophy) and Fazio-Londe atrophy. Werdnig-Hoffmann disease (infantile muscular atrophy) is an anterior horn cell disease of infancy that runs a rapid course; it begins in the first year of life with death resulting in several months to years. Sometimes the clinical picture is more slowly progressive. The disorder is autosomal recessive. The infant's mother may have noted diminished fetal movements in the last trimester. At birth the child is limp and flaccid and cries feebly. The child's reflexes are unobtainable, and feeding is difficult because of the child's weakness. Tongue fasciculations may be found. Eye movements are intact, giving the child an alert appearance despite the widespread weakness. The laboratory and pathologic findings resemble those found in ALS.

A progressive bulbar palsy of childhood is known as Fazio-Londe atrophy. There is no known treatment for this disorder nor for Werdnig-Hoffmann disease.

Kugelberg-Welander disease (juvenile progressive spinal muscular atrophy). Kugelberg-Welander disease, or juvenile progressive spinal muscular atrophy, is an anterior horn cell disease of childhood or adolescence. It is slowly progressive and, although usually beginning in the first or second decade of life, may not be diagnosed until the patient is 30 years of age or older. The disorder has been recognized more frequently in recent years. Some of these cases may represent infantile

muscular atrophy with a long survival. A male preponderance is noted in the juvenile group. Weakness begins in the lower extremities, with the hip flexors affected first. Patients may have atrophy at this stage or only much later. The proximal weakness may lead to difficulty in rising from a low chair or walking up stairs. When the disease is established in the lower extremities, the patient may also have proximal upper extremity weakness, and there may be some bulbar involvement. The distribution of the weakness may easily lead the physician to diagnose myopathy or dystrophy, especially facioscapulohumeral and limb-girdle muscular dystrophy. Most patients have fasciculations. Electromyography and a muscle biopsy also support the diagnosis of a neuropathic process and exclude primary muscle disease. Muscle enzymes are sometimes elevated.

Other chronic spinal muscular atrophies. A variety of other chronic spinal muscular atrophies of adult onset occur either sporadically or with varied patterns of inheritance and different distributions of muscle wasting and weakness. Those with proximal involvement, such as facioscapulohumeral and scapulohumeral muscular atrophy, may be confused with muscular dystrophy. Scapuloperoneal spinal muscular atrophy involves the face, neck, and shoulder girdle, as well as footdrop. A neuronal rather than a neuropathic form of Charcot-Marie-Tooth disease can be categorized with the spinal muscular atrophies. Unlike other forms of Charcot-Marie-Tooth disease, the nerve conduction velocity is normal to borderline, and hypertrophic neuropathy is not found on sural nerve biopsy.

SYNDROMES OF PROGRESSIVE HEREDITARY ATAXIA

The progressive hereditary ataxias constitute a significant proportion of the chronic disorders seen by neurologists. A scientifically based classification is not possible at this time because the cause of these disorders is not known in most instances. The clinical symptoms are diverse, and the pathologic findings can vary from a discrete degeneration of one neuronal system and tract to multifocal and multisystem degeneration. Eponyms are still used to describe a few of these disorders in spite of some clinical and pathologic heterogeneity. Although the site of disease in the hereditary ataxias is basically the cerebellum and its pathways, classifications often include disorders that involve other neural systems because they can be found in the same kinships. The various syndromes demonstrate clinical or pathologic evidence of involvement of the following systems: spinocerebellar tracts, cerebellum, retinal ganglion cells or optic nerve, basal ganglia, midbrain, pons, olives, cochlea, dorsal columns, cortiospinal tracts, ventral horn cells, and peripheral nerves. The cerebral hemispheres, especially the cortical neurons, are involved in some instances. There is often an array of associated musculoskeletal abnormalities, including kyphoscoliosis and pes cavus, and cardiac lesions, including myocarditis and cardiac rhythm disturbances. Epilepsy, mental retardation, and dementia may occur. Endocrine abnormalities are seen in some cases. The following are the better known syndromes.

FRIEDREICH'S ATAXIA. Friedreich's ataxia is the best characterized of all the hereditary ataxias, with degeneration involving posterior and lateral columns of the spinal cord and the cerebellum. The common form of inheritance is autosomal recessive, and the symptoms begin soon after the first decade. Another atypical pattern, in which the pattern of inheritance is dominant, has been described with the onset at about 20 years of age. Cases of Roussy-Lévy syndrome and Charcot-

Marie-Tooth disease have been reported in families with Friedreich's ataxia.

Pathology. The conspicuous pathologic conditions are in the spinal cord, which is visibly shrunken. The fiber loss in the fasciculus gracilis is complete, and the fasciculus cuneatus is affected less intensely. The pyramidal tracts show progressive attentuation as they descend caudally in the spinal cord. Degeneration is constant in the posterior spinocerebellar tracts and common in the anterior spinocerebellar tracts. The cerebellar cortex is normal or shows some loss of Purkinje cells, but the white matter is gliotic and the dentate nuclei show severe cell loss. The vestibular nuclei are also shrunken and gliotic. Nerve fiber loss may be noted in the optic tract and when severe is accompanied by corresponding abnormalities in the lateral geniculate body. The cerebral cortex is usually normal. Myocardial muscle may sow degeneration and replacement by macrophages and fibroblasts.

Clinical manifestations. Ataxia of the lower extremities is almost always the first symptom; the trunk and upper extremities are affected later. Antecedent injury and infection may sometimes be noted. The incoordination that occurs is caused by lesions in both the cerebellum and its pathways. Lesions in the posterior columns result in a Romberg's sign with a profound loss of position and vibratory senses. Later there may be some impairment of spinothalamic sensory modalities. The hands usually become clumsy after the gait disturbance is well developed. Dysarthric speech usually follows the development of appendicular and truncal ataxia. Sometimes the patient has prominent head titubation and side-to-side movements, called choreiform by some, which are probably caused by combined sensory and motor disturbances. The mentation is usually normal. Muscle atrophy is uncommon unless there is associated neuropathy of the peroneal muscular atrophy type. The stretch reflexes are lost early, but flexor spasms and extensor plantar responses occur as manifestations of corticospinal (pyramidal) tract involvement. The superficial abdominal reflexes usually are maintained. Ocular abnormalities are found when the disease is established. Horizontal, rotary, vertical, and periodic alternating nystagmus may occur. Optic atrophy, pigmentary degeneration of the retina, and extraocular nerve palsies may develop. A syndrome of progressive external ophthalmoplegia has been described with Friedreich's ataxia. Deglutition may be impaired later in the disease. Cardiac rhythm disturbances and respiratory disease are important causes of morbidity and mortality.

Laboratory findings. The diagnosis is apparent from the characteristic clinical picture. No laboratory abnormality is diagnostic. A disturbance of pyruvate metabolism occurs, but it is not known how this may be related to the nervous manifestations. Overt diabetes or chemical diabetes mellitus may be found. Electrocardiograms may be abnormal; echocardiography may demonstrate evidence of asymmetric septal hypertrophy. Sensory action potentials are absent or markedly reduced in amplitude at an early stage of the disease. In contrast, motor nerve conduction velocities remain normal or decrease only slightly with disease progression. The prominent alteration of sensory action potentials reflects involvement of large myelinated nerve fibers and neurons in dorsal root ganglia.

Differential diagnosis. In the differential diagnosis various other hereditary and sporadic disorders may be considered, including congenital spastic paraplegia, muscular dystrophies, tabes dorsalis, multiple sclerosis, and the olivopontocerebellar degenerations. Bassen-Kornzweig syndrome (abetalipoproteinemia), a familial disorder with posterior and lateral column degeneration, pes cavus, and cardiac abnormalities, may mimic Friedreich's ataxia but is associated with abnormalities in the peripheral blood smear (acanthocytosis) and in blood lipids.

Management. No specific treatment for Friedreich's ataxia exists. An exercise program, especially hydrotherapy, is important. Orthopedic correction of the symptomatic skeletal disorders should be carried out. Infection, arrhythmia, heart failure, and diabetes are treated in the usual way. Acetazolamide, physostigmine, and ketogenic diets are undergoing evaluation for treatment of the ataxic components of this disease, but the benefits appear questionable or short lived.

ROUSSY-LÉVY SYNDROME. Roussy-Lévy syndrome is an autosomal dominant disorder that usually begins in childhood, but there are instances in which the disorder begins later in life. Features of this neuropathy include skeletal disorders such as clubfoot and kyphoscoliosis, wasting of the muscles of the lower extremity and the small hand muscles, generalized areflexia, unsteady gait, and tremor of the hands resembling intention tremor. Other cerebellar signs are absent. Cataracts and deafness may occur. Sensory disturbance is generally absent, although in some instances posterior column modalities are greatly impaired, thus linking this disorder with the spinocerebellar ataxias. Roussy-Lévy syndrome has been viewed by some as intermediate between Friedreich's ataxia and Charcot-Marie-Tooth disease (see Chapter 192). Demyelination and onion bulb formation (layering secondary to proliferation of Schwann cells and fibroblasts) are seen pathologically. Nerve conduction velocities are prolonged. The disease runs a slowly progressive course.

REFSUM'S DISEASE. Refsum's disease is a rare disorder with an autosomal recessive pattern of inheritance, which may resemble Charcot-Marie-Tooth disease (see Chapter 192). The cardinal disturbances are retinitis pigmentosa with night blindness, chronic sensorimotor polyneuropathy, and cerebellar ataxia. In most instances deafness and cardiomyopathy occur. Other reported occurrences include pupillary abnormalities, cataracts, anosmia, skeletal abnormalities, ichthyosis, and palpably enlarged nerves. The age of onset varies from early childhood to the second and third decades of life. The disorder is slowly progressive, and in some instances striking exacerbations and then remissions without obvious cause have occurred. Sometimes the deficits are static. Findings of laboratory studies are normal, but the serum phytanic acid level is markedly elevated. The CSF protein concentration may be significantly elevated. Pathologically, peripheral nerves are hypertrophied and onion bulb formation is seen. Loss of myelin and some axonal loss are demonstrable. Administered early in the course of the disease, vitamin A may reverse or delay some of the retinal manifestations of this disease. Similarly, dietary exclusion of phytol and phytanic acid may be beneficial, but information is not adequate at this time.

BASSEN-KORNZWEIG SYNDROME (ABETALIPOPROTEINEMIA). Bassen-Kornzweig syndrome (abetalipoproteinemia) is a rare autosomal recessive disorder characterized by the triad of malabsorption, acanthocytosis, and neurologic abnormalities. Patients are unable to synthesize an apolipoprotein required for the formation and transport of very low–density and low-density lipoproteins and chylomicrons. Malabsorption results in bulky, foul-smelling stools, and a small intestine biopsy shows prominent vacuolation of epithelial cells. With appropriate stains these vacuoles can be shown to contain fat. Malabsorption of fat-soluble vitamins leads to deficiencies of vitamins A and E. Acanthocytes are present in all patients with this syndrome. They are thought to result from abnormal lipid being incorporated into the red cell membrane. Neurologic abnormalities are manifest usually in the first decade of life. Psychomotor retardation with weakness and areflexia may be noted. Later, dysarthria, ataxic gait, intention tremor, and posterior column signs become apparent. Retinal abnormalities occur in all patients with visual disturbances, usually beginning in adolescence. The retinal abnormalities may stabilize or return to normal with administration of parenteral vitamin A in large doses. Musculoskeletal abnormalities include equinovarus foot deformity and scoliosis. Myocardial fibrosis with heart failure and rhythm disturbances have been observed. Pathologic studies may demonstrate demyelination in the posterior columns and the spinocerebellar tracts, loss of neurons in the cerebellum and spinal cord, and demyelination of some peripheral nerves. No therapy is available at this time, but parenteral vitamin supplements may delay the deterioration of visual function.

OTHER HEREDITARY ATAXIAS. Soon after Friedreich's studies of hereditary ataxia, a number of reports appeared describing individuals and families with features of Friedrich's ataxia but with more extensive pathologic changes in the cerebellar cortex, inferior olivary nuclei, brainstem, and in some cases the basal ganglia and cerebral cortex. These patients with olivopontocerebellar atrophy have a predominance of spasticity and hyperreflexia over sensory findings in the lower extremities.

Another type of predominantly spinal ataxia, which occurs with spasticity in contrast to Friedreich's ataxia, is Sanger Brown spinal ataxia. Menzel described a patient with many of the pathologic features typical of Friedreich's ataxia but also with conspicuous atrophy involving mainly the middle cerebellar peduncle, the pontine nuclei, and the olivary nuclei. A sporadically occurring disorder was described by Dejerine and Andre-Thomas, differing from the Menzel form pathologically in that the spinal cord was spared. Late cortical cerebellar atrophy was described by Marie, Foix, and Alajounine. The Ramsay Hunt syndrome, in which dentatorubral atrophy occurs, is characterized clinically by myoclonus and cerebellar ataxia. Many of these syndromes may be accompanied by manifestations of disease above the brainstem, including mental retardation, dementia, seizures, movement disorders, optic atrophy, and pigmentary retinal degeneration. The diagnosis of these disorders is based on the clinical features, and no consistent diagnostic test is available, although visual and brainstem evoked potentials, electromyography, and MRI may be helpful.

SYRINGOMYELIA

Syringomyelia (from *syrinx,* meaning tube) refers to a tubular dilation of the spinal cord extending over many segments. Syringobulbia sometimes occurs in association with syringomyelia and refers to a cavitation extending above the foramen magnum but usually not extending above the medulla. This disease has a serious morbidity, its cause is still in dispute, and a consensus does not exist on management.

PATHOPHYSIOLOGY. Syringomyelia may be divided into the following categories:

1. *A form communicating with the fourth ventricle.* This is seen most commonly in association with developmental abnormalities of the craniospinal junction such as Arnold-Chiari malformation. It may occur with acquired disease such as arachnoiditis, tumors, and cysts. It has been suggested that syringomyelia develops as a result of blockage of the outlet of the fourth ventricle, combined with gradual downward pulsations of CSF into the central canal.
2. *An accompaniment of spinal cord tumors, especially those that*

are intramedullary in location, such as ependymoma and hemangioblastoma. Some studies report intramedullary tumors in 25% of all cases of syringomyelia. Cavitation also may occur in association with an extramedullary tumor.
3. *As a sequel to spinal cord trauma, including traumatic paraplegia and quadriplegia.* The injury is usually serious, but it has been reported to follow minor trauma.
4. *Not associated with any of these circumstances.*

PATHOLOGY. Externally at surgery or autopsy the spinal cord may appear swollen and tense. The syrinx is most apparent at the cervical region but may extend infrequently to involve the lumbrosacral enlargement. When the lesion is large, it may appear to occupy the entire cross section of the spinal cord, sparing only the peripheral islands of nervous tissue. Typically the gray matter is most damaged. The cavity fluid is commonly a clear, slightly yellowish liquid. If the cavity is lined by ependyma, the term "hydromyelia" may be used.

CLINICAL MANIFESTATIONS. Syringomyelia in its classic form is a progressive disorder of young people, especially those in their second and third decades of life. It is characterized by muscle atrophy, dissociated anesthesia, and paraparesis with neurotrophic changes, including neurogenic arthropathy and kyphoscoliosis. The age of onset varies between 10 and 60 years, but cases have also been seen at the extremes of life. The precise clinical manifestations depend on the location of the cavity. Since the cavity is usually most obvious initially in the cervical enlargement, the initial signs reflect disease there. The disease may be unilateral or monosymptomatic at the outset but usually becomes characteristic with time.

Involvement of the ventral horns of the spinal cord leads to weakness of the hand and the forearm muscles and striking atrophy, scoliosis, and a characteristic loss of lumbrical and interosseous function with resulting clawhand and main en griffe deformities. Deep reflexes in the upper extremity are lost early in the course of the disease. Interruption of the spinothalamic fibers (which decussate just anterior to the central canal) before cavitation extends into the dorsal columns induces dissociated anesthesia, with impairment of temperature and pain sensations but retention of light touch and proprioceptive sensibilities. Spastic paraparesis results from the lateral extension of the cavitation to affect the corticospinal tracts. The paraparesis starts asymmetrically but ultimately becomes symmetric with the development of clonus, extensor plantar responses, and a loss of superficial abdominal reflexes. Spinchter involvement is late. Cavitation at the first dorsal (thoracic) segment leads to ipsilateral Horner's syndrome. Extension of the disease into the medulla leads to weakness and wasting of the tongue, dissociated fifth nerve sensory loss, palatal weakness, and nystagmus. Pain in the neck and shoulder occurs, mimicking radicular pain. In advanced cases the disease is recognizable, but in the early stages it must be differentiated from other disorders such as intramedullary cord tumors and the central cord syndrome that may result from trauma and hematomyelia. If the onset is asymmetric with sensory complaints, root compression must be excluded. Demyelinating disease, tumors of the spinocranial junction, and arachnoid cysts may be considered in some instances. Muscle wasting and fasciculations require that motor neuron disease be considered.

LABORATORY FINDINGS. The confirmation of the diagnosis of syringomyelia requires roentgenographic studies. Myelography demonstrates an enlargement of the spinal cord and narrowing of the subarachnoid space. Air myelography accurately demonstrates the diameter of the spinal cord and may identify tonsillar herniation if present. By manipulation of the air and fluid at myelography, changes in the collapsibility of a syrinx may be demonstrated and thus the syrinx can be differentiated from a tumor. CT scanning of the spinal canal combined with a contrast study of the subarachnoid space also permits a good visualization of syrinx anatomy, but MRI may be all that is necessary.

MANAGEMENT. The optimal treatment for syringomyelia has not been established. A number of procedures have been advocated. These include posterior fossa decompression with or without plugging of the obex, myelotomy, and sectioning the filum terminale. A shunt also may be placed between the cavity and the spinal subarachnoid space. The variety of procedures suggests that none is optimal for every patient, and repeat surgery may be necessary.

COMBINED SYSTEM DISEASE (VITAMIN B₁₂ DEFICIENCY)

(See also Chapter 61.)

Combined system disease primarily affects the lateral and dorsal columns of the spinal cord and is related to vitamin B_{12} deficiency. Vitamin B_{12} is a nonsynthetic coenzyme that is derived from foodstuffs, the best sources being liver, kidney, meat, and milk. Plants contain no vitamin B_{12}. In the United States the average daily diet contains 15 to 39 μg of vitamin B_{12} of which perhaps 5 μg is absorbed in the ileum with the aid of intrinsic factor, a glycoprotein from gastric secretions. The most important cause of vitamin B_{12} deficiency in humans is pernicious anemia, a presumed autoimmune disease associated with atrophic gastritis and the absence of intrinsic factor necessary for vitamin B_{12} absorption. Inadequate dietary intake and malabsorption syndromes also rarely may lead to neurologic involvement.

PATHOLOGY. The pathologic condition is confined to the white matter of the spinal cord and occasionally involves the cerebrum and optic nerve. Disturbances in L-Methylmalonyl coenzyme A may lead to abnormalities of myelin. The earliest lesion is a separation of the myelin lamellae and the formation of intramyelin vacuoles, leading eventually to complete destruction of myelin. As in wallerian degeneration, numerous lipophages appear and come to lie within the perivascular spaces of blood vessels. Axonal degeneration occurs later. The result is a severe depletion of myelin and damage to axons. These changes give the tissue a spongy, vacuolated appearance. Marked gliosis ensues with time. The lesions, which are spotty initially and later become confluent, begin in the posterior columns and move forward into the lateral columns. Scattered lesions, however, are seen in the other tracts of the spinal cord, including the spinothalamic tracts. Lesions are sometimes found in the optic nerve and cerebral white matter.

CLINICAL MANIFESTATIONS. Parathesias of all four extremities are usually the first manifestation. The lower extremities are sometimes the first to show symptoms. Motor manifestations, predominantly increased fatigue, weakness, and stiffness, then occur in the lower extremities. The motor signs, combined with the prominent defect in postural sensation resulting from dorsal column disease, lead to a unsteadiness of gait and falling episodes. Behavior change and intellectual alterations may be prominent. Rarely, visual impairment with centrocecal scotomas and later optic atrophy may occur, apparently sometimes in isolation, as a manifestation of vitamin B_{12} deficiency. The clinical findings demonstrate a loss of vibration and position senses. The muscle tone of the lower extremities is increased, with extensor plantar responses and clonus. If treatment has been delayed, spastic paraplegia may be noted. In most instances the stretch reflexes are exaggerated,

but occasionally they are diminished or absent, returning with treatment. Distal impairment of pain, light tough, and temperature may be found, suggesting a peripheral neuropathic process. In infants born to vegetarian mothers, florid encephalopathy, anemia, hyperpigmentation, and methylmalonic aciduria may develop in the first year of life.

LABORATORY FINDINGS. The neurologic picture may mimic other metabolic, inflammatory, and degenerative diseases of the spinal cord. The hematologic picture may be normal. A consistent finding is methylmalonic aciduria. The serum vitamin B_{12} level is reduced. The Schilling test establishes the diagnosis of intrinsic factor deficit; since it involves a flushing dose of vitamin B_{12}, treatment begins at the time of the test. The disease should be considered for an infant who was born to a vegetarian mother and has an obscure and unexplained encephalopathy. Visual evoked responses may be abnormal in amplitude and velocity in patients without obvious damage to the optic system.

MANAGEMENT. Treatment involves administering one of the various preparations of vitamin B_{12} intramuscularly and continuing for life, usually monthly (see Chapter 61). Generally all the manifestations respond, but the extent of the response depends on the duration of symptoms. Patients who have had gait disturbance for less than 6 months show the best response. Improvement may continue for months and sometimes years.

NEUROCUTANEOUS SYNDROMES

The neurocutaneous syndromes, or phakomatoses, are congenital conditions, usually dominantly inherited and characterized by various cutaneous, ocular, neurologic, and mesenthymal abnormalities. The term "phakomatoses" is descriptive and has no causal or pathogenetic basis. The syndromes are remarkable for the wide spectrum of individual variation in clinical expression among members of the same affected family; for example, neurofibromatosis may be represented by a few café au lait spots in one family member and by generalized neurofibromatosis with cutaneous, neuroectodermal, and mesenchymal abnormalities in another.

Neurofibromatosis (von Ricklinghausen's disease)

Neurofibromatosis is the most common of the phakomatoses. The disorder has autosomal dominant transmission with variable penetrance. The cutaneous hallmark of this disease is café au lait spots; these are brownish, pigmented macules that may be found on any part of the skin surface. Some suggest that any person with more than six café au lait spots, each greater than 1 cm in broadest diameter, may be presumed to have the disease. Freckles in the axillae are particularly significant. Cutaneous and subcutaneous hard and soft fibromas and lipomas also occur. A variety of associated abnormalities are involved, including bony abnormalities such as spinal fusion defects, posterior orbital roof defects, basilar impression (see Chapter 186), syringomyelia, and pheochromocytoma. Schwannomas and neurofibromas are common. Parenchymal brain tumors occur, of which astrocytoma is the most common. There is a high incidence of optic nerve glioma, acoustic neuroma (which may be bilateral), and meningiomas (which may be multiple). The clinical abnormalities reflect these diverse lesions. Mental retardation occurs in 10% of patients, and seizures occur with the same frequency. Optic nerve glioma may lead to papilledema, visual field disturbance, proptosis, optic atrophy, and blindness. Tumors of the eighth cranial nerve are manifested by mild vestibular symtpoms and progressive hearing loss. Brainstem and cerebellar symptoms and signs may result, as well as obstructive hydrocephalus. Tumors of other cranial nerves are less common.

Neurofibromas may involve the entire extent of multiple roots and peripheral nerves, causing pain, disfigurement, paresis, and sometimes spinal cord compression. The diagnosis is suggested by the skin lesions. Every patient with such lesions and neurologic symptoms should be screened for intracranial mass lesions. This is now aided by MRI. MRI has superseded all other radiographic procedures to demonstrate tumors of the eighth nerve, brain, or spinal cord in this disorder. The CSF protein concentration is almost always elevated with spinal neurofibroma and with acoustic tumors.

Von Hippel-Lindau disease

Von Hippel-Lindau disease is an autosomal dominant disorder, but the expression of the disease varies reatly between and among families. The range of onset of ocular and neurologic signs extends from the first to the fifth decade of life. The syndrome includes retinal, neurovascular, and visceral components. The first manifestations are usually referable to retinal hemangiomas, which are sometimes multiple and are bilateral in one third of these cases. Examination of the fundus reveals dilated, tortuous arteries entering the lesion and enlarged draining veins. Bleeding from the lesion may lead to retinal detachment, glaucoma, cataract, uveitis, and blindness. Enucleation is sometimes necessary because of pain. Photocoagulation is useful in controlling the vascular lesion. Cerebellar hemangioblastoma occurs in 10% to 20% of the affected patients and may appear in the absence of retinal lesions. The first symptom of this tumor is often headache, followed by manifestations of obstructive hydrocephalus (vomiting and papilledema) and cerebellar symptoms, usually gait and speech disturbance. These tumors are readily operable. They are usually benign but may recur and may be multiple. Abnormalities associated with cerebellar hemangioblastoma include syringomyelia, hemangioma of the brainstem, spinal cord angioblastic tumors, polycythemia, and pheochromocytoma. The visceral manifestations of von Hippel-Lindau disease include angiomas and cysts of various organs. A serious associated lesion is renal cell carcinoma, which may be bilateral.

Ataxia-telangiectasia

Ataxia-telangiectasia is a relatively rare autosomal recessive disorder, the cardinal manifestations of which are progressive cerebellar ataxia, oculocutaneous telangiectasia with oculomotor apraxia, a tendency to frequent sinopulmonary infection, lymphoreticular malignancy, and other malignancies. The ataxia begins early, but the bulbar telangiectases are not evident until the third to eighth years of life; they first appear on the bulbar conjunctivae as horizontal symmetric streaks and give the eyeball a blood shot appearance; later they may spread to include the eyelid, face, and neck. Unlike Sturge-Weber syndrome and other neurocutaneous syndromes, the talengiectases do not involve the CNS. The finding of choreoathetosis may be so striking that it overshadows the cerebellar disturbance. Patients surviving until adolescence may develop features of spinocerebellar disease and clinical and electromyographic features of peripheral neuropathy. With time, intellectual impairment occurs in more than one third of patients. Endocrine disorders, especially female hypogonadism, and signs of premature aging of skin and graying of hair are found. Immunologic disturbance is prominent, manifested by frequent infection, especially sinopulmonary infection, a profound deficiency or absence of IgA and sometimes IgE, thymic hypoplasia or aplasia, and depressed cellular and humoral im-

munity. Lymphopenia is found in 30% of patients. The incidence of all types of tumors, especially lymphoid tumors, is at least 10%; there is also an increased incidence of all tumor types in relatives. The α-fetoprotein serum concentration is elevated and serves as a marker for this disease. The increased levels of this protein may reflect a defect of hepatic maturation.

Two remarkable features of ataxia-telangiectasia are exquisite radiosensitivity and a tendency toward violent transfusion reactions (related to infusion of IgA, to which the patient can make antibodies). Chromosome anomalies may be one factor predisposing the patient to oncogenesis. The most striking pathologic findings are in the cerebellum, where there is almost selective cortical cerebellar degeneration, especially affecting Purkinje cells and to a lesser extent granular cells and basket cells. Neuronal degeneration is also common in the vermis and in the dentate and olivary nuclei. Demyelination with variable axonal loss is common in the dorsal columns. Minor changes, including gliosis and gliovascular malformations, may be found in the cerebral hemispheres.

Sturge-Weber syndrome

The hallmark of Sturge-Weber syndrome is a unilateral facial nevus that predominantly involves the upper face, especially the upper eyelid, and is associated with a thin-walled vascular nevus on the surface of the ipsilateral cerebral cortex. The nevus is flat or only slightly elevated, unlike the common cutaneous, cavernous strawberry hemangioma. Involvement of the face by the nevus in the absence of involvement of the upper eyelid may be confidently used to exclude a diagnosis of Sturge-Weber syndrome. Other features of this disorder include buphthalmos, epilepsy, hemiparesis, hemianopsia, and progressive intellectual disturbance. The diagnosis of Sturge-Weber syndrome should be suspected in all children with the typical facial nevus and neurologic symptoms, especially focal motor seizures and hemiparesis. Skull roentgenograms may show "tram-track" calcification in the cerebral cortex. Calcification is rarely demonstrated on roentgenograms before patients are 2 years of age but is apparent earlier with CT scanning. Histologic examination shows excessive vascularization of the pia, usually in the parietal and occipital regions. Gliosis and calcium concretions are found in the underlying cortex. Management should involve early commencement of anticonvulsant therapy because intellectural decline seems to result partly from intractable seizures. Consideration should be given to early ablative surgery (for example, lobectomy) to control intractable seizures and halt intellectual decline.

Tuberous sclerosis (Bourneville's disease)

Seizures and mental retardation are the most common neurologic manifestations of tuberous sclerosis (Bourneville's disease). The earliest cutaneous lesions are multiple, dull white depigmented macules, leaf shaped and increasing in size with age. Ultraviolet light helps in recognizing them in fair-skinned persons. The other common skin manifestations are adenoma sebaceum, a nodular facial eruption resembling acne but without pustules; shagreen patches, which are indurated excrescences usually over the sacrum; and café au lait spots. Seizures and mental retardation become apparent in the first decade of life. The seizures may precede the characteristic skin lesions by many years. A funduscopic examination may disclose nodules that histologically are formed from retinal ganglion cells, fibroblasts, and glial cells. Nodules also occur in the parenchyma of the brain or on the surface; they may also line the surface of the ventricles to create the "candle guttering" commonly mentioned in descriptions of this disease. Other tumors, including vascular malformations, meningiomas, gliomas, and hamartomas, are also recognized.

Incontinentia pigmenti (Bloch-Sulzberger syndrome)

Incontinentia pigmenti, or Bloch-Sulzberger syndrome, an uncommon disorder in which epilepsy and mental and motor retardation are prominent, is occasionally familial. The majority of reported cases have been in females, and it has been suggested that the condition in males is fatal in utero. In the early days of life widespread erythematous and bullous lesions appear, becoming crusted and indurated; this is followed by persistent secondary pigmentation with linear streaks over the trunk, arms, and legs. These disappear by the end of the second decade of life. Eye lesions, suggesting dysplasia or glioma, may occur and may be mistaken for retrolental hyperplasia. Local application of steroids is helpful in treating the skin lesions.

BIBLIOGRAPHY

Adams RD and Victor M: Principles of neurology, ed 4, New York, 1989, McGraw-Hill Inc.

Callen JP and Meckler RJ, editors: Neurocutaneous disorders, vol 5, Philadelphia, 1987, Neurologic Clinics, WB Saunders Co.

Hallpike JF, Adams CWM, and Tourtellotte WW, editors: Multiple sclerosis: pathology, diagnosis and management, London, 1983, Chapman & Hall.

Jacob E and Herbert V: Vitamin B$_{12}$ and the nervous system. In Kumar S, editor: Biochemistry of brain, New York, 1980, Pergamon Press Inc.

Koetsier JC: Demyelinating disease. In Vinken PJ, Brwyn GW, and Klawans HL, editors: Revised series 3, Amsterdam, 1985, Elsevier Science Publishers.

Logue V and Edwards MR: Syringomyelia and its surgical treatment—an analysis of 75 cases, J Neurol Neurosurg Psychiatry 44:273, 1981.

Rubinstein LJ et al: Disseminated necrotizing leukoencephalopathy: a complication of treated nervous system leukemia and lymphoma, Cancer 35:291, 1975.

149·ABNORMALITIES OF THE CRANIOVERTEBRAL JUNCTION

Paul L. Schraeder

Disorders of the craniovertebral junction, including platybasia, basilar impression, basilar invagination, Arnold-Chiari malformations, and Klippel-Feil syndrome, occur in varying degrees of severity. They may be clinically asymptomatic but can have associated signs and symptoms that range from subtle to severe as a result of the involvement of the brainstem, cerebellum, cranial nerves, spinal cord, or nerve roots. Although each can occur singly, various combinations of these abnormalities are often found in the same patient.

PLATYBASIA AND BASILAR IMPRESSION

Platybasia is a flattening of the base of the skull in which, on a lateral skull roentgenogram, the angle created by lines connecting the nasion, tuberculum sellae, and the anterior margin of the foramen magnum is greater than 143 degrees. The term is often incorrectly used synonymously with basilar impression, since these anomalies commonly coexist. In basilar impression one half or more of the odontoid process of the axis protrudes above Chamberlain's line (a line drawn from the back of the hard palate to the posterior margin of the foramen magnum). These deformities are usually congenital and can be associated with varying degrees of atlantooccipital assimilation, Klippel-Feil syndrome, and Arnold-Chiari mal-

formations. Basilar invagination, also defined by Chamberlain's line, consists of an upward herniation of the margin of the foramen magnum and is acquired in diseases in which the bones of the skull are softened, such as rickets, osteomalacia, Paget's disease, and osteogenesis imperfecta.

The clinical findings are variable and more likely to be associated with the congenital anomalies. Often the patient has only a short neck with limited motion. In more severe cases abnormalities of the lower cranial nerves, cerebellum, and motor and sensory long tracts are found. A syrinx of the cervical spinal cord and medulla or an Arnold-Chiari malformation may be present. The importance of considering craniovertebral junction anomalies in the differential diagnosis of multiple sclerosis and foramen magnum tumors cannot be overemphasized, since the diagnosis can usually be based on a technically adequate plain skull roentgenogram. The degree of CNS structural involvement can be documented by magnetic resonance imaging (MRI). Surgical decompression is indicated if symptoms are progressive.

ARNOLD-CHIARI MALFORMATIONS

Arnold-Chiari malformations include several congenital hindbrain anomalies, the most important of which are the displacement of the cerebellum and an elongated medulla through the foramen magnum into the cervical spinal canal (type 2) and the displacement of the cerebellar tonsils into the cervical canal (type 1). Basilar impression is often present. Hydrocephalus, aqueductal stenosis, and anomalies of the cerebral hemispheres, such as the absence of the septum pellucidum and heterotopias, may occur.

The patient with the type 2, or infantile, form usually has communicating hydrocephalus early in life; the downward displacement of posterior fossa structures probably interferes with cerebrospinal fluid (CSF) flow. It is most commonly associated with a spinal midline defect such as spina bifida, meningocele, or myelomeningocele in the lumbosacral region. Myelomeningocele is a saccular, soft mass covered with friable skin, weaping CSF, and containing elements of the spinal cord and cauda equina. The patient usually is paraplegic and subject to recurrent bacterial meningitis originating from the lumbosacral defect. The treatment involves shunting procedures for the hydrocephalus and repair of the myelomeningocele. However, the latter procedure is performed only to prevent infection because the paraplegia almost invariably persists after surgery. Diagnosis of this disorder in utero is possible via ultrasound, roentgenograms of the fetus, and amniocentesis to determine whether the α-fetoprotein concentration is increased.

The type 1, or adult, form is often asymptomatic until adulthood. The symptoms and signs include varying degrees of dysfunction of the cerebellum, motor and sensory long tracts, and cranial nerves. If present, a particularly helpful sign of medullary dysfunction is downbeat nystagmus (a nystagmus in the primary position of gaze, with the fast phase beating downward). Syringomyelia of the cervical cord and medulla is often present, as are associated bony abnormalities such as fusion of cervical vertebrae. Hydrocephalus is less common than in type 2. Foramen magnum tumors must be considered in the differential diagnosis. The diagnosis depends on a high index of suspicion. The common finding of basilar impression on the plain skull roentgenogram and the characteristic findings of a herniated cerebellum and brainstem on cervical myelography confirm the diagnosis. MRI of this abnormality provides an excellent view. Treatment in the form of decompression by an upper cervical laminectomy and by a suboccipital craniectomy may be helpful for patients with progressive symptoms.

KLIPPEL-FEIL SYNDROME

In Klippel-Feil syndrome an asymptomatic congenital fusion of two or more cervical vertebrae is not uncommon. In the more extreme situation a congenital fusion of the second to sixth cervical vertebrae in association with a narrow spinal canal may be found. The patient has a short, squat neck, with the head appearing to rest on the shoulders and significant limitation of movement of the head and neck. This deformity is commonly associated with basilar impression, Arnold-Chiari malformations, and an undescended scapula (Sprengel's deformity). Evidence of spinal cord compression (that is, hyperreflexia, an extensor plantar response, and loss of position and vibration senses) is an indication for obtaining MRI or myelogram and performing cervical cord decompression.

BIBLIOGRAPHY

Adams JH, Corsellis JAN, and Duchen LW, editors: Greenfield's neuropathology, New York, 1984, John Wiley & Sons Inc.
Adams RD and Victor M: Principles of neurology, ed 2, New York, 1985, McGraw-Hill Inc.
Ramsey RG: Neuroradiology, Philadelphia, 1987, WB Saunders Co.

150 · BASAL GANGLIA DISORDERS AND RELATED CONDITIONS

Roger Duvoisin *and* Arthur S. Walters

PARKINSONISM

DEFINITION. Parkinsonism is a distinctive symptom complex comprised of tremor, muscular rigidity, bradykinesia, and characteristic alterations of posture and attitudes of the limbs. The tremor is usually a resting tremor, that is, most marked when the affected part is at rest. Muscular rigidity refers to a hypertonicity of the musculature that can be noticed during passive manipulation of the limbs, as a uniform resistance to movement. It differs from spasticity, which is more marked in the antigravity muscles (for example, the flexor muscles of the arm and the extensor muscles of the leg), and gives way, often suddenly, in the "clasp-knife" phenomenon during sustained stretching of the muscles. Bradykinesia comprises a slowness of all bodily movement, a loss of automatic motor activity such as eye-blinking and swallowing, a loss of associated movements such as the swing of the arms on walking, hesitation on initiating a motor act, and rapid fatigue during continuing or repetitive motor actions.

ETIOLOGY. The most common cause of parkinsonism encountered today is Parkinson's disease, also referred to as idiopathic parkinsonism or paralysis agitans. Most authorities believe that Parkinson's disease represents a specific morbid entity, although, its cause is not currently known. Iatrogenic parkinsonism closely resembling Parkinson's disease may be induced by various drugs, principally the major tranquilizers or, rarely, methyldopa, α-methyl-para-tyrosine, reserpine, and other agents that interfere with the synthesis or the storage of dopamine or that block the striatal dopamine receptors. Drug-induced chemical parkinsonism is always reversible, usually within 1 or 2 weeks after the offending agent is discontinued. A form of parkinsonism occurring as a sequela of *encephalitis lethargica* (von Economo's disease), termed "postencephalitic parkinsonism," was common in the years 1920 to 1940 but subsequently declined in incidence and is now rare. Parkin-

sonism may also occur as part of the clinical manifestation of several distinct degenerative disorders of the nervous system such as olivopontocerebellar atrophy, striatonigral degeneration, and progressive supranuclear palsy. Juvenile parkinsonism may on rare occasions represent an unusually early onset of Parkinson's disease but more often represents Wilson's disease.

EPIDEMIOLOGY. Parkinson's disease occurs throughout the world in all racial and ethnic groups. Differences in prevalence in different groups are difficult to assess because of the differences in medical practice. Population surveys have shown a prevalence of about 130:100,000 standard population. Parkinson's disease is uncommon in people under 40 years of age; the mean age at onset is about 60 years and the prevalence increases with age. Approximately 1% of the population older than 60 years of age has Parkinson's disease. Although genetic factors have long been suspected of playing a significant role in causing Parkinson's disease, little evidence exists proving familial concentrations of the disease. Family studies show that only about 2% of the adult siblings of patients with Parkinson's disease also have the disease. Reports of families with multiple cases usually represent another disorder, most commonly olivopontocerebellar atrophy, which can often mimic Parkinson's disease and occurs in both recessive inheritance and dominant inheritance patterns.

PATHOGENESIS. Parkinsonism is currently regarded as a pathophysiologic state reflecting primarily a dysfunction of the brain dopamine neuronal systems. The most consistent pathologic feature found at autopsy is a degeneration of the pigmented neurons of the substantia nigra. These neurons contain a melanin pigment that can be seen during a gross inspection of sections cut through the midbrain of normal human specimens. This pigment is lost in Parkinson's disease because of a neuronal degeneration of the substantia nigra. Any morbid process that produces a degeneration of these neurons is associated with a parkinsonian state.

The substantia nigra projects its axons principally to the striatum (the caudate nucleus and the putamen), which normally contains dopamine. The concentration of dopamine in the striatum is significantly reduced in Parkinson's disease and in experimental animals with lesions of the substantia nigra. The hypothalamus has important dopamine neurons. The degeneration of these neurons in Parkinson's disease may be correlated with autonomic dysfunctions such as seborrhea, excessive sweating, orthostatic hypotension, and anorexia. The dopaminergic neurons of the substantia nigra also extend to the limbic lobe, especially to the medial temporal lobe. The involvement of these neurons may account for behavioral changes typical of the disease. The sympathetic neurons of the spinal cord and the peripheral autonomic ganglia may also degenerate in Parkinson's disease, contributing to the orthostatic hypotension and other autonomic dysfunctions.

The cause of the neuron degeneration of Parkinson's disease is unknown. Because of the high degree of selective involvement of widely dispersed neuron groups, the disorder is classified as a system degeneration, and many physicians believe it may have a metabolic or viral cause. The recent discovery that a meperidine analog 1-methyl-4-phenyl 1,2,3,6-tetrahydropyridine (MPTP) can cause permanent parkinsonism in humans has lead to increased speculation that there is an environmental cause of Parkinson's disease.

CLINICAL MANIFESTATIONS. The most common initial symptoms are a slight weakness and a tendency to tremble, usually appearing in one hand or less often in one foot. Often the patient has some slowness or awkwardness in using the affected limb, a tendency to posture the arm flexed at the elbow, some loss of facial expression, and a deliberate quality of speech even though complaining only of the tremor. The symptoms at first are mild and may persist with little change for 1 to 2 years. However, gradually they become more marked, and similar manifestations appear on the opposite side of the body. Subsequently, the posture becomes less erect and the patient stands gently stooped and walks with a shuffling gait without swinging the arms. With further progression of the disease, all movement becomes slow gradually, walking becomes difficult, and the tremor and rigidity become generalized. The patient may have tremors in the lips, tongue, jaw, and facial muscles, as well as in the limb muscles and axial muscles. In general, the rigidity is most marked in the spinal musculature.

As bradykinesia becomes gradually more severe, all movement is marked by abrupt interruptions. Thus the patient's feet suddenly seem to stick to the floor when walking, and there is inability to move them for a moment. The patient may also suddenly walk with short shuffling steps that become progressively shorter and faster, a phenomenon termed "festination." During festination the patient's trunk may lean farther and farther with each step, and the patient may fall. The patient seems to be pushed forward by an unseen force or to be chasing after his center of gravity. This phenomenon is termed "propulsion." Similar backward stepping is termed "retropulsion" and similar sidewise stepping is termed "lateropulsion." These occurrences are usually associated with the loss of the normal "righting" of the body to sudden displacement and with an impairment of equilibrium. The patient may fall and be injured. Because these patients not only lack the normal postural responses to an impending fall but also lack protective movements, they fail to raise their hands to protect themselves and may suffer blows to the head and face.

In advanced stages of the disease the patients are largely immobile, are confined to a bed or wheelchair, and require assistance in the acts of daily living. Impaired deglutition results in the pooling of saliva in the fauces, drooling, weight loss because of the difficulty in ingesting adequate amounts of food, and the risk of aspiration and secondary bronchopneumonia. The failure of the cricopharyngeal muscles to relax appears to delay swallowing. The patient may point to the larynx and explain that the food remains stuck at that point.

In approximately one third of patients with Parkinson's disease the later course of the illness is complicated by gradual dementia. Initially the patient may be forgetful and have a tendency to develop minor confusional episodes that may be ascribed to medication. Reducing the dosage of anticholinergic drugs or discontinuing them entirely may result in a clearing of these symptoms, but gradually the symptoms reappear. The patient may be confused and irritable and have paranoid ideas. Many patient have a typical pattern of complex visual hallucinations. The patient may see strange people wandering about or may claim to have seen a deceased relative. Initially the patient may be aware that the hallucinations are unreal. With the advent of dementia, however, the patient reacts to the hallucinations, often with paranoia. The patient may have frank delirium. Drugs with anticholinergic properties, including not only the antiparkinsonian drugs but also antihistamines, tricyclic antidepressants, and many tranquilizers, may induce the patient's hallucinations and increase confusion. The drug-induced exacerbation of dementia usually clears in several days after the offending agent is withdrawn.

Typically, the patient with Parkinson's disease speaks rapidly in a soft monotone. The patient loses the normal rhythm of speech and runs syllables together without pause or inflection. The first few words may be spoken clearly, but then the voice becomes softer, articulation becomes slurred, and the patient utters words with increasing speed (tachyphemia). Voice amplitude may dwindle rapidly to a whisper and speech may cease altogether. The patient's handwriting shows analogous changes; the letters become progressively smaller (micrographia) and tremulous until the patient ceases writing, the hand apparently frozen for a moment before resuming the task.

The stooped posture characteristic of Parkinson's disease may be marked in some patients, yet it disappears when the patient sits back in a reclining chair or lies down. Many patients also have a mild scoliosis with the thoracic spine gently curving in most cases away from the side of the initial symptoms. In some cases the patient leans to one side, with a lateral tilt of the trunk of as much as 10 to 15 degrees from the vertical while standing. Usually the tilt is more pronounced in the sitting position and the patient tends to slump to one side. Patients are often unaware of these postural aberrations.

Characteristic changes in the attitude of the hands occur in parkinsonism, even in the drug-induced form. The patient holds the fingers extended with the metacarpophalangeal joints flexed about 30 degrees. The abnormal attitude of the fingers abruptly disappears when the patient grasps an object with the hand but reappears when the hand is at rest. Patients often have flexion of the toes with dorsiflexion of the proximal phalanges. Sometimes the first toe assumes a constant dorsiflexed position simulating the position of the first toe in the Babinski sign.

Symptoms of autonomic dysfunction are very common. Increased secretion of sebum (seborrhea) is evident in an oiliness of the skin, especially of the face. When seborrhea is marked, the patient has a scaly erythematous eruption of the skin, especially along the nasolabial folds, behind the ears, at the eyebrows, and in the scalp. Some patients have intermittent, sometimes profuse, bouts of diaphoresis. Chronic constipation with reduced bowel motility is a ubiquitous feature of Parkinson's disease. Mild impairment of micturition with urgency and hesitation is common, especially in elderly male patients. A small percentage of patients have orthostatic hypotension. These patients complain of dizziness on standing up or on suddenly arising from a sitting position. Such patients may have Shy-Drager syndrome, in which peripheral autonomic failure is coupled with extrapyramidal manifestations.

LABORATORY FINDINGS. Laboratory findings may include a mild microcytic anemia in some cases, presumably representing a nonspecific feature of chronic illness. Chest roentgenograms may show a slight scoliosis. Skull roentgenograms and computed tomographic (CT) brain scans should be normal. Patients with dementia, however, may have some cortical atrophy and ventricular enlargement. The electroencephalogram (EEG) is either normal or shows minimal slowing and disorganization. Such changes, however, may be the result of drug therapy, especially therapy involving anticholinergic agents. The EEG of patients with marked bradykinesia and those with dementia may show moderate to marked slowing and diffuse disorganization.

Cineradiographic studies of swallowing often reveal an abnormal pattern caused by a delayed relaxation of the cricopharyngeal muscles. Contrast radiography of the gastrointestinal tract commonly reveals hypomotility of the intestines, delayed stomach emptying, and varying degrees of distention of the large bowel. A megacolon may rarely be found in patients with severe constipation.

DIAGNOSIS. The diagnosis of parkinsonism is based primarily on the clinical manifestations. The presence of the triad of tremor, rigidity, and bradykinesia, as well as the characteristic postural changes, the seborrhea, and the monotone tachyphemic speech, forms a distinctive clinical picture. In early cases with minimal physical findings a diagnosis may be difficult to make, and the physician may need to do a reevaluation after a period. The differential diagnosis comprises a wide variety of disorders. The clinical setting helps make the diagnosis easier. Thus parkinsonism in a young patient should suggest Wilson's disease. One should consider the possibility of arteriosclerotic cerebrovascular disease in an elderly patient. The patient who has suffered several minor strokes and has mild bilateral hemipareses may have what is termed "arteriosclerotic parkinsonism." Dementia is more common in such cases. The patient's speech is slurred rather than monotone and tachyphemic. The lower extremities are more involved than the upper extremities. Mild spasticity rather than a rigidity should occur. The plantar reflexes may be extensor. No seborrhea is present. Despite all these distinctive features, however, differentiation in individual cases may be difficult. The CT scan or MRI may be helpful in showing evidence of multiple previous cerebral infarcts.

Rarely patients with brain tumors may have symptoms resembling Parkinson's disease. More commonly, patients with Parkinson's disease may also coincidentally have brain tumors. The appropriate thyroid function tests can exclude hypothyroidism. Hypoparathyroidism may on rare occasions mimic parkinsonism. Thus one should check serum calcium levels, especially in patients with a history of a thyroidectomy in the past.

Differentiating among the various parkinsonian syndromes may be difficult in early cases. A patient with a history of encephalitis lethargica (in lay terms, "sleeping sickness") and of oculogyric crises (uncontrollable uprolling of the eyes) may have postencephalitic parkinsonism. Signs of cerebellar dysfunction in addition to parkinsonian features suggest an olivopontocerebellar atrophy. Cerebellar atrophy is seen on CT scans or MRI. A history of treatment with tranquilizers or of psychiatric care should arouse a suspicion of drug-induced parkinsonism. Patients having a primarily bradykinetic syndrome with little or no tremor and a poor or paradoxic response to levodopa therapy may have striatonigral degeneration. CT scans or MRI shows striatal atrophy affecting particularly the putamen. The diagnosis of striatonigral degeneration can be established with reasonable certainty only on postmortem examination. Impairment of ocular motility, especially for vertical downgaze, is characteristic of progressive supranuclear palsy.

COURSE. The course of Parkinson's disease is one of slow gradual progression for many years. There is great variability from one patient to another; some have unilateral symptoms for 10 years or more, whereas others may reach a stage of significant disability within 10 years. Before the introduction of levodopa therapy the life expectancy of patients with Parkinson's disease was significantly reduced. With current treatment, life expectancy has approached the norm. Patients with advanced disease may succumb to intercurrent infections, but Parkinson's disease is not generally fatal.

MANAGEMENT. The most effective treatment available today is levodopa, which is the immediate metabolic precursor of dopamine. The rationale for this treatment is to replenish the cerebral stores of dopamine. Levodopa may be given alone but is most commonly given in combination with an inhibitor of dopa decarboxylase to protect the levodopa from decarbox-

ylation to dopamine in the kidney, bowel, and other extracerebral tissues and to permit a larger proportion of the levodopa taken by mouth to reach the brain. The decarboxylase inhibitor alphamethyldopa hydrazine (carbidopa) is generally employed in a combination tablet (Sinemet) containing levodopa and carbidopa in a 10:1 ratio. The inhibitor does not cross the blood-brain barrier and so does not prevent the conversion of levodopa to dopamine in the brain. One must carefully adjust the dosage and the dosing schedules to the individual patient to obtain optimal results. The average dosage is 25 mg of alphamethyldopa hydrazine in combination with 250 mg of levodopa three times daily. The major dose-limiting side effect of this treatment is the induction of choreiform involuntary movements. If these are excessive, the dosage should be reduced. Orthostatic hypotension and sinus tachycardia may occur and may require special measures. The patient may have agitation, insomnia, nightmares, and rarely hallucinations and even frank delirium. A long-acting combination of carbidopa and levodopa that is now in the experimental stage was developed with the hope of lessening some of the side effects and response fluctuations that patients with Parkinson's disease experience with the shorter action of Sinemet.

A variety of drugs possessing central anticholinergic properties may be of use as an initial treatment in mild cases or as an adjunct to levodopa therapy. These include trihexyphenidyl (Artane), benztropine (Cogentin), and amantadine (Symmetrel). The tricyclic antidepressant drugs imipramine (Tofranil) and amitryptyline (Elavil) are useful for patients with depression complicating the parkinsonism. The phenothiazines and haloperidol should be avoided because they block the desired actions of levodopa therapy.

Stereotactic surgery to produce a small lesion in the ventrolateral nucleus of the thalamus can effectively alleviate tremor and rigidity on the opposite side of the body. To alleviate symptoms on both sides, bilateral operations are required. The risk of the second operation is considerably greater than that of a single unilateral procedure. About 15% of patients who have had a bilateral thalamotomy have suffered a significant pseudobulbar palsy. Bradykinesia, speech impairment, disturbances of gait and equilibrium, and other features are not altered by surgery, nor has the progression of the disease been modified. Levodopa therapy has largely supplanted the surgical treatment of parkinsonism. Surgery may still be useful, however, in carefully selected patients who have a unilateral tremor as their major problem and who have failed to respond to drug treatment. A new surgical technique is in the experimental stage. Transplantation of adrenal medullary tissue to the brain in patients with Parkinson's disease has been performed to provide the striatum with a new cellular source of catecholamines. Initial results indicate that some clinical improvement results.

Recently a new class of drugs that act directly at dopamine receptor sites was investigated for the treatment of parkinsonism. These dopamine receptor agonists were shown to have substantial therapeutic efficacy, comparable in some instances to that of levodopa. One of the agents, bromocriptine (Parlodel), is available for this use. Deprenyl, a monoamine oxidase inhibitor, prevents the breakdown of dopamine. It is without the usual hypertensive side effects, is used extensively in Europe, and seems to be a helpful adjunctive therapy when used with levodopa.

Physical therapy and a sensible program of exercise are useful in maintaining patient mobility and general well-being. Attention to maintaining good bowel habits is needed to counter the chronic constipation so common among parkinsonian patients.

ESSENTIAL TREMOR

DEFINITION. Essential tremor is a benign hereditary condition characterized by a postural tremor usually affecting the hands, the head, and often the voice. Other terms for this condition are "benign essential tremor," "familial tremor," and "senile tremor."

ETIOLOGY. Essential tremor is a genetic trait transmitted in an autosomal dominant pattern with considerable variation in its severity. Curiously, families harboring this trait appear to enjoy unusual longevity. There are no observable pathologic lesions, and the nature of the underlying neural dysfunction is a subject of speculation.

CLINICAL MANIFESTATIONS. The patient has a tremor of the hands, perhaps best described as a trembling, with a frequency of about 8 to 10 Hz symmetrically in both upper extremities. The patient is usually an adult, but rarely the disorder may appear in childhood or adolescence. In some members of affected families the tremor may not appear until the patient reaches advanced age and it may then be termed "senile tremor." At first the tremor may only appear during periods of stress, and the patient feels it as a transient "nervousness." Unlike the tremor of parkinsonism, it tends to disappear at rest and is most noticeable when the hands are held up with the arms outstretched or when the patient attempts to hold a fixed posture for a moment; hence its description as a postural tremor. The tremor diminishes during movement and consequently in most cases causes relatively little disability. There is no rigidity or bradykinesia as in parkinsonism and no loss of coordination as in the intention tremor of multiple sclerosis or cerebellar disease.

Patients commonly have a rhythmic bobbing of the head. The tremor may also involve the thorax, diaphragm, and abdomen resulting in a vocal tremor. Rarely the tremor may involve the lower extremities.

The tremor is more marked during stressful moments and may be absent when the patient is relaxed. It is often most prominent when the patient arises in the morning and diminishes somewhat during the day. When the tremor is severe, it may interfere with tasks requiring dexterity and steadiness. Patients with this tremor tend to write rapidly and in large letters to minimize the trembling.

Aside from the tremor there are no abnormalities of nervous function. A slight hypotonia of the musculature and a slight hyperextensibility of the joints may occur in many cases.

DIAGNOSIS. The diagnosis rests on observing the tremor, noting its distribution in the body and the lack of any other neurologic abnormality. Also helpful is the family history. The condition is often mistaken for parkinsonism, especially in elderly patients. Differentiation may be made readily by noting the absence of the bradykinesia, rigidity, and postural aberrations of parkinsonism. The micrographic handwriting of the parkinsonian patient is conspicuously absent. In contrast to the parkinsonian patient, the patient with essential tremor has a lively facial expression, a normal speed and spontaneity of body movement, and normal associated movements.

In parkinsonism there may be a tremor of the lips, jaw, tongue, and facial muscles but not a rhythmic tremor of the entire head.

The evolution of essential tremor also helps in making the diagnosis. The patient who has had a symmetric tremor of the hands for many years, with no other stigmata of parkinsonism, almost certainly has essential tremor. The tremor of Parkinson's disease, moreover, usually has a unilateral onset, whereas essential tremor develops in both upper extremities simultaneously and more or less symmetrically.

The differential diagnosis of essential tremor includes the tremor of hyperthyroidism, chronic alcoholism, anxiety, and cerebellar degeneration. The absence of associated features should exclude these conditions.

COURSE. The tremor increases slowly in severity and bodily distribution for many years. Most patients with essential tremor live a normal life with little or no disability.

MANAGEMENT. Patients with essential tremor are frequently aware that an alcoholic beverage temporarily suppresses the tremor. Alcohol often induces a rebound effect, however, with increased tremor a few hours later or the following day. Various sedatives and minor tranquilizers such as the benzodiazepines are commonly employed in attempts to control the tremor. Although the tremor may be significantly reduced, it is never completely abolished. Propranolol (Inderal) is the most effective treatment, but it has significant side effects and should be employed cautiously. It may lower the blood pressure, slow the pulse, and provoke congestive heart failure. Propranolol may induce bronchospasm and should not be given to patients with a history of asthma. Recently it was shown that the anticonvulsant primidone (Mysoline) is effective in controlling essential tremor.

Stereotactic thalamotomy can effectively abolish essential tremor in the contralateral limbs, but the condition is rarely disabling enough to warrant brain surgery.

CHOREA

The term "chorea," derived from the Greek word for "dance," is applied to a state of motor hyperactivity in which the speed, amplitude, and frequency of body movement are abnormally increased. Given that there is a broad range of normality, it is understandable that minor degrees of chorea may pass unnoticed or be taken simply as nervousness or fidgetiness. Careful observation, however, may reveal brief twitches of the hands, fleeting facial grimaces, and a slight irregularity of movement. In overt chorea, brief irregular jerky movements of the limbs, head, trunk, face, and tongue are observed. The patient has a sudden flexion and extension of a limb, inappropriate gestures, exaggerated blinking, involuntary protrusions of the tongue, and abrupt contractions of major muscle groups. When these phenomena are mild, the patient may be unaware of them or regard them as normal voluntary movements. The automatic movements that are normally outside awareness are particularly affected. Thus the patient may walk with an excessive armswing. Normal gestures become flamboyant. Stepping is exaggerated. The patient appears "loose jointed" and moves excessively rapidly. In severe cases all movement is distorted and impaired by violent involuntary jerks and twitches. High stepping, flinging movements of the arms, sudden starts and stops, bowing, and turning abruptly reduce walking to a caricature of the norm. Respiration may be irregular, with hyperventilation, deep sighs, and panting breaths occurring in a random sequence. Speech becomes slurred with an explosive quality. Choreic patients may also be emotionally labile, impulsive, and aggressive. The common underlying feature of chorea appears to be disinhibition.

The patient with chorea has difficulty maintaining a fixed posture for more than a fleeting moment. For example, a handgrip cannot be maintained; the grip is relaxed intermittently, producing an effect picturesquely termed "milkmaid's grasp." The patient cannot keep the mouth open steadily. Instead, the mouth opens and closes at irregular intervals, and the tongue relaxes and protrudes in rapid darting movements while the patient is constantly changing position, seeming to squirm in the seat. When attempting to stand still, the patient constantly shifts weight from one foot to the other, and a continuous motion of the legs and feet causes a swaying and rocking back and forth.

Chorea is a pathophysiologic state reflecting a dysfunction of the basal ganglia that may be regarded as the opposite of parkinsonism. Chorea occurs in association with a variety of disorders; the motor disturbances are similar, although the clinical settings may differ. All choreas show similar pharmacologic responses. Postulations include increased sensitivity of striatal dopamine receptors or hyperactivity of striatal dopaminergic systems. The major tranquilizing drugs, which interfere with dopaminergic function, induce parkinsonism but reduce chorea. In contrast, drugs useful in treating parkinsonism, notably levodopa, induce or exacerbate chorea. The major side effect of levodopa in the treatment of parkinsonism is the induction of choreiform involuntary movements.

Huntington's chorea

DEFINITION. Huntington's chorea, or Huntington's disease, is a chronic progressive hereditary disorder of adult life characterized by choreic involuntary movements, behavioral changes, and dementia.

ETIOLOGY AND PATHOGENESIS. Huntington's chorea is transmitted in an autosomal dominant pattern with virtually complete penetrance. The gene is located on the short arm of chromosome 4. There are no formes frustes, nor does the condition skip generations. The disease may be expected to develop in half of the offspring of an affected parent. Unfortunately, the initial symptoms usually do not appear until after the patient is 40 years of age, which ensures the continued prevalence of the disease.

The abnormality is confined to the brain, which in advanced cases shows an extensive atrophy of the basal ganglia. The caudate nucleus and putamen are particularly affected and may be reduced to thin layers of gliotic tissue. There is severe and widespread loss of neurons and nerve fibers. The cause of the neuron degeneration is unknown.

Postmortem biochemical investigations have shown a selective loss of γ-aminobutyric acid (GABA) in the caudate nucleus and putamen. GABA is a prominent and widespread neurotransmitter in the brain, and its loss appears to result from the degeneration of the striatal neurons that normally synthesize and store it. A decrease in angiotensin, acetylcholine, substance P, and dynorphin also is noted in the striatum. On the other hand, increased levels of somatostatin and neuropeptide Y are found in the striatum of Huntington patients, since the neurons that synthesize these substances are spared.

EPIDEMIOLOGY. Huntington's chorea occurs throughout the world in all ethnic and racial groups. The prevalence varies from 4 to 7:100,000 standard population. In certain communities the prevalence is much higher.

CLINICAL MANIFESTATIONS. The main clinical manifestations are a gradual development of choreic phenomena and mental deterioration. Considerable variations in symptoms, age of onset, and rate of progression may be noted. Mental disturbances may precede the chorea by a number of years. Behavior changes marked by impulsive or antisocial acts, depression, or withdrawal suggestive of schizophrenia may be the initial manifestations. Conversely, some patients may exhibit chorea for a number of years before mental changes become apparent. In such cases severe involuntary movements of the face, tongue, and head may profoundly limit speech and render a clinical evaluation of the mental state difficult. Rarely, the disease may become symptomatic in childhood or adolescence. Juveniles tend to have a rigid bradykinetic syndrome instead of the more usual chorea. The rigid form of Huntington's chorea may resemble Parkinson's disease.

Mild at first and sometimes dismissed as mannerisms, the chorea gradually becomes more severe. Violent flinging movements, rapid darting movement of the tongue, sudden jerking of the head, irregular respiration, contortions of the trunk, and thrashing and kicking of the limbs combine to create a dramatic clinical picture. Falls and injuries may result from the violent involuntary motor activity; physical exhaustion from the constant and excessive activity contributes to the death of patients with advanced disease.

The mental changes are usually those characteristic of organic brain disease. Impairment of memory, a gradual decline in intellectual capacity, apathy, and a disregard for personal hygiene are seen as in other organic dementias. Patients may also be irritable or have sudden bursts of aggressive behavior, fits of depression, and impulsive behavior. Because of the prominence of mental changes, many patients must be committed to a psychiatric facility. Some patients may be hospitalized for psychotic reactions, and only much later, when the chorea appears, is the correct diagnosis established.

LABORATORY FINDINGS. Laboratory findings include an EEG that is most often diffusely abnormal. A CT scan may show enlargement of the lateral cerebral ventricles with a "butterfly" appearance on coronal sections, especially in advanced cases. Plasma growth hormone levels are elevated, and an exaggerated response to insulin-induced hypoglycemia is usually found. GABA levels in the spinal fluid are reported to be reduced.

DIFFERENTIAL DIAGNOSIS. The diagnosis rests primarily on clinical findings. With the combination of mental disturbance, the choreic involuntary movements, and a positive family history, it is usually easy to make the diagnosis. In the absence of one of these elements, diagnosis may be difficult. In the absence of a family history, the diagnosis must remain presumptive and alternatives must be considered. Patients with Alzheimer's disease have similar mental changes and occasionally may have involuntary movements. The involuntary movements are never a prominent feature, however, and other neurologic deficits may be found. Cerebrovascular disease may lead to chorea, but usually the involvement is unilateral, acute or subacute in onset, and associated with other neurologic abnormalities. Lupus erythematosus can be a cause of chorea and may result in behavior changes and psychotic reactions. Usually the nervous system is involved late in the course of the lupus after the diagnosis has been established. Rarely, thyrotoxicosis and hyperparathyroidism may induce choreic manifestations and behavior changes. Sydenham's chorea differs because it affects mainly children and adolescents and is not associated with dementia. Occasionally, psychiatric patients who have undergone long-term neuroleptic therapy and have tardive dyskinesia may have abnormal movements that strikingly resemble those of Huntington's chorea. With these patients the predominance of oral dyskinesia and the lack of progression with time should help distinguish this disorder from Huntington's chorea.

COURSE. The severity of the chorea and dementia gradually increases for 10 to 20 years or more. Patients with advanced disease are disabled, are largely confined to a bed and chair, and may need to be placed in a chronic care facility. In terminal stages the chorea may be replaced by widespread muscular rigidity.

MANAGEMENT. Only symptomatic therapy is available. Dopamine receptor blocking agents such as haloperidol and the phenothiazines may reduce the chorea, but it is rarely possible to suppress the involuntary movements completely. Dopamine depleting agents such as reserpine also are fairly effective. The major tranquilizers may help control the psychotic behavior. Minor tranquilizers such as the benzodiazepines sometimes help control mild agitation of hyperactivity. Genetic and family counseling are of great value.

PREVENTION. The main hope of preventing Huntington's chorea lies in genetic counseling. All offspring of patients with this disease should be advised of its genetic character and offered adequate counseling. The recent localization of a marker for the Huntington gene to chromosome 4 raises the possibility that prenatal and presymptomatic clinical testing soon will become generally available.

Hemichorea

DEFINITION. Unilateral chorea, usually termed "hemichorea" or "hemiballism," is an uncommon disorder of acute or subacute onset, commonly occurring in association with cerebrovascular disease.

ETIOLOGY AND PATHOGENESIS. Postmortem studies in patients with hemichorea have usually shown a vascular lesion, either an infarct or a hemorrhage in the internal capsule damaging the subthalamic nucleus or its connections to the globus pallidus. Unilateral chorea also may occur as a consequence of an infarction of the head of the caudate nucleus resulting from atherosclerotic vascular disease.

CLINICAL MANIFESTATIONS. Hemichorea usually develops subacutely for weeks and sometimes for several months after recovery from a cerebrovascular accident (posthemiplegic chorea). It begins insidiously with mild adventitious involuntary movements of the hand, slowly progressing to involve the entire upper extremity, the face, and to a lesser extent the lower extremity of the same side. In the most severe cases the patient's movements are violent and flinging; the resemblance to throwing movements has led some neurologists to prefer the term "hemiballism" for severe hemichorea. In these cases the movements are disabling, and the exhaustion resulting from the continuous motor activity may hasten the patient's death.

Some cases of hemichorea develop in the absence of a previous cerebrovascular accident, although the manifestations are otherwise similar. Hemichorea also has occurred as a complication of stereotactic brain surgery used to treat parkinsonism.

COURSE. In patients surviving the cerebrovascular accident responsible for the hemichorea, the activity usually stabilizes and in most cases gradually subsides spontaneously. The patient may then be left with a residual hemiparesis.

MANAGEMENT. The major tranquilizing drugs can suppress or greatly reduce hemichoreic movements, although often only at dosages producing some degree of parkinsonism on the opposite side.

Sydenham's chorea

DEFINITION. Sydenham's chorea, the most important form of chorea in childhood and adolescence, is associated with rheumatic fever. Sydenham's chorea, carditis, migratory polyarthritis, subcutaneous nodules, and erythema marginatum compose the major clinical manifestations of rheumatic fever.

ETIOLOGY AND PATHOGENESIS. The association of Sydenham's chorea with rheumatic fever is clear, but the nature of the underlying cerebral disorder is uncertain. The chorea is not fatal, and opportunities for studying the neuropathology of rheumatic chorea are few. A mild diffuse vasculitis has been found, presumably reflecting the widespread involvement of connective tissue characteristic of rheumatic fever. Some degenerative changes in the neurons in the cerebral cortex, basal ganglia, and cerebellum also have been described. Evidence exists indicating that patients with rheumatic chorea have antibodies to streptococcal antigens that react with neurons of the subthalamic nuclei and the caudate nuclei. Thus the chorea, as in other manifestations of rheumatic fever, may be related to immune mechanisms triggered by streptococcal infections.

EPIDEMIOLOGY. Sydenham's chorea has become rare with the significant decline of rheumatic fever since the advent of antibiotics. It is almost exclusively confined to patients 7 to 14 years of age, the peak incidence being at 8 years of age. It is rare after puberty. Girls are affected more frequently than boys. It sometimes occurs in association with pregnancy in the patient's late teens or early twenties. Seasonal variation paralleling that of rheumatic fever is noted; cases of chorea are uncommon in the summer.

CLINICAL MANIFESTATIONS. The onset is usually insidious; "nervousness" develops in a child who was previously well. Some stressful incident may be thought responsible for the change in behavior, but as the condition worsens, emotional lability, aimless involuntary movements, impaired coordination, and muscular weakness appear. The weakness may be so marked that the child is unable to get up out of bed, walk unassisted, or even sit up unsupported. The child drops things, fumbles, and has difficulty speaking. Involuntary movements of the tongue, mouth, and palate give the child's speech a slurred, explosive quality. Facial grimacing, sudden jerks of the head, and flinging movements of the limbs complete the picture of generalized chorea. In some cases the chorea may be more pronounced on one side of the body, but bilateral involvement is usual. There is great variability in the severity of the involuntary movements, which usually become much more pronounced when the affected child is disturbed and under stress.

Muscle tone is reduced, and the reflexes are sometimes pendular. At times delayed relaxation results in a "hung-up" reflex. Mental changes are commonly present. The child usually is irritable and is sometimes listless and apathetic.

The child may have other signs of rheumatic fever such as a cardiac murmur. Concurrent arthritis is unusual, but arthritis may precede or follow an attack of the chorea.

DIFFERENTIAL DIAGNOSIS. The acute onset of choreiform involuntary movements in a child or an adolescent should immediately bring to mind the possibility of Sydenham's chorea. Acute chorea also may be a manifestation of various drug intoxications, jimsonweed poisoning, or a complication of anticonvulsant therapy with phenobarbital, phenytoin, or ethosuximide. Acute chorea has been associated with pertussis, encephalitis, lupus erythematosus, and Schönlein-Henoch purpura. The presence of tics and habit spasms occasionally may make the differential diagnosis difficult. They should be distinguished by a more chronic course and by their stereotyped character.

LABORATORY FINDINGS. Laboratory findings may include a mild anemia and a slight eosinophilia. Leukocytosis and an elevated erythrocyte sedimentation rate usually indicate cardiac involvement. Studies of the cerebrospinal fluid (CSF) are within normal limits in most cases. A mild pleocytosis has been reported. Serum titers of streptococcal antibodies may be elevated.

The EEG usually shows some diffuse slowing and disorganization. In the rare case of unilateral chorea the EEG abnormalities may be greater over the opposite cerebral hemisphere. Radionuclide brain scans and CT scans show no abnormalities.

COURSE. Sydenham's chorea is a benign condition that usually subsides within 1 to 2 months. Minor choreic phenomena may persist up to 6 months, but complete recovery is the norm. Recurrences are common and have been observed in about one third of cases after several months and even after several years. Long-term follow-up studies have suggested that neurotic personality traits may persist indefinitely.

MANAGEMENT. The traditional treatment of having the patient rest in a darkened room may suffice in mild cases. Involuntary movements may be reduced to some extent by sedating the patient with barbiturates, chloral hydrate, or mild tranquilizers. The phenothiazines or haloperidol can effectively control the chorea and should be recommended when the involuntary movements are severe.

Sydenham's chorea is considered a major diagnostic sign of rheumatic fever and an indication to initiate prophylactic antibiotic therapy to prevent the subsequent development of other manifestations of rheumatic fever.

TORSION DYSTONIAS

The torsion dystonias are a heterogeneous group of disorders characterized by slow, involuntary turning and twisting movements of the neck, trunk, and limbs produced by forceful muscle contractions and culminating in sustained abnormal postures. The manifestations may be confined to one body part (for example, the neck in torticollis), or the process may be generalized. Several clinical types of the disorder are distinguished by the body distribution of the movements and postures, the clinical manifestations, the pattern of the disorder's progression, a familial history, and other clinical features. Some of these clearly represent distinct entities, but the nosologic identity of many of these disorders remains uncertain, and the classification of individual cases may often be speculative. The most important syndromes are spasmodic torticollis, primary idiopathic torsion dystonia, and dystonic writer's cramp. Additional entities are oromandibular dystonia and blepharospasm either alone or in combination (Meige syndrome) and spasmodic dysphonia.

Spasmodic torticollis

DEFINITION. Spasmodic torticollis is the most familiar type of torsion dystonia, characterized by a deviation of the head to one side. The spasm begins with a slow, usually tremulous or jerky movement producing a turning of the head to one side and elevation of the shoulder. Contractions of the sternocleidomastoid muscle and the trapezius muscle bring the ear close to the shoulder of the same side. The deviation of the head is maintained for 1 to 2 minutes and then a period of relaxation follows, with the head returning toward the normal midline position but not reaching it.

CLINICAL MANIFESTATIONS. The torticollis comprises both a slow, involuntary movement and a sustained abnormal posture. The movement often can be momentarily overcome by an effort of will or by sensory contact. The patient may temporarily arrest the spasm simply by stroking the cheek with a finger. Many patients also have a rhythmic nodding head tremor and a postural tremor of the hands similar to essential tremor. Inspection and palpation reveal hypertrophy of the sternocleidomastoid muscle.

ETIOLOGY. In most cases the cause is completely unknown. In some cases spasmodic torticollis may represent the initial manifestation or an oligosymptomatic expression of primary idiopathic torsion dystonia. In many cases the patient may have a history of trauma to the head or neck that appears to have precipitated the symptoms. The significance of such trauma is unclear.

PATHOGENESIS. Little is known of the pathogenesis of idiopathic spasmodic torticollis. An analysis of the lesions producing similar posture abnormalities of the head in animals suggests that the involvement of various structures in the brainstem can cause spasmodic torticollis. An abnormal response to vestibular stimuli is postulated as one explanation. Thus far, no consistent pathologic lesions have been found. On occasion, torticollis and other focal or segmental dystonias can be late manifestations of treatment with neuroleptics such as the phenothiazines or haloperidol (tardive dystonia). The involuntary movements of tardive dystonia are sustained longer than the usual movements of tardive dyskinesia.

LABORATORY FINDINGS. Electromyography of the involved muscles shows rhythmic discharges and increased activity on the abnormal side.

COURSE. Spasmodic torticollis may begin in childhood but more commonly makes its appearance in adult life. It increases in severity gradually for many years and may remain stable and essentially unchanged throughout a normal life span. A mild scoliosis and later some tortipelvis may be noted in many cases. As the spasms become more severe, they may be painful. Secondary osteoarthritic changes may occur in the cervical spine. During periods of emotional stress the intensity of the spasms often increases.

MANAGEMENT. No satisfactory treatment is currently available. Various tranquilizing drugs are commonly employed and often yield some relief for painful spasms. Diazepam, baclofen, and related drugs have been most frequently used for this purpose. Amantadine, alone or in combination with haloperidol, has been recommended by some clinicians. Anticholinergic agents such as trihexyphenidyl (Artane) in high doses may help, especially in younger patients who can tolerate the large doses required. Psychotherapy may help alleviate secondary neurotic reactions, especially during periods of stress.

Surgical denervation of the cervical musculature may reduce the torticollis. However, the diffuse and variable involvement of the neck muscles generally limits the benefits of limited denervation, whereas more extensive denervation produced by sectioning all the upper cervical motor nerve roots is disfiguring. Stereotactic lesions of the thalamus are made as a last resort, but the results often are transitory and bilateral procedures are required to yield a significant benefit. Dramatic initial benefits are reported, but because of the common recurrence of the spasms and the significant incidence of complications of the bilateral operation, thalamotomy is now rarely performed for spasmodic torticollis.

Physical therapy emphasizing range-of-motion exercises and training the patient to become more aware of the head position has been useful in some cases. Supplemented with biofeedback monitoring techniques, such exercises sometimes have proved disappointing.

Primary idiopathic torsion dystonia

DEFINITION. Idiopathic torsion dystonia is a chronic, slowly progressive disorder beginning in childhood or adolescence and characterized by slow, involuntary twisting movements of the limbs, neck, and trunk culminating in fixed abnormal postures.

ETIOLOGY AND PATHOGENESIS. The disorder is inherited; two genetic patterns are recognized. One occurs almost exclusively in patients of Ashkenazi Jewish descent. It appears to be associated with high intelligence. The other major form is an autosomal dominant disorder with an extremely variable expression. A rare sex-linked form occurring only in females in which dystonic spasms are induced or exacerbated by exercise was recently recognized. Despite the inexorable progression for years that results in severe disability, no morbid anatomic alteration of the nervous system in idiopathic torsion dystonia has yet been found. Postmortem studies have revealed no consistent abnormality. The pathogenesis of this disorder is also unknown. From the evidence of cases of torsion spasms associated with brain tumors, various encephalopathies, and hepatolenticular degeneration (Wilson's disease), a lesion in the lateral putamen appears to be present.

CLINICAL MANIFESTATIONS. A tendency to invert the foot while walking is the most common initial symptom of idiopathic torsion dystonia, especially in children. Minimal at first and perhaps regarded as a mannerism, the phenomenon gradually becomes more pronounced with exaggerated stepping movements lending the gait a bizarre quality. The child may step squarely on the lateral border of the foot. Abnormal posturing of the arm in internal rotation and extension may then appear. Within a few years the process becomes generalized with torticollis, retrocollis, tortipelvis, kyphoscoliosis, and athetoid posturing of the hands. The wrists become hyperflexed, and the fingers become extended. Although at the outset the abnormal movements occur only as adventitious muscle contractions superimposed on and altering the pattern of normal voluntary movement, the torsion spasms in time become sustained and result in abnormalities of posture that become fixed and constant. Patients with long-standing cases have extraordinary contortions and skeletal deformities. All voluntary movement becomes slow, awkward, and laborious. Dysphagia and dysarthria may occur at an advanced stage of the disease. Many patients also have a postural tremor similar in appearance to essential tremor.

LABORATORY FINDINGS. Concentrations of serum dopamine β-hydroxylase (DBH) are reported to be elevated in the autosomal recessive form of idiopathic torsion dystonia, but this finding has not been confirmed. Routine hematologic and blood chemistry studies are normal.

DIAGNOSIS. Torsion spasms may be symptomatic of Wilson's disease, cerebral birth injury, encephalitis, and rarely brain tumor. The development of the torsion spasms and abnormal postures in childhood, in the absence of evidence for another cause, leads to the diagnosis of primary torsion dystonia. Evidence of a similar disorder in other members of the family may help establish the diagnosis. Some individuals in a given family may have only a mild scoliosis of which they may be unaware. Thus an examination of the parents and siblings, even if they deny having symptoms, may be useful. The bizarre nature of the initial symptoms and their marked fluctuation in intensity has often led physicians to suspect that they are psychogenic or "hysterical." This may delay the establishment of the correct diagnosis and result in inappropriate therapy. Differentiation from focal forms of dystonia may be difficult early in the course of the disease until the generalized nature of the affliction becomes evident.

A distinctive dystonia occurring in childhood or adolescence with dystonic gait and marked by diurnal fluctuation, exacerbation with exercise, and a dramatic therapeutic response to levodopa has recently been recognized and named "dopa-responsive dystonia." Parkinsonian features may appear later in the course.

MANAGEMENT. No fully satisfactory treatment is available. Diazepam and related drugs may diminish the intensity of the spasms and the consequent pain. Anticholinergic drugs such as trihexyphenidyl (Artane) and benztropine (Cogentin) in high doses are the most effective therapy available today. Doses of trihexyphenidyl as high as 40 to 60 mg/day are required. Carbamazepine (Tegretol) also has been effective in certain cases.

A stereotactic thalamotomy may induce a partial alleviation of distressing symptoms for a few years. Bilateral surgery is usually necessary, and the subsequent progression of the disease may require another operation to maintain the initial benefit. Surgery does not alter the course of the disease. Reports of benefit from electrical stimulation of the cervical spinal cord have been controversial.

Writer's cramp

The term "writer's cramp" refers to spasms of the muscles of the forearm and hand provoked by attempts to perform fine movements such as writing, buttoning, or working with small tools. It has been regarded as an occupational neurosis, and many varieties have been described in different occupational settings, such as instrumentalist's cramp and violin player's cramp. Psychologic factors have often been implicated. Some cases represent a highly localized dystonic process that very slowly increases to involve the entire upper extremity after many years. Its cause and pathogenesis are entirely unknown. There is no known effective treatment. Training the patient to use the opposite unaffected hand may help.

Oromandibular dystonia and blepharospasm (Meige syndrome)

Oromandibular dystonia is a condition characterized by spasms of the jaw muscles and has been described as a form of focal dystonia. Patients with this disorder suffer from a slow, involuntary forceful opening of the mouth and a deviation of the jaw with a protrusion of the tongue. The phenomenon is somewhat similar to the acute dystonic reactions that may be provoked by the phenothiazines. Several features typical of other dystonias may be observed. For example, the patient may be able to abort a spasm by stroking his chin with his hand. Spasms can be sufficiently forceful to dislocate the jaw and fracture the teeth.

The cause and pathogenesis of this remarkable disorder are unknown. There is no satisfactory treatment. As in other dystonias, diazepam, baclofen, and anticholinergic agents may yield partial relief.

When patients have sustained and forced involuntary closure of the eyelids, they are defined as having blepharospasm. Blepharospasm can occur by itself or with other entities. Blepharospasm with oromandibular dystonia is termed "Meige syndrome." When patients have unilateral blepharospasm with unilateral spasm of the lower facial muscles, independent of the jaw muscles, they have hemifacial spasm. Botulinum toxin (which blocks acetylcholine release from the nerve terminals) injected locally recently was found to be highly successful in the treatment of all these types of blepharospasm. Botulinum toxin also is being used experimentally for other types of focal dystonia. Blepharospasm has also been treated by surgically interrupting the branch of the facial nerve responsible for eye closure.

GILLES DE LA TOURETTE'S SYNDROME

DEFINITION. Gilles de la Tourette's syndrome (Tourette's syndrome) is the syndrome of multiple tics including corprolalia (uttering frequent obscenities) and impulsive behavior, named after the neurologist who gave the first full description of this remarkable disorder.

ETIOLOGY. The cause of Tourette's syndrome is unknown, but genetic factors are suspected. A biochemical defect in purine metabolism, presumably genetically determined, has been suggested as the cause at least in some cases. Psychologic factors were formerly considered causally significant.

PATHOGENESIS. The underlying pathogenesis is unknown. The effectiveness of major tranquilizers in controlling many of the symptoms, however, has suggested an abnormal predominance of brain dopaminergic neural systems. In support of such an hypothesis is the possible alteration of CSF levels of the dopamine metabolite homovanillic acid (HVA) in patients with Tourette's syndrome. A dysfunction of other transmitter systems, notably serotonin, γ-aminobutyric acid, and dynorphin, has been suggested, but a clear model of neurotransmitter imbalance comparable to that available for parkinsonism is not yet established.

CLINICAL MANIFESTATIONS. Tourette's syndrome usually starts in childhood with minor involuntary movements, chiefly frequent eye-blinking, facial twitches, and grunting, or "clearing the throat," noises. These may be disregarded as mannerisms or ascribed to an irritation of the eyes or the throat by allergies or other factors for some time before they are recognized as tics. Hyperactive behavior is commonly noted and may be the initial manifestation in some children. Later in the course of the disease, shrugs of the shoulders, sudden jerks of the head, and sudden inappropriate vocalizations appear. After several years the abrupt jerking movements spread from the muscles of the neck and shoulders to the arms and legs. Subsequently, the patient may constantly make repetitive vocalizations, grunts, barks, and cooing noises and ultimately may utter frequent obscenities. The impulsive behavior, vocalizations, and coprolalia understandably interfere with the patient's social adjustment and frequently prevent regular attendance at school. The involuntary nature of the tics and vocalizations is often unrecognized, and disciplinary measures are applied inappropriately. Self-mutilation such as lip biting and gnawing the tips of the fingers is noted in some cases.

COURSE. Tourette's syndrome has a variable course. Usually the progression is gradual, from one or two tics in childhood to the full-blown syndrome in adolescence or young adulthood. Some patients have spontaneous remissions that may rarely be of long duration, but in general the disorder persists essentially unchanged through adult life.

DIFFERENTIAL DIAGNOSIS. The syndrome is so remarkable and distinctive that, when all the elements are present, the correct diagnosis is usually not difficult to make. Some individuals may suffer only one or two tics throughout life, never having coprolalia or other features. The major difficulty in diagnosis has been the tendency to consider the motor and behavior abnormalities as expressions of a psychologic disorder. Many such patients are thought to be psychotic or hysterical. The motor disturbances are sometimes similar to those of chorea but differ in their stereotyped character. Characteristically, the patient experiences a sense of inner pressure and frustration when attempting to control the tic by an effort of will and a sense of relief when allowing the tic to occur. This sense of release does not accompany choreic movements. The vocalizations and coprolalia clearly distinguish Tourette's syndrome from the choreas.

MANAGEMENT. The major tranquilizing drugs are remarkably effective in suppressing the tics, impulsive behavior, vocalizations, and coprolalia. In contrast, amphetamines and levodopa may exacerbate the tics. Haloperidol and pimozide are most commonly used today. The dosage and the therapeutic response may be limited by sedation and drug-induced parkinsonism to a level yielding only a partial control of the tics. The noradrenalin receptor-blocker clonidine (Catapres) is effective in mild cases of Tourette's syndrome.

WILSON'S DISEASE

DEFINITION. Wilson's disease is a genetic disorder characterized by the signs and the symptoms of basal ganglia dysfunction and hepatic cirrhosis described in 1912 by Wilson, who named it hepatolenticular degeneration.

ETIOLOGY AND PATHOGENESIS. Wilson's disease is a familial disorder occurring in an autosomal recessive pattern. Only homozygous autosomes produce symptoms. The pathogenesis involves an abnormality of copper metabolism. There is a failure of synthesis of the serum copper-binding protein ceruloplasmin. As a result, copper accumulates gradually in the tissues, ultimately producing pathologic changes in the brain, liver, kidney, and other organs. In a sense the disease is a form of copper poisoning caused by a defect in the transport of copper that renders patients unable to handle trace amounts of copper normally present in the diet. The accumulation of copper in the liver in abnormal amounts can be detected in infancy. Ultimately the concentration of copper in the liver reaches levels hundreds of times greater than normal and induces a form of cirrhosis. The accumulation of copper in the brain results in degenerative changes involving mainly the basal ganglia but also the cerebral cortex, cerebellum, and other parts of the nervous system. In severe cases necrosis and cavitation of the globus pallidus and putamen may occur. Copper deposits in the cornea result in a golden-brown ring of pigment visible at the outer margin of the cornea.

EPIDEMIOLOGY. Wilson's disease is relatively rare. Its prevalence is estimated at 30:1 million standard population. It has been estimated that as many as 1% of the inmates of chronic mental hospitals have this disorder. Neurologic manifestations develop in most cases in adolescence or early adulthood. Its onset as early as 4 years of age and as late as the fifth decade of life is reported.

CLINICAL MANIFESTATIONS. Many cases are diagnosed in children when they have the signs and symptoms of hepatic disease. If proper treatment is instituted at this time, neurologic manifestations may never appear. With improved diagnosis in recent years, many cases have been identified in the neonatal period or in early childhood before the appearance of clinical manifestations.

The first manifestation of nervous system involvement is usually a decline in intellectual function. Deterioration in schoolwork is a frequent early sign. The patient may then become depressed and withdrawn and exhibit some slowness of movement, loss of facial expression, and slurring of speech. A tendency to keep the mouth open constantly is often noted. Voluntary movement becomes abnormal, with athetoid posturing of the arms and hands. Involuntary movements may develop such as slow, writhing movement of the limbs, a tremor similar to that of Parkinson's disease, and wing-beating movements of the arms. Patients who first have symptoms in childhood tend to have dystonic and athetoid features, whereas those who first have symptoms after childhood have dysarthria and a tremor of the hands. Muscular rigidity and bradykinesia may then develop, leading to a clinical picture resembling that of Parkinson's disease; Wilson's disease is an important cause of juvenile parkinsonism. There is considerable variability, and many cases show features of both the childhood and adult forms.

The Kayser-Fleischer ring, a golden-brown ring of pigmentation at the outer margin of the cornea, is almost always present in patients with neurologic manifestations. This ring may easily be seen when the iris is lightly pigmented; in dark-eyed patients it can be seen with slit-lamp examination. Convulsions, unexplained periods of coma, and mental changes simulating psychosis or affective disorders may occur rarely.

LABORATORY FINDINGS. If the cirrhosis is sufficiently severe, the results of liver function tests may be abnormal. The serum uric acid level is often decreased and may be a useful clue to the correct diagnosis. CT scans and MRI usually show the hepatic cirrhosis and may show lytic lesions in the basal ganglia. Reduced signal in the lenticular nucleus caused by the paramagnetic effect of copper may be seen with MRI.

DIAGNOSIS. The childhood cases of Wilson's disease are apt to be confused with cerebral palsy and rarely with primary idiopathic torsion dystonia. Cases with a later onset are often erroneously classified as juvenile parkinsonism. Patients with prominent mental changes may be thought to have schizophrenia. The possibility of Wilson's disease should always be kept in mind when a young patient shows chronic progressive mental changes and extrapyramidal features. A history of a previous hepatic disorder, possibly diagnosed at the time as a form of hepatitis, may be a helpful clue. Finding a low serum uric acid level in the routine chemistry profile may be another helpful clue. The diagnosis can be established with considerable confidence by finding the Kayser-Fleischer ring in the cornea. If it cannot be seen by direct visual inspection, the patient should be referred to an ophthalmologist for a slit-lamp examination of the cornea. If Wilson's disease is suspected, the serum ceruloplasmin level should be determined. A low serum ceruloplasmin level, less than 20 mg/dl, is usually confirmatory. Further confirmation of the diagnosis is made by finding an elevated urinary excretion of copper, 200 μg/day and an elevated liver copper level more than 250 μg/g, measured in a liver biopsy specimen. Defective incorporation of ^{64}Cu in leukocytes may also confirm the diagnosis. Because specially prepared copper-free containers, tubes, needles, and glassware must be used, these chemical tests should be performed only in a center experienced in the diagnosis and treatment of Wilson's disease.

COURSE. In the absence of treatment the clinical course of the disease is one of gradual decline culminating in advanced cases in severe rigidity, ataxia, and dementia. Ultimately the patient dies of inanition and intercurrent infection. Some patients die of the hepatic disease or of the complications of cirrhosis such as a hemorrhage from ruptured esophageal varices.

MANAGEMENT. Specific treatment should begin as soon as the diagnosis is established, even in asymptomatic cases. The goal of therapy is to remove the copper from the tissues and to prevent its reaccumulation. Copper removal is achieved with chelating agents such as penicillamine (usually 1 g/day) and the reaccumulation of copper is prevented by maintaining the patient on a copper-poor diet and administering potassium sulfide to reduce copper absorption. Chelating agents must be given in dosages adequate to produce a copper diuresis. The 24-hour urinary excretion of copper is measured during the treatment to ensure that an adequate diuresis is achieved. The potassium sulfide is given by mouth (20 mg three times daily as sulfurated potash) following meals to precipitate copper in the bowel in the form of the highly insoluble copper disulfide. Penicillamine may cause a pyridoxine deficiency; to prevent this, a pyridoxine supplement (50 mg/day) is usually given in conjunction with the chelating agent. Improvement of the neurologic manifestations, fading of the Kayser-Fleischer rings, and improvement of the hepatic dysfunction can be expected. Even severe manifestations may be markedly or completely reversed. Treatment must, however, be continued indefinitely. Recently zinc sulfate was found effective in some cases of Wilson's disease in a dosage of 50/mg three or four times daily. Liver transplantation performed for relief of life-threatening cirrhosis reverses the ceruloplasmic deficit and alleviates the neurologic features of the disease.

IDIOPATHIC ORTHOSTATIC HYPOTENSION

DEFINITION. Orthostatic hypotension reflecting an insufficiency of the autonomic nervous system occurs in diabetes mellitus, polyneuritis, Parkinson's disease, the hereditary ataxias, and other disorders of the nervous system. It may also occur after the administration of tranquilizers, antidepressants, antihypertensives, and other drugs. In a small group of patients orthostatic hypotension develops (usually in middle-age) without other clinical manifestations of a nervous system dysfunction. These are designated idiopathic orthostatic hypotension or primary orthostatic hypotension. Nearly all patients with this disorder, however, subsequently have impotence, anhidrosis, and an atonic bladder; many also have parkinsonism and ataxia. Patients exhibiting such evidence of diffuse involvement of the nervous system have been designated as having Shy-Drager syndrome following the description by Shy and Drager of the postmortem findings in a typical patient. It remains uncertain whether idiopathic orthostatic hypotension with or without manifestations of the additional involvement of the nervous system represents a distinct morbid entity.

ETIOLOGY. Idiopathic orthostatic hypotension is a degenerative disorder of the nervous system of unknown cause. It may be grouped among the multiple system atrophies of the central nervous system, including striatonigral degeneration and Parkinson's disease.

PATHOLOGY. The most common feature found during postmortem examination is a degeneration of the intermediolateral cells of the spinal cord. In some cases intracytoplasmic inclusion bodies (Lewy bodies) are found in these cells and also in the paravertebral sympathetic ganglia. Neuron degeneration and Lewy bodies may also be found in the substantia nigra, the locus ceruleus, various cranial nerve motor nuclei, and the olivary nuclei. In some cases the cerebral cortex may show atrophic change.

CLINICAL MANIFESTATIONS. Light-headedness, faintness, or even a loss of consciousness on standing is the major clinical symptom of this disorder. Initially the patient may have only weakness, dizziness, and faintness when suddenly standing up from a seated or supine position, as in rising from bed in the morning. If questioned, the patient may report more subtle symptoms including impaired sexual performance in men (with an inability to maintain penile erection and delayed ejaculation), loss of sweating, urinary urgency, and urinary frequency. The orthostatic hypotension may become so severe after several years that the patient cannot assume the upright position and remains confined to a bed and chair. When the patient stands up, the blood pressure drops precipitously, and syncope usually occurs when the blood pressure falls below 80/50 mm Hg. Such a drop can be appreciated by palpating the radial pulse. The heart rate fails to increase in response to the fall in pressure. The pallor and sweating that normally occur in response to hypotension fail to occur in these patients because of the dysfunction of the peripheral autonomic nerves.

The autonomic deficiency can be demonstrated by studying the response to Valsalva's maneuver. Hypotension is readily produced, but tachycardia during the maneuver, hypertension on conclusion of the maneuver, and subsequent bradycardia (all observed in normal subjects) do not occur.

In patients with the Shy-Drager syndrome the signs and symptoms of central nervous system involvement also develop. Usually these include a parkinsonian state with bradykinesia, mild rigidity, tremor, monotone speech, ataxia, and dysarthria. Distal wasting of the limb muscles may also be found. Shy and Drager noted atrophy of the iris in their cases.

COURSE. The course of orthostatic hypotension is one of gradual progression. Patients with advanced disease are usually confined to bed by the severe hypotension. Ultimately the patients may succumb to myocardial infarction, cerebral infarction, inanition, or intercurrent infections. Sleep apnea complicating the late course of the illness has been implicated as a cause of death in some cases.

MANAGEMENT. Orthostatic hypotension may be treated symptomatically with sodium chloride supplements or with fludrocortisone (0.1 to 1 mg daily titrated gradually) to increase blood volume. Wearing elastic hose and abdominal binders may help prevent the pooling of large volumes of blood in the legs and in the splanchnic circulation in the erect position. Ephedrine (25 mg three times a day) and phenylephrine administered orally may also be helpful. The combined use of a monoamine oxidase inhibitor with hydroxyamphetamine, methylphenidate, tyramine, or levodopa is described by some investigators. The levodopa may help relieve the parkinsonian symptoms occurring in many cases but when used alone usually aggravates the orthostatic hypotension. Some investigators have recommended the use of indomethacin.

BIBLIOGRAPHY

Aaron AM, Freeman JM, and Carter S: The natural history of Sydenham's chorea, Am J Med 38:83, 1965.
Backlund EO and others: Transplantation of adrenal medullary tissue to striatum in parkinsonism: first clinical trials, J Neuro Surg 62:169, 1985.
Ballard PA, Tetrud JW, and Langston JW: Permanent human parkinsonism due to 1-methyl-4-phenyl-1,2,3,6-tetrahydropyridine (MPTP): seven cases, Neurology 35:949, 1985.
Battista AF: Surgical approach to blepharospasm: nerve thermolysis. In Marsden CD and Fahn S, editors: Movement disorders, London, 1982, Butterworth Scientific.
Bird MT, Palkes H, and Prensky AL: A follow up study of Sydenham's chorea, Neurology 26:601, 1976.
Birkmayer W and Birkmayer GD: Effect of (−) deprenyl in longterm treatment of Parkinson's disease: a 10 year experience, J Neural Transm (Suppl) 22:219, 1986.
Caine ED: Gilles de la Tourette's syndrome: a review of clinical and research studies and consideration of future directions for investigation, Arch Neurol 42:393, 1985.
Calne DB: Parkinsonism, London, 1969, Butterworth, Inc.
Chase T, Wexler NJ, and Barbeau A, editors: Huntington's disease, New York, 1979, Raven Press.
Costero I: Cerebral lesions responsible for death of patients with active rheumatic fever, Arch Neurol Psychiatry 62:48, 1949.
Critchley M: Observations on essential (heredofamilial) tremor, Brain 72:113, 1949.
Diess A and others: Long-term therapy of Wilson's disease, Ann Intern Med 75:57, 1971.
Duvoisin RC: Clinical diagnosis of the dyskinesias, Med Clin North Am 56:1321, 1972.
Duvoisin RC: Parkinsonism: a guide for patient and family, New York, 1978, Raven Press.
Eldridge R: The torsion dystonias: literature review and genetic and clinical studies, Neurology 20(suppl):1, 1970.
Gorman WP and others: A comparison of primidone, propranolol, and placebo in essential tremor, using quantitative analysis, J Neurol Neurosurg Psychiatry 49:64, 1986.
Haber SN and others: Gilles de la Tourette's syndrome: a postmortem neuropathological and immunohistochemical study, J Neurol Sci 75:225, 1986.
Herz E and Glaser GH: Spasmodic torticollis: clinical evaluation, Arch Neurol Psychiatry 61:227, 1949.
Hoogenraad TV, Van der Hamer CJ, and Van Hattum J: Effective treatment of Wilson's disease with oral zinc sulphate: two case reports, Br Med J (Clin Res) 289(6440):273, 1984.
Hughes RO, Cartlidge NEF, and Millac P: Primary neurogenic orthostatic hypotension, J Neurol Neurosurg Psychiatry 33:363, 1970.
Kang UJ, Burke RE, and Fahn S: Natural history and treatment of tardive dystonia, Movement Disorders 1:193, 1986.
Marsden CD: Dystonia: the spectrum of the disease, Res Publ Assoc Res Nerv Ment Dis 55:351, 1976.
Marsden CD and Harrison MJG: Idiopathic torsion dystonia (dystonia musculorum deformans), Brain 97:703, 1974.
Martin JB and Gusella JF: Huntington's disease: pathogenesis and management, N Engl J Med 315:1267, 1986.
Martin JP and Alcock NS: Hemichorea associated with a lesion of the corpus luysii, Brain 57:504, 1934.
Mauriello JA: Blepharospasm, Meige syndrome, and hemifacial spasm: treatment with botulinum toxin, Neurology 35:1499, 1985.
Nygaard TG and Duvoisin RC: Hereditary dystonia—parkinsonism syndrome of juvenile onset, Neurology 36:1424, 1986.
Schirger A and others: A new agent in the management of idiopathic orthostatic hypotension and Shy-Drager syndrome, Mayo Clin Proc 56:429, 1981.
Shapiro AK and others: The Gilles de la Tourette's syndrome, New York, 1977, Raven Press.
Shy GM and Drager GA: A neurological syndrome associated with orthostatic hypotension: a clinical-pathologic study, Arch Neurol 2:511, 1960.
Sternlieb I and Scheinberg IH: Penicillamine therapy for hepatolenticular degeneration, JAMA 189:146, 1964.
Sternlieb I and Scheinberg IH: Prevention of Wilson's disease in asymptomatic patients, N Engl J Med 278:352, 1968.
Strickland GT and Leu M-L: Wilson's disease, Medicine 54:113, 1975.
Waltz JM and Davis JA: Cervical cord stimulation in the treatment of athetosis and dystonia, Adv Neurol 37:225, 1983.
Wilson SAK: Progressive lenticular degeneration: familial nervous disease associated with cirrhosis of the liver, Brain 34:295, 1912.
Yahr MD and Duvoisin RC: The drug treatment of parkinsonism, N Engl J Med 287:20, 1972.

151 · VIRAL AND SLOW VIRAL INFECTIONS OF THE CENTRAL NERVOUS SYSTEM

Francisco Gonzalez-Scarano

A viral infection of the central nervous system (CNS) is usually the by-product of a systemic infection with that virus and represents a small percentage of all infections caused by that particular virus. Among all viruses that infect humans, those with the potential for causing infections of the nervous system are called neurotropic. To invade the nervous system, a neurotropic virus usually replicates in peripheral tissue, such as muscle or the lymphatic system, before entering the nervous system either via the bloodstream or directly through peripheral nerves.

Viral infections of the nervous system are named by the specific compartment affected; many involve only the meninges (meningitis), and some involve the meninges and neural parenchyma (meningoencephalitis). The spinal cord is preferentially involved in poliovirus infections (poliomyelitis), and herpes zoster, the etiologic agent of varicella (chickenpox) and zoster dermatitis, infects the sensory ganglia (ganglionitis).

Although most infections of the nervous system are acute with development and resolution occurring over days to weeks, an important group of infections that have a subacute or chronic course exists. Among such infections are those caused by unconventional agents (slow viruses or prions) and those caused by conventional viruses with long incubation periods (human immunodeficiency virus). Because of their chronic course and their diffuse nature, they are usually considered encephalopathies. Autoimmune causes have been postulated for encephalopathies that occur after a systemic infection has cleared.

ASEPTIC MENINGITIS

DEFINITION. Aseptic meningitis, the most common CNS infection, is a relatively benign, nonpurulent infection of the meninges. Meningitis is defined by the presence of cerebrospinal fluid (CSF) pleocytosis; aseptic meningitis indicates negative bacterial cultures (on occasion the aseptic meningitis syndrome is caused by fungi or cancer cells).

ETIOLOGY AND PATHOGENESIS. Many episodes of aseptic meningitis are unrecognized, and the etiologic factors of others is often not clear. Mumps and lymphocytic choriomeningitis viruses, as well as a variety of viruses that affect the alimentary tract, are common causes of meningitis in the United States. The specific cause can be established by culturing the offending virus from either the throat or stools (CSF viral cultures are rarely positive) or by establishing seroconversion in association with the syndrome. This latter is, by definition, a retrospective diagnosis.

CLINICAL MANIFESTATIONS AND COURSE. The patient with aseptic meningitis has acute onset of headache, photophobia, and fever, sometimes with nausea and vomiting. The classical signs of meningitis (stiff neck) are present in a minority of adult cases. Aseptic meningitis does not affect the brain or spinal cord parenchyma, and therefore there should be no neurologic abnormalities nor changes in the level of consciousness. The course of aseptic meningitis is self-limited, and the recovery is complete within 1 to 2 weeks.

LABORATORY FINDINGS. The most important laboratory findings in the diagnosis of aseptic meningitis are the CSF cell count, which is elevated and predominantly lymphocytic, and the bacterial culture, which is negative. Early in the course of infection, polymorphonuclear leukocytes may predominate in the CSF. The CSF glucose level is normal except in rare instances, and the CSF protein level is normal or modestly elevated (less than 150 mg/dl). Serologic tests are usually necessary to identify the offending virus, but in some instances stool and throat cultures can identify the agent. CSF viral cultures are rarely positive.

DIAGNOSIS AND MANAGEMENT. The syndrome of aseptic meningitis may be a manifestation of partially treated bacterial infection, tuberculous and fungal infection, or carcinomatous invasion of the meninges. Parameningeal bacterial infections (brain abscess and cerebritis) may present a similar picture. All cases of aseptic meningitis require exhaustive examination of the CSF including fungal stains, antigen assays, and fungal cultures. Computed tomography (CT) or magnetic resonance imaging (MRI) may be necessary to exclude abscess. When the diagnosis is uncertain, treatment for bacterial infection should be instituted. Treatment for viral meningitis is supportive.

ENCEPHALITIS

Encephalitis is a nonpurulent inflammatory disease of the brain that may be diffuse or focal, depending on the virus. Most encephalitides are accompanied by a meningeal reaction, with characteristics similar to those of aseptic meningitis. Encephalitis also produces neurologic changes that range from somnolence and lethargy to deep coma. In addition to fever and headache, the patient with encephalitis may develop convulsions, hemiparesis, aphasia, and alterations in behavior. Infection with some agents has a high mortality. Although certain clinical characteristics can suggest a specific virus as the cause in a case of encephalitis (see discussion of rabies and herpes simplex in this chapter), in most instances the diagnosis is based on serologic tests, viral cultures, and brain biopsy.

Arbovirus encephalitis

DEFINITION. Arbovirus (arthropod-borne) encephalitis is an epidemic encephalitis transmitted by arthropods, usually mosquitoes and sometimes ticks.

ETIOLOGY AND PATHOGENESIS. Arboviruses exist in a complex cycle that involves vertebrate and invertebrate hosts. Mosquitoes acquire the virus either by biting an infected mammal or by vertical transmission. Humans enter the cycle infrequently, and usually only as recipients, becoming infected by a virus from the saliva and feces of an infected mosquito. Arboviral infections are thus associated with outdoor activities and are most common in the late summer and early fall. Most arboviral infections are systemic, and even in areas where the invertebrate hosts are common, encephalitis occurs infrequently.

In the United States the virus responsible for most cases of encephalitis is La Crosse virus (California encephalitis), followed by St. Louis, western equine, and eastern equine encephalitis viruses. The vectors responsible for transmission of each of these diseases are different, as is the usual age of infection. The necessity for specific vectors (mosquito strains) accounts for the geographic localization of arboviral infections, since mosquito strains occur in different ecologic niches.

CLINICAL MANIFESTATIONS AND COURSE. As with most encephalitides, headache and other minor symptoms may be the only clinical manifestations. The disease may progress to convulsions and focal neurologic deficits and may eventually result in coma and death. California encephalitis affects children, and although it is seldom the cause of permanent deficits, it tends to cause severe convulsions in the acute phase. On the other hand, St. Louis encephalitis affects the elderly more severely. Eastern equine encephalitis is the most severe of the North American arboviral encephalitides.

LABORATORY FINDINGS. The CSF findings are similar to those of aseptic meningitis, but in some instances of eastern equine encephalitis the CSF may be hemorrhagic. The diagnosis is based on serologic tests.

DIAGNOSIS AND MANAGEMENT. The epidemiologic pattern is helpful in the identification of the specific virus involved. As with other brain infections, treatable entities must be excluded. Patients with arboviral encephalitis are supported with intravenous fluids and anticonvulsants when necessary.

Herpes simplex encephalitis

DEFINITION. Herpes simplex encephalitis is the most common sporadic, or nonepidemic, encephalitis.

ETIOLOGY AND PATHOGENESIS. Adult cases of herpes encephalitis are most commonly caused by type 1 herpes simplex virus (HSV), whereas infant encephalitis is most commonly caused by type 2 HSV. HSV type 1 is commonly present in a latent state in the trigeminal ganglion of adults, and reactivation is responsible for mucosal and labial lesions. The pathogenesis of encephalitis is unclear but may result from reactivation of the latent virus and invasion of the brain parenchyma. The virus has a propensity for endothelial cells, causing a severe hemorrhagic necrosis, and tends to attack the temporal lobes, leading to aphasia and behavioral changes.

CLINICAL MANIFESTATIONS AND COURSE. Headache, fever, and symptoms of meningeal involvement occur early in the course of this disease. Severe convulsions, aphasia, behavioral changes, and coma may occur. In the absence of treatment, death or survival with severe neurologic deficit is the most common outcome.

LABORATORY FINDINGS. The CSF may be hemorrhagic, in addition to demonstrating the findings of aseptic meningitis, and the glucose level may be less than normal. MRI and, less frequently, CT show focal abnormalities.

DIAGNOSIS AND MANAGEMENT. In the appropriate clinical setting the diagnosis is based on biopsy of the brain, which demonstrates antigen present in cells, and from which virus may be grown in tissue culture cells. Acyclovir, an antiviral agent, is used after tests are performed to firmly establish the diagnosis.

Cytomegalovirus

Until recently, cytomegalovirus encephalitis was a disease of children, occurring in association with cytomegalic inclusion disease. In this generalized disease, tissue changes are characterized by enlarged cells with intranuclear inclusion bodies. The brain involvement in these affected children can range from a fatal encephalitis to mental retardation and can lead to microcephaly.

Systemic cytomegalovirus infections in adults are associated with the immunodeficient state and occur particularly commonly after transplantation. Systemic and neurologic infections caused by cytomegalovirus also develop in individuals with acquired immunodeficiency syndrome (AIDS). The latter are frequently complicated by direct neurologic involvement by the AIDS virus, as noted later in this chapter, and it is difficult to delineate a specific clinical picture.

Several experimental drugs are being used in the treatment of systemic cytomegalovirus infection.

Rabies

Although human rabies is a rare disease in the United States, it is still an important problem worldwide. Moreover, the incidence of wildlife rabies in the United States has increased raising the possibility that more humans may become affected in the future. Rabies usually develops after the bite of an infected animal, since the virus is present in saliva. Rabies virus travels up the involved peripheral nerve to the CNS. The incubation period depends on the location of the bite; bites in the distal extremities lead to a longer incubation. The virus attacks neurons and has a preference for those in the brainstem. This produces characteristic spasms during swallowing (hydrophobia) and increased lacrimation and salivation. Consciousness is preserved initially. After the virus replicates within the CNS it spreads centrifugally to salivary and lacrimal glands. Rabies virus has been transmitted by corneal transplantation.

A significant minority of patients with rabies do not exhibit the usual findings and may present a paralytic picture that can be confused with the Guillain-Barré syndrome.

DIAGNOSIS AND MANAGEMENT. Diagnosis of rabies is based on its characteristic clinical features, the history of exposure to a rabid animal or of occupational exposure, and specialized tests such as immunofluorescence of corneal smears. Once encephalitis has developed, rabies is usually fatal. Fortunately, postexposure immunization is highly effective, since the incubation period is long. Recent vaccines have few of the side effects that complicated the use of the first two generations of vaccines (see the discussion of acute disseminated encephalomyelitis in this chapter).

POLIOMYELITIS

DEFINITION. Poliomyelitis is an inflammation of the motor neurons of the spinal cord and brainstem caused by poliovirus, a commonly occurring enteric virus.

ETIOLOGY AND PATHOGENESIS. Poliovirus is an enteric pathogen with three main antigenic subtypes that vary in their neurotropism. Before widespread vaccination, poliovirus occurred in epidemics in which enteric and respiratory disease was the main manifestation. In a small percentage of individuals the virus spreads hematogenously to the gray matter of the spinal cord and brainstem, causing flaccid paralysis of muscles, including respiratory muscles. Fatalities are due to respiratory paralysis. Some recovery occurs, although focal paralysis of the lower extremities is a common sequela to paralytic polio. Most cases of polio in the United States occur in the few unvaccinated individuals or in vaccinated patients with unrecognized immunodeficiency. Since the attenuated live vaccine virus can spread among members of a family, immunodeficient relatives of vaccine recipients and occasionally other susceptible adults can contract vaccine-associated polio.

LABORATORY FINDINGS. The virus can be cultured from the throat and stool. In paralytic polio the CSF formula is similar to that of aseptic meningitis or meningoencephalitis.

DIAGNOSIS AND MANAGEMENT. Treatment is supportive.

HERPES ZOSTER

DEFINITION. Herpes zoster (shingles) is a sporadic painful eruption of the skin in an area supplied by one or more adjacent sensory nerve roots.

ETIOLOGY AND PATHOGENESIS. Varicella-zoster or herpes zoster virus causes varicella (chickenpox), as well as zoster dermatitis. Primary infection with this virus causes the common childhood exanthem and occasionally a mild cerebellitis. The virus is thought to remain latent in the dorsal root ganglia of the spinal cord (or the trigeminal ganglion of the brainstem) where reactivation by unknown stimuli leads to the development of dermatitis. The eruption is vesicular, and the fluid within the vesicles contains giant cells, which are diagnostic.

CLINICAL MANIFESTATIONS AND COURSE. The area supplied by the affected nerve root develops a lancinating pain followed by the eruption, which is self-limited. Postherpetic pain that is sometimes disabling is a common sequela, particularly in elderly patients. Other sequela include corneal scarification (in trigeminal zoster), encephalitis, myelitis, and a vasculitis on the affected side in trigeminal zoster that can lead to cerebral infarction. A generalized zoster eruption similar to varicella may occur in patients who are immunosuppressed particularly in patients with AIDS.

LABORATORY FINDINGS. Herpes zoster virus may be isolated from the skin lesions early in their course. The fluid within the vesicles also contains giant cells, which can be an important diagnostic finding.

DIAGNOSIS AND MANAGEMENT. The dermatomal involvement of the herpetic lesions, the vesicular eruption, and the burning pain are characteristic enough to allow for clinical diagnosis of herpes zoster in most instances. Many clinicians advocate the use of oral acyclovir or steroids for the prevention of a postherpetic neuralgia. Herpes zoster involving the ophthalmic division of the trigeminal nerve can lead to severe corneal problems, and an ophthalmologic evaluation is recommended. If intractable postherpetic neuralgia develops, the pain may be treated with nerve blocks, pharmacologic analgesia similar to that for trigeminal neuralgia, or other surgical procedures (see Chapter 146).

ACUTE DISSEMINATED ENCEPHALOMYELITIS

DEFINITION. Acute disseminated encephalomyelitis (ADEM) is an acute demyelinating disease that follows a viral infection or vaccination.

ETIOLOGY AND PATHOGENESIS. Antecedent viral illnesses such as measles, mumps, and respiratory infections have been implicated as precipitating causes of ADEM. Recent work in postmeasles ADEM suggests that autoimmunity against myelin components may be responsible for the development of this syndrome. Immunity against components of myelin was also thought to cause development of ADEM after vaccination with the original rabies vaccine, which contained CNS tissue. Neuropathologic examination demonstrates an acute inflammatory reaction with destruction of myelin around blood vessels in the brain and spinal cord.

CLINICAL MANIFESTATIONS AND COURSE. The clinical manifestations vary depending on the affected region of the CNS. Neurologic deficits appear after the initial infection has reached its peak and are usually severe, with paralysis, changes in consciousness, and coma.

LABORATORY FINDINGS. In patients with ADEM the CSF is inflammatory, has an increase in the total protein level and lymphocyte count, and, in the most severe cases, may be hemorrhagic. MRI and CT may be useful in delineating the extent of white matter involvement and the degree of breakdown of the blood-brain barrier.

DIAGNOSIS AND MANAGEMENT. The diagnosis is based on the history and laboratory data as outlined previously in this chapter. Since an autoimmune etiology has been postulated, steroids have been used in some situations, but no data exist suggesting that steroids alter the course of this disease. Therefore treatment is generally supportive.

DISEASES WITH LONG INCUBATION PERIODS

Some infectious diseases of the nervous system have prolonged incubation periods—months to years. Some of these diseases are caused by conventional viruses, others by defective forms of conventional viruses, and one group of diseases, the spongiform encephalopathies, by unconventional agents whose nature is still being actively investigated.

HIV encephalopathy (AIDS-dementia complex)

DEFINITION. A constellation of neurologic findings consisting of mental changes, focal signs, and seizures are associated with infections by the type 1 human immunodeficiency virus (HIV-1).

ETIOLOGY AND PATHOGENESIS. A number of neurologic symptoms, beginning with mild memory deficits, progressing to a global dementia, and accompanied by focal neurologic signs and sometimes seizures, are associated with AIDS. Although patients with AIDS have a propensity to acquire a number of secondary bacterial, viral, and parasitic infections, this particular syndrome is associated with specific nervous system involvement by HIV. The neuropathologic changes are largely in the white matter and consist of multinucleated giant cells with minimal inflammatory changes. Many patients with HIV infections also develop axonal and demyelinative polyneuropathies (Guillain-Barré syndrome). Primary infections with HIV are sometimes associated with aseptic meningitis.

CLINICAL MANIFESTATIONS AND COURSE. Changes in memory and other cognitive functions have been identified in patients with HIV infection who have yet to show signs of AIDS. It is not clear whether all of these patients progress to full-blown dementia, or whether the neurologic problems signify that the systemic disease is likely to develop soon. Full-blown dementias have a poor prognosis and are commonly associated with AIDS.

LABORATORY FINDINGS. MRI shows changes in the white matter of the brain. The CSF may show a few inflammatory cells and usually shows evidence of intraaxial synthesis of antibody directed against the virus. Viral antigen is detectable in the CSF of many HIV-infected patients, but it is not yet clear whether this is necessarily associated with the development of HIV encephalopathy. Other conditions frequently associated with AIDS, such as toxoplasmosis and progressive multifocal leukoencephalopathy and cytomegalovirus infections, must be excluded, usually with CT and MRI. The diagnosis of HIV encephalopathy may require brain biospy.

DIAGNOSIS AND MANAGEMENT. In the evaluation of HIV encephalopathy, treatable infections and brain lymphoma must be excluded and brain biospy may be required. There is information that suggests that encephalopathic patients treated with one antiviral drug, zidovudine or azidothymidine (AZT), have improved mental function.

Spongiform encephalopathies (kuru and Creutzfeldt-Jakob disease)

Kuru is a progressive, uniformly fatal disease first seen in a group of natives in the eastern highlands of New Guinea. The disease started with cerebellar ataxia, eventually led to inanition and death, and was thought to be transmitted by ritualistic endocannibalism. Since the disappearance of cannibalism the disease has decreased in frequency, and the average incubation period is estimated to be about 7 years but can range from 2 to 20 years.

Creutzfeldt-Jakob disease (CJD) is a rare condition with a worldwide distribution, occurring primarily in middle-aged persons. Most patients show symptoms of a progressive dementia, which is accompanied by other neurologic deficits and characteristically includes myoclonus, rapid jerks of the trunk and limbs. Some patients may manifest CJD as cortical blindness, and others as cerebellar ataxia, similar to kuru.

Both diseases have a characteristic neuropathology that consists of spongiform changes throughout the gray and white matter. The disease can be transmitted to chimpanzees and other subhuman primates by intracerebral inoculation of diseased tissues. The mode of transmission of CJD is not established, but human-to-human transmission has occurred with corneal transplantation and with inadequately sterilized neurosurgical instruments.

Identification of the agent that causes CJD, kuru, and the animal counterparts of these diseases is being pursued by several large laboratories. It may represent an entirely new class of pathologic organisms composed primarily of protein and referred to as prions.

Subacute sclerosing panencephalitis

Subacute sclerosing panencephalitis is a rare sequela of measles infection or, even less frequently, of vaccination with live attenuated measles virus. The patient, usually a child, has an insidious deterioration of mental function followed by myoclonic jerks, muscle weakness, seizures, and severe dementia. In most cases the disease is fatal within 1 year of onset. The CSF shows high levels of antibody against measles virus, but the virus persists in the neuraxis despite this immune response. A defective measles virus or an immune response not directed against all the viral components may be responsible for the development of this disease. Widespread vaccination has decreased the incidence of measles to a point where subacute sclerosing panencephalitis is usually seen in the United States only in foreign-born children.

Progressive multifocal leukoencephalopathy

Progressive multifocal leukoencephalopathy (PML) is a white matter disease caused by a papova virus termed the "JC virus." Most adults have antibodies against the JC virus, indicating that asymptomatic infections are common. The virus attacks oligodendrocytes, which make and maintain myelin in the CNS. The disease therefore causes extensive demyelination that can be detected by CT and MRI. PML occurs with immunodeficiency and until recently was seen only in patients with renal transplants or systemic lymphoma. It is now common, since it occurs in patients with AIDS. No specific diagnostic tests are available, but MRI and CT can in many instances point to the correct diagnosis. Specific therapy is not available.

BIBLIOGRAPHY

Bryson YJ and others: Treatment of first episodes of genital herpes simplex virus infections with oral acyclovir: a randomized double-blind controlled trial in normal subjects, N Engl Med 308:916, 1983.
Diener TO: Prp and the nature of the scrapie agent, Cell 49:719, 1987.
Gonzalez-Scarano F and Tyler K: Molecular pathogenesis of neurotropic viral infections, Ann Neurol 22:565, 1987.
Itoyama Y and others: Distribution of papovavirus myelin-associated glycoprotein and myelin basic protein in progressive multifocal leukoencephalopathy lesions, Ann Neurol 11:398, 1982.
Navia BA and others: The AIDS dementia complex. I. Clinical features, Ann Neurol 19:517, 1986.
Portenoy RK, Duma C, and Foley KM: Acute herpetic and postherpetic neuralgia: clinical review and current management, Ann Neurol 20:651, 1986.
Whitley RJ and others: Vidarabine versus acyclovir therapy in herpes simplex encephalitis, N Eng J Med 314:144, 1986.

152 · VASCULAR DISEASES OF THE CENTRAL NERVOUS SYSTEM

Rosalie A. Burns

Various diseases of the cerebral vessels set the stage for what is commonly known as a stroke or a cerebrovascular accident (CVA). CVA is the third leading cause of death in the United States and a major cause of disability. The general term "cerebrovascular accident" is so broad, however, that it is insufficient as a diagnosis. More specific and meaningful diagnostic categories to which therapy can be related include cerebral infarction caused by either an arterial thrombosis or an embolus; transient cerebral ischemia or transient ischemic attacks (TIAs); cerebral hemorrhage, either subarachnoid or parenchymal; and infarction and hemorrhage caused by a venous thrombosis.

The diagnosis for a patient who has sustained a CVA cannot rest with a description of the presumed pathophysiologic conditions alone. An attempt to localize the lesion in the central nervous system, thereby suggesting which cerebral vessel is involved, is important for both therapy and prognosis. An example is the situation in which prophylactic surgery on extracranial cerebral vessels is contemplated. The cause of the vas-

cular wall abnormality must be considered. For example, a cerebral thrombosis can be superimposed on a vessel showing atherosclerotic change, or it may be associated with a vasculitis. In an older patient, vascular disease frequently occurs in conjunction with diabetes or hypertension. Hypertension is a frequent cause of underlying cerebrovascular disease, producing hyalinization, a fibrinoid change of the arterioles, and Charcot-Bouchard microaneurysms. A history of hypertension is frequently obtained in patients with a cerebral thrombosis, is commonly present in patients with an intracerebral (parenchymal) hemorrhage, and is usual for patients with the lacunar state (état lacunaire). Severe hypertension may lead to hypertensive encephalopathy. For the older patient, temporal arteritis should be considered as a cause of CVA. For a younger patient, less common but pertinent causes of CVA that must be considered include collagen-vascular disease, infections such as meningovascular syphilis, drug ingestion (for example, cocaine, alcohol, amphetamines, or LSD), hyperlipidemia, migraine headache, fibromuscular dysplasia, dissection, mitral valve prolapse, atrial myxoma with emboli, homocystinuria, polycythemia vera, sickle cell disease, hyperviscosity syndromes, various coagulopathies, pregnancy, the use of oral contraception, and moyamoya disease.

Finally, hemodynamic causes of ischemia, which may be superimposed on a compromised cerebral circulation, should be considered. These would include, for example, various causes of hypotension. The clinical manifestations of cerebrovascular disease are characterized by a sudden onset, in contrast to the gradual downhill progression of a cerebral tumor, an abscess, or a subdural hematoma. In most instances a clinical diagnosis can be made on the basis of a thorough history and physical examination, but 5% to 20% of seemingly straightforward CVAs turn out on further study to warrant an alternative diagnosis. Thus it is important that all patients with a presumed CVA undergo a basic diagnostic workup.

ANATOMY AND PHYSIOLOGY OF THE CEREBRAL CIRCULATION

The flow of blood to the brain, approximately 50 ml/100 g of brain each minute, is normally regulated by a process called autoregulation. This mechanism operates through alterations in the caliber of the cerebral arterioles and the small arteries. This intrinsic myotonic blood vessel reactivity maintains the cerebral blood flow at a relatively constant level between the mean arterial blood pressures of approximately 60 mm Hg and 150 mm Hg in the normal individual. In the hypertensive patient with arteriolar wall thickening, normal blood flows are maintained at higher mean pressures. Autoregulation is transiently disturbed by an acute cerebral insult such as a seizure, head trauma, or a CVA. Without autoregulation the cerebral blood flow passively follows the blood pressure.

The cerebral circulation is commonly divided into the extracranial circulation, referring to the major vessels originating from the aortic arch and traversing the neck to the base of the skull, and the intracranial circulation, referring to the intracranial portions of the internal carotid and the vertebral arteries and their branches (Fig. 152-1). extracranial arteries arising from the aortic arch are the innominate artery, giving rise to the right common carotid artery and the right subclavian artery, and the separate left common carotid and subclavian arteries. The vertebral arteries are the first branches of each subclavian artery. As they ascend, the vertebral arteries pass through the foramina in the transverse processes of the upper six cervical vertebrae and then turn around the atlas to enter the skull

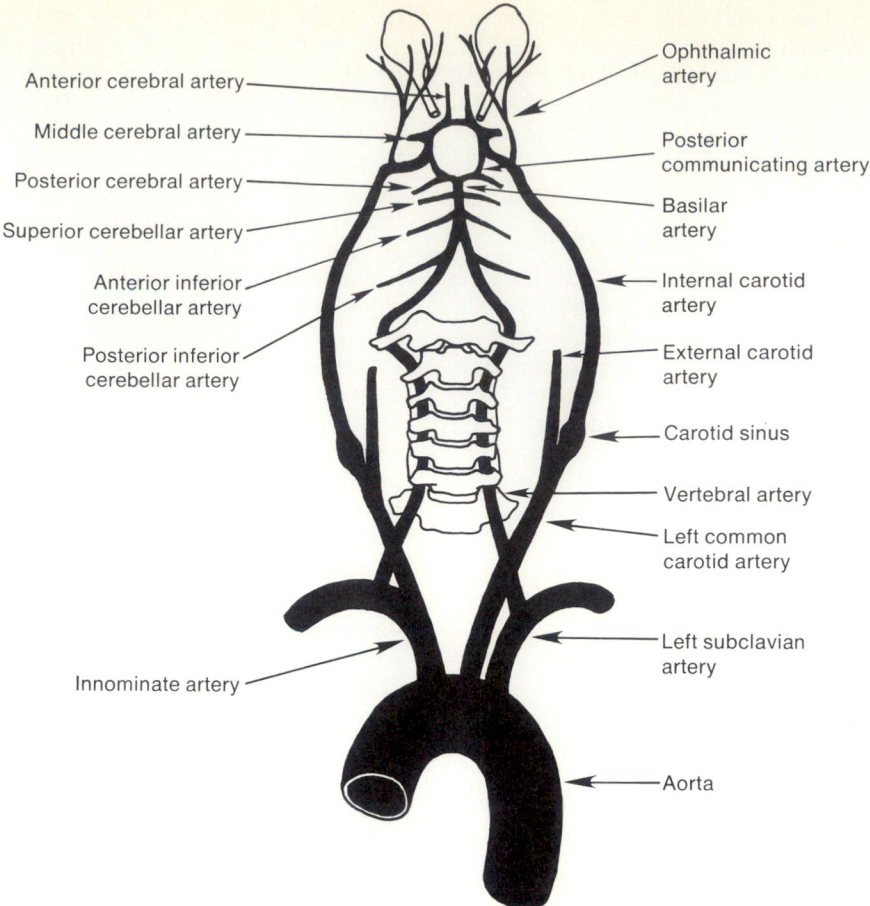

Fig. 152-1 Cerebral circulation.

through the foramen magnum. Intracranially the vertebral arteries unite to form the basilar artery. The basilar artery divides into the two posterior cerebral arteries that join the circle of Willis.

The common carotid arteries bifurcate in the neck into the external carotid artery and the internal carotid artery, with the internal carotid artery continuing intracranially through the base of the skull. The portion of the internal carotid artery that is just distal to the bifurcation of the common carotid artery is the carotid sinus. The ophthalmic artery arises from the internal carotid artery intracranially and proximal to the origin of the anterior cerebral artery, the middle cerebral artery, and the posterior communicating artery. The posterior communicating branch of the internal carotid artery forms a major connection through the circle of Willis with the posterior basilar-vertebral circulation. The intracranial arteries may receive collateral blood flow, bypassing occluded vessels, by means of communication with the extracranial vessels or with other intracranial vessels. An example of the communication with the extracranial vessels is the retrograde blood flow that may occur through the ophthalmic branch of the internal carotid artery by way of external carotid vessel anastomoses. Intracranially, distal anastomoses occur between the subarachnoid arterial branches of the various cerebral arteries. The circle of Willis also provides a means of collateral blood flow; for example, the circle of Willis unites the carotid arterial system with the basilar-vertebral arterial system through the posterior communicating artery. Frequent anomalies of the circle of Willis make the adequacy of this source of collateral circulation unpredictable.

INFARCTION OF THE BRAIN

PATHOGENESIS. In an infarction of the brain a localized drop in cerebral blood flow results in permanent structural change to a focal area of the brain. Vessel occlusion may be caused by a thrombosis with an underlying vessel wall disease or by an embolus. Sites of predilection for underlying atherosclerosis include the carotid sinus in the neck, the intracranial internal carotid artery at the siphon (near the origin of the ophthalmic artery), the middle cerebral artery at its first major bifurcation, the vertebral arteries at their entrance to the cranial cavity and at their junction forming the basilar artery, the basilar artery itself, the posterior cerebral arteries at their origin, and the anterior cerebral arteries as they bend around the genu of the corpus callosum. In hypertensive patients, arteriosclerosis and thrombosis occur in the smaller cerebral arteries.

Infarctions may be pale or hemorrhagic. Pale infarctions involve tissue softening, liquefaction, and eventual glial scarring and cavity formation. Hemorrhagic infarctions are usually caused by an embolus and show abundant petechial hemorrhages.

In an infarction caused by an embolus, the embolic material may arise from an intracardiac mural thrombus following a myocardial infarction, from the diseased valves of rheumatic heart disease, from prosthetic valves, from mitral valve prolapse, from the heart in atrial fibrillation, as a complication of cardiac surgery, or from plaques in the extracranial cerebral arterial system. Infrequently, an embolus from a peripheral vein may reach the brain by way of an atrial septal defect, a so-called paradoxical embolus. Septic emboli can arise from vegetations of acute and subacute bacterial endocarditis. Emboli may arise from an atrial myxoma or from the nonbacterial valvular vegetations of Libman-Sacks endocarditis in lupus erythematosus.

The neurologic deficits that occur with a brain infarction are directly related to the functional anatomy of the disturbed region. The acute symptoms of a cerebral infarction may be magnified by local cerebral edema, and improvement may occur with time as the edema subsides and collateral circulation develops. An area of remaining encephalomalacia persists, and clinically the patient has a residual deficit of varying degree that warrants efforts at physical rehabilitation.

CLINICAL MANIFESTATIONS. In an infarction caused by a thrombosis the onset is sudden and the neurologic deficit commonly appears abruptly; the patient may simply awaken with the deficit. In some instances the infarction may progress for hours, in which case the term "thrombosis in evolution" is appropriate, or there may be a stuttering onset with small increments of increasing deficit that may occur for days to weeks. The patient may have had previous TIAs. Symptoms associated with a cerebral thrombosis at its onset may include headache or, for a small percentage of patients, seizures.

The onset of an infarction caused by an embolus is sudden, commonly even more abrupt than with an infarction caused by thrombosis. Because small branches may become occluded, neurologic deficits may be confined to the distribution of single branches, and monoparesis, for example, would not be unusual. A cortical localization in the cerebrum is common. A higher incidence of seizures at onset is noted than with a thrombosis or with a hemorrhage. Because the emboli may dissolve or move further downstream, blood may gain access to a previously occluded vessel, resulting in a hemorrhagic infarction. Identifying a site of origin is one of the more useful criteria for differentiating an embolus from a thrombosis. Additional differentiating features are the presence of multiple occlusions in the peripheral arteries and the arteries supplying the brain, as in the showering of multiple emboli, and an absence of cerebral atherosclerosis.

In contrast to the progressive course expected with a tumor, an abscess, a subdural hematoma, or a massive intracerebral hemorrhage, the patient with an accomplished cerebral infarction caused by a thrombosis or by an embolus commonly reaches a plateau period of stabilization, followed by improvement. Mortality early in the disease is approximately 15%. There is a substantial recurrence rate for cerebral infarction in the first several years, ranging from approximately 20% to 40%.

LABORATORY FINDINGS. Laboratory studies for patients with an accomplished cerebral infarction are aimed at detecting the small but significant percentage of nonvascular central nervous system disorders that may masquerade as an infarction (mainly a brain tumor or a subdural hematoma). For the most part this can be accomplished with screening studies such as computed tomographic (CT) scanning with and without injecting contrast material, magnetic resonance imaging (MRI) and serial electroencephalograms (EEGs).

The CT scan of a cerebral infarction may show an area of decreased density (decreased attenuation) as early as 8 hours after the onset, but it is more often positive approximately 72 hours after the onset. The detection of lesions depends on the timing of the study in relation to the onset of the illness and on the resolution of the equipment used. After approximately 7 days the injection of contrast material may show an enhancement suggesting a tumor. Interpreting such a finding may require coordinating clinical and laboratory data with repeated observations of the clinical course and the performance of serial

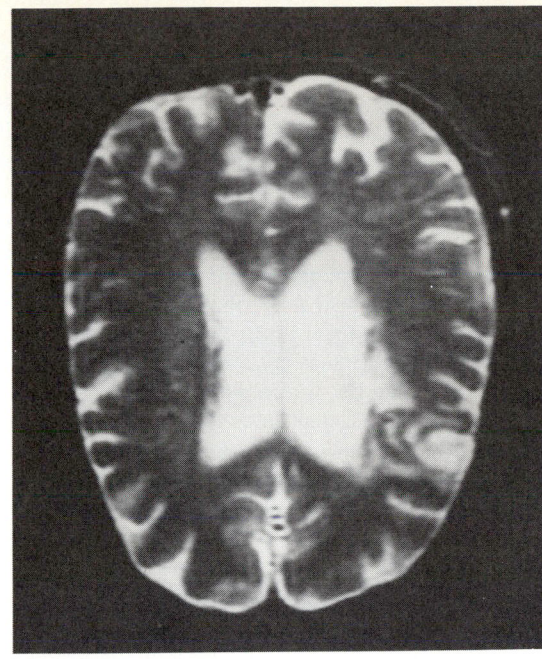

Fig. 152-2   Magnetic resonance demonstrating hyperintensity of old infarction *(left)* on proton density image.

roentgenographic studies. In an embolic infarction the CT scan may show single or multiple areas of decreased attenuation, earlier contrast enhancement than with a thrombotic infarction, and evidence of a hemorrhage after 3 to 5 days if the lesion evolves from a pale infarction to a red infarction. With MRI, cerebral infarctions can be detected much earlier (even within hours) and with greater sensitivity than with CT scanning. Lacunar and brainstem strokes are examples of infarctions that are more readily detected. On T_2 weighted images, the increased water content in the area of the infarction appears as an area of hyperintensity (Fig. 152-2), eas on the T_1 weighted images, there may be a slight hypointensity.

Cerebral infarctions may produce focal slow wave activity on the EEG. Serial testing may be required to differentiate them from mass lesions because it is common for the EEG abnormality to improve with infarctions but not with tumors. Infarctions of the brainstem or cerebellum are unlikely to produce EEG changes. Other diagnostic tests that aid in determining the cause of a CVA include blood and cerebrospinal fluid (CSF) serologic tests for syphilis, blood lipid tests for hyperlipidemia, and antinuclear antibody tests for vasculitis. The possibility of a silent myocardial infarction should be investigated by performing electrocardiography and cardiac enzyme tests early and then later in the course of the disease. In infarction, the CSF obtained by lumbar puncture may reveal a small increase in white blood cells and protein. A total protein level greater than 100 mg/dl suggests a cerebral neoplasm. Hemorrhagic fluid may be found after 24 or 48 hours in instances of a hemorrhagic infarction seen with an embolus.

MANAGEMENT AND PREVENTION. The treatment of a patient with an accomplished infarction caused by a thrombosis is generally supportive. Any associated cardiac disease must be treated to improve and maintain the cerebral blood flow, but no attempt should be made to lower hypertensive blood pressure levels to less than 110 mm Hg diastolic pressure in the first several weeks. Because the baseline range of autoregulation is elevated in hypertensive patients, and because autoregulation is impaired following a CVA, the cerebral blood flow is vulnerable to the lowering of the systemic blood pressure. An adequate fluid balance should be maintained, but the treatment of cerebral edema with steroids or hyperosmolar agents has not been routinely beneficial. Although the infarction resulting from a cerebral embolus is treated similarly, consideration should be given to using anticoagulants to prevent the production of further emboli if no evidence exists to suggest a hemorrhagic infarction and if no other major medical contraindication such as blood dyscrasia, severe hypertension, severe liver disease, or gastrointestinal bleeding is present. In this situation a continuous intravenous infusion of heparin (5000 units initially followed by approximately 1000 units an hour, extending the partial thromboplastin time to one and one half to two times the control level) may be used after a 24-hour period of observation, with the use of the CT scan to exclude hemorrhage. Warfarin (Coumadin) should be initiated and maintained so that the prothrombin time is approximately one and one half times the control level. Heparin may then be discontinued. Surgery may be a possible option for removing the source of the embolic material, as in valvular disease. To treat a patient with thrombosis in evolution, after excluding hemorrhage, the physician should consider the urgent use of heparin to prevent the presumed propagation of a thrombus or an embolization from a thrombus. If heparin cannot be given, an alternative is the use of the antiplatelet agent, aspirin (300 mg a day).

Syndromes of the cerebral arteries

The neurologic deficits in cerebral occlusive vascular disease are generally related to the functional anatomy of the disturbed region. An infarction in the distribution of the middle cerebral artery, supplying the motor and sensory regions of the cerebral convexity, may result in hemiparesis and hemisensory disturbance (the arm more involved than the leg) with various forms of aphasia when the dominant cerebral hemisphere speech centers are involved. An occlusion of the middle cerebral artery may be indistinguishable from a thrombosis of the internal carotid artery and commonly results from an embolus from this extracranial vascular source. An occlusive vascular retinopathy may occur with occlusion of the internal carotid artery of with emboli from the internal carotid artery to the retinal arteries. With an infarction of the medial surface of the cerebral hemisphere, supplied by the anterior cerebral artery, the motor weakness and sensory deficit are more apparent in the leg than in the arm, in contrast to the situation with a middle cerebral artery disturbance. The patient may have gait apraxia. The involvement of the paracentral lobule on the medial surface of the hemisphere may produce urinary incontinence.

Decreased blood flow through the posterior cerebral artery, which supplies the occipital lobe, results in homonymous hemianopsia, and the involvement of its thalamic branches can produce hemisensory deficits. These deficits are associated at times with a persistent and disagreeable sensation known as thalamic pain. The syndrome of Déjérine-Roussy consists of a transient motor deficit, a hemisensory impairment, spontaneous pain, and abnormal involuntary movements of a choreoathetoid type, all developing contralateral to the lesion. An infarction of the left calcarine cortex and the splenium of the corpus callosum results in a right homonymous hemianopia, a difficulty in identifying colors, and alexia (difficulty in reading) without agraphia (difficulty in writing). When both posterior cerebral arteries are involved, cortical blindness may result, and if patients are unaware of this blindness, they are said to have Anton's syndrome. A persistent amnesia may result from

a bilateral infarction of the hippocampal gyri with an occlusion of both posterior cerebral arteries.

The involvement of a perforating thalamic branch of the posterior cerebral artery to the subthalamic nucleus may result in contralateral hemiballismus. The involvement of the branches to the paramedian midbrain (also supplied by small rostral paramedian branches of the basilar artery) may result in Weber's syndrome, in which a third nerve palsy is present on the side of the infarction with contralateral upper motor neuron signs. When the third nerve nucleus is involved, because of its midline configuration, a contralateral superior rectus palsy also appears. Both internal ophthalmoplegia (dilated and fixed pupil) and ptosis, when present because of the involvement of the third nerve nucleus, are bilateral. In Benedikt's syndrome, in addition to the features of Weber's syndrome, the involvement of the regions of the red nucleus and the medial lemniscus results in chorea and hemisensory deficits on the opposite side.

Upward gaze paralysis may occur from unilateral infarctions involving the posterior commissure in the midbrain or from the bilateral involvement of the pretectum, the posterior commissure, or the dorsal midbrain tegmentum. Downward gaze paralysis may result from bilateral involvement dorsal and medial to the red nuclei. Bilateral lesions of the rostral pontine tegmentum and the midpontine tegmentum may also cause a paralysis of either upward or downward gaze in some cases. The involvement of branches of the posterior cerebral artery may produce isolated manifestations of these various syndromes.

Syndromes of the basilar artery and its branches

In the basilar arterial system there may be an occlusion of the small paramedian vessels supplying the medial pontine structures, involvement of the short circumferential branches involving the lateral pons and the long circumferential branches producing involvement of the cranial nuclei and the nerves as in the superior cerebellar artery syndrome and the anterior inferior cerebellar artery syndrome, or involvement of the basilar artery itself, commonly with a loss of consciousness caused by lesions of the reticular formation. These brainstem syndromes are commonly partial or incomplete because of the overlapping distribution of the arterial supply. It is common for a patient to have bilateral brainstem signs when a drop in the blood flow through the basilar arterial system affects branches on both sides of the brainstem.

The descriptive term "locked-in syndrome" is applied to the situation occurring with a lesion in the caudal basis pontis in which the patient is quadriplegic or quadriparetic, with a retention of consciousness and vertical eye movements. In this de-efferented state the patient is mute and uncommunicative unless communication can be achieved by response with the retained eye movements to appropriate questioning.

A jerky conjugate movement of the eyes in the vertical plane, occurring spontaneously in a patient with a pontine infarction or a hemorrhage, is known as ocular bobbing.

The involvement of the paramedian branches of the basilar artery to the medial and superior pons can produce an internuclear ophthalmoplegia (the syndrome of the medial longitudinal fasciculus with paralysis of adduction on the side of the lesion and nystagmus in the abducting eye), an ipsilateral ataxia, and a contralateral hemiparesis. The involvement of the dentato-rubro-thalamo-olivary pathway in the brainstem may be followed after a period of time by the development of continuous rhythmic movements of the palate, called palatal myoclonus. The patient may also have an associated rhythmic titubation of the head and nystagmus.

When paramedian branches of the basilar artery to the medial inferior pons are affected, there may be a combination of an involvement of the abducens nucleus, the seventh nerve as it curves around this nucleus, and the corticospinal pathways, producing Millard-Gubler syndrome. Patients with this syndrome have a paralysis of the lateral rectus muscle, a peripheral facial palsy on the side of the infarction, and a contralateral hemiparesis.

Pontine lesions involving the pontine paramedian reticular formation (PPRF) are characterized by a paralysis of conjugate horizontal gaze to the side of the lesion (Foville's syndrome). If the medial longitudinal fasciculus should also be involved on the same side, the so-called 1½ syndrome may result from the additional paralysis of adduction on the side of the lesion. The resulting condition is a paralysis of abduction and adduction in the eye on the side of the lesion, and a paralysis of adduction in the opposite eye. Ipsilateral ataxia and contralateral paresis of the arm and leg may also be noted in the medial pontine syndromes at the midpons and the inferior pons.

In an occlusion of the short circumferential branches of the basilar artery, an infarction occurs in the lateral midpons and is manifested by ipsilateral incoordination or ataxia. The patient may have impaired facial sensation and a paralysis of the muscles of mastication on the side of the lesion. Contralateral hemianesthesia may occur.

Involvement of the long circumferential branches of the basilar artery produces the syndromes of the superior cerebellar artery and the anterior inferior cerebellar artery. The superior cerebellar artery supplies the lateral area of the caudal midbrain and the rostral pons in its course to the cerebellum. An infarction in this distribution produces a syndrome involving ipsilateral involuntary movements and ataxia. A sensory deficit for pain and temperature may involve the entire contralateral body. Horizontal nystagmus may be associated with an ipsilateral paresis of conjugate gaze. The patient may have partial deafness, Horner's syndrome, bulbar myoclonus, and dysarthria. Horner's syndrome consists of miosis, ptosis, and decreased sweating on the ipsilateral face and may be partial. It is caused by an interruption of the sympathetic nervous system pathways in the brainstem.

In the syndrome of the anterior inferior cerebellar artery (Fig. 152-3), vertigo occurs, as well as sudden ipsilateral deafness, facial paralysis, Horner's syndrome, ipsilateral cerebellar ataxia, nystagmus, nausea, vomiting, paresis of conjugate lateral gaze, ipsilateral loss of touch sensation on the face, possible contralateral hemisensory impairment of pain and temperature perception, and hemiplegia. With an occlusion of the internal auditory artery, which supplies the structures of the inner ear, ipsilateral sudden deafness also may occur, along with tinnitus and vertigo. A syndrome of an occlusion of the labyrinthine branch of the internal auditory artery may be recognized clinically, producing only vertigo and a diminished ipsilateral labyrinthine response to caloric stimulation.

Syndromes of the vertebral arteries

An occlusion of the vertebral artery can result in the syndrome of the posterior inferior cerebellar artery or can produce the medial medullary syndrome. The syndrome of the posterior inferior cerebellar artery (Fig. 152-3) is also known as Wallenberg's syndrome or the lateral medullary syndrome. The pathologic condition involves the inferior portion of the vestibular nuclei, and vertigo is a significant symptom. Other signs include ipsilateral facial hypesthesia for pain and temperature,

paralysis of the palate, pharynx, and larynx with dysphagia and dysarthria, cerebellar ataxia, Horner's syndrome, and contralateral hypesthesia for pain and temperature.

In the medial medullary syndrome the hypoglossal nerve is involved in the medulla with weakness and atrophy of the tongue on the same side. The patient has a paresis of the arm and leg on the contralateral side, but the face is spared. Because of the involvement of the medial lemniscus, the patient has a loss of position and vibratory perception on the contralateral side.

An infarction of the cerebellum is often not suspected while the patient is alive. It is caused most often by a vertebral artery occlusion. Its signs may be overshadowed by those brainstem deficits that occur with a decreased blood flow in the long circumferential branches supplying both the brainstem and the cerebellum. An acute onset is associated with vomiting, dizziness or vertigo, gait ataxia, dysmetria, dysarthria, and nystagmus. Progressive neurologic deterioration may occur after a latent interval of 24 to 96 hours. A cerebellar hemorrhage or an expanding mass lesion in the posterior fossa must be considered in the differential diagnosis; a CT scan or MRI can help in this differentiation. If accompanied by significant edema, infarctions of the cerebellum may become life threatening through compression of the brainstem. If signs of progressive brainstem dysfunction develop, there should be an immediate decompression of the infarcted cerebellar hemisphere or shunting of the CSF.

Lacunar syndromes

The lacunar syndromes occur mostly in hypertensive patients and are the result of small infarctions (0.5 to 15 mm) called lacunes (état lacunaire). Lacunes characteristically occur in the corona radiata, basal ganglia, internal capsule, or pons and result in several discrete syndromes. In the pure motor stroke the lacune may be located in the internal capsule or the pons. Sensory, speech, or visual deficits are not noted. In the pure sensory syndrome the thalamus is implicated, and the deficit, as the descriptive name implies, is confined to the sensory system. In the syndrome of homolateral ataxia with crural paresis the lesion is thought to involve corticopontine pathways in the corona radiata. Contralateral ataxia and weakness are found (both on the same side of the body), with the leg more involved than the arm. The dysarthria–clumsy hand syndrome suggests a pontine lacune and is manifested mainly by a marked dysarthria and difficulty with fine movements of the hand contralateral to the lesion. Contralateral central facial weakness and finger-to-nose wavering are also present, along with a deviation of the protruded tongue away from the side of the lesion and some dysphagia. In the lacunar syndromes each episode tends to have a good prognosis, but multiple episodes may develop in time, resulting in a pseudobulbar palsy. In a pseudobulbar palsy the involvement of the bilateral corticobulbar fibers results in dysarthria and dysphagia. The patient may also lose control over emotional outbursts such as laughing and crying (emotional incontinence) and may have a gait with small steps (marche à petits pas). Multiple lacunes or multiple infarcts may result in dementia (multiinfarct dementia).

Because the lacunar syndromes are commonly caused by the hyalinization of intracerebral arterioles, evaluating for large vessel disease with arteriography is not usually necessary.

Dissection of arteries

Dissection of arteries supplying the brain is being recognized more frequently and may account for 5% of ischemic strokes occurring in young adults. Subintimal dissections of intracra-

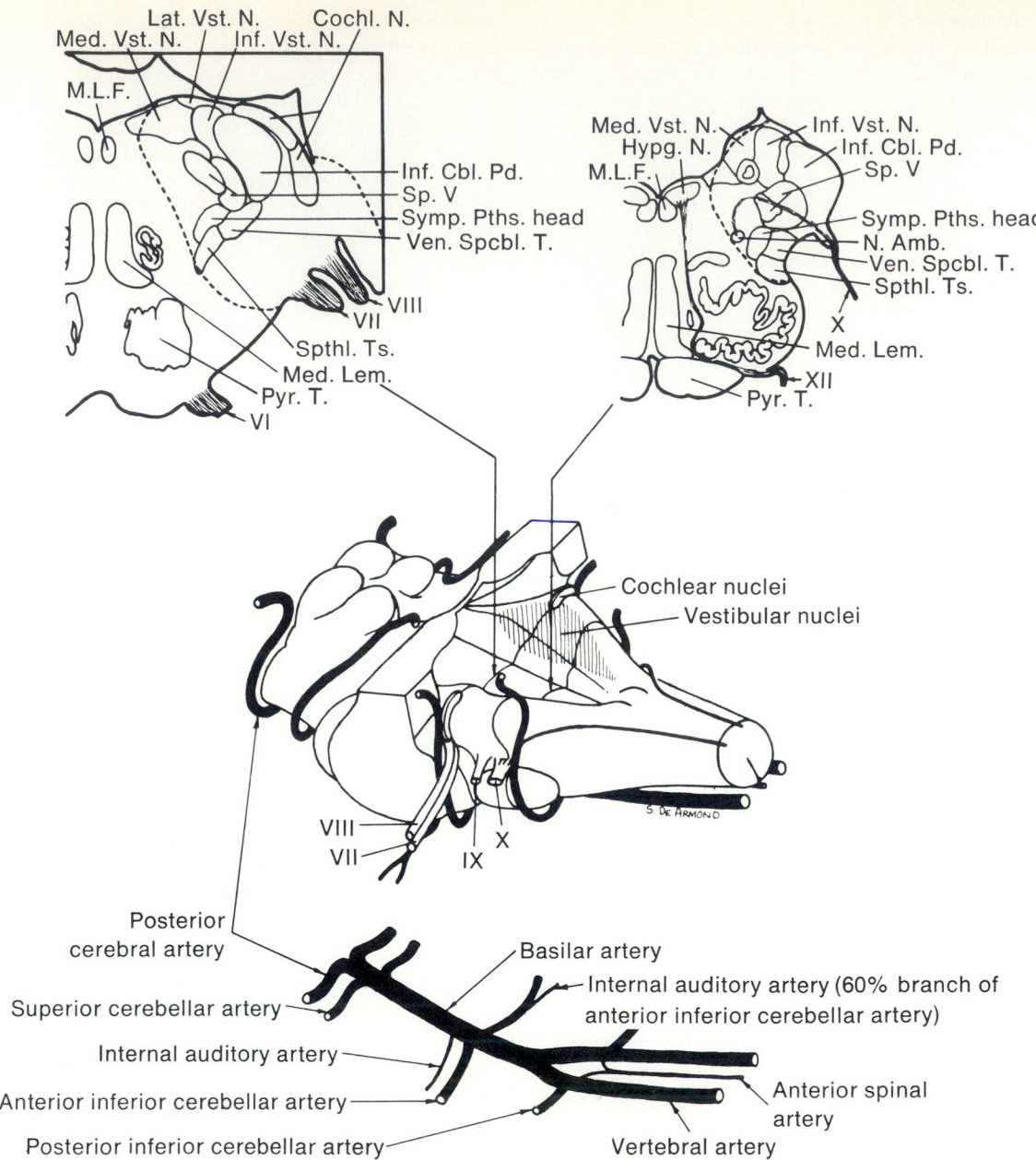

Fig. 152-3   Anatomy of brainstem showing cross sections at level of blood supply by anterior cerebellar artery *(upper left)* and posterior inferior cerebellar artery *(upper right);* longitudinal view of cochlear and vestibular nuclei and relation of blood vessels to brainstem *(middle);* and a view of long circumferential branches of basilar-vertebral artery system *(below).* Regions of cochlear and vestibular nuclei are cross-hatched. Dotted lines in cross sections *(top)* outline sites of ischemia in syndrome of anterior inferior cerebellar artery *(upper left)* and posterior inferior cerebellar artery *(upper right). Cochl. N.,* dorsal and ventral cochlear nuclei; *Hypg. N.,* hypoglossal nucleus; *Inf. Cbl. Pd.,* inferior cerebellar peduncle; *Inf. Vst. N.,* inferior vestibular nucleus; *Lat. Vst. N.,* lateral vestibular nucleus; *M.L.F.,* medial longitudinal fasciculus; *Med. Lem.,* medial lemniscus; *Med. Vst. N.,* medial vestibular nucleus; *N. Amb.,* nucleus ambiguus; *Pyr. T.,* pyramidal tract; *Sp. V.,* Spinal tract and nucleus of the fifth cranial nerve; *Spthl. Ts.,* lateral and ventral spinothalamic tracts; *Symp. Pths. head,* pathways controlling sympathetic outflow to head; *Ven. Spcbl. T.,* ventral spinocerebellar tract. (From Burns RA: Otolaryngol Clin North Am, 6:287, 1973.)

nial arteries of unknown cause may develop in otherwise healthy individuals with a mean age of 25 years. Spontaneous or traumatic dissection of the major extracranial cerebral arteries occurs most often in patients younger than 50 years. In dissection of the internal carotid artery, ipsilateral head, face, and neck pain, Horner's syndrome, and focal ischemic cerebral signs may occur. In cervical vertebral artery dissection, the lateral medullary syndrome is common and pain occurs high in the neck.

INFARCTION OF THE SPINAL CORD

The blood supply to the spinal cord consists of one anterior spinal artery, which supplies the anterior two thirds of the cord, and two posterior spinal arteries, which supply the dorsal root entry zones and the posterior columns. These vessels originate superiorly from the branches of the vertebral arteries, but they receive major contributions in their course along the length of the spinal cord from the radicular arteries, which derive from branches of the vertebral arteries and subclavian arteries, the aorta (intercostal and lumbar branches), and the iliac arteries. A major contributing branch is the great anterior medullary artery of Adamkiewicz, which is a branch of the aorta supplying the spinal cord at approximately its first or second lumbar levels.

The spinal cord is particularly vulnerable to an infarction at the watershed area in the midthoracic cord, where ascending and descending branches meet and where a decrease in the blood flow in one of the major contributing branches would be most likely to produce symptoms.

The syndrome of the anterior spinal artery is most commonly the result of a proximal vascular occlusion such as occurs with a dissecting aneurysm of the aorta, or an occlusion of the artery of Adamkiewicz (iatrogenic at surgery or with catheterization in aortography). Atherosclerosis of the anterior spinal artery is uncommon. In the spontaneous disorders, back pain is common initially. The sudden onset of quadriplegia (with cervical cord lesions) or paraplegia (with the more common thoracic or lumbar lesions) may be associated in the early stages with spinal shock (flaccidity and decreased reflexes). Ultimately, spasticity and increased deep tendon reflexes (corticospinal tract signs or pyramidal tract signs) prevail. Sensory signs reflect the bilateral involvement of the spinothalamic tracts with a decrease in pain and temperature sensations. Position sense, vibration sense, and variable degrees of touch sense remain intact because of the preservation of the posterior columns. The patient becomes incontinent. The prognosis for the recovery of function is poor, and myelography may be necessary to determine that there is no spinal cord compression.

The syndrome of the posterior spinal artery is uncommon. Because the findings reflect the relatively small area of the spinal cord involved (the posterior horns and the posterior columns), deficits are not striking. Ipsilateral proprioceptive deficits may be present, and some physicians have noted hemiparesis.

TRANSIENT ISCHEMIC ATTACKS

DEFINITION. Transient ischemic attacks (TIAs) are syndromes in which focal neurologic deficits develop abruptly and last for either a period of minutes or up to an arbitrary maximal duration of 24 hours. They are a common forerunner of a CVA. The transient symptoms or signs reflect focal areas where the decreased cerebral blood flow temporarily is unable to satisfy the metabolic requirements but where an accomplished infarction has not occurred. Although most TIAs last only minutes and are completely reversible, there can be borderline situations with a more prolonged or persistent residual deficit of a minimal degree such as a reversible ischemic neurologic deficit (RIND) or transient ischemic attacks with incomplete recovery (TIA-IR). The focal ischemic symptoms generally occur in either the distribution of the carotid arterial system or the basilar-vertebral arterial system. Symptoms of involvement in the carotid arterial system include ipsilateral monocular blindness (amaurosis fugax), contralateral motor deficits or sensory deficits, aphasia when the dominant hemisphere is involved, and headache. These symptoms reflect an ischemia in the distribution of the branches of the internal carotid artery: the ophthalmic artery, the anterior cerebral artery, and the middle cerebral artery. Patients may describe amaurosis fugax, or fleeting blindness, either as a curtain ascending or descending in front of one eye or as merely monocular blurring. Funduscopic examination in some patients shows cholesterol emboli, platelet-fibrin emboli, or calcific retinal emboli such as Hollenhorst plaques (refractile cholesterol deposits) seen at the retinal arterial bifurcations. Unilateral visual blurring in combination with contralateral motor signs or sensory signs is highly suggestive of carotid artery disease. Symptoms of disease in the basilar-vertebral arterial system reflect its supply to the brainstem, the inferior temporal lobe, the occipital lobe, and the cerebellum. Because of the compact nature of the structures in the brainstem, isolated symptoms are unusual. Symptoms of TIAs in the basilar-vertebral arterial system include vertigo, visual disturbances, dysarthria, facial paresthesias, headache, disorders of equilibrium, vomiting, dysphagia, alternating weakness of the opposite sides of the body, loss of consciousness, drop attacks, and transient global amnesia. A drop attack is a sudden fall without a loss of consciousness. Transient global amnesia describes a brief episode of difficulty with short-term memory that may result from a bilateral hippocampal ischemia in the distribution of the posterior cerebral arteries. Vertigo is the most common symptom of an insufficiency of the basilar-vertebral arterial system, although vascular disease accounts infrequently for the complaint of dizziness, and isolated vertigo without other brainstem symptoms is more often labyrinthine in origin. The physician should also consider other diagnoses, such as myasthenia gravis and drug toxicity, in the presence of isolated and recurrent dysarthria or diplopia.

ETIOLOGY AND PATHOGENESIS. Approximately 70% of patients with TIAs have atherosclerotic lesions of the extracranial cerebral vessels, with the region of the carotid sinus being a major site. These vessels can be stenotic, occluded, or patent but containing an ulcerating atheroma. Stenotic lesions must narrow the vessel lumen by 90% to decrease the flow significantly. Platelet-fibrin aggregates or cholesterol emboli from these atheromatous lesions are probably a major factor in producing attacks. Microembolic material may produce only a temporary occlusion, with symptoms resolving as the microemboli disintegrate or disappear or as the collateral channels open. Emboli derived from the heart are more likely to result in an infarction. Decreased cardiac output resulting in a decreased cerebral perfusion pressure does not result in focal neurologic symptoms (TIAs) unless this hemodynamic change is superimposed on significantly narrowed cerebral vessels. For example, syncope caused by a decreased cardiac output is not a TIA. In the basilar-vertebral arterial system, emboli are less easily demonstrated and hemodynamic causes may be more significant. Mechanical compression by skeletal or muscular structures may be responsible for the blood flow changes in some cases. Occasionally no apparent basis for TIAs can be found.

CLINICAL MANIFESTATIONS. In the face of a negative neurologic examination or one with minimal residual signs, the general physical examination, particularly the cardiac evaluation, becomes particularly important. Cardiac murmurs and arrhythmias should be sought. The blood pressure should be measured for evidence of hypertension, orthostasis, or a difference in systolic pressure of 20 mm Hg or more in the two arms. The difference in systolic pressure, although uncommon, suggests an occlusion of a proximal subclavian artery resulting in a reversal of the blood flow down the vertebral artery and producing brainstem symptoms (subclavian steal syndrome). The neurovascular examination includes palpating the carotid, superficial temporal, and radial artery pulses. Auscultation for bruits is performed with the bell of the stethoscope over the carotid bifurcations, the supraclavicular areas, and the orbits. A bruit caused by stenosis at the carotid bifurcation, heard best at the angle of the mandible, is generally not prominent over the more proximal common carotid artery, where murmurs that are transmitted from the heart may be heard.

LABORATORY FINDINGS. Laboratory studies include those described for an accomplished infarction, but other tests are aimed at guiding a course for CVA prevention. Studies to determine a cardiac source of embolism include performing a 24-hour Holter monitor and echocardiography. Noninvasive screening tests for extracranial cerebrovascular disease such as ultrasound of the carotid arteries, supraorbital directional Doppler scanning, ophthalmodynamometry, and oculoplethysmography can provide gross information about the presence of a carotid artery stenosis or occlusion (see Chapter 100). These techniques do not identify the patient with an ulcerated plaque or a small plaque, do not reveal intracranial disease, and are not useful in evaluating the basilar-vertebral arterial circulation. They are a safe means of confirming a suspicion of extracranial carotid vascular disease, but they do not establish the pathogenesis because atherosclerosis is common. On occasion, when the noninvasive diagnostic screening tests are not sufficiently helpful to satisfy clinical suspicion or when they point to the need for further study, cerebral angiography may be warranted. Because this procedure carries a mortality of approximately 0.1% and can result in a 0.6% incidence of permanent severe focal neurologic deficit, it should not be undertaken lightly and is not needed to confirm the diagnosis of TIA.

Cerebral angiography is the most definitive method of localizing a vascular lesion, although it does not prove the vascular nature of the symptoms. Aortic arch studies do not show the intracranial vessels satisfactorily, and selective filling of nondiseased carotid arteries may be indicated for a more complete evaluation. These procedures should be performed only when the diagnosis is in doubt and the determination would significantly alter patient management or when prophylactic surgery for a remediable lesion is contemplated. Since MRI can demonstrate the blood vessel lumen without the need for contrast material and is able to do so in various planes, it is likely that MRI will be used more in the noninvasive evaluation of extracranial cerebral vascular disease, including dissection.

COURSE. Because somewhere between 25% and 40% of patients who have TIAs have a CVA within 3 to 5 years, the goal in identifying them is prophylactic and is intended to prevent the development of an accomplished infarction. These patients most often die of cardiac disease.

MANAGEMENT. No unanimity exists about the best treatment. The methods of treatment can be directed toward correcting the hemodynamic and cardiac irregularities, regulating the blood clotting mechanisms, or repairing the arterial vessel wall. There is statistical support for the effect of aspirin in decreasing platelet aggregability. Doses of 300 mg a day are recommended. Other antiplatelet agents that are used but lack the same statistical clinical validation include sulfinpyrazone (Anturane) (100 to 200 mg twice a day) and dipyridamole (Persantine) (50 mg three times a day). Frequent recent TIAs warrant a brief course of intravenous heparin if there are no contraindications such as a diastolic blood pressure of 110 mm Hg or greater, blood in the CSF or apparent on the CT scan, blood dyscrasia, gastrointestinal bleeding, or severe liver disease (see discussion of "Management and prevention" on p.729 for dosages).

The acute period is not the time for vigorous antihypertensive management, which may decrease the cerebral blood flow. The diastolic blood pressure, however, should be gradually lowered to 110 mm Hg. For patients who are good candidates for surgery and who are willing to have surgery, a carotid endarterectomy should be considered for eroded plaques or for stenoses of 70% or more. The best surgical response with occlusive disease is in unilateral carotid stenosis. Investigation with cerebral angiography, including the aortic arch, is necessary. When performed by an experienced surgeon, carotid surgery has a mortality of 1% and a morbidity for transient or permanent neurologic deficits of approximately 1% to 2%. Vertebral stenoses are rarely treated surgically. The proximal subclavian artery is surgically accessible for treating the subclavian steal syndrome.

For patients in whom standard extracranial surgical techniques are ruled out by completely occluded lesions or by inaccessible lesions, microsurgical cerebral revascularization to bypass the occluded vessel has been attempted. These procedures, such as the superficial temporal artery to middle cerebral artery (STA-MCA) bypass, involving an anastomosis of the small extracranial arteries to the cortical arteries, have not proven beneficial. An alternative course of treatment is a 3- to 6-month maintenance course of warfarin (Coumadin) if no contraindications are present. Warfarin has been shown to decrease TIAs, at least in the first several months of use, although no consensus exists regarding its role in preventing thrombosis and an accomplished infarction. The prothrombin time should be maintained between one and one fifth and one and one half times the control levels, and there should be no contraindications such as blood dyscrasia, evidence of blood on a CT scan or in the CSF, severe hypertension, liver disease, or patient noncompliance.

CEREBRAL HEMORRHAGE

PATHOGENESIS. Intracerebral hemorrhage or parenchymal hemorrhage occurs with increased frequency in hypertensive patients. The bleeding into the substance of the brain is caused by a rupture of microaneurysms of the arteriolar vessels (Charcot-Bouchard aneurysms), the result of hypertensive vascular disease. The most common site for these hemorrhages, accounting for about 60% of cases, is in the area of the putamen. Other common locations, with an incidence of about 10% each, are the thalamus, the tegmentum of the pons, the cerebellum, and the cerebral white matter.

When an intracerebral hemorrhage occurs in the absence of hypertension, it is appropriate to consider other sources of bleeding: a cerebral aneurysm, an arteriovenous malformation (AVM), a hemorrhage into a tumor, arteritis, an obscure angiopathy, a blood dyscrasia, anticoagulation, or the rupture of a mycotic aneurysm in bacterial endocarditis.

Bleeding may occur into the substance of certain brain tumors, either as the patient's initial problem or during the course of the tumor. Tumors with a predilection for hemorrhage include glioblastoma multiforme, hemangioblastoma, pituitary tumors (pituitary apoplexy), renal cell carcinoma, melanocarcinoma, and choriocarcinoma. The physician may suspect a tumor as an underlying cause of an intracerebral hemorrhage from a history of progressive symptoms preceding the hemorrhagic event, from findings on a CT scan, or if the hemorrhagic CSF reveals an elevation in total protein concentration exceeding the 1 mg/dl for each 1000/mm³ red blood cells normally occurring from blood alone.

Arteritides that may result in a hemorrhage include tuberculous arteritis and lupus erythematosus. An infrequently described amyloid angiopathy occurs in the cortex of nonhypertensive older patients and may result in a lobar hemorrhage.

CLINICAL MANIFESTATIONS. The clinical manifestations of an intracerebral hemorrhage are characterized by an abrupt onset, often said to develop during a period of activity rather than during rest. Headache is common at the onset. Seizures are infrequent, occurring in about 10% of patients. With a massive intracerebral hemorrhage, a loss of consciousness in the ictal period is common and the course is rapidly downhill, the intracerebral hematoma acting as a mass lesion and causing cerebral herniation. The neurologic deficit at onset depends on the location and amount of bleeding. Small hemorrhages in the cerebral hemisphere may mimic a cerebral infarction. Bleeding into the basal ganglia is associated with varying degrees of hemiparesis, hemisensory deficit, and homonymous hemianopsia. Conjugate deviation of the eyes toward the side of the lesion can be overcome by ice-water labyrinthine stimulation. If the hemorrhage is massive, bilateral pyramidal tract signs develop early, with respiratory irregularities and pupillary changes reflecting brainstem compression from herniation. Thalamic hemorrhages are commonly associated with medial and downward deviation of the eyes. Pontine hemorrhages are associated with a rapid loss of consciousness, flaccid quadriplegia, miotic but still reactive pupils, ocular bobbing, abnormalities of conjugate lateral gaze that persist during a doll's head (or eye) reflex and ice-water caloric testing, and at times hyperpyrexia. The patient with a cerebellar hemorrhage may have an occipital headache, gait ataxia, a paralysis of lateral gaze, seventh nerve palsy, and lateralized incoordination on the side of the hemorrhage. The patient's condition often progresses rapidly to coma and death as pressure causes further brainstem compromise.

The prognosis for a patient with a massive intracerebral hemorrhage is exceedingly grave. The mortality is 90%. Since the advent of CT scanning, smaller intracerebral and brainstem hemorrhages can be differentiated from infarctions, and the overall prognosis for patients with a cerebral hemorrhage is more optimistic than previously realized.

LABORATORY FINDINGS. Among the most important laboratory studies is the CT scan, which clearly shows the increased attenuation of acute intracerebral blood. MRI also demonstrates hemorrhage and, contrary to the CT scan, will do so for an indefinite period of time. The appearance of hemorrhage on MRI scanning varies depending on how much time has passed since the hemorrhage occurred, as well as on the imaging sequence. This is related to the different intensities created by the progressive conversion of oxyhemoglobin to deoxyhemoglobin, then to the paramagnetic substance methemoglobin, and finally to the appearance of hemosiderin-laden macrophages in the periphery of the hematoma. A lumbar puncture is unnecessary to document the bleeding, may introduce a danger of cerebral herniation, and may not detect deep noncommunicating bleeding in 15% of the cases.

MANAGEMENT. The treatment is mainly supportive. Dehydrating agents such as mannitol (0.25 to 1.5 g/kg body weight in a 20% solution given rapidly intravenously) may be tried for the prevention of herniation. Corticosteroids are commonly used (10 mg dexamethasone intravenously followed by 4 mg every 6 hours, tapering the dosage after 7 days) but are of questionable value for this disorder unless vasogenic edema is present. Surgical evacuation of large intracerebral hematomas has not proved generally beneficial with the exception of a hemorrhage in the cerebellum. The cerebellar hematoma is more accessible, and early surgical intervention, either the evacuation of the hematoma or the placement of an intraven-

tricular shunt, is essential. The intraventricular shunt is also of use when a cerebellar infarction is associated with local edema and increased intracranial pressure.

SUBARACHNOID HEMORRHAGE AND OTHER MANIFESTIONS OF VASCULAR ANOMALIES

Trauma is probably the most common cause of a subarachnoid hemorrhage. A spontaneous subarachnoid hemorrhage, however, which accounts for 5% of CVAs, is caused by a rupture of a berry aneurysm or an arteriovenous malformation directly into the subarachnoid space.

Aneurysms

BERRY ANEURYSMS. Berry aneurysms are believed to arise from areas of congenital weakness in the vessel wall at bifurcations of the major branches of the circle of Willis in the subarachnoid space. They usually do not appear in childhood, and only rarely do they produce neurologic signs by a local nonhemorrhagic compression of the adjacent structures (paralytic aneurysms). The occurrence of a spontaneous subarachnoid hemorrhage from a ruptured berry aneurysm correlates best with aneurysmal size, being most likely with aneurysms 1 cm or greater in diameter.

The majority of berry aneurysms are found on the anterior circle of Willis. They occur, for example, at the first major bifurcation of the middle cerebral artery, at the origin of the anterior cerebral artery, adjacent to the anterior communicating artery, and at the junction of the posterior communicating artery and the internal carotid artery. These posterior communicating aneurysms are commonly associated with signs of a third nerve palsy, including pupillary dilatation, ptosis, and extraocular palsies, because the third nerve is in close anatomic proximity.

FUSIFORM ANEURYSMS. Fusiform aneurysms appear to be dilatations of the entire circumference of a vessel for several centimeters, returning at each end to the vessel's normal caliber. These rarely rupture, although they may compress nearby structures. Most often patients with them are asymptomatic. Although they are commonly attributed to atherosclerosis and are more common in hypertensive patients, their presence in some younger patients has suggested a congenital abnormality.

CLINICAL MANIFESTATIONS. The initial clinical manifestation of a subarachnoid hemorrhage from a ruptured aneurysm is of sudden onset with a severe and commonly generalized headache that the patient may describe as feeling "like the top of my head is coming off." The initial bleeding is associated with sudden collapse and death in many instances. However, a patient coming to an emergency room with a severe headache from a subarachnoid hemorrhage may have no focal neurologic deficits during the clinical examination. Focal signs are present if the arterial bleeding also produces an intracerebral hemorrhage. Blood in the subarachnoid space also may be associated with cerebral vasospasm, which may produce ischemia with focal signs. The pressure of arterial bleeding directly into the subarachnoid space may produce preretinal subhyaloid hemorrhages (that appear as large, boat-shaped hemorrhages). Subhyaloid hemorrhages seen on the funduscopic examination suggest the diagnosis. Nuchal rigidity and Kernig's sign (restriction of straight leg raising as a result of meningeal irritation) are common.

LABORATORY FINDINGS. A diagnosis of a spontaneous subarachnoid hemorrhage can be suspected clinically and confirmed with either a CT scan, which may show subarachnoid blood in the first several days, or a lumbar puncture, which shows bloody CSF with a xanthochromic supernatant fluid in essentially all instances. A reliable method of distinguishing a subarachnoid hemorrhage from blood introduced into the CSF by a traumatic lumbar puncture is to compare an accurate count of red blood cells in the first and last tubes of fluid collected. The number should not decrease in the pathologic situations. The opening pressure is also likely to be elevated in a subarachnoid hemorrhage. Calcification in the wall of an aneurysm may allow it to be seen on plain skull roentgenograms or CT scans even before a subarachnoid hemorrhage. Cerebral angiography is commonly used to demonstrate the location of a cerebral aneurysm. More recently, aneurysms may be seen with MRI, and their patency or the presence of thrombosis within them, assessed. MRI does not demonstrate blood in the cerebrospinal fluid in acute subarachnoid hemorrhage. However, with massive subarachnoid hemorrhage from a ruptured berry aneurysm, localized clots may be demonstrable in the perianeurysmal area. Because berry aneurysms may be multiple, a complete angiographic study of the intracranial circulation usually is required before surgical intervention. At that time one should obtain appropriate roentgenograms of the kidney to look for commonly associated polycystic kidneys. Coarctation of the aorta may also be associated.

PROGNOSIS AND MANAGEMENT. A significant percentage of initial subarachnoid hemorrhages result in sudden death. Of those patients who survive, approximately 30% rehemorrhage within a 2-week period and again have a significant mortality. The preferred treatment for a patient who is a good candidate for surgery is one of a variety of techniques that attempt to clip the aneurysm or to decrease the blood flow through it. Experience shows that, despite the urgency, these procedures often are best deferred for a period of stabilization, usually from 10 days to 2 weeks, because cerebral vasospasm is common during this early period. During the stabilization period, blood-volume expansion is recommended.

Another complication of a subarachnoid hemorrhage is the development of a communicating hydrocephalus with ventricular enlargement, because the subarachnoid blood may obstruct the absorption of CSF. Normal pressure hydrocephalus may result, and shunt procedures may be required.

Arteriovenous malformations

Arteriovenous malformations (AVMs) are abnormal direct communications between the arterial and venous systems, occuring both within and on the surface of any portion of the central nervous system. These are congenital abnormalities in which venous channels contain blood under arterial pressure, so a rupture is a common problem. They account, however, for only 0.1% of cases of subarachnoid hemorrhage. The hemorrhage may occur at any time in life and may be associated with signs of a subarachnoid hemorrhage or with all the clinical manifestations of an intracerebral hemorrhage. Since a seizure disorder may be the initial symptom and may begin at any age, AVMs should be considered in the diagnostic evaluation of seizure problems. The patient may have a history of headaches. The abnormal shunting of blood is said to steal blood from other cerebral regions, producing ischemic symptoms on rare occasions.

AVMs may be associated with a cranial bruit, audible with the bell of the stethoscope applied to the skull. Calcification may be noted on skull roentgenograms or a CT scan. The CT scan with injection of contrast material may indicate the presence of an abnormal blood flow or a pooling of blood. Angiography is, however, often required for delineation. Small, ruptured AVMs may be so disrupted by a hemorrhage that they may not be detected even by an angiogram. At times, delayed or repeat studies, performed when the hemorrhage has resolved show a malformation not previously seen. More recently, MRI has proved invaluable in the diagnosis of arteriovenous malformations, since they can be imaged directly without the aid of contrast materials. Through MRI many more occult cerebrovascular malformations, such as the cavernous hemangioma (occult angioma), are being detected.

Treatment of AVMs is primarily surgical when they are accessible and is aimed at preventing a further hemorrhage after the initial episode of bleeding. Interventional roentgenographic techniques, with embolization or acrylic injections of the malformation, may be tried for nonresectable lesions.

Arteriovenous fistulas

Arteriovenous fistulas, which can occur between the internal carotid artery and the cavernous sinus (through which the artery passes), are most often caused by cranial trauma and basilar skull fracture, although they can occur spontaneously or develop from rupture of aneurysms. Blood enters the venous system under high pressure, resulting in proptosis, chemosis, blindness, extraocular muscle palsies, and a local cranial bruit.

SPINAL CORD HEMORRHAGE

A spinal cord hemorrhage may be subarachnoid or intramedullary. A primary spinal cord subarachnoid hemorrhage is an infrequent occurrence and is caused most often by a ruptured spinal AVM. Back pain is common and headache, mimicking that of a ruptured intracranial berry aneurysm, may occur as blood circulates in the subarachnoid space. Intramedullary hemorrhage (hematomyelia) may also occur as a result of an AVM, trauma, or blood dyscrasia, with the patient having severe back pain and sudden paraplegia.

The diagnosis of spinal AVM is difficult to make, and these lesions are often mistaken for herniated discs or spinal tumors. There is nothing absolutely characteristic about their natural history, which is often that of progressive spinal cord disease, thought possibly to be caused by compression. Less often there is a sudden onset caused by a subarachnoid or intramedullary hemorrhage. Progression followed by regression and repeated subsequent events is common. Pain, weakness (with combined upper and lower motor neuron signs), sensory deficits, and early micturition difficulties are frequent. Males are affected more often than females. Symptoms may occasionally vary with posture, exercise, and the menstrual cycle.

The majority of lesions occur in the midthoracic and lower thoracic and thoracolumbar cord, and their length can be extensive. Occasionally cutaneous angiomas are present on the back, making it possible to localize the spinal AVM to the same segment. Less often an audible bruit may be heard over the spine, defining an otherwise undiagnosed myelopathy. The CSF is commonly but nonspecifically abnormal. Laboratory investigation includes spinal MRI and may require performing roentgenographic contrast studies such as myelography (with a visualization of the posterior surface of the cord) or arteriography for a definitive diagnosis. The surgical excision of some localized AVMs is possible.

VENOUS THROMBOSIS

A thrombosis may occur in the cortical veins or in any of the dural venous channels draining blood into the internal jugular veins, such as the superior sagittal, transverse, or cavernous sinuses. Infection is a common predisposing cause, as with underlying chronic otitis media, mastoiditis, or cellulitis of the face or neck, and it is associated with dehydration, cachexia, congestive heart failure, shock, and sepsis. Other associations include the postpartum or postoperative period, debilitation, thrombocytopenia, cryofibrinogenemia, disseminated intravascular coagulation, hemolytic anemia, paroxysmal nocturnal hemoglobinuria, leukemia, diabetic ketoacidosis, ulcerative colitis, polycythemia, or sickle cell disease. The use of oral contraceptives may be a predisposing factor. A tumor may also invade the venous sinuses.

The patient's initial symptoms vary with the site of the thrombosis, but headache, increased intracranial pressure, and seizures are not uncommon. Papilledema may be present. With a thrombosis of the sagittal sinus the patient has intracranial hypertension resulting from an obstruction of CSF reabsorption and may have jacksonian seizures. Motor weakness may be greater in the legs than in the arms, and either a lower extremity monoparesis or a paraparesis may develop. With a thrombosis of the cavernous sinus and an obstruction of the ophthalmic veins the patient has proptosis, chemosis, and frequent involvement of the third, fourth, and sixth cranial nerves (resulting in ophthalmoplegia) and the sympathetic nerves that also traverse this sinus. Focal features including seizures are characteristic of a primary cortical vein thrombosis.

Pathologic findings include various combinations of infarction, hemorrhage, and associated cerebral edema. In regard to diagnostic studies, MRI is extremely helpful in venous occlusive disease, demonstrating a lack of the usual flow void in the venous sinuses and hyperintensity (methemoglobin) in the intraluminal clot in the subacute phase. A prolonged serial cerebral angiogram has not been needed since the advent of MRI. A CT scan without the injection of contrast material may show a dense sinus early and with the injection of contrast material may demonstrate the so-called delta sign, in which a triangular filling defect is visible in the sagittal sinus. The treatment of a venous thrombosis is directed at any known infection, and anticoagulation is often considered when a hemorrhage is not demonstrated by a CT scan or lumbar puncture. Fever and peripheral leukocytosis are indications for a lumbar puncture to exclude meningitis if the CT scan does not show an intracranial mass effect.

HYPERTENSIVE ENCEPHALOPATHY

(See Chapter 87.)

Infrequently the systemic blood pressure may rise to an extent that overcomes the ability of the cerebral arterioles to maintain the cerebral blood flow within a normal range. With this breakdown in autoregulation, cerebral edema develops and multiple small infarctions and petechial hemorrhages occur. This situation is seen in patients with severe malignant hypertension, acute glomerulonephritis, and eclampsia.

Clinically the patient with hypertensive encephalopathy has severe hypertension, headache, vomiting, confusion, obtundation, and often seizures. The course is subacute and can be reversed dramatically by appropriate antihypertensive therapy. Hypertensive retinopathy is usually present, and papilledema is common. The CSF pressure is elevated, and the protein levels may be high. Focal signs may be found, in which case care must be taken to determine whether a cerebral infarction has occurred. This differentiation is particularly important because a marked lowering of the blood pressure is contraindicated in an infarction with its associated disturbance of autoregulation.

UNCOMMON VASCULAR DISEASES OF THE CENTRAL NERVOUS SYSTEM

Arteritis caused by collagen-vascular disease can result in infarction and less frequently in hemorrhage. The collagen disorder most commonly implicated is lupus erythematosus, in which the central nervous system signs may be the patient's initial problem. Polyarteritis nodosa also, but less frequently, involves the cerebral vessels. Determination of the erythrocyte sedimentation rate (ESR) is a valuable screening test for collagen disorders. Cerebral angiography may show evidence of arteritic changes in the cerebral vessels.

In the older patient, temporal arteritis, a giant cell arteritis affecting the cranial vessels and associated with polymyalgia rheumatica, may result in headache, occlusion of retinal arteries, and occasionally cerebral infarction. The ESR is significantly elevated in temporal arteritis. Cerebral angiography may show evidence of arteritic changes in the superficial temporal artery and scattered areas of involvement in other branches of the external carotid artery. The intracranial cerebral arteries are rarely involved by the pathologic process, although the vertebral arteries and the cavernous portion of the internal carotid arteries may be affected. If temporal arteritis is suspected, a biopsy of a lengthy portion of the superficial temporal artery may establish the diagnosis, and corticosteroid therapy is urgently warranted, particularly to prevent blindness.

A giant cell arteritis described originally in young Oriental women is known at Takayasu's disease or pulseless disease. This disorder affects major branches of the aortic arch with, for example, carotid and subclavian artery stenosis, and may produce cerebral infarction. The sedimentation rate is increased in this disorder. Patients may have cataracts and retinal atrophy.

Granulomatous arteritis involves the small and medium-sized cerebral vessels, may have an autoimmune basis, and at least in some instances may be related to infection with herpes zoster ophthalmicus. The CSF in granulomatous arteritis shows a moderate mononuclear pleocytosis and an elevation of the total protein concentration, frequently exceeding 100 mg/dl. Women are affected somewhat more commonly than men, and the disorder may occur at any age with the majority of patients being affected in the fifth to eighth decades of life. A leptomeningeal biopsy should be considered before therapy with prednisone if the diagnosis is obscure.

Inflammatory changes in the cerebral blood vessel walls may occur with a variety of meningeal infections. In meningovascular lues, a secondary form of syphilis, the cerebral blood vessels in the subarachnoid space are affected by meningitis. This is reflected by the meningeal response noted in the CSF, with pleocytosis and an elevated total protein concentration.

Mucormycosis is an opportunistic fungal disease. The fungus gains access to the central nervous system through the nose and sinuses in debilitated diabetic patients and those with blood dyscrasias, causing cerebral thromboses. Pyogenic and tuberculous arteritides occur infrequently, and other rare causes of infarction are typhus, schistosomiasis, falciparum malaria, and trichinosis.

The term "vasospasm" should be avoided except in specific situations. Vasospasm does occur in the presence of a subarachnoid hemorrhage. It is *not* a cause of transient cerebral ischemia, with the exception of the vasoconstrictive phase of migraine headaches. During this vasoconstrictive phase the patient may have a variety of focal signs, including visual field defects and unilateral motor and sensory deficits, the so-called hemiplegic migraine. On a rare occasion such deficits may not reverse and may result in an infarction. Platelet hyperaggregability may contribute to a thrombosis in patients with migraine headaches.

Fibromuscular dysplasia is an infrequent nonatheromatous vascular disorder involving an intimal and medial fibroplasia of the extracranial internal carotid and vertebral arteries, as well as other large systemic vessels such as the renal arteries.

Cerebral angiography shows a beaded appearance of the vessel caused by segmental sections of narrowing alternating with areas of dilatation. The intracranial arteries are usually not involved. This disorder is far more common in women than in men, and its cause is poorly understood. It is most often discovered as an incidental angiographic abnormality, and occasional symptoms of progressive cerebral ischemia may warrant the use of anticoagulants, vascular bypass surgery, endarterectomy, or intraarterial dilation.

Mitral valve prolapse (see Chapter 94) caused by a myxomatous degeneration is a common cardiac disorder that may account at times for the development of cerebral platelet-fibrin emboli.

Atrial myxomas are tumors of endothelial or subendothelial origin with myxoid degenerative changes. These tumors arise most often from the left side of the heart's atrial septum, but they also may be present on the right side or in the ventricles. They most commonly occur in the middle years of life, with cardiac, systemic, and embolic effects. The patient may have a recent history of the rapid development of heart failure, weight loss, fatigue, and fever. An embolus from an atrial myxoma should be suspected in any patient with a cerebral embolus who has a normal sinus rhythm and no evidence of bacterial endocarditis. On auscultation of the heart the findings of rheumatic mitral valve disease may be suggested, or a characteristic tumor plop may be detected. There may be a variability in the auscultatory findings with position change on different examinations. The histologic characteristics of the embolus can be useful in making the diagnosis.

The more definitive diagnostic tests include two-dimensional ultrasonic cardiac imaging and angiocardiography. A long-term neurologic follow-up is warranted after myxoma removal because there may be a delayed invasion of a previously embolized vessel wall leading to aneurysm formation or metastatic tumor growth.

Homocystinuria (see Chapter 195) is an inborn error of metabolism in which there is an increased incidence of arterial and venous thrombosis. Other stigmata such as a Marfan's-like appearance and dislocated ocular lenses should suggest this diagnosis. Other features include generalized osteoporosis, mental retardation, and bony abnormalities such as scoliosis and chest deformity. The diagnosis can be substantiated by urinary testing for homocystine and by measuring a low level of cystathionine synthetase in a skin tissue culture or a liver biopsy specimen.

Various hematologic disorders have been associated with cerebrovascular disease. Hyperviscosity syndromes associated with other systemic diseases may result in small vessel occlusion and multiple areas of infarction or hemorrhage. Various neoplasms may be associated with disseminated intravascular coagulation and cerebral infarction. In polycythemia the increased blood viscosity may predispose the patient to cerebral arterial thrombosis, venous thrombosis, and small hemorrhages. A venous sinus thrombosis may occur, and the retinal veins may become occluded. Sickle cell disease should be suspected in young black patients who have had multiple episodes of neurologic disturbance. In sickle cell disease, dural sinus thrombosis and cerebral arterial or venous occlusion may occur. There may be an associated hemorrhage. A vasculopathy occurs in sickle cell disease, involving arterial vessels in the anterior part of the circle of Willis. Repeated transfusions aimed at keeping hemoglobin S levels below 30% can decrease the incidence of recurrent CVA.

Patients with thrombotic thrombocytopenic purpura have a characteristic triad of thrombocytopenic purpura, hemolytic anemia, and neurologic symptoms; the neurologic symptoms may be the first manifestation or the main manifestation. Patients may have alterations in mentation, seizures, and focal neurologic deficits. The small cerebral vessels show hyperplasia and platelet thrombi. The treatment of this disorder is generally unsatisfactory.

An association with pregnancy or the postpartum period is noted in approximately 35% of young women with a CVA in the carotid system. Researchers speculate that known alterations of clotting factors in pregnancy such as a decrease in fibrinolysins and an increase in fibrinogen, as well as other clotting factors, may be significant. Venous sinus thrombosis and cortical vein thrombosis are associated with both the postpartum period and the use of oral contraceptives. Consumptive coagulopathies resulting in a CVA have been reported with abruptio placentae, septic abortion, intrauterine fetal death, amniotic fluid embolism, uterine rupture, saline abortion, hydatidiform mole, placenta accreta, transfusion reaction, eclampsia, and severe preeclampsia. The low platelet count is the single most important finding in the diagnosis of a consumptive coagulopathy complicating one of these gynecologic situations. Thrombotic thrombocytopenic purpura occurs with increased frequency during pregnancy, and the renal dysfunction with hematuria and proteinuria may suggest the diagnosis of eclampsia.

The association of oral contraceptives with an increased risk of CVA appears well established. Several multiinstitutional controlled studies have noted that women who use oral contraceptives have a significantly increased relative risk of a thrombotic CVA and a lesser risk of a hemorrhagic CVA. The risks are increased with age and hypertension. Smoking is a risk factor for hemorrhage; preparations higher in estrogen and probably progestin content are associated with a greater risk of thrombosis.

Moyamoya disease is a condition in which there are occlusions of one or more cerebral vessels in and around the circle of Willis with the development of a telangiectatic network in the lenticulostriate and thalamoperforating arteries. This telangiectatic network acts as a source of collateral circulation to circumvent the occluded vessels and has the angiographic appearance of a haze or a puff of smoke. The Japanese name "moyamoya" is derived from this description. A rete mirabile is also commonly seen, which is a transdural anastomotic network of small vessels between the external and internal carotid arterial branches. This was originally described as a syndrome in young Orientals, but a similar syndrome may occur in children and in some adults with a slowly progressive occlusive disease of the circle of Willis from any cause. Both cerebral infarction and hemorrhage may occur. Cerebral angiography is necessary to establish this diagnosis.

BIBLIOGRAPHY

Buonanno F and Toole JF: Management of patients with established ("completed") cerebral infarction, Stroke 12:7, 1981.

Committee on Cerebro-Vascular Disease: A classification and outline of cerebrovascular diseases II, Stroke 6:565, 1975.

Easton JD and Sherman DG: Management of cerebral embolism of cardiac origin, Stroke 11:433, 1980.

Gomori JM and others: Intracranial hematomas: imaging by high-field MR, Radiology 157:87, 1985.

Gomori JM and others: Occult cerebral vascular malformations: high field MR imaging, Radiology 158:707, 1986.

Grotta JC: Medical progress: current medical and surgical therapy for cerebrovascular disease, N Engl J Med 317:1505, 1987.

Oral contraception and increased risk of cerebral ischemia or thrombosis, N Engl J Med 288:871, 1973.

Sundt TM Jr and Whisnant J: Subarachnoid hemorrhage from intracranial aneurysms, surgical management and natural history of disease, N Engl J Med 299:116, 1978.

153 · EFFECTS OF PRIMARY AND METASTATIC TUMORS ON THE CENTRAL NERVOUS SYSTEM, AND PSEUDOTUMOR CEREBRI

Gary Rea *and* **George Paulson**

BRAIN TUMORS

Brain tumors include both malignant and benign space-occupying lesions. These tumors produce symptoms by local destruction, by irritating surrounding structures, and by producing increased intracranial pressure. The term "benign" generally refers to tissue type, but unfortunately, benign tumors may be lethal ultimately because of their location and the inability to remove them completely and safely. Brain tumors may be found in patients of any age group and in any part of the central nervous system (CNS) or its surrounding structures. Growth rates vary but range from the explosive growth of glioblastomas to the desultory and almost imperceptible changes of some meningiomas. To understand and predict the effect of a tumor on a patient, the histopathology, location, signs, and symptoms of that neoplasm must be known.

CLASSIFICATION AND PATHOLOGY. Tumor taxonomy for the primary neoplasms is traditionally based on the presumed cell of origin, often with specific comments or titles reflecting regional and anatomic factors. The taxonomy often seems confused, and there may be uncertainty regarding the cell of origin or only an indefinite linkage of the cell type with the prognosis for an individual case. The location of the tumor may be as relevant as the cell type. Some neoplasms, for example, a pinealoma, originate from specific areas, in this case the pineal gland; classification reflects origin. The vast majority of CNS tumors arise from glial cells (astrocytomas grade I to IV, oligodendrogliomas, and ependymomas), the leptomeninges (meningiomas), Schwann cells (Schwannomas), ganglion cells (medulloblastomas), embryonal cell remnants (dermoids, teratomas, and craniopharyngiomas), or metastatic deposits.

Astrocytic tumors originate from the astrocytes and can be partially defined by location (for example, a cerebellar astrocytoma). Astrocytic neoplasms are the most common of the primary tumors (40% to 50%), and the group includes several cell types that represent a transformation of the normal stellate astrocytes into a more fibroblastic appearance. Cavities or pseudocysts may form, and some astrocytomas may become more malignant with time. Astrocytomas are graded histologically from I to IV; grade I suggests a relatively slow-growing neoplasm.

The astrocytoma grade IV, also called glioblastoma multiforme, is the most anaplastic and malignant form. The tissue reveals evidence of marked dedifferentiation. In glioblastoma multiforme the nuclear/cytoplasmic ratio is increased and mitoses are common, with prominent cellular necrosis and changes in the surrounding blood supply. Frequently, more than one lobe of the brain is involved. Glioblastomas are the most common gliomas, with a peak incidence in the productive fifth and sixth decades of life. They are not completely resectable, and death usually occurs within 18 months. Between grades I and IV there are numerous astrocytic variants, and differences in the clinical state depend largely on the tumor's location in the brain.

The astrocytic neoplasms of the cerebellum deserve particular note when discussing the importance of tumor location. Patients with astrocytomas may have classic cerebellar symptoms, morning vomiting, and cranial nerve signs (particularly involving the sixth cranial nerve). The tumor is often cystic with a tumor nodule in the cyst wall. Unlike patients with cerebral astrocytomas, in patients with cerebellar astrocytomas, surgery, and adjunctive therapy can lead to prolonged survival and, in the cystic tumors, a total remission. The pontine astrocytoma, which is common in childhood, responds poorly to radiation therapy and cannot be removed surgically.

The oligodendroglioma originates from oligodendroglial cells and is composed of small, round cells with spherical nuclei. It usually evolves slowly and often can be detected on a routine skull roentgenogram because intracranial calcification may occur. The clinical pattern of an oligodendroglioma is indistinguishable from that of a benign astrocytoma and reflects the tumor location. Surgery can be curative, or the disease may continue for decades.

Ependymal cell tumors include the ependymomas, choroid plexus papillomas, and, according to some pathologists, colloid cysts. Microscopically, ependymomas can be identified by their characteristic formation of rosettes. These tumors originate from the walls of the ventricular system, usually occur in children, and may invade CNS tissue or obstruct the ventricles. They can be treated surgically and with radiation therapy but are rarely cured. Death usually occurs within 5 to 7 years. Unlike the ependymomas, the choroid plexus papillomas and the colloid cysts do not invade tissue. They produce symptoms by exerting local pressure on surrounding neural elements or by causing hydrocephalus. For example, a patient with a colloid cyst of the third ventricle, which at times blocks the foramen of Monro, can have hydrocephalus, variable confusion, and intermittent headache. Choroid plexus papillomas and colloid cysts can be totally removed surgically, although this is sometimes difficult.

Tumors that arise from the meninges assume an importance beyond their incidence because of their insidious onset and their potential for total removal. These meningiomas grow slowly but can be exceedingly vascular, and removal is not always possible when the tumor has invaded critical structures. They include several cell types, and differences in prognosis may be postulated on the basis of the cellular variety. The cells are often uniform and may form characteristic whorls. The meningiomas, along with cholesteatoma and metastatic disease, often affect the skull. Although they are histologically benign, meningiomas may involve structures such as the cavernous sinus, the carotid artery, the cranial nerves, the brainstem, or the sagittal sinus, so they cannot always be completely removed. In these cases a significant debulking may allow the patient long-term relief of symptoms.

Tumors arising from Schwann cells develop in association with the cranial nerves, most commonly with the eighth nerve. The fifth, ninth, and tenth cranial nerves are much less frequently involved. These benign tumors are well encapsulated. The symptoms they produce depend on their location. For example, an acoustic neuroma can cause not only tinnitus and hearing loss, but also signs of pressure on the seventh or fifth cranial nerves or even cerebellar symptoms resulting from pressure on nearby pathways. Depending on their size and involvement of surrounding elements, tumors occurring secondary to Schwann cells can be surgically cured.

If the histologic pattern of the cerebellar tumor is that of a medulloblastoma, it is considered to have developed from a primitive cell in the cerebellum. In a child the midline signs of truncal ataxia and vomiting may be the initial symptoms of medulloblastoma, and later the nerve roots may also be involved because these tumors often seed along the spinal canal. Medulloblastomas cannot be cured by surgery, radiation, or chemotherapy, but with aggressive treatment the patient may survive longer than 5 years.

Some tumors seem congenital and by their natural history invoke the concept of "cell rests." Examples are the giant cell astrocytoma or gemistocytic astrocytoma of tuberous sclerosis and the colloid cyst in the area of the foramen of Monro. In these conditions abnormal cells have presumably been present since birth but begin to grow in early adolescence. The tumors linked with von Recklinghausen's disease include acoustic neuroma and fibromas on the nerve roots or on the peripheral nerves. Granulomas, chromaffin-cell tumors, or tumors of vascular origin are rare enough to be only an infrequent consideration. Occasionally tumors are seen that are even more obviously congenital than the astrocytomas of tuberous sclerosis. Dermoid tumors and teratomas, for example, can be found in the midline posteriorly or at the base of the skull and may include evidence of primitive cell types.

Metastatic disease is one of the most frequent causes of brain tumor in adults. The most common sources of metastatic disease are lung tumors in men and breast tumors in women. Intracranial metastases occur most often with headaches, seizures, and sometimes focal neurologic deficits. The metastatic tumors may be multiple or solitary, and in favorable locations some transient benefit may follow removal of the solitary lesions. Otherwise the treatment of intracranial metastases is radiation therapy and chemotherapy. Patients with tumors at the base of the skull may have face pain or numbness. Nasopharyngeal growths, which include carcinoma, can be difficult to diagnose, but roentgenograms of the base of the skull or computed tomographic (CT) scans can be helpful. Some patients require a nasopharyngeal biopsy.

Other intracranial masses occur in addition to the brain tumors just reviewed. An abscess may have the same symptoms as a tumor. Abscesses can be characterized both by the systemic symptoms such as fever and by increased pressure, but they may be indistinguishable from neoplasia until surgery is performed. Young patients with subdural hematomas may have focal weakness and headache, but an aged patient may only remain in bed with no local signs apparent.

In meningeal carcinomatosis a diffuse infiltration of the meninges by tumor cells takes place. Pleocytosis, a low value for cerebrospinal fluid (CSF) glucose, and an elevated value for protein in CSF are common in these patients. The syndrome may be overlooked when the presence of generalized cancer is unknown. Patients may have cranial nerve signs such as facial numbness or diplopia, back pain, neck ache, or the infiltrating sheets of cancer cells can produce generalized weakness with areflexia in the legs. The treatment of meningeal carcinomatosis consists of irradiation of the region of maximal involvement, as well as intrathecal chemotherapy.

PATHOPHYSIOLOGY. The skull is filled with incompressible substances, and a tumor may produce effects by an increase in pressure, by regional edema, or by destroying tissue. Regardless of the pathologic type, the location of the tumor is of great importance. Supratentorial tumors often involve the motor or sensory systems, and many patients have seizures. A substantial percentage of patients have an adult onset of seizures as the initial manifestation of an infiltrative tumor. The traditional triad of papilledema, projectile vomiting, and headache occurs late in the course of the disease and results from the increased intracranial pressure. The diagnosis is usually possible before this stage, and in modern medicine few patients are seen with this triad as the initial clinical manifestation of a supratentorial tumor. Instead, focal seizures in an adult, changes in mental function, dull, inexplicable headaches, and a slowly progressive weakness may be among the first recognizable features. It is not recognized sufficiently that tumors may fluctuate in their manifestations through partial and abortive seizures, small hemorrhages, shifts in intracerebral pressure, or vascular involvement. Some patients seem to have transient ischemic attacks, although a neoplasm is eventually discovered. The memory can be defective, particularly when the frontal or temporal lobes are involved. Extracerebral structures such as the first cranial nerve can be involved when meningiomas are present, and these more slowly growing tumors often have few initial signs. Glioblastomas, on the other hand, are likely to begin with changes over a matter of weeks or months, and commonly the patient is obviously ill when first seen.

Infratentorial tumors are much more subtle in their effect and are relatively more common in childhood when the history is more difficult to obtain. When the cerebellopontine angle is involved, as in adult acoustic neuroma, the patient shows cerebellar dysfunction, difficulty with hearing and with the vestibular system, or complex disturbances in eye movements. Pressure on the sixth cranial nerve may produce diplopia.

Hydrocephalus, the dilatation of the ventricular system by the obstruction of CSF pathways, can result from tumors. It may occur independent of a neoplasm, for example, with congenital aqueductal stenosis, even during adult life. Hydrocephalus following the obstruction of the subarachnoid space by blood or a previous meningitis can produce a mixed clinical picture, with an initial improvement after the insult and then late deterioration. Signs of hydrocephalus include leg weakness or spasticity, presumably resulting from stretching of the long periventricular fibers arising from the parasagittal region, or symptoms of increased intracranial pressure plus a generalized cerebral dysfunction.

SYMPTOMS THAT SIGNAL THE POSSIBILITY OF TUMOR

Progressive focal neurologic disturbance. Whereas cerebrovascular disease can have a stepwise or stuttering onset, a sudden catastrophic insult, or a transient defect with a complete recovery, the brain tumor commonly has a more insidious onset. Punctuated by gradually increasing weakness, by a subtle sensory loss, or by adult-onset seizures that are not always relieved by medications, the progressive nature of the decline from a tumor generally becomes obvious when the history is adequate. Often the findings and the complaints are less obvious for patients with a tumor than for patients with cerebrovascular accidents (CVAs) or degenerative disease.

Mentation. A personality change and an insidious decrease in mentation may occur. Frontal lobe disease in particular is associated with striking behavior changes, including facetiousness or inappropriate comments. Depression, or the appearance of a loss of joy of life, is common with brain tumors, and a few patients with infiltrative tumors may have a striking deficit in their memory or judgment.

Onset of seizures in adult life. The onset of seizures in adult life always raises the specter of a tumor unless alcoholism or another logical explanation is readily apparent. Even when the diagnostic workup does not document a tumor, a follow-up may reveal a more ominous diagnosis later. The patient who most needs an evaluation and a follow-up by a neurologic specialist is the patient who has unexplained seizures beginning in adulthood.

Change in the character of headaches. Many patients with vascular headache have repetitive headaches throughout their life with a diminution in the middle years, whereas patients with brain tumors may have persistent, steady, or intractable dull pain rather than intermittent severe episodes. Consistently unilateral pain, or a pain that changes in character for a few weeks, suggests a need for an additional workup. Intermittent sharp pains in the head or the face as with tic douloureux and dull facial pains are only rarely associated with tumors, and then more often with growths at the base of the skull than with growths in the brain. Stress-induced headaches (for example, pain resulting from cough, sneeze, or strain, and even repetitive headache that results from routine exercise) may require a more intensive evaluation for a tumor than is necessary for nonspecific headaches. This is particularly true if the headache is severe and persistently triggered by exercise or cough and even more so if the pain is unilateral. A dull headache that occurs in the morning seems to be more common with tumors than a headache that occurs at other times of the day. The headache caused by a brain tumor may respond to aspirin.

Signs and symptoms of increased intracranial pressure. Besides local symptoms produced by tumor, there are signs and symptoms caused solely by the diffuse increase in intracranial pressure. The classic triad suggesting this increase in intracranial pressure includes headache, vomiting, and papilledema. Further symptoms reflect the effects of pressure on vital centers in the diencephalon and the hindbrain and damage to the cranial nerves. With the compression of the third nerve by the herniation of the uncus of the temporal lobe over the tentorial edge, the pupil dilates and may not react reflexly by constriction to light, and eventually the lid droops. In many instances mydriasis is a late sign, and pupillary dilation resulting from increased intracranial pressure is often an indication that something should have been done already to reduce the pressure. Because 10% of normal people have slightly unequal pupils, a minimal asymmetry in pupil size is often irrelevant. Although not every dilated pupil implies an increase in intracranial pressure, dilation, especially with an impaired pupillary reflex and decreasing consciousness, remains a time-honored and valuable sign of an impending cerebral herniation. The cerebellar tonsils may herniate through the foramen magnum, and such a herniation may produce a stiff neck or a tilting of the head caused both by the reflex tonic neck responses and by the conscious efforts of the patient to prevent pain whenever the neck is flexed. With these patients a search for papilledema is desirable, but papilledema is not present in every patient with increased intracranial pressure. A loss of venous pulsations at the optic disc is usual with markedly increased pressure, but some unaffected people have retinal venous pulsations that are difficult to see, and a few patients have no visible pulsations

even when the CSF pressure is normal. A loss of previously observed pulsations can, however, signify a recent increase in pressure. In the assessment of increased pressure it is often a change from the result of the previous examination that is of the greatest consequence.

Unfortunately, occasional patients, particularly if their changes have developed slowly, may have almost no signs of increased intracranial pressure until the disease is in a dangerously late stage. Most neurologists have seen patients in whom papilledema was an incidental finding or in whom the only complaint was diplopia caused by third nerve pressure, or patients with repetitive morning vomiting followed by an abrupt herniation. The clinician must remain alert to detect this kind of patient, who is often potentially treatable. There is no substitute for informed clinical suspicion to detect a cerebral herniation.

In some instances, such as benign intracranial hypertension (pseudotumor cerebri) or lead encephalopathy, there is increased pressure in the absence of a tumor.

DIFFERENTIAL DIAGNOSIS. CVAs are likely to have a different temporal pattern than a brain tumor, although either can sometimes have a stepwise or episodic onset. Patients with brain tumors occasionally have a sudden deterioration in function of the CNS, particularly if there is a change in pressure, a seizure, or a hemorrhage into the tumor, but sudden changes are more typical of vascular disease. Patients with subdural hematomas can have moderate hemiparesis and headache, but they can also have only apathy and an apparently depressed state with few other symptoms. Fortunately, the current techniques of CT and MRI can distinguish subdural hematomas from brain tumors. Multiple sclerosis, particularly when its course lacks classic remissions and exacerbations, can be confused with a brain tumor, and a brain tumor at the base of the skull or in the area of the foramen magnum can be falsely labeled as a case of multiple sclerosis. When in doubt the physician should perform ancillary diagnostic techniques. Dementia of the type seen in Alzheimer's disease often leads to an evaluation to rule out a tumor of the frontal or temporal lobe. The severe cortical dementia with intact motor and sensory systems that is so characteristic of Alzheimer's disease is in fact uncommon with brain tumors. Brain tumors often affect mentation but rarely lead to severe dementia in early stages. Patients with Alzheimer's disease may have profound memory deficits with intact social graces and no motor or sensory deficits. As mentioned earlier, for the diagnosis of a brain tumor, lesser and more subtle signs can be particularly significant. Extreme dementia is more common in patients with Alzheimer's disease than in patients with a brain tumor; complete hemiparesis is more common in CVAs than in brain tumors; and severe ataxia is more commonly seen with a degeneration of the cerebellum than with brain tumors. Epilepsy can be an initial complaint of patients with brain tumors and deserves a detailed evaluation and a close follow-up. In some cases only time may clarify the diagnosis. With abscesses the clinical manifestations can resemble those of a subacute tumor, and the diagnosis may be apparent only during surgery. In fact an abscess is a "tumor" in the sense of swelling, and it may manifest any of the clinical features of neoplastic disease. Meningeal infections and tumors of the CNS are rarely confused. But unfortunately, tonsillar herniation from a tumor can lead to a stiff neck just as with meningitis. The differentiation is imperative, since diagnosis of meningitis requires a spinal tap, whereas a lumbar puncture in a patient with tonsillar herniation can be fatal.

LABORATORY FINDINGS. Skull roentgenograms are usually performed when increased pressure is suspected so that an erosion of the posterior clinoid processes may be viewed. An erosion of the posterior clinoid processes or the presence of intracranial calcifications may confirm the need for further laboratory studies. However, plain roentgenograms are of little benefit in detecting a brain tumor as a rule, and in fact a chest roentgenogram to look for a primary lung tumor or metastatic disease is more valuable. On the other hand, CT has revolutionized the management of patients in whom a brain tumor is suspected. This test is especially useful with contrast enhancement to identify the presence of the more vascular tumors. Changes in ventricle size and shifts of the midline structures also are readily apparent with CT. Radioisotope scanning is useful for the detection of infections such as herpes simplex encephalitis, and even for abscess. Both isotope and CT scans can often detect a tumor when the patient is first seen. The appearance of a lesion with an infarction may be anatomically more consistent with the distribution of a major vessel and, although possibly normal immediately after a major CVA, within a week is usually positive. The most recent advance in neuroradiologic imaging is magnetic resonance imaging (MRI). Based on the reaction of hydrogen protons in a strong magnetic field, it can give more anatomic detail than the CT scan. MRI is sensitive to changes in water content; thus the cerebral edema is highly visible. Because of MRI's ability to produce sagittal images, it also gives improved views of spinal cord tumors. Electroencephalography is still a desirable test, particularly because it is a harmless screening technique. Slow-growing tumors may produce no change in the electroencephalogram (EEG) or may result in focal epileptic discharges. Rapidly developing tumors and abscesses generate marked focal slowing in the EEG. With increased intracranial pressure, rhythmic, periodic, and high-voltage slowing may be noted, particularly frontally. Examination of CSF for protein and cytologic analysis is of value in selected cases, but a lumbar puncture is not usually necessary and may be harmful to patients with rapidly growing tumors. In the presence of a mass, downward herniation may occur when pressure is suddenly reduced from below. If increased pressure is discovered inadvertently during a lumbar puncture, the immediate use of antiedema agents such as steroids or mannitol should be considered and the patient must be monitored carefully. The fluid available in the manometer should be studied even though the additional amount removed must be limited. The purposes of performing the lumbar puncture should be met and cultures should be obtained as needed, since the problems after a lumbar puncture in this situation appear to be related to the further flow of CSF from the sustained subarachnoid puncture site and not the CSF removed for study.

MANAGEMENT. Surgical therapy for brain tumors depends on the type of lesion and its location, and ranges from decompression for the palliation of headaches to total removal. Cases must be considered individually, and even in the therapy for metastatic tumors each patient deserves careful evaluation to avoid fruitless surgery or nihilistic neglect. Although total surgical removal is currently the best hope for curing tumors of the CNS, the use of debulking surgical procedures, adjunctive radiation therapy, and chemotherapy can prolong the life of patients with unresectable neoplasms. Radiation treatment to multifocal, intracranial neoplasms is the treatment of choice after a tissue diagnosis is made. A new technique that combines the therapeutic effectiveness of local irradiation on rapidly dividing neoplastic cells with the anatomic imaging capability of either MRI or CT scan is being evaluated. This brachytherapy consists of stereotactically placing highly radioactive seeds into the tumor for short periods. Brachytherapy may obviate the need for craniotomy and perhaps for whole brain irradiation. A variety of other chemotherapeutic and immunotherapeutic approaches are also being evaluated for brain tumor treatment and are being compared to current surgical therapy. The future value of these modalities requires further investigation.

In addition to treatment that is directed at the tumor itself, patients who have brain tumors often require anticonvulsants, antiedema agents such as steroids, and aggressive pain control agents. Their families should not be neglected, since they are dealing not only with the specter of death, but also with possible alteration in the patient's personality. Support groups can be helpful in this area.

The management of tumors or of a new growth of the skull is similar to that of any other bony structure, and in fact the skull often is surgically more accessible than other bony areas. With the exception of a massive thickening such as with Paget's disease, the intracranial contents usually are not affected by an overgrowth of bone. The cranial nerves are impinged on in some cases, and if the outflow tracts for the CSF are compromised in the foramen magnum area by thickened bone or meninges, hydrocephalus can result.

Patients with tumors of the pituitary gland often have a hormone imbalance and disturbances in their visual fields. These tumors may require a combination of surgical, radiation, and endocrinologic management. Pituitary microadenomas can be detected with high-resolution CT scans. These small tumors produce endocrinologic symptoms without neurologic signs. They may be treated medically (for example, with bromocriptine) or surgically.

NEUROLOGIC COMPLICATIONS OF CANCER THERAPY

It is increasingly apparent that necrosis resulting from radiation occurs in the brain tissue and its supportive tissues and that the late effects of radiation can be extremely insidious in onset. Vulnerability to the effects of radiation varies from person to person, and the precise limits of therapy are uncertain, but any patient whose brain receives more than 4000 rad may have secondary effects. It seems likely that chemotherapy has an additive effect. Radiation-induced spinal cord lesions are particularly common after therapy for pulmonary or breast lesions. Brown-Séquard syndrome, spasticity, and a moderate elevation in CSF protein concentration are among the clinical observations in these cases. No useful therapy exists for radiation-induced changes in the CNS, but steroids may slow the progressive course of what seems to represent not only a deterioration of neural tissue but also scarring and a breakdown in the local blood supply to the nerve tissue. At times radiation effects may even appear as a tumorous swelling and may require surgery for adequate diagnosis. Whenever there is a recurrence of symptoms in an area of previous radiation therapy, the possibility of radiation-induced symptoms must be considered.

Almost all chemotherapeutic agents are potentially neurotoxic when used in large doses. The most common toxic effect from these chemicals is a peripheral neuropathy with paresthesias, weakness, and sensory loss. The paresthesias reflect the type and amount of drug used, as well as the duration of the therapy. The use of vincristine in particular is almost universally associated with some degree of neuropathy. Intrathecal injections of methotrexate may cause catastrophic generalized weakness, paresthesias, or severe cerebral irritation. Periventricular gliosis also can result from using intrathecal injections of methotrexate, which is nevertheless often the best available agent to treat meningeal carcinomatosis.

EFFECTS OF REMOTE TUMORS ON THE NERVOUS SYSTEM

The nervous system can react to the presence of a tumor in numerous ways, and immunologic or toxic factors associated with a tumor are difficult to separate from the direct effects of local metastases. Nevertheless, in some patients who have no local metastasis a cerebellar syndrome develops, with a slowly progressive deterioration in balance and coordination. A few patients without a focal spread of the cancer have combined muscle and nerve disease (neuropathy and myopathy) that appears as paresthesias, sensory loss, and a weakness in the proximal musculature. Classic polymyositis can also be linked to a tumor, again without any obvious metastatic nodules in the muscle. These entities may be mixed in complex clinical patterns and can be confused at times with the overlapping and direct effects from metastatic foci. For example, in rare cases a mild dementia may be linked to the presence of a tumor outside the brain, although an unrecognized depression or a local metastatis is a more common explanation for the mental change with neoplasia. The syndrome of a remote effect of cancer, particularly the sensory neuropathies, is most often seen with carcinoma of the lung, but cancer of the breast, ovary, or stomach also is associated with remote effects on the central nervous system. The syndrome of inappropriate antidiuretic hormone (ADH) secretion also is reported secondary to carcinoma and appears in the usual fashion with usually only a mild hyponatremia.

Another paraneoplastic syndrome is the tendency in the late stage of carcinoma, particularly after treatment with radiation therapy or chemotherapy, for a patient to have superimposed infections. These infections may consist of an easily recognized bacterial meningitis, but in addition, subtle fungal infection such as with *Cryptococcus* often are noted in patients with neoplasia. The involvement of the brain tissue by the papovavirus in the syndrome of progressive multifocal leukoencephalopathy (occurring primarily in patients with leukemia, lymphoma, or immunosuppression) produces mental deterioration, motor deterioration, and death within weeks.

PSEUDOTUMOR CEREBRI, OR BENIGN INTRACRANIAL HYPERTENSION

Pseudotumor cerebri, or benign intracranial hypertension, involves increased intracranial pressure in the absence of an intracranial mass lesion, obstructive hydrocephalus, meningitis, hypertensive encephalopathy, or any other demonstrable structural lesion. The patient has an intractable headache and papilledema associated with a measurable increase in intracranial pressure but is alert and nonsomnolent and has no focal neurologic signs, in contrast to the patient with a lesion. The patient may have a sixth nerve palsy. The major physical threat posed by pseudotumor cerebri is a potential decrease in visual acuity or a defect in the visual fields, so these clinical signs must be carefully monitored. Pseudotumor cerebri may occasionally appear without papilledema. The syndrome is more common in women than in men, and although it can occur at any age, it has a peak age incidence in the third decade of life.

Although the pathogenesis of pseudotumor cerebri is not formulated well, this disease is found in association with a number of other disorders, including Addison's disease, steroid treatment or withdrawal, pregnancy, the use of oral contraceptives, hypoparathyroidism, hypervitaminosis A, hypovitaminosis A, the administration of drugs (tetracycline, nalidixic acid, or the phenothiazines), the time of the menarche or the menopause, and commonly in young obese women with menstrual irregularities. The increased intracranial pressure associated with a thrombosis of the venous sinuses is often included as a cause of benign intracranial hypertension. This form is known as otitic hydrocephalus because of an association with otitis media in some cases, although hydrocephalus is not present.

The differential diagnosis of pseudotumor cerebri includes considering midline ventricular tumors, tumors of the nondominant, silent frontal lobe, malignant hypertension with retinopathy, and variations of the optic fundi (pseudopapilledema).

The definitive diagnostic tests for pseudotumor cerebri include a CT scan to exclude a mass lesion and a lumbar puncture to record the pressure and also to eliminate the possibility of a chronic meningeal process such as sarcoid or fungal meningitis by an analysis of the CSF. The CT reveals small or normal-sized ventricles without a shift in their location, and without any focal abnormality. The CSF should be normal.

The treatment of an uncomplicated pseudotumor cerebri includes using diuretics (for example, furosemide, 40 mg four times a day, or acetazolamide, 500 mg twice a day) and weight reduction when appropriate. Repeated lumbar puncture with the removal of CSF is often recommended. Steroids (dexamethasone, 16 mg daily in a divided dosage, or prednisone, 60 to 80 mg a day for short courses) are used. Immediate and aggressive surgical treatment such as a lumboperitoneal shunting of CSF, and rarely a subtemporal decompression, should be considered when the patient's vision is threatened. Although pseudotumor cerebri is considered a relatively self-limited condition, chronic elevations of CSF pressure are described and patients may have acute recurrences.

BIBLIOGRAPHY

Armstrong RM: Effects upon the nervous system from remote tumors. In Goldensohn ES and Appel SH, editors: Scientific approaches to clinical neurology, vol I, Philadelphia, 1977, Lea & Febiger.

Burger PC and Vogel FS: Surgical pathology of the nervous system and its coverings, New York, 1976, John Wiley & Sons Inc.

Wilkins R and Rengarchary S, editors: Neurosurgery, vol 3, New York, 1985, McGraw-Hill Inc.

154 · NUTRITIONAL DISORDERS OF THE NERVOUS SYSTEM

Stanley R. Schiff*

Vitamins, which are important cofactors for enzyme function, are required for the normal metabolism of nerve tissue. In the early 1900s investigators noted characteristic neurologic syndromes associated with diets that are deficient in unique elements. The most common nutrition disorders of the nervous system are caused by vitamin deficiencies, often by deficiencies of the B complex vitamins. The clinical manifestations of vitamin deficiencies can be variable because many patients have multiple deficiencies of varying degrees and the lack of even one vitamin may adversely affect the use of others. The vitamin

*Material in this chapter is based in part on the first edition, written by David P. Dunn.

deficits produce an abnormal metabolism and eventual structural defects. For complex and often poorly understood reasons, multiple levels of the neuraxis are involved in these disorders, often in highly specific ways. Deficiencies are apt to arise as the result of many situations such as fad diets, starvation, malabsorption problems, antagonism by drugs, neoplasia, and other debilitating disease. In North America a nutritional disorder of the nervous system most commonly occurs when a chronic alcoholic forsakes a normal diet. In addition, some suggest that alcohol may interfere with gastrointestinal absorption of various vitamins including thiamine.

BERIBERI (NUTRITIONAL POLYNEUROPATHY)

DEFINITION. Beriberi results from thiamine-poor diets. It is a subacutely evolving, symmetric polyneuropathy involving the distal peripheral nerves, with sensory symptoms predominating.

ETIOLOGY AND PATHOGENESIS. Beriberi is usually associated with a subsistence diet of thiamine-deficient rice, but it also has occurred in Western populations during famines. Although emphasis is placed on the lack of thiamine in alcoholic polyneuropathy and many patients respond to administration of thiamine, most alcoholic nutritional neuropathies are found in patients who have a mixed deficiency state. The cell bodies of the motor and sensory neurons are affected metabolically, resulting in an axonal degeneration that involves the distal parts of the neurons.

CLINICAL MANIFESTATIONS AND COURSE. Clinical manifestations include sensory deficits, muscle weakness, and atrophy that are more prominent in the legs than in the arms, start in the distal regions of the legs, and progress proximally and symmetrically. Symptoms (for example, numbness, paresthesia, dysesthesia) are out of proportion to the objective findings. Diverse sensory symptoms begin insidiously in the feet and calves. Patients complain of numbness, coldness, pain, aches, burning sensations, a "dead" sensation in the feet, and just not feeling right. One patient complained of a sensation that felt "like a thousand ants with cold and hot feet marching around" his legs. As the disease progresses, the hands may become similarly affected. The involved areas are often extremely tender, and even the pressure of bedsheets can cause pain. Stroking the sole of the foot can feel like a hot knife to patients, almost causing them to leap from the bed. Eventually a complete sensory loss may develop in a stocking and glove distribution. Muscle numbness and atrophy usually occur later in this disease. Weakness ranges from slight to so severe that the patient cannot stand or walk. As the disease progresses, the muscle weakness increases. The deep tendon reflexes, especially the ankle jerks, disappear early in the course of the disease.

LABORATORY FINDINGS. Underlying causes of malnutrition such as malabsorption must be evaluated with the appropriate laboratory tests. Nerve conduction velocities may be preserved in nutritional neuropathies, as opposed to other common neuropathies in which the myelin sheath around the axon is primarily involved.

DIAGNOSIS AND MANAGEMENT. The diagnosis of neuropathy may be suggested by the patient's history, but it is confirmed by neurologic findings during a clinical examination. An accurate history is essential to identify the cause more specifically as a nutritional deficit related to alcoholism or to eliminate other possible causes of neuropathy. The possibility of toxins found in illegally distilled liquor causing or contributing to a neuropathy should be kept in mind. Treatment consists of abstinence from alcohol, vitamin therapy (especially

with B complex vitamins), and a nutritious diet. The use of other drugs that interfere with the metabolism of vitamins should be carefully evaluated. The carbohydrate load found in some intravenous solutions can precipitate further problems in a patient who is thiamine deficient.

WERNICKE'S ENCEPHALOPATHY AND KORSAKOFF'S PSYCHOSIS

DEFINITION. Wernicke's encephalopathy is an acutely evolving disease manifest as confusion, a wide-based stumbling walk (gait ataxia), and disturbances of eye movement, among which involuntary oscillations (nystagmus) are the most common. Korsakoff's psychosis, primarily a disturbance of the ability to form new memories, frequently evolves in the course of the disease and is usually resistant to treatment. The patient has a loss of recent memory with the rest of the cognitive functions left intact. The overwhelming majority of patients with this combination are chronic alcoholics.

ETIOLOGY AND PATHOGENESIS. Vitamin B_1 deficiency is central to the production of this syndrome. Ingested thiamine is phosphorylated to form the coenzyme cocarboxylase, which is essential in energy-producing pathways of carbohydrate metabolism. Cocarboxylase is necessary to the activity of the enzyme pyruvate decarboxylase in the initial reaction of the tricarboxylic acid cycle and to the function of the enzyme transketolase in the hexose monophosphate shunt. Exactly how the metabolic abnormalities produce the various lesions in this disorder is unknown. Presumably those regions of the brain that have the most enzyme activity at risk are the most involved. Some patients have a genetic abnormality of transketolase. With a normal diet such a patient has no problems, but when the diet is thiamine deficient, the disease develops. It is important to always give thiamine to guard against the possible precipitation of Wernicke's encephalopathy whenever glucose is administered to an alcoholic or comatose patient. It can take as little as 7 weeks for thiamine reserves to be exhausted in alcoholism. Tissue necrosis and blood vessel changes are produced in the hypothalamus, especially the mammillary bodies, the central gray matter of the brainstem, and the thalamus. Atrophy occurs in the cerebellum. The abnormalities of the eye movements are caused by the brainstem lesions, the gait ataxia is caused by the cerebellar atrophy, and the memory defects have been linked to the involvement of the thalamus.

CLINICAL MANIFESTATIONS AND COURSE. Although nystagmus is the most common ocular manifestation, the eye muscles that cause each eye to move laterally, the lateral recti, are often partially or completely paralyzed. The patient may be unable to move the eyes conjugately up and down and horizontally. When thiamine is administered, the eye abnormalities may start to improve in a matter of hours. Nystagmus may be a permanent sequela. The gait ataxia does not improve as quickly as do the ocular manifestations, and often the improvement is incomplete. The disorder of mentation initially consists of a quiet state of disorientation, memory loss, apathy, decreased concentration, and misperceptions of people and objects, described as the global confusional state. Some patients have delirium tremens in which agitation, hallucinations, and tremors are prominent.

Treatment may reverse all the mental changes. The persistence of a memory loss as the other signs return to normal indicates the presence of Korsakoff's psychosis. The patient cannot remember recent events but retains older pieces of information. When patients cannot remember an object or a number after 5 minutes, they have difficulty learning new information. Confabulation is often used to fill in the gaps of information. One patient, when asked where he was in the morning, although actually in the hospital, responded with a detailed description of the boarding house where he had lived for several years. The reponse of the memory loss to thiamine is poor. Most patients do not recover completely, and the intellectual deficits persist to varying degrees.

The majority of patients have an associated nutritional polyneuropathy and a plethora of other diseases. Death can occur after treatment has started and is probably related to the severity of the lesions in the brainstem.

LABORATORY FINDINGS. Laboratory findings include increased levels of blood pyruvate, but the increase is not specific for this disorder. The blood transketolase assay is the preferred test. The activity of transketolase is markedly decreased when thiamine is deficient.

DIAGNOSIS AND MANAGEMENT. The clinical manifestations in a malnourished alcoholic patient should lead to a correct diagnosis. Laboratory tests and the response to thiamine can confirm the diagnosis. Treatment includes immediate parenteral administration of 100 mg of thiamine. This dosage should be continued daily in the acute phase of the disease. Rapid administration of thiamine can lead to resolution of the syndrome within 2 to 5 hours, and may prevent the development of Korsakoff's psychosis. Once developed, its response to thiamine is much less evident. Other associated diseases must be sought and treated. Because of the general nutritional depletion, these patients require more than just thiamine replacement, and both a good diet and multivitamin therapy must be instituted.

NUTRITIONAL AMBLYOPIA

Nutritional amblyopia, a characteristic type of amblyopia (decreased vision), is found in undernourished individuals. The patient complains of a slowly progressive, usually bilateral, visual loss for close work or reading. An examination of the central visual fields reveals decreased vision corresponding to the point of fixation or extending from it to the blind spot (central scotoma or centrocecal scotoma). The peripheral vision is intact, and unless the disease is far advanced, the optic nerve appears normal. The amblyopia is caused by the involvement of the papillomacular bundle, which carries the nerve fibers for central vision. No single vitamin deficiency is implicated as the cause of this disorder. In the past tobacco and alcohol were suggested as causal agents, but a good diet and vitamin B therapy result in the return of vision even with the continuation of smoking and drinking. Amblyopia is found in association with other vitamin deficiency syndromes and is present in undernourished patients who did not use alcohol and tobacco. Strachan syndrome is a disorder characterized by amblyopia, painful neuropathy, and orogenital dermatitis. It has been found in malnourished populations in tropical countries and in prisoners of war confined in the Far East and Middle East during World War II.

PELLAGRA

The prevalence of pellagra, which includes cutaneous, alimentary, and neurologic symptoms, has greatly diminished since niacin enrichment of bread became a general practice in 1940. In North America the disease is still seen in alcoholics. The neurologic symptoms can begin with subtle mental change, including insomnia, nervousness, fatigue, and depression. The cerebral symptoms can progress to an acute confusional psychosis.

Niacin deficiency, pellagra, can cause a wide spectrum of neurologic deficits in the central nervous system. Mental change is an early symptom; the patient may appear anxious, confused, and even frankly psychotic. Without treatment the brain damage may result in a permanent dementia. A weaknss of the legs and a loss of position sense in the feet with resulting unsteadiness in walking are indicative of the spinal cord involvement, which clinically mimics vitamin B_{12} deficiency. Peripheral nerve abnormalities are less common and may be caused by associated vitamin deficits and protein deficits. Niacin deficiency first causes the neurons to swell, but if it is persistent, they eventually disintegrate. Niacin therapy reverses the neurologic defects, but because other concurrent deficiencies are common, B complex vitamins should also be given.

CEREBELLAR CORTICAL DEGENERATION

Although cerebellar cortical degeneration is usually found in chronic alcoholic patients, it has occurred in nonalcoholic patients with severe malnutrition. The anterior superior cortex of the cerebellar vermis, the central region of the cerebellum, becomes atrophic with a selective loss of Purkinje cells. This regional atrophy causes gait ataxia. The anterior lobes of the lateral hemispheres may be involved, but not as much as the vermis. Thiamine is essential to some of the nerve cell transmitters in the cerebellum. The role of the other nutritional factors and their relation to thiamine are unknown. A transient cerebellar syndrome, responsive to thiamine, has been described and presumably represents a stage of reversible biochemical abnormality that precedes the pathologic lesion in the course of the disease.

VITAMIN B_{12} DEFICIENCY (PERNICIOUS ANEMIA)

(See Chapter 148.)

The most commonly recognized neurologic defect in vitamin B_{12} deficiency is a demyelination of the posterior and lateral columns of the spinal cord, known as subacute combined degeneration (SCD). Less commonly recognized is the cerebral involvement producing a progressive dementia. The peripheral and optic nerves can be demyelinated. Usually the neurologic manifestations are concurrent with pernicious anemia. It must be strongly emphasized, however, that the neurologic manifestations can be present in the absence of anemia. There is usually a disorder of vitamin B_{12} absorption. In addition to patients who have a lack of gastric intrinsic factor, those who have had a gastrectomy, disease of the gastric tract, a dietary deficiency (in strict vegetarians), and rare genetic disorders of vitamin B_{12} transport of proteins and enzymes can have a failure of vitamin absorption as a sequela. Abuse of nitrous oxide is reported to produce both the hematologic and neurologic manifestations of vitamin B_{12} deficiency.

SCD starts with numbness and tingling in the toes and fingers followed by an unstable gait and stance. Position sense is lost in the feet. The deep tendon reflexes are lost when the fibers of the reflex arc are damaged in the cord. Babinski's sign (upgoing great toe on stroking the sole of the foot) reflects the lateral column involvement that eventually causes muscle weakness. Dementia can be mild or severe depending on the tissue damage in the cerebrum. Some loss of pain distally in the extremities indicates a neuropathy. The Schilling test is often required for diagnosis, since as many as 25% of patients may have normal serum B_{12} levels (see Chapter 148). Cyanocobalamin therapy may reverse the deficits completely depending on the severity of the disease. Treatment (see Chapter 61) should begin immediately after vitamin B_{12} blood levels are determined, since complete recovery is possible in mild cases. The Schilling test results are not altered by exogenously administered vitamin B_{12}. Neurologic recovery is slow and often progressive for 1 year. Continued intramuscular administration of vitamin B_{12} is needed for life in cases of pernicious anemia.

BIBLIOGRAPHY

Victor M, Adams RD, and Collins GH: The Wernicke/Korsakoff syndrome, Philadelphia, 1971, FA Davis Co.

155·PROBLEMS OF NERVE AND MUSCLE

Hiroshi Mitsumoto *and* Theodore L. Munsat

STRUCTURE AND FUNCTION

Anterior horn cells (α motor neurons) are located in the anterior horn gray matter of the spinal cord (Fig. 155-1). Their motor axons leave the spinal cord via the anterior roots, form large mixed peripheral nerves with other motor and sensory axons, and finally reach the innervated muscle through the independent motor nerves. The anterior horn cell and the totality of muscle fibers innervated by it are called a motor unit. The synaptic region between the nerve and the muscle is the neuromuscular junction. At this synapse acetylcholine is released from the presynaptic motor terminal and initiates the excitation-contraction events.

Muscle contraction is monitored by the muscle spindles (intrafusal fibers) and the Golgi tendon organs through large sensory fibers. These sensory fibers return to the spinal cord through the posterior roots. Their cell bodies are located in the dorsal root ganglion. Cutaneous sensation is transmitted by small sensory fibers. Voluntary and involuntary control of muscle contraction is mediated by pyramidal and extrapyramidal systems in the central nervous system (CNS). The muscle fiber is a long, cylindric, syncytial cell connected to a tendon at each end. It contains numerous myofibrils running parallel to the muscle fiber. Myofibrils are composed of regularly oriented repeating units, sarcomeres, which appear histologically as cross-striations and consist of a series of alternating dark (A) and light (I) bands containing the fundamental contractile proteins. The I band consists of thin myofilaments, which contain actin and which penetrate the A band as well. The A band consists of the thick filaments, which contain myosin, in addition to the ends of the thin filaments. When muscle fibers contract isotonically, thin filaments on either side of the A band move toward each other, between thick filaments. Thus the I band, the sarcomeres, and the total length of the muscle shorten by the interdigitation of these contractile elements.

The contraction is triggered by calcium ions released from the sarcoplasmic reticulum, an intracellular cistern that stores calcium and is adjacent to the myofibrils. At the neuromuscular junction acetylcholine molecules are released from the presynaptic motor terminal and reach the receptor site of the postsynaptic membrane, resulting in a depolarization of the sarcolemma. The depolarization is rapidly transmitted to the entire muscle fiber through a tubular (T) system that is a direct extension of the outer sarcolemma. The T system makes contact with the sarcoplasmic reticulum at the A-I band junction, forming a so-called triad. Calcium ions are then resequestered into the sarcoplasmic reticulum, and the contraction is ended.

There are basically two fiber types in human muscle, present in roughly equal proportions. Each human skeletal muscle is composed of random admixtures of both fiber types. The type I fibers have high oxidative activity and are slow-twitch fibers physiologically. The type II fibers have low oxidative capac-

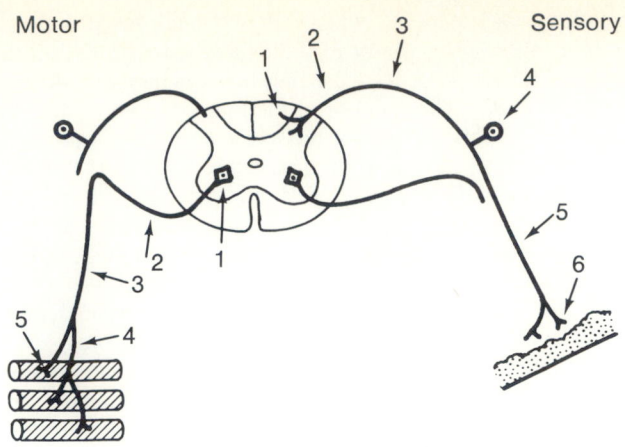

Fig. 155-1   Motor system: *1*, anterior horn cells; *2*, anterior root; *3*, peripheral nerve; *4*, motor nerve terminal; *5*, neuromuscular junction. Sensory system: *1*, posterior horn and posterior column, *2*, root entry zone; *3*, posterior root; *4*, dorsal root ganglion; *5*, peripheral nerve; *6*, sensory nerve terminal (cutaneous). (From Bradley W G: Disorders of peripheral nerves, Oxford, 1974, Blackwell Scientific Publications.)

ity and high anaerobic activity and are fast-twitch fibers physiologically.

SIGNS AND SYMPTOMS

Weakness is the cardinal manifestation of neuromuscular disorders. It can occur in any muscle group such as the limb, trunk, ocular, swallowing, or respiratory muscles. Weakness involving primarily proximal muscles is seen in myopathies. A characteristic maneuver of using the arms on the thighs while arising from the floor (Gowers' sign) is typically seen in Duchenne-type muscular dystrophy. Vertebral column alterations are common in advanced neuromuscular disorders that begin in childhood. Increased lumbar lordosis is often seen in the ambulatory child with Duchenne-type muscular dystrophy. Specific distributions of muscle weakness and atrophy are seen in certain neuromuscular disorders such as peroneal atrophy, facioscapulohumeral muscular dystrophy, and limb-girdle muscular dystrophy. Increased muscle size in a weak muscle is known as pseudohypertrophy and is particularly characteristic of Duchenne-type muscular dystrophy. Fasciculations are visible, discrete, rapid, spontaneous muscle twitches typically seen in motor neuron diseases. Muscle tone is generally decreased in myopathies and neuropathies but is increased in amyotrophic lateral sclerosis (ALS). The deep tendon reflexes are lost early in neuropathies and late in myopathies. Muscle contracture is a common sequela of unused muscle in advanced neuromuscular disorders, especially myopathies. Aches, cramps, and pains may be an early complaint in neuromuscular disorders. Sensory symptoms such as numbness and paresthesias are manifestations of peripheral (sensory) neuropathies. Graded loss of sensation in the distal part of the extremities (stocking and glove distribution) is typical of peripheral neuropathies. Sensory loss in the distribution of a specific single peripheral nerve is seen in a mononeuropathy. Loss of pain, touch, and temperature sense is a result of small sensory fiber involvement, whereas loss of vibration and position sense is a result of large sensory fiber involvement.

PATHOPHYSIOLOGY
Pathology

Investigating morphologic changes is of prime importance for the correct diagnosis of neuromuscular disorders. The tissue must be properly processed and interpreted, however, by an experienced neuromuscular morphologist.

The pathologic changes of muscle basically consist of those resulting from denervation in which muscle fibers undergo atrophy, at times in groups, and myopathies in which muscle fibers undergo random degeneration and often regeneration. Certain myopathies can be diagnosed correctly only with histochemical techniques that involve processing muscle quick-frozen at the time of the biopsy. A small piece of frozen muscle specimen is also used for biochemical diagnosis of specific enzyme deficiency myopathies.

Electrophysiology

The measurement of nerve conduction velocities (NCVs) of individual peripheral nerves and the needle electrode examination of muscle (electromyography, EMG) provide valuable pathophysiologic data on neuromuscular disorders. NCVs are normal in myopathies but are impaired in many neuropathies. When the myelin sheath surrounding the axon is damaged (demyelinating neuropathies), nerve conduction is markedly delayed in contrast to nerve conduction in axonal neuropathies, which is not delayed as regularly or to the same degree. The loss of nerve fibers (axonal neuropathies) results in markedly diminished or even absent evoked potentials in sensory nerve fibers (sensory neuropathies) and motor fibers (motor neuropathies).

In disorders of nerve and muscle the EMG may demonstrate changes in the motor unit potentials, alterations in the recruitment of motor units on increased voluntary contraction, and spontaneous muscle fiber activities at rest (whereas a normal EMG is entirely silent when the tested muscle is at rest). In myopathies, motor unit potentials are decreased in amplitude and are polyphasic because of the scattered loss of muscle fibers. In active denervation, as seen in acute and subacute axonal motor neuropathies, the remaining motor units may be normal. In chronic motor neuropathies, however, they become polyphasic, broadened, and of high amplitude because of reinnervation. Recruitment is prominent and rapid with low-level voluntary muscle contraction in myopathies but is diminished in neuropathies. A normal EMG is entirely silent when the muscle is at rest. Spontaneous fibrillation potentials and positive waves occur at rest in active denervation and in some necrotizing myopathies. Spontaneous fasciculations are most often present in motor neuron disease. Myotonic discharge sounding like a racing car when the audio is amplified represents muscle membrane instability and is characteristic of the myotonic disorders. The function of the neuromuscular junction can be studied by the repetitive stimulation of a motor nerve at various rates and by recording the motor response.

Clinical enzymology

Serum enzymes such as creatine kinase (CK), lactic dehydrogenase (LDH), serum glutamic-oxaloacetic transaminase (SGOT), and aldolase have increased levels in necrotizing myopathies, particularly in Duchenne-type muscular dystrophy, polymyositis, and muscle necrosis associated with myoglobinuria. These sarcoplasmic enzymes are released from the muscle cells because of necrosis or leakage through the sarcolemma. In denervated muscle CK is generally normal but may occasionally be mildly elevated. The level of CK elevation helps differentiate Duchenne-type muscular dystrophy, when it is high, from other myopathies of young children. A study of CK isoenzymes can detect their origin (that is, muscle, heart, or brain). The CK enzyme level is sometimes markedly elevated after physical exertion, particularly in those with neuromuscular disorders. Thus CK level should be measured after reasonable rest for at least a day.

PERIPHERAL NEUROPATHIES
Nutritional deficiencies

ALCOHOLIC NEUROPATHY. Alcoholic neuropathy is one of the most common neuropathies. Clinically, the patient has a painful and predominantly sensory symmetric polyneuropathy that may have a subacute or chronic course. Paresthesias of the feet are often disturbing, and in advanced cases motor impairment with footdrop prevents successful ambulation. It is generally believed that alcoholic neuropathy is caused by nutritional deficiency. However, recent evidence suggests that alcohol itself may be neurotoxic. Vitamin replacement therapy rarely results in complete recovery.

VITAMIN B$_{12}$ DEFICIENCY (PERNICIOUS ANEMIA). (See Chapters 61, 148, and 154.) Vitamin B$_{12}$ deficiency affects the nervous system at several levels. Cerebral involvement results in dementia, spinal cord damage results in defective motor and sensory pathways (combined system disease), and peripheral nerve damage causes a symmetric motor and sensory neuropathy with prominent paresthesias. There is often a marked loss of vibration and position sense with upper motor neuron signs such as spasticity and increased reflexes. Folic acid therapy may improve the hematologic findings, but the neurologic manifestations continue or may even worsen. Vitamin B$_{12}$ should be given parenterally. This often results in a dramatic improvement within a few days.

OTHER NUTRITIONAL POLYNEUROPATHIES. Other nutritional polyneuropathies occur with pyridoxine and niacin deficiency. A peripheral neuropathy may also occur with the malabsorption syndrome.

Toxic and metabolic neuropathies

HEAVY METALS. Acute arsenic poisoning causes a rapidly progressive polyneuropathy and an acute encephalopathy. In more chronic arsenic toxicity a mixed sensory-motor peripheral neuropathy develops. The nails may show white transverse lines (Mees' lines). Lead poisoning typically results in a pure motor neuropathy in the arms. Radial nerve palsy is common. Lead encephalopathy is common in children and rare in adults. Toxic levels of arsenic are best detected in the hair or nails, and toxic levels of lead are best detected in the serum and urine. These neuropathies are potentially reversible depending on the degree of damage. The source of toxic exposure should of course be eliminated. Dimercaprol treatment is used for both arsenic and lead poisoning. Penicillamine is particularly effective for the treatment of lead neuropathy.

ORGANIC COMPOUNDS. Various organic solvents, insecticides, and herbicides are neurotoxic. Triorthocresylphosphate and acrylamide may produce a mixed sensory-motor polyneuropathy. The pathologic changes are primarily those of axonal damage. These neuropathies are usually associated with industrial or accidental exposures. Glue sniffing (n-hexane) can result in a severe axonal neuropathy.

DRUG-INDUCED NEUROPATHIES. Anticonvulsants (phenytoin), chemotherapeutic agents (isoniazid, nitrofurantoin), and antineoplastic drugs (vinca alkaloids, cisplatin, nitrogen mustard) may produce a chronic mixed sensory-motor neuropathy. Vitamin B$_6$ (pyridoxine) should always be given with isoniazid therapy because isoniazid interferes with pyridoxine metabolism. A severely painful, predominantly sensory polyneuropathy along with myelopathy is reported with the recreational abuse of nitrous oxide. Cases of nitrous oxide neuropathy are found among dentists and dental technicians who abuse nitrous oxide.

Megavitamin B₆. Massive vitamin B_6 consumption (a daily oral intake of 1 g or more for more than 2 months) may cause a painful, purely sensory polyneuropathy. Those who develop vitamin B_6 toxic neuropathy usually consume an unusually large amount of other vitamins and health food supplements. As little as 150 mg/day is reported to cause this neuropathy. EMG shows an axonal sensory polyneuropathy. The neuropathy usually resolves slowly after vitamin B_6 is discontinued.

DIABETIC NEUROPATHY. Diabetes mellitus is one of the most common causes of neuropathy. Although its presentation may vary greatly, there are three main clinical presentations. The first is a distal, symmetric, predominantly sensory neuropathy that is primarily demyelinating. The pathogenesis of this diffuse symmetric polyneuropathy is not clear. However, possibilities include a direct effect of hyperglycemia on the peripheral nerves, a hyperglycemia-induced depeletion of myoinositol resulting in increased metabolism of the sorbitol pathway, and a diffuse microangiopathy. Although the true incidence of diabetic neuropathy is not known, approximately 5% of all diabetic patients have a significant clinical neuropathy. A larger number have electrophysiologic abnormalities. The damage is greater with poorly controlled diabetes of long duration. Thus it is generally believed that better diabetic control leads to a better prognosis of diabetic neuropathy. Second, there may be proximal acute mononeuropathies (in the form of lumbosacral radiculoplexopathy) characterized by a painful motor deficit. An occlusion of the vasa nervorum is probably the cause of this form of neuropathy. These diabetic mononeuropathies are generally self-limited, and the symptoms disappear slowly in most cases. Finally, autonomic neuropathy is the least common type but may be disturbing to the patient. Impotence in males, diarrhea, and orthostatic hypotension are a result of autonomic dysfunction.

UREMIC NEUROPATHIES. Patients with chronic renal disease often have a predominantly sensory axonal polyneuropathy characterized by burning paresthesias. This neuropathy may develop or worsen in patients undergoing hemodialysis, although hemodialysis usually results in a modest benefit. Renal transplantation is usually beneficial. Objective neurologic improvement is often delayed many months. The pathogenesis remains uncertain.

ACUTE INTERMITTENT PORPHYRIA. Acute intermittent porphyria is a dominantly inherited metabolic disorder that is associated with decreased levels of urobilinogen I synthetase. It results in a proximal sensory-motor polyneuropathy, prominent emotional disturbances, constipation, abdominal pain, nausea, and vomiting. The neuropathy is of an axonal type. Acute attacks may be precipitated by barbiturates, alcohol, and sulfonamides. Acute attacks of porphyric neuropathies can be treated with intravenously administered hematin.

OTHER METABOLIC NEUROPATHIES. Chronic mixed sensory-motor polyneuropathies occur in certain patients with hepatic cirrhosis, serum hepatitis, hypothyroidism, and hypoglycemia.

Systemic disorders

POLYARTERITIS NODOSA. Of all patients with polyarteritis nodosa, 20% to 30% have peripheral nerve lesions, usually appearing as an acute mononeuritis multiplex. Necrotizing vasculitis involves the nutrient vessels of individual large nerves, resulting in actual nerve infarction. Later in the course of the disease, after many individual nerves have been damaged, the clinical manifestation is a distal symmetric sensory-motor neu-

ropathy. In this case, small blood vessels in the epineurium are involved. Muscle biopsy is also helpful in making the diagnosis. The neuropathy of polyarteritis nodosa responds poorly to corticosteroid therapy and requires more aggressive immunosuppressive therapy.

RHEUMATOID NEUROPATHY. Patients with seropositive rheumatoid arthritis commonly manifest four types of neuropathy. Acute lesions of the major nerves of the upper and lower extremities comprise about 40% of all rheumatoid neuropathies. These lesions result from nerve compression by joint effusion or osteophytes. The lateral popliteal nerve at the fibular head is a common site. Local corticosteroid injection or surgical decompression is the preferred treatment. The second type of neuropathy is an occlusion of the small digital arteries resulting in a digital neuropathy manifest as distal sensory loss in one finger. A distal symmetric sensory polyneuropathy of insidious onset is also seen, but less frequently. Distal symmetric mixed sensory-motor neuropathy is the least common type of the rheumatoid neuropathies. This type is usually more severe and has a poor prognosis. Immunologically mediated arteritis is the cause of this diffuse neuropathy, and it is usually found in nerve or muscle biopsies.

SYSTEMIC LUPUS ERYTHEMATOSUS. In systemic lupus erythematosus peripheral nerve lesions are relatively uncommon. A diffuse neuropathy may occur and a vascular occlusion of the vasa nervorum may produce a mononeuritis multiplex.

MONOCLONAL GAMMOPATHY. Chronic polyneuropathies associated with paraproteinemia (plasma cell dyscrasia) occur in patients with Waldenström's macroglobulinemia, lymphoproliferative disorders, multiple myeloma, or osteosclerotic myeloma. Recent studies indicate that as many as 10% of patients with chronic polyneuropathy of undetermined cause may have abnormal serum proteins. The usual clinical presentation is a chronic mixed sensory-motor polyneuropathy. In some patients, antibodies reacting against nerve fibers are identified. Patients with IgM-K monoclonal proteins, which react against a myelin antigen called myelin-associated glycoprotein (MAG), may develop a unique demyelinating neuropathy characterized by widening and separation of myelin lamellae visible with electron microscope examination. However, in most polyneuropathies associated with paraproteinemia, the pathologic process is less clear. Some neuropathies are predominantly axonal, whereas others are predominantly demyelinating. Cryoglobulins, which precipitate in serum at low temperatures, are associated with painful sensory-motor polyneuropathy with or without a detectable underlying disorder. In this neuropathy, immune deposits are found in small nerve vessels. Perineurial inflammation (perineuritis) or true vasculitis is seen in neuropathy associated with cryoglobulin. A search for such monoclonal gammopathy is important in patients with idiopathic polyneuropathies. Although treatment depends on the nature of the paraproteinemia, corticosteroids and antineoplastic drugs are useful. Plasma exchange may have a beneficial effect.

PRIMARY AMYLOIDOSIS. (See Chapter 76.) Sporadic primary amyloidosis is characterized by light chain—immunoglobulin deposits, whereas familial amyloidosis has prealbumin deposits in the tissue. Polyneuropathy occurs in only 10% of sporadic primary amyloidosis but much more frequently in the familial forms. Three main types of familial amyloidosis have been described: the Andrade type, which is a peripheral neuropathy characterized by prominent pain with distal ulcer formation and prominent autonomic manifestations; the Rukavina type, which is a progressive, distal, large fiber polyneuropathy; and the Van Allen type, which is a painful, distal, symmetric sensory-motor neuropathy. Neuropathy is rarely seen in secondary amyloidosis.

Infectious and parainfectious neuropathies

ACUTE IDIOPATHIC POSTINFECTIOUS POLYRADICULONEUROPATHY (GUILLAIN-BARRÉ SYNDROME)

Definition. Guillain-Barré syndrome is an acute, monophasic polyneuropathy often following a nonspecific infectious process.

Etiology. More than 50% of patients with Guillain-Barré syndrome have had a prior nonspecific infection, usually 10 to 14 days before the onset of the neuropathy. Guillain-Barré syndrome is an immune-mediated disease in which cellular immune mechanisms play a dominant role. Experimental allergic neuritis provides a putative animal model that appears to reproduce many of the important features of Guillain-Barré syndrome. However, recent studies suggest that plasma factors may also be important in the pathogenesis of both experimental allergic neuritis and Guillain-Barré syndrome.

Clinical manifestations. The annual incidence is 0.6 to 1.9:100,000 standard population. This amounts to more than 2000 cases every year in the United States. The neurologic illness usually starts with limb paresthesias. Occasionally patients have severe pain, particularly in the back and limbs. The most characteristic feature is weakness. In 50% of the patients weakness is diffuse from the onset, whereas in the other 50% it spreads upward from the lower limbs to sequentially involve the upper limbs, the respiratory muscles, and then the bulbar muscles in the most severe cases. The neuropathy usually peaks at 3 to 4 weeks. Tracheostomy and mechanical respiratory support are necessary in the most severe cases. The cerebrospinal fluid (CSF) findings are helpful. The CSF protein level increases within a few weeks after the onset, but CSF cells remain normal. The EMG commonly shows conduction block (manifest as the diminution of compound motor action potentials without slowing of conduction velocities when the longer nerve segment is tested), a marked slowing of nerve conduction consistent with the demyelination, or both. A nerve biopsy may reveal active demyelination and perivenular lymphocytic infiltration, but biopsy is rarely necessary to establish the diagnosis. Improvement usually starts within 5 to 6 weeks after the onset and continues slowly. The recovery may be prolonged, lasting several months or even a few years. The mortality is about 10%. Most patients recover satisfactorily.

Management. During the acute phase the patient should be watched closely for respiratory impairment, which can develop quickly. Respiratory assistance should be instituted early. Proper positioning and passive stretching of the limbs are essential for preventing bedsores and contractures. The benefit of corticosteroid therapy has not been proved. Plasmapheresis appears beneficial, particularly when begun within 7 days of onset or when given before respiratory failure. Furthermore, younger patients who have only peripheral nerve conduction block seem to have more beneficial results than older patients with nerve conduction slowing.

IDIOPATHIC RECURRENT POLYNEUROPATHY. The first attack of idiopathic recurrent polyneuropathy may be similar to that of the Guillain-Barré syndrome. Its course is more subacute in evolution, however, and it reaches its maximal severity months after the onset. It is characterized by recurrent similar attacks spaced many months or even years apart. Patients with this neuropathy often respond well to steroid therapy or plasmapheresis.

DIPHTHERITIC NEUROPATHY. Demyelination caused by the diphtheria neurotoxin is usually delayed for 15 to 40 days after the onset of a pharyngitis. Paralysis often begins in the palate but then rapidly spreads to all the nerves, both motor and sensory. The patient may require a tracheostomy and artificial respiration. Recovery usually occurs rather quickly (within 15 to 30 days). With adequate immunization this neuropathy is rarely seen today.

LEPROSY. (See Chapter 50.) In lepromatous leprosy the skin lesion is the most dominant feature. The nerves, however, are frequently affected. The neuropathy, when it occurs, is distal, symmetric, and predominantly sensory. In the tuberculoid form there is a mononeuritis multiplex with severe anesthesia in the involved distribution.

HERPES ZOSTER (SHINGLES). (See the discussion of "Viral infections of the central nervous system" in Chapter 37.) This is a neurocutaneous manifestation of the varicella-zoster virus. The patient usually has a severe girdlelike pain on one side lasting 3 or 4 days. This is followed by a vesicular eruption in the same dermatomal distribution. The virus is thought to remain dormant in the dorsal root ganglia for many years following an episode of varicella (chickenpox). The reactivation of the virus then leads to the clinical symptoms. Herpes zoster often occurs with an underlying illness such as a tumor or in patients who have been immunosuppressed. The infection may spread to the spinal roots, the leptomeninges, and the spinal cord, producing muscle weakness and spasticity. Acyclovir, an antiviral agent, administered intravenously may hasten recovery and shorten the duration of pain in acute herpes zoster. When patients who are developing herpes zoster are also immunosuppressed, the use of this antiviral agent may be justified. Early corticosteroids may prevent postherpetic neuralgia. Postherpetic neuralgia is one of the most difficult types of pain to control. Recent therapies include using membrane stabilizers such as phenytoin or carbamazepine, transcutaneous nerve stimulation, and a combination of antidepressant and phenothiazine.

HUMAN IMMUNODEFICIENCY VIRUS INFECTION. Human immunodeficiency virus (HIV) infection in acquired immunodeficiency syndrome (AIDS) is associated with a wide variety of central and peripheral nervous system and muscle disorders. Various types of peripheral neuropathy have been reported. Acute polyradiculoneuropathy, clinically indistinguishable from Guillain-Barré syndrome, may occur with HIV infection. In contrast to the usual Guillain-Barré syndrome, these patients have an increased number of lymphocytes in the CSF, as well as an increased CSF protein level. Other clinical presentations include a slowly progressive motor-sensory polyneuropathy, predominantly sensory neuropathy, brachial or lumbosacral plexopathies, and mononeuritis multiplex. With the increasing frequency of HIV infection, more of these cases will undoubtedly be seen.

Hereditary neuropathies

CHARCOT-MARIE-TOOTH DISEASE (PERONEAL MUSCULAR ATROPHY). Charcot-Marie-Tooth disease is the most commonly encountered hereditary neuropathy. Both autosomal dominant and recessive inheritance occurs, although the latter is infrequent. The genetic defect is now traced to chromosome 1. The disease may start in the first or second decade of life or later, with slowly progressive weakness and wasting in the distal legs. This results in a "reversed champagne bottle" appearance. The sensory involvement is considerably less than the motor deficit, but a decrease in position and vibration sense is usual. In the demyelinating form, enlarged peripheral nerves may become palpable. The EMG is characterized by a marked slowing of NCVs. A nerve biopsy reveals segmental demyelination and an onion-bulb formation that results from recurrent demyelination and remyelination. In the axonal form the NCVs may be relatively normal despite prominent muscular weakness.

HYPERTROPHIC NEUROPATHY (DÉJÉRINE-SOTTAS DISEASE). Déjérine-Sottas disease, an autosomal recessive neuropathy, usually starts with progressive sensory and motor neuropathy in the first few years of life. There is a marked onion-bulb formation and severe segmental demyelination. The nerves are prominently enlarged.

HEREDITARY SENSORY NEUROPATHY. The hereditary sensory neuropathies are a group of progressive neuropathies that are characterized by the severe loss of various sensory modalities. Both dominant and recessive forms of inheritance are described. The clinical characteristics include distal ulcers and mutilation of the hands and feet.

REFSUM'S DISEASE. Refsum's disease is a metabolic neuropathy with increased serum levels of phytanic acid. Retinitis pigmentosa, ataxia, cutaneous lesions (ichthyosis), and a hypertrophic sensory-motor polyneuropathy develop. Improvement follows use of a special diet excluding phytols. Plasmapheresis may be effective.

Carcinomatous (paraneoplastic) neuropathies

Neoplasms can affect the peripheral nerves in a variety of ways. Neuropathies can result from a direct tumor infiltration or from compression, chemotherapeutic agents, or malnutrition. However, neuropathies unrelated to these definable causes (that is, paraneoplastic neuropathies) also are seen. Carcinomatous (paraneoplastic) neuropathy occurs in 4% to 5% of all cancer patients. Both a mixed sensory-motor axonal neuropathy and a subacute pure sensory axonal neuropathy occur. The subacute pure sensory axonal neuropathy is caused by degeneration of the dorsal root ganglia. Pulmonary, ovarian, breast, and stomach carcinomas are the major tumors found. This neuropathy often precedes the detection of cancer. However, if after 2 years of observation, a cancer is still not found in a patient who has pure sensory neuropathy, it is unlikely that one will be found.

NEUROMUSCULAR JUNCTION DISORDERS
Myasthenia gravis

DEFINITION. Myasthenia gravis (MG), first described by Willis in 1675, is characterized by weakness and abnormal fatigability. It most commonly affects the facial, oculomotor, laryngeal, pharyngeal, and respiratory muscles. Partial recovery characteristically follows rest and therapy with anticholinesterase drugs.

ETIOLOGY. The fundamental abnormality in MG is at the neuromuscular junction. There is a reduction of acetylcholine (ACh) receptors on the muscle because of autoimmune damage. Elevated serum antibodies to the ACh receptor are found in most patients. The origin of the autoimmune process is still poorly understood. Of these patients 75% have thymic abnormalities with hyperplastic glands or an actual thymoma. The thymoma is rarely malignant. The role of the thymus in the pathogenesis is unclear, but it is suggested that primitive myoid cells found in the gland serve as the initiating antigenic stimulus.

CLINICAL MANIFESTATIONS. The incidence of MG is approximately 1:20,000 standard population. The female to male ratio is 3:2. The most characteristic clinical features are pathologic fatigability and weakness, worsened by exertion and improved by rest. When patients are first seen, 50% of them have ocular palsies, 33% have bulbar weakness, and 20% have limb muscle weakness. Ptosis and diplopia are common symptoms of ocular muscle involvement; in fact, MG may be limited to the ocular muscles. Facial weakness often produces a typical snarl expression when the patient smiles. The voice becomes nasal and indistinct. Severe respiratory distress is seen in the advanced stages. The limb weakness differs from that of other neuromuscular diseases by the abnormal fatigability and the absence of wasting. Fluctuations in the severity of the disease are common and occur unpredictably. The weakness may be intensified by an increasing dosage of anticholinesterase agents, aminoglycoside antibiotics, membrane stabilizers (such as quinine, procainamide, and phenytoin), and infections. Intravenous administration of edrophonium (Tensilon) in a test dose of 2 mg followed by 8 mg is used for diagnostic purposes. A rapid but temporary improvement of the weakness should result. A saline control should always be used.

LABORATORY FINDINGS. The repetitive stimulation of a motor nerve provides the most useful diagnostic information. The amplitude of the evoked muscle contraction declines with both slow and fast stimulation. A single fiber EMG can be of additional diagnostic help. A roentgenogram and preferably a computed tomographic (CT) scan of the chest may demonstrate the presence of a thymoma. A muscle biopsy generally reveals nonspecific changes and is less useful. The ACh receptor antibodies, which provide important evidence of autoimmunity, are found in about 90% of patients and are helpful in establishing a diagnosis. Only a fair correlation exists between the severity of the illness and the titer of the ACh receptor antibody.

MANAGEMENT. The treatment of MG consists of administering the anticholinesterase agents neostigmine (Prostigmin) (15 mg three times daily initially) or pyridostigmine (Mestinon) (60 mg three times daily initially) for early and mild cases. The dosage should be carefully adjusted to avoid excessive levels that might block the neuromuscular junction. Corticosteroids suppress the autoimmune process, and their therapeutic benefit is clearly demonstrated. A single-dose, alternate-day program is preferred, using the smallest effective dosage. Azathioprine (Imuran) is being used more frequently when additional immunotherapy is required or when the patient cannot tolerate corticosteroids. Early thymectomy is indicated for most patients. At least 75% of patients improve after a thymectomy, and many have remission of MG. Plasmapheresis has a significant beneficial effect in controlling acute exacerbations of MG. Plasmapheresis is an important addition to the therapeutic armamentarium of this disease.

Eaton-Lambert (myasthenic) syndrome

The Eaton-Lambert (myasthenic) syndrome is a unique and uncommon defect of neuromuscular transmission, occurring in association with small cell carcinoma of the lung (75%) and less frequently with other cancers. The male to female ratio is 5:1. More than two thirds of males with myasthenic syndrome have malignancy, whereas only 25% of females with this disorder have cancer. Myasthenic syndrome without malignancy is associated with other autoimmune disorders. There is much information suggesting that myasthenic syndrome is caused by an autoimmune process against the presynaptic axon terminal. The defect of the neuromuscular transmission is caused by a decreased number of ACh packets released at the presynaptic nerve terminals. Clinically, the weakness differs from that of MG in being particularly prominent soon after the patient arises in the morning. Exercise may help briefly. Patients often complain of a dry mouth. Deep tendon reflexes are usually absent. Repetitive nerve stimulation (10 to 50 Hz) produces a marked facilitation of the amplitude of the muscle contraction, which is in contrast to the declining amplitude seen in true MG. Treatment of the underlying cancer may result in improvement. Guanidine and 4-aminopyridine, which facilitate ACh release at the neuromuscular junction, may be of benefit in some patients. Immunotherapy with corticosteroids or azathioprine is the treatment of choice. Plasmapheresis may provide an additional benefit.

Botulism

(See the discussion of "Botulism" in Chapter 41.)

Botulism results from the ingestion of the exotoxin of *Clostridium botulinum*. The illness is characterized by progressive descending bulbar and skeletal muscle paralysis. Botulinum toxin is the most powerful neurotoxin known. It interferes with the release of ACh by blocking exocytosis at the motor nerve terminal.

The illness often starts with a blurring of vision, diplopia, and difficulty in chewing and swallowing. The weakness becomes generalized rapidly, and respiratory failure often develops quickly. Intensive respiratory care, including a tracheostomy and assisted respiration, is mandatory. The effectiveness of botulinum antitoxin has not yet been proved. Guanidine facilitates ACh release at the neuromuscular junction and is effective in certain patients; the dosage is 20 mg/kg of body weight daily in three divided doses.

DISORDERS OF MUSCLE
Muscular dystrophies

DEFINITION. The diagnosis of muscular dystrophy rests on clinical, genetic, and histologic features. It has been suggested that the term "muscular dystrophy" be reserved for cases of progressive, genetically determined, primary, degenerative myopathy. It has been further suggested that only X-linked recessive types (Duchenne and Becker types) are clinically, genetically, pathologically, and biochemically homogeneous enough to warrant the term "dystrophy."

X-LINKED DYSTROPHIES

Duchenne-type muscular dystrophy. Duchenne-Type muscular dystrophy (DMD) is the most uniform clinical entity among the muscle disorders. The disease, when inherited, is transmitted by a defective X chromosome in the asymptomatic female carrier. It is clinically expressed only in males. About one third of cases of DMD, however, appear to be caused by spontaneous mutations and are not inherited. The incidence of DMD is estimated at from 20 to 30:100,000 live-born males. The incidence in the general population is approximately 3:100,000.

Pathogenesis. The location of a defective gene for DMD has been recently identified on the middle of the short arm of the X chromosome (X_p21). This is a major breakthrough in a long search for the pathogenesis in this little understood muscle disease. It is now demonstrated that the macroprotein dystrophin is specifically absent in muscle. Dystrophin is present at the sarcolemma and at the junctional portion of the T-system. Defects resulting from abnormal dystrophin is suspected to increase calcium inside the muscle cell leading to poor muscle contraction and subsequent degeneration.

Clinical manifestations. The patient shows symptoms at 2 to 4 years of age of clumsiness, weakness, and occasional falling. He often walks on his toes because of heel cord contractures. He has pseudohypertrophy, particularly of the calves, with accentuated lumbar lordosis. He requires increasing amounts of hand support to attain an upright posture (Gowers' sign).

The disease progresses inexorably, confining the patient to a wheelchair at 9 to 11 years of age. At this stage, scoliosis and multiple contractures ensue and respiratory difficulty develops. Patients inevitably die by their late twenties.

The ocular muscles are rarely involved. Verbal intelligence is often impaired. Most patients have cardiomyopathy but have symptoms only in the late stages of DMS.

Laboratory findings. The serum CK determination is one of the most valuable tests for DMD. Before the patient is 10 years of age, the serum CK level is dramatically elevated, often more than 200-fold. Usually the CK level falls later in life and may approach normal by the time the patient is 20 years of age. In fact, a significant CK elevation is a prerequisite for the diagnosis of DMD before the patient is 10 years of age. The electrocardiogram shows a tall R wave in the anterior precordial leads in about 70% of patients. The EMG shows the classic changes of myopathy. A muscle biopsy reveals large hyalinized muscle fibers, groups of regenerating fibers, profound connective and fat tissue proliferation, and other histologic features of myopathy. A specific test to identify an absent dystrophin in muscle tissue will become available for suspected patients.

Carrier detection. Reliable carrier detection is now available using genetic linkage studies with increasingly effective probes. All families should receive genetic counseling. The serum CK level is the most sensitive indicator of the carrier state. It tends to fall, however, after patients are 20 years of age. Carrier detection therefore should be carried out early. Attempts to identify an affected male fetus prenatally have been unsuccessful. Prenatal sex determination, however, can often be of help to a pregnant carrier.

A specific carrier detection technique will be available in the near future by using the sensitive dystrophin methods.

Management. DMD is an incurable disease. Incurable and untreatable are not synonymous terms, however, and much can be done to make these patients' lives more rewarding and comfortable. Proper management is best carried out by a team consisting of the neurologist, pediatrician, orthopedic surgeon, physiotherapist, occupational therapist, and social worker. Supportive therapy has prolonged a useful life into the third decade in many instances. In the very near future, therapeutic trials with human dystrophin will be available.

Becker-type muscular dystrophy. Becker-type muscular dystrophy is a milder form of dystrophy that also is inherited as an X-linked recessive trait. The clinical signs and symptoms are much less severe than with DMD, and patients survive well into adult life. Recently it was shown that muscle fibers in Becker-type muscular dystrophy do contain dystrophin as compared to DMD in which dystrophin is absent. In Becker-type muscular dystrophy, dystrophin is abnormal either in quality or quantity.

FACIOSCAPULOHUMERAL MUSCULAR DYSTROPHY. Facioscapulohumeral (FSH) muscular dystrophy is an autosomal dominant disorder of multiple pathologic types. The affected patient has symptoms by the end of the first decade or during the second decade of life. Facial weakness usually appears first. Gradually a weakness of the upper arms and shoulders develops; later the weakness may involve the hip muscles. The neck and shoulder muscles become atrophied, but the trapezius muscle is preserved. Scapular winging is prominent. The muscles of the upper arms are atrophied out of proportion to those of the forearms. Some features are only minimally expressed, and spontaneous arrest occurs in certain patients. The laboratory investigation should include serum enzyme studies, EMG, and a muscle biopsy. The CK concentration may be slightly elevated but is more often normal. The muscle biopsy may show various types of abnormality, including inflammation, denervation, lipid storage or necrotizing myopathy, in patients with identical clinical deficits.

LIMB-GIRDLE MUSCULAR DYSTROPHY. In limb-girdle muscular dystrophy, an autosomal recessive condition, weakness involves the proximal muscles of all limbs and the muscles of the shoulder and hip girdles. The condition is pathologically heterogeneous. The CK concentration may be slightly elevated but is more often normal. Identical clinical manifestations occur with anterior horn cell disease (spinal muscular atrophy), storage diseases, metabolic diseases, and mitochondrial myopathies.

OCULAR MYOPATHY AND OCULOPHARYNGEAL DYSTROPHY. In ocular myopathy and oculopharyngeal dystrophy, ptosis is the first symptom and progresses insidiously with or without an external ophthalmoplegia. Later, proximal muscle weakness may occur in the arms or even in the legs. In ocular myopathy the symptoms begin in early adulthood and the inheritance is autosomal dominant.

Oculopharyngeal dystrophy occurs with high frequency in patients of French-Canadian origin. This condition begins in late adult life with slowly progressive ptosis and dysphagia. It is almost always inherited as an autosomal dominant trait. Muscle biopsy shows scattered, small, angular fibers and rimmed vacuoles. Yet another group of disorders is characterized by progressive ophthalmoplegia of the external ocular muscles and is associated with proximal muscle weakness, dysphagia, and other systemic signs. Kearns' syndrome is a sporadic disease consisting of a triad of progressive external ophthalmoplegia, heart block, and retinal pigmentary changes, often with other systemic abnormalities. In these patients morphologic and biochemical abnormalities are present in muscle mitochondria. The pathogenesis of these conditions is unclear, and the classification is unsettled. The CK level occasionally is elevated in the ocular myopathies.

Inflammatory myopathies

POLYMYOSITIS AND RELATED CONDITIONS. Polymyositis is characterized by a noninfectious, nonsuppurative inflammation of the striated muscle (polymyositis) and the skin (dermatomyositis). Progressive muscle weakness is the paramount sign (see Chapter 19 for details).

POLYMYALGIA RHEUMATICA. Polymyalgia rheumatica occurs almost exclusively in patients older than 60 years of age. Females are affected twice as often as males. The chief symptoms are severe, proximal muscle pains and stiffness without weakness. Approximately 20% of patients with polymyalgia rheumatica also have a temporal arteritis that may result in acute blindness. Almost all patients have a high erythrocyte sedimentation rate. If there is any hint of temporal arteritis, a temporal artery biopsy may be helpful and corticosteroids should be administered. The EMG and muscle biopsy findings are normal (see Chapter 23 for details).

TRICHINOSIS. Muscle infestation with the larvae of *Trichinella spiralis* produces severe muscle pain and frequently weakness. Early symptoms consist of periorbital edema or a skin rash with petechiae. Pain while attempting to open the jaw or with chewing is common because of the masseter muscle involvement. Eosinophilia is characteristic. The muscle biopsy reveals numerous larvae and inflammation (see Chapter 55 for details).

Metabolic myopathies

HYPOTHYROID MYOPATHY. In adults hypothyroidism is associated with a slowness of movement, cramps, muscle hypertrophy, and weakness. In congenital cretinism the infant may appear robust, but the muscle is actually hypotonic and weak. Myoedema (mounding of the muscle on percussion) and a delayed relaxation of the muscle stretch reflex are commonly present.

MALIGNANT HYPERPYREXIA OR MALIGNANT HYPERTHERMIA. Malignant hyperpyrexia or hyperthermia is a rare but potentially fatal condition often triggered by halogenated anesthetic agents or succinylcholine. It occurs in 1:14,000 to 75,000 patients who undergo anesthesia. When inherited, it is transmitted as an autosomal dominant trait. Patients may have signs of myopathy such as muscle hypertrophy, lumbar lordosis, mild hip weakness, and percussion myotonia. On exposure to anesthetic agents, (particularly halothane or succinylcholine), the patient demonstrates fasciculations and increased muscle tone, particularly of the masseter muscle. Jaw clenching during the induction of anesthesia is a typical early sign. The body muscles become rigid, and excessive body heat is produced. Marked lactic acidosis, muscle necrosis, and cardiovascular collapse ensue.

The anesthesia should be discontinued, oxygen should be administered, and the patient should be cooled. Intravenously administered dantrolene sodium has a therapeutic effect. Renal failure can occur as a result of massive myoglobinuria. A diagnostic test called in vitro halothane/caffeine contracture test is available in some centers.

MITOCHONDRIAL MYOPATHIES. A series of myopathies resulting from abnormal mitochondrial enzymes has been identified. The initial clinical symptoms of these myopathies are proximal muscle weakness, exercise intolerance, and muscle pain. Muscle biopsy may show abnormal accummulation of mitochondria, termed "ragged-red fibers," on Gomori's one-step trichrome stain. Occasionally these myopathies are familial and often show a maternal inheritance, since mitochondria are derived from the mother (mitochondria contain their own DNA strand). A series of enzyme deficiencies, particularly cytochrome C deficiency, has been identified. These myopathies are often associated with systemic mitochondrial disease manifest as lactic acidosis, seizures, encephalopathy, ocular palsy, endocrinopathy, cardiac myopathy, or retinopathy. Mitochondrial biochemical analyses are required to identify such specific enzyme deficiencies.

PERIODIC PARALYSES

Definition. Periodic paralyses are rare muscle disorders and are characterized by episodes of weakness usually associated with alterations of serum potassium levels. These attacks of weakness are classified according to whether the serum potassium level is low or high during an attack. The so-called normokalemic periodic paralysis is most likely a variant of hyperkalemic periodic paralysis.

Hypokalemic periodic paralysis. In hypokalemic periodic paralysis the serum potassium level may be as low as 1.5 mEq/L during an attack. The weakness affects the limb and trunk muscles but not the respiratory, bulbar, or ocular muscles. The inheritance is autosomal dominant. Attacks usually begin in the second decade of life. Rest after exercise or after heavy carbohydrate meals may precipitate an attack. Potassium salts, in doses of 5 to 10 g of oral potassium chloride, can terminate an attack. Acetazolamide (250 mg or more daily as needed) is the preferred therapy for prevention.

Hyperkalemic periodic paralysis. Hyperkalemic period pa-

paralysis is also autosomal dominant in its form of inheritance. Attacks of weakness begin shortly after exercise and are generally brief compared to those in the hypokalemic form. There is often a symptomatic myotonia that is best demonstrated by a slowness of eye opening after tight closure. The serum potassium level may be elevated or normal during an attack. Acute attacks usually require no treatment. Acetazolamide is effective prophylactically in this form of periodic paralysis.

GLYCOGEN STORAGE DISEASE

Acid maltase deficiency (glycogenosis type II). Acid maltase is a lysosomal enzyme that splits the terminal glucose from glycogen. Its absence results in a marked glycogen accumulation in the lysosome and in the sarcoplasm. The infantile form of acid maltase deficiency is the most severe. Generalized glycogen accumulation, cardiopulmonary failure, and severe generalized weakness result in early death. The later infantile and juvenile forms may resemble muscular dystrophy, and their courses are more benign. Adult-onset acid maltase deficiency may mimic limb-girdle muscular dystrophy or polymyositis. Acid maltase deficiency is autosomal recessive in its inheritance.

McArdle's disease (glycogenosis type V). The enzyme myophosphorylase that degrades glycogen in anaerobic glycolysis is defective in this muscle disease. Typical clinical manifestations include postexertional muscle cramps and myoglobinuria. Patients usually first have symptoms in the second decade of life. The failure of lactic acid to rise with ischemic exercise is a diagnostic indicator, as is an absence of phosphorylase detected with histochemical studies. Similar clinical manifestations are seen in fructokinase deficiency (glycogenosis type VII).

Debranching enzyme deficiency. In the case of debranching enzyme deficiency myopathy (glycogenosis type III), muscle weakness is often in the distal muscles and no lactate is produced with ischemic exercise.

LIPID STORAGE DISEASES

Carnitine deficiency myopathy. Carnitine deficiency myopathy is caused by a deficiency of carnitine that helps transfer fatty acids into the mitochondria for β-oxidation. Patients have slowly progressive proximal muscle weakness. A biopsy shows increased fat droplets in the muscle fibers. Because of the hepatic involvement no ketone is produced during fasting. A biochemical analysis of muscle carnitine is required to confirm the diagnosis.

Carnitine palmityl transferase (CPT) deficiency. CPT is an enzyme that facilitates oxidative metabolism of fatty acids. In this myopathy, postexertional muscle cramps and myoglobinuria are typical symptoms. A muscle biopsy shows no significant fat accumulation, unlike carnitine deficiency, and often is normal. Therefore biochemical analysis of the muscle specimen is required to confirm the diagnosis.

ALCOHOLIC MYOPATHIES. Acute alcoholic myopathy is characterized by muscle tenderness, rhabdomyolysis, and myoglobinuria and occurs with both high blood alcohol levels and acute protein depletion and vitamin depletion. Acute renal tubular necrosis may be a serious complication. Chronic alcoholic myopathy occurs infrequently and is largely related to malnutrition. It is characterized by proximal muscle weakness, particularly in the legs. Chronic neurogenic muscle atrophy is the basic process in this condition. In acute alcoholic myopathy, muscle enzyme levels may be elevated 300-fold, whereas in the chronic form they may be elevated only threefold to fourfold.

Myotonic disorders

MYOTONIC DYSTROPHY. Myotonic dystrophy is an autosomal dominant disease characterized by myotonia, distal muscle wasting, cataracts, testicular atrophy, and other polysystemic abnormalities. The cause is unknown, but recent evidence suggests a generalized membrane abnormality. The genetic defect has been traced to chromosome 19.

The incidence is estimated at 3 to 5:100,000 standard population. Myotonic dystrophy is manifest in adolescence or early adult life. The patient's face is expressionless, and there are temporal muscle wasting and frontal balding. Myotonia can be elicited with direct percussion or with the voluntary contraction of the muscle. The EMG shows typical myotonic discharges with myopathic changes. Besides the neuromusclar abnormalities the patient has cataracts, testicular atrophy, abnormal glucose tolerance, cardiac conduction blocks, and pulmonary hypoventilation. Myotonic dystrophy may appear in neonates born to affected mothers. In this case prominent signs are severe hypotonia and facial paralysis, but the myotonia is mild.

The muscle histologic findings are characterized by type I (high-oxidative) fiber atrophy and marked central nucleation. The treatment is with membrane stabilizers such as quinine, procainamide, and especially phenytoin. Genetic counseling is important to prevent unwanted affected offspring.

MYOTONIA CONGENITA (THOMSEN'S DISEASE). Myotonia congenita (Thomsen's disease) is transmitted as an autosomal dominant trait. The muscles are stiff, but with continued exercise they loosen and movement becomes almost normal. Muscle hypertrophy may be present, but weakness does not occur. Exposure to cold worsens the symptoms. The Becker-type of myotonia congenita is autosomal recessive, and muscle wasting and weakness may occur.

Congenital myopathies

The congenital myopathies are characterized clinically by hypotonia and a slowly progressive proximal weakness with or without a family history. They are a pathologically heterogeneous group. Peculiar structural alterations of the muscle have been observed.

CONGENITAL FIBER TYPE DISPROPORTION. In congenital fiber type disproportion, the type I muscle fibers are less numerous and smaller than type II (low-oxidative) fibers. This condition is occasionally inherited as an autosomal dominant trait. One third of the patients have congenital hip dislocation. Weakness may improve or worsen with time.

CENTRAL CORE DISEASE. The weakness in central core disease usually progresses slowly throughout life. Mitochondria and oxidative enzyme activity are deficient in the center of the muscle fiber, and the central portion of the muscle fiber is abnormal histologically. Skeletal deformities are a result of the early onset of the muscle disease. Malignant hyperthermia has been reported in some patients with central core disease.

NEMALINE MYOPATHY. Nemaline myopathy, a congenital myopathy, is characterized by the presence of small, rodlike inclusions in the oxidative (type I) muscle fibers. There may be type I fiber predominance and atrophy. The rods are composed of α-actinin similar to Z-band material. Both inherited and sporadic cases have been described. Adult-onset nemaline myopathy has been reported.

CENTRONUCLEAR (MYOTUBULAR) MYOPATHY. In myotubular myopathy the term "myotubular" refers to the similarity of these fibers to fetal myotubes. The nuclei are central rather than peripheral in location. The inheritance varies. There may be extraocular muscle involvement, cardiopulmonary failure, and EEG abnormalities.

Myoglobinuria

Myoglobin is the reddish brown respiratory pigment that transports and stores oxygen in muscle fiber. A breakdown of the muscle fiber results in the release of myoglobin into the serum. Excessive myoglobin in the serum may produce renal tubular necrosis and renal failure.

PRIMARY MYOGLOBINURIA. Primary myoglobinuria is a sudden-onset myoglobinuria of unkown cause, often precipitated by sepsis or exercise. Apparently, myoglobinuria may occur in otherwise normal people after unusually exhausting exercise.

SECONDARY MYOGLOBINURIA. Metabolic myopathies such as McArdle's disease, phosphofructokinase deficiency, and carnitine palmityl transferase deficiency often appear with postexertional myoglobinuria. In malignant hyperthermia massive myoglobinuria may occur. Other causes of myoglobinuria include a crush injury, excessive long-term ethanol intake, a lightning injury, and drug reactions.

A striking elevation of serum muscle enzymes almost always accompanies myoglobinuria. In cases of severe myoglobinuria, renal function should be carefully monitored. Diuresis should be maintained with fluid replacement, diuretics, and mannitol, and the urine should be kept alkaline.

DISORDERS OF THE SPINAL ROOTS, BRACHIAL PLEXUS, AND SPINAL CORD
General signs and symptoms

SPINAL ROOTS. Damage to the spinal anterior (ventral) root results in segmental weakness, whereas posterior spinal root damage produces dermatomal sensory loss of all modalities and radicular pain in the same distribution. An examination reveals weakness and wasting only in the muscles belonging to the root in question with a corresponding sensory loss. This specific distribution of the muscle weakness and sensory change can distinguish a root lesion from a plexus or nerve lesion. When multiple roots are involved, however, localization becomes difficult. In such situations the EMG becomes an important ancillary test.

SPINAL CORD. Damage to the spinal cord produces a loss of neuron function at the level of the lesion, resulting in paralysis and atrophy of the muscles in the territory of the damaged motor neurons. Sensory function is also lost in the territory of the dermatome belonging to the segment of the lesion. The lesion also interrupts the ascending and descending spinal cord tracts. Damage to the ascending tracts results in a loss of sensation of all modalities below the level of the lesion. Damage to the descending tracts (corticospinal tracts) produces a paralysis followed by spasticity and pathologic reflexes below the level of the lesion. Sphincter disturbances result from interrupted descending tracts controlling the bladder and bowel. The signs vary depending on the size of lesion, whether it is intrinsic or extrinsic, and the rapidity of damage. For example, a small tumor arising in the center of the cervical spinal cord at the fifth segmental level (C5) produces a loss of cutaneous sensation in the fifth cervical dermatome. If the lesion is larger, the muscles belonging to the nerve roots at this level become weak and atrophied. Fasciculations may appear. When the lesion is even larger, the white matter fiber tracts are affected. The muscles below the level of the fifth cervical spinal segment become spastic with brisk and pathologic reflexes. A sensory examination in the early stages may show only a loss of sensation in the legs because of the topographic arrangement of the nerve fibers. Later sensory loss is complete below C5.

Specific disorders

DEGENERATIVE VERTEBRAL OSTEOARTHRITIS (SPONDYLOSIS). Common neurologic sequelae of spondylosis include shoulder and neck pain (cervical spondylosis) and low back pain (lumbosacral spondylosis). There may be no objective neurologic deficit in the early stages. In advanced spondylosis neurologic damage may occur. Compression of the spinal roots at the intervertebral foramen and of the spinal cord because of narrowing of the spinal canal are major complications. Root compression produces radicular pain, muscle weakness, and wasting in the territory of the root. Spinal cord compression occurs most commonly at the cervical level and produces slow progressive spastic paraparesis (spondylitic cervical myelopathy). A narrowing of the spinal canal at the lumbosacral level results in lumbosacral canal stenosis, causing intermittent exercise-induced leg pain. When physical therapy and other conservative measures do not help and neurologic deficits are progressive, surgical decompression is indicated.

DISC DISEASE. When the intervertebral disc undergoes degenerative changes, its soft nucleus pulposus may extrude and compress the nerve root laterally. It also may compress the spinal cord anteriorly at the cervical and thoracic levels. Disc herniation is often a result of sudden or excessive movement in the cervical or lumbar regions. Severe radicular pain develops in the distribution of the compressed root. The nerve roots most commonly compressed are the fifth and sixth cervical roots, the fifth lumbar root, and the first sacral root. Stretching the lumbar and sacral nerve roots by straight leg raising or increasing spinal canal pressure by sneezing may precipitate severe radicular pain. The diagnosis of disc disease can be confirmed by myelography. Conservative treatment consists of prescribing bed rest, analgesics, and traction for cervical radiculopathy. When conservative measures are unsuccessful, surgical treatment is often necessary.

SPINAL CORD TUMOR. Expanding lesions within the spinal canal can compress the nerve roots and spinal cord. The most common intramedullary tumor is a glioma. Intraspinal extramedullary tumors also produce a compression of the spinal roots and the spinal cord. These tumors include schwannomas, neurofibromas, and meningiomas. Epidural masses may be associated with the bony destruction of the adjacent vertebral bone and are commonly caused by metastatic carcinoma. Lymphoma may produce an epidural mass without any bony destruction. A sudden onset of paraplegia, fever, and localized tenderness over the spinal column suggests an epidural abscess. Cauda equina lesions may be caused by tumors or herniated discs. Sphincter disturbances are common with these masses.

BRACHIAL PLEXOPATHY (NEURALGIC AMYOTROPHY). Brachial plexopathy is an unusual neuropathy involving only the brachial plexus. It may occur in association with infection, trauma, immunization, or surgery. Males are four times more frequently affected than females. Occasionally familial occurrence is seen. The cause is unknown. The disease is characterized by a severe pain in one or both shoulders that may last for 1 day to 3 months. Motor symptoms occur, and the affected muscle rapidly becomes paralyzed and atrophied. One cord of the brachial plexus or a single nerve root may be involved. The patient usually recovers function in 6 months to 2 years.

BIBLIOGRAPHY

Bradley WG: Disorders of peripheral nerves, Oxford, Eng, 1974, Blackwell Scientific Publications Inc.

Brooke MH: A clinician's view of neuromuscular diseases, Baltimore, 1985, Williams & Wilkins.

Chad D, Munsat LL, and Adelman LS: Diseases of muscle. Rosenberg R, editor: Clinical neurosciences, New York, 1984, Churchill Livingstone Inc.

Dyck PJ and others, editors: Peripheral neuropathy, Philadelphia, 1984, WB Saunders Co.

Engel AG and Banker BQ, editors: Myology basic and clinical, New York, 1986, McGraw-Hill Inc.

Layzer RB, editor: Neuromuscular manifestations of systemic disease, Philadelphia, 1985, FA Davis Co.

Lisak RP and Barchi RL, editors: Myasthenia gravis, Philadelphia, 1982, WB Saunders Co.

Munsat TL: The classification of human myopathies. In Vinken PJ and Bruyn GW, editors: Handbook of clinical neurology, vol 40, Amsterdam, 1979, Elsevier Science Publishing Co Inc.

Walton SJ, editor: Disorders of voluntary muscles, Edinburgh, 1988, Churchill Livingstone Inc.

Dental correlations

Joel B. Epstein*

SLEEP DISORDERS
Nocturnal bruxism

Excessive nonfunctional grinding and clenching of the teeth is considered an important cause of periodontal disease, tooth wear, pulpal damage, fracture of restorations, and temporomandibular joint (TMJ) dysfunction. The intensity and duration of a muscle contraction during sleep and their association with a specific phase of the sleep cycle suggest that nocturnal bruxism is separate from bruxism that occurs during waking hours and may require different considerations in management.

Nocturnal bruxism (Fig. 1) occurs in association with REM sleep and usually accompanies movements of the limbs

---

*Material in "Dental correlations" is based in part on the first edition, written by Vernon J. Brightman.

and periods of increased heart rate. REM sleep represents a state of partial arousal. Usually the patient is unaware of nocturnal bruxism, and attention is drawn to it only by a partner or parent or if the patient wakes with the teeth tightly together or jaw fatigue. Like other occurrences associated with REM sleep, nocturnal bruxism may be instigated by any stimulus, external, internal, physical, or emotional, that disturbs sleep. A familial pattern has been described. It is often a transient and inconsistent occurrence. There is no evidence to associate psychologic abnormality or brain lesions with nocturnal bruxism, and the sleep electromyogram (EMG) records of affected individuals are normal.

Alcohol is an important stimulus of nocturnal bruxism. Alcohol may act as a stimulant of the reticular activating system rather than as a central nervous system (CNS) depressant, resulting in an increase in the frequency and duration of nocturnal bruxism. The intensity and duration of masseter muscle contraction during a period of nocturnal bruxism cannot be achieved by conscious activity.

MANAGEMENT. The majority of recommended treatments have not been tested in a sleep laboratory, which is essential for the study of nocturnal bruxism. A full-arch maxillary occlusal splint, or night guard, when tested under these conditions, reduces the level of masseter muscle EMG activity in about 50% of patients. Changing the vertical dimension of the appliance results in reduced masseter muscle EMG levels. The occlusal appliance is an effective treatment modality for some patients with this problem. Skeletal muscle relaxants used before sleep may also be a useful adjunct in management of nocturnal bruxism.

Sleep apnea syndrome

In patients with sleep apnea syndrome considered secondary to upper airway obstruction, the possibility that mandibular retrognathism is the cause should be considered. Such obstruction may be secondary to mandibular fractures, ankylosis of the TMJ, or developmental malposition of the man-

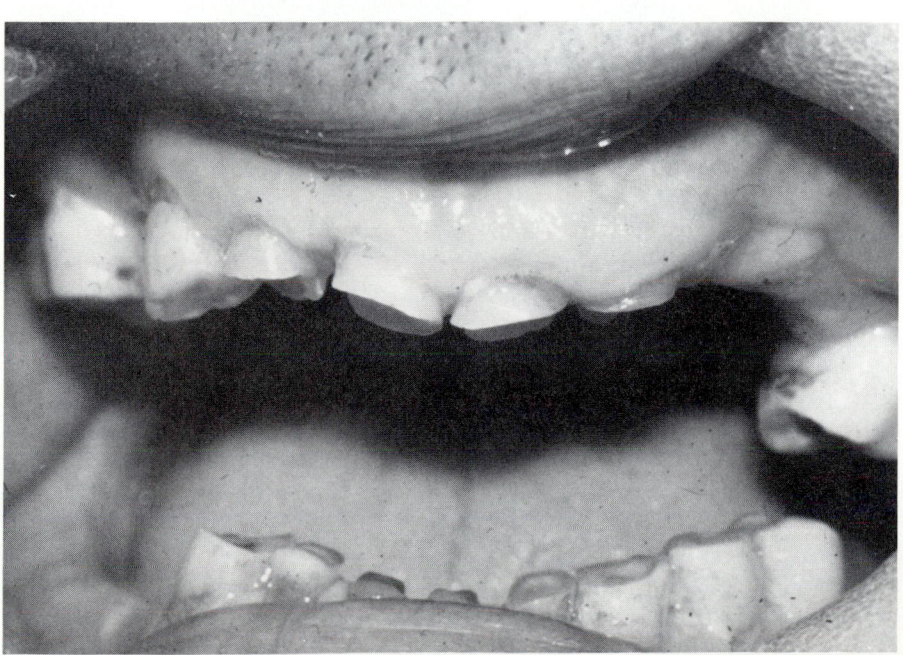

Fig. 1 Severe attrition of dentition in patient with long-standing nocturnal bruxism.

dible. Cure of sleep apnea has occurred in a number of patients who have had surgical correction of mandibular retrognathism.

Sleep disturbance associated with depression

Unrecognized and untreated depression may complicate the diagnosis and treatment of a number of oral problems. Depression may be associated with otherwise unexplained oral symptoms such as burning tongue, dysgeusia, and atypical facial pain. Although disturbances of sleep pattern are not specific for depression, they are often a major concern and may be the dentist's first clue that suggests considering psychiatric factors in the differential diagnosis of an oral complaint. Disturbances of sleep patterns are often so distressing to patients, particularly older patients, that they accept psychiatric consultation even when they reject this as a cause.

BIBLIOGRAPHY

Bear SE and others: Sleep apnea syndrome: correction with surgical advancement of the mandible, Oral Surg 38:543, 1980.

Beck FE and others: Recognition and management of the depressed dental patient, Oral Health 71:25, 1981.

Clarke NG and others: Bruxing patterns in man during sleep, J Oral Rehabil 11:123, 1984.

Clarke NG and others: Distribution of nocturnal bruxism in man, J Oral Rehabil 11:529, 1984.

Rugh JD and others: Experimental occlusal discrepancies and nocturnal bruxism, J Prosthet Dent 51:548, 1984.

Sheikholeslam A and others: A clinical and electromyographic study of the long-term effects of an occlusal splint on the temporal and masseter muscles in patients with functional disorders and nocturnal bruxism, J Oral Rehabil 13:137, 1986.

Suzuki JB: Etiology of parafunction: a brief of psychological and occlusal genesis, Periodont Abst 27:48, 1979.

ALCOHOLISM AND DRUG ABUSE

Alcoholism (Fig. 2) and drug abuse are associated with behavior changes and oral and systemic tissue changes that can be of considerable significance in dental treatment. A variety of psychotic and unpredictable behaviors are seen in association with substance abuse. These behaviors may reflect a drug's effect on the CNS, as well as underlying behavior problems that become more prominent with drug use. Awareness of some characteristic alcoholic and drug abuse behaviors can assist dentists when they encounter these problems. Failure to keep appointments, elaborate explanations for not undertaking dental treatment or home care, garrulous or argumentative speech, obtunded behavior, and consistent alcoholic breath odor suggest continuing substance abuse.

The dentist must also be aware of narcotic addicts who use dental pain as an excuse for obtaining drugs. The dosages of narcotics or other drugs that are usually prescribed may be relatively ineffective for the habituated or addicted patient. Addictive behavior should be suspected when a patient consults several practitioners for drugs, when a patient requests a specific opiate such as Percodan because it's "the only medication that works," or when a patient postpones dental or surgical treatment indefinitely. Addicts devise elaborate and convincing stories to obtain narcotics and other abused substances. Drug addiction is seen in all classes of society, and physicians, nurses, and dentists perpetrate some of the more elaborate ruses on their colleagues.

The dentist who keeps prescription pads with a preprinted narcotic license number or limited stocks of barbiturates or narcotics is at greater risk of burglary. Employee abuse of nitrous oxide may also occur. Repeated, heavy use of nitrous oxide is associated with myeloneuropathy. Access to nitrous oxide should be strictly controlled.

Numerous publications document the effects of narcotic addiction on the oral cavity. Rampant dental caries, especially involving the gingival third of teeth, is described in heroin addicts and may relate to opiate-induced xerostomia. Poor oral hygiene is characteristic of all addicts and contributes to rampant caries and gingival and periodontal disease, including acute necrotizing ulcerative gingivitis. Excessive occlusal wear and other evidence of bruxism are common and probably relate to central effects of drugs; similar phenomenon may occur in response to alcohol ingestion (see the discussion of "Nocturnal bruxism" in this chapter).

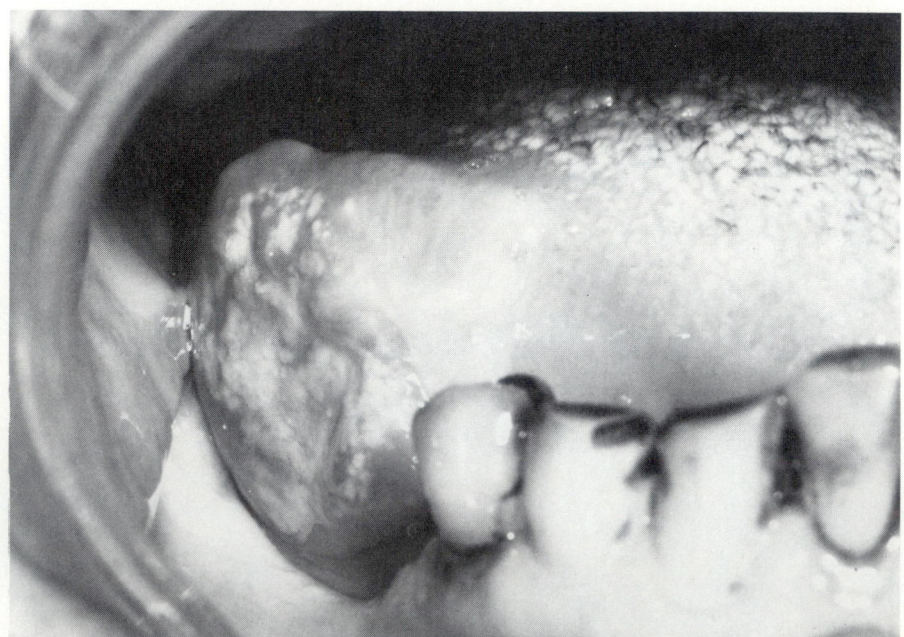

Fig. 2 Patient with chronic alcoholism, demonstrating poor hygiene, dental neglect, generalized mucosal erythema, and indurated ulceration of lateral border of tongue, which proved to be squamous cell carcinoma.

It should be recognized that drug abusers often use more than one drug. Surveys show that more than 20% of alcoholics abuse a number of substances besides alcohol. Potentiation of the various substances frequently occurs and may account for more than 20% of drug-related accidental and suicidal deaths each year. The U.S. surgeon general reports that abuse may involve haphazard prescriptions of sedatives, hypnotics, narcotics, antidepressants, tranquilizers, and antihistamines. It is important that the dentist who prescribes drugs in these categories take an adequate history of alcohol use, review the drug interactions of the drugs prescribed, restrict the quantities of the drugs prescribed, and estimate the likelihood the patient will comply with precautions regarding a drug's use, including limitations on alcohol consumption.

Maxillofacial trauma is common in addicts and alcoholics and frequently draws the attention of the oral surgeon and hospital dental service. Diminished smell and taste sensation often occurs, particularly as a result of cocaine or volatile chemical use or as a result of CNS damage from alcohol and other abused toxic substances. These symptoms and other oral sensory disturbances may be the patient's first complaint.

MANAGEMENT. The dentist must be aware of multiple systemic diseases that may occur in alcoholics and drug addicts. Toxic damage to the liver from continued alcohol abuse leads to cirrhosis, and intravenous use of other drugs puts addicts at a high risk of hepatitis. If the cirrhosis is severe, the hepatotoxicity may seriously compromise the formation of intrinsic blood coagulation factors and impair detoxification of prescribed drugs. The deficiencies in clotting factors may be reversed by administration of vitamin K. Decreased detoxification of estrogens in the compromised liver results in the formation of arterial spiders on the skin. These spiders should be distinguished from petechial hemorrhages. Multiple petechiae may be caused by platelet deficiency that can occur as a result of the toxic effects on the bone marrow. Hypoalbuminemia and anemia caused by toxic effects of alcohol on the liver and bone marrow or by an associated nutritional deficiency may occur and complicate hospital management and the administration of general anesthetic agents. Obstructive pulmonary disease occurs with prolonged heroin abuse and may be the basis of dyspnea and wheezing in these individuals. These patients usually have abnormal pulmonary function tests but often have normal auscultatory and radiographic chest examinations. The nephrotic syndrome (with raised blood urea nitrogen level, proteinuria, and generalized edema) and cardiac arrhythmias are also described in association with narcotic addiction.

Administration of a general anesthetic to a narcotic addict or an alcoholic poses special problems. Withdrawal of the abused drugs and substitution of a defined medication (such as methadone or diazepam) may control withdrawal symptoms. Sedation before general anesthesia must take into account the recent history of drug abuse. Hypotension and respiratory depression secondary to narcotic abuse along with concerns regarding additional liver toxicity make general anesthesia more hazardous than usual. Patients with these conditions need carefully selected anesthetic agents and adequate monitoring during anesthesia. The postoperative period must also be managed specially to control pain and establish methadone maintenance without significant withdrawal problems.

Intravenous drug abuse increases risk of infection by agents such as hepatitis B, delta hepatitis, human immunodeficiency virus, other viral agents and bacterial agents such as *Neisseria gonorrhoeae, Treponema pallidum,* and *Mycobacterium tuberculosis.* Hepatitis B infection may result in acute or chronic active hepatitis with persistent hepatitis B antigenemia. The management of any patient who is at risk requires adequate infection control procedures and personal protection that includes up-to-date immunizations, barrier precautions, and sterilization.

Methods for measuring the commonly abused substances in blood and urine are available from most diagnostic laboratories that provide toxicologic assays. Confirmation of suspected drug abuse and monitoring of blood levels are possible and often desirable before major surgery and general anesthesia.

BIBLIOGRAPHY

American Dental Association: Chemical dependency: the road to recovery, J Am Dent Assoc 115:17, 1987.

Centers for Disease Control: Recommended infection control practices for dentistry, MMWR 35:237, 1986.

Centers for Disease Control: Recommendations for prevention of HIV transmission in health care settings, MMWR 36(suppl):2s, 1987.

Epstein JB and Mathias RG: Infection control in dental practice: demands of the 1980's, J Can Dent Assoc 52:695, 1986.

Gotta AW and others: Anesthetic management of the narcotic addict. II. Preoperative evaluation, J Hosp Dent Pract 11:13, 1977.

Gotta AW and others: Anesthetic management of the narcotic addict. II. Intraoperative and post-operative care, J Hosp Dent Pract 12:17, 1978.

Gutman L and others: Nitrous oxide–induced myelopathy-neuropathy; potential for chronic misuse by dentists, J Am Dent Assoc 98:58, 1979.

Jaffe L and Schuckit MA: The importance of drug use histories in a series of alcoholics, J Clin Psychiatry 42:224, 1981.

Novak A and others: The deliberate inhalation of volatile substances, J Psychedelic Drugs 12:105, 1980.

SYNCOPE

Syncope is due to a sudden fall of blood pressure or failure of the cardiac systole, resulting in cerebral anemia and subsequent loss of consciousness. The cause of a syncopal episode may vary from patient to patient, but an increased catecholamine level as a result of anxiety and pain is frequently the immediate cause of reduction in cerebral blood flow. Syncopal episodes are sometimes mistaken for allergic or toxic reactions to local anesthetic agents when they follow infiltration or regional block anesthesia. It is important that a record of any reaction be noted and the true nature of the episode be established. Data useful in establishing the differential diagnosis include pulse and blood pressure recordings during the episode and a history of the events and any unusual symptoms that immediately precede the episode. Review of the patient's medications may identify a potential cause of postural hypotension such as use of an antihypertensive drug. Measurement of the blood pressure in the recumbent and standing positions and measurement of blood glucose level at a subsequent appointment may help identify postural hypotension. Consultation with a physician may be required to establish the diagnosis and to make recommendations that may help prevent syncope in the future.

MANAGEMENT. Most patients in syncope respond to being placed in a supine position with the legs elevated (Trendelenburg's position). An upright position in a chair may cause prolonged cerebral ischemia, which can precipitate complications of syncope including convulsions and nausea. The proper positioning of the patient is important, since the majority of clinical manifestations arise from inadequate flow of cerebral blood. Manipulation and movement of the extremities increase the return of blood from the periphery. Tight or restrictive clothing, such as a necktie or belt, should be loosened. Placing a cold towel on the patient's forehead may be soothing.

Establishing a patent airway is the next step in treatment. Frequently the head-tilt position is sufficient to stimulate respiration. It is also advisable to administer oxygen. If the patient is not responding rapidly to these measures, a respiratory stimulant, such as aromatic spirits of ammonia, should be used.

During syncope, vital signs, including blood pressure, pulse, and respiration, must be monitored. They must be compared with the patient's baseline values to determine the severity and progression of the emergency. A temporary drop in blood pressure usually occurs, and the pulse may be rapid and thready or slow and steady. Dilated but reactive pupils, pale skin, excessive perspiration, nausea, and vomiting may occur. If a peripheral pulse cannot be detected, cardiac failure should be considered and cardiopulmonary resuscitation should be administered. However, recovery from a syncopal episode usually occurs promptly after cerebral circulation is regained and without residual complication. On rare occasions patient may remain hypotensive for a more extended period after syncope and may require administration of phenylephrine or other vasopressor substance to counteract peripheral vasodilation.

The patient should remain seated until vital signs are stable and all discomfort and anxiety pass. The patient should not be allowed to stand quickly or walk unattended. Dental treatment should be discontinued, and the practitioner should attempt to discover the syncopal precipitant so that future therapy may be modified to prevent recurrence.

EPILEPSY

Epilepsy is a common disorder that affects 0.5% of the North American population. The dentist needs to reduce the risk of seizure during the dental visit. It is also important to know how to manage a patient if a seizure occurs. The other concern of the dentist is to minimize and treat the oral side effects of long-term administration of phenytoin.

Although it is true that seizures may occur at times with no or only minimal warning, this is rare for the majority of treated, noninstitutionalized epileptic persons. Dental care for many epileptic individuals can be provided safely by the general practitioner using the following guidelines.

An accurate record of the patient's seizure history is essential. The seizure history should be corroborated if possible by the patient's physician or by a family member. A history of recent seizure activity (frequency, when, where, and what happened) should be taken. A description of the events associated with the onset of the seizure (failure to take medication, side effects of additional medications, alcohol consumption, association of seizures with sleep, menstrual cycle, fever, stress, or other events) should be recorded. Any prodromal symptoms should be noted.

The oral examination of an epileptic patient may show the results of trauma (Fig. 3) that occurs during seizure activity and may demonstrate effects of anticonvulsive-drug therapy. Laboratory study of serum anticonvulsive drug levels may be indicated when control of seizures is poor and additional medication is being considered before dental treatment.

Gingival hyperplasia induced by phenytoin (DPH) affects at least 40% to 50% of those who use phenytoin for more than 3 months. The more severe effects may not develop until after several years of continual use of the drug. Both the drug and the local irritation from plaque, calculus, restorations, or appliances are causative factors. The pathogenesis of the gingival changes caused by this drug indicate that the gingival lesion does not represent hypertrophy, hyperplasia, or fibrosis but is an uncontrolled growth of connective tissue of apparently normal cell and fiber composition.

The clinical appearance of phenytoin-induced gingival hyperplasia is usually characteristic. The clinical appearance can vary depending on the location of the lesion and the extent of secondary inflammatory changes. Diagnosis is based on the history of phenytoin use and the clinical appearance of the lesions. With rare exceptions the hyperplasia is restricted to the gingivae and after extraction of teeth and excision of the hyperplastic tissue, there is no recurrence.

MANAGEMENT. Treatment of phenytoin-induced gingival hyperplasia should emphasize excellent oral hygiene and elimination of local gingival irritants. The patient's physician may be consulted to determine whether other medications may replace phenytoin. The patient with menarche frequently begins a period of difficult management because of the increased frequency of seizures that may occur at this time. Some physicians advocate avoidance of phenytoin in treating female adolescents to prevent both gingival hyperplasia and hirsutism. The epileptic patient's medication should be reviewed before orthodontic treatment is begun.

Surgical removal of hyperplastic gingivae, root planing, and removal of local irritants are needed after hyperplasia has developed. Hyperplasia does not resolve by removal of local gingival irritants. Good oral hygiene and interdental massage may reduce the rate of recurrence of hyperplasia. Topically applied medications, including antiplaque agents such as chlorhexidine, may be useful in reducing the microbial irritation and may be an adjunct in prevention of recurrence of gingival hyperplasia.

A mentally retarded epileptic patient presents a difficult management problem, particularly if good oral hygiene is not maintained. In such cases the value of surgery should be considered when the gingival overgrowth interferes with function or is a source of severe halitosis or hemorrhage.

Routine dental local anesthetic procedures are not associated with increased risk of seizures and do not interact with the commonly used anticonvulsant medications. Seizures have been reported when lidocaine is administered intravenously for the treatment of cardiac arrhythmias, but the amount contained in dental local anesthetic agents is unlikely to cause a seizure, particularly if the dentist aspirates before injection. General anesthesia, including nitrous oxide sedation, may induce seizures, and local anesthesia is preferred. General anesthetic agents also may precipitate anticonvulsant drug toxicity, and some anesthetics, such as ketamine, are known to produce high-frequency EEG activity and convulsions. Although diazepam is frequently administered intravenously to control persistent seizures and is considered a relatively safe drug for this purpose, cardiopulmonary arrest may occur when it is administered with barbiturates.

Since emotional upsets may induce seizures in some patients medication to control anxiety is often prescribed for epileptic patients before dental treatment. An additional 10 to 20 mg of phenobarbital for epileptic individuals who are already using this drug routinely 1 or 2 hours before the dental appointment is usually well tolerated and does not produce significant drowsiness. In patients who are not using barbiturates, diazepam may be a useful antianxiety agent before dental procedures. Temporary increase in the dose of other anticonvulsive agents (phenytoin, carbamazepine, primidone, and ethosuximide) for prophylactic control of seizures in the dental office is usually not recommended.

Poorly retained crowns, bridges, and partial dentures, as well as loose and grossly carious teeth, are a hazard for the epileptic patient because of risk of aspiration during a seizure. Dentures should be fabricated to include a radiopaque marker in the event that radiographic examination is needed to rule out aspiration after a seizure.

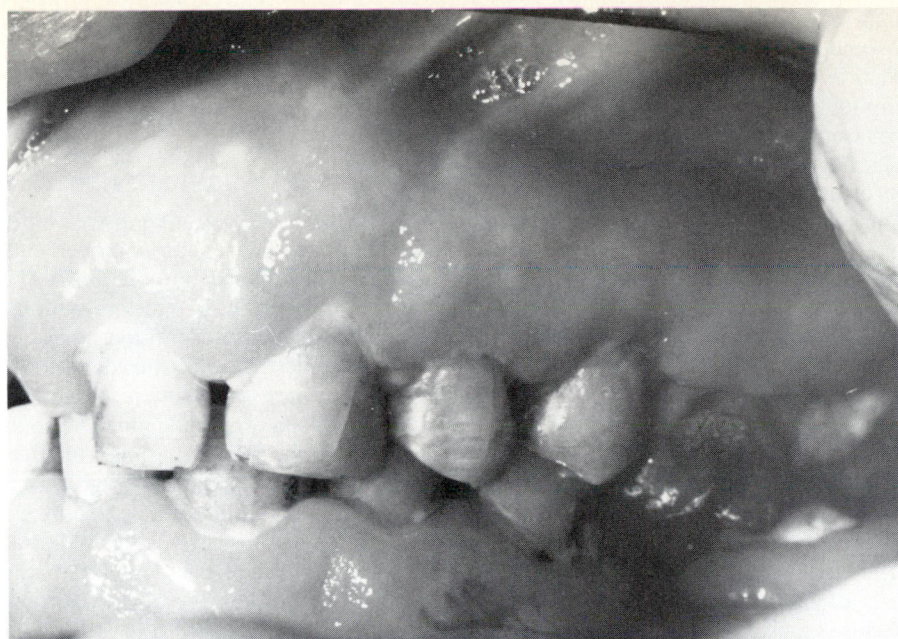

Fig. 3 Patient with gingival hyperplasia caused by phenytoin and poor oral hygiene affecting intradental and facial gingivae. Gingival hyperplasia is fibrotic but with peripheral inflammatory component associated with poor plaque control.

MANAGING A PATIENT HAVING A SEIZURE. The majority of seizures are brief, self-limited events that result in no permanent ill effects, provided patients are prevented from harming themselves while unconscious. Patients who are subject to frequent seizures should be closely observed during the dental visit. Partial seizures, manifest as impairment of consciousness, ictal automatism, and inappropriate speech or sounds, usually pass in a few minutes and leave the patient confused and tired, but otherwise unaffected. Restraint is not needed in these cases and may at times produce a violent defensive response.

If a partial or generalized seizure occurs in the dental chair, the patient should be placed in a supine position either in the chair or on the floor. The patient's head should be placed to the side so that saliva and vomitus can exit and the possibility of aspiration is reduced. Efforts should be made to maintain a patent airway by the use of the head-tilt position, and secretions should be suctioned from the patient's mouth to prevent aspiration. Occasionally during a seizure there are periods of apnea. At times oxygen administered through a face or nose mask may be helpful. Patients' extremities should be gently restrained from uncontrolled movements to prevent them from injuring themselves. Placing objects between a patient's teeth during a seizure is generally not recommended. Improper intraoral placement of any device may result in greater damage to oral and dental structures. The device could be broken and aspirated during the seizure.

During the postictal phase the patient must be carefully observed so that respiratory depression or airway obstruction does not occur. The emergency situation is not over until all vital signs are normal and the patient is alert and oriented. The patient should not be discharged from the dental office unaccompanied. It is recommended that the patient relax for the remainder of the day and not carry on any strenuous activity, since the potential for a subsequent seizure exists.

If a patient suffers more than one seizure without regaining consciousness, status epilepticus should be considered and an emergency team should be summoned. A 50% dextrose solution should be administered intravenously. If the dentist is experienced in administering diazepam intravenously, a dose not exceeding 10 mg may be given over 2 minutes, and the dose should be repeated in 20 to 30 minutes if convulsions continue. Barbiturates administered intravenously may also terminate a convulsion, but when they are given with diazepam, they may cause respiratory depression. Barbiturates are not advised unless an electrocardiograph is available. An antiepileptic drug such as phenytoin may be given intravenously after diazepam has stopped the seizure, but it is not used as the primary drug.

BIBLIOGRAPHY

Evans DEN: Anesthesia and the epileptic patient—a review, Anesthesia 30:34, 1975.
Hassel TM and others: Summary of an international symposium on phenytoin-induced teratology and gingival pathology, 99:652, 1979.
Livingstone S, editor: The medical treatment of epilepsy, Pediatr Ann 8:110, 1979.
Smith QT: Gingival fibrosis during phenytoin-ingestion, Northwest Dent 57:23, 1978.

OTOLOGIC SYMPTOMS ASSOCIATED WITH TEMPOROMANDIBULAR JOINT DYSFUNCTION

Otalgia (pain in and around the ear) and other aural complaints are frequently included among the symptoms of TMJ dysfunction. Otalgia is the predominant aural symptom, but other symptoms of TMJ dysfunction may include fullness in the ears, dizziness, vertigo, tinnitus, and hearing loss. Otologic consultation may not identify pathosis to account for the patient's symptoms, and the patient's symptoms may be ascribed to dental problems or TMJ dysfunction. Other health-care workers and the media have described a broad concept of TMJ dysfunction. This includes orofacial symptoms and ear, neck, shoulder, and even more distant musculoskeletal and sensory abnormalities caused by TMJ dysfunction.

Otalgia appears convincingly established as a symptom of

TMJ dysfunction, and may occur in more than three fourths of patients according to some studies. Despite a long history of association between TMJ dysfunction and dizziness, beginning with Costen's description in the 1930s, there is still little data to support this correlation. Researchers believe that otologic problems and TMJ problems often occur together because of the shared innervation of masticatory, tensor tympani, and tensor palati muscles. Thus, if these muscles go into spasm, it could lead to eustachian tube dysfunction and concomitant aural symptoms. In addition, the stapedius muscle, which is innervated by the facial nerve, may have effects on hearing and other otologic symptoms. However, careful evaluation in a recent study of patients with both TMJ dysfunction and aural symptoms led to the conclusion that the correlation between TMJ dysfunction and aural symptoms, excluding otalgia, may be coincidental.

In one sense the otologic symptoms associated with TMJ dysfunction are a restatement of Costen's syndrome, in which spasm within the masticatory muscle system has replaced mechanical impingement of the condyle on the glenoid fossa, ear canal, and related nerves, as the development of symptoms. Spasm within the masticatory muscles is currently well accepted and experimentally established as an explanation for jaw pain, mandibular deviation, and joint dysfunction. However, spasm of the tensor tympani and tensor palati have not been convincingly demonstrated. Other abnormalities, such as vasomotor swelling of the eustachian tube and other changes in the inner ear, could conceivably account for the dizziness, tinnitus, and hearing loss in some patients who have other signs of TMJ dysfunction.

MANAGEMENT. Treatment of TMJ dysfunction is the same whether aural symptoms are present or not. Therapy may include care in use of the jaw, a soft diet, heat applied to the masticatory muscles, antiinflammatory agents, muscle relaxants, interocclusal bite appliances, physiotherapy, and biofeedback relaxation. These treatment modalities are effective in acute TMJ dysfunction, and are also helpful in more chronic forms of the disorder. There is no evidence to support suggestions that structural changes (occlusal or orthognathic) are mandatory in the management of TMJ dysfunction, as most studies report an 80% to 90% long-term success rate, regardless of whether structural changes were completed or not. When organic intrinsic joint disease involving bone or cartilage is present, joint surgery may be considered part of patient care after nonsurgical therapy has been thoroughly assessed. The objective of treatment is to reduce painful muscle spasm, trismus, mandibular deviation, pathologic joint sounds, and tenderness and sensory abnormalities experienced over the joint and surrounding areas. Symptoms of fullness in the ear, tinnitus, and dizziness may not improve with any certainty.

BIBLIOGRAPHY

Appelberg DB and others: TMJ disease: result of a 10 year study, Postgrad Med 65:167, 1979.
Appleberg DB and others: Otological manifestations in TMJ dysfunction, J Oral Rehabil 7:249, 1980.
Brookes GB and others: "Costen's syndrome"—correlation or coincidence: a review of 45 patients with temporo-mandibular joint dysfunction, otalgia and other aural symptoms, Clin Otolaryngol 5:23, 1980.
Costen JB: Neuralgias and ear symptoms associated with disturbed function of the temporomandibular joint, J Am Med Assoc 107:252, 1936.
Greene CS and Laskin DM: Long term evaluation of treatment for myofascial pain-dysfunction syndrome: a comparative analysis, J Am Dent Assoc 107:235, 1983.
Greene CS and Marbach JJ: Epidemiologic studies of mandibular dysfunction: a critical review, J Prosthet Dent 48:184, 1982.
Jonck LM: Ear symptoms in TMJ disturbance, S Afr Med J 54:782, 1978.
Laskin D and others: The president's conference on the examination, diagnosis and management of TMJ disorders, Chicago, 1982, American Dental Association.
Lipton JA and Marbach JJ: Predictors of treatment outcome in patients with myofascial pain-dysfunction syndrome and organic temporomandibular joint disorders, J Prosthet Dent 51:387, 1984.

INVOLUNTARY JAW MOVEMENTS

A variety of degenerative diseases of the CNS are associated with abnormal and repetitive movements of the jaws and facial muscles. The majority of these problems appear with advancing age and may seriously interfere with denture function. In patients with a natural dentition, these involuntary jaw movements may destroy both the dentition and the periodontium. In addition, these jaw movements may be associated with TMJ dysfunction and orofacial pain. The conditions most commonly discussed in the dental literature include senile tremor, parkinsonism, tardive dyskinesias (Fig. 4), and the destructive ruminative jaw movement seen in some decerebrate patients. In some patients with these problems, effective drugs that reduce the tremor and facilitate dental care are available. In others a means of controlling the abnormal movements is not possible because of unacceptable side effects of an otherwise effective drug or the lack of effective therapy.

Intention tremors of the jaws and head are often worse when a patient is required to perform specific jaw movements such as bite registration for dentures. These tremors may be less severe when the patient is more relaxed. Loss of proprioceptive jaw sensation through extraction of teeth often worsens a tremor. Repetitive tongue movements and muscle tonus within the tongue may result in trauma to the lingual mucosa and abrasion and ulceration of the tongue. Patients with increased muscle activity may also complain of burning sensations in the tongue that appear to be caused by repetitive trauma, constant muscle tension in the tongue, or both.

The development of rigidity in some affected muscle groups may occur in Parkinson's disease and may prove as great a problem for dental treatment as the presence of tremor. When rigidity of one or more facial and masticatory muscle groups is present, completion of a prosthesis may be limited in extension and retention in the areas of muscle activity or rigidity.

A number of medications used in the treatment of Parkinson's disease, either alone or in combination with levodopa, are strongly anticholinergic and produce considerable inhibition of salivary flow. Benztropin mesylate (Cogentin), trihexyphenidyl (Artane), cycrimine (Pagitane), biperiden (Akineton), procyclidine (Kemadrin), and amantadine (Symmetrel) all possess this property. The tricyclic antidepressants and the antihistamines may also cause xerostomia. The xerostomic effects of these drugs may be useful in controlling sialism seen in many of these patients. However, the anticholinergic effect often predominates and contributes to dryness and soreness of the tongue and oral mucosa. Xerostomia may contribute to burning mouth, increase difficulties with denture use, and increase development of root surface and recurrent caries. Infections that may occur in patients with drug-induced xerostomia include candidiasis and suppurative parotitis.

The main side effects of levodopa that concern dentists are the possibility of postural hypotension and the development of choreiform and dystonic movements of the head and jaws. Burning sensations of the tongue and bitter taste are also side effects of this medication.

Tardive dyskinesia describes a broad group of extrapyramidal motor disorders that have been observed as long-term side effects of the administration of some neuroleptic drugs. Med-

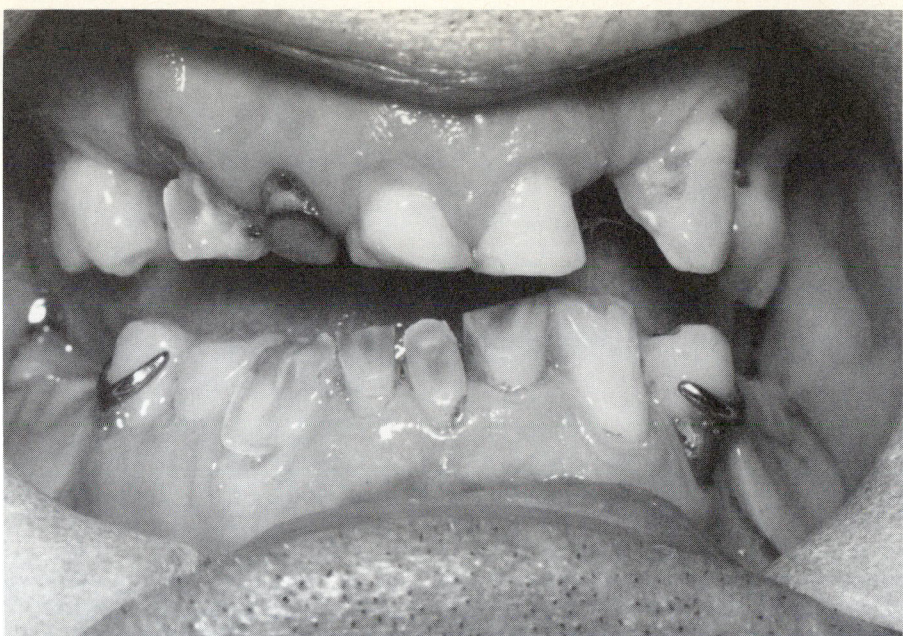

Fig. 4 Severe attrition of dentition. Dental fractures can be seen in individual with severe abnormal extra-pyramidal motor disorder (tardive dyskinesia). Patient's maxillary partial denture was fractured by excessive forces on appliance.

ications that are associated with dyskinesias include phenothiazines such as trifluoperazine (Stelazine), thioridazine (Mellaril), and chlorpromazine (Thorazine); butyrophenone tranquilizers such as haloperidol (Haldol); and reserpine derivatives such as Serpasil. The dyskinetic side effects of these medications are believed to result from hypersensitivity of the basal ganglia to dopamine. The minor benzodiazepine tranquilizers (chlordiazepoxide, diazepam, and lorazepam) are free of this side effect.

Although the manifestations of tardive dyskinesia are not limited to the head and neck, a characteristic syndrome has been described in which there are rhythmic involuntary movements of the tongue, face, mouth, and jaws. Involuntary mouthing, lip tremor, chewing or puckering of the lips, and fasciculation or darting movements of the tongue are all described as part of this syndrome. Other manifestations may include agitation or jitteriness, dystonic problems, such as spasm of the neck muscles, trismus, swallowing difficulties, and protrusion of the tongue, or Parkinson-like symptoms.

The risk of tardive dyskinesia is higher for elderly women taking large drug doses. Symptoms frequently persist after the offending drug is discontinued. Some control of the symptoms is usually possible, with the various medications used to treat other basal ganglia abnormalities. Such dyskinetic symptoms usually prevent the wearing of dentures and attempts at controlling them should be made for this reason, as well as to alleviate the patient's suffering. The incidence of tardive dyskinesia is not accurately known. The majority of cases are seen in persons in institutions, where similar symptoms may be attributed to psychiatric and neurologic mannerisms and to senile dyskinesias.

MANAGEMENT. In some patients, diazepam or other muscle relaxants administered before the dental visit may produce greater relaxation during treatment. In severely affected patients, intravenously administered sedatives supplemented with nitrous oxide and oxygen may control tremors. In some cases construction of dentures may entirely eliminate a jaw tremor,

just as resting the hands on a table or in pockets may alleviate mild tremors in patients with Parkinson's disease. Construction of acrylic night guards, modification of existing appliances, or use of muscle relaxant medications may be helpful in controlling such symptoms. Because of the complex interaction of all elements of the masticatory system, correction of occlusal disharmonies and other dental defects can sometimes alleviate tremors and related sensory complaints.

In entirely different categories of cause and management are the powerful ruminatory (circular grinding) movements of the mandible seen in essentially decerebrate patients as a result of injuries to the cerebral cortex, trigeminal nuclei, and hypothalamus. Lack of tongue coordination, and lip and cheek movements with the jaw movements leads to severe self-inflicted wounds of the oral cavity. The majority of dental appliances cannot withstand these forces, and special stents, which may be ligated to the molar teeth, may be needed to minimize the self-inflicted damage. Spasm of the masseter muscles usually complicates the problem, and an oral examination including dental impressions can usually be performed on these patients only after the administration of curare or succinylcholine to eliminate the spasm.

BIBLIOGRAPHY

Bassett A and others: Tardive dyskinesia: an unrecognized cause of orofacial pain, Oral Surg 61:570, 1986.

Cohen CI: A case report; periodontal surgery in parkinsonism utilizing intravenous sedation, NY State Dent J 44:19, 1978.

Delwaide PJ and others: Spontaneous bucco-linguo-facial dyskinesia in the elderly, Acta Neurol Scand 56:256, 1977.

Fielding ML: Case report: construction of complete dentures for Parkinson patient, Dent Survey 53:36, 1977.

Hanson GE and others: A tongue stent for prevention of oral trauma in the comatose patient, Crit Care Med 3:200, 1975.

Pratrap-Chand R and others: Bruxism: its significance in coma, Clin Neurol Neurosurg 87:113, 1985.

Richmond G and others: Survey of bruxism in the institutionalized mentally retarded population, Am J Ment Defic 4:418, 1984.

Simpson GM and Kline NS: Tardive dyskinesia: manifestations, incidence,

etiology and treatment. In Yahn MD, editor: The basal ganglia, Res Publ Assoc Res Nerv Ment Dis 55:427, 1976.
Sunden-Kuronen B and others: Oral tardive dyskinesia, Acta Odontol Scand 41:343, 1983.

STROKE

Cerebrovascular accidents (CVAs or strokes) are a leading cause of death and disability. The majority of strokes in the older population occur because of failure of blood vessels that have been previously compromised by diabetes or hypertension. Detection of abnormal blood glucose levels and elevated blood pressure during dental office visits contributes to the effort to control this problem.

In general the untoward effects of hypertension on the cerebral vasculature are long term and include degenerative changes and weakening of the walls of cerebral arterioles that predispose patients to thrombosis, microaneurysms, and hemorrhage. Hypertension also leads to changes in the endocardium, aorta, and carotid tree that may contribute emboli to the cerebral vasculature. Patients who have chronic untreated elevations of the diastolic pressure which may lead to a variety of arteriosclerotic changes, have most CVAs.

Vascular changes underlying transient ischemic attacks and CVAs are not restricted to the cerebral vasculature. Similar changes may be present in the carotid artery system. An occlusion in any vessel of the carotid system may have a significance beyond any associated local symptoms. Patients with these occlusions should be referred to an appropriate practitioner for more detailed examination of the carotid system. Excessive calcification of the oral or superficial facial branch of the external carotid may be detected in radiographs. Swelling and bruits noted over the major carotid vessels in the neck should suggest the possibility of more extensive carotid artery problems that could predispose a patient to a stroke. Doppler pulsed ultrasonography is used in stroke patients to screen the branches of the carotid system, including the lingual artery, for irregularities of pulse rhythm and periodic reductions of the flow in the lingual arteries.

ORAL MANIFESTATIONS. Oral symptoms and functional disability of varying degrees may develop as a result of a stroke. The character of the problems depends on the location and extent of cerebral damage. Oral sensory dysfunction, ranging from mild dysesthesia to pain requiring analgesics and even neurosurgery, may occur. Patients who are mildly affected usually accept these problems as part of the complex of symptoms that results from the stroke. These oral complaints are often not reported, since a more severely handicapping hemiplegia exists. Alternatively, the dentist may be consulted about oral sensory dysfunction by stroke patients who hope that dental treatment will assist with a persistent and annoying oral symptom. Thorough evaluation of such patients to rule out other possible oral or dental causes for these symptoms is indicated, although in most cases cerebral damage is the cause of the problem.

Patients occasionally have taste abnormalities after a stroke. Painful cerebral damage may occur from obstruction of vessels supplying areas of the CNS. The pain is usually intractable and poorly localized. Facial pain caused by CVAs (Wallenberg's syndrome) is frequently associated with other neurologic abnormalities.

Some degree of oral motor dysfunction usually accompanies oral dysesthesia that is secondary to a stroke. Motor dysfunction affecting the muscles of mastication, deglutition, and facial expression (Fig. 5) contributes to the unfortunate effects of stroke on the orofacial area. Problems with speech (articulation

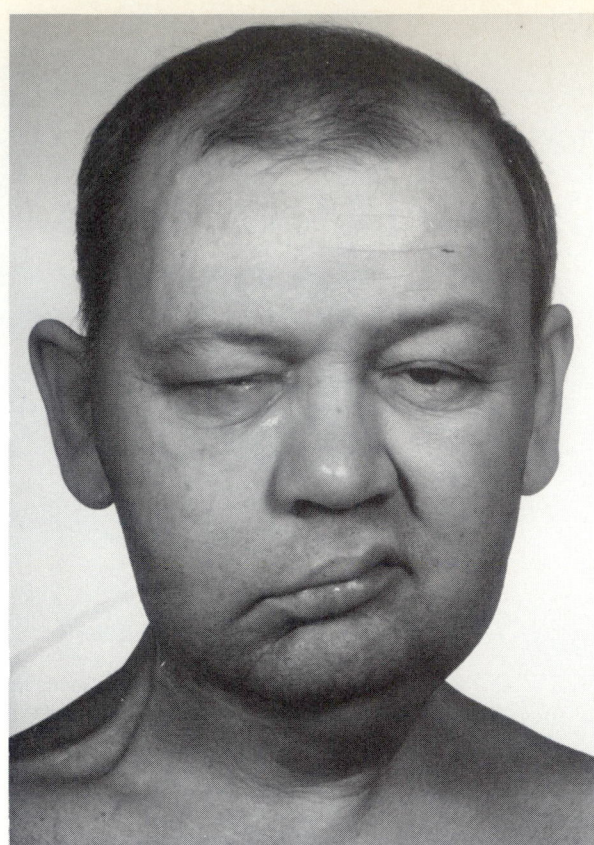

Fig. 5   Patient demonstrates right-sided facial paralysis with ptosis, loss of nasolabial fold, and drooping of corner of mouth following a cerebrovascular accident.

in particular), dribbling of saliva, difficulties in swallowing, choking episodes, and nasal regurgitation of fluids may occur. Lack of muscle tone and inability to control the muscles of mastication limit retention of dentures and clearing of a bolus from the buccal and lingual sulci. Plaque and food debris are retained around the teeth, and weakness or paralysis of the hand, arm, and shoulder may significantly reduce the effectiveness of oral hygiene measures.

Malformations of the cerebral vasculature may occur in various angiomatous syndromes. Some of these syndromes, such as Sturge-Weber and von Hippel-Lindau syndromes, also involve the face and oral tissues with a visible hemangiomatous birthmark or phacomatosis. Neurologic changes secondary to cerebral angiomatosis are common complications of these syndromes. Orofacial hemangiomatosis in patients who have evidence of focal neurologic disease should be considered part of one of these phacomatoses until an alternative explanation for the neurologic problem is established. Surgical treatment of an orofacial hemangioma in such a patient should be attempted only after the extent of the vascular malformation and its collaterals is adequately defined.

Cerebral venous thromboses, including cavernous sinus thrombosis, are serious, rare complications of facial and jaw fractures, dental infection with facial cellulitis, and surgical procedures, particularly those performed in the anterior maxillary and pterygoid plexus regions. The infection is spread via connections between the intracranial and extracranial venous circulations in these locations. Cerebral venous thrombosis is not a cause of cerebral infarction and stroke, although small emboli may reach the cerebral arterial circulation through arteriovenous anastomoses, confusing the signs and symptoms characteristic of cerebral venous thrombosis.

Arteritis is a rare cause of cerebral infarction or hemorrhage that may be generalized throughout the carotid system or may manifest as localized tenderness over temporal or facial arteries or as chronic pain in the areas supplied by those vessels. These vascular problems and migraine are considered in more detail in Chapter 146.

MANAGEMENT. The patient who has hemiplegia or another major physical disability often presents a management problem for the dentist. The treatment facility must allow access for the physically handicapped.

The practice of deferring elective dental treatment for patients whose blood pressure is constantly more than 160/95 mm Hg is designed to encourage patients to obtain and follow an antihypertensive therapeutic regimen. In general the blood pressure reading alone is a poor predictor of the likelihood of a CVA occurring at a given time. Spasm of the cerebral arterioles is detected as a response to peak elevations of systolic blood pressure in patients with malignant hypertension. This probably contributes to the cerebral edema, petechial hemorrhages, and small infarctions that underlie the syndrome of hypertensive encephalopathy. Besides these patients, however, the risk that dental procedures will trigger transient cerebral ischemic attacks, cerebral hemorrhage, or any other type of CVA in a patient with a markedly elevated blood pressure is unknown. Precautions usually are taken to allay nervousness, limit the length of a visit, prevent intravascular injection of anesthetics with vasoconstrictors, and monitor the blood pressure during dental treatment. The wisdom of such management remains unquestioned, but its contribution to the prevention of strokes may be minimal.

A number of oral prosthetic devices have been designed to address some of the problems faced by patients after a stroke. Success with these appliances depends on the willingness of the dentist and the patient to experiment and persist with use and on the ingenuity of the prosthetic device design (Fig. 6). Initially patient comfort should be improved by prophylaxis, polishing of dentures, institution of a regular program of denture and oral hygiene, and relining of poorly retentive dentures.

Retention of large amounts of food debris, particularly in the buccal sulcus of the affected side is a common problem in stroke patients. Processing of an acrylic extension to the buccal flange of the lower denture may aid in controlling this problem and may also assist in the retention of the denture by lax muscles. Bite splints or night guard appliances may protect the tongue and buccal mucosa from irregularities in the dental arch and from dental trauma. These irritants can aggravate lingual dysesthesias and glossodynia, particularly in patients with hyperactive lingual musculature. A wire or acrylic palatal extension added to the posterior edge of an upper denture can improve control over swallowing and reduce nasal regurgitation and certain types of speech defects after a stroke. An electronically controlled visual speech aid unit has been developed in association with the palatal extension to help coordinate palatal movements. In the stroke patient who still has natural teeth, an electric toothbrush and a water irrigating device may facilitate oral hygiene. A number of devices have been fabricated to aid the physically handicapped patient who has weak or poorly controlled hand and arm movement with oral hygiene. Oral antiplaque and antiseptic rinses may be useful in patients who can manage rinsing but have difficulty with mechanical oral hygiene methods.

BIBLIOGRAPHY

Fardal O and Turnbull RS: A review of the literature on use of chlorhexidine in dentistry, J Am Dent Assoc 112:863, 1986.
Myers DE and others: Evaluation of lingual artery hemodynamics in stroke patients using Doppler ultrasound, J Oral Surg 51:252, 1981.
Selley WG: Dental help for stroke patients, Br Dent J 143:409, 1977.
Tatoian JA and others: Meningitis and temporal lobe abscess of dental origin: report of a case, J Oral Surg 30:423, 1972.

DEMYELINATION AND DEGENERATION OF THE CENTRAL NERVOUS SYSTEM

Amyotrophic lateral sclerosis (ALS or Lou Gehrig's disease) and multiple sclerosis (MS) are of interest because they may be infectious. These diseases should be compared with those that are more certainly associated with slow viral infection. The evidence for an infectious cause is still obscure in MS and ALS, but transmissible infectious agents have been demonstrated in nervous tissue from patients with kuru and Creutzfeldt-Jakob disease. These diseases have been transmitted to both humans and experimental animals by viral agents.

An adult who acquires rapidly progressive dementia but who does not have a space-occupying intracranial lesion may have Creutzfeldt-Jakob disease. Because of potential hazards associated with the infectious agent of Creutzfeldt-Jakob disease, it is prudent to use the precautions recommended for patients with other infectious diseases. Barrier precautions to reduce percutaneous exposure to blood and nervous tissue are suggested. However, there is no evidence to indicate that MS or ALS can be transmitted in this manner.

Multiple sclerosis

MS is the most common of the demyelinating diseases and usually runs a protracted course. The problems in providing dental care are similar to those encountered in treating patients with physical handicaps. Dental care requires assessment of a patient's ability to maintain adequate oral hygiene. Other considerations in individuals with MS include loss of facial and masticatory muscle tonicity (Fig. 7), inability to support the head, development of muscle spasms and rigidity, and involuntary movements of the jaws.

The sensory abnormalities characteristic of MS, including localized paresthesias, numbness, and pain, may affect the oral cavity, jaws, and face. Physicians have paid particular attention to trigeminal neuralgia and atypical facial pain in patients with MS. Sensory impairment over the distribution of the trigeminal nerve occurs in 1% to 4% of patients with MS. Researchers at the Mayo Clinic have shown that 2% of patients with trigeminal neuralgia have MS. Autopsy studies suggest that plaquelike lesions at the point of entry of the roots of the fifth cranial nerve into the pons are the source of the neuralgic pains in these cases, although the disseminated character of the intracerebral lesions of MS leaves this uncertain in some cases. MS should always be considered in the differential diagnosis of unexplained orofacial pain, especially if the pain is accompanied by symptoms of numbness or other sensory abnormality.

Amyotrophic lateral sclerosis

ALS is an insidiously progressive disease with severe effects on respiration and deglutition. ALS ultimately results in death. It is important that the dentist, through adequate history taking and consultation, be aware of the patient's diagnosis and prognosis and plan dental care appropriately.

Syringomyelia

Syringomyelia is a rare disease that affects the CNS. It can result in intractable jaw and face pain of central origin, which

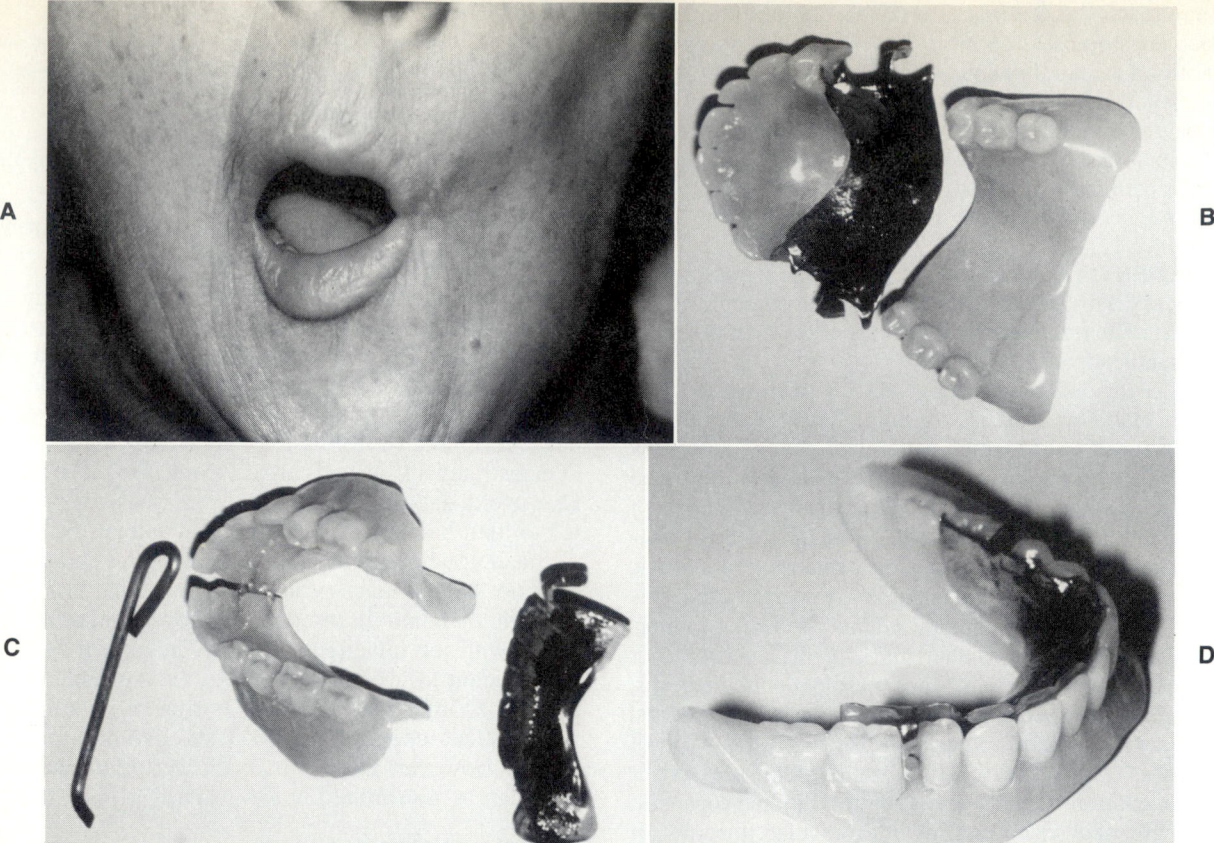

Fig. 6 **A,** Patient demonstrates some unique difficulties encountered both in prosthetic management associated with motor dysfunction and with limited labial aperture. **B** and C, Complete dentures were fabricated in sections and placed as individual portions into oral cavity. **D,** Dentures assembled in mouth to form single rigid appliance that functions as complete upper and lower dentures. (Courtesy of Dr. P. Stevenson-Moore).

is distinct from pain of peripheral or neuropathic origin. During progress of the disease, areas of the body, including the face and jaws, may become anesthetic, and injuries to these areas that result in scar formation may occur.

Vitamin B₁₂ deficiency

See Chapter 154.

Phacomatoses

Oral or facial manifestations of a number of conditions may occur in conditions that include neurofibromatosis, tuberous sclerosis, Sturge-Weber syndrome, ataxia telangiectasia, and incontinentia pigmenti. Neurofibromatosis and tuberous sclerosis are of special interest because of their association with predisposition to malignancy in the nervous system.

Multiple neurofibromatosis is an inherited disorder that has a frequency of 1:2000 to 4000 live births. Multiple neurofibromatosis is characterized by the presence of patchy areas of melanin deposition (café au lait spots) and multiple neurofibromas. The diagnosis of neurofibromatosis is based on the presence of multiple macules or nodules, café au lait spots, and family history. As many as 10% of the patients with neurofibromatosis have well-developed oral lesions. The tongue is the most common oral site of neurofibroma, which may result in macroglossia. The lesions are generally asymptomatic and are frequently discovered on routine oral examination.

The characteristic skin lesions of tuberous sclerosis (ade-

noma sebaceum) occur over the nose in a "butterfly distribution," in the nasolabial folds and on the chin and forehead. The lesions appear either as telangiectatic lesions or small, firm, yellow, gray, or red elevated nodules. Similar lesions may occur intraorally. Fibromas and enlargement of the gingivae are described even when patients have not received phenytoin to control seizures. A pitting of the labial and buccal enamel of the permanent dentition, which is characteristic of tuberous sclerosis, is reported, as are other miscellaneous oral abnormalities, including hyperkeratosis, jaw cysts, facial asymmetry, high palate, cleft lip and palate, and retarded eruption.

Oral changes occur in about one third of patients with Sturge-Weber syndrome (Fig. 8). These changes may include massive growths of the gingiva, asymmetric jaw growth, and altered dental eruption. The change in tooth eruption sequence is thought to be caused by differential blood flow to the affected area. It is important to differentiate angiomatous lesions of the jaw from other causes of gingival hyperplasia, especially if surgery is planned in the area of tissue change. Classically the intraoral lesions in Sturge-Weber syndrome occur on the same side of the body as the other angiomas the patient exhibits.

Patients with ataxia telangiectasia have fine, symmetric, bright red streaks in the conjunctiva. These lesions usually extend with age to the "butterfly" area of the face and neck, as well as to the extremities. These changes may also be manifest on the hard and soft palate and throughout the nasal mucosa. Small stature, thin, sad face, and stooping shoulders,

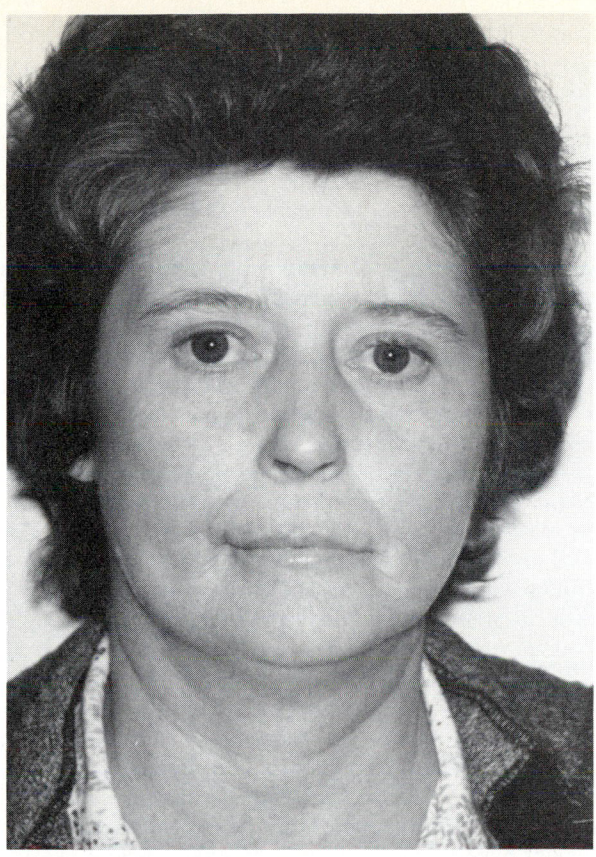

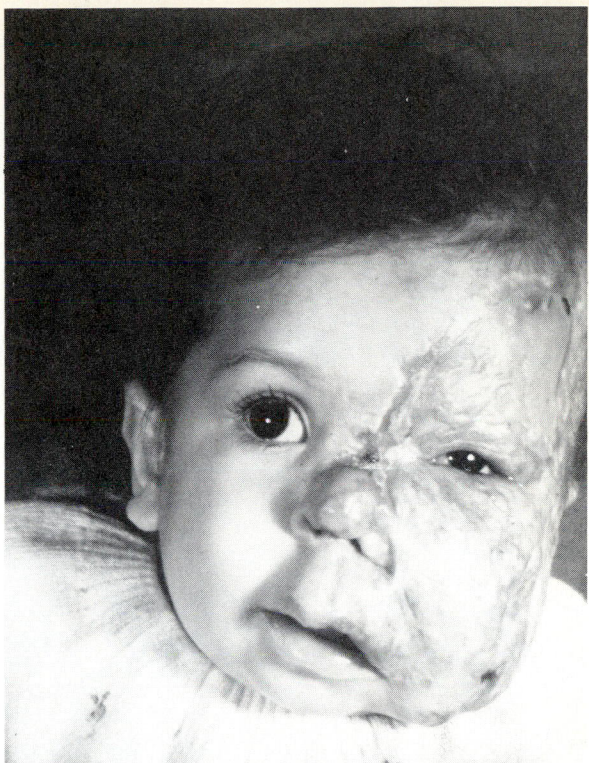

Fig. 8 Child with Sturge-Weber syndrome, showing extensive facial lesion.

Fig. 7 Patient with multiple sclerosis, demonstrating loss of facial muscle tone resulting in flat, expressionless face.

along with excessive drooling and poor quality of speech, are considered characteristic of the syndrome.

The oral changes of incontinentia pigmenti are limited to the dentition, which exhibit delayed eruption and missing or peg-shaped teeth. These anomalies affect both deciduous and permanent dentitions and occur with a familial distribution.

BIBLIOGRAPHY

Brightman VJ: Benign tumors of the oral cavity. In Lynch MAL, editor: Burket's oral medicine, Philadelphia, 1977, JB Lippincott Co.

Cohen L: Disturbance of taste as a symptom of multiple sclerosis, Br J Oral Maxillofac Surg 2:184, 1965.

Epstein JB, Schubert MM, and Hatcher DC: Multiple neurofibromatosis, Oral Surg Oral Med Oral Pathol 56:560, 1983.

Gajdusek DC and others: Precautions in medical care of, and handling materials from patients with transmissible virus dementia (Creutzfeldt-Jakob disease), N Engl J Med 297:1253, 1977.

Gorlin RJ and Pindborg JJ: Syndromes of the head and neck, ed 2, New York, 1979, McGraw-Hill Inc.

Mulder DW, editor: The diagnosis and treatment of amyotrophic lateral sclerosis, Boston, 1980, Houghton Mifflin Co.

Pisanti S: Burn injuries in a patient with syringomyelia—case report, J Oral Med 32:104, 1977.

Roller NW and others: Amyotrophic lateral sclerosis, J Oral Surg 37:46, 1974.

Rushton JG and Olafson RA: Trigeminal neuralgia associated with multiple sclerosis, Arch Neurol 13:383, 1965.

Scully C: Orofacial manifestations in tuberous sclerosis, J Oral Surg 44:706, 1977.

Vinken P and Bruyn GW: Handbook of clinical neurology. Vol. 9. Multiple sclerosis and other demyelinating disorders, Amsterdam, 1970, North-Holland Publishing Co.

NEUROMUSCULAR DISEASE

The masticatory and facial muscles may exhibit evidence of neuromuscular disease at the same time other regional muscle groups are affected, or they may be the location of the first complaint in some neuromuscular disorders. Patients who complain of difficulties with speaking and swallowing, those who can no longer manage full dentures, and those with trismus and TMJ dysfunction may have complaints caused by neuromuscular disease. These patients should be evaluated for signs of unequal masticatory muscle strength, facial muscle palsy, unexplained deviation on opening the mouth, and muscle tremors and fasciculations. The technique for evaluating facial and masticatory muscle function is fully described by Bosma. In the majority of patients, isolated spasms affecting one or more masticatory muscles explain the abnormal function observed, but on occasion, evidence of masseter or pterygoid muscle weakness is detected.

When evidence of orofacial neuromuscular dysfunction is noted, either as a presenting complaint suggesting a neuromuscular disorder or along with other previously diagnosed problems, the dentist should consult with the patient's physician. In a number of circumstances, treatment of the neuromuscular problem greatly assists in managing the patient's dental problems.

With the exception of EMG recording of the masticatory cycle, little work has been done recording the various parameters currently available as clinical measurements of limb muscles. Nerve conduction studies of the branches of the facial nerve may be used as part of the management of a facial palsy, but in general, data on orofacial neuromuscular function of current clinical usefulness are minimal.

Myasthenia gravis

The primary signs and symptoms of myasthenia gravis occur in the orofacial-pharyngeal area. A flat, expressionless face, drooping corners of the mouth, paresis of the orbicularis oris

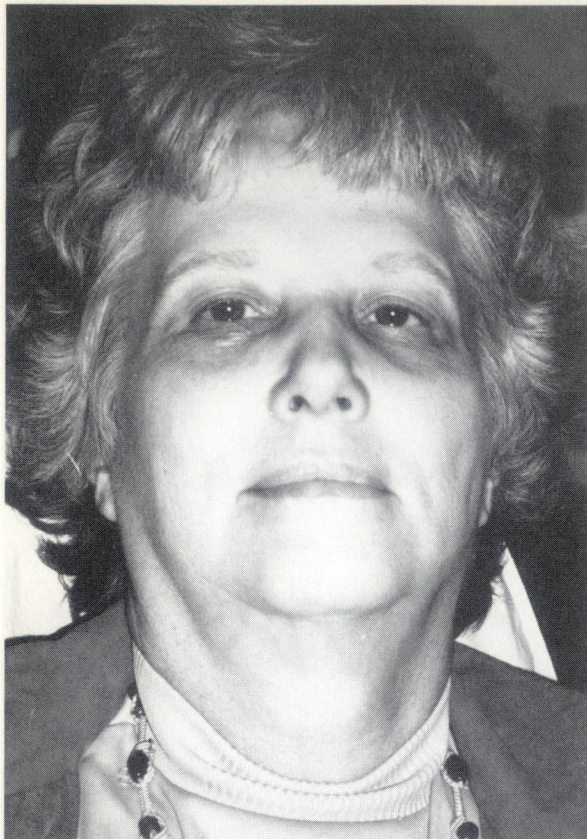

Fig. 9 Patient demonstrates loss of facial muscular tone resulting in expressionless face. Patient complained of general fatigue, depression, and weak voice, as described in myasthenia gravis.

and oculi muscles, weakness of the neck muscles, general fatigue and depression, and a flat, weak voice are characteristic of myasthenia gravis (Fig. 9). An incorrect diagnosis of depression is sometimes made. Protrusive movements of the tongue appear weak and limited. Stertorous breathing and dyspnea may also be apparent even with the patient at rest. The soft palate hangs motionless, and the cheeks hang closely along the buccal surfaces of the teeth. Dysphagia and regurgitation of food into the mouth are common. Masticatory, facial, and neck muscles are often among those primarily affected, leading to inability to keep the jaws closed without guiding and holding the mandible in place by hand. The anticholinesterase drugs may stimulate saliva production as a side effect, and the patient may have difficulty handling the saliva if swallowing and masticatory and facial muscle function are weak.

MANAGEMENT. The ability to manage full dentures may be compromised in patients with myasthenia gravis because of inability to maintain a peripheral seal or retain the lower denture by muscular control. Construction of a thin peripheral border to the denture is recommended, and maximum extension of the denture is desirable. The laxity of the buccinator and masseter muscles brings them in close contact with the sides of the upper denture and may block the flow of parotid saliva or cause it to accumulate under the upper denture and dislodge it.

Infections, including dental abscesses, and stress may induce a crisis in patients with myasthenia gravis. Ideally, in the patient subject to repeated crises, dental care should be provided in a hospital dental center or other location where facilities for intubation and artificial respiration are available. Excessive saliva often needs to be controlled by keeping patients upright and using effective aspiration during dental treatment.

Inflammatory myopathies

Myofascial dysfunction affecting the muscles of mastication (TMJ) may be the result of localized inflammatory changes in one or more of these muscles as a result of trauma, excessive movement under stress, or minor ruptures in ligaments or muscle fibers. Localized inflammatory changes occurring in these muscles can lead to symptoms indistinguishable from those of TMJ dysfunction. Polymyalgia rheumatica and trichinosis are possible causes of an inflammatory myopathy of the masticatory muscles. Appropriate screening tests (sedimentation rate and eosinophil count, respectively) may be required to rule out these possibilities. On occasion muscle biopsy is required.

MANAGEMENT. Management of an inflammatory myopathy of the masticatory muscles is the same as that used for control of TMJ dysfunction. A routine of local applications of heat, antiinflammatory agents, rest of the jaw and associated muscles, occlusal appliances, and physiotherapy may be used.

Malignant hyperthermia

Malignant hyperthermia during general anesthesia continues to be associated with a high mortality. The problem persists largely because the disease is often not diagnosed until widespread and irreversible cellular damage has occurred. The history may help identify risk if any of the following are noted: malignant hyperthermia during a previous general anesthesia, a positive family history of malignant hyperthermia, serum biochemical abnormalities (for example, elevated creatinine phosphokinase [CPK] levels), and musculoskeletal disease in the patient or a relative. Unfortunately, only about one third of patients manifest malignant hyperthermia as a musculoskeletal abnormality, so the presence of muscle disease is a useful guide only when one or more of these conditions are also present. Of those who have malignant hyperthermia, many display skeletal muscle rigidity as part of their neuromuscular problem. The presence of elevated CPK levels is also nonspecific for this condition, raised levels being found in a number of conditions such as coronary thrombosis, severe neuromyopathies, myxedema, and late pregnancy. Where available, muscle biopsy with evaluation of the in vitro response to halothane remains the most accurate predictor of susceptibility.

BIBLIOGRAPHY

Bigot C and others: Dental and periodontal incidence in two systemic diseases: Friedrich's ataxia and Duchenne de Boulogne's disease, Inform Dent 59:23, 1977.

Bond WS: Detection and management of the neuroleptic malignant syndrome, Clin Pharm 3:302, 1984.

Bosma JF: Sensorimotor examination of the mouth and pharynx, Fronti Oral Physiol 2:78, 1976.

Bottomley WK and others: Management of patients with myasthenia gravis who require maxillary dentures, J Prosthet Dent 38:609, 1977.

Hawada T and others: Masticatory function in the patient with Kugelberg Welander disease, J Hiroshima Univ Dent Soc 8:216, 1975.

Hawada T and others: Roentgenocephalometric analysis of open bite in patients with progressive muscular dystrophy, J Hiroshima Dent Soc 8:55, 1976.

Hawada T and others: Masticatory performance in patients with progressive muscular dystrophy, J Hiroshima Dent Soc 8:61, 1976.

Kamiiski H and others: Correction of myopathic face associated with myotonic muscular dystrophy, J Maxillofac Surg 5:48, 1977.

Kent JN and others: Correction of severe dentofacial deformity associated with myotonia congenita, J Oral Surg 36:129, 1978.

Nissen RL and others: Malignant hyperthermia, Laryngoscope 92:1183, 1982.

Pollock RA and others: Malignant hyperthermia in the head and neck surgery patient: an update and review, Laryngoscope 93:318, 1983.

Sessler DI: Malignant hyperthermia, J Pediatr 109:9, 1986.

NEUROLOGIC CONDITIONS

DIAGNOSIS OF OROFACIAL PAIN. Accurate diagnosis of orofacial pain is essential if effective therapy is to be provided. In this section pain is used as an inclusive term to describe sensory complaints that may include burning, paresthesia, hyperesthesia, anesthesia, and pain.

The mouth and face are probably the most common sites of pain in the body. The head, neck, and oral regions represent common sites of chronic and referred pain. Pain is a multidimensional phenomenon including sensory-discriminative, affective, cognitive, and motivational dimensions. It is also related to temporal and spatial summation of sensory input. Sensory input can arise from any tissue including muscular, skeletal, vascular, or neurologic tissues, or combinations of them. This input can be due to physical-chemical stimuli caused by trauma, tumors, inflammation, and infection and to alteration in function of the neurologic input. Modulation of input is due to CNS function at the spinal, midbrain, and cortical levels. Chronic pain most often has multiple causes. Atypical facial pain is due to multiple factors and may include local or regional conditions, as well as central neurologic conditions and the affective and psychologic factors of the pain experience. Thus therapy must often involve multiple considerations and multidisciplinary therapy. General concepts useful in understanding facial pain are shown in the following:

Concepts in pain:

  I. Etiology (agent)
    A. Inflammatory
    B. Trauma
    C. Tumor
    D. Infection
    E. Neurologic
    F. Pressure
    G. Traction
  II. Tissue (site)
    A. Nerve
    B. Vascular
    C. Muscular
    D. Bone
    E. Neurologic
      1. Central
      2. Peripheral
      3. Deafferentation
  III. Pain experience/expression
    A. Sensory input
    B. Psychologic (emotional)
    C. Cultural
    D. Familial
    E. Learned (operant)
    F. Descending inhibition
      1. Brainstem
      2. Cortex

Common facial pain conditions are discussed in this section and are outlined in Table 1.

BIBLIOGRAPHY

Alexander JM: Radionuclide bone scanning in the diagnosis of lesions of the maxillofacial region, J Oral Surg 34:249, 1976.
Epstein JB and others: Bone scintigraphy of fibro-osseous lesions of the jaw, Oral Surg 51:346, 1981.
Epstein JB and Ruprecht A: Bone scintigraphy: an aid in diagnosis and management of facial pain associated with osteoarthrosis, Oral Surg 53:37, 1982.
Tow DE and others: Bone scan in dental disease, J Nucl Med 19:845, 1976.

Peripheral neuropathy

Symptoms of burning tongue, unexplained orofacial pain (especially atypical pain), and other oral sensory deficits are frequently attributed to peripheral neuropathy affecting the trigeminal nerve. The diagnosis of peripheral neuropathy of the trigeminal nerve is usually tacitly accepted in a diabetic individual who has well-documented evidence of peripheral neuropathy elsewhere. Dental literature emphasizes a causative role for diabetes in some oral dysesthesias, but little direct evidence exists to implicate diabetic peripheral neuropathy as the pathologic change underlying these symptoms. There is also some question whether the long stated relationship between burning tongue, atypical facial pain, and other oral dysesthesias is valid. Screening tests for diabetes carried out on dental patients with these symptoms at times reveal mild glucose intolerance or even undiagnosed frank diabetes. These results justify medical consultation and treatment.

Burning mouth syndrome

Burning mouth syndrome (BMS) is a well-known symptom disorder characterized by a burning sensation of the tongue and occasionally the lips, gingiva, and palate. BMS may be accompanied by complaints of taste disturbance. Occasionally, local tissue inflammation or lesions may be seen. Many causes are suggested, including local irritation, candidiasis, iron deficiency, vitamin deficiency (folate or B_{12}), anemia, hormonal changes, immunologic abnormalities, xerostomia, and diabetes. However, in many cases no organic pathosis is identified. Psychologic factors are considered important in the cause of BMS. Psychologic conditions may include anxiety reactions and depressive disorders. Studies have found a depressive or anxiety disorder in approximately 50% of patients with BMS, but a purely psychologic disorder cannot be inferred in all cases. In a study of taste and tactile and thermal sensory functions in patients with BMS, specific changes in peripheral or central sensory function was suggested rather than a psychogenic origin. BMS without local cause and without an underlying medical cause is more common in postmenopausal women.

MANAGEMENT. Local oral infection, other oral conditions, or underlying medical conditions should be ruled out. Vitamin B−complex deficiency is identified as the cause in some patients. When identified, replacement may be useful in as many as one third of the deficient patients. If management can be directed at an identified probable cause, the prognosis is improved. Various treatment trails including librium (15 to 30 mg/day), treatment of xerostomia (sialagogues and discontinuing medications causing dry mouth), topical antifungals, and tricylic antidepressants have been recommended.

BIBLIOGRAPHY

Browning S and others: The association between burning mouth syndrome and psychosocial disorders, Oral Surg 64:171, 1987.
Gorsky M and others: Burning mouth syndrome: a review of 908 cases, J Oral Med 42:7, 1987.
Grushka M: Clinical features of burning mouth syndrome, oral Surg 63:30, 1987.
Grushka M and Sessle BJ: Burning mouth syndrome: a historical review, Clin J Pain 2:245, 1987.
Grushka M and others: Pain and personality profiles in burning mouth syndrome, Pain 28:155, 1987.
Grushka M and others: Psychophysical assessment of tactile, pain and thermal sensory functions in burning mouth syndrome, Pain 28:169, 1987.
Lamey PJ and Allam BF: Vitamin status of patients with burning mouth syndrome and the response to replacement therapy, Br Dent J 160:81, 1986.
Main DMG and Basker RM: Patients complaining of a burning mouth, Br Dent J 154:206, 1983.

Table 1   Characteristics of facial pains

Characteristics of pain	Tic douloureux	Atypical facial pain	Vascular facial pain	Myofascial pain or TMJ dysfunction
Frequency	Abrupt on-off, intermittent, pain free	Constant	Intermittent or clustered	Constant or fluctuating
Manifestations	Stabbing, sharp, electric	Burning, aching, occasional jabs	Throbbing, burning, pulsing	Aching, with jaw use, radiating
Spread	Unilateral	Unilateral or bilateral, often nonanatomic	Unilateral	Primarily unilateral
Location	Trigeminal nerves	Trigeminal or upper cervical nerves	Mid or upper face	Lateral facial or cervical nerves
Sensory changes	Minimal—no sensory change	Frequent sensory complaints	No sensory changes	No sensory changes
Precipitant	Triggered by nonpainful stimulus	Rarely triggered	No trigger	No trigger
Facial expression	Facial grimace	Often depressed effect	Facial flushing, lacrimation	No facial flushing
Tenderness	No local tenderness	Dysesthesia, rare local tenderness	Rare local mild tenderness	Tender over TMJ and muscles

Van der Ploeg HM and others: Psychological aspects of patients with burning mouth syndrome, Oral Surg 63:664,1987.

Zegarelli DJ: Burning mouth: an analysis of 47 patients, Oral Surg 58:34, 1984.

Trigeminal neuralgia

Tic douloureux (trigeminal neuralgia) is characterized by electric shock–like, stabbing pain of abrupt onset and short duration. The pain is unilateral in each episode, and there are pain-free episodes between attacks. Nonnoxious stimulation triggers the pain. There is no or only minimal sensory loss in the region of pain. The pain most often involves the second and third divisions of the trigeminal nerve, although other nerves, including the glossopharyngeal, nervus intermedius, and vagus nerves, may also be involved. Deviations from the classic description occur. Aching or burning pain may continue between attacks. Significant sensory loss mandates evaluation for pathologic processes such as tumor or infection. Tic douloureux is a disease of the elderly, with peak incidence between 50 and 70 years of age. Pain may be triggered by light touch, exposure to cold, or complex actions such as brushing teeth, chewing, and swallowing. The trigger is usually ipsilateral to the pain. Patients often complain of pain in the area of the dentition. Thus the dentist must always be confident of a pathologic diagnosis before beginning therapy. Since patients often complain of pain in the jaws, dental procedures, including endodontics and extractions, are often completed without change in the pain. If a dental cause of the pain is ruled out with appropriate diagnostic tests, no irreversible therapy should be begun and consultation should be sought.

The majority of patients with trigeminal neuralgia have mechanical compression of the trigeminal nerve by the superior cerebellar artery where it emerges from the pons. The region of impingement of the vessel corresponds with the region of facial pain. A small percentage of patients may have MS and the pain syndrome caused by a demyelinating plaque in the trigeminal root. Ratner and others proposed an etiologic theory that trigeminal neurolgic pain is caused by foci of abscess and bone resorption in bone cavities of the maxilla and mandible. This theory is not supported in treatment studies by others, and its conditions are seen in people with no pain. However, dental irritants such as abscess or other pathoses in orofacial structure can act as a triggering stimulus for tic douloureux. Physicians and dentists often think that something must be wrong where the pain is, and this may lead to unnecessary multiple dental procedures without a specific diagnosis.

MANAGEMENT. Therapy involves trials of anticonvulsant medications but may lead to neurosurgical procedures in patients who do not respond to medical therapy or do not tolerate the medications. Treatment of any local irritant in the distribution of the nerve may assist in reducing the frequency of the pain by reducing nerve input and reducing the spatial and temporal summation that may contribute to the episodes of pain.

BIBLIOGRAPHY

Calvin WH and others: A neurophysiological theory for the pain mechanism of tic douloureux, Pain 3:147, 1977.

Jannetta PJ: Microsurgical approach to the trigeminal nerve for tic douloureux, Prog Neurol Surg 7:180, 1976.

Loeser JD: Tic douloureux and atypical facial pain, J Can Dent Assoc 12:917, 1985.

Loeser JD: Tic douloureux and atypical facial pain. In Wall PD and Melzack R, editors: Textbook of pain, Edinburgh, 1985, Churchill Livingstone Inc.

Ratner EJ and others: Jawbone cavities and trigeminal and atypical facial neuralgias, Oral Surg 48:3, 1979.

Deafferentation pain

Pain is not simply a function of the amount of body damage, but is influenced by attention, anxiety, suggestion, other psychologic variables, and alteration in function of the neurologic processes. Pain signals are modulated as described in the gate-control theory by concurrent somatic input and by descending central influences. Deafferentation, the suppression, alteration, or removal of afferent nerve impulses, has received attention as a possible cause of chronic pain. Deafferentation caused by disease, injury, or other lesions of the periphery or CNS may lead to a hypersensitivity and an increased probability of chronic or referred pain.

Researchers have found that areas of the brainstem exert powerful inhibitory influences over the sensory system. Psychologic modulation of pain is also well documented. Some therapeutic pain management techniques, including transcutaneous electric stimulation (TENS), massage, acupuncture, relaxation, operant conditioning, biofeedback, and other psychologic techniques, take advantage of these mechanisms.

The potential mechanisms in deafferentation pain are described based on altered afferent input and alteration in the CNS, which has been demonstrated in the spinal cord, brainstem, and cortex. Deafferentation has been specifically studied in the trigeminal system. The findings of studies of deafferentation, in which pulpectomies were performed in animals, may be of particular relevance to so-called atypical facial pain. A useful analogy is phantom limb pain. This pain is thought to be caused by deafferentation and by changes in the dorsal horn, the thalamus, and the cortex. These changes may lead to pattern-generating mechanisms that can produce pain. Once this pattern-generating mechanism becomes established, any input may act as a trigger of pain or it may be self-generating without specific trigger. Deafferentation may result in hyperesthesia, dysesthesia, and paresthesia in the area of the neurologic change.

Several chronic pain conditions are linked to deafferentation. These include causalgia, neuralgia, and sensory neuropathy. Deafferentation may occur with damage to a limb, resulting in phantom limb pain, or damage to dental nerves during dental procedures such as pulpectomy, extraction, or other surgical procedures. Morphologic and physiologic changes are seen in deafferentation in the somatosensory system in the oral region. The changes may be due to alteration in receptive fields caused by unmasking of existing afferent or sprouting collateral nerves or reduction in inhibition of spinal dorsal horn neurons, which leads to a decrease in afferent-induced inhibition. Peripheral nerve lesions lead to degeneration of peripheral nerves and their central projections in the brainstem. Abnormal activity of peripheral and brainstem neurons with spontaneous firing and hyperactivity have been seen and may be the cause of pain. In the development of chronic pain, multiple events, such as inflammation leading to changes in neural function that result in summation of events that produce chronic pain, may be required in addition to deafferentation. Extensive convergence of peripheral afferents may explain some of the clinical findings of referred pain in acute and chronic pain states.

Deafferentation may occur more frequently in the head, neck, and oral region than any other body area. It is possible that deafferentation may be significant in many facial pain complaints. The nature of the pain attributed to deafferentation is chronic, aching discomfort, frequently with a burning quality. Deafferentation may be involved in the pathogenesis of symptoms described as atypical facial pain, BMS, and other pain states.

MANAGEMENT. Management of deafferentation pain includes treatment of all regional pathosis so that peripheral neurologic input is reduced and any spatial or temporal summation and referral of symptoms that may be part of the pain state are affected. Medical therapy that has been used includes tricyclic antidepressant drugs and in some cases phenothiazines. Tricyclics that have analgesic effects include amitriptyline, imipramine, clomipramine, and doxepin. The mechanism of action in pain relief may be due to reduction in depressive symptoms and local anesthetic effects, and possible anticonvulsant effects may suppress neuronal firing. There may be a common biochemistry underlying pain and depression. Low levels of serotonin may lead to hypersensitivity to pain. Tricyclics inhibit neuronal uptake and increase synaptic serotonin, noradrenaline, and dopamine, which are all transmitters that may be involved in pain. These neurotransmitters may enhance the effects of endogenous opiates. The pain-relieving effects appear to be independent of the antidepressant effects. The most frequently used medication is amitriptyline (25 to 150 mg at bedtime). Some physicians have used a tricyclic with a phenothiazine such as fluphenazine (1 mg three times per day). The onset of symptom relief is variable, and therapeutic trials may be required at adequate dosages for as long as 4 weeks.

BIBLIOGRAPHY

Biggs JT and Miranda FJ; Dental causalgia: a chronic oral pain syndrome, Quintessence Int 14:595, 1983.

Dubner R and Bennett GJ: Spinal and trigeminal mechanisms of nociception, Annu Rev Neurosci 6:381, 1983.

Feinmann C: Pain relief by antidepressants: possible modes of action, Pain 23:1, 1985.

Kaas JH and others: The reorganization of somatosensory cortex following peripheral nerve damage in adult and developing mammals, Annu Rev Neurosci 6:325, 1983.

Loeser JD: Tic douloureux and atypical face pain. In Wall PD and Melzack R, editors: Textbook of pain, London, 1984, Churchill-Livingstone Inc.

Melzack R: Recent concepts of pain, J Med 13:147, 1982.

Melzack R and Wall PD: Pain mechanisms: a new theory, Science 150:971, 1965.

Pilowsky I and others: A controlled study of amitriptyline in the treatment of chronic pain, Pain 14:169, 1982.

Roberts AM and others: Further observations on dental parameters of trigeminal and atypical facial neuralgias, Oral Surg 58:121, 1984.

Roberts WJ: A hypothesis on the physiological basis for causalgia and related pain, Pain 24:297, 1986.

Runmore MM and Schlichting DA: Clinical efficacy of antihistaminics as analgesics, Pain 25:7, 1986.

Sessle BJ: The neurobiology of facial and dental pain: present knowledge, future directions, J Dent Res 66:962, 1987.

Sessle BJ and others: Convergence of cutaneous, tooth pulp, visceral, neck and muscle afferents onto nociceptive and non-nociceptive neurones in trigeminal subnucleus caudalis (medullary dorsal horn) and its implications for referred pain, Pain 24:219, 1986.

Tasker RR: Deafferentation, In Wall PD and Melzack R, editors: Textbook of pain, London, 1984, Churchill-Livingstone Inc.

Taub A and Collins WF: Observations on the treatment of denervation dysesthesia with psychotropic drugs: postherpetic neuralgia, anesthesia dolorosa, peripheral neuropathy, Adv Neurol 4:309, 1974.

Wall PD: The gate control theory of pain mechanisms: a re-examination and re-statement, Brain 101:1, 1978.

Walsh TD: Antidepressants in chronic pain, Clin Neuropharmacol 6:271, 1983.

VASCULAR HEADACHE AND FACIAL PAIN

Pain of vascular origin often is described as aching with a pulsing periodicity. Vascular headaches have been described in detail and may appear as classic migraine or any of its variants, including cluster headache (see Chapter 146). Although these vascular headaches are recognized, variants may occur more localized to the face. These facial vascular pains must be differentiated from other causes to determine an effective therapy.

Vascular pain may be associated with other pain syndromes, resulting in a vascular component to the pain. This may occur in severe muscular pain such as that associated with whiplash injury. The flexion and extension that result in whiplash can affect the masticatory system, resulting in TMJ dysfunction and pain. The vascular component of pain may be noted when the muscular pain is severe and leads to symptoms that are associated with vascular pain such as throbbing, avoidance of bright lights and noises, nausea, and vomiting. There is a continuum of pain from those that are primarily muscular to those that are primarily vascular.

MANAGEMENT. Effective treatment depends on recognition of the components of the pain complaint and treatment of the primary factors leading to the continuing pain. Treatment may require diet modification and use of therapeutic or prophylactic antimigraine medications.

BIBLIOGRAPHY

Bakal DA and Kaganov JA: Muscle contraction and migraine headache: psychophysiologic comparison, Headache 17:208, 1977.

Blau JN and Diamond S: Dietary factors in migraine precipitation: the physicians' view, Headache 24:184, 1984.

Featherstone HJ: Migraine and muscle contraction headaches: a continuum, Headache 25:194, 1985.

Gunderson CH: Management of the migraine patient, Am Fam Physician 33:137, 1986.

Jensen K and others: Classic migraine: a prospective recording of symptoms, Acta Neurol Scand 73:359, 1986.

Kaganov JA and others: The differential contribution of muscle contraction and migraine symptoms to problem headache in the general population, Headache 21:157, 1981.

Mathew NT: Prophylaxis of migraine and mixed headache: a randomized controlled study, Headache 21:105, 1981.

Olesen J: Some clinical features of the acute migraine attack: an analysis of 750 patients, Headache 18:268, 1978.

Tfelt-Hansen P and others: Prevalence and significance of muscle tenderness during common migraine attacks, Headache 21:49, 1981.

SECTION TWELVE

SKIN DISEASES AND THEIR ORAL MANIFESTATIONS

Edited by **Bernard A. Kirshbaum** *and* **Robert N. Arm**

This section is intended to acquaint the dentist with some dermatologic conditions that may be encountered during routine examination.

ORAL MANAGEMENT OVERVIEW

Although each disease represents individual management problems, many have similar precautions. Specific precautions are covered for each disease.

The two major problems encountered in treating a patient with oral lesions are relieving the symptoms and maintaining dental preventive therapy. Symptomatic relief generally can be obtained by avoiding irritating agents and using topical anesthetics. Spicy or acid food and alcoholic drinks and solutions, including most mouthwashes, may bring added discomfort to a patient with oral lesions. A bland diet is preferable when symptoms are severe. A patient with severe pain may require a diet of blenderized purées or soft foods.

For mouth rinsing, a mixture of 1 tablespoon of baking soda in 8 oz of warm water may be best. New, nonalcoholic mouth rinses can be used and may be especially helpful for dental health if they contain fluoride. A solution of 0.12% chlorhexidine gluconate (Peridex), which is available for control of plaque and gingivitis, has been reported to be effective for treatment of oral mucositis and for oral hygiene.

Many agents can be applied for topical relief. Some, such as emollient mixtures (Orabase), provide a protective barrier. Others provide anesthetic relief as well. For single lesions or those in a limited area, 5% lidocaine ointment can be used. For longer action an anesthetic in an emollient base may be helpful. For diffuse mucosal involvement a rinse may be best. Viscous lidocaine, although commonly used, is often disliked because of its texture and taste. Complications to lidocaine overdose have been reported in a pediatric population. A solution of 0.5% dyclonine (Dyclone) or 0.5% aqueous diphenhydramine (Benadryl) provides excellent relief. Combinations of equal amounts of these two solutions have been reported to be even more effective. Generally, 1 teaspoon (5 ml), either alone or on crushed ice, is swished in the mouth; this can be used every hour if needed. Since both these agents are antihistamines, they produce slight sedation if swallowed. These solutions are not readily available and must be made by the pharmacy. The pharmacy sometimes substitutes commercially available 0.5% diphenhydramine elixir (Benadryl Elixir) for convenience. This should be avoided, since the elixir can cause a severe burning sensation; it can be used if the patient can tolerate it.

In some diseases patients have sialorrhea or xerostomia. Increased salivation should be explained to the patient, but generally no treatment is needed. A synthetic saliva solution may help a xerostomic patient. The many commercially available products for xerostomia include atomized sprays (Salivart), pump sprays (Xero-lube, Moi-stir), solutions (Sal-eze), and swabs (Moi-stir). One can also make a 2% methylcellulose solution or solution of 5% glycerin, 1% methylcellulose, flavoring agent, and buffered to a pH of 7 with sodium bicarbonate. For severe xerostomia a fluoride mouth rinse or gel should be included in the treatment.

Once the patient is comfortable, mouth care is easier. Comprehensive treatment should be avoided during acute flare-ups. Oral hygiene should always be stressed, since it prevents secondary infections, allows lesions to heal faster, and prevents dental breakdown. If toothbrushing, even with a small brush, is not possible, a 4 × 4 gauze may be used to clean the mouth. If tolerated, a sponge with baking soda (Toothette) may be useful. The lemon glycerin swabs provided in many hospitals for oral hygiene may irritate the lesions and, if used for a long period, may cause enamel decalcification because of the acidity. Some toothpastes irritate lesions because of their flavoring agents. The use of a bland toothpaste or plain baking soda is recommended.

156 · CONGENITAL DISEASES

Bernard A. Kirshbaum *and* **Robert N. Arm**

ECTODERMAL DYSPLASIAS

Ectodermal dysplasias have been divided into two broad categories, hypohidrotic ectodermal dysplasia and anhidrotic ectodermal dysplasia. The major difference between these two groups is the patient's ability to sweat. More than 60 separate diseases have been reported in these dysplasias.

Anhidrotic ectodermal dysplasia is a rare familial disorder characterized by scanty hair, thin dry skin, and dental abnormalities. The hair is thin, sparse, and dry on the scalp, eyebrows, eyelashes, bearded areas, axillae, and pubic areas. Eccrine and sebaceous glands are almost absent, so no sweating or sebum production occurs and skin is dry. The nails may also be absent or malformed. Ophthalmologic abnormalities, sensorineural hearing losses, and mental deficiencies have been reported. The characteristic facies is suggestive of congenital syphilis, with frontal bossing, saddle nose (depressed nasal bridge), prominent supraorbital ridges, and pointed chin. The lips, especially the upper, are often thickened, and furrows, especially at the buccal commissures, may give a pouting expression. The cheekbones are characteristically high and wide with narrowing of the lower half of the face. The eyebrows are scanty with the outer two thirds usually absent; the eyes slant upward producing a somewhat Oriental appearance. The cheeks may have telangiectasia and small papules simulating milia and adenoma sebaceum. These patients are often short.

Nail dystrophy, hyperkeratosis of volar skin, genital anomalies, and cleft lip and palate may be present. Hypoplasia of glands in the oral, pharyngeal, and tracheobronchial tree has been reported. This hypoplasia makes the patient susceptible to bronchitis and pneumonia. Mild defects in immunologic systems have also been reported.

Anhidrotic ectodermal dysplasias are familial, and the most common form is probably transmitted by an X-linked recessive gene, with only males fully expressing the disorder. Female carriers have milder abnormalities involving teeth and breasts and have diminished ability to sweat. Autosomal recessive and dominant forms have been reported. In these other forms, females may have more characteristics of the disorder.

Since these patients do not sweat, they are uncomfortable in hot weather because of elevated body temperature. With exertion they experience fatigue and asthenia. Many tolerate infections poorly and die of complications from bacterial and viral illnesses. Unexplained pyrexia in infancy should include ectodermal dysplasia in a differential diagnosis.

Diagnosis is often based on noninvasive techniques for detecting sweat glands. This may be done by direct visualization, using a loupe to examine the palmar fingertip skin. Other techniques include making impressions of the skin by the starch iodine method and the bromphenol blue method. Because the heterogeneous nature of this disease may make diagnosis difficult, a palmar skin biopsy to check the eccrine sweat glands has been recommended.

No specific treatment exists for anhidrotic ectodermal dysplasia. To function relatively normally, patients must modify their living conditions to avoid the dangers of increased temperatures. Management of these patients in infancy is highly specialized, and stringent methods to prevent hyperthermia must be used. Because of possible hypoplasia of tracheobronchial glands, the complications of pneumonia must be prevented. The hyperthermia can lead to mental retardation or early death.

Early diagnosis may be a problem because of difficulty recognizing early dental, hair, and facial changes at birth. Cystic fibrosis must be included in a differential diagnosis. Genetic counseling is indicated for patients with this condition, as well as those who have a family history and may be carriers of this trait.

Early manifestations of hypohidrotic ectodermal dysplasia are similar to those of the anhidrotic type and include high fever, pulmonary complications, and diminished sweating. Patients with the hypohidrotic type generally have normal dentition and facies. The classic clinical presentation is via an X-linked genetic transmission. An autosomal recessive variant associated with hypothyroidism and its complications has been reported.

Congenital ectodermal dysplasias are pathogenetic developmental defects found primarily in structures derived from ectoderm at the embryologic level but may affect other tissues

as well. In addition to the X-linked recessive type, a large, heterogeneous group of syndromes is characterized by manifestations in at least two structures (hair, teeth, nails, and sweat glands) with or without other signs. The degree of anhidrosis, hypohidrosis, or hidrosis, as well as the manifestations in other involved tissues, determines the nosologic classification.

ORAL MANIFESTATIONS. Patients with anhidrotic ectodermal dysplasia have oligodontia or anodontia. The remaining teeth are affected by delayed eruption pattern and developmental abnormalities ranging from conical or peg-shaped teeth to teeth with hypoplastic hypocalcified enamel. Some reports suggest that these teeth may be more vulnerable to carious lesions. The tongue may also appear enlarged, filling the edentulous areas. Oligondontia and alveolar aplasia give the patient's face an older appearance. Cleft lip and palate may be present. Secondary fungal infections may occur in a child receiving long-term antibiotic therapy for pulmonary complications.

DENTAL MANAGEMENT. The dentist plays a major role in psychologic management of the child by providing a normal-appearing mouth and thus enhancing the child's self-image. The maintenance of natural teeth is vital for a successful prosthesis. Edentulous patients may have a problem retaining prosthetic devices because of frequent occurrence of aplasia. Success with complete dentures has been reported in some cases. Microbial infection must be prevented, since hyperthermia may develop during the fever. Careful oral hygiene must be maintained. Supplemental hygiene aids such as 0.12% chlorhexidine gluconate and artifical salivas may be useful.

BIBLIOGRAPHY

Bartlett RC, Eversole LR, and Adkins RJ: Autosomal recessive hypohidrotic ectodermal dysplasia: dental manifestations, Oral Surg 33:736, 1972.

George DI and Escobar VH: Oral findings of Clouston's syndrome (hydrotic ectodermal dysplasia), Oral Surg 57:258, 1984.

Giansanti JS, Long SM, and Rankin JL: The "tooth and nail" type of autosomal dominant ectodermal dysplasia, Oral Surg 37:576, 1974.

Goepferd SJ and Carroll CE: Hypohidrotic ectodermal dysplasia: a unique approach to esthetic and prosthetic management, J Am Dent Assoc 102:867, 1981.

Lambert WC and Bilinski DL: Diagnostic pitfalls in anhidrotic ectodermal dysplasia: indications for palmar skin biopsy, Cutis 31:182, 1983.

Nakata M and others: a genetic study of anodontia in X-linked hypohidrotic ectodermal dysplasia, Am J Hum Genet 32:908, 1980.

Pike MG and others: A distinctive type of hypohidrotic ectodermal dysplasia featuring hypothyroidism, J Pediatr 108:109, 1986.

Pinheiro M and Friere-Maia N: Dermoodontodysplasia: an eleven-member, four generation pedigree with an apparently hitherto undescribed pure ectodermal dysplasia, Clin Genet 24:58, 1983.

Pinheiro M, Pereira LC, and Friere-Maia N: A previously undescribed condition: tricho-odonto-onycho-dermal syndrome: a review of the tricho-odonto-onychial group of ectodermal dysplasias, Br J Dermatol 105:371, 1981.

Reed WB, Lopez DA, and Landing B: Clinical spectrum of anhidrotic ectodermal dysplasia, Arch Dermatol 102:134, 1970.

Saunder KD: Consideration in dental treatment of children with ectodermal dysplasia, J Am Dent Assoc 93:1177, 1976.

Sofaer JA: A dental approach to carrier screening in X-linked hypohidrotic ectodermal dysplasia, J Med Genet 18:459, 1981.

Solomon LM and Keuer EJ: The ectodermal dysplasias: problems of classification and some newer syndromes (review article), Arch Dermatol 116:1295, 1980.

Witkop CJ, Brearley LJ, and Gentry WC: Hypoplastic enamel, onycholysis, and hypohidrosis inherited as an autosomal dominant trait: a review of ectodermal dysplasia syndromes, Oral Surg 39:71, 1975.

EPIDERMOLYSIS BULLOSA DYSTROPHICA

Epidermolysis bullosa dystrophica is a hereditary vesiculobullous disorder that involves both skin and mucosa. Several diseases are included under this name, including autosomal dominant and recessive forms. Lesions may occur spontaneously but often arise from trauma.

In the simplex form, lesions generally appear shortly after birth at frictional sites and heal without scarring. One fifth of the patients have affected nails. The condition improves as the child grows, especially after puberty. Lesions are generally caused by trauma and are exacerbated by increased temperature. Transmission is autosomal dominant. The blister forms intraepidermally.

In the junctional form of epidermolysis bullosa, the blister forms below the epidermis but above the basal lamina. The spectrum of severity in this form ranges from mild to life threatening. In one type the teeth are severely affected and dysplastic. Retardation and secondary anemia are common. Pyloric atresia rarely occurs. Junctional epidermolysis bullosa is transmitted in an autosomal recessive mode.

The dominant dystrophic form is transmitted as an autosomal dominant trait. Bullae, generally of the toes, ankles, knees, fingers, hands, and elbows, form and then heal, leaving scars. The nails may be thick and dystrophic. One fifth of the patients have onset of lesions by 1 year of age, and they may improve with age. Mucous membranes may be involved. Bullae, vesicles, and erosions may be found on the tongue, buccal mucosa, palate, pharynx, and esophagus. Angular contractures may be present at the gingivolabial sulcus. Faucial and pharyngeal scarring with associated hoarseness and dysphagia may occur. The teeth are normal, and the conjunctiva is usually not involved. Other changes include partial alopecia of the scalp, absence of body hair, dwarfism, and contractures with formation of clawlike hands, pseudosyndactylism, and atrophy of phalangeal bones.

The recessive dystrophic form resembles the dominant form but often is more severe and involves the conjunctiva and cornea. It is an autosomal recessive disorder. The bullae arise at any pressure or trauma site; rupture easily, leaving raw, denuded areas; and heal leaving scars and pigment changes. The scarring can lead to clawhand. Nails are absent or dystrophic. Nikolsky's sign is present. Scarring of the esophageal mucosa can lead to stenosis and dysphagia.

The letalis form is most severe, causing death during the first few months of life. No scarring or pigment changes are noted. Shortly after birth, lesions appear and nails may be shed. The entire body except the palms and soles may be involved. Vesicular changes may occur in other organ systems.

Diagnosis can be difficult on a plain microscopic examination. Total evaluation must include clinical, genetic, microscopic, electromicroscopic, and laboratory studies. To help distinguish the disorder microscopically from pemphigus and pemphigoid, an electron microscope is used. Immunofluorescent staining is also helpful. Prenatal diagnosis has been possible with fetoscopy and a biopsy of fetal skin.

Squamous cell carcinoma has been reported in patients with epidermolysis bullosa. Whether this is incidental or related is unknown. Patients with congenital esophageal atresia and Crohn's disease also have been reported.

The disease is rare, occurring in approximately 1 of 50,000 births and in the severe form in only 1 of 500,000.

Therapy is generally directed toward the symptoms. Systemic and topical steroids and vitamin ointments may be of some benefit. Unnecessary trauma should be prevented. The patient should be instructed to wear loose-fitting clothing and soft, well-ventilated leather shoes. Blisters may be treated with saline compresses and topical antibiotic ointments to minimize secondary infection. Because of problems with increased temperature, a cool environment is helpful. If esophageal problems occur, a soft, blenderized diet may be important. Therapy with the anticonvulsant phenytoin has decreased blistering; in one study more than half the patients showed a 40% decline in number of blisters.

ORAL MANIFESTATIONS. Oral involvement varies depending on the form of the disease. In the dominant simplex form, only 2% of the patients have oral lesions. A biopsy shows cleavage through the basal layer. The bullae heal without scars.

In the dominant dystrophic form, patients more commonly have oral involvement with resulting scarring. No odontogenic changes have been noted.

In the recessive dystrophic form, 16% of the patients have oral involvement. Some mucosal lesions appear soon after birth, possibly from the sucking reflex, and leave scars. On histologic examination a cleavage may be seen below the basement membrane. Enamel hypoplasia has been reported together with a pockmarked appearance of the teeth. The dentin appears uninvolved. Other reported changes include maxillary atrophy with mandibular prognathism.

All patients with the letalis form have oral lesions. When these lesions are examined microscopically, cleavage may be noted between the cell membrane of the epidermal and dermal layers. The bullae are most often present at the junction of the hard and soft palates. Severe alterations of enamel formation, as well as microscopic dentinal changes, have been reported. Gardner and Hudson believe that the enamel problems arise from ameloblastic dysfunction.

Caries and periodontal disease may occur because pain in oral lesions and severe effects in the hands make effective oral hygiene impossible.

DENTAL MANAGEMENT. Dental management must be aimed at preventing oral disease and trauma to the tissues. Atraumatic sponges or soft toothbrushes can be used for daily debridement. Palliative oral treatment with topical anesthetics may aid in the total systemic management. Supplemental rinses with baking soda or chlorhexidine may help prevent diseases.

The entire body must be protected when treating a patient with generalized involvement. The chair, headrest, operating table, and head ring should be covered with padding; sheepskin or synthetic sheepskin bedding is recommended. The body should be lightly covered or protected in a burn tent. In all reported dental management cases, patients were treated in the operating room. Adhesives were not used. Electrocardiographic leads, stethoscope, and intravenous lines were either wrapped lightly with gauze or protected by a thin layer of Gamgee tissue. The concern of causing a lesion from placement of a throat pack has been mentioned. No laryngeal or pharyngeal problems have been reported. The procedure followed employs a well-lubricated laryngoscope, preferably a MacIntosh, to prevent trauma. After the endotracheal tube is situated, it is inflated sightly. Lubricated gauze is then gently placed to protect the oral cavity; the suggested lubricant was a hydrocortisone cream.

In a study by James and Wark, administration of 309 general anesthetizations in 33 patients was successfully completed without laryngeal problems. The authors reported that 51% of the patients had microstomia or gross dental problems that would interfere with intubation.

Patients have tolerated restorations, prophylaxis, and extractions well. Although some have tolerated prosthodontic treatment, others have not because of trauma that created new lesions. A denture with a topical steroid cream might prevent these problems.

BIBLIOGRAPHY

Block MS and Gross BD: Epidermolysis bullosa dystrophica recessive: oral surgery and anesthetic considerations, J Oral Maxillofac Surg 40:753, 1983.

Buchbinder LH and others: Severe infantile epidermolysis bullosa simplex, Arch Dermatol 122:190, 1986.

Carroll DL, Stephan MJ, and Hays GL: Epidermolysis bullosa—review and report of case, J Am Dent Assoc 107:749, 1983.

Cooper TW and Bauer EA: Epidermolysis bullosa: a review, Pediatr Dermatol 1:181, 1984.

Doi O and others: A case of epidermolysis bullosa dystrophica with congenital esophageal atresia, J Pediatr Surg 21:943, 1986.

Eady RAJ and Tidman MJ: Diagnosing epidermolysis bullosa, Br J Dermatol 108:621, 1983.

Endruschat AJ and Keenan DS: Anesthetic and dental management of a child with epidermolysis bullosa dystrophica, Oral Surg 36:667, 1973.

Gardner DG and Hudson CD: The disturbances in odontogenesis in epidermolysis bullosa hereditaria letalis, Oral Surg 40:483, 1975.

Gorlin RJ: Epidermolysis bullosa, Oral Surg 32:760, 1971.

Howden EF and Oldenburg TR: Epidermolysis bullosa dystrophica: report of two cases, J Am Dent Assoc 85:1113, 1972.

James I and Wark H: Airway management during anesthesia in patients with epidermolysis bullosa dystrophica, Anesthesiology 56:323, 1982.

Johnston DE, Koehler RE, and Balfe DM: Clinical manifestations of epidermolysis bullosa dystrophica, J Dig Dis Sci 26:1144, 1981.

Kero M and Niemi KM: Epidermolysis bullosa, Int J Dermatol 25:75, 1986.

Raab B and others: Epidermolysis bullosa acquisita and inflammatory bowel disease, JAMA 250:1746, 1983.

Song IC and Dicksheet S: Management of squamous cell carcinoma in a patient with dominant-type epidermolysis bullosa dystrophica: a surgical challenge, Plast Reconstr Surg 75:732, 1985.

Tomlinson AA: Recessive dystrophic epidermolysis bullosa, Anesthesia 38:485, 1983.

Wright JT: Epidermolysis bullosa: dental and anesthetic management of two cases, Oral Surg 57:155, 1984.

NEUROFIBROMATOSIS (VON RECKLINGHAUSEN'S DISEASE)

Neurofibromatosis is a form of inherited neuroectodermal dysplasia with manifestations in the skin, soft tissues, bone, and central nervous system. It is one of four major neurocutaneous syndromes; the others are tuberous sclerosis, Sturge-Weber syndrome, and Klippel-Trenaunay-Weber syndrome. The skin lesions include neurofibromas, café au lait spots, freckling in the axillary, neck, and perianal areas (Crowe's sign), and bronzing (diffuse hyperpigmentation) of the skin. There may be associated nevus anemicus, pigmented hairy nevi, sacral hypertrichosis, cutis verticis gyrata (deep furrows and folds of skin and subcutaneous tissues extending vertically over the scalp), and short stature. Osseous findings include spina bifida, dislocations, and fractures but are mainly erosive changes producing kyphosis, lordosis, kyphoscoliosis, and pseudarthrosis. Neuromas of the spinal nerves occasionally cause paralyses. Tumors of the cranial nerves, as well as brain tumors, epilepsy, mental retardation, and dementia, also occur in von Recklinghausen's disease.

Optic gliomas have been found in approximately 14% of patients, mostly before 10 years of age. After age 10, acoustic neuromas and meningiomas have been reported in 3% and 1% of patients, respectively. In one study from Denmark approximately 45% of the patients had malignant or benign central nervous system tumors, most of which were gliomas.

The cutaneous neurofibromas (fibroma molluscum) are tumors that vary in size from pinhead to large, pendulous, flabby masses; the skin over these is usually coarsened and may become deeply pigmented. Many of the soft tumors are pedunculated, and an underlying cutaneous defect can be felt as a ring or buttonhole at the base of the lesion. Plexiform neuromas are subcutaneous neurofibromas that form along the course of peripheral nerves in large, irregular beaded masses. Neurofi-

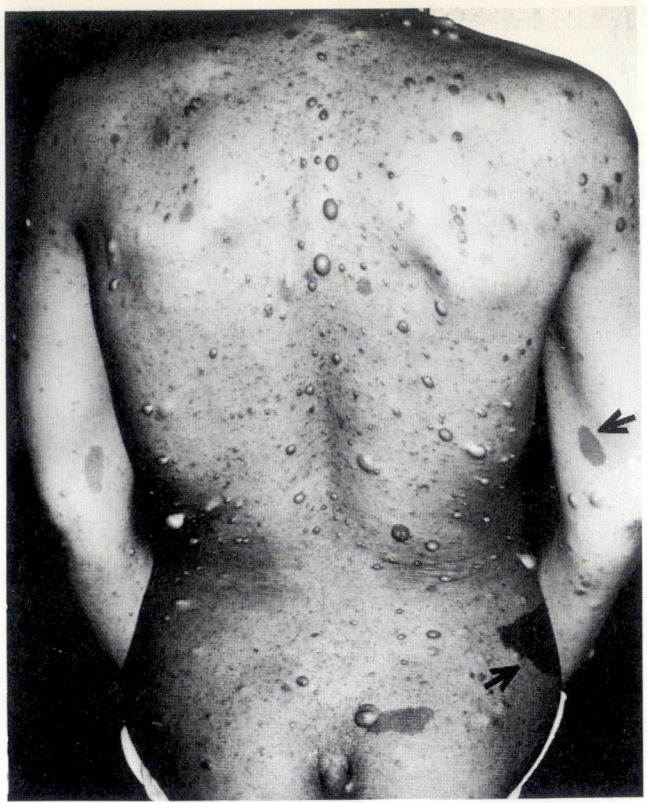

Fig. 156-1 Neurofibromatosis. Note café au lait spots (arrows) and multiple neurofibromas.

bromas may be found on any part of the skin surface, although usually not on the palms and soles.

Café au lait spots are brownish macules, often round to oval, varying from 0.5 to 15 cm or more in diameter. Some believe the presence of six or more café au lait spots 1.5 cm or more in diameter is sufficient to establish the diagnosis of neurofibromatosis even in the absence of tumors (Fig. 156-1). However, café au lait spots are not pathognomonic of von Recklinghausen's neurofibromatosis. Although they may vary in appearance, these spots can be seen in the orbital glioma syndrome (which may have neurofibromas), Albright's syndrome, Silver syndrome, and tuberous sclerosis. In Albright's syndrome (polyostotic fibrous dysplasia and precocious puberty) the café au lait spots generally have a more irregular outline, often called "coast of Maine" appearance. Silver syndrome can be recognized by the patient's triangular face, which is caused by a disproportionately large head for a small facial mass (pseudohydrocephaly) tapering to a narrow jaw, short stature, and significant asymmetries. The patient may have syndactylism of the second and third toes and a short, incurved fifth finger; about one third of patients are retarded. Turned-down corners of the mouth have also been reported.

Many other organ systems may be involved in neurofibromatosis. Endocrine disorders, such as acromegaly, cretinism, hyperparathyroidism, myxedema, precocious puberty, and growth retardation, have been described. From 5% to 10% of patients with pheochromocytomas have neurofibromatosis. Retinal tumors (phakomas) may also be found.

In approximately 90% of patients with von Recklinghausen's neurofibromatosis, pigmented hamartomas of the iris (Lisch nodules) occur. These usually asymptomatic nodules increase with age and are the basis for diagnosis.

Neurofibromatosis is an autosomal dominant inherited disease without sex linkage; it does not skip generations. It occurs in approximately 1 in 2500 to 3300 births. The disease is found in approximately 1 in 200 patients with mental retardation. About 50% of the cases are sporadic, involve no family history of the disease, and probably represent new spontaneous mutations. Once established, the disorder is transmitted in a mendelian dominant pattern, but in succeeding generations the defect may show incomplete penetrance and can vary from café au lait spots to extensive neurofibromas. The basic defect explaining the tendency of the neural sheath (Schwann cells and endoneurial fibroblasts) to form tumors is unknown.

The diagnosis of neurofibromatosis is based on the clinical findings and is simplified by the presence of typical lesions and café au lait spots. It can be confused with other diseases involving pigmented spots (see preceding discussion). Often the parents first notice the disease because of skin changes or delayed development. In mild forms, difficulty in school associated with poor motor coordination, hyperactivity, and possible seizures may be the initial findings. Electroencephalographic changes have been noted in 18% of patients; approximately 12% were associated with seizures and 7% with retardation.

Another syndrome often confused with neurofibromatosis is the multiple endocrine neoplasia disorder known as Sipple's syndrome. The patient may have neuromas or neurofibromas and pheochromocytomas. The neuromas are generally mucosal and histologically resemble traumatic neuromas. The major characteristic of Sipple's syndrome is thyroid nodules, which generally become medullary thyroid carcinoma. *Any* thyroid nodule in this syndrome should be treated with aggressive surgery. Often multiple parathyroid adenomas occur. There may be associated intracranial hemorrhages, Cushing's disease, and diabetes.

Although neurofibromatosis is generally a benign, disfiguring disease, death may occur from associated meningiomas and gliomas, as well as from sarcomatous degeneration of the lesions. Malignant degeneration has been reported in 2.5% to 16% of patients. Excision of disfiguring superficial lesions remains the only available treatment, but this can be a formidable task when neurofibromas are numerous.

Genetic counseling is indicated for patients with von Recklinghausen's disease to ensure all options are understood. Careful periodic examinations are needed to prevent complications.

ORAL MANIFESTATIONS. Neurofibromatosis can often be recognized by multiple neurofibromas of the face. The nodules may also appear in the mouth. They are nonulcerated, mucosa-covered masses or pendulous polyps most often located on the tongue and lips. Plexiform neurofibromas in the tongue can lead to macroglossia. Neurofibromas have also been reported in the floor of the mouth, buccal mucosa, edentulous alveolar ridges, gingiva, and palate. Although generally benign, neurofibromas can undergo malignant transformation. A biopsy is indicated for diagnosis, especially when the lesions change appearance.

Maxillary and mandibular bone abnormalities with resulting facial asymmetry have been reported. Some of these abnormalities are related to osteoclastic resorption by pressure atrophy from tumor growth. A radiolucent area is visible on roentgenograms. Stimulation of bone growth, resulting in hyperplasia with focal hypoplasia caused by restructuring, has been reported. Hypoplasia of the mandibular ramus may occur. Muller and Slootweg reported radiolucencies of the ascending ramus in the area of the sigmoid notch, as well as an increased depth of the notch with exostosis of the zygoma. At surgery the radiolucencies proved to be neurofibromas. Some of the

lytic lesions have been known to disappear spontaneously.

Reports of oral manifestations vary from 6% to 72% of patients. Macroglossia, especially if no lesions are seen, must be carefully evaluated to detect thyroid problems. Some patients may not know they have neurofibromatosis despite the classic appearance. A maxillary tuberosity enlargement diagnosed as neurofibroma was reported in a patient with a family history of lesions but no prior diagnosis of neurofibromatosis.

DENTAL MANAGEMENT. Early recognition and biopsy are important. The asymmetries resulting from neurofibromatosis may lead to major occlusal problems and reconstructive difficulties. Orthognathic surgical intervention and removal of lesions that interfere with function may help. Removing all lesions is almost impossible, and careful periodic observation is indicated to rule out malignant change. Once removed, the lesion may recur, and continued changes in the soft tissue and bone may develop, making prosthetic construction difficult.

The systemic problems in von Recklinghausen's disease greatly affect dental treatment. Many patients have seizures and may be taking anticonvulsants (see Chapter 145). Pheochromocytomas may cause intermittent headaches that may often be mistaken for temporomandibular joint problems. More importantly, the labile hypertension must be closely monitored. Mental retardation may make oral hygiene more difficult. Multiple alterations in the skeleton, especially the arms and hands, also may affect hygiene. One must determine whether mobility of the teeth is caused by periodontal disease or by lesions. Diagnosis and management of lesions displacing impacted teeth is required to rule out neurofibromas. Neurofibromas should be considered in the diagnosis and management of lesions causing displacement of impacted teeth.

BIBLIOGRAPHY

Barone DA: Neurofibromatosis, a clinical review, Postgrad Med 66:73, 1979.
Bartlett RC and others: A neuropolyendocrine syndrome: mucosal neuromas, pheochromocytomas and medullary thyroid carcinomas, Oral Surg 31:206, 1971.
Blatt J and others: Neurofibromatosis and childhood tumor, Cancer 57:1225, 1986.
Brady GL and others: Solitary neurofibroma of the maxilla, J Oral Maxillofac Surg 40:453, 1982.
Brasfield RD and DasGupta TK: Von Recklinghausen's disease: a clinico-pathological study, Ann Surg 175:86, 1972.
Casino AJ and others: Oral facial manifestations of the multiple neoplasia syndrome, Oral Surg 51:516, 1981.
Crawford AH and Bagamery N: Osseous manifestations of neurofibromatosis in childhood, J Pediatr Orthop 6:72, 1986.
Gorlin RJ and others: Multiple mucosal neuromas, pheochromocytomas and medullary carcinoma of the thyroid—a syndrome, Cancer 22:293, 1968.
Johnson BL and Charneco DR: Café au lait spots in neurofibromatosis and in normal individuals, Arch Dermatol 102:442, 1970.
Muller H and Slootweg PJ: Maxillofacial deformities in neurofibromatosis, J Maxillofac Surg 9:89, 1981.
Nelson AM: Small bowel adenocarcinoma associated with neurofibromatosis, Am J Gastroenterol 77:149, 1982.
Papadopoulos H and others: Neurofibroma of the mandible, review of the literature and report of a case, Int J Oral Surg 10:293, 1981.
Riccardi VM: Von Recklinghausen neurofibromatosis, N Engl J Med 305:1617, 1981.
Rittersma J and others: Neurofibromatosis wth mandibular deformities, Oral Surg 33:718, 1972.
Shapiro SD and others: Neurofibromatosis: oral and radiographic manifestation, Oral Surg 58:493, 1984.
Sorensen SA and others: Long-term follow-up of von Recklinghausen neurofibromatosis, N Engl J Med 314:1010, 1986.
Vincent SD and Williams TP: Mandibular abnormalities in neurofibromatosis, Oral Surg 55:253, 1983.
Watts PG and Theaker JM: A rare case of maxillary tuberosity enlargement: von Recklinghausen's neurofibromatosis, Br J Oral Maxillofac Surg 24:452, 1986.
Westerhof W and others: Neurofibromatosis and hypertelorism, Arch Dermatol 120:1579, 1984.

White AK and others: Head and neck manifestations of neurofibromatosis, Laryngoscope 96:732, 1986.

TUBEROUS SCLEROSIS: ADENOMA SEBACEUM; EPILOIA (BOURNEVILLE-PRINGLE SYNDROME)

Tuberous sclerosis is a triad of symptoms that includes adenoma sebaceum, mental retardation, and epilepsy. Rayer first described the disorder in 1835, and von Recklinghausen made the first microscopic descriptions in 1862. Bourneville first described the entire syndrome in 1880, including the waxy or translucent papular eruptions on the nose, cheeks, and forehead; mental retardation; epilepsy; and brain and kidney tumors. In 1890 Pringle described in detail the dermatologic manifestations. Often the term "Bourneville-Pringle syndrome" is used synonymously for tuberous sclerosis. The term "epiloia" was used in 1911 by Sherlock as an acronym for the triad of *epi*lepsy, *lo*w *i*ntelligence, and *a*denoma sebaceum. The term "epiloia" is no longer commonly used as a synonym for tuberous sclerosis.

The primary cutaneous finding in tuberous sclerosis is adenoma sebaceum, characterized by mostly pinhead-sized, yellowish red, translucent waxy papules on the face. These are located mainly in the rostral and paranasal areas, circumoral regions, and on the nose, cheeks, and chin in a symmetric distribution. The papules often are distributed in a butterfly-shaped pattern. The forehead is usually less involved, and periorbital lesions are generally minimal (Fig. 156-2). Although the papules remain discrete, they may form large aggregates in the affected areas; they persist indefinitely and may increase in number. They usually appear after early childhood, with 90% present by 4 years of age. Other findings may include subungual fibromas, shagreenlike patches on the skin in approximately 20% of patients, hypopigmented white leaf-shaped macules, poliosis (depigmented hair), café au lait spots, and oral fibrous papules. Subungual fibromas are small, digitate, asymptomatic fibromatous tumors that may be found protruding from beneath the fingernails and toenails. Shagreen patches are irregular areas of knobby skin ranging from 1 to 8 cm and may occur on the trunk, most often in the lumbosacral area. They are a form of connective tissue nevi. White, lanceolate,

leaflike macules are present in 15% to 50% of the patients. They may be the only manifestation of this condition and are often the first sign of tuberous sclerosis in the newborn. These lesions are not vitiligo but are hypomelanotic macules containing less melanin in the melanocytes. Depigmented eyelashes or eyebrows (poliosis) may occur as the result of leukoderma affecting the hair follicles. Café au lait spots may also be present, but not as frequently as in neurofibromatosis.

Mental deficiency is usually observed early in life and varies from slight to profound mental impairment. Some reports show that the deficiency may occur in only 60% of patients. Epilepsy is also variable, ranging from minimal to severe; myoclonic seizures may occur early in life. The seizures are usually discernible as infantile spasms (salaam, or nodding, spasms). These repetitive myoclonic muscle spasms last for seconds, occur in groups of 10 to 50, and involve the neck, trunk, and limbs. Although other causes exist for these infantile spasms, approximately 25% of children with them eventually develop tuberous sclerosis within a few years. In later life up to 93% of these patients develop grand mal seizures. Abnormal electroencephalographic changes have been reported in almost 90% of the cases. Both neurologic and mental changes have been associated with tumor formations and tuber-shaped areas of sclerosis that alter normal cerebral convolutions. Often they resemble potatolike nodules in the brain. Roentgenographic examination may reveal intracranial calcifications ("brain stones") in the region of the basal ganglia or in the cortex. These occur in 14% of patients at 1 year of age and increase to approximately 60% by 10 years of age. Malignant astrocytomas have been reported in approximately 6% of cases.

Other organ systems may be involved. Cortical thickening and sometimes osteoporosis may occur in long bones, sclerotic lesions in the skull and vertebrae, and cystic changes (pseudocysts, similar to those of sarcoidosis and hyperparathyroidism) in the phalanges. Renal hamartomas and cardiac tumors, as well as cystic changes in the lungs, have been reported. Retinal tumors (phakomas) similar to those occurring in von Recklinghausen's disease, have been reported in 3% to 100% of patients.

Tuberous sclerosis is an inherited disease with an autosomal

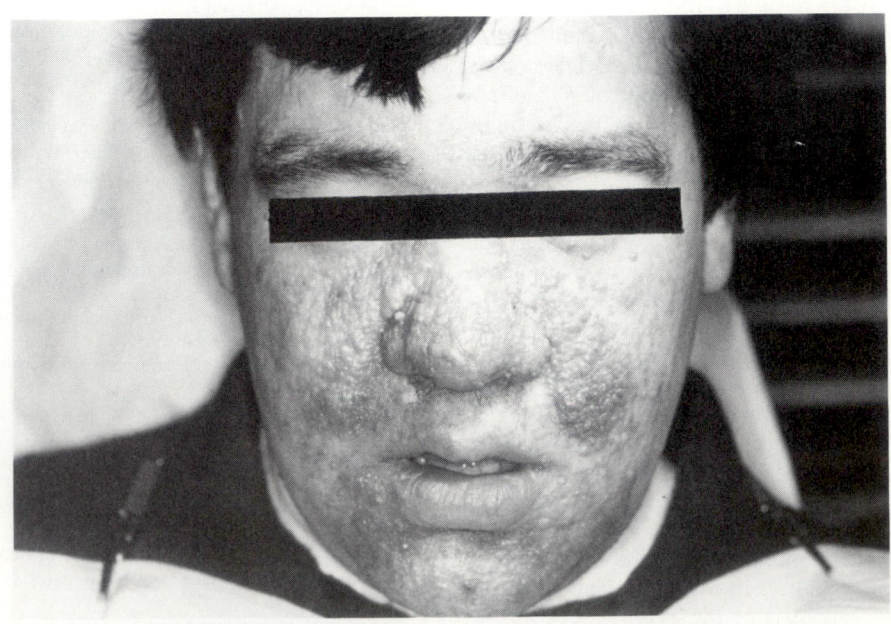

Fig. 156-2   Tuberous sclerosis in mentally retarded young adult.

dominant pattern, equal sex distribution, and varied expression in successive generations. Some individuals only have skin lesions; others have epilepsy or other manifestations. Although most facial lesions appear by late childhood, in rare cases the patient has no facial lesions. The reproductive capacity of these individuals is low, and an estimated 50% to 80% of cases occur as spontaneous mutations. A defective gene has been reported in 1 in 10,000 to 300,000 persons. In a population of institutionalized mentally retarded patients, the incidence of this gene has been reported as 1 in 100 to 300. The mechanism by which the disease causes its effects is unknown.

The term "adenoma sebaceum" for the skin lesions is a misnomer; they are neither adenomas nor of sebaceous origin. Histologically, they are essentially vascular and connective tissue tumors (angiofibromas), with giant cells, hyperplasia of the hair follicles, and nervelike structures. The retinal tumors (phakomas) are gliomas, renal hamartomas may be angiomyolipomas, and cardiac tumors are rhabdomyomas.

The course of tuberous sclerosis varies with the degree of involvement. Patients with few symptoms may lead fairly normal lives. The skin lesions do not undergo malignant change. Spontaneous pneumothorax may occur in those with pulmonary involvement, and hematuria and renal failure may occur in those with kidney lesions. Mental deficiency and seizures may be severe, and the patients may die in the third or fourth decade of life as a result of progressive neurologic deterioration.

Patients with facial lesions of adenoma sebaceum have been treated with dermabrasion, but regrowth has been reported after months or years. Liquid nitrogen cryosurgery, electrocautery and curettage, and excisions have been attempted with varying results. Recently, argon and carbon dioxide lasers have been used with good results.

Management of seizures and other neurologic manifestations is a major therapeutic concern. Often these patients require anticonvulsant therapy. No known gene marker is useful in prenatal diagnosis. Genetic counseling is important for those who manifest any clinical traits, but this probably does not affect the incidence of new cases, since more than half arise from spontaneous mutations.

ORAL MANIFESTATIONS. The most common oral manifestation is a fibrous growth, generally found on the anterior gingiva but also reported on the lips, buccal mucosa, and tongue (Fig. 156-3). Although generally mucosa covered, these growths may also be bluish, red, or yellowish. Gingival hyperplasia may be caused by phenytoin (Dilantin) therapy used to control the epilepsy. Stirrups and Inglis reported a patient with gingival hyperplasia that could not be explained by drug therapy or poor oral hygiene. We have seen fibrous growth in an edentulous patient awaiting dentures and in a young male, neither of whom was taking anticonvulsants. Periodontitis caused by poor oral hygiene is common in retarded individuals.

Hyperostosis, which caused alveolar enlargements, high vaulted palate, and cystic mandibular lesions, has been reported. Teeth with a delayed eruption pattern have been noted. Hoff and co-workers reported enamel hyperplasia, which they believed was caused by defective amelogenesis.

Since the descriptive information on oral lesions varies, biopsy should be performed and all tissue, including gingivectomy specimens, submitted for histopathologic study.

DENTAL MANAGEMENT. Patient management is frequently difficult; 75% of patients have neurologic involvement, including retardation and epilepsy. Pulmonary problems alter management if general anesthesia is required. Many patients have progressive dyspnea from lung involvement and are susceptible to spontaneous rupture of pulmonary cysts, which leads to pneumothorax and may compromise treatment.

In the edentulous patient from whom we removed a fibrous tumor, no regrowth has occurred in 3 years, and the patient has tolerated dentures well. However, careful follow-up is necessary to check for additional tumor growths.

BIBLIOGRAPHY

Cassidy SB: Tuberous sclerosis in children: diagnosis and course, Compr Ther 10:43, 1984.
Cassidy SB and others: Family study in tuberous sclerosis: evaluation of apparently unaffected parents, JAMA 249:1302, 1983.
Hoff M and others: Enamel defects with tuberous sclerosis, Oral Surg 40:261, 1975.
Hunt A: Tuberous sclerosis: a survey of 97 cases. II. Physical findings, Dev Med Child Neurol 25:350, 1983.
Lagos JC and Gomez MR: Tuberous sclerosis: reappraisal of a clinical entity, Mayo Clin Proc 42:26, 1967.
Mackler SB and others: Tuberous sclerosis with gingival lesions, Oral Surg 34:619, 1972.
Marshall D, Saul GB, and Sachs E: Tuberous sclerosis, N Engl J Med 261:1102, 1959.
Morimoto K and Mogami H: Sequential CT study of subependymal giant-cell astrocytoma associated with tuberous sclerosis, J Neurosurg 65:874, 1986.
Morisaki I and others: Epulis in a child with tuberous sclerosis, J Pedodontics 11:386, 1987.
Nickel WR and Reed WB: Tuberous sclerosis, Arch Dermatol 85:209, 1962.
Reed WB, Nickel WR, and Campion G: Internal manifestations of tuberous sclerosis, Arch Dermatol 87:715, 1963.
Rushton MA: Some less common bone lesions affecting the jaws, tuberous sclerosis with jaw lesions, Oral Surg 9:289, 1956.
Scully C: Oral mucosal lesions in association with epilepsy and cutaneous lesions: the Pringle-Bourneville syndrome, Int J Oral Surg 10:68, 1981.
Stirrups DR and Inglis J: Tuberous sclerosis with non-hydantoin gingival hyperplasia, Oral Surg 49:211, 1980.
Weits-Binnerts JJ and others: Dental pits in deciduous teeth, an early sign in tuberous sclerosis, Lancet 2:1344, 1982.
Weston J and others: Carbon dioxide laserbrasion for treatment of adenoma sebaceum in tuberous sclerosis, Ann Plast Surg 15:132, 1985.
Wiederholt WC and others: Incidence and prevalence of tuberous sclerosis in Rochester, Minnesota, 1950 through 1982, Neurology 35:600, 1985.
Williams R and Taylor D: Tuberous sclerosis, Surv Ophthalmol 30:143, 1985.

STURGE-WEBER SYNDROME (ENCEPHALOTRIGEMINAL ANGIOMATOSIS)

Sturge-Weber syndrome is a congenital anomaly consisting of craniofacial angiomatosis, meningeal hemangioma, and cerebral calcification. The cutaneous vascular nevus (port-wine stain, or nevus flammeus) may be large or small and is present at birth, usually located along the course of the superior and middle branches of the trigeminal nerve (Fig. 156-4). An associated meningeal hemangioma occurs on the same side, with calcifications and cortical atrophy of the adjacent brain tissue. A possible etiologic factor is the altered circulation in the cerebral cortex underlying the hemangioma, which leads to degeneration that can result in focal or generalized contralateral jacksonian convulsions, contralateral hemiplegia, sensory deficit, and mental retardation. Convulsive disorders in up to 80%, mental retardation in more than 50%, and hemiplegia in approximately 30% of patients have been reported.

The nevus flammeus is usually unilateral with a sharp border but may be bilateral or midline. The oral mucous membranes may be affected on the same side. The most commonly involved areas are the lips, cheek, palate, gingiva, tongue, and floor of the mouth.

Ocular disorders have been reported in more than 30% of patients. Glaucoma and choroidal angiomatosis may be present in the ipsilateral eye.

Characteristic calcifications in the outer layers of the cerebral cortex may be seen in roentgenograms of the skull as sinuous, double-contoured lines ("tram lines") that follow the convo-

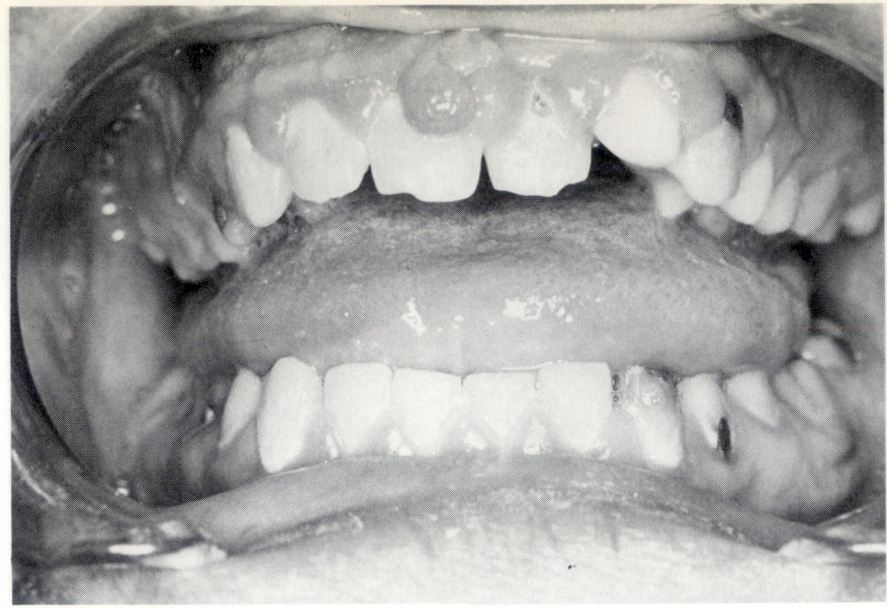

Fig. 156-3   Tuberous sclerosis with fibrous gingival growth in patient not being treated with anticonvulsive therapy.

lutions of the cerebral cortex on the affected side. Calcification of the gyri reported by Weber in 1922 are associated with atrophic areas of the cerebral cortex. Similar calcifications also occur in the Klippel-Trenaunay-Weber syndrome and in childhood leukemia.

Sturge-Weber syndrome is a congenital disorder possibly related to faulty embryologic development of the ectoderm and mesoderm. The cause is unknown. Almost all cases have been sporadic, affecting both sexes equally. Although occasionally more than one family member is affected, this disorder does not seem to be inherited. At present no preventive measures seem to be available, and the disease cannot be determined before birth. Usually the seizures begin between 3 and 9 months after birth. The cortical calcifications are generally not seen until later by routine roentgenography. Computed tomography has been used to detect these lesions earlier in life.

Treatment is generally directed at the neurologic manifestations. Phenytoin (Dilantin) is generally used to control the seizures.

Confusion in literature often occurs between Sturge-Weber syndrome and Klippel-Trenaunay-Weber syndrome (angioosteohypertrophy). Although they can sometimes occur together, they are separate entities. Klippel-Trenaunay-Weber syndrome consists of hypertrophy of the soft tissues and bone secondary to increased vascular supply, with cutaneous and bony hemangiomas. It is often associated with varicose veins in the long bones. The orofacial region may be involved with or without concurrent Sturge-Weber syndrome, although the hemangiomas more often occur on the trunk and extremities. Arteriovenous fistulas and visceral hemangiomas have also been reported. Klippel-Trenaunay-Weber syndrome usually does not show paralysis, epilepsy, the intracranial calcifications, mental retardation and congenital glaucoma seen in Sturge-Weber syndrome.

ORAL MANIFESTATIONS. Hemangiomas of the face and mucosa are readily seen. Generally a cutaneous vascular nevus (port-wine stain) occurs over an area of the face innervated by the trigeminal nerve. Oral involvement occurs in about 40% of patients and consists of a bluish red lesion that blanches on pressure and is found most often on the buccal mucosa and lips. Less common lesions involve the gingiva of the ipsilateral maxilla and palate. The mandibular gingiva, floor of mouth, and tongue are rarely involved. The lesions resemble a vascular hyperplasia or large, tumorlike mass. Microscopic examination reveals thin-walled vessels similar to those in a cavernous hemangioma. Pyogenic granuloma and possibly early eruption of teeth have been reported from increased vascularity. More than 80% of patients have epilepsy and may be taking phenytoin (Dilantin). Gingival problems caused by phenytoin are common. Since more than 50% of patients are mentally retarded, oral hygiene problems typically occur. Hemiplegia, seen in 30% of patients, may also lead to oral hygiene problems. One report indicated that the gingival hyperplasia may not be caused by phenytoin, poor hygiene, or angiomas but by a true hyperplasia.

In Klippel-Trenaunay-Weber syndrome, vascular lesions involve the bone. Bony hypertrophy and early eruption have been reported.

DENTAL MANAGEMENT. The major problem in patients with Sturge-Weber syndrome is possible hemorrhage from the angiomas. If the involved area is treated, a complete workup may be indicated, including angiographic studies. Hospitalization of the patient with standby pressure splints and blood may also be required. For general anesthesia, oral intubation may be safer so that unseen hemangiomas are not traumatized. All dental treatment must be done with extreme care. Forms of treatment of the vascular areas have included sclerosing solutions, freezing by application of solid carbon dioxide, liquid nitrogen, and electrodesiccation. Use of a carbon dioxide laser has been reported to avoid problems during a gingivectomy related to the phenytoin hyperplasia.

Problems with epilepsy and retardation must be addressed. Special hygiene aids may help the patient, especially if hemiplegia is present.

In Klippel-Trenaunay-Weber syndrome, bone hypertrophy can lead to occlusal problems or tilting of the teeth. The bony shape also can create problems with prosthesis. The bony angiomas create difficult and possibly life-threatening bleeding

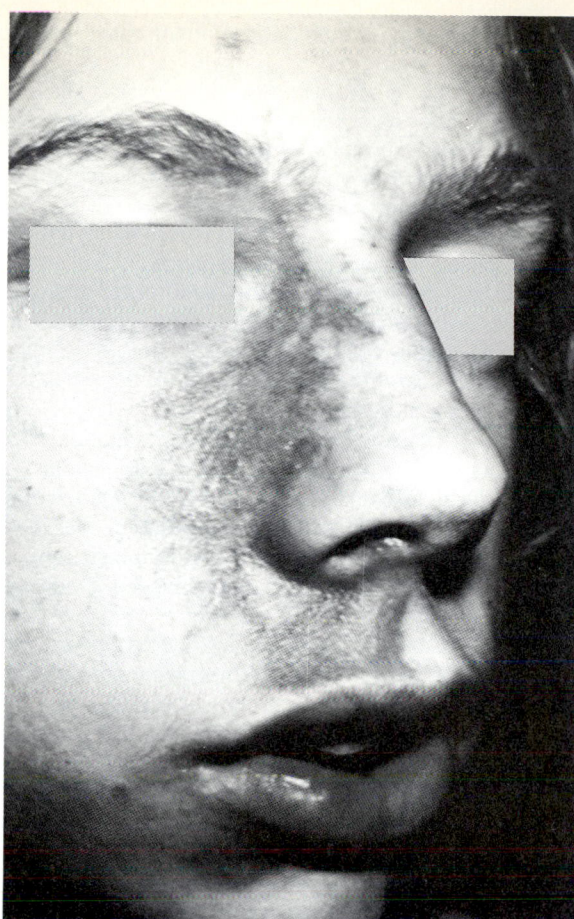

Fig. 156-4 Encephalotrigeminal angiomatosis (Sturge-Weber syndrome) in mentally retarded adolescent. Color of lesion is that of port wine.

problems during surgery. Patients may have thrombocytopenia because of chronic hemorrhage of the vascular lesions. The presence of arterial insufficiency with secondary heart disease caused by arteriovenous fistulas may alter the treatment plan.

BIBLIOGRAPHY

Alexander GL and Norman RM: The Sturge-Weber syndrome, Bristol, UK, England, 1960, John Wright & Sons, Inc.

Bendl BJ and others: Sturge-Weber syndrome, Cutis, 31:286, 1983.

Crinzi RA and others: Management of a dental infection in a patient with Sturge-Weber disease, J Am Dent Assoc 101:798, 1980.

Farman AG and Wilson S: Diagnostic imaging in Sturge-Weber syndrome, Dentomaxillofac Radiol 14:97, 1985.

Hylton RP: Use of CO_2 laser for gingivectomy in a patient with Sturge-Weber disease complicated by Dilantin hyperplasia, J Oral Maxillofac Surg 44:646, 1986.

Kouskoukis CE and Kanitakis CJ: The Sturge-Weber syndrome, J Dermatol Surg Oncol 8:47, 1982.

Schofield D and others: Klippel-Trenaunay and Sturge-Weber syndromes with renal hemangioma and double inferior vena cava, J Urol 136:442, 1986.

Wilson S and others: Angiography, gingival hyperplasia and Sturge-Weber syndrome: report of case, J Dent Child 55:283, 1986.

Ykna RA, Cassingham RJ, and Carr RF: Periodontal manifestations and treatment in a case of Sturge-Weber syndrome, Oral Surg 47:408, 1979.

BLOOM'S SYNDROME

Bloom's syndrome is a rare hereditary disorder characterized by telangiectatic erythema in the "butterfly" area of the face, sunlight sensitivity, and dwarfism. The skin changes of the face and hands consist of erythematous patches resembling lupus erythematosus. There may also be bullous, crusted lesions on the lips. These manifestations usually develop in the first months or few years of life, and sunlight exacerbates them in the summer months. The infants are generally of low birth weight and because of immunodeficiencies may be in overall poor health. If they are kept indoors, often the skin lesions may not be seen and diagnosis may be delayed. Eczematization and vesiculation of the involved areas can result in atrophy, mainly on the face. In addition, café au lait spots, acanthosis nigricans, ichthyosis, prominent ears, hypospadias, cryptorchidism, syndactyly, and hypertrichosis may occur. These individuals show a pituitary type of retarded height and weight in early life. The skeletal frame is small; the body is delicate but well proportioned. Growth may resume later in life, and these patients may eventually have a normal stature. Intelligence and sexual maturation are normal.

Bloom's syndrome is characterized by its high frequency of chromosome breaks and rearrangements. The incidence of both myotatic chiasmata and sister chromatid exchanges increases. The syndrome is caused by an autosomal recessive gene, and a high rate of homozygosity is present. In addition, it occurs more often in Jews of Eastern European origin, with a high incidence in Russian Jews. Bloom's syndrome also occurs in other ethnic and racial groups, especially in which inbreeding or consanguinity are found.

The differential diagnosis of Bloom's syndrome includes the Rothmund-Thompson syndrome (poikiloderma congenitale), lupus erythematosus, ataxia-telangiectasia (Louis-Bar syndrome), and Cockayne's syndrome (trisomy 10). One quarter of the patients with Bloom's syndrome develop malignancies, most often leukemias and lymphomas. Other patients may have carcinomas, Wilms' tumor, and meningiomas. These conditions may result from the chromosomal structural changes and resulting malignant transformation or from the impaired immunologic defenses. Another major complication is repeated infections because of the patient's altered immunity.

No specific therapy exists for Bloom's syndrome, only treatment directed at the symptoms and avoidance of sunlight to prevent exacerbation of lesions. Genetic counseling is indicated for those who have the defective gene. The patient should be closely watched for development of malignancies.

ORAL MANIFESTATIONS. Intraoral lesions have not been found in patients with Bloom's syndrome, but delayed eruption and absence of maxillary lateral incisors have been reported. The patient may have the erythematous rash on lips in addition to the butterfly facial eruption. Manifestations of malignancy, particularly the leukemias, may be first seen in the mouth, and a potential increase in oral infections may occur.

Since these patients are sensitive to sunlight, long-term or high-powered light sources should be advoided.

DENTAL MANAGEMENT. The major management problem centers on related systemic disease because of the decreased immunoglobulins predisposing the patient to infections. Oral hygiene should be stressed, and supplemental aids to avoid infection should be used. The other major systemic problem involves the development of malignancies and their treatment. (See Chapter 9 on immunodeficiency diseases and Chapter 73 on leukemia for further details.)

BIBLIOGRAPHY

Bloom D: Congenital telangiectatic erythema resembling lupus erythematosus in dwarfs, Am J Dis Child 88:754, 1954.

Bloom D: The syndrome of congenital telangiectatic erythema and stunted growth, J Pediatr 68:103, 1966.

German J, Bloom D, and Passarge E: Bloom's syndrome. VII. Progress report for 1978, Clin Genet 15:361, 1979.

German J, Bloom D, and Passarge E: Bloom's syndrome. XI. Progress report for 1983, Clin Genet 25:166, 1984.

Goodman RN and Gorlin RJ: Atlas of the face in genetic disorders, St Louis, 1977, The CV Mosby Co.

Kuhn EM and Therman E: Cytogenetics of Bloom's syndrome, Cancer Genet Cytogenet 22:1, 1986.

Vanderschueren-Lodeweyckx M and others: Bloom's syndrome, possible pitfalls in clinical diagnosis, Am J Dis Child 138:812, 1984.

BASAL CELL NEVUS SYNDROME (NEVOID BASALIOMA SYNDROME; NEVOID BASAL CELL CARCINOMA SYNDROME; GORLIN'S SYNDROME)

Basal cell nevus syndrome is a hereditary disorder characterized by multiple basal cell carcinomas, pitted depressions on the patient's palms and soles, bony abnormalities of the ribs and spine, multiple cysts including odontogenic keratocysts, and abnormalities of the nervous system and other organs.

The usually multiple basal cell epitheliomas may number in the hundreds and may appear early in life. They can occur on any part of the body but tend to affect the central facial area (eyelids, periorbital areas, nose, cheeks, and around the lips). In addition to the usual characteristics, the epitheliomas may be nodular or pigmented or may resemble nevi or seborrheic keratosis, but microscopic examination reveals the typical appearance of basal cell carcinomas. They can occur with calcifications or osteoid formation. From puberty onward, the newer lesions grow more rapidly with the true invasive character of basal cell carcinoma. Metastasis, especially to the brain and lung, can occur. Rarely the basal cell carcinomas may be unilateral.

Pitting of the hands and feet occurs in about 70% of patients. The pitting often does not develop until the second decade of life or later, becoming more apparent with advancing age. The pits are characterized by partial or complete absence of the stratum corneum. The pits are discrete, shallow, 1 to 2 mm depressions found on the palms and soles.

Other skin manifestations include milia and cysts, especially of the limbs. Webbing of the neck has also been reported.

Various skeletal abnormalities may occur in up to 75% of patients with basal cell nevus syndrome. Approximately 65% of these abnormalities involve the spine and vertebrae, with scoliosis, cervical and upper thoracic fusion (lack of segmentation), and kyphoscoliosis. The ribs show bifurcation, splaying, synostosis, and partial agenesis or rudimentary cervical ribs. Spina bifida occurs in more than 40% of patients. Approximately one third of them have shortened metacarpal, usually the fourth or the fifth, and metatarsal bones.

Calcification of the dura, especially in the falx cerebri and cerebelli and basal ganglia, occurs in up to 80% of patients and may be seen on skull roentgenograms. Mental retardation and neurologic abnormalities may be encountered, as well as medulloblastomas, meningiomas, and other brain tumors. An increased incidence of schizophrenia seems to occur.

The characteristic facial appearance includes hypertelorism, lateral displacement of the medial canthi, frontal and temporal parietal bossing, accentuated supraorbital ridges, and a broad nasal root.

Eye problems have been reported in many patients, including dystopia canthorum, congenital blindness, nystagmus, and occasionally glaucoma. Endocrine problems have included ovarian fibromas and male hypogonadism associated with a female pubic hair pattern and scanty facial hair. Mammary fibromas and calcifications may occur. Some patients have pseudohypoparathyroidism.

Patients with the syndrome often have cysts. These cysts include superficial cysts of the limbs, multiple jaw keratocysts, median brain cysts, lymphatic mesenteric cysts, and renal cysts. Cholesteatomas that resemble the aggressive jaw keratocysts have been reported.

This genetic disorder has an autosomal dominant pattern with up to 95% penetrance and variable expression. Not every patient exhibits all the features of this syndrome, and varying formes frustes are often seen. It occurs mainly in whites; males and females are about equally affected.

If the basal cell carcinomas are untreated, the invasive, aggressive nature of this disorder may result in large, eroding ulcerations and occasional metastases. Curettage and electrofulguration may be sufficient therapy for most lesions; some may require surgical excision, including the microscopically controlled Mohs' surgical technique. Radiation therapy may be indicated for a few lesions, but because of the great numbers that develop, cumulative dose effects make this modality impractical.

Careful total systemic examination is necessary to rule out multiple complications of basal cell nevus syndrome. Cardiac problems must be treated aggressively. Complications of the multiple cysts must be evaluated. Renal problems can lead to hypertension, and cholesteatomas can result in deafness. Therapy is aimed at treatment of the symptoms.

Because of the genetic nature of the syndrome, careful genetic counseling is necessary, together with a review of the family history to determine any possible complications from incomplete penetrance.

ORAL MANIFESTATIONS. Usually the first clinical sign is the development of the multiple basal cell carcinomas of the face. Another early finding is orofacial clefting, which occurs more often in patients with this syndrome than in the normal population. A mild mandibular prognathism can also be seen but is often missed.

Approximately 75% of patients have multiple jaw keratocysts, which can be detected early on a panoramic roentgenogram. The lesions are multiple, multilocular, radiolucent cystlike areas that may resemble soap bubbles. Pathologically, they are odontogenic keratocysts. They can occur in young children, and in 50% of cases the keratocysts may be the first sign of basal cell nevus syndrome. They are painful lesions that drain into the oral cavity, possibly leading to pathologic fracture. The keratocysts may be associated with unerupted teeth and may displace erupted teeth as well, particularly the premolars. The mandible is affected twice as often as the maxilla. Unfortunately, they may be diagnosed simply as jaw cysts instead of the clinically significant keratocysts. Other reported findings include the frontal bossing, hypertelorism, and possible oligodontia.

DENTAL MANAGEMENT. The patient may have pain, swelling, trismus, and fever secondary to an infected keratocyst. The complete roentgenograms are necessary to delineate fully the area involved. A computed tomographic (CT) scan may be helpful. The cysts should be treated because the keratocysts tend to be more aggressive than other cysts. Surgical removal should be complete to avoid possible recurrence, generally caused by a "daughter" cyst. To avoid deformity, reconstruction must be considered as part of the surgical treatment plan. Maintenance of remaining teeth may be important for prosthetic retention. The facial basal cell carcinomas can also be aggressive and lead to deformity, thus creating a need for a facial prosthesis.

In addition, care must be taken to evaluate systemic involvement because these patients may have central nervous system, behavioral, cardiac problems, and hypertension.

BIBLIOGRAPHY

Barnes DA, Borns P, and Pizzutillo PD: Cervical spondylolisthesis associated with the multiple nevoid basal cell carcinoma syndrome, Clin Orthop 162:26, 1982.

Camisa C: The nevoid basal-cell carcinoma syndrome, simultaneous extirpation of numerous basal-cell carcinomas on the face by curettage and electrodesiccation under general anesthesia, J Dermatol Surg Oncol 7:893, 1981.

Correl TW: Bilateral cysts of the jaw occurring with multiple skin lesions, J Am Dent Assoc 101:978, 1980.

deBoer EM and Bruynzell DP: Basal cell nevus syndrome and webbed neck, Dermatologica 173:245, 1986.

de la Plaza R, Rodriguez E, and Castillo E: Two cases of nevoid basal cell carcinoma syndrome, Plast Reconstr Surg 71:114, 1983.

Ellis DJ and others: Nevoid basal cell carcinoma syndrome: report of a case, J Oral Surg 30:851, 1972.

Gorlin RJ and others: The multiple basal cell nevi syndrome, Cancer 18:89, 1965.

Gutierrez MM and Mora RG: Nevoid basal cell carcinoma syndrome, J Am Acad Dermatol 15:1023, 1986.

Howell JB and Anderson DE: Commentary: the nevoid basal cell carcinoma syndrome, Arch Dermatol 118:813, 1982.

Howell JB and others: Identification and treatment of jaw cysts in the nevoid basal cell carcinoma syndrome, J Oral Surg 25:129, 1967.

Jones KL and others: The Gorlin syndrome: a genetically determined disorder associated with cardiac tumors, Am Heart J 111:1013, 1986.

Lindeberg H and others: The nevoid basal cell carcinoma syndrome: oto-neurological aspects, J Laryngol Otol 100:1181, 1986.

Miller AS and others: Nevoid basal cell carcinoma syndrome, Oral Surg 36:533, 1973.

Naguib MG and others: Central nervous system involvement in the nevoid basal cell carcinoma syndrome: case report and review of the literature, Neurosurgery 11:52, 1982.

Olson RAJ and others: Nevoid basal cell carcinoma syndrome: review of the literature and report of a case, J Oral Surg 39:308, 1981.

Owens SC and others: Gorlin's basal cell nevus syndrome, Arch Otolaryngol Head Neck Surg 112:773, 1986.

Pritchard LJ and others: Variable expressivity of the multiple nevoid basal cell carcinoma syndrome, J Oral Maxillofac Surg 40:261, 1982.

Santis HR and others: Nevoid basal cell carcinoma syndrome associated with renal cysts and hypertension, Oral Surg 55:127, 1983.

Scully RE and others: Case records of the Massachusetts General Hospital, case 10—1986, N Engl J Med 314:700, 1986.

VanDijk E and Neering H: The association of cleft lip and palate with basal cell nevus syndrome, Oral Surg 50:214, 1980.

PSEUDOXANTHOMA ELASTICUM (GRÖNBLAD-STRANDBERG SYNDROME)

Pseudoxanthoma elasticum (Grönblad-Strandberg syndrome) is a rare, inherited disorder of elastic tissue involving the skin, retina, and blood vessels. Of the four variations, two are autosomal dominant and two are autosomal recessive. The most common form is an autosomal recessive trait. Women are affected more frequently than men; the incidence is approximately 1 in 160,000 persons.

The skin lesions are small, yellowish papules that initially form parallel to the skin lines and then coalesce. They are usually found in flexural areas: the sides of the neck, axillae, antecubital fossae, abdomen, groin, thighs, and perineum. The lesions have the appearance of plucked chicken skin or yellowish goose flesh. They are often found in early childhood but may be overlooked. They generally appear by the second decade of life. The skin becomes lax and redundant and may resemble that of a basset hound. Gastric, rectal, and vaginal lesions may also occur.

Retinal lesions called angioid streaks are the result of tearing of the elastic tissue in Bruch's membrane and are found radiating along the vessels outward from the optic disc. Retinal hemorrhages and exudates also occur as a result of changes in the elastic tissue of the retinal vessels, leading to varying degrees of blindness.

Arterial involvement can result in epistaxis and hematemesis. Peripheral vascular calcification may produce intermittent claudication. Hypertension, cerebral hemorrhage, and myocardial infarction may occur, contributing to patients' morbidity and mortality. Skin lesions do not appear to bleed excessively. Because idiopathic gastrointestinal bleeding rarely occurs in young children, one should rule out pseudoxanthoma elasticum when bleeding occurs.

Although the primary defect is not known, it involves degeneration of elastic fibers throughout the body. No specific test exists for this degeneration, but a skin biopsy shows the characteristic frayed, fragmented, irregularly clumped retractile fibers in the middle to lower third of the dermis. They appear to be altered elastic tissue, as confirmed with special stains.

Rare cases of the disease occurring along with either Marfan's or Ehlers-Danlos syndrome have been reported. D-penicillamine can induce a pseudoxanthomatous elasticum—like reaction.

No specific treatment exists; vitamin E (tocopherol) may be helpful. Plastic surgery for cosmetic reasons may be attempted. Major complications have been reported in pregnancy; in one study five of seven pregnant patients had major gastrointestinal bleeding or congestive heart failure.

ORAL MANIFESTATIONS. Yellowish white patches of the mucosa have been reported in about 5% of patients with pseudoxanthoma elasticum. These patches resemble Fordyce granules when seen on the buccal mucosa but are not sebaceous glands. They may also occur on the labial mucosa, soft palate, and lips.

DENTAL MANAGEMENT. Although the lesions present no problem, the systemic involvement resulting from arterial elastic fiber degeneration may cause difficulties. Arterial breakdown and rupturing may cause gastrointestinal bleeding and arterial occlusion, which may result in myocardial and cerebral infarction. Arterial calcifications have been noted on roentgenograms. Hypertension is also a common problem. Caution should be used in treatment of the patient, especially because of the vascular alterations. (See Chapter 87 on cardiovascular disease for management of hypertensive patient.)

BIBLIOGRAPHY

Berde C and others: Pregnancy in women with pseudoxanthoma elasticum, Obstet Gynecol Surv 38:339, 1983.

Fasshauer K and others: Neurological complications of Grönblad-Strandberg syndrome, J Neurol 231:250, 1984.

Goette DK and Carpenter WM: The mucocutaneous marker of pseudoxanthoma elasticum, Oral Surg 51:68, 1981.

Gorlin RJ and Goldman HM: Thoma's oral pathology, St Louis, 1970, The CV Mosby Co.

Light N and others: Collagen and elastin changes in D-penicillamine-induced pseudoxanthoma elasticum—like skin, Br J Dermatol 114:381, 1986.

Morgan AA: Recurrent gastrointestinal hemorrhage: an unusual cause, Am J Gastroenterol 77:925, 1982.

Nickoloff BJ, Noodleman FR, and Abel EA: Perforating pseudoxanthoma elasticum associated with chronic renal failure and hemodialysis, Arch Dermatol 121:1321, 1985.

O'Holleran M and Merrell RC: Pseudoxanthoma elasticum and polyposis coli, Arch Surg 116:476, 1981.

Premalatha S, Yesudian P, and Thambiah AS: Perumbilical pseudoxanthoma elasticum with transepidermal elimination, Int J Dermatol 21:604, 1982.

Scully RE and others: Case records of the Massachusetts General Hospital, case 10—1983, N Engl J Med 308:579, 1983.

Turck M: Recurrent hematemesis and diffuse 'gooseflesh,' Hosp Pract 19:133, 1984.

157·ENDOCRINE AND METABOLIC DISORDERS

Anthony V. Benedetto *and* Robert N. Arm

DIABETES MELLITUS

The skin changes found in patients with diabetes mellitus can be related to infection, arteriosclerosis, neuropathy, microangiopathy, long-term insulin therapy, and metabolic abnormalities. About 30% of diabetic patients have cutaneous manifestations.

Most of the other skin conditions of diabetic patients are not necessarily related to or dependent on control of the blood glucose level.

Pruritus is common in diabetic patients. It is often localized to the lower extremities but may be generalized. Frequently the skin is dry (xerotic). When the anogenital region is involved, a fungal infection may be the cause of the pruritus. Treatment of generalized pruritus includes infrequent bathing, the use of mild soaps, and the topical application of moisturizing lotions containing menthol, camphor, phenol, or pramoxine, with or without hydrocortisone. Fungal infections are treated with the various available topical imidazole agents or other topical antifungal preparations. For severe infections, systemic antifungal agents are needed.

Diabetic dermopathy, also known as diabetic shin spots, occurs on the lower extremities and resembles traumatic scars. The lesions appear as small, depressed, pigmented scars that may have a superficial scale (Fig. 157-1). The hyperpigmentation is caused by deposition of hemosiderin in the upper dermis. These spots are a useful skin marker, but they show no relationship to the severity of the diabetes or to its complications. Controversy surrounds whether shin spots are related to diabetic microangiopathy. No specific treatment exists.

Patients with diabetes mellitus often are chronic carriers of nasal *Staphylococcus aureus* infection. They are more susceptible to styes, pyodermas, furuncles, and carbuncles. Treatment for this is directed toward control of the infection, which can alter insulin requirements. Recurrent infections may be related to uncontrolled blood glucose levels.

Monilia (Candida) infections are typically associated with diabetes mellitus. Vaginitis, pruritus ani, paronychia, interdigital infections, intertrigo, and balanitis can occur. These entities should suggest possible diabetes, especially if no other reasons exist for their occurrence.

Superficial fungal infections (dermatophytosis) involving the groin and feet require prompt therapy, since bacterial infection may supervene.

Papular eruptive xanthomas can occur. They appear as firm, pinkish yellow nodules and papules, symmetrically located on elbows, knees, buttocks, and dorsa of the hands and feet. Less than 1% of diabetic patients, usually young men, have them.

Bullosis diabeticorum is most often associated with peripheral neuropathy and is very rare. Painless blisters develop rapidly on the hands, feet, toes, fingers, and forearms. They are slow to heal and generally leave no scar. Treatment is usually conservative and directed to the symptoms.

Granuloma annulare consists of pale yellow to salmon pink papules. There are two forms. A localized annular form, found most often on the extremities, is not as closely associated with diabetes mellitus as is the disseminated form, which consists of diffuse, small, confluent annular lesions. This usually occurs on sun-exposed areas of older adults. The localized form is

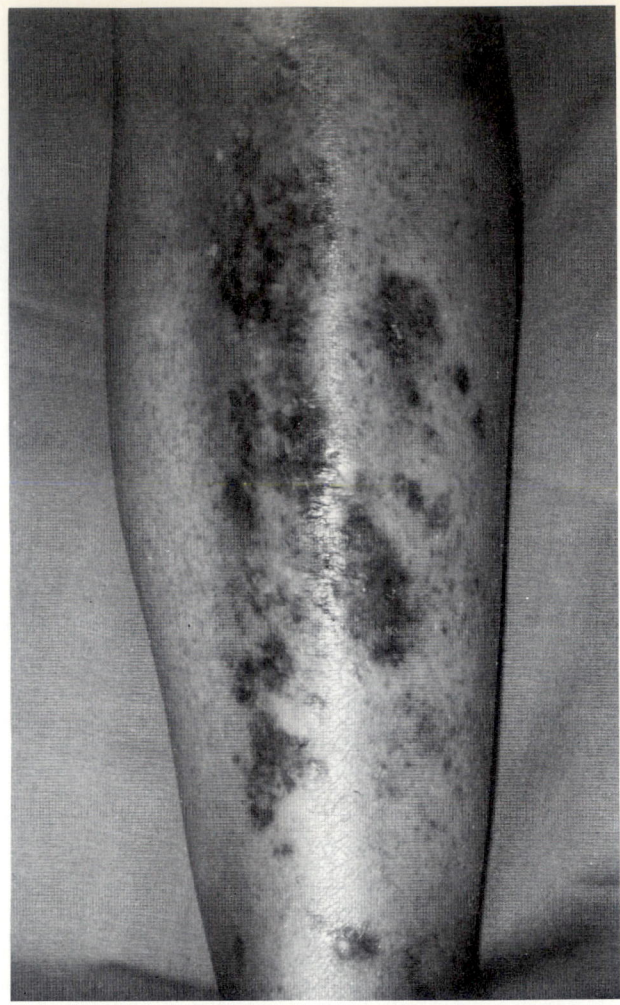

Fig. 157-1   Diabetic dermopathy (shin spots).

more common in children. Screening for diabetes should be done in both cases.

Necrobiosis lipoidica diabeticorum is similar histologically, but not clinically, to granuloma annulare. It is the best-known cutaneous marker for diabetes, but its relationship to the clinical disease is unclear. It is found in only 3 in 1000 patients with established diabetes. However, the lesions also may occur in the absence of diabetes; in these cases there is often a strong family history of diabetes, steroid-induced hyperglycemia, or previously abnormal blood sugar levels in the absence of overt diabetes. Diabetes eventually develops in some of these patients. Most patients with necrobiosis lipoidica diabeticorum are women.

The development of necrobiosis lipoidica diabeticorum does not appear to be altered by control of the diabetes. The lesions are characteristic in the fully developed state: oval or irregular indurated plaques with a glazed surface, central atrophy, yellow-orange discoloration, and prominent telangiectases, surrounded by a violaceous border. The lesions usually occur on the lower extremities, but in 15% of patients they are found on the arms, hands, trunk, and scalp (Fig. 157-2). Atypical forms also occur.

The progression of necrobiosis lipoidica diabeticorum is slow. Ulceration and variable scarring occur. Topical or intralesional administration of corticosteroids sometimes may help, but these agents should be used carefully because they also induce atrophy.

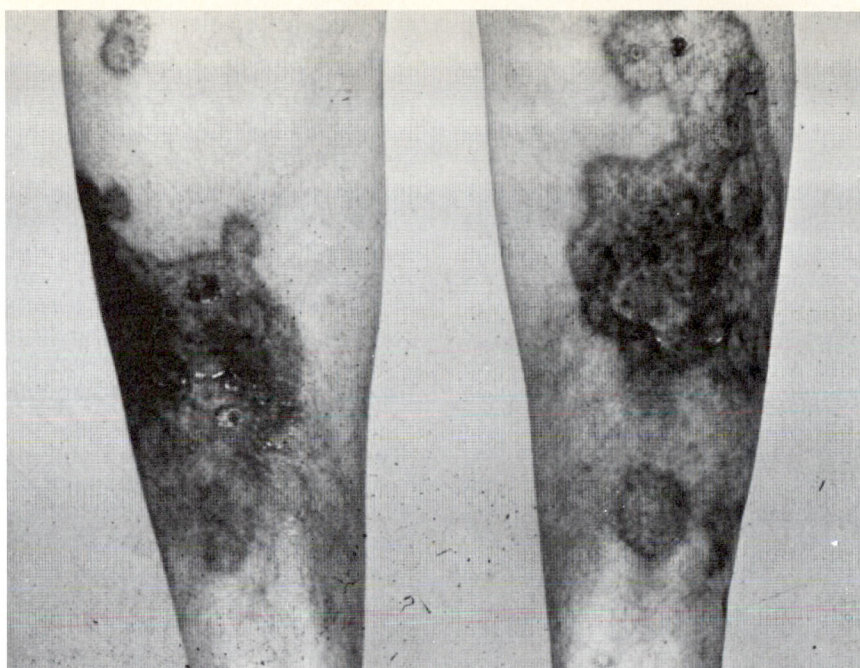

Fig. 157-2   Necrobiosis lipoidica diabeticorum. Lesions are initially paler and atrophic. In advanced stages, as here, there is marked atrophy with hyperpigmentation.

ORAL MANIFESTATIONS AND DENTAL MANAGEMENT.
The oral manifestations of diabetes mellitus include xerostomia, glossopyrosis, dysgeusia, gingival tenderness, gingivitis, and periodontitis, which are thought to result from peripheral neuropathy and diabetic microangiopathy. Poor wound healing and lowered resistance to infection, especially to candidiasis, are also frequently seen. (See Chapter 19 on diabetes.)

THYROID DISEASE
Hyperthyroidism

In hyperthyroidism the patient's skin is warm and moist because of increased cutaneous blood flow and sweating. The skin feels soft and is described as being "fine." This connotes its texture and does not imply thinness, since studies show the skin to have normal thickness. Palmar erythema and onycholysis (separation of the nail distally from the nail bed; also known as Plummer's nail) may be seen in some patients with hyperthyroidism, but neither sign is specific for this condition. The scalp hair may be fine and friable and may shed diffusely during active hyperthyroidism, but it regrows when the disease is controlled.

An addisonian type of pigmentation, generally sparing the buccal mucosa, is occasionally noted in chronic cases of active hyperthyroidism. This may be caused by increased secretion of melanocyte-stimulating hormone (MSH) by the pituitary. Vitiligo occurs in about 7% of thyrotoxic individuals. Other skin conditions found in association with hyperthyroidism include diffuse thinning of scalp hair, hypertrophic osteoarthroppathy, acropachy, and, infrequently, chronic urticaria and generalized pruritus.

Perhaps the most striking complication of hyperthyroidism is the syndrome of pretibial myxedema, which consists of thickened nodules and plaques on the anterior tibial surfaces of the legs.

The nodules and plaques on the shins have a waxy, translucent appearance and may be flesh colored to pink or violaceous. They are formed by the deposition of acid mucopolysaccharides, which cause dilation of the follicular orifices as the material accumulates, resulting in a peau d'orange appearance. It may be accompanied by exophthalmos and does not necessarily improve after surgical or radioactive iodine therapy for thyrotoxicosis.

Hypothyroidism

In primary myxedema caused by insufficiency of the thyroid gland, the patient's skin becomes rough and dry, mainly on the extensor surfaces of the extremities, and sometimes appears ichthyotic. The skin of the face becomes puffy, especially around the eyes and on the cheeks. The facial features become coarsened, with a broad, thick nose; fat lips; and a large, clumsy, smooth, red tongue; the patient has a dull expression. The oral mucous membranes also become thickened. The feet and hands may become swollen, but this is a nonpitting brawny edema caused by the deposition of mucin. The swelling is not to the extent found in pretibial myxedema (see the preceding discussion on hyperthyroidism). The skin may develop a yellowish tint as a result of carotenemia, and the skin temperature falls below normal. The hair becomes universally sparse, dry, and thin and is lost from the outer third of the eyebrows. The nails are brittle, show striations, and break readily at the edges. When hypothyroidism develops as a result of pituitary failure, the skin and hair changes are milder than those found in patients with primary myxedema.

ORAL MANIFESTATIONS AND DENTAL MANAGEMENT.
See Chapter 187 on thyroid disease.

PITUITARY DISEASE
Acromegaly

Acromegaly is usually the result of a benign eosinophilic pituitary adenoma secreting excessive amounts of somatotropin, or growth hormone (GH). In the adult this results in the enlargement of bone and cartilage of the skull, hands, and feet, since the epiphyses of the long bones have already closed. In children, whose epiphyses are not yet closed and are therefore capable of linear bone growth, excessive secretion of GH results in gigantism.

In acromegaly, GH causes an increase in mucopolysaccharides and collagen in the skin, which results in water retention and a thickened, doughy appearance of the skin. This is most noticeable over the face and distal extremities, where the skeletal changes are also most prominent; thus the name acromegaly. The skin can become so thickened on the scalp that furrows and ridges result, producing cutis verticis gyrata. Facial features enlarge and are accentuated, creating the characteristic facies of hypertrophic frontal bosses and supraorbital ridges; edematous eyelids; an exuberant, elongated nose; an enlarged lower jaw (prognathism) with widely spaced teeth; and a protruding lower lip. Macroglossia is usually also present, along with enlarged ears. The hands and feet become abnormally prominent. The skin becomes coarse and leathery, often with excessive sweating and oiliness. The body hair is coarse and increased in amount. Hyperpigmentation of the skin develops, probably as a result of increased melanocyte stimulating hormone secretion. Hypothyroidism may develop when the normal pituitary tissue is destroyed.

ORAL MANIFESTATIONS AND DENTAL MANAGEMENT.
See Chapter 186 on pituitary disease.

ADRENAL DISEASE
Adrenal insufficiency (Addison's disease)

Deficiency of glucocorticoid production by the adrenal glands occurs primarily when the adrenals are destroyed by surgical removal, infections (tuberculosis, viral infections, histoplasmosis), metastatic malignancies, or autoimmune diseases. Secondary adrenal deficiency occurs when pituitary corticotropin, or adrenocorticotropic hormone (ACTH), is insufficiently secreted.

One of the skin manifestations of Addison's disease is the gradual onset of diffuse hyperpigmentation, which ranges from brown to black and is more pronounced on exposed areas of the body. It is also found on the tongue, gums, buccal mucosa, areolae, genitalia, and areas of friction, such as the knees, elbows, knuckles, and belt line. Scars, pigmented nevi, and hair may become darker, with brunettes showing deeper pigmentation than blonds. The oral pigmentation develops in spots, rather than diffusely, and may be pale to dark brown, blue, or black. It is usually seen on the buccal mucosa bilaterally and eventually involves the entire mucosal lining, including the gingiva. Vitiligo develops in 15% of the individuals with Addison's disease.

The diffuse hyperpigmentation is induced by an increased secretion of β-MSH from the pituitary, which occurs because adrenal cortisol is not present to function in the feedback system of hypothalamic-pituitary-adrenal control. The differential diagnosis must include other sources of hyperpigmentation such as scleroderma, lupus erythematosus, chronic renal and hepatic diseases, hemochromatosis, melanemia, thyrotoxicosis, and the ingestion of busulfan, actinomycin D, and arsenic. Replacement therapy with corticosteroids can reduce the pigmentation gradually.

ORAL MANIFESTATIONS AND DENTAL MANAGEMENT.
See Chapter 188 on adrenal disease.

Adrenocortical hyperplasia (Cushing's syndrome; hypercortisolism)

Excessive amounts of circulating glucocorticoid hormones can result in Cushing's syndrome when a functioning benign or malignant adrenal cortex tumor is present. More common, however, is Cushing's disease, which results when a pituitary

gland microadenoma inappropriately hypersecretes ACTH, causing bilateral adrenal hyperplasia. Nonpituitary neoplasms such as pulmonary oat cell carcinoma and pancreatic carcinoma can result in hypercortisolism by secreting ectopic ACTH; this is known as the ectopic ACTH syndrome. The clinical findings are similar in the various types of hypercortisolism. These patients characteristically have a "moon" facies, with telangiectasia over the cheeks and often a dusky, plethoric flush. The hair of the face is increased, with thinning scalp hair more noticeable in females, as well as hypertrichosis of the body and extremities. Excessive deposits of fat over the clavicles and back of the neck result in the characteristic "buffalo hump."

Acneiform lesions of the face, consisting of perifollicular papules and pustules, can occur, but this "steroid acne" does not produce the comedones and deep cystic lesions seen in adolescent acne vulgaris.

Some patients have an addisonian-like, brownish hyperpigmentation because of the increased secretion of β-MSH from the pituitary. Acanthosis nigricans may develop in intertriginous areas of the neck, axillae, and groin. With loss of dermal collagen and elastin, the skin becomes thin, dry, and fragile. Because of resultant atrophic skin and decreased vascular tone, blood vessels appear more prominent, producing cutis marmorata (marblelike mottling of the skin), especially of the lower extremities. Blood vessels have less support, and vascular fragility increases. This appears in patients as purpura and ecchymoses caused by minor trauma to the extremities and other areas of the body. Broad, purple, atrophic striae appear on the trunk and the extremities.

Patients with Cushing's syndrome are more susceptible to superficial fungal infections such as *Trichophyton rubrum* and tinea versicolor (caused by *Pityrosporum orbiculare*). Although *T. rubrum* is an organism commonly found in fungal involvement of the feet, inguinal area, and nails, in Cushing's syndrome the infection becomes disseminated over the trunk and buttocks. These superficial infections often clear spontaneously after the patient is cured.

ORAL MANIFESTATIONS AND DENTAL MANAGEMENT.
See Chapter 188 on adrenal disease.

Acanthosis nigricans

The lesions of acanthosis nigricans are hyperpigmented, velvety textured, or slightly verrucous plaques occurring in the patient's axillae, sides and back of the neck, anogenital region, groin and other flexural surfaces, and submammary, umbilical, and even palmar-plantar regions (Fig. 157-3). The lips and mucosae are rarely involved.

There are five types of acanthosis nigricans. *Benign acanthosis nigricans* can occur in association with a variety of endocrinopathies, such as insulin-resistant diabetes mellitus, acromegaly and gigantism, Cushing's disease and syndrome, hyperandrogenic states, Addison's disease, polycystic ovaries (Stein-Leventhal syndrome), pituitary adenomas, hypothyroidism, hyperthyroidism, hepatolenticular degeneration (Wilson's disease), and lipodystrophy with hyperlipidemia. Acanthosis nigricans is often permanent and improves in only a few patients after the endocrinopathy is successfully treated.

Hereditary benign acanthosis nigricans may be found in several non-endocrine-related disorders, including an autosomal dominant inherited trait that appears during childhood or puberty and persists throughout adulthood. Flexural surfaces (axillae and neck) are involved to a limited extent, and no association exists with underlying disease.

Drug-induced acanthosis nigricans has been found after high-dose nicotinic acid or diethylstilbesterol administration in

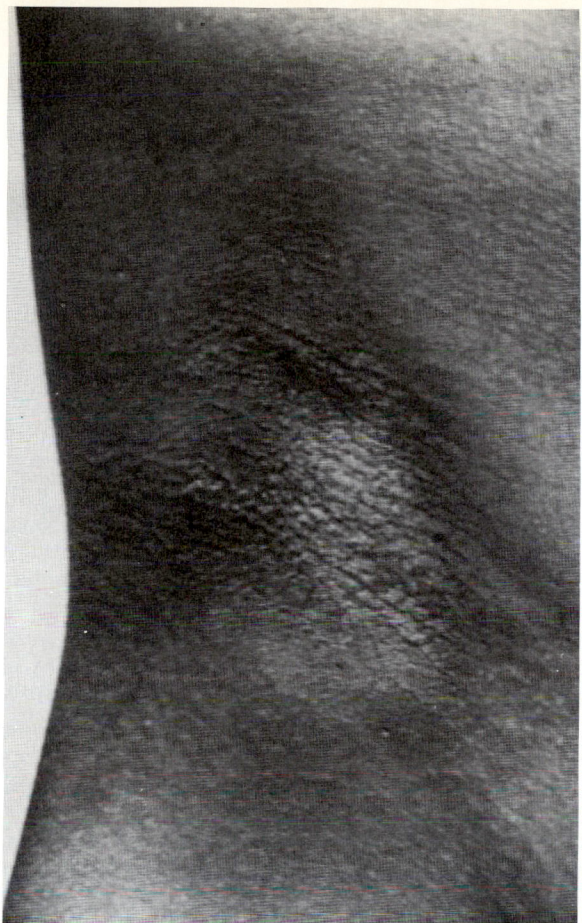

Fig. 157-3 Acanthosis nigricans in axilla. It is hyperpigmented and papular.

young men and as a side effect of oral contraceptive therapy. One report cited a skin reaction caused by insulin injection, which resulted in a lesion resembling acanthosis nigricans. In these patients the acanthosis nigricans generally resolves when the drug is discontinued.

Pseudo–acanthosis nigricans is seen in obese, dark-skinned patients. In these individuls no obvious genetic predisposition or clinically evident endocrine disorder exists, but the obesity probably produces insulin resistance and hyperinsulinemia, which in turn is the suspected mechanism for acanthosis nigricans. Ordinarily, weight reduction leads to diminution of the lesions.

Whichever of the previous four types of acanthosis nigricans are present, most authorities believe that insulin resistance with hyperinsulinemia is the main, unifying feature in most patients with acanthosis nigricans. One must understand, however, that even though insulin resistance is the predominant mechanism, most patients do not require insulin treatment and many do not even have diabetes mellitus. Rather, they are discovered to have hyperinsulinemia when circulating insulin levels are measured.

Malignant acanthosis nigricans is not a malignant condition, but is acanthosis nigricans found in those patients who have a known or an occult malignancy, usually an adenocarcinoma but at times even a lymphoma. (See Chapter 164 on cutaneous signs of internal malignancy.)

ORAL MANIFESTATIONS. Oral lesions of acanthosis nigricans have been seen in up to half of patients. They generally occur on the lips and tongue, appearing as verrucous plaques. The tongue may be hypertrophic, have elongated papillae, and resemble a fissured tongue. Other mucosal lesions have been reported on the palate and buccal mucosa. All forms—benign, "malignant," pseudo, hereditary, and drug-induced—can occur in the mouth, although the patient with the pseudo form rarely has oral lesions. All forms have the same histopathologic signs, consisting of a papillary surface with hyperkeratosis. Widening of the prickle cell zone along with slight acanthosis and atrophy and occasional hyperpigmentation are also noted. At times, edema and even hypertrophic, inflamed verrucous and papillomatous mucosae are seen. The buccal mucosa in particular can have a velvety verrucous, diffuse unevenness.

DENTAL MANAGEMENT. The "malignant" form is of the most concern because the clinician must realize that although the biopsy of the oral mucosa is benign, an underlying malignancy may exist. The malignancy is in the gastrointestinal tract in more than 70% of patients, especially in the stomach (about 55%). Approximately one fifth of the lesions of acanthosis nigricans occur before the malignancy is diagnosed.

Generally, no treatment of the lesion other than surgical shaving is needed. Topical steroids have helped some patients.

Other problems in dental management have resulted from the underlying systemic diseases, whether endocrine or malignant, and the subsequent therapy for them. (Refer to the chapter on the particular disease for treatment.)

PORPHYRIA

The porphyrias are a group of inherited and acquired disorders of porphyrin metabolism. Except for acute intermittent porphyria, all patients with the variations show photosensitivity reactions, which usually appear as vesiculobullous eruptions on sun-exposed areas. Subsequent cigarette paper–like scars, milia, hyperpigmentation, and hypertrichosis may develop.

The porphyrins are products of hemoglobin and myoglobin synthesis. These compounds absorb sunlight in the ranges of 400 to 410 nm (Soret band) and 500 to 600 nm. Problems occur as a result of overproduction of porphyrin precursors. Both liver and bone marrow may be involved.

In *erythropoietic porphyrias* the blood and bone marrow fluoresce. The disorders are all inherited. The rare autosomal recessive variant, congenital erythropoietic porphyria (Günther's disease), has mutilating photosensitivity. Shortly after birth, vesicles and bullae appear on sun-exposed areas of the infant's skin. Healing is poor and often results in scarring. Milia, hypertrichosis, scarring alopecia, ectropion, loss of nasal cartilages, loss of the terminal phalanges, and erythrodontia eventually occur. Frequently an associated hemolytic anemia with splenomegaly is seen. Sunlight avoidance is mandatory; β-carotene has been reported to be of some help. Splenectomy may ameliorate the hemolytic anemia as well as photosensitivity and porphyrin excretion.

Erythropoietic protoporphyria is inherited as an autosomal dominant disorder. The disease begins in childhood with burning and tingling on sun exposure. Urticarial plaques and eczematous areas develop, together with a papular thickening of the skin having a cobblestone appearance. Sunlight through window glass can also precipitate symptoms. Micronodular cirrhosis has been reported as part of the syndrome. Minimal hypertrichosis, scarring, and hyperpigmentation develop. Frequently the disease improves after the first decade of life. Protection from sunlight by using an opaque sunscreen and oral administration of β-carotene are useful. *Erythropoietic coproporphyria* is clinically similar to erythropoietic protoporphyria.

The *hepatic porphyrias* are both inherited and acquired. *Acute intermittent porphyria* is an autosomal dominant form that often appears initially with signs of an acute surgical abdomen. The disease appears to be more common in females than males and more often in Scandinavian, Anglo-Saxon, or German populations. Most often it develops in the third or fourth decade of life but can occur earlier. Clinical manifestations also include psychotic episodes and neurologic abnormalities similar to lead poisoning. The neurologic abnormalities may include seizures and insomnia. Skin changes occur in most patients. Treatment includes a special high-carbohydrate diet. These patients do not seem to be affected by the sun. A screening of psychiatric patients noted an increased incidence of porphyria.

Porphyria variegata is similar to acute intermittent porphyria, with acute attacks and an autosomal dominant transmission. Patients with this form have photosensitivity reactions. This disease usually begins in young adults. Vesicles develop on the dorsa of the hands, face, and neck on exposure to sun. Tissue-paper scars, milia, plaques of lichenfied skin, hypertrichosis, and hyperpigmentation occur. These patients have fragile skin and often appear older than their chronologic age. Exposure to sunlight must be minimized, sunscreens may be useful, and trauma to the extremities should be avoided.

Porphyria cutanea tarda is an acquired variant; patients have cutaneous manifestations similar to those of porphyria variegata. Alcohol, hexachlorobenzene, chlorinated hydrocarbons (polychlorinated biphenyl and dioxin), iron, and estrogens can all precipitate attacks. The onset is in later adult life. Photosensitivity occurs in the late summer and autumn. Vesicles, milia, tissue-paper scars, and sclerodermoid skin changes are found. Treatment includes the use of sunscreens (minimal help), avoidance of alcohol and other substances that may provoke an attack, and very low doses of chloroquine. Phlebotomy, at intervals of 2 to 4 weeks with removal of 500 ml of blood each session, is helpful. The phlebotomy induces anemia and a low serum iron level, which helps prevent symptoms from developing. In many instances, the cautious introduction of oral chloroquine therapy is effective following phlebotomy. Porphyria cutanea tarda has been reported with increased incidence of lymphoma and renal failure. In patients with renal failure, urine testing is not helpful and diagnostic blood tests must be used. Neuropathies have also been reported.

ORAL MANIFESTATIONS. The most remarkable manifestations of the porphyrias in the patient's oral cavity is a reddish brown tooth discoloration. This erythrodontia shows red fluorescence in ultraviolet light. Other signs may occur in various forms and include vesiculobullous lesions that heal slowly on sun-exposed surfaces of the face. The patients may also develop deformed ears, noses, and eyelids as a result of bullae rupturing and healing. Because the patients may be placed on a special high-carbohydrate diet, an increased incidence of caries and periodontal disease may be noted.

DENTAL MANAGEMENT. Dental esthetics presents a problem because of the severe tooth discoloration with porphyrias. Various forms of esthetic coverage may be tried. A tooth veneering system using composite resins should be attempted, but no results have been published to date. Because of the patient's photosensitivity, night appointments are recommended. The use of facial protection, as with a mask, may be beneficial if bright light is used.

The systemic involvement varies with the type of porphyria; thus consultation is mandatory. Problems reported include hemolytic anemia, neurologic disturbances, behavioral disorders, and fluid imbalance. The neurologic involvement can vary from epileptiform convulsions to a uniplegia or paraplegia. Behavioral problems can include emotional disturbances and overt psychosis. The fluid problems may lead to need for fluid restriction despite signs the patient may be dehydrated. This fluid problem may lead the physician to request improvement of masticatory capabilities.

Some medications may exacerbate or precipitate the porphyria or may affect involved organs. Barbiturates, muscle relaxants, sulfonamides, tetracycline, antileptics, and anticonvulsants may precipitate porphyria. In extreme cases, use of the medications can lead to death. Additional caution must be taken because of liver and hematopoietic problems.

Oral hygiene should be stressed to these individuals because of their special diets. Dietary recommendations in the dental office should be checked carefully, and consultation with a dietician or physician may be necessary to achieve appropriate carbohydrate and fluid balance.

HYPERLIPIDEMIAS

Xanthomas are papular or nodular yellow-orange lesions that develop as the result of deposition of lipid in cells (xanthoma cells). They generally appear in association with disorders of lipid metabolism but may occasionally occur without any evidence of abnormal lipids or lipoproteins in the blood. The importance of xanthomatous lesions is their connection to possible systemic disease with cardiovascular complications. Approximately 40% of patients have elevated cholesterol levels.

The hyperlipoproteinemias (hyperlipidemias) are classified into five major types on the basis of electrophoresis and ultracentrifuge separation of serum. The manifestations vary with type. The manifestations of hyperlipoproteinemia type I are eruptive cutaneous xanthomas; type II, tuberous, tendinous, palpebral (xanthelasma), and childhood xanthomas; type III, tuberous and tendinous xanthomas, xanthoma palmaris (xanthomas along the palmar creases), and sometimes palpebral and eruptive xanthomas; type IV, generally no external manifestations, but when present, eruptive xanthomas (usually on the buttocks) are characteristic skin findings; type V, eruptive xanthomas and, rarely, tuberous xanthomas.

Most lesions develop in adulthood, except for hyperlipoproteinemia type II, which may appear in childhood. In type II a strong predisposition exists to atherosclerotic coronary artery disease. Eruptive xanthomas are pinhead- to pea-sized, reddish yellow papules. They occur in crops and may be pruritic. Extensor and pressure surfaces are involved. The lesions may ulcerate and sometimes may regress. They indicate elevated triglyceride levels and may vary as the triglyceride levels fluctuate. These lesions are seen in types I, II, IV, and V.

Eruptive xanthomas also may occur as a result of insulin-dependent diabetes mellitus (xanthoma diabeticorum). When the diabetes is brought under control, the patient's triglyceride levels are lowered and the lesions involute. Weight reduction and carbohydrate intake restriction are mandatory.

Tendinous xanthomas occur as nontender nodules on tendons, fascia, and periosteum. The Achilles tendon and extensor tendons of the fingers are most often involved.

Tuberous xanthomas are located on the knees, elbows, knuckles, and other extensor surfaces. They are yellowish red plaques or patches of papules that do not ulcerate and, once developed, are stable. Tendinous and tuberous xanthomas are usually associated with types II and III.

Planar xanthomas occur in various areas of the body, but when they appear on the ocular palpebra, they are also known as xanthelasma. Planar xanthomas are always soft, yellow, and macular, but at times may be slightly elevated. Xanthelasma can occur on the upper or lower eyelids, often bilaterally, and are the most commonly found xanthomas. In two thirds of patients with xanthelasma, no lipid abnormality can be found. When an abnormality is present, usually in young adults, it is type II or III. Other forms of planar xanthomas are those seen on the face, neck, upper trunk, and arms and are associated with the secondary hyperlipidemias found in various paraproteinemias and in obstructive hepatobiliary disease (xanthomatous biliary cirrhosis). In these diseases, serum levels of phospholipids and cholesterol are increased. The triglyceride levels are elevated, and the plasma is clear, showing no chylomicrons. Hepatomegaly is present, and pruritus is severe. Xanthoma palmaris, in which yellow planar xanthomas occur in the creases of the palms and volar aspect of the fingers, may also be present.

Xanthoma disseminatum is rare, and characteristic yellow-red papulonodular lesions are found in the flexural areas of the patient's neck, antecubital fossae, and groin. Yellowish pink to orange xanthomatous nodules can be found scattered over the mucous membranes of the mouth, tongue, pharynx, larynx, and even the bronchi. With upper respiratory tract involvement, the patient can have dysphagia, laryngeal obstruction with hoarseness, and dyspnea. Diabetes insipidus results from xanthomatous lesions in the area of the sella turcica and pituitary gland. Usually found in adults, xanthoma disseminatum most often has a benign course and rarely invades bone or other internal organs. In xanthoma disseminatum the serum lipid levels are normal and therefore the disease is thought to result from the proliferation of non–X histiocytic cells with secondary accumulations of lipid (cholesterol).

Xanthomatosis in myxedema is caused by an increase of pre-β-lipoproteins. These eruptions respond to treatment with thyroid medication.

In chronic pancreatitis the lipoprotein concentrations are increased, with elevated triglyceride and cholesterol levels. Xanthoma disseminatum is seen among these patients with an increase in pre-β-lipoprotein, which responds only when the pancreatitis is controlled. Maculopapular lesions and cutaneous nodules occur in the flexural creases, conjunctiva, and mucous membranes. The nephrotic syndrome may also be associated with eruptive xanthomas and occasionally with chylomicronemia.

Cerebrotendinous xanthomatosis is a rare autosomal recessive disease. The patient typically has tendon xanthomas, cataracts, and neurologic dysfunction. Because the blood lipid levels are normal, authorities have debated whether this is possibly related to histiocytic proliferation.

If the patient has isolated xanthelasma, generally no workup besides a serum cholesterol level and preprandial and postprandial glucose concentrations is needed. Other forms of xanthomas require evaluation of serum cholesterol and triglyceride levels, examination of serum turbidity, and lipoprotein electrophoresis. Evaluation of cardiovascular function may be needed because of the atherosclerotic coronary artery disease in type II and the ischemic heart disease and peripheral vascular disease in type III.

ORAL MANIFESTATIONS AND DENTAL MANAGEMENT. See appropriate chapters on lipidemias and cardiovascular disease.

HEMOCHROMATOSIS

Hemochromatosis (bronze diabetes) is characterized by the triad of hyperpigmentation, diabetes mellitus, and hepatic cirrhosis. Increased iron deposition is found in the skin, liver, heart, pancreas, and endocrine organs, with impairment of their function. Hyperpigmentation is generalized and is more prominent on the face, flexural creases, and exposed areas. Pigmentation of the oral mucosae occurs in approximately 15% of the affected patients. This pattern of hyperpigmentation is similar in appearance to that of Addison's disease, but adrenal insufficiency cannot be demonstrated. The conjunctivae and lid margins are pigmented in 20% of patients. The spectrum of pigmentation can vary from brown to slate gray, and these colors may be present simultaneously. The increased pigmentation is usually caused by melanin rather than iron deposition in the skin.

Hereditary hemochromatosis is transmitted as an autosomal recessive trait. There is partial biochemical expression in the heterozygote. The classic triad of skin pigmentation, hepatomegaly, and diabetes occurs late in approximately the fifth or sixth decade of life. Often the initial symptoms are weakness and joint pain.

Patients with hemochromatosis tend to have dry, scaly skin. The disorder occurs in men more frequently than women and usually develops between the ages of 40 and 60 years. In addition to diabetes mellitus and hyperpigmentation, these individuals also have hepatic cirrhosis with accompanying features of spider angiomas, sparse body hair, ecchymoses, and gynecomastia. In addition to treating the underlying disease, it is important to remove excessive body iron by repeated phlebotomy.

ORAL MANIFESTATIONS AND DENTAL MANAGEMENT. See Chapter 69.

BIBLIOGRAPHY

Alaupovic P: Apoproteins and lipoproteins, Atherosclerosis 13:141, 1970.

Bang G: Acanthosis nigricans maligna, paraneoplasia with oral manifestations, Oral Surg 29:370, 1970.

Bartz WM: On the control of cholesterol synthesis, Metabolism 22:1507, 1973.

Beamish MR and others: Transferrin iron, chelatable iron and ferritin in idiopathic hemochromatosis, Br J Haematol 22:219, 1974.

Benedetto AV and Taylor JS: Porphyria cutanea tarda: update 1978, Cutis 21:483, 1978.

Benedetto AV and others: Porphyria cutanea tarda in three generations of a single family, N Engl J Med 298:358, 1978.

Bernstein JE and others: Bullous eruption of diabetes mellitus, Arch Dermatol 115:324, 1979.

Braverman IM: Skin signs of systemic disease, ed 2, Philadelphia, 1981, WB Saunders Co.

Brenner DA and Bloomer JR: The enzymatic defect in variegate porphyria, N Engl J Med 302:765, 1980.

Brodie MJ and others: Hereditary coproporphyria, Q J Med 46:229, 1977.

Bromley GS and Goulian D: Xanthoma disseminatum: an unusual cause of facial and limb deformity, Plast Reconstr Surg 72:552, 1983.

Brown T and Winkelmann RK: Acanthosis nigricans: a study of 90 cases, Medicine 47:33, 1968.

Caravati CM and others: Cutaneous manifestations of hyperthyroidism, South Med J 62:1127, 1969.

Chevrant-Breton M and others: Cutaneous manifestations of idiopathic hemochromatosis: study of 100 cases, Arch Dermatol 113:161, 1977.

Chremos SN: Relentless localized myxedema, with exophthalmos, clubbing of the fingers and hypertrophic osteoarthropathy: observations on an unusual case, Am J Med 38:954, 1965.

Christianson HB: Cutaneous manifestations of hypothyroidism including purpura ecchymoses, Cutis 17:45, 1976.

Cohenour W and Gamble JW: Acanthosis nigricans: review of literature and report of case, J Oral Surg 29:48, 1971.

Cripps DJ and others: Porphyria turcica, Arch Dermatol 16:46, 1980.

Cunliffe W and others: Vitiligo, thyroid disease and autoimmunity, Br J Dermatol 80:135, 1968.

Curth HO and others: The site and histology of the cancer associated with acanthosis nigricans, Cancer 15:433, 1962.

Deacon SP: Pituitary dependent Cushing's disease, Br Med J 1:1409, 1977.

Dean G: The porphyrias, Philadelphia, 1963, JB Lippincott Co.

DeLeo VA and others: Erythropoietic protoporphyria, Am J Med 60:8, 1976.

Dietschy JM and Wilson JD: Regulation of cholesterol metabolism, N Engl J Med 282:1128, 1179, 1241, 1970.

Doughaday WH: Cushing's disease and basophilic microadenomas, N Engl J Med 298:798, 1978.

Fleischmajer R: Cutaneous and tendon xanthomas, Dermatologica 128:113, 1965.

Flier JS: Insulin receptors and insulin resistance, Annu Rev Med 34:145, 1983.

Flier JS: Metabolic importance of acanthosis nigricans, Arch Dermatol 121:193, 1985.

Freinkel RK and Freinkel N: Hair growth and alopecia in hypothyroidism, Arch Dermatol 106:349, 1972.

Gordon DA and others: Acromegaly: a review of 100 cases, Can Med Assoc J 87:1106, 1962.

Gouterman IH and Sibrach LA: Cutaneous manifestations of diabetes, Cutis 25:45, 1980.

Grace ND and Powell LW: Iron storage disorders of the liver, Gastroenterology 64:1257, 1974.

Gross ME and others: Porphyria cutanea tarda: clinical features and laboratory findings in 40 patients, Am J Med 67:277, 1979.

Harber LC and Bickers DR: The porphyrias: basic science aspects, clinical diagnosis and management. In Malkinson F and Pearson R, editors: Yearbook of dermatology, Chicago, 1975, Year Book Medical Publishers, Inc.

Harlan SL and Winkelmann RK: Porphyria cutanea tarda and chronic renal failure, Mayo Clin Proc 58:467, 1983.

Havel RJ and others: Role of specific glycopeptides of human serum lipoproteins in the activation of lipoprotein lipase, Circ Res 27:595, 1970.

Holt PJA and Marks R: Epidermal architecture, growth and metabolism in acromegaly, Br Med J 1:496, 1976.

Holt PJA and Marks R: The epidermal response to change in thyroid states, J Invest Dermatol 68:299, 1977.

Huntley AC: The cutaneous manifestations of diabetes mellitus, J Am Acad Dermatol 7:427, 1982.

Izumi AK and Richman SP: Ectopic adrenocorticotropic hormone syndrome associated with metastatic skin tumors and Cushing's syndrome, Arch Dermatol 102:556, 1970.

Kahn CR and others: The syndrome of insulin resistance and acanthosis nigricans, insulin receptor disorders in man, N Engl J Med 294:739, 1976.

Kanis JA and others: Clinical and laboratory study of acromegaly: assessment before and one year after treatment, G J Med 43:409, 1974.

Katz DA and others: Peripheral neuropathy in cerebrotendinous xanthomatosis, Arch Neurol 42:1008, 1985.

Lai CL and others: Case report of symptomatic porphyria cutanea tarda associated with histiocytic lymphoma, Cancer 53:573, 1984.

MacKechnie HL: Hyperthyroid induced urticaria, South Med J 75:740, 1982.

Matsuoka LY and others: Acanthosis nigricans, hypothyroidism, and insulin resistance, Am J Med 81:58, 1986.

Mendelsohn S and Verbov J: Diabetes and the skin—a review, Br J Clin Pract 37:85, 1983.

Mishkel MA and others: Xanthoma disseminatum, Arch Dermatol 113:1094, 1977.

Moschella SL: Cutaneous xanthomatoses: a review and their relationship with the current classification of the hyperlipoproteinemias, Lahey Clin Found Bull 19:106, 1970.

Mostofi RS and others: Oral malignant acanthosis nigricans, Oral Surg 56:372, 1983.

Muller SA: Dermatologic disorders associated with diabetes mellitus, Mayo Clin Proc 41:689, 1966.

Mullin GE and Eastern JS: Cutaneous consequences of accelerated thyroid function, Cutis 37:109, 1986.

Nerup J: Addison's disease—a review of some clinical pathological and immunological features, Dan Med Bull 21:201, 1974.

Ober KP: Acanthosis nigricans and insulin resistance associated with hypothyroidism, Arch Dermatol 121:229, 1985.

Orth DN and Liddle GW: Results of treatment in 108 patients with Cushing's syndrome, N Engl J Med 285:243, 1971.

Parker F: Normocholesterolemic xanthomatosis, Arch Dermatol 122:1253, 1986.

Perdrup A and Poulsen H: Hemochromatosis and vitiligo, Arch Dermatol 90:34, 1964.

Reed WB and others: Erythropoietic protoporphyria: a chemical and genetic study, JAMA 214:1060, 1970.

Roberts WC and others: Hyperlipoproteinemia: a review of the five types with first report of necropsy findings in type III, Arch Pathol 90:46, 1970.

Schnall AM and others: Pituitary function after removal of pituitary microadenomas in Cushing's disease, J Clin Endocrinol Metab 47:410, 1978.

Scoggins RB and Harlan WR Jr: Cutaneous manifestations of hyperlipidemia and uremia, Postgrad Med 41:537, 1967.

Scully RE and others: Case records of the Massachusetts General Hospital, case 39—1984, N Engl J Med 311:839, 1984.

Sekula SA and others: The porphyrias, Am Fam Physician 33:219, 1986.

Sibbold RG and Schachter RK: The skin and diabetes mellitus, Int J Dermatol 23:567, 1984.

Strakosch DR and Gordon RD: Early diagnosis of Addison's disease: pigmentation as sole symptom, Aust N Z J Med 8:189, 1978.

Tasjian D and Jarratt M: Familial acanthosis nigricans, Arch Dermatol 120:1351, 1984.

Tishler PV and others: High prevalence of intermittent acute porphyria in a psychiatric patient population, Am J Psychiatry 142:1430, 1985.

Tyrrell JB and others: Selective trans-sphenoidal resection of pituitary microadenomas, N Engl J Med 298:753, 1978.

Valbeg LS and Ghent CN: Diagnosis and management of hereditary hemochromatosis, Annu Rev Med 36:27, 1985.

Warnock GR and others: Multiple asymptomatic yellowish-white nodules on the free gingiva, J Am Dent Assoc 114:367, 1987.

Witbeck E: Acute intermittent porphyria: clinical management and report of a case, Spec Care 8:27, 1985.

158 · GASTROINTESTINAL DISORDERS WITH CUTANEOUS LESIONS

Shelley S. Schuler and **Robert N. Arm**

GARDNER'S SYNDROME

Gardner's syndrome is a hereditary autosomal dominant disorder believed to result from disturbance at a single genetic locus with a 100% penetrance but varied expressivity. The disease is characterized by adenomatous polyps of the colon and rectum that commonly undergo malignant degeneration and is associated with cutaneous, osseous, and dental lesions. The incidence ranges from 1 in 8300 to 16,000 births.

The skin manifestations consist of large sebaceous or epidermoid cysts located mainly on the patient's face and scalp but also occurring on the trunk, scrotum, and extremities. They may be present at birth or appear early in childhood, many years before the intestinal polyps develop. Often, they are small and go unnoticed by the patients. In some cases the epidermoid cysts are very large and disfiguring. Simple fibromas and lipomas may be noted. Other fibrous tumors called desmoids can arise from the connective tissue of muscle or scars and can be deeply invasive.

The osteomas of the skull, maxilla, or mandible may be palpable in the skin or may be found only on roentgenographic examination. The long bones are seldom involved.

Dental abnormalities include odontomas, multiple sclerotic changes, dentigerous cysts, and unerupted and supernumerary teeth.

The polyps are uncommon in childhood, but half the patients with this syndrome have adenomatous polyps by the age of 20 years, which is often when the malignant changes begin. Carcinomatous degeneration of polyps develops in up to 100% of these individuals. If untreated, the malignancies invariably are fatal. Lymphoid hyperplasia of the terminal ilium and mesenteric fibrosis have also been reported.

Other tumors reported include adrenal carcinoma, thyroid carcinoma, ovarian tumors, melanoma, carcinoid tumors, and leiomyomas of the gastrointestinal tract and retroperitoneum.

Ocular manifestations of pigmented ocular fundus lesions recently have been reported. More than 90% of the patients with Gardner's syndrome have some form of pigmented ocular fundus lesion. Studies have suggested that the presence of one or two large lesions in one or both eyes would indicate

Gardner's syndrome. One or two small lesions are inconclusive.

The treatment consists primarily of removal of sebaceous cysts (particularly if they are large or disfiguring), appropriate correction of the dental abnormalities, and extirpation of involved sections of the large bowel and rectum. Genetic counseling is important, and prophylactic surgery before malignant change has been recommended.

ORAL MANIFESTATIONS AND DENTAL MANAGEMENT.
See Chapter 184.

BIBLIOGRAPHY
Gardner EJ and Richards RC: Multiple cutaneous and subcutaneous lesions occurring simultaneously with hereditary polyposis and osteomatosis, Am J Hum Genet 5:139, 1953.
Gordon WC Jr and others: Gardner's syndrome, Ann Surg 155:538, 1962.
Gorlin RJ and Chaudry AP: Multiple osteomatosis, fibromas, lipomas and fibrosarcomas of the skin and mesentery, epidermoid inclusion cysts of the skin, leiomyomas, and multiple intestinal polyposis, N Engl J Med 263:1151, 1962.
Marshall KA and others: Excision of multiple epidermal facial cysts in Gardner's syndrome, Am J Surg 150:615, 1985.
Thomas JG and others: Gardner's syndrome, Oral Surg 51:213, 1981.
Traboulsi EI and others: Prevalence and importance of pigmented ocular fundus lesions in Garnder's syndrome, N Engl J Med 316:661, 1987.
Whitson E and others: Orbital osteoma in Gardner's syndrome, Am J Ophthalmol 101:236, 1986.

PEUTZ-JEGHERS SYNDROME (MELANOSIS-POLYPOSIS)

Peutz-Jeghers syndrome is a hereditary autosomal dominant disorder but has up to 40% occurrence in sporadic, noninherited cases. Penetrance is variable, with certain individuals exhibiting either pigmentation or intestinal polyposis alone.

The skin manifestations of Peutz-Jeghers syndrome are characterized by pigmentation. The pigmentation consists of brown to bluish or black macules on the patient's lip, especially the lower lip, which appear in early childhood or may be present at birth. Macular lesions may also occur elsewhere on the face, perinasally and periorbitally, but mainly circumorally. Slate gray to brown lesions may be found on the oral mucosa, tongue, palate and gingiva. Associated macules have been occasionally noted on the hands, feet, and elbows or scattered diffusely across the surface of the skin. The macules are irregular and may vary in size from 1 mm to 1 cm; they range from relatively light to dark. In later years of life the facial pigmentation may fade or disappear completely, but the mucosal pigmentation persists. The oral pigmentation resembles that normally found in blacks and individuals with adrenal insufficiency. Some biopsies have shown an increased number of melanocytes with long dendrites filled with melanosomes. In one patient the skin pigmentation occurred in areas of psoriatic plaques. Skin fibroblasts in Peutz-Jeghers syndrome reportedly have five times more chance to have malignant transformation when exposed to murine sarcoma virus.

Polyps can be found in many locations, and each patient may have multiple locations. In 70% of patients, polyps are found in the small intestine (especially in the ilium, 36%, and the duodenum, 27%); 35% of patients have polyps in the stomach, 25% in the colon, and 12% in the rectum. These polyps are hamartomatous. Previous reports indicated they rarely underwent malignant transformation. Now, malignant transformations have been reported in up to 10% of patients. These occur especially in the gastric areas, as well as in colonic and rectal areas. Biopsies of the polyps also have shown dysplasia and carcinoma in situ.

Other lesions, particularly in the genital region, have been reported. Up to 20% of female patients have ovarian granulosa cell lesions, which have caused precocious puberty in some females. Several cases of male Sertoli cell tumors have been reported related with gynecomastia. Additional tumors found in females include cervical adenocarcinoma and increased incidence of breast malignancies.

Treatment consists of prevention of malignant changes by closely watching the polyps, as well as genetic counseling.

ORAL MANIFESTATIONS AND DENTAL MANAGEMENT.
See Chapter 184.

BIBLIOGRAPHY
Banse-Kupin LA and Douglass MC: Localization of Peutz-Jeghers macules to psoriatic plaques, Arch Dermatol 122:679, 1986.
Jeghers H and others: Generalized intestinal polyposis and melanin spots of the oral mucosa, lips, and digits, N Engl J Med 241:993, 1961.
Johnson M and others: Gastrointestinal polyposis associated with alopecia, pigmentation and atrophy of fingernails and toenails, Ann Intern Med 56:935, 1962.
Lower NJ: Peutz-Jeghers syndrome with pigmented oral papillomas, Arch Dermatol 111:503, 1975.
Rodu B and Martinez MG: Peutz-Jeghers syndrome and cancer, Oral Surg 58:584, 1984.
Solh HM and others: Peutz-Jeghers syndrome associated with precocious puberty, J Pediatr 103:593, 1983.
Tovar JA and others: Peutz-Jeghers syndrome in children: report of two cases and review of literature, J Pediatr Surg 18:1, 1983.
Wilson DM and others: Testicular tumors with Peutz-Jeghers syndrome, Cancer 57:2238, 1986.

CRONKHITE-CANADA SYNDROME

Cronkhite-Canada syndrome is a rare disorder possibly caused by impaired immunity. It consists of generalized gastrointestinal polyposis and ectodermal changes, including alopecia, onychodystrophy, and hyperpigmentation. The onset is often marked in patients by sudden abdominal cramps and diarrhea, with loss of albumin and electrolytes, steatorrhea, and sometimes melena. Hypoproteinemia, anemia, edema, tetany, and weight loss result, which can lead to death.

The associated ectodermal changes include alopecia of the scalp, eyebrows, and axillary, pubic, and other body hair; as well as frecklelike hyperpigmentation of the hands, arms, face, body folds, palmar creases, and occasionally buccal surfaces. The nails become brittle and atrophic and may be shed.

Benign adenomatous polyps of the stomach, small bowel, colon and rectum, as well as cystic glandular dilation, have been described. The abdominal symptoms are a major part of this syndrome and lead to the electrolyte imbalance and hypoproteinemia.

Patients are usually middle aged to elderly. Other diseases reported with Cronkhite-Canada syndrome have been severe erosive arthritis associated with gastrointestinal symptoms and systemic lupus erythematosus (SLE).

Treatment is directed toward treating the enteropathy causing the protein loss and includes use of corticosteroids. In the patient with SLE, complete resolution of all the gastrointestinal symptoms has been reported during the steroid therapy. Hair may regrow and pigmentation may disappear with treatment. Occasionally a bowel resection of the involved segments has led to improvement. Spontaneous remission has also been reported.

ORAL MANIFESTATIONS AND DENTAL MANAGEMENT.
See Chapter 184.

BIBLIOGRAPHY
Cronkhite LW and Canada WJ: Generalized gastrointestinal polyposis: an unusual syndrome of polyposis, pigmentation, alopecia and onychotrophia, N Engl J Med 252:1011, 1955.
Kubo T and others: Canada-Cronkhite syndrome associated with systemic lupus erythematosus, Arch Intern Med 146:995, 1986.

Sanders KM and others: Erosive arthritis in Cronkhite-Canada syndrome, Radiology 156:309, 1985.

Utsunomiya J and others: Peutz-Jeghers syndrome: its natural course and management, John Hopkins Med J 136:71, 1975.

HEREDITARY HEMORRHAGIC TELANGIECTASIA (RENDU-OSLER-WEBER DISEASE)

Hereditary hemorrhagic telangiectasia is characterized by telangiectases of the skin of the face, fingers and toes, mucous membranes, and gastrointestinal tract. The face and nasal mucosa are involved in more than 60% of patients, with frequent nosebleeds that often require transfusion in almost 80% of these patients. Gross or occult blood is often reported in the bowel. The lesions may look punctiform, spiderlike, or nodular with colorations from red to purple. The small, dilated capillaries mainly occur in the mouth, nasal mucosa, ears, palms, fingertips, nail beds, and feet.

Arteriovenous malformations and fistulas of the lungs have been reported in 65% of patients and generally develop later in life. These may lead to spontaneous pulmonary hemorrhages and hemothorax. Bleeding may also occur in the kidneys, bladder, liver, meninges, and brain and can be life threatening. Histologically, these malformations appear as dilated, thin-walled vessels lined by a single layer of endothelial cells. The vascular walls appear to be formed of poor connective cells and seem to lose their elastic fibers. This leads to an inability to contract, which causes continuous bleeding.

The telangiectases usually appear at puberty and tend to increase in number in middle age. Epistaxis is the most frequent and persistent sign, especially in childhood. The disease is inherited as an autosomal dominant trait and most often affects people of Jewish ancestry.

A major complication is pulmonary microemboli, which may lead to brain abscesses and result in a 40% mortality. Because of the pulmonary arteriovenous malformations, septic microemboli are allowed to escape the pulmonary capillary filter. They enter directly into the circulation, are carried to the brain, and cause abscess.

Treatment of the telangiectasia by dermatoplasty, surgical resection, local destruction, and sclerosing agents has been tried. Attempts to control the bleeding tendencies have included estrogen and steroid therapy. Because of possible problems from the pulmonary alterations, pulmonary evaluation may be indicated.

ORAL MANIFESTATIONS. Telangiectasia can be seen throughout the patient's oral cavity. They appear as dilated capillaries or spiders that blanch on pressure. The lips and tongue are most commonly involved, followed by the gingiva. The number of lesions increases with age. The patient may have poor oral hygiene and periodontal problems; they may avoid brushing because possible rupturing of the vascular lesions of the gingiva leads to bleeding.

DENTAL MANAGEMENT. Dental treatment may be done normally as long as trauma to lesions is avoided. Major complications arise from the systemic involvement, including pulmonary and cerebral hemorrhages. Although telangiectases are easy to recognize, the family history is helpful but not always positive. These patients tend to exhibit hemorrhaging gingiva with both spontaneous bleeding and bleeding secondary to trauma. This often makes home care and periodontal therapy difficult. Splints, pressure packs, and hemostatic agents are beneficial to control bleeding after periodontal or oral surgical procedures. Telangiectasia is often treated similar to hemangiomas with sclerosing solutions and cautery. Often a gingival vascular area must be eliminated for the patient to maintain good periodontal health. Dental prostheses have caused rupture of vascular lesions, necessitating their removal or elimination of the vascular abnormality. One prosthesis was made with a relief chamber to allow the nodule to stay without irritating it. In some cases the prosthesis acted as a pressure splint to treat the bleeding, and one patient had spontaneous regression of lesions beneath the denture. Multiple lesions may make prosthetic devices difficult for the patient to tolerate. The patient should be warned about the possible inability to wear a prosthesis and also that a prosthesis may help.

BIBLIOGRAPHY

Harrison DFN: Familial haemorrhagic telangiectasia: 20 cases treated with systemic oestrogen, Q J Med 33:25, 1964.

Hashimoto K and Pritzker MS: Hereditary hemorrhage telangiectasia—an electron microscopic study, Oral Surg 34:751, 1972.

Hattler AB and Summers RB: Hereditary hemorrhagic telangiectasia—report of case and clinical consideration, J Am Dent Assoc 103:421, 1981.

Hodgson CH and others: Hereditary hemorrhagic telangiectasia and pulmonary arteriovenous fistula, N Engl J Med 261:625, 1959.

Olson JW and others: Hereditary hemorrhagic telangiectasia: prosthetic management and considerations, J Prosthet Dent 50:767, 1983.

Press OW and Ramsey PG: Central nervous system infections associated with hereditary hemorrhagic telangiectasia, Am J Med 77:86, 1984.

Shashy SS and others: Spontaneous hemothorax in a patient with Osler-Weber-Rendu disease, South Med J 78:1393, 1985.

Ulso C and others: Long-term results of dermatoplasty in the treatment of hereditary haemorrhagic telangiectasia, J Laryngol Otol 97:223, 1983.

Weber FP: Some telangiectasic and other anomalous vascular groups, especially those of dysplastic origin, Med Press 210:219, 1943.

ACRODERMATITIS ENTEROPATHICA

Hereditary and acquired forms of acrodermatitis enteropathica exist. The syndrome, resulting from zinc deficiency, is characterized by a distinctive dermatitis located around the body orifices and extremities; the patient has alopecia, diarrhea, and mental changes. Clinical symptoms are marked by exacerbations and remissions.

The patient's eczematous skin eruptions consist of symmetric, grouped vesiculobullous lesions on a bright-red erythematous base around the mouth, nose, eyes, ears, genitalia, perineum, and buttocks, as well as on the elbows, knees, hands, feet, and scalp. The vesiculobullous lesions progress to crusted, seborrhea-like and psoriasiform patches with exudates. The lesions become altered by bacterial and fungal (Candida) infections (Fig. 158-1). Healing occurs without atrophy or scarring.

The fingers and toes may show severe redness and swelling of the paronychial areas, with subungual thickening and transverse grooving of the nails. Blepharitis and photophobia often occur. These patients have an increased susceptibility to candidal and bacterial infections.

Alopecia involves not only the scalp but also the eyebrows, eyelashes, and sometimes the rest of the body hair. The alopecia is usually reversible when the disease is controlled by appropriate treatment.

Diarrhea is found in most patients, and at times severe malabsorption may occur. Children often have stunted body growth and personality and mental changes. These children are apathetic and depressed and appear mentally dull.

The hereditary form of this disease is inherited as an autosomal recessive trait and begins in early infancy. Cutaneous manifestations usually develop shortly after breast feeding is stopped or can occur up to 2 years of age (rare cases may occur as late as 10 years). An insidious onset usually occurs; the affected child fails to thrive and develops erythematous, scaling, pustular lesions around body orifices. The zinc deficiency is probably related to malabsorption.

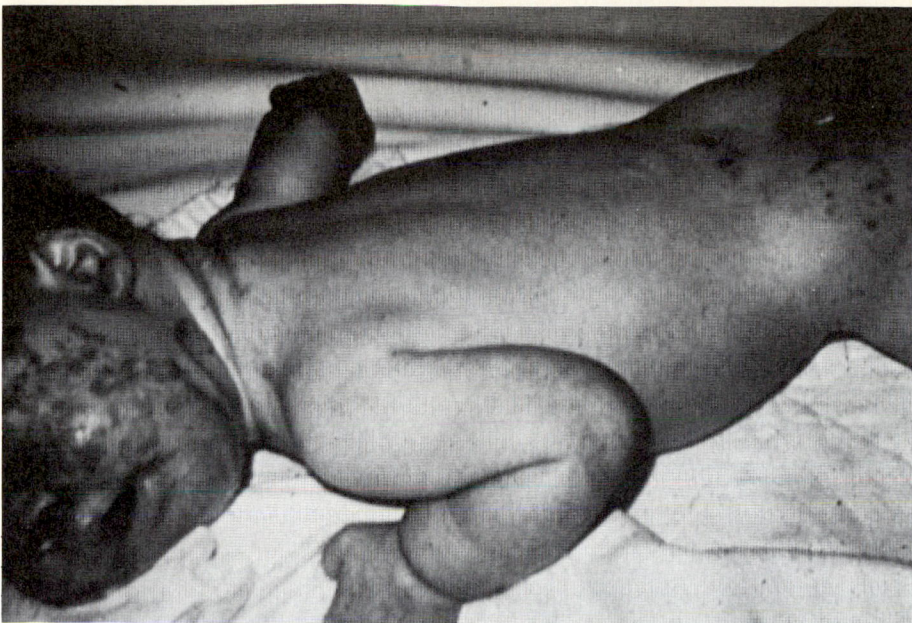

Fig. 158-1   Acrodermatitis enteropathica in infant. Note perioral and perianal lesions appearing as exudates on erythematous base.

The acquired form of acrodermatitis enteropathica most often occurs in patients receiving total parenteral nutrition (intravenous hyperalimentation) when zinc supplements have not been added to the nutritional fluid. Many of these patients have inflammatory bowel disease and a partial zinc deficiency at the onset. Patients with the acquired form develop seborrhea-like and candidal eruptions in the groin and orbital and circumoral regions. Eczema with dry, brittle, fissured skin may appear. Angular stomatitis, alopecia, and chronic paronychia have been noted. Frequently the eruption is mistaken for *Candida* or other fungal infections, eczema, or seborrheic dermatitis. The symptoms can also be confused with acquired immunodeficiency syndrome (AIDS).

Treatment for both the hereditary and the acquired forms of this disease is zinc replacement, either by oral or intravenous routes. The response is dramatic and rapid. In the inherited form, replacement therapy must be lifelong.

ORAL MANIFESTATIONS. Perioral vesiculobullous lesions surrounded by bright-red erythematous zones are common. Perleche, glossitis, and stomatitis have been reported. The patient's tongue and buccal mucosa may have white patches of varying sizes. Secondary infection with *Candida* organisms alters the appearance, and a coated tongue may be seen. Classic candidal lesions of the mucosa leave a raw erythematous area after rubbing off the white surface.

DENTAL MANAGEMENT. Elective dental treatment should be delayed when acute lesions are present. The vesiculobullous lesions resolve after zinc therapy. The stomatitis and glossitis may be relieved by using bland mouth rinses and avoiding alcoholic rinses.

The major therapy must be aimed at treating the *Candida* infection by using antifungal agents. Allowing a nystatin troche to dissolve slowly two to four times a day gives better results than the oral suspension. The use of a clotrimazole troche (Mycelex) five times a day or ketoconazle (Nizoral) once a day appears to provide excellent results. One must remember to treat dental prostheses with antifungal soaks.

Bright dental light may affect the patient, who has photophobia. Reported depression in adults may create management problems.

BIBLIOGRAPHY

Bernstein B and Leyden J: Zinc deficiency and acrodermatitis after intravenous hyperalimentation, Arch Dermatol 114:1070, 1978.

Brazin S and others: The acrodermatitis enteropathica–like syndrome, Arch Dermatol 115:597, 1979.

Danbolt N: Acrodermatitits enteropathica, Br J Dermatol 100:37, 1979.

Gorlin RJ and Goldman HM: Thoma's oral pathology, St Louis, 1970, The CV Mosby Co.

Graves K and others: Hereditary acrodermatitis enteropathica in an adult, Arch Dermatol 116:562, 1980.

Hirsh FS and others: Gluconate zinc in acrodermatitis enteropathica, Arch Dermatol 112:475, 1976.

Moynahan EJ: Acrodermatitis enteropathica: a lethal inherited human zinc deficiency disorder, Lancet 2:399, 1974.

Nelder KH and others: Acrodermatitis enteropathica, Int J Dermatol 17:380, 1978.

Tong TK and others: Childhood acquired immune deficiency syndrome manifestations as acrodermatitis enteropathica, J Pediatr 108:426, 1986.

ULCERATIVE COLITIS WITH PYODERMA GANGRENOSUM AND PYOSTOMATITIS VEGETANS

Skin and oral lesions occur in approximately one third of the patients with ulcerative colitis. Two types of oral lesions are aphthous stomatitis and pyostomatitis vegetans. Dermatologic lesions include erythema nodosum, which may develop during the acute phase, and pyoderma gangrenosum (vegetans).

Pyoderma gangrenosum appears mainly on the legs but occasionally on the trunk and upper extremities; it appears in up to 10% of the patients with active ulcerative colitis, who often also have associated oral lesions. Minor trauma may precipitate lesions. In addition to ulcerative colitis, these lesions also occur less commonly in Crohn's disease, leukemia, acute active hepatitis, carcinoid tumor, paraproteinemia, and polyarthritis. The lesions are characterized by an irregular ulcer with a raised inflammated, dusky red or purple border and a boggy necrotic base; they develop rapidly, almost explosively. The lesion begins as an erythematous papulovesicle or pustular nodule that quickly becomes necrotic and ulcerates. The ulcers have rolled edges surrounded by an erythematous halo (Fig. 158-2). Sat-

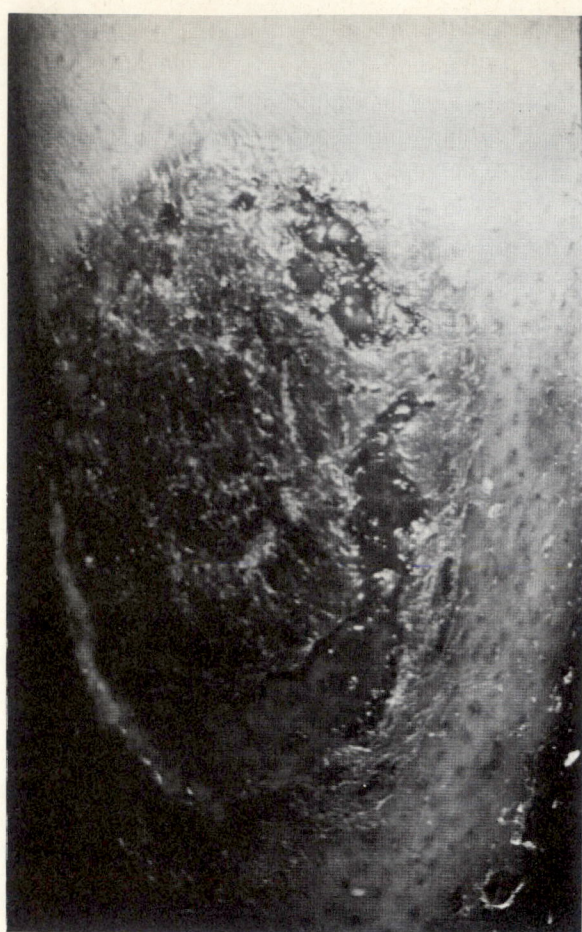

Fig. 158-2   Pyoderma gangrenosum on anterior surface of leg. There is ulceration with rolled, undermined edges and purulent (but sterile) drainage.

ellite lesions may develop, break down, and fuse to form large, phagedenic ulcerations that extend peripherally. When healing occurs, a thin atrophic scar forms. The histologic findings are nonspecific inflammation in the dermis and around the vessels, with ulceration of the epidermis; there is no evidence of necrotizing angiitis. Despite the term "pyoderma," bacterial cultures from these ulcers are frequently sterile. The patients may have acute high fever with the onset of the lesions.

Other dermatologic findings associated with ulcerative colitis include perianal abscesses and fistulas (reported in 10% to 20% of patients), palmar erythema, and clubbing of fingers. Thrombophlebitis (in up to one third of patients) and arterial thromboses also occur; a hypercoagulable state is apparently associated with ulcerative colitis.

Exacerbation of the bowel disease may correlate with worsening of the skin lesions. Therefore control of the ulcerative colitis with systemic steroids may help to heal the ulcers. Dosages higher than necessary to control the bowel disease component or even suprapharmacologic doses (pulse therapy) may be required to halt progressive pyoderma gangrenosum.

Intralesional steroids, sulfa drugs, clofazimine, and immunosuppressive agents have been useful in selected patients. Appropriate topical care is mandatory.

ORAL MANIFESTATIONS. Oral manifestations of pyoderma gangrenosum (vegetans) were initially reported in two of the five cases described by Hallopeau. He was describing the dermatitis vegetans that has often been related to pemphigus.

Although cutaneous involvement is generally present, McCarthy in 1949 reported several cases of oral involvement only and used the term "pyostomatitis" vegetans. In one of his patients the oral involvement was the first sign of disease. Pyostomatitis vegetans is a rare oral lesion. About 75% of the patients with oral involvement also have gastrointestinal problems, primarily colitis and occasionally Crohn's disease. The oral lesions are often asymptomatic and start as small, red, inflamed areas less than 5 mm in size. They have a yellowish gray, necrotic surface that can be rubbed off easily, leaving a raw exposed surface. The lesions are generally ovoid, well delineated, and slightly raised. They resemble papillomatous projections with minute ulcerations and pockets of pus at the tips. They may be numerous and form aggregates or coalesce. They are commonly found on the buccal mucosa, mucobuccal fold, labial gingiva, palate, and lips. A cerebriform tongue has been reported. The lesions follow the course of the underlying colitis. Males seem to be affected 3:1 over females.

A biopsy usually is needed and shows various patterns. An early lesion resembles an epithelial abscess with eosinophils. Areas of intraepithelial separation are similar to the acantholysis of pemphigus. Older lesions generally have ulcerated surfaces and fewer eosinophils. In both an infiltrate of lymphocytes and prominent cells occur in the connective tissue. Although histopathologically the oral lesions can resemble pemphigus, many differences exist. The inflammatory infiltrate includes eosinophils and more lymphocytes. The clinical difference includes painless lesions and follows a course similar to the gastrointestinal disease. Clinically, pyostomatitis vegetans may be a separate entity from pemphigus and is best classified either separately or with the associated gastrointestinal problem (See discussion on pemphigus in Chapter 168.)

DENTAL MANAGEMENT. Systemic management is indicated for the diffuse disease. Antibiotics, radiation therapy, surgery, and topical steroids seem to be ineffective. Systemic treatment with corticosteroids appears to help. The oral lesions follow a similar course as the gastrointestinal disease with periods of spontaneous remission. Although topical steroids do not cure the problem, they may be useful in treating the oral lesions, especially if pain is present. Topical anesthetics also ease the pain. A gastrointestinal workup as part of a complete physical examination may be indicated with referral to a physician. Unfortunately, little is reported concerning the treatment of periodontal lesions, and nothing on the prognosis of the dentition or future prosthetics has been mentioned. Because pain (although rare) may occur, oral hygiene may be affected and should be reinforced to the patient.

BIBLIOGRAPHY

Basler RSW: Ulcerative colitis and the skin, Med Clin North Am 64:941, 1980.
Cataldo E and others: Pyostomatitis vegetans, Oral Surg 52:172, 1981.
Hansen LS and others: The differential diagnosis of pyostomatitis vegetans and its relation to bowel disease, Oral Surg 55:363, 1983.
Johnson RB and Lazarus GS: Pulse therapy, therapeutic efficacy in the treatment of pyoderma gangrenosum, Arch Dermatol 118:76, 1982.
McCarthy FP: Pyostomatitis vegetans: report of 3 cases, Arch Dermatol Syph 60:750, 1949.
McCarthy P and Shklar G: A syndrome of pyostomatitis vegetans and ulcerative colitis, Arch Dermatol 88:281, 1963.
McGarity WC and others: Pyoderma gangrenosum at the parastomal site in patients with Crohn's disease, Arch Surg 119:1186, 1984.
Yusuf H and Ead RD: Pyoderma gangrenosum with involvements of the tongue, Br J Oral Maxillofac Surg 23:247, 1985.

REGIONAL ENTERITIS (CROHN'S DISEASE)

Crohn's disease is a granulomatous regional enteritis. Multiple skin and oral findings have been reported, including perianal fistulas, erythematous nodular (erythema nodosum–like), and ulceronodular skin lesions. Pyoderma gangrenosum and pyostomatitis vegetans both occur in Crohn's disease, but the prevalence is much lower than in ulcerative colitis. Local and "metastatic" extension of the granulomatous disease to involve perianal tissue and distant skin sites has been reported.

Patients have facial alterations with lip changes, including chronic granulomatous cheilitis causing an enlarged lip. Melkersson-Rosenthal syndrome has been reported related to Crohn's disease and involved facial palsy and fissured tongue. One study reported oral lesions in 62 of 700 patients.

Crohn's disease can lead to malabsorption and possibly perforation. There appears to be an increased incidence of gastrointestinal malignancy. Skin changes are caused by the malabsorption.

Other systemic findings have included rosacea-like eruptions and digital clubbing. One report cited malignant transformation of an anal skin tag into a squamous cell carcinoma. This was not related to drug therapy.

The skin lesions and oral lesions tend to respond to the same therapy as the gastrointestinal problem.

ORAL MANIFESTATIONS AND DENTAL MANAGEMENT.
See Chapter 184.

BIBLIOGRAPHY

Brook IM and others: Chronic granulomatous cheilitis and its relationship to Crohn's disease, Oral Surg 56:405, 1983.

McCallum DI and Kinmont PD: Dermatological manifestations of Crohn's disease, Br J Dermatol 80:1, 1968.

Mesa M and others: Diagnostic problems between oral lesions of Crohn's disease and Melkersson-Rosenthal syndrome/cheilitis granulomatosa, Clin Prev Dent 7:23, 1985.

Somerville KW and others: Malignant transformation of anal skin tags in Crohn's disease, Gut 25:1124, 1984.

Sutphen JL and others: Metastatic cutaneous Crohn's disease, Gastroenterology 86:941, 1984.

Verbov JL: The skin in patients with Crohn's disease and ulcerative colitis, Trans St Johns Hosp Dermatol Soc 59:30, 1973.

DERMATITIS HERPETIFORMIS (DUHRING'S DISEASE)

Dermatitis herpetiformis is a chronic, recurrent, intensely pruritic disease usually appearing as grouped, angular, or gyrate erythematous vesicles. The eruption is polymorphous and may include urticarial, maculopapular, papulovesicular, and rarely bullous lesions with a generally symmetric distribution. The lesions most commonly affect the scapular, extensor surfaces of the arms and legs, sacral regions, and buttocks, although any area of the body can be affected. Postinflammatory hyperpigmentation and occasional scarring may remain when the lesions regress. Pruritus, often described by patients as having a concomitant burning sensation, can be severe at times. The onset may be sudden, with no associated constitutional symptoms, although many patients have an associated gluten sensitivity.

The disease is relatively uncommon. The onset occurs generally between the second and fifth decades of life and mainly in the second and third. Children may rarely be affected. The incidence is twice as frequent in men as women; it is found in all races. There appears to be no familial incidence. Genetic transmission has been studied and an increased relationship seems to exist with human lymphocyte antigen (HLA) B8 and HLA-DW3 tissue types. The incidence of dermatitis herpetiformis appears to be approximately 11 in 100,000. Patients often have severe emotional stress, although differentiating between cause and effect is sometimes difficult. The disease has also been related to hormonal changes and vaccination, but the true cause remains unknown. A direct relationship to gluten in the diet exists, and a gluten-free diet has eliminated symptoms. Occasionally, the severe bullous form has been associated with internal malignant disease, usually regressing after the carcinoma has been successfully treated. Conversely, there is no increased risk of malignancy in patients with dermatitis herpetiformis.

Direct immunofluorescent staining shows the presence of immunoglobulins, particularly IgA, at the dermoepidermal junction in uninvolved perilesional skin. There seems to be two major patterns: (1) granular IgA deposits at the dermal papillary tips along with C_3 and (2) to a much lesser extent IgG and linear IgA deposits along the basement zone unassociated with other immunoglobulins.

Most, if not all, patients with dermatitis herpetiformis and granular IgA deposits have an associated gastrointestinal abnormality caused by gluten sensitivity. This is similar to celiac disease (nontropical sprue) but fortunately is less severe. This gluten-sensitive enteropathy is seen more frequently in dermatitis herpetiformis patients associated with HLA-DW3 and HLA-B8 tissue types. Patients with linear IgA deposits have no evidence of the enteropathy and have a normal prevalence of HLA-DW3 and HLA-B8. Also included in differential diagnosis must be the ulcerative bullous diseases, IgA disease, pemphigus, pemphigoid, and erythema multiforme.

In patients with gluten-sensitive enteropathy, strict adherence to a gluten-free diet has been helpful and been reported to clear the lesions in the skin and gastrointestinal system. On adding gluten to the diet, the lesions return. The disease has also been reported to respond dramatically to dapsone, sulfoxone, and sulfapyridine. Systemic steroids may be required when the disease is severe. The side effects of each of these modalities must be considered when treatment is undertaken with any of them. Topical steroids and oral antipruritic agents may be important adjuncts.

ORAL MANIFESTATIONS. The oral cavity is generally reported to be involved in 1% to 10% of patients. In one study up to 70% of the patients had oral manifestations. It is unknown whether the increased number is caused by better identification, or identification of other entities, not dermatitis herpetiformis. The lesions generally appear after the skin lesions. The lesions are usually asymptomatic, but patients may have a burning sensation. When the lesions appear, they are generally reddish brown bullae that undergo degeneration and ulcerate. The common locations are the buccal mucosa, soft palate, and tongue. The lesions occur less frequently on the lips, alveolar ridge, and gingiva. In addition, atrophy of the filiform and fungiform papillae of the tongue has been reported. The disease has also been reported in association with Sjögren's disease. Definitive diagnosis of the lesions is done through biopsy, which shows an eosinophilic infiltrate and an IgA deposit on immunofluorescence.

DENTAL MANAGEMENT. The oral lesions respond to the same treatment as the skin lesions, including a gluten-free diet. They also respond to sulfapyridine treatment, but caution must be used with long-term use because of its toxicity. For oral hygiene, alkaline rinses (bicarbonate) or saline rinses may help.

Sensitivity of patients to halogens has been reported, which may contraindicate the use of fluorides and certain antiseptic rinses and preparations containing iodine.

BIBLIOGRAPHY

Economopoulo P and Laskaris G: Dermatitis herpetiformis: oral lesions as an early manifestation, Oral Surg 62:77, 1986.

Fraser NG and others: Dermatitis herpetiformis and Sjögren's syndrome, Br J Dermatol 100:213, 1979.

Fry L and others: The small intestine in dermatitis herpetiformis, J Clin Pathol 27:811, 1974.

Gawkrodger DJ and others: Dermatitis herpetiformis: diagnosis, diet and demography, Gut 25:151, 1984.

Hietanen J and Reunala T: IgA deposits in the oral mucosa of patients with dermatitis herpetiformis and linear IgA disease, Scand J Dent Res 92:230, 1984.

Katz SI: Dermatitis herpetiformis: clinical, histologic, laboratory and therapeutic clues, Int J Dermatol 17:529, 1978.

Marks JM and others: Small bowel changes in dermatitis herpetiformis, Lancet 2:1280, 1966.

Russotto SB and Ship II: Oral manifestations of dermatitis herpetiformis, Oral Surg 31:42, 1971.

Sachs JA and others: Different HLA associated gene combinations contribute to susceptibility for coeliac diseases and dermatitis herpetiformis, Gut 27:515, 1986.

MALIGNANT ATROPHIC PAPULOSIS (DEGOS' DISEASE)

Malignant atrophic papulosis is a fatal cutaneointestinal syndrome of unknown cause, characterized by endovasculitis of the skin, gastrointestinal tract, and sometimes other viscera. It is a rare disorder, occurring chiefly in men between 20 and 40 years of age. The average survival is 2 years, but a few patients have lived for 6 years or more.

Clinically the manifestations consist of a discrete, asymptomatic, pale rose to erythematous rounded edematous papules measuring 2 to 10 mm, which are generally discrete but may coalesce. The eruption is mainly on the trunk, more often involving the back, with an average of 30 lesions. Sometimes hundreds of lesions may be present. Other areas of the skin may be affected, but the face, palms, and soles are spared. The lesions evolve slowly over weeks to months, becoming umbilicated with a central depression. The periphery becomes livid red and telangiectatic. An atrophic porcelain-white scarred center is the unique and diagnostic identifying feature. There may be successive crops of lesions, with a few new ones appearing at intervals over several years. Urticaria-like, ulceropustular, and gummatous nodular lesions have been described.

Abdominal complaints that are the result of anemic infarcts of the intestines generally develop a few months after the onset of skin lesions. The gastrointestinal symptoms include nausea, vomiting, hematemesis, epigastric and abdominal pain, colic, diarrhea, malabsorption, ileus, and melena. Occasionally these symptoms may precede the skin lesions. Death generally ensues within a few months from hemorrhage and multiple perforations of the intestine, leading to fulminant peritonitis.

Other viscera that may be involved are the heart, pericardium, kidneys, and bladder. White plaques similar to those in the skin and gastrointestinal tract may involve the cerebral cortex. Neurologic symptoms in this disease include headache, numbness in the extremities, ataxia, and diplopia. Retinal and scleral plaques and microaneurysms of the bulbar conjunctival vessels may also occur.

The basic pathogenetic mechanism is vascular obliteration from endovasculitis and thrombosis with resultant ischemic infarction of the involved tissues. Histologically, small arterial endothelial swelling and proliferation occurs with fibrinoid necrosis of the intima and thrombosis, producing wedge-shaped infarcts resulting from the obliteration of small arteries and arterioles. Direct immunofluorescent studies have failed to demonstrate a consistent pattern of immunoreactant depositions. No effective therapy is known; the administration of corticosteroids is usually of no value. Heparin, dipyridamole, and aspirin have been of value, as reported anecdotally.

ORAL MANIFESTATIONS. Lesions of the oral cavity are rare. The few that occur resemble the cutaneous lesions. Erythematous papules may change to lesions with a white atrophic center and an erythematous border. The lips are most likely to be involved. A biopsy is indicated.

DENTAL MANAGEMENT. Management must be directed at the symptomatic relief of the limited oral involvement in the patient with this rare cutaneous disease. No adequate therapy is known, although steroids have been tried. Systemic involvement is fatal. Consultation is indicated to learn the extent of organ involvement before treatment. Management must be directed at complications from the organs involved. Topical pain control may be useful.

BIBLIOGRAPHY

Gorlin BJ and Goldman HM: Thoma's oral pathology, St Louis, 1970, The CV Mosby Co.

May RE: Degos' syndrome, Br Med J 1:161, 1968.

Roenigk HH Jr and Farmer RG: Degos' disease (malignant papulosis), JAMA 206:1508, 1968.

Shwayder TA: Scaly papules with atrophy: Degos' disease or malignant atrophic papulosis, Arch Dermatol 122:90, 1986.

Stahl D and others: Degos' disease treated with platelet-suppressive drugs, Lancet 2:46, 1977.

Strole WE Jr and others: Progressive arterial occlusive disease (Kohlmeier-Degos), N Engl J Med 276:195, 1967.

159 • LIVER DISORDERS

Shelley S. Schuler

The cutaneous signs of liver disease are related to the severity of the underlying condition.

Urticaria, as well as fever and arthralgias, may be part of the prodrome of hepatitis B. A scarlatiniform eruption limited to the patient's trunk and proximal portions of the extremities, without affecting the face, may be present at the onset; this usually fades within a week.

Pruritus may occur if biliary obstruction is present. Pruritus may be caused by retained bile salts. This is confirmed if the patient finds relief using agents such as cholestyramine that bind bile acids and their metabolites in the intestinal lumen to prevent their absorption.

Jaundice, or icterus, is the generalized yellow (faint golden to deep greenish yellow) discoloration of the skin, mucous membranes, and other body tissues caused by the binding of bile pigment bilirubin to connective tissue. Jaundice is a primary sign of liver disease and always requires careful evaluation. The intensity of clinical jaundice often fails to reflect accurately the concurrent serum bilirubin concentration. A rise in serum bilirubin concentration may precede the development of jaundice by several days and persist despite the concentration of bilirubin decreasing or returning to normal.

Xanthomatous lesions (planar xanthomas) may appear on the face, extremities, and trunk in patients with obstructive biliary disease such as biliary cirrhosis.

Spider angiomas, which consist of a central vascular punctum and radiating telangiectatic "legs," occur commonly in chronic liver disease. They may also appear during the acute stage of viral hepatitis and regress after the illness is over. However, spider angiomas are not pathognomonic signs of liver disease; they are also often seen in pregnant women, patients with other hyperestrogen states, and otherwise normal young adults and children.

Palmar erythema ("liver palms"), a blotchy erythema on the thenar and hypothenar eminences and fingertips, may occur in persons who exhibit spider angiomas. A similar erythema may be noted in pregnant women and is also associated with rheumatoid arthritis, thyrotoxicosis, and malnutrition. In lupus erythematosus the palmar erythema tends to be more violaceous and discrete.

ORAL CONSIDERATIONS AND DENTAL MANAGEMENT.
See section on liver diseases in Chapter 184.

BIBLIOGRAPHY

Braverman IM: Skin signs of systemic disease, Philadelphia, 1981, WB Saunders Co.
Fitzpatrick TB and others: Dermatology in general medicine, ed 3, New York, 1987, McGraw-Hill Book Co.
Sarkany I: The skin lesions associated with liver disease, Prog Dermatol 4:1, 1969.

160 · RENAL DISORDERS

Shelley S. Schuler *and* **Robert N. Arm**

Various hereditary syndromes affect the skin and may also show renal involvement. These include, among others, hereditary hemorrhagic telangiectasia (Osler-Weber-Rendu disease) with vascular anomalies; pseudoxanthoma elasticum (Grönblad-Strandberg syndrome) with vessel changes and calcium renal stones; angiokeratoma corporis diffusum (Fabry's disease) with glomerular and tubular glycolipid storage; tuberous sclerosis (Bourneville's disease) with hamartomas and angiomyolipomas; neurofibromatosis (von Recklinghausen's disease) with tumors in the kidney; von Hippel-Lindau disease with cystic kidneys and hypernephroma; and sickle cell disease with hematuria, isosthenuria, renal infarcts, and the nephrotic syndrome.

Patients with vasculitides (Schönlein-Henoch anaphylactoid purpura and "allergic" vasculitis) may have both skin and glomerular effects. The connective tissue diseases (systemic lupus erythematosus, progressive systemic sclerosis, polyarteritis nodosa, and Wegener's granulomatosis) may produce profound changes in the skin and the kidneys.

Metabolic diseases can cause significant alterations in the kidneys' function and structure as well as cutaneous changes, although not always simultaneously in the same patient. Thus diabetes mellitus produces nodular intercapillary glomerulosclerosis (Kimmelstiel-Wilson disease), diabetic dermopathy, and necrobiosis lipoidica diabeticorum. Gout may result in nephritis caused by tophi in interstitial tissue of the renal pyramids and tophaceous deposits in subcutaneous tissues. Systemic amyloidosis causes amyloid deposition in glomeruli, blood vessels, and interstitial tissue around tubules and also results in cutaneous deposits in the dermis and subcutis. Dysproteinemic states (paraproteinemia and cryoglobulinemia) cause glomerulonephritis and purpura, livedo reticularis, Raynaud's phenomenon, acrocyanosis, and ulceration of the skin. "Metastatic" calcinosis produces deposition of calcium in the tubular epithelium and the cutis.

Some neoplasms that affect the skin can also infiltrate the kidney, including Kaposi's sarcoma, urticaria pigmentosa (mastocytoma), leukemia, lymphoma, and multiple myeloma.

Patients with advanced renal failure have various skin disorders. Uremic frost is caused by a greatly increased concentration of urea in the sweat and its subsequent precipitation on the skin. This is rarely seen today, but is a serious prognostic sign when it occurs. Dry scaly skin (xerosis), itching, and excoriations more frequently occur. They may be associated with linear purpura and secondary pyoderma. The pruritus may be intractable; ultraviolet therapy has sometimes been successful. Dialysis may help relieve the intense itching. Secondary hyperparathyroidism has been implicated in renal pruritus. Burning, painful paresthesias of the dorsal or plantar surfaces of the feet is a common early sign of peripheral neuropathy.

Soft tissue calcification in uremia results mainly from hyperphosphatemia. Calcinosis cutis may be present in the skin and subcutaneous tissues as infiltrated plaques, firm white papules, and nodules filled with a milky substance. Calcinosis may also occur in the conjunctiva and cornea, periarticular tissue, arteries, and viscera. Patients may have a hemorrhagic diathesis caused by a platelet defect and increased capillary permeability, resulting in easy bruisability, bleeding from the gums and nasal mucosa, and purpura and ecchymoses. Pallor of the skin, mucous membranes, and nail beds is the result of anemia. The accumulation of urinary pigments gives the skin a sallow complexion. A brownish discoloration of the skin may be caused by the deposition of hemosiderin from repeated transfusions and hemodialysis. Patients may lose hair on the extremities. Poor wound healing is attributed to the connective tissue changes, an increase in dermal elastic fibers with decreased collagen turnover.

Uremic onychopathy is of two types: a brown arc spanning the distal part of the nail proximal to the line of its separation from the nail bed and the "half-and-half nail," characterized by a whiteness proximally and a dark brown or reddish discoloration of the distal portion.

A bullous eruption similar to porphyria cutanea tarda (PCT) occurs in 16% of long-term dialysis patients. They have the eruption on the dorsa of the hands, as well as pruritus, skin fragility, and possibly hemorrhagic bullae on areas exposed to sunlight. However, facial hirsutism and milia formation do not occur. Histologically the bullae are subepidermal and are indistinguishable from those of PCT. True PCT occurs in hemodialysis patients at a higher rate than expected. However, plasma uroporphyrin concentrations are very high in dialysis patients with true PCT and normal in those with the PCT-like syndrome. A possible photosensitizer has been postulated but not yet proved as the cause.

Kyrle's disease, or hyperkeratosis follicularis et parafollicularis has affected increasing numbers of hemodialysis patients. This is accompanied most frequently by diabetes mellitus and end-stage renal disease. Kyrle's disease is characterized by hyperpigmented, often pruritic, papules and nodules with a central keratin plug, scattered across the skin surface.

In patients undergoing immunosuppressive therapy for renal disease, fungal and viral infections occur more frequently and are more extensive. *Candida* infection, herpes simplex, molluscum contagiosum, and warts are more persistent in these patients and may respond to therapy only when the dosages of the immunosuppressive drugs are reduced for a short period. Steroid-induced acne has also been noted in patients undergoing prolonged therapy.

ORAL MANIFESTATIONS AND DENTAL CONSIDERATIONS. See Section 8 on renal disease.

BIBLIOGRAPHY

Bergfeld W and Roenigk HH Jr: Cutaneous complications of immunosuppressive therapy, Cutis 22:169, 1978.
Bluefarb SM and Caro WA: Cutaneous manifestations of renal diseases, Mod Med 37:159, 1969.
Fitzpatrick TB and others: Dermatology in general medicine, ed 3, New York, 1987, McGraw-Hill Book Co.
Gilchrist B and others: Relief of uremic pruritus with ultraviolet light therapy, N Engl J Med 297:136, 1977.
Gilcrest BA and others: Bullous dermatosis of hemodialysis, Ann Intern Med 83:480, 1975.
Gruskin SE and others: Oral manifestations of uremia, Minn Med 53:495, 1970.

Lindsay PG: The half and half nail, Arch Intern Med 119:583, 1967.

Massey SG and others: Intractable pruritus as a manifestation of secondary hyperparathyroidism, N Engl J Med 279:697, 1968.

Parfitt PM: Soft tissue calcification in uremia, Arch Intern Med 124:544, 1969.

Poh-Fitzpatrick M and others: Porphyria cutanea tarda associated with chronic renal disease and hemodialysis, N Engl J Med 116:191, 1980.

Scoggins RB and Harlan WR Jr: Cutaneous manifestations of hyperlipidemia and uremia, Postgrad Med 41:537, 1967.

Stone RA: Kyrle-like lesions in two patients with renal failure undergoing dialysis, J Am Acad Dermatol 5:707, 1981.

161 · HEMATOLOGIC DISORDERS

Shelley S. Schuler *and* **Robert N. Arm**

Most hematologic disorders have both dermatologic and oral manifestations, some of which are severe. The chapter on hematologic diseases presents a detailed review of diagnosis, treatment, oral manifestations, and management. Only specific dermatologic manifestations are presented here.

POLYCYTHEMIA VERA

The skin changes in polycythemia vera are caused primarily by an increase of red blood cells. Patients have vascular engorgement of the viscera and skin. The distended cutaneous vessels ultimately produce an intense red color, mainly on the face, neck, and distal extremities. Because facial erythema with superimposed telangiectasia occurs, rosacea may be mistakenly diagnosed. Not all patients with polycythemia vera are deeply erythematous, and the intensity of color can vary from day to day. Sometimes erythema may persist after normal hematocrit values have been achieved, a result of vascular distension.

Minor injury to a patient's skin may cause petechiae and ecchymoses. Intramuscular injections may result in hematomas. Cyanosis also may be present.

Pruritus may be severe in patients with polycythemia vera, especially after a hot shower or bath, when burning sensations may persist far longer than in persons with eczema and ichthyosis. The intense pruritus and burning paresthesias are associated with increased histamine levels and with the overdistention of cutaneous vessels that are unable to respond to localized heating by further vasodilation.

Acne urticata is a chronic, severely pruritic eruption of pale red, wheallike papules sometimes surmounted by vesicles and appearing in crops on the face and extensor aspects of the extremities. They often result in scarring and hyperpigmentation following excoriations. Although acne urticata is considered a specific sign of polycythemia vera, it has also been found in patients with lymphomas and carcinomas.

Erythromelalgia (erythermalgia) is a peculiar vascular response with sensations of burning accompanying erythematous swelling of the legs. This may develop after a person exercises or is exposed to heat or if the legs have been in a dependent position for a long time. Elevation and cooling of the legs help to alleviate the symptoms. Leg ulcers and cold sensitivity result from increased blood viscosity produced by the increased red cell mass.

ORAL MANIFESTATIONS. The vessels of oral mucosa are also dilated in patients with polycythemia vera. The tongue, pharynx, and tonsils may be a deep reddish blue. The engorgement may cause macroglossia. Bleeding gums and epistaxis frequently occur. As on the skin, mild trauma may produce petechiae and ecchymoses on the gums, especially after injec-

tions. Patients have not reported the burning skin sensation in the oral cavity, but this may occur. Occasionally cyanosis may be present.

SICKLE CELL DISEASE

Cutaneous ulcerations are found in 25% to 75% of patients with sickle cell anemia and 2.6% of heterozygotes (patients with sickle cell trait). The sickled red blood cells become trapped in capillaries, which leads to further stasis, deoxygenation, decreased pH, and increased sickling. Packing of these cells in small vessels causes thrombosis and infarction. This results in "punched-out," sharply marginated, painful ulcers that tend to be unilateral and generally occur around the malleoli. The ulcers may be deep or shallow; their severity is out of proportion to the initial trauma. The ulcers are chronic and indolent and heal slowly, with atrophic scars that readily break down again. The scars are often hypopigmented with a peripheral zone of hyperpigmentation. Patients with sickle cell disease usually have long, slender extremities (asthenic habitus). The mucous membranes, nail beds, and palms are pale; the conjunctivae are icteric; and the lower areas of the legs show residual hyperpigmentation, often because of hemosiderin deposition.

THROMBOCYTOPENIA AND OTHER PLATELET ABNORMALITIES

Purpura is caused by extravasation of blood into the skin or mucous membranes, usually resulting from rupture of the capillary walls. It appears as distinctive macules that may vary from bright red to brownish, rust colored, or purple. The lesions may be petechiae—superficial, pinhead-sized (less than 3 mm), round, hemorrhagic macules—or ecchymoses ("black and blue marks"), which form flat, irregular-shaped, bluish purple patches that signify deep and more extensive interstitial hemorrhages. They gradually assume a yellowish hue as they fade.

Purpura caused by thrombocytopenia may be the result of decreased platelet production or increased destruction. Purpura may also be caused by various thrombopathies, including hereditary thrombasthenia; by a phospholipid defect; by metabolic states (uremia or liver disease); and by dysproteinemias (cryoglobulinemia, macroglobulinemia, or hyperglobulinemia). In addition, purpura may result from an increase in platelets (thrombocythemia), as in myeloproliferative disorders.

LEUKEMIAS
Specific lesions

The lesions of leukemia are the same as those found in the malignant lymphomas and consist of macules, papules, nodules, tumors, and plaquelike infiltrations that range in color from pink to reddish brown to purple (violaceous to plum colored). The solid lesions are firm but not stony hard and are composed of leukemic infiltrates. These lesions may rarely appear before the disease is found in the bone marrow or peripheral blood. Patients may have leukemic infiltrates at sites of trauma, including intramuscular injections, recent surgical scars, burns, herpes zoster, and herpes simplex. Leukemia cutis may resemble mycosis fungoides by forming arciform lesions and plaques, with massive infiltration occasionally producing a leonine facies, especially in patients with chronic lymphocytic leukemia. Sometimes the facial involvement may resemble rosacea or lupus erythematosus; subcutaneous periarticular nodules may simulate juxtaarticular nodes; and ulcerations in genital areas may mimic venereal disease. Infiltration of erectile tissue may produce priapism.

Patients with lymphocytic leukemia have leukemic infiltrates consisting of discrete nodules and tumors, wtih occasional widespread diffuse swelling and infiltration accompanied by erythroderma. Leonine facies is more often found in patients with chronic lymphocytic leukemia. Infiltrates may begin as one or more discrete, bluish red or plum-colored, painless, rubbery nodules in the skin or as nodular subcutaneous infiltrations under otherwise normal skin.

Tumors and plaques may become ulcerated, especially on the genitalia. Patients may have a diffuse infiltrated erythroderma as a generalized swelling and redness of the skin with intense pruritus. The skin surface may vary from smooth to lichenfied, slightly scaly, eczematous, or severely exfoliative.

Granulocytic leukemia may be associated with chloroma. Chloroma, named for its green color, is the only lesion that is pathognomonic in any of the leukemias. It is a granulocytic sarcoma and is the only cutaneous tumor that is green. The green pigment is caused by the enzyme myeloperoxidase (verdoperoxidase), which fades in a few hours after the cut tumor is exposed to air. Chloroma is rare and occurs mainly in childhood; it is caused by the infiltration of immature granulocytic cells in the periosteum, primarily of the orbital and cranial bones, although the sternum, vertebrae, pelvis, and long bones may be involved. Chloromas can expand epidurally and subdurally, causing compression of the brain, cranial nerves, and spinal cord. Chloroma may develop at the same time as acute granulocytic leukemia or may precede it by as much as 1 year.

The cutaneous nodules occurring in patients with leukemia tend to involve the trunk but may also affect the face and extremities. They may be firm or elastic and livid red to mahogany in color.

Patients with monocytic leukemia may have two types of cutaneous lesions. The macular form may resemble an acute exanthem or secondary syphilis; these lesions subsequently turn from pink to slate blue. The second type consists of pale, discrete papules deep in the skin; these may later soften and undergo necrosis, forming multiple small ulcerations. Acute monocytic leukemia tends to have more florid oral lesions than the other forms of leukemia.

ORAL MANIFESTATIONS. Oral lesions are predominant findings in patients with acute leukemias but also may occur in those with chronic leukemia. Leukemic infiltrates often produce hyperplasia of the gums that sometimes completely covers the teeth. This occurs in more than one third of patients with acute myelocytic leukemia but in only about 5% of those with acute lymphocytic leukemia. The red, friable gingival tissue bleeds spontaneously or after minimal trauma. The gums and buccal mucosa frequently ulcerate, producing a necrotic appearance. These ulcerations affect approximately one third of patients. Secondary infection, particularly with yeast, may occur in up to one half, and petechiae and ecchymotic areas also affect about half of patients.

Nonspecific lesions

Leukemids are nonspecific cutaneous eruptions found in leukemia. They are polymorphous and may resemble urticaria, bullae, and erythema multiforme, as well as papulonecrotic and eczematous lesions. Diffuse erythroderma, hemorrhagic exanthems, and ulcerations frequently occur in patients with all types of leukemias.

Pruritus is probably the most common nonspecific manifestation of leukemias, especially the lymphocytic type. Patients may have prurigo-like papules that are pale, edematous, and surmounted by minute vesicles. In patients with exfoliative erythroderma, pruritus may become unbearably severe.

Herpes zoster especially occurs with lymphocytic leukemia and also with Hodgkin's disease and myeloma; it may become hemorrhagic or gangrenous and sometimes generalized. Bullae may form in the mouth, simulating pemphigus.

Other nonspecific cutaneous findings commonly found in patients with leukemias include pallor caused by anemia, purpura and hemorrhage of the skin and mucous membranes caused by thrombocytopenia, and the general wasting resulting from malignant disease.

MULTIPLE MYELOMA

The skin lesions in patients with multiple myeloma are usually either direct extensions or metastatic from bone lesions. They are reddish blue, subcutaneous nodules, 1 to 2 cm in diameter, generally occurring on the trunk and consisting of collections of malignant plasma cells. The lesions usually appear after the diagnosis of multiple myeloma has already been established through other findings. Primary cutaneous plasmacytomas unrelated to bony lesions are rare. No characteristic clinical features enable a diagnosis without a histologic examination. Patients may have the lesions for years before other evidence of multiple myeloma appears.

Amyloidosis is found in 10% of patients with myeloma. The lesions are generally located on the skin, mucosal surfaces, tongue, gastrointestinal tract, heart, blood vessels, and muscle. On the buccal, nasal, conjunctival, vaginal, and anal mucosa, patients may have yellowish to pale red papules or plaques where purpura may occur after minor trauma. A biopsy of these sites confirms the presence of amyloid.

Amyloid in the skin presents as translucent, waxy, yellow to pink, superficial and slightly elevated lesions varying from 1 mm to several centimeters. The lesions occasionally occur on the eyelids, nasolabial folds, and around the mouth, as well as on the neck, axillae, chest, periumbilical areas, and perineum. Because of their shiny, translucent quality, they may appear vesicular but are solid papules. The lesions develop purpura when rubbed or pinched because amyloid deposited in the vessel walls makes them fragile. When an area of skin is diffusely involved, it may have a sclerodermal appearance. Rarely, bullae that may be hemorrhagic develop as a result of cleavage through dermal or subepidermal amyloid deposits. Infiltration of the face may resemble myxedema; patients may have coarse features and a rigid expression. Alopecia may develop when hairy sites (scalp, eyebrows, axillae, pubic areas) become infiltrated. Patients with this form of amyloidosis generally have no pruritus.

Cryoglobulinemia is found in about 5% of patients with multiple myeloma. The clinical findings are blotchy cyanosis following exposure to cold, Raynaud's phenomenon (sometimes causing digital gangrene), purpura, and necrosis. Hemorrhagic bullae may occur and lead to cutaneous ulcers (especially on the ankles, hands, and ears), bleeding gums, epistaxis, and cold urticaria that becomes hemorrhagic on rewarming.

Severe hyperlipoproteinemia may result from dysproteinemia of multiple myeloma, with the formation of cutaneous and visceral xanthomatosis. Normolipemic patients may have diffuse, flat xanthomas that appear before diagnosis of systemic myelomatosis.

Nonspecific skin findings associated with myeloma include pruritus, pallor (caused by anemia), ichthyosiform dermatitis, pemphigoid, dermatomyositis, uremic frost (when severe renal impairment develops), and disappearance of the nails' lunulae.

Purpura occurs as a result of thrombocytopenia, amyloidosis

of cutaneous vessels, and hyperglobulinemia. The incidence of herpes zoster infections increases in these patients.

ORAL MANIFESTATIONS. Amyloidosis may involve patients' oral mucosa. When affected, the gingiva appears spongy, thickened, and nodular and bleeds readily following minor trauma. Amyloid deposited diffusely in the tongue produces induration, usually painless macroglossia with uniform enlargement, and sometimes protrusion of the tongue. The surface of the tongue may be smooth, pale, and atrophic. If the involvement is spotty, erythematous nodules and papules occur. Patients may have yellowish to pale red papules or plaques on the buccal mucosa. Often the dentist may be asked to do a gingival biopsy to confirm the diagnosis of amyloidosis associated with myeloma.

Another possible oral finding is purpura from the thrombocytopenia. Minor trauma may produce purpura in vascular areas affected by amyloidosis.

Solitary plasmacytomas also have been reported in the oral cavity. Panoramic and lateral skull roentgenograms may show the classic "punched-out" radiolucent lesions of multiple myeloma.

MALIGNANT LYMPHOMA

Cutaneous manifestations occur during the course of the disease in about 50% of patients with lymphomas. The morphology of specific cutaneous lesions and nonspecific eruptions is similar in leukemia and lymphoma. Malignant lymphoma of the skin is usually metastatic from some internal organ but may occasionally be a primary skin lesion.

The specific lesions with the characteristic malignant cells include papules, nodules, and tumors; infiltrations; and plaques, ulcerated lesions, and erythroderma. The most distinctive specific lesions are violaceous to plum-colored papules or subcutaneous firm nodules of various sizes. Patients may have a solitary nodule, especially on the scalp, for years before it causes symptoms. These tumors are firm but not stony hard (unlike metastatic carcinoma), have a rubbery consistency, and may vary from dusky red to a dark violet color. The specific lesions can occur anywhere on the body surface or in the oral cavity, the conjunctivae, and the genitalia. They may have a general distribution, may form clusters or circinate or arciform patterns, or may coalesce into large plaques. Nodules and ulcerations may occur on the tonsils, palate, tongue, and nasopharynx. Symmetric swelling of the lacrimal, orbital, and salivary glands may result from infiltration with malignant cells. The lymph nodes may become necrotic, resulting in the formation of sinus tracts with ulcerations of the overlying skin.

Any of the lymphomas can occasionally begin with skin lesions, which may remain localized for months or years before visceral involvement occurs. Generally, however, the reverse is true; by the time specific lesions are found on the skin, the diagnosis of lymphoma has usually been made. In patients with Hodgkin's disease, skin lesions usually appear in the late stages and indicate widespread involvement with a poor prognosis.

The nonspecific manifestations of lymphoma include pruritus, prurigo-papular eruptions, pigmentation, erythema multiforme, erythema nodosum, and urticaria. Eczematous and psoriasiform dermatitis, exfoliative dermatitis, and bullous lesions may also occur. Patients may be pale when anemia develops and may have purpura when thrombocytopenia occurs. In addition, skin infections may supervene as a patient's immune state becomes compromised. These infections can be bacterial, superficial or deep fungal, or viral (herpes simplex or herpes zoster).

The nonspecific lesions mentioned previously are more commonly associated with Hodgkin's disease, whereas more specific lesions occur more frequently with non-Hodgkin's lymphoma. Generalized pruritus and excoriations may be the only manifestation of Hodgkin's disease for years before other evidence of the disease appears. Exfoliative dermatitis is likewise associated mainly with Hodgkin's disease and infrequently with non-Hodgkin's lymphoma. It may begin as an erythrodermic patch that becomes generalized with pronounced scaling. Pruritus may become intense, and patients feel chilly because of the heat loss resulting from vasodilation and increased blood flow in the skin. The nails may become dystrophic and are shed, and the hair may fall out. Exfoliative dermatitis is associated with lymphomas or leukemias in up to 25% of patients. Acquired ichthyosis may occur in association with lymphomatous diseases, more often with Hodgkin's disease than the other lymphomas. Ichthyotic patients may have mildly dry skin or extreme fishlike scales, as well as hyperkeratosis of palms and soles. The ichthyosis may subside when the lymphoma is in remission.

CUTANEOUS T-CELL LYMPHOMA (MYCOSIS FUNGOIDES)

Cutaneous T-cell lymphoma (CTCL) is a neoplasm of helper-T cells that first appears as a skin disease. After a variable time the malignant T cells invade the lymph nodes, peripheral blood, and visceral organs. This process frequently results in death. CTCL encompasses classic mycosis fungoides, Sézary syndrome (the exfoliative erythrodermic phase), and lymphoma cutis.

Mycosis fungoides occurs more often in men than women; it may develop as early as adolescence but is diagnosed most often in patients 40 to 60 years of age. Its duration may be 1 year or several decades, when it becomes progressively more severe. The average course is about 10 years, but when the tumor stage develops, survival is usually less than 3 years.

Three phases of the disease are recognized: (1) a premycotic phase consisting of erythematous, eczematous, and psoriasiform lesions, usually accompanied by intense pruritus; (2) an infiltrated plaque phase; and (3) a tumor phase. These phases do not always follow in sequence; the disease may begin with any of these forms, and one may exist without the others. Generally, however, the onset is insidious, with the premycotic phase lasting from months to many years. Pruritus, at times intense, may be the sole initial manifestation, or it may accompany various clinical presentations resembling seborrheic dermatitis, psoriasis, eczema, neurodermatitis, parapsoriasis, and erythema multiforme, as well as urticarial lesions and scaly patches. The eruptions may be transitory or persistent; they may remit spontaneously and recur later. In many patients with parapsoriasis en plaques (pale, erythematous, fingerlike to palm-sized patches) and poikiloderma (diffuse variegated erythema) of the trunk, mycosis fungoides eventually may develop.

The configuration of lesions may be bizarre; arciform, large ring, crescent, and ribbonlike forms occur. The color is often vivid, predominantly shades of red such as scarlet, salmon, rose, and crimson, sometimes with a bluish or yellowish tinge. Erythroderma and exfoliative dermatitis may develop and become generalized. The universal redness (l'homme rouge) and scaling are accompanied by edematous and thickened skin, with leonine facies, ectropion, scanty hair, and dry ridged nails. Patients may have enlarged spleen and lymph nodes (dermatopathic lymphadenopathy).

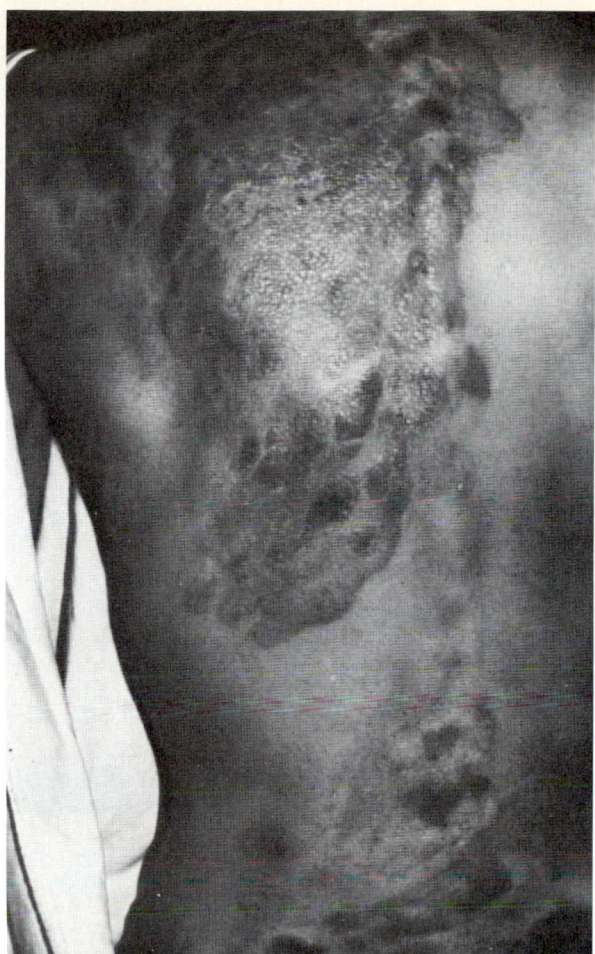

Fig. 161-1 Mycosis fungoides on back. Plaque stage with beginning early tumor formation is shown. Lesions are erythematous and slightly infiltrated.

In the plaque stage (Fig. 161-1) the premycotic lesions become infiltrated, sometimes resulting in a pebbly surface. Induration may initially be present in only a few of the lesions, and infiltrated plaques may arise in previously uninvolved areas. These lesions also assume bizarre shapes, and the pruritus continues; the color varies from shades of red to brownish or purple. The infiltration becomes progressively more severe, leading to extensive plaques that coalesce to produce widespread involvement, interspersed with some patches of normal skin. Eventually almost the entire skin surface may become infiltrated, resulting in a universal erythroderma with thickened skin. Patients may have exceedingly painful superficial and sometimes large ulcerations.

The tumor stage is characterized by nodules and tumefactions of varying sizes and shapes that develop in the infiltrated plaques, in the erythrodermic areas, or on previously uninvolved surfaces. These tumors most often occur on the trunk, but they may occur anywhere on the skin and occasionally in the mouth or upper respiratory tract. The colors are those seen in the plaques, often a dusky bluish red. The tumors tend to break down and form deep necrotic ulcers with rolled edges. Despite this, and even with extensive involvement, patients at first do not seem gravely ill, and the pruritus tends to diminish somewhat with the onset of the tumor stage. Occasionally tumors spontaneously regress and disappear, as the lesions in

the premycotic and infiltrative (plaque) stages sometimes do, but recurrence and progression are inevitable. Lesions of all three stages may be present at the same time.

The d'emblée form of mycosis fungoides refers to the disorder when large tumors appear de novo without the first two stages of the disease. This may sometimes be a manifestation of a malignant lymphoma. The Sézary syndrome is simply a variant manifestation of mycosis fungoides. It is an erythrodermic phase of mycosis fungoides in which a peculiar atypical monocytic cell is found in the circulating blood, as well as in the lymph nodes and the cutaneous infiltrate. The Sézary cell is considered to be a giant abnormal lymphocyte with a large convoluted nucleus and a narrow rim of cytoplasm. The nucleus is cerebriform with lobulations and indentations; the cytoplasm is vacuolated. Sézary syndrome is characterized by severe pruritus accompanying a generalized erythroderma that is often fiery red. Patients have a leonine facies, with edema of the eyelids and ectropion, diffuse alopecia, hyperkeratosis of palms and soles, dystrophic nails, splenomegaly, and diffuse superficial lymphadenopathy. Generally a leukocytosis occurs in the range of 20,000 cells/mm^3 with an absolute lymphocytosis, up to 19% eosinophils, and the abnormal Sézary cell. This has led to the belief that the Sézary syndrome may be a leukemic phase of mycosis fungoides.

Human T-lymphotrophic virus type I (HTLV-I) is associated with a particularly aggressive form of T-cell malignancy. This form often affects young patients and may be associated with hypercalcemia, leukemia, organomegaly caused by infiltration, and widespread skin lesions. The malignant cells in these patients are phenotypically helper/inducer-T cells such as those in classic CTCL. However, they often have in vitro functional properties of suppressor-T cells, which differs from those in classic CTCL. These patients have a very poor prognosis.

The therapy for mycosis fungoides is based on the disease stage. Drug therapy includes topical, intralesional, and systemic administration of corticosteroids; topical administration of nitrogen mustard and nitrosourea; intralesional administration of nitrogen mustard and bleomycin; immunotherapy with BCG vaccine, levamisole, and other agents; and chemotherapy with cytotoxic or immunosuppressive agents including azaribine, methotrexate, procarbazine, and bleomycin. Physical agents include ultraviolet light and grenz-ray therapy in the early stages. Electron beam therapy, teleroentgen therapy, and conventional radiation therapy are used in the later stages. Ultraviolet light (320 to 400 nm) and psoralen therapy (PUVA) alone or in combination with the retinoids (isotretinoin or etretinate) have also been useful.

ORAL MANIFESTATIONS. The tumors of mycosis fungoides may occur in the mouth, most often on the tongue, palate, buccal mucosa, and gingiva. As on the skin, the tumors may have a bluish red color and often break down.

BIBLIOGRAPHY

Amorosi EL and Ultmann JE: Thrombotic thrombocytopenic purpura; report of 16 cases and review of the literature, Medicine 45:139, 1966.

Beacham BE and others: Bullous amyloidosis, J Am Acad Dermatol 3:506, 1980.

Braverman IM: Skin signs of systemic disease, ed 2, Philadelphia, 1981, WB Saunders Co.

Broder S and others: NIH Conference: T cell lymphoproliferative syndrome associated with human T cell leukemia/lymphoma virus, Ann Intern Med 100:543, 1984.

Burg G and others: Monocytic leukemia: clinically appearing as "malignant reticulosis of the skin," Arch Dermatol 114:418, 1978.

Cyr CP and others: Mycosis fungoides, Arch Dermatol 94:558, 1966.

Domonkos AN and others: Andrew's diseases of the skin, ed 7, Philadelphia, 1982, WB Saunders Co.

Edelson RL and others: Preferential cutaneous infiltration by neoplastic thymus-derived lymphocytes, Ann Intern Med 80:685, 1974.

Ellis CN and Voorhees JJ: Etretinate therapy, J Am Acad Dermatol 16:267, 1987.

Fitzpatrick TB and others: Dermatology in general medicine, ed 3, New York, 1987, McGraw-Hill Book Co.

Fromer JL and Geokas MC: Cutaneous manifestations in lymphomas, NY J Med 63:3222, 1963.

Hegde UM and others: Platelet antibodies in thrombocytopenic patients, Br J Haematol 35:113, 1977.

Karayalcin G and others: Sickle cell anemia: clinical manifestations in 100 patients and review of the literature, Am J Med Sci 269:51, 1975.

Michaud M and others: Oral manifestations of acute leukemia in children, J Am Dent Assoc 95:1145, 1977.

Mikhail GR and others: Malignant plasmacytoma cutis, Arch Dermatol 101:59, 1970.

Ratz JL and Bailin PL: Cutaneous amyloidosis: a case report of the tumefactive variant and a review of the spectrum of clinical presentations, J Am Acad Dermatol 4:21, 1981.

Sergeant GR: Leg ulceration in sickle cell anemia, Arch Intern Med 133:690, 1974.

Waldenstrom J: Diagnosis and treatment of multiple myeloma, New York, 1970, Grune & Stratton, Inc.

Willemze R and DeGraff-Reitsma CB: Characterization of T cell subpopulation in skin and peripheral blood of patients with cutaneous T cell lymphomas and benign inflammatory dermatoses, J Invest Dermatol 80:60, 1983.

Wright JM and others: Mycosis fungoides with oral manifestations, Oral Surg 51:24, 1981.

Yoder FW and Schuen RL: Aleukemic leukemia cutis, Arch Dermatol 112:367, 1976.

162 · CONNECTIVE TISSUE DISORDERS

Bernard A. Kirshbaum and **Robert N. Arm**

LUPUS ERYTHEMATOSUS

Lupus erythematosus (LE) appears in two basic forms: a purely cutaneous form called discoid lupus erythematosus (DLE) and systemic lupus erythematosus (SLE). A lupuslike syndrome occurs with the use of certain medications and is called drug-induced LE. This resembles the basic forms.

The cutaneous lesions of DLE are usually discrete, heliotropic colored plaques with disklike and irregular configurations. They heal centrally with slight scaling and usually a moderate amount of scarring (Fig. 162-1). In active lesions the borders remain edematous and scaly with telangiectasia contributing to the lesion's bright red color. Patulous follicular orifices may contain dry, horny keratinous plugs that resemble carpet tacks when removed. Atrophy usually is accompanied by depigmentation and hyperpigmentation. Darker-skinned patients are more severely affected with leukoderma. Typically the lesions occur on the exposed areas of the face, ears, and scalp but can also be found on the neck, shoulders, trunk, forearms, and legs. Single lesions may be localized to a small area of the body, usually the face, where it often appears as the "butterfly" lesion over the bridge of the nose and flush areas of the cheeks. Some patients have a generalized distribution of discoid lesions. SLE is more likely to develop in individuals with widespread lesions. About 5% of patients with DLE eventually develop SLE.

Patients with SLE have various dermatologic disorders. These include a classic malar erythema (butterfly rash), which occurs in approximately 50% of patients. Light exposure generally exacerbates this rash, but not in all patients. Periorbital edema with erythema and periungual erythema occurs, along

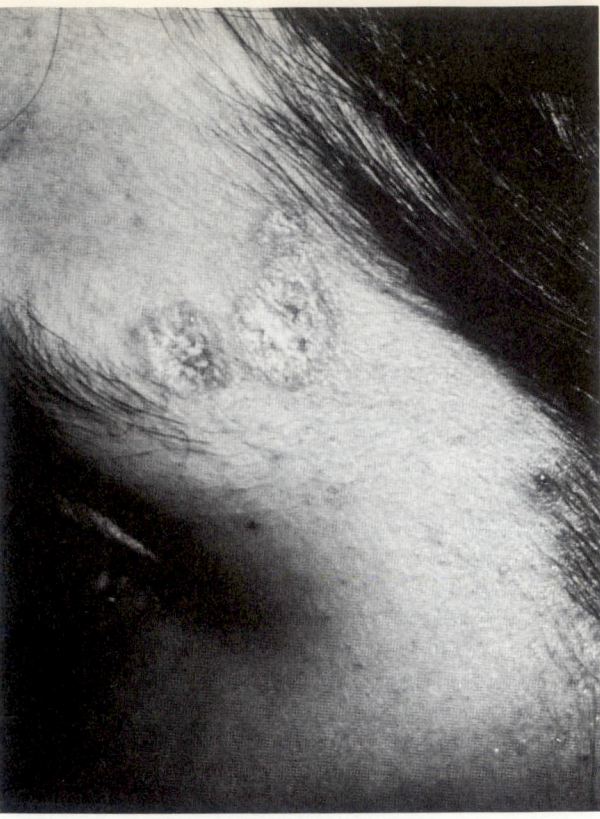

Fig. 162-1   Lesions of chronic discoid lupus erythematosus. Note scarring. Lesions are surrounded by erythema. (Courtesy of Department of Dermatology, The Cleveland Clinics.)

with telangiectasia; both conditions resemble dermatomyositis. Patients also may have alopecia, purpura and petechiae, recurrent urticaria, digital gangrene, and leg ulcers.

The diagnosis of LE is covered in more detail in Chapter 16. It is based on the 1982 American Rheumatologists Association's standards, where 4 of 11 criteria must be met.

The cause of LE is unknown, but sunlight and local physical trauma precipitate the lesions. Women are affected more than men in a 2:1 ratio for overall LE and 9:1 for SLE. Blacks have SLE 3:1 over whites. The incidence is approximately 1 in 400 to 2000.

The results of laboratory tests are generally normal for patients with DLE. Conversely, patients with SLE frequently have abnormalities, including false positive serologic tests for syphilis, antinuclear antibodies, positive rheumatoid factor, elevated erythrocyte sedimentation rate, and abnormal serum globulins, anti-DNA antibody tests, and complement deficiencies. Direct immunofluorescence testing of tissue sections is usually positive in DLE, with IgG and complement located at the dermal-epidermal junction.

The treatment of skin lesions of LE consists of avoiding precipitating causes (heat, light, cold, physical trauma, emotional stress). Intralesional and topical administration of corticosteroids and oral chloroquine, quinacrine, or hydroxychloroquine is usually effective. Therapy with these agents should be undertaken only with due regard to ocular and other potential side effects. Drug-induced LE often resolves after patients stop administration of the causative agent.

ORAL MANIFESTATIONS. Oral lesions occur in 25% to 50% of patients with DLE. These lesions often begin with an irregular whitish area that extends peripherally. A centrally depressed red area may erode or superficially ulcerate, whereas the border expands and remains white, elevated, and hyperkeratotic. An erythematous, hyperemic halo or bluish red inflammatory zone may surround this border. If the central portion or the entire area heals, a slightly atrophic scar may remain.

Oral ulcerations occur in 7% to 25% of patients with SLE and occur more frequently as the disease worsens. About 90% of the lesions appear on the hard palate. More than half the lesions are painless. Occasionally patients have pain associated with the lesion or with ischemia caused by vasculitis. Patients with SLE appear to have more bleeding and purpura than those with DLE.

DENTAL CONSIDERATIONS. See Chapter 34 for a detailed review.

BIBLIOGRAPHY

Callen JP: Systemic lupus erythematosus in patients with chronic cutaneous (discoid) lupus erythematosus, J Am Acad Dermatol 12:278, 1985.

Callen JP and others: Subacute cutaneous lupus erythematosus, J Am Acad Dermatol 15:1227, 1986.

Clark SK: Cutaneous lupus erythematosus: recognition of its many forms, Postgrad Med 79:195, 1986.

Feldman S and Kaplan D: The patient with systemic lupus erythematosus, Prim Care 5:123, 1978.

Haymes SR and others: Lupus erythematosus, Dermatol Clin 4:267, 1986.

Stevens MB: Systemic lupus erythematosus, clinical issues, Springer Semin Immunopathol 9:251, 1986.

Urman JD and others: Oral mucosal ulceration in systemic lupus erythematosus, Arthritis Rheum 21:58, 1978.

Zysset MK and others: Systemic lupus erythematosus: a consideration for antimicrobial prophylaxis, Oral Surg 64:30, 1987.

SCLERODERMA

Scleroderma is a hardening of the skin characterized by circumscribed or diffuse, hard, smooth, ivory-colored areas that are immobile over the underlying tissues. Patients have progressive fibrotic changes in the dermal collagen and the connective tissue of other involved organs. A classic hidebound skin occurs. The disease may be localized (morphea) or systemic (progressive systemic sclerosis) and has an insidious course. The cause is unknown, but an autoimmune mechanism probably is involved. Sclerotic collagen generally increases, together with pronounced thickening and condensation of the connective tissue, and increased collagen-bound hexosamine. Sclerosis also occurs in the subcutaneous tissues.

Laboratory findings in scleroderma may include an elevated erythrocyte sedimentation rate and mild anemia. Immunologic changes consist of a frequently positive rheumatoid factor and occasionally a false positive serologic reaction for syphilis. Antinuclear antibodies are present in about half these patients but are usually of low titer compared to those in SLE. The LE cell test is seldom positive. Hypergammaglobulinemia with a particular increase of IgG may occur, and antithyroid antibodies have been noted.

The treatment of scleroderma generally has poor results. Spontaneous recovery from scleroderma, especially the minor forms, often occurs, especially in children. Treatment consists mainly of physiotherapy (warmth, massage, exercise, and baths) to prevent ankylosis, contractural deformities, and immobility. The various therapeutic modalities attempted include para-aminobenzoic acid, chelating agents, penicillamine, dimethyl sulfoxide, and azathioprine. Some have been highly recommended but none has been totally effective. Vasodilators are helpful, and sympathectomy may temporarily improve the cutaneous circulation. Systemic corticosteroids reduce joint symptoms and give patients a feeling of well-being, but ultimately do not offer any lasting benefit.

Morphea (circumscribed scleroderma); linear scleroderma

Morphea is a localized form of scleroderma. It may occur as multiple guttate lesions mainly on the chest and neck or as oval or linear plaques of hard, dry, smooth skin primarily on the chest, face, or scalp. These lesions are often ivory colored or white with a faint violaceous border. Band-like lesions may form along the course of a rib, on the long axis of an extremity, or vertically on the forehead. Solitary linear lesions that develop on the scalp and forehead are called en coup de sabre ("saber stroke") because of their appearance and are sometimes associated with facial hemiatrophy. Linear scleroderma usually develops in the first decade of life. The localized forms of scleroderma occur in females twice as often as males and rarely lead to the generalized forms. No satisfactory treatment exists, but some lesions reach an end point beyond which the sclerosis does not progress, and many undergo spontaneous resolution, especially in children and adolescents.

ORAL MANIFESTATIONS. The elastic qualities of the lip are lost in patients with morphea, which often causes a stricture. A localized white scar may also occur on the lip. The alveolar ridges, gingiva, and mucosa underlying the affected area may be involved as well. A roentgenogram of the involved bone reveals a radiolucency. This absence of bone is caused by fibrosis. Teeth in the area may have enamel defects. In one patient a cleft developed after shedding of the teeth.

In the en coup de sabre form, hemifacial atrophy can lead to esthetic and functional problems.

Although thickening of the periodontal ligament is reported more often in progressive systemic sclerosis, it has been seen in localized scleroderma.

DENTAL MANAGEMENT. The direct effect on the periodontium may not be as severe as in progressive systemic sclerosis, but problems still may occur in linear scleroderma because of limited access of the oral cavity. This access problem and pain may lead to poor hygiene, causing increased caries and periodontal disease. Lip strictures may also make placement of a removable prosthesis impossible. A "hinge" may allow for flexibility needed to place the appliance. This may be especially useful in progressive systemic sclerosis. Widening of the periodontal ligament has been reported in localized scleroderma, but this thickening is not as common as in progressive systemic sclerosis, where it has been reported in up to 100% of patients. This change occurs in all teeth, but often the posterior teeth seem to be more involved. Biopsy review of the periodontal ligament area shows a loss of normal arrangement of collagen fibers and thickening of the wall with narrowing of the lumina of the periodontal membrane's blood vessels.

The bone deformities may be corrected by surgery, but this may be difficult because of the overlying skin problem. The resorption of bone, particularly the posterior and inferior angle of the mandible, coronoid process, and condyle, as occurs in progressive systemic sclerosis, has not been reported in patients with localized scleroderma.

Progressive systemic sclerosis

Progressive systemic sclerosis appears in two forms: acrosclerosis and diffuse scleroderma. The onset is generally in late adolescence and the early twenties and is diagnosed between the ages of 30 and 50 years. Approximately 4.5 in 1 million persons have the disease, with females affected 3:1 over males.

Acrosclerosis

Acrosclerosis, which accounts for 95% of all cases of scleroderma, is characterized by cutaneous sclerosis of the digits (sclerodactyly) and Raynaud's phenomenon, but visceral involvement often occurs. Young women, usually in late adolescence or early adult life, are mainly affected. Acrosclerosis begins with Raynaud's phenomenon, and arthralgias or symptoms resembling those of rheumatoid arthritis. In the early phases, transient and recurrent erythema and edema occur, especially of the hands and fingers; sometimes the onset is insidious without edema. The sclerodermatous changes and atrophy shortly supervene; the skin becomes yellowish, smooth, shiny, and firm, and retraction occurs so that skin is bound to the underlying structures. The face becomes expressionless and appears drawn and taut with a loss of normal lines. The mouth cannot be opened to its full width, and the forehead cannot be wrinkled. The patient may have a fixed stare, and the lips form a permanent grimace. Movement of the mouth is impeded, and mastication is difficult. The hands become clawlike, with sclerodactyly, tapered fingers, and shiny, hidebound skin. Contractures of the fingers occur, not only from the tight skin, but also from fibrosis of muscles, sclerosis of the synovia, and disuse atrophy. The fingers become semiflexed and immobile. Gradual resorption of bone occurs in the terminal phalanges, with shortening of the fingers. A progressive increase of induration extends from the fingertips to the hand and forearm.

Raynaud's phenomenon, which is almost universally present in acrosclerosis, varies from mild vasospasm to severe attacks of vascular insufficiency resulting in gangrene. Small, pitted scars and ulcerations on the fingertips are characteristic. Trophic ulcers of the knuckles, toes, and ankles occur from the combination of trauma and chronic vascular insufficiency. Changes in the feet and toes are similar to those in the hands and fingers but are generally less severe.

Roentgenograms may show small areas of calcification at the base and borders of the ulcers. Calcium is also deposited around major joints and in the fingers. The skin over these firm, whitish nodules sometimes erodes, and bits of calcium are discharged at the surface; this is often accompanied by cellulitis and secondary bacterial infection. Calcinosis cutis (Thibierge-Weisenbach syndrome) develops relatively late in the course of scleroderma, whereas it appears earlier and is more disabling in dermatomyositis.

Telangiectatic lesions typically appear on the face, lips, buccal mucosa, and hands of patients with scleroderma. The lesions range from dusky to bright red or pink and from 1 to 5 mm. They are oval to square or multiangular with sharp or indistinct borders. Although telangiectasia is also seen in the other collagen diseases, these "telangiectatic mats" with their characteristic shapes occur most commonly in scleroderma. Linear telangiectases are also found on the posterior nail fold in scleroderma and the other connective tissue diseases.

The combination of *c*alcinosis, *R*aynaud's phenomenon, *e*sophageal dysfunction, *s*clerodactyly, and *t*elangiectasia forms the acronym called the CREST syndrome. This is a relatively benign form of scleroderma in which visceral involvement is uncommon or minimal.

Conversely, visceral scleroderma without cutaneous sclerosis is known to occur. Patients with this condition usually have Raynaud's phenomenon and some telangiectasia that may be overlooked.

Cutaneous pigmentary changes occurring in scleroderma are of three types:

1. Hyperpigmentation and hypopigmentation, which are postinflammatory changes appearing in areas of sclerosis
2. Patches of perifollicular pigmentation developing in sites of complete pigment loss and resembling repigmenting vitiligo
3. A generalized hyperpigmentation, especially of exposed areas and mucous membranes, which mimics the pigmentation of adrenal insufficiency, but in which no adrenal insufficiency exists

Diffuse scleroderma

Diffuse scleroderma is an uncommon form of scleroderma. It begins with edema and subsequent hardening of the skin over the chest and spreads rapidly to the head and extremities. The sclerotic areas appear yellowish brown and waxy. The visceral involvement resembles acrosclerosis; however, Raynaud's phenomenon does not occur, and sclerodactyly does not develop because this disease is rapidly fatal. Visceral involvement affects mainly the gastrointestinal tract and the lungs, followed by the cardiovascular and renal systems, but all internal organs may be involved. Fibrosis of internal organs occurs, with loss of smooth muscle and parenchymal tissue and progressive loss of visceral function. Women are affected more than men in a ratio of 3:1, with increasing incidence in older persons that peaks in those over 65 years of age.

ORAL MANIFESTATIONS AND DENTAL MANAGEMENT. See Chapter 172 on collagen vascular disorders.

BIBLIOGRAPHY

Connolly SM: Scleroderma: therapeutic options, Cutis 34:274, 1984.
Cunningham PH and others: Scleroderma: developments from Osler to the present, South Med J 73:770, 1980.
Marmary Y and others: Scleroderma: oral manifestations, Oral Surg 52:32, 1981.
Piette WW, Dorsey JK, and Foucar E: Clinical and serologic expression of localized scleroderma, J Am Acad Dermatol 13:342, 1985.
Rowell NR and Hopper FE: The periodontal membrane in systemic sclerosis, Br J Dermatol 96:15, 1977.
Saad MN and Khoo CTK: Localized scleroderma of the premaxilla and upper lip, Br J Plast Surg 33:245, 1980.
Singsen BH: Scleroderma in childhood, Pediatr Clin North Am 33:1119, 1986.
Velayos EE and others: The "CREST" syndrome: comparison with systemic sclerosis (scleroderma), Arch Intern Med 139:1240, 1979.
White SC and others: Oral radiographic changes in patients with progressive systemic sclerosis (scleroderma), J Am Dent Assoc 94:1178, 1977.

DERMATOMYOSITIS

Dermatomyositis is a necrotizing inflammatory disease of unknown cause that affects striated muscles, skin, and subcutaneous tissue. Muscle weakness is the major symptom. Although myositis is sometimes found in association with SLE, scleroderma, rheumatoid arthritis, and rheumatic fever, it is not a prominent finding in these conditions. When muscle involvement occurs without skin changes, it is known as polymyositis. Dermatomyositis is a relatively rare condition. Although adults are affected most frequently, about 15% of cases develop in children and young adolescents; it may occur as early as 1 year of age or as late as 70 years of age. Females are twice as frequently affected as males. No racial or geographic predilection exists. Dermatomyositis follows a variable course. It may be acute and intense, ending fatally within a year, or there may be long periods of remission and recurrence with the disease progressing slowly for a decade or more. Permanent remission occurs in a few patients. The disease has been noted following infection, physical trauma, immunization, and drug administration. It is not caused by any of these but is probably a hypersensitivity reaction or the result of an autoimmune mechanism. The presence of malignancy has frequently been associated with dermatomyositis, which may appear before the signs and symptoms of carcinoma. Patients with dermatomyositis should be examined carefully to rule out visceral cancer.

Patients may have a vague prodrome or a febrile episode, followed by muscle inflammation and degeneration associated with edema and dermatologic changes. Erythema, telangiectasia, and pigmentary changes occur; ultimately interstitial calcinosis may develop. The classic initial manifestation is a pinkish violet erythema and puffy swelling of the eyelids and face (the characteristic heliotrope eruption), which may also involve the upper part of the trunk, with or without edema. This stage may last for months but is eventually superseded by skin changes akin to those in SLE, affecting not only the face but also the neck, shoulders, arms, and chest. This is accompanied by deep tenderness and a firm, slightly pitting brawny edema over the shoulder girdle, arms, and neck. Linear telangiectases are noted on the cuticles and fingernail folds in dermatomyositis as in the other collagen diseases, and occasionally ulceration of the fingertips may occur, although this is not a regular feature as in scleroderma. Gottron's papules are a pathognomonic sign; these are flat-topped, faintly violaceous lesions on the dorsa of the fingers over the interphalangeal joints. They occur relatively late in the disease in about one third of the patients. When they regress, atrophy, telangiectasia, and hypopigmentation remain in these sites. At this stage patients have intermittent fever, malaise, anorexia, and severe weight loss.

Some of the early signs of dermatomyositis may be transient violaceous blotchy lesions on the trunk, extremities, and face, which may be accompanied by a fine scale. In this stage the disease may be diagnosed as seborrheic dermatitis, contact dermatitis, or an allergic reaction. Occasionally urticarial lesions, vesicular and bullous lesions and erythema multiforme–like lesions may occur, as well as photosensitivity. Sun-exposed areas develop a confluent violaceous, telangiectatic, slightly scaling eruption, which becomes fixed as minute hyperpigmented and hypopigmented macules with telangiectasia and atrophy. This speckled appearance of the skin, called poikiloderma atrophicans vasculare, occurs in the late stages of dermatomyositis, rarely in SLE, and not at all in scleroderma. Poikilodermatomyositis is the name given to this stage of the disease.

Vasomotor disturbances (Raynaud's phenomenon) occur in less than one third of patients; alopecia of the scalp may also be seen. Erythematous patches and telangiectases of the face and upper chest may be present for months or years with occasional flare-ups eventually subsiding into brown pigmentation. When the disease regresses, a bronze discoloration develops that mimics the hyperpigmentation of adrenal insufficiency, and hypertrichosis may occur in the sites of previous cutaneous involvement. The skin, subcutaneous, and muscle involvement occurs mainly on the upper half of the body around the shoulder girdle, elbows, and hands. Sometimes the pelvic girdle is involved. Sclerodactyly, diffuse sclerodermoid changes in the skin, hyperpigmentation, and hypopigmentation develop in about 25% of patients. The term "sclerodermatomyositis" has been applied to this condition, which may appear in 6 months to 3 years after the onset of the myositis. When the sclerodermatous features become prominent, the myositis is usually less active.

No relation exists between the extent of skin lesions and the degree of muscle involvement in dermatomyositis. The skin lesions may be minimal with pronounced myositis, or conversely, the patient may have extensive cutaneous disease with relatively little muscle involvement.

The earliest symptoms of dermatomyositis are soreness and weakness of muscles sometimes accompanied by swelling and tenderness. It is symmetric and affects primarily the shoulder girdle and pelvic region, as well as the neck and proximal muscles of the arms. Patients have difficulty raising their arms, rising from chairs, and walking up stairs. The muscles initially feel doughy, later firm, and ultimately become atrophic and fibrotic with calcification, especially in children. Dysphagia and dysphonia result from involvement of the striated muscles of the pharynx, palate, and esophagus. Esophageal motility changes may be seen on roentgenographic examination. Cardiac muscle may also become involved, ultimately with cardiac failure.

Calcinosis cutis occurs in dermatomyositis; it tends to be more diffuse and appears earlier than in scleroderma. It is found in the subcutaneous tissue, dermis, and muscle and is demonstrable roentgenographically. Unlike scleroderma, it rarely affects the fingers. Calcification develops in children more frequently than in adults.

Laboratory findings include an increased erythrocyte sedimentation rate. Proteinuria and hematuria are commonly present, along with increased urinary excretion of creatine. Urinary creatinine is decreased. Serum levels of aldolase, creatinine, and phosphokinase are elevated, and serum glutamic oxaloacetic transaminase (SGOT) is also increased. Leukocytosis may be present in patients with acute disease, and subsequently leukopenia may occur. Patients with chronic dermatomyositis have anemia with low serum iron concentration. One third of patients have antinuclear antibodies; serum α_2- and γ-globulin levels may be elevated. Rheumatoid factor is present in 10% of patients. Electromyographic studies are useful to distinguish this disease from other myopathies and neuropathy.

Treatment for dermatomyositis consists of the administration of corticosteroids and supportive therapy. Corticosteroids help control the inflammatory process and induce remissions but do not appreciably alter the ultimate course of the disease. Prednisone should be used with regard to all its potential side effects. Methotrexate and azathioprine are also effective. Testosterone proprinate may be given in the convalescent stages to recover muscle mass. If an associated internal malignancy exists, its removal will clear the signs of dermatomyositis in many patients. Bed rest, warmth, and analgesics are essential for patients with acute forms of the disease; physiotherapy is necessary to prevent contractures. The disease tends to be progressive with remissions.

ORAL MANIFESTATIONS. A diffuse stomatitis and pharyngitis are nonspecific clinical findings in dermatomyositis. Facial edema and erythema generally occur; 20% of patients may have lesions on the palate, tongue, and buccal mucosa. They appear as erythema, papules, shallow ulcers, and white patches. These lesions are often similar to those seen in lupus erythematosus.

The muscle involvement can affect facial and jaw muscles, making it difficult for patients to speak and eat and preventing normal facial expression. The muscle dysfunction can lead to alteration of the temporomandibular joint, and myofascial pain syndrome may develop. Calcinosis, especially in the tongue, may occur, and the tongue may become large and immobile. Roentgenograms may show the calcified masses in the soft tissue. Telangiectatic lesions of the lips and cheeks have been reported. Altered tooth morphology may occur, especially shortened roots, calcified pulp chambers, and pulp stones. An increased incidence of tooth fracturing during extraction indicates dentinal involvement. Infections may be masked by the edema and may spread faster because of treatment with systemic steroids.

DENTAL MANAGEMENT. Because of their poor response to therapy, patients may be difficult to manage. Often, little can be done to benefit them. Care must be taken to avoid infection, with careful examinations and detail to oral hygiene instruction. Once infection starts, it may be diagnosed late and progress rapidly. A patient with Ludwig's angina leading to death has been reported. Care must be taken in removal of teeth because they tend to fracture.

Careful consultation to find the extent of systemic disease should be done. Particular attention should be paid to possible cardiopulmonary involvement. Muscle involvement may lead to lack of control of the neuromuscular mechanism of the head and neck. The drugs patients are receiving should be evaluated for their side effects and their role in dental treatment.

BIBLIOGRAPHY

Barnes B: Dermatomyositis and malignancy, Ann Intern Med 84:68, 1976.
Bohan A and Peter JB: Polymyositis and dermatomyositis, N Engl J Med 292:344, 1975.
Callen JP: Dermatomyositis, Int J Dermatol 18:423, 1979.
Callen JP and others: The relationship of dermatomyositis and polymyositis to internal malignancy, Arch Dermatol 116:295, 1980.
Cunningham JD and others: Head and neck manifestations of dermatomyositis-polymyositis, Otolaryngol Head Neck Surg 93:673, 1985.
Fridrich KL and others: Dermatomyositis presenting with Ludwig's angina, Oral Surg 63:21, 1987.
Sanger RG and Kirby JW: The oral and facial manifestations of dermatomyositis with calcinosis, Oral Surg 35:476, 1973.
Tymms KE and others: Dermatopolymyositis and other connective tissue diseases, J Rheumatol 12:1140, 1985.
Vesterager L and others: Dermatomyositis and malignancy, Clin Exp Dermatol 5:31, 1980.

MIXED CONNECTIVE TISSUE DISEASE (OVERLAP SYNDROME)

Mixed connective tissue disease (MCTD), or overlap syndrome, is seen in patients, mostly female, who have features of SLE, dermatomyositis, and scleroderma.

The most common symptom is joint pain. The cutaneous manifestations include nonscarring alopecia, discoid LE, swelling of the hands with sclerodactyly, and pigmentary abnormalities. The pigmentary changes, resembling those seen in scleroderma, are a "salt and pepper" discoloration caused by retention of pigment in the follicles. Raynaud's phenomenon also occurs. Patients have fever, splenomegaly, lymphadenopathy, hypergammaglobulinemia, impaired esophageal motility, pulmonary fibrosis, violaceous suffusion of the eyelids, proximal muscle weakness, pain, and tenderness.

The fluorescent antinuclear antibody (FANA) test based on the pattern of nuclear fluorescence and the dilution titer of the serum to produce fluorescence is an excellent diagnostic procedure. Patients with MCTD have high titers to ribonucleoprotein (RNP) antigen, which persist through periods of remission. Patients usually respond to administration of corticosteroids (prednisone). The prognosis is generally good, with long periods of remission.

BIBLIOGRAPHY

Joshi RM and others: Polymyositis associated with overlap syndrome, J Postgrad Med 32:39, 1986.
LeRoy EC and others: Undifferentiated connective tissue syndromes, Arthritis Rheum 23:341, 1980.
Sharp GC and others: Current concepts in the classification of connective tissue diseases: overlap syndromes and mixed connective tissue disease (MCTD), J Am Acad Dermatol 2:269, 1980.
Tan EM: Mixed connective tissue disease—an evolving clinical syndrome, West J Med 132:350, 1980.

RHEUMATOID ARTHRITIS

Rheumatoid nodules occur in 20% to 30% of patients with rheumatoid arthritis. They are associated with the more severe forms of the disease, higher levels of rheumatoid factor, more severe joint manifestations, and vasculitis. Nodules are rarely the initial symptom; more often they develop during the course of the disease. They appear over bony prominences, especially the olecranon and its vicinity; they are also found on the heels, ears, knuckles, and ischial tuberosities. Ulceration and breakdown of the nodules may occur. The nodules persist and may recur after excision.

Patients with nodules may have linear subcutaneous bands. These are fixed, subcutaneous bands, 3 to 5 mm wide and several centimeters long. They are nontender and are located on the trunk.

Pyoderma gangrenosum occurs rarely, manifested by an ulceration surrounded by violaceous discoloration. The lesions may appear as "punched-out" draining areas with a bluish red rim. The response to systemic corticosteroid therapy is often dramatic.

Rheumatoid vasculitis, which is slightly more common in men, involves the venules and small and medium-sized arteries. Deposition of IgG, IgM, and the third component of complement (C3) is present. Ulcerations, livedo reticularis, Raynaud's phenomenon, ecchymoses, and gangrene may occur. Painful ulcerations develop on patients' legs and ankles. They heal slowly and may be preceded by ecchymoses and palpable purpura. Peripheral neuropathy is often associated with the vasculitis.

Small infarctions occur in the paronychial areas. These are asymptomatic, last only 3 to 4 days, and heal leaving a residual brown macule. Necrosis of the digits occurs more frequently in patients with high titers of rheumatoid factor. Painful nodules may develop in the digital pulp, sometimes in crops, healing with scars, hyperkeratosis, and brown discoloration.

Patients undergoing long-term corticosteroid therapy are susceptible to steroid-induced purpura and ecchymoses.

ORAL MANIFESTATIONS AND DENTAL MANAGEMENT. See Chapter 34.

BIBLIOGRAPHY

Bjarnason D and others: Early rheumatoid arthritis: approach to diagnosis and treatment, Postgrad Med 79:46, 1986.
Harris ED Jr: Pathogenesis of rheumatoid arthritis, Am J Med 28:80, 1986.
Hughes GR: Rheumatoid arthritis, Br J Hosp Med 21:584, 1979.
Kaye BR and others: Rheumatoid nodules, Am J Med 76:279, 1984.
Littman H and others: Medical and dental coordination in juvenile rheumatoid arthritis, Ann Dent 44:32, 1985.
Ogden GR: Complete resorption of the mandibular condyles in rheumatoid arthritis, Br J Dent 160:95, 1986.
Sanders B and others: Psoriasis and rheumatoid arthritis: their relationship in TMJ ankylosis, J Oral Med 34:4, 1979.
Silman AJ: Recent trends in rheumatoid arthritis, Br J Rheumatol 25:328, 1986.

WEGENER'S AND LYMPHOMATOID GRANULOMATOSIS
Wegener's granulomatosis

Cutaneous lesions are present in about half of the patients with Wegener's granulomatosis. They appear as ulcerated, nodular, petechial, papulovesicular, pyoderma gangrenosum–like, or urticarial lesions. The lesions are often bilateral and nonspecific. Histologically they are similar to the generalized findings of a necrotizing vasculitis.

The classic triad of Wegener's granulomatosis includes the type of changes occurring with a necrotizing granuloma, particularly of the nose, paranasal sinuses, and lungs; vasculitis of small arteries and veins, especially in the lungs; and necrotizing glomerular nephritis. Often the clinical features include sinusitis, nasal obstruction or rhinorrhea, otitis media, and pulmonary findings often concurrent with the polyvasculitis and glomerular nephritis. Histologic examination usually shows a necrotizing vasculitis with thrombosis; occasionally a granulomatous reaction occurs with an inflammatory infiltrate. Hemorrhagic granulomatous lesions that persist and often are crusted occurring around the nose, nasal septum, pharynx, trachea, or larynx should alert one to consider the diagnosis of Wegener's granulomatosis.

Treatment relies mainly on cyclophosphamide (Cytoxan). Azathioprine (Imuran), methotrexate, and prednisone are also beneficial.

ORAL MANIFESTATIONS. About 40% of patients have oropharyngeal lesions. The gingival lesion is pathognomonic. This is often a painful, proliferative, granular gingivitis that can start on intradental papillae and coalesce rapidly. It is exophytic and hyperplastic, with an ulcerative to granular surface and a bright red color suggestive of strawberries. This "strawberry" gingivitis generally persists despite periodontal therapy. Occasionally it is limited to one papilla but often is generalized and florid. The gingiva appears to improve as the systemic disease improves. The histologic examination reveals an acute vasculitis and an inflammatory infiltrate containing plasma cells, eosinophils, and neutrophils. A necrotizing vasculitis generally must be confirmed by microscopy. Superficial biopsies may fail to show the vasculitis because small to medium-sized arteries are needed. The gingival lesions occur in approximately 15% of patients. Tongue lesions, especially ulcerations, have the same incidence.

DENTAL MANAGEMENT. When one sees the strawberry gingivitis, biopsy should be performed to confirm the diagnosis of Wegener's granulomatosis. This may be the initial finding of the disease and may lead to appropriate diagnosis. To help control the gingivitis, careful oral hygiene and periodontal therapy must be provided and often supplemented with mouth rinses, particularly chlorhexidine. Care must be taken because of the systemic manifestations and immunosuppressive therapy required in this disease.

BIBLIOGRAPHY

Batsakis JG: Wegener's granulomatosis and midline (nonhealing) "granuloma," Head Neck Surg 1:213, 1979.

Hansen LS and others: Limited Wegener's granulomatosis: report of a case with oral, renal and skin involvement, Oral Surg Oral Med Oral Pathol 60:524, 1985.

Horan RF and others: Recent onset of gingival enlargement, Arch Dermatol 122:1436, 1986.

Isrealson H and others: The hyperplastic gingivitis of Wegener's granulomatosis, J Periodont 52:81, 1981.

Kornblut AD and others: Wegener's granulomatosis, Laryngoscope 90:1453, 1980.

Raustia AM and others: Ultrastructural findings and clinical follow-up of "strawberry gums" in Wegener's granulomatosis, J Oral Pathol 14:581, 1985.

Lymphomatoid granulomatosis

Lymphomatoid granulomatosis is a severe systemic disease with a necrotizing pulmonary angiitis as the major feature. The cutaneous lesions are nonspecific and may precede the lung lesions. Erythematous or purplish nodules and plaques may ulcerate or may mimic panniculitis.

Therapy usually consists of systemic steroids. In approximately 12% of patients the disease progresses to lymphoma. The mortality rate is high.

BIBLIOGRAPHY

Brodell RT and others: Cutaneous lesions of lymphomatoid granulomatosis, Arch Dermatol 122:303, 1986.

Chanda JJ and Callen JP: Necrotizing vasculitis (angiitis) with granulomatosis, Int J Dermatol 23:101, 1984.

Gross PR: Lymphomatoid granulomatosis, Cutis 25:305, 1980.

Gupta S and others: Lymphomatoid granulomatosis of the oropharynx, Ear Nose Throat J 59:152, 1980.

Rosen T and others: Lymphomatoid granulomatosis, Int J Dermatol 18:497, 1979.

Wood ML and others: Cutaneous lymphomatoid granulomatosis: a rare cause of recurrent skin ulceration, Br J Dermatol 110:619, 1984.

BEHÇET'S DISEASE

Behçet's disease is a progressive, systemic, multisystem disease of unknown cause. A genetic predisposition has been suggested, since in some countries patients have a three to four times increased frequency of HLA-B5 antigen; however, this does not occur in the United States or England. Others report an increase in HLA-B12 antigen, and in England an increase in HLA-B27 (also seen in Reiter's syndrome) has been reported. A predilection for the disease seems to occur in the Mediterranean basin, Middle East, and Japan. In Japan the incidence appears to be 1 in 10,000 persons, whereas in England (Yorkshire) the incidence is only about 1 in 150,000. In most countries males apparently are affected more often, up to 5:1 over females. In Northern America, Britain, and Australia more females seem to be affected, as in aphthae. Behçet's disease generally affects those between the ages of 15 and 45 years, but most commonly occurs in the third decade.

Hippocrates first recorded the disease as he described patients with aphthous ulcers in the mouth, discharge and sores about the genitalia, watery inflammation of the eyes, and loss of sight in some patients. This described the classic triad of iritis and oral and genital ulcerations. Other problems may include pyoderma, erythema nodosum–like lesions, polyarthritis, and central nervous system, cardiac, renal, pulmonary, and intestinal involvement.

Behçet's disease is thought to be related to vasculitis, with 60% of patients having an increased erythrocyte sedimentation rate and about 80% having dysproteinemia. Others believe an autoimmune mechanism exists, with both total complement and C_9 increased. C_2, C_3, and C_4 are decreased before an attack of the uveitis. Biopsy of the oral ulcers has revealed C_3 and C_9 in blood vessel walls with C_9 increased in the basement membrane. In addition, lymphocytes show a cytotoxicity to homogenates of oral mucosa. Some studies suggest a viral etiologic factor, but most do not.

The initial manifestations generally are oral or genital ulcers. Mucosal lesions resemble recurrent aphthae. The genital ulcers occur on the scrotum and penis in men and the labia in women. The genital ulcers appear small, punched out, and deeper than those in the oral cavity, and patients generally have more pain.

Ocular manifestations include photophobia, conjunctivitis, iritis, uveitis, neuritis, hypopyon, and vitreous opacification. Eye involvement is a major cause of disability and can lead to blindness.

About 80% of patients with Behçet's disease have skin lesions that consist of follicular and perifollicular pustules, inflamed dermal nodules, cellulitis, and furunculosis. These develop on the trunk, limbs, and flexural areas, and may clear up in 2 weeks. Sterile pustules or erythematous edema often occur in 24 to 48 hours at the sites of venipuncture or injections.

This pathergy or skin hyperreactivity should alert the physician to the possibility of Behçet's disease.

The diagnosis is based on clinical findings because no pathognomonic laboratory test exists. A list of major and minor criteria has been developed to aid in the diagnosis. The major criteria include recurrent aphthous stomatitis, recurrent genital ulcerations, eye lesions (recurrent uveitis, chorioretinitis), and skin lesions (cutaneous vasculitis, thrombophlebitis, skin hyperreactivity). The minor criteria include arthralgia, intestinal ulcers, central nervous system involvement (meningoencephalitis, brainstem involvement, psychologic changes), and orchitis or epididymitis. Definitive diagnosis is made if all four major criteria are present.

Since often the diagnosis is not definitive, one must include Stevens-Johnson syndrome, Reiter's syndrome, SLE, and aphthous ulcers in the differential diagnosis.

Systemic symptoms of malaise, fever, and arthralgias are variable. Thrombophlebitis, which may be superficial or deep, occurs in 20% to 65% of patients; this can include vena cava obstruction. With thrombosis of the hepatic vein, a Budd-Chiari syndrome exists. Central nervous system involvement may be fatal. The arthralgias affect up to 50% of patients, who have joint pain, erythema, and swelling. Approximately 50% have gastrointestinal symptoms, including ulcers, vomiting, abdominal pain, flatulence, and diarrhea or constipation.

The prognosis varies. The disease can wax and wane with spontaneous remissions and exacerbations, often even after 60 years. One organ system involvement may remain active, whereas others may be in remission. In general, however, the disease activity diminishes and finally ceases after many years.

ORAL MANIFESTATIONS. Oral ulcerations are often the initial sign of Behçet's disease (75% of patients) and eventually are present in more than 95% of patients. The lesions are almost indistinguishable from aphthae. They occur on non–bone-bound tissues. The lesions appear circular and red during the early stages. In the first day or two a shallow, round, or oval ulcer approximately 2 to 10 mm with discrete erythematous borders develops. Eventually this has a whitish or yellowish necrotic pseudomembrane. The ulcer generally heals in 10 to 14 days without scarring. One or many ulcers may occur at irregular intervals. They commonly affect the buccal vestibule, tongue, floor of mouth, and lips. The extent of the lesions varies, and often spontaneous exacerbation or remission occurs after years. They can also erode into deep submucosa and heal very slowly. Patients may have persistent lesions for years, often with fetid breath, dysphagia, and pain. In severe cases the palate, pharynx, and esophagus are also affected.

The distinguishing feature of aphthous ulcers in Behçet's disease is that 65% of patients with oral ulcerations also have genital ulcers and about 80% have iritis. Other typical associations are skin lesions (80% of patients) and arthritis (60%). The arthritis may affect the temporomandibular joint. Trauma may exacerbate the lesions. Sepsis and thrombosis have been reported at venipuncture sites and may occur in the mouth. The lesions appear to worsen after patients eat certain foods, especially English walnuts.

DENTAL MANAGEMENT. Dental management of the lesions in patients with Behçet's disease may be difficult, and various forms of treatment have had variable results in different patients. Topical steroids, especially a fluorinated steroid such as Lidex, applied three to five times daily may be beneficial. A solution is necessary to treat multiple lesions, but dexamethasone elixir may give a burning sensation; a tablet dissolved in water may be tried. Tetracycline seems to help; a 250 mg capsule is dissolved in 5 ml of water, and four times a day patients swish this in the mouth for at least 2 minutes and then swallow. Chlorhexidine used twice a day has assisted somewhat in avoiding secondary infections and maintaining periodontal health.

Local treatment of the lesions with corticosteroids has been beneficial, but allowing the physician to treat the entire systemic disease may be preferable. If the oral lesions are the major findings, 4 mg of prednisone daily may be useful initially. Up to 60 mg of prednisone have been administered daily in acute exacerbations of the disease. For patients in relapse, azathioprine, chlorambucil, and corticosteroids have been used singly or in combination. For systemic lesions, colchicine also has been tried. Occasionally, intralesional injection of steroids may help.

Besides managing the oral lesions, one must be cautious with the use of systemic medications and possible systemic involvement. If the pain caused by lesions increases periodontal disease and caries because of a patient failing to care for the gingiva, a soft toothbrush with a bland toothpaste such as baking soda may be used and supplemented with chlorhexidine.

REITER'S SYNDROME

Reiter's syndrome is a symptom complex consisting of nongonococcal urethritis, conjunctivitis, arthritis, and dermatitis. A predisposition to this complex is strongly associated with the HLA-B27 antigen. Two forms of the syndrome exist: postinfectious and venereal. Some patients have no initiating event they can document.

The postinfectious variant occurs after dysenteric infections caused by *Shigella, Salmonella, Campylobacter,* and *Yersinia* organisms. The venereally transmitted form affects men 15 to 50 times more often than women; no specific etiologic agent has been substantiated, but *Chlamydia* and *Mycoplasma* organisms have been suggested as possible causes. In one study about 60% of all patients with Reiter's syndrome had evidence of chlamydial infection. All strains of a given species may not produce the syndrome. Although in most patients the onset is 8 to 28 days after sexual activity or dysentery, some have suggested a delayed onset of up to 2 years after the ureterogenital infection. As with other infectious diseases, one must rule out infections with such organisms as *Gonococcus* and *Staphylococcus* and their related postinfection syndromes.

Reiter's syndrome is variable and recurrent. Often it is chronic with multiple relapses, but it is self-limiting. The onset is usually abrupt, often with no prodromal symptoms, generally a few weeks after sexual exposure. The subjects are generally 25 to 35 years of age. Diarrhea, especially of the enteric form, may be the first sign. Often, heel and ankle pain and polyarthritis causes the patient to seek professional care. Initial constitutional symptoms of fever, weakness, anorexia, weight loss, and anemia may be present along with a purulent urethral discharge. The bilateral catarrhal conjunctivitis rarely has a purulent exudate and is generally not painful. Keratitis may occasionally develop with painful ulcerations. The eye symptoms may clear spontaneously in a few days or weeks or may progress to iridocyclitis.

Keratoderma blenorrhagicum refers to the hyperkeratotic, scaling, serpiginous lesions that develop on the palms, soles, legs, and scalp of patients with Reiter's syndrome. Lesions on the abdomen and buttocks tend to be psoriasiform. This eruption develops about 1 month after the onset of urethritis and follows the appearance of the arthritis; it is self-limited and may last weeks to months. Nail and paronychial involvement may be severe and can lead to onycholysis, nail thickening,

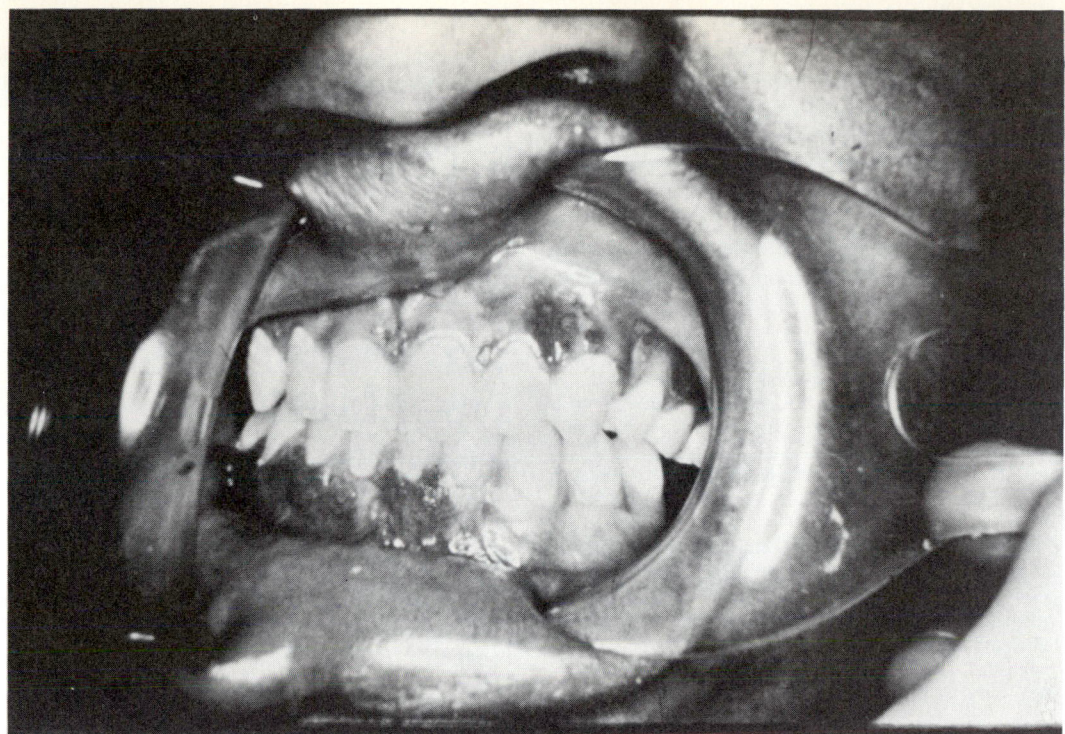

Fig. 162-2   Erythematous areas and shallow ulcerations of gingiva in patient with Reiter's syndrome.

and dystrophy. Penile lesions occur in 25% of male patients; balanitis is the most common manifestation. Painless, shallow erosions with keratotic margins occur near the corona of the glans penis. Dry scaling of the glans penis may occur, and scaling, erosive plaques may appear on the scrotum. Rarely an exfoliative dermatitis may develop; this may be fatal in severely ill patients who have protracted disease. As with psoriasis, the skin lesions are treated with tar and topical steroid creams.

The arthritis is an inflammatory polyarthritis often resembling rheumatoid arthritis. The lower extremities are more commonly involved, especially the knees, heels, and ankles. The arthritis can be disabling. Occasionally, only one joint may be involved. Classic treatment for rheumatoid arthritis has been tried but is not as successful.

Systemic complications may include urethral stricture, prostate vesiculitis, and less commonly, neurologic and cardiac manifestations. A cervical or lumbar radiculopathy and seizure disorder have been reported. Patients with widespread dermatitis may have a polyneuritis. Aortic insufficiency and first-degree atrioventricular heart blocks may occur after initial onset of Reiter's syndrome.

ORAL MANIFESTATIONS. Although Reiter's syndrome also involves eyes, mouth, and genitals, the lesions are different from Behçet's disease. Oromucosal lesions occur in differing percentages of patients, affecting 15% to 80% depending on the report. Often the lesions are missed because of mild symptoms or their brief appearance; the oral lesions last only a few days. They usually are concomitant with other classic manifestations but may be the initial sign. The generally painless lesions can occur anywhere but more often on the buccal mucosa, tongue, gingiva, palate, and tonsillar pillars (Fig. 162-2). The lesions are psoriasiform. They initially exhibit a vesicular area with an erythematous border and quickly form a shallow ulcer. Confluence of the patches of denuded papillae may look similar to migra-

tory glossitis (geographic tongue) (see Chapter 168). Some patients have reported a slight burning, loss of taste, and pain.

DENTAL MANAGEMENT. Aimed at symptomatic relief, the therapy for Reiter's syndrome is similar to that for Behçet's disease. If pain occurs, topical anesthetic ointment (5% lidocaine) applied to each lesion or a rinse of 0.5% aqueous diphenhydramine (Benadryl) or 2% viscous lidocaine for multiple lesions is beneficial. To avoid pain when eating, patients should eat a bland diet with no citrus fruits. A neutral mouth rinse (sodium bicarbonate; calcium bicarbonate for hypertensive patients) or a peroxide rinse keeps the mouth clean. Chlorhexidine, generally twice a day, helps prevent secondary infection and gingivitis caused by the potential lack of oral hygiene. The patient should avoid mouth rinses, elixirs, and beverages containing alcohol.

Multiple therapies have been tried without success; none cures the patient. As with Behçet's disease, the most favorable results have resulted from use of tetracycline ointment or a 250 mg capsule dissolved in water, held in the mouth as long as possible, and swallowed four times a day. Topical corticosteroids, especially fluorinated steroids such as Lidex, have been beneficial. Other modalities have included administering acidophilus tablets and zinc. Trials with levamisole, a drug affecting the immune system, have shown little promise. Although cauterizing agents such as phenol or silver nitrate may initially decrease the pain, they enlarge the lesions and prolong healing.

Vitamins have helped in some patients with vitamin deficiency. Some researchers suggest determining folate, iron, and vitamin B_{12} levels routinely, since one study showed 15% of patients with Reiter's syndrome had low levels of all three. Although the patients were treated only for the deficiency, 60% were cured. Other studies have demonstrated only a 5% to 7% rate of vitamin deficiency.

A complete medical history before dental treatment is required because of the effect of generalized involvement and drug therapy on treatment. Generalized involvement can include cardiac, central nervous system, vascular (thrombophlebitis in up to 20% of patients with Reiter's syndrome probably requiring anticoagulants), and various autoimmune diseases. (For management, see Chapter 34.)

Drug therapy may also alter treatment. Treatment of arthritis with aspirin may alter patients' platelet function. Phenylbutazone, also used in arthritis, may cause aplastic anemia. If long-term steroids are administered, the increased risk of shock and infection must be evaluated.

BIBLIOGRAPHY

Arnet CF: Reiter's syndrome: report of a case, J Oral Surg 38:382, 1980.

Baker H: Reiter's disease. In Rook A, Wilkinson DS, and Ebeling FJG, editors: Textbook of dermatology, ed 3, Oxford, 1979, Blackwell Scientific Publications.

Bengtsson A and others: Reiter's syndrome—a comparative study of patients with the complete and the incomplete syndrome, Clin Rheumatol 5:70, 1986.

Callen JP: The spectrum of Reiter's disease, J Am Acad Dermatol 1:75, 1979.

Catterall RD: Clinical aspects of Reiter's disease, Br J Rheumatol 22(suppl 2):151, 1983.

Chajek T and Fainaru M: Behçet's disease: report of 41 cases and review of the literature, Medicine 54:179, 1975.

Cohen L: Etiology, pathogenesis and classification of aphthous stomatitis and Behçet's syndrome, J Oral Pathol 7:347, 1978.

Ersoy F and others: HLA antigens associated with Behçet's disease, Arch Dermatol 113:1720, 1977.

Esguep A and others: Behçet's syndrome: report on five cases, J Oral Med 42:25, 1987.

Fox R and others: The chronicity of symptoms and disability in Reiter's syndrome, Ann Intern Med 910:190, 1979.

Francis TC: Recurrent aphthous stomatitis and Behçet's disease, Oral Surg 30:476, 1970.

Good AE: Reiter's disease, Postgrad Med 61:153, 1977.

Good AE: Reiter's disease: a review with special attention to cardiovascular and neurologic sequelae, Semin Arthritis Rheum 3:253, 1979.

Good AE: Reiter's disease, Cutis 24:514, 1979.

Graykowski EA and Hooks JJ: Summary of workshop on recurrent aphthous ulcers, South Med J 70:559, 1977.

Haim S and others: Clinical and laboratory criteria for the diagnosis of Behçet's disease, Br J Dermatol 102:361, 1980.

Ingram GJ and Scher RK: Reiter's syndrome with nail involvement: is it psoriasis? Cutis 37:37, 1985.

Is Reiter's syndrome caused by chlamydia? Lancet, 2:317, 1985, (editorial).

Jorizzo JL: Behçet's disease: an update based on the 1985 international conference in London, Arch Dermatol 122:556, 1986.

Kousa M and others: Frequent association of chlamydial infection with Reiter's syndrome, Sex Transm Dis 5:57, 1978.

Lehner T: Progress report: oral ulceration and Behçet's syndrome, Gut 18:491, 1977.

Marks JS and others: The natural history of Reiter's disease—21 years of observations, Q J Med 60:685, 1986.

Merchant H and others: Zinc sulfate supplementation for treatment of recurrent aphthous ulcers, South Med J 70:559, 1973.

Meyer J and others: Levamisole in aphthous ulcers, evaluation of three regimes, Br Med J 1:671, 1977.

Miller MF and others: A retrospective study of the prevalence and incidence of recurrent aphthous ulcers in a professional population, Oral Surg 43:532, 1977.

Miller MF and others: The inheritance of recurrent aphthous stomatitis, Oral Surg 49:409, 1980.

Nally FF: Behçet's syndrome with autoimmune findings, Oral Surg 25:357, 1968.

Nicholas KD and others: Periadenitis mucosa necrotica recurrens, J Oral Surg 33:65, 1975.

Pruessner HT and others: Diagnosis and treatment of chlamydial infections, Am Fam Physician 34:81, 1986.

Rosenberg AM and Petty RE: Reiter's disease in children, Am J Dis Child 133:394, 1979.

Sander HM and Randle HW: Use of colchicine in Behçet's syndrome, Cutis 29:344, 1986.

Sharp JT: Reiter's syndrome, Curr Prob Dermatol 5:157, 1973.

Ship II and others: Recurrent aphthous ulcers, Am J Med 32:32, 1962.

Silverman S and others: Recurrent aphthous stomatitis: current status of etiology and treatment, J Calif Dent Assoc 5:38, 1977.

Stanley HR: Management of patients with persistent recurrent aphthous stomatitis and Sutton's disease, Oral Surg 35:174, 1973.

Walden CA: Psoriasiform lesions of the oral mucosa, Oral Surg 37:872, 1974.

Wilkey D and others: Budd-Chiari syndrome and renal failure in Behçet's disease, Am J Med 75:541, 1983.

Wong RC and others: Behçet's disease, Int J Dermatol 23:25, 1984.

Wray D and others: Nutritional deficiencies in recurrent aphthous ulcers, J Oral Pathol 7:418, 1978.

Yli-Kerttula UI: Clinical characteristics in male and female uro-arthritis or Reiter's syndrome, Clin Rheumatol 3:351, 1984.

Zizic TM and Stevens MB: The arthropathy of Behçet's disease, John Hopkins Med J 136:243, 1975.

163 · MISCELLANEOUS SKIN DISORDERS

Anthony V. Benedetto *and* **Robert N. Arm**

MASTOCYTOSIS

Mastocytosis is an uncommon disorder characterized by aggregates of mast cells in the skin and, occasionally, the internal organs.

Urticaria pigmentosa

Urticaria pigmentosa is the accumulation of mast cells in pigmented lesions of the skin that appear as yellowish brown to reddish brown macules and papules and, occasionally, as nodules. The lesions may be few or numerous, scattered discretely or forming large coalescent areas. Sometimes they are present at birth, but they appear usually within the first year of life, infrequently later in childhood, and rarely after puberty. The condition clears spontaneously, and pigmentation disappears in most cases by midadolescence but sometimes may persist into adult life. When lesions appear for the first time in adult life, they are less likely to undergo spontaneous regression. The lesions of urticaria pigmentosa are located mainly on the trunk, but they also occur on the extremities and to a lesser extent on the head and neck. The palms and soles are not involved, and lesions are rarely found on mucous membranes.

Firm stroking or rubbing of the lesions causes them to urticate (Darier's sign). Vesicles and bullae containing clear fluid may develop at sites of mast cell infiltrates in the skin of children. This tendency for vesiculation may persist for a few years but is not found in older people with urticaria pigmentosa.

Mastocytoma

Mastocytoma is a mast cell infiltrate occurring usually as a solitary nodule in infancy. Sometimes a few lesions may appear on the trunk, neck, or forearm. Rubbing the lesion sometimes produces systemic symptoms (flushing and colic) caused by the release of histamine. Mastocytomas may occur in bones of adults (see systemic mastocytosis).

Telangiectasia macularis eruptiva perstans

Telangiectasia macularis eruptiva perstans (TMEP) is a rare presentation of mastocytosis that occurs primarily in adults and seldom in children. Numerous hyperpigmented telangiectatic macules appear mainly on the trunk and sometimes on the extremities. Telangiectasia is notable in the lesions, and severe erythema occurs. Dermatographism and urtication on rubbing (Darier's sign) are present along with pruritus. Patients with TMEP may have an increased incidence of peptic ulcer disease, and at times bone lesions may be caused by focal collections of mast cells.

Diffuse infiltrative cutaneous mastocytosis

Diffuse infiltrative cutaneous mastocytosis (DICM) is a rare condition in which almost the entire skin is infiltrated with mast cells, giving a doughy, boggy, thickened appearance. The leathery and lichenified skin is caused by enormous aggregates of small papules on the surface of the skin. A diffuse erythroderma may involve the entire body. Mild trauma produces blistering, and generalized intense pruritus and flushing may occur.

Systemic mastocytosis (extracutaneous)

Systemic mastocytosis implies infiltrates of mast cells occurring in organs other than the skin. It is most often associated with urticaria pigmentosa and DICM, but in rare instances it may occur without cutaneous lesions. Bone, liver, spleen, and the gastrointestinal tract are most often involved; the brain and central nervous system are not affected. Bone involvement is uncommon in children but occurs in up to 30% of older patients with systemic mastocytosis. It is seen roentgenographically as osteoporosis and osteosclerosis. Mastocytomas account for approximately 25% of bone lesions; there may be associated bone pain. Mast cell infiltrates of the liver generally do not cause symptoms, but hepatomegaly and fibrosis may occur. Splenomegaly may also be caused by collections of mast cells. Infiltration of mast cells in the small bowel is not usually associated with symptoms but occasionally may result in malabsorption.

Most patients with mastocytosis are asymptomatic; about one third have pruritus or flushing. The degranulation of mast cells in large quantities with a release of histamine may result in symptoms of headache, flushing, pruritus, dizziness, diarrhea, nausea and vomiting, cardiac palpitations and tachycardia, hypotension, syncope, and even shock. This can be induced in several ways, including vigorous rubbing of skin; extremely hot or cold baths; exercise; ingesting spicy foods, cheese, or alcohol; and ingesting or injecting certain drugs, including codeine, morphine, aspirin, atropine, polymyxin B, and radiopaque dyes. Heparin release from mast cells may account for the purpuric appearance of some of the skin lesions. Rare instances of mast cell leukemia or lymphoma have been reported.

Mastocytosis occurs in all races, but most cases reported have been in whites; males and females are equally affected. Because some cases have appeared in familial patterns, heritable factors have been suggested, but most instances of mastocytosis are single events and genetic transmission is therefore unlikely.

Since most cases of mastocytosis regress spontaneously, the need for intervention is minimal. Solitary mastocytomas may be excised if troublesome to patients. Systemic mastocytosis tends to persist. The management is usually symptomatic, with reliance on antihistamines, antiserotonin agents, and the avoidance of foods, drugs, and activities that may produce pruritus and flushing.

ORAL MANIFESTATIONS. Mucosal lesions are rare and cannot be definitely diagnosed without a biopsy. If the patient has systemic signs, especially skin lesions, one may assume the diagnosis. The lesion generally appears pigmented, suggesting a hematoma. Lesions more often appear on the face.

In systemic mastocytosis a facial flush may suggest systemic involvement. Patients may report histamine headache, which they may confuse as being of dental origin. Bone lesions may occur throughout the skeleton, especially in marrow spaces. Roentgenographically, lesions appear stippled with areas of sclerotic and lytic changes. Generalized osteoporosis and os-

teosclerosis and pathologic fractures have been reported. Although involvement of the skull has been mentioned, no specific findings in the jaws have been reported, and a biopsy is indicated. Histopathology of bone lesions shows rapid bone turnover with a mast cell infiltrate (mostly round cells but some spindle and stellate forms), amorphous material, and a woven bone pattern under polarized light. Eosinophilia has also been reported. Lymph node involvement may confuse the diagnosis and can suggest myelofibrosis, myeloproliferative process, or malignancy.

DENTAL MANAGEMENT. Once a diagnosis is made, the major problem may be the patients' hypotension and headaches associated with systemic involvement. Antihistamines may help control the headaches. Caution should be used with drugs that may precipitate histamine release, such as codeine (meperidine appears safe) and aspirin. Events such as extreme temperature changes should be monitored. Careful roentgenographic analysis can reveal possible complications to surgical procedures. Although such complications are unlikely, the surgeon and anesthesiologist must be aware of them. Histamine release, even in patients with asymptomatic cutaneous disease, has been reported to cause severe reactions, including cardiovascular collapse and death. No evidence of inhalation anesthesia causing histamine release has been found, but halothane may increase the hypotension. Prophylactic antihistamine therapy has been suggested for trauma procedures and surgery.

BIBLIOGRAPHY

Brogan H and others: Urticaria pigmentosa (mastocytosis), Acta Med Scand 163:223, 1959.

Caplan RM: Urticaria pigmentosa and systemic mastocytosis, JAMA 194:1077, 1965.

Cryer PE and Kissane JM: Systemic mastocytosis, Am J Med 61:671, 1978.

Demis DJ: The mastocytosis syndrome: clinical and biochemical studies, Ann Intern Med 59:194, 1963.

Fine JD: Mastocytosis, Int J Dermatol 19:117, 1980.

Fishman RS, Fleming CR, and Li CY: Systemic mastocytosis: with review of gastrointestinal manifestations, Mayo Clin Proc 54:51, 1979.

Gagnon JH and others: Mastocytosis—unusual manifestations: clinical and radiologic changes, Can Med Assoc J 112:1329, 1975.

Gerrard JW and Ko C: Urticaria pigmentosa: treatment with cimetidine and chlorpheniramine, J Pediatr 94:843, 1979.

Hills E and others: Bone metabolism in systemic mastocytosis, J Bone Joint Surg 63A:665, 1981.

Klaus SN and Winkelman RK: Course of urticaria pigmentosa in children, Arch Dermatol 86:68, 1962.

Leder LD: Subtle clues to diagnosis by histochemistry in mast cell disease, Am J Dermatopathol 1:261, 1979.

Lennert K and Parwaresch MR: Mast cell neoplasia: a review, Histopathology 3:349, 1979.

Roberts LG II and others: Shock syndrome associated with mastocytosis: pharmacologic reversal of the acute episode and therapeutic prevention of recurrent attacks, Adv Shock Res 8:145, 1982.

Sagher F and Evan-Paz Z: Mastocytosis and the mast cell, Chicago, 1967, Year Book Medical Publishers, Inc.

Soter NA and Austen FA: The diversity of mast cell derived mediators: implications for acute, subacute, and chronic cutaneous inflammatory disorders, J Invest Dermatol 67:313, 1976.

Soter NA and others: Oral disodium cromoglycate in the treatment of systemic mastocytosis, N Engl J Med 301:465, 1979.

Turk J and others: Intervention with epinephrine in hypotension associated with mastocytosis, J Allergy Clin Immunol 71:189, 1983.

Webb TA and others: Systemic mast cell disease: a clinical and hematopathologic study of 26 cases, Cancer 49:927, 1982.

Yam LT and others: Eosinophilia in systemic mastocytosis, Am J Clin Pathol 73:48, 1980.

SARCOIDOSIS

Sarcoidosis (Boeck's sarcoid) is a granulomatous (reticular) disorder of unknown cause that involves the skin and internal organs, including the lungs, mediastinal and peripheral lymph nodes, myocardium, liver, spleen, kidneys, central nervous system, eyes, lacrimal and parotid glands, and phalangeal bones.

The disease usually has its onset in early adult life, progressing insidiously, and generally following a persistent course marked by remissions and relapses. The typical patient in the United States is a black female 20 to 40 years of age. The cutaneous manifestations are diverse; papules, nodules, plaques, and tumors may appear anywhere on the skin surface. The lesions are usually multiple, firm but slightly elastic to the touch, and involve the entire dermis. The overlying epidermis is somewhat thinned with red to purple or brownish discoloration. Alopecia has been associated with scalp lesions.

In generalized sarcoidosis a number of papules or small nodules may occur on the face, eyelids, neck, and shoulders. They may be lichenified and show central pitting; this is known as miliary sarcoid. Over time these papules may gradually involute into faint macular lesions. They must be differentiated from syringoma, trichoepithelioma, xanthelasma, and lichen planus.

Moderately large plaques, called Hutchinson's plaques, typically appear symmetrically on the arms, shoulders, thighs, and buttocks. These plaques are slightly elevated with a flat, nodular, or lobulated surface.

Lupus pernio is characterized by persistent smooth, shiny, violaceous plaques that may appear on the forehead and cheeks and other acral areas, including the nose, ears, toes, and fingers. Lupus pernio seems to have a predilection for women over 40 years of age and is associated with chronic fibrotic sarcoidosis of various other organ systems. Lupus pernio is also frequently associated with sarcoidosis of the upper respiratory tract and granulomas of the bones, which are seen roentgenographically as "punched-out" cysts, especially in the distal phalanges. Patients often have nasal ulcerations and septal perforations, lacrimal gland involvement, chronic uveitis, and advanced intrathoracic pulmonary disease progressing to chronic fibrotic pulmonary sarcoidosis.

When polyarthralgias or polyarthritis, erythema nodosum, bilateral hilar adenopathy, and occasionally uveitis either precedes or accompanies cutaneous lesions of sarcoidosis, this combination of findings is known as Löfgren's syndrome. It frequently occurs in young women, especially during pregnancy or in puerperium. The tender, red nodules generally appear on the face, extensor surfaces of the upper and lower extremities, and upper part of the back. Fever, weight loss, fatigue, and malaise may accompany these findings.

Ocular involvement, mainly as granulomatous uveitis, occurs in approximately 35% of patients. Patients may also have nodular lesions of the iris (keratotic "mutton fat" precipitates) and lesions of the sclera, retina, choroid, and optic nerve. The lacrimal gland may show painless, nodular swelling unilaterally or bilaterally. There may be associated involvement of the submaxillary salivary glands or the parotid glands (Sjögren-like syndrome or Mickulicz's syndrome). Uveitis with fever and enlargement of the parotid gland (and other salivary glands) along with facial nerve palsy (Bell's palsy) is known as uveoparotid fever or Heerfordt's syndrome. This may last from 2 to 6 months and frequently occurs with pulmonary hilar lymphadenopathy and central nervous system sarcoidosis.

Only 25% of patients have visible conjunctival lesions of sarcoidosis; however, conjunctival sarcoidal granulomas may be present without clinically evident conjunctival disease. Many authorities now believe that a biopsy of the conjunctiva is a safe outpatient procedure with low morbidity and high diagnostic yield even with no clinical evidence of conjunctival sarcoidosis. This makes biopsy a readily available diagnostic tool, especially in patients difficult to diagnose.

Sharply delineated plaques with psoriasiform scaling may occur on the trunk and extremities. Sarcoid lesions resembling keloids may develop in old scars of various causes (burns, surgery, or trauma). No pathophysiologic explanation exists for this scar phenomenon, but it may be the manifestation of the hypersensitivity state found in patients with sarcoidosis and an indication of circulating immune complexes. Subcutaneous calcium deposits, prurigo, alopecia, and erythema multiforme also have been associated with sarcoidosis.

Deep-seated nodules 1 to 3 cm in diameter may occur on the trunk and extremities. They are subcutaneous but are attached to the overlying skin, which may be slightly violaceous. This form is known as Darier-Roussy sarcoid.

The characteristic histologic finding is a "naked tubercle" consisting of large, pale-staining epithelioid cells, with histiocytes, lymphocytes, and Langhans' giant cells but without evidence of caseation. In longstanding lesions, the cellular inclusions (Schaumann's and asteroid bodies) occur. Neither is specific for sarcoidosis, but both are found within the giant cells. Schaumann's bodies are concentric, laminated, basophilic, aggregated spherules, and asteroid bodies appear as a central core surrounded by radiating spicules ("open umbrella frame").

Immunologic abnormalities of sarcoidosis are of two types: a depressed in vivo cell-mediated immunity (CMI) and a significant hyperreactivity of humoral immunity.

Delayed hypersensitivity (CMI) reactions are impaired, causing skin test anergy to various intradermal allergens (*Trychophyton* and *Candida*, mumps, pertussis, PPD tuberculin) and an inability to induce contact sensitization to potent sensitizers such as dinitrochlorobenzene (DNCB). This effect is also shown in the high helper-T–cell/suppresor-T–cell activity in sarcoid-affected tissue. Other associated features are the increased activity of killer (K) and natural killer (NK) lymphocytes and the possible correlation between K-cell activity and elevated serum angiotensin I–converting enzyme (SACE) levels and lysozyme activity. Used as a prognostic parameter and not for diagnosis, SACE is elevated in approximately 60% of patients with active sarcoidosis and about 10% with other diseases. Therefore one can monitor a patient's therapeutic progress by measuring SACE levels because it fluctuates with disease activity.

A delayed granulomatous response to intracutaneous injection of sarcoidosis tissue extracts occurs; this is the basis of the Kveim test. After 4 to 6 weeks the inoculated area is excised and examined microscopically. In patients with active sarcoidosis, typical epithelioid "naked" granulomas are seen in the previously inoculated tissue; however, with persistent and chronic sarcoidosis, the Kveim test becomes less sensitive and granulomas are difficult to discern. Because of false positive and false negative reactions, and the difficulty in obtaining and processing the Kveim antigen, this test has been abandoned in the routine diagnostic workup of suspected sarcoidosis.

The other immunologic aspect of sarcoidosis is its ability to enhance humoral immunity with elevated immunoglobulin levels and a nonspecific increase in circulating antibody titers, an indication of chronic, persistent sarcoidosis. This hypergammaglobulinemia is present in at least 80% of patients with sarcoidosis, with elevated IgG, IgA, and IgM most often found. Therefore, immediate-type reactions are usually unimpaired.

Circulating immune complexes recently have been found in more than 50% of patients with acute sarcoidosis, especially those who also have erythema nodosum, uveitis, polyarthritis, bilateral hilar lymphadenopathy, and an elevated erythrocyte sedimentation rate (ESR). These immune complexes are thought to activate the complement system, which is reflected in decreased levels of serum complement. Moreover, elevated levels of ESR may be an indicator of immune complex activity.

The treatment of the systemic disease is with judicious use of corticosteroids. The skin lesions typically respond to topical and intralesional corticosteroid administration. Occasionally, systemic corticosteroid therapy may be required for extensive or disfiguring skin lesions.

ORAL MANIFESTATIONS. The usual finding in the head and neck of patients with sarcoidosis is involvement of salivary glands and lymph nodes. Although oral lesions have been reported, few have been proved. In one review, only 12 mucosal lesions and 16 intraoral minor salivary gland lesions were documented. Mucosal lesions resemble lesions of other granulomatous processes and often mimic cancer. They are often slightly raised, maculopapular lesions varying in color from pale to reddish, often nontender, occasionally coalescing into a plaque, and possibly ulcerated. They are typically located on the hard palate, uvula, and faucial pillars.

The salivary gland lesions appear more often in the major glands, as mentioned earlier. Bilateral involvement may occur. Glandular involvement may lead to various degrees of xerostomia. Mucosal dryness, atrophy, and burning may follow in severe cases of xerostomia. Parotid and lacrimal involvement is part of Heerfordt's syndrome.

Although bone lesions are not common, they do occur. They are generally cystlike lytic areas with intact periosteum and thinning of medullary trabecular areas. They often appear diffuse without obvious cause and with loss of lamina dura. The lesions may cause tooth mobility and delayed or abnormal healing at extraction sites. Resolution may occur after the patient is treated systemically.

DENTAL MANAGEMENT. The major concerns during dental treatment are the effect of steroid therapy and the extent of systemic involvement. Supplemental steroids may be needed during treatment, and any alterations in the tissue response must be watched. Topical steroids may benefit patients with rare symptomatic lesions. In those with severe xerostomia an artificial saliva solution is helpful, especially when removable prosthetics are indicated. The clinician should avoid endodontics and extractions if the teeth are asymptomatic and vital despite lytic areas because the cystic areas may be of sarcoid origin. Nonspecific oral lesions should be confirmed by a biopsy.

BIBLIOGRAPHY

Austen KD: Biologic implications of the structural and functional characteristics of the chemical mediators of immediate hypersensitivity, Harvey Lect 73:93, 1979.

Betten B and Koppany HS: Sarcoidosis with mandibular involvement of the mandibular condyle, J Oral Surg 34:1026, 1976.

Caruthers B and others: Sarcoidosis: a comparison of cutaneous manifestations with chest radiographic changes, J Natl Med Assoc 67:364, 1975.

Cohen C and others: Systemic sarcoidosis: report of two cases with oral lesions, J Oral Surg 39:613, 1981.

Crystal RG and others: Pulmonary sarcoidosis: a disease characterized and perpetuated by activated lung T-lymphocytes, Ann Intern Med 94:73, 1981.

Daniele RR and others: Immune complexes in sarcoidosis, Chest 74:261, 1978.

Delaney P: Neurological manifest actions in sarcoidosis, Ann Intern Med 87:336, 1977.

Fanburg BL and others: Elevated serum angiotensin I converting enzyme in sarcoidosis, Am Rev Respir Dis 114:525, 1976.

Fong KF and Israel CW: Conjunctival biopsy in the diagnosis of sarcoidosis, South Med J 72:124, 1979.

Goodwin JS and others: Suppressor cell function in sarcoidosis, Ann Intern Med 90:169, 1979.

Greer KE, Harman LE, and Kayne AL: Unusual cutaneous manifestations of sarcoidosis, South Med J 70:666, 1977.

Hamner JE and Scofield HH: Cervical lymphadenopathy and parotid gland swelling in sarcoidosis: a study of 31 cases, J Am Dent Assoc 74:1224, 1967.

Israel HL: The treatment of sarcoidosis, Postgrad Med J 46:537, 1970.

Israel HL: Sarcoidosis, malignancy and immunosuppressive therapy, Arch Intern Med 138:907, 1978.

James DG and Jones WW: Immunology of sarcoidosis, Am J Med 72:5, 1982.

James DG and Jones WW: Sarcoidosis and other granulomatous disorders, Philadelphia, 1985, WB Saunders Co.

James DG and Neville E: Pathobiology of sarcoidosis, Pathobiol Annu 7:31, 1977.

James DG, Neville E, and Walker A: Immunology of sarcoidosis, Am J Med 59:388, 1975.

James DG and others: A worldwide review of sarcoidosis, Ann NY Acad Sci 278:321, 1976.

Kantor FS, Dwyer JM, and Mangi RJ: Sarcoid, J Invest Dermatol 67:470, 1976.

Lieberman J: Elevation of serum angiotensin-converting-enzyme (ACE) level in sarcoidosis, Am J Med 59:365, 1975.

Mayock RL and others: Manifestations of sarcoidosis: analysis of 145 patients with a review of nine series selected from the literature, Am J Med 35:67, 1963.

Neville E, Carstairs LS, and James DG: Sarcoidosis of bone, Q J Med 46:215, 1977.

Neville E and others: Sarcoidosis of the upper respiratory tract and its association with lupus pernio, Thorax 31:660, 1976.

Nosal A and others: Angiotensin-I-converting enzymes and gallium scan in noninvasive evaluation of sarcoidosis, Ann Intern Med 90:328, 1979.

Obenauf CD and others: Sarcoidosis and its ophthalmic manifestations, Am J Ophthalmol 86:648, 1978.

Orlian AI and Birnbaum M: Intra-oral localized sarcoid lesion, Oral Surg 49:341, 1980.

Scadding JG and Mitchell DN: Sarcoidosis, ed 2, London, 1985, Chapman & Hall.

Sharma OP: Sarcoidosis: a clinical approach, Springfield, Ill, 1985, Charles C Thomas, Publisher.

Siltzbach LE: Sarcoidosis: clinical features and management, Med Clin North Am 51:483, 1967.

Siltzbach LE and others: Course and prognosis of sarcoidosis around the world, Am J Med 57:847, 1974.

Solomon DA and others: The diagnosis of sarcoidosis by conjunctival biopsy, Chest 74:271, 1978.

Studdy PR and others: Biochemical findings in sarcoidosis, J Clin Pathol 33:528, 1980.

Thomas RG and Merkow L: Sarcoidosis with involvement of the mandibular condyle, J Oral Surg 34:1026, 1976.

Tillman HH and others: Sarcoidosis of the tongue: report of a case, Oral Surg 21:190, 1966.

Wurm K and Rosner R: Prognosis of chronic sarcoidosis, Ann NY Acad Sci 278:732, 1976.

ANGIOKERATOMA CORPORIS DIFFUSUM UNIVERSALE (FABRY'S DISEASE)

Angiokeratoma corporis diffusum universale (Fabry's disease) is characterized by minute, black to bluish black ectatic vascular papules varying from pinpoint size to 3 or 4 mm and sometimes surmounted by a fine keratotic scale. The lesions may be flat or slightly raised, but they do not blanch with pressure. They are generally concentrated between the umbilicus and the knees, usually in clusters of variously sized papules. The angiokeratomas appear in the thousands and tend to aggregate in the lumbosacral region; on the hips, buttocks, thighs, and knees; in the umbilicus; and on the scrotum and penis. Groups of punctate angiectatic lesions may occur on the lips, gingiva, buccal mucosa, palate, and conjunctiva, as well as on the lower extremities and around the elbows and nails. Patients also have involvement of the gastrointestinal, respiratory, and genitourinary tracts. The face, scalp, and ears are not affected.

Fabry's disease, inherited as an X-linked disorder of glycosphingolipid metabolism, is the result of the defective activity of the lysosomal enzyme, α-galactosidase A (ceramide trihexosidase). Because of this enzymatic defect, two neutral glycosphingolipids, designated as globotriaosyl ceramide (Gal-Gal-Glc-Cer) and galabiosyl ceramide (Gal-Gal-Cer), gradually accumulate in most visceral tissues and body fluids. They affect smooth, striated and cardiac muscle fibers; renal tubules and glomeruli; connective tissue cells of the cornea; ganglion and perineural cells of the autonomic nervous system; histiocytes; and vascular endothelial cells. This lysosomal storage in vascular endothelium, mainly of the ceramide trihexoside Gal-Gal-Glc-Cer, causes clinical disease when its accumulation leads to luminal narrowing with resultant organ ischemia and infarction. The deposits of glycosphingolipids are birefringent and demonstrate a "Maltese cross" configuration when examined under polarized light.

Because Fabry's disease is an X-linked familial disorder, the complete expression of the disease spectrum occurs only in the hemozygous male. The characteristic angiectatic lesions of angiokeratomas usually begin to appear in late childhood or early adolescence. The onset of pain, the hallmark of Fabry's disease, occurs at about the same time but may be delayed until the second or third decade of life. The hemozygous male may experience two types of pain. The episodic type of agonizing, burning pain initially begins in the palms and soles, then radiates proximally and to other parts of the body. This "Fabry crisis" can last from a few minutes to several days. Fabry crisis may be triggered by emotional stress, exercise, and fatigue, or rapid changes in temperature and humidity and may produce acute abdominal or flank pain or even renal colic. These crises may be accompanied by a low-grade fever and an elevated ESR.

The other type of pain experienced by most patients with Fabry's disease is a constantly burning, tingling paresthesia of the hands and feet. These acroparesthesias may occur daily and exacerbate later in the day.

Patients with Fabry's disease also have diminished sweating with heat intolerance; cataracts and corneal opacities; tortuous retinal and conjunctival vessels with sausage-link constrictions and dilations; diarrhea and proctocolitis; fever; signs of central nervous system involvement that are sometimes transient, such as tremor, paresis, paresthesias, unconsciousness, and aphasia; occasionally arthritis of the distal interphalangeal joints; and edema of the ankles. Death generally results from renal insufficiency with uremia; other causes are hypertension, cerebrovascular accidents, and cardiac disease with congestive heart failure. Death usually occurs in the fourth or fifth decade of life.

Heterozygous females, as carriers of the disease trait, have only mild or no features of the disease; they sometimes have skin lesions or cataracts and usually a normal life span.

Laboratory findings include albuminuria. The urinary sediment reveals large "mulberry cells" containing doubly refractile glycolipid granules. Polaroscopy reveals the characteristic birefringent Maltese cross lipid globules. These findings may also occur in the bone marrow.

No specific treatment is known. Therapy is usually supportive, aimed at relieving pain and treating associated renal, cardiac, and cerebrovascular problems. Recently, diphenylhydantoin alone or in combination with carbamazepine has been beneficial in alleviating some of the pain experienced by the affected hemozygous males and the symptomatic heterozygous females.

ORAL MANIFESTATIONS. Lesions may occur on the lips, buccal mucosa, and soft palate. They appear as punctate lesions or bluish red linear and reticular telangiectases. No oromucosal involvement has been reported in the female carrier. Individual angiokeratomas unrelated to Fabry's disease have been reported; one was a large, spontaneously regressing angiokeratoma of the palate.

DENTAL MANAGEMENT. Although the vascular lesions may resemble the telangiectases seen in hereditary hemorrhagic telangiectasia, they present no major problem if caution is taken to prevent hemorrhage. Treatment is similar to that for hemangiomas with use of sclerosing solutions and cautery. Hypertension is common, as are vascular effects in the kidney and heart, which lead to uremia and possible heart disease. Central nervous system involvement may cause tremors and paresthesia.

BIBLIOGRAPHY

Archard HO and Brindley HP: Ultrastructural observations of the oral mucosa in Anderson-Fabry disease, J Oral Pathol 4:273, 1975.

Arm RN and others: A recurrent intraoral vascular lesion: abstract presentation, Am Assoc Oral Pathol April 1975.

Calhoun DH and others: Fabry disease: isolation of a CDNA clone encoding human α-galactosidase A, Proc Natl Acad Sci USA 82:7364, 1985.

Danehower CC and Moyer DG: Angiokeratoma corporis diffusum, Arch Dermatol 94:628, 1966.

DeGroot WP: Angiokeratoma corporis diffusum Fabry, Dermatologica 128:321, 1964.

Desnick RJ and Sweely C: Fabry's disease: defective α-galactosidase A. In Standbury JB and others, editors: Metabolic basis of inherited disease, ed 5, New York, 1983, McGraw-Hill Book Co.

Desnick RJ and others: Enzymatic diagnosis of hemozygotes and heterozygotes: Fabry's disease, J Lab Clin Med 81:157, 1973.

Desnick RJ and others: Enzyme therapy. XII. Enzyme therapy in Fabry's disease: differential enzyme and substrate clearance kinetics of plasma and splenic α-galactosidase isozymes, Proc Natl Acad Sci USA 76:5326, 1979.

Gorlin RJ and Goldman HM: Thoma's oral pathology, St Louis, 1970, The CV Mosby Co.

Gorlin RJ and Sedano HO: Stomatologic aspects of cutaneous diseases: angiokeratoma corporis diffusum (Fabry's syndrome), J Dermatol Surg Oncol 5:180, 1979.

Hayen DO: Thrombosed angiokeratoma simulating malignant melanoma, Arch Dermatol 93:358, 1966.

Johnson DL and Desnick RJ: Molecular pathology of Fabry's disease: physical and kinetic properties of alpha galactosidase A in cultured human endothelial cells, Biochem Biophys Acta 538:195, 1978.

Kint JA: Fabry's disease, α-galactosidase deficiency, Science 167:1268, 1970.

Lockman LA and others: Relief of pain of Fabry's disease by diphenylhydantoin, Neurology 23:871, 1973.

Orpitz JM and others: The genetics of angiokeratoma corporis diffusum (Fabry's disease) and its linkage relations with the X_2 locus, Am J Hum Genet 17:335, 1965.

VonGemmingen GR and others: Angiokeratoma corporis diffusum (Fabry's disease), Arch Dermatol 91:206, 1965.

Wise D and others: Angiokeratoma corporis diffusum: a clinical study of 8 affected families, QJ Med 31:177, 1962.

164 · CUTANEOUS SIGNS OF INTERNAL MALIGNANCY

Shelley S. Schuler

Numerous signs occur in the skin that can alert the practitioner to the possibility of internal malignancy. These range from direct cutaneous metastases to remote effects of the tumor or paraneoplastic syndromes. The more common signs are discussed here.

Cutaneous metastases occur with several internal malignancies; lung, gastrointestinal, breast, and ovarian carcinomas and melanomas are the most frequent. The metastatic lesions may be nodular, papular, or plaquelike; they may be single or multiple. Usually they are identified by performing a biopsy when the diagnosis of the skin condition is in question. The lesions may overlie the tumor or occur at a distant site. Breast cancer is the most common underlying malignancy, followed by cancer of the stomach, lung, uterus, and kidney.

Acquired ichthyosis is most frequently associated with lymphomas and Hodgkin's disease, but it has been reported with multiple myeloma, carcinoma of the breast and cervix, and oat cell carcinoma of lung. Ichthyosis may appear as generalized dryness or may resemble the fish scales of the inherited ichthyosis vulgaris. Liver damage with subsequent impairment of vitamin A metabolism may contribute to the ichthyosis.

Intense, generalized, recalcitrant pruritus is a well-recognized symptom of Hodgkin's disease. Severe pruritus may indicate a poor prognosis. Intractable itching of the nose has been reported in patients with brain tumors.

Paget's disease of the nipple and areola is a well-known indicator of underlying breast cancer. It appears as an eczematous area that does not respond to therapy. An underlying breast tumor is always found in the ipsilateral breast and occasionally in the contralateral breast as well.

Extramammary Paget's disease of the genital area is also associated with malignancies, usually in nearby anatomic sites, such as the prostate, apocrine glands, rectum, uretha, Bartholin's glands, and cervix.

Acquired hypertrichosis lanuginosa, "malignant down," is linked to internal malignancy such as carcinoma of the bronchus, gallbladder, colon, rectum, uterus, or urinary bladder. It is characterized by the sudden appearance of fine, silky, lanugo-like hair on the face and eventually the whole body. The development of the hair may precede the malignancy by several years.

The Leser-Trélat sign is the relatively sudden development of numerous seborrheic keratoses with pruritus. This sign, which occurs with gastrointestinal malignancies, is very rare and requires careful interpretation, since multiple seborrheic keratoses commonly develop in the absence of cancer.

Erythema gyratum repens may resemble a wood grain or knotty pine. It is associated with carcinoma of the breast and oat cell tumors of the lung. Festooned lesions appear on the trunk and extremities.

Migratory thrombophlebitis is linked to carcinoma of the pancreas and other types of malignancies.

Torre's syndrome (sebaceous adenomas) should suggest an underlying gastrointestinal malignancy, usually of the colon. The lesions are multiple, occurring on the trunk as smooth, elevated, pedunculated tumors. These patients have a good prognosis, considering that many of them have multiple primary cancers. These cancers are usually low grade malignancy and often respond well to radiation therapy. Whenever a sebaceous adenoma is removed, a more complete history and a further search are needed to rule out visceral disease.

The so-called malignant form of acanthosis nigricans is always associated with an underlying malignancy. Adenocarcinomas of the stomach, gastrointestinal tract, lung, ovary, breast, and prostate have been found. It has also been seen in patients with lymphoma and Hodgkin's disease. The lesions in the malignant form are severe and widespread. Patients may have palmar thickening. Mucosal involvement occurs in more than 50% of patients. Lesions may precede the finding of malignancy by several years. Treatment of the underlying cause leads to resolution of the acanthosis nigricans.

Subcutaneous nodular fat necrosis occurs in 2% to 3% of patients with pancreatitis and pancreatic carcinoma. Subcutaneous nodules develop in the pretibial regions and rarely on the scalp, arms, and face. The nodules may be asymptomatic. Liquefaction degeneration may occur with resultant discharge of an oily liquid. Synovitis of the small joints, causing poly-

arthritis, has been reported. The syndrome is probably caused by the release of pancreatic lipases that reach the fat by way of lymphatics.

In the glucagonoma syndrome, necrolytic migratory erythema is associated with a pancreatic α-islet cell tumor that secretes glucagon. The skin manifestations consist of gyrate and circinate erythemas that involve the trunk, groin, perineum, and limbs and undergo necrosis with scarring. Perioral erythema and crusting and a red tongue are also present. New lesions develop as old lesions heal. Weight loss, diabetes, refractory anemia, diarrhea, and venous thrombosis are other features of the syndrome. Most patients are postmenopausal women. The condition responds to removal of the tumor. It is important to recognize this disease, since the tumor is potentially curable.

BIBLIOGRAPHY

Andree VC and Petkov I: Skin manifestations associated with tumors of the brain, Br J Dermatol 92:675, 1975.

Binnick A and others: Glucagonoma syndrome, Arch Dermatol 113:749, 1977.

Braverman IM: Skin signs of systemic disease, Philadelphia, 1981, WB Saunders Co.

Brownstein MH and Helwig EB: Metastatic tumors of the skin, Cancer 29:1298, 1972.

Brownstein MH and Helwig EB: Patterns of cutaneous metastases, Arch Dermatol 105:862, 1972.

Curth HO and others: The site and histology of the cancers associated with malignant acanthosis nigricans, Cancer 15:364, 1962.

Feiner AS and others: Prognostic importance of pruritus in Hodgkin's disease, JAMA 240:2738, 1978.

Holt P and Davis M: Erythema gyratum repens, Br J Dermatol 96:343, 1977.

Leonard DD and Deaton WR: Multiple sebaceous gland tumors and visceral carcinomas, Arch Dermatol 110:917, 1974.

Liddel K and others: Seborrheic keratoses and carcinoma of the large bowel, Br J Dermatol 92:449, 1975.

Mallinson CN and others: A glucagonoma syndrome, Lancet 2:1, 1974.

Rosenberg FW: Cutaneous manifestations of internal malignancy, Cutis 20:227, 1977.

Roulon DB and Helwig EB: Multiple sebaceous neoplasms of the skin, Am J Clin Pathol 60:745, 1973.

Sibrack LA and Gouterman IH: Cutaneous manifestations of pancreatic disease, Cutis 21:703, 1978.

Swanson K and others: The glucagonoma syndrome, Arch Dermatol 114:224, 1978.

165 · NEOPLASMS OF THE SKIN

Anthony V. Benedetto *and* **Robert N. Arm**

Cutaneous neoplasia can be categorized as benign, premalignant, and malignant. Often the manifestations and prognosis are different when the lesions occur on the skin as opposed to the mucous membranes. The neoplasia of the mouth are presented separately from their associated skin lesions.

BENIGN NEOPLASMS

Benign neoplasms are isolated new growths consisting of normal cells. There are many different types of benign neoplastic lesions; their nomenclature depends on their tissue of origin: epidermis, dermis, and dermal appendages; fibrous, vascular, fatty, muscular, osseous, and neural tissues; and the pigmented cells. The following represents only a brief listing of the most frequently encountered benign cutaneous neoplasms, many of which occur on the head and neck.

Seborrheic keratosis

Of the many benign cutaneous tumors, seborrheic keratosis occurs most often. Without any tendency for malignant de-

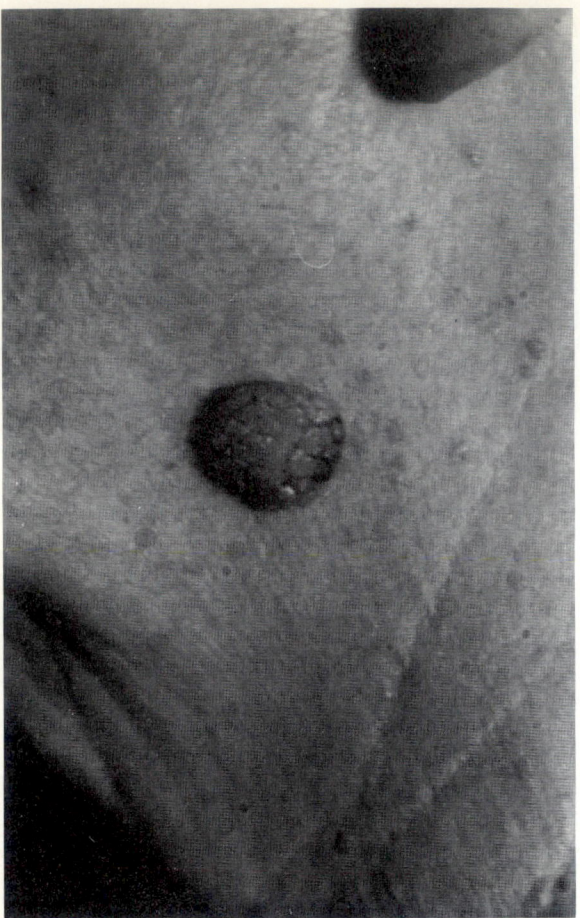

Fig. 165-1   Seborrheic keratosis of neck. Lesion is elevated and nodular with waxy crenated surface.

generation, seborrheic keratosis usually appears as a hyperpigmented, firm but soft, sessile tumor. It may feel waxy, manifesting numerous furrows and keratin-filled, follicle-like openings scattered over its surface, which contributes to its overall verrucous character (Fig. 165-1). The tumor may also appear to be "stuck onto" the surface of the skin, demonstrating distinct margins and a flat surface. These "stucco keratoses" are more often found on patients' distal extremities and occasionally on the trunk and can easily be scraped off with little or no bleeding. The larger sessile type of seborrheic keratosis occasionally yields to the slightest amount of picking or lifting, resulting in moderate bleeding and delayed regrowth.

Seborrheic keratoses more commonly occur in older persons, with equal distribution in males and females. These tumors have little tendency to disappear spontaneously.

Dermatosis papulosa nigra, a variant of seborrheic keratosis, usually appears as multiple lesions over the face and neck in dark skinned individuals and generally affects persons at a younger age than those with seborrheic keratosis. An estimated 35% of all adult blacks have dermatosis papulosa nigra, which seems to be a family trait.

Leser-Trélat sign occurs when a profuse number of pruritic seborrheic keratoses appear rapidly over months, heralding the presence of possible occult malignancy, most often in the gastrointestinal tract.

Seborrheic keratoses are treated with superficial surgical procedures such as cryosurgery, curettage, and chemical cautery or electrocautery. Unnecessary deep surgery should be avoided to ensure the best cosmetic results.

Skin tag

Acrochordon, fibroepithelial papilloma, or soft fibroma—also known as the skin tag—is another common epidermal tumor appearing most frequently in the intertriginous areas of the neck, axillae, and groin. Usually skin colored but occasionally pigmented, these tiny (1 to 5 mm), pedunculated projections of skin are soft but fibrous. Because of their location, they often become traumatized and irritated. Women are affected more often, and these lesions also seem to appear among family members. Frequently occurring with seborrheic keratoses, a skin tag may bleed profusely when severed from its stalk or base. Treatment should be conservative and superficial: snipping with scissors or light electrocauterization.

Epidermal cyst

These slowly growing cysts composed of an epithelial lining may occur anywhere on the body intradermally or subcutaneously. Rarely seen in children, the cyst is filled with a cheesy appearing, often putrid-smelling, keratinous material. Commonly called a "sebaceous cyst" by laypersons, it is also referred to as a "wen" if it affects the scalp. The sebaceous cyst found in various areas of the body (epidermal cyst) can be differentiated microscopically from the sebaceous cyst or wen of the scalp (trichilemmal cyst). The difference between epidermal versus trichilemmal cyst is in the histologic morphology of their cyst walls; clinically they are indistinguishable. Complete excisional extirpation of the cyst sac and its contents is the recommended treatment.

Milium

Milia are tiny (1 to 3 mm), firm, whitish globoid epidermal cysts usually occurring on the face. They are found subepidermally and usually appear and frequently disappear spontaneously. At times surgical extirpation may be necessary. They also may result from trauma or occur as sequelae of various types of subepidermal blistering disease or desquamating processes, such as on the hands in epidermolysis bullosa and porphyria cutanea tarda, as a result of second-degree burns, or after a facial dermabrasion.

Favre-Racouchot syndrome

Nodular yellow elastosis with cysts and open black comedones of Favre-Racouchot may occur over the lateral malar prominences and lateral ocular canthi, especially in elderly men who have been outdoors much of their lives. These hard "blackheads," which are difficult to express, are black because of melanin embedded within the cyst as laminated horny material of lipoid substance, similar to sebum. Yellowish, skin-covered papules, 1 to 5 mm in size, occur among these comedones. Both papules and comedones appear after many years of constant sun exposure, which produce the elastotic changes that occur in the dermis. Treatment is by surgical extirpation of the cyst contents.

Sebaceous hyperplasia

The soft, yellowish pink, flattopped and umbilicated tiny papules (1 to 3 mm) that appear on the forehead and cheeks in middle-aged patients are called sebaceous hyperplasia. These are the result of hamartomatous overgrowth of one or a few sebaceous glands, which, when they appear in large numbers, can be cosmetically disconcerting. Treatment is best accomplished by lightly electrodesiccating the lesions.

Syringoma

Soft, fleshy, skin-colored or slightly yellowish pink flat-topped papules (1 to 5 mm) that appear around the eyelids, especially the lower lids and upper part of the cheeks, mainly in young women are called syringomas. These are thought to be adenomas of the epidermal eccrine ducts, which develop in the upper to middermis. Because of their location within the dermis, complete extirpation with minimal scarring is difficult. However, electrocautery can produce good cosmetic results.

Nevus araneus

The "spider nevus," or nevus araneus, usually appears as a red, slightly raised or flat punctum with several tiny, tortuous blood vessels radiating from its center. Spider nevi most often occur on the face and usually appear spontaneously or as the result of minor trauma, such as a superficial abrasion, ruptured comedonal cyst, or an insect bite. However, other conditions can precipitate their appearance, most notably pregnancy or cirrhosis of the liver. These spider angiomas may then occur on the trunk, usually from the waist up, and on the upper extremities. When they occur during pregnancy, many disappear spontaneously months later. Treatment is best achieved by electrocautery of the central punctum, which causes the remaining radiating vessels to disappear as well.

Granuloma pyogenicum

Usually occurring as a singular, beefy red, soft but firm, slightly pedunculated raised papule, the pyogenic granuloma, or granuloma pyogenicum, may occur anywhere on the body but most often affects the fingers and face. The oral cavity is a common site for this benign tumor, and when it appears on the gingiva during pregnancy, it is known as granuloma gravidarum (pregnancy tumor). Histopathologic studies have shown this lesion to be a capillary hemangioma. Treatment should be surgical excision and electrodesiccation of the base.

Venous lake

Venous lakes appear as dark blue to black, slightly raised and occasionally fluctuant, smooth-surfaced papules 1 to 6 mm in size, which occur most commonly in older patients on exposed skin, especially on the ears and lips. Their cystic contents of blood usually can be drained; if their endothelial lining is destroyed, they disappear without scarring and with minimal therapeutic effort. Venous lakes are not true hemangiomas but a collection of venous blood in dilated vascular spaces.

Lipoma

Lipomas can occur singly or as multiple, subcutaneous nodular growths, which are soft, movable, and usually nontender. The overlying skin is usually normal in appearance. Lipomas vary in size from 1 to 10 cm and even larger when left untreated for many years. They may occur anywhere on the body but more frequently develop on the neck, shoulders, proximal extremities, and trunk. Their presence generally seems not to have any systemic significance. Complete surgical excision is the treatment of choice, especially when a lipoma is enlarging.

Melanocytic neoplasia

Benign melanocytic tumors are composed of one of three types of cells: nevus cells, epidermal melanocytes, or dermal melanocytes.

The nevus cell basically is a melanocyte, the pigment-bearing cell of the skin. Histologically, however, nevus cells can be differentiated from melanocytes when they (1) are grouped in clusters or "nests," (2) demonstrate no dendritic processes (intercellular attachments), and (3) appear morphologically as large, oval or elongated cells that contain a homogeneous cytoplasm with little or no melanin and a large, well-formed nucleus.

The benign neoplasms of the nevus cell are the nevocellular (nevocytic) nevi. Depending on where they are located in the skin, nevocellular nevi are classified as *junctional nevi* (nevus cells at the border of the dermis and epidermis), *compound nevi* (within both the epidermis and the dermis), and *intradermal nevi* (entirely within the dermis).

Nevocytic nevi vary considerably in their clinical presentation, and in general one cannot identify their histopathologic identity by gross clinical examination; only light microscopy can achieve this. Clinically, however, nevi are well circumscribed, round or oval, highly pigmented or skin colored, flat or raised, pedunculated or verrucous, and sessile or papillomatous. Most nevi appear during early childhood, some may be present at birth, and others may develop in adult life. They may occur on any area of the body, even the mucous membranes. Nevi appear as small, pigmented "beauty marks" with or without hair growing out of their center, or they can be so large as to cover half the body surface (giant pigmented hairy nevi). Most congenital and acquired nevocellular nevi are benign; at the first sign of change, however, whether in color, shape, or size, the individual should see a skin specialist promptly.

Epidermal melanocytes are dendritic cells found within the epidermis that biochemically manufacture pigment within their cytoplasm. This elaborate and complicated process, of which melanin is the end product, gives the skin its characteristic color.

The benign neoplasms of the epidermal melanocyte include lentigines, ephelides (freckles), and café au lait spots (see Chapter 156 for discussion of von Recklinghausen's neurofibromatosis and Albright's syndrome).

Ephelides (freckles) are small, hyperpigmented macules on the light-exposed areas of the skin. First seen in very young children after sunlight exposure, freckling intensifies with each subsequent exposure. No treatment is necessary.

Lentigines are benign hyperpigmented macules occurring in the elderly over the sun-exposed areas of the face and extremities, especially the dorsa of the hands. They appear as single or multiple, uniformly brown pigmented lesions with irregular borders, which slowly increase in size with age. Rarely seen before the fourth or fifth decade of life, 90% of all octogenarians have at least one lentigo senilis, or solar lentigo. They vary in size from a few millimeters to centimeters, but malignant degeneration does not occur. This differs from lentigo maligna (see page 816). Commonly referred to as "liver spots," flat seborrheic keratoses (stucco keratoses) and solar lentigines closely resemble each other and only can be differentiated with light microscopy. Treatment is electrodesiccation, chemical cauterization, or superficial cryosurgery with liquid nitrogen.

The benign neoplasms of the dermal melanocyte include the nevi of Ota and Ito and the blue nevus.

The nevi of Ota and Ito are bluish or slate gray to brown, speckled hyperpigmentations usually occurring unilaterally over the face (nevus of Ota) or over the supraclavicular, scapular, and deltoid areas (nevus of Ito). Differing only by location, these dermal melanocytic hyperpigmented nevi may be present at birth or may appear at a later age. They occur bilaterally. Malignant degeneration in these lesions is extremely rare, but patients with malignant melanoma involving the eye and associated with the nevus of Ota have been reported. Along with bluish brown discoloration of the forehead, nose, temple, and periorbital and malar areas, patients may also have a patchy bluish pigmentation of the sclera, cornea, conjunctiva, and retina of the ipsilateral eye. Occasionally the oral and nasal mucosae are similarly hyperpigmented. No effective treatment exists.

The blue nevus is a rare, well-circumscribed, dome-shaped blue to blue-black papule 1 to 10 mm in size. Usually occurring on the extremities, the blue nevus also appears on other parts of the body, including the face, scalp, oral mucosa, vagina, uterine cervix, and prostate. An uncommon variant, the cellular blue nevus, occurs more frequently on the buttocks and may become malignant and metastasize. Treatment consists of prophylactic surgical excision.

PREMALIGNANT LESIONS

Although the cytology of the individual cells that comprise the premalignant lesions is morphologically atypical and malignant, the fact that these atypical cells remain within the surface epidermis makes them biologically benign. Once the atypical cells of these carcinomas in situ breach the epidermal-dermal junction and invade the dermis, they become biologically malignant, thus the term "premalignant."

Of the premalignant lesions common to the skin, actinic keratoses (solar keratoses) occur most frequently. Given a sufficient amount of time and the necessary host response, many of these lesions undergo malignant transformation into invasive epidermoid (squamous cell) carcinoma. Actinic keratoses (formerly designated as senile keratoses) are adherent, hyperkeratotic lesions found on exposed, sun-damaged skin, usually on an erythematous base. They are most often seen in multiple numbers in light-skinned individuals who have obvious weather-beaten (solar elastotic) skin. These lesions have a fine, white scale on their surface that is easily detached from their less well-defined erythematous base, producing punctate areas of bleeding. Histologically the actinic keratosis appears as numerous atypical and dyskeratotic cells with many mitoses in the epidermis. The presence of actinic keratoses is predicated on how much radiation and physicochemical damage an individual's skin has sustained during a lifetime, in addition to the relative susceptibility of the tissues exposed. The total cumulative effect of prolonged and sustained exposure to ultraviolet light is essential in the development of actinic keratoses; other causative but less frequently encountered agents include exposure to ionizing radiation, radiant heat, and pitch and other coal and petroleum distillate by-products.

Because of their tendency to transform into malignant lesions, actinic keratoses should be treated. If there is no invasion of the dermis, treatment by superficial destruction is all that is necessary. This can be accomplished with cryosurgery, curettage, and chemical cautery or electrocautery. Topical application of 5-fluorouracil has proved useful in treating multiple lesions over a large surface area. Prophylaxis can be accomplished by avoidance of excessive and persistent sunbathing and by the routine use of topical sunscreening agents with a sun-protective factor (SPF) of 15 or higher.

Bowen's disease is a less frequently seen type of intraepidermal squamous cell carcinoma in situ. It can occur as a single lesion or as multiple lesions. The possibility of prolonged exposure to arsenicals should be suspected when numerous lesions of Bowen's disease are found, especially if they involve the palms and soles. The lesions occur in areas of the skin not usually exposed to the sun, including the genitalia and perineum. Lesions of Bowen's disease are somewhat more well defined, more hyperkeratotic, and often larger than actinic ker-

atoses but occur much less often. After the keratotic roof is removed from a lesion, the base is usually redder and thicker than that of lesions in actinic keratosis; the lesions may even appear plaquelike or verrucous.

When similar changes of Bowen's disease occur on the male genitalia, particularly the glans penis, the lesion usually is referred to as erythroplasia of Queyrat. This erythroplasia generally appears as a well-circumscribed, erythematous, velvety, often moist and shiny patch or plaque. An excisional biopsy with histologic examination is the only definitive way to differentiate Bowen's disease from other lesions similar in appearance, such as those in Paget's disease or invasive carcinoma, especially when the genitalia are involved.

At one time authorities thought that systemic malignancies occurred more often in patients who had multiple lesions of Bowen's disease, but this concept has been abandoned.

Treatment of Bowen's disease is complete surgical excision, best accomplished by Mohs' technique. In the past, when surgery other than the Mohs' technique was used to treat Bowen's disease, there was a high rate of recurrence. This recurrence in Bowen's disease can be attributed to the frequent involvement of the epithelium of the follicular apparatus, through which the intraepithelial dysplastic changes are carried deep into the dermis instead of remaining relatively superficial.

Melanocytic lesions

Atypical epidermal melanocytes are potentially more aggressive and dangerous and may occur as in situ carcinomas. These include lentigo maligna, superficial malignant melanoma in situ, acral lentiginous malignant melanoma in situ, and congenital melanocytic nevi.

Lentigo maligna is an in situ melanoma appearing on exposed areas of the skin in elderly persons. Usually it appears as an irregularly outlined, macular lesion of various shades of light and dark brown and most often occurs on the face and rarely on the extremities. After many long years of slow development, invasion into the dermis and transformation into a lentigo maligna melanoma are signalled by the appearance of darker brown to black foci of induration. These typically appear when the lentigo maligna has been present for 10 to 15 years and has reached the size of 4 to 6 cm. Invasion also may occur with more recent, smaller lesions. It is postulated that one third of all lentigo malignas develop into lentigo maligna melanoma. The treatment of choice for lentigo maligna is simple excision. Care must be taken with larger lesions, since frequently atypical melanocytes occur deep within the dermis along the basal layer of the external root sheath of hair follicles. For this reason the more precise microscopically controlled excision of the Mohs' micrographic surgical technique is preferred. Curettage and electrodesiccation can be counterproductive. Since superficial radiation therapy has resulted in recurrences of lentigo maligna and in some cases the development of lentigo maligna melanoma, this form of therapy is not recommended.

In contrast, superficial spreading malignant melanoma (SSMM) in situ is found on exposed and unexposed skin in younger adults. It is usually a smaller lesion, less than 2.5 cm, and may be slightly raised. It also has an irregular outline and appears in various shades of brown, black, pink, blue, and gray. Invasion into the dermis occurs more quickly, usually after a few months to years of growth, and this is seen as a developing nodule or ulceration. When found during the very early stages of development, a SSMM in situ may be misdiagnosed as a nevocellular nevus.

Acral lentiginous melanoma in situ is found on the hairless skin of the palms and soles, mucous membranes, and in the ungual and periungal regions. Invasion is particularly aggressive and occurs more rapidly after a short period of in situ growth. More frequently seen in blacks and Orientals, these lesions also occur in the nail matrix, causing longitudinal pigmented bands in the nail bed and plate. They also may appear as macular or slightly nodular lesions on the oral and nasal mucosa or on the mucocutaneous areas of the anogenital region.

Another, although rare, precursor lesion to melanoma is the congenital nevus. There are two types: the giant hairy nevus and the smaller congenital melanocytic nevus. Since both have a tendency to transform into a melanoma at an early age, usually before puberty, extirpation of any changing congenital melanocytic nevus, no matter what size, is recommended.

Recently the dysplastic nevus has been identified as an important marker for malignant melanoma. It is a peculiar-appearing melanocytic nevus, larger (5 to 15 mm) than the average benign melanocytic nevus with an eccentric shape and irregular borders along with an admixture of the colors brown, black, tan, and pink, occurring in various family members of patients with malignant melanoma. On microscopic examination this melanocytic nevus usually is found to be a compound nevus in which many of the individual melanocytes possess atypical nuclei. It was subsequently discovered that many of these "dysplastic nevi" developed into malignant melanoma. Initially designated as the B-K mole syndrome, then the familial atypical multiple mole–melanoma (FAMMM) syndrome, now it is known as the dysplastic nevus syndrome. Dysplastic nevi may continue to appear throughout adult life on covered and exposed areas of the body, and each individual lesion has the potential to transform into malignant melanoma. Not only has the dysplastic nevus been recognized as a marker for an autosomally inherited syndrome, but now it also is recognized as appearing spontaneously in those patients who have had a malignant melanoma or in those at high risk of developing a malignant melanoma. The dysplastic nevus can also be found in normal individuals, who may never develop a malignant melanoma.

Treatment of all precursor or melanoma in situ lesions is complete excision.

MALIGNANT NEOPLASMS

Malignant neoplasms are fast growing, aggressive, locally invasive aberrations of normal tissue growth. Malignant neoplasms can be differentiated from benign neoplasms by various histopathologic characteristics. Malignant tumors are composed of cells that are atypical, with nuclei that vary in size and shape (pleomorphic) and are hyperchromatic and anaplastic. Typically these cells demonstrate a lack of orderly architectural alignment, or a loss of polarity, and the presence of normal and abnormal mitoses.

Basal cell and squamous cell carcinomas and malignant melanomas constitute most malignant neoplasms of the skin. Basal cell carcinoma is the most commonly occurring cutaneous carcinoma, accounting for 85% of skin malignancies; it rarely metastasizes. Squamous cell carcinomas comprise approximately 10% of all skin malignancies and occasionally become aggressive and metastasize. Malignant melanoma, representing 4% to 5% of skin malignancies, is the most lethal and devastating of all skin tumors.

Squamous cell carcinoma

Squamous cell carcinoma (invasive epidermoid carcinoma) is a keratinizing epithelial neoplasm with a potential for me-

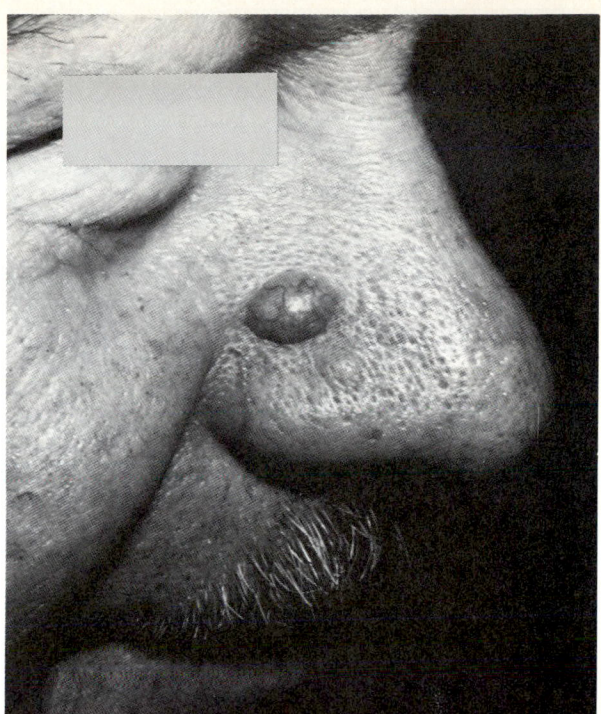

Fig. 165-2 Early basal cell carcinoma. Populonodular lesion with pearly surface and telangiectasia. (Courtesy of Department of Dermatology, The Cleveland Clinics.)

tastases. Long-term ultraviolet light (sun) exposure, ionizing radiation (repeated small doses of roentgen rays), chemical carcinogens (arsenicals and coal distillate by-products), chronic trauma, and ulcerations (previous burns and longstanding granulomatous lesions, as with tuberculosis, lupus erythematosus, and osteomyelitis) are the main causes for squamous cell carcinoma. These are associated with a more favorable prognosis, since all de novo cutaneous squamous cell carcinomas and those of the mucous membranes have a more aggressive biologic behavior that more frequently results in treatment failures and metastases. Dark-skinned individuals show less tendency to form these skin cancers than do lightly pigmented individuals.

Clinically, lesions of squamous cell carcinoma, whether occurring early or late, are diverse in appearance, appearing initially as a nonhealing papular or verrucous lesion. Eventually, as the tumor enlarges in depth and breadth, it becomes fixed to underlying structures, and the center usually becomes ulcerated.

Histologically, the more undifferentiated a tumor appears, the more malignant is its behavior. The higher the grade of malignancy, the lesser is the tendency for keratinization by the individual cells and usually the deeper the tumor extends within the dermis.

Treatment includes any of the various techniques of radiation therapy, excision, and electrothermic destruction, as long as the tumor's complete extirpation is ensured. An adaptation of standard excisional surgery is the Mohs' technique, now called Mohs' micrographic surgery, which entails a complete histologic examination of all excised cancerous tissue. This definitively establishes the complete removal of the skin cancer. Mohs' surgery is preferred for more aggressive tumors. Topical chemotherapeutic agents should not be used in the treatment of invasive squamous cell carcinoma.

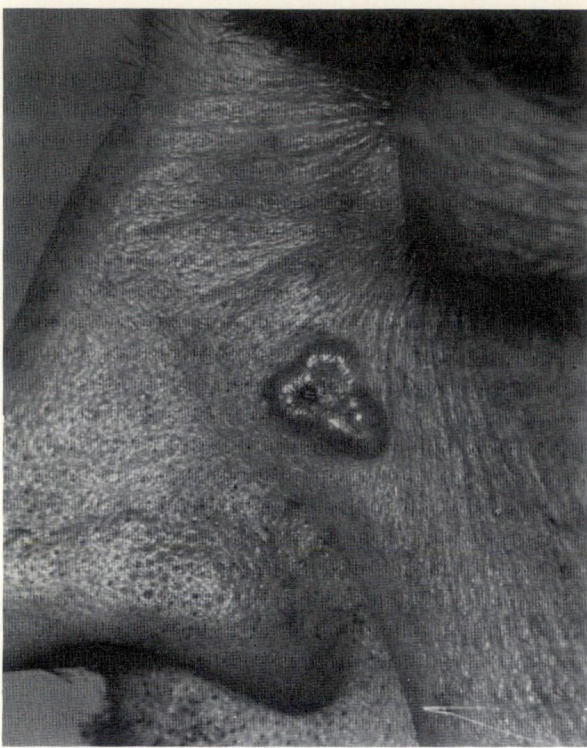

Fig. 165-3   More advanced basal cell carcinoma than in Fig. 165-2 with rolled pearly borders, depressed center, and early ulceration. (Courtesy of Department of Dermatology, The Cleveland Clinics.)

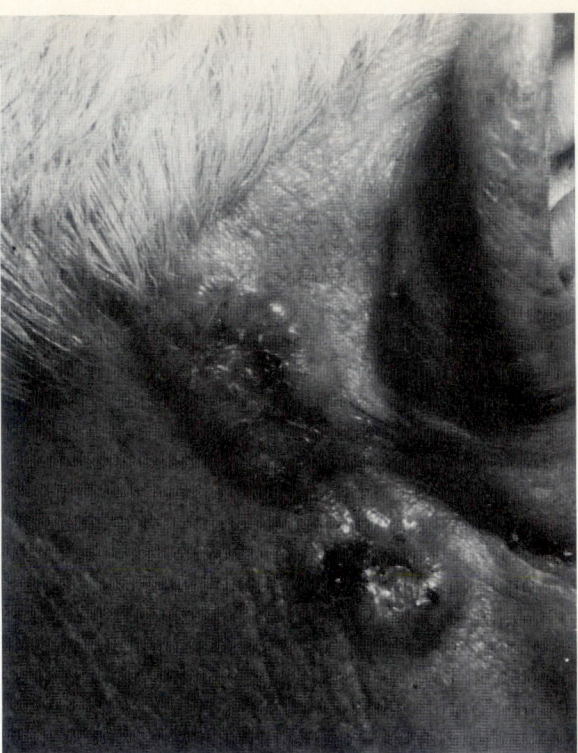

Fig. 165-4   Basal cell carcinoma at slightly more advanced stage than in Fig. 165-3 (rodent ulcer). (Courtesy of Department of Dermatology, The Cleveland Clinics.)

Basal cell carcinoma

Basal cell carcinoma is the least malignant but the most common of all skin cancers. A basal cell carcinoma is an epithelial cutaneous tumor arising from the basal cell layer of the epidermis and its appendages; it is composed of cells resembling the immature cells of these structures.

Basal cell carcinoma occurs in younger adults as well as in elderly persons, usually in cutaneous areas damaged by ultraviolet and ionizing radiation; thus it appears less often in darkly pigmented individuals. Increased exposure to chemical carcinogens probably also contributes to its pathogenesis. Clinically the basal cell carcinoma takes on a characteristic appearance. Usually a small, smooth-surfaced papule appears over an area that might show evidence of actinic damage (Fig. 165-2). Eventually the papule becomes friable and bleeds with slight trauma. The tumor slowly enlarges, developing a depressed, slightly sclerotic center that subsequently may ulcerate. At this point the borders of the tumor thicken, giving the appearance of the edges being rolled upon themselves (Fig. 165-3). Basal cell carcinoma also can be pigmented, making differentiation from melanoma sometimes difficult.

A basal cell carcinoma can show variations in its clinical presentation. Some of the more troublesome types of basal cell carcinoma, which may be recurrent and sometimes relatively resistant to therapy, include the following.

1. Superficial basal cell carcinoma may resemble a papulosquamous lesion clinically but occurs in multifocal islands in the papillary dermis, some of which are clinically inapparent.
2. Morpheiform (sclerotic) basal cell carcinoma simulates a superficial cicatrix whose borders may not be distinct. Histologically, small nests of tumor cells are trapped in a fibrous tissue stroma.

3. Metatypical or basosquamous cell carcinoma is characteristically ulcerated, conforming to the former description of the "rodent ulcer" (Fig. 165-4). In this type, elements of squamous cell carcinoma are seen interspersed among islands of basal cell carcinoma, and occasionally the biologic behavior is that of an aggressive squamous cell carcinoma rather than that of a basal cell carcinoma.

Treatment is either surgical excision or radiation therapy. Mohs' micrographic surgery is preferred for the more aggressive types of basal cell carcinoma or those resistant to other forms of therapy. Cryosurgery has been used in the treatment of basal cell carcinoma; however, many believe that it is just a temporary palliative procedure, since it sometimes does not fully obliterate the tumor. For total extirpation, considerable freezing of the deep tissues is necessary. Prophylaxis can be accomplished by consistently using sunscreens and by avoiding any form of direct radiation to the skin.

Patients with the basal cell nevus syndrome (formerly nevoid basal cell carcinoma) have various ectodermal defects, as well as many basal cell carcinomas over the the entire body, which appear as early as the first decade of life (see discussion of basal cell nevus syndrome in Chapter 156).

Malignant melanoma

Malignant melanoma is a potentially aggressive, metastasizing tumor that develops from atypical melanocytes. The pigmented premalignant and precursor lesions already discussed have the potential to develop into the following types of malignant melanoma: lentigo maligna melanoma, superficial spreading malignant melanoma, acral lentiginous malignant melanoma, nodular malignant melanoma, and, rarely, a malignant melanoma developing within the dermis from a preex-

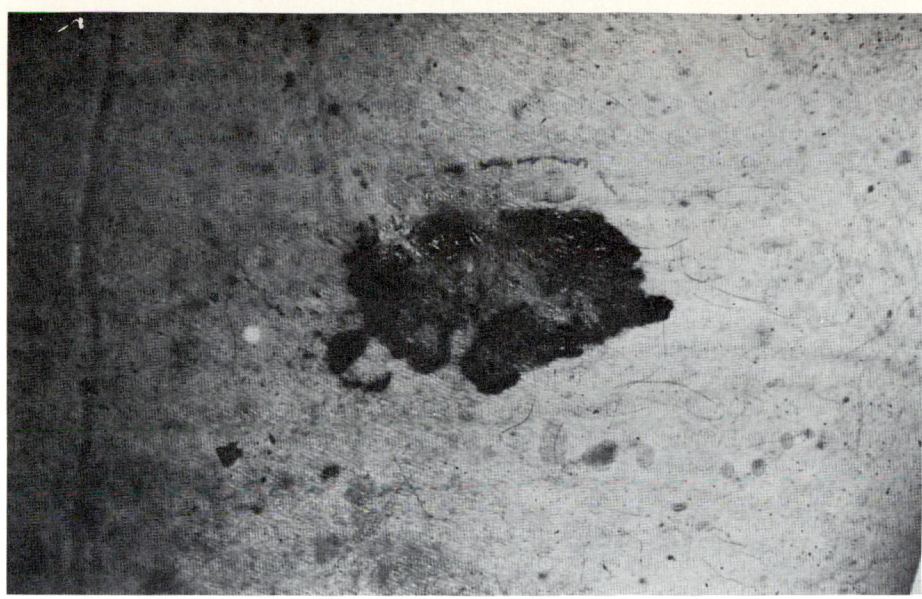

Fig. 165-5   Malignant melanoma, superficial spreading type, with mottled blue-black pigmentation.

isting congenital melanocytic nevus or intradermal nevus.

In the past decade the incidence of melanoma has increased in the United States. Some of the contributing factors for this increased prevalence are more leisure time spent out in the sun and the increase in population in the South and Southwest. Worldwide increased incidence of melanoma has been reported. In most large series the sex ratio of occurrence approximates 1:1. The occurrence of melanomas in whites is six to seven times greater than that in blacks in the same geographic localities, and the incidence ranges from 4 to 8:100,000 population annually. Melanomas in whites occur anywhere on the body, with the sun-exposed areas affected most frequently. However, blacks and Orientals tend to have melanomas of the palms, soles, nail beds, and mucous membranes.

The most common type of melanoma is the superficial-spreading melanoma, which constitutes 70% of all melanomas. It usually occurs as a slightly elevated, irregularly shaped, arciform notched lesion with variations in color (brown, blue, black, pink, and gray) (Fig. 165-5). It is thought to undergo a lateral (radial) growth phase for 1 to 7 years before nodular formation and vertical growth begin.

About 15% of all melanomas appear as nodular forms. This probably arises as an invasive nodule de novo, demonstrating both horizontal and vertical growth from the beginning; histologically the epidermis is the last layer involved in such melanomas. Nodular melanomas are blueberry shaped with variations in color ranging from black to gray (Fig. 165-6). They are the quickest of all the melanomas to grow and metastasize.

Lentigo maligna melanoma develops over many years from a lentigo maligna and is usually slow to metastasize, which accounts for the high survival rate among patients. Its malignant transformation is evident clinically when a darker brown or bluish black intradermal, nodular induration occurs within the macular lentigo maligna.

A fourth type of melanoma recently identified is the acro-lentiginous, or palmar-plantar subungual-mucosal, melanoma. This type is similar in appearance to a lentigo maligna melanoma (a macule with variegate pigmentation), but it is much more aggressive. It occurs most often on the hands, feet, oral

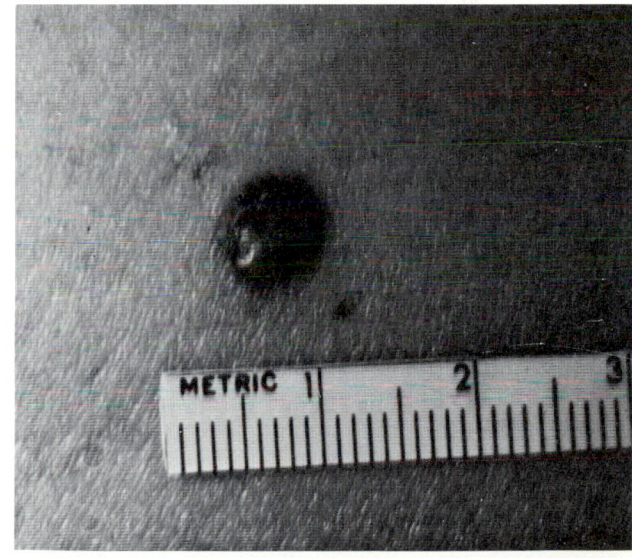

Fig. 165-6   Nodular malignant melanoma. This was an intensely blue-black lesion.

mucous membranes, and genitalia of blacks and Orientals and rarely in whites.

Two microscopic measurements have helped to predict the biologic behavior, and thus the prognosis, of the various types of melanoma. Prognosis is determined by an estimation of the depth of invasion of the tumor cells within the skin. This classification is referred to as Clark's levels of invasion, and no diagnosis of melanoma should be made without it. Clark's level I indicates that tumor cells still lie within the epidermis (in situ carcinoma); level II tumor cells are within the papillary dermis but do not fill it; in level III the papillary dermis is filled with tumor cells; in level IV tumor cells have entered the reticular dermis; and in level V the tumor has penetrated the subcutaneous fat. In the second (Breslow) classification, the thickness of a malignant melanoma is measured by estimating the distance between the granular cell layer of the epidermis and the deepest tumor cell down to wherever it has reached in the skin. This is accomplished with the aid of a calibrated ocular micrometer mounted in the eyepiece of a microscope. Lesions less than 0.75 mm deep are associated with a 5-year patient survival rate of almost 100%; patients with tumors extending to 1.5 mm in depth have a 75% to 80% survival rate in 5 years; but those with tumors deeper than 3 mm have a guarded prognosis.

The controversy of prophylactic lymph node dissection continues. The overall 5-year patient survival for disease involving the regional nodes is approximately 30%. Whether removal of lymph nodes containing microscopic foci of tumor ultimately improves survival is debatable. In addition, melanomas from the BANS region (upper *b*ack, posterolateral *a*rm, posterior and lateral *n*eck, and posterior *s*calp) may be more aggressive and metastasize more readily, even at a 0.89 to 1.69 mm thickness. Of nonpalpable regional nodes, 15% to 20% show tumor involvement. Surgical excision is the treatment of choice. Malignant melanoma has a relatively high spontaneous regression rate (15% total and 13% partial). Moreover, following removal of the primary tumor, there can be a delay in invasion and metastases of up to 35 years.

An additional prediction of prognosis and survival is the clinical staging of the patient with malignant melanoma. In stage I no clinical evidence of metastases exist. In stage II only regional lymph node metastases exist. In stage III disseminated metastases are present.

Level I lesions require only wide local excision. For level II lesions less than 0.75 mm thick, the Melanoma Clinical Cooperative Group recommends a wide local excision with a 3 to 5 cm border and primary closure using a split-thickness skin graft. For lesions of levels III, IV, V, and thicker than 1.5 mm, a wide local excision with graft is followed by lymph node dissection, whether the nodes are palpable or not. For isolated local recurrence, wide local excision is also recommended. Frederic E. Mohs, who developed micrographic surgery, advocates using zinc chloride paste fixation along with his microscopically controlled excisions. In his series the 10-year cure rate was at least 30% better in all levels of tumor invasion; however, the concept of measuring tumor thickness with a micrometer was unknown at the time of his study.

Adjuvant chemotherapy is usually reserved for metastatic melanoma. In the past, single-drug therapy has been shown to be as effective as combination chemotherapy. Current drugs of choice are dimethyltriazenoimidazolecarboxamide (DTIC), the nitrosoureas (CCNU and methyl CCNU), cisplatin, and bleomycin. Chemotherapy along with immunotherapy with intralesional injection of bacille Calmette-Guérin (BCG) or vaccinia and other immune stimulators, such as interleukin II, are currently under investigation.

NEOPLASMS OF THE MOUTH

The clinician may see various lesions of the face and mouth that may cause difficulty with the diagnosis. Basal cell carinoma of the face has many forms and may appear benign. In the mouth many white hyperkeratotic lesions or speckled erythroplakias appear, and diagnosis is often difficult. Often, diagnostic biopsy is the only way to make a definitive diagnosis.

In a massive screening of more than 23,000 caucasian Americans, over 10% had at least one oral lesion. Almost 3800 lesions were found in approximately 2800 people. Thus, two or more lesions often occur in the same person, making di-

agnosis difficult. The clinical diagnosis of "leukoplakia" was reported in approximately 30 per 1000 people. This clinical white patch did not imply anything more than a change in color. Inflammation was present in approximately 17 in 1000 persons and irritation fibroma (connective tissue hyperplasia) was found in 12 in 1000. Carcinoma occurred in less than 1 per 1000 people.

Benign lesions

KERATOSIS. Seborrheic keratosis and actinic keratosis occur on the face, generally in older people. Actinic keratosis appears frequently on the lips and is called actinic cheilitis. It is usually seen in conjunction with a ruddy, weather-beaten complexion resulting from exposure to ultraviolet radiation from the sun. The lips appear dry, scaly white, and hyperkeratotic with surrounding erythema. Histologically the epithelium is thickened with dysplasia and keratin formation. The underlying connective tissue is generally inflamed. There is often extensive collagen degeneration, which is similar to that of senile elastosis. Because of the possible malignant transformation, surgical treatment is indicated. This usually consists of a superficial lip "shave." If severe dysplasia or malignancy has occurred, surgical excision may be necessary. A sunscreen such as zinc oxide or PABA may prevent further irritation. Careful follow-up is needed.

FORDYCE'S SPOTS. Fordyce's spots, or granules, may appear as groups of discretely minute (1 mm or less), yellowish globoid lesions at the vermillion border, usually of the lower lip or on the adjacent buccal mucosa. Affecting the elderly more often, Fordyce's spots represent clusters of ectopic sebaceous glands, not a neoplasm.

PAPILLOMA. The clinical papilloma occurs in approximately 4 per 1000 people and is a true benign epithelial neoplasm. It appears as a mucosal white-colored, elevated lesion with a papillary surface. Treatment consists of total excision of the lesion.

KERATOACANTHOMA. The keratoacanthoma is a confusing lesion that is often difficult to differentiate from squamous cell carcinoma. Although keratoacanthomas are thought to arise from epidermal cells of skin appendages, they also occur in the mouth. They appear as nodules with raised, rolled, indurated borders and a central keratin plug. This plug often sequestrates, leaving a central crater. Histologically the nodules show prolific acanthosis and hyperkeratosis and parakeratosis. Often a well-delineated border from the adjacent stratified epithelium exists. When dysplastic features occur, distinguishing keratoacanthoma from a well-differentiated squamous cell carcinoma is often extremely difficult. The lesion is usually a self-healing epithelioma, and 80% of all the skin keratoacanthomas appear on the head and neck region, particularly on the cheek, nose, and lips. They generally grow rapidly for several weeks and then involute spontaneously within several months. This rapid growth gives the appearance of carcinoma. The etiologic factors are unkown but have been suggested to be hereditary, viral, chemical, or secondary to sunlight. The treatment is usually excision, and there is a very low recurrence rate. Although keratoacanthomas do heal spontaneously, some undergo malignant change and act aggressively.

PIGMENTED LESIONS. Pigmented lesions also occur in the nouth. Pigmentation may appear as normal racial pigmentation or may be caused by tumors, syndromes (such as Peutz-Jeghers), endocrine problems (such as Addison's disease), drugs (such as antimalarials), systemic disease (such as jaundice), foreign bodies (such as amalgam tatoo), and organisms (such as black hairy tongue). One must often determine whether the pigmentation is intrinsic or extrinsic.

True pigmented nevi occur in the oral cavity less commonly than on the skin. On the skin, some estimate that approximately 15 skin nevi occur per caucasian patient. This is not the case orally. The lesions are generally small, asymptomatic, and easily confused with amalgam tattoos. Oral nevi have been reported in patients 10 to 80 years of age, although mostly in persons in their third and fourth decades. Unlike skin nevi, which occur equally in males and females, oral nevi more frequently affect females. Approximately two-fifths are found on the hard palate. Less frequently, nevi occur on the labial mucosa, gingiva, vermillion border of the lips, and buccal mucosa. Lesions are small, generally between 0.1 and 3.0 cm, slightly raised, and sessile. About 80% are pigmented and range from blue to gray, brown, or black. They appear well circumscribed and superficial, often similar to normal racial pigmentation. All nevi types have been reported, but their ratios of occurrence are unlike those of nevi involving the skin. More than half are intradermal, and over one-third are blue nevi. Together, compound and junctional nevi account for less than 10%. Although other nevi occur about equally on the hard palate and buccal mucosa (25% each), the blue nevus occurs mostly on the hard palate (60%) and the labial mucosa (20%). The blue nevus is generally a light to deep blue color.

Whether a benign nevus can transform into a malignant lesion is not clear. A high ratio of melanoma to nevi in the mouth exists, and often distinguishing a nevus from a melanoma in early stages may be impossible. Removal of pigmented lesions is suggested, even if they are asymptomatic.

A related entity appearing in the oral cavity is the melanotic macule (ephelis, melanosis, or lentigo). It generally occurs in the sixth decade of life, although persons 4 to 80 years of age are affected. It is reported in approximately 1 per 1000 patients. The macules occur twice as frequently in females. They are generally singular, 0.1 to 2 cm, and brownish, blue, black, or gray macules. They are usually well-circumscribed lesions located on the vermillion border of the lower lip (30%), gingiva (23%), and buccal mucosa (16%). Up to 20% are nonpigmented but have the same histology as the pigmented macules.

Amalgam tattoos often look the same as melanotic macules and nevi and are often confused with them. Roentgenograms sometimes show amalgam fragments. Because of diagnostic problems, pathologists recommend removal of pigmented lesions if no diagnosis is known.

Premalignant lesions

Oral dysplasias often resemble malignancies and require biopsies for definitive diagnosis. Multiple entities have been reported to be "malignant." The proof is mostly speculative. One of the main problems centers around the clinical diagnosis of "leukoplakia." In general use, this refers to a clinical white patch and does not imply diagnosis. It can range from a clinical benign hyperkeratosis to a malignant carcinoma in situ. Unfortunately, this confusion has resulted in it being called a "premalignant" lesion. We believe that a white patch should be called a "white patch" to avoid inference of premalignancy when it is not meant.

Problems in evaluating dysplastic lesions are common. A study by Pindborg and co-workers in 1985 showed a wide range of diagnoses from examination of the same specimens. The diagnoses from one specimen ranged from mild dysplasia to frank squamous cell carcinoma. This variation may account for some of the incidence of malignant transformation. A com-

pounding factor is the confusion caused by secondary infections, particularly with *Candida* organisms. *Candida* infection can turn normal lesions into dysplasia, but these may be completely reversible with antimycotic therapy.

Syphilitic glossitis, changes from radiation therapy, and "field" changes in patients with diagnosed malignancy are generally considered premalignant. The most common is syphilitic glossitis, with reports of 20% to 50% malignant transformation. The field change is in the diagnosed cancer patient who often develops a second primary site. Radiation therapy, immunosuppressive drugs, and other agents (tobacco, especially chewing tobacco; snuff; alcohol) can increase the likelihood of malignant change. Debatable premalignant relationships have been reported in lichen planus and unlikely relationships in nicotine stomatitis, epulis fissuratum, and lesions caused by trauma. Patients should be carefully examined at routine dental checkups, and biopsies should be done when any clinical changes are seen.

A 7-year study of more than 250 patients with "leukoplakia" revealed that higher risk of malignant transformation occurred in those with erythroplasia (erythroleukoplakia) and a clinical verrucous-papillary hyperkeratotic pattern.

A special type of "leukoplakia" has been reported, not associated with malignant transformation but with another serious fatal disease. "Hairy leukoplakia," or oral condyloma planus, has been reported in patients positive for the human immunodeficiency virus (HIV) and is now considered one of the classic signs of acquired immunodeficiency syndrome (AIDS). Histologically, candidiasis is prevalent, as is atypia. Ultrastructural studies revealed the presence of an encapsulated herpeslike virus. The hairy leukoplakia occurs on the lateral borders of the tongue and resembles a white, hyperkeratotic, corrugated patch that does not rub off. The patient usually has no symptoms but may report occasional soreness. With the serious implications of AIDS, one must evaluate the lateral border of the tongue carefully and perform a biopsy when suspicion arises.

Malignant lesions

The most common skin malignancy, basal cell carcinoma, is rare in the mouth. The most common oral malignancy is squamous cell carcinoma. Since some believe basal cell carcinomas to be associated with epidermal adnexal structures, they say such carcinomas cannot occur in the mouth. Histologically proven malignant lesions have been reported on the gingiva, lower lip, and palate. They are slightly raised, grayish or white, with a pebbly surface and hyperemic surroundings. Circumferential induration has been reported. Most patients are more than 60 years of age and are asymptomatic. Most have a history of cutaneous basal cell carcinomas. Some debate has surrounded whether the gingival lesions represent a surface ameloblastoma because of the similar histology. Treatment involves total wide excision.

Squamous cell carcinoma is the most common oral malignancy and generally occurs on the posterolateral borders of the tongue and floor of the mouth. However, it can occur anywhere in the oral cavity. Carcinomas have varied appearances, are generally red or white and speckled, and are often indurated or ulcerated. A suspicious, nonhealing, undiagnosed lesion should be biopsied. Treatment includes surgery and radiation therapy, possibly with chemotherapy. Advances in chemotherapy have greatly reduced the size of the lesions but not the need for additional therapy. Verrucous carcinoma is a variant often related to tobacco use. It appears as a thick, hyperkeratotic area, usually with a verrucoid surface. Biopsy generally shows an almost benign appearance. Often a second biopsy and careful review with the pathologist are needed to confirm the diagnosis of this slowly growing malignancy.

Malignant melanomas of the mouth represent less than 2% of all melanomas. Most are pigmented, and the patient may have bleeding but no pain. The prognosis is poor because most lesions have already metastasized by the time of diagnosis. The cure rate of oral melanomas is less than that of cutaneous lesions. Oral melanomas have been reported more frequently in males (2:1), unlike oral nevi, which occur more often in females. Metastases from the skin have also been reported. Treatment depends on the tumor's staging.

DENTAL MANAGEMENT. All treatment modalities of malignancy can cause difficulties during dental treatment, which necessitates consultation and collaboration. Radiation therapy probably presents the most serious problem. All patients should have a thorough dental evaluation before radiation therapy. This therapy may cause xerostomia, radiation caries (severe cervical caries), and slow or absent healing. After radiation therapy, extractions can and generally do lead to osteoradionecrosis with possible sloughing of parts of the jaws, especially the mandible because of decreased vascularity. All teeth in poor or debatable condition or in a poorly motivated patient should be extracted before radiation therapy. Some recommend extraction of all molars because these teeth may cause the most difficulty in endodontics and extractions and with oral hygiene. Those teeth saved must be treated daily with fluoride. Fluoride gel in a tray is best and easiest to use; 0.4% stannous fluoride is often recommended. An artificial saliva solution may benefit the xerostomic patient. A topical anesthetic such as 0.5% aqueous diphenhydramine (Benadryl) or 2% viscous lidocaine helps relieve radiation stomatitis or an erythematous "burn" of the mucosa. Frequent dental visits with close scrutiny of oral hygiene is necessary. The addition of bland mouth rinses such as baking soda or the use of chlorhexidine may be beneficial. Any future extractions must be done with consultation and careful evaluation; the patient must be warned of possible consequences. High-dose antibiotic therapy has been recommended to prevent any infection, but this may not help.

The patient undergoing chemotherapy may present difficulties because of alterations in bone marrow, painful oral ulcerations, or secondary infections. The dentist can help prevent problems by limiting oral infection before chemotherapy, removing sharp cusps, and helping to maintain patients' oral hygiene. Many major centers are rquiring routine dental consultations before and during chemotherapy. Improved oral hygiene has decreased the incidence of ulcerations, helped prevent systemic infection, and allowed the patient to maintain a better life-style. Careful attention to oral hygiene is necessary. Oral rinses with baking soda and chlorhexidine may be beneficial. Decreased stomatitis in patients using nonsteroidal antiinflammatory drugs has been reported.

Patients undergoing cancer surgery of the head and neck may require reconstruction with oral prostheses. This may be necessary at surgery to prevent facial deformities and to close oral-antral communications. These patients must be closely watched for any recurrent disease. The teeth must be maintained in good condition, and hygiene must be stressed.

The most important factor in dental management is maintaining a team concept. The earlier the diagnosis of the malignancy is made and the sooner all potential complications are removed, the healthier the patient will be.

Such a team must include physicians (head and neck surgeon, radiation therapist, oncologists), dentists (oral and maxiofacial surgeon, general dentist, prosthodontists), support personel (speech therapist, dietician, social worker) and the patient and his family.

BIBLIOGRAPHY
Premalignant lesions and malignant neoplasms

Amonette RA and others: Metastatic basal cell carcinoma, J Dermatol Surg Oncol 7:397, 1981.

Andersen SL, Nielsen H, and Raymann F: Relationship between Bowen's disease and internal malignant tumors, Arch Dermatol 108:367, 1973.

Andrade R and others, editors: Cancer of the skin, ed 2, Philadelphia, 1976, WB Saunders Co.

Arons MS and others: Scar tissue carcinoma. I. A clinical study with special reference to burn scar carcinoma, Ann Surg 161:170, 1965.

Bleehen SS: Pigmented basal cell epithelioma, Br J Dermatol 93:361, 1975.

Boncinelli U, Fornieri C, and Muscatello U: Relationship between leukocytes and tumor cells in precancerous and cancerous lesions of the lip: a possible expression of immune reaction, J Invest Dermatol 71:407, 1978.

Borel DM: Cutaneous basosquamous carcinoma: review of the literature and report of 35 cases, Arch Pathol 95:293, 1973.

Brownstein MH and Rabinowitz AD: The precursors of cutaneous squamous cell carcinoma (review), Int J Dermatol 18:1, 1979.

Callen JP and Headington J: Bowen's and non-Bowen's squamous intraepidermal neoplasia of the skin, Arch Dermatol 116:422, 1980.

Cataldo E and Doki HC: Solar cheilitis, J Dermatol Surg Oncol 7:989, 1981.

Cutler B, Posalaky Z, and Katz I: Cell processes in basal cell carcinoma, J Cutan Pathol 7:310, 1980.

Dvoretzky I, Fisher BK, and Haker O: Mutilating basal cell epithelioma, Arch Dermatol 114:239, 1978.

Epstein E and others: Metastases from squamous cell carcinomas of the skin, Arch Dermatol 97:245, 1968.

Epstein W and Kligman AM: The pathogenesis of milia and benign tumors of the skin, J Invest Dermatol 26:1, 1956.

Farmer ER and Helwig EB: Metastatic basal cell carcinoma: a clinicopathologic study of 17 cases, Cancer 46:748, 1980.

Freeman RG: Histopathologic considerations in the management of skin cancer, J Dermatol Surg 2:215, 1976.

Gorlin RJ: Bowen's disease of the mucous membrane of the mouth: a review of the literature and a presentation of six cases, Oral Surg 3:35, 1959.

Graham JH and Helwig EB: Premalignant cutaneous and mucocutaneous diseases. In Graham JH, Johnson WC, and Helwig EB, editors: Dermal pathology, New York, 1972, Harper & Row, Publishers, Inc.

Graham JH and others: Solar keratosis with squamous cell carcinoma: a new biologic concept, Am J Pathol 55:26a, 1969.

Hairston MA Jr, Reed RJ, and Derbes VJ: Dermatosis papulosa nigra, Arch Dermatol 89:655, 1964.

Hashimoto K and Lever WF: Histogenesis of skin appendage tumors, Arch Dermatol 100:356, 1969.

Helm F: Cancer dermatology, Philadelphia, 1979, Lea & Febiger.

Indianer L: Controversies in dermatopathology, J Dermatol Surg Oncol 5:321, 1979.

Jacobs GH, Rippey JJ, and Altini M: Prediction of aggressive behavior in basal cell carcinoma, Cancer 49:533, 1982.

James MP, Wells GC, and Whimster IW: Spreading pigmented actinic keratosis, Br J Dermatol 98:373, 1978.

Kimura S: Trichilemmal cysts, Dermatologica 157:164, 1978.

Kobayasi T: Dermo-epidermal junction in invasive squamous cell carcinoma, Acta Derm Venereol (Stockh) 49:445, 1969.

Luderschmidt C and Plewig G: Circumscribed sebaceous gland hyperplasia: autoradiographic and histoplanometric studies, J Invest Dermatol 70:207, 1978.

Lund HZ: How often does squamous cell carcinoma of the skin metastasize? Arch Dermatol 92:635, 1965.

Martin H, Strong E, and Spiro RH: Radiation-induced skin cancer of the head and neck, Cancer 25:61, 1970.

McGravran MH and Binnington B: Keratinous cysts of the skin, Arch Dermatol 94:49, 1966.

Mehregan AH: Lentigo senilis and its evolutions, J Invest Dermatol 65:429, 1975.

Mehregan AH and Pinkus H: Intraepidermal carcinoma: a critical study, Cancer 17:609, 1964.

Mohs FE: Chemosurgery: microscopically controlled surgery for skin cancer, Springfield, Ill, 1978, Charles C Thomas, Publisher.

Moller R, Reymann F, and Hou-Jensen K: Metastases in dermatological patients with squamous cell carcinoma, Arch Dermatol 115:703, 1979.

Neoplasms of the skin and malignant melanoma: a collection of papers presented at the Twentieth Annual Clinical Conference on Cancer, 1975,

University of Texas Cancer Center, M.D. Anderson Hospital and Tumor Institute, Houston, Chicago, 1976, Year Book Medical Publishers, Inc.

Olson R, Nordquist R, and Everett MA: Dyskeratosis in Bowen's disease, Br J Dermatol 81:676, 1969.

Pinkus H: "Sebaceous cysts" are trichilemmal cysts, Arch Dermatol 99:544, 1969.

Rahbari H and Mehregan AH: Basal cell epithelioma (carcinoma) in children and teenagers, Cancer 49:350, 1982.

Ronchese F: Keratoses, cancer and the sign of Leser-Trélat, Cancer 18:1003, 1965.

Sanderson KV: The structure of seborrheic keratoses, Br J Dermatol 80:588, 1968.

Sedlin ED and Fleming JL: Epidermal carcinoma arising in chronic osteomyelitic foci, J Bone Joint Surg 45:827, 1963.

Strayer DS and Santa Cruz DJ: Carcinoma in situ of the skin: a review of histopathology, J Cutan Pathol 7:244, 1980.

Totten JR: The multiple nevoid basal cell carcinoma syndrome, Cancer 46:1456, 1980.

Willoughby C and Soter NA: Stucco keratosis, Arch Dermatol 105:859, 1972.

Winkelmann RK and Muller SA: Sweat gland tumors, Arch Dermatol 89:827, 1964.

Melanocytic neoplasms and melanomas

Alper J and others: Birthmarks with serious medical significance: nevocellular nevi, sebaceous nevi, and multiple café-au-lait spots, J Pediatr 95:696, 1979.

Breslow A: Thickness, cross-sectional areas and depth of invasion in the prognosis of cutaneous melanoma, Ann Surg 172:902, 1970.

Clark WH Jr and others: The histogenesis and biologic behavior of primary human malignant melanomas of the skin, Cancer Res 19:705, 1969.

Clark WH Jr and others: Human malignant melanoma, New York, 1979, Grune & Stratton, Inc.

Day CL Jr and others: Cutaneous malignant melanoma: prognostic guidelines for physicians and patients, CA 32:113, 1982.

Day CL Jr and others: Predictors of late deaths among patients with clinical stage I melanoma who have not had visceral or bony metastases within the first 5 years after diagnosis, J Am Acad Dermatol 8:864, 1983.

Greene MH and others: Acquired precursors of cutaneous malignant melanoma, the familial dysplastic nevus syndrome, N Engl J Med 312:91, 1985.

Guiliano AE and others: Melanoma from unknown primary site and amelanotic melanoma, Semin Oncol 9:442, 1982.

Kopf AW and others: Congenital nevocytic nevi and malignant melanoma, J Am Acad Dermatol 1:123, 1979.

Kopf AW and others, editors: Malignant melanoma, New York, 1979, Masson Publishing USA, Inc.

Lanier VA and others: Congenital giant nevi: clinical and pathological considerations, Plast Reconstr Surg 58:48, 1976.

Lee JAH: Melanoma and exposure to sunlight, Epidemiol Rev 4:110, 1982.

Lew RA and others: Sun exposure habits in patients with cutaneous melanoma—a case control study, J Dermatol Surg Oncol 12:981, 1983.

McGovern VJ: The classification of melanoma and its relationship with prognosis, Pathology 2:85, 1970.

Michalik EE and others: Rapid progression of lentigo maligna to deeply invasive lentigo maligna melanoma: report of two cases, Arch Dermatol 119:831, 1983.

Mihm MC Jr and others: The clinical diagnosis, classification and histogenetic concepts of the early stages of cutaneous malignant melanomas, N Engl J Med 284, 1078, 1971.

Mihm MC Jr and others: Early detection of primary cutaneous malignant melanoma: a color atlas, N Engl J Med 289:989, 1973.

Reed RJ: Acrolentiginous melanoma. In Reed JR: New concepts in surgical pathology of skin, New York, 1976, John Wiley & Sons, Inc.

Reimer RR and others: Precursor lesions in familial melanoma, JAMA 239:744, 1978.

Rhodes AR and others: The malignant potential of small congenital nevocellular nevi: an estimate of association based on a histologic study of 234 primary cutaneous melanomas, J Am Acad Dermatol 6:230, 1982.

Schreiber MD and others: Malignant melanoma in southern Arizona, Arch Dermatol 117:6, 1981.

Neoplasms of the mouth

Bouquot JE: Common oral lesions found during a mass screening examination, J Am Dent Assoc 112:50, 1986.

Buchner A and Hansen LS: Melanotic macule of the oral mucosa, Oral Surg 49:55, 1980.

Chaudhry AP and others: Primary malignant melanoma of the oral cavity, Cancer 11:923, 1958.

Devildos LR and Langlois CC: Intramucosal cellular nevi, Oral Surg 52:162, 1981.

Dummett CV and Barnes G: Oromucosal pigmentation: an updated literary review, J Periodontol 42:725, 1971.

Eversole LR and others: Oral condyloma planus (hairy leukoplakia) among homosexual men: a clinicopathologic study of thirty-six cases, Oral Surg 61:249, 1986.

Gazi MI: Unusual pigmentation of the gingiva, Oral Surg 62:646, 1986.

Girard KR and Hoffman BL: Actinic cheilitis, Oral Surg 50:21, 1980.

Greenspan D and others: Oral "hairy" leukoplakia in male homosexuals: evidence of association with both papillomavirus and a herpes-group virus, Lancet 2:831, 1984.

Hatziotis JC and Mylona-Hatziotis AJ: Blue nevi of the oral cavity: review of the literature and report of two cases, J Oral Surg 31:772, 1973.

Jackson D and Simpson HE: Primary malignant melanoma of the oral cavity, Oral Surg 39:553, 1975.

Liroff KP and Zeff S: Basal cell carcinoma of the palatal mucosa, J Oral Surg 30:730, 1972.

Marlett RH: Generalized melanoses and non-melanotic pigmentations of the head and neck, J Am Dent Assoc 90:141, 1975.

Mosby EL and others: Gingival and pharyngeal metastasis from a malignant melanoma, Oral Surg 36:6, 1973.

Pindborg JJ and others: Subjectivity in evaluating oral epithelial dysplasia, carcinoma in situ and initial carcinoma, J Oral Pathol 14:698, 1985.

Silverman S and others: Junction nevus of the oral mucosa, Oral Surg 39:259, 1975.

Silverman S and others: Oral leukoplakia and malignant transformation, Cancer 53:563, 1984.

Teles JCB and others: The labial melanotic macules, Oral Surg 42:196, 1976.

Whyte AM and others: The intraoral keratoacanthomas: a diagnostic problem, Br J Oral Maxillofac Surg 24:438, 1986.

Young SK and others: Generalized eruptive keratoacanthoma, Oral Surg 62:422, 1986.

Malignant lesions and dental management

Beume J and others: Radiation complications in edentulous patients, J Prosthet Dent 26:193, 1976.

Carl W and others: Oral surgery and the patient who has had radiation therapy for head and neck cancer, Oral Surg 36:651, 1973.

Cox FL: Endodontics and the irradiated patient, Oral Surg 42:679, 1976.

Curtis TA and others: Complete denture prosthodontics for the radiation patient, J Prosthet Dent 36:66, 1976.

Daly TE and Drane JB: The management of teeth related to the treatment of oral cancer, Seventh National Cancer Conference Proceedings, Head Neck Cancer, 1973.

Greenberg MS and others: The oral flora as a source of septicemia in patients with acute leukemia, Oral Surg 53:32, 1982.

Karmioi M and Walsh RF: Dental caries after radiotherapy of the oral regions, J Am Dent Assoc 91:838, 1975.

Montgomery S: Endodontic complications in an irradiated patient, J Endodont 3:277, 1977.

Nakamoto RY: Use of a saliva substitute in postradiation xerostomia, J Prosthet Dent 42:539, 1979.

Pappas GL: Bone changes in osteoradionecrosis, Oral Surg 27:622, 1969.

Schofield IDE and others: Osteoradionecrosis of maxillae, Oral Surg 45:692, 1978.

Shannon IL and others: A saliva substitute for use by xerostomic patients undergoing radiotherapy to the head and neck, Oral Surg 44:656, 1977.

KAPOSI'S HEMORRHAGIC SARCOMA

In the last few years the clinical picture of Kaposi's sarcoma has changed dramatically from a rare disease seen late in life, with patients having an average survival of 10 years, to a disease related to AIDS, affecting any age group, and associated with an early death.

Kaposi's idiopathic hemorrhagic sarcoma is a neoplastic disease characterized by abnormal proliferation of lymphoreticular and endothelial cells. It develops primarily in the skin, but multicentric visceral involvement usually follows to a variable degree. In classic Kaposi's sarcoma the initial sites are usually the feet, toes, and legs; dark reddish blue to purplish, sharply demarcated macular, papular, or other nodular lesions appear. Sometimes a reddish brown component occurs that later becomes bluish. Lesions may sometimes appear first on the hands, forearms, ears, nose, or genitalia, but most often occur

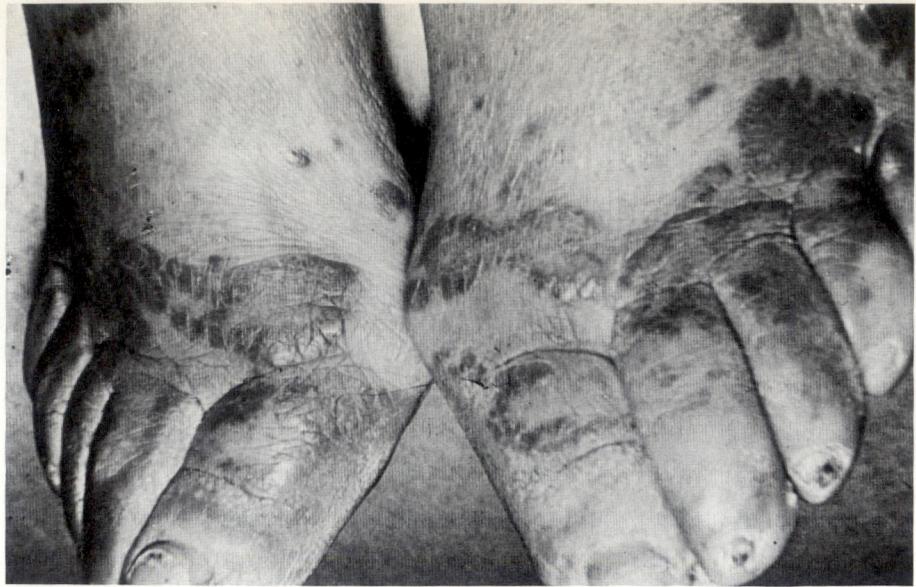

Fig. 165-7   Kaposi's hemorrhagic sarcoma with plaque lesions on dorsa of feet and toes.

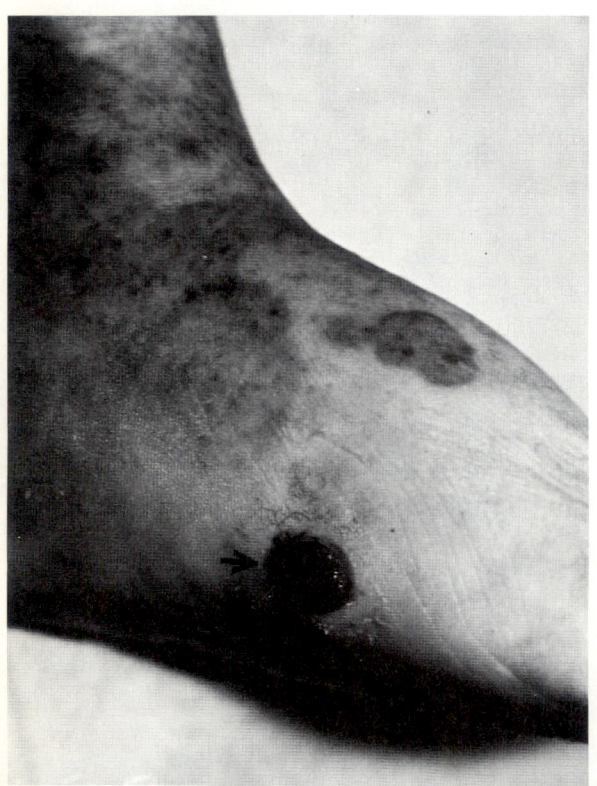

Fig. 165-8   Kaposi's hemorrhagic sarcoma with nodular and plaque lesions. Nodule *(arrow)* is dusky and erythematous. Plaques are infiltrated and reddish brown.

in these locations after the appearance of lesions on the lower extremities. The macular and papular lesions may coalesce to form infiltrated plaques from which nodules may develop (Fig. 165-7). Nodules may occasionally be the initial lesion, appearing as a dusky violaceous angioma with a firm rubbery consistency (Fig. 165-8). Patients often have a brawny edema of the affected extremity with subsequent development of lymphedema. Elephantiasis may affect the legs, and verrucuous ichthyotic lesions may develop on the feet, ankles, and lower

half of the legs as a result of the chronic edema and stasis. Ulcers are uncommon and occur from trauma rather than spontaneous necrosis.

The gastrointestinal tract is the most common extracutaneous site of classic Kaposi's sarcoma. Characteristic bluish nodules may occur on the tongue, palate, pharynx, and esophagus and throughout the intestinal tract and may lead to internal hemorrhage as the most serious complication. The respiratory tract is the next most frequently involved area. Lesions may occur in the lungs, pleura, and larynx, but bleeding from these sites is uncommon. Kaposi's sarcoma has been reported in every organ, including the heart, liver, spleen, kidneys, adrenal glands, testes, and lymph nodes; however, these lesions are generally not clinically significant.

Occasionally, periods of spontaneous remission of the lesions may occur, especially early in the disease. Kaposi's sarcoma has been associated with other neoplastic diseases, such as mycosis fungoides, Hodgkin's disease, lymphosarcoma, leukemia, and multiple myeloma. Histologically, Kaposi's sarcoma consists of masses of spindle cells, fibroblasts, and proliferating capillaries. Its behavior is that of a multifocal proliferative and reactive process originating in the reticuloendothelial system.

Death infrequently is the direct result of the disease and in the classic form is attributed to the disease only when it progresses rapidly and acts as a true sarcoma. If the course is more prolonged, death may be from other causes, such as hemorrhage, intestinal perforation with peritonitis, septicemia, or bronchial pneumonia.

The disease is found worldwide, but the classic form occurs predominantly in Europe (central and eastern European countries and Italy). In the United States the classic form mainly affects Jews of Galician, Polish, or Russian extraction and southern Italians, with some cases occurring in blacks. In Western countries the peak incidence is in the sixth and seventh decades of life. The duration of the classic disease is approximately 10 years, but death may occur 3 to 50 years after onset. Another form of Kaposi's sarcoma has been described in equatorial and southern Africa, primarily among Bantus. In Africa it tends to affect a much younger age group. In the 1960s the incidence of Kaposi's sarcoma in the United States was 0.02

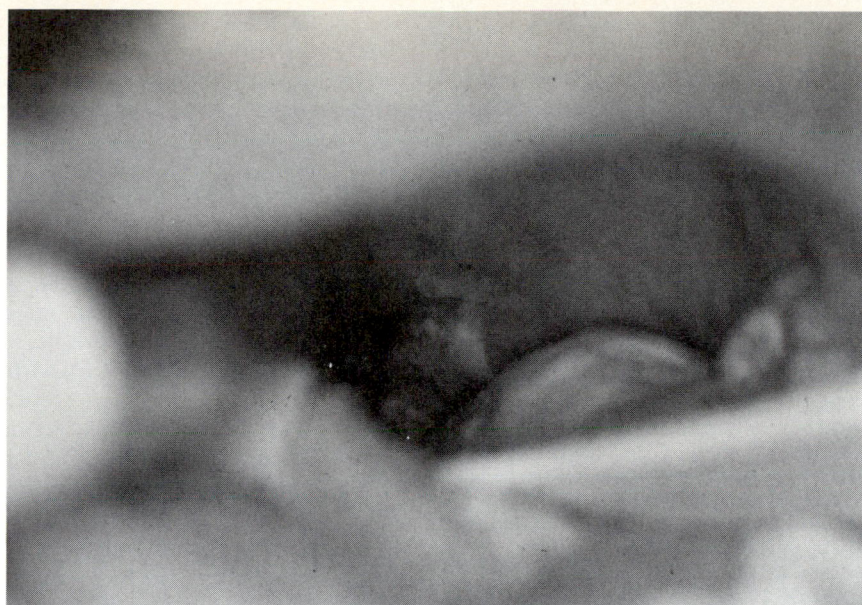

Fig. 165-9   Plaque-like lesion in soft palatotonsillar area in young man who eventually died of pneumocystis pneumonia. Histologic examination of reddish-blue lesion with areas of white necrosis revealed it to be Kaposi's sarcoma.

to 0.06 per 100,000 population; but in Africa, especially Uganda, it composed 9% of all cancers. In the late 1960s the geographic distribution of Kaposi's sarcoma in equatorial and southern Africa was reminiscent of Burket's lymphoma, and some suggested a potentially infectious origin. As early as 1960, a high incidence with generalized lymph node involvement and rapid death was reported. Males are affected more than females in a ratio of 10 to 15:1.

In early studies of Kaposi's sarcoma, familial involvement was infrequent, and cases occurred in which no consanguinity existed, which suggested against a hereditary origin. Because of the clustered distribution, infections and environmental factors were discussed. In 1978, Giraldo and associates reported electromicroscopic studies that demonstrated a herpes-type virus in tissue culture cell lines from African patients with Kaposi's sarcoma. They postulated a childhood form of Kaposi's with lymphadenitis that reflected an unidentified impairment of the immune system.

Immunosuppressed patients, because of corticosteroid therapy and other forms of immunosuppression and particularly after renal transplantations, have a higher incidence of Kaposi's sarcoma, including mouth lesions.

The additional documentation of AIDS has shown that Kaposi's sarcoma is one of the key findings in this disease. The finding of Kaposi's sarcoma in young male homosexuals, intravenous drug users, and debilitated patients must suggest the diagnosis of AIDS. In AIDS the initial lesions may appear anywhere on the body, and dissemination to the skin and internal organs occurs rapidly. The pathogenesis seems to be related to the impaired cellular immunity caused by the virus. The human T-lymphotrophic virus type III (HTLV-III), now called the HIV virus, has been isolated from patients with AIDS. The disease is associated with oral candidiasis and hairy leukoplakia. Death is often associated with a secondary opportunistic infection, particularly cytomegalovirus (CMV) or with *Pneumocystis carinii*.

ORAL MANIFESTATIONS. Oral lesions may occur without skin lesions, but generally skin lesions appear either before or

during oral manifestations. Several cases of primary oral malignancy have been reported. They most often involve the palate but can occur on the alveolar ridges, lips, and tongue. They appear as a raised, reddish to mucosal-colored mass similar to pyogenic granuloma. In the classic form the patient is generally 50 years of age or older. Secondary infection and hemorrhage of the lesions often occur from trauma.

In AIDS, oral manifestations including candidiasis and hairy leukoplakia, may be early signs of the disease. Once Kaposi's sarcoma occurs with the oral lesions possibly being the first sign, the diagnosis of AIDS can be made (Fig. 165-9).

DENTAL MANAGEMENT. Biopsy of the lesion is the key to early diagnosis. The classic form of Kaposi's sarcoma can be cured. Since Kaposi's sarcoma occurs frequently in patients undergoing immunosuppressive therapy, as well as in patients with AIDS, complications of dental therapy may arise because of the drugs as well as the disease. Care must be taken, since these patients are extremely prone to infection; reverse isolation may be necessary. Careful barrier technique is necessary to protect the clinician. Although uncommon, potential transmission to the clinician may occur.

Oral hygiene must be stressed to patients, and adjuncts such as chlorhexidine, baking soda rinses, and topical fluoride may benefit them. Unless patients require reverse isolation, where all dentistry may be precluded except to eliminate infection, care may be rendered in a private office using barrier techniques.

BIBLIOGRAPHY

Ackerman LV and Murray JF: Symposium on Kaposi's sarcoma, New York, 1962, S Karger.

Boldogh I and others: Kaposi's sarcoma. IV. Detection of CMV DNA, CMV RNA, and CMV NA in tumor biopsies, Int J Cancer 28:469, 1981.

Centers for Disease Control: Kaposi's sarcoma and pneumocystis pneumonia among homosexual men—New York and California, Morbid Mortal Weekly Rep 30:305, 1981.

Centers for Disease Control: Update on acquired immune deficiency syndrome (AIDS)—U.S., Morbid Mortal Weekly Rep 31:507, 1982.

Davis J: Kaposi's sarcoma: present concept of clinical course and treatment, NY J Med 68:2067, 1968.

Durack DT: Opportunistic infections and Kaposi's sarcoma in homosexual men, N Engl J Med 205:1465, 1981.

Dutz W and Stout AP: Kaposi's sarcoma in infants and children, Cancer 13:684, 1960.

Farman AG and Uys PB: Oral Kaposi's sarcoma, Oral Surg 39:288, 1975.

Friedman-Kien AE and others: Disseminated Kaposi's sarcoma in homosexual men, Ann Intern Med 96:693, 1982.

Giraldo G, Beth EL, and Henle W: Antibody patterns to herpes virus in Kaposi's sarcoma: serological association of American Kaposi's sarcoma with cytomegalovirus, Int J Cancer 72:126, 1978.

Holecek MJ and Harwood AR: Radiotherapy for Kaposi's sarcoma, Cancer 41:1733, 1978.

Howard WR and others: Kaposi's hemorrhagic sarcoma, Cutis 21:503, 1978.

Johnson R, Horwitz SN, and Frost P: Disseminated Kaposi's sarcoma in a homosexual man, JAMA 247:1739, 1982.

Klepp O and others: Association of Kaposi's sarcoma and prior immunosuppressive therapy, Cancer 42:2626, 1978.

Lo TCM and others: Radiotherapy for Kaposi's sarcoma, Cancer 45:684, 1980.

Lozada F and others: Oral manifestations of tumor and opportunistic infections in the acquired immunodeficiency syndrome (AIDS): findings in 53 homosexual men with Kaposi's sarcoma, Oral Surg 56:491, 1983.

Nickles GB and others: Kaposi's sarcoma in a patient with acquired immune deficiency syndrome, J Oral Maxillofac Surg 42:56, 1984.

Nisce LZ and others: Once weekly total and subtotal skin electron beam therapy for Kaposi's sarcoma, Cancer 47:640, 1981.

Safai B and Good RA: Kaposi's sarcoma: a review and recent developments, Clin Bull 10:62, 1980.

Safai B and others: Association of Kaposi's sarcoma with secondary primary malignancies: possible etiopathogenic implications, Cancer 45:1472, 1980.

166 · ERYTHEMAS

Shelley S. Schuler and Robert N. Arm

ERYTHEMA MULTIFORME

Erythema multiforme is an acute inflammatory syndrome that involves the skin, mucous membranes, and in the more severe forms, various internal organs. As the name "multiforme" implies, the lesions appear in many varieties, including macular, papular, nodose, vesicular, and bullous. They may be iris shaped (resembling a target or bull's-eye), annular, or circinate (Fig. 166-1). Patients may also have purpura, urticarial lesions, vesicles, and bullae. The lesions are not only polymorphous but variable in color as well, sometimes with exudation. Most often the lesions are found on the face, neck, forearms, and legs (especially the extensor surfaces), and the dorsa of hands and feet (palms and soles), frequently with a symmetric distribution. Mucous membranes are also occasionally involved. The onset of the eruption is usually fairly rapid, developing within 12 to 24 hours after a short prodromal period. Recurrent attacks may appear at regular intervals; the lesions usually heal without scarring.

The disease more commonly occurs in the spring and fall and seldom in summer. More cases are noted during viral epidemics. Although erythema multiforme may occur at any age, it mainly affects persons 10 to 40 years of age. The severe bullous form more often occurs in adolescents and young adults. The disease is rare in children less than 3 years of age and adults over 50. When it affects adults of the older age group, the possibility of an occult carcinoma must be considered.

Although the exact cause of erythema multiforme is unknown, it is generally considered to be a toxic or hypersensitivity syndrome. Circumstantial evidence exists for an immune complex etiologic factor for at least some cases. Different types of skin lesions may be produced by the same causative agent, and conversely, different causative agents may evoke similar clinical reactions on the skin and mucous membranes. Erythema multiforme has been associated with several viral and chlamydial infections (herpes simplex virus, coxsackievirus B-5, influenza virus type A, Epstein-Barr virus (mononucleosis), and echovirus infection; mumps; psittacosis; and lymphogranuloma venereum), viral immunizations (vaccination and poliovirus), deep fungal infections (histoplasmosis and coccidioidomycosis), bacterial infections (typhoid fever, leprosy, *Mycoplasma pneumoniae* infection, tularemia, tuberculosis, and *Yersinia* infection); BCG vaccination, collagen diseases (dermatomyositis, allergic vasculitis, lupus erythematosus, and polyarteritis nodosa), malignancies (carcinoma and lymphoma), following radiation therapy, and as a result of drug reactions (penicillins, sulfonamides and related compounds, iodides, bromides, phenytoin, phenolphthalein, salicylates, sulindac, minoxidil, and barbiturates). The eruptions in children and young adults are more often related to infections, whereas in older persons they are associated with drugs and malignancies. Shelley reported that 15% of patients had herpes before the erythema multiforme. Other studies show that herpes may occur before the syndrome, but little evidence shows a direct causal relationship; it may be a hypersensitivity reaction. No cause is found in many patients.

A wide clinical spectrum occurs among patients with erythema multiforme, with gradations from a relatively localized minor eruption on the skin and mucous membranes to a major multisystem disorder with a potentially fatal outcome. The maculourticarial form usually occurs on the extremities, especially extensor surfaces, dorsa of hands, nail folds, and mucous membranes. The eruptions tend to be grouped over the elbows and knees and less frequently on the palms and soles. The characteristic target (iris) lesion is urticarial with a dusky center that sometimes forms a vesicle surrounded by a brighter erythematous ring; fine petechiae may occur. The trunk may be affected, but usually this follows severe involvement of the extremities. Careful examination of the skin reveals a sun-exposed distribution of skin lesions. The skin lesions also tend to occur at sites of physical trauma (isomorphic or Koebner's phenomenon). Lesions usually appear in crops for a few weeks, healing in about 1 week and leaving residual hypopigmentation or hyperpigmentation but no scarring. The vesiculobullous form may develop in preexisting lesions; this form often involves mucous membranes more than the skin and sometimes affects mucous membranes alone. Recurrences are more common in patients with the vesiculobullous type than in those with the maculourticarial form.

The severe form of erythema multiforme is often called erythema multiforme major or Stevens-Johnson syndrome. In this severe form a prodrome of 1 day to 2 weeks may variably consist of fever, malaise, sore throat, rhinitis, cough, chest pain, arthralgias, myalgias, vomiting, and diarrhea. A neutropenia may occur. Following this prodrome, bullae abruptly erupt on the skin and mucous membranes, including those of the conjunctivae, nose, lips, mouth, tongue, esophagus, respiratory tract, genitalia, and rectum. The bullae rupture and become erosions and ulcerations, sometimes with hemorrhagic crusting and pseudomembranous coverings. Eye involvement includes bullae, catarrhal or purulent conjunctivitis, corneal ulcerations, anterior uveitis, and occasionally panophthalmitis, sometimes with resultant corneal opacities and blindness. Vulvovaginitis may cause fibrotic bands or stenosis of the vagina; balanitis may result in adhesion of the prepuce to the glans. Shedding of the nails may also occur.

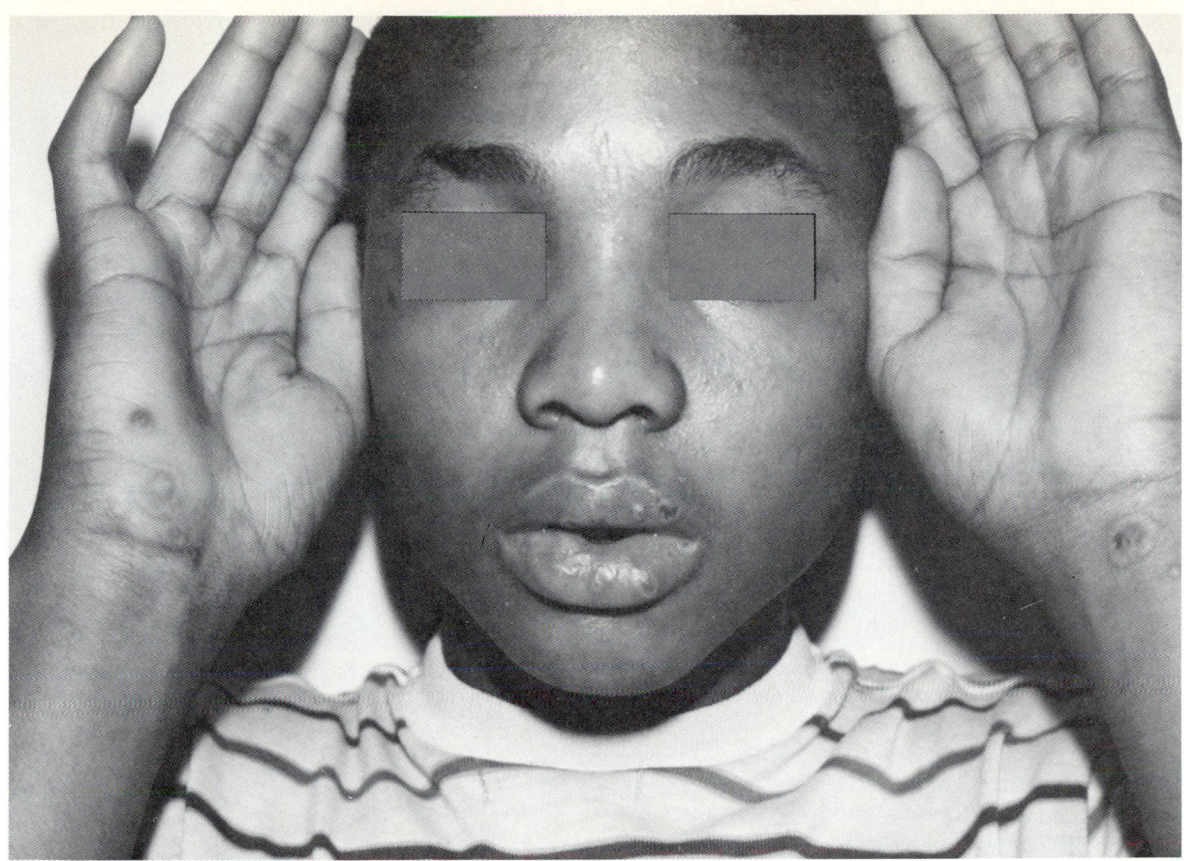

Fig. 166-1   Erythema multiforme. Lesions on lips are ruptured vesicles, and those on hands are vesicles and iris lesions.

Staphylococcal scalded skin syndrome (SSSS) may be confused with Stevens-Johnson syndrome, but patients with SSSS usually have a very high fever. Toxic epidermal necrolysis can also be confused with Stevens-Johnson syndrome.

The roentgenographic changes in the lung are seen as patchy infiltrates, resembling the pattern of atypical pneumonia. Lymphadenopathy may be present, and proteinuria, hematuria, tubular necrosis, and progressive renal failure have been noted. Mortality in the severe forms of erythema multiforme (Stevens-Johnson syndrome) is 5% to 25% of patients.

Mild cases of erythema multiforme usually clear in a few weeks and require only local symptomatic treatment to allay symptoms of burning and itching and to drain bullae. Removal of underlying causes, when these are known, is important in both minor and major forms of the disease. Patients with severe forms require systemic administration of corticosteroids, along with supportive therapy that includes mouthwashes and oral hygiene, eye irrigations, mydriatics, lubricants, and local antibiotics to prevent secondary infection. Antihistamines are sometimes useful, but in general, drugs (laxatives, analgesics, and sedatives) should be avoided because these drugs may cross-react with those responsible for the eruption. Intravenous fluid replacement may be needed.

ORAL MANIFESTATIONS. When clinicians hear the name erythema multiforme, they envision blood-encrusted lips, but this does not always occur. The variable features of this disease can present a diagnostic challenge. Often skin and oral lesions are independent of each other and may vary from mild to severe. The mild lesions, if found only intraorally, present the most difficult problem for diagnosis, with a differential diagnosis ranging from recurrent aphthous stomatitis and primary herpes to pemphigus in older patients. When limited to the oral cavity, the disease is often self-limiting and resolves after a time, often 2 to 4 weeks. If lesions remain, a biopsy may help rule out other disease. Biopsy features of erythema multiforme are not pathognomonic. The histopathology generally shows a nonspecific inflammatory infiltrate, mild acanthosis, and occasionally a perivascular chronic inflammatory cell infiltrate. A study of Lozado reported 24% of patients with oral lesions only, 38% with oral and lip lesions, and 38% with oral, lip, and skin lesions.

The lesions generally develop rapidly, beginning as an erythematous area where vesicles form, break down, and quickly ulcerate. Often the lesions coalesce, forming a grayish white pseudomembrane and leaving a yellowish white exudate (Fig. 166-2). During the lesion formation the patient may complain of sialorrhea and dysphasia. A mild fever and lymphadenitis may accompany the lesions.

In Stevens-Johnson syndrome, the severe form of erythema multiforme, visceral lesions also occur in addition to cutaneous, oral, ocular, and genital mucosal lesions. The oral lesions generally appear more necrotic and the skin rash more maculopapular than the classic target lesions of erythema multiforme. It is not uncommon for oral lesions to precede the others, often starting during a prodromal period that may resemble a common respiratory infection.

DENTAL MANAGEMENT. In the mild form of erythema multiforme, treatment is directed at the symptoms. The severe form requires systemic steroid therapy.

The patient generally is most concerned about the pain and inability to eat and drink. Decreased fluid intake can lead to dehydration, for which the young patient especially may need

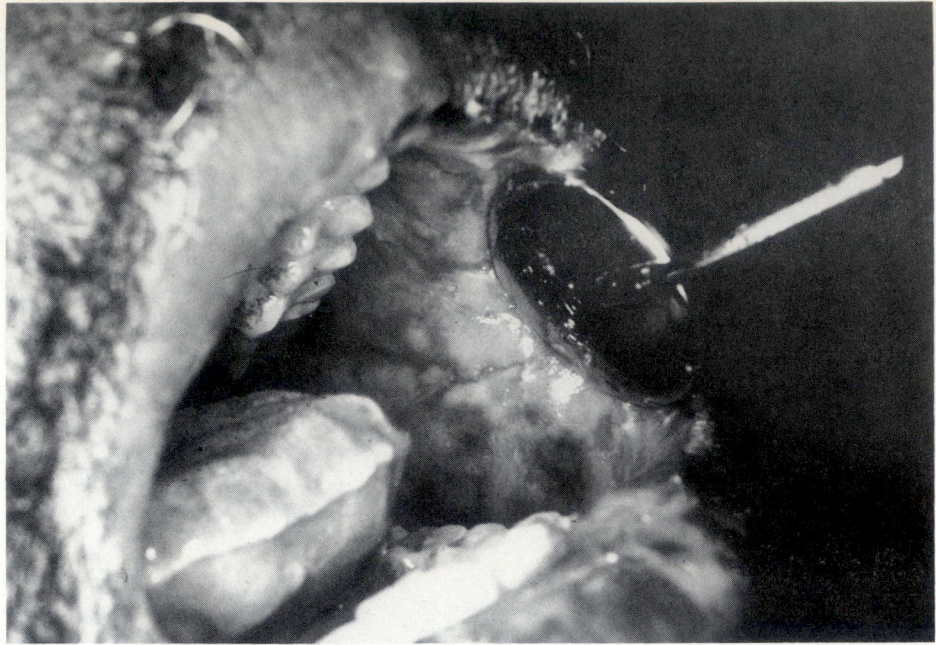

Fig. 166-2 Large ulcerative lesions with pseudomembrane of tongue and buccal mucosa in patient with recurrent erythema multiforme.

intravenous therapy. Systemic corticosteroids are the treatment of choice, and the disease begins to resolve within days. Therapy directed at the symptoms includes topical anesthetics, neutral mouth rinses, and a switch to a liquid and then a soft, bland diet.

Patients should be instructed to avoid alcohol-containing mouth rinses and trauma to the mucosa. They should use a soft, sponge-type toothbrush or gauze.

A recent study of a patient with erythema multiforme showed that prophylactic use of acyclovir, 200 mg five times a day for 7 days, and then maintenance therapy three times a day, helped in preventing recurrent herpes labialis. During this treatment the patient developed no recurrent erythema multiforme.

BIBLIOGRAPHY

Araujo OE and Flowers FP: Stevens-Johnson syndrome, J Emerg Med 2:129, 1984.

Bianchine JR and others: Drugs as etiologic factors in Stevens-Johnson syndrome, Am J Med 44:390, 1968.

Edmond BJ and others: Erythema multiforme, Pediatr Clin North Am 30:631, 1983.

Fulghum DD and Catalano PM: Stevens-Johnson syndrome from clindamycin, JAMA 223:318, 1973.

Green JA and others: Post-herpetic erythema multiforme prevented with prophylactic oral acyclovir, Ann Int Med 102:632, 1985.

Helligren L and Hersle K: Erythema multiforme: statistical evaluation of clinical and laboratory data in 224 patients and matched healthy controls, Acta Allergol 21:45, 1965.

Kalb RE and others: Stevens-Johnson syndrome due to mycoplasma pneumonia in an adult, Am J Med 79:541, 1985.

Lozado F and Silverman S: Erythema multiforme, Oral Surg 46:628, 1978.

Meyers W: Erythema multiforme, Arch Dermatol 101:707, 1970.

Mok CH and Stevens FRT: Stevens-Johnson syndrome, Med J Aust 2:591, 1964.

Naz MM and Ranalli DN: Stevens-Johnson syndrome, Oral Surg 53:263, 1982.

Nesbit SP and Gobetti JP: Multiple recurrence of oral erythema multiforme after secondary herpes simplex: report of a case and review of literature, J Am Dent Assoc 112:348, 1986.

Shelley WB: Herpes simplex virus as a cause of erythema multiforme, JAMA 201:153, 1967.

Shklar G: Oral lesions of erythema multiforme: histologic and histiochemical observations, Arch Dermatol 92:495, 1965.

Webster GM and Simon JF: Erythema multiforme limited to the oral cavity: report of case, J Am Dent Assoc 83:1106, 1971.

ERYTHEMA NODOSUM

Erythema nodosum is a transitory syndrome of acute inflammatory erythematous nodules in the skin that are generally limited to the extensor surfaces of the extremities, especially the legs. It is not a specific entity but represents a hypersensitivity reaction to several infectious and other systemic processes and drug reactions; it most often occurs in relation to group A β-hemolytic streptococcal infections (pharyngitis, tonsillitis, and scarlet fever) and tuberculosis infections, as well as sarcoidosis. Other infections associated with this syndrome include bacterial infections (*Yersinia* species), deep fungal infections (blastomycosis, histoplasmosis, and coccidioidomycosis), superficial fungal infections (tinea capitis in the kerion formation stage), and chlamydial and viral infections (psittacosis, cat-scratch fever, and lymphogranuloma venereum). The eruption appears in relation to deep mycoses and tuberculosis when skin tests for these diseases show conversion to a positive reaction. Other noninfectious conditions in which erythema nodosum may occur include ulcerative colitis, regional enteritis (occasionally), Behçet's syndrome, leukemia, Hodgkin's disease, and following radiation therapy of pelvic malignancies. Occasionally, erythema nodosum may occur in patients receiving medication, especially sulfonamides, iodides, bromides, and contraceptive pills.

Erythema nodosum occurs most often in the spring and fall and least often in the summer. The greatest incidence is found in patients 20 to 35 years of age; the disease is rare after age 50. It occurs three times more often in women than in men. The incidence has been diminishing as the result of the control of many infectious diseases. Prodromal symptoms may include fever, chills, malaise, and arthralgia. The lesions consist of tender nodules, 1 to 5 cm in diameter, mainly on the anterior tibial surfaces; around the knees and ankles; occasionally on the thighs, forearms, and face; and rarely on the trunk. Episcleral nodules may develop in the palpebral fissures bilaterally. The cutaneous nodules are initially bright red, and the skin is smooth and shiny. Later the color may go through changes similar to those of a bruise (erythema contusiformis). Usually a few nodules are present, but dozens may occur, sometimes coalescing into larger plaques and producing induration and edema in affected areas, resembling erysipelas. The usual duration of erythema nodosum is 3 to 6 weeks, but sometimes it may last for months. During healing a fine scale may evolve, but neither suppuration nor resultant scarring ensues.

Hilar adenopathy may appear on chest roentgenograms if erythema nodosum is caused by sarcoidosis. Löfgren's syndrome, associated with sarcoidosis, consists of fever, erythema nodosum skin lesions, periarticular swelling of the ankles, and bilateral hilar enlargement.

Histologically, septal panniculitis occurs. Patients have inflammation of the blood vessels of the fibrous septum between the subcutaneous fat lobules, with perivascular infiltrate of neutrophils, lymphocytes, histiocytes, and eosinophils. Occasionally the lesion may appear granulomatous but with no caseation. Special studies reveal complement deposition, which suggests a possible immune mechanism.

The treatment of erythema nodosum is directed mainly at the underlying cause (sarcoidosis, tuberculosis, or drug reaction) of the eruption. Bed rest and intralesional cortisone are sometimes beneficial. Nonsteroidal antiinflammatory agents (aspirin, indomethacin, and naproxen) and systemic corticosteroid therapy can give temporary relief from symptoms, although they may not shorten the course of the eruption. Supersaturated potassium iodide may also relieve the symptoms. Recurrences sometimes arise after withdrawal of corticosteroids, and these agents should be used only when no evidence of an underlying infectious process exists.

ORAL MANIFESTATIONS. Erythema nodosum is often a secondary finding of an underlying systemic disease. Although the lesions are generally located on the extremities, intraoral lesions related to underlying disease may occur. If patients report erythematous lesions on the extensor surfaces of the arms or legs, a careful history must be taken and referral for diagnosis made to determine the underlying cause. Cases of erythema nodosum have been reported before the onset of Behcet's syndrome.

BIBLIOGRAPHY

Bodansky HJ: Erythema nodosum and infectious mononucleosis, Br Med J 2:1263, 1979.

Fine RM and Meltzer HD: Erythema nodosum: form of allergic cutaneous vasculitis, South Med J 61:680, 1968.

Fine RM and Meltzer HD: Chronic erythema nodosum, Arch Dermatol 100:33, 1969.

Frayha RA and Nasr FW: Erythema nodosum—arthropathy complex as an initial presentation of Behçet's disease: report of 5 cases, J Rheumatol 5:244, 1978.

Soderstrum RM and Krull EA: Erythema nodosum: a review, Cutis 21:806, 1971.

Tierney LM and Schwartz RA: Erythema nodosum, Am Fam Physician 30:227, 1984.

Weinstein L: Erythema nodosum, DM 6:1, 1969.

ERYTHEMA CHRONICUM MIGRANS; LYME DISEASE

Erythema chronicum migrans (ECM) is an annular, expanding erythematous lesion caused by a spirochetal infection resulting from a tick bite (family Ixodidae). The lesion begins as a papule and gradually expands peripherally to form a

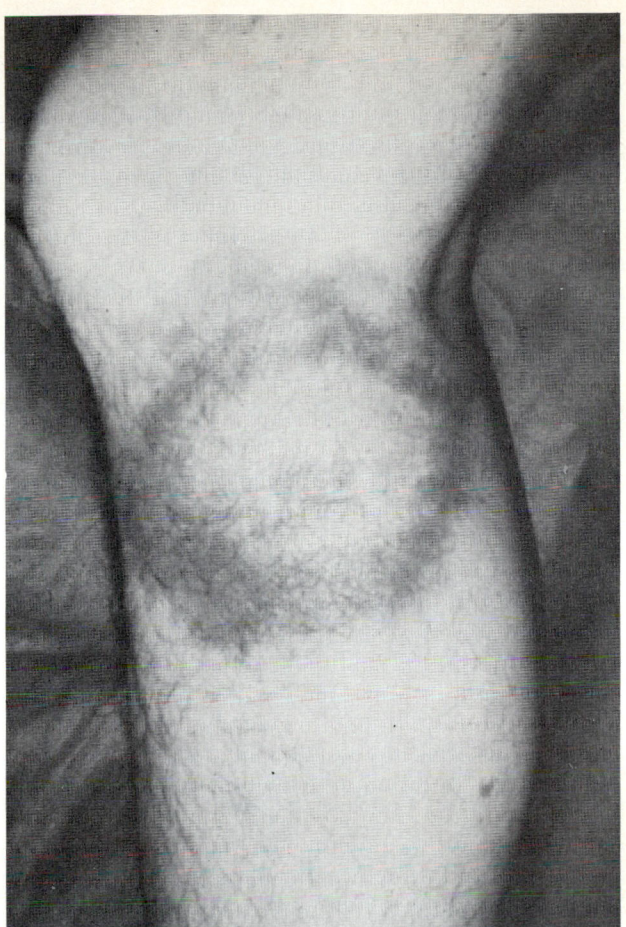

Fig. 166-3 Erythema chronicum migrans. Note central clearing. (Courtesy of Westwood Pharmaceuticals.)

palpable ring with an edematous border, trailing scales and then central clearing (Fig. 166-3). Regional lymphadenopathy may occur. The lesion may persist several months without therapy.

ECM is one of the manifestations of Lyme disease (named after Lyme, Conn., where a clustering of the disease occurred). The earliest signs are ECM, fever, headache, and myalgias (flulike symptoms). About 1 month later a transient, asymmetric arthritis appears, usually affecting only a few joints but usually the knees. These attacks last about 1 to 4 weeks and often recur. The central nervous and cardiac systems may also be affected in Lyme disease with Bell's palsy, encephalomeningitis, and varying degrees of atrioventricular block. These last approximately 2 months. Lyme arthritis is caused by a spirochete (Borrelia burgdorferi). In a study on Lyme's disease, 37% of patients had ECM alone and 63% had signs of disseminated infection, most often affecting the brain or meninges, other skin sites, lymph nodes, and joints.

The cause of ECM is a spirochete, *Borrellia burgdorferi*, living within the gut of ticks. The tick *Ixodes dammini* has been implicated. Cultures on patients have seldom identified organisms. Often, the diagnosis must be based on the clinical picture. Antibody titers of convalescent serum have been positive. The arthritis is probably mediated by an immune complex. Patients often have specific antispirochetal titers.

ECM responds readily to antibiotics, especially tetracycline and penicillin. Erythromycin is also beneficial. Tetracycline may prevent development of the major later sequelae of the joints, central nervous system, and heart. Therefore, tetracycline, 250 mg four times daily for 10 days, is the drug of choice. Later, if necessary, high doses of intravenous penicillin are administered. Improvement in patients taking potassium iodide has been reported.

A major complication of Lyme disease has been seen during pregnancy. In one study, 5 of 19 pregnant women had fetal complications, including syndactyly, blindness, rashes, intrauterine fetal death, and prematurity.

ORAL MANIFESTATIONS. A review of the literature fails to reveal oral involvement in erythema chronicum migrans. It does not appear to be related to erythema migrans (geographic tongue, migratory glossitis) for which no proven etiology has been found. (See section on psoriasis, p. 842).

More than 80% of patients with Lyme disease may have head and neck complaints, including headache and stiff neck. Patients may seek dental care because of these headaches. Cranial or spinal neuropathies, especially unilateral or bilateral Bell's palsy, have been reported. Neuropathies and lesions of the erythema chronicum migrans suggest a diagnosis of Lyme disease.

BIBLIOGRAPHY

Centers for Disease Control: Lyme disease—United States, 1980, MMWR 30:489, 1981.
Eichenfield AH and others: Childhood Lyme arthritis: experience in an endemic area, J Pediatr 109:753, 1986.
Gross GP and others: Erythema chronicum migrans with purpura and polymorphonuclear infiltrate, Arch Dermatol 115:873, 1979.
Hardin JA and others: Immune complexes and the evolution of Lyme arthritis, N Engl J Med 301:1358, 1979.
Markowitz LE and others: Lyme disease during pregnancy, JAMA 255:3394, 1986.
Mast WE and Burrows WM: Erythema chronicum migrans in the United States, JAMA 236:859, 1976.
Reik L and others: Neurologic abnormalities in Lyme disease without erythema chronicum migrans, Am J Med 81:73, 1986.
Shrestha M and others: Diagnosing early Lyme disease, Am J Med 78:235, 1985.
Smith RL and others: Erythema chronicum migrans, Cutis 17:962, 1976.
Steere AC and others: Erythema chronicum migrans and Lyme arthritis, Ann Intern Med 86:685, 1977.
Steere AC and others: Treatment of early manifestations of Lyme disease, Ann Intern Med 99:22, 1983.

167·INFECTIONS

Bernard A. Kirshbaum *and* **Robert N. Arm**

Viral infections

Bernard A. Kirshbaum *and* **Robert N. Arm**

HERPES SIMPLEX

Herpes simplex virus (HSV) infects humans, who are its only natural host. Antibodies to HSV can be detected in 50% to 100% of certain childhood and adult populations based on group selections. The virus is spread by direct contact and is very contagious. Most primary infections occur in children, and many are subclinical. HSV-1 was formerly associated almost exclusively with oral, mucosal, and skin lesions above the waist; HSV-2 usually caused genital and skin lesions below the waist. Conversely, oral mucosal lesions may be caused by HSV-2 and genital lesions may be caused by HSV-1, which is undoubtedly associated with more liberal sexual practices.

The HSV infections can be divided into primary and recurrent. The incubation period for the primary infection is 4 to 5 days but can be as long as 12 days. Several forms of primary infection exist.

Primary herpes

GINGIVOSTOMATITIS. Gingivostomatitis is the most common form of primary herpes, occurring usually in children but sometimes in adults. It may be asymptomatic, but generally there is a prodrome of fever, malaise, restlessness, and drooling. Vesicles that promptly ulcerate appear and may become widespread on the buccal and gingival mucosa, tongue, palate, tonsils, and pharynx. Patients have regional lymphadenopathy and considerable pain in oral tissues, along with foul breath and loss of appetite. Dehydration and acidosis may occur, especially in young children, because the oral pain makes even fluid intake difficult. Recovery is complete in about 2 weeks.

GENITAL HERPES. In genital herpes a circumscribed patch of vesicles on an erythematous base appears on the glans or shaft of the penis, labia, clitoris, vaginal wall, or cervix. The primary infection may be very painful, with urinary retention caused by dysuria resulting from urethral involvement. Milder cervical or vaginal wall infection may go unnoticed. Lesions may also occur on the thighs and perianally. Regional lymphadenopathy is present.

KERATOCONJUNCTIVITIS. HSV can cause a purulent conjunctivitis and a very painful dendritic keratitis. Autoinoculation of the eye may occur from another site on the body by way of the fingers. An ophthalmologist should be consulted when eye involvement is suspected. Topical antiviral agents that are effective in the eye include idoxuridine and adenosine arabinoside.

INOCULATION HERPES. Inoculation herpes can occur when an abrasion in the skin comes in contact with HSV. The most common sites are the index and middle fingers. Medical and dental personnel are at higher risk of this "herpetic whitlow," which is extremely painful. Swelling, erythema, and vesiculation of the fingertip or finger pad occur. This is often confused with a pyogenic infection, but incision, drainage, and antibiotics are of no help in the herpes infection.

Recurrent herpes

Recurrent HSV infection occurs in up to 40% of patients. The virus persists in the local nerve ganglia, from which recurrent invasion of the skin occurs. Sunlight, menses, fever, infection, debilitation, stress, trauma, and pregnancy can trigger recurrence. Many times no initiating factor can be identified. The lesions are often painful.

The most common type of recurrence is the "fever blister" or "cold sore," also known as herpes labialis. The lesions recur at almost the identical site each time. A tingling or burning sensation generally precedes the development of the lesion. This prodrome may last from a few hours to 2 days; then vesicles erupt for 2 to 4 days but rupture quickly if trauma occurs. These vesicles evolve into crusts lasting 8 to 11 days. Healing follows, without scarring unless secondary bacterial infection supervenes. The lesions remain infectious for varying periods, and thus patients should be told that the lesions are infectious until the crusts fall off.

Recurrent HSV infections may also occur intraorally on the hard palate (bound oral tissue) or other areas such as the buttocks. The same prodrome occurs. Circumscribed vesicles on an erythematous base develop and evolve as already described.

Recurrent genital HSV infection is an escalating problem. The recurrent infection is often shorter in duration and less symptomatic than the primary infection but very contagious. Particularly important are the devastating effects that genital HSV infections have on the neonate and the developing fetus. Cesarean birth is needed for delivery of the infant if active vaginal herpes infection is present.

In patients with atopic dermatitis, a condition of disseminated cutaneous infection called eczema herpeticum can develop. Severe disseminated herpes infection can also occur in patients receiving immunosuppressive agents and in those with certain malignancies.

No permanent cure for recurrent HSV infections exists at present. However, acyclovir (Zovirax), both as topical ointment and oral capsules, is effective in mitigating the active eruption. Acyclovir is also available for intravenous administration in patients with severe disseminated herpes infection, which may occur in immunosuppressed patients. Local compresses and medications to relieve pain are beneficial. Patients must understand the infectious nature of the disease.

BIBLIOGRAPHY

Corey L and others: Infections with herpes simplex viruses, N Engl J Med 314:686, 1986.
Harger JH and others: Current understanding of genital herpes simplex infections, J Reprod Med 31:365, 1986.
Kaufman RH: Clinical features of herpes genitalis, J Reprod Med 31:379, 1986.
Marlowe SI: Medical management of genital herpes, Arch Dermatol 121:467, 1985.
Saginur R and others: Herpes simplex in the dental office, Can Dent Assoc J 52:700, 1986.
Strauss SE and others: NIH conference—herpes simplex virus infection: biology, treatment, and prevention, Ann Intern Med 103:404, 1985.
Zakay-Rones Z and others: Hypothesis: the gingival tissue as a reservoir for herpes simplex virus, Microbiologica 9:367, 1986.

HERPES ZOSTER

Herpes zoster, also called "shingles" or zoster, is caused by the reactivation of varicella (chickenpox) virus that remains dormant in the sensory ganglia. The disease is characterized by groups of vesicles on an erythematous base in a dermatomal arrangement. Zoster occurs only in persons who previously have had chickenpox. It is infectious for a person who has not had chickenpox, that is, a person who has not had varicella can receive the infection from someone with zoster, but a patient with chickenpox cannot transmit zoster to another individual.

The frequency of herpes zoster increases with age. Two thirds of the patients are over 45 years of age. It is rare in children, and the incidence is thought to be 2:1000 in the general population. Increased frequencies of zoster are found in association with Hodgkin's disease, other lymphomas, leukemia, and renal transplantation because of immunosuppression. Antineoplastic agents, corticosteroids, and radiation therapy have also been implicated in the induction of zoster, as well as its dissemination.

The prodrome usually consists of painful burning, tingling, itching, or tenderness along one or more contiguous sensory nerves. The dermatomes affected are along thoracic nerves (50%), cervical nerves (20%), lumbosacral nerves (10%), and trigeminal nerves (10% to 15%). Bilateral involvement is rare. Two to 4 days after the initial symptoms, grouped papulovesicles erupt along the involved nerve. These evolve into pustules, which later are crusted. Regional lymphadenopathy

may occur. Once the eruption appears, the symptoms may decrease, but not in all patients. In young adults the lesions resolve in 2 to 3 weeks, whereas in older patients it may take longer. A few scattered vesicles or pustules outside the involved dermatome may appear.

Cutaneous dissemination, occurring 6 to 10 days after the onset of dermatomal lesions, develops in about 2% of patients. However, cutaneous and systemic dissemination may occur in 25% of patients with Hodgkin's disease, other lymphomas, or leukemia and in those receiving corticosteroids or immunosuppressive agents. Systemic zoster may involve the gastrointestinal tract, myocardium, lungs, and central nervous system. The patients most susceptible to zoster meningoencephalitis are those with ophthalmic zoster, that is, involvement of the ophthalmic division of the fifth cranial nerve. If the nasociliary branch is affected, with lesions on the side of the nose, vesicles and ulceration may develop on the cornea. Adenosine arabinoside has recently been used to treat disseminated zoster as well as acyclovir intravenously.

Postherpetic neuralgia is a complication of herpes zoster. Patients have intractable, disabling pain in the area of the healed zoster. This occurs in about 30% of patients over 40 years of age. These patients frequently have a more aggressive form of dermatomal zoster, with deeper, more necrotic lesions and at times very severe pain during the zoster attack.

The treatment includes analgesics for the pain, drying lotions and compresses, and topical corticosteroid sprays. When the possibility of eye involvement exists, an ophthalmologist should be consulted.

BIBLIOGRAPHY

Cobo LM and others: Oral acyclovir in the treatment of acute herpes zoster ophthalmicus, Ophthalmology 93:763, 1986.
Friedman-Kien AE and others: Herpes zoster: a possible early clinical sign for development of acquired immunodeficiency syndrome in high-risk individuals, J Am Acad Dermatol 14:1023, 1986.
Fueyo MA and Lookingbill DP: Herpes zoster and occult malignancy, J Am Acad Dermatol 11:480, 1984.
Garty BZ and others: Tooth exfoliation and osteonecrosis of the maxilla after trigeminal herpes zoster, J Pediatr 106:71, 1985.
Harnisch JP: Zoster in the elderly: clinical, immunologic and therapeutic considerations, J Am Geriatr Soc 32:789, 1984.
Liesegang TJ: The varicella-zoster virus: systemic and ocular features, J Am Acad Dermatol 11:165, 1984.
Newton-John H and others: Herpes zoster, Aust Fam Physician 15:1343, 1986.

WARTS

Warts (verrucae) are viral-induced benign tumors of the epidermis and mucous membranes. They are caused by papovaviruses and occur at some time in 80% of the population; at any given time 10% of children and 5% of adults have warts. There are several varieties of warts: vulgaris (common), plantar (sole of the foot), flat (facial and other body areas), periungual, and condyloma acuminatum (genital or perirectal). It has been shown recently that many different types of human papovaviruses induce these various forms. Some of the viruses in this group are oncogenic, particularly those found in the genital areas and on the cervix.

Antibodies to warts develop, and many believe that this is responsible for partial immunity to recurrence. Patients with active warts often have low titers of IgM antibody. During regression of warts, either spontaneous or induced, wart antibody titers rise, and both IgG and IgM antibodies develop. Among patients with recurrence, 25% have IgG antibodies.

Warts can regress spontaneously. One third of warts are

usually gone within 6 months, and two-thirds disappear within 2 years. However, some lesions may persist for many years.

Patients who are pregnant, are immunosuppressed, or have immunodeficiency states show a higher rate of wart infection, and the warts are often extensive and recalcitrant to treatment. This includes renal transplant patients, those with acquired immunodeficiency syndrome (AIDS), patients undergoing immunosuppressive therapy for other diseases, and those with lymphomas, Hodgkin's disease, chronic lymphocytic leukemia, and Wiskott-Aldrich syndrome.

Many treatments for warts are available. It is best to begin conservatively because of the benign nature of the condition. Irritants (salicyclic acid compounds), carbolic and trichloroacetic acid, liquid nitrogen freezing, and podophyllin solutions (best for condyloma acuminatum) are established therapies. Surgery (curettage and electrodesiccation) is useful for isolated or persistent lesions. Laser destruction may become necessary for recalcitrant warts.

Immunotherapy with dinitrochlorobenzene should be avoided because it results in permanent sensitization of the skin. Local injection of bleomycin may be effective but carries potential risks. The clearing of warts is often enhanced by suggestion therapy.

BIBLIOGRAPHY

Adler-Storthz K and others: Identification of human papillomavirus in oral verruca vulgaris, J Oral Pathol 15:230, 1986.
Giullet GY and others: Cutaneous and mucosal warts: clinical and histopathological criteria for classification, Int J Dermatol 21:89, 1982.
Jenson AB and others: Frequency and distribution of papilloma virus structural antigens in verrucae, multiple papillomas, and condylomata of the oral cavity, Am J Pathol 107:212, 1982.
Lutzner MA: The human papilloma viruses, Arch Dermatol 119:631, 1983.
Lutzner MA and others: Different papilloma viruses as the cause of oral warts, Arch Dermatol 118:393, 1982.
Mroczkowski TF and others: Warts and other human papilloma virus infections, Postgrad Med 78:91, 1985.

MOLLUSCUM CONTAGIOSUM

Mulluscum contagiosum is caused by a pox virus. It is spread by direct contact and occurs most often in children. However, the lesions can develop in adults, often through sexual contact. Patients with atopic dermatitis may be susceptible to widespread, generalized infection.

The virus infects the skin, and lesions are probably spread by autoinoculation. The incubation period ranges from 14 to 50 days. The lesions appear as dome-shaped, umbilicated papules that are translucent or whitish. They occur most often on the face, neck, arms, inner aspect of the thighs, pubic area, and buttocks. Some lesions involute spontaneously, but many persist for months to years. Occasionally a giant molluscum occurs, requiring surgical excision.

The skin lesions are benign and should be treated delicately. A curette can be used to shell out the molluscum body (which is the central core), or the body can be expressed and the central cavity cauterized with carbolic acid. Freezing with liquid nitrogen is also effective.

ORAL MANIFESTATIONS AND DENTAL MANAGEMENT. See section on viral infection in Chapter 58.

BIBLIOGRAPHY

Brown ST and others: Molluscum contagiosum, Sex Transm Dis 8:227, 1986.
Felman YM: Molluscum contagiosum, Cutis 33:113, 1984.
Laskaris G and Sklavounou A: Molluscum contagiosum of the oral mucosa, Oral Surg 58:688, 1984.
Lynfield YL and Laude TA: Molluscum contagiosum: an unusual presentation, Cutis 30:321, 1982.

Pierard-Franchimont C and others: Growth and regression of molluscum contagiosum, J Am Acad Dermatol 9:669, 1983.

ACQUIRED IMMUNODEFICIENCY SYNDROME

Toby Shawe and Bernard A. Kirshbaum

The acquired immunodeficiency syndrome (AIDS) is caused by a retrovirus previously designated as human T-cell leukemia (lymphotropic) virus type III (HTLV-III/LAV). This virus has recently been renamed human immunodeficiency virus (HIV).

The nonspecific manifestations of this infection include fatigue, malaise, night sweats, fever, diarrhea, weight loss, and generalized persistent nontender lymphadenopathy. This is the AIDS-related complex (ARC). The more specific manifestations of AIDS include opportunistic infections and Kaposi's sarcoma. The diagnosis is confirmed by detecting antibodies to HIV antigens by means of enzyme-linked immunosorbent assay (ELISA) and immunoblotting techniques. It is also important to examine general hematologic parameters in these patients because of anemia and leukopenia (lymphopenia), as well as to perform T-lymphocyte subset determinations, since the retrovirus directly attacks and lyses T cells (T4), causing a diminution in the helper/suppressor (T4/T8) ratio. This inversion of the ratio is pathognomonic of the disease and is a marker of the individual's vulnerability to infections. Associated polyclonal rise in IgG and skin anergy to delayed hypersensitivity testing occur.

The skin and mucous membrane manifestations of AIDS include certain opportunistic infections that are more virulent in these patients, Kaposi's sarcoma and squamous cell carcinoma, and several nonspecific skin diseases associated with or apparently enhanced by AIDS.

Herpes simplex is among the infectious diseases that more frequently occur. Patients with HIV disease often have a history of recurrent, severe anogenital herpes simplex infection, often with a chronic course. These individuals may sometimes have pronounced attacks of oral herpes simplex lesions that commonly extend to and involve esophageal and tracheobronchial mucosa. Mucocutaneous herpes simplex usually responds promptly to a 7- to 10-day course of intravenous acyclovir. Viral shedding ceases within several days, and the lesions reepithelialize. Continuous administration of oral acyclovir may control these recurrences.

Molluscum contagiosum has also been reported in these immunosuppressed patients, often resulting in hundreds of molluscum lesions, which recur almost as promptly as they are removed. Langerhans' cells, which have the antigen on their surface, represent the first step in the dermatoimmunologic cascade. Not only are helper-T lymphocytes diminished, but Langerhans' cells also are decreased in patients with AIDS. This immunologic defect may permit the molluscum contagiosum virus to continue infecting keratinocytes, thereby causing many lesions.

Herpes zoster is another viral disease associated with immunosuppressed conditions, and in patients with AIDS this runs a more virulent course. Cytomegalovirus may also be responsible for atypical oral infections, and cutaneous lesions consisting of localized ulcers and maculopapular rash with terminal petechial and pruritic papuloulcerative eruptions have been noted. Hyperpigmented, indurated cutaneous plaques have been reported as heralding a disseminated cytomegalovirus infection. Concurrent infections of herpes simplex and cytomegalovirus have been described. Biopsy and culture of suspicious lesions are recommended. Trimethoprim combined with sulfamethoxazole is used to treat cytomegalovirus infection. Papova virus (warts) and papilloma virus have been associated with this syndrome because of the profound defect in cell-mediated immunity.

A unique new oral lesion named oral "hairy leukoplakia" has been described. These thickened, whitish, poorly demarcated patches are usually found on the lateral border of the tongue and rarely on the dorsal and ventral surfaces of the tongue, with extension to the buccal mucosa. The lesion is usually solitary but may be bilateral and measures from a few millimeters to 3.5 cm. They are usually asymptomatic but may be sore. These lesions do not rub off and do not regress spontaneously. Electron microscopy has shown the presence of two viruses in the epithelial cells of hairy leukoplakia: papilloma virus and Epstein-Barr virus (EBV); the cells contain EBV deoxyribonucleic acid (DNA) and viral capsid antigen. The lesions usually have a superficially invasive fungal organism.

Several fungi associated with AIDS have been reported, including histoplasmosis, which may appear as widespread erythematous maculopapular eruptions on the trunk and proximal extremities; a mild folliculitis; and papules with central keratinous plugs. *Histoplasma capsulatum* is a dimorphic fungus endemic in eastern and central parts of the United States. This disease should be suspected in AIDS patients from these areas.

Cryptococcus neoformans has been isolated from lesions resembling molluscum contagiosum, and *Acanthamoeba castellani* has also been cultured from a papule of a patient with disseminated infection with this organism.

Extensive infection with *Trichophyton rubrum* is an important sign in immunodepressed HIV-positive patients. However, the most common infection in AIDS, although not diagnostic of the disease, is oral candidiasis. Candidiasis is present in all high-risk groups, and all homosexual/bisexual men with AIDS have oral manifestations. Oropharyngeal candidiasis responds to antifungal treatment with nystatin liquid or clotrimazole applied every 4 hours. Oral ketoconazole or intravenous amphotericin B may be required to resolve highly resistant cases. However, oral candidiasis recurs in most patients soon after treatment is stopped, and these patients must receive oral ketoconazole or nystatin maintenance therapy indefinitely. When esophagoscopy reveals candidal infection affecting the gastrointestinal tract, in combination with HIV seropositivity, the patient is classified as having AIDS.

Because of the high level of sexual activity as well as orogenital contact, homosexual AIDS patients are at an increased risk for oral lesions of syphilis, gonorrhea, and atypical oral infections, such as with *Escherichia coli*.

Mycobacterium avium-intracellulare is a Runyon group III, nonchromagenic, niacin-negative species of mycobacteria. It is a common environmental contaminant, especially in the Southwest United States. Cellular immunity defects predispose AIDS patients to infection with this organism, and the clinical findings are indistinguishable from infection with *M. tuberculosis*. In disseminated infection with *M. avium-intracellulare*, patients may have oral lesions, and samples of palatal gingiva show a granulomatous histiocytic process. Acid-fast stains reveal clusters of mycobacteria within the cytoplasm of the histiocytes. These infections are usually resistant to isoniazid, rifampin and other commonly used antitubercular agents. Patients with *M. avium-intracellulare* infection usually die.

Chronic, initially pustular acneiform folliculitis has been described as an early warning skin sign in AIDS and ARC patients. These occur in two forms, a relapsing folliculitis concentrated around the axillae and a diffusely scattered eruption on the face, back, chest, and buttocks. In these infections a severe, mixed perifollicular infiltrate with lymphocytes, poly-

morphonuclear leukocytes, plasma cells, and granulomatous inflammation occur. Treatment with local steroids and emollients and systemic antibiotics are only partly successful because relapses are frequent. A rare eosinophilic pustular folliculitis has also been described in AIDS and ARC patients. This may be associated with hypersensitivity of the skin to dermatophytes and *Demodex folliculorum* infection.

Tinea versicolor caused by *Pityrosporum* tends to be more prominent in patients with immunosuppressed disease.

The most common malignancy associated with AIDS is Kaposi's sarcoma. These lesions are significantly different in location and configuration from the rare type of Kaposi's sarcoma occurring in Eastern European men. The lesions seen in HIV-infected patients are generally smaller, moderately infiltrated, reddish blue to brownish papules and plaques located mainly on the upper part of the trunk and face, including the nose as well as the upper extremities. These lesions may vary from solitary brownish macules and larger red-brownish papules to widespread violaceous tumors covering parts of the trunk and extremities. Kaposi's sarcoma in the oral cavity occurs in 5% to 50% of patients with AIDS. Although the oral lesions usually occur in AIDS patients in whom the tumor is widely disseminated, it can be the first site in which these lesions appear. Multifocal, often symmetric oromucosal lesions occur most often on the hard and soft palate but have been reported on all mucosal surfaces. Kaposi's sarcoma is a multicentric vascular angiosarcomatous neoplasm. As with its cutaneous counterparts, the oral lesions begin as poorly circumscribed, erythematous macules on nonkeratinized mucosal lining or as irregular, pinkish, pebbly looking papules about 0.5 cm in diameter on keratinized mucosa. The macules increase in size (to 2 cm or more) and in number. As they mature, hemosiderin is progressively deposited within the lesions, forming reddish, bluish, purplish, or brownish nodular vegetating plaques, which reveal the lesions' vascular sarcomatous nature. These lesions can be confused with gingivitis, pyogenic granuloma, vascular malformations (including hematoma, hemangioma, lymphangioma, angiofibroma, and hemangiopericytoma), and foci of ecchymoses caused by trauma. Histologically, they reveal the proliferation of slitlike vascular channels lined by decreased numbers of endothelial cells containing enlarged nuclei and the spindle-shaped neoplastic cells in the connective tissue that are the hallmark of Kaposi's sarcoma. The connective stroma contains scattered macrophages with both hyaline and eosinophilic granules.

Treatment includes radiation therapy and single-agent chemotherapy as well as combination chemotherapy employing vincristine, bleomycin, dactinomycin, adriamycin, carmustine (BCNU) and cyclophosphamide, as well as podophyllotoxin and parenterally administered α-interferon. Unfortunately, chemotherapeutic regimens aggravate the patient's immunosuppressed state, and most AIDS patients with Kaposi's sarcoma die of overwhelming opportunistic infections and irreversible cachexia and wasting. It has not been established whether successful treatment of Kaposi's sarcoma increases an individual's survival. The development of this tumor is an ominous sign, since death invariably follows in a few months to a few years following the initial diagnosis.

An increase in incidence of oral squamous cell carcinoma has been reported in association with AIDS patients.

Among the nonspecific manifestations related to AIDS, the development or aggravation of seborrheic dermatitis has been noted frequently. The appearance may vary from mild to extensive reddening and scaling of the face in these patients. It has been suggested that this may be associated with more intense infection with *Pityrosporum* yeasts, and some of these cases may be tinea faciale. To confirm this, scrapings should be examined with potassium hydroxide preparations or fungal cultures. *D. folliculorum* may also be present in greater numbers than in normal patients.

Vasculitis eruptions may also occur in patients with AIDS, appearing as purpuric lesions with histologic evidence of leukocytoclastic vasculitis and deposition of complement factors. Epithelioid agiomatosis, an unusual cutaneous vascular neoplasm distinct from Kaposi's sarcoma, has also been reported. The cutaneous lesions are solitary or multiple papulles and nodules. In some patients the lesions also affect internal organs. Histologically the neoplasms are composed of proliferating blood vessels and cells with epithelioid. In some patients the lesions gradually disappear, but in some instances, they may be the cause of death from disseminated intravascular coagulation or laryngeal obstruction by the tumor. Erythema elevatum diutinum has also been reported, as well as other types of atypical lymphoreticular neoplasms. Acquired ichthyosis and xeroderma, as well as yellow nail syndrome have been reported in patients with AIDS. Recalcitrant psoriasis has been observed among patients infected with HIV.

Drug eruptions in AIDS patients receiving antibiotics for opportunistic infection also is common. Patients receiving sulfamethoxazole-trimethoprim for *Pneumocystis carinii* develop extensive macular rashes. An extensive eczematous skin eruption in an AIDS patient treated with systemic spiramycin for toxoplasmosis also has been reported. An exanthematic eruption mimicking syphilitic roseola has been reported. There is no scaling in these lesions, which helps to differentiate this eruption from pityriasis rosea. Other viral exanthems (EB virus, cytomegalovirus, hepatitis B virus) must be considered in the differential diagnosis. These individuals are more susceptible to xerostomia, recurrent aphthae, and precocious peridental disease. Acrodermatitis enteropathica has been reported as occurring in childhood AIDS. Profound alterations in hair patterns have been reported in some black men 2 to 3 years after the first symptoms of AIDS. The hair became longer, lighter, softer, silky, and occasionally discolored.

BIBLIOGRAPHY

Anneroth G and others: Acquired immunodeficiency syndrome (AIDS) in the U.S. in 1986: etiology, epidemiology, clinical manifestations, and dental implications, J Oral Maxillofac Surg 44:956, 1986.

Chernosky ME and Finley VK: Yellow nail syndrome in patients with acquired immunodeficiency disease, J Am Acad Dermatol 13:731, 1985.

Cockerell CJ and others: Epithelioid agiomatosis: a distinct vascular disorder in patients with the aquired immunodefiency syndrome or AIDS-related complex, Lancet 2:654, 1987.

Conant MA and others: Squamous cell carcinoma in sexual partner of Kaposi's sarcoma patient, Lancet 1:286, 1982.

Eversol LR and others: Oral Kaposi's sarcoma associated with acquired immunodeficiency syndrome among homosexual males, J Am Dent Assoc 107:248, 1983.

Farthing CF and others: Skin disease in homosexual patients with acquired immune deficiency syndrome (AIDS) and lesser forms of human T cell leukemia virus (HTLV-III) disease, Clin Exp Dermatol 10:3, 1985.

Freidman-Kien AE and others: Herpes zoster: a possible early clinical sign for development of acquired immunodeficiency syndrome in high-risk individuals, J Am Acad Dermatol 14:1023, 1986.

Greenspan D and others: Oral "hairy" leukoplakia in male homosexuals: evidence of association with both papillomavirus and a herpes-group virus, Lancet 2:831, 1984.

Greenspan JS and others: Replication of Epstein-Barr virus within the epithelial cells of oral "hairy" leukoplakia: an AIDS associated lesion, N Engl J Med 313:1564, 1985.

James WD and others: A papular eruption associated with human T cell lymphotropic virus type III disease, J Am Acad Dermatol 13:563, 1985.

Johnson TM and others: AIDS exacerbates psoriasis, N Engl J Med 313:1415, 1985.

Kalter DC and others: Maculopapular rash in a patient with acquired immunodeficiency syndrome, Arch Dermatol 121:1455, 1985.

Klein RS and others: Oral candidiasis in high-risk patients as the initial manifestation of the acquired immunodeficiency syndrome, N Engl J Med 311:354, 1984.

Leonidas JR: Hair alteration in black patients with the acquired immunodeficiency syndrome, Cutis 39:537, 1987.

Lombardo PC: Molluscum contagiosum and the acquired immunodeficiency syndrome, Arch Dermatol 121:834, 1985.

Lozado F and others: Oral manifestations of tumor and opportunistic infections in acquired immunodeficiency syndrome (AIDS): findings in 53 homosexual men with Kaposi'a sarcoma, Oral Surg 56:491, 1983.

Martin J: Acquired immunodeficiency syndrome and Kaposi's sarcoma, Int J Dermatol 23:483, 1984.

Mayoral F and Penneys NS: Disseminated histoplasmosis presenting as a transepidermal elimination disorder in an AIDS victim, J Am Acad Dermatol 13:842, 1985.

Montilla P and others: Lymphomatoid granulomatosis and the acquired immunodeficiency syndrome (letter), Ann Intern Med 106:166, 1987.

Muhlemann MF and others: Early warning skin sign in AIDS and persistent generalized lymphoadenopathy, Br J Dermatol 114:419, 1986.

Penneys NS and Hicks B: Unusual cutaneous lesions associated with acquired immunodeficiency syndrome, J Am Acad Dermatol 13:845, 1985.

Perniciaro C and Peters MS: Tinea faciale mimicking seborrheic dermatitis in a patient with AIDS, N Engl J Med 30:315, 1986.

Sindrup JH and others: Skin manifestations in AIDS, HIV infection, and AIDS-related complex, Int J Dermatol 26:267, 1987.

Soeprono FF and Schinella RA: Eosinophilic pustular folliculitis in patients with acquired immunodeficiency syndrome, J Am Acad Dermatol 14:1020, 1986.

Tong TK and others: Childhood acquired immune deficiency syndrome manifesting as acrodermatitis enteropathica, J Pediatr 108:426, 1986.

Volberding P: Therapy of Kaposi's sarcoma in AIDS, Semin Oncol 11:65, 1984.

Volpe F and others: Oral manifestations of disseminated mycobacterium avium intracellulare in a patient with AIDS, Oral Surg Oral Med Oral Pathol 60:567, 1985.

Warner LC and Fisher BK: Cutaneous manifestations of AIDS, Int J Dermatol 25:337, 1986.

Wofford DJ and Miller RI: Acquired immunodeficiency syndrome (AIDS): disease characteristics and oral manifestations, J Am Dent Assoc 111:258, 1985.

FUNGAL INFECTIONS

Bernard A. Kirshbaum *and* **Robert N. Arm**

Superficial fungal infections, also known as tineas and dermatophyte infections, are limited to the keratin layer of the skin. There are several forms: tinea corporis (ringworm of the body), tinea pedis (athlete's foot), tinea capitis (ringworm of the scalp), tinea cruris (jock itch), and onychomycosis (fungal infection of the nails). These infections are caused by a number of fungi, the most common being *Trichophyton rubrum, T. mentagrophytes, Microsporum canis, M. audouini,* and *Epidermophyton floccosum.* The topical antifungal agents miconazole, clotrimazole, and cyclopyroxolamine, econozole and other imidazole derivatives, and the systemic agent griseofulvin are used for therapy. Ketoconazole is a newer systemic agent that is effective in some resistant cases.

Tinea corporis affects all ages. *T. rubrum, T. mentagrophytes,* and *M. canis* are the fungi most commonly isolated in this infection. The classic "ringworm" of the glabrous skin is an annular, erythematous, scaling patch with a spreading, active border and central clearing (Figs. 167-1 and 167-2). Lesions may be located on the face, trunk, and extremities, as well as intergluteally. The lesion tends to be pruritic. An eczematous form with vesicles, pustules and oozing may also be encountered; this is most often caused by *T. mentagrophytes.* These infections respond well to topical antifungal agents. When infection is severe, extensive, or prolonged, griseofulvin or ketoconazole may be required to control the lesions.

Tinea pedis may be a persistent and disabling problem. A

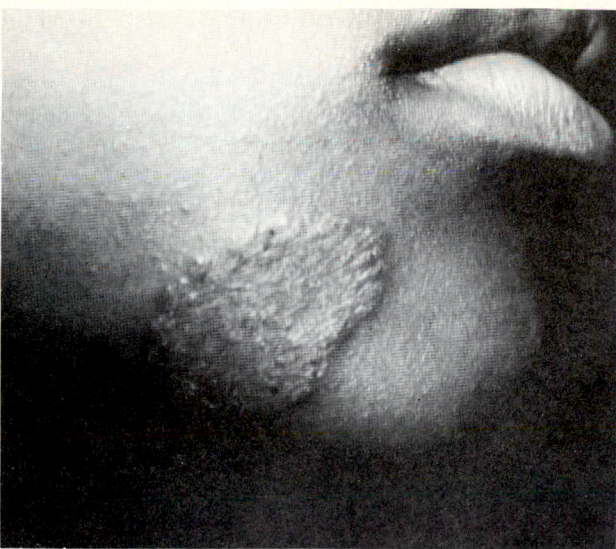

Fig. 167-1 Tinea on face of child. Lesion is slightly elevated with sharply demarcated erythematous border.

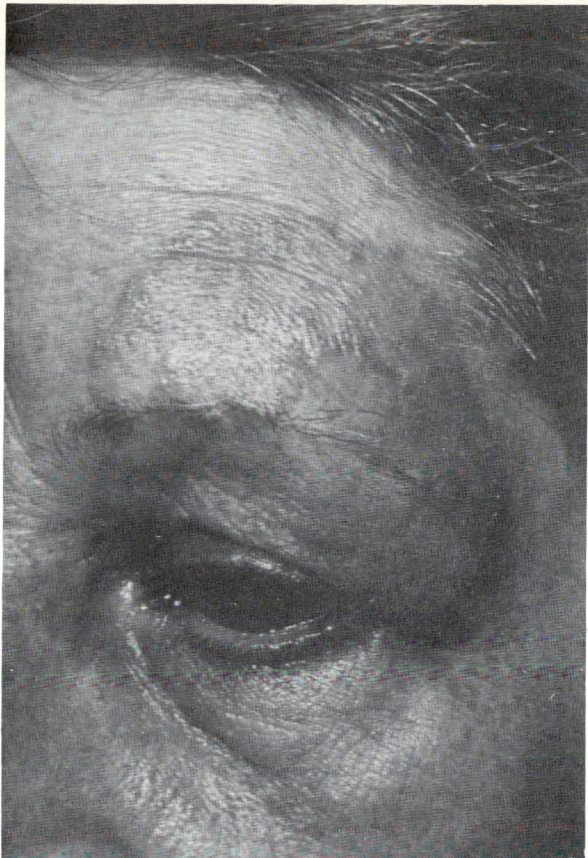

Fig. 167-2 Tinea on face of adult is less elevated and less inflamed than in children. (Courtesy of Department of Dermatology, The Cleveland Clinics.)

chronic, fine, dry scaling in the "moccasin distribution" on the feet is common in both men and women; the infecting agent characteristically is *T. rubrum*. An inflammatory, pustular, and vesicular variant occurring on the plantar surfaces is caused by *T. mentagrophytes*. Interdigital infections usually involve the third and fourth interspaces but may also be found in the other toe spaces. These areas commonly become secondarily infected, and antibiotic therapy may be required in addition to topical (or, if needed, systemic) antifungal agents.

Tinea capitis is almost exclusively a disease of children. In addition to the classic ringworm, it may appear as a diffuse, dandrufflike scaling, as an alopecic patch, as black dots on the scalp, or as a boggy, tender, oozing mass with crusts and alopecia. The form described last is called a kerion and is a hypersensitivity reaction to the fungal infection. Many species of superficial fungi (mainly in the *Microsporum* and *Trichophyton* groups) can cause tinea capitis. Scalp dermatophyte infections usually require griseofulvin therapy, since topical antifungal agents do not penetrate the follicles sufficiently.

Tinea cruris is an erythematous, scaling, pruritic eruption involving the groin. It is more common in men and tends to occur in warmer months. *E. floccosum* and *Candida albicans* are the usual causative agents in women, who seldom have the condition. When tinea crusis occurs in women, diabetes and obesity are among the contributing factors. *T. rubrum* and *T. mentagrophytes* are usually responsible for the infection in men. Topical antifungal therapy is indicated, and sometimes systemic agents (griseofulvin or ketoconazole) may be needed. Healing occurs with residual hyperpigmentation that fades slowly. Because of the thinness of scrotal skin and its inability to support an environment for fungal growth, the scrotum is usually not involved.

Onychomycosis is dermatophyte infection of the nails. The nails become thickened and discolored with subungual debris. Usually only one or a few nails are involved. Toenails do not respond as well as fingernails to therapy, which includes oral griseofulvin (or ketoconazole), which sometimes must be administered for many months before clearing. Topical antifungal agents are distinctly less effective in the treatment of onychomycosis. Surgical avulsion of the nails also may be beneficial, especially if followed by griseofulvin and topical therapy.

ORAL MANIFESTATIONS AND DENTAL MANAGEMENT. See section on fungal infections in Chapter 58.

BIBLIOGRAPHY

Faergemann J and Fredriksson T: Tinea versicolor: some new aspects on etiology, pathogenesis and treatment, Int J Dermatol 21:8, 1982.

Griffith ML and others: Superficial mycoses: therapeutic agents and clinical applications, Postgrad Med 79:151, 1986.

Honig PJ and Smith LR: Tinea capitis masquerading as atopic or seborrheic dermatitis, J Pediatr 94:604, 1979.

Jones HE: Therapy of superficial fungal infection, Med Clin North Am 66:873, 1982.

Krowchuk DP and others: Current status of the identification and management of tinea capitis, Pediatrics 72:625, 1983.

Lee SC and others: Psoriasis with tinea corporis, Cutis 26:159, 1980.

Safer EF and others: Tinea facei coexistent with discoid lupus erythematosus, Arch Dermatol 117:121, 1981.

Zinberg M and others: Recurrent fungal infection of the face: diagnostic pitfalls, Cutis 33:180, 1984.

YEAST *(CANDIDA)* INFECTIONS

Infections with the yeast *Candida albicans* are also known as moniliasis (from the former genus name for *Candida*). They may appear as monilial intertrigo and may be found in chronic paronychia. Factors predisposing patients to *Candida* infection include obesity, diabetes mellitus, and other endocrine disorders such as hypothyroidism, hypoparathyroidism, and hypoadrenalism. Iron deficiency anemia, zinc deficiency, pregnancy, use of oral contraceptives or broad-spectrum antibiotics, chronic debilitating illness, cancer chemotherapy, and deficiencies in cell-mediated immunity also predispose patients to the infection.

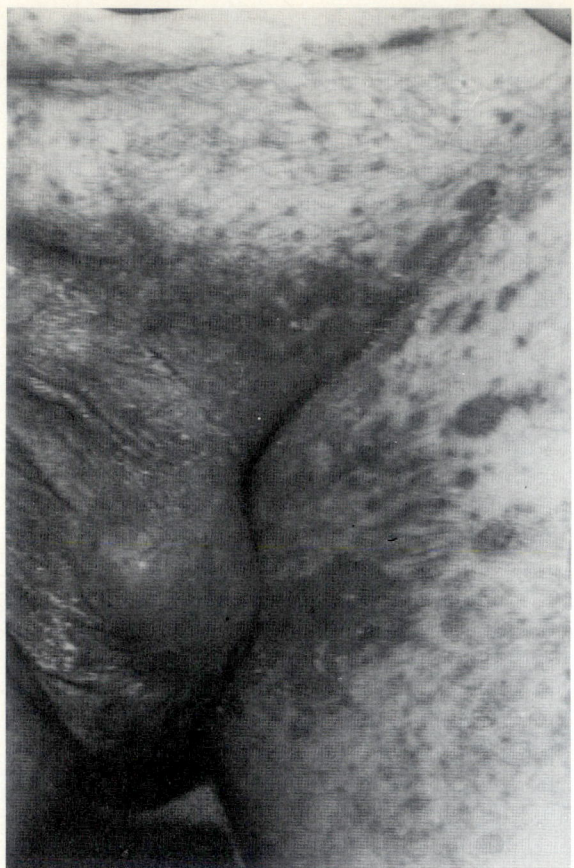

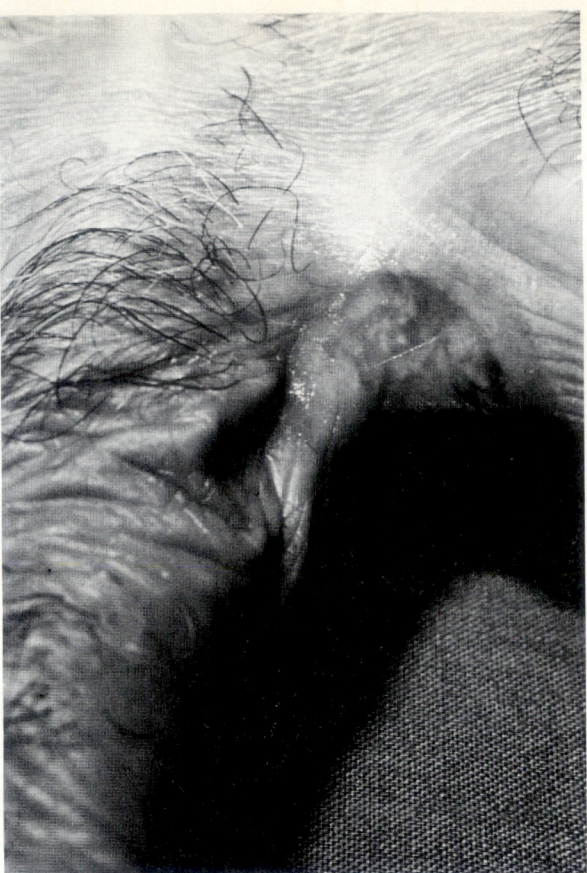

Fig. 167-3 Candidiasis of finger web (erosio interdigitale blastomy-cetica). Lesion is moist and erythematous and occurs in patients, such as bartenders, whose hands are continually wet. (Courtesy of Department of Dermatology, The Cleveland Clinics.)

Fig. 167-4 Genital intertrigo in candidiasis. This is a moist and ery-thematous eruption. Note satellite lesions, highly suggestive of *Candida* organisms. (Courtesy of Department of Dermatology, The Cleveland Clinics.)

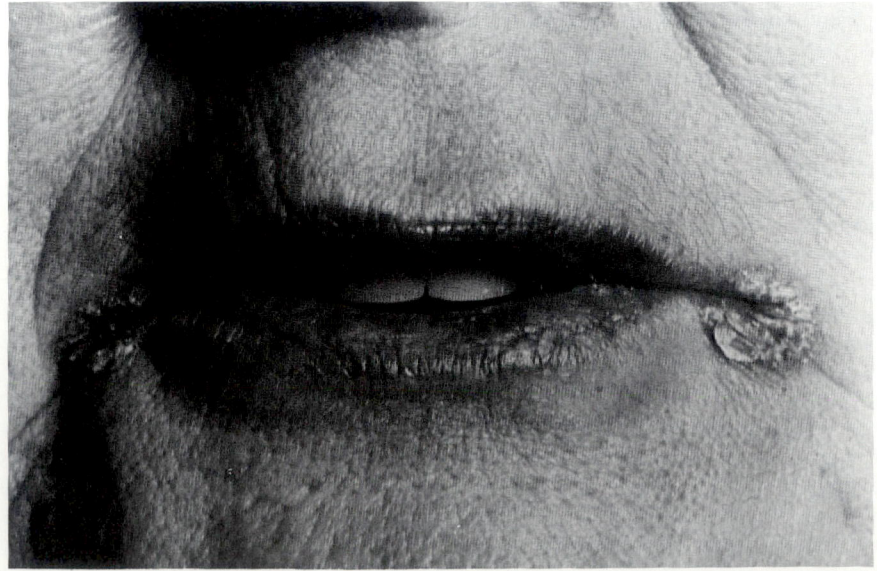

Fig. 167-5 Angula cheilitis in candidiasis. Note white scale on erythematous base. (Courtesy of Department of Dermatology, The Cleveland Clinics.)

Thrush, which is the name given to *Candida* infection of the mouth and throat, occurs most often in infants and in adult patients receiving antibiotics or immunosuppressive drugs. The buccal mucosa, tongue, and gums become red and may have clumps of white material that are easily scraped off. Cultures of these patches reveal *Candida* organisms. The treatment includes local topical anesthetics and nystatin rinses or troches. Zinc is an important adjunct when there is an accompanying deficiency (see discussion of acrodermatitis enteropathica in Chapter 158).

Vaginal moniliasis (candidiasis) can be passed back and forth between sexual partners. *C. albicans* is a common inhabitant of the vaginal tract; overgrowth of the organism may lead to the clinical manifestations. Women have a curdy, white discharge, as well as severe burning and itching. Men may have only a persistent erythematous patch on the penis or scrotum, which may be asymptomatic. Fungal infection involving the penis is almost invariably monilial. The predisposing factors are the same as for other forms of *Candida* infection.

Monilial intertrigo appears as a fiery red, burning, itching, uncomfortable groin rash in adults or as a "diaper" rash in infants. Other areas of involvement are under pendulous breasts or abdominal folds and intergluteally. Characteristic "satellite" lesions usually occur at the periphery of the eruption (Fig. 167-4). Candidiasis intertrigo may also occasionally develop in the finger webs of persons who do "wet work," primarily bartenders and household workers (Fig. 167-3). Mucocutaneous candidiasis is a spectrum of diseases, all of which are chronic, recurrent, and recalcitrant (Figs. 167-3 to 167-5). Topical antiyeast agents (nystatin, ketoconazole, and amphotericin B) and drying compresses are used in treatment.

ORAL MANIFESTATIONS AND DENTAL MANAGEMENT. See section on yeast infection in Chapter 58.

BIBLIOGRAPHY

Collins JR and Van Sickels JE: Chronic mucocutaneous candidiasis, J Oral Maxillofac Surg 41:814, 1983.

Holmstrup P and Bessermann M: Clinical therapeutic and pathogenic aspects of chronic oral multifocal candidiasis, Oral Surg 56:388, 1983.

Klein RS and others: Oral candidiasis in high-risk patients as the initial manifestation of the acquired immunodeficiency syndrome, N Engl J Med 311:354, 1984.

Owens NJ and others: Prophylaxis of oral candidiasis with clotrimazole troches, Arch Intern Med 144:290, 1984.

Rodu B and others: Oral candidiasis in cancer patients, South Med J 77:312, 1984.

168 · SKIN DISEASES

Shelley S. Schuler *and* **Robert N. Arm**

TOXIC EPIDERMAL NECROLYSIS (LYELL'S DISEASE); STAPHYLOCOCCAL SCALDED SKIN SYNDROME

Toxic epidermal necrolysis (Lyell's disease) is an extensive, blistering disease. Patients have a toxic erythema of the skin with necrosis and peeling, which gives a scalded appearance. Initially, this can clinically resemble staphylococcal scalded skin syndrome (SSSS; see later discussion). Histologically, however, the cleavage plane is at the dermoepidermal junction. This full-thickness loss of epidermis results in massive fluid loss and loss of protection from infections. This results in dehydration, electrolyte imbalance, and scarring. Mortality is high despite the best supportive care.

The disease is caused by a hypersensitivity reaction to a wide variety of drugs, most notably sulfa drugs, barbiturates, hydantoins, and allopurinol. Other implicated agents are infections, including viral (herpes simplex, varicella-zoster virus) and bacterial; *Aspergillus* organisms; neoplasia such as lymphomas and leukemias; quinine in tonic water; and radiation therapy.

Adult disease

Onset is abrupt with nonspecific prodromal symptoms, including burning, skin tenderness, fever, fatigue, diarrhea and vomiting, malaise, and arthralgias. The condition may become grave within hours. A morbilliform rash or urticarial lesions appear predominantly on the face and extremities and lead to an erythroderma. Vesicles then appear that rapidly become confluent, producing large flaccid bullae leading to full-thickness epidermal denudation over large areas of the body. The epidermis may peel off in large sheets, leaving a raw, red, scalded-appearing skin surface (Fig. 168-1). Nikolsky's sign (dislodging of the epidermis adjacent to and surrounding a bullous lesion by sliding pressure applied with a finger) is usually present. Mucous membranes, including lips, buccal mucosa, and conjunctivae, may be severely affected, and onycholysis of fingernails and toenails may occur. Patients may also have purpuric and hemorrhagic manifestations in the skin. The extensive sloughing of epidermis causes extensive plasma loss, resulting in fluid and electrolyte imbalance. Other associated systemic complications are fever, liver damage, renal failure, and shock.

Histopathologic examination of early lesions shows vacuolization and bulla formation at the basal cell layer. Little or no inflammatory infiltrate appears in the dermis. Later, subepidermal bullae form. Dermal vessels show endothelial swelling, but no necrosis or vasculitis.

The treatment is usually systemic corticosteroids in high doses, adequate replacement of fluids and electrolytes, topical and systemic antibiotics, and skilled nursing care. The mortality is approximately 30%. In patients who recover, symblepharon and ectropion, trichiasis, corneal opacities, alopecia, and anonychia may result from the scarring.

Staphylococcal scalded skin syndrome

SSSS is usually linked to infection with group 2 phage types of *Staphylococcus aureus*, usually type 71. Only colonization is required to cause the syndrome without overt infection. A staphylococcal exotoxin (epidermolysin) is responsible. Children and newborns up to 3 months are frequently affected by SSSS, also called Ritter's disease. It generally develops in children less than 5 years of age and rarely occurs in adults.

SSSS usually occurs in a child or an infant with severe purulent conjunctivitis, otitis media, or nasopharyngeal infection who develops a faint yellow-amber eruption with circumoral predilection. The child may complain of skin tenderness and have fever and irritability. A generalized macular erythema develops. Within 24 to 48 hours there is a positive Nikolsky's sign, and large bullae develop over massive areas of the body (Fig. 168-2). Sheets of epidermis wrinkle and separate easily, leading to loss of plasma and body heat. The fluid loss may subside quickly, followed by dry desquamation within the first week. Mucous membrane involvement is rare, and cultures taken from intact bullae are usually sterile.

A histologic examination shows noninflammatory epidermal splitting within the middle to upper epidermis just beneath the stratum corneum. Bullae contain acantholytic cells with no dermal reaction. This is unlike the toxic epidermal necrolysis

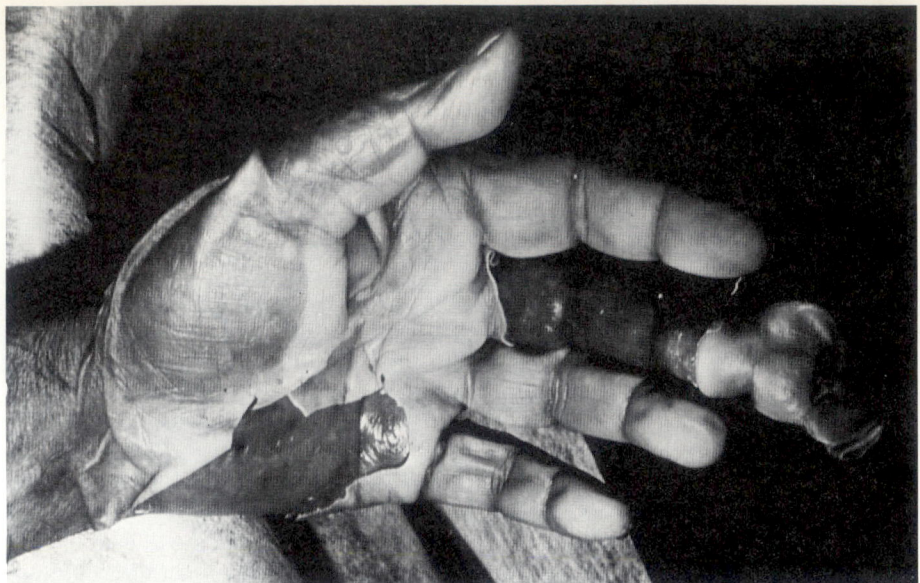

Fig. 168-1 Toxic epidermal necrolysis showing extensive exfoliation. (Courtesy of American Academy of Dermatology.)

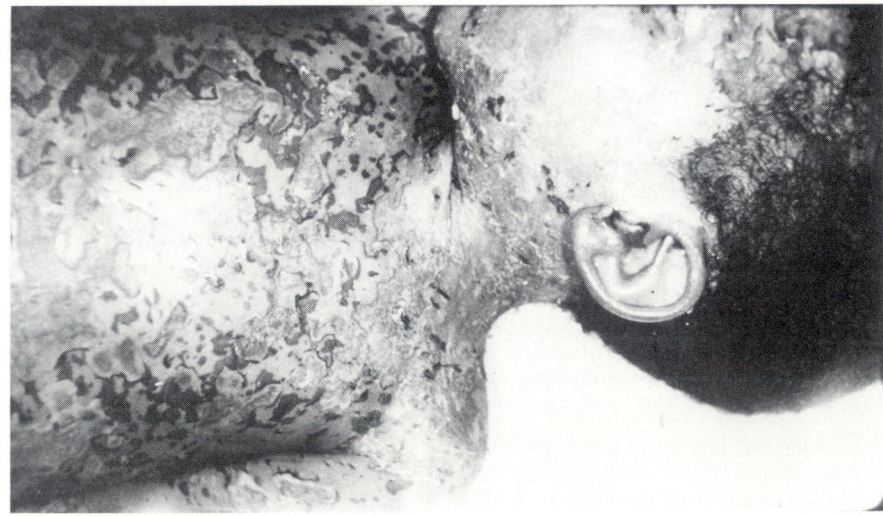

Fig. 168-2 Large areas of ruptured bullae with denudation in this infant with SSSS led to fluid loss and death.

of adults, in which the bullae develop at the basal layer or the basement membrane zone.

Treatment with appropriate antibiotics has greatly reduced associated mortality unless severe underlying infection is present. The prognosis is good, with rapid reepithelialization because of the superficial level of desquamation.

ORAL MANIFESTATIONS. The mucosa can be extensively involved with vesiculobullous lesions in toxic epidermal necrolysis. Patients with SSSS have less frequent oral involvement. The lesions resemble those of major erythema multiforme (Stevens-Johnson syndrome). When lesions are present, Nikolsky's sign is usually demonstrable. In a short time the mucosal lesions erode.

Increased severity of the disease process leads to excessive pain, especially when patients attempt to eat or drink.

DENTAL MANAGEMENT. Although systemic management is indicated for definitive treatment, patients should be made as comfortable as possible. Topical anesthetic solutions, such as 0.5% aqueous diphenhydramine (Benadryl), are highly beneficial in relieving patients' sensitivity. The lesions may worsen with rough cusps and restorations. All elective dental treatment should be deferred.

With increased use of nonsteroidal antiinflammatory drugs in dentistry, one should note that ibuprofen (Motrin) and sulindac hypersensitivities have been related to toxic epidermal necrolysis syndrome resembling Stevens-Johnson syndrome.

BIBLIOGRAPHY

Hansen RC: Staphylococcal scalded skin syndrome, toxic shock syndrome and Kawasaki disease, Pediatr Clin North Am 30:533, 1983.

Levitt L and Pearson RW: Sulindac induced Stevens-Johnson–toxic epidermal necrolysis syndrome, JAMA 243:1262, 1980.

Ossoff R and Giunta JL: The staphylococcal scalded skin syndrome versus erythema multiforme, Oral Surg 40:126, 1975.

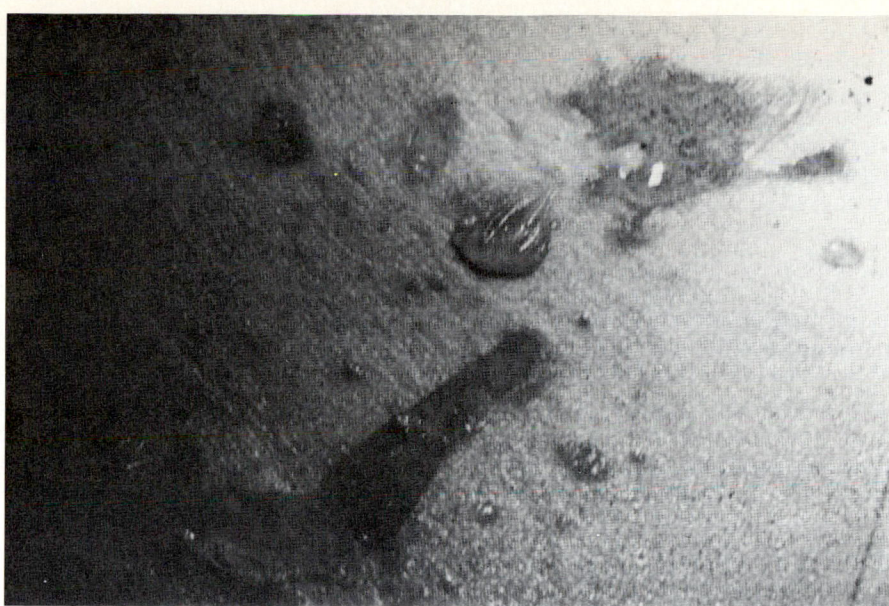

Fig. 168-3 Flaccid bullae in pemphigus vulgaris. There is no erythema around lesions (lesions arise from uninflamed skin).

PEMPHIGUS AND PEMPHIGOID

The most important group of bullous dermatoses in terms of morbidity and mortality is the pemphigus/pemphigoid group. In pemphigus, autoantibodies appear within the epidermis. In the diseases of the pemphigoid group, autoantibodies occur beneath the epidermis at the basement membrane zone. In both conditions bullae appear de novo with no surrounding erythema (Fig. 168-3).

Pemphigus vulgaris

Pemphigus vulgaris is reported to have a higher incidence in Jews but occurs in populations throughout the world. Persons 40 to 60 years of age are most often affected. It may remain localized for some months, often in the mouth, with the bullae being small and flaccid. If bullae persist, erosions and ulcers may occur, and the disease may progress to widespread skin and mucosal distribution, including the nose, pharynx, larynx, esophagus, vulva, penis, and anus. Secondary bacterial infections with crusting may occur and account in part for the characteristic mousy odor. Lesions that heal spontaneously or with therapy do not leave scars. Pemphigus vulgaris appears to be autoimmune associated and has been related to myasthenia gravis and thymoma, penicillamine therapy, and an undiagnosed systemic malignancy.

Histologically, a primary acantholysis with intraepidermal splitting and bulla formation occurs. A positive Nikolsky's sign is present in the blistered and adjacent normal-appearing skin. If the condition is left untreated, patients steadily deteriorate and eventually die; the average survival time is about 14 months (Fig. 168-3).

The treatment of all forms of pemphigus depends on the severity. Treatment includes hospitalization for intensive local skin care and high doses of corticosteroids. Immunosuppressive agents such as methotrexate, azathioprine, and cyclophosphamide may be administered for their adjunct corticosteroid-sparing effects. Pemphigus has been reported to coexist with malignancy, but the types of malignancy are so varied that no specific causal relationship has been established.

ORAL MANIFESTATIONS. Pemphigus is found in the mouth in 80% to 90% of patients. As noted previously, it is often localized in the mouth in many patients, and frequently the mouth may be the initial site of involvement in up to two thirds of patients. Most common sites include the buccal mucosa, palate, lips, and gingiva. The lesions are vesicobullous in nature, often weeping, and may produce painful ulcers. The rupturing generally occurs immediately after vesicle formation resulting from trauma, unlike the skin lesions, which can remain intact for days. The ulcerations vary in size, are often covered with a yellowish gray pseudomembrane, and may be confused with other lesions.

Differential diagnosis of pemphigus includes aphthous ulcers, lichen planus, benign mucous membrane pemphigoid (which may resemble early mucosal lesions of pemphigus vulgaris), and major erythema multiforme (Stevens-Johnson syndrome), which appears clinically similar, but pemphigus has a more abrupt onset and acute febrile course. Other blistering diseases such as toxic epidermal necrolysis, dermatitis herpetiformis, and bullous erythema multiforme (minor), candidiasis, and desquamative gingivitis should also be considered.

Examination should include testing for Nikolsky's sign; however, if Nikolsky's sign is positive, it is not pathognomonic becase it may also be positive for other disorders. Cytologic diagnosis may help if the pathologist is familiar with the cytology of pemphigus. The cytologic diagnosis based on Tzanck cells (acantholytic cells) and immunofluorescent cytology showing pericellular and intercellular deposition of IgG. Biopsy is often needed for definitive diagnosis. Early lesions that have not undergone degenerative changes should be selected for biopsy, especially if a vesicle is present. If pemphigus is included in the differential diagnosis, arrangements for immunofluorescence should be made before biopsy. Although oral cytologic study may suggest a diagnosis, it cannot really replace the biopsy. Care must be taken in doing the biopsy, since the surface may slough and ruin pathologic diagnosis.

DENTAL MANAGEMENT. The treatment for pemphigus is generally systemic, but topical oral corticosteroids may be beneficial for patients with severe lesions or if the disease is limited to the oral cavity. For prolonged gingival contact, steroids may be applied beneath a splint or denture. Topical anesthetics, especially a rinse of 0.5% aqueous diphenhydramine (Benadryl), alleviate the pain. Hygiene can be promoted by use of a neutral mouth rinse or peroxide rinse. Chlorhexidine solution helps promote oral hygiene. Occasionally, antibiotics may be needed for secondary infection.

Of major concern to the dentist is the systemic use of corticosteroids and immunosuppressants, which may lead to increased infection and delayed healing. Supplemental antibiotics may be needed before treatment.

Pemphigus vegetans

Pemphigus vegetans is a variant of pemphigus vulgaris that occurs in patients with increased resistance to the disease. Two types of pemphigus vegetans occur. The Neumann type begins with flaccid bullae resembling pemphigus vulgaris, most often found in the intertriginous areas. These bullae become eroded, forming fungoid vegetations and papillomatous proliferations. The onset may sometimes be insidious, with lesions found in the nose, mouth, axillae, genitalia, perineum, or umbilicus. After the bullae erupt, they develop verrucous vegetations on their moist bases, covered by crusts and a surrounding inflamed border. These lesions may coalesce into larger patches or form irregular patterns. Initially the symptoms are mild with long periods of spontaneous remission of the disease. Later, patients may have febrile episodes with other constitutional symptoms. The terminal phases are similar to those of pemphigus vulgaris, with intercurrent infection aggravated by the use of corticosteroid therapy.

The Hallopeau type (dermatitis vegetans, pyodermite vegetans) follows a more benign course, and the lesions are pustules rather than bullae. Large areas of exuberant granulation tissue and moist verrucous vegetating plaques form, become crusted, and exude serum and pus with a distinctive foul odor. They may break down and form central ulcerations with vesicles and pustules at the periphery of the plaques. Characteristic development of large granulomatous masses in the intertriginous areas of the axillae and groin occurs. Occasionally, single lesions may be localized to the ankles, but disseminated lesions may develop as vegetating masses and multiple ulcerations on various parts of the body and mucous membranes, including those of the lips, buccal mucosa, and vagina. This form of the disease may be an abnormal tissue reaction to various infectious processes, including viral-bacterial symbiosis, in persons who are immunologically deficient. Although it tends to follow a chronic, prolonged course, the Hallopeau type may resemble pemphigus vulgaris and terminate fatally.

ORAL MANIFESTATIONS. Oral lesions of pyodermite vegetans were reported in two of the five first cases described by Hallopeau. Although cutaneous involvement is generally present, McCarthy reported several patients with oral involvement only and used the term "pyostomatitits vegetans." Many patients with oral involvement also have gastrointestinal problems, and often the lesions follow a similar course to gastrointestinal disease, with periods of spontaneous remission. A biopsy is usually needed for diagnosis.

cAlthough the oral lesions resemble pemphigus, many differences exist, including the presence of eosinophils, generally painless lesions, and often underlying gastrointestinal problems. Clinically, pyostomatitis vegetans may be a separate entity or is best classified as part of the gastrointestinal disease syndrome, instead of with pemphigus. (See section on pyostomatitis vegetans, pp. 791-792.)

DENTAL MANAGEMENT. The main problem in dental management is maintenance of oral hygiene; careful instruction and supplements, including chlorhexidine, may be necessary. Other major problems deal with systemic therapy, including immunosuppressive agents patients may be receiving.

Treatment of the disease generally must be done through systemic management. Symptoms of oral lesions may be lessened with application of topical corticosteroids and topical anesthetics.

Referral for systemic workup, including a possible gastrointestinal workup, as part of the total physical examination may be indicated. Antibiotics seem to be of limited value when pustules occur in pyostomatitis vegetans.

Pemphigus foliaceus and pemphigus erythematosus

Pemphigus foliaceus and pemphigus erythematosus are considered to be variant forms of pemphigus vulgaris. Epidemiologically, pemphigus foliaceus occurs worldwide without any racial or ethnic prevalence but is endemic in Brazil, where it is known as fogo selvagem. It usually occurs in adults 30 to 60 years of age, except in Brazil, where adolescents and young adults in a family, especially women, are affected. It begins locally and insidiously, usually on the scalp and face, advancing to flaccid bullae with prominent scaling and crusting of the scalp, face, and upper areas of the trunk. The mucous membranes are usually not affected. Histologically, there is acantholysis and a subcorneal split with bulla formation high within the epidermis. Autoantibodies occur at the site of bulla formation. Pemphigus foliaceus, other than that in Brazil, tends to present a more generalized exfoliative dermatitis with similar histologic and immunologic findings. The prognosis is relatively good, but the response to corticosteroid therapy is less favorable than in the non-Brazilian form.

Pemphigus erythematosus (Senear-Usher syndrome) clinically resembles a mixture of pemphigus vulgaris, seborrheic dermatitis, and lupus erythematosus. Red, greasy, crusted, eroded lesions occur in the malar and sternal areas, on the scalp, and occasionally in the mouth. The course is more chronic than that of pemphigus vulgaris.

The lesions of pemphigus foliaceus and pemphigus erythematosus are caused by an intraepidermal blister associated with a neutrophilic infiltrate and the presence of many eosinophils. The blisters are small, flaccid, and easily broken. In addition to the clinical similarity to lupus erythematosus, the patient may manifest antinuclear antibodies and deposition of immunoglobulins at the dermoepidermal junction in addition to the more typical immunofluorescence findings of pemphigus (see following discussion). Histologically, in both pemphigus foliaceous and pemphigus erythematosus, the acantholysis develops subcorneally, which is more superficial than in pemphigus vulgaris and vegetans.

In all types of pemphigus, immunofluorescence studies demonstrate IgG antibody fixed in vivo within the epidermal intercellular space. Serum from patients with these diseases also contains this IgG antibody. An increase in this antibody precedes clinical flares of the disease. Lesions are produced when this antibody binds to a specific antigen on the epidermal cell membrane, causing release of one or more proteases and a resultant separation of the epidermal keratinocytes. Immunologically this mechanism is unique, in that neither complement nor an influx of inflammatory cells is required for the development of lesions.

Hailey-Hailey disease (benign familial chronic pemphigus)

Hailey-Hailey disease, or benign familial pemphigus, is a rare hereditary disorder characterized by recurrent vesicular and bullous eruptions most commonly appearing on the neck, axillae, upper part of the trunk, and groin. It is caused by an irregular dominant gene in 70% of patients. An epidermal defect appears to involve a fault in synthesis or maturation of the tonofilament and desmosome complex or a fault in the synthesis of intercellular substance. External agents such as friction, freezing, and ultraviolet irradiation may precipitate acantholysis. Infection (especially with *Candida albicans* and staphylococci) is another important precipitating factor. Histologically, Hailey-Hailey disease appears very similar to pemphigus vulgaris except for the following characteristics: Hailey-Hailey disease has more extensive acantholysis but less damage to the acantholytic cells with a few intercellular bridges remaining so that neighboring cells still adhere loosely to one another, giving the appearance of a dilapidated brick wall. Clinically, groups of small vesicles erupt on normal or erythematous skin with initially clear contents that soon become turbid. The lesions extend peripherally, and the center may heal or show soft, flat, moist vegetations. Sweating and heat usually aggravate this condition, whereas cold may cause regression of the lesions. The diseases to be considered in the differential diagnosis include chronic bacterial intertrigo, mycotic infections, infectious eczematoid dermatitis, and impetigo.

The treatment includes topical and systemic antibiotics, corticosteroid preparations, and the removal of external precipitating factors when possible. Grenz-ray therapy has been used with some success. Dapsone has been reported to be effective. Excision of localized areas of involvement, followed by split-thickness grafting, has been successfully performed. Some patients do not have recurrences of the disease, whereas in others the process continues at the periphery of the graft.

Pemphigoid

BULLOUS PEMPHIGOID. Bullous pemphigoid occurs worldwide with no racial or sexual prevalence. It usually affects those over 60 years of age, beginning as areas of erythema lasting several days or weeks, followed by the development of large, tense, tough bullae that remain intact or, if ruptured, heal rapidly. It predominates on the limbs and trunk and seldom affects mucous membranes. This disease may undergo spontaneous remission, but recurrent attacks occur. Death may occur from complications.

Histologically a subepidermal bulla formation occurs without acantholysis. Autoantibodies are localized to the lamina lucida of the basement membrane zone. The subepidermal bullae contain a neutrophilic infiltrate, often with eosinophils. Direct immunofluorescence of the skin shows linear or tubular IgG (sometimes IgA or IgM) in the basement zone. Often C1q, C3, C4, and C5, properdin, and factor B are present. The specific IgG antibody combines with a basement membrane antigen and fixes complement by the classic pathway, attracting neutrophils to the dermal-epidermal junction, thus initiating release of proteolytic enzymes and tissue destruction. The alternate pathway of complement may also be activated. Electron microscopy shows IgG binding to the lamina lucida of the basement membrane in the region of the anchoring filaments. Complement components are decreased in the blister fluid of the bullous pemphigoid.

Differential diagnosis includes eczematous eruptions and pemphigus vulgaris. Patients with pemphigus vulgaris, however, have severe mucosal lesions and small, flaccid, easily broken bullae rather than the tense, tough, large bullae of pemphigoid. There is no Nikolsky sign. The treatment consists of corticosteroids and immunosuppressive agents. Major complications may occur with secondary infection of the lesions or may result from the immunosuppressive agents, which causes secondary infections, particularly herpes.

Benign mucosal pemphigoid (cicatricial pemphigoid, ocular pemphigus). Benign mucosal pemphigoid is a disabling but nonfatal vesiculobullous eruption of the mucous membranes, especially the conjunctivae. Ocular lesions occur in 10% to 80% of patients in various studies. The lesions include symblepharon, corneal opacifications, and ankyloblepharon. The disease is not really "benign" because of the blindness and scarring that may occur. Only about one quarter to one third of patients have skin lesions. The disease is mainly seen in individuals between 40 and 65 years of age, often occurring in patients over 65. Women are affected two to five times as often as men. The cause is unknown. Histologically, the formation of subepidermal bullae without acantholysis occurs. Immunofluorescence studies have shown IgG deposits in the lamina lucida of the oral, conjunctival, and epidermal lesions, identical to that found in bullous pemphigoid. Circulating antibodies reactive to the basement zone are occasionally found with indirect immunofluorescence.

Constant care by an ophthalmologist is necessary to relieve eye problems. Combined treatment with corticosteroids and immunosuppressive agents may be helpful, and sulfapyridine may give temporary relief, but therapy is generally ineffective.

The two striking clinical features are the bullae on the mucous membranes of the conjunctivae, mouth, nose, larnyx, pharynx, esophagus, penis, vulva, vagina, and anus and the formation of scars. Koebner's phenomenon (development of new lesions in traumatized areas) is often seen. Pemphigoid must be differentiated from pemphigus vulgaris and ulcerative lichen planus.

Oral manifestations. In bullous pemphigoid, oral lesions occur in 8% to 31% of patients. Skin lesions are generally always the first sign. In patients with benign mucous membrane pemphigoid, almost 100% have oral lesions. This nonfatal, painful, chronic disease may resemble vesiculobullous lesions of pemphigus and other similar diseases. Unlike pemphigus, the bullae have thicker walls and remain visible for a longer time. The sloughed mucous membranes are raw and bleed but heal in about 2 weeks. They also may scar. Gingival lesions are common in benign mucous membrane pemphigoid and resemble a desquamative gingivitis with an erythematous appearance.

Because of local trauma, the gingival lesions may remain for a long time. A biopsy using immunofluorescent studies is necessary for definitive diagnosis.

After the lesion heals, scarring may occur. This may cause decreased vestibular depth, leading to later problems with dental prostheses.

Dental management. Since the disease is often limited to the oral cavity, the dentist may have to make the diagnosis and provide local management. The easy sloughing of the mucosa leads to a nondiagnostic tissue specimen, and care must be taken during the biopsy to avoid this. Once the diagnosis is established, treatment can include systemic steroids or intralesional injections. Use of splints may help topical steroids stay in place. Oral hygiene is a problem and may be supplemented by topical steroids to control lesions, peroxide solutions, and other bland rinses such as baking soda. The use of chlorhexidine or oral tetracycline rinses may help control secondary infection. A topical anesthetic may be beneficial for patients with the painful lesions. Studies seem to show that the best topical steroid is fluocinonide ointment (0.05% Lidex).

Since prosthetic devices may be difficult to place because of the lesions and scarring, maintenance of the dentition must be stressed to patients. One study has shown successful use of a split-thickness skin graft to gain vestibular depth. The patient successfully used a full denture. One should note, however, that grafting has had limited success on the skin and is a difficult procedure.

BIBLIOGRAPHY

Armin A and others: Pemphigus vulgaris and malignancy, Int J Oral Surg 14:376, 1985.

Asboe-Hansen G: Diagnosis of pemphigus, Br J Dermatol 83:81, 1970.

Aufdermorte TB and others: Modified topical steroid therapy for the treatment of oral mucous membrane pemphigoid, Oral Surg 59:256, 1985.

Berger RS and others: Familial benign chronic pemphigus: surgical treatment and pathogenesis, Arch Dermatol 104:380, 1971.

Cataldo E and others: Pyostomatitis vegetans, Oral Surg 52:172, 1981.

Correll RW and Schott TR: Multiple painful vesiculoulcerative lesions in the oral mucosa, J Am Dent Assoc 110:765, 1985.

Coscia-Porrazzi L and others: Cytodiagnosis of oral pemphigus vulgaris, Acta Cytol 29:746, 1985.

Eversole LR and others: Oral lesions as the initial signs in pemphigus, Oral Surg 32:354, 1972.

Ferguson CP and Taybos GM: Diagnosis and treatment of pemphigus, Quint Int 7:473, 1985.

Grattan CEH and others: Oral herpes simplex infection in bullous pemphigoid, Oral Surg 61:40, 1986.

Hasler JF: The role of immunofluorescence in the diagnosis of oral vesiculobullous disorders, Oral Surg 33:362, 1972.

Jordon RE and others: Direct immunofluorescent studies of pemphigus and bullous pemphigus, Arch Dermatol 103:486, 1971.

Laskaris G: Juvenile pemphigus vulgaris, Oral Surg 51:415, 1981.

Lever WF and Hashimoto K: The etiology and treatment of pemphigus and pemphigoid, J Invest Dermatol 53:373, 1969.

McCarthy FP: Pyostomatitis vegetans: report of 3 cases, Arch Dermatosyph 60:750, 1949.

McCarthy P and Shklar G: A syndrome of pyostomatitis vegetans and ulcerative colitis, Arch Dermatol 88:281, 1963.

McCarthy PL: Benign mucous membrane pemphigoid, Oral Surg 33:75, 1972.

Mostofi RS and others: Possible role of Koebner's phenomenon in the development of mucous membrane pemphigoid, J Prosthet Dent 55:589, 1986.

O'Hara PB and others: Split thickness graft for treatment of oral benign mucous membrane pemphigoid, Oral Surg 49:487, 1980.

Perry HO and Brunsting LA: Pemphigus foliaceous, Arch Dermatol 91:9, 1965.

Pinckney RCN: Bullous pemphigoid: a case report, Br J Oral Maxillofac Surg 23:167, 1985.

Pisanti S and others: Pemphigus vulgaris incidence in Jews, Oral Surg 38:382, 1974.

Shklar G, Meyer I, and Zacarian SA: Oral lesions in bullous pemphigoid, Arch Dermatol 99:663, 1969.

Urbanek VE and Cohen L: Benign mucous membrane pemphigoid, Oral Surg 31:772, 1971.

Wright ET, Epps RL, and Newcomer VD: Fluorescent antibody studies in pemphigus vulgaris, Arch Dermatol 93:562, 1966.

Zegarelli D: Pemphigus, Oral Surg 44:384, 1977.

PSORIASIS

Psoriasis is a chronic, papulosquamous skin disease characterized by systemic lesions of fine, silvery white scales over a thickened erythematous base (Fig. 168-4). It involves all areas of the body, including glabrous skin, scalp, and mucous membranes. The major areas of involvement are the extensor surfaces of the extremities and the scalp.

The age of onset can be from infancy to late adult life, with no predilection to sex. Psoriasis may affect various family members without conformity to the laws of mendelian genetics. With the recent emphasis of HLA typing, B locus antigens HLA-B13 and HLA-BW17 have been observed to be significantly increased in psoriasis. HLA-BW17 portends early onset of the disease, and patients possessing HLA-BW16 and HLA-BW17 probably will demonstrate a more severe form of the disease.

The etiology of psoriasis is unknown. Pathophysiologically, epidermal cell turnover rate is increased, resulting in a more rapid growth rate of the epidermal cells. The usual 28 days required for basal cells to become skin surface cells can be telescoped into 2 to 5 days. This helps to account for the clinical appearance of thickened epidermis with persistent and exuberant scaling and for the elevated serum uric acid levels because of the consequent increased nucleic acid degradation.

When the semiadherent scale is lifted off a plaque of psoriasis, minute punctate bleeding is often found (Auspitz sign). This characteristic feature of psoriasis, although not exclusively associated with this disease, can be supported by the histologic findings of increased capillary vascularization in the dermal papillae just beneath the thickened (acanthotic), rapidly proliferating areas of the epidermis.

Another interesting feature of psoriasis (again, not exclusive for this disease) is Koebner's, or isomorphic, phenomenon—the appearance of morphologically identical skin lesions over normal skin areas that have been recently traumatized. This isomorphic response may be elicited by trauma such as scratching or rubbing, sunburn, or surgery involving the skin.

Many descriptive terms are used to identify the various configurations of the erupting lesions of psoriasis. For instance, guttate (droplike) psoriasis most commonly occurs in children and young adults following an upper respiratory tract infection with group A β-hemolytic streptococci or following acute emotional trauma or physical trauma such as sunburn. Linear lesions of psoriasis are characteristic of Koebner's reactions following scratching. Exfoliative erythroderma (total body involvement with scaling and hyperemia) is an acute, uncontrolled flare-up usually following a severe illness or toxic reaction to medication. Exfoliative erythroderma occurs under comparable circumstances in many other papulosquamous diseases such as various forms of eczema, atopic dermatitis, and pityriasis rubra pilaris. Exfoliative erythroderma is a serious medical emergency and results in severe morbidity and occasionally mortality because of the excessive heat loss and fluid and electrolyte imbalance.

Approximately 50% to 75% of patients with psoriasis have some form of nail dystrophy, which varies from minor pitting on the surface of the nail bed to onycholysis with partial and incomplete nail growth.

Pustular psoriasis

The two forms of pustular psoriasis are the localized and the generalized. In either case, sterile pustules, in groups or singly, appear in psoriatic plaques or in previously uninvolved sites. No pyogenic organisms have been implicated as the causative agents of either the localized or the generalized form of pustular psoriasis. Localized pustular psoriasis may have varying manifestations. Groups of pustules may be localized on the palms, soles, or periungual areas, with or without associated lesions of psoriasis elsewhere on the body; this is known as palmoplantar pustulosis. Pustular lesions may or may not be symmetric and may cover very large areas. Onycholysis may occur because lakes of pus beneath the nail lift it from the nail bed.

Generalized pustular psoriasis of von Zumbusch is an acute generalized eruption of superficial sterile pustules associated with high fever, leukocytosis, lymphopenia, heat and fluid loss, electrolyte imbalance, hypocalcemia, and hypoalbuminemia. Bacteremia and cardiopulmonary decompensation may result. The mortality may be appreciable. Pustules appear episodically over generalized erythroderma. The cause is unknown, but the disorder sometimes occurs during treatment of psoriasis with or after withdrawal of systemic corticosteroids, occasionally in association with extremely potent topical corticosteroids, or after indiscreet use of irritating topical therapy.

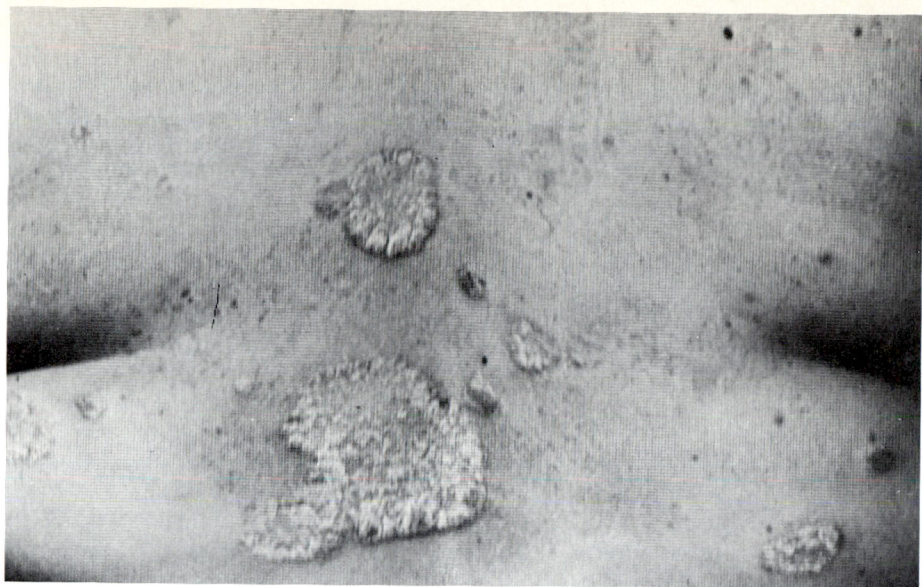

Fig. 168-4   Psoriasis. Note scaly surface of patches. (Courtesy of Department of Dermatology, The Cleveland Clinics.)

Psoriatic arthritis

The arthritis associated with psoriasis is usually seronegative, polyarticular erosive joint disease, characteristically involving the small joints, especially the distal interphalangeal joints. When psoriatric arthritis is present, some form of nail dystrophy usually exists. With progressive disease, skin and joints may flare simultaneously. Patients with spinal involvement have a high incidence of HLA-B27 tissue type. Approximately 15% of all patients with psoriasis may have psoriatic arthritis.

MANAGEMENT. The safest treatment for psoriasis, which is as old as the disease, is ultraviolet light. This may be in the form of natural sunlight or ultraviolet light treatment.

Photochemotherapy, the combined use of ultraviolet light and medication, may be administered topically or systemically. Topical photochemotherapy may include topical tar preparations or topical corticosteroids with ultraviolet light. Systemic photochemotherapy has been developed and combines oral ingestion of 8-methoxypsoralen and exposure to ultraviolet light. The combination of light and medication works synergistically, whereas individually they would be less effective.

Other effective therapy includes topical corticosteroids (with or without occlusion), topical anthralin and tars, and systemic methotrexate for severe skin and arthritic disease. Systemic corticosteroids are usually contraindicated because they can precipitate pustular psoriasis and rebound phenomenon when they are discontinued.

Treatment of localized pustular psoriasis is varied and not very effective. Topical corticosteroids, grenz-ray therapy, Dapsone, tars, or ultraviolet light may result in remission. The treatment for generalized pustular psoriasis includes intravenous methotrexate, supportive measures, and etretinate, which is now considered the drug of choice.

ORAL MANIFESTATIONS. Psoriasis of the face and mouth is rare. Some deny the existence of oral psoriasis and believe it may be another entity, but histologically proven lesions have shown the same remission and exacerbation pattern as the skin lesions. These lesions may occur on the buccal mucosa, lips, palate or tongue, gingiva, and floor of the mouth. Their appearance varies, ranging from sharply demarcated plaques that are gray to yellowish white to ring-shaped striae. Raised, beefy red lesions and elevated ulcerated masses have been reported. Two major studies involving 100 patients and 200 patients have examined the incidence of oral disease. In the larger study, none of the 200 patients was aware of the oral lesions, but 11.5% had lesions. The lesions have included angular cheilosis (3.5% to 11%), fissured tongue (6% to 9.5%; a controlled study reported 6.5% fissured tongue in normal persons), geographic tongue (1% to 5%), and smooth tongue (1%). Reports of *Candida* infections and desquamative gingivitis have appeared. Increased lip lesions caused by Koebner's phenomenon as a result of trauma from protrusion of the maxillary incisors have been reported.

Biopsies of geographic tongue lesions (migratory glossitis, erythema migrans) and lesions of Reiter's syndrome appear similar to those of psoriatic lesions. All these diseases may be related.

Arthritis in psoriasis generally affects the fingers, but the temporomandibular joint may also be involved. The hands may be involved with both psoriatic skin lesions and arthritis affecting patients' ability to perform oral hygiene and leading to gingivitis. Increased efforts at oral hygiene should be tried.

DENTAL MANAGEMENT. Usually the lesions are asymptomatic and require no therapy, but sore mouths have been reported, especially during mastication. Symptomatic relief can be obtained with topical anesthetics. Intralesional steroid injections may eliminate discrete lesions but are impractical for diffuse lesions; topical steroids may help. Neutral rinses and a bland diet prevent some of the soreness.

Although no dental therapy is contraindicated, there have been reports of problems in obtaining a clear incision line during periodontal surgery. Lesions seem to flare up if traumatized. Patients have tolerated prosthetic appliances. Arthritis in the temporomandibular joint may be a problem and may be difficult to treat, but antiinflammatory drugs and injections of steroids may help. Special hygiene aids may be needed for patients with severe hand problems.

Systemic involvement may also present a problem. Diabetes, myopathia, ulcerative colitis, and *Candida* infections may affect oral treatment. The *Candida* infections may be treated with nystatin or ketoconazole. Systemic effects of drug therapy (steroids, methotrexate) alter working conditions, and patients taking steroids may require supplemental steroids and may have altered healing. Methotrexate may alter bone marrow function and cause oral ulcerations.

BIBLIOGRAPHY

Baker H: Psoriasis: a review, Dermatologica 150:16, 1975.
Baker H and Ryan TJ: Generalized pustular psoriasis: a clinical and epidermiological study of 104 cases, Br J Dermatol 80:771, 1968.
Brenner S and others: Psoriasis of the lips: the unusual Koebner phenomenon caused by protruding upper teeth, Dermatologica 164:413, 1982.
Buchner A and others: Oral lesions in psoriatic patients, Oral Surg 41:327, 1976.
Cram DL: Psoriasis: current advances in etiology and treatment, Am Acad Dermatol 4:1, 1981.
DeGregori G, Pippon R, and Davies E: Psoriasis of the gingiva and tongue: report of a case, J Periodontol 42:97, 1971.
Doben DI: Psoriasis of the attached gingiva, J Periodontol 47:38, 1976.
Ellis CN and Voorhees JJ: Etretinate therapy, J Am Acad Dermatol 16:267, 1987.
Farber EM and Cox AJ, editors: Psoriasis: proceedings of the second international symposium, New York, 1977, Yorke Medical Books.
Farber EM and Nall ML: The natural history of psoriasis in 5600 patients, Dermatologica 148:118, 1974.
Fischman SL, Barnett ML, and Nisengard, RJ: Histopathologic, ultrastructural and immunologic findings in oral psoriatic lesions, Oral Surg 44:253, 1977.
Hietanen J and others: Study of the oral mucosa in 200 consecutive patients with psoriasis, Scand J Dent Res 92:50, 1984.
Jones LE and others: Desquamative gingivitis associated with psoriasis, J Periodontol 42:35, 1972.
Pisanty S and Ship II: Oral psoriasis, Oral Surg 30:351, 1970.
Salmon TN and others: Oral psoriasis, Oral Surg 28:48, 1974.
Svejgaard A and others: HL-A in psoriasis vulgaris and in pustular psoriasis: population and family studies, Br J Dermatol 91:145, 1974.
White DK, Lewis HJ, and Miller AS: Interoral psoriasis associated with widespread dermal psoriasis, Oral Surg 41:174, 1976.

ERYTHEMA MIGRANS

Erythema migrans (geographic tongue, benign migratory glossitis) has the histopathology of a psoriatic lesion. Some believe that it is often overlooked because patients fail to complain about it or do not report it. Incidence in normal subjects ranges from 0.3% to 15%; in most studies the average is approximately 1% to 2.5% of the population. The difference supposedly is whether one considers entire tongue involvement necessary, or only subtle changes. The cause is not known, but geographic tongue is often related to other diseases. Associations have been found with psoriasis, fissured tongue, dermatitis (lichen planus, possibly pyoderma gangrenosum), Reiter's syndrome, infectious agents, gastrointestinal disturbances, nutritional alteration, allergies (atopy, asthma), hormonal problems (diabetes, pregnancy, or psychosomatic processes). Although many thought the process was commonly limited to the tongue, it has been reported in other areas, including the buccal mucosa, vestibular area, lips, and rarely the gingiva. When it occurs throughout the mouth, it has been called stomatitis areata migrans or migratory stomatitis. Clinically the lesions of stomatitis or glossitis migrans appear to migrate daily, with margins changing shape. They appear as well-circumscribed areas of red, depapillated, desquamative epithelium with a yellow-white border and slightly raised in comparison to surrounding areas. The process is self-limited and may remain present in some form for long periods or at times may completely resolve. No racial or age predilection seems to exist. Many report an equal ratio of males and females, but some studies suggest an increased incidence in females, up to 2:1 over males. Suggestion of a genetic predisposition has been made in studies using the HLA group. Marks and Czarny found an increased level of HLA-B15 (now called HLA-BW62 and HLA-BW63) in patients with geographic tongue and atopy. In patients with geographic tongue without atopy, the HLA levels appear to be no different than those in normal subjects. Wysocki and Daley also found an increased level in patients with juvenile insulin dependent diabetes and geographic tongue.

More than a threefold increase in geographic tongue was found in patients with atopy in the study by Marks and Czarny. Using a broad definition of geographic tongue, they found 14% of a normal population had geographic tongue, but 46% of patients with atopy and more than 50% of those with intrinsic asthma had the finding. A fourfold increase of geographic tongue in patients with juvenile diabetes was reported by Wysocki and Daley; using a narrow definition, however, they found 2% incidence of geographic tongue in their control population, but 8% in the diabetic population.

DENTAL MANAGEMENT. No treatment is indicated for geographic tongue or stomatitis, except rare palliative treatment for burning, pain, or itching. This includes eating a bland diet, avoiding spicy and acid foods, and applying topical anesthetics in extreme cases.

BIBLIOGRAPHY

Hume WJ: Geographic stomatitis: a critical review, J Dent 3:25, 1975.
Marks MB: Recognizing the allergic person, Am Fam Physician 16:72, 1977.
Marks R and Czarny D: Geographic tongue: sensitivity to the environment, Oral Surg 58:156, 1984.
Rahaminoff P and Muhsam HV: Some observations on 1246 cases of geographic tongue, Am J Dis Child 93:519, 1957.
Ralls SA and Warnock GR: Stomatitis areata migrans affecting the gingiva, Oral Surg 60:197, 1985.
Redman RS and others: Psychological component in the etiology of geographic tongue, J Dent Res 45:1403, 1966.
Sapiro SM and Shklar G: Stomatitis areata migrans, Oral Surg 36:28, 1973.
Weathers DR and others: Psoriasiform lesions of the oral mucosa (with emphasis on "ectopic geographic tongue"), Oral Surg 37:872, 1974.
Wysocki GP and Daley TD: Benign migratory glossitis in patients with juvenile diabetes, Oral Surg 63:68, 1987.

LICHEN PLANUS

Lichen planus is a complex entity. It may be composed of several variants or possibly different diseases, because of the statistical variation from oral and dermatologic diseases. This variation may result from the clinical referral pattern reported by various authors. Lichen planus is generally considered an unique eruption of symmetrically distributed, flattopped, polyhedral, violaceous papules, usually involving the flexural surfaces and mucous membranes either as a single lesion or in groups. No racial predilection seems to exist. Many studies have suggested a female predominance of approximately 60%, but occasional reports show male dominance. In the overall populaton, 0.9% to 1.2% appear to have lichen planus. In a general dental clinic population, only 0.6% have been reported to have lichen planus. The disease occurs most often after the third decade of life, affecting persons 30 to 70 years of age. The youngest patient reported was a 6-month-old infant. Males seem to develop the disease approximately 10 years before females. More than 35% of all patients are above 50 years of age.

The cause is unknown, but the occasional finding of immunoglobulins at the dermal-epidermal interface has led many to hypothesize an immune pathogenesis for this disease. A genetic predisposition has been suggested, with some studies finding HLA-A28 and others, HLA-A3 or HLA-B7. Because of these various findings some have suggested that different diseases are present. Emotional stress, as a potential etiologic factor, has been investigated thoroughly. Some reports state that the appearance of lichen planus, or at least the symptoms,

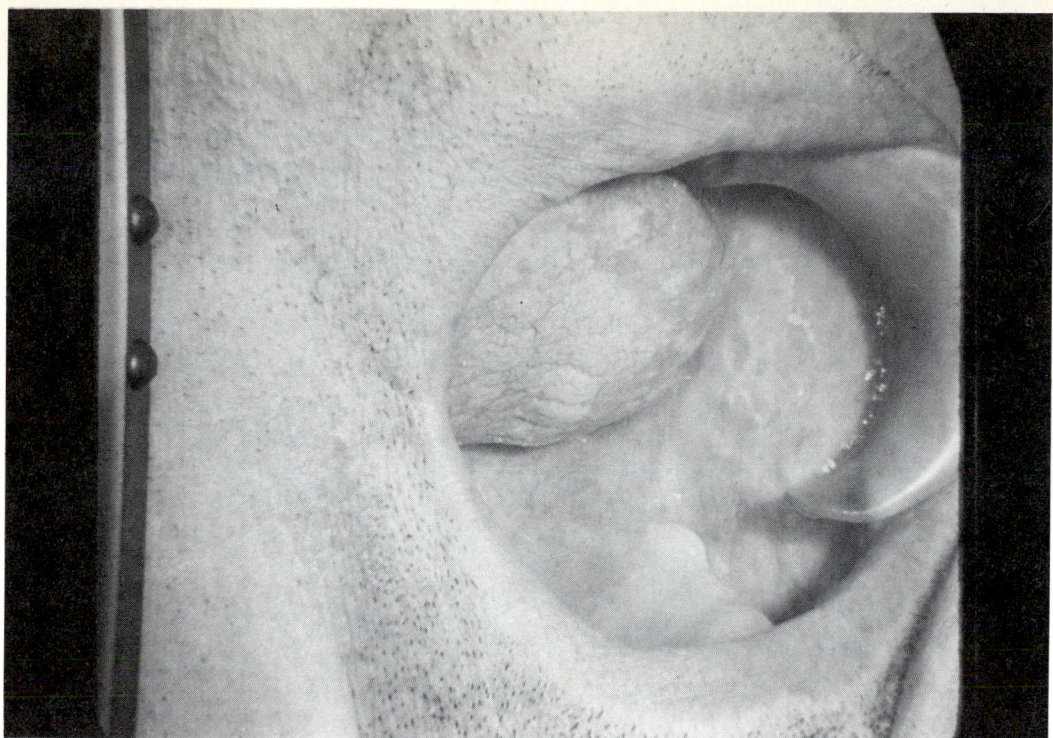

Fig. 168-5   Reticular form of oral lichen planus with white, lacy Wickham's straie.

often occurs 1 to 2 weeks after a stressful event. A study by Allen and co-workers, however, suggested no greater tendency toward anxiety or stressful life events exists in patients with lichen planus. Lichen planus has been associated with other dermatologic entities, including pemphigus, pemphigoid, dermatitis herpetiformis, and alopecia areata, as well as with various systemic diseases, including diabetes (6% to 85%), liver disease, ulcerative colitis, and myasthenia gravis. Theories of possible viral etiologic factors are no longer accepted.

Lesions of the oral mucosa occur in 65% to 75% of all patients with lichen planus of the glabrous skin. One report found only a 35% incidence. This large variation may suggest more than one entity, a different referral pattern, or different diagnostic criteria for oral lesions. Many pattern variations exist, of which the most frequent are annular lesions, most commonly found on the genitalia; hypertrophic lesions occurring over the distal lower extremities; follicular or cicatricial alopecia of lichen planopilaris, occurring in the hair-bearing regions; and the typical pterygia of lichen planus found on the nail plate.

Histopathologically, characteristic changes distinguish lichen planus from other disease entities. These include surface changes of hyperorthokeratosis, changes at the junction of the dermis and epidermis with "saw-toothing" and dystrophic changes, and an infiltrate of lymphocytes near the epidermis.

Treatment is usually directed toward the symptoms. The most common therapies include topical, intralesional, and systemic corticosteroids, depending on the severity of the lesions. Other treatments have been antipruritics, tranquilizers, and vitamin A metabolites. In about two thirds of most patients the lesions resolve spontaneously within 8 to 12 months. Up to 90% of the lesions resolve within 2 years, but some cases may last up to 15 years before disappearance. Relapses are common and occur often and are reported in 20% of patients. Oral lesions respond differently.

ORAL MANIFESTATIONS. As mentioned, oral lesions occur in about two thirds of all patients with skin lesions, but these represent only about half the patients with oral lichen planus. In various reports, only 20% to 50% of patients with oral lichen planus may have skin lesions. In one report, only 4% had skin lesions. This may again point to either different variations of the disease occurring or the diagnostic criteria varying from author to author. The incidence of oral lichen planus has been reported as 1.2 per 100 population. The sexual predilection ranges from 67% for females to 60% for males. Many suggest an equal predilection. Most lesions appear in the fifth decade of life. Some studies suggest the onset has no relationship to family history, tobacco, or *Candida* infection, but others report an increased incidence for smokers and an even greater incidence for those who chew tobacco. This may indicate that a lichenoid response may be occurring and confused with lichen planus. The most common location is the buccal mucosa (80% of lesions). They are generally located opposite the molars and often bilaterally. Lesions may also occur on the gingiva, tongue, lips, and palate.

The classic lesion is the recticular form. This has been described as a slightly raised, radiating, bluish white or gray, lacy, velvety, threadlike papule in a linear, annular, or netlike arrangement. These lines are called Wickham's striae (Fig. 168-5). This is the most common form and also has the highest degree of spontaneous resolution (up to 40%).

Occasionally the lesions coalesce to a larger plaque with radiating striae. This plaquelike form is described as slightly raised, coarsely textured white plaques. They often may occur as solitary lesions and may have radiating striae (Fig. 168-6). Remissions are less common (about 7%). Another form, the papular type, consists of small, raised, white papules, 0.5-1.0 mm in size, that appear in clusters, forming a pebbly appearance, or may start coalescing, resembling the plaquelike lesion.

A more severe form of lichen planus is the erosive or vesicular (bullous) form. These patients may seek care more frequently because of increased symptomatology, including

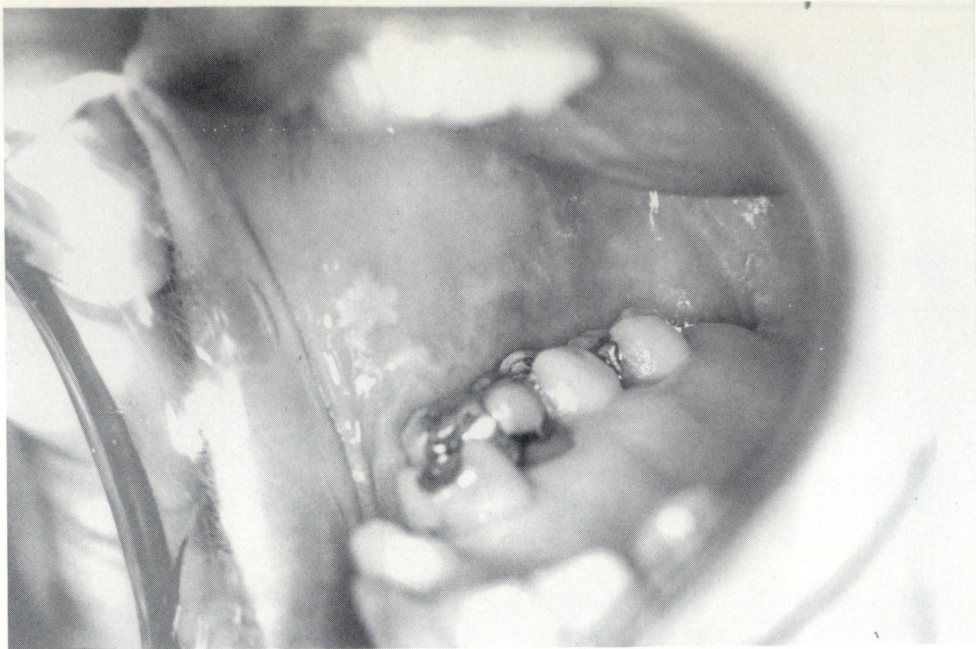

Fig. 168-6   Plaque form of lichen planus with large white plaque and radiating straie.

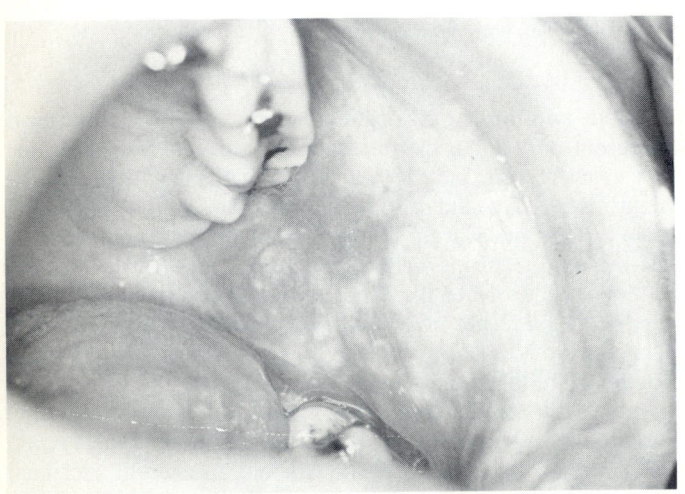

Fig. 168-7   Erosive form of lichen planus with raw erythematous area and some white plaque and straie.

pain and discomfort. The erosive type appears as ulcerative mucosa, often surrounded by striae; whereas in the bullous type, small bullae or vesicles of varying sizes from millimeters to centimeters occur. These can rupture and leave a raw, red erosion of irregular shape and size (Fig. 168-7). The chief complaint may be a burning sensation. Occasionally a pseudomembrane may cover the lesion. Spontaneous remission is rare, with reports generally averaging less than 5%. On the gingiva, lichen planus may resemble desquamative gingivitis. Often these erosive lesions may be confused with pemphigoid, pemphigus, or lupus erythematosus.

Another form of lichen planus is the atrophic type. The lesion appears as a reddened zone resulting from atrophy. Striae at the periphery often occur. The lesion has poorly defined margins and frequently appears on the tongue. Patients with these lesions often have symptoms that include a burning sensation.

A biopsy may be needed for diagnosis. As with the skin, the histopathology is diagnostic and show "saw-toothed" rete ridges, a subepithelial bandlike infiltrate of lymphocytes, liquefaction degeneration (hydropic) of the epithelial basement membrane, and hyperorthokeratosis or hyperparakeratosis. Yeast infection occurs in 47% of patients with lichen planus. When the multiple lesions were checked in one study, the yeast infection had been found in only 37% of the lesions. Careful review of histologic criteria or repeat biopsies may be necessary, since often the lichen planus may appear as nonspecific "leukoplakia" lesions.

DENTAL MANAGEMENT. The lesions are generally asymptomatic, especially in the reticular form. In the atrophic and erosive forms, up to two thirds of the patients may complain of discomfort and burning. Symptomatic relief may be obtained with topical anesthetics. This may include a topical lidocaine ointment or an aqueous diphenhydramine (Benadryl) rinse. The use of neutral mouth rinses (baking soda) and avoidance of alcoholic solutions are recommended. Bland food and avoidance of extreme temperatures in food may also benefit patients. Because most of these lesions do not resolve as skin lesions do, treatment may be necessary. One of the more successful treatments has been topical steroids, especially fluocinonide (Lidex). This topical steroid can be applied as an ointment or gel. Other steroids such as betamethasone and triamcimolone have also been used. Intralesional steroids for small areas have been beneficial. Steroid rinses may help diffuse areas, as may systemic therapy. Because of possible yeast infection, the antifungal agent griseofulvin has been tried. Results have varied from improvement, no effect, or worsening of the lesions. Topical vitamin A, both acid and analog forms, has been tried with debatable results. Occasionally, systemic low doses of vitamin A have been helpful. Treatment with systemic isotretinoin has resulted in slight improvement in some patients, but none wanted retreatment because of the side effects.

Oral hygiene must be stressed and the patient assisted, especially when erosive gingival lesions are present. The use of a chlorhexidine solution seems to promote oral hygiene and helps improve the lesions. Topical steroids administered along the gingival margin may also help heal the gingival lesions.

Prostheses may be a problem for some patients. Removable prostheses and contact with lesions may provide a mechanical irritation and exacerbate the lesions, especially on ulcerative areas. A fixed prosthesis has been recommended. The use of topical steroids beneath the removable appliance may help. The creation of an appliance that is a carrier of topical steroids may help when palatal lesions are present. Again, oral hygiene must be stressed.

The most severe problems are found in the patient who is "high strung," emotional, and overanxious. Some of these patients may be "cancer phobic," and a biopsy may help "treat" the patient's fear. Often these patients have been described as "mirror watchers." A study by Allen and associates suggested no significant difference existed in anxiety levels between patients with lichen planus and controls. One management concern is the possible incidence of cancer in lichen planus. Most reports of cancer have occurred in erosive lesions. Most likely the incidence of cancer is less than 1%, especially eliminating inappropriate cases. In most studies the range of cancer incidence is 0.3% to 3.0%, with one study reporting 10%. In a review of the literature, multiple problems have been reported in the documentation of cancer in lichen planus. These have included insufficient evidence of documented lichen planus, the cancer being in a remote site unrelated to the lichen planus, inadequate history to rule out carcinogenic agents, whether the cancer preceded the lichen planus, or whether the lesion is true lichen planus or just a lichenoid response. Kritchkoff reviewed 223 patients with lichen planus in whom cancer was reported. He stated only 15 of those probably had a true occurrence of both lichen planus and cancer. Eight of these 15 had other carcinogenic factors. Although the incidence of cancer in lichen planus may be no more than expected for normal patients, this debate suggests that the patient's course should be followed closely.

A medical history is necessary because lichen planus has been reported in various systemic diseases, especially diabetes. Some research shows no increased incidence, but a report by Howell and Rick suggests an incidence of diabetes in 13% of patients with lichen planus and in 20% of those with erosive lichen planus.

Another problem in management of patients with lichen planus is that lichenoid lesions may closely resemble lichen planus and are treated differently. These lichenoid lesions have been reported after patients used many different drugs, including nonsteroidal antiinflammatory drugs, antimalarials, methyldopa, and others. There have been reports of lichenoid responses from a galvanic reaction from copper in dental restorations and occasionally from mercury. In a study by Potts and co-workers, 17% of all patients with lichen planus and 30% of patients with severe erosive lichen planus were receiving nonsteroidal antiinflammatory drugs (9% for controls). Many improved when the medication was stopped.

BIBLIOGRAPHY

Allen CM and others: Relation of stress and anxiety to oral lichen planus, Oral Surg 61:44, 1986.

Al-Ubaidy SS and Nally FF: Oral lichen planus—a clinical evaluation of 120 cases over a 12 year period, J Int Dent Assoc 20:257, 1974.

Bagan JV and others: Treatment of lichen planus with griseofulvin, Oral Surg 60:608, 1985.

Boozer CH: Benign migratory glossitis associated with lichen planus, J Oral Med 29:58, 1974.

Bouqot JE and Gorlin RJ: Leukoplakia, lichen planus, and other keratoses in 23,616 white Americans over the age of 35 years, Oral Surg 61:373, 1986.

Camisa C and Allen CM: Treatment of oral erosive lichen planus with systemic isotretinoin, Oral Surg 62:393, 1986.

Christensen E: Arterial blood pressure in patients with oral lichen planus, J Oral Pathol 6:139, 1977.

Christensen E: Glucose tolerance in patients with oral lichen planus, J Oral Pathol 6:143, 1977.

Doyle JL and others: Diagnosis and treatment of erosive lichen planus, J Oral Med 40:18, 1985.

Erpenstein H: Periodontal and prosthetic treatment in patients with oral lichen planus, J Clin Periodontol 12:104, 1985.

Fellner MJ: Lichen planus—a review, Int J Dermatol 19:71, 1980.

Greenspan JS: Oral lichen planus—a double blind comparison of treatment with betamethasone valerate aerosol and pellets, Br Dent J 144:83, 1978.

Holmstrup P: The frequency of Candida in oral lichen planus, Scand J Dent Res 82:584, 1974.

Howell FV and Rich GM: Oral lichen planus and diabetes: a potential syndrome, J Calif Dent Assoc 1:58, 1973.

Jolly M: Lichen planus and its association with diabetes mellitus, Med J Aust 1:990, 1972.

Kaplan B and Barnes L: Oral lichen planus and squamous carcinoma, Arch Otolaryngol 111:543, 1985.

Kritchkoff DJ: Oral lichen planus: evidence regarding potential malignant transformation, J Oral Pathol 7:1, 1976.

Krogh P and others: Yeast species and biotypes associated with oral leukoplakia and lichen planus, Oral Surg 63:48, 1987.

Murti PR and others: Yeast species and biotypes associated with oral leukoplakia and lichen planus, Oral Surg 63:48, 1987.

Murti PR and others: Malignant potential of oral lichen planus: observations in 722 patients from India, J Oral Pathol 15:71, 1986.

Potts AJC and others: The medication of patients with oral lichen planus and the association of non-steroidal anti-inflammatory drugs with erosive lesions, Oral Surg 64:541, 1987.

Randell S: Erosive lichen planus, management of oral lesions with intralesional corticosteroid injections, J Oral Med 29:88, 1974.

Reisman RJ: The malignant potential of oral lichen planus—diagnostic pitfall, Oral Surg 38:227, 1974.

Saman PD: Lichen planus: an analysis of 300 cases, Trans St Johns Hosp Dermatol Soc 46:36, 1961.

Scully C and El-Kom M: Lichen planus: review and update on pathogenesis, J Oral Pathol 14:431, 1985.

Silverman S and others: A prospective follow-up study of 570 patients with oral lichen planus: persistence, remission and malignant association, Oral Surg 60:30, 1985.

Zegarelli DJ: Multimodality steroid therapy of erosive and ulcerative oral lichen planus, J Oral Med 38:127, 1983.

DISORDERS OF THE DIGESTIVE SYSTEM

Edited by **Walter Rubin**

169·THE STRUCTURE AND FUNCTION OF THE DIGESTIVE SYSTEM

Walter Rubin

OVERVIEW

The gut is a long, muscular tube that propels ingested food and accumulated secretions caudad from its origin at the bottom of the hypopharynx to the rectum and anus, where its contents are evacuated during defecation. The major role of the gut is to assimilate from the diet adequate calories and the nutrients that are essential for good health: proteins, fats, carbohydrates, vitamins, minerals, and water. The normal assimilation of most ingested proteins, fats, and carbohydrates depends on (1) the intraluminal digestion or hydrolysis of large, nonabsorbable molecules into smaller ones, a process mediated largely by digestive enzymes secreted into the lumen of the gut, and (2) the transport or absorption of digested substances by the lining epithelial cells from the lumen of the gut into its wall, from which they are transported by the blood and lymphatic vessels to the liver and other organs of the body. Normally almost all dietary calories, proteins, carbohydrates, lipids, and water are assimilated, with the exception of cellulose, some oligosaccharides, and other dietary fiber and roughage that cannot be digested.

The gut is divided into several anatomic divisions—esophagus, stomach, small intestine, and large intestine—each of which performs certain specialized functions. The esophagus serves merely as a conduit to move food from the hypopharynx to the stomach. The stomach serves primarily as a secretory organ and a reservoir. It secretes acid (to kill swallowed bacteria), mucus, and pepsinogen (a proteolytic enzyme that helps digest dietary protein), but the stomach's only essential secretion is intrinsic factor, a glycopeptide that permits adequate absorption of dietary vitamin B_{12}. The reservoir function of the stomach also is important. The stomach collects food that is hurriedly swallowed and empties it slowly into the duodenum, the proximal small intestine, so that its acidity can be rapidly neutralized, its osmolality quickly made isotonic, and its nutrients comfortably digested and absorbed. This proximal region of the small intestine is the principal site of digestion and absorption and therefore is the most important region of the gut. When chyme enters the duodenum, it stimulates the pancreas to secrete sodium bicarbonate into the duodenum, which neutralizes the gastric acid, and more important, to se-crete many digestive enzymes that are essential for the normal digestion of food. Chyme in the duodenum also stimulates the gallbladder to contract and discharge stored bile through the common bile duct and the relaxed distal Oddi's sphincter into the duodenum. Although most nutrients are absorbed in the proximal small bowel, vitamin B_{12} is absorbed predominantly in the distal small intestine (ileum), which contains receptors for the vitamin B_{12}–intrinsic factor complex. The bile acids that promote fat absorption in the proximal small intestine are themselves also reabsorbed primarily in the distal small bowel, returned to the liver, and resecreted into the bile, to be brought once again into the duodenum; this process is called entero-hepatic circulation.

A large amount of water and electrolytes is transported across the gut. Each day about 9 L of fluid enters the upper small intestine: about 2 L from the diet, 1.5 L from saliva, 2.5 L from gastric secretion, 1.5 L from the pancreas, 0.5 L from bile, and 1 L from intestinal secretions. Most of this fluid, about 8 L, is absorbed in the small intestine; only about 1 L enters the large intestine, whose major role is to extract most of the remaining water, store the feces in the rectum and sigmoid colon, and evacuate them when desired. About 100 to 200 g of feces is normally defecated daily. Diarrhea is present by definition when more than 300 g or 300 ml of stool is defecated in a day. If more than approximately 2 L of fluid enters the large bowel each day, even a normal colon cannot absorb enough water to reduce the daily fecal weight to less than 300 g. Thus diarrhea may result from a failure of either the small or large intestine to function normally. Net absorption is the net result of influxes into and outfluxes from the gut lumen. Thus diarrhea may result either from a failure of true absorption (outflux) or from excessive secretion (influx). The tremendous diarrhea associated with cholera, for example, results from extraordinary secretion in the small bowel. Cyclic adenosine monophosphate (AMP) in intestinal epithelial cells promotes their secretion, and thus any cause of elevated intestinal cyclic AMP promotes secretory diarrhea.

Although the histology of the gut is fundamentally similar in all its segments, there are variations, especially of the epithelial cells, that reflect the specialized functions of each of the divisions. The basic histologic structure of the gut wall consists of four layers, or tunicae. The innermost layer, the mucosa, consists of a surface epithelium resting on a layer of loose connective tissue (lamina propria) that is delimited below by a narrow layer of smooth muscle (muscularis mucosae). In most regions of the gut the epithelial cells extend from the surface into the lamina propria—and sometimes even below, as in the duodenum—to form a network of glands. Below the muscularis mucosae, the second layer, the submucosa, consists of a denser connective tissue through which numerous larger arteries, veins, and lymphatics traverse. The third layer, the muscularis externa, which is largely responsible for the contractile or motor activity of the gut, is a thick layer of smooth muscle formed in most regions by an inner layer of circumferentially oriented fibers and an outer layer of longitudinally oriented fibers. In the proximal third of the esophagus and distal rectum and anus, the smooth muscle is replaced in part or entirely by skeletal (voluntary) muscle, thus subjecting these areas to diseases that affect skeletal rather than smooth muscle. The fourth or outermost layer of gut, the adventitia, consists of a narrow layer of connective tissue and contains many larger traversing vessels. Along much of its length this layer is covered by a flat epithelium or mesothelium (mesentery) and in such areas is referred to as the serosa.

The epithelial cells that line the gut and form its glands are the most important constituent cells because they largely determine most of the specialized functions characteristic of each segment and play an important protective role in each. These cells are continually turning over; they die, are desquamated into the lumen of the gut, and are replaced through the replication, differentiation, and migration of undifferentiated epithelial cells located within the glands or, in the esophagus, at the base of the epithelium. This process is extremely important for the maintenance of normal populations of epithelial cells and therefore for the structural and functional integrity of the gut. Impairment of this process in the stomach, for example, by some forms of experimental stress can lead to ulceration of the surface. In celiac disease the rapid death of mature epithelial cells and their inadequate replacement through an increased rate of replication and differentiation lead to atrophy of the surface lining and malabsorption. Normally the cells lining the surface of the gut are completely renewed approximately every 3 to 7 days. Many of the cells in the glands, however, have a much longer life span; the parietal cells in the stomach, for example, are thought to live for many weeks.

Most of the gut epithelial secreting cells are exocrine cells; that is, they secrete mucus, digestive enzymes, acid, or other substances directly into the lumen of the gut or into the duct of a gland. The gut is also, however, the largest endocrine organ in the body and contains many different morphologic types of endocrine epithelial cells that secrete in a basal direction into the lamina propria. These cells produce polypeptide hormones and biogenic amines such as 5-hydroxytryptamine (serotonin). Some of these polypeptide hormones have been identified, and many of their apparent physiologic functions are understood: for example, secretin, the first hormone discovered, and cholecystokinin-pancreozymin (CCK-PZ), both from the proximal small intestine, and gastrin from the distal stomach and the proximal small intestine. Many other gut hormones and putative hormones have been discovered only recently, however, and their physiologic roles have yet to be defined. This group includes somatostatin; enteroglucagon; gastric inhibitory polypeptide (GIP); vasoactive intestinal polypeptide (VIP), probably located in nerves; bombesin; motilin; and enkephalin, also in nerves. When released, these substances may act locally rather than at distal sites; that is, they may serve "paracrine" rather than endocrine functions. The gut endocrine cells exhibit many morphologic and cytochemical characteristics of neurons, synthesize and secrete many polypeptides and amines also found in the nervous system, and have been considered a possible part of a neuroendocrine system. There are many similarities among different polypeptide and amine-synthesizing endocrine cells in the body. Although

these cells once were thought to arise embryologically from neural ectoderm (neural crest), they indeed develop from entoderm. These cells have been named APUD (amine precursor uptake decarboxylation) cells, and tumors derived from them have been called apudomas.

The gut also is an important immunologic organ, active in both cell-mediated and humorally mediated immunologic processes. Lymph follicles are present along its length and are most prominent in the submucosa and mucosa, particularly in the distal ileum, where they often form visible aggregates called Peyer's patches, and in the appendix and large intestine. Special epithelial cells, called "M-cells," reside in the surface over Peyer's patches; they can transport macromolecules and antigens from the intestinal lumen into the patches. Gut lymphocytes are recirculated: they drain from the gut back into the systemic circulation through the intestinal lymphatics and thoracic duct. Disease processes that block the drainage of lymph and lymphocytes from the gut into the systemic circulation, such as Whipple's disease and lymphangiectasia, characteristically reduce the number of lymphocytes observed in peripheral blood counts. The lamina propria of the gut normally contains numerous plasma cells that produce all classes of immunoglobulins but predominantly IgA (see Chapter 3). Much of this IgA, sometimes called secretory IgA, can be found within the gut lumen; much is along the surface of the lining epithelium in the form of a dimer bound to a glycopeptide, which is produced by the epithelial cells and has been called secretory piece and transport piece. The secretory piece is thought to help transport the IgA across the lining epithelial cells into the lumen of the gut. The gut may be the site of primary immunizations; secretory IgA and local immunologically competent cells are thought to play important roles in protecting the gut and body from potentially harmful substances, microorganisms, and other agents that enter the body by the intestinal route. It also is thought that immunologic processes occurring in the gut may go awry and cause some poorly understood inflammatory diseases, such as ulcerative colitis and granulomatous ileocolitis.

The gut has millions of intrinsic neurons whose cell bodies are arranged largely within two plexuses: the myenteric (Auerbach's) plexus, located between the circular and transverse muscle layers of the muscularis externa, and the submucous (Meissner's) plexus, located along the submucosa. Much of the motor activity of the gut is intrinsic, regulated in large measure by this intrinsic nervous system. It is also modulated in part, however, by the innervation of extrinsic nerves—the classic postganglionic sympathetic (thoracolumbar) and preganglionic parasympathetic (craniosacral) nerves—and by humoral agents. Parasympathetic stimulation classically has been thought to have excitatory effects on the gut and sympathetic stimulation inhibitory effects, but this view is proving to be much too simplistic. The extrinsic nerves, particularly the vagus, are mixed nerves containing numerous afferent as well as efferent fibers and releasing many neurohumoral mediators, with varying physiologic effects. In general, gut contractility, secretion, and blood flow vary together. Whenever the motor activity of the gut is stimulated, its secretory activity and blood flow are also usually increased. Eating is the usual physiologic stimulus that activates the digestive system.

ESOPHAGUS AND SWALLOWING

The esophagus, the first part of the gut, extends from the hypopharynx, where the cricopharyngeus muscle forms its upper esophageal sphincter, through the posterior aspect of the chest to join the stomach just below the diaphragm. The lower esophageal sphincter is a nonanatomic, physiologic high-pressure zone that extends along the last few centimeters of the esophagus and normally prevents the regurgitation of the gastric contents, including acid, back into the esophagus. The esophagus is the least sophisticated part of the gut; it serves only as a conduit to bring swallowed food and saliva from the hypopharynx to the stomach. Thus it is lined by a stratified squamous epithelium to protect against "wear and tear."

Swallowing is a complex physiologic process integrated through a swallowing center in the medulla oblongata. After food is chewed into small pieces and lubricated with the alkaline mucous saliva, which also contains amylase and some lipase enzymatic activities, the tongue moves a bolus of food back into the pharynx to initiate swallowing. The pharyngeal muscles contract and the soft palate is elevated, occluding the passage between the pharynx and nasopharynx and preventing the regurgitation of food into the nose. The glottis closes and the epiglottis folds over it, preventing the aspiration of food into the respiratory passages. The contraction of the pharyngeal muscles moves the food into the hypopharynx, and the upper esophageal sphincter relaxes, permitting the bolus to enter the esophagus. A primary peristaltic wave is initiated in the upper esophagus, which with the aid of gravity moves the bolus down the esophagus. Finally, the lower esophageal sphincter relaxes, permitting the bolus to enter the stomach, the fundus of which relaxes (receptive relaxation) to receive it. Each of these processes—the blockage of the nasopharynx and respiratory tract, the relaxation of the sphincters, and the initiation of the primary peristalsis—is independently initiated by deglutition and is integrated through the swallowing center. Impairment of any of these processes, for example, by a neurologic or muscular disorder, can result in serious consequences while eating, such as the aspiration of food into the lungs, the regurgitation of food through the nose, or the inability of food to enter the esophagus. If the esophagus is distended, for example, by a piece of food that is stuck or regurgitated from the stomach, a secondary peristaltic wave is initiated at a level just above the distention to move the piece down into the stomach.

STOMACH

The stomach, the short second segment of gut, is a secretory organ and more usefully functions as a reservoir. However, its secretion of the glycoprotein intrinsic factor, which is necessary for the adequate absorption of dietary vitamin B_{12}, is actually its only essential function. Intrinsic factor and essentially isotonic hydrochloric acid are secreted by the parietal (oxyntic) cells, a major constituent of the gastric glands throughout most of the gastric mucosa. Pepsin, a proteolytic enzyme secreted as the proenzyme pepsinogen, which is activated by acid and pepsin itself, is produced by the chief cells, the second major constituent of the same gastric glands, although immunologically identifiable pepsinogens also are produced by gastric mucous cells. The surface of the stomach and the numerous pits (foveolae) that connect the surface with the gastric glands below are lined by mucous cells. These are largely responsible for the neutral mucus or glycoprotein that coats and lubricates the surface of the stomach and is thought to play some protective role as well. The glands in the pyloric antrum, the most distal portion of the stomach, and also in the cardia, a narrow segment of stomach encircling the esophagogastric junction, are lined by a different type of mucous cell (pyloric gland cell) and contain few if any parietal or chief cells. Also present within the gastric glands, although these are usually not apparent in routine hematoxylin- and eosin-stained histologic sections, are at least four morphologic types of endocrine cells.

The G cells, located in pyloric glands, produce the hormone gastrin; the D cells produce somatostatin; and the EC cells produce serotonin (5-hydroxytryptamine); the product of the ECL cells has not yet been identified. The replicating undifferentiated cells that maintain the populations of the differentiated epithelial cells are located in the upper regions (necks) of the glands.

The surface of the stomach is quite impermeable to water and ions, a property probably resulting largely from the tightness of the junctions between the adjoining epithelial cells. As a result, hypotonic and hypertonic solutions can be maintained for some time within the gastric lumen. The impermeability of the surface to ions permits an electric potential of about -40 to -60 mV, possibly generated largely by a parietal Cl^- pump, to be maintained between the luminal and serosal surfaces of the mucosa. The impermeability to H^+—the so-called mucosal barrier to acid back-diffusion—plays an important protective role by preventing the acid secreted into the lumen from diffusing back into the mucosa. When this barrier is broken, for example, by agents such as aspirin and ethanol, acid can diffuse back into the mucosa, often causing erosions, ulceration, and even hemorrhage. This is thought to be the mechanism by which alcohol and aspirin cause erosive gastritis. Damage to the mucosal barrier can be detected by a decrease in or loss of the normal transmucosal potential difference. In recent years certain prostaglandins have been discovered to possess cytoprotective properties; by some poorly understood mechanism, these seem to protect the stomach and maintain its structural and functional integrity.

During the interdigestive (fasting) period the stomach is usually inactive; it exhibits little motor activity and secretes little fluid, most of which resembles an ultrafiltrate of plasma and little of which is thought to arise from the parietal cells. In fact, the normal fasting person secretes only about 2 to 5 mEq acid an hour. The act of eating or even hunger, the thought of food, or the desire to eat stimulates gastric motor and secretory activity; a normal meal usually stimulates this activity for about 3 to 4 hours. Although the stimulated secretions contain mucus from mucous cells and pepsinogen from chief cells, most of the volume is probably produced by the parietal cells, which secrete intrinsic factor and approximately isotonic hydrochloric acid. Thus the composition of gastric juice secreted during a meal approaches that of the parietal cells, and its pH may approach 1 (100 mEq H^+/L) or even lower. Many substances stimulate the parietal cells to secrete, including Ca^{++} and caffeine, but acetylcholine, gastrin, and histamine are probably the most potent and physiologically important stimulants. The parietal cell membrane seems to have receptors for each of these three stimulants, and the effect produced by one seems to be related to the actions of the other two. If the receptor for histamine is blocked by a histamine H_2-receptor blocking drug (for example, cimetidine) or if the muscarinic effects of acetylcholine are reduced with atropine or a vagotomy, the responsiveness of the parietal cells to the other two respective agents is markedly reduced. That is the reason, for example, why acid secretion can be almost abolished with cimetidine even though this agent in essence only eliminates the "histamine tone" on the parietal cell. Second messengers, such as cyclic AMP and Ca^{++} play a role, but the final secretion of H^+ at the cell membrane depends on a K^+, H^+-ATPase that promotes an exchange of H^+ for K^+. The secreted H^+ comes from carbonic acid formed from the reaction of carbon dioxide and water, which is mediated by the enzyme carbonic anhydrase. Thus for every H^+ molecule secreted, a HCO_3^- molecule is released into the lamina propria, thus accounting for the alkaline venous blood, or alkaline tide, that flows from the stomach during a meal.

Although a meal stimulates gastric secretion for 3 to 4 hours, the maximum rate of acid secretion is reached in about 1 hour. Monitoring the acidity of the gastric contents during a meal often reveals a rather precipitous fall in the pH after about 1 hour. During the first hour the secreted acid is usually well buffered by the ingested food, especially by the protein. After this hour, however, much of the food has left the stomach and much of the buffering capacity of the retained food has been exhausted; the acid that is now being secreted at about its maximal rate can no longer be adequately buffered and the pH usually falls toward 1, where it generally remains for several additional hours. Thus patients with peptic ulcers often have immediate symptomatic relief by eating because the food buffers the gastric acid, but their pain often returns 1 or more hours later because of the presence of unbuffered gastric acid produced by the very food they may have originally ingested to relieve their pain. The dietary protein, the greatest buffer of gastric acid, is also the major stimulus of its secretion.

The stimulation of gastric secretion and motor activity by a meal traditionally is divided into three phases: cephalic, gastric, and intestinal. The cephalic phase is the stimulation before the food even reaches the stomach. Feeling hungry, thinking of eating, smelling food, hearing the dinner bell (as with Pavlov's dogs), chewing, tasting, and swallowing all stimulate gastric secretion. The efferent limb of this stimulation is mediated by the vagus nerves, which stimulate secretion largely by their release of acetylcholine in the wall of the stomach, which in turn stimulates the parietal cells not only directly but possibly indirectly by stimulating a release of gastrin from the antral G cells. The cephalic phase of gastric secretion can be eliminated by a vagotomy or reduced by anticholinergic drugs or by the traditionally bland, unseasoned diets that make eating tasteless and unattractive. The gastric phase of gastric secretion is initiated by the presence of food in the stomach. This stimulation is mediated by gastrin, whose release is stimulated by dietary constituents such as peptide and Ca^{++}; by intrinsic and extrinsic nerves, which are activated at least in part by gastric distention and which lead again to the release of acetylcholine; and by dietary substances such as caffeine and Ca^{++}, which directly stimulate the parietal cells. The intestinal phase of gastric secretion is stimulated by the entrance of the chyme into the small intestine and is mediated probably again by both neural and humoral factors and at least in part by the release of gastrin from the duodenum. In all three phases the three major stimulants at the site of the parietal cells are probably acetylcholine, gastrin, and histamine, released from cholinergic nerve terminals, endocrine cells, and mast cells, respectively.

The control of acid secretion is very complex; in fact, humoral and neural feedback mechanisms tend to reduce its secretion. For example, when secreted acid bathes the antrum, it suppresses the secretion of gastrin, inhibiting it completely when the pH is reduced to approximately 1. When acid enters the duodenum, it also tends to reduce gastric acid secretion, perhaps in part through its stimulation of the release of secretin and possibly other enterogastrones, humoral agents (hormones) released from the small intestine that inhibit gastric activity.

The acid secretory function of a patient's stomach can be assessed clinically. A nasogastric tube is passed into the subject's stomach while he is fasting, and the gastric secretions are continually aspirated and titrated to neutrality with sodium hydroxide. In this way the basal acid output (BAO), the rate of acid secretion during fasting, is determined. The patient then receives a stimulant of gastric secretion—usually histamine, histalog, or more commonly pentagastrin, a synthetic pentapeptide containing the active tetrapeptide of gastrin—in a dose to elicit a maximal secretory response from the patient's stomach. The aspirates are collected during four subsequent 15-minute periods and again titrated. The largest amount of acid secreted in a period, usually during the second or third period, multiplied by four gives the maximal acid output (MAO) or peak acid output (PAO), that is, the maximal rate at which that patient's stomach can secrete acid. The MAO is actually a measurement of the number of parietal cells in a subject's stomach: the more parietal cells, the more acid the stomach can secrete when maximally stimulated. The values obtained vary somewhat among different laboratories, but the BAO of most normal subjects is about 2 to 5 mEq acid an hour, and the MAO is about 20 to 30 mEq acid an hour. Patients with atrophic changes in their stomachs (atrophic gastritis or gastric atrophy) and therefore with diminished numbers of parietal cells secrete smaller amounts, whereas patients with duodenal ulcer disease as a group secrete more acid than normal subjects in both the basal and stimulated states, findings that indicate these patients have more parietal cells and are less successful in reducing acid secretion during the basal (fasting) state. The marked hypersecretory characteristics observed in patients with gastrinomas (Zollinger-Ellison syndrome) are discussed in Chapter 173.

As already noted, in the interdigestive period the stomach exhibits little motor activity as well. Even then the stomach is thought to contain an electrogenic pacemaker, located high on the greater curvature of its body, which emits myoelectric waves at a rate of about 3 waves a minute. These waves are conducted along the outer longitudinal muscle layer. They produce few muscle depolarization spikes and contractions. When motor activity is stimulated by eating or by hunger (hunger pangs probably result from gastric peristalsis, possibly initiated through the vagus by a low or falling blood sugar), peristaltic contractions arise in the mid to distal body of the stomach at the same pacemaker rate and sweep caudad through the antrum toward the muscular pyloric sphincter, which forms the junction between the distal stomach and duodenum. The rate at which the gastric contents are emptied into the duodenum probably depends not only on the physical nature of the contents (liquids and solids of varying size and consistency) but also on the completion of the peristaltic waves, the force of antral contractions, the squeeze and tension in the pyloric sphincter, the pressure generated in the proximal duodenum (bulb), and the interrelationships of these ever-changing factors. This motor activity that regulates the rate of gastric emptying is in turn controlled by the intrinsic and extrinsic nerves, humoral agents, and locally released, active paracrine substances, the same factors that affect gastric secretion.

As noted previously, a major physiologic function of the stomach is to act as a reservoir. Although meals may be eaten in only a few minutes and the food passes rapidly through the esophagus, the food is stored in the stomach, is churned in the antrum by its motor activity, and is slowly emptied into the proximal small intestine, the major site of digestion and absorption. The regulation of gastric emptying is extremely important in avoiding impaired absorption and the unpleasant symptoms commonly produced when the gastric contents are rapidly emptied or dumped into the small intestine (dumping syndrome). These symptoms are often observed in patients who have undergone gastric surgery, usually for ulcer disease or tumors.

Many factors affect the rate of gastric emptying: the amount and physical state of the gastric contents and the pH, osmolality, lipid content, and caloric content of the chyme being emptied into the duodenum. These factors presumably affect gastroduodenal motor activity largely through the neural and hormonal mechanisms already mentioned. The greater the gastric content and distention, the more rapid gastric emptying tends to be. Liquids are emptied more rapidly than solids, and small solids more easily than large ones. The greater the acidity, hyperosmolality (and in part hypoosmolality), fat content, and caloric content of the chyme entering the duodenum, the stronger is the feedback from the duodenum to slow down the rate of gastric emptying. These feedback regulatory processes initiated in the duodenum permit the acid chyme to be rapidly neutralized and made isotonic within the duodenum and the fat and other nutrients to be more leisurely and adequately digested and absorbed in the proximal small intestine, as described more fully in the following section.

SMALL INTESTINE, PANCREAS, AND LIVER

The small intestine, about 6 m in length, comprises the duodenum, jejunum, and ileum. The duodenum, the short first segment, consists of the bulb, just beyond the stomach, and the descending, transverse, and ascending portions, which are retroperitoneal and partially encircle the head of the pancreas. At the ligament of Treitz, where the duodenum assumes a mesenteric covering and penetrates into the peritoneal cavity at the base of the mesentery, it becomes the jejunum, the proximal half of the remaining small intestine; the distal half is the ileum. The junction between the two halves is arbitrary and involves no structural or functional demarcation. The ileum ends at the ileocecal valve, the muscular sphincter between the small and large intestines.

The surface area of the small intestine is enhanced by the presence of many visible folds (plicae circulares) and numerous finger-shaped projections of the mucosa, the intestinal villi, which can be seen with a magnifying glass or low-power microscope. The villi are lined by tall columnar epithelial cells (differentiated villous epithelial cells) that have numerous tall apical microvilli, seen with a light microscope as a prominent striated (brush) border. These are the most important cells in the gut, because they are responsible for the absorption of digested nutrients from the bowel lumen into the lamina propria; many of the important enzymes and carrier systems for this transport are associated with the brush border membrane. At the base of the villi, the epithelium forms glands, or crypts, that extend into the lamina propria to the muscularis mucosae. The crypts are lined predominantly by undifferentiated cells but also contain, especially at their bases, serous cells, the Paneth's cells, that contain prominent apical secretory granules, the nature and function of which have yet to be clearly defined. Goblet cells, mucous cells that secrete an acid mucus and that resemble brandy goblets when distended with mucus, are located along the crypts and villi. Again, several morphologic types of endocrine cells are present, predominantly in the crypts, but these usually are not apparent in routinely stained sections.

The pancreas is a retroperitoneal gland whose head is encircled by the duodenum and whose body and tail extend to the left and upward, behind the stomach and lesser sac, to the hilus of the spleen. The pancreas actually is a dual organ. Its islets of Langerhans, which are more numerous in its body and tail, are aggregates of at least four types of endocrine cells that secrete insulin, glucagon, somatostatin, and pancreatic polypeptide. Most of the organ, however, functions as an exocrine gland whose acinar cells synthesize, store, and secrete many digestive enzymes, which flow through small ducts into the main duct of Wirsung or the accessory duct of Santorini and through the ampulla of Vater and Oddi's sphincter into the descending segment of the duodenum. The secretion from the acinar cells contains relatively little water in volume but is rich in the digestive enzymes, as follows:

1. *The proteolytic enzymes trypsinogen, chymotrypsinogen, procarboxypeptidase, proaminopeptidase, and elastase.* The trypsinogen is activated in the duodenum to trypsin by means of enterokinase, an enzyme in the brush border of the epithelial cells. In turn, trypsin activates trypsinogen and the other proenzymes to change to their active moieties.
2. *Amylase.* Amylase catalyzes the hydrolysis of α-1,4-glucosidic bonds and thereby converts dietary starch and glycogen to glucose, short straight-chain oligosaccharides (maltose and the like), and isomaltose.
3. *Lipolytic enzymes.* These are lipase, which hydrolyzes the 1 and 3 bonds of triglycerides, mechanically assisted by another secreted protein, colipase; phospholipases A_1 and A_2, which hydrolyze phospholipids, including the conversion of lecithin to lysolecithins; and other lipases that hydrolyze cholesterol esters and water-soluble esters of fatty acids.
4. *Ribonuclease and deoxyribonuclease*

Besides the acinar secretion, the duct cells secrete a large volume of alkaline water that is rich in sodium bicarbonate.

The liver also is an endocrine and exocrine organ. Bile, its exocrine secretion, is secreted by the hepatocytes (liver parenchymal cells) into the canaliculi, the small excretory channels formed by adjacent hepatocytes. Bile drains into the bile ductules and ducts, which like the pancreatic ducts are lined by cells that secrete alkaline water rich in sodium bicarbonate into the bile. The bile flows from the left and right main hepatic ducts into the common hepatic duct and common bile duct. In the interdigestive (fasting) state, when Oddi's sphincter at the distal end of the common bile duct is closed, little bile enters the duodenum; most of it flows back through the cystic duct into the gallbladder, where it is stored and concentrated by the absorption of water and electrolytes by the lining epithelial cells. During a meal, however, the gallbladder is stimulated to contract and Oddi's sphincter to open, thereby permitting both stored and newly formed bile to flow into the duodenum.

Bile contains bile pigment, predominantly bilirubin diglucuronide, which gives bile its yellow color. Bile also contains bile acids, lecithin, and cholesterol; the detergent bile acids and lecithin serve to solubilize insoluble cholesterol by incorporating it into mixed micelles. The bile acids are synthesized in the liver from cholesterol and are conjugated largely with glycine and taurine to form the principal primary bile acids: glycocholic, taurocholic, glycochenodeoxycholic, and taurochenodeoxycholic acids. These are stored mainly in the gallbladder bile during the fasting state and are released into the duodenum when the gallbladder empties during eating. They aid fat absorption mainly by solubilizing the fatty acids and monoglycerides produced by the digestion of dietary fat, thereby bringing them more rapidly to the surface of the absorbing intestinal epithelial cells. Although this physiologic function is performed predominantly in the proximal small intestine, the bile acids themselves are absorbed primarily in the distal ileum, returned to the liver, resecreted into the bile, and returned to the duodenum or gallbladder. In this way an individual bile acid molecule may be returned two or three times to the proximal small intestine during a single meal to aid in the absorption of the ingested lipid. This enterohepatic circulation helps to maintain the body's bile acid pool of 2 to 4 g. Only about 15% of this pool is lost in the feces each day, and this amount is readily restored by the synthesis of new bile acid in the liver. If the fecal loss of bile acid is increased because of disease, surgical removal, or a bypass of the distal ileum, hepatic synthesis also increases in an effort to maintain a normal pool of bile acid. The enhanced synthesis can compensate satisfactorily for a moderate loss of bile acid, but a greater rate of fecal loss results in a significant reduction in the bile acid pool.

The rate of bile secretion by the liver cells is greatly influenced by the rate at which the hepatocytes secrete bile acid, which in turn is influenced largely by the enterohepatic circulation and the rate at which bile acid is returned to the liver. In the fasting state, when most of the bile acid pool is stored in the gallbladder (or possibly in the intestine if there is no gallbladder), the liver cells usually make little bile. This bile also is often lithogenic; that is, it contains too much cholesterol in relation to its bile acid content, such that the bile is supersaturated in respect to cholesterol. The composition of this hepatic bile usually is corrected, however, when it enters the gallbladder and mixes with the stored bile there or when the contents of the gallbladder and its stored bile acids are emptied into the intestine during a meal, thereby causing the bile acids to move through the enterohepatic circulation and thus increase the rate of hepatic bile formation. Some individuals, however, especially those with diseased or absent terminal ileums and therefore reduced bile acid pools and those who have some metabolic derangement of hepatic function, secrete a more persistent lithogenic bile, making them more susceptible to the formation of cholesterol gallstones in the gallbladder.

DIGESTION, ABSORPTION, AND MOTILITY IN THE SMALL INTESTINE

When chyme enters the small intestine (duodenum), it initiates many rapid physiologic processes functioning principally to promote efficient and rapid digestion and absorption. Although the stomach can retain hyperosmolar and hypoosmolar solutions, these rapidly are rendered isotonic when introduced into the duodenum. This occurs through active absorption, rapid fluxes of water across the mucosa, and dilution with the isotonic secretions of the pancreas, bile, and intestine. If much hypertonic solution is rapidly dumped into or produced during digestion in the small intestine, as may occur when the reservoir function of the stomach is impaired by gastric surgery, rapid fluxes of water from the blood into the intestinal lumen may quickly deplete the blood volume and lead to the symptoms of dumping syndrome (weakness, light-headedness, faintness, palpitations, sweating, and diarrhea).

When gastric acid enters the duodenum, it stimulates a quantitative release of the hormone secretin from the wall of the duodenum, which in turn stimulates the epithelium of the pancreatic and biliary ducts to secrete a large volume of their alkaline juices into the duodenum. In this way the acidic chyme is neutralized, the feedback slowing of the gastric emptying of acid in the duodenum permitting a more rapid and complete neutralization within the proximal duodenum. The neutralization of acid chyme within the proximal intestine is essential for normal absorption, because an acid pH impairs the bile acids' ability to solubilize the fatty acids and monoglycerides and also impairs the digestive action of the pancreatic enzymes. Lipase may be irreversibly denatured by an acid pH.

When chyme enters the duodenum, it stimulates the release of another hormone, CCK-PZ, largely because of its content of fatty acid. CCK-PZ in turn stimulates the gallbladder to contract, the pancreatic acinar cells to secrete their enzyme-rich juice, and Oddi's sphincter to open, thereby permitting

bile and pancreatic secretions to enter the duodenum easily. CCK-PZ and secretin are synergistic, each augmenting the physiologic activity of the other. Even before chyme enters the duodenum, the act of eating produces some stimulation, especially of pancreatic secretion, through the cephalic and gastric phases; vagal cholinergic fibers and released gastrin, which structurally resembles CCK-PZ and engages in some of the same activity, stimulate some acinar secretion.

The pancreatic enzymes are essential for normal digestion. Salivary amylase, active at a neutral or alkaline pH, and gastric pepsin, active at an acid pH, play a digestive role but are unnecessary. Within the proximal small intestine the pancreatic enzymes digest dietary protein into amino acids and small peptides; starch and glycogen into glucose, maltose, other short-chain straight oligosaccharides, and isomaltose; and triglycerides (neutral fat) into fatty acids and 2-monoglycerides. These products of digestion, together with other dietary substances such as the disaccharides lactose from milk and milk products and sucrose (table sugar), must then be transported by the lining intestinal epithelial cells from the intestinal lumen into the lamina propria.

As already noted, the fatty acids and monoglycerides, as well as fat-soluble vitamins and cholesterol, are solubilized in mixed micelles by the bile acids so that they can move rapidly through the unstirred water layer to the surface membrane of the lining cells, which they penetrate passively. Within the epithelial cells most of the fatty acids and monoglycerides are resynthesized into triglyceride, which in turn is converted into chylomicron particles with the addition of phospholipid and β-lipoprotein to the surface. The chylomicrons are secreted into the lamina propria and drained by the lacteals (lymphatics) through the thoracic duct into the systemic circulation. Short- and medium-chain triglycerides, containing more soluble fatty acids with fewer than 10 and 10 to 14 carbon atoms, respectively, are more rapidly hydrolyzed within the intestine. They do not require solubilization within micelles, and most of their absorbed fatty acids are drained directly into the vascular capillaries of the portal circulation. The bile acids also aid fat digestion by promoting and stabilizing emulsions of fat particles within the intestinal lumen and by stabilizing and protecting lipase and colipase.

The amino acids are actively transported by the epithelium to the lamina propria. Some small peptides are hydrolyzed by peptidases in the brush border and cytosol of the epithelial cells, and the resultant amino acids are also transported across. A few small peptides cross the epithelial cells intact. All these products derived from dietary protein are absorbed mainly into the portal circulation.

Glucose and galactose are also actively absorbed by the lining epithelium. Several disaccharidase enzymes, located in the brush border of these lining cells, are also essential for the normal absorption of dietary carbohydrate. For example, luminal maltose and isomaltose, produced from the digestion of starch and glycogen, must be split by brush border maltase and isomaltase before their contained glucose can be satisfactorily transported across these cells. Similarly, milk sugar lactose must be split by lactase and sucrose by sucrase (invertase) to ensure normal absorption of their component hexoses, glucose-galactose and glucose-fructose, respectively. A deficiency of intestinal lactase, a common clinical occurrence, may result in the malabsorption of ingested lactose, the fermentation of lactose by intestinal bacteria, especially in the colon, and cramps and osmotic diarrhea if appreciable milk or dairy products are ingested.

The active absorption of glucose, galactose, and amino acids is coupled with the absorption of Na^+. Thus in certain secretory diarrhea states such as cholera, in which large amounts of body water and salt are lost by their voluminous secretion into the gut (because of activation of adenylate cyclase), the absorption of Na^+ and water can be promoted and partially restored by the oral administration of isotonic Na^+-containing fluids that also contain glucose or sucrose (which is split to glucose and fructose). The intestinal epithelial cells also contain a sodium pump that extrudes Na^+ from the cell into the interstitial fluid and thereby provides for the active absorption of Na^+ from the intestinal lumen. The absorption of the products of digestion and of Na^+ also provides for the secondary passive absorption of water from the lumen. The intestine can also absorb Cl^- actively, coupled in the jejunum and ileum with HCO_3^- secretion, and thus the chyme contains a higher concentration of HCO_3^- and becomes more alkaline toward the distal ileum.

The absorption of most vitamins (except B_{12}), iron, and calcium also is maximal in the proximal small intestine; the absorption of some is complex and is still not entirely understood. Calcium absorption is promoted by vitamin D, possibly because of its effects on binding protein, whereas iron absorption is enhanced by the presence of anemia.

The motor activity of the small intestine, quiescent during the interdigestive state, is aroused by eating, an effect also mediated by intrinsic and extrinsic nerves and hormones. The small intestine exhibits little peristaltic activity but rather has prominent multiple segmental contractions that squirt the chyme forward and backward, thereby mixing it with the digestive enzymes and other secretions and promoting digestion and absorption. Because these contractions are more frequent in the proximal than in the distal small bowel, the net effect is to propel the chyme forward toward the large intestine. When the distal ileum contracts, the ileocecal sphincter is stimulated to relax, permitting the chyme to be squirted into the cecum of the large intestine. An increased pressure in the cecum, produced by distention or contractions of the cecum, for example, in turn stimulates the ileocecal sphincter to contract to prevent the contaminated cecal contents from regurgitating back into the ileum. The normal small intestine is practically sterile, largely because its motor activity effectively propels the chyme forward, but the large intestine, which is essentially a large, stagnant loop, contains high titers of bacteria. Whenever the contents of the small intestine are in stasis because of either impaired motor activity or a mechanical blockage, abnormal numbers of bacteria proliferate in the stagnant small intestine and may lead to malabsorption of fat and vitamin B_{12} (bacterial overgrowth or stagnant loop syndrome).

LARGE INTESTINE

The colon, or large bowel, is divided into several segments: (1) the cecum, the blind pouch into which the ileum empties and from which the small rudimentary appendix extends, (2) the ascending colon, (3) the hepatic flexure, (4) the transverse colon, (5) the splenic flexure, (6) the descending colon, (7) the sigmoid colon, (8) the rectum, and (9) the anus. The ascending colon, descending colon, rectum, and anus are extraperitoneal and relatively fixed. In contrast the cecum (usually), transverse colon, and sigmoid colon are invested with a mesentery, are located within the abdominal cavity, and are much more movable. The rectum begins where the sigmoid colon exits from the abdominal cavity, a point about 16 cm from the anal orifice. The anus, or anal canal, comprises the distal 2 to 3 cm of the large bowel, from the point where the columnar epithelium of the rectum becomes stratified squamous epithelium to the anal orifice where the anus joins the skin.

The outer longitudinal muscle of the colon does not form a complete layer but rather is organized into three longitudinal bands, the taeniae coli. The final muscular sphincter at the end of the large bowel, which is ultimately responsible for fecal continence, is actually a dual sphincter: the internal anal sphincter, prominent smooth muscle that is continuous with the muscularis externa, and the external anal sphincter, a surrounding sheath of skeletal or voluntary muscle (the levator ani) that is innervated by neurons emanating from sacral segments of the spinal cord and allows for voluntary control of defecation. The parasympathetic innervation of the proximal two thirds of large bowel is received through the vagus nerves from the "cranial outflow," whereas the parasympathetic innervation of the distal third, including the internal anal sphincter, is derived from the "sacral outflow" and sacral nerves.

The mucosal surface of the large intestine is relatively flat, because there are no villi and the folds are relatively inconspicuous, with the exception of three semicircular folds in the rectum, the so-called rectal valves, which can serve as landmarks during proctoscopy, and several short longitudinal folds at the rectum-anus junction, the so-called rectal columns of Morgagni. The surface of the colon is lined by tall columnar epithelial cells with a narrow brush border. Long, straight crypts of Lieberkühn extend from the surface to a prominent muscularis mucosae. The undifferentiated cells are located predominantly in the lower halves of the crypts, which also contain numerous goblet cells, differentiated columnar cells along the upper portions, and endocrine cells. Paneth's cells usually are not present in the normal large bowel. The lamina propria usually contains more connective tissue cells than other parts of the gut, and lymph nodules are relatively abundant in the mucosa and submucosa. The mucosal and submucosal veins in the distal rectum and anus—the internal and external hemorrhoidal plexus—are especially prominent and subject to becoming distended, varicose, and thrombosed.

The small appendix, the blind-ending evagination of the cecum, is lined by columnar epithelium. Its crypts are less regular in shape and length and contain a relatively large number of endocrine cells, which probably give rise to the relatively common carcinoid tumors (argentaffinomas) that develop in the appendix. The muscularis mucosae is poorly developed, and numerous lymph nodules and lymphocytes fill much of the mucosa and submucosa.

The major role of the large intestine is to receive the ileal effluent, about 1 L a day, to absorb most of its water and salt to produce about 100 g of solid feces, and to store and evacuate the feces. The colon actively absorbs Na^+ and Cl^- and along with them passively absorbs water. The colon also secretes HCO_3^- and K^+, some of the K^+ in exchange for Na^+ under the control of aldosterone. Because of the small amount of stool normally evacuated, relatively little K^+ is lost, but with diarrhea appreciable quantities of body K^+ can be lost.

The motility of the colon is extremely slow and sluggish. It exhibits several short segmental contractions, some contractions of larger segments, and occasional peristaltic activity. In the interdigestive state the colonic contents are thought to be forwarded at a net rate of only about 5 cm an hour, but when colonic motility is stimulated by eating, this net rate is approximately tripled. This enhanced motility often moves feces into the rectum and initiates a defecation reflex. Whenever the rectum is distended, usually by the addition of new feces, the rectal muscle is stimulated to contract and the internal sphincter to relax, and the subject experiences an urge to defecate. The tension in the external sphincter, however, is reflexly increased by tension in its muscle spindles, thereby preventing the evacuation of feces. A person who does not wish to defecate can voluntarily maintain the tension in the external sphincter, and in this case the contraction and tension in the rectal muscles are decreased reflexly, the tension in the internal sphincter is increased, and the urge to defecate is abated until additional feces distend the rectum even further. If the person wishes to defecate, the defecation reflex can be facilitated voluntarily by sending neural impulses from the cerebral cortex to the defecation center in the medulla. Impulses from the center largely to sacral segments of the spinal cord result in the relaxation of the external sphincter and other perineal muscles, the continued relaxation of the internal sphincter, further contraction of the rectal and sigmoid muscles, and finally the evacuation of the feces. Defecation is assisted by increasing intraabdominal pressure through Valsalva's maneuver and contraction of abdominal muscles.

SPLANCHNIC BLOOD FLOW

The motor activity, secretory activity, and blood flow of the digestive system generally vary together. Thus eating also increases the splanchnic blood flow such that it constitutes a larger percentage of an enhanced cardiac output. The enhanced perfusion of the digestive organs is essential to provide the water and electrolytes necessary for secretion, to provide the nutrients and oxygen to support the increased metabolic activity and work of the cells involved, and to transport the absorbed nutrients from the intestine into the portal and systemic circulation. The control of the splanchnic circulation and local perfusion is not clearly defined but is influenced by intrinsic neural, hormonal, and metabolic factors as well as by the extrinsic autonomic nervous system and humoral agents. The increased cardiac output associated with eating results sometimes in postprandial angina pectoris in patients with coronary artery disease. The increased oxygen required by the activated gut during and following a meal has been considered responsible for the postprandial abdominal pain (intestinal angina) occasionally experienced by patients with intestinal vascular disease and thought to be caused by intestinal ischemia.

BIBLIOGRAPHY

Fawcett D: Textbook of histology, ed 11, Philadelphia, 1986, WB Saunders Co.

Johnson L: The physiology of the gastrointestinal tract, ed 3, New York, 1987, Raven Press.

Rubin W: The epithelial "membrane" of the small intestine, Am J Clin Nutr 24:45, 1971.

Rubin W and others: The normal human gastric epithelia: a fine structural study, Lab Invest 19:598, 1968.

170 · MANIFESTATIONS OF DISORDERS OF THE DIGESTIVE SYSTEM

Walter Rubin

NATURE AND SYMPTOMS OF DIGESTIVE DISORDERS AND APPROACH TO EVALUATING PATIENTS

Disorders of the digestive system are among those most commonly encountered in clinical medicine. They produce a multitude of symptoms, including pain and discomfort, alterations in bowel habit such as with diarrhea and constipation, nausea, vomiting, abdominal distention, dysphagia, hemorrhage, anemia, gaseousness, edema, jaundice, alterations in mental status, arthritis and arthralgias, rashes, visual disturbances, and constitutional symptoms such as fever, malaise, weakness, anorexia, and weight loss. Digestive system disorders are associated with a variety of etiologic agents and pathologic alterations: infections with viruses, bacteria, and parasites; toxins such as alcohol and lead; many drugs (most prescribed drugs may produce gastrointestinal symptoms); benign and malignant neoplasms; acute, chronic, and granulomatous inflammatory processes; acute and chronic ulcerations; primary neurologic, muscular, or vascular disorders; connective tissue diseases; congenital and acquired enzyme deficiencies; and allergic and immunologic disorders.

However, in many patients—probably more than half of those with chronic or recurrent symptoms—the symptoms are not associated with any identifiable cause, pathology, or overt pathophysiologic process. The disorders of such patients have been labeled "functional bowel disease," "irritable bowel syndrome," "functional dyspepsia," and other similar names; that is, these have been considered psychosomatic disorders whose symptoms are the somatic results of life's stresses. Such disorders are better considered as having an unknown cause or probably many causes, some of which may be related at least in part to emotional factors. For example, many patients with chronic cramps and diarrhea whose conditions were diagnosed a few years ago as irritable bowel syndrome today are recognized as having a lactase deficiency and lactose intolerance. This condition has been appreciated for only about 20 years and is easily treated if correctly diagnosed. In addition to common gastrointestinal symptoms without recognizable causes, symptoms associated with recognized pathologic processes often are not clearly understood; for example, the pain or discomfort produced by peptic ulcers and gastroesophageal reflux. Finally, the causes of many pathologic processes involving the digestive system such as peptic ulcer disease, ulcerative colitis, and granulomatous ileocolitis still are unknown or not well understood.

When evaluating patients with gastrointestinal disorders, as with many other diseases, a careful history and physical examination are essential. Many digestive disorders can be tentatively diagnosed, or at least the diagnostic possibilities can be greatly narrowed, by means of a good history in itself. The physician must have a clear picture of the patient's symptoms: their nature, characteristics, location, onset, duration, and temporal relationships; their relationships to body postures, movements, functions, and stresses; and their associated symptoms and systemic manifestations such as fever, malaise, anorexia, and weight loss. Are the symptoms acute or chronic, persistent or intermittent, progressive or remittent? How are they elicited and how are they relieved? When do they occur? Do they wake the patient at night? How are they affected by eating, belching, defecating, and passing flatus and by body postures, movements, and respirations? Because eating stimulates the digestive system into action—the gut to increase its motor activity, the gallbladder to contract, the stomach and pancreas to secrete, and the splanchnic circulation to increase—symptoms resulting from gastrointestinal disorders often are precipitated or enhanced by eating. Are the symptoms affected by particular foods? What drugs is the patient receiving? Is there a family history of the same or similar symptoms or related diseases? The complete physical examination should include careful abdominal, rectal, and, with most females, pelvic examinations. A careful search should be made for direct and rebound abdominal tenderness, spasm, masses, organomegaly, hernias, distention, ascites, abnormal bowel sounds, and bruits, and any findings should be carefully characterized.

The symptoms and physical signs associated with specific diseases are discussed at length in the following chapters describing specific disorders of the digestive system. This chapter, however, briefly discusses a few of the common manifestations of digestive disorders such as pain, diarrhea, constipation, nausea and vomiting, gastrointestinal bleeding, protein-losing enteropathy, gaseousness, dysphagia, and distention, and some of the common systemic manifestations such as fever, anorexia, satiety, weight loss, rash, and arthralgia.

PAIN

Pain and various kinds of discomfort are common symptoms of disorders of the digestive system. The sensory fibers to the abdominal viscera are carried with the sympathetic (first thoracic to second lumbar) and parasympathetic nerves. The mechanisms by which the abdominal viscera generate pain are not fully understood. Stretching of the hepatic or splenic capsules, distention or tension of the gut wall smooth muscle, and traction on the mesenteric attachment each stimulate sensory fibers and produce pain. The discomfort produced by peptic ulcers and peptic esophagitis, however, is not well understood, because the mucosa of most of the gut is anesthetic. Such tissue can be removed in a biopsy, for example, without causing discomfort to the patient. Perhaps the pain generated by mucosal ulcerations or inflammations is produced by associated muscle tensions or spasms, its threshold having been lowered by the inflammation. However, the quality of pain produced by esophageal spasm (often a severe, angina-like pain) usually is distinctly different from that produced by reflux esophagitis (often a burning or gnawing pain). Visceral pain tends to be deep, not clearly localized, central or bilateral, and aching, dull, burning, or vague in quality, often producing more suffering or discomfort than actual sharp pain. In contrast, somatic (parietal) pain such as that produced by inflammation or irritation of the parietal peritoneum usually is well localized, lateral, sharp, and discrete. Visceral pain usually is referred to the somatic dermatomes corresponding to the spinal levels from which its sensory fibers emanate. As mentioned, however, it may not be clearly localized and often includes a few spinal segments about and/or below the level from which its major innervation originates. Thus pain arising from the esophagus usually is referred to the chest; stomach, duodenal, biliary, and pancreatic pain to the upper abdomen above the umbilicus; pain in the small intestine to the periumbilical area; and colonic pain to the lower abdomen. Pain arising from the central portions of the diaphragm usually is referred to the ipsilateral shoulder. Severe pain, especially when associated with acute inflammation of the parietal peritoneum, commonly leads to a reflex spasm of the musculature innervated by the same spinal segments; this is the involuntary abdominal spasm or guarding that should be carefully sought in the physical examination.

As discussed previously, a careful history often reveals the probable cause of discomfort or at least restricts the likely causes. The following descriptions of classic symptoms associated with some common gastrointestinal disorders demonstrate the value of the history in establishing or suggesting the nature of these disorders.

Heartburn (pyrosis) resulting from gastroesophageal reflux usually is perceived as a recurrent retrosternal or high epigastric burning, gnawing, or heaviness and is usually brought on by eating or recumbency, is accompanied by the regurgitation of sour juice (gastric acid) or a sour taste, and is relieved by antacids. Odynophagia, or retrosternal discomfort occurring when food is swallowed, usually suggests inflammation (esophagitis) or occasionally neoplasia of the esophagus. The diagnosis of esophageal spasm is suggested by severe, persistent, retrosternal pain that often recurs and frequently mimics the pain of myocardial infarction, sometimes even radiating to the neck and arms and often relieved by nitroglycerin; esophageal spasm also is associated with dysphagia with both liquids and solids. The more serious disorders such as myocardial infarction, coronary insufficiency, dissecting aneurysm, and perhaps pulmonary embolus should be excluded from the diagnosis.

Peptic ulcer disease classically produces an epigastric burning, aching, or gnawing discomfort recurring 1 or more hours after eating or during sleep and relieved immediately by eating or ingesting an antacid; the pain occurs in the presence of unbuffered gastric acid and is relieved by its neutralization.

Gallbladder disease, usually cholelithiasis in which a gallstone obstructs the cystic duct, is suggested by recurrent attacks of persistent epigastric or right upper quadrant pain that sometimes radiates to the tip of the right scapula, is often promoted by eating, commonly lasts ½ to 2 hours, and frequently is associated with nausea and belching. Choledocholithiasis, the presence of a stone in the common duct, may cause similar symptoms although it may also cause left upper quadrant or left chest pain. If the pain persists, especially if it is associated with fever and tenderness in the right upper quadrant, the probable diagnosis is acute cholecystitis.

Persistent upper abdominal or periumbilical pain that is usually severe and lasts many hours, that often radiates straight through to the back and is commonly relieved by bending forward (jackknifing or assuming a fetal position), and that commonly is accompanied by nausea and vomiting suggests acute pancreatitis, especially in an alcoholic patient. Similar symptoms can be produced by a posterior penetrating ulcer. If this type of pain arises and persists in an otherwise healthy middle-aged or older person, especially if it is associated with weight loss, a diagnosis of pancreatic carcinoma is likely.

Pain associated with biliary tract disease as described previously has been called biliary colic. The terms "colic" and "colicky pain" generally have been used in two senses. When used to describe pain associated with biliary tract disease or with the passage of a kidney-ureteral stone (renal colic), these terms generally refer to a severe persistent discomfort during which the patient can find no comfortable position or relief and usually keeps moving around attempting to escape the pain. Renal colic usually is a severe, persistent pain in the lumbar area or flank that often radiates into the groin, testis, or penis and is commonly accompanied by nausea and vomiting. The second and more accurate usage of the term refers to a rhythmic recurring pain, each recurrence usually starting mildly and increasing in severity to be followed by an interval of little or no discomfort. Such pain, like that occurring during labor, is characteristic of a hollow muscular viscus contracting recurrently against an obstruction. This colicky abdominal pain is characteristic of an intestinal obstruction, especially an early obstruction before any strangulation or embarrassment of the intestinal circulation has occurred. It usually is associated with abdominal distention, audible borborygmi, nausea and vomiting, and the inability to pass feces or gas. Milder and more common forms of this type of colicky pain are commonly called cramps.

In contrast to the restlessness of the patient with renal colic, when the parietal peritoneum is inflamed or irritated in acute peritonitis, the patient lies perfectly still, because any movement of the peritoneum results in extreme aggravation of the pain. The physician need only tap the side of the bed lightly or percuss or palpate the abdomen gently to elicit marked superficial or rebound tenderness. The acute, catastrophic onset of abdominal pain followed by peritonitis suggests the perforation of a viscus, such as a peptic ulcer; a similar but somewhat less acute pain in an older patient with vascular disease might suggest a vascular catastrophe such as an embolus or acute occlusion of the superior mesenteric artery.

Upper abdominal discomfort that is subsequently localized in the right lower quadrant and is accompanied by focal superficial and rebound tenderness (focal peritoneal signs) and fever is of course classically symptomatic of acute appendicitis. Similar symptoms and signs in the left lower quadrant in an older person suggest diverticulitis, but similar symptoms and signs can be produced by other disorders such as a twisted ovarian cyst or mittelschmerz in a younger woman. Therefore a careful rectal and pelvic examination is needed in addition to a full history and routine physical examination.

An acutely swollen liver such as may be produced by congestive failure, hepatitis, alcoholic hepatitis, metastatic cancer, and fatty infiltration commonly produces persistent upper abdominal pain that often is more pronounced on the right side and sometimes is worsened by body movements and even respirations; the detection of a large, tender liver during the physical examination reveals the origin of the pain.

Abnormalities of the abdominal wall such as hernias may cause recurrent or persistent (as with an incarcerated or strangulated hernia, abdominal wall hematoma, or myositis) abdominal pain that is often intensified by movement and straining and by contracting the abdominal musculature. The cause of this pain is confirmed by eliciting focal tenderness in the abdominal wall that is increased when the supine patient lifts his head and thereby contracts his rectus sheath and, when applicable, by demonstrating a hernia at the site of tenderness.

Abdominal pains of primary *neural* origins sometimes pose diagnostic problems. Pain of *radicular* origin often is sharp and shooting, usually is worsened by movements of the spine or by coughing, sneezing, and straining, and often is accompanied by tenderness over the spine. Tabes dorsalis and diabetic neuropathy can lead to severe, recurrent, puzzling pains. Pain resulting from herpes zoster usually is diagnosed by its dermatomic distribution and classic skin lesions, but when it occurs without a rash or after a rash has been forgotten, it can be puzzling. The recurrent pains of porphyria usually are severe, persistent, deep, visceral-like pains that mimic acute visceral disease such as gallbladder disease.

Acute severe abdominal pain accompanied by minimal physical findings suggests an ischemic episode to the gut resulting from a vascular catastrophe or strangulation of a portion of the gut caused by an internal hernia or twisting of a loop of gut or vascular pedicle. Puzzling recurrent postprandial periumbilical pain that sometimes is associated with diarrhea, especially in an older person with vascular disease, suggests a more insidious chronic vascular insufficiency, the rare intestinal angina.

Chronic recurrent abdominal pain, commonly in a young or middle-aged woman who previously has consulted many physicians and has undergone many studies with negative results and who may have undergone an operation such as cholecystectomy or the lysis of adhesions, suggests functional bowel disease. This pain often is associated with other gastrointestinal symptoms such as constipation or less commonly diarrhea; sometimes alternating constipation and diarrhea; gaseousness with eructations, borborygmi, or flatulence; nausea; and abdominal distention. The pain usually is worsened by eating and is relieved somewhat by a bowel movement, belching, or passing flatus. These symptoms rarely interrupt a sound sleep. The symptoms often are promoted or aggravated by periods of emotional stress, and the patient often exhibits other neurotic symptoms. Evidence of depression should be carefully sought in the history of patients suspected of having functional symptoms; constipation often is associated with depression. If the history suggests that abdominal cramps often accompanied by diarrhea, flatulence, and distention are produced by the ingestion of milk, ice cream, and other dairy products, a diagnosis of lactase deficiency and lactose intolerance is suggested.

The onset of abdominal pain in previously healthy middle-aged and elderly patients should be treated with great respect. The onset of functional symptoms in these patients is not common in the absence of depression. An organic cause of the pain should be suspected and sought, with due concern for the high incidence of malignancy in these circumstances. The physician should elicit a complete drug history from all patients, because drugs are common causes of gastrointestinal disturbances, including pain.

Finally, it should be remembered that referred abdominal pain may be produced by disease affecting other organ systems: the lungs, heart, and genitourinary tract. Thus pneumonia, pulmonary infarction, and myocardial infarction occasionally produce pain in the upper abdomen and sometimes, surprisingly, even tenderness. The careful history, physical examination, and laboratory tests usually reveal the correct cause of the pain. Pain arising in the pelvis, such as that produced by pelvic inflammatory disease, or in the bladder, such as that produced by acute urinary retention, commonly is perceived in the lower abdomen. Pain originating in the kidney, such as with acute pyelonephritis, commonly is felt in the lumbar and flank region but also may be perceived more anteriorly in the abdomen.

DIARRHEA

Acute diarrhea and chronic diarrhea are common manifestations of gastrointestinal disorders. When a patient complains of diarrhea, the physician should elicit a careful history to determine exactly what the patient means, including the number of bowel movements each day; whether they wake the patient at night; the patient's usual bowel habits; whether the symptoms are acute, recurrent, or chronic; the presence of associated symptoms; and a clear description of the character of the stools, including their approximate volume and consistency and whether they contain blood, mucus, pus, or fat. An estimate of the daily volume of stool may be helpful; an accurate weight should be obtained in cases of chronic diarrhea of puzzling cause. Diarrhea to one patient may mean passing a single somewhat soft or mushy stool each day, whereas to another it may mean the "runs," sitting on the toilet often and passing numerous large volumes of water.

The normal bowel habit varies tremendously among individuals. Most people comfortably pass about one formed stool each day, whereas others may pass two or three, and still others may defecate only every 2, 3, or 4 days. As discussed in Chapter 169, the average person puts out approximately 100 to 200 g of stool each day, about 70% of which is water. Diarrhea, defined as the passage of more than 300 g of stool each day, may result from a disorder of either the small or large bowel, owing to an impairment of absorption or secretion in either.

The normal ileal effluent introduced into the colon is approximately 1 to 1.5 L each day. If it exceeds approximately 2 to 3 L, diarrhea ensues. Excessive ileal effluent may result from a disease of malabsorption, an inflammatory disease of the small intestine, or excessive secretion in the small intestine, which commonly is produced by a number of toxins, hormones, and other humoral substances, some of which seem to act by stimulating adenylate cyclase and elevating epithelial cyclic adenosine monophosphate (AMP) levels. Among such agents are numerous bacterial toxins such as cholera toxin and those of toxigenic *Escherichia coli;* certain prostaglandins as may be produced by medullary carcinomas of the thyroid; and vasoactive intestinal polypeptide and possibly gastrin, hormones produced in excessive amounts by some non-β islet cell tumors of the pancreas.

Several factors can impair the colon's net absorption of water and its ability to form solid stool: a reduced colonic mucosa from previous surgery, a diseased mucosa from inflammatory disease, and a rapid transit through the colon caused by enhanced motor activity, especially peristaltic activity. In addition, increased fatty acids in the colon, particularly the hydroxylated acids, resulting from a malabsorption syndrome, or excessive bile salts in the colon resulting from ileal resection or disease reduce the net absorption of salt and water and cause diarrhea. Osmotic diarrhea may be produced by the presence in colonic chyme of increased amounts of nonabsorbable, soluble, osmotically active substances such as salt cathartics or the bacterial metabolites of the unabsorbed lactose ingested by patients with lactase deficiency. A villous adenoma, a tumor that often secretes much water, mucus, and potassium, occasionally causes diarrhea, especially in older individuals. The presence of increased nondigestible and nonabsorbable hydrophilic roughage and fiber in the diet (as is found in the normal diets of many nonwesternized societies such as in rural Africa) results in the passage of more stool and water each day. Thus a fecal output normal in many parts of the world would be considered diarrhea in Americans.

Diarrhea caused by dietary factors, as is the case with diseases of malabsorption and with the osmotic diarrhea produced by lactose in patients with lactase deficiency, may be eliminated or markedly reduced by fasting. In contrast, a secretory diarrhea caused by a bacterial enterotoxin or hormone usually is affected little by fasting. A choloretic diarrhea produced by excessive bile salts in the colon also tends to improve with fasting, because most of the bile salts are then retained in the unstimulated gallbladder.

Acute diarrhea is extremely common. When it occurs in otherwise healthy individuals who are not under stress or taking some recently initiated medication, it most often is produced by infectious agents. Most of these agents formerly were thought to be viruses, because routine stool cultures generally were negative, but with improved culture techniques and recognition of more bacterial pathogens, bacteria now are known to be more common causes. Bacteria cause diarrhea either by producing enterotoxins that cause secretory diarrhea or by directly invading the mucosa, predominantly in the distal ileum and colon, or by both mechanisms. Organisms that predominantly invade and ulcerate the mucosa, such as *Shigella* organisms, often produce a dysentery-like symptomatology, including fever, constitutional symptoms, and blood and pus (leukocytes) in the stools. In contrast, the enterotoxin forms of diarrhea such as those produced by cholera and staphylococcal enterotoxin usually are associated with little fever and few constitutional symptoms. *Clostridium perfringens* and *Bacillus cereus* are predominantly enterotoxin producers, whereas *Yersinia enterocolitica, Vibrio parahaemolyticus,* and *Campylobacter* organisms are predominantly invaders. Many bacteria can both invade and produce toxins, their relative abilities varying among strains. Most cases of *E. coli* diarrhea in the United States and those contracted by American tourists in Mexico are produced by predominantly toxigenic strains, but

some cases are caused by strains that mainly invade. Even some strains of *Shigella,* the classic invader, produce toxins. Although *Salmonella* strains may produce toxins, they predominantly invade; these usually affect the distal small bowel, rarely ulcerating the mucosa, and thus they do not usually produce the ulcerative dysenteric picture commonly produced by *Shigella* organisms (see discussion of "Shigellosis" in Chapter 41). *Clostridium difficile,* the usual cause of the pseudomembranous colitis that may follow antibiotic therapy, also produces toxin and inflammatory changes of the colonic mucosa.

Acute diarrheas also may be produced by protozoan parasites, especially by *Giardia lamblia* and *Entamoeba histolytica.* The incidence of parasitic diarrheas varies, of course, among populations and geographic areas.

Patients with acquired immunodeficiency syndrome (AIDS), who frequently suffer from both acute and chronic diarrhea, often have gastrointestinal infections, not only with the common pathogens but also unusual ones such as cytomegalovirus and the protozoa *Cryptosporidium* and *Isospora.*

A careful history should be elicited from the patient with acute diarrhea, not only for clues to possible noninfectious causes but also to determine whether other close associates are similarly affected and thus whether a common food or water source can be implicated as the cause. Acute diarrhea, especially in children, often is seen when an intestinal disease, presumably caused by a virus, is known to be prevalent.

Most cases of acute diarrhea are self-limited, usually last from 1 to a few days, and often are accompanied by variable other symptoms such as abdominal cramps, nausea, vomiting, anorexia, fever, myalgia, and headache. These cases often are viral. The physician probably should perform few diagnostic tests, especially if the case is mild, there is no blood in the stool, and the patient looks well. If the patient does not look well, however, and has profound diarrhea, dehydration, prominent constitutional symptoms, bloody stools, or the symptoms of dysentery, proctoscopy should be performed and the stools should be examined for blood, leukocytes, and parasites and should be cultured. Most patients should be treated supportively with fluids, electrolytes, restricted activity, and probably an antidiarrheal agent such as an opiate or diphenoxylate. However, some recent studies have suggested that infectious diarrhea resulting from bacterial agents such as *Shigella* organisms may be worsened by antiperistaltic agents, presumably because they retard intestinal elimination of the organisms. Fluids and electrolytes usually can be replaced orally, possibly with the addition of glucose or sucrose to salt solutions for secretory diarrhea. This replacement should be performed parenterally if patients are markedly depleted or cannot take oral medications.

Whereas acute diarrhea usually is self-limited and requires little diagnostic effort, chronic diarrhea must be evaluated more aggressively to establish an accurate diagnosis and to institute proper therapy. Again a complete, careful history and physical examination and routine laboratory tests are essential to discover evidence of inflammatory bowel disease, a malabsorption syndrome, an endocrine disturbance, and previous illnesses or surgical procedures that might be relevant. The history should include any travel by the patient, fever, abdominal pain, tenesmus, rectal urgency, distention, blood or fat in the stools, nausea, vomiting, anorexia, weight loss, anemia, rashes, allergies, arthralgias, arthritis, and eye symptoms. All medications should be stopped, if possible. The workup of such patients usually should include examination of the stool for blood, leukocytes, eosinophils, mucus, fat, and ova and parasites, especially *Giardia* organisms and *E. histolytica* but also others such as *Strongyloides* and *Schistosoma* organisms. The stool should be cultured, although bacteria are not expected to be the cause of chronic diarrhea. The patient usually should undergo proctosigmoidoscopy, a rectal biopsy in most cases, a barium enema examination, and a gastrointestinal and small bowel series.

If the diagnosis is still unclear, the presence of steatorrhea, indicating a disease of malabsorption, should be sought by a quantitative determination of fecal fat. If a malabsorption syndrome is present, the specific disease should be diagnosed as outlined in Chapter 174. Lactase deficiency as a possible cause of the patient's diarrhea can be determined by performing a lactose tolerance test and/or by assessing the response to a lactose-free diet. The presence of a functioning carcinoid tumor as the cause of the diarrhea can usually be detected by means of a urinary 5-OH-indole acetic acid (5-HIAA) determination. The possible existence of other endocrine abnormalities such as hyperthyroidism and adrenal insufficiency should be determined by additional appropriate tests.

The history, physical examination, routine laboratory tests, elimination of medications, and other diagnostic tests and procedures suggested usually should detect or strongly suggest the cause of the patient's chronic diarrhea. They should reveal or suggest the presence of most cases of ulcerative colitis; granulomatous ileocolitis; diverticulitis; other, rarer intestinal inflammatory diseases such as tuberculosis, fungal infections, some cases of eosinophilic gastroenteritis, and amyloidosis; villous adenomas, lymphomas, carcinoid tumors, and other intestinal tumors; diseases causing the malabsorption syndrome; choleretic diarrhea; partial intestinal obstruction; fecal impaction with overflow diarrhea; parasitic diseases; lactase deficiency; drug-induced diarrhea, including pseudomembranous enterocolitis (usually acute); endocrinopathies such as hyperthyroidism, adrenal insufficiency, and hypoparathyroidism; uremic colitis; and pellagra. A diagnosis of ischemic bowel disease or ischemic colitis usually is suggested by the presence of "thumbprinting" or other roentgenographic intestinal changes and often by fecal blood, usually in an older person with vascular disease, congestive failure, and often abdominal bruits. The diabetic patient with diarrhea resulting from a visceral neuropathy also usually exhibits peripheral neuropathic signs and other evidence of a visceral neuropathy such as postural hypotension. Diabetic patients also have malabsorption resulting from bacterial overgrowth or celiac disease, which has a higher incidence in diabetes. A diagnosis of functional bowel disease is suggested by a history of chronic diarrhea in an otherwise healthy young or middle-aged patient (usually a woman) when tests are negative, other neurotic manifestations are present, and stress frequently aggravates the symptoms.

If the diagnosis still is uncertain, especially in patients who do not seem to have a functional disorder, the search should be continued and additional tests should be performed. The daily fecal weight should be measured to determine whether the diarrhea is of large or small volume; large volumes suggest a secretory diarrhea. The fecal Na^+, K^+, and osmolality concentrations should be determined to detect the presence of a significant quantity of unidentified osmotically active substances, indicating an osmotic diarrhea. The normal stool usually is moderately hyperosmolar, averaging 375 mOsm, because of the presence of organic substances produced by colonic bacteria. The effects of fasting on the fecal output can be assessed, as noted previously, to help determine the nature of the diarrhea. Surreptitious diarrhea resulting from the inges-

tion of laxatives should be suspected in puzzling cases, especially in patients exhibiting neurotic or psychotic symptoms. Alkalinization of the stool can reveal the presence of phenolphthalein by its red color, and the presence of melanosis coli on proctosigmoidoscopy suggests the use of anthraquinone laxatives. Melanosis coli is a benign, brown-black discoloration of the colonic mucosa that results from the presence of pigment-laden macrophages in the lamina propria. The pigmentation is associated with constipation and the habitual use of anthraquinone laxatives and may disappear when the laxatives are discontinued.

If the cause still is not evident, more unusual types of endocrine abnormalities that cause secretory diarrhea should be considered. Watery diarrhea syndrome (pancreatic cholera), often caused by a tumor that secretes vasoactive intestinal polypeptide (VIP) (vipoma) in the pancreas and occasionally in neural or other organs, is suggested by secretory diarrhea usually associated with hypokalemia and gastric hypochlorhydria (hyposecretion). Serum VIP levels can be determined by an immunoassay at certain medical centers. Serum gastrin levels should be determined to detect a *gastrinoma*, because about 10% of such tumors initially are associated with diarrhea rather than with the more classic manifestations of the Zollinger-Ellison syndrome. Serum calcitonin levels should also be determined to detect the presence of a medullary carcinoma of the thyroid. Abnormal prostaglandin secretion has been implicated as the cause of diarrhea in cases of medullary thyroid carcinoma and in other cases of obscure, puzzling secretory diarrhea. Immunoassays of serum prostaglandins should become increasingly available in the future. If prostaglandins are suspected of being the cause of a puzzling case of secretory diarrhea, the effects of inhibiting prostaglandin synthesis with indomethacin or some other agent can be determined.

Food allergies may be the cause of puzzling diarrhea, commonly in children but occasionally also in adults. This diarrhea often is accompanied by abdominal pain and other gastrointestinal symptoms. These patients often have a family history of allergy, exhibit eosinophilia and elevated IgE levels, and also have allergic reactions of other organs, such as hives, eczema, rhinitis, and asthma, that may be initiated by the same dietary antigen. About 20% of patients with eosinophilic gastroenteritis are found to have an allergy to a dietary antigen and improve after it is eliminated. This poorly defined syndrome, which often produces diarrhea, is characterized by inflammation of portions of the gut, predominantly with eosinophils, and usually is accompanied by peripheral eosinophilia and often fever. When the mucosa is predominantly involved, diarrhea and varying degrees of malabsorption, protein-losing enteropathy, and occult or gross blood loss are the usual manifestations. Predominant involvement of the tunica muscularis, especially of the stomach and upper intestine, often results in obstructive symptoms. Involvement of the serosa and peritoneum can lead to ascites. The gastrointestinal series may reveal no apparent abnormality or may show changes suggestive of Crohn's disease, a malabsorption syndrome, or a focal tumor or nodules. When a food allergy is suspected as the cause of diarrhea, skin testing may be of some help, but usually the elimination of milk and other dietary proteins must be empirically assessed.

The proper treatment of patients with diarrhea depends on establishing an accurate diagnosis of the specific disorder. The following chapters describe in greater detail the diseases that cause diarrhea and their pathology, clinical manifestations, physical and laboratory abnormalities, method of diagnosis, and specific therapy. General supportive therapy of these patients should include assessment of water, electrolyte, and nutritional losses and deficiencies and their repletion. General supportive therapy for mild diarrheas that are not controlled by a specific therapy also has included agents such as opiates and anticholinergics that inhibit gut motility and sometimes also hydrophilic bulk agents such as psyllium seed preparations that absorb water and harden the stools.

CONSTIPATION

Constipation, both actual and perceived, is a common gastrointestinal complaint. It is a cause of chronic discomfort and concern and a major focus of attention of thousands of people, especially those in middle and old age. As discussed previously, the normal bowel habit varies tremendously among individuals; some apparently normal, asymptomatic people evacuate only once every 2 or 3 days or even less frequently without any appreciable difficulty. True constipation should therefore be judged not solely by the frequency of evacuation but by the character of the feces and evacuation. If the stools are so dehydrated and hard that evacuation is difficult or painful or cannot be attained without mechanical or therapeutic assistance, the person can be said to be constipated. Constipation may cause abdominal pain and cramps and even intestinal obstruction as a result of fecal impaction. Many constipated individuals complain of sluggishness, dullness, weakness, malaise, fatigue, anorexia, and headaches. The extent to which such symptoms are functional in nature or are caused, perhaps in part, by the constipation is unclear. By metabolizing feces, colonic bacteria produce "toxins" such as ammonia and short-chain fatty acids that can dull the sensorium and impair the intellect. These toxins are normally drained, however, into the portal circulation and to the liver, where they are metabolized. Only with liver disease, when this metabolism is impaired or when the toxins are shunted from the portal circulation to the systemic circulation, are sufficient quantities of these substances thought to reach the systemic circulation and central nervous system to produce appreciable effects such as hepatic encephalopathy, which clearly is promoted or aggravated by constipation, presumably because of the increased toxin production. Whether constipation can affect the brain of an otherwise normal person has not been established.

Because of the marked variability of the normal stooling habit and the uncertainty of symptoms attributed to constipation, it often is difficult for a physician to decide whether an individual truly is constipated and should be treated. One asymptomatic young woman, for example, always defecated with firm but not hard or voluminous stools, once every 2 weeks without difficulty. Her workup, including a rectal examination, proctosigmoidoscopy, barium enema, and thyroid studies, was normal. It was not clear if she was constipated or if she should have been treated to promote more frequent evacuations. In contrast, many patients, often middle-aged or older women, feel sluggish, weak, and dull or have headaches unless they have at least one complete movement each day. These patients often believe they cannot completely evacuate their stool. Regardless of whether these individuals have ever been truly constipated, they often have become so habituated to the use of laxatives, suppositories, or enemas that it has become almost impossible for them to defecate satisfactorily without assistance.

Most cases of chronic constipation are thought to be functional in nature and thus have been given names such as spastic colon, spastic colitis, functional constipation, and functional bowel syndrome. The pathogenesis of functional constipation is unclear. Perhaps some of these patients had so successfully learned to suppress their defecation reflex at the time of rigorous toilet training that at times of rectal distention they no longer recognize the urge to defecate and unconsciously inhibit the reflex. Some of these patients have alternating periods of constipation and diarrhea. Patients with functional constipation often pass small, hard fecal pellets similar to those produced by rabbits. Many of these patients are bothered most by abdominal cramps and pain. Studies in recent years have demonstrated that patients with chronic constipation and pain often exhibit abnormal, severe contractions or spasms of their sigmoid colons that cause the pain. Some of these patients have learned to control these spastic contractions through operative conditioning and thereby have been relieved of their pain. The abnormal sigmoid contractions observed in these patients are similar to those associated with colonic diverticulosis, and it is now thought that these patients, because of the abnormal colonic pressures, are prone to diverticulosis.

Almost everyone has become acutely constipated at some time, an experience often promoted by travel and being away from familiar bathrooms, diet, and habits, by an intercurrent illness, by hospitalization, by a period of unaccustomed inactivity, by some unusual emotional stress, by a medication, by the development of a perianal condition that makes defecation painful, or by an injury or illness that impedes Valsalva's maneuver and the ability to increase intraabdominal pressure and thereby defecate. Most of these experiences last only a short time and the cause of the constipation usually is evident; the individual usually requires little more than a mild laxative to prevent fecal impaction. Some cases of acute constipation or obstipation are of course more serious, such as an intestinal obstruction or an ileus resulting from a severe acute illness, but the primary underlying disorders in these instances usually are readily recognizable.

If constipation of recent onset persists, however, or if a patient with chronic constipation has never been fully evaluated, a more thorough investigation is warranted to determine the cause of constipation. Most patients should receive a complete history and physical examination, including careful neurologic, rectal, and pelvic examinations; the usual laboratory tests; and proctoscopy, a barium enema, and usually a gastrointestinal and small bowel series. What cause is considered most likely for the altered bowel habit depends largely on the age of the patient and clinical setting. Causes that should be considered include medications; inactivity; an emotional disorder, especially an inapparent depression; a metabolic disorder such as hypothyroidism, hypercalcemia, or in rare cases porphyria or lead poisoning; a mechanical obstruction, especially a rectal or colonic carcinoma in a middle-aged or older person; diverticulitis; an ileus or an intestinal pseudoobstruction such as a motor abnormality of the gut, usually resulting from a disease involving the nerves or muscle, such as scleroderma; megacolon; a neurologic or muscular disorder that impairs the ability to perform Valsalva's maneuver successfully and to defecate; and laxative abuse that may impair a person's ability to defecate normally, perhaps by damaging the enteric nerves of the bowel and its motility. The habitual use of irritant laxatives may in fact also alter the roentgenographic appearance of the colon, producing the so-called cathartic colon which shows a loss of haustra and an effacement of the mucosal pattern, especially on the right side, and occasionally even a megacolon. These roentgenographic features may erroneously suggest the presence of ulcerative or granulomatous colitis or other diseases.

In most cases of chronic constipation no correctable underlying cause can be identified. In the management of these patients the physician's goal is to promote a regular, comfortable bowel habit with minimal concern, effort, and laxative assistance, to divert the patient's attention and energies to more important and enjoyable matters, and to promote the patient's emotional and psychologic well-being. A caring, devoted physician should lend sympathetic support. Serious emotional or psychologic problems such as depression should be identified and treated, with the aid of a psychiatrist if necessary. The patient should be encouraged to exercise regularly, to maintain good hydration with a liberal fluid intake, and to increase the fiber and roughage of his diet. He should be encouraged to eat vegetables and fruits, including prunes, figs, and prune juice. Bran and/or a hydrophilic bulk laxative such as a psyllium seed preparation should be added to the diet. The patient should be taught about the defecation reflex in terms he can understand. He should be encouraged to sit relaxed in a comfortable familiar bathroom with pleasant reading material one to three times each day at the same time and after the same meal(s). If additional therapy is necessary, the smallest necessary amount of the mildest laxatives should be used.

NAUSEA AND VOMITING

Nausea and vomiting often are manifestations of gastrointestinal disorders but also commonly result from diseases of other organs. A vomiting center located in the medulla oblongata is responsible for the integrated act of vomiting. Outflow from this center causes a sensation of nausea, a spasm of the duodenum and gastric antrum, relaxation of the body and fundus of the stomach and the lower esophageal sphincter, and forceful contractions of the abdominal muscles and diaphragm that force the gastric contents into the esophagus. Slow deep inspirations with a partially closed glottis reduce intrathoracic pressure and promote the reflux of the gastric contents into the esophagus, which are then swept back into the stomach by secondary peristalsis. Repetition of this process constitutes retching. Vomiting ensues when strong contractions of the abdominal muscles force the diaphragm up, the intrathoracic pressure increases, the upper esophageal sphincter opens, and the esophageal contents are propelled out the mouth. Vomiting commonly is accompanied by autonomic manifestations such as salivation, sweating, pallor, and tachypnea. The vomiting center receives afferent impulses from many areas including the cortex, the eighth nerve (labyrinth mechanism), abdominal and other viscera, and a chemoreceptor trigger zone nearby in the medulla that may be stimulated by substances in the circulation, for example, drugs such as apomorphine. Thus nausea and vomiting may be initiated by stimuli from all over the body, including the cortex (with willful vomiting), the labyrinth (as in motion sickness, labyrinthitis, and Meniere's disease), and a host of chemical and metabolic irritants. Nausea and vomiting may accompany many acute illnesses of many organ systems such as myocardial infarction, pyelonephritis, and meningitis. Nausea and vomiting also commonly accompany many acute illnesses of the digestive system such as gastroenteritis, appendicitis, pancreatitis, cholecystitis, peritonitis, and viral and alcoholic hepatitis.

A number of patients have acute, subacute, recurrent, or chronic nausea and vomiting without such obvious associated acute illnesses. The possibility of pregnancy, a common cause of nausea and vomiting in susceptible patients, should be excluded before any roentgenographic studies are performed. Drug toxicity, metabolic disorders such as uremia or hypercalcemia, and increased intracranial pressure also must be considered and eliminated as possible causes.

Abnormalities of the digestive system, especially obstructing lesions, are in such patients common causes of nausea and vomiting and also regurgitation, which may be mistaken for vomiting but which is usually unaccompanied by nausea, abdominal contractions, and associated autonomic symptoms. A careful description of the vomitus or regurgitated material may reveal something about the nature and location of the disorder. If the vomitus contains bile—if it is yellow and tastes bitter—then an obstructing lesion of the esophagus, stomach, or duodenal bulb is unlikely. If the material contains acid—tastes sour—then an obstructing lesion of the esophagus is unlikely. Identifiable food that is regurgitated probably comes from either the esophagus or stomach; if it is expelled many hours after it was ingested, obviously the esophagus or stomach is not emptying normally. Thus if the patient's problem is in the esophagus (an obstructing lesion such as a tumor or stricture, a motor disorder such as achalasia, or a diverticulum that catches and retains the food), the regurgitated material often contains food but usually not acid or bile. If the stomach fails to empty because of an obstructing peptic ulcer or cancer or because of a motor disorder such as a diabetic gastric atony, the vomitus usually contains acid (if the patient's stomach can secrete it) and food but no bile. A distended stomach usually can be suspected by the finding of a succussion splash in the physical examination (the splash heard with a stethoscope over the stomach when the patient is shaken from side to side). Active ulcers may cause vomiting without obstructing the stomach, but an obstruction should be suspected in known ulcer patients. The regurgitation commonly associated with an incompetent lower esophageal sphincter and gastroesophageal reflux (often with heartburn) usually contains acid and therefore tastes sour, but it also may contain bile. If an obstruction exists high in the intestine but below the ampulla of Vater, bile usually is prominent in the vomitus, and the patient may exhibit little distention. If an obstruction exists lower in the small intestine or in the large intestine, distention usually is prominent and the vomitus is more apt to be feculent or putrid, the result of bacterial metabolism of intestinal contents. Intestinal obstructions, especially mechanical obstructions, usually are associated with prominent abdominal cramps and pain as well. With obstructions, especially those that are high in the gut, the vomiting often is marked after eating. In metabolic abnormalities such as pregnancy, early uremia, and alcoholic toxicity, the vomiting often is prominent in the morning.

Evaluation of patients with persistent or recurrent nausea and vomiting usually includes a flat plate roentgenogram of the abdomen (after excluding the possibility of a pregnancy), passage of a nasogastric tube and aspiration of gastric contents (if an obstruction is suspected), and barium studies of the esophagus, stomach, and intestines. A functional cause of chronic vomiting is not unusual, but possible gastrointestinal, metabolic, drug-related, and other organic causes should first be excluded from the diagnosis of these patients. Vomiting may be the sole symptom in patients with a functional disorder or may be associated with other manifestations of a functional bowel syndrome. As discussed previously, the physician should attempt to make a positive diagnosis rather than a diagnosis based solely on exclusion by correlating the symptoms with periods of stress and identifying other abnormal emotional and psychologic symptoms. A severe emotional disorder must be identified and treated with psychiatric assistance. Vomiting, especially in young women, may be a manifestation of bulimia or atypical anorexia nervosa.

Management of nausea and vomiting depends on the cause being identified. Significant dehydration and electrolyte and metabolic derangements must be recognized and corrected as rapidly as necessary. Severe acute hypokalemic metabolic alkalosis can result from losses of potassium and gastric acid. Vomiting, especially by intoxicated patients, may also lead to aspiration pneumonia. Severe retching may lead to a mucosal tear, usually near the esophagogastric junction (Mallory-Weiss syndrome) with resultant bleeding, or even to an esophageal rupture (Boerhaave's syndrome) with mediastinitis and serious consequences.

GASTROINTESTINAL BLEEDING

Bleeding from the gastrointestinal tract, revealed as either an acute hemorrhage or occult blood in the stool, is a common manifestation of gastrointestinal disease. A gastrointestinal hemorrhage is a serious, potentially lethal medical emergency. The patient usually has hematemesis, the vomiting of red blood or a dark material resembling coffee grounds, and/or the passage through the rectum of red blood (hematochezia) or black, tarry, sticky stools (melena). The coffee-ground material results from the conversion of hemoglobin to hematin by the acid in the stomach, whereas a melenic stool results from the alteration of at least 50 ml of blood in the gut, usually requiring several hours and probably bacterial action. Hematemesis usually means the bleeding is at a site proximal to the ligament of Treitz; continual vomiting or nasogastric aspiration of large amounts of red blood from the stomach usually suggests that the stomach or esophagus is the site of the hemorrhage, the duodenum being a less likely possibility. Melena also suggests the upper gastrointestinal tract as the site of bleeding, although bleeding from the jejunum, ileum, or even the right side of the colon can produce melena if the transit is slow. The passage of red blood through the rectum suggests that the bleeding site is distal to the ligament of Treitz, usually in the colon or rectum, but brisk bleeding from the upper gut with rapid intestinal transit also produces red rectal blood.

Even before a hemorrhage is apparent, bleeding patients often have symptoms of acute blood loss, the severity of which depends on the rate and magnitude of loss. Such symptoms include weakness, malaise, dyspnea, palpitations, faintness, sweating, and even syncope.

The physician's first concern with bleeding patients should be for the vital signs and the perfusion of the vital organs: the heart, brain, and kidneys. An acute blood loss of less than 500 ml or 10% of the blood volume rarely affects the vital signs significantly. A loss of more than 2 L or 35% to 40% usually produces frank hypovolemic shock. A loss of 1 to 2 L or 15% to 35% usually produces tachycardia and decreased blood pressure (pulse greater than 100 and systolic blood pressure less than 110 mm Hg) and "tilting" (when the patient rises from the prone position, the systolic blood pressure falls more than 10 mm Hg, the pulse increases more than 20 beats, and the patient often feels faint or light-headed). Blood should be drawn immediately for a hemoglobin and hematocrit determination and type and cross-match; a large-bore intravenous needle should be inserted immediately and an infusion begun; and if the patient shows signs of shock, he should immediately receive saline or preferably a colloidal volume expander (plasma or dextran), to be replaced with blood as soon as it can be obtained. The patient should receive only enough blood to maintain satisfactory blood pressure, pulse, and perfusion of the brain, heart, and kidneys. His mind should be clear, he should not feel faint, he should be free of angina and ischemic electrocardiographic changes, and he should be excreting good volumes of urine.

In addition to treating shock and observing and maintaining the patient's vital signs, circulation, and vital functions, the physician's goal is to diagnose the cause of bleeding, to control it, and to treat the underlying lesion. A surgeon and gastroenterologist, if available, should be consulted to help in the workup and management and to perform endoscopy or surgery if necessary. A history, physical examination, and laboratory tests should be performed as quickly and thoroughly as the patient's condition permits. All pertinent historical data should be elicited, including previous known diseases and bleeding and any use of drugs or toxins that can cause gastrointestinal bleeding (such as aspirin, alcohol, and antiinflammatory agents) or impair clotting (such as anticoagulants). The nose and throat should be examined as possible sites of the bleeding. If there is any question of actual bleeding having occurred, the presence of blood in the stool, vomitus, or gastric aspirate should be confirmed by a guaiac or benzidene test. The ingestion of iron, bismuth, or licorice can turn the stools dark (although not sticky), and beets can make them red. The hemoglobin and hematocrit determinations obtained soon after a hemorrhage do not reflect the severity of blood loss but continue to decline over many hours as the plasma volume is reexpanded by the addition of interstitial fluid. The finding of hypochromic, microcytic red cells suggests that the blood loss is chronic as well as acute. The finding of marked anemia in a patient with a good blood pressure and pulse also suggests a chronic slow loss of blood or antecedent anemia. Soon after bleeding the patient usually exhibits moderate leukocytosis and thrombocytosis and, if the bleeding site is in the upper gut, usually an elevation of blood urea nitrogen, even when renal function is normal.

The site of bleeding should be determined. A nasogastric tube should be passed, and the gastric contents aspirated. The presence of blood in the gastric contents (or a history of hematemesis) indicates that the site of bleeding is proximal to the ligament of Treitz; the absence of blood means either that the bleeding has stopped or that the site is not in the esophagus or stomach. If bile but no blood is recovered with continuous aspiration, there is no active bleeding in the proximal duodenum. If blood is recoverd from the stomach, the stomach should be washed with ice-cold saline or water in an effort to stop or slow the bleeding. If lower gastrointestinal bleeding is suspected because of the rectal passage of red blood and the absence of hematemesis and blood in the stomach, usually anoscopy and proctoscopy should be performed to determine if the rectum or anus is the site of bleeding or if the blood is coming from above these areas.

Common causes of acute severe upper gastrointestinal hemorrhage include peptic ulcers, erosive gastritis, esophageal and gastric varices, esophagitis, Mallory-Weiss tears, and less commonly polyps, benign and malignant tumors, vascular malformations, ruptured aneurysms, hematobilia, inflammatory bowel disease, and diverticula. Stress erosions or ulcerations are common causes of hemorrhage in patients susceptible to them because of severe trauma, severe illness, burns, central nervous system trauma or operations, and sepsis and other severe infections. Common causes of acute lower gastrointestinal hemorrhage include hemorrhoids and, in patients over 50 years of age, colonic diverticulosis and angiodysplasia. Less common causes include inflammatory bowel disease, colonic polyps, other benign and malignant tumors, gut ischemia, and radiation enteritis. Inflammatory bowel disease, including proctitis, is a relatively common cause of hematochezia or bloody diarrhea but an uncommon cause of severe hemorrhage. A Meckel's diverticulum is a relatively common site of gastrointestinal bleeding in young patients. Patients with impaired clotting resulting from anticoagulants or thrombocytopenia may have gastrointestinal bleeding; the less impaired the clotting, the more likely is an underlying lesion such as an ulcer whose bleeding was promoted by the anticoagulation.

The initial diagnostic procedures and therapy depend on the likely diagnosis derived from the history, the physical examination, the routine laboratory results, and the probable site of bleeding. A patient who has ingested aspirin or alcohol may very well be bleeding from erosive gastritis. If the patient has a history of ulcer disease and has ulcer symptoms, a peptic ulcer is most likely the cause of upper gastrointestinal bleeding. If the patient has cirrhosis as established by the history or physical examination, varices may be the cause; alcoholics, however, even with established cirrhosis and varices, commonly bleed because of other causes such as erosive gastritis, a peptic ulcer, esophagitis, and Mallory-Weiss tears. A patient, especially an alcoholic, who has hematemesis after much retching and initial vomiting of nonbloody material is likely to be bleeding from a Mallory-Weiss tear. A patient who is taking anticoagulant drugs or who is found to have petechiae, ecchymoses, or blood in the urine probably has a bleeding diathesis causing or contributing to the gastrointestinal hemorrhage. The physical finding of abnormal pigmentation or vascular lesions of the hands, face, lips, or mouth may reveal the presence of a Peutz-Jeghers syndrome or Osler-Weber-Rendu disease, respectively, as the cause of the bleeding.

In general, if the bleeding is from the upper gut, an emergency or early endoscopy (esophagogastroduodenoscopy) should be performed if the technique is available and the patient's condition permits. Although studies have not yet clearly demonstrated that emergency endoscopy alters the outcome of patients with gastrointestinal bleeding, the procedure usually establishes a rapid diagnosis for bleeding in the esophagus, stomach, or duodenum and permits proper therapy to be initiated immediately. Even if the bleeding is too brisk to permit complete visualization, the site of bleeding usually can be determined, and some diagnostic possibilities such as varices and diffuse erosive gastritis can be excluded. Endoscoy is especially helpful in patients such as alcoholics who are likely to have many possible causes for their bleeding. Their varices may be demonstrable by an esophagogram, but endoscopy usually is required to determine these as the source of the bleeding rather than gastritis or some other lesion. Endoscopy is usually required to identify many lesions, such as erosive gastritis, esophagitis, duodenitis, a Mallory-Weiss tear, or small vascular lesions such as occur in patients with Osler-Weber-Rendu disease. Therapeutic procedures such as the use of laser beams and electrocautery may be used with endoscopes to control some types of bleeding. Angiography is helpful in some cases of upper gastrointestinal bleeding, especially if the bleeding site cannot be successfully demonstrated by endoscopy or if a vascular anomaly is the cause of bleeding. Angiography or radioactive scans can demonstrate the bleeding site usually when the bleeding is arterial and occurs at a rate of 0.5 ml/min or more. The dye or radioactive material can be seen collecting in the gut lumen. Esophagography and gastrointestinal series are performed in many cases, but once barium has been introduced into the stomach in an emergency study, it impedes subsequent endoscopic and especially angiographic examinations for some time. A patient who has a classic history suggesting peptic ulcer disease and who apparently has stopped bleeding may require only a gastrointestinal series.

If brisk lower gastrointestinal bleeding continues and arises at a level above the reach of the proctoscope, angiography or a radioactive scan usually is the procedure of choice. If the bleeding site cannot be found in the colon, it should be sought in the small intestine and even in the stomach. Emergency barium enemas and small bowel series usually are less determinative in patients with severe lower gastrointestinal bleeding, especially older patients in whom diverticulosis and angiodysplasia, a vascular lesion usually of the right side of the colon, are common causes of such bleeding. In at least 50% of the cases of brisk diverticular bleeding the bleeding site is on the right side of the colon even though diverticula are much more common on the left. If the bleeding is not brisk, especially in a patient under 45 years of age and especially if polyps, a neoplasm, or inflammatory bowel disease is suspected, a barium enema and small bowel series may be performed before angiography is considered. Colonoscopy usually cannot be successfully performed when the bleeding is appreciable but may be used after the bleeding has ceased, ideally after a period of bowel preparation (see Chapter 171).

Therapy for gastrointestinal bleeding, in addition to general supportive measures, depends on the specific cause and often must be individualized according to the condition and associated medical problems of the patient. If the bleeding is so brisk that an adequate blood volume and adequate perfusion of vital organs cannot be maintained, usually emergency surgery must be performed to control it. Even if vital signs and functions can be maintained by means of transfusions, the physician should try to avoid the need for massive transfusions of 15 units or more, to avoid the attendant complications and increased possibility of death. Acid-peptic related disorders such as ulcers, gastritis, and esophagitis are usually treated by controlling gastric acidity with antacids, H_2-receptor blocking drugs, or constant gastric suction, although it usually is advisable not to leave nasogastric tubes in patients with gastric or esophageal lesions. Patients with bleeding varices should receive intravenous vasopressin (Pitressin) in an effort to reduce the splanchnic blood flow and portal pressure and perhaps endoscopic sclerosis or tamponade with the Sengstaken-Blakemore tube. Some physicians do not use the tamponade because of the attendant risks, and still others advocate early surgery, especially in low-risk patients. The local arterial perfusion of vasopressin has been used in many medical centers to reduce local blood flow and persistent bleeding. It is perfused into a branch of the superior mesenteric artery or inferior mesenteric artery to control colonic diverticular bleeding or into the left gastric artery to control bleeding from erosive gastritis, a gastric ulcer, or a Mallory-Weiss tear. Some angiographers occlude local arterial branches to a persistently bleeding site by injecting an autologous clot or gelatin sponge (Gelfoam). Some angiographers have even been able to introduce catheters into the portal circulation and inject bleeding varices with sclerosing agents. These latter procedures are available in relatively few medical centers and should still be viewed as experimental. With the remarkable capabilities of angiographers to introduce catheters into increasingly more vessels, however, new angiographic as well as therapeutic endoscopic techniques will become available for rapidly controlling gastrointestinal bleeding and thereby avoiding surgery.

The slow, inapparent loss of blood from the gastrointestinal tract is another common manifestation of gastrointestinal disorders. These patients often have iron deficiency anemia or an occult fecal blood loss detected by routine testing of the stool with guaiac or benzidene. These tests usually are positive if the daily blood loss is at least 5 ml. The benzidene test is more sensitive but less specific, and thus in some weakly positive cases dietary meat may have to be restricted to be certain the test is positive. Many gastrointestinal lesions have been alleged to produce occult blood loss and hypochromic microcytic anemia, the more common of which are cancers of the colon, stomach, ampulla of Vater or pancreas, and esophagus; colonic and gastric polyps; peptic ulcers; and gastritis, usually produced by drugs such as aspirin. Colon cancer in particular tends to produce occult blood loss, and thus the examination of three stool specimens for occult blood with the Hemoccult test has been advocated as a yearly screening test for the detection of early colon cancer in people over 40 years of age. Other lesions thought to produce occult blood in the stools and iron deficiency anemia include almost all other known gastrointestinal lesions, including hiatus hernia and diverticulosis. These two conditions are very common and certainly may be associated with acute hemorrhage. Their presence should not be accepted, however, as a cause of occult blood loss. Patients found to have occult fecal blood or unexplained iron deficiency anemia should usually undergo proctoscopy, an air-contrast barium enema, esophagography, and a gastrointestinal and small bowel series. If the cause still has not been satisfactorily determined, colonoscopy and esophagogastroduodenoscopy should be performed as well.

PROTEIN-LOSING ENTEROPATHY

Lesions of the gut may result not only in a loss of blood but also in an abnormal loss of plasma proteins in excess of the small amounts normally leaked each day into the lumen of the gut. Bleeding lesions such as an ulcer or inflammatory bowel disease obviously cause a loss of plasma as well as red blood cells, but the resultant anemia or diminished blood volume and consequent symptoms are more likely to attract the patient's and physician's attention than a low level of serum albumin and possible edema. In contrast, some diseases of the gut result in an excessive loss of albumin and other plasma proteins with relatively little or no appreciable loss of blood cells. If the loss of albumin cannot be satisfactorily replaced by new synthesis in the liver, hypoalbuminemia and possibly edema result. If the patient does not have the nephrotic syndrome, liver disease, malnutrition, or some other apparent condition to explain a low level of serum albumin, the presence of protein-losing enteropathy can be demonstrated by injecting chromated Cr 51 serum albumin or iodinated I 131 serum albumin intravenously and demonstrating a markedly decreased half-life of the albumin and the recovery of much of the radioactivity in the stools.

Many diseases that obstruct the intestinal lymphatics, produce mucosal ulceration, or involve the mucosa even without apparent ulceration produce an abnormal enteric loss of plasma protein. Diseases often associated primarily with hypoalbuminemia and edema include (1) Menetrier's disease, a form of hypertrophic gastritis characterized by giant gastric folds and/or nodules, especially in the body and fundus of the stomach, marked hyperplasia of the surface and pit mucous cells, atrophy of the normal glandular cells, hypersecretion of mucus, and hyposecretion of acid; (2) primary or secondary lymphangiectasia, a blockage of the intestinal lymphatics secondary to some recognizable inflammatory or neoplastic disease, such as tuberculosis or lymphoma, or primarily resulting from their malformation (a form or part of Milroy's disease) and usually also associated with some degree of malabsorption and diarrhea and a depletion or reduction of circulating lymphocytes; (3) some cases of eosinophilic gastroenteritis, a poorly defined entity related in some cases to an apparent food allergy and often also producing pain, diarrhea, and blood loss; and (4) some gut lymphomas. Many other diseases may be associated with significant enteric protein loss, hypoalbuminemia, and edema, but other manifestations of the diseases usually are more prom-

inent and usually attract more attention. These disorders include Crohn's disease, ulcerative colitis, intestinal lymphomas, Whipple's disease, celiac disease, tropical sprue, gastric ulcer, gastric cancer, acute infectious enteritides, constrictive pericarditis, severe right-sided heart failure, and some cases of hypersecretory hypertrophic gastropathy such as may be associated with the Zollinger-Ellison syndrome.

The workup of patients suspected or demonstrated to have protein-losing enteropathy should include roentgenograms of the gastrointestinal tract. The need for additional studies depends on the findings of the history, physical examination, laboratory examination, and roentgenograms. The treatment of patients with protein-losing enteropathy depends on the cause. For example, patients with demonstrated focal lesions may require surgery; those with lymphangiectasia may benefit from the replacement of dietary lipid with short- and medium-chain triglycerides; those with inflammatory bowel disease may benefit from steroids; and those with eosinophilic gastroenteritis may benefit from elimination diets or steroids.

GASEOUSNESS

Gaseousness is a common gastrointestinal complaint resulting in excessive belching, abdominal bloating or distention associated with cramps and pain, or excessive flatulence.

Gas usually can be observed in the stomach and large intestine of the normal person, about 50 ml in the stomach and 100 ml in the intestine. The gas in the gut is derived from swallowed air, nitrogen therefore usually forming a large percentage of the gas, from the rapid fluxes of gases between the bowel lumen and blood, and from gas prodcued in the lumen. Carbon dioxide is formed in the duodenum from the neutralization of gastric acid and fatty acids by the secreted sodium bicarbonate, 22.4 ml of carbon dioxide resulting from each mEq of acid neutralized. In the colon hydrogen and carbon dioxide are produced largely from the bacterial fermentation of nonabsorbed food or, in the case of carbon dixoide, in part from the reaction of secreted HCO_3 with fatty acids produced by the bacteria. About one third of adults also have bacteria that produce methane, but it is produced independently of food ingestion and persists even when fasting. The hydrogen and methane formed in the colon are absorbed in part into the circulation and cleared effectively in the lungs, and thus the rates of colonic formation of these gases can be estimated by analyzing expired breath. Trace amounts of malodorous gases also are formed in the colon and account for the repugnant odors of flatus.

The gas in the stomach is largely swallowed air with the addition of some carbon dioxide. When a person is erect, the gastric air bubble accumulates in the upper part of the stomach near the esophagogastric junction, and much of it can be readily eructated. When a person is supine, however, most of the air accumulates in the antrum,and the esophagogastic junction is covered with gastric fluid; thus little of the swallowed air is eructated, and most of it passes into the duodenum. Because of its low viscosity, gas moves rapidly through the small intestine. The large volume of carbon dioxide produced in the duodenum, about half or more of the duodenal gas after a meal, is rapidly absorbed in the small intestine. The hydrogen, carbon dioxide, and methane formed in the colon occasionally account for over half of the colonic gas and flatus in some patients, although in most patients nitrogen usually accounts for 50% to 90%. Little oxygen is found in the colon or flatus because of its rapid utilization by bacteria. The amount of flatus and its content of hydrogen and carbon dioxide are appreciably increased when the amounts of fermentable substrates entering the colon are increased, for example, by increasing undigestible dietary substances such as the oligosaccharides found in beans and other roughage and fiber, in the presence of a malabsorption syndrome, or by the ingestion of lactose by a person with lactase deficiency.

About 2 to 3 ml of air is thought to enter the stomach with each swallow; the occasional eructation following a meal or the drinking of a carbonated beverage emanates from the gastric air bubble. On the other hand, patients who have frequent recurrent belching usually have been observed to swallow or aspirate air before each belch. Most of this air moves only partway down the esophagus before being expelled (esophageal eructations). Thus chronic excessive belching usually is a functional habit that often is promoted or aggravated by emotional stress rather than the result of excessive gas formation in the stomach or intestine. The mechanism and functional nature of the eructations should be explained to these patients, whose symptoms often improve with the reassurance that no significant disease exists.

Many patients complain of chronic abdominal bloating and cramps or pain attributed to the presence of excessive intestinal gas. These patients have in the past been thought to have excessive aerophagia—the swallowing of too much air with meals or when swallowing saliva—which leads to excessive gas. Recent studies have shown, however, that such patients have normal amounts of intestinal gas and that when their intestines are perfused with volumes of gas tolerated by normal subjects, the abdominal pain is reproduced. Thus it appears that these patients have some sort of motor disorder or that they are abnormally sensitive to the usual distentions of the gut. These patients also benefit from the reassurance that they do not have a serious disease. Because they react even to normal quantities of intestinal gas, it should be reduced if possible. They should be warned against repetitive belching, because some of the swallowed or aspirated air may reach the stomach. They should remain erect after meals to promote eructation of gastric gas and to minimize the amount passing into the intestine. The amount of carbon dioxide produced in the duodenum can theoretially be reduced by neutralizing or inhibiting gastric acid secretion (with antacids or inhibitors) and by reducing dietary fat. The amount of gas produced in the colon can be decreased by reducing the intake of nondigestible foods such as beans, roughage, fiber, and lactose, especially with patients with lactase deficiency. Finally anticholinergics and antispasmodics may be tried, although their efficacy in reducing this pain has not been established.

An effort can also be made to reduce the intestinal gas of patients complaining of excessive flatus. In some medical centers the amount of flatus can be measured, or a sample of colonic gas can be more easily collected for analysis with a syringe and rectal tube. If the gas is predominantly nitrogen, the problem is excessive aerophagia and the patient can be advised accordingly. On the other hand, if hydrogen and carbon dioxide are major constituents (hydrogen can also be detected in expired breath), the major problem is the colonic presence of excessive nonabsorbed fermentable substrates; the major therapeutic thrust then should be to reduce dietary beans, other roughage and fiber, and lactose (especially with patients with lactase deficiency) and to exclude the possibility of a malabsorption syndrome.

OTHER MANIFESTATIONS OF GASTROINTESTINAL DISORDERS

Many other symptoms, which are discussed in greater detail in subsequent chapters, may be the initial or associated manifestations of disorders of the digestive system. Jaundice is a common manifestation of hepatic or biliary disease and pancreatic cancer. Abdominal distention may result from gaseous intestinal distention (such as that resulting from an intestinal obstruction or ileus), ascites, an abdominal mass, a hernia, or organomegaly such as a large liver, spleen, or uterus. Dysphagia, the sensation of food or drink sticking when swallowed, is a common manifestation of disorders of the esophagus. Fever in a patient with a gastrointestinal disorder suggests an inflammatory or, less commonly, a neoplastic process. Anorexia commonly accompanies obstructive, neoplastic, and inflammatory processes, especially of the liver, and must be differentiated from early satiety, the loss of appetite and the feeling of fullness after eating little. Satiety may occur with a milder form of anorexia but is also often experienced with obstructing, infiltrating, or exophytic lesions of the stomach, usually neoplasms, that prevent its normal filling. An appreciable weight loss commonly accompanies inflammatory and neoplastic processes of the digestive system as well as diseases of malabsorption. Rashes, arthralgias, or arthritis may accompany digestive diseases, especially acute and chronic hepatitis and inflammatory bowel disease.

BIBLIOGRAPHY

Greenberger NJ: Gastrointestinal disorders: a pathophysiologic approach, ed 3, Chicago, 1986, Year Book Medical Publishers, Inc.
Sleisenger MH and Fordtran JS: Gastrointestinal disease, ed 5, Philadelphia, 1988, WB Saunders Co.

171·SPECIAL TECHNIQUES FOR DIAGNOSING DISORDERS OF THE DIGESTIVE SYSTEM

William O. Frank and **Harvey B. Lefton**

The purpose of this chapter is to discuss the various specialized diagnostic tests available to detect pathologic conditions in various segments of the gastrointestinal tract. For the sake of clarity the gastrointestinal tract is considered in the following segments: esophagus, stomach, small bowel, colon (large bowel), liver, hepatobiliary tree, and pancreas. For each of these segments the appropriate specialized diagnostic tests are discussed. The indications for their use are emphasized, their technical aspects are briefly discussed, and when applicable, modifications being made to permit therapeutic intervention are described. New tests and instruments for the diagnosis and treatment of digestive disorders are being developed almost daily; a few of the more promising new ones are included, even though they may not yet be routinely available or their value clearly established. Finally, abdominal sonography, computed tomography, and angiography are discussed.

ESOPHAGUS

A battery of tests is available for evaluating the competence of the lower esophageal sphincter, esophageal peristaltic activity, and esophageal mucosal inflammation or masses. Esophageal mucosal inflammation and masses are diagnosed directly by esophagoscopy, biopsy, and cytologic specimens. (Endoscopy is discussed under "Stomach.") Other diagnostic tests include the Bernstein test, esophageal manometry, pH probe test, and esophageal scintigram. As mentioned in other chapters, these tests are used in a select group of patients with reflux esophagitis or in whom an esophageal motility disorder is suspected.

Bernstein test

The Bernstein test endeavors to reproduce the patient's symptoms by perfusing the esophageal mucosa with acid to determine whether the symptoms originate from the esophagus, presumably from reflux esophagitis.

In this test a tube is positioned in the upper third of the esophagus with its opening 30 cm from the teeth. A Y-tube is connected to the other end of this tube, which in turn is connected to reservoirs of 0.1N HCl and saline. After an initial drip of saline, the acid solution is permitted to flow until symptoms appear or until 30 minutes has elapsed. If the patient's usual symptoms are reproduced, the drip is switched back to saline. If the symptoms vanish within 3 to 4 minutes, redripping the acid reproduces them rapidly if they result from an esophageal lesion.

Superficially, this test appears to be easy to interpret. In some patients, however, the acid perfusion of the esophagus elicits discomfort or pain different from the patient's original pain. It has not been clearly determined whether these patients should be considered to have a positive Bernstein test result. In addition, the test results may be negative in patients with an esophageal stricture caused by reflux esophagitis. Despite these limitations, this test is an invaluable clinical tool for diagnosing reflux esophagitis.

Esophageal manometry

Esophageal manometry is a technique used to assess the functioning of the upper and lower esophageal sphincters and the motor activity of the body of the esophagus. A bundle of catheters is passed into the esophagus. The open tips of the catheters are separated from one another by a known distance. By means of pumps, water is infused through each catheter at a constant rate. Another arm of each catheter is connected to a low-volume displacement transducer to record pressures on a calibrated recorder. When the outflow of water from a catheter is impeded by the contraction of esophageal muscle or by the tightening of a sphincter, the event is recorded as an increase in pressure occurring at the tip of that catheter. In this way the resting pressures of the sphincters and the degree of their relaxation after swallowing can be determined, as well as the amplitude, velocity, and coordination of the peristaltic waves in the body of the esophagus. The test is performed on patients suspected of having esophageal motor disorders. In achalasia, for example, the test reveals a hypertonic lower esophageal sphincter that fails to relax normally on swallowing and the absence of peristaltic waves in the body of the esophagus. Diffuse esophageal spasm is detected by the simultaneous recording of high-pressure contractions in several catheters at the same time.

pH probe test for reflux

In the pH probe test a pH electrode attached to a manometric catheter is positioned 5 cm above the lower esophageal sphincter, which is located by its high pressure recorded by the catheter. The pH in the esophagus normally is about 6, but if acid is refluxed from the stomach, it falls to 4 or lower. The patient is asked to perform certain maneuvers that tend to promote reflux (Valsalva's maneuver, vigorous sniffing, and elevation of the legs). If no reflux is demonstrated, the catheter is passed into the stomach, 300 ml or 0.1N HCl is infused into the stomach, the catheter assembly is withdrawn to the same location in the esophagus, and the maneuvers are repeated. Be-

cause the stomach clearly now contains acid, reflux should readily be detected by observing an acid pH of 4 or lower in the esophagus. Occasionally pH probes may be left in the esophagus for several hours, for example, during sleep or for 24 hours, to record the frequency of reflux and the rate at which refluxed acid is cleared from the esophagus.

Gastroesophageal scintigram

Of all the tests discussed in the preceding paragraphs, none actually demonstrates reflux of gastric juice into the esophagus. The demonstration of the reflux of a radioactive isotope, technetium, into the esophagus during scanning of the esophagogastric area documents reflux of gastric contents. This test is a recent development but is proving to be a simple, reliable test for reflux.

Esophagoscopy

Esophagoscopy is discussed in the following section on endoscopy.

STOMACH

Several tests are available for evaluating pathologic lesions in the stomach, for measuring gastric emptying of solids and liquids, and for evaluating the physiology of a stomach altered by surgery. Upper endoscopy permits the gastroenterologist to directly inspect superficial mucosal disease, masses, and ulcers in all areas of the stomach. The measurement of gastric emptying of solids or liquids provides an indirect measure of gastric motility. A scintigraphic technique to assess enterogastric reflux also detects altered gallbladder emptying and simultaneously measures gastric emptying. Each of these tests is discussed in the following sections.

Endoscopy

UPPER ENDOSCOPY. The flexible fiberoptic endoscope is a diagnostic tool used to detect pathologic conditions in the esophagus, stomach, and duodenum. These instruments are forward viewing, have a flexible tip that can be deflected 180 degrees in any direction, and have channels to permit the passage of biopsy foceps, cytology brushes, irrigating or injecting cannulas, and snares or cautery equipment for operative procedures. The examination of the upper gastrointestinal tract with an endoscope permits the physician with direct vision to inspect and perform a biopsy in all portions of the esophagus, stomach, and duodenum. The procedure can be easily performed with little risk and discomfort to the patient, although serious complications such as perforation have been known to occur.

Because upper endoscopy is a common procedure, the indications for its use are important. Most gastroenterologists agree that upper endoscopy should be performed in patients with (1) upper gastrointestinal hemorrhage, (2) an abnormal roentgenographic appearance of the upper gastrointestinal tract, (3) unexplained chest or abdominal pain and negative upper gastrointestinal roentgenographic studies, and (4) unexplained symptoms and a history of previous upper gastrointestinal surgery.

An endoscopic examination of a patient with upper gastrointestinal hemorrhage is a rapid and accurate way to determine directly the site of bleeding. Upper endoscopy should probably be the first diagnostic test for evaluating most patients with upper gastrointestinal hemorrhage, for reasons based on several important observations. It is now recognized that upper gastrointestinal roentgenographic studies commonly do not reveal superficial mucosal lesions such as erosions or inflammation.

Furthermore, several potential sites of gastrointestinal bleeding sometimes coexist in the same patient, and roentgenograms cannot determine which site is bleeding. Upper endoscopy circumvents these problems. Upper endoscopy should be performed within the first 24 to 48 hours after the episode of bleeding, however, because superficial mucosal lesions may heal within 48 hours. Thus the advantages of upper endoscopy over upper gastrointestinal roentgenograms are (1) superficial mucosal lesions are routinely detected, (2) the clinician is able to determine the site of hemorrhage rapidly and accurately in virtually all patients, including patients with multiple potential sites of bleeding, and (3) a rapid, accurate diagnosis enables the clinician to render appropriate medical or surgical therapy.

When upper gastrointestinal series have detected filling defects, masses, ulcers, and strictures in the esophagus, stomach, and duodenum, upper gastrointestinal endoscopy should be performed (except for duodenal ulcers). A major advantage of an endoscopic study in these patients is that biopsy and cytology specimens can also be obtained from lesions or suspicious areas of the gut for pathologic study, which enables the clinician to differentiate malignant from benign disease. If the mass is intramural or extrinsic to the gut and no mucosal break is present, however, an appropriate biopsy sample cannot be obtained using conventional endoscopic biopsy techniques.

An upper gastrointestinal series may not reveal ulcers in the upper gastrointestinal tract and, as mentioned previously, commonly does not detect superficial mucosal lesions. Because these lesions may produce symptoms referable to either the thorax or abdomen, upper endoscopy should probably be performed in patients with unexplained chest or abdominal pain and negative gastrointestinal roentgenograms.

Contrast studies of the upper gastrointestinal tract often are difficult to interpret after operations. The gastric emptying time and gastrointestinal transit time are commonly dramatically altered. Therefore good air-contrast studies may be unobtainable, and it may be difficult to differentiate postoperative changes from intrinsic disease. For these reasons the upper gastrointestinal series may not be satisfactory, and careful endoscopic evaluation may be necessary in such postoperative cases.

THERAPEUTIC ENDOSCOPY. The use of upper endoscopy in diagnosing upper gastrointestinal pathologic conditions is well accepted. In addition to its diagnostic capabilities, a therapeutic and operative role for upper endoscopy is now being rapidly developed. Because upper gastrointestinal lesions commonly are associated with bleeding, it would seem appropriate to combine the diagnostic and therapeutic roles of upper endoscopy. Specialized equipment and double-channel upper endoscopes are available to control gastrointestinal hemorrhage by laser cautery, heater probe, electrocautery, and injecting and sclerosing bleeding varices. Other therapeutic roles for endoscopy include removal of polyps and foreign bodies, dilation of strictures, and insertion of prosthetic tubes to relieve an obstruction. Endoscopic laser therapy permits debulking of esophageal and gastric cancers.

Gastric motility studies

Research into the electromechanical events of gastric motility has shown that the stomach can be divided into two distinct physiologic segments, the proximal and distal portions. The proximal stomach serves as a reservoir. This portion relaxes to receive food boluses from the esophagus—a phenomenon called *receptive relaxation*—and adapts to increasing volumes with little change in pressure, a phenomenon called *accommodation to distention*. These two phenomena maintain a low

intragastric pressure as the stomach fills. The distal stomach acts as the gastric mixer and grinder. Peristaltic waves, progressive circular rings of contraction, begin in the corpus and sweep down the stomach to the pylorus. The terminal antrum contracts forcefully and the pylorus closes tightly. This electromechanical activity causes propulsion, squeezing, and retropulsion of the gastric contents and thoroughly mixes, grinds, and triturates gastric solids. It also permits a slow passage of chyme into the small bowel.

Because disturbances of gastric motility alter gastric emptying, tests to measure the gastric emptying of solids and liquids can detect disturbances of gastric motor function. Several techniques have been devised to measure gastric emptying. The classic clinical test is to use a nasogastric or Ewald tube to measure the volume of food and secretions retained in the stomach at a given time after a meal. Newer, more sophisticated tests of gastric emptying include monitoring the emptying of roentgenographic contrast agents, of a saline load, of labeled nonabsorbable markers, or of plastic spheres. A promising new method monitors the rate of disappearance of radioactive-labeled food from the stomach using a gamma camera or scintillation deflector.

Abnormal gastric motility and therefore abnormal gastric emptying are found in at least two groups of patients: those with diabetes mellitus and those who have had gastric surgery. With the advent of new prokinetic drugs such as metoclopramide that promote gastric emptying, it is especially important to differentiate such disorders from mechanical obstructions and other disorders that may require surgery.

Scintigraphic technique to measure enterogastric reflux

The reflux of bile and digestive enzymes from the small bowel into the stomach has been described in patients with postsurgical alkaline gastritis (Billroth II surgery), gastric ulcers, reflux esophagitis, and functional dyspepsia; it is unclear what role enterogastric reflux plays in the pathogenesis and symptomatology of these patients. Recently a new scintigraphic technique has been developed to measure enterogastric reflux.

The test is performed in the following manner. ^{99m}Tc-HIDA $(N,N^l - [2,6$-dimethylphenylcarbamoylmethyl]iminodiacetic acid) is administered intravenously. This agent is excreted by the hepatobiliary tree, and when counts are maximal over the gallbladder, the patient drinks a liquid test meal mixed with indium 111 and DTPA (diethylenetriamine pentaacetic acid). Windows are set for each of these radioactive-labeled agents, which are counted over a specified time interval. In essence the small bowel contents become labeled with ^{99m}Tc-HIDA and the gastric contents with ^{111}In-DTPA. Reflux of ^{99m}Tc-HIDA into the stomach therefore reflects enterogastric reflux. This test is still experimental but may prove to be an important clinical test for the groups of patients listed previously. The test also measures rates of gallbladder and gastric emptying.

SMALL BOWEL

Diseases of the small bowel, apart from peptic ulcer disease of the duodenum and some acute infectious disorders, are relatively uncommon. Abdominal pain, diarrhea, and intestinal obstruction are common symptoms produced by disorders of the small intestine. Barium-contrast roentgenograms (small bowel series) generally are the most useful tests for diagnosing diseases of the small bowel, especially neoplasms and inflammatory disorders such as regional enteritis. Endoscopy undoubtedly will play a larger role in the future. At the present time the distal ileum can be directly viewed with the colonoscope and at least the duodenal bulb and descending duodenum with the duodenoscope. Undoubtedly new endoscopes that are introduced orally or rectally will in the future permit the direct viewing of and the biopsy of more portions of the small bowel. In certain patients suspected of having a parasitic infection such as giardiasis or an abnormal growth of bacteria in the small bowel, a thin tube can be passed into the small intestine to obtain intestinal aspirates for microscopic examination and appropriate culture studies. In many patients with a malabsorption syndrome diagnosed by the detection of excessive fat in the stool (steatorrhea), a peroral biopsy of small intestine mucosa is necessary for diagnosing the specific cause of the malabsorption.

Small bowel biopsy

The available instruments for a relatively safe peroral biopsy of the small intestine include (1) the *multipurpose biopsy tube* (also called the Rubin or Quinton tube), which obtains one to four mucosal samples with one passage; (2) the *Crosby capsule*, which obtains one large mucosal sample; and (3) the *hydraulic suction biopsy tube,* which obtains several samples during a single passage. These tubes are passed under fluoroscopic control through the mouth and the stomach to the ligament of Treitz, the duodenojejunal junction. Obtaining biopsy tissue samples from this site permits histologic comparisons of the mucosa among patients and in the same patient at different times.

To be definitive and free of artifacts, peroral biopsy samples must be obtained, processed, and interpreted correctly. For a small bowel biopsy to have maximal diagnostic value, (1) the biopsy site must be precisely radiologically localized, (2) the biopsy samples must be properly oriented and promptly fixed, (3) the gross specimen should be examined with a dissecting microscope or a low-power microscope, mainly to determine the presence or absence of normal villi, and (4) serial sections cut perpendicular to the lumen and extending to the muscularis mucosae to include the full width of the mucosa should be examined microscopically.

This procedure has a relatively low morbidity and mortality. Complications include perforation and hemorrhage at the biopsy site. The diseases that may be diagnosed by means of an intestinal biopsy include adult and childhood celiac disease, tropical sprue, giardiasis, Whipple's disease, congenital β-lipoprotein deficiency, hypogammaglobulinemic enteritis, and occasionally lymphangiectasia, eosinophilic gastroenteritis, amyloidosis, and intestinal lymphoma.

COLON

The colon (large bowel) is the most common site for cancer. In addition other diseases of the colon such as polyps, diverticulosis and diverticulitis, inflammatory bowel disease (ulcerative colitis and Crohn's disease), and bacterial and parasitic infections are common. Because colonic disease is prevalent, there has been a strong impetus to improve diagnostic techniques. The double-contrast roentgenographic method (introduction of barium followed by air insufflation) is superior to the former single-contrast method and postevacuation roentgenograms for detecting colonic lesions. Colonoscopes now permit direct inspection of the entire colon from the anus to the cecum.

Rectal exam and occult blood testing

The initial test for suspected colonic disease is digital examination of the rectum. This allows the clinician to assess anal sphincter tone, hemorrhoidal disease, rectal masses, coc-cygeal pain, and the prostate (in men) or the cervix (in women). Stool is obtained, which is smeared on a guaiac-impregnated slide. A drop of hydrogen peroxide solution is put on the slide, and occult blood is noted by the presence of a blue color. This may be the first and only warning of blood loss from an occult gastrointestinal lesion. A false positive result can occur in patients on iron or those eating red meat or peroxidase-rich fruits and vegetables (beets, cantelope, cauliflower). False negative results can occur in patients taking vitamin C or mineral oil. This test indicates blood loss but does not give a clue to cause or site in the gastrointestinal tract.

Colonoscopy

Colonoscopes are flexible fiberoptic instruments 160 to 180 cm long. They have one or two channels for the passage of biopsy forceps, cytology brushes, snares, and electrocautery equipment. In addition there are channels for suction and air insufflation.

Considerable skill is required, but an experienced colonoscopist can reach the cecum in approximately 90% of patients. The colon can be inspected thoroughly as the colonoscope is slowly withdrawn from the cecum. Biopsy samples are taken from suspicious areas of mucosa, and polyps are removed using snare and electrocautery equipment. Successful colonoscopy requires proper colonic preparation (involving a residue-free diet and use of laxatives or enemas) to eliminate fecal residue. Emergency endoscopy often is unsuccessful, because the suction capacity of present colonoscopes is inadequate to remove the usual fecal contents or blood satisfactorily.

Colonoscopy should be performed in (1) patients in whom barium enemas reveal abnormalities, (2) patients who have iron deficiency anemia and Hemoccult-positive stools but whose gastrointestinal tract has a normal roentgenographic appearance, (3) selected patients with inflammatory bowel disease or diverticulosis, and (4) patients with colonic polyps. The indications for colonoscopy are obvious in the first group of patients. Patients in the second group commonly have colonic lesions such as polyps despite a normal barium enema examination. Patients with inflammatory bowel disease often have abnormalities revealed by barium enemas. Patients with chronic idiopathic ulcerative colitis have increased risk of colon cancer; these patients should routinely undergo colonoscopy. Colonoscopy should usually be deferred, however, in patients with severe, acute inflammation because of the increased risk of perforation. Colonic polyps are considered premalignant lesions, and the larger the polyp the greater the likelihood of malignant transformation. If colonic polyps removed by colonoscopic polypectomy are found to have carcinoma that does not extend into the stalk, their removal can be considered a cure. This important technical advance underlies the significance of this diagnostic tool.

Colonoscopy is not a benign procedure, but it is associated with a low morbidity and mortality. The complications include perforation and bleeding, especially after polypectomy, that may require surgical intervention. A barium enema study should not be performed for at least 2 to 3 days in patients who have had biopsies, especially after a polypectomy, because the high intraluminal pressures generated during a barium enema theoretically may cause perforation at the site of a mucosal biopsy or polypectomy.

Fiberoptic sigmoidoscopy

Fiberoptic sigmoidoscopy is currently being used in place of rigid sigmoidoscopy. A fiberoptic sigmoidoscope is a flexible endoscope with channels similar to those of the colonoscope but is only 35 cm to 65 cm long. This instrument allows a more comfortable examination of the rectum and sigmoid colon than does the rigid sigmoidoscope.

LIVER

A liver biopsy often is necessary for diagnosing liver disease, because the symptoms, signs, and results of liver function tests often do not allow for reliable discrimination among various liver diseases. A definitive diagnosis of liver disease therefore is commonly based on characteristic histologic findings. For example, a liver biopsy is required to distinguish chronic active hepatitis from chronic persistent hepatitis and may be necessary to detect hepatic tuberculosis, sarcoidosis, or metastases. A liver biopsy may be performed blindly or under direct vision during laparoscopy (peritoneoscopy); either procedure is acceptable. A major advantage of peritoneoscopy, however, is that the liver, peritoneal cavity, and other organs (spleen, stomach, and gallbladder) can also be inspected. In the following sections the transthoracic (blind) liver biopsy and laparoscopy are discussed separately.

Transthoracic liver biopsy

In a transthoracic liver biopsy, liver dullness first is localized through percussion at the anterior axillary line in the right ninth, tenth, or eleventh intercostal space during inspiration and expiration. The site is marked and anesthetized, and a small incision is made. During expiration, a biopsy needle (such as the Vim-Silverman, Menghini, or Jamshuti needle) is directed toward the liver. As the needle approaches the liver capsule, suction is applied to the glass syringe, and the needle is passed into the liver and rapidly withdrawn. The procedure may be performed using ultrasound guidance if a solitary lesion is present.

The procedure has a low morbidity and mortality. Associated complications are intrahepatic or peritoneal hemorrhage, bile leakage and bile peritonitis, the creation of traumatic arteriovenous shunts, and vasovagal shock. Before a liver biopsy is performed, the patient's platelet count and prothrombin time should be checked. A liver biopsy can be performed if the platelet count is higher than $50,000/mm^3$ and the prothrombin time is less than 3 seconds more than normal. Contraindications to a liver biopsy are an uncooperative patient, an extrahepatic biliary tract obstruction existing longer than 2 months, a low platelet count, prolonged prothrombin time, significant ascites, and the suspected presence of ascending cholangitis.

Laparoscopy

Laparoscopy permits direct inspection of the peritoneal cavity and intraabdominal organs and thus is a valuable and safe technique for diagnosing intraabdominal pathologic conditions. A state of pneumoperitoneum is produced with carbon dioxide or nitrous oxide using a Verres needle inserted through the anterior abdominal wall into the peritoneal cavity, usually in a lower abdominal quadrant. A small incision then is made in the skin, usually at the inferior margin of the umbilicus. The laparoscope trocar and cannula are introduced through this incision into the peritoneal cavity; the trocar then is withdrawn and replaced by the laparoscope.

Many manipulating and operating instruments can be safely introduced into the peritoneal cavity through a second smaller trocar under direct visual guidance. These are used for palpation, manipulation, and exposure of intraabdominal organs. Insulated instruments capable of applying a high-frequency cutting or coagulating current are used for hemostasis, lysis of adhesions, and procedures such as tubal sterilization. Biopsy forceps and combined suction coagulation instruments can be used for safe and accurate tissue sampling as indicated.

Laparoscopy is indicated (1) to evaluate liver disease, (2) to solve abdominal diagnostic problems, and (3) to determine the stage of a malignant disease. Liver biopsies performed under direct vision using the laparoscope are superior to blind liver biopsies in diagnosing and ascertaining the stage of chronic liver disease, primary and metastatic hepatic cancer, and lymphomas. In addition, laparoscopy is a valuable technique for performing certain invasive roentgenographic procedures.

Hepatic radionuclide imaging

Disease within or adjacent to the liver is often difficult to detect and is even more difficult to localize accurately. Hepatic radionuclide imaging is a fairly sensitive noninvasive technique for detecting and localizing a pathologic condition within or adjacent to the liver. Several available radioactive-labeled colloids are taken up by the liver after being injected intravenously. Rose bengal sodium I 131 is concentrated in hepatocytes and is excreted through the biliary tract. In contrast, gold Au 198, iodinated I 131 human serum albumin aggregated, and technetium Tc 99m sulfur colloid are sequestered by the reticuloendothelial cells (Kupffer's cells). Hepatic lesions that replace or displace normal liver tissue usually appear as an area of diminished activity (Fig. 171-1). A lesion must be at least 2 cm before it can be detected and larger if it is located deep within the hepatic parenchyma.

Hepatic scans are useful for detecting a hepatic tumor (primary or secondary) (Fig. 171-1), abscess, or traumatic injury to the liver. In addition, with hepatic scans the clinician can follow such lesions at various intervals to evaluate the response to appropriate therapy. The liver scan is a poor test for detecting hepatic involvement in systemic disease, however, because the results are unreliable in this context. The scan is of little value in patients with cirrhosis because it often exhibits many small filling defects; it may be useful, however, in demonstrating a change in the liver or the presence of splenomegaly. Hepatic scans are probably indicated in patients suspected of having hepatomegaly or splenomegaly.

A filling defect noted on a liver scan does not indicate whether the lesion is solid or cystic or whether it is an abscess, tumor, or area of trauma. Liver scanning with gallium citrate Ga 67 can distinguish a primary tumor from a secondary tumor because it is taken up by viable hepatoma cells but not by metastatic tumor cells. In addition, a pyogenic hepatic abscess concentrates Ga 67, but an amebic abscess does not.

HEPATOBILIARY TREE

Obstruction of the hepatobiliary tree (biliary tract) by either malignant or benign disease commonly requires surgical intervention. The aim of the clinician is to determine the presence, location, and cause of an extrahepatic biliary obstruction, which often cannot easily be differentiated from cholestatic (medical) jaundice by its symptoms, signs, or liver function tests. Roentgenographic studies such as the oral cholecystogram or intravenous cholangiogram cannot achieve a complete view of the biliary tree when the serum bilirubin exceeds a certain level, even if no obstruction is present. The ideal diagnostic test should therefore differentiate patients with cholestatic jaundice from those with extrahepatic biliary tract obstruction, should accurately detect the site of obstruction, and should achieve a complete view of the biliary tree even in the presence of high serum bilirubin levels. Ultrasonography and computed tomography, discussed in later sections, may demonstrate the presence of dilated intrahepatic and extrahepatic ducts, a di-

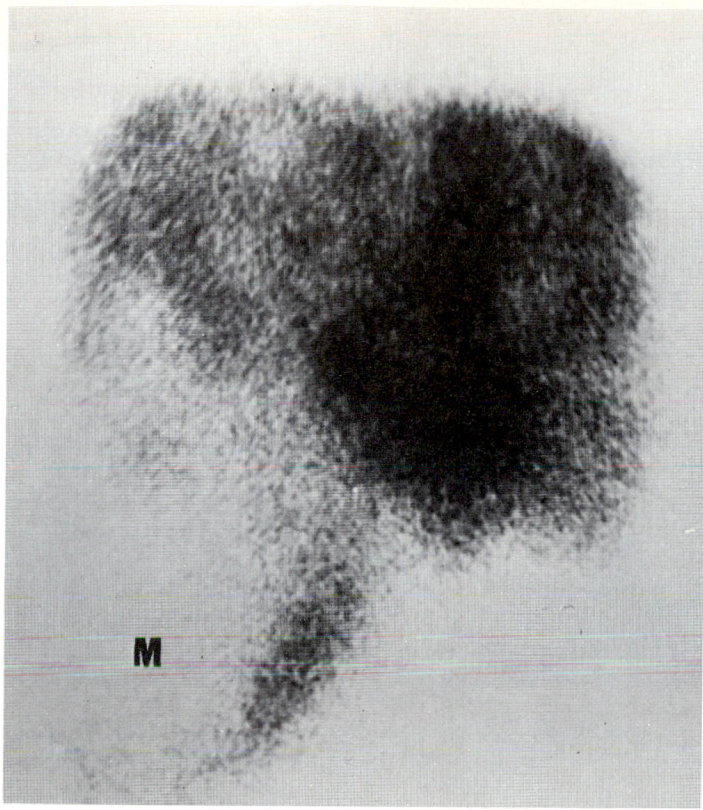

Fig. 171-1   Liver scan with technetium Tc 99m sulfur colloid reveals multiple defects owing to metastatic colon carcinoma. Large metastatic mass *(M)* has replaced much of right lobe. (Courtesy of George Popky, MD.)

lated gallbladder, gallstones, and enlargement of the head of the pancreas, but the usefulness of these techniques often is limited.

Diagnostic tests that fulfill the above criteria have recently become available. The transhepatic cholangiogram using the very fine Chiba needle and endoscopic retrograde cannulation of the pancreaticobiliary tree (ERCP) are especially useful. In addition ^{99m}Tc-HIDA and ^{99m}Tc-PIPIDA (paraisopropyl iminodiacetic acid) scans, which permit noninvasive radionuclide imaging of the hepatobiliary tree, are helpful in many cases.

Transhepatic cholangiography with the Chiba needle

Transhepatic cholangiography using the Chiba needle is performed with fluoroscopic guidance. The needle is passed into the liver and is slowly withdrawn while contrast dye is slowly injected through it. When a biliary duct is visualized, the rest of the contrast dye is injected rapidly until the entire biliary tree is opacified, and then the needle is rapidly withdrawn.

This procedure allows visualization of the biliary tract even in the presence of deep jaundice. Other advantages are that it does not require specialized equipment or extensive clinical experience, it is readily available in most hospitals, and it commonly identifies the site and type of obstruction. Before the procedure is performed, the patient's coagulation profile should be satisfactory (as is required for a liver biopsy). The procedure's complication rate (of bleeding, bile peritonitis, and perforation of the gallbladder) is at least 10%. Most gastroenterologists consider this test a preoperative procedure and before performing it consult with a surgeon and prepare an operating room.

In addition to its diagnostic value, several innovative ther-

apeutic applications of the procedure have been developed recently. These include the decompression of the biliary tree in patients who have a malignant obstruction, the insertion of endoprostheses for internal biliary tract drainage, and dislodgment of stones from the common duct.

Endoscopic retrograde cannulation of the biliary tree

Endoscopic retrograde cannulation of the pancreaticobiliary tree is performed with a side-viewing endoscope. This is passed into the duodenum, and the ampulla of Vater is visualized. A cannula is passed via the endoscope through the ampulla into the common duct, and contrast dye is injected through the cannula while fluoroscopy detects and monitors the opacification of the biliary and pancreatic ducts (Fig. 171-2). When the ductal systems of the pancreas and biliary tract have been amply opacified, the cannula is withdrawn, the endoscope is removed, and roentgenograms are obtained. This technique demands considerable expertise and sophisticated equipment.

A therapeutic role for the procedure has been developed. Side-viewing endoscopes now have been refined to permit the endoscopist to remove stones from the common duct after performing a sphincterotomy. Also, stents can be placed endoscopically in the common duct to relieve obstruction or strictures.

HIDA and PIPIDA imaging

^{99m}Tc-HIDA *N,N'*-[dimethylphenylcarbamolymethyl]iminodiacetic acid) and ^{99m}Tc-PIPIDA (paraisopropyl iminodiacetic acid) have recently been used for imaging of the hepatobiliary tree. These agents are taken up by the hepatocytes and excreted into the biliary tree where they are concentrated and thus can

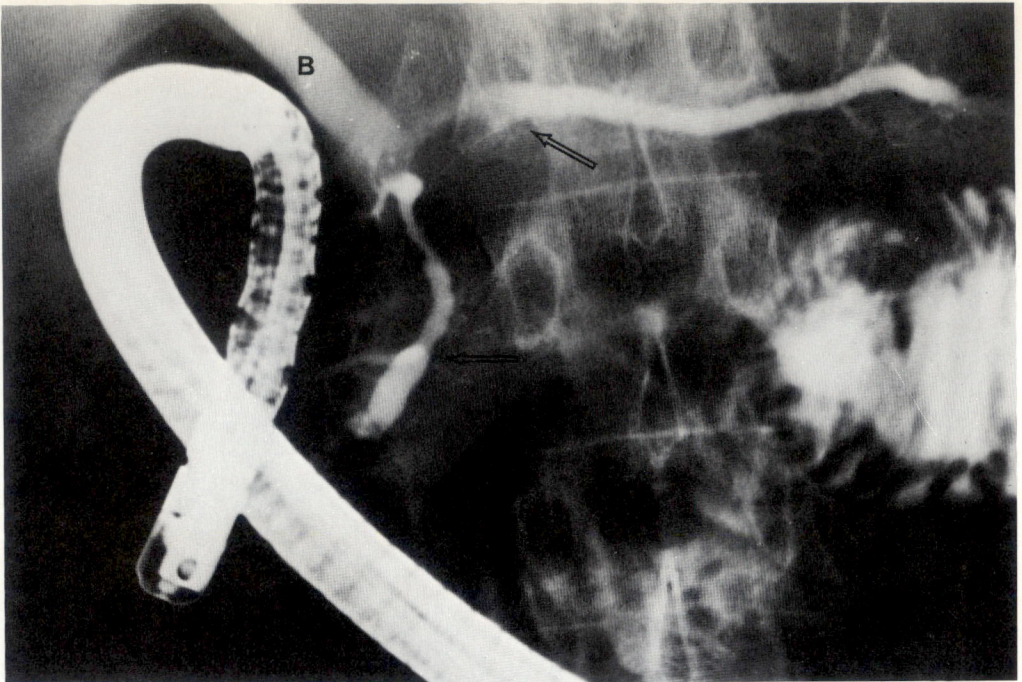

Fig. 171-2   ERCP reveals infiltration and displacement of main pancreatic duct *(between arrows)* by carcinoma of pancreas. *B* denotes partially emptied common bile duct. (Courtesy of Harvey Lefton, MD.)

detect a site of obstruction. This test enables the clinician to distinguish between intrahepatic and extrahepatic jaundice by noninvasive techniques and is an excellent means of diagnosing cystic duct obstruction in patients suspected of having acute cholecystitis.

PANCREAS

Until recently it has been difficult to study the pancreas without resorting to invasive tests such as angiography. Ultrasonographic examination and computed tomography are noninvasive tests currently available for assessing pancreatic disease. The pancreatic ducts also can be studied directly with the endoscopic retrograde cannulation technique outlined previously, and the very fine Chiba needle can be passed transabdominally under fluoroscopic control into the pancreas to obtain tissue for cytologic analysis.

Endoscopic retrograde cannulation of the pancreatic ductal tree

Endoscopic retrograde cannulation can be performed with the main pancreatic duct in the same manner as with the common bile duct (Fig. 171-2). In addition, some endoscopists have advocated flushing the pancreatic ductal system with saline to obtain secretions for cytologic analysis and to determine carcinoembryonic antigen levels, but the results have been disappointing. ERCP has a greater degree of specificity than computed tomography scan in detecting pancreatic structural abnormalities of the pancreatic duct.

Pancreatic biopsy

In the literature pancreatic biopsy is said to be dangerous and unreliable even though morbidity and mortality figures have not been cited. Some surgeons recommend resecting an apparent pancreatic malignancy after surgical inspection and palpation alone, even though 3% to 25% of such lesions turn out to be benign. Because the mortality for pancreatic resection is approximately 22% and the 5-year survival rate after surgery for pancreatic carcinoma is less than 1%, the operative risk does not seem justified if there is no histologic proof of malignancy.

The diagnosis of pancreatic cancer and the choice of appropriate therapy require histologic confirmation. Noninvasive diagnostic tests such as computed tomography and ultrasonography and invasive diagnostic tests such as angiography and endoscopic retrograde cholangiopancreatography can locate disease and masses in the pancreas and may suggest their malignant nature, but these tests do not provide histologic proof.

Preoperative pancreatic biopsy tissue can be obtained during endoscopic retrograde cholangiopancreatography or by percutaneous fine needle aspiration using an imaging technique. In the former technique, material can be aspirated from the pancreatic duct through the cannula, or a brush can be inserted into the pancreatic duct to obtain cytologic specimens. The yield with this technique appears to be good, and the technique is quite safe. In the fine needle aspiration techinque, the mass is located by an imaging technique such as endoscopic retrograde cholangiopancreatography, angiography, ultrasonography, or computed tomography. A point on the skin perpendicular to the lesion is identified, and a thin needle (20 to 23 gauge) 10 to 15 cm long is introduced through this site after appropriate local preparation. This needle is then passed transabdominally into the mass. Cytologic specimens are aspirated by applying suction to the attached syringe while moving the needle up and down in the mass. The yield from this technique is good, and the procedure is relatively safe. Several authors suggest that endoscopic retrograde cholangiopancreatography and fine needle aspiration should be used in patients with suspected cancer in the tail or body of the pancreas because these patients do not require a bypass operation. For patients with suspected cancer in the head of the pancreas, however, the

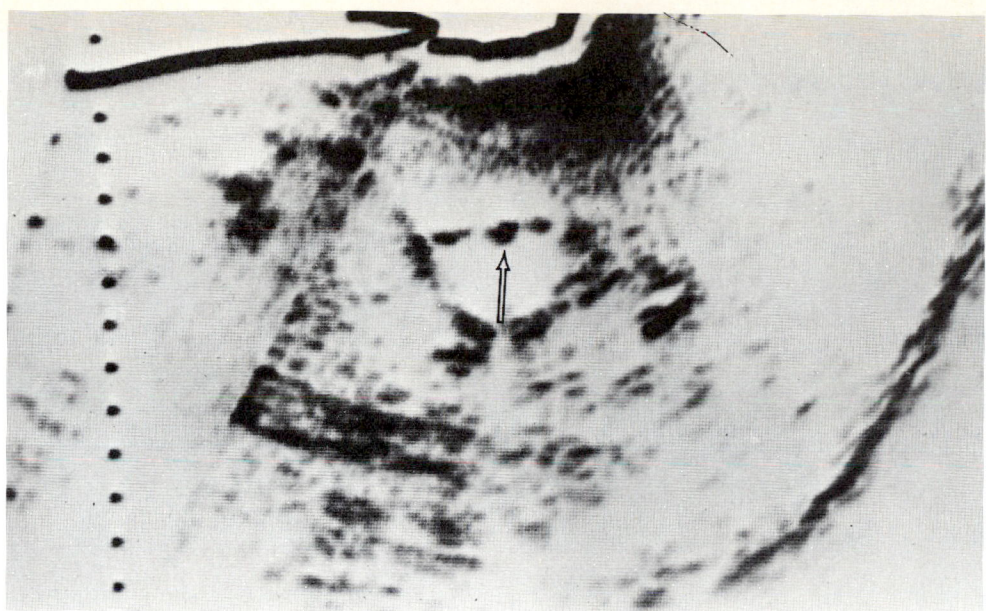

Fig. 171-3 Ultrasonography of gallbladder reveals presence of three "floating" gallstones *(arrow)*. (Courtesy of George Popky, MD.)

intraoperative biopsy technique is more applicable because these require a bypass procedure.

OTHER DIAGNOSTIC METHODS

The use of ultrasonography, computed tomography, and angiography in the past decade has greatly improved the roentgenographic diagnosis of digestive disorders; such diagnosis is far superior to that achieved with conventional barium studies alone.

Abdominal ultrasonography

Ultrasound is a mechanical vibration of a frequency in the range above human hearing (greater than 20,000 Hz) produced by applying an electrical pulse to a transducer. When a pulse of ultrasonic energy is reflected from an interface in the abdomen to the transducer, a minute voltage change is produced that is amplified, processed, and converted into an image on the screen of an ultrasonic scanner. A tissue interface occurs between tissues of different composition. Ultrasonic imaging does not require organ function, and thus a nonfunctioning organ can be visualized as adequately as a functioning one. Because gas and barium sulfate strongly reflect sound, an ultrasonogram cannot be made of a gas- or barium-filled bowel.

ULTRASONIC DIAGNOSIS OF PANCREATIC DISEASE. A normal pancreas often cannot be visualized by ultrasonography. The area of the pancreas, however, can be defined precisely because of its close relationship to the splenic and portal veins, which are visible with ultrasonography in most patients. In acute pancreatitis an enlarged and edematous pancreas is visible ultrasonically as an almost echo-free band running across the abdomen 2 cm anterior to the aorta and inferior vena cava. A pancreatic pseudocyst may be shown as a single or multilocular echo-free area. Serial ultrasonograms are a noninvasive means of detecting the rupture, migration, or resolution of the pseudocyst. An ultrasonogram showing chronic pancreatitis is similar to that showing acute pancreatitis except when fibrosis or calcification is present and obscures the ultrasonic outline of the pancreas. Pancreatic carcinoma appears as a localized enlargement with few internal echoes, a ragged margin, and the attenuation or obliteration of retropancreatic organs such as the aorta. Ultrasonography can reveal only carcinomas at least 2 to 3 cm in size. An ultrasonogram of the pancreas can usually differentiate pancreatitis from pancreatic carcinoma.

ULTRASONIC DIAGNOSIS IN THE LIVER AND BILIARY TREE. Ultrasonography of the gallbladder is performed after an overnight fast because the gallbladder is then at its maximal size. Once the gallbladder has been ultrasonographically identified, its long axis is scanned. Gallstones, detected in over 90% of patients with cholelithiasis, are characterized by strong linear echoes near the posterior wall and a marked attenuation of the sound beam posterior to them (Fig. 171-3). Dilated intrahepatic and extrahepatic biliary tracts, including the common bile duct, are visualized as enlarged echo-free areas on ultrasonograms. Intrahepatic mass lesions such as cysts, primary or metastatic malignancy, and cirrhosis can be demonstrated by ultrasonograms, but ultrasonography probably is not the best diagnostic tool for this purpose.

ULTRASONIC DIAGNOSIS OF INTRAABDOMINAL ABSCESSES. Ultrasonic examination of the abdomen is an excellent method for diagnosing intraabdominal abscesses; ultrasonography demonstrates abscesses directly and has a level of accuracy over 95%. The abscess appears as an echo-free zone with sharply defined walls. In addition its relationship to other organs and the skin surface can be plotted, and its size can be measured in three dimensions. Abscesses must be distinguished, however, from normal fluid-filled structures, especially the gallbladder.

ULTRASONIC DETECTION OF ASCITES AND OTHER INTRAPERITONEAL FLUIDS. Ascites, except when it is loculated by intraperitoneal adhesions, collects in dependent portions of the peritoneal cavity, especially in the hepatorenal space. The depth of the fluid layer in the most dependent part of the abdomen can be measured by an ultrasonogram; layers of fluid as little as 1 cm deep can be detected by this method. Other free intraperitoneal fluids, however, such as peritoneal

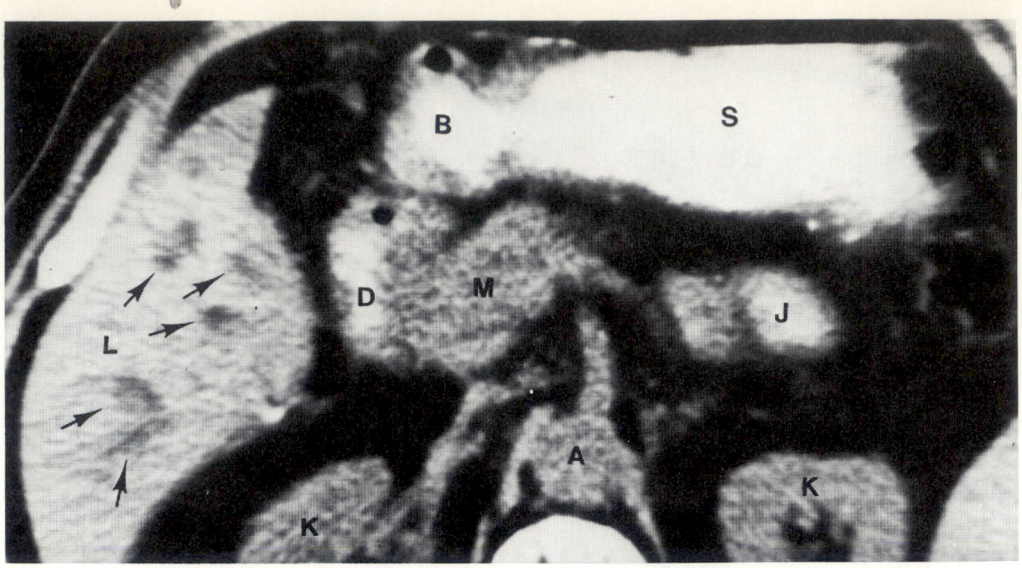

Fig. 171-4   CT scan of abdomen in jaundiced patient reveals large mass *(M)* in head of pancreas and probably dilated ducts *(arrows)* within liver *(L)*. Also identifiable are contrast-filled stomach *(S)*, duodenal bulb *(B)*, descending duodenum *(D)*, loop of jejunum *(J)*, aorta *(A)*, and kidneys *(K)*. (Courtesy of George Popky, MD.)

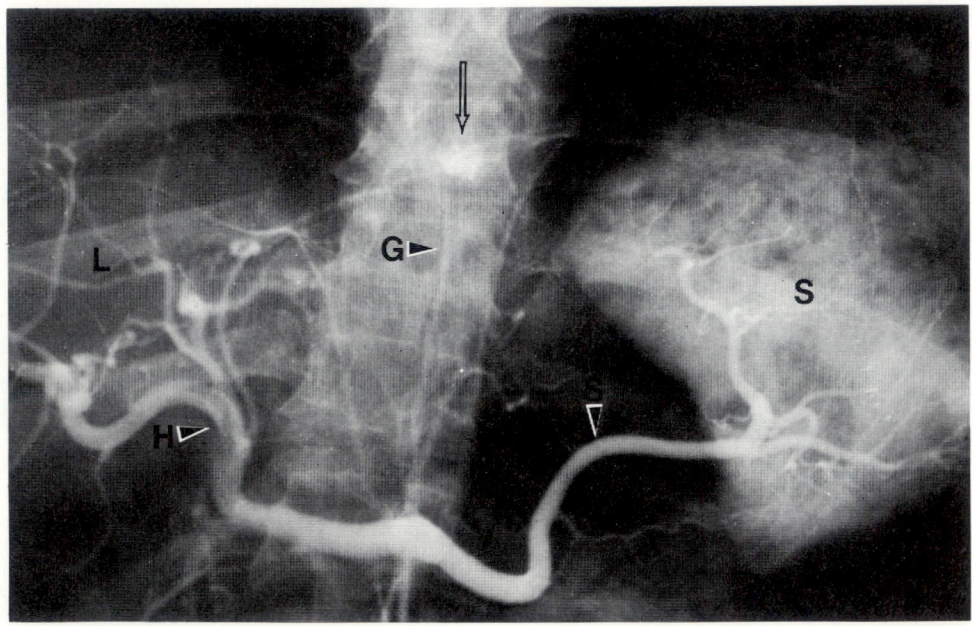

Fig. 171-5   Angiography performed through celiac axis of patient with gastrointestinal bleeding reveals intraluminal collection of contrast material *(upper arrow)* that arises from left gastric artery *(arrow at G)* and accumulates at esophagogastric junction. Hemorrhage at this site was due to Mallory-Weiss tear. Splenic artery is denoted by arrow at *S,* hepatic artery by arrow at *H,* spleen by S, and liver by *L.* (Courtesy of Linda Griska, MD.)

dialysates and blood, cannot be distinguished from ascites by their ultrasonic properties.

OTHER INDICATIONS FOR ULTRASONOGRAPHY. Ultrasonography can be used to localize lesions accurately for needle aspiration and radiotherapy planning and to estimate an organ's volume.

Computed tomography

Computed tomography (CT scanning) is a roentgenographic technique that records minor differences in roentgen ray ab-

sorption and records an image by computer processing of roentgen rays transmitted through the body. Anatomic definition by CT scanning is more precise than that achieved by ultrasonography, but the equipment is extremely expensive and the radiation dose is substantial. Intestinal gas does not interfere with abdominal CT scanning, but the absence of fat impairs the quality of the scan. CT scans are used in the detection of (1) liver metastases, cysts, and abscesses, (2) pancreatitis and pancreatic carcinoma (Fig. 171-4), and (3) biliary tract obstruction. Parenchymatous disease of the liver cannot be defined clearly by CT scanning. In many cases CT scanning and ultrasonography are complementary diagnostic examinations. CT scanning can identify intraabdominal and extraperitoneal masses. It can also locate intraabdominal abscesses and guide percutaneous drainage and stent placement.

Visceral angiography

The ability to perform selective catheterization and the subsequent magnification of intraabdominal blood vessels has dramatically improved the diagnostic capability of visceral angiography (Fig. 171-5). Therapeutic capabilities have been developed for visceral angiography as well. The selective occlusion of vessels can be accomplished through an arterial catheter for the control of gastrointestinal bleeding, preoperative devascularization of tumors, and treatment of arteriovenous malformations. Techniques of pharmacoangiography, the injection of drugs through an arterial catheter, can be used to enhance opacification, differentiate between normal and tumor vessels, control gastrointestinal bleeding, and treat hepatic metastases.

With the introduction of ultrasonography and CT scanning it has been necessary to reevaluate the role of visceral angiography in the diagnosis of tumors of the pancreas and liver. Visceral angiography of the pancreas cannot readily differentiate pancreatic carcinoma from chronic pancreatitis or detect pancreatic carcinoma in a curable stage. Ultrasonography and CT scanning are superior to pancreatic visceral angiography in these conditions. On the other hand, hepatic visceral angiography is superior to ultrasonography and CT scanning in the diagnosis of vascular tumors of the liver such as angiomas, hemangioendotheliomas, benign hepatic adenomas, and most primary hepatomas. Metastatic disease involving the liver, however, is better diagnosed by radionuclide scanning, ultrasonography, or CT scanning. In such instances angiography should be reserved for special situations in which the results from the other tests cannot determine the diagnosis. Although visceral angiography is an excellent method for diagnosing splenic and hepatic ruptures, peritoneal lavage should be performed to detect intraperitoneal bleeding before visceral angiography; peritoneal lavage often eliminates the need for angiography. Visceral angiography, like endoscopy of the gastrointestinal tract, is indicated for both localization and therapy in the management of patients with acute gastrointestinal bleeding. The intraarterial infusion of vasopressin is effective in controlling gastric mucosal bleeding, bleeding esophageal varices, and colonic diverticular bleeding.

BIBLIOGRAPHY

Bruguera M, Bordas JM, and Rodes J: Atlas of laparoscopy and biopsy in the liver, Philadelphia, 1979, WB Saunders Co.
Bureharth F, Jensen LI, and Olesen K: Endoprosthesis for internal drainage of the biliary tract: technique and results in 48 cases, Gastroenterology 77:133, 1979.
Chaudhurt TK: Gastrointestinal imaging with radionuclides. In Freeman LM and Weissman HS, editors: Nuclear medicine annual, New York, 1983, Raven Press.
Demling L: Recent advances in gastrointestinal endoscopy, Am J Gastroenterol 69:533, 1978.
Gudjonsson B and Spiro HM: Biopsy techniques in the diagnosis of pancreatic cancer, Gastroenterology 75:726, 1978.
Kreek JMJ and Balint JA: "Skinny needle" cholangiography: results of a pilot study of a voluntary prospective method for gathering risk data on new procedures, Gastroenterology 78:598, 1980.
Malmud LS and Fisher RS: Scintigraphic evaluation of disorders of the esophagus, stomach, and duodenum, Med Clin North Am 65:1291, 1981.
Ogoshi K and others: Endoscopic pancreaticocholangiography in the evaluation of pancreatic and biliary disease, Gastroenterology 64:210, 1973.
Perrault J and others: Liver biopsy: complications in 1000 patients and outpatients, Gastroenterology 74:103, 1978.
Sleisenger MJ and Fordtran JS: Gastrointestinal disease, ed 2, Philadelphia, 1978, WB Saunders Co.
Tolin RD and others: Enterogastric reflux in normal subjects and patients with Billroth II gastroenterostomy: measurements of enterogastric reflux, Gastroenterology 77:1027, 1979.
Wolff WL and others: Colonofiberoscopy: a new and valuable diagnostic modality, Am J Surg 123:130, 1972.

172 · DISORDERS OF THE ESOPHAGUS

Harris R. Clearfield

CLINICAL ANATOMY

The esophagus is a muscular tube that propels the contents of the pharynx to the stomach. It has no significant secretory or absorptive functions. Sphincters surround the pharyngoesophageal and gastroesophageal junctions and normally are closed until swallowing occurs. The distance from the incisor teeth to the upper esophageal sphincter in the adult is approximately 15 to 18 cm. The distance from the incisor teeth to the lower esophageal sphincter varies with the individual's height; it averages 40 cm in men and 37 cm in women. The esophageal diameter usually is 1.5 to 2.5 cm. Pressure on the esophagus may occur from structures in close proximity such as the thyroid gland, aortic arch, tracheal bifurcation, and left atrium. These relationships can be important, since an aneurysm of the descending aorta can push the esophagus anteriorly and enlargement of the left atrium can force the esophagus posteriorly.

The musculature of the upper third of the esophagus is striated, the middle third has variable amounts of striated and smooth muscle, and the lower third is entirely smooth muscle. This muscle distribution determines the expression of certain diseases. Scleroderma, for instance, involves only the smooth muscle of the middle and distal thirds.

Ordinarily the esophagus is lined with squamous epithelium, which extends to the esophagogastric junction, where it joins the columnar epithelium of the stomach approximately 1 to 2 cm above the diaphragm. This junction is easily seen endoscopically, since the pale color of the squamous epithelium forms a sharply demarcated line with the salmon-colored columnar epithelium. Chronic reflux esophagitis can result in proximal migration of the columnar epithelium, producing a condition known as Barrett's esophagus. In contrast to the rest of the gastrointestinal tract, the esophagus lacks a serosal layer, thus giving rise to the difficulties with esophageal surgery such as anastomotic leaks.

PHYSIOLOGY OF THE ESOPHAGUS
Swallowing

For a liquid or solid bolus to be swallowed, the airway must be protected and the upper esophageal sphincter (UES), which normally is closed, must open synchronously to accept the transfer. The sphincter is a high-pressure zone between the pharynx and the body of the esophagus. Although a discrete muscular sphincter cannot be identified, it appears to correlate closely with the cricopharyngeus muscle. Once past the UES the bolus is propelled by a peristaltic wave that begins at the cricopharyngeus and travels distally at a rate of approximately 3 to 5 cm/sec. The lower esophageal sphincter (LES) relaxes with the initiation of swallowing and is prepared for the passage. A dry swallow initiates the same series of events. Coordination of the muscular activity in the pharynx and UES responsible for swallowing is controlled by impulses from the ninth and tenth cranial nerves. If central or peripheral pathology interferes with the neurologic control, choking or coughing can result from deviation of the pharyngeal contents into the airway. Primary peristalsis refers to the peristaltic wave initiated by swallowing, whereas secondary peristalsis, which also propels the bolus distally towards the stomach, originates in the esophagus at a point where food or liquid has not been totally propelled by the initial peristaltic event or has refluxed back into the esophagus from the stomach.

Lower esophageal sphincter

Although no specific band of circular muscle can be identified anatomically or histologically as the LES, certain circular muscle fibers at the lower end of the esophagus have specialized physiologic and pharmacologic responses. The function of this sphincter is measured by manometric techniques, which involve placing perfused polyethylene tubes at 5 cm intervals and measuring the pressure changes above, below, and in the sphincteric area. In resting conditions the LES remains closed and is seen as a high-pressure zone that separates the fundic pressure, slightly positive when compared to the atmospheric pressure, from the intraesophageal body pressure, which is slightly negative in relation to atmospheric pressure. Normal LES pressures are between 10 and 20 mm Hg. The LES relaxes with swallowing but rebounds after the peristaltic wave reaches the sphincter, resulting in a return to baseline pressure. The LES resting pressure seems to be largely determined by the intrinsic muscle tone, which in turn is influenced by distinct responses from adjacent fibers of the esophageal body or gastric fundus and by neural cholinergic impulses. There also may be a role for modification of postprandial LES pressure by gastrin and other hormones.

SYMPTOMS OF ESOPHAGEAL DISEASE

Because the esophagus is inaccessible for physical examination, the history is important in establishing a diagnosis. Fortunately, the symptoms usually are quite helpful in localizing the pathology and estimating the severity of the disorder, as best shown with dysphagia and heartburn.

Dysphagia

Dysphagia is a compelling symptom, since it always requires investigation and refers to difficulty in swallowing. If the patient localizes the holdup of the solid or liquid bolus to the lower sternum, the pathology probably is in the distal third of the esophagus. Cervical and midsternal dysphagia may represent pathology in the upper or mid esophagus, but lower third abnormalities also may induce proximal symptoms resulting from motility disturbances.

The symptom reflects inability of a bolus to move easily from the esophagus into the stomach. A patient who has difficulty with steak or apples but can eat softer food has mild to moderate dysphagia. One who can tolerate only liquids has severe dysphagia. The progression from mild to severe dysphagia is seen in disorders in which the lumen is slowly narrowed, such as in carcinoma and reflux esophagitis, whereas the acute onset of severe dysphagia suggests esophageal spasm or a lower esophageal ring.

Odynophagia refers to painful swallowing. The cause can be obvious, such as acute tonsillitis, but esophagitis of any cause can induce substernal pain upon swallowing. It is en-

countered in patients receiving antibiotics, radiation, or chemotherapy, and moniliasis should always be considered in these settings.

Heartburn

Heartburn would seem to be a symptom easily recognized by the general public and medical professionals alike. Unfortunately, the symptom often is misinterpreted by both. Heartburn refers to epigastric or low substernal pain that is often but not always burning in character and that radiates upward into the chest. It occurs most often after meals or when recumbent, bending over, straining at stool, or coughing. Patients frequently describe indigestion (localized epigastric discomfort without chest radiation) as heartburn, whereas physicians may interpret localized substernal pain as heartburn. The symptom frequently generates humorous comments, but recurrent heartburn is a serious matter, since reflux esophagitis with its attendant bleeding and dysphagia is not a minor problem.

Chest pain

Esophageal motility disorders such as esophageal spasm can produce anterior chest pain that could easily be confused with cardiac disease. Approximately 15% of patients with clinical angina pectoris are not found to have cardiac pathology, and esophageal disorders should be considered in this group. Esophagitis also can produce chest pain, but the relationship to meals and relief with antacids usually makes the differentiation less difficult.

Globus hystericus

Patients may complain of a "lump" or "tightness" in the throat, localizing these symptoms to the cervical area. The discomfort usually is caused by spasm of the cricopharyngeus muscle at the superior esophageal sphincter. Dysphagia does not occur, the patient does not cough or vomit while eating, and the symptom usually can be seen as a reflection of an anxiety reaction. Appropriate diagnostic studies should be done, however, to rule out organic disease and reassure the patient.

Bad taste in the mouth

Patients may complain of a persistent "bad" or bitter taste in the mouth. If examination of the mouth reveals no organic disease and if drugs known to produce a disagreeable taste (metronidazole, anticholinergic therapy) can be excluded, a psychogenic cause should be considered. It is uncommon for esophageal reflux to cause this symptom, but the clinician also should consider the rare patient with a Zenker's diverticulum who may complain of a bad taste before dysphagia occurs.

DIAGNOSTIC STUDIES
Barium upper gastrointestinal roentgenogram

The barium upper gastrointestinal roentgenogram provides an appraisal of the esophageal, gastric, and duodenal mucosa. The ability to detect superficial esophageal erosions and inflammation previously was limited, but currently double-contrast techniques (barium and air) provide more detailed mucosal assessment. This type of roentgenogram is excellent for demonstrating hiatal hernias and obstructing lesions and may provide useful information about peristalsis and esophageal spasm. Gastroesophageal reflux, if moderate to severe, can be detected during the examination. A skilled radiologist is needed to perform the study properly. The barium upper gastrointestinal roentgenogram does not distinguish benign from malignant obstructing lesions and has poor sensitivity for demonstrating early esophagitis, Barrett's esophagus, and motility disorders.

Upper gastrointestinal endoscopy

The fiberoptic endoscope provides direct visualization of the esophagus, stomach, and duodenum. Biopsies of abnormal areas are easily obtained, and early esophagitis can be detected. The procedure cannot demonstrate esophageal spasm or other motility disorders and is not helpful for demonstrating gastroesophageal reflux. In general, it provides more definitive mucosal information, and many would suggest that it be the procedure of choice for investigating substernal pain, heartburn, and dysphagia. The procedure costs approximately twice as much as the barium roentgenogram, and there is a small risk of complications such as esophagogastric perforation or adverse cardiopulmonary events. The decision on endoscopy versus roentgenogram should be based on a thorough clinical evaluation; for example, a barium study could suffice for a patient with troublesome heartburn, whereas endoscopy should be considered if heartburn is associated with dysphagia.

Esophageal motility

The esophageal motility study provides information about peristalsis, spasm, and sphincter function. As previously noted, it is performed by measuring pressures in the esophagus and stomach as sensed through perfused polyvinyl tubes positioned 5 cm apart. The examination is best used in patients with unexplained substernal chest pain, searching for evidence of esophageal spasm and its variants, and when achalasia or scleroderma is suspected. Although the lower esophageal sphincter pressure can be measured, the study is not particularly useful in evaluating gastroesophageal reflux disease. Esophageal motility studies have considerable research value in the investigation of esophageal physiology and the effects of various drugs on the normal and diseased esophagus.

Acid perfusion test

The instillation of 0.1N HCl into the body of the esophagus produces no symptoms in the normal patient. If the perfusion reproduces the patient's substernal discomfort, a diagnosis of esophagitis is likely. The impression is strengthened if the acid-induced pain is abolished by saline infusion and recurs when acid is readministered. The test is useful for distinguishing between esophageal spasm and inflammatory conditions.

Acid reflux recordings

The esophagus normally has a pH of approximately 7, but acid reflux from the stomach can lower the pH quickly and dramatically. If a diagnosis of gastroesophageal reflux disease is uncertain, a pH probe can be placed through the nose into the body of the esophagus and a continuous recording of esophageal pH can be obtained over a period of several hours up to 24 hours, usually with changes in body position noted. This study usually was performed in a hospital setting because of the need for proximity to the recording device, but the recent availability of small, self-contained digitalized monitors worn around the neck and attached to narrow-caliber catheters extending through the nose into the esophagus permits ambulatory recording of continuous pH readings during activity and sleep. This currently is the most accurate appraisal of gastroesophageal reflux.

ESOPHAGEAL INFECTIONS
Viral esophagitis

Viral esophagitis rarely is encountered in the otherwise normal adult, but herpes simplex virus (HSV) may cause the sudden onset of self-limited substernal chest pain and odynophagia in young adults, sometimes associated with herpes labialis. Patients who are immunocompromised from acquired immunodeficiency syndrome (AIDS), radiation, immunosuppressive treatment for organ transplant, chemotherapy, or corticosteroid therapy are at much greater risk for viral esophagitis. HSV and cytomegalovirus (CMV) are most commonly encountered and result in odynophagia. Double-contrast barium studies generally show discrete shallow ulcers that are diffusely scattered. Upper gastrointestinal endoscopy is a more sensitive diagnostic tool and may also show considerable hemorrhage and exudation in more severe cases. The histologic diagnosis of HSV depends on biopsy evidence of ballooning degeneration, multinucleated giant cells, and intranuclear inclusion bodies. In the absence of viral cultures, the diagnosis of CMV infection depends on finding individual cells bearing typical intranuclear and cytoplasmic inclusions. It is important to distinguish if possible between CMV and HSV esophagitis, since the latter responds to the drug acyclovir. Untreated HSV esophagitis in the immunocompromised patient is progressive and may lead to herpetic pneumonia. There is no effective therapy for CMV esophagitis.

Monilia esophagitis

Monilia esophagitis generally does not occur unless the patient harbors a malignancy, is immune suppressed by drugs or AIDS, or has been treated with antibiotics. Although oropharyngeal candidiasis usually is asymptomatic, unless severe disease is present, esophageal involvement is accompanied by odynophagia, substernal discomfort, and perhaps bleeding. The pharynx of susceptible patients should be inspected routinely for the characteristic whitish plaques, but only half of the patients with candida esophagitis have oral involvement. Esophageal involvement can be reasonably suspected by the "shaggy" muscosal appearance seen by barium upper gastrointestinal roentgenogram, but a more secure diagnosis can be achieved with upper gastrointestinal endoscopy, at which time biopsies and brushings of the involved mucosa show the mycelial growth and invasion.

Patients generally respond rapidly to mycostatin oral suspension (500,000 to 1 million units four times daily). Patients resistent to this therapy may benefit from ketoconazole, recognizing that occasional hepatotoxicity has been reported, or amphotericin B. Monilia esophagitis occurring in the presence of antibiotic therapy presents few problems with appropriate therapy, but immune-suppressed patients must be treated intensively, since mucosal invasion and systemic candidiasis may occur.

MOTILITY DISORDERS
Oropharyngeal dysphagia

A variety of degenerative and inflammatory disorders of striated musculature can interfere with the pharyngeal swallowing mechanism. These disorders include dermatomyositis, muscular dystrophy, and myasthenia gravis. Central and peripheral nervous system diseases that also may lead to oropharyngeal dysphagia include cerebrovascular accidents, Parkinson's disease, Huntington's chorea, brainstem tumors, and multiple sclerosis. Some patients have no known associated disease and are said to have cricopharyngeal spasm.

This disorder may occur in association with Zenker's diverticulum.

CLINICAL MANIFESTATIONS. Patients describe difficulty in moving food from the mouth into the cervical esophagus and may experience aspiration if liquid (more commonly than solids) "spills" over into the trachea. Patients who experience coughing during eating should be suspected of this disorder. Asthma, chronic bronchitis, and aspiration pneumonia may occur.

DIAGNOSIS. The initial procedure should be a barium upper gastrointestinal roentgenogram. This may reveal evidence of local pathology such as a Zenker's diverticulum, upper esophageal stricture (benign or malignant), or aspiration, since barium refluxes from the closed cricopharyngeus muscle into the trachea.

An esophageal motility examination should be considerd if the barium roentgenogram is unremarkable. This study may reveal incoordination in the relaxation of the upper esophageal sphincter. Unfortunately, technical problems in the manometric study of the upper sphincter may lead to questionable findings.

MANAGEMENT. Symptoms secondary to systemic disease require treatment of the underlying problem. For instance, myasthenia gravis patients symptomatically improve with appropriate treatment. Unfortunately, many of the diseases that lead to oropharyngeal dysphagia are not easily remedied. Mild symptoms usually are treated symptomatically, but cricopharyngeal myotomy should be considered for patients with evidence of aspiration. Tracheotomy has been used when myotomy cannot be performed or when the result is unsatisfactory.

Diffuse esophageal spasm

Diffuse esophageal spasm (DES), a disorder of middle or older age, can produce substernal pain that may be indistinguishable from angina pectoris. The discomfort is described as "squeezing" or "pressure" and may radiate to the back. Dysphagia may be associated with the pain or may occur independently, and complete obstruction can occur. A barium upper gastrointestinal roentgenogram may demonstrate sacculations and areas of spasm throughout the esophagus ("corkscrew" esophagus); however, asymptomatic patients may show similar findings, whereas individuals with significant symptoms may show no abnormality by roentgenogram (Fig. 172-1). An esophageal motility examination may show high amplitude, nonperistaltic waves. Unfortunately, the symptoms and motility abnormalities often are intermittent, thus a study that reveals no symptoms does not exclude the diagnosis. Provocative tests such as intravenous edrophonium have been tried in an effort to reproduce the pain and motility aberrations, but unfortunately, these efforts succeed in only about one third of patients with DES. Pharmacologic measures currently available such as calcium channel blockers may be helpful to some but are of no benefit to many others. Esophageal dilation and even longitudinal esophageal myotomies have been tried with varying degrees of success. Reassurance and the knowledge that the symptoms usually are intermittent may have to suffice for some patients. If it is difficult to distinguish the symptoms of DES from cardiac disorders, the cardiac evaluation should take precedence.

Nutcracker esophagus

Some patients with midsternal chest pain are found to have peristaltic waves of much higher amplitude than normal in the esophagus. This "nutcracker" phenomenon produces discomfort indistinguishable from DES, and the treatment is similar.

Hypertensive lower esophageal sphincter

High pressure in the lower esophageal sphincter is rare; when it occurs it leads to substernal chest pressure as previously described.

Achalasia

Achalasia is a motility disorder that affects esophageal smooth muscle and the LES. Peristaltic contractions are absent, and the LES fails to relax adequately, leading to dysphagia and its attendant nutritional sequelae. Chest pain is not a dominant symptom but may occur. Dysphagia leads to vomiting and thus to the risk of pulmonary complications secondary to aspiration.

ETIOLOGY. The cause of achalasia is unknown, but neurogenic etiologic factors seem likely. A vagal denervation process has been described and is supported by a decrease (or absence) of ganglion cells in the distal esophagus.

DIAGNOSIS. The diagnosis is suggested by the history of gradually increasing dysphagia, vomiting, and weight loss. An upper gastrointestinal barium examination usually shows absent peristalsis, varying degrees of esophageal dilation (depending on the chronicity of the process), and a narrowed terminal esophagus (Fig. 172-2). If the patient swallows the barium while recumbent, the liquid will remain in the esophagus until the patient sits or stands, at which time it will slowly empty through the narrowed segment. An upper gastrointestinal endoscopy should be performed in all patients with dysphagia. The findings in achalasia are most striking at the lower esophageal sphincter, since gentle pressure with the tip of the fiberscope usually permits entrance into the stomach. The endoscopy also should be performed to exclude the possibility of carcinoma of the distal esophagus or proximal stomach. An esophageal motility examination demonstrates absent peristalsis and a hypertensive LES that relaxes insufficiently with swallowing.

TREATMENT. Pharmacologic efforts to reduce lower esophageal sphincter pressure with calcium channel blocking agents such as nifedipine have had limited success. The most useful approach to uncomplicated achalasia usually is forceful (pneumatic) dilation of the LES with an inflated balloon. The rapid distension is performed to rupture circular muscle fibers and thus reduce the high pressure in the LES. Approximately 50% of patients have a good or excellent response to this approach. A second dilation is offered when the response is inadequate. Patients who derive little benefit from this approach are advised to undergo a Heller-type myotomy, a longitudinal muscle-splitting procedure that begins in the distal esophagus and is carried through the LES into the proximal stomach. Reflux of gastric contents often occurs after dilation and esophageal myotomy.

Scleroderma

Scleroderma is a multiple-system disorder that affects the esophagus in at least 75% of these patients. The esophageal symptoms and peristaltic abnormalities occasionally precede the cutaneous findings. Scleroderma is a fibrosing disease, and in the esophagus it leads to replacement of smooth muscle with collagenous tissue in the mid and distal segments. The LES pressure is decreased and peristalsis is absent in the body of the esophagus. Gastroesophageal reflux secondary to the hypotensive LES occurs. Symptoms include dysphagia and heartburn. The diagnosis is suggested by knowledge of

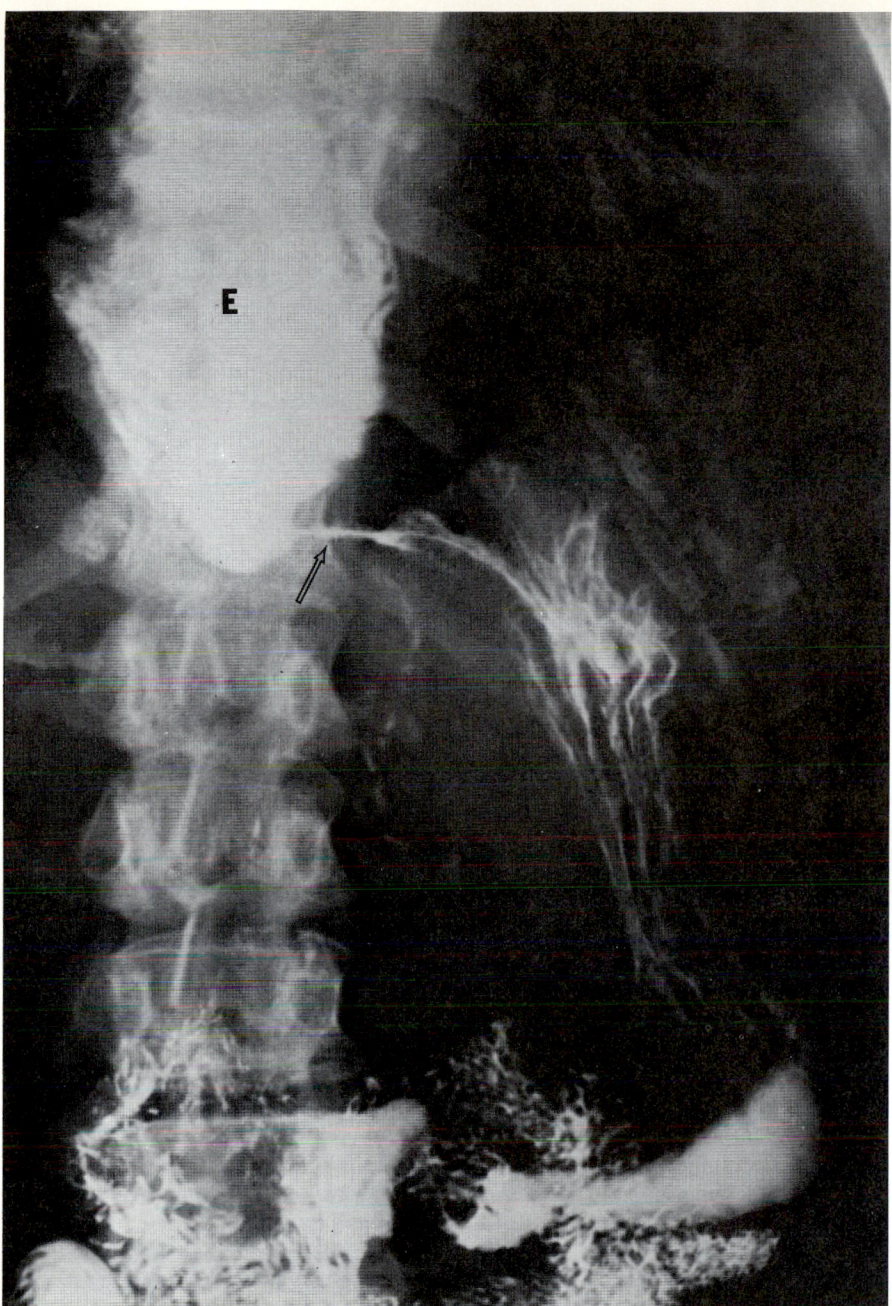

Fig. 172-1 Gastrointestinal series from 72-year-old man with achalasia. Note markedly dilated esophagus *(E)* with retained barium, food, and secretions and symmetrically narrowed distal esophagus *(arrow)*. (Courtesy of George Popky, MD.)

the multiple-system features, the symptoms, an upper gastro-intestinal barium roentgenogram showing absent peristalsis, and a motility examination demonstrating the peristaltic and LES abnormalities outlined above. Unfortunately, there is no effective therapy for scleroderma, but the incidence of reflux esophagitis is sufficiently high that symptomatic patients should be placed on maintenance histamine-2 receptor antagonist therapy.

STRUCTURAL DISORDERS OF THE ESOPHAGUS
Zenker's diverticulum

Pressure builds within the pharynx during the act of swallowing. The cricopharyngeus, playing the dominant role of the superior esophageal sphincter, relaxes to accommodate the bolus. A slight delay in relaxation of the sphincter leads to sufficient pressure in some patients to herniate the mucosa posteriorly between the cricopharyngeus and the inferior constrictor. This beginning diverticulum usually enlarges gradually and descends along the left side of the cervical spine. The enlarging diverticulum may exert pressure on the esophagus, thus narrowing the lumen and producing dysphagia. Regurgitation from the diverticulum may occur hours after the meal, and the undigested nature of the food should suggest the cause. A bad taste and unpleasant breath may occur when food ferments in large diverticula. The diagnosis is best established by an upper gastrointestinal barium roentgenogram. Endoscopy without knowledge of the disorder could lead to perforation. Small asymptomatic diverticula that are detected incidentally

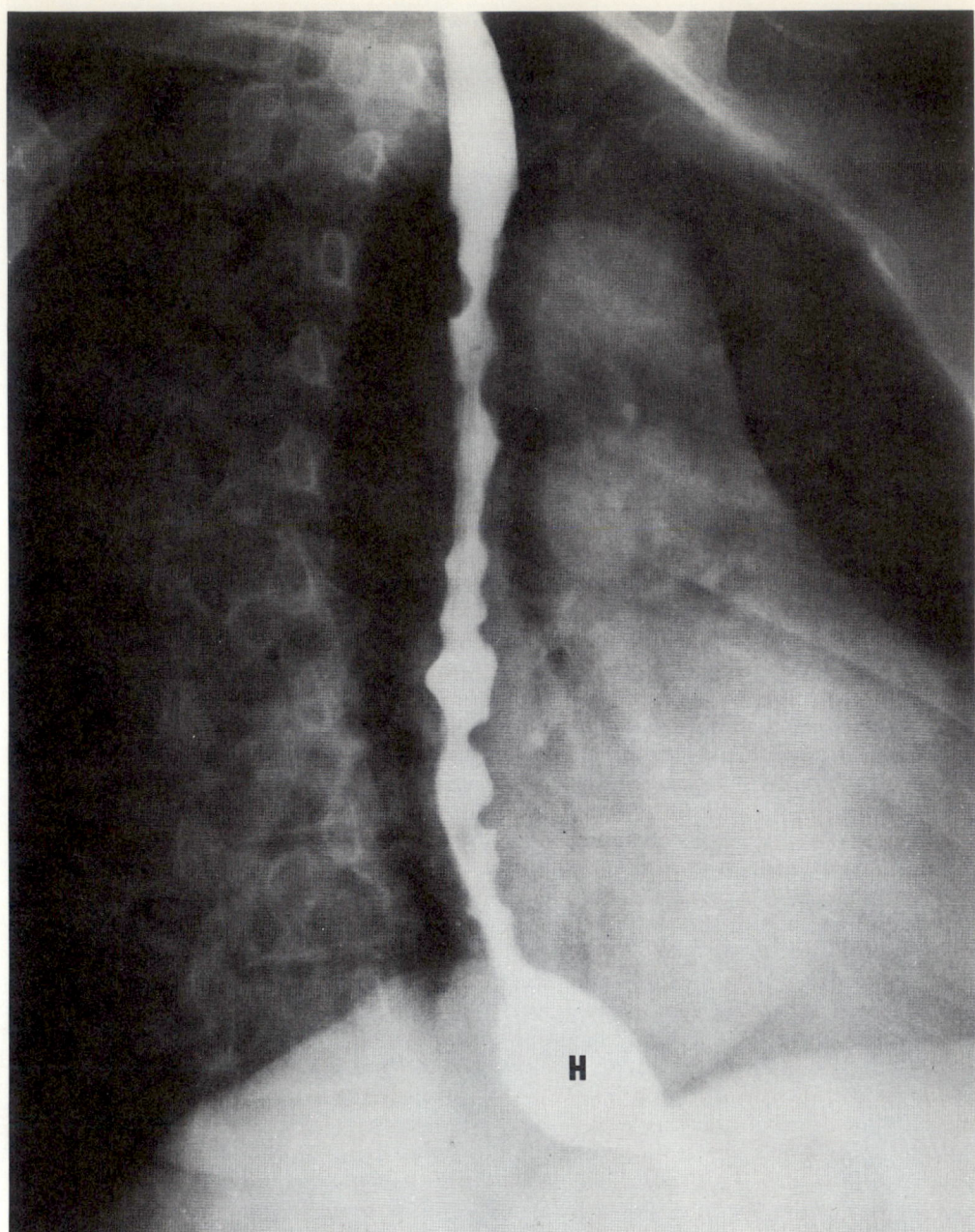

Fig. 172-2 Patient with recurrent episodes of chest pain and dysphagia exhibits "corkscrew" appearance, sacculations, and pseudodiverticula of esophagus, findings indicative of esophageal spasm. He also has hiatus hernia *(H)*. (Courtesy of George Popky, MD.)

by roentgenogram do not require therapy. Symptomatic diverticula can be removed surgically. The excision sometimes is combined with a myotomy of the cricopharyngeus to prevent recurrence.

LOWER ESOPHAGEAL RING

A lower esophageal ring (Schatzki ring) is a circumscribed narrowing usually located at the squamocolumnar junction proximal to a hiatal hernia. It contains little muscle; its interior is composed mainly of lamina propria. Patients with a ring of 20 mm or wider usually have few symptoms. Dysphagia is intermittent when the ring measures between 12 and 20 mm and is more persistent when the lumen is less than 12 mm. The dysphagia usually begins with solid foods, sometimes requiring endoscopic removal of an impacted food bolus. Pro-

gressive narrowing of the ring may reduce the patient to a liquid diet. The diagnosis is best established by an upper gastrointestinal roentgenogram. Upper gastrointestinal endoscopy often is done to search for evidence of esophagitis and to rule out neoplasm, particularly when dysphagia is present. Asymptomatic rings require no treatment, but dysphagia is best managed with esophageal dilation.

GASTROESOPHAGEAL REFLUX DISEASE

Gastroesophageal reflux disease (GERD) refers to inflammation of the esophageal mucosa caused by regurgitation of gastric contents into the esophagus. The symptoms of reflux are common, with one study finding that 7% of normal individuals experienced heartburn daily, twice that number noticed it weekly, and about one third had the symptoms at least once a month. Although attention had been directed toward the presence or absence of a hiatal hernia, it became apparent that the lower esophageal sphincter (LES) and other factors were more important than whether a portion of the proximal stomach had herniated into the chest.

Factors contributing to reflux

1. *LES weakness* (a baseline pressure less than 10 mm Hg) often is found in patients with severe GERD. However, this is not a good predictor for disease, since many patients reflux with normal LES pressures, whereas others with lower pressures may not reflux.

2. *Impaired esophageal clearance* (a delay in peristaltic response to the refluxed gastric contents) allows longer contact time.

3. *Increased volume and acidity of gastric contents* puts acid hypersecretors who reflux at greater risk for mucosal damage.

4. *Increased intraabdominal pressure* caused by constricting garments, obesity, chronic coughing, or straining at stool can influence reflux.

Esophageal histology

Biopsies from normal individuals show that the dermal pegs extend less than 50% of the full thickness of the epithelum and that the basal layer is relatively thin, constituting less than 15% of the mucosal thickness. Patients with reflux show dermal pegs that extend toward the epithelial surface, thickening of the basal epithelial layer, and varying degrees of infiltration of neutrophils.

Symptoms

Heartburn is the dominant symptom. It frequently occurs after meals and with activities such as lying in bed, bending forward, lifting weights, straining, or heavy exertion. It also may be associated with belching. Regurgitation occurs less frequently than heartburn but under similar circumstances. A sour or bitter taste results as gastric contents reflux back into the mouth. A narrowing of the lumen secondary to fibrosis occurs in advanced GERD and may lead to dysphagia. The patient usually experiences symptoms with solids initially, but the process becomes gradually more frequent and severe if untreated. Substernal pain may occur with swallowing (odynophagia) or during periods of reflux. The discomfort may be difficult to distinguish from coronary artery disease. Patients with GERD may experience pulmonary symptoms, particularly at night, if aspiration complicates the reflux process. Asthma, bronchitis, or pneumonia may occur. The ulcerations that may occur with GERD may lead to upper gastrointestinal bleeding. It may present as melena or iron deficiency anemia, but major hemorrhage can occur.

Diagnosis

The history can be sufficiently convincing to establish the diagnosis. Unfortunately, the symptoms may be vague and may present problems in distinguishing them from gastric ulcer, esophageal motility disorders, and cardiac disease. If cardiac disease cannot be excluded on the basis of a history and physical examination, investigation of this possibility takes precedence over esophageal studies.

Upper gastrointestinal barium roentgenogram

The barium roentgenogram may show reflux of barium (and presumably acid) from the stomach into the esophagus, but failure to show this does not exclude GERD. The procedure also can demonstrate moderate to severe degrees of esophagitis, including ulcerations and stricture, but milder degrees of esophagitis often are undetected (Fig. 172-3).

Esophageal pH monitoring

There is little need for esophageal pH monitoring if the symptoms of reflux are convincing, but the test can be quite helpful when the chest symptoms are atypical and the presence of reflux is uncertain. Ambulatory pH monitoring units permit assessment of (1) the number of reflux episodes, (2) how long the acid remains in the esophagus, (3) the relation of the episodes to meals and sleep, and (4) the relation of reflux to symptoms.

Radionuclide scintiscanning

The pH monitoring techniques are the most sensitive for detecting reflux, but they are inconvenient and time-consuming. The barium roentgenogram is convenient and inexpensive but insensitive. The radionuclide scintiscanning technique offers a reasonable compromise, although it does have limitations. The procedure requires graded increases in the pressure within an abdominal binder with interval esophageal imaging to assess reflux. However, the artificial increase in intraabdominal pressure may be a provocative strategy that may not reflect day-to-day events.

Esophageal acid infusion test

The esophageal acid infusion test (Bernstein test) was introduced to determine whether substernal discomfort is related to acid reflux. If substernal pain can be reproduced following infusion of dilute HCl and can be abolished with saline infusion, this reasonably supports esophagitis as the causative mechanism. GERD, however, is not the only cause for esophagitis, since viral, fungal, and chemical esophagitis can produce similar responses.

Esophageal motility examination

The esophageal motility examination generally is not a valuable procedure for clinical study of GERD. The correlation between LES pressures and reflux is not sufficient to justify routine use of the procedure.

Upper gastrointestinal endoscopy

Upper gastrointestinal endoscopy should be considered (1) for patients with moderate to severe symptoms related to GERD, (2) when the diagnosis of GERD is uncertain, and (3) when complications such as stricture or ulceration are present. The procedure also should be performed for the diagnosis and surveillance of Barrett's esophagus. Besides visualizing the pathology, biopsies can be obtained for the diagnosis of esophagitis or malignancy or both.

Barrett's esophagus

Barrett's esophagus refers to either the extension of gastric columnar mucosa into the esophagus or islets of columnar mucosa found in the lower esophagus. This type of mucosal "misplacement" once was thought to be of congenital origin, but it has become clear that it is mainly acquired as a result of reflux esophagitis that leads to proximal extension of gastric epithelium. The columnar epithelium appears to be less able to withstand the chemical and thermal challenges of ingested food, resulting in the full spectrum of esophagitis. The clinical features that distinguish Barrett's esophagitis from GERD are the proximal location of strictures and ulceration,

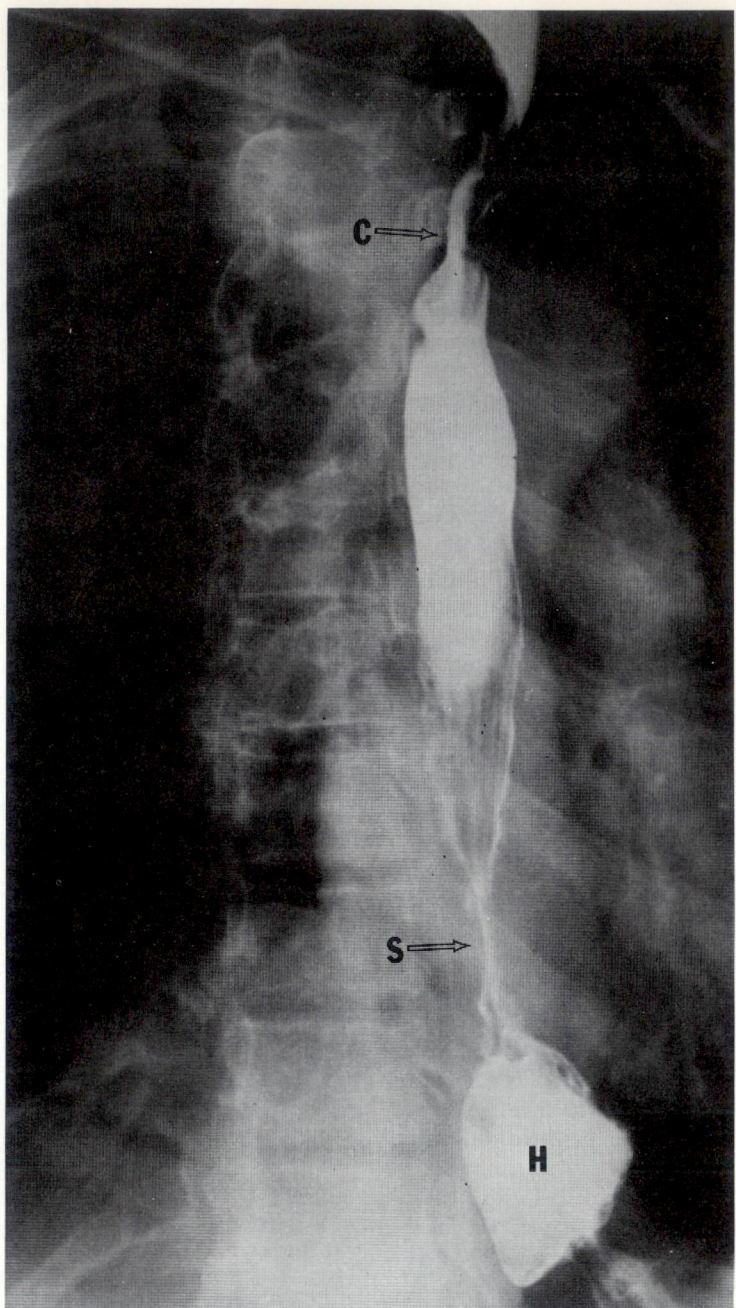

Fig. 172-3.   Patient with dysphagia has peptic stricture *(arrow at S)* located above hiatus hernia *(H)*. Of graver consequence, he is also found to have constricting carcinoma in upper esophagus *(arrow at C)*. (Courtesy of George Popky, MD.)

which are usually 3 to 5 cm above the esophagogastric junction.

Barrett's epithelium has a higher risk of adenocarcinoma, perhaps because dietary carcinogens can penetrate more easily into the mucosa or because of the nonspecific carcinogenic effect of chronic inflammation. Yearly endoscopic testing is recommended to detect severe dysplastic change or early carcinoma.

Upper gastrointestinal endoscopy is required for the diagnosis of Barrett's esophagitis, since the proximal location of the inflammatory reaction can be identified and biopsies can be obtained at varying levels to determine whether columnar epithelium is located at least 3 cm above the esophagogastric junction.

Barrett's esophagitis is treated in the same way as GERD.

Although the inflammatory reaction usually improves or subsides, there is no convincing evidence that the risk of carcinoma is eliminated. Antireflux surgical procedures also are effective in treating the esophagitis associated with Barrett's epithelium, but there is no apparent benefit in terms of cancer prevention.

TREATMENT OF REFLUX ESOPHAGITIS
Nonpharmacologic measures

DIET. Patients are advised to avoid eating large meals to reduce the volume of liquids taken at mealtime, since overdistention and intermittent relaxation of the LES induced by swallowing or meals clearly contribute to reflux. Carbonated beverages, sucking on hard candies, and chewing gum should be avoided, because these lead to gastric distension with air. Smaller meals and weight reduction can be beneficial for obese patients, since intraabdominal pressures may be excessive in such individuals. Foods that lower LES pressure such as mints, chocolate, fat, and spicy tomato drinks are best avoided. Orange juice and very hot or cold liquids may be uncomfortable for certain patients.

POSTURAL MANEUVERS. Patients should be advised to avoid lying down for at least 2 hours after meals and to refrain from snacking for at least 2 hours before retiring, since reflux is more likely to occur when the patient is recumbent. Patients with frequent reflux also should be advised against bending at the waist and certain fitness exercises that increase intraabdominal pressure. Chronic coughing and constipation should be treated, since they also lead to increased intraabdominal pressure. Elevating the head of the bed by 4 to 6 inches is extremely important for patients with GERD, since nocturnal reflux clearly plays an important role, and gravity can be used to prevent the process.

SMOKING AND ALCOHOL. Smoking and alcohol have been shown to reduce LES pressure. In addition, alcohol has a direct irritating effect on the inflamed mucosa.

AGGRAVATING MEDICATIONS. Medications that relax the LES or inhibit salivation such as anticholinergics and tricyclic antidepressant drugs should be avoided if possible. Patients with esophageal strictures should be extremely careful about using drugs that have a locally corrosive effect on the mucosa such as potassium chloride tablets, quinidine, tetracycline, and aspirin.

Agents that neutralize gastric acid

ANTACIDS. The buffering capacity of a standard meal is sufficient to keep the gastric pH above 3.5 for approximately 1 hour. The gastric pH subsequently decreases secondary to acid secretion stimulated by the gastric contents. Antacids can be taken as necessary for occasional heartburn, but the correct timing for therapy of esophagitis is 1 hour after the meal, 3 hours after the meal, and at bedtime. An antacid-alginic acid combination is an alternative to other antacid preparations. This medication forms a highly viscous solution of sodium alginate, which layers on the surface of the gastric contents and may make initial contact with the esophageal mucosa if reflux occurs. Antacids are most effective for intermittent use, since patient compliance is poor for the seven-dose regimen, and complications can be significant, including diarrhea, hypermagnesemia in patients with renal insufficiency, and adsorption of coadministered drugs.

Agents that inhibit gastric acid secretion

Cimetidine, the first histamine-2 receptor antagonist, was introduced for clinical use in 1977. It has revolutionized the treatment of peptic disorders. It can reduce basal acid secretion by 90% and food-stimulated secretion by 70% for several hours. It can be given in dosages of 300 mg four times a day, 400 mg twice a day, or 800 mg each night to treat peptic ulcer. Cimetidine has a less dramatic effect on the healing of GERD, but endoscopic and histologic improvement does occur. However, cimetidine can interfere with cytochrome P-450 system in the hepatocyte, thus delaying metabolism of such drugs as warfarin, phenytoin, diazepam, and theophylline. Elderly patients occasionally experience confusional episodes during cimetidine therapy, particularly if associated renal or hepatic disease is present.

Ranitidine, the second histamine-2 receptor antagonist, was introduced in 1983. It has a longer active duration and no significant effect on cytochrome P-450. It can be given as 150 mg twice a day or 300 mg each night. Famotidine, a more potent histamine-2 receptor antagonist recently introduced, has the same healing effect on peptic ulcer disease as the preceding agents.

The histamine-2 receptor antagonists apparently are equally valuable as therapy for GERD. The nocturnal dose is the most important, since reflux during sleep is not neutralized by food or salivation.

Drugs that increase LES pressure and/or enhance upper gastrointestinal motility

METOCLOPRAMIDE. This drug is a derivative of procainamide, without the antiarrhythmic effects. It has both dopamine-inhibiting and cholinergic properties. LES pressure is increased, and gastric emptying is enhanced with metoclopramide, features of value for patients with GERD. There is also a central antiemetic effect that is helpful for patients with nausea associated with other upper gastrointestinal symptoms. Approximately 10% of patients complain of fatigue or other central nervous system symptoms, probably because of the inhibition of dopamine.

BETHANECHOL. This is a cholinergic agent that also increases LES pressure but does not have a significant effect on gastric emptying or nausea. Side effects include diarrhea, mild crampy discomfort, and urinary frequency.

Metoclopramide and bethanechol should be reserved for patients who fail to respond adequately to dietary, postural, and H$_2$-receptor antagonist therapy. Metoclopramide and bethanechol usually are given in conjunction with the histamine-2 receptor antagonists.

Esophageal dilation

Esophageal strictures can be dilated by the passage of weighted rubber bougies under fluoroscopic control. The bougies are sized so that each successive dilation is accomplished with a larger dilator. Tight strictures may require the passage of a wire through the stricture into the stomach, with the dilators passed over the guide. More recently balloons have been placed within the stricture and inflated to expand the lumen. The results from these procedures often are satisfactory, and the risk of complications such as perforation or bleeding is acceptably low.

Antireflux surgery

More effective surgical procedures have been available for the past several decades, although they are less commonly used since the advent of histamine-2 receptor antagonist therapy. Although several techniques are described, they share the aim of securing several centimeters of esophagus below the diaphragm by wrapping the fundus of the stomach around the distal esophagus. These procedures succeed in preventing reflux, although some tightness of the LES may occur, requiring postoperative dilations for some patients.

TUMORS OF THE ESOPHAGUS

See Chapter 180.

ESOPHAGITIS RESULTING FROM CAUSTIC AGENTS

The ingestion of strong acids or alkalis occurs accidentally in children and generally as a suicide attempt in adults. The pharynx should be inspected when caustic ingestion is suspected. Burns in the hard or soft palate confirm the diagnosis but do not indicate whether the esophagus is involved. The absence of burns does not exclude caustic ingestion, since rapid swallowing may spare the pharynx. Cautious endoscopy can be done in such cases to confirm the diagnosis. A chest roentgenogram to evaluate for mediastinitis or aspiration pneumonia is essential. Therapy usually consists of antibiotics, intravenous fluids, and general supportive care. Some physicians prefer to start corticosteroid therapy to prevent strictures, whereas others begin prophylactic dilations after the acute inflammatory process has subsided. There is no consensus on the value of these early approaches. Esophageal stricture is the major chronic sequela of caustic ingestion and generally requires esophageal dilations. Carcinoma has been described as a long-term complication of caustic ingestion.

BIBLIOGRAPHY

Agha FP and others: Herpetic esophagitis: a diagnostic challenge in immunocompromised patients, Am J Gastroenterol 81:246, 1986.

Dodds WJ and others: Pathogenesis of reflux esophagitis, Gastroenterology 81:376, 1981.

Goldman LP and Weigert JM: Corrosive substance ingestion: a review, Am J Gastroenterol 79:85, 1984.

Mathieson R and Dutta SK: Candida esophagitis, Dig Dis Sci 28:365, 1983.

Ott DJ and others: Radiological evaluation of dysphagia, JAMA 256:2718, 1986.

Richter JE and Castell DO: Diffuse esophageal spasm: a reappraisal, Ann Intern Med 100:242, 1984.

Robinson RG: Management of reflux esophageal disease, Am J Med 77:106, 1984.

Sprechler SJ and Goyal RK: Barrett's esophagus, N Engl J Med 315:362, 1986.

Wesdorp ICE: Results of conservative treatment of benign esophageal strictures: a follow-up study in 100 patients, Gastroenterology 82:487, 1982.

173 · ACID-PEPTIC DISEASES

Walter Rubin

This chapter focuses on several disorders whose pathogenesis is not well understood but depends at least in part on the secretion of acid by the stomach. These conditions include peptic ulcer disease, Zollinger-Ellison syndrome, stress erosions, and some varieties of gastritis. Gastroesophageal reflux disease, another common acid-related disorder, is discussed in Chapter 172. Additional types of gastritis and other disorders of the stomach unrelated to acid secretion are included at the end of this chapter.

PEPTIC ULCER DISEASE

A peptic ulcer is a benign (nonmalignant) ulceration in the mucosal surface of the gut. Most peptic ulcers are located in the stomach (gastric ulcer) or duodenal bulb (duodenal ulcer), the first part of the small intestine just beyond the stomach. Duodenal ulcers are three times as common as gastric ulcers. On occasion ulcers develop just beyond the bulb in the duodenum (postbulbar ulcer) or in rare cases even more distally in the duodenum or jejunum (jejunal ulcer). Peptic ulcers occasionally occur in the esophagus of patients with esophagitis from gastroesophageal reflux. When patients or physicians refer to ulcers or ulcer disease, they usually are referring to a duodenal or gastric ulcer. Ulcers usually occur singly, but occasionally two or even more may be present at the same time.

The incidence of peptic ulcer disease seems to be declining in the United States, but it is still a common disorder, developing at some time in approximately 10% of the population. Because ulcers may cause no symptoms and their presence therefore may not be apparent, their incidence may be even greater. Most victims of ulcer disease, however, have recurrent pain and consult their physicians time and again for relief of the symptoms and with the hope of preventing the recurrences that most of these patients inevitably have. About 10% to 20% of these patients at some time have a life-threatening complication: a hemorrhage, perforation, or obstruction. Failure to assess and manage these patients properly on these occasions can be tragic.

New techniques, drugs, and knowledge have in the past few years modified the methods of diagnosing and treating ulcer disease. The development of better and more tolerable flexible fiberoptic endoscopes has enlarged the role of endoscopy in diagnosing and sometimes treating disease in communities where this technique is available. The development of an immunoassay test for serum gastrin has made the diagnosis of Zollinger-Ellison syndrome much easier. The use of dietary and anticholinergic therapy has been losing favor, whereas a better understanding of the proper use of antacids has been developed. Finally, a new class of drugs, the histamine H_2-receptor blockers, has become the most effective practical means for controlling gastric acidity and treating ulcer disease.

ETIOLOGY AND PATHOGENESIS. Despite much research, the causes and pathogenesis of peptic ulcers and their associated symptoms are still poorly understood. Genetic and psychosomatic factors and a failure of the mucous membrane to maintain its integrity and normal resistance have been thought to play possible roles in causing peptic ulcers, but the acid secreted by the stomach is still believed to play a major role and still receives the most attention. Patients who secrete no acid, such as those with pernicious anemia, rarely if ever have benign peptic ulcers, whereas patients who secrete huge amounts of acid, such as those with Zollinger-Ellison syndrome, have a marked tendency to develop ulcers and associated complications. Patients with ulcers often have pain when there is unbuffered acid in their stomachs, and characteristically this pain often is rapidly relieved when that acid is neutralized or diluted with antacid, food, or even water. Acid secretion seems to play an especially large role in the pathogenesis of duodenal ulcers, which are statistically associated with the production of large amounts of acid; however, many individual patients with duodenal ulcers secrete normal quantities. In contrast, patients with benign gastric ulcers commonly exhibit atrophic changes of the stomach and secrete normal or even decreased amounts of acid.

The role that diet, such as a diet of spicy foods, and drugs play in producing peptic ulcers remains unclear. Antiinflammatory agents such as aspirin, steroids, and the nonsteroidals probably promote peptic ulceration, especially of the stomach. An increased incidence of ulcer disease is associated with cigarette smoking, but its association with alcohol ingestion, which clearly causes gastritis, has not yet been established.

Emotional stress also has been thought to play a possible role in the development of ulcers. Strong emotional reactions such as anxiety, anger, or frustration seem to activate ulcers or produce symptoms in many patients with ulcer disease. Obviously, emotional stress cannot be a sole cause of ulcers, because most people under stress do not have them.

Recently a bacterium has been suggested as a possible pathogenic factor in at least some patients with duodenal and gastric ulcers. A *Campylobacter*-like organism, which has been called *Campylobacter pylori* and is associated with antral gastritis, can be identified in the antrum of probably most patients with duodenal and gastric ulcers and in many patients with dyspepsia, but it is found in fewer normal individuals. The significance of this infection remains to be clarified.

CLINICAL MANIFESTATIONS. Peptic ulcers may be asymptomatic. The most common symptoms of an uncomplicated ulcer is pain, most often in the epigastrium but sometimes in one or both upper quadrants, and less commonly in the back, lower abdomen, or chest. The pain often is perceived as a burning or gnawing sensation but also may be described as a hunger pain, a heaviness, an ache, a cramp, or even a sharp pain. The pain characteristically occurs when the stomach is empty or when not enough of a meal remains in the stomach to buffer adequately the secreted acid stimulated by the meal. Therefore it often begins 1 or more hours after eating and at night when the patient is asleep. The pain is characteristically relieved, usually within a few minutes, by buffering or diluting the gastric acid with the ingestion of an antacid, milk, food, or even water; the pain returns some time later, presumably when the gastric acidity has again increased. Most duodenal ulcers produce classic symptoms, whereas the pain of gastric ulcers tends to be somewhat atypical; pyloric channel ulcers classically produce pain when the patient eats.

Because peptic ulcers recur in most patients, many have a history of similar recurrent pains lasting a few days or weeks. Some patients, especially those with duodenal ulcers, experience seasonal attacks of pain in the spring or autumn. Sometimes patients can correlate episodes of pain with precipitating factors such as emotional stress, an alcoholic binge, or some dietary indiscretion such as eating particularly spicy foods.

Nausea and vomiting may be associated with uncomplicated ulcer disease, but these symptoms in a patient with an ulcer suggest the presence of an obstruction, in which case the vomitus usually is nonbilious. When an ulcer perforates, the patient usually has sudden, severe abdominal pain, becomes acutely ill, may even go into shock, and develops signs of peritonitis. When an ulcer hemorrhages, the patient often vomits gross blood or material with the appearance of coffee grounds (hematemesis) and usually notes that his stools have become black (melena) or sometimes grossly bloody if the bleeding is brisk and intestinal transit is rapid. Because of a rapid loss of blood he may feel weak, light-headed (especially on standing), and short of breath; he may have palpitations and may even faint or go into shock. A slower chronic rate of bleeding may produce iron deficiency anemia and symptoms of chronic anemia.

The physical examination of ulcer patients usually is not very helpful in reaching a diagnosis. It commonly reveals some nonspecific abdominal tenderness, usually in the epigastrium. Especially in patients with duodenal ulcer, the tenderness is often localized. Occasionally a patient with an obstruction may exhibit a succession splash produced by the retained food and secretions in the stomach. A specimen of feces should be obtained in the rectal examination and examined for the presence of gross or occult blood.

DIAGNOSIS. The diagnosis of a peptic ulcer is not difficult in most patients. A careful history alone suggests the correct diagnosis with most patients, especially those with duodenal ulcer disease. Many patients with ulcers have atypical symptoms, however, and many patients with typical ulcer symptoms (epigastric pain that begins 1 or more hours after eating and is relieved by antacids) have no demonstrable abnormality or less commonly have some other disease. Thus a diagnosis of a peptic ulcer must be confirmed in every new patient by appropriate laboratory tests, particularly a gastrointestinal series or endoscopy if it is available. Patients who have well-established duodenal ulcer disease with typical recurrent symptoms may be treated and followed to be certain that the expected response is obtained without repeating the roentgenographic and endoscopic studies each time.

Many disorders can cause upper abdominal pain possibly suggestive of ulcer disease. Gallbladder disease may cause recurrent pain in the epigastrium rather than in the right upper quadrant or over the right scapula, but this pain commonly is brought on by eating and is not usually relieved by the ingestion of food or antacid; however, the use of an antacid and the concomitant belching occasionally produce some relief. Biliary colic is more often accompanied by nausea and vomiting than is pain resulting from a peptic ulcer. When the gallbladder is acutely inflamed (acute cholecystitis), there usually are right upper quadrant tenderness, fever, and leukocytosis.

Heartburn (reflux esophagitis), caused by the reflux of gastric acid into the esophagus, usually is perceived by the patient as a burning, gnawing, or heaviness behind the sternum or sometimes high in the epigastrium. Although the discomfort may wake the patient at night or may be relieved by antacids, the symptoms commonly are felt while eating or soon after eating, often are worse when the patient is lying down, and frequently are accompanied by regurgitation of food or acid (marked by its sour taste) into the throat (pyrosis). It should be noted, however, that a significant number of patients with ulcer disease also have reflux and heartburn.

The pain of acute pancreatitis usually occurs in the upper abdomen but characteristically lasts many hours and is a persistent, severe pain usually accompanied by nausea and vomiting and unrelieved by food or antacid. The pain commonly radiates directly through to the back, and patients often seek relief by assuming a flexed fetal position. A posterior peptic ulcer penetrating into the pancreas may produce identical symptoms and may even be associated with elevated serum amylase levels, presumably a result of the pancreatitis it has caused.

Diseases above the diaphragm such as myocardial infarction, pulmonary embolus, and pneumonia sometimes produce abdominal pain, but a careful history, physical examination, and appropriate laboratory tests should readily differentiate these conditions from ulcer disease.

The first symptom of acute appendicitis often is an epigastric pain that might suggest ulcer disease, but the more classic symptoms and abdominal findings of appendicitis usually develop within a few hours, and the temperature and white blood cell count usually are elevated.

Vascular disease sometimes produces acute or even recurrent upper abdominal pain (intestinal angina), but this pain is not relieved by antacids and may characteristically be produced or intensified by eating.

Functional bowel disease (functional dyspepsia) is the most common imitator of ulcer disease. Its symptoms, however, often are produced or worsened by eating, often are associated with much belching resulting from aerophagia, and tend to be more persistent.

An acutely swollen liver associated with congestive failure, metastatic cancer, fatty infiltration, hepatitis, or alcoholic hepatitis can produce upper abdominal pain, but eating usually has little effect on this symptom. The liver usually is found to be tender by palpation, and a careful history and physical examination usually reveal a probable cause for the acutely enlarged liver.

Cancers of the digestive system, especially of the stomach and pancreas, may produce upper abdominal pain, but this pain usually is more persistent and unaffected or increased by eating.

Many drugs commonly cause dyspepsia-like symptoms. Any drugs suspected of causing such symptoms should be discontinued in symptomatic patients.

When abnormalities of the abdominal wall such as hernias cause upper abdominal pain, the pain usually is unaffected or occasionally is worsened by eating and usually is intensified

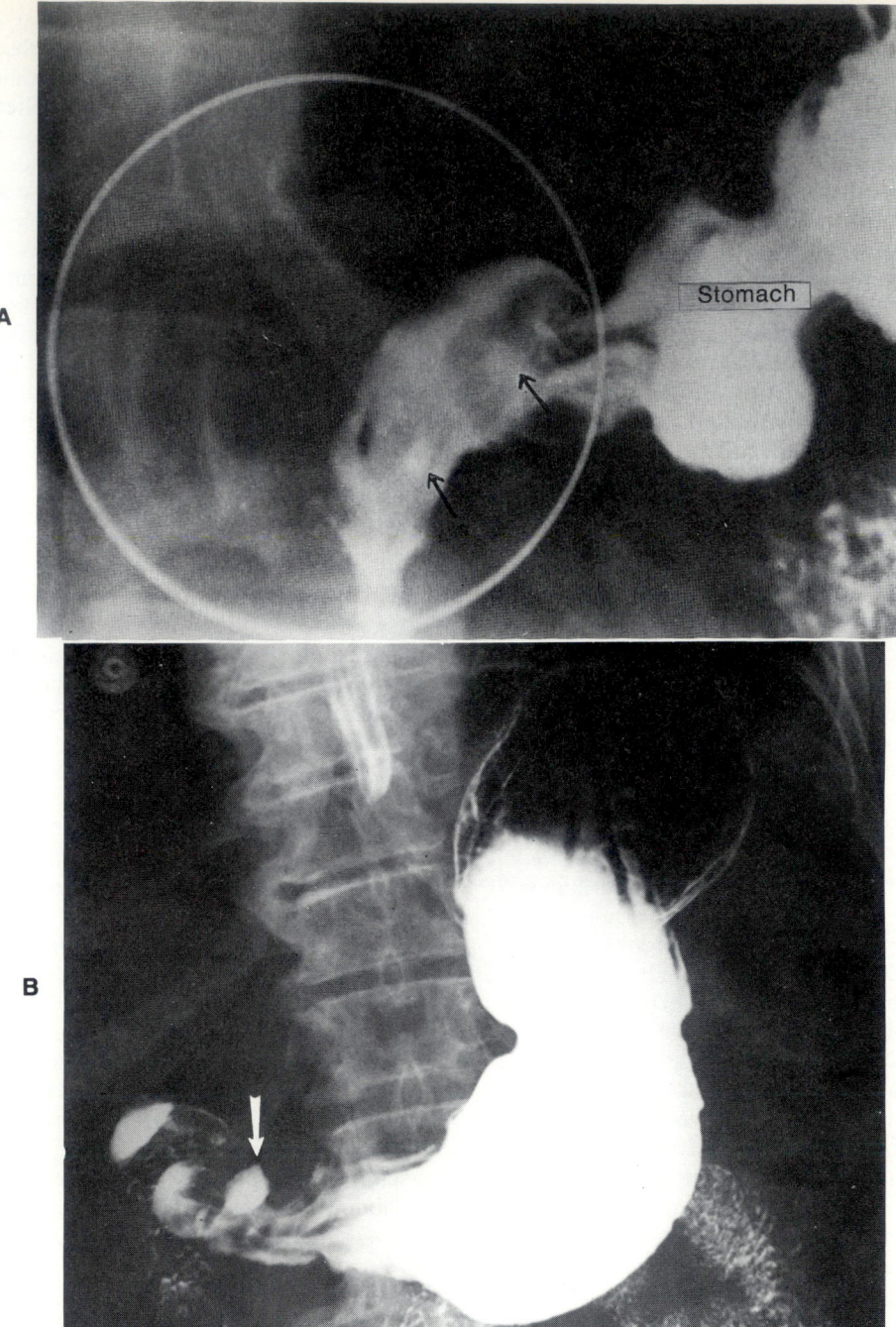

Stomach

Fig. 173-1   Gastrointestinal series demonstrates **A,** duodenal and **B,** gastric ulcers. Barium is collected in ulcer craters or niches *(arrows).* (Courtesy of George Popky, MD.)

by straining (increasing intraabdominal pressure) or by contracting the abdominal musculature, and the focal tenderness usually is increased when the reclining patient lifts his head (flexes his neck) and contracts his rectus muscles.

LABORATORY FINDINGS. The usual laboratory tests should include a complete blood count for detecting anemia and leukocytosis, an examination of the stool for occult blood, and a serum calcium test for detecting an occasional elevation resulting from an associated hyperparathyroidism or more likely from multiple endocrine tumors with Zollinger-Ellison syndrome. The serum gastrin level also should be determined if the test is available, especially if the patient also has chronic diarrhea, atypical or multiple ulcers, or severe ulcer disease—manifestations suggesting Zollinger-Ellison syndrome.

The diagnosis of a peptic ulcer usually is confirmed by a gastrointestinal series, which demonstrates the presence of the ulcer crater in 80% to 90% of patients with a peptic ulcer (Fig. 173-1). In some cases of duodenal ulcer the roentgenogram may fail to demonstrate the crater's presence but may show some deformity or spasm of the duodenal bulb and thus suggest the presence of an ulcer or at least scarring from previous ulcer disease. If the gastrointestinal series fails to reveal an ulcer despite a suggestive history, a gastroenterologist (if available) should be consulted, and endoscopy should be performed (esophagogastroduodenoscopy) to examine the mucosal surfaces directly. This procedure identifies some ulcers and even other lesions sometimes not apparent on the gastrointestinal roentgenograms and occasionally reveals duodenitis, an inflammation of the duodenal bulb without frank ulceration, a condition that may produce symptoms similar to those of an ulcer. If both the gastrointestinal series and endoscopy fail to reveal an ulcer or other cause for the patient's symptoms, other appropriate tests such as ultrasonography of the gallbladder should be performed to detect the cause.

If the gastrointestinal series demonstrates the presence of a duodenal ulcer, endoscopy is unnecessary and proper therapy can be instituted or continued. If, however, a gastric ulcer is revealed, further tests must be performed to eliminate the possibility that the lesion is one of the 3% to 8% of gastric ulcers that actually are ulcerated cancers. A gastric secretory study should be performed to confirm that the patient can secrete acid, and a gastroenterologist should be consulted to perform a gastroscopy to observe the lesion, take multiple biopsy samples along its circumference for pathologic examination, and obtain brush specimens of its surface for cytologic examination. If the patient can secrete acid and all the other tests suggest a benign disease, vigorous medical therapy should be instituted, and a gastrointestinal series (and endoscopy in some cases) should be repeated at later dates to confirm normal healing of the ulcer.

If an obstruction of gastric outflow is suspected, a nasogastric or Ewald tube should be passed into the stomach to detect, measure, and evacuate any retained food and secretions. A gastrointestinal series and endoscopy should be performed after evacuation, but often these procedures, especially roentgenography, reveal only an obstruction to the outflow of the stomach but not the cause. In this instance these procedures have to be repeated after a period of treatment with nasogastric suction. In patients with an obstruction the degree of dehydration should be immediately assessed, and the levels of serum electrolytes, blood urea nitrogen, and creatinine should be determined.

Bleeding ulcers must be differentiated from other causes of upper gastrointestinal hemorrhage while the patient's vital signs are monitored and while he is being given blood necessary for maintaining satisfactory blood pressure and adequate perfusion of the heart, brain, and kidneys. If the patient has blood in the stools but not hematemesis, the stomach should be aspirated with a nasogastric tube to determine whether blood is present and thereby to confirm the upper gastrointestinal tract as the site of bleeding. If the patient's condition is reasonably stable and the bleeding indeed seems to be arising from the upper gastrointestinal tract, a gastroenterologist (if available) should be consulted, and emergency endoscopy should be performed to establish a diagnosis and institute proper therapy as soon as possible. Endoscopy is especially helpful in patients who are likely to have many possible causes for their bleeding. Alcoholics, for example, especially those with liver disease, have bleeding commonly caused not only by ulcers but also by esophageal or gastric varices, gastritis, esophagitis, and Mallory-Weiss tears of the esophagus or stomach. Endoscopy often makes a rapid, specific diagnosis possible. If the bleeding is very brisk and thus prevents complete visualization, at least the site of the bleeding usually can be determined and some causes such as varices and diffuse erosive gastritis usually can be excluded from diagnostic possibilities.

If a perforation is suspected, a plain roentgenogram of the abdomen should be obtained for the detection of free air in the peritoneal cavity.

Other laboratory tests such as routine chest roentgenograms and electrocardiograms usually are helpful with most patients, especially if a disease of the chest or heart is suspected. If other diseases are strongly suspected or if the diagnosis of an ulcer cannot be made, other pertinent laboratory tests should be performed such as a serum amylase test if acute pancreatitis is suspected, liver function tests if liver disease is suspected, or cholecystography if gallbladder disease is suspected.

COURSE. Peptic ulcer disease must be viewed as a chronic illness. Most ulcers heal by themselves and become asymptomatic but then recur at a later time. Indeed, approximately 50% to 75% of patients whose duodenal ulcers heal have a reactivation of their ulcers within 1 year of healing. About 10% to 20% of ulcer patients at some time have a life-threatening complication such as a hemorrhage, perforation, or obstruction.

MANAGEMENT

Uncomplicated ulcers. There are four goals in treating the patient with uncomplicated ulcer disease: (1) to alleviate symptoms, (2) to promote healing, (3) to prevent recurrences, and (4) to prevent complications. Achieving the first two goals is not difficult in most cases, especially because ulcers usually heal by themselves, although they recur later. Good medical therapy, however, is designed primarily to reduce gastric acidity by inhibiting acid secretion or by neutralizing secreted acid and thus alleviating symptoms more rapidly and hastening healing. Preventing recurrences and complications has been a more difficult problem, and physicians generally have been unable to resolve this problem with medical therapy. Long-term use of the histamine H_2-receptor blockers such as cimetidine, however, promises perhaps to be a practical and effective way of reducing ulcer recurrences and complications.

Patients traditionally are encouraged to get adequate rest, relaxation, and sleep. Anxiety and anger should be reduced as much as possible by whatever practical means seem effective, such as instructing the patient, encouraging him to let out his feelings, manipulating his environment, encouraging participation in sports, using tranquilizers, and so on. Drugs thought to be ulcerogenic, such as aspirin, should be avoided or replaced with alternatives. Smoking and alcohol ingestion should be minimized or eliminated if possible.

The role of diet in the treatment of peptic ulcers has been extensively debated in recent years. The traditional restrictive bland diets eaten in frequent small meals are unnecessary or possibly even harmful. Patients should eat just three regular meals a day and avoid highly seasoned and spicy foods or any foods noted to cause symptoms. Caffeine-containing beverages such as regular coffee, tea, and colas also may be restricted. The frequent meals traditionally advocated are not only inconvenient but also continually stimulate the secretion of acid they are intended to reduce. The traditional bedtime snack is especially harmful, because it stimulates acid secretion for about 4 hours while the patient is asleep and unable to take an antacid. The traditional bland diets are not only unattractive to patients but generally contain much milk sugar lactose, which causes abdominal cramps, gas, and even diarrhea in many patients who have lactose intolerance (lactase deficiency). The bland diet also tends to be high in calories and, because of its high fat content, possibly atherogenic.

Anticholinergic drugs long have been used to reduce gastric acid secretion in ulcer patients, but because of their limited effectiveness and disturbing side effects they are losing favor. When taken in the optimal dosage, four times a day (½ hour before each meal and at bedtime), they reduce meal-stimulated acid secretion by only about 30% to 50%. They do not significantly reduce acid secretion without producing at least some dryness of the mouth and commonly other more disturbing side effects such as urinary retention, constipation, heartburn, tachycardia, drying of bronchial secretions, visual disturbances, and precipitation or aggravation of glaucoma.

The agents recommended for the control of gastric acidity in ulcer patients are the long-used antacids, which neutralize secreted acid, or the new histamine H_2-receptor blockers (cimetidine, ranitidine, and famotidine), which effectively inhibit acid secretion. Because these two classes of drugs work differently, they may be used together if desired.

The antacids are effective, relatively safe drugs when used properly, but the physician should be aware of the problems they may cause. Absorbable antacids such as sodium bicarbonate can produce an appreciable alkalosis, especially in patients with renal disease, and if appreciable amounts are taken along with much calcium (from calcium carbonate or a large quantity of milk products), occasionally the very rare but serious milk-alkali syndrome (hypercalcemia and alkalosis) may develop. The antacids containing calcium have been losing favor not only because they can cause hypercalcemia and renal impairment but also because they are thought to stimulate acid secretion. The aluminum antacids, when used in large amounts, occasionally can cause phosphate depletion (by forming insoluble precipitate in the gut) and thereby anorexia, weakness, and bone pain. Antacids must be used especially carefully in patients with renal failure, because the cations (calcium, magnesium, or aluminum) can cause toxicity. The aluminum antacids tend to cause constipation, whereas the magnesium antacids tend to produce diarrhea; thus the physician may have to change preparations or use more than one type in accordance with the effects on the inidividual patient. Some antacids, especially the aluminum antacids, may bind various drugs such as tetracyclines within the gut and thereby affect their absorption. The physician must be aware of this phenomenon and check the effects of the antacids on the absorption of other medications the patient takes. If a patient requires a salt-restricted diet, a low-sodium antacid must be used.

Antacids must be used in adequate amounts and at proper times to ensure satisfactory acid neutralization. Different preparations vary in terms of potency, the rate of neutralizing acid, and the length of time they remain effective in the stomach. If taken when the stomach is empty, most antacids rapidly leave the stomach and therefore are effective for only 10 to 20 minutes. When taken an hour after a meal, however, when the acid secreted in response to the meal is no longer adequately buffered by the food remaining in the stomach, the antacid usually is effective for 2 to 3 hours. The amount of antacid required depends not only on the potency of the preparation used but also on the amount of acid the individual patient secretes; this of course usually is difficult for the physician to know without performing secretory tests, which are neither always available nor usually desirable. The physician should be aware, however, that if a patient's symptoms are not responding satisfactorily, that patient might require more antacid. The solid chewable antacid preparations are much less effective than their liquid counterparts and should not be used.

If antacid therapy is the choice, the physician usually should prescribe about 100 mEq of a liquid aluminum and magnesium antacid (usually about 1 oz [30 ml] of the more potent antacids or 2 or 3 oz [60 or 90 ml] of the weaker ones) to be taken 1 hour and 3 hours after each of the three meals and every 2 hours thereafter. If symptoms are not well controlled by this regimen, the antacid can be taken more frequently, even every hour. The physician must consider whether a low-salt antacid should be used and whether the chosen antacid might interfere with the absorption of other durgs the patient requires. It may be necessary to change or alternate preparations if diarrhea or constipation develops.

The histamine H_2-receptor antagonists effectively inhibit the gastric acid secretion stimulated by histamine. Histamine long has been known to be a powerful stimulant of acid secretion, but the conventional antihistamines used to treat allergic patients block only the histamine H_1-receptors and have essentially no effect on gastric acid secretion. When the histamine H_2-receptor blockers are taken as prescribed, they effectively reduce gastric acidity in most patients by inhibiting about 70% or more of the acid normally secreted. Of particular importance, the dose taken at bedtime inhibits most nocturnal acid secretion during the period when the patient is asleep and unable to take antacids. Because the drugs are eliminated mainly through the kidneys, the dosage should be reduced in patients with renal disease. The histamine H_2-receptor blockers generally are well tolerated, although they occasionally may cause side effects and drug interactions.

Sucralfate (Carafate), another new effective agent for treating peptic ulcer disease, does not affect acid secretion or gastric acidity but rather seems to bind with the proteinaceous base of the ulcer, protecting it from further injury (by some poorly understood mechanism) and thus permitting it to heal. The drug is considered a "cytoprotective" agent, that is, an agent that protects the mucosa and promotes its integrity. Because little of the drug is absorbed, it has few side effects.

Treatment with antacids, histamine H_2-receptor blockers, or sucralfate should be continued for 6 to 8 weeks. The pain in most patients usually is controlled within the first week of therapy, and most ulcers heal by the sixth week. When pain does occur during the early period of therapy, antacids may be taken for relief.

Special aspects of gastric ulcers. If gastrointestinal roentgenograms or endoscopy suggests a malignancy, if the stomach cannot secrete acid even after maximal stimulation with histamine, betazole (Histalog), or pentagastrin, or if the pathologic or cytologic specimens reveal malignancy, a surgeon should be consulted and an appropriate resection performed if possible. If all these tests suggest a benign disease, the vigorous medical therapy outlined previously should be instituted. The gastrointestinal series or preferably endoscopy should be repeated in 3 weeks to confirm that the ulcer is healing and again at 6 weeks (if it is not healed at 3 weeks), at which time the ulcer should be healed or at least reduced in size by 90%. Another gastrointestinal series should be performed at 12 weeks to confirm complete healing. If the series at any time reveals a possibility of malignancy or if the ulcer is not healing by 3 weeks, not almost healed by 6 weeks, or not completely healed by 12 weeks, surgery probably should be recommended if the patient is a reasonable candidate. Some large benign ulcers with craters wider than 2.5 cm may require more than 12 weeks to heal. If such an ulcer appears benign and seems to be healing well, medical therapy can be continued beyond 12 weeks and a follow-up gastrointestinal series, endoscopy, or both, can be performed in a few weeks to confirm complete healing.

Surgery. Surgery for peptic ulcer disease should be reserved mainly for patients with the complications of perforation, recurrent significant hemorrhage or an acute severe or persistent hemorrhage, or an obstruction that fails to open satisfactorily despite good medical therapy. Gastric ulcers suspected of being carcinomas or that fail to heal satisfactorily with medical therapy also should be treated surgically. The poorest indication for surgery is apparent intractability, that is, persistent or very frequent recurrent symptoms despite good medical therapy.

Such patients should be carefully evaluated, even with endoscopy if necessary, to make sure that their symptoms result from active ulcers, that they are following their prescribed therapy, and that they do not have Zollinger-Ellison syndrome.

The results of surgery vary with the talent of the individual surgeon, the hospital where it is performed, and the selection of patients; the overall mortality is about 1% to 2% (lower in some medical centers), and the recurrence rate probably well below 10%. The two most widely used procedures in the United States are truncal vagotomy with a drainage procedure (usually a pyloroplasty) and truncal vagotomy with a gastric resection and gastrojejunostomy (Billroth II procedure). The former procedure probably has a somewhat lower mortality and morbidity, whereas the latter procedure probably results in a somewhat lower incidence of recurrent disease.

Although surgery seems to prevent recurrent disease in most cases, it unfortunately also causes postoperative symptoms (postgastrectomy syndrome) in up to 50% of patients. Patients selected for surgery should be warned that they may be exchanging their ulcer symptoms for other discomforts. Although these symptoms usually are most prominent during the months immediately after the operation, many patients suffer chronic symptoms for years. Common postoperative complaints include diarrhea, weight loss, weakness, early satiety, and postprandial distress.

Some patients have a postprandial syndrome consisting of light-headedness, weakness, sweating, palpitations, nausea, and diarrhea. When these symptoms occur an hour or later after eating, they usually are the result of reactive hypoglycemia. More often they occur during the meal or soon afterward; this is known as dumping syndrome. The syndrome probably results from a rapid emptying of the stomach, causing the accumulation of hypertonic chyme in the small intestine, and the rapid flux of water from the blood into the intestinal lumen, causing a rapid reduction of blood volume.

Complications. When a patient with ulcer disease has a perforation, hemorrhage, or obstruction, he should be hospitalized and a surgeon and ideally a gastroenterologist should be consulted immediately. A patient with a perforation usually requires immediate surgery. A patient with an obstruction should be treated with continuous nasogastric suction, intravenous fluids and electrolytes, and intravenous histamine H_2-receptor blocker. After 3 days of suction the nasogastric tube should be withdrawn and the patient put on a liquid diet and antacids. If intravenous histamine H_2-receptor blocker cannot be continued, a full antacid regimen should be employed, as outlined previously. The stomach should be aspirated at least once a day, about 1 hour after a meal. If the outlet obstruction seems to be improving, that is, if the retention is less than 500 ml and progressively improves, the medical therapy can be continued and the diet advanced to include soft food. If the obstruction does not improve, if a low-grade chronic obstruction persists, or if the patient has a history of recurrent obstruction, surgery is recommended. If the diagnosis of a mechanical outlet obstruction could not be confirmed by the gastrointestinal series or endoscopy when the patient was first seen, these procedures should be repeated after the period of nasogastric suction, especially if surgery is contemplated. A mechanical outlet obstruction must be differentiated from gastric atony, a motility disturbance that may result from diabetic gastroparesis, other severe diseases, drugs, or unknown causes.

Patients with bleeding ulcers should receive blood, usually whole blood, to maintain a satisfactory blood pressure and the adequate perfusion of the heart, brain, and kidneys and should be treated with antacids and/or a histamine H_2-receptor blocker (intravenously if necessary). Most patients with bleeding ulcers require no blood or only a few units. If bleeding persists, control may be accomplished by endoscopic coagulation. If the bleeding remains so brisk and persistent that vital signs cannot be easily maintained or if 6 or more units of blood are required during the first 24 hours, surgery probably should be performed if the bleeding continues even then. If brisk bleeding is permitted to continue such that the patient requires massive transfusions (10 or more units over a 24- or 48-hour period), the mortality risk increases considerably. Such patients therefore should be identified as soon as possible so that surgery can be performed and the arterial bleeder ligated before the patient needs massive amounts of blood and serious complications develop. If a patient continues to bleed for more than 3 days, even if his blood requirements are not great, surgery probably should be recommended as well. The decision must be made individually for patients, however, and the decision of whether to operate often is affected by the patient's clinical condition and the presence or absence of associated diseases.

PREVENTION. Recurrent ulcer disease and its complications are difficult if not impossible to prevent. The patient who has only occasional short attacks of active disease is unlikely to follow any prescribed prophylactic regimen even if a practical effective one could be devised. The patient who suffers more frequent attacks, especially if they are precipitated by recognizable factors, can be educated to avoid the precipitating circumstances or to institute a medical program prophylactically whenever such circumstances arise or as soon as the first symptoms appear. Thus if the patient finds himself under undue stress, if he ingests an excessive amount of alcohol or too much spicy food, or if he must take some drug thought to be ulcerogenic, he can begin taking antacids frequently, a histamine H_2-receptor blocker, or sucralfate and a tranquilizer if necessary in the hope of preventing or aborting a recurrence of symptoms. The patient with frequent or continual ulcer symptoms should be encouraged to follow an intensive long-term medical program to determine whether the symptoms can be controlled and prevented. Patients who have disease apparently uncontrollable with good medical treatment should be carefully evaluated to determine whether their symptoms indeed result from active ulceration (with endoscopy if the gastrointestinal series does not definitely reveal an ulcer) and to make sure they understand and are following the prescribed medical program. If they are found to have active ulcer disease, they should be carefully tested for Zollinger-Ellison syndrome by determining their serum gastrin level. Many truly intractable ulcers are found to be penetrating ulcers (extending beyond the wall of the stomach) and may require surgery.

It is difficult to maintain patients on long-term antacid therapy, especially in quantities adequate to control gastric acidity most of the time. However, a histamine H_2-receptor blocker taken in proper dosage each day at bedtime is an effective prophylactic treatment for patients who suffer frequent recurrent duodenal ulcer disease. In controlled clinical studies, duodenal ulcers were found to recur in about 50% to 75% of patients within 1 year after healing, whereas the prophylactic use of a histamine H_2-receptor blocker reduced the recurrence rate to about 20%.

ZOLLINGER-ELLISON SYNDROME

DEFINITION AND ETIOLOGY. Zollinger-Ellison syndrome, thought to be present in fewer than 1% of ulcer patients, usually is caused by a non-β islet cell tumor of the pancreas, a gastrinoma, that continually secretes the hormone gastrin and produces high blood levels. Gastrin causes hyperplasia of the acid-secreting parietal (oxyntic) cells in the stomach and continually stimulates them to secrete, and thus the patient produces large amounts of acid even when fasting. As a result, almost all of these patients eventually have ulcer disease that usually is severe.

The tumors of the pancreas tend to be small and difficult to find. About 50% of these patients have two or more tumors in the pancreas, and about 10% to 20% of patients have multiple endocrine adenomatosis type I syndrome with additional adenomas, hyperplasia, or carcinomas in the parathyroid, pituitary, or adrenal glands. In about 5% of patients with Zollinger-Ellison syndrome the gastrinoma is located in the proximal duodenum, and in another 5% the tumor is in the stomach, hilus of the spleen, or some other organ. About two thirds of gastrinomas are malignant, usually low-grade malignancies that metastasize slowly to the duodenum, local lymph nodes, and eventually the liver and other organs. In the past, however, when the diagnosis and treatment of the syndrome often were unsatisfactory, the patients usually died of the complications of ulcer disease rather than the malignancy. Gastrinomas are apudomas, tumors arising from a group of endocrine cells, the amine precursor uptake decarboxylation (APUD) cells, that synthesize polypeptide hormones and biogenic amines. Some gastrinomas also produce other polypeptides and amines, such as corticotropin (ACTH), glucagon, insulin, vasoactive intestinal polypeptide, and serotonin. In rare cases Zollinger-Ellison syndrome may result from a hyperplasia of the gastrin-producing cells (G cells) in the antrum of the stomach rather than from a gastrinoma.

CLINICAL MANIFESTATIONS. In about 75% of patients with Zollinger-Ellison syndrome, ulcers develop in the duodenal bulb or occasionally in the stomach, whereas in the rest ulcers develop more distally in the duodenum or in the jejunum. The ulcers usually are single but may be multiple. Patients usually have a virulent form of ulcer disease. They commonly have intractable ulcers causing pain that is unusually resistant to traditional medical therapy. These patients have a high incidence of ulcer complications, especially perforations and hemorrhages, and they commonly require surgery because of these complications or the intractability. If the syndrome is not recognized and a conventional ulcer operation is performed, ulcers and their complications usually continue to develop even after surgery. Because of the virulence of the disease, if it is not diagnosed and managed properly, many patients will die, primarily from a complication.

About 40% of patients with Zollinger-Ellison syndrome have diarrhea, and in about 10% the diarrhea precedes the ulcer disease. Several causes of the diarrhea have been proposed: (1) the large volumes of water and acid secreted by the stomach, (2) malabsorption resulting from an acid pH in the proximal small intestine and the consequent inhibition of the pancreatic digestive enzymes, especially lipase, and of the ability of the bile acids to form micelles, (3) acid damage to the proximal small intestinal mucosa, (4) impaired salt and water absorption in the small intestine, and (5) altered intestinal motility. Regardless of the precise cause, if the voluminous secretion of the stomach is stopped or prevented from entering the small intestine by nasogastric suction, surgery, or the use of a histamine H_2-receptor blocker, the diarrhea usually ceases.

DIAGNOSIS. Zollinger-Ellison syndrome should be suspected in any patient with severe or intractable disease, post-bulbar or jejunal ulcers, multiple ulcers, recurrent ulcers after surgery, ulcers associated with chronic diarrhea, hypercalcemia

(possible type I syndrome), or prominent gastric or small intestinal folds incidentally discovered by roentgenography or endoscopy. If the syndrome is suspected, the diagnosis is not difficult to establish. Gastric secretory studies usually reveal markedly elevated fasting and stimulated acid outputs. The basal acid output usually is at least 10 mEq/hr, and in about half the cases it is at least 60% of the maximal acid output, the maximal rate the stomach can secrete when stimulated with histamine, betazole (Histalog), or pentagastrin. The diagnosis is confirmed by demonstrating a very high serum gastrin level by immunoassay. In questionable cases the serum gastrin level can be induced to rise even higher (by 50% or 400 pg/ml) by infusing calcium or injecting secretin. The secretin injection test is especially helpful because in patients who do not have Zollinger-Ellison syndrome secretin usually depresses serum gastrin levels or has little effect. The rare cases of antral G-cell hyperplasia can be differentiated from the syndrome by the secretin injection test (with a normal response) or by feeding the patient a standard meal. Postprandial serum gastrin levels usually rise more than 50% above fasting levels in normal individuals and in those with G-cell hyperplasia but not in patients with gastrinomas, which are usually little affected by eating. Zollinger-Ellison syndrome also can be differentiated from other conditions that may be associated with high serum gastrin levels, such as pernicious anemia, atrophic gastric mucosa, or a retained gastric antrum following a Billroth II operation. The patients with pernicious anemia and atrophic gastritis secrete no gastric acid or reduced amounts, and patients with a retained antrum probably can be differentiated by their normal response to secretin. About 20% to 40% of gastrinomas can be demonstrated by arteriography, and some by computed tomography.

Because the ulcers associated with Zollinger-Ellison syndrome can be very mild and because the immunoassay for serum gastrin is now simple and readily available, some physicians suggest obtaining a routine serum gastrin determination for all patients with peptic ulcer disease.

MANAGEMENT. Because most of the tumors and their local metastases cannot be found or satisfactorily removed by surgery and because conventional ulcer surgery usually is not adequate in controlling the disease, total gastrectomy has become the conventional therapy. In perhaps 10% to 20% of patients a discrete solitary pancreatic tumor can be identified, often in the duodenum, and can be entirely removed, making gastric resection unnecessary. Such patients should be followed postoperatively with serum gastrin and gastric secretory studies. In the past few years long-term histamine H_2-receptor blocker therapy has been shown to be an effective alternative to total gastrectomy for patients with Zollinger-Ellison syndrome. Patients with this treatment, however, should be carefully followed and their gastric secretion monitored, since they often require higher dosages of the drugs for the control of the gastric acidity and symptoms. The addition of an anticholinergic drug often permits satisfactory control in patients whose symptoms cannot be controlled with a reasonable dose-age of histamine H_2-receptor blocker alone. Newer, even more potent antisecretory drugs such as the experimental K,H-ATPase inhibitors (omeprazole, for example) promise to be even more effective agents for medical treatment of these patients. The basal rate of acid secretion should be maintained below 10 mEq H^+ per hour.

Perhaps every patient with Zollinger-Ellison syndrome should be explored after a careful preoperative search for a resectable tumor. If such a tumor cannot be found during surgery, even with the use of operative sonography, then a conventional ulcer operation probably should be performed to permit easier subsequent medical control of gastric acid secretion. As noted previously, about two-thirds of gastrinomas are malignant, although usually of very low grade. Whereas most patients in the past died of complications of severe ulcer disease, with the newer methods of diagnosis and treatment most patients in the future probably will live longer and eventually die of their malignancy.

STRESS EROSIONS

Acute erosions or superficial ulcerations commonly develop in the stomach and/or duodenum of patients under conditions of severe stress such as shock, severe trauma, burns, sepsis, surgery, and renal, respiratory, or hepatic failure. The lesions are characteristically superficial, limited to the mucosa, and often multiple. The so-called Cushing's ulcer, associated with trauma to the head, brain surgery, or increased intracranial pressure resulting from a brain tumor or other cause, commonly is located high on the lesser curvature of the stomach, whereas the so-called Curling's ulcer, associated with burns, characteristically is located in the duodenum. The lesions develop rapidly, often within 24 to 48 hours of the stressful episode, and if clinically apparent usually cause gastrointestinal bleeding resulting in either hematemesis or melena. Less commonly lesions cause significant epigastric pain, nausea, or vomiting. Since they are superficial, they usually are not detectable by a routine gastrointestinal series, but they more often are demonstrable by double-contrast techniques. They are best diagnosed by endoscopy, which also reveals their number and the extent of gastric involvement with erosive changes.

The pathogenesis of stress erosions remains unclear. Although the presence of gastric acid seems necessary, only in the case of Cushing's ulcer has gastric hypersecretion been demonstrated. In some types of stress ulceration a breakage of the gastric mucosal barrier to acid back-diffusion seems to occur, thereby permitting luminal acid to gain access to and perhaps damage the mucosa. This postulated mechanism, however, does not account for duodenal erosions or for cases apparently associated with intact mucosal barriers. In some experimental animal models the applied stress seems to interfere with the normal process of epithelial replication, which maintains normal populations of surface cells. Evidence in recent years, however, suggests that stress erosions may be caused by mucosal ischemia, a result of altered mucosal blood flow.

The best therapy for stress erosions is prevention. Continual maintenance of the gastric pH level above 3.5 or preferably 5 by means of antacids and/or histamine H_2-receptor blockers markedly reduces the incidence of these erosions in identified high-risk patients. This preventive therapy is increasingly being adopted in intensive care units. If erosions and bleeding develop, the patient should undergo diagnostic endoscopy and his stomach should be lavaged with ice-cold saline or water in an effort to control the bleeding. The patient should receive blood as needed (see Chapter 170) and antacids and/or histamine H_2-receptor blockers to control gastric acidity. If the stomach is the site of persistent bleeding, infusion of vasopressin (Pitressin) into the left gastric artery may be considered in institutions where this technique is available; endoscopic coagulation of bleeding sites is another alternative. If these measures fail, however, surgery may be necessary, even though these patients usually are in poor condition and thus have a high surgical risk and often develop additional ulcers after surgery. The patient with a single pumping erosion, who may require only ligation or local resection, usually is a better surgical candidate than one with many diffuse erosions involving much of the stomach and occasionally requiring a total gastrectomy.

GASTRITIS

Acute and chronic inflammations of the gastric mucosa are common pathologic processes.

Acute erosive gastritis, if symptomatic, usually causes hematemesis and/or melena but may also cause abdominal pain, nausea, and vomiting. The acute erythema, friability, and erosions may be limited to a small area of the gastric mucosa or may be more diffuse, sometimes involving the entire stomach. The cause of the gastritis may be inapparent but commonly is alcohol, which is thought to act by breaking the mucosal barrier to acid back-diffusion, or antiinflammatory agents, which also break the barrier or inhibit prostaglandin synthesis. Aspirin is the most prominent of these agents, but phenylbutazone, indomethacin, corticosteroids, and others have also been incriminated as causes. These same antiinflammatory agents also have been thought by some to promote ulcer formation.

The management of acute erosive gastritis is similar to that of stress erosions discussed previously. The general measures for gastrointestinal bleeding should be instituted (see Chapter 170). The stomach should be lavaged with ice-cold saline or water in an effort to stop or retard bleeding. Endoscopy should be performed to establish the diagnosis and to ascertain the extent of gastric involvement. Gastric acidity should be controlled with antacids, a histamine H_2-receptor blocker, or both. If significant bleeding continues, the infusion of vasopressin into the left gastric artery or endoscopic coagulation may be considered if these techniques are available. If significant bleeding continues despite these measures, surgery must be considered. However, surgery for acute gastritis, especially a diffuse gastritis, is not very satisfactory, and the procedure of choice is unclear. Most surgeons first attempt to control the bleeding with a vagotomy and pyloroplasty or a vagotomy and antrectomy and resort to a total gastrectomy only if these more conservative procedures fail. Some surgeons, however, advocate early total gastrectomy for diffuse involvement that cannot be successfully managed with vigorous medical therapy.

Acute necrosis and inflammation of the stomach that often are severe can be caused by corrosive agents (corrosive gastritis) or in rare cases by an acute pyogenic infection of the wall of the stomach (phlegmonous gastritis). The ingestion of a strong alkali or acid, usually in an attempted suicide, can cause necrosis of the stomach wall as well as burns of the mouth and esophagus. The necrosis may lead to perforation and peritonitis, hemorrhage, or a later stricture formation. (See Chapter 172 for the management of such patients.)

Chronic gastritis, the chronic inflammation of the gastric mucosa, occurs commonly, especially in older people. Because this condition usually is asymptomatic, its presence often is discovered when an associated gastric lesion such as an ulcer, polyp, or cancer leads to a biopsy or resection of the stomach. The classification of types of chronic gastritis has been somewhat arbitrary and controversial. Superficial gastritis is an inflammation in which acute and chronic inflammatory cells are largely limited to the upper portions of the mucosa between the gastric pits. In atrophic gastritis the inflammation extends deeper to involve the glands, and there is a concomitant loss of normal glandular cells and their variable replacement with intestinal types of cells (intestinal metaplasia) and pyloric gland cells (pseudopyloric metaplasia). The progressive loss of parietal cells is accompanied by a comparable reduction in their ability to secrete acid and intrinsic factor. The loss of most of the parietal cells is associated with achlorhydria, inadequate absorption of dietary vitamin B$_{12}$ (measured by the Schilling test), and the possible eventual development of pernicious anemia. When such severe atrophy is associated with little or no inflammation, the lesion is called gastric atrophy.

Chronic gastritis often is limited solely or largely either to the area of the stomach that contains the fundic or gastric glands (chronic fundal gland gastritis) or to the area of the pyloric glands (antral gastritis). The causes of these forms of chronic gastritis are unknown, but the frequent association between atrophic fundal gastritis and certain immunologic phenomena suggests a possible role of immunologic processes in its pathogenesis. About 60% of patients with atrophic fundal gastritis and 90% of those with pernicious anemia have antibodies to parietal cells in their circulation. Most patients with pernicious anemia also have antibodies to intrinsic factor and, along with many others who also have severe atrophic fundal gastritis, have high serum gastrin levels, a result of increased numbers of pyloric G cells and the absence or reduction of acid secretion to inhibit G-cell secretion.

In contrast, predominant antral gastritis is not usually associated with parietal cell antibodies, elevated serum gastrin levels, or such reduction in acid secretion unless the process has extended proximally to involve much of the body and fundus of the stomach. Antral gastritis commonly is observed in patients with peptic ulcer disease and has been thought by some to result form the reflux of bile and bile acids from the duodenum into the stomach. More recently, chronic infection with *Campylobacter pylori* has been thought to be a common cause of antral gastritis. In patients who have undergone a gastrojejunostomy and thereby have regular reflux of bile through the anastomosis into the stomach, gastritis regularly develops around the stoma (stomal gastritis). Stomal gastritis usually is asymptomatic, but it occasionally has been considered the possible cause of epigastric pain, nausea, and vomiting and is sometimes the source of gastrointestinal bleeding. After a partial gastric resection and especially after a Billroth II procedure, atrophic gastritis with a loss of parietal and chief cells often develops in the gastric remnant. The pathogenesis of this alteration is unclear, but the reflux of bile and the elimination of the antral G cells and the trophic effects of their gastrin have been suggested as playing a role. These gastric remnants appear to have an increased risk of developing carcinoma 15 years or more after the operation, and some physicians thus have advocated following these patients with regular endoscopic examinations.

A biopsy or resection performed because of the presence of gastric ulcers, polyps, or cancer usually reveals atrophic gastritis, and stomachs known to have atrophic gastritis seem to have an increased risk of developing these lesions. It remains unclear whether the presence of gastritis predisposes or leads to the development of ulcer, polyps, and cancer or whether the gastritis is an unrelated result of pathologic gastric processes that independently lead to the development of these lesions.

The term "hypertrophic gastritis" or gastropathy usually refers to the presence of thickened gastric mucosa and enlarged gastric folds, which often are difficult to differentiate roentgenographically and endoscopically from lymphomas and infiltrating carcinomas. Menetrier's disease is characterized by giant gastric folds, nodules, or both especially in the body of the stomach, as well as marked hyperplasia of the surface and pit mucous cells, atrophy of the normal glandular cells, the hypersecretion of mucus, and the hyposecretion of acid. It is one of the causes of protein-losing enteropathy, and patients sometimes have edema resulting from a low serum albumin level (see Chapter 170) but more commonly experience epigastric pain. The diagnosis may be determined by endoscopy and biopsy, but sometimes a laparotomy and full-thickness mucosal biopsy are required. Patients with Zollinger-Ellison syndrome often have large gastric folds, an increased thickness of the mucosa, and hyperplasia of the fundic glands, especially of the parietal cells. These changes result from the trophic effects of the elevated levels of circulating gastrin, and of course, these patients exhibit marked hypersecretion of gastric acid rather than the hypochlorhydria usually found in patients with Menetrier's disease. Hypersecretory hypertrophic gastropathy involves changes that resemble the gastric changes associated with Zollinger-Ellison syndrome, with large gastric folds and thickened fundic mucosa, mainly because of an increased number of parietal and chief cells. These patients, however, do not have gastrinomas, elevated serum gastrin levels, or the markedly elevated acid secretions associated with that syndrome. Their acid secretions are often elevated, however, and the condition seems to be associated with an increased incidence of duodenal ulcer disease. These patients sometimes may exhibit an abnormal enteric loss of plasma proteins and, as in patients with Menetrier's disease, hypoalbuminemia sometimes may develop.

OTHER GASTRIC DISORDERS

Several other disorders of the stomach are discussed in other chapters, such as the common benign and malignant neoplasms (Chapter 180), the rare Crohn's disease (Chapter 175), eosinophilic gastroenteritis (Chapter 170), and motor disturbances such as pseudoobstruction and diabetic gastroparesis (Chapter 177).

Acute gastric dilation

Acute gastric dilation is an acute motor disturbance in which the stomach fails to empty and therefore accumulates food and secretions in an enlarging "third space." It may be produced by drugs such as anticholinergics but is more commonly associated with many, often severe illnesses such as trauma, surgery, pneumonia, myocardial infarction, and sepsis. The condition can be recognized by the presence of a succussion splash and by means of an abdominal roentgenogram or nasogastric aspiration and must be differentiated from a mechanical obstruction. The patient must be placed on constant nasogastric suction while the resultant fluid and electrolyte disturbances are corrected.

Adult hypertrophic pyloric stenosis

Adult hypertrophic pyloric stenosis, an unusual hypertrophy of the phyloric muscle, causes symptoms of pyloric obstruction in adults: nausea, vomiting, and gastric retention. The gastrointestinal series and endoscopy reveal a symmetric narrowing of the pylorus and an "umbrella defect" in the base of the duodenal bulb. The lesion must be differentiated from an infiltrating carcinoma, from the scarring or inflammation of peptic ulcer disease, and from inflammatory processes such as Crohn's disease, eosinophilic gastroenteritis, and tuberculosis or tertiary syphilis, which rarely affect the stomach. Surgery may be required to relieve the symptoms or occasionally to determine the definitive diagnosis.

Gastric volvulus

Gastric volvulus (torsion), a rare acute or chronic twisting of the stomach, may cause severe upper abdominal pain and the regurgitation of saliva rather than gastric contents. The abdominal roentgenogram usually demonstrates the diagnosis. Surgery may be required if an acute volvulus does not subside but progresses to strangulation or if a chronic volvulus produces repeated symptoms.

Gastric diverticula

Gastric diverticula are rare lesions that occur most commonly just below the cardia on the posterior wall near the lesser curvature. They usually can be diagnosed by a gastrointestinal series, but occasionally endoscopy is required to differentiate them from an ulcer. They usually are asymptomatic and require no treatment except in the rare cases of bleeding, perforation, or severe pain that therefore may require surgery.

Bezoars

Bezoars, aggregates of organic and/or inorganic matter, occasionally develop in the stomach, especially in a gastric remnant after a partial gastrectomy. They often cause anorexia, satiety, nausea, and vomiting. These usually large masses can be differentiated from tumors by gastrointestinal roentgenograms and endoscopy. Often bezoars can be fragmented at the time of the endoscopy and removed by repeated lavage. Some phytobezoars (composed of vegetable matter) may be partially digested with the aid of cellulase and/or papain and then successfully removed with lavage. Trichobezoars (composed of hair) are more resistant to digestion. In rare cases aggregates of inorganic substances are found. If the bezoars cannot be successfully removed by lavage after mechanical or enzymatic fragmentation, surgery may be necessary. Other swallowed foreign bodies occasionally lodged in the stomach also may be gripped and removed at the time of endoscopy.

BIBLIOGRAPHY

Sleisenger MH and Fordtran JS: Gastrointestinal disease, ed 5, Philadelphia, 1988, WB Saunders Co.

174 · DISORDERS OF ABSORPTION—THE MALABSORPTION SYNDROME

Gerald H. Escovitz *and* Geoffrey L. Braden

Malabsorption is the inability to absorb dietary foods. It may be caused by maldigestion (deficiency or inactivation of pancreatic enzymes and bile salts) or by a disease of the small intestine that results in a mucosal barrier to absorption. Pancreatic insufficiency is discussed more extensively in Chapter 182. This chapter focuses on diseases of the small intestine.

NORMAL PHYSIOLOGY

Most people in the United States and other developed countries ingest 50 to 100 g of fat in their daily diet. Normally less than 5 g of fat can be recovered from the stool daily, and the excretion of more than 7 g is considered abnormal. The lipids in the normal diet are primarily triglycerides that contain long-chain fatty acids usually 16 and 18 carbon atoms in length. After ingestion, the first important action occurs when triglyceride, a large water-insoluble molecule, is hydrolyzed into free fatty acids (FFA) and a β-monoglyceride (β-MG) by the action of the pancreatic enzyme lipase (Fig. 174-1). The FFA and β-MG formed are also water insoluble but are readily solubilized by the detergent properties of bile salts, which are synthesized in the liver and excreted into the bile.

Bile salts, detergents with special physicochemical properties, are amphipaths; that is, they have both hydrophilic and hydrophobic regions. They are synthesized from cholesterol precursors and conjugated to glycine and taurine. In the intestine they mix with lipase, dietary triglyceride, FFA, and β-MG. The bile salts aggregate into water-soluble particles called "micelles" by aligning themselves so that their hydrophilic regions align at the aqueous surface and their hydrophobic regions cluster away from the aqueous solution. The bile salts solubilize the FFA and β-MG by incorporating them within their hydrophobic regions to form mixed micelles. This formation occurs when the concentration of bile salts is greater than the critical micellar concentration (CMC) of 2 to 5 mM, when the medium is at a proper pH, and when the bile salts are conjugated to taurine or glycine.

This solubilization of fat is apparently essential for its absorption at normal rates, possibly by making the fat more accessible to the epithelial cells lining the small intestine. At this stage the large, water-insoluble fat particles have been transformed into smaller water-soluble particles. The fat-soluble vitamins (A, D, E, and K) also are incorporated in the interior part of the micelles.

FFA and β-MG dissociate from the bile salts at the intestinal surface and diffuse passively into the epithelial cells of the upper small intestine. There are four stages in the passage of lipids from the intestinal lumen to the circulation: (1) their uptake into the mucosal cells, (2) the reesterification of FFA and β-MG into triglycerides, (3) the formation of chylomicrons, and (4) the secretion of chylomicrons into the lymphatic circulation.

The first stage of the passage is the passive, non-energy-dependent transport of FFA and β-MG through the lipophilic membrane of the brush border. Intracellular passage is facilitated in the aqueous medium of the cell by a small protein that binds the FFA and the β-MG. In the smooth endoplasmic reticulum FFA and β-MG are resynthesized into triglycerides, with each step requiring a different activating enzyme. The resulting triglyceride molecules coalesce into larger particles that are coated with a lipoprotein. These larger particles, chylomicrons, exit from the base of the cell and enter the lymphatic circulation. The lipoprotein coating is necessary for the normal departure of the triglyceride from the intestinal cell.

The bile salts themselves are not absorbed with the lipids they solubilize but pass on to the distal ileum, where they are actively absorbed. They are then returned to the liver via the portal circulation, are resecreted into the bile, and are used again in the formation of micelles. Thisi enterohepatic circulation preserves the total body pool of bile salts at approximately 4 G. Only about 15% of the bile salt pool, or about 600 mg, is lost in the stool each day, and the loss is readily replaced by hepatic synthesis of new bile salts.

Triglycerides whose FFA is of shorter length (from 6 to 10 carbon atoms) are called medium-chain triglycerides (MCT) and are able to bypass steps in absorption that are necessary for triglycerides with longer FFA. MCT require lower concentrations of lipase to be hydrolyzed from triglyceride, form micelles at concentrations of bile salts below the CMC, are absorbed intact, and inside the cell are released directly into the portal circulation. MCT thus avoid the normal process of intracellular reesterification and formation of chylomicrons. These properties of MCT make it an effective therapeutic agent in a variety of conditions that cause malabsorption.

PATHOPHYSIOLOGY

Disorders that interfere with any of the steps necessary for normal digestion may produce steatorrhea. The several clinical entities that cause pancreatic insufficiency cause steatorrhea

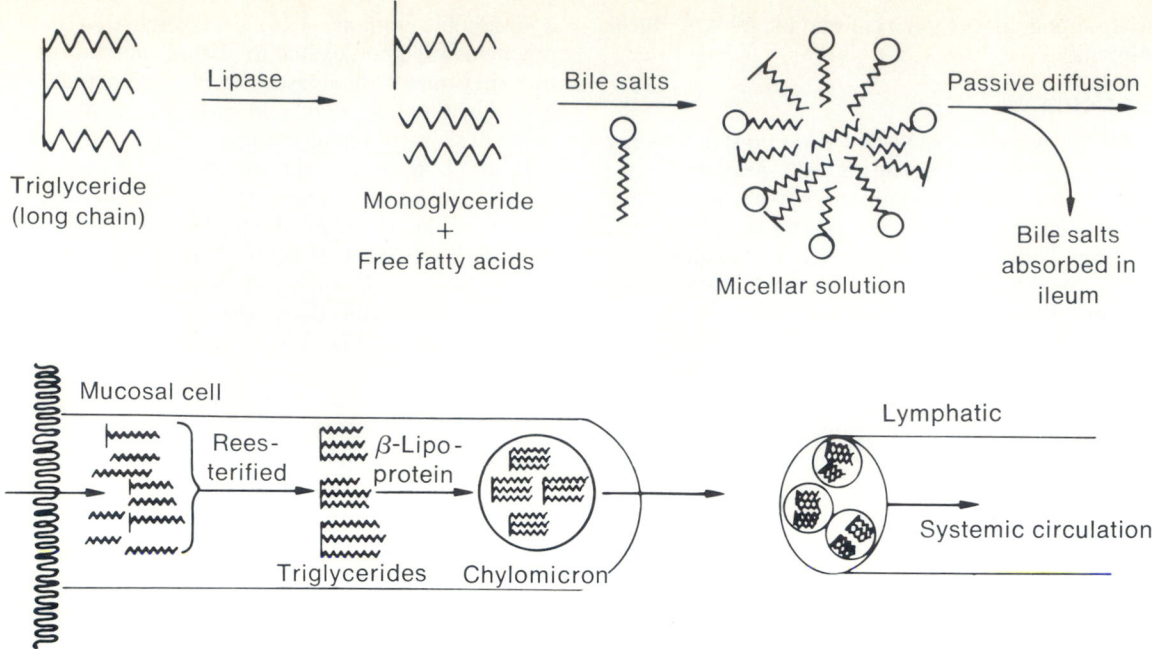

Fig. 174-1   Sequence of steps in normal absorption of dietary lipids. Malabsorption may result when any of these essential steps is disturbed by disease processes. See text for details.

consisting mainly of undigested triglycerides. Impaired micelle formation caused by bile salt deficiency, altered pH, or deconjugation of bile salts also leads to impaired fat absorption. Many disorders directly affect the small bowel mucosa and thereby inhibit fat absorption. These clinical entities include intestinal resection, which simply eliminates part of the bowel; a wide variety of muscosal diseases such as celiac sprue that inhibit the transport of FFA and β-MG across the mucosal cell; disease processes that selectively impair the normal metabolism within the mucosal cell, such as congenital β-lipoprotein deficiency; specific defects of the transport of chylomicrons into the lymphatics, such as lymphangiectasia; and disease processes that involve several steps, such as the malabsorption that occurs after a Billroth II gastric resection, in which there may be bacterial overgrowth in a stagnant loop and/or relative pancreatic insufficiency because of an inadequate mixing of ingested lipids with pancreatic secretions.

In addition, a wide variety of metabolic defects may accompany fat malabsorption. Protein-losing enteropathy is caused by an abnormal protein loss through diseased mucosa. This commonly occurs in patients with celiac sprue, eosinophilic gastroenteritis, radiation enteritis, diffuse ileojejunitis, and Crohn's disease and causes hypoproteinemia. Severe malabsorption may produce both hyponatremia and hypokalemia. Hypocalcemia and hypomagnesemia, both of which may contribute to muscle irritability and even tetany, may occur in patients with chronic diseases of the mucosa such as celiac sprue, after intestinal resection, and in other conditions causing significant malabsorption such as pancreatic insufficiency. Hypocalcemia may be made more severe by vitamin D malabsorption. Anemia often is present. Mucosal diseases such as celiac sprue may lead to several types of anemia with deficiencies of iron, folate, and vitamin B_{12}. Vitamin B_{12} absorption also may be decreased in diseases that cause bacterial overgrowth, because it may be metabolized by the bacteria and thus not be absorbed. Vitamin B_{12} absorption may also be decreased as a result of diseases or surgical resection involving

the terminal ileum, the site of vitamin B_{12} absorption. A tendency toward bleeding in cases of vitamin K deficiency is seen both in diffuse mucosal disease and in conditions that affect micelle formation.

In general, disorders that involve minimal fat malabsorption have fewer metabolic side effects than those with more severe malabsorption. Mucosal diseases usually have the most severe accompanying metabolic disorders; the steatorrhea of pancreatic insufficiency is next in severity.

CLINICAL PRESENTATION

Patients with the malabsorption syndrom may have symptoms of general malabsorption or symptoms caused by the deficiency of a specific substance such as vitamin A, D, or K, calcium, magnesium, iron, or folate. The patient with malabsorption syndrome classically has bulky, oily, malodorous stools associated with significant weight loss, muscle wasting, weakness, edema, anemia, ecchymoses, abnormal bleeding, a smooth tongue, hyperkeratosis of the skin, skeletal pain, and even tetany. The oral cavity manifestations of malabsorption occur when vitamin deficiencies are part of the clinical presentation. These may include reddening and ucleration of the oral mucosa (stomatitis), swelling and burning of the tongue (glossitis), and fissuring of the corner of the mouth (cheilosis), all of which are associated with vitamin B deficiencies. If vitamin B_{12} deficiency is prominent, atrophy of the tongue may be present.

In the United States dramatic symptoms of malabsorption syndrome are rare, and the physician must be alert to more subtle symptoms. Stools may be water, and occasionally a patient may be constipated. Weight loss may be slight. There may be abdominal pain. Symptoms of deficiencies of vitamins A, K, D, and iron may occur as isolated phenomena. Edema caused by hypoalbuminemia and the glossitis, stomatitis, or neuropathy related to vitamin B deficiencies may also occur as isolated phenomena.

An unexplained laboratory finding may also be the first clue to the presence of malabsorption syndrome, such as an unexplained anemia, hypocalcemia, hypocholesterolemia, hypoalbuminemia, hypoprothrombinemia, or a flat glucose tolerance curve.

In many patients the diagnosis of the clinical condition causing malabsorption is readily apparent from the history, such as with patients who have had a massive small bowel resection, abdominal irradiation, or a pancreatic resection. The symptoms of malabsorption are also not difficult to interpret in patients with a history of alcoholism and recurrent pancreatitis, in patients from a geographic area where tropical sprue is endemic, in patients taking one of the medications associated with malabsorption, in patients with the obvious skin findings of scleroderma or dermatitis herpetiformis, and in patients with diabetes mellitus and severe peripheral neuropathy.

In many cases, however, the history is not helpful in diagnosing the cause of malabsorption, either because there is no significant history or because the symptoms are nonspecific. Abdominal pain and distention, often associated with conditions causing malabsorption, also occur in a number of conditions not associated with malabsorption. The causes of diarrhea, weight loss, anorexia, anemia, and so on are many, and these symptoms can be taken only as clues to be evaluated in the context of other findings.

The results of the physical examination of patients with malabsorption vary greatly. Some patients appear essentially normal or even overweight. However, there may be signs of weight loss, muscle wasting, or of the specific nutritional deficiencies just described. Hypotension and tachycardia may be present. Pallor, skin atrophy, hyperkeratosis, ecchymoses, clubbing, cheilosis, glossitis, and peripheral edema all may be present. The abdomen may be protuberant, with loops of small intestine visibly distended. Peripheral neuropathy or findings of combined system disease are occasionally observed.

CLINICAL APPROACH

Several steps must be taken when evaluating a patient suspected of having malabsorption syndrome:

1. Objective confirmation of malabsorption
2. Diagnosis of the specific disorder responsible for the syndrome
3. Institution of specific and supportive therapy
4. Evaluation of the patient's responses to the therapy, since in many conditions that cause malabsorption the therapeutic trial is also a diagnostic step

OBJECTIVE CONFIRMATION OF STEATORRHEA. A quantitative analysis of fecal fat is the best single test for confirming the presence of steatorrhea. Stools should be collected for at least 3 consecutive days while the patient is ingesting at least 70 g (ideally, 100 g) of fat daily. The excretion of more than 7 g daily confirms the diagnosis of fat malabsorption.

A qualitative estimate of fat malabsorption may be made with a Sudan III stain of a stool sample. A slide is prepared with a mixture of stool and Sudan III and examined microscopically for the presence of fat globules. Finding such globules correlates with moderate to severe steatorrhea, usually with more than 20 g of fat excretion a day. This test is insensitive for steatorrhea between 7 and 20 g a day. The oral ^{14}C-triolein breath test is also useful. ^{14}C-labeled glycerol esterified to triolein is administered orally. After absorption the ^{14}C-labeled glycerol is metabolized to $^{14}CO_2$ and then exhaled. The repiratory excretion is measured over 6 hours. A decrease is seen with fat malabsorption.

Other tests such as the serum carotene test, the vitamin A absorption test, and the urinary indican test are not sufficiently specific or reliable and should not be used.

DIAGNOSIS OF THE SPECIFIC DISORDER RESPONSIBLE FOR MALABSORPTION SYNDROME. Once the diagnosis of malabsorption syndrome has been confirmed, the selection of subsequent tests is determined by the physician's suspicion of a cause based on the history and physical examination. Many tests or procedures may be used, but the following are the most reliable and most widely used.

Secretin test. A tube placed in the second portion of the duodenum is used to aspirate fluid, bicarbonate, and enzymes secreted by the pancreas after the intravenous administration of secretin. Classic pancreatic insufficiency severe enough to cause malabsorption usually produces abnormal results on the secretin test with a marked decrease of fluid volume, bicarbonate concentration, and enzyme concentration. This test usually becomes positive when pancreatic enzyme activity is reduced 60% to 75%. (For a description of this test, see Sleisenger and Fordtran in the bibliography.)

More recent studies indicate that the secretions of pancreatic fluid and bicarbonate in patients with chronic pancreatitis may not differ significantly from normal secretions. Thus when there is a suspicion of pancreatic insufficiency and the test results are equivocal, the patient's response to pancreatic enzyme therapy should be viewed as part of the confirmatory diagnostic evaluation.

Bentiromide test. This test is based on chymotrypsin hydrolysis of an oral dose of a synthetic tripeptide, benzolytyrosyl-paraaminobenzoic acid. The paraaminobenzoic acid released is absorbed and excreted into urine by the kidneys. A 6-hour urine collection is obtained, and the amount of paraaminobenzoic acid is calculated. Uriniary excretion of paraaminobenzoic acid correlates with chymotrypsin activity. This test is insensitive for mild pancreatic enzyme deficiency.

Bile acid–breath test. When bile salt deconjugation is suspected as a cause of malabsorption, the simple and reliable bile acid–breath test may be used. Bile acids conjugated to radioactive carbon (^{14}C) glycine or ^{14}C taurine are administered orally, and the patient's breath is analyzed for radioactive carbon dioxide. The taurine or glycine normally remains conjugated to the bile salt, and the molecule recirculates via the enterohepatic circulation. In patients with bacterial overgrowth, however, the glycine or taurine is deconjugated from the bile acid and metabolized. The resulting radioactive carbon dioxide diffuses in a high concentration across the intestinal wall, into the venous circulation, and thence to the lungs to be discharged.

D-Xylose test. D-Xylose, a 5-carbon sugar, does not require intact pancreatic function for its absorption. Therefore if D-xylose given orally is not found to have been discharged in the urine in normal amounts, this is presumptive evidence of intestinal mucosal disease. Abnormal results may be misleading in patients with inadequate hydration, vomiting, delayed gastric emptying, ascites, and bacterial overgrowth, but the test is quite reliable when meticulously performed.

Small bowel biopsy. Suction biopsy of the small intestine is a safe and reliable procedure when performed by an experienced gastroenterologist. Several specific small bowel disorders such as celiac disease, Whipple's disease, abetalipoproteinemia, lymphoma, lymphangiectasia, and giardiasis may be diagnosed in this manner.

Small bowel roentgenograms. Roentgenograms of the small bowel may reveal the nonspecific findings of dilation, coarsening of the folds, flocculation, segmentation, and clumping or may show specific disorders such as Crohn's disease, multiple diverticula, stricture, blind loops, lymphoma, and carcinomatosis.

Schilling test. The Schilling test evaluates vitamin B_{12} absorption. If impaired absorption results from deficient gastric secretion of intrinsic factor, the usual cause of pernicious anemia, the Schilling test results may be improved by adding intrinsic factor to the oral dose of radioactive vitamin B_{12}. If impaired vitamin B_{12} absorption results from bacterial overgrowth, then the test results may be improved by pretreating the patient with antibiotics. If, however, the impaired absorption results from a resection or disease of the terminal ileum, the site of vitamin B_{12} absorption, neither the addition of intrinsic factor nor pretreatment with antibiotics significantly improves the vitamin B_{12} absorption measured by the test.

Other tests. A small bowel aspiration and culture are helpful in guiding the therapy for bacterial overgrowth. The aspirate may be analyzed for impaired micelle formation in patients suspected of having this problem. Aspiration of the small bowel for parasites when the stool examination is negative is especially useful for *Giardia lamblia* and *Strongyloides stercoralis*. In patients suspected of having malabsorption syndrome, it is also important to delineate nutritional deficiencies by measuring the levels of serum sodium, potassium, calcium, phosphate, magnesium, iron, folate, vitamin B_{12}, albumin, cholesterol, and carotene, as well as the prothrombin time. If anemia is present, its specific nature should be determined.

INSTITUTION AND EVALUATION OF SPECIFIC THERAPY. When the test results are equivocal or in instances in which tests are unavailable, the initiation and evaluation of the patient's response to a specific therpy should be viewed as a diagnostic test. Even in patients whose diagnosis appears to have been objectively confirmed, a poor therapeutic response should lead the physician to reconsider the accuracy of the diagnosis. This principle is discussed in greater detail in the following sections.

SPECIFIC DISORDERS CAUSING MALABSORPTION
Pancreatic insufficiency

In the United States chronic pancreatitis (usually caused by alcoholism) is the most common cause of pancreatic insufficiency. In such cases the patient usually has a lengthy history of recurrent episodes of pancreatitis with progressive, persistent, debilitating pain. The malabsorption in these patients generally is severe (measured fecal fat greater than 30 g daily) and is accompanied by weight loss, vitamin and mineral deficiencies, and often diabetes mellitus. The secretin test is rarely necessary in these patients. The response of the patient with malabsorption to commercial preparations of pancreatic digestive enzymes (often given with supplementary histamine H_2-receptor blockers) is usually excellent, including a resultant weight gain and the correction of metabolic abnormalities. The pancreas has tremendous physiologic reserve. Pancreatic insufficiency does not usually cause clinically significant steatorrhea until 90% of enzyme output is lost. Diabetes results from destruction of the islets of Langerhans as the pancreas becomes more fibrotic. Concomitant glucagon deficiency from the pancreas contributes to brittle diabetes in these patients. When diabetes is caused by chronic pancreatitis, diabetic retinopathy and nephropathy are less common.

Other, less common causes of pancreatic insufficiency are a pancreatic resection for either chronic pancreatitis or pancreatic cancer, a pancreatic carcinoma that blocks the main pancreatic duct at the head of the pancreas, cystic fibrosis occurring in children or young adults, and in rare cases insufficiency caused by the gastric hypersecretion occurring in patients with Zollinger-Ellison syndrome or by a massive small bowel resection, which inactivates pancreatic enzymes by lowering the duodenal pH.

Patients with these less common causes of pancreatic insufficiency show a malabsorption pattern similar to that of chronic pancreatitis. Patients with cystic fibrosis, however, may have milder symptoms. The secretin test often is helpful in confirming the diagnosis in these cases. The D-xylose test, bile acid–breath test, and small bowel roentgenogram, all of which are normal in these patients, are useful in ruling out other possible causes. In some patients the diagnosis of pancreatic insufficiency can be made only after a successful response to a therapeutic trial of pancreatic enzymes. This approach to diagnosing pancreatic insufficiency is valid when the more specific measures already described are not helpful or when they are unavailable to the physician.

Disorders of bile salts; bacterial overgrowth

QUANTITATIVE CHANGES. Quantitative disorders, that is, a decrease in the amount of intraluminal bile salts below the CMC, include hepatocellular disease, intrahepatic cholestasis or extrahepatic obstruction, and resection, bypass, or disease of the distal ileum. Hepatocellular disease leads to inadequate synthesis of bile salts. Intrahepatic or extrahepatic cholestasis prevents bile salts from reaching the gut lumen. Resection, bypass, or disease of the terminal ileum such as Crohn's disease all lead to an increased fecal excretion of bile salts with a subsequent reduction of the bile salt pool.

The patient's history, physical examination, and gastrointestinal roentgenograms usually suggest the diagnosis. The secretin test, the D-xylose test, and a small bowel biopsy all have normal results. Although it is possible to analyze aspirates of the small bowel for their concentration of bile salts, this procedure is not generally available or usually necessary.

Patients who have quantitatively deficient intraluminal bile salts usually have moderate steatorrhea (15 to 25 g daily) and rarely have the severe metabolic defects such as anemia, hypoproteinemia, and vitamin and mineral deficiencies found in patients with pancreatic insufficiency or mucosal disease. Once the specific diagnosis is made, reversible causes such as an extrahepatic obstruction or ileitis can be treated. In irreversible instances such as an ileal resection, therapy with MCT should be initiated because exogenous bile salts are generally not effective.

QUALITATIVE CHANGES FROM BACTERIAL OVERGROWTH. Qualitative changes occur in bile salts when they are deconjugated by an overgrowth of intestinal bacteria, as occurs in patients with multiple intestinal diverticula, blind loops, strictures, and some motility disorders such as scleroderma. The common denominator in these disorders is a condition of stasis that permits bacterial overgrowth. The bacteria deconjugate bile salts, which are then unable to form micelles. In addition, the mucosa is damaged, with focal villous blunting and flattening. The exact cause of this is unknown, but it may be secondary to chemical irritation by deconjugated bile salts or bacterial toxins and enzymes. Bacterial overgrowth also may bind the vitamin B_{12}–intrinsic factor complex and may metabolize D-xylose, both of which may lead to confusing laboratory results.

The diagnosis of bacterial overgrowth is suspected from the clinical presentation. The malabsorption associated with bacterial overgrowth is mild to moderate (7 to 20 g daily of fecal fat) and usually involves no serious metabolic side effects.

Bacterial overgrowth may be confirmed indirectly with the breath test using bile salts labeled with ^{14}C taurine and directly by analyzing a small bowel aspirate for its bile salt content and the adequacy of micelle formation; the aspirate may also be cultured for a quantitative analysis of aerobic and anaerobic bacteria. A culture also is useful in determining the antibiotic sensitivity of the bacteria for therapeutic intervention. It is important to look for a surgically correctable cause such as diverticula or a stricture. Antibiotic therapy is indicated with causes such as scleroderma that cannot be treated with surgical therapy.

Mucosal disease

CELIAC DISEASE. Celiac disease (celiac sprue, or gluten enteropathy) is a prototype of the malabsorption syndrome. Its cause is unknown, but the therapeutic response to the elimination of gluten from the diet indicates that this protein, through either a direct toxic effect or an immunologic reaction, is the major contributing factor. Gluten is a high-molecular-weight protein found in wheat, rye, barley, oats, and other grains but not in corn or rice. The protein triggers an inflammatory response in the mucosa that leads to damage of villi and impaired absorption on a cellular level. Eventually villi are destroyed, with loss of mucosal absorptive area. Cell-mediated immunity with infiltration and activation of T lymphocytes is an important cause of the damage. The importance of genetic factors is demonstrated by the high incidence of histologic abnormalities of the intestinal mucosa in asymptomatic relatives of patients with celiac disease and the high incidence of HLA-8 or DW3 tissue antigens in these patients. Many patients also have a history compatible with childhood celiac disease.

Steatorrhea in these patients often is moderate to severe (25 to 40 g daily) and often is accompanied by hypoproteinemia, hypocalcemia, hypomagnesemia, hypokalemia, and anemia. In some patients an occult anemia, ecchymoses, osteomalacia, or tetany may be symptoms. In patients with celiac sprue the D-xylose test results are abnormal, and small bowel roentgenograms usually show nonspecific findings of dilation, coarsening of the folds, flocculation, and clumping of barium. Because the disease is most severe in the upper small bowel and relatively spares the terminal ileum, the vitamin B$_{12}$ absorption test results may be normal. These patients often have a secondary lactose intolerance.

No single test is specific for the diagnosis of celiac sprue. The abnormal D-xylose results and roentgenograms only indicate an intestinal mucosal disease, which have many possible causes. A small bowel biopsy must be performed; the typical findings with celiac disease are flattened villi and increased infiltration of inflammatory cells. Even then, because celiac sprue is not the only condition that causes this histologic picture, a therapeutic response to a gluten-free diet is necessary to confirm the diagnosis absolutely. Most patients with gluten enteropathy respond to a gluten-free diet with both clinical and histologic improvement, although in raare cases a very ill patient may require supplemental therapy with corticosteroids. The response to the gluten-free diet usually is observed within 1 or 2 weeks but occasionally only after many weeks of therapy. A lack of response to a gluten-free diet should cause the physician to reconsider the diagnosis, since this therapeutic trial is an important part of the diagnostic evaluation. However, the diet should be reviewed carefully, since inadvertent gluten ingestion is a common cause of apparent therapeutic failure. Endomysial antibodies have been reported to be elevated in most patients, and this may aid in the diagnosis of sprue.

DISEASES THAT MAY BE CONFUSED WITH CELIAC DISEASE
Tropical sprue

Tropical sprue causes histologic findings similar to those of gluten enteropathy, but these, as well as the malabsorption and metabolic abnormalities, often are less severe. Macrocytic anemia usually is present. This condition is endemic in certain tropical and subtropical regions such as Southeast Asia, the Indian subcontinent, and the Caribbean. When this condition appears in a temperate climate, the patient usually has previously resided in an endemic area. The cause of this condition is unknown, but it has been postulated that an infectious bacteria damages the mucosa. Patients usually respond to broad-spectrum antibiotics, folate, and parenteral vitamin B$_{12}$. Some patinets may require up to 6 months of therapy before a significant clinical response is seen. Antibiotic and folic acid administration should be continued as long as the clinical and laboratory improvement continues.

Collagenous sprue. Collagenous sprue is similar to celiac sprue in many ways, but biopsy reveals a dense band of collagen in the lamina propria. These patients do not respond to a gluten-free diet. The prognosis for theese patients is grim, and death is almost certain.

Intestinal lymphoma. An intestinal lymphoma may be either a secondary development in patients with long-standing gluten enteropathy or a primary condition that may be confused with celiac sprue. Patients with malabsorption caused by intestinal lymphoma usually have severe, persistent abdominal pain, fever, and severe malabsorption; their small bowel biopsy results are similar to those of celiac sprue, and the patients fail to respond to a gluten-free diet. Whereas celiac sprue is most severe in the upper small intestine, lymphoma affects the entire small bowel. Diffuse intestinal lymphoma is common in patients from the Mideast and is most often seen in young adults and teenagers.

Treatment of patients with diffuse intestinal lymphoma associated with malabsorption syndrome generally is ineffective. In one series of nine patients, none survived beyond 4 years.

Dermatitis herpetiformis. Two thirds of the patients with dermatitis herpetiformis have histologic changes that are revealed by small bowel biopsy. Some of these changes are identical to the findings with classic celiac sprue, whereas in other patients the changes may be less severe and less specific. In patients with dermatis herpetiformis, steatorrhea, and histologic abnormalities of the small intestine, the malabsorption responds to a gluten-free diet with no effect on the skin disease. On the other hand, the skin disease responds to dapsone or sulfapyridine with no effect on the malabsorption. Thus these appear to be two separate diseases that may often coexist. The patient with dermatitis herpetiformis should be evaluated for malabsorption in the manner previously described.

Crohn's disease. Crohn's disease is an idiopathic inflammatory disease of the small intestine and colon. The most common site of involvement is the terminal ileum and adjacent ascending colon. Often the bowel is involved with skip areas in between. Several factors contribute to malabsorption. Loss of absorptive area results from inflammation, resection, or fistulas between loops of bowel causing a mechanical bypass. Loss of bile salts from disease or resection of the terminal ileum contributes to steatorrhea. Bacterial overgrowth from stasis or a stricture inactivates bile salts, also causing steatorrhea.

IATROGENIC CAUSES. Malabsorption of mucosal origin often is caused by therapy applied for other conditions. Such therapies include an intestinal resection or bypass, radiation therapy, and medications.

Surgical resection. Resection of 50% or more of the small intestine usually results in significant malabsorption. Resection of a smaller portion of small bowel in the distal ileum also may lead to significant steatorrhea. Patients who have had a significant resection of small bowel should be carefully evaluated for steatorrhea, which often is severe, and for all of the other metabolic abnormalities associated with a severe malabsorption syndrome. Bile salts are selectively reabsorbed in the distal 90 cm of terminal ileum. A resection of 60 cm or more can result in significant steatorrhea.

In these patients hypoproteinemia and vitamin and mineral deficiencies and their sequelae are the rule and must be evaluated and treated vigorously.

Radiation enteritis. Patients with a known history of radiation therapy to the abdomen who have any of the symptoms of malabsorption should be evaluated for malabsorption syndrome. The symptoms may occur soon after the therapy or after months or even years have elapsed. The mechanism for malabsorption in these patients may be direct and generalized damage to the small bowel mucosa. If this damage includes the distal ileum, a quantitative deficiency of bile salts may result and contribute to the malabsorption, whereas if there is a stricture, the resulting stasis may lead to bacterial overgrowth and the deconjugation of bile salts.

The malabsorption may be severe, especially when severe mucosal damage occurs. The therapy should be directed to the specific cause: surgery for a stricture, MCT for a damaged terminal ileum, and so on. A diet free of gluten, lactose, and milk protein may be of value.

Medications. Colchicine therapy may result in mild steatorrhea and abnormal results on the D-xylose test. The mechanism of action appears to be an inactivation of mucosal intracellular enzymes that resynthesize triglyerides from FFA and β-MG. Neomycin also causes mild malabsorption by a direct toxic effect on mucosal enzymes, by inhibiting lipase action, by precipitating bile salts, or by some combination of these. Cathartic agents may cause mild malabsorption, perhaps because of an increase in motility and intestinal transit time. Malabsorption occurs only in habitual users of relatively large amounts of cathartic agents. Podophyllin, bisacodyl, colocynth, and jalap have been found to cause malabsorption under these conditions. Cholestyramine often is used to decrease the diarrhea associated with bile salt malabsorption, that is, choleretic enteropathy. Although the cholestyramine mitigates diarrhea in these cases, it further diminishes the bile salt pool and may exacerbate the malabsorption. The extent of malabsorption in these patients generally is related to the dosage of cholestyramine. Paraaminosalicylic acid also may cause malabsorption if given in a high dosage.

In all of these conditions malabsorption is generally mild and stops when the medication is discontinued.

MISCELLANEOUS CAUSES OF MALABSORPTION OF MUCOSAL ORIGIN
Whipple's disease

Whipple's disease is an uncommon disease that causes moderate to severe malabsorption and its associated with a wide spectrum of systemic manifestations that may include arthritis, arthralgia, fever, an increase in skin pigmentation, pleuritis, pericarditis, central nervous system symptoms, and anemia. The classic histologic finding for this disease is an infiltration of the lamina propria with macrophages that stain red with periodic acid–Schiff stain. Over the years many observers have

described small rodlike structures detected in biopsies, and electron microscopy clearly shows the presence of small bacilli (0.25 μm wide and 2 μm long). These, however, have not yet been cultured successfully.

Patients with Whipple's disease generally are ill from both the malabsorption and the systemic involvement and in the past have almost invariably died. Treatment with antibiotics, however, has completely altered this grim prognosis, and most patients become asymptomatic within several weeks. Trimethoprim-sulfamethoxazole for 1 year is the treatment of choice. Penicillin and tetracycline also have been effective agents.

Abetalipoproteinemia. Abetalipoproteinemia is a rare genetic disorder in which there is an absence of the lipoprotein that joins to triglycerides within the mucosal cell to form chylomicrons. The result is an accumulation of triglycerides within the mucosal cell and malabsorption.

Because this is a congenital disorder, it usually appears as malabsorption in infants. The clinical picture also includes neurologic symptoms (of which ataxia is the most prominent), retinitis pigmentosa, and acanthocytosis. Other than malabsorption, none of the symptoms has been well explained.

These patients have low levels of serum cholesterol and triglycerides. Serum electrophoresis reveals either an absence or minute amounts of β-lipoprotein. Malabsorption is moderate and, in infants with only malabsorption, may be confused with celiac disease or cystic fibrosis. A small bowel biopsy is necessary to confirm the diagnosis; it reveals villi that are normal in shape, have excessive amounts of fata droplets in mucosal cells, and have almost no fat in the lacteals.

The therapy for the malabsorption is the administration of MCT, which decreases the excretion of fat and leads to a weight gain and increased strength. It may be necessary to supplement MCT with the fat-soluble vitamins. This treatment does not appear to arrest the neurologic component of the disease, which tends to progress. Because this disease was described relatively recently, the long-term natural history after treatment with MCT is not clearly known.

Small intestinal ischemia. Although malabsorption associated with small bowel ischemia is rare, the increase in life expectancy in the United States and the resultant increase in visceral ischemia undoubtedly will lead to an increased incidence of this disorder. Malabsorption that is usually mild may be seen with diffuse arteriosclerosis, vasculitis, polycythemia vera, and Kohlmeier-Degos disease (necrotic skin lesions and vasculitis of the small bowel). Therapy is directed at the underlying disorder. Malabsorption usually results from surgical resection of intestine.

Eosinophilic gastroenteritis. Eosinophilic gastroenteritis, which has been considered an allergy to foods, is characterized by an increase in eosinophils both in the lamina propria and in the peripheral blood and may be accompanied by malabsorption of fat and protein-losing enteropathy. Patients with this condition usually have an increased incidence of allergic disorders and often a dramatic increase in symptoms when certain foods are ingested. The objective of therapy is to eliminate foods from the diet in a sequential manner, but usually the long-term use of corticosteroids also is required.

Amyloidosis. Both primary and secondary amyloidosis may be associated with malabsorption, which usually is moderate but may be associated with protein-losing enteropathy. The infiltration of amyloid protein may cause a motility disorder, and a bacterial overgrowth also may occur. Encroachment on the vascular supply may cause ischemia, with resultant pain and diarrhea.

The small bowel biopsy may or may not reveal the amyloid

deposits. For that reason, a rectal biopsy is often performed to confirm the presence of amyloidosis in patients with suspected amyloidosis and malabsorption.

There is no treatment for amyloidosis; the disease usually is relentless and fatal.

Disorders of lymphatic transport

INTESTINAL LYMPHANGIECTASIA. Intestinal lymphangiectasia is a rare disorder characterized by abnormally dilated lacteals that may distort the villous architecture. The cause of this disorder is unknown, but it leads to the accumulation of chylomicrons between the intestinal cells and the lamina propria as a result of an inability to transport the chylomicrons into the lacteals. Malabsorption is moderate and is associated with protein-losing enteropathy, hypoproteinemia, lymphocytopenia, and peripheral edema. The disease usually affects children and young adults.

The diagnosis usually can be made with a small bowel biopsy. The specific therapy uses MCT, which not only corrects the fat malabsorption but also improves the intestinal protein loss and its sequelae. The prognosis with early diagnosis and treatment is good.

A clinical picture similar to that of lymphangiectasia may be seen in patients whose adominal lymphatics are blocked by disseminated carcinoma or lymphoma.

Miscellaneous causes of malabsorption

PARASITIC DISEASES. (See Chapters 55 and 56.) A variety of parasitic diseases may be associated with malabsorption, including giardiasis *(Giardia lamblia),* strongyloidiasis *(Strongyloides stercoralis),* hookworm disease, coccidiosis *(Isospora belli),* and capillariasis *(Capillaria philippinensis).* In the United States the last three diseases are extremely rare and strongyloidiasis also is rare, but giardiasis is increasingly common. Giardiasis may cause malabsorption, often in patients with IgA deficiency but also in patients with normal immunoglobulins. A severe *Strongyloides* infestation usually is seen in patients whose immune system has been compromised either by chemotherapy for cancer or by corticosteroids. In these instances malabsorption may be more severe, and the patient may be very ill.

When a parasitic origin is suspected for a patient's malabsorption, the stool examination may reveal the parasite. Duodenal aspiration and a small bowel biopsy may be necessary, however, to confirm the diagnosis. Because the ingestion of barium may "wash out" the parasite, it should be delayed in patients suspected of having a parasitic infestation until the aspiration and biopsy have been performed.

Parasitic conditions generally respond well to specific therapy (metronidazole for *Giardia* organisms and thiabendazole for *Strongyloides* srains), leading to the remission of malabsorption and other symptoms of the infestation.

DIFFUSE ILEOJEJUNITIS. Diffuse ileojejunitis is a rare, poorly defined inflammatory disease of the small bowel. Patients often have fever, malaise, abdominal cramps, diarrhea, and malabsorption. The diagnosis usually requires an exploratory laparotomy and biopsies of the inflamed bowel. The intestinal mucosa may exhibit patchy areas of villous atrophy resembling that of celiac disease. Some patients respond to steroid therapy, but for most the prognosis is poor. The mortality is high.

VIRAL AND BACTERIAL GASTROENTERITIS. Mild to moderate fat malabsorption may be found in patients with acute viral gastroenteritis. The malabsorption is generally self-limited. Metabolic complications other than transient electro-lyte changes do not occur. Gastroenteritis caused by *Shigella* organisms, *Escherichia coli,* cholera, *Clostridium* species, staphylococci, and *Yersinia* strains also may have an associated self-limited malabsorption.

DIABETES MELLITUS. Malabsorption associated with diabetes mellitus usually occurs in patients who have peripheral and autonomic neuropathy. Malabsorption usually is mild to moderate, but a persistent, frequent, watery diarrhea that causes patients considerable annoyance is common. It is assumed that the diarrhea and malabsorption are caused by an enteric neuropathy. Recently a deficiency of α_2-adrenergic tone at the level of the enterocyte has been described. α_2-Adrenergic stimulation increases fluid and electrolyte absorption. This tone can be partially restored by the drug clonidine, an α_2-agonist. Bacterial overgrowth occasionally is present, and some patients have been found by the small bowel biopsy to have flattened villi. Most patients, however, have neither bacterial overgrowth nor histologic changes in the small bowel.

The treatment is symptomatic and directed at reducing the frequency of stools. The malabsorption may make the control of the diabetic patient's blood sugar difficult and may lead to episodes of both hyperglycemia and hypoglycemia. In these patients a complete reversal of diarrhea and malabsorption is rare.

MALABSORPTION ASSOCIATED WITH ENDOCRINE DISEASE. Malabsorption that is usually mild has been reported in cases of hyperthyroidism, adrenal insufficiency, hypoparathyroidism, carcinoid, and systemic mast cell disease. In all of these conditions the endocrinopathy is usually obvious and severe, and the malabsorption is a rather unimportant aspect of the patient's problem. The malabsorption responds to the treatment of the primary disease.

Somewhat more common is the malabsorption occurring in patients with Zollinger-Ellison syndrome. In these patients the disorder probably results from the excessive gastric secretion and consequent acid pH in the proximal small bowel, which inactivates pancreatic enzymes and damages the mucosa. Malabsorption in these patients always responds to treatment of the primary problem.

SCLERODERMA. The smooth muscle fibrosis of scleroderma also may involve the small bowel, with a resultant dilation of bowel, decreased motility, and stasis. Although originally reported in patients with obvious skin manifestations, small bowel involvement with scleroderma may occur in patients with minimal skin changes or none at all. The malabsorption usually is mild to moderate and often is the result of bacterial overgrowth caused by intestinal stasis. The malabsorption usually responds to antibiotic therapy with a total or partial remission.

MALABSORPTION ASSOCIATED WITH DISORDERED IMMUNOGLOBULINS

Hypogammaglobulinemia. Hypogammaglobulinemia, especially IgA deficiency, may be associated with malabsorption. Although the presence of flattened villi and the response of the disorder to a gluten-free diet once were assumed to imply an interrelationship of IgA deficiency and celiac sprue, it is now known that *G.lamblia* infestation is the usual cause of malabsorption in these patients. Treatment of the giardiasis usually reverses the malabsortpion.

α-Chain disease. Malabsorption may be seen in α-chain disease, a rare disorder characterized by proliferation of cells producing homogeneous, partially complete heavy chains of IgA. The malabsorption is severe and accompanied by hypoproteinemia, anemia, hypocalcemia, and hypomagnesemia. The lamina propria of the entire small bowel is infiltrated with round cells, and the mucosa is thickened and distorted. The diagnosis is confirmed by immunoelectrophoresis followed by specific immunologic tests. Although tetracycline therapy has helped some patients, the disease generally progresses to overt lymphoma and death.

Macroglobulinemia. Waldenström's macroglobulinemia, an IgM gammopathy, sometimes may cause malabsorption. The probable cause is an infiltration of the lamina propria with proteinaceous material and a distention of the villi. The diagnosis is made with immunoelectrophoresis. This disease is not as relentless as α-chain disease and may respond to chemotherapy.

POSTGASTRECTOMY SYNDROME. Postgastrectomy malabsorption may be seen in patients who have had a gastric resection such as the Billroth II operation. The malabsorption usually is mild to moderate, but it can be severe. Because of the relatively rapid gastric emptying the patient also may have bloating and symptoms referable to dumping of reactive hypoglycemia. Symptoms related to decreased vitamin D and calcium absorption are common, as is iron deficiency anemia.

The principal cause of the malabsorption seems related to the rapid gastric emptying, which results in inadequate mixing of ingested food with bile salts and pancreatic enzymes. In rare cases, bacterial overgrowth may be present in a stagnant afferent loop.

Patients with a stagnant afferent loop and bacterial overgrowth usually require corrective surgery. For others, a trial of several small feedings with supplemental pancreatic enzymes may mitigate all or most of the malabsorption. Patients whose malabsorption is serious and fails to respond to these measures may need surgical revision. Many patients with gastric resection, even those without malabsorption, may require supplemental vitamins and minerals, especially vitamin D, calcium, and iron. These needs are even more intense when malabsorption is present.

DISORDERS OF CARBOHYDRATE ABSORPTION
Normal physiology

Most carbohydrates are ingested as starch and glycogen and to a lesser extent as the disaccharides lactose and sucrose. In the intestinal lumen the starch and glycogen are digested by α-amylase secreted by the salivary glands and pancreas, to form oligosaccharides of 2 to 10 glucose molecules. These molecules are further broken down at the brush border–lumen interface by oligosaccharidases, which are located on the outer surface of the intestinal brush border. These enzymes hydrolyze the glucose α-dextrins to glucose. Specific brush border enzymes act on lactose to form glucose and galactose (lactase) and on sucrose to form glucose and fructose (sucrase). The monosaccharides are then transported across the intestinal epithelium by specific active transport systems that are energy dependent.

As is the case with fat malabsorption, conditions that inhibit any of these steps can lead to malabsorption of sugars. The intraluminal phase rarely is a clinical problem in carbohydrate malabsorption, because amylase rarely is so reduced in quantity that it becomes a clinical problem. Thus disorders of carbohydrate absorption result either from a deficiency or absence of oligosaccharidases located at the brush border or from a defect in one or more specific transport systems.

When any of these disorders exist, unabsorbed disaccharides or monosaccharides remain in the intestinal lumen, where they have an osmotic effect. The net flow of water into the intestinal lumen results in bloating, increased intestinal transit, and

crampy abdominal pains. The unabsorbed sugars are fermented by colonic bacteria and create an acid pH that appears to inhibit the absorption of water and electrolytes in the colon. In addition, the bacterial fermentation produces gas, which adds to the abdominal cramping. The net result, depending on the severity of the problem, is diarrhea, crampy abdominal pain, flatulence, and bloating.

There are several specific disorders of carbohydrate malabsorption, but lactase deficiency (lactose intolerance) is by far the most common and is clinically the most important.

Lactose intolerance (lactase deficiency)

Although a premature infant may have transient lactase deficiency, lactase activity usually is very high in the neonatal period. This activity declines in childhood, however, and much of the world's population over 10 years of age has a lactase deficiency. This is called acquired lactase deficiency. Whites of Northern European ancestry are an exception to this acquired deficiency, but even in this group up to 20% may have this deficiency. An acquired deficiency therefore may be considered normal. Certain racial groups, notably blacks, Asians, and Eskimos, have an incidence as high as 70% to 95%. The deficiency of lactase is minimal in some individuals and more severe in others of the same race, and thus there is wide individual variation in the ability to absorb lactose even with a "pure" racial group. In the United States there is clearly a major difference in incidence between whites of Northern European origin and all others.

It has been demonstrated that lactase deficiency is inherited as an autosomal recessive condition. It has been postulated that the decrease in intestinal lactase seen in adults (the acquired form) is secondary to the decrease in mild ingestion after childhood and the subsequent lack of enzyme stimulation by ingested lactose. This hypothesis, however, is not supported by evidence. There also has been controversy about the extent to which milk proteins or other constituents contribute to the symptoms. Recent evidence supports the theory that lactose—and lactose alone—is responsible for symptoms in lactase-deficient individuals.

In the congenital form of lactose intolerance, virtually no lactase is present at birth, and the reaction to ingested lactose is immediate and severe. Whereas the acquired form of lactase deficiency has been viewed as a genetic (autosomal recessive) defect in enzyme regulation, the congenital form has been regarded as a structural change in the gene itself. More recent studies of patients with the congenital form, however, reveal minute quantities of lactase that is qualitatively indistinguishable from normal lactase. Thus the congenital form of this disorder may be just one end of a spectrum of the defect in enzyme regulation.

The third form of lactase deficiency is secondary lactase deficiency, that is, a deficiency that occurs in association with other diseases and is resolved when the primary disease is treated. Secondary lactase deficiency is most common in conditions that affect large areas of small bowel mucosa, such as sprue, acute gastroenteritis, and bowel ischemia. Postgastrectomy diarrhea often is caused by rapid gastric emptying in which ingested lactose does not have adequate time to make contact with intestinal lactase. Lactose intolerance has also been found to be the cause of some cases of so-called spastic colon; patients thus diagnosed may in fact have occult lactose intolerance. In these patients a lactose-free diet eliminates the symptoms of the irritable colon syndrome.

DIAGNOSIS. In most instances a history of the symptoms described occurring 1 to 4 hours after the ingestion of milk or milk products suggests the diagnosis of lactase deficiency. Many patients are aware of this association and inform the physician of it, but many others are not and with these the burden of diagnosis rests with the physician. The usual diagnostic test is the lactose tolerance test, in which 50 g of lactose is given orally and the clinical response noted. In more than 90% of patients with lactase deficiency who are given this test, abdominal cramps and diarrhea develop. It is also possible to measure the blood glucose in these patients, as with a glucose toelrance test, because those with lactase deficiency have a flat curve. However, patients with a normal lactase content, also may have a flat curve. A simpler and more accurate confirmation of the diagnosis can be obtained with a lactose breath test. A standard amount of lactose is ingested. The malabsorbed portion passes into the colon, where it is metabolized with release of CO_2 and H_2. The hydrogen is absorbed by the colon and excreted by the lungs, where it can be measured. Lactose malabsorption results in increased breath hydrogen excretion. The diagnosis also can be made from a tissue assay of lactase enzyme activity from a small bowel biopsy.

MANAGEMENT. Treatment consists of removing lactose from the diet, a regimen that may not be as simple as it seems, because many foods, such as all milk products, bakery goods made with milk, and canned and frozen fruits and vegetables, contain lactose. In time both the physician and the patient will learn just how much lactose the patient can tolerate and in what form. Because the degree of lactase deficiency varies from patient to patient, the extent to which each patient can tolerate lactose also varies. For this reason the dietary restrictions should be individualized.

Other disorders of carbohydrate absorption

The other disorders of carbohydrate absorption are rare. The deficiency of sucrase is associated with low levels of isomaltase as well. The primary form of this disease is a genetic defect that results in a virtual absence of enzymes. Symptoms develop in the neonatal period, and the disorder can be diagnosed definitively with a biopsy and enzyme assay. Patients respond well to withdrawing sucrose from the diet. A secondary form of sucrase deficiency occurs with the same disease entities associated with lactase deficiency.

Glucose-galactose malabsorption is the result of selectively impaired intestinal transport of glucose and galactose. The symptoms appear almost immediately after birth as low blood sugar levels and, if the condition is not treated, dehydration. These patients respond well to a diet that contains fructose as the only carbohydrate.

BIBLIOGRAPHY

Benson GD, Kowlessar OD, and Sleisenger MH: Adult celiac disease with emphasis upon response to the gluten free diet, Medicine 43:1, 1964.

Bond JH and Levitt MD: Use of breath hydrogen (H_2) in the study of carbohydrate absorption, Am J Dig Dis 22:379, 1977.

Cooper BT and others: Celiac disease and malignancy, Medicine (Baltimore) 59:249, 1980.

Finlay JM, Hogarth J, and Wightman KJR: A clinical evaluation of the D-xylose tolerance test, Ann Intern Med 61:411, 1964.

Fromm H and Hofmann AF: Breath test for altered bile-acid metabolism, Lancet 2:621, 1971.

Gray GM: Congenital and adult intestinal lactase deficiency, N Engl J Med 294:1057, 1976.

Howdle PD and others: Cell-mediated immunity to gluten within the small intestinal in coeliac disease, Gut 23:115, 1982.

Newcomer AD and others: Triolein breath test. A sensitive and specific test for fat malabsorption, Gastroenterology 76:6, 1979.

Ochner RK and Isselbacher KJ: Recent concepts of intestinal fat absorption, Rev Phsiol Biochem Pharmacol 71:107, 1974.

Rubin CE and Dobbins WO III: Peroral biopsy of the small intestine: a review of its diagnostic usefulness, Gastroenterology 49:676, 1965.

Sleisenger MH and Fordtran JS: Gastrointestinal disease, ed 3, Philadelphia, 1983, WB Saunders Co.

Spiro H: Clinical gastroenterology, New York, 1983, Macmillan Publishing Co.

175 · INFLAMMATORY DISEASES OF THE INTESTINES

Harvey B. Lefton

INFLAMMATORY BOWEL DISEASE

DEFINITION. Inflammatory bowel disease is a general classification of inflammatory processes affecting the large and small intestines. Ulcerative colitis is one such inflammatory condition involving the mucosa and submucosa of the colon. The disease may inflame part or all of the large intestine. Occasionally when the entire colon is involved, 5 to 10 cm of the most distal terminal ileum is inflamed; this is referred to as backwash ileitis. A milder form of ulcerative colitis may affect only the rectum and sigmoid; this is called proctosigmoiditis. This inflammatory process also is limited to the mucosa and submucosa.

Crohn's disease is an inflammatory condition involving all layers of the gut. The disease may inflame segments of the colon or small intestine. Although ulcerative colitis usually is continuous, beginning in the rectum and extending retrograde to involve various portions of the colon, Crohn's disease usually is segmental, with normal intestine between areas of inflammation. Most commonly, the terminal ileum and right colon are involved. The colon may be affected and the rectum not affected. Lesions also have been reported in the esophagus, stomach and duodenum.

In the past 20 years a greater effort has been made to differentiate the histologic and clinical course of patients with ulcerative colitis and Crohn's disease. The approach to treatment is based on this differentiation. Despite an improved understanding of these diseases, the inflammation in about 10% of patients is still indeterminate because it shares features of both processes.

ETIOLOGY. Possible causes of inflammatory bowel disease have been investigated since these conditions were first recognized. Infectious agents have been considered as causes. Bacillary dysentery was not distinguished from idiopathic ulcerative colitis until about 100 years ago.

Sophisticated techniques have been used in the search for infectious agents. Speculation has centered around L-forms of *Pseudomonas* species, viruses, and atypical bacteria. Using homogenates of diseased colon, investigators have produced granulomas in the foot pads of mice and inflammatory lesions in the small intestine of rabbits. These lesions are nonspecific and have not been uniformly reproduced in different laboratories. The evaluation of gut flora has shown increased numbers of anaerobes in patients with regional enteritis. Advocates of a "slow virus" hypothesis have isolated an agent with the physical characteristics of an RNA-like picornavirus, and animal transmission studies have been conducted with varying results. The question of whether this virus is the pathogen of inflammatory bowel disease or is an innocent passenger has not been resolved. No one has been able to fulfill the requirements of Koch's postulates.

Immunologic factors have been cited as a possible cause of inflammatory bowel disease. Hypersensitivity reactions characterized by increased mast cell degranulation have been studied. An increased incidence of allergic reactions in colitis patients with asthma, hay fever, and eczema has also been noted. The presence of extraintestinal lesions in patients with inflammatory bowel disease has also been cited as evidence of immunologic changes in patients with inflammatory bowel disease. Colon antibodies have been found in the sera of patients with inflammatory bowel disease, but these have not been demonstrated on the colonic epithelium, suggesting that the antibodies are caused by the inflammatory process rather than initiating agents. These antibodies also have been found in the sera of patients with pernicious anemia, collagenopathies, and colon cancer.

Prostaglandins have been implicated in the pathogenesis of inflammatory bowel disease. These agents are the principal mediators of the inflammatory process throughout the body. Elevated prostaglandin levels have been found in rectal biopsy tissues from patients with ulcerative colitis and infectious diarrhea. Although no evidence as yet suggests that this is the cause of inflammatory bowel disease, prostaglandins appear to play a role in propagating the inflammatory response. Drugs that have been found to inhibit prostaglandins play a major role in the treatment of inflammatory bowel disease.

Inflammatory bowel disease can occur in several members of the same family. Although no genetic mode of inheritance has been determined, one fifth of the patients with the disease have a familial history of inflammatory bowel disease. No evidence exists that a single dominant gene is involved. An increased incidence of inflammatory bowel disease in monozygous twins has been shown; when one twin has the disease, the sibling has an increased risk. Several studies have shown that high numbers of Ashkenazi Jews have the disease in the United States and South Africa. Similar studies in Tel Aviv, however, indicate a much lower than predicted incidence in the same group in Israel, an observation that emphasized the difficulty in separating hereditary from environmental factors. The lack of a higher than normal incidence of the disease in spouses of patients with inflammatory bowel disease is evidence against environmental factors. The association between ankylosing spondylitis, a classic genitically determined disease, and inflammatory bowel disease further supports a genetic role in its cause. It has been reported that in some families that share histocompatibility antigens, several members have inflammatory bowel disease. A major concern in these family studies is whether true genetic forces have a role or whether the common environment plays a role.

Much has been written about psychologic factors associated with inflammatory bowel disease. The "colitis personality" distinguished by feelings of helplessness, deependency, anxiety, and despair is not unique to patients with inflammatory bowel disease but characterizes a common response to any chronic debilitating disease. That many people have these personality traits without having the disease is further evidence against this association. In fact, one study of the emotional profile of patients with inflammatory bowel disease showed that they had less life stress than patients with irritable bowel syndrome. Although the onset of symptoms may be associated with a major life crisis, the emotional stress itself is not a causative factor.

Whatever the cause of Crohn's disease may be, the disease seems to be relatively new, to be increasing in its incidence, and to be three to five times more common in whites and two to three times more common in Ashkenazi Jews.

Chronic ulcerative colitis

PATHOLOGY. The hallmark of chronic ulcerative colitis is an inflammatory reaction of the mucosa and submucosa. The disease begins in the rectum and involves the bowel contiguously.

Macroscopically, the mucosa may have a granular appearance if the disease is mild. Ulcers and hemorrhage occur in the active phase. When fulminant the disease may include the stripping of the mucosa with actual areas of sloughing; normal mucosa may remain between these areas. When the healing phase is completed, these islands of normal mucosa may be pushed up by surrounding fibrous tissue, giving a polypoid appearance to this normal tissue that is referred to as pseudopolyps. Marked hyperemeia is present in ulcerative colitis, accounting in part for the bleeding that occurs when the mucosa is swabbed or stool passes over it. As healing occurs, submucosal scarring may develop and give rise to residual pitting of the mucosa. This may be the only sign remaining after a mild attack. The submucosal fibrosis may also cause the rectal valves to lose their contours and have a blunted or rounded appearance. Perianal disease is uncommon but may cause a hyperpigmentation of the perianal skin that remains after an attack. Shallow rectal fissures are occasionally present.

Microscopically, changes related to the activity of disease can be observed. In severe disease there is loss of goblet cells and marked vascular congestion. The submucosa and lamina propria may contain mononuclear cell infiltrates. Collections of neutrophils may occur in the epithelial crypts and give rise to crypt abscesses that usually penetrate the mucosa and drain into the bowel lumen. Burrowing ulcers do not occur unless there is necrosis of the myenteric plexus, such as occurs with toxic megacolon. With healing the epithelial lining of the bowel is restored, and the inflammatory infiltrate is diminished. Complete healing observed macroscopically is usually reflected microscopically in the diminished numbers of crypts and in the presence of some degree of submucosal fibrosis. Pseudopolyps appear in areas of normal mucosa, and the numbers of goblet cells are diminished. Vascular congestion appears to be an early finding in the inflammatory picture. Rectal biopsies of patients with quiescent disease may reveal vascular congestion as a harbinger of recurrent inflammation. The rectal biopsy is also important in detecting precancerous changes in the colon. The loss of goblet cells, severe dysplasia in the absence of an inflammatory process, and glandular elements in the submucosa may serve as the first signs of malignant degeneration. The recognition of such changes is important because colonic cancers are often multifocal, flat, infiltrative lesions that are metastatic by the time they have been recognized.

CLINICAL MANIFESTATIONS. The hallmark of ulcerative colitis is rectal bleeding and diarrhea. The frequency of bowel movements and the amount of blood present reflect the activity of the disease. Scant bleeding and a minimal change of consistency of stools may occur in patients with mild disease or inflammation limited to the rectosigmoid. Moderate to severe disease is characterized by more frequent bleeding. The patient may experience tenesmus with rectal pressure, the urge to have repeated bowel movements, and the passage of scant amounts of bloody mucoid material. Abdominal cramps may precede each episode and may be only partially relieved by defecation. Along with the change in the pattern of bowel movements, the patient may have nocturnal diarrhea. Although patients may not recognize a minor change in daytime stool habits, nocturnal symptoms are quite troublesome. Abdominal bloating and gas may accompany bloody diarrhea. Fatigue and malaise may result from anemia caused by rectal bleeding. In patients with severe disease a decrease in serum albumin levels can occur and lead to edema. Profuse mucoid diarrhea also can cause an electrolyte imbalance. Fever and tachycardia may accompany severe exacerbations and are especially prominent when toxic dilation of the colon (toxic megacolon) occurs. In patients with toxic megacolon the abdominal wall is tender. Large, dilated loops of bowel are palpable, and tympany is noted with percussion.

Extraintestinal manifestations may be prominent. Skin manifestations may include erythema nodsum, characterized by red, swollen nodules usually on the thighs and legs. A severe form of ulcerating skin disease with a purulent discharge (pyoderma gangrenosum) may occur on the arms or legs. Cultures from these lesions reveal only normal skin flora. Healing usually occurs when the colon inflammation comes under control.

Pyoderma gangrenosum may also occur in the mouth in the form of deep uclers that sometimes ulcerate through the tonsillar pillar. Pyostomatitis vegetans, a purulent inflammation of the mouth, also may occur; inflammatory vegetations usually are sterile lesions like those in pyoderma gangrenosum and respond not to local therapy but rather to control of the disease. Aphthous stomatitis, gingivitis, and oral *Candida* infections also may occur.

Eye changes, such as episcleritis, uveitis, corneal ulcers, and retinitis, may cause eye pain or photophobia.

Joint symptoms occur in up to 20% of patients with the disease. "Colitic arthritis" usually affects the ankles, knees, and wrists. Ankylosing spondylitis and sacroiliitis are common findings in patients with colitis. Conversely, the incidence of colitis is increased in patients with these arthritic disorders. Ankylosing spondylitis occurs 20 times more commonly in patients with colitis than in the general population. Patients with colitis who have backache should have a careful roentgenographic search for narrowing of the sacroiliac joints, osteophytes, and calcification of paraspinal ligaments. The arthritic disease may not improve with control of the colitis. Patients with spondylitis and colitis are HLA-B27 positive, whereas those with only peripheral arthritis do not have this histocompatibility antigen.

Perhaps the most pernicious complication of ulcerative colitis is liver disease. Pericholangitis may occur with an intense inflammation of portal areas. Fatty infiltration of the liver, bile duct carcinomas, sclerosing cholangitis, chronic active liver disease, granulomatous hepatitis, and primary biliary cirrhosis occasionally have been noted in these patients. Although the other extraintestinal manifestations usually undergo remission with medical or surgical control of the colon inflammation, liver disease may continue and progress to cirrhosis, liver failure, and death.

Thrombophlebitis is a serious complication in patients with colits. Hypercoagulable states occur in patients with severe disease and may promote thrombosis of major veins throughout the abdomen, thighs, and legs.

LABORATORY FINDINGS. Anemia is commonly associated with inflammatory bowel disease. It may be caused by iron deficiency, chronic disease, or severe bleeding. Leukocytosis occurs in active disease, but a white blood cell count higher than 15,0000/mm³ is rare and usually is a sign of intraabdominal abscess or toxic megacolon. Hypoalbuminemia may occur along with an electrolyte imbalance. Low serum magnesium and potassium levels often are found during profuse diarrhea. Smears of stool specimens show many red blood cells, neutrophils, and eosinophils. The sedimentation rate also is elevated.

Table 175-1   Comparison of inflammatory bowel diseases

Site and symptoms	Ulcerative colitis	Crohn's colitis
Usual location	Rectosigmoid and left colon	Right colon
Small bowel involvement	Rare "backwash ileitis"	Common
Area of spread	Contiguous	Noncontiguous segments
Fistulas	Uncommon	Common
Abscesses	Uncommon	Common in fistulas
Rectal bleeding	In most patients	In 50% of patients
Ulcers	Small mucosal ulcers	Large deep ulcers
Strictures	Rare	Common
Pseudopolyps	Common	Never occurs
Carcinoma	Risk increases 10% with each decade	Increased risk

DIAGNOSIS. A careful history and physical examination are important in establishing the presence of inflammatory bowel disease, and they may help exclude gonorrheal proctitis, ischemic colitis, and irritable bowel syndrome. A full evaluation is necessary to exclude Crohn's colitis (Table 175-1). The presence of abdominal tenderness and a dilated colon may indicate toxic dilation. The rectal examination reveals bleeding. Pseudopolyps also may be palpable in the rectal examination.

Sigmoidoscopy should precede roentgenographic studies. The presence of diffusely inflamed rectal mucosa along with discrete ulcers and mucus indicates active disease. During the healing phase or with quiescent disease the mucosa may have a granular appearance, and friability can be confirmed by swabbing the mucosa. The rectal valves usually are blunted in this stage, indicating submucosal edema. A rectal biopsy may be helpful in distinguishing between ulcerative colitis and Crohn's disease.

Stool cultures should be obtained to rule out the possibility of shigellosis and *Campylobacter* infection. A stool examination also should be performed to exclude the possibility of amebiasis, and the stool should be tested for *Clostridium difficile* toxin.

A barium enema examination can help determine the extent of the disease and rule out a carcinoma (Fig. 175-1). It is imperative that patients with inflammatory bowel disease be gently prepared for roentgenography. Harsh cathartics aggravate an electrolyte imbalance and may cause shock. Saline enemas help cleanse the colon and allow for suitable roentgenograms. A severely ill patient should not undergo any contrast study, however, until the condition is stabilized and improved. The barium enema may show the disease limited to the rectosigmoid, as in proctosigmoiditis, in which there is a widening (greater than 2 cm) of the space between the sacrum and the barium-filled rectum, as shown on lateral films. The amount of the colon involved also can be measured with the barium study. A granular appearance, along with small ulcerations, is characteristic. With severe disease a loss of haustra occurs. As healing proceeds, marked narrowing and shortening of the colon develop, giving the colon a tubular appearance. Intense spasm may occur, and areas may mimic strictures. Residual pseudopolyps may be present from previous attacks. Care must be taken to evaluate these areas closely, and any area of narrowing must be considered a carcinoma until proven otherwise. Often agents that relax the colon open up these areas. Barium studies should not be performed on patients who

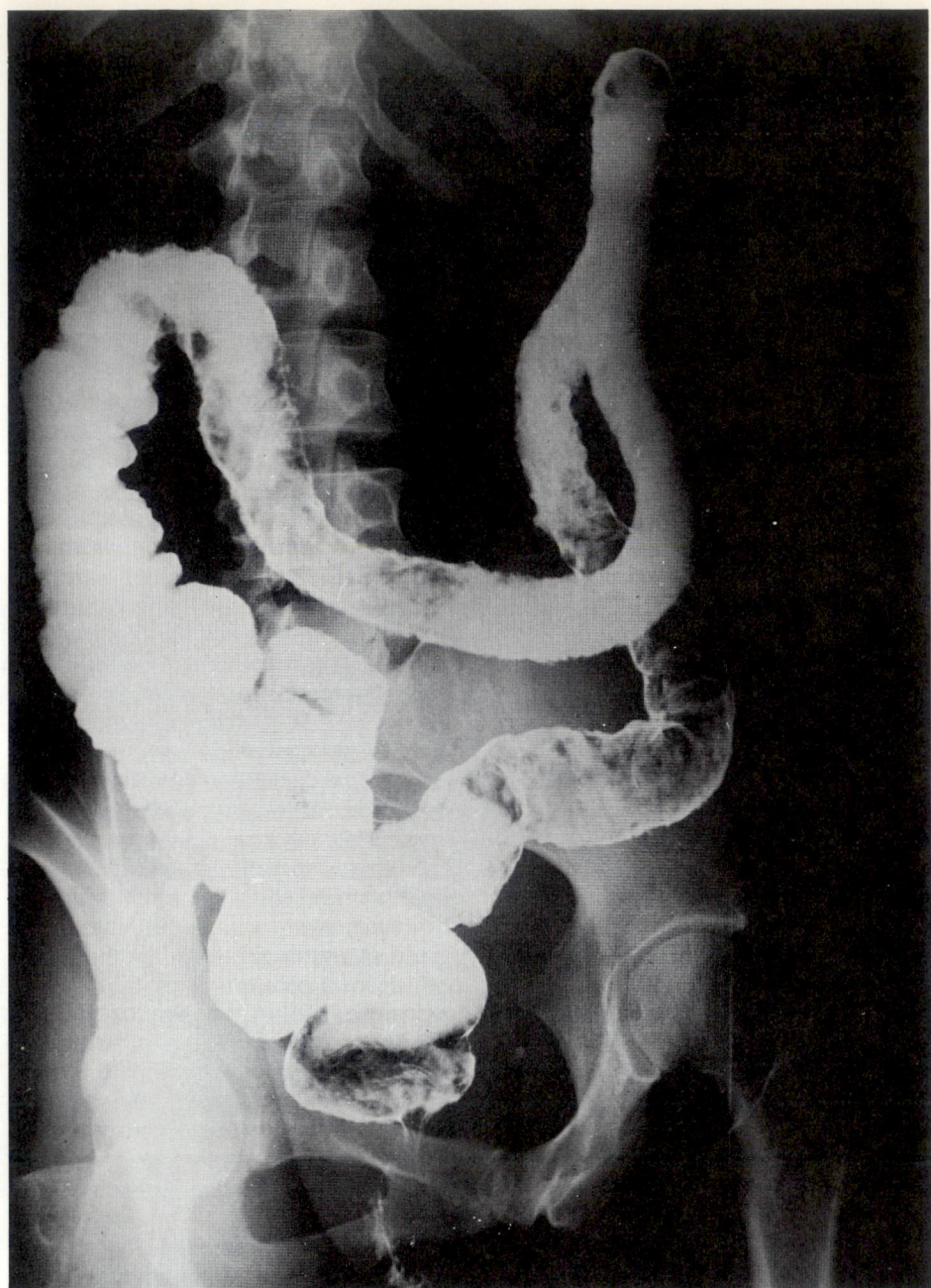

Fig. 175-1 Barium enema in 34-year-old woman with bloody diarrhea reveals classic changes of diffuse ulcerative colitis. Note loss of normal mucosal pattern, loss of haustra, and diffuse ulcerations along surfaces.

are severely ill, but a plain roentgenogram of the abdomen may reveal air in the the bowel outlining irregular mucosa. A plain roentgenogram of the abdomen should be made with patients who have abdominal pain and distention to confirm a diagnosis of megacolon. A transverse colon greater than 6.5 cm in diameter indicates such a process, which should be watched closely because surgical intervention may be necessary.

Persistently narrowed areas should be evaluated with colonoscopy and biospy. A colonoscopy should also be performed on patients with normal roentgenograms and persistent symptoms. These patients usually are found to have proctosigmoiditis or mild inflammatory bowel disease. Colonoscopy can make a more accurate determination of the extent of colon involvement. Colonscopy should be performed by a skilled

endoscopist, in patients with colitis, especially in ill patients with acutely inflamed colons, because the risk of perforation is significantly increased.

COURSE. Ulcerative colitis is a chronic disease that may be characterized by acute attacks and remissions, a continual lower degree of activity, or an initial episode followed by quiescent disease. Those who have the disease during childhood are a major concern, because they often fail to grow and develop normally. They have a risk of developing carcinoma that increases by 10% each decade after the first 10 years of disease. Up to 75% of patients have only one or two attacks that can be quickly controlled by medical therapy; the remainder have recurrent exacerbations and require further treatment. Patients may have increased flare-ups during the first trimester of pregnancy or after delivery, but during the second and third trimester the disease usually is quiescent. Patients with frequent active disease have a higher incidence of massive hemorrhage, perforations, and colon cancer and have an increased risk of dying of a disease complication or developing amyloidosis. Statistical analysis of patients with inflammatory bowel disease reveals that those with severe disease have an annual mortality of 14%, whereas quiescent disease is associated with a 2% to 4% mortality. The mortality of the first attack is much higher for patients over 60 years of age.

Patients with proctosigmoiditis have the best outlook; in 90% of these patients the disease is limited to this area of the bowel. Usually inflammation subsides over 3 to 5 years, and residual scarring is minimal. These patients do not appear to have an increased risk of cancer.

The incidence of colon carcinomas is increased in patients with a long history of colitis. The major problem is that a carcinoma often is metastatic by the time it is symptomatic. There is also an increased incidence of multifocal neoplasms that are not revealed by roentgenography. The monitoring of these patients should be strict and should consist of yearly roentgenography or annual colonscopy with biopsy. Any suspicious area revealed on a roentgenogram should be evaluated colonoscopically. Some authors have advocated alternating barium enemas with colonscopy and biopsy at 6-month intervals for the better detection of early cancers. Measurements of the carcinoembryonic antigen (CEA) may be helpful in spotting the early development of cancers. A rising CEA titer in a patient should trigger a search for neoplastic disease.

MANAGEMENT. The therapy for ulcerative colitis is aimed at reducing the inflammation and correcting the effects of the disease. Patients with weight loss and dehydration may require intravenous electrolyte replacement. Transfusion is required if the patient has severe anemia. The dietary treatment may include low-residue, high-nitrogen prepared supplements. A bland diet may be most easily tolerated during exacerbations. Dietary restrictions occasionally have been imposed automatically rather than with good logic, but this approach should be avoided because the aim is to provide calories and amino acids in the most palatable form. High-residue foods, caffeinated beverages, and spices stimulate peristalsis and should be avoided. Milk products may contribute to diarrhea because of either a long-standing lactose intolerance or a newly acquired lactase deficiency.

Medical treatment is directed to reducing inflammation. Sulfasalazine is used to initiate and maintain a remission in ulcerative colitis. Its active moiety, 5-aminosalicylate, has a direct antiinflammatory effect in dosages of 2 to 8 g a day. Although the colon flora are not altered by sulfasalazine, colon bacteria are required to split the drug. Patients can be maintained in remission by doses of 1 to 2 g a day. The drug is not without side effects. Nausea and abdominal distress may result but can be ameliorated by the use of enteric-coated tablets that dissolve in the small bowel. Severe skin reaction also may occur, including exfoliative dermatitis and photosensitive reactions. Because hemolytic anemia, agranulocytosis, pancytopenia, and thrombocytopenia also may occur, frequent blood counts are mandatory. Although most side effects of the drug develop within the first month of thereapy, delayed skin and hematologic reactions have been reported in patients who had taken the medication for 1 to 2 years. Sulfasalazine interferes with folate metabolism, and supplemental folic acid may be needed in the treatment. Recently trials have been carried out with 5-aminosalicylate moieties in Europe. These agents hold the promise of having the same antiinflammatory effects of

sulfasalazine without the side effects and risk of sulfa allergy. They are being tested in tablet and enema form. An enema form of 5-aminosalicylate, Rowasa, is now available for use in patients with left-sided colitis.

Corticosteroids and corticotropin (ACTH) should be used in patients with severe disease or in those who have not responded satisfactorily to sulfasalazine. These steroids have an antiinflammatory effect on the bowel. They are administered in high dosages that are adjusted as the patient improves. Therapy is initiated with 40 to 80 units of ACTH by intramuscular or intravenous injection or with 40 to 60 mg of oral prednisone each day. Maintenance therapy consists of 20 to 40 units of ACTH or 10 to 20 mg of prednisone daily. Alternate-day therapy with eventual discontinuance of the medication is indicated when the patient goes into remission. Often steroids can be discontinued and remission maintained by sulfasalazine. Anemia, electrolyte imbalance, and negative protein states should be treated because patients may not respond to the steroid treatment until these problems are corrected. Several studies have suggested that patients receiving steroids have a higher risk of complications requiring surgery. Analysis of these reports, however, indicates that it is the patient with severe disease who receives steroids and that the complications are related to the severity of disease rather than to the treatment. Patients with proctosigmoiditis may benefit from the instillation of steroids in specially prepared enemas. These preparations may induce a remission by themselves or in conjunction with oral steroids. Because at least 25% of rectally administered steroids are absorbed, systemic effects may occur. The use of steroid suppositories and steroid rectal foams should be avoided in patients with active disease. These agents contain small amounts of steroids and have a minimal area of penetration.

Many side effects are associated with the use of ACTH and steroids. The development of cushingoid facies, fluid retention, hypokalemia, and muscle cramps may be troublesome. Emotional instability and severe depression or hypermania may also develop but usually subside promptly when the drug is discontinued. Hypertension and diabetes are serious side effects that may require treatment or discontinuance of the steroid therapy. Long-term therapy may cause osteoporosis and vertebral compression fractures as well as cataracts. Steroid-induced myopathy characterized by quadriceps wasting may be debilitating and may impair the patient's ability to climb stairs. Steroids increase the patient's susceptiblity to many infections, including oral candidiasis. Young patients undergoing steroid treatment may have growth failure or alterations in the menstrual cycle. Patients undergoing surgery require increased doses of steroids before and after the operation because their own adrenal response to stress is blunted. Patients treated with ACTH should have their therapy maintained and react to the stress of surgery without difficulty. Patients requireing long-term steroid treatment should be closely evaluated for a possible colectomy because the risks of steroid side effects and carcinoma associated with active long-term disease may be greater than those of surgery. Tixocortol pivalate is a steroid that is devoid of systemic effects. It is being studied in enema and liquid form. Initial results are encouraging for the use of this agent in healing colonic inflammation.

Immunosuppressive medications such as azathioprine have been used as treatment for ulcerative colitis with varying results. Some authors have reported that lower steroid dosages are effective when azathioprine is given concomitantly. To date there has been no good study to support the efficacy of immunosuppressive agents. The risk of hematologic suppression and superinfection is increased in patients taking these medications, and therefore they should be reserved for patients who have not responded to more traditional medical therapy.

Surgery for ulcerative colitis is indicated in patients with intractable disease. Patients with severe recurrent diarrhea and bleeding that have not responded to medical therapy require surgery. The presence of a perforation, intraabdominal abscess, stricture, or premalignant biopsy changes is an indication for surgery. Patients with toxic megacolon must be followed closely; if there is evidence of further colonic dilation or if the patient does not improve in 24 to 72 hours, surgery is required.

Proctocolectomy along with the construction of a permanent ileostomy is the usual operative procedure. The timing of surgery is important, because the mortality of elective surgery is less than 5% but rises to 15% to 20% if emergency surgery becomes necessary. If the patient is very ill, the surgeon may elect to perform a subtotal colectomy and ileostomy initially and to remove the rectal stump at a later time. If the rectum is in good condition, an ileorectal anastomosis may be performed in rare cases, but the rectal segment still has a risk of developing recurrent disease and carcinoma. The English experience with this procedure has been better than the American. Proctectomy may impair the sexual function in men if the parsympathetic nerves are not carefully removed from the rectal serosa. A patient with toxic megacolon may undergo a decompression cecostomy initially and a proctocolectomy later after the patient's condition improves. There has been much concern about the psychologic implications for patients after an ileostomy. With the new disposable ileostomy equipment available today, however, patients find they can enjoy athletics, perform strenuous work, and have normal sexual activity despite the operation. Women can have normal pregnancies. Patients who are relieved of much suffering and disability find ileostomy acceptable. Proctocolectomy combined with ileostomy is a curative procedure for ulcerative colitis; most patients can look forward to a normal life expectancy after successful surgery.

Crohn's disease

PATHOLOGY. Crohn's disease is an inflammatory disease of the small or large intestine. The inflammation involves all the layers of the gut, and thus the term "transmural colitis" has been used to describe this disease in the colon. Gross examination may reveal mucosal ulceration: aphthous ulcers within mucosa that appears normal, deep ulcers within areas of swollen mucosa, or long linear serpiginous ulcers. Punctate areas of mucosal hemorrhage may alternate with areas of gross hemorrhage. If edema is pronounced in the submucosa, ballooning of the mucosa may give rise to a cobblestone-like appearance of the intestinal surface. Perianal fistulas may occur with either colonic or small bowel disease and produce copious drainage of purulent and fecal material. The perianal region may have scarring and darkening of the surrounding skin as a result of severe inflammation.

With the involvement of either the colon or small intestine in Crohn's disease, microscopic examination reveals inflammatory infiltrate in all layers of affected bowel, with plasma cells and lymphocytes predominating in the lamina propria. The serosa may be congested. Deep ulcers may extend into the muscularis, and fistulous tracts may extend from the ulcers, through the bowel wall, and into adjoining segments of intestine. Granulomata composed of epithelioid multinuclear cells are observed in almost 60% of cases. They may be present in areas of severe inflammation or in relatively normal-appearing intestine far removed from other areas of inflammation; they often occur near the lymph channels in the intestine. Granulomas also have been found in bone marrow and muscle tissue. The intestinal muscularis often is hypertrophied and may remain thickened even after the inflammation subsides. Fibrosis may occur in the submucosa and serosa, but the degree of bowel shortening that occurs in ulcerative colitis is not present in Crohn's disease. Dense areas of fibrosis may produce a narrowing or stricturing of the intestinal lumen. Regional lymph nodes often are enlarged in cases of intense inflammation and may contain granulomata. The mesentery may be edematous, and mesenteric nodes may be matted together.

CLINICAL MANIFESTATIONS. Although bleeding is a prominent feature of ulcerative colitis, it is present in only 50% of patients with transmural colitis. Bleeding is rare in cases of small bowel Crohn's disease. Diarrhea is the most common feature in both large and small bowel disease. Patients with disease limited to the terminal ileum may have a tender right lower quadrant mass and obstructive symptoms of pain, nausea, vomiting, and distention. Weakness, fatigue, anorexia, and fever are common symptoms of active disease. An intraabdominal abscess or enterocutaneous fistula may be the initial manifestation of the disease or may develop during its course.

The disease is solely perianal in 5% of cases. More often, however, perianal disease accompanies ileocolitis or colonic disease. Severe perianal disease, sometimes occurring with numerous fistulous tracts, may lead to an undermining and sloughing of the entire perineum. Enterovesical fistulas may occur and produce stool in the urine and pneumaturia. Compression of the right ureter by an inflamed terminal ileum may lead to hydronehprosis and pyelonephritis.

Other manifestations depend on the location of the disease. Inflammation of the small intestine may impair its absorption of vital nutrients. Calcium, iron, and folate are absorbed in the duodenum, and disease in this region may lead to malabsorption and deficiencies of theses substances. Disease in the terminal ileum may interfere with the absorption of bile salts and vitamin B_{12}, although marked malabsorption of these substances more commonly follows surgical resection of the distal ileum. The malabsorption of bile salts may result in their introduction in increased amounts into the colon and the production of choleretic diarrhea. More severe malabsorption, as occurs usually after the resection of at least 100 cm of terminal ileum, can lead to a critical reduction of the bile salt pool and the malabsorption of dietary fat and fat-soluble vitamins. An impaired ileal absorption of bile salts also may cause the bile to become lithogenic (containing too much cholesterol in respect to bile salts), thereby increasing the incidence of gallstones. Ileal disease or resection has also been associated with hyperoxaluria and an increased incidence of oxalate kidney stones. It is not clear whether this association results from an enhanced intestinal absorption of oxalic acid caused by the intraluminal binding of calcium by malabsorbed fatty acids or from the ileal malabsorption of glycine-conjugated bile salts, their conversion into glyoxalate by colonic bacteria, and the subsequent conversion of absorbed glyoxalate into oxalate. Inflammation of the small or large intestine may impair the intestinal absorption of salt and water and also may cause excessive intestinal protein loss, hypoalbuminemia, and possibly pedal edema.

Extraintestinal manifestations also develop in Crohn's disease, usually in association with colonic involvement. Arthritis, pyoderma gangrenosum, erythema nodosum, uveitis, and liver disease have all been reported. In patients with long-standing disease, amyloidosis may develop, often first indicated by the presence of proteinuria or hepatosplenomegaly.

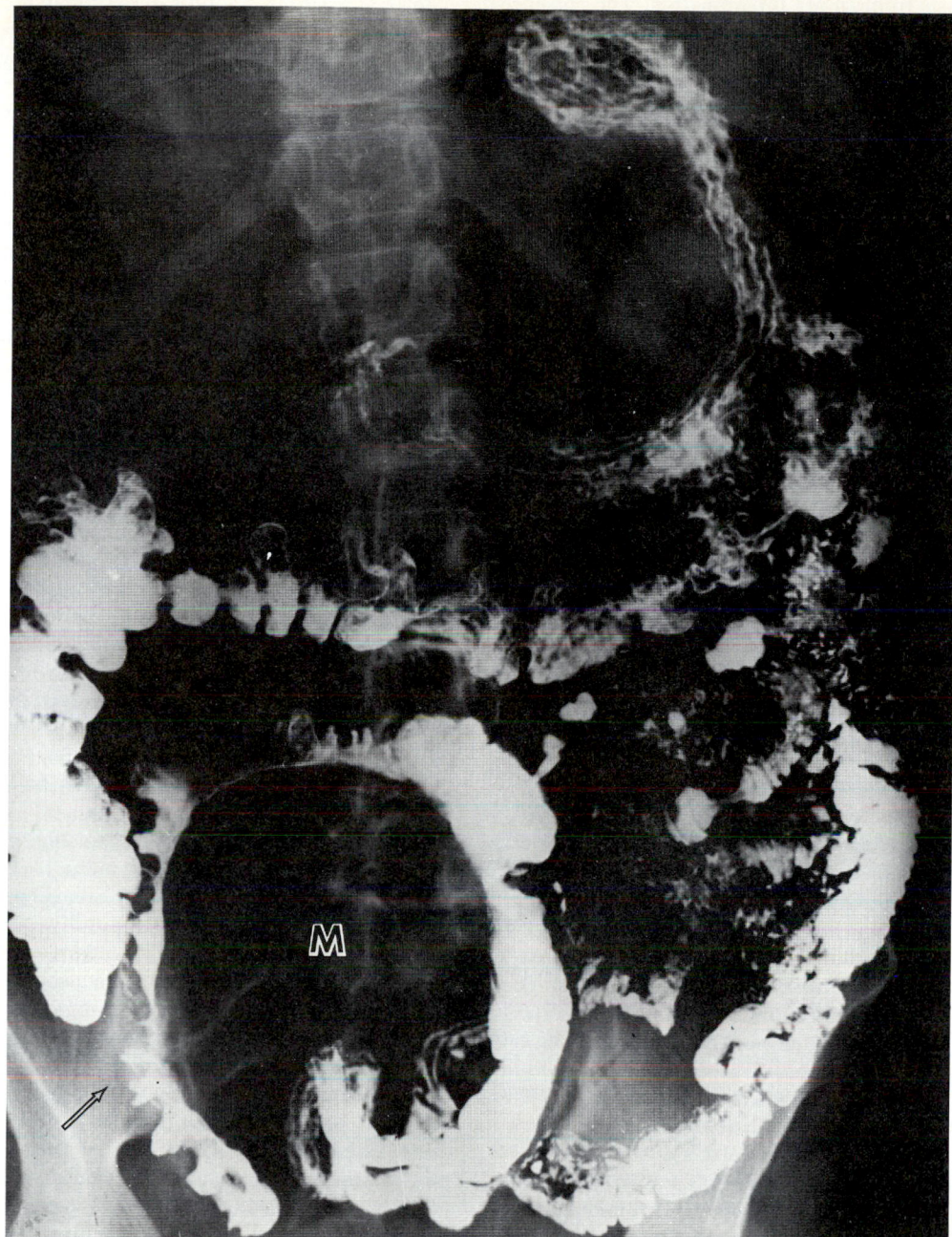

Fig. 175-2 Small bowel series reveals irregularity and nodularity of diseased distal ileum *(arrow)* and extrinsic pressure and displacement of distal small bowel by large inflammatory mass *(M)*. These changes are due to regional ileitis.

Many patients initially have the symptoms and signs of acute appendicitis, and the diagnosis of Crohn's disease is made at the time of laparotomy. An incidental appendectomy should not be performed at this time because of an increased risk of postoperative fistula formation.

The physical findings reflect the involvements just described, including the presence of an abdominal tenderness, mass, and distention. The rectal examination may reveal perianal complications, rectal tenderness, blood, or narrowing and induration.

LABORATORY FINDINGS. The absorptive function of the small bowel is more likely to be altered in patients with Crohn's disease than in those with ulcerative colitis. Electrolyte abnormalities and low albumin levels commonly occur in cases of severe disease. Anemia, usually resulting from an iron or

sometimes a folate deficiency, also may be present. Leukocytosis may be present, but white blood cell counts greater than $15,000/mm^3$ suggest an abscess or perforation. Stool specimens may show red blood cells and eosinophils. Cultures are negative for enteric pathogens. Fresh stool specimens should also be examined for ova and parasites.

DIAGNOSIS. The diagnosis of Crohn's disease depends on effective barium studies. As with ulcerative colitis, caution must be exercised to avoid the use of cathartics. A barium enema accompanied by filling of the terminal ileum and a small bowel series (Fig. 175-2) help determine the extent of the disease. In ileitis there is classically a narrowing of the terminal ileum with ulcerations and cobblestoning of the mucosa. The classic "string sign" indicates a luminal narrowing of the distal ileum produced either by the inflammation and edema of active disease or by fibrosis from an old inflammation. The presence of ulcers helps identify this as active disease. The barium study may reveal an abnormality of the terminal ileum in cases of tuberculosis, lymphoma, actinomycosis, periappendiceal abscess, and cecal cancer. The history should help to distinguish the disease from these entities, but a lymphoma may be difficult to differentiate from inflammatory bowel disease. Long intestinal segments usually are involved in lymphomas, and regional adenopathy may be present. Lymphomas are more common in middle-aged men and may be associated with symptoms of malabsorption. Because Crohn's disease can occur in any part of the bowel, there may be fibrosis, ulcers, and cobblestoning in the duodenum, jejunum, or colon as well as the ileum. Fistulas between segments of bowel are common, as are sinus tracts, especially extending from the large bowel to the perineum. In older patients diverticulitis and ischemic bowel disease must also be differentiated from Crohn's disease. Associated arteriosclerotic cardiovascular disease and atrial fibrillation make a diagnosis of ischemic disease of the large or small bowel more likely. Diverticulitis may be suspected if there is the appearance of local disease in the sigmoid colon on roentgenograms.

Sigmoidoscopy may be helpful in determining the presence of proctitis and sigmoiditis but usually cannot differentiate granulomatous colitis from ulcerative colitis. A rectal biopsy may be helpful in diagnosing Crohn's disease, especially if it reveals granulomas. Colonoscopy may be helpful in a patient who has diarrhea, weight loss, or bleeding but no roentgenographic signs, by demonstrating typical aphthous ulcerations in the colon.

COURSE. Crohn's disease is a protean illness characterized by exacerbations and remissions. It is estimated that 5% to 10% of affected patients die of the illness. The initial location of the disease may provide some clue to its probable course. Life tables indicate that up to 80% of patients require surgery within 20 years. Patients who undergo surgery appear to have a 60% chance of requiring additional surgery. Patients whose initial disease is ileocolic have a 73% surgical rate; if the initial site is the colon or small intestine, the rate is 50%. Ileocolic disease in at least 50% of patients eventually "burns out," causing minimal symptoms.

The incidence of carcinomas of the small bowel is increased in patients with Crohn's disease. Whereas most small bowel tumors occur within 20 cm of the ligament of Treitz, in Crohn's disease most cancers develop in involved segments of small intestine. There is also an increased risk of colon cancer in patients with transmural colitis, but the incidence is much less than with ulcerative colitis. Although there are good statistical data indicating rates of carcinomas in patients with ulcerative colitis, none is available for patients with Crohn's disease of the colon.

About 25% of patients who have Crohn's disease before the age of 21 experience growth failure. The risk of severe disease requiring several operations also is greater in this group.

Assessing recurrent disease after surgery is problematic. Because the surgeon cannot be sure he has removed all of the diseased area, and because the pathologist often finds microscopic disease in normal-appearing portions of gross specimens, much of what has been called recurrent disease probably is residual disease not appreciated during the operation. Although some maintain that the disease does not extend along the intestine unless surgery is performed, an accuratee natural history of the disease cannot be ascertained until more sensitive methods are developed for the detection of all areas of affected bowel.

MANAGEMENT. Crohn's disease may recur and remit without the patient receiving any treatment. Certainly some patients in later life have been incidentally found by barium enema to have the classic narrowed terminal ileum. If carefully interviewed, such patients may indicate that they have had episodes of diarrhea and cramps during their life but that the symptoms were never severe enough for them to seek medical attention. Indeed, many patients may reveal that they have seen their doctor over the years for cyclic bouts of what was considered intestinal flu. It is therefore easy to understand that most reports of treatment have been anecdotal. It was not until the National Cooperative Crohn's Disease Study (NCCDS) was completed that some firm facts about the modalities of treatment emerged. The goal of this multiple-center study was to establish quantitative estimates about the disease's activity and to measure the responses of patients to various treatments. The study showed that prednisone was effective in inducing remission in 78% of patients during the 4 months of study. Prednisone was most effective in patients with disease of the small intestine and in reducing arthritic symptoms. Ileocolic and colonic disease responded well to sulfasalazine, but small intestinal disease did not, probably because colonic bacteria are needed to break sulfasalazine into its active component 5-aminosalicylate and the inactive sulfapyridine moiety. The study showed that the antimetabolite azathioprine was no more effective than a placebo but that it was the most toxic of the drugs used in the treatment of Crohn's disease. The drug had to be discontinued in 12% of the patients receiving it; pancreatitis developed in half of these patients. Of the patients taking a placebo, 30% achieved remission during the study.

Thus there are effective drugs for the treatment of Crohn's disease. Sulfasalazine in a daily dosage of 4 to 8 g is used to treat ileocolic and colonic disease, and there is evidence that perianal disease and fistulas respond well to this medication. Sulfasalazine therapy can be tapered off when remission occurs and eventually discontinued. Unlike the situation with ulcerative colitis, the remission of transmural colitis does not appear to be sustained by sulfasalazine; the NCCDS report seems to indicate that no drug is effective in maintaining remission. Prednisone and ACTH have a role in suppressing the symptoms of the disease. Prednisone initially is given in oral dosages of 40 to 80 mg daily. ACTH may be given intravenously in a soluble form or intramuscularly in a gel in a daily dosage of 40 to 80 units. An observable response to this therapy may appear only after 2 to 4 weeks. The patient's sense of well-being and appetite often are restored before the diarrhea and abdominal cramps are controlled. Once remission is achieved, this drug therapy should be tapered off. Giving the drug only every other day can reduce the side effects. As already noted, the NCCDS report indicates that steroids do not maintain remissions of Crohn's disease. Some patients have recurrent symptoms when the drug is discontinued and respond again when it is reinstituted in a small dosage. It seems unwise to discontinued the drug in these patients. This observation underscores the need to individualize the therapy. Recent studies have suggested that metronidazole in dosages of 1 to 2 g daily may help heal perineal fistulas.

Symptomatic and supportive treament is important in Crohn's disease in the large and small intestines. Diarrhea and cramping may be controlled by loperamide in a dosage of 2 mg four times daily or diphenoxylate in a dosage of 2.5 to 5 mg up to four times a day. Atropine analogs may also be helpful in reducing abdominal spasm when used alone or in conjunction with these other drugs. Patients with severe disease involving the terminal ileum and those who have had surgical removal of the distal ileum may have diarrhea resulting from bile salt malabsorption rather than from inflammation. In these patients the bile salts pass unabsorbed into the colon, where they exert a cathartic effect. With the administration of the bile salt resin cholestyramine in dosages of 4 to 12 g daily, bile salts are bound and the diarrhea is diminished. Because Crohn's disease frequently affects the small intestine, malnutrition is often a major problem, as may be reflected by a moderate weight loss or cachexia with hypoalbuminemia. In patients with symptoms of partial obstruction a low-residue elemental diet supplying 1500 to 2400 calories daily helps maintain a positive nitrogen balance. Dietary supplements have the advatange of being absorbed in the upper bowel and thereby reducing the flow of material through diseased distal segments of the intestine. Reducing the residue in the diet and thereby the solid material flowing through the ileum may prove helpful even for patients with less severe disease. Some patients with ileal disease develop a lactase deficiency and become intolerant of dietary lactose. If such patients avoid milk and dairy products, their cramps and diarrhea may be reduced.

Some patients do not respond well to dietary changes or are too ill to take in adequate oral nutrition. These patients benefit from a therapy of total parenteral nutrition, which involves the continuous infusion of fluid rich in elemental amino acids and hypertonic glucose through a catheter in the subclavian vein. Fat solutions also are available for this therapy. This technique has the advantage of removing all absorptive requirements from the bowel and putting it at rest. Reports have indicated that a positive nitrogen balance is achieved, that patients gain weight, and that the drainage through fistulas decreases. This technique may allow patients who are resistant to steroids to correct their negative nitrogen and caloric balance and to respond to therapy. Parenteral alimentation has also been used to improve patients' nutritional status before major surgery. In patients who have had an extensive resection of bowel, the absorptive surface of the small intestine may be so reduced that adequate oral nutrition will never be possible. In these individuals total parenteral nutrition administered on an outpatient basis has been successful. Parenteral alimentation is not without risk, however. Infection at the intravenous site, sepsis, and the development of fatty liver and a phosphorus deficiency are some of the more common complications.

As in ulcerative colitis, anemia in Crohn's disease should be corrected with oral administration of iron and folate and if necessary with blood transfusions. Because vitamin B_{12} is absorbed in the terminal ileum, a deficiency may occur if severe disease occurs in the terminal ileum or if there has been a resection of more than about 60 cm of this region. Monthly injections of 1000 µg of cyanocobalamin are indicated in such patients. Electrolyte abnormalities should be corrected by intravenous replacements. Serum magnesium levels may fall in severe disease, causing secondary hypocalcemia that should be corrected by intravenous replacement. If a loss of bile salts leads to a malabsorption and deficiency of the fat-soluble vitamins (K, D, A, and E), causing clotting disturbances, bone resorption, and possibly even visual problems, these vitamins must be replenished, preferably with water-soluble analogs.

Surgery is not curative in Crohn's disease as it is in ulcerative colitis. Therefore surgery is reserved for patients who have not responded to medical treatment or who have disorders such as an abscess, free perforation, or unremitting obstruction that do not respond to medical management. Several series have shown that patients do better postoperatively if their disease had been brought under control by medical treatment before surgery.

The most common procedure for ileocolic disease is the segmental removal of the distal ileum and right colon. In the past a simple bypass procedure creating an anastomosis between the ileum and the transverse colon commonly was performed, but its common failure to control the disease activity has put this procedure in disrepute. A small area of intestinal disease may be treated by resection of as much diseased area as is feasible, but the removal of large areas of small intestine may lead to serious malabsorption problems and cause serious nutritional problems for patients. Such patients may require long-term parenteral nutrition, as already discussed. Patients with enteroenteric fistulas may benefit from resections that eliminate the short circuit of nutrients from the upper to lower small intestine. Enterocutaneous fistulas that occur from the small bowel to the abdominal wall or from the rectum to the perineum are best treated medically along with surgical drainage of any local abscesses that form. The disease occasionally involves the duodenum, and a gastric outlet obstruction may occur; these patients often do well with a simple gastrojejunostomy, leaving the diseased segment in place. Patients with colonic disease pose a different problem. Strictures may cause obstruction in the large bowel; occasionally these can be resected. Severe colonic disease may be treated with a colectomy. If the rectum is not diseased, a subtotal colectomy along with the creation of an ileorectal anastomosis may be performed, but at least one third of these patients then require proctectomy within 3 years for subsequent rectal disease that cannot be adequately managed medically. If the total colon is diseased, the patient requires proctocolectomy and ileostomy. Unlike patients with ulcerative colitis, however, about one third to half of these patients experience recurrent disease in the remaining ileum. A significant number of patients have inflammation of the ileostomy stoma, which can often be treated with topical steroids. Patients who have inactive disease and those in whom ileal disease does not develop are able to live normal productive lives despite the ileostomy.

APPENDICITIS AND APPENDICEAL ABSCESS

DEFINITION. The appendix is an anatomic remnant of the base of the cecum. Inflammation and perforation of this structure can occur, causing an abscess, generalized peritonitis, and death. Although appendicitis is a disease of decreasing incidence, it still is the most common cause for abdominal surgery in patients 10 to 20 years of age.

EPIDEMIOLOGY. Like diverticular disease, appendicitis is most prevalent in industrialized urban communities. Whether the diet is a precipitating factor is still conjectural. This disease occurs most commonly in communities where low-fiber diets are the standard and a high meat intake is common. The incidence of disease is markedly lower in vegetarians and in rural cultures that have high-fiber diets.

PATHOGENESIS. Most commonly the symptoms arise from the occlusion of the appendiceal lumen by stool. Occasionally food particles or barium sulfate may obstruct the lumen. An obstruction of the lumen does not always cause inflammation; asymptomatic calcified concretions (fecaliths) are often seen in abdominal roentgenograms. In children the appendiceal lumen may be obstructed by hyperplasia of lymphatic follicles, a mechanism possibly accounting for the increased association of appendicitis with viral respiratory and enteric infections in children. The appendix may occasionally be occluded by pinworms, ascarides, or other parasites. In older patients a carcinoma of the cecum may obstruct the appendiceal orifice. Patients with collagen vascular disease occasionally have arteritis of the appendix leading to necrosis and perforation.

Occlusion of the appendiceal lumen leads to edema and congestion of the wall, pain, and ulceration and necrosis of the mucosa. The appendix fills with pus, swells, and ruptures, leading to a localized abscess, peritonitis, or septicemia.

CLINICAL MANIFESTATIONS. The patient usually notes the onset of generalized mild abdominal pain or cramping, symptoms often confused with the presence of a mild intestinal flu. Anorexia and nausea with emesis may occur. The patient may or may not have a low-grade fever. As the inflammation increases in the appendix, especially when it extends to the adjoining parietal peritoneum, the generalized pain subsides and localized right lower quadrant pain and tenderness develop, classically at McBurney's point (2 to 5 cm from the iliac crest on the line between the iliac crest and umbilicus). If the appendix is retrocecal, back pain may occur. If the cecum is low-lying and the appendix is in the pelvis, tenderness may be elicited only by a digital examination of the rectum or a pelvic examination. Patients with malrotation of the cecum may have pain in the right upper quadrant or periumbilically, and the examining physician may note tenderness and guarding in the right upper quadrant. Tenderness may occur when the patient flexes the right hip if the inflamed appendix is resting on the psoas muscle; pain is also elicited when the examiner forcibly extends the right hip (the psoas sign). As the inflammation progresses, or if perforation occurs, the patient's fever rises and tachycardia and lethargy may become prominent. In elderly patients the symptoms often are minimal up to the time of perforation. Diffuse abdominal pain, diffuse peritoneal signs, and the absence of bowel sounds suggest that perforation has occurred.

LABORATORY FINDINGS. The leukocyte count is mildly elevated early in the disease. A leukocytosis of more than $15,000/mm_3$ along with a marked shift to the left signals severe inflammation. In elderly or debilitated patients leukopenia may occur. The sedimentation rate is elevated but is not a basis for the diagnosis.

DIAGNOSIS. The clinical history and physical examination are the most important factors in making the diagnosis of appendicitis. A plain roentgenogram of the abdomen may reveal an ileus, but usually roentgenograms are not helpful. The use of a barium enema can be carefully considered for undiagnosed patients who are stable. Appendicitis may cause perforation and peritoneal soilage, but more commonly edema occurs at the tip of the cecum without filling of the appendix. Regional enteritis may be discovered by the barium enema; occasionally a small bowel roentgenogram is needed to fill the terminal ileum and show disease in this region. A careful history may reveal that the symptoms of a patient in the middle of her menstrual cycle are the result of ovulation (mittelschmerz symptoms). Other causes of pelvic disease in women should be considered, such as salpingitis, an ectopic pregnancy, or a twisted ovarian cyst. In older patients the possibility of a perforating cecal cancer should be considered. Diabetic ketoacidosis in children may cause abdominal pain, but proper urine and blood tests should reveal its presence. Hematuria or pyuria with bacilluria should alert the physician to the possibility of a renal calculus or infection as the cause of the pain. Right-sided diverticulitis in an adult may appear clinically identical to acute appendicitis.

COURSE. The mortality of surgery for nonperforative appendicitis is less than 3%. Most deaths result from pneumonia, embolism, or myocardial infarction. Patients with an abscess formation have a much greater risk of death. Generalized peritonitis and miliary liver abscesses are serious complications with a mortality up to 50%. Pylephlebitis (pus in the portal vein) may lead to portal thrombosis and liver abscesses. Anaerobic bacteria and Enterobacteriaceae have a major role in these infections. These patients have chills, fever, and jaundice. Broad-spectrum antibiotics can help control the infection, but surgical drainage of liver abscesses may be needed. An intestinal obstruction caused by adhesions may be a late complication of surgery in patients with acute appendicitis or an appendiceal abscess.

MANAGEMENT. The preferred treatment is the surgical removal of the appendix, which should be carried out as soon as the diagnosis seems certain and the patient is stabilized. Dehydration should be corrected preoperatively. Gastric or intestinal intubation should be initiated preoperatively in patients with obstructive symptoms. The removal of the appendix and drainage of an abscess, if present, help to decrease postoperative complications. If a perforation has occurred, it may be impossible to identify the appendix; surgical drainage of the abdomen is then indicated. In this situation there is an increased incidence of colocutaneous fistulas, which require later surgical resection. Appendicitis may complicate a pregnancy, but most surgeons agree that appendectomy is indicated regardless of the risk to the fetus. Nonoperative therapy has occasionally been advocated in cases of acute nonperforative appendicitis. The patient fasts and is treated with large dosages of antibiotics and intravenous fluids to allow the inflammatory process to subside. This therapy should be considered only when surgical treatment is not available or when the general condition of the patient is so poor that surgery is contraindicated.

DIVERTICULAR DISEASE OF THE COLON

DEFINITION. Diverticulosis is a disease in which small sac-like outpouches of mucosa and submucosa are present in any or all regions of the colon, most often in the sigmoid colon. Patients may be asymptomatic, have recurrent episodes of pain, have bleeding, or develop inflammation from an intramural, pericolic, or intraabdominal perforation.

EPIDEMIOLOGY. Diverticulosis is a disease of urban society; studies have shown a lower incidence among rural populations. The incidence increases as well in those people who have moved from the country to industrialized centers. Decreased fiber in the diet is strongly correlated with the incidence of diverticulosis. Indeed, studies have shown diverticular disease to be one fourth as common in vegetarians as in age-matched controls on standard diets. There is a low incidence of colonic disease in Africans on high-fiber diets and an increased incidence of diverticular disease in those Africans on Western diets. The consumption of refined sugar, wheat, and much meat is correlated with a tendency to diverticulosis. Colonic diverticula are rare in patients under 40 years of age, but thereafter the incidence in the United States increases to include about 50% of patients at age 80.

PATHOGENESIS. The motor activity of the colon—the contractions of colonic muscle—gives rise to segments of high pressure. If the stool lacks residue and bulk, higher colonic pressures are generated, especially in the sigmoid colon, as a result of the decreased caliber of the lumen (Laplace's law). The colonic wall is weakened in areas where the nutrient vessels penetrate the wall along the mesenteric border, and the increased pressure causes ballooning of the mucosa through these areas to form saccular outpouches. Marked hypertrophy of the colonic muscle also occurs and further increases these pressures.

CLINICAL MANIFESTATIONS. Most patients with diverticulosis remain asymptomatic. As a result of the abnormal spasm or pressure of the sigmoid colon, however, some patients have recurrent left lower quadrant pain and during the physical examination may be found to have a tender loop of sigmoid colon. The diverticula may perforate the wall of the bowel, producing inflammation or diverticulitis. Perforation beyond the wall may lead to a pericolic or more distant abscess or even to frank peritonitis. The abdominal wall may be rigid and marked guarding may be present if there is severe inflammation or abscess formation. Fever may occur, and a high fever with shaking chills signals the perforation of a diverticulum along with an abscess or peritonitis. The inflammation may cause an intestinal obstruction or diarrhea. An extended inflammation in the bladder or left ureter may cause a urinary tract infection, hydronephrosis, or even fistula between the colon and bladder. Diverticula are a common cause of lower gastrointestinal bleeding in patients over 50 years of age, usually unaccompanied by active inflammation, pain, or fever. The bleeding usually is self-limited, but massive blood loss and shock may occur, in which case the site of bleeding is often in the right side of the colon.

LABORATORY FINDINGS. Patients with mild disease may have an elevated leukocyte count. A high leukocyte count with a marked shift to the left is associated with severe inflammation and abscess. Anemia may be present if bleeding has occurred. If anemia is present in the absence of overt bleeding, a search should be made for a neoplasm or another inflammatory process, although diverticula too have been alleged to be a source of occult blood loss.

DIAGNOSIS. The diagnosis of diverticular disease depends on a good history, physical examination, and barium study. If active inflammation is present, the barium enema may be deferred to avoid the risk of perforating the bowel or soiling the peritoneal cavity through a perforation already present. Sigmoidoscopy usually has negative results in these patients. The barium enema may not resolve the possibility of a neoplasm being present. Indeed, a carcinoma may occur in areas of diverticular narrowing. In addition, the muscular hypertrophy that occurs in patients with diverticulosis may appear as luminal narrowing. Colonoscopy and biopsy may be helpful in making the diagnosis of cancer in these areas. Great care must be exercised during colonoscopy, because an overdistention with air may cause diverticular perforation. If an abscess formation is suspected, colonoscopy should be deferred. Colonoscopy may be helpful in differentiating Crohn's disease and ischemic bowel disease from diverticular disease.

MANAGEMENT. Recurrent attacks of left lower quadrant pain may be treated with bed rest and a bland diet. Severe pain requires hospitalization and administration of meperidine or pentazocine. These agents decrease colon spasms and do not increase intraluminal pressure. The use of anticholinergics is controversial, although many physicians use them to decrease spasms. Intravenous glucagon has also been used for this purpose with some success.

Bulk agents such as psyllium seed preparations have also been used to reduce spasms and prevent attacks. These agents cause water retention in the feces and increase their size, thus reducing colonic pressure so that less force is exerted during defecation. Studies have shown that a higher contraction pressure is required for the expulsion of small stools and a lower pressure for bulky bowel movements. Patients who find bran unpalatable may use psyllium or methylcellulose preparations in a glass of water at bedtime. These patients may note some abdominal distention and increased flatus initially with these bulk agents, because they are partially digested by colonic bacteria. The addition of fruit and vegetables to the diet also helps to increase the dietary fiber. The long-term preventive effects of bran and fiber are still conjectural.

Patients who have bleeding should be monitored closely, because transfusion may be necessary, but bleeding is often self-limited. If a patient's bleeding is vigorous or unremitting, angiography may be helpful in identifying the bleeding site and allows the selective infusion of vasopressin (Pitressin), which may be helpful in controlling the bleeding. If bleeding recurs, surgical resection is indicated.

Patients suspected of having a perforated diverticulum should receive intravenous antibiotics. If the patient's condition does not improve in 24 to 48 hours, surgical intervention is probably necessary. The draining of abscess material and a diverting colostomy are indicated. When the infection has been controlled, the patient may undergo a resection of the involved area, along with anastomosis of the bowel and closure of the colostomy.

For patients with severe pain, an elective sigmoid resection can be helpful. In rare cases a subtotal colectomy along with an ileorectal anastomosis is needed for extensive colonic diverticular disease.

PSEUDOMEMBRANOUS ENTEROCOLITIS AND ANTIBIOTIC-INDUCED DIARRHEA

DEFINITION. Diarrhea may occur in patients receiving antibiotic therapy as a result of an alteration of the fecal flora. Often this condition is mild and subsides when the antibiotic therapy is discontinued. Occasionally a severe disease results with the development of thick mucosal exudate that has the appearance of a membrane. This condition is extremely serious and demands aggressive treatment.

ETIOLOGY. When diarrhea develops while an individual is receiving antibiotics, the cause of the altered bowel habit usually is evident. Because this symptom also may occur several days or even weeks after the antibiotic is discontinued, however, a careful history must be obtained. Pseudomembranous enterocolitis commonly has been associated with the use of clindamycin but also occurs in association with amoxicillin, cephalosporins, ampicillin, and other agents. Patients who are debilitated or have renal failure or low-output syndromes seem to have a higher risk of contracting the disease. Pseudomembranous enterocolitis has been reporteed as a complication of major abdominal surgery, but most of these patients had been receiving antibiotics, which can be implicated as a cause of superinfection. Many early reports of pseudomembranous enterocolitis, especially of postoperative cases of the disease, stressed the finding of *Staphylococcus aureus* in the stool, but the role played by this organism remains unclear at present. Recent studies have shown a major role for *Clostridium difficile* in the pathogenesis of antibiotic-produced pseudomembranous enterocolitis. This bacterium has been found in the stool of many patients with the disease, and an identified cytopathic toxin of the *Clostridium* strain also has been found in the stool of patients with pseudomembranous enterocolitis. This toxin also has been found in up to 25% of patients with milder forms of antibiotic-related diarrhea. When antibiotics are administered, presumably the normal colonic flora are inhibited, allowing *C. difficile* to proliferate (especially if it is resistant to the antibiotic) and produce toxin.

PATHOLOGY. The gross appearance of the bowel affected by antibiotic-related diarrhea can vary greatly. Mild hyperemia and granularity may occur. In fully developed cases of pseudomembranous enterocolitis, raised yellow plaques of exudate can be seen coalescing to form a membrane. This can occur throughout the gut and may be patchy. The underlying mucosa may be edematous and hyperemic and sometimes necrotic and ulcerated. The microscopic examination shows that the membrane contains leukocytes, mucus, and fibin, and the muscosa exhibits edema, congestion, inflammation, and occasionally ulceration and necrosis.

CLINICAL MANIFESTATIONS AND DIAGNOSIS. A careful history of patients with diarrhea is needed to determine whether they have received antibiotics. Bowel movements may occur every 15 to 20 minutes, but the severely ill patient may be unaware of them. The patient may describe his stool as mucoid, usually without blood, and a greenish brown liquid mucoid material may be detected in the rectum in the absence of solid stool. The patient may be febrile and may have lost considerable fluid, electrolytes, and protein. Sigmoidoscopy may reveal mild or severe inflammation along with yellow raised membranous plaques of exudate. Carefully performed colonoscopy may be helpful in demonstrating these lesions if sigmoidoscopy does not. A barium enema examination may reveal nodular filling defects in the colon, but often the patient is too ill to undergo this study. Stool cultures may demonstrate the presence of *C. difficile* if appropriate anaerobic cultures are made, but more commonly the stool is tested for *C. difficile* enterotoxin.

MANAGEMENT. Pseudomembranous enterocolitis is a life-threatening disease with up to a 50% mortality. Patients must be placed in isolation to avoid danger of the infection spreading to others. Infected individuals must be treated aggressively with massive fluid and electrolyte replacement. Potassium supplements may be needed, and intravenous sodium bicarbonate may be required to correct acidosis. Intravenous albumin may be necessary to improve the patient's plasma protein levels and to prevent shock. Vancomycin given orally is effective in a dosage of 125 to 500 mg four times daily for 10 to 14 days. Shorter courses of therapy are associated with a high relapse rate. Metronidozole hydrochloride (Flagyl), in doses of 250 to 500 mg three times daily is an effective and less expensive alternative to vancomycin. Cholestyramine, a bile acid–binding resin, also may be given to bind the toxin of *C.difficile* and to help reduce the diarrhea. Antispasmodics have been used cautiously but may increase the risk of megacolon.

RADIATION ENTERITIS

DEFINITION. Radiation injury to the bowel occurs after pelvic or abdominal radiation therapy for a malignant disease. The disease appears more commonly in patients who also have had previous pelvic surgery or an abdominal inflammation that gives rise to adhesions that cause the fixation of loops of bowel. Radiation injury rarely results with radiation doses of less than 3000 rad but is very common when more than 4500 rad is given. Symptoms may occur immediately or be delayed for several years after treatment.

PATHOGENESIS. Radiation damage is greatest in tissues that have a rapid cell turnover, since cells undergoing differentiation and growth are more sensitive than cells that have matured. Because cell renewal is constant in the gut, this area is very sensitive to radiation effects. Mucosal cells are most susceptible to radiation effects, and severe sloughing of the mucosa may result if the radiation is intense. The small arterioles of the gut also are very sensitive to radiation and may become inflamed and degenerate; this process may occur soon after treatment or be a late effect. Fibrosis of the arterioles occurs along with resultant ischemia, which may lead to intestinal necrosis and ulceration. Patients with an underlying arteriolar disease are most susceptible to these effects. Severe fibrosis of the gut, along with stricture formation, is a late effect of radiation injury. The histologic findings are marked inflammation, arteriolar narrowing or thrombosis, and foam cells in the submucosa. If present, ulcers may be deep, giving rise to the formation of abscesses or fistulas.

CLINICAL MANIFESTATIONS. Nausea is a common symptom of a radiation injury in the gut, probably resulting from a central nervous system effect of radiation, as nausea can occur in patients undergoing radiotherapy in other parts of the body. A change in bowel habits, abdominal cramping, and diarrhea may occur. If the damage is severe, a bloody mucoid diarrhea may develop. Abdominal distention, along with diarrhea, may result from the late effects of stricture formation. Malabsorption may occur if a severe small bowel disease, stasis (with bacterial overgrowth), or significant enteroenteric fistulas are present. Malabsorption is manifested by severe diarrhea and weight loss. Obstipation occurs if strictures develop in the rectosigmoid.

LABORATORY FINDINGS. If bleeding or malabsorption occurs, anemia and hypoalbuminemia may result. Pyuria or stool in the urine develops if the fistulization extends into the bladder.

DIAGNOSIS. Sigmoidoscopy should be performed in all patients suspected of having radiation colitis. Erythema, friability, and cyanosis of the mucosa may be present. Occasionally ulcers occur. If sigmoidoscopy is unrevealing, a barium enema should be performed; this may demonstrate ulceration, stricture formation, internal fistulas, or areas of abscess. Colonoscopy is helpful in delineating ulceration, but care must be exercised to avoid perforating inflamed segments. Small bowel roentgenograms are necessary to demonstrate the disease in the small intestine.

MANAGEMENT. Patients with inflammatory radiation disease may respond to steroid enemas. No studies have demonstrated the efficacy of oral steroids in treating this disease. If stagnant loops of bowel are present and give rise to bacterial overgrowth, antibiotics may reverse the associated diarrhea and malabsorption. If the patient has abdominal cramping, antispasmodics and bulk agents should be given. Low rectal strictures can be dilated with rubber dilators. Strictures elsewhere often are asymptomatic or cause occasional abdominal cramps and diarrhea. Long, symptomatic strictures require surgical resection. A diverting colostomy may be needed for low colonic strictures.

INTESTINAL ULCER

Isolated intestinal ulcers, although unusual, have been found in the cecum, sigmoid colon, and rectum. The presenting symptoms are related to the ulcer's location. Cecal ulcers have been found incidentally in autopsies or in patients with right lower quadrant pain that mimics that of appendicitis. Sigmoid ulcers may cause no abdominal pain and may develop into a perforation. Unlike solitary ulcers elsewhere, rectal ulcers are usually asymptomatic and have been discovered incidentally by sigmoidoscopy, but they occasionally cause rectal bleeding. The cause of these lesions is unknown. They usually range in diameter from 5 mm to 5 cm, and occasionally the ulcers are multiple. The histologic findings are necrosis, inflammatory exudate, and an increased number of fibroblasts in the submucosa. These findings are nonspecific and give no clues about the cause of the lesions. Barium roentgenograms may reveal a solitary ulcer with surrounding edema. Rectal lesions may be followed by sigmoidoscopy, and some have been reported to remain static for years. The advent of colonoscopy allows the examination, removal of biopsy samples, and following of sigmoid and cecal ulcers under direct vision; previously when these ulcers were deteced on roentgenograms, they were often surgically resected because carcinoma was suspected. The methods of treatment that have been used for rectal ulcers include steroid enemas, electrocoagulation, topical sclerosing agents, and antibiotics. None of these therapies has been successful, leaving surgery as the only consistently successful measure for treating symptomatic intestinal ulcers.

OTHER DISEASES OF THE INTESTINES
Endometriosis

Endometriosis, the presence of islets of endometrial tissue in extrauterine sites, may affect the small and large intestine as well as other intraabdominal and pelvic sites. Subserosal intestinal implants, which are most common in the rectosigmoid and in women 30 to 40 years of age, usually are asymptomatic but may produce abdominal or rectal pain and occasionally bowel obstruction. Intestinal implants may be discovered incidentally during an abdominal operation; they may appear as intramural or extrinsic lesions in barium roentgenograms of the small or large bowel; or the presence of rectosigmoid lesions may be suggested by the finding of tender, irregular indurated nodules in the cul-de-sac during a pelvic examination. For the diagnosis to be definitive, laparoscopy or even a surgical exploration may be necessary. The lesions usually do not require therapy, but when symptomatic they may necessitate the use of analgesics, sedatives, or antispasmodics and, when more severe, hormonal therapy or occasionally even excisional surgery.

Pneumatosis cystoides intestinalis

Pneumatosis cystoides intestinalis, the presence of several gas-filled cysts in the submucosa or subserosa of the small and large bowel and sometimes in the mesentery and omentum, almost always is associated with another underlying disease. Chronic obstructive pulmonary disease and obstructing peptic ulcer disease are common associated disorders. Pneumatosis has also been associated with inflammatory bowel disease, mesenteric vascular occlusion, necrotizing enterocolitis, intestinal lymphoma, perforated diverticula, collagen-vascular disease, Whipple's disease, and intestinal parasites; pneumatosis has also been seen following abdominal trauma, the ingestion of caustic agents, recent surgical bowel anastomosis, and sigmoidoscopy or colonoscopy. Pneumatosis cystoides intestinalis usually is asymptomatic, although it has been thought at times to produce abdominal pain, diarrhea, rectal bleeding, tenesmus, or partial obstruction. The cysts may rupture into the peritoneal cavity and produce pneumoperitoneum, but unless the bowel wall is infected, they usually do not cause peritonitis. Pneumatosis usually is detected incidentally in an abdominal roentgenogram, during an abdominal operation, or in sigmoidoscopy when protruding soft, pale bluish masses are noted. The condition rarely requires the specific therapy of decompression of the cysts by extracting their nitrogen with inhalation oxygen therapy or of surgical resection. Rather, the treatment usually is directed toward the associated disorder.

Colitis cystica superficialis and profunda

Colitis cystica superficialis and profunda are benign conditions of the colon characterized by the presence of mucus-filled cysts. In the superficialis variety the small cysts are located in the mucosa and may be observed on the mucosal surface as small, gray blebs from which mucus can be drained. The condition usually is associated with pellagra, and often the patient has diarrhea. Both the lesions and the symptoms usually respond to niacin or tryptophan therapy.

In the profunda variety the epithelial-lined cysts are located below the mucosa and must be differentiated form mucus-producing adenocarcinomas. Associated symptoms include lower abdominal cramps, rectal tenesmus, and mild diarrhea with fecal mucus and blood. The pathogenesis of the lesions is not clear; perhaps they develop during the healing process of a previous colonic inflammation. The cysts most often are located on the anterior rectal wall within 12 cm of the anal verge and may be palpated in the rectal examination as firm, rubbery, sessile, or polypoid nodules. In sigmoidoscopy the overlying mucosa may appear normal, edematous, congested, ulcerated, or umbilicated; a biopsy should clarify the diagnosis. A barium enema may reveal only some nodular irregularity of the bowel wall. Local surgical excision has been the conventional therapy.

BIBLIOGRAPHY

Banks B, Zetzel L, and Richter H: Morbidity and mortality in regional enteritis: report of 168 cases, Am J Dig Dis 14:369, 1969.

Bartlett JG and others: Antibiotic-associated pseudomembranous colitis due to toxin-producing clostridia, N Engl J Med 298:531, 1978.

Block GE: Surgical management of Crohn's colitis, N Engl J Med 302:1068, 1980.

DeCosse JJ and others: The natural history and management of radiation induced injury of the gastrointestinal tract, Ann Surg 170:369, 1969.

Devrode GJ and others: Cancer risk and life expectancy of children with ulcerative colitis, N Engl J Med 285:17, 1971.

Fawaz KA and others: Ulcerative colitis and Crohn's disease of the colon: a comparison of the longterm postoperative course, Gastroenterology 71:372, 1976.

Gennaro AR and Rosemond GP: Diverticulitis of the colon, Dis Colon Rectum 17:74, 1974.

Gitnick GL: Etiology of inflammatory bowel diseases: are we making progress? Gastroenterology 78:1090, 1980.

Glotzer DJ and others: Comparative features and course of ulcerative and granulomatous colitis, N Engl J Med 282:582, 1970.

Kirsner JB and Shorter RG, editors: Inflammatory bowel disease, Philadelphia 1989, Lea & Febiger.

National cooperative Crohn's disease study, Gastroenterology 77:825, 1979.

Painter NS and Burkitt DP: Diverticular disease of the colon: a disease of Western civilization, Chicago, 1970, Year Book Medical Publishers, Inc.

176 · VASCULAR DISEASES OF THE GASTROINTESTINAL TRACT

Harvey M. Licht

The intraabdominal gastrointestinal tract receives its blood supply from three major arteries branching from the abdominal aorta: the celiac axis, superior mesenteric artery, and the inferior mesenteric artery. The celiac axis divides into the left gastric artery, the splenic artery, and the hepatic artery, each of which has extensive collateral channels with the others. These vessels supply the stomach, duodenum, pancreas, spleen, and liver. The superior mesenteric artery supplies the small intestine distal to the duodenum as well as the right colon to the proximal transverse colon. There is a rich collateral anastomosis with branches of the celiac axis and the inferior mesenteric artery. The inferior mesenteric artery supplies the rectum, sigmoid, descending colon, and distal transverse colon and also has collateral anastomosis with the superior mesenteric artery and with a branch from the internal iliac artery that supplies the distal rectum.

Systemic or localized diseases may affect the vascular tree

and circulation of the gut and lead to ischemic syndromes of the intestinal tract. These may be divided into occlusive and nonocclusive causes of ischemia, and these syndromes may present as chronic or acute catastrophic illness. The most common and usually the most serious cases of intestinal ischemia result from involvement of the superior mesenteric artery.

OCCLUSIVE VASCULAR DISEASE OF THE GASTROINTESTINAL TRACT

The major types of occlusive diseases affecting the gastrointestinal vascular tree include atherosclerosis, thrombosis, embolus, and vasculitis with focal involvement of vessels.

Acute occlusion of the superior mesenteric artery is an abdominal catastrophe with a mortality reportedly as high as 90%. The most frequent cause of the acute occlusion is an embolus, less commonly a de novo arterial thrombosis, a complication of atherosclerosis. Most emboli orginate from the heart, and patients who are predisposed to this include those with valvular heart disease, patients with recent myocardial infarction and mural thrombus, and patients with atrial fibrillation. The superior mesenteric artery is the vessel most commonly occluded by embolus because of its large diameter and because it makes an oblique angle as it originates from the aorta.

The patient with acute mesenteric ischemia usually manifests abdominal pain, which often is diffuse, persistent, and severe. It may last for several hours and may be associated with nausea and vomiting and occasionally with diarrhea, which may be bloody or at least may contain occult blood. The patient usually appears acutely ill and often has signs of intravascular depletion, which is secondary to third spacing of fluid in the mesentery and affected bowel. Early in the course the patient may exhibit few abdominal findings, although he often is distended and may have some tenderness. If the disease is allowed to progress without intervention, within hours to 1 to 2 days the ischemia may progress to transmural infarction with attendant fever and the physical findings of peritonitis such as guarding and rebound tenderness. Early in the course of the illness laboratory data are nonspecific. There may be hemoconcentration secondary to third spacing, and there may be a nonspecific rise in the serum amylase or the serum phosphorus. Leukocytosis and metabolic acidosis characteristically develop with infarction. A roentgenogram of the abdomen also is nonspecific. There may be signs of ileus or perhaps focal, dilated, edematous loops of bowel, or even "thumb-printing." Late roentgenographic findings such as air in the bowel wall or in the portal venous system suggest the onset of gangrene and transmural infarction, and at this point survival is unlikely.

The diagnosis of acute mesenteric ischemia should be considered when a patient in a group at high risk such as one with valvular or atherosclerotic heart disease, arrhythmia, or congestive heart failure develops severe, persistent abdominal pain and the physical examination, laboratory data, and flat plate of the abdomen are consistent with the findings of this disorder. Arteriography should be done after initial resuscitation and may show evidence of thrombosis or embolus or may show signs of vasospasm of the arteries consistent with nonocclusive ischemic disease. Aggressive management with intraarterial infusion of a vasodilator such as papaverine or prostaglandin E₁ is initiated, and the patient is taken to surgery to assess the viability of the intestine as well as to perform vascular reconstructive surgery if indicated. The mortality without such an aggressive approach is 90%, but it may be reduced by half with early diagnosis and aggressive management.

Atherosclerosis of the superior mesenteric artery rarely causes symptoms, perhaps because of the rich collateral circulation of the gut. However, an occasional patient does experience chronic recurrent abdominal pain, characteristically occurring 15 to 30 minutes after a meal. Because of the association between eating and pain, most patients reduce their food intake and lose weight. This symptom complex is called intestinal angina and is analogous to cardiac angina. Because of the atherosclerotic narrowing of the vessels, the blood supply apparently cannot be increased adequately to meet the increased metabolic demands of the postprandial intestine. It is not known how many patients with this uncommon syndrome eventually develop acute mesenteric ischemia with thrombosis. The diagnosis of intestinal angina is confirmed by angiography, and treatment includes surgical vascular repair. Recently attempts have been made at percutaneous transluminal angioplasty.

Occlusive disease of the celiac axis is rare. A controversial syndrome, celiac axis compression syndrome has been thought to be a rare cause of vague abdominal pain, supposedly from the compression of the celiac axis by the median arcuate ligament.

Acute colonic ischemia resulting from thrombosis or embolism of the inferior mesenteric artery and producing an acute clinical picture similar to that of acute occlusion of the superior mesenteric artery is also rare. However, atherosclerotic narrowing of the inferior mesenteric artery undoubtedly contributes to the occasional cases of ischemic colitis. The inferior mesenteric artery actually can be sacrificed during surgery, with ischemic colitis subsequently occurring in only 1% of cases.

A less common and often more focal cause of occlusive disease affecting the splanchnic circulation is vasculitis, which also may affect the systemic vessels. This may be seen in polyarteritis nodosa, systemic lupus erythematosus, Henoch-Schönlein purpura, and rheumatoid arthritis. The vasculitis of the splanchnic arteries may cause abdominal pain, gastrointestinal bleeding, and other manifestations of intestinal ischemia and occasionally acute cholecystitis, pancreatitis, or serositis. "Obstruction" of splanchnic arteries and attendant manifestations of intestinal ischemia also may be produced by use of vasoconstricting drugs such as vasopressin or ergot alkaloids.

NONOCCLUSIVE VASCULAR DISEASE OF THE GUT

Nonocclusive ischemic disease of the bowel is caused by a low flow state. This may be secondary to decreased cardiac output with congestive heart failure, an arrythmia, or myocardial infarction. It also may occur in patients with hypovolemia, for example, in patients with gastrointestinal hemorrhage or extensive burns. As a compensatory mechanism to maintain systemic blood pressure in such a setting, there is vasoconstriction of the mesenteric bed, leading to reduced blood flow to the gut. Animal studies have documented that vasoconstriction may persist after the initial insult is relieved and thus flow to the gut may still be diminished for several hours or even days after correction of the systemic problem. Use of medications such as digoxin or vasopressor drugs may aggravate the intestinal vasoconstriction.

The symptoms, clinical signs, and pertinent laboratory and roentgenographic findings of patients with nonocclusive mesenteric ischemia are similar to those in patients with occlusive disease. Patients with nonocclusive disease also often exhibit findings of severe vascular disease and low cardiac output. Although these usually are very sick, high-risk patients, the high mortality (90% to 100%) in untreated patients with bowel infarction warrants the same aggressive approach as recommended in the management of patients with occlusive disease, including early angiography, local instillation of vasodilators, and early surgery if needed. Vigorous treatment of the underlying conditions causing decreased cardiac output and diminished splanchnic perfusion may prevent critical intestinal ischemia from developing or perhaps may revert early symptomatic ischemia so as to prevent bowel infarction and the attendant high mortality seen even with aggressive management.

ISCHEMIC COLITIS

Ischemia of the colon has become recognized more commonly as a cause of acute and chronic bowel syndromes. Colonic ischemia may affect any part of the colon. The areas most susceptible to ischemia are the "watershed" areas, which are sites of anastomosis between two major arterial supplies. Some examples of this are the splenic flexure, where the superior mesenteric artery anastomoses with the inferior mesenteric artery, and the rectosigmoid, where the inferior mesenteric artery anastomoses with a branch of the internal iliac artery.

The patient, who often is elderly, characteristically has crampy abdominal pain associated with localized tenderness and diarrhea, which may be grossly bloody. In contrast to patients with acute mesenteric ischemia, the patient usually does not appear acutely ill. He may exhibit no apparent predisposing factors or may reveal signs of atherosclerosis or a low flow state.

Colonic ischemia usually is a self-limited process initially causing submucosal hemorrhage, which may be seen as "thumb-printing" on a barium enema. This may then progress to mucosal necrosis and manifest as segmental colitis, which often heals in several days to weeks. However, the ischemia may follow a chronic course that may mimic idiopathic ulcerative colitis. In about one third of patients the ischemia affects the muscularis propria, leading to fibrosis and stricture. A small number of patients progress acutely to transmural infarction, gangrene, and even peritonitis and require surgery for this severe complication.

In 10% of cases colonic ischemia may be associated with a lesion that obstructs the lumen of the colon. The obstruction leads to colonic distention, increased intraluminal pressure, decreased blood flow in the colonic wall, and ischemia. A barium enema generally reveals the underlying obstructing lesion.

MESENTERIC VENOUS THROMBOSIS

Mesenteric venous thrombosis is a less common cause of acute intestinal ischemia and accounts for only 5% of patients with this disorder. There may be predisposing factors leading to venous thrombosis such as stasis secondary to portal hypertension with cirrhosis; intraabdominal infection; the postoperative state; and hypercoagulable states associated with antithrombin III deficiency, protein C deficiency, polycythemia vera, neoplastic disease, or use of oral contraceptives. These patients may have abdominal pain for several weeks before the acute illness. The pain usually is not associated with weight loss. The acute pain of the ischemic event often is associated with nausea and vomiting; however, gastrointestinal bleeding is uncommon. Arteriography often is not diagnostic, and the diagnosis usually is made by laparotomy. There is a high risk of recurrent thrombosis, perhaps as high as 30%, if anticoagulation is not started in the immediate postoperative period.

OTHER VASCULAR DISORDERS

Vascular malformations are a common cause of gastrointestinal bleeding. These malformations vary from hereditary telangiectasia, seen in Rendu-Osler-Weber syndrome, to angiodysplasia, found in elderly individuals without a family history of the disorder. The common presentation is painless gastrointestinal bleeding that may vary from severe life-threatening hemorrhage to occult bleeding that manifests as anemia. Since barium contrast roentgenograms are not helpful, angiography or endoscopy usually is required to establish a diagnosis and the site of bleeding, but even these procedures may fail to detect the lesions.

HEREDITARY HEMORRHAGIC TELANGIECTASIA

Rendu-Osler-Weber syndrome, which is inherited as an autosomal dominant trait, is characterized by the presence of multiple telangiectasias in the skin and mucous membranes of the nose and mouth and throughout the gastrointestinal tract, most commonly in the stomach and duodenum. Occasionally the disease skips a generation. Patients commonly have epistaxis, whereas gastrointestinal bleeding usually occurs later in life. In one study the initial episodes of epistaxis occurred at the mean age of 11 years, and the first gastrointestinal hemorrhage at 55 years of age. The lesions, which are composed of dilated, convoluted venules and capillaries, appear as flat, red, well-defined vascular lesions usually less than 3 mm in diameter. When viewed endoscopically, the lesions in the gastrointestinal tract have the same appearance as those on the skin.

Treatment usually is supportive, although estrogens have been used with some success for epistaxis. The gastrointestinal lesions are best treated by electrocoagulation or ablation by laser therapy or with a heater probe. Surgery should be done only as a last resort, because the lesions tend to be numerous and scattered throughout the gut.

ACQUIRED ANGIODYSPLASIA

Angiodysplasia, commonly referred to as vascular ectasia or arterial-venous malformation, is a localized dilation of submucosal veins and capillaries without true arterial venous communication. The lesion is most commonly diagnosed in elderly individuals at an average age of 65 years, and it most often is found in the cecum and ascending colon. Angiodysplasia initially was thought to be rare, but since the widespread use of angiography in the 1970s, it has become recognized as a major cause of gastrointestinal bleeding; together with colonic diverticula, it accounts for most cases of massive lower gastrointestinal bleeding in patients over 40 years of age. The bleeding typically is painless and tends to be recurrent. The diagnosis may be made endoscopically by seeing a localized flat, red lesion or with angiography by noting early venous filling during the arterial phase, a vascular tuft in the arterial phase, or delayed emptying of a dilated vein in the venous phase. Treatment may be with surgical resection or endoscopic obliteration by electrocoagulation or thermal injury. In a few patients these lesions may be numerous and present in the left colon or upper gastrointestinal tract, thus accounting for recurrent episodes of bleeding after initial surgical or ablative therapy of the right colonic angiodysplasia.

Angiodysplasia also has been associated with aortic stenosis, and there have been anecdotal reports of cessation of bleeding and disappearance of the vascular lesions following aortic valve surgery. Angiodysplasia also is commonly noted in people with chronic renal failure, and is a common cause of gastrointestinal bleeding in this subgroup of patients. The pathogenesis of the angiodysplasia in elderly individuals or in association with aortic stenosis and renal failure currently is unknown.

BIBLIOGRAPHY

Boley S, Brandt L, and Veith F: Ischemic disorders of the intestine, Curr Probl Surg 15:6, 1978.
Boley S and others: Persistent vasoconstriction—a major factor in nonocclusive mesenteric ischemia, Curr Top Surg Res 3:425, 1971.
Boley S and others: Initial results from an aggressive roentgenological and surgical approach to acute mesenteric ischemia, Surgery 82:848, 1977.

177 · INTESTINAL OBSTRUCTION

Robert R. Atkins

MECHANICAL OBSTRUCTION AND ILEUS

DEFINITION. An intestinal obstruction is a process that prevents the normal progress of intestinal contents through the gut. The process causing obstruction may be mechanical or neurogenic.

ETIOLOGY. Intestinal obstruction may be classified in several ways. One such classification is by cause, that is, mechanical obstruction or neurogenic obstruction. Mechanical occlusion of the bowel lumen may be further classified into three types of abnormalities: (1) an obturation obstruction, (2) an intrinsic bowel lesion, and (3) an extrinsic bowel lesion. Obturation obstructions can be caused by gallstones, foreign bodies, bezoars, meconium, and fecal impaction. Intrinsic bowel lesions include congenital and acquired stenosis and atresia. Acquired narrowing may be secondary to neoplastic lesions or inflammatory conditions such as regional enteritis, diverticulitis, ischemic stricture, or radiation enteritis. An extrinsic obstruction may result from occlusion by adhesions, internal and external hernias, extrinsic masses, and volvulus.

Mechanical obstruction also may be classified by the level of obstruction, as small bowel obstruction or large bowel obstruction. Knowing the level of obstruction facilitates both diagnosis and management. Small bowel obstructions most commonly are caused by adhesions (70%), internal and external hernias (8%), and cancer (9%). In the large intestine, adhesive bands are an uncommon cause of obstruction, whereas carcinoma (67%), volvulus (9%), and diverticulitis (7%) are the most common causes.

In neurogenic obstruction or nonmechanical obstruction the intestinal contents do not progress through the bowel because of intestinal paralysis, the cause of which is one of several neurohumoral defects. Also called adynamic ileus, it commonly is seen after abdominal surgery and may follow any peritoneal insult. Adynamic ileus also is associated with a variety of other extragastrointestinal conditions, including fractures of the spine or pelvis, retroperitoneal hemorrhage, trauma, pyelonephritis, and ureteral stone. Diseases in the chest such as pneumonia, myocardial infarction, and rib fractures may be associated with adynamic ileus. It also is caused by metabolic abnormalities such as uremia and especially hypokalemia. Sepsis is a common cause of adynamic ileus, whereas intestinal ischemia is a less common cause.

PATHOPHYSIOLOGY. An obstruction to the normal flow of intestinal contents results in distention of the bowel with gas and fluid. Most of the retained gas is swallowed air and thus is predominantly nitrogen, which is poorly absorbed by the intestines. The accumulation of ingested matter and the daily 7 to 10 L of gastrointestinal secretion adds to the distention. Large amounts of fluid are lost from the intravascular space as a result of vomiting and inhibition of absorption caused by the obstruction. After 24 hours of obstruction, there is net secretion of water and electrolytes into the lumen, further compounding the distention and fluid loss. In addition to hypovolemia and loss of electrolytes, an obstruction causes dramatic rises in intraluminal pressure, especially in closed-loop obstruction, the obstruction of a loop of intestine at both ends, such as is caused by a hernia or adhesive band. A form of closed-loop obstruction may result from a colonic obstruction when the ileocecal valve is competent. Impairment of mucosal blood flow results from the effects of distention, torsion, or extrinsic pressure, resulting in ischemia, necrosis, bacterial invasion, and eventually perforation and peritonitis.

CLINICAL MANIFESTATIONS. A mechanical obstruction of the small bowel is manifested by mid abdominal, paroxysmal, colicky pain, abdominal distention, and vomiting. The higher the obstruction the more frequent and severe are the paroxysms of pain. Between these episodes the patient may be relatively comfortable. Vomiting occurs early with high intestinal obstruction, and the vomitus may be profuse and contain bile. With distal small bowel obstruction vomiting is delayed and the vomitus may contain feculent material resulting from the action of bacteria on the retained intestinal contents. In the case of colonic obstruction, vomiting may even be absent. With continued distention the pain may gradually diminish, probably because of an impairment of motility. The development of a continuous, localized pain may signal the onset of strangulation, but it usually is not possible to differentiate the symptoms of strangulation from those of a simple obstruction. Early in the course of an obstruction some loose stools or flatus may be passed, but complete obstipation and failure to pass gas ensue.

The physical examination begins with a search for scars of previous surgery. Early in the course of a small bowel obstruction the distention may be minimal. With prolonged obstruction, particularly of the distal small bowel, the abdomen becomes distended and tympanic. Bowel sounds characteristically are heard coincident with the onset of pain, are hyperactive and high pitched, and often have a musical or tinkling quality. Late in the course of an obstruction or when strangulation occurs, these findings may be absent. Tenderness and rigidity usually are minimal, as is fever. Unless a sausagelike abdominal mass can be palpated, the physical findings of strangulation may be no different from those of a nonstrangulating obstruction. Shock, fever, rigidity, and rebound are late findings and usually indicate peritoneal soilage.

In cases of adynamic ileus the patient's most prominent complaints are distention and obstipation. Colicky pain is not present, and vomiting, although frequent, usually is not profuse. Distention and tympany may be prominent in the physical examination, but tenderness and rigidity are absent. Bowel sounds usually are absent.

Mechanical obstruction of the colon is manifested by a more prominent distention than occurs with a small bowel obstruction. Pain may be colicky and tends to localize in the hypogastric area in cases of left colonic lesions or in the epigastrium and right upper quadrant in cases of right-sided lesions. In cases of colonic obstruction, pain tends to have a more delayed onset and is less severe than with a small bowel obstruction. Vomiting occurs late and, surprisingly, is rarely feculent. A history of blood in the stool or a recent change in bowel habits is common, resulting from the underlying cause of the obstruction. Although the patient may pass small amounts of stool and gas early in the course of colonic obstruction, obstipation and a failure to pass gas rapidly follow. On physical examination the abdomen is found to be distended and tympanitic. Bowel sounds are less frequent and lower pitched than in small bowel obstruction. The rectal examination may demonstrate a fecal impaction, mass, or blood or if the obstruction is above the rectum, the rectum may be essentially empty.

In all forms of obstruction dehydration and hypovolemia ensue and are manifested by a fall in urine output and eventually shock.

LABORATORY FINDINGS. The loss of fluids and electrolytes leads to hemoconcentration, a fall in the levels of serum chloride and potassium, and a rise in the level of blood urea nitrogen. Although the hemoglobin level may rise initially with hemoconcentration, prolonged obstruction leads to severe congestion of the intestine and a loss of blood into the lumen. A significant loss of blood may result in a fall in the level of hemoglobin. The leukocyte count may be normal early in the course of obstruction but may rise appreciably with a shift to the left, particularly if strangulation ensues. The level of serum amylase occasionally rises as it diffuses from the obstructed lumen into the circulation.

Roentgenograms of the abdomen are extremely helpful in confirming the clinical diagnosis and determining the point of obstruction. Repeated roentgenograms are needed to assess the patient's progress. In cases of a mechanical small bowel obstruction, loops of distended small bowel arranged in a step-ladder pattern may occur in a central location. Air-fluid levels can be seen on roentgenograms made with the patient erect. Little or no gas is seen in the colon. In cases of strangulating obstruction a single distended loop may occur, but in at least 50% of these cases roentgenograms are not helpful.

The colon is distinguished from the small bowel by the haustral markings, which do not traverse the entire diameter of the bowel, whereas in a distended small bowel the valvulae conniventes can be seen encircling the entire lumen. In cases of colonic obstruction with a competent ileocecal valve, distended loops of colon can be seen arrayed along the perimeter of the abdominal cavity. In cases of colonic obstruction with an incompetent ileocecal valve, the roentgenographic appearance may resemble that of a partial small bowel obstruction with distended loops of small and large intestine. When fecal impaction causes obstruction, masses of feces usually can be seen in the rectum and extending proximally.

Adynamic ileus is manifested by the dilation of all levels of the intestinal tract, commonly including the stomach. Air-fluid levels may be seen on lateral and upright films.

Barium should never be given by mouth to determine the point of obstruction until the possibility of colonic obstruction has been excluded. Barium may become inspissated above a colonic obstruction and aggravate the situation. A colonic obstruction can be ruled out by performing a barium enema; once it has been ruled out, barium can safely be given orally, since it does not become inspissated above a small bowel obstruction.

MANAGEMENT. With a few exceptions a mechanical obstruction is treated surgically. Before surgery, electrolyte and fluid balances should be restored and intestinal decompression with nasogastric suction or a long intestinal tube should be attempted. Decompression may lessen the symptoms but should not give the physician a false sense of success. Surgery should not be delayed unless there is unequivocal evidence that the obstruction has resolved. Broad-spectrum antibiotics are given while awaiting surgery. The choice of surgical procedure is dictated by the site of the obstruction and the surgeon's experience.

Certain situations can be managed nonsurgically. Adynamic ileus, particularly following an abdominal operation, is treated with decompression with a long intestinal tube. Sigmoid volvulus may be treated by decompression with a colonoscope or sigmoidoscope. Intussusception in children may be treated with

hydrostatic reduction; however, in adults it should be treated surgically. An obstruction caused by Crohn's disease may abate with supportive care and decompressive therapy. When fecal impaction causes obstruction, disimpaction may be accomplished by gently breaking up and removing feces digitally or with a proctoscope or by means of water, saline or oil retention enemas.

IDIOPATHIC INTESTINAL PSEUDOOBSTRUCTION

Idiopathic intestinal pseudoobstruction is a chronic disease characterized by recurrent episodes of intestinal obstruction without demonstrable mechanical obstruction of the bowel lumen. In some patients this condition occurs secondary to an underlying disorder such as systemic sclerosis, amyloidosis, diabetes, myxedema, or myotonic dystrophy. Even when these disorders are excluded, however, there remains a group of patients with no cause for the illness. In these patients the abnormality is thought to be related to a defect in the propulsive ability of the intestine. Other areas of the gastrointestinal tract such as the esophagus commonly demonstrate motility disorders. Although their cause is unknown, defects in the ganglion cells of the intestine have been found in some patients. Another group of patients has been shown to have a degeneration of the gut smooth muscle. The disorder may be familial in some instances.

Patients often have pseudoobstruction early in life and suffer recurrent bouts of obstruction associated with crampy abdominal pain, vomiting, distention, diarrhea, and occasionally steatorrhea. The physical exam reveals distention with minimal tenderness and a reduction in bowel sounds. Abdominal roentgenograms reveal distended loops of bowel. The barium swallow examination reveals a marked dilation of the small bowel and delayed transit.

Colonic pseudoobstruction also can occur, and as in the other forms of pseudoobstruction, no mechanical blockage can be demonstrated. The disease in the colon, however, usually is associated with an acute severe illness, electrolyte disorder, or narcotic therapy and is self-limited. This problem may be better classified as an isolated colonic ileus rather than pseudoobstruction.

The treatment of pseudoobstruction is mainly supportive and includes nasogastric suction and intravenous fluids. Some of the newer agents that stimulate gut motility have shown some promise in the management of this problem; however, more research is needed. Unfortunately, these patients commonly have undergone exploratory surgery before the diagnosis of pseudoobstruction is made.

MEGACOLON

Megacolon is characterized by the massive enlargement of the diameter of all or a portion of the colon. Megacolon usually is accompanied by severe constipation or obstipation. It may result from acquired or congenital abnormalities.

Congenital megacolon, or Hirschsprung's disease, is a disorder of intestinal motility usually manifested in infancy by intractable constipation. The disease is familial, is more common in males, and results from a congenital absence of myenteric ganglion cells in the colonic wall. The defect usually is confined to the distal colon but occasionally may involve long segments of colon. The aganglionic segment is unable to relax; that is, it is tonically contracted. This segment acts as a functional obstruction, and the portion of colon proximal to it becomes massively dilated. Roentgenographic examination with a barium enema reveals colonic dilation proximal to a narrowed segment. The diagnosis is made by detecting an absence of ganglion cells in a surgical biopsy specimen of the involved segment. Surgical excision of the abnormal segment with a "pull-through" and anastomosis of normal colon to the rectal stump is the procedure of choice.

Psychogenic megacolon, a common disorder of childhood, results from chronic stool holding. Its onset occurs later in childhood than Hirschsprung's disease, but it must be differentiated from that disease by means of a barium enema and rectal biopsy. The treatment involves changing the toilet habits and giving large doses of mineral oil and enemas. A similar condition may occur in adults, particularly in psychotic patients being treated with phenothiazines.

Acquired megacolon may result from a number of infections, metabolic, and neuromuscular disorders. Chagas' disease, commonly found in South America, results from an infection with *Trypanosoma cruzi* and is manifested by megacolon, megaesophagus, megaduodenum, and/or megaureter. It is caused by the destruction of Auerbach's plexus by a tissue reaction to the parasite. Chronic megacolon also may occur in association with scleroderma, amyloidosis, lead poisoning, and myxedema. Neurologic disorders associated with megacolon include parkinsonism, multiple sclerosis, spinal cord lesions, and diabetic visceral neurophathy. Narcotic, anticholinergic, and phenothiazine drugs may cause severe constipation and dilation. Habitual laxative abuse has been associated with megacolon. Any chronic partial obstruction of the distal colon may cause megacolon. The treatment is that for the underlying disorder.

Acute toxic megacolon may result from any inflammatory disorder of the colon but most commonly is associated with chronic ulcerative colitis or Crohn's disease of the colon (see Chapter 126).

BIBLIOGRAPHY

Cohn L and Atik M: Strangulation obstruction: closed loop studies, Ann Surg 153:94, 1961.
Cope Z: The early diagnosis of the acute abdomen, ed 14, London, 1972, Oxford University Press.
Ehrenpreis T: Hirschsprung's disease, Chicago, 1970, Year Book Medical Publishers, Inc.
Faulk DL and others: Chronic intestinal pseudoobstruction, Gastorenterology 74:922, 1978.
Miller LD and others: The pathophysiology and management of intestinal obstruction, Surg Clin North Am 42:1285, 1962.
Silen W and others: Strangulation obstruction of the small intestine, Arch Surg 85:121, 1962.

178 · FUNCTIONAL BOWEL DISEASE

Julian Katz

DEFINITION. Functional bowel disease is a group of clinical features probably best viewed as a syndrome rather than a disease. There are no demonstrable anatomic abnormalities and a variety of causes. The recognition in recent years of lactase deficiency in some patients previously thought to have functional symptoms suggests that additional "organic" abnormalities will be identified in the future in some of these patients, leading to the development of more specific therapies.

Functional bowel disorders are heterogeneous, but the symptoms include abdominal pain, excessive borborygmi, abdominal bloating, and alterations in stool frequency. A morphologically demonstrated organic disease such as a peptic ulcer, celiac disease, ulcerative colitis, or a bowel tumor may produce the same symptoms. Distention, relief of pain with a bowel movement, and more frequent and looser stools, along with the onset of pain, are significantly more common with functional bowel disease than with organic disease. Other symptoms of functional bowel syndrome are notable mucus in the stool and a sensation of incomplete evacuation. Most patients have abdominal discomfort, but painless, runny stools are another symptom of functional bowel disease. Different terms have been used to describe the syndrome. *Spastic colitis* emphasizes the disturbed bowel motility that may be present, but in functional disorders there is no mucosal inflammation. *Psychophysiologic gastrointestinal reaction* emphasizes that certain patients have an altered physiologic response to stress, often with lower pain thresholds. *Irritable bowel or colon* is another commonly used term.

ETIOLOGY. Intestinal motility studies suggest that there may be abnormal motor patterns in patients who have the irritable bowel syndrome of pain and problems with bowel movements. These differences are evident in the basal state and in response to physiologic and pharmacologic stimuli. On the right side of the colon segmental contractions normally result in retrograde and forward mixing and churning movements, with a periodic mass movement of the stool into the left colon. In the left colon normal segmental contractions retard the passage of the stool into the rectum. Manometric studies demonstrate that the segmental contractions of the sigmoid colon are increased in frequency and amplitude in patients with irritable bowel syndrome, particularly during periods of symptoms. Abdominal cramps are correlated with increased intraluminal pressures and with the contraction of the circular layer of smooth muscle. In patients with painless diarrhea, the activity of sigmoid segmental contractions decreases.

Control and coordination of the contractile patterns of the colon are related to intrinsic myoelectric activity. Pacemakers are located in the circular muscle of the colon, and a basic electrical rhythm can be recorded. Patients with irritable bowel syndrome have abnormal myoelectric patterns demonstrable by intraluminal mucosal electrodes. These patients have an increased percentage of slower frequency waves, and altered motility of the small intestine can be demonstrated in some cases.

Bowel contractions are affected by many factors, including food intake, the autonomic nervous system, physical activity, and psychologic states. Altered responses to meals, cholinergic and anticholinergic drugs, humoral agents, and emotional stresses occur in patients who have an irritable bowel syndrome. In patients with notable postprandial symptoms, the normal increase in segmental contractions following eating is exaggerated. Cholecystokinin and gastrin, which are released in the gut in response to eating, also exaggerate the increase in colonic muscular activity. Patients with abdominal pain and constipation often respond to stress with increased amplitude and frequency of sigmoid segmental contractions, and contractile activity decreases in patients with diarrhea. Increased fluid transport into the bowel may be a major factor when patients have painless diarrhea with large stool volumes.

The syndrome includes clinical symptoms that patients attribute to intestinal gas. These include belching, bloating, and excessive flatus. Bowel gas is 99% composed of odorless gases: nitrogen, oxygen, hydrogen, carbon dioxide, and in about 30% of adults, methane. Intestinal gas derives from swallowed air, gases produced within the colon, and gases that diffuse from the blood into the gut lumen. Air is swallowed as part of food, in association with eating and drinking, and by the habit of aspirating air into the esophagus. Eructation occurs in some people as an annoying but benign response to air swallowing. Further gas is produced in the intestine as acid reacts with bicarbonate to form carbon dioxide. An additional important source of gas production is the fermentation by colonic bacteria of carbohydrates that are not entirely absorbed in the small intestine. Lactose intolerance is a common cause of bloating and flatulence. The milk sugar lactose is a disaccharide composed of glucose and galactose; if the small intestine has insufficient lactase to digest the carbohydrate into its two component sugars, the lactose is used by colonic bacteria, resulting in the release of hydrogen, carbon dioxide, and organic acids that react with bicarbonate to produce additional carbon dioxide. Lactase insufficiency is genetically determined and very common in certain ethnic groups such as Orientals and American blacks. Other carbohydrates not digested by enzymes in the intestine such as the oligosaccharides in beans are fermented by colonic bacteria.

Abdominal discomfort and bloating, particularly after meals, have been attributed to excessive gas. Yet the total volume of intestinal gas in patients with these clinical gas syndromes is not increased over the normal volume, either in the fasting state or following a large meal. Rather, these patients show a retarded passage of gas through the intestine and a retrograde movement of gas in the gut. The introduction of gas into the intestine in an amount tolerated by normal subjects provokes pain in these patients. Thus these problems are related to a motility disturbance in the small intestine and an increased perception of distention of the bowel.

EPIDEMIOLOGY. Of all patients seen by gastroenterologists, 20% to 40% have functional bowel symptoms. A survey of apparently healthy people showed that 30% had recurrent abdominal pain and alterations in bowel habits. Epidemiologic studies have suggested that the fiber content of the diet may play a role in the pathogenesis of functional bowel disease, but other factors besides the type of fiber may cause patients to complain of bowel problems. East Europeans and rural Africans both consume large amounts of fiber, but Europeans are more troubled by functional bowel distress.

No environmental or emotional stress pattern, personality type, sex, age group, or psychiatric disturbance is correlated with functional bowel syndrome. The alterations in colonic motility and myoelectric activity that occur in patients with irritable bowel syndrome can be found in many patients who are not bothered by gastrointestinal symptoms. Patients' response to the motility disturbance is determined by their attitude, conditioning, and cultural background. Some patients have a definite lower pain threshold to distention of the gut.

CLINICAL MANIFESTATIONS AND COURSE. Different functional syndromes have been described that may have disparate mechanisms and that would therefore respond to different treatment programs. Usually the symptoms can be expected to return, often provoked by changes in the patient's life pattern or psychologic stress. In 20% of an otherwise well population, abdominal pain occurs more than six times a year. Pain below the navel that is relieved by defecation or the passage of flatus is a characteristic of irritable bowel syndrome. Some patients may have painless diarrhea, whereas others have straining at stool and obstipation, culminating in ill-formed stools. There may be another pattern of upper abdominal distress with features suggesting acid-peptic disease but without readily demonstrable mucosal inflammation.

DIAGNOSIS. The diagnosis should not merely be made by excluding other disorders. A history compatible with a bowel motility disorder is necessary for a diagnosis of an irritable bowel syndrome. Roentgenographic studies show no specific abnormalities. Diverticulosis of the colon may be present, however; it has been associated with similar increased sigmoid pressures and abdominal pains such as occur in irritable bowel syndrome. Endoscopic examination of the gastrointestinal tract is unrevealing in the evaluation of dyspeptic symptoms. Perhaps most important, the circumstances that contribute to an enhanced physiologic bowel response to varied stresses should be identified. The recent onset of seemingly functional symptoms without obvious precipitating causes or a nocturnal prominence of these symptoms should mandate a more vigorous search for an organic origin, such as pancreatic carcinoma. Often the best test, after the preliminary evaluation, is a therapeutic trial, as discussed in the following section.

MANAGEMENT. The scientific basis of most dietary regimens for the treatment of functional bowel syndrome is questionable. Vigorous dietary restriction of the composition and consistency of the diet is not helpful. Regular balanced meals that are moderate in nonabsorbed spices and food temperatures are a sufficient recommendation. The elimination of specific dietary carbohydrates is helpful in treating distention, cramps, and flatulence in some patients; a decrease in foods that contain large amounts of nonabsorbable carbohydrates such as beans and cabbage reduces gas production in the gut. Lactose is not completely absorbed even by patients without an obvious lactase deficiency, and a diet limited in milk, ice cream, and soft cheeses might be tried. A low-fat diet may reduce carbon dioxide production in the upper small intestine.

The role of added dietary fiber in the treatment of functional bowel symptoms is controversial. In a high-fiber diet stool weight increases and the transit time of the stool probably decreases; a reduction in intraluminal pressures in the sigmoid colon also has been described. Symptomatic relief has not been clearly demonstrated with such a diet, however, and large amounts of fiber must be ingested for alterations in bowel function to occur. Supplementary mucilloid bulk agents probably should be tried as a means of adding measured amounts of fiber.

Convincing studies of the efficacy of anticholinergic agents are lacking. Some such drugs do cause the myoelectric patterns of the irritable bowel to become more normal. A trial of one of these drugs for a few weeks is justified. Antidiarrhea agents such a diphenoxylate, loperamide, or even codeine may give confidence to the patient who suffers from diarrhea. Endorphin blockers, pharmaceutical agents involved in prostaglandin and other hormone metabolism, and drugs in development may be effective. Recent work with the operant conditioning (biofeedback) of colonic motility shows some positive results. The use of psychotherapeutic modalities of therapy may often be necessary, but reassurance, education, and careful and compassionate follow-up are most important.

BIBLIOGRAPHY

Almy TP and Rothstein RI: Irritable bowel syndrome: classification and pathogenesis, Annu Rev Med 38:257, 1987.

Burns TW: Colonic motility in the irritable bowel syndrome, Arch Intern Med 140:247, 1980.

Drossman DA: Diagnosis of the irritable bowel syndrome, Ann Intern Med 90:431, 1979.

Levitt MD and Bond JH: Flatulence, Annu Rev Med 31:127, 1980.

Thompson WG and Heaton KW: Functional bowel disorders in apparently healthy people, Gastroenterology 79:283, 1980.

179·ANORECTAL DISORDERS

Harvey B. Lefton

DEFINITION. Disease in the anorectal region may result from infectious, inflammatory, or neoplastic processes. Pain is a common feature of disease of the lower anus, whereas bleeding, difficulty with defecation, and rectal fullness characterize disease in the upper canal and rectum.

ANATOMY. Location of the pathologic process determines the symptoms. The perianal region and lower anal canal are lined with squamous epithelium and innervated by somatic nerves with pain receptors. Venous drainage is to the inferior vena cava, and lymphatics drain to the inguinal nodes. The pectinate line is the beginning of the portion of the upper anus lined with mucous membrane. The upper anal canal is innervated by sympathetic nerve fibers that do not carry pain impulses. Lesions in this area produce discomfort by triggering spasms of the rectum or by pressuring the surrounding musculature. Venous drainage in the upper anus is to the portal system, and the lymphatics drain to the lumbar nodes. At the pectinate line are epithelial bulges called papillae (Fig. 179-1). Proximal to this line are the rectal columns of Morgagni—mucosal folds separated by crypts.

The anal canal has an internal sphincter consisting of rectal smooth muscle and an external sphincter that joins with the puborectal muscles, the levator ani coccyx. The internal sphincter is under autonomic control and relaxes as stool is propelled against it. The external sphincter is controlled voluntarily once toilet training is completed. Although cutting the internal sphincter does not produce symptoms, chronic inflammation or surgical injury of the external sphincter results in soilage and incontinence.

The ischiorectal and perirectal spaces contain large deposits of fatty tissue. When an infection invades this region from the anus or rectum, large, painful abscesses can develop.

SKIN DISORDERS

The most common symptom of anal disease is pruritus, which may result from psoriasis, atopic dermatitis, seborrhea, or lichen planus of the anal canal. Infection with *Trichophyton organisms* or *Candida albicans* may also produce anal pruritus. Surgical injury to the anal canal, hemorrhoids, and recurrent anal infection can cause incontinence resulting in chronic soilage with alkaline rectal contents and eventually producing intense pruritus and hyperpigmentation of the perianal skin. *Enterobius vermicularis* (pinworm) infestation may cause nocturnal anal pruritus, especially in children.

Commonly no identifiable dermatologic or inflammatory process is present. In some patients a severe emotional upset may precede the onset of pruritus; these patients benefit from treatment with mild tranquilizers. Improvement in anal hygiene alleviates the discomfort related to soilage. If the patient has anal incontinence and incomplete rectal emptying, the administration of a tap water enema after defecation can remove the alkaline rectal fluid; this should be followed by drying the perineum. The use of medicated pads substituted for toilet paper also reduces perianal irritation. Mild tranquilizers or sleeping aids should be administered if anxiety accompanies incontinence.

In rare cases pruritus may be associated with anal condylomas caused by a papovavirus infection, a condition common in homosexual patients. Treatment with a podophyllin solution may eradicate these anal warts. Occasionally surgery or cautery is necessary.

HEMORRHOIDS

Hemorrhoids are varicose veins occurring in the anus. Precipitating factors include pregnancy, prolonged sitting, straining at stool because of constipation, recurrent diarrhea, and portal hypertension. The incidence of hemorrhoids increases with advancing age, and 70% of people over 50 years of age have hemorrhoids.

External hemorrhoids are covered by skin. They become symptomatic when the vessels become thrombosed, causing the surrounding tissues to swell and become painful. Initially the patient notes a palpable anal mass and marked rectal throbbing. Anoscopy reveals soft bluish masses covered by skin. Often these lesions remit with treatment of sitz baths, emollients, and stool softeners; complete resorption of the clot usually occurs in 2 to 4 weeks. Severe pain may necessitate surgical removal of the clot, however, leaving an open wound that is subject to a secondary infection. Occasionally spontaneous healing produces a prolapsed skin tag. These markers of healed hemorrhoids are usually asymptomatic and do not require surgical excision.

Internal hemorrhoids are varicosities covered by mucous membrane that cause rectal bleeding. Because this region lacks sensory innervation, pain is not a common feature. Patients may have the sensation of rectal fullness if hemorrhoids are large. The prolapse of swollen internal hemorrhoids may cause anal pruritus and soilage. Prolapsed internal hemorrhoids also may become strangulated by the anal sphincter, producing pain (Fig. 179-2). The most important aspect of the treatment of uncomplicated internal hemorrhoids usually involves reassuring the patient that a rectal cancer is not present. Local anesthetics, cortisone suppositories, and sitz baths help promote healing. Sclerosing agents can be injected into the hemorrhoid to promote fibrosis. More recently the ligation of internal hemorrhoids with rubber bands has been performed to cause a sloughing of the lesion; this procedure is associated with few problems. Surgical excision is indicated when significant bleeding develops or hemorrhoids remain prolapsed. Laser vaporization and infrared photocoagulation have been used in place of surgery but offer minimal advantages.

FISSURES

A break in the lining of the anal canal causes a painful ulceration. Such a break develops in the posterior midline of the anal canal as a result of a paucity of muscular support fibers in this region and the high pressure of defecation. The pain from an anal fissure often is so severe that administration of opiates is required. Topical anesthetics must be used before digital examination or anoscopy. The examiner may see a sentinel skin tag resulting from anal thickening. Because of the repeated trauma of defecation, untreated fissures do not heal. Surgical treatment is necessary to resolve this lesion. Anal stenosis is a late feature of an untreated fissure or an improper surgical resection.

FISTULAS

Burrowing infections of the anal crypts and altered anal immunologic mechanisms are thought to play a role in the development of anal fistulas. Infections may drain to the perianal region or burrow internally to adjacent areas in the bowel, bladder, or vagina. Patients may have a history of recent anal abscesses or may note pus or fecal soilage on their underclothing. Fistulas also may occur in patients with Crohn's disease, tuberculosis, carcinoma, or lymphogranuloma venereum. Fistulas not associated with inflammatory bowel disease should be surgically probed and resected. In patients with Crohn's

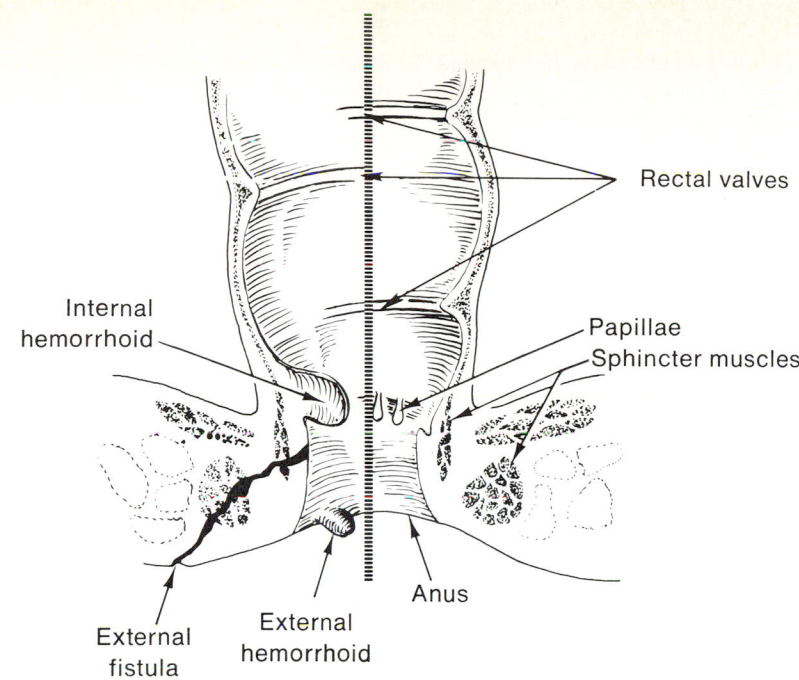

Internal
hemorrhoid

Rectal valves

Papillae
Sphincter muscles

Anus

External
fistula

External
hemorrhoid

Fig. 179-1   Normal and abnormal findings of anorectal region.

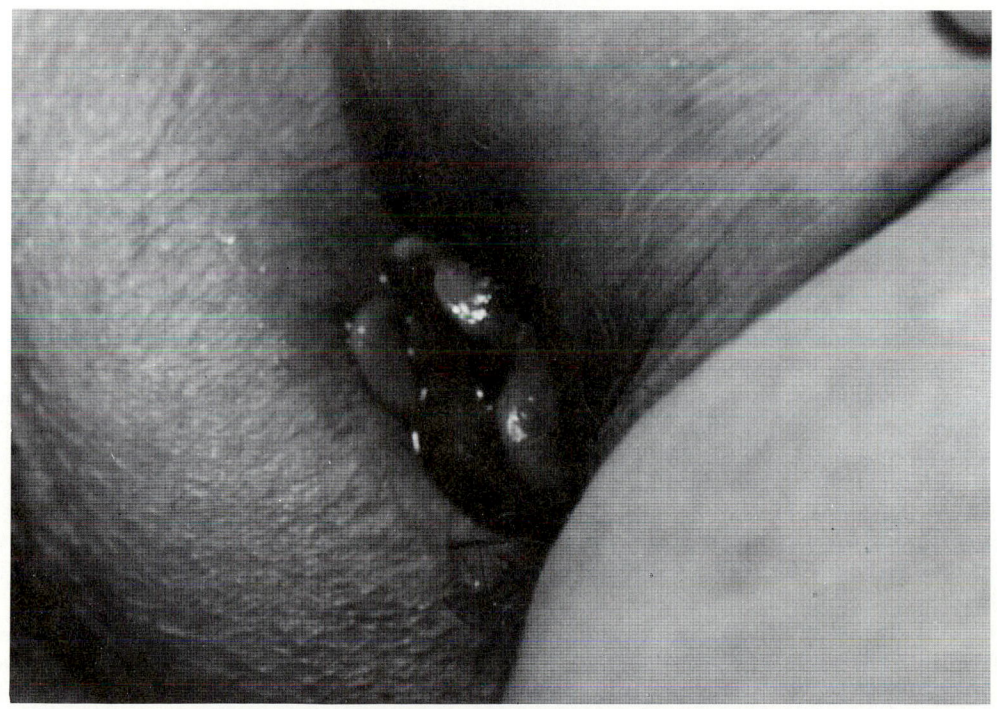

Fig. 179-2   Prolapsed thrombosed internal hemorrhoids.

disease, surgical resection often leads to indolent ulcers. Such patients should have abscesses drained and should be treated with oral sulfasalazine or metronidazole. A recurrent anal abscess leads to anal stenosis.

TUMORS

Malignant tumors are rare in the anus. An epidermoid carcinoma may originate as a small mass that goes on to ulcerate and cause pain. This is a slow-growing tumor that is locally invasive and spreads through the lymphatics. The treatment consists of abdominoperineal resection. When the inguinal nodes are involved, the prognosis is poor, but radiation therapy may have palliative value for these patients.

Several other tumors may occur in the anus. A basal cell carcinoma of the anus may develop as an anal nodule in elderly patients. This is a superficial cancer that responds well to excisional therapy. Bowen's disease (intraepithelial squamous cell carcinoma) of the anus first appears as a draining reddish anal plaque; this also responds to excisional therapy. Malignant melanoma is a very aggressive lesion of the anus that appears as a tender bluish nodule. The lesion may have the appearance of a hemorrhoid but on palpation is very hard. The mortality with malignant melanoma is high even with the most radical surgical procedures. A cloacogenic carcinoma may occur in the transitional epithelium of the proximal anus; this extensive carcinoma requires abdominoperineal resection and is associated with a high mortality.

BIBLIOGRAPHY

Fazio VJ, editor: Anorectal disorders, Clinics in Gastroenterology, vol. 16, Philadelphia, 1987, WB Saunders Co.

180 · TUMORS OF THE GUT

Paul B. Weisberg

Gastrointestinal neoplasms are a common cause of morbidity and mortality throughout the world. The relative incidence of some types of tumors varies widely, however, among different populations according to geographic location and dietary habits. Both benign and malignant lesions may arise in any level of the gastrointestinal tract, and any of the cell types found there can be the source of tumor formation. Most, however, originate in the mucosa. With the exception of certain colonic polyps, benign neoplasms do not pose clinical problems as commonly as malignant tumors. With the current advances in diagnostic and therapeutic technology, particularly endoscopy, the diagnosis and management of this group of disorders should become increasingly successful.

ESOPHAGEAL NEOPLASMS
Benign tumors

LEIOMYOMAS. Leiomyoma, a smooth muscle tumor, is the most common of the benign esophageal neoplasms, but its incidence is less than 10% of that of malignant tumors. Leiomyomas usually are clinically silent; about half of the reported cases are found in autopsy studies. When large they may produce dysphagia by causing a partial obstruction, but only rarely do they ulcerate and bleed as gastric leiomyomas do. The diagnosis usually is made with a barium roentgenogram, in which the lesion appears as a smooth, constant filling defect. Endoscopy reveals a mass with normal overlying mucosa, and for this reason an endoscopic biopsy usually is not helpful in determining the diagnosis. The only treatment is surgical enucleation of the tumor.

OTHER BENIGN TUMORS. Other benign tumors are extremely rare in the esophagus and usually are present as polyps. A long pedicle is characteristic of the fibrovascular polyp. Other lesions that have been reported include lipomas, fibromas, squamous papillomas, neurofibromas, lymphangiomas, and cysts.

Malignant tumors

EPIDERMOID CARCINOMA. Carcinoma arising in the squamous epithelium is the most common of the esophageal tumors. Epidemiologic data show that the incidence of such carcinomas is much higher in some populations than in others. Men in certain regions of the Soviet Union, Iran, and China have an incidence 10 to 30 times that of American white males. American black males have an incidence almost 4 times that of American white males—15.6 compared to 4:100,000—and males in general have a higher incidence than females. A number of causative associations have been identified. The incidence of carcinoma is increased among patients with a history of alcohol abuse, cigarette smoking, lye stricture, exposure to ionizing radiation, achalasia, and Plummer-Vinson syndrome.

Clinical manifestations. Epidermoid carcinomas usually occur in middle-aged or older people. The most common initial symptom is progressive dysphagia (first with solids, then with soft foods, and finally with liquids), which results from gradual narrowing of the esophageal lumen. Odynophagia also occurs but is less common. As the obstruction becomes marked, food and secretions may be retained, resulting in symptoms of tracheal aspiration. A constant substernal or back pain is a poor prognostic sign, because it usually signifies a local extension of the tumor outside the esophagus. Gross hemorrhage is unusual, but occult bleeding is common, and these patients commonly become anemic as a result of iron deficiency. Anorexia and weight loss also accompany the illness. If advanced the tumor may erode into adjacent organs, leading to the development of a tracheoesophageal fistula or in rare cases an aortoesophageal fistula. The physical examination may reveal nonspecific findings such as evidence of weight loss, anemia, supraclavicular adenopathy or hepatomegaly resulting from metastases, and signs of aspiration pneumonitis.

Diagnosis. When a carcinoma of the esophagus is suspected, the diagnostic procedure of choice is the barium swallow examination with an upper gastrointestinal series. The usual finding is of a localized, often circumferential luminal narrowing with irregular or shelflike boundaries and mucosal destruction. Occasionally the tumor may appear to involve only one side of the lumen or may appear as a smooth tapered lesion, in which case it is difficult to differentiate a carcinoma from a benign stricture. When feasible, fiberoptic endoscopy should be performed after roentgenography in an effort to determine the extent of the lesion and to confirm the diagnosis with biopsy and brush cytology. When both biopsy and brush cytology are performed, the diagnostic accuracy approaches 96%. When endoscopy cannot be performed, an exfoliative cytologic examination may be made of gastric aspirates and washings taken from the region of the tumor through a nasogastric tube; this method has a diagnostic accuracy only slightly less than that of endoscopic studies. Computed tomography of the mediastinum also can be of value in selected cases to determine the extent of the lesion. Newer techniques of radioisotope scanning with materials that are preferentially picked up by squamous cell carcinomas are under investigation.

Management. The two major therapeutic modalities available are radiation therapy and surgical extirpation, performed either alone or in combination. The choice of therapy for a given patient depends on many factors, the most important of which is the location of the lesion in the esophagus. Lower-third lesions (50%) are most accessible to surgical removal, middle-third lesions (30%) are somewhat more difficult, and upper-third lesions (20%) are technically very difficult to remove surgically. For this reason, high-dose radiation therapy traditionally has been used for most upper- and middle-third tumors and less commonly for lower-third lesions. Any patient with evidence that the tumor has spread probably should be treated with radiation rather than resection, regardless of the location. The symptoms can be palliated with either modality, and the overall 5-year survival rate, approximately 5%, is the same with both therapies. Recent studies using a combination of preoperative radiation and surgical excision, however, have shown that this approach may significantly increase the survival rate for selected patients. For symptomatic palliation at any stage of the disease, esophageal dilation, insertion of a prosthetic tube, or destruction of the tumor with laser or thermal techniques can be performed.

ADENOCARCINOMA. The true incidence of primary adenocarcinomas of the esophagus is difficult to determine, because many of these lesions originate in the columnar epithelium of the stomach and grow upward in the esophageal wall. An adenocarcinoma in an otherwise normal esophagus accounts for less than 1% of all esophageal malignancies. If patients with Barrett's esophagus are included, the rate increases to 3% to 7%. The columnar epithelium in Barrett's esophagus is considered by many to be a premalignant lesion because of its strong association with esophageal adenocarcinoma.

This disease is most common in the same age-group as epidermoid carcinomas and usually appears in a similar fashion, with dysphagia as one of the earliest and most prominent symptoms. Other clinical manifestations are likewise very similar. The diagnosis can be established with the same approach, using roentgenographic and endoscopic techniques.

Because conventional radiation therapy is relatively ineffective in treating patients with an adenocarcinoma, surgery for the palliation of obstructive symptoms or a curative resection should be performed on those who are operative candidates. The routine resection of the lesion results in a 9% 5-year survival rate.

OTHER MALIGNANT TUMORS. Malignant tumors of the esophagus other than squamous cell carcinomas and adenocarcinomas are extremely rare. Other types that have been reported include carcinosarcomas, pseudosarcomas, verrucous carcinomas, melanomas, and argyrophil cell carcinomas. Metastatic lesions of the esophagus are also distinctly uncommon, but the contiguous spread of tumors from adjacent organs does occur, particularly from the lungs and the thyroid gland.

GASTRIC NEOPLASMS
Benign tumors

GASTRIC POLYPS. Benign gastric polyps are relatively rare lesions; their incidence revealed by autopsies is about 0.5%. Histologically, they are either hyperplastic (80%) or adenomatous (20%), but the two types may coexist. Villous adenomas are rare. Achlorhydria occurs in 95% of patients with benign gastric polyps and in virtually all patients with multiple polyps, although no causal relationship has been proved. Only 2% of all achlorhydric patients develop polyps. Polyps are present in 5% of patients with pernicious anemia. Gastric polyps are important primarily because of their association with malignancy; 25% to 35% of patients with polyps also have a gastric carcinoma. True hyperplastic polyps never contain malignancy, but 20% to 40% of adenomatous polyps are cancerous. In addition, 30% to 60% of patients with adenomatous polyps have a coexisting cancer. The rate is much lower for patients with hyperplastic lesions. Polyps that are sessile and larger than 2 cm in diameter are much more likely to be malignant than lesions that are stalked and less than 1 cm in diameter. Gastric polyps also have been found in association with several of the intestinal polyposis syndromes such as Gardner's, Peutz-Jeghers, and Cronkhite-Canada syndromes and familial polyposis coli.

Clinical manifestations. Most patients with gastric polyps are over 50 years of age, and the disease shows no sex predilection. Many patients are asymptomatic, but others describe a vague upper abdominal discomfort that is usually not related to eating. Gross bleeding is rare, but occult blood loss producing iron deficiency anemia and the attendant symptoms is common. Occasionally a large antral polyp may prolapse into the pylorus and produce a transient gastric outlet obstruction.

The physical examination usually reveals little except for the signs of iron deficiency anemia or pernicious anemia. Likewise the laboratory evaluation is nonspecific, showing some form of anemia and, if gastric analysis is performed, total achlorhydria in 95% of these patients.

Diagnosis. The upper gastrointestinal series, particularly an air contrast study, reveals most lesions as round, translucent filling defects. Gastroscopy is somewhat more sensitive than roentgenography in detecting small lesions and has the added advantage of allowing the direct removal of biopsy and brush cytology tissue samples. Exfoliative cytology also may be useful.

Management. If a polyp is thought to be the cause of symptoms or complications, or if it is sessile or larger than 2 cm in diameter, it should be removed. Removal should be performed through the gastroscope with a snare-cautery if possible. Otherwise, surgical excision is indicated. If an associated malignancy can be excluded from the diagnosis, patients with small or even several polyps can be observed instead.

LEIOMYOMAS. Leiomyomas are the most common benign tumors of the stomach. They usually are found incidentally during surgery or an autopsy; they rarely produce clinical symptoms unless they are larger than 3 cm in diameter. When large, they have a tendency to ulcerate and may cause gross hemorrhage. On roentgenograms they appear as large, smooth, filling defects that may have a central ulceration. Gastroscopy shows a mass with normal overlying mucosa and the ulcer if one is present. Because the lesion is intramural, an endoscopic biopsy and brush or exfoliative cytology usually cannot establish the diagnosis preoperatively. Symptomatic lesions as well as those found incidentally during surgery should be excised.

OTHER BENIGN TUMORS. Very few other benign tumors of the stomach occur. About 25% of ectopic pancreatic tissue occurs in the stomach, usually on the greater curvature of the distal antrum. Rarely larger than 2 cm in diameter, about half of these lesions produce vague abdominal symptoms. Roentgenographically and endoscopically, they appear as smooth submucosal masses with a central umbilication that represents the duct. Symptomatic lesions are treated by a distal gastrectomy. Other rare tumors that have been reported include lipomas, fibromas, and tumors of vascular and neural origin.

Malignant tumors

ADENOCARCINOMA. Gastric carcinoma is one of the most insidious and lethal of all malignancies and accounts for most gastric malignancies. Fortunately, its incidence in the United States has been declining over the last several decades, and the 5-year survival rate has increased to 9%. A comparison of the relative incidences of gastric carcinoma among various populations around the world reveals that there are marked differences. The reason for this is unknown, but it is probably related to genetic or, more likely, environmental factors. In all populations mostly older individuals are affected, males are affected more often than females, and nonwhites are affected more often than whites.

Gastric carcinomas have been associated with a number of factors that are thought to be predisposing influences. Genetic factors undoubtedly operate in certain situations, such as in kindreds in which the incidence of gastric malignancy is unusually high. People with blood group A have a 10% higher risk than others, and there is a vague relationship of gastric carcinoma with the secretion of the Lewis substance in the saliva. In addition to genetic factors, several disease states are associated with a higher incidence of gastric cancer, such as acanthosis nigricans, in which the associated malignancy commonly develops in the stomach, and dermatomyositis. Certain pathologic and physiologic changes in the gastric mucosa also are known to be related to malignancy; these abnormalities are hypochlorhydria, achlorhydria, atrophic gastritis, and chronic gastritis. A causative role for these disorders, however, has not been established. Gastric polyps, pernicious anemia, hypertrophic gastropathy (Menetrier's disease), and gastric resection with gastroenterostomy are also associated with higher rates of cancer; the incidence of cancer in the last of these usually does not begin to rise until many years after surgery. In the past a chronic benign gastric ulcer was thought to be a predisposition to cancer, but it is extremely doubtful that such a relationship exists. A malignant degeneration of benign gastric ulcers probably does not occur.

Clinical manifestations. The gross morphologic form of a gastric adenocarcinoma can be of several different types: a sessile or pedunculated polypoid mass; a superficial spreading plaque that may be elevated, flat, or depressed; an ulcerated lesion with or without a mass effect; or an infiltrating intramural tumor (linitis plastica). Regardless of the growth pattern of the tumor, the early stages of the disease when it is limited to the mucosa and submucosa are generally symptom free. The lesion eventually grows out of the confines of the stomach, extends locally into adjacent organs, and metastasizes via the lymphatic and hematogenous routes to distant organs such as the liver, lung, bones, and central nervous system. By the time symptoms appear, the tumor is usually in an advanced stage, but distant metastases are not necessarily present.

The symptoms of gastric carcinoma are nonspecific, but some are encountered regularly. Pain occurs in 70% to 90% of patients and usually is an early symptom. It is generally vague and may or may not be affected by meals or medications such as antacids. Pain is sometimes worsened by meals in contradistinction to that caused by benign peptic ulcer disease. Anorexia and early satiety occur in almost two thirds of patients and nausea and vomiting in half, with weight loss having occurred in most by the time other symptoms are present. Additional symptoms include weakness, easy fatigability, abdominal bloating, fever, and changes in bowel habits. Although gross hemorrhage may occur, occult bleeding is more common and leads to iron deficiency anemia.

The physical findings in patients with an advanced gastric carcinoma are related to the local spread and metastases of the tumor and to its systemic effects. About half have a palpable abdominal mass, but only 20% have tenderness. The liver may be enlarged, but unless it is nodular, the presence of metastases cannot be assumed. Metastatic lesions may occur as Virchow's node (left supraclavicular node), as pelvic metastases revealed as Blumer's shelf in the rectal examination, and as Krukenberg's tumor in the ovary. Physical signs of anemia are common, but severe cachexia occurs in only about 20% of these patients.

The laboratory findings are nonspecific and usually show an anemia of the iron deficiency type, macrocytic type (if the patient has pernicious anemia or folate deficiency), combined type, or normochromic and normocytic type. There usually is occult blood in the stool, and many patients are hypoproteinemic. In patients with hepatic metastases, the bilirubin and alkaline phosphatase levels may be elevated. A gastric analysis may be performed, and if no acid is secreted with maximal stimulation and there is an ulcerating lesion of the stomach, a malignancy is almost certainly present; no conclusions can be drawn, however, if any acid at all is present. In 25% of patients with gastric cancers achlorhydria is present. Varying amounts of acid are secreted in the remaining 75%.

Diagnosis. The diagnostic procedure of choice when gastric carcinoma is suspected is a barium roentgenographic study (Fig. 180-1). The double-contrast study is preferred to the traditional study because the latter is not as sensitive in detecting small lesions; this is especially true for small superficial spreading tumors and small polypoid masses. Large intraluminal tumors and ulcerating masses can generally be detected with either study. A tumor infiltrating the wall of the stomach (linitis plastica) usually appears only as a nondistensible, poorly motile organ with no apparent mass. Although roentgenographic criteria alone can correctly identify a gastric lesion as benign or malignant in 80% of cases, there are many false positive and false negative results. For this reason endoscopy is of great value in the differential diagnosis of gastric lesions. With the questionable exception of very small gastric ulcers that appear benign on roentgenograms, most lesions in the stomach should be examined endoscopically, and tissue samples should be obtained for biopsy and cytologic examination. The diagnostic accuracy for carcinomas when this approach is applied is 96% to 98%. An exfoliative cytologic examination can also be used to confirm the diagnosis of malignancy. This technique has a 90% accuracy rate and a false positive rate of 1% to 2%. The time-honored approach of obtaining serial roentgenograms to document the healing of gastric ulcerating lesions as an indication of benignity is inappropriate because malignant ulcerations also may seem on roentgenograms to heal. Computed tomography may be helpful in selected cases.

Management. Patients with an untreated gastric carcinoma have a 5-year survival rate of about 1% or less. The surgical removal of the entire tumor mass offers the only hope for a cure, but this is possible in only a small number of patients. Any patient in whom a spread of the tumor outside the stomach cannot be shown, however, should undergo surgery. A partial or subtotal gastrectomy is usually performed, except for lesions high in the cardia, in which case a total gastrectomy is almost always performed. Attempts at more extensive resections commonly result in a higher operative mortality. Occasionally palliative surgery alone must be performed for a complication such as an obstruction, hemorrhage, or perforation.

Metastatic disease is managed with a combination of chemotherapy, radiation therapy, and immunotherapy, all of which result in only a small lengthening of the patient's life span.

MALIGNANT LYMPHOMA. Malignant lymphomas account for about 5% of all gastric malignancies in the United States. Lymphomas of all cell types have been reported, and the gastric involvement may be the primary tumor or a manifestation of more diffuse disease, as is seen in 40% of patients with a disseminated lymphoma. A gastric lymphoma may occur in patients at a younger age than does gastric carcinoma, but the clinical manifestations are otherwise very similar. Most patients have abdominal pain, and many have weight loss, nausea, vomiting, and constitutional symptoms. When the lymphoma is confined to the stomach, the physical examination is usually unremarkable. In cases of disseminated disease hepatosplenomegaly and peripheral adenopathy may occur. Occasionally signs of iron deficiency anemia are found. A gastric analysis usually shows an acid-secreting capability.

The roentgenographic findings in patients with gastric lymphoma commonly mimic the appearance of other benign and malignant gastric lesions. A marked enlargement of the rugal folds may be more indicative of a lymphoma. It is also impossible to differentiate a lymphoma from a carcinoma endoscopically by its gross appearance. An endoscopic biopsy and brush cytologic examination may be of some value in making the diagnosis. An exfoliative cytologic examination is consid-

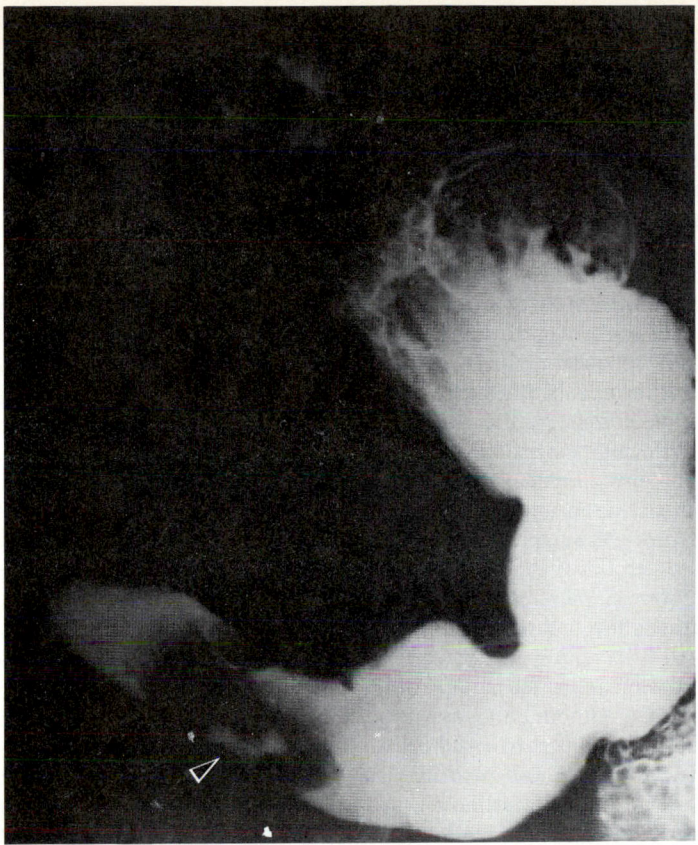

Fig. 180-1   Ulcerating mass *(arrow)* in antrum of this barium-filled stomach is adenocarcinoma. Patient also has hiatus hernia. (Courtesy of Georgy Popky, MD.)

ered by some to be the best way to establish the diagnosis preoperatively.

The treatment of a localized gastric lymphoma consists of the surgical excision of the tumor followed by postoperative radiation therapy. With this regimen the 5-year survival rate is more than 50%. Chemotherapy is indicated for patients with a disseminated lymphoma or diffuse intraabdominal disease.

LEIOMYOSARCOMA. Leiomyosarcomas comprise 1% of all gastric cancers. They tend to occur in patients at a younger age than carcinomas but result in the same kinds of symptoms. Ulceration and gross hemorrhage are more common than with other gastric malignancies. Of these patients, 75% have a palpable epigastric mass that may be tender. Roentgenograms show a round, intramural mass that may have a central ulceration. The endoscopic findings are similar, but with these studies it is usually not possible to differentiate a leiomyosarcoma from a benign leiomyoma, although the larger it is, the more likely it is that the tumor is a sarcoma. Exfoliative cytology has reportedly been helpful in making a preoperative diagnosis. The only treatment is surgical resection, which is curative in more than 50% of these cases.

SMALL BOWEL NEOPLASMS
Benign tumors

Small bowel tumors account for fewer than 5% of all gastrointestinal neoplasms; about 40% of small bowel tumors are malignant. Of the benign tumors, the most commonly occurring type is the adenoma, which may consist of ectopic islet cell tissue or Brunner's gland hyperplasia or may be a true neoplasm similar to adenomatous polyps that occur elsewhere in the gastrointestinal tract. Juvenile polyps also occur but usually are part of an inherited polyposis syndrome. Leiomyomas occur less commonly than adenomas but are more likely to cause symptoms. Lipomas are still less common and occur most often in the distal ileum and ileocecal valve area. Hemangiomas are very rare but are important in that 70% of these patients have gross hemorrhage from the lesion.

Most patients with benign small bowel tumors are over 50 years of age, and the symptoms are usually related to obstructive phenomena, intussusception, or gross or occult bleeding. The physical examination rarely reveals a palpable mass. The diagnosis generally must be made with roentgenographic studies such as small bowel barium contrast roentgenography, arteriography, or computed tomography. Fiberoptic enteroscopy may be available in some medical centers. The treatment of symptomatic benign small bowel tumors is surgical removal.

Malignant tumors

In order of decreasing incidence, adenocarcinomas, lymphomas, and leiomyosarcomas are the most common small bowel malignancies. Adenocarcinomas occur in the older age-groups and are almost always found within 20 cm on either side of the ligament of Treitz, usually in the duodenum. Several disease states have been associated with an increased incidence of enteric carcinoma: celiac sprue, dermatitis herpetiformis, chronic regional enteritis, and the Peutz-Jeghers syndrome. Abdominal pain, bleeding, constitutional symptoms, and occasionally acute small bowel obstructions are the usual presenting symptoms. An ulcerating lesion may sometimes be confused on roentgenograms with atypical peptic ulcer disease. The therapeutic approach is surgical.

A lymphoma of the small bowel may be a primary lesion or secondary to disseminated disease. The involvement of the bowel may also be localized or diffuse. Patients with a lymphoma are generally younger than those with other gastrointestinal malignancies. Abdominal pain and bleeding are common symptoms, and when the involvement is focal, a tender abdominal mass commonly can be palpated. Hepatosplenomegaly and peripheral adenopathy occur in disseminated disease. In some cases of diffuse primary intestinal lymphomas, malabsorption is significant and the disease may closely resemble celiac sprue. The disease can be suspected on the basis of small bowel roentgenograms and confirmed by the examination of tissue obtained by biopsy or surgery. Focal lesions are treated with surgery and radiation and/or chemotherapy. Surgery is of no value if the involvement is diffuse except to treat complications such as an obstruction, perforation, or hemorrhage.

Leiomyosarcomas are usually large tumors and tend to occur in the jejunum and ileum. Pain and bleeding are common symptoms, and perforation may occur but is not as common as with lymphosarcomatous lesions. A palpable abdominal mass is common. Surgical removal is the only effective therapy.

Carcinoid tumors are lesions arising from the enterochromaffin cells of the gastrointestinal tract. Although these tumors may occur anywhere, they are usually found between the duodenum and the transverse colon, and the highest incidence is in the appendix. Metastases may occur, but the tumor is considered a very low-grade malignancy. Most lesions are asymptomatic except when hepatic metastases have occurred, in which case the carcinoid syndrome results. This complex of symptoms includes abdominal cramps and diarrhea, cutaneous flushing, cyanosis, bronchospasm, telangiectasia, pellagra-like skin lesions, and valvular lesions of the heart. These manifestations result from the secretion by the tumor tissue of a number of biogenic amines and other substances, the most characteristic of which is serotonin. When a carcinoid tumor is suspected on clinical grounds, the diagnosis may be established by the finding of elevated levels of 5-hydroxyindoleacetic acid (5-HIAA) in the urine. Barium contrast studies of the gastrointestinal tract may show filling defects, and arteriography also has been used to determine the diagnosis. Radionuclide scanning, ultrasonography, and computed tomography may document hepatic lesions that are accessible for a needle biopsy. Symptomatic and incidentally discovered lesions may be removed surgically if the patient does not have the carcinoid syndrome. If the disease is metastatic, the therapy is symptomatic and includes the special use of serotonin antagonists. Chemotherapy has also been successful in alleviating symptoms, but survival data are inconclusive because few patients actually die as a direct consequence of their disease.

COLONIC AND RECTAL NEOPLASMS
Benign tumors

EPITHELIAL POLYPS. Benign polyps of the large bowel are a common medical problem occurring in up to 8% of the population. Their clinical significance lies not only in the symptoms they may produce but also in their relationship to colorectal cancer. This association of epithelial polyps with malignancy has been reported in terms of several descriptive categories, including size, location, number, presence or absence of a stalk, and histologic characteristics. The histologic classification seems the most important. Four major types have been described: (1) hyperplastic polyps, which are simply overgrowths of normal colonic cellular elements, account for 25%

of all polyps but constitute the majority of smaller polyps, especially those under 5 mm in size; they are not associated with malignancy; (2) adenomatous polyps, which are neoplasms that consist of abnormal glandular tissue that may show varying degrees of dysplasia from a mild atypia to a carcinoma in situ; they may undergo malignant degeneration or may be found concurrently with or in proximity to a frank carcinoma (sentinel polyp); (3) villous adenomas, characterized by multiple frondlike projections, which arise from cells at the base of the crypts of Lieberkühn; 25% to 50% of these lesions undergo malignant change; and (4) mixed villoglandular polyps, also described as adenovillous or tubulovillous polyps, which contain components that are both adenomatous and villous and therefore are considered likely to be premalignant lesions.

A polypoid lesion has an increased probability of containing carcinoma if it is large, especially over 2 cm in size, if it is present in a greater number, if it lacks a pedicle, and perhaps if it is located in the left side of the colon, because most polyps and most carcinomas occur there. These relationships do not preclude the likelihood that a carcinoma may develop de novo without going through an adenomatous stage.

Clinical manifestations. Most polyps occur in middle-aged and older patients, and most are asymptomatic. The most common symptom is gross or occult bleeding. A change in bowel habits or pain may also occasionally be reported, the pain usually resulting form intussusception or an obstruction caused by a large lesion. Villous adenomas have been associated with the passage of large amounts of protein-rich mucus, which rarely may lead to hypoproteinemia and hypokalemia.

Diagnosis and management. A diagnosis of polyps in most patients being evaluated either because they have symptoms or for screening purposes can be made with routine sigmoidoscopy and/or a barium enema. Flexible fiberoptic sigmoidoscopy and an air-contrast barium enema can detect more and smaller lesions, however. Fiberoptic colonoscopy has also come to play an important role in the diagnosis and management of polypoid colonic lesions. A colonoscopic examination of the whole colon commonly detects lesions not detectable with other techniques. In addition, most polyps can be removed endoscopically by means of snare cautery, even if they are large or sessile. Laparotomy is indicated for only those lesions that cannot be removed endoscopically or, in the case of malignant polyps, if the possibility of residual cancer exists. As a rule, most colonic polyps should be removed, regardless of their size and even if they are asymptomatic, because of their association with cancer. Lesions less than 1 cm, however, have an incidence of malignancy of only about 1%.

After polypectomy, periodic follow-up examinations are mandatory. The stool guaiac test, flexible sigmoidoscopy, an air-contrast barium enema, and colonoscopy should all be part of the program. Though there is no generally accepted protocol for these studies, stool guaiac tests and sigmoidoscopy should probably be performed yearly, whereas the air-contrast barium enema and colonoscopy can be alternated every 2 to 3 years. Patients who have had several polyps or polyps with foci of carcinoma and who otherwise have a high risk of carcinoma should have full evaluations annually.

OTHER BENIGN TUMORS. Benign lesions of the colon other than epithelial polyps are rare. Juvenile polyps are large, pedunculated hamartomas that usually occur in childhood, most commonly in the rectum. They may bleed, may cause a rectal prolapse or intussusception, and commonly autoamputate. They also occur as a part of several inherited multiple polyposis syndromes. Pseudopolyps consist of inflammatory and normal elements and usually occur in conjunction with ulcerative colitis, but they may occur in any inflammatory disease of the colon. Lipomas are sometimes found in the cecum near the ileocecal valve. Leiomyomas rarely occur in the colon but when present may ulcerate and cause hemorrhage much as they do in the stomach and small bowel.

Malignant tumors

ADENOCARCINOMA. Colorectal cancer is one of the most common causes of death resulting from a malignancy; it constitutes almost half of the gastrointestinal cancers in the United States. Adenocarcinomas account for over 95% of all colorectal malignancies. As is the case with many other tumors, the incidence of colon cancer varies greatly among different populations around the world. As a rule, the more industrialized nations have a significantly higher incidence than less industrialized societies. Many explanations have been proposed to account for this difference. In industrialized societies the relatively high-fat, low-residue diet, food additives, ingested carcinogens, and less frequent bowel movements have all been postulated as possible causative factors. A high-fiber diet, frequent stools, and lack of exposure to industrial carcinogens and additives are thought by some to explain the lower incidence in less industrialized cultures. Because none of these relationships has been proved, they remain interesting but speculative factors.

A number of medical conditions, however, have a definite association with the development of colon cancer, including the presence of adenomatous, villous, or mixed polyps, familial multiple polyposis and Gardner's syndrome, Peutz-Jeghers syndrome, Turcot's syndrome, and chronic ulcerative colitis, especially universal colitis beginning before adulthood or of more than 10 years' duration. Long-standing Crohn's colitis also has been shown to be associated with a higher incidence of colon carcinoma. Genetic factors are probably associated in many cases as well, as is apparent both in cases of multiple polyposis, in which the development of carcinoma is virtually certain, and in data showing that the chances of having colon cancer are increased for family members of patients with the disease. In addition there is evidence that a "cancer family" syndrome exists in which many members are affected.

Adenocarcinomas may occur anywhere in the colon, but approximately 75% occur in the sigmoid colon or rectum. Fewer than 15% occur proximal to the hepatic flexure, and the rest are in the transverse or descending colon. Four types of growth patterns have been described: ulcerating, polypoid, colloid, and scirrhous. Except for possible differences in the presenting symptoms, there is no practical importance in this classification.

Clinical manifestations. The symptoms of adenocarcinomas vary depending on their gross morphologic form and location in the colon. Abdominal pain is a common complaint in most patients with lesions proximal to the peritoneal reflection but occurs in only about 25% of those with rectal tumors. Most colon cancers bleed, but gross blood in the stool is more common with left-sided lesions. Iron deficiency anemia, sometimes profound, is more common in cecal and ascending colon tumors. Changes in bowel habits commonly occur, especially with left-sided lesions. Patients may complain of recent constipation, diarrhea, or a change in the timing, frequency, consistency, or caliber of the stools. Weight loss occurs in 25% to 50% of patients. Other nonspecific symptoms such as anorexia or malaise also may occur. Colloid tumors commonly cause large amounts of mucus to appear in the stool. The more common ulcerating and scirrhous types occasionally may appear more catastrophically, causing an intestinal obstruction or confined or free perforation, particularly with left-sided tumors.

The physical examination may reveal signs of anemia, evidence of recent weight loss, an enlarged and nodular liver or jaundice if there are hepatic metastases, or, less commonly, ascites if peritoneal seeding has occurred. An abdominal mass can be palpated in many patients, particularly those with right-sided lesions. A mass can be palpated directly or through the bowel wall in the rectal examination of many patients with tumors of the rectum or rectosigmoid. A Blumer's or rectal shelf resulting from a pelvic spread also may be detected. Fecal masses proximal to partially obstructing lesions sometimes are present, but a more acute obstruction is accompanied by abdominal distention, tympany, abnormal or absent bowel sounds, and other signs. Localized or diffuse peritonitis is found if perforation has occurred.

The laboratory findings in patients with colonic cancer are nonspecific. Most of these patients show evidence of anemia, usually of the iron deficiency type. Many also have positive results on the stool guaiac test, although some lesions may bleed intermittently, occasionally causing negative results. In patients with liver metastases the serum alkaline phosphatase level may rise, but some tumors can themselves produce an alkaline phosphatase isoenzyme. When the hepatic involvement is extensive, the level of serum bilirubin usually is elevated. The peripheral leukocyte count may be elevated in the presence of inflammatory complications such as tumor necrosis and perforation. Carcinoembryonic antigen is present in most patients with a colorectal carcinoma, but the diagnostic value of this determination is unproved, because it is also found in patients with other gastrointestinal malignancies and in some benign disorders of the alimentary tract, liver, and lung. The serum level of carcinoembryonic antigen may be of prognostic value, however, in proven cases of colon and rectal cancer.

Diagnosis. Any patient whose clinical presentation even remotely suggests the possibility of colorectal cancer should be evaluated for this disease. The initial studies should include a stool guaiac test, a digital rectal examination, sigmoidoscopy, and a barium enema. With flexible fiberoptic sigmoidoscopy about 50% to 75% of colon tumors can be seen. With endoscopy the lesions appear as friable, stalked, or sessile polypoid intraluminal masses; as circumferential, constricting lesions that partially or completely occlude the lumen; or as localized areas of inflamed, ulcerated tissue. On roentgenograms colon cancer can appear as an intraluminal, polypoid filling defect; as an abrupt localized stenosis, sometimes with overhanging edges giving it an apple core appearance; or just as an area of focal mucosal irregularity and stiffness. It is very difficult to differentiate benign from malignant polyps on roentgenograms except to ascertain probabilities. In general, almost half of all lesions larger than 2 cm in diameter contain malignancy, about 10% of lesions between 1 and 2 cm in diameter are malignant, and only 1% of polyps less than 1 cm in size contain cancer. As is true with upper gastrointestinal barium contrast studies, an air-contrast barium enema detects more and smaller lesions than the conventional procedure.

Fiberoptic colonoscopy should also be used as a complement to the barium enema in the workup of most patients. Because about 3% of colon cancers occur with a second synchronous malignancy and also because the incidence of other simultaneous benign neoplasms is increased, colonoscopy is appropriate even in cases in which a lesion has already been detected by sigmoidoscopy or a barium enema. It is certainly indicated when there is a strong clinical suspicion and other studies are negative or inconclusive. Colonoscopy is most productively used to determine the nature of roentgenographically or clinically suspected lesions by direct visualization, by snare-cautery removal of polypoid masses when possible, and by biopsy and cytologic studies of nonremovable lesions. Several benign diseases may mimic carcinoma of the colon very closely. The diagnosis must differentiate an adenocarcinoma from other diseases such as a colonic stricture resulting from inflammatory disease such as ulcerative colitis or granulomatous colitis, lymphogranuloma venereum, an ischemic stricture, and diverticulitis. Cecal involvement with an appendiceal abscess, tuberculosis, an amebic granuloma, or actinomycosis may also be difficult to distinguish roentgenographically from carcinoma. Colonic sarcomas, although rare, must also be differentiated.

Management. The only potentially curative therapy for colorectal cancer is surgical extirpation of the tumor. Colonoscopic snare-cautery removal of malignant pedunculated polyps is probably curative if the malignancy does not extend below the muscularis mucosae. In most other circumstances laparotomy is advised. Lesions above the peritoneal reflection usually can be handled by a wide resection and end-to-end anastomosis. Lesions below this level may require an abdominoperineal resection. The patient's level of carcinoembryonic antigen should be obtained before surgery for reference in the follow-up period. A preoperative evaluation to detect local and distant spread may be performed with a computed tomography or radionuclide scan of the liver, perhaps supplemented by a liver needle biopsy if it is indicated. If these studies have positive results, attempts at curative surgery should not be made, but palliative procedures should not be avoided to correct or even prevent complications such as an obstruction, hemorrhage, or perforation. Rectal lesions in patients who are not surgical candidates can be managed with laser or thermal destruction or local excision. Radiation therapy and chemotherapy have been tried in combination with and without surgery, resulting in an increased length of survival.

Prognosis. Although the overall 5-year survival rate for patients with colorectal carcinoma treated with surgery is about 37%, the prognosis in individual cases depends on several factors. In general, the survival rate is negatively correlated with an increasing degree of penetration by the tumor through the bowel wall, increasing numbers of positive regional lymph nodes, and the degree of histologic dedifferentiation. In 3% of these patients a second primary colon cancer develops, and in most the primary tumor recurs within 5 years after surgery. For this reason a program of follow-up care should be instituted that includes periodic physical examination, stool guaiac tests, liver function tests, sigmoidoscopy, and an air-contrast barium enema or colonoscoy. If a higher preoperative level of carcinoembryonic antigen decreases significantly after surgery, periodic determinations of its level have prognostic value because a tumor recurrence may be signaled by a rise toward the preoperative level.

Other malignancies

Lymphomas rarely occur as a primary colorectal lesion. When present, a lymphoma commonly causes abdominal pain and gross bleeding or may result in intussusception. A lymphoma usually appears similar to an adenocarcinoma on roentgenograms but may mimic ulcerative colitis. The treatment is a combination of radiation therapy and surgery. Leiomyosarcomas are also rare but almost always involve the rectum or sigmoid colon, producing pain, bleeding, and constipation. Carcinoid tumors of the colon are most common in the rectum and rarely produce the carcinoid syndrome. Epidermoid car-

cinomas of the anus account for about 2% of large bowel cancers and usually cause local pain and a bleeding mass. The rare mucinous adenocarcinoma of the anal glands may appear as recurrent anorectal fistulas. Malignant melanoma has also been reported to arise in the anal skin.

GASTROINTESTINAL POLYPOSIS SYNDROMES

The gastrointestinal polyposis syndromes are a group of interesting but exceedingly rare disorders that have in common the presence of large numbers of polyps in the alimentary tract and that are with one exception of genetic origin. They are differentiated from one another on the basis of histopathologic findings, the distribution of lesions, patterns of inheritance, and extraintestinal manifestations. At least six different syndromes have been described.

Familial polyposis coli

Familial polyposis coli is the most common of the polyposis syndromes. It is characterized by the appearance in childhood or early adulthood of adenomatous polyps that usually are confined to the colon but have also been reported in several patients in the stomach and small intestine. The lesions may be pedunculated or sessile, and they generally remain small. With time, however, they increase in number until literally hundreds of polyps may be carpeting the colon from the rectum to the cecum. The disease is transmitted as an autosomal dominant trait.

The symptoms, when they occur, consist of abdominal pain, diarrhea with or without blood, and occasionally weight loss. Some patients remain asymptomatic, and their disease is diagnosed only because they are known to be members of an affected kindred. Early diagnosis of this disease is extremely important, because the incidence of adenocarcinoma of the colon approaches 100%, usually developing between the ages of 20 and 40 years.

The diagnosis usually can be made with a barium enema, sigmoidoscopy, or colonoscopy and biopsy. Because of the almost universal tendency of familial polyposis coli to develop into carcinoma, the preferred management is early total proctocolectomy.

Gardner's syndrome

Gardner's syndrome is characterized by multiple polyposis of the colon in association with bony and soft tissue tumors. The colonic lesions are adenomatous polyps similar to those occurring in familial polyposis coli but may not be as numerous. They may also occasionally be found in the small intestine, particularly the ileum and in the stomach. The disease is inherited as an autosomal dominant trait, and the clinical features related to the colon are the same as in familial polyposis coli.

The extraintestinal manifestations of Gardner's syndrome usually precede the appearance of the colonic lesions by many years. The most common bony lesions are osteomas, which have a tendency to affect the mandible and facial bones, leading to a noticeable deformity. There may also be multiple exostoses and a thickening of the cortices of the long bones. The soft tissue lesions affect mostly cutaneous and subcutaneous tissues but may also affect other areas of the body. The most common abnormalities are epidermoid cysts, lipomas, fibromas, and connective tissue tumors. In addition there is a tendency for masses of fibrous tissue hyperplasia to form, leading to keloids in scars, adhesions after surgery in the abdomen, and fibrous tumors of the retroperitoneum and peritoneal space.

The potential of these intestinal lesions to become malignant is the same as in familial polyposis coli. The preferred management is an early total colectomy.

Peutz-Jeghers syndrome

Peutz-Jeghers syndrome is defined by the association of generalized gastrointestinal polyposis with mucocutaneous pigmentation. It is transmitted as a single pleiotropic gene that has a high degree of penetrance. The histologic examination reveals that these polyps are hamartomas or juvenile polyps with a prominent smooth muscle component. They occur most often in the small intestine, particularly in the jejunum and ileum, but may affect the stomach and colon as well. Polyps also have been reported in the respiratory and urinary tracts. The lesions appear in childhood and may produce symptoms related to the polyps such as hemorrhage, intestinal obstruction, intestinal infarction resulting from torsion, or intussusception.

Mucocutaneous pigmentation occurs in Peutz-Jeghers syndrome as hairless melanin spots usually found on the lips, buccal mucosa, face, forearms, hands, soles, digits, and the perianal region. Other associated findings include ovarian cysts and tumors, exostoses, and digital clubbing. Not all features of the syndrome are present in every patient.

The incidence of gastrointestinal carcinomas in this syndrome is about 2% to 3%, an incidence greater than that in the general population. The only treatment for the disorder, however, is aimed at management of the complications; preventive surgery is not indicated.

Turcot's syndrome

Turcot's syndrome is a very rare disorder consisting of the presence of polyposis coli in association with malignant central nervous system tumors. The colonic lesions may be both adenomatous and villous and have a great potential for malignant change. The central nervous system tumors are usually medulloblastomas or glioblastomas of the brain or spinal cord, which lead to death in most patients. The disease is transmitted as an autosomal recessive trait.

Cronkhite-Canada syndrome

Cronkhite-Canada syndrome is rare and is the only polyposis syndrome that does not appear to have a genetic base. It is characterized by generalized gastrointestinal polyposis, alopecia, onychodystrophy, and cutaneous hyperpigmentation. The histologic examination reveals that the gastrointestinal lesions are juvenile polyps, which occur most commonly in the stomach and colon although the small intestine and the esophagus also may be involved. The gastric mucosa usually is markedly hypertrophic and may resemble that occurring in patients with Menetrier's disease. About half of these patients have cutaneous hyperpigmentation, which occurs as brown macules on the face, upper extremities, back, and soles.

The average age of the patient at the onset of symptoms is 60. The usual symptoms are anorexia, weight loss, abdominal pain, diarrhea, anemia, and hypoproteinemia with peripheral edema. Males and females are affected equally. Although remissions occur, about half of these patients undergo a rapid downhill course of the disease and die because of an electrolyte imbalance, hemorrhage, or other complications.

Juvenile polyposis

Two forms of juvenile polyposis, a heritable disorder, have been recognized: juvenile polyposis coli and generalized juvenile polyposis. The histologic examination reveals that the lesions are hamartomas that differ from the Peutz-Jegher polyp in lacking smooth muscle components but that are histologi-

cally the same as those found in the Cronkhite-Canada syndrome. The disease typically develops in childhood, but the polyps may also be found in adults in the same families. It is thought to be transmitted as an autosomal dominant trait.

Regardless of whether the polyps are limited to the colon or are distributed throughout the gastrointestinal tract, the symptoms are usually the result of a complication such as hemorrhage or intussusception. It is not unusual with sigmoidoscopy or colonoscopy to find stalks without tumors as a result of autoamputation. Juvenile polyps are not considered to be premalignant, but various carcinomas have occurred in nonaffected members of some kindreds. Some patients have had congenital anomalies, but the ectodermal abnormalities seen in Cronkhite-Canada syndrome do not occur. There is no treatment except for management of complications.

BIBLIOGRAPHY

Brooks JJ and Enterline HT: Primary gastric lymphomas: a clinicopathologic study of 58 cases with long-term follow-up and literature review, Cancer 51:701, 1983.

Dworkin DM and Winawer SJ: Neoplastic colonic polyps: a review, Curr Concepts Gastroenterol 10:3, 1985.

Eisenberg B and others: Carcinoma of the colon and rectum: the natural history reviewed in 1704 patients, Cancer 49:1131, 1982.

Gastrointestinal and hepatobiliary malignancies, Surg Clin North Am 66:673, 1986.

Lawrence W JR: Gastric carcinoma, CA 36:216, 1986.

Parker EF and others: Carcinoma of the esophagus, Ann Surg 6:195, 1982.

Sherlock P: *Epidemiology and pathogenesis of colorectal cancer*. In Stearns WW Jr, editor: Neoplasms of the colon, rectum and anus, New York, 1980, John Wiley & Sons, Inc.

Skudder PA Jr and Schwartz SI: Primary lymphoma of the gastrointestinal tract, Surg Gynecol Obstet 160:5, 1985.

Thorson AG and others: The role of colonoscopy in the assessment of patients with colorectal cancer, Dis Colon Rectum 29:306, 1986.

Winawer SJ: Detection and diagnosis of colorectal cancer, Cancer 51:2519, 1983.

181 · DISEASES OF THE PERITONEUM AND MESENTERY

William O. Frank

ANATOMY AND PHYSIOLOGY

ANATOMY. The peritoneal cavity and the organs it contains are lined by a serous membrane, the peritoneum. The visceral peritoneum encases the abdominal organs and forms the mesenteries from which they are suspended. The parietal peritoneum lines the anterior, lateral, and posterior walls of the abdominal cavity. Retroperitoneal organs such as the duodenum, ascending and descending colon, and portions of the pancreas, kidneys, and adrenal glands are lined anteriorly by the parietal peritoneum.

BLOOD SUPPLY. The majority of the peritoneal surface and mesentery is supplied by the splanchnic arteries and drained by the splanchnic and portal venous system. A much smaller portion of the peritoneal surface is supplied by the intercostal, subcostal, lumbar, and iliac arteries and drained by the lumbar and iliac veins that enter the inferior vena cava.

INNERVATION. The innervation of the parietal peritoneum differs from that of the visceral peritoneum. Twigs from the spinal nerves that supply the abdominal wall innervate the respective areas of the parietal peritoneum. An irritation of the parietal peritoneum thus gives rise to afferent stimuli transmitted via the intercostal nerves and is perceived as *somatic pain*. In contrast, an irritation of the visceral peritoneum gives rise to afferent stimuli transmitted via the distribution of the respective visceral sympathetic nervous system. The diaphragmatic peritoneum has a double innervation: the phrenic nerves innervate its central portion and the intercostal nerves its peripheral portion. A pathologic condition involving the visceral peritoneum has a more precise pain localization and more definite physical signs than a pathologic condition involving the visceral peritoneum because the parietal peritoneum is innervated by somatic afferent nerves. An irritation of the diagphragmatic peritoneum may refer pain to the shoulder (phrenic innervation) or to the thoracic and abdominal wall (intercostal innervation).

PHYSIOLOGY. The movement of fluid and both high– and low–molecular weight solutes across the peritoneal membrane occurs by means of simple passive diffusion. Peritoneal lymphatics remove the solid and liquid material from the peritoneal cavity. The intercellular gaps between the mesothelial cells that line the peritoneal cavity and the endothelial cells of the terminal lymphatics permit this passive passage of fluid and solutes.

The clearance of peritoneal fluid from the abdominal cavity is biphasic; a rapid initial clearance is followed by a slower constant clearance phase. Studies in humans using intraperitoneal saline and radioactive-labeled albumin indicate that an equilibration of saline between the serum and peritoneal fluid occurs within 2 hours, after which fluid is absorbed at a relatively constant rate of 33 ml an hour. In the initial 2 hours the rate of absorption varies with the osmolar gradient and becomes consant after equilibration.

DIAGNOSIS OF PERITONEAL DISEASE

HISTORY AND PHYSICAL EXAMINATION. The cardinal manifestations of peritoneal disease are abdominal pain and ascites. Direct tenderness, rebound tenderness, and involuntary spasm of the anterior abdominal musculature are the major signs of peritoneal irritation.

ROENTGENOGRAPHY. Ascites may reflect the presence of peritoneal disease. Large amounts of fluid are detected on plain abdominal roentgenograms as abdominal haziness, an increased density shifting to the pelvis on upright films, a separation of bowel loops, and the obliteration of the psoas muscle shadows. Smaller amounts of fluid (800 to 1000 ml) are detected by an obliteration of the hepatic angle, an increased thickness between the air-filled bowel lumen and extraperitoneal fat layer, and a widening of the flank strip (the line formed by the lateral colonic wall and peritoneum). A sonographic examination and CT scan of the abdominal cavity can also detect ascites.

Other specialized roentgenographic techniques are available for detecting peritoneal disease, such as the introduction of pneumoperitoneum for demonstrating nodules on the parietal peritoneum. Barium contrast studies of the gastrointestinal tract may demonstrate bizarre angular patterns of the intestinal loops, rigidity of the bowel along with diminished peristalsis, or altered mucosal patterns along with filling defects or flattened folds that indirectly reflect the visceral peritoneal involvement of the small bowel.

ABDOMINAL PARACENTESIS. Diagnostic paracentesis for the detection of obvious or suspected ascites can be easily performed at the bedside with the patient sitting or supine after having emptied the bladder. The midline area located midway between the umbilicus and pubis is anesthetized, and a needle or catheter is inserted using a sterile technique. The aspirated fluid is evaluated by gross inspection and the following examinations: the determination of specific gravity, a cell count and differential cell count, a Gram stain, a bacterial culture and cultures for tuberculosis and fungi, a cytologic examination, a Suda stain evaluation, and determinations of protein, glucose, amylase, lactic dehydrogenase, and lipid concentrations.

PERITONEAL BIOPSY. Cope's needle or the Vim-Silverman needle can be used to perform a biopsy of the peritoneum. With this technique hemorrhage is the major complication, usually from enlarged intra-abdominal veins, but a perforation or infection may also occur. Adequate tissue for histologic study can usually be obtained with either needle, but the diagnostic yield with the blunt-ended Cope's needle is probably higher.

PERITONEOSCOPY. With peritoneoscopy the clinician can directly inspect the peritoneum or abdominal organs and perform a biopsy of a suspected pathologic lesion under direct vision. The technique is described more fully in Chapter 171.

ASCITES

PATHOPHYSIOLOGY. Ascites is the accumulation of fluid within the peritoneal cavity. The mechanisms of this accumulation have not been exactly defined, but the development of ascites is associated with several abnormal physiologic factors. Alterations in the portal venous pressure, colloidal osmotic pressure, hepatic lymph formation, splanchnic lymphatic drainage, sodium metabolism, and subperitoneal capillary permeability have been thought to contribute to ascitic fluid accumulation.

An elevated portal venous pressure increases the hydrostatic pressure in the splanchnic capillary bed and increases the filtration pressure. The elevated filtration pressure is balanced by the plasma colloidal osmotic pressure, which primarily reflects the albumin concentration. According to the Frank-Starling law, a rise in the portal venous pressure or a fall in the plasma albumin concentration leads to ascites formation. In addition, an increased hepatic lymph formation and decreased splanchnic lymphatic reabsorption may cause an ascitic fluid accumulation, especially in patients with cirrhosis. Renal sodium retention leads to an expansion of plasma volume and secondarily to ascites because of an overflow phenomenon. Renal sodium retention may occur in patients with cirrhosis for a number of reasons, including an impaired hepatic inactivation of aldosterone or renin, a hepatic production of the humoral stimulator of aldosterone secretion, or a deficiency of an unknown natriuretic hormone. Alterations in renal hemodynamics in cases of cirrhosis, particularly an intrarenal vasoconstriction that reduces cortical perfusion, may also cause renal sodium retention. Excessive sodium reabsorption and impaired water diuresis at the proximal or distal tubules may possibly also account for the increased sodium retention in cases of cirrhosis. Finally, an increased permeability of the subperitoneal capillaries in patients with inflammatory and neoplastic diseases of the peritoneum may cause ascites formation. The relative importance of these possible mechanisms, however, undoubtedly varies according to the underlying disorder and the individual patient, and the mechanism remains uncertain in most cases.

CLINICAL AND LABORATORY FINDINGS. Abdominal distention is the major symptom of ascites, and when a large amount of fluid is present, the patient may also complain of dyspnea and abdominal discomfort. In the physical examination the flanks can be seen to bulge, and a fluid wave may be elicited. If 1.5 to 2 L of fluid is present, a shifting dullness can usually be detected. Placing the patient on the hands and knees and percussing the flatness over the dependent abdomen (puddle sign) may detect as little as 300 to 400 ml of fluid.

A laboratory evaluation of the peritoneal fluid is essential. Exudative and transudative ascitic fluid are differentiated by their protein concentrations and specific gravity. Peritoneal fluid with protein concentrations greater than 3 g/100 ml or a specific gravity greater than 1.016 is classified as an exudate; peritoneal fluid with values below these is designated as a transudate. *Transudative ascites* is usually associated with congestive heart failure, an inferior vena cava obstruction, the Budd-Chiari syndrome, hypoalbuminemia, cirrhosis, Meigs' syndrome, and vasculitis. *Exudative ascites* is usually found in cases of a peritoneal malignancy, tuberculosis peritonitis, myxedema, pancreatic ascites and bacterial peritonitis, although exudative ascites may also occur in cases of uncomplicated congestive heart failure or cirrhosis. Glucose concentrations less than 60 mg/dl suggest a neoplastic effusion. Amylase or lipase levels are increased in patients with pancreatic ascites. Triglyceride levels are higher in the peritoneal fluid than in the plasma in patients with chylous ascites. Bloody ascites usually indicates a neoplasm, particularly a hepatoma or ovarian carcinoma. A leukocyte count of 250 cells/mm^3 or more in the ascitic fluid is an indication of a peritoneal irritation caused by an infection, inflammation, or tumor infiltration. The white blood cell differential count is important. Polymorphonuclear leukocytes reflect an acute bacterial infection, whereas mononuclear cells characterize a chronic inflammatory disease. A cytologic examination to detect a malignancy is valuable; it has positive results in 60% to 90% of these cases.

DIFFERENTIAL DIAGNOSIS. Ascites may be found in patients with or without direct involvement of the peritoneum. Portal hypertension and hypoalbuminemia are common causes of ascites in patients without direct involvement.

PORTAL HYPERTENSION

Cirrhosis. Cirrhosis is the most common cause of ascites in North America. The causes of cirrhotic ascites involve many factors including portal hypertension, hypoalbuminemia, alterations in lymph flow, and the renal retention of sodium and water. Ascites in patients with cirrhosis is discussed in Chapter 183.

Cardiac causes of portal hypertension. A mechanical or functional impedance to hepatic venous flow is often associated with ascites. Cases of congestive heart failure, particularly right-sided and constrictive pericarditis, are included in this category. Constrictive pericarditis should be considered in cases of ascites of obscure origin, and appropriate diagnostic tests should be performed, including cardiac catheterization if necessary.

Inferior vena cava and hepatic vein obstruction. Inferior vena cava and hepatic vein obstructions characteristically cause ascites and hepatomegaly (the Budd-Chiari syndrome). This syndrome occurs when thrombi, venous fibrosis, anomalous venous valves, or a tumor occludes the hepatic venous outflow. Thrombosis may result from polycythemia vera (and other causes of hyperviscosity or thrombocytosis) or from hemoglobinopathies such as sickle cell disease or may be associated with the use of oral contraceptives. An idiopathic membranous obstruction of the inferior vena cava, a surgically correctable condition, has been reported in Japan.

The clinical presentation and course of this disorder may be acute, subacute, or chronic. The signs and symptoms include abdominal pain with ascites and tender hepatomegaly. Splenomegaly and jaundice are much less common, and the results of liver function tests are often not dramatically abnormal. The diagnostic workup commonly shows an elevated femoral venous pressure along with normal pressures in the superior vena cava, and a liver biopsy reveals centrilobular necrosis and congestion and/or centrilobular fibrosis and occasionally cirrhosis. Hepatic venography may show a vena cava obstruction or a narrow, occluded main hepatic vein with a network pattern of neighboring veins.

HYPOALBUMINEMIA. Approximately 12% of patients with the nephrotic syndrome have ascites. These patients almost invariably have a level of serum albumin lower than 2.5 g/dl and usually lower than 1.5 g/dl. Protein-losing enteropathy and malnutrition are rare causes of hypoalbuminemic ascites in North America.

OTHER ASCITES. Ascites may occur in patients with myxedema or ovarian disease or in the form of pancreatic ascites, bile ascites, or chylous ascites.

Myxedema. Patients with myxedema often have significant exudative ascites that responds poorly to diuretics. The peritoneal fluid is yellow and gelatinous and has a protein concentration greater than 4 g/dl; the protein electrophoresis of ascitic fluid is similar to that of the serum. This ascites is thought to result from an increased capillary permeability and an escape of protein-rich fluid. The ascites is rapidly cleared after the start of thyroid therapy.

Ovarian disease. Ovarian carcinoma, Meigs' syndrome, and the ovarian overstimulation syndrome are causes of ascites in female patients. Meigs' syndrome consists of ascites and hydrothorax associated with ovarian fibromas or cystadenomas. *Strauma ovarii* is a rare, unilateral ovarian teratoma that contains thyroid tissue. Patients may have the symptoms of hyperthyroidism, ascites, or an ovarian mass. The diagnosis should be suspected if abdominal roentgenograms demonstrate ovarian calcification and if iodine 131 uptake is localized in the abdomen. After treatment with clomiphene citrate and human menopausal gonadotropin, the ovarian overstimulation syndrome may occur, leading to massive ascites, pleural effusions, and hypovolemia with enlarged ovaries.

Pancreatic ascites. Ascites may develop in patients with acute pancreatitis, chronic pancreatitis, or a pancreatic carcinoma. Occasionally a massive, intractable, exudative ascites develops in patients with chronic pancreatitis. This pancreatic ascites usually results from a leaking pseudocyst or a break in the pancreatic duct. The leaking pancreatic juice in either case causes a chemical peritonitis with elevated levels of protein, amylase, and lipase in the ascitic fluid. These patients rarely respond to conventional medical management and often require surgical intervention to correct the pancreatic pathologic condition before the ascites resolves.

Bile ascites. Bile ascites, which results from the leakage of bile from the hepatobiliary tree, usually occurs in patients who have had bile duct surgery. Its onset may be delayed until 2 months after the surgery. The magnitude and severity of the ascites usually reflect the magnitude of the leakage. A peritoneal tap reveals bile in the fluid, and the diagnosis can virtually be made on this basis. Occasionally the bile ascites resolves after the paracentesis, but the majority of patients require surgical correction of the leaking biliary tree.

The acute leakage of bile into the peritoneal cavity, as is sometimes observed after a percutaneous liver biopsy, may result in acute severe peritonitis (bile peritonitis) and the rapid progression of the patient into shock; such cases may require immediate surgical intervention to drain the peritoneal cavity and repair the hepatic or biliary tear.

Chylous ascites. Acute or chronic chylous ascites occurs when there is accumulation of lipid-rich lymph in the peritoneal cavity. Malignant or benign neoplasms are the cause in 80% of the chronic cases. These patients usually have weight loss, hypoproteinemia, and inanition but not abdominal pain. The cause of acute chylous ascites may be an obstruction, trauma, or rupture of chyle-containing cysts, but in the majority of patients no cause is found. These patients have an abrupt onset of crampy abdominal pain, usually after a heavy meal and usually localized in the right lower quadrant.

The peritoneal fluid in patients with chylous ascites is turbid, separates into lipid and aqueous layers on standing, and stains positively for fat. The fluid is sterile and has an elevated lymphocyte count and a high lipid content (the triglyceride levels exceed those of plasma). *Pseudochylous ascites* is also opalescent but contains phospholipid-protein material from degnerating cells rather than large amount of triglycerides.

The cause of chylous ascites is often discovered only with laparotomy. Intravenous hyperalimentation or the administration of medium-chain triglycerides may be helpful. Acute or idiopathic cases usually clear spontaneously, but chronic cases usually lead to progressive debilitation and death, depending on the underlying neoplasm.

TREATMENT OF ASCITES. The successful treatment of ascites often depends on the treatment of the underlying disease. In patients with cirrhotic ascites the mainstays of medical therapy are sodium restriction (250 to 500 mg/day) and diuretics. Judicious use of this medical regimen should not cause complications. Some patients with a refractory ascites that does not respond to conventional medical therapy may be candidates for peritoneovenous (LeVeen) shunt which continuously infuses the ascitic fluid into the patient's systemic venous circulation (see Chapter 183).

INFECTIONS OF THE PERITONEUM
Tuberculous peritonitis

Tuberculous peritonitis, one of the most important diseases involving the peritoneum, is an unusual form of tuberculosis. The incidence is approximately 0.5%. Tuberculous peritonitis may commonly be mistaken for a neoplastic disease or for ascites caused by cirrhosis. Cirrhosis in fact predisposes the patient to tuberculous peritonitis.

PATHOGENESIS. A tubercle bacillus infection of the peritoneum may occur as the result of (1) an activation of a long-latent tuberculous focus in the peritoneum, (2) a primary focus in the lung or elsewhere, (3) infected mesenteric lymph nodes, (4) a contamination from tuberculous enteritis, and (5) tuberculous salpingitis. Although an extraperitoneal site of infection is present in the majority of patients, it is often not clinically apparent. The extraperitoneal site of infection may be active or inactive. In fact, many patients with tuberculous peritonitis appear to have a reactivation of a latent peritoneal focus established at the time of earlier hematogenous spread from a primary focus, usually in the lung. A hematogenous spread from active pulmonary tuberculosis or diffuse miliary tuberculosis can, however, also cause active tuberculous peritonitis.

EPIDEMIOLOGY. Tuberculous peritonitis is most commonly found in an inner-city population in which cirrhosis is common and many patients are poorly nourished and debilitated. There is no sex or age predilection, but 80% to 90% of the patients in previously reported clinical series were black.

CLINICAL MANIFESTATIONS. Tuberculous peritonitis should be suspected in patients with ascites, fever, and unexplained constitutional symptoms with or without diffuse abdominal pain or tenderness. Symptoms are usually constitutional and nonspecific. The majority of patients have an insidious onset and have constitutional symptoms for several months before the diagnosis: fever, anorexia, weakness, malaise, and weight loss are present in 80% of these patients. Abdominal pain is usually described as being vague, dull, and diffuse but

is present in only one half of the patients. Rarely, tuberculous peritonitis may appear as an acute condition of the abdomen. Vomiting, diarrhea, and constipation are variable symptoms. The physical examination reveals the presence of ascites along with diffuse abdominal tenderness in approximately 70% of these patients. Hepatomegaly or a palpable mass caused by loculated fluid or inflamed mesentery is present in one fourth of these patients. A lymphadenopathy may be present, but the classic doughy abdomen is rare. The "dry" form of tuberculous peritonitis involves little or no ascites, but extensive peritoneal adhesions are present.

LABORATORY FINDINGS. Routine blood studies are usually normal, including the white blood cell and differential cell counts and hemoglobin and hematocrit values. The tuberculin skin test is positive in most patients. If the disease is generalized, other studies may prove useful. A chest roentgenogram shows pulmonary infiltrates in about 15% of patient with tuberculous peritonitis and pleural effusions in 40%. Contrast studies of the gastrointestinal tract, pyelograms, and salpingograms are rarely useful. A transthoracic liver biopsy or lymph node biopsy may show caseating granulomata but does not prove that there is also peritoneal involvement. Less than one half of these patients have evidence of disease outside the peritoneum.

The most important initial diagnostic test is an examination of the peritoneal fluid. In patients with tuberculous peritonitis the protein concentration is greater than 2.5 g/dl and the count of leukocytes, predominantly mononuclear, is greater than 250 cells/mm^3. Acid-fast stains of the peritoneal fluid have positive results in less than 5% of patients and cultures in only 40%; however, if 1 L of ascitic fluid is removed and centrifugally concentrated before being cultured, the yield is increased to 80%. A peritoneal biopsy shows granulomata in 70% of these patients, but the culture yield from peritoneal biopsies is not well known. Peritoneoscopy or laparotomy is probably the best method for diagnosing tuberculous peritonitis. Peritoneoscopy should be performed first, however, and laparotomy then only if the results of peritoneoscopy are inconclusive and the diagnosis is still suspected.

PROGNOSIS AND MANAGEMENT. Before appropriate chemotherapy was available, the mortality of tuberculous peritonitis was approximately 60%. With the introduction of antituberculous chemotherapy, the disease is now curable. After chemotherapy begins, the constitutional symptoms should resolve within 1 to 2 weeks, and fever should disappear by the fourth week. The role of steroids in the treatment of tuberculous peritonitis to reduce the incidence of late fibrotic complications is unclear.

Spontaneous bacterial peritonitis

Spontaneous or "primary" peritonitis is an acute or subacute bacterial infection of the peritoneum not associated with any of the usual causative factors such as a bowel perforation. Laparotomy must usually be performed because this condition often cannot be differentiated from an acute peritonitis that is a surgical emergency. This diagnostic possibility should be considered preoperatively in (1) patients with previous ascites, such as nephrosis, who have fever or changing abdominal signs and symptoms; (2) patients with a focus for bacteremia such as an indwelling catheter, cellulitis, or a urinary, biliary, or pulmonary infection; and (3) patients with a decreased immunologic competence.

SPONTANEOUS BACTERIAL PERITONITIS IN CIRRHOTIC PATIENTS. Spontaneous bacterial peritonitis occurs in almost 10% of cirrhotic patients with portal hypertension and overt ascites. The offending organisms in these patients are predominantly of enteric origin, usually *Escherichia coli*. Pneumococci and streptococci are also common organisms in this infection. Anaerobic organisms are rarely found. The pathogenesis of spontaneous bacterial peritonitis in these patients is unknown.

Clinical manifestations and laboratory findings. For practical reasons, any deterioration in a chirrhotic patient with ascites should alert the clinician to the possibility of bacterial peritonitis. Fever is usually present but may be absent. Patients with decompensated alcoholic liver disease and bacterial peritonitis often cannot be distinguished from cirrhotic patients without bacterial peritonitis. Paracentesis is the diagnostic procedure with which to differentiate between these two diseases. Bacterial peritonitis can be excluded fom the diagnostic possibilities only with sterile cultures of the ascitic fluid. A leukocyte count of 300 cells/mm³ or greater in the ascitic fluid and a 25% or higher proportion of polymorphonuclear cells suggests but does not determine a diagnosis of bacterial peritonitis, since similar values may be found in patients with sterile ascites. A Gram stain of the ascitic fluid has a positive result in only half of these patients.

Prognosis and management. Once the diagnosis has been established, an appropriate antibiotic therapy is initiated and continued for 10 to 14 days. A cephalosporin is commonly used in combination with an aminoglycoside. Antibiotic concentrations in the ascitic fluid in patients with peritonitis rapidly achieve bactericidal levels, and therefore the intraperitoneal injection of antibiotics or the drainage of peritoneal fluid is unnecessary. Delayed recognition and treatment, however, adversely affect the outcome.

Intraabdominal abscess

Abscesses in the abdomen are usually caused by anaerobic bacteria (particularly *Bacteroides fragilis* and gram-positive cocci) mixed with enteric gram-negative bacilli. The most common locations are in and around the liver, around the appendix, and in the area of the distal colon. Abscesses usually follow a spontaneous perforation of the bowel (such as from a diverticulum or the appendix), surgery on the large bowel, or infection in the biliary tract. From an abscess in the abdomen the infection may spead to the liver via the lymphatics, the venous channels, or the arterial system or by direct extension. Certain anaerobic bacteria are likely to cause septic phlebitis along with resultant septic emboli carried to the liver through the portal system or to the lungs through veins draining the lower rectum or pelvis. (See discussion of "Infections caused by nonsporeforming anaerobes" in Chapter 49.)

Patients with intra-abdominal abscesses have fever with or without symptoms or signs related to the abdomen. Although a patient may have pain, tenderness, or a mass, there may be no physical findings or complaints referable to the abdomen. Leukocytosis is usually present along with a shift to the left in the white cell series. Blood cultures may have a positive result. The abscess may be demonstrable with ultrasonography, a liver-spleen scan, computed tomography, or a gallium scan (gallium is concentrated in pus).

The therapy consists of surgical drainage and treatment with antibiotics directed against the likely bacteria for at least 2 weeks.

NEOPLASMS OF THE PERITONEUM
Primary mesothelioma

Primary mesotheliomas, which are rare, arise from the epithelial and mesenchymal components of the mesothelium. The majority of patients with primary mesotheliomas have a history of asbestos exposure and pathologic evidence of pulmonary asbestosis. Although asbestos appears to play a role in the pathogenesis of mesothelioma, the exact pathophysiologic mechanism is unknown. The tumors usually involve the visceral and parietal peritoneum extensively, but the histologic characteristics are quite variable. Patients with mesotheliomas have abdominal pain, nausea, vomiting, weight loss, abdominal distention, and commonly ascites. A peritoneal biopsy or cytologic examination of the peritoneal fluid may suggest the diagnosis, but an exploratory laparotomy is usually required, often to rule out some other primary neoplasm. Systemic and intraperitoneal chemotherapy and radiation have been tried as therapeutic methods but have not proved helpful. The prognosis is poor, and most patients survive less than 2 years after the diagnosis is made.

Secondary carcinomatosis

Metastatic cancer or the extension of a neighboring primary tumor is a common cause of peritoneal disease. Approximately 80% of these cases are metastatic adenocarcinomas; other metastatic tumors are extremely rare. One third of the patients with leukemia or a lymphoma, however, have an infiltration into the peritoneum. Patients with peritoneal carcinomatosis have diffuse abdominal pain, weight loss, nausea, and vomiting and commonly have ascites. The pathophysiologic mechanism by which peritoneal metastases induce ascites is unknown. The ascitic fluid may be either a transudate or an exudate and often contains red cells or gross blood. Peritoneal carcinomatosis is diagnosed by a cytologic examination of ascitic fluid, a peritoneal biopsy, or peritoneoscopy. The long-term prognosis is poor; however, cytotoxic agents, radioactive implants, or quinacrine instillation leads to a good response in about 50% of these patients.

Pseudomyxoma peritonei

Pseudomyxoma peritonei is a rare form of mucinous ascites, usually associated with mucinous cystadenomas or cystadenocarcinomas of the ovary or mucoceles of the appendix. Mucinous ascites is also associated with ovarian fibromas or teratomas, uterine carcinomas, and carcinomas of the bile ducts, but these are rare causes. Patients with pseudomyxoma peritonei primarily have an increasing abdominal girth and few systemic complaints. Laparotomy or peritoneoscopy reveals that the mucinous material lies free in the abdomen or is firmly attached to the peritoneum. Nests of columnar cells are located in the peritoneum, but whether these cells are malignant is a controversial issue. Because the tumor may be benign or of low-grade malignancy, it rarely metastasizes, and the clinical course of the disease is often long and drawn out. Death usually results from an intestinal obstruction or fistulas. The treatment of choice is surgical removal of the ovaries, appendix, peritoneal nodules, and omentum along with evacuation of the mucin and instillation of an alkylating agent.

FAMILIAL PAROXYSMAL POLYSEROSITIS
ETIOLOGY AND PATHOLOGY. Familiar paroxysmal polyserositis, or familial Mediterranean fever, is an inherited disease characterized by recurrent, acute, self-limited attacks of fever associated with signs of peritonitis, pleuritis, and arthritis. The cause of familial Mediterranean fever is unknown, but it appears to be inherited as a single autosomal recessive trait and is found predominantly in patients of Mediterranean or Middle Eastern origin. During an acute at-

tack inflammatory changes occur in the serosa that are reversible; however, repeated attacks may lead to secondary inflammatory adhesions. The major complication in these patients is an increased susceptibility to amyloidosis; amyloid is deposited in the intima and media of arterioles and the subendothelial area of venules. There is a characteristic pattern of parenchymal distribution of amyloid and an extensive involvement in the renal glomeruli, adrenal glands, spleen, and pulmonary alveolar septa but usually a sparing of the liver sinusoids and heart muscle (see also Chapter 15).

CLINICAL MANIFESTATIONS. The first attack usually begins when patients are in their first or second decade. The acute attacks are of relatively short duration, 24 to 48 hours, and are unpredictable. Between attacks these patients are completely asymptomatic. An interesting, recently recognized phenomenon is that attacks do not occur during pregnancy. An acute attack is associated with a high fever and the classic signs of peritonitis, pleuritis, and arthritis. The symptoms and signs of peritonitis are virtually universally present in all patients. The disease sometimes cannot easily be differentiated from an acute abdominal catastrophe, and therefore laparotomy occasionally must be performed. An injudicious use of narcotics by these patients may result in drug addiction. Laboratory findings are nonspecific.

DIAGNOSIS. When the characteristic clinical pattern of recurrent self-limited attacks is present in a person of the appropriate ethnic background, the diagnosis is not difficult. Occasionally, however, there is a failure to consider the possibility of this disease, and as a result the patient is subjected to one or more unnecessary laparotomies before the diagnosis is made. Abdominal attacks must be differentiated from acute abdominal disorders such as appendicitis, pancreatitis, cholecystitis, perforations, and intestinal obstructions. In addition, porphyria and hyperlipidemia with acute abdominal symptoms must be excluded from diagnostic possibilities.

MANAGEMENT. The treatment of choice is colchicine therapy. Controlled trials have shown that the prophylactic use of colchicine reduces the frequency of attacks in most patients with familial Mediterranean fever. Furthermore, if colchicine is administered at the onset of the prodrome, attacks may be aborted. The mechanism by which colchicine affects this disease is uncertain, but it is postulated to interfere with the cellular phase of the inflammatory response. Because long-term colchicine therapy may cause azoospermia and chromosomal abnormalities, a course of intermittent therapy should be tried.

PROGNOSIS. If amyloidosis or drug addiction does not develop, the prognosis is excellent and normal longevity can be expected.

OTHER DISEASES OF THE PERITONEUM
Peritoneal vasculitis

The autoimmune vascular diseases such as systemic lupus erythematosus and periarteritis nodosa, as well as the allergic vasculitis associated with Schönlein-Henoch purpura, are rare causes of isolated peritonitis. Both categories of these vasculitis syndromes, however, more commonly involve the arteries of the gut and therby may cause a hemorrhage, ulceration, perforation, obstruction, or infarction of the gastrointestinal tract. Laparotomy may be the only way to distinguish isolated peritonitis from a gastrointestinal complication in these groups of patients. Cases of isolated peritonitis usually resolve with steroid therapy.

Granulomatous peritonitis

Sarcoidosis, Crohn's disease, and foreign bodies may cause noncaseating granulomata in the peritoneum, which may be associated with ascites. Tuberculous peritonitis must be excluded from the diagnostic possibilities in these patients by means of appropriate cultures and tests.

DISEASES OF THE MESENTERY AND OMENTUM
Mesenteric inflammatory disease

Mesenteric inflammatory disease is a poorly defined pathologic condition ranging from inflammatory to fibrotic lesions of the mesentery. It is commonly called mesenteric panniculitis or retractile mesenteritis, depending on its predominant pathologic features.

ETIOLOGY AND PATHOGENESIS. Trauma, infection, or ischemia is the causative agent that initiates the pathologic sequence. It is postulated that the underlying pathogenetic defect involves an excessive growth of normal fat tissue that undergoes degeneration, necrosis, and xanthogranulomatous inflammation. Abnormal lipid material is released from the degenerating lipocytes and causes granulomatous inflammation that progresses to fibrotic scarring.

CLINICAL MANIFESTATIONS. Patients with mesenteric panniculitis have recurrent episodes of localized or generalized crampy abdominal pain, weight loss, nausea, vomiting, and low-grade fever. In certain patients mesenteric panniculutis progresses to retractile mesenteritis. These patients have the same symptoms but in addition may have a bowel obstruction, mesenteric thrombosis, and an intestinal obstruction. Roentgenographic evaluation of the gastrointestinal tract may reveal displacement, extrinsic pressure deformities, separation, and a distortion of mucosal patterns of intestinal segments.

PATHOLOGY. Laparotomy in patients with mesenteric panniculitis reveals a thickened mesentery root, usually limited to the small bowel mesentery. In patients with retractile mesenteritis the mesentery is thickened, fibrotic, retracted, and studded with pale gray plaques. The histologic examination reveals varying degrees of mesenteric fat, inflammation, and fibrosis.

PROGNOSIS AND MANAGEMENT. Because mesenteric panniculitis is a rare disease, its prognosis and the most appropriate therapy have not been established.

Mesenteric cysts

Mesenteric cysts are usually chylous lymphatic cysts. These cysts are sequestrations of lymph vessels that may or may not communicate with the lymphatic system. The cause of these mesenteric cysts is unknown. They are usually asymptomatic but may produce symptoms that are usually related to their site and size. When they are symptomatic, surgical excision or enucleation is required.

Mesenteric tumors

Mesenteric tumors are rare but may arise from any of the cellular elements of the mesentery.

Mesenteric hernias

Various forms of herniation of the mesentery result from an anomalous intestinal rotation along with fusion of the mesentery and parietal peritoneum during embryonic development.

Omental torsion and infarction

Torsion of the omentum is an acute surgical condition that may mimic acute appendicitis or acute cholecystitis. Cases of omental infarction have a similar clinical picture.

BIBLIOGRAPHY

Berkowitz HD and others: Improved renal function and inhibition of renin and aldosterone secretion following peritoneovenous (LeVeen) shunt, Surgery 84:120, 1978.

Dinarello CA and others: Colchicine therapy for familial Mediterranean fever: a double-blind trial, N Engl J Med 291:934, 1974.

Dineen P, Homan NP, and Grafe WR: Tuberculous peritonitis: 43 years' experience in diagnosis and treatment, Ann Surg 184:717, 1976.

Donowitz M, Kerstein MD, and Spiro HM: Pancreatic ascites, Medicine 53:183, 1974.

Gregory PB and others: Complications of diuresis in the alcoholic patient with ascites: a controlled trial, Gastroenterology 73:534, 1977.

Sleisenger MH and Fordtran JS: Gastrointestinal disease, ed 5, Philadelphia, 1988, WB Saunders Co.

Tavill AS and others: The Budd-Chiari syndrome: correlation between hepatic scintigraphy and the clinical, radiological and pathological findings in nineteen cases of hepatic venous outflow obstruction, Gastroenterology 68:509, 1975.

182 · DISORDERS OF THE PANCREAS

Ralph M. Myerson

The pancreas has both endocrine and exocrine functions. Although this chapter deals primarily with the exocrine pancreas, it is important to recognize that the pancreas plays an important neuroendocrine role, acting as both the producer of certain gastrointestinal polypeptide hormones and as the target for the action of others.

ENDOCRINE PANCREAS

The endocrine component of the pancreas, the islets of Langerhans, are composed of specialized cells that secrete several polypeptide hormonal products. Cells designated as B or β-cells secrete *insulin,* whereas A or α-cells secrete *glucagon.* The effects of these hormones on glucose metabolism and their role in the pathophysiology of diabetes mellitus are discussed in Chapter 105. Glucagon also appears to inhibit pancreatic secretion in humans. D or δ-cells, along with specialized cells in the gastric antrum, secrete *somatostatin,* a polypeptide that inhibits secretion of gastric acid. Somatostatin also appears to have antitrophic effects and an inhibitory effect on secretion of pancreatic protein, an action that may be mediated by an inhibitory effect on the pituitary. Other specialized islet cells produce *vasoactive intestinal polypeptide (VIP), pancreatic polypeptide (PP),* and possibly *gastrin.* Normally none of these hormones is secreted in any substantial quantity. The endocrine cells are commonly referred to as APUD (amine precursor uptake and decarboxylation) cells. Functional tumors referred to as apudomas may develop from these cells leading to characteristic clinical syndromes. Insulinomas, glucagonomas, somatostatinomas, and vipomas have been described. The pancreas is also a common site for a gastrinoma, a gastrin-producing tumor responsible for Zollinger-Ellison syndrome.

EXOCRINE PANCREAS

The exocrine component of the pancreas is composed of small groups of acini separated into lobules by connective tissue stroma. Each acinus drains into a small pancreatic duct. These ducts unite to form a herringbone pattern, eventually draining into the major excretory ducts of Wirsung and Santorini.

The general function of the exocrine pancreas is twofold: secretion of enzymes important for the digestion of dietary fat, carbohydrates, and protein, and secretion of water and bicarbonate to create an alkaline medium within the pancreatic ducts

and the duodenum. Acid inactivates pancreatic enzymes.

The pancreatic enzymes, which are synthesized by the acinar cells, play an important role in intraluminal digestion by hydrolyzing food substances into a form that can be absorbed. Four classes of pancreatic digestive enzymes have been identified. *Amylase* acts to hydrolyze starch into maltose and has properties similar to those of salivary amylase. Pancreatic juice contains at least three *lipolytic enzymes:* lipase to hydrolyze triglycerides into monoglycerides and fatty acids, a phospholipase to hydrolyze phospholipids, and a carboxylesterase. The pancreas also synthesizes a number of *proteolytic enzymes* in the form of inactivity zymogens that are rapidly activated on their entrance into the duodenum. The major proteolytic enzymes thus formed are trypsin, chymotrypsin, elastase, and carboxypeptidase A and B. In essence these enzymes act by cleaving the peptide bonds of ingested dietary proteins, thus forming smaller protein fractions. The nucleolytic enzymes constitute the fourth group of pancreatic enzymes. These are ribonuclease and deoxyribonuclease, which act to hydrolyze the phosphodiesterase bonds that unite mononucleotides in nucleic acids.

The bicarbonate present in pancreatic juice is secreted by the cells of the pancreatic ducts by a complex process not yet completely understood. The origin of the bicarbonate excretion appears to be extracellular, and its pH, its bicarbonate concentration, and the partial pressure of carbon dioxide seem to be important variables. Carbonic anhydrase is present in ductular epithelium.

PHYSIOLOGY OF PANCREATIC SECRETION

Pancreatic secretion is controlled by a complex interaction of neural and hormonal influences. Vagal stimulation results in an increase in the volume, bicarbonate concentration, and enzyme content of pancreatic juice. A number of gastrointestinal polypeptide hormones also influence pancreatic secretions. Gastrin, secreted by specialized cells in the gastric antrum, stimulates the secretion of pancreatic enzymes. The intestinal enzyme bombesin, or gastrin-releasing peptide (GRP), also stimulates pancreatic enzymes, possibly by its stimulatory effects on gastrin and cholecystokinin-pancreozymin (CCK-PZ). The latter hormone, also secreted by the small intestine, is a potent stimulant of pancreatic enzyme but only a weak stimulant of pancreatic bicarbonate secretion. On the other hand, secretin, another hormone secreted by the small intestine, plays little or no role in the secretion of pancreatic enzymes but is a potent stimulant of bicarbonate secretion by the pancreatic ducts.

The so-called *cephalic phase* of pancreatic secretion occurs when a person sees, smells, or chews food. It is mediated by the vagus nerve, which stimulates pancreatic secretion directly and also indirectly by causing the secretion of gastrin and acid in the stomach.

Once food reaches the stomach, the *gastric phase* of gastric and pancreatic secretion takes place. The distention of the stomach stimulates gastrin release, probably by vagal reflexes. The release of gastrin also is stimulated by products of protein digestion and by certain substances such as calcium. The released gastrin and neural reflexes stimulate the gastric parietal cells to secrete acid and the pancreas to secrete its enzymes.

The *intestinal phase* of pancreatic stimulation, which accounts for most of the pancreatic secretion, is initiated when acid enters the duodenum. Secretin is released when the pH of the duodenal contents falls to 4.5 or lower. Its action in stimulating the pancreatic ducts to secrete bicarbonate is essential in maintaining the alkaline pH of the duodenum. Another component of the intestinal phase of pancreatic secretion is stimulation of the secretion of CCK-PZ by certain food substances. Fatty acids, especially those with long chains (16 to 18 carbon atoms), are particularly potent stimulants of CCK-PZ. Certain amino acids and some polypeptides also stimulate the secretion of CCK-PZ. There is evidence that CCK-PZ and secretin potentiate each other's actions.

DISORDERS OF THE PANCREAS

The disorders of the exocrine pancreas may be classified in the following categories: congenital abnormalities, acute pancreatitis, chronic pancreatitis, and tumors.

Congenital abnormalities

Primary congenital abnormalities of the pancreas may be of an anatomic or a functional nature.

Numerous *anatomic anomalies* of the pancreas exist, but with the exception of the annular pancreas and ectopic pancreas, they are rarely of clinical significance. In cases of annular pancreas a ring of pancreatic tissue arising from the head of the pancreas encircles the descending part of the duodenum. This tissue ring is one of the causes of obstructive vomiting in the neonate, and surgical correction is required. Most cases are accompanied by other congenital anomalies such as Down's syndrome and congenital heart disease.

An ectopic pancreas results from the dislocation of pancreatic tissue from the primitive endodermal buds and its migration to another site during embryologic development. The most common sites for an ectopic pancreas are the distal stomach, duodenum, and jejunum. The roentgenographic and endoscopic findings are those of an intramural lesion with a central umbilication. In most instances the lesion is asymptomatic and is discovered serendipitously. In rare cases bleeding may occur from superficial ulceration.

Congenital cysts usually are asymptomatic. They may occur as part of a polycystic disease in many organs, including the liver and kidney. They are clinically insignificant, in contrast to acquired cysts that occur as the result of a carcinoma or parasitic infection. Pseudocysts, an important complication of pancreatitis, are discussed in a later section.

Pancreas divisum is a condition in which the dorsal and ventral pancreatic buds fail to fuse. The duct of Wirsung and the accessory duct of Santorini empty into the duodenum independently. Pancreas divisum has been associated with acute relapsing pancreatitis. This has been attributed by some investigators to a functional ductular stenosis related to an inadequacy of drainage of the orifice of the accessory papilla.

Functional anomalies include congenital deficiencies in any or all of the pancreatic secretions; these are quite rare. Cystic fibrosis, or more properly, mucoviscidosis, is an autosomal recessive disorder that affects the function of many exocrine glands, including the exocrine pancreas, the mucous glands of the bronchi, the salivary and sweat glands, and others. The disease is characterized by an increased viscosity of the mucus in these glands. As a result the pancreatic ducts become obstructed by inspissated material, producing dilation of the ducts, retention cyst formation, and atrophy and fibrosis of the pancreas. Pancreatic insufficiency along with a resultant weight loss and poor growth and maturation follow. The involvement of the respiratory tract in cystic fibrosis leads to recurrent infections, pansinusitis, and pulmonary insufficiency. The involvement of the sweat glands results in an inability to conserve sodium, potassium, and chloride. Measuring the sodium or chloride content in sweat is the basis of a diagnostic test for

cystic fibrosis. The treatment consists of replacement therapy with pancreatic enzymes and prophylaxis and therapy of respiratory infections.

Acute pancreatitis

ETIOLOGY AND PATHOGENESIS. Acute pancreatitis is characterized by varying degrees of enzymatic autodigestion of the pancreas. The following list illustrates the many causes of acute pancreatitis:

> Alcohol
> Biliry tract disease
> Trauma
> Contagious spread of an infection or a penetrating duodenal ulcer
> Hyperlipidemia
> Hyperparathyroidism and hypercalcemia
> Viral causes, for example, mumps
> Familial disorders
> Drugs
> Idiopathic and miscellaneous cause

It is difficult to ascribe a common pathophysiologic defect to this wide and varied group of causes. Currently, the most widely accepted view is that acute pancreatitis is caused by hypertension in the pancreatic duct. In animal models, pancreatitis can be produced by dietary manipulation using a choline-deficient diet supplemented by ethionine (the CDE diet), or by stimulation of the pancreas by secretogoges such as CCK-PZ.

Alcohol is known to stimulate the secretion of pancreatic juice and at the same time may produce an obstruction to the flow within pancreatic ducts. Alcohol also appears to have a direct toxic effect in the acinar cell, disrupting its integrity and allowing the escape of pancreatic enzymes into pancreatic tissue.

In patients with biliary tract disease pancreatitis is most often associated with passage of a gallstone from the common duct through the ampulla of Vater into the duodenum. A common distal channel for both the bile and pancreatic ducts, as occurs in many cases, presumably causes a predisposition for the reflux of bile into the pancreatic duct, resulting in pancreatitis. In addition, refluxed bile may contain altered components that are especially harmful, such as biliary lecithin, which may be converted to lysolecithin by pancreatic phospholipase, and deconjugated bile, which may occur in the presence of bacteria in the common bile duct and duodenum. Both lysolecithin and deconjugated bile produce pancreatitis in experimental animals when refluxed into the pancreatic duct.

The mechanisms by which hypercalcemia, hyperparathyroidism, and hyperlipidemia produce pancreatitis are unclear. In hyperparathyroidism, pancreatic calcification may occur, but its presence is not essential for pancreatitis to develop. Types I, IV, and V hyperlipidemia may predispose a patient to pancreatitis, and it appears that chylomicronemia may be responsible by a mechanism not yet understood.

Contiguous infections occurring postoperatively or as a consequence of an abdominal catastrophe such as a perforated viscus may produce pancreatitis by direct spread of the inflammatory process to the pancreas. A penetrating duodenal ulcer also may produce pancreatitis. Mumps virus has a predilection for the pancreas, a phenomenon related to the histologic and functional similarities between the salivary glands and the pancreas.

A number of drugs have been implicated in the development of pancreatitis. A causal relationship has been most convincingly demonstrated for azathioprine, thiazides, sulfonamides, furosemide, estrogens, and tetracycline. There is suggestive evidence as well for a causative role played by L-asparaginase, chlorthalidone, corticosteroids, ethacrynic acid, phenformin, and procainamide. Little is known about the pathogenesis of drug-induced pancreatitis.

CLINICAL MANIFESTATIONS. There are no specific or pathognomonic features that distinguish pancreatitis with certainty from other diseases. Pancreatitis involves a wide spectrum of clinical patterns, ranging from clinically inapparent involvement to fulminant cases that rapidly lead to death.

The clinical picture is correlated with the pathophysiologic process. Milder cases usually are associated with edema of the pancreas, more severe cases are associated with hemorrhage and suppuration, and the most severe cases are associated with pancreatic necrosis and necrosis of adjacent and occasionally distant adipose tissue.

Abdominal pain is by far the most common symptom of acute pancreatitis and is present in almost all of these cases. The pain usually is epigastric and commonly radiates through to the back. The pain is steady and is made worse by eating and helped somewhat by sitting upright or leaning forward. As inflammation spreads throughout the pancreas and is accompanied by exudation and peritonitis, the pain spreads and becomes generalized throughout the abdomen. Nausea and vomiting are symptoms in most patients.

In milder cases abdominal tenderness is confined to the epigastrium and usually is not accompanied by fever or tachycardia. In severe cases the abdominal findings are more impressive and include marked tenderness, abdominal wall spasm, and the absence of peristaltic sounds. There may be abdominal distention, and the findings may mimic those of peritonitis resulting from a perforated viscus. If there has been hemorrhage into the peritoneal cavity, ecchymoses may be present in the flanks (Turner's sign) or periumbilically (Cullen's sign). Tachycardia is present, and a temperature of 100° to 102° F (37.8° to 38.9° C) is common. The patient may be restless or lie motionless and may be confused or semiconscious. If the cause is alcohol, the clinical picture may be complicated by the findings of acute alcoholic intoxication or an alcoholic withdrawal syndrome such as delirium tremens.

The patient may have accompanying shock and hypotension if there has been significant pancreatic exudation and loss of fluid into the peritoneal space. The extremities may be cold and clammy, and signs of dehydration may be present. Renal insufficiency and a left pleural effusion may accompany acute pancreatitis. Some of the pathophysiologic events occurring in cases of pancreatitis are thought to be initiated and mediated by vasoactive substances released into the peritoneal cavity and subsequently absorbed into the bloodstream or passing directly into the blood from their pancreatic origin.

The examiner may get a clue as to the cause of the pancreatitis from the associated physical findings such as biliary tract disease, an alcoholic syndrome, parotid swelling, band keratopathy, eruptive xanthoma, and so on.

LABORATORY FINDINGS. The most reliable laboratory test for the diagnosis of acute pancreatitis is the serum amylase test. An elevated level of serum amylase, although not pathognomonic for acute pancreatitis, is very strong supportive evidence of the diagnosis when the clinical presentation is compatible. This elevation occurs rapidly as a result of a disruption of the integrity of the acinar cell wall and an escape of amylase into the blood. The increased serum amylase level is reflected in the urine as well as in the ascitic or pleural fluid that may accompany acute pancreatitis. Amylase originating from the pancreas is filtered by the kidney at a faster rate than amylase from other sources. A reliable method of documenting an increased urinary amylase is to simultaneously determine the renal clearances of amylase and creatinine. The ratio of the clearance of amylase to the clearance of creatinine is normally 1% to 5%; in cases of acute pancreatitis it is over 5%.

Although the amylase level may become elevated within hours of an attack, elevation of the serum lipase level occurs later in the course of the disease and persists for a longer period of time. Serum lipase elevations occur much less commonly than hyperamylasemia. Leukocytosis is common, and the hemoglobin may be elevated because of a loss of fluid into the abdomen. Subsequent drops in the hemoglobin and hematocrit may be associated with a hemorrhage into the pancreas or the peritoneal cavity. Hyperglycemia and glycosuria commonly accompany acute pancreatitis, even in nondiabetic patients. The impairment in glucose metabolism is related to the involvement of the contiguous islets of Langerhans. Renal failure caused by acute tubular necrosis resulting from shock may accompany acute pancreatitis.

Signs of an extrahepatic biliary obstruction in pancreatitis are common because of inflammatory changes in the head of the pancreas in the region of the papilla of Vater. Serum alkaline phosphatase and bilirubin elevations commonly occur. Alcoholic liver disease may contribute to these abnormalities.

Lactescent serum resulting from hyperlipidemia involving triglycerides and/or chylomicrons may accompany acute pancreatitis. Inasmuch as hyperlipidemia may produce acute pancreatitis, it is important that the levels of serum lipids are followed through the patient's recovery and convalescent period so that the cause can be differentiated from its effects.

Hypocalcemia is a fairly common laboratory finding in cases of acute pancreatitis. It has been attributed to the precipitation of ionized calcium in areas of fat necrosis. Hypercalcemia or a normal serum calcium level in the presence of acute pancreatitis raises the distinct possibility of underlying hyperparathyroidism. Hypomagnesemia also has been observed in cases of acute pancreatitis, and it too has been attributed to the deposition of magnesium in areas of fat necrosis, although alcoholism may contribute to its presence.

Abdominal roentgenograms may be helpful in establishing a diagnosis of acute pancreatitis. Opaque biliary calculi may appear, suggesting the possibility that the pancreatitis may have occurred in association with biliary tract disease. Calcifications within the pancreas indicate that the patient has previously had damage to the pancreas.

Several roentgenographic findings are considered suggestive of acute pancreatitis although they are by no means pathognomonic. Most commonly observed is the so-called sentinel loop, a localized segment of small bowel ileus usually involving the jejunum. The transverse colon may be spastic as a consequence of irritation caused by pancreatic exudation. The ascending colon and hepatic flexure proximal to the area of spasm may become distended, suggesting the presence of an obstructing lesion. This finding is referred to as the colon cutoff sign. Widening of the duodenal loop caused by the pressure of an edematous head of the pancreas may be seen on a plain roentgenogram of the abdomen or with a barium meal examination. The stomach may be anteriorly displaced. The use of ultrasonography and computed tomography (CT) in diagnosing mass lesions is well established. Recently several investigators have evaluated the use of ultrasonography in acute pancreatitis. Its chief value lies in the detection of gallstones, at which its accuracy is over 95%. The pancreas may be visualized in only 65% to 75% of patients, and when it is, there is poor correlation between pancreatic enlargement caused by acute pancreatitis and that caused by other factors. Ultrasonography has been helpful in detecting pancreatic pseudocysts.

Most observers feel that computed tomography is better than ultrasonography in both correlating the clinical findings with the clinical type of acute pancreatitis and in diagnosing the complications of acute pancreatitis.

DIFFERENTIAL DIAGNOSIS. It may be difficult to differentiate acute pancreatitis from other acute abdominal disorders. The emphasis should be on excluding from the diagnostic possibilities an acute surgical emergency, especially a perforated peptic ulcer. The patient with a perforated peptic ulcer usually assumes an immobile supine position with knees tightly flexed. Signs of generalized peritonitis commonly develop more quickly when there is a perforation. The presence of free air in the abdomen is, of course, a valuable aid in differentiating the two conditions. In patients with acute biliary tract disease the localization of the discomfort in the right upper quadrant is a helpful finding. The serum amylase level usually is normal or only slightly elevated. The use of radionuclide imaging (HIDA and PIPIDA scans) may be helpful in the differential diagnosis.

Other conditions to be differentiated from acute pancreatitis include alcoholic hepatitis, an expanding or dissecting aortic aneurysm, mesenteric vascular occlusion, and volvulus of the bowel. Rarer conditions to be excluded from the diagnostic possibilities include a sickle cell crisis, tabetic crisis, porphyria, Schönlein-Henoch purpura, and lead poisoning.

The presence of an elevated level of serum amylase caused by acute pancreatitis must be differentiated from macroamylasemia, in which abdominal discomfort may occur. The diagnosis of macroamylasemia is confirmed by the presence of a low or normal rather than elevated urinary amylase.

MANAGEMENT. Because of the complexities involved and the monitoring required, patients with severe pancreatitis may require treatment in an intensive care unit. There is no specific or definitive therapeutic modality for acute pancreatitis. Every effort should be made to put the pancreas at rest, presumably because continuing pancreatic secretion may perpetuate the process. Because of the stimulating effect of gastric acid on the pancreas, efforts have been made to control acidity. Gastric suction and the administration of the histamine H_2-receptor antagonist and antacids have been employed therapeutically for this purpose. In addition, the patient is given nothing orally, so that the gastric phase of acid secretion is slowed. The results of these measures to combat gastric acidity are equivocal in terms of altering the course of acute pancreatitis. There is little doubt that nasogastric suction is beneficial, but its benefit may be derived from its decompressing effects rather than from its removal of gastric acid. There is as yet no convincing evidence about the benefits of antacids or cimetidine and especially of any benefit of anticholinergics, which have been used in the past.

The profound hemodynamic and electrolyte disturbances that accompany pancreatitis make it mandatory that the patient's fluid and electrolyte balances and urinary output be closely monitored. The central venous pressure should be employed for this purpose in a severely compromised patient. Colloid infusions may be necessary, as well as occasionally blood transfusions, if there has been significant hemorrhage. If endoscopic retrograde cholangiopancreatography (ERCP) is considered, the procedure should be deferred until the acute pancreatitis has subsided, since the procedure may cause a flare-up of the process. Total parenteral nutrition (TPN) improves nitrogen balance and places the pancreas at rest.

Alleviation of pain is an important component of this therapy. The decompression of the stomach with a nasogastric tube helps ease the pain of distention. Morphine should be avoided because of its tendency to constrict Oddi's sphincter. Small doses of meperidine may be administered as needed. The tendency for patients with pancreatitis, particularly chronic pancreatitis, to become dependent on narcotics is noteworthy, and the physician should be on guard for addicted patients who may be adept at feigning the signs and symptoms of acute pancreatitis.

Acute pancreatitis in itself does not require the use of antibiotics, but when this condition is accompanied by acute cholecystitis, cholangitis, a pancreatic abscess, or an infection contiguous to the pancreas, antibiotics are indicated. Ampicillin and/or one of the cephalosporins, along with an aminoglycoside such as gentamicin, is most commonly employed.

Pulmonary and cardiac complications should be treated appropriately. Respiratory aid may be required in the form of oxygen and intermittent positive pressure. Complicating pulmonary infections should be treated promptly. Patients with cardiac disease may require the administration of digitalis and diuretics.

Various agents have been tried empirically as treatments for acute pancreatitis without noteworthy success. Steroids have not proved helpful, nor has the use of aprotinin (Trasylol), a polypeptide that inhibits trypsin and kallikrein.

Surgery may be necessary for acute pancreatitis in certain circumstances. Surgical intervention in the case of gangrene or empyema of the gallbladder may abort the occurrence of secondary pancreatitis. Surgery is also recommended for the drainage of a pancreatic abscess, but differentiating an abscess with certainty from a phlegmonous infiltration of the pancreas or from a pseudocyst of the pancreas is extremely difficult. These conditions may mimic one another, even in their appearance, with ultrasonography and computed tomography. A meticulous individualization of each patient that correlates clinical findings with the results of special studies is required.

Peritoneal lavage in the treatment of acute pancreatitis has received favorable reports but is not yet generally accepted as a therapeutic modality.

Once the acute pancreatitis has subsided, surgery has an important role in cases in which biliary tract disease or hyperparathyroidism has been demonstrated as the underlying causative mechanism.

PROGNOSIS AND COMPLICATIONS. The prognosis of patients with acute pancreatitis depends largely on the severity of the inflammatory response. In mild edematous pancreatitis the mortality is less than 5%, but the mortality rises to above 50% in cases in which there is hemorrhage and/or necrosis. Shock, renal failure, infection, bleeding, and respiratory failure increase the mortality.

The complications of an acute episode of pancreatitis were discussed previously. The potential late complications include pseudocyst formation, abscess, pancreatic ascites, recurrence, and chronicity.

LATE COMPLICATIONS
Pseudocyst. A pseudocyst of the pancreas is a nonepithelialized cavity containing blood, serum, panncreatic secretions, and inflammatory exudate. Pseudocysts that develop as a complication of acute pancreatitis are almost invariably of alcoholic origin. With the continuing secretion of pancreatic juice into the pseudocyst, a pseudocyst may expand to a considerable

size, producing pain, a palpable and sometimes tender mass, and evidence of impingement on the stomach, duodenum, or other abdominal organs. A pseudocyst may cause nausea and vomiting and occasionally obstructive jaundice. Leakage or an overt rupture into the peritoneal cavity may occur, often with dire consequences. A rupture into the stomach or intestine sometimes occurs, often causing gastrointestinal bleeding. Pseudocysts usually are present singly but may be multiple; their size varies. They may occur within the pancreatic tissue or may be located within the lesser peritoneal sac, within the mesentery, behind the peritoneum, or as far distant as the mediastinum.

The diagnosis of a pseudocyst should be suspected in a patient in whom pain persists after acute alcoholic pancreatitis subsides and in whom the elevation of the level of serum amylase or lipase persists. The pseudocyst may be palpable and is commonly demonstrable as a mass lesion with a barium meal or enema examination. An extrinsic pressure on or a displacement of the gastrointestinal tract or left kidney suggests the presence of a pseudocyst. Ultrasonography and computed tomography are helpful in establishing the diagnosis. The major dangers of a pancreatic pseudocyst are rupture and bleeding; both are uncommon.

Evidence is accumulating that many pseudocysts regress spontaneously, but those that are symptomatic should be approached surgically. The procedure of choice is a cystenterostomy into an adjacent portion of the stomach or intestine. The results of surgery generally are quite satisfactory.

Pancreatic abscess. A pancreatic abscess is a rare complication of acute pancreatitis. It usually occurs within a few weeks of an acute episode and is characterized by a high fever and a tender abdominal mass. Leukocytosis is common. Enteric organisms and probably anaerobes such as *Bacteroides fragilis* usually are responsible for the inflammatory reaction, but occasionally *Staphylococcus aureus* or a species of *Streptococcus* is involved. If surgical drainage is not performed, the mortality is high.

Pancreatic ascites. Persistent ascites may develop after a bout of acute pancreatitis, especially in cases of a poorly walled-off pseudocyst. Abdominal paracentesis reveals ascitic fluid with a high amylase content, which differentiates pancreatic ascites from ascites caused by cirrhosis of the liver. Drainage of the fluid may result in a lasting remission, but many cases are resistant to conservative therapy and may require surgery.

Relapsing acute pancreatitis

In some cases when the underlying cause of pancreatitis remains, as in patients with alcoholism or cholelithiasis, attacks of acute pancreatitis may recur. Recurrences may result in chronic pancreatitis, especially if the underlying causative mechanism is not remedied.

Chronic pancreatitis

When the pancreas is subjected to repeated bouts of pancreatitis, regardless of the cause, it may undergo irreversible inflammatory changes, fibrosis, and eventual calcification. Alcohol is the most common cause of chronic pancreatitis, either because of a specific toxic effect of alcohol or because pancreatitis associated with biliary tract disease is more amenable to corrective therapy.

The clinical course is characterized by recurrent attacks of pain and disability, although in some patients chronic pancreatitis may occur without preceding pain. In fully developed cases of chronic pancreatitis, especially when there is pancreatic calcification, pain may be steady and unrelenting, suggesting a mechanical cause, or it may be intermittent. The pain is boring and poorly localized and tends to radiate to the midback. Characteristically it is relieved when the patient sits upright and bends forward. Other symptoms are caused by the endocrine and exocrine pancreatic insufficiency that develops.

Glucose intolerance is common in these patients, and the diabetes may be brittle, although an insulin requirement above 40 units a day is uncommon. Diabetic complications such as retinopathy, glomerulosclerosis, and peripheral vascular disease are uncommon, perhaps because of the shorter duration of the diabetic state in patients with chronic pancreatitis. Diabetic ketoacidosis, however, is a distinct threat. Peripheral neuropathy is fairly common, probably because of the contributing factors of alcoholism and malnutrition.

Steatorrhea is common in chronic pancreatitis and often is disabling. Its presence signifies the destruction of at least 80% of the gland. Fecal fat losses in excess of 50% of the oral intake may result from a deficiency in pancreatic lipase. Weight loss and multiple nutritional deficiencies, particularly of the fat-soluble vitamins, result as a consequence of steatorrhea.

Chronic pancreatitis is usually not difficult to diagnose. The clinical history and the finding of pancreatic calcification in the presence of endocrine and/or exocrine pancreatic insufficiency are a sufficient basis for the diagnosis. The diagnosis is supported by tests of the pancreatic capacity to secrete enzymes, fluid, and bicarbonate. The secretin test, a measure of the ability of the pancreas to respond to an intravenous dose of secretin, is most commonly used for this purpose. With a duodenal tube the baseline and serial levels of bicarbonate concentration are measured.

Gross and microscopic examinations of the stool to detect excess quantities of fat are helpful in determining the presence of steatorrhea, but a 3-day quantitative fecal fat analysis is preferable. Steatorrhea resulting from chronic pancreatitis must be appropriately differentiated from that resulting from other causes. The D-xylose test, small bowel barium meal examination, and small bowel biopsy have normal results in cases of chronic pancreatitis and thus help to distinguish this steatorrhea from that produced by a mucosal disorder of the small intestine.

Selective angiography and endoscopic retrograde cholangiopancreatography may prove helpful in establishing the diagnosis (Fig. 182-1).

The treatment is directed to the endocrine and exocrine insufficiency. Diabetes mellitus should be treated appropriately. Steatorrhea should be treated with pancreatic extracts. Additional therapy with antacids or the histamine H_2-receptor antagonist may be helpful in protecting the pancreatic extracts because pancreatic enzymes are readily inactivated at a pH below 4.5. Vitamin supplements are indicated to correct any deficiencies. Satisfactory absorption and nutrition should be restored with the proper use of this therapy, but the caloric intake can be enhanced if necessary by adding easily absorbed medium-chain triglycerides to the diet.

Various surgical procedures have been used to try to reestablish pancreatic drainage. These may be effective in cases in which a segmental obstruction of the pancreatic ducts can be demonstrated. In most cases, however, acinar destruction has occurred, prohibiting surgical correction.

Pain frequently is disabling in chronic pancreatitis. Because addiction is fairly common among these patients, a program of analgesia should be carefully planned. The value of neu-

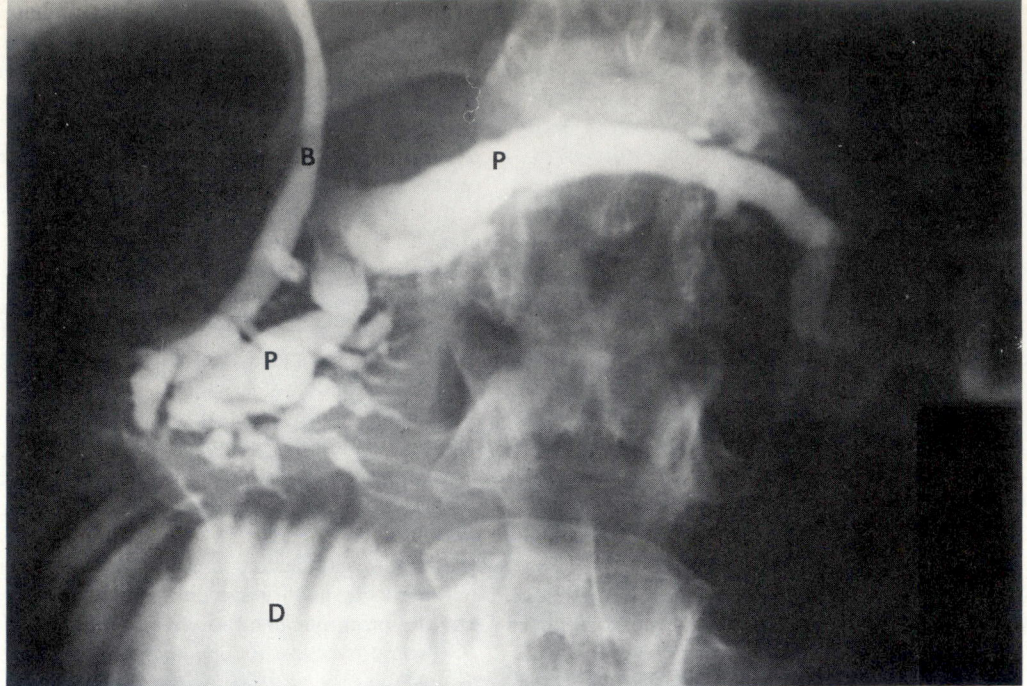

Fig. 182-1   Endoscopic retrograde cholangiopancreatography reveals marked dilation, irregularity, and "clubbing" of pancreatic ducts, changes found in chronic pancreatitis. *B,* Common bile duct; *D,* duodenum; *P,* main pancreatic duct. (Courtesy of Harvey Lefton, MD.)

rosurgical procedures such as a dorsal root interruption or celiac axis ganglionectomy is debatable. More radical and dangerous surgery such as a subtotal pancreatectomy may have to be attempted in selected cases in an effort to control unremitting pain.

Tumors of the pancreas

Benign tumors of the exocrine pancreas may arise from acinar cells (adenomas and cystadenomas) or from supporting tissues (lipomas, neuromas, hemangiomas, fibromas, myxomas, and lymphangiomas). Benign tumors are rare and not usually of clinical significance. Neoplasms also may arise in the endocrine pancreas. Gastrinomas and insulinomas are the most common of these, but glucagonomas, somatostatinomas, and VIP-secreting tumors also occur rarely. These may be benign or malignant. These endocrine tumors are not discussed in this chapter.

Carcinomas of the pancreas originate most commonly from ductal epithelial and occasionally from acinar tissue. Because of the inaccessibility of the pancreas and the insidious and nonspecific nature of symptoms related to carcinomas of the pancreas, the disease is rarely diagnosed early in its course. Pancreatic carcinomas are increasing in incidence and currently rank second to colonic carcinomas as the most common cause of death among carcinomas originating in the gastrointestinal tract. Alcoholism, chronic pancreatitis, and diabetes mellitus have been mentioned as possible predisposing factors, but the evidence for these is inconclusive.

CLINICAL MANIFESTATIONS. Most patients with a pancreatic carcinoma have abdominal discomfort. The pain usually is not disabling, is nonspecific, and is confined to the epigastrium or right upper quadrant when the head of the pancreas is involved. When the tumor arises in the body or tail of the pancreas, the pain tends to be located in the midline or left upper quadrant. In its most characteristic form the pain radiates

straight through to the back, is intensified when the patient is in the supine position, and is relieved by maneuvers that flex the spine, such as sitting up or lying on the side with the knees flexed.

Anorexia and weight loss are almost universal symptoms and may be extreme. Obstructive jaundice is present in at least 90% of patients with a carcinoma of the pancreatic head and is commonly the presenting complaint. Jaundice is a late manifestation of carcinomas of the body or tail of the pancreas and indicates the spread of the disease to the head of the pancreas or the liver.

Less common clinical symptoms and signs include fever and chills related to a biliary tract obstruction and/or tumor necrosis, nonbacterial thrombotic endocarditis, migratory thrombophlebitis, and psychiatric symptoms.

DIAGNOSIS. The diagnosis of a carcinoma of the head of the pancreas is strongly suggested by the appearance of relatively painless jaundice in an older patient along with a weight loss. Except for the jaundice and weight loss the results of the physical examination may be completely negative. Occasionally a distended gallbladder may be palpated (Courvoisier's sign). A metastatic spread to the liver results in a palpable enlargement of the organ, usually accompanied by irregularity and an increase in its consistency. Laboratory tests are helpful in confirming the presence of obstructive jaundice. Relatively high elevations of the levels of alkaline phosphatase, leucine aminopeptidase, 5'-nucleotidase, and γ-glutamyl transpeptidase in the presence of moderate elevations of serum transaminase values (serum glutamic-oxaloacetic transaminase and serum glutamic-pyruvic transaminase) of less than 300 units strongly suggest an obstructive process. There may be an impairment of glucose tolerance if there has been sufficient destruction of pancreatic islet cells.

The diagnosis is much more difficult to make in cases of carcinomas of the body or tail of the pancreas. The physical examination and routine laboratory studies usually are within normal limits until the process is advanced.

The conventional barium meal examination may reveal evidence of extrinsic pressure on the stomach and duodenal loop. This usually is first manifested as a widening of the duodenal loop and an encroachment on the lumen of the duodenum. An extrinsic pressure or actual invasion of the greater curvature of the gastric antrum may also occur. Hypotonic duodenography may provide a more detailed picture of this area.

An increasing number of special studies that have become available during the last decade are helpful in detecting mass lesions of the pancreas. Angiographic visualization of the pancreas has been improved through the capability of introducing the contrast material into smaller arteries (superselective angiography) and through the use of magnification techniques. Characteristic features of carcinomas, such as the encasement of blood vessels, have been recognized.

An improved visualization of the biliary tree in cases of a suspected obstruction has resulted from a refinement of the techniques of percutaneous (Chiba fine needle) transhepatic cholangiography and endoscopic retrograde cholangiopancreatography.

Ultrasonography and computed tomography have been helpful in detecting mass lesions of the pancreas as well as in disclosing the presence of a dilated gallbladder or bile ducts. These relatively simple, noninvasive techniques are often employed early in the diagnostic process to confirm the suspected presence of obstructive jaundice or a pancreatic carcinoma.

Pancreatic scanning using selenomethionine has not proved sufficiently reliable in differentiating pancreatic carcinomas from pancreatitis and other nonneoplastic conditions.

MANAGEMENT. The abdomen should be surgically explored in suspected cases of carcinomas of the pancreas, especially when the head of the pancreas is thought to be involved. If there is no evidence of local or distant metastases, a radical pancreaticoduodenectomy (Whipple's operation) may be attempted in the hope of a cure. In the presence of metastatic spread, a palliative bypass procedure such as cholecystojejunostomy may be performed to relieve the obstructive jaundice and its attendant problems.

In patients with a carcinoma of the body and tail of the pancreas a curative operation is rarely performed, because a metastatic spread of the tumor has almost invariably already taken place.

The medical management of patients with a carcinoma of the pancreas is aimed at the palliation of symptoms, such as the relief of pain, maintenance of nutrition, and treatment of complications. Chemotherapy and radiation have little or no influence on the primary lesion but may be helpful in the relief of pain.

The prognosis is extremely poor. Generally the 5-year survival rate is below 2%. Most patients are dead within 1 year, regardless of the form of treatment. Patients with carcinomas that arise from the ampulla of Vater have a much better prognosis and a 5-year survival rate of up to 25%.

BIBLIOGRAPHY

Bank S, Wise L, and Gersten M: Risk factors in acute pancreatitis, Am J Gastroenterol 78:637, 1983.

Blamey SL and others: The early identification of patients with gallstone-associated pancreatitis using clinical and biochemical factors only, Ann Surg 198:574, 1983.

Foley WD and others: Computed tomography, ultrasonography and endoscopic retrograde pancreatography in the diagnosis of pancreatic disease. A comparative study, Gastrointest Radiol 5:29, 1980.

Hill MC and others: Acute pancreatitis. Clinical vs. CT findings, Am J Radiol 139:263, 1981.

Lang P and Pedersen T: Initial treatment of acute pancreatitis, Surg Gynecol Obstet 157:332, 1983.

Mallory A and Kern F: Drug-induced pancreatitis: A critical review, Gastroenterology 78:813, 1980.

Sankaran S and Walt AJ: The natural and unnatural history of pancreatic pseudocysts, Br J Surg 62:37, 1975.

Sarles JC and others: Surgical treatment of chronic pancreatitis: report of 134 cases treated by resection or drainage, Am J Surg 144:317, 1982.

Weinstein BJ and Weinstein DP: Ultrasonographic evaluation of the pancreas, CRC Crit Rev Diagn Imaging 18:81, 1982.

183 · DISEASES OF THE LIVER
Graham H. Jeffries

CLINICAL MANIFESTATIONS OF HEPATIC DISEASE
Jaundice

Jaundice (icterus) is a yellow discoloration of the skin or sclerae caused by an excessive level of bilirubin; this is usually detected when the serum level of bilirubin exceeds 2 to 3 mg/dl.

BILIRUBIN METABOLISM

Production. The major proportion of excreted bilirubin (80% to 90%) is derived from the catabolism of red cell hemoglobin by reticuloendothelial cells. Senescent red cells sequestered in the spleen are ingested by macrophages, and intracellular lysosomal enzymes separate iron and globin from the hemoglobin, open the tetrapyrrol ring, and catabolize the molecule through several intermediates (including biliverdin) to bilirubin. The color changes of a bruise reflect a similar degradation of hemoglobin by tissue macrophages. Small amounts of bilirubin are formed by the breakdown of other hemoproteins (myoglobin and cytochromes), particularly in the liver, or from hemoglobin synthesized by bone marrow cells but not incorporated into mature peripheral red cells.

Transport. The bilirubin released from reticuloendothelial cells is relatively nonpolar and poorly soluble in an aqueous solution; albumin, which has the capacity to bind two molecules of bilirubin on each protein molecule, is the major carrier of bilirubin in plasma and determines the distribution of the pigment. The high affinity between albumin and bilirubin limits the diffusion of bilirubin into cells (except in the liver) unless the plasma concentration exceeds the albumin binding capacity (see discussion of "Jaundice from impaired hepatic conjugation of bilirubin" later in this chapter). The albumin-bilirubin complex is not filtered in the glomeruli, and thus unconjugated pigment is not excreted in the urine.

Hepatic uptake. The uptake of bilirubin by liver cells is facilitated by the permeability of the hepatic sinusoids, which permits albumin-bilirubin to diffuse rapidly into Disse's space in contact with the liver cell membrane, and by binding proteins (Y and Z proteins), which concentrate bilirubin in the cytoplasm of liver cells; the displacement of bilirubin from albumin-binding sites requires the presence of a high-affinity carrier protein at the liver cell membrane.

Hepatic conjugation. In the liver cells bilirubin is conjugated to form bilirubin diglucuronide (conjugated bilirubin) by a microsomal enzyme system, glucuronyl transferase in the presence of uridine diphosphate glucuronic acid; this reaction converts nonpolar bilirubin to a water-soluble organic anion that is excreted in bile. Conjugation is a prerequisite for the biliary secretion of bilirubin.

Hepatic secretion. The secretion of conjugated bilirubin into the bile canaliculi is an active process that probably is carrier mediated; this is normally the rate-limiting step in bilirubin excretion. Organic anions, including bilirubin and bile acids, are secreted into the bile canaliculi by independent mechanisms; in Dubin-Johnson syndrome an impaired hepatic excretion of conjugated bilirubin and other organic anions is associated with a normal bile acid excretion. The rate of bilirubin secretion in bile nevertheless appears to be modulated by bile acid secretion.

Intestinal degradation. In the gut the conjugated bilirubin is deconjugated and converted to colorless urobilinogens by bacterial enzymes. The urobilinogen may be excreted in the stool or may be reabsorbed to undergo biliary or renal excretion.

PATHOPHYSIOLOGY OF JAUNDICE. Patients with jaundice can be divided into two groups. In cases of unconjugated hyperbilirubinemia there may be an excessive bilirubin production, an impaired hepatic uptake of bilirubin, or a depressed hepatic conjugation. Conjugated hyperbilirubinemia may result from the impaired hepatic excretion of bilirubin diglucuronide. The term "cholestasis" refers to abnormalities of hepatic excretion involving reduced bile flow and impaired hepatobiliary excretion; cholestatic jaundice results from intrahepatic lesions (intrahepatic cholestasis) or extrahepatic lesions obstructing the biliary system (extrahepatic cholestasis).

Jaundice from excessive bilirubin production. Increased red cell destruction *(hemolysis)* and ineffective erythropoiesis (as in cases of thalassemia and pernicious anemia) lead to excessive bilirubin production. The normal capacity of the liver to excrete bilirubin is such that the serum level of unconjugated bilirubin rarely exceeds 3 to 5 mg/dl in patients with chronic hemolytic disease. When acute or chronic liver disease reduces the hepatic excretion of conjugated bilirubin, an increased bilirubin load caused by hemolysis contributes to an increase in the serum level of conjugated bilirubin.

Jaundice from reduced hepatic uptake of bilirubin. In *Gilbert's disease* plasma clearance of unconjugated bilirubin is reduced, resulting either from impaired uptake at the liver cell membrane or from altered transport within the cell; this is a common cause of mild unconjugated hyperbilirubinemia without other abnormalities of liver cell function. In some cases an increase in the bilirubin load (hemolysis) accentuates the patient's jaundice. Patients with a portal-systemic shunt may also exhibit mild unconjugated hyperbilirubinemia caused by a decreased plasma clearance of unconjugated bilirubin.

Jaundice from impaired hepatic conjugation of bilirubin. Unconjugated hyperbilirubinemia commonly occurs in the neonatal period, particularly in premature infants with a relatively immature transport and conjugating system for bilirubin. In Crigler-Najjar syndrome a partial or complete lack of the enzyme systems for conjugating bilirubin leads to marked unconjugated hyperbilirubinemia. When the serum level of pigment exceeds the albumin binding capacity, diffusion of lipid-soluble bilirubin into the brain causes metabolic injury (kernicterus).

Jaundice from impaired excretion of conjugated bilirubin. In Dubin-Johnson syndrome and Rotor's syndrome a metabolic defect in the hepatic transport of organic anions leads to conjugated hyperbilirubinemia. Patients with a liver cell injury, regardless of whether it is metabolic (such as hypoxia), toxic (such as carbon tetrachloride or ethanol toxicity), viral (such as hepatitis type A or B), or the result of other causes (such as bacterial endotoxin), commonly have jaundice caused by the impaired excretion of conjugated bilirubin. Damage to bile ductules within the portal triads (such as occurs in primary biliary cirrhosis) and infiltration of the liver (such as by a granuloma or neoplasm) also lead to intrahepatic cholestasis. An extrahepatic ductal obstruction may result from gallstones, a stricture, or a neoplasm; these are the more common causes of "surgical" obstructive jaundice (extrahepatic cholestasis).

Cutaneous manifestations

PRURITUS. Both intrahepatic and extrahepatic cholestasis are commonly associated with generalized itching; in some patients with chronic cholestasis (such as primary biliary cirrhosis), this symptom may precede the onset of jaundice, whereas patients with severe hepatocellular failure and deep jaundice may remain free of pruritus. This symptom may interfere with a patient's sleep and may lead to a severe skin excoriation with bleeding or infection. Although it has been suggested that retained bile acids cause the stimulation of skin receptors, the severity of pruritus is only weakly correlated with the concentration of bile acids in peripheral blood plasma or skin. The decrease in pruritus with cholestyramine therapy, which was formerly attributed to bile acid chelation with a lowering of plasma bile acid levels, may result from the chelation of some other agent that accumulates in patients with cholestasis.

SKIN RASHES. In patients with acute type B hepatitis a skin rash may precede or coincide with the episode of acute hepatitis; the rash is commonly an acute erythema with edema (hives) or may be maculopapular and purpuric, particularly on the legs. This rash results from vascular injury caused by circulating immune complexes and often coincides with arthralgias or overt acute arthritis.

PIGMENTATION. Chronic cholestasis with jaundice leads to an increase in the melanin pigmentation of the skin. In patients with primary or secondary hemochromatosis the skin may have a bronze or slate-gray color that varies with the deposition of melanin or iron; hypogonadism in these patients causes the skin to be soft in texture with a loss of axillary and pubic hair. Patients with porphyria cutanea tarda may have an increase in fine facial hair, particularly in the periorbital area; photosensitivity resulting from uroporphyrin retention may cause bullous skin lesions in areas exposed to the sun, along with secondary scarring and depigmentation.

SPIDER ANGIOMAS. Spider angiomas (vascular spiders) are arteriovenous anastomoses that vary in size from 1 to 10 mm in diameter, are usually concentrated on the face, neck, upper thorax, and arms, and typically have a pulsating central arteriole with radiating vessels. Although small spider angiomas may appear during the course of acute hepatitis, multiple large lesions are usually observed in patients with chronic progressive liver disease. Similar arteriovenous anastomoses have been demonstrated in the lungs. The pathogenesis of spider angiomas remains obscure. The appearance of small lesions during pregnancy suggests that they may be related to hormonal changes in chronic liver disease; alternatively, their development may be initiated by the same factors that cause palmar erythema and the increase in cardiac output in cirrhotic patients.

PALMAR ERYTHEMA. Erythema of the thenar and hypothenar eminences and the distal fingers is a common feature of chronic liver disease and is related to local vasodilation.

XANTHOMAS. The hepatic synthesis and secretion of a plasma high-density lipoprotein (lipoprotein X) containing cholesterol and phospholipid are greatly increased in patients with cholestasis. Deposits of lipoprotein in aggregates of macrophages in the skin are correlated with serum cholesterol levels in excess of 450 mg/dl. Flat yellow plaques (xanthelasma) are most common on the eyelids, in skin creases on the neck and palms, and in recent scars. Nodular xanthomas may develop over pressure areas.

NAIL CHANGES. Clubbing of the nails is relatively common in patients with chronic cholestasis; the pathogenesis is uncertain. White nails with a loss of lunulae are associated with hypoproteinemia in patients with chronic liver failure; in rare cases local copper deposition in patients with Wilson's disease may cause the lunulae to appear blue.

Oral manifestations

FETOR HEPATICUS. Fetor hepaticus is a sweetish, musty odor on the breath of patients with liver failure and/or an extensive portal systemic shunting of blood. The odor has been attributed to the excretion of mercaptans (methyl mercaptan and dimethylsulfide) that are produced by the bacterial degradation of methionine in the gut and that accumulate in the peripheral circulation because of impaired hepatic detoxification or shunting past the liver.

LESIONS RESULTING FROM NUTRITIONAL DEFICIENCIES. Heavy alcohol ingestion often is accompanied by an inadequate diet; deficiencies of the B vitamins, vitamin C, folic acid, and zinc may cause oral lesions. Glossitis and cheilosis (resulting from B vitamin deficiency), a smooth tongue (folate deficiency), loosening of the teeth along with gingivitis and bleeding (vitamin C deficiency), and a crusting vesicular eruption around the mouth (zinc deficiency) are features that may accompany liver disease in alcoholic patients.

MUCOSAL BLEEDING. Depressed plasma levels of the clotting factors synthesized by the liver (causing a prolonged prothrombin time and partial thromboplastin time) result from malabsorption of vitamin K in patients with obstructive jaundice or from impaired hepatic protein synthesis in patients with liver failure. This may cause gingival bleeding or postoperative hemorrhage following the extraction of a tooth. Thrombocytopenia in patients with hypersplenism adds to the risk of bleeding, particularly when platelet function is depressed by aspirin.

Changes in liver size or consistency

Liver enlargement usually indicates liver disease and may reflect changes in the parenchymal cells (infiltration with fat or glycogen), intrahepatic or extrahepatic cholestasis, venous congestion (heart failure, constrictive pericarditis, or hepatic vein occlusion), diffuse inflammation (toxic and viral hepatitis), pyogenic or amebic abscess formation, a cellular infiltration that is either diffuse (macrophages in Gaucher's disease or hematopoietic cells in extramedullary hematopoiesis) or focal (granuloma or neoplasm), cyst formation (polycystic liver or hydatid disease), or fibrosis with regeneration nodules (cirrhosis in alcoholics).

A small, shrunken liver in patients with acute liver failure indicates massive or multilobular necrosis with collapse of the parenchyma; in patients with macronodular cirrhosis the liver often is shrunken and impalpable.

Hepatic tenderness suggests inflammation (acute hepatitis, an abscess, or cholangitis) or an acute stretching of the liver capsule (congestion or acute infiltration). Palpation is often helpful in detecting the induration associated with infiltration or fibrosis and the nodules associated with cirrhosis or a tumor; bimanual palpation may detect hepatic pulsation in patients with tricuspid insufficiency. Vascular bruits indicate arteriovenous fistulas, vascular neoplasms (particularly hepatomas), or an aortic compression caused by liver enlargement; the latter can be excluded from the diagnostic possibilities by positioning the patient. Friction rubs may be heard over superficial necrotic tumor nodules or in patients with acute perihepatitis.

Portal hypertension

Normally approximately 25% of the cardiac output of blood flows through the liver; the hepatic artery contributes approximately 0.5 L/min and the portal vein approximately 1 L/min. The pressure gradient across the sinusoidal bed between portal and hepatic veins fluctuates with the respiratory cycle between 0 and 5 mm Hg. In patients with portal hypertension this pressure gradient is increased in excess of 10 to 12 mm Hg either by an increase in the splanchnic blood flow or by an increase in resistance to the blood flow through the liver.

PATHOGENESIS OF PORTAL HYPERTENSION

Conditions that increase splanchnic blood flow. Portal hypertension resulting from increased splanchnic blood flow is relatively uncommon in the United States. Splenic, hepatic, or mesenteric arteriovenous fistulas may result from trauma or the rupture of congenital or acquired aneurysms. Massive splenomegaly usually is accompanied by an increase in the splenic blood flow; an increase in hepatic vascular resistance caused by cellular infiltration of the hepatic sinusoids increases portal pressure in some patients with hematologic disorders (such as agnogenic myeloid metaplasia). Although arteriovenous shunts have been demonstrated in the splenic circulation of some patients with cirrhosis, changes in the splanchnic blood flow probably play a minor role in the pathogenesis of portal hypertension in these patients.

Conditions that increase hepatic vascular resistance. The lesions that may obstruct the liver's blood flow are clinically separable into the following four groups, each with different manifestations and prognoses.

Extrahepatic obstruction of the portal system. Portal vein thrombosis usually is a complication of an infection, inflammation, neoplasm, or clotting disorder. Umbilical sepsis in infancy may cause thrombosis of the portal vein at the porta hepatis. An intraabdominal abscess complicating a ruptured appendix or diverticulum may lead to pylephlebitis. Acute hemorrhagic pancreatitis or neoplasms of the pancreas commonly cause thrombosis or obstruction of the splenic vein; this may be confined to the splenic vein, causing localized splenic hypertension, or may extend to involve the portal vein. Portal vein thrombosis has been described as a complication of polycythemia vera, paroxysmal nocturnal hemoglobinuria, antithrombin III deficiency, and the use of oral contraceptive hormones—conditions that increase the risk of venous thrombosis. In patients with established cirrhosis and portal hypertension, local venous stasis, hepatoma, or shunt surgery may be complicated by portal vein thrombosis.

Presinusoidal obstruction of portal vein radicles. Fibrosis of the portal triads in patients without cirrhosis can cause an obstruction in the portal venous system without increasing the hydrostatic pressure within the hepatic sinusoids. This fibrosis may be idiopathic in some patients with noncirrhotic portal hypertension or may be caused by schistosomiasis, chronic arsenic or vinyl chloride toxicity, congenital hepatic fibrosis, granulomatous disease (such as sarcoidosis), or neoplastic infiltration. In the absence of cirrhosis or hepatic infiltration, these patients usually maintain normal liver function.

Sinusoidal and postsinusoidal obstruction. Obstruction to the blood flow at the level of the sinusoidal bed and hepatic vein tributaries is the most common mechanism of portal hypertension in patients with cirrhosis. Fatty infiltration and inflammation contribute to reversible portal hypertension in patients with acute alcoholic hepatitis, but progressive fibrosis, particularly pericentrally in the hepatic lobule (central sclerosis), and nodular regeneration cause irreversible changes in blood flow. In patients with venoocclusive disease, toxic plant alkaloids initiate an inflammatory reaction around small tributaries of the hepatic veins and central veins, leading to subsequent fibrosis and thrombosis; a similar lesion may complicate radiation injury to the liver.

Hepatic venous obstruction (Budd-Chiari syndrome). The major hepatic veins may be occluded by congenital webs, by thrombosis, or by a neoplasm such as a hepatoma or lymphoma.

MANIFESTATIONS OF PORTAL HYPERTENSION

Portal-systemic venous collateral circulation. In response to the increased pressure gradient between the portal and systemic venous systems, venous collaterals are established in areas where these systems communicate. The most common and clinically significant collateral circulation is formed by anastomotic veins in and around the esophagus; a retrograde flow in the left gastric and gastroepiploic veins drains portal blood from the portal vein and spleen through gastric and esophageal varices into the azygos system. These collaterals may also communicate with bronchial veins in the mediastinum. In the falciform ligament, umbilical or paraumbilical veins drain from the left branch of the portal vein to the anterior abdominal wall at the umbilicus; the prominent collateral system radiating from the umbilicus to the epigastric, lateral thoracic, and saphenous veins is a *caput medusae*. The abdominal wall collaterals, which are best demonstrated when the patient is standing, must be distinguished from the ascending collaterals of an inferior vena caval obstruction. Turbulent blood flow at the umbilicus may establish a venous hum or palpable venous thrill. Hemorrhoidal vessels become more prominent as collaterals between the inferior mesenteric and the iliac venous systems. Spontaneous collaterals also develop between splenic and renal veins or in vascular adhesions between visceral and parietal areas of peritoneum.

Splenomegaly. Although portal hypertension leads to congestive splenomegaly, there is a poor correlation between splenic size and the severity of portal hypertension in patients with cirrhosis. The most significant problems relating to splenomegaly in patients with portal hypertension are an increased risk of traumatic rupture of the spleen and an increased splenic sequestration of blood cells contributing to anemia, leukopenia, and thrombocytopenia.

Ascites. Portal hypertension is the major factor determining the selective accumulation of fluid in the peritoneal cavity of patients with liver disease. The increased hydrostatic pressure in the splanchnic bed and in the relatively permeable hepatic sinusoids increases the transudation of lymph; when lymph formation exceeds the capacity of the lymphatic system to drain fluid from the abdomen, ascites accumulates. In the absence of sinusoidal congestion (as in patients with schistosomiasis or portal vein thrombosis), ascites is unusual; splanchnic congestion alone is insufficient to precipitate ascites. The lowered intravascular colloidal osmotic pressure in patients with hypoproteinemia contributes to the development of both ascites and peripheral edema. Patients with cirrhosis and ascites exhibit secondary hyperaldosteronism with increased rates of aldosterone secretion and excretion and elevated plasma hormone levels. The precise mechanism of the increased aldosterone secretion in these patients is not well defined, although it has been attributed to the splanchnic pooling of blood and a decrease in the systemic pool.

A right pleural effusion often accompanies tense ascites; this fluid has the same characteristics as the ascitic fluid and may result either from the direct leakage of ascitic fluid through the diaphragm or from the passage of lymph from the liver through the diaphragm.

Hepatic coma and precoma

Hepatic coma is a metabolic encephalopathy manifested by disturbances in higher integrative functions, fluctuating changes in the level of consciousness, psychiatric changes, impaired motor coordination along with increased reflexes, a flapping tremor and variable rigidity, and hyperventilation with respiratory alkalosis. Electroencephalography shows that high-amplitude slow waves (2 to 3 Hz) replace the normal α-waves. These neuropsychiatric abnormalities are observed in patients with metabolic encephalopathy from a variety of causes; patients with hepatic encephalopathy usually have overt clinical signs of liver disease and/or a major portal-systemic shunt (either spontaneous or surgically created). A marked hepatic fetor is usually present, particularly when portal-systemic shunting is a significant causal factor.

PATHOGENESIS OF HEPATIC COMA. Failure of the liver to detoxify exogenous substances such as depressant drugs or endogenous substances such as ammonia, coupled with a variable shunting of portal venous blood directly into the peripheral circulation, exposes the central nervous system to elevated blood levels of agents that are potentially toxic. Both clinical and experimental evidence suggest that ammonia may play a significant role in patients with chronic encephalopathy. Intestinal bacteria in the distal small bowel and colon generate ammonia by deamination of amino acids and hydrolysis of urea; a decrease in the rate of hepatic urea synthesis from ammonia increases the peripheral blood concentration of ammonia. The blood-brain barrier is relatively permeable to ammonia but limits the diffusion of ammonium ions; the pK of this weak alkali is such that a mild alkalosis reduces ionization and increases the ammonia diffusion. In experimental studies it has been shown that ammonia inhibits oxidative phosphorylation in the brain; this reversible metabolic change may be the biochemical basis for the disturbance of brain function.

In addition to ammonia, other products of bacterial metabolism can also accumulate and modify brain function; biogenic amines such as octopamine may act as false neurotransmitters.

In patients with liver disease, encephalopathy may also be precipitated by a variety of other metabolic stresses; those of particular clinical importance include the action of sedative agents or narcotics, disturbances of acid-base, fluid, and electrolyte balances (particularly hypokalemic alkalosis during diuretic therapy), infections, hypoxia, and hypoglycemia. Patients with cirrhosis may enter a deep coma following the administration of standard doses of a depressant drug, resulting in part from a decreased hepatic drug metabolism and in part from an increased brain sensitivity.

Impaired hepatic detoxification

The liver plays a central role in the detoxification and excretion of many endogenous and exogenous substances. Microsomal enzymes of the smooth endoplasmic reticulum participate in oxidative, hydrolytic, or conjugating reactions that modify organic substances and facilitate their excretion in either the bile or the urine. The activity of these enzyme systems may be genetically variable (for example, normal subjects may exhibit a slow or rapid acetylation of drugs) or may be stimulated by agents such as phenobarbital that induce hyperplasia of the smooth endoplasmic reticulum. The metabolism of individual compounds is influenced by hepatic blood flow, transport, and concentration in the liver cell and by enzyme activity;

other agents that are similarly metabolized may competitively inhibit the metabolism of a given substance.

CHANGES IN DRUG METABOLISM IN LIVER DISEASE. The distribution and metabolism of drugs can be affected by several mechanisms in patients with acute or chronic liver disease. Hypoalbuminemia resulting from impaired plasma protein synthesis modifies the distribution and action of drugs by decreasing drug binding in plasma. A reduced hepatic blood flow or portal-systemic shunting reduces the plasma clearance of agents with a high rate of extraction during a single pass through the liver; conversely, agents with a low single-passage clearance are unaffected by changes in the hepatic blood flow. A decrease in the number of liver cells (cirrhosis) or the activity of liver cells (acute hepatitis) usually decreases the capacity for metabolizing drugs. Cholestasis in patients without liver cell damage is associated with a decrease in the hepatic excretion and enterohepatic circulation of many agents and thus modifies the route of their excretion without depressing their metabolism.

In alcoholic patients several variables may modify the action and metabolism of drugs. Chronic alcoholics usually have an increased central nervous system tolerance to sedative agents that parallels their tolerance to ethanol. When such a patient has elevated blood levels of ethanol, the metabolism of drugs is usually depressed, whereas chronic alcoholics withdrawn from ethanol usually exhibit an increased activity of hepatic microsomal enzymes along with an increased metabolism of drugs. Finally, in patients in whom alcoholism has caused acute or chronic liver disease the metabolism of drugs is again depressed.

Although the hepatic metabolism of exogenous agents usually produces nontoxic metabolites, this process varies. Some drug metabolites such as propranolol metabolites remain therapeutically active, whereas others are hepatotoxic, such as the intermediates in the metabolism of acetaminophen (see discussion of "Toxic and drug-induced liver disease" later in this chapter).

CHANGES IN HORMONE METABOLISM. The endocrine abnormalities occurring in patients with liver disease may be only indirectly related to the liver disease or may result from changes in the distribution and metabolism of hormones by the liver.

Thyroid function in liver disease. There is an increased incidence of hypothyroidism and autoimmune thyroid disease in patients with idiopathic chronic active hepatitis and primary biliary cirrhosis. In alcoholic patients with liver disease there may be signs that suggest hyperthyroidism, such as a tremor, restlessness, hypermetabolism, tachycardia, and peripheral vasodilation; althogh altered levels of thyroid binding protein may modify the results of T_3 uptake tests, the serum thyroxine levels are usually normal.

Gonadal function in liver disease. *Hypogonadism* with testicular atrophy, impotence, and gynecomastia is particularly common in patients with cirrhosis. Malnutrition causes an endocrine dysfunction, and ethanol directly inhibits spermatogenesis. In cases of hemochromatosis, iron accumulation depresses the pituitary secretion of gonadotropins. Gynecomastia is associated with depressed levels of free testosterone and normal levels of estrogens. In women, chronic liver disease may suppress ovulation or lead to delayed menarche, oligomenorrhea, or amenorrhea.

Adrenal function in liver disease. A reduced plasma clearance of aldosterone contributes to the hyperaldosteronemia of patients with cirrhosis. Although liver disease may reduce the conjugation and excretion of glucocorticoids, normal regula-

tory mechanisms maintain normal plasma levels of free hormones.

Changes in nutrition and metabolism

MALNUTRITION. Malnutrition in patients with chronic liver disease may be caused by anorexia, a deficient diet, malabsorption. or increased catabolism. The diet of patients with alcoholic liver disease often is deficient in protein, folic and ascorbic acids, B vitamins, and minerals such as potassium, zinc, and magnesium; specific deficiencies in these patients may be accentuated by impaired utilization, such as the inhibition of folic acid utilization by ethanol, or by increased gastrointestinal or urinary losses of minerals. Chronic cholestasis increases the risk of a deficiency of the fat-soluble vitamins that require bile salt micelles for their intestinal absorption. In patients with liver failure the restriction of dietary protein for the control of hepatic encephalopathy accelerates muscle wasting and protein malnutrition.

CARBOHYDRATE METABOLISM. Because of the central role of the liver in regulating blood sugar levels by its uptake and conversion of monosaccharides to glycogen when carbohydrates are ingested and by the release of glucose from glycolysis or gluconeogenesis during fasting, it might be expected that liver disease would impair blood glucose homeostasis. Life-threatening hypoglycemia may complicate acute liver failure in patients with massive or multilobular hepatic necrosis (toxic or viral hepatitis with coma) or may be caused by impaired gluconeogenesis in alcoholics who drink after a period of fasting and in patients with Reye's syndrome or tetracycline toxicity. Hypoglycemia in patients with glycogen storage disease is the result of a genetically determined lack of the enzymes that control glycogenolysis. In some patients with a hepatocellular carcinoma (hepatoma), hypoglycemia results from a poor intake and glucose utilization by the neoplasm, whereas in others glycogen storage with impaired glucose release appears to play a major role.

Diabetes mellitus in patients with cirrhosis is the coincidental occurrence of two common diseases or may be causally related (as in cases of hemochromatosis or chronic pancreatic insufficiency in the alcoholic with cirrhosis). Liver biopsies in diabetic patients usually demonstrate fatty infiltration, but in some diabetic patients the pathologic features of acute alcoholic hepatitis—pericentral fibrosis and alcoholic hyalin—have been described; these patients may be at risk for the development of cirrhosis. A glucose load in a cirrhotic patient often leads to hyperglycemia resulting from a delayed uptake of glucose; fasting glucose levels, however, are normal in nondiabetic patients.

NITROGEN METABOLISM. The functions of the liver in the metabolism of amino acids and proteins include synthesis of nonessential amino acids, synthesis of liver and plasma proteins, catabolism of amino acids and proteins, and conversion of ammonia to urea. The plasma levels of amino acids and proteins are regulated by hepatic synthesis, secretion, and uptake.

In patients with acute liver disease, impaired plasma protein synthesis is quickly reflected by a fall in the concentration of proteins that have a short half-life—the clotting factors—rather than those with a long half-life such as albumin. A prolonged prothrombin time resulting from severe acute liver disease and impaired synthesis must be distinguished from decreased synthesis caused by malabsorption of vitamin K associated with cholestasis; if the prothrombin time does not become normal after parenteral vitamin K injection, the impaired synthesis is caused by liver failure. In comatose patients with acute hepatitis, a fall in the level of blood urea nitrogen, an increase in the level of ammonia in the blood, and increased plasma and urinary levels of amino acids reflect severe impairment of nitrogen metabolism. In patients with chronic liver disease a decrease in the concentration of plasma proteins synthesized by the liver may reflect protein malnutrition, depressed hepatic synthesis and secretion, or an expanded volume of distribution (with ascites). In stable patients with cirrhosis, reduced plasma protein synthesis is partially compensated for by decreased plasma protein catabolism.

FATTY ACID AND TRIGLYCERIDE METABOLISM. Fatty infiltration of the liver, evident histologically as membrane-bound triglyceride droplets in the parenchymal cells, either reflects an increase in stored triglyceride as in obese patients or results from derangements in liver cell metabolism. An excessive peripheral mobilization of triglyceride (in cases of uncontrolled diabetes mellitus) or impaired hepatic metabolism of fatty acids, derived from either the diet or fat depots (in cases of liver injury resulting from carbon tetrachloride, ethanol, or tetracycline), increases the hepatic level of triglyceride.

CHOLESTEROL, LIPOPROTEIN, AND BILE ACID METABOLISM. Cholesterol synthesis in the liver is regulated by the activity of the rate-limiting enzyme β-hydroxy-β-methylglutaric CoA reductase; the concentration of the primary bile acid, chenodeoxycholic acid, returning to the liver from the gut as it undergoes enterohepatic recirculation, appears to modulate enzyme activity. Newly synthesized hepatic cholesterol is incorporated into liver cell membranes, converted to the primary bile acids (cholic acid and chenodeoxycholic acid), secreted into bile or utilized in the synthesis of plasma lipoproteins that are secreted by the liver.

The normal processes that regulate plasma lipoprotein synthesis and degradation are only partly understood; both genetic and dietary factors play a role in regulating plasma levels of both low-density and high-density lipoproteins. In patients with liver disease, cholestasis increases the hepatic synthesis and secretion of a high-density lipoprotein rich in cholesterol and phospholipid; the plasma remains clear despite markedly elevated cholesterol levels. Conversely, when hepatic synthesis is impaired, serum cholesterol and lipoprotein levels are depressed, and a reduced fraction of esterified cholesterol in the plasma reflects the decreased plasma levels of the enzyme lecithin cholesterol acyl transferase (see later discussion of "Enzymes reflecting hepatic synthesis"). The taurine and glycine conjugates of the primary bile acids, cholic and chenodeoxycholic acid, serve two important detergent functions in the enterohepatic circulation; in bile they form mixed micelles with phospholipid and solubilize cholesterol, and in the upper jejunum they form mixed micelles with long-chain fatty acids and monoglyceride and facilitate the intestinal absorption of fat and fat-soluble vitamins (A, D, and K). The role of altered bile acid and cholesterol secretion in the pathogenesis of cholesterol gallstones is discussed in detail in Chapter 135; the role of altered bile acid metabolism in the pathogenesis of malabsorption is discussed in Chapter 125. Normally there is a highly efficient clearance of bile acids from portal blood as it passes through the hepatic sinusoids; thus most of the bile acid pool is retained within the enterohepatic circulation, and peripheral blood levels are low, rising only transiently after meals. Cholestasis, liver cell dysfunction, and portal-systemic shunting each decrease the hepatic clearance of bile acids and elevate peripheral blood levels, particularly after meals. An increased concentration of bile acid in the peripheral blood is a very sensitive but nonspecific index of liver disease.

Hematologic abnormalities

ANEMIA. Chronic anemia in patients with liver disease is usually mild and results from a variable shortening of the survival of red blood cells caused by an accelerated splenic sequestration of cells coupled with a suppression of erythropoiesis. Peripheral blood cells are usually normochromic and normocytic but may have macrocytic indices; the reticulocyte count is usually low. The plasma haptoglobin level may be depressed because of both increased red cell breakdown and reduced protein synthesis. Factors other than protein depletion and ethanol that depress erythropoiesis in cases of liver disease remain undefined. In alcoholic patients folate deficiency causing severe anemia and megaloblastic erythropoiesis responds dramatically to folate therapy. Severe hemolytic anemia may be associated with hyperlipidemia in some patients with acute alcoholic hepatitis or is precipitated by acute viral hepatitis in patients with glucose-6-phosphate dehydrogenase deficiency; brisk hemolysis in patients with liver disease usually causes a dramatic increase in serum bilirubin levels. Acute viral hepatitis rarely may be complicated by aplastic anemia.

Acute bleeding is a life-threatening complication of ruptured esophageal varices. Recurrent blood loss is an obvious cause of iron deficiency anemia in patients with cirrhosis. Lesions other than esophageal varices—gastroesophageal tears, erosive gastritis, ulcer disease, and neoplasm—must be considered in the differential diagnosis of upper gastrointestinal bleeding in patients with cirrhosis.

LEUKOPENIA AND THROMBOCYTOPENIA. Hypersplenism in patients with cirrhosis often causes a modest reduction in peripheral white cells and platelets, but this reduction is rarely responsible for infection or bleeding. Thrombocytopenia coupled with altered platelet function and gastric erosions caused by the ingestion of aspirin in patients with portal hypertension increases the risk of massive gastric mucosal hemorrhage.

CLOTTING ABNORMALITIES. The increased risk of bleeding in patients with depressed synthesis and plasma concentrations of clotting proteins can usually be corrected by a prophylactic infusion of fresh-frozen plasma; patients with liver disease who are bleeding massively also require the appropriate replacement of clotting proteins with fresh blood or fresh-frozen plasma. In severe cases of acute liver disease (hepatitis with coma) or decompensated cirrhosis complicated by septicemia, disseminated intravascular coagulation is often a terminal complication.

Immunologic manifestations

In patients with acute type A or B viral hepatitis, serologic changes reflect the immune response to the viral agents (see later discussion of "Acute viral hepatitis").

In patients with chronic liver disease, particularly chronic active hepatitis, idiopathic cirrhosis, and primary biliary cirrhosis, polyclonal hypergammaglobulinemia is often accompanied by serologic abnormalities. In patients with autoimmune chronic active hepatitis, serologic tests for antinuclear antibody, rheumatoid factor, and antimitochondrial and smooth muscle antibodies as well as LE cell tests are often positive. In primary biliary cirrhosis, immunologic abnormalities include increased plasma levels of IgM, a high titer of antimitochondrial antibodies and circulating immune complexes.

The role of immunologic mechanisms in the pathogenesis of these diseases of the liver is discussed in later sections describing individual diseases.

Circulatory and renal manifestations

Peripheral vasodilation, with a wide pulse pressure, and a precordial ejection systolic murmur are clinical signs of an increase in cardiac index that often accompanies liver failure. Vasoactive intestinal peptide, a duodenal hormone of the secretin group, may be responsible for these changes; with liver failure, the hormone escapes hepatic degradation, and peripheral blood levels increase.

Arterial oxygen saturation can be depressed in patients with cirrhosis and portal hypertension; when oxygen therapy does not correct this abnormality, the presence of vascular shunts that bypass pulmonary alveoli is suggested. These may be intrapulmonary arteriovenous shunts or portal-pulmonary shunts.

The total blood and plasma volumes are usually normal or slightly increased in patients with untreated cirrhosis. Portal hypertension, however, increases the relative volume of blood in the splanchnic bed. With the onset of ascites the renal blood flow and glomerular filtration remain normal, but tubular reabsorption of sodium is maximally stimulated by high aldosterone levels, and the urine is low in volume, is concentrated, and has a low sodium and an increased potassium content. With progressive liver failure, patients with terminal liver disease and ascites usually exhibit a decreasing creatinine clearance with progressive renal failure. This process is not a result of hypovolemia or decreased total renal blood flow but appears to be related to the intrarenal shunting of blood from the cortex to the medulla; the pathogenesis of this intrarenal circulatory change is unexplained. The term "hepatorenal syndrome" refers to this renal failure that complicates terminal liver disease.

CLINICAL AND LABORATORY ASSESSMENT OF PATIENTS
Assessment of liver function

The biochemical tests that are commonly performed in the evaluation of patients with liver disease do not provide a quantitative measure of liver function. These tests, however, are of value in establishing a differential diagnosis, in following the clinical course of patients with liver disease, and in determining their prognosis. In respect to any single liver disease the tests lack specificity (for example, elevations of the level of serum bilirubin are observed in patients with a wide range of liver diseases) and vary in their sensitivity (for example, jaundice develops in a minority of patients with acute viral hepatitis).

SERUM BILIRUBIN. In the van den Bergh reaction, formerly used to measure plasma levels of bilirubin, the amounts of diazopigment formed in the absence and presence of ethanol (direct and total reacting bilirubin) provided a measure of conjugated and total bilirubin concentrations. It is unfortunate that several of the methods that have been adapted for use by the autoanalyzer overestimate the levels of the conjugated fraction, particularly in patients with mild unconjugated hyperbilirubinemia.

In the absence of hemolysis an elevated serum bilirubin level is specific for liver disease but may result from impaired uptake or conjugation, parenchymal cell injury, or intrahepatic or extrahepatic cholestasis. Fractionation of the serum bilirubin level into conjugated and unconjugated fractions is of particular value in distinguishing patients with unconjugated hyperbilirubinemia caused by hemolysis or Gilbert's disease. Serial measurements of the total serum bilirubin are more accurate than the clinical evaluation of the degree of jaundice in following the course of icteric liver disease.

The serum bilirubin test is insensitive for liver disease. Many patients with acute hepatitis, cirrhosis, or extensive infiltrative disease may not have jaundice because of the high capacity of the liver to excrete conjugated bilirubin.

SERUM BILE ACIDS. Serum bile acid concentrations are measured by chromatographic and radioimmunoassay methods that are expensive and difficult to adapt for the routine clinical laboratory; these factors limit their clinical use. Fasting and/or postprandial levels of serum bile acids are usually elevated in patients with liver disease without jaundice; changes in the hepatic blood flow, parenchymal cell injury, or cholestasis reduces the hepatic clearance and excretion of bile acids. Serum bile acid measurements may be of particular value in the early detection of liver disease in patients exposed to potential hepatotoxins, such as occurs during methotrexate therapy for psoriasis; other liver tests have not been of value in detecting early progressive liver disease.

SULFOBROMOPHTHALEIN CLEARANCE. Sulfobromophthalein (BSP) is an organic anion that binds to albumin following intravenous injection and is subsequently concentrated by liver cells and secreted in bile partly as a glutathione conjugate. The plasma clearance of BSP, measured as the residual plasma concentration 30 or 45 minutes after an intravenous injection of the dye (5 mg/kg body weight), is a sensitive test for liver disease in patients without jaundice. The clinical value of this test has been offset by other diagnostic procedures and by the risk of local tissue necrosis if the agent is injected extravascularly, as well as by the rare occurrence of anaphylactic reactions.

SERUM ENZYMES
Enzymes reflecting liver cell injury. Enzymes present in high concentrations in liver cells are released with acute liver cell injury or necrosis; the levels of transaminases and lactic dehydrogenase are measured routinely, but many other enzymes have similar patterns of serum activity following acute liver injury. In patients with liver disease, serum transaminase levels in excess of 500 units (normally less than 40 units) indicate acute liver cell injury; values in a lower range are observed in patients with cholestasis and are of little value in a differential diagnosis. The serum glutamic-oxaloacetic transaminase may also originate from cardiac and skeletal muscle, as well as other sources. There is a poor correlation between the serum enzyme levels and the severity of liver cell necrosis revealed by liver biopsy; the enzyme has a relatively short half-life in the blood, and the time of sampling may not coincide with the period of maximal liver cell injury.

Enzymes reflecting cholestasis. Cholestasis, regardless of whether it is intrahepatic or extrahepatic, causes an increase in the serum activity of alkaline phosphatase, 5'-nucleotidase, leucine aminopeptidase, and γ-glutamyl transpeptidase. An elevation of the level of serum alkaline phosphatase is not a specific sign of liver disease because this enzyme may also arise from bone (with increased osteoblastic activity), from the gut, from the placenta during pregnancy, and from certain tumor cells (such as carcinoma of the lung); the site of the origin of the increased serum enzyme can be analyzed by isoenzyme patterns or can be more simply determined by measuring enzymes that are liver specific, such as γ-glutamyl transpeptidase. The mechanism causing the enzyme level elevation in patients with cholestasis appears to be an increase in enzyme synthesis and release into the plasma rather than reduced excretion; thus there is no correlation between serum levels of conjugated bilirubin and elevated enzyme levels.

Enzymes reflecting hepatic synthesis. The enzyme lecithin-cholesterol acyl transferase, which determines esterification of cholesterol in plasma, is synthesized by liver cells and secreted into the plasma. Depressed enzyme levels, as well as a reduced fraction of esterified cholesterol in the plasma, reflect an impaired hepatic protein synthesis in patients with liver failure. This enzyme is not measured routinely, but similar clinical information can be gained from other tests that measure protein synthesis in the liver (prothrombin time).

PLASMA PROTEINS

Albumin. Although a depressed level of serum albumin may reflect impaired hepatic protein synthesis, particularly in patients with chronic liver disease, other factors may also lower plasma levels; these include malnutrition, changes in the volume of distribution (with ascites), increased protein losses (with proteinuria, massive hemorrhage, or recurrent paracentesis), and hypercatabolism (with infections).

Globulins. The globulins are a large number of heterogeneous plasma proteins produced by the liver (α- and β-globulins) or by lymphoid cells (immunoglobulins). An electrophoretic or immunologic analysis of the concentration of individual globulins may be of diagnostic value. Lowered α_1-globulin levels occur in cases of α-1-antitrypsin deficiency, whereas extreme hypergammaglobulinemia occurs in patients with chronic active hepatitis.

Blood clotting factors. Depressed levels of blood clotting factors that are synthesized by the liver are reflected by changes in the prothrombin time. In patients with acute viral hepatitis a marked prolongation of the prothrombin time (greater than 20 seconds) is an early reflection of severe liver disease.

URINARY AND FECAL EXCRETION OF BILE PIGMENTS.

In patients with unconjugated hyperbilirubinemia the urine remains free of conjugated bilirubin (that is, the jaundice is *acholuric*); the binding of lipid-soluble unconjugated bilirubin to albumin does not permit glomerular filtration. At low plasma levels, conjugated bilirubin is excreted in the urine and therefore a darkening of the urine is an early symptom of cholestasis.

An excessive bilirubin production by hemolysis or ineffective erythropoiesis increases pigment excretion and is quantitatively reflected by the 24-hour fecal excretion of urobilinogen. The urine may contain higher concentrations of urobilinogen in patients with increased fecal pigment or in patients with parenchymal liver disease and an impaired hepatic excretion of absorbed urobilinogen. Liver disease increases the urinary excretion of uroporphyrin and coproporphyrin, which are normally excreted in bile; in patients with Dubin-Johnson syndrome there is a characteristic increase in the urinary excretion of coproporphyrin I.

Assessment for occult liver disease

Patients known to have a high risk for developing liver disease may benefit from an early recognition of liver involvement before the onset of the clinical illness.

GENETICALLY DETERMINED DISEASES.

In families with idiopathic hemochromatosis, those individuals most likely to be affected can be identified by HLA typing. Measurements of the serum levels of ferritin and iron and of the total iron-binding capacity provide evidence of excessive iron storage. The removal of excessive tissue iron by phlebotomy prevents parenchymal disease in the liver, endocrine system, and heart. Similarly, the early identification of patients with asymptomatic Wilson's disease by measurements of the plasma ceruloplasmin levels and the serum and urinary copper levels permits the use of chelation therapy and prevents progressive disease.

HEPATITIS B CARRIERS.

With the advent of the routine serologic screening of blood donors for hepatitis B infection, many hepatitis B carriers have been identified. Patients without signs of liver disease and with repeatedly normal serum transaminase levels have normal liver biopsies. Those with elevated levels of serum transaminases and hypergammaglobulinemia require a liver biopsy to document or exclude a diagnosis of chronic active hepatitis.

TOXIC HEPATITIS.

Patients who receive therapeutic agents that have a potential for causing liver disease not only should be informed of that risk but also if possible should be screened for the development of liver disease. In patients receiving isoniazid or methyldopa, a mild increase in the levels of serum transaminases precedes the onset of more severe, symptomatic, and potentially fatal acute hepatitis; high-risk patients receiving one of these agents should be screened with serial enzyme tests.

Not all patients with drug-related liver disease exhibit early changes demonstrated by the routine liver tests. In patients undergoing long-term methotrexate therapy for psoriasis, progressive hepatic fibrosis may develop that is not reflected by changes in the levels of serum enzymes; these patients require repeated liver biopsies at intervals of 6 to 12 months to prevent irreversible liver injury.

OCCUPATIONAL EXPOSURE TO POTENTIALLY TOXIC AGENTS.

Occupational exposure to the vinyl chloride monomer in the manufacturing of polyvinylchloride is associated with an increased risk of hepatic fibrosis or an angiosarcoma of the liver. The most appropriate prophylactic measures against liver disease in these patients are environmental measures to prevent exposure; biochemical abnormalities may be absent during the period of exposure.

NEOPLASMS INVOLVING THE LIVER.

The presence of metastatic disease in the liver may modify the patient's treatment and prognosis. The earliest biochemical changes preceding detectable liver enlargement are an increase in the levels of the serum enzymes associated with cholestasis (alkaline phosphatase, 5'-nucleotidase, and γ-glutamyl transpeptidase). Isotopic liver scanning and computed tomography of the liver are probably as sensitive as determinations of enzyme level elevations for establishing the presence of metastases in the liver; selective biopsies may be performed on lesions thus localized to provide a tissue diagnosis. The cost-benefit ratio for many of the relatively expensive scanning procedures used in the search for metastatic disease has not been established in prospective studies; such studies will be necessary to prevent the overuse of these procedures.

Assessment of the patient with jaundice

In most patients with jaundice the correct diagnosis can be determined from the medical history and physical examination; confirmation of this diagnosis may require additional studies. In other patients the diagnosis can be based only on diagnostic tests.

Biochemical studies usually support the clinical data base in differentiating four groups of patients: (1) those with unconjugated hyperbilirubinemia, (2) those with acute liver cell injury (hepatitis), (3) those with chronic parenchymal liver disease (cirrhosis), and (4) those with intrahepatic or extrahepatic cholestasis. The further evaluation of each of these groups is discussed in the following sections.

UNCONJUGATED HYPERBILIRUBINEMIA.

In adult patients hemolytic diseases and Gilbert's disease are the most common causes of unconjugated hyperbilirubinemia (see later discussion of "Disorders of bilirubin metabolism"). The patient with primary hemolytic disease usually is anemic and has an increased reticulocyte count and an increased fecal excretion of urobilinogen (see Chapter 67). Patients with Gilbert's disease exhibit fluctuating, mild jaundice with unconjugated hyperbilirubinemia but without anemia or other clinical or biochemical evidence of liver disease; they may need reassurance but require no further diagnostic studies.

ACUTE HEPATITIS. A diagnosis of acute drug-related or viral hepatitis is usually confirmed by a marked elevation of the levels of serum transaminases. A history of the use of a potentially toxic drug provides presumptive evidence of a drug-related illness; when the disorder is a hypersensitivity response, peripheral eosinophilia provides additional support for the diagnosis. The clinician usually must be satisfied with the patient's recovery following drug withdrawal; rechallenge with the drug to confirm the diagnosis unequivocally involves a high risk of death. In patients with viral hepatitis, serologic tests for hepatitis A antibody and the hepatitis B antigens may confirm the diagnosis (see later discussion of "Acute viral hepatitis"). A liver biopsy cannot differentiate between hepatitis caused by drugs or by viral agents; a needle biopsy is often of value, however, in the diagnosis of hepatitis with predominant cholestasis (see discussion of "Cholestasis").

CHRONIC PARENCHYMAL DISEASE (CIRRHOSIS). The cirrhotic patient with jaundice usually has other clinical signs of chronic liver disease and often exhibits other evidence of liver failure. When acute alcoholic hepatitis is responsible for jaundice with or without established cirrhosis, the ratio of the levels of serum transaminases in plasma (SGOT/SGPT) is usually in excess of 2:1. Ultrasonographic studies of the gallbladder, biliary tree, and pancreas are of value in excluding gallstones or an extrahepatic biliary obstruction from the diagnostic possibilities. A liver biopsy should be performed to confirm the diagnosis unless it is contraindicated by an increased risk of bleeding caused by a prolonged prothrombin time.

CHOLESTASIS. Biochemical tests are of minimal value in differentiating intrahepatic cholestasis from extrahepatic cholestasis. To document the cause of cholestasis the clinician must seek anatomic evidence of biliary tract obstruction. An ultrasonographic study of the biliary system usually documents the presence or absence of gallstones in the gallbladder and shows dilated intrahepatic and common bile ducts in patients with a complete extrahepatic obstruction of more than 10 days' duration. Computed tomography provides similar information about the biliary tree (at higher cost) but gives a better definition of pancreatic lesions. In patients without evidence of a biliary tract obstruction, a liver biopsy can be performed with minimal risk of bile peritonitis; this may confirm the presence of an intrahepatic lesion or may suggest an extrahepatic obstruction when the portal triads are edematous and infiltrated with polymorphonuclear cells. Patients with evidence of a biliary obstruction (dilated ducts shown by ultrasonography) usually can be examined preoperatively by transhepatic (Chiba fine needle) and/or retrograde cholangiography.

DISEASES OF THE LIVER
Disorders of bilirubin metabolism

GILBERT'S DISEASE. Gilbert's disease is a familial disorder of bilirubin transport, probably is inherited as an autosomal dominant trait, and is the most common cause of chronic, mild, unconjugated hyperbilirubinemia in adults.

Pathogenesis. A decrease in the rate of clearance of labeled bilirubin from the plasma of patients with Gilbert's disease suggests a hepatic uptake defect that requires a higher plasma level of unconjugated bilirubin to maintain the normal total bilirubin clearance. Compensated hemolysis accentuates the unconjugated hyperbilirubinemia in many patients. It has been reported that the activity of glucuronyl transferase is reduced in homogenates of liver obtained by a liver biopsy from patients with Gilbert's disease; it is possible that the same defect that impairs the bilirubin clearance from plasma also decreases the interaction between substrates and the enzyme system in vitro.

Clinical manifestations. Gilbert's disease is usually diagnosed in healthy young adults; if an intercurrent illness has led the patient to seek health care, the possibility of viral hepatitis is often considered. Concentrations of unconjugated bilirubin are usually less than 3 mg/dl (the normal level is less than 1 mg/dl) with exacerbations during febrile episodes or periods of fasting. Jaundice and unconjugated hyperbilirubinemia resolve completely when the subject is given a drug such as phenobarbital that stimulates hepatic microsomal drug metabolism.

Laboratory findings. The only laboratory abnormalities in patients with Gilbert's disease are an increase in unconjugated hyperbilirubinemia and possibly changes caused by mild compensated hemolysis: reticulocytosis and a lowered level of serum haptoglobin unaccompanied by anemia.

Differential diagnosis. Other causes for unconjugated hyperbilirubinemia must be considered; these include hemolytic disease, excessive bilirubin production without hemolysis, impaired hepatic uptake of bilirubin caused by drugs such as novobiocin, and parenchymal liver disease. Unconjugated bilirubinemia has been described during recovery from viral hepatitis (but may have resulted from coincidental Gilbert's disease) and also results from a delayed bilirubin clearance in cirrhotic patients with portacaval anastomoses.

Management. The mechanism causing jaundice should be explained to the patient, with reassurance concerning the benign nature of this disorder

CRIGLER-NAJJAR SYNDROME. Crigler-Najjar syndrome is a congenital, nonhemolytic, unconjugated hyperbilirubinemia associated with hepatic glucuronyl transferase deficiency.

Pathogenesis. The two types of Crigler-Najjar syndrome differ in their inheritance and in the severity of the metabolic defect. Patients with type I have an autosomal recessive defect that causes a complete lack of glucuronyl transferase activity in the liver; their serum bilirubin levels range from 25 to 31 mg/dl, and their bile is colorless. Patients with type II have an autosomal dominant defect causing a low level of hepatic glucuronyl transferase activity; their bilirubin levels are lower than those in patients with the type I defect, and the administration of phenobarbital decreases their jaundice by increasing hepatic conjugation and excretion of bilirubin.

Clinical manifestations. Patients with type I Crigler-Najjar syndrome usually die of severe kernicterus in infancy. Those with type II disease may have kernicterus in childhood but may also survive to adulthood without central nervous system damage. Deep acholuric jaundice may be the only clinical feature.

Differential diagnosis. There are no other causes for severe, chronic unconjugated hyperbilirubinemia in adults.

Management. Adult patients should receive genetic counseling with respect to the risk of transmitting the defect. Treatment with phenobarbital decreases jaundice in the adult but may require sedative doses. With infants, vigorous measures to prevent kernicterus may improve the chances of survival in patients with type II disease.

DUBIN-JOHNSON SYNDROME. Dubin-Johnson syndrome is an autosomal recessive disorder of hepatic transport of conjugated bilirubin and other organic anions into bile.

Pathogenesis. Patients with Dubin-Johnson syndrome have a normal hepatic uptake and conjugation of bilirubin but an impaired secretion of the conjugated pigment into the bile canaliculus; conjugated bilirubin returns to the plasma and is excreted in the urine. The transport defect is not confined to conjugated bilirubin; the biliary excretion of other organic anions, both endogenous (coproporphyrin I and metanephrine glucuronide) and exogenous (iopanoic acid [Telepaque], BSP, and indocyanine green), is also reduced. The striking black pigmentation of the liver that increases with the age of the patients with this syndrome has been attributed to the conversion of retained metanephrine glucuronide to melanin pigments. The impaired excretion of iodinated compounds, such as iopanoic acid, used in contrast roentgenography explains why the gallbladder is not seen on oral cholecystograms. The enterohepatic circulation of bile acids is normal in these patients, suggesting a dual transport mechanism for the organic constituents of bile.

Clinical manifestations. Patients with Dubin-Johnson syndrome usually have mild jaundice that is often first noted during pregnancy when the excretion of bilirubin may be further impaired by increased hormone levels. Dark urine reflects the excretion of conjugated bilirubin. Unlike patients with cholestasis, these patients do not have pruritus, and the liver is normal in size. Intermittent and usually mild right upper quadrant discomfort has been described in some patients; this is unexplained.

Laboratory findings. Biochemical studies typically show mild to moderate elevations of conjugated bilirubin (usually lower than 10 mg/dl) with normal levels of serum alkaline phosphatase, transaminase, and serum proteins. Fasting and postprandial serum bile acid levels are normal. BSP excretion is atypical of patients with cholestasis; BSP retention is accompanied by a late increase in plasma BSP levels caused by the appearance of conjugated dye. There is a selective increase in the urinary excretion of coproporphyrin I that differs from the pattern of increased coproporphyrin III excretion in patients with cholestasis.

The diagnosis of Dubin-Johnson syndrome is confirmed by the presence of dark pigment in the liver cells, particularly in the centrilobular areas.

Differential diagnosis. Intrahepatic or extrahepatic cholestasis can be differentiated from this syndrome by the elevation of the levels of serum enzymes, alkaline phosphatase, 5'-nucleotidase, or γ-glutamyl transpeptidase, by the presence of pruritus and elevated serum bile acid levels, and by the morphologic or anatomic lesions causing cholestasis.

Management. The patient should be educated and reassured about the benign nature of this syndrome. No treatment is indicated.

ROTOR'S SYNDROME. It was formerly thought that Rotor's syndrome was a variant of Dubin-Johnson syndrome; there are, however, significant biochemical and morphologic differences. In patients with Rotor's syndrome retention of conjugated bilirubin is not accompanied by hepatic pigmentation, oral cholecystography usually has normal results, and urinary excretion of coproporphyrin I is not increased.

BENIGN RECURRENT INTRAHEPATIC CHOLESTASIS. Benign recurrent intrahepatic cholestasis is a rare, often familial disorder characterized by recurrent episodes of unexplained intrahepatic cholestasis. The first attack may occur during childhood, and the onset of each episode is usually acute and accompanied by variable nausea and vomiting; pruritus with dark urine and light stools accompanies the jaundice for periods of several months. A liver biopsy reveals the changes of intrahepatic cholestasis—bile stasis in dilated canaliculi—and mononuclear infiltration of the portal triads. Between attacks both liver function and hepatic morphology are normal.

Acute viral hepatitis

Viral hepatitis is an infectious disease caused by several hepatotropic viruses; these include hepatitis A virus (HAV), hepatitis B virus (HBV), non-A, non-B agents, and the hepatitis delta virus (HDV). HAV infection formerly was called infectious hepatitis or short-incubation hepatitis. HBV infection previously was called serum hepatitis, homologous serum jaundice, posttransfusion hepatitis, or long-incubation hepatitis. HAV and HBV infections are now based on immunologic rather than clinical or epidemiologic information. Infection by NANB agents cannot be defined by serologic studies at this time; an NANB viral agent is assumed when serologic tests exclude injection with other agents. HDV infection is associated with HBV infection; the delta agent is a defective RNA virus that requires HBV infection for its expression.

ETIOLOGY. HAV is a 27-nm DNA enterovirus of a single serotype. Acute HAV infection is associated with the presence of virus in the liver, bile and stool during the preicteric period of illness. Infection is associated with an early immunologic response with the appearance of IgM anti-HAV during the acute illness. The later IgG anti-HAV response provides lifelong immunity to further infection.

HBV is a capsulated DNA virus. Infection is associated with the appearance of high concentrations of viral antigen in the blood; 22-nm particles present as spheres or filaments correspond to the surface coat of the virus and are referred to as the hepatitis B surface antigen (HB_sAg); 42-nm particles of intact virus (Dane particle) are present in smaller numbers and consist of an outer surface coat (HB_sAg) and a 27-nm virus core. Antigens associated with the virus core have been designated as core antigen (HB_cAg) and e-antigen (HB_eAg); DNA polymerase activity is also associated with the virus core. Antibodies to core antigen (anti-HB_c) appear soon after the onset of acute hepatitis but do not appear to limit that infection; anti-HB_c in the IgM fraction suggests recent infection. Antibodies to surface (anti-HB_s) and e-antigen (anti-HB_e) usually are associated with resolution of HBV infection.

Non-A, non-B hepatitis agents have not been identified serologically. Epidemiologic studies suggest that there are at least two viral agents. One is transmitted parenterally with a long incubation period, and the other has been implicated in short-incubation outbreaks of waterborne hepatitis.

The HDV agent is a defective RNA virus that is infective in man and in experimental primates only in association with hepatitis B surface antigen.

EPIDEMIOLOGY

Acute type A viral hepatitis. Hepatitis A may occur as a sporadic illness or in epidemic outbreaks. The virus is excreted in a high titer in the stool of acutely infected patients for a period of several days at the onset of the acute illness. The virus usually is transmitted by the fecal-oral route. Epidemic outbreaks have been traced to contaminated drinking water and to the ingestion of contaminated shellfish that filter and concentrate the virus; the virus may not be inactivated by steaming bivalves. Male homosexual subjects have an increased risk of infection, and primate handlers have a high risk of infection from animals with an anicteric infection. Hepatitis A virus infection results in lasting immunity with high circulating titers of anti-HAV antibody. In underdeveloped areas with poor sanitation, infection is most common in the young; in areas with optimal sanitation older age-groups remain susceptible.

Acute type B viral hepatitis. Transmission of hepatitis B virus usually is related to the high titer of the virus that may be present in the blood of patients with acute or chronic illness or in healthy carriers. The following modes of transmission have been well documented.

Parenteral transmission. Epidemics of hepatitis B infection have been associated with the use of vaccines containing pooled human serum, such as with yellow fever vaccine during World War II, and the recurrent use of inadequately sterilized tattoo needles or syringes and needles, such as in early venereal disease clinics using intravenous arsenicals. Recipients of blood transfusions, particularly of several units obtained from paid donors, in the past were very likely to have an acute infection. With the routine use of sensitive screening tests for HB_sAg, the healthy carrier of HBV has been virtually eliminated from the donor pool, and the transmission of the virus by blood transfusion is now rare. There are certain blood fractions, however, that still contain significant titers of virus; pooled plasma, fibrinogen, and factor VII concentrates may transmit infection. Parenteral drug abuse with shared, unsterilized needles is a major cause of infection in the young adult and adolescent population.

Vertical transmission. The risk of HBV transmission from mother to infant is greatest when the mother has an acute hepatitis B infection during the last trimester of pregnancy or immediately after delivery; although HB_sAg has been detected in some samples of cord blood, the highest risk of infection appears to occur during delivery. Maternal HBV carriers who have high titers of HB_sAg, who are HB_eAg positive, and who have previous children with serologic evidence of infection are most likely to transmit hepatitis B in subsequent pregnancies. The high incidence of the hepatitis B carrier state in several African and Asian populations may be related to the vertical transmission of the disease; most infected infants become carriers.

Nonparenteral transmission. Many patients with a serologically documented HBV infection do not have a history of parenteral exposure by a transfusion or needle. Although epidemiologic studies in a closed population of mentally defective children provided evidence for the nonparenteral transmission of hepatitis B, possibly by fecal-oral exposure, such transmission may require intimate contact. The familial clustering of hepatitis B infections may result in part from vertical transmission and in part from nonparenteral transmission. The possibility that the infection can be transmitted venereally is supported by the high incidence of HBV infections among homosexual males (30% to 50% have either HB_sAg or anti-HB_s), but the incidence of infection among the spouses of HB_sAg-positive carriers is no greater than among family members.

Nosocomial transmission. Surgeons, dental surgeons, and hospital personnel who have direct contact with blood (operating room, dialysis, and laboratory staff) have an increased risk of accidental parenteral exposure to HBV; the evidence of a past infection among these health care personnel demonstrates an incidence (16.8%) twice that in a matched population. Transmission from unrecognized carriers is probably more common in these personnel than that from patients with a known hepatitis infection. The relatively high rate of infection among health care personnel raises the question of whether HBV might be transmitted to patients. One epidemiologic study concluded that an inhalation therapist with a severe exudative dermatitis on both hands transmitted hepatitis B to two patients in an intensive care unit. There have also been well-documented outbreaks of hepatitis B among patients treated by oral surgeons who were subsequently found to be HB_sAg-positive. Serologic studies comparing the incidence of past HBV infections among the patients of HB_sAg-positive and HB_sAg-negative surgeons provide no additional evidence of this hepatitis B transmission. The potential risk of hepatitis B transmission occurring during dental surgery may be reduced by the routine use of operating gloves.

Acute non-A, non-B viral hepatitis. Serologic studies of patients with posttransfusion hepatitis have documented the presence of transmissable agent(s) serologically distinct from hepatitis A and B viruses. Non-A, non-B infections have become the most common cause of posttransfusion hepatitis, particularly in patients receiving several units of blood. A chronic carrier state has been identified in one patient following an acute infection.

The sporadic occurrence of non-A, non-B hepatitis not associated with a transfusion or accidental inoculation is evidence of nonparenteral transmission; a recent epidemic of waterborne hepatitis serologically distinct from hepatitis A and B provides strong evidence for the fecal-oral transmission of another viral agent. The further characterization of non-A, non-B agents awaits the development of serologic methods to identify these viruses and their antibodies.

HDV agent. Acute HDV infection may be concurrent with acute HBV infection or may be superimposed on chronic HBV infection. The routes of infection parallel those for HBV. HDV infection may be responsible for severe, acute exacerbations of hepatitis in patients with chronic HBV infection.

CLINICAL MANIFESTATIONS. The clinical manifestations of acute hepatitis resulting from viruses A, B, and non-A, non-B are similar. Differences in the incubation period following exposure have been well documented in experimental studies but usually cannot be defined in a clinical setting. Thus the diagnosis of the causative viral agent is usually based on serologic tests. The varying clinical pattern of infection with the hepatitis virus appears to be influenced by the age, nutrition, and immune status of the patient; the factors that affect the severity of the illness are not well defined.

The clinical spectrum of acute viral hepatitis includes the following typical and atypical patterns of the disease. The first three are typical patterns; the last two are atypical patterns.

1. Infection without clinical evidence of hepatitis
2. Anicteric hepatitis
3. Icteric hepatitis
4. Cholestatic viral hepatitis
5. Fulminant viral hepatitis

Infection without clinical evidence of hepatitis. Many subjects exposed to the hepatitis viruses remain well without evidence of liver disease. A transiently positive test for HB_sAg or a rising titer of IgM antibodies to the hepatitis agents (anti-HA or anti-HB_s) provides immunologic evidence of infection. Serum transaminase levels may be increased for a variable period.

Anicteric hepatitis. Patients with anicteric hepatitis usually exhibit the prodromal symptoms of a viral illness (malaise, anorexia, nausea and vomiting, headache, and fever); abdominal discomfort may focus the physician's attention on a mildly enlarged tender liver. Although the patient remains anicteric, the urine may become dark because of the excretion of conjugated bilirubin. In infants and young children, HAV infection often is associated with diarrhea. The symptomatic illness is usually of brief duration and coincides with the onset of elevated serum transaminase levels. Although patients with anicteric hepatitis usually recover completely, a significant percentage of those with a hepatitis B or non-A, non-B infection have late sequelae; chronic persistent hepatitis, chronic active hepatitis, or a chronic carrier state.

Icteric hepatitis. The *preicteric* or prodromal phase of icteric hepatitis may be abrupt in onset (usually in type A) or may develop insidiously (often in types B and non-A, non-B) with symptoms common to many viral illnesses. Fever usually is maximal at the onset of the illness and may persist until the onset of jaundice. Malaise, weakness, headache, and myalgia are relatively common, and gastrointestinal symptoms including nausea, vomiting, and anorexia, along with right upper quadrant abdominal pain, are prominent complaints; there may also be a striking loss of taste for cigarettes. During the preicteric period patients with an HBV infection may exhibit the clinical manifestations of circulating immune complexes, which include maculopapular, urticarial, or petechial skin rashes, arthralgias, or acute arthritis. Late in the preicteric period hepatic enlargement and tenderness are usual, and the urine becomes dark before jaundice develops.

The *icteric phase* is one of increasing jaundice, with peak serum bilirubin levels usually less than 10 mg/dl within 10 to 14 days, followed by a slower decline to normal levels. The patient's symptoms usually improve within a few days of the onset of jaundice, although anorexia may persist for a longer period and pruritus increases in those with progressive cholestasis. The liver may remain enlarged through the icteric period, but tenderness usually declines during the early icteric phase. Splenomegaly may be noted during the acute illness.

The *convalescent phase* following the disappearance of jaundice may be brief but may extend over several months, accompanied by complaints of malaise, early fatigue, particularly after an unaccustomed activity, and mild hepatic tenderness. During this period the levels of serum transaminases may remain mildly elevated.

Cholestatic viral hepatitis. Cholestatic viral hepatitis is a relatively uncommon clinical pattern of HAV infection in which fairly typical icteric hepatitis passes into a more prolonged cholestatic phase with deep jaundice, marked pruritus, and prominent biochemical features of intrahepatic cholestasis. Despite the deep jaundice, which may persist over several weeks, the patient usually feels relatively well and does not appear to be seriously ill. Liver enlargement with minimal tenderness often persists during the period of jaundice. Diarrhea in these patients results from the cathartic action of fatty acids that are poorly absorbed with low intestinal concentration of bile acids.

Fulminant viral hepatitis. In patients with fulminant viral hepatitis (viral hepatitis with coma), extensive hepatic necrosis causes acute hepatic failure with coma and commonly leads to death. This is a rare complication of acute hepatitis (1% of icteric patients) caused by viruses A, B, non-A, non-B, or D. Clinically, the preicteric period may be brief and accompanied by severe abdominal pain, vomiting, and a high fever that persist despite bed rest. A sudden decrease in liver size, the early development of drowsiness, irritability, insomnia, or confusion, a marked prolongation of the prothrombin time that is not corrected by the parenteral administration of vitamin K, and signs of fluid retention are clinical features that suggest a fulminant course. The progression of hepatic failure leads to deepening hepatic encephalopathy accompanied by hyperventilation and respiratory alkalosis, convulsions (particularly in children), progressive stupor, and coma. Clinical problems that can be anticipated in these patients include hypoglycemia, severe bleeding caused by a deficiency in clotting factor synthesis, aspiration pneumonia or septicemia, lactic acidosis, cardiac arrhythmias or arrest, and renal failure.

LABORATORY FINDINGS. Liver cell damage and necrosis are reflected by an increase in serum levels of the transaminases; elevation of enzyme levels during recovery indicates persistent

disease activity (see later discussions of "Chronic persistent hepatitis" and "Chronic active hepatitis"). In icteric patients, both conjugated and unconjugated serum bilirubin levels become elevated; the increase in conjugated bilirubin is caused by impaired liver cell excretion of the conjugated pigment or intrahepatic cholestasis. Serum alkaline phosphatase levels rise during the icteric period and reach their peak values later than the peak values of transaminase; the most marked elevation occurs in patients with severe cholestasis. In patients with typical icteric hepatitis, serum albumin may fall slightly late in the clinical course. Hypoprothrombinemia indicates liver failure or a vitamin K deficiency in deeply jaundiced patients. During the recovery period a slight increase in serum γ-globulin levels is consistent with uncomplicated disease; marked elevations suggest the possibility of chronic active hepatitis.

Hematologic findings early in acute illness may include leukopenia along with relative lymphocytosis or the presence of atypical mononuclear cells. A mild anemia often develops during the course of the illness, resulting from a reduced bone marrow response to repeated blood drawing. In rare cases the acute illness may be complicated by severe thrombocytopenia, hemolytic disease (particularly in patients with glucose-6-phosphate dehydrogenase deficiency), or aplastic anemia.

Serologic tests. In patients with acute type A hepatitis, anti-HA antibodies usually develop during the period of jaundice; the early immune response produces a high titer of IgM antibody followed by rising titers of IgG antibody. Patients with hepatitis B usually exhibit the viral antigens HB_sAg, HB_eAg, and DNA polymerase during the preicteric and early icteric phases. The hepatitis B antibodies anti-HB_s and anti-HB_e usually appear in the early icteric period when the antigens are cleared from the blood. In patients who recover but remain in a carrier state and in patients with chronic persistent or chronic active hepatitis, the hepatitis B antigens usually persist along with anti-HB_e but not anti-HB_s or anti-HB_e. Patients with HDV infection may exhibit IgM anti-D antibody in low titer during acute infections; chronic infection is associated with both IgM and IgG anti-D antibodies in high titer.

PATHOLOGY. In patients with typical viral hepatitis, regardless of whether it is asymptomatic, anicteric, or icteric, a liver biopsy shows evidence of parenchymal cell degeneration or necrosis, infiltration with inflammatory cells with proliferation of Kupffer's cells, and evidence of cell regeneration. Damaged parenchymal cells enlarge with ballooning of their cytoplasm or may undergo hyaline degeneration to form acidophilic bodies with pyknotic nuclei (Councilman's bodies); these degenerating cells are scattered focally throughout the liver lobule. Cell necrosis usually is balanced by cell regeneration that can be recognized by the presence of mitotic figures or multinucleated cells. Within the liver lobule, hyperplastic Kupffer's cells accumulate cell debris as an acid-fast pigment, lipofuscin, and foci of mononuclear cells collect at sites of cell necrosis.

In the portal tracts there are variable edema and an infiltration of inflammatory cells that are predominantly mononuclear. There may be evidence of ductular epithelial injury with cell vacuolation and later ductular proliferation. The inflammatory infiltrate expanding the portal triads usually persists into the later convalescent period when signs of parenchymal cell injury have resolved. A complete histologic recovery is the usual outcome.

Patients with cholestatic hepatitis usually exhibit varying degrees of parenchymal cell necrosis and inflammatory infiltration. In addition, the intrahepatic cholestasis is reflected histologically by the presence of bile plugs in dilated bile canaliculi, particularly in the central zones, and increased bile staining of parenchymal cells and Kupffer's cells.

In patients with fulminant hepatitis, liver biopsies performed early in the acute illness usually show multilobular zones of necrosis with the collapse of the reticulum framework of the normal lobule. Autopsies have shown that massive necrosis leads to a shrunken, bile-stained liver (acute yellow atrophy) with extensive areas of lobular collapse, few mononuclear inflammatory cells, and residual liver cells only in some areas adjacent to the preserved portal triads. In patients who survive fulminant hepatitis, normal lobular structure of the liver regenerates completely without fibrosis.

Some patients with typical icteric hepatitis, particularly those with a more prolonged course of severe disease, may have bridging or multilobular necrosis demonstrated by a liver biopsy rather than the typical focal necrosis. Clinically, these patients may recover without sequelae, or the disease may progress rapidly to fulminant hepatitis; chronic active hepatitis with progressive fibrosis and cirrhosis is more likely to develop in these patients than in patients with focal necrosis alone.

MANAGEMENT. There are no specific measures that significantly modify the course of typical acute viral hepatitis. The symptomatic patient usually feels better with bed rest, but progressive ambulation should be permitted as the patient improves and feels well. The patient should be encouraged to eat a normal diet of foods that appeal to him; specific restrictions are unnecessary. When anorexia or nausea is prolonged and the patient's caloric intake is not optimal, oral or intravenous supplements may be necessary. Most patients can be treated at home; hospitalization is indicated for high-risk patients—pregnant, diabetic, or elderly patients and those with complicating disease—and for those who are judged to be severely ill and are vomiting or have an elevated prothrombin time. Although corticosteroid therapy may accelerate the patient's biochemical improvement, the duration of the illness is not shortened, and a relapse appears to be more likely when the therapy ends; corticosteroid therapy is thus not indicated.

When the diagnosis has been established, further laboratory tests should be performed as necessary to monitor the patient's progress. When the patient is acutely ill, a daily measurement of the prothrombin time after a vitamin K injection (10 mg intramuscularly) is of value in detecting a sudden deterioration in liver function. Measurements of the levels of serum bilirubin and enzymes at intervals of several days during the acute illness and at longer intervals during recovery provide objective data on the patient's course.

Drugs should be given cautiously to the acutely ill patient; the reduced activity of hepatic microsomal drug metabolizing enzymes may lead to a delayed plasma clearance of many sedative agents. Oxazepam (Serax) is an ideal sedative for patients with acute hepatitis, because the volume of distribution, plasma binding, clearance, and excretion of this agent are not modified in acute hepatitis.

In patients with prominent cholestasis and severe itching, cholestyramine (up to 4 g three times a day) may provide symptomatic relief; this agent increases the malabsorption of fat-soluble vitamins and precipitates a vitamin K deficiency unless vitamin K is replaced parenterally.

Patients with fulminant hepatitis require intensive nursing care and support. A comatose patient requires a cuffed endotracheal tube and assisted ventilation, if necessary, to prevent aspiration and to ensure adequate ventilation. Continuous intravenous administration of glucose is necessary to provide calories and to prevent hypoglycemia in the absence of glycogen stores or gluconeogenesis. Bleeding may be controlled by infusions of fresh-frozen plasma to replace clotting factors, and measures to eliminate the ammonia production by intestinal bacteria should include cleansing enemas, the intragastric instillation of neomycin (4 to 6 g daily), and dietary protein elimination. Gastric neutralization achieved with antacids or intravenously infused histamine H_2-receptor blocking drugs reduces the risk of massive bleeding from stress erosions in the stomach. Therapy with high doses of corticosteriods has been shown to increase the mortality of patients with severe viral hepatitis; the earlier use of these drugs was based on uncontrolled observations. Many measures have been proposed for eliminating potential toxins normally removed by the liver, in the hope that this would reverse the coma and improve the survival rate; these measures include hemodialysis, plasmapheresis or an exchange transfusion, cross-perfusion with a human volunteer or primate, and charcoal hemoperfusion. Although these procedures may temporarily restore the patient's consciousness, they have not increased the survival rate of patients with fulminant hepatitis. In adult patients, whose chance of survival from deep coma is limited (hepatic regeneration is less active in adults than in children), orthotopic liver transplantation should be considered.

PROGNOSIS. Most patients recover completely from typical viral hepatitis. Some patients, however, have benign or serious sequelae. Early recovery from acute hepatitis may be followed by a relapse. A chronic carrier state without liver disease, chronic persistent hepatitis lasting for more than 6 months, or chronic active hepatitis may follow an acute infection with HBV or non-A, non-B viruses.

Relapsing acute hepatitis. The relapse of acute hepatitis is usually milder than the initial episode but has similar clinical, laboratory, and pathologic features. The acute exacerbation may occur during the convalescent period or following complete clinical and biochemical recovery. The possibility that late relapses result from an infection by a different viral agent usually has not been excluded by serologic tests. At the onset of a relapse the patient usually notes a decrease in appetite with malaise and fatigue, and the liver again becomes enlarged and tender. The prognosis for full recovery following a relapse does not differ from that of the initial attack, and in the absence of clinical, biochemical, or histologic evidence of chronic active hepatitis the patient can be reassured.

Chronic hepatitis B carrier state. Following recovery from acute hepatitis B, regardless of whether it is asymptomatic, anicteric, or icteric, some patients fail to clear the hepatitis B antigens from the blood and remain carriers for a long period. The incidence of the chronic carrier state following infection is greatest in infancy and early childhood, possibly because of a greater immune tolerance, and in patients undergoing immunosuppressive therapy or long-term renal dialysis. The hepatitis B carrier may exhibit no clinical, biochemical, or pathologic evidence of liver disease, may be asymptomatic with minor elevations of serum transaminase levels, or may have progressive chronic active hepatitis.

The major considerations in the management of the hepatitis B carrier are to define the presence or absence of progressive liver disease and to prevent the transmission of the disease. Patients with normal levels of serum enzymes demonstrated by repeated testing do not require further diagnostic assessment; liver biopsies do not show evidence of liver disease. Patients with elevated levels of serum transaminases may have chronic persistent hepatitis (a benign process) or chronic active hepatitis (a progressive disease); the latter is particularly likely if γ-globulin levels are elevated. A liver biopsy is indicated in patients with abnormal liver function to differentiate these disorders.

The hepatitis B carrier with a low titer of HB_sAg and a negative test result for HB_eAg with anti-HB_e probably has a low risk of transmitting the disease. The risk of the nonparenteral transmission of hepatitis is minimized with careful practice of personal hygiene. Some experimental studies have indicated that the use of interferon can terminate the carrier state, but this treatment is not currently clinically available.

Chronic persistent hepatitis. Chronic persistent hepatitis is a benign form of chronic hepatitis B or non-A, non-B that follows an acute infection. The patient may be asymptomatic or mildly symptomatic and may have lethargy, weakness, and mild hepatic tenderness; jaundice if present is mild, with a minimal, fluctuating elevation of serum transaminase levels and mild changes of acute hepatitis demonstrated by a liver biopsy. The disease often persists for months or years, but complete recovery is the final outcome. (Chronic active hepatitis is discussed in a later section.)

PROPHYLAXIS
General measures. Good personal hygiene is a major factor in reducing the fecal-oral transmission of the hepatitis viruses. Enteric precautions should be maintained with hospitalized patients who have acute hepatitis during the symptomatic period of early illness; the fecal excretion of hepatitis A virus does not extend into the later icteric phase (after 1 to 2 weeks of icterus) when the patient is recovering. Contact with infected blood should be avoided through the use of gloves, the careful disposal of needles, and the appropriate labeling and handling of blood specimens.

Prevention of transfusion-associated hepatitis. The use of sensitive tests for hepatitis B antigens has greatly reduced the incidence of posttransfusion hepatitis B. The risk of the transmission of hepatitis B virus by concentrates of antihemophilic globulin has been decreased experimentally by the addition of hepatitis B immune globulin (HBIG). Serologic tests to screen for carriers of non-A, non-B hepatitis are not yet available commercially; the risk of this infection may be decreased by excluding commercial donors and those with elevated serum transaminase levels.

Cleaning and sterilizing instruments and equipment. Instruments should be cleaned by a person wearing protective gloves and if possible should be sterilized by autoclaving before being used again. When heat sterilization is not possible, such as with fiberoptic endoscopes, effective cold sterilizing procedures should be used.

Prevention by passive immunization. Two preparations of γ-globulin are commercially available for hepatitis prophylaxis. Normal serum globulin (ISG) contains high titers of anti-HA and low titers (1:80) of anti-HB_s. Hepatitis B immune globulin (HBIG) prepared from specific immune sera has high titers of anti-HB_s. The recommendations of the U.S. Public Health Service for hepatitis prophylaxis are as follows.

Hepatitis A. Preexposure prophylaxis is recommended for travelers planning to visit tropical or developing countries; a single injection of 2 ml of ISG (in adults) is recommended for those staying less than 3 months and 5 ml for those staying 3 or more months, followed by repeated ISG injections at 4- to 6-month intervals. A similar schedule of ISG prophylaxis is recommended for those who handle recently imported primates.

Postexposure prophylaxis with ISG (0.02 ml/kg) is recommended within 2 weeks of exposure for those in close personal contact with a person who has hepatitis A, such as contact occurring within a household. Prophylaxis is of value for contacts within institutions when there is evidence of a hepatitis A outbreak; the risk of an institutional spread of the infection appears to be particularly high among those in contact with children under the age of 2 years who have anicteric infection.

Hepatitis B. Postexposure prophylaxis with HBIG (0.05 ml/kg) currently is recommended immediately after a single acute parenteral (needle) or oral exposure to infected blood, and at the time of delivery in infants of mothers who are HB_sAg carriers or who have suffered from HBV infection during the third trimester (0.13 ml/kg). HBIG should be followed by hepatitis B vaccination to establish active immunity.

The value of immune prophylaxis for non-A, non-B hepatitis has not yet been determined.

Active immunization. Plasma-derived or recombinant HB vaccine given in three doses over a 6-month period is effective in establishing active immunity (anti-HB_s) in over 95% of healthy adults and 99% of children. A poorer response (64%) has been reported in hemodialysis recipients. Preexposure vaccination is recommended for the following individuals: healthcare workers with exposure to blood or potential needle stick; patients and staff of institutions for the developmentally disabled; hemodialysis patients; homosexually active men; users of illicit injectable drugs; recipients of clotting factor concentrates; household and sexual contacts of HBV carriers; and members of any other group defined as being at high risk. In individuals with a particularly high risk of HB infection, initial serologic testing for evidence of HBV infection may be cost effective in selecting for vaccination those without previous exposure.

HEPATITIS RESULTING FROM OTHER VIRAL AGENTS
Infectious mononucleosis. When a patient has infectious mononucleosis, the liver usually is involved. Jaundice is relatively uncommon, but when it occurs it usually is cholestatic unless there is brisk hemolysis, and the liver may be slightly enlarged and tender; biochemical signs of mild cholestasis (elevated levels of serum alkaline phosphatase, 5'-nucleotidase, and γ-glutamyl transpeptidase) commonly accompany portal infiltration with mononuclear cells. The prognosis for complete recovery is excellent; no patients with infectious mononucleosis have had fulminant hepatitis or documented chronic liver disease.

Other viral infections in immunocompromised patients or neonates. *Congenital rubella* infections are commonly associated with an enlargement of the liver and spleen; the clinical pattern of liver disease ranges from cases of mild hepatitis along with minimal necrosis and inflammation to severe, fatal cases of giant cell hepatitis.

Herpes simplex (types 1 and 2) may cause severe hepatitis in patients with a generalized herpetic infection; in neonates the type 2 infection is more common, although either agent may be responsible for a generalized infection in malnourished or immunosuppressed patients. Diffuse hepatocellular necrosis may lead to liver failure.

Cytomegaloviruses are responsible for a spectrum of liver disease that varies with the age and susceptibility of the patient. The infection in healthy children or adults usually is subclinical. A neonatal infection may be mild and subclinical or may cause hepatomegaly with cholestatic jaundice. In adults the clinical syndrome of cytomegalic mononucleosis occurs spontaneously or follows a massive transfusion; the histologic picture is similar to that of viral hepatitis. In immunocompromised patients, hepatomegaly and liver dysfunction may accompany the more serious pulmonary infection.

Bacterial infection and liver disease

Gram-negative bacterial infection. Cholestatic jaundice is a relatively common complication of gram-negative sepsis in infants; an infection of the urinary tract is the most common source. In adults jaundice is a less common complication of a severe infection, which is usually intraabdominal and associated with septicemia. Pathologic changes in the liver include bile stasis with dilated bile canaliculi containing bile plugs, Kupffer's cell hyperplasia, and nonspecific cellular infiltration. The pathogenesis of cholestasis in patients with gram-negative sepsis may be related to the direct invasion of the liver by organisms or to the effects of bacterial toxins on the liver cell; experimental studies have shown that the endotoxins of *Escherichia coli* and *Salmonella enteritidis* reduce bile flow and organic anion excretion in isolated perfused rat livers.

Typhoid fever is accompanied by jaundice in up to 25% of the patients. The liver usually is enlarged and tender, and serum alkaline phosphatase and transaminase levels are moderately elevated (two to five times normal levels). Focal liver cell necrosis with marked mononuclear cell infiltration and Kupffer's cell hyperplasia is the usual hepatic lesion, which resolves within 2 weeks after the initiation of therapy; intrahepatic cholestasis may be mild.

Pneumococcal infection. Before antibiotics came into use, jaundice was reported as a complication in up to 30% of patients with lobar pneumonia; biochemical studies to determine the mechanism of this jaundice were not available at that time. In more recent clinical experience jaundice has been an uncommon feature of pneumococcal pneumonia. Cholestasis caused by hepatocellular injury is the most likely mechanism of jaundice, but the specific cause for this injury has not been determined; in some patients hemolysis may accentuate the jaundice.

Gonococcal infection. Gonococcal perihepatitis, causing the symptoms of right upper quadrant abdominal pain and guarding, may complicate gonococcal pelvic inflammatory disease in the female. Localized tenderness and a friction rub over the liver area are signs of local peritonitis. Liver tests may show a minimal elevation of the levels of serum transaminases without hyperbilirubinemia, and a liver biopsy demonstrates an acute inflammatory infiltration of the capsule and subcapsular liver parenchyma.

Spirochetal infection. A leptospiral infection may cause hepatocellular injury and jaundice. Usually jaundice in these patients is accentuated by a more severe renal lesion that limits the urinary excretion of conjugated bilirubin. The hepatic lesion is minimal and involves focal necrosis, Kupffer's cell hyperplasia, periportal infiltration, and cholestasis in deeply jaundiced patients.

Syphilis causes a diffuse hepatitis that may lead to pericellular fibrosis and cirrhosis in infants with congenital infection. Adults with early secondary syphilis may exhibit evidence of hepatitis with mild jaundice and elevated levels of serum enzymes; miliary granulomas and focal infiltrations with polymorphonuclear and mononuclear cells are the typical hepatic lesions.

Tuberculosis of the liver is discussed in the later section, "Granulomatous and infiltrative diseases."

Pyogenic liver abscess

A pyogenic liver abscess is a complication of cholangitis, portal pyemia, or septicemia. Biliary tract disease caused by an infection with gram-negative and anaerobic enteric organisms is now the most common recognized cause of acute liver abscesses; an infection extending from the biliary tree usually produces multiple lesions. Infections via the portal system, formerly a more common complication of umbilical sepsis in infancy or acute appendicitis, now have a lower incidence with the earlier diagnosis and therapy of the primary lesions; intraabdominal sepsis may be followed by hepatic lesions, usually in the right lobe. Abscesses resulting from a staphylococcal infection may occur without a clinically detectable focus of the infection or may complicate an obvious focus at a distant site.

CLINICAL MANIFESTATIONS. The clinical features of a liver abscess are those of sepsis and a space-occupying lesion within the liver. The patient usually has fever and chills and polymorphonuclear leukocytosis with a shift to the left. Abdominal symptoms include anorexia, nausea, vomiting, and epigastric or right upper quadrant pain; these features may be of minimal diagnostic value in patients with preexisting abdominal disease. The right diaphragm often is elevated, and pleural effusion is caused by local inflammation. Jaundice may result from the predisposing biliary tract obstruction but is a late clinical manifestation of the liver abscess itself; it is associated with a high mortality. Hepatic enlargement and tenderness are commonly observed.

LABORATORY FINDINGS. In patients without biliary tract disease, liver tests often show only a minimal elevation of levels of serum alkaline phosphatase or transaminases; enzyme levels may remain normal. Hypoalbuminemia occurs commonly in these severely ill patients; both impaired synthesis and increased catabolism are its probable causes. Blood cultures have positive results in up to 50% of these patients. With isotope scanning of the liver, a focal area or areas of decreased uptake indicate the site of the hepatic lesion(s). A gallium scan may show a corresponding area of enhanced uptake. Ultrasonography or computed tomography may be of value in differentiating abscesses from solid space-occupying lesions.

DIAGNOSIS. Unless the clinician strongly suspects that the patient has a liver abscess, the lesion may not be diagnosed during life. This diagnosis must be considered in any patient with biliary tract disease complicated by sepsis and in patients with other foci of intraabdominal sepsis that do not respond promptly to surgical drainage and antibiotic therapy. Pyogenic abscesses must be differentiated from amebic abscesses (see discussion of "Amebic liver abscess").

MANAGEMENT. Surgical drainage is the recommended treatment for pyogenic liver abscesses associated with biliary obstruction or some other intraabdominal pathologic disorder. Conservative therapy using parenteral antibiotics may be appropriate for patients without another abdominal disease; a percutaneous needle aspiration of the abscess is of benefit in decompressing the abscess cavity and in providing pus for identification of the organism(s) by a Gram stain and aerobic and anaerobic cultures.

Amebic liver abscess

Invasive *Entamoeba histolytica* may cause single or multiple liver abscesses, usually in the right lobe. A past or recent history of amebic dysentery suggests a diagnosis of a liver abscess, but most patients with a liver abscess have not had symptomatic amebic colitis and do not have trophozoites in their stools. The clinical features of amebic abscesses and pyogenic liver abscesses are indistinguishable. The onset of the illness may be gradual or sudden and accompanied by fever, sweats, malaise, weight loss, and hepatic pain, enlargement, and tenderness. Scanning techniques provide evidence of a focal lesion(s) in the liver. The diagnosis is established by serologic tests, by the recovery of amebic pus ("anchovy sauce") that may contain trophozoites on needle aspiration, or by a response to specific antiamebic therapy (see Chapter 54). Tests of liver function are of no value in diagnosis, because they may remain normal or show only a minimal elevation of enzyme levels. A positive response to therapy is symptomatic improvement, a decrease in liver size and tenderness, and a gradual decrease in the size of the hepatic lesion shown by serial liver scans over several months.

Hepatic schistosomiasis

Hepatic schistosomiasis results from the inflammatory response to ova that are filtered out of the portal blood by the small branches of the portal vein within the portal triads. Acute schistosomiasis, following the infestation and maturation of the parasites and the deposition of ova (2 to 8 weeks after the infection), is accompanied by fever, diarrhea, intense eosinophilia, and hepatic enlargement with tenderness. A transient mild increase in the levels of hepatic alkaline phosphatase and transaminases in the serum reflects the early acute reaction to the parasite. In patients with chronic schistosomiasis, progressive fibrosis of the portal triads leads to a presinusoidal portal obstruction and portal hypertension. The liver may be of normal size or slightly enlarged and firm, and portal hypertension leads to splenomegaly and a collateral venous circulation. Bleeding from esophageal varices is the major complication. Patients with portal hypertension caused by schistosomiasis usually maintain normal liver function and do not develop hepatic encephalopathy with episodes of variceal bleeding. Ascites is uncommon in patients with schistosomiasis because the pressure in the hepatic sinusoids is normal.

A diagnosis of hepatic schistosomiasis in patients with portal hypertension is suggested by the presence of ova in the stools or in rectal mucosal biopsy specimens; this diagnosis is confirmed when ova are identified in "squash" preparations of liver biopsy specimens.

Toxic and drug-induced liver disease

Clinical and experimental evidence suggests that liver injury caused by toxic agents or drugs may be mediated by covalent binding of the agent or metabolite in the liver (toxicity) or by an immunologic reaction (hypersensitivity). Hepatotoxic reactions cause a predictable liver injury in both experimental animals and humans; the liver disease is related to the dose of the toxic agent or drug and usually is observed after a short latent period, such as occurs with carbon tetrachloride liver injury. Conversely, hypersensitivity reactions are uncommon and unpredictable and have not been observed in experimental animals; these reactions are unrelated to the drug dose, occur at variable intervals following exposure to the drug (decreasing with subsequent exposure), and may be accompanied by other signs of a hypersensitivity reaction, such as eosinophilia. These distinctions between hepatotoxic and hypersensitivity reactions have been blurred by an increasing knowledge of the hepatic metabolism of individual drugs. Individual variations in drug metabolism may be responsible for some hepatotoxic drug reactions that formerly were thought caused by hypersensitivity; that is, an individual "hypersensitivity" may be metabolic in some patients rather than immunologic.

TOXIC DRUG REACTIONS

Carbon tetrachloride. Carbon tetrachloride is a typical hepatotoxin that is metabolized by the liver to form toxic intermediates that bind to microsomal protein and cause liver cell necrosis. Its toxicity is increased by phenobarbital and ethanol, which increase the production of labile intermediates in the liver.

Carbon tetrachloride exposure by inhalation or ingestion usually occurs accidentally or as a suicide attempt. After an early period of variable central nervous depression with drowsiness, dizziness, headache, and nausea, there may be a period of 2 to 4 days before the onset of liver and renal disease. Jaundice and liver enlargement result from diffuse fatty degeneration and centrilobular necrosis; massive or bridging necrosis is relatively rare. The changes in liver function are similar to those caused by acute viral hepatitis with an extreme elevation of levels of serum transaminases in both anicteric and icteric patients. Although severe liver failure may cause death in hepatic coma during the first week of the illness, after that time renal failure is the dominant clinical problem. The supportive therapy for patients with fulminant viral hepatitis is appropriate also for patients with severe toxic hepatitis; renal dialysis may be necessary for the management of acute renal failure. After a single exposure to carbon tetrachloride, survivors have normal liver function and structure, but repeated exposure (usually occupational) can cause hepatic fibrosis and cirrhosis.

Ethanol. Ethanol is a direct hepatotoxin in humans as well as experimental animals. The acute ingestion of intoxicating doses causes a fatty liver that may be accompanied by a minimal serum transaminase elevation. In baboons the chronic ingestion of ethanol with an adequate diet leads to the spectrum of pathologic changes that have been documented in alcoholic patients (see later discussion of "Alcoholic cirrhosis").

Acetaminophen. In recommended doses acetaminophen is a safe analgesic agent for healthy subjects; potentially toxic metabolites are rapidly conjugated with glutathione to form nontoxic compounds. With the ingestion of an excessive dose (usually in a suicide attempt), hepatic glutathione is depleted, and toxic metabolites that bind microsomal protein accumulate in the liver. A latent, asymptomatic period of up to 24 hours following the ingestion precedes evidence of severe liver cell necrosis that may cause fatal liver failure. With an early diagnosis of a suicidal overdosage, treatment with N-acetyl cysteine within 12 hours of ingestion protects against liver injury by providing a source of glutathione for drug detoxification.

Isoniazid. The high incidence (10% to 20%) of mild elevations of serum transaminase levels (usually less than 100 units) among patients receiving isoniazid suggests that this agent is mildly hepatotoxic. Icteric liver disease occurring with the clinical, biochemical, and pathologic features that mimic acute viral hepatitis has been reported in approximately 1% of older patients receiving therapy with this drug. Severe isoniazid hepatitis was formerly thought to be a hypersensitivity (immunologic) reaction to the drug, but more recent metabolic studies in experimental animals document the formation of toxic metabolites, particularly when drug metabolism is stimulated by phenobarbital.

The minor elevations of serum transaminase levels during isoniazid therapy are usually transient and disappear with continued drug administration. Overt hepatitis is more common during the first 12 weeks of therapy but may be delayed; jaundice is usually preceded by anorexia, nausea, vomiting, and abdominal discomfort.

The prophylactic use of isoniazid should be restricted when possible to low-risk patients, those under 35 years of age who do not drink alcohol. When this agent is used in patients with a high risk of hepatitis, clinical and biochemical monitoring (SGOT tests at 2- to 4-week intervals) may provide earlier evidence of acute liver disease; severe, fatal hepatitis (occurring in 10% of icteric patients) may thus be reduced. Transient elevated levels of SGOT and SGPT occur in 10% to 20% of all patients taking isoniazid, however, and thus are not necessarily an indication for discontinuing this therapy.

Sex hormones. The synthetic androgens, methyltestosterone and carbon 17 alkyl-substituted steroids cause a reversible, dose-related intrahepatic cholestasis. Clinical features include jaundice, a slight liver enlargement, and variable conjugated hyperbilirubinemia with elevated levels of alkaline phosphatase, 5'-nucleotidase, and γ-glutamyl transpeptidase. Liver biopsies show cholestasis without liver cell necrosis.

Prolonged therapy with anabolic steroids, usually in patients with aplastic anemia, has been associated with the development of peliosis hepatis, in which dilated sinusoids or blood-filled cystic spaces replace normal liver cords. In these patients liver enlargement usually precedes changes in liver function.

Intrahepatic cholestasis appearing in the third trimester of pregnancy and manifested as pruritus gravidarum or cholestatic jaundice with pruritus appears to result from an exaggeration of the mild biochemical cholestasis that is normal in late pregnancy. Patients with recurrent cholestasis of pregnancy have normal estrogen levels and normal hormone metabolism; following pregnancy liver function is normal unless they are challenged with exogenous estrogens. In these patients cholestatic jaundice may follow the administration of oral contraceptive hormones. The relation of oral contraceptive hormone therapy to the development of hepatic adenomas is discussed in the later section on "Neoplastic diseases."

HYPERSENSITIVITY DRUG REACTIONS

Chlorpromazine. Chlorpromazine is one of many drugs that may induce jaundice and intrahepatic cholestasis as the result of a sensitivity reaction. Up to 50% of patients taking this drug may exhibit minimal increases in levels of serum enzymes (alkaline phosphatase and serum transaminase), which may be caused by the binding of drug metabolites to proteins in the canalicular membrane. Cholestatic jaundice, occurring in 1% to 2% of treated patients, often is preceded by fever, skin rash, lymphadenopathy, and eosinophilia. A liver biopsy reveals intrahepatic cholestasis with minimal centrilobular cell necrosis and a portal infiltration of mononuclear cells and eosinophils. After the administration of the drug is discontinued, the jaundice usually subsides within a few weeks; in rare cases the condition may progress to a clinical picture of chronic intrahepatic cholestasis resembling primary biliary cirrhosis. With subsequent exposure to the drug the onset of recurrent liver disease usually is more rapid.

The treatment of chlorpromazine jaundice includes discontinuing the drug, parenteral administration of vitamin K to correct for its malabsorption, and use of cholestyramine (up to 4 g with each meal) to reduce pruritus.

Fluorinated anesthetic agents. The use of halothane and methoxyflurane, particularly with repeated exposures, rarely is associated with acute hepatitis. Clinical and serologic studies have excluded hypoxia and acute viral hepatitis as causes of liver necrosis in many patients with this anesthetic exposure. Although metabolic injury remains a possible cause, the presence of an immunologic mechanism is supported by in vitro studies that demonstrate circulating antibodies in the patient's sera that bind to the surface membrane of liver cells from rabbits previously exposed to halothane. It is clinically observed that patients usually have an unexplained fever during the week after surgery, followed by anicteric hepatitis with a marked elevation of levels of serum transaminases or by hepatitis with jaundice. A liver biopsy reveals that liver cell necrosis is centrilobular in distribution and is accompanied by a mononuclear cell infiltration and Kupffer's cell hyperplasia. Massive necrosis with fulminant hepatitis is relatively common

(50% of these patients). Patients with an unexplained fever or hepatic dysfunction following the use of fluorinated anesthetic agents should not be reexposed to these agents; a recurrent episode of drug hepatitis is more likely to be severe and fatal.

Methyldopa. Methyldopa may cause a drug-related acute hepatitis that resembles acute viral hepatitis. The onset of liver disease occurs usually within 4 weeks of the initiation of the therapy, and jaundice often is preceded by fever, malaise, anorexia, nausea, or vomiting and elevated serum transaminase levels. Early discontinuation of the drug before the onset of jaundice usually is followed by prompt recovery, but continued or recurrent drug therapy may lead to jaundice with massive liver necrosis and hepatic failure. Careful clinical follow-up with serum transaminase determinations during the first 8 weeks of therapy has been recommended to prevent severe acute liver disease.

Methyldopa therapy has also been associated with the development of chronic active hepatitis (see later discussion of "Chronic active hepatitis").

Fatty liver

The normal liver contains small amounts of fat (about 5% of its weight), which includes phospholipid, cholesterol and cholesterol esters, triglycerides, and fatty acids in cell membranes or in membrane-enclosed lipid droplets (liposomes) of stored fat or of lipoprotein. This normal lipid can be seen with a light microscope only when special lipid stains are used. As fat accumulates in the liver, the triglyceride content increases to up to 50% of liver weight, and large droplets of triglyceride distend the liver cells.

PATHOGENESIS. The mechanisms of triglyceride accumulation in the liver include (1) an increased amount of triglyceride or fatty acid presented to the liver either from the peripheral adipose tissue or from the diet, (2) an increased synthesis of fatty acid and triglyceride by the liver, and (3) a decreased hepatic oxidation of fatty acids or secretion of lipoprotein. These three mechanisms play varying roles in different clinical situations.

In cases of obesity the fatty liver reflects the general increase in triglyceride stores resulting from an excessive caloric intake. In cases of diabetes mellitus and starvation there is an increase in the mobilization of peripheral fat; the hepatic uptake of fatty acids in excess of oxidation and lipoprotein secretion leads to fatty liver. The fatty liver commonly present in alcoholics is caused by the hepatic accumulation of dietary or peripheral lipid when the hepatic oxidation of fatty acid is impaired by alcohol; the hepatic synthesis of fatty acid may also be increased. The severe derangement of protein metabolism in patients with protein malnutrition, in some patients with a toxic liver injury such as that caused by carbon tetrachloride, phosphorus poisoning, or tetracycline toxicity, or in patients with Reye's syndrome is accompanied by a fatty liver resulting from the impaired oxidation of fat and decreased lipoprotein synthesis and secretion.

CLINICAL MANIFESTATIONS AND LABORATORY FINDINGS. Enlargement of the liver is the most common clinical manifestation of fatty liver; associated hepatic tenderness varies with the rate of liver enlargement and the presence of inflammation or cell necrosis. Fatty liver often causes no impairment of liver function; a minor elevation of serum alkaline phosphatase or transaminase levels (less than twice the normal levels) is consistent with fatty liver but may reflect a toxic liver cell injury such as alcoholic hepatitis. When fatty liver is only one manifestation of a severe liver injury, patients exhibit features of hepatitis (see earlier discussions of "Carbon tetrachloride" and "Alcoholic hepatitis") or acute hepatic encephalopathy (fatty liver of pregnancy, tetracycline toxicity, or Reye's syndrome). Reye's syndrome is a fulminant illness in children (at a mean age of 11 years) that commonly follows an influenza B infection; the acute encephalopathy is caused in part by cerebral edema and in part by ammonia toxicity. In the liver there is histologic evidence of glycogen depletion, mitochondrial injury, and fatty infiltration; impaired gluconeogenesis and the depletion of glycogen precipitate hypoglycemia, the reduced levels of urea cycle enzymes impair urea synthesis and elevate the blood ammonia levels, and the cell membrane injury permits leakage of liver cell enzymes into the plasma.

MANAGEMENT AND PROGNOSIS. Fatty liver may be decreased by treatment of the underlying cause, including weight reduction, alcohol withdrawal, and improved diabetic control. Patients with liver failure require appropriate supportive care (see earlier discussion of "Fulminant viral hepatitis"). Milder degrees of fatty liver may persist for long periods without changes in liver structure. In patients with severe fatty liver, including diabetics, those with a short bowel syndrome or a jejunoileal bypass (as a treatment of massive obesity), and those undergoing long-term methotrexate therapy for psoriasis, histologic changes that mimic those occurring in alcoholic hepatitis (cell degeneration with hyaline inclusions and centrilobular fibrosis) sometimes progress to cirrhosis and liver failure; these changes are not revealed by liver function tests and require a liver biopsy for their early identification.

Liver disease resulting from hepatic congestion and/or decreased perfusion

CONGESTIVE HEART FAILURE. Right upper quadrant discomfort and liver enlargement and tenderness are common clinical features of heart failure; an expansile pulsation of the liver with corresponding pressure changes in the neck veins suggests tricuspid insufficiency. In patients with constrictive pericarditis an enlargement of the liver and spleen and abdominal distention with ascites sometimes mimic cirrhosis of the liver. The congested liver exhibits distended central veins and congested centrilobular sinusoids; the centrilobular liver cell necrosis usually is caused by decreased perfusion and hypoxia. Alterations in liver function include a mild elevation of enzyme levels or cholestasis; changes in the metabolism of drugs and protein synthesis may dramatically modify the patient's response to anticoagulant therapy.

SHOCK. Acute hypotension in patients with cardiovascular disease (such as occurs during open heart surgery or with cardiac arrest) followed by subsequent recovery is associated with hypoxic necrosis of centrilobular liver cells; this leads to a clinical and biochemical picture of acute hepatitis with a marked elevation of levels of serum transaminases followed by variable jaundice. With complete cardiovascular recovery, hepatic regeneration restores normal liver lobules; with repeated injury, centrilobular fibrosis replaces liver cells.

HEPATIC VEIN OCCLUSION. The causes of a hepatic venous obstruction (Budd-Chiari syndrome) include congenital webs, venous thrombosis (such as occurs in myeloproliferative disease, in paroxysmal nocturnal hemoglobinuria, and in pregnancy or with oral contraceptive use), neoplastic disease (such as a hepatoma or lymphoma), or endophlebitis with fibrosis complicating venoocclusive disease and hepatic radiation therapy. An acute hepatic venous occlusion causes marked liver congestion, central zonal necrosis, and abdominal distention with a rapid accumulation of ascites. The clinical picture varies from an acute illness with dramatic abdominal pain, liver and abdominal enlargement, shock, and early death to a more

chronic illness with features of portal hypertension including ascites, venous collaterals, and bleeding from esophageal varices. The diagnosis is supported by a centrilobular pattern of congestion and hemorrhagic necrosis revealed by a liver biopsy and is confirmed by roentgenographic studies of the inferior vena cava and hepatic veins. A liver scan often shows a diffuse decrease in the hepatic uptake of the isotope and a relative concentration of the isotope in the caudate lobe, which has an independent hepatic venous drainage into the inferior vena cava. The prognosis of a patient with the acute Budd-Chiari syndrome is poor; obstruction caused by congenital webs can be relieved surgically, but removal of clots usually is unsuccessful. The relief of portal hypertension by a portacaval shunt may extend the life of some patients.

Chronic active hepatitis

Chronic active hepatitis is a chronic disease process resulting from varying causes in which a continued destruction of liver cells, usually in a periportal distribution, is associated with inflammation and a progressive fibrosis that replaces liver parenchyma and ultimately leads to cirrhosis.

ETIOLOGY. The important causative factors of chronic active hepatitis are infection by hepatitis B and non-A, non-B viruses, autoimmune liver injury, and hypersensitivity reactions to certain drugs (usually following recurrent or continued exposure to methyldopa, isoniazid, oxyphenisatin, and halothane). Patients with Wilson's disease and primry biliary cirrhosis may also have the clinical, biochemical, and pathologic features of chronic active hepatitis.

PATHOGENESIS. Humoral or cellular immunologic mechanisms or both probably play a major role in the pathogenesis of chronic active hepatitis, regardless of the primary cause. The evidence in support of an immunologic pathogenesis is as follows.

1. Patients with idiopathic or autoimmune chronic active hepatitis have an increased incidence of other diseases that may have an autoimmune basis, including Sjögren's syndrome, chronic thyroiditis, and pulmonary fibrosis. The higher incidence of the HLA-B8 antigen in these patients and an increased incidence of autoimmune diseases in close relatives suggest that genetic factors play some role.
2. Hypergammaglobulinemia in patients with chronic active hepatitis often is extreme, often parallels the disease activity, and often is accompanied by positive results on serologic tests for multiple autoantibodies that lack organ specificity; these include antinuclear, anti-DNA, antimitochondrial, and anti–smooth muscle antibodies as well as positive tests results for lupus erythematosus (LE) cells. These immunologic phenomena are uncommon in patients with hepatitis B–related chronic active hepatitis.
3. Periportal areas adjacent to the liver lobule are heavily infiltrated with plasma cells and lymphocytes.
4. Immunologic phenomena that may play a specific role in liver cell injury have been reported to occur with chronic active hepatitis. Chronic active hepatitis in patients who are HB_sAg positive is associated with the localization of HB_sAg on the surface membrane of liver cells; liver cell injury may be caused by lymphocytes with Fc receptors that bind anti-HB_s and react with membrane-bound antigen. Specific lipoprotein antigen on the liver cell membrane has been suggested as the target for sensitized lymphocytes in cases of autoimmune chronic active hepatitis.

Although these immunologic phenomena provide an explanation for the chronic liver injury, the specific factors that regulate the development of the disease have not been determined.

CLINICAL MANIFESTATIONS. The clinical spectrum of chronic hepatitis is broad. A large proportion of patients with mild disease may remain well and asymptomatic, and in these the only evidence of a slowly progressive liver disease might be mild fluctuations in levels of serum transaminase and hyperglobulinemia; this asymptomatic course would explain the late development of cirrhosis many years after a hepatitis B infection. Alternatively, patients with a more active and rapidly progressive disease exhibit symptoms suggestive of an acute hepatitis of insidious onset; malaise, lethargy, anorexia, arthralgias, a low-grade fever, and right upper quadrant discomfort are relatively common. Jaundice with dark urine and pruritus is a feature of severe exacerbations. In young women with autoimmune disease, amenorrhea is common. The physical findings are related in part to hepatic inflammation (liver enlargement, tenderness, and cholestasis) and in part to chronic liver injury and/or cirrhosis (spider angiomas, splenomegaly, ascites, and collateral abdominal veins).

PATHOLOGY. In early chronic active hepatitis the normal lobular architecture of the liver is preserved. The portal areas are expanded and may be joined by fibrous septa, and the liver cell plates adjacent to the portal areas are disrupted; individual cells exhibit hyaline (piecemeal) necrosis, and other cells are separated from the normal cords by proliferating mesenchymal cells or acute and chronic inflammatory cells, particularly lymphocytes, plasma cells, and eosinophils. Regenerating liver cells from rosettes on the periphery of the lobule, and proliferation within the portal areas increases the number of bile ductules. Within the hepatic lobules, parenchymal cell necrosis and infiltration are minimal. Bile stasis may be noted in patients with jaundice.

As chronic active hepatitis progresses, the increasing fibrosis extending from portal areas into the lobule distorts the normal architecture, and regeneration nodules result in cirrhosis.

Either a spontaneous remission or treatment with corticosteroids decreases the parenchymal cell necrosis and inflammatory cell infiltration, leaving portal fibrosis or inactive cirrhosis.

DIFFERENTIAL DIAGNOSIS. A history of drug ingestion, evidence of a hepatitis B infection, or the potential exposure to non-A, non-B hepatitis through a transfusion, as well as high titers of autoantibodies, usually distinguishes patients with chronic active hepatitis caused by drugs, a hepatitis infection, or an autoimmune disease, respectively. Determining the causal agent is of clinical importance, because cessation of drug therapy usually is followed by remission, whereas patients with a hepatitis B infection are more likely to respond poorly to corticosteroid therapy.

In patients with prominent cholestasis, a high titer of antimitochrondrial antibodies suggests a diagnosis of primary biliary cirrhosis; these patients are more likely to have a decreased number of smaller bile ducts as well as damage to larger bile ducts within the portal areas. In young patients Wilson's disease must be considered and excluded from diagnostic possibilities by measuring serum ceruloplasmin and serum and urinary copper levels.

MANAGEMENT AND PROGNOSIS. Controlled clinical trials have shown that patients with severe autoimmune chronic active hepatitis respond to treatment with prednisone or a combination of prednisone and azathioprine; 80% of symptomatic patients with severe biochemical changes (SGOT levels more than 10 times normal or five times normal along with γ-globulin levels twice the normal) treated with prednisone (60 mg daily initially, reduced to a maintenance dosage of 20 mg daily), or prednisone (30 mg daily initially, reduced to a maintenance dosage of 10 mg daily) and azathioprine (50 mg daily) have entered clinical, biochemical, and histologic remission. This remission usually is maintained by continued prednisone therapy, but slow withdrawal of drug therapy after 6 months of sustained remission is followed by a relapse in up to 50% of patients. A symptomatic and biochemical relapse requires further steroid therapy. Alternate-day prednisone therapy reduces the side effects of the treatment but appears to be less effective than daily doses of steroids in maintaining histologic remission.

Although symptomatic patients with severe autoimmune disease clearly benefit from drug therapy, the benefit of this treatment in patients who are asymptomatic and have less active disease remains uncertain; in patients with a slowly progressive disease, the side effects of drug therapy may offset any benefit that results from a decrease in the disease activity.

Patients with chronic active hepatitis caused by HBV or non-A, non-B infection respond poorly to corticosteroid therapy. The use of antiviral agents or interferon in these patients may be effective in terminating the viral infection; however, this therapy remains experimental.

Cirrhosis of the liver

DEFINITION. In cirrhosis of the liver the normal lobular architecture of the liver is disrupted by fibrosis and regenerative nodules.

ETIOLOGY AND CLASSIFICATION. Cirrhosis is the end stage of chronic liver injury resulting from various causes, some of which are well defined wheras others are poorly understood. Despite the current limitations in our understanding of the mechanisms of cirrhosis, the following etiologic classification is most useful clinically:

I. Idiopathic or posthepatic cirrhosis
II. Alcoholic cirrhosis
III. Metabolic cirrhosis
    A. Hemochromatosis
    B. Wilson's disease
    C. α-1-Antitrypsin deficiency
    D. Other metabolic disorders
IV. Biliary cirrhosis
    A. Primary
    B. Secondary
V. Congestive (cardiac) cirrhosis

IDIOPATHIC OR POSTHEPATIC CIRRHOSIS

Pathogenesis. The development of cirrhosis following hepatitis B or non-A, non-B infection has been well documented by serial liver biopsies. Bridging necrosis during the acute infection and chronic active hepatitis (regardless of the cause) are recognized precursor lesions. Many patients with established cirrhosis do not give a history of alcoholism or a preceding hepatitis infection and do not exhibit the features of chronic active liver disease; these patients with idiopathic cirrhosis may have the end stage of asymptomatic, undiagnosed chronic active hepatitis.

Pathology. The liver in patients with idiopathic or posthepatic cirrhosis is more likely to have large irregular nodules and broad intervening bands of scarring (macronodular cirrhosis) than small regular nodules (micronodular cirrhosis); the liver is typically shrunken in patients with end-stage disease. In the earlier phase of active cirrhosis the microscopic features of chronic active hepatitis are present in addition to cirrhotic scarring and nodular regeneration. In the late stage, regenerative nodules often formed by double cords of liver cells are separated by dense fibrous bands containing proliferating bile ducts and sparse inflammatory cells.

Clinical manifestations. The clinical features of active idiopathic cirrhosis are those of chronic active hepatitis coupled with variable manifestations of the cirrhosis itself: portal hypertension with splenomegaly and hypersplenism, ascites, portal-systemic collaterals, and hepatic encephalopathy. Patients with compensated cirrhosis and normal liver function may show splenomegaly and hypersplenism; patients with decompensated cirrhosis are more likely to have ascites and edema, bleeding from esophageal varices, or hepatic encephalopathy.

Management and prognosis. Patients with chronic active hepatitis and established posthepatic cirrhosis may benefit from corticosteroid therapy (see earlier discussion of "Chronic active hepatitis"); the desired result of treatment is a compensated cirrhosis that is no longer progressive. The complications of cirrhosis require appropriate supportive therapy (see later discussion of "Management of complications of cirrhosis"). In young patients with advanced idiopathic cirrhosis and liver failure, orthotopic liver transplantation may prolong survival.

ALCOHOLIC CIRRHOSIS

Pathogenesis. The development of cirrhosis in chronic alcoholics is related to the amount of alcohol consumed and the duration of alcohol abuse; although undetermined factors may modify the development of liver disease in individual patients, cirrhosis is the usual outcome in those who have a liquor intake in excess of 1 pint a day for 15 years. Former hypotheses that various nutritional deficiencies associated with alcoholism are responsible for the development of cirrhosis are not supported by experimental studies with baboons; when carbohydrates were replaced by ethanol in an otherwise complete diet, these animals showed the pathologic spectrum of acute alcoholic hepatitis and cirrhosis occurring in patients who abuse alcohol. This evidence provides the strongest support for the current hypothesis that alcohol is a direct hepatotoxin.

Pathology. The earliest hepatic lesion observed following excessive alcohol consumption is a fatty liver without fibrosis or liver cell necrosis. With progressive injury the fatty liver may be accompanied by evidence of parenchymal cell injury; when examined with a light microscope, damaged cells exhibit eosinophilic inclusions (alcoholic hyalin) that correspond to collections of fibrillar material detected with electron microscopy. Cell organelles also exhibit degenerative changes. An infiltration with polymorphonuclear cells and early fibrosis, particularly within the lobule adjacent to the central veins, complete the pathologic picture of acute alcoholic hepatitis. Although the relationship of fatty liver, alcoholic hepatitis, and cirrhosis requires further clarification, the development of progressive scarring and cirrhosis following continued alcohol abuse is more rapid in patients who exhibit centrilobular fibrosis or sclerosis; indeed, patients with severe acute alcoholic hepatitis and central hyaline sclerosis progress rapidly to decompensated cirrhosis. End-stage cirrhosis in alcoholics is usually a micronodular cirrhosis with regular small regenerative nodules. The pathologic cause is manifested only in the lesions of continued alcoholic injury—fatty infiltration and alcoholic hyalin; these cellular changes may be nonspecific.

Clinical manifestations. The earliest indication of alcoholic liver disease often is an enlarged liver detected on a routine physical examination. Minor changes in serum enzyme levels reflect liver cell injury. The initial episodes of symptomatic hepatic decompensation accompanied by anorexia, nausea or vomiting, abdominal swelling, right upper quadrant abdominal pain, or jaundice are often precipitated by the superimposition of acute alcoholic hepatitis on hepatic fibrosis or cirrhosis from earlier injury. The patient with acute decompensation caused by alcoholic hepatitis is usually febrile, is often malnourished, and exhibits signs of both acute hepatitis and a more chronic liver disease, which may include an enlarged and tender liver, spider angiomas, gynecomastia, jaundice, ascites, and ethanol intoxication or withdrawal signs. Jaundice with conjugated hyperbilirubinemia, elevated levels of serum enzymes (with the SGOT level more than twice that of SGPT), and a prolonged prothrombin time reflect acute liver injury; in some patients cholestasis is predominant.

The clinical features of alcoholic cirrhosis without acute alcoholic hepatitis vary with the severity of the disease and its complications. A firm enlargement of the liver and spleen and normal results on routine tests of liver function are consistent with compensated alcoholic cirrhosis. Patients with decompensated cirrhosis usually exhibit signs of liver failure and have the complications of ascites, hepatic encephalopathy, and bleeding from esophageal varices as well as biochemical evidence of an impaired hepatic synthetic function (hypoproteinemia, prolonged prothrombin time, and an elevated level of ammonia in the blood).

Differential diagnosis. In patients with acute alcoholic hepatitis, sepsis and other causes of acute hepatitis must be considered. The causes of hepatic decompensation in patients with cirrhosis are discussed in subsequent sections on the management of portal hypertension, ascites, and encephalopathy. A percutaneous liver biopsy is of value in pathologically confirming the diagnosis of acute or chronic liver disease caused by alcohol and in assessing the prognosis of these patients.

Management and prognosis. Early withdrawal from alcohol is the only major factor that significantly modifies the course of alcoholic hepatitis and cirrhosis and prolongs the patient's survival. In patients with acute alcoholic hepatitis who stop drinking, the liver disease is reversible unless central hyaline sclerosis or cirrhosis is already present. Patients with end-stage cirrhosis and portal hypertension have irreversible lesions that progress despite the withdrawal from alcohol.

Nutritional support for the malnourished alcoholic patient should include oral protein supplements to restore the nitrogen balance (unless a high protein intake is contraindicated by the presence of hepatic encephalopathy), vitamin supplements to correct deficiencies of B vitamins, folic acid, and ascorbic acid, and supplements of potassium and trace metals such as zinc in patients with deficiencies.

Chlordiazepoxide (Librium) is recommended in the treatment of the manifestations of alcohol withdrawal; the parenterally administered doses should be adjusted to meet the individual needs of the patient.

Treatment of the complications of cirrhosis is discussed in sections on portal hypertension, ascites, and coma.

METABOLIC CIRRHOSIS

Hemochromatosis. Hemochromatosis results from an excessive deposition of iron in the liver and other organs. The disease may be genetically determined (idiopathic hemochromatosis) or may result from excessive iron absorption and storage in patients with diseases that modify iron metabolism, such as occurs with thalassemia or following portacaval shunting. The factors that cause an excessive intestinal absorption of iron in patients with either idiopathic hemochromatosis or secondary hemochromatosis are currently undetermined.

Idiopathic hemochromatosis is inherited as an autosomal defect that is either dominant with a varying expression or recessive; affected family members often have an HLA profile similar to that of the patient with the disease, and the incidence of the HLA-A3 gene is higher in patients with this disease.

Pathology. In patients with hemochromatosis, stored iron is increased from a normal level of 3 to 4 g to amounts in excess of 20 to 40 g; this excess iron is deposited in the parenchymal cells of many organs as well as in the reticuloendothelial system.

The earliest hepatic lesion in asymptomatic young relatives of parents with established hemochromatosis is an increase in both parenchymal and reticuloendothelial hepatic iron without fibrosis. Progressive iron overload leads to increasing portal fibrosis and the development of fibrous septa between lobules; a micronodular or occasional macronodular cirrhosis finally results. Parenchymal cells, Kupffer's cells, and the cells of proliferating bile ducts are heavily infiltrated with iron.

In the pancreas the iron deposits lead to fibrosis and degeneration of the islet cells. In the heart, infiltrated myocardial cells undergo degeneration with subsequent fibrosis. In the endocrine system, iron storage is particularly prominent in the thyroid, parathyroid, and anterior pituitary glands and in the zona glomerulosa of the adrenal gland; this storage does not lead to fibrosis. Testicular atrophy is associated with minimal iron deposition and probably results from pituitary dysfunction. Iron deposits in the chief cells of the gastric mucosa and in salivary glands do not impair secretion. In the larger joints the deposition of iron in the synovium is often accompanied by chondrocalcinosis, which may cause arthritic symptoms.

Clinical manifestations. Skin pigmentation, diabetes mellitus (usually insulin dependent), cirrhosis of the liver, hypogonadism, and cardiac arrhythmias or failure are the more common features of idiopathic hemochromatosis. Abdominal pain, usually in the right upper quadrant, is a prominent initial symptom. The liver usually is enlarged and firm, and splenomegaly is common. Liver function is well preserved in most patients; others exhibit a mild elevation of levels of serum transaminases (usually less than twice the normal level). Severe impairment of liver function most often is observed in patients with heart failure or with late development of a hepatocellular carcinoma.

Diagnosis. In patients with early or late hemochromatosis, excessive body iron stores are associated with a greatly increased saturation of serum transferrin (usually near 100%) and elevated serum levels of ferritin. A liver biopsy provides the most reliable evidence of the iron overload.

Management. Phlebotomy is the most effective means of removing iron from the body (250 mg iron/500 ml of blood); weekly phlebotomy usually is tolerated well by patients with idiopathic hemochromatosis; 1 to 2 years of treatment may be necessary to remove excess iron stores. When iron stores are depleted, the serum ferritin level usually falls below 3 μg/dl, the serum transferrin level rises and the iron saturation falls, and normal hemoglobin levels are no longer maintained. To maintain the depletion of iron stores, patients with idiopathic hemochromatosis require phlebotomy two to six times each year; their serum ferritin levels should be maintained below 20 μg/dl. In patients with secondary hemochromatosis and anemia, phlebotomy may not be possible; intravenous infusions of desferrioxamine are of minimal benefit.

Heart failure, diabetes mellitus, and other endocrine disorders require appropriate therapy.

Prognosis. In the past patients with hemochromatosis who went untreated often died of cardiac complications. With phlebotomy, patients with established cirrhosis are more likely to live longer but have an increased incidence of hepatomas. Patients with idiopathic hemochromatosis who are diagnosed and treated before hepatic fibrosis or cirrhosis develops have a normal life expectancy.

Wilson's disease. Wilson's disease is an autosomal recessive defect of copper metabolism. An excessive body accumulation of copper probably results from a decreased biliary excretion of the metal. The hepatic manifestations of established disease are chronic active hepatitis and cirrhosis. The liver contains an excessive amount of copper, usually more than 50 μg per gram of wet weight (the normal amount is 4 to 8 μg per gram). Nonhepatic manifestations of Wilson's disease include Kayser-Fleischer corneal rings, neurologic disease (causing tremor, rigidity, ataxia, and changes in mentation), acute hemolytic disease, renal tubular dysfunction, and bone demineralization.

The possibility of Wilson's disease should be considered in any young patient with chronic active hepatitis or cirrhosis of unknown cause. Kayser-Fleischer rings detected in a split-lamp examination of the cornea and depressed serum levels of the copper protein ceruloplasmin are usually present. An elevated level of urinary copper excretion after a test dose of penicillamine or a direct measurement of hepatic copper content confirms the diagnosis. The treatment of Wilson's disease is penicillamine therapy (500 mg three times daily).

α-1-Antitrypsin deficiency. The plasma protease inhibitor system, α-1-antitrypsin (the major α_1-globulin), is relatively deficient in patients with the Pi^{ZZ} phenotype (the normal phenotype is Pi^{MM}); these patients appear to have a defect in the hepatic secretion of α_1-globulin, which accumulates in membrane-bound vacuoles in the liver cells. Homozygous (Pi^{ZZ}) patients usually have cholestasis during their first year of life or progressive hepatomegaly and cirrhosis in later childhood. There is no specific therapy for this disorder; hepatic transplantation offers hope for the future.

BILIARY CIRRHOSIS

Primary biliary cirrhosis. Primary biliary cirrhosis, the cause of which has not been determined, is characterized clinically by chronic intrahepatic cholestasis and pathologically by chronic inflammation and fibrosis of portal triads with destruction of smaller bile ducts.

Pathogenesis. The current hypothesis is that primary biliary cirrhosis is an autoimmune disease in which small bile ducts are damaged or destroyed by immunologic mechanisms.

Pathology. The earliest hepatic lesions observed in biopsies of patients with mild asymptomatic cholestasis (an elevated level of serum alkaline phosphatase without jaundice) appear to be a mononuclear inflammatory reaction that expands the portal triads and an associated loss of smaller bile ducts or evidence of damage to the epithelium of larger bile ducts. The bile ducts may terminate in areas of heavy mononuclear cell infiltration or in granulomas. Initially the fibrosis is minimal, and the hepatic lobules are normal. As the disease progresses, piecemeal necrosis of liver cells adjacent to the portal areas disrupts liver cell plates, fibrosis extends to adjacent portal areas, and centrilobular cholestasis reflects the onset of jaundice. In the late stage of the disease a macronodular cirrhosis with prominent cholestasis often is present. Lipid-laden macrophages accumulate along the hepatic sinusoids in patients with extreme hyperlipidemia.

Clinical manifestations. The incidence of primary biliary cirrhosis is highest in women 40 to 60 years of age; males are rarely affected. Asymptomatic disease has been diagnosed by serologic tests and liver biopsies in patients with isolated elevations of the level of serum alkaline phosphatase; these patients often remain well without progression of their disease over long periods. Pruritus and jaundice are the most common presenting symptoms in patients with progressive disease. Chronic intrahepatic cholestasis leads to fat malabsorption with diarrhea in some patients, hypercholesterolemia with the development of xanthomas, and an increased risk of duodenal ulcer disease (probably related to a decreased duodenal neutralization of acid). In the early cholestatic phase of the illness the liver synthetic function is well preserved, and albumin levels remain normal. Later manifestations of cirrhosis in patients with a poor prognosis include the development of portal hypertension with bleeding from esophageal varices, ascites, and encephalopathy; these complications of cirrhosis are unusual presenting signs. Osteomalacia caused by malabsorption of vitamin D and of 25-hydroxycholecalciferol that is normally cycled through the enterohepatic circulation is a common cause of severe bone demineralization and pathologic fractures of the spine and ribs.

Diagnosis. Primary biliary cirrhosis usually is associated with extremely high titers of antimitochondrial antibodies (lower titers are observed in patients with chronic active hepatitis). This serologic test combined with a liver biopsy usually is sufficient to establish the diagnosis in patients with prominent cholestasis. Transhepatic Chiba fine needle or endoscopic retrograde cholangiography is sometimes necessary to rule out an extrahepatic biliary tract obstruction in patients who may have gallstones.

Management. There is no specific treatment for primary biliary cirrhosis; these patients do not respond to corticosteroid or azathioprine therapy. The symptomatic and supportive treatment includes use of oral cholestyramine (4 g up to three times a day) to relieve the itching and daily supplementary fat-soluble vitamins to prevent deficiencies of vitamins K, A, and D; the recommended daily oral dosages are 5 to 10 mg of vitamin K_1, 10,000 units of vitamin A, and 100 to 299 μg of 25-hydroxycholecalciferol (vitamin D).

Prognosis. The average life expectancy of symptomatic patients is 5 years after the onset of jaundice. Increasing jaundice and the complications of cirrhosis indicate a poor prognosis. Recent rials of penicillamine therapy designed to prevent the copper accumulation that might accelerate liver disease have shown that this agent is of minimal benefit. Patients with advanced primary biliary cirrhosis should be considered for orthotopic liver transplantation; this procedure prolongs survival in these patients.

Secondary biliary cirrhosis. An extrahepatic biliary obstruction with or without cholangitis leads to progressive portal fibrosis; true cirrhosis in these patients is rare. The clinical features are those of cholestasis with late hepatic failure and intermittent episodes of cholangitis. Pathologically, the early lesions are those of an extrahepatic obstruction with bile stasis, ductular proliferation, and the dilation of larger bile ducts. Bile infarcts and bile lakes, the foci of liver cells that have undergone necrosis with bile extravastion, usually are located at the periphery of lobules adjacent to the portal tracts. The portal tracts are edematous, have concentric fibrosis around the bile ducts, and are infiltrated with mononuclear and polymorphonuclear cells. In cases of advanced secondary biliary cirrhosis, regenerative nodules are surrounded by condensed fibrous tissue containing proliferating bile ducts.

MANAGEMENT OF COMPLICATIONS OF CIRRHOSIS
Portal hypertension and upper gastrointestinal bleeding.
The immediate management of patients with cirrhosis and massive upper gastrointestinal bleeding has four objectives: (1) to restore the circulating blood volume and to stabilize the patient, (2) to control the bleeding, (3) to define the site of bleeding, and (4) to anticipate and prevent or treat other complications of liver disease.

The patient usually requires intensive care monitoring and an immediate transfusion of whole blood. Measures that are effective in providing temporary control of variceal bleeding include intravenous or selective mesenteric arterial infusion of vasopressin, which induces splanchnic vasoconstriction and lowers portal venous pressure; insertion of a Sengstaken-Blake-

more esophageal tube to provide balloon tamponade of the varices, and endoscopic injection of varices with a sclerosing agent. Massive uncontrolled bleeding from esophageal or gastric varices may require the use of the Sengstaken-Blakemore esophageal tube; in inexperienced hands this method involves a high risk of esophageal erosion, esophageal perforation, and pulmonary aspiration. Patients with cirrhosis, portal hypertension, and esophageal varices may have bleeding from a variety of esophageal, gastric, and duodenal lesions. Bleeding is more likely to be from esophageal varices in patients whose cirrhosis is relatively compensated, whereas in patients with decompensated cirrhosis the bleeding commonly is from acute gastric erosions. Esophagogastroduodenoscopy provides the most accurate assessment of the bleeding site; alternatively, if the bleeding continues to be massive, selective arteriography with an injection of contrast dye may localize the site of the blood loss into the gut. Cirrhotic patients with massive bleeding are likely to develop ascites or hepatic coma; the measures for reducing these problems include the restriction of salt and measures that clear blood from the gastrointestinal tract and reduce bacterial action (see discussion of "Hepatic encephalopathy").

Measures aimed at reducing the risk of recurrent bleeding from esophageal varices have included drug therapy with propranolol, endoscopic sclerotherapy to obliterate the varices, and surgical decompression of the portal venous system. Treatment with propranolol in doses sufficient to reduce the resting pulse rate by 25% has been reported to reduce the frequency of both initial and recurrent bleeding in patients with cirrhosis. Repeated injection sclerotherapy currently is the preferred method to control bleeding; when varices have been obliterated by repeated sclerosis, the frequency of bleeding is decreased. Sclerotherapy may be complicated, however, by esophageal ulceration and stricture. It has not been established that this procedure prolongs the survival of patients with advanced cirrhosis.

Surgical decompression of the portal system with a splenorenal, mesocaval, or portacaval anastomosis usually is effective in lowering the portal pressure and in the long-term control of variceal bleeding; patient survial may not be prolonged. These procedures have a high operative mortality in patients with hepatic decompensation and increase the risk of postoperative hepatic encephalopathy. The procedure of choice in low-risk patients may be a distal splenorenal shunt that selectively decompresses esophageal varices without significantly decreasing the mesenteric blood flow to the liver; progressive liver failure is less likely after this procedure. When evaluating patients for shunt surgery, it is necessary to demonstrate that the splenic, portal, and/or renal veins are patent by selective splenic arteriography or transhepatic or transsplenic portal venography. Measurements of the wedged hepatic venous pressure and the inferior vena cava pressure indicate the pressure gradient across the liver and differentiate a presinusoidal obstruction from cirrhosis.

Ascites. When ascites is present, it is important to determine the precipitating cause as well as to promote a safe diuresis. Causes for ascites other than liver disease must be considered, including heart failure, constrictive pericarditis, acute pancreatitis with a pancreaticoperitoneal fistula, bacterial peritonitis, and neoplastic infiltration of the peritoneal cavity. In patients with established cirrhosis and portal hypertension, ascites may be precipitated by bleeding (with an increase in secondary hyperaldosteronism), by an increase in salt intake, by peritoneal infection with enteric organisms or tubercle bacilli, by further hepatic decompensation, by the development of a hepatoma, or by thrombosis of hepatic or portal veins; the precipitating factor in the patient should be determined. An initial diagnostic paracentesis with examination of the ascitic fluid to detect bacteria, enzymes (lactate dehydrogenase and amylase), malignant cells, and inflammatory cells is of particular value in the diagnosis of peritonitis and neoplastic disease. The following management program provides an effective and safe diuresis in the majority of patients with cirrhosis and ascites:

1. The dietary sodium intake is restricted to less than 2 g daily; the fluid intake also may have to be restricted to 1000 ml daily in patients who exhibit a decrease in the serum sodium concentration below 130 mEq/L.
2. The diuretic program must provide aldosterone blockade to prevent severe hypokalemia. Initially over a period of several days an increase in the dosage of spironolactone from 100 mg to 400 mg daily is recommended; when the urinary sodium excretion exceeds that of potassium, the addition of hydrochlorothiazide (50 mg daily) or furosemide (40 mg daily) increases the sodium excretion without promoting potassium loss.
3. The weight loss in patients without peripheral edema should not exceed 0.5 kg daily; a more rapid diuresis at a rate that exceeds the rate of fluid mobilization from the peritoneal cavity increases the risk of hypovolemia.
4. Patients with severe hypoproteinemia should receive daily intravenous infusions of salt-poor albumin (25 to 50 g) to restore the plasma oncotic pressure and to maintain the plasma volume.
5. The patient's weight, renal function, serum electrolyte concentrations, and mental status should be monitored regularly to reduce complications of azotemia, electrolyte imbalances, and encephalopathy.
6. The goal of therapy should be not to eliminate all ascitic fluid but to reduce ascites and permit normal function.

Hepatic encephalopathy. In patients with cirrhosis, hepatic encephalopathy may be precipitated by gastrointestinal bleeding; by a fluid, electrolyte, or acid-base imbalance, particularly hypokalemic alkalosis or water intoxication; by infection; by the use of depressant drugs such as sedatives, tranquilizers, or narcotics; or by other metabolic insults including azotemia, hypoxia, hypoglycemia, and an increase in dietary protein intake. Precipatating causes should be identified and eliminated. In all patients with a chronic or intermittent hepatic encephalopathy, measures that lower the level of blood ammonia are of value in improving the patient's mental function; these measures include restriction of dietary protein to a level that can be tolerated by the patient, enemas and cathartics to empty the colon, and orally administered neomycin or lactulose to reduce the formation and absorption of ammonia in the colon.

Granulomatous and infiltrative diseases

Hepatic granulomas have been described in association with a large number of local and systemic diseases. The most common causes of hepatic granulomata include sarcoidosis, pulmonary and miliary tuberculosis, histoplasmosis, brucellosis, primary biliary cirrhosis, Hodgkin's disease, and hypersensitivity reactions. The liver usually is enlarged and may be tender. The most common abnormalities in liver function are elevated levels of serum alkaline phosphatase and related enzymes; levels of serum transaminases are slightly elevated in patients with acute disease. The presence of hepatic granulomas is demonstrated by needle biopsy; the determination of the primary cause of hepatic granulomatous disease usually requires other clinical data, although the presence of caseating necrosis strongly suggests that miliary tuberculosis is the cause. Hepatic granulomas usually heal with fibrosis without long-term sequelae; rarely they may cause portal hypertension resulting from hepatic fibrosis.

Infiltrative disease of the liver such as that caused by metastatic carcinoma (see the following section), amyloidosis, or even fat also characteristically produces hepatic enlargement, possible tenderness, and elevations of the levels of serum alkaline phosphatase and related enzymes.

Neoplastic diseases

The liver may be involved in a variety of benign and malignant primary and metastatic neoplasms including carcinomas, lymphomas, hemangiomas, and angiosarcomas, the last of which may result from exposure to vinyl chloride. If large, a tumor produces hepatic enlargement sometimes accompanied by pain or tenderness. The mass may be demonstrated by means of radionuclide scanning, ultrasonography, computer tomography, or angiography. Malignant lesions often produce early and disproportionate elevations of the levels of serum alkaline phosphatase and related enzymes. Because of their clinical importance and incidence and the current interest in them, hepatic adenomas, primary carcinomas, and metastatic carcinomas are discussed in more detail below.

HEPATIC ADENOMAS. The development of large hepatic adenomas has been associated with the use of oral contraceptive steroids. Patients with these lesions may have abdominal pain, acute intraperitoneal bleeding and shock, or a palpable abdominal mass. Most of these lesions have been resected, but conservative treatment with withdrawal from hormone therapy has led to a regression of the tumor in some patients. Hepatic adenomas occurring in patients not receiving oral contraceptive steroids are usually small and do not cause symptoms.

HEPATOCELLULAR CARCINOMA (HEPATOMA). The factors that predispose a patient to the development of primary carcinomas of the liver include cirrhosis (particularly hemochromatosis and idiopathic cirrhosis), chronic HBV infection, and the exposure to high levels of aflatoxin in the diet. The high incidence of HBV infections and the contamination of food with aflatoxin might contribute to the high incidence of hepatomas in certain populations in Asia and Africa.

The major clinical features of a hepatoma are sudden hepatic decompensation in a patient with previously stable cirrhosis (usually caused by a tumor invasion or thrombosis of portal or hepatic veins), gastrointestinal bleeding, rapid development of ascites (often containing blood or malignant cells), sudden enlargement of the liver with local pain and a vascular bruit or friction rub, hypoglycemia, and increased plasma levels of α-fetoprotein. In patients without cirrhosis, a hepatic lobectomy or hepatic resection with transplantation occasionally provides a cure; in patients with cirrhosis, the development of a hepatoma usually leads to death; chemotherapy is of limited value in prolonging the patient's survival.

SECONDARY CARCINOMAS OF THE LIVER. The common primary carcinomas that metastasize to the liver are lesions of the lung, breast, and gastrointestinal tract (stomach, pancreas, and colon). The earliest clinical sign of hepatic involvement is usually mild cholestasis with an elevation of the levels of serum alkaline phosphatase, 5'-nucleotidase, and γ-glutamyl transpeptidase. Elevated levels of carcinoembryonic antigen indicate the presence of metastatic disease, and filling defects may be detected by liver scanning. Nodular hepatic enlargement and jaundice are later features of hepatic involvement. In rare cases metastatic deposits at the porta hepatis may cause extrahepatic cholestasis; this obstruction may be determined by transhepatic cholangiography and may be relieved by local radiotherapy.

BIBLIOGRAPHY

Gitnick G: Non-A, non-B hepatitis: etiology and clinical course, Annu Rev Med 35:265, 1984.

Jacobson IM and Dienstag JL: Viral hepatitis vaccines, Annu Rev Med 36:241, 1985.

Schiff L and Schiff ER: Diseases of the liver, ed 6, Philadelphia, JB Lippincott Co.

Shafritz DA and Lieberman HM: The molecular biology of hepatitis B virus, Annu Rev Med 35:219, 1984.

Sherlock S: Diseases of the liver and biliary system, ed 7, Oxford, England, 1985, Blackwell Scientific Publications, Inc.

Zimmerman HJ: Hepatotoxicity, New York, 1978, Appleton-Lange.

184 · DISEASES OF THE BILIARY TRACT

Roger D. Soloway

Unparalleled recent progress in understanding the pathogenesis of the most common biliary tract disease, cholesterol and pigment cholelithiasis, the continued expansion of knowledge concerning bile secretion and the enterohepatic circulation of bile salts, and the development of endoscopic retrograde cholangiopancreatography from hepatic catheterization of the gallbladder and extracorporeal shock wave lithotripsy (ESWL), along with manometry and thin needle cholangiography, have combined to improve our understanding of biliary diseases and to underline their importance.

BILE SECRETION AND COMPOSITION

BIOCHEMISTRY. Cholesterol is an essential component of all biomembranes. Exogenous cholesterol originates in the diet and is a minor source of the cholesterol used. The liver is the major endogenous source of cholesterol; the small intestine and skin also contribute. The endogenous synthesis is in a complex balance with the intake and enterohepatic recirculation of cholesterol. The rate-limiting enzyme for cholesterol synthesis is hydroxymethylglutaryl-coenzyme A (HMG-CoA) reductase.

A knowledge of the characteristics of bile flow and composition is important for an understanding of gallstone formation and dissolution. Bile salts are the major end product of cholesterol metabolism and are formed via a large number of intermediates only in the liver. The enzyme, $7\text{-}\alpha$-hydroxylase, which adds a hydroxyl group to the cholesterol molecule in the $7\text{-}\alpha$ position of the steroid molecule, is the rate-limiting enzyme for bile acid synthesis and determines that the resultant compound can only be converted to bile acids.

Chenodeoxycholic acid (hydroxyl groups at the $3\text{-}\alpha$ and $7\text{-}\alpha$ positions on the sterol nucleus) and cholic acid (hydroxyl groups at the $3\text{-}\alpha$, $7\text{-}\alpha$, and $12\text{-}\alpha$ positions) are the two primary bile acids produced by the liver from cholesterol. They are conjugated with taurine and glycine before their secretion into the bile; unconjugated bile acids are not excreted into the bile in appreciable quantities. Bile acids are reabsorbed from the jejunum and colon by passive transport and from the distal 100 cm of ilium by active transport. Most are reabsorbed unchanged and return to the liver via the portal vein, where they are efficiently taken up by the liver and resecreted into the bile. Bile acids entering the colon or otherwise exposed to bacteria undergo deconjugation and/or dehydroxylation. Thus some unconjugated primary bile acids return to the liver, where they are reconjugated before resecretion. Other primary bile acids are transformed by colonic bacterial dehydroxylation into secondary bile acids. Cholic acid is dehydroxylated at the $7\text{-}\alpha$ position into deoxycholic acid, a major component of fecal bile acids. Deoxycholic acid is also extensively reabsorbed by passive diffusion and conjugated in the liver and excreted into the bile. In contrast, chenodeoxycholic acid is dehydroxylated into lithocholic acid, which is poorly reabsorbed and is the other principal fecal bile acid. Chenodeoxycholic acid is also partially dehydrogenated by intestinal bacteria at the $7\text{-}\alpha$ position and rehydrogenated after reabsorption by the liver, forming either chenodeoxycholic acid or its $7\text{-}\beta$ epimer, ursodeoxycholic acid (2% to 3%). These are the major steps in the enterohepatic circulation of bile acids that result in the preservation of 90% of the bile acids secreted each day.

Cholesterol and phospholipids require bile salts for their biliary secretion, and their secretion increases along with increasing bile salt secretion. At a high rate of bile salt secretion, bile is likely to be undersaturated with cholesterol.

PHYSICAL CHEMISTRY. Cholesterol is minimally soluble in water but is carried in bile micelles that are about 50 Å in diameter. Micelles are spherical or biplanar aggregates of phospholipids and bile salts that have their charged portions facing outward into the surrounding polar water environment and their nonpolar portions facing inward, creating a microenvironment suitable for the transport of nonpolar compounds such as cholesterol. Alone, bile salts form small micelles capable of solubilizing relatively small amounts of cholesterol. Phospholipids are poorly soluble in water, but when present in mixed micelles with bile salts, they greatly expand micellar size, permitting the solubilization of a much greater quantity of cholesterol. The relationship of these three compounds can be plotted using triangular coordinates so that any point in the resultant triangular graph represents a mixture of these lipids. The use of in vitro mixtures of lipids has demonstrated the boundaries of a small micellar zone in which mixtures of cholesterol, bile salts and phospholipids are transparent, because all the compounds are in solution. Cholesterol does not precipitate from such solutions, even after standing for a long time. Mixtures supersaturated with cholesterol, even though initially clear, quickly demonstrate the formation of cholesterol crystals. The series of mixtures between the micellar and supersaturated zones delineates the metastable zone. In this zone the mixtures also develop cholesterol crystals, only slowly. However, gallbladder bile samples taken from a control group and from patients with stones have not conformed closely to the behavior of in vitro mixtures. Thus the formation of cholesterol microcrystals does not follow closely the predictions developed from the in vitro systems. Additional factor affecting cholesterol nucleation time such as the presence of protein accelerators or inhibitors are essential for cholesterol stone formation.

Bilirubin, the end product of heme catabolism and the major component of pigment stones, is secreted into the bile at a rate of 300 mg daily after conjugation with glucuronic acid. Even though partial deconjugation occurs within the intestine, less than 10% of biliary bilirubin is reabsorbed unaltered for resecretion into the bile; the remainder is converted into various urobilinogens and stercobilinogens, which undergo a separate metabolism and excretion in urine or feces.

Little is known about the metabolism of the other components of pigment stones. Calcium is secreted into hepatic bile, perhaps as a cation for the anionic bile acids, and also is actively secreted by the gallbladder, especially in response to an obstruction. The mechanisms by which phosphate and carbonate are secreted into the bile are unknown, but because the pH of bile varies between 6.5 and 8, the concentration of these anions, which are significant components of some pigment stones, must be extremely small. Furthermore, the mechanism by which they reach high concentrations in stones is unknown. One theory suggests that some proteins act as a stone skeleton, upon which stone components precipitate, while other proteins facilitate or inhibit stone formation, perhaps through alteration of the various solubility products for calcium salts.

PHYSIOLOGY. Bile salts are actively secreted into the canaliculus. The volume and electrolyte content of the canalicular flow are further modified as it passes through the ductular system. During fasting the normal gallbladder concentrates hepatic bile rapidly, at a rate of 16% of the volume present every hour. The average pressure of Oddi's sphincter during fasting is 20 to 30 mm Hg, which is greater than the pressure in the common duct. Some hepatic bile enters the intestine, but bile salts are reabsorbed and resecreted into bile. Because of this amplification process the gallbladder contains 80% to 95% of the bile acid pool after a 16-hour fast. In response to a meal containing fats or proteins, cholecystokinin, a polypeptide hormone, is released from cells in the intestinal wall, especially in the duodenum, and together with other hormones causes the relaxation of Oddi's sphincter and the coordinated contraction of the gallbladder. Over the following 2 to 3 hours the gallbladder remains contracted, and the bile acid pool circulates two to three times. The sphincter then returns to its resting level, and the gallbladder relaxes, again permitting a partial sequestration of the bile acid pool within the gallbladder before its release in response to the next meal.

The bile acid pool normally is 3 to 5 g. It circulates about eight to ten times daily. The pool does not circulate constantly but rather goes out in waves stimulated by postprandial hormone release and changes in motility. The fecal losses are balanced by the hepatic synthesis of about 300 to 500 mg daily. Thus at any time about 90% of the hepatic bile acids secreted are derived from recirculation. Because in humans the synthesis can replace only a 10% pool loss, efficient bile acid reabsorption is essential for preservation of the bile acid pool.

About 1 g of cholesterol is secreted by the liver each day, and 50% of this is reabsorbed. The conversion of cholesterol into bile salts enables more cholesterol to be excreted. These steps are the only means by which the body can excrete cholesterol. Phospholipids are hydrolyzed by pancreatic phospholipase, and the components are reabsorbed and synthesized into the triglycerides and phospholipids by the intestinal mucosal cells.

CHOLELITHIASIS AND CHOLECYSTITIS

DEFINITION. Cholelithiasis is the presence of gallstones within the gallbladder. Choledocholithiasis is the presence of stones in the common duct resulting from their passage from the gallbladder or their primary formation in the common duct. Intrahepatic stones may reflux into the intrahepatic ducts from the common duct or may form there primarily. In the United States stones rarely form outside the gallbladder, but this is common in the Orient. In postcholecystectomy patients in Western countries there is a 15% incidence of choledocholithiasis.

Cholesterol stones

ETIOLOGY. Cholesterol stones are 50% to 99% cholesterol and are formed in the gallbladder when currently unclear factors permit the nidation of cholesterol and some calcium bilirubinate, followed by the growth of the stone through the addition of cholesterol crystals. The cholesterol concentration must exceed its solubility in bile for precipitation to occur; in addition, sufficient time must elapse. Except in rare instances hepatic bile does not contain cholesterol crystals, and in more than

98% of these cases cholesterol stones form only in the gallbladder. The growth of stones results from an imbalance of the factors accelerating and inhibiting cholesterol precipitation or binding to protein. This complex system currently is the focus of investigation.

EPIDEMIOLOGY. Approximately 20 million people in the United States have gallstones. Of these stones 75% are predominantly cholesterol and 25% predominantly pigment. The incidence of cholesterol stones is three times as high in females as in males; they are uncommon in patients before puberty and begin to become significantly more common after 20 years of age, reaching a peak incidence in the eighth decade, an age at which most of the population has stones. The incidence and type of stones vary greatly among countries. Many European nations have an incidence comparable to that in the United States. Indian tribes throughout the United States and in parts of Latin America, where they have been studied, have an extraordinarily high incidence of gallstones, approaching 100% of the population in old age. In Bolivia 100% of the stones are of the cholesterol type. In contrast, among the Masai people in Africa, all types of gallstones are rare. In the Orient, pigment gallstones predominate except in urban Japan, where the westernization of the diet has been accomplished by a steady increase in cholesterol stones, which now equals the incidence in the United States (75%).

Obese patients are more likely to develop cholesterol stones because, like Indians, they have a higher secretion of biliary cholesterol and a lower secretion of bile acids. In obese patients the level of biliary cholesterol reverts to normal with a weight loss approaching the patient's ideal weight. In general, hypercholesterolemic patients do not have an increased secretion of biliary cholesterol and do not have an increased incidence of cholesterol stones.

PATHOGENESIS. The mechanism of the formation of supersaturated hepatic bile is still a matter of debate. Early attention focused on the increase in HMG-CoA reductase and the decrease in 7-α-hydroxylase in these patients as compared to a control group, suggesting that the cause of the biliary lipid abnormalities was an imbalance between the formation of cholesterol and bile acids. Further investigation disclosed that chenodeoxycholic acid could suppress the secretion of biliary cholesterol in less than 1 hour, indicating that this effect could occur without a change in the hepatic enzymatic content. It has been hypothesized that the types of bile acids being secreted determine at least in part the amount of cholesterol secreted into the bile and that the activity of HMG-CoA reductase and 7-α-hydroxylase results from this differential effect at the site of the formation of biliary micelles. The arrangement of lecithin and cholesterol within the micelle resembles the lipid structure of a membrane, but the origin of biliary lipids is still unknown.

Although the secretion of bile supersaturated with cholesterol is a prerequisite for the formation of cholesterol stones, it is not sufficient for the formation of stones. Recent studies have demonstrated that biliary cholesterol nucleation time is much more rapid for cholesterol gallstone formers than for patients with pigment stone or nonstone formers. Proteins have been identified that both accelerate and inhibit cholesterol stone formation. Although bile may remain lithogenic for cholesterol after cholecystectomy, cholesterol stones rarely form in the ducts and cholesterol crystals cannot be identified in the bile. Time is needed for the growth of a stone, and this is provided by sequestration within recesses in the gallbladder, especially if the gallbladder does not empty completely in response to a meal. Gallbladder mucus or desquamated epithelium together with small amounts of calcium bilirubinate provides an excellent nidus for stone formation. Many small nidi and microcrystals are probably evacuated by the gallbladder before a stone reaches a clinically significant size.

Chronic cholecystitis invariably accompanies chronic cholelithiasis, but it is unclear whether it is an initiating or a perpetuating feature in cholelithiasis because acalculous cholecystitis is observed in 5% of patients undergoing biliary tract surgery. Perhaps cholecystitis will be found to be an initiator, causing gallbladder obstruction resulting from edema and causing excessive mucus secretion. This would provide the nidus for the formation of a gallstone and the stasis needed for gallstone growth.

The operative incidence of cholelithiasis increases with the age of the patient; whether this occurs because over a longer time it is more likely that a random event will occur or because of the aging process is not clear. Females have an incidence of cholesterol cholelithiasis three times higher than that of males. Studies of pregnant women using realtime ultrasonography have demonstrated that during the third trimester the gallbladder is dilated and is less responsive to a standard contractile force. In addition, the increased levels of estrogens secreted at this time are associated with an increased cholesterol saturation and cholestasis. The incidence of cholelithiasis is higher in certain families. In addition, groups such as the American Indians have a dual biochemical defect, a higher hepatic secretion of cholesterol and a smaller bile salt pool with a lower secretion of bile salts. Obese patients also have this dual defect until their weight returns to the ideal range. The effects of diet on cholelithiasis are being studied. Low-cholesterol, low-fat diets lower the level of cholesterol in bile by 20%, but the effects are complex because bile acid metabolism is also affected. Any disease reducing the conservation of circulating bile acids and therefore reducing the return of bile acids to the liver through the enterohepatic circulation results in a decreased secretion of bile acids into bile. In such diseases cholesterol secretion is virtually unchanged, and thus bile becomes supersaturated with cholesterol. Regional enteritis involving the terminal ileum, an ileojejunal bypass, cystic fibrosis, and small intestinal resection have been associated with a higher incidence of cholelithiasis caused by this mechanism. Various drugs have been implicated in the formation of stones, including oral contraceptives, estrogens, and clofibrate (a systemic cholesterol-lowering agent that increases the biliary secretion of cholesterol while decreasing the bile salt pool).

CLINICAL MANIFESTATIONS. Ultrasonographic surveys indicate that 90% of patients have gallstones for their entire adult life without developing symptoms. Because of this long period of latency, it is not possible to know when the formation of symptomatic stones may have begun. Gallstones rarely cause symptoms in patients under 20 years of age; the peak incidence occurs in patients 40 to 60 years of age.

Flatulence, bloating, eructation, fatty food intolerance, and nonspecific abdominal discomforts have been ascribed to cholelithiasis. Such symptoms are present with the same incidence in patients without stones, however, and these symptoms are not resolved by a cholecystectomy. The symptoms of cholelithiasis result from the passage or impaction of stones in the gallbladder or at Oddi's sphincter. The classic and most common symptom is pain caused by the impaction of stones in the ampulla of the gallbladder. Typically this occurs 4 to 6 hours after an evening meal and awakens the patient from sleep. The pain is steady, builds in intensity, lasts from 15 minutes to 6 hours, and may require administration of narcotics for relief. It usually stops when the stone returns to the body of the gallbladder. Typically such episodes are separated by symptom-free periods of months to years. Biliary pain is most commonly located in the epigastrium (28% of these patients) or subcostaly in the right upper quadrant (22%) but also may be located any place within the abdomen, such as substernally (11%) or over the right or left lower rib cage or back (10%).

When pain occurs with each meal, it may be caused by the impaction of a stone in the cystic duct; the pain results from the contraction of the gallbladder behind the stone, increasing the gallbladder pressure. A similar syndrome may be caused by the impaction of a stone in Oddi's sphincter, but this condition usually is accompanied by constant pain, hyperamylasemia, and jaundice.

Stones that pass through the cystic duct and Oddi's sphincter without impaction do not cause further problems and are eliminated in the feces. However, severe pancreatitis may result from stone passage. Although pancreatitis that occurs because of passage of stones is not common, it is generally much more severe than alcoholic pancreatitis and more commonly leads to the formation of pseudocysts and pancreatic abscesses.

When an inflamed gallbladder attaches to the first or second portion of the duodenum, a fistula may result. Large gallstones can then pass into the intestine and become impacted at the ileocecal valve, the narrowest area between the fistula and the anus. This impaction may cause a progressive intestinal obstruction leading eventually to gallstone ileus.

In almost all cases of chronic cholecystitis in the United States, gallbladder bile and stones are not infected. When stones are infected, however, it is unlikely that they will become sterilized because of their labyrinthine structure. Thus any subsequent obstruction to a gallbladder containing infected stones often results in the development of an acute infection, causing bacteremia. Bacterial infection occurs more commonly in association with acute cholecystitis but is not necessary for its development.

When the bile is infected, cholangitis occurs following an obstruction of Oddi's sphincter. Once cholangitis develops, repeated episodes are likely along with the subsequent passage of stones because of the persistent infection of the glands lining the ductular system. Stenosis of Oddi's sphincter also may result, leading to the formation of common duct and hepatic stones. Stones in these locations are associated with additional cholangitis and intrahepatic abscesses.

The chronic obstruction of the gallbladder neck by a stone or by fibrosis and/or swollen lymph nodes leads to the concentration of biliary calcium and to increased secretion of calcium and mucus, along with resorption of biliary lipids. If the gallbladder continues to secrete, it may become very enlarged, a condition called hydrops that is more commonly visualized than palpated. This is the exception to Courvoisier's law that a palpable gallbladder in patients with obstructive jaundice indicates the likelihood of an obstructing tumor of the common duct rather than a stone. In cases of hydrops there is no evidence that the bile duct is obstructed because the levels of bilirubin and alkaline phosphatase are normal. If there is a significant secretion of calcium carbonate, the bile becomes radiopaque (so-called limy bile). If this condition is demonstrated on a plain roentgenogram of the abdomen, it is proof that the gallbladder is chronically obstructed. Calcification in the wall of the gallbladder, called porcelain gallbladder, is an indication for cholecystectomy, because such gallbladders are more susceptible to development of a carcinoma.

LABORATORY FINDINGS AND DIAGNOSIS. Gallbladder disease is rarely associated with changes in the results of liver blood tests unless the bile duct is obstructed. Acute cholecystitis, however, may affect the liver surrounding the gallbladder bed, causing a rise in the levels of aminotransferases and alkaline phosphatase. This elevation also occurs if the gallbladder is intrahepatic in location. In cases of an obstruction of the bile duct or a postoperative stricture formation, the level of alkaline phosphatase is usualy elevated, often with an elevated level of serum bilirubin.

Oral cholecystograms obtained following administration of six iopanoic acid (Telepaque) tablets on 2 successive days allow for adequate visualization of more than 95% of normal gallbladders. Cholesterol stones, which usually are radiolucent, appear as filling defects in the opacified gallbladder. In 95% of the cases in which the gallbladder cannot be seen on the cholecystogram, this indicates the presence of gallbladder disease.

If the symptoms are typical of biliary pain and no stone is demonstrated, biliary drainage should be performed. Small stones and sludge can be demonstrated by the microscopic examination of bile collected through a duodenal tube following the administration of magnesium sulfate or cholecystokinin, which causes the gallbladder to contract. The presence of cholesterol crystals usually indicates the presence of a stone, sludge, or cholesterolosis. Cholesterol crystals occur in stacks; they are flat and rectangular with one corner commonly missing (resembling the state of Utah). The presence of these crystals can be confirmed by demonstrating birefringence using a polarizing light stage on the microscope.

An alternative method of diagnosis that avoids the use of radiation is an ultrasonographic examination of the gallbladder. This is more accurate than oral cholecystography for 1 to 2 mm stones and is currently the method of choice for screening patients in whom stones are suspected. However, the technique does not allow accurate measurement of the size of a stone and does not determine whether the patient may undergo medical dissolution, because it cannot establish gallbladder function.

In cases of severe abdominal pain, failure of the gallbladder to concentrate intravenous technetium 99m PIPIDA (paraisopropyl iminodiacetic acid), which is rapidly excreted into the biliary system, suggests the presence of acute cholecystitis or a blockage of the cystic duct.

Common duct stones cannot usually be effectively diagnosed by means of ultrasonography. In 20% of the cases of choledocholithiasis the common bile duct is not dilated, and in this situation either percutaneous transhepatic cholangiography (which may require 15 to 20 passes in the patient with a nondilated biliary tract) or endoscopic retrograde cholangiopancreatography is the procedure of choice. The contract obtained in these procedures is so superior to that of intravenous cholangiography that the latter procedure has been abandoned.

MANAGEMENT. Cholecystectomy currently is the treatment of choice for symptomatic gallstones and is the standard against which all other treatments should be measured. The indications for cholecystectomy in patients with asymptomatic stones are debatable. The mortality of this procedure in patients under 60 years of age is about 0.5% to 1% in medical centers. The mortality and morbidity are higher if the surgeon is unfamiliar with the wide variety of vascular and biliary tree anomalies that occur in this region. The most common mistake is an inadvertent ligation or transection of the common bile duct. Nonetheless, a successful cholecystectomy results in a permanent cure in 95% of these patients, and there is also no measurable change in digestion.

Patients, especially those with concomitant illnesses that increase the risk of surgery, may prefer an attempt at medical dissolution of gallstones using chenodeoxycholic acid. Bile acids act by reducing cholesterol secretion into bile and by increasing the size of the bile acid pool. Because of their possible teratogenicity, these drugs are not administered to patients under 40 years of age. These agents do not dissolve calcified cholesterol stones or stones in patients whose gallbladder cannot be visualized by oral cholecystography. The efficacy of the agents also is reduced in patients with stones larger than 1 cm in diameter and in obese patients, and these agents do not dissolve radiolucent pigment stones. Thus, dissolution occurs successfully in about 70% to 80% of cases after a 2-year course. In approximately 50% of these patients stones reform after this dissolution. The long-term regimen for such patients may include repeated courses of bile acids. Several alternative forms of treatment show early promise because of their rapid action (within 24 hours): transhepatic catheterization of the gallbladder with instillation of methyl tert-butyl-ether and extracorporeal shock wave lithotripsy.

Acute cholecystitis should be treated with an appropriate antibiotic coverage for intestinal flora, such as with ampicillin and gentamicin. Surgeons now tend to prefer performing a cholecystectomy promptly when the toxicity is controlled.

PREVENTION. Because heredity plays a major role in the formation of stones, there seems to be little that can be done to prevent stone formation. However, maintaining the patient's weight in the ideal range and avoiding prolonged fasts or drugs known to cause alterations in biliary lipid composition seem important. Eating frequent small meals and a snack just before bedtime to keep bile circulating for the longest possible time during the day should be helpful in keeping the bile undersaturated with cholesterol during the greatest portion of the day.

NEOPLASTIC DISEASE
Carcinoma of the gallbladder and extrahepatic biliary ducts

DEFINITION, ETIOLOGY, AND EPIDEMIOLOGY. Although other tumors may metastasize to the gallbladder, the predominant tumors are adenocarcinomas of the gallbladder and cholangiocarcinomas of the extrahepatic biliary ducts. The causes of these tumors are unknown. The incidence of gallbladder cancer is about 3:200,000 people in the United States. Bile duct cancer has a lower incidence. The incidence of gallbladder cancer is 3.4 times higher in females than in males, which parallels the incidence of gallstones. In contrast, the incidence of cancer of the biliary tract is equal in males and females. The incidence of cholelithiasis among patients with cancer of the gallbladder is at least 75%, whereas it is significantly less (32%) among those with biliary tract cancer. Patients in both groups have an average age of 63 to 65 years at the onset of the disease. In Japan the incidence of carcinoma is highest in patients with black stones (3.4%), intermediate in those with cholesterol stones (1%), and lowest in those with bilirubinatepalmitate stones (0.16%). Cancer of the gallbladder is much more common in Amerind populations and is the most common gastrointestinal tumor in Amerind women.

Cholangiocarcinomas have been associated with chronic intrahepatic cholangitis, hepatolithiasis, ulcerative colitis, and infections with *Opisthorchis sinensis*. The incidence of bile duct tumors is higher in patients with choledochocele after undergoing choledochoduodenostomy. Half of these tumors develop within 4 years of the operation, suggesting an interaction between biliary and intestinal components.

CLINICAL MANIFESTATIONS. Cancer of the gallbladder has been detected incidentally during elective cholecystectomy for gallstones, but unfortunately even these patients have a very poor survival rate. Patients with a clinically evident carcinoma usually have a palpable mass or right upper quadrant pain caused by peritoneal involvement. The disease commonly is unresectable. Cancer of the bile duct usually is detected at an earlier stage, because even a slight growth causes a bile duct obstruction. Cancer of the left or right hepatic duct does not cause symptoms until it has reached a large size, since complete obstruction of one duct does not cause jaundice because the unobstructed lobe can handle the increased biliary secretion. The level of alkaline phosphatase, however, may be considerably elevated. A tumor at the bifurcation of the left and right hepatic ducts, called a Klatskin tumor, causes early jaundice.

LABORATORY FINDINGS. Because of the bile duct obstruction, the level of alkaline phosphatase may be elevated as much as 20 to 40 times the normal level. Serum levels of carcinoembryonic antigen (CEA) and CA-19-9 are frequently elevated.

DIAGNOSIS. Ultrasonography may identify a gallbladder mass or a dilated intrahepatic duct. The diagnosis may be made with a fine-needle biopsy and/or with percutaneous fine-needle cholangiography or retrograde cholangiography. Fine-needle cholangiography is preferred for the diagnosis of intrahepatic lesions because percutaneous transhepatic catheters may be placed, depending on the patient, as a definitive procedure or as a decompressive measure before surgery, irradiation, or chemotherapy.

COURSE. Although bile duct tumors may be discovered at an early stage, patients with such tumors have a poor 5-year survival rate, and there is no evidence that radical surgical procedures extend the life expectancy. In patients with extensive disease the morbidity may be reduced by placement of percutaneous biliary catheters with multiple side-holes through the tumor. These tubes can eventually be clamped so that bile can drain internally from above to below the lesions and into the intestine. Alternatively, stents can be placed through the tumor via Oddi's sphincter by endoscopy. When bile can pass freely into the intestine, jaundice and pruritis can clear and the patient's appetite may increase. Various chemotherapeutic regimens have been tried without any striking success. Radiotherapy has been reported to increase the survival rate, but no controlled trials have been reported to date.

Carcinoma of the ampulla of Vater

Cancer arising from the ampulla of Vater is more common than cancer of the extrahepatic bile ducts but less common than cancer of the gallbladder. Patients with ampullary carcinoma usually have obstructive jaundice that must be differentiated from other types of extrahepatic obstruction such as that caused by carcinoma of the pancreas or the bile ducts, choledocholithiasis, a stricture of the common bile duct, and sclerosing cholangitis; this carcinoma must also be differentiated from intrahepatic cholestasis caused by drugs, primary biliary cirrhosis, and numerous other hepatic disorders. Ampullary carcinomas commonly produce occult blood in the feces but rarely bleed grossly. The diagnosis is probably best determined by endoscopic retrograde cholangiopancreatography (ERCP), which often permits a direct visualization of the lesion, and a biopsy, as well as roentgenographic visualization of the pancreatic and biliary ducts. If necessary, percutaneous fine-needle cholangiogrphy, ultrasonography, or computed tomography may also be helpful in demonstrating dilated biliary ducts and an obstructing extrahepatic lesion. Patients with ampullary carcinoma have the best prognosis among those with biliary and pancreatic carcinomas; the 5-year survival rate after a radical pancreaticoduodenectomy (Whipple's procedure) may be as high as 25% to 50%.

BIBLIOGRAPHY
Cholelithiasis

Admirand WH and Small DM: The physicochemical basis of cholesterol gallstone formation in man, J Clin Invest 47:1043, 1968.

Allen MJ and others: Rapid dissolution of gallstones by methyl tert-butyl-ether: preliminary observations, N Engl J Med 312:217, 1985.

Grundy SM: Factors affecting biliary lipid composition. In Cohen S and Soloway RD, editors: Contemporary issues in gastroenterology, vol 4, New York, 1985, Churchill Livingstone, Inc.

Holtzbach RT and Kibe A: Pathogenesis of cholesterol gallstones. In Cohen S and Soloway RD, editors: Contemporary issues in gastroenterology, vol 4, New York, 1985, Churchill Livingstone, Inc.

Holzbach RT and others: Cholesterol solubility in bile: evidence that supersaturated bile is frequent in healthy man, J Clin Invest 52:1467, 1973.

Sauerbruch T and others: Fragmentation of gallstones by extracorporeal shock waves, N Engl J Med 314:818, 1986.

Smith BF and LaMont JT: Gallbladder mucin and gallstone formation. In Cohen S and Soloway RD, editors: Contemporary issues in gastroenterology, vol 4, New York, 1985, Churchill Livingstone, Inc.

Soloway RD and Trotman BW: Pigment gallstones. In Ostrow JD, editor: Bile pigments and jaundice: molecular, metabolic and medical aspects, New York, 1985, Marcel Dekker, Inc.

Wagner CI and others: Kinetic analysis of biliary lipid excretion in man and dog. J Clin Invest 57:473, 1976.

Carcinoma and the gallbladder

Strom BL and others: Carcinoma of the gallbladder. In Cohen S and Soloway RD, editors: Contemporary issues in gastroenterology, vol 4, New York, 1985, Churchill Livingstone, Inc.

Carcinoma of the ampulla of Vater

Soloway RD, Balistreri WF, and Trotman BW: The gallbladder and biliary tract. In Bouchier IAD, editor: Recent advances in gastroenterology, ed 4, New York, 1980, Churchill Livingstone, Inc.

Dental correlations

Michael E. Pliskin, Barry H. Hendler, Barbara J. Steinberg, *and* **Louis F. Rose***

DISEASES OF THE ESOPHAGUS

Although pathologic manifestations vary widely, the primary clinical symptom of all esophageal disorders is dysphagia. This symptom can have a number of causes, including the following:

1. Mechanical obstruction such as a malignant esophageal tumor
2. Uncoordinated contraction reflex of the swallowing musculature because of neurologic disease
3. Plummer-Vinson syndrome, which results in muscular degeneration or stenosis
4. Collagen vascular disease (scleroderma or progressive systemic sclerosis), which causes increased rigidity of the esophageal wall
5. Infections, particularly with *Candida* organisms, which can cause retrosternal burning and esophageal spasm

From a diagnostic standpoint, the dentist should be aware that although patients frequently associate dysphagia with dental problems, this symptom usually indicates serious underlying systemic disease. Therefore, when all possible dental causes (for example, space-occupying infection) have been ruled out, diagnostic efforts immediately should turn to a complete evaluation through medical consultation.

Plummer-Vinson syndrome occurs most frequently in women in the fourth and fifth decades. The primary cause of the syndrome is iron deficiency, and the main symptom, dysphagia, results from muscular degeneration in the esophagus and stenoses or webs of the esophageal mucosa.

---

*Material in this chapter is based in part on the first edition of which Shirley Brown was a contributing author.

In addition to dysphagia, Plummer-Vinson syndrome has many other clinical manifestations that are significant in dental practice. Patients often have a thinned vermillion border of the lips, angular cheilitis, and reduced width of the mouth. The oral mucosa is thin, atrophic, inelastic, dry, and glazed, and the tongue often becomes red and painful and appears smooth because of loss of papillae.

The atrophic mucosal changes of Plummer-Vinson syndrome appear to predispose these individuals to leukoplakia and in some cases oral and pharyngeal carcinoma. (In a study of 250 patients with carcinoma of the mouth and upper respiratory tract, 70% had a history of Plummer-Vinson syndrome.)

MANAGEMENT. The management of patients with Plummer-Vinson syndrome includes the following:

1. Patients are encouraged to eat a well-balanced diet, which at first consists of semiliquid or soft foods.
2. Treatment of the oral pain may include the use of viscous 2% lidocaine or diphenhydramine hydrochloride and dyclonine HCl (Benadryl-Dyclone solution). (Dyclone 0.5% and Benadryl 5 mg/ml mixed with equal parts of Maalox or Milk of Magnesia. The solution must be used and not the more common elixir, because the latter contains alcohol, which will burn the tissues.)
3. The patient must be followed closely for development of red and/or white lesions that may represent dysplastic or carcinomatous lesions. A biopsy and pathologic examination should be done on these lesions.

Progressive systemic sclerosis (PSS, or scleroderma) is a chronic collagen vascular disease of possible autoimmune origin. It is characterized by diffuse scleroses of the skin, gastrointestinal tract, heart muscle, lungs, and kidneys and most commonly affects women between 20 and 50 years of age. A recent study has shown that head and neck manifestations occur in 80% of scleroderma patients. These include dysphagia because of esophageal involvement; thinning and rigidity of the lips; narrowing of the oral aperture; loss of skin-folds around the mouth, giving a masklike facies; hardness and rigidity of the tongue; and xerostomia, all of which may render speech extremely difficult. Mandibular movement sometimes is restricted when the muscles of mastication are affected by the disease and become rigid. Dental roentgenograms commonly reveal a uniform thickening of the periodontal membrane space, especially around posterior teeth.

Progressive systemic sclerosis presents several problems unique to dentistry. Since the oral aperture may be narrowed and the face rigid, access to the teeth and periodontium is impaired. This may limit the scope of treatment and necessitate special prosthetic techniques. In addition, since these patients frequently suffer from sclerotic "clawing" of the hands (sclerodactyly) (Fig. 1), which diminishes manual dexterity, toothbrushing and flossing may be difficult or impossible. These patients therefore require constant comprehensive oral care and frequent professional oral prophylaxis.

CREST syndrome refers to calcinosis, Raynaud's phenomenon, esophageal dysfunction, sclerodactyly, and telangectasia. The disease is characterized by its slow evolution over decades, lack of visceral involvement, anti-Scl 70, and anti-centromere/kinetochore antibodies. These autoantibodies may be regarded as serologic markers for scleroderma and CREST syndrome. The incidence in the former is only 15% to 20%, whereas it is 70% to 90% in the latter. Long-standing CREST can involve severe pulmonary hypertension because of the marked sclerosis of small pulmonary arteries.

Candida infections of the esophagus usually occur when the mouth and pharynx also are involved, a condition known as "candidal oropharyngoesophagitis." The disease is caused by

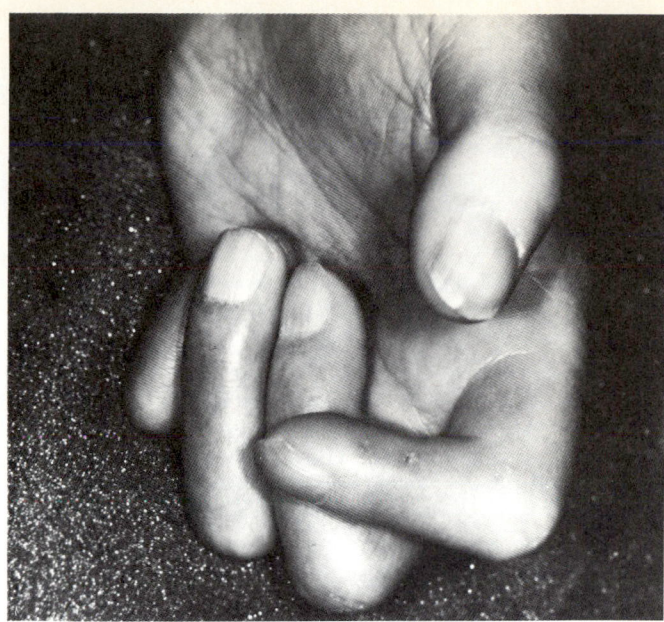

Fig. 1   Sclerodactyly in 55-year-old man with scleroderma.

an overgrowth of the hyphal form of *Candida albicans* and may occur in individuals with malignant disease or endocrine or immunologic disorders such as acquired immunodeficiency syndrome (AIDS) and in patients undergoing antibiotic, corticosteroid, or immunosuppressant therapy. These patients usually complain of chronic dysphagia, oropharyngeal soreness of varying intensity, and occasional retrosternal burning. The appearance of the candidal lesions is distinctive, characterized by soft, white, slightly elevated "curdlike" plaques that, when stripped from the tissue, leave a bleeding mucosal surface.

MANAGEMENT. The management of patients with *Candida* infections includes the following:

1. Consultation with patients' physician to determine underlying medical problems
2. Local treatment with nystatin rinses, clotrimazol troches, or ketoconazole tablets
3. Meticulous cleansing of dentures

PEPTIC ULCER DISEASE

The dental patient with peptic ulcer disease requires special consideration in three general areas of treatment: drug therapy, stress management protocol, and oral surgery.

MANAGEMENT. The management of patients with peptic ulcer disease includes the following:

1. Possible drug interactions and adverse during effects must be evaluated
2. The patient must avoid aspirin, all aspirin-containing analgesics, phenylbutazone, steroids, and nonsteroidal antiinflammatory drugs
3. Acetaminophen or any of its compounds (acetaminophen-codeine combinations) or propoxyphene hydrochloride is the analgesic of choice
4. Anticholinergics used to treat patients with peptic ulcer disease may cause xerostomia, increasing the caries rate and decreasing retention of dentures. The former may be treated by daily home use of fluorides, and the latter with adhesives or artificial saliva.
5. Antacids generally contain calcium, magnesium, or aluminum salts, which will bind to orally administered antibiotics such as erythromycin and particularly tetracycline. Because this binding action causes a decrease of as much as 80% in the absorption

of these antibiotics, they should not be taken within 1 hour of the antacid.

6. Penicillin V should be given instead of penicillin G because of the resistance of the former to gastric acid. This should be a general rule for all patients but is particularly important for patients with peptic ulcer disease.
7. Stress should be reduced by having shorter dental visits and by using appropriate sedation techniques such as nitrous oxide or tranquilizers.
8. Because the patient with peptic ulcer disease may have occult bleeding with chronic anemia, the dentist should obtain a complete blood count and hematocrit and hemoglobin levels before extensive oral or periodontal surgery.

In oral diagnosis the dentist can benefit from results of studies performed on a large number of hospitalized patients with and without peptic ulcer disease. The studies revealed that certain vascular formations of the lips occur about 25% more frequently and at an earlier age in patients with a history of peptic ulcer than in groups without ulcers. However, the cause of the formations is not clearly understood at this time. These vascular formations were seen more often in men than in women and were of three types:

1. *Microcherry*. This is a sharply circumscribed red dot, usually smaller than 1 mm in diameter. It is most commonly found on the inner surface of the lower lip but may be seen on the vermilion border and on the upper lip as well. Microcherries may occur singly, or there may be several that are widely separated.
2. *Glomerulus*. This formation is a 1 to 2 mm aggregate of tortuous, thin-walled red vessels that resemble the glomerulus of the kidney. When pressure is applied to the glomerulus, it blanches; as the pressure is released, it may pulsate.
3. *Venous lake*. This is a dilated portion of a submucosal vein that resembles a small varicosity. The venous lake is a single bluish mound that collapses on slight pressure and does not pulsate. It often is found at the inner surface of the labial commissures and less commonly along the vermilion border of the lip.

TUMORS AND VASCULAR AND INFLAMMATORY DISEASES OF THE GASTROINTESTINAL TRACT

This important group of gastrointestinal diseases has dental significance in two areas: oral lesions and physical evaluation of the dental patient. From the standpoint of oral lesions, the dentist should be conversant with the signs of each syndrome, ranging from fibrous tumors of the facial bones associated with Gardner's syndrome to the specific and nonspecific oral lesions of Crohn's disease. The dentist also should be aware that metastatic lesions of gastrointestinal tumors such as gastric adenocarcinoma can occur intraorally.

Proper dental management requires that the dental practitioner fully understand the medical management of these patients and obtain medical consultation so that the side effects of medical treatment can be adequately differentiated from other systemic problems affecting oral health. The effects of common drug regimens such as steroid therapy can affect dental treatment, and in many cases drugs used in dentistry such as aspirin compounds are contraindicated for use in these patients.

Because chronic gastrointestinal bleeding is a hazard in many of these syndromes, patients often may be anemic and thrombocytopenic. They also may undergo changes in red and white blood cell counts secondary to the immunosuppressive drugs that are commonly used. As a general rule, therefore, the dentist should routinely obtain hematocrit and hemoglobin values and a complete blood cell count with differential before performing any oral surgical procedure.

TUMORS OF THE GASTROINTESTINAL TRACT
Adenocarcinoma of the stomach

Malignant gastric tumors can metastasize to the head and neck region as a tumor mass or manifest as hyperpigmentation of the dermis and oral mucosa. Only a few cases of metastatic oral lesions from gastric adenocarcinoma have been reported. Of clinical importance is the fact that metastatic lesions involving the oral or perioral structures may be the first evidence of malignant disease arising from a distant origin. These lesions may produce a variety of signs and symptoms, including swelling, pain, looseness of teeth, and paresthesia. In many cases the patient is asymptomatic, and the lesion is discovered during routine oral examination. The mandible is affected more frequently than the maxilla by metastatic tumor. For example, Clausen and Poulsen found that 82% of these tumors were in the mandible, whereas 85% of the cases reported by Meyer and Shklar were the mandible. The molar area is predominantly involved, presumably because of the rich hematopoietic tissue in this region. This mechanism of metastasis has been discussed by Stockdale, who described the extreme significance of the plexus of vertebral veins, or Batson's plexus, as the pathway of dissemination. The physiologic importance of this plexus has been described in detail by Eckenhoff.

Roentgenographically, the metastatic lesions are not pathognomonic, producing more frequently osteolytic lesions but occasionally presenting as osteoplastic foci. The lesions may be well demarcated and confined, or they may exhibit diffuse, poorly outlined involvement of a large portion of the bone. Pathologic fracture may result from the large destruction of bone and may on occasion be the presenting complaint. Metastasis to the oral soft tissues also may occur and may be similar in clinical appearance to connective tissue hyperplasia under an ill fitting denture. It is clear, therefore, that after obtaining a careful medical history and performing a clinical and roentgenographic examination, a biopsy must be done on all suspicious lesions.

The association between occult malignancy and acanthosis nigricans (focal or diffuse hyperpigmentation of the dermis) is well established. More than 50% of patients over 30 years of age who have acanthosis nigricans eventually develop a malignancy, usually adenocarcinoma of the stomach. Acanthosis nigricans appears as velvety, hyperpigmented, hyperkeratotic varicosities, usually in the skin-folds of the neck, axillae, groin, anogenital regions, and other flexural surfaces. Oral manifestations occur in 30% to 40% of patients, primarily on the tongue and lips. The papillae on the dorsum of the tongue become elongated and hypertrophic, producing deep furrows. The labial mucosa and vermilion border may become thickened and covered with papillomatous tumors and cracks. Papillomatous growths also may appear on the tongue, gingiva, and the buccal and palatal mucosa. In addition, leukoedema of the buccal mucosa may occur.

Adenocarcinoma of the colon and rectum

Although cases of metastatic adenocarcinoma to the head and neck region have been well documented, such cases arising from a primary site in the colon and rectum are rare. Moffat reported a lesion that began as a bony metastasis in the mandible with subsequent epulis formation. The patient appeared for treatment with a hard, ulcerated nodule 1.2 by 1 cm, arising from the alveolar margin.

Lee reported a case of adenocarcinoma of the colon with metastasis to the lip. The lesion was a single, round, indurated pinkish gray nodule 1 cm in diameter at the vermilion border of the lower lip.

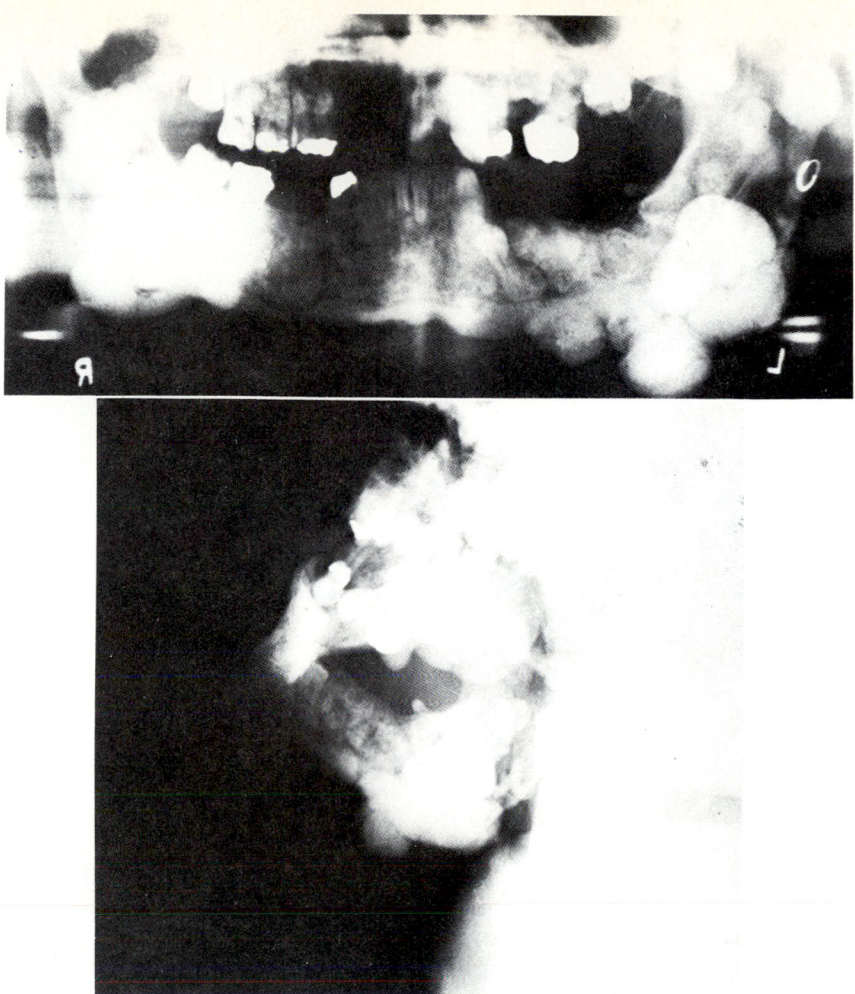

Fig. 2 Osteomas in 17-year-old man with Gardner's syndrome.

Cases of metastasis from the rectum to the parotid gland, palate, and gingiva, although rare, also have been noted in the literature.

Gastrointestinal polyposis syndromes

Both Gardner's syndrome and Peutz-Jeghers syndrome, which are representative of this group of disorders, generally are identified through the family medical history, since they are both inherited as autosomal dominant conditions. Both syndromes demonstrate cutaneous, gastrointestinal, and orofacial manifestations.

In Gardner's syndrome epidermoid or sebaceous cysts of the skin may occur on the face, trunk, and extremities. Fibrous tumors of the skin (fibromas and desmoids) also may occur, the latter most notably seen on surgical scars of the abdomen. Multiple polyps of the colon and rectum with a high malignant potential also are characteristic of this syndrome, which generally develops during or after the second decade.

Manifestations in the head and neck region, in addition to the epidermoid cysts previously mentioned, include multiple asymptomatic osteomas that are scattered throughout the craniofacial skeleton (Fig. 2). These tumors generally appear at puberty and may involve the frontal bone, mandible, maxilla, and sinuses. The long bones also may show involvement. Odontomas, dentigerous cysts, bony exostoses, hypercementosis, supernumerary teeth, and permanent impacted teeth are other common oral findings associated with Gardner's syndrome.

Because of the high level of orofacial involvement in Gardner's syndrome, the dentist can have an important role in its diagnosis. Early diagnosis of the disease is essential, since malignancy rates in untreated individuals appear to be as high as 50% to 100%. Treatment usually involves surgery of the lower intestinal tract to remove the polypoid lesions and any adjacent normal tissue that is likely to undergo malignant transformation.

Peutz-Jeghers syndrome is an autosomal dominant disease characterized by hamartomatous polyps of the gastrointestinal tract and by mucocutaneous melanin deposits. The melanin pigmentations usually are discrete brown or bluish black macules ranging in size from 1 to 10 mm. They are seen most frequently about the perioral, perinasal and periorbital orifices and also may occur on the hands, feet, and trunk. In the mouth the buccal mucosa and lips usually are affected, and pigmentation also may occur on the palate, gingiva, and, less often, the tongue. Intraoral lesions are round, oval, or irregular brown macules 1 to 5 mm in diameter (Fig. 3).

Both mucosal and skin pigmentations first appear shortly after birth in individuals with Peutz-Jeghers syndrome. Since the skin pigmentations fade during adulthood, oral mucosal pigmentation remains the most constant feature of this syndrome. Dermabrasion for cosmetic treatment of the pigmented spots on the lips and oral mucosa occasionally has been at-

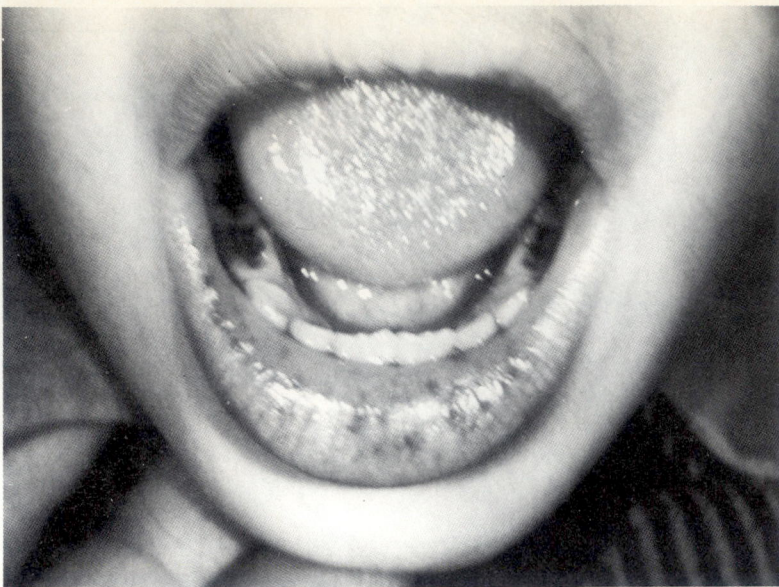

Fig. 3   Pigmentations in 9-year-old girl with Peutz-Jeghers syndrome.

tempted, with generally disappointing results. Recent studies indicate that the pigmentation can now be treated successfully with argon and ruby lasers.

The hamartomatous polyps have been thought to have a very low potential for malignancy and the disease was believed to have a relatively benign course. However, several studies have recently associated the syndrome with gastrointestinal carcinoma, malignant tumors of the breast, and unusual tumors such as ovarian sex-cord tumors and the rare Sertoli cell tumor of the ovary. Other investigators have emphasized the young age of patients at the development of malignant tumors of the pancreas and breast. Giardiello and associates studied the incidence of cancer in 31 patients with Peutz-Jeghers syndrome and found that 48% developed cancer—nongastrointestinal carcinoma in 10 patients, gastrointestinal carcinoma in four, and multiple myeloma in one. In addition, adenomatous polyps of the stomach and colon occurred in three other patients. According to a relative risk analysis, the observed development of cancer in these Peutz-Jeghers patients was 18 times greater than expected in the general population. These results suggested that patients with Peutz-Jeghers syndrome have an increased risk of developing both gastrointestinal and nongastrointestinal cancer. Therefore, the dentist should be aware of cancer development in patients with this syndrome.

VASCULAR DISEASE OF THE GASTROINTESTINAL TRACT
Hereditary hemorrhagic telangiectasia

Hereditary hemorrhagic telangiectasia (HHT) was first described by Osler in 1901, and it frequently bears his name (Rendu-Osler-Weber syndrome). It is a disorder of the capillaries and small blood vessels and is transmitted by simple autosomal dominant inheritance. A deficiency in elastic fibers produces abnormally thin vascular walls, resulting in vascular dilation and spontaneous ruptures. These telangiectases, which occur on cutaneous, visceral, and mucosal surfaces, commonly appear before puberty or after menopause or the male climacteric. They appear as nonpulsating, red or purple, spiderlike or nodular lesions, and pressure causes blanching that does not completely disappear.

Oral lesions of HHT develop most frequently on mucosal surfaces of the lips and on the tip and dorsum of the tongue, although the palate, gingiva, and buccal mucosa also may be affected. The early oral lesion is a cherry red macule ranging from 1 to 3 mm in diameter. Biopsies are rarely indicated, since the syndrome is easily diagnosed from the pathognomonic skin and oral lesions and from the family history.

In addition to the obvious telangiectases, HHT is characterized by spontaneous bleeding, more frequently from mucous membranes than from the skin. The most common site of such bleeding in nearly all HHT patients is the nasal mucosa, with bleeding from oral telangiectases second in frequency to epistaxis. The gastric mucosa also may bleed chronically, as evidenced clinically by hematemesis and melena. The resultant anemia and thrombocytopenia may lead to facial pallor, fatigue, and generalized weakness. Although deaths from severe hemorrhage in HHT patients have been reported, the disease is seldom life threatening.

Treatments to eliminate telangiectatic areas include irradiation and surgical excision. Aminocaproic acid may be applied topically for severe epistaxis. Estrogens have been administered systemically to reduce the frequency and severity of bleeding, with varying degrees of success. For good preventive treatment, a low-roughage diet and avoidance of drugs such as aspirin with erosive and anticoagulant properties are recommended for the patient with HHT, and living quarters should be well humidified to reduce irritation of the oral and nasal mucosa.

MANAGEMENT. The management of patients with HHT includes the following:

1. The dentist should be aware that episodes of bleeding from oral lesions may occur in these individuals with or without traumatic insult.
2. The patient with gingival telangiectases should be advised to brush the teeth gently to minimize trauma to the lesions.
3. Protheses should be kept away from telangiectic areas.
4. Hemorrhages, should they occur, may be controlled by applying direct pressure or by cauterizing the lesions.
5. Prophylaxis of bleeding can be done using a sclerosing agent such as morrhuate sodium or sodium tetradecyl sulfate injected into the lesion.

6. Dental surgical procedures should be performed after obtaining a hemoglobin, hematocrit, platelet count, and medical consultation.

Encephalotrigeminal angiomatosis

Encephalofacial or encephalotrigeminal angiomatosis (Sturge-Weber syndrome) is characterized by the combination of venous angioma of the leptomeninges over the cerebral cortex with ipsilateral angiomatous lesions of the face and occasionally of the skull, jaws, and oral soft tissues. The facial angiomatoses (portwine nevi) may follow the dermatomes of one or more of the trigeminal divisions. A second common feature is the presence of intracranial calcifications resulting in spastic hemiplegia with or without mental retardation. Oral changes occur in about a third of the patients and consist of angiomatous lesions of the gingiva, buccal mucosa, and tongue.

MANAGEMENT. The management of patients with encephalotrigeminal angiomatosis includes the following:

1. The dentist must avoid traumatizing the oral soft tissue angiomatous lesions.
2. Since patients may be taking phenytoin (Dilantin) to control seizures, a distinction must be made between gingival hyperplasia caused by phenytoin and that caused by angiomatous changes, particularly if gingival surgery is anticipated.

INFLAMMATORY BOWEL DISEASE

Some of the diseases included in this group have specific oral manifestations, which in certain cases are the initial signs of the diseases.

Ulcerative colitis

In addition to gingivitis and oral candidiasis, four oral lesions occur frequently in patients with ulcerative colitis: recurrent aphthous ulcerations, pyoderma gangrenosum, pyostomatitis vegetans, and hemorrhagic ulcers of the oral mucosa and skin.

RECURRENT APHTHOUS ULCERATIONS. Of patients with ulcerative colitis 4% to 20% exhibit aphthous ulcers that appear spontaneously and in most cases concurrently with other major symptoms of the disease. The ulcers usually are less than 10 mm in diameter and occur on the nonkeratinized mucosa of the lips, cheeks, oral vestibule, and margins of the tongue. They appear as round or oval ulcers surrounded by a bright red halo and covered by a grayish white, fibrinous exudate (Fig. 4). These painful lesions may persist for 4 to 14 days and generally heal without scarring. A very severe type of aphthous ulceration, referred to as periadenitis mucosa necrotica recurrens, or major aphthous ulcer, may accompany ulcerative colitis. These lesions are more painful and larger than those previously described and may be as large as 30 mm in diameter. They appear as large necrotic areas with indurated borders surrounded by redness and edema (Fig. 5). Requiring between 10 and 40 days to heal, these lesions leave a fibrous retractile scar.

PYODERMA GANGRENOSUM. Pyoderma gangrenosum is a severe, sometimes life-threatening complication of ulcerative colitis characterized by spreading ulcer of the extremities, abdomen, and perineum. The ulcers have a granulating base and deeply undermined edges and are surrounded by a striking blue-red areola. Very painful oral ulcerations also may develop over the 4- to 8-week period when bowels symptoms are present. These irregularly shaped ulcerations of 10 to 20 mm in diameter have grayish bases and rolled margins.

PYOSTOMATITIS VEGETANS. This unusual lesion of the

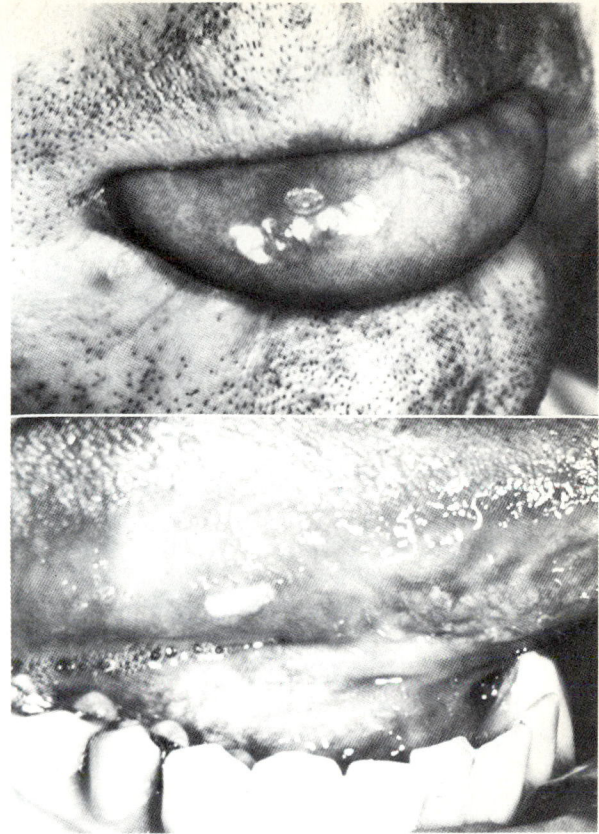

Fig. 4   Recurrent aphthous ulcerations associated with ulcerative colitis.

oral mucous membranes seems to occur only in the individual with ulcerative colitis. Possibly the result of an autoimmune mechanism, the vegetative purulent lesions develop over a period of 6 to 8 weeks and tend to parallel the bowel symptoms in severity. They usually are sterile, resistant to local therapy, and best controlled by effectively treating the colitis. In addition to these lesions, the patient with pyostomatitis vegetans may have pyrexia and submandibular lymphadenopathy.

HEMORRHAGIC ULCER OF ORAL MUCOSA AND SKIN. Irregularly shaped hemorrhagic ulcer of various sizes may occur on the oral mucosa and skin of the cheeks and the inner aspect of the thighs, buttocks, and lower abdomen in patients with ulcerative colitis. The lesions develop within 1 to 3 days, starting as hemmorrhagic bullae that subsequently burst to become ulcers.

These four types of oral lesions associated with ulcerative colitis generally do not respond to local treatment until the colitis is controlled by medical or surgical therapy. Local treatment consists of topical 2% viscous lidocaine application to relieve pain and topical steroids to reduce the severity of mucosal inflammation.

Crohn's disease

Crohn's disease, or regional enteritis, is characterized chiefly by granulomatous lesions of the intestinal tract that may fistulate onto the external surface of the abdomen.

Oral lesions have been found in approximately 6% to 20% of patients with Crohn's disease. They can occur at any time during the course of the disease and may be present before intestinal involvement is demonstrable. These lesions may re-

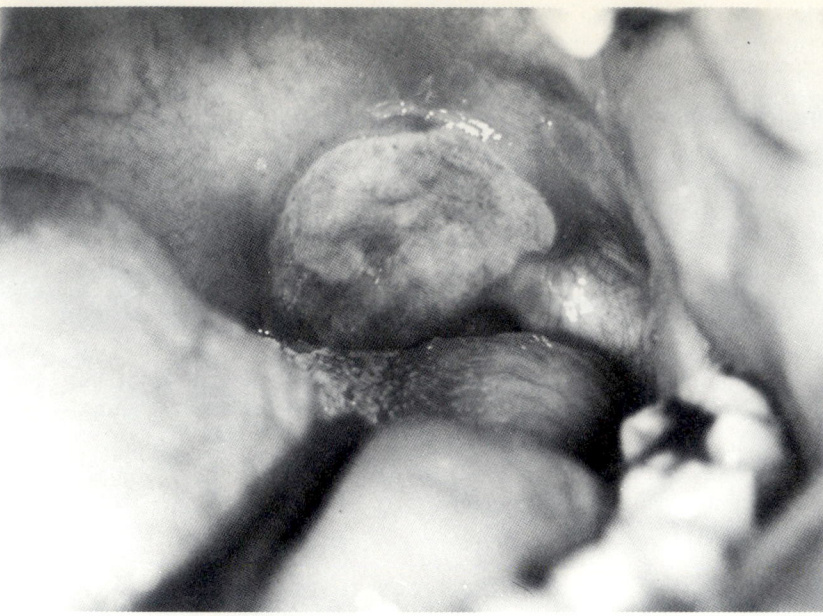

Fig. 5   Major aphthous ulcerations associated with ulcerative colitis.

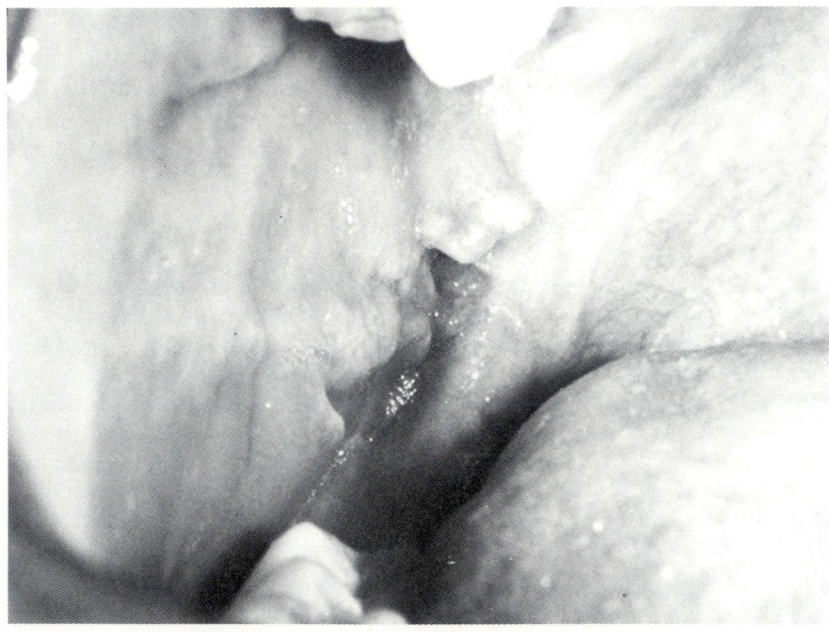

Fig. 6   Polypoid lesion in 14-year-old girl with Crohn's disease.

cur in various forms and in different locations in the same patient and may or may not be correlated with the exacerbation and remission of intestinal symptoms. Oral lesions occur more commonly in patients with colonic disease than in those with disease confined to the small bowel. Patients with extraintestinal manifestations of Crohn's disease, such as skin and joint lesions, have a greater chance of developing oral lesions as well.

The oral lesions seen in patients with Crohn's disease are either "specific" or "nonspecific," as differentiated by clinical and histologic features. The specific oral lesions are histologically similar to the intestinal lesions of the disease. They most commonly occur in the mucobuccal fold or buccal mucosa, where they are described as having a lobulated, hypertrophic,

fissured appearance, with or without linear ulcerations. The diffuse buccal lesions have a "cobblestone" appearance that is characteristic of Crohn's disease. Lesions on vestibular and retromolar mucosa are indurated and polypoid, often resembling denture-induced connective tissue hyperplasia (epulis fissuratum) (Fig. 6). Specific lesions of the gingiva, alveolar mucosa, and lips appear as areas of diffuse red swelling, sometimes accompanied by angular cheilitis.

Nonspecific lesions are the recurrent aphthous-type ulcers and are probably the most common oral lesions of Crohn's disease. The onset of these ulcers, which generally are widespread and severe, may be concurrent with bowel symptoms. The cause is not certain, but it is suspected that since measurably lower IgA secretion rates have been found in patients with active Crohn's disease, the oral mucous membranes may be more likely to undergo an immunologic reaction to exogenous oral antigens, resulting in these lesions.

The oral lesions generally regress when intestinal symptoms are brought under control. Local steroids may reduce inflammation in some patients, and 2% viscous lidocaine rinses are prescribed to reduce pain. Surgical excision of a severe lesion occasionally may be necessary.

A possible association between Crohn's disease and periodontal disease has been reported in the literature. Segal and Loewe reported altered neutrophil function, and Koldkjaer and associates reported enhanced lysozyme activity in patients with Crohn's disease. These two findings also may be seen in certain forms of rapidly progressive periodontal disease. Further research in this area may provide new approaches to treating these conditions.

MANAGEMENT. The management of patients with inflammatory bowel disease includes the following:

1. A medical consultation must be obtained regarding the severity of the disease.
2. Stress must be reduced with shorter appointments and judicious use of sedation.
3. Patients on immunosuppressive therapy require complete blood counts and differential.
4. Anemia may be present secondary to chronic blood loss; therefore, hematocrit and hemoglobin must be obtained before extensive oral surgical procedures.
5. Patients on corticosteroid therapy may have hyperglycemia, peptic ulcers, and osteoporosis, all of which may have adverse effects on dental therapy.
6. Steroid supplements may be required if the patient is taking or has been treated with corticosteroids.

A number of protocols can help determine the necessity of steroid supplementation. A reasonable general rule to follow is to supplement if the patient has received corticosteroid therapy. Supplementation consists of a dose of 5 mg or more of prednisone or its equivalent daily for a contiuous 2-week period or longer within the past year. The dosage of steroid supplementation depends on the corticosteroid dose the patient is taking and the amount of stress the procedure causes (see box).

DISEASES OF THE LIVER

Diseases that affect the liver are of interest to the dentist for several reasons. Obviously, the dental practitioner has the unique opportunity to function as primary diagnostician by using an accurate medical history or by recognizing the varied oral manifestations of hepatic disease or dysfunction. These manifestations run the gamut from fector hepaticus, a sweetish musty odor on the breath of patients with liver failure or extensive portal systemic shunting of blood, to jaundice of the oral mucosa or sclera. In addition, enlargement of the parotid glands secondary to increased parotid salivary flow in patients with alcoholic cirrhosis, lesions caused by nutritional deficiency, and bleeding secondary to depressed plasma levels of clotting factors synthesized by the liver may be readily evident in patients having dental therapy. Also, since the hepatitis virus is transmitted via blood and other body fluids through accidental needle punctures, open wound contact, accidental ingestion, or splashing of mucous membranes, the dentist and auxillary personnel are at increased risk of exposure, making it mandatory to take specific and careful precautions when dealing with patients known to be carriers of the virus.

DENTAL MANAGEMENT FOR STEROID SUPPLEMENTATION (GENERAL GUIDELINES)

I. Patients present by taking steroids
  A. No increase in corticosteroid medication is required in the adrenally suppressed patient undergoing periodontal probing, simple alloy restorations, scaling or prophylaxis unless the patient has a high level of anxiety.
  B. For moderately stressful procedures done under local anesthesia such as several extractions, third molar impactions, periodontal surgery, extensive restorative procedures, or incision and drainage of an abscess, double the daily dose up to a maximum of 60 mg prednisone. Taper 50% dose/day over 2 to 3 days to maintenance dose.
  C. Major dental procedures under general anesthesia such as treatment of acute facial trauma, orthognathic surgery, or management of severe oral infections require parenteral administration of corticosteroids in a hospital setting.
II. Patients on alternate-day steroid therapy
  A. Treat on day the patient is taking steroid and use protocol I with the following exceptions:
    1. On day 2 following the procedure, reduce steroid level to maintenance dose.
    2. On day 3, resume alternate-day schedule.
III. Patients who have a past history of steroid usage
  A. If the patient has been off the steroids for the past 12 months, treat normally.
  B. Patient formerly on 5 mg of prednisone or more for at least 2 weeks within the past 12 months
    1. Day of treatemnt: 20 to 60 mg of prednisone, depending on the stress of the procedure.
    2. Reduce by 50% on day 2.
    3. Off steroids on day 3.

Hepatitis B

The major features of hepatitis B are summarized as follows:

Major characteristics of hepatitis B

Frequency	Approximately 40% of cases of hepatitis
Transmission	Blood
	Semen
	Saliva
	Percutaneous
Mode of transmission	50% oral
	50% parenteral
	Most cases of post transfusion hepatitis are non A, non B
Incubation	6 weeks to 6 months
Symptoms	Approximately 50% of cases are subclinical
Death rate	1% to 3% of jaundiced patients
Carrier state	Become infectious 20 to 100 days after exposure; remain infectious up to 4 months; 5% to 10% become chronic carriers
Preexposure immuno-prophylaxis	Hepatitis B vaccine
Postexposure immuno-prophylaxis	Hepatitis B immuno globulin (HBIG) plus vaccination should be given within 1 week of needle stick injury and up to 14 days after sexual exposure

EPIDEMIOLOGY. In an epidemiologic study of 1245 dentists, evidence of hepatitis B infection was reported to be 13.6%. However, among oral surgeons the prevalence of hepatitis B is even greater. In a survey among 650 oral surgeons, the prevalence of hepatitis, as determined by serologic markers, was reported to be 29.3%. Current information dictates that a patient who has a history of hepatitis A may indeed be a carrier of hepatitis B.

A patient who has fully recovered from hepatitis A is not infectious. Therefore, positive identification of hepatitis A or B becomes important to the dentist in determining which patients represent a danger to dental personnel and the other patients. The discovery of hepatitis B surface antigen (HB$_s$Ag) made testing possible so that patients could be indentified who are classified as chronic carriers. HB$_s$Ag may be detected approximately 1 month before and 1 to 2 months after the development of the icteric or jaundiced phase of the disease.

The estimated lifetime risk of type B infection in the United States varies from almost 100% for groups at the highest risk to approximately 5% for the population as a whole. An estimated 200,000 individuals are infected each year and a fourth of them become jaundiced. More than 10,000 patients are hospitalized with hepatitis B each year, and an average of 250 die of fulminant disease. Between 5% and 10% of patients with type B infection become carriers. A carrier is defined as a person who is HB$_s$Ag positive on at least two occasions at least 6 months apart. The United States currently contains an estimated pool of 400,000 to 800,000 infectious carriers. A particularly high carrier rate is found in prostitutes, male homosexuals, patients with a history of lymphoma, individuals with Down's syndrome, or patients receiving renal dialysis or immunosuppressive drugs. Also, patients should be considered as carriers of hepatitis B when, in addition to having a history of hepatitis, they abuse drugs or are in a generally debilitated state of health. Chronic acfjtive hepatitis develops in more than 25% of carriers (100,000 to 200,000) and often progresses to cirrhosis. Furthermore, recent studies have demonstrated an association between the type B carrier state and the occurrence of liver cancer. It is estimated that 4000 persons die of hepatitis B–related liver cancer.

MODES OF TRANSMISSION

Saliva. HB$_s$Ag has been detected in 76% of salivary samples from carriers and can be transmitted by kissing or in children by sharing food and toys.

Nasopharyngeal secretions. Nasopharyngeal secretions have been shown to be 40% antigen positive and may represent a source of potential transmission. Transmission by droplet spray, however, has not been adequately documented.

Semen. Semen was found to be positive in approximately 50% of carriers. Studies have shown increased evidence of hepatitis B among male homosexuals, prostitutes, and promiscuous individuals, suggesting a sexual mode of transmission.

Urine. The antigen has been detected in a small percentage of serum-positive patients, and this may be a source of infection, especially in incontinent individuals.

Feces. The presence of antigen in feces has not been adequately documented. Fecal transmission seldom occurs.

Various parts of the world have a high incidence of hepatitis B, and patients from these countries present a potential risk of infectious disease in the dental office. In addition, people from certain groups at high risk need to be identified regarding their carrier status of hepatitis B. It is recommended that patients in the following categories be routinely tested for the presence of HB$_s$Ag:

Hemophiliacs
Hemodialysis patients and staff (data on HB^{5}Ag status usually is available from the hemodialysis unit)
Patients who have received a renal transplant

Patients who have been institutionalized for mental treatment or penal service for over 6 months; staff of the same institutions
Patients on methadone or similar replacement therapy for narcotic addiction
Patients with a history of or showing evidence of parenteral drug abuse such as multiple forearm scars
Patients who have lived "off base" for longer than 6 months in Mediterranean, Middle Eastern, tropical, and southeast Asian countries, as well as other areas or countries (for example, Alaskan Eskimos, Haitians), where the incidence of hepatitis B is known to be high; also immigrants or refugees from southeast Asia, Japan, China, Hong Kong, and the countries previously listed
Patients having close contact with a known hepatitis B carrier, morticians, promiscuous male homosexuals, bisexuals, and female prostitutes

Interpretation of the serologic markers for hepatitis B is summarized in the following list. If the patient is in the acute or carrier phase of the disease, dental care can be done only with vigorous infection control precautions.

Interpretation of the serologic markers for hepatitis B

Serologic marker	Interpretation
HB$_c$Ag	Acute infection or chronic carrier state; becomes positive about 6 weeks after exposure
Anti-HB$_c$Ag	Shows past infection to HB$_c$Ag; denotes immunity and generally remains positive for life
HB$_e$Ag	When present indicates that HB$_s$Ag-positive patients are highly infectious
Anti-HB$_e$Ag	Indicates that the HB$_s$Ag patient probably will develop anti-HB$_s$Ag and recover
Anti-HB$_c$Ag	This is an antibody to the core antigen and means that the patient has been exposed to the hepatitis B virus; does not denote immunity or infectious state; included in epidemiological studies to determine infection

Cirrhosis

Patients with liver cirrhosis present the dentist with two major management considerations: (1) bleeding tendencies and (2) inability to metabolize and detoxify certain drugs. Listed below are some of the signs of advanced liver disease that the dentist should be able to recognize.

Signs associated with advanced liver disease and cirrhosis.

Jaundice (skin and/or sclera)
Ascites
Edema of ankles
Sexual dysfunction
Gynecomastia
Hepatosplenomegaly
Esophageal varices
Parotid gland enlargement
Ecchymosis/petechiae
Spontaneous gingival bleeding
Spider angiomas

Listed below are some of the abnormal laboratory findings in cirrhotic patients.

Laboratory findings seen in patients with cirrhosis

Hypoprothrombinemia
Hypoalbuminemia
Elevated transaminase levels
Thrombocytopenia
Leukopenia
Hyperbilirubinemia

MANAGEMENT. The management of patients with liver disease includes the following:

1. Consult with the physician to determine the extent and severity of liver disease.
2. Question the patient thoroughly about bleeding history.
3. Obtain preoperative prothrombin time, partial thromboplastin time, and bleeding time.
4. Obtain complete blood count differential, and platelet count.
5. If coagulation studies are abnormal, consult with a hematologist before any dental therapy is begun.
6. Oral surgical procedures should be done as atraumatically as possible using topical thrombin, sutures, and packing of surgical sites.
7. Minimize drugs metabolized in the liver such as local anesthetics, analgesics (aspirin, acetaminophen, nonsteroidal antiinflammatory agents, codeine), sedatives (Valium, barbiturates) and antibiotics, especially ampicillin and tetracycline.

Using the above management guidelines, it should be possible to properly evaluate and treat the patient with liver disease. For example, nonsurgical, simple extractions, scalings, and gingival curettage can be done in the patient with mild prolongation of the prothrombin time (less than one and a half times control value). Patients undergoing more advanced surgical procedures such as multiple extractions, flap surgery, gingivectomy, bony impactions and apicectomy may require hospitalization. Patients with platelet counts of 50,000 to 100,000/mm^3 should have their counts raised to within normal range before any invasive dental treatment. Physician consultation is mandatory before any treatment is begun on the hematologically compromised patient.

Liver dysfunction can significantly reduce the metabolism and biliary excretion of drugs. Unfortunately, liver function tests have little value in predicting the biotransformation of drugs. Patients with significant cirrhosis may have a small amount of metabolic deficits, whereas others may demonstrate a marked hyperactivity to therapeutic doses of drugs. Also, there may be significant variability within the same individual. The mechanism for drug hyperreactivity seems to be twofold. First, hypoalbuminemia alters drug binding. Second, cirrhosis, with its destruction of the liver, significantly impairs blood flow through the liver, retarding the metabolism of lidocaine and like drugs. Every effort should be made to use drugs not metabolized in the liver or at least to reduce the dosage, depending on the extent of liver damage.

DISEASES OF THE PANCREAS

Extensive investigation of the dental manifestations of patients with diseases of the pancreas has been limited. Nevertheless, there are two primary areas in which a basic understanding of pancreatic disease and its oral manifestations are invaluable to both dentists and physicians. The first involves dental correlations of patients with cystic fibrosis, and the second focuses on the testing of parotid saliva in the diagnosis of pancreatic disorders.

Cystic fibrosis

Cystic fibrosis, fibrocystic disease of the pancreas, was first recognized in 1938 and is a genetically carried mendelian disease that occurs in approximately one out of every 2000 live births in whites. Pancreatic function may become severely impaired, thereby producing a malabsorption syndrome. The exocrine glands throughout the body are affected, leading to changes in secretions, which become viscid. Thickened mucus brings about obstructions of glands, with consequent dilation,

and manifestations are particularly evident in the pulmonary and digestive tracts. In children, mucous plugs occur in small airways and cause obstruction, with recurrent infection and eventually chronic bronchitis and bronchiectasis. The throat often is secondarily infected with streptococci, coagulase-positive staphylococci, pneumococci, and *Pseudomonas* organisms. Digestion is impaired, and therefore growth may be severely retarded. In the digestive tract, pancreatic secretions are insufficient, and newborns may develop intestinal obstructions because of luminal impaction of inspissated bile. Sweat glands, too, are often affected and the high sodium content of the secretions provides an important diagnostic tool.

ORAL MANIFESTATIONS. Patients with cystic fibrosis may show occlusion of the nasal cavity and maxillary sinus after recurrent infections. This results in chronic mouth breathing and a higher incidence of open bite malocclusions and a high palatal vault.

The submaxillary gland is usually enlarged and has been found to have highly turbid secretions. In the submaxillary saliva the values of total protein and many of the enzymes, as well as calcium and phosphorus, are elevated, whereas sodium chloride and potassium concentrations are within normal limits. With regard to minor salivary glands, eosinophilic plugs frequently are found in the ducts of the labial salivary glands. Weisman and others suggest that in reality, it is the secretion of the minor salivary glands scattered throughout the oral cavity in the buccal and labial mucosae, and hard and soft palates that have higher sodium values in patients with cystic fibrosis; these values, in fact, are considerably higher than those for parotid or submaxillary secretions.

Most salivary studies have involved the parotid gland and its relation to patients with cystic fibrosis. Several investigators have reported that patients with cystic fibrosis exhibited increased rates of flow of parotid saliva when the secretion was collected without stimulation. When the parotid secretion was reflexly stimulated, a higher flow rate was noted in one investigation. The results of two concurrent studies show that in a control group there was no significant difference in the resting state with a graded reflex stimulus of increasing intensity. There was a tendency for electrolyte levels of parotid saliva to be higher in a group of patients with cystic fibrosis than in a control group of comparable age and sex. Only in the case of inorganic phosphorus, however, was this elevation statistically significant. Also, the glycoproteins of parotid saliva were not found to be significantly altered either in amount or proportion in those patients.

The teeth of patients with cystic fibrosis often are discolored. The discoloration is more pronounced at the cervical and middle third of the clinical crown and is first seen at the cementoenamel junction where the enamel layer is thinnest. Tetracycline administration often has been implicated in this staining, since the drug has often been used to combat recurrent pulmonary infections. In addition to a relatively high prevalence of tetracycline discolorations, enamel defects also have been found in approximately 10% of these patients; however, the amount of dental caries has not been significantly elevated.

The possibility for delayed formation and consequent eruption of the teeth in patients with cystic fibrosis was suggested in light of the reported delay in other maturational processes. However, only an insignificant trend in dental age retardation was found in a study by Primosch when compared to chronologic age. A significant skeletal age retardation was noted, but its deviation was not as severe as previously indicated. The magnitude of the skeletal age retardation over dental age supports the concept that skeletal development is more vulnerable than tooth formation. It is therefore doubtful, based on the findings of this study, that any evaluation of dental age in patients with cystic fibrosis will be of diagnostic value to the clinician.

DIAGNOSTIC TESTING FOR PANCREATIC DISORDERS BY EXAMINATION OF PAROTID SALIVA. Several results have been obtained from studies of parotid saliva in patients with pancreatic disorders, specifically chronic pancreatitis. First, the salivary output and the maximum bicarbonate concentration and amylase content in parotid saliva of patients with pancreatic disorders were significantly less than those of patients with nonpancreatic disorders. Second, an abnormal saliva test was found in 83% of patients with pancreatic disorders. Third, a comparison was made of the parotid saliva with the pancreozymin secretion test in regard to diagnostic reliability in both pancreatic and nonpancreatic disorders. These data indicated that an abnormal parotid saliva test was 88.6% accurate in diagnosing pancreatic disorders, whereas the positive pancreozymin secretion test was only 65.9% positive.

NUTRITIONAL DISORDERS
Julian Katz

Earlier in this century, certain significant diseases were shown to be states of nutritional deficiency. These readily recognized entities, such as scurvy, beriberi, and pernicious anemia, were cured by the administration of specific chemical substances that could be isolated and identified. This was an exciting time for nutritional research, because curable diseases were being increasingly uncovered. For example, just 50 years ago many patients in psychiatric institutions in the United States had the curable and preventable illness pellagra. The availability and distribution of foods, education, and dietary fortification and enrichment eradicated this cause of mental disease. The physician or dentist today rarely sees the classic vitamin-deficiency diseases and considers nutritional problems concerns of those involved with public health and food technology. Educational, social, and economic failures are the major causes of clear-cut nutritional deficiencies. Yet obesity is a form of malnutrition, and certain diseases may be related to a chronic unsatisfactory diet. Diseases resulting from multiple-factor causes, such as cardiovascular disease and bowel cancer, also may be related to an individual's susceptibility to certain foods and nutrients.

Nutritional disorders affect the entire body, although they may manifest initially in a limited area. The most common of these areas is the oral cavity, one of the most sensitive indicators of the body's nutritional status. The dentist is in a unique position to encounter early signs of nutritional deficiency among dental patients, since oral soft tissue changes frequently are significant in these metabolic derangements.

The components of good nutrition include carbohydrates, fats, proteins, amino acids, vitamins, water, and many elements that are required in small amounts. Carbohydrates are most quickly and easily digested by the body to meet its energy needs. Fats have twice the energy value of most other foods and are used in the transport and absorption of fat-soluble vitamins. Proteins provide the body with energy and are important constituents, through their component amino acids, of additional body proteins and an array of nitrogen-containing compounds needed by the body. Minerals form a part of many important compounds active in metabolism, and deficiencies in some of these essential minerals may have profound systemic effects. Vitamins are essential for the body to carry out many metabolic processes needed for growth and the maintenance

of life. Water, which accounts for more than 60% of total body weight is needed for absorption and elimination of materials, for maintenance of body temperature, and as a medium in which many important chemical and physical reactions take place.

A state of chemical and physical equilibrium is maintained only when the necessary nutrients are supplied in suitable amounts. The specific requirement for any one substance is related to the overall composition of the diet and compensatory metabolic changes that can accommodate for quantitative fluctuation of each nutrient in the diet. When the limits of any nutritional requirement are violated because of either an inadequate or excessive supply, then the body's equilibrium can no longer be adequately maintained and clinical problems may occur.

Individuals may develop a nutritional deficiency when consuming an inadequate diet or when the absorption and utilization of ingested foods are satisfactory but other physical conditions increase the nutritional requirements.

General malnutrition

Primary malnutrition can be defined as undernutrition because of environmental lack of essential foodstuffs. It is especially prevalent in underdeveloped countries where the food supply is uncertain because of famine, drought, or other disasters or where nutritional education is limited and farming techniques are inadequate.

In secondary malnutrition, adequate food is available, but the individual is unable to make full use of it for other reasons.

ALTERED EATING BEHAVIORS. Altered eating behaviors include the anorexia from chronic disorders such as advanced malignant disease, infection, renal failure, depression, and anorexia nervosa. Chronic anorexia with nutritional deficiency also is particularly common in alcoholics and can be induced by some drugs as an unwanted side effect. Food fads are common in adolescents, and some dietary constituents may be proscribed by certain ethnic or religious practices. These can cause general malnutrition as well.

OBESITY. Obesity is the most common form of malnutrition in the developed nations. The incidence of obesity in adults in North America may be 15% to 20%. Obesity is an excess of adipose tissue and is not the same as overweight, which is defined in terms of age, height, sex, and body frame tables. Adipose tissue can be evaluated practically with a caliper measurement of the skin-fold thickness, but an individual who is 15% to 20% overweight can be considered obese.

Although an obese person ingests more calories than required by the body for energy, the cause of obesity is not that obvious. Many obese people ingest no more or fewer calories than lean people. In few patients can well-defined causes of obesity be found, such as hypothalamic tumors, rare genetic disorders, and endocrine diseases. Most obesity, however, is related to psychologic, genetic, behavioral, and social factors. The fat cells of obese people contain more fat than those of lean subjects, and in cases of greater obesity there are more adipocytes in the body. The number of fat cells does not remain stable from childhood but actually may increase in adulthood.

Metabolic abnormalities are associated with obesity, apparently as the consequence of becoming obese. A relative resistance to the metabolic effects of insulin occurs, and the growth hormone response to various stimuli is blunted. The production of cortisol and the excretion of 17-hydroxysteroids are altered, and some studies have shown differences in the metabolism of thyroid hormones.

Epidemiologic studies show an association of certain diseases with obesity and an increased mortality in obese individuals. There are difficulties in interpreting these data, especially when several factors coexist. For example, although the incidence of arteriosclerotic coronary artery disease increases as weight increases, obesity alone does not seem to be associated with an increased risk of myocardial infarction. However, obesity does increase the incidence of angina and sudden death. When obese people achieve and maintain a desirable weight, the mortality falls.

The treatment of obesity is difficult. Over 90% of fat patients who successfully lose weight return to or surpass their initial weight within 5 years. Behavior modification is required. A diet reduced by 3500 to 7000 calories a week will provide a weekly loss of 1 to 2 pounds of adipose tissue. More drastic programs, such as fasting with protein supplements, result in a more rapid weight loss that may initially be caused by loss of muscle mass with accompanying water, but these drastic diets rarely provide longlasting weight loss. Physical activity is not very effective in losing weight, but moderate activity usually is accompanied by a decrease in caloric intake. The calories lost in 1 hour of vigorous tennis are about equal to those in a slice of cherry pie. Frequency of meals may be as important as diet composition; regular balanced meals are associated with weight control despite alterations in caloric intake. Most obese people eat little or no breakfast. Intestinal bypass surgery has been used for the treatment of morbid obesity, but there are considerable hazards associated with these procedures, such as electrolyte, vitamin, and mineral deficiencies and severe liver disease.

DISORDERS INTERFERING WITH INGESTION. Oropharyngeal disease is the cause of most ingestion disorders. Painful lesions, such as oral ulceration and glossopharyngeal neuralgia, neurologic syndromes interfering with the act of swallowing, such as bulbar palsy and myasthenia gravis, and mechanical obstruction from a neoplasm or esophageal stricture may all cause dysphagia, with reduced food intake leading to general malnutrition.

Problems of dental origin can certainly interfere with ingestion. These include poorly functioning partial or complete dentures, pain associated with periodontal disease, and decayed or poorly restored teeth. Masticatory insufficiency also can result from temporomandibular joint disease and occlusal abnormalities associated with maxillary and mandibular growth abnormalities, particularly those which cause severe prognathism, micrognathism, and apertognathia.

DEFECTIVE ABSORPTION. A wide range of gastrointestinal disorders have been related to malabsorption of single or multiple dietary constituents. The most common of these are as follows:

1. Pancreatic failure and steatorrhea because of hepatobiliary disease. These are frequently associated with malabsorption of fat and fat-soluble vitamins such as retinol and calciferol.
2. Intestinal mucosal disorders, especially gluten-induced enteropathy and sprue. On occasion, these disorders present evidence of nutritional deficiency only, without symptoms of gastrointestinal disease.
3. Failure of special adaptive mechanisms for the absorption of individual dietary constituents, such as lack of intrinsic factor in vitamin B_{12} deficiency.
4. Rapid intestinal transmission of food after gastrectomy or vagotomy.
5. Bacterial colonization and overgrowth in various areas of the gut, resulting in steatorrhea.

Certain disorders may cause malabsorption through several different mechanisms. For example, regional ileitis or enteritis (Crohn's disease) leads to fat malabsorption by interfering with the recycling of bile salts, vitamin B_{12} deficiency by preventing specific ileal absorption of the vitamin B_{12} intrinsic factor complex, and general malabsorption of all nutrients if involvement of the gut is widespread.

EXCESSIVE LOSS OF NUTRIENTS. Losses from the body for which intestinal absorption cannot compensate may lead to a deficiency in individual nutrients. Chronic blood loss, for example, is a major cause of iron deficiency, and protein-deficient states may result from severe proteinuria or from various enteropathies.

INCREASED REQUIREMENTS. During certain periods of life a more "normal" dietary intake may become inadequate in the face of increased requirements. Such relative malnutrition may arise in pregnancy and during periods of rapid growth in infancy and adolescence. Two mechanisms exist to offset the effects of some nutritional deficiencies, such as negative nitrogen balance. First, many nutrients exist in storage forms in the body, and these can be mobilized for a limited time to compensate for deficiencies in intake. Second, for certain deficiencies larger proportions of the individual nutrient can be absorbed from the diet.

Specific nutritional deficiencies

Energy is provided by dietary carbohydrates, fats, and proteins. One gram of carbohydrate yields 4 calories; 1 g of fat, 9 calories; and 1 g of protein, 4 calories. Ethanol has significant caloric value, providing 7 calories in 1 g. Energy requirements decline as adults grow older, but pregnancy and lactation require additional calories and protein. Carbohydrates, particularly plant foods, provide most of the calories in the diet, and fat provides highly concentrated energy. The body is not totally efficient in deriving energy from the three major nutrients, however, and there are individual differences in metabolic activity and physical activity. The following section is a discussion of essential nutrients and the effects of deficiency in each case, particularly as manifested in the oral cavity.

PROTEINS. Protein is a vital constituent of the diet, since it is the only source of essential amino acids, that is, those not produced by the body. Ingested protein is hydrolyzed in the intestine to the various component amino acids, which are subsequently absorbed by the bloodstream. Of the 20 amino acids found in food protein, only 8 (isoleucine, lysine, methionine, phenylalanine, tyrosine, threonine, tryptophan, and valine) are essential for adults, since they cannot be synthesized by the human body. During active growth in infancy histidine and arginine are also necessary in larger amounts and hence are considered by some to be semiessential amino acids. Since humans have no pool for storage of essential amino acids other than their own body protein, removal of just one of these essential amino acids can rapidly lower the level of protein synthesis. This is critical if it occurs during growth periods when metabolic demands require protein synthesis.

The effects of protein calorie deficiency in children may vary from mild growth retardation to general starvation or protein malnutrition (kwashiorkor). Infants in starvation characteristically remain alert, and reutilization of amino acids liberated from the child's own tissues allows synthesis of serum albumin to continue. In cases of protein malnutrition, generalized edema usually occurs because of a decrease in serum albumin. These individuals are characteristically lethargic and apathetic. Flaky dermatosis and pigmentary changes are also common.

Oral evidence of protein malnutrition includes edema of the tongue, with scalloping of the lateral margins from pressing against the teeth. The dorsum of the tongue may also appear smooth and erythematous because of papillary atrophy. Angular cheilitis and fissuring around the lips may appear, in addition to changes in lip pigmentation that are particularly noticeable in dark-skinned individuals. Sialosis and xerostomia are other features of kwashiorkor, and the resulting dry oral mucosa is particularly vulnerable to trauma and infection.

FATS. Two fatty acids, linoleic acid and linolenic acid, are essential dietary constituents that are necessary for the biosynthesis of prostaglandins. Although all other lipids can be manufactured in the body and thus are nonessential ingredients of the diet, their consumption does assist in the absorption of fat-soluble vitamins, such as retinol, calciferol, tocopherol, and vitamin K.

Prostaglandins are widely distributed in the tissues and apparently are synthesized from fatty acids stored within cellular membranes. Their role of action is complex and includes a role in mediating the inflammatory response and in regulating a number of metabolic reactions. It is possible that prostaglandins act directly at several sites in the cell or indirectly by regulating the rate of cyclic AMP production. Deficiency of essential fatty acids is uncommon, virtually confined to infants being fed parenterally or on restricted diets. A dry, flaky dermatosis often develops. No oral manifestations of essential fatty acid deficiency have been documented in humans, although dentinogenesis has been altered in experimental animals.

CARBOHYDRATES. Carbohydrates satisfy the major energy needs of the human body. The dietary switch from natural to refined carbohydrates in the United States has been widespread and may have significant effects on overall health status. High intake of sticky carbohydrate foods can increase caries incidence in the susceptible person.

MINERALS. The essential need for any mineral can be determined by observing altered functions when the diet is deficient only in that element, demonstrating a response with the administration of the supplementary mineral, and then correlating the deficiency state with a low level of the mineral in blood or tissue. Minerals function as structural components of the skeleton and soft tissue and as solutes in body fluids.

Iron. Iron plays a vital role in cellular respiration. There are only 3 to 4 g of iron in the body. About 70% is in hemoglobin, both in circulating erythrocytes and in the normoblasts of the bone marrow. Twenty percent of the iron is in storage form (ferritin or hemosiderin) in the macrophages of the liver, spleen, and other organs. Another 5% of body iron is in the myoglobin of skeletal muscle, and a small; but functionally important, quantity is in iron-containing enzymes such as cytochromes A, B, and C; cytochrome oxidase catalase; peroxidase; and iron flavoproteins.

There are no excretory mechanisms for iron, although about 1 mg/day is lost passively through cell desquamation from the skin and intestines and through growth of nails and hair. In menstruating women fluid loss of around 30 ml further depletes iron by 0.5 mg daily, and additional deficits result from pregnancy and lactation. Children also have a high need for iron because of rapid growth and expansion of the blood volume.

The body iron content is thus determined almost entirely by absorption, the physiologic control of which is complex and mediated through events in the mucosal cells of the gastrointestinal tract. The average American diet contains 15 to 20 mg of iron per day of which the body requires around 10%. Since only about 5% to 10% of dietary iron is actually absorbed, this may be a marginal amount for individuals with a greater need for the substance. Although normal men and postmenopausal women need about 10 mg of iron in the diet daily, women with menstrual loss need about 18 mg/day, and an additional 1.5 mg/day of iron is needed during pregnancy for the tissues of the fetus and expansion of the maternal blood volume.

If iron is depleted through the chronic blood loss of certain diseases or if dietary iron absorption is impaired, a negative iron balance results, and the pathologic tissue changes of iron deficiency occur. Iron deficiency can cause changes in the tissues that are not related to the hematologic effects. In a large sample of patients with iron deficiency anemia, atrophic glossitis was found in 39% and angular cheilitis in 14%. These changes are caused by tissue depletion of iron and may appear before the development of anemia. The severity of glossitis does not approach that seen in vitamin B_{12} or folic acid deficiency. In mild cases there is some discomfort and redness associated with flattening of the papillae around the margin of the tongue. In more severe cases there is redness and atrophy of the filiform and fungiform papillae. Angular cheilitis is a less specific abnormality and the absence of teeth and wearing ill-fitting dentures may favor its development.

Another result of iron deficiency is dysphagia caused by postcricoid esophageal stricture, originally described by Kelly and Patterson in 1919. Plummer-Vinson syndrome occurs in about 7% of iron-deficient subjects and an esophageal web can be found in a number of such cases. The web consists of a fold of normal mucosa or a stricture with chronic inflammation of the muscle layers of the esophagus. The syndrome occurs most frequently in middle-aged women and commonly is accompanied by glossitis and angular cheilitis. In most cases glossitis improves quite rapidly after the commencement of iron replacement, with regeneration of the filiform papillae within 3 weeks. Angular cheilitis responds more slowly, probably because of concurrent infection.

Iodine. Iodine is needed for the production of thyroid hormones, thyroxine (T_4) and triiodothyronine (T_3). The adult human body contains about 40 mg of iodine, about half of which is located in the thyroid gland. Dietary sources include iodized salt, seafood, and foods grown in soil with adequate iodine content. Iodine deficiency may lead to goiter, a swelling of the thyroid gland caused usually by iodine deficiency, which is endemic in regions away from the sea and where soil content of iodine is low. The decreased level of iodine causes the pituitary to release thyroid-stimulating hormone (TSH), which induces the thyroid to produce additional thyroid hormones. When this occurs over a significant length of time the gland gradually enlarges. The patient with a thyroid goiter may be hyperthyroid, hypothyroid, or euthyroid (normal functioning gland). Local pressure from thyroid swelling may lead to coughing, voice changes, and breathing difficulty.

The levels of circulating thyroid hormone, particularly T_3 and T_4, can be measured easily to determine the thyroid status of the patient. Children of parents with iodine deficiency may be born with cretinism (congenital hypothyroidism). The child may look normal at birth but eventually develops slowly and is small for his age, with a large tongue, late eruption of teeth, saddle depression of the nose, and possible mental retardation. Early administration of thyroid hormone can prevent these complications.

Since the metabolic rate is generally elevated in hyperthyroidism, administration of epinephrine to these individuals, such as in local anesthetics, should be avoided.

Calcium and phosphorus. Calcium and phosphorus are the most abundant minerals in the body. The bones and teeth can store about 99% of the body's calcium and 75% of the body's phosphorus, with the rest found in blood, soft tissue, and extracellular fluid. The main function of calcium is to provide rigidity and strength to bones and teeth. Since it is also necessary for proper muscle contraction, blood clotting, and nerve irritability, a low serum calcium level can lead to muscle cramps and tetany. Serum calcium is particularly important in maintaining viable cardiac muscle contractility. Phosphorus contributes to bone and teeth rigidity and plays a major role in the quick release of energy from adenosine triphosphate (ATP) and adenosine diphosphate (ADP) molecules. It is also an essential constituent of nucleic acids and nucleoproteins that are involved in DNA and RNA synthesis. Phosphorus aids in the absorption and metabolism of carbohydrates, such as glucose and glycogen, and, as a constiuent of phospholipid, promotes emulsification and transportation of fats and fatty acids. Finally, phosphates have an important buffering function in blood and saliva.

Diseases associated with calcium and phosphorus deficiencies include osteoporosis, rickets, and osteomalacia. Osteoporosis is an abnormal rarefaction of bone resulting from failure of the osteoblasts to lay down bone matrix. The generalized form is associated with calcium and hormonal deficiencies, whereas the localized form is caused by disuse or immobilization. Rickets is a disturbance in normal mineralization of the osteoid matrix characterized by bending or distortion in bones. This is caused by a decreased absorption of calcium or phosphorus or both in calciferol-deficient children. Osteomalacia is an adult condition characterized by softening of the bone with pain and tenderness, which is caused by deficiency of calcium and phosphorus or of calciferol. Osteoporosis is treated with high-calcium diets, sex hormones, and fluorides. Rickets and osteomalacia are treated with calciferol and high-calcium diets.

Sodium and potassium. The greatest concentration of sodium in the body is in extracellular fluid. It is necessary for muscle contractility, nerve impulse conduction, maintaining equilibrium between the extracellular and intracellular fluid compartments, and maintaining the pH level of blood. The average daily intake of sodium in the United States is about 5 g, about five times the daily physiologic requirement. Excessive sweating can lead to salt depletion and result in symptoms of nausea, vomiting, cramps, exhaustion, or respiratory failure. Patients with severe vomiting and diarrhea can also develop rapid salt depletion.

Potassium is the main cation of the cell. Since it is present in many foods, a varied diet supplies an adequate amount of this mineral. Potassium deficiency results in muscle weakness and excess potassium can lead to cardiac irritability and arrhythmias. The most common causes of potassium deficiency are infectious or nutritional diarrhea and excess water loss from diuretic agents without potassium supplementation.

Magnesium. Magnesium is required for the proper action of enzymes responsible for energy transformation of phosphate bonds. The bones provide the body with magnesium stores; they contain around 70% of the magnesium in the average adult. Most vegetables contain useful amounts of the mineral, of which the average adult daily requirement is 300 to 350 mg. A greater amount of magnesium is required during pregnancy. Deficiency of this mineral can result in a condition similar to hypocalcemic tetany.

Copper. Copper is utilized in the body for the formation of hemoglobin and production of viable erythrocytes. No evidence of ill health resulting from dietary deficiency of copper has been reported.

Sulfur. Sulfur is present in all protein material but most abundantly in the amino acids methionine and cystine. It is also biologically active in the vitamins thiamine and biotin, in

Table 3 Recommended adult daily dietary allowance of vitamins

	Men	Women*
FAT-SOLUBLE VITAMINS		
Retinal (A)	5000 IU	4000 IU
Calciferol (D)	400 IU	400 IU
Tocopherol (E)	15 IU	12 IU
WATER-SOLUBLE VITAMINS		
Ascorbic acid (C)	45 mg	45 mg
Niacin†	20 mg	14 mg
Riboflavin†	1.8 mg	1.4 mg
Thiamine†	1.5 mg	1.1 mg
Pyridoxine	2 mg	2 mg
B$_{12}$	3 µg	3 µg
Folic acid	400 µg	400 µg

*The allowances of all vitamins except calciferol are higher during pregnancy and lactation.
†The allowance decreases after age 22.

the cell as sulfate ion, such as chondroitin sulfate in bone and cartilage, and in the sulfhydryl (—SH) group of certain enzymes. Little is known regarding the sulfur requirement or deficiency in humans.

Fluoride. Fluorude has a more definite role in the prevention of caries; the safety and efficacy of fluoridated water have been demonstrated. Fluoride replaces some of the hydroxyl ions in hydroxyapatite, lessening the solubility of dental enamel. If excessive fluoride is ingested during tooth formation, mottled enamel occurs. A role for fluoride in preventing osteoporosis has not been established.

Trace elements. Zinc, manganese, molybdenum, cobalt, and selenium are needed by the body in small amounts. The balanced diet usually supplies these trace elements adequately. Little is known about their requirements or deficiency states in humans.

VITAMINS. Vitamins may be defined as essential organic dietary factors that are incapable of being synthesized within the body. Although they are required by the body in relatively small amounts, their absence often results in pathologic conditions. The daily dietary allowance of vitamins recommended for adults is given in Table 3. Numerous vitamins exist and are classified as either water- or fat-soluble as follows:

Fat-soluble vitamins	Water-soluble vitamins
Retinol (A)	Thiamin (B$_1$)
Calciferol (D)	Riboflavin (B$_2$)
Tocopherol (E)	Pyridoxine (B$_6$)
K	B$_{12}$
	Folic acid
	Pantothenic acid
	Biotin (H)
	Nicotinic acid (niacin)
	Ascorbic acid (C)

Retinol (vitamin A). Retinol is a long-chain, high-molecular-weight alcohol that is abundant in leafy green vegetables, animal fats, particularly certain fish liver oils, and milk. Carotenes, which form the yellow pigments of most fruits and vegetables, essentially consist of two molecules of retinol.

The main storage site of retinol is the liver, and sufficient reserves normally exist for as long as 1 year. For this reason there is no justification for including retinol in supplemental vitamin preparations if the individual is consuming a well-balanced diet.

Other than its action on the retina, where it serves as a

precursor for rhodopsin (visual purple), the precise role that retinol plays in general metabolism is less clear. Retinol is essential for the maintenance of the structure and function of epithelial glandular tissue. There is a range of metabolic steps that appear to be influenced by retinol, in which epithelial cells are particularly sensitive. The effect of this vitamin on the membrane stability of plasma cells and lysosomes may account for its observed action in regulating keratinization. Endocrine function is also influenced by the availability of retinol, with thyroxine and steroid synthesis being sensitive to deficiencies. There may be some relationship between retinol and the vitamin B complex and ascorbic acid, since typical signs of vitamin B and ascorbic acid deficiency have occurred experimentally in animals under conditions of retinol deprivation.

In retinol deficiency the eyes are among the first sites to be affected; night blindness, xerophthalmia, and conjunctival ulcerations occur, in addition to photophobia and, in some cases, permanent blindness. The skin becomes dry and scaly because of an increase in keratinization. Since the body is unable to excrete large doses of the substance, disease states develop in individuals who have ingested excessive amounts. In hypervitaminosis A, alopecia, peeling of the skin, coarsened hair, and generalized bone pair occur.

Oral signs of retinol deficiency include increased keratinization of the oral mucosa and keratinization of formerly nonkeratinized tissues. The resultant hyperkeratotic areas may appear as white patches. Metaplasia of the salivary ductal epithelium has been reported, sometimes causing xerostomia and altered taste and smell. Although the relationship between retinol and enamel formation has been studied extensively, there is little convincing evidence that retinol causes any significant dental changes in humans.

Oral manifestations of hypervitaminosis A include atrophy of the oral mucosa, gingival inflammation, and scaling of the lips.

The keratin-decreasing property of retinol has been employed successfully in the management of certain hyperkeratotic lesions of the skin and oral mucosae.

Calciferol (vitamin D). Calciferol is the general name for a group of steroids possessing antirachitic activity. Their primary action is to increase the plasma calcium and phosphate concentration by stimulating intestinal absorption of these minerals and resorption of bone. Calciferol thus is utilized primarily in the absorption of calcium and phosphorus from the intestinal tract and in the formation and maintenance of the skeletal system and teeth. Fish liver oils are extremely rich in calciferol, as are all dairy products. Pasteurized milk is enriched to contain 400 IU of calciferol per quart, and many other foodstuffs, such as bread and cereals, are irradiated to increase their calciferol content. There is no evidence to suggest that increased calciferol intake has any beneficial action on the formation or eruption of teeth, nor does it render any caries protection. Calciferol deficiency leads to rickets in children and osteomalacia in adults.

Rickets. Rickets usually appears during the first 24 months of life. The chief manifestations are seen in the bones, where defects in the mineralization of the organic matrix occur. Soft areas in the skull are frequently the earliest evidence of this disease. The rachitic child may have large prominent frontal bones, which give the head an enlarged appearance. Bowed legs and enlarged wrists and ankles are common signs of the disease, as are spontaneous fractures in severe cases.

In calciferol-sensitive rickets, a form of disease that responds to calciferol administration, there are surprisingly few oral manifestations. Since most of these children show no evidence of dentin or enamel hypoplasia, the level of calciferol does not seem to be critical in either amelogenesis or dentinogenesis. Calciferol-resistant rickets, a form of the disease that is due to renal tubular disorders, usually is more severe. These children reportedly develop dental abnormalities that include changes in the pulp horns and dentin. Eruption of the teeth may be delayed and roentgenographic signs, such as reduced density of the alveolar lamina dura and loss of crestal bone, are common.

Osteomalacia (adult rickets). Osteomalacia, or adult calciferol deficiency, is almost nonexistent in the United States. The disease is characterized by an irregular increase in the thickness of the cortex and trabeculation of bones. These tissues are poorly calcified and contain fibrous bone marrow and islands of osteoid tissue. The diagnosis of calciferol deficiency may be confirmed by abnormally low serum calcium and phosphate and elevated alkaline phosphatase levels.

Tocopherol (vitamin E). Tocopherol is a fat-soluble vitamin and a component of grains, vegetable oils, and green vegetables. Diets lacking tocopherol have been known to produce thrombocytosis, hemolytic anemias, and dermatologic changes in children, particularly premature infants. Symptoms are far less notable in adults, but there may be alterations in the formation of erythrocytes. Dental or oral changes have not been noted in humans with tocopherol deficiency, although some minor alterations have been recorded in the periodontium and teeth of laboratory animals.

Vitamin K. Vitamin K is a water-soluble, heat-stable substance formed from phylloquinone and farnoquinone vitamin K_1 and K_2) and is required for hepatic synthesis of coagulation factors II (prothrombin), V, VII, IX (Christmas factor), and X (Stuart-Power factor). Normal hepatic function and adequate dietary supplies of vitamin K are needed for successful production of these proteins. Phylloquinone is derived from leafy green vegetables, whereas farnoquinone is synthesized by intestinal bacteria.

Deficiency of vitamin K leads to inadequate production of the coagulation factors just listed and hence to significant hemorrhagic diathesis. In the adult, the most frequent cause of vitamin K deficiency is malabsorption, usually from steatorrhea or obstructive jaundice.

The oral manifestations of vitamin K deficiency include gingival bleeding and excessive postextraction hemorrhage. Therefore, to evaluate the magnitude of vitamin K deficiency in an individual before commencing a surgical procedure, a prothrombin time (PT) should be obtained. The surgical procedure should be postponed if the PT is less than 50% of control. Administration of intramuscular doses of vitamin K usually has a therapeutic effect in 8 to 12 hours, as reflected in a repeat PT that indicates adequate coagulability.

Vitamin B complex. Vitamin B complex is composed of many separate biologic factors; the exact chemical composition and significance in human nutrition are yet to be determined. The factors that make up the vitamin B complex are all water soluble but their solubility rates vary considerably. The clinically important B complex vitamins are thiamine (B_1), riboflavin (B_2), pyridoxine (B_6), folic acid, pantothenic acid, nicotinic acid (niacin), and biotin.

Thiamine (vitamin B_1). The function of thiamine is to form the coenzyme thiamine pyrophosphate, which is required for oxidative decarboxylation of pyruvate and α-ketoglutarate. In thiamine deficiency, therefore, lactate and pyruvate build up and interfere with carbohydrate metabolism. This deficiency state is exacerbated by large amounts of carbohydrate in the diet. Affected individuals may become irritable and experience loss of appetite, nausea, and vomiting, in addition to chronic diarrhea and inflammatory lesions of the intestines. As the deficiency state worsens, cardiac dilation may occur, leading to congestive heart failure.

Preventive measures such as the enrichment of flour and other foods and the avoidance of polished rice as the primary food staple have limited the incidence of thiamine deficiency. This deficiency now occurs primarily in alcoholics. Disorders that prevent the ingestion and absorption of food and those which accelerate the metabolic rate can lead to a thiamine deficiency. Thiamine is lost in the urine in cases of profound diuresis, and glucose loading may provoke symptoms in individuals in whom thiamine stores are marginal. Few foods are rich in thiamine, but beans, nuts, whole grain, meats, fish, and eggs are good sources.

The syndromes caused by thiamine deficiency are beriberi, polyneuritis, Wernicke's encephalopathy, and Korsakoff's syndrome. The heart failure that occurs with a thiamine deficiency is a type of high-output failure occurring with clear lungs, an enlarged heart, a normal sinus rhythm, dependent edema, and an elevated venous pressure. Beriberi heart disease is associated with an insufficiency of other B vitamins when the diet has been grossly lacking in thiamine for over 4 months. The early symptoms of neuritic (dry) beriberi include numbness of the legs and paresthesias. Muscle weakness develops gradually and may cause quadriceps weakness along with a difficulty in rising from a squatting position. Paralysis occurs along with advanced polyneuritis. Wernicke's encephalopathy is characterized by apathy, confusion, occasionally delirium, and cerebellar ataxia. Eye signs are always present, including nystagmus and paralysis of the external rectus and other extraocular muscles. Patients with Korsakoff's syndrome have a defect in memory, particularly of recent events, as well as confabulation. The mortality of Wernicke's syndrome is quite high, but parenteral thiamine therapy and the institution of a good diet can lead to a complete recovery; however, the features of Korsakoff's syndrome may persist.

The oral lesions associated with thiamine deficiency are rarely severe enough for the patient to seek professional help. Some of these manifestations include hypersensitivity of the teeth and oral mucosa and enlargement of the fungiform papillae of the tongue. Small vesicles or "cracks" may appear in the vermilion border of the lips and commissures of the mouth. Therapeutic doses of approximately 100 mg daily are commonly administered to alcoholics and other thiamine-deficient individuals.

Riboflavin (vitamin B₂). Riboflavin is found within cells in combination with specific enzymes of cellular oxidation reactions. The biochemical role of riboflavin is to form the two flavoprotein coenzymes, flavin adenine dinucleotide and flavin mononucleotide. Riboflavin deficiency leads to the development of seborrheic dermatitis and corneal vascularization. Anemia also may develop, and this may be related to disturbance of folate utilization, since the flavoprotein enzymes are involved in its metabolism.

Severe and varied lesion of the oral mucosa and circumoral tissues occur in riboflavin deficiency. Angular cheilosis, characterized by painful lesions in commissures of the mouth, is considered a specific manifestation of riboflavin deficiency, although it may also occur in deficiencies of panthothenic acid and pyridoxine hydrochloride. The pseudocheilotic areas associated with decreased vertical dimension and loss of intermaxillary space usually slant downward and outward, whereas the cheilotic lesions associated with ariboflavinosis are more horizontal. These fissures commonly become encrusted because of secondary infection. Glossitis is another reported effect of riboflavin deficiency, and enlargement of the fungiform papillae gives the dorsum of the tongue a granular appearance. There also may be complete atrophy of the filiform papillae. The vermilion border of the lips and, to a lesser extent, the buccal mucosa may acquire a purplish hue that resembles cyanosis. Individuals with chronic prolonged B complex deficiency have been known to develop bullous lichen planus and painful periodontitis.

Pyridoxine (vitamin B₆). Pyridoxine is a white crystalline substance that is soluble in water and alcohol. The three forms of the vitamin, all of which are derivatives of pyridine, are pyridoxine, pyridoxal, and pyridoxamine. The first is found in plants and the remaining two in animal products. Their wide distribution in nature makes dietary deficiency a rarity. The active forms of this vitamin are the coenzymes pyridoxal phosphate and pyridoxamine phosphate, which circulate in the plasma bound to albumin. They participate in several reactions of amino acid metabolism, including decarboxylation, transamination, and racemization. Pyridoxine may also be involved in antibody formation.

Clinical deficiency states of pyridoxine are most frequently associated with malnutrition secondary to alcoholism. Generalized dermatitis and neurologic disturbances, especially peripheral neuropathy, are common signs of deficiency. The oral changes in pyridoxine deficiency are relatively nonspecific and include angular cheilitis, glossitis, and generalized stomatitis. Papillary atrophy of the dorsum of the tongue may also develop. These oral changes are virtually identical to those found in iron deficiency, and it has been suggested that the oral changes of iron deficiency are related to coexisting changes in pyridoxine utilization. Simple deficiency states can be corrected with a daily dose of 50 to 150 mg of pyridoxine administered orally.

Vitamin B₁₂. Vitamin B₁₂ is the generic term for a group of cobalt-containing vitamins (cobalamins) that participate as coenzymes in a diverse group of metabolic reactions. Of the vast amount of biochemical work on their actions that has been conducted using bacteria, the two reactions proven to occur in humans are methylmalonate-succinate isomerization and methylation of homocysteine to cysteine, which occur in the synthesis and repair of DNA.

Vitamin B₁₂ arises almost solely from bacterial sources; it is not found in plants and cannot be manufactured by higher animals. Humans are totally dependent on dietary vitamin B₁₂, the principal sources of which are animal products, especially meat, liver, kidney, egg yolk, and milk. Since the absorption rate is only 70%, 7 to 8 μg must be ingested daily to satisfy the metabolic requirement of 2 to 5 μg.

Vitamin B₁₂ is stored in the liver in quantities sufficient to sustain requirements for many years. Successful absorption of dietary vitamin B₁₂ from the gut depends on its binding to a gastric mucoprotein intrinsic factor (IF) secreted into normal gastric juice by the parietal cells. The B₁₂-IF complex so formed is carried down the small bowel and is absorbed in the ileum, where the mucosal cell membranes have specific receptors for this complex. Splitting of the complex occurs at the brush border of the cell and vitamin B₁₂ is then absorbed. Most deficiency states are caused by an absorptive defect, most frequently from lack of IF. This can result from primary gastric mucosal atrophy or gastrectomy.

Pernicious anemia is by far the most common effect of vitamin B₁₂ deficiency, and the term should be reserved for this disease complex. The gastric mucosal lesion responsible for this disease is probably autoimmune, since these patients also have a high incidence of other organ-specific autoimmune disorders, such as Hashimoto's thyroiditis. In addition, there is a high incidence of antigastric parietal cell antibody and anti-intrinsic factor antibody in the sera of patients with pernicious anemia. Glossitis and stomatitis have long been observed in all forms of vitamin B_{12} deficiency. Glossitis occurs in 50% to 60% of patients with pernicious anemia and characteristically fluctuates in severity. Initially, an active inflammatory reaction occurs; the extreme tenderness, rawness, and edema usually interfere with eating. This inflammation regresses and is followed by progressive atrophy of the filiform and fungiform papillae. Recurrent oral ulceration without angular cheilitis is another feature of the disease.

Within 48 hours after specific B_{12} replacement therapy, the symptoms of pernicious anemia are often relieved, and regeneration of the tongue papillae may be evident within a week.

Since most defects are absorptive in nature, vitamin B_{12} replacement must be administered by injection. Initially, six to ten injections of 1000 μg of hydroxycobalamin is usually given in preference to cyanocobalamin, since the former is more efficiently retained. At the rate of one injection daily, this is usually sufficient to produce a therapeutic response and to reconstitute depleted body stores.

Folic acid. This B complex vitamin is present in a wide variety of naturally occurring foodstuffs, especially liver, yeast, and green vegetables. Since folic acid is heat labile, large portions of food folate are lost during cooking. The daily requirement varies from 5 to 50 μg. Body stores are smaller than those of vitamin B_{12} and normal metabolism can only be sustained for a few months once folate is no longer included in the diet.

Dietary folate deficiency is especially common in alcoholics, the elderly, and the malnourished. Significant folic acid deficiency almost invariably occurs with malabsorption syndrome from widespread gastric mucosal disease, such as gluten enteropathy and tropical sprue. Increased body requirements of folic acid occur during pregnancy and in the presence of rapidly growing tumors or other processes characterized by rapid cell turnover. Antifolate cytotoxic drugs and anticonvulsant drugs, such as phenytoin, may also cause folate deficiency.

The clinical and hematologic effects of folic acid deficiency are virtually indistinguishable from those of vitamin B_{12} deficiency. The oral manifestations are also similar to those found in B_{12} deficiencies, with severe oral ulcerations as the predominant clinical sign. These lesions respond promptly to therapeutic folate administration. Oral therapy (usually consisting of 5 mg three times daily) is suitable for most patients, even those with malabsorption syndromes. Although vitamin B_{12} administration is harmless, folic acid should be administered to certain patients with caution. The potential hazards include precipitation of subacute combined degeneration of the spinal cord in patients who actually have vitamin B_{12} deficiency rather than folate deficiency and an increase in the growth rate of folate-dependent tumors. An accurate diagnosis of folic acid deficiency is thus vitally important.

Pantothenic acid. Pantothenic acid is used by the body in conjunction with folic acid and biotin. The body requires 10 to 15 mg daily of pantothenic acid for synthesis of coenzyme A. Deficiency of pantothenic acid in laboratory animals has produced adrenocortical deficiency, malformation and resorption of the roots of teeth, resorption of supporting tissues, and varying degrees of osteoporosis. It is not clear, however, whether deficiency syndromes exist in humans; there has been no clinical evidence that pantothenic acid deficiency in humans is associated with any particular lesion or syndrome.

Nicotinic acid (niacin). Lean meats, liver, potatoes, and vegetables are good sources of nicotinic acid. In general, animal tissues contain the vitamin in the form of the amide, whereas plants contain it in the form of acid. Nicotinic acid is converted by the body into its amide, nicotinamide, which is then used for the production of nicotinamide adenine dinucleotide (NAD) and nicotinamide adenine dinucleotide phosphate (NADP). As such, it is involved as an acceptor and donor in oxidation and reduction reactions.

Deficiency in nicotinic acid results in pellagra, a condition characterized by symmetric, red scaly dermatitis of the stocking and glove areas that may darken and subsequently desquamate. These lesions are aggravated by sunlight and heat and often are accompanied by diarrhea, numbness and burning sensations, vertigo, nervousness, progressive weakness, and anorexia. The prominent oral lesion of pellagra is generalized erythema of the mucosa with papillary atrophy of the tongue, which causes considerable discomfort. Fibrin-covered ulcerations may develop subsequently, the tongue may become fiery red, and shallow ulcerations may be noted on the dorsum and along the lateral margins. Secondary ulceronecrotic gingivostomatitis is also a finding in patients with pellagra, along with herpes labialis and angular cheilosis.

The treatment for pellagra consists of high therapeutic doses of niacinamide, usually 150 to 300 mg daily. Excess amounts do not cause serious side effects and are readily eliminated in the urine.

Biotin. Biotin functions as a coenzyme in carboxylation reactions. Egg white contains the substance avidin, which has a high binding affinity for biotin. Therefore when an individual ingests an abnormally large amount of raw egg whites, there is a tendency to bind the biotin from the diet and prevent its absorption. The only general effect of biotin deficiency known is a scaly dermatitis. Oral manifestations of biotin deficiency are infrequent and consist primarily of atrophy of the lingual papillae.

Ascorbic acid (Vitamin C). Ascorbic acid is a water-soluble vitamin found in citrus fruits and fresh vegetables, such as cabbage, cauliflower, and tomatoes. The ascorbic acid content of these foods varies considerably, depending on freshness and the method of storage. Comparatively little is lost in the usual cooking procedures. Ascorbic acid is a potent reducing agent and, together with dihydroascorbic acid, forms a redox system. Its primary function in humans is in the hydroxylation of proline.

In the extreme deficiency state, known as "scurvy," the collagen in connective tissue, osteoid, and dentin is functionally defective and leads to widespread clinical pathologic conditions of the supporting tissues of blood vessels, bones, and teeth. A hemorrhagic tendency caused by capillary fragility is another characteristic effect, probably attributable to poor collagenous support of these vessels. Skin petechiae occur about the hair follicles and skin of the lower extremities and arms. Subperiosteal hemorrhages are characteristic findings and may be demonstrated on roentgenograms. Anemia often results, both from chronic bleeding and from hemolysis. Mild deficiency states of ascorbic acid are more common than scurvy, resulting from any condition that increases the metabolic demand in the absence of increased intake of the vitamin. Such imbalance may be manifested by impaired wound healing, hyperkeratosis, petechiae, and chronic gingivitis, with a tendency to hematoma formation.

In both mild ascorbic acid deficiency and scurvy, oral tissue pathologic conditions are significant. Gingivitis is one of the early manifestations, with bleeding at the gingival margins, swelling and ulceration. As the deficiency becomes more accute, the gingiva becomes grossly inflamed and bleeds on the slightest pressure or probing. In this state the oral tissues are highly susceptible to secondary infection, particularly those caused by Vincent's organism *(Borrelia vincentii)*. Local factors such as calculus, poor oral hygiene, and malocclusion further aggravate the effects of the deficiency state.

Recent studies now offer the first concrete evidence that subclinical ascorbic acid deficiency significantly increases susceptibility to periodontal disease. One report demonstrates that the periodontal tissues of animals fed a diet marginally deficient in ascorbic acid are more susceptible to breakdown when challenged by experimentally induced dental plaque than are control animals. In another report, a host defense factor was altered by an acute dietary deficiency of ascorbic acid. Animals fed diets with no ascorbic acid experienced an increase in the permeability of the gingival lining that could have contributed to the development of spontaneous scorbutic gingivitis.

A conclusive determination of the need for ascorbic acid intake above that required for general nutrition has not been made. It has also not been shown that ascorbic acid intake above that which is required for tissue saturation produces any preventive or therapeutic effects on the periodontium. At this time the requirement of ascorbic acid for wound healing and tissue repair is the only indication for its use in the treatment of oral lesions other than those associated with clinical scurvy. The usual therapeutic dose ranges from 300 to 500 mg daily, in divided doses.

Nutritional therapy

Patients in need of nutritional support require amino acids for protein synthesis and nonprotein calories to provide energy, as well as essential vitamins and minerals. If the gastrointestinal tract is functional, enteral feeding is preferable. Nutrition can be supplied with natural foods and with preparations in which nutritional components are added to produce a defined mixture. The available preparations generally provide 1 calorie/ml and serve as supplements and meal replacements. The carbohydrate source is usually corn syrup, sucrose, or lactose, but lactose-free products are best for patients with milk intolerance. When patients have problems with the digestion or absorption of fat, medium-chain triglycerides are a better source of calories than the usual long-chain triglycerides. Protein is usually derived from egg albumin, milk solids, and plant protein. Diets that supply amino acids and protein hydrolysates rather than intact proteins are termed "elemental diets." Elemental diets are used for nutritive support and therapeutic benefit in a variety of disorders, but the efficacy of these expensive diets has not been proved.

Parenteral nutrition involves the intravenous administration of protein nitrogen and calories, usually with a central superior vena cava catheter. Nonprotein calories must be administered for the synthesis of proteins; hypertonic dextrose usually is used. Fat may be equivalent to carbohydrates in its utilization for calories, and it also supplies essential fatty acids. Protein hydrolysates and crystalline amino acid mixtures are used as a source of nitrogen. Branched-chain amino acids have special properties and may be increasingly used in situations such as severe stress and liver failure in which they are less likely to provoke portal-systemic encephalopathy. The availability of synthetic amino acids makes it possible to vary the amino acid components of the solution. Parenteral hyperalimentation is effective in maintaining the nitrogen balance and promoting a weight gain and is used when enteral feeding cannot be used, in such conditions as enterocutaneous fistulas, a short bowel, and a prolonged ileus. Parenteral hyperalimentation has also

been used in patients with renal failure, cancer, and extensive burns. Complications include sepsis and metabolic disorders such as hyperglycemia and deficiency states, particularly those involving trace elements. Vitamin deficiencies are rare, because their replacement in the alimentation fluid is adequate. The home use of parenteral nutrition is becoming increasingly available.

DIETARY GOALS. Dietary goals for the United States have been set by a congressional committee after consultation with many experts. The reaction from nutritional scientists, physicians, and the community has been widespread and diverse, and the value of dietary change remains controversial. There is no assurance that an altered diet provides protection from disease.

The first goal is to avoid becoming overweight. Moderation in caloric intake may be the single most important dietary practice the public could observe, but certainly many other risk factors are implicated in the probability of disease. Other goals are to increase the consumption of complex carbohydrates and to reduce the use of refined simple sugars. An advantage of this recommendation is that such a diet has a higher intake of dietary fiber, the nondigestible component of plant foods. High-fiber diets are epidemiologically associated with a lower incidence of colon cancer, diverticular disease, and hyperlipidemia. No firm evidence has implicated sugar as a cause of arteriosclerosis or diabetes, but controlled human studies have established that the incidence and prevalence of dental caries can be diminished by reducing sugar consumption.

Many studies have shown that blood lipid levels can be altered by reducing the amount of saturated fat in the diet. Whether this alteration can achieve the purpose of preventing arteriosclerotic heart disease is not certain. The association of a total fat intake with certain cancers also supports the goal of a reduction of the total fat in the diet rather than an increased intake of polyunsaturated fats. Obesity might also be effectively treated by decreasing the fat intake. A reduction in the consumption of cholesterol has also been proposed, yet dietary cholesterol may not be nearly as important as weight control and inherent metabolic processes in achieving beneficial lipid levels.

The goal to reduce the intake of salt has been set even though the optimal requirement for sodium has not been established. Sodium chloride may have an effect on the elevation of the blood pressure in some individuals, but many others are not susceptible.

To implement these goals most Americans would need to change their eating patterns. These recommendations are aimed at the prevention of diseases that have multiple causes but may involve an interaction with the diet. These goals should probably be recognized at this time as prudent, but tentative.

BIBLIOGRAPHY
Gastrointestinal disorders

Amato AE and Small EW: Oral manifestations of Gardner's syndrome: report of a case, J Oral Surg 28:458, 1970.

Astacio JN and Alfar C: Oral mucosa metastasis from gastric adenocarcinoma, Oral Surg 28:859, 1969.

Babin RW, Ceilley RI, and DeSanto LW: Oral hyperpigmentation and occult malignancy: report of a case, J Otolaryngol 7:389, 1978.

Basu MK and others: Oral manifestations of Crohn's disease, Gut 16:249, 1975.

Bernstein ML and McDonald JS: Oral lesions in Crohn's disease: report of two cases and update of the literature, Oral Surg 46:234, 1978.

Biedlingmaier JF, Blanchard CL, and Masi J: Necrotizing sialometaplasia of the palate and adenocarcinoma of the esophagus, Ear Nose Throat J 59:222, 1980.

Blacharsh C: Dental aspects of patients with cystic fibrosis: a preliminary clinical study, J Am Dent Assoc 95:106, 1977.

Caldwell TA, Schweber SJ, and Lucchesi FJ: Resection of tongue lesion associated with hereditary telangiectasia (Osler-Weber-Rendu disease), J Oral Surg 28:299, 1970.

Carr D: Granulomatous cheilitis in Crohn's disease, Br Med J 4:636, 1974.

Croft CB and Wilkinson AR: Ulceration of the mouth, pharynx, and larynx in Crohn's disease of the intestine, Br J Surg 59:249, 1972.

Crumley RL: Synchronous carcinomas of the parotid and colon, Ear Nose Throat J 57:31, 1979.

Eccles JD: Erosion of teeth by gastric contents, Lancet 2:479, 1978.

Eisenbud L, Katzka I, and Platt N: Oral manifestations of Crohn's disease, Oral Surg 34:770, 1972.

Everett FG and Hahn CR: Hereditary hemorrhagic telangiectasia with gingival lesion, J Periodontol 47:295, 1976.

Ferguson MM and others: Coeliac disease associated with recurrent aphthae, Gut 21:223, 1980.

Fraser NG, Kerr NW, and Donald D: Oral lesions in dermatitis herpetiformis, Br J Dermatol 89:439, 1973.

Gius JA and others: Vascular formations of the lip and peptic ulcer, JAMA 183:725, 1963.

Glazer RI, Spatz SS, and Catone GA: Viral hepatitis: a hazard to oral surgeons, J Oral Surg 31:504, 1973.

Golding PL, Smith M, and Williams R: Multisystem involvement in chronic liver disease, Am J Med 55:772, 1973.

Gorlin RJ and Goldman HM: Thoma's oral pathology, ed 6, St Louis, 1970, The CV Mosby Co.

Harrison PV, Scott DG, and Cobden I: Buccal mucosa immunofluorescence in coeliac disease and dermatitis herpetiformis, Br J Dermatol 102:687, 1980.

Hashimoto K and Pritzker MS: Hereditary hemorrhagic telangiectasia: an electron microscopic study, Oral Surg 34:751, 1972.

Hicks KA and Dickie WR: Amyloidosis: report of case presenting with macroglossia, Br J Plast Surg 26:274, 1973.

Howden GF: Erosion as the presenting symptom in hiatus hernia, Br Dent J 131:455, 1971.

Hurst PS, Lacey JH, and Crisp AH: Teeth, vomiting and diet: a study of the dental characteristics of seventeen anorexia nervosa patients, Postgrad Med J 53:298, 1977.

Jones JH and Mason DK: Oral manifestations of systemic disease, Philadelphia, 1980, WB Saunders Co.

Kakizaki G and others: A new diagnostic test for pancreatic disorders by examination of parotid saliva, Am J Gastroenterol 65(5):437, 1976.

Keith DA: Oral features of primary amyloidosis, Br J Oral Surg 10:107, 1972.

Kelley ML Jr: Purulent mucocutaneous lesions associated with ulcerative colitis, Med Radiogr Photogr 44:39, 1968.

Kutscher AH and others: Parotid saliva in cystic fibrosis, Am J Dis Child 110:643, 1965.

Lamster I and others: An association between Crohn's disease, periodontal disease and enhanced neutrophil function, J Periodontol 49:475, 1978.

Lee BM: Metastasis of colon carcinoma to the lip, Arch Dermatol 105:608, 1972.

Levy B and Smith WK: A jaw metastasis from the colon, Oral Surg 38:769, 1974.

Little JW and Falace DA: Dental management of the medically compromised patient, St Louis, 1980, The CV Mosby Co.

Lowe NJ: Peutz-Jeghers syndrome with pigmented oral papillomas, Arch Dermatol 3:503, 1975.

Lund BA, Moertel CG, and Gibelisco JA: Metastasis of gastric adenocarcinoma to oral mucosa, Oral Surg 25:805, 1968.

Lynch MA, editor: Burket's oral medicine, ed 7, Philadelphia, 1977, JB Lippincott Co.

Mandel ID and others: Parotid saliva in cystic fibrosis, Am J Dis Child 110:646, 1965.

Marmer J, Barbero GJ, and Sibinga MS: The pattern of parotid gland secretion in cystic fibrosis of the pancreas, Gastroenterology 50:551, 1966.

Matthews N and others: Buccal biopsy in diagnosis of Crohn's disease, Lancet 1:500, 1979.

Merck, Sharp & Dohme, Division of Merck & Co Inc, West Point, Pa, Package insert for Heptavax B, May 1982.

Moffat DA: Metastatic adenocarcinoma of the rectum presenting as an epulis: a case report, Br J Oral Surg 14:90, 1976.

Nugent FW and Bulan MB: Extracolonic manifestations of ulcerative colitis, Am Fam Phys 5:68, 1972.

O'Brien KT, Saunders DR, and Templeton FE: Chronic gastric erosions and oral aphthae case report, Dig Dis 17:447, 1972.

Ohsiro T and others: Treatment of pigmentation of the lips and oral mucosa in Peutz-Jeghers syndrome using ruby and argon lasers, Br J Plast Surg 33:346, 1980.

Pindborg JJ: Atlas of diseases of the oral mucosa, ed 3, Philadelphia, 1980, WB Saunders Co.

Primosch RE: Tetracycline discoloration, enamel defects, and dental caries in patients with cystic fibrosis, Oral Surg 50(4):301, 1980.

Redding SW, Carr RF, and Foti CE: Gardner's syndrome: report of a case, J Oral Surg 39:50, 1981.

Rimland D and others: Hepatitis B outbreak traced to an oral surgeon, N Engl J med 296:953, 1977.

Ritter SB and Petersen G: Esophageal cancer, hyperkeratosis and oral leukoplakia: follow-up family study, JAMA 236:1844, 1976.

Russotto SB and Ship II: Oral manifestations of dermatitis herpetiformis, Oral Surg 31:42, 1971.

Schwartz HC and Olson DJ: Amyloidosis: a rational approach to diagnosis by intraoral biopsy, Oral Surg 39:837, 1975.

Snyder MB and Cawson RA: Oral changes in Crohn's disease, J Oral Surg 34:594, 1976.

Stanback JS and Peagler FD: Primary amyloidosis, Oral Surg 26:774, 1968.

Taylor VE and Smith CJ: Oral manifestations of Crohn's disease without demonstrable gastrointestinal lesions, Oral Surg 39:58, 1975.

Uthman AA: Plummer-Vinson syndrome, Oral Surg 20:449, 1965.

Walker JEG: Possible diagnostic test for Crohn's disease by use of buccal mucosa, Lancet 2:759, 1978.

Weisman RA and Calcaterra TC: Head and neck manifestations of scleroderma, Ann Otolaryngol 87:332, 1978.

White DK, Hayes RC, and Benjamin RN: Loss of tooth structure associated with chronic regurgitation and vomiting, J Am Dent Assoc 97:833, 1978.

Wiesmann UN, Boat TF, and diSant'Agnese PA: Sodium concentration in unstimulated parotid saliva and on oral mucosa in normal subjects and in patients with cystic fibrosis, J Pediatr 76:444, 1970.

Zambito R: Hospital dental practice: a manual, Garden City, NY, 1978, Medical Examination Publishing Co, Inc.

Nutritional disorders

Bigaouette J and Howard L: Nutrition-related disorders, Int J Dermatol 16:605, 1977.

Caddell JL: Magnesium in the therapy of orofacial lesions of severe protein-calorie malnutrition, Br J Surg 56:826, 1969.

Delgado H and others: Nutritional status and the timing of deciduous tooth eruption, Am J Clin Nutr 28:216, 1975.

Falconer DT: Scurvy presenting with oral symptoms, Br Dent J 146:313, 1979.

Gigliotti R and others: Familial vitamin D refractory rickets, J Am Dent Assoc 82:383, 1971.

Hjorting-Hansen E and Bertram U: Oral aspects of pernicious anemia, Br Dent J 125:266, 1968.

Hood J, Burns CA, and Hodges RE: Sjögren's syndrome in scurvy, N Engl J Med 282:1120, 1979.

Marks SC, Lindahl RL, and Bowden JW: Dental and cephalometric findings in vitamin D resistant rickets, J Dent Child 32:259, 1965.

Millard HD and Gobetti JP: Nonspecific stomatitis—a presenting sign in pernicious anemia, Oral Surg 39:562, 1975.

Nakamoto T and Mallek HM: Significance of protein-energy malnutrition in dentistry: some suggestions for the profession, J Am Dent Assoc 100:339, 1980.

Protein deficiency and tooth and salivary gland development, Nutr Rev 32:24, 1974.

Sapiro SM: Folic acid deficiency preceding nontropical sprue, J Oral Med 32:106, 1977.

Soni NN and Marks SC: Microradiographic and polarized light study of dental tissues in vitamin D–resistant rickets, Oral Surg 23:755, 1967.

ENDOCRINOLOGY

Edited by **Doris G. Bartuska**

185 · INTRODUCTION TO THE DISEASES OF THE ENDOCRINE SYSTEM AND THE MECHANISM OF ACTION OF HORMONES

Mary B. Dratman

Endocrine disorders are often slow in onset and subtle in presentation. They decrease longevity and erode the quality of life. Therefore early identification and treatment of these disorders bring great benefit to the patient, as well as professional gratification to the physician. In recent years the chances of successfully treating previously unsuspected endocrinopathies have been greatly improved by the availability of sensitive techniques for measuring hormones and their metabolites and for measuring their effects on the individual patient. In addition to these biochemically based approaches, a diversity of new imaging techniques make it possible to look inside the body and observe structural and functional changes even in small endocrine glands. In spite of these advances, endocrine disorders often remain undiagnosed and therefore untreated for many years after their onset. However, when the attentive medical practitioner is closely following the patient and has a high level of consciousness regarding the possibility of an endocrine disorder, even early changes in endocrine status can be detected.

The material presented in this section is intended to augment and sustain this level of consciousness. It emphasizes the great importance of physical diagnosis in endocrinology and stresses the features of the clinical presentation that signal the presence of early hormonal dysfunction. Throughout this section, attention is given to the important influence of genetic endowment, developmental processes, and previous life history on the clinical picture. This provides a basis for detecting the presence of masked or unusual presentations of endocrine disorders. Great stress is also laid on the requirement for studying the patient with well-established chemical, functional, and imaging methods and for using appropriate endocrine challenge methodologies to substantiate the diagnosis.

In addition to establishing an organ-and-system-oriented approach to endocrine problems of patients in clinical practice, the responsiveness of endocrine systems is delineated at different stages of life and in patients with a variety of nonendocrine diseases. When appropriate, the basic role of hormones in maintaining health and defending against disease is considered. However, discussion of the biochemical mechansims of endocrine functions and dysfunctions is necessarily limited. Therefore some current problems in basic endocrinology are mentioned to set the stage for the clinical discussions that follow.

CHANGING CONCEPTS OF THE NATURE AND DOMAIN OF ENDOCRINE SUBSTANCES. As a result of recent advances in the technology as well as the philosophy of hormone research, seemingly inviolate tenets of endocrinology have been reexamined. The endocrine gland can no longer be considered the sole source and guardian of its secretions. Nonendocrine cells such as neurons may produce hormones. Even individual cells dispersed among a variety of tissues may produce, store, or release such diverse information-transmitting substances as serotonin, norepinephrine, gastrointestinal peptides, calcitonin, glucagon, endorphins, and somatostatin. Whereas hormones were once thought to be disseminated only via the bloodstream, it is now evident that they travel by a variety of routes. Many do indeed reach their targets through the general circulation, but some are first secreted into a portal circulation and reach selected tissues in high concentration before they enter the mainstream. Some tissues receive high concentrations of hormones through innervation by neuroendocrine cells. For example, pituicytes in the neurohypophysis are rich in vasopressin delivered by nerve terminals from perikarya in the supraoptic and paraventricular nuclei. This is a hormone-conserving device, since the effect of receiving a small number of potent molecules directly into the specialized extracellular space constituting a synaptic cleft or neuroeffector junction is far greater than the effect produced by receiving them through the general circulation. The so-called parahormones may actually percolate from the hormone-synthesizing cell to an adjacent target cell, with the result that maximal concentrations are made available locally before there is any dilution whatsoever within the vascular compartment. This process is thought to operate, for example, among the different cells of the islets of Langerhans.

ROLE OF CELLULAR AND TISSUE RESPONSIVITY TO CHEMICAL MESSENGERS: IMPORTANCE OF THE RECEPTOR CONCEPT. Hormone effects are now known to be limited not only by their rate, route, efficiency of dissemination, and their half-life in extracellular fluids, but also by conditions prevailing at their cellular destination. The outer cell membrane is functionally and morphologically complex. It acts as a responsive barrier to the passage of nutrients to and from the extracellular fluid via its multiplicity of gates and channels. It also bears specialized structures serving as recipients for and transducers of molecular information arriving at the surfaces of cells, or as receptors mediating internalization of chemical messages (hormones) through the medium of endocytosis. The most thoroughly studied hormone-sensing and information-transducing cell membrane structures include the adenosine triphosphate (ATP)–cyclic adenosine monophosphate (AMP) generating system, linked to the guanosine triphosphate–guanosine monophosphate (GTP-GMP) regulatory systems; the prostaglandin-forming systems; and the phospholipase C, diacylglycerol, inositol phosphate, calcium ion–dependent protein kinase C generating system.

Receptors may be present in any part of the cell and are defined in terms of their special properties relevant to the molecules received. They are specific in that they differentiate (have discriminatory recognition sites) among closely related molecular species. At the same time they are capable of interacting with a wide variety of analogous substances that may block, feebly mimic, or occasionally produce even more potent effects than the reference ligands. Receptor capacity for a given class of compounds is limited, and the apparent kinetics of receptor-ligand interaction are susceptible to measurement and specification. It is now customary to define properties of hormones in terms of their "specific" binding, that is, their participation in limited-capacity, high-affinity binding interactions with proteins on or within cells or subcellular organelles.

CELLULAR MECHANISMS OF HORMONE ACTION. Experiments based on the receptor concept have led to impressive ongoing discoveries of molecular mechanisms of hormone action. According to present formulations, peptide hormones and biogenic amines are detained at the cell surface because of their size, water solubility, or spatial properties. There they encounter and bind to highly specialized regions of the plasma membrane (receptor regions), causing, for example, excitation of catalytic units at the cytoplasmic interface, culminating in a burst of intracellular second-messenger activity and a cascade of integrated molecular responses that acutely alter cellular function for self-limited periods.

Whereas peptide hormones are detained rather than excluded from entry into cells, the plasma membrane apparently does not block the passage of steroid hormones and their metabolites into the cell sap. Upon entry, they are either recognized and avidly bound by receptors in the cells, or they diffuse back out again. Changes in transcription, messenger ribonucleic acid (mRNA), and protein synthesis occur promptly following steroid hormone administration to adrenalectomized animals. These results are thought to stem from the formation of steroid hormone–receptor complexes in the nucleoplasm of hormone-sensitive cells. Thereupon, alterations in gene transcription result from well-defined interactions between regions of the hormone-activated receptor and specific elements of the genome.

Strong evidence has accumulated in support of a nuclear site of triiodothyronine action. In addition to the nuclear receptor, there is also considerable interest in the role of membrane, mitochondrial, cytosol, and synaptosome high-affinity binding sites for triiodothyronine, thyroxine, or both. Variants of the c-erb-A protooncogenes are reported to code for the nuclear receptors for a large "superfamily" of hormones, including thyroid, steroid, vitamin D, and retinol hormones.

IMPORTANCE OF HORMONE METABOLISM IN DETERMINING ROUTES OF HORMONE ACTION. Some once confusing aspects of the actions of hormones have been clarified by recognizing that hormone actions and hormone metabolism are often highly interdependent processes. Not all hormone metabolites are generated in all tissues, and not all receptive tissues are responsive to the same metabolite. These principles have been most dramatically illustrated by recent observations relevant to differences in testosterone and dehydrotestosterone action and to the actions of another steroid hormone, cholecalciferol. The latter molecule is either synthesized in the skin or derived from the diet (on which basis it was long considered to be a vitamin). It is then transported to several different tissues (such as liver and kidney), where it is differently metabolized and remetabolized by each of them; the metabolites are then transported once again to distant sites (bone, gut, and renal tubule), where they produce coordinated but different effects on calcium metabolism. The ultimate actions of these metabolites vary according to the state of the responding tissue and the presence or absence of other naturally occurring synergists and antagonists.

HORMONES AND THE NERVOUS SYSTEM. A serious new look is being taken at the functional consequences of hormone action in the nervous system. The discovery that a specific portion of a long-known pituitary hormone (β-lipotropin) exhibits the same amino acid sequence as a putative neurotransmitter (the methionine enkephlin portion of β-endorphin, mediating endogenous morphine-like actions) has created a stir in the field of psychoneuroendocrine relationships. In addition, several recent observations suggest that not only biogenic amines but thyroid hormones, hypothalamic and gastrointestinal peptides, and steroid hormones are concentrated and metabolized within neurons and actively implicated in nervous system development and adult nervous system function. It therefore seems evident that further knowledge of the metabolism and fate of hormones in the brain, and their relationship to other chemical transformations occurring in the nervous system, may help to elucidate obscure aspects of the functions of both systems.

Ultimately, such knowledge will be crucial in the management of patients, not only as they require treatment for endocrine diseases, but also as they undergo hormonal changes in response to developmental, psychophysiologic, and aging processes throughout the course of their lives.

BIBLIOGRAPHY

Axelrod, J: Relationships between catecholamines and other hormones, Recent Prog Horm Res 31:1, 1975.

Barker, JI: Peptides: roles in neuronal excitability, Physiol Rev 56:435, 1976.

Cuatrecasas, P, and others: Hormone receptor complexes and their modulation of membrane function, Recent Prog Horm Res 31:37, 1975.

DeLuca, HF: Recent advances in the metabolism and function of vitamin D, Fed Proc 28:1678, 1969.

Dratman, MB: On the mechanism of action of thyroxine, an amino acid analog of tyrosine, J Theor Biol 46:255, 1974.

Hoch, FL: Metabolic effects of thyroid hormones, Handbook Physiol Sect 7(3):391, 1974.

Irvine, CHG: A four compartment model of thyroxine metabolism. In Harland, WA, and Orr, JS, editors: Thyroid hormone metabolism. New York, 1975, Academic Press, Inc.

Kuhlenbeck, H: The central nervous system of vertebrates: a general survey of its comparative anatomy with an introduction to the pertinent fundamental biologic and logical concepts, vols 1-4, New York, 1967-1975, Academic Press, Inc.

Loh, HH, and others: β-Endorphin is a potent analgesic agent, Proc Natl Acad Sci USA 73:2895, 1976.

Mashio, Y, and others: High affinity 3,5,3'-L-triiodothyronine binding to synaptosomes in rat cerebral cortex, Endocrinology 110:1257, 1982.

Oppenheimer, JH, and Samuels, H, editors: Molecular basis of thyroid hormone action, New York, 1983, Academic Press.

Sterling, K: Thyroid hormone action at the cell level, NEJM 300:117-123 and 173, 1979.

Weinberger, C, and others: The c-erb-A gene encodes a thyroid hormone receptor, Nature 234:641, 1986.

186 · HYPOTHALAMIC AND PITUITARY DISORDERS

Calvin Ezrin

ENDOCRINE HYPOTHALAMUS

The hypothalamic-pituitary relationship is the most important in neuroendocrinology. The hypothalamus, a complicated

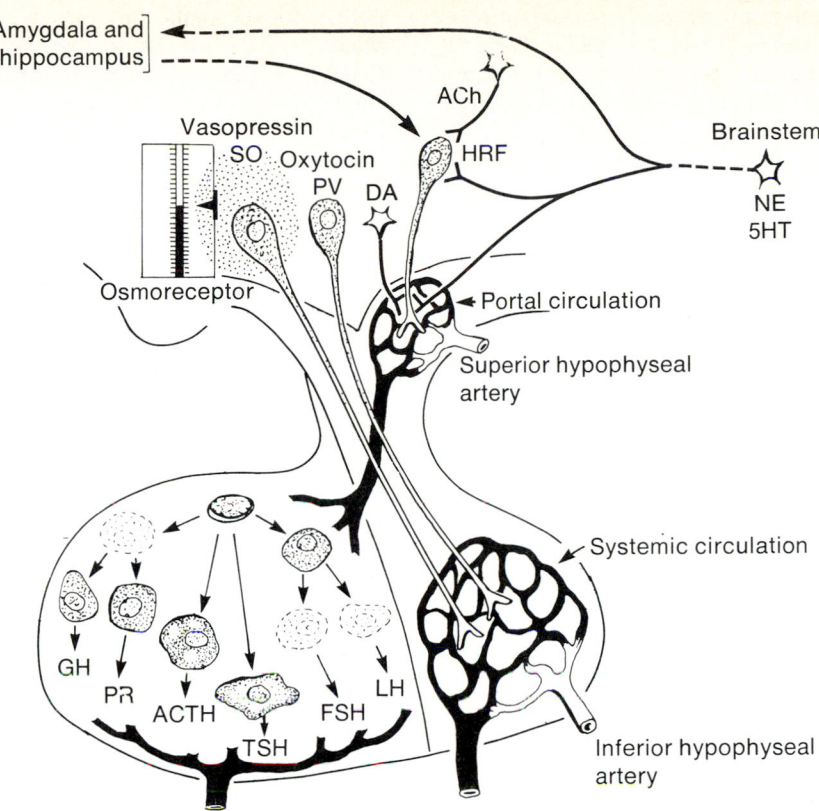

Fig. 186-1 "Endocrine hypothalamus" (see text). *SO,* supraoptic nuclei; *PV,* paraventricular nuclei; *HRF,* hypothalamic releasing factor; *DA,* dopamine; *NE,* norepinephrine; *5HT,* 5-hydroxytryptamine; *Ach,* acetylcholine; *GH,* growth hormone; *PR,* prolactin; *ACTH,* adrenocorticotropin; *TSH,* thyroid-stimulating hormone; *FSH,* follicle-stimulating hormone; *LH,* luteinizing hormone. (From Ezrin C, Godden JO, and Volpé R: Systematic endocrinology, ed 2, New York, 1979, Harper & Row, Publishers.)

collection of nerve cells and fiber tracts, participates in the regulation of many autonomic functions and body rhythms. The hypothalamus also contains cells that combine neural and secretory activity. This portion is difficult to define anatomically, but since it produces hormones, it may accurately be designated as the "endocrine hypothalamus." The hormones it produces are delivered to the pituitary gland (Fig. 186-1). The endocrine hypothalamus is composed of cells that are typical neurons capable of being excited to conduct action potentials and releasing specific substances at their terminals. However, unlike typical neurons, which release neurotransmitters into synaptic clefts, neurosecretory cells release their products into perivascular spaces.

The first neurosecretory cells to be recognized were those of the supraoptic and paraventricular nuclei of the hypothalamus, whose cell bodies and axon process color intensely with specific stains. Neurophysins, specific carrier proteins for vasopressin and oxytocin, are responsible for this intense staining. The axons of these neurons terminate in the posterior pituitary adjacent to capillaries. Depolarization of the axon terminal causes a release of hormone by a process called stimulation-secretion coupling, which occurs only in the presence of adequate calcium.

Many clinical and experimental observations have shown that anterior pituitary secretion is largely dependent on the hypothalamus. Certain neurons of the medial basal hypothalamus are believed to synthesize and secrete specific hypothalamic adenohypophysiotropic hormones, or regulatory factors, that stimulate or inhibit the secretion of anterior pituitary cells. Axons of these neurons terminate directly in the perivascular zone surrounding the primary capillary network of the pituitary portal circulation in the median eminence, from which they travel via the pituitary portal veins to the anterior lobe. Neurotransmitters, such as norepinephrine, 5-hydroxytryptamine, and acetylcholine, influence the secretion of hypothalamic-regulating hormones and factors and thus indirectly affect anterior pituitary function. One major exception to this rule is dopamine, which has a direct inhibitory action on the release of prolactin from the pituitary.

CONTROL OF ANTERIOR PITUITARY SECRETION

The adenohypophysis produces six distinct hormones: *thyrotropin* (thyroid-stimulating hormone), *corticotropin* (adrenocorticotropic hormone), two *gonadotropins* (follicle-stimulating hormone and luteinizing hormone), *prolactin,* and *somatotropin* (growth hormone). Morphologic studies have shown that the adenohypophysis contains at least five different cell types, each producing one or two closely related hormones. Thus the anterior pituitary may be regarded as a confederation of several relatively independent endocrine glands grouped together anatomically, probably to permit the hypothalamus to efficiently exert higher control. Consideration of the function of each of the anterior pituitary hormones and their regulation leads to a better understanding of the entire endocrine system.

Thyrotropin, or thyroid-stimulating hormone (TSH)

The hypothalamic *thyrotropin-releasing hormone* (TRH) stimulates the release of TSH, which in turn acts on the thyroid to increase the output of its two hormones: tetraiodothyronine, or thyroxine (T_4), and triiodothyronine (T_3). The role of TRH in maintaining the narrow normal range of concentration of the circulating thyroid hormones is probably relatively minor. It seems to mediate thyroid activation that results from prolonged exposure to cold and also appears to be involved in the thyroid adaptation of the newborn to the relatively cold extrauterine environment. The increased serum T_4 level in the newborn represents a true hyperthyroid state that is self-correcting.

Hypothyroidism caused by thyroid insufficiency leads to increased secretion of TSH in an attempt to restore normal levels of circulating thyroid hormones. Increased serum TSH is the most sensitive test for primary hypothyroidism.

Corticotropin, or adrenocorticotropic hormone

Adrenocorticotropic hormone (ACTH), a polypeptide, regulates the growth and function of the adrenal cortex. It is especially important in controlling the production and release of glucocorticoid hormones such as cortisol, which is made by the zona fasciculata. The zona glomerulosa, which produces the important mineralocorticoid aldosterone, is largely controlled by the renin-angiotensin system. The production of sex steroids by the zona reticularis is governed by a mechanism that is still unclear. Cells containing ACTH account for no more than 10% of the anterior pituitary cell population. The pituitary "corticotroph" is the most basophilic and PAS-positive of all the pituitary cells. It undergoes a limited loss of granulation in a characteristic crescentic pattern under the influence of prolonged excessive levels of circulating cortisol, such as occurs in Cushing's syndrome, which may result from various causes (see Chapter 188). It seems that ACTH and β-lipotropin, a parent molecule of several polypeptide neurotransmitters, are both produced by the same basophil subtype. They probably share a common precursor.

The release of ACTH appears to be governed by at least three independent mechanisms:

1. *Negative feedback.* Cortisol, the principal adrenal glucocorticoid, inhibits ACTH release when its level rises higher than normal. If the cortisol level falls, ACTH secretion is stimulated through a negative feedback; the cortisol level rises again and turns off the ACTH.
2. *Diurnal rhythm.* In human beings ACTH secretion is maximal in the early morning hours with a gradual fall after 8 AM. Consequently, afternoon plasma cortisol levels (which closely reflect ACTH release) are only about one half of the 8 AM value. This diurnal rhythm may be abolished by certain central nervous system lesions. It is also lost in Cushing's syndrome and may be absent in some emotionally depressed patients.
3. *A stress-activated mechanism.* Stressful stimuli, such as trauma, hypoglycemia, or pyrogens, increase the delivery of corticotropin-releasing factor (CRF) to the adenohypophysis. This stress mechanism, stimulating the corticotrophs, may override the negative feedback and diurnal rhythm control systems. The greater the stress, the more ACTH is secreted.

Gonadotropic hormones—follicle-stimulating hormone and luteinizing hormone

Immunostaining reveals that follicle-stimulating hormone (FSH) and luteinizing hormone (LH) arise from the same subtype of pituitary basophil cell. These gonadotropins play major roles in ovarian and testicular functions.

OVARIAN FUNCTION. FSH, a glycoprotein, enlarges a ripening ovarian follicle to the point of rupture. Under FSH influence the follicular cells secrete estrogen. Ovulation, in midcycle, results from an additional surge of secretion of another glycoprotein, LH. Both gonadotropins are released by a hy-

pothalamic hormone designated gonadotropin-releasing hormone (GnRH) or luteinizing hormone–releasing hormone (LHRH or LRH). When the fertilized ovum is implanted, chorionic gonadotropin is secreted to maintain the corpus luteum beyond its normal life span of 2 weeks. Normal menstruation results from a falling level of progesterone.

The ovarian steroids, estrogen and progesterone, exert a negative feedback effect on both FSH and LH secretion. After physiologic ovarian failure (menopause) or destruction or removal of the ovaries, FSH and LH secretion rise considerably.

TESTICULAR FUNCTION. The gonadotropic control of testicular maturation and function is complex. FSH is necessary for the development of LH receptors to permit the full action of LH. FSH stimulates the production of androgen-binding protein, which transports testosterone into the seminiferous tubule where it helps to stimulate spermatogenesis. The testicular interstitial, or Leydig, cells are driven to produce testosterone by LH or, as it is known in the male, by interstitial cell–stimulating hormone (ICSH). In male patients with primary hypogonadism, as in females, the serum gonadotropin levels increase, suggesting that there is a negative feedback between the testes and the pituitary. When it is administered therapeutically, testosterone inhibits ICSH but not FSH. FSH secretion is probably normally inhibited by a nonsteroid substance (designated "inhibin") made by the tubules. In some aging men testosterone production falls and ICSH (LH) levels increase. Thus in men there may be a late menopause, but it has received little clinical attention because impotence and reduced performance in elderly men can usually be ascribed to other factors.

Prolactin

The recognition of prolactin as a separate human hormone was delayed for some time because of the considerable similarity in molecular structure of prolactin and growth hormone. These two hormones arise from separate subtypes of pituitary acidophils. Prolactin is one of the group of hormones necessary for sufficient breast development to permit milk secretion. When the breast has developed under the influence of estrogen, progesterone, and prolactin during pregnancy, milk secretion appears to depend on an additional postpartum pituitary secretion of prolactin. During the last trimester of pregnancy, when circulating levels of prolactin are high because of estrogen-induced prolactin cell hyperplasia, the breast is prevented from secreting milk by the accompanying increased levels of estrogen. Lactation ensues soon after delivery, which causes a rapid decrease in estrogen levels.

Breast-feeding raises serum prolactin levels and delays resumption of menses. Hyperprolactinemia may interfere with ovulation by decreasing the manufacture or release of GnRH. It may also decrease the responsiveness of the gonadotrophs to LRH or the ovaries to gonadotropins.

The manufacture and release of prolactin are under the control of a hypothalamic inhibitor, prolactin-inhibiting factor (PIF), which may be dopamine.

Somatotropin, or growth hormone

Somatotropin, a protein hormone consisting of 191 amino acids, is produced by a subtype of an acidophil cell. It stimulates protein anabolism, releases free fatty acids by lipolysis, and induces hyperglycemia by interfering with glucose use. Circulating levels of growth hormone fluctuate rapidly in response to nutritional and psychic events, to sleep, and to muscular exercise. This fluctuation occurs as a result of hypothalamic influences via intermittent stimulation by growth hormone–releasing hormone and tonic inhibition by somatostatin. Hyperglycemia inhibits the release of growth hormone, whereas hypoglycemia stimulates its output.

Some of the effects of growth hormone are mediated by serum peptides of hepatic origin, somatomedins, whose levels are dependent on growth hormone. To achieve normal adult body size in the first two decades of life, a person needs somatotropin. When a child lacks this hormone, growth is severely retarded. Growth hormone–deficient children respond to human growth hormone with a substantial increase in growth rate. Species specificity is seen in the clinical use of growth hormone and gonadotropins but not with any of the other pituitary hormones.

CLINICAL PITUITARY DISORDERS

The major disease processes involving the pituitary are tumor, infarct, and granuloma. In addition, congenital selective hypofunction may result from hypothalamic deficiency. Diseases of the pituitary may have many different presentations. Local compressive effects from expanding tumors and manifestations of endocrine imbalance are the most common events that bring a patient to clinical attention.

The optic chiasm and hypothalamus are the most important superior relations of the pituitary fossa. The pituitary gland lies above the sphenoid sinus, into which downward-growing pituitary tumors may project. The internal carotid arteries (as well as the third and sixth cranial nerves) are in the cavernous sinuses, which are lateral to the pituitary gland and may occasionally be compressed by pituitary tumors. Mistaking a carotid aneurysm for a pituitary tumor may lead to a fatal surgical outcome.

Hyperpituitary syndromes

Clinically significant pituitary hypersecretion usually results from tumors, some of which may not be readily apparent. Hyperplasia of specific cell types may result from target gland failure (such as primary hypothyroidism) or from alteration of normal hypothalamic regulatory mechanisms. Prolactin cell hyperplasia may result from suprahypophyseal lesions or drugs such as phenothiazines that interfere with the production and delivery of PIF to the pituitary.

ACROMEGALY. Acromegaly, the syndrome of adult growth hormone excess, and gigantism, its counterpart beginning in childhood, are the result of growth hormone–secreting tumors, some of which have an accompanying prolactin cell component. Acromegaly is characterized by enlargement of the extremities, coarsening of the facial features, and a high incidence of impaired sugar tolerance (Fig. 186-2). The pituitary tumor may reduce vision by compressing the visual pathway. Gigantism begins when the limb bones are still capable of further longitudinal growth. Pituitary giants may reach a height of 8 feet (240 cm) and weigh more than 300 pounds (135 kg). These individuals usually have some associated acromegalic features.

The symptoms and signs result from either local compression by the tumor or its metabolic effects. Headache, which may vary from mild to severe, usually results from the expanding tumor pressing on the sensitive walls of the sella turcica; it may also be the product of hormonal influences. Pressure upward on the optic chiasm most commonly produces a bitemporal hemianopia, but other visual field defects also occur.

The frequent association of diabetes mellitus with acromegaly indicates that somatotropin and insulin are antagonistic with respect to blood sugar levels. The bony and soft tissue overgrowth of acromegaly is an expression of the increased anab-

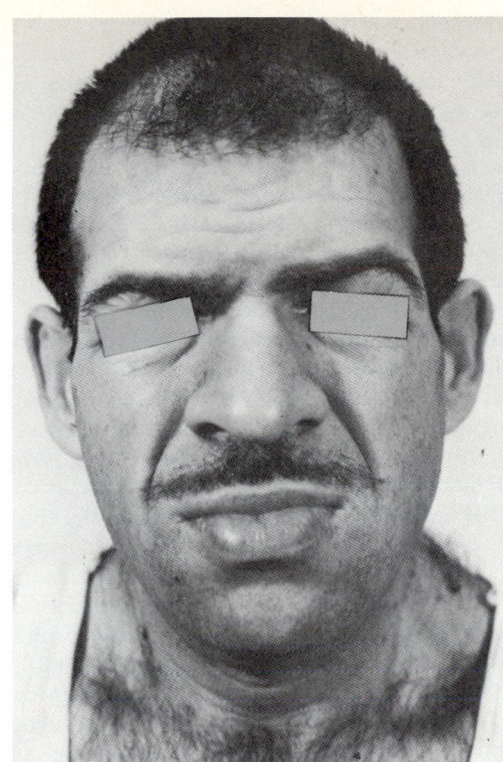

Fig. 186-2 This 36-year-old man had acromegaly owing to pituitary adenoma hypersecreting growth hormone (see text). (From Ezrin C, Godden JO, and Volpé R: Systematic endocrinology, ed 2, New York, 1979, Harper & Row, Publishers.)

olism that characterizes this disorder. Hypermetabolism with heat intolerance and excessive perspiration is found in about one third of patients with acromegaly, whereas hyperthyroidism occurs in less than one twentieth of cases. Hyperparathyroidism may also accompany acromegaly, sometimes as a feature of multiple endocrine adenomatosis, which may be familial and include pancreatic islet tumors. Some patients with acromegaly have galactorrhea, usually because the tumor consists of both prolactin- and growth hormone–producing cells.

Although conventional roentgenographic views of the sella turcica may sometimes miss a small adenoma causing acromegaly, computerized tomography or magnetic resonance imaging rarely do. Besides the usual finding of considerable sellar distortion, roentgenograms often reveal enlargement of the accessory nasal sinuses, prognathism, thickening of the inner table of the skull, spinal osteoporosis, and tufting of the terminal phalanges. Increased thickness of the skin may be demonstrated by measuring the heel pad for the subcutaneous fat layer by roentgenography.

For the laboratory confirmation of acromegaly, circulating growth hormone levels should be measured by immunoassay. Normally the administration of glucose inhibits the secretion of growth hormone. In acromegaly this inhibition does not occur, and sustained elevations of growth hormone or even increased levels are observed when the samples are taken during a glucose tolerance test. Impaired glucose tolerance is found in at least one third of patients with acromegaly, and one sixth have diabetes mellitus requiring treatment. Elevation of the fasting serum inorganic phosphate (greater than 4.5 mg/dl) is an indirect measure of growth hormone secretion. Often the administration of TRH raises growth hormone levels in patients with acromegaly, a response not seen in normal subjects.

Therapy for acromegaly usually involves transsphenoidal pituitary adenomectomy, with drugs or radiation as adjuvants. Irradiation, either with conventional high voltage or proton beams, has also been used as primary therapy in acromegaly, but slowness of response and high incidence of hypopituitarism are disadvantages. A dopaminergic agent bromocriptine has also been used to treat acromegaly. It blocks the release of growth hormone for adenoma cells, but the doses required are higher than those needed to control hyperprolactinemia. Bromocriptine is useful when waiting for the effects of conventional radiation therapy to appear. An octapeptide, Sandostatin analog (SMS 201-995), if administered subcutaneously has successfully lowered growth hormone levels in acromegaly. Accompanying transient insulin deficiency and hyperglycemia were not considered sufficient drawbacks to block further studies of this mode of treatment.

CUSHING'S SYNDROME. Because most of the clinical features of Cushing's syndrome are a direct consequence of adrenocortical hyperfunction, it is discussed in Chapter 188.

PROLACTINOMA. Patients with prolactin-secreting tumors may have amenorrhea or galactorrhea. Because prolactin is antigonadotropic and to some extent antiandrogenic, prolactinoma should be considered in any man complaining of impotence. The tumors vary in size from microadenomas that do not distort the seller outline to macroadenomas that may exert considerable pressure on surrounding structures. These tumors most often arise in the interior portions of the gland and by downward extension may erode the floor of the sella into the sphenoid sinus. Thus cerebrospinal rhinorrhea or meningitis may rarely be the presenting feature of such a tumor. Prolactinomas may not be associated with endocrine symptoms or signs in some patients and may be discovered on a skull roentgenogram taken for other reasons. Nonfunctioning pituitary tumors may induce excess prolactin secretion from the surrounding normal gland by interfering with the delivery of PIF. The final diagnosis of prolactinoma rests on the immunochemical demonstration of prolactin in tumor tissue supplemented by electron-microscopic identification of the cardinal features of the characteristic fine structure of this tumor.

Serum prolactin should be measured in every patient with prolonged amenorrhea, primary or secondary. Serum prolactin (normal upper limit in both sexes is 18 ng/ml) tends to be higher with larger tumors. Levels greater than 200 ng/ml are usually diagnostic of tumor. Intermediate levels may be caused by hyperplasia or tumor. In patients with normal sellar tomography and moderate prolactin excess, a failure to respond to TRH is strong evidence of tumor rather than hyperplasia. However, in some cases of prolactinoma there is a brisk response to TRH, perhaps from hyperplastic cells in the non-tumorous portions of the gland.

Male patients usually do not have galactorrhea and only rarely show gynecomastia. Their most common symptom is impotence, sometimes with normal circulating levels of testosterone. In some cases of impotence with androgen deficiency, testosterone replacement does not help until the serum prolactin levels are lowered.

The antiprolactin drug bromocriptine has been very successful in reducing greatly elevated prolactin levels, sometimes to normal. In such cases the galactorrhea ceases, menses return, and fertility results. The usual effective dose is between 5 and 10 mg/day in two doses. The most prominent side effect is nausea, which diminishes as therapy is continued. Postural hypotension may also be troublesome, but it can be minimized by starting treatment with low doses such as 1.25 mg/day until

tolerance is developed. Although there is no evidence that bromocriptine is teratogenic, the drug should be discontinued once pregnancy is diagnosed. Bromocriptine now seems to have significant antitumor effect, which is sometimes apparent shortly after treatment is begun. In most cases the prolactin level rises after therapy is withdrawn, but sometimes not to its former level.

Progressive tumor growth, particularly with optic chiasmal compression, is a clear indication for surgery. Most of these tumors, even those of considerable size, can be handled by a transsphenoidal approach. In patients with slow-growing tumors extending downward, resection may lead to complications of cerebrospinal fluid rhinorrhea or meningitis. In these cases a more conservative approach may be warranted, particularly in the elderly.

Resection of a microadenoma in an infertile woman may restore normal ovulatory cycles and remove the risk of aggravating tumor growth by the resulting estrogen excess of pregnancy. In a large series studying bromocriptine-treated infertile women with prolactinomas, several normal pregnancies resulted, with evidence of mild pituitary enlargement in some cases. These patients did not receive prepregnancy irradiation, which has been recommended as a means of inhibiting the estrogen-stimulated overgrowth of a prolactinoma in pregnancy. In no case was there sufficient growth of the tumor during pregnancy to warrant surgery. However, there have been instances of rapid advancement of tumors in pregnancy requiring decompression of the visual pathway or reinstitution of bromocriptine therapy in the last trimester, which seemed to produce an antitumor effect.

There is little experience with irradiation as the sole treatment of prolactinomas. Persistent hyperprolactinemia following tumor removal calls for either a course of irradiation or the use of bromocriptine.

THYROTROPIN-SECRETING ADENOMA. The uncommon diagnosis of a TSH-secreting pituitary adenoma can be considered when the serum TSH levels are elevated in association with increased serum T_4. If the serum TSH were measured routinely in patients with hyperthyroidism, more cases might be diagnosed. After treating the hyperthyroidism with antithyroid drugs and radioiodine, the pituitary tumor may be dealt with by surgery and, if necessary, postoperative irradiation.

Anterior pituitary insufficiency

The clinical picture in anterior pituitary insufficiency may vary greatly, depending on the patient's age at onset and the number of anterior pituitary hormones affected. Failure of a single anterior pituitary hormone may be the result of congenital hypothalamic deficit or, less commonly, selective pituitary failure. Hypogonadotropic hypogonadism with anosmia *(Kallman's syndrome)* is a relatively common example of a neurologic defect resulting in pituitary underactivity. These patients show delayed puberty and a eunuchoid habitus. Serum gonadotropin levels are low but respond to LRH, although sometimes only after repeated doses. Growth hormone lack is often caused by a hypothalamic defect.

Assessment of pituitary hormone reserve in patients with hypothalamic-pituitary disease can be performed in a few hours on an outpatient basis. The test involves the rapid sequential administration of TRH (200 μg), GNRH or LRH (100 μg), CRH_1 and GRH (1 μg/kg of body weight). These four stimuli do not interfere with each other. TSH, prolactin, FSH, LH, ACTH (or cortisol), and GH are measured before the injections, and then 30 minutes and 60 minutes afterwards. This combined test has proved useful in screening patients for possible anterior pituitary insufficiency, but the expense of the many hormone assays involved makes it less suitable for routine use than selectively employing individual stimulation tests as suggested by clinical and routine laboratory findings.

The pituitary gland is really a confederation of several relatively independent endocrine glands grouped in close relation to the hypothalamus, which exerts considerable governing control. To encourage an organized approach to the clinical problems arising from insufficient pituitary function, each of the subglands of the pituitary should be considered separately in every case of pituitary disease.

GONADOTROPIC HORMONES. If gonadotropin (FSH and LH) production fails before sexual maturity, puberty does not take place. In growing males who lack androgenic hormone, the epiphyses remain unfused, and if the secretion of growth hormone is adequate, the long bones continue to grow. The arms and legs become disproportionately long, and the individual's arm span exceeds his height (normally they are equal). These eunuchoid patients may have osteoporosis, presumably because testicular androgens have not produced their protein anabolic effect. The penis remains small, the scrotum does not develop mature rugae, the testes are tiny, and the prostate is underdeveloped. These patients do not develop libido or become potent. Congenital absence of gonadotropin leads to poor gonadal development with hypoplastic testes, which are often undescended.

Girls with isolated hypogonadotropism have amenorrhea and poor sexual development. However, because pubic and axillary hair is also under the control of adrenal androgens, they do have a small amount of hair in these regions (if they have more severe disease with associated deficiency of corticotropin, pubic and axillary hair is completely absent). The epiphyses do not fuse at the normal time, and a eunuchoid habitus develops. Some patients have a partial congenital deficiency of hypothalamic stimulation of gonadotropic function, with sufficient basal output of estrogen to induce secondary sexual characteristics but no menses.

The manifestations are similar when gonadotropin deficiency develops in adult life, except that these patients do not have a eunuchoid habitus. Men have loss of libido and testicular atrophy. Pubic and axillary hair is decreased, and there is usually some loss of facial hair with decreased frequency of shaving. When testicular androgen production fails, hair may grow again on previously bald areas. In female patients secondary amenorrhea develops, usually with some regression of secondary sexual characteristics.

In general there are two types of hypogonadism. The first, caused by gonadal failure, is called primary hypogonadism. It is associated with elevated levels of pituitary gonadotropic secretion through failure of the normal negative feedback control of gonadal steroids on the pituitary. Secondary or hypogonadotropic hypogonadism is the result of pituitary or hypothalamic disease. GnRH is a 10–amino acid linear polypeptide that stimulates the release of both LH and FSH. Response to LRH (100 µg in a single intravenous injection) with a rise in serum LH and FSH indicates that the pituitary is not at fault; however, some patients with hypothalamic failure leading to hypogonadotropic hypogonadism respond only after a series of injections. In addition, some patients with only pituitary disease may be hypogonadotropic because of the failure of endogenous LRH to reach the gonadotrophs. In these cases relatively large doses of exogenous LRH may stimulate the gonadotrophs. Thus the response to hypothalamic releasing hormones is not always a reliable method of distinguishing between hypothalamic and pituitary pathology. A serum prolactin level should be determined in every patient with acquired hypogonadotropic hypogonadism because hyperprolactinemia can interfere with hypothalamic-pituitary-gonadal function in a variety of ways.

Male hypogonadism of testicular, pituitary, or hypothalamic origin may be treated by replacing the androgen, which may be given as an intramuscular compound such as testosterone propionate or testosterone enanthate. The usual replacement dose is 400 mg monthly. Oral androgens are available, but in some individuals these produce hepatocellular jaundice. The most useful oral agent is fluoxymesterone, a fluorinated derivative of methyltestosterone. A daily dose of 2 to 10 mg usually suffices. To restore spermatogenesis requires administering human gonadotropic preparations containing both FSH and ICSH. Such treatment usually must continue at least 3 months to produce a full quantitative restoration of spermatogenesis.

In adult women sequential estrogen and progestational agents restore secondary secondary sexual characteristics and produce regular withdrawal menses. Infertility is treated by the sequential administration of human FSH followed by human chorionic gonadotropin, which induces ovulation. This treatment may be complicated by the production of ovarian cysts that may rupture and cause serious consequences. It may also produce multiple pregnancy.

Clomiphene citrate, an estrogen analog that blocks estrogen receptor sites, stimulates the hypothalamus to release LRH and thereby induces ovulation. An ovulatory response may be determined by careful basal body temperature readings or by the serum progesterone level, which rises greatly in the luteal phase.

THYROTROPIN. Pituitary hypothyroidism, resulting from a deficiency of thyrotropin (TSH), may produce all the characteristic signs of myxedema: lethargy, cold intolerance, bradycardia, excessive dryness, and myxedematous infiltration of the skin. Serum thyroxine and T_3 resin uptake are decreased. The radioimmunoassay of TSH clearly distinguishes between primary myxedema and that arising from pituitary or hypothalamic failure. In primary hypothyroidism the serum TSH is usually substantially elevated. In "hypothalamic hypothyroidism" serum TSH is virtually undetectable until TRH is administered, following which there is a substantial rise in the serum TSH. In pituitary hypothyroidism TSH is usually undetectable before and after the administration of TRH. Thyrotropin deficiency rarely exists alone; it is usually accompanied by latent insufficiency of corticotropin and obvious hypogonadism.

CORTICOTROPIN. Lack of corticotropin (ACTH) is usually manifested by nausea, the earliest symptom of cortisol deficiency. Hypotension, loss of pubic and axillary hair in females (under adrenal androgen control), and hypoglycemia are other clues suggesting ACTH deficiency. These episodes of adrenal insufficiency are often precipitated by infection and other stress. Serum electrolyte levels are usually normal, although hyponatremia may sometimes be found, especially in patients who have been vomiting.

Most patients who have severe anterior pituitary insufficiency have pallor out of proportion to the moderate degree of anemia present. This pallor probably reflects a deficiency of the portion of the corticotropin molecule that has melanocyte-stimulating properties. Patients with primary adrenal insufficiency usually have increased pigmentation. These two conditions can be differentiated by the intravenous ACTH (Cortrosyn) test and the resultant response of plasma cortisol levels or of urinary excretion products of cortisol, that is, 17-hydroxycorticoids or urinary free cortisol (see Chapter 188). The ACTH reserve of the anterior pituitary can be assessed with metyrapone, which acts on the adrenal cortex by blocking the

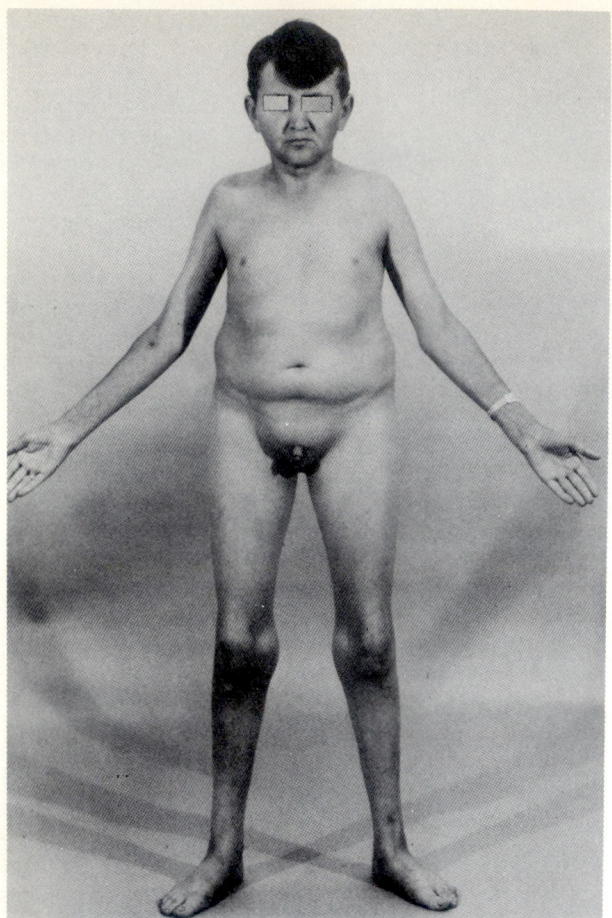

Fig. 186-3   This 47-year-old man with congenital pituitary dysplasia has deficient production of growth hormone, gonadotropins, and ACTH (see text). (From Ezrin C, Godden JO, and Volpé R: Systematic endocrinology, ed 2, New York, 1978, Harper & Row, Publishers.)

conversion of 11-desoxycortisol to cortisol and thus markedly reducing the normal cortisol inhibition of ACTH output. If the pituitary can respond by increasing its secretion of ACTH, urinary and plasma desoxycortisol increases along with 17-hydroxycorticoids derived from its metabolic degradation. In diseases of the endocrine hypothalamus, which affect the production of CRF, or pituitary disease, which involves the corticotrophs, there is no significant increase in desoxycortisol or 17-hydroxycorticoids.

Insulin-induced hypoglycemia has been used as a stress test of the responsiveness of the endocrine hypothalamus and the pituitary corticotrophs and somatotrophs. During hypoglycemia, plasma cortisol levels (a reflection of ACTH secretion) normally rise appreciably, as do growth hormone levels.

SOMATOTROPIN. If somatotropin is lacking, growth is severely retarded. If the patient is also hypogonadal with open epiphyses, slow growth will continue for several decades (Fig. 186-3).

Growth hormone seems to produce many of its effects via somatomedins, which are growth-promoting polypeptides made in the liver under its influence. Since fasting plasma growth hormone levels are frequently undetectable in normal children, the measurement of somatomedin-C by radioimmunoassay is a practical screening test for growth hormone deficiency. Other useful tests are vigorous exercise for 20 minutes to increase circulating growth hormone levels or administration of estrogen, such as 0.02 mg of ethinyl estradiol daily for three

days. Somatotropin secretion may be provoked by L-dopa (10 mg/kg body weight by mouth) or arginine (0.5 gm/kg given intravenously). These agents produce peak concentrations of more than 5 ng/ml of growth hormone in most normal children. Insulin-induced hypoglycemia (0.1 unit/kg of body weight intravenously) normally results in significant somatotropin secretion with a maximum from 30 to 60 minutes. This test should be used with extreme caution since prolonged reduction of blood sugar may cause permanent intellectual impairment or even death.

Clinically, the earliest recognizable endocrine deficiency in patients with progressive pituitary failure is hypogonadism. Lack of growth hormone response to various stimuli may also be an early manifestation of pituitary hypofunction.

Selective failure of growth hormone production has been reported in some members of certain families. These patients mature sexually somewhat later than usual, with androgenic hormone limiting further growth by inducing epiphyseal closure. Growth hormone–deficient children, diagnosed on the basis of a blunted GH secretory response after two or more provocative stimuli, should be treated with human growth hormone (HGH) (approximately 0.1 unit/kg intramuscularly) three times per week. A successful response appears to be a growth rate of about three inches (7.5 cm) per year, or at least a doubling of the pretreatment growth rate. The older, taller, and heavier the children, and the more advanced their bone age, the less they respond to growth hormone treatment. Only human growth hormone is effective in such patients.

Until recently, human pituitary GH had been extracted from human cadaver pituitaries. Early in 1985, four young adults who had been treated years earlier with it, were reported to have died of Creutzfeldt-Jakob disease, a "slow virus" infection of the brain. Because of the concern that the disease might have resulted from human pituitary tissue contaminated with the infectious agent, such preparations are no longer used in the United States. Recently, a new method of producing human growth hormone by recombinant DNA technology has produced unlimited quantities of what was previously a scarce medication, with the additional advantage of being free from any viral contamination. Some patients develop antibodies to the hormone, but only rarely does this significantly decrease the therapy's effectiveness. Hypothyroidism, which develops in some patients, blunts the growth-promoting effect of growth hormone. Therefore, thyroid hormone levels should be determined about twice a year during treatment to detect any deficiency and correct it by appropriate thyroxine replacement. Glucocorticoid dosage in patients with multiple pituitary deficiencies should be kept as low as possible to minimize adverse effects on growth.

PROLACTIN. The sustained estrogen excess of pregnancy induces such a marked prolactin cell increase that at term the weight of the gland has nearly doubled. This enlarged pituitary seems especially vulnerable to ischemic infarction following severe postpartum hemorrhage. After postpartum shock sufficient to produce extensive pituitary necrosis, a woman does not lactate, presumably because of inadequate prolactin secretion. Such patients are deficient in other anterior pituitary hormones as well. Prolactin deficiency may be verified by the failure of TRH to induce a sharp increase in serum levels of prolactin.

General investigation of pituitary problems

VISUAL FIELD DEFECTS. Because the optic chiasm lies above the diaphragma sellae, an upward-extending pituitary tumor often produces a visual defect by pressure on this part of the visual pathway. This defect, usually a bitemporal hemianopia, results from compression of the crossing central fibers of the chiasm; the uncrossed lateral fibers are spared. A wide variety of visual field defects have been observed in such patients, but the usual earliest changes are enlargement of the blind spot, loss of color vision (especially for red), and a wedge-shaped area of decreased vision in the upper temporal quadrant that gradually enlarges to occupy the full temporal field. Most patients with extensive visual defect have primary optic atrophy. Although papilledema is rare, it may develop with large tumors that cause increased intracranial pressure. If the pressure in the visual pathway is relieved early enough, the visual fields may return to normal, often dramatically a few hours after surgery.

ROENTGENOGRAPHY OF PITUITARY TUMORS. An intrasellar tumor slowly expands the pituitary fossa and destroys or distorts the clinoid processes. Calcification in the suprasellar region is common in craniopharyngiomas, and thickening of the tuberculum sellae may result from a suprasellar meningioma. Computed tomography (CT) has been a major advance in evaluating pituitary adenomas, clearly showing the degree to which a tumor has become suprasellar. Such scans also have their shortcomings, including a failure to detect many microadenomas (pituitary tumors less than 1 cm in diameter). They also fail to define the anatomic relationship of an adenoma to the optic chiasm, and they do not visualize cavernous sinus invasion very well. Magnetic resonance imaging (MRI) is equally as sensitive as CT and has the further advantage of providing more information about the relationship between the adenoma and optic chiasm. MRI more precisely defines the extent of the tumor and can even detect invasion of the cavernous sinus. MRI seems to be more sensitive than computerized tomography for evaluating microadenomas. It is also better for detecting hemorrhage and cyst formation within the pituitary gland.

The subarachnoid space may expand into the pituitary fossa if there is a defect in the diaphragma sellae. Thus the pituitary fossa may gradually enlarge and simulate a tumor, even producing a visual field defect by herniation of the optic chiasm and nerves into the sella. In this event, even though the pituitary gland is compressed from above, there is usually no pituitary insufficiency. CT or MRI can usually detect the presence of cerebrospinal fluid in the pituitary fossa, which is characteristic of this empty-sella syndrome. An aneurysm of the internal carotid artery may also expand the pituitary fossa within. Carotid angiography may be required to exclude an aneurysm or meningioma.

Treatment of patients undergoing pituitary surgery

Before a patient with a pituitary tumor is operated on, accompanying adrenal or thyroid hypofunction must be treated. A typical protocol includes 100 mg of hydrocortisone intramuscularly 1 hour before surgery. Intraoperatively and postoperatively, 100 mg of hydrocortisone as the water-soluble hemisuccinate or phosphate in 1 L of 5% glucose is given intravenously at a rate of approximately 100 ml/hour. The usual total dose is 300 mg over the first 24 hours. On subsequent days the glucocorticoid dosage can be reduced and given intramuscularly (50 mg of hydrocortisone every 6 hours on the second day and 25 mg every 6 hours on the third day). By the fourth day the patient can be given hydrocortisone (10 mg every 6 hours orally) and by the fifth day (if there have been no complications) maintenance with hydrocortisone (20 to 30 mg) in divided doses can be instituted.

The safest way to assess postoperative pituitary function is to compare serum thyroid hormone determinations with the preoperative values. If the operation has not produced hypothyroidism, pituitary resection has probably spared at least one fourth of the gland. If thyroid studies remain normal, adrenal steroid supplementation can probably be withdrawn, but this should be done cautiously, since selective corticotropin deficiency may be present.

It is essential that the patient with permanent hypopituitarism be convinced of the importance of properly treating the adrenal insufficiency accompanying anterior pituitary failure. Patients should obtain a Medic-Alert bracelet showing that they are taking hydrocortisone or prednisone because of pituitary insufficiency. Adjustment of steroid dosage to meet increased requirements during illness, stress, or surgery should be emphasized. The first symptom of relative adrenal insufficiency is nausea, which calls for a doubling of the usual steroid dosage until the situation is clarified. A portable injection kit of soluble hydrocortisone should be obtained for emergency use. Through such adjustments patients with pituitary insufficiency can lead vigorous lives.

Conditions simulating hypopituitarism

ANOREXIA NERVOSA. Because of superficial similarities and their respective clinical features, anorexia nervosa and adiposogenital dystrophy may be mistaken for organic pituitary disease. Anorexia nervosa is seen chiefly in psychoneurotic adolescent girls and is characterized by amenorrhea and extreme emaciation in the absence of any organic disease (Fig. 186-4). Until the patient is close to starvation, she remains active and hostile. When the syndrome is well developed, the body temperature is often subnormal and the pulse rate and blood pressure are low. Serum T_3 levels are reduced because of a decreased peripheral deiodination of T_4. An increase in reverse T_3 indicates a deflection of the normal peripheral disposal of T_4.

Amenorrhea is largely the result of hypothalamic dysfunction and may also be perpetuated by malnutrition. Resumption of normal menses usually does not occur until the patient's weight has returned to a sufficient level.

Effective treatment is based on the concept that the disorder is primarily psychiatric with secondary endocrine and metabolic manifestations. Psychotherapy to reduce conflict with the environment should be attempted only after extreme emaciation has been overcome, which sometimes requires duodenal or parenteral feeding. During the period of refeeding, the patient may become edematous. In general young patients respond more quickly with sympathetic, supportive handling. The older the patient and the longer she has had her symptoms, the more difficult and unsatisfactory is the treatment. There is an appreciable mortality rate in this condition from infection and suicide. Anorexia nervosa also occurs in males, although rarely.

ADIPOSOGENITAL DYSTROPHY. A more common form of emotionally engendered nutritional disturbances in males is adiposogenital dystrophy. It is seen in obese boys who have moderately delayed puberty. Less often, a similar clinical picture is produced by a tumor in the suprasellar region that causes hypogonadism and that by pressure on the hypothalamus produces hyperphagic obesity.

In the functional type of adiposogenital dystrophy the obesity is usually associated with psychologic maladjustment. Evidence of thyroid or adrenal insufficiency should strongly suggest organic disease. In obese adolescent boys the genitalia often seem unduly small because the phallus is partly hidden by suprapubic fat (Fig. 186-5). They usually require only ca-

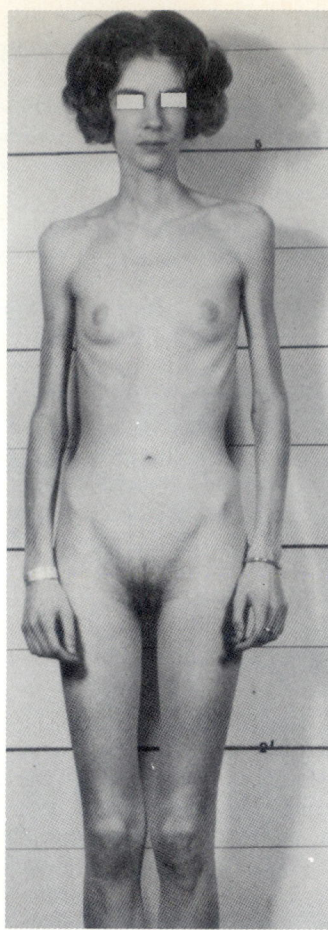

Fig. 186-4   Nineteen-year-old female with anorexia nervosa (see text). (From Ezrin C, Godden JO, and Volpé R: Systematic endocrinology, ed 2, New York, 1979, Harper & Row, Publishers.)

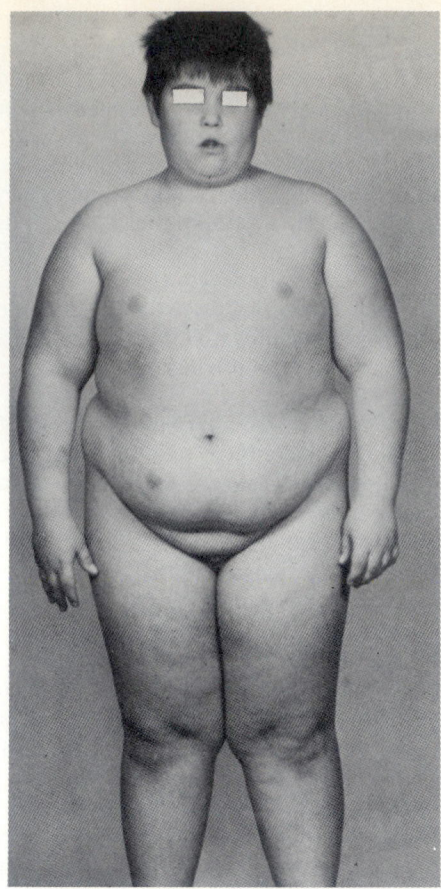

Fig. 186-5   Adiposogenital dystrophy in 16-year-old male (see text). (From Ezrin C, Godden JO, and Volpé R: Systematic endocrinology, ed 2, New York, 1979, Harper & Row, Publishers.)

loric restriction supplemented by a structured exercise program. Most of these boys later mature into normal fertile men, with the obesity often disappearing spontaneously.

Diseases of the posterior pituitary—diabetes insipidus

The antidiuretic hormone vasopressin is required to maintain the normal osmotic pressure of plasma. Increased plasma osmolality associated with dehydration stimulates "osmoreceptors" in the anterior hypothalamus, causing the neurohypophyseal terminals of the supraopticohypophyseal tract to release vasopressin into the general circulation. In the kidney vasopressin acts on the distal renal tubules and collecting ducts to increase reabsorption of water. Deficiency of or unresponsiveness to vasopressin causes diabetes insipidus, characterized by water diuresis and secondary polydipsia. It is usually associated with neurohypophyseal disease but also may arise from hypothalamic disorders.

ETIOLOGY. The known causes of diabetes insipidus can be divided into hereditary, traumatic (including postsurgical), inflammatory, and degenerative. A large number of cases appear to be idiopathic. Hereditary diabetes insipidus, a rare disorder, is thought to be caused by the failure of the supraoptic nuclei to develop sufficiently to produce adequate amounts of antidiuretic hormone. Another rare inherited variant, nephrogenic diabetes insipidus, results from the failure of the kidney to respond to vasopressin. With head injury the pituitary stalk

may be torn without any associated skull fracture. Metastatic lesions in the hypothalamus or neurohypophysis may interfere with the production or delivery of vasopressin. Lithium and the antibiotic demeclocycline may produce a type of nephrogenic diabetes insipidus. A similar end-organ resistance to vasopressin accounts for the polyuria that may be seen with hypercalcemia and hypokalemia.

Chest and bone roentgenograms help diagnose sarcoid and eosinophilic granulomata, important causes of diabetes insipidus. The most useful diagnostic test is the serum osmolality, determined after 8 hours of fluid deprivation. Normal subjects successfully maintain their osmolality in spite of the challenge of dehydration. A random measurement of serum osmolality may give significant diagnostic information, since patients with psychogenic polydipsia may have a slight degree of water intoxication, whereas subjects with diabetes insipidus may be somewhat behind in their fluid replacement and therefore have a slightly higher than normal serum osmolality.

MANAGEMENT. A nasal spray of lsyine-vasopressin may relieve polyuria for a few hours, but the limited effect of this therapy is a considerable drawback. The synthetic, long-acting vasopressin analog 1-deamino-8-D-arginine vasopressin (DDAVP), given intranasally twice daily, provides good control of diuresis. This drug appears to be the treatment of choice. A less convenient therapy is the intramuscular administration of long-acting vasopressin in oil; 1 ml (containing 5 units) usually is given about three times a week.

In both nephrogenic and ordinary diabetes insipidus, thiazide diuretics paradoxically may act as antidiuretics. Additional potassium may be required to prevent hypokalemia in these patients. Vasopressin-responsive diabetes insipidus can also be treated with chlorpropamide, carbamazepine, or clofibrate, which either release small amounts of residual vasopressin or amplify the action of antidiuretic hormone at the renal level. The dosage of chlorpropamide varies from 125 to 500 mg daily; hypoglycemia may complicate this treatment, particularly in patients with associated anterior pituitary disease.

Injudicious overtreatment resulting in too much water retention can be dangerous and sometimes fatal, particularly postoperatively with the production of serious cerebral edema.

PINEAL GLAND

The pineal gland may play a role in neuroendocrine control of the pituitary gland and in some circadian rhythms. There are important photic stimuli to the pineal gland; the visual information in the retina travels through the midbrain and reaches the pineal gland via sympathetic fibers. Darkness activates the sympathetic nerves and periods of light lead to a decrease in sympathetic activity. The pineal hormone, melatonin (5-methoxy-N-acetyl tryptamine), is produced during periods of darkness. The function of the pineal gland is unknown, but of clinical importance is the possibility of pineal calcification and tumor formation. Tumors that destroy the pineal gland can cause precocious puberty, and melatonin-synthesizing tumors may inhibit gonadal function.

BIBLIOGRAPHY

Bishop PM: Clomiphene, Br Med Bull 26:22, 1970.
Blackwell RE and Guillemin R: Hypothalamic control of adenohypophyseal secretions, Annu Rev Physiol 35:357, 1973.
Bloch HJ and Joplin GF: Some aspects of radiological anatomy of the pituitary gland and its relationship to surrounding structures, Br J Radiol 32:527, 1959.
Cohen R and others: Pituitary stimulation by combined administration of four hypothalamic releasing hormones in normal men and patients, J Clin Endocrinol Metab, 6262:892, 1986.
Crooke AC: Induction of ovulation with gonadotropins, Br Med Bull 26:17, 1970.
Ezrin C: Hypophysis (pituitary gland), illustrated by Netter FH In Endocrine system and selected metabolic diseases, Ciba Collection of Medical Illustrations 4(1):3, 1965.
Ezrin C, Horvath E, and Kovacs K: Anatomy and cytology of the normal and abnormal pituitary gland. In De Groot LJ, editor: Endocrinology, vol 1, New York, 1979, Grune & Stratton, Inc.
Ezrin C, Kovacs K, and Horvath E: Hyperprolactinemia: morphologic and clinical considerations, Med Clin North Am 62:393, 1978.
Guyda HJ, and others: Medical Research Council of Canada therapeutic trial of human growth hormone: first 5 years of therapy, Can Med Assoc J 112:1301, 1975.
Hardy J: Transsphenoidal surgery of hypersecreting pituitary tumors. In Kohler PO and Ross GT, editors: Diagnosis and treatment of pituitary tumors, New York, 1973, American Elsevier Publishers Inc.
Hershman JM: Use of thyrotropin-releasing hormone in clinical medicine Med Clin North Am 62:313, 1978.
Kreiger DT, Amarosa K, and Linick F: Cyproheptadine-induced remission of Cushing's disease, N Engl J Med 293:893, 1975.
Lamberts SWJ: A guide to the clinical use of the somatostatin analogue SMS 201-995 (Sandostatin), Acta Endocrinol 116:54, 1987.
Lawrence A, Pinsky SM, and Goldfine ID: Conventional radiation therapy in acromegaly: review and reassessment, Arch Intern Med 128:369, 1971.
McGregor AM and others: Reduction in size of a pituitary tumor by bromocriptine therapy, N Engl J Med 300:291, 1979.
Mortimer CH and others: Gonadotropin releasing hormone therapy in hypogonadal males with hypothalamic pituitary dysfunction, Br Med J 4:617, 1974.
Robinson AG: DDAVP in the treatment of central diabetes insipidus, N Engl J Med 294:507, 1976.
Rogol AD and others: Growth hormone release in response to human pancreatic tumor growth hormone-releasing hormone-40 in children with short stature, J Clin Endocrinol Metab 59:580, 1984.
Spark RE, Dickstein G, and Pallotta J: Complete remission of acromegaly with medical treatment, JAMA 241:573, 1979.
Tolis G and others: Pituitary hyperthyroidism, Am J Med 64:177, 1978.
Tyrrell JB and others: Cushing's disease: selected transsphenoidal resection of pituitary microadenomas, N Engl J Med 298:573, 1978.
Veldhuis JD and Hammond JM: Endocrine function after spontaneous infarction of the human pituitary: report, review, and reappraisal, Endocr Rev 1:100, 1980.

187 · THE THYROID GLAND

Thomas F. Nikolai

ANATOMY

The thyroid gland (Fig. 187-1) is a relatively small structure lying low in the anterior neck. It is H or butterfly shaped, containing two lobes connected by an isthmus. The isthmus usually lies over the second and third rings of the trachea with the lobes lying along the anterolateral and lateral aspect of the trachea, although frequently it may be much lower in the neck and occasionally it may be partially substernal. A pyramidal lobe juts upward from the isthmus in about 25% of individuals. The size of the thyroid in North Americans is substantially smaller now than 20 to 30 years ago, probably as a result of the increase in iodine in the diet. In adults the thyroid weighs 16.7 ± 6.9 g, and the lobes measure 2 to 2.5×2 to 2.5 cm in width and thickness and 3.5 to 4 cm in height. The thyroid in females is larger than that in males by 5% to 10%. The child's thyroid weighs about 1.5 g at birth and reaches adult size by 15 to 19 years of age. There are minor differences in size and shape among normal thyroids (Fig. 187-2). The normal thyroid tissue is soft to slightly firm in consistency. Its surface is usually smooth, slightly lobulated, covered by a thin, fibrous capsule, and attached to adjacent structures by loose connective tissue.

The blood supply, which is extremely rich (4 to 6 ml/min g of thyroid tissue, about twice as much blood per gram as the kidney tissues receives), comes from the right and left superior thyroid arteries off the common carotid artery and the inferior thyroid arteries off the subclavian artery. Venous drainage occurs through the thyroid veins into the jugular system. An extensive lymphatic vascular system is also present. Innervation is supplied by the adrenergic and cholinergic autonomic nervous systems arising from the cervical sympathetic ganglia and following the arteries into the thyroid and the vagus nerves through the superior and inferior laryngeal nerves. The main function of the nerve supply of the thyroid is to regulate blood flow. The adrenergic fibers terminate at the basement membrane and may directly affect function of the follicular cell through the release of bioactive amines.

The four parathyroid glands (Fig. 187-1) lie on the back side of the thyroid, two near the superior poles and two near the inferior poles. They sometimes lie inside the capsule of the thyroid and occasionally are actually embedded within the thyroid tissue, not being visible on gross examination of the thyroid. The recurrent laryngeal nerve also lies on the posterior or medical posterior side of the thyroid lobes alongside the trachea, although its location may vary considerably.

HISTOLOGY

The lobes and isthmus of the thyroid are composed of numerous lobules, each with its own blood, lymphatic, and nerve supply and each further divided into 20 to 40 follicles. Interspersed among the follicles are perifollicular light or

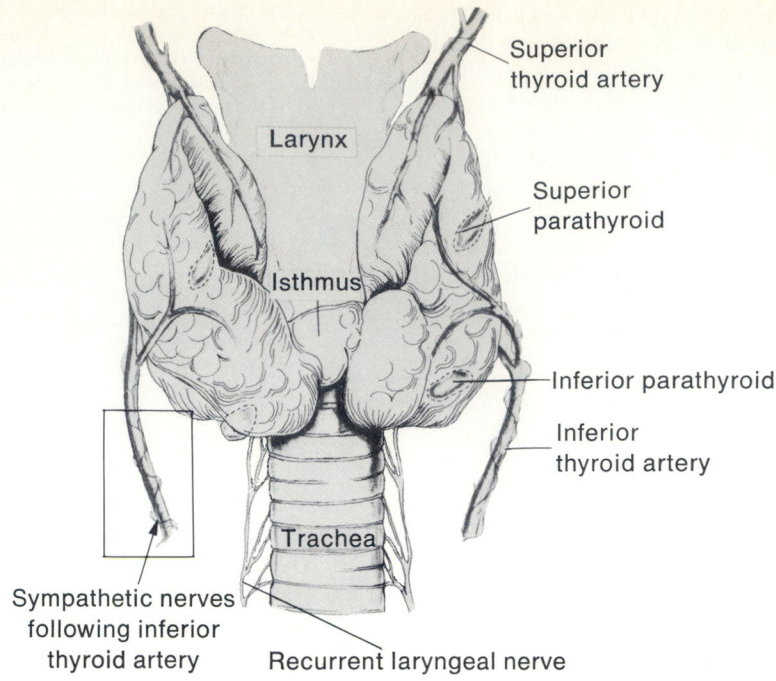

Fig. 187-1   Normal thyroid anatomy.

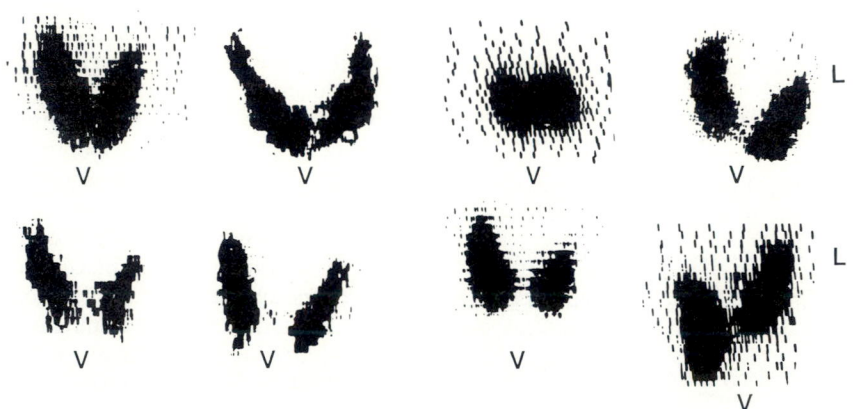

Fig. 187-2   Variation in size and shape of normal human thyroid by radioactive iodine (^{131}I) scanning.

"C" cells that produce calcitonin. They constitute only about 5% of the total cell population of the thyroid. Recently cells that produce somatostatin have been identified in the thyroid. The follicles are the main functional units, producing thyroxine (T_4) and triiodothyronine (T_3). They are spheroidal structures surrounded by follicle cells, about 200 to 300 μm in size, and filled with pink-staining colloid that is almost all stored thyroglobulin (TG). The size of the follicle and the amount of colloid present in each follicle are inversely related to the activity of the gland. The individual follicle cell tends to be small and cuboidal or somewhat flattened when less active and elongated from base to apex when stimulated. Electron microscopy has shown the relationship between the synthetic sequence of thyroid hormone and the anatomy of the follicle cell. Biosynthesis of noniodinated TG protein occurs in the ribosome. The TG then enters the ergastoplasmic vesicles and is transported to the Golgi apparatus where the carbohydrate moiety is added. Next it is transported in secretory droplets to the microvilli where it is released in the colloid.

CHEMISTRY

The thyroid gland's role in the body is to produce thyroid hormone in quantities sufficient to meet the needs of the whole organism. It produces two biologically active hormones: the iodothyronines (L-triiodothyronine [T_3] and L-thyroxine [T_4]) and the iodotyrosines (monoiodotyrosine [MIT] and diiodotyrosine [DIT]). The structures of these compounds and closely related compounds and metabolic products are shown in Fig. 187-3.

The iodothyronines are composed of two ether-linked benzene rings with a hydroxyl group at position 4' and an alanine side chain at position 1. T_4 has four iodine atoms. Deiodination at position 5 is the reaction that produces the majority of T_3. Tetrac (3,5,3',5'-tetraiodothyroacetic acid) and triac (3,5,3'-triiodothyroacetic acid) are produced by peripheral metabolism of thyroid hormones and have slight biologic activity, with more in some species than in others. Another compound produced in the thyroid and containing three iodine atoms, 3,3',5'-triodothyronine (reverse T_3, RT_3), is metabolically inactive. Many similar compounds that have organic or halogen substi-

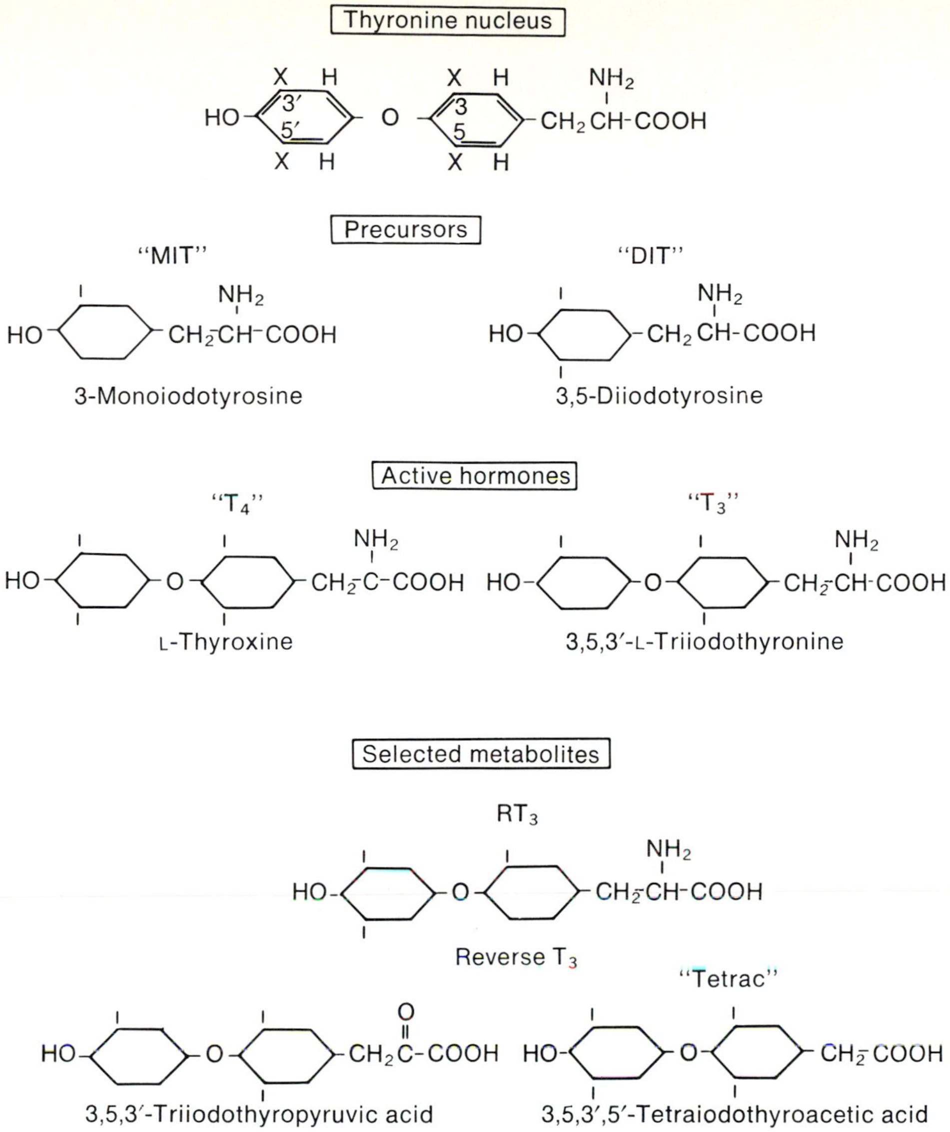

Thyronine nucleus

Precursors

"MIT"   "DIT"

3-Monoiodotyrosine   3,5-Diiodotyrosine

Active hormones

"T₄"   "T₃"

L-Thyroxine   3,5,3'-L-Triiodothyronine

Selected metabolites

RT₃

Reverse T₃

                                        "Tetrac"

3,5,3'-Triiodothyropyruvic acid   3,5,3',5'-Tetraiodothyroacetic acid

Fig. 187-3   Thyroid hormones and related compounds.

tutions on the benzene ring or fatty acid substitutions for the end alanine have been synthesized and have biologic activity ranging from 1% to 617% of that of T_4.

Extrathyroidal iodine metabolism

Iodine is unique to the thyroid because it is the only substrate needed for hormone production that is not used by other tissues. Approximately 50 μg of iodine daily is needed to maintain normal thyroid hormone biosynthesis. In recent years the iodine content of American diets has greatly increased so that the average person is ingesting 300 to 500 μg each day (much more in countries such as Japan where seafood is a major portion of the diet). Therefore, iodine deficiency does not exist today in most of the world, except for many of the third world countries where people do not eat much seafood. Iodine is rapidly and efficiently absorbed from the gastrointestinal tract with little lost in the stool. The normal thyroid contains a large reserve (about 10 mg) of iodine, sufficient to provide iodine supplies for up to 6 months if none is ingested. Ninety-five percent of the thyroid iodine is present in colloid stores. In the plasma, iodine is present in two forms, as inorganic iodide not bound to serum proteins (1 to

1.5 μg/dl) and as iodothyronines (T_4 and T_3) that are mainly bound to plasma proteins (4 to 8 μg/dl) and are hormonally active.

The thyroid extracts iodine from the serum by an efficient trapping mechanism that normally concentrates iodide up to a 20:1 gradient between the thyroid and plasma. This trapping mechanism is stimulated by thyroid-stimulating hormone (TSH), is dependent on sodium, potassium, and magnesium ions, is blocked by thiocyanate, perchlorate, and iodides, and is slowed by hypopituitarism. Although iodide trapping also occurs to a much lesser extent in the salivary glands, stomach, breasts, and choroid plexus, iodothyronine synthesis does not occur in these tissues except for a minimal amount by mammary tissue. Most iodine not taken up by the thyroid, and that diffusing from the thyroid gland, is promptly lost in the urine. About the same amount of iodide absorbed is excreted in the urine each day except for 3% to 5% excreted in the stool, sweat, and expired air. Substantially more may be excreted by lactating women or in certain disease states such as those associated with heavy proteinuria or gastrointestinal malabsorption.

The kidney and the thyroid readily clear most of the ingested

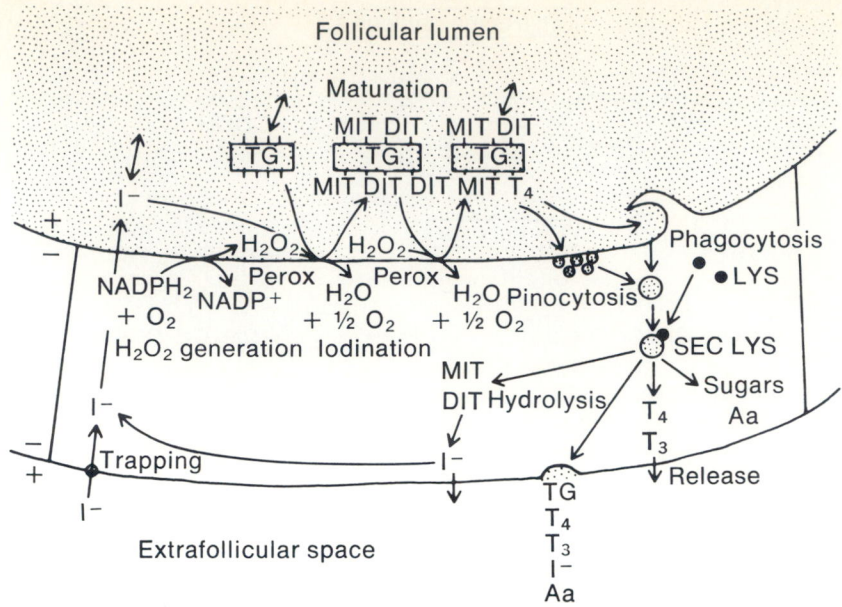

Fig. 187-4   Model of iodine metabolism in thyroid follicle. Follicular cell is shown facing follicular lumen (stippled area) and extra cellular space (lower part). Sequence of events shown has been largely documented. However, the possibility of active iodine transport at apex of cell or of intracellular iodination and the relative roles of pinocytosis verses phagocytosis and of diffusion versus secretion of thyroid hormones remain controversial. *Perox,* peroxidase; *TG,* thyroglobin; *MIT,* monoiodotyrosine; *DIT,* diiodotyrosine; *LYS,* lysosome; *SEC LYS,* secondary lysosome; *Aa,* amino acids; + and −, electric charge of membranes (see text). (From Van Herle AJ and others. Reprinted by permission of the New England Journal of Medicine, 301: 239, 1979.)

and recycled iodide from the serum. The renal clearance is about twice that of the thyroid.

Synthesis of thyroid hormones

The synthesis of thyroid hormones involves the uptake and use of iodine and amino acids to form the iodothyronines T_4 and T_3 and the receptor protein TG. The sequence of synthesis of thyroid hormones is shown schematically in Fig. 187-4.

Iodine circulating in plasma is concentrated at the follicle cell surface by the iodide trapping mechanism against an electrical gradient and then is transported into the cell. The energy required to concentrate iodine is supplied by high-energy phosphate bonds. In the follicle cell the iodine is oxidized to a higher energy state by hydrogen peroxide–generating system that uses nicotinamide adenine dinucleotide phosphate (NADPH) as a coenzyme. In this very reactive state the iodine readily reacts with the amino acid tyrosine, which is attached to TG, and the iodotyrosyl compounds MIT and DIT, which are formed under the influence of peroxidase enzyme. Whether the initial iodination of the tyrosine-TG complex occurs in the follicle cell lumen in the apex of the microvilli adjacent to the colloid or after exocytosis into the colloid is unknown. Oxidative coupling of MIT and DIT molecules attached to TG occurs to form T_3, T_4, and minute amounts of RT_3, probably catalyzed by the same peroxidase. Approximately 120 molecules of MIT, DIT, T_3, and T_4 are attached to TG at this point. The iodide trapping mechanism is influenced by multiple factors of which TSH seems to be the most important. TSH enhances iodide trapping by the thyroid, and hypophysectomy decreases it. Marked increases in the thyroid/plasma iodide ratio up to several hundred–fold have been reported in diffuse toxic goiter and in animal glands highly stimulated by TSH. Iodide trapping is inhibited by thiocyanate and perchlorate ions that in high concentrations also inhibit organic binding. The

iodination of tyrosine also is stimulated by TSH and reduced by hypophysectomy. The antithyroid drugs propylthiouracil and methimazole block iodination of tyrosine, as well as the coupling of MIT and DIT to form the iodotyrosines. An internal autoregulatory control of iodine metabolism called the Wolff-Chaikoff effect causes a block in the thyroid peroxidase system when excess iodide is present.

Storage and secretion of thyroid hormones

The colloid provides the organism with a large hormone reservoir that would last 3 to 4 months if no more thyroid hormone were made. If the thyroid is completely blocked by antithyroid agents, it takes as long as 2 weeks for any noticeable decrease in serum T_4 and an increase in TSH to occur. T_4 accounts for about 35% of the organic iodine content of the thyroid, and T_3 accounts for 5% to 8%. TG is the storage form of thyroid hormone. Secretion of thyroid hormone begins when colloid droplets are taken up by the follicular cell by phagocytosis. These colloid droplets are digested by proteases present in lysosomes. Once freed from TG, T_4, T_3, and RT_3 are secreted into the plasma and the MIT and DIT are deiodinated and recirculated. The TG molecule is broken down, first by reduction of disulfide bonds by glutathione and then by proteolysis. The iodine and tyrosine are reused in the metabolic cycle of the follicular cell. Microtubules are apparently involved in the secretory process, since inhibitors of these, namely colchicine and vincristine, block secretion of T_4 and T_3. Microsomal iodotyrosine dehalogenase is responsible for the separation of iodide from MIT and DIT and thus prevents these compounds from appearing in plasma. Very small amounts of TG leak out of the thyroid through the lymphatic system in normal individuals, and increased amounts occur in the plasma of patients with nontoxic goiter, hyperthyroidism, certain congenital goiters, thyroid malignancy, radiation thyroiditis, and subacute thyroiditis and from manipulation during thyroid surgery. Lysis of TG and secretion of T_4 and T_3 are inhibited by iodine and lithium.

There is little else in the colloid other than TG, a 19S glycoprotein containing about 10% carbohydrate. It has a molecular weight of 660,000. Each TG molecule contains approximately 120 molecules of MIT (17% to 28%), DIT (24% to 42%), T_4 (35%), and T_3 (5% to 8%). Natural TG is distinctly heterogeneous between different species and to some extent even within the same animal species. Under the control of TSH, synthesis of TG occurs in the rough endoplasmic reticulum of the follicular cell, where the carbohydrate portion is also added. It then moves through the Golgi apparatus to the apex of the cell in the microvilli and into the colloid by exocytosis. A different iodoprotein has been found in very small quantities in normal thyroids and in larger quantities in thyroid disorders such as hyperthyroidism, nontoxic goiters, endemic goiter, and Hashimoto's thyroiditis. This protein has electrophoretic mobility similar to that of serum albumin. Congenital defects of TG synthesis lead to deficient thyroid hormone production and goiters.

Peripheral binding, metabolism, and physiologic effects of thyroid hormones

BINDING. On entering the blood, T_4 and T_3 are largely bound to the serum proteins thyroxine-binding globulin (TBG), thyroxine-binding prealbumin (TBPA), and thyroxine-binding albumin (TBA) in a reversible association. TBG and TBA bind both T_4 and T_3, but TBPA binds only T_4 (possibly a minor amount of T_3). Because of extensive binding of thyroid hormone by these proteins, the serum levels of thyroid hormone fluctuate with the levels of the proteins.

Both TBG and TBPA have only one binding site for T_4 on each molecule. Barbital, salicylate, penicillin, and 2,4-dinitrophenol inhibit thyroid hormone binding to TBPA. TBA poorly binds both T_4 and T_3. The functions of the thyroid-binding proteins are multiple. In combination with T_4 and T_3 they achieve a macromolecular size that results in little renal excretion of T_4 and T_3, providing a large metabolically inert reservoir. The interaction between thyroid-binding proteins and thyroid hormone is expressed by TBG and T_4 as follows:

$$T_4 + TBG \rightleftarrows T_4 - TBG$$

Since interaction strongly favors the bound form (T_4—TBG), only 0.02% to 0.03% of T_4 exists in a free form. Because T_3 has less affinity for TBG, 0.3%, or about 10 times more than T_4, exists in the free form. Only the free thyroid hormones are available to the peripheral tissues because the T_4-TBG complex is too large to leave the vascular system. Therefore the metabolic effects of thyroid hormone are due to the small amount of unbound or free hormone. As is discussed later in the chapter, there are numerous factors and disease states that affect the concentration of thyroid-binding proteins.

METABOLISM. T_4 and T_3 are deiodinated to inactive metabolites in the liver and kidney and probably in many other body tissues as well. It is generally agreed that the majority of T_3 in the blood comes from peripheral conversion of T_4 and that very little is synthesized within the thyroid itself. Since T_3 and RT_3 have more rapid clearance rates than T_4, their serum concentrations are much lower than that of T_4. Most T_3 and RT_3 is derived from extrathyroidal deiodination of T_4. Hypothyroid patients receiving T_4 replacement only and unable to produce any thyroid hormone of their own maintain near normal serum ratios of T_4, T_3, and RT_3, indicating indirectly that

the amount of T_3 and RT_3 coming from the thyroid is relatively small.

LOW T_3 SYNDROME. Abnormalities of peripheral T_4 and T_3 metabolism have been labeled the low T_3, reverse T_3, or sick euthyroid syndrome. The deiodination of T_4 to T_3 is depressed in certain situations, including total starvation, semistarvation (carbohydrate and protein but not lipid), acute infection, stress, many chronic diseases (pulmonary, cardiac, hepatic, renal, and neoplastic), and use of certain drugs. This results in decreased peripheral T_3 production and frequently lowers the serum T_3 concentration to subnormal levels. A gradual corresponding rise in the RT_3 concentration occurs as more T_4 is deiodinated through the T_4-to-RT_3 pathway. Not infrequently with this fall in serum T_3, the serum T_4 concentration slowly rises above normal, sometimes giving the false impression that the patient has hyperthyroidism. This phenomenon occurs within 36 to 48 hours of the start of acute starvation or illness and rapidly returns to normal with feeding or recovery.

This same change occurs in the full-term fetus and also is found in the cord blood at birth, probably related to immature deiodinating enzyme systems in the fetus and the neonate. Within a few hours after birth the serum T_3 rises by 200% to 400% and the T_4 by 25% to 50%, and the RT_3 declines very slightly, apparently as a result of a transient increase in TSH. A number of drugs block the conversion of T_4 to T_3. They include corticosteroids, propranolol, propylthiouracil, sodium iopanate, sodium ipodate, and amiodarone. Interestingly, corticosteroids, propranolol, and propylthiouracil are used to treat severe thyrotoxicosis and thyrotoxic crisis, and this newly discovered effect of suppression of T_4-to-T_3 conversion contributes further to their pharmacologic effect. They also have other effects on thyroid function that are discussed later.

The low serum T_3 concentration occurring at birth, from acute and chronic illness, and from starvation is probably a normal response of the organism to these states and leads to a down regulation of body metabolism. Since serum levels of hormones do not reflect their intracellular or nuclear concentration, the serum changes cannot be assumed to reflect what is happening at the cellular level where hormonal action is manifested.

ACTION OF THYROID HORMONES. It is impossible to relate all the effects of thyroid hormones to a single mechanism. At the present time their effects can best be explained by multiple mechanisms induced by the free thyroid hormone levels presented to the target issues. Most of the metabolic effects of the thyroid hormones are due to T_3, since T_4 is primarily a prohormone. The free thyroid hormone diffuses easily into the extracellular fluid and enters the cells where it is reversibly bound to sites on the cell surface and to proteins within the cells.

Table 187-1 summarizes the possible mechanisms of action of thyroid hormone. The occupancy of nuclear binding receptors is a prerequisite for many of the actions of T_3. The T_3-occupied nuclear receptor promotes synthesis of messenger ribonucleic acid (mRNA), which is a rate-limiting factor in protein synthesis. Fasting decreases nuclear receptors for T_3, suggesting a physiologic down-regulation of cellular metabolism. T_3 receptors are also located on the inner mitochondrial membrane in thyroid hormone–responsive tissues and are absent in tissues not responding to thyroid hormone such as brain and testes. With T_3 binding, uncoupling of oxidative phosphorylation, increased oxygen consumption, and adenosine 5'-triphosphate (ATP) generation occur in isolated mitochondrial vesicles.

Table 187-1   Sites and mechanisms of actions of thyroid hormones

Site	Action
Cell nucleus	Stimulates mRNA synthesis
	Increases target cell protein synthesis
Mirochondria	Increases α-glycerophosphate dehydrogenase
	Promotes uncoupling of oxidative phosphorylation
	Increases ATP generation
	Increases O_2 consumption
Cell membrane	Stimulates Na^+,K^+, ATPase ("sodium pump")
Adrenergic receptor pathway	Increases number of receptors
	Amplifies β-adrenergic signal
Tyrosine metabolic pathway	Modifies metabolic pathway
	Acts as precursor for alternate adrenergic neurotransmitters

It has been long noted clinically that many manifestations of hyperthyroidism resemble excessive adrenal medullary or epinephrine-like activity and that the β-adrenergic blocking agent propranolol blocks these effects. However, increased catecholamine secretion from the adrenal medulla is not present. The proposed mechanism of this effect of thyroid hormone is an increase in the number of β-adrenergic cellular receptors, an amplification of the β-adrenergic signal at the cell membrane, or both. Another possible mode of action of thyroid hormone is that it functions as amino acid analogs of tyrosine. These analogs enter into and modify metabolic pathways in tyrosine metabolism and act as precursors for alternate adrenergic neurotransmitters. In the nervous system, T_3 is concentrated in peripheral adrenergic nerves and in certain areas of the brain.

Many other effects on the body are noted in thyroid disease states and probably result from the actions already discussed. The actions and metabolism of other hormones, including 21-carbon corticosteroids, cortisol, aldosterone, epinephrine, parathyroid hormone, and glucagon, are modulated by T_3. Temperature regulation is also affected by thyroid hormone; myxedematous animals die readily with cold exposure. Growth retardation in hypothyroid children and animals is readily reversed by thyroid hormone. Hyperglycemia is produced by excessive thyroid hormone, and hyperthyroidism depletes liver and muscle glycogen. Marked hypercholesterolemia with increase in phospholipids and total lipids occurs in hypothyroidism. Vitamin deficiencies are sometimes associated with hyperthyroidism, probably owing to increased requirements. Osteoporosis and osteomalacia occur in long-standing hyperthyroidism as a result of increased bone resorption and decreased vitamin D–potentiated intestinal absorption of calcium.

ANTITHYROID AGENTS. Goitrogens are chemicals that inhibit thyroid hormone synthesis or release, leading to compensatory increases in TSH and thyroid enlargement. These chemicals occur naturally in certain foods such as cabbage, turnips, kohlrabi, and rutabagas, which are rarely eaten in quantities sufficient to cause a problem. They contain some thiocyanate and progoitrogens (thioglucosidases) that must be activated by intestinal bacteria.

The antithyroid agents generally encountered in clinical practice are those used to treat hyperthyroidism and drugs used for other purposes that also affect thyroid function. Drugs used to treat hyperthyroidism manifest their effect in two ways. Monovalent anions such as thiocyanate and perchlorate block iodine trapping by the thyroid, which is overcome by excessive amounts of iodides. They are rarely used today because of significant toxic effects such as irreversible aplastic anemia.

The second group of drugs blocks intrathyroidal iodination of tyrosine and the coupling reaction. A wide variety of these agents is known, but the only two used in the United States are the thioureas, methimazole and propylthiouracil.

Drugs such as iodides and lithium that are commonly used for the treatment of other diseases may affect thyroid function. Iodides under certain conditions block intrathyroidal hormone synthesis and lead to thyroid enlargement and hypothyroidism. Goiters and hypothyroidism develop in 20% to 30% of patients undergoing long-term lithium therapy, owing to depression of hormone release from the thyroid.

THE THYROID IN PREGNANCY. The rise in estrogen level that occurs in the first month of pregnancy causes increased liver synthesis of TBG. This results in increased binding and concentrations of T_4 and T_3, although the free concentrations of both hormones remain essentially unchanged. These estrogen-induced effects return to normal or nonpregnant levels in 3 to 4 weeks after delivery.

The thyroid gland may enlarge by 25% to 50% during pregnancy, and occasionally a bruit is heard over it reflecting increased blood flow. This effect is due to iodine deficiency caused by an increased renal iodide clearance in pregnancy. It is much less frequent in recent years owing to the increased amount of iodine in the American diet.

T_3, T_4, and TSH do not cross the placental barrier. Therefore thyroid failure in the mother or fetus is not prevented by transplacental transfer of T_4 and T_3. However, the thioureas do cross the placental barrier and can cause fetal hypothyroidism if administered in inappropriately high doses to the mother. The thyroid-stimulating immunoglobulin (TSI) present in Grave's disease also crosses the placental barrier and can cause temporary hyperthyroidism in the fetus at birth (neonatal hyperthyroidism.) More recently a thyrotropin-binding inhibiting immunoglobulin (TBII) has been found to trigger hypothyroidism in some patients. This immunoglobulin also crosses the placenta to the fetus and may cause temporary hypothyroidism in the newborn.

TESTS OF THYROID FUNCTION AND CONCENTRATION AND BINDING OF THYROID HORMONES

Several methods exist for measuring thyroid function. Careful clinical assessment for thyroid disease should precede thyroid testing except in specific circumstances where testing will uncover abnormalities that are not obvious clinically. There are several diseases of the thyroid affecting different measures of thyroid function, as well as frequently associated changes in peripheral binding and metabolism of thyroid hormones, and no one test can consistently measure all these changes. In addition, many drugs affect thyroid function and the thyroid tests. Interpretation of the test results should be made in light of these factors before a diagnosis is made and treatment is begun.

RADIOACTIVE IODINE UPTAKE. The radioactive iodine uptake (RAIU) test directly measures the accumulation of iodine by the thyroid. Two radioactive isotopes of iodine (^{131}I and ^{123}I) are now in common use. ^{123}I has the advantages of a shorter half-life and lower levels of radiation. The thyroid is unable to distinguish between stable iodine (^{127}I) and its radioactive isotopes. The RAIU test is used in the diagnosis of hypothyroidism, hyperthyroidism, thyrotoxicosis factitia, biosynthetic defects of the thyroid, and thyroiditis. In recent years new factors have appeared that have diminished the usefulness of this test. Improved measurements of thyroid hormone concentrations by radioimmunoassay and better knowledge of the peripheral metabolism and binding of thyroid hormones give more precise information than the RAIU. Even more important, the increasing content of iodine in the diet, primarily owing to food preservatives, has caused a progressive decline in the normal value of the RAIU. The normal uptake of RAIU at 24 hours was 25% to 50% 15 to 20 years ago and now is only 10% to 25%, but this varies considerably in different areas of the United States and the world, primarily because of the differing dietary iodine content.

The RAIU is dependent on the daily iodine intake, the serum inorganic iodide concentration, the rate of iodine turnover in the thyroid, and the urinary clearance of iodine. When ^{131}I is used, the uptake is measured by scintillation counter over the thyroid at 24 hours. However, measurements at 2, 4, and 6 hours are sometimes useful, especially in hyperthyroidism. The value obtained is the percentage of the dose, administered orally or intravenously, that is counted in the thyroid. Each institution performing this test must establish its own range of normal values.

The RAIU is increased in 80% to 90% of the cases of hyperthyroidism. The uptake at 2, 4, or 6 hours frequently is more diagnostic of hyperthyroidism because the uptake, conversion, and excretion of iodine may be so rapid in this disease that the amount of isotope retained in the thyroid at 24 hours is less than at the shorter intervals. The RAIU is sometimes increased in the failing thyroid gland (Hashimoto's thyroiditis), in iodine deficiency, in pregnancy (relative iodine deficiency owing to increased renal iodine clearance), immediately after recovery from thyroiditis, in congenital intrathyroidal enzyme defects, and in nephrosis (as a result of excessive loss of thyroid-binding proteins). It is decreased or suppressed by elevated concentrations of inorganic iodine, in hypothyroidism, in thyroiditis, and by exogenous thyroid hormone intake. An increase in the inorganic iodide pool decreases the RAIU by a dilutional effect in the serum and by the inhibitory effects of increased intrathyroidal iodine, as discussed previously. Measuring the 24-hour urinary iodine excretion can help establish the presence of excessive body iodide stores, since levels greater than 1 to 1.5 mg strongly suggest increased intake of iodine.

The RAIU used alone is a poor test for hypothyroidism, and this test must be combined with TSH stimulation to be of value. In thyroiditis (either subacute or lymphocytic) the RAIU may be quite variable depending on the degree to which the thyroid is affected and the stage of the disease. It is suppressed when exogenous thyroid is taken in physiologic or greater quantities unless autonomous thyroid function exists. Organic iodides such as those used in roentgenographic dye also suppress the RAIU for varying periods of time relative to their rates of deiodination and excretion. Dyes administered for renal studies are usually excreted in 3 to 5 days, whereas those used for cholecystography may persist from 3 weeks to 3 months.

Measurement of the 24-hour absolute iodine uptake (AIU) does make the RAIU much more sensitive, although it needs to be used only infrequently. The AIU is calculated as follows:

$$AIU = \frac{\text{24-hour urinary iodide } (\mu g/24 \text{ hr}) \times \% \text{ RAIU}}{\% \text{ 24-hour urine RAI content}}$$

The normal thyroid takes up 70 to 75 μg of iodine each day. Values greater than this tend to indicate hyperthyroidism and reduced values indicate hypothyroidism.

THYROID SCAN. The thyroid scan provides useful information concerning localization, size, shape, and uniformity of function of the thyroid. The thyroid gland is first labeled with a radioactive isotope (^{123}I or technetium 99). Following this a scanner makes a visual image or graphic representation of the uptake of the isotope in the thyroid tissue. The principal values of the thyroid scan are to provide (1) localization and function of nodules present within the thyroid and (2) localization of functioning thyroid tissue present in ectopic locations such as the lingual area, neck nodes, substernal area, and metastatic foci in bone, liver, lung, ovaries, and so forth.

Although most techniques are incapable of localizing areas of dysfunction less than 1 cm in size, a new technique called the pinhole thyroid scan gives resolution of functional areas as small as 2 to 3 mm.

THYROID ULTRASONOGRAPHY. The thyroid and surrounding structures are easily and quickly identified by ultrasound techniques. New real time high-resolution ultrasound transducers can now detect lesions 1 to 2 mm in size. The predominant use of ultrasound is to distinguish solid nodules from cystic nodules, to accurately measure thyroid size and volume, and to guide needles for aspiration of thyroid cysts and of cystic and solid lesions to provide cells for cytologic examination.

T$_4$ TEST. Several methods have been developed in the past 15 years to measure serum T$_4$ concentrations more precisely. These include column chromatography, competitive protein-binding analysis, and radioimmunoassays. Since the column chromatography method does not afford complete separation of T$_4$ when high concentrations of iodine are present, it has generally been discarded. The competitive protein-binding assay is much more precise because of the specificity of the interaction between T$_4$ and TBG that is the basis of the test procedure. However, because it requires 3 to 4 hours and several different steps, it has essentially been replaced by the radioimmunoassay for T$_4$, which is performed in one step in about 1½ hours. The normal values are 5 to 12 μg/dl. T$_4$ concentrations increase in hyperthyroidism and elevated TBG states and decrease in hypothyroidism and low TBG states.

T$_3$ TEST. The T$_3$ assay procedure is quite similar to the T$_4$ radioimmunoassay. The normal values are 100 to 184 ng/dl. T$_3$ levels have been shown to decrease by about one third by 70 to 80 years of age. T$_3$ concentrations usually parallel T$_4$ changes in hypothyroidism and hyperthyroidism and with TBG change. As previously described, in the low T$_3$ syndrome T$_3$ levels decrease owing to a block in the peripheral T$_4$-to-T$_3$ metabolism. This may be caused by many acute and chronic illnesses and certain drugs. In T$_3$ thyrotoxicosis the thyroid gland overproduces only T$_3$, resulting in an elevated serum T$_3$ with a normal T$_4$ concentration.

FREE T$_4$ AND FREE T$_3$ TESTS. Since the free or unbound concentrations of T$_4$ and T$_3$ are correlated with their biologic effect, ways to measure the free levels have been sought. However, their concentrations are too low to be measured directly, and therefore an indirect dialysis method using radioactive-labeled T$_4$ or T$_3$ has been developed. Since the free T$_4$ (FT$_4$) test is relatively expensive and somewhat complicated and time consuming, its use in clinical medicine is not yet widespread. The free T$_3$ (FT$_3$) test is available only in research laboratories.

T$_3$ UPTAKE TEST. The T$_3$ uptake (T$_3$U) test measures the number of binding sites on the thyroid-binding proteins (TBG, TBPA, and TBA) that are unoccupied and serves as an index of the proportion of FT$_4$. Radioactive-labeled T$_3$ (T$_3$ ^{131}I) is added to a serum sample and allowed to saturate all the free binding sites present. An absorbent material such as a resin sponge is next added to take up the excess labeled T_3. The percentage of labeled T_3 attached to the absorbent material is calculated. T_3 uptake by the resin method gives normal values of 34% to 46%.

Excess binding sites are present in hypothyroidism because the T_4 is low and the TBG is less saturated. Therefore the T_3U is decreased, since more labeled T_3 can attach to TBG binding sites. The opposite occurs in hyperthyroidism. When elevated concentrations of TBG are present, as occurs in pregnant or estrogen-stimulated women, more unbound TBG sites are present and take up more labeled T_3, resulting in a low T_3U. Opposite changes occur with decreased TBG concentrations.

TBG TEST. Abnormalities in the concentration of TBG are frequently encountered in clinical practice, leading to substantial changes in the T_4, T_3, and T_3U test results. This can result in a false diagnosis of thyroid disease. The TBPA concentration is much less variable and rarely leads to abnormalities in these tests. Although a radioimmunoassay has been developed for TBG, the usual method of assay is to measure the T_4 binding capacity of this protein. There are many factors other than thyroid disease that can alter levels of TBG. They include the following:

Increase	Decrease
Estrogens	Chronic illness (e.g., diabetes, liver disease, renal disease)
Pregnancy	
Oral contraceptives	
Neonatal state	Androgens
Acute hepatitis	Other anabolic steroids
Genetic (X-chromosome linked)	Glucocorticoid (large dose)
	Genetic (X-chromosome linked)
Acute intermittent porphyria	Idiopathic
Idiopathic	Starvation
Fluorouracil	
Marijuana abuse	

The most common cause of low TBG is chronic disease states such as diabetes mellitus, liver disease, and renal insufficiency. The usual case of an increased TBG is a hyperestrogen state such as pregnancy, oral contraceptive therapy, or estrogen replacement therapy. However, it is rarely necessary in clinical practice to assess TBG-binding capacity, since typical changes in the T_4 and T_3U occur from TBG increase or decrease. Simply stated, when hyperthyroidism or hypothyroidism is present, the T_4 and T_3U are elevated or depressed together, respectively. When TBG increase is present, a reciprocal change occurs (T_4 increases and T_3U decreases), and the reverse is true for TBG decrease (T_4 decreases and T_3U increases). Knowledge of these changes has resulted in the development of the free thyroxine index.

FREE THYROXINE INDEX. Since the free concentrations of T_4 and T_3 determine their biologic activity, their measurement is helpful, especially when abnormalities in the concentration of TBG are present as noted previously. Since the FT_4 method is expensive and cumbersome, an indirect method of calculating the free T_4 concentration called the free thyroxine index (FT_4I) has been developed. The FT_4I equals the product of the T_4 and T_3U. The normal values are 1.5 to 5.5. The FT_4I may be the easiest and cheapest measurement of the free T_4 level. Studies have shown that this index remains normal when the T_4 is elevated or decreased as a result of TBG changes because of the reciprocal changes that occur in the T_3U. A similar calculation can be used to determine the free triiodothyronine

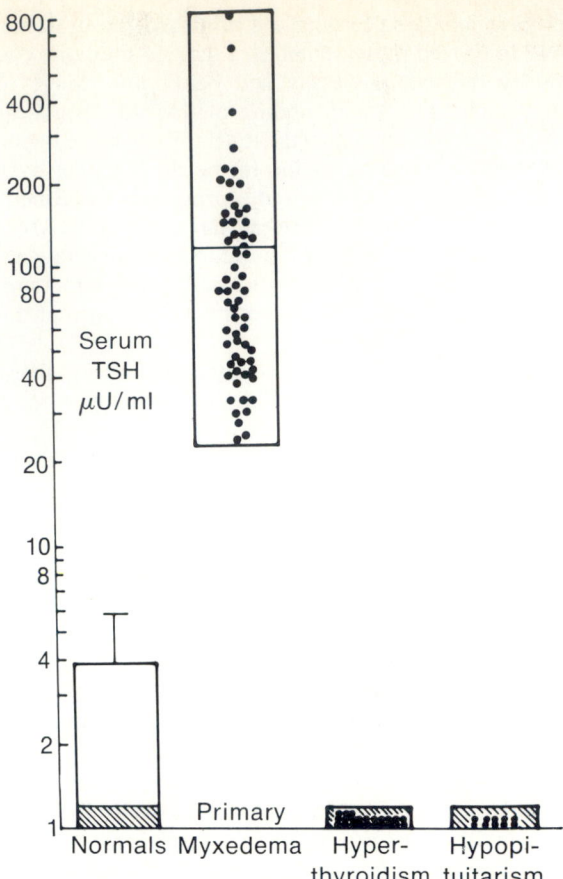

Fig. 187-5 Serum thyrotropin *(TSH)* in normal individuals (vertical bar shows standard deviation) and those with primary myxedema, hyperthyroidism, and hypothyroidism resulting from hypopituitarism. (From Hershman JM and Pittman JA, Jr: Ann Intern Med 74:482, 1971.)

index (FT_3I) from the product of the T_3 concentration and the T_3U.

TESTS THAT MEASURE THYROID-REGULATING FACTORS

TSH measurement and TRH stimulation test. The measurement of TSH or thyrotropin by radioimmunoassay is common in most medical centers and reflects the level of pituitary TSH stimulation of the thyroid. Normal TSH values are 0 to 8 µU/ml. The pituitary output of TSH responds inversely to the serum thyroid hormone levels and is stimulated by thyrotropin-releasing hormone (TRH) under negative feedback control through the hypothalamus and pituitary. There is no diurnal rhythm of TSH. High levels are seen in the neonate during the first 72 hours after birth and in primary hypothyroidism. In certain thyroid diseases such as lymphocytic thyroiditis, in goiter resulting from iodine excess or deficiency, or in the gland reduced in size by surgery or radioactive iodine therapy, elevations of serum TSH are present even when serum T_4 and T_3 concentrations are still normal because excess stimulation of the gland is required to maintain normal thyroid function. The TSH assay can be useful to the clinician in three ways. First, the TSH is helpful in distinguishing primary hypothyroidism (high levels of TSH) from pituitary or hypothalamic hypothyroidism (decreased levels) (Fig. 187-5). In this situation it has largely replaced the TSH stimulation test. Second, in primary hypothyroidism it is used to assess the adequacy of thyroid replacement, since elevated TSH levels should return to normal with proper replacement.

Lastly, the TSH assay is used to assess the response to TRH stimulation. TRH stimulation is helpful in (1) directly assessing pituitary TSH reserve; (2) detecting suppressed pituitary TSH resulting from excess serum thyroid hormone concentrations; and (3) differentiating between pituitary and hypothalamic hypothyroidism. From 200 to 500 μg of TRH is given intravenously, and the output of TSH is measured before and at different time intervals after the TRH is given. The maximal or peak response is usually seen between 20 and 40 minutes after TRH administration but can be delayed up to 60 minutes in hypothalamic disease. There is a gradual decline in the TSH response to TRH with age in men but not in women. Increased responses are seen in patients with with hypothyrodism, and decreased responses are seen in hyperthyroidism. This test is very sensitive to slight increases in the T_4 and T_3 serum concentrations. Partial to complete suppression of the TSH response to TRH occurs with T_4 and T_3 levels within the normal range, although slightly in excess of what is normal for that individual.

TSH stimulation test. The TSH stimulation test detects the thyroid's ability to respond to TSH by an increase in the RAIU and the output of T_4 (and T_3). As usually performed, a 5- to 10-unit dose of TSH is injected intramuscularly after measurement of the RAIU, and the RAIU is measured again 24 hours later. The TSH stimulation dose is sometimes repeated 2 or 3 days in a row to ensure that maximal stimulation of the thyroid has occurred. The 1-day test dose is adequate in most instances. This test is useful in (1) detecting a decrease in thyroid reserve that occurs in the failing thyroid gland, (2) differentiating the suppressed thyroid resulting from increased concentrations of thyroid hormone from the damaged thyroid present in different forms of thyroiditis, and (3) differentiating primary hypothyroidism from pituitary and hypothalamic hypothyroidism caused by TSH deficiency. This test requires considerable time and may be dangerous in the elderly patient, and it is used much less frequently today because measurement of TSH and the TRH stimulation test give similar information as discussed previously.

Highly sensitive TSH test. Most TSH tests currently in use do not accurately measure low concentrations of TSH below 0.5 μU/ml. Recently a new TSH assay called the highly sensitive TSH (HS-TSH) test has become available in many medical centers and reference laboratories. This assay accurately measures low concentrations of TSH down to 0.04 μU/ml. The new HS-TSH assay is helpful in accurately measuring suppressed levels of TSH in hyperthyroidism (except in rare cases of TSH producing a pituitary tumor or in the syndrome of pituitary resistance to thyroid hormone) and in cases in which therapeutic suppression of TSH levels is very important, such as in the treatment of thyroid carcinoma. The HS-TSH test probably should be performed in all cases of hyperthyroidism that are not obviously Grave's disease.

In addition, the new HS-TSH assay has displaced the TRH test for measuring suppressed pituitary TSH secretion. With the advent of the HS-TSH assay, the TRH test's main diagnostic value is in differentiating hypothalamic hypothyroidism (TRH deficiency) from pituitary hypothyroidism (TSH deficiency). The HS-TSH assay also is replacing both the T_3 and T_4 suppression tests.

T_3 suppression test. Thyroid hormone given in physiologic or pharmacologic quantities completely suppresses the normal thyroid by suppressing the hypothalamic pituitary axis, causing decreased TSH secretion. This can be measured by a decrease in the RAIU and the serum T_4 concentration (if T_3 is the suppressor used). This phenomenon forms the basis of the thyroid suppression test in which 75 to 100 μg of T_3 is given orally for 7 to 10 days and the RAIU or the T_4 or both are measured before and after the T_3 is taken. Failure of suppression of the thyroid indicates autonomous function of the thyroid gland. This autonomy may be due to the thyroid stimulating immunoglobulin (TSI) present in Grave's disease or residing in the thyroid in nontoxic and toxic uninodular and multinodular goiter. The chief value of this test lies in its help in sorting out the different presentations of Graves' disease, such as the euthyroid form with exophthalmos, and in testing for the suppressability in nontoxic goiter. Since the TRH stimulation test gives similar information, the T_3 suppression test is used much less frequently today.

THYROID AUTOANTIBODIES. Six types of thyroid autoantibodies have been identified: thyroglobulin antibody, microsomal antibody, colloid antibody, antinuclear antibody, thyrotropin receptor antibody (TSI), and thyrotropin-binding inhibitor immunoglobulin (TBII).

The antithyroglobulin and antimicrosomal methods are the two tests for these antibodies generally used. Low titers of antibodies occur in about 6% of normal individuals without evidence of thyroid disease. There is a gradual increase in frequency with age. A relatively high percentage of individuals with Graves' disease (35% to 50%), primary hypothyroidism (45% to 80%), and Hashimoto's thyroiditis (71% to 92%) have positive test results for thyroid autoantibodies, and these are all considered to be autoimmune thyroid diseases. The antimicrosomal antibodies are more likely to be present in higher concentration in these diseases. Very high titers usually occur in patients with Hashimoto's thyroiditis and are probably diagnostic. Antibodies to the TSH receptor (TSI) stimulate the follicular cells in the same fashion as TSH. Another TSH receptor antibody (TBII) blocks the TSH receptor and causes hypothyroidism. Thyroid autoantibodies are discussed further under "Diffuse toxic goiter." Their presence must be interpreted in the light of the whole clinical picture; their presence alone is rarely meaningful unless other clinical or laboratory abnormalities of thyroid disease are present.

THYROID BIOPSY AND ASPIRATION CYTOLOGY. Thyroid tissue obtained by small open biopsy or percutaneous needle biopsy may be extremely valuable in establishing the correct diagnosis of a thyroid disorder. It is helpful in distinguishing between the different types of thyroiditis, between benign and malignant thyroid neoplasms, and between different types of nontoxic goiter.

The percutaneous needle biopsy is relatively easily accomplished with the patient under local anesthesia. A Vim-Silverman-Franklin or True-Cut needle is used. The needle biopsy can be performed as an outpatient procedure and has a minimal morbidity risk. A small open biopsy can be performed with the patient under local or general anesthesia and generally is the preferred method because a larger, more representative tissue specimen is obtained.

Aspiration of thyroid nodules suspected of harboring malignancy is increasingly frequent. The advocates of this procedure state that it has reliable diagnostic accuracy, does not spread cancer, and results in much less thyroid surgery. A small-gauge needle is passed into the nodule, and cells from the nodule are obtained by aspiration. Guidance of the biopsy needle by ultrasonography increases the accuracy of placement. The cells are classified by the cytologist as nonmalignant, malignant, or indeterminate. Only patients with malignant or indeterminate cytology are subjected to thyroid surgery. The result is that two thirds of the patients who ordinarily would have had thyroid surgery are shown to have benign disease and can be treated with thyroid suppression therapy.

CLINICAL ASSESSMENT OF THYROID FUNCTION

Thyroid disease usually is manifest by typical systemic symptoms and signs and/or by enlargement or irregularity of the thyroid gland with or without associated local neck symptoms. A carefully taken history and close examination are the starting point of clinical assessment. Suspected or obvious thyroid disease can be substantiated by appropriate thyroid function studies.

Hypothyroidism

Hypothyroidism is a clinical disease state occurring when insufficient thyroid hormone is available to tissue sites of action. The severity of the hormone deficiency and the length of time it is present determine the extent of the clinical disease. Myxedema is a severe form of hypothyroidism. Cretinism results from severe hypothyroidism in the fetus or neonate.

ETIOLOGY. Hypothyroidism can be classified by the patient's age at onset and by etiologic factors. Separation of patients according to age is important because the clinical presentation varies substantially among infant, juveniles, and adults. Hypothyroidism in infants includes all cases in neonates until 4 to 5 years of age when brain development is complete. The juvenile period encompasses the 5- to 18-year age-group until growth and sexual maturation are complete. All cases thereafter are classified as adult hypothyroidism. Endemic iodine deficiency, which previously was the most common cause of hypothyroidism in all age-groups throughout the world, is still present in certain parts of the world but rarely occurs in the developed nations owing to iodine supplementation. The causes and incidence of hypothyroidism in the infant have been clearly established by mass screening of neonates. In 1977 the Newborn Screening Committee of the American Thyroid Association, after reviewing a number of screening studies, noted that 166 cases of permanent congenital hypothyroidism were found in 730,000 newborn infants studied for an incidence of 1 in 4400 births. About 85% of the affected infants had thyroid agenesis, about 10% had thyroid dysplasia with only a remnant of thyroid tissue in normal or ectopic location, and most of the rest had TSH deficiency owing to a sporadic or familial hypothalamic-pituitary disorder. In the same studies additional cases of decreased thyroid reserve resulting from low normal serum T_4 and elevated TSH concentrations were found in euthyroid infants. These averaged one case for every four or five cases of hypothyroidism. They are believed to represent mild defects in thyroid hormone synthesis or decreased tissue response to TSH or thyroxine. An occasional infant has hypothyroidism and goiter at birth as a result of maternal drug ingestion, usually methimazole or propylthiouracil taken for treatment of hyperthyroidism.

The causes of hypothyroidism are usually similar in juveniles and adults. The most frequent of these are idiopathic atrophy, chronic lymphocytic thyroiditis, and loss of tissue owing to thyroidectomy or radioactive iodine treatment. The incidence in juveniles is between 4 and 12 per 10,000. In adults the incidence is 5 to 8 cases per 1000 new patients. The causes are idiopathic atrophy or chronic lymphocytic thyroiditis in 60% to 70% of patients and tissue loss from radioactive iodine therapy or thyroid surgery in about 30%. Between 50% and 80% of patients with thyroid atrophy have significantly elevated thyroid antibody titers, suggesting that chronic lymphocytic

thyroiditis is a factor in the thyroid failure. Less than 10% of cases are related to hypothalamic pituitary disease from Sheehan's syndrome, pituitary adenoma, craniopharyngioma, empty-sella syndrome, head trauma, and hypothalamic disease. TSH deficiency usually occurs in association with other pituitary hormone deficiencies. TRH deficiency as a cause of hypothyroidism is quite rare. It may occur as an isolated defect or in association with defects of other hypothalamic releasing hormones, secondary to intracranial neoplasms, serious head trauma, or central nervous system infection. Rare cases of hypothyroidism are due to ingestion of goitrogens (found in cabbage and some other vegetables). Iodine and lithium ingestion result in goiter and hypothyroidism in a few individuals. Hypothyroidism from iodine results from the inability to escape from iodine's inhibiting effects on organic binding. Lithium works by blocking secretion of thyroid hormone from the follicle cell. Patients with chronic lymphocytic thyroiditis, Graves' disease, and radiation thyroiditis are more susceptible to this effect.

Females are more susceptible to almost all thyroid diseases. The neonatal screening programs have shown a 4:1 female to male preponderance. In juveniles and adults two to six females are affected for every male. Certain types of hypothyroidism such as that caused by chronic lymphocytic thyroiditis are inherited or occur with high frequency in some families. Peripheral resistance to thyroid hormone and intrathyroidal enzyme defects usually occur by autosomal recessive inheritance.

CLINICAL MANIFESTATIONS. At all ages the initial manifestations of hypothyroidism are very subtle and may be clinically nonevident or easily overlooked. The signs and symptoms listed below progress gradually in relation to the severity of the thyroid hormone deficiency.

General

Coarse or hoarse voice
Decreased growth (juvenile)
Weight gain (slight)
Psychomotor slowing
Hypokinesia
Somnolence
Cold sensitivity
Fluid retention
Mental retardation (infant)
Cretinoid facies (infant)

Skin and appendages

Decreased sweating
Decreased sebaceous activity
Thickened skin with hyperkeratosis
Coarse hair
Diffuse hair loss
Thick tongue

Cardiovascular

Bradycardia
Increased diastolic blood pressure
Narrow pulse pressure
Decreased cardiac output
Peripheral vasoconstriction
Enlarged heart

Respiratory

Hypoventilation

Gastrointestinal

Constipation
Decreased stooling rate
Abdominal distention
Increased gaseousness

Endocrine

Menorrhagia
Hypomenorrhea or amenorrhea
Decreased fertility
Impotence and oligospermia
Galactorrhea

Hematopoietic

Anemia

Neuromuscular

Weakness
Muscle cramps
Paresthesias
Peripheral neuropathy
Hypotonia
Ataxia
Incoordination

When thyroid hormone is withheld from athyreotic individuals, signs and symptoms of hypothyroidism may begin within 2 weeks and are present in all within 3 or 4 weeks. Frank myxedema is present within 6 to 8 weeks. Usually, however, the progression of hypothyroidism is much slower and more insidious so that the patient can seldom give an approximate

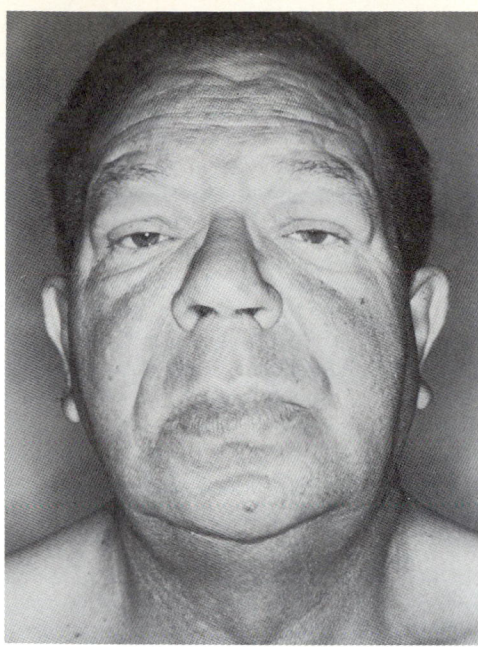

Fig. 187-6   Patient with classic features of myxedema. Note pale edematous appearance of facies with thick lips and puffy eyelids.

date for the onset of symptoms. In patients with a history of previous radioactive iodine therapy or thyroid surgery or with fatigue, myalgias, arthralgias, weight gain, hypersomnolence, cold intolerance, hoarseness, constipation, normochromic and normocytic anemia, growth retardation, delayed puberty, menstrual abnormalities, and mental sluggishness, hypothyroidism should be suspected.

In infants typical characteristics gradually develop. These infants feed poorly, are lethargic and hypersomnolent, and move infrequently. Severe constipation and abdominal distention are almost always present. Hypoventilation, episodes of cyanosis, and choking are common. A large tongue may add to frequent respiratory difficulties. The skin is dry and coarse. An umbilical hernia is sometimes found. Carotenemia and prolonged icterus neonatorum occur. Hypothermia, bradycardia, and low pulse pressure are present. A goiter occurs if thyroid tissue and excess TSH are present. Within a few months of birth these signs and symptoms progress rapidly. Linear growth failure, delayed closure of the fontanelles, muscular hypotonia, and delayed relaxation of the deep tendon reflexes develop. All developmental stages are delayed. Intellectual retardation begins. The typical appearance of short stature with increased trunk-to-limb ratio; large head; broad, flat nose with widely set eyes; sparse, coarse hair; thick, dry skin; enlarged, protruding tongue; protuberant abdomen; and mental deficiency develops with time, resulting in the classic picture of cretinism.

In juveniles the principal features of hypothyroidism different from those found in adults are the development of growth retardation with increased trunk-to-limb ratio and delay in sexual maturation. These children become lethargic and less active. Although some mental sluggishness may develop, intellectual deterioration does not occur. When hypothyroidism is severe, linear growth and bone development essentially stop.

As hypothyroidism progresses at all ages, almost all areas of the body are affected with progression to full-blown myxedema (Fig. 187-6). This consists of mental sluggishness, sallow complexion, edematous-appearing facies, coarse voice with slow speech, and very dry, coarse skin. A goiter may or may not be present. If present it usually indicates excess TSH secretion and primary thyroid failure. The thyroid tissue that is present, whether of normal size or enlarged, is frequently substantially firmer than normal and bosselated, which is very suggestive of chronic lymphocytic thyroiditis. The speech is thick, slow, and sometimes slurred. The skin becomes dry, coarse, and cool. Marked pallor may develop as a result of associated anemia. Sweating and sebaceous activity are decreased. The lips appear puffy, pale, and dry. The pulse is slow and regular with decreased pulse pressure. Hypertension occasionally develops. Increased heart size may occur as a result of pericardial effusion. There may be abdominal distention, flatulence, and constipation, sometimes leading to fecal impaction. Mental sluggishness with poor memory, drowsiness, and personality changes gradually develops. Occasionally an organic psychosis (myxedema madness) results. Peripheral neuropathy, manifest by paresthesias and pain (usually having a burning character) in the extremities associated with ataxic gait, occurs. Although obese patients are often referred to endocrinologists for evaluation of possible hypothyroidism, not more than two thirds of hypothyroid patients gain weight and the weight gain is rarely more than 10 or 15 pounds.

Menstrual disorders sometimes occur in hypothyroid women. Most commonly, prolonged excessive bleeding results, but irregular menstrual periods, amenorrhea, and hypomenorrhea can also occur. Muscle aching and stiffness frequently occur. Galactorrhea with hyperprolactinemia is being reported with increasing frequency. Muscles sometimes appear hypertrophic and are quite firm and inelastic. Delayed relaxation of the deep tendon reflexes develops. Occasionally, if the diagnosis is overlooked for months, hypoventilation and extreme lethargy result. The patient must be stimulated to respond. Patients with severe myxedema eventually lapse into coma and die if untreated.

LABORATORY FINDINGS. The finding of a low T_4 level is common in all forms of hypothyroidism unless an elevated TBG concentration is present. In this instance the FT_4I ($T_4 \times T_3U$) will correct for the TBG change and show a low T_4. The FT_4 is also low. The level of protein-bound iodine (PBI) is usually low but may be normal or elevated if abnormal iodinated materials are present in the serum from exogenous sources or from diseases such as chronic lymphocytic thyroiditis in which abnormal iodinated proteins are released from the damaged thyroid into the blood.

The TSH should invariably be determined in hypothyroidism. In the majority of instances it is elevated, confirming primary hypothyroidism. If the TSH is normal or low, pituitary or hypothalamic (secondary or tertiary) hypothyroidism must be considered. While the old TSH test did not distinguish between normal and low values, the new HS-TSH does and is helpful in these cases.

The TRH stimulation test can distinguish between primary, secondary, and tertiary forms of hypothyroidism. In primary hypothyroidism the elevated serum TSH excessively responds to intravenously administered TRH (200 to 500 µg). In contrast, in pituitary hypothyroidism the normal or low serum TSH does not respond to TRH administration. In hypothalamic hypothyroidism the low or normal TSH responds normally, although sometimes sluggishly. The maximal response in the TSH may not occur until 1 hour after TRH administration, whereas normally the peak TSH response occurs at 20 to 30 minutes.

The RAIU test may be depressed to below 10% in hypothyroidism, but its diagnostic accuracy is not good enough to be used as a test for hypothyroidism. However, the RAIU does not respond to TSH stimulation in primary hypothyroidism because the thyroid is already being maximally stimulated by endogenous TSH. In pituitary TSH deficiency and hypothalamic TRH deficiency the RAIU responds to TSH stimulation and thus can be used to differentiate from primary hypothyroidism. However, in recent years, because of the availability of TRH and the ease of the TRH stimulation test, this test has largely replaced the TSH stimulation test in the diagnosis of hypothyroidism.

As previously noted, thyroid autoantibody titers are elevated in a high percentage of patients with idiopathic thyroid atrophy and in a higher percentage of patients with hypothyroidism and chronic lymphocytic thyroiditis. Other tests formerly used, the basal metabolic rate (BMR) and the Achilles reflex time, have been replaced by the more precise tests described above.

Anemia, which is usually normocytic and normochromic but occasionally macrocytic, occurs in about half of the advanced cases. When macrocytic anemia is present, the coexistence of pernicious anemia must also be considered. The serum cholesterol level is frequently elevated above 300 mg/dl, but this is of little diagnostic value because it is often elevated from other causes.

The electrocardiogram frequently shows bradycardia, low voltage, and inverted or low T waves. In severe myxedema, enzymes from muscle tissue such as creatinine phosphokinase (CPK), aldolase, and serum glutamic-oxaloacetic transaminase (SGOT) may be elevated. Hyperprolactinemia, occasionally in the presence of galactorrhea, is not uncommon but usually is not measured. A low serum iron level, decreased iron-binding capacity, elevated uric acid level, rapid sedimentation rate, and carotemia may be present. The serum proteins show minor changes such as slightly elevated β-globulin levels, slightly decreased albumin and γ-globulin levels, and slightly increased TBG binding capacity.

DIFFERENTIAL DIAGNOSIS. On occasion severe anemia, nephrotic syndrome, or Cushing's syndrome may have superficial resemblance to myxedema. In nephrosis the T_4 may be low because of abnormal metabolism of T_4, as well as excessive urinary excretion of TBG-T_4 complex. Measurements of the T_3 uptake, FT_4I, and TSH are needed for differentiation of these two diseases, and occasionally the TRH stimulation test may be necessary. Patients with neurasthenia and anorexia nervosa frequently are quite hypometabolic, and thyroid failure must be ruled out by multiple thyroid function tests. Liver disease also may cause hypometabolism and decreased or elevated serum proteins, resulting in decreased or elevated TBG levels and abnormal T_4 serum concentrations. Low-T_4 syndrome occurs in severely ill patients and can result from a number of factors such as low TBG and decreased metabolism, liver clearance, and production of T_4. It does not respond to thyroid replacement.

MANAGEMENT. Several preparations are available for replacement therapy in hypothyroidism. These medications include pure T_3, mixtures of T_3 and T_4, and pure T_4 (Table 187-2). They all are rapidly absorbed and relatively inexpensive. They do not cause allergic reactions and have no side effects except hypermetabolic symptoms if excess amounts are given. Dosage requirements increase with body size, as noted in Table 187-2, which also shows equivalent doses of the different preparations. In adults 1.6 μg of T_4/kg of body weight is adequate in over 90% of patients with hypothyroidism.

The need for thyroid hormone may decrease slightly with age and increase somewhat with stress and infection, although rarely is it necessary to adjust the dosage under these circumstances. The amount of thyroid hormone given to restore euthyroidism varies among individuals but the amounts noted in Table 187-2 are usual. The level at which replacement therapy should be started and the rate at which it should be increased vary depending on the severity and duration of the hypothyroidism and associated illnesses. Infants can be given a full replacement dose immediately. If a patient has had hypothyroidism for a short time and otherwise is young and healthy, replacement also can start at full dosage immediately. However, in those with hypothyroidism of moderate severity of many months' duration, initial dosage should be about one-fourth to one-third full dosage (25 to 50 μg of T_4) and increased by one fourth to one third at 10- to 14-day intervals until euthyroidism is achieved. In the elderly and those with associated serious disease, only about 12.5 to 25 μg of T_4 should be given initially and then the dosage should be increased by the same amount at 2- to 3-week intervals. The patient should be monitored carefully for aggravation of underlying disease or new problems each time before the dosage is increased.

Adequacy of replacement therapy is judged by several criteria. Although clinical judgment is very subjective, most clinicians continue to increase the amount of thyroid hormone until all signs and symptoms of the hypothyroid state have disappeared. More reliable criteria are the restoration of the T_4 to normal (usually 8 to 10 μg/dl) and suppression of the elevated TSH to normal.

In infants it is important to start thyroid replacement within the first few weeks of life to prevent mental retardation. Recent studies have demonstrated that if thyroid hormone is started by 3 months of age, mental retardation is unlikely. Retardation does occur and is progressive if treatment is delayed longer than 3 to 6 months. In the juvenile, treatment results in catch-up growth and normal physical and sexual development, although some decrease in stature may be the outcome if hypothyroidism has been present longer than 2 or 3 years.

In the past the most commonly used preparation of thyroid hormone was desiccated thyroid. Desiccated thyroid (thyroid extract) is an extract of animal thyroid gland and is standardized according to iodine content (0.2%). Thyroglobulin is a purified porcine protein whose biologic activity is measured by its ability to inhibit propylthiouracil-induced goiter in rats. It has been shown that the iodine content of these animal preparations varies considerably and does not reflect the T_4 and T_3 content well. In addition, the proportion of T_4 to T_3 varies among the different batches of the extracted hormone.

When synthetic T_3 and T_4 combinations became available, they were used frequently. However, there is no need to give T_3 and T_4 together, since there is substantial peripheral metabolism of T_4 to T_3 and steady serum T_4 and T_3 levels are easily maintained in the normal range throughout the day with adequate T_4 replacement alone. Furthermore, T_4 and T_3 combinations cause the serum T_3 level to peak substantially above normal each day between 2 and 8 hours after the daily dose is given. Thus it appears that the pure T_4 preparations are preferable for replacement therapy.

TRANSIENT HYPOTHYROIDISM. Transient hypothyroidism is not infrequent, and if it is unrecognized, lifelong thyroid replacement therapy may be given inappropriately. It occurs on recovery from subacute thyroiditis and following discontinuation of thyroid hormone that has been given to a patient with a normal thyroid gland for obesity, fatigue, or other reasons. Transient hypothyroidism can be the presenting feature of lymphocytic thyroiditis. It also can follow recovery from silent thyroiditis and postpartum thyroiditis, therapy with radioactive iodine and total thyroidectomy for treatment of Graves' hyperthyroidism, and iodine or lithium therapy. The

Table 187-2   Thyroid hormones preparations

	Preparation	Composition	Equivalent dose	Usual daily requirement	Absorption (%)
T_3	L-Triiodothyronine	Pure T_3	25 μg	50-75 μg	85
	Desiccated thyroid	20-30 μg T_4, 7-11 μg T_3	60 mg	120-180 mg	50-75
T_3-T_4 combination	Thyroglobulin	20-30 μg T_4, 7-11 μg T_3	60 mg	120-180 mg	50-75
	Synthetic liotrix (two products)	50 μg T_4 and 12.5 μg T_3; 60 μg T_4 and 15 μg T_3	1 tablet	2-3 tablets	70-80
T_4*	L-Thyroxine	Pure T_4	50 mg	75-150 mg	50-80

*Infants' and children's T_4 dosage should be calculated by body weight as follows:
  0-1 yr: 9 μg/kg/day   6-10 yr: 4 μg/kg/day
  1-5 yr: 5 μg/kg/day   11-20 yr: 3 μg/kg/day

hypothyroidism in most of these patients is mild, and spontaneous recovery occurs within 6 to 8 weeks. Therefore patients with mild degrees of hypothyroidism should be observed for several months before instituting therapy, or treatment should be limited to 3 to 6 months.

MYXEDEMA COMA. Myxedema coma is frequently fatal and must be treated promptly and aggressively. It usually occurs in elderly patients with prolonged hypothyroidism. Infection, cold exposure, trauma, and central nervous system depressants are frequent predisposing factors. Untreated hypopituitarism may mimic this condition. The clinical state varies from extreme lethargy, hypersomnolence, and impaired consciousness to deep coma. It is characterized by subnormal temperature (as much as 14° F [10° C] below normal at times), bradycardia, hypotension, and hypoventilation. Laboratory tests usually reveal a very low T_4 and FT_4I, elevated TSH, depressed arterial PO_2, and elevated PCO_2. Severe dilutional hyponatremia similar to the inappropriate antidiuretic hormone (ADH) syndrome is not uncommon. Therapy should be started promptly with T_4 (500 μg intravenously) to replace the severe peripheral thyroid hormone deficit. Because relative adrenal insufficiency may be present owing to severe myxedema, hydrocortisone (100 mg intravenously) is given initially and repeated in doses of 25 to 50 mg every 6 hours thereafter. Hypertonic intravenous fluids and glucose are needed, but the fluids should be given judiciously to avoid fluid overload and resultant congestive heart failure. Assisted respiratory support with oxygen therapy is usually necessary. Further heat loss should be prevented by the use of blankets, but victims should not be rewarmed rapidly. Intravenous T_4 (50 to 150 μg daily) should be continued until the patient is responding and can take it orally. The initial response to this type of treatment program begins within 24 hours with increase in body temperature and improvement in the vascular state.

Hyperthyroidism

Hyperthyroidism is a clinical hypermetabolic disorder produced by excessive secretion of thyroid hormone and its effect on peripheral tissues. The term "thyrotoxicosis" is frequently used interchangeably with hyperthyroidism, although technically thyrotoxicosis includes other states in which excessive thyroid hormone levels and action are present from sources other than the thyroid such as exogenous thyroid hormone intake. The following is a classification of thyrotoxicosis:

I. With elevated RAIU
  A. Diffuse toxic goiter (Graves' disease)
  B. Toxic multinodular goiter (Plummer's disease)
  C. Toxic uninodular goiter (toxic adenoma)
  D. Excess TSH production
    1. Pituitary tumor
    2. Autonomous pituitary function
    3. Excessive TRH secretion
  E. Tumor-producing thyroid stimulators
    1. Hydatidiform mole and choriocarcinoma of uterus owing to excess human chorionic gonadotropin
    2. Embryonal carcinoma of testes
    3. Other malignancies
II. With suppressed RAIU
  A. Excess exogenous intake of thyroid hormone
    1. Factitious hyperthyroidism
    2. Iatrogenic hyperthyroidism
  B. Thyroiditis with transient hyperthyroidism
    1. Subacute thyroiditis
    2. Lymphocytic thyroiditis
  C. Iodide-induced hyperthyroidism (Jod-Basedow disease)
  D. Metastatic follicular carcinoma of the thyroid
  E. Struma ovarii

Diffuse toxic goiter, toxic multinodular goiter, toxic uninodular goiter, lymphocytic thyroiditis (a transient thyrotoxicosis), and the thyrotoxicosis secondary to excessive exogenous intake of thyroid hormone given for thyroid suppression or replacement therapy account for 98% to 99% of all cases of hyperthyroidism. When there is a clinical impression or suspicion of hyperthyroidism, this should be substantiated by elevated serum T_4 and T_3 concentrations, a high T_3U, and elevated free thyroid indices (FT_4I and FT_3I). Hyperthyroidism is associated with an excess of both T_4 and T_3 except in three situations: (1) the occasional patient with T_3 hyperthyroidism, (2) hyperthyroidism associated with low T_3 syndrome, and (3) hyperthyroidism associated with low TBG. T_3 thyrotoxicosis with normal T_4 levels has been found in diffuse toxic goiter, toxic multinodular goiter, and toxic uninodular goiter. It appears that in some of these patients the onset of hyperthyroidism is first manifested by T_3 overproduction, but only after several weeks or months does excessive T_4 production occur. In one study T_4 and T_3 elevations were found in 87.5% of hyperthyroid patients, with the rest having only elevated T_4 levels. A normal serum T_3 concentration may be due to reduced peripheral T_4-to-T_3 conversion owing to associated acute and chronic illness. The HS-TSH test or the TRH test may be used to help identify this form of hyperthyroidism. Low TBG concentration, if present with hyperthyroidism, may result in normal T_4 and T_3 concentrations, but this association can be determined easily by noting a very high T_3U and elevated FTI.

Once the diagnosis of thyrotoxicosis appears established by the clinical impression and the finding of elevated serum concentrations of T_4 and T_3, the specific cause should be sought so that appropriate therapy can be given. An RAIU test should be performed in all patients except pregnant women to determine whether they have high or low RAIU, as outlined previously. Further differentiation is outlined later in the chapter as the individual disease entities are discussed.

CLINICAL MANIFESTATIONS. The severity of the illness caused by thyrotoxicosis is related to the severity and duration of the hormone excess, the age of the patient, and the presence or absence of other disease. Like hypothyroidism, hyperthyroidism affects almost all body systems, as listed below:

General

Weight loss
Irritability
Anxiety
Emotional lability
Hyperkinesia
Insomnia
Fatigue
Heat intolerance
Apathy
Decreased attention span
Psychosis

Skin and appendages

Onycholysis
Excessive diaphoresis
Increased sebaceous activity
Thinning of hair
Palmar erythema
Infiltrative dermopathy
Acropachy

Cardiovascular

Tachycardia
Increased systolic blood pressure
Wide pulse pressure
Increased cardiac output
Peripheral vasodilation
Systolic heart murmur

Pulmonary

Exertional dyspnea
Weakened respiratory msucles

Gastrointestinal

Increased stooling
Diarrhea
Nausea and vomiting
Anorexia
Polyphagia

Endocrine

Hypomenorrhea
Decreased fertility
Decreased potency and libido
Gynecomastia
Abnormal liver function

Hematopoietic

Decreased neutrophils
Increased lymphocytes

Neuromuscular

Weakness
Muscle wasting
Tremor
Hyperactive deep tendon reflexes

Optic

Infrequent blinking
Lid lag and retraction
Widened palpebral fissures
Decreased upward gaze
Photosensitivity
Proptosis
Increased tearing
Lid edema
Weakness of convergence
Infiltrative ophthalmopathy
Extraoculomotor paresis

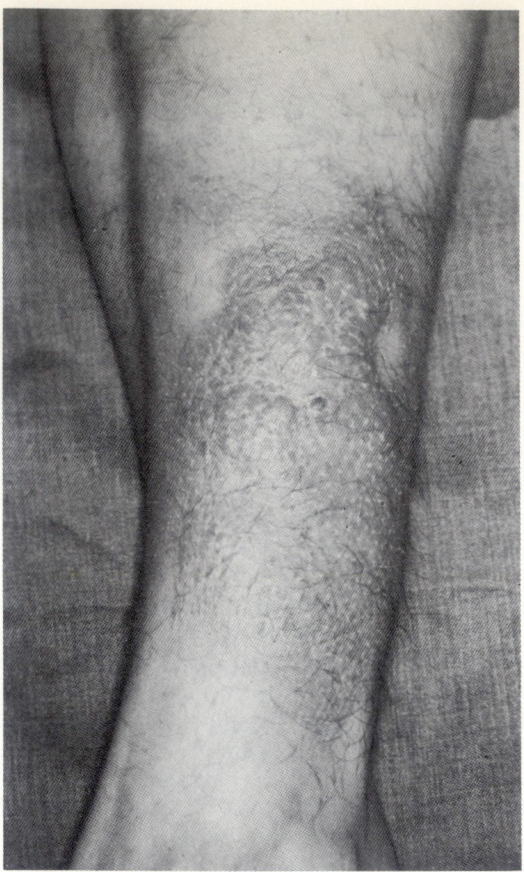

Fig. 187-7   Infiltrative dermopathy of Graves' disease, demonstrating typical plaque of pretibial myxedema.

The skin is warm, smooth, and thinned with loss of much of the keratin layer. Heat intolerance, excessive sweating, palmar erythema, fine soft hair, and onycholysis (Plummer's nails) frequently are present. Infiltrative dermopathy, commonly known as pretibial myxedema (Fig. 187-7), an infiltration of the skin and subcutaneous tissue with a mucopolysaccharide substance, occurs only in Graves' disease. It most commonly occurs in association with infiltrative ophthalmopathy. It is seen most often over the lower and middle one third of the pretibial areas, but it may also involve the ankles and feet and rarely the thighs and other parts of the body as well. Lesions appear as a painless, violaceous induration of the skin and subcutaneous tissue in irregular single or multiple plaques, most often in an asymmetric pattern. At times the skin changes are so mild that they are found only by careful inspection and palpation, and occasionally they are so severe that they resemble elephantiasis. Clubbing of the fingers with swelling and erythematous changes in the soft tissues at the base of the nails called thyroid acropachy develops occasionally in patients with Graves' disease, who usually also have infiltrative ophthal-

mopathy and dermopathy. Periosteal new bone formation may occur in association with these acral changes.

Optic manifestations. The characteristic eye changes (Fig. 187-8) that occur in thyrotoxicosis are referred to as an ophthalmopathy and are usually classified as (1) the benign (noninfiltrative) changes associated with most forms of thyrotoxicosis, and (2) the infiltrative forms seen only in Graves' disease. Forward protrusion or proptosis (exophthalmos) usually occurs only with Graves' disease. The noninfiltrative changes are generally related to increased adrenergic stimulation and consist of infrequent blinking (Stellwag's sign), widened palpebral fissures (Dalrymple's sign), lid lag (von Graefe's sign), decreased upward motion of the eye with associated decreased wrinking of the forehead on upward gaze (Joffroy's sign), and weakness of convergence (Möbius' sign). The severe infiltrative form is characterized by exophthalmos owing to increased retroorbital edema, infiltration of fat, mucopolysaccharides and fibrous tissue, and hypertrophic weakened extraocular muscles. Lid edema, diplopia, ophthalmoplegia, increased tearing, irritation, and photosensitivity accompany these infiltrative changes. Occasionally, visual impairment occurs owing to corneal ulceration, optic neuritis, retinal hemorrhage, and orbital or bulbar infection. These complications result from constant exposure of the cornea and from excessive traction on the optic nerve because of the severe proptosis.

Cardiovascular manifestations. The excess thyroid hormone causes a hyperdynamic cardiovascular response by direct stimulation of adenylate cyclase (cyclic AMP system) and by augmentation of adrenergic activity. This results in tachycardia

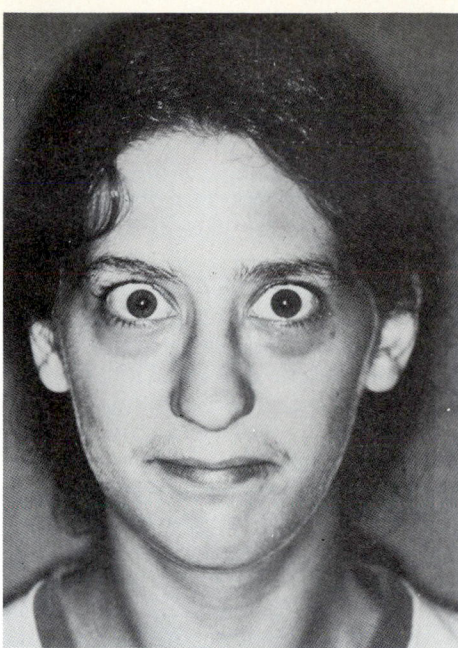

Fig. 187-8   Ophthalmopathy of Graves' disease. Patient has typical noninfiltrative changes (stare with marked upper and lower lid retraction).

even in the resting and sleeping states, widened pulse pressure, hyperdynamic precordial activity, increased cardiac output, peripheral vasodilation leading to prominent, bounding, peripheral arterial pulses, and warm erythematous extremities. Cardiac arrhythmias sometimes occur, especially in the elderly and in those with preexisting cardiac disease. The most common are atrial fibrillation that is poorly responsive to digitalis, premature ventricular contractions, and occasionally paroxysmal supraventricular tachycardia. Congestive heart failure may develop in the elderly and those with associated heart disease. Breathlessness is common, and occasionally mild hypoventilation results from weakness of respiratory muscles.

Gastrointestinal manifestations. Weight loss occurs in the majority of cases in spite of a marked increase in appetite and food intake. However, in about 10% no weight change is noted and in another 10% weight gain occurs. Severe thyrotoxicosis may result in anorexia, especially in the aged and in those with associated serious disease. Intestinal hypermotility with increased stooling is common. Frank diarrhea, nausea, vomiting, and abdominal pain may occur. In some cases the gastrointestinal symptoms predominate so that serious gastrointestinal disease is suspected. Occasionally hepatomegaly with abnormal liver function develops.

Neuromuscular and psychiatric manifestations. General manifestations include fatigue, increased irritability, increased emotional lability, restlessness, nervousness, and short attention span. Purposeless movements may be so severe at times that chorea is suspected. Speech may be very rapid. Teachers may note that affected children cannot concentrate and do poorly in schoolwork. Occasionally apathy, lethargy, and depression may predominate, and frank psychosis can occur. A fine tremor of the tongue, of the slightly closed lids, and of the fingers is usually present with hyperactive deep tendon reflexes. Muscle weakness occurs only after months of hyperthyroidism and is most prominent in the proximal muscles. Patients note difficulty in stair climbing, getting up from the squatting position, or holding the legs outstretched from a

sitting position for more than 15 to 20 seconds (the healthy person can do this for up to 60 seconds). Muscle atrophy occurs in severely affected patients and frequently appears more severe than it actually is because of the associated subcutaneous fat atrophy from weight loss. Prolonged hyperthyroidism may lead to increased severity of osteoporosis or osteopenia already present and may result in compression fractures of vertebrae.

Genitourinary manifestations. Increased urinary frequency occurs as a result of increased renal blood flow and glomerular filtration. This is probably aggravated by nervousness and restlessness. Menstrual abnormalities, usually hypomenorrhea and occasionally amenorrhea, occur in about 50% of women. Infertility is common, especially in severe thyrotoxicosis. In men mild gynecomastia, decreased libido, and impotence have been reported.

DIFFUSE TOXIC GOITER (GRAVES' DISEASE). Diffuse toxic goiter or Graves' disease is the most common form of hyperthyroidism, accounting for 40% to 60% of all cases of thyrotoxicosis. It is characterized by a combination of (1) hyperthyroidism, (2) infiltrative ophthalmopathy, (3) infiltrative dermopathy, and (4) thyroid acropachy. Hyperthyroidism occurs alone in about 50% of the cases and with infiltrative ophthalmopathy in the other 50%. Infiltrative dermopathy develops in about 5% to 10% of patients with infiltrative ophthalmopathy. Thyroid acropachy occurs in 1% to 2%, usually those with infiltrative ophthalmopathy. About 5% to 10% of patients with infiltrative ophthalmopathy are euthyroid or hypothyroid when first seen. These patients usually have associated chronic lymphocytic thyroiditis that prevents the overstimulated thyroid from oversecreting thyroid hormone. The thyroid gland is symmetrically enlarged (30 to 80 g) in most cases of Graves' disease, but it is normal in about 10% and very large (over 100 g) in others. It is slightly firmer than normal and nontender. Vascularity is markedly increased so that a bruit is frequently heard over the thyroid. Microscopic examination shows marked hyperplasia and hypertrophy of the follicular epithelium. This disease occurs most often between the ages of 30 and 50 and affects females about seven times more frequently than males. There is an increased incidence in some families, suggesting autosomal recessive inheritance. Graves' disease is associated frequently with chronic lymphocytic thyroiditis and occasionally with rheumatoid arthritis, pernicious anemia, vitiligo, systemic lupus erythematosus, myasthenia gravis, premature menopause, and Addison's disease.

Etiology. The cause of Graves' disease is the body's production of an abnormal thyroid stimulator different from TSH. Severe physical or emotional trauma such as an automobile accident, death of a loved one, or divorce appears to be an inciting cause in about 50%. A marked increase in frequency occurred in Denmark during the German occupation from 1941 to 1945. A long-acting thyroid stimulator (LATS) is found in the blood of about 60% of patients with Graves' disease. This substance is characterized simply by its longer duration of action in stimulating the mouse thyroid compared to TSH. LATS is a 7S IgG immunoglobulin produced by B lymphocytes. It is capable of inducing thyroid hyperplasia and iodine accumulation in the thyroid independent of the pituitary gland. Before the discovery of LATS the pituitary gland and TSH were considered possible causes of Graves' disease. With the advent of the radioimmunoassay for TSH, TSH levels were found to be uniformly reduced in Graves' disease, further negating a pituitary role. Another IgG protein, LATS-protector (LATS-P), was subsequently found. It could stimulate only the human thyroid (not the mouse thyroid) but in addition prevented

LATS from being neutralized in thyroid tissue assay systems. Subsequently, newly developed assay systems have shown multiple effects of these thyroid stimulating immunoglobulins (TSIs), as they are now called. These effects include (1) stimulation of endocytosis of colloid, which is a prerequisite for the release of thyroid hormone from follicular cells; (2) stimulation of the intrathyroidal adenylate–cyclic AMP system; and (3) displacement of radioactive-labeled TSH from TSH cellular membrane receptors. Therefore at this time Graves' disease is believed to be an autoimmune disease caused by TSIs, which are autoantibodies to TSH receptors on the follicular cell membrane and as such compete with TSH for these receptors. In addition, once TSIs attach to the receptors, they act exactly like TSH and activate the intracellular enzyme cascade system. Nearly all patients with diffuse toxic goiter have evidence of TSIs by these different assays.

The pathologic mechanism for stimulating B lymphocytes to start producing TSI is unknown. That it is a hereditary defect is suggested by (1) its strong concordance in monozygotic twins, (2) a frequent familial occurrence, (3) a frequent occurrence of other autoimmune diseases in associated family members, and (4) the increased prevalence in those with HLA-B8 (whites) and HLA-BW35 (Japanese) white cell antigens.

The natural history of Graves' disease was noted early in the twentieth century when effective treatment was unavailable. The severity of the hyperthyroidism was found to be variable with remissions and exacerbations and a tendency to resolve spontaneously in months or years. However, severe disability often resulted from the persistence of the hyperthyroidism, and death occurred in 10% to 20% of affected individuals. With the advent of effective treatment, death is infrequent and severe disability is unusual.

Diagnosis. The diagnosis is frequently obvious in the patient who has clinical hyperthyroidism with associated ophthalmopathy and pretibial myxedema or thyroid acropachy. In patients without other signs of Graves' disease, the presence of clinical hyperthyroidism with elevated serum levels of T_4 and T_3 and elevated RAIU is enough to confirm the diagnosis. The thyroid scan is usually not indicated in this disease but sometimes is helpful in differentiating diffuse toxic goiter from toxic multinodular goiter. The measurement of TSI or LATS is not routinely performed but is indicated in diagnostic problems and probably will become routine as the TSI assay becomes readily available.

Management

Surgery. Except in a few centers, surgery is the treatment of choice only in selected patients, usually children and adolescents, especially if their hyperthyroidism is difficult to control with antithyroid drug therapy. The patient must be prepared with an antithyroid drug before surgery. Usually propylthiouracil or methimazole is administered for several weeks before surgery to render the patient euthyroid. Following this, inorganic iodine is given in addition for 7 to 10 days to reduce the marked vascularity of the gland caused by the thioureas. More recently, propranolol alone, given for 5 to 7 days before surgery, has been an effective means of controlling hyperthyroidism. During the surgical procedure, 90% to 98% of the thyroid tissue is removed. Immediate postoperative complications include local hemorrhage, tracheal compression, and transient hypoparathyroidism. Permanent hypoparathyroidism and vocal cord paralysis owing to injury of the recurrent laryngeal nerve occur in less than 0.5% of patients. Permanent postoperative hypothyroidism occurs in 30% to 50% of patients with extensive thyroid resection. With less extensive thyroid resection, hypothyroidism is much less frequent but the incidence of postoperative recurrence of the hyperthyroidism, sometimes as long as 20 to 30 years later, is substantially higher (15% to 20%).

Radioactive iodine. [131]I therapy is the most common mode of treatment for Graves' disease in adults. It is contraindicated in children and adolescents and in pregnant women with hyperthyroidism. The main form of radiation from ^{131}I is the β-particle, which accounts for about 90% of its activity. Since these β-rays travel only about 2 mm within the thyroid gland, large doses can be directed to the thyroid gland without giving significant radiation to other structures. The usual dose is 5 to 15 mCi, which is generally calculated so that about 100 μCi is given per gram of thyroid tissue. The first effects of radioactive iodine begin to occur in about 1 month, and 80% of the patients achieve euthyroidism within 2 to 3 months. The rest require more than one dose. The only significant adverse effect from radioactive iodine therapy is hypothyroidism; between 20% and 50% of patients are hypothyroid within 1 year. Those who do not become hypothyroid should be followed indefinitely because most follow-up studies have shown a 2% to 5% incidence of hypothyroidism per year after the first year.

There has been no evidence of other hazards from the effects of radiation on the body such as increased incidence of malignancy such as leukemia or of congenital abnormalities in the offspring of treated patients. Even in children, in whom other forms of radiation have been shown to be a major cause of thyroid carcinoma, the use of ^{131}I has not caused increased incidence of malignancies. The incidence of thyroid carcinoma is lower in patients treated with radioactive iodine than in the general population.

Thiourea therapy. Two drugs, propylthiouracil and methimazole, are used in the treatment of hyperthyroidism. These drugs ameliorate hyperthyroidism by inhibiting the peroxidase enzyme system, thus preventing oxidation of trapped iodine, iodination of tyrosines, and coupling of iodotyrosines. In addition, propylthiouracil but not methimazole inhibits the peripheral conversion of T_4 to T_3. The usual daily dosage of propylthiouracil is 400 to 600 mg in three or four divided doses. The equivalent dose of methimazole is about one-tenth that of propylthiouracil. Experience has shown that patients with severe hyperthyroidism may require larger dosages, so starting daily dosages of 800 to 1000 mg are sometimes used in severely ill patients. Clinical improvement with a fall in the T_4 and T_3 levels occurs within 2 or 3 weeks, and the majority of patients are rendered euthyroid within 6 to 8 weeks. The dosage is gradually reduced at that time. A maintenance dosage of 100 to 200 mg daily is usual. The thyroid gland also usually decreases in size with effective treatment. If it enlarges during therapy, progressive uncontrolled disease or the onset of hypothyroidism should be suspected. The main drawbacks of therapy with thioureas are their side effects and the length of time they must be given. Granulocytopenia occurs in less than 1% of patients, and leukocytosis, liver dysfunction, skin eruptions, arthralgias, myalgias, and lymphadenopathy occur in up to 5%. Initially, monthly monitoring of the T_4, white blood cell counts, and liver function tests is indicated. With control of the hyperthyroidism after 2 or 3 months, monitoring should take place every 2 or 3 months. Most physicians continue thiourea therapy for 1 to 2 years. After discontinuing the medication, the recurrence rate of hyperthyroidism is about 50% to 60%, most often in the first 2 years. A recent report suggests that treatment can be discontinued after 3 or 4 months but the recurrence rate is higher. There is no method that predicts accurately whether a patient will have a recurrence when thiourea therapy is stopped. Recent investigations, however, suggest that the disappearance of TSI during thiourea therapy may indicate permanent remission. There is no evidence that antithyroid drugs alter the course of the disease, even though they suppress the production of thyroid hormone.

TOXIC MULTINODULAR GOITER. Toxic multinodular goiter is also known as Plummer's disease. It usually occurs in patients with long-standing nontoxic multinodular goiter resulting from autonomous or semiautonomous function of slowly growing nodules. It accounts for 10% to 20% of the cases of thyrotoxicosis and occurs most often in individuals over 50 years of age. The nodules probably synthesize thyroid hormone less efficiently than normal thyroid tissue so that substantially more nodular tissue must be present before overproduction and thyrotoxicosis occur. Usually 75 to 100 g or more of thyroid tissue is present when hyperthyroidism develops. The thyroid scan reveals localization of the iodine in the nodules with suppressed function in the intervening thyroid tissue. TSH stimulation activates the suppressed areas of function but stimulates the autonomous and semiautonomous functioning nodules only slightly or not at all because they have lost much of their responsiveness to TSH. Hyperthyroidism present in some patients with multinodular goiter may be a form of Graves' disease, since the thyroid tissue between the nodules is hyperplastic whereas the nodule tissue has large, relatively inactive follicles and does not accumulate iodine. The hyperthyroidism present with toxic multinodular goiter is usually mild, but because this disease occurs most often in patients over the age of 50 who frequently have other illnesses, severe disability can occur. It is much more frequent in women than in men. The symptoms and signs are similar to those seen in Graves' disease, but cardiac problems such as atrial fibrillation and congestive heart failure are much more common in this older age group. Infiltrative ophthalmopathy and dermopathy do not occur. The thyroid gland is quite nodular and varies greatly in size and contour.

Diagnosis. The elevation of the serum levels of T_4 and T_3 is usually mild, substantially less than in most cases of Graves' disease, and the RAIU may be elevated. The scan shows varying degrees or patchy areas of uptake. T_3 toxicosis, the low-T_3 syndrome, and a low TBG sometimes confuse the laboratory studies. The HS-TSH is suppressed, and TSIs are not present. In patients with only borderline elevation of T_4 and T_3 levels and in those with the low T_3 syndrome, HS-TSH or TRH testing may be indicated. Suppressed HS-TSH or lack of TSH response to TRH stimulation indicates excessive levels of thyroid hormone.

Management. The usual treatment recommended for elderly patients with toxic multinodular goiter is radioactive iodine. Because the RAIU is usually lower than in Graves' disease, substantially more radioactive iodine is needed. The average dose is at least 15 mCi and may be 30 mCi or more. Thyroidectomy is indicated if significant tracheal and esophageal obstruction is present or simply to debulk an extremely large goiter, which usually has considerable amounts of fibrous tissue. An occasional patient may choose thyroidectomy over radioactive iodine therapy for cosmetic reasons; the goiter rarely returns to normal size after radioactive iodine therapy. Thiourea therapy is used infrequently for this type of hyperthyroidism except as preparation for surgery or as interim therapy until radioactive iodine is effective.

TOXIC UNINODULAR GOITER. Toxic uninodular goiter is an autonomous functioning follicular adenoma of the thyroid that produces thyrotoxicosis, although in rare instances it can be due to a follicular carcinoma. It causes 3% to 5% of the cases of thyrotoxicosis. It appears usually as a single nodule

or rarely as two or three nodules. Hyperthyroidism seldom occurs while the autonomous functioning nodule is less than 2.5 to 3 cm, since nodules do not produce thyroid hormone as efficiently as normal tissue. TSH is suppressed and TSIs are not present in this disease. Slow progressive growth with increasing hormone production and suppression of normal thyroid tissue gradually occurs over many years. Most autonomous functioning thyroid nodules or hot nodules never produce hyperthyroidism.

Elevation of the serum T_4 and T_3 concentrations and the RAIU is usually present, although an occasional patient may have only T_3 toxicosis. The thyroid scan reveals uptake only in the nodule with suppression of the rest of the gland. TSH stimulation may occasionally be necessary to show areas of suppressed normal thyroid tissue. Radioactive iodine therapy (usually 20 to 30 mCi or more) and surgery (simple excision of the nodule) are equally effective treatments. After removal of the nodule by radioactive iodine therapy or surgery, the suppressed normal thyroid tissue functions again. A small residual nodule may remain after radioactive iodine treatment.

HYPERTHYROIDISM CAUSED BY EXCESS TSH. Excessive TSH production is an extremely rare cause of hyperthyroidism. It can be caused by a TSH-producing pituitary tumor, by excess pituitary production of TSH from hypothalamic dysfunction resulting from excess TRH secretion, or from partial pituitary resistance to thyroid hormone in which the pituitary set point for negative feedback control appears to be higher than normal. It is usually suspected only if the serum TSH is inadvertently found to be elevated or if visual field impairment or other signs and symptoms suggesting pituitary disease occur in a patient with hyperthyroidism. The presence of an elevated serum TSH concentration and the confirmation of the pituitary tumor and pituitary and hypothalamic dysfunction are necessary to confirm the diagnosis. The TSH level is normal or low in all other forms of hyperthyroidism.

HYPERTHYROIDISM CAUSED BY TUMORS. The clinical hyperthyroidism associated with choriocarcinoma or hydatidiform mole is rare and generally mild in spite of sometimes greatly increased T_4 and T_3 concentrations. The presence of a high concentration of human chorionic gonadotropin (HCG), a weak thyroid stimulator, appears to be the cause of thyroid hyperfunction. Hyperthyroidism caused by other tumors producing thyroid stimulators is infrequent and poorly understood. Control of the tumor causes a reduction in the thyroid stimulators and cures the hyperthyroidism.

THYROTOXICOSIS CAUSED BY THYROIDITIS. Subacute thyroiditis (discussed later in this chapter in detail) is sometimes associated with transient thyrotovicosis owing to a release of substantial amounts of stored thyroid hormone from the damaged thyroid gland. The diagnosis is usually obvious; the patient has a firm, very tender, slightly enlarged thyroid with a mild to moderate degree of thyrotoxicosis. Subacute thyroiditis is frequently associated with a systemic illness manifested by malaise, diffuse aches and pains, and low-grade fever. It is sometimes preceded by a viral respiratory illness.

Silent thyroiditis has been reported with increased frequency in recent years and now accounts for 10% to 20% of the cases of thyrotoxicosis. The thyroid gland is slightly enlarged in 50% of cases of lymphocytic thyroiditis and is usually firm and nontender. This disease is frequently confused with diffuse toxic goiter and is first suspected only when a suppressed RAIU is found. Percutaneous needle or open biopsy of the thyroid may be necessary to confirm the diagnosis. The hyperthyroidism usually lasts 6 to 12 weeks and requires treatment with sedatives, propranolol, or corticosteroids in patients with moderate or severe disease.

IODINE-INDUCED HYPERTHYROIDISM. Iodine-induced hyperthyroidism (Jod-Basedow disease) apparently was much more common when iodine prophylaxis was in vogue 20 or more years ago. Its present incidence is unknown. It usually occurs in a patient with a nontoxic multinodular goiter who has taken iodine for prophylaxis or treatment of other diseases or for roentgenographic studies. It also has been reported to occur in patients with a normal thyroid and those with other thyroid diseases. A disturbance or failure in the intrathyroidal control of iodine metabolism probably causes this disease. It is usually transient, lasting 2 to 4 months. Iodine-induced hyperthyroidism should be suspected in any patient with hyperthyroidism and a depressed RAIU, and such patients should be questioned about recent inorganic or organic iodine intake. Excessive inorganic iodine intake or roentgenographic iodine-containing dyes may also depress the RAIU in patients with diffuse or toxic multinodular goiter. In this circumstance the suppressed RAIU becomes elevated within a few days after the inorganic iodine or renal roentgenographic dyes are excreted (although excretion may take up to 6 to 8 weeks to occur after cholecystographic contrast material is given). In contrast, the RAIU stays suppressed during the duration of the hyperthyroidism with Jod-Basedow disease. At times it may be necessary to measure the 24-hour urinary iodide concentration to determine whether excessive iodide ingestion is present. Levels greater than 2000 to 2500 µg confirm this.

THYROTOXICOSIS CAUSED BY EXOGENOUS THYROID HORMONE INTAKE

Thyrotoxicosis factitia. Thyrotoxicosis factitia is a form of thyrotoxicosis without hyperthyroidism. Thyrotoxicosis factitia owing to surreptitious self-administration of thyroid hormone is quite rare. It most often occurs in individuals with underlying psychiatric problems who have paramedical training and access to thyroid hormone. Most will vehemently deny intake of thyroid hormone. The diagnosis should be suspected in patients who meet the clinical criteria described previously and who have a suppressed uptake and a nonpalpable or small thyroid. TSH stimulation will produce function in the suppressed thyroid tissue.

Iatrogenic thyrotoxicosis. Iatrogenic thyrotoxicosis, which is usually mild, results when an excessive amount of thyroid hormone is administered to a patient with hypothyroidism or to a patient being given suppressive thyroid hormone therapy for a multinodular goiter that has developed some autonomous function. In a multinodular goiter the combination of the exogenous thyroid hormone intake and the persistent endogenous hormone production results in thyroid hormone excess and sometimes in mild thyrotoxic symptoms and signs. The diagnosis is usually obvious, and all that is needed is to discontinue administration of thyroid hormone or reduce the amount given.

DIFFERENTIAL DIAGNOSIS OF THYROTOXICOSIS. Patients with psychoneurosis may have sweating, tremor, stare, tachycardia, weakness, fatigue, weight loss, and purposeless movements suggestive of thyrotoxicosis. Hypermetabolism associated with pheochromocytoma may produce severe sweating, tachycardia, tremor, and weight loss. Weight loss, fatigue, and other symptoms associated with occult malignancy, anemia, diabetes, hyperparathyroidism, cardiac disease, and myasthenia may suggest possible hyperthyroidism. Luft's syndrome, a rare abnormality caused by overgrowth and excessive function of skeletal muscle mitochondria, produces severe hypermetabolism and mimics hyperthyroidism. With many of these diseases there is an increased association of hyperthyroidism. In most instances, however, the available thyroid tests should easily prove or disprove the presence of hyperthyroidism.

SPECIAL ASPECTS OF HYPERTHYROIDISM

Hyperthyroidism in the infant, child, and adolescent. Neonatal hyperthyroidism is usually the result of transplacental transfer of TSI from the mother to the infant. Hyperthyroidism is present at birth and usually lasts for only 1 or 2 weeks until all the TSI has been metabolized and cleared from the neonate's blood. The mother almost always has a history of recent or remote Graves' disease.

Most other types of thyrotoxicosis seen during childhood and adolescence are due to Graves' disease. There is still controversy about the best mode of treatment. The majority of centers treat patients with thioureas initially, but a substantial number still recommend subtotal thyroidectomy. Radioactive iodine has been given as the initial treatment, but most physicians worry about its use because of the increased incidence of thyroid cancer in infants and children who have had head and neck irradiation. Children having toxic reactions to the thiourea compounds or not responding well to them are usually treated with subtotal thyroidectomy and occasionally with radioactive iodine.

Hyperthyroidism in pregnancy. Hyperthyroidism in pregnancy is almost always due to Graves' disease and is associated with an increased incidence of spontaneous abortion and stillbirths. Radioactive iodine should never be given to pregnant women because it crosses the placental barrier and the fetal thyroid concentrates iodine after the twelfth week of gestation. Propranolol also is contraindicated for treatment of hyperthyroidism because it may possibly cause intrauterine growth retardation, fetal distress, low Apgar scores, postnatal depression, hypoglycemia, bradycardia, and prolongation of labor. Subtotal thyroidectomy following preparation with thioureas is frequently performed during the first half of pregnancy. Most physicians only use thioureas. Since these drugs cross the placenta and accumulate in the fetal thyroid, substantially reduced dosages are used, less than 300 mg of propylthiouracil each day to keep the T_4 level in the upper range of normal. T_4 and T_3 do not cross the placenta, so adding T_4 to the mother's treatment to prevent hypothyroidism in the infant does not work.

Thyrotoxic crisis. Thyrotoxic crisis (thyroid storm) is relatively rare and is precipitated in the hyperthyroid patient by infections, trauma, surgery, and withdrawal from antithyroid drugs (especially in patients with very large thyroids). It is a life-threatening condition manifested by marked restlessness, agitation, extreme tachycardia (130 to 160 beats/min), high fever (104° to 106° F [40° to 41° C]), prostration, dehydration, nausea, vomiting, diarrhea, delirium, and psychosis. Treatment must be instituted promptly as follows: (1) propylthiouracil, 800 to 1200 mg/day in four divided doses; (2) propranolol, 160 to 240 mg/day in four divided doses orally or 1 to 2 mg intravenously every 1 to 2 hours; (3) potassium iodide, 500 mg orally every 6 hours, or sodium iodide, 0.5 g by intravenous drip every 8 hours; (4) intravenous fluid therapy; (5) mechanical treatment of hyperthermia; *and* (6) corticosteroids in high doses if the patient does not show prompt response to the other treatment in 12 to 24 hours. Patients not responding to this regimen can be treated with peritoneal dialysis, exchange transfusion, or plasmapheresis to rapidly lower thyroid hormone levels.

Infiltrative ophthalmopathy. The course of infiltrative ophthalmopathy seen with Graves' disease is unpredictable. It usually occurs with hyperthyroidism but it can occur alone before, or within a few months or years after the hyperthyroidism. In the majority of cases it follows a relatively benign course with progressive proptosis over a period of months and then a slow, spontaneous remission over many weeks and months, sometimes leaving a small but significant residual proptosis. Although the benign noninfiltrative eye changes disappear when the hyperthyroidism leaves, the severe changes generally follow an independent course. Typically bilateral, symmetric eye involvement with some restriction of extraocular muscle motion is seen on initial examination. However, in some cases the involvement may be unilateral or asymmetric, and the patient may be euthyroid or hypothyroid. At times a firm goiter is present. This indicates chronic lymphocytic thyroiditis, which is the cause of hypothyroidism or at least prevents hyperthyroidism as a result of the persistent effect of TSI. Diagnostic evaluation includes tests to exclude the possibility of orbital tumor and other orbital disease and to confirm that Graves' disease is really present. Orbital roentgenography, tomography, computed tomography, or orbital ultrasonography can be used to check for orbital tumor. The presence of Graves' disease can be demonstrated in four ways. Two methods are the HS-TSH test and the TRH stimulation tests, indicating suppression of the hypothalamic pituitary axis. The third is the T_3 suppression test (previously discussed), which in most cases show a nonsuppressive thyroid. Finally, the presence of TSI also supports the diagnosis of Graves' disease. However, in some cases of Graves' ophthalmopathy, one, two, or all of these tests may be normal.

The treatment of infiltrative ophthalmopathy depends on the severity of the ocular involvement. In most mild cases, sleeping with the head of the bed elevated and using diuretics helps reduce periorbital and lid edema. One percent methylcellulose drops in each eye as needed helps relieve the gritty sensation that many patients experience. If diplopia is present, prism fitting helps correct the visual abnormality, but if it persists, extraocular muscle surgery may be necessary to restore binocular vision. When the corneas remain uncovered much of the time, tarsorrhaphy and/or section of Müller's muscle in the upper lid may be necessary to prevent recurrent corneal ulceration and orbital infection. Severe inflammatory changes can be treated with retrobulbar injections of corticosteroids or large oral doses of corticosteroids, which usually should be continued for several months. If this fails or if the proptosis is rapidly progressive and optic neuritis develops with visual loss, surgical orbital decompression is indicated. Supervoltage orbital radiation therapy is also effective sometimes if given within the first year after severe eye changes occur.

Nontoxic goiter

Nontoxic goiter is defined as any enlargement of the thyroid not associated with hypothyroidism or hyperthyroidism. The following is a classification of the causes of nontoxic goiter:

I. Nontoxic diffuse goiter
  A. Iodine deficiency
  B. Biosynthetic or enzmatic defects
  C. Goitrogens
  D. Thyroiditis
  E. Tissue resistance to thyroid hormone
II. Nontoxic multinodular goiter
  A. Long-standing nontoxic diffuse goiter
III. Nontoxic uninodular goiter
  A. Neoplasms
    1. Benign
    2. Malignant
  B. Cysts
  C. Thyroiditis
  D. Hemorrhage

This classification helps sort out the different goiters according to their physical characteristics, so that a logical diagnostic workup and treatment can be determined. The most frequent causes of nontoxic goiter are minor intrathyroidal biosynthetic defects, thyroiditis, neoplasms, cysts, and hemorrhage. The others are found relatively infrequently.

NONTOXIC DIFFUSE GOITER. The exact cause of most cases of nontoxic goiter in the United States is not known. Possible causes include minor intrathyroidal biosynthetic defects and excessive thyroid stimulation by growth factors from the pituitary or immune system. These goiters are sporadic and acquired in some, hereditary and familial in others. Nontoxic diffuse goiter is believed to represent a compensatory increase in thyroid size owing to minor degrees of decreased thyroid hormone synthesis, probably resulting from multiple causes such as minor intrathyroidal acquired enzyme defects. The slight decrease in serum thyroid hormone levels results in increased TSH stimulation of the thyroid. This returns thyroid hormone levels to normal but does not correct the underlying primary defect. Although increased TSH levels are not usually demonstrated, minor increases of TSH within the normal range are found and probably are sufficient to produce the thyroid enlargement. The role of TSH in initiating and maintaining the goiter is substantiated by the rapid regression of some goiters with suppressant doses of thyroid hormone, an action mediated only by the suppression of TSH production. The exact intrathyroidal defect or defects are thought to be subtle and minor in degree. Whether they are acquired or congenital and why there is an extremely high female-to-male ratio (7 to 9:1) are unknown. Minor degrees of iodine deficiency and intake of weak goitrogens in drugs or food may further aggravate the intrathyroidal defect. Genetic factors probably play an important role, since similar goiters or other thyroid disease is found in 30% to 40% of these patients' relatives. Abnormal growth factors or excessive production of growth factors by the pituitary may be involved in other cases.

Although iodine deficiency is still common in some undeveloped areas of the world, it is no longer prevalent in North America owing to iodine salt supplementation for the past 60 to 70 years and to iodine compounds used to preserve foods in more recent years. Goitrogens in water, foods, and drugs occasionally cause minor outbreaks or isolated cases of goiter. It is not known whether ingestion of small amounts of weak goitrogens contributes to the generation of goiters in those with a genetic tendency, minor biosynthetic defects, or mild degrees of iodine deficiency. Established types of intrathyroidal enzyme defects are due to autosomal recessive inheritance. They occur most often in infants and children and frequently lead to hypothyroidism. Nontoxic diffuse goiter also has been reported in the rare syndrome of tissue resistance to thyroid hormones. Thyroiditis as the cause of goiter is discussed as a separate entity later in this chapter.

Diagnosis. The diagnosis of the types of nontoxic diffuse goiters discussed thus far is usually established by the history and physical findings. The RAIU and the serum concentrations of T_4, T_3, and TSH are normal except in the occasional patient whose defect is severe enough to cause hypothyroidism. Low titers of thyroid autoantibody may be present in some of these patients but do not help to clarify the diagnosis. Percutaneous needle or small open thyroid biopsy is helpful in establishing the pathologic diagnosis but is used infrequently, since the diagnosis is usually based on the clinical features. The use of sophisticated tests to check for intrathyroidal enzyme defects or for minor degrees of iodine deficiency is not indicated. The patient should be questioned about the use of drugs and foods that have goitrogenic activity, but this is rarely rewarding.

Management. Thyroid suppression is the principal mode of treatment of nontoxic diffuse goiters unless iodine deficiency or intake of goitrogens is found. Thyroid hormone in the form of T_4 (Table 187-2) is given in physiologic doses. It gradually suppresses TSH and thyroid hormone production and reduces the goiter to normal or near normal size within 2 to 6 months. Thyroid surgery is not indicated in this type of goiter except to help establish the diagnosis or reduce the bulk of very large goiters. Surgery should always be followed by thyroid suppression therapy, since removal of thyroid tissue only aggravates the defect and since hyperplasia and regrowth of the residual thyroid tissue or frank hypothyroidism usually occurs with time. Iodine prophylaxis is not indicated unless iodine deficiency is established because it may induce Jod-Basedow disease or hypothyroidism.

Thyroiditis

ACUTE SUPPURATIVE THYROIDITIS. Acute thyroiditis is also known as suppurative or bacterial thyroiditis. The usual causative organisms are *Staphylococcus, Streptococcus,* and *Pneumococcus.* They gain entry to the thyroid from infected contiguous structures or from hematogenous spread from a distant focus. The onset is usually abrupt with fever, localized or diffuse swelling and pain radiating upward in the anterior lateral neck to the jaw and ear, localized erythema, increased heat, and painful swallowing. The condition is quite rare and must be differentiated from inflammation and infection from bacteria and fungi such as *Actinomyces,* usually in lymph nodes. Thyroid function studies are usually normal, but the thyroid scan shows decreased function in the suppurative area. Prompt antibiotic therapy causes rapid resolution in a few days, but an abscess can develop and surgical drainage may be necessary.

SUBACUTE THYROIDITIS (DE QUERVAIN'S THYROIDITIS). Subacute thyroiditis (de Quervain's, granulomatous, or giant cell thyroiditis) is a localized or diffuse, nonsuppurative inflammation of the thyroid characterized by multiple types of inflammatory cells (polymorphonuclear leukocytes and mononuclear cells), noncaseating granuloma formation with multinucleated giant cells, and disruption of thyroid follicles. The cause is considered to be an immunologic response to a viral infection, since it frequently occurs several weeks after a viral upper respiratory tract infection. This disorder is uncommon. There is a female predominance (3 to 4:1), and it occurs most often between the ages of 25 and 50 years.

The initial complaint is usually a sore throat or earache of several weeks' duration, which is frequently misdiagnosed as pharyngitis or otitis media. The thyroid gland is usually diffusely enlarged with mild to severe localized tenderness, although there may be a localized area of enlargement and tenderness and infrequently a single nontender nodule. The thyroid tenderness may be exquisite, causing the patient to withdraw rapidly when thyroid palpation is attempted. In 10% to 20% of cases there are severe signs and symptoms of systemic disease and hyperthyroidism. These include fever, tachycardia, chills, sweats, malaise, severe dysphagia, and headache. The hyperthyroidism results from the release of excessive quantities of stored thyroid hormone from damaged thyroid follicles. Even in severe cases the diagnosis is frequently overlooked

and the disease is misdiagnosed as fever of unknown origin (FUO), dental abscess, pharyngitis, otitis media, or influenza. The disease is self-limited, lasting 1 to 3 months. Other causes of tenderness in the thyroid area that may be confused with subacute thyroiditis include local hemorrhage into thyroid cysts, acute thyroiditis, acute inflammation or spasm of neck muscles, abscess of adjacent structures and lymph nodes, and tender carotid arteries. Laboratory studies are frequently normal in mild cases. In moderate or severe inflammation laboratory abnormalities may include (1) elevated sedimentation rate; (2) mild leukocytosis and occasionally mild anemia; (3) a depressed RAIU except in localized disease, in which the thyroid scan shows decreased uptake in the involved area; (4) elevated serum T_4 and T_3 concentrations in severely affected patients; and (5) the presence of low titers of thyroid autoantibodies in about 50% to 60% of patients. Thyroid biopsy may be needed in some cases, but the diagnosis is usually obvious on the basis of clinical criteria and laboratory studies.

Mild and moderate cases should be treated with analgesics such as aspirin and acetaminophen. The patient should be assured that the disease is self-limited and usually clears within 1 to 2 months. In severe cases, especially those with thyrotoxicosis, more potent antiinflammatory agents should be used. Corticosteroids provide prompt relief of symptoms and tenderness within 24 to 48 hours and should be continued for 3 to 4 weeks. The usual starting dose of prednisone is 30 to 50 mg daily, with gradual reduction by 5 to 10 mg every 4 to 7 days. About 10% of patients have a recurrence after 3 or 4 weeks of corticosteroids and require a second course of therapy. Following recovery from moderate and severe episodes a transient hypothyroidism lasting 1 to 3 weeks may occur in 30% to 50% of patients. Thyroid damage leading to permanent hypothyroidism rarely develops in this disease.

CHRONIC LYMPHOCYTIC THYROIDITIS (HASHIMOTO'S THYROIDITIS). Chronic lymphocytic thyroiditis (Hashimoto's or autoimmune thyroiditis) is believed to be an autoimmune disease with development of multiple types of thyroid autoantibodies to thyroid proteins. It is a common disorder, accounting for over 90% of nontoxic diffuse goiter in children and over 50% in adults. It is far more frequent in women than in men and occurs most commonly between the ages of 20 and 50 years. A family history is present in over 70%, and Graves' disease also is common in affected families. There is an increased incidence of chronic lymphocytic thyroiditis in patients with other autoimmune disorders such as pernicious anemia, Addison's disease, reumatoid arthritis, systemic lupus erythematosus, Sjögren's syndrome, and chronic hepatitis and in relatives of patients with these diseases. The pathologic changes in the thyroid vary from mild inflammation to total destruction and atrophy. Initially a focal or diffuse infiltration of lymphocytes occurs with gradual destruction of follicle cells and disruption of follicles. Intrafollicular macrophages appear in the disrupted follicles and fibrosis begins. Typical oxyphilic cytoplasmic changes occur in follicle cells, which are called Askanazy or Hürthle cells and are considered almost pathognomonic of the disease. With time, extensive fibrosis and destruction of thyroid follicles occur, not infrequently leading to hypothyroidism, thyroid atrophy, and nodularity of the remaining thyroid tissue.

The initial clinical feature is usually a small or medium-sized, nontender (very slightly tender in about 10%), diffuse goiter that is slightly firmer than normal or rubbery in consistency. The goiter gradually enlarges over several years and becomes firmer, more bosselated, and somewhat nodular, but the nodules are usually of similar consistency and indistinct.

About 20% of the patients initially have hypothyroidism. In children about 50% have spontaneous recovery after several months. A significant number of patients with lymphocytic (silent) thyroiditis have transient hypothyroidism. Occasionally, localized lymphadenopathy, vocal cord paralysis, and compression of the trachea and esophagus occur, especially with large goiter. In these cases malignancy must be ruled out by biopsy or surgical excision.

The diagnosis is established by the combination of clinical features and laboratory studies. The finding of a firm, diffusely enlarged thyroid is frequently the main criterion used to make the diagnosis. The T_4 and T_3 levels are usually normal, but the PBI may be elevated owing to the release of nonhormonal iodoproteins from the damaged thyroid follicles. In euthyroid patients, 10% to 20% have elevated baseline levels of TSH and up to 50% have lack of thyroid reserve shown by an excessive TSH response to TRH stimulation. The RAIU may be normal or increased, suggesting hyperthyroidism, but TSH stimulation does not increase the RAIU further. These responses to TRH and TSH stimulation indicate lack of thyroid reserve and an already maximally stimulated thyroid. Further confirmation of the diagnosis is made by the finding of high titers of thyroid antibodies; however, in 30% to 50% of patients antibody test results are negative or titers are low and thus nondiagnostic. Needle biopsy leads to definitive histologic diagnosis and should be used in problem cases or in index cases in families with a history of goiter. Differentiation of chronic lymphocytic thyroiditis from other types of diffuse goiter by clinical and laboratory tests without biopsy is accurate in only 70% to 80% of cases. However, further clarification of the diagnosis is unnecessary, since the treatment is the same, that is, suppressive doses of thyroid hormone. Differentiation from thyroid carcinoma is usually not difficult because thyroid carcinoma occurs as a single, hard nodule and chronic lymphocytic thyroiditis occurs as a firm, rubbery, diffusely enlarged thyroid.

SCLEROSING THYROIDITIS (REIDEL'S THYROIDITIS). Sclerosing thyroiditis (Reidel's thyroiditis) is an extremely rare form of thyroiditis characterized by extensive fibrosis and fixation of the thyroid to adjacent structures. It is often associated with mediastinal and retroperitoneal fibrosis and frequently causes symptoms by compressing adjacent structures such as the trachea, esophagus, and recurrent laryngeal nerves. The thyroid is slightly or moderately enlarged and nontender but strikingly hard and fixed, suggesting carcinoma. The presence of associated mediastinal and retinal peritoneal fibrosis should prompt suspicion of the disease. Biopsy is usually performed to establish the diagnosis. Thyroid tests are usually normal, but hypothyroidism does occur. Surgery may be necessary to relieve local obstruction and nerve compression.

Adenomas

Adenomas of the thyroid are benign neoplasms classified according to their histologic characteristics (embryonal, fetal, microfollicular, macrofollicular, papillary cystadenoma, and Hürthle cell). They usually grow slowly and almost imperceptibly over years. They frequently have a well-developed capsule and do not invade blood vessels or the capsular structure. The rest of the thyroid is normal, unlike the thyroid in nontoxic multinodular goiter. Most follicular adenomas retain some ability to concentrate iodine and synthesize thyroid hormone. Hyperthyroidism may occur when the nodule is 2.5 to 3 cm or greater. Thyroid function tests are usually normal. The thyroid scan shows a cold area in the nonfunctioning adenomas and an increased uptake of iodine in the functioning nodules. The cold nodules require needle biopsy, aspiration cytology, or surgical excision to exclude malignancy. The presence of a functioning nodule is usually evidence against thyroid malignancy, since functioning follicular carcinomas of the thyroid rarely concentrate iodine well. The functioning nodules may simply be observed, but because a few may grow slowly with time and produce hyperthyroidism, surgical excision or ablation with radioactive iodine can be done.

THYROID CYSTS. Thyroid cysts and hemorrhage into thyroid cysts or thyroid parenchyma account for the majority of the nonmalignant single nodules in the thyroid. These lesions usually arise from thyroid adenomas or from the nodules in nontoxic multinodular goiter. Some adenomas contain single or multiloculated cysts. Acute hemorrhage into the thyroid cyst or into the thyroid parenchyma probably occurs as the result of rupture of the fragile new blood vessels in these lesions. Hemorrhage into the thyroid may develop suddenly as a painful nodule, but most often appears as an asymptomatic nodule found by the patient, a relative, or the physician. These hemorrhagic nodules may be discovered first at the time of aspiration of a nodule for cytology or by ultrasonography. They may slowly resolve spontaneously. Occasionally necrosis of the center of a malignant nodule occurs, forming a cyst. Sometimes a single asymptomatic thyroid nodule that is cold on the thyroid scan is found to be due to subacute or granulomatous thyroiditis on surgical biopsy.

Carcinoma of the thyroid

Thyroid cancer is rare and accounts for less than 1% of all malignancies. Its annual incidence is about 25 cases per million people. In autopsy series as many as 0.1% of thyroids are found to have small or microscopic papillary cancers that are of low-grade malignancy and questionable clinical significance. Malignant neoplasms of the thyroid are usually of four types: papillary or papillary-follicular, follicular, anaplastic, and medullary, although occasionally a primary lymphoma, lymphosarcoma, or sarcoma of the thyroid is found as well as metastatic malignancy from other areas of the body. The degree of malignancy varies considerably among these different thyroid tumors. Thyroid carcinomas usually occur as single nodules.

PAPILLARY CARCINOMA. Papillary and papillary-follicular carcinoma are considered to be the same kind of tumor. This relatively benign form of malignancy accounts for 50% or more of the cases of carcinoma of the thyroid and for nearly all the thyroid cancer that occurs in children and young adults. In recent years an epidemic of papillary carcinoma of the thyroid has occurred in young adults 5 to 20 years after they received radiotherapy of the head, neck, or chest for multiple reasons such as enlarged thymus, birthmarks, enlarged tonsils, and acne vulgaris. Papillary carcinoma usually occurs as an asymptomatic nodule in the normal thyroid and occasionally spreads to other areas of the thyroid or to the adjacent lymph nodes. It tends to be more malignant in those over 50 years of age. Distant metastases are unusual. The tumor may or may not be encapsulated. Histologic examination reveals masses of columnar epithelial cells arranged in papillary projections, with a significant number having some follicular structural features. These tumors do not accumulate radioactive iodine to any extent.

FOLLICULAR CARCINOMA. Follicular carcinoma accounts for about 25% of the cases of thyroid carcinoma. It generally occurs between 40 and 60 years of age. Its degree of malignancy varies considerably, but it is usually more malignant than the papillary type. It has a tendency for hematogenous spread via invasion of blood vessels to the lung, liver, and bone. The usual initial clinical feature is as a slow-growing, asymptomatic nodule in the thyroid like the papillary carcinoma, but occasionally metastatic lesions to bone or lung are found initially. Follicular carcinoma is generally more malignant in older people. The tumor is usually encapsulated and the histology varies greatly. At times histologic features appear completely benign to the pathologist and malignancy is proved only by the finding of distant metastases. These tumors sometimes accumulate radioactive iodine and synthesize thyroid hormone so that thyrotoxicosis occurs when bulky masses of the tumor are present, although this is rare.

ANAPLASTIC CARCINOMA. Anaplastic carcinoma of the thyroid accounts for about 10% of thyroid malignancies. It most often occurs in patients over 50 years of age and is slightly more common in females. The malignancy usually is a rapidly growing lesion invading adjacent structures and metastasizing throughout the body. The tumors are unencapsulated and composed of anaplastic small or large cells with numerous mitoses. The clinical course is one of rapid growth of a neck mass that is sometimes painful and tender. Involvement of local structures occurs early in the course, causing hoarseness, tracheal obstruction, and difficulty in swallowing. There are also problems from distant metastases in brain, liver, and lung. The tumor mass is usually extremely hard and fixed. A rapid downhill course usually occurs, leading to death within 3 to 6 months.

MEDULLARY CARCINOMA. Medullary carcinoma arises from the C cells of the thyroid. It accounts for 5% to 10% of thyroid carcinoma and is more malignant than follicular carcinoma. It usually spreads by lymphatic channels within the thyroid to adjacent lymph nodes. It is sporadic in about half the cases and is caused by autosomal dominant inheritance in the rest. The hereditary variety, multiple endocrine neoplasia type IIA (MEN IIA), Sipple's syndrome), is associated with pheochromocytoma, parathyroid adenoma, carcinoid syndrome, and Cushing's syndrome. A syndrome called MEN IIB is similar to MEN IIA but also includes mucosal neuromas and marfanoid appearance. These tumors secrete calcitonin, which can be used to monitor results of treatment. C-cell hyperplasia precedes the appearance of the medullary carcinoma in the hereditary variety and can be detected by finding elevated baseline serum calcitonin concentrations or an excessive response of the serum calcitonin to pentagastrin or calcium infusion. Family members of patients with medullary carcinoma of the thyroid should be checked every 1 to 2 years with these tests for occult carcinoma or C-cell hyperplasia. These tumors tend to be multicentric in the hereditary form but not in the sporadic variety. The finding of large amounts of amyloid material in histologic sections aids in the diagnosis.

DIAGNOSIS AND MANAGEMENT. The main concern in the patient with the single nodule is to determine if it represents thyroid cancer. There are certain clinical features and laboratory tests that help differentiate cancerous nodules from other lesions and point out those that are more likely to be carcinoma. Since most benign single nodules occur in patients over 40 years of age and in women, the presence of a nodule in a patient of either sex under 40 years of age and in a man at any age makes carcinoma more likely. Also, anyone with a thyroid nodule and a history of irradiation of the head, neck, or chest in infancy or childhood should be considered to have carcinoma unless proved otherwise. Fixation of the thyroid, vocal cord paralysis, and enlarged anterior neck lymph nodes also increase the possibility of thyroid malignancy, as does nonfunction of the nodule on the thyroid scan. Some characteristics make a nodule less likely to be malignant. These in-

clude (1) presence in a multinodular gland (unless in a child); (2) thyroid cysts; (3) ability to concentrate iodine on the thyroid scan; (4) presence for years without growth; (5) nodules shown to be calcified on roentgenographic examination; and (6) benign classification on the basis of aspiration or needle biopsy cytology.

For years needle biopsy of thyroid nodules was believed to be contraindicated because of the chance of spreading cancer cells. However, in recent years needle biopsy and needle aspiration of single thyroid nodules have been increasingly reported and appear to be helpful in deciding if a nodule is malignant or benign. The tissue and cells obtained by these techniques are classified as benign, malignant, or indeterminant.

Treatment of the uninodular goiter consists of surgical excision of all nodules that fit the clinical criteria for increased malignancy or those classified as malignant or indeterminant by needle biopsy and aspiration. Either a near total thyroidectomy or removal of the lobe and isthmus is done unless there is local spread, which dictates more radical neck surgery to remove all cancerous tissue. If carcinoma is found and there is evidence of iodine accumulation, large doses (100 to 150 mCi) of ^{131}I are given except with the anaplastic and medullary varieties. Thyroid suppression therapy is also instituted postoperatively in maximal physiologic doses sufficient to keep the T_4 in the upper range of normal, to suppress the TSH to below normal, and to inhibit TSH response to TRH. In the patient with follicular carcinoma of the thyroid, large doses of ^{131}I are given postoperatively to ablate any remaining thyroid tissue and, if possible, to eradicate any residual malignancy. The long-term survival of those with papillary and follicular carcinoma of the thyroid is excellent and exceeds 80% at 10 years in most studies.

The primary mode of treatment of medullary carcinoma of the thyroid is total thyroidectomy. This is also done in family members documented to have increased levels of calcitonin and/or excessive calcitonin response to calcium or pentagastrin infusion, since they are usually found to have C-cell hyperplasia or occult carcinoma. Metastatic disease may respond to some types of chemotherapy.

Anaplastic carcinoma of the thyroid rarely responds to any form of treatment. Usually needle or open biopsy is done to establish the diagnosis, and postoperative radiotherapy may give short-term relief. Chemotherapy should be considered.

When a thyroid cyst is suspected, this can be confirmed by diagnostic ultrasonography or by aspiration, which eradicates most of the mass in addition to obtaining cells for cytologic diagnosis. If the cyst recurs after the first aspiration, this can be repeated three to five times at 1- to 2-month intervals. If the cyst reccurs after three to five aspirations surgical excision is an option, but observation at 6- to 12-month intervals also can be done.

In women over 40 years of age who have nodules of the thyroid but do not have criteria for malignancy, thyroid suppression is begun and follow-up examinations are made at 3- to 6-month intervals. If there is evidence of growth of the lesion during suppression therapy, surgical excision is indicated.

BIBLIOGRAPHY

Brown J and others: Autoimmune thyroid diseases—Graves' and Hashimoto's, Ann Intern Med 88:379, 1978.

Butch RS, Simeone JF, and Mullen PR: Thyroid and parathyroid ultrasonography, Radiol Clin NA 23:57, 1985.

Caplan RH and Kujak R: Thyroid uptake of radioactive iodine: a reevaluation, JAMA 215:916, 1971.

Caplan RH, Pagliara AS, and Wickus G: Laboratory diagnosis of hyperthy-roidism: a reappraisal, Postgrad Med 66:75, 1979.

Chopra IJ: An assessment of daily production and significance of thyroidal secretion of 3,3′5′-triiodothyronine (reverse T₃) in man, J Clin Invest 58:32, 1976.

DeGroot LJ: Thyroid carcinoma, Med Clin North Am 59:1233, 1975.

Dratman MB: The mechanism of thyroxine action. In Li CH, editor: Hormonal proteins and peptides, New York, 1978, Academic Press, Inc.

Grove AS, Jr: Evaluation of exophthalmos, N Engl J Med 292:1005, 1975.

Hamburger JI, Miller JM, and Kini SR: Clinical-pathological evaluation of thyroid nodules—handbook and atlas, Detroit, 1979, private publication.

Hamilton CR, Jr and Maloof F: Unusual types of hyperthyroidism, Medicine 52:195, 1973.

Hollander CS and others: Clinical and laboratory observations in cases of triiodothyronine toxicosis confirmed by radioimmunoassay, Lancet 1:609, 1972.

Ingbar SH and Braverman LE: Werner's the thyroid, ed 5, Philadelphia, 1986, JB Lippincott Co.

Ingbar SH and Woeber KA: The thyroid gland. In Wilson JD, editor: Williams' textbook of endocrinology, ed 7, Philadelphia, 1985, WB Saunders Co.

Mackin JF, Canary JJ, and Pittman CS: Thyroid storm and its management, N Engl J Med 291:1396, 1974.

Miller JM: Plummer's disease, Med Clin North Am 59:1203, 1975.

Mochizuky Y, Mowafy R, and Pasternack B: Weights of human thyroids in New York City, Health Phys 9:1299, 1963.

Nadler NJ: Iodination of thyroglobulin in the thyroid follicle. In Cassano C and Andreoli M, editors: Current topics in thyroid research, New York, 1965, Academic Press, Inc.

Nikolai TF and others: Lymphocytic thyroiditis with spontaneously resolving hyperthyroidism (silent thyroiditis), Arch Intern Med 140:478, 1980.

Ross DD: New sensitive immunoradiometric assays for thyrotropin, Ann Intern Med 104:718, 1986.

Royce PC: Severely impaired consciousness in myxedema—a review, Am J Med Sci 261:46, 1971.

Schimmel M and Utiger RD: Thyroidal and peripheral production of thyroid hormones: review of recent findings and their clinical implications, Ann Intern Med 87:760, 1977.

Solomon DH and others: Identification of subgroups of euthyroid Graves' ophthalmopathy, N Engl J Med 296:181, 1977.

Sterling K: Thyroid hormone action at the cell level, N Engl J Med 300:117, 173, 1979.

Van Herle AJ, Vassart G, and Dumont JE: Control of thyroglobulin synthesis and secretion, N Engl J Med 301:239, 307, 1979.

Volpé R: The role of autoimmunity in hypoendocrine and hyperendocrine function: with special emphasis on autoimmune thyroid disease, Ann Intern Med 87:86, 1977.

Zellmann HE: Iatrogenic and factitious thyroidal disease, Med Clin North Am 63:329, 1979.

188 · THE ADRENAL CORTEX

Francis H. Sterling and Ernest M. Gold*

INTRODUCTION

Diseases related to the hormones of the adrenal cortex present special problems in dental practice. Although disorders of the adrenal glands themselves are uncommon, the therapeutic use of adrenal steroid hormones (glucocorticoids) is quite common and recognition of the consequences is not always easy. Although it is routine practice to inquire about medications before initiating dental procedures, patients often do not think of ointments and skin creams, nose drops, and sinus preparations, as drugs. Any of these may contain potent glucocorticoids that not only depress immunity, wound healing, and hemostasis but also enhance bone loss. Used occasionally, these preparations present no problem, but continuous use for many weeks can result in Cushing's syndrome. Rapid withdrawal of steroids may cause adrenal insufficiency.

---

*Deceased.

It is the purpose of this chapter to review the anatomy, biochemistry, physiology, and pathophysiology of the adrenal cortex, emphasizing those features of special importance in dentistry.

STRUCTURE AND FUNCTION

The adrenal gland is best thought of as a group of glands juxtaposed for special function. The adrenal medulla, whose major products are the catecholamines, epinephrine (adrenalin), and norepinephrine (noradrenalin), is enveloped by the adrenal cortex, whose major products are steroid hormones—glucocorticoid, mineralocorticoid, and androgen. The only physiologic glucocorticoid in humans is cortisol (hydrocortisone) and the major mineralcorticoid is aldosterone.

The blood supply to the adrenal glands is unusual. Unlike the kidney with its single artery and single vein, each adrenal gland, nestled on top of the kidney just under the diaphragm, has 30 or 40 arterioles perforating its capsule. These arise from three arteries: the inferior diaphragmatic, the aorta, and the renal arteries. Anastomoses just under the capsule allow the blood to percolate through the cortex to the medulla, thereby delivering a concentration of cortisol not achieved anywhere else in the body. This high concentration induces the enzyme that converts norepinephrine to epinephrine. Each adrenal gland has only one adrenal vein, which empties into the inferior vena cava on the right and the renal vein on the left.

The adrenal cortex has three zones. The outermost zona glomerulosa produces the salt hormone (mineralocorticoid) aldosterone, which causes the kidney (and some other tissues) to retain sodium and excrete potassium and hydrogen ions. The major clinical problems arising from too much or too little aldosterone are levels of serum potassium that are too low or too high, respectively. The zona glomerulosa has a complex regulation but for clinical purposes the major stimuli to the zona glomerulosa are the peptide angiotensin II and potassium.

The zona fasciculata and the innermost zona reticularis can be thought of as a single gland controlled by adrenocorticotropic hormone (ACTH) from the pituitary, which stimulates both cortisol and androgen production. Evidence indicates another pituitary androgen-stimulating hormone exists but it seems to be of minor clinical importance.

BIOSYNTHESIS OF STEROID HORMONES. Steroid hormones are modified cholesterol molecules produced in the nonpregnant adults principally by the adrenal cortex and gonads. (An exception would be vitamin D, which is in fact a steroid hormone.) The placenta also produces large quantities of steroids. The usual source of cholesterol for the adrenal cortex is the circulating low-density lipoprotein complex, although when necessary the adrenal cells can make cholesterol from acetate. The receptor-mediated "ingestion" of the circulating lipoprotein complex by adrenal cells makes feasible radionuclide scans of the adrenal area by injecting radioactive cholesterol.

As noted in Figure 188-1, cholesterol is converted to pregnenolone by two steps. The first step is removing the side chain from cholesterol after two hydroxylations. The 21 carbon–steroid pregnenolone can give rise to mineralocorticoid, glucocorticoid, or androgen. The second step removes hydrogen and transposes a double bond to produce progesterone. Progesterone is made in all zones of the adrenal, as well as the gonads. In the inner zones of the adrenal gland, progesterone is successively hydroxylated on positions 17, 21, and 11 to become cortisol, the only physiologic glucocorticoid in humans. In the zona glomerulosa, it is hydroxylated at positions 21 and 18 and then reduced at position 18 to become aldosterone, the most important mineralocorticoid. In the inner zones

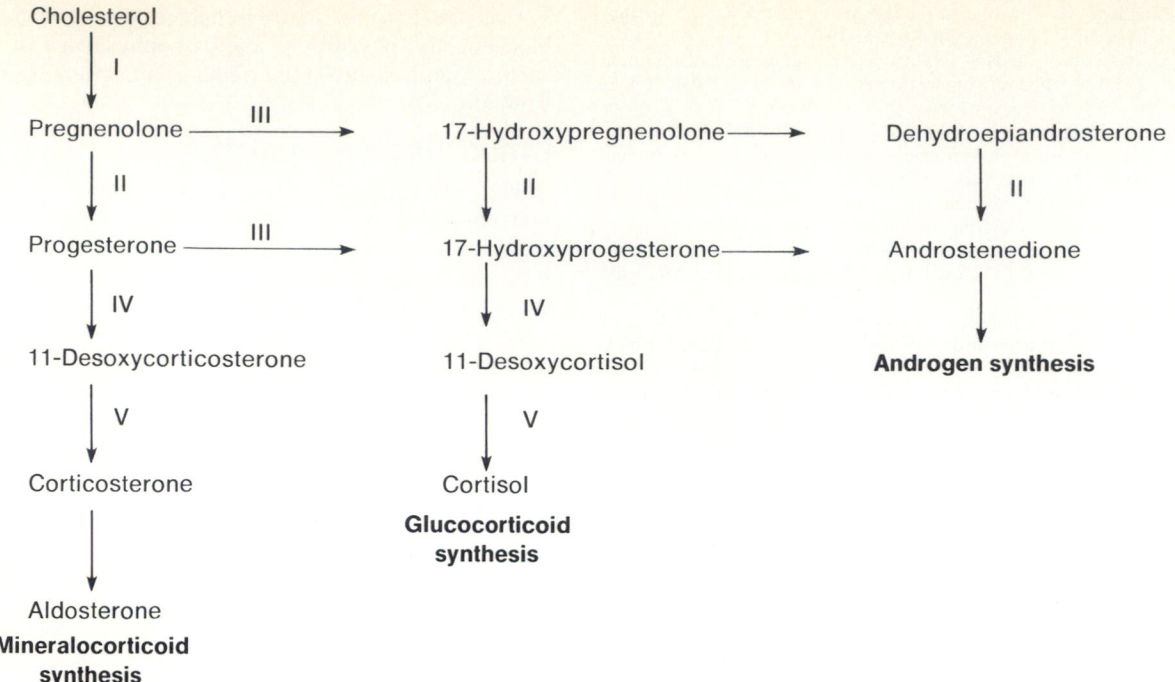

Fig. 188-1   Pathways of steroid biosynthesis, *I*, 20 and 22 hydroxylases, 20, 22 desmolase; *II*, 3-β-OH dehydrogenase; *III*, 17-α-hydroxylase; *IV*, 21-hydroxylase; *V*, 11-β-hydroxylase.

of the adrenal gland, as in the gonad, progesterone can be converted to androgen. Unlike the gonad, the adrenal does not normally convert the androgens to estrogens via aromatization. If there is a deficiency or imbalance of any of these enzymatic steps, either because of congenital enzyme deficiency or tumors of the adrenal, a number of diseases can result from various combinations of excesses or deficiencies of glucocorticoid, mineralocorticoid, or sex hormones. These adrenogenital syndromes are discussed below.

METABOLISM AND TRANSPORT. When steroid hormones are released into the circulation, they associate with carrier proteins produced mainly by the liver. Although these proteins have names such as cortisol-binding globulin (CBG) and sex hormone–binding globulin (SHBG), it is unwarranted to conclude that transport is their only, or even their major, function. They are clinically important because an increase or decrease in the binding protein alters plasma hormone levels and suggests endocrine disease when none is present, since it is the unbound or free hormone level that correlates best with disease. The most common cause of a high plasma cortisol level is pregnancy or birth control pill use, since estrogen markedly increases synthesis of any binding protein. However, the free plasma cortisol level is normal in these circumstances. Similarly, men treated with female hormones for prostate cancer routinely have plasma cortisol levels twice the upper limit of normal, but there is no adrenal disease. Again, the free hormone level is normal.

All steroids are metabolized by reduction of double bonds (hydrogenases or reductases), thereby inactivating the steroid. They then are conjugated to make them water soluble (usually to sulfate or glucuronide) so that the kidney can excrete them. Nearly all steroids are excreted in the urine.

Disease, especially liver disease, and drugs may alter the metabolism of steroids. This becomes a problem when patients are taking exogenous steroids for replacement or therapy. For example, 30 mg of hydrocortisone is the usual replacement

dose for a healthy adult. It might, however, be inadequate in an alcoholic whose rate of degradation of drugs often is accelerated. Similarly, the use of anticonvulsants or certain antibiotics accelerates the nonspecific degradative hepatic enzymes so that the normal dose of 30 mg might be insufficient.

CELLULAR ACTION. There is little evidence for active transport of steroid hormones into cells. They enter all cells, not because they are fat-soluble but because they are water-insoluble. Steroid molecules that are not bound to transport proteins are "pushed out" of the water in the plasma into the water in the cell. They pass through the phospholipid bilayer of the cell membrane as light passes through a window pane and on through the similar membranes of the various organelles in the cell until an equilibrium is achieved. Various steroid hormones more often enter some tissues than others, because if the cell contains receptor proteins, the steroid is effectively removed from the aqueous phase. The steroid receptor proteins are especially concentrated in the nucleus. The union of steroid and receptor protein changes the shape of the latter so that it "fits" and can interact with a particular part of the DNA to effect the production of specific mRNA (transcription). The particular mRNA then moves to ribosomes to initiate production of a unique protein (translation). For example, one of the numerous roles of cortisol is initiating the synthesis of each enzyme required for gluconeogenesis. This contributes to the elevation of the blood sugar by this "sugar hormone" or glucocorticoid.

PHYSIOLOGIC ACTION. In considering the actions of hormones, it is important to distinguish the effect of a physiologic quantity given to an individual who lacks the hormone from that of a pharmacologic amount given to a normal person. For example, a patient who lacks adrenal glands is generally ill, loses weight, and becomes immunologically impaired. Physiologic daily replacement doses of steroids equivalent to 30 mg of cortisol or 7.5 mg of prednisone restore good health, weight, and immunity. 7.5 mg of prednisone daily has little effect on the immune system of a normal person. However, the doses of prednisone used to treat autoimmune disease, (60 mg/day) are severely immunosuppressive and often lead to life-threatening infections. Until the advent of the acquired immune deficiency syndrome (AIDS) epidemic, pharmacologic doses of glucocorticoids were the major cause of immunodeficiency diseases.

The physiologic role of cortisol is to enable adaptation to a stressful environment via complex interactions with a number of other hormones. The best way to appreciate the physiologic role of cortisol is to consider the consequences of cortisol deficiency. In general, cortisol helps to maintain blood pressure, blood volume, blood sugar levels, appetite, and a feeling of well-being.

The role of mineralocorticoid is better defined. Aldosterone, in conjunction with many other hormones, helps to maintain blood volume, and it is the major regulator of serum potassium. The hormone causes reabsorption of sodium in exchange for potassium or hydrogen ions in the distal nephron, as well as in some nonadrenal tissues, such as salivary glands and the colon. Most potassium present in the urine is there because of the effect of aldosterone on the distal nephron.

PHYSIOLOGIC REGULATION. Cortisol, the most vital adrenal hormone, is regulated by ACTH produced in the corticotroph of the anterior pituitary. ACTH, a 39 amino acid peptide, is regulated in turn by several neurohormones produced in the hypothalamus just above the pituitary. The most important of these is a 41 amino acid peptide called corticotropin-releasing factor or hormone (CRF or CRH). The capillary blood perfuses this median eminence of the hypothalamus, which hangs like a nipple above the pituitary, and then runs down the pituitary stalk venules to deliver the tiny but highly concentrated quantities of CRF (the hypothalamic-pituitary portal system). ACTH is then released into the general circulation where its major target is the adrenal cortex.

There is a true diurnal variation in the secretion of ACTH and cortisol. The highest values occur early in the morning and the lowest values late at night. Cortisol feeds back on both the pituitary and the brain to inhibit ACTH. Excess glucocorticoid administration suppresses both the pituitary and hypothalamic hormones, but physiologic increases in cortisol, such as the early morning peaks, do not suppress corticotroph. Stress easily overrides any suppression of the corticotroph by quantities of glucocorticoids that are within the physiologic range. In addition, ACTH stimulates androgen production by the adrenal, but there is new evidence for another pituitary peptide that has a more specific effect on adrenal androgen production.

ACTH also has some minor influence on mineralcorticoid production. ACTH injection is a powerful, acute but not chronic stimulus to the zona glomerulosa and causes a prompt rise in aldosterone. If a patient remains supine all day, the diurnal variation of aldosterone parallels that of cortisol, that is, it is highest before arising in the morning and lowest at night. But the physiologic regulation of aldosterone production is mainly accomplished by the renin-angiotensin system and by serum potassium. Because this system is triggered by standing, aldosterone is higher 4 hours after arising in the morning. Aldosterone defends against low blood volumes and hyperkalemia.

In response to real or perceived (heart failure) low blood volume, the kidneys secrete an enzyme called renin from the juxtaglomerular apparatus into the general circulation. Angiotensinogen, an α_2-globulin manufactured in the liver and cleaved by plasma proteases, is shortened to a substrate for renin. Renin cleaves the renin substrate to result in a 10 amino acid peptide called angiotensin I. This is shortened again to an 8 amino acid peptide, angiotensin II, by an aminopeptidase called the angiotensin-converting enzyme (ACE) found in highest concentration in the pulmonary capillaries. Angiotensin II in the circulation has two important functions. It is a powerful arteriolar vasoconstrictor, raising blood pressure; it also is the major regulator of the secretion of aldosterone, which helps maintain blood volume by retaining sodium. As blood volume is restored, renin secretion is suppressed.

If the serum potassium level rises, it directly stimulates the zona glomerulosa to release aldosterone. Aldosterone in turn causes the distal nephron to secrete potassium (or hydrogen ion) in exchange for sodium. As the potassium is excreted, aldosterone secretion returns to normal.

One might expect that, if the renin-angiotensin-aldosterone system were activated by hypovolemia, hypokalemia would be a consequence. This does not happen for reasons discussed below (see "Hyperaldosteronism"). The renin-angiotensin system as described above is the circulating system for the regulation of aldosterone. However, angiotensinogen, renin, and the converting enzyme are also produced in the brain where angiotensin II regulates the sympathetic outflow from the area postrema. The whole system also operates in the walls of certain blood vessels, thereby regulating the microcirculation. These and other "micro" systems are unrelated to aldosterone secretion.

GLUCOCORTICOID DEFICIENCY SYNDROMES

Deficiency of glucocorticoid can result from:

1. Destruction of the adrenal cortex with or without destruction of the adrenal medulla (Addison's disease)
2. Lack of stimulation of the adrenal cortex by ACTH resulting from disease of the pituitary or hypothalamus (or chronic suppression of the pituitary and hypothalamus by exogenous steroid followed by sudden steroid withdrawal)
3. Defective hormonogenesis as a result of congenital or acquired enzyme deficiencies (including adrenogenital syndromes)

DEFINITIONS. *Primary adrenal failure*, or Addison's disease, is the term applied to destruction of the adrenal cortex. Addison's 1855 description is as valid today as ever: "general languor and debility, remarkable feebleness of the heart's action, irritability of the stomach, and peculiar change in the color of the skin." The feebleness of the heart's action reflects hypotension and hypovolemia, the irritability of the stomach indicates chronic vomiting and inability to sustain nutrition, and the altered skin color results from hypersecretion of ACTH and related pituitary peptides. Since the patients lack both glucocorticoid and mineralocorticoid, death usually occurs unless steroids are administered.

Secondary adrenal failure is a consequence of ACTH deficiency. These patients are rarely as ill as patients with Addison's disease for several reasons. Pituitary insufficiency is often partial; associated hypothyroidism decreases the amount of cortisol necessary for maintenance; and most important, these patients have aldosterone, which prevents severe hypotension and hyperkalemia. Although they suffer from weakness and languor, patients with hypopituitarism often live undiagnosed for decades. They survive until infection or other stress intervenes.

Special mention must be made regarding patients who recently have been treated with pharmacologic doses of glucocorticoids, such as 20 mg of prednisone or more daily. When the dose of prednisone is abruptly reduced to a physiologic amount, these patients may appear normal, but their hypothalamic pituitary adrenal axis is still suppressed. Therefore if

Table 188-1 Causes of adrenal failure

Type	Cause
Primary adrenal failure (Addison's disease)	AIDS Idiopathic atrophy—autoimmune adrenalitis Infectious diseases—tuberculosis, overwhelming bacteremia Infiltrative diseases—amyloidosis, carcinoma Vascular disorders—hemorrhage, infarction, anticoagulant therapy Iatrogenic—surgical ablation
Secondary adrenal failure (ACTH deficiency)	Pituitary disorders—tumors, necrosis Hypothalamic disorders—tumors, trauma, granulomatous disease, iatrogenic—surgery, steroid therapy

steroids are suddenly withdrawn or if stress such as dental surgery is superimposed, these patients may develop an adrenal crisis unless steroids are augmented to at least twice the usual daily replacement dose.

Defective hormonogenesis results in cortisol deficiency, usually as a result of a congenital enzyme dificiency. In the case of a partially deficient enzyme, cortisol tends to be low and ACTH high, since feedback inhibition by cortisol is minimal. The adrenals became large. Depending on which enzyme is missing, androgen or mineralocorticoid may accumulate. (See below.)

ETIOLOGY AND PATHOGENESIS. Table 188-1 lists the causes of adrenal failure. Worldwide, infections are the most common cause. Addison's original patients suffered from tuberculosis of the adrenal gland. With the control of infectious disease, Addison's disease became rare. Although autoimmune destruction of the adrenal cortex became the most common cause in the United States for some time, this is no longer the case. The recent epidemic of AIDS has spurred a resurgence of adrenal insufficiency from tuberculosis, histoplasmosis, and a variety of other infections. Autoimmune adrenal destruction follows the infiltration of the adrenal cortex with lymphocytes presumably directed against adrenal antigens. The cause is unknown but probably is multifactorial. Autoimmune adrenal deficiency may be associated with other endocrine deficiencies as well, such as autoimmune hypothyroidism and type I diabetes mellitus. Infiltrative diseases rarely cause adrenal insufficiency, since more than 90% of the gland must be destroyed before symptoms occur. Metastases to the adrenal gland occur commonly in certain cancers such as lung cancer. Again, adrenal insufficiency rarely is diagnosed. Hemorrhage into both adrenal glands is a well-known complication of anticoagulant therapy.

Secondary adrenal insufficiency can occur from any destructive lesion of the anterior pituitary gland or the hypothalamus and usually is associated with abnormalities of other pituitary hormones. Rarely isolated deficiency of ACTH occurs. Pituitary disease in the adult often is due to tumors which result not only in deficient ACTH and cortisol but can lead to excessive amounts of other hormones. For example, a tumor could secrete thyroid-stimulating hormone and trigger hyperthyroidism but also compress the normal pituitary to cause loss of ACTH. The most common cause of secondary adrenal insufficiency is cessation of exogenous steroid therapy of usually longer than 3 weeks.

CLINICAL MANIFESTATIONS. Adrenal failure occurs as either an acute or chronic syndrome. Acute adrenal failure may result from acute destruction of the adrenal gland from bilateral hemorrhage or necrosis (anticoagulant therapy, trauma, or sep-

sis-induced coagulopathy); however, it is more likely to occur as the result of acute stress (infection and even minor surgery) in a patient who already has partial adrenal insuffficiency. Either way, the clinical features are those of shock. There may be fever or even hypothermia if the blood sugar level is low. Because the findings are in no way specific for adrenal failure and because of the life-threatening situation, this is one of the few times in medicine that the patient is treated first and diagnosed later. (See below.)

Chronic adrenal failure may be insidious and develop over months or years. Depending on the degree to which the glands have been destroyed, the patients may be profoundly weak and wasted with hypotension, especially when standing, or they may function fairly normally and experience weakness and inanition only when under some stress. The patients tend to become hypoglycemic because of impaired gluconeogenesis. Weight loss and hyperpigmentation are almost universal features of chronic adrenal insufficiency. The pigmentation is a function of excess ACTH and related peptides secreted by the pituitary as well as the baseline coloration of the skin. The hyperpigmentation may be less striking in a very fair patient than in an olive-skinned patient, and black individuals may become intensely black. Parts of the skin that are normally dark such as the areola of the breast, the genitalia, freckles and moles, and pressure points such as the elbows and knees are likely to show prominent pigmentation. New scars that form while the plasma ACTH is elevated are likely to be hyperpigmented. The dentist may notice diffuse or speckled pigmentation in the mouth, especially the dentate margin of the gums and the lips, tongue, and buccal mucosa. Pigmentation in the mouth is quite normal in dark complexioned individuals such as Indians and blacks but is distinctly unusual in patients who are normally fair skinned.

DIAGNOSIS. The diagnosis of adrenal insufficiency is based on the demonstration of the adrenal gland's inability to secrete enough cortisol in response to synthetic ACTH (cosyntropin) to raise the plasma cortisol to the level usually seen in stress. In the morning, the plasma cortisol normally is between 5 and 25 μg/dl, but during periods of extreme stress it may rise to 50 or 60 μg/dl. Symptoms of adrenal insufficiency are rare in patients whose levels rise to 20 μg/dl, but there are exceptions. Patients with only partial destruction of the glands who maintain the plasma level in the mid-normal range fare well in normal circumstances but not under stress.

There are various protocols for ACTH stimulation tests. A simple screening test involves measuring plasma cortisol 30 minutes after intramuscular injection of 0.25 mg cosyntropin. There is normally an increase of at least 7 μg/dl and the absolute cortisol rises above 18 μg/dl. To definitely rule out adrenal insufficiency, however, it must be demonstrated that the plasma cortisol can rise above the upper limit of normal. If this simple test results in a plasma cortisol above 25 μg/dl, it is highly unlikely that the patient's symptoms are a consequence of adrenal insufficiency. If the values are equivocal, a more definitive test is needed to rule out partial adrenal insufficiency.

To do this it is not necessary to increase the quantity of cosyntropin; the same 0.25 mg should be given intravenously over a more prolonged period, such as 8 hours. Patients whose adrenal glands have atrophied because of chronic ACTH deficiency may require even more prolonged stimulation, such as infusions every 8 hours for 3 days. Plasma cortisol increases stepwise on each day, eventually resulting in a plasma cortisol level greater than 25 μg/dl.

The standard test for diagnosing secondary adrenal insufficiency is the metyrapone test. Metyrapone blocks the last step in the synthesis of cortisol—the addition of a hydroxyl group at the 11 position. As the plasma cortisol falls, the normal response of the pituitary gland is to secrete ACTH, thereby stimulating the adrenal gland to secrete cortisol lacking that hydroxyl group (11 desoxycortisol). Both cortisol and 11 desoxycortisol should be measured before and after administration of the drug to ascertain that cortisol production was inhibited.

Metyrapone has traditionally been given in dosages of 750 mg every 4 hours for six doses. Because the duration of action of metyrapone is short, it is more reliable to administer 500 mg every 2 hours for 12 doses. Patients with active hepatic metabolism (alcoholics or patients on anticonvulsants, for example), may require even higher doses.

A rise in the plasma 11 desoxycortisol above 10 µg/dl indicates that the hypothalamic pituitary adrenal axis is intact. A poor response to metyrapone and an adequate response to exogenous ACTH indicates hypothalamic or pituitary disease. If the etiologic factors are not obvious, hypothalamic or pituitary disease could be identified by measuring plasma ACTH following administration of corticotropin-releasing hormone, but this is rarely necessary.

MANAGEMENT

Acute adrenal insufficiency. Although adrenal insufficiency is a rare cause of hypotensive illness, a patient who develops manifestations suggesting acute adrenal insufficiency should be given hydrocortisone without waiting for test results to confirm the diagnosis. Physiologic—not pharmacologic—doses of hydrocortisone for a few days (until the diagnosis is clarified) will not cause immunosuppression, impair wound healing, or cause complications and will be life-saving if there is adrenal insufficiency.

The amount of glucocorticoid for addisonian crisis is three times the usual 30 mg replacement dose. Generally 100 mg of hydrocortisone is administered intravenously, along with hydration and other supportive measures. If the patient is extremely ill, this dose may have to be repeated in 8 hours. There is a tendency to overtreat the patient with addisonian crisis; since there is no test to monitor the adequacy of therapy in Addison's disease, the clinical response must be relied on.

No mineralocorticoid therapy is necessary in a patient who receives more than 60 mg of hydrocortisone per day because cortisol also has some mineralocorticoid effect.

Chronic adrenal insufficiency. The usual replacement dose is 20 mg of cortisol in the morning and 10 mg in the evening. This is an attempt to mimic the diurnal variation. The dose varies somewhat from one individual to another. Measuring plasma or urinary cortisol is useless in assessing efficacy of treatment since the hormone rapidly enters cells. The dose is increased in patients who have postural hypotension, weakness, anorexia, and inability to secrete a water load; the dose is decreased in patients with plethora, weight gain, muscle weakness, or hypertension. During periods of stress such as fever, patients should double the dosage for several days if the illness is transient and seek medical supervision if it persists. Since the cortisol must be administered parenterally if the patient is unable to eat, the patient should wear a Medic Alert bracelet and both the patient and his family must be given appropriate instructions.

Only one oral mineralocorticoid is commercially available, 9 α-fluoro-hydrocortisone (Florinef). The usual dose is 0.1 mg/day. Not all patients require mineralocorticoid, but hyperkalemia is the principal manifestation of mineralocorticoid deficiency. The only parenteral mineralocorticoid is 11 desoxycorticosterone, but parenteral mineralocorticoid is rarely required.

In hypopituitarism, mineralocorticoid is unnecessary since aldosterone production is independent of ACTH.

For patients with adrenal insufficiency who undergo routine dental procedures, the dose of hydrocortisone should be doubled on the day of the procedure. If general anesthesia is required, higher doses should be given under medical supervision.

GLUCOCORTICOID EXCESS SYNDROMES

DEFINITION

Pituitary Cushing's syndrome. When the glucocorticoid excess is caused by excess ACTH of pituitary origin clinicians have traditionally called this Cushing's *disease*. All other clinical conditions have been referred to as Cushing's syndrome. The pathologic condition in the pituitary gland may be an ACTH-secreting neoplasm or hyperplasia of the ACTH-secreting cells (corticotrophs). Regardless of the cause, the corticotrophs generally behave like a turned-up thermostat. That is, they are not truly autonomous but require a higher than normal amount of cortisol to suppress ACTH secretion. The plasma ACTH level may be only slightly elevated but the usual diurnal variation and the normal decrease in steroid production in the evening and night do not occur. Only a small amount of ACTH is necessary to maintain these hyperplastic glands.

If adrenal hyperfunction is due to ACTH, clinical effects of excess androgen, glucocorticoid, and mineralocorticoid will be present. The mineralocorticoid effect is due to cortisol, not aldosterone. Since ACTH stimulates aldosterone only acutely, the renin-angiotensin-aldosterone system tends to be suppressed.

Iatrogenic Cushing's syndrome. Iatrogenic Cushing's syndrome is due to exogenous steroid administration. Since the usual steroids used to treat inflammatory disease, such as prednisone, have little mineralocorticoid activity, the iatrogenic syndrome has less hypokalemia and no clinical manifestations of androgen or ACTH (pigmentation) effect.

Adrenal Cushing's syndrome. Adrenal Cushing's syndrome results from an adrenal tumor that may be benign or malignant. Not all adrenal tumors secrete hormones, but those that do, especially if malignant, tend to secrete relatively more androgen. The virilization is therefore more striking than that seen in pituitary Cushing's syndrome.

Ectopic ACTH production. Although many kinds of tumors can secrete ACTH, the most common source is lung cancer. Generally the diagnosis of cancer is obvious and the patients are very ill. The tumors can sometimes be occult. As a rule the ACTH level in the plasma is much higher than in pituitary Cushing's syndrome, as is the plasma cortisol level. The reason is that ACTH production by a tumor usually is truly autonomous, unlike that in pituitary Cushing's syndrome. Accordingly, the protein catabolic state and hypokalemia are much more striking in ectopic ACTH syndrome.

CLINICAL MANIFESTATIONS. The clinical manifestations of pituitary Cushing's syndrome are those of excess cortisol, excess androgen, excess ACTH, and only rarely those of a pituitary mass, since often the tumors are small. Patients are often obese with a round face, red complexion (plethora), hypertension, and diabetes. Women tend to have hirsutism (Table 188-2).

Glucocorticoid effects

Carbohydrate, protein, and fat metabolism. Cortisol excess results in relentless gluconeogenesis: production of glucose from the breakdown of protein. The patients tend to be diabetic

Table 188-2   Clinical manifestations of Cushing's syndrome

Manifestation	Occurrence (%)
Obesity	90
Red face (plethora)	75
Hypertension	75
Hirsutism	65
Muscle weakness	60
Menstrual disorders	60
Acne	45
Bruising	40
Mental disorders	40
Backache (osteoporosis)	40

despite very high insulin levels, since glucose utilization is also impaired. Not even elevated insulin prevents the breakdown of protein throughout the body (especially in the muscles). The high insulin level leads to fat deposition everywhere. Muscle wasting causes the girth of the arms and legs to diminish despite fat deposition, contributing to the impression of a redistribution of body fat. Moon facies, buffalo hump, and supraclavicular fat pads are also present.

Hematopoietic system. A leucocytosis of about 12,000 with an increase in mature polymorphonuclear leukocytes, lymphopenia, and eosinopenia is often present. The neutrophils do not leave the circulation and thereby contribute to the immune deficiency. Very high white blood cell counts are rare.

Immune system. High-dose glucocorticoid therapy is a more common cause of an acquired immune deficiency disorders than the AIDS virus. There is marked depression of delayed hypersensitivity and antibody production is also abnormal. Infection or heart failure usually causes death if the cortisol excess is not corrected.

Cardiovascular system. Both glucocorticoid and mineralocorticoid hypertension are present. Cortisol increases peripheral resistance by a different mechanism than does mineralocorticoid and is independent of sodium intake. In addition, cardiomyopathy combined with hypertension can lead to heart failure.

Musculoskeletal. In addition to proximal myopathy, protein breakdown in bone leads to severe osteoporosis, especially in the vertebrae. It is not unusual for patients with Cushing's syndrome to lose 3 or 4 inches in height. Calcium is excreted in the urine and can lead to kidney stones. Intestinal absorption of calcium is impaired by steroids further contributing to the negative calcuim balance in these patients.

Skin, hair, and appendages. The skin becomes very thin. In addition to plethora, patients experience easy bruisability, especially in the elderly. Stretch marks (striae) (especially on the lower abdomen, thighs, and shoulders) appear in patients who gain weight. Thinning and loss of head hair occurs, and lanugo hair, a fine downy baby-type hair appears on the face and body. In women, hair growth characteristic of men often occurs.

Eyes. Cataracts result from excess glucocorticoid. Signs of diabetic retinopathy in longstanding cases may also be present.

Central nervous system. Mental changes ranging from insomnia and mild personality changes to frank psychosis are common in Cushing's disease. The type of mental change seems to depend on the underlying personality, since repeated courses of steroid therapy for an inflammatory disease tend to produce the same change in a given individual. One patient may become depressed and another euphoric.

DIAGNOSIS. The diagnosis of Cushing's syndrome is established by detection of high plasma or urinary cortisol levels, loss of diurnal variation, and lack of normal suppression of cortisol by exogenous glucocorticoid in a patient who has clinical evidence of cortisol excess. The history and physical examination are a bioassay that is just as important as the chemical assays. The pattern of cortisol secretion seen in mild Cushing's disease can also appear in psychiatric depression, but depressed patients do not manifest signs of cortisol excess for reasons that are still unclear.

Cushing's disease may be intermittent, requiring repeated measurements. Unfortunately, no single test currently yields a foolproof diagnosis.

Screening test. In patients who lack a strong clinical picture of Cushing's syndrome, the best screening test is to measure plasma cortisol 8 hours after administering 1 mg of the powerful glucocorticoid dexamethasone at midnight. The plasma cortisol should fall below the lower limit of normal for the laboratory. In addition to patients with Cushing's syndrome (except for rare cases who cannot metabolize dexamethasone), certain patients with psychiatric depression, morbid obesity, or states of stress such as alcohol withdrawal will not exhibit suppression.

Classical tests

Baseline measurements

PLASMA CORTISOL IN THE AM AND PM. Because patients with Cushing's syndrome lose the normal diurnal variation, measuring cortisol levels in the morning and late evening is useful. Levels are highest in the early morning, and the nadir is about 10 or 11 PM. For outpatient collections, blood is often drawn at 4 PM although this is less than ideal. Because of the intermittent secretion of cortisol, urinary measurements are more reliable.

24-HOUR URINARY FREE CORTISOL. Patients with Cushing's syndrome have values in excess of 100 μg/day. Mildly elevated baseline values also appear in patients with unipolar depression and those under stress.

Dexamethasone suppression tests. The purpose of the suppression tests is twofold. The low-dose test should distinguish patients who have Cushing's syndrome from patients who are merely suspected of having the syndrome because of hypertension and obesity. The high-dose test should distinguish patients with pituitary Cushing's syndrome from those with ectopic ACTH production or adrenal tumors.

Low-dose (2 mg) suppression test. A dosage of 2 mg of dexamethasone (given as 0.5 mg every 6 hours for 2 days) is more than twice the replacement dosage and should suppress cortisol production even in depressed and obese patients. Urinary free cortisol is collected on each day and normally should be less than 30 μg/24 hours. Patients with pituitary Cushing's syndrome do not usually exhibit suppression unless the dexamethasone dosage is much higher.

High-dose (8 mg) dexamethasone suppression test. This test has been used to distinguish pituitary Cushing's syndrome from ectopic ACTH production and adrenal tumors. Patients with pituitary Cushing's usually exhibit suppression to less than 50% of the baseline. Adrenal and ectopic Cushing's patients usually do not experience suppression at all.

Other tests

ACTH stimulation test. Patients with Cushing's disease tend to show an exaggerated response to ACTH because the adrenal glands are large and the ACTH is usually high-normal, that is, the glands are not maximally stimulated. Patients with ectopic ACTH respond poorly because they actually are stimulated maximally. Those with an adrenal adenoma respond poorly because the adenoma itself does not respond and the normal adrenal gland is atrophied. The same results are seen with metyrapone, which blocks steroidogenesis and causes an endogenous ACTH stimulation test. Patients with pituitary Cushing's syndrome show marked increases in both ACTH and 11 desoxycortisol.

Localization procedures. Because occasional exceptions to each test exist, it is important to examine the adrenal glands using computerized tomograms or magnetic resonance imaging. Adrenal tumors large enough to cause Cushing's syndrome are almost always visible, enabling the surgeon to approach the proper side.

If there is no tumor, both adrenal glands usually look enlarged, or at least plump. It then becomes important to localize the source of ACTH. Current radiologic techniques must be further refined to diagnose pituitary adenomas, since these are often quite small. Selective venous sampling with measurement of ACTH can be useful in determining the source of the ACTH.

MANAGEMENT

Pituitary Cushing's syndrome. Unfortunately, the cure for pituitary Cushing's syndrome often creates other disorders. If pituitary Cushing's syndrome is due to a pituitary adenoma and if the adenoma can be removed without too much damage to the remaining pituitary tissue, the patient is cured. However, if the disease is due to hyperplasia of the corticotrophs, removing the abnormal cells without damage to the normal pituitary is unlikely. Recurrence of Cushing's disease after hypophysectomy is common.

Bilateral adrenalectomy quickly corrects hypercortisolism but leaves the pituitary problem untreated. Five percent to twenty percent of patients develop an enlarged pituitary gland and require hypophysectomy or irradiation (Nelson's syndrome). These patients develop intense hyperpigmentation. Drug therapy with metyrapone may successfully correct the effects of hypercortisolism (for instance, immunosuppression, hypertension, and diabetes) and buy time for patients who are too ill to immediately undergo surgery. Mitotane (ortho para DDD), which is widely used in chemotherapy for inoperable adrenal carcinoma because of its necrotic effect on the inner zones of the adrenal cortex, has also been used in low dosages to treat pituitary Cushing's syndrome. However, it is extremely toxic. Pituitary irradiation has limited efficacy. In the future, hormonal therapy for Cushing's syndrome may be possible with drugs that are cortisol antagonists (such as RU 486) and with congeners of corticotropin-releasing hormone (CRH) that may block the effect of CRH on the pituitary gland.

Adrenal adenomas. Cushing's disease caused by an adrenal adenoma is cured permanently by resection. The suppressed normal adrenal gland recovers function and the patient's condition becomes normal.

Malignant tumors of the adrenal gland are inefficient in steroidgenesis and hence are generally large at the time of diagnosis. If they have metastasized, the hypercortisolism may be treated with metyrapone or ketoconazole (which blocks cortisol synthesis), RU 486 (which blocks cortisol action), or mitotane (which damages adrenal tissue). Only the last decreases the tumor size, but it does not greatly improve chances of survival.

Ectopic ACTH syndrome. Although most of these cases are due to very malignant tumors such as lung cancer, some result from slow-growing or even quite benign tumors such as bronchial carcinoids, islet cell adenomas, pheochromocytomas, and other tumors with a good prognosis. If the tumor site is not obvious a careful search must be made.

MINERALOCORTICOID DEFICIENCY SYNDROME (HYPOALDOSTERONISM)

DEFINITION. Isolated aldosterone deficiency with normal cortisol production can be due to a congenital deficiency of enzyme activity peculiar to the zona glomerulosa (18 hydroxylase, 18 dehydrogenase) or an acquired disease of the zona glomerulosa or impairment of renin production. Congenital enzyme deficiency is quite rare but acquired aldosterone deficiency is common in patients with diabetic nephropathy. Originally it was proposed that destruction of the juxtaglomerular apparatus in the kidney, the site of renin production, was the only cause (hyporeninemic hypoaldosteronism). It now appears that there is more than one cause: renin may not be activated or there may be no adrenal response to angiotensin II. Because hyperkalemia and hyperchloremia are involved, these syndromes are termed "type IV renal tubular acidosis."

CLINICAL MANIFESTATIONS. The major manifestations of hypoaldosteronism are those of hyperkalemia in adults. Infants with aldosterone deficiency may have hyponatremia, but this is minimal in adults because of increased proximal tubular sodium reabsorption. The two most important hormonal regulators of potassium are aldosterone and insulin; insulin moves potassium into cells. If a patient has both aldosterone and insulin deficiency (most of these patients are diabetic), dramatic elevations of potassium occur as the blood glucose rises. Heart block and arrhythmias may lead to syncope.

DIAGNOSIS. The hyporeninemic variety of hypoaldosteronism is diagnosed by finding low levels of plasma aldosterone and renin after appropriate stimulation consisting of a low (10 mEq daily) sodium diet and 40 mg of furosemide daily for 3 days. On the third day, blood is drawn after the patient has been upright for 4 hours. These three stimuli—sodium restriction, a diuretic, and upright posture—normally trigger marked increases in renin and aldosterone. If both remain low, this establishes the diagnosis of hyporeninemic hypoaldosteronism. If the renin is elevated, however, while the aldosterone remains low, an ACTH stimulation test using 0.25 mg cosyntropin intramuscularly is performed. Thirty minutes after injection, blood is drawn for cortisol and aldosterone determinations. A rise in cortisol levels but no change in aldosterone levels demonstrates a diagnosis of disease of the zona glomerulosa.

MANAGEMENT. Acute elevations of serum potassium are best treated by infusing insulin (with glucose unless the serum glucose is already elevated). Chronic hyperkalemia can be managed with the mineralocorticoid 9 α-fluoro-hydrocortisone (Florinef), usually in a dose of 0.1 mg daily, but diabetic patients with hypertension sometimes can be managed with potassium-wasting diuretics alone (furosemide or thiazides).

MINERALOCORTICOID EXCESS SYNDROME (HYPERALDOSTERONISM)

DEFINITION. *Primary hyperaldosteronism* is a syndrome resulting from excess production of aldosterone because of either a solitary autonomous adenoma (Conn's syndrome) or hyperplasia of the zona glomerulosa (that is, not the result of activation of the renin-angiotensin system [idiopathic hyperaldosteronism]). The distinguishing features of primary hyperaldosteronism are elevated plasma aldosterone and suppressed plasma renin. Most patients have an adenoma. Of those with hyperplasia, a minority show abnormal sensitivity to ACTH and can achieve suppression with glucocorticoid. The stimulus for the hyperplasia in most patients is obscure. There is evidence for other stimuli to the zona glomerulosa, including a pituitary peptide other than ACTH. Regardless of the etiologic factors, the clinical hallmarks of primary hyperaldosteronism are hypertension and hypokalemia.

Secondary hyperaldosteronism is a condition of hyperplasia of the zona glomerulosa resulting from a renin-angiotensin system activated by poor renal perfusion. This is most commonly seen in heart failure, hepatic failure, and nephrotic syndrome. In these three conditions, there is hypokalemia but no hypertension.

PATHOGENESIS AND PATHOPHYSIOLOGY. Aldosterone's principal action is to increase the excretion of potassium and hydrogen in the distal nephron and collecting duct in exchange for sodium. If sodium is not present in the distal nephron, aldosterone is not effective and potassium accumulates in the body. Potassium that has filtered through the glomerulus is almost completely absorbed in the proximal nephron. Most of the potassium that appears in the urine is the result of aldosterone's effect distally.

Aldosterone's effect on sodium is clinically less important than its impact on potassium. Most sodium that is filtered by the glomerulus is also reabsorbed in the proximal nephron and in the loop of Henle. A number of hormones influence sodium reabsorption, including atrial natriuretic hormone and endogenous digitalis. Whenever the blood volume expands, these natriuretic hormones come into play. In primary hyperaldosteronism, the autonomous secretion of aldosterone causes the distal tabule sodium absorption and potassium and hydrogen ion secretion. Hypokalemia and alkalosis result. There is little increase in the serum sodium or blood volume, however, because as soon as the volume increases, sodium reabsorption in the proximal nephron decreases because of natriuretic hormones. This in turn makes ample sodium available to the distal nephron for exchange. Naturally, there is no edema. Hypertension depends on an adequate sodium intake. Limiting sodium intake ameliorates hypertension, and the resultant decrease in blood volume removes the stimulus to the natriuretic factors; hence sodium is reabsorbed proximally. If sodium is not delivered to the distal nephron, the aldosterone becomes ineffective and hypokalemia corrects.

In secondary hyperaldosteronism, even though the measured blood volume may be normal, there is less "effective" blood volume. In cirrhosis, for example, there is loss of vascular tone, the patients tend to be hypotensive, and neither the kidney nor the brain is well perfused. The brain's response to decreased effective volume is to secrete antidiuretic hormone, whereas the kidney reacts by secreting renin and reabsorbing sodium proximally as natriuretic factors diminish. The aldosterone production may increase 10-fold. The net result is salt and water retention, edema, and low serum sodium concentration despite high total–body sodium. Since the sodium is reabsorbed proximally and not delivered to the distal nephron, the serum potassium is only slightly low. Administering diuretics that block sodium reabsorption, both proximally and in the ascending limb of Henle's loop, delivers sodium to the site of action of aldosterone and leads to severe hypokalemia.

CLINICAL MANIFESTATIONS. Hypokalemia is responsible for most of the clinical manifestations of primary hyperaldosteronism. Hypertension is not malignant and its usual complications, such as retinopathy and cardiac hypertrophy, generally do not occur. Headache may be prominent. Hypokalemia causes muscle weakness and occasionally paralysis. Tetany may result from alkalosis. Nephrogenic diabetes insipidus also results from hypokalemia. Because of impaired insulin release, mild glucose intolerance is present.

DIAGNOSIS OF PRIMARY HYPERALDOSTERONISM. The diagnosis of primary hyperaldosteronism is suspected in patients with hypertension and hypokalemia. Most hypokalemia is due to diuretic therapy rather than to hyperaldosteronism. The hallmark of primary hyperaldosteronism is elevated and nonsuppressible plasma aldosterone and low nonstimulatable plasma renin.

Renin secretion is normally stimulated by volume contraction after 3 days of a low (10 mEq) sodium diet and 40 mg of furosimide daily. An elevated plasma renin level rules out primary hyperaldosteronism.

If the plasma renin level remains suppressed, the aldosterone level is measured. Usually a high (100 mEq) sodium diet is administered for 3 days with or without 0.1 mg fluorohydrocortisone daily. Alternatively, saline may be infused intravenously for a more rapid test. If the aldosterone is low, the 11 desoxycorticosterone (DOC) should be measured because tumors may secrete this mineralocorticoid (although this is rare).

Once the diagnosis of nonsuppressible aldosterone with nonstimulatable renin is confirmed, it is necessary to distinguish an aldosteronoma from hyperplasia. The blood pressure of hyperplastic patients does not improve after surgery, and they should not undergo surgery.

Localization. Computerized tomographic scanning or magnetic resonance imaging can localize the tumor, as can imaging with radioactive idocholesterol after suppressing adrenocortical function by administering steroids. These procedures have markedly improved diagnostic accuracy.

MANAGEMENT. Primary hyperaldosteronism caused by an aldosteronoma is managed best by removing the adrenal gland containing the tumor. The hypokalemia corrects immediately although the hypertension may require several months to correct. Patients who are too ill to undergo surgery can be treated with spironolactone, a steroid analog that blocks both aldosterone and testosterone receptors. This is obviously more acceptable in women. Men are likely to develop gynecomastia and may become infertile and impotent. As noted earlier, severe sodium restriction ameliorates the effects of aldosterone but such diets are poorly tolerated.

Primary hyperaldosteronism caused by bilateral hyperplasia should not be managed surgically. A minority of these patients may be glucocorticoid suppressible. The others often respond, contrary to expectation, to angiotensin-converting enzyme inhibitors such as captopril or enalapril maleate.

CONGENITAL ADRENAL HYPERPLASIA

DEFINITION. Adrenocortical hyperplasia during fetal development results from inborn errors in cortisol biosynthesis. Compensatory overproduction of ACTH by the fetus to overcome cortisol deficiency produces hyperplastic but inefficient adrenal cortices. Congenital adrenal hyperplasia (CAH), sometimes called the adrenogenital syndrome, was first described more than 100 years ago in association with anomalies of genital development. It is now appreciated that deletions of discrete enzymes produce these unique, often bizarre syndromes as a result of deficiencies and excesses of selective adrenocortical hormones. CAH occurs in about 1 of every 5000 births, indicating a current prevalence of 50,000 cases in the United States. The most common enzyme deletion is 21-hydroxylase deficiency.

PATHOGENESIS. CAH is the common result of deficiencies in any one of five enzyme systems that transform cholesterol to cortisol (Table 188-3). These enzymes, primarily hydrox-

Table 188-3   Congenital adrenal hyperplasia syndromes

Enzyme deficiency	Precursor steroid	Sodium balance*	Androgen excess†
20-Hydroxylase	Cholesterol	—	—
3-βB-OH-dehydrogenase	Dehydroepiandrosterone (DHA)	—	Female only
17-α-Hydroxylase	Progesterone	+ (Corticosterone excess)	—
21-Hydroxylase	17-Hydroxyprogesterone	—	+
11-β-Hydroxylase	11-Desoxycortisol	+ (Desoxycorticosterone excess)	+

*—, Sodium loss; +, retention.
†—, Androgen deficiency; +, excess.
‡ Development of female (F) or male (M) genitalia.
§Genetic male with (XY) sex chromosomes.
||Genetic female with (XX) sex chromosomes.

ylases, are only relatively specific so that a single enzyme such as 21-hydroxylase is essential not only for cortisol biosynthesis but also for aldosterone formation. Each enzyme deficiency is marked by consequences that uniquely identify the deficient step—steroid substrates *after* the block are decreased and steroid precursors *before* the block are increased.

The biologic implications of CAH depend entirely on the specific enzymatic step involved and the quantitative extent of the deficiency. All five of the common inborn errors share three features: (1) they are associated with varying degrees of (usually latent) cortisol deficiency; (2) they are accompanied by a compensatory increase in ACTH production, thereby producing adrenal hyperplasia; and (3) the biologically active precursors that accumulate produce diverse anatomic and physiologic aberrations responsible for the typical clinical manifestations of each syndrome. If the defects are quantitatively severe, these manifestations may be detected in the newborn. Subtle defects, however, may not become apparent until adult life in some patients.

Deficient or excessive androgen production is the usual cause for genital anomalies associated with CAH. When genetic males (46,XY) cannot produce testosterone, their genitalia do not differentiate from the basic female external phallus, a situation described as male pseudohermaphroditism. This occurs in three of the five CAH syndromes associated with deficient production of either 17-hydroxyprogesterone or its precursors, all essential for androgen production (Table 188-3). By contrast, the other two CAH syndromes are accompanied by excessive androgen production and therefore result in early masculinization of males or "precocious puberty." Genetic females (46,XX), on the other hand, are exposed to excess androgens in three of the five syndromes, thereby resulting in masculine-appearing genitalia (for example, clitoral hypertrophy) at birth.

This condition, termed female pseudohermaphroditism, can result in mistaken sex identification and sometimes tragic gender maladjustments later in life. Milder degrees of the same enzyme deficiencies may not be recognized until adulthood, and in the female these may appear simply as hirsutism. Two of the five syndromes are associated with deficient androgen and estrogen production in genetic females, and despite normal external genitalia, such women do not mature sexually; they come to medical attention in adult life because of a failure to menstruate (primary amenorrhea) or because of infertility.

Deficient or excessive mineralocorticoid production is the other major clinical problem associated with CAH syndromes. Three of the five common enzymatic defects lower the production of aldosterone as well as other potent mineralocorticoids. This results in failure to maintain sodium balance, a potentially lethal problem unless these "salt-losing" forms of CAH are detected early in infancy. The opposite situation, excessive mineralocorticoid production, occurs in the other two forms of CAH. In neither case is aldosterone responsible, although it is the normal end product of mineralocorticoid biosynthesis. In one case, 17-hydroxylase deficiency, weak salt-retaining hormone, corticosterone, and the potent salt-retaining hormone 11-desoxycorticosterone (DOC) accumulate; in the other, 11-hydroxylase deficiency, excessive production of 11-desoxycorticosterone alone is responsible.

The occurrence of adult-onset CAH has also been described. It is still unclear if the late-onset form is acquired or is a mild form of the classic congenital type. Clinically, the onset of virilization is seen around the time of the menarche. Adult-onset CAH has many of the signs and symptoms of the polycystic ovarian syndrome, such as hirsutism, menstrual irregularity, and occasionally clitoral enlargement, and cannot be easily distinguished on physical examination.

Both the adrenal glands and gonads require some of the same enzymes for steroidogenesis, and in the mild forms of CAH it is necessary to stimulate the adrenal glands with ACTH and measure steroid hormones to be certain of the abnormality.

There are several reports of hydroxysteroid dehydrogenase deficiency in older males in whom hypospadias was present at birth and gynecomastia developed at puberty.

CLINICAL MANIFESTATIONS. The distinctive clinical features of the CAH syndromes result from inappropriate production of both sex steroids and mineralocorticoids.

Genital abnormalities are the major clue to excessive androgen production in infant girls. When this is accompanied by dehydration and hyponatremia, suggesting salt loss, 21-hydroxylase deficiency or the less common 3-β-OH-dehydrogenase deficiency syndrome should be suspected. However, virilized female children with hypertension and hypokalemia raise consideration of only one defect, 11-β-hydroxylase deficiency. Similarly, males with prematurely developed genitalia should be evaluated for salt-losing defects (21-hydroxylase deficiency), whereas if they retain excessive salt, 11-β-hydroxylase deficiency should be considered. Finally, a salt-losing syndrome in a phenotypic female may require determination of chromosomal sex to define a defect such as 20-hydroxylase deficiency.

In summary, the combination of sexual disorders with disorders of sodium and potassium balance should raise suspicion of CAH.

DIAGNOSIS. Diagnosis of CAH syndromes involves determination of genetic sex by chromosomal studies and measurement of selected adrenocortical steroids to establish the enzymatic defect in cortisol biosynthesis. In the presence of appropriate clinical findings, unusual elevations in selected steroid precursors in blood or urine can confirm the diagnosis with precision.

MANAGEMENT. The treatment of the CAH syndromes is much the same as that for adrenocortical failure. In all cases this involves lifelong replacement of cortisol in physiologic doses. In syndromes with mineralocorticoid deficiency, daily maintenance doses of fluorocortisone are necessary. Genital ambiguities in the female are not reversible, and plastic surgery procedures are often required. Most important, cortisol not only provides replacement therapy but also suppresses excessive ACTH, ends further adrenal hyperplasia, and stops the overproduction of precursors responsible for all the physiologic aberrations associated with CAH.

BIBLIOGRAPHY

Arteaga E, Klein R, Biglieri EG: Use of the saline infusion test to diagnose the cause of primary aldosteronism, Am J Med 79:722, 1985.

Atkinson AB, Kennedy AL, Carson DJ and others: Five cases of cyclical Cushing's syndrome, Br Med J 291:1453, 1985.

Avgerinos PC and others: The corticotropin-releasing hormone test in the postoperative evaluation of patients with Cushing's syndrome, J Clin Endocrinol Metab 65:906, 1987.

Gallant C, Kenny P: Oral glucocorticoids and their complications, J Am Acad Dermatol 14:161, 1986.

Gold PW and others: Abnormal hypothalamic-pituitary-adrenal function in anorexia nervosa: pathophysiologic mechanisms in underweight and weight-corrected patients, N Engl J Med 314:1335, 1986.

Gold PW and others: Responses to corticotropin-releasing hormone in the hypercortisolism of depression and Cushing's disease: pathophysiologic and diagnostic implications, N Engl J Med 314:1329, 1986.

Howlett TA and others: Diagnosis and management of ACTH-dependent Cushing's syndrome: Comparison of the features in ectopic and pituitary ACTH production. Clin Endocrinol (Oxf) 24:699, 1986.

Larsen JL, Cathey WJ, Odell WD: Primary adrenocortical nodular dysplasia, a distinct subtype of Cushing's syndrome, Am J Med 80:976, 1986.

Petersen P and Jacobsen SEH: Cushing's disease presenting with severe osteoporosis, Acta Endocrinol 111:168, 1986.

Schteingart DE and others: Cushing's syndrome secondary to ectopic corticotropin-releasing hormone-adrenocorticotropin secretion, J Clin Endocrinol Metab 63:770, 1986.

Scott HW Jr, Abumrad NN, and Orth DN: Tumors of the adrenal cortex and Cushing's syndrome, Ann Surg 201:586, 1985.

Taylor AL and Fishman LM: Corticotropin-releasing hormone, N Engl J Med 319:213, 1988.

White PC, New MI, and Dupont B: Congenital adrenal hyperplasia (first of two parts), N Engl J Med 316:1519, 1987.

White PC, New MI, and Dupont B: Congenital adrenal hyperplasia (second of two parts), N Engl J Med 316:1580, 1987.

Wulffraat NM and others: Immunoglobulins of patients with Cushing's syndrome due to pigmented adrenocortical micronodular dysplasia stimulate in vitro steroidogenesis, J Clin Endocrinol Metab 66:301, 1988.

Zimmerman M and Coryell W: Review: The dexomethasone suppression test in healthy controls, Psychoneuroendocrinology 12:245, 1987.

Zovickean J and others: Usefulness of inferior petrosal sinus venous endocrine markers in Cushing's disease, J Neurosurg 68:205, 1988.

189 • PHEOCHROMOCYTOMA

Norman H. Ertel

Pheochromocytomas are chromaffin cell tumors derived from neuroectoderm. They are not common; in 15,984 consecutive autopsies performed at one clinic, there were 15 cases with adrenal pheochromocytoma, an incidence of less than 0.1%. However, when patients with hypertension are screened for curable forms of this disease, 0.1% to 0.7% are found to have pheochromocytoma. Since hypertension, the most common chronic disease in the United States, affects 15% of the adult population, discovery of a curable form is most important.

Several important advances in the past decade have made the diagnosis and treatment of pheochromocytoma much easier:

(1) the standardization and widespread use of accurate methods to determine urinary catecholamines and metabolites, as well as the recent development of sensitive and specific methods for measuring plasma catecholamines; (2) effective localization of tumors by selective adrenal angiography, ultrasound, I-131 meta-iodobenzylguanidine (MIBG) scintography, computerized tomography (CT), and particularly, magnetic resonance imaging (MRI); (3) widespread knowledge of proper preoperative and intraoperative care of patients, particularly the need for adrenergic blockade, attention to blood volume, and safe anesthetic agents.

PATHOLOGY. Pheochromocytomas are benign or malignant tumors composed of chromaffin cells that are derived from neuroectoderm, darken on exposure to chromium salts, and synthesize and secrete catecholamines. On electron microscopy both normal and neoplastic cells have characteristic granules that are similar to the chromaffin granules of the normal adrenal medulla. These electron-dense vesicles are about 100 to 300 nm in size and are key subcellular structures in the synthesis, storage, and secretion of the catecholamines. Although approximately 85% of the catecholamine in the normal adrenal medulla is epinephrine, norepinephrine secretion usually predominates in pheochromocytomas, possibly because tumor cells are not exposed to the high adrenal coticosteroid concentrations provided to the normal adrenal medulla by the portal blood supply from the adrenal cortex. The enzyme that converts norepinephrine to epinephrine, phenylethanolamine-N-methyltransferase (PNMT), is inducible by high levels of glucocorticoids. Less than 10% of pheochromocytomas are malignant. Histologic criteria, such as cellular atypia, increased mitotic figures, or invasion of blood vessels, are not helpful in predicting metastatic disease. However, malignant tumors are common in children and in patients excreting large amounts of dopamine or its major metabolite, homovanillic acid (HVA). Large tumors are likely to be malignant.

In nonfamilial cases about 80% of the tumors are located within the adrenal glands and are unilateral, about 10% are intraadrenal and bilateral, and about 10% are extraadrenal. Fortunately, most extraadrenal tumors (paragangliomas) are found within the abdomen, occurring either in the superior paraaortic area or at the bifurcation of the aorta. They are rarely found in the posterior mediastinum, neck, or bladder. Significant epinephrine secretion as determined by fractionation of urinary catecholamines greatly increases the likelihood of intraadrenal tumor, although in rare instances intrathoracic pheochromocytomas have been able to secrete epinephrine. Intraadrenal pheochromocytomas may range in size from less than 1 cm to palpable masses larger than the kidney, and may weigh from 2 to 2000 g. However, the average tumor is usually less than 10 cm in diameter and weighs about 100 g.

FAMILIAL PHEOCHROMOCYTOMA. Pheochromocytoma is familial in up to 10% of patients. There are at least five syndromes (see following paragraphs), all characterized by an increased incidence of bilateral disease (more than 50% of cases). Adrenal medullary hyperplasia has been described both as a precursor of tumor and in association with early symptomatic disease. When genetic studies are adequately described, the familial disease is inherited as an autosomal dominant trait.

Simple familial pheochromocytoma. It is not known whether some of these families were unrecognized multiple endocrine neoplasia or adenoma (MEN or MEA) kindreds. There is a syndrome of familial extraadrenal pheochromocytoma, however.

Multiple endocrine neoplasia type II (MEN II or IIA, Sip-

ple's syndrome). The components of this syndrome include medullary carcinoma of the thyroid (MCT), pheochromocytoma or adrenal medullary hyperplasia, and parathyroid adenoma and hyperplasia. In a member of an affected family one or more of these manifestations may predominate. However, the other components may be present but asymptomatic. The early diagnosis of pheochromocytoma in such patients is particvularly important, since the asymotomatic patient is still at risk for sudden death during a paroxysmal hypertension episode, particularly associated with surgery. As many as 30% of deaths in MEN II may be attributed to pheochromocytoma. Therefore screening of family members is important. In such patients total urinary catecholamines or catecholamine metabolites may be normal, and specific determination of urinary epinephrine may be necessary to make an early diagnosis.

Multiple endocrine neoplasia type III (MEN IIB or III, mucosal neuroma syndrome). Multiple endocrine neoplasia type III consists of multiple mucosal neuromas, MCT, and pheochromocytoma; hyperparathyroidism is uncommon. In a review of 41 such patients, oral neuromas occurring in the lips, tongue, and buccal mucosa were most common (37 patients). Additional findings are thickened eyelids and lips ("bumpy lips"), a marfanoid habitus, and a variety of gastrointestinal disturbances, including persistent diarrhea, constipation, and megacolon, related to diffuse intestinal ganglioneuromatosis. An interesting physical finding in all patients examined is thickening of the corneal nerves.

Pheochromocytoma and von Recklinghausen's neurofibromatosis. Less than 1% of patients with neurofibromatosis have pheochromocytoma, but about 5% of patients with pheochromocytoma have neurofibromatosis. However, the latter may be subtle, with multiple café au lait spots, isolated neurofibromas, or skeletal abnormalities.

Von Hippel-Lindau disease. Pheochromocytoma occurs in from 10% to 25% of patients with retinal-cerebellar hemangioblastomatosis and may be diagnosed only by roentgenographic techniques in a significant proportion of cases.

CLINICAL MANIFESTATIONS. Most patients with pheochromocytoma are detected as a result of screening patients with sustained hypertension or a history of paroxysms. The paroxysm is dramatic and the triad of severe headache, sweating, and palpitations occurs in the majority of attacks. Other common features of the paroxysm include pallor, nausea and vomiting, tremor, chest pain, epigastric pain, dyspnea, weakness, and severe anxiety (feelings of "impending doom"). Paroxysmal hypertension with return to normal blood pressure between attacks is present in only about 25% of patients. About 10% of patients have no demonstrable evidence of hypertension, and the remaining 65% have permanent hypertension. Of the patients with permanent hypertension, approximately 50% have had paroxysmal episodes but frequently are unaware of the significance of such symptoms. Only a few physicians recommend screening all newly diagnosed hypertensive patients for pheochromocytoma. Abnormal glucose tolerance is common, in part related to α-adrenergic suppression of insulin release by the increased circulating catecholamines. However, clinical diabetes mellitus appears in less than 10% of patients. The following clinical clues signal the possibility of a potentially life-threatening tumor:

1. Patients with untreated essential hypertension have no change or a rise in blood pressure when they stand up. A fall in blood pressure on standing is seen in the majority of patients with pheochromocytoma; this is thought to be a form of autonomic dysfunction secondary to circulating high catecholamine levels.
2. A history of hypertension, palpitations, or flushing during or

after parturition, surgery, or general anesthesia is suggestive of pheochromocytoma.
3. A paradoxical hypertensive response to antihypertensive drugs, such as methyldopa, reserpine, or guanethidine, strongly suggests pheochromocytoma, since such drugs either displace catecholamines from storage sites or inhibit uptake at the sympathetic nerve endings. Hypertension following hydralazine hydrochloride, thyroid-releasing hormone (TRH) testing, imipramine, desipramine, saralasin, or metoclopramide are other clinical clues.
4. Paroxysmal attacks provoked by a change in position, palpation of an abdominal mass, compression of the abdomen, or a hot or cold shower are of diagnostic value.
5. Even in patients without spontaneous or provoked paroxysms, the presence of unexplained sweating, fever, weight loss, or tachycardia, along with sustained hypertension, suggests the possibility of pheochromocytoma.

When a paroxysm is provoked by micturition or swallowing, the presence of a pheochromocytoma in the bladder or posterior mediastinum, respectively, should be suspected. Physical signs, other than hypertension and those already noted, are uncommon. In patients whose pheochromocytoma is part of a familial MEN syndrome, the signs and symptoms of the associated disease, such as the enlarged thyroid and diarrhea associated with MCT, may predominate.

COURSE. Frequency of paroxysms can range from once in several months to 25 times a day and last from 30 seconds to 1 week. They usually last less than 15 minutes but characteristically become more frequent with time. During a paroxysm the blood pressure often exceeds 250/150 and may be so high as to be unrecordable by the sphygmomanometer. Although patients with sustained hypertension may be susceptible to any of the complications of severe essential hypertension, including nephropathy, stroke, cardiac failure, or retinopathy, patients who are normotensive between paroxysms are relatively free of such disorders. Thus the latter group usually has normal fundi, whereas more than 50% of the patients with persistent hypertension have grade 3 or 4 hypertensive retinopathy. During the paroxysm the patient is in grave danger of sudden severe retinopathy, pulmonary edema with or without congestive heart failure, lactic acidosis, and cerebral hemorrhage. The paroxysmal form of the disease may evolve into sustained hypertension. Persistent rather than paroxysmal hypertension is seen more often in children and patients with malignant or multiple tumors. Pheochromocytoma occurring during pregnancy is unusually dangerous for both mother and child. It is frequently not recognized because the obstetrician may attribute the hypertension and other symptoms to toxemia of pregnancy. Although catastrophic episodes can occur at any time, shock, severe hyperpyrexia, arrhythmias, pulmonary edema, and cerebral hemorrhage are most frequently noted soon after delivery.

DIAGNOSIS. Measuring urinary catecholamines and their major metabolites is the principal laboratory method for the diagnosis of pheochromocytoma. An abbreviated diagram of the biosynthesis and metabolism of the biologically active catecholamines is shown in Fig. 189-1. The major metabolites of norepinephrine are normetanephrine and vanillylmandelic acid (VMA); those of epinephrine are metanephrines and VMA; and the major one of dopamine is HVA. The most commonly used tests are for the urinary total catecholamines, metanephrines, and VMA. Any one of these tests will be elevated in more than 90% of patients with pheochromocytoma. A second assay will raise the yield to 95%. The urinary metanephrine assay is the most reliable of the three tests in separating patients

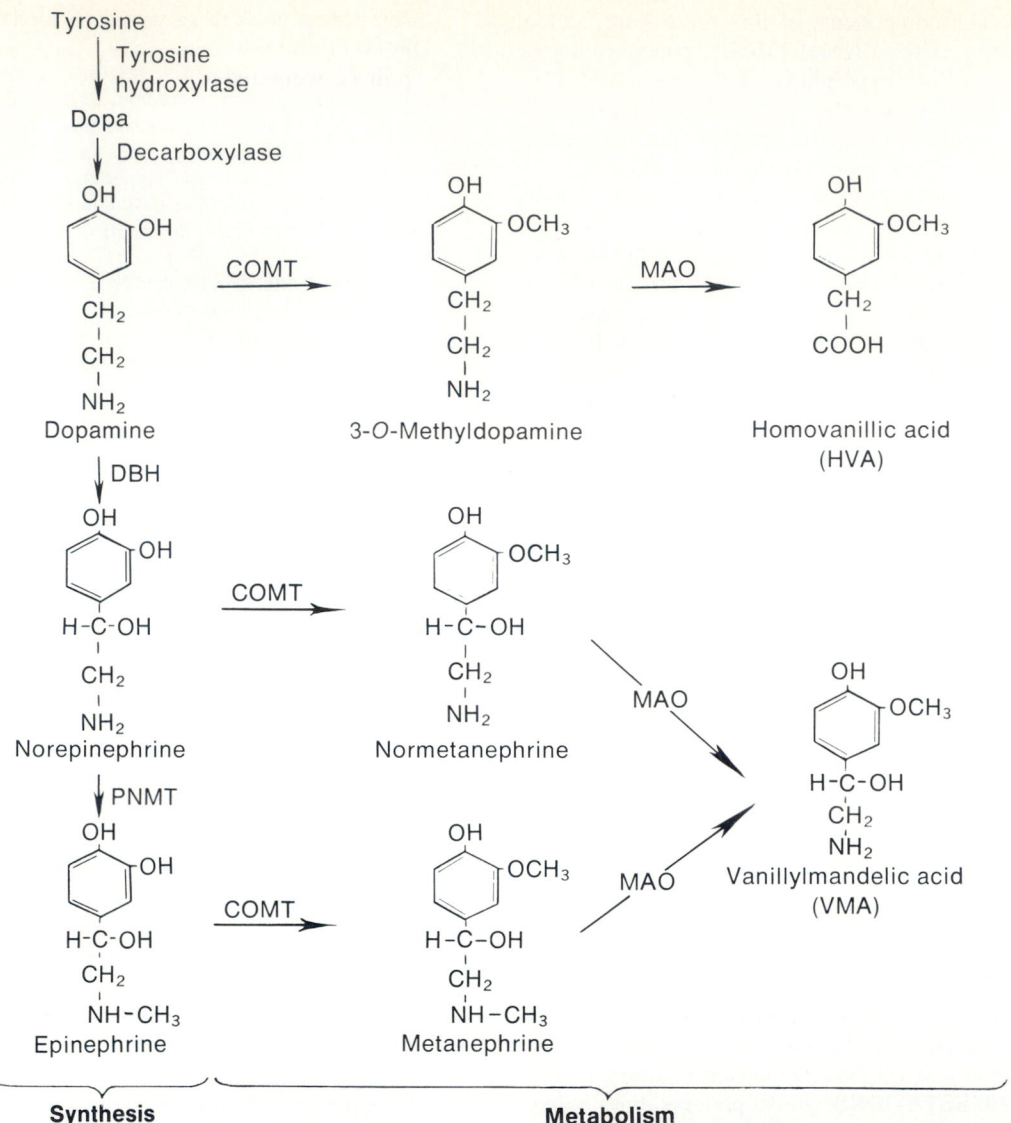

Fig. 189-1　Simplified scheme for biosynthesis and metabolism of major catecholamines. There are other routes of metabolism that are variably used, depending on tissue and species. *Dopa,* dihydroxyphenylalanine; *DBH,* dopamine-β-hydroxylase; *PNMT,* phenylethanolamine-*N*-methyltransferase; *COMT,* catechol-*O*-methyltransferase; *MAO,* monoamine oxidase.

with pheochromocytoma from other hypertensives. When a normal value is found in a patient who is thought on clinical grounds to have this tumor, further workup should include repeated assays, fractionation of total catecholamines (to epinephrine and norepinephrine) in the event that epinephrine secretion predominates, hourly collection of urine samples during and immediately after an attack, or plasma catecholamine determinations. Normal values for 24-hour excretion of catecholamines and metabolites and a list of the drugs that interfere with determinations are shown in Table 189-1. Methyldopa (Aldomet) presents particular difficulties when measuring urinary catecholamines because it is frequently given to patients with hypertension and may lead to abnormally high results for a prolonged period after its discontinuance.

Recent studies suggest that plasma catecholamines may be as useful as, and possibly more useful than, urinary determinations in the diagnosis of pheochromocytoma (Fig. 189-2). In using plasma levels, the physician must be careful to eliminate other physiologic and pathologic causes of catecholamine elevation. Thus, although the upper limits for plasma norepi-

nephrine and epinephrine in the resting, supine state are 400 and 70 ng/L, respectively, these values may be considerably elevated by cigarette smoking, exercise, hypoglycemia, or a stressful illness such as myocardial infarction or ketoacidosis. A plasma-free catecholamine value greater than 2000 ng/L is diagnostic of pheochromocytoma. Values greater than 1000 ng/L are abnormal but may overlap with those seen in some hypertensive patients; at this juncture, a clonidine test is helpful. Clonidine, a centrally acting α-adrenergic agonist, has been administered in an oral dose of 0.3 mg 2 or 3 hours before obtaining plasma for catecholamine measurements in an attempt to eliminate stress-related increases in plasma catecholamines. This drug does not affect the release of these hormones from an adrenal tumor, so a plasma catecholamine value greater than 500 ng/L after clonidine indicates pheochromocytoma. However, false positive and false negative results do occur. It has been suggested that platelet catecholamine levels, markedly elevated in patients with pheochromocytoma, are normal in patients with neurogenic hypertension accompanied by raised plasma catecholamine values.

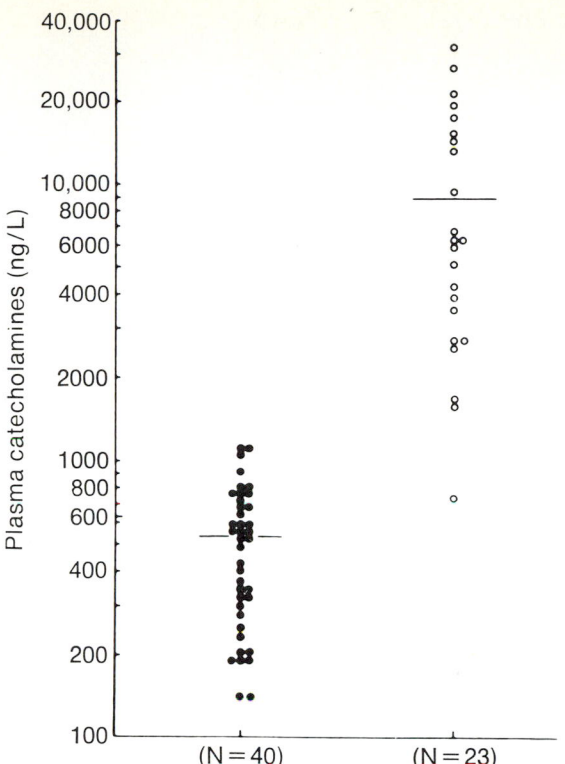

Fig. 189-2 Plasma catecholamines in 23 patients with proven pheochromocytoma and in 40 patients with suspected (but without) pheochromocytoma. (From Bravo EL and others. Reprinted, by permission of the New England Journal of Medicine 301:682, 1979.)

Table 189-1 Urinary catecholamines and metabolites

Test	Normal range (mg/24 hr)	Interfering drugs*
Free catecholamines	<0.15	Methyldopa, levodopa, isoproterenol, caffeine, theophylline, quinine, quinidine, labetolol
Norepinephrine	<0.08	
Epinephrine	<0.02	
Dopamine	<0.4	
Metanephrines	<1.3	MAO (monoamine oxidase) inhibitors, caffeine, chlorpromazine, roentgenographic contrast media containing methylglucamine†
Vanillylmandelic acid	<6.8	MAO inhibitors†, clofibrate†, nalidixic acid, disulfiram

*Cause a real or apparent increase in urinary values, except as indicated by †.
†Cause a real or apparent decreased in urinary values.

Imaging techniques. An abdominal flat-plate roentgenogram locates the tumor in only 15% of patients, and less than 50% of tumors can be localized by intravenous pyelography with nephrotomography. The introduction of CT scanning was a major advance in the localization of both intraadrenal and extraadrenal pheochromocytomas. Since more than 70% of pheochromocytomas can be detected by unenhanced CT, the risk of hypertensive crisis associated with intravenous injection of a contrast medium is avoided. However, MRI also has this advantage, and recent data from the National Institutes of Health indicate that MRI may become the imaging procedure of choice, particularly when prior surgery makes the CT scan difficult to interpret. MRI of the adrenal glands provides tissue characterization not attainable with CT. Pheochromocytomas light up in T2-weighted imaging (long TE, or echo delay time; long TR, or relaxation time) and are easily differentiated from other adrenal masses because of their very high signal intensity (Fig. 189-3). Because it does not use ionizing irradiation, MRI is ideal when diagnostic imaging is required during pregnancy. It must be emphasized that although MRI is the preferred localization procedure at the present time, a biochemical diagnosis must be achieved before attempting anatomic localization. Ultrasonography is also useful for localizing pheochromocytoma (Fig. 189-4). Invasive procedures, such as aortography, selective adrenal arteriography, venography, and vena caval catheterization for plasma catecholamines, are hazardous and often misleading in the localization of tumors. Such procedures should be reserved for the patient who has had an unsuccessful exploration or who has recurrent disease. Such patients must be pretreated with phenoxybenzamine to prevent crisis.

Scintography with MIBG, a radiopharmaceutical that concentrates in adrenergic vesicles, has also been useful in localizing pheochromocytomas, particularly when they occur in unusual extraadrenal sites such as the pericardium. Specificity is greater than 95% and the false negative result rate is about 13%. More recent use of I-123 MIBG promises to improve image quality and reduce the false negative result rate. This technique may identify adrenomedullary hyperplasia, an early stage of pheochromocytoma not detectable by CT. Other endocrine tumors, such as carcinoid and medullary thyroid carcinoma, may yield a positive image.

Pharmacologic tests, such as lowering blood pressure with phentolamine or raising it with histamine, tyramine, or glucagon, were useful in the past but have little or no use at present. The intravenous glucagon (1 mg) stimulation test is the safest of these and has been made more specific by measuring plasma catecholamines. A value greater than 2000 ng/L or a threefold increase 1 to 3 minutes after glucagon is a positive result. Intravenous phentolamine may be useful as both a diagnostic and therapeutic measure when a patient is seen in hypertensive crisis or with malignant hypertension.

MANAGEMENT. With the rare exception of patients with metastatic disease or those with severe illness preventing surgery, operative removal is the treatment of choice for pheochromocytoma. In the past such surgery was associated with mortality rates of up to 50%, mainly because of hypertensive crisis, congestive heart failure, and cardiac arrhythmias occurring during anesthesia or surgery. Fortunately, such complications have largely been eliminated by newer developments in preoperative and intraoperative management.

Medical therapy. In patients with norepinephrine-secreting tumors, the long-acting α-adrenergic blocking agent phenoxybenzamine (Dibenzyline) in divided doses of 20 to 150 mg orally per day reduces the blood pressure to normal. Most physicians use this drug in all cases for preoperative control. Although generally well tolerated, this agent may cause nasal stuffiness, gastrointestinal distress, and orthostatic hypotension. Metyrosine (α-methyl-L-tyrosine), a recently introduced drug, blocks the initial and rate-limiting step of catecholamine biosynthesis when given orally in a dose of 250 to 1000 mg four times a day. Urinary excretion of catecholamines and metabolites is decreased up to 80%, with accompanying improvement in the clinical status of the patient. However, side effects including diarrhea, sedation, and anxiety are prominent; therefore this drug is best reserved for the rare patient not adequately controlled by phenoxybenza-

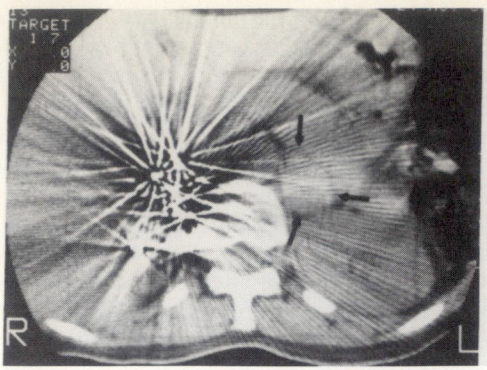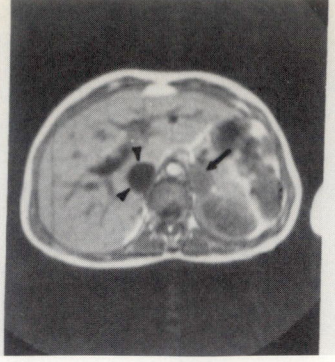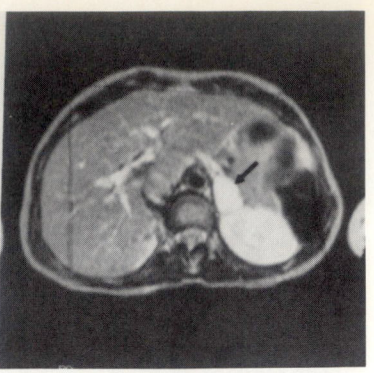

Fig. 189-3 Series of films from patient with MEN II, medullary carcinoma of thyroid, and previous right adrenalectomy for pheochromocytoma. **A,** CT scan. Left adrenal mass visible *(arrows),* but immense clip artifacts from previous right adrenalectomy compromise study. **B,** MRI–T1-weighted image. Clip artifacts *(two arrowheads on left)* appear as area of absence signal. Right adrenal mass *(arrow)* is easier to see on MRI than on CT because there are no clip artifacts. **C,** MRI–T2-weighted image. Very bright right adrenal mass *(arrow)* classic for MRI of pheochromocytoma. (Courtesy of John L Doppman, National Institutes of Health.).

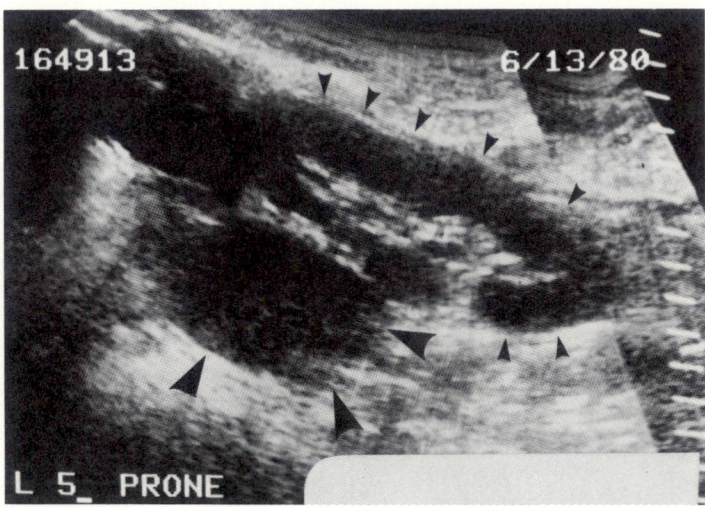

Fig. 189-4 Ultrasonogram demonstrating the same tumor *(large arrows)* near kidney *(small arrows)* as in Fig. 189-3.

mine or for patients with metastatic pheochromocytoma. Prazosin (Minipress), a postsynaptic α-adrenergic blocker, and labetolol, an agent with both α- and β-adrenergic blocking activity, have been used to treat pheochromocytoma medically. Labetol should be used with caution because it has been reported to elicit a hypertensive response in patients with this tumor.

β-Adrenergic blockade is not used routinely. Indications for this therapy include recurrent arrythmias or persistent tachycardia. Patients with pheochromocytoma may be extremely sensitive to propranolol, and the starting dose should not exceed 10 mg three times a day. In patients with predominantly epinephrine-secreting tumors, propranolol is the initial treatment, but close observation for unopposed α-adrenergic blockade is mandatory. It should be emphasized that propranol should not be started before adequate α-adrenergic blockade is achieved in norepinephrine secretors because resulting unopposed α-adrenergic effects may result in death owing to hypertensive crisis or coronary artery spasm. Patients with pheochromocytoma are often hypovolemic, but adequate sympathetic blockade corrects this problem by the time of surgery. Angiotensin-converting enzyme inhibitors (captopril, enala-

pril) and calcium-channel blockers (nifedipine) have been reported to lower blood pressure in patients with pheochromocytoma, but their role, if any, in the management of such patients is unclear.

Long-term medical therapy is always required in patients with functioning metastatic pheochromocytomas. In such patients, if the malignancy is discovered at surgery, it is important to remove as much of the tumor as possible, since these tumors do not respond well to radiotherapy or currently available cytotoxic agents (streptozotocin, I-131 MIBG). Malignant pheochromocytomas are frequently slow-growing; survival beyond 5 years is not unusual, although 50% of patients die within 2 years despite adequate adrenergic blockade. Long-term medical therapy may also be necessary in patients with major medical contraindications to surgery, such as severe cardiomyopathy or recent myocardial infarction. Phenoxybenzamine has been the agent of choice for long-term administration, but metyrosine may also prove to be an effective agent.

PHEOCHROMOCYTOMA IN PREGNANCY. Pheochromocytoma in pregnancy is rare but important to manage because in undiagnosed cases maternal mortality approaches 50%.

Treatment includes adrenergic blockade and, if the pregnancy is near term, cesarean section with subsequent search for the tumor.

BIBLIOGRAPHY

Bravo EL and Gifford EW: Pheochromocytoma: diagnosis, localization, and management, N Engl J Med 311:1298, 1984.

Chatal JF and Charbonnel B: Comparison of iodobenzylguanidine imaging with computed tomography in locating pheochromocytoma, J Clin Endocrinol Metab 61:769, 1985.

Doppmann JL and others: Differentiation of adrenal masses by magnetic resonance imaging, Surgery 102:1018, 1987.

Ertel NH and Gutkin M: Pheochromocytoma. In Conn HF and Conn RB Jr, editors: Current diagnosis, Philadelphia, 1980, WB Saunders Co.

Ertel NH and Modlinger R: Pheochromocytoma. In Conn HF, editor: Current therapy, Philadelphia, 1981, WB Saunders Co.

Fink IJ and others: MR imaging of pheochromocytomas, J Comput Assist Tomogr 9:454, 1985.

Hauptman JB, Modlinger RS, and Ertel NH: Pheochromocytoma resistant to α-adrenergic blockade, Arch Intern Med 143:2321, 1983.

Hauss GM, Van Aken H, and Lawin P: Anesthetic management in patients with pheochromocytoma, Cardiology 72(suppl 1):174, 1985.

Khairi MRS and others: Mucosal neuroma, pheochromocytoma and medullary thyroid carcinoma: multiple endocrine neoplasia type 3, Medicine 54:89, 1975.

Lynn MS and others: Pheochromocytoma and the normal adrenal medulla: improved visualization with I-123 MIBG scintography, Radiology 156:789, 1985.

Manger WM and Gifford RW Jr: Pheochromocytoma, New York, 1977, Springer-Verlag, Inc.

Spergel G, Bleicher SJ, and Ertel NH: Carbohydrate and fat metabolism in patients with pheochromocytoma, N Engl J Med 278:803, 1968.

Taylor HC, Mayes D, and Anton AH: Clonidine suppression test for pheochromocytoma: examples of misleading results, J Clin Endocrinol Metab 63:238, 1986.

Zweifler AJ and Julius S: Increased platelet catecholamine content in pheochromocytoma: a diagnostic test in patients with elevated catecholamines, N Engl J Med 306:890, 1982.

190 · THE TESTES

Elaine German *and* **Leslie I. Rose**

EMBRYONIC DEVELOPMENT

Normal development of the testes and accessory sexual structures depends on (1) genetic determination—fertilization of the ovum by sperm carrying the Y chromosome, and (2) the activity of three testicular hormones—testosterone, dehydrotestosterone (DHT), and müllerian regression factor (MRF).

The primitive urogenital (UG) ridge, formed during the fourth to sixth weeks of fetal life, is capable of differentiation into either ovary or testis. Sex determination depends on the chromosomal composition of the primordial germ cells that migrate to the UG ridge from the yolk sac. Presence of the Y chromosome causes differentiation of testicular cords, which contain precursors of Sertoli cells and sperm. The H-Y antigens, one of a number of male-specific cell surface histocompatibility antigens, may play a major role in male gonadal differentiation and development.

Sertoli cells may produce MRF, which causes involution of the müllerian ducts, the precursors of female genital organs. Leydig cells, probably stimulated by chorionic gonadotropin, synthesize testosterone in the fetus at 7 to 8 weeks.

Testosterone, which is converted to DHT after entering the effector cell, is necessary for development and differentiation of the wolffian ducts into epididymis, vas deferens, seminal vesicles, and ejaculatory ducts. Development of male external genitalia also depends on testosterone activity. Fetal phallus, glans, and scrotal folds are identifiable by the ninth week, and testicular descent into the scrotum via the inguinal canal begins by the twelfth week.

At birth each testis measures 1.4 to 2 cm in length, 0.7 cm in width, and 1 cm in thickness and weighs approximately 0.5 g. Leydig cells become quiescent until puberty and hormone levels (gonadotropins, androgens, and estrogens) remain low throughout childhood. During adolescence the testis grows under the stimulation of pituitary FSH and locally produced androgens. The fully developed testis measures 3.5 to 5.5 cm in length, 2.1 to 3.2 cm in width, and 3 cm in anteroposterior diameter, and weights 15 to 20 g. Testes have two primary functions: production of sperm and secretion of androgens and estrogens.

Spermatogenesis and hormonal synthesis become active at puberty. This major event is controlled by the central nervous system (Fig. 190-1). Gonadotropin-releasing hormone (GnRH), a decapeptide synthesized in the hypothalamus, stimulates the release of two gonadotropin hormones, produced by special cells in the pituitary: luteinizing hormone (LH), also called interstitial cell–stimulating hormone (ICSH), and follicle-stimulating hormone (FSH). LH stimulates the testicular Leydig cells to produce and secrete androgens and estrogens. FSH induces development and maturation of sperm in the seminiferous tubules.

If gonadal tissue does not develop (as in gonadal dysgenesis, genotypes XO, X isochromosome, and XY deleted) or if testosterone is absent or inactive before differentiation of the genital ducts occurs, both internal and external genitalia will be female even though the genetic sex is male (XY). As is true with many other hormones, the androgens and estrogens produced as a result of gonadotropic stimulation act to suppress further gonadotropin release when certain systemic levels are reached (negative feedback).

Testosterone primarily inhibits LH, whereas estrogens appear to have more effect on FSH. In addition, a nonsteroidal substance produced by Sertoli cells, inhibin, suppresses FSH secretion. All testicular hormones—testosterone, Δ^4 androstenedione, DHT, estradiol, and estrone—are synthesized from cholesterol. Approximately 7.5 mg of testosterone is produced daily by a normal man; 95% of this is made by the testes and the remaining 5% by the adrenal glands. The testes produce two thirds of the male's estrogen. The rest is produced by the adrenal glands and from conversion of testosterone and androstenedione to estrogen in peripheral tissues.

Abnormalities of the testes and testicular function can result from chromosome abnormalities, enzyme defects, end-organ hormone resistance, hormone deficiencies and excess, and unknown causes. These can be broadly classified under syndromes of *hypogonadism (decreased* androgen production and/or spermatogenesis) and *hypergonadism (increased* androgen production.) Hypogonadism occurs more frequently and is the more important group.

HYPOGONADISM

Primary hypogonadism may be present at birth as a genetic or embryologic defect or may occur at any time later in life as a result of infections, trauma, roentgen rays, or drugs. Secondary hypogonadism results from failure of the hypothalamus to elaborate GnRH or the pituitary to produce LH/FSH.

I. Primary hypogonadism
  A. Developmental abnormalities
    1. Anorchia
    2. Cryptorchidism

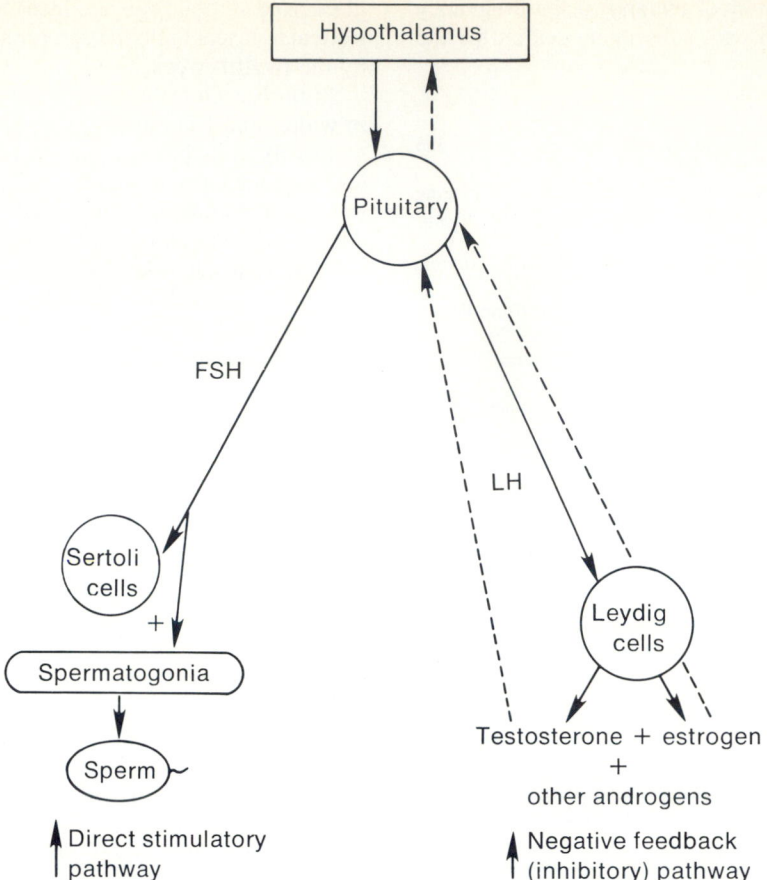

Fig. 190-1   Hypothalamic-pituitary-testicular feedback mechanisms (see text).

3. Klinefelter's syndrome
4. Male Turner's syndrome
5. Complete testicular feminization
6. Incomplete testicular feminization (male pseudoher-maphroditism)
   a. Reifenstein's syndrome
   b. Rosewater's syndrome
   c. Adrenal enzyme deficiency syndromes
   d. Testicular enzyme deficiency syndromes
7. Sertoli-cell-only syndrome
8. XYY karyotype

B. Postpubertal abnormalities
1. Varicoceles
2. Spinal cord damage
3. Infections
4. Hypothyroidism and hyperthyroidism
5. Malnutrition
6. Heavy metal toxicity
7. Drugs
8. Myotonia dystrophica
9. Physical factors
10. Trauma
11. Castration

II. Secondary hypogonadism
A. Kallman's syndrome (isolated gonadotropin deficiency)
B. Isolated LH (ICSH) deficiency (fertile eunuch)
C. Panhypopituitarism
D. Drugs
E. Laurence-Moon-Biedl syndrome
F. Stress
G. Delayed puberty

The clinical picture of hypogonadism relates to the time at which androgen deficiency first occurs. Prepubertal deficiency

results in infantile genitalia, female axillary and pubic hair distribution, absence of acne and seborrhea, and absence of vocal changes. Growth continues at a slower rate and without the adolescent spurt. Since epiphyseal closure depends on sex steroids, these patients develop a eunuchoid habitus—long arms and legs and an arm span that is 2 inches (5 cm) greater than height. Gynecomastia, wide hips, and girdle obesity may also be present, and muscle mass is diminished.

Hypogonadism occurring after puberty usually produces less dramatic changes. However, in young men beard and hair growth may be diminished, genitalia may become smaller, and libido may be reduced or absent. Gynecomastia may occur; the voice remains deep. There may be fewer changes or none in older men.

Primary hypogonadism
DEVELOPMENTAL ABNORMALITIES

Anorchia (disappearing testis). Although phenotypically and genetically males, men with anorchia have small penises and no detectable gonadal tissue. Testes with androgen and MRF production must have been present in early fetal life to initiate male development and disappearance of female structures. However, for unknown reasons they are reabsorbed before external genitalia have completely developed. Virilization at puberty does not occur since adrenal glands alone cannot produce sufficient testosterone. Lack of negative feedback raises LH and FSH levels. Testosterone, given parenterally, is used in treatment to achieve maximal development of stature and secondary sexual characteristics.

Cryptorchidism. Failure of either one or both testes to descend into the scrotum occurs in about 10% of males at time of birth. However, by the time puberty has occurred, only 0.3% to 0.4% still have undescended testes. Unilateral cryptorchidism is five times more frequent than the bilateral form. The undescended testes lie within either the inguinal canal or the abdomen. These testes are very prone to develop malignancies (40 times more frequently than normal testes) and are nonfunctional in their undescended positions. Orchiopexy is indicated at an early age to preserve testicular function and make observation for malignant changes feasible. Even after orchiopexy the previously undescended testis remains at increased risk for malignant change.

Uncorrected bilateral cryptorchid testes result in a functionally castrated male, presenting with a clinical picture of prepubertal hypogonadism. Correction usually results in normal virilization, although spermatogenesis is often impaired, even when orchiopexy is performed before puberty. In patients with unilateral cryptorchidism, the scrotal testis is frequently abnormal with reduced fertility.

Recently intranasal gonadotropin-releasing hormone has been used effectively to produce testicular descent in 30% to 40% of boys with undescended testes.

Klinefelter's syndrome (seminiferous tubule dysgenesis). Klinefelter's syndrome is one of the most common genetic abnormalities, occuring in 1:500 newborn males. Classically, the chromosomal constitution is XXY, but multiple variants, including XY, exist. Moderate mental retardation and personality disorders are common. Testes are small and firm and histologically show hyalinization of the seminiferous tubules. Serum testosterone levels are low to low-normal, whereas gonadotropin levels are elevated.

Diabetes mellitus, chronic bronchitis, emphysema, autoimmune disorders, thyroid abnormalities, and malignancies occur frequently in these men.

Male Turner's syndrome (Noonan's syndrome). Males with male Turner's syndrome have a phenotypic appearance similar to females with Turner's syndrome (XO chromosome)—short stature, webbed neck, low-set ears, shieldlike chest, cubitus valgus, ptosis, ocular anomalies, mental retardation, cardiovascular anomalies, cryptorchidism and/or small fibrous testes, gynecomastia, and lymphedema of hands and feet. However, the chromosomal karyotype is usually XY. Treatment with testosterone is appropriate.

Complete testicular feminization. Individuals with complete testicular feminization have an XY karyotype but appear in adulthood as well-developed, often handsome women. The external genitalia are feminine, but the vagina is shallow and ends in a blind pouch. Axillary and pubic hair is absent.

The testes, which are prone to malignancy, are located in the labia majora, inguinal canal, or abdomen. Testosterone levels often are similar to those of normal males, indicating that the target tissues are unresponsive to androgens.

The testes should be removed as soon as the diagnosis is made. Since these individuals are psychologically and physically female, it is advisable to avoid all reference to male genetic sex and to inform parents and patient only of the need to remove abnormal gonadal tissue because of potential malignancy. Once the testes are removed, combination estrogen-progesterone therapy should be instituted.

Incomplete testicular feminization (male pseudohermaphroditism). Incomplete testicular feminization represents a number of conditions resulting from defective androgen synthesis or partial resistance of target tissues to androgens. Patients have an XY genotype with widely variable sexual abnormalities. Genitalia are often ambiguous because of hypospadias and unfused scrotal folds. Gynecomastia may also be

present. If hypospadias is severe, individuals are usually reared as females, necessitating removal of the testes and treatment with estrogen at puberty; if mild, reconstructive surgery may be possible.

Reifenstein's syndrome. Reifenstein's syndrome is a hereditary sex-linked recessive testicular disorder. Individuals have hypospadias, gynecomastia, eunuchoidism, and postpubertal testicular atrophy. The chromosomal constitution is normal.

Rosewater's syndrome. Rosewater's syndrome consists of familial hypogonadism and gynecomastia, probably caused by genetic mutation. Testosterone levels are normal; gonadotropin levels are normal or high. Estrogens are also elevated, resulting in gynecomastia.

A number of enzyme deficiencies in testes or adrenal glands resulting in defective androgen synthesis produce similar sexual abnormalities.

Adrenal enzyme deficiency syndromes. Adrenal enzyme deficiency syndromes resulting in hypogonadism include the following:

1. 3-β-Hydroxysteroid dehydrogenase deficiency produces mineralocorticoid and glucocorticoid defects, resulting in salt-losing patients with pseudohermaphroditism.
2. 17-Hydroxylase deficiency produces hypertension along with varying degrees of male pseudohermaphroditism because of deficits in androgens, estrogen, and cortisol. These patients also lack pubic and axillary hair.
3. A patient with C-21-hydroxylase deficiency virilizes early but usually has small testes and an abnormally pigmented scrotum (females are virilized).
4. C-11-hydroxylase deficiency results in mild sexual abnormalities in the male (females appear virilized) accompanied by hypertension owing to increased production of 11-deoxycorticosterone.

Testicular enzyme deficiency syndromes. The testicular enzyme deficiency syndromes resulting in hypogonadism include the following:

1. 17-β-Hydroxysteroid oxidoreductase deficiency results in impaired androstenedione conversion to testosterone. Germinal elements are absent. Males have ambiguous genitalia, gynecomastia, and cryptorchidism.
2. 5-α reductase deficiency blocks the conversion of testosterone to DHT, resulting in hypospadias. These patients are usually reared as females until puberty, when virilization occurs.

Sertoli-cell-only syndrome. Germinal cells are completely absent in the testes. Leydig cells are present and testosterone is produced, but levels are somewhat lower than normal. These men are virilized but infertile.

XYY karyotype. The XYY karyotype occurs with a frequency of 0.01% to 0.02% among males. Patients are tall and have pustular acne. Spermatogenesis may be impaired in spite of normal gonadotropin and testosterone levels.

POSTPUBERTAL ABNORMALITIES

Varicoceles. Varicoceles are often associated with decreased motility and sperm count, thought to result from abnormal venous drainage or temperature control. Improvement occurs after surgical correction.

Spinal cord damage. Cord damage may elevate testicular temperature resulting in decreased sperm production. The ability to ejaculate is lost if lesions are located between the sixth thoracic and the third lumbar vertebrae.

Infections. Orchitis develops in 15% to 25% of males with parotitic mumps. Permanent damage to the seminiferous tubules may result if infection occurs during puberty or afterward.

The full effect may not become apparent for 15 to 20 years.

Gonorrhea, leprosy, tuberculosis, brucellosis, syphilis, and disease caused by other organisms may also cause sufficient damage to produce infertility.

Hypothyroidism and hyperthyroidism. Oligospermia and low testosterone levels may occur in hypothyroidism. Severe hyperthyroidism may decrease sperm count and motility.

Malnutrition. Starvation, fad diets, chronic illness, or malignancy may lower production of sperm and androgens because of malnutrition. Gonadotropin levels also decrease.

Heavy metal toxicity. Testicular necrosis is caused by cadmium and to a lesser extent by bismuth, mercury, aluminum, platinum, lithium, silver, tin, nickel, uranium, boron, and lead.

Drugs. Methadone produces a 50% decrease in ejaculate volume, with low levels of prostatic and seminal vesicle fluid. It also decreases testosterone levels and greatly reduces sperm motility. Various cytotoxic agents (alkylating agents, periwinkle, and alkaloids) inhibit spermatogenesis by direct toxic action on the germinal cells.

Myotonia dystrophica. Myotonia dystrophica is a genetic syndrome in which lenticular opacities, frontal baldness, and myotonia coexist with testicular atrophy. Testosterone levels are low and gonadotropins elevated. Patients with cystic fibrosis and other congenital conditions such as Laurence-Moon-Biedl syndrome (see discussion on "Secondary hypogonadism") also have failure of seminiferous tubule function.

Physical factors. Elevating testicular temperature by 4° to 5° F (2° to 3° C) for only 30 minutes to 3 hours can diminish spermatogenesis. The temperature increase can result from fever, hot baths, and saunas. Very low temperatures, below 23° F (-5° C), for prolonged periods can also impair sperm production, probably as a result of diminished blood flow.

Permanent damage to germinal cells in adults also may occur with single exposure of radiation of 600 rads or more. Spermatogonia are the most radiation sensitive, whereas Leydig cells are more resistant. Irreversible damage to prepubertal testes occurs at doses of 2400 to 3000 rads. Genitals should be shielded from roentgen rays during childhood, puberty, and adulthood when fertility is desired. People working with roentgenographic equipment and radioisotopes should also take precautions.

Men living at altitudes of 4270 feet (1280 M) or higher for more than 40 days have been found to have decreased sperm numbers and motility, as well as poor-quality semen. Space flight also alters spermatogenesis.

Some men in later years have diminished function of Leydig cells resulting in hot flashes, irritability, inability to concentrate, decreased libido with impotence, and depression, symptoms indicative of male climacteric. Interruption of vascular supply to the testes may be the cause.

Secondary hypogonadism

Decrease in the production or release of the gonadotropic hormones LH (also known as ICSH) and FSH will result in hypogonadism. The etiologic factors may lie in the hypothalamus, with decreased or ineffective secretion of GnRH, or because of a lesion in the pituitary gland itself. The absence of serum and urinary gonadotropins after adolescence in patients with decreased gonadal function is diagnostic.

KALLMAN'S SYNDROME (ISOLATED GONADOTROPIN DEFICIENCY). Hypogonadism caused by decreased gonadotropins owing to hypothalamic dysfunction, associated with absence of sense of smell because of olfactory lobe agenesis, characterizes Kallman's syndrome. Other pituitary functions are intact. This syndrome occurs in both males and females.

Patients are eunuchoid and may have midline abnormalities such as harelip and clef palate. It may be associated with X-linked recessive or male limited-dominant inheritance or with no chromosomal abnormality at all.

ISOLATED LUTEINIZING HORMONE (INTERSTITIAL CELL–STIMULATING HORMONE) DEFICIENCY (FERTILE EUNUCHS). Patients with isolated LH deficiency show gynecomastia and eunuchoid stature. LH and testosterone levels decrease, but FSH secretion is normal. Spermatogenesis is feasible if testes are sufficiently mature. Testosterone should be administered. Human chorionic gonadotropin (HCG) may be administered to promote full testicular development.

PANHYPOPITUITARISM. Failure of the pituitary gland to elaborate any of its tropic hormones (such as thyroid-stimulating, adrenocorticotropic, leutinizing/follicle-stimulating, and growth hormones) can result from tumors, histiocytosis, granulomata (such as tuberculoid and sarcoid), cysts, central nervous system infections, trauma, and vascular lesions, or may be idiopathic. Hypothalamic lesions may lead to absent or diminished secretion of releasing hormones, thereby decreasing pituitary hormonal production. Patients with panhypopituitarism starting in childhood are short and have high-pitched voices and small external genitalia. They require lifelong replacement with thyroid hormone, cortisone, and testosterone. Adult hypopituitarism usually results from chromophobe adenomas but may also be related to trauma, metastatic tumors, infections, and so on. Involvement of the posterior pituitary with resultant diabetes insipidus may also occur.

DRUGS. Chlorpromazine, carbon tetrachloride, and estrogens all block gonadotropin secretion. This produces testicular hypofunction resulting in hypogonadism.

LAURENCE-MOON-BIEDL SYNDROME. Obesity, mental deficiency, hypogenitalism, retinitis pigmentosa, and polydactyly characterize the Laurence-Moon-Biedl syndrome, which is inherited as a recessive trait. Hypogonadism may be of either primary (testicular aplasia) or secondary (hypothalamic) origin. Patients with suspected secondary hypogonadism require complete evaluation of growth, thyroid, adrenal, and antidiuretic hormones.

STRESS. Major surgery, trauma, or burns and severe emotional stress may be sufficient to suppress gonadotropin secretion with a resultant drop in testosterone production.

DELAYED PUBERTY. Puberty, which occurs normally between 9 and 16 years of age, is occasionally delayed until ages 20 to 22. Slow development of the hypothalamus is believed to be responsible. Differentiation from hypogonadotropic eunuchoid patients is difficult. This disorder can be familial.

Evaluation and management

Patients with hypogonadism initially have developmental abnormalities, impotence, or infertility.

Important history will include age, occupation, past medical illness (especially tuberculosis, mumps, venereal disease, cryptorchidism, previous abdominal surgery, and hernia repair), smoking habits, ethanol use, medications, and sexual habits.

The physical examination should include special attention to body build, height, arm span, muscle development, hair distribution, external genitalia, sense of smell, palate, and lips.

Laboratory studies will depend on abnormalities found during the physical examination. Evaluation of the pituitary-hypothalamic-testicular axis requires determining LH, FSH, and testosterone levels. Fertility evaluation requires sperm analysis. A GnRH stimulation test may also be helpful.

Testosterone replacement should be given to patients with

androgen deficiency. Long-acting parenteral preparations (testosterone cypionate, propionate, and so on) are recommended for patients under middle age when rapid prostatic enlargement will not produce problems with obstruction. Short-acting preparations (oral 17-α-methylated testosterone) are used in older men.

In patients who have germinal epithelium in their testes, fertility may be possible if spermatogenesis and androgen production can be stimulated by exogenous gonadotropins. HCG, which acts like LH to stimulate Leydig cells, plus human menopausal gonadotropin, which, like FSH, stimulates spermatogenesis, may be effective. However, therapy is protracted, expensive, and too often unsuccessful.

Recently, GnRH analogs have been used therapeutically. GnRH is normally secreted in a pulsatile fashion by the hypothalamus. Long-term, low-dose pulsatile therapy by infusion pump has been effective in inducing puberty in boys with isolated gonadotropin deficiency. Long-term, intermittent, subcutaneous injections of GnRH have triggered spermatogenesis in hypogonadotropic men. Continuous infusion of GnRH ultimately suppresses gonadotropin after a short transient period of stimulation. This can suppress testosterone in patients with prostatic carcinoma and in hypergonadotropic hypergonadism.

HYPERGONADISM

Hypergonadism in the male is caused by excess androgens. Children show all the manifestations of precocious puberty: growth of axillary and pubic hair, enlargement of phallus and testes, deepening of voice, acne, and so on. Testicular tumors and tumors in the region of the third ventricle (pinealoma, teratoma, astrocytoma, hamartoma, and craniopharyngioma) may be the cause. Familial precocious sexual development as well as hypergonadism from adrenal-androgen excess may also occur.

TESTICULAR TUMORS

Neoplasms of testes occur in approximately 1:100,000 normal men and are the most common tumors in the 24- to 35-year-old group. The frequency is much higher (1:2000) in cryptorchidism, even after surgical orchiopexy.

Testicular tumors in order of frequency are (1) seminoma; (2) teratocarcinoma; (3) embryonal carcinoma (chorioepithelioma and others); (4) teratoma; (5) interstitial cell (Leydig cell) tumor; (6) fibroma, lipoma, adrenoma, myxoma; and (7) unclassified neoplasms. Lymphomas, plasmacytomas, leukemia, and metastatic carcinomas may also occur. Embryonal carcinomas, particularly chorioepitheliomas and teratocarcinomas, may secrete gonadotropins, resulting in syndromes of hyperestrogenism. Interstitial cell tumors may produce hypergonadism, such as precocious puberty in children.

DIAGNOSIS. A mass is usually present, although some tumors are so small that they can be identified only on multiple microscopic sections. Urinary excretion of 17-ketosteroids, estrogens, or gonadotropins is helpful in diagnosis when these are present. Serum α-fetoprotein may be elevated.

MANAGEMENT. Surgical removal combined with radiotherapy and chemotherapy has proved effective.

BIBLIOGRAPHY

Bunick EM and Rose LI: Testicular syndromes. I. Abnormalities of childhood and adolescence, Compr Ther 3:62, 1977.
Bunick EM and Rose LI: Testicular syndromes. II. Adult abnormalities, Compr Ther 3:69, 1977.
Ingbar S, editor: Contemporary endocrinology I, New York, 1979, Plenum Publishing Co.
Lipshultz LI and Howards SS, editors: Infertility in the male, Edinburgh, 1983, Churchill Livingstone.
Silvers WK and Wachtel SS: H-Y antigen: behavior and function, Science 195:956, 1977.

191 • THE OVARY

Leonore C. Huppert

The human ovary is a small, bilateral ovoid structure located on either side of the uterus adjacent to the lateral pelvic walls. The mature ovary measures approximately 2.5 to 5 cm in length, 1.5 to 3 cm in width, and 0.5 to 1.5 cm in thickness. The combined weight of both ovaries during the reproductive years is 10 to 20 g. Blood vessels and nerves enter the ovary via the mesovarium, a thin fold of tissue adherent to the posterior aspect of the broad ligament. In addition to the mesovarium, the ovary receives support from the infundibulopelvic and utero-ovarian ligaments.

HISTOLOGY AND EMBRYOLOGY

Histologically, the ovary is composed of follicles, which contain germ cells surrounded by specialized hormonally active tissue, and fibrous tissue stroma. Tissue that will eventually develop into an ovary is identifiable within the human embryo by 4 weeks after fertilization. At this stage in development the germ cells, containing the genetic information for the next generation, are located outside the embryo. During the next month of embryogenesis the germ cells migrate into the embryo and colonize the primitive ovary. The original 1000 to 2000 germ cells undergo rapid proliferation or mitosis to form about 600,000 oogonia by the end of the second month of intrauterine life. During the fourth month of gestation certain oogonia transform into primary oocytes by initiating the process of meiosis or reductional chromosomal division. These cells are arrested in an early stage of meiosis that will not be completed until many years later when the ovum is finally ovulated and fertilized. Because of continued mitosis and meiosis, at 5 months the ovary contains about 2 million oogonia and 5 million primary oocytes. During the remainder of fetal life many of these cells degenerate, so that at birth the ovary contains approximately 2 million oocytes and no oogonia.

The developing primary oocyte is surrounded by a thin layer of flattened granulosa cells forming the primordial follicle. Certain primordial follicles further differentiate after birth into primary follicles, characterized by an increase in the numer of granulosa cells and the development of a surrounding concentric arrangement of stromal cells destined to become the theca interna of the mature follicle. Follicular development up to this stage is independent of gonadotropin stimulation by the pituitary gland. Further follicular maturation, however, requires the action of gonadotropins.

FOLLICULAR GROWTH AND DEVELOPMENT

The ovaries grow steadily from birth until puberty. The prepubertal rise in gonadotropins permits further follicular maturation, with a resultant increase in ovarian estrogen (the most potent of which is estradiol [E_2]) production by the granulosa cells. The secondary, or graafian, follicle is characterized by increased numbers of granulosa cells surrounding a large, fluid-filled antral cavity into which the ovum projects. The concentrically arranged thecal cells surrounding the follicle further differentiate into theca interna and theca externa. The theca interna is highly vascular and can produce hormones.

In the pubertal female a number of follicles in each cycle, under the influence of cyclic gonadotropin stimulation from the pituitary gland, are stimulated to the stage of the graafian follicle. Further interaction between the ovary and the pituitary leads to the continued growth of usually two follicles. One of these tertiary follicles grows until it reaches a diameter of about 1 mm and then undergoes atresia. The follicle ultimately destined to ovulate reaches a diameter of 1.5 to 2 cm and migrates to the periphery of the ovary. Responding to the appropriate signal from the pituitary gland, ovulation takes place. Ovulation is not an explosive event but rather is characterized by a slow ooze of material from the follicle. Prostaglandins, whose levels increase within the follicle before rupture, probably mediate the ovulation process.

Immediately after release of the egg, follicular collapse and hemorrhage ensue. This is followed by hypertrophy of granulosa and theca interna cells. Morphologic and biochemical alterations in these cells lead to the formation of the corpus luteum, which replaces the original follicle. The granulosa cells, which previously were avascular, are penetrated by blood vessels. The corpus luteum can produce both estrogen and progesterone and has a self-limiting life span of approximately 12 to 14 days. As the corpus luteum regresses, it becomes fibrous and hyalinized. The remaining structure, called the corpus albicans, forms approximately 70 days after ovulation.

The postmenopausal years are heralded by a decline in the number of ova and follicles within the ovary. Ultimately, the combined processes of ovulation and atresia consume all remaining germ cells in the ovary, thus ending the endocrine and reproductive function of this organ. The postmenopausal ovary acquires a wrinkled surface appearance and shrinks to less than one third of its former active size.

ENDOCRINE EVENTS OF THE MENSTRUAL CYCLE

The adult menstrual cycle represents a delicate interaction of many components of the reproductive system. The ultimate target of the fluctuating hormone levels is the uterus, whose lining undergoes cyclic changes in response to the steroid hormones estrogen and progesterone, produced by the ovary. The ovary in turn produces its hormones and prepares an egg for ovulation under the influence of the pituitary gonadatropins follicle-stimulating hormones (FSH) and luteinizing hormone (LH). The regulation of gonadotropin secretion appears to be under the dual control of the hypothalamic hormone gonadotropin-releasing hormone (GnRH) and the local steroid hormone milieu.

Menstruation usually occurs every 25 to 30 days, although cycles of 21 to 42 days' duration may also be normal. The fixed portion of the menstrual cycle is the postovulatory phase, which usually lasts approximately 13 days. Variations in the length of the preovulatory phase therefore determine the overall length of the menstrual cycle.

A new menstrual cycle begins with the onset of menstruation when estrogen and progesterone levels are at a nadir (Fig. 191-1). The earliest hormonal event in the new cycle is an increase in pituitary FSH, which actually begins the day before the onset of menses. This hormone then stimulates the development of the graafian follicle. FSH specifically causes hyperplasia and hypertrophy of the granulosa cells and also induces more of its own receptors. There is also a rise in LH levels at the start of each cycle, which is probably necessary to maintain the low levels of steroidogenesis within the ovary. LH-stimulated androgenic steroid precursors from the theca interna diffuse into the avascular granulosa, where they convert into estrogen. Continued follicular stimulation by FSH

leads to significant estrogen production by the granulosa cells approximately 1 week before ovulation. This rise in estrogen enhances the FSH-mediated increase in FSH receptors and together with FSH induces LH receptors on the granulosa cells. An adequate complement of LH receptors ensures normal ovulation and eventual corpus luteum formation. The ability of the granulosa to respond directly to LH during the immediate preovulatory period permits for the first time in the cycle the production of significant intrafollicular levels of progesterone.

As estrogen production by the ovary increases, the amount of FSH produced by the pituitary declines. The mechanism involved in this interaction is called negative feedback and is described in the next section. Before ovulation a large proportion of the estrogen being produced comes from those few follicles continuing to grow. The high local estrogen concentrations within these follicles augment their responsiveness to FSH by increasing their numbers and affinity to FSH receptors. The smaller follicles that produce significantly less estrogen, on the other hand, have a lesser response to FSH and eventually undergo atresia.

The rapid, late follicular rise in estrogen stimulates the pituitary gland to release a large burst of gonadotropin. The principal gonadotropin released at this time is LH, although a modest rise in FSH also occurs. Estrogen levels rapidly decline as LH levels start to rise. Ovum release occurs within 24 hours of the LH peak.

The newly formed corpus luteum produces large amounts of progesterone, with peak levels occuring 8 to 9 days after ovulation. Lesser but still significant amounts of estrogen are also produced. These high levels of estrogen and progesterone secretion by the ovary maintain FSH and LH production by the pituitary gland at a minimum level. Even though LH levels are low at this time, some continued LH stimulation is necessary to support the corpus luteum for its normal life span. Unless pregnancy occurs, the corpus luteum starts to degenerate 9 to 11 days after ovulation. There is a rapid decline in progesterone and estrogen levels, which ultimately reach the point at which they can no longer maintain the endometrium, and menstruation ensues.

CONTROL MECHANISMS OF THE HYPOTHALAMIC-PITUITARY-OVARIAN AXIS

The interactions between the pituitary gland and ovary are controlled by negative and positive feedback mechanisms. The predominant mechanism throughout the cycle is the negative feedback effect of ovarian steroids on gonadotropin secretion. The most pronounced inhibitory effect is that of estrogen on FSH secretion, although low levels of estrogen may also inhibit tonic LH secretion. The midcycle LH surge, however, is controlled by positive feedback. The rapidly rising estrogen levels are fed back on the pituitary gland, leading to the large burst of LH release. Both the amount of estrogen produced and the duration of the estrogen peak appear to be important in activating the positive feedback mechanism.

Synthesis and release of gonadotropins by the pituitary gland does not occur without stimulation by hypothalamic GnRH in a pulsatile fashion. Frequency and amplitude of GnRH pulses are, in turn, influenced by hypothalamic neurotransmitters and by steroid hormone feedback. In general, norepinephrine appears to stimute GnRH secretory neurons, whereas dopamine inhibits them. Endogenous opiods such as the endorphins and enkephalin may inhibit GnRH by activating dopaminergic neurons.

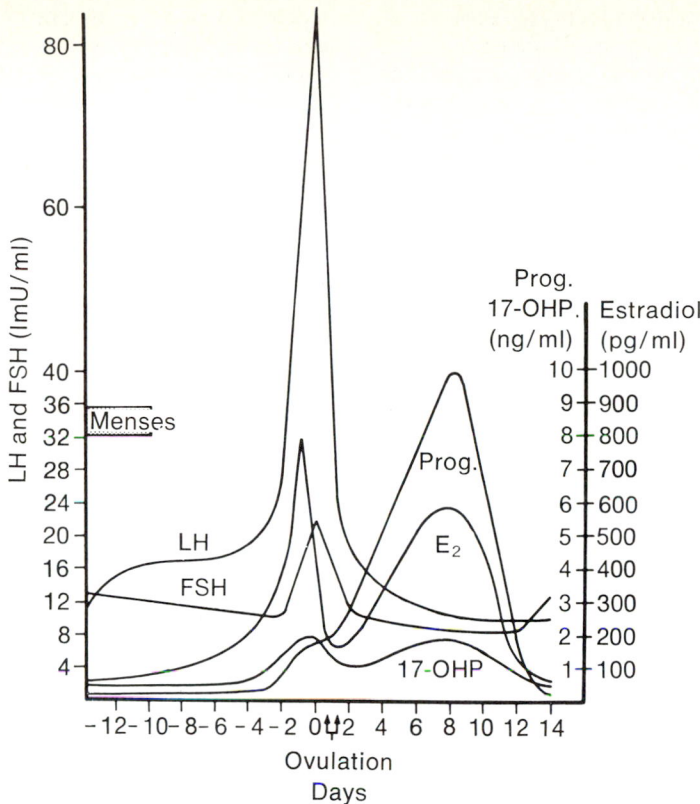

Fig. 191-1 Plasma hormone fluctuations during the human menstrual cycle. *LH,* luteinizing hormone; *FSH,* follicle-stimulating hormone; *Prog.,* progesterone; *E_2,* estradiol; *17-OHP,* 17-hydroxyprogesterone. (From Speroff L and Vande Wiele RL: Am J Obstet Gynecol 109:234, 1971.)

PITUITARY-OVARIAN RELATIONSHIPS FROM BIRTH TO MENOPAUSE

FSH and LH are first detected within the human fetal pituitary gland by 10 weeks of gestation. GnRH is also detectable within the fetal hypothalamus during the first trimester. Gonadotropin levels increase until midgestation, at which point they sharply decline and remain low until birth. The midpregnancy FSH surge is temporarily related to and may be responsible for the differentiation of oogonia to primary oocytes. The decline in gonadotropin levels probably results from negative feedback by high fetal estrogen levels derived from placental conversion of fetal and maternal precursor hormones. This interaction represents the first appearance of the negative feedback system.

Immediately after birth and delivery of the placenta, the precipitous drop in estrogen levels induces a surge of FSH in the neonate. By this time the hypothalamus and pituitary gland exhibit an exquisite sensitivity to the negative feedback effect of estrogen. The small amounts of estrogen produced by the ovary during childhood keep gonadotropins at a low level. Gonadotropin production starts to rise between the ages of 8 and 10, signaling the approach of puberty. Although the exact mechanism of the prepubertal gonadotropin rise is unknown, it is believed to result from the acquisition of pulsatile GNRH release and from a loss in sensitivity of the hypothalamus to negative feedback inhibition by estrogen. A characteristic nocturnal elevation of FSH and LH occurs during the peripubertal years and disappears once the adult pituitary-ovarian relationship establishes itself. Finally, before ovulatory cycles can occur, the hypothalamus and pituitary must develop their ability to respond in a positive manner to high levels of estrogen in order to produce the ovulatory surge of LH.

The approach of the menopause, on the other hand, is heralded by a small diminution in estrogen levels and a rise in FSH levels. This alteration is probably the consequence of decreased numbers of follicles present within the ovary, as well as of an impaired ability by the remaining follicles to produce estrogen.

Elevated FSH levels may be present in women who are still menstruating normally, but nonetheless herald subtle alterations in the ovarian-pituitary axis which precede menopause. An elevated FSH is a poor prognostic sign when ovulation induction is being considered. As estrogen levels further decline, the ability to generate a midcycle estrogen surge is lost and ovulation ceases. Cycles become more irregular and anovulatory bleeding occurs. Ultimately, estrogen levels decline to the point at which they are no longer sufficient to cause endometrial proliferation and the final menstrual flow or menopause occurs. As ovarian estrogen production ceases, gonadotropin levels continue to rise and finally reach stable postmenopausal values 1 to 3 years after the menopause. FSH levels are consistently higher than LH levels in postmenopausal women.

THE ABNORMAL OVARY

Ovarian disease may be divided into functional and neoplastic disorders.

Functional disorders—amenorrhea

Ovarian dysfunction often becomes apparent when the target organ, the endometrium, no longer functions appropriately. Thus amenorrhea (failure to menstruate) or abnormal uterine bleeding is often the clinical sign that prompts an investigation of ovarian function. Precocious or delayed pubertal development, as well as premature onset of the menopause, also suggests a functional abnormality of the ovary. Although in some instances ovarian dysfunction is intrinsic to the ovary, failure of normal ovarian function more frequently results from improper stimulation. More rarely, menstrual failure is caused by disease or absence of the uterus or abnormalities in the outflow tract.

PRIMARY AMENORRHEA. Extragonadal problems account for 40% of cases of primary amenorrhea. Outflow abnormalities include absence or obstruction of the vagina or cervix. Imperforate hymen is probably the most common cause of obstructed flow. Congenital absence of the vagina, aplasia of the vagina, and complete transverse vaginal septum are less frequent findings. Very rarely, severe cervical stenosis can prevent menstruation. Absence of the upper two thirds of the vagina together with absence of the uterus and fallopian tubes is classified as müllerian agenesis, also known as *Rokitansky-Kuster-Hauser syndrome*. A small, blind vaginal pouch is present in these patients. Ovarian function is completely normal, accounting for normal pubertal development.

Another group of patients with the same clinical picture, including blind vaginal pouch, absent uterus, and normal secondary sex characteristics, are those with *testicular feminization*. These patients, although phenotypically female, are genetic males with an XY karyotype. They have normal testes producing normal male amounts of testosterone. The abnormality in this condition is an end-organ insensitivity to testosterone that prevents the formation of male internal and external genitalia. It is important to obtain a karyotype in all females with a blind vaginal pouch and absent uterus, since phenotype females with a Y chromosome in their karyotypes have a high risk of gonadal malignancy and should undergo gonadectomy. Vaginal dilation or reconstructive surgery is occasionally required to ensure a functioning vagina. In addition to absence of the uterus, amenorrhea may result from damage to the endometrium, rendering it unable to respond to normal cyclic stimulation. Intrauterine synechiae (scar tissue), a condition known as *Asherman's syndrome*, may occur following curettage after birth or at the time of abortion. The basal layer of endometrium from which subsequent endometrium regenerates becomes scarred and no further proliferation, secretion, or menstruation will occur. Curettage for the purpose of removing the scar tissue followed by high-dose estrogen therapy occasionally results in endometrial regeneration. The endometrium can also become incompetent following infection. This is exceedingly rare in the United States and may be due to tuberculosis or schistosomiasis.

Abnormal ovaries resulting from an abnormal sex chromosome complement account for approximately one third of cases of primary amenorrhea. The most common chromosomal abnormality is the absence of one X chromosome, producing a 45,XO karyotype and streak ovaries without ova or follicles. This condition, known as *Turner's syndrome*, is characterized by various somatic abnormalities, including short stature, webbed neck, shield chest, widely spaced nipples, an increased carrying angle of the arms, and occasionally coarctation of the aorta. Affected individuals fail to experience spontaneous puberty but do respond to hormone replacement therapy with breast development and menstruation. Occasionally, one individual may have multiple cell lines with different sex chromosome complements (for example, XO/XX and XO/XY). These mosaic conditions are also associated with streak gonads. Somatic abnormalities are much less frequent in these conditions than in pure Turner's syndrome. The presence of a Y chromosome in the karyotype of a phenotypic female dictates

removal of the gonads because of an increased incidence of malignant degeneration.

SECONDARY AMENORRHEA. Less frequently, the ovary can cause secondary amenorrhea, or interruption of menstruation once it has already been established. One of the more common ovarian causes of secondary amenorrhea, however, is the *polycystic ovarian syndrome*. This condition, also known as *Stein-Leventhal syndrome*, is characterized by amenorrhea, obesity, and hirsutism. Instead of the regular cyclic events of the normal menstrual cycle, hormones are produced in a steady state fashion. Typically, the ovary produces abnormal levels of weak androgenic hormones, which presumably interfere with the normal pituitary-ovarian feedback interaction. The pattern of gonadotropin secretion from the pituitary gland is characterized by low to low-normal levels of FSH and elevated LH levels. In addition to abnormal steroidogenesis within the ovary, there may also be a hypothalamic defect responsible for the elevated LH levels. The ovaries in this condition are enlarged and smooth, with no evidence of recent ovulatory activity. The smooth, shiny appearance of these ovaries is probably caused by anovulation rather than the disease process itself. Patients with this condition are good candidates for the induction of ovulation with clomiphene citrate if they wish to conceive.

Rarely, women in the reproductive years may undergo premature menopause. Symptomatically and endocrinologically, this condition is indistinguishable from the normal physiologic event of the menopause. Occasionally, this premature menopause may result from chromosomal mosaicism, which was mentioned earlier. A small number of patients who appear to be prematurely menopausal may have the *resistant ovary syndrome*. In this condition the ovary is refractory to gonadotropin stimulation. Little estrogen is produced and gonadotropin levels rise. Small follicles, however, are present, distinguishing this condition from the menopause.

The most common cause of secondary amenorrhea is an abnormality in the hypothalamic-pituitary axis leading to improper ovarian stimulation. Gonadotropin secretion from the pituitary may be compromised as a result of compression from intrinsic or extrinsic pituitary tumors or vascular lesions. Pituitary necrosis resulting from obstetric hemorrhage (Sheehan's syndrome) may also lead to amenorrhea. In these conditions surgery or hormonal replacement therapy is provided as needed.

Not infrequently, small pituitary tumors that produce abnormally large amounts of prolactin are identified. Patients with this condition often have amenorrhea and galactorrhea. Occasionally, no tumor can be demonstrated roentgenographically when prolactin levels are elevated. This suggests the presence of a tumor too small to be detected by current roentgenologic means or abnormal prolactin secretion caused by improper hypothalamic control. When prolactin levels return to normal, either surgically or medically with bromocriptine, menstruation will resume. Other hormonally active pituitary tumors such as those producing excess corticotropin (Cushing's disease) and abnormal amounts of growth hormone (acromegaly) may also interfere with menstrual function. Rarely, a condition may be seen known as the *empty-sella syndrome*, characterized by an enlarged sella turcica containing cerebrospinal fluid that displaces and compresses the pituitary gland.

Failure to uncover a pituitary disorder leads to the diagnosis of hypothalamic amenorrhea. Hypothalamic dysfunction is the most frequent cause of secondary amenorrhea. Essentially, it is a diagnosis of exclusion after uterine, ovarian, or pituitary abnormalities have been ruled out. No obvious endocrinopathy may be identified, but cyclic reproductive function ceases. Stress, extremes of weight, prior history of oral contraceptive use, and serious systemic illness are often associated factors. Inducing periodic menstruation with an oral progestogen is indicated to prevent continuous estrogen stimulation of the endometrium. Often patients with hypothalamic amenorrhea resume menstruation spontaneously.

DIAGNOSIS. Although the causes of amenorrhea vary, the diagnostic approach to these patients is straightforward. Once anatomic abnormalities have been ruled out, progesterone should be administered. Since progesterone will provoke menstruation only when the endometrium has been primed by estrogen, bleeding following withdrawal of progesterone rules out abnormalities of the outflow tract, uterus, and ovary other than polycystic ovarian disease. Measurement of serum androgens and an LH determination help detect polycystic ovaries. The prolactin level must be determined in all patients to exclude a pituitary microadenoma.

If a patient does not bleed in response to progesterone, either she is hypoestrogenic because of ovarian, pituitary, or hypothalamic dysfunction, or she has an unresponsive endometrium. The latter possibility may be discounted if the patient can be induced to bleed by combined estrogen and progesterone therapy. Further evaluation of the hypoestrogenic patient must include a determination of gonadotropin levels. Elevated gonadotropin levels indicate ovarian failure, and a karyotype should be ordered. Low or normal gonadotropin levels suggest pituitary or hypothalmic disease. Patients should be examined carefully for pituitary tumor and reevaluated as long as they remain amenorrheic.

THERAPY. Induction of ovulation is indicated in amenorrheic or anovulatory women desirous of pregnancy. Currently five ovulatory agents are of clinical usefulness. Bromocriptine mesylate (Parlodel), a dopamine agonist, is used to lower prolactin levels specifically in the hyperprolactinemic patient. It is effective whether there is a tumor or not. Patients who have prolactin-secreting adenomas must be cautioned that there is a small chance the tumor will enlarge during pregnancy. Clomiphene citrate (Clomid and Serophene) is a nonsteroidal estrogen available in oral form. It appears to induce ovulation by attaching to hypothalamic and pituitary estrogen receptors, thus displacing endogenous hormones. Since clomiphene is essentially devoid of estrogenic activity in humans, the pituitary perceives a hypoestrogenic state and elaborates gonadotropin, thereby initiating follicular development. Successful ovulation induction requires an intact hypothalamic-pituitary-ovarian axis and some endogenous estrogen. Clomiphene is a very safe drug with a low rate of multiple births (4% to 8% twins). Pergonal (combined FSH/LH) or Metrodin (pure FSH) are injectable agents used to induce ovulation in patients who lack endogenous gonadotropins or who fail to respond to clominphene. These drugs are administered on an individualized basis and ovarian response should be monitored by means of serum estradiol levels and ultrasounds for follicular development. Pergonal and Metrodin are potent drugs with the potential for a significant number of multiple gestations (25%) and ovarian hyperstimulation. For the patient with an intact pituitary but deficient GnRH stimulation, ovulation can be induced by means of a GnRH agonist administered subcutaneously or intravenously in a pulsatile fashion via an infusion pump. However, this technique is not widely used, since it is cumbersome and somewhat costly. In addition, some multiple pregnancies have ocurred.

Ovarian neoplasm

Malignant ovarian tumors are a significant cause of morbidity and mortality in women. Of all diseases unique to women, cancer of the ovary ranks as the foremost cause of death. Ovarian neoplasms are rare in children, but if they should occur, the risk of malignancy is high. The chances of an ovarian neoplasm being malignant are lowest during the reproductive years. During these years true neoplasms must be distinguished from functioning cysts, which derive from the follicle or corpus luteum and often spontaneously regress. As women pass into the fifth and sixth decades of life, the risk of an ovarian neoplasm being malignant once again increases.

The most frequent clinical features in patients with ovarian neoplasms are abdominal swelling and discomfort. Often, however, ovarian neoplasms are asymptomatic and are detected only at the time of pelvic examination. The differential diagnosis of an enlarged ovary includes bowel lesions such as diverticulitis or carcinoma, an enlarged fallopian tube resulting from infection or ectopic pregnancy, or a pedunculated uterine leiomyoma. In young women ultrasonography is occasionally useful in distinguishing small, functional cysts from neoplastic tumors. In children or older women, however, the clinician usually proceeds directly to laparotomy. Findings at the time of surgery dictate either a conservative or a radical operative approach. Because ovarian carcinoma has usually metastasized by the time of diagnosis, surgery is frequently followed by chemotherapy.

Ovarian neoplasms are often classified according to their histologic type—60% to 70% of all ovarian neoplasms derive from the coelomic epithelium that surrounds each ovary; 15% to 20% of all neoplasms originate in germ cells; another 5% to 10% derive from the stroma; and only 5% are metastatic in origin. Ovarian tumors may also be classified according to their degree of malignancy and hormonal activity.

BIBLIOGRAPHY

DiSaia DJ, Morrow CP, and Townsend DE: Synopsis of gynecologic oncology, New York, 1975, John Wiley & Sons, Inc.

Erickson GF: Normal ovarian function, Clin Obstet Gynecol 21:31, 1978.

Givens JR: Normal and abnormal androgen metabolism, Clin Obstet Gynecol 21:115, 1978.

Speroff L and VandeWiele RL: Regulation of the human menstrual cycle, Am J Obstet Gynecol 109:234, 1971.

Speroff L, Glass RH, and Kase NG: Clinical gynecologic endocrinology and infertility, ed 3, Baltimore, 1983, The Williams & Wilkins Co.

Styne DM and Grumbach MM: Puberty in the male and female, its physiology and disorders. In Yen SSC and Jaffe RB, editors: Reproductive endocrinology: physiology, pathophysiology, and clinical management, Philadelphia, 1978, WB Saunders Co.

Winter JSD, Faiman C, and Rayes FI: Normal and abnormal pubertal development, Clin Obstet Gynecol 21:67, 1968.

Yen SCC: The human menstrual cycle. In Yen SCC and Jaffe RB, editors: Reproductive endocrinology: physiology, pathophysiology, and clinical management, Philadelphia, 1978, WB Saunders Co.

192 • HUMORAL SYNDROMES ASSOCIATED WITH NEOPLASMS

Doris G. Bartuska *and* **Helen Feit**

Clinical signs and symptoms resulting from hormonal production by nonendocrine cancers have been called paraneoplastic syndromes, humoral syndromes associated with cancer, or ectopic hormone syndromes. The availability of sensitive assay techniques has led to the elucidation of a wide variety of these syndromes. It is probable that all cancers elaborate humoral substances, but clinically only those that secrete biologically active materials are recognized. Examples of these "humors" include peptide hormones, precursors of peptide hormones, prostaglandins, fetal proteins, and enzymes. At least 50 hormones or their precursors have been shown to be produced by cancers, most of which are protein or peptide (see the following incomplete list).

Humoral substances produced by nonendocrine neoplasms

Hypercalcemia of malignancy factor
Osteoclast-activating factor
1,25 Dihydroxyvitamin D
Proopiomelanocortin (POMC); adrenocorticotropic hormones (ACTHs); melanocyte-stimulating hormone (MSH)
β-endorphin; lipotropins; corticotropin-like intermediate lobe peptide (CLIP)
Vasopressin (antidiuretic hormone [ADH])
Gonadotropins (human chorionic gonadotropin [HCG] and its subunits)
Hypoglycemia-producing factors (insulin-like growth factors [IGF] I and II)
Gastric peptides: gastrin, glucagon, secretin, bombesin, vasoactive intestinal peptide, cholecystokinin
Erythropoietin
Hypophosphatemia-producing factor
Growth factors; growth hormone; growth hormone–releasing hormone (GHRH)
Corticotropin-releasing hormone (CRH)
Prolactin
Kinins
Prostaglandins
Calcitonin
Renin
Placental lactogen
Cachectin
Somatostatin

Many of the symptoms and signs that appear in the patient with cancer results from endocrine or metabolic activities of the tumor itself. Several theories have been advanced to explain the phenomenon of humoral secretion by neoplasms. Cells contain genetic material coded with the same information; it is possible that gene derepression accompanies neoplastic transformation. Another hypothesis involves tissue dedifferentiation; this implies a return to more primitive gene expression and reversal of tumor tissue differentiation. Additional evidence shows that specific types of tumors elaborate specific types of hormones and that the cells from the different tumors producing the same hormone are similar in morphologic, histochemical, and ultrastructural characteristics and in embryologic origin. A unified theory of polypeptide hormone production by these tumor cells suggests that they are caused by dysplasia of neural ectoderm. A common embryologic ancestry probably accounts for their shared endocrine potential. These cells have been designated APUD (amine precursor uptake and decarboxylation) cells to highlight their common ability to synthesize and store biogenic amines.

Current data suggest that all peptide hormones begin in the preprohormone form, which contains methionines, the universal codon for protein synthesis, plus a variable-length additional amino acid sequence. The preprohormone degrades to the prohormone, which is generally biologically inactive. It is then enzymatically degraded to the bioactive hormone. After being secreted into the blood, it degrades further into the carboxy fragment, which is biologically inert, and the amino fragment, which may have biologic activity.

Physicians should be aware of these syndromes so that a correct diagnosis can be established. Humoral secretions by the neoplasm may precede other clinical evidence of the tumor by weeks or months. In addition, humoral production can be used to localize the tumor and to assess response to chemotherapy, surgery, or radiation therapy. The reappearance of the circulating "humor" can be used as a "marker" to detect a recurring neoplasm.

This chapter is concerned with some of the more common endocrine manifestations of malignancy.

Table 192-1 lists a spectrum of the endocrine syndromes associated with malignancy and the involved hormones. It has been estimated that one of these syndromes will be present in 15% to 50% of patients with cancer and that 75% of cancer patients will manifest some aspect of a paraneoplastic syndrome during their life span.

HYPERCALCEMIA AND NEOPLASMS

Hypercalcemia is the most common recognizable endocrine abnormality associated with neoplasia. It occurs in about 0.3% of patients in a general hospital; of these about 20% have cancer and about 5% have hyperparathyroidism. It has been estimated that 10% to 20% of patients with cancer will have hypercalcemia at some time.

Symptoms of hypercalcemia are subtle and nonspecific. The earliest manifestations are polyuria, nocturia, anorexia, nausea, vomiting, constipation, lethargy, weakness, dry mouth, or behavioral changes. Persistent progressive hypercalcemia results in severe dehydration, azotemia, mental confusion, coma, cardiovascular collapse, and death. The serum calcium level is usually between 12 and 16 mg/dl. Patients with primary hyperparathyroidism usually have only a modest elevation of serum calcium (up to 12 mg/dl). Hypercalcemia can be worsened by dehydration, immobilization, thiazide administration, adrenal insufficiency, hyperthyroidism, and vitamin D intake.

Hypercalcemia is common with some cancers such as those of the lung and breast. It occurs rarely with other tumors such as colon or uterine cancers. Breast cancer is the most common tumor associated with hypercalcemia, which usually indicates metastases to bone. Other solid tumors such as squamous cell carcinoma of the lung, esophagus, kidney, pancreas, and ovary cause hypercalcemia by producing a humoral factor (humoral hypercalcemia of malignancy). Patients exhibit biochemical changes similar to those found in hyperparathyroidism, such as hypercalcemia, hypophosphatemia, and elevated nephrogenous cyclic AMP excretion. This was thought to be secondary to production of PTH or a PTH-like substance. However, recent research reported by Burtis has shown this to be a different protein (see Chapter 193). Other humoral substances such as prostaglandins, vitamin D sterols, and tumor growth factors may be responsible.

MANAGEMENT. Patients with hypercalcemia are usually dehydrated. *Hydration* is the most urgent objective and can be accomplished by giving intravenous isotonic saline (3 to 10 L/day) to correct the fluid depletion and induce calcium diuresis. The amount of fluid and its composition are determined by the cardiopulmonary, renal, and electrolyte status of the patient. After initial volume repletion, forced diuresis with furosemide, 40 to 80 mg intravenously, results in appreciable calcium diuresis. Furosemide inhibits tubular reabsorption of sodium with a concomitant increase in calcium excretion. Careful attention must be given to electrolyte losses and replacement. Thiazide diuretics are contraindicated because they may decrease urinary excretion of calcium.

Reversal of hypercalcemia and hypercalciuria can be achieved

Table 192-1   Endocrine syndromes associated with malignancy

Syndrome	Hormone	Tumor sites
Hypercalcemia	Osteolytic factors	Lung (squamous), kidney, ovary, many squamous sites
Cushing's	ACTH CRH POMC	Lung (oat cell, bronchial adenoma), thymus, pancreas, thyroid (medullary), stomach, ovary
Inappropriate antidiuresis	ADH	Lung (oat cell)
Zollinger-Ellison	Gastrin	Pancreas (non−β-islet-cell adenomas)
Gynecomastia	Gonadoctropins (HCG, α-, or β-subuntis)	Lung (large cell) testes
Precocious puberty	Gonadotropins (HCG, α-, or β-subunits)	Liver, lung (bronchogenic), teratoma
Erythrocytosis	Erythropoietin	Cerebellum (hemangioblastoma), liver, uterus, kidney
Hypoglycemia	IGF-2	Retroperitoneal or intrathoracic fibrosarcomas, liver, adrenal glands
Galactorrhea	Prolactin	Kidney (hypernephroma)
Pigmentation	ACTH/MSH, lipotropin	Bronchus (oat cell)
Hyperthyroidism	β-HCG	Choriocarcinoma, testis, lung
Others	Serotonin, histamine, insulin, growth hormone, prostaglandins, kinins, secretin, HPL, gastric peptides	Various

with plicamycin (Mithracin) in doses considerably lower than those recommended for use in the treatment of tumors. This drug has a direct effect on bone by inhibiting resorption of calcium from bone. The recommended dose is 25 μg/kg body weight diluted in 1 L of 5% glucose in water and administered by slow intravenous infusion over 4 hours. Intravenous bolus injection has been used by some physicians. This reverses hypercalcemia in 24 to 48 hours, and the effect may last several days. Additional therapy may be given in 2 or 3 days, and subsequent therapy at intervals of 1 week will maintain serum calcium at normal or near-normal levels. Thrombocytopenia and abnormalities in clotting factors can appear when the drug is used habitually, especially with the higher antitumor dosage.

Corticosteroids are effective in treating hypercalcemia associated with myeloma and some breast cancers but less reliable in treating hypercalcemia associated with other malignant neoplasms. Steroids may cause decreased bone resorption, decreased gastrointestinal absorption of calcium, and increased urinary excretion of calcium; they also have a direct action on bone by blocking the action of osteoclast-activating factor. Prednisone, 60 to 100 mg in divided doses orally, or hydrocortisone, 100 to 300 mg intravenously, every 24 hours has been used. The risks of regular steroid use are osteoporosis and the metabolic and electrolyte abnormalities of the cushingoid state.

Calcitonin has a direct inhibitory action on bone and reduces osteoclastic resorption. Renal effects and gastrointestinal actions have also been described. Calcitonin lowers the elevated serum calcium of patients with carcinoma, multiple myeloma, and primary hyperparathyroidism. The recommended starting dose is 4 MRC (Medical Research Council) units/kg body weight every 12 hours subcutaneously or intramuscularly (50 to 400 units). The calcium-lowering response occurs about 2 hours after the injection and lasts for 6 to 8 hours.

Neutral phosphates are effective, but the risk of ectopic calcifications must be recognized because phosphate combines with calcium and deposits in bone and body tissues. Intravenous phosphate, 1.5 to 2 g, should be given slowly over 8 hours. Large amounts of phosphate given rapidly can cause hypocalcemia and shock and should be used only when other methods are not available.

When calcium is lowered to normal or near normal levels, oral phosphate, 1 to 3 g/day in divided doses, is helpful for regular use. A divided dose of 1.5 g/day is reliable and prevents the side effect of diarrhea that is seen with a larger dose of 5 g/day.

Indomethacin, a prostaglandin synthetase inhibitor, has been used with some positive results, as have diphosphonates, estrogen, and progestins.

Primary treatment of the tumor with surgery, irradiation, or cytotoxic agents removes the source of other calcium-elevating substances and lower serum calcium. Adjunctive measures such as increasing body activity, avoiding immobilization, and providing hydration should be used whenever possible.

CUSHING'S SYNDROME

The secretion of large amounts of ACTH is associated with carcinoma of the lung (oat cell type). Lung cancer accounts for 60% of the cases; bronchial carcinoids, epithelial tumors of the thymus, medullary carcinoma of the thyroid, pancreatic tumor, pheochromocytoma, neuroblastoma, and other tumors may be other possible causes.

Tumors associated with this syndrome have also been associated with an increase in POMC; however, human β-MSH has been shown to be an artifact of extraction methods. Most purification methods split β-MSH from a larger peptide, which appears to be β-lipotropin (LPH). It has been found in more than 90% of tumor extracts from a variety of carcinomas and is elevated in 60% of patients with untreated lung cancer who do not have clinical Cushing's syndrome.

The clue to Cushing's syndrome is hypokalemic alkalosis. Any patient with a low serum potassium level, elevated blood sugar level, marked weakness, edema, hypertension, behavioral changes, and increased pigmentation should be studied. Confirmation is obtained by finding high levels of plasma cortisol with loss of the normal diurnal variation, increased urinary 17-hydroxycorticoids or free urinary cortisol, plasma ACTH greater than 200 pg/ml, and failure of suppression with exogenous glucocorticoids. Occult tumors can be localized by finding elevated ACTH levels in selected venous samples.

Surgical removal of the tumor, irradiation, or chemotherapy results in remission of the symptoms resulting from cortisol excess. Treatment with metyrapone, an enzyme blocker, may be used as a temporary measure to reduce cortisol production. Mitotane also suppresses the synthesis of adrenal steroids but requires several weeks of treatment before it is effective.

INAPPROPRIATE ANTIDIURESIS

The continued secretion of antidiuretic hormone (ADH, or vasopressin) inappropriate to the body's needs causes hyponatremia, overhydration, decreased serum osmolality, and concurrent inappropriately elevated urine osmolality. The resulting hypervolemia leads to irritability, drowsiness, lethargy, mental confusion, convulsions, and coma.

Treatment of this syndrome is directed against the tumor itself in the form of surgery, irradiation, or chemotherapy. Oversecretion of vasopressin is only associated with symptoms when excess water is given. Treatment consists of water restriction. Other forms of treatment include drugs that prevent the renal response to vasopressin, such as demeclocyline and lithium carbonate.

HYPOGLYCEMIA

Spontaneous hypoglycemia can occur in patients with nonpancreatic neoplasms. The majority of these are large, mesenchymal tumors such as retroperitoneal or intrathoracic fibrosarcomas, neurofibromas, hepatomas, and adrenocortical carcinomas. Symptoms include sweating, tachycardia, flushing, hunger, drowsiness, convulsions, and coma.

The cause of the hypoglycemia is uncertain. Suggested mechanisms include production of a nonsuppressible, insulin-like material (IGF-2), excessive glucose use by the tumor, and impaired gluconeogenesis. Surgical removal of the tumor alleviates the symptoms. When this is impossible, drug treatment is an option; glucocorticoids in high doses have been used, as well as glucagon and streptozotocin. Continuous intravenous administration of 10% to 20% glucose can be an interim measure.

ECTOPIC GONADOTROPINS

Gynecomastia or precocious puberty results from the ectopic secretion of gonadotropins by neoplasms. These gonadotropins are similar to HCG. HCG-like material is present in normal tissue; however, there appear to be biochemical differences in the HCG that is elaborated with cancer. The ectopic production of the α- and β-subunits of HCG has also been described. The treatment includes surgery, irradiation, or chemotherapy, directed at the tumor.

BIBLIOGRAPHY

Bartuska D: Humoral manifestations of neoplasms, Semin Oncol 2:405, 1975.
Baylin SB and Mendel JG: Ectopic (inappropriate) hormone production by tumors: mechanisms involved and the biological and clinical implications, Endocr Rev 1:45, 1980.
Canfield R, editor: Etidronate Disodium: a new therapy for hypercalcemia of malignancy: proceedings of a symposium, Am J Med 82(2A):1, 1987.
Mundy GR and others: The hypercalcemia of cancer: clinical implications and pathogenetic mechanisms, N Engl J Med 310:1718, 1984.
Mundy GR: Ectopic humoral syndromes in neoplastic disease, Hosp Pract 22:179, 1987.
Simpson EL and others: Absence of parathyroid hormone messenger RNA in nonparathyroid tumors associated with hypercalcemia, N Engl J Med 309:325, 1983.

193 • MINERAL METABOLISM AND METABOLIC BONE DISEASE

William J Burtis *and* **Howard Rasmussen**

PHYSIOLOGY OF BONE

To understand the pathophysiology of the disease states discussed in this chapter, an understanding of both skeletal and mineral homeostasis is needed. Bones support the body, provide sites of muscular attachment for movement, and protect fragile tissues such as the lungs and central nervous system.

Skeletal homeostasis refers to the process of responding to changing demands for mechanical strength while maintaining skeletal integrity. In addition, bone serves an important biochemical role as a calcium reservoir. Mineral homeostasis refers to the process of maintaining serum calcium and phosphate levels within physiologic limits. Before discussing bone disease, it is necessary to review briefly the structure and turnover of bone and the hormonal regulation of mineral metabolism.

Structure and turnover of bone

Bone is a functional, dynamic tissue with approximately 30,000 living cells/cubic mm. These cells, interconnected by long processes running through tiny bone canaliculae, and the envelope of cells that surrounds bone mediate the processes of skeletal and mineral homeostasis. Bone can respond rapidly to changes in mineral and hormone concentrations. Through the complex process of remodeling, all skeletal tissue is destroyed and rebuilt with a half-life of about 20 months. Throughout adult life, bone retains an extraordinary capacity for morphologically accurate regeneration following injury.

Bone is a tissue with two components: an organic matrix made up largely of collagen and proteoglycans and a solid mineral phase. This mineral phase is not completely homogeneous but consists of several different types of calcium phosphate salts. The predominant type is small crystals of hydroxyapatite ($Ca_{10}[PO_4]_6[OH]_2$). There is a lesser content of amorphous calcium phosphate characterized by a lower calcium/phosphate ratio than that of crystalline hydroxyapatite. Regardless of which form exists in a particular region of bone, the essential fact is that matrix formation always precedes bone mineral deposition. This means that it is the amount and organization of the matrix that determine the size and shape of the bone. The mineral component is deposited in close apposition to the collagen fibrils. It is this intimate relationship that confers on bone its unique mechanical and tensile properties.

At the tissue level there are two types of bone, cortical and trabecular. The cortical bone forms the solid component of the shafts of long bones and the tabular surfaces of the flat bones of the face, pelvis, and vertebrae. This bone is dense and solid except where it is penetrated by haversian canals. The trabecular or spongy bone fills the layer between the tables of flat bones and vertebrae and also the distal ends of the shafts of long bones. It is, as its name implies, a spongy lacework of tiny interlocking trabeculae.

There are two types of bone formation, endochondral and intramembranous. In the former, growth occurs on the surfaces of the vertebral bodies and at specialized epiphyseal plates at the end of long bones. At these sites the growth event is a proliferation of cartilage cells, which then lay down an extracellular organic matrix. The deposition of this new matrix actually extends the length of the bone. Following this phase the cartilage cells hypertrophy and partially resorb the new matrix. The remaining matrix then calcifies to create primary bone. Once formed, this primary bone undergoes successive remodeling cycles of resorption and redeposition of true bone (intramembranous bone).

At the periosteal surface of all long bones, as well as the bones of the face, the process of bone formation does not involve the formation of primary cartilaginous bone but occurs by direct bone deposition consisting of collagen synthesis, extracellular organization of the collagen into distinct lamellae, and mineralization of these lamellae. This type of bone formation is known as modeling, in contrast to remodeling (see discussion that follows). Since it continues at a slow rate throughout life, the total cortical diameter of the long bones increases slightly with age and the shape of the facial bones undergoes continued change. Although not usually influenced by changes in hormone concentration within the physiologic range, this bone is sensitive to excess amounts of growth hormone and parathyroid hormone. The former causes the rate of its formation to increase, accounting for the increase in glove and shoe size and the prognathism characteristic of acromegaly.

Cessation of longitudinal growth depends on the disappearance of the growth or epiphyseal plates. The rates of their maturation and growth vary independently, and both are under hormonal control. Thyroid hormone deficiency causes a delay in both, testosterone increases both, and growth hormone increases growth rate without altering maturation.

Once a human reaches adulthood the epiphyseal bone growth stops, but the skeleton continues to undergo constant remodeling throughout life. This remodeling is of two types: the haversian remodeling of cortical bone and the surface remodeling of trabecular bone. In the first type a group of bone-resorbing cells enters the cortical bone perpendicular to the long axis of the bone and then, after penetrating a variable distance, turns at right angles and cuts out a cylindric core of bone. This resorptive phase is followed by a quiescent phase and then a phase of new bone formation that fills or nearly refills the cylindric core except for a small canal, the haversian canal, containing blood vessels and nerve fibers. It is obvious that in this compact cortical bone, a remodeling sequence in one of these bone remodeling units (BMUs) must start with resorption of old bone followed by formation of new within the resorption cavity. Thus haversian remodeling is a sequential process. A group of cells is activated to become *osteoclasts* that resorb bone, followed by a resorptive phase during which the osteoclasts remove old bone, followed by a reversal phase in which resorption has stopped and the bone surface is lined with mononuclear cells but no formation is occurring, followed by a phase of formation of new bone matrix by *osteoblasts*, followed finally by the mineralization of bone by *osteoid osteocytes*.

A clarifying comment concerning the processes of bone formation and resorption is necessary. As noted previously, the formation of either type of bone is a two-step process: (1) the elaboration of an organic matrix and (2) subsequent mineralization of that matrix. However, when bone is resorbed, both matrix and mineral are removed simultaneously. Hence unmineralized bone, so-called osteoid, results from a failure of normal mineralization rather than from selective removal of the mineral from the matrix of old, previously mineralized bone.

Trabecular bone remodeling, a surface rather than an internal remodeling process, also follows this sequence of activation → resorption → reversal → formation → mineralization. The only difference, aside from the geometric one of internal versus surface remodeling, is that the process is more rapid in trabecular bone than in cortical bone.

After 20 to 25 years of age the amount of both trabecular and cortical bone removed during the resorption phase is not quite replaced during the phase of subsequent formation within each remodeling site, or BMU. This means there is a slow but progressive loss of skeletal mass at an annual rate of 0.5%. In men this continues at a more or less constant linear rate throughout life. In women, however, beginning at menopause (45 to 55 years of age), the net loss of bone is accelerated significantly for 4 to 7 years, so that in many women over 60 the mass of bone is critically reduced and vertebral and hip fractures are common. This condition, known as postmenopausal osteoporosis, will be discussed later in this chapter.

In a variety of other conditions changes in the rates of remodeling and the balance between resorption and formation can occur. The major hormones involved in regulating the various steps in bone remodeling are presented in Fig. 193-1.

To fully understand the remodeling process and the diseases associated with it, its cellular basis must be considered. As previously mentioned, osteoclasts are responsible for resorption and osteoblasts for bone formation. However, recent work has shown that these cells arise from separate precursor pools. Osteoclasts arise from bloodborne cells, probably a subclass of monocytes, and osteoblasts derive from bone tissue cells. In most situations in which an increase in the rate of activation of new BMUs occurs, there is a concomitant increase in both resorption and subsequent formation. For example, in most patients with mild hyperparathyroidism there is a significant increase in the rate of bone remodeling without a change in bone mass. This observation implies some type of close *coupling* between the number and activity of osteoclasts and the number and activity of the osteoblasts that will subsequently appear at a remodeling site.

In other words, by some means not yet understood, osteoclasts and osteoblasts must "communicate" so that bone resorption and subsequent bone formation remain linked. Parathyroid hormone (PTH) is a potent stimulus that activates bone remodeling. PTH receptors are known to be present on osteoblasts but have never been demonstrated on osteoclasts. Two theories have been postulated to explain how PTH might initiate osteoclastic bone resorption. One theory holds that under the influence of PTH, the envelope of inactive osteoblasts lining the bone surface separates to expose calcified bone tissue directly to osteoclasts, which then begin the bone resorption process. The other theory, for which there is some recent evidence, holds that under the influence of PTH, osteoblasts produce a "paracrine" chemical mediator which in turn stimulates osteoclasts to start bone resorption. In some bone diseases, to be discussed later in the chapter, the link between bone resorption and formation is deficient, resulting in osteoporosis or, less commonly, osteopetrosis.

Mineral metabolism

It is convenient to consider mineral metabolism in terms of two ions, calcium and phosphate; three organs, kidney, gut, and bone; and three hormones, vitamin D and its metabolites, PTH, and calcitonin (CT). The first of these hormones is a group of sterols and the other two are peptides.

CALCIUM METABOLISM. There are two critical aspects of calcium metabolism. The first is that the plasma ionized calcium concentration is a major regulator of all types of cellular functions, most notably neuromuscular excitability. When this concentration falls, neuromuscular excitability increases and a condition of tetany with spontaneous muscle contractions may ensue. When full blown, the syndrome of tetany is characterized by muscle stiffness and cramps, carpal or pedal spasm, circumoral paresthesias, bronchospasm, laryngospasm, and, particularly in young children, grand mal seizures. Two useful clinical clues in the diagnosis of tetany are Chvostek's sign (contractions of the facial muscles in response to a light tapping of the facial nerve) and Trousseau's sign (carpal spasm induced by occluding the circulation to the forearm and hand with a blood pressure cuff). A lengthening of the QT_c interval of the electrocardiogram can also signal hypocalcemia.

Hypercalcemia results in depressed neuromuscular excitability, anorexia, drowsiness, nausea, constipation, and often polyuria and polydipsia because of a direct effect of the high plasma calcium level on the concentrating ability of the kidney.

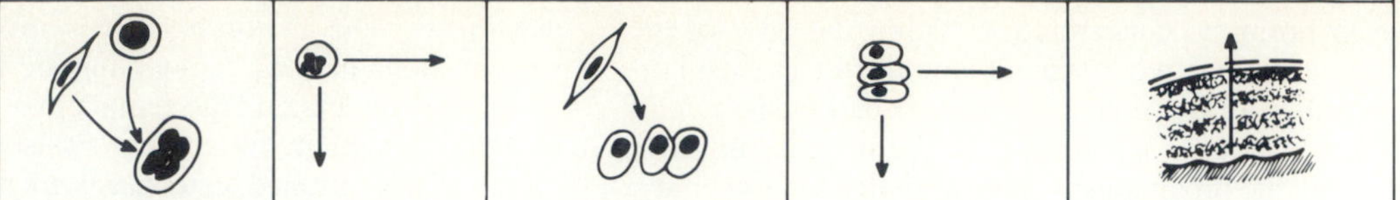

Phase	Activation	Resorption	Reversal	Formation	Mineralization
Cell or cellular event	Osteoprogenitor → Osteoclast	Osteoclast	Osteoprogenitor$_{II}$ → Osteoblast Osteoclast → ?	Osteoblast	Osteoid osteocyte
Control factors Positive	PTH↑ TH↑ Ca^{2+}↑ Paget's factor↑	PTH↑ TH↑ Ca^{2+}↑ 1,25(OH)$_2$D$_3$↑	CT↑ Estrogen↑ Phosphate↑	Fluoride↑ Phosphate↑ 25(OH)D$_3$?	Phosphate↑ $\begin{cases}1,25(OH)_2D_3 \\ 24,25(OH)_2D_3\end{cases}$↕ 25(OH)D$_3$↑
Negative	CT↓ Estrogen ?↓	CT↓ EHDP↓ Fluoride↓	Cortisol↓ Immobilization↓ Age↓	Immobilization↓ Age↓ Cortisol↓ EHDP↓	Fluoride↓ EHDP↓

Fig. 193-1   Ionic and hormonal control of the bone remodeling process. Process is a sequential one of activation → resorption → reversal → formation → mineralization. Factors listed in lower half of the figure are thought to regulate the respective steps, *PTH*, parathyroid hormone; *TH*, thyroid hormone; *CT*, calcitonin; *EHDP*, disodium ethane-1 hydroxy-1 diphosphonate.

Because of calcium's many effects on cell function and its critical role in maintaining normal neuromuscular excitability, an elaborate system has developed to maintain the plasma calcium concentration within a very narrow range of 9.5 to 10.5 mg/dl of total calcium or 3.8 to 4.8 mg/dl of ionized calcium. The difference between these values depends on the fact that approximately 60% of the serum calcium is bound, largely to albumin but also to a minor degree to organic anions. Only the ionized component of the serum calcium is biologically important in terms, for example, of neuromuscular excitability. However, in routine clinical practice it is usually the total calcium that is measured. In most cases when total calcium is increased or decreased, there is a corresponding increase or decrease in ionized calcium. However, there are conditions in which there is an increase or decrease in the total protein or anion content of the serum, and this is associated with an increase or decrease in total calcium but no change in ionized calcium.

The second feature of calcium metabolism is that the serum calcium concentration is maintained despite fluctuating demands of the skeleton. Therefore, even in periods of rapid skeletal growth, a fall in serum calcium concentration does not occur. It seems, in other words, that the growing skeleton communicates its need to the intestine.

Figure 193-2 is a schematic representation of calcium metabolism. There is 1.5 to 2 kg of calcium in the average adult. Over 97% of this is in the skeleton, a small amount (5 to 10 g) is in the cells, and 1 to 2 g is in the plasma and extracellular fluids. In a normal young adult there is a constant exchange of calcium between the plasma and the bone, kidney, and intestine. When the daily dietary calcium intake is 1000 mg, there is a net absorption of approximately 200 mg and a total intestinal absorption of 350 mg because of an endogenous secretion of 150 mg. There is a net accretion of approximately 500 mg of calcium into new bone each day and a net removal of approximately 520 mg from old bone. The kidney filters 7000 mg daily and reabsorbs all but 220 mg, which is excreted

into the urine. The bulk of the filtered calcium is reabsorbed in the proximal tubule, and this process is probably not regulated by hormones. The remainder, 700 to 1050 mg, is reabsorbed distally in a process controlled by PTH. A small amount of calcium is lost each day in shedding of the skin.

From the data represented in Fig. 193-2, it is apparent that the intestine and kidney are vital in helping the organism maintain a normal or positive calcium balance. If the functions of these organs are integrated properly, a normal calcium balance can be maintained. The intestine normally absorbs only a small percentage of the ingested calcium. This percentage is obviously greater in growing children. The major hormone regulating this process of intestinal calcium absorption is the active metabolite of vitamin D, 1,25-dihydroxyvitamin D$_3$. However, since intestinal and renal adaptation to a low calcium intake is not completely efficient, individuals with a daily dietary intake of less than 300 mg may be in negative calcium balance, even though they absorb as much as 30% of the ingested amount. Furthermore, it is likely that this adaptation becomes less efficient with advancing age. Under these circumstances the only source of calcium for the maintenance of a normal serum level is the calcium in bone mineral. Hence, dietary calcium lack leads to a progressive loss of bone mass.

PHOSPHATE METABOLISM. The normal adult contains approximately 1 kg of elemental phosphorus present as free inorganic phosphate ($HPO_4^=$, $H_2PO_4^-$, or $PO_4^{\equiv}$), as inorganic phosphate as part of the mineral lattice of bone mineral, or in a variety of organic phosphate esters ranging from deoxyribonucleic acid (DNA), ribonucleic acid (RNA), and adenosine triphosphate (ATP) to the glycolytic intermediates and phospholipid. Approximately 85% of the total is in bone, 0.008% in plasma and extracellular fluids, and the remainder in cells. As illustrated in Fig. 193-3, there is a constant turnover of phosphate in the body. A typical daily diet provides approximately 1000 mg of phosphate phosphorus. Between 65% and 80% is absorbed. The plasma and extracellular fluids contain only 800 mg. Following a normal meal, the plasma phosphate

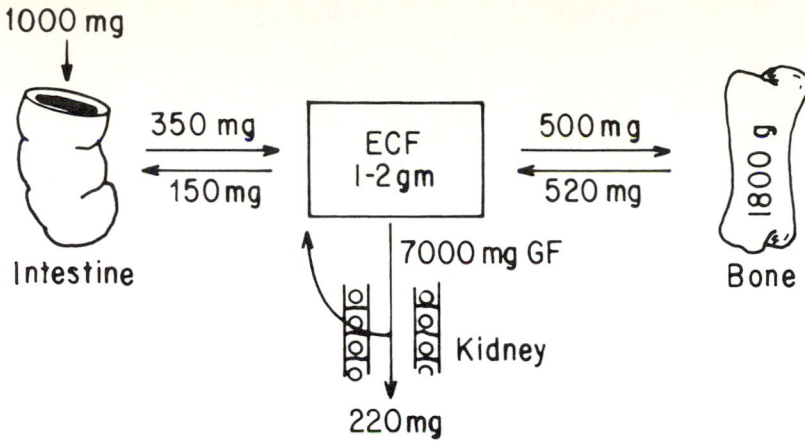

Fig. 193-2   Schematic representation of human calcium metabolism (see text). *ECF*, extracellular fluid; *GF*, glomerular filtration.

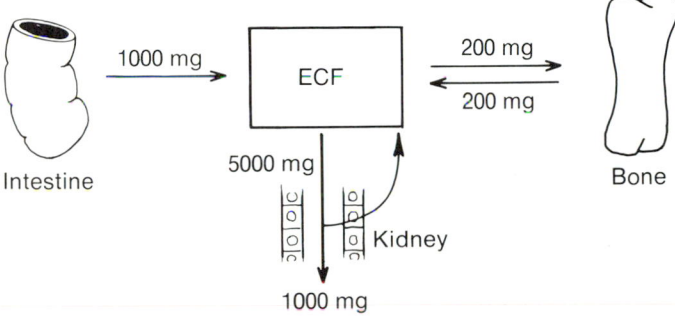

Fig. 193-3   Schematic representation of human phosphate metabolism.

concentration of 2.8 to 4 mg/dl (as phosphorus) rises as much as 1 mg/dl. However, the kidney filters approximately 5000 mg each day, of which approximately 1000 mg is excreted and the remainder is reabsorbed. Reabsorption occurs in both the proximal and distal tubules and is inhibited at both sites by PTH. CT also inhibits proximal tubular reabsorption of phosphate. The effect of vitamin D metabolites is controversial. There is evidence that 25-hydroxyvitamin D may stimulate proximal tubular phosphate reabsorption. Finally, there is the accretion of approximately 200 mg of phosphate into new bone each day and the removal of a slightly greater amount from the resorption of old bone.

A comparison of the scheme of calcium metabolism illustrated in Fig. 193-2 with that of phosphate metabolism shown in Fig. 193-3 reveals one important difference. The intestine plays the major role in determining the availability of the calcium ion. In the case of phosphate, the kidney plays the dominant role. This can be dramatically illustrated by the changes that occur in vitamin D deficiency. The active metabolite, $1,25(OH)_2D_3$, regulates the intestinal absorption of both calcium and phosphate. When the plasma concentration of $1,25(OH)_2D_3$ falls, the intestinal absorption of both ions decreases. However, calcium absorption may rapidly decrease to none and because of endogenous fecal excretion of calcium may lead to a net loss of calcium from the body. On the other hand, phosphate absorption, although it may diminish, will still lead to a net absorption of several hundred milligrams. Thus under most circumstances the plasma phosphate concentration is determined by the renal threshold for phosphate ex-

cretion (renal tubular maximum phosphate reabsorption/glomerular filtration rate, TmP/GFR), and not by the dietary intake. From this difference it is easy to see why phosphate accumulation and hyperphosphatemia commonly occur in chronic renal disease.

VITAMIN D METABOLISM. The natural source of vitamin D in humans is the skin, where under the influence of ultraviolet irradiation from the sun the provitamin 7-dehydrocholesterol is converted to vitamin D_3 (Fig. 193-4). This compound is biologically inert, at least in normal physiologic concentrations, and must undergo further metabolism before exerting its biologic effect. In city-dwellers who live in northern climates, work indoors, and go about fully clothed, the rate of vitamin D synthesis in the skin may be insufficient to supply the body's need. In this case what was once a hormone derived from skin becomes an essential dietary trace substance, a vitamin. This dietary need can be supplied by either synthetically prepared vitamin D_3 or vitamin D_2 (irradiated ergosterol). As far as is known, vitamin D_2 and vitamin D_3 are equipotent and are metabolized in the same way, although they have a difference in side chain structure.

Vitamin D_3 is considered a prohormone, not a hormone. It is normally made in the skin and either stored in adipose tissue or bound to a sterol-binding protein in the plasma. The first step in its metabolic conversion is to 25-hydroxyvitamin D_3 $(25[OH]D_3)$. This conversion takes place in the liver microsomes and is probably regulated by a number of factors. However, in general the higher the amount of D_3 made in the body, the higher the amount of circulating $25(OH)D_3$. This compound is stored largely in the plasma, bound to the same sterol-binding protein as vitamin D_3. Its normal concentration in human plasma is 20 to 50 ng/ml. It has a direct action on bone by increasing bone resorption. It is less effective on a molar basis in this regard than is $1,25(OH)_2D_3$, but since it is present in considerably higher concentrations than $1,25(OH)_2D_3$, it may play a physiologic role in regulating bone resorption. In addition, $25(OH)D_3$ serves as the substrate for the further metabolic conversions to 1,25-dihydroxyvitamin D_3; 24,25-dihydroxyvitamin D_3; and 25,26-dihydroxyvitamin D_3 (Fig. 193-4). Very little work has been done on the biology and possible clinical relevance of $25,26(OH)_2D_3$. Of the other two metabolites, $1,25(OH)_2D_3$ is the more important and more fully studied and is used clinically. Both it and $24,25(OH)_2D_3$ are made in the kidney mitochondria from $25(OH)D_3$. There is evidence that $24,25(OH)_2D_3$ is also made elsewhere, particularly in bone.

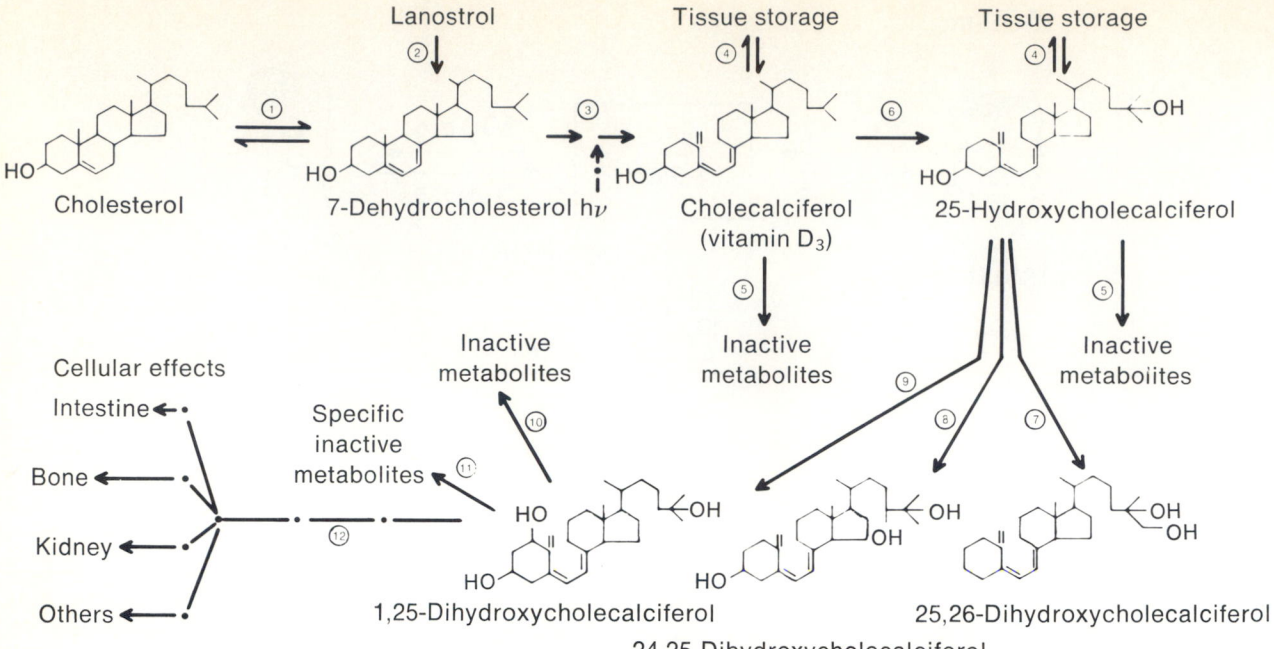

Fig. 193-4   Vitamin D metabolism. Vitamin D can come from diet or be synthesized in skin from cholesterol. Cholesterol is converted first to 7-dehydrocholesterol *(1)*. This compound is activated by sunlight *(3)* and gives rise to vitamin D_2. Vitamin D can be stored *(4)*, catabolized *(5)*, or converted in liver to 24-hydroxycholecalciferol (25-hydroxyvitamin D_3) *(6)*. This metabolite can be converted into one of three dihydroxymetabolites *(7, 8, and 9)*. Little is known of $25.26(OH)_2D_3$. The $24.25(OH)_2D_3$ may have a function. The most studied and most active metabolite, $1.25(OH)_2D_3$, is made in kidney. It acts on intestine, bone, and possibly kidney.

However, the kidney appears to be the major source of $1,25(OH)_2D_3$ in humans. The plasma concentration of $24,25(OH)_2D_3$ is usually about one-tenth that of $25(OH)D_3$, and little is known about the factors that regulate its synthesis. A striking fact about its metabolism is that its rate of catabolism is slow, with a turnover time of days rather than hours, unlike $1,25(OH)_2D_3$.

The renal biosynthesis of $1,25(OH)_2D_3$ is highly regulated. Its concentration in normal human plasma is 35 to 60 pg/ml, or approximately 0.1% of the concentration of $25(OH)D_3$. The major factors known to control its rate of synthesis are PTH and plasma phosphate. An increase in PTH or a fall in plasma phosphate will stimulate $1,25(OH)_2D_3$ synthesis. However, other factors are obviously important too because not all patients with primary hyperparathyroidism or acquired hypophosphatemia have high values of plasma $1,25(OH)_2D_3$.

The intestine and bone are the major sites of action of $1,25(OH)_2D_3$. Its major effect on the intestine is to stimulate the active absorption of both calcium and phosphate. Its effect on bone is to stimulate the resorption of bone, thereby liberating both calcium and phosphate from old bone. In addition to these well-established effects, it is clear that $1,25(OH)_2D_3$ and the other metabolites of vitamin D have a direct action on muscle. A major sign of vitamin D deficiency is profound proximal muscle weakness. Recent evidence suggests that $1,25(OH)_2D_3$ also exerts a negative feedback effect on the parathyroid gland. Conversely, when the $1,25(OH)_2D_3$ level is low, it stimulates synthesis of PTH. This may be part of the reason that secondary hyperparathyroidism develops in renal failure, which is associated with impaired ability to synthesize $1,25(OH)_2D_3$.

The site(s) of action of $24,25(OH)_2D_3$ is still a matter of controversy, but this metabolite seems to exert two physiologically important effects: it suppresses PTH secretion and stim-

ulates bone mineralization. To understand the possible significance of these actions, it is necessary to consider the consequences of vitamin D deficiency.

The most dramatic results of vitamin D deficiency are rickets and osteomalacia. These are failures of mineralization of endochrondal and membranous bone, respectively. As mentioned previously, bone formation is a two-step process of initial matrix formation followed by its mineralization; osteomalacia or rickets results from a delay in the mineralization process. In severe vitamin D deficiency the absolute rate of matrix synthesis also decreases, but there is always a greater relative decrease in the mineralization rate so that increasing amounts of unmineralized osteoid appear. There continue to be two schools of thought concerning the pathogenesis of the osteomalacia of vitamin D deficiency. One school holds that a deficiency of $1,25(OH)_2D_3$ alone is sufficient to explain the process. In this view the two effects of $1,25(OH)_2D_3$—increasing absorption of calcium and phosphate from the gut and increasing resorption of calcium and phosphate from old bone—are sufficient to raise the serum concentrations of calcium and phosphate to normal and thereby ensure appropriate mineralization of bone. Thus the mineralization process proceeds normally as long as the ion product $(CA^{++} \times HPO_4^=)$ in plasma is normal. The other school, while not disputing that $1,25(OH)_2D_3$ exerts these effects, points out that there are conditons in which the mineral ion product and the plasma $1,25(OH)_2D_3$ are normal, but the $25(OH)D_3$ and $24,25(OH)_2D_3$ concentrations are low and osteomalacia is present. On the basis of this and other experimental data, they argue that $25(OH)D_3$ and $24,25(OH)_2D_3$ directly effect bone mineral metabolism.

PARATHYROID HORMONE (PTH) METABOLISM. PTH is a straight-chain polypeptide of 84 amino acids. It is unusual because it undergoes peripheral metabolism (Fig. 193-5), lead-

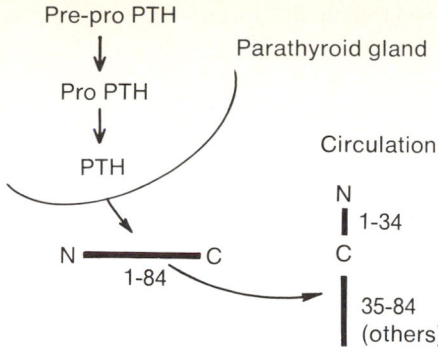

Fig. 193-5   Synthesis and metabolism of parathyroid hormone. PTH is made as larger precursor (pre-pro PTH) in parathyroid gland. This is processed (pro PTH) eventually to peptide containing 84 amino acid residues. This is major secretory product of gland. It is metabolized in periphery to N-terminal fragment (amino acids 1 to 34), which is biologically active, and C-terminal one, which is not.

ing to the appearance of multiple fragments in normal plasma. Not all of these are biologically active, and some of them may come from partial degradation of the native hormone in the gland before its release into the circulation. These multiple types of circulating fragments lead to considerable difficulty in making a direct correlation between immunoreactive PTH, that measured by radioimmunoassay, and the biologically active hormone in plasma.

The major peripheral conversion is from the original molecule of 84 amino acids to a C-terminal fragment of amino acids 35 to 84 and an N-terminal fragment of amino acids 1 to 34. Both the parent 84 amino acid molecule and the N-terminal fragment are biologically active. It is not known with any certainty whether the conversion from the parent molecule to the N-terminal fragment is a necessary step before this hormone exerts its effects. Some believe that this is the case and that the 84 amino acid molecule is actually a prohormone. However, the data supporting this view are incomplete, and it remains possible that only some of the physiologic effects, such as those on the kidney, are exerted by the N-terminal hormone, whereas other actions, such as those on bone, result from the 84 amino acid hormone. Alternatively, the peripheral conversion may represent a purely catabolic process and the pathway of hormone degradation. Against this view are the facts that synthetic human N-fragment possesses all the biologic actions of the 84 amino acid molecule and that peripheral conversion of the parent molecule to the N-terminal fragment is controlled by Ca^{++}. In any case there is very little N-terminal fragment normally present in plasma, and its half-life is a matter of minutes. On the other hand, there is considerably more of the 35 to 84 amino acid fragment and other C-terminal fragments derived from it. These are biologically inactive and persist for longer periods in the circulation.

Radioimmunoassay is a commonly used method of measuring the concentration of a hormone in plasma or serum. In theory this is a simple technique in which an antibody to the particular hormone is raised in a suitable animal. This antibody is then used as a reagent to measure the amount of the hormone in blood. The fact that PTH undergoes peripheral metabolism makes it difficult to develop an assay that measures the biologically active hormone in plasma. Different antibodies against the bovine 84 amino acid molecule recognize different antigenic determinants on this molecule, and when used in a radioimmunoassay they measure different mixtures of intact

84 amino acid molecule and C-terminal fragments. Hence, different assays yield different absolute results on the same sample of plasma. Furthermore, since an absolute standard and human 84 amino acid molecules are not available, the standard employed in different assays is not the same. It is usually a serum from a patient or patients with hyperparathyroidism. To further complicate the issue, the kidney is a major site for the disposal of the C-terminal fragments. Hence, in chronic renal disease the level of immunoreactive PTH is high both because of phosphate retention and hypocalcemia leading to secondary hyperparathyroidism and because of a decreased rate of catabolism of C-terminal fragments.

PTH has two major functions: maintaining the plasma calcium concentration and regulating the rate of bone remodeling. There is a negative feedback relationship between the plasma calcium concentration and the rate of PTH secretion; a fall in calcium concentration stimulates secretion and a rise suppresses it. This basic control system is augmented by two other factors: catecholamines stimulate PTH secretion and $24,25(OH)_2D_3$ suppresses it. The physiologic significance of these subsidiary modulators is unknown.

The major effects of PTH are exerted on two organs, bone and kidney. The hormone acts on all bone cell types: preosteoclasts, osteoclasts, osteoblasts, and osteocytes. The physiologic consequences of its actions depend on the calcium balance of the organism. When dietary calcium is adequate, the actions of PTH on kidney (directly) and gut (indirectly) are the major factors in determining mineral homeostasis. In this case an increase in PTH does not lead to a net loss of bone mineral but only to an increase in the rate of bone remodeling. This occurs because PTH is a potent inducer of the activation step of the remodeling process (Fig. 193-1). However, in calcium deficiency states an increase in PTH leads to a net loss of bone mineral because, in addition to an enhanced rate of bone remodeling, there is an imbalance between bone resorption and subsequent formation. Under these circumstances the bone and kidney become the major organs determining plasma calcium concentration. Thus prolonged calcium deficiency leads to bone loss and osteoporosis.

PTH exerts three major effects on the kidney at three anatomically distinct tubular sites. It inhibits proximal tubular phosphate reabsorption; it stimulates $1,25(OH)_2D_3$ synthesis at a proximal tubular site; and it stimulates the distal tubular reabsorption of calcium. Since $1,25(OH)_2D_3$ is the major hormonal regulator of intestinal calcium absorption, the PTH-mediated synthesis of $1,25(OH)_2D_3$ coordinates events in the intestine with those in the kidney. However, for the system to function correctly, the various renal tubular effects of PTH must be integrated. An imbalance between these renal effects can lead to hypercalciuria (excess urinary calcium excretion) and thereby to renal stones.

At the cellular level PTH has two effects. It increases the uptake of calcium, and it stimulates the enzyme adenylate cyclase. The latter effect is of practical significance because, as a consequence of cyclase activation in proximal renal tubular cells, the content of cyclic adenosine 3'5'-monophosphate (cyclic AMP) in the cell increases. Some of this leaks out of the cell across the luminal membrane and appears in the urine. Although other hormones such as vasopressin acting in other parts of the nephron also activate adenylate cyclase in their target cells, only in the case of PTH does this increase the content of cyclic AMP in the urine. By measuring the creatinine clearance, the total urinary cyclic AMP, and the plasma cyclic AMP, it is possible to calculate the amount of cyclic AMP filtered at the glomerulus and thus obtain a value known as the *nephrogenous cyclic AMP.* This is the total urinary cyclic AMP minus the filtered cyclic AMP. It is reported in relation to renal mass, in terms of nmoles per 100 milliliters glomerular filtrate (GF). The normal values are 0.5 to 2.5 nmoles/100 ml GF. They fall to 0 in hypoparathyroidism and range from 2.6 to 10 in hyperparathyroidism. The measurement of nephrogenous cyclic AMP is therefore an in vivo assay of biologically active PTH in man. It is a better discriminator between normal individuals and patients with hyperparathyroidism than are the usual radioimmunoassays for PTH. However, as will be discussed, there is another clinical condition that may be associated with hypercalcemia and high nephrogenous cyclic AMP: so-called humoral hypercalcemia of malignancy. Other tests can distinguish this condition from primary hyperparathyroidism.

CALCITONIN METABOLISM. Calcitonin (CT) is a single-chain peptide hormone containing 32 amino acid residues. In contrast to PTH, the entire molecule of CT appears necessary for the hormone to exert its biologic effect. Also unlike PTH, there is no evidence that CT, once secreted, undergoes any peripheral metabolism other than that of rapid degradation.

CT is secreted by the parenchymal or "C" cells of the human thyroid gland. These cells are distinct in function and embryologic origin from the classic cells that synthesize, store, and secrete thyroid hormones. The latter do not produce CT, whereas the parenchymal cells produce CT but not thyroid hormones. Thus within the thyroid there are two distinct endocrine tissues.

As with PTH secretion, there is a feedback relationship between the secretion rate of CT and the plasma calcium concentration. However, in the case of CT secretion, the relationship is the opposite to that found with PTH. A rise in plasma calcium concentration stimulates CT secretion, and a fall causes secretion to cease. In addition, gastrin and possibly other gastrointestinal hormones enhance CT secretion. Following the ingestion of a meal containing calcium, CT secretion increases before a detectable increase in plasma calcium concentration is observed.

One of the problems in defining the function of CT is that, in contrast to most other hormones, no clinical syndrome attributable to CT deficiency is yet known. Patients after total thyroidectomy do very well with only thyroid hormone replacement, and no significant changes in calcium or bone metabolism occur. A clinically recognizable syndrome involving CT excess is medullary carcinoma. Even in these cases it is abnormalities other than the effect of CT on mineral metabolism that bring the patients to the attention of a physician. The most interesting speculation is that CT is a calcium storage hormone. Its secretion is stimulated by calcium ingestion, and its action on bone produces a net uptake of calcium by the skeleton during times of calcium surplus. Simultaneously, it minimizes any postprandial rise in plasma calcium concentration.

The target organs for CT are bone and kidney. In the kidney, CT (like PTH) inhibits proximal tubular phosphate reabsorption, but unlike PTH it increases rather than decreases urinary calcium excretion. It has two effects on bone. The first is a rapid suppression of osteoclastic bone resorption and a shortening of osteoclast lifetime. The second, less rapid result is a suppressed activation of new bone remodeling units (BMUs). In this regard the effects of CT on bone remodeling are the opposite of those of PTH (Fig. 193-1).

In addition to acting on kidney and bone, CT also increases fluid and electrolyte secretion in the intestine. The physiologic significance of this is unknown.

COORDINATE CONTROL OF MINERAL METABOLISM. To clarify the nature of the feedback system controlling plasma calcium concentration, it is worthwhile to describe the physiologic consequences of deficiencies in calcium, PTH, phosphate, and vitamin D.

In the case of dietary calcium deficiency, reduced intestinal calcium absorption leads to a fall in the serum calcium concentration. This stimulates PTH secretion. The PTH acts on the distal nephron to increase the renal retention of calcium and on the proximal nephron to increase the synthesis of $1,25(OH)_2D_3$. The increased $1,25(OH)_2D_3$ acts on the intestine to stimulate intestinal calcium absorption, but this is relatively ineffective in cases of dietary calcium deficiency. In addition, the PTH and $1,25(OH)_2D_3$ act together to stimulate net removal of calcium from bone. By these direct or indirect effects on the three organs, PTH serves to maintain a normal serum calcium concentration at the expense of the net skeletal mineral balance. PTH also alters phosphate metabolism. At the level of both bone and intestine, the greater flow of calcium into the extracellular fluids is accompanied by an increased transfer of phosphate. These effects would be expected to raise the serum phosphate concentration, but this does not occur. In fact, a slight fall in plasma phosphate concentration actually occurs because the increased circulating PTH blocks phosphate reabsorption in the proximal renal tubules.

In the case of a sudden PTH deficiency, the lack of effect of PTH on bone would reduce delivery of both calcium and phosphate to the extracellular fluids. The loss of the renal effects would lead to an increase in renal calcium loss, a decrease in phosphate loss, and a decrease in $1,25(OH)_2D_3$ synthesis. A lack of the vitamin D hormone would decrease intestinal absorption of calcium and phosphate. Because of all these changes the serum calcium concentration would fall from its normal value of 9.5 to 10.5 mg/dl to the range of 5 to 6 mg/dl. On the other hand, the plasma phosphate concentration would rise from 3 to 4.5 mg/dl to a value of 7 to 9 mg/dl. This would occur despite decreased delivery of phosphate from bone and intestine because of the profound change in the renal threshold (TmP/GFR) for phosphate excretion that occurs in the absence of PTH.

Phosphate deficiency from simple dietary lack is nearly unheard of, but a state of phosphate deficiency can result if a low phosphate intake is combined with the administration of phosphate binders such as aluminum hydroxide (Amphojel). It may also occur in patients with diabetic ketoacidosis or alcoholism, particularly during the treatment of these conditions. A deficiency of phosphate lowers plasma phosphate concentration. This stimulates the renal synthesis of $1,25(OH)_2D_3$ (independent of PTH action). The increased $1,25(OH)_2D_3$ stimulates intestinal calcium and phosphate absorption and the net removal of these ions from bone. These events cause a rise in the serum calcium concentration and hence a fall in PTH secretion. This decreases distal tubular reabsorption of calcium, thereby enhancing the rate of disposal of calcium in the urine so that marked hypercalcemia does not occur. However, hypercalciuria is found because of the increased delivery of calcium from gut and bone. The excretion of phosphate in the urine declines to undetectable values because of both a lack of PTH effect on the proximal tubule and the direct impact that phosphate deficiency exerts on the renal tubular phosphate transport system.

Vitamin D deficiency is the most complicated of the deficiency states discussed in this chapter. Deficiency of vitamin D does not have any immediate consequence because the body stores a considerable amount of this prohormone, which may be sufficient to supply the body's needs for several months. Eventually, however, the concentrations of $25(OH)D_3$

and $24,25(OH)_2D_3$ begin to fall. This leads to a decrease in bone resorption, which in turn causes a fall in the serum calcium concentration. As a result the rate of PTH secretion is increased, leading to renal retention of calcium, increased synthesis of $1,25(OH)_2D_3$, and accelerated renal phosphate loss. The biochemical findings at this point are a nearly normal plasma calcium concentration and a low plasma phosphate concentration. The low concentrations of plasma phosphate, $25(OH)D_3$, and $24,25(OH)_2D_3$ decrease the rate of bone mineralization so that osteomalacia develops. As the bone surface becomes increasingly covered with osteoid, less bone mineral is released. Furthermore, as the degree of vitamin D deficiency progresses, the plasma $1,25(OH)_2D_3$ level falls, leading to a decrease in intestinal calcium absorption and the plasma calcium concentration, and therefore to more severe secondary hyperparathyroidism. At this point the plasma calcium concentration is approximately 7 mg/dl and the phosphate concentration is 1.5 to 2 mg/dl. Profound muscle weakness develops, and the plasma alkaline phosphatase level rises.

The plasma alkaline phosphatase derives from several organs, most notably liver and bone. Its concentration in blood increases in liver disease (particularly obstructive liver disease) and in a variety of metabolic bone diseases. Increased bone alkaline phosphatase activity occurs in bone diseases in which bone formation rates are high, such as Paget's disease and primary hyperparathyroidism, and in most states in which there is a mineralization defect, such as osteomalacia and vitamin D deficiency.

HYPERCALCEMIC DISORDERS OF MINERAL HOMEOSTASIS

A convenient way to classify disorders of mineral homeostasis is by the prominent pathophysiologic change seen in the serum calcium level. A large number of conditions are associated with hypercalcemia, as outlined below:

Primary hyperparathyroidism
  Parathyroid adenoma
  Diffuse hyperplasia
  Multiple endocrine neoplasia
  Parathyroid carcinoma
Familial hypocalciuric hypercalcemia
Malignancy-associated hypercalcemia
  Local osteolytic hypercalcemia
  Humoral hypercalcemia of malignancy
Granulomatous diseases
  Sarcoidosis
  Tuberculosis
  Fungal diseases
  Berylliosis
  Silicone-induced granulomatosis
Endocrinopathies
  Hyperthyroidism
  Adrenal Insufficiency
  Pheochromocytoma
Medications
  Thiazide diuretics
  Lithium
  Vitamins D or A
  Milk-alkali syndrome
Immobilization

This section focuses on four disease states in which elevated serum calcium plays a major role. Primary hyperparathyroidism is the most common cause of hypercalcemia in the out-

patient setting. Familial hypocalciuric hypercalcemia is a recently recognized, related disorder. Malignancy-associated hypercalcemia is the most common diagnosis in hospitalized patients with hypercalcemia, and sarcoidosis and other granulomatous diseases are sometimes accompanied by hypercalcemia, apparently produced by unregulated production of $1,25(OH)_2D_3$.

Primary hyperparathyroidism

DEFINITION. Primary hyperparathyroidism is a disorder of mineral and bone metabolism caused by increased secretion of parathyroid hormone (PTH) by the parathyroid glands.

ETIOLOGY. In most cases (85%), primary hyperparathyroidism is associated with a hyperfunctioning adenoma of a single parathyroid gland. The cause of the adenoma is unknown. In unusual cases (less than 5%), primary hyperparathyroidism results from parathyroid carcinoma. In the remaining 10% to 15% of cases, it is associated with diffuse hyperplasia of all four glands. In patients with parathyroid hyperplasia, the condition is sometimes familial and may be part of a syndrome of multiple endocrine neoplasia (MEN). MEN-1 includes neoplasia of the pituitary, pancreatic islets, and parathyroids, while MEN-2 consists of the triad of pheochromocytoma, medullary carcinoma of the thyroid, and parathyroid hyperplasia. Recent evidence indicates a circulating parathyroid mitogenic factor in MEN-1, which may be responsible for the parathyroid hyperplasia.

Secondary hyperparathyroidism develops in response to chronic hypocalcemia, as in chronic renal disease, calcium malabsorption, or vitamin D deficiency. With prolonged hypocalcemia the hyperplastic glands may become relatively autonomous; that is, they may become overactive and cause hypercalcemia. This tertiary hyperparathyroidism is difficult to distinguish from the primary form.

PATHOGENESIS. Elevated PTH levels act directly on bone and kidney, and indirectly (via $1,25(OH)_2D_3$) on the intestine to cause hypercalcemia. It is important to realize that PTH production by a parathyroid adenoma is not entirely autonomous. Rather, the adenoma appears to function at an elevated set point, but hormone secretion is usually still under some feedback control. This means that if the serum calcium is transiently raised even further above the set point, some suppression of PTH secretion ensues, tending to return the serum calcium to its (elevated) baseline level.

In some patients with primary hyperparathyroidism, initial clinical features of the disease are renal stones. In these patients $1,25(OH)_2D_3$ levels are markedly elevated, resulting in intestinal hyperabsorption of calcium. Serum calcium in these patients is often only mildly elevated, but urine calcium is excessive, resulting in calcium oxalate or calcium phosphate nephrolithiasis. In these patients, it seems that PTH exerts a proportionally greater effect on the proximal renal tubule (1α-hydroxylase activity) than on the distal renal tubule (calcium resorption), but the exact details of pathogenesis are unclear.

In other patients, primary hyperparathyroidism first appears clinically as bone disease. Osteitis fibrosa cystica, the classical bone lesion, involves a pronounced increase in both bone resorption by osteoclasts and formation of osteoblasts. This accelerated bone remodeling results in the appearance of subperiosteal resorption, marrow fibrosis, and bone cysts (so-called brown tumors). Currently, with earlier diagnosis of hyperparathyroidism, bone disease more commonly consists of a moderate increase in bone turnover with some net resorption, causing accelerated osteoporosis. In general, patients with bone disease have higher serum calcium but lower serum

$1,25(OH)_2D_3$ and lower urine calcium than patients with renal stones. Whether this variation in clinical presentation results from differences in PTH metabolism, or from quantitative or qualitative differences in PTH receptors in different tissues, remains unknown.

CLINICAL MANIFESTATIONS. The diagnostic rate of primary hyperparathyroidism is steadily improving with routine blood chemistry screening, as milder cases are detected. It is the most common cause of hypercalcemia among outpatients, with about 100,000 new cases diagnosed in the United States each year. Primary hyperparathyroidism is twice as common in women as in men, with a peak incidence between 40 and 60 years of age.

The classic clinical features of patients with primary hyperparathyroidism are "stones, bones, and groans." The renal stone symptoms are obvious, consisting of recurrent episodes of low back pain radiating to the groin (renal colic), hematuria, and passage of stones or gravel. The bone symptoms include pain and tenderness in areas of markedly increased turnover (often prominent over the tibial periosteum), pathologic fractures as a consequence of bone cysts, or simply the usual symptoms of osteoporosis (recurrent back pain from vertebral compression fractures and progressive kyphosis).

The "groans" refer to the protean symptoms resulting from hypercalcemia itself. These may include polyuria and polydipsia, anorexia, constipation and abdominal pain, pruritis, headache, weakness (particularly in the proximal muscles), fatiguability, emotional lability, and loss of mental acuity. The degree of mental disturbance correlates with the elevation in serum calcium and is wholly reversible. Personality changes characterized by listlessness, depression, and loss of spontaneity and initiative are common with moderate hypercalcemia, whereas acute psychoses manifested by delirium, disorientation, confusion, paranoid ideation, or hallucinations commonly occur with severe hypercalcemia. If hypercalcemia has been present for a long time, the portion of the cornea not covered by the eyelids (band keratopathy) may calcify and be visible on routine exam or more commonly, on slit-lamp examination. With severe hypercalcemia, weight loss, anemia, arrhythmias, marked proximal muscle weakness, psychosis, extreme mental obtundation, coma, and death may ensue.

As multiphasic screening uncovers less severe cases of primary hyperparathyroidism, more asymptomatic patients or patients with only mild symptoms are seen. Whether such nonspecific symptoms as depression, headache, decreased mental acuity, or constipation actually result from mild hyperparathyroidism is often difficult to determine. Hypertension is common in patients with either primary or secondary hyperparathyroidism, but the mechanisms underlying its pathogenesis are not yet understood. There may also be a somewhat increased incidence of peptic ulcer disease and pancreatitis among patients with hyperparathyroidism.

LABORATORY FINDINGS. The two biochemical hallmarks of primary hyperparathyroidism are hypercalcemia and hypophosphatemia. Serum calcium is most often in the range of 10.5 to 12.5 mg/dl but may be higher. Particularly in patients with renal stones, the elevation in serum calcium may be subtle and intermittent. Serum phosphate is generally low or low-normal, and the renal phosphate threshold (TmP/GFR) is usually below 2.7 mg/dl as a result of PTH's phosphaturic action on the proximal renal tubule. Other laboratory findings may include mild metabolic acidosis, anemia, elevated alkaline phosphatase, and higher sedimentation rate. Urine calcium may be low, normal, or high, depending on dietary factors and on the clinical variant of hyperparathyroidism as discussed above.

High quality roentgenograms of the hands may demonstrate subperiosteal resorption on the phalanges, but only in a minority of cases.

Radioimmunoassays of PTH have been difficult to perfect, largely because PTH undergoes extensive peripheral metabolism, as discussed above. The biologically active fragments (largely N-terminal) have a half-life of minutes, whereas the many inactive fragments (largely C-terminal) clear much more slowly. Thus immunoreactive PTH (iPTH) levels depend critically on the antisera and trace fragment used in the assay. Currently, most clinically useful PTH assays employ C-terminal antisera, which tend to provide an integrated measure of PTH activity, except in renal failure where concentrations of iPTH are elevated by impaired renal clearance of the C-terminal fragments. Other laboratories offer midregion assays, N-terminal assays, or all three assays. In most cases, iPTH is above normal in hyperparathyroidism, but for the above reasons it is crucial to use a reliable laboratory that documents its experience in differentiating various diagnoses.

An alternative to directly measuring iPTH is to perform an assay of its biological activity. As mentioned, this can be done by measuring total urinary cyclic AMP (UcAMP), of which approximately 50% is contributed by the action of PTH on the proximal renal tubule. For increased accuracy, specifically the PTH-dependent nephrogenous component (NcAMP) may be calculated by subtracting the contribution of filtered cAMP (plasma concentration $\times$ glomerular filtration rate) from the measured total UcAMP. Nephrogenous cyclic AMP is almost always elevated in hyperparathyroidism, but may increase as well in patients with humoral hypercalcemia of malignancy (see below). Levels of $1,25(OH)_2D_3$ are usually in the high-normal range or frankly elevated in primary hyperparathyroidism. In subtle cases of hyperparathyroidism with intermittent hypercalcemia, a condition common in patients with renal stones, 1 week on a low calcium diet followed by an oral calcium tolerance test may be necessary to make the diagnosis.

DIAGNOSIS. The approach to the definitive diagnosis of the condition causing hypercalcemia depends on the degree of hypercalcemia. With plasma calcium concentrations greater than 12.5 to 13 mg/dl, the hypercalcemia should be treated immediately. Once the plasma calcium level has been lowered, definitive diagnostic procedures can begin. If, on the other hand, a patient with nonspecific symptoms is discovered by multiphasic screening to have a plasma calcium concentration between 10.6 and 12.5 mg/dl, a logical approach to the differential diagnosis can be followed (Fig. 193-6). The first step is to establish the validity of the measurement by repeating it. If two out of three consecutive measurements of fasting plasma calcium concentration are greater than 10.5 mg/dl, hypercalcemia exists. The next step, or one that can be carried out at the time the second blood sample is collected, is to obtain a spot urine sample for simultaneous measurement of plasma and urine calcium, phosphate, and creatinine. From these data it is possible to calculate the TmP/GFR, a measure of the renal threshold for excretion. If this value is greater than 3.0, it virtually rules out humoral hypercalcemia of malignancy and primary hyperparathyroidism. If less than 2.7, it makes one of these two diagnoses very likely. Values between 2.7 and 3.0 are of borderline significance. The nephrogenous cyclic AMP can be measured at the same time. If a high nephrogenous cyclic AMP is found in conjunction with either a low or borderline TmP/GFR, either primary hyperparathyroidism or humoral hypercalcemia of malignancy exists. A low nephrogenous cyclic AMP with a normal or high TmP/GFR rules out these conditions. In an occasional equivocal case, a patient

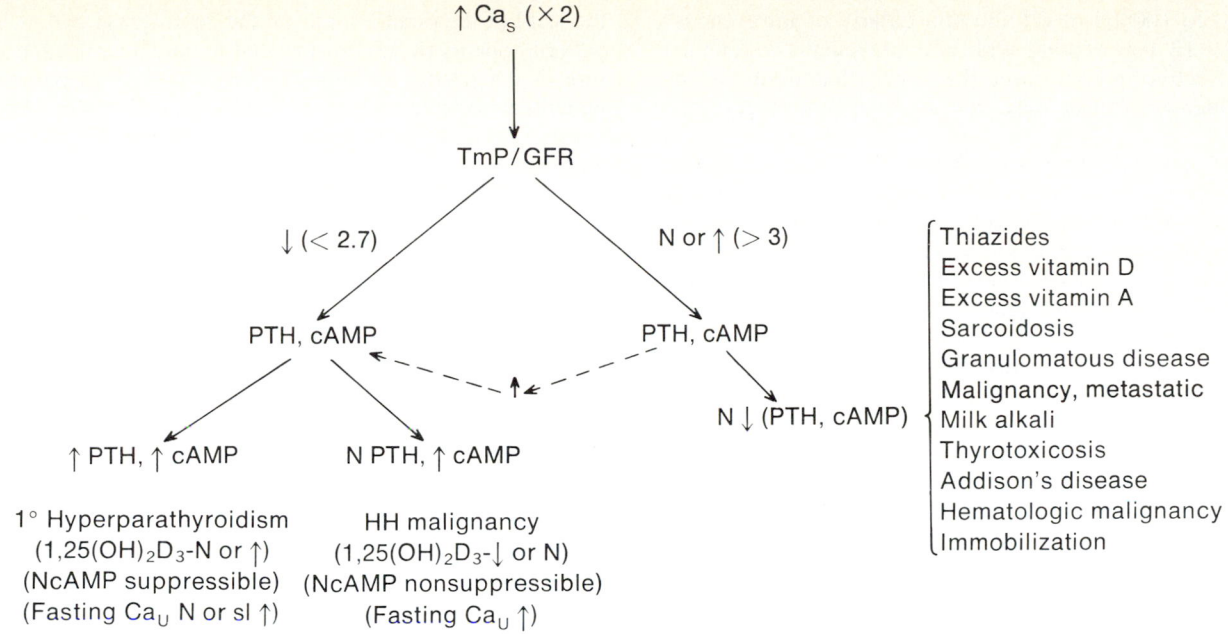

Fig. 193-6   Flow diagram of laboratory approach to differential diagnosis of hypercalcemia. Once presence of hypercalcemia is established, measurement of renal tubular maximum phosphate reabsorption/glomerular filtration rate (TmP/GFR), immunoreactive PTH, nephrogenous cyclic AMP, and in some cases plasma 1.25(OH)$_2$D$_3$ allows differentiation of various causes of hypercalcemia. *PTH,* parathyroid hormone; *cAMP,* cyclic AMP; *Ca$_s$,* serum calcium; *CA$_u$,* urinary calcium; *HH,* humoral hypercalcemia; *N,* normal; *NcAMP,* nephrogenous cyclic AMP.

may have a high normal nephrogenous cyclic AMP and a borderline TmP/GFR. In such a patient further diagnostic procedures are necessary.

Differentiating between primary hyperparathyroidism and humoral hypercalcemia of malignancy is usually not difficult. In the majority of patients with the latter condition the presence of tumor is obvious by the time the hypercalcemia develops. An occasional case may be difficult to detect, but the diagnosis can usually be determined by measuring the plasma immunoreactive PTH and 1,25(OH)$_2$D$_3$ concentrations. These are usually high or high-normal in primary hyperparathyroidism and low or low-normal in humoral hypercalcemia of malignancy.

COURSE. Primary hyperparathyroidism is often a chronic disease. It is common for mild, asymptomatic hypercalcemia to persist for years with little if any progression. Some patients insidiously develop symptoms attributable to the disease, whereas others experience recurrent episodes of nephrolithiasis, or slowly progressive osteoporosis. In general, patients with more severe bone symptomatology show a more rapidly progressive course than those presenting with stones or "groans."

Occasionally superimposed on this chronic natural history may be an episode of acute hypercalcemia, a so-called parathyroid crisis. This life-threatening situation may be triggered by intercurrent illness, dehydration, or immobilization. Calcium-induced diabetes insipidus exacerbates dehydration and hypovolemia-induced renal retention of calcium exacerbates hypercalcemia, thus creating a vicious cycle of deterioration. Serum calcium in such cases may climb rapidly over several days to levels of 15 to 20 mg/dl or higher.

MANAGEMENT. Severe hypercalcemia from any cause constitutes a medical emergency, and therapy to reduce the serum calcium concentration should be instituted promptly. The first and most important step is prompt intravenous rehydration with normal saline. Once this has been accomplished, it is essential to evaluate the renal and cardiac status before proceeding further. If urine output is deemed adequate and cardiac function is normal, combined infusion of normal saline, 2 L every 6 hours, and furosemide, 40 mg every 6 hours, should be given. Since Ca^{++} and Na$^+$ reabsorption occurs predominantly in the proximal renal tubule, this therapy increases the filtered load of calcium. When proximal Na$^+$ reabsorption is blocked, Ca^{++} reabsorption is also inhibited, producing marked calcium diuresis. This therapy alone may lower the plasma calcium concentration by 1.5 to 2 mg/dl. However, it is difficult to maintain this form of therapy for more than a few days because of the complicated problems with K$^+$ and Na$^+$ balances.

As soon as the patient is able to take substances orally, treatment with inorganic phosphate in doses of 0.25 to 0.5 g every 4 hours should be instituted. Before beginning this therapy, it is important to assess renal function and measure plasma phosphate. Most patients with severe hypercalcemia have low plasma phosphate concentrations. However, patients with hypercalcemia resulting from excess vitamin D have high levels of plasma phosphate. Phosphate therapy is contraindicated in this situation. Otherwise, in the typical patient with hypercalcemia who has normal renal function and a low plasma phosphate concentration, oral phosphate therapy is a safe and effective treatment that can be continued for days or weeks.

On the other hand, intravenous use of phosphate in the immediate treatment of hypercalcemia is highly controversial. Infusion of phosphate under these circumstances can lead to massive ectopic calcification, marked and rapidly developing hypocalcemia, and sudden death. This indicates that this form of therapy should not be used to treat hypercalcemia.

Although less widely used than several other agents, CT can be very effective in treating acute hypercalcemia. This is particularly true if increased bone resorption contributes significantly to the hypercalcemia. CT treatment is especially effective when combined with oral phosphate therapy. Administration of 50 to 100 IU of CT intramuscularly or intravenously every 8 to 12 hours along with oral phosphate treatment is usually effective in controlling the hypercalcemia until a definitive diagnosis can be made and more specific therapy can begin.

Another class of drugs that may be employed is the glucocorticoids. They are particularly effective in treating the hypercalcemias of vitamin D excess, sarcoidosis, myeloma, and leukemias. Mithramycin, a potent antitumor agent, is also especially effective in the treatment of the hypercalcemia of malignancy. The use of these agents will be discussed in relation to specific conditions.

Surgery is the definitive treatment for hyperparathyroidism because currently there is no satisfactory chronic medical treatment. A history of renal stones, progressive bone disease, symptoms attributable to hypercalcemia, or serum calcium greater than 12 to 12.5 mg/dl clearly indicates parathyroidectomy. In less severe cases the potential for increased bone loss, slight mental impairment, or the increased risk of parathyroid crisis with advancing age must be weighed against the expense and risk of surgery, and management of such cases is controversial. There is currently a need for controlled studies regarding the optimal management of mild, asymptomatic cases of primary hyperparathyroidism.

Although it is a truism that all surgery should be performed only by qualified and experienced surgeons, this is particularly the case with parathyroid surgery. It is essential that the initial procedure be as successful as possible. This requires both surgical skill and a detailed knowledge of the anatomic variability in the location of the parathyroid glands. It is also vital to determine whether the disease is due to adenoma or hyperplasia. In theory this should be easy, but in practice it may be exceedingly difficult and requires close cooperation between the surgeon and the surgical pathologist. When a suspected adenoma is removed, biopsy of at least one other "normal" gland is necessary. If there is any question as to its anatomic structure, all four glands should be identified.

In cases of hyperplasia of all four glands, the surgical rule has been the removal of three and one half of the four glands. However, complete removal of parathyroid tissue in the neck with autotransplantation of a small amount of parathyroid tissue into the forearm muscle is being explored currently as a way to manage this disease.

Attempts to localize the parathyroid tumor preoperatively include computed tomography, ultrasonography, nuclear subtraction scans, and selective venous catheterization with determination of iPTH. All of the imaging techniques have limited sensitivity (70% to 80%) and specificity (80% to 90%), whereas selective catheterization is expensive, requires specific expertise, and is associated with some morbidity. Thus localization attempts are usually reserved for patients in whom hyperparathyroidism persists after an unsuccessful parathyroid exploration.

Familial hypocalciuric hypercalcemia

DEFINITION. Familial hypocalciuric hypercalcemia (FHH), also known as familial benign hypercalcemia, is a distinct variant of primary hyperparathyroidism notable for its benign natural history.

PATHOGENESIS. The etiologic factors of this familial, presumably genetic syndrome are unknown. Renal tubular resorption of divalent cations, both calcium and magnesium, is inappropriately high for the level of PTH. The resultant mild hypercalcemia, however, does not suppress PTH secretion as would be expected. Hence there appears to be a lesion both at

the level of the renal tubule and the parathyroid cell. A similar pattern appears in lithium-induced hypercalcemia, but the nature of the lesion is unknown. The parathyroid pathology in patients who have undergone surgery resembles chief cell hyperplasia, although the total mass of parathyroid tissue is often little greater than normal.

CLINICAL MANIFESTATIONS. This syndrome has only recently been recognized as a distinct clinical entity. The incidence of FHH appears to be less than 5% of that of typical hyperparathyroidism. Inheritance is autosomal dominant with a high degree of penetrance by age 20. Affected offspring frequently experience mild neonatal hypercalcemia, which is clinically benign (although rarely they may have severe neonatal hyperparathyroidism). Within the first two decades of life most affected individuals become hypercalcemic; hence FHH has an onset that is distinctly earlier than that of primary hyperparathyroidism. However, these patients do not go on to develop renal stones or parathyroid bone disease. There does appear to be a somewhat higher rate of pancreatitis, chondrocalcinosis, and arthralgias. However, most patients are totally asymptomatic or have nonspecific complaints of headache, abnormal mentation, or fatigue.

LABORATORY FINDINGS. Mild to moderate hypercalcemia and hypermagnesemia are present. Fractional excretion of both calcium and magnesium are low, resulting in relative hypocalciuria and hypomagnesuria. However, 24-hour urine calcium excretion overlaps substantially with that seen in sporadic hyperparathyroidism, so while a high value (greater than 300 mg/day) may exclude FHH, a low or normal value is not diagnostic. Immunoreactive PTH, nephrogenous cyclic AMP, and $1,25(OH)_2D_3$ levels are high-normal to elevated.

MANAGEMENT. The principal importance of diagnosing FHH lies in its singular lack of response to parathyroid surgery. In one study series, for example, 21 of 27 patients remained hypercalcemic following one or more neck explorations whereas five patients developed symptomatic hypoparathyroidism. Thus the clinical challenge is to distinguish FHH from hyperparathyroidism (on the basis of familial association, early onset, and benign course with supportive biochemical evidence) to avoid ineffective and potentially hazardous surgery.

Malignancy-associated hypercalcemia

DEFINITION. The course and management of various types of malignancy are frequently complicated by the development of hypercalcemia, occurring by one of several mechanisms, as discussed below.

PATHOGENESIS. Malignancy-associated hypercalcemia falls into two broad categories, local osteolytic hypercalcemia (LOH) and humoral hypercalcemia of malignancy (HHM). In LOH, hypercalcemia results from locally excessive bone resorption associated with primary or metastatic tumor involving the bone itself. In HHM, a tumor remote from the bone releases a substance into the circulation that causes hypercalcemia by generalized bone resorption or, in a minority of cases, by increased intestinal calcium absorption. The nature of the hypercalcemic substance or substances is currently a matter of some debate.

Local osteolytic hypercalcemia occurs frequently in malignancies such as multiple myeloma, lymphoma involving bone, or metastic breast carcinoma. Bone biopsies display marked osteoclastic activity, but the precise mechanism by which these and other tumors accelerate local bone resorption is not clear. Tissue culture medium that has been exposed to bone marrow aspirates from hypercalcemic patients with myeloma or lymphoma contains a substance or substances that stimulate osteoclasts. Originally called osteoclast-activating factor (OAF), this substance is currently thought to be not a single protein but several cytokines (including interleukin-1) produced by lymphocytes and macrophages. The prostaglandin PGE-2 appears to mediate production of these factors, although there is no systemic increase in prostaglandin levels. The sensitivity of myeloma-associated hypercalcemia to glucocorticoids probably reflects the inhibited production of these osteoclast-activating cytokines. With breast carcinoma, osteoclast activity increases locally, but cultured breast carcinoma cell lines are capable of directly resorbing even irradiated (osteoclast-depleted) bone.

Humoral hypercalcemia of malignancy is most common with squamous (lung, esophagus, and so forth), renal, or urothelial carcinomas. Bone biopsies display increased resorption by osteoclasts, decreased formation by osteoblasts, and no marrow involvement by tumors. When the primary tumor is resected the hypercalcemia resolves, demonstrating that the hypercalcemia is a paraneoplastic syndrome mediated by a tumor-derived substance. Patients with HHM are typically hypophosphatemic with elevated nephrogenous cyclic AMP excretion, suggesting that the responsible factor may be PTH; indeed, in the past the syndrome was referred to as ectopic hyperparathyroidism. However, PTH cannot be isolated from such tumors; mRNA coding for PTH has not been detected in such tumors; serum iPTH levels are not elevated; and $1,25(OH)_2D_3$ levels are usually low. Recent evidence indicates that the tumor-derived hypercalcemic factor in these patients is a novel protein with partial homology to PTH. A similar factor appears to be present in medium from cultured normal keratinocytes, suggesting that it plays an unknown paracrine role in the normal physiology of squamous epithelia.

A number of other substances have been proposed as mediators of humoral hypercalcemia of malignancy. Prostaglandins have been postulated to cause HHM but are rarely elevated systemically. Recently attention has focused on tumor-derived transforming growth factors (TGFs), which can be extracted from virtually all malignant tumors and possess potent bone-resorbing activity in vitro. Indeed, partially purified tumor extracts containing the PTH-like factor discussed above also have been shown to possess TGF-like activity. Whether both activities might reside in a single protein and/or contribute to the hypercalcemia will have to await further characterization of the PTH-like factor.

One unusual, recently recognized humoral mechanism for hypercalcemia appears in a small subset of patients with lymphoma. These patients have been shown to have elevated levels of $1,25(OH)_2D_3$, with hypercalcemia on the basis of intestinal hyperabsorption of calcium (and probably also $1,25(OH)_2D_3$-mediated bone resorption). Patients with rare HTLV-1–associated T-cell leukemias usually have hypercalcemia, the cause of which is still unknown.

EPIDEMIOLOGY. Malignancy-associated hypercalcemia is the most common source of elevated calcium levels in hospitalized patients and the second most common cause (after hyperparathyroidism) in outpatients. LOH is particularly common with multiple myeloma and metastatic breast carcinoma, but may also appear with many other tumors involving bone. HHM occurs most often in cases of squamous cell carcinoma but also is seen frequently in renal cell, ovarian, bladder, and breast carcinoma and in pheochromocytoma. HHM is distinctly uncommon in gastrointestinal tumors and (unlike ectopic ADH or ACTH syndromes) in oat cell carcinoma of the lung.

CLINICAL MANIFESTATIONS. The clinical features are those of hypercalcemia per se, modified by the underlying malignancy. In multiple myeloma or lymphoma, bone pain from osteolytic lesions or symptoms caused by hypercalcemia may be the initial clinical signs of the malignancy. In LOH with metastatic disease and in most cases of HHM, hypercalcemia usually occurs relatively late in the course of the disease. Patients may develop pruritis, constipation, anorexia, polyuria, renal insufficiency, arrythmias, and deteriorating mental status progressing to coma as a result of the hypercalcemia. Onset of these symptoms is usually quite rapid (weeks to months) in malignancy-associated hypercalcemia, in contrast to the more gradual onset of hypercalcemic symptoms (months to years) in most cases of primary hyperparathyroidism. The rapid development of hypercalcemic symptoms results both from the aggressive nature of the malignancy itself, and from reduced feedback control of the factors causing the hypercalcemia.

LABORATORY FINDINGS. Laboratory results reflect the pathogenesis of the hypercalcemia. Laboratory evidence for multiple myeloma includes an elevated sedimentation rate, Bence-Jones proteins in the urine, a monoclonal spike in serum immunoglobulins, or a combination of these. A bone marrow biopsy may be necessary to diagnose lymphoma. In LOH, hypercalcemia attributable to excessive bone resorption results in suppressed to low-normal iPTH levels, suppressed nephrogenous cyclic AMP (NcAMP) excretion, and low $1,25(OH)_2D_3$ levels, with marked fasting hypercalciuria. In HHM caused by the newly identified PTH-like factor, the renal phosphate threshold decreases and urinary (or nephrogenous) cAMP excretion increases as in hyperparathyroidism, but serum iPTH levels are not elevated. Additional differences from hyperparathyroidism are that $1,25(OH)_2D_3$ concentrations are usually low-normal in HHM; fasting calcium excretion is higher; and on bone biopsy (unnecessary in the clinical setting), there is no increase in bone formation to compensate for accelerated osteoclastic resorption. Furthermore, as mentioned above, the hypercalcemia generally has a subacute onset in HHM, whereas in primary hyperparathyroidism the serum calcium level usually climbs much more gradually because most parathyroid adenomas retain some feedback control. In the uncommon variety of HHM seen with rare cases of lymphoma, $1,25(OH)_2D_3$ levels are high and parathyroid function tests are appropriately suppressed.

COURSE AND PROGNOSIS. Malignancy-associated hypercalcemia is readily controlled on an acute basis with intravenous (IV) medications and fluids but is more difficult to treat in the outpatient setting unless effective therapy is available for the tumor itself. The prognosis depends partially on that of the underlying neoplasm, but in general, hypercalcemia signals a relatively advanced stage of malignancy. Particularly in HHM associated with squamous cell cancer, hypercalcemia is a grave prognostic sign with survival typically less than 6 months. On the other hand, in multiple myeloma and some lymphomas, hypercalcemia is occasionally the initial clinical sign of a malignancy that can be completely reversed by successful antitumor therapy.

MANAGEMENT. With moderate to severe hypercalcemia (greater than 13 mg/dl), the first step is to administer IV saline at rates of 150 to 200 cc/hr (as hemodynamically tolerated), which induces a brisk calciuresis. Once the patient is intravascularly repleted, loop diuretics such as furosemide (20 mg IV every 6 hours) may be added to prevent pulmonary venous congestion and to augment calcium excretion. Further treatment depends on the pathogenesis of the hypercalcemia. In cases with elevated $1,25(OH)_2D_3$, as in some lymphomas, a low calcium diet and treatment with glucocorticosteroids can lower intestinal absorption of calcium. In the more common cases of hypercalcemia resulting from excess bone resorption, such as LOH or HHM, agents that inhibit bone resorption are indicated. These include calcitonin, diphosphonates, placamycin, and less specifically, prostaglandin synthetase inhibitors and glucocorticosteroids.

A reasonable choice of agent to accompany the initial saline diuresis is calcitonin (50 to 400 units subcutaneously every 12 hours), which has little toxicity and may lower serum calcium by an additional 1 to 2 mg/dl. Clinically, however, patients usually develop tachyphylaxis to the hypocalciuric effects of calcitonin after a few weeks, so this agent cannot be a chronic treatment. Often this is true even with human calcitonin and even when calcitonin is combined with glucocorticosteroids as some researchers recommend. It is not clear what mediates this resistance to calcitonin. However, sometimes oral phosphate therapy can prolong its effectiveness (see below).

The chemotherapeutic agent plicamycin (formerly mithramycin) in low doses (15 to 25 μg/kg IV over several hours) quite reliably lowers serum calcium by inhibiting bone resorption. The peak effect of a single dose is seen at about 36 hours, with control of hypercalcemia lasting from several days to over a week. Unfortunately, plicamycin requires IV infusion and is relatively toxic, potentially causing renal insufficiency, hepatotoxicity, and clotting abnormalities.

The diphosphonate ethane–1-hydroxydiphosphonate (EHDP, etidronate) recently was released for IV use in hypercalcemia of malignancy. In dosages of 7.5 mg/kg given as daily infusions over several hours, it is usually well tolerated, at least for the short term. Unfortunately, this diphosphonate is poorly absorbed orally and impairs bone mineralization. It leads to osteomalacia if given chronically in oral doses, making it less useful for outpatient therapy. Other diphosphonates, equipotent in inhibiting bone resorption but less effective on mineralization, have been used successfully in Europe for oral treatment of malignancy-associated hypercalcemia. However, these are currently unavailable in the United States.

Long-term outpatient therapy for cancer-related hypercalcemia is often difficult with the agents currently available. Clearly, treatment of the malignancy itself is most important and may also be the most effective means to control the hypercalcemia. Mobilization of the patient and good oral hydration are important but frequently overlooked adjuncts for maintaining normocalcemia. Oral phosphate can be used if the serum phosphorus is closely monitored and kept below about 4 mg/dl. Chronic calcitonin, prostaglandin synthetase inhibitors, or glucocorticosteroids are given frequently with variable degrees of success. Often, however, the patient must periodically receive IV therapy to adequately control hypercalcemia.

Sarcoidosis and other granulomatous diseases

DEFINITION. Hypercalcemia, hypercalciuria, or both may be clinical features of sarcoidosis and other granulomatous diseases.

PATHOGENESIS. Hypercalcemia occurs in these diseases by a unique mechanism that has only recently been elucidated. Macrophages within the granulomas themselves appear to cause the hypercalcemia by secreting $1,25(OH)_2D_3$. Early observations noted that hypercalcemia in tuberculosis patients often worsened after improved diet and sunlight exposure in a sanitorium, whereas in sarcoidosis patients hypercalcemia frequently grew worse in the summer or developed after small doses of vitamin D, suggesting a hypersensitivity to vitamin D causing hyperabsorption of dietary calcium. An unexpected development was the report of an anephric patient with sarcoidosis who developed hypercalcemia with elevated levels of

$1,25(OH)_2D_3$, despite the fact that the normal crucial step in the conversion of vitamin D to this active metabolite occurs in the kidney. Recently, in patients with sarcoidosis, it has been demonstrated that lymph node homogenates, themselves, contain the enzyme 1α-hydroxylase, enabling them to synthesize $1,25(OH)_2D_3$ in situ. Presumably this synthesis, unlike that in the kidney, is autonomous and impervious to feedback inhibition, resulting in hypercalcemia whenever vitamin D substrate levels are high. Even more recently it has been shown that *normal* pulmonary macrophages, after stimulation with mitogens, also express 1α-hydroxylase activity. Together with other reports indicating effects of $1,25(OH)_2D_3$ on the immune system, these observations suggest that this metabolite normally may play a paracrine role in the immune response.

CLINICAL MANIFESTATIONS. Hypercalcemia occurs in approximately 10% of patients with sarcoidosis, whereas hypercalciuria appears in about 20%. These figures are lower than in older study series, presumably reflecting earlier diagnosis and improved treatment. Hypercalcemia also occurs in patients with active tuberculosis, berylliosis, histoplasmosis, coccidioidomycosis, and rarely with eosinophilic granuloma, candidiasis, and silicone-induced granulomatosis.

Because the parathyroid axis remains intact in these diseases, most of the excess intestinally absorbed calcium is excreted in the urine, making hypercalciuria even more common than hypercalcemia. Thus these patients are particularly susceptible to nephrolithiasis. Otherwise the clinical features are those of the underlying disease.

LABORATORY FINDINGS. The diagnosis of sarcoidosis is often suggested by a chest roentgenogram showing enlarged paratracheal lymph nodes. An elevated angiotensin-converting enzyme (ACE) level is supporting evidence. Tissue biopsy revealing noncaseating granulomas may be necessary to confirm the diagnosis. The most common derangement of mineral homeostasis is a pattern of mild, intermittent hypercalcemia with sustained hypercalciuria. Levels of $1,25(OH)_2D_3$ are elevated, whereas parathyroid function tests (iPTH or NcAMP) show appropriate suppression. Levels of 25-hydroxyvitamin D usually remain normal. These disturbances of calcium metabolism mimic those seen in absorptive hypercalciuria, a common diagnosis in patients with recurrent renal stones, and these cases may pose a difficult diagnostic challenge as the roentgenographic and other manifestations of sarcoidosis may be subtle and easily overlooked.

MANAGEMENT. Hypercalcemia (or hypercalciuria with renal stones) is one of the indications for steroid therapy in sarcoidosis. The elevated levels of $1,25(OH)_2D_3$ in this condition are exquisitely sensitive to glucocorticoids, and even low doses of prednisone usually result in normocalcemia. In advanced sarcoidosis, however, renal impairment caused by hypercalcemic nephropathy may occur. In granulomatous infections, successful antimicrobial treatment normalizes serum and urine calcium levels.

HYPOCALCEMIC DISORDERS OF MINERAL HOMEOSTASIS

Hypocalcemia, although less common than hypercalcemia, can also be life threatening. From the preceding discussion of the physiology of mineral metabolism, it is evident that hypocalcemia can develop (1) as a consequence of PTH deficiency or end-organ refractoriness to the actions of this hormone; (2) as a result of vitamin D deficiency; or (3) as a consequence of a marked increase in the serum phosphate concentration as seen in uremia, following chemotherapy for leukemia or phosphate infusion. Hypocalcemia also may accompany acute pan-

Table 193-1 Differential diagnosis of tetany

Cause	Serum*				Urine nephrogenous cyclic AMP*
	Ca	P	pH	PTH	
Hypoparathyroidism	↓	↑	N	↓	↓
Mg deficiency	↓	N	N	↓	↓
Pseudohypoparathyroidism	↓	↑	N	↑	↓ N
Vitamin D deficiency	↓	↓	N	↑	↑
Alkalosis					
Respiratory	N	N	↑	N	↑ N
Metabolic	N	N	↑	N	N

* ↓, Decreased; ↑, increased; N, normal.

creatitis, probably because free fatty acids, which are released by the action of pancreatic lipase on retroperitoneal fat and perhaps by agents that stimulate calcium uptake into muscle and other tissues, precipitate calcium soaps. Hypocalcemia uncommonly occurs in prostate and other malignancies in which uncontrolled osteoblastic bone formation characterizes bone metastases. Conditions associated with hypocalcemia include:

Hypoalbuminemia (ionized calcium normal)
Hypoparathyroidism
  Idiopathic
  Surgical
  Transient postoperative
  Magnesium deficiency
Pseudohypoparathyroidim
Vitamin D disorders
  Viatamin D deficiency
  Intestinal malabsorption
  Vitamin D resistance
Hyperphosphatemia
  Renal insufficiency
  IV phosphate therapy
  Chemotherapy (cell lysis syndrome)
Calcium disposition
  Acute pancreatitis
  Osteoblastic metastases

"False hypocalcemia," that is, low albumin-bound and total serum calcium with normal ionized calcium, is common among chronically ill, hospitalized patients with hypoalbuminemia. A rough approximation for the decrease in total serum calcium that may result from decreased serum albumin is 0.8 mg/dl decrease in calcium per 1 gm/dl decrease in albumin. In individual patients this formula frequently is inaccurate, and direct measurement of ionized calcium may be necessary.

"True hypocalcemia," that is, decreased ionized calcium (which may produce severe symptoms of neuromuscular excitability), is less common but much more significant clinically. This section focuses on two conditions in which hypocalcemia plays a major role in the clinical picture. Hypoparathyroidism may be chronic but more often is transient following neck surgery or as a result of magnesium depletion. Pseudohypoparathyroidism with end-organ resistance to PTH is an uncommon but physiologically interesting cause of hypocalcemia. Vitamin D deficiency and renal failure, in which the hypocalcemia is at least partially compensated by secondary hyperparathyroidism, are discussed in the section on disorders of skeletal homeostasis.

Hypoparathyroidism

DEFINITION. Hypoparathyroidism is a disorder of mineral metabolism caused by insufficient activity of the parathyroid glands.

PATHOGENESIS. Autoimmune destruction of the parathyroid glands is probably the most common cause of idiopathic hypoparathyroidism. It is sometimes familial and may be associated with other autoimmune endocrine deficiencies, including adrenal insufficiency and chronic mucocutaneous candidiasis. Rarely, it results from primary hypoplasia of the parathyroid glands, which in Di George's syndrome is accompanied by congenital absence of the thymus. Permanent hypoparathyroidism also may occur in about 2% of cases from neck surgery such as total thyroidectomy or extensive parathyroidectomy. Very rarely, it results from infiltrative disease, such as hemochromatosis or metastatic cancer, or from irradiation.

Transient postoperative hypoparathyroidism with mild hypocalcemia accompanied by few if any symptoms is very common and must be distinguished from permanent iatrogenic hypoparathyroidism. It occurs after thyroid, parathyroid, or laryngeal surgery as a consequence of both impaired production of and increased demand for PTH. Transiently impaired PTH production may result from ischemic damage to the parathyroids during surgery even if no parathyroid tissue is removed. Increased demand for PTH (the "hungry bones syndrome") occurs when calcium is redeposited in bones demineralized from previous hyperthyroidism or hyperparathyroidism.

Hypomagnesemia is an important source of reversible hypoparathyroidism in alcoholics with chronic malnutrition, individuals with malabsorption syndromes, or patients treated with medications (cis-platinum, aminoglycosides, and amphotericin) that cause a renal magnesium leak. Whereas mild hypomagnesemia stimulates PTH production, severe cases (serum levels less than about 1 mg/dl) are associated with depleted intracellular magnesium, resulting in impaired PTH secretory capacity. In addition, there appears to be a component of target organ resistance to PTH. Hence magnesium depletion leads to functional hypoparathyroidism with hypocalcemia.

PTH deficiency causes hypocalcemia because it decreases intestinal absorption of calcium, bone resorption, and distal renal tubular reabsorption of calcium. In the absence of PTH the renal phosphate threshold increases, resulting in phosphate retention. Serum levels of 1,25$(OH)_2D_3$ are low, and bone turnover decreases markedly.

CLINICAL MANIFESTATIONS. Hypoparathyroidism typically begins insidiously, with slowly increasing episodic symptoms dominated by increased neuromuscular irritability. Paresthesias in the fingers, toes, and perioral region are typical. Muscle cramps may occur in the lower back, legs, or elsewhere. Children often experience syncopal episodes or seizures, whereas mental lassitude, impaired memory, or psychoneurotic behavior are common central nervous system manifestations of hypocalcemia in adults. Often these symptoms are attacks precipitated by physical or emotional stress and exacerbated by the alkalosois of hyperventilation. Life-threatening tetany with laryngospasm may occur in severe cases (Table 193-1). With longstanding hypocalcemia, subcapsular cataracts and calcified basal ganglia may develop.

A physical exam may reveal hypocalcemic muscle twitching; skin and hair are often dry and teeth may be hypoplastic. Eliciting Chvostek's or Trousseau's signs demonstrate latent tetany. Chvostek's sign is a twitching of the corner of the mouth, which is produced by tapping lightly on the facial nerve about one inch anterior to the ear. Trousseau's sign is carpal spasm (involuntary flexure of the wrist and metacarpal joints) following inflation of a blood pressure cuff on the upper arm to about 150 mmHg for 3 minutes.

With postoperative hypoparathyroidism, the symptoms and signs are similar. The nadir of serum ionized calcium typically occurs 2 to 4 days after neck surgery, so patients should be carefully observed for signs of latent tetany at that time.

LABORATORY FINDINGS. In hypoparathyroidism, total serum calcium may fall as low as 5 mg/dl and phosphorus may increase to 8 mg/dl or more. Immunoreactive PTH levels may be undetectable or at least inappropriately low for the degree of hypocalcemia. Nephrogenous cAMP and serum $1,25(OH)_2D_3$ levels are low. The renal phosphate threshold (TmP/GFR) is elevated, and the electrocardiogram may show a prolonged Q-T interval.

The serum magnesium level must be measured in any patient with hypocalcemia to rule out hypomagnesemia as a treatable cause of hypoparathyroidism. Patients experiencing malabsorption frequently have low albumin and 25-hydroxyvitamin D levels, which contributes to hypocalcemia. Antiparathyroid antibodies appear in many idiopathic cases of chronic hypoparathyroidism, but the test for this is usually unavailable.

MANAGEMENT. Emergency treatment of tetany requires that a distinction be made between hyperventilation with respiratory alkalosis (which only requires reassurance and having the patient breathe slowly several times into a paper bag) and hypocalcemia. True hypocalcemic tetany requires prompt treatment to (1) overcome the patients' discomfort and fear; (2) prevent the occurrence of fatal laryngospasm; and (3) prevent the occurrence of seizure. Initial medical management involves infusing calcium gluconate or chloride intravenously at a rate of 1 to 2 mg/kg over 15 to 20 minutes. A maintenance dose of 10 to 15 mg/kg every 6 to 12 hours usually maintains a normal or low-normal serum calcium concentration until diagnosis and definitive treatment begin.

The parathyroid glands are often destroyed in patients with idiopathic chronic hypoparathyroidism, making these patients even more difficult to manage than permanent postoperative patients, in whom some residual parathyroid function usually remains. PTH itself is not available for replacement therapy, so treatment consists of oral calcium supplements plus vitamin D. Clearly this regimen cannot respond to minute-by-minute changes in metabolic demands. Furthermore, without the distal renal tubular action of PTH, normocalcemia usually results in marked hypercalciuria. Therefore a therapeutic balance must be found between minimizing hypocalcemic symptoms and triggering hypercalciuria with its risks of nephrolithiasis and nephrocalcinosis. Unpredictable episodes of vitamin D intoxication with hypercalcemia may occur even in patients on a previously stable regimen, so frequent biochemical monitoring is essential.

Standard therapy is oral calcium (1 to 2 gm/day) together with some form of vitamin D. The calcium may be given as carbonate so long as stomach acidity is adequate to allow absorption; otherwise it must be given as lactate or gluconate. Vitamin D was previously given as 40,000 to 100,000 units/day, but the recent introduction of $1,25(OH)_2D_3$ (calcitriol) as a therapeutic agent has lowered the risk of vitamin D intoxication because it acts more quickly and has a shorter duration. The usual dosage of calcitriol is 1 to 2 µg/day, but some patients require less and others require as much as 12 µg/day while recovering from severe hypocalcemia. The goal in therapy is to maintain the serum calcium concentration between 8 and 9 mg/dl to prevent symptomatic hypocalcemia. As discussed above, to decrease the risk of hypercalciuria, nephro-

lithiasis, and episodic vitamin D intoxication, normocalcemia is best avoided.

Transient postoperative hypoparathyroidism is usually mild and can be managed with oral or intravenous calcium supplements. If severe bone disease is present, hypocalcemia may be prolonged and administration of $1,25(OH)_2D_3$ in a dosage of 1 to 3 µg/day along with oral calcium may be necessary. Most patients with postoperative hypoparathyroidism recover normal parathyroid function with full resolution of any hypocalcemic symptoms by 1 to 4 weeks after surgery. Occasionally, many years after neck surgery, patients with incomplete recovery of the PTH axis may develop hypocalcemia resulting from progressive fibrosis of the parathyroid glands or increased demand for PTH.

The prognosis of hypocalcemia in cases of magnesium deficiency depends on that of the underlying disease. Parenteral followed by oral magnesium replacement usually restores parathyroid function fairly quickly.

Pseudohypoparathyroidism

DEFINITION. Pseudohypoparathyroidism (PHP) refers to a group of uncommon syndromes resulting from target organ resistance to the actions of PTH.

PATHOGENESIS. The first hormone resistance syndrome ever to be postulated (by Fuller Albright in 1942), PHP is still not completely understood. PTH resistance may result from target organ lesions at the level of the PTH receptor, the adenylate cyclase complex, or beyond. At least three biochemical variants of PHP have been described. *Type Ia*, the first recognized and most familiar, has a characteristic pathognomonic phenotype called Albright's hereditary osteodystrophy (see discussion of clinical manifestations) in most affected patients. These patients have chronic hypocalcemia and hyperphosphatemia despite elevated iPTH levels. They show little increase in nephrogenous cAMP excretion or phosphaturia in response to exogenous PTH. They may also display varying degrees of resistance to other peptide hormones including TSH, LH, and FSH.

Recently it has been demonstrated that patients with PHP type Ia have a defect in the stimulatory regulatory subunit (Gs) of the adenylate cyclase complex in erythrocytes and various other tissues. Specifically, Gs activity is about 50% lower in PHP type Ia compared to controls. Presumably, incomplete transmission of the hormonal binding signal to the intracellular "second messenger" accounts for the observed lack of response. Why PTH resistance dominates the clinical picture over other cAMP-mediated hormones and whether Gs deficiency accounts for the phenotypical appearance is not clear at this time. Some patients with PHP type Ia have osteitis fibrosa cystica, and many show increased hydroxyproline excretion in response to exogenous PTH, suggesting at least partial skeletal responsiveness to PTH (it is not known to what degree the effect of PTH on bone depends on cAMP). Finally, some patients, often from type Ia families, bear the phenotypic expression of Albright's hereditary osteodystrophy without being hypocalcemic (so-called pseudopseudohypoparathyroidism, or PPHP). How this attenuated syndrome relates to PHP is also unclear, but some individuals progress from PPHP to PHP type Ia or vice versa.

Patients with the variant known as *PHP type Ib* again exhibit PTH resistance, with a blunted increase in nephrogenous cAMP excretion or phosphaturia in response to exogenous PTH. However, Gs activity is normal, other hormonal systems are generally intact, and most patients do not display Albright's hereditary osteodystrophy. Presumably, these patients have a defect at the level of the PTH receptor.

Finally, patients with the less common variant known as *PHP type II* also have hypocalcemia and hyperphosphatemia with elevated iPTH levels. While they do not show increased phosphaturia in response to exogenous PTH, they do display an appropriate increase in nephrogenous cAMP excretion. Therefore the defect leading to PTH resistance in PHP type II may lie distal to both the PTH receptor and the adenylate cyclase complex.

EPIDEMIOLOGY. All of the PHP variants are uncommon, although their precise incidence is unknown. In familial cases various modes of inheritance have been described; other cases are sporadic. Females are more often affected than males.

CLINICAL MANIFESTATIONS. Patients with PHP, at least of the Ia type, show a constellation of phenotypic abnormalities referred to as Albright's hereditary osteodystrophy. Affected individuals are short (often less than 5 feet tall), with a stocky build and round face. Shortening of the metacarpal joints, particularly the fourth and fifth, is characteristic. When the patient makes a fist, the affected metacarpal joints have dimples rather than knuckles. Roentgenographic examination often reveals shortened metatarsals and a thickened calvarium. Ectopic ossifications may be palpated as hard, nontender nodules in the regions of the large joints. Mental retardation, usually mild, is typically but not always present. Symptoms caused by hypocalcemia usually bring the patient to medical attention.

LABORATORY FINDINGS. Hypocalcemia with hyperphosphatemia and normal renal function suggests hypoparathyroidism. In patients with PHP, however, immunoreactive PTH levels are elevated rather than low. The diagnosis is established most reliably by demonstrating a blunted urinary cAMP response to exogenous PTH (the Ellsworth-Howard test). In the uncommon type II patients, diagnosis requires blunted phosphaturic response to exogenous PTH, but this test is subject to borderline results unless performed under strict protocol conditions. Unfortunately, preparations of PTH for human use are currently unavailable on a commercial basis.

COURSE AND MANAGEMENT. The short stature and phenotypic appearance often do not appear until the preteenage years. Likewise, even in congenital cases, symptoms of hypocalcemia rarely are present in infancy and have an average age of onset of 8½ years. Hypocalcemia and hyperphosphatemia are usually milder than in idiopathic hypoparathyroidism, and some patients may be only intermittently hypocalcemic, presumably reflecting incomplete peripheral resistance to PTH. Symptomatic hypocalcemia should be managed as described in the section on hypoparathyroidism.

DISORDERS OF SKELETAL HOMEOSTASIS

There are a number of diseases of mineral metabolism in which clinical repercussions are felt mainly at the level of bone. These so-called metabolic bone diseases are accompanied by varying degrees of impaired mineral homeostasis, which is discussed later.

Osteoporosis

DEFINITION. Osteoporosis is by far the most prevalent metabolic bone disease in this country, affecting some 20 million older Americans and causing over one million fractures per year. It is a condition characterized by a reduction in both bone protein and bone mineral per unit volume, in other words,

decreased bone density with the composition of the remaining bone being essentially normal. Skeletal homeostasis is impaired to such an extent that minimal trauma or stress can fracture the bone.

ETIOLOGY. Osteoporosis is exceedingly common in postmenopausal women but can occur for a variety of reasons in other age-groups or in men. No single etiologic factor is to blame in most cases, but a number of risk factors have been identified as follows:

    I. Hormonal
        A. Low estrogen or androgen
        B. Cushing's syndrome
        C. Thyrotoxicosis
        D. Hyperparathyroidism
        E. Diabetes (?)
    II. Nutritional
        A. Calcium deficiency
        B. Postgastrectomy
        C. High protein diet (?)
        D. High phosphate diet (?)
    III. Drugs and toxins
        A. Alcohol
        B. Cigarettes
        C. Glucocorticosteroids
        D. Anticonvulsants
    IV. Miscellaneous
        A. Female sex
        B. Caucasian race
        C. Family history
        D. Lack of exercise
        E. Low body weight
        F. Aging

PATHOGENESIS. In most cases the pathogenesis of osteoporosis is not clear. Humans usually attain peak bone mass about age 35, followed by gradual loss of bone mass at an approximate rate of 0.5% per year. Superimposed on this natural history are other risk factors (see outline), the most important of which in postmenopausal women is almost certainly estrogen withdrawal (Fig. 193-7). Lack of estrogen appears to sensitize bone osteoclasts to PTH, and this decreases the coupling of bone formation with resorption. The small net shift of calcium out of bone suppresses parathyroid activity and lowers plasma $1,25(OH)_2D_3$ with consequent decreased dietary calcium absorption, increased renal phosphate threshold, and higher urinary calcium excretion. It should be emphasized that all of these changes are small, so laboratory parameters usually remain well within the normal range.

Several other hormonal conditions are associated with osteoporosis, often at a relatively early age. Hypercortisolism, whether from Cushing's syndrome or from chronic glucocorticosteroid therapy, augments osteoclastic bone resorption while inhibiting intestinal calcium absorption and osteoblastic bone formation, leading to a rapid loss of skeletal tissue. Hyperthyroidism increases the metabolic rate of bone, increasing bone turnover with some net bone resorption. Hyperparathyroidism, if severe, may cause osteitis fibrosa cystica, but today is more often associated with accelerated osteoporosis. Hypogonadism from any cause (gonadal dysgenesis, pituitary tumor, oophorectomy, premature menopause) decreases bone mass.

CLINICAL MANIFESTATIONS. The usual finding in patients with osteoporosis is the sudden onset of back pain in the thoracic or lumbar spine brought on by physical activity. Roentgenography may reveal crush, wedge-shaped fractures of one or more vertebral bodies. The amount of pain

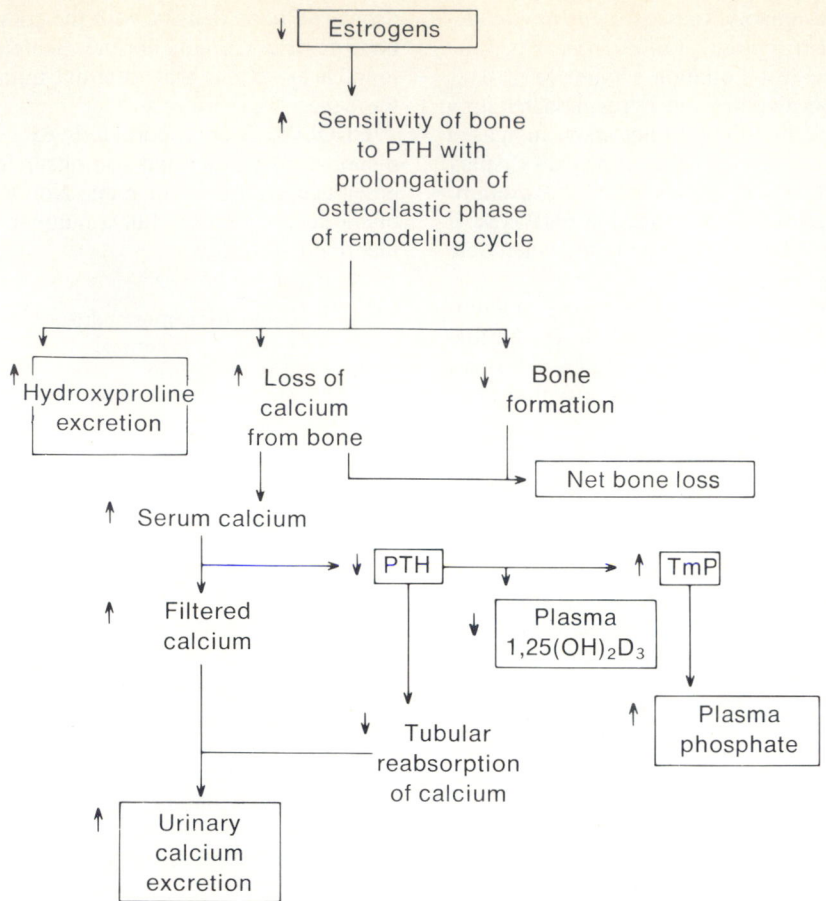

Fig. 193-7   Pathogenesis of postmenopausal osteoporosis (see text).

varies enormously; some women have reduced stature and a history of chronic back pain, and others have a dramatic onset of severe pain. The pain following any fracture ameliorates with time but is usually followed by persistent dull, aching pain. Once osteoporosis has begun, the subject usually suffers multiple fractures over a period of several years. In some cases the disease is manifested by a Colles' fracture of the wrist or a femoral neck fracture after minimal trauma.

DIAGNOSIS. The diagnosis is usually relatively easy. It is necessary to rule out known endocrine causes. In an occasional older woman, hyperparathyroidism may be manifested by osteoporosis. The possibilities of thyrotoxicosis, Cushing's syndrome, or hypogonadism should be considered. Vertebral fractures may also occur in patients with myeloma, leukemia, or metastatic carcinoma. In postmenopausal osteoporosis, all laboratory findings are usually normal.

COURSE. The course of osteoporosis is highly variable. One patient may have several fractures within a year, whereas others may have fractures separated by several years. However, the disease is usually progressive, and eventual loss of stature, persistent back pain, and kyphosis are common.

MANAGEMENT. At present there is no generally accepted specific therapy of osteoporosis once it has developed. General measures such as adequate dietary intake of calcium, phosphate, and vitamin D, specific back exercises, and appropriate physical activity should be encouraged. Immobilizing the spine in a cast, brace, or corset is usually not helpful and may, in fact, accelerate the rate of bone loss. Various programs of calcium and vitamin D with or without fluorides, or a

combination of estrogens and androgens, have been suggested but are not able to reverse the bone loss. Treatment with $1,25(OH)_2D_3$ has also been advocated, but its efficacy remains unknown. CT has been employed, but the results are highly variable.

PREVENTION. The question of how to prevent osteoporosis is the subject of considerable controversy. However, with the advent of more precise ways of estimating bone mass in patients by noninvasive means, considerable evidence shows that administration of estrogens following surgically induced or natural menopause will prevent the loss of bone mineral and bone mass, as well as the other changes commonly seen. This strongly suggests that estrogen prophylaxis can prevent or greatly reduce the occurrence of osteoporosis. However, there are several problems with the use of estrogens. First, if therapy is continued for several years and then stopped, the rate of bone loss promptly increases. The implication of this finding is that prophylaxis should be lifelong to be effective. Second, although all women show a phase of rapid bone loss in the immediate postmenopausal period, not all lose sufficient bone to lead to osteoporosis and fractures. It is not known what factors determine which women in a particular population will have clinically evident disease, nor is there any method currently available to identify the patients most likely to have the disease. Third, estrogen therapy is attended with several potentially serious side effects, in particular, a greater risk of thromboembolic disease and endometrial carcinoma. However, modern low-dose estrogen replacement given cyclically for 3 weeks each month has decreased these risks considerably.

Osteomalacia

DEFINITION. Osteomalacia is a defect in the mineralization of bone matrix leading to an accumulation of nonmineralized or poorly mineralized osteoid. Rickets, its counterpart in children, involves a failure in the mineralization of epiphyseal growth-plate cartilage.

ETIOLOGY. A wide number of conditions can lead to osteomalacia or rickets, as shown by the following outline:

    I. Vitamin D deficiency
   II. Vitamin D malabsorption
      A. Sprue syndrome
      B. Postgastrectomy–blind loop syndrome
      C. Small bowel resection or bypass
      D. Pancreatic insufficiency
      E. Exudative enteropathy
      F. Laxative abuse
      G. Bile salt deficiency
      H. Lactose intolerance
  III. Impaired 25-hydroxylation (liver)
      A. Neonatal hepatitis
      B. Cirrhosis of liver
      C. Microsomal enzyme induction
         1. Phenytoin
         2. Barbiturates
         3. Glutethimide
  IV. Impaired 1α-hydroxylation (kidney)
      A. Genetic enzyme defect (vitamin D-dependent rickets, type I)
      B. Chronic renal failure
   V. Resistance to 1,25(OH)$_2$D$_3$ (vitamin D-dependent rickets, type II)
  VI. Phosphate depletion and hypophosphatemia
      A. Negative phosphorus balance (antacids)
      B. Familial hypophosphatemic rickets
      C. Hereditary hypophosphatemic rickets with hypercalciuria
      D. Oncogenic osteomalacia
      E. Primary hypophosphatemic bone disease
      F. Fanconi syndrome
 VII. Hypophosphatasia
VIII. Renal osteodystrophy

Most of these conditions are related either to a deficiency or malabsorption of vitamin D, or to some metabolic alteration in its metabolism. In addition, phosphate deficiency (which commonly accompanies vitamin D deficiency) may itself lead to osteomalacia. Hypophosphatasia and renal osteodystrophy are discussed under separate headings.

PATHOGENESIS. As the outline shows, quite disparate pathophysiologic mechanisms may lead to undermineralized bone, rickets, and osteomalacia. Simple dietary lack of vitamin D is much less common today than in the past, but occasionally appears (particularly in late winter) in breast-fed infants not given vitamin supplements, in vegetarians, and in elderly shut-ins. Disorders causing malabsorption of vitamin D are more likely to cause osteomalacia. Because of the extensive entero-hepatic circulation of vitamin D and its metabolites, vitamin D$_3$ production in the skin frequently cannot compensate for intestinal malabsorption, as even this component may be lost in the stool.

It is often stated that 1,25(OH)$_2$D$_3$ is the only active metabolite of vitamin D$_3$ and therefore in cases of dietary lack, malabsorption, or phenytoin-induced catabolism of vitamin D, serum 1,25(OH)$_2$D$_3$ concentration should be reduced. Some patients with these conditions do have low values, but many have normal or high values at a time when serum 25(OH)D$_3$ values are low and both osseous and biochemical evidence indicates the presence of osteomalacia. Based on this infor-

mation, it would seem that several metabolites of vitamin D are normally active. The possible roles of changes in the metabolism of different vitamin D metabolites in the pathogenesis of osteomalacia are shown in Fig. 193-8. In this scheme a deficiency of vitamin D$_3$ leads first to a decreased serum concentration of 25(OH)D$_3$, 24,25(OH)$_2$D$_3$, and 1,25(OH)$_2$D$_3$. These changes cause a decrease in bone resorption, bone mineralization, and intestinal calcium absorption. Bone serum calcium and phosphate concentrations tend to fall. The fall in serum calcium concentration stimulates PTH secretion so that secondary hyperparathyroidism develops. This leads to a further fall in the serum phosphate concentration and so to a further delay in mineralization. It also leads to a stimulation of the renal production of 1,25(OH)$_2$D$_3$ so that levels of this metabolite rise to the normal or even supranormal range. However, this alone is insufficient to enhance bone resorption, and it also causes a further decrease in 25(OH)D$_3$ levels. As the 25(OH)D$_3$ is depleted, the serum 1,25(OH)$_2$D$_3$ concentration also falls.

There are several clearly defined syndromes of inherited rickets and osteomalacia. One rare disorder is the so-called vitamin D-dependent rickets, type I, which is usually inherited as an autosomal recessive trait. It is caused by a partial deficiency of the renal enzyme (1α-hydroxylase) responsible for catalyzing the conversion of 25(OH)D$_3$ to 1,25(OH)$_2$D$_3$. A variant of this syndrome, vitamin D-dependent rickets, type II, is associated with normal levels of the enzyme but partial resistance to the action of 1,25(OH)$_2$D$_3$. The names for these syndromes were chosen before their pathogenesis was understood and reflect the fact that their cure depends on both adequate ultraviolet light exposure and pharmacologic doses of vitamin D.

A second major pathogenetic category of rickets and osteomalacia comprises disease states associated with hypophosphatemia. Even with normal vitamin D metabolism, phosphate depletion (as seen in patients ingesting large amounts of phosphate-binding antacids, for example) can cause osteomalacia. Hypophosphatemia triggers a prompt fall in renal phosphate excretion and normally increases 1,25(OH)$_2$D$_3$ production by the proximal renal tubule. Elevated 1,25(OH)$_2$D$_3$ levels result in greater intestinal calcium absorption and less PTH secretion with secondary hypoparathyroidism. The hypophosphatemia, elevated 1,25(OH)$_2$D$_3$ levels, and depressed PTH levels all contribute to inhibited bone formation and a net shift of phosphate from the skeleton into the bloodstream.

Familial hypophosphatemic rickets (FHR) is currently the single most prevalent cause of rickets in the United States. Also called vitamin D-resistant rickets, it is usually inherited as an X-linked dominant trait. The disease appears to result from a primary disorder of proximal renal tubular function, causing a marked renal phosphate leak. Despite severe hypophosphatemia, an associated impairment in the proximal tubular enzyme 1α-hydroxylase leads to inappropriately low levels of 1,25(OH)$_2$D$_3$ with intestinal malabsorption of calcium and phosphate. Hereditary hypophosphatemic rickets with hypercalciuria is a recently described variant of FHR in which 1α-hydroxylase activity remains intact so that 1,25(OH)$_2$D$_3$ levels are appropriately elevated for the degree of hypophosphatemia. Oncogenic osteomalacia is a syndrome similar to FHR that occasionally develops in adults with benign mesenchymal tumors. There tumors, which are usually small and may be occult, produce an unknown humoral factor causing a severe renal phosphate leak. As in FHR, the renal phosphate leak is apparently accompanied by inhibited 1α-hydroxylase, as 1,25(OH)$_2$D$_3$ levels are usually in the low-normal range.

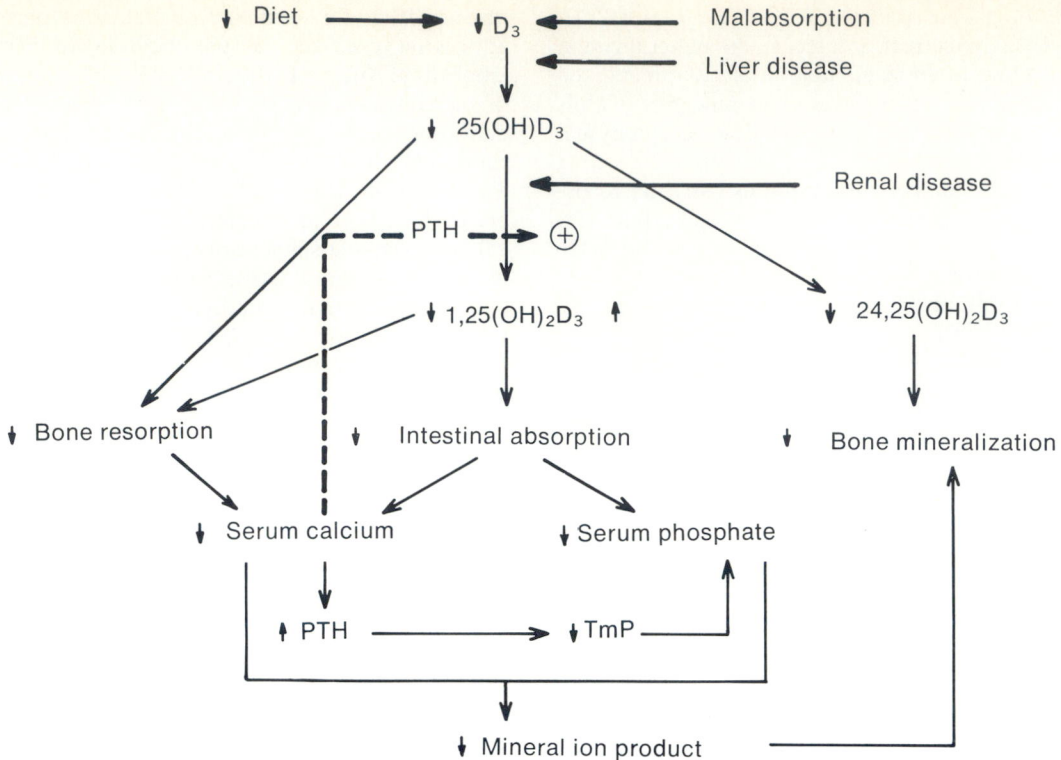

Fig. 193-8   Pathogenesis of osteomalacia of vitamin D deficiency (see text).

When the tumor is resected, the hypophosphatemia and osteomalacia resolve.

Muscle weakness is often a prominent manifestation of these states. Its development is probably a consequence of phosphate deficiency or the deficiency of one or more vitamin D metabolites. There is evidence that vitamin D and its metabolites act directly on muscle, but the metabolite involved and its precise function are unknown.

CLINICAL MANIFESTATIONS. The most dramatic effect of vitamin D deficiency in children is rickets, characterized clinically by femoral and tibial bowing, growth retardation, a rachitic rosary (enlarged costochondral metaphases), and other bone deformities. A striking initial clinical feature is often profound proximal muscle weakness, leading to a characteristic waddling gait, inability to climb stairs, and difficulty in rising from a sitting position. Hypocalcemic seizures or tetany may occur, and dentition frequently is delayed.

In adults, osteomalacia results in bone pain and tenderness that may be diffuse, localized in the back, or elicited by pressure over the anterior tibial surface. Again, proximal muscle weakness is often a major complaint. Latent tetany may be elicited, but seizures are rare in adults with vitamin D deficiency. If the cause is intestinal malabsorption, signs and symptoms range from marked steatorrhea with passage of numerous, foul-smelling stools, bloating, and abdominal pain to few or no symptoms of gastrointestinal malfunction.

Familial hypophosphatemic rickets shows symptoms at an early age with short stature and the typical bone deformities of rickets but without seizures, tetany, or muscle weakness. Affected males tend to have more severe disease than females. Later in life, bone pain persists and bone overgrowth may occur around the large joints and at sites of muscle attachment. Hereditary hypophosphatemic rickets with hypercalciuria is similar in the few cases that have been described, with occasional hematuria or renal colic resulting from kidney stones.

LABORATORY FINDINGS. Typically, adults with osteomalacia have a slightly reduced serum calcium concentration (7.5 to 8.5 mg/dl), a low serum phosphate concentration (1.5 to 2.5 mg/dl), an elevated alkaline phosphatase level (>120 IU), and reduced concentrations of $25(OH)D_3$ in the serum. The serum $1,25(OH)_2D_3$ level may be low, normal, or high. Secondary hyperparathyroidism with elevated nephrogenous cyclic AMP, low TmP/GFR, and high iPTH is the rule. Although these are the usual findings, some patients early in their disease may have a normal or high serum phosphate concentration in spite of secondary hyperparathyroidism. Urinary calcium excretion is low and intestinal calcium absorption is reduced. Creatinine clearance is normal.

In patients with osteomalacia on the basis of phosphate depletion, including those with familial hypophosphatemic rickets, the laboratory findings are somewhat different. Hypophosphatemia and elevated bone alkaline phosphatase are still characteristic, but unlike osteomalacia caused by vitamin D deficiency, serum calcium is usually normal and no secondary hyperparathyroidism is present. In patients with hypophosphatemia caused by dietary deficiency or intestinal malabsorption, the 24-hour urine phosphate is low, and while the renal phosphate threshold and serum $1,25(OH)_2D_3$ level are elevated. In patients with hypophosphatemia caused by a renal phosphate leak, the renal phosphate threshold (TmP/GFR) is low, and $1,25(OH)_2D_3$ levels are inappropriately low (in FHR and oncogenic osteomalacia).

Roentgenographic examination usually reveals skeletal demineralization and in severe cases pseudofractures or Looser's zones, which are linear areas of undermineralization perpendicular to the long axis of the bones. They usually are symmetric and occur at the axillary margin of the scapula, interior arches of the femoral neck, pubic and ischial rami, ribs, and metatarsals.

DIAGNOSIS. In the typical case, diagnosis is easy once suspected. When it has been confirmed by clinical, laboratory, and roentgenographic examination, the problem is to identify why the metabolism of vitamin D has changed. Such an evaluation includes a careful dietary history, a history of possible drug use, and a family history. Evaluating renal, hepatic, and/or gastrointestinal function may be necessary. Often the history alone suggests the diagnostic approach to pursue. Rarely, biochemical vitamin D deficiency with muscle weakness occurs without apparent evidence of renal, hepatic, or intestinal disease. If dietary lack is clearly not involved, usually an occult malabsorption syndrome is found.

COURSE. If left untreated, the deficiency progresses to severe and incapacitating weakness, skeletal pain, and debility.

MANAGEMENT. In most instances osteomalacia can be treated by increased oral doses of vitamin D_3. If malabsorption is present and can be corrected by a gluten-free diet, bile salts, or pancreatic enzymes, absorption of the vitamin will improve; doses ranging from 5000 to 10,000 units/day are sufficient. Similar doses are usually effective in patients with the postgastrectomy blind loop syndrome. In these cases bacterial infection within the loop may be responsible for catabolism of vitamin D_3, necessitating antibiotic therapy in addition to vitamin D_3. In some patients with a marked decrease in the amount of small bowel, for example, following resection for Crohn's disease, larger doses of vitamin D may be required. In these cases administering the more polar $25(OH)D_3$ in doses of 50 to 75 μg/day may be more effective. In cases of phenytoin or phenobarbital ingestion in which continued administration is necessary to control a seizure disorder, 5000 to 10,000 units of vitamin D_3 per day are usually sufficient to prevent vitamin D deficiency.

Familial hypophosphatemic rickets is unresponsive to vitamin D_3 even in large doses but can be successfully treated with a combination of oral phosphate (0.25 to 0.75 g four times/day) and $1,25(OH)_2D_3$ (0.25 to 4 μg/day depending on the age and size of the patient and the severity of the disease). In many patients this program almost completely heals the rickets and restores a nearly normal growth rate. However, to be effective, it must be continued throughout the entire growth period. The appropriate dose of $1,25(OH)_2D_3$ must be judged by giving amounts sufficient to prevent phosphate-induced secondary hyperparathyroidism but not high enough to induce hypercalciuria and its attendant risk of renal damage. Although the manifestations of the disease lessen somewhat after skeletal growth stops and the serum alkaline phosphatase concentration returns to normal, most adults with this condition have persistent muscle and skeletal pains, fatigability, and moderate to marked osteomalacia on bone biopsy. These patients benefit significantly from combined phosphate and $1,25(OH)_2D_3$ therapy, but longterm studies of this therapy have not been reported.

Renal osteodystrophy

DEFINITION. Renal osteodystrophy is the bone disease that develops with chronic renal failure. It includes a spectrum of osseous changes, ranging from almost pure osteomalacia to nearly pure osteitis fibrosa cystica (that is, hyperparathyroid bone disease). It is associated with a variety of changes in mineral and vitamin D metabolism and parathyroid function.

PATHOGENESIS. Multiple factors are involved in the development of renal osteodystrophy. As renal function declines, a point is reached when phosphate clearance decreases. This leads to a rise in serum phosphate concentration and a decline in serum ionized calcium, causing secondary hyperparathyroidism. The increase in IPTH increases renal phosphate clear-

ance so that for a time the serum phosphate may not rise significantly but secondary hyperparathyroidism with increased bone turnover may be evident. Further decline in renal function leads to progressive phosphate retention, hyperphosphatemia, and progressively more marked secondary hyperparathyroidism. In addition, with renal failure renal conversion of $25(OH)D_3$ to $1,25(OH)_2D_3$ is impaired, leading to a fall in serum $1,24(OH)_2D_3$ levels and intestinal calcium absorption. Recent evidence suggests that a low serum $1,25(OH)_2D_3$ level itself may stimulate PTH synthesis. For all of these reasons, secondary hyperparathyroidism with parathyroid hyperplasia usually accompanies chronic renal insufficiency. The excessive PTH produces progressively more marked osteitis fibrosa cystica.

The osteomalacia component of renal osteodystrophy was until recently more difficult to explain. Theories explaining the inhibition of bone mineralization included metabolic acidosis and resistance to the actions of vitamin D. However, recent evidence suggests that the most important factor causing osteomalacia in renal failure is aluminum toxicity. Aluminum, whether from dialysis water, aluminum hydroxide–containing phosphate-binding gels taken to control hyperphosphatemia, or other sources, accumulates in renal failure and may reach toxic levels in the bone. Special aluminum staining of bone biopsy specimens reveals a line of aluminum deposition at the mineralization front in patients with osteomalacic renal osteodystrophy. In addition, aluminum may inhibit PTH release or action, decreasing bone turnover and allowing further accumulation of aluminum.

CLINICAL MANIFESTATIONS. Eventually some type of bone disease appears in most patients with chronic renal failure, whether treated conservatively or by chronic hemodialysis. Clinical features may include profound proximal muscle weakness similar to that seen in vitamin D deficiency, lethargy, fatigability, weight loss, anemia, pruritus, bone pain and tenderness, fractures, and soft tissue calcification. The presentation varies from patient to patient.

LABORATORY FINDINGS. The serum phosphate concentration is usually high, particularly in untreated cases, and is associated with a marked decrease in creatinine clearance. The serum calcium concentration may be low, normal, or high, but the ionized portion is usually low. However, if prolonged secondary hyperparathyroidism has been present, one or more of the hyperplastic glands may undergo an adenomatous transformation leading to the appearance of *tertiary* hyperparathyroidism with hypercalcemia. The serum $1,25(OH)_2D_3$ concentration is low to undetectable, and the $25(OH)D_3$ may also be moderately low, whereas alkaline phosphatase activity is usually higher. Increased iPTH is the rule. However, there is no simple correlation between the elevation of iPTH and the degree of hyperparathyroidism. This is because PTH undergoes peripheral metabolism (Fig. 193-5). As a result, C-terminal, biologically inactive, but immunologically measurable peptides are generated. The kidney is a major site for the disposal of these peptides, so in progressive renal failure these inactive PTH fragments accumulate. Also, because with severe renal failure the measurement of nephrogenous cyclic AMP no longer indicates parathyroid function, there is no way to accurately measure the amount of biologically active parathyroid hormone.

MANAGEMENT. The management of this frequent and often debilitating complication of chronic renal failure and dialysis is far from ideal. Neither from the history, clinical symptoms, serum chemistries, nor hormone levels is it possible to determine with confidence whether renal osteodystrophy results from hyperparathyroidism, osteomalacia, or both. Plasma or urine aluminum levels do not accurately reflect either the total body accumulation of aluminum or the degree of osteomalacia. Bone biopsies are the most reliable means of determining the type of osteodystrophy in these patients. It is not unusual for a patient suffering renal osteodystrophy to have different histology on successive bone biopsies. In particular, progression from predominant hyperparathyroid bone disease, through a mixed phase, to predominant osteomalacia is common.

The traditional treatment, even early in renal insufficiency, has been to reduce serum phosphate to the normal range if possible to prevent secondary hyperparathyroidism. Antacids containing aluminum hydroxide (such as Basaljel) bind dietary phosphate and decrease its intestinal absorption. While these phosphate-binding gels are poorly absorbed, recent evidence indicates that with chronic use enough aluminum is absorbed to cause bone toxicity and osteomalacia. Therefore the current trend is toward using less aluminum hydroxide, and preventing severe hyperphosphatemia by dietary or other means. In addition, other approaches to controlling secondary hyperparathyroidism can be attempted. These include maintaining a normal or even slightly elevated level of serum calcium using vitamin D therapy. In particular, replacing $1,25(OH)_2D_3$ (commercially available as Calcitriol) appears helpful and may have the added benefit of direct feedback inhibition of PTH synthesis, as mentioned previously. However, caution is vital with this approach to avoid the complications of severe hypercalcemia, hyperphosphatemia, and soft tissue calcification. Subtotal parathyroidectomy is only rarely indicated in renal failure to control medically intractable hypercalcemia, as increased bone pain from osteomalacia often ensues.

Patients with the osteomalacia type of renal osteodystrophy respond poorly to any form of vitamin D or other conventional therapy. Recently, the chelating agent deferoxamine mesylate has been given intravenously in an attempt to remove aluminum from the bone in these patients. This treatment appears to benefit some patients, especially those who have not previously undergone parathyroidectomy.

Paget's disease of bone

DEFINITION. Paget's disease of bone (osteitis deformans) is a primary, focal bone disease, in which mineral metabolism may be secondarily affected. Bone involvement is asymmetric, with the femur, pelvis, vertebrae, skull, and tibia most often involved. The disease is common, affecting 2% to 3% of persons over 40 years of age of Anglo-Saxon origin. Involved bone may be asymptomatic, or may become painful or deformed.

PATHOGENESIS. From recent evidence, the most likely etiologic factor in Paget's disease appears to be a slow virus infection of bone. Viral-like inclusion bodies appear in osteoclasts of affected bone, antibodies raised against paramyxoviruses react with these osteoclasts, and recently nucleic acid probes directed against measles virus RNA have been demonstrated to bind to pagetic bone cells but not to normal bone. Whether the agent is measles virus, respiratory syncytial virus, or some other paramyxovirus is unclear at present.

Bone involved in Paget's disease is highly cellular, with many giant osteoclasts containing up to 100 nuclei and with large numbers of active osteoblasts. This results in high bone turnover, but the new bone is laid down in an atypical fashion resulting in a mosaic pattern characteristic of the disorder. Early in the course of the disease there may be a lytic phase, in which bone resorption exceeds bone formation. Later, bone formation tends to exceed resorption, resulting in the characteristically enlarged cotton-wool appearance of involved bones on roentgenographs.

CLINICAL MANIFESTATIONS. About two thirds of patients with Paget's disease of bone are asymptomatic, with the disease appearing on only roentgenographic examination or by an elevated alkaline phosphatase level on routine blood screening. The skin overlying involved bone may be warm, reflecting the increased blood flow caused by the bone's intense metabolic activity. Pain is the most common complaint in symptomatic patients. It may be localized over involved bone, especially at sites of incomplete transverse fractures, which are common in the femur and tibia. Even more common is joint pain in the hip, knee, or lower back, resulting from involvement of adjacent bone or from osteoarthritis. A less common but still important source of pain in Paget's disease is nerve root compression by bone overgrowth at the vertebral foramina.

Skeletal deformity is not uncommon in longstanding Paget's disease and may be severe. Anterolateral bowing of an involved femur, tibia, or both is frequent. There may be protrusio acetabuli into an involved pelvic bone. Pathologic transverse "chalk stick" fractures of the long bones may occur; rarely they may result in permanent separation. The skull may be enlarged, occasionally resulting in "leonine facies." Rarely, the cervical vertebrae protrude into the base of the skull, potentially resulting in brainstem herniation.

Hearing loss is the most common neurologic complication of Paget's disease, occurring in 50% of patients with skull involvement. Usually the deficit is sensorineural resulting from distortion of the chochlea or, less often, from compression of the eighth nerve. Other cranial nerve compression syndromes occasionally cause diplopia, dysphagia, or dysarthria.

Bone tumors are more frequent in pagetic bone, but remain rare. Giant cell tumors (relatively benign) may develop in the skull or facial bones. Osteosarcomas (highly malignant) occur in less than 1% of patients, usually with involvement of the long bones.

Increased cardiac output can occur in patients with extensive bone involvement, but high-output cardiac failure is uncommon. Extramedullary hematopoesis can appear, resulting form obliteration of the bone marrow cells by fibrous tissue and bone cells.

LABORATORY FINDINGS. The most characteristic laboratory finding in Paget's disease of bone is an elevated serum alkaline phosphatase, reflecting increased osteoblastic bone formation. Hydroxyproline is a modified amino acid unique to bone matrix protein. The 24-hour urine hydroxyproline level may be high, reflecting increased osteoclastic bone resorption. The roentgenographic appearance of Paget's disease of bone, as mentioned earlier, is a "cotton-wool" pattern with uneven contours, overall enlargement of the bone, and loss of the normal trabecular pattern. Bone scan, in which radionuclide is taken up by new bone laid down by osteoblasts, is more sensitive but less specific than roentgenograms for detecting Paget's disease.

The diagnosis of Paget's disease almost always depends on the clinical presentation and roentgenographic appearance of bone. Bone biopsy is rarely indicated and is relatively hazardous because the increased metabolic activity of the bone predisposes to focal hemorrhage. The extent of the disease and response to therapy are best monitored by bone scan and the alkaline phosphatase level.

Normally, mineral metabolism homeostasis remains intact in patients with Paget's disease of bone. Although involved bone turns over much more rapidly than normal, formation and resorption remain closely coupled, so there is no large net movement of mineral into or out of bone at any given time. The hormones maintaining mineral homeostasis are fully able to compensate for the small net mineral transport that does occur. However, if a patient with Paget's disease is immobilized (for example, following a fracture), hypercalcemia is common. Normal weight-bearing stimulates bone formation: without it, there is a temporary state of excess bone resorption. In normal bone this effect is relatively small, but in Paget's disease and other states of high bone turnover (such as adolescence, hyperparathyroidism, and multiple myeloma), immobilization with a temporary uncoupling of bone resorption and formation leads to rapid loss of calcium from bone, frequently resulting in hypercalcemia.

MANAGEMENT. Asymptomatic patients with Paget's disease require no treatment. Patients who have pain, deformity, or neurologic symptoms attributable to Paget's disease usually derive benefit from medications designed to slow the rate of bone turnover. Calcitonin in pharmacologic doses inhibits osteoclast activity, slowing the pagetic process. Unfortunately, it has several drawbacks: it is expensive, it must be given parenterally as subcutaneous injections, and a significant number of patients develop tolerance to the hormone (often but not always with formation of anticalcitonin antibodies). Side effects of salmon calcitonin include nausea, a metallic taste in the mouth, and flushing. It was hoped that the recent introduction of synthetic human calcitonin would obviate many of the drug's disadvantages, but side effects appear to be just as common and some patients still develop resistance by unknown mechanisms.

Other potentially beneficial medications are the diphosphonates. These analogs of pyrophosphate also inhibit osteoclastic bone resorption and slow down the pagetic process. The only diphosphonate presently available in the United States is etidronate. Unfortunately, this has a major disadvantage: it impairs bone mineralization to a greater extent than other diphosphonates, so osteomalacia is a dose-limiting toxicity. Etidronate is given orally in low doses and only at 6-month intervals to avoid this complication. Some patients may actually develop increased pain and pathologic fractures of pagetic bone, presumably as a result of osteomalacia, particularly at higher doses of etidronate. Other diphosphonates have been used to treat Paget's disease in Europe with fewer apparent complications and may become available in the United States in the future.

Orthopedic procedures, including hip replacement or osteotomy to correct severe bowing of the leg bones, are sometimes indicated in Paget's disease. Before any elective orthopedic procedure, medication (usually calcitonin) should be given for several months to slow the activity of the disease. This decreases the vascularity of the bone and overlying tissue, thus facilitating otherwise difficult surgery. Pretreatment also lowers the risk of the patient developing hypercalcemia as a complication of immobilization.

PRIMARY DISORDERS OF SKELETAL HOMEOSTASIS
Osteogenesis imperfecta

Osteogenesis imperfecta is a hereditary disorder of collagen metabolism that varies in severity. It is characterized by a propensity to bone fractures following minimal trauma, hyperextensible joints, blue sclerae, and eventual deafness. Specific defects in type 1 collagen synthesis in which osteo-

blasts are unable to create normal bone matrix protein, have recently been identified in some cases. There is no known available treatment. Other hereditary conditions associated with osteopenia resulting from impaired matrix formation include the Ehlers-Danlos syndrome, Marfan's syndrome, Menkes' syndrome, homocystinuria, and Hutchinson-Gilford progeria.

Osteopetrosis

Osteopetrosis, or marble bone disease, is a rare hereditary condition in which the normal process of bone remodeling is deficient because of abnormal osteoclasts that appear incapable of resorbing bone. Thus bone density increases with time, leading to a reduced marrow cavity, anemia, compressed cranial nerves, synostoses, and often death in early childhood. A milder, dominantly inherited form presents in adolescence. Recently, in experimental case reports, early bone marrow transplant has apparently cured the disease by replacing the defective hematopoietic precursor of the osteoclast.

Hypophosphatasia

Hypophosphatasia is a familial disease in which the skeletal deformities of rickets and osteomalacia develop despite the presence of normal metabolism of vitamin D, parathyroid hormone, and bone mineral. It is inherited as an autosomal recessive trait and may appear in infancy, childhood, or adulthood. The cardinal features of the disease are rickets and/or osteomalacia of variable severity with a low serum and bone alkaline phosphatase and the excretion of excessive amounts of phosphoethanolamine in the urine. On bone biopsy, rickets and osteomalacia are seen. The primary defect is thought to be a lack of the normal amount of alkaline phosphatase in bone matrix vesicles, which delays or inhibits nucleation of bone mineral crystals. There is no definitive treatment, but continuous high phosphate intake has been reported to lead to an improvement in some cases.

BIBLIOGRAPHY

Bijvoet OLM: Kidney function in calcium and phosphate metabolism. In Avioli LV and Krane SM, editors: Metabolic bone disease, vol 1, New York, 1977, Academic Press Inc.

Broadus AE: Nephrogenous cAMP as a parathyroid function test, Nephron 23:136, 1979.

Broadus AE and others: The importance of circulating 1,25-dihydroxyvitamin D in the pathogenesis of hypercalcemia and renal stone formation in primary hyperparathyroidism, N Engl J Med 302:421, 1980.

Broadus AE and others: Humoral hypercalcemia of cancer: identification of a novel parathyroid hormone-like peptide, N Eng J Med 39:556, 1988.

Habener JF and Potts JT, Jr: Biosynthesis of parathyroid hormone, N Engl J Med 299:580, 635, 1978.

Haussler MR and McCain TA: Basic and clinical concepts related to vitamin D metabolism and action, N Engl J Med 297, 974, 1977.

Heath H, Hodgson SF, and Kennedy MA: Primary hyperparathyroidism: Incidence, morbidity, and potential economic impact in a community, N Engl J Med 302:189, 1980.

Insogna KL and others: Sensitivity of the parathyroid hormone-1,25-dihydroxyvitamin D axis to variations in calcium intake in patients with primary hyperparathyroidism, N Engl J Med 313:1126, 1985.

Juan D: Hypocalcemia: differential diagnosis and mechanisms, Arch Int Med 139:1166, 1979.

Law WM and Heath H: Familial benign hypercalcemia (hypocalciuric hypercalcemia): clinical and pathogenetic studies in 21 families, Ann Int Med 102:511, 1985.

Lee DBN, Zawada ET, and Kleeman CR: The pathophysiology and clinical aspects of hypercalcemic disorders, West J Med 129:278, 1978.

Levine MA and others: Activity of the stimulatory guanine nucleotide-binding protein is reduced in erythrocytes from patients pseudohypoparathyroidism and pseudopseudohypoparathyroidism: biochemical, endocrine and genetic analysis of Albright's hereditary osteodystrophy in six kindreds, J Clin Endocrinol Metab 62:497, 1986.

Mason RS and others: Vitamin D conversion by sarcoid lymph node homogenate, Ann Int Med 100:59, 1984.

Mundy GR and others: The hypercalcemia of cancer: clinical implications and pathogenic mechanisms, N Engl J Med 310:1718, 1984.

Nordin BEC: Metabolic bone and stone disease, Baltimore, 1973, The Williams & Wilkins Co.

Pak CYC: Calcium urolithiasis, New York, 1978, Plenum Publishing Corp.

Parfitt AM: Equilibrium and disequilibrium hypercalcemia: new light on an old concept, Metab Bone Dis Rel Res 1:279, 1979.

Rasmussen H and Bordier P: The physiological and cellular basis of metabolic bone disease, Baltimore, 1974, The Williams & Wilkins Co.

Rasmussen H and Bordier P: Vitamin D and bone, Metab Bone Dis Rel Res 1:7, 1978.

Riggs BL and Melton LJ: Involutional osteoporosis, N Engl J Med 314:1676, 1986.

Stewart A and others: Biochemical evaluation of patients with malignancy associated hypercalcemia: evidence for humoral and non-humoral groups, N Engl J Med 303:1377, 1980.

Dental correlations

S. Gary Cohen and **Barbara J. Steinberg**

PITUITARY GLAND DISORDERS
Hypothalamic-hypopituitary disorders

ORAL MANIFESTATIONS. Several craniofacial malformations are associated with hypothalamic-pituitary disorders. The most common is that of a single maxillary deciduous and permanent dental incisor; cleft lips and cleft palates have also been reported. Other craniofacial manifestations include hypotelorism and other facial dysmorphologies.

Hyperpituitarism

Adult hyperpituitarism—acromegaly. The most striking feature in patients with acromegaly is the gradual proliferation of osseous and soft tissue of the acral parts of the body, especially the hands, feet, and face. The ears, nose, and lips are enlarged, which contributes to the typically coarse, acromegalic facial expression. Localized areas of hyperpigmentation are often seen along the nasolabial folds.

The tongue may enlarge disproportionately from the mouth, with marked papillary hypertrophy, and either protrude somewhat or develop indentations around the lateral margins from pressing against the teeth. The lingual enlargement appears to result both from increased diameter of the muscle fibers, especially those in the anterior half, and from thickened epithelium and subepithelial connective tissue.

In acromegaly there is marked thickening of the cranium including the facial bones and paranasal sinuses, with pronounced bony ledging and massive frontal bossing.

This disorder stimulates the mandibular growth centers, especially the condyle. Exaggerated condylar growth causes a mesial shift in the occlusion and increased prominence of the chin. The width of the mandible is also increased. Recent studies indicate that a large proportion of acromegalic patients have an Angle Class III malocclusion with complete or partial crossbite. Overdevelopment of the mandible and pressure from the enlarged tongue on the alveolar processes can lead to a relative mandibular prognathism with flaring and spacing of the teeth. The size of the teeth is unchanged, but increased cementum deposition is common.

Advanced periodontal disease is usually a feature of acromegaly, especially when the malocclusion is severe. Metabolic disturbance of the jaws and oral soft tissues may also contribute to periodontal breakdown.

An increase in the size of the larynx causes the voice to deepen.

Juvenile hyperpituitarism—gigantism. The clinical features of acromegaly are rare in children suffering from gigantism. It is commonly assumed that these changes do not occur while longitudinal growth is taking place. During puberty, the changes associated with hyperpituitarism are confined chiefly to the mandible and, to a lesser extent, the maxilla. These changes consist of thickening of the cortical bone of the mandible and enlargement of the paranasal sinuses. On occasion, periosteal ossifications are seen at the sites of muscle and tendon attachments.

The overdevelopment of the mandible and face begin to produce the pathognomonic facies of adult hyperpituitarism. Roentgenographically the bones are seen to be poorly calcified and have large trabeculae. Individuals with gigantism manifest accelerated dental development, including early eruption of the teeth. Mineralization of the teeth, however, is not affected by the excess in growth hormone.

DENTAL MANAGEMENT. Diabetes and hypertension are the significant complications most often associated with hyperpituitarism. The dentist must be familiar with the treatment and management of patients with these disorders. (Refer to appropriate sections in this text).

Acromegaly. Unfortunately, correcting abnormal growth-hormone dynamics does not reverse the skeletal deformities associated with acromegaly. Surgical correction may be necessary after the growth hormone is normalized.

Soft tissue deformities generally regress when acromegaly is controlled by appropriate therapy. Therefore the tongue should become smaller. If this does not take place and marked dysarthria occurs, a partial glossectomy may be indicated.

Hypopituitarism

ORAL MANIFESTATIONS. There is a marked effect on both facial and dental development in children with hypopituitarism. The condition disturbs facial growth, retarding mandibular development and leading to malocclusion with excessive crowding of the teeth. Although the teeth are normal in size, the crowns are not always completely erupted and roots tend to be shortened. There is delayed and incomplete eruption of the teeth along with an even greater delay in skeletal development. Slower dental development begins with delayed shedding of deciduous teeth with unresorbed roots. In addition, permanent teeth take longer to erupt and show incomplete roots and closure of the apical foramen.

When pituitary destruction occurs, regardless of the cause, there appears to be hypofunction of the salivary glands with resultant xerostomia. Decreased salivary flow increases the incidence of caries and periodontal disease.

DENTAL MANAGEMENT. Since these individuals experience a higher incidence of caries and gingival inflammation, frequent dental checkups are important. Patients with destruction of the pituitary gland may be on maintenance replacement therapy, including steroids. It is therefore important for the dentist to understand the management of the patient on exogenous steroids (see discussion of adrenal cortex).

DISORDERS OF THYROID GLAND
Hyperthyroidism

ORAL MANIFESTATIONS. The hyperthyroid patient presents with facial skin that is warm, moist, and often flushed. Excessive melanin pigmentation may occur on the skin and the patient's hair may be fine and friable.

Eye signs are a prominent feature of the condition and easily recognized by the dentist. These include infrequent blinking, dilated pupils, protruding eyeballs (exophthalmus), and lid-lag caused by spasm of the muscles of the upper eyelid, which exposes the sclera above the corners when the patient is looking downward. In addition, weakness of the extrinsic muscles of the eyes occurs because of lymphocytic infiltration, which may cause squinting and double vision (diplopia).

Clinical examination of the thyroid can reveal a gland of normal size or as much as four times larger. Usually the gland is symmetrically involved and feels rather firm and lobulated. A systolic bruit may be heard over the thyroid because the gland's vascular supply has engorged.

Children with hyperthyroidism experience premature loss of deciduous teeth and early eruption of permanent teeth, though the teeth and jaws are usually well formed and present no unusual irregularities. Infants born of hyperthyroid mothers have been reported to have several teeth erupted at birth.

There is a tendency toward osteoporosis of the alveolar bone in the hyperthyroid patient. These patients also appear to develop caries and periodontal disease at a rapid rate, possibly from consuming excessive amounts of sugars to satisfy increased caloric demands.

A few patients with hyperthyroidism have been found to have thyroid tissue in the tongue below the area of the embryonic thyroglossal duct. These patients should be evaluated by a physician for the presence of a normal thyroid gland before the mass is surgically removed.

DENTAL MANAGEMENT. In hyperthyroid individuals, emotional stress, infection, trauma, and surgery can precipitate a thyroid crisis or "storm," which may be fatal. Therefore palpation and inspection of the thyroid gland should be included in the routine head and neck examination performed by the dentist. If thyroid enlargement is noted, even in a patient who appears to be euthyroid, or if the dentist suspects hyperthyroidism, either from the medical history or from readily discernible clinical signs, the patient should be referred for medical consultation and management before dental treatment begins. Once medical treatment has been instituted and the patient is euthyroid, there is no contraindication to dental treatment.

In the event of a dental emergency in a hyperthyroid patient, such as an acute oral infection, the dentist must consult with the physician concerning management of the emergency. Often conservative treatment, consisting of antibiotics and analgesics, is advisable. If dental therapy must be rendered immediately, the controlled environment of a hospital operating room is optimum. The physician should bring the patient to a euthyroid state before any surgery. Local anesthetics without epinephrine or other pressor amines should be used, if needed, since the myocardium in these patients is highly sensitive to epinephrine and its use can precipitate severe arrhythmias, tachycardia, and/or chest pain.

Many hyperthyroid patients take propylthiouracil to inhibit the excessive synthesis of thyroid hormone. Because this drug may cause agranulocytosis, hypoprothrombinemia, and bleeding, a complete blood count with differential and prothrombin time must be obtained before surgery.

The dentist should recognize the symptoms of thyroid storm and be able to manage this potentially fatal crisis. It has an abrupt onset with symptoms of extreme restlessness, nausea, vomiting, and abdominal pain. Shortly thereafter, fever, profuse sweating, tachycardia, pulmonary edema, and congestive heart failure develop. If the patient develops severe hypertension and becomes comatose, death may occur. Immediate treatment consists of large doses (600 to 1000 mg) of propylthiouracil given intravenously, along with medication to diminish the metabolic effects of thyroid hormones. One of these, propranolol hydrochloride, is a β-adrenergic blocking agent and the drug of choice to reverse the cardiac and psychomotor

effects of thyrotoxicosis when given intravenously at a rate of 1 mg/min until the crisis is controlled (usually 2 to 10 minutes), with the total dose not to exceed 10 mg. Proper treatment should also include general supportive measures such as replacing fluids, glucose, electrolytes, and vitamin B complex and applying wet packs, cool air, and ice packs to control temperature.

Hypothyroidism
ORAL MANIFESTATIONS
Cretinism. The skin of the face is coarse, thick, dry, and wrinkled. The lips are enlarged, puffy, and pale, and the patient frequently holds his mouth partially open, probably caused in part to an enlarged tongue.

In cretinism, the base of the skull is foreshortened, the face wide and short, the mandible underdeveloped, and the maxilla overdeveloped. The bridge of the nose is retracted and fontanelle closure is delayed, resulting in an unusually large head. The gingiva is spongy, and deciduous teeth erupt and exfoliate later than normal. Permanent teeth may erupt later as well. There is a high frequency of enamel hypoplasia in deciduous teeth; the permanent dentition is also hypoplastic, but to a lesser degree. Thus malocclusion is relatively frequent in cretinism because of the faulty patterns of growth and development. A widening of the dental arch with flaring and spacing of the teeth may be observed. An open bite, receding chin, and enlarged protruding tongue lead to mouth breathing, which eventually results in drying and breakdown of gingival tissues.

Juvenile myxedema. Juvenile myxedema has the same clinical picture as cretinism, but the symptoms are less severe. The oral changes consist of retarded tooth eruption and defective formation of the jaws. There is delayed shedding of the primary teeth, which retards secondary dentition development; that is, the completion of the roots of the permanent teeth slows and delays the eruption rate. The teeth are poorly formed and enamel hypoplasia is common. In the deciduous dentition the hypoplasia is limited to those portions of teeth that mineralize in fetal life and infancy. In the permanent dentition, minor enamel hypoplasia dating from infancy and early childhood appears on incisors and first molars, but very rarely in premolars and second molars. In some seriously affected patients, dentin apposition is markedly delayed and pulp chambers are larger than normal. The dental age of hypothyroid children is many years younger than their chronologic or bone age.

Adult myxedema. In adult hypothyroidism, the skin and lips are pale and their texture is dry and scaly. Even more striking, however, is the puffy, myxedematous appearance of the entire face, with the nose, ears, and lips especially enlarged. The hair is dry and brittle and the eyebrows thin or entirely absent.

Generalized swelling may affect the tongue, causing difficulty in speech and scalloping around the margins from constant pressure against the teeth. This swelling of the tongue, coupled with swelling of the vocal cords, produces a characteristic husky, low-pitched voice. Since dental development is complete before the onset of the condition, there is no effect on the teeth and supporting tissues. However, gingivitis and rampant caries frequently occur, due in part to mouth breathing that accompanies the tongue enlargement. Hypothyroidism has been associated with an impairment in the normal immune response, and patients may develop chronic mucocutaneous candidiasis.

DENTAL MANAGEMENT. The dentist may be the first person to suspect hypothyroidism by recognizing the typical orofacial changes. Early detection and medical management can prevent permanent mental retardation in very young individuals, as well as the oral complications of delayed eruption of teeth, malocclusion, enlargement of the tongue, and skeletal retardation.

In general, there is probably no danger in providing dental care for the patient with mild symptoms of untreated hypothyroidism. However, there is still the slight risk that the patient will develop myxedema coma. This risk markedly increases in the elderly patient with very severe hypothyroidism, especially during the winter months.

A myxedema coma can be precipitated by infections, surgery, and the use of central nervous system (CNS) depressants. It is extremely important that the dentist be aware that the hypothyroid patient is hypersensitive to drugs. This is a result of the lowered metabolic rate and CNS depression. Extreme care should be exercised when administering analgesics, anesthetics, barbiturates, hypnotics, and tranquilizers. A standard adult dose of morphine or meperidine (Demerol), for example, is contraindicated in the hypothyroid patient since the cardiovascular system and kidneys may be unable to eliminate excess medication, thus causing prolonged CNS depression. It is prudent to seek medical evaluation and treatment before dental treatment. Emergency dental care for oral infections that can precipitate a crisis should be limited to conservative measures.

The dentist should be able to recognize and manage the initial stages of myxedema coma. The condition is characterized by hypothermia, bradycardia, severe hypotension, and epileptic seizures. Approximately 300 μg thyroxine should be administered intravenously and 100 to 200 μg given daily therafter, with monitoring of the plasma thyroid hormone blood levels. Hypothermia is best treated by covering the patient with warm blankets and allowing endogenous body heat to raise the temperature gradually. Artificial respiration is necessary if the patient shows signs of respiratory distress. If there is any suggestion of adrenal steroid insufficiency, 100 to 200 mg hydrocortisone should be given intravenously.

Acute nonsuppurative (subacute) thyroiditis

ORAL MANIFESTATIONS. An upper respiratory infection or a sore throat usually precedes subacute thyroiditis. Patients frequently complain of a sore throat and pain on swallowing. The tenderness is not in the posteior pharynx but is localized to the thyroid area. Examination of the thyroid shows localized tenderness, and often the intense pain makes palpation of the gland impossible. Localized nodules may persist as sequelae of subacute thyroiditis.

DENTAL MANAGEMENT. Initially, patients with subacute thyroiditis have clinical evidence of mild thyrotoxicosis. Hypothyroidism may result from recurrent subacute thyroiditis, but permanent destruction of the gland is extremely rare. Before starting any dental treatment, the dentist should consult the physician regarding patients' thyroid status if they have subacute thyroiditis or have had it in the past. (Refer to the recommendations in the sections on hyperthyroidism and hypothyroidism.)

Chronic thyroiditis
HASHIMOTO'S THYROIDITIS
Oral manifestations. The thyroid gland is usually enlarged, nontender, and extremely firm and indurated.

Dental management. Refer to the section on hypothyroidism, since Hashimoto's thyroiditis is the most common cause of hypothyroidism in the adult.

RIEDEL'S THYROIDITIS
Oral manifestations. The thyroid is stony-hard and is bound firmly to the trachea and to the cervical strap muscles. Pre-

senting symptoms generally include dyspnea, dsyphagia, or hoarseness caused by localized pressure in the neck.

Dental management. Hypothyroidism may occur with Riedel's thyroiditis. See the section on dental management of the hypothyroid patient.

DISORDERS OF ADRENAL GLAND
Hyperadrenocorticism—Cushing's syndrome
Michael Glick

ORAL MANIFESTATIONS. Patients with Cushing's syndrome develop a facial appearance that is plethoric and round (moon face) with a ruddy color that simulates glowing health. Hirsutism and acne are also present. Overall growth and development, including skeletal and dental age, are retarded in long-standing Cushing's syndrome. Osteoporosis, although rare, may occur in the jaws and the gingiva may enlarge.

A recent study reveals that some patients with Cushing's syndrome have altered oral sensation. Thresholds for light touch detection and two-point discrimination on the hands and in the mouth, as well as oral and manual stereognosis, were measured in patients with untreated Cushing's syndrome and in normal volunteers. Results indicate that patients with Cushing's syndrome displayed decreased two-point discrimination on the tongue and palate and decreased oral stereognosis.

DENTAL MANAGEMENT. The dentist should be aware that serious conditions may accompany Cushing's syndrome, including hypertension, heart failure, diabetes mellitus, osteoporosis, impaired healing, and emotional depression or psychosis. Evaluation and dental management of patients with these disorders are included in the appropriate sections of this text.

Hypoadrenocorticism—Addison's disease (primary adrenal insufficiency)
Michael Glick

ORAL MANIFESTATIONS. An early manifestation of Addison's disease is unusual pigmentation of the skin, especially at pressure points and on the oral mucous membranes. This results from stimulation of pituitary melanotrophic activity.

The oral pigmentations appear as irregular spots that may vary in color and intensity, ranging from pale brown to gray or even black. They occur most frequently on the cheek but may be found on the gingiva, palate, tongue, and lips.

Administration of corticosteroids is the usual treatment for Addison's disease and often leads to suppression of the individual's immune response. Consequently, patients receiving steroid therapy are more prone to developing chronic mucocutaneous candidiasis and oral infections that may be difficult to treat with conventional therapy.

Secondary adrenal insufficiency is a condition caused by chronic administration of corticosteroids for a variety of conditions. This results in the suppression of endogenous steroid secretion.

DENTAL MANAGEMENT. Primary and secondary adrenal suppression are managed identically. This involves knowing the dose and duration of medication, along with the proposed dental therapy.

Patients who are taking steroids present two potential problems to the dentist: increased susceptibility to infection and the possibility of adrenal crisis.

Dental patients taking corticosteroids are at increased risk of developing severe dental infection, since corticosteroids alter the host's normal inflammatory response. The chance of infection can be minimized by employing atraumatic and aseptic techniques and by adequate antimicrobial therapy. Some authors recommend that patients take bactericidal broad-spectrum antibiotics on the day of oral surgery and for 5 days thereafter.

Stress induced by infection, trauma, surgery, anesthesia, and the like may lead to adrenal crisis in any patient with primary or secondary adrenal insufficiency. In these patients there is adrenal atrophy with inhibited production of cortisol caused by suppression of the pituitary-adrenal feedback system. Physical or emotional stress increases the metabolic demand for corticoids. Since this demand cannot be met by the adrenal cortex, the dosage of exogenous corticoids may need to be increased.

The risk of adrenal crisis generally increases with the severity and duration of acute stress. Prophylactic supplementation during periods of stress is effective. Adequate prophylaxis is based on ensuring the presence of glucocorticoid in at least the amount that the normal individual would produce in response to similar stress. But which patients need prophylaxis and how much corticosteroid is necessary is open to debate. Even more controversial is the question of how long steroids can be administered before suppressing adrenal activity and, more importantly, impairing stress response.

Currently, protocols for managing adrenal-suppressed patients during dental procedures are based on conservative evaluation of the level of adrenal suppression rather than on the patient's ability to respond to stressful stimuli. Pharmacologic doses of glucocorticosteroids are administered to patients with suspected adrenal insufficiency to avoid episodes of hemodynamic instability and cardiovascular collapse during surgery. However, although physiologic glucocorticosteroid replacement is necessary for surgical stress to be tolerated, there is no hemodynamic advantage to supraphysiologic replacement. The major stressors during surgery are the reversal of and recovery from anesthesia and endotracheal extubation rather than the surgical trauma itself. Over 200 surgical events reviewed in the medical literature, including both major and minor surgery in which patients received the equivalent of 20 to 300 mg per day of hydrocortisone for 6 days up to 20 years, were performed uneventfully without supplemental glucocorticosteroids. This indicates that even when adrenal insufficiency is present, the stress response is not suppressed.

Basically, there are two types of stress that stimulate ACTH secretion: neurogenic stress (caused by stimuli such as skin incisions) that is carried by neuropathways to the hypothalamus and systemic stress (caused by hypertension, hypoglycemia, hypoxia, and exercise) that is transported to the hypothalamus via the circulatory system. The latter does not depend on intact nerve cell transmission. The stress response, which is the ability to cope with the threat of change to the homeostasis or metabolic balance of the body, is determined by mechanisms independent of those that control normal plasma cortisone levels. Although the feedback mechanism can take up to 12 months to recover, the body's disrupted equilibrium usually returns to normal within 30 days. Thus the initial administration of local anesthetics is the only surgical traumatic stimuli present. During general anesthetic surgical procedures, local anesthetics are still used, thus blocking the neuropathways. But systemic stress, caused by general anesthetic procedures, still elicits a stress response.

With this information, newer protocols for managing patients on corticosteroids must be devised. Studies have shown no adrenal suppression with low-dose corticosteroids (30 mg/D of hydrocortisone or its equivalent), even when administered for a month or longer. Therefore no prophylactic supplementation should be necessary before any dental procedure for those patients on low-dose steroids.

Most alternate-day regimens cause minimal suppression and do not require supplementation, particularly if treatment is performed on the day steroids are not taken. Even with short-term daily high-dose corticosteroids, impaired stress response is transitory (returning in 14 to 30 days). Thus supplementation is unnecessary for routine dental care if at least 30 days have passed since cessation of corticosteroid therapy.

Patients on daily high-dose (supraphysiologic) glucocorticoid should be managed as if completely suppressed. Moreover, even after the medication is stopped, recovery of the pituitary-adrenal mechanism may be delayed for up to 12 months (note that maximum output equals 300 mg/day).

All elective treatment, with or without supplementation, should be scheduled in the morning. Long-acting local anesthetic agents should be combined with good postoperative pain management through medication. Sedation can be helpful to allay psychologic factors.

No general increase or supplementation is necessary for short, minor procedures that involve minimal stress, for instance, routine restorations, small biopsies, simple extractions, denture appointments, and prophylaxis. This level of stress approximates that of daily life. These patients should be monitored during the procedure and a postoperative call later that day should be made for follow up. Procedures or extensive anxiety that may cause moderate stress can be managed by increasing the usual dose (up to a maximum 300 mg of hydrocortisone or its equivalent) 1 to 2 hours before treatment. This dose is usually tapered to the patient's daily dose over the next several days. Dental procedures that are likely to be very stressful require higher dosages and their procedures might best be performed in the hospital. In general, an intravenous infusion of 200 mg hydrocortisone and 150 mg cortisone is administered on the day of surgery and gradually tapered over a period of 5 to 7 days to the patient's usual dose.

Despite all precautions an acute adrenal crisis may occur, and the dentist should be able to recognize and initially manage the condition. Symptoms of crisis include hypotension, weakness, nausea, vomiting, headache, and fever. Immediate treatment consists of 100 mg hydrocortisone administered intravenously or intramuscularly. The patient should be transported to a medical facility as soon as possible.

PHEOCHROMOCYTOMA

ORAL MANIFESTATIONS. Patients with pheochromocytoma as a manifestation of those disorders in which multiple endocrine glands hyperfunction or hypofunction may show oral manifestations. In multiple endocrine neoplasia (MEN) type II (Sipple's syndrome), patients may develop pheochromocytoma, medulary thyroid carcinoma, parathyroid hyperplasia, oral signs of hypercalcemia, and particularly, parathyroid hyperplasia. (See section on parathyroids.) Multiple endocrine neoplasia (MEN) Type IIb (mucosal neuroma syndrome) includes a constellation of conditions such as medullary thyroid carcinoma, parathyroid adenoma, pheochromocytoma, mucosal neuromas, and somatic abnormalities. Large, thick, nodular lips and thick, often everted upper eyelids form a distinct facies pathognomonic of this syndrome. Mucosal neuromas, which are microscopically composed of enlarged tortuous nerves, are a valuable clinical marker, since they appear in childhood and generally antedate clinical presentation of the thyroid and adrenal neoplasms. The neuromas produce a characteristic diffuse or nodular involvement of the anterior dorsum of the tongue, the lips, the buccal mucosa adjacent to the oral commissures, and occasionally the palate and mandible. They are asymptomatic and benign but may require surgical correction for aesthetic reasons. The oral and labial neuromas usually appear by 10 years of age. Because mucosal neuromas also may occur in the conjunctiva, the dentist should examine this area as well.

DENTAL MANAGEMENT. The potential risk of sudden hypertensive crisis and related cardiovascular complications makes pretreatment preparation necessary, particularly if extensive surgical treatment is considered. The mainstay of preparation is α-adrenergic blockade, with or without β-blockade, and with plasma volume expansion. One preoperative protocol involves α-adrenergic blocking agents beginning 4 to 10 days before the procedure to expand plasma volume and control hypertension. To increase plasma volume, an albumin-starch expander such as hetastarch (Hespan) is the treatment of choice unless there is severe anemia present. In this case, 1 to 2 units of whole blood are administered. Expanding plasma volume with blood or fluid is preferable to using pressor agents for this purpose.

For outpatient surgery it is important to minimize stress; sedation is beneficial. Other prudent measures include monitoring blood pressure and pulse throughout the procedure and preparing an intravenous line with medications (such as direct-acting vasodilators and α-adrenergic blocking agents) to manage increased blood pressure if necessary.

MINERAL METABOLIC AND METABOLIC BONE DISEASE

Hyperparathyroidism

S. Gary Cohen

ORAL MANIFESTATIONS. The clinical signs and symptoms of hyperparathyroidism (HPTH) primarily reflect the pathophysiology of hypercalcemia. Whitlock summarizes them as "stones, bones, abdominal groans and psychic moans." However, an elevated serum calcium level may also be seen in sarcoidosis, vitamin D intoxication, multiple myeloma, and carcinoma of the lung. The serum calcium level in these diseases is lowered by administering 100 mg hydrocortisone/day (or its equivalent) for 10 days, whereas calcium levels remain unchanged in hyperparathyroidism.

Bone and dental changes are late manifestations of hyperparathyroidism. Dependable radiographic changes only appear after a 30% loss of bony mineral content. In addition to increased serum calcium level, an elevated alkaline phosphatase level reflects the amount of bony alteration. Alkaline phosphatase levels below 13 KA units rarely correlate with radiographic changes, while bony changes are evident with levels greater than 20 KA units.

Generalized osteoporosis with cortical resorption is the most common bone lesion. Dental roentgenographic signs include rarefactions, loss of trabeculation, ground-glass appearance, total or partial loss of lamina dura, lytic lesions, and metastatic calcifications.

The rarefaction is secondary to the generalized osteoporosis. The finer trabeculae disappear later, leaving a coarser pattern. Small lytic lesions may occur that histologically prove to be giant cell tumors. The compact bone of the jaws may thin and eventually disappear. This may be evident as loss of the lower border of the mandible, the cortical margins of the inferior dental canal and floor of the antrum, and lamina dura. Spontaneous fractures may occur with the thinning of these areas of compact bone.

Although the skeleton may undergo decalcification, this does not directly affect fully developed teeth. However, with significant skeletal decalcification the teeth appear more radiopaque.

The loss of lamina dura is neither pathognomonic nor a consistent sign of hyperparathyroidism. A similar loss of lamina dura may also occur in Paget's disease, osteomalacia, fibrous dysplasia, sprue, Cushing's syndrome, and Addison's disease. Various studies indicate lamina dura changes in only 40% to 50% of known hyperparathyroid patients.

The lesions of hyperparathyroidism are called brown tumors because they contain areas of old hemorrhage and clinically appear brown. As the tumor increases in size it may involve the cortex with resultant expansion. The cortex is eventually destroyed. Although the tumor rarely breaks through the periosteum, gingival swelling may result.

The brown tumor lesion contains an abundance of multinucleated giant cells, fibroblasts, and hemosiderin. This histologic appearance is also consistent with central giant cell tumor and giant cell reparative granuloma. Associated bone changes consist of a generalized osteitis fibrosa with patches of osteoclastic resorption on all bone surfaces. This is replaced by a vascular connective tissue that represents an abortive formation of coarse-fibered woven bone. This histologic picture is also present in fibrous dysplasia, giant cell reparative granuloma, osteomalacia, and Paget's disease.

All giant cell and osteoporotic lesions should be further investigated to rule out hyperparathyroidism. This should include a direct parathormone assay.

Other clinical manifestations of hyperparathyroidism include tooth mobility, malocclusion, and metastatic soft tissue calcifications. Cementifying fibromas of the jaws are associated with familial hyperparathyroidism. Increasing mobility and drifting of teeth with no apparent pathologic periodontal pocket formation may be seen. Periapical radiolucencies and root resorption may also be associated with this gradual loosening of the dentition. The teeth may be painful to percussion and mastilation. However, a positive thermal and electric pulp test response will be elicited. Splinting is a useful adjunct to prevent pain and further drifting. The splint should be maintained until treatment of the hyperparathyroidism results in bone remineralization.

Malocclusion may result from the increased mobility and drifting of the dentition. Extreme demineralization and collapse of the temporomandibular and paratemporomandibular bones may also lead to malocclusion.

Metastatic calcifications, while rare, may occur in the oral mucosa and associated paraoral soft tissues including blood vessels. These calcifications are visible roentgenographically.

Since hyperparathyroidism may display a myriad of oral signs and symptoms the dentist is in an important position to recognize and diagnose this condition. Correlation of clinical, laboratory, radiographic, and histologic data is necessary for the definitive diagnosis. Early detection is imperative to circumvent potential irreversible kidney damage.

DENTAL MANAGEMENT. Generally, routine dental treatment involves no modifications unless there are associated medical complications present. In any phase of hyperparathyroidism before complete remineralization the dentist should take care to avoid iatrogenic jaw fractures during surgical procedures.

Following corrective parathyroid surgery all bone lesions tend to regress spontaneously, although rather slowly at times. The skeleton recalcifies and serum calcium levels return to normal. Surgical intervention of existing giant cell lesions is not necessary except to correct gross deformity or to extract displaced or resorbed teeth.

Hypoparathyroidism
S. Gary Cohen

Hypoparathyroidism is a metabolic abnormality characterized by hypocalcemia and consequent neuromuscular symptoms. Muscular and peripheral nerve irritability often increase, causing a clinical picture that can be mistaken for a seizure disorder. These phenomena form the basis for the Chvostek's and Trousseau's signs. In frank tetany, painful muscular spasms occur that may involve oral and laryngeal musculature. Oral and dermatologic findings may precede hypocalcemia. Soft tissue calcifications and ectopic development of true bone may occur, particularly in pseudohypoparathyroidism, as a result of the related hyperphosphatemia. An abnormal response to parathyroid hormone, ectopic calcifications, and other skeletal abnormalities may indicate a number of conditions, such as idiopathic hypoparathyroidism, pseudohypoparathyroidism, pseudopseudohypoparathyroidism, basal ganglion calcification syndrome, basal cell nevus syndrome, Turner's syndrome, and Gardner's syndrome.

Aberrant developmental patterns may occur if hypoparathyroidism occurs during tooth development (particularly ages 6 months to 3 years). Parathyroid hormone influences the eruption rate and affects both matrix formation and calcification. This may present as enamel hypoplasia, with single or parallel horizontal bands and poorly mineralized dentin. Histologic investigations show that dentinal arrest lines appear simultaneously with the onset of clinical signs of hypocalcemia. It may be that the histologic picture of the dentin may act as a permanent, nonerasable record of disturbances in calcium metabolism. Malformed teeth, anodontia, short blunt root apices (particularly molars), elongated pulp chambers (often occluded by pulp stones even in primary teeth), multiple impacted teeth, and mandibular exostoses may be present. Replacement therapy at the appropriate time can prevent many of these developmental problems.

Acute or chronic hypoparathyroidism does not affect erupted dentition. However, the maxilla and mandible may become abnormally dense despite a lowered serum calcium level. The trabeculae increase in number and are unusually well calcified. Surgically induced hypoparathyroidism does not cause oral problems except for occasional vague mouth discomfort that is relieved with normalization of serum calcium.

Idiopathic hypoparathyroidism may occur singly or as part of an autoimmune polyendocrinopathy syndrome that can include any combination of superficial mucocutaneous candidiasis, hypoadrenocorticism, keratoconjunctivitis, intestinal malabsorption, pernicious anemia, diabetes mellitus, thyroiditis, and mental retardation.

Acute and chronic oral candidiasis is the most consistent manifestation of the polyendocrinopathy syndrome. The enamel hypoplasia associated with the polyendocrinopathy syndrome is not solely the result of a lowered serum calcium but may manifest more generalized ectodermal involvement.

Hypoparathyroidism should be included in any differential diagnosis of chronic or unresponsive candidiasis. Clinical and roentgenographic evaluation of dentition (in children) is helpful in diagnosing a polyendocrinopathy syndrome definitively. Early hormonal replacement can prevent the development of the more serious complications of these syndromes.

Frequent oral evaluations are essential in the patient with any form of hypoparathyroidism. Hypoplastic teeth are caries prone; meticulous oral hygiene should be stressed. Periodic roentgenographic evaluations help detect dentigerous cysts that can form at the sites of impacted teeth.

Before dental treatment the patient's serum calcium level should be monitored and should be above 8 mg/100 ml to prevent the possibility of cardiac arrhythmias, generalized convulsions, laryngospasm, or bronchospasm.

Hypophosphatasia

ORAL MANIFESTATIONS. Dental abnormalities are noted only in the juvenile type of hypophosphatasia, of which the first clinical symptom is often premature loss of primary teeth. These teeth show little sign of resorption. The teeth most frequently lost are the primary mandibular central and lateral incisors, followed by the maxillary incisors and, less commonly, the posterior teeth. Additional signs of juvenile hypophosphatasia are loss of anterior alveolar bone, lack of periodontal attachment fibers, and reduced or complete absence of cementum.

Roentgenographic evidence of the disorder consists of enlarged pulp chambers and root canals, sometimes giving the tooth a shell-like appearance; reduced thickness of the dentin and irregular dentin formation with large dentinal tubules and many areas of interglobular dentin; enamel hypoplasia; and irregular calcifications and lesions in the alveolar bone. The histologic features of the jaw bones are similar to those of rickets and osteomalacia.

Dental Management. If the dentist observes these signs, the patient should be referred for medical management. Caution is vital during dental procedures to avoid jaw fractures in hypocalcified areas. The oral manifestations of hypophosphatasia usually resolve with treatment of the disorder.

Familial hypophosphatemic vitamin D-resistant rickets

ORAL MANIFESTATIONS. Characteristic oral findings are often the first clinically noticeable signs of this disorder. These include multiple gingival and periapical abscesses not associated with caries or trauma, resulting from disturbances in calcium and phosphate metabolism during tooth development. Histologically, the dentin is thin and consists of globules of abnormally calcified dentin. Dentinal clefts, tubular defects, or voids in the calcified matrix of dentin occur in the region of the pulp horns. These defects usually extend to the dentin-enamel junction. Small fissures in the surface enamel that are exposed by abrasion, minimal decay, or restorative procedures may extend into the pulp. Through these defects oral microorganisms can enter pulpal tissues, causing the teeth to abscess. Additionally, a reported absence of secondary dentin formation may contribute to the early invasion of the pulp by oral microorganisms.

The histologic appearance of enamel is usually normal. Enamel hypoplasia has been cited, but it does not occur consistently. Both the cementum and periodontal ligament are often absent. Roentgenographic examination usually reveals a thin dentinal layer and unusually large pulp chambers with the pulp horns projecting to the dentin-enamal junction. Other findings include indistinct lamina dura, thinning cortical plates, and lacy trabeculation.

DENTAL MANAGEMENT. Controlling the existing infection and preventing further pulp exposure are the primary goals of treatment. The functional tooth surface can be protected with composite resins or glass ionomer cements. These wear quickly, however, necessitating constant surveillance. Acrylic splints can prevent wear in patients with evidence of bruxism. Prophylactic stainless steel crowns on primary teeth and cast crowns for permanent teeth with minimal tooth reduction also protect teeth. Diet counseling, oral hygiene instruction, and systemic and topical fluorides must be provided regularly to these patients.

Pseudohypophosphatasia

DEFINITION. This is a variation of hypophosphatasia that involves a normal serum alkaline phosphatase level in the presence of an elevated urinary phospoenthanolamine level.

ORAL MANIFESTATIONS. The primary oral symptom is premature loss of the anterior deciduous teeth, which often appear translucent. The other oral manifestations are similar to those of hypophosphatasia.

Osteomalacia

ORAL MANIFESTATIONS. Although there seem to be no radiologic or chemical changes in the teeth of patients with osteomalacia, there are definite roentgenographic changes in the jawbones. There is evidence of generalized demineralization of bone with bony deformities containing excess osteoid and fibrous connective tissue and diminished or absent cortical bone shadows. These changes may affect the alveolar lamina dura, the outlines of the sinuses, the inferior dental canal, and the lower border of the mandible. In cancellous bone the trabeculae are thinner and may be absent on roentgenograms.

Other oral aspects of osteomalacia include loosened teeth and weakened jawbones that are predisposed to fractures.

DENTAL MANAGEMENT. The dentist should observe for signs of tetany caused by low serum calcium levels, such as involuntary twitching of the facial muscles. When performing dental procedures the dentist must be careful to avoid a jaw fracture. The jaw manifestations associated with osteomalacia generally respond to treatment of the underlying deficiency.

Osteoporosis

ORAL MANIFESTATIONS. Alveolar bone is highly susceptible to osteoporosis, particularly in patients who have lost teeth and developed disuse atrophy. In the edentulous patient, especially one without a prosthetic replacement, disuse atrophy results in loss of normal trabeculation, as well as general loss of contour in the alveolar process. The alveolar bone often loses its cortical layer; the residual ridges are sharp and covered with spicules from uneven resorption. In some cases so much alveolar bone is lost that the mandibular and maxillary ridges become flat. This loss of vertical dimension manifests as a decrease in facial height. There is a significant correlation between skeletal osteopenia and residual ridge and alveolar bone density, so any therapeutic measures that affect osteoporosis could effect residual ridge density.

In addition, other local factors may modify bone density. Posttraumatic osteoporosis may occur, resulting from disuse and from interference with the blood supply. Immobilizing bone for long periods invariably leads to osteoporosis. Irradiation of bone, hyperemia of traumatic or inflammatory origin, and neurogenic disturbances, particularly those involving the sympathetic nervous system, may result secondarily in vascular changes that interfere with adequate nutrition to the involved bone, thus causing osteoporosis.

The decreased bone mass, with reduced density and enlarged bone spaces, makes the bone porous and fragile, which increases the risk of mandibular fracture. This may occur spontaneously or during dental treatment.

The roentgenographic changes of osteoporosis consist of increased radiolucency of the bone with fine, indistinct trabeculae and thinning of the cortex. Fatty marrow replaces the bone trabeculae that are resorbed. In senile or postmenopausal osteoporosis, the lamina dura of tooth sockets is thinner but still discernible, whereas in the osteoporosis of Cushing's syndrome the lamina dura may be completely obliterated. In roentgenograms of osteoporotic jaws, teeth are sharply distinct in contrast to the more lucent bone. Osteoporosis of the maxilla is accompanied by an increase in the size of the paranasal sinuses, often with marked thinning of the bone. In dentulous patients this results in the maxillary antrum extending deeply between the roots of the teeth. The canals, in which the branches of the superior dental nerves usually run, are lost and the nerves may lie in the antral lining. In such cases inflammation in the antrum is likely to cause referred pain in the maxillary teeth. The extension of the maxillary antrum weakens the bone and increases the likelihood of tuberosity fracture during extraction of maxillary molars.

DENTAL MANAGEMENT. The relationship between dietary calcium and phosphorus and alveolar bone resorption in edentulous patients is under investigation. Studies comparing diets of subjects who have minimal bone resorption with diets of those who have severe alveolar bone loss indicate a direct cause-and-effect relationship between low calcium intake, calcium phosphorus imbalance, and severe ridge resorption. Another study demonstrates that ingestion of calcium and vitamin D dietary supplements reduces the degree of postextraction alveolar bone resorption by 36%. Investigators administered 750 to 1000 mg calcium and 375 to 4000 units of vitamin D daily to patients with a low calcium or a high phosphorus intake. They concluded that these dietary supplements increase the resistance of the alveolar bone to both mechanical and nutritional biochemical stresses. Sodium fluoride, (25 mg/dl) also is prescribed to increase the strength of the hydroxyapatite crystal matrix of the bone.

The supporting mucosa in osteoporotic individuals who wear dentures may become sensitive to trauma from the denture base material. Therefore bases should be relined with a soft material extending over the entire support area, and the occlusion carefully balanced.

Osteopetrosis

ORAL MANIFESTATIONS. The roentgenographic findings are the most striking. The maxilla and mandible may show a diffuse, symmetric sclerosis, with thickened cortices and medullary cavities that have been replaced by bone to create a "bone-within-bone" appearance. At times, the roots of the teeth cannot be distinguished from the supporting bone. Abnormal development of teeth is characterized by delayed eruption (caused by increased sclerosis of the bone), enamel hypoplasia, malformations of the crowns and roots, narrowing or obliteration of the dental pulp chambers, and increased caries. Increased sclerosis narrows the foramens and may compress the cranial nerves, leading to visual loss, deafness, facial palsies, and neuralgias. Additionally, some patients show limited mandibular opening, secondary to bilateral thickening of the coronoid processes and malar bones.

DENTAL MANAGEMENT. The most frequent problems relate to teeth extraction and to periapical infection. With the abnormal bone density, there is greater risk of root fractures during extraction. Also, because of its avascularity the bone is fragile, increasing the possibility of iatrogenic jaw fractures during extraction. Osteomyelitis is another complication that can result from tooth extraction, usually affecting the mandible. Susceptibility to osteomyelitis is due to both abnormal neutrophil function and to decreased vascularity of the bone.

Management of the osteomyelitis includes conventional antibiotics, sequestrectomy, and hyperbaric oxygen treatments. Use of a vasoconstrictor containing local anesthetic is questionable, since the area is already vascularly compromised. Also, because antibiotics cannot reach necrotic areas easily, they should be given only in the presence of acute infection rather than prophylactically.

Pyknodysostosis

A variation of osteopetrosis is a syndrome known as pyknodysostosis. These patients also have fragile bones and are prone to osteomyelitis. The most distinct characteristic is dwarfism. Facially, patients show hyperplastic rami, obtuse mandibular angle, and micrognathia.

SEX HORMONAL ALTERATIONS
Ovaries

There are four periods of life during which there is an imbalance of female sex hormones. Puberty, menstruation, pregnancy, and menopause bring rapid changes in the sex hormone balance as the body accommodates to developmental and growth changes. These periods of imbalance may show early but definite tissue changes that are manifest in the mucous membranes of the oral cavity. Similar changes may appear in women taking oral contraceptives. These changes do not necessarily result from direct hormonal action on the tissues but are perhaps best explained as the effects of local traumatic factors on tissues conditioned to change by hormonal activity.

PUBERTY

Oral manifestations. During puberty there may be a noticeable rise in the incidence of gingivitis associated with the commencement of sex hormone secretion. The gingivitis may exist before detectable colonization by spirochetes or black-pigmented *Bacteroide* organisms. The hormonal events of puberty do not seem to foster the colonization of those pathogens implicated in adult periodontics.

Clinically during puberty there may be a nodular hyperplastic reaction of the gingiva in areas where food debris, materia alba, plaque, and calculus are deposited. The inflamed tissues are deep red and may be lobulated, with ballooning distortion of the interdental papillae. Bleeding may occur when patients chew food or brush their teeth. Histologically the tissue appearance is consistent with inflammatory hyperplasia.

Dental management. Local preventive care, including a vigorous program of good oral hygiene, is vital. Periodontal therapy also may be necessary in the individual with puberty gingivitis.

MENSTRUATION. Oral changes that may accompany the menses include swollen, erythematous gingival tissues; herpes labialis; aphthous ulcers; prolonged hemorrhage following oral surgery; and swollen salivary glands.

In some women, postoperative hemorrhage occurs more frequently during the menses than at other times. There are no significant hematologic findings accompanying this, other than a slightly reduced platelet count and a small increase in clotting time.

Swelling of the salivary glands, particularly the parotid, occurs occasionally during menses. There is an associated increase in gynecologic complaints, though the cause is unclear.

Recurrent aphthous ulcerations occur in some women in a pattern that seems related to their menstrual cycle. The ulcers appear during the luteal phase of the cycle and heal following menstruation. Oral contraceptives, high doses of estrogens, and synthetic progesterones can help to resolve these lesions.

PREGNANCY

Oral manifestations. The popular notion that pregnancy causes tooth loss ("a tooth for every pregnancy") and that calcium is withdrawn in significant amounts from the maternal dentition to supply fetal requirements has no histologic, chemical, or roentgenographic evidence to support it. On the other hand, calcium is readily mobilized from bone to supply these demands, and demineralization of the alveolar processes can result.

The relationship between dental caries and pregnancy is not well defined. The more comprehensive clinical studies suggest that pregnancy does not contribute directly to the carious process. It is most likely that when an increase in caries activity is noted, it can be attributed to an increase in local cariogenic factors.

Another condition that may influence the pregnant patient's teeth is acid erosion, which may be caused by repeated regurgitation of gastric contents associated with morning sickness or esophageal reflux.

Periodontal disease occurs in 50% to 100% of all pregnant women and is thus the most consistent oral manifestation. Gingival changes occur most frequently in association with poor oral hygiene and local irritants, especially bacterial plaque. However, the hormonal and vascular changes that accompany pregnancy often exaggerate the inflammatory response to these local irritants. The high levels of progesterone, for example, have a direct effect on the microvasculature of the gingiva. Hormonal changes also disturb the nutrition, function, and metabolism of the cells in the supporting tissues of teeth. Gingival changes are most noticeable from the second month of gestation, reaching a maximum in the eighth month. They occur earlier and more frequently in the anterior dental quadrants than in posterior areas.

Clinically, the appearance of inflamed gingiva during pregnancy is characterized by a fiery red color of the marginal gingiva and interdental papillae. The tissue is edematous, with a smooth, shiny surface texture, loss of resiliency, and a tendency to bleed easily. The interdental papillae may hypertrophy and form pseudopockets.

In addition to generalized gingival changes, pregnancy may also cause single, tumorlike growths, usually on the interdental papillae or other areas of frequent irritation. This localized area of gingival hypertrophy is referred to as a "pregnancy tumor," "epulis gravidarum," or "pregnancy granuloma." The last term is preferred since the histologic appearance is similar to the pyogenic granuloma. The reported frequency of pregnancy granuloma varies from none to 5%. The lesion occurs most frequently on the buccal aspect of the maxillary anterior region during the second trimester. It often grows rapidly, although it seldom becomes larger than 2 cm in diameter. Pregnancy granuloma classically starts to develop in an area afflicted by inflammatory gingivitis. Poor oral hygiene invariably is present, and often there are deposits of plaque or calculus on the teeth adjacent to the lesion. The gingiva becomes hyperplastic and enlarges in a nodular fashion to give rise to the clinical mass. The fully developed pregnancy granuloma is a sessile or pedunculated lesion that is usually painless. The color varies from purplish red to deep blue, depending on the vascularity of the lesion and the degree of venous stasis. The surface of the lesion may be ulcerated and covered by a yellowish exudate, and gentle manipulation of the mass easily induces hemorrhage. Bone destruction is rarely observed around pregnancy granulomas.

Most of these lesions regress spontaneously several months after the termination of pregnancy. If chewing causes hemorrhage from the enlarged hyperemic gingival tissue or if ulceration has occurred, the growth should be removed surgically during pregnancy, ideally in the second trimester.

An additional oral finding that may be seen in the pregnant patient is generalized tooth mobility. This change is probably related to the degree of gingival disease and disturbance of the attachment apparatus, as well as to mineral changes in the lamina dura. This condition usually reverses after delivery.

Dental management. Dental evaluation of the pregnant patient, as with all others, begins with a thorough medical history. The history should note any complications the patient has encountered in the pregnancy to date and record any previous miscarriages, recent cramping, spotting, or pernicious vomiting. If at all possible, the next step is to contact the patient's obstetrician or physician to discuss her medical status and dental needs and the proposed treatment plan. The most important objectives in planning dental treatment for the pregnant patient are to establish a healthy oral environment and to obtain optimum oral hygiene levels. These are achieved by means of a good preventive dental program consisting of nutritional counseling and rigorous plaque control measures in the dental office and at home.

The quality of the diet affects caries formation, pregnancy gingivitis, and oral infections. Diet is also important for the developing dentition during fetal gestation because it influences chemical composition, eruption time, malocclusion, and susceptibility to caries.

The pregnant patient should maintain a good plaque control program to minimize the exaggerated inflammatory response of the gingival tissues. The heightened tendency for gingival inflammation should be clearly explained to the patient so that acceptable oral hygiene techniques may be taught, reinforced, and monitored throughout the pregnancy. Scaling, polishing, and root planing may be performed whenever necessary.

Other than good plaque control, no elective dental care should be undertaken during the first trimester or last half of the third trimester. The first trimester is the period of organogenesis, when the fetus is highly susceptible to environmental influences. In the last half of the third trimester there is a hazard of premature delivery because the uterus is very sensitive to external stimuli. Prolonged chair time should be avoided, since supine hypotensive syndrome may occur. In a semireclining or supine position, the great vessels, particularly the inferior vena cava, are compressed by the gravid uterus. By interfering with venous return, this compression will cause hypotension, decreased cardiac output, and eventual loss of consciousness. Supine hypotensive syndrome can usually be reversed by turning the patient on her left side, thereby removing pressure on the vena cava and allowing blood to return from the lower extremities and pelvic area.

The second trimester is the safest period for providing routine dental care. Even so, it is advisable to limit care to minimal treatment such as simple operative procedures. The emphasis is on controlling active disease and eliminating potential problems that could arise in late pregnancy. Extensive reconstruction procedures and major oral or periodontal surgery should be postponed until after delivery. Emergency dental care may be rendered at any time during pregnancy, after consultation with the patient's physician.

One controversial area in the treatment of the pregnant patient involves taking dental roentgenograms. Only serious dental emergencies require roentgenographic evaluation, especially during the first trimester when the developing fetus is particularly susceptible to the effects of radiation. Routine roentgenograms should be avoided and taken only when necessary therapy would otherwise be seriously compromised. The patient must wear a protective lead apron to reduce the amount of radiation emitted to the abdominal area. Excess scatter and secondary radiation can be avoided by periodic inspection of roentgenographic units to ensure proper beam collimation and filtration. High-speed film should be used to minimize exposure.

Another area of controversy involves drug therapy, since any drugs given to the pregnant patient can affect the fetus by diffusion across the placenta. Dentists should be particularly cautious when administering drugs of any kind to the pregnant patient (see Table 1). Most pharmaceutical houses caution against using many of their products during pregnancy because of the lack of well-controlled research on human subjects. In cases of pressing emergency appropriate drug therapy can be instituted, but overprescribing should be avoided. Most of the drugs commonly used in dental practice appear to be relatively safe. Nevertheless, documented consultation with the patient's physician before drug administration is recommended. It is considered safe practice to use local anesthetics with a vasoconstrictor (1:100,000). Analgesics, including acetaminophen and aspirin (excluding the third trimester, when bleeding problems can occur during or after delivery) are also safe. Antibiotics, including penicillin, cephalosporins, and erythromycin, appear relatively safe for both mother and fetus.

There are certain drugs commonly prescribed by dentists that are known to cause complications in pregnancy and are therefore best avoided. These include: diazepam (Valium), chlordiazepoxide (Librium), flurazepam (Dalmane), meprobamate (Miltown), streptomycin, and tetracycline. It is prudent to avoid using nitrous oxide during organogenesis, and general anesthesia or intravenous sedation should be avoided throughout the pregnancy.

The practice of giving a pregnant patient fluoride to prevent

Table 1   Dental drug administration during pregnancy

Drug	1st Trimester	2nd & 3rd Trimester
Local anesthetics		
Lidocaine	Yes	Yes
Mepivacaine	Yes	Yes
Analgesics		
Aspirin	Yes	Yes, but avoid in late third trimester
Acetaminophen	Yes	Yes
Codeine ·	Yes	Yes
Phenacetin	No	No
Antibiotics		
Penicillin	Yes	Yes
Erythromycin	Yes	Yes
Tetracycline	No	No
Streptomycin	No	No
Sedatives/hypnotics		
Nitrous oxide with 50% oxygen	No	Yes
Diazepam	No	No
Barbiturates	No	No

Adapted from Platzker ACD and others: Drug "administration" via breast milk, Hosp Pract **15**:111-117, 1980; and Warheit A: Dental roentgenology in the obstetric patient, Clin Obstet Gynecol **9**:71, 1966.

Table 2 Drug use in breast feeding

Drug	Compatible with breast feeding
Local anesthetics	
Lidocaine	Yes
Mepivacaine	Yes
Analgesics	
Aspirin	Yes, but only in occasional therapeutic doses
Acetaminophen	Yes
Codeine	Yes
Antibiotics	
Penicillin	Yes; however, development of sensitivity should be considered; may affect gastrointestinal flora
Erythromycin	Yes; however, development of sensitivity should be considered; may affect gastrointestinal flora
Tetracycline	No; may cause dental discoloration; may affect gastrointestinal flora
Streptomycin	No; may cause deafness
Cephalosporins	Yes; however, development of sensitivity should be considered; may affect gastrointestinal flora
Sedatives	
Nitrous oxide	Yes
Diazepam	Yes, but only in small, occasional doses
Barbiturates	Yes

Adapted from Platzker ACD and others: Drug "administration" via breast milk, Hosp Prac **15:**111, 1980.

future caries in the child has long been a controversy with inconclusive results. There is insufficient information regarding the efficacy of prenatal fluoride. Generally, researchers agree that fluoride supplements are not necessary for those who live in optimally fluoridated communities. The patient who does not reside in a fluoridated community should be informed of the desirability of giving fluoride to a newborn to offer caries protection to the permanent dentition.

Another perplexing problem for the dentist arises when a nursing mother requires a drug during dental treatment. There is a risk that the drug can enter the breast milk and be transferred to the nursing infant, in whom exposure could have adverse effects. Unfortunately, there is little conclusive information about drug dosage and effects via breast milk; however, retrospective clinical studies and empiric observations coupled with known pharmacologic pathways allow recommendations to be made. Significantly, the amount of drug excreted in breast milk is usually not more than 1% to 2% of the maternal dose; therefore it is highly unlikely that most drugs have any pharmacologic significance for the infant.

A few drugs, or categories of drugs, are definitely contraindicated for nursing mothers. These include lithium, anticancer drugs, radioactive pharmaceuticals, phenindione, chloramphenicol, and isoniazid. Table 2 compiles recommendations regarding administration of commonly used dental drugs during breast feeding. These recommendations are general guidelines only; as with drug use in pregnancy, individual physicians may wish to modify these suggestions.

In addition to choosing drugs carefully, it is desirable for the mother to take the drug just after breast feeding and then to avoid nursing for 4 hours or more if possible. This markedly decreases the drug concentration in breast milk. After nursing, mothers should wipe the child's teeth to prevent the milk from adhering to tooth structures and causing decay.

Interestingly, breast feeding may help straighten children's

teeth because breast-fed babies use different tongue patterns than bottle-fed infants. In bottle feeding the infant's tongue must move forward while swallowing to stop the flow of milk; this forward thrust can easily become a habit. Breast feeding requires infants to use their mouth muscles more vigorously but does not force them to push their tongues forward. Children who have been breast fed for more than 1 year have the least risk of malocclusion.

MENOPAUSE

Oral manifestations. During the menopausal years, women appear to experience an increase in oral symptoms that may result from endocrine disturbances (reduced estrogen), calcium and vitamin deficiencies, and various underlying psychologic factors. They may experience flushing ("hot flashes"), sweating, headaches, and depression. They may also complain of dry mouth because of decreased salivary secretion, as well as burning sensations of the mouth and tongue. Taste sensations may alter, causing a frequent complaint of salty or "metallic" taste.

The gingival mucosa of menopausal women may atrophy, in a manner similar to that of the vaginal mucosa. This gingival condition, termed "desquamative gingivitis," is noted for diminished surface keratinization and epithelial detachment from the subjacent connective tissue corium, followed by bullous lesion formation and epithelial desquamation. The corium is left exposed to the oral environment and undergoes a diffuse inflammatory response characterized by marked redness, shiny edema, increased dryness, burning pain, and hypersensitivity to tactile, chemical, and thermal stimuli.

Postmenopausal osteoporosis manifests in the oral cavity as osteopenia. It results in inadequate amounts of bone in the mandible, loss or mobility of teeth, edentulism, and poorly fitting dentures. It is observable roentgenographically with diminished bone mass in the mandibular angular cortex, loss of lamina dura, and diminished alveolar crest.

Dental management. Postmenopausal osteoporosis can be prevented and treated by sound dietary control with adequate levels (1200 mg/day) of dietary calcium or with calcium supplements, hormonal therapy (estrogen replacement), and exercise programs. The condition is becoming more prevalent because of dietary inadequacies of young women and could become an important issue in dental care for postmenopausal women.

Many of the symptoms and complaints of the menopausal patient, such as abnormal taste sensations, glossodynia, and desquamative gingivitis, respond favorably to estrogen supplement therapy. In addition, counselling may be indicated for some patients, and it is most appropriate for the dentist to refer the menopausal patient for medical evaluation and treatment to optimize the benefits of dental treatment.

ORAL CONTRACEPTIVES. The number of women taking oral contraceptives has reached an estimated 8 to 10 million in the United States and 50 million worldwide. As a result of such widespread use, many systemic and oral side effects have appeared.

Among the undesirable systemic effects associated with the use of oral contraceptives are an increased incidence of thromboembolic events, increased risk of myocardial infarction, and, in certain instances, a significant elevation in blood pressure.

Oral manifestations. One of the most common effects on the oral mucous membranes in those individuals taking oral contraceptives is gingival inflammation. Many such women have an exaggerated gingival inflammatory response to local irritants, characterized by fiery red, enlarged, and hemorrhagic gingival tissues. There are several mechanisms that may contribute to this exaggerated gingival response, including an alteration in microvasculature caused by elevated serum levels of sex hormones. This leads to increased vascular permeability and resultant edema of the perivascular tissue with a significant increase in gingival fluid. Recent investigation has shown that the addition of sex hormones to gingival tissue can cause a significant rise in the synthesis of prostaglandin E_2. Since E-type prostaglandins are potent mediators of inflammation, this may be another mechanism whereby sex hormones increase inflammation. Another factor under consideration is intake disruption of the gingival mast cells, liberating stores of histamine and proteolytic enzymes and thus aggravating the inflammation produced by local irritants.

Women taking oral contraceptives demonstrate a significant increase in the number of *Bacteroides* species in the gingival microflora. Increased female sex hormones substituting for the naphthoquinones required by certain *Bacteroides* species most likely are responsible for this rise. This suggests that estrogens and progesterone can alter the subgingival microflora, thereby further mediating the increase in gingival inflammation observed in these individuals.

Although there appears to be no correlation between the severity of inflammation and the particular type of progesterone or estrogen in the various brands of oral contraceptives, there may be a direct relationship between the severity of inflammation or periodontal destruction and the duration of hormone therapy; this suggests that oral contraceptives may have a cumulative effect in altering host resistance. A roentgenographic change related to oral contraceptives is an increased number of punctate radiopaque areas in the mandible. The opacities are thought to result from thickened endosteal plates of bone, a result of the parathyroid-stimulating effect of the estrogen in oral contraceptives. This effect is one of bone apposition, which could account for a denser and more radiopaque endosteum.

Measurable changes have been observed in the saliva of women taking sex hormones, including a decrease in concentrations of protein, sialic acid, hexosamine, fucose, hydrogen ions and total electrolytes.

Because another side effect of oral contraceptives is spotty melanotic pigmentation of the skin, this suggests a relationship between the use of oral contraceptives and the occurrence of gingival melanosis in fair-skinned individuals.

The dental literature reports that women taking oral contraceptives experience a twofold to threefold increase in the incidence of localized osteitis following extraction of mandibular third molars. The higher incidence of osteitis in these patients may be attributed to the effects of oral contraceptives and estrogens on blood clotting factors. Because a patient's coagulation and fibrinolytic factors are cyclic when taking oral contraceptives, there may be a temporary shift, increasing the fibrinolytic components in relation to clotting factors. If this shift occurs while a patient is recovering from a third molar extraction, the loss of surgical clot may result. Another mechanism to be considered is the presence of tissue activators after teeth are removed, which may cause high fibrinolytic activity and consequent lysis of clots.

Dental management. The dentist should be aware of the systemic and oral side effects of oral contraceptives. A comprehensive medical history and assessment of vital signs, particularly blood pressure, are extremely important in this group of patients. Treatment of gingival inflammation exaggerated by oral contraceptives includes establishing an oral hygiene

program and eliminating all local predisposing factors. Periodontal surgery may be indicated if there is inadequate resolution after initial therapy (scaling, root planing, and curettage).

It is recommended that any teeth extractions (especially of third molars) be performed on nonestrogenic days (days 23 to 28) of the pill cycle, to reduce the risk of a postoperative localized osteitis.

The dentist must also consider possible antibiotic-oral contraceptive interactions which could decrease contraceptive efficacy. Certain antibiotics—including penicillins, tetracyclines, sulfonamides, and rifampin—interact with the contraceptive steroids indirectly by suppressing the intestinal flora, thus diminishing the availability of hydrolytic enzymes to regenerate the parent steroid molecule. Consequently, plasma concentrations of the contraceptive steroids are abnormally low and the steroid clears more rapidly from the body than under normal circumstances. Although such interactions occur in only a small percentage of patients taking both drugs concurrently, there is at present no method for determining those individuals at greatest risk.

Other drugs known to reduce the effectiveness of oral contraceptives include barbiturates, phenylbutazone, and phenytoin sodium. When prescribing a drug that can decrease oral contraceptive efficacy, the dentist should advise the patient to use an additional method of contraception during the period of concurrent drug use.

THE ABNORMAL OVARY

Turner's syndrome (45, X females). When comparing patients with Turner's syndrome to normal adult women, significant differences in craniofacial size and morphology are evident. The calvarium maxilla, and mandible are smaller in Turner's syndrome patients and the cranial base is shorter and flattened. The maxilla and the mandible are retrognathic and posteriorly inclined in relation to the cranial base, with greater sagittal jaw relationship and overjet. Total or partial loss of an X chromosome, as seen in Turner's syndrome, seems to influence both the size and shape of specific craniofacial structures. Much of the alteration in facial prognathism can be explained by size and shape differences of the cranial base rather than by differences in jaw position.

Recent studies indicate that 45,X women have a lower incidence of caries than do normal women. The difference is more pronounced in the incisor region than in premolar and molar teeth. This indicates that the basic chromosomal disorder alters caries susceptibility, but at this time the factors that are responsible remain unknown.

Testes

Gingival changes in pubertal males have been reported in association with increased secretion of both adrenal and testicular androgens. This may cause a diffuse gingival inflammatory lesion, which is exacerbated by local irritation.

There have been several reported cases of primary tumors of the testes metastizing to the oral cavity. Metastatic lesions have appeared on the alveolar ridge, gingivobuccal sulci, alveolar mucosa, palate, and gingiva. In some instances the histologic appearance of the metastatic lesion is quite different from that of the primary testicular tumor.

KLINEFELTER'S SYNDROME (47, XXY). Patients with Klinefelter's syndrome have a slender face and marked malocclusion. Mandibular prognathism, a flat palate, and maxillary hypoplasia are common as well. A cleft palate may occur in the individual with a 47,XXY karyotype. The permanent teeth tend to be larger than normal in males with this syndrome, indicating that the presence of an extra X chromosome has a growth-promoting effect that begins at an early age.

TESTICULAR FEMINIZATION SYNDROME. Although 46, XY females have a generally female phenotype, their teeth resemble those of a normal male. The large teeth in 46, XY females may result from modified endocrine function, or perhaps there is a gene (or genes) on the Y chromosome that increases teeth size.

BIBLIOGRAPHY

Ackerman GL and Nolan CM: Adrenocortical responsiveness after alternate-day corticosteroid therapy, N Eng J Med 278(8):405, Feb 1968.

Albert TW and Howerton DW: Pheochromocytoma: case report and review of diagnosis and treatment, J Oral Maxillofac Surg 44:657, 1986.

Baab DA and others: Laboratory studies of a family manifesting premature exfoliation of deciduous teeth, J Clin Periodontal 13:677, 1986.

Bahn SL: Glucocorticosteroids in dentistry, J Am Dent Assoc 105:476, Sept 1982.

Bainton R: Interaction between antibiotic therapy and contraceptive medication, Oral Surg 61(5):453, 1986.

Barnett ML: Inhibition of oral contraceptive effectiveness by concurrent antibiotic administration, J Periodontal 56(1):18, 1985.

Bedi R, Brook AH: Changes in general, craniofacial and dental development in juvenile hypothyroidism, Br Dent J 157:58, 1984.

Bercovici B, Gron S, and Pisanty S: Vaginal and oral cytology of the menopause, Acta Cytol 29(5):805, 1985.

Boue DC and others: Turner's syndrome: controlling facial growth. Report of a case, J Int Asso Dent Child 14:21, 1983.

Brenna MD and others: Multidisciplinary management of acromegaly and its deformities, JAMA 253(5):682, 1985.

Chiodo GT and Rosenstein DI: Dental treatment during pregnancy: a preventive approach, J Am Dent Assoc 110(3):365, 1985.

Crosher R: Advanced dental development in cerebral gigantism, Br Dent J 161:374, 1986.

Dahllof G and others: Enamel disturbances in congenital hypopituitarism: report of a case, J Dent Child 50:451, 1983.

Danowski TS and others: Probabilities of pituitary-adrenal responsiveness after steroid therapy, Ann Intern Med 61(1):11, 1964.

Davies R and Saha S: Osteoporosis, Am Fam Physician 32:107, 1985.

DeBoom GW, Jensen JL, and Correll RW: Diffuse, increased radiodensity of the maxilla and mandible, J Am Dent Assoc 110(3):381, 1985.

Estep HL and others: Pituitary-adrenal dynamics during surgical stress, J Clin Endocrinol Metab 23:419, 1963.

Ferguson MM, Carter J, and Boyle P: An epidemiological study of factors associated with recurrent aphthae in women, J Oral Med 39(4):212, 1984.

Fung DE: Hypophatasia, Br Dent J 154:49, 1983.

Gier RE and Janes DR: Dental management of the pregnant patient, Dent Clin N Am 27(2):419, 1983.

Glenn FB, Flenn WD III, and Duncan RC: Prenatal fluoride tablet supplementation and improved molar occlusal morphology: part V, J Dent Child 51:19, Jan-Feb 1984.

Glenn FB, Glenn WD III, Duncan RC: Prenatal fluoride table supplementation and the fluoride content of teeth: part VII, J Dent Child 51:344, Sept-Oct 1984.

Glick M: Glucocorticosteroid replacement therapy: literature review and suggested replacement therapy, Oral Surg 67:614, 1989.

Graber AL and others: Natural history of pituitary-adrenal recovery following long-term suppression with corticosteroids, J Clin Endocrinol Metab 25:11, 1965.

Gupta DS, Gupta MK, and Borle RM: Osteomyelitis of the mandible in marble bone disease, Int J Oral Maxillofac Surg 15:201, 1986.

Heaton BW and McClendon JL: Childhood pseudohypophosphatasia: clinical and laboratory study of two cases, Texas Dent J 103:4, 1986.

Herbert FL: Hereditary hypophosphatemia rickets: an important awareness for dentists, J Dent Child 53:223, 1986.

Herrmann HJ II and Myall WT: Observations on the significance of the thyroid gland to the dentist, Spec Care Dent 3(1):13, 1983.

Huseman CA and others: Sexual precocity in association with septo-optic dysplasia and hypothalamic hypopituitarism, J Pediatr, 92(5):748, 1984.

Jensen BL: Craniofacial morphology in Turner syndrome, J Craniofac Genet Dev Biol 5:327-340, 1985.

Kata J, Benumof J, and Kadis LB: Anesthesia and uncommon diseases. Pathophysiologic and Clinical Correlations, ed 2, Philadelphia, WB Saunders Co, 1981.

Kinirons MJ and Glasgow JFT: The chronology of dentinal defects related to medical findings in hypoparathyroidism, J Dent 13(4):346, 1985.

Kleinmann RE and others: Anterior neck abscess masquerading as acute suppurative thyroiditis, J Nucl Med 20(10):1051, 1979.

Klinefelter H, Winkenwerder WL, and Bledsoe T: Single daily dose prednisone therapy, JAMA 241(25):2721, 1979.

Kribbs PJ, Smith DE, and Chestnut CH III: Oral findings in osteoporosis. Part II; relationship between residual ridge and alveolar bone resorption and generalized skeletal osteopenia, J Prosthet Dent 50(5):719, 1983.

Lamey PJ, Carmichael F, and Scully C: Oral pigmentation, Addison's disease and the results of screening for adrenocortical insufficiency, Br Dent J 158:297, 1985.

Littner MM and others: Management of the pregnant patient, Quintessence Int 2(2):253, 1984.

Mahfouz SA and Sherif HAH: A study of the lysosomal activity of human gingivae during pregnancy, Egyptian Dent J 31(1):83, 1985.

Meurman JH and Hakala PE: Cranial manifestations of hypophosphatasia in childhood nephrotic syndrome, Int J Oral Maxillofac Surg 13:249, 1984.

Miller D and Robblee JA: Perioperative management of a patient with a malignant pheochromocytoma, Can Anaesth Soc J 32:278, 1985.

Morris HG and Jorgensen JR: Recovery of endogenous pituitary-adrenal function in corticosteroid-treated children, J Pediatr 79(3):480, 1971.

National Health and Medical Research Council Statement: Guidelines for dental treatment; dentistry and pregnancy, Aust Dent J, 29(4):265, 1984.

Noren JB and Alm J: Congenital hypothyroidism and changes in the enamel of deciduous teeth, Acta Paediatr Scand 72:485, 1985.

Osborn R and others: Osteomyelitis of the mandible in a patient with malignant osteopetrosis, J Oral Med 40(2):76, 1985.

Ozkan S, Ucok Z, and Alagol F: Dental manifestations of familial hypophosphatemic vitamin D-resistant rickets: report of case, J Dent Child 51:448, 1984.

Pangrazio-Kulbersh V: Hypothyroidism in orthodontic practice. Case report, JCO XVII(11):771, 1983.

Peake RL: Thyroiditis, Postgrad Med 57(7):95, 1975.

Renner RP, Boucher LJ, and Kaufman HW: Osteoporosis in postmenopausal women, J Prosthet Dent 52(4):581, 1984.

Rothwell BR, Gregory CEB, and Sheller B: The pregnant patient: considerations in dental care, Spec Care Dent 7:124, 1987.

Sadeghi-Nejad A and Senior B: Autosomal dominant transmission of isolated growth hormone deficiency in iris-dental dysplasia (Rieger's syndrome), J Pediatr 85(5):644, 1977.

Seow WK: X-Linked hypophosphatemic vitamin D-resistant rickets, Aust Dent J 29(6):371, 1984.

Shapiro S and others: Postmenopausal osteoporosis: dental patients at risk, Gerodontics 1:220, 1985.

Sones AD, Wolinsky LE, Kratochvil FJ: Osteoporosis and mandibular bone resorption: a prosthodontic perspective, J Prost Dent. 56:732, 1986.

Svoboda, P.J., Mendieta, C., Reeve, C.M., "Albers-Schonberg Disease Complicated With Periodontal Disease" J Periodontal 54(10):592, 1983.

Takala I and others: Caries prevalence in Turner's syndrome (45, X females), J Dent Res 64(2):126, 1985.

Townsend GC and Alvesalo L: The size of permanent teeth in Klinefelter (47,xxy) syndrome in man, Arch Oral Biol 30(1):83, 1984.

Vittek J and others: Salivary concentrations of steroid hormones in males and in cycling and postmenopausal females with and without periodontitis, J Periodont Res 19:545, 1984.

Volpe R, Row VV, and Ezrin C: Circulating viral and thyroid antibodies in subacute thyroiditis, J Clin Endocrinol Metab 27:1275, 1967.

Warnakulasuriya S, Markwell BD, and Williams DM: Familial hyperparathyroidism associated with cementifying fibromas of the jaws in two siblings, Oral Surg 59(3):269, 1985.

Wiesenfeld D and others: Salivary gland dysfunction following radioactive iodine therapy, Oral Pathol 55(2) 1:38, 1983.

Winstock D and Warnakulasuriya S: Partial glossectomy for macroglossia in an elderly acromegalic. A case report, Int J Oral Maxillofac Surg 15:629, 1986.

Winter WE and others: Solitary central maxillary incisor associated with precocious puberty and hypothalamic hamartoma, J Pediatr 101(6):965, 1982.

Yanover L and Ellen RP: A clinical and microbiologic examination of gingival disease in parapubescent females, J Periodontol 57(9):562, 1986.

Zachariades N and Koundouris I: Maxillofacial symptoms in two patients with pyknodysostosis, J Oral Maxillofac Surg 42:819, 1984.

Zachariades N and others: Osteopetrosis: report of a case with maxillary and mandibular involvement, J Oral 112:97, 1987.

Zuppinger KA and others: Cleft lip and chorioideal coloboma associated with multiple hypothalamo-pituitary dysfunctions, J Clin Endocrinol Metab 33:934, 1971.

GENETICS AND METABOLISM

Edited by **Doris G. Bartuska**

194·HUMAN GENETICS

Kathleen Toomey

BASIC PRINCIPLES
Gene concept and single gene inheritance

The human genome is contained in the cellular component deoxyribonucleic acid (DNA), which is located within the nucleus of each cell, and in the as yet ill-defined "extranuclear" elements of inheritance. The DNA molecule is composed of two chains, with a repeating backbone of sugar-phosphate groups coiled and bound by the affinity of complementary attached base pairs (adenine-thymine and guanine-cytosine), the order of which determines the sequence of amino acids ultimately produced from any given segment of the molecule (Fig. 194-1). Each sequence of three base pairs, a codon, is capable of being transcribed into a complementary strand of messenger ribonucleic acid (mRNA), a molecule differing from DNA in sugar composition (ribose instead of deoxyribose) and in the substitution of uracil for thymine as a complement to adenine. The 20 amino acids are coded for by one or more of the 64 triplet possibilities, and so-called genetic code (Table 194-1). The mRNA transcription of the DNA code attaches to a ribosome located in the cytoplasm, where transfer RNA–amino acid complexes are assembled in line, peptide bonds are formed between amino acids, and a protein molecule is produced—the translation process (Fig. 194-2). The beginning and ending triplet codons are specialized messages of initiation and termination of the translation process. The protein products are enzymes, structural proteins, or regulator proteins. The entire process is undoubtedly under control mechanisms, many of which have yet to be elucidated. Certainly, one method of control is "feedback inhibition," in which the accumulation of the product itself turns off the process through interaction of the product with the gene itself or with some intermediary compounds.

Errors in the genetic code take the form of alterations in base composition. These may be point mutations in which a single base is changed or deletions of one or more bases from the sequence. As can be seen from Table 194-1, there are potential mutations that will not alter the ultimate product. In general these involve the third member of the triplet; for example, glycine is coded for by DNA sequences CCA, CCG, CCT, or CCC. Arginine and leucine allow more room for error because they are coded for by six possible codons each, whereas the codes for methionine and tryptophan leave no room for error, having one specific codon each.

Depending on the position of the error, the new product may be clinically indistinguishable from the normal product and may or may not be ascertained biochemically. These are usually

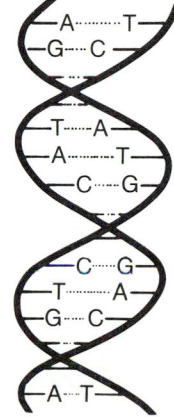

Fig. 194-1   Schematic representation of DNA molecule. Sugar (deoxyribose)-phosphate backbones in double helical configuration with *purines*, adrenine, *A*, and guanine, *G*, attached by hydrogen bonds to *pyrimidines*, thymine, *T*, and cytosine, *C*, respectively. RNA molecule differs in sugar composition (ribose for deoxyribose) and one pyrimidine (uracil for thymine).

termed normal protein polymorphisms. A mutation may significantly alter the status of the protein product, making it less efficient or totally nonfunctional. Such changes are at the root of many of the inborn errors of metabolism or disorders involving a generalized alteration in a structural protein. Finally, a mutation may alter both the functional properties and the antigenicity of the product.

Errors in the genetic code also occur in the form of deletions of base pairs. Such errors result either in a "frameshift" of the code, if one or two bases are deleted, or in the deletion of an amino acid, if the deletion involves an entire triplet codon.

The human hemoglobins are replete with examples of each of these types of errors. Point mutations account for hemoglobins S, C, and E; frameshifts for hemoglobins Tak, Wayne, and Cranston; and triplet deletions for hemoglobins Freiburg, Tochigi, Leiden, Lyon, and Tours. Elongation of the hemoglobin chain because of an error in the termination sequence accounts for hemoglobin Constant Spring and others.

MENDEL'S LAWS AND THE MEIOTIC PROCESS. During interphase the human genome is dispersed throughout the nucleus. During mitosis and meiosis the genome becomes recognizable as 22 distinct and identifiable chromosome pairs called autosomes and two sex chromosomes—XX in females and XY in males. These 46 chromosomes each contain hundreds or thousands of gene loci. The corresponding genes on two homologous (like) chromosomes are called alleles. If the two alleles are identical, the individual is said to be homo-

Table 194-1   The genetic code

Amino acid	DNA triplet codons
Alanine	CGA, CGG, CGT, CGC
Arginine	GCA, GCG, GCT, GCC, TCT, TCC
Asparagine	TTA, TTG
Aspartic acid	CTA, CTG
Cysteine	ACA, ACG
Glutamic acid	CTT, CTC
Glutamine	CTT, GTC
Glycine	CCA, CCG, CCT, CCC
Histidine	GTA, GTG
Isoleucine	TAA, TAG, TAT
Leucine	AAT, AAC, GAA, GAG, GAT, GAC
Lysine	TTT, TTC
Methionine	TAC
Phenylalanine	AAA, AAG
Proline	GGA, GGG, GGT, GGC
Serine	AGA, AGG, AGT, AGC, TCA, TCG
Threonine	TGA, TGT, TGC, TGG
Tryptophan	ACC
Tyrosine	ATA, ATG
Valine	CAA, CAG, CAT, CAC
Chain end	ATT, ATC, ACT

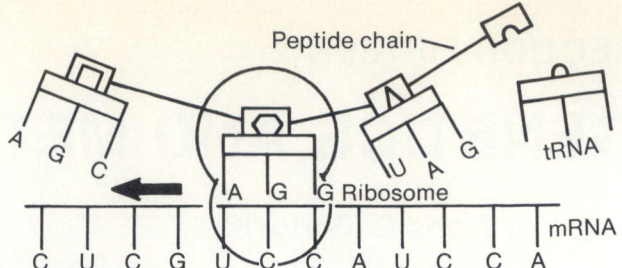

Fig. 194-2   Protein synthesis: mRNA chain is attached to ribosome in cytoplasm where amino acid–tRNA complexes are assembled as corresponding triplet is positioned at assembly sites. Peptide bond is formed between amino acids, tRNA separates from chain of amino acids, and protein molecule is released into cytoplasm, *A*, adenine; *G*, guanine; *C*, cryosine; *U*, uracil.

Table 194-2   Mating possibilities: autosomal dominant (A) and recessive (a) allelic pairs

Mating type	Parental genotypes	Gametes	Genotypes of offspring
1	AA × AA	All A × all A	All AA
2	AA × Aa	All A × 1a:1a	1AA:1Aa
3	AA × aa	All A × all a	All Aa
4	Aa × Aa	1A:1a × 1A:1a	1AA:2Aa:1aa
5	Aa × aa	1A:1a × all a	1Aa:1aa
6	aa × aa	All a × all a	All aa

zygous at that locus; if they are not alike, they are termed heterozygous alleles. Chromosomal behavior during meiosis explains the observations of Mendel that resulted in his laws of segregation and independent assortment. Further knowledge of chromosomal structure and behavior also explains apparent exceptions to these laws.

Each gamete contributes a haploid (n = 23) set of chromosomes to the zygote. This reduction of the chromosome number from the somatic diploid (2n) number of 46 is achieved by the process of meiosis. The meiotic process is preceded by a replication of the entire genome. Each chromosome is composed of two chromatids (sister chromatids), which in turn are each a single DNA, double helical structure. During the early stages of meiosis the DNA-protein threads condense, become visible, and align themselves into pairs of homologous chromosomes. This "synaptonemal complex" is thus composed of four chromatids (two homologous pairs of sister chromatids). They further condense, and exchanges of segments of DNA between homologous but *nonsister* chromatids take place. This is called chiasma formation. This process allows for crossing-over DNA segments and further variation in the inheritance of combinations of genetic traits. By the end of the first meiotic division the paired chromosomes are aligned along the metaphase plate, chiasmata have disappeared, and one member of each pair of homologous chromosomes segregates randomly into one or the other of two daughter nuclei. The second meiotic division is a further division of each segregated chromosome without further replication of DNA. Thus each of four daughter nuclei receives a haploid set of chromosomes that have twice segregated at random into daughter nuclei. This process explains Mendel's law of segregation; that is, a parent transmits one and only one allele for a given trait via the germ cell of the offspring.

Mendel's law of independent assortment relies on the genes for traits studied being discontinuous and located on different chromosomes or very far apart on the same chromosome. Thus, when following the transmission of two or more such traits, the offspring manifest combinations of traits in predictable ratios based on random segregation of chromosomes. The obvious exception to this law involves two traits, the loci for which are located close together on the same chromosome and are said to be "linked." The genes at such loci do not assort

independently as predicted but at some other ratio that is nonetheless predictable on the basis of their distance apart on the chromosome (map unit distance). The closer two loci are, the more often they can be predicted to segregate together, and the farther apart they are, the more often they will be separated during the process of crossing-over. The assortment ratios of linked loci will not reach the randomness observed between unlinked genes.

AUTOSOMAL DOMINANT INHERITANCE. The genotype of an individual is the composition of alleles at a given locus. One may or may not be able to ascertain this directly in the laboratory. In the case of hemoglobin it is possible to separate the products of each allele during hemoglobin electrophoresis and to know the genotype. If such precise determination cannot be made, other manifestations of gene expression are used. An individual's phenotype may be ascertained by enzyme activity, physical appearance, or a measure of some other biologic function. If an individual is heterozygous at a given locus, that trait manifesting itself phenotypically is said to be the dominant trait. The alternative allele is termed recessive. Only one allele for a dominant trait need be present for an individual to manifest that phenotype. For many dominant traits one cannot tell by examining the individual's phenotype whether they are homozygous or heterozygous at the locus.

For matings involving a given dominant trait, A, in one or both parents, five possibilities exist (mating types 1 to 5, Table 194-2). If dominant trait A is extremely common, most matings will be of genotypes 1 and 2. If, however, A is rare, most will be of type 5. If for some reason dominant trait A, although rare, results in a phenotype that causes mates to be attracted to each other, matings of types 1, 2, or 4 may be most frequent.

Autosomal dominant inheritance (the gene is located on 1 of the 22 autosomal pairs) is characterized by two additional features: males and females express the trait equally, and male-to-male transmission may be observed.

AUTOSOMAL RECESSIVE INHERITANCE. A recessive allele for a given characteristic segregates in the same manner as does a dominant allele. For a recessive allele to manifest itself fully, however, an individual is nearly always homozygous for the allele. Whereas physical examination may not reveal the heterozygous state of a recessive allele, some measure of biochemical activity may uncover a difference between either of the homozygous states (AA or aa) and the heterozygote, Aa, which is *phenotypically* indistinguishable from AA.*

Most abnormal recessive genes are rare in the population, although all persons carry a certain number of them. Although estimates vary, it is believed that all humans carry one or two recessive alleles (in the heterozygous state) for traits that are lethal in the homozygous state. It is also thought that humans may carry another five or six that, when present in the double dose, are in some way deleterious to our well-being or reduce the "perfect functioning" of some body pair or system. Although not much is known about this phenomenon, it appears that genes that manifest as abnormal in the homozygous state (abnormal recessive genes) are genetic messages for enzymes or subunits of enzymes and that the *normal* message for an enzyme is most often the dominant allele. On the other hand, *abnormal* dominant alleles appear to involve structural proteins, which may account for the greater likelihood of an abnormal dominant gene being manifest in the heterozygous state as opposed to requiring laboratory aids. (There are, of course, exceptions to these generalizations.)

Matings involving the presence of a recessive allele, a, in one or both parents are shown in Table 194-2, matings 2 to 6. If the recessive allele is common, most matings will be of type 4, 5, or 6. If the recessive allele is lethal in the homozygous state, there will be virtually no matings of types 3, 5, and 6, and few (depending on the frequency of the gene in the population) of type 4; most matings involving a rare recessive gene will be of type 2.

PSEUDODOMINANCE. The inheritance of recessive gene (a) may be difficult to distinguish from dominant inheritance when it appears in both parent and child, as in matings 5 and 6. In the case of rare recessive genes, this may occur when a homozygous recessive individual mates with a relative who is a carrier of the same gene—mating 5. The resultant transmission from parent to child in this case is called pseudodominance.

HARDY-WEINBERG LAW. If the population incidence of the homozygous state for a recessive trait or disease is known, the frequency of carriers (heterozygotes) can be determined by applying the Hardy-Weinberg law. For any two alleles at a given locus, the frequency of genotypes AA, Aa, and aa will be equal to p^2, $2pq$, and q^2, respectively, where $p^2 + 2pq + q^2 = 1$, p equals the frequency of A and q equals the frequency of a in that population, and $p + q = 1$.

X-LINKED INHERITANCE. Just as the autosomes segregate randomly into daughter nuclei, so do the sex chromosomes. However, unlike gene pairs located on autosomes, genes located on the X chromosome have two alleles in the 46,XX female and only one in the 46,XY male. Identical loci on the X and Y chromosomes are not thought to exist. The male is said to be hemizygous for the locus, whereas a female may be homozygous or heterozygous. Because there is only one set of

X chromosome loci in the male, his phenotype behaves as though he were homozygous for the alleles present on his X chromosome. Unlike autosomal inheritance, there is sex distribution difference among the phenotypes for a given trait. Mating possibilities for dominant (B) and recessive (b) X-linked genes are given in Table 194-3.

It can be seen that, if the *recessive* allele is lethal, there will be no matings of types 3, 4, 5, and 6, since females who are homozygous will be eliminated (3 and 6), as well as hemizygous males (4, 5, and 6). Heterozygous females, however, will in general be phenotypically normal, and matings of types 1 and 2 will be most common.

On the other hand, if the *dominant* allele is lethal, the only mating that may occur is type 6.

If the X-linked trait in question is dominant but lethal only in the hemizygous X^BY or homozygous X^BX^B state, mating of types 1 to 4 will not occur and only matings of 5 and 6 will be seen. The heterozygous female for such a gene may or may not be phenotypically detectable.

LYON HYPOTHESIS. At about 16 days of gestational age in female embryos, a process known as random inactivation of the X chromosome occurs. On the average the X of maternal origin is inactivated in 50% of the cells.* This inactivated X chromosome can be detected in the interphase nucleus as a clump of darkly staining chromatin known as a Barr body. In most circumstances all but one X chromosome in a given cell are inactivated, and the total number of X chromosomes equals one plus the number of Barr bodies. Once either the maternal or paternal X chromosome is inactivated in a given nucleus, all daughter cells derived from that cell will have the same X chromosome inactivated. Since inactivation is a random process, the actual distribution of inactivated maternal and paternal X chromosomes fits a standard distribution curve so that there will be a few females at either end of the curve in whom a greater percentage of one or the other X chromosomes remain active. This is one explanation for a few heterozygous females manifesting an X-linked recessive trait. Two other explanations for such a manifestation are homozygosity at the locus, such as may result from matings 4 or 6, and the presence of only one X chromosome in females with karyotypes 45,XO, who would behave at that locus as hemizygous males.

The key difference between X-linked inheritance and autosomal inheritance is the failure of father-to-son transmission in the case of X-linked traits. It may appear to have been transmitted from father to son if the mother is heterozygous at the locus for which the father is hemizygous, and the mother is phenotypicaly normal, whereas the father is not.

Y-LINKED (HOLANDRIC) INHERITANCE. There are undoubtedly genes on the Y chromosome that could be transmitted from father to son. Investigation into the presence of the HY antigen and a testis determining factor (Tdf) is currently under way. The role of this or other male determining genes in sexual differentiation is not fully understood.

VARIABLE EXPRESSIVITY, INCOMPLETE PENETRANCE, AND AGE OF EXPRESSION. It must be remembered that the ability to detect the presence of a given gene depends on the availability of specific biochemical assays and the knowledge of the total spectrum of the gene's expression. The term "variable expressivity" refers to the phenomenon whereby a presumably identical gene possessed by two individuals is accompanied by apparently different manifestations. This is common

---

*One can argue with the application of the word "phenotype." In general it has come to mean the physical and mental status of an individual determined by the usual means of examination and some laboratory aids. As more sophisticated means of examination become readily available, the definition of the word may change.

---

*There is now evidence that a small portion of both X chromosomes is never inactivated.

Table 194-3   Mating possibilities: X-linked dominant (B) and recessive (b) allelic pairs

Mating type	Parental genotypes		Gametes		Genotypes of offspring	
	m	f	m	f	m	f
1	X^BY	$\times$ X^BX^B	$1X^B:1Y$	$\times$ all X^B	All X^BY	All X^BX^B
2	X^BY	$\times$ X^BX^b	$1X^B:1Y$	$\times$ $1X^B:1X^b$	$1X^BY:1X^bY$	$1X^BX^B:1X^BX^b$
3	X^BY	$\times$ X^bX^b	$1X^B:1Y$	$\times$ all X^b	All X^BY	All X^BX^b
4	X^bY	$\times$ X^BX^B	$1X^b:1Y$	$\times$ all X^B	All X^BY	All X^BX^b
5	X^bY	$\times$ X^BX^b	$1X^b:1Y$	$\times$ $1X^B:1X^b$	$1X^BY:1X^bY$	$1X^BX^b:1X^bX^b$
6	X^bY	$\times$ X^bX^b	$1X^b:1Y$	$\times$ all X^b	All X^bY	All X^bX^b

among autosomal dominant genes. A grandparent and grandchild may clearly possess a certain dominant gene, yet the intervening parent (who must have transmitted the gene from parent to child) may show only some features of the trait or genetic disorder. If evidence for the gene's expression in such an individual is totally undetectable, or if this obligate person has not reached or did not live until the *age of expression* for the trait, the gene is said to demonstrate *incomplete penetrance*. As more is learned about genetic diseases and traits, previous cases of incomplete penetrance may be reclassified as new variation in expressivity.

MULTIPLE ALLELES. Thus far only two alternative alleles at any given locus have been considered. On occasion a locus has multiple alleles. In this case the number of genotypes and phenotypes depends on the number of different alleles and their respective dominance or recessivity. An example of this is the locus for the ABO blood group in human beings for which there are three possible alleles, which of course are present only two at a time.

CODOMINANCE. Codominance refers to the equal expression of two alleles at a given locus, whether they are present in the homozygous or heterozygous state. In some cases this depends on the method of observation. The MN blood groups are the classic examples of codominance. When parents of types M and N are mated, their children may be M, N, or MN when studied immunologically. Electrophoretically, hemoglobins A and S (sickle cell hemoglobin) are codominant. Phenotypically, A is dominant and S recessive, since the homozygous SS genotype is required for a person to have sickle cell anemia. On the other hand, in the laboratory the S gene may be made to express itself in the heterozygous (AS) individual's blood cells (sickle cell trait). Under such conditions S acts as the dominant allele. The conditions under which observations were made must always be considered when investigating the mode of inheritance of a given characteristic.

Chromosome structure and abnormalities

STRUCTURE AND NOMENCLATURE. The human chromosome complement is discussed and described as the chromosomes appear during or close to the metaphase portion of the mitotic process. It is at this time that the 22 autosomal pairs and two sex chromosomes are condensed and consist of two chromatids joined together at a dense constriction known as the centromere (Fig. 194-3). Each chromosome consists of a short arm (p) and long arm (q). By convention (Paris Conference, 1971) they are oriented with the short arm above the long arm below the centromere, from largest to smallest, and are grouped according to the relative lengths of the long and short arms.

Chromosomes 1, 2, and 3 belong to the A group, are the largest, and are *metacentric;* that is, the long and short arms

are nearly equal in length. Chromosomes 4 and 5 (B group) are *submetacentric*, with the short arms easily recognizable. The C group consists of chromosomes 6 to 12 and the X chromosome. Before 1971 and the application of staining techniques that gave each chromosome a characteristic banding pattern, it was difficult to distinguish one member of this group from another. They could be separated as a group, however, from the D group (13 to 15) because the C group are metacentric and submetacentric and larger than the *acrocentric* D group. This latter group consists of three chromosomes that often appear to have only a long arm and centromere. There may be a short arm of varying staining quality and additional polymorphic variants known as satellites. These structures are connected to the short arms of the acrocentric chromosomes by thread-like stalks of varying length. Satellites are singular or double and stain with varying intensity from person to person. The E (16 to 18) and F (19 to 20) groups of chromosomes are quite small but can be easily distinguished by their size, centromere location, and banding patterns. Chromosomes 21 and 22 (G group) are the smallest acrocentrics and like the D group may possess short arm and satellite variants. The Y chromosome is often grouped with the G group based on size. It is, however, easily distinguishable from them by the more densely stained long arm and the more nearly parallel alignment of the long arms. Q-banding (discussed in the following) stains the Y chromosome a bright fluorescence, which is not shared with any other chromosome.

STAINING OF CHROMOSOMES. Chromosome preparations may be made from virtually any actively dividing cell line. Most commonly, peripheral blood, skin biopsies, bone marrow, and amniotic fluid fetal cells are used. The cells are allowed to grow and divide until a sufficient quantity are available for analysis. The time required to achieve this number is approximately 72 hours in the case of peripheral blood and 2 to 3 weeks in the case of fibroblast cultures derived from a skin biopsy or amniotic fluid aspirate. Bone marrow cells are already actively dividing cells. The culture is then treated with Colcemid for varying periods of time to half the mitotic process at metaphase. Cells are then subjected to hypotonic treatment and fixation and dropped onto slides for staining.

With the introduction of a method for *consistently* reproducing a pattern of light and dark areas on chromosomes by Caspersson and Zech in 1968, it became necessary to standardize the nomenclature used in designating these areas (Fig. 194-4). Periodically, cytogeneticists update the first standardization, which was constructed during the Paris Conference in 1971. In general a routine preparation of banded metaphase chromosomes does not clearly show every band identified in the ideal preparation. A number of staining techniques have been devised that can be used to highlight areas of chromosomes not easily examined by the other techniques.

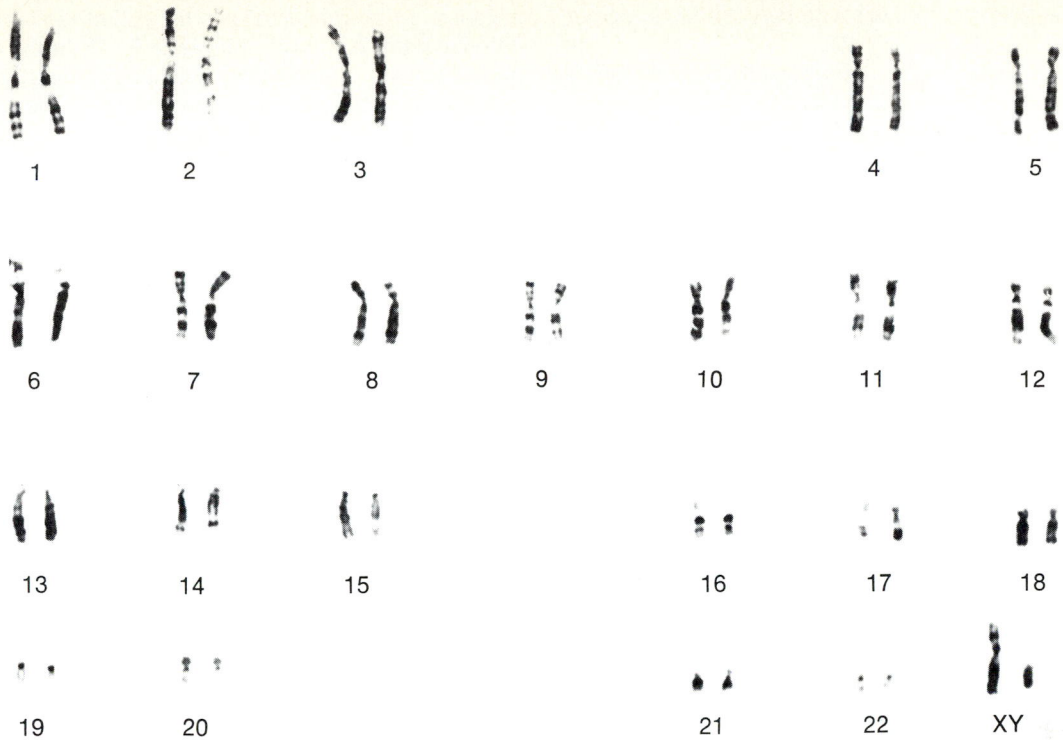

Fig. 194-3   Giemsa-banded male karyotype. Chromosomes are arranged in pairs from largest to smallest. Centromeres are positioned on drawn lines. *Metacentric* chromosomes have nearly equal long (q) and short (p) arms. The difference in length between q and p arms in *submetacentric* chromosomes is easily seen on inspection. In *acrocentric* chromosomes, there may be no p arm or only a very small one.

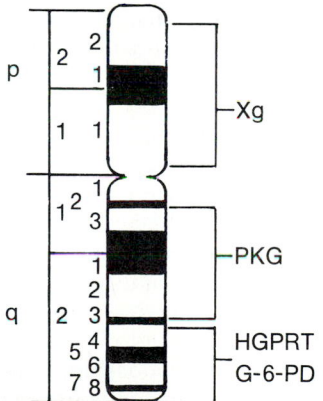

Fig. 194-4   Idealized banding pattern for X chromosome. Long, *q,* and short, *p,* arms are divided into large regions *1* and *2* by largest dark bands. Some longer chromosomes have three such regions. Both light and dark bands within each region are numbered consecutively from centromere distally. This system allows room for further band identification. A band is then designated by a notation including arm (*p* or *q*), region (*1, 2,* or *3*), and band number (such as p 12, q 24). Notation to right indicates regional localization of loci for *Xg,* and enzymes *PGK, HGPRT,* and *G-6-PD.* Over 100 loci have been mapped to X chromosome.

Table 194-4   Chromosomal abnormalities

Type	Manifestations
Abnormalities of number	Aneuploidy—trisomy, monosomy, tetrasomy
	Mosaicism
	Fragments
	Polyploidy—triploid, tetraploid
Structural abnormalities	Deletions
	Inversions—paracentric, pericentric
	Rings
	Translocations (balanced or unbalanced)—robertsonian, reciprocal
	Isochromosomes—short arm, long arm

ABNORMALITIES. Abnormalities of the human chromosome complement involve either the number or the structure of chromosomes (Table 194-4).

The human karyotype is designated 46,XX or 46,XY. Chromosome number is followed by the sex chromosome complement, which is then followed by the appropriate designation for any variants or abnormalities. Errors in the *number* of chromosomes are either *aneuploidy* or *polyploidy.* Aneuploidy usually involves only one, but sometimes two, chromosomes that may be either missing (monosomy) or present in additional numbers (trisomy, tetrasomy, and so on). Aneuploidy may arise during meiosis in either the ovum or the sperm. Meiotic nondisjunction refers to the failure of a chromosome pair to segregate into daughter cells, with both members remaining in one cell and no member of the pair entering the second. In most cases the only surviving gamete is the one with the extra chromosome. The fertilized product of a normal gamete and one that has had a nondisjunctional event is then said to be trisomic for the chromosome involved, such as in trisomy 21. It is written 47,XX (or XY), + 21. If both chromosomes 21 and 18 failed to segregate, the product would be 48,XX (or XY), + 18, + 21.

If nondisjunction occurs some time after fertilization or during mitosis, the result may be mosaicism for two or more cell lines, depending on the ability of the abnormal cell lines to reproduce. The karyotype may then appear as 46,XX/

47,XX, + 21, indicating a female with two cell lines, one of which is trisomic for chromosome 21.

Nondisjunction may also involve the sex chromosomes. Resulting karyotypes may be 45,X/47,XXY/47,XYY and 47,XXX, or mosaicism such as 45,X/46,XX and 45,X/46,XX/47,XXX.

Polyploidy refers to the presence of additonal haploid (n) sets of chromosomes. There are 69 chromosomes in a triploid and 92 in a tetraploid cell. This may arise by retention of a polar body during meiosis (triploidy) or by failure of separation of dividing chromosomes into two separate nuclear membranes (tetraploidy).

The most common *structural aberrations* of chromosomes are those involving one or more breaks on a single chromosome (deletions, inversions, rings, isochromosomes) and those involving breaks and/or fusions on two different chromosomes.

Deletions of a portion of a chromosome result from either one break, in which case the entire segment distal to the break is lost, or two breaks, in which case the proximal and distal chromosome parts may rejoin. In either case the cell is then monosomic for the lost fragment. If two breaks occur the intevening segment is reversed in direction and rejoins at the breakpoints, an *inversion* results. If the breaks are both on the same side of the centromere, the inversion is paracentric. If the centromere is between the breakpoints, it is a pericentric inversion. In such aberrations one is usually unable to detect any deleted chromosome material. If two breaks occur near the ends of the long and short arms of a chromosome, the two deleted ends may join to form a *ring* chromosome. The amount of deleted material depends on the sites of the breaks, but it will involve the most distal ends of the chromosomes. Finally, if there is a horizontal break through the centromere of a chromosome, an *isochromosome* may form. One (rarely both) of the resulting fragments retains a functional amount of the centromere. The new structure then consists of either two short arms or two long arms and is termed an isochromosome. The resulting nucleus is trisomic for the remaining arm and monosomic for the lost arm.

Translocations between chromosomes may be either balanced, with no apparent loss of chromosome material, or unbalanced, in which there is deleted or trisomic material. Translocations resulting from the attachment of two acrocentric (13 to 15, 21 and 22) chromosomes at or near the centromere are termed robertsonian translocations, and those involving any other chromosome segments are termed reciprocal. The designation 45,XY,rob(14q21q) indicates that there are only 45 different structures in this male karyotype and that there has been a fusion of the long arms of chromosomes 14 and 21 without identifiable loss of chromosome material. (One assumes, however, that there is some loss of material in all rearrangements involving breaks. In many cases it appears to be clinically insignificant.) If a sperm from the "translocation carrier" contains the translocated chromosome (14q21q) as well as the paternal chromosome 21 and fertilizes an egg containing one 21 and one 14, the result is an unbalanced translocation and is designated 46,XX, − 14, + rob(14q21q). The zygote is trisomic for chromosome 21.

When fragments of chromosome arms are translocated, the karyotype nomenclature usually designates at what bands the breaks are thought to have occurred. For example, the karyotype 46,XY,rcp(3;13)(p24;q31) indicates that this is a male karyotype with a balanced reciprocal translocation. It arose when a fragment resulting from a break on the short arm (p) of chromosome 3 at band 24 attached to the long arm (q) of chromosome 13 at breakpoint 31, and the fragment of chromosome 13 from band q31 to the end of the long arm attached to breakpoint p24 of chromosome 3. As in the case of robertsonian translocations, such "balanced carriers" may form germ cells with "unbalanced" contents. The zygote may be normal, a balanced carrier, or an unbalanced carrier, being either trisomic for 3p beyond point 24 and monosomic for 13q beyond point 31, or monosomic for the 3p and trisomic for the 13q fragments.

Chromosome fragments resulting from a single break near the end of a chromosome arm are usually lost to subsequent generations of cells. However, the consistent presence of fragments has been reported in both normal and abnormal individuals. Occasionally, gaps and breaks without loss of material are found in preparations of human chromosomes. They may be related to inherent chromosome instability or the effects of drugs. The significance of such findings is under investigation. Several disorders have been described that are associated with increased chromosome instability. These are Bloom's syndrome, ataxia-telangiectasia, and Fanconi's anemia, which are quite dissimilar clinically. The highest degree of instability is seen in Bloom's syndrome, in which there is a 30% incidence of lymphoproliferative disease.

Multifactorial inheritance

Early eugenicists failed to outline the single gene mode of inheritance, undoubtedly because they selected traits that were not only determined by a number of different genes, or *polygenic*, but by nongenetic factors as well, or *multifactorial*. Most common traits of man, as well as a few common birth defects (congenital heart disease, dislocated hip, and cleft lip and palate) are inherited in this manner. It is supposed that everyone possesses a certain liability (number of genes) for a given multifactorial characteristic. An individual's liability may exceed the threshold beyond which the trait becomes evident, either on the basis of the number of genes alone or because some other factor (radiation, drug, virus, and so on) has pushed his liability beyond the threshold. Such traits are heritable, but to a lesser degree than traits determined by single genes. First-degree relatives of an only affected individual will share the trait 3% to 5% of the time. Unlike single gene inheritance, the greater the number of related individuals who share the trait, the greater is any other relative's liability over that of the general population. This liability depends on the number of relatives affected and their relationship to the person in question. Other factors are of varying importance for different multifactorial traits or disorders. For example, neural tube defects (spina bifida and anencephaly) have a higher incidence in populations of the British Isles than those of North America, cleft lip and palate is seen more frequently among Orientals than other groups, congenital dislocation of the hip affects females more often than males, and pyloric stenosis affects more males than females. For these latter two examples, if the proband is of the least often affected sex, his or her relatives are at a greater liability than if the proband is of the sex most often affected. Tables based on empiric data have been constructed for many of the traits and disorders and should be consulted on an individual basis.

CLINICAL GENETICS

Diagnosis of genetic disease requires an appreciation of the etiologic heterogeneity of seemingly similar disorders. Without this, errors in diagnosis may lead to erroneous counseling regarding prognosis, recurrence risks, and available therapeutic and reproductive options. Allowing an individual or family to be guided through the decision-making process with an ac-

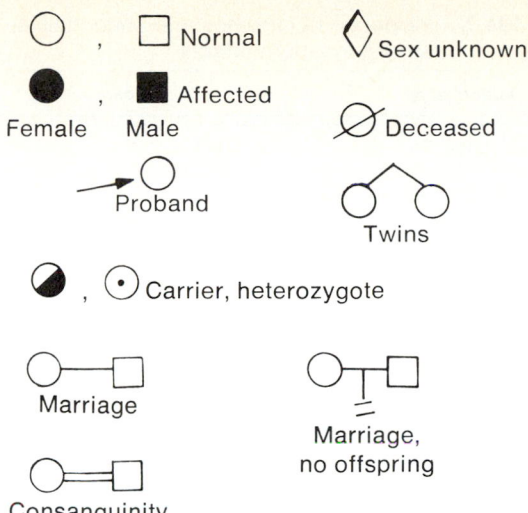

Fig. 194-5   Pedigree symbols.

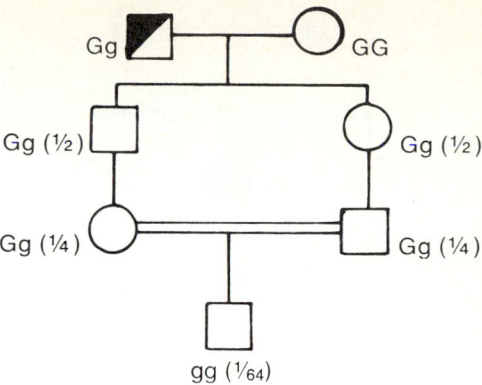

Fig. 194-6   Common grandfather in first-cousin mating is known to be heterozygote for recessive gene g. Mating is at 1/64 risk of producing child homozygous gg.

Table 194-5   Inbreeding coefficients of consanguineous matings

Mating	Inbreeding coefficient
Parent-child	1/4
Sibling-sibling	1/4
Uncle-niece	1/8
First cousin	1/16
Second cousin	1/64
First cousin once removed	1/32

curate data base and assisting them in implementing *their* decision should be the goal of the genetic counseling team. As more individuals are trained in this process, genetic counseling will become a routine component in the practice of the medical arts.

Pedigree construction and analysis

The purposes of constructing the family history are (1) to determine the pattern of inheritance of a given trait or disease within any given family, *despite* the diagnosis; (2) to use the pattern of inheritance to narrow diagnostic possibilities; and (3) to determine other individuals at risk among extended family members.

The pedigree is constructed using the symbols depicted in Fig. 194-5. The individual who has come to attention is known as the proband and those seeking information are the consultands. The proband may or may not be the consultand. The sexes and ages of siblings, parents, grandparents, aunts, uncles, and cousins are indicated in the pedigree. If a pattern of abnormalities emerges from this investigation, it should be extended through appropriate family lines. Authors of a pedigree may designate affected individuals by their own symbols, although a few conventional symbols are indicated in the figure. Additional information includes occurrence of unexplained infertility, early childhood deaths, stillbirths, and miscarriages.

Often, simple examination of the pedigree reveals a pattern of inheritance. It cannot be too strongly emphasized that all aspects of the condition in question must be considered before providing definitive information to the patient and family. Most common genetic disorders have been well described and their patterns of inheritance established; however, in any given family the possibility of a new variant, a previously unrecognized mode of inheritance of a given disorder, or nongenetic factors resulting in a phenocopy of a genetic disorder may be discovered.

CONSANGUINITY. Matings involving related individuals are termed consanguineous and are of particular interest when dealing with rare autosomal recessive diseases. Everyone "carries" at least one or two rare recessive "lethal" genes. These genes are derived from hundreds of possibilities, and the chance of any two unrelated individuals being carriers of the same recessive gene (heterozygotes) is the square of the frequency of carriers in the population. For even the most common of

such genes, cystic fibrosis (CF), where the carrier frequency is 1 in 20 in the Caucasian population, the chance that two randomly mated persons share the CF gene is $(\frac{1}{20})^2$, or $\frac{1}{400}$, and the chance that any random couple will have a child with CF is $\frac{1}{400} \times \frac{1}{4} = \frac{1}{1600}$. If two individuals are closely related and it is known that a common ancestor carries a specific recessive gene either through carrier testing or birth of an affected child, the related couple will be at a predictable increased risk of both being carriers. In the mating depicted in Fig. 194-6, first cousins whose grandfather is known to be a carrier of a recessive lethal gene, g, each have a ¼ chance of also carrying the gene, and there is a 1/16 chance of both being carriers. Any given pregnancy is therefore at a $(\frac{1}{16} \times \frac{1}{4}) = \frac{1}{64}$ risk of being homozygous for that gene, gg. The kinship coefficient of this mating is 1/16. The inbreeding coefficient of the offspring is the same, 1/16. The inbreeding coefficient of any product of a consanguineous union is the probability that two alleles at a given locus are identical by virtue of descent. Inbreeding coefficients for the most commonly encountered consanguineous matings are listed in Table 194-5. In Fig. 194-7 both common grandparents are assumed to be heterozygotes for the recessive gene, g, because of the birth of an affected child. The siblings of this child, who are themselves unaffected, have a ⅔ chance of being heterozygotes (two of the remaining three possibilities once the homozygous affected state is excluded). If there is no further consanguinity, the chance that both first cousins are heterozygotes is therefore $(\frac{2}{3} \times \frac{1}{2})(\frac{2}{3} \times \frac{1}{2}) = \frac{1}{9}$, and their risk of having an affected child is $(\frac{1}{9} \times \frac{1}{4}) = \frac{1}{36}$.

Such calculations are necessary only when there is no means of carrier detection. If the diagnosis of an affected family member is known, it may be possible to determine the heterozygote state among unaffected relatives. It is always important to include carrier testing of the "obligate" heterozygotes in the

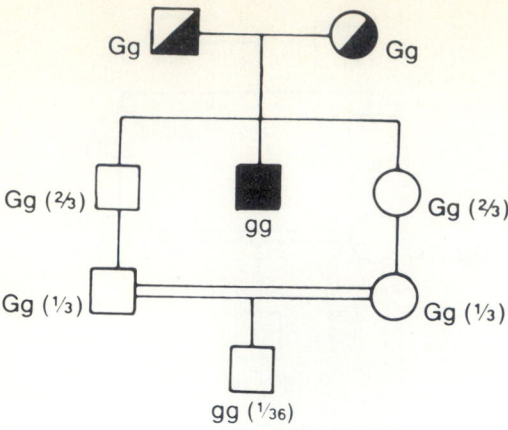

Fig. 194-7 Both common grandparents to first-cousin mating are known to be heterozygotes for g by virtue of affected child with gg genotype. Mating is at 1/36 risk of producing child homozygous gg.

Table 194-6 Genetic diseases demonstrating ethnic differences in frequency

Genetic disorder	Ethnic group with relatively high frequency
β-Thalassemia	Italians, Greeks
α-Thalassemia	Chinese
Adrenal hyperplasia	Eskimos
Tay-Sachs disease	Jews (Ashkenazi)
Familial dysautonomia	Jews (Ashkenazi)
Aspartylglycosaminuria	Finns
Neural tube defects	Irish

family to eliminate the possibility of an unusual biochemical variant that may not be detected by the usual means.

ETHNICITY. The family history should also include information with regard to the ethnic origins of ancestors. There are now a number of genetic disorders known to occur in higher frequency among certain populations. An abbreviated list is found in Table 194-6. Such information is important both in searching for prospective disorders, especially when dealing with consanguineous matings, as well as in establishing diagnostic possibilities in individuals with rare diseases. Determination of such high-risk populations is also useful in implementing heterozygote detection programs. The prototype of such programs is the Tay-Sachs Disease–Carrier Screening Program. The desirable criteria for such programs are met in this disease in the following ways:

1. An identifiable population is at high risk. Individuals of Eastern European (Ashkenazi) Jewish descent have a heterozygote frequency of approximately 1/27, compared to non-Ashkenazi Jews with a carrier frequency of 1/300.
2. Carrier detection is possible. The biochemical defect resulting in this lethal neurodegenerative disease is known to be a deficiency of the enzyme hexosaminidase A. Detection of the enzyme's activity may be performed on a blood sample or fibroblast cultures. Heterozygotes will demonstrate approximately 50% of normal activity.
3. Prenatal diagnosis is available.

The ultimate fourth criterion, treatment, is not yet possible for this disease.

Table 194-7 Incidence of chromosome abnormalities among live-born infants

Abnormality	Incidence
Trisomy 21	1:660
Trisomy 13	1:7000
Trisomy 18	1:7000
47,XXY	1:700 (males)
45,X	1:2500-1:5000 (females)
47,XYY	1:700 (males)
47,XXX	1:2000-1:4000 (females)

Clinical cytogenetic disorders

Generally, aberrations in the amount of chromosome material are associated with malformation syndromes of varying complexity. Typically, chromosome abnormalities result in physical defects of many body parts; for instance, mental retardation, growth delay, congenital heart disease, renal abnormalities, and variations of development of ears, nose, fingers are noted with increased frequency in nearly every syndrome. Additionally, there are such endless possibilities for deletions and trisomies that is it practical to mention only the most commonly occurring (Table 194-7).

TRISOMY 21 (DOWN'S SYNDROME). Trisomy 21 is the most frequent autosomal trisomy among children, occurring in 1 in every 600 to 700 live births. Ninety-five percent of cases result from nondisjunction, whereas the other 5% are divided between mosaics and unbalanced translocations. Neonates with Down's syndrome may be recognized by a characteristic facial appearance consisting of flattened facial profile, flat nasal bridge, creases over the inner canthi of the eyes (epicanthal folds), small, low-set ears, increased folds of skin at the nape of the neck, hypoplastic irides (Brushfield's spots), hypotonia, and microcephaly. There may also be a single palmar crease, hypoplasia of the midphalanx of the fifth digit with an incurving of the fifth finger (clinodactyly), congenital heart disease (in about 40%), and duodenal atresia (in about 25%). There is an increased risk of childhood leukemia, and life expectancy is generally reduced depending on accompanying medical problems. Recurrent ear infections, as well as a probable congenital sensorineural hearing loss, result in hearing deficits.

There is an increased incidence of Down's syndrome and other aneuploidies with advanced maternal age. However, *all* infants with Down's syndrome should be karyotyped to rule out the possibility of translocation, in which case other family members (parents first, followed by others as necessary) should be studied. The recurrence risk for a chromosomally abnormal child after the birth of the first is 0.5% to 1% in the case of nondisjunction and may be 10% to 15% in the case of familial robertsonian translocations. If a parent is a carrier of a balanced translocation involving both chromosomes 21, the risk of recurrence for trisomy 21 is 100%. (The only gametes such a parent can produce have either no chromosome 21 or the translocation 21/21.)

TRISOMY 13 AND TRISOMY 18. Both trisomy 13 and 18 result in children with much more severe malformations than those with trisomy 21. There is a high frequency of severe congenital heart disease, neurologic and mental impairment, renal abnormalities, and growth retardation. Trisomy 13 can be distinguished by the presence of microphthalmia, polydactyly, and cleft lip and palate. Although these latter abnormalities may occur in infants with trisomy 18, they are less frequent. More often these infants demonstrate prominent heels (rocker-bottom feet), flexion deformities of the fingers, small, round heads, and fingerprints (dermatoglyphics) consisting of 10 (or a majority) simple arch patterns. Life expectancy is severely reduced to weeks or months, although a number with only mild cardiac or renal anomalies may survive longer. Again, even though a diagnosis may be clinically obvious, karyotyping should be performed to confirm the diagnosis and to rule out the presence of a translocation.

As already stated, the potential exists for many other clinical cytogenetic abnormalities. In general any individual with multiple malformations, especially if mental retardation is present, deserves a chromosome analysis. Syndromes accompanied by monosomy for a portion of chromosome material are usually more devastating than trisomy for the same material. Several chromosome abnormalities are seen almost exclusively in products of spontaneous abortion. No doubt these aberrations are associated with defects so severe as to interfere with even intrauterine survival.

ABNORMALITIES OF THE SEX CHROMOSOMES. Unlike aneuploidies of the autosomes, the phenotypic features of sex chromosome abnormalities are not generally as severe. Intelligence is often (if not usually) normal, and major disturbances of development concern the gonads. Many of the changes in physiognomy are secondary to malfunctioning ovaries or testes.

The most common sex chromosome abnormalities are Klinefelter's syndrome (47,XXY), Turner's syndrome (45,X), males with 47,XXY constitution, and 47,XXX females.

Klinefelter's syndrome. Males with an additional X chromosome have a positive buccal smear. Phenotypically, they are characterized by tall stature, decreased development of male secondary sex characteristics, a eunuchoid habitus, mild mental retardation, gynecomastia, and hypergonadotropic hypogonadism, with testicular atrophy demonstrating tubular sclerosis and Leydig cell hyperplasia on biopsy. Klinefelter's syndrome is often not suspected until adolescence or later, when the patient may be seen with a complaint of infertility.

Turner's syndrome. Among spontaneous abortuses of 12 weeks' gestation or less, 15% of chromosome abnormalities are 45,X. This is indeed intriguing, since survivors with Turner's syndrome are certainly not severely physically nor mentally impaired. The phenotypic features of live-born girls with Turner's syndrome are lymphedema of hands and feet at birth (which later resolves), short stature in childhood and adolescence, and failure of development of secondary sex characteristics, with ovarian dysgenesis and usually infertility. Girls are also described as having a broad, "webbed" neck, an increased carrying angle of the arms (cubitus valgus), the appearance of widely spaced nipples and a "shield chest," multiple-pigmented nevi, and hyperconvex fingernails. Intellectually, girls with Turner's syndrome may exhibit a perceptual handicap but are not mentally retarded as a part of the syndrome. Coarctation of the aorta is seen in approximately 15%. It is interesting to speculate that the females known to have Turner's syndrome actually manifest a mild form of the more usual phenotype, which is so severe that it accounts for the large number of 45,X karyotypes among abortuses. Such fetuses have been shown to have severe lymphedema and cystic hygromas, as well as hypoplastic left-heart syndrome, which is incompatible with life.

Mosaicism is common among girls with Turner's syndrome. The physical and developmental features vary depending on the exact chromosome constitution. Mosaics may be 45,X/ 46,XX; 45,X/46XX$_{iq}$; 45,X/46XX$_{ip}$; and 45,X/46,XY. A mosaic karyotype containing a 46,XY cell line is of particular importance. Dysgenetic gonads containing an XY cell line should be removed because of the high frequency of malig-

nancy. Fertility has been reported in mosaics and rarely in a few females in whom only a 45,X cell line could be detected.

Females with Turner's syndrome may be expected to attain an adult height of approximately 4 feet 10 inches. Hormonal replacement is begun sometime during the adolescent years. Timing of such therapy depends on both physical and psychologic parameters; however, discussion of the need for such therapy should begin with the parents during the early years.

XYY males and XXX females. The XYY male was originally detected among a group of incarcerated men and unfortunately came to be associated with a picture of a tall, aggressive, retarded male with severe acne. In fact, this karyotype is probably more common than previously appreciated and is associated with few if any physical or mental abnormalities and not with infertility.

The poly-X female may demonstrate mental deficiency (33%) and some minor dysmorphic features. XXX females may be fertile. The more X chromosomes there are in a male or female karyotype, the more severe are the physical abnormalities and the higher the incidence of mental retardation.

Single gene disorders

Those genetic diseases and variants that are inherited in the mendelian modes now number close to 3000. As it is not possible to adequately summarize all these disorders, several broad categories are considered here. The reader is referred to more comprehensive reviews and to other chapters in this volume for further consideration.

LYSOSOMAL STORAGE DISEASE (LSD). Lysosomal enzymes (acid hydrolases) are responsible for the catabolism of various cellular materials. Their impaired function results in the accumulation of substrate within vacuoles, a process that may itself be toxic to the cell or that may result in accumulation of other cellular substances and limit cellular functioning in general. For any given enzyme deficiency, those tissues that engage in the highest rate of substrate turnover are most severely affected by the alteration in biochemical activity, whereas other tissues are affected to a lesser degree.

In general, lysosomal storage diseases are progressive, often fatal, and diagnosable biochemically or pathologically by the presence of stored material in characteristic configurations: myelin figures, "zebra bodies," Gaucher's cell, onionskin lesions, and so on.

AMINOACIDOPATHIES AND DISORDERS OF PURINE METABOLISM. Many of the disorders involving errors in amino acid metabolism are associated with mental retardation, seizure disorders, and failure to thrive in infancy. The nonspecificity of many of the symptoms has led to the use of the "amino acid screen" in infants and children with poorly defined illness. An astute practitioner is able to clinically narrow the diagnostic possibilities. Table 194-8 lists the disorders to be suspected when one or more clinical signs or symptoms are particularly prominent.

Early recognition of an aminoacidopathy permits the prompt institution of an appropriate diet and in some cases the amelioration of the effects of the disorder. In addition, several aminoacidopathies are responsive to vitamin supplementation.

Phenylketonuria (PKU), the best-known disorder of amino acid metabolism, if untreated, is characterized by the development of mental retardation, seizures, eczema, and associated light pigmentation when compared to family members. PKU was the first inborn error of metabolism subjected to newborn screening attempts. Several states have now mandated the screening of every neonate for a panel of inborn errors of metabolism as well as congenital hypothyroidism. Optimally,

Table 194-8 Signs and symptoms suggestive of some inborn errors of metabolism (all more common causes of the presenting finding must be ruled out)

Clinical sign or laboratory finding	Associated disorders
Failure to thrive	Almost all
Vomiting	Many
Diarrhea	Cystic fibrosis, galactosemia, Wolman's disease, congenital lactic acidosis
Jaundice	Galactosemia, Wolman's diseae, Crigler-Najjar syndrome, carbamyl phosphate synthetase deficiency, hypothyroidism
Dislocated lens	Homocystinuria
Hypotonicity or hypertonicity	Almost all
Seizures	Amino acid disorders, glycogen storage disease
Coarse facial features	GM_1, GM_3, MPS, mucolipidosis II
Metabolic acidosis	Renal tubular acidosis, organic acid disorders
Hypoglycemia	Glycogen storage disease
Hyperammonemia	Urea cycle defects, hyperlysinemia
Thrombocytopenia	Organic acid disorders
Malodorous urine	Tyrosinemia, phenylketonuria (musty), maple syrup urine disease (maple sugary), methionine malabsorption (malts), isovaleric acidemia (cheesy)

Adapted from Burton BK and Nadler HJ: Pediatrics 6:398, 1978.

disorders to be screened should be ascertained as early as possible and be amenable to some form of treatment.

A recently recognized problem is the case of the adult female who is no longer on a restricted diet and has a treated aminoacidopathy; most notable is PKU. During pregnancy the low phenylalanine diet must be reinstituted to prevent high levels of the amino acid crossing the placenta and affecting the fetus, even though there is little likelihood of the fetus having the same genetic defect as the mother.

Not all of the inborn errors are necessarily manifested in infancy or childhood. Homocystinuria should be suspected in adults with dislocated lenses, early thromboembolic events, mild mental retardation, or schizophrenia. Renal calculi or disease may be present in cystinuria, hyperprolinemia, and cystinosis. An immunodeficiency state is associated with adenine deaminase deficiency and purine nucleoside phosphorylase deficiency. Hypoxanthine-guanine phosphoribosyltransferase (HGPRT) deficiency (Lesch-Nyhan syndrome) is associated with hyperuricemia, retardation, choreoathetosis, and self-destructive behavior. It is an X-linked disease.

HEMOGLOBINOPATHIES. Hemoglobin variants result from those mutations of the genetic code that have caused alterations in the amino acid sequence of one or more of the subunits of the hemoglobin molecule. The most common variants result from amino acid substitutions at a single point in the globin chain. Most of these variants have no clinical consequence and are usually only detected if the substitution changes the electrophoretic properties of the molecule.

Clinically, five main types of hemoglobin disease are recognized: (1) unstable hemoglobins, usually owing to substitutions that affect the helical turns of the subunits, resulting in hemoglobin instability; (2) rapid hemoglobin oxidation, resulting in methemoglobinemia; (3) abnormal oxygen affinity, usually caused by inner chain substitutions; (4) sickle cell diseases, with instability of the red cell membrane; and (5) the thalassemias, in which there is diminished or absent synthesis of a hemoglobin chain. All of these mutations can be expressed

in some way in the heterozygote state, although the homozygous state is required for severe clinical disease in the sickle cell anemias. Thalassemia pathology is more complex.

DISORDERS OF COAGULATION. The most common heritable disorders of coagulation are hemophilia A and B and von Willebrand's disease. Hemophilia A and B result from deficiencies of clotting factors VIII and IX, respectively, and are X linked. There is marked variability in the clinical pictures depending on the level of circulating factor. Males with up to 2% factor VIII levels are severely affected, those with 2% to 5% of normal are moderately affected, and those with 5% to 20% levels may encounter problems only with severe trauma or surgery. Because this is an X-linked gene, female carriers are subject to the effects of the Lyon hypothesis. About 70% of female carriers have low levels of factor VIII (20% to 70% of normal) and may show mild symptoms. Unless a female has two affected sons, an affected brother and son, or an affected father, one cannot be certain that she is a carrier. An isolated case may represent a new mutation. Carrier testing is difficult and requires measurement not only of factor VIII but also of factor VIII–related antigen. These values must be plotted with well-established controls to determine the likelihood of any female being a carrier. In equivocal cases the entire family history must be analyzed and bayesian principles applied. By weighing the probabilities of various combinations of affected and unaffected relatives, a more precise determination of the "carrier" may be made.

Factor IX disease is similar to factor VIII deficiency in mode of inheritance and clinical manifestations. Carrier testing is less reliable than that for hemophilia A, and an in-depth family history is the best assessment of carrier probabilities.

Von Willebrand's disease is an autosomal dominant disorder in which there is an alteration in bleeding time. The von Willebrand factor is under autosomal control and serves as a substrate for an X-linked factor. Blood from a patient with hemophilia A will correct bleeding in a von Willebrand's patient; however, the reverse is not true. Diagnosis is made by demonstrating low factor VIII, decreased platelet adhesiveness, and prolonged bleeding time. An affected individual (male or female) is at 50% risk of passing the gene on to any given offspring.

Complex genetic syndromes

There are now recognized to be complex malformation syndromes inherited in an autosomal dominant, a recessive, or an X-linked manner in addition to those that result from chromosome abnormalities. The diagnosis of such syndromes is usually in the hands of the experienced dysmorphologist or clinical geneticist. Many believe it is only a matter of time before a new technique demonstrates the chromosome aberration or biochemical error responsible for these syndromes. Until then, counseling with regard to mode of inheritance must rely on data acquired from affected individuals and families.

In any given individual one defect or symptom may dominate the clinical picture. A search for other anomalies or symptoms may reveal that the dominant feature is not isolated but rather is only one component of a syndrome complex. Realizing the presence of such combinations allows the examiner to direct a search for related defects or symptoms. Accurate diagnosis is necessary to provide adequate management and counseling regarding recurrence risks.

The currently recommended terminology for patterns of morphologic defects includes the terms "sequence," "syndrome," "association," and "field defect."

A *sequence* refers to a given malformation and its secondary deformations. This term would apply, for example, to the former Pierre Robin syndrome (micrognathia and cleft palate). The primary malformation may be isolated or accompanied by other malformations (with their secondary deformations) and therefore would be part of a *malformation syndrome*. A group of anomalies (defects, primary malformations) that are thought to be pathogenetically and etiologically related is a syndrome. Syndromes are often of single gene inheritance or result from chromosome abnormalities. A few are caused by definite environmental agents such as alcohol, phenytoin, and rubella. An *association* is a nonrandom occurrence of several defects in more than one individual; however, no sequence or syndrome can be identified. For many patterns of malformation, association is a temporary designation until such time that a syndrome or sequence can be identified. A *field defect* is defined as the result of disturbed development in all or part of a morphogenic field. It differs from a sequence in that there are no disruptive forces at work and the primary defect no doubt traces back to an early germ layer.

Multifactorial disease

Most common diseases of man, as well as a few specific birth defects, of which cleft lip and palate is one, fall into the category of multifactorial inheritance. That is, the inheritance of the disease or trait is determined by the action of many genes (polygenic) interacting with a variety of environmental factors. Most traits that demonstrate continuous variation (height, weight, intelligence, and so on) in a population are multifactorial. Some seemingly discontinuous traits (one either does or does not possess the trait or the disease, such as diabetes, hypertension, or cleft lip and palate) may be considered to have a continuously distributed liability and a threshold for liability beyond which a specific trait is expressed.

The increased risk for relatives of an index case varies directly with the closeness of the relationship. In cleft lip and palate, which has a population incidence of 1:1000, first-degree relative risk is 40:1000, second-degree is 7:1000, and third-degree is 3:1000. In disorders in which there is an unequal sex distribution, relatives of the more rarely affected sex are at a greater risk. Such sex differences exist for pyloric stenosis (more males affected than females) and congenital dislocation of the hip (more females affected than males). The more severe the malformation (bilateral versus unilateral cleft lip), the greater the risk of recurrence, and the recurrence risk increases with increasing numbers of affected relatives. In general, after the birth of one affected individual, the risk for a second affected person is 3% to 5%; after two affected, 10%; and after three, 14%. It can be seen that a family with many affected individuals approaches the risks of single gene disorders (25% and 50%).

It is extremely important to eliminate the possibility that the individual possesses a complex malformation syndrome, of which the defect under consideration is only a part. Failure to do so may result in errors in counseling regarding recurrence risks or other associated features. For example, cleft lip and palate accompanied by lip pits or cysts is a dominantly inherited syndrome (van der Woude syndrome), and relatives without obvious clefts should be examined for the presence of lip pits to determine individuals at risk.

The human gene map, linkage, and association

Family studies and somatic cell hybridization techniques have been used to locate specific gene sequences to individual chromosomes. To date more than 150 loci have been localized to specific human autosomes, with over 100 of these pinpointed to the X chromosome. The loci may be quite biochemically specific (such as ABO blood group, various enzymes, and structural proteins) or as yet nonspecific, such as nail-patella syndrome (chromosome 9), testis determining factor (Y chromosome), and hereditary spherocytosis (chromosome 12). It is possible in a few instances to use linkage information in determining risk of disease, even through the specific biochemical abnormality of the disease in question is unknown. The genetic locus for the disease and the locus for a biochemical marker that can be measured must be closely linked. For example, the locus controlling the expression of blood types in tissues and fluids (saliva) other than blood, the secretor locus, has been used in the prenatal prediction of myotonic dystrophy (MD), an autosomal dominant disorder in which the specific metabolic error is unknown. By determining the genotypes of both parents with regard to secretor status and provided the mating is genetically informative, the secretor status of the fetus may be used to predict the likelihood of the occurrence of MD. (Informative refers to the arrangement of alleles for MD and secretor status in the parents. Ideally, the affected parent is a double heterozygote at the two loci.)

Not to be confused with linkage is association. Linkage refers to genes located on the same chromosome within some small distance of one another; association implies that there is a higher than random occurrence of a gene and a specific trait. Neither a direct causal relationship nor linkage is implied.

The HLA complex is located on chromosome 6. It can be said to be linked to the other loci on chromosome 6. Much confusion has arisen over the HLA-associated diseases. For the most part these are multifactorial diseases, and many are autoimmune diseases with familial aggregation. Five mechanisms of HLA disease associations have been considered: (1) HLA specificity at the cell surface acting as a receptor for a virus or pathogenic agent, (2) a weakening of immunologic tolerance occurring as a result of a cross-reaction of an HLA antigen with a viral or bacterial antigen, (3) linkage disequilibrium within the HLA locus itself, (4) mutations of genes linked to the HLA complex, and (5) immune response genes closely linked to the HLA locus that also demonstrate linkage disequilibrium. Mechanisms 1 and 5 are not mutually exclusive, and it may be that more than one of these will apply in various diseases.

DNA technology

The ability to synthesize and clone DNA has led to the production of multiple biologic products, as well as the use of specific DNA sequences as probes in the identification of genetic mutations.

The first step in DNA analysis is the isolation of DNA from the nuclei of patients' leukocytes, tissue, or cultured fibroblasts. After preparation this genomic DNA is subjected to restriction endonuclease digestion. Each of the many restriction endonucleases that can be used has a specific nucleotide recognition sequence. An enzyme cleaves the DNA at predictable sites and, as a result, produces specific fragments of DNA of reproducible size. The number and size of the fragments are determined by the number and locations of recognition sequences for that endonuclease within the DNA. Following digestion, agarose gel electrophoresis is used to separate the DNA fragments by size. The DNA is then transferred from the gel by Southern blotting and fixed to a nitrocellulose filter by baking. Hybridization with radiolabeled sequences of DNA occurs before the filter is washed to remove unhybridized radioactivity and is autoradiographed. DNA fragments containing sequences that hybridize with the radioactive probe appear as bands on the developed film. The size of the DNA fragments within a band is determined by comparison with the location of known molecular weight markers in the same gel.

These techniques (isolation, cloning, and hybridization) permit the identification of genotypes whose implications are already known, and they provide the basis for exploring many other traits and characteristics of individuals.

The most reliable genetic diagnostic tests become possible when the gene for the disease locus has been cloned. There is already a considerable list of such cloned genes although a listing at any point in time is by definition incomplete as new entries may be made daily. The diagnosis of genetic disorders utilizing DNA technology involves either the identification of the mutation in a given person's DNA sequence or the identification of a closely linked marker gene which a high percentage of the time segregates with the locus of interest from generation to generation.

These diagnostic techniques may be applied to any tissue from which DNA can be isolated, including material extracted from chorionic villous sampling, amniocytes, fibroblasts, leukocytes, tumors, bacteria, and viruses.

In addition to diagnostic applications, DNA technology has found application in virtually every aspect of science. These include prenatal diagnosis of single gene disorders; diagnostic agents for bacterial, viral, and parasitic infection; production of therapeutic agents (for instance, hormones and interferon); vaccines, blood products; completion of the human gene map; gene replacement; and understanding of the regulation of human development from fetal life to aging.

Prenatal diagnosis

Reference has been made to the availability of prenatal diagnostic studies for various genetic disorders. The most widely used techniques are fetal ultrasound and amniocentesis. Grayscale and real-time ultrasound are routinely used to determine gestational age by measuring the fetal biparietal diameter, trunk and crown-rump length, and placenta size and location. In a pregnancy at risk the same instruments may be used to examine in greater detail the bony and dense soft tissue structures of the fetus. Meningoceles, occipital encephaloceles, anencephaly, absent kidneys, and anomalous limbs may be diagnosed in this manner. Amniocentesis in prenatal diagnosis involves the insertion of a needle into the amniotic cavity at the sixteenth to seventeenth week of gestation. Approximately 30 ml of fluid is removed under sterile conditions and referred to the genetics laboratory for appropriate analysis. A portion of the fluid may be separated and analyzed for α-1-fetoprotein (AFP), while the cell button (cells of fetal origin) is dispersed into flasks containing growth media. These cells are grown for approximately 2 to 3 weeks, by which time there is usually a sufficient number of actively dividing cells to perform a chromosome analysis or biochemical studies.

AFP is 100 times greater in concentration in fetal blood than adult blood. It was found to be elevated in the amniotic fluid of pregnancies affected with a variety of birth defects, including anencephaly, other open neural tube defects, congenital nephrosis, esophageal atresia, and omphalocele, as well as in fetal demise and twin pregnancies.

Measuring AFP in maternal serum between the fourteenth and seventeenth week of gestation is now used as a screening test in many obstetric practices. Elevated AFP levels in maternal serum samples warrant a repeat sample and persistent elevation is followed by ultrasonography and amniocentesis. Low levels of AFP have been associated with an increased incidence of chromosome abnormalities. Low levels are de-

termined by individual laboratories and expressed as values of so many multiples of the mean or as a fraction. Tables have been constructed that alter the age-related risk figures for a chromosomally abnormal fetus based on the AFP value obtained. Application of such statistical tables results in a corrected risk figure based on maternal age and AFP value. If this newly derived risk figure warrants further investigation by amniocentesis, the parents should be informed.

Chorionic villous sampling (CVS), or biopsy, is the process of removing small amounts of tissue of fetal origin located at the site of the developing placenta between the ninth and eleventh week of gestation. The procedure is usually performed transvaginally but may be transcutaneous and is always conducted under ultrasound guidance. Because this tissue is in a vigorous mitotic state, it may be processed immediately for the production of metaphase chromosomes. Combined with the early timing of the procedure, this allows a result to be available within the first trimester in most cases. Risk figures for this procedure are yet to be firmly established; however, the rate is expected to be 1% to 2% in specialized centers. Tissue from CVS may also be subjected to biochemical analysis and molecular studies. This technique is rapidly becoming the method of choice for prenatal diagnosis.

Fetal blood sampling and fetoscopy (fetal visualization) are performed in only a limited number of centers. Fetal blood sampling has been used primarily in the diagnosis of hemophilia and the hemoglobinopathies. With the advent of DNA diagnosis of these disorders, however, fetal blood sampling is rarely needed. Fetoscopy may accompany fetal blood sampling or may be used alone to diagnose various structural malformations, such as polydactyly (as a sign of a more complex syndrome), cleft lip, and neural tube defects. Currently, fetal skin biopsy is being investigated as a means of diagnosing serious disorders via skin pathology.

Indications for prenatal counseling include:

1. Drug ingestion during gestation
2. Radiation exposure
3. Chemotherapy
4. Family history of nonmetabolic, nonchromosomal genetic disorder
5. More than two previous unexplained miscarriages
6. As part of infertility workup

Indications for amniocentesis and prenatal counseling include:

1. Advanced maternal age (woman over 35 years of age)
2. Previous child with trisomy or other aneuploidy
3. Previous child with multiple anomalies about which nothing more is known
4. Previous child with neural tube defect
5. Carrier X-linked disorder
6. Translocation carrier
7. Carrier of autosomal recessive disorder for which biochemical testing is available (ascertained through either previously affected child or voluntary screening program)

BIBLIOGRAPHY

Antenatal diagnosis, US Department of Health and Human Services, US Public Health Service, National Institutes of Health Pub No 79-1973, Bethesda, MD, April 1979.
Emery EH and Rimoin DL, eds: Principles and practice of medical genetics, Edinburgh, 1983, Churchill Livingstone Inc.
McKusick VA: Mendelian inheritance in man, ed 7, Baltimore, 1986, The Johns Hopkins University Press.
Murphy EA and Chase GA: Principles of genetic counseling, Chicago, 1975, Year Book Medical Publishers.
Smith DW: Recognizable patterns of human malformation vol 7, Major problems in clinical pediatrics, ed 3, Philadelphia, 1982, WB Saunders Co.

Vogel F and Motulsky AG: Human genetics, problems and approaches, New York, 1979, Springer-Verlag New York Inc.

Weatherall DJ: DNA in medicine: implications for medical practice and human biology, Lancet 2:1440, 1984.

195 · INHERITED METABOLIC DISORDERS

Adam J. Jonas *and* William A. Horton

The ramifications of a single mutant gene usually involve multiple organ systems. Since most genes code for proteins, the generalized nature of most genetic diseases is due to the widespread distribution of nearly all of these proteins, whether they provide structural support or catalyze metabolic reactions. Thus in most cases, if a protein is absent or defective, all tissues in which that protein has a function may be damaged. In addition, if a metabolic pathway is blocked, all the cells in the body may be exposed to high levels of toxic precursor metabolites or deficiencies of vital end products. Hence genetic diseases cannot be broken down by organ systems but rather must be considered in broad categories. In this chapter disorders are grouped according to whether they are of lysosomal storage, amino acid metabolism, nucleic acid metabolism, metal metabolism, or connective tissue.

DISORDERS OF LYSOSOMAL STORAGE
Glycosphingolipidoses

Glycosphingolipidoses are disorders of glycosphingolipid catabolism. The compounds are membrane lipids composed of a backbone of ceramide (sphingosine plus a long-chain fatty acid) to which various substances are attached. When the attached substance is a simple sugar or group of sugars, the compound is called a cerebroside. If it is a sialic (neuraminic) acid, the term "ganglioside" is used. When phosphocholine is attached, sphingomyelin is produced. Sphingomyelin and sulfatide (galactose and sulfate added in turn to ceramide) are the major lipids in myelinated nervous system membranes. Glycosphingolipids are normally degraded by the stepwise removal of the terminal sugar or other residue by lysosomal acid hydrolases (Fig. 195-1). When the pathway is blocked because of an enzyme deficiency, the precursor molecules accumulate in lysosomes causing enlargement, interruption of normal function, and eventually death of the cell. Clinically this is reflected by progressive neurologic deterioration with or without visceral involvement depending on the distribution of the stored glycosphingolipids, that is, cerebrosides in neuronal and extraneuronal tissues, gangliosides essentially in central nervous system gray matter, and sulfatides in central nervous system white matter. There is considerable variation in the age of onset and the rate of progression of disease even in disorders in which the same enzyme deficiency is found. This presumably reflects the degree of in vivo enzyme deficiency, which is not necessarily the same as that measured in vitro. In general there is no treatment for these disorders, but in many cases prenatal diagnosis is possible by measuring the activity of the enzyme in question in amniotic fluid cells. The major glycosphingolipidoses are labeled in Fig. 195-1 and listed in Table 195-1.

Two forms of *GM₁ gangliosidoses* (generalized gangliosidosis) are known. In the infantile form (type 1, *Landing's disease*) the initial manifestations are usually seen soon after birth. These include psychomotor degeneration, seizures, coarse facial features, enlargement of the tongue and alveolar processes, cherry-red spot of the retina, hepatosplenomegaly, and the bone changes of dysotosis multiplex (see "Mucopolysaccharidoses" later in this chapter). Death usually occurs by 2 years of age. The activity of the enzyme GM_1 β-galactosidase is reduced to between 1% and 5% of normal, and massive amounts of its substrate, GM_1 ganglioside, are found in the brain and viscera. Other galactose-containing substrates, including mucopolysaccharides (glycosaminoglycans), polysaccharides, and glycoproteins, are found in increased amounts in the liver, spleen, and bone.

In the less common juvenile (type 2) GM_1 gangliosidosis, development is normal during the first year. Progressive psychomotor deterioration accompanied by seizures, ataxia, and spasticity begins soon afterwards, and death usually ensues by 10 years of age. These children lack the retinal cherry-red spot, coarse facial features, and visceromegaly of type 1, and the bone changes are mild. The histologic features are similar to those of type 1, except that there is little visceral storage of the GM_1 ganglioside. GM_1 β-galactosidase activity is absent as with type 1, and the two disorders are thought to be allelic. Adult forms (type 3) have been recognized in patients presenting with dysarthria and abnormalities of gait.

Tay-Sachs disease (GM_2 gangliosidosis I, infantile amaurotic idiocy) occurs primarily in Ashkenazi Jews, whose carrier rate for this autosomal recessive trait is approximately 1 in 30 persons. The disease is due to a deficiency in hexosaminidase A, one of the two main forms of the enzyme found in human tissues. GM_2 ganglioside is stored in the brain, but there is no visceral or bone involvement. The first symptoms of psychomotor deterioration appear at 6 to 9 months, and there is a rapid downhill course with blindness, deafness, seizures, and decerebrate rigidity over the next 2 or 3 years. Macrocephaly and a retinal cherry-red spot are commonly observed. Death occurs by 4 years of age.

GM₂ glangliosidosis II (Sandhoff's disease) is clinically almost identical to Tay-Sachs disease. It results from a deficiency of both hexosaminidases A and B. In addition to the storage of GM_2 ganglioside in the brain, these children also have accumulation of globoside in neuronal and visceral tissues; hexosaminidase B catalyzes the first step in globoside breakdown. This disorder has no particular ethnic predilection.

Trihexosyl ceramidosis (Fabry's disease, angiokeratoma corporis diffusum) has an X-linked inheritance; it is the only sphingolipidosis not transmitted as an autosomal recessive trait. In the hemizygous male, corneal opacities and burning pain in the lower extremities develop during early childhood. Raised red-purple skin lesions (angiokeratomas) distributed over the lower trunk and upper thighs usually appear during the second decade. Pinpoint spots may also be seen on the lips of some patients. Kidney failure is the most foreboding manifestation during adulthood, but cardiac disease may occur as well. Patients usually die in their forties. The clinical picture is variable in the hererozygote female; corneal lesions are often observed together with varying degrees of the other features. Trihexosyl ceramide is found in large amounts in nearly all tissues, as well as in the plasma and urine. This accumulation is due to a deficiency of trihexosyl α-galactosidase A.

Gaucher's disease (glucosyl ceramidosis) is the most common of the sphingolipidoses. There are three distinct forms that differ in the age of onset and degree of central nervous system involvement. They are all characterized by varying degrees of marked splenomegaly, hepatomegaly, osteoporotic erosion of the skeleton, anemia, thrombocytopenia, and accumulation of lipid in cells of the reticuloendothelial system. Type I, the adult or chronic nonneuronopathic type, is by far

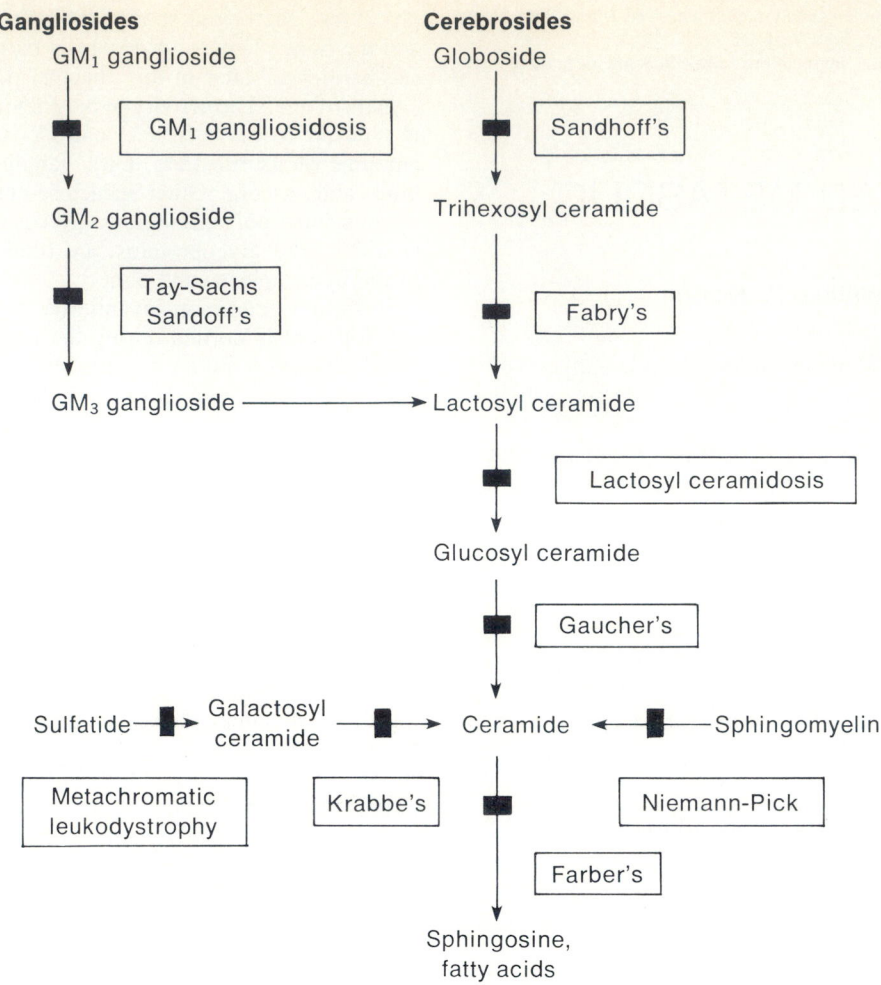

Fig. 195-1   Glycosphingolipid metabolism.

Table 195-1   Glycosphingolipidoses

Disorder	Common name	Inheritance*	Enzyme defect
GM₁ gangliosidosis	Landing's diseae	AR	β-Galactosidase
GM₂ gangliosidosis I	Tay-Sachs disease	AR	Hexosaminidase A
GM₂ gangliosidosis II	Sandhoff's disease	AR	Hexosaminidase A, B
Trihexosyl ceramidosis	Fabry's disease	XL	α-Galactosidase A
Glucosyl ceramidosis	Gaucher's disease	AR	β-Glucosidase
Sphingomyelinosis	Niemann-Pick disease	AR	Sphingomyelinase
Sulfatide lipidosis	Metachromatic leukodystrophy	AR	Arylsulfatase A
Globoid cell leukodystrophy	Krabbe's disease	AR	β-Galactosidase
Lipogranulomatosis	Farber's disease	AR	Ceramidase

*AR, autosomal recessive; XL, X-linked recessive.

the most common and is seen primarily in Ashkenazi Jews. It appears during late childhood or early adulthood with splenomegaly, bone pain, and easy bruising. In adults the major problems are related to skeletal involvement (for example, pain and fractures) and hemorrhagic episodes. Lung involvement may predispose patients to pneumonia, a frequent cause of death. However, the disease is compatible with a normal life span.

Type 2, the acute neuronopathic or infantile form of Gaucher's disease, appears during infancy with loss of neurologic function, spasticity, and enlargement of the liver and spleen. Psychomotor deterioration progresses, and death usually ensues by 2 years of age. The even rarer type 3 juvenile or subacute neuronopathic form has many of the same features as type 2, but the course is more protracted. The onset is usually during the latter part of the year, and death occurs near the end of the first decade.

The clinical features in all forms of Gaucher's disease result from the widespread deposition of glucosyl ceramide owing to a deficiency of glucocerebroside β-glucosidase (glucocerebrosidase). In contrast to most other glycosphingolipidoses, the degree of enzyme deficiency correlates with the severity of the disease. Patients with type 2 have less than 10% normal activity, those with type 3 about 15%, and those with type 1 up to 40%.

Sphingomyelin lipidosis (Neimann-Pick disease) is a group

of disorders characterized by the storage of sphingomyelin and other lipids throughout the body. Although five types have been identified, over 80% of patients have type A. In this acute neuronopathic form, hepatosplenomegaly and central nervous system dysfunction are evident by 6 months of age. The cherry-red spot of the retina is often seen, as are anemia, thrombocytopenia, osteoporosis, and a brownish yellow discoloration of the skin. Death usually occurs by 3 years of age.

In type B, the chronic nonneuronopathic type, symptoms develop somewhat later and the course is more protracted. There is no neurologic impairment, but pulmonary infiltration is common. Type C, the chronic neuronopathic form, resembles type A, but the onset usually occurs during the second year and the children live to between 5 and 15 years of age. Type D is similar to type C, but all patients with type D have a common ancestry in Nova Scotia. The adult form, type E, is characterized by a later onset and mild chronic symptoms without neurologic involvement.

Pathologically there is an accumulation of sphingomyelin throughout the reticuloendothelial system in all types and in the brain in the neuronopathic forms. Cholesterol and other glycolipids may also be stored. A deficiency of sphingomyelinase has been demonstrated in types A, B, and C, but the defect remains unknown in types D and E.

Sulfatide lipidosis, often called *metachromatic leukodystrophy* (MLD), comprises three closely related disorders that are characterized by the accumulation of sulfur-containing glycosphingolipids. The most common is the late infantile form in which gait disturbances and incoordination develop during the second year. Seizures, spasticity, optic atrophy, incontinence, and dementia are seen subsequently, and death intervenes by 10 years of age. The juvenile form appears during the second decade with personality changes and mental deterioration. Many of the features of the infantile form eventually develop, and death usually comes during the thirties. The adult onset of psychosis and dementia with the late appearance of neurologic signs characterizes the very rare adult type of MLD.

In all three forms sulfatide is stored in the liver, gallbladder, kidney, peripheral nerves, and especially the central nervous system white matter. Histologically it is seen as metachromatically staining cytoplasmic inclusions. The urinary sediment also stains metachromatically. In addition, there is diffuse demyelination and gliosis in both the central and peripheral nervous systems. The sulfatide storage is due to a deficiency of arylsulfatase A, one of two lysosomal arylsulfatases. Interesting, the other, arylsulfatase B, is deficient in the Maroteaux-Lamy syndrome (muopolysaccharidosis type VI), which has clinical features quite distinct from MLD. There is also a condition known as multiple sulfatase deficiency (mucosulfatidoses) in which both arylsulfatases A and B and a microsomal arylsulfatase C are deficient. This condition has features of both MLD (late infantile form) and the mucopolysaccharidoses (see the following discussion).

Krabbe's disease (globoid cell leukodystrophy) affects primarily central nervous system white matter. The clinical picture is that of progressive psychomotor retardation, rigidity, seizures, and optic atrophy beginning between 4 and 6 months of age, with death occurring before 2 years of age. At autopsy almost total absence of myelin, severe gliosis, and the abundance of "globoid cells" are found in the cerebral white matter. The absence of activity of galactocerebroside β-galactosidase has been observed.

Farber's disease (lipogranulomatosis) is due to the deficiency of ceramidase. It is apparent during infancy and is manifested by hoarseness, painful and swollen joints, subcutaneous and periarticular nodules, growth retardation, pulmonary infiltration, and progressive neurologic dysfunction. The involved tissues show infiltration by macrophages and foam cells that form granulomas. There is also lipid storage in neurons.

Mucopolysaccharidoses

The mucopolysaccharidoses (MPS) are a heterogeneous group of disorders characterized by the widespread accumulation of mucopolysaccharides (glycosaminoglycans) throughout the body. Attached to a core protein, these substances normally comprise the so-called ground substance of connective tissue matrix. They consist of polymers of repeating disaccharide units composed of alternating uronic acid and hexosamine (often sulfated) residues. Four major mucopolysaccharides are found in human tissues: chondroitin sulfate (CS), dermatan sulfate (DS), heparan sulfate (HS), and keratan sulfate (KS). In normal tissues degradation of the polymyers proceeds by the sequential removal of the terminal residue by lysosomal exoglycosidases and sulfatases. If one of the enzymes is missing, degradation is blocked and the substance accumulates within the lysosomes. Since the enzymes are specific for particular residues that are frequently components of different mucopolysaccharides, more than one of these compounds often accumulates from such a block. There is, however, some partial breakdown of these polymers into smaller fragments by lysosomal endoglycosidases such as hyaluronidase; it is these fragments that are excreted in the urine.

The recognized mucopolysaccharidoses are listed in Table 195-2. Despite the variety of different enzyme deficiencies that are responsible for these disorders, there is a considerable overlap of clinical features. This is due to the ubiquitous nature of these substances in the body. The differences between the disorders, however, probably reflect in part the different distribution of the individual mucopolysaccharides (for example, KS is found predominantly in cartilage) and therefore the location of greatest tissue damage. Most patients with mucopolysaccharide storage disease exhibit varying degrees of coarsening of the facies, enlarged tongue, wide-spaced teeth, limitation of joint motion, and skeletal changes known as dysotosis multiplex (enlarged or J-shaped sella turcica, widened ribs, beaking of the lumbar vertebrae, and short, broad, poorly modeled tubular bones of the limbs). Corneal clouding, mental retardation, and liver and spleen enlargement are common. Except for Hunter's syndrome (MPS II), which is X linked, all of these disorders are transmitted as autosomal recessive traits. Although there is no successful treatment for any of the conditions, prenatal diagnosis is available for most of them.

MPS I implies a deficiency of α-L-iduronidase and the resultant tissue storage and urinary excretion of DS and HS. Two clinical forms are recognized. *MPS I H, Hurler's syndrome,* is the prototype of the mucopolysaccharidoses. Large size, stiff joints, thoracolumbar kyphosis, and mild coarsening of facial features are noted between 6 and 12 months of age. During the second year, liver and spleen enlargement, corneal clouding, cardiac murmurs, macrocephaly, umbilical hernia, dwarfism, and grotesque facial features appear. Skeletal roentgenograms show the typical changes of dysostosis multiplex. Beyond 2 years of age mental and physical deterioration progresses, and death occurs between 6 and 10 years of age.

In the mild variety *MPS I S, Scheie's syndrome,* corneal clouding with retinal degeneration and glaucoma, clawhand, carpal tunnel syndrome, and frequently aortic regurgitation develop in midchildhood. The facies are moderately coarse and intelligence is normal. Life expectancy is well into adulthood

Table 195-2   Mucopolysaccharidoses

Designation	Eponym	Inheritance*	Urinary excretion†	Enzyme defect
MPS I H	Hurler	AR	DS, HS	α-L-Iduronidase
MPS I S‡	Scheie	AR	DS, HS	α-L-Iduronidase
MPS I H/S	Hurler-Scheie	AR	DS, HS	α-L-Iduronidase
MPS II severe	Hunter	XL	DS, HS	Iduronate sulfatase
MPS II mild	Hunter	XL	DS, HS	Iduronate sulfatase
MPS III A	Sanfilippo A	AR	HS	Heparan-N-sulfatase
MPS III B	Sanfilippo B	AR	HS	N-Acetyl-α-D-glucosaminidase
MPS III C	Sanfilippo C	AR	HS	Acetyl CoA: α-glucosaminide-N-acetyltransferase
MPS III D	Sanfilippo D	AR	HS	N-acetyl-α-D-glucosaminade-6-sulfatase
MPS IV A	Morquio	AR	KS	Galactosamine-6-sulfate sulfatase
MPS IV B	Morquio	AR	KS	β-galactosidase
MPS V	Vacant			
MPS VI severe	Maroteaux-Lamy	AR	DS	Arylsulfatase B
MPS VI intermediate	Maroteaux-Lamy	AR	DS	Arylsulfatase B
MPS VI mild	Maroteaux-Lamy	AR	DS	Arylsulfatase B
MPS VII	Sly	AR	DS, HS	β-Glucuronidase

*AR, autosomal recessive: XL, X linked.

†DS, dermatan sulfate; HS, heparan sulfate; KS, keratan sulfate.

‡Scheie's syndrome was originally designated MPS V. When the defective enzyme was found to be the same as in Hurler's syndrome, the designation was changed to MPS I S.

and may be normal. A few patients have been described with the biochemical features of MPS I and a clinical phenotype of intermediate severity. They are thought to be genetic compounds, having the combination of Hurler and Scheie genes at the α-L-iduronidase locus (MPS I H/S).

Mild and severe forms of *MPS II, Hunter's syndrome*, are recognized. Both are due to a deficiency of iduronate sulfatase and are X-linked. Boys with the severe form closely resemble children with Hurler's syndrome except that they usually lack corneal clouding and tend to live into the second decade. In addition, deafness is more common. In mild Hunter's syndrome, survival is well into adulthood and intelligence is relatively well preserved.

MPS III, Sanfilippo's syndrome, is a phenotype consisting of severe mental retardation, mild to almost absent physical features of the mucopolysaccharidoses, minimal visceral and skeletal involvement, and excretion of HS in the urine. The screening test for mucopolysacchariduria may be borderline or even negative. Four distinct enzyme deficiencies that produce this phenotype have been identified (Table 195-2). They can be distinguished only by biochemical means. Sanfilippo A syndrome resulting from a deficiency of heparan-N-sulfatase is the most common.

The features of *MPS IV, Morquio's syndrome*, initially resemble those of the other mucopolysaccharidoses, but by mid-childhood a distinct clinical picture emerges. It consists of corneal clouding, severe dwarfism, protruding chest with kyphoscoliosis, gait disturbance, genu valgum, and flat feet. Instability of the cervical spine owing to the combination of hypoplasia of the odontoid process and ligamentous laxity is common, as is aortic regurgitation. Intelligence is probably unaffected, and life expectancy is into the forties.

In general *MPS VI, Maroteaux-Lamy syndrome*, resembles Hurler's syndrome except for delayed onset, longer survival, normal intelligence, and the excretion of only DS. Three clinical forms are recognized. Striking dwarfism, corneal clouding, valvular heart disease, joint stiffness, and contractures, especially involving the hip and knee, characterize the severe form, which becomes apparent between 2 and 4 years of age. Odontoid hypoplasia may be a problem, and death usually supervenes in the third decade. The mild form is manifested by mild skeletal abnormalities, joint stiffness, corneal clouding, aortic stenosis, and survival into adulthood. As expected, the intermediate form shows a phenotype of intermediate severity, and it may represent a genetic compound between the severe and mild forms.

MPS VII, Sly's syndrome, is characterized by mental retardation, visceromegaly, dysostosis multiplex, and a deficiency of β-glucuronidase.

Glycoproteinoses

Glycoproteins are widely distributed cellular components present in neuronal tissues. Neurologic damage may ensue if the lysosomal degradation of glycoproteins is impaired. Sialidosis, fucosidosis, mannosidosis, and aspartylglycosaminuria are examples of disorders resulting from defective glycoprotein degradation. All are quite rare and are thought to be inherited as autosomal recessive traits.

Sialidosis is due to a deficiency of sialidase (neuraminidase). Pathologically there is an accumulation of sialic acid–containing substances. Two clinical forms have been observed. Sialidosis type 1 appears between 8 and 15 years of age with decreasing vision, retinal cherry-red spot, neuropathy, seizures, and progressive myoclonus. These children may have normal intelligence and lack the typical somatic features of lysosomal storage diseases. The patients survive into adulthood. In sialidosis type 2 the phenotype is variable but resembles that seen in children with Hurler's syndrome, that is, corneal clouding, coarse facies, visceromegaly, short stature, joint stiffness, and the roentgenographic changes of dysostosis multiplex. The retinal cherry-red spot is found, and ataxia and mental retardation are common. The onset of this dysmorphic type may occur during the infantile or juvenile period.

Fucosidosis occurs in two forms: type 1, which has a clinical picture similar to Hurler's syndrome, and a milder type 2. Angiokeratomas of the skin similar to those seen in Fabry's disease occur in patients with the latter type. In both types, α-L-fucosidase is deficient and fucose-containing glycolipids are stored in lysosomes. The disorder is rare, and many of the patients have been Italian. Mannosidosis is clinically similar to fucosidosis. Mannose-containing glycolipids are found in many tissues, and the enzyme α-D-mannosidase is deficient. It has both infantile (type I) and milder forms (type II).

Aspartylglycosaminuria is due to a deficiency of aspartylglycosaminidase and is more common in Finland than the United States. The central nervous system is affected, resulting in mental deterioration and ataxia beginning at about 5 years of age. Somatic involvement is mild, and patients may have normal life spans.

Mucolipidosis II (ML II, I-cell disease) and *Mucolipidosis III (ML III, pseudo-Hurler polydystrophy)* are grouped with the glycoproteinoses. Actually they are severe (ML II) and milder (ML III) defects in lysosomal enzyme processing. Deficient activity of UDP-*N*-acetylglucosamine: glycoprotein-*N*-acetylglucosaminyl-phosphotransferase results in the failure to add mannose-6-phosphate to synthesized lysosomal hydrolases. Without this recognition marker, the hydrolases are not incorporated within lysosomes. Since a variety of enzymes are affected, these disorders have features of many storage diseases. In general, ML II resembles Hurler's syndrome and ML III resembles Maroteaux-Lamy syndrome.

Transport disorders

It is recognized that the products of lysosomal degradative processes exit the lysosome via transport systems. Defects in transport result in the accumulation of small molecular weight substances. Cystinosis is the best studied of these disorders in which defective amino acid transport results in the lysosomal storage of cystine. Cystinosis is autosomal recessive and has a spectrum of severity. The most severe form is characterized by growth failure, photophobia, retinopathy, hypothyroidism, renal Fanconi's syndrome, and progressive glomerular damage resulting in renal failure by the end of the first decade of life.

AMINOACIDOPATHIES

The aminoacidopathies result from deficient activity of enzymes that catalyse the normal interconversion and degradation of amino acids. In most cases the disease processes result from the toxic effects of substances that accumulate before the metabolic block. Sometimes, however, a deficiency of the product of the blocked reaction is responsible. In general these disorders are rare, are inherited as recessive traits, and may be diagnosed prenatally. Specific treatment is often possible.

Aromatic amino acid disorders

Disorders of aromatic amino acid metabolism are shown in Fig. 195-2. *Phenylketonuria* (PKU) is the most common aminoacidopathy, occurring at a rate of approximately 1 in 15,000 live births. It has an autosomal recessive inheritance and results from reduced activity of hepatic phenylalanine hydroxylase. Phenylalanine accumulates in the plasma, and its keto acid metabolites (such as phenylpyruvic acid) spill over into the urine. Infants are normal at birth, but if they are untreated, vomiting, poor growth, seizures, and mental retardation develop. Pigmentation is usually reduced because melanin is deficient, and eczema is common. The treatment consists of a diet low in phenylalanine. If instituted early and strictly adhered to, this allows normal development.

In addition to classic PKU, several variants have been identified. Some children have persistent mildly elevated plasma phenylalanine levels. Others show only a transient elevation in phenylalanine levels; this is thought to reflect immaturity of the normal hydroxylating enzyme system. Normal development without treatment can be expected in patients with these variant conditions.

Some children with the characteristic features of PKU have been found to have progressive neurologic deterioration despite adequate dietary treatment. These children have defects in the synthesis of tetrahydrobiopterin, a cofactor for phenylalanine

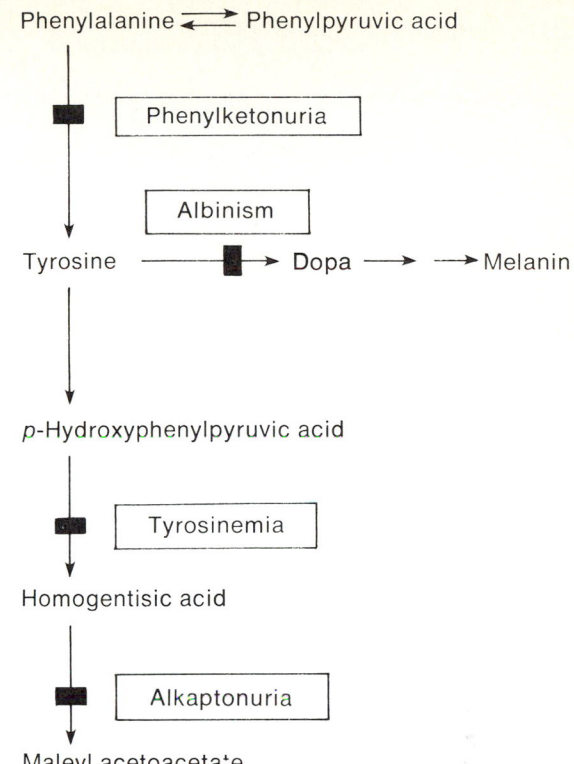

Fig. 195-2 Aromatic amino acid metabolism.

hydroxylase. Tetrahydrobiopterin is a cofactor for a number of hydroxylation reactions, and its absence leads to inadequate neurotransmitter levels. Therapy consists of replacement of these neurotransmitters and phenylalanine restriction.

Disturbances of tyrosine metabolism occur in at least three conditions. Thirty percent of premature infants and 10% of term infants suffer from a transient elevation of tyrosine (and phenylalanine) in the neonatal period. This is thought to be due to immaturity of the enzyme parahydroxyphenylpyruvic acid oxidase. Treatment with high doses of vitamin C, a cofactor for this enzyme, may be helpful.

Oculocutaneous tyrosinemia (tyrosinemia II) is characterized by elevated tyrosine levels, skin rashes, corneal irritation and ulceration, behavioral disturbances, and, frequently, mental retardation. The disorder is a consequence of defective hepatic tyrosine aminotransferase. Hepatorenal tyrosinemia (tyrosinemia I) is marked by progressive hepatic damage and impaired renal proximal tubular function (renal Fanconi's syndrome). Decreased activity of fumaryl acetoacetate hydrolase appears to be responsible. The disorder causes either early death from hepatic failure or a pattern of progressive hepatic cirrhosis. Both forms of tyrosinemia are treated with diets low in phenylalanine and tyrosine.

Alkaptonuria is an autosomal recessive disorder that results from deficient activity of the enzyme homogentisic acid oxidase. The manifestations (degenerative arthritis of the spine, knees, hips, and shoulders) result from the deposition of blue-black ochronotic pigment (a polymer of homogentisic acid) in connective tissues, especially cartilage. The pigment can be seen in the cornea, nasal cartilage, and pinna.

Sulfur-containing amino acid disorders

Although the finding of homocystine in the urine occurs in several disorders, including the deficiency of *N*-5, 10-methylene tetrahydrofolate reductase and defects in the ab-

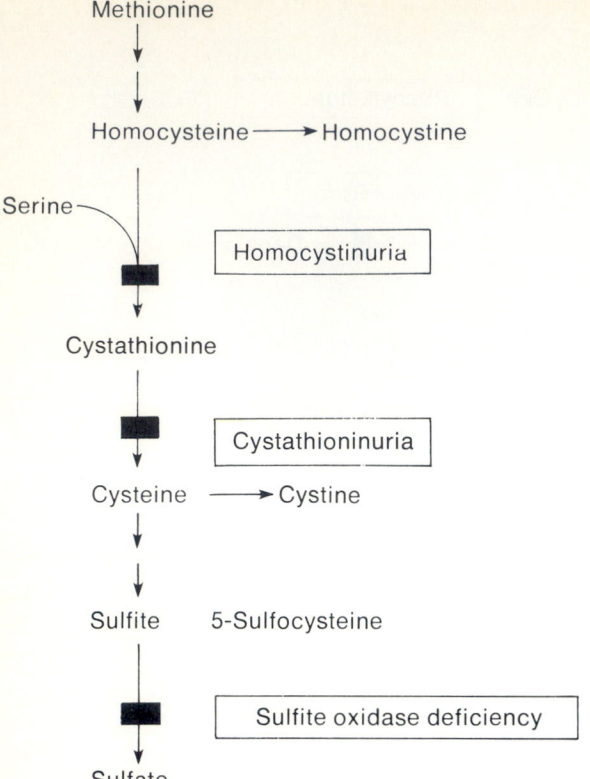

Methionine

Homocysteine ⟶ Homocystine

Serine

Homocystinuria

Cystathionine

Cystathioninuria

Cysteine ⟶ Cystine

Sulfite   5-Sulfocysteine

Sulfite oxidase deficiency

Sulfate

Fig. 195-3   Sulfur-containing amino acid metabolism.

sorption and metabolism of vitamin B_{12}, the term "homocystinuria" usually refers to a specific autosomal recessive condition resulting from a deficiency of the enzyme cystathionine synthetase. The patients resemble those with Marfan's syndrome because of their tall stature, kyphoscoliosis, pectus excavatum, and dislocated lenses, but they lack joint laxity and valvular heart disease. Moreover, osteopororsis, mental retardation, and recurrent thromboembolic phenomena occur frequently in homocystinuria. The enzyme defect interferes with conversion of methionine to cystine and results in the accumulation of homocystine (Fig. 195-3). The majority of the clinical manifestations of homocystinuria are thought to result from the disruptive effects of homocystine on collagen cross-linking.

Cystathioninuria is another rare autosomal recessive disorder of sulfur-containing amino acids. It is due to the deficiency of cystathionase and is characterized by the presence of large amounts of cystathionine in the urine and plasma. The clinical features are variable. In most affected individuals the metabolic abnormalities are corrected by high doses of vitamin B_6.

Sulfite oxidase deficiency has been observed in a child with severe developmental delay, dislocated lenses, and the excretion of large amounts of the amino acid 5-sulfocysteine in the urine.

Branched-chain amino acid disorders

A number of disorders involve defective breakdown of branched-chain amino acids (Fig. 195-4). All are characterized by the accumulation of organic acids. Their clinical features are quite similar and include ketoacidosis (often with hyperammonemia) vomiting, flaccidity (sometimes spasticity), seizures, coma, leukopenia, thrombocytopenia, and mental retardation. All are inherited as autosomal recessive traits, and prenatal diagnosis is available for many.

Maple syrup urine disease (MSUD) is the most common. It results from defective decarboxylation of the keto derivatives of leucine, isoleucine, and valine; these substances spill over into the urine, imparting a distinctive odor. The infants usually become symptomatic and often die during the first week of life unless a diet restricted in these amino acids is imposed. In milder forms the symptoms occur episodically and survival is prolonged at least into childhood; one type shows a dramatic response to thiamine, the cofactor for the decarboxylase enzyme.

Propionic acidemia results from a deficiency of propionyl-CoA carboxylase. Usually infants have an overwhelming illness that follows protein feeding and is characterized by severe ketoacidosis, hyperammonemia, and hypoglycemia. The latter two metabolic derangements are thought to result from interference with ureagenesis and gluconeogenesis. In a few children, however, acidosis is intermittent and is brought on by acute infection or excessive dietary protein. Rarely patients show clinical improvement following the administration of biotin.

The conversion of L-methylmalonyl CoA to succinyl CoA requires the participatioon of methylmalonyl CoA mutase and 5-deoxyadenosyl cobalamin, an active metabolite of vitamin B_{12}. *Methylmalonic acidemia* is due to a defect in this conversion. Some forms respond to treatment with high doses of vitamin B_{12}, others are treated with protein restriction.

As noted in Fig. 195-4, several other defects in branched-chain amino acid degradation have been described. They are rare, and genetic heterogeneity has been observed in most. They include isovaleric acidemia owing to isovaleryl CoA dehydrogenase deficiency, β-methylcrotonylglycinuria resulting from β-methylcrotonyl CoA carboxylase deficiency, and α-methyl-β-hydroxybutyric and α-methylacetoacetic aciduria owing to α-methylacetoacetyl CoA β-ketothiolase deficiency.

UREA CYCLE DISORDERS

The urea cycle is responsible for removing of ammonia that results from protein degradation. Inherited deficiencies of enzymes in this cycle have been identified (Fig. 195-5). Hyperammonemia is common to all disorders. In general all the syndromes exhibit neurologic dysfunction and protein intolerance; however, the severity may range from an overwhelming illness with seizures, stupor, and coma occurring after the beginning of milk feeding to episodic symptoms associated only with acute infections or high dietary protein intake. Mental retardation and hepatomegaly are common in these survivors, however. Therapy consists of dietary protein restriction, arginine supplementation when appropriate, and the exploitation of alternative routes of nitrogen excretion using sodium benzoate.

Argininosuccinic aciduria is the most common of the urea cycle disorders. It is due to a deficiency of the enzyme argininosuccinase. Three clinical forms have been established: a neonatal form with lethargy, seizures, and early death; an infantile form with vomiting, hepatomegaly, failure to thrive, and an onset during the first few weeks of life; and a chronic form with seizures, ataxia, mental retardation, and peculiar short, brittle, friable hair. All three are inherited as autosomal recessive traits and are probably allelic mutations.

The deficiency of ornithine transcarbamylase (OTCD) is an X-linked disorder that is lethal in boys. The features are variable in affected girls; some demonstrate the usual neurologic symptoms and others are essentially asympto-

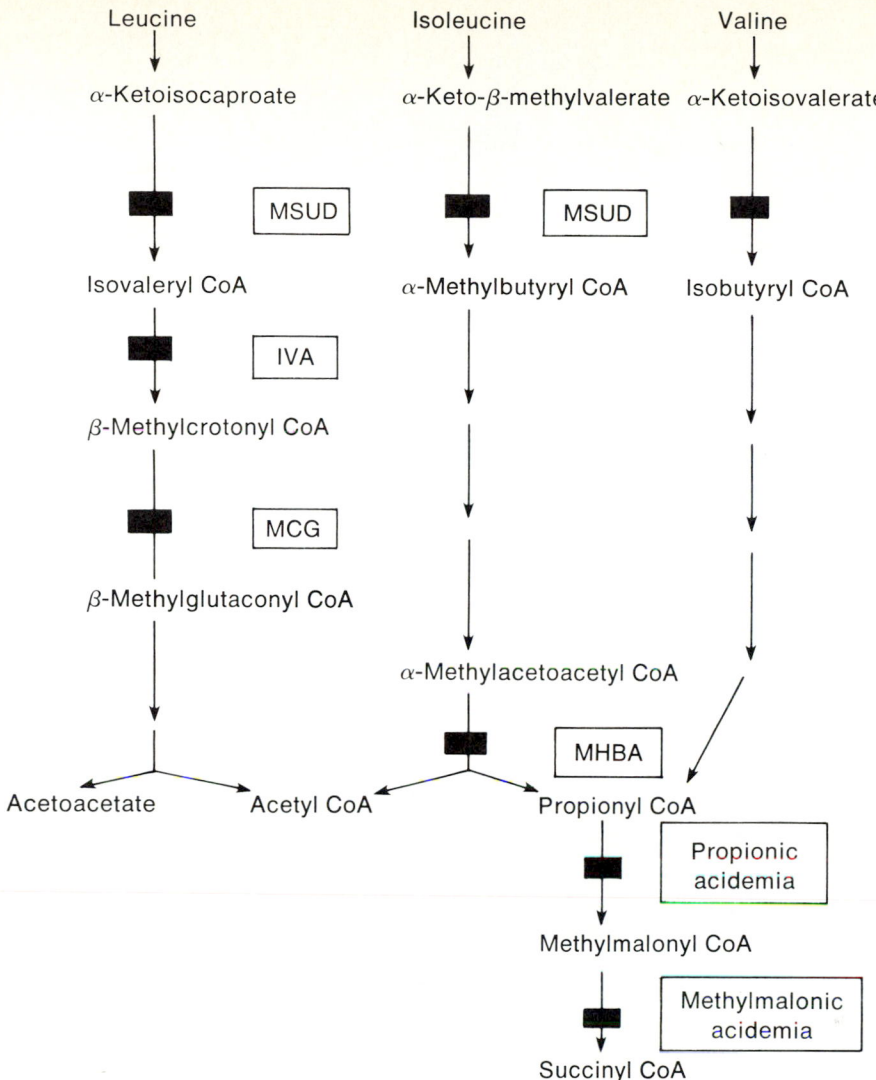

Fig. 195-4   Branched-chain amino acid metabolism. *MSUD*, maple syrup urine disease; *IVA*, isovaleric acidemia. *MCG*, methylcrotonylglycinuria; *MHBA*, methylhydroxybutyric and methylacetoacetic aciduria.

matic except during periods of stress or high protein intake.

At least three varieties of citrullinemia are recognized. The first is lethal in the neonatal period. Neurologic symptoms, hepatomegaly, and osteoporosis develop during the first year of life in the second. The third is apparently benign. They are ue to a deficiency of argininosuccinic acid synthetase and have an autosomal recessive inheritance.

A few patients have been reported to have deficiencies of carbamyl phosphate synthetase and arginase. The first enzyme is responsible that trapping free ammonia and the other for cleaving urea from arginine to produce ornithine. Both deficiencies are autosomal recessive conditions.

Several biochemical defects in amino acid metabolism have been identified that appear to be of little clinical importance. In each case the precursors to the metabolic blocks accumulate in the blood and often are found in the urine. The disorders in this category include histidinemia owing to a lack of histidinase, hyperprolinemia owing to a deficiency of either proline oxidase or β-1-pyrroline-5-carboxylic acid dehydrogenase, hydroxyprolinemia resulting from the absence of hydroxyproline oxidase, and possible lysinuria owing to a deficiency of lysine ketoglutarate reductase. All of these are autosomal recessive traits.

DISORDERS OF NUCLEIC ACID METABOLISM

The *Lesch-Nyhan syndrome* is an X-linked disorder of purine metabolism. Affected boys are normal at birth, but within a few months progressive choreoathetosis, spasticity, mental retardation, and a peculiar tendency toward self-mutilation develop. Patients have increased production of uric acid and may exhibit all the clinical features of gout including hyperuricemia, gouty arthritis, tophi, urinary tract stones, crystalluria, and nephropathy. Death usually comes during adolescence. The disorder is due to a deficiency of hypoxanthine-guanine phosphoribosyltransferase (HGPRT), the enzyme that normally catalyzes the transfer of 5-phosphoribosyl-1-pyrophosphate (PRPP) to guanine and hypoxanthine to form their respective ribonucleotides. The deficiency of HGPRT is associated with a high level of intracellular PRPP, which contributes to increased de novo purine synthesis and ultimately to increased uric acid production. Treatment with allopurinol reduces uric acid production and its sequelae but has little effect on the central nervous system abnormalities. Measurement of HGPRT activity in hair follicles (which are largely clonal in origin with regard to the X chromosome) has been successful for detecting carrier females.

Another disorder of purine metabolism is *xanthinuria*, an

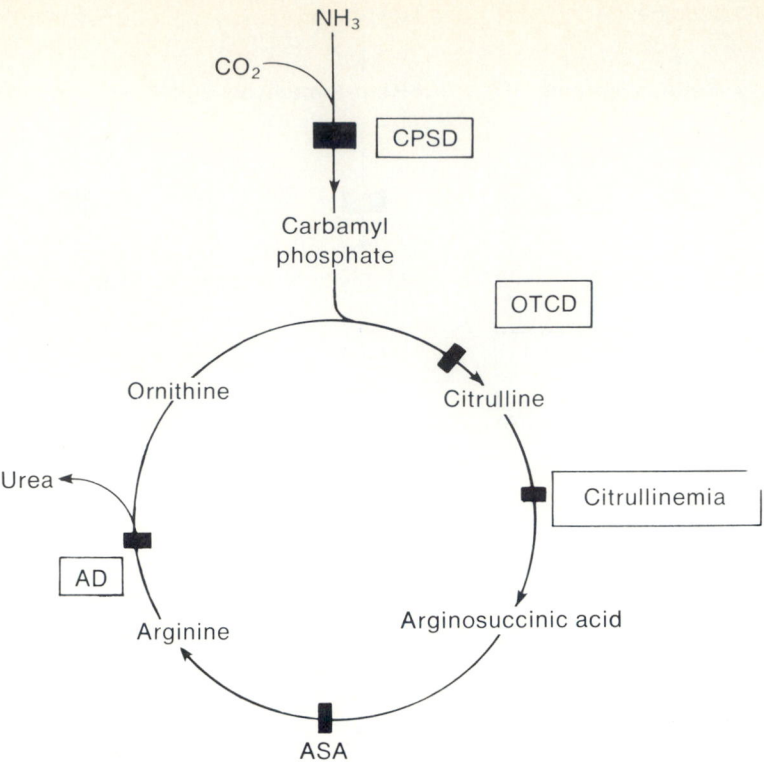

Fig. 195-5 Urea cycle. *CPSD*, carbamyl phosphate synthetase deficiency; *OTCD*, ornithine transcarbamylase deficiency; *ASA*, arginosuccinic aciduria; *AD*, arginase deficiency.

autosomal recessive disorder caused by a deficiency of xanthine oxidase. This enzyme is responsible for the last two steps in purine breakdown, the oxidation of hypoxanthine to xanthine and of xanthine to uric acid. In most patients the disorder is benign and is characterized by low levels of uric acid in the serum and urine and a high urinary excretion of hypoxanthine and xanthine. The latter may result in xanthine stones, in which case high fluid intake to maintain a large urinary volume is indicated.

Immune deficiency is associated with reduced activity of at least two enzymes involved in purine metabolism. In both cases the trait shows autosomal recessive inheritance and the mechanisms responsible for the immunodeficiency are not understood. Children with *adenosine deaminase deficiency* have profound lymphopenia and absent or very low levels of immunoglobulins, and in general they show evidence of combined B- and T-cell dysfunction. Some of these patients also have skeletal abnormalities resembling those seen in certain types of dwarfism, suggesting a common link between proliferating cartilage and lymphoid cells. If untreated, these children die of overwhelming infection; however, repeated transfusions with frozen red blood cells (as a source of the enzyme) or more recently histocompatibility-matched bone marrow transplantation has met with success in some patients.

Impaired immunity restricted primarily to T-lymphocyte dysfunction is associated with a deficiency of purine *nucleoside phosphorylase*. The infections tend to be less severe and most often involve viruses.

Orotic aciduria is an autosomal recessive disorder of pyrimidine metabolism. It is characterized by growth failure, hypochromic anemia associated with megaloblastic changes in the bone marrow, and the excessive urinary excretion of orotic acid. Two clinically identical forms can be distinguished biochemically. Type 1 results from the deficiency of two sequential enzymes involved in the conversion of orotic acid to uridine-

5-phosphate. The enzymes are orotate phosphoribosyl transferase and orotidine 5′-phosphate decarboxylase. In type 2 only the decarboxylase is deficient. Both are inherited as autosomal recessive traits. Treatment with uridine results in hematologic remission, improvement in growth, and a decrease in urinary orotic acid excretion.

DISORDERS OF MINERAL METABOLISM

Wilson's disease is an autosomal recessive disorder of copper metabolism. The clinical manifestations usually develop during adolescence or early adulthood but may not appear until the forties. Nearly half the patients have neurologic symptoms such as spasticity, rigidity, dysarthria, tremor, and psychiatric disturbances, and about 40% have hepatic abnormalities such as hepatomegaly, cirrhosis, and hepatic failure. In addition, renal tubular dysfunction often develops during the course of the disease. Plasma levels of copper and its binding protein ceruloplasmin are low. In contrast, an excess of copper is found in the brain (especially in the basal ganglia), liver, kidney, and cornea (Kayser-Fleischer rings). The basic defect is unknown. If untreated, Wilson's disease is fatal, but therapy to reduce total body copper is often successful. The mainstay of treatment is penicillamine, which enhances urinary copper excretion.

Menkes' kinky hair syndrome is another disorder of copper metabolism. It is transmitted as an X-linked recessive trait and is characterized by sparse kinky hair that microscopically shows pili torti, progressive neurologic degeneration, metaphyseal irregularities of the long bones, hypothermia, and generalized arterial occlusive disease.

CONNECTIVE TISSUE DISORDERS

The so-called connective tissues of the body, including skin, bone, teeth, cartilage, ligament, tendon, fascia, joint capsule, sclera, and elements of the heart and blood vessels, are affected by many inherited disorders. In some conditions such as ami-

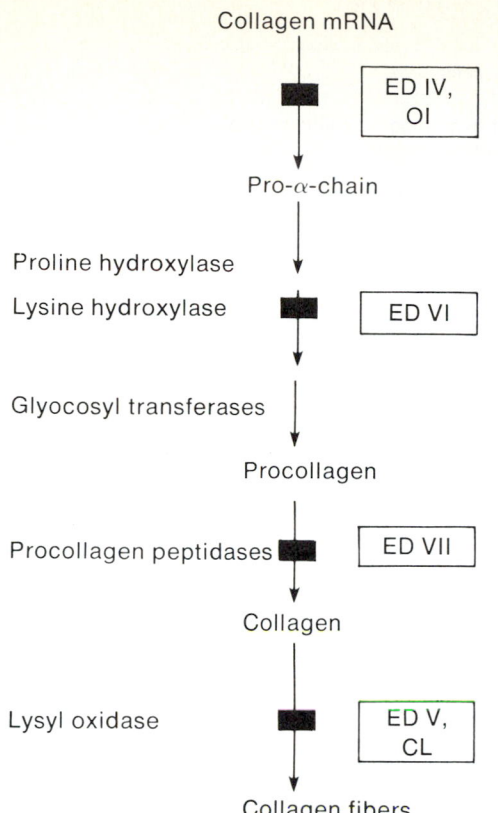

Fig. 195-6   Type I collagen synthesis. *EDS*, Ehlers-Danlos syndrome; *OI*, osteogenesis imperfecta.

noacidopathies, connective tissue metabolism is altered as part of a generalized metabolic derangement. In other disorders such as mucopolysaccharidoses and mucolipidoses, it is disturbed by the lysosomal storage of material in connective tissue cells. In yet other situations primary defects in connective tissue metabolism have been identified or at least strongly suspected. Of those found, most have involved the biosynthesis of collagen, one of the three major components of connective tissue matrices. Collagen and the other two components, elastic fibers and mucopolysaccharides ("ground substance," glycosaminoglycans), are elaborated by a number of cells including fibroblasts, osteoblasts, odontoblasts, and chondroblasts.

Collagen is actually a family of genetically distinct fibrous proteins that provide tensile strength and other attributes to connective tissues. Each collagen type has its own distinct composition and tissue distribution. For example, type I is found in skin, bone, tendons, fascia, and dentin; types II, IX, and X in cartilage; type III in blood vessels and skin; type IV in basement membrane, and types V and VI in most interstitial tissues. The biosynthesis of the collagens is complex. In general it involves the synthesis of a precursor molecule (pro α chain), which is sequentially modified by hydroxylation of many proline and lysine residues, glycosylation of certain hydroxylysines, and folding of these chains to form a triple helical structure (procollagen). Short segments are removed from both ends of the helix as the procollagen is secreted from the cell to become collagen. Additional modifications lead to the formation of intramollecular and intermolecular cross-linkages that characterize the polymeric forms of collagen found in tissues. Variations in this posttranslational modification scheme contribute to the diversity of organization and function displayed by collagens in different tissues. The biosynthesis of type I collagen is best understood, and several abnormalities

in the scheme have been identified (Fig. 195-6). Clinical abnormalities of connective tissues can result from abnormalities in other constituents such as elastin, but in these situations the disease process is not nearly as well understood.

Marfan's syndrome is the prototype of inherited connective tissue disorders. It is an autosomal dominant trait and occurs in all races. Tall stature with disproportionately long, thin limbs, especially distally (arachnodactyly), is the major skeletal feature, but dolichocephaly, pectus excavatum, pigeon breast, high-arched palate, and prognathism also occur. Laxity of joint capsules, ligaments, tendons, and fascia results in generalized joint hypermobility and kyphoscoliosis. The major ocular manifestations are myopia, retinal detachment, and ectopia lentis.

Nearly two thirds of patients with Marfan's syndrome have evidence of cardiovascular involvement. Areas receiving the greatest hemodynamic pulsatile stress, such as the aortic ring and ascending aorta, show the most damage. Usually aortic ring dilation occurs first, producing aortic regurgitation. It is soon followed by progressive widening of the ascending aorta, often accompanied by dissection and even rupture. Aortic dilation and its complications lead to death in 80% of patients dying of the syndrome. Mitral regurgitation owing to redundancy of the chordae tendineae is very common and may contribute to congestive heart failure. These patients have an increased susceptibility to bacterial endocarditis.

The phenotypic expression of Marfan's syndrome varies widely. Some patients exhibit the "classic findings" of the syndrome, whereas others are only very mildly affected. At the present time it is not clear if the syndrome is a single entity or more like several similar but distinct disorders. The basic defect remains unknown, although an abnormality in either collagen or elastin is suspected. Treatment consists of prophylactic antibiotics for dental extraction, hormonal induction of premature puberty to lessen the kyphoscoliosis, and possibly catecholamine-blocking agents such as propranolol to diminish left ventricular contractility and thus reduce the hemodynamic stress on the ascending aorta.

The *Ehlers-Danlos syndromes* (EDS) are a group of conditions characterized by hypermobility of joints, hyperextensibility of skin, and increased tissue friability. EDS are currently classified into nine types, and heterogeneity is recognized within several of the types (Table 195-3). The gravis type, EDS I, is characterized by generalized severe joint hypermobility. Musculoskeletal deformities such as pes planus may occur. Skin hyperextensibility and easy bruising are severe, and the increased fragility leads to skin splitting and subsequent "cigarette-paper" scarring, particularly on the forehead, elbows, knees, and shins. Excessive bleeding after dental extraction is not uncommon. Varicose veins are frequent, as are molluscoid pseudotumors and subcutaneous calcified spheroids. Generalized tissue friability may complicate postsurgical or posttraumatic wound healing, as reflected by the premature rupture of fetal membranes.

The mitis type, EDS II, resembles EDS I but is milder. Joint laxity is often limited to the hands and feet, and cutaneous involvement is minimal. There is a slight tendency to bruising but little scar formation. Varicose veins are uncommon and tissue friability is rare. Severe hypermobility of all joints, usually without musculoskeletal deformities, characterizes EDS III, the benign hypermobility type. Skin changes are minimal. The arterial, ecchymotic, or Sack's type, EDS IV, is the most malignant owing to the tendency to spontaneous rupture of large and intermediate arteries and bowel perforation. The skin is very thin and bruises easily; underlying veins are prominent, but stretchability is not a major feature.

Table 195-3   Ehlers-Danlos syndromes

Classification	Type	Inheritance*	Clinical features	Basic defect
I	Gravis	AD	Generalized severe joint hypermobility, skin hyperextensibility, easy bruisability, molluscoid pseudotumors, subcutaneous spheroids, poor wound healing, premature rupture of fetal membranes	Unknown
II	Mitis	AD	Similar to EDS I but milder, joint laxity limited to hands and feet, little cutaneous involvement and tissue friability	Unknown
III	Benign hypermobility	AD	Severe hypermobility of all joints	Unknown
IV	Arterial, ecchymotic, Sack's	AD/AR	Spontaneous rupture of large arteries, perforation of bowel, thin skin with prominent underlying veins	Reduced synthesis of type III collagen
V	X linked	XL	Marked hyperextensibility of skin, minimal joint hypermobility	Deficiency of lysyl oxidase
VI	Ocular	AR	Severe scoliosis, moderate joint involvement, ocular fragility with scleral rupture or retinal detachment or both	Deficiency of lysyl hydroxylase
VII	Arthrochalasis multiplex congenita	AR	Short stature, generalized joint hypermobility with multiple subluxations, abnormal facies	Defective cleavage of collagen propeptides
VIII	Periodontal	AD	Mild to moderate skin hyperextensibility and joint hypermobility, marked skin friability, generalized periodontitis	Unknown
IX	Vacant			
X	Fibronectin defect	AR	Skin hyperextensibility, joint hypermobility, easy bruisability, petichiae, striae, defective platelet aggregation	Unknown
XI	Vacant			

*AD, autosomal dominant; AR, autosomal recessive; XL, X linked.

Table 195-4   OI syndromes

Type	Age at presentation	Inheritance*	Features
I	Newborn to adult	AD	Bone fragility, blue sclerae, deafness (dentinogenesis imperfecta uncommon)
II	Newborn	AD	Usually lethal in neonatal period
III	Newborn to childhood	AD/AR	Progressive deformities of spine and limbs, normal sclerae, dentinogenesis imperfecta relatively common
IV	Newborn to adult	AD	Bone fragility, normal sclerae, dentinogenesis imperfecta (deafness uncommon)

*AD, autosomal dominant; AR, autosomal recessive.

The X-linked type, EDS V, manifests only minimal joint hypermobility in contrast to marked hyperextensibility of the skin. Cutaneous bruisability and fragility are moderately increased. The ocular type, EDS VI, is characterized by severe scoliosis and ocular fragility in addition to moderate joint and skin involvement. Corneoscleral rupture or retinal detachment may occur after minor trauma. Short stature and generalized joint hypermobility are characteristic of EDS VII. Subluxations of hips, knees, elbows, and feet are common, and affected infants are floppy. Skin stretchability and bruisability are moderately increased. Abnormal facies, including hypertelorism, epicanthic folds, and scooped-out midfacies, may be part of the disorder. The major features of EDS VIII include generalized severe periodontitis in addition to mild to moderate skin hyperextensibility and joint hypermobility and marked skin friability. EDS X is characterized by soft hyperextensible skin, easy bruisability, joint hypermobility, dystrophic scarring,

striae distensae, and petechiae. The designations EDS IX and XI are no longer used because it has been determined that the disorders for which these terms were originally used do not exhibit the cardinal features of the syndrome. Specific abnormalities in collagen biosynthesis have been identified in EDS IV, V, VI, and VII. In EDS IV, which seems to be inherited as an autosomal dominant trait in some families but in an autosomal recessive fashion in others, type III collagen synthesis is diminished. There is reduced activity of lysyl oxidase in EDS V, lysyl hydroxylase in EDS VI, and procollagen peptidase in some patients with EDS VII. A structural defect at the cleavage site of type I collagen for procollagen peptidase has been demonstrated in other cases of EDS VII. Abnormal platelet aggregation, which is corrected with fibronectin, has been identified in EDS X, but it is not known if this is the primary defect. The basic defects have not been identified in EDS I, II, III, and VIII.

The treatment varies according to the type. In general, patients should avoid trauma and wear protective padding over bony prominences. Particular care should be taken during surgical, dental, and obstetric procedures.

Cutis laxa is characterized by excessive loose skin over the entire body. The skin is extensible, but in contrast to EDS it does not return to place on release, nor is there increased bruisability or friability. Joint hypermobility is usually not a feature. Both autosomal dominant and recessive forms are reported. Hernias, pulmonary emphysema, and diverticuli of the gastrointestinal and genitourinary tracts leading to early death occur in the recessive type, whereas in the dominant form involvement is limited to the skin.

Two related disorders of copper transport have been identified. The *occipital horn syndrome* is a rare X-linked disorder that has been previously called EDS IX and X-linked cutis laxa. Its features include bony protuberances in the occipital region, hypermobile joints, osteomalacia, chronic diarrhea, and bladder diverticulae. Decreased serum copper and ceruloplasmin levels have been observed. *Menkes' syndrome* is characterized by lax skin, joint hypermobility, vascular rupture,

Table 195-5   Partial list of chondrodysplasias

Disorder	Inheritance*	Age at diagnosis	Major clinical features	Oral manifestations	Complications
Achondroplasia	AD	Birth	Short limbs, bowed legs, stubby fingers, bulging forehead, sunken face	Malocclusion, overcrowding	Hydrocephalus (infant), spinal cord compression
Hypochondroplasia	AD	Childhood	Similar to achondroplasia but milder (may approach normality)	None	Usually none
Multiple epiphyseal dysplasia†	AD	Childhood to young adulthood	Short limbs	None	Precocious osteoarthritis‡
Spondyloepiphyseal dysplasia congenita	AD	Birth	Short trunk, barrel chest, myopia	Cleft palate	Subluxation of cervical spine owing to odontoid hypoplasia, retinal detachment, precocious osteoarthritis‡
Spondyloepiphyseal dysplasia tarda	XL	Childhood	Short trunk (mild)	None	Precocious osteoarthritis‡
Spondylometaphyseal dysplasia	AD	Infancy	Short trunk, barrel chest, bowed legs	None	Usually none
Metaphyseal chondrodysplasia, Schmid type	AD	Childhood	Short limbs, bowed legs	None	Usually none
Metaphyseal chondrodysplasia, McKusick type (cartilage-hair hypoplasia)	AR	Late infancy	Severe shortening of trunk and limbs, sparse blond hair, light complexion, immune deficiency	None	Squamous cell carcinoma of skin, complications of viral infections
Metatropic dwarfism	AR	Birth	Short limbs, severe progressive kyphoscoliosis, large joints, joint limitation	None	Usually none
Kniest syndrome	AD	Birth	Short limbs, kyphoscoliosis, large joints, contractures, myopia	Cleft palate	Retinal detachment, precocious osteoarthritis‡ with contractures
Pseudoachondroplasia	AD	Early childhood	Short trunk and limbs, ligamentous laxity, bowing of long bones (forearm)	None	Precocious osteoarthritis,‡ flexion contractures at knees
Diastrophic dwarfism	AR	Usually birth	Short limbs, kyphoscoliosis, joint contractures, clubfoot, hitchhiker thumb, cauliflower ear	Cleft palate	Precocious osteoarthritis‡ with contractures
Ellis–van Creveld syndrome	AR	Birth	Short limbs, polydactyly, congenital heart disease	Midline cleft upper lip; buccolabial frenula; natal, conical, and missing teeth	Usually none
Trichorhinophalangeal syndrome	AD	Childhood	Mild short stature, sparse hair, prominent nose, short hands	Malocclusion, supernumerary incisors	Usually none

*AD, autosomal dominant; XL, X-linked inheritance; AR, autosomal recessive.
†Two types: Fairbanks, which involves most epiphyses, and Ribbing, which is milder and often involves only capital femoral epiphyses.
‡Precocious arthritis involves weight-bearing joints, particularly the hips.

central nervous system dysfunction, and abnormal hair. It is thought to be due to abnormal attachment of copper to intracellular metallothionine.

Osteogenesis imperfecta (OI) is a generalized disorder of the skeletal, ocular, cutaneous, otic, dental, and vascular tissues. Four clinical types are recognized (Table 195-4), but there is considerable heterogeneity among each type. All appear to reflect abnormalities of type I collagen. OI type I, which is the most common and the prototype of OI, is characterized by osseous fragility that varies from minimal to moderately severe (for instance, fractures at birth), blue sclerae, and the onset of hearing loss in adults. The frequency of fractures tends to decrease with age, especially after puberty. Roentgenographs demonstrate generalized osteopenia and excessive callus formation at fracture sites. Vertebral bodies exhibit a typical codfish-like appearance, and skull films usually reveal wormian bones. Some families exhibit opalescent dentin (dentinogenesis imperfecta). Intrauterine fractures, roentgenographs that demonstrate crumpled long bones and beaded ribs, and perinatal death typify OI type II, the lethal perinatal form. Contrary to

the earlier view that the inheritance pattern is autosomal recessive, most cases of OI type II appear to result from new dominant mutations. Gonad mosaicism has been reported. Patients with OI type III exhibit moderately severe to severe osseous fragility, usually accompanied by deformities of the spine and limbs and growth deficiency. Their sclerae are blue during infancy but become gray white with time. OI type IV is characterized by bone fragility with severe bony deformities with white sclerae.

Therapy in OI is limited primarily to orthopedic surgical management of skeletal deformities. Immobilization may aggravate osteopenia and should be avoided.

Pseudoxanthoma elasticum (PXE) is a generalized connective tissue disorder that affects primarily the eyes, skin, and cardiovascular system. PXE has been tentatively classified into two autosomal dominant and two autosomal recessive types. The dominant type I is characterized by a subcutaneous yellow, raised rash over flexure sites, particularly the neck, axillae, groin, and cubital area, severe chorioretinitis, and complications of arterial degeneration (hypertension, angina pectoris, and intermittent claudication). Dominant type II is milder, showing only a macular rash, stretchable skin, retinal angioid streaks, myopia, high-arched palate, and blue sclerae. Recessive type I is manifested by skin changes similar to those of the dominant type I, plus angioid streaks and a predisposition to gastrointestinal hemorrhage. In the rare recessive type II there are no eye or vascular changes, but there is generalized lax skin infiltrated with degenerative elastic fibers. In general, PXE is thought to result from defective elastic fibers. There is no definitive treatment.

The *Winchester syndrome* is an autosomal recessive disorder characterized by coarse facial features, dwarfism, joint contractures, corneal opacities, osteoporosis, and carpal tunnel osteolysis. The destructive joint changes resemble rheumatoid arthritis. Although the basic defect is unknown, there is pathologic replacement of bone and cartilage by dense fibrous tissue, and structurally abnormal fibroblasts have been seen.

Clinical features of *fibrodysplasia ossificans progressiva*, an autosomal dominant disorder, include progressive ossification of fascia, tendons, ligaments, and aponeuroses. The process usually begins in childhood and leads to severe disability. Microdactyly, particularly of the first digits, is frequent. The basic defect remains unknown.

The combination of short stature, brachydactyly, limited joint mobility, myopia, and small spherical lenses that often dislocate characterizes the *Weill-Marchesani syndrome*. It is inherited as an autosomal recessive trait, although heterozygotes may have short stature.

The *chondrodysplasias* are a subgroup of connective tissue disorders that involve cartilage, especially cartilage growth (endochondral ossification). Since most of the skeleton develops embryologically and grows subsequently by this process, abnormalities are reflected by reduced skeletal growth, often with deformities. Membranous ossification may also be involved in the pathogenetic process. Although dwarfism usually dominates the clinical picture, extraskeletal problems are often present and abnormalities of dental development are common. There are over 100 recognized *chondrodysplasias*, most of which are very rare. The diagnosis rests on the combination of clinical, genetic, roentgenographic, and histologic features. With a few exceptions the basic defects have not been identified in these disorders. Abnormalities of type II collagen have been observed in cases of spondyloepiphyseal dysplasia congenita. There is no treatment to stimulate skeletal growth. However, many of the nongrowth-related problems can be managed effectively. The salient features of several of these disorders are listed in Table 195-5.

BIBLIOGRAPHY

Aleck KA and Shapiro LJ: Genetic-metabolic considerations in the sick neonate, Pediatr Clin North Am 25:431, 1978.
Bloskovics ME: Phenylketonuria and other phenylalaninaemias, Clin Endocrinol Metabol 3:87, 1974.
Cheah KS: Collagen genes and inherited connective tissue disease, Biochem J 229:287, 1985.
Dorfman A and Matalon R: The mucopolysaccharidoses: a review, Proc Natl Acad Sci USA 73:630, 1976.
Frimpter GW: Aminoacidurias due to inherited disorders of metabolism (in two parts), N Engl J Med 289:835, 895, 1973.
Gompertz D: Inborn errors of organic acid in metabolism, Clin Endocrinol Metabol 3:107, 1974.
Hirschorn R and Weissman G: Genetic disorders of lysosomes, Prog Med Genet 1:49, 1976.
Hollister DW, Byers PH, and Holbrook KA: Genetic disorders of collagen metabolism, Adv Hum Genet 12:1, 1982.
Horton WA: Bone dysplasias. In Kelly V, editors: Practice in pediatrics, vol 7, New York, 1983, Harper & Row, Publishers Inc.
Horton WA: Heritable connective tissue disorders. In Jackson LG and Schimke RN, editors: Clinical genetics: a source book for physicians, New York, 1979, John Wiley & Sons Inc.
Kelly TE: The mucopolysaccharidoses and mucolipidoses, Clin Orthop 114:116, 1976.
Palmar SH: Metabolic aspects of immunodeficiency disease, Semin Hematol 17:30, 1980.
Pyeritz RE: Marfan syndrome. In Emery A and Rimoin D, editors: Principles and practice of medical genetics, Edinburgh, 1983, Churchill Livingstone Inc.
Sass-Kortsak A and Bearn A: Hereditary disorders of copper metabolism. In Stanbury JB, Wyngaarden JB, and Frederickson DS, editors: The metabolic basis of inherited disease, ed 4, New York, 1978, McGraw-Hill Inc.

196 · THE PORPHYRIAS

Karl E. Anderson, Shigeru Sassa, *and* Attallah Kappas

The porphyrias are a group of inherited and acquired disorders characterized by abnormalities in the activities of specific enzymes of the heme biosynthetic pathway (Fig. 196-1). Disturbances of porphyrin-heme biosynthesis can also be evoked by a wide variety of chemicals.

HEME BIOSYNTHETIC PATHWAY

Heme is probably synthesized in all aerobic cells because it is required for vital cellular hemoproteins, including mitochondrial respiratory cytochromes. More heme is made in the bone marrow and liver than in other organs. In the bone marrow, heme is utilized primarily to make hemoglobin, which is a transport protein for molecular oxygen, whereas in liver most newly formed heme is used for synthesis of cytochrome P-450. This cytochrome is a key component of the microsomal mixed-function oxidase system, which oxidizes a variety of drugs and endogenous steroids. Since the bone marrow and liver synthesize more heme than other tissues, it is not surprising that diseases of porphyrin metabolism should be expressed particularly in erythroid cells and in the liver.

In the synthetic pathway for heme, the first and the last three enzymes are mitochondrial, whereas the intermediate enzymes are found in the cytosol. The first enzyme of the pathway is δ-aminolevulinic acid (ALA) synthase, which catalyzes the condensation of glycine and succinyl CoA to form ALA. This enzyme requires pyridoxal $5'$-phosphate as a cofactor. ALA is a δ- rather than an α-amino acid and therefore does not participate in protein synthesis. It is, however, an obligate precursor for porphyrin and heme formation. Two molecules of ALA are condensed to form a monopyrrole, porphobilinogen (PBG), by a cytosolic enzyme, ALA dehydratase. PBG deaminase, also known as uroporphyrinogen (UROgen) I synthase, converts four PBG molecules to a linear tetrapyrrole, hydroxymethylbilane. UROgen III cosynthase then reverses one of the four pyrroles and catalyzes ring closure to form UROgen III. The type I isomers of UROgen and coproporphyrinogen (COPROgen) are normally produced in insignificant amounts, and there are no known heme compounds derived from these type I porphyrinogens.

A cytosolic enzyme, UROgen decarboxylase, removes four carboxyl groups from four acetic acid side chains of UROgen III in a stepwise fashion, yielding COPROgen III (which contains four methyl groups rather than the four acetic acid groups). COPROgen III is oxidatively decarboxylated to PROTOgen IX by a mitochondrial enzyme, COPROgen oxidase. Thus PROTOgen IX contains two vinyl groups replacing two of the propionic acid groups in COPROgen III.

PROTOgen oxidase then removes six hydrogen atoms to yield protoporphyrin (PROTO) IX. Finally, ferrous iron (Fe^{2+}) is inserted into PROTO IX by the action of ferrochelatase to form heme. Outside the reducing environment of the cell, porphyrinogens are largely autooxidized to porphyrins and then excreted in urine or bile. Porphyrinogens are colorless and nonfluorescent, whereas porphyrins are aromatic compounds that are reddish and fluoresce bright red in ultraviolet light.

The rate of heme synthesis in the liver is thought to be controlled primarily by ALA synthase. ALA synthase activity in normal liver is very low. In response to various chemicals, drugs, and hormones, liver ALA synthase can be markedly induced (in experimental systems by 50-fold or more), indicating that this enzyme can greatly increase in amount when greater hepatic heme synthesis is required.

Hepatic ALA synthase is regulated by heme, the end product of the pathway. Repression of enzyme synthesis rather than inhibition of activity is the principal regulatory action of heme on ALA synthase in the liver.

Control of heme biosynthesis in erythroid cells appears to occur by a somewhat different mechanism than in the liver. Heme biosynthesis in erythroid cells is not necessarily regulated by ALA synthase. Drugs and foreign chemicals that induce ALA synthase in the liver and produce hepatic porphyria experimentally do not induce this enzyme or stimulate porphyrinogenesis in erythroid cells.

Very little is known about the control of ALA synthase and heme biosynthesis in cell types other than liver and erythroid cells, but available evidence suggests that, as in the bone marrow, it may be different from the liver.

CLASSIFICATION AND DIAGNOSIS OF THE HUMAN PORPHYRIAS

Porphyrias are classified as either erythropoietic or hepatic depending on the primary organ in which overproduction of porphyrins or precursors take place (Table 196-1). They are also characterized on the basis of clinical features and patterns of excretion of porphyrins and their precursors. As will be apparent, the two most important clinical features of the porphyrias are (1) neurovisceral manifestations in acute intermittent porphyria and other types of porphyria in which there is excess accumulation and excretion of porphyrin precursors (that is, ALA and PBG) and (2) cutaneous photosensitivity in those porphyrias in which excess porphyrins accumulate in blood and skin.

Because the human porphyrias differ greatly in their clinical manifestations and management, for proper therapy it is important to establish precisely which type of porphyria is present in a patient. In the inherited types it is important to study family members as well. For example, relatives of patients with the hereditary hepatic porphyrias should be screened, and those found to have clinically latent porphyria should be advised to avoid factors, including drugs such as barbiturates and sulfonamides, that can produce life-threatening neurologic attacks. Certain treatments for porphyria cutanea tarda (for example, phlebotomy and chloroquine) are not useful for other porphyrias. β-Carotene and sunscreens are useful for preventing photosensitivity mainly in erythropoietic protoporphyria.

Congenital erythropoietic porphyria

In humans congenital erythropoietic porphyria (CEP) is characterized biochemically by the excessive production and excretion in urine of type I isomers of uroporphyrin (URO) and coproporphyrin (COPRO). CEP is transmitted in an autosomal recessive fashion and is extremely rare. Only 60 authentic cases

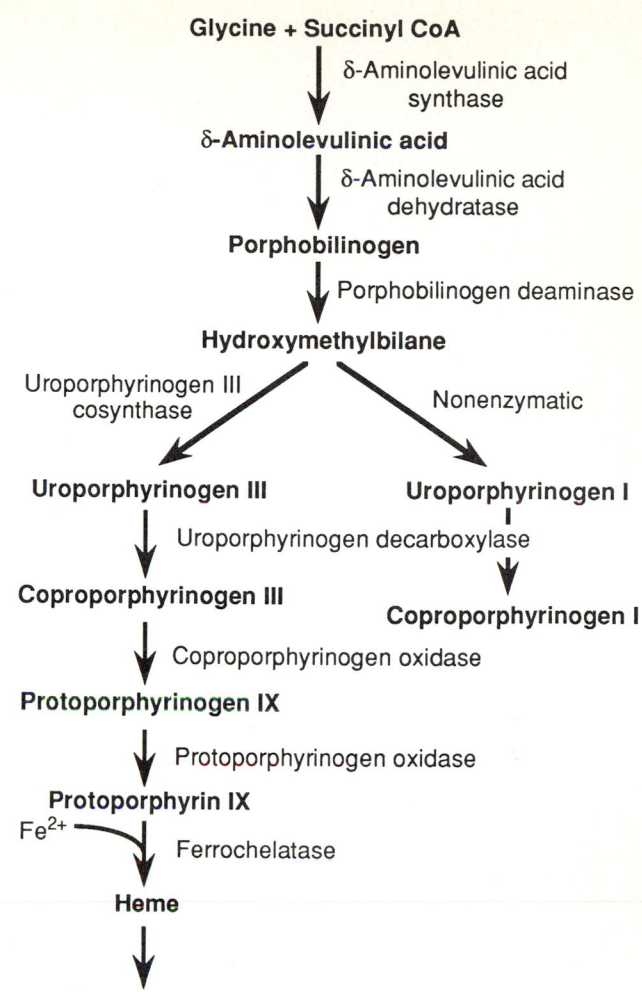

Fig. 196-1 Intermediates *(bold)* and enzymes of heme biosynthetic pathway. A form of porphyria has been associated with deficiencies of each of these enzymes, with the exception δ-aminolevulinic acid synthase.

were reported up to 1978. The earliest sign of the disorder is massive excretion of URO, which may be evident in the neonate or young child as reddish or pink urine. CEP can also be recognized in utero by finding increased porphyrins in amniotic fluid. The disease appears to have no preferential population distribution.

CLINICAL MANIFESTATIONS. The major clinical characteristics are photosensitivity and hemolytic anemia, usually beginning in infancy. Reddish urine is also an early sign. Neurologic symptoms are not observed. Skin lesions resulting from photosensitivity are usually extensive and severe. Vesicular and bullous skin lesions are present on the exposed portions of the body and occur more frequently in the summer months. Lesions may become infected and ulcerate, and this further promotes scarring and deformity. Severe deformities with loss of the nails, terminal phalanges, nasal and auricular tissue, and eyelids can occur. Hypertrichosis, hyperpigmentation, and hypopigmentation are very common. Both deciduous and permanent teeth may show brownish staining (erythrodontia) with intense red fluorescence under ultraviolet light, as is characteristic of porphyrins. Porphyrin deposited in the teeth and in bone is mainly URO, probably owing to its affinity for calcium phosphate.

Mild to severe hemolytic anemia is common, with associated

Table 196-1 Classification and major features of the clinical porphyrias

| Classification | Deficient enzyme | Autosomal inheritance | Major presenting symptoms* | | | Excess excretion of ALA, PBG, porphyrins*† | |
			Photo-sensitivity	Neurovisceral	Increased red cell porphyrins†	Urine	Stool
Erythropioetic							
Congenital erythropoietic porphyria	UROgen III co-synthase	Recessive	+ (severe)	−	*URO I,* COPRO I	*URO I,* COPRO I	
Erythropoietic protoporphyria	Ferrochelatase	Dominant	+	−	*PROTO*	−	PROTO
Hepatic							
Acute intermittent porphyria	PBG deaminase	Dominant	−	+	−	ALA, *PBG*	
Hereditary coproporphyria	COPROgen oxidase	Dominant	+	+	−	ALA, PBG, *COPRO*	*COPRO*
Variegate porphyria	PROTOgen oxidase	Dominant	+	+	−	ALA, PBG, *COPRO*	COPRO, *PROTO*
Porphyria cutanea tarda	UROgen decarboxylase	‡	+	−	−	*URO*	*ISOCOPRO*

* +, Present; −, absent; UROgen, uroporphyrinogen; COPROgen, coproporphyrinogen; PROTOgen, protoporphyrinogen; URO, uroporphyrin; COPRO, coproporphyrin; PROTO, protoporphyrin; ALA, δ-aminolevulinic acid; PBG, porphobilinogen; ISOCOPRO, isocoproporphyrin.
† Findings of major diagnostic importance are italicized.
‡ Dominant inheritance has been documented in some families but not others.

erythroid hyperplasia in the bone marrow, reticulocytosis, circulating normoblasts, and increased fecal urobilinogen. Multiple transfusions may be required. Anemia may be improved by splenectomy in some patients with CEP. The anemia of CEP may also result in part from ineffective erythropoiesis in the bone marrow.

The mechanism of hemolysis in CEP is not fully understood. Photohemolysis of CEP red cells can be demonstrated in vitro, but the extent of hemolysis in vivo is not clearly correlated with exposure to light. Splenic destruction of porphyrin-laden erythrocytes is an important factor in the hemolytic process and explains why some patients with this disorder respond at least partially to splenectomy.

LABORATORY FINDINGS. Large amounts of URO and COPRO are excreted in urine, whereas ALA and PBG excretion is normal. The color of the urine varies from faint pink to dark red depending on the porphyrin content. The amount of COPRO is usually less than that of URO, which can sometimes reach 500 mg/day. Smaller amounts of the less carboxylated porphyrins (that is, 7-, 6-, and 5-carboxylated) are also excreted. Most of the urinary URO and COPRO is type I, but smaller increases in type III URO and COPRO are also found. Feces contain large amounts of COPRO, less URO, but little or no increase in protoporphyrin (PROTO). Fecal COPRO is mainly type I. Plasma also contains URO and COPRO, whereas porphyrins are virtually undetectable in normal plasma. Circulating erythrocytes contain large amounts of URO I and lesser although still excessive concentrations of COPRO I. For reasons that are not clear, PROTO may increase and become the major porphyrin in erythrocytes in some patients with CEP.

UROgen III cosynthase is decreased to about one-tenth to one-third the normal level in erythrocytes. The basic abnormality may be a structural gene defect for UROgen III cosynthase.

MANAGEMENT. Therapy for this severe condition is difficult and often only marginally successful. Photopathic damage to the skin can result in scarring, and patients should be shielded from sunlight as much as possible. Sunscreens and β-carotene may be somewhat beneficial. Splenectomy or blood transfusions may improve anemia and decrease the production of red cells and porphyrins by the bone marrow.

Erythropoietic protoporphyria

Erythropoietic protoporphyria (EPP) is an inherited disease that is also characterized clinically by cutaneous photosensitivity, but this is generally much less severe than in CEP. Patients with EPP have marked increases in PROTO in erythrocytes, plasma, and feces but no increased porphyrins in urine. EPP is much more common than CEP, and more than 300 cases have been reported. EPP is an autosomal dominant disorder with a variable degree of clinical expression. In fact, it can be completely latent. In contrast to the hereditary hepatic porphyrias, which are also autosomal dominant disorders, latent EPP has not been found to be activated clinically by exposure to chemicals, drugs, or hormones.

CLINICAL MANIFESTATIONS. Signs and symptoms, usually beginning in childhood, follow exposure to sunlight. Burning and itching of the skin, often very soon after sun exposure, can be accompanied by edema and erythema. Vesicles and residual scarring are usually not prominent. Cholelithiasis can also be present, and liver function tests may be abnormal. Fluorescence of the teeth is not found. Hemolysis is usually absent or mild in EPP.

LABORATORY FINDINGS. Urine porphyrins and porphyrin precursors are normal. Increases of PROTO in erythrocytes and feces are striking, and significant amounts of PROTO are present in plasma. In EPP the increased erythrocyte PROTO is, for unknown reasons, not complexed with zinc, as it is in other conditions associated with excess red cell PROTO, such as lead poisoning and iron deficiency.

PROTO accumulation occurs in late normoblasts, and the PROTO level is much higher in reticulocytes than in mature red cells of patients with EPP. Much of the porphyrin diffuses out of red cells into plasma as red cells mature. In contrast, in lead poisoning the increased erythrocyte zinc PROTO declines only slightly with cell aging. Therefore plasma PROTO is elevated in EPP but not in lead poisoning. Loss of PROTO from red cells in EPP has been estimated to be 40% of the total PROTO content of the circulating erythrocytes each day. This loss, combined with the additional loss from bone marrow normoblasts and reticulocytes, could readily account for most of the daily PROTO excretion in feces in this disorder without postulating a major extraerythropoietic source of PROTO formation, such as the liver. Nevertheless, there is evidence that excess PROTO may also be produced by the liver in EPP.

There is an inherited deficiency of ferrochelatase in EPP, probably in all tissues. It is likely that this deficient enzyme becomes rate limiting for heme formation in erythroid cells in the marrow and possibly in the liver as well. Patients with clinically manifest EPP, as well as completely latent gene carriers of the EPP defect (with normal red cell porphyrins), can be identified by assessing ferrochelatase activity in cultured cells such as mitogen-stimulated lymphocytes.

MANAGEMENT. Tolerance to sun exposure can be significantly increased by oral β-carotene in many patients with EPP. This treatment can produce a yellow or yellow-orange skin coloration, but it is seldom a major cosmetic problem. Liver dysfunction and considerable protoporphyrin deposition in the liver develop in a minority of patients with EPP. Other causes of liver disease should be sought and treated in such patients, and consideration should be given to cholestyramine therapy, which may increase fecal excretion of PROTO.

Acute intermittent porphyria

Acute intermittent porphyria (AIP), an autosomal dominant disease, is probably the most common type of the hereditary hepatic porphyrias (that is, AIP, hereditary coproporphyria, and variegate porphyria). In AIP the basic defect is an inherited deficiency of PBG deaminase (Fig. 196-1). Clinical manifestations rarely occur before puberty. AIP has been referred to as the Swedish type of porphyria, and it is perhaps most common in Scandinavia and the British Isles. The incidence of AIP was previously estimated on the basis of urinary ALA and PBG determinations to be 1.5 per 100,000 in Sweden. Since urinary ALA and PBG are not necessarily increased in a gene carrier of this disorder, this is clearly an underestimate. More recently it was estimated that the incidence of AIP in the population 15 years of age or older in Sweden is 7.7 per 100,000. The highest incidence has been observed in Lapland (100 per 100,000), and all latent and expressed cases in that region appear to be related to a single family. Assays for erythrocyte PBG deaminase can detect almost all gene carriers regardless of age or clinical severity. Such assays, when used to screen large numbers of relatives of AIP patients, may increase the apparent incidence of the gene carrier state for AIP by as much as 10-fold.

CLINICAL MANIFESTATIONS. The clinical symptoms of AIP, hereditary coproporphyria (HCP) and variegate porphyria (VP), are very similar, except that HCP and VP may also be associated with photosensitivity, which does not occur in AIP. All symptoms in AIP can be related to neurologic disturbances involving especially the autonomic nervous system. Thus "neurovisceral" symptoms such as abdominal pain, vomiting, and constipation are thought to result from metabolic disturbances in autonomic nerves in the abdomen.

The severity of symptoms, frequency of acute episodes, and age at onset of the clinical expression of AIP are highly variable. In the great majority of gene carriers the disorder remains clinically latent throughout their lives. This and the fact that the degree of PBG deaminase deficiency is not correlated with disease activity make it evident that additional factors including drug, nutritional, and hormonal influences are important in the

clinical expression of AIP. Many drugs that are hazardous to patients with AIP cause the induction of ALA synthase in the liver.

Because the deficiency of PBG deaminase is inherited in an autosomal dominant fashion, it is transmitted as commonly to males as to females. Symptoms develop after puberty more frequently in women than in men, and they often occur in the luteal phase of the menstrual cycle and sometimes during pregnancy. However, pregnancy is usually well tolerated.

Acute episodes usually begin with abdominal pain. Because there is no peritoneal inflammation, the findings on physical examination are often not impressive. Ileus with rather diffuse small bowel dilation may be evident on a roentgenographic film of the abdomen. Leukocytosis and fever may be absent even when there is severe pain from AIP, although either or both may sometimes accompany an AIP attack. Hypertension and tachycardia occur frequently and are probably due to autonomic dysfunction. Peripheral neuropathy, mood changes, and other psychiatric manifestations can also occur in AIP. Other central nervous system complications may include seizures and hypothalamic involvement with inappropriate ADH secretion. Hyponatremia, which is not uncommon in patients with acute symptoms, may be caused by salt depletion from nausea and vomiting or by hemodilution owing to inappropriate ADH secretion. Neuropathy can progess over days or weeks and lead to muscle paralysis, quadriplegia, and death from respiratory paralysis. Such severe fatal attacks are quite rare unless porphyria is recognized late and the patient is treated with harmful medications before diagnosis. The mortality rate from AIP appears to be declining as better diagnostic methods become widely employed and as more relatives of known AIP patients are screened for the disease before the onset of symptoms.

Chronic symptoms including pain and depression occur between attacks in some patients with AIP. Management is difficult, and because AIP is characterized by acute rather than by long-term painful symptoms, other causes of pain should be sought carefully. Patients with AIP may have acute illnesses of other kinds, including appendicitis, and it should not be assumed that abdominal pain in a patient with AIP always is due to porphyria.

LABORATORY FINDINGS. PBG deaminase deficiency is the primary genetic defect in AIP. Decreased PBG deaminase activity has been described not only in the liver but also in erythrocytes, cultured skin fibroblasts, cultured amniotic cells, and mitogen-stimulated lymphocytes. This enzyme deficiency (about 50% of the normal level) is found regardless of the presence or absence of clinical symptoms. It is inherited as an autosomal dominant trait.

AIP is characterized also by the excretion of large amounts of ALA and PGB in urine. PBG is detected with Ehrlich's aldehyde reagent, with which it combines to form a complex with a reddish color (as in the Watson-Schwartz test). The Watson-Schwartz test may give false positive results. A preferred method is the column chromatographic method of Mauzerall and Granick, which is specific for PBG and is also quantitative. ALA in urine is usually increased in AIP but to a lesser degree than PBG.

Urinary PBG may decrease during clinical remissions of AIP, but usually it remains increased for a prolonged period. Many gene carriers of AIP who have low PBG deaminase activity in erythrocytes but never have symptoms excrete normal amounts of PBG throughout their lives, but some excrete very large amounts of ALA and PBG. Thus it is useful to measure and follow urine ALA and PBG excretion in AIP gene carriers, although this does not provide an absolute indication of when symptoms may occur.

Porphyrin concentrations may be increased in freshly voided urine from patients with AIP in remission and in relapse, presumably because of spontaneous cyclization of PBG to form porphyrins (especially URO). This nonenzymatic porphyrin formation is facilitated by prolonged storage of urine, an acidic urine pH, and light.

Both ALA and PBG have been detected in the plasma and cerebrospinal fluid of patients with AIP. ALA is chemically similar to γ-aminobutyric acid (GABA) and may interfere with normal GABA neurotransmitter functions. It is not clear, however, that symptoms of AIP are caused by a direct effect of ALA on the central nervous system.

Metabolic factors associated with clinical activation of AIP include the onset of puberty, hormonal variations in the menstrual cycle, exposure to a variety of drugs and environmental chemicals, changes in dietary carbohydrate or fat, and reduced caloric intake. Drugs known to be harmful to patients with acute intermittent porphyria, hereditary coproporphyria, and variegate porphyria include barbiturates, sulfonamides, meprobamate, glutethimide, methaqualone, anticonvulsants (phenytoin and others), griseofulvin, oral contraceptives, and alcohol. Narcotic analgesics (morphine and others), phenothiazines (chlorpromazine and others), chloral hydrate, aspirin, and penicillin are known to be safe for use by these patients. Information on the effect of most other drugs in these disorders is inadequate. Metabolites of gonadal and adrenal steroid hormones (such as androgens and progesterones) can induce ALA synthase. Estrogens and their metabolites appear to have less porphyrinogenic properties, and adrenal glucocorticoids have none.

Acute exacerbations of the hereditary hepatic porphyrias may occur after a reduced intake of calories and may be ameliorated by increases in carbohydrate ingestion or by infusions of large amounts of glucose. The salutary effect of glucose in the treatment of hereditary hepatic porphyrias has an experimental analogy, termed the "glucose effect," in the use of glucose to prevent chemically induced porphyria. Glucose administration can block the induction of hepatic ALA synthase by a number of porphyria-inducing drugs.

MANAGEMENT. When a diagnosis of AIP is established in an acutely ill patient, all drugs known to exacerbate the disease should be discontinued. An adequate caloric intake, preferably high in carbohydrates, should be ensured, if necessary by intravenous infusion of at least 300 g of glucose daily. In patients with hyponatremia owing to inappropriate ADH secretion, caution should be exercised to avoid a further excess in water in the form of intravenous solutions. Although glucose infusions in acute attacks of porphyria are not always beneficial, such treatment remains an important mode of therapy.

Pain is most effectively treated with morphine, meperidine, or codeine, and nausea with a phenothiazine such as chlorpromazine. The latter is often useful for sedation as well. Insomnia can be treated with chloral hydrate. Continued treatment between attacks is seldom needed, and there is no clear evidence that chlorpromazine or other drugs have a preventive action.

A more recently developed treatment is intravenous hematin infusion. Hematin, which can be given only intravenously, is effective in lowering urinary output of ALA and PBG and probably shortens the duration of an acute attack. The daily administration of a luteinizing hormone-releasing hormone (LH-RH) analogue to suppress cyclical ovarian hormone production has been reported recently to be effective in preventing frequent premenstrual attacks of AIP.

Hereditary coproporphyria

Hereditary coproporphyria (HCP) is similar to AIP and variegate porphyria in its clinical symptoms. Unlike patients with AIP, however, those with HCP may also display cutaneous photosensitivity. Acute attacks of HCP are provoked by the same drugs that precipitate acute attacks of AIP. The disorder is inherited in an autosomal dominant fashion, the clinical expression and severity are quite variable, and as in AIP, latent carriers are common. HCP is generally less severe than AIP. As in AIP, acute attacks occur more commonly in females than in males.

LABORATORY FINDINGS. The predominant biochemical finding in clinically expressed HCP is marked elevation of COPRO III excretion in urine and stool. During acute attacks urinary ALA and PBG concentrations are also increased. In some patients with HCP, greater than 95% of urinary porphyrins are COPRO, whereas in others URO is also increased to a degree similar to AIP. Feces contain large amounts of COPRO. Fecal PROTO may also be increased, but always much less than COPRO.

GENE DEFECT. COPROgen oxidase has recently been shown to be approximately 50% deficient in patients with HCP. Since COPROgen oxidase is a mitochondrial enzyme, the enzyme assay must be carried out in cells other than circulating erythrocytes, and for this purpose cultured skin fibroblasts, cultured lymphocytes, and leukocytes have been employed.

A 50% COPROgen oxidase deficiency in HCP still provides a level of activity for this enzyme that is far in excess of normal UROgen I synthase activity in the liver. Thus normally low activity of PBG deaminase relative to that for COPROgen oxidase may explain the excessive excretion of ALA and PBG during acute attacks of HCP. As in AIP, attacks occur when ALA synthase is increased by drugs, hormones, or other factors. Attacks occur less readily in HCP than in AIP, and HCP is a less severe disease, presumably because UROgen I synthase activity is normal in HCP whereas it is decreased by 50% in AIP. Severe homozygous HCP has been described.

Variegate porphyria

Variegate porphyria (VP) is another of the autosomal dominant types of hereditary hepatic porphyria. It is characterized by symptoms very similar to those of AIP and HCP. VP is sometimes called protocoproporphyria hereditaria or South African porphyria, since it is most common in the white population in South Africa. The disease is called "variegate" porphyria because it can be manifested by an acute attack with neurovisceral symptoms or by cutaneous photosensitivity or both, and it can also be completely latent clinically. The neurovisceral symptoms are essentially the same as in AIP and HCP.

BIOCHEMICAL FINDINGS. Most patients with VP excrete large amounts of PROTO in feces, with lesser increases of COPRO, a pattern generally not observed in AIP, HCP, and porphyria cutanea tarda. As in HCP, urine PBG is elevated during acute attacks, but it is often normal during remission of the disease. In AIP, in contrast, normal levels of urinary PBG are less common once the disorder has become clinically apparent.

GENE DEFECT. The enzyme defect in VP is 50% deficiency of PROTOgen oxidase. Homozygous cases of VP have been reported.

δ-Aminolevulinic acid dehydrase porphyria

The cases of three unrelated males with a newly recognized form of porphyria called δ-aminolevulinic acid dehydrase

(ALAD) porphyria have been reported in Germany and Sweden. These patients developed symptoms in childhood or their teens, including severe neuropathy, resembling AIP. Excretion of ALA was markedly increased, and erythrocyte ALA dehydratase was decreased to less than 2% of normal. Family studies indicated that their disease is autosomal recessive and results from an inherited deficiency of ALA dehydratase.

Porphyria cutanea tarda

Porphyria cutanea tarda (PCT) is characterized by skin photosensitivity and excessive excretion of porphyrins in urine and feces. In contrast to the hereditary hepatic porphyrias (AIP, HCP, and VP), acute attacks of neurovisceral symptoms do not occur. Drugs known to precipitate acute attacks of hereditary hepatic porphyrias probably have no effect in PCT.

PCT is probably the most common type of porphyria. Many patients with PCT are considered to have an acquired disorder. However, a hereditary form of the disease, with symptoms very similar to those of the acquired form, also occurs. Furthermore, a PCT-like syndrome can occur in normal subjects after exposure to certain chemicals, particularly halogenated hydrocarbons such as hexachlorobenzene, tetrachlorodibenzo[p]dioxin (TCDD), methyl chloride, and vinyl chloride.

CLINICAL MANIFESTATIONS. Skin lesions often begin with erythema and can progress to vesicular and bullous lesions that may eventually ulcerate. Chronic skin changes include hyperpigmentation, hypopigmentation, scarring, hypertrichosis, and sclerodermoid changes. Unlike EPP, the rapid development of painful erythema after exposure to light is usually not seen in PCT.

Liver dysfunction with or without cirrhosis is common among patients with PCT, and this is often, although not always, associated with excess alcohol intake. Liver biopsy frequently reveals siderosis, although not often to the degree found in hereditary hemochromatosis. The extent to which liver injury is essential to the development of PCT is unclear, but PCT is not found in the majority of patients with liver damage resulting from alcohol or other causes.

Iron overload is another factor contributing to PCT. Iron removal by repeated phlebotomy is known to be highly effective in the treatment of PCT. Although total iron-binding capacity in serum is usually normal, there is an increase in the saturation of serum transferrin with iron in most patients with PCT. The serum ferritin concentration may be a better index of iron overload and response to phlebotomy in PCT.

PCT sometimes appears in men treated with estrogens for prostatic carcinoma and in women given estrogen-progestin combinations for birth control or estrogens alone for the treatment of menopausal symptoms. The time of onset of the PCT syndrome after beginning estrogen therapy is variable, ranging from a month to years.

Chloroquine administration to a patient with PCT results in acute hepatocellular damage, fever, malaise, nausea, and vomiting. This adverse reaction to chloroquine, which does not occur in nonporphyric individuals, is associated with a large amount of URO excreted in the urine. The apparent explanation is that chloroquine becomes concentrated in lysosomes and mitochondria where porphyrins also accumulate and forms a complex with the porphyrins. This is then released from hepatocytes and excreted in urine. The pathogenesis of the transitory liver cell injury is not understood but may result from release of proteolytic enzymes from lysosomes into the cytosol of hepatocytes.

LABORATORY FINDINGS. Urine porphyrins are increased in PCT. The main urinary porphyrins are URO and 7-carboxylic porphyrin with lesser increases of 6- and 5-carboxylic porphyrins, and COPRO. URO in urine is approximately 70% type I isomer, whereas the 7- and 6-carboxylic porphyrins are about 90% type III, and 5-carboxylic porphyrin and COPRO are about equally types I and III. The isomer distribution in the hepatic and fecal porphyrins is similar to that in the urinary porphyrins. The liver contains large amounts of porphyrins, but concentrations in erythrocytes and bone marrow are normal. Urinary excretion of PBG is normal and urine ALA is normal or only slightly increased.

Fecal porphyrins are also increased and consist mostly of COPRO and isocoproporphyrins. The isocoproporphyrin series is normally present in stool in small amounts, but it is increased markedly in PCT as a result of a deficiency of UROgen decarboxylase activity in the liver. Isocoproporphyrin may also be found in urine.

The laboratory diagnosis of PCT should include porphyrin analysis in both urine and feces. Erythropoietic porphyrias should be excluded by demonstrating that red cell porphyrin content is normal. The presence of large amounts of isocoproporphyrin in feces appears to be quite specific for PCT, although urine porphyrins should also be shown to have a pattern consistent with this disorder. Either thin-layer or high-pressure liquid chromatographic methods are most suitable for identification and quantitation of the individual porphyrins in urine and stool.

ENZYMATIC ABNORMALITY. There appear to be two distinct types of PCT, a sporadic type and a familial form that can occur in several members of the same family. The sporadic type, which appears to include the majority of patients with PCT, is characterized by decreased UROgen decarboxylase activity in the liver but not in other tissues including erythrocytes. In familial PCT the deficiency of UROgen decarboxylase probably occurs in all cells and not just the liver. The mode of inheritance of erythrocyte UROgen decarboxylase deficiency in familial PCT is consistent with an autosomal dominant trait.

MANAGEMENT. PCT is the most readily treated form of porphyria. Exposure to agents that contribute to clinical activation, such as alcohol, estrogens, and excess iron, should be discontinued. A repeated phlebotomy regimen to reduce excess hepatic iron content is usually very effective. An alternative approach, with which there is less experience, is a low-dose chloroquine regimen that gradually removes porphyrins from the liver. The transient hepatocellular reaction that occurs in PCT patients with standard doses of chloroquine is minimal with this low-dose regimen.

Hepatoerythropoietic porphyria

This rare disorder resembles CEP but has some biochemical features of PCT (excess excretion of URO, 7-carboxylate porphyrin, and isocoproporphyrin). Erythrocyte PROTO is also increased. As in CEP, cutaneous photosensitivity begins in infancy or childhood. Erythrodontia, mutilation of facial features, hemolysis, and liver damage are less common. UROgen decarboxylase is markedly deficient in the tissues of these patients, which indicates that this disease is the homozygous form of familial PCT.

Porphyria associated with other disorders

HEREDITARY TYROSINEMIA. Hereditary tyrosinemia is an inborn error of metabolism characterized by hepatic cirrhosis in early childhood, renal tubular defects, and hypophosphatemic rickets. The derangement in tyrosine metabolism is associated with low activity of fumarylacetacetate hydrolase, the enzyme that catalyzes formation of succinylacetacetate from fumarylacetacetate. Some patients with tyrosinemia have symptoms similar to those in AIP, such as severe abdominal pain, nausea, vomiting, fever, hypertension, tachycardia, and pain and weakness in the lower extremities. As in AIP, urine ALA is increased; however, urine PBG is normal. Urine from patients with tyrosinemia also contains succinylacetone, a by-product of the deranged amino acid metabolism in this disorder and an extremely potent inhibitor of ALA dehydratase. ALA dehydratase activity is markedly reduced in erythrocytes and livers of patients with tyrosinemia. Production of succinyl-acetone therefore explains the excess urinary ALA excretion, which in turn may be related to the AIP-like symptoms in this disorder. The clinical symptoms of patients with tyrosinemia and elevated urinary excretion of ALA are remarkably similar to those observed in AIP or in lead poisoning. The prepubertal onset of symptoms and the normal levels of urinary PBG in tyrosinemia distinguish it from AIP. Lead poisoning can be excluded by measuring blood lead and erythrocyte protoporphyrin levels.

PORPHYRIA CUTANEA TARDA OCCURRING WITH OTHER DISORDERS. There have been reports of skin blistering in patients undergoing hemodialysis for chronic renal failure. Most cases have been termed "pseudoporphyria" or "chronic bullous dermatosis of hemodialysis" because of the absence of elevated porphyrins in plasma, urine, or feces, but some have been associated with significant increases of porphyrins in urine, plasma, or blister fluid and marked excess of isocoproporphyrin in feces. This apparent association between hemodialysis and PCT is unexplained.

PCT has been reported to occur in some patients with immunologic disorders such as systemic lupus erythematosus and Felty's syndrome and the acquired immunodeficiency syndrome (AIDS). AIP also has been reported in association with systemic lupus erythematosus. The reasons for these associations have not been established.

Porphyrin-producing hepatocellular tumors occur rarely. Hepatocellular carcinomas have been reported to occur quite frequently in some series of patients with PCT, but presumably these are mostly complications of chronic liver disease or chemical exposure and are not porphyrin-producing tumors.

BIBLIOGRAPHY

Anderson KE and others: Prevention of cyclical attacks of acute intermittent porphyria with a long-acting agonist of luteinizing hormone-releasing hormone, New Eng J Med 311:643, 1984.

DeLeo VA and others: Erythropoietic protoporphyria: 10 years experience, Am J Med 60:8, 1976.

Elder GH: Differentiation of porphyria cutanea tarda symptomatica from other types of porphyria by measurement of isocoproporphyrin in feces, J Clin Pathol 28:601, 1975.

Kappas A, Sassa S, and Anderson KE: The porphyrias. In Stanbury JB and others, editors: The metabolic basis of inherited disease, ed 5, New York, 1983, McGraw-Hill Inc.

Tschudy DP and Lamon JM: Porphyrin metabolism and the porphyrias. In Bondy PK and Rosenberg LE, editors: Metabolic control and disease, ed 8, Philadelphia, 1980, WB Saunders Co.

197·METABOLIC AND DIRECT TOXIC EFFECTS OF ETHANOL

Ralph Myerson

Ethanol exerts its effects on tissues and organs either directly by its action on enzymes and structural components of the cell

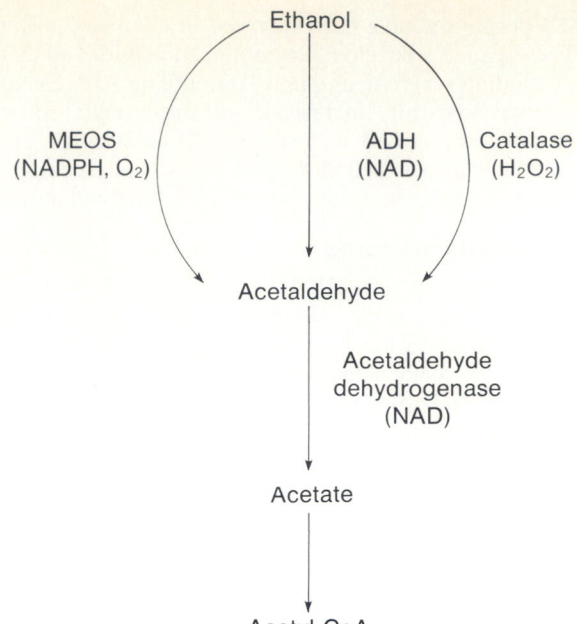

Fig. 197-1   Pathways in metabolism of alcohol. Ethanol is metabolized to acetaldehyde by three enzyme systems: (1) alcohol dehydrogenase (ADH) with nicotinamide adenine dinucleotide (NAD) as cofactor; (2) catalase in presence of H_2O_2; and (3) microsomal ethanol oxidizing system (MEOS) that requires presence of reduced nicotinamide adenine dinucleotide phosphate (NADPH) and O_2. Acetaldehyde is metabolized to acetate in presence of NAD. Acetate is then converted to acetyl coenzyme A (CoA).

or indirectly through changes induced during the metabolism of ethanol.

ETHANOL METABOLISM

Ethanol is a weakly charged molecule that passes easily through cell membranes, rapidly equilibrating between blood and tissues. Its absorption occurs principally from the proximal portion of the small intestine, although modest amounts are absorbed from the stomach and colon.

Ethanol is metabolized predominantly by the liver. The first step in its metabolism is its oxidation to acetaldehyde, and this reaction can be catalyzed by at least three different enzyme systems: alcohol dehydrogenase (ADH), catalase, and a microsomal ethanol oxidating system (MEOS) (Fig. 197-1).

The central and major mechanism of ethanol oxidation is a reaction with the cytoplasmic enzyme ADH with nicotinamide adenine dinucleotide (NAD) as a cofactor. This reaction leads to the production of reduced NAD, NADH.

The enzyme catalase plays a neglible role in ethanol metabolism. Hydrogen peroxide is required, and again acetaldehyde is produced.

The third enzyme system, MEOS, is formed in the smooth endoplasmic reticulum of the hepatocyte. A number of drugs that are metabolized by the microsomal systems may show altered metabolism in alcoholics. Increased rates of metabolism of tolbutamide, warfarin, phenytoin, and certain sedative and anesthetic drugs have been reported in alcoholics during non-drinking periods. On the other hand, the metabolism of these drugs may be decreased when they are given concomitantly with ethanol. This may lead to drug intoxication. MEOS may serve as a reserve mechanism, acting in the presence of excess ethanol that ADH is incapable of metabolizing.

As already noted, the formation of acetaldehyde is the first step in the metabolism of ethanol. Acetaldehyde has been closely scrutinized for evidence that it is responsible for the toxic actions of alcohol. Acetaldehyde, however, is itself very rapidly metabolized into acetate by the enzyme acetaldehyde dehydrogenase. As a result of the speed of this reaction, only minute amounts of acetaldehyde accumulate in the blood—too little to produce toxicity. Disulfiram (Antabuse) blocks the action of the enzyme acetaldehyde dehydrogenase, allowing significant levels of acetaldehyde to accumulate if ethanol is consumed. The so-called aldehyde reaction results. This consists of intense flushing, sweating, and hypotension caused by vasodilation. Disulfiram has been widely used as therapy to condition alcoholics against the use of ethanol. Acetaldehyde dehydrogenase also requires NAD as a substrate to accept hydrogen. This reaction, as well as the metabolism of ethanol to acetaldehyde, results in a depletion of NAD, an increase in NADH, and a change in the NAD/NADH ratio.

The final steps in ethanol metabolism involve the conversion of acetaldehyde to acetate and acetate to acetyl-CoA. The carbon skeleton of ethanol eventually becomes incorporated into a variety of metabolic products.

METABOLIC EFFECTS OF ETHANOL

A variety of effects have been ascribed to the abnormalities produced by the metabolism of ethanol (see following outline). Some of these are the results in the change that occurs in the NAD/NADH ratio during alcohol metabolism. In essence, the excess NADH requires the presence of H receptors to restore NAD and the NAD/NADH ratio to normal.

Effects produced by ethanol metabolism
I. Carbohydrate metabolism
  A. Decrease in gluconeogenesis, producing hypoglycemia if glycogen depletion exists
  B. Inhibition of galactose metabolism
II. Protein metabolism
  A. Increased synthesis of lipoproteins (at high ethanol concentrations the opposite occurs)
  B. Decreased synthesis of albumin and other proteins
III. Lipid metabolism
  A. Increase in liver lipids (fatty liver)
  B. Increase in serum triglycerides
IV. Increase in lactate production
  A. Lactic acidosis
  B. Decrease in uric acid secretion and resultant hyperuricemia
V. Other effects
  A. Decreased serum levels of magnesium and phosphate
  B. Interference with citric acid cycle activity
  C. Increased catecholamine release
  D. Increased oxygen consumption

Some of these metabolic effects have clinical expressions that are of significance. A rare but serious effect is the development of *hypoglycemia* resulting from depression of gluconeogenesis by ethanol. This is manifest when there has been glycogen depletion by starvation.

The increase in NADH resulting from the metabolism of ethanol causes an increase in the reduction of pyruvate to lactate. The resultant *hyperlactacidemia* results in a decrease in urate excretion and *hyperuricemia*. Hyperlactacidemia may also result in an increase in urinary magnesium excretion and *hypomagnesemia*.

The profound effects of ethanol on lipid metabolism are apparently the result of several pathogenic mechanisms. Lipid accumulation in the liver is related primarily to increased hepatic lipid synthesis. The increase in NADH results in increased tissue levels of reduced metabolites, such as L-glycerophos-

phate, which provides the three-carbon skeleton for the synthesis of triglycerides. Mobilization of fat from peripheral deposits to the liver and decreased lipid oxidation in the liver by a decrease in the activity of the citric acid cycle are other mechanisms by which ethanol produces a *fatty liver*.

Alcoholism in nondiabetic patients can result in *ketoacidosis*. The typical history is one of heavy chronic ethanol intake and a recent binge of several days that is followed by anorexia, abdominal pain, and decreased food intake. There is subsequent vomiting, which leads to cessation of food and alcohol intake. The patients usually show symptoms 24 to 72 hours after their last intake and are dehydrated and tachypneic and have mental obtundation. The blood sugar concentration is usually less than 400 mg/dl and indeed can be near normal. There is a metabolic acidosis caused primarily by hyperketonemia, low bicarbonate levels, and possible lactic acidosis.

DIRECT TOXIC EFFECTS OF ETHANOL

Ethanol exerts direct effects on practically all organs and body systems, and many of these effects are expressed by clinical manifestations.

NERVOUS SYSTEM. Both the central and the peripheral nervous systems display a myriad of effects, both acute and chronic, that are directly or indirectly related to ethanol ingestion. The mechanisms of these effects are complex and hypothetical in most instances, but the evidence suggests that these manifestations are predominantly direct effects of ethanol. Ethanol is a central nervous system (CNS) depressant that decreases neuronal activity, although some behavioral stimulation is seen at low blood levels.

There is evidence that ethanol affects a variety of nervous tissue parameters, including ion transfer across membranes, energy metabolism, the action potential of nerves, and neurotransmitter function and metabolism. Ethanol also has effects on neuroamine metabolism.

In addition to these direct effects of ethanol, there are indirect consequences of excessive ethanol intake, such as the propensity for trauma, infections, and vitamin and nutritional deficiency.

Acute effects of ethanol on the central nervous system include acute alcoholic intoxication, acute hallucinosis, and seizures ("rum fits"). Intoxication usually appears as blood ethanol levels of 100 to 200 mg/dl. With blood ethanol levels greater than 400 mg/dl, stupor and/or coma appear, and those greater than 500 mg/dl are often fatal. Seizures may also occur as a result of ethanol withdrawal, although delirium tremens is the most common of the withdrawal syndromes. Some tolerance to ethanol usually develops after repeated exposure to the drug. Several mechanisms exist for the development of this tolerance—increased ethanol metabolism, the development of cellular and pharmacodynamic tolerance, or behavioral tolerance may occur. These mechanisms may operate even in the presence of unchanging blood ethanol concentrations.

Chronic alcoholism may result in a slowly progressive process of global dementia. Other chronic processes include *cerebellar degeneration, central pontine myelolysis, Korsakoff's psychosis,* and *Marchiafava-Bignami disease. Wernick's encephalopathy* is believed to be closely related to an associated deficiency in thiamine chloride.

Peripheral neurologic syndromes include alcoholic polyneuritis and traumatic neuropathies, such as Saturday night palsy, which is secondary to radial nerve compression. Myopathy has also been described in alcoholics. The acute process may be severe enough to produce myoglobin-induced acute tubular necrosis of the kidney. In most instances overt manifestations of the myopathy are minimal or minor. Repeated bouts, however, may lead to a chronic disabling myopathy involving primarily proximal musculature.

In all central nervous disorders seen in alcoholics, the possibility of head trauma must be considered. Alcoholics have a propensity for skull fractures, cerebral contusions, and subdural hematomas.

LIVER. It has been demonstrated that in addition to effects exerted indirectly on the liver by the metabolism of ethanol, ethanol exerts a direct effect on the liver, readily producing demonstrable morphologic changes in both animals and human beings. When severe, these changes may give rise to overt clinical manifestations such as acute alcoholic hepatitis or the "fatty liver syndromes." *Mallory's bodies* (intracytoplasmic eosinophilic clumps), cellular infiltration, and hepatocyte necrosis are the hallmarks of acute alcoholic hepatitis. Although clinically inapparent in most instances, this acute hepatitis may be manifest as a serious and possibly fatal clinical condition.

It is likely that repeated bouts of acute alcoholic hepatitis lead to the development of portal fibrosis and Laënnec's cirrhosis. Other factors, however, obviously play important roles, since cirrhosis develops in only about 10% of chronic alcoholics. It is not clear what factors predispose a person to or prevent the development of cirrhosis, but genetic factors, androgen/estrogen imbalance, collagenase activity, heavy metals, and a host of others have been cited.

HEART—ALCOHOLIC MYOCARDIOPATHY. There is convincing clinical, laboratory, and experimental evidence to show that ethanol exerts a direct toxic effect on the myocardium. In vivo and in vitro experiments in human beings and animals have demonstrated that ethanol depresses myocardial function by decreasing myocardial contractility. Elevated end-diastolic ventricular pressure and cardiac failure result. Several factors contribute to these hemodynamic changes, including a loss of the inotropic effects of myocardial catecholamines and a decrease in oxidative enzymes. Mitochondrial changes are noted early after ethanol administration, followed by lipid accumulation and myofibrillar disruption. Changes in membrane permeability may be the basic mechanism causing these manifestations. Clinically, a low-output, chronic type of cardiac failure results, which may be difficult to differentiate from other cardiomyopathies.

In rare instances beriberi heart disease has been reported in alcoholics (occidental beriberi). This is a hyperkinetic, high-output failure, in contrast to the low-output cardiac failure characteristic of alcoholic cardiomyopathy.

HEMATOLOGIC EFFECTS. A variety of hematologic abnormalities have been described following excessive intake of ethanol. Many result from the complications of alcoholism—cirrhosis of the liver with hypersplenism, gastrointestinal bleeding, and nutritional, folic acid, and vitamin deficiencies. However, evidence has shown that ethanol itself exerts a direct effect on the formed elements of the blood.

Reversible vacuolization of red blood cell and white blood cell precursors in the bone marrow has been noted. These changes resemble those seen with chloramphenicol toxicity. They occur in the absence of nutritional and vitamin deficiencies and have developed despite the concomitant administration of large doses of folic acid.

A reversible type of sideroblastic anemia associated with ringed sideroblasts in the iron-stained bone marrow has been reported following excessive ingestion of ethanol. The changes can be reversed by treatment with parenteral administration of pyridoxal phosphate and are thought to result from the effects of ethanol on vitamin B_6 metabolism.

Stomatocytic changes of erythrocytes have been described in alcoholism and respond to withdrawal of ethanol.

Thrombocytopenia often accompanies acute alcoholic excess. There is usually a fairly rapid return to normal or near normal platelet counts following ethanol withdrawal. Leukopenia and reduced leukocyte bone marrow reserve have also been noted in alcoholics. This is probably related to the action of ethanol as a folate antagonist.

Ethanol has also been shown to produce a depression of leukocyte mobilization into areas of trauma in nutritionally normal individuals. A decrease in the bactericidal activity of serum in vitro has been reported to follow ethanol ingestion. These phenomena may help to explain the increased susceptibility of alcoholics to infection.

GASTROINTESTINAL TRACT

Esophagus. Esophagitis is common after ethanol ingestion, occurring as a result of both irritations of the esophageal mucosa and the reflux of gastric contents. Heavy drinking associated with retching and vomiting may produce a tear in the mucosa at the gastroesophageal function—the Mallory-Weiss syndrome. Esophageal and gastric varices can develop as a result of cirrhosis-induced portal hypertension.

Stomach. Alcoholic gastritis is an extremely common complication of ethanol ingestion and a frequent cause of hemorrhage. The evidence that ethanol is a secretagogue of gastric acid is not convincing. Most studies indicate that ethanol-induced damage to the gastric mucosa results from interference with the gastric mucosal barrier. This allows for back diffusion of hydrogen ions from the gastric lumen, with resultant histologic changes in the form of hemorrhage, edema, and cellular infiltration. The changes are variable and seem to be dependent on the concentration and amount of ethanol consumed. There is also evidence that nutritional status may play a role and that gastric mucus contributes a protective action.

Pancreas. The pancreas is a prime target for the effects of ethanol in certain individuals. Ethanol produces an increase in pancreatic secretion, apparently by stimulating the acid-secretin mechanism. Resection of the parietal cell mass abolishes the pancreatic response to ethanol.

There is also evidence that ethanol causes an increase in pancreatic duct pressure, apparently by a contraction of the sphincter of Oddi. The increased intrapancreatic pressure produced by a combination of increased pancreatic secretion and elevated intraductal pressure may be the cause of acinar rupture, leading to ethanol-induced pancreatitis.

Chronic pancreatitis is a common complication of alcoholism and may result from repeated attacks of acute pancreatitis. There is also evidence that qualitative and quantitative changes occur in pancreatic secretion following long-term use of ethanol. The role, if any, of these changes in the production of pancreatitis remains unsettled. Malnutrition may play a role in the pancreatic insufficiency seen in chronic alcoholics.

ENDOCRINE SYSTEM. A variety of hormonal changes have been reported in association with the acute and chronic intake of ethanol. With acute intake, ethanol appears to have a stimulatory effect on the adrenal cortex, producing an increase in blood cortisol levels. This response does not occur in hypophysectomized animals, suggesting that ethanol stimulates adrenocorticotropic hormone (ACTH) release.

Increases in the excretion of urinary catecholamines have been reported during chronic ethanol intake, and alcoholic withdrawal symptoms have been attributed to persistent elevations of catecholamine levels. The diuretic effect of ethanol has been attributed to its inhibitory effect on the secretion of antidiuretic hormone (ADH). However, in the presence of falling blood ethanol concentrations, there is an increase in vasopressin excretion, so that most alcoholics are slightly overhydrated. Ethanol effects in the thyroid are minimal; modest decreases in thyroxine (T_4) and triiodothyronine (T_3) have been noted.

Acute modest ethanol intake with blood levels of 100 mg/dl or less may increase libido in men but simultaneously decrease erectile capacity. In chronic alcoholism, even in the absence of liver impairment, there is a significant incidence of testicular atrophy, oligospermia, azoospermia, and infertility. Hypoandrogenism and an imbalance of the estrogen/androgen relationship may occur with resultant feminization. In women, the repeated intake of ethanol may result in amenorrhea, spontaneous abortions, and sterility.

Fetal alcohol syndrome (FAS) may result from ethanol intake during pregnancy, although the specific amount of ethanol required and the period of vulnerability during pregnancy have not been defined. The clinical signs and symptoms in the neonate with FAS include a mixture of abnormalities: prominent epicanthal eye folds, poorly formed ears, small teeth with faulty enamel, atrial or ventricular septal defects, aberrant palmar creasing, limitations of joint motion, and microcephaly with mental retardation.

Increased risk of cancer

Cancer is second only to cardiovascular disease as a cause of death in alcoholics. The rate of carcinoma is 10 times that expected in the general population. The sites with the greatest increase of cancer occurrence over expected rates include the oral cavity and neck, esophagus, stomach, liver, and pancreas.

BIBLIOGRAPHY

Cicero TJ: Neuroendocrinological effects of alcohol, Ann Rev Med 32:123, 1981.
Frank D and Raichi RF: Alcohol-induced liver disease, Alc: Clin Exp Res 9:66, 1985.
Israel Y: Cellular effects of alcohol: a review, Q J Stud Alcohol 31:293, 1970.
Isselbacher KJ: Metabolic and hepatic effects of alcohol, N Engl J Med 296:612, 1977.
Lieber C: To drink (moderately) or not to drink? N Engl J Med 310:846, 1984.
Mendelson JH and Mello NK: Biologic concomitants of alcoholism, N Engl J Med 301:912, 1979.
Myerson RM: Metabolic aspects of alcohol and their biological significance, Med Clin North Am 57:925, 1973.
Van Thiel DH: Gastrointestinal and hepatic manifestations of chronic alcoholism, Gastroenterology 81:594, 1981.

198·PATHOGENESIS AND DIAGNOSIS OF DIABETES MELLITUS*

Oliver E. Owen *and* Charles R. Shuman

Diabetes mellitus is a chronic systemic disorder of diverse etiologic factors characterized by disturbances in glucose, lipid, and protein metabolism. It is caused by a decreased availability or reduced activity of insulin, which is required for regulation of metabolic homeostasis. The heterogeneity of the diabetic syndromes is expressed in a variety of clinical presentations, ranging from asymptomatic states in patients with mild insulin deficiency to debilitating conditions of weakness, weight loss,

*This work was supported in part by the United States Public Health Service Research Grant RR00349, General Research Centers Branch, National Institutes of Health.

thirst, polyuria, dehydration, and coma in those with severe insulin deprivation. In the chronic course of diabetes, progressive and characteristic complications occur in the retina, kidneys, peripheral nervous system, connective tissue, and major arteries.

Diabetes is a disease of global distribution, affecting individuals of all ages. Peak incidence in the United States occurs in the fifth decade of life. Among younger groups, both sexes are equally affected; in older groups, the disease is seen more frequently in females. In some populations, epidemiologic studies have shown an increased frequency related to changes in life-style: urbanization, dietary changes, obesity, and stress are putative factors in this propensity for glucose intolerance and diabetes mellitus. In the United States an estimated 2% to 3% of the population have abnormally high blood glucose concentrations, and about half of this group has diabetes mellitus. The prevalence of insulin-dependent, ketosis-prone diabetes mellitus is estimated to be 0.2% of the population. The incidence of non-insulin-dependent, ketosis-resistant diabetes mellitus is three to five times more frequent than the insulin-dependent type of diabetes. A growing prevalence of diabetes has been related to the greater longevity of the population because the incidence increases with aging.

Heredity has long been considered a primary pathogenetic factor of diabetes, as denoted by the disorder's familial occurrence. However, genetic studies have been hampered by the difficulty in demonstrating specific "markers" for the transmission of the disease and by the recognition of environmental factors, which appear to increase predisposition. Important contributions to knowledge of the inheritance of diabetes have been made by the study of its transmission in twins. Analysis of data on monozygotic twins has shown that the concordance rates for those in whom the index twin develops diabetes after 40 years of age is nearly 100%. When the index twin developed diabetes before 40 years of age, concordance was seen in less than 40%.

Insulin and macronutrient metabolism

Insulin is synthesized in the β-cells of the islets of Langerhans as a single-chain polypeptide. The first precursor is preproinsulin. This precursor is converted to proinsulin by microsomal proteases within minutes of its synthesis. Proinsulin is transferred from the rough endoplasmic reticulum to the Golgi apparatus, where it is packaged into microvesicles. Within the Golgi complex and continuing in the accumulated secretory granules, proinsulin is cleaved in equal molar amounts of insulin and C-peptide following β-cell stimulation with nutrients. The mature secretory granules migrate to and become incorporated in the plasma membrane for extrusion of insulin and C-peptide into the extracellular space.

Insulin is a polypeptide hormone that circulates in the blood and travels through the extracellular fluids as a water-soluble molecule. During starvation, about 10 units of insulin are released from the β-cells per day, whereas during the usual nutritional state, about 40 units of insulin are released per day from the β-cells. In the basal state the concentration of insulin in peripheral blood oscillates at 10 to 12 minute intervals around mean values of about 6 to 12 μU/ml and about 18 to 36 μU/ml of serum plasma in lean and obese humans, respectively. The amplitude of the oscillations is 2 to 3 μU/ml. The pulsatile periods of insulin secretion are disturbed in diabetes, and insulin responses to meals or glucose challenges are absent in type I and diminished in type II diabetes. After an oral load or mixed meal the circulating insulin concentrations increase 10- to 20-fold in lean humans and 20- to

Table 198-1   Insulin action

	Anticatabolic effects	Anabolic effects
Liver	Decreased glycogenolysis, gluconeogenesis, and ketogenesis	Increased glycogen synthesis and fatty-acid synthesis
Adipose tissue	Decreased lipolysis	Increased glycerol synthesis and fatty-acid synthesis
Muscle	Decreased protein catabolism and amino acid output	Increased amino acid uptake, protein synthesis, and glycogen synthesis

40-fold in obese humans. The rise in serum plasma insulin concentrations parallels the rise in blood glucose concentrations; however, the fall in insulin concentrations is not as low as the glucose decline following oral intake. During the postchallenge period, oxidative- and nonoxidative-glucose (amino acids) disposal rates increase severalfold, depending on the quantity of carbohydrate (protein) administered. There is a reciprocal depression of fat oxidation when glucose oxidation is augmented during the postprandial period. These acute changes in the nature and quantities of oxidized or stored macronutrients are absent in type I diabetes and decreased in type II diabetes.

Insulin travels freely through the extracellular fluids and binds to receptors on the plasma membranes of certain tissues to initiate the transduction of its signals. When insulin attaches to its unique site on the plasma membrane, it forms a receptor-ligand complex. Within milliseconds, this complex triggers short-lived chain reactions, leading to subsequent cellular anabolic responses. Insulin is the principal hormone responsible for promoting macronutrient storage in the form of protein, triglycerides, and glycogen. It enhances proteogenosis, lipogenesis, and glycogenesis and suppresses proteolysis, lipolysis, gluconeogenesis, and glycogenolysis (Table 198-1). By promoting the translocation of glucose from the extracellular to the intracellular space and by decreasing the availability of free fatty acids, insulin also augments glucose oxidation.

The insulin receptor consists of two α- and two β-subunits. The α-subunits are on the external surface of the plasma membrane and serve as the binding sites for insulin. The β-subunits cross the plasma membrane and extend into the interior surface where they rapidly transmit the insulin signals. The insulin receptor is controlled by one gene and is produced as a single-chain precursor in a manner similar to preproinsulin synthesis. The receptor-precursor protein matures into a tetrameric structure and becomes incorporated into the plasma membrane. When insulin is linked to its receptor, the tyrosine residues of the receptor are phosphorylated; thus the insulin receptor is in part an insulin-dependent tyrosine kinase. Many signals are transmitted from the insulin-receptor complex to promote the activities of several plasma membrane–transport systems (permeases) and cytoplasmic anabolic enzymes. For example, the insulin-receptor complex rapidly stimulates the translocation of glucose from the extracellular fluids to the cytoplasm of many tissues. Vesicles with many glucose permeases are located just beneath the plasma membrane. The insulin-receptor complexes stimulate cells, causing the glucose-rich permease vesicles to fuse the plasma membrane and increase glucose transport manifold. In addition, the insulin-receptor complex causes a fall in the intracellular concentrations of cyclic adenosine monophosphate (AMP). However, glucagon counteracts the roles of insulin. Both glucagon and epinephrine activate

adenylate cyclase at the inner surface of the plasma membrane (Fig. 198-1). Adenylate cyclase converts adenosine 5'-triphosphate (ATP) to cyclic AMP, a water-soluble second messenger that diffuses throughout the cell, activating protein kinases that in turn phosphorylate other intracellular proteins, especially enzymes. In general, these phosphorylated enzymes are energized proteins that stimulate catabolism, mobilizing glucose from glycogen and perhaps, free fatty acids from triglycerides and amino acids from proteins.

Additional members of the receptor-ligand second messenger unit are interlinking stimulatory and inhibitory G proteins. G proteins, so-called because they bind guanine nucleotides, act as transducers of information across the cell membrane. They differ in that one G protein interconnects the stimulating hormones (glucagon and epinephrine) and the other interconnects the inhibitory hormones (prostaglandins and adenosine) to adenylate cyclase. Cyclic AMP can also be regulated by undergoing degradation via phosphodiesterases. These degrading phosphodiesterases are responsive to the intracellular concentrations of calcium.

Among the regulators of cell behavior are the inositol phospholipid metabolites arising from precursor phosphoinositides located in the cell membrane. These metabolies function as intracellular messengers transmitting signals within the cytosol, activating protein kinase C, and mobilizing intracellular calcium.

Clearly, insulin and its metabolic effects are deficient in diabetes mellitus. Many of the other hormonal abnormalities may be secondary phenomena. Abnormal insulin mutants that bind ineffectively to the receptor are a rare cause of diabetes. Defective receptors have been described, but such disorders are poorly understood. In some cases immunoglobulins compete with insulin for the binding sites on the receptors, but these anomalies are uncommon.

Classification of diabetes

Before 1980 a variety of descriptive terms were used to classify the various types of diabetes mellitus. Confusing terminology and lack of uniformity in the definitions of types of disease created problems in the assessment of data concerning the course, management, and complications of diabetes. Utilizing epidemiologic data and the emerging evidence concerning immunologic phenomena, the National Diabetes Data Group (NDDG), sponsored by the National Institutes of Health (NIH) and the Expert Committee on Diabetes Mellitus of the World Health Organization (WHO), developed a classification of diabetes mellitus and other disorders with impaired glucose tolerance that has received wide acceptance by the leading diabetic associations.

The major clinical categories are type I, or insulin-dependent diabetes mellitus (IDDM), and type II, or non-insulin-dependent diabetes mellitus (NIDDM). These two types encompass the overwhelming majority of patients in the temperate zones of the world. A third category is termed "other types of diabetes mellitus," which includes a variety of disorders associated with glucose intolerance and formerly was known as secondary diabetes. A separate category of gestational diabetes mellitus (GDM) was devised for those patients with diabetes developed during pregnancy. In 1985 the WHO Expert Committee created an additional category termed "malnutrition-related diabetes mellitus" (MRDM) to include a large population of patients in tropical and developing countries. The clinical classification of diabetes mellitus and impaired glucose tolerance as revised in the WHO Technical Report 727, 1985, is shown in Table 198-2.

Table 198-2 Classification of diabetes mellitus and glucose intolerance

Diabetes mellitus (DM)
  Insulin-dependent diabetes mellitus (IDDM)
  Non-insulin-dependent diabetes mellitus (NIDDM)
    Nonobese DM
    Obese DM
  Malnutrition-related diabetes mellitus (MRDM)
  Other types of diabetes mellitus (associated with certain conditions
    or syndromes)
    Pancreatic disease–associated DM
    Hormonally associated DM
    Drug- or chemical-induced DM
    Abnormalities related to insulin or its receptors
    DM caused by certain genetic syndromes
    Miscellaneous DM

Impaired glucose tolerance (IGT)
  Nonobese DM
  Obese DM
  DM associated with certain conditions

Gestational diabetes mellitus (GDM)

Statistical risk classes
  Previous abnormality of glucose tolerance (Prev AGT)
  Potential abnormality of glucose tolerance (Pot AGT)

Reproduced from Shuman CR: Diabetes mellitus. In Nutrition and metabolism in patient care, Philadelphia, 1988, WB Saunders Co.

Type I: insulin-dependent diabetes mellitus

IDDM is the most frequent form of diabetes seen in young patients, but it may occur at any age and accounts for approximately 20% of the total diabetic population. It usually is characterized by an abrupt onset of symptoms although present evidence indicates that IDDM develops through an antecedent latent period of autoimmune damage to pancreatic β-cells. The immunologic markers include the presence of islet cell antibodies and certain human lymphocyte antigen (HLA) groups (DR_3/DR_4). IDDM is associated with a progressive decline in the insulin secretory response to intravenously administered glucose (but not initially to orally administered glucose). Type I diabetes is thought to be initiated in the genetically susceptible individual by environmental factors such as viral, toxic, or chemical agents that damage pancreatic β-cells, resulting in the formation of altered protein components. This material is a foreign antigen to the immune system, establishing the basis for an autoimmune reaction against the cell of origin, the β-cell. At present the identity and nature of the β-cell antigen is unknown.

A decisive factor in the autoimmune hypothesis was the description by Gept in 1965 of insulitis, an inflammatory mononuclear cell infiltration of pancreatic islets in patients with newly diagnosed diabetes. Subsequently, sera of diabetic patients was shown to contain antibodies reactive with islet cells. Antibodies of several types have been described and demonstrated in nearly all patients with initially onsetted type I diabetes. Islet cell antibodies (ICAs) can be present for many months or years before clinical diabetes is apparent. Not all patients with ICAs progress to frank diabetes. The role of ICAs in the pathogenesis of diabetes is not clear, but their presence is a possible predictor of type I diabetes.

A viral cause for diabetes has been suggested. However, epidemiologic studies of mumps, coxsackie B, and rubella indicate this is an improbable cause. The long prodromal period required for the evolution of type I diabetes and the failure to detect viruses in islets of diabetic patients suggests that these infections, as well as other environmental factors (such as chemical or toxins), represent precipitating agents rather than the cause of β-cell destruction.

During the early 1970s a relationship between certain HLA antigens in the A and B loci (A_1A_2, B_8B_{15}) diabetes was found simultaneously in Denmark and England in studies of juvenile diabetic patients. Further investigation by workers in these countries and in the United States demonstrated a more profound association between juvenile diabetes and HLAs in the D locus (DR_3 and DR_4). In these studies 97% of children manifested one or the other of these antigens. Those possessing both DR_3 and DR_4, with one antigen inherited from the father and one from the mother, comprised half of the diabetic children studied. The relative risks for diabetes were shown to be 5 for DR_3 and 6.8 for DR_4; for the heterozygous state of DR_3 and DR_4, the risk advanced to 14.3. Associations with B locus antigens appear to break the linkage between B_8 and DR_3 and between B_{15} and DR_4. These genetic and immunologic features, including the presence of islet cell antibodies, established a basis for the pathogenesis of juvenile-onset diabetes, distinguishing it from adult-onset diabetes.

A reasonable hypothesis incorporating the observed immunologic and genetic data in type I diabetes suggests that a foreign antigen is produced by the β-cytotoxic effect of viral infection. The foreign antigen is engulfed and processed by macrophage cells, which insert the processed antigen into the cell membrane in propinquity to class II molecules (HLA-DR, HLA-DP, or HLA-DQ). This immunogenic complex is recognized by specific receptors of helper-T lymphocytes activated by cell-to-cell interaction and by the influence of interleukin 1, a soluble lymphokine released by the macrophage cells. The activated helper-T lymphocytes produce interleukin 2, which causes their proliferation and activates cytotoxic T lymphocytes. The latter cells are responsible for the cell-mediated immune reactions directed against the foreign antigens. In addition, helper-T cells activate B lymphocytes with interleukin 4, a growth factor, stimulating an antigen-specific response programmed to increase antibodies against the foreign antigen. The clones (of B lymphocytes activated by immune receptors and B-cell growth factors) divide into plasma cells, which become the effector system for antibody production. These responses are modulated by suppressor-T cells, which regulate the expansion of antigenic stimulation. The suppressor system in type I diabetes is thought to be deficient. In the sequence of cell-mediated and humoral autoimmunity, pancreatic β-cells become positive for class II molecules through transfer of these antigens from lymphocytes or endothelial cells in the islets. Thus β-cells possess the autoimmune complex leading to the appearance of islet-cell antibody and providing the target for cytotoxic lymphocyte destruction of the cells.

Strong support for these concepts is provided by observations on the sequential transplantation of pancreatic tissue from a nondiabetic individual to his identical twin with type I diabetes. In this transplantation, the pancreas from the discordant twin rapidly lost its function and displayed evidence of insulitis with invasion of cytotoxic lymphocytes, indicating that the autoimmune response for β-cells was preserved in this patient. The absence of a significant response in ICA in the graft recipients indicates a subsidiary role for the humoral limb of autoimmunity.

A major concern arising from these observations is the need to develop methods for halting the autoimmune reactions leading to β-cell destruction. Early observations of the reaction of immunosuppressive drugs, particularly cyclosporin A, support the view that autoimmunity represents a basic factor in the

Table 198-3 Comparison between IDDM and NIDDM

	IDDM	NIDDM
Former names	Juvenile, growth-onset, ketosis-prone	Adult, maturity-onset, ketosis-resistant
Age of onset	Usually under 30 years of age; occurs at any age	Peak incidence—5th decade; may occur at younger ages
Symptoms	Usually abrupt; thirst, polyuria, weight loss	Frequently none or thirst, fatigue, visual blurring, vascular or neural complications
Nutritional status	Usually monobese	60% to 80% obese
Coma syndrome	Diabetic ketoacidosis	Hyperosmolar state; ketosis rarely with infection or stress
Endogenous insulin and C-peptide	Negligible to absent	Normal levels, but low in relation to blood sugar
Lipid abnormalities	Frequent cholesterol and LDL elevations; hyperlipidemia in ketoacidosis	Triglyceride (VLDL) and LDL cholesterol increased
Insulin	All patients dependent on insulin	Required for 20% to 30%
Sulfonylurea	No response	Effective for majority
Diet	Mandatory	Mandatory; diet alone may control blood sugar

Reproduced from Shuman CR: Diabetes mellitus. In Nutrition and metabolism in patient care, Philadelphia, 1988, WB Saunders Co.

pathogenesis of type I diabetes. Nonetheless, knowledge pertaining to the pathogenesis of type I diabetes mellitus is incomplete and controversy exists.

Type II: non–insulin-dependent diabetes mellitus

Two groups of patients with NIDDM are recognized by different body composition—obese and nonobese. The former comprises approximately 80% of individuals with NIDDM in most populations. In addition, a third group has been described among blacks in whom an initial form of insulin-requiring diabetes progresses to NIDDM that responds to sulfonylurea treatment. A small subgroup of patients within the NIDDM category has IDDM or latent type I diabetes mellitus. They are detected by the presence of islet cell antibodies and HLA-DR$_3$/DR$_4$, with manifestations of slowly progressive β-cell loss and a long latency period for the evolution of type I disease. Their response to sulfonylurea therapy indicates there are sufficient numbers of surviving β-cells to sustain partial glycemic control. The distinctions between the two major clinical categories of overt diabetes are shown in Table 198-3.

Type II diabetes has strong genetic determinants as demonstrated in studies of familial transmission and of identical twins, the latter showing a concordance of nearly 100% among twins with this disease. Although the precise nature of the inherited defect is unknown, it appears to involve a reduced ability to secrete insulin normally in response to a rising concentration of plasma glucose. Pathophysiologic alterations in type II diabetes involve progressive decreases in the insulin secretory response to glucose and in tissue sensitivity to circulating insulin.

Although longitudinal studies of type II diabetes are not available, epidemiologic data indicate that glucose intolerance manifests initially as a rise in postprandial plasma glucose concentrations with normal fasting glycemia. With advancing glucose intolerance, hyperglycemia in the fasting state develops and is associated with a progressive reduction in serum insulin concentration. During the early periods of development the rising blood glucose concentration induces greater fasting levels of serum insulin concentration in the patient with type II diabetes. Simultaneously there is a reduction in the response to insulin by target tissues. This reduction is related to a decrease in insulin-receptor number following insulin-receptor down-regulation. Concurrently, postreceptor defects develop. Both the reduction in receptor number and postreceptor defects induce insulin resistance or insensitivity. An additional factor is the utilization of fatty acid as fuel, which suppresses glycolysis (Randle's glucose–fatty acid cycle) leading to hyperglycemia. This may be of special importance in the patient with type II diabetes. Obesity can be viewed as an important environmental factor in the causation of type II diabetes. Insulin resistance or insensitivity and augmented lipolysis are probably epiphenomena secondary to β-cell dysfunction.

The condition of patients with type II diabetes is frequently improved by weight reduction, dietary management, exercise, and sulfonylurea medication. A decrease in body fat stores is accompanied by increased insulin secretory responses and decreased insulin resistance in liver, muscle, and adipose tissues. Sulfonylurea medication acts on the pancreatic β-cells to increase calcium mobilization and to partially restore insulin secretory responses to rising blood glucose levels. In addition, evidence of the stimulating influence of sulfonylurea on insulin activity in liver and muscle tissues has accumulated. It has also been suggested that this drug has a direct action on these tissues. These observations indicate a reversal of the basic pathophysiologic disturbances of type II diabetes mellitus caused by sulfonylurea. During periods of hyperglycemia unresponsive to diet, exercise, and sulfonylurea, human insulin is used singly or in combination with the oral drug.

Other types of diabetes mellitus

The class of diabetes termed "other types of diabetes mellitus" (formerly termed "secondary diabetes mellitus") is a heterogeneous group of disorders associated with hyperglycemia or glucose intolerance. Included are the diseases affecting the pancreas such as hemachromatosis, pancreatitis, and adenocarcinoma. The relatively uncommon endocrinopathies, including Cushing's disease, acromegaly, pheochromocytoma, aldosteronoma, and thyrotoxicosis, are associated with diabetes in approximately 15% to 25% of cases and with impaired glucose tolerance in 50% or more. Certain drugs, such as diuretic agents, β-adrenergic blockers, and Dilantin, can impair insulin secretion and cause diabetes or serve as a detection device for latent diabetes. Genetic or acquired defects in insulin receptors represent rare but specific causes of diabetes with insulin resistance. Similar conditions occur in the presence of antibodies to insulin receptors found rarely in patients with lupus erythematosus or other autoimmune states. A list of the subdivisions of this class of diabetes and representative examples are found in Table 198-2.

Gestational diabetes mellitus

In approximately 2% of pregnant women, gestational diabetes mellitus (GDM) occurs early or by the 24th to 28th week of gestation. Among the factors responsible for reduced maternal glucose utilization are hormonal changes involving the gonadal hormones estrogen-progesterone, placental lactogen, hypercortisolism, and hyperthyroxinosis, resulting in increased resistance to insulin activity. The sparing of glucose metabolism in the maternal tissues provides greater amounts of glucose for the developing conceptus. If the insulinogenic gravid state exceeds the β-cell–insulin secretory capacity, diabetes mellitus results. When unrecognized, GDM increases the risk of perinatal morbidity and mortality for the newborn.

Glucose abnormalities frequently disappear following parturition. However, these patients are known to have an increased risk of diabetes in later years. After 10 to 15 years, nearly 50% of patients with GDM develop diabetes mellitus, usually type II.

Impaired glucose tolerance

The term "impaired glucose tolerance" (IGT) has replaced the former designations of subclinical, chemical, or latent diabetes mellitus, thereby avoiding the psychologic, social, and economic disadvantages related to the term "diabetes." Individuals within this category have plasma glucose concentrations between normal and those diagnostic of diabetes mellitus. Over variable time periods they may progress to overt diabetes with worsening glucose tolerance. However, for the majority, glucose intolerance does not progress, and in some, serial testing may reveal a reversion to normal.

IGT also is distinguished from diabetes by the absence of microvascular complications such as retinopathy and nephropathy. Patients in this category have been found in several studies to have a higher prevalence of macrovascular disease than is found in control populations but less than is observed in those with diabetes. Because of these observations and to retard progression to diabetes, patients are given advice concerning dietary control of obesity, treatment of hypertension and hyperlipidemia, and elimination of smoking.

Malnutrition-related diabetes mellitus

Malnutrition-related diabetes mellitus (MRDM) has been described in tropical and developing countries as a commonly encountered form of diabetes mellitus. It has not been described in developed countries or in the temperate zones, although the J-type of diabetes found in Jamaica may be a variant of MRDM.

The WHO Technical Report published in 1985 describes two subgroups of MRDM, including calcareous pancreatic diabetes and protein-deficiency diabetes. The role of protein deficiency in reducing insulin secretory activity of the pancreatic β-cells requires further study to determine the pathogenesis of this disorder. In some patients on a low protein diet the ingestion of the cassava root appears to induce pancreatic calcification with the gradual evolution of a diminished insulinogenic capacity and diabetes.

Statistical risk classes

For purposes of metabolic data accumulation and analysis, two classes of statistical risks for diabetes and IGT have been recognized. These designations are not used in medical records as clinical states but are reserved for research or investigative purposes.

1. *Previous abnormality of glucose tolerance (Prev AGT)*. Patients who have had diabetes in the past or have manifested IGT and in whom current tests exhibit normal results are said to have Prev AGT. Most frequently, this category includes former gestational diabetic patients whose metabolic impairment subsided post partum. Other rare examples include stress-induced and drug-induced diabetes, which may disappear on withdrawal of the provoking agent. It is believed that these individuals are at increased risk for diabetes under conditions of weight gain, stress exposure, or illness.

Table 198-4   Criteria for diagnosis of diabetes mellitus and impaired glucose tolerance

	Plasma		Whole blood	
	Venous	Capillary	Venous	Capillary
DIABETES MELLITUS				
Fasting glucose*	≥ 140 (7.8)	≥ 140 (7.8)	≥ 120 (6.7)	≥ 120 (6.7)
2 hr post glucose†	≥ 200 (11.1)	≥ 220 (12.2)	≥ 180 (10.0)	≥ 200 (12.2)
IMPAIRED GLUCOSE TOLERANCE				
Fasting glucose*	< 140 (7.8)	< 140 (7.8)	< 120 (6.7)	< 120 (6.7)
2 hr post glucose†	140-200 (7.8-11.1)	160-220 (8.9-12.2)	120-180 (6.7-10.0)	140-200 (7.8-11.1)

GESTATIONAL DIABETES

WHO criteria are the same as those given for diabetes mellitus. O'Sullivan and Mahan criteria: Using a 100 g glucose load, two or more of the following values must be met or exceeded:

Venous plasma glucose*

Fasting—105 (5.8)	1 hr—190 (10.6)	2 hr—165 (9.2)	3 hr—145 (8.1)

Reproduced from Shuman CR: Diabetes mellitus. In Nutrition and metabolism in patient care, Philadelphia, 1988, WB Saunders Co.
*mg/dl (mmol/L)
†Oral glucose challenge is 75 g/kg for adults and 1.75 g/kg to 75 g/kg for children. Diagnostic criteria for children are same as those for adults.

2. *Potential abnormality of glucose tolerance (Pot AGT)*. Individuals at greater risk of diabetes than the general population are placed in the category of Pot AGT, previously designated as potential diabetes or prediabetes. Included in this category are those with normal glucose tolerance who are first-degree relatives of diabetic patients, an identical twin of a type I or type I proband, an HLA identical sibling of a diabetic patient, or an individual with positive islet cell antibody determination. In addition, individuals with android obesity and hypertension and those with an adverse pregnancy record, spontaneous abortions, or large infants (9 lb or greater) are at potential risks for diabetes. Interest in this category is whetted by the concept of immunoprevention of type I diabetes that depends on reliable markers for the development of this disease.

Diagnostic criteria of diabetes mellitus

In 1980 revised standard values for the diagnosis of diabetes mellitus and IGT were presented by the NDDG sponsored by the NIH and by the Expert Committee on Diabetes of the WHO (Table 198-4). These diagnostic criteria were developed after analysis of epidemiologic studies that suggested previous standards for blood, plasma and serum glucose concentrations were inappropriately low. The higher plasma glucose concentrations promulgated in the revised criteria provide a more reliable value for predicting diabetes than the formerly recommended United States Public Health Service criteria. International acceptance of these diagnostic standards has been helpful in providing a basis for uniformity in research and therapeutic assessments.

Diabetes is a common disease, and its diagnosis is not difficult if the physician remains attentive to the possibility. Symptoms of fatigue, thirst, polyuria, weight loss, and recurrent infection are encountered in patients with fully developed diabetes. Diabetic proneness is considered in the android obese, individuals with a positive family history of diabetes, and in those with unfavorable obstetric histories, premature arterio-sclerosis, neuropathy, or glycosuria. Urine glucose determinations are often used as a screening test but are never acceptable for diagnosis.

Determinations of glucose concentrations in properly obtained blood samples are the only reliable criteria for the diagnosis of diabetes. Plasma or serum glucose measurements using the glucose analytic method are preferred over those of whole blood because there is less interference with equipment and differences in hematocrit and water distribution are eliminated. Specific laboratory enzymatic or colorimetric techniques are the preferred methods to measure glucose concentrations in biological fluids. The measurement of blood glucose with reagent strips and reflectance meters is generally too unreliable to unequivocally establish the diagnosis of diabetes mellitus. The glucose concentrations obtained from venous plasma are roughly comparable to those obtained using arterial whole blood or capillary blood, although venous plasma glucose determinations are preferred for standardization of results.

FASTING PLASMA GLUCOSE. Normal plasma glucose concentrations vary slightly depending on the reagents used by individual laboratories but do not exceed 115 mg/dl (Table 198-4). Diabetes can be diagnosed with confidence if the fasting plasma glucose (GPG) concentrations are greater than 140 mg/dl on two separate occasions. Immediate confirmation of the diagnosis is provided by demonstrating an elevation of glycosylated hemoglobin (Hb A_{1c}) greater than normal in association with elevated FPG. An elevated Hb A_{1c} is indicative of an increase in blood glucose above normal for several weeks or more. Since the Hb A_{1c} determinations are not standardized and are subject to error, this measurement cannot serve as a sole diagnostic determinant. Advantages of FPG are several, including standardization of conditions for the test and for obtaining the blood sample and the absence of the effects of age, previous diet, or activity. Disadvantages are related to the late occurrence of fasting hyperglycemia in the diabetic syndrome; postcibal hyperglycemia with normal FPG is an earlier phase, during which treatment of type II disease can arrest its progression.

TESTING OF VENOUS PLASMA GLUCOSE CONCENTRATIONS AFTER GLUCOSE OR FOOD. A standardized test of glucose tolerance is required to detect diabetes in an early phase of metabolic abnormality. Such a procedure is found in the 2-hour determination of venous plasma glucose after the administration of 75 g of glucose in 300 ml of water (which may be flavored) taken over a period of 3 minutes in fasting conditions of 10 hours. Patients for whom the procedure is scheduled should consume a proper diet of normal or elevated carbohydrate content (150 g or more) for 3 days, should rest, and should refrain from smoking. The results of the test can be affected by certain medications (such as diuretics and glucosteroids), illness, surgery, or stress.

Venous plasma glucose determinations are normally values less than 140 mg/dl 2 hours after the glucose load. Diabetes mellitus is diagnosed if the 2-hour value is equal to or greater than 200 mg/dl. Values between 140 mg/dl and 200 mg/dl are classified as impaired glucose tolerance. Confirmation (with a second determination) of one abnormal value is required to confirm the diagnosis.

An elevated FPG correlates well with a corresponding rise in the plasma glucose after a meal or a glucose challenge. An elevated postcibal plasma glucose, however, may not be accompanied by an elevated FPG.

ORAL GLUCOSE TOLERANCE TEST. Traditionally, the oral glucose tolerance test (OGTT) has provided the final decision concerning the diagnosis of diabetes. This test can be seriously misleading, however, if scrupulous care is not exerted in its performance. Preparation of the patient and precision in the timing of blood sampling are required to obtain reliable results. The test is not required for diagnostic purposes when the FPG is unequivocally elevated; it is inadvisable if hyperglycemia (300 mg/dl) is present because the rapid rise in blood sugar following glucose administration may induce hyperosmolarity and cardiac arrhythmia.

With the current criteria for the diagnosis of diabetes based on FPG and 2-hour post-glucose-load determination of plasma glucose (2-hour PG), the OGTT is rarely required. In our experience this test is used only in questionable conditions of glucose intolerance, for example, when the FPG concentration is less than 140 mg/dl but postchallenge values are anticipated to be elevated. It is used most frequently as a 5-hour test for the detection of idiopathic hypoglycemia. There is a poor correlation in the plasma glucose concentrations between the OGTT and response after a meal. Equally discordant are the signs and symptoms compatible with hypoglycemia and chemically detectable hypoglycemia in plasma.

The recommended procedures for the OGTT are the same as those outlined for the 2-hour PG test. These include a balanced diet of increased or normal carbohydrate intake for 3 days with a 75 g glucose load in 300 ml of beverage given in 3 to 5 minutes after an overnight 10- to 12-hour fast. This test should not be performed in patients who are hospitalized, ill, or taking medications that will interfere with the results. After a fasting blood sample is taken to measure the plasma glucose concentration, the patient remains quiet without smoking or taking additional beverages until 2 hours have passed, at which point a blood sample is taken to measure the plasma glucose concentration. Previous recommendations for blood samples taken at ½, 1, and 1½ hours have been removed by the WHO, since there is no evidence that these values contribute to the diagnosis of diabetes or to other aspects of the disorder and its management.

The diagnosis of diabetes mellitus should be made when the 2-hour PG value is greater than 200 mg/dl. This applies to all age-groups, as do the criteria for IGT. IGT is diagnosed when the FPG is less than 140 mg/dl and the 2-hour PG is between 140 and 200 mg/dl.

There are two different criteria recommended for the diagnosis of GDM (Table 198-4). The NDDG has advocated the criteria established in 1964 by O'Sullivan and Mahan based on an extensive survey of OGTTs performed during pregnancy. These lower values reflect the reduced glycemic levels found during normal pregnancies. The OGTT performed for the detection of gestational diabetes differs from the customary test by using a 100 g glucose load and by obtaining blood samples at 1-hour intervals for 3 hours after oral administration of glucose.

The second criterion used by the WHO for the diagnosis of GDM is the same as that applied to the nonpregnant population. The OGTT is performed in the conventional manner using 75 g of glucose as the loading dose, with blood samples taken in the fasting state and 2 hours after glucose ingestion.

DIABETES SCREENING DURING PREGNANCY. Screening procedures for GDM are recommended at the outset of pregnancy and between the 24th and 28th weeks of pregnancy if the initial screening is normal. Of particular importance is screening of pregnant patients with one or more of the following: obesity, family history of diabetes, glycosuria, history of previous pregnancy with spontaneous abortion, hydramnios, preeclampsia, large baby (9 lb or more), or elevated plasma glucose concentrations.

A practical and convenient screening procedure is the oral administration of a 50 g glucose load with a single blood sample taken at 1 hour for venous plasma glucose. If the screening test is positive (plasma glucose concentration greater than 150 mg/dl), an OGTT should be performed.

DIABETES SCREENING FOR THE NONPREGNANT INDIVIDUAL. Unless well-planned and carefully constituted, community-wide screening for diabetes serves only to obtain publicity for the sponsoring organization. These efforts have been discredited because of the following: poor followup; failure to rescreen positive or borderline results; false positive results causing psychic trauma or incorrect treatment; and adverse cost/benefit ratio.

Selective screening is recommended for patients in high-risk groups, including those with hypertension, cardiac disease, or pregnancy. Physicians should routinely screen patients in the office, with particular attention to the elderly, the obese, those with positive family history of diabetes, and those with hyperlipidemia, gout, or arteriosclerosis. Patients can be screened with a FPG determination or with a plasma glucose determination 2 hours after administration of a 75 g glucose load as described above. A less accurate but useful procedure is to obtain a plasma glucose determination 2 hours after a meal containing an estimated 75 g of carbohydrate. Because the latter test is not standardized, a positive result requires additional testing with the conventional OGTT.

Additional diagnostic procedures

Serum insulin determinations are not useful in the diagnosis of diabetes mellitus. Attempts to distinguish type I from type II diabetes using serum insulin radioimmunoassay have not proved fruitful, since some patients with type II manifest reduced serum insulin concentrations. On the other hand, elevated serum insulin values are observed in obese type II diabetic patients and in other patients with insulin-resistant states (acanthosis nigricans with insulin resistance).

Determinations of serum insulin are not accurate in patients previously treated with exogenous insulin because of the likelihood of insulin antibody production. However, measurements of total insulin and antibody-bound insulin provide a potentially useful determination of the free insulin concentration.

CONNECTING PEPTIDE RADIOIMMUNOASSAY. The connecting peptide (C-peptide) radioimmunoassay is useful when information is needed concerning endogenous insulin secretions, particularly in patients who are likely to have insulin antibody present in their serum (which precludes accurate insulin assays).

C-peptide is the amino acid sequence within the proinsulin molecule joining the α- and β-chains of insulin. This peptide is cleaved from proinsulin and packaged in secretory granules with insulin so that it is released in equimolar concentrations in the secretory process. Because C-peptide is not terminally metabolized in its passage through the liver, determinations of its plasma or urinary concentrations have provided useful information concerning rates and amounts of insulin secretion. Fasting or stimulated C-peptide determinations or both have been examined in type I and type II patients. Stimulation with glucagon injection (1 mg) or Sustacal feeding has been used but has not yielded information superior to that obtained from fasting C-peptide measurements alone.

Studies of type I patients suggest that a small residual C-peptide secretory capacity (endogenous insulin present) denotes a more stable form of IDDM than the labile type I diabetes

seen in the total absence of C-peptide. In type II diabetes, C-peptide can be normal or reduced depending on insulinogenic potential, which can change significantly during the treatment of this condition.

In patients with factitious hypoglycemia produced by surreptitious insulin administration, C-peptide levels are low to absent. In contrast, patients whose hypoglycemia is caused by covert self-administration of sulfonylurea manifest elevated serum C-peptide (and insulin) concentrations.

Glycosylated hemoglobin

Glycosylated hemoglobin (Hb A_{1c}) is an adduct of glucose to hemoglobin at specific amino acid residues terminal valine of the β-chain and to the α-amino lysine side chains. It is produced in a two-step biochemical nonenzymatic reaction. An initial rapid Schiff base reaction forms a labile, reversible aldimine form, which then undergoes an intramolecular Amadori rearrangement to become a stable, irreversible ketoamine formation. The concentration of this compound is directly related to the rise in blood glucose over an interval of time. The normal concentration of Hb A_{1c} varies depending on the method employed for its determination and on the individual laboratory techniques, since there are no standard preparations or methodology. There is a linear rise in Hb A_{1c} as the blood sugar increases in diabetic patients. Since the life span of the erythrocyte is 120 days, a change in Hb A_{1c} concentration can be observed only after several weeks if the ambient blood sugar concentration is changed. In general, an ambient plasma glucose level of 120 mg/dl is equivalent to a Hb A_{1c} value of approximately 6%, and a plasma glucose level of 250 mg/dl is reflected in a Hb A_{1c} value of 12%. A number of methods are available, including chromatographic techniques, radioimmunoassay, and isoelectric focusing, that give comparable but not interchangeable results. False high or low values are found in the presence of hemoglobinopathies, azotemia, and certain drugs. There is evidence that the measurement of the stable ketoamine form of glycohemoglobin can be standardized with the use of a thiobarbituric acid reagent.

Presently Hb A_{1c} is not used as a diagnostic study for diabetes because of lack of standardization of test procedures, problems with quality control, and overlapping values between normal and diabetic persons. The test may be used for screening or for corroboration of the diagnosis provided by a plasma glucose determination. Currently Hb A_{1c} is extremely useful for the assessment of glycemic control over 6- to 12-week periods in patients with either type I or type II diabetes mellitus. Further clinical studies will define the role of Hb A_{1c} or other glycosylated proteins (such as fructosamine and glycoalbumin) in the diagnosis and management of diabetes and will provide a tool for the investigation of the complications of diabetes.

Physiologic and physiopathologic production of glucose and ketone bodies by liver

When the usual hepatic production rate of glucose (about 0.86 mmol/min/1.73 m²) occurs in the presence of hyperglycemia, the liver is metabolizing inappropriately. Hyperglycemia occurs because insulin action on the extrahepatic tissue and on the liver is diminished. However, in the overnight fasting periods, the hyperglycemia compensates for the low insulin action, and normal rates of glucose oxidation occur, provided that the plasma free fatty-acid concentrations are not elevated.

During the usual postabsorptive fasting state when hepatic

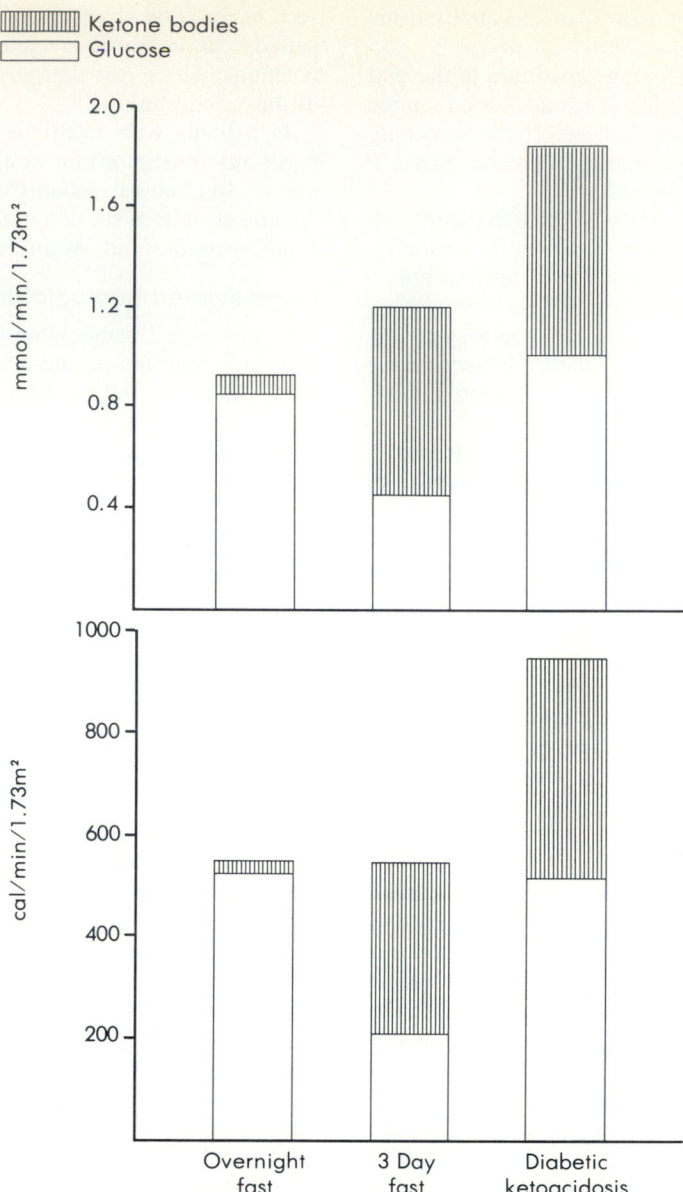

Fig. 198-1   Hepatic glucose and ketone body production rates and caloric equivalents for glucose (corrected for lactate and pyruvate recycling) and ketone bodies (acetoacetate and β-hydroxybutyrate).

glucose production is high, ketone-body production is low. During starvation, when hepatic glucose production is low, ketone-body production rate is high (Fig. 198-1). These reciprocal changes in hepatic delivery of glucose and ketone bodies, coupled with the appropriate release and oxidation of amino acids and free fatty acids, maintain fuel homeostasis during brief and prolonged periods of caloric deprivation. The loss of these related and reciprocal processes, coupled with flooding the bloodstream with an excess of free fatty acids and localized heightened oxidation of amino acids, leads to metabolic decompensation.

The degree of insulin deficiency correlates with the subsequent loss of fuel homeostasis. Once 90% of the β-cell insulin secretory capacity is lost, hyperglycemia occurs during the fasting state and becomes grossly accentuated postprandially. The decrease in insulin sensitivity with a reduced rate of glucose uptake per given blood glucose concentration in most tissues, especially in muscle with its gross mass, becomes coupled with an abnormal hepatic glucose production

rate, causing the fasting and postprandial elevated glucose concentrations. However, with this limited loss of insulin secretory capacity, glucose oxidation and storage is indistinguishable from normal. Thus the combination of low serum insulin concentrations coupled with high blood glucose concentrations results in normal extrahepatic glucose disposal rates (Fig. 198-2). In addition, during this mild state of insulin insufficiency, lipolysis is normal. With progressive losses of insulin secretory capacity, greater degrees of metabolic decompensation develop. Initially the ability to augment glucose storage during postprandial hyperglycemia develops and is accompanied by glycosuria. Diminished glucose oxidation is superimposed on the inability to dispose of glucose via nonoxidative pathways. With greater loss of insulin action, postprandial anabolism fails and eventually catabolism prevails in all states of nutrition. Ketonemia develops and ketonuria follows. Finally, nonsensible catabolism develops with fulminant proteolysis and lipolysis, resultant augmented gluconeogenesis and ketogenesis, inducing dehydrating hyper-

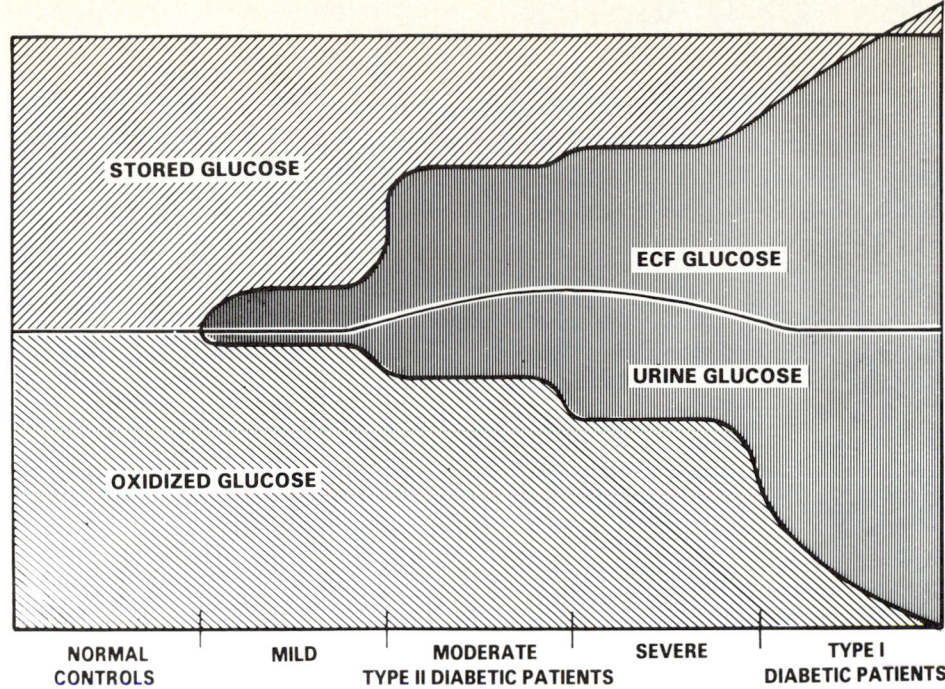

Fig. 198-2   Schematic presentation of glucose disposal rates in normal controls and patients with various degrees of deterioration. (Reproduced from Owen OE and others: Resting and postprandial fuel utilization in normal and diabetic humans. In Clinical nutrition and metabolic research. Basel, 1986, S Karger.)

glycemia and ketoacidosis. Without corrective therapy, death occurs.

Conclusion

In summary, diabetes mellitus is a global disease affecting all facets of metabolism. The incidence of diabetes increases as the population ages. It is a disease of insulin insufficiency forming a spectrum from hyperglycemia to fulminant ketoacidosis. The understanding of the pathogenesis of diabetes is advancing rapidly. It is hoped that molecular biological and immunologic knowledge will soon allow not only full characterization of various types of diabetes mellitus but also corrective therapy.

BIBLIOGRAPHY

Bosi E and others: Mechanisms of autoimmunity: relevance to the pathogenesis of type I (insulin-dependent) diabetes mellitus, Diabetes Metab Rev 3(4):893, 1987.

Bottazzo GF and others: Evidence for a primary autoimmune type of diabetes mellitus, Br Med J 2:1253, 1978.

Bottazzo GF and others: Complement-fixing islet cell antibodies in type I diabetes; possible monitors of active β-cell damage, Lancet 1:668, 1980.

Bunn HF: Nonenzymatic glycosylation of protein: relevance to diabetes. In Skyler JS and Cahill GF Jr, editors: Diabetes mellitus, New York, 1981, Yorke Medical Books.

Craighead JE: Current views on the etiology of insulin-dependent diabetes mellitus, N Engl J Med 229:1439, 1978.

DeFronzo RA, Ferrannini E, and Koivisto V: New concepts in the pathogenesis and treatment of non-insulin-dependent diabetes mellitus, Am J Med 74(suppl 1A):52, 1983.

Eisenbarth GS: Type I diabetes mellitus: a chronic autoimmune disease, N Engl J Med 314:1360, 1986.

Fentrain G and others: Cyclosporin increases the rate and length of remissions in insulin-dependent diabetes of recent onset: results of a multicentre double-blind trial, Lancet 1:119, 1986.

Flier JS, Kahn CR, and Roth J: Receptors, antireceptor antibodies and mechanisms of insulin resistance, N Engl J Med 300:413, 1979.

Gorsuch AN and others: Evidence for a long prediabetic period in type I (insulin-dependent) diabetes mellitus, Lancet 11:1363, 1981.

Harris MI and others: International criteria for the diagnosis of diabetes and impaired glucose tolerance, Diabetes Care 8:562, 1985.

Kolterman OG and others: Mechanisms of insulin resistance in human obesity: evidence for receptor and postreceptor defects, J Clin Invest 65:1272, 1980.

Kuzuya H and others: Clinical significance of circulating C-peptide in type I and type II diabetes. In Melchionda N, Horwitz DL, and Schade DS, editors: Recent advances in obesity and diabetes research, New York, 1984, Raven Press.

Learnmark A and others: Islet-specific immune mechanisms, Diabetes/Metab Rev 3(4):959, 1987.

Michelsen B and Lernmark A: Molecular cloning of a polymorphic DNA endonuclease fragment associates insulin-dependent diabetes mellitus with HLA-DQ, J Clin Invest 79:1144, 1987.

National Diabetes Data Group: Classification and diagnosis of diabetes mellitus and other categories of glucose intolerance, Diabetes 28:1039, 1979.

O'Sullivan JB and Mahan CM: Criteria for the oral glucose tolerance test in pregnancy, Diabetes 13:278, 1964.

Owen OE and others: Human splanchnic metabolism during diabetic ketoacidosis, Metabolism 26:381, 1977.

Owen OE and others: Effects of therapy on the nature and quantity of fuels oxidized during diabetic ketoacidosis, Diabetes 29:365, 1980.

Owen OE and others: Hepatic, gut, and renal substrate flux rates in patients with hepatic cirrhosis, J Clin Invest 68:240, 1981.

Owen OE and others: Resting and postprandial fuel utilization in normal and diabetic humans. In Dietze G and others, editors: Clinical nutrition and metabolic research, Basel, 1986, S Karger.

Owen OE and others: A reappraisal of the caloric requirements of men, Am J Clin Nutr 46:875, 1987.

Owen OE: Regulation of energy and metabolism. In Kinney JM and others, editor: Nutrition and metabolism in patient care, Philadelphia, 1988, WB Saunders Co.

Owen OE: Obesity. In Kinney JM and others, editors: Nutrition and metabolism in patient care, Philadelphia, 1988, WB Saunders Co.

Stiller CR and others: Effect of cyclosporin immunosuppression in insulin-dependent diabetes mellitus of recent onset, Science 223:1363, 1984.

Unger RH, Dobbs RE, and Orci L: Insulin, glucagon, and somatostatin secretion in the regulation of metabolism, Annu Rev Physiol 40:307, 1978.

WHO Expert Committee: Second report on diabetes mellitus, Technical report series No. 646, Geneva, Switzerland, 1980.

WHO Study Group: Technical report series No. 727, Geneva, Switzerland, 1985.

199 · TREATMENT OF DIABETES MELLITUS

Harry Gottlieb

The concentration of blood glucose reflects a balance between glucose absorption, production, and utilization. Insulin promotes anabolic processes such as hepatic glycogen synthesis, amino acid incorporation into protein, and fat deposition. Glucagon and other hormones such as epinephrine, glucocorticoids, and growth hormone stimulate glucose production, lipolysis, and gluconeogenesis. The central nervous system participates in maintaining that glucose concentration by triggering counterregulatory and neural responses to hypoglycemia. Insulin release is stimulated by glucose, amino acids, ketones, free fatty acids, neural stimuli, and gastrointestinal hormones. Insulin release is inhibited by somatostatin, epinephrine, and low blood glucose.

During feeding, increased insulin and decreased glucagon secretion favor glycogen synthesis and contribute to diminished hepatic glucose output. During fasting, most of these metabolic processes are reversed—blood insulin falls and glucagon rises. These changes, typified by increased gluconeogenesis, glycogenolysis, and lipolysis, result in a rise in blood glucose concentration.

The relationship between hyperglycemia, via its pathophysiologic and biochemical consequences, and the acute and chronic complications of diabetes mellitus remains a subject of debate among specialists in diabetes. It is clear that hyperglycemia directly or as a result of insulin deficiency can be associated with increased intracellular concentrations of sorbitol (such as in the lens of the eye), elaboration of minor hemoglobin components (such as the glycosylated hemoglobin A_{IC}), an increase in platelet aggregation, and changes in basement membrane composition. Although no available prospective study provides irrefutable proof, convincing data suggest that persistent hyperglycemia may be the requisite milieu or at least the "trigger" for the chain of events responsible for the development of microvascular and macrovascular changes associated with the complications of diabetes mellitus. The diabetes control and complications trial (DCCT), a multicentered study sponsored by the National Institutes of Health, is attempting to provide a definitive answer to this question. In addition to possible long-term benefits, good control is important in preventing diabetic ketoacidosis, inhibiting bacterial infection, accelerating wound healing, decreasing maternal and fetal morbidity and perinatal mortality, and promoting normal growth and development in the young diabetic.

The diabetic patient should aim to achieve a normal fasting blood glucose level and a 2-hour postprandial serum or plasma glucose level of 140 mg/dl or lower. These glucose levels, however, must be achieved without frequent or severe hypoglycemia and must be consistent with the patient's ability to function productively. Although these blood glucose levels can be routinely achieved in the patient with type II diabetes, they are more difficult to obtain in the ketosis-prone, hypoinsulinemic (type I) diabetic patient. Even multiple injections of regular insulin alone or in combination with long-acting insulin or the use of the open-loop insulin pump cannot duplicate the constant endogenous spurts of insulin that normal β-cell insulin secretion provides. Only the perfection of a glucose electrode in a closed-loop insulin pump or successful transplantation of β-cells or of the total pancreas can provide this type of insulin

secretion, that is, immediate response by the β- or α-cell to minimal increases or decreases in blood glucose with bursts of insulin or glucagon release.

DIET

Diet remains the cornerstone of diabetic therapy. The objectives of a proper diet are to promote proper growth and development in children, provide proper nutrition with an appropriate balance of protein, carbohydrate, and fat (saturated and unsaturated), provide appropriate nutrition, and normalize weight. The diet proportions must be tailored to the type of insulin used and to the individual's activity to normalize blood sugars while preventing hypoglycemia. The following principles are of utmost importance in diet treatment:

1. Approach the diet to be used as a prescription. When using the exchange diet lists provided by the American Diabetes Association and the American Dietetic Association, the prescriber *must* be familiar with the contents of those lists. A team approach—using the individual expertise of physician, dietitian, and nurse, and enlisting other family members when appropriate—can provide the best possible background for diet education and subsequent patient compliance.
2. Obtain a dietary history, including height, weight, type of work, food preferences, and activity patterns, including exercise.
3. Individualize the diet prescription.

Calculate the ideal weight of the patient as follows: for women, 100 lb for the first 5 feet of height, 5 lb for each additional inch; for men, 106 lb for the first 5 feet of height, 6 lb for each additional inch. Subtract 10% for a small frame and add 10% for a large frame. The total calories required are the basal calories of the patient plus activity needs. Basal calories are 10 calories for each pound of ideal body weight. Add 30% of basal calories to the diet prescription for a sedentary individual, 50% of basal calories for a moderately active individual, and 100% of basal calories for a strenuously active individual. Add or subtract 3500 calories from the diet for the patient to gain or lose 1 lb. Therefore, subtract 500 calories a day from the total caloric prescription for the patient to lose 1 lb/wk, and add 500 calories a day to the diet prescription for the patient to gain 1 lb/wk.

The current recommended distribution for the diet components of the American Diabetes Association are carbohydrate, 50% to 60% of the total calories; fat, 30% of the total calories; and protein, 12% to 18% of the total calories. Most insulin-requiring diabetic patients (whether insulin-dependent or non-insulin-dependent) who are taking multiple dose regular insulin, intermediate-acting insulin, or both, depending on the type of diabetes (that is, type I or type II) and the patient's specific insulin regimen, do well on the following distribution of calories: 20% of the total daily calories at breakfast time, 30% at lunch, 10% for a midafternoon snack, 30% at dinner, and 10% for an evening snack. Some active type I diabetic patients may require a midmorning snack. Presently it is recommended that the diet have no more than 10% of the total calories as saturated fats, with the remainder of the fats being nonsaturated.

Although the recommended total carbohydrate intake has been increased, simple sugars are still restricted. Crapo and co-workers have shown that simple and complex carbohydrates produce varying elevations in the plasma glucose that are characteristic for the specific source and form of that carbohydrate. Jenkins has popularized the term "glycemic index," which describes the effect of equivalent amounts of simple or complex carbohydrates on the plasma glucose by comparing the effect of these foods with that of a standard amount of glucose. For instance, a white potato gives a glycemic response similar to that of glucose. Rice, on the other hand, produces a much lower glycemic response. Presently the general recommendation emphasizes the use of complex carbohydrates and restricts the use of simple sugars to approximately 5% of the calories. Fructose has been recommended as a sweetener in diabetic diets. Plasma glucose response to fructose ingestion is much smaller than with glucose. However, patients who ingest large amounts of fructose, which is readily taken up by the liver where it is metabolized, must take its caloric content into consideration. The ingestion of these large amounts can result in abdominal discomfort and diarrhea. The level of plasma triglyceride also limits the amount of carbohydrate in a diet prescription for certain individuals, since genetically predisposed individuals may exhibit a rise in plasma triglyceride with an increase in carbohydrate. Cholesterol should be limited to 300 mg/day or less. The diet should contain foods high in fiber. High fiber diets have been associated with lower postprandial blood plasma glucose elevation. This has been shown in non-insulin-dependent type II diabetic patients, as well as in non-diabetic patients. The decrease in plasma glucose excursion is attributed to a decrease in absorption. Individuals can achieve high fiber in their diet by including dishes made of dry beans, a variety of vegetables, whole grain cereals, and bran. Alcohol can be taken in moderation by some patients. Its caloric content, namely 7 kcal/g must be included in a day's allowance and should be substituted for with fat exchanges. It must be made clear to diabetic patients that, for individual diabetic patients on insulin or hypoglycemic agents, alcohol may increase the risk of hypoglycemia; thus these patients and patients with hypertriglyceridemia should avoid alcohol.

Programmed physical exercise has been shown to improve fitness and to provide a generous sense of well-being. For many people, physical training improves several of the factors prominent in the development of cardiovascular disease. During exercise, if there is no insulin in the type I diabetic patient's system, that patient may experience hyperglycemia as a result of the catecholamine surge that occurs. Insulin-requiring type II diabetics have demonstrated an increase in insulin sensitivity and a decrease in insulin requirements during exercise. A major risk exists in type I and type II diabetic patients with peripheral neuropathy; they may undergo soft tissue and joint injury during exercise programs. Diabetic patients who have autonomic neuropathy can experience a decreased cardiovascular response to dehydration. Patients with unstable proliferative retinopathy could exacerbate their condition with exercise and that exercise could be associated with vitreous hemorrhage and retinal detachment.

In summary, the diet should be flexible and understandable to both patient and physician. For the obese patient, weight loss alone may decrease insulin requirements. Efficacy of the diet is determined by whether the patient achieves the intended result—proper growth and development and normalization of weight—in a normal work or school setting without hyperglycemia or hypoglycemia.

ORAL HYPOGLYCEMIC AGENTS

Although diet therapy remains the foundation of treatment of diabetic patients, some diabetic patients require drugs in addition to diet to normalize their blood sugar. This may be either the result of the patient's inability to comply fully with the diet or of the patient's hypoinsulinemia, for which diet therapy alone cannot compensate. In the controversial multi-centered University Group Data Project study sponsored by the National Institutes of Health, the investigators concluded that tolbutamide was no more effective than diet alone in the treatment of diabetes and that patients so treated had a significant increase in cardiac-related deaths. This controversy is now dormant after heated debate in the early 1970s. Currently many physicians use first and second generation sulfonylurea drugs to treat type II non-insulin-dependent diabetic patients with residual β-cell-secreting capacity and varying degrees of insulin resistance. Many physicians who use sulfonylureas in the treatment of certain patients who have maturity-onset diabetes believe them to be safe drugs. The new, second generation sulfonylurea drugs are glyburide (Micronase and DiaBeta) and glipizide (Glucotrol). Their major actions, similar to the first generation drugs, are to increase insulin secretion initially, to increase insulin receptors on the cell membrane, and to decrease insulin resistance by its action at the postreceptor level. Several studies indicate that even in those patients in whom the drugs are effective initially, there is a 25% secondary failure rate, although some patients are able to use these drugs for long periods. There is no available hard data to show these drugs to be harmful in patients who maintain normal fasting glucose levels and 2-hour postprandial plasma glucose levels less than 150 mg/dl.

Drugs currently used in the United States are first generation sulfonylurea drugs, tolbutamide (Orinase), acetohexamide (Dymelor), tolazamide (Tolinase), and chlorpropamide (Diabinese). The second generation sulfonylurea drugs are glyburide (Micronase and Diabeta) and glipizide (Glucotrol). Glyburide has a biological plasma half-life of approximately 6 hours. Glipizide has a plasma half-life of 2 to 4 hours. Both have hypoglycemic action up to 24 hours. The sulfonylureas initially act by stimulating insulin secretion. Many studies demonstrate that these agents promote their biological effect later by increasing insulin receptor numbers and affinity of insulin to receptors in adipose tissue, skeletal muscle, and liver cells. Glyburide is usually given once a day, but as one approaches the maximum dose (20 mg), it may need to be given twice a day. Its action decreases markedly after 12 hours. Tolbutamide, with a duration to 6 hours, is short acting. Tolazamide, lasting about 10 hours, and acetohexamide, acting about 12 to 14 hours, are intermediate-acting sulfonylureas, whereas chlorpropamide acts up to 72 hours. All of the sulfonylureas are metabolized to some degree in the liver. Tolazamide and particularly acetohexamide have metabolites with hypoglycemic action. In addition, chlorpropamide has antidiuretic and disulfiram-like effects.

Metabolites of the remaining compounds do not produce active metabolites as a result of their liver metabolism. The amount of tolbutamide excreted in the urine is 100%; chlorpropamide, 80% to 90%; tolazamide, 85%; glipizide, 68%; acetohexamide, 60%; and glyburide, about 50%. Chlorpropamide has antidiuretic and disulfiram-like effects. The selection of the specific sulfonylurea drug is determined by the duration of action, nature and severity of side effects, danger of hypoglycemia, drug interactions, and preexistence of hepatic or renal disease. The second generation sulfonylurea drugs are excreted through the bowel and the urine and have less interaction with other drugs in view of its anionic binding. The daily dosage range of these drugs is as follows: tolbutamide, 0.5 to 3 g; acetohexamide, 0.25 to 1.5 g; tolazamide, 0.1 to 1 g; chlorpropamide, 0.1 to 0.5 g; glibenclamide, 2.5 to 20 mg; glyburide 2.5 to 20 mg; and glipizide 2.5 to 40 mg. The starting dose of tolbutamide is 0.5 g twice daily, and there is rarely any advantage in using more than 1.5 g/day. The starting dose for the second generation sulfonylureas is 2.5 mg for glyburide and glipizide. The dose is increased at weekly intervals. Hypoglycemic reactions with sulfonylureas, although less common than with insulin, can be quite severe and last for several days, particularly with long-acting chlorpropamide in patients with renal insufficiency. For reasons of metabolism and excretion, sulfonylureas are contraindicated for patients with hepatic and renal insufficiency. In using sulfonylureas, special attention must be given to drug interactions, as with acetylsalicylic acid, phenytoin, propranolol, barbiturates, ethanol, clofibrate, phenylbutazone, and acetaminophen, all of which can potentiate or inhibit the hypoglycemic activity of first generation sulfonylureas.

The other class of oral hypoglycemic drugs is the biguanides. These drugs presumably act by decreasing glucose uptake from the gastrointestinal tract and inhibiting gluconeogenesis. Because phenformin, the only biguanide used in the United States, was associated with death from lactic acidosis, it is no longer used.

In summary, sulfonylureas are used with diet and exercise in the treatment of some patients with non-insulin-dependent (type II) diabetes. They are not prescribed for patients with hypoinsulinemic, insulin-dependent type I diabetes nor, by most physicians, during pregnancy or major surgery. When the disorder is not controlled with these agents, control is sought with insulin therapy.

INSULIN THERAPY

The object of diabetic management is to keep the patient symptom free and to prevent complications while the individual pursues a normal life-style. Since there appears to be a positive relationship between control and complications, normalization of intermediary metabolism is recommended. Although an appropriate diet prescription is the most important part of diabetic management, insulin is the most important medication for the hypoinsulinemic, type I patient.

Insulin is used primarily for the hypoinsulinemic, ketosis-prone type I diabetic patient, as well as for the insulin-requiring, insulin-resistant, overweight type II diabetic patient with hyperglycemia resulting from noncompliance with the prescribed diet. Insulin treatment can be initiated for short periods in some patients during pregnancy, severe infection, and stress. At present, highly purified beef, pork, mixtures of beef and pork, and human insulin are available. Human insulin is made available by Lilly, with the use of a recombinant DNA technique, and by Novo and Nordisk, through a process in which threonine is substituted for alanine at position 30 of the B chain in their highly purified porcine insulin preparations. Antibodies are produced by all of the insulins. There are less antibodies produced by pork insulin than by beef insulin, and human insulin produces the least antibodies. Short-acting insulins (regular and semilente), intermediate-acting insulins (Nuetral Protomine Hagedorn [NPH] and lente), and long-acting insulins (protamine zinc and ultralente) are available in single-peak and monocomponent forms. One manufacturer's highly purified preparation has a proinsulin level of less than 0.0001%; other purified insulins have less than 0.001% proinsulin. Insulin allergy is greatest with beef insulin or beef-pork insulin mixtures. Allergy occurs much less with pork insulin and even less with human insulin. There is no demonstrated need for transferring patients who are well controlled on beef, pork, or beef-pork mixture insulin to purified pork or human insulin. As with any change in insulin therapy, some patients changing to highly purified or human insulin or to a different type of insulin may require either a decrease or an increase of insulin dose by 10% to 20%. Most patients use the same dose as previously. The action times of the currently used insulins are listed in Table 199-1.

Human insulin or purified pork insulin is recommended for intermittent insulin therapy for newly diagnosed type I insulin-dependent patients, for newly diagnosed insulin-requiring type II patients with potentially long life spans, for pregnant patients who develop gestational diabetes, and for patients with insulin allergy, insulin antibody–mediated resistance, or lipodystrophy. The efficacy of human and pork insulin are equivalent, but human insulin is less immunogenic than the least immunogenic animal insulin. The human and highly purified insulins are noted in Table 199-1. The human insulins are available now in an NPH and regular mixture, and in NPH, lente, or regular alone. The effect of insulin is a result of various factors, namely absorption, insulin resistance, and factors such as infection and stress. The urine glucose currently is not used to assess the patient's insulin needs. Instead, fingerstick blood sugars are done using enzyme-impregnanted sticks that elicit a color change that is compared to a color chart; these strips can also be used with some glucose measuring device. There are many companies that put out strips, or glucose measuring devices, or both. The devices are getting smaller and less expensive and are generally comparable.

In stabilizing a new diabetic patient, the physician can begin with 10 to 20 units of an intermediate-acting insulin (NPH or lente), using the blood glucose level as a guide. The morning dose of insulin is not usually increased by more than 5 to 10 units/day except in acute situations. As stabilization proceeds, regular short-acting insulin can be added to the regimen in the morning; intermediate- and short-acting insulins can be used in the evening also.

Using another approach, the physician can prescribe multiple doses of regular insulin before meals and bedtime or later if necessary, using the blood glucose level to determine the dose of insulin required: 5 units of short-acting insulin for a blood glucose level of 200 to 250 mg/dl, 10 units for 250 to 300 mg/dl, and 15 units for 300 to 350 mg/dl. If the patient refuses multiple doses of regular insulin, once the blood sugar levels have stabilized, two thirds to three fourths of the total dose of regular insulin can be given as an intermediate-acting insulin before breakfast. Regular insulin is added to this dose in the same syringe if there is morning postprandial hyperglycemia. The majority of type I diabetic patients control their disorder with injections of both short- and intermediate-acting insulins given at both 8 am and 5 to 6 pm daily. When the morning dose of intermediate-acting insulin exceeds 40 units, it may be necessary to split the dose because wide swings in blood glucose levels can occur, resulting in a low sugar level at peak insulin action followed by reactive hyperglycemia (called the "Somogyi effect"). This is caused by the action of counterregulatory hormones (catecholamines, glucagon, cortisol, and growth hormone). Usually two thirds of the total insulin dose is given in the morning and one third in the afternoon. Patients who have the so-called dawn phenomenon have hyperglycemia on rising in the morning. This has been attributed to growth hormone effect, decreased effective insulin available, or both. One of the techniques utilized for patients who have marked hypoglycemia in the early morning is to give the long-acting dose late at night or before bedtime in late evening. Increasing numbers of type I diabetic patients use multiple doses of regular insulin with self-monitoring blood glucose in an attempt to achieve better control.

Glucose monitoring at home is achieved by placing a drop of blood (obtained by pricking the finger) on a glucose oxidase reagent strip that develops a color corresponding to the blood

Table 199-1   Insulin preparations

Product	Manufacturer	Form	Strength
Rapid acting (onset ½-4 hours, duration 5-16 hours*			
Humulin Regular	Lilly†	Human	U-100
Humulin Regular (buffered regular) (for insulin pumps only)	Lilly	Human	U-100
Novolin R (regular) (formerly Actrapid Human)	Squibb/Novo	Human	U-100
Velosulin (regular)	Nordisk-USA	Human	U-100
Iletin II Regular	Lilly	Beef	U-100
Iletin II Regular	Lilly	Pork	U-100, U-500
Purified Pork R (regular) (formerly Actrapid)	Squibb/Novo	Pork	U-100
Velosulin (regular)	Nordisk-USA	Pork	U-100
Purified Pork S (Semilente) (formerly Semitard)	Squibb/Novo	Pork	
Iletin I Regular	Lilly	Beef/Pork	U-40, U-100
Regular	Squibb/Novo	Beef/Pork	U-100
Iletin I Semilente	Lilly	Beef/Pork	U-40, U-100
Semilente	Squibb/Novo	Beef	U-100
Intermediate-acting (onset 1-4 hours, duration 16-28 hours)*			
Humulin L	Lilly	Human	U-100
Humulin NPH	Lilly	Human	U-100
Insulatard + (NPH)	Nordisk-USA	Human	U-100
Novolin L (lente) (formerly Monotard Human)	Squibb/Novo	Human	U-100
Novolin N (NPH)	Squibb/Novo	Human	U-100
Iletin II Lente	Lilly	Beef	U-100
Iletin II NPH	Lilly	Beef	U-100
Iletin II Lente	Lilly	Pork	U-100
Iletin II NPH	Lilly	Pork	U-100
Insulatard (NPH)	Nordisk-USA	Pork	U-100
Purified Pork Lente (formerly Monotard)	Squibb/Novo	Pork	U-100
Purified Pork N (NPH) (formerly Protaphane)	Squibb/Novo	Pork	U-100
Iletin I Lente	Lilly	Beef/Pork	U-40, U-100
Iletin I NPH	Lilly	Beef/Pork	U-40, U-100
NPH	Squibb/Novo	Beef	U-100
Long acting (onset 4-6 hours, duration 36 hours)*			
Iletin II PZI	Lilly	Beef	U-100
Iletin II PZI	Lilly	Pork	U-100
Purified Beef U (Ultralente) (formerly Ultratard)	Squibb/Novo	Beef	U-100
Iletin I PZI	Lilly	Beef/Pork	U-40, U-100
Iletin I Ultralente	Lilly	Beef/Pork	U-40, U-100
Ultralente	Squibb/Novo	Beef	U-100
Mixtures			
Mixtard + 30% (30% Regular, 70% NPH)	Nordisk-USA	Pork	U-100
Nevolin 70/30	Squibb/Novo	Semi Synthetic Human (Pork)	U-100

Modified from Diab Forecast, March 1986.

*Onset and duration are rough estimates. They can vary greatly within the range listed and from person to person.

†Nordisk's and Squibb/Novo's human insulins are converted from pork insulin. Lilly's human insulins are made by recombinant DNA technology.

glucose level. The intensity of the color is compared to a color chart or read in a glucose measuring device. Much evidence is accumulating that suggests that good metabolic control can delay or prevent microvascular complications in patients with diabetes. The level of Hb A_{1c} can also be used to monitor control. A glycosylated hemoglobin is glucose level dependent and is produced by the nonenzymatic glycosylation of the hemoglobin with glucose. Glucose can also attach to other proteins and nucleic acids in addition to hemoglobin. The glycosylation of glucose with proteins is being evaluated in the pathogenesis of diabetic complications. Thus the glycohemoglobins reflect time-averaged blood glucose levels during preceding weeks to months, forming an irreversible end product of glycosylated protein after passing through a stage that is initially reversible. Since most current techniques measure the reversible (as well as the irreversible) product, the limits of the particular test being used to measure glycosylated hemoglobin must be known to the physician using the test. Glycosylated hemoglobin is normally 3% to 6% of the total hemoglobin but is elevated when diabetes is out of control. It rarely exceeds

15%. Since Hb A_{1c} is present during the life of the red blood cell, it can be used as a reflection of glucose control over a prolonged period.

INSULIN MANAGEMENT IN SPECIAL SITUATIONS

SURGERY. With minor procedures under local anesthesia there is no change in the oral hypoglycemic or insulin regimen. However, with major procedures a variety of methods are necessary, including the following: An intravenous drip of 1000 ml of 5% glucose in water is started preoperatively. One third to one half of the usual morning intermediate-acting insulin dose is administered preoperatively and the remainder is given postoperatively. Regular insulin is given as needed postoperatively. Another practice is to use a low-dose continuous infusion of regular insulin during surgery. The drip consists of 100 units of regular insulin added to 500 ml of 0.5% normal saline solution. Albumin or blood is not used in the insulin drip. One hundred milliliters of infusion mixture is allowed to run rapidly through the tubing before connecting it to the patient to minimize adherence of insulin to the bottle or tubing. A bolus of 2 to 4 units of regular insulin is given intravenously, and a continuous drip of 2 to 3 units of regular insulin is then continued every hour. Blood glucose levels are measured every half hour. The dose of the insulin drip is raised or lowered as needed. In this way intraoperative hypoglycemia is avoided and a smoother postoperative course is ensured.

The patient should have a full liquid exchange diet (equal calories of carbohydrate, protein, and fat composition). If only a clear liquid diet can be retained, the diet can be isocaloric and purely carbohydrate in content. If vomiting occurs, the physician should be notified to alter the regimen. Regular insulin is ordered every 4 hours as needed postoperatively once the insulin drip is discontinued until the patient is eating. Then the patient is eased back into the usual insulin regimen.

INFECTIONS AND EXERCISE. Infections increase the need for insulin, and exercise decreases the need in type II diabetic patients. Type I diabetic patients need some basal insulin in their systems so as not to become ketotic or hyperglycemic. Therefore the insulin dose should be raised in response to infections and lowered with increased exercise in patients who have endogenous or exogenous insulin secretion.

HYPOGLYCEMIA. The patient must be instructed to be aware of untoward symptoms at the time of peak insulin action. Short-acting insulins are more likely to produce catecholamine-type symptoms of tachycardia, hunger, circumoral pallor, and sweating. The longer-acting insulins are more likely to yield psychiatric, neurologic, or central nervous system symptoms such as bizarre behavior, lethargy, nausea, vomiting, stupor, or coma. Hypoglycemic symptoms are myriad but usually are repeated in a given individual. The importance of eating on time, including snacks, and making allowances for extreme activity needs to be emphasized. Recommendations should be individualized. The insulin-dependent patient should be instructed to have sugar or hard candy available if hypoglycemic symptoms occur. Concentrated glucose preparations such as Glutose are available. The glucagon kit is available for those patients unable to take sugar or a glucose preparation. This can be injected intramuscularly by a member of the family to raise the blood sugar. It has a short-term effect and needs to be followed by some concentrated carbohydrate.

INSULIN ALLERGY. Allergic reactions can occur within 15 to 20 minutes, or a delayed reaction can occur at least 4 hours after an injection. Both can be local or systemic. The local reaction is manifested by swelling, redness, or hives and usually subsides after a week. If it persists, human insulin should be substituted if that insulin has not been used previously. If anaphylactoid or vasculitis (systemic) type of reactions occur in a patient who is insulin-dependent, desensitization to insulin is necessary. The patient should not receive insulin for at least 12 hours before the attempted desensitization procedure. Epinephrine (1:1000) should be available to be given in doses of 0.1 to 0.3 ml subcutaneously if needed. Insulin is given at half-hour intervals in increasing doses and 0.001, 0.002, 0.004, 0.01, 0.02, 0.04, 0.1, 0.2, 0.5, 1, 2, 4, and 8 units of regular insulin as long as there are no untoward reactions. The first three insulin doses are given intradermally, and the remainder can be given subcutaneously. In addition to an allergy to the insulin itself, allergy to the vehicle or preservative may exist.

LIPOATROPHY. Lipoatrophy is an indication for highly purified or human insulin preparations. Improvement of lipoatrophy often occurs when insulin is injected directly into the atrophic area.

INSULIN RESISTANCE. Insulin antibodies of the IgG type can appear within 6 to 8 weeks after the initiation of insulin therapy but do not necessarily result in resistance. Resistance has been defined as a need for more than 200 units of insulin a day; realistically, it should refer to any diabetic patient taking more insulin than a nondiabetic person requires to maintain normoglycemia (40 to 50 units/day). For the majority of these patients, switching to human insulin can ameliorate the condition. For others, corticosteroids may be needed. It is clear that the category of insulin resistance covers a myriad of entities. Some of these are receptor abnormalities, such as obesity with decreased insulin receptors, whereas others have their causes at the receptor and postreceptor level, namely insulin-resistant states such as the diseases associated with acanthosis nigricans and lipodystrophic states.

INSULIN DELIVERY. Research continues on oral types of insulin. Currently there has been no success in producing them. However, nasal and rectal short-acting insulins have been tested in Europe and are almost ready for distribution.

Portable open-loop insulin devices preprogrammed to provide continuous basal low-dose insulin infusion and insulin boluses before meals and at bedtime are available. For most patients these devices have no advantage over multiple-dose regular insulin regimens. Their use in the treatment of type I diabetes is limited by their lack of response to changing blood glucose concentrations. On the horizon is improved insulin delivery mimicking normal β-cell secretion. This awaits the availability of a portable closed-loop system with an implantable glucose electrode that can release insulin in response to changing blood glucose concentrations or the successful transplantation of β-cells or the entire pancreas.

DIABETIC KETOACIDOSIS

Diabetic ketoacidosis (DKA) is the ultimate result of absolute insulin deficiency and glucagon excess. Increased insulin need can be precipitated by infection or stress or result from the contrainsulin effects of glucagon, catecholamines, steroids, and growth hormone. The resultant hypoinsulinemia permits increased glucose production by the liver and decreased end-organ utilization. The increasing hyperglycemia produces glycosuria and associated water and electrolyte loss as a result of solute diuresis. The decreased insulin and increased glucagon output result in increasing lipolysis, gluconeogenesis, and increased activity of carnitine acyltransferase. This enzyme system controls the transfer of fatty acids to the mitochondria for fatty-acid oxidation and ketogenesis. Thus there is increased production of β-hydryxobutyric acid, acetoacetic acid, and other organic ketogenic acids. With the increased production of these acids by the liver, ketoacidosis results, since the amounts of ketoacids produced are in excess of the peripheral tissues' capacity to use them, and the renal and respiratory compensatory mechanisms that were stimulated eventually fail to maintain a normal pH.

The time interval from the onset of hyperglycemia to the development of DKA is variable. The signs and symptoms most commonly seen are polyuria, polydipsia, polyphagia, weakness, weight loss, signs of dehydration (particularly sunken eyeballs, decreased skin turgor, and dry mucous membranes), tachycardia, hypotension, vomiting, Kussmaul respirations, flaccid reflexes, abdominal tenderness and distention, lipemia retinalis, fever, depressed sensorium, and coma. The degree of obtundation seems to correlate more closely with the hyperosmolality present than with the blood sugar level or degree of acidosis.

DKA must be suspected in any diabetic patient with a changing sensorium. Hypoglycemic coma, lactic acidosis, alcoholic ketoacidosis, and drug intoxication (such as with salicylates or ethylene glycol) must be part of the differential diagnosis. Initial studies usually include a complete blood count, a urinalysis, and a capillary glucose test using a glucose oxidase reagent strip for a rapid estimate of the blood glucose level. In addition, a blood glucose determination, serum acetone with dilutions, serum electrolytes (sodium, potassium, carbon dioxide, and chloride), blood urea nitrogen, serum calcium and phosphorus, arterial blood gas (for pH, P_{CO_2}, P_{O_2}), electrocardiogram, chest roentgenogram, and cultures from blood, urine, stool, or other indicated sites are essential. Bacterial infection is the most common documented precipitating factor in DKA but usually the specific cause is obscure. Therefore a careful history and a meticulous physical examination are important in directing studies and treatment. Flow sheets that include all laboratory data, intake and output of fluids, serum ketones, urinary glucose and ketones, insulin therapy, and electrolyte replacement are useful tools. Blood glucose should be checked hourly after the onset of therapy. Electrolytes and serum acetone should be checked approximately every 4 hours, and blood gases every 4 to 6 hours depending on the clinical response.

Successful treatment of DKA requires normalization of the metabolic state, replacement of fluids and electrolyte deficits, and treatment of the initiating cause, such as infection, acute myocardial infarction, or pancreatitis. Individualization of patient treatment with careful monitoring by the physician remains the key to decreased mortality.

Most medical centers currently use some variation of continuous low-dose intravenous insulin infusions in the treatment of DKA. It is clear that nearly maximal insulin effect is achieved with plasma insulin levels of 20 to 200 μU/ml. In most cases plasma insulin levels within that range result in a decrease in blood glucose of 70 to 100 mg/dl/hr. These plasma levels can be achieved with infusion of regular insulin at a rate of 2 to 10 units/hr. These plasma insulin levels can also be achieved by giving an intramuscular injection of 10 units of regular insulin initially and then 5 units of regular insulin hourly intramuscularly. Intramuscular treatment is not recommended in severe DKA, since there is marked dehydration and decreased tissue perfusion with resultant decreased uptake of intramuscularly or subcutaneously injected insulin.

These low-dose regimens result in less hypoglycemia and hypokalemia. Since continuous low-dose regimens are not 100% effective, it is recommended that 10 units of regular insulin by intravenous bolus be administered, followed by 10 units of regular insulin in each hour, initially by continuous infusion. The dose is then increased or decreased depending on the effect on the blood glucose. The solution usually contains 100 units of regular insulin in 500 ml of normal saline; 100 ml of this solution is allowed to run through the tubing before connecting it to the patient. More concentrated insulin solutions are made when larger hourly insulin doses are infused. Once acidosis and dehydration are corrected, regular insulin can be given subcutaneously.

Fluid therapy is promptly instituted with normal saline to increase intravascular volume. The first 1 or 2 L can usually be given rapidly in the first hour while monitoring the patient's cardiovascular status. Since the water deficit is usually more marked than the electrolyte deficit, a switch is made to half-normal saline after 1 or 2 L of normal saline is infused, depending on the severity of dehydration, intravascular volume depletion, and hypotension. Hypotension is usually corrected by normal saline solution, except in certain critical clinical situations such as concomitant gram-negative bacillary bacteremia or an acute myocardial infarction. Volume expanders

such as albumin are rarely necessary. At the onset of therapy, gastric contents are aspirated to prevent aspiration by the patient and the nasogastric tube is removed. Intake and output are monitored throughout therapy. A central venous line may be necessary to monitor fluid therapy. When the blood glucose level drops to 250 mg/dl, 5% glucose in water, normal saline, or half-normal saline, depending on the clinical situation at the time, is added to the fluid therapy.

Total body potassium depletion is always present initially in DKA. Intravascular volume contraction and potassium shift from inside cells to the extracellular fluid give falsely high values of serum potassium at the onset of therapy for the ketoacidotic state. Serum potassium usually reaches its low point 2 to 4 hours after the onset of therapy as a direct result of rehydration and potassium shift into cells. During the time the ketoacidotic state is being reversed, potassium is driven into the cell in exchange for hydrogen and sodium. If sodium bicarbonate is used in therapy, it will further increase potassium influx into the cell and decrease the serum value even more. With pH levels at 7.1 or below, sodium bicarbonate is usually given intravenously. This is of debatable value since the increase in blood pH shifts the oxyhemoglobin dissociation curve and decreases delivery of oxygen to tissues. If the serum potassium level is low at the onset of therapy (below 4 mEq/dl), replacement potassium therapy is initiated immediately in the form of chloride or phosphate salts (40 mEq/L of intravenous solution). If the serum potassium is 4 mEq/L or higher, the physician can wait 1 to 2 hours before introducing potassium therapy.

Phosphate deficit is usually present at the onset of therapy. Repletion of phosphate can be part of the initial potassium replacement and be given as potassium phosphate. Serum calcium and phosphorus levels must be measured before replacement, and further monitoring of these levels is important if phosphate therapy is initiated. If phosphorus levels become elevated, phosphate complexing with calcium could be disastrous, producing interstitial calcifications and hypocalcemia that could result in arrhythmias and respiratory paralysis. Phosphorus levels below 1 mEq/dl should be treated judiciously. Once the patient can accept oral feeding, adequate phosphorus can be provided in the diet to make up the deficit.

In summary, DKA is a medical emergency that requires urgent attention, with therapy directed to correcting the metabolic deficits, expanding intravascular volume to increase tissue perfusion, and treating any identifiable precipitating cause.

HYPERGLYCEMIC, HYPEROSMOLAR, NONKETOTIC COMA

Although hyperglycemic, hyperosmolar, nonketotic coma can occur in any type of diabetic patient, it usually occurs in those with diet or oral agent–controlled maturity-onset (type II) diabetes and rarely occurs in those with type I diabetes. The absence of significant ketosis in combination with the hyperglycemia is related to the presence of enough insulin secretion to inhibit lipolysis. There is severe osmotic diuresis with loss of water and electrolytes. Water is lost in excess of electrolytes and serum osmolality may be elevated above 350 mOsm/kg water. Sodium levels routinely are greater than normal, sometimes in the range of 170 to 180 mEq/L. High sodium levels signify extreme dehydration and volume contraction. The plasma glucose level may be very high, usually 600 to 1000 mg/dl or higher. With increasingly high osmolalities, neurologic signs appear, ranging from lethargy and confusion to coma. Hemoconcentration can precipitate thrombotic events. Although there is the typical diabetic triad of polyuria, polydipsia, and polyphagia at the onset, eventually central nervous system stimulation of the thirst mechanism is impaired as the succeeding events of progressive dehydration, volume contraction, and coma ensue.

The treatment is intravascular volume expansion. Initially, normal saline solution is given. The first 2 L is given in 2 to 3 hours. Subsequent to these initial intravenous fluids and as the intravascular fluid space is expanded, half-normal saline solution is substituted. As the blood glucose approaches 250 mg/dl, 5% dextrose can be used in saline, half-normal saline, or water as required by the clinical situation. Electrolytes must be replaced, as in diabetic ketoacidosis. Either a small amount of insulin or no insulin is necessary for the treatment of these patients. Low-dose continuous insulin infusions in the range of 0.5 to 2 units of regular insulin in each hour have been used initially. A central venous pressure line may be needed to monitor fluid therapy. It is important to treat the precipitating cause if identifiable. Infection, dialysis (because of the large amounts of glucose infused), and drug therapy with thiazides, intravenous phenytoin, high-dose corticosteroids, and propranolol (which impair insulin secretion or glucose disposal) have been implicated as factors precipitating hyperglycemic, hyperosmolar, nonketotic coma.

ALCOHOLIC KETOACIDOSIS

Alcoholic ketoacidosis occurs in the chronic ethanol abuser who has had decreased ethanol intake for several days. Since vomiting is a frequently associated symptom, food and ethanol intake is limited. Ethanol levels are usually low at the time of admission to the hospital. In contrast, alcoholic hypoglycemia is generally associated with high ethanol levels and is due to inhibition of gluconeogenesis. Blood sugars in alcoholic ketoacidosis are usually less than 400 mg/dl, and plasma insulin levels are decreased. The β-hydroxybutyrate/acetoacetate ratio is often 2 to 2½ times higher than in diabetic ketoacidosis. Acidosis is usually not profound, and these patients generally respond to small doses of insulin and dextrose infusion.

COMBINED KETOACIDOSIS AND LACTIC ACIDOSIS

The combination of ketoacidosis and lactic acidosis exists in clinical settings such as anoxic states and shock that predispose diabetic patients to lactic acidosis. If extreme metabolic acidosis is present with hyperglycemia and negative serum acetone, lactic acidosis should be suspected. β-Hydroxybutyric acid is not measured by the nitroprusside reagent, Acetest, which is the most commonly used qualitative reagent to measure plasma or serum ketones, although this reagent does measure acetoacetic acid and acetone. β-hydroxybutyric acid production is favored in lactic acidosis. Serum lactate and pyruvate levels should be obtained for diagnostic purposes when combined β-acidosis and lactic acidosis is suspected. Treatment of the primary disease producing the lactic acidosis, in addition to the treatment of the diabetic ketoacidosis, is of prime importance. Phenformin, no longer used in the United States, has been implicated in several reports in the ketoacidosis–lactic acidosis syndrome.

DIABETES IN PREGNANCY

Each year 10,000 babies are born to diabetic women. Type I diabetes is present in 0.1% to 0.3% of all pregnant women. Before 1922 and the discovery of insulin, fetal mortality was almost 100%. Currently total mortality for children born to pregnant diabetic women is approaching those born to nondiabetic women.

The profile of the gestational diabetic woman is of onset of diabetes in the second or third trimester, a family history of diabetes, previous babies that weigh more than 4 kg, and a history of stillbirth. Screening is recommended between 24 and 28 weeks of gestation. However, we recommend it at the first visit for women with a high risk of developing gestational diabetes. The screening test is a 50 g glucose load. Those who have positive screening tests (a 1 hour postprandial glucose level over 150 mg/dl) need glucose tolerance testing. Pre-pregnancy counseling of the young diabetic woman who wishes to become pregnant should be conducted. Since major organogenesis is completed by the sixth or seventh week of gestation, pre-pregnancy counselors should stress that normal levels of glycosylated hemoglobins and blood glucose at conception will significantly reduce congenital malformations.

Currently there is no dispute about the desirability of keeping maternal blood glucose as close as possible to nondiabetic levels in the insulin-dependent diabetic patient. Consensus dictates that such efforts should be initiated before conception. Whether optimal diabetes control is achieved by intensive insulin treatment or by an insulin pump, no difference to perinatal outcome has been demonstrated.

Insulin requirements usually decrease in the first trimester, level off during the first part of the second trimester, and increase in the second half of pregnancy. Insulin requirements decrease early in the pregnancy as a result of the demand of the fetus for glucose and amino acids from the maternal circulation in the first half of the pregnancy. The elaboration of significant amounts of human placental lactogen, increased free cortisol, and increased insulin degradation by the placenta in the second half of pregnancy increase insulin requirements. Generally, by the third trimester most women who were insulin-dependent before pregnancy require a morning and late afternoon dose of both intermediate insulin (lente or NPH) and short-acting insulin (semilente or regular).

During pregnancy, fasting blood glucose levels should be kept to less than 100 mg/dl without the development of hypoglycemia. This correlates with increased fetal survival and decreased perinatal morbidity. It is important to be aware of the rise in insulin requirements coincident with the increasing elaboration of placental contrainsulin factors. Failure to make immediate and sometimes dramatic insulin dose adjustments could lead to diabetic ketoacidosis.

Dietary management is as important for the pregnant patient as for the nonpregnant patient. There is one major difference in the goal of the diet prescription in the pregnant diabetic woman: no attempt is made to normalize maternal weight to avoid starvation ketosis. Instead, it is best to aim for a weight gain of 24 to 26 lbs during the pregnancy. A diet of 16 calories for each pound of body weight is prescribed. The distribution of total calories into carbohydrate, protein, and fat is individualized for each patient. The diet of the pregnant diabetic patient, as recommended by the American Diabetes Association in 1987, should include 50% to 60% of the total calories in the form of carbohydrate and 12% to 20% in the form of protein. The remaining calories are supplied as fats; 20% of the total calories should be in the form of polyunsaturated fatty acids.

When feasible, delivery is attempted vaginally. In patients whose obstetric or medical circumstances dictate early delivery, cesarean section may be required. Fetal well-being during pregnancy is monitored by stress tests, nonstress tests, amniocentesis, and ultrasound. Currently, estriol determinations and human placental lactogen levels are rarely used. When it is important to consider early delivery, the lecithin/sphingomyelin ratio is obtained through amniocentesis. This ratio can be a factor in the decision to delay delivery when the ratio is less than 2.5:1 and the other parameters of fetal and maternal well-being are stable. However, a major fall (one-third) in insulin requirements, an increase in maternal toxemia, or fetal distress may force immediate delivery even with lower lecithin/sphingomyelin ratios.

Delivery requires prospective recognition of the postpartum loss of contrainsulin factors mentioned previously. To compensate for this, a low-dose continuous regular insulin drip of 0.5 to 2 units/hr following a 1- to 2-unit bolus injection can be administered. There is usually a postpartum decrease in insulin requirements. There can be a total loss of insulin need for as long as 10 days. This phenomenon is thought to result from inhibition of growth hormone by human placental lactogen during gestation.

In summary, management of the pregnant diabetic woman requires a team approach involving an internist, obstetrician, and pediatrician who pay careful attention to the unique pathophysiologic demands of the fetus and mother during pregnancy and who tailor insulin, dietary, obstetric, and delivery decisions to meet these demands.

BIBLIOGRAPHY

Bogardus C and others: Effects of physical training and diet therapy on carbohydrate metabolism in patients with glucose intolerance and non–insulin-dependent diabetes mellitus, Diabetes 333:311, 1984.

Brownlee M: Nonenzymatic glycosylation and the pathogenesis of diabetic complication, Ann Intern Med 101:527, 1984.

Buchanan TA and others: Medical management of diabetes in pregnancy, Clin Perinatol 12(3):625, 1985.

Coustan DR: Randomized clinical trial of insulin pump vs. intensive conventional therapy in diabetic pregnancy, JAMA 255:631, 1986.

Crapo PA and others: Postprandial hormone responses to different types of complex carbohydrate in individuals with impaired glucose tolerance, Am J Clin Nutr 33:1723, 1980.

Felig P: Diabetes mellitus. In Burrow GN and Ferris TF, editors: Medical complications during pregnancy, Philadelphia, 1975, WB Saunders Co.

Galloway JA and Bressler R: Insulin treatment in diabetes mellitus, Med Clin North Am 62:663, 1978.

Gerich JD: Potential future modes of therapy in diabetes mellitus, Minn Med 62:46, 1979.

Gliedman MD and others: Long-term effects of pancreatic transplant function in patients with advanced juvenile-onset diabetes, Diabetic Care 1:1, 1978.

Jenkins DJA: The glyaemic index of foods tested in diabetic patients, Diabetologia 24:257, 1983.

Kidson W and others: Treatment of severe diabetes mellitus by insulin infusion, Br Med J 2:691, 1974.

Krall LP and Chabot VA: Oral hypoglycemic agent update, Med Clin North Am 62:681, 1978.

Kreisberg RA: Diabetic ketoacidosis, Ann Intern Med 88:681, 1978.

Layer P and others: Effect of a purified amylase inhibitor on carbohydrate tolerance in normal subjects and patients with diabetes mellitus, Mayo Clin Proc 61:422, 1986.

Lebovitz HE: Oral hypoglycemic agents. In The diabetes annual: 1984, Amsterdam, 1984, Elsevier Publishing.

Mandarino L and others: Mechanism of hyperglycemia and response to treatment with an inhibitor of fatty-acid oxidation in a patient with insulin resistance due to antiinsulin receptor antibodies, J Clin Endocrinol 59:658, 1984.

Matas AJ and Sutherland ER: Current states of islet and pancreatic transplantation in diabetes, Diabetes 25:785, 1976.

Miller RE: Pancreatic neuroendocrinology: peripheral neural mechanisms in the regulation of the islets of Langerhans, Endocr Rev 2(4):471, 1981.

Ney D and Hollingsworth DR: Nutritional management of pregnancy complicated by diabetes, Diabetes Care 4:647, 1981.

Page MM and others: Treatment of diabetic coma with continuous low-dose infusion of insulin, Br Med J 2:687, 1974.

Santiago JF and others: Open-loop and closed-loop devices for blood glucose control in normal and diabetic subjects, Diabetes 28:71, 1979.

Schneider S and others: Studies on mechanism of impaired glucose control during regular exercise in type II diabetes, Diabetologia 28:355, 1984.

Semple PF, White C, and Manderson WF: Continuous intravenous infusion of small doses of insulin in treatment of diabetic ketoacidosis, Br Med J 2:694, 1974.

Skyler JS and Cahill GF Jr, editors: Symposium on diabetes mellitus, Am J Med 70:101, 325, 579, 1981.

200 · CHRONIC COMPLICATIONS OF DIABETES MELLITUS

Robert L. Lavine

With the discovery of insulin and with improved therapy, patients having diabetes mellitus are living longer. With increased longevity the occurrence of chronic complications of this disease has become a major concern. These chronic complications correlate in large part with the duration of the disordered carbohydrate metabolism; whether they also correlate with the degree of metabolic abnormality remains debatable. An in-depth discussion of this controversy is beyond the scope of this chapter. However, one common bias is that there is a correlation—the worse the control of the diabetic state or the worse the metabolic abnormality, the worse the complication and the earlier it is seen in the course of the diabetes. Data are accruing to support this viewpoint. The purpose of this chapter is to describe the various chronic complications of diabetes mellitus in order to give the reader an overview of the widespread and varied systemic involvement that can occur in this disease.

ARTERIOSCLEROTIC COMPLICATIONS

Arteriosclerotic complications occur at least twice as frequently in diabetic patients as in nondiabetic patients. Diabetes mellitus seems to accelerate the arteriosclerotic process, but how it does this is unknown. It is possible that glycosylation of the low-density lipoprotein receptor of the arterial wall plays a role. It is likely that the severe and widespread arteriosclerotic involvement in the diabetic patient differs from arteriosclerosis in the nondiabetic patient only in degree and severity and does not represent an arteriosclerotic process unique to diabetes mellitus. Arteriosclerosis observed in diabetic patients occurs at an earlier age, is more diffuse, involves smaller arteries as well as larger ones, progresses at a more rapid rate, is as common in women (even in premenopausal women) as in men, demonstrates an increased incidence of medial sclerosis of the arteries (the pathogenic significance of which is unknown), and is associated with a poorer prognosis. Major arteriosclerotic complications occur in the coronary arteries, cerebral arteries, and peripheral arteries.

Coronary artery disease

Coronary artery disease results from accumulation of fat and cholesterol deposits in the media of the coronary arteries. These deposits can coalesce to become plaques (atheroma), which can become calcified and fibrotic and lead to narrowing and obstruction of the vessel. The plaques can also ulcerate, resulting in thrombus formation that can cause partial or complete occlusion of the vessel. Complete occlusion leads to myocardial ischemia, which results in myocardial infarction with loss of heart tissue. Partial occlusion can result in the exertional chest pain of angina pectoris.

In diabetic patients the incidence of coronary artery disease is greater than in nondiabetic individuals, and survival after myocardial infarction, especially long-term survival, is shorter.

As in the nondiabetic patients, most diabetic patients with myocardial infarction have a crushing, burning, substernal chest pain that may radiate down the arms and up the neck. This pain is associated with profound fatigue, nausea, and sweating. However, 10% of diabetic patients have little or no pain during a myocardial infarction. There may be a higher incidence of ventricular tachyarrhythmias following myocardial infarction in diabetic patients; however, the course is no different than in nondiabetic patients, except that myocardial infarction deteriorates diabetic control and can cause diabetes in a previously nondiabetic patient. Whereas hypoglycemia must be avoided because it may precipitate arrhythmias, control of the diabetes must continue during and after infarction because the elevation of free fatty acids that accompanies uncontrolled diabetes can adversely affect myocardial function.

Cerebrovascular disease

As a result of arteriosclerotic involvement of the cerebral arteries, thrombotic cerebrovascular accidents (CVAs) are frequently observed in diabetic patients. The CVA syndromes are similar to those observed in nondiabetic patients; however, there seems to be a higher incidence of CVAs involving the branches of the vertebrobasilar system of the brain. In evaluating a diabetic patient with a CVA, it must be kept in mind that hypoglycemia and hyperosmolar, hyperglycemic, nonketotic coma can produce similar neurologic dysfunction that can be reversed with appropriate treatment. However, when these disorders have been ruled out, treatment of a diabetic patient with a CVA is similar to treatment of a nondiabetic patient with a CVA plus treatment of the diabetes.

Peripheral vascular disease

Seventy percent of all non–trauma-induced amputations in the United States are the result of diabetes mellitus. Involvement of peripheral arteries by the accelerated arteriosclerosis of diabetes leads to claudication (exertional muscle pain caused by muscle ischemia when blood flow is adequate at rest but inadequate with exercise) or loss of the extremity when blood flow is totally inadequate. Peripheral pulses are usually absent. In 20% of diabetic patients, however, palpable pulses are present, but signs of peripheral vascular disease are observed. This results from involvement of smaller arteries without significant large arterial involvement. Since both small and large arteries are affected in diabetes, it is common to first see small distal areas (tip of a toe or heel) involved before large areas (foot or leg). In the nondiabetic patient large areas (foot or leg) are usually involved at the outset because large arteries are mainly affected. Why peripheral vascular disease is symptomatically a disease of the lower extremities in both diabetic and nondiabetic patients is unknown. However, it may be related to the higher pressures normally observed in lower extremity arteries than those of the upper extremities.

Although surgical removal of atheromatous plaques and occlusions (endarterectomy) or the use of bypass procedures is of help in nondiabetic peripheral vascular disease, these procedures are less likely to help the diabetic patient because the arteriosclerotic process is more diffuse and also involves smaller arteries. However, in selected cases arteriography and endarterectomy or bypass is of value. In other selected cases balloon angioplasty is helpful. This procedure involves expanding the constricted arterial segment from within using an arterial catheter containing an expandable segment. If the procedure is successful, more aggressive surgical intervention can be avoided. Unfortunately, amputation is frequently the only feasible procedure if adequate blood flow cannot be restored.

THE "DIABETIC FOOT"

The "diabetic foot" is the complex result of several processes, ending in foot ulceration, infection, gangrene, and tissue loss and leading to loss of locomotion. A deficiency in blood flow caused by peripheral vascular disease plays an important role. Another process involves thickening of the basement membrane of the arterioles. Diabetic peripheral neuropathy (see "Neuropathy" later in this chapter), which causes decreased sensation and foot deformity and thereby leads to trauma, also plays a role. Finally, a fourth pathologic process, infection, can turn this condition into an emergency.

In all patients it is important to make a clinical judgment as to whether the foot lesion has resulted predominantly from ischemia or neuropathy. Although both conditions are present to some degree and almost all are complicated by infection, this differentiation is important, since healing can occur when the lesion is primarily neuropathic, whereas the prognosis is extremely bad when the lesion is predominantly ischemic. A patient with decreased sensation in the feet who has little pain despite an infected foot lesion and who has loss of position and vibratory senses, wasting of the interosseous muscles of the feet, loss of the ankle jerk, and a warm foot with good pulses has a predominantly neuropathic lesion. This patient has a good chance of healing and therefore must be treated aggressively. If osteomyelitis is present, the prognosis becomes poor. A patient with a painful lesion, with or without absent pulses, who exhibits dependent rubor, a cool foot, and poor venous filling (in the absence of varicose veins) and who also has other evidence of ischemia, such as thickened nails and hair loss on the foot and leg, has a much poorer prognosis for healing.

The objectives of treatment are to heal the foot lesion and preserve tissue. If this is not feasible, amputation is necessary. All patients with significant foot lesions should be hospitalized and treated with bed rest, antibiotics (after appropriate cultures), local therapy with whirlpool, debridement, and drainage. The last two procedures must be done in an extremely conservative fashion in the patient with a predominantly vascular lesion, since the ability to heal this type of lesion is questionable. Roentgenograms are helpful to determine whether osteomyelitis is present or not. However, films must be interpreted cautiously, since neuropathy can produce osteoporotic "washed out" bones and can be confused with osteomyelitis. If healing cannot be accomplished, adequate amputation must be carried out. Finally, diabetes must be well controlled to maximize the patient's ability to heal and combat the infection.

One of the most important aspects to consider when discussing the diabetic foot is prevention. Many of the events that lead to eventual amputation are preventable. Therefore the patient must be educated regarding proper care and attention to the feet.

EYE COMPLICATIONS—CATARACTS AND RETINOPATHY

A leading cause of blindness in the United States is diabetes mellitus. Uncontrolled diabetes can be accompanied by reversible blurred vision, which can become worse as diabetes is initially controlled. This is caused by swelling of the lens, a result of the accumulation of fructose and sorbitol that increases the osmolality within the lens. If this process continues or is frequent, lens protein is denatured and cataracts form. Two types of cataracts are seen: (1) metabolic or juvenile cataracts, which may be observed in children and young adults who have grossly uncontrolled diabetes, and (2) senile cataracts, which are more common than metabolic cataracts. These cataracts are similar to the senile cataracts of nondiabetic patients but tend to occur at a younger age.

A major eye problem is diabetic retinopathy. This problem is typically observed 10 to 15 years after the onset of diabetes. Diabetic retinopathy is classified into three categories:

1. Background retinopathy consists of microaneurysms, intraretinal hemorrhages (blot, dot, and flame hemorrhages), retinal edema, and hard, waxy exudates.
2. Maculopathy consists of hard exudates, edema, and less often hemorrhage in the macula yielding a marked deficit in visual acuity.
3. Proliferative retinopathy (malignant retinopathy) consists of new blood vessel formation, glial scars, and preretinal and vitreous hemorrhages that lead to vitreous opacity and retinal detachment. Sixty percent of the patients discovered to have this form of diabetic retinopathy are blind in that eye within 5 years, whereas patients having only background retinopathy do not become blind unless maculopathy or proliferative retinopathy supervenes.

The cause of diabetic retinopathy is thought to be related to retinal ischemia resulting from the metabolic abnormalities of the diabetic state. The increased blood coagulability, increased blood viscosity, increased red blood cell clumping, and increased platelet adhesiveness that are present in diabetes can reduce blood flow in the retinal capillaries and cause ischemia. In addition, the elevated levels of hemoglobin A_{1c} observed in diabetes can add to the ischemia, since this hemoglobin less readily gives up oxygen to the tissues. It is postulated that ischemic areas of the retina release a blood vessel–stimulating factor leading to new blood vessel formation not only in the retina but also in the anterior chamber of the eye and iris. Repeated hemorrhage into the anterior chamber can lead to glaucoma.

No treatment is indicated for background retinopathy at present except for diabetic control. Therapy using the xenon arc or the argon laser has been demonstrated to be beneficial in proliferative retinopathy and maculopathy and is now the treatment choice. Vitrectomy is helpful in selected cases. Pituitary ablation is no longer indicated in most cases.

NEPHROPATHY

Diabetic nephropathy is a clinical syndrome of progressive renal dysfunction leading to hypertension, varying degrees of the nephrotic syndrome, and renal failure. Although most patients having diabetes for 20 years have some histopathologic evidence of diabetic renal involvement, only 50% of patients have the clinical syndrome, usually observed 10 to 15 years after the onset of diabetes.

Typically, proteinuria is the first manifestation of the syndrome; it increases with time. Later, progressive renal failure is evidenced by increasing urea nitrogen and creatinine levels. By the time the patient is excreting a significant amount of protein (2 to 3 g/24 hr), life expectancy is decreased to 6 years. When urea nitrogen and creatinine are elevated, life expectancy drops to 3 years. During this latter period hypertension appears or becomes severe and difficult to control. This not only increases the renal damage but also markedly increases the retinal deterioration; almost all patients with nephropathy have retinopathy.

Death is inevitable unless dialysis and renal transplantation are employed. In the past many centers would not accept diabetic patients for either long-term dialysis or renal transplant programs because of poor results, but fortunately this is changing. Chronic renal failure from diabetic nephropathy is the most common renal disease treated in many renal failure treatment centers.

None of the histopathologic changes observed in the kidneys of diabetic patients is specific for diabetes mellitus. However, the widespread changes and the variety of lesions observed strongly suggest diabetes. Typical lesions include glomerular capillary basement membrane thickening along with deposits of basement membrane–like material in the mesangial areas (diffuse glomerulosclerosis), thickening of the arteriolar basement membrane (arteriolosclerosis), nodular accumulations of basement membrane–like material in the mesangium, the so-called Kimmelstiel-Wilson lesion (nodular glomerulosclerosis), and cellular infiltrates and scarring of the renal interstitium (interstitial disease). Other common lesions include the capsular drop and hyaline cap ("exudative lesions") and glycogen deposition in the renal tubules. Usually all the lesions are present to varying degrees. However, the lesion that seems to correlate best with the clinical picture is the lesion of diffuse glomerulosclerosis.

In addition to proper therapy for diabetes, treatment consists of finding and treating any other entity that causes deterioration of renal function, such as hypertension, urinary infection, urinary obstruction, and nephrotoxic drugs. As renal function deteriorates, the patient should be evaluated for entrance into renal dialysis and transplantation programs and for the appropriate time to place an access arteriovenous fistula. When terminal renal failure appears, insulin requirements may need to be drastically reduced; however, some insulin is usually necessary.

NEUROPATHY

The nervous system is affected by diabetes mellitus in many ways. Diabetic neuropathy refers to abnormalities of the function of peripheral nerves (and certain cranial nerves) in diabetes mellitus. Although diabetic neuropathy can be the initial symptom of diabetes mellitus, more typically the clinical signs of the neuropathies are observed about 10 years after the onset of the disease. The neuropathies can be classified according to the nervous tissue element involved.

Peripheral neuropathy

Peripheral neuropathy is a metabolic disorder of the peripheral nerves possibly caused by increased sorbitol and decreased myo-inositol levels in the nerve fibers. This leads to a decrease in the conduction velocity of the nerve impulse. This disorder affects the distal segments of the nerves before the proximal segments and affects the nerves in the lower extremities to a greater degree than those of the upper extremities. The dysfunction results in a "stocking-glove" distribution of the symptoms and signs. Both motor and sensory functions are affected, resulting in numbness, dysesthesia, loss of position and vibratory sensation, muscle wasting, and deformity of the foot. Peripheral neuropathy leads to two serious problems: (1) trauma to the feet and trauma to and deterioration of joints (Charcot's joint), with ultimate production of the diabetic foot and loss of locomotion; and (2) incapacitating pain syndrome. This syndrome is associated with depression, weight loss, and markedly uncontrolled diabetes.

Mononeuropathy

Mononeuropathy is caused by infarcts of a single nerve or different single nerves (mononeuropathy multiplex). The onset is relatively rapid and is accompanied by loss of motor and sensory function of the involved nerve. There can be severe pain in the distribution of the nerve and a positive Tinel's sign (shooting pain along the nerve when percussed). If this process occurs in the cranial nerves of the eye (nerves III, IV, or VI), it is termed "cranial neuropathy." Cranial neuropathy most frequently involves the third cranial nerve. Symptoms include ophthalmoplegia, ptosis, unilateral headache, and a dilated pupil with a spared pupillary light reflex. The major condition to be considered in the differential diagnosis is aneurysm of the circle of Willis. However, third nerve palsy caused by aneurysm is usually associated with loss of the pupillary light reflex.

Radiculopathy

Radiculopathy is caused by infarction of the nerve root. This yields a sensory syndrome whose symptoms and signs are present in the distribution of the nerve root. Patients complain of pain in a root distribution, which may be aggravated with coughing or straining. A classic presentation is intercostal neuritis. Certain cases of upper abdominal pain in the diabetic patient result from involvement of the lower thoracic nerve roots. This must be kept in mind when evaluating a diabetic patient with abdominal pain.

Amyotrophy

Amyotrophy is characterized by asymmetric wasting and weakness of the muscles of the pelvic girdle. There may be pain and loss of reflexes or, occasionally, increased reflexes. Fasciculations are sometimes observed. In contrast to the other neuropathies, this type of neuropathy is usually seen in middle-aged or older men who have diabetes of recent onset or newly diagnosed diabetes.

The cause of this lesion is disputed. Some consider it to be secondary to infarction of the lumbar plexus, whereas others consider it to be secondary to a metabolic abnormality of the nerve terminals. Although biopsy is usually unnecessary, muscle biopsy reveals noninflammatory degeneration of single muscle fibers. Electromyography reveals changes of denervation but no evidence of primary muscle disease.

Autonomic neuropathy

Any autonomic function can be affected by diabetes mellitus. Patients with autonomic neuropathy usually have had long-term diabetes with other major complications. The role of autonomic neuropathy in the morbidity and mortality of diabetes mellitus is more widely appreciated. The various autonomic neuropathies are listed in the following outline. Treatment is mainly symptomatic. However, metoclopramide has been successfully used for gastroparesis, and broad-spectrum, nonabsorbable antibiotics can be helpful in treating some cases of diabetic diarrhea.

Types of autonomic neuropathy

I.   Pupillary abnormalities
II. Cardiovascular abnormalities
     A. Persistent tachycardia
     B. Persistent bradycardia
     C. Cardiac denervation syndrome (loss of sympathetic and parasympathetic nerve function)
     D. Abnormalities in Valsalva's maneuver
     E. Abnormal beat-to-beat variation
     F. Postural hypotension
III. Gastrointestinal abnormalities
     A. Esophageal motility disorders
     B. Gastroparesis (gastric atony)
     C. Gallbladder motility abnormalities
     D. Diabetic diarrhea
     E. Colonic motility problems (constipation, "megacolon")

IV. Genitourinary abnormalities
     A. Atonic bladder
     B. Impotence
     C. Retrograde ejaculation
V.   Abnormalities of sweat gland and sebaceous gland function
     A. Hyperhidrosis
     B. Hypohidrosis
     C. Deficient sebum production

Diabetic pseudotabes

The term "diabetic pseudotabes" is sometimes used to denote a disorder caused by the signs and symptoms of the various diabetic neuropathies that together resemble the disorder tabes dorsalis. It does not denote another form of diabetic neuropathy. Diagnosis rests with evaluation of serum and spinal fluid serologic tests for syphilis. The level of spinal fluid protein is not of diagnostic help, since elevated levels are observed in diabetic neuropathy.

DERMOPATHY

Patients with diabetic dermopathy may have pigmented atrophic lesions over the shins ("shin spots"). These lesions are thought to be related to trauma. Another chronic skin manifestation of diabetes is necrobiosis lipoidica diabeticorum. This lesion is usually observed in young diabetic women whose diabetes started in childhood. Typically, these lesions are noted on the anterior shin (the process is usually bilateral, but not symmetric). The lesions have a pink to tan border and a waxy-looking and waxy-feeling depressed central area in which telangiectatic vessels are observed. Histologically, the lesions reveal necrosis and loss of the subcutaneous fat, capillaries with thick basement membranes, and granuloma formation.

Both dermopathy and necrobiosis are usually of no medical consequence. However, necrobiosis can be a cosmetic problem and does respond to intralesional injection of corticosteroids. This lesion occasionally ulcerates and requires skin grafting.

BIBLIOGRAPHY

Bradley WE, editor: Aspects of autonomic neuropathy, Ann Intern Med 92:293, 1980.
Bunick EM and Lavine RL: The role of hyperglycemia in the development of complications in the diabetic patient. In Coodley EL and others: Internal medicine update: 1979-1980, New York, 1979, Grune & Stratton, Inc.
Jarrett J: Diabetes and the heart: coronary heart disease, Clin Endocrinol Metab 6:389, 1977.
Kohner EM and Oakley NW: Diabetic retinopathy, Metabolism 24:1085, 1975.
Levin ME: The diabetic foot, J Am Podiatry Assoc 66:825, 1976.
Pirart J: Diabetes mellitus and its degenerative complications: a prospective study of 4400 patients observed between 1947 and 1973, Diabetes Care 1:168, 252, 1978.
Raskin P and Rosenstock I: Blood glucose control and diabetic complications, Ann Intern Med 105:254, 1986.
Watkins PJ, editor: Long-term complications of diabetes, Clin Endocrinol Metab 15:715, 1986.
West KM, editor: Symposium of epidemiology of diabetes and its macrovascular complications, Diabetes Care 2:63, 1979.

201 · HYPOGLYCEMIA AND HYPOGLYCEMIC DISORDERS

Clinton W. Young *and* **John H. Karam**

Symptomatic hypolglycemia occurs when the central nervous system is deprived of sufficient glucose to meet its metabolic needs. It is usually seen when the blood glucose level drops below 40 mg/dl.

PATHOPHYSIOLOGY. Numerous mechanisms serve to

maintain blood glucose within a narrow range (80 to 100 mg/dl). The postprandial rise in blood glucose stimulates the pancreatic β-cells to secrete insulin, which promotes the uptake of glucose into liver, muscle, and adipose tissue, thus normalizing the blood glucose level within 2 hours. Overstimulation of the β-cells postprandially, as a result of accelerated glucose absorption after rapid gastric emptying, can result in a too rapid disposal of ingested glucose and consequent hypoglycemia 2 to 5 hours after eating (postprandial or reactive hypoglycemia).

By 5 to 8 hours after eating (the postabsorptive state), circulating nutrients of exogenous origin have returned to premeal levels. At this time glucose must arise endogenously from hepatic glycogenolysis and gluconeogenesis to provide sufficient fuel for proper functioning of the central nervous system. An adequate rate of hepatic glucose production depends primarily on an appropriate decline in circulating insulin levels with fasting and, to a lesser extent, on a rise in glucagon, growth hormone, and cortisol levels. These hormonal changes program the hepatic enzymatic steps necessary for glycogenolysis and gluconeogenesis. Any condition that impairs hepatic glucose production (for example, hyperinsulinism; deficiency of cortisol, glucagon, or growth hormone; severe hepatic parenchymal disease; or hepatic enzymatic deficiencies) can result in fasting hypoglycemia.

The causes of hypoglycemia are outlined as follows:

Reaction to exogenous insulin
Postprandial (reactive) hypoglycemia
   Early hypoglycemia (alimentary)
      Gastrectomy
      Increased vagal tone (functional)
   Late hypoglycemia (occult diabetes)
Fasting hypoglycemia
   Without hyperinsulinism
      Endocrine or enzymatic disorders
      Severe hepatic dysfunction
      Extrahepatic tumors
   With hyperinsulinism
      Pancreatic β-cell tumor
      Surreptitious administration of insulin or sulfonylureas
        (factitious hypoglycemia)
Alcohol hypoglycemia

ETIOLOGY

Reaction to exogenous insulin. Insulin reaction, the most commonly seen hypoglycemic disorder, results from insulin overdosage in the diabetic patient. This usually occurs when the patient fails to eat adequately or engages in strenuous physical activity without an appropriate reduction in insulin dosage.

Postprandial (reactive) hypoglycemia. Postprandial hypoglycemia can be classified as early (within 2 to 3 hours of a meal) or late (3 to 5 hours after eating). Early, or alimentary, hypoglycemia occurs when there is a rapid discharge of ingested carbohydrate into the small bowel, followed by rapid glucose absorption and hyperinsulinism. It may be seen after gastrointestinal surgery, particularly in association with the "dumping syndrome" after gastrectomy; more commonly it is functional and can result from overactivity of the parasympathetic nervous system mediated via the vagus nerves. Late hypoglycemia (occult diabetes) is caused by a delay in early insulin release, which results in exaggeration of the initial hyperglycemia during a glucose tolerance test. In response to this hyperglycemia, an exaggerated insulin response produces late hypoglycemia.

Fasting hypoglycemia. Fasting hypoglycemia can occur spontaneously in certain endocrine diseases (such as hypopituitarism, Addison's disease, or myxedema), in disorders causing severe hepatic dysfunction, or as a consequence of inborn metabolic diseases of childhood such as glycogen storage disease. These conditions are usually obvious, with hypoglycemia being only a secondary feature. When fasting hypoglycemia is a primary manifestation in an adult without a clinically apparent endocrine or hepatic disorder, the principal causes are (1) hyperinsulinism owing to either pancreatic β-cell tumors or surreptitious administration of insulin or sulfonylureas, and (2) non-insulin-producing extrahepatic tumors.

Alcohol hypoglycemia. Alcohol hypoglycemia can occur after a period of fasting or within several hours after drinking ethanol in combination with mixes containing sugar. In either case the blood ethanol level may be considerably below legal standards for intoxication.

CLINICAL MANIFESTATIONS. Regardless of the cause of hypoglycemia, it is characterized by Whipple's triad, which comprises a history of hypoglycemic symptoms, an associated blood glucose level of 40 mg/dl or less, and immediate recovery following administration of glucose.

Acute hypoglycemia. A precipitous fall in blood glucose to hypoglycemic levels is often heralded by symptoms of adrenergic discharge (sweating, palpitations, anxiety, and tremulousness). Syncope or convulsions can also occur. These symptoms and signs are more commonly associated with an insulin reaction or postprandial reactive hypoglycemia than with fasting hypoglycemia.

Subacute and chronic hypoglycemia. Neuroglycopenic symptoms are the principal manifestation of slowly developing hypoglycemia. They evidence a lack of glucose in the central nervous system and can include blurred vision or diplopia, headache, feelings of detachment, slurred speech, and weakness. Personality and mental changes vary from anxiety to psychotic behavior. These symptoms and signs are more commonly associated with the disorders producing fasting hypoglycemia.

MANAGEMENT. Prolonged hypoglycemia can cause permanent brain damage, convulsions, and death. Prompt recognition and treatment are therefore mandatory. If the patient is conscious and able to swallow, sugar, glucose, candy, or orange juice should be given. If the patient is unconscious, the danger of aspiration necessitates reliance on one of two methods: the intravenous administration of 50 ml of 50% dextrose over 1 to 2 minutes (the treatment of choice) or the intravenous or intramuscular administration of 1 mg glucagon if the hepatic glycogen reserve is adequate. When consciousness is restored, oral feeding can begin.

Prevention of recurrent hypoglycemic attacks depends on proper diagnosis and management of the underlying disorder.

POSTPRANDIAL (REACTIVE) HYPOGLYCEMIA

Postgastrectomy alimentary hypoglycemia. Treatment of postgastrectomy alimentary hypoglycemia involves more frequent feedings with small portions of rapidly assimilated carbohydrate and larger portions of slowly absorbed fat and protein. Occasionally, anticholinergic drugs such as propantheline (15 mg orally four times daily) can be useful in reducing vagal overactivity.

Functional alimentary hypoglycemia. Early alimentary-type reactive hypoglycemia in a patient who has not undergone surgery is classified as functional. It is most often associated with chronic fatigue, anxiety, irritability, weakness, poor concentration, decreased libido, headaches, hunger after meals, and tremulousness. However, most patients with these symptoms do not have hypoglycemia. Furthermore, even in those with documented early hypoglycemia, it is likely to be only a secondary manifestation of their nervous imbalance, with consequent vagal overactivity causing increased gastric emptying and early hyperinsulinism.

Indiscriminate use and overinterpretation of glucose tolerance tests have led to an unfortunate tendency to overdiagnose functional hypoglycemia. As many as one third or more of normal subjects have hypoglycemia with or without symptoms during a 5-hour glucose tolerance test; thus the nonspecificity of this test makes it a highly unreliable tool for evaluating patients with suspected episodes of postprandial hypoglycemia. Accordingly, to increase diagnostic reliability, hypoglycemia should be documented at the time of a spontaneous symptomatic episode during routine daily activity. Personality evaluation suggestive of hyperkinetic compulsive behavior in thin, anxious patients, supports this diagnosis in those with a compatible history.

With documented functional postprandial hypoglycemia, there is no harm and occasional benefit in reducing or eliminating the refined sugar content in the patient's diet while increasing the frequency and reducing the size of meals. However, it should not be expected that these maneuvers will cure the neurasthenia, since the reflex response to hypoglycemia is only one component of a generalized primary nervous hyperactivity. Supportive counseling and mild sedation should be the mainstays of therapy, with dietary manipulation only an adjunct. Oral anticholinergic drugs have helped in certain advanced cases.

Late hypoglycemia (occult diabetes). Patients with late hypoglycemia are usually quite different from those with early hypoglycemia. They are more phlegmatic and often obese and frequently have a family history of diabetes mellitus. In obese patients treatment is directed at reduction to ideal weight. These patients often respond to reduced carbohydrate intake with multiple, spaced, small feedings that are high in protein. They should be considered early diabetic patients and advised to have periodic medical evaluations.

HYPOGLYCEMIA CAUSED BY PANCREATIC β-CELL TUMORS. Fasting hypoglycemia in an otherwise healthy adult is most commonly due to an adenoma of the islets of Langerhans (insulinoma). Ninety percent of such tumors are single and benign, but multiple adenomas can occur, as well as malignancies with functional metastases. (β-Cell hyperplasia as a cause of fasting hypoglycemia is not well documented in adults.) Adenomas can be familial and have been found in conjunction with tumors of the parathyroid glands and the pituitary gland (multiple endocrine adenomatosis, type 1).

Clinical diagnosis. The signs and symptoms of tumor-related hypoglycemia are those of subacute or chronic hypoglycemia. Permanent and irreversible brain damage can occur. Delayed diagnosis has often resulted in prolonged psychiatric care or treatment for psychomotor epilepsy. In chronic cases obesity can result as a consequence of overeating to relieve symptoms. These often develop in the early morning or after missing a meal, and they occasionally occur after exercise. Typically they begin with evidence of glucose deficiency in the central nervous system. Sweating and palpitations may not occur with subacute hypoglycemia until a profound degree of hypoglycemia develops.

Laboratory diagnosis. β-Cell tumors do not reduce secretion in the presence of hypoglycemia, and a serum insulin level of 15 μU/ml or more with a concomitant blood glucose value below 40 mg/dl suggests an insulinoma. Other causes of hyperinsulinemic hypoglycemia must be considered, however, such as surreptitious administration of insulin or sulfonylureas.

Prolonged fast. Demonstration of hypoglycemia with in-appropriate fasting hyperinsulinism during a prolonged, hospital-supervised fast remains the most reliable diagnostic maneuver for insulinoma. In normal men the blood glucose value will not fall below 55 mg/dl during a 72-hour fast; in some normal women, however, the value can fall to as low as 22 mg/dl and lower limits have not been established. (These women remain asymptomatic despite this degree of hypoglycemia, probably because ketogenesis is able to provide sufficient fuel for the central nervous system.) Ratios of insulin (in microunits per milliliter) to glucose (in milligrams per deciliter) are therefore essential. Nonobese, normal subjects maintain a ratio of less than 0.3. Obese subjects may have an elevated ratio, but hypoglycemia does not occur. Virtually 100% of patients with insulinomas have an abnormal insulin-to-glucose ratio during prolonged fasting.

Oral glucose tolerance testing. Oral glucose tolerance testing has *not* been a valuable diagnostic tool because the variable responsiveness of insulinomas to glucose gives confusing results. Most insulinomas respond poorly to glucose, and a diabetic oral glucose tolerance curve results. In the rare tumors that release insulin in response to glucose, a "flat" curve can be seen. However, flat curves are also seen in normal subjects.

Stimulation tests. Demonstration of an exaggerated insulin response to intravenous tolbutamide (insulin level >200 μU/ml within 15 minutes) or glucagon (insulin level >135 μU/ml) can be helpful in documenting insulinoma. However, this response is seen in only 50% to 80% of patients with insulinomas and many false positive results occur (for example, in obesity or hepatic disease). In addition, these tests can produce prolonged, hazardous hypoglycemia in patients with insulinomas.

Suppression test. Suppression of C-peptide during insulin-induced hypoglycemia is the basis of a recently developed diagnostic test for insulinoma. This small peptide, connecting the A and B chains of insulin, is released in equimolar quantities with endogenous insulin and thus reflects endogenous insulin secretion, which cannot be directly monitored during insulin infusion. Whereas in normal subjects C-peptide levels will be suppressed to 50% or less of baseline levels during hypoglycemia induced by 0.1 unit of insulin/kg body weight/hr, absence of suppression suggests the presence of an autonomous insulin-secreting tumor.

Roentgenography. Pancreatic arteriography can occasionally locate tumors preoperatively; however, because of the small size of β-cell adenomas (1 cm or less in most cases), the accuracy rate is only 50% and the false positive rate is about 5%. Computed tomography and magnetic resonance imaging have not proved helpful because of their inability to distinguish small tumors within the pancreas. Percutaneous transhepatic pancreatic vein catheterization with insulin assay has proved useful as a means of localizing insulinomas but is a painful, poorly tolerated procedure.

Documentation of factitious hypoglycemia. Surreptitious insulin or sulfonylurea administration can be difficult to prove. A suspicion of self-induced hypoglycemia is strengthened if the patient is associated with the health professions or has access to insulin or sulfonylurea drugs taken by a diabetic family member. The triad of hypoglycemia, high insulin levels and low C-peptide immunoreactivity is pathognomonic of exogenous insulin administration. Demonstration of circulating antibodies to insulin supports this diagnosis in suspected cases. When sulfonylurea abuse is suspected, a chemical test of the plasma to detect the presence of these drugs will distinguish factitious hypoglycemia from insulinoma.

Management

Surgical measures. Surgery is the treatment of choice,

preferably by a surgeon experienced in removing insulinomas and capable of mobilizing the pancreas and adequately exploring the posterior surface of the head, body, and tail. Blood glucose should be monitored throughout surgery, and 10% dextrose in water should be infused at a rate of 100 ml/hr or faster. In cases in which the diagnosis has been established but no adenoma is located, intraoperative ultrasound may localize a small nonpalpable tumor. If this is not successful, subtotal pancreatectomy is usually indicated, including the entire body and tail of the pancreas. Total pancreatectomy is seldom required in view of the efficacy of long-term therapy with diazoxide in most patients.

Diet and chemotherapy. In patients with inoperable functioning islet cell carcinoma or in patients in whom subtotal removal of the pancreas has failed to produce a cure, reliance on frequent feedings is necessary. Since most tumors are not responsive to glucose, carbohydrate feedings every 2 to 3 hours will usually prevent hypoglycemia, although obesity can become a problem. Glucagon should be available for emergency use. Certain drugs, such as diazoxide (300 to 600 mg/day orally), have been useful. (To control the sodium retention characteristic of diazoxide, thiazides should be given. In patients who do not tolerate diazoxide because of its side effects (gastrointestinal upset, hirsutism, or water retention) the calcium channel blocker verapamil has been beneficial in preventing hypoglycemia by inhibiting insulin release from insulinoma cells. Streptozotocina cytotoxic drug, has been found to be especially useful in decreasing insulin secretion in islet cell carcinomas, and effective doses have been achieved without the undue renal toxicity that characterized early experience with the drug.

Prognosis. When insulinoma is diagnosed early and cured surgically, complete recovery is likely—although brain damage following severe hypoglycemia is not reversible. A significant increase in the survival rate has been shown in streptozotocin-treated patients with islet cell carcinoma, with reduction in tumor mass as well as decreased hyperinsulinism.

HYPOGLYCEMIA CAUSED BY EXTRAPANCREATIC TUMORS. In rare cases hypoglycemia can be caused by extrapancreatic tumors, including mesenchymal tumors (retroperitoneal sarcomas, hepatomas, and adrenocortical carcinomas) and miscellaneous epithelial-type tumors. They are frequently large and readily palpated or visualized on urograms.

Laboratory diagnosis depends on the demonstration of fasting hypoglycemia associated with serum insulin levels generally below 10 µU/ml. None of these tumors has ever been reported to release immunoreactive insulin, and the mechanism of their hypoglycemic effect remains obscure. Release of insulin-like growth factors by the tumors has recently been reported as a cause of the hypoglycemia.

The prognosis is generally poor, and surgical removal should be attempted when feasible. Dietary management of the hypoglycemia is the mainstay of medical treatment, since diazoxide is usually ineffective.

ALCOHOL HYPOGLYCEMIA
Fasting hypoglycemia after alcohol ingestion. After 18 to 24 hours of fasting, hepatic glycogen reserves become depleted and continued hepatic glucose production becomes totally dependent on gluconeogenesis. Under these circumstances a blood concentration of ethanol as low as 45 mg/dl (considerably below most states' legal level of intoxication of 100 mg/dl) can produce profound hypoglycemia by blocking gluconeogenesis. Neutroglycopenic symptoms in a patient whose breath smells of alcohol can be mistaken for alcoholic stupor.

Adequate food intake during alcohol ingestion prevents this type of hypoglycemia.

Reactive hypoglycemia after alcohol ingestion. When soft drinks containing sugar are used as mixers to dilute alcohol in beverages (gin and tonic, rum and cola), insulin release appears to be greater than when the soft drink alone is ingested, and there is a greater tendency for a late hypoglycemic overswing 3 to 4 hours later. This can be prevented by avoiding the use of sugar mixers when drinking alcohol or ensuring supplementary food intake to provide sustained absorption.

BIBLIOGRAPHY

Axelrod L and Ron D: Insulin-like growth factor II and the riddle of tumor-induced hypoglycemia, N Eng J Med 319:1477, 1988.
Berger M and others: Functional and morphologic characterization of human insulinomas, Diabetes 32:921, 1983.
Cho KJ and others: Localization of the source of hyperinsulinism: percutaneous transhepatic portal and pancreatic vein catheterization with hormone assay, Am J Radiology 139:237, 1982.
Cryer PE: Glucose counterregulation in man, Diabetes 30:261, 1981.
Daggett PR and others: Is preoperative localisation of insulinomas necessary? Lancet 1:483, 1981.
Dons RF and others: Anomalous glucose and insulin responses in patients with insulinoma: caveats for diagnosis, Arch Intern Med 145:1861, 1985.
Isselbacher KJ: Metabolic and hepatic effects of alcohol, N Engl J Med 296:612, 1977.
Johnson DD and others: Reactive hypoglycemia, JAMA 243:1151, 1980.
Jordan RM, Kammer H, and Riddle MR: Sulfonylurea-induced factitious hypoglycemia: a growing problem, Arch Intern Med 137:390, 1977.
Karam JH and others: Feedback-controlled dextrose infusion during surgical management of insulinomas, Am J Med 66:675, 1979.
LeQuesne LP and others: The management of insulin tumors of the pancreas, Br J Surg 66:373, 1979.
Rifkin MD and Weiss SM: Intraoperative sonographic identification of nonpalpable pancreatic masses, J Ultrasound Med 3:409, 1984.
Rizza RA and others: Pathogenesis of hypoglycemia in insulinoma patients; suppression of hepatic glucose production by insulin, Diabetes 330:377, 1981.
Scarlett JA and others: Factitious hypoglycemia: diagnosis by measurement of serum C-peptide immunoreactivity and insulin-binding antibodies, N Engl J Med 297:1029, 1977.
Service FJ, editor: Hypoglycemic disorders: pathogenesis, diagnosis and treatment, Boston, 1983, GK Hall.
Ulbrecht JS and others: Insulinoma in a 94-year-old woman: long-term therapy with verapamil, Diabetes Care 9:186, 1986.

202 · DISORDERS OF LIPOPROTEIN METABOLISM

David M. Capuzzi

Overwhelming evidence assembled over the past 30 years indicates a strong association between elevations of plasma lipid levels (hyperlipidemia) and the premature development of atherosclerotic coronary heart disease (CHD). Plasma lipoproteins function as water-soluble vehicles that transport lipids in the bloodstream. Hyperlipidemia can result from an increased rate of synthesis, a decreased rate of clearance of the circulating lipoproteins, or both. All the major plasma lipids (cholesterol, triglycerides, and phospholipids) are transported in the circulation bound noncovalently to proteins, and a rise in circulating lipid levels is always associated with an elevation of plasma lipoproteins. Several prospective large-scale epidemiologic studies have demonstrated a link between elevated serum or plasma cholesterol levels and the accelerated progression of atherosclerosis. Recent results of clinical intervention trials have shown that a sustained reduction in elevated plasma lipoprotein cholesterol levels can decelerate or even reverse the atherogenic process in some patients. Some forms

Table 202-1   Human plasma lipoproteins

Lipoprotein class	Density (d) g/ml	Electrophoretic mobility	Apoprotein content	Major lipids
Chylomicrons and chylomicron remnants	d < 1.006	Remain at origin	A-I, A-II, B-48, C-I, C-II, C-III, E	Exogenous triglycerides
Very low density lipoproteins (VLDL)	d < 1.006	Pre-β	B-100, C-I, C-II, C-III, E	Endogenous triglycerides
Intermediate density lipoproteins (IDL)	d < 1.019	Between β and pre-β	B-100, E	Endogenous triglycerides, cholesterol esters
Low density lipoproteins (LDL)	1.019 < d < 1.063	β	B-100	Cholesterol esters, free cholesterol
High density lipoproteins (HDL)	1.063 < d < 1.21	α	A-I, A-II	Cholesterol esters, phospholipids

of hyperlipidemia can cause episodes of acute pancreatitis. Significant elevations of plasma lipids can lead to formation of xanthomas, deposits of lipids in the skin and tendons. Rational treatment of elevated lipoprotein levels (hyperlipoproteinemia) requires some understanding of the structure and function of lipoproteins and their dynamic interactions in vivo. Over the past decade there have been dramatic advances in fundamental knowledge of the function and metabolism of lipoproteins and in defining pathophysiologic and genetic factors underlying the various lipoprotein disorders. The application of this growing information should bring about significant improvements in diagnostic and therapeutic approaches. For routine clinical purposes emphasis has been placed on determinations of plasma or serum levels of lipids, particularly cholesterol and triglycerides, and on estimates of elevations of specific lipoprotein classes by sample inspection and electrophoretic separations. These methods have been useful for the broad classification of several phenotypic patterns of lipid transport, but the hyperlipoproteinemias are varied and heterogeneous in origin and result from a complex interplay of environmental and genetic factors. The general phenotypic categories of hyperlipoproteinemia are types I, II, III, IV, or V, depending on the specific lipoprotein class or classes elevated. A given type of hyperlipoproteinemia may reflect a diversity of underlying metabolic abnormalities, and conversely a specific disease of lipoprotein transport can display different phenotypic patterns on lipoprotein electrophoretic analysis.

Increasing emphasis in plasma lipoprotein studies has been placed on monitoring the circulating levels, kinetics, and disposal sites for metabolic removal of the apoprotein constituents of the lipoproteins or apolipoproteins. These investigations have led to the discovery of a number of apolipoprotein abnormalities. The development of refined techniques for determination of plasma apolipoprotein levels ensures that these measurements will be widely applied for more definitive delineation of specific lipoprotein disturbances.

PLASMA LIPOPROTEINS

The circulating lipoproteins are classified by their density characteristics, by ultracentrifugal flotation, and by their electrophoretic mobility. The plasma lipoproteins contain small amounts of carbohydrates covalently bound to the apoproteins in addition to a large complement of noncovalently bound lipid. Nonpolar lipids such as triglyceride and cholesterol esters form the oily core of the lipoprotein molecule, whereas unesterified cholesterol, phospholipids, and apoproteins comprise the surface components. Five major classes of plasma lipoproteins can be separated by ultracentrifugal and electrophoretic means (Table 202-1). The larger and lighter lipoproteins contain a higher percentage of lipid, especially triglyceride, and a lower

percentage of protein than the smaller and denser lipoproteins. In order of decreasing size and increasing density, the lipoprotein families are chylomicrons, very low density lipoproteins (VLDL), intermediate density lipoproteins (IDL), low density lipoproteins (LDL), and high density lipoproteins (HDL). By ultracentrifugal analysis, these lipoprotein families can be classified according to density (d) as follows: chylomicrons, d<1.006; VLDL, d<1.006; IDL, d<1.019; LDL, 1.0l9<d<1.063; and HDL, 1.063<d<1.21. After electrophoretic separation of lipoproteins on paper or agarose gel at pH 8.6, chylomicrons remain at the origin, VLDL has pre-β-mobility, LDL has β-mobility, and HDL has α-mobility. IDL forms a broad band between the pre-β-and β-regions. Each major lipoprotein class contains a complement of each major lipid class, but the proportions differ. Lipoprotein triglycerides represent the transport cargo of triglyceride-rich lipoproteins (chylomicrons and VLDL); the other lipids probably serve to stabilize the structure of the circulating aggregate and to facilitate its solubility in plasma.

PLASMA APOLIPOPROTEINS

Several methods have been developed for the preparation, isolation, and characterization of the apolipoproteins, and the amino acid sequences of several have been determined. Each plasma lipoprotein density class contains a characteristic distribution of apoproteins, and many of these apoproteins are present in more than one lipoprotein density class. The A apoproteins (apo A-I and apo A-II) comprise about 90% of human HDL protein, with an apo A-I to A-II ratio of about 3:1 by weight. Apo A-I and apo A-II are also present in small amounts in chylomicrons and in trace amounts in VLDL. Apo A-I is synthesized by both the liver and intestine, whereas apo A-II is synthesized mainly by the liver. Apo A-I is an activator of the enzyme lecithin-cholesterol acyltransferase (LCAT), which catalyzes the transfer of a fatty acyl moiety from the position 2 of lecithin to the position 3 of cholesterol in HDL, forming cholesterol esters and lysolecithin in plasma. Apo A-II can inhibit the activity of LCAT, activate the hepatic triglyceride lipase, or both.

Apoprotein B (apo B) is a heterogeneous protein that exists primarily in two forms: apo B-100 and apo B-48. Apo B-100, synthesized in the liver, is the major apoprotein of human VLDL and LDL. Apo B-100 constitutes more than 95% of the LDL apoproteins and about 25% of the total LDL mass. Apo B-48 is a major apoprotein constituent of the chylomicrons and of the chylomicron remnants that result from catabolic depletion of their core triglycerides.

A group of small-molecular-weight apoproteins (approximately 10,000 daltons), the C apoproteins (apo C), consists of at least three distinct proteins: apo C-I, apo C-II, and apo Cat least three distinct proteins: apo C-I, apo C-II, and apo C-III. The C apoproteins are the major protein constituents of chylomicrons and VLDL. Small amounts of apo C are found in HDL and trace amounts in LDL. Apo C-II is the specific cofactor necessary for triglyceride hydrolysis by lipoprotein lipases (LPLs) of extrahepatic origin and hence plays a crucial role in the metabolism of chylomicrons and VLDL. Apo C-III, the most abundant of the C apoproteins, has been found in three polymorphic forms containing respectively no (apo C-III-0), one (Apo C-III-1), or two (apo C-III-2) sialic acid residues. Although apo C-III can activate LCAT and inhibit activation of LPL, the specific functions of its heterogeneous forms are currently unclear.

Apo E is a constituent of all the circulating lipoproteins except LDL and is found in several polymorphic forms. The complex pattern reflects the presence of multiple alleles for apo E at a single gene locus and varying degrees of sialylation. The liver is the major site of apo E synthesis, but macrophages and other extrahepatic cell types have also been shown to produce this apoprotein. Apo E plays a central role in the hepatic removal of remnants of triglyceride-rich lipoproteins from the circulation through an interaction with specific plasma membrane receptors. Apo E levels are greatly elevated in the VLDL remnants isolated from subjects with type III hyperlipoproteinemia. Apo E enrichment also occurs in the abnormal lipoproteins (remnants and HDL_c) isolated from the plasma of cholesterol-fed animals.

In addition to the apolipoproteins already discussed, others, such as apo A-III, apo A-IV, apo D, apo F, and Lp(a), can be detected in the circulation in small concentrations. However, little is known about these apoproteins, and additional work is required to delineate their structure, function, metabolism, and clinical importance.

DYNAMICS OF LIPID TRANSPORT BY LIPOPROTEINS

The circulating lipoproteins transport hydrophobic core lipids, mainly triglycerides and cholesterol esters, to their sites of utilization, directed by the interactions between constituent apoproteins, enzymes, and cell surface receptors. Before use by the cells, triglycerides and cholesterol esters must be hydrolyzed to liberate, respectively, fatty acids and free cholesterol. Fatty acids are taken up by adipose tissues and muscle for storage or for oxidation for energy. Unesterified sterols are used by all cells as structural components of membranes and are also used for the production of steroid hormones and bile acids.

The various circulating lipoproteins are all interrelated, and lipid transport in the plasma must be considered a complex metabolic process regulated by a variety of dietary and hormonal controls. Triglycerides are quantitatively the major lipids transported in plasma, since about 70 to 150 g of triglyceride enter and leave the plasma daily; only about 1 g of cholesterol or phospholipid traverses the plasma compartment. In addition to triglyceride transport, the plasma lipoproteins can remove cholesterol esters from tissues, provide cholesterol for membrane and steroid hormone synthesis, and transport carotenoids and fat-soluble vitamins. Increasing evidence indicates that plasma lipoproteins and apolipoproteins have other significant, although as yet unknown, functions.

Conceptually, lipoprotein metabolism can be divided into exogenous and endogenous pathways that transport lipids of dietary and hepatic origin, respectively. The largest quantities of lipoproteins are involved in the transport of dietary fat. Exogenous dietary triglycerides enter the circulation as chylomicrons; endogenous triglycerides are released as hepatic VLDL. Chylomicrons are synthesized by the intestinal mucosal cells following a triglyceride-containing meal. The fatty acids and monoglycerides derived from the intraluminal action of pancreatic lipase on exogenous long-chain glycerides are emulsified by bile salts to form micellar aggregates that are absorbed by jejunal mucosal cells and reesterified to triglycerides intracellularly. Chylomicrons are thus formed with triglycerides as their major constituent (90% to 95%) and with minor amounts of cholesterol, phospholipids, and apoproteins. These particles (800 to 5000 Å in diameter) are secreted into the intestinal lymphatics and reach the bloodstream via the thoracic duct.

Apo B-48 constitutes about one fifth of the apoprotein complement of chylomicrons; apo C constitutes most of the remaining four-fifths. Since only minor amounts of the C apoproteins are synthesized in intestinal mucosal cells, their presence in the lymph is largely due to a transfer of apo C from lipoproteins of hepatic origin. The intestinal mucosa produces VLDL and HDL both in the fasting state and during lipid absorption. In abetalipoproteinemia apo B, which is considered critical for the secretion of triglyceride-rich lipoproteins, is completely absent from the plasma. Apparently because of a failure of cells to release apo B, intracellular glycerides accumulate in the intestine and liver, and the plasma is devoid of chylomicrons, VLDL, and LDL.

LPL is fixed to the luminal surface of the endothelial cells that line the capillaries of adipose tissues, muscle, and other tissues. Activated by apo C-II bound to chylomicrons, LPL hydrolyzes the triglyceride cargo to fatty acids and monoglycerides. The fatty acids traverse the endothelial cells and enter the underlying adipocytes, muscle, or other cells, where they become reesterified to triglycerides or oxidized. As the core triglycerides become depleted, the chylomicron shrinks and dissociates from the capillary endothelium. Also during chylomicron catabolism, some surface cholesterol, phospholipids, and apoproteins are transferred to HDL_3. HDL_3 and LCAT interact in a concerted fashion to remove these surface compounds and thereby remodel the chylomicrons so that LPL can continue to split the triglyceride core. The lecithin phospholipids and free cholesterol that are transferred to HDL_3 interact with LCAT to form esterified cholesterol and lysolecithins as HDL_3 undergoes conversion to HDL_2. The net result is conversion of the chylomicron to a chylomicron remnant particle that is enriched in cholesterol esters, apo B-48, and apo E. The C apoproteins and apo A-I are transferred to HDL. The triglyceride-depleted remnants are then released back into the circulation and pass on to the liver, so entering a second removal stage.

Chylomicron remnants are taken up efficiently by the hepatocyte as a unit by a receptor-mediated process. This uptake is mediated by the binding of remnant apoproteins to specific apo E receptors or so-called chylomicron remnant receptors on the hepatocyte surface. The surface-bound remnants are then internalized and degraded within lysosomes by a process called receptor-mediated endocytosis. The net effect of this overall process is the delivery of dietary triglycerides to extrahepatic tissues and of cholesterol to the liver. The cholesterol reaching the liver can have several fates, including (1) reesterification for storage as cholesterol esters, (2) direct excretion into the bile, (3) conversion to bile acids followed by biliary excretion, (4) utilization for membrane production, and (5) repackaging into secretory lipoproteins, particularly VLDL and HDL for use by other tissues of the body. The production and removal of the circulating lipoproteins are shown schematically in Figs. 202-1 and 202-2.

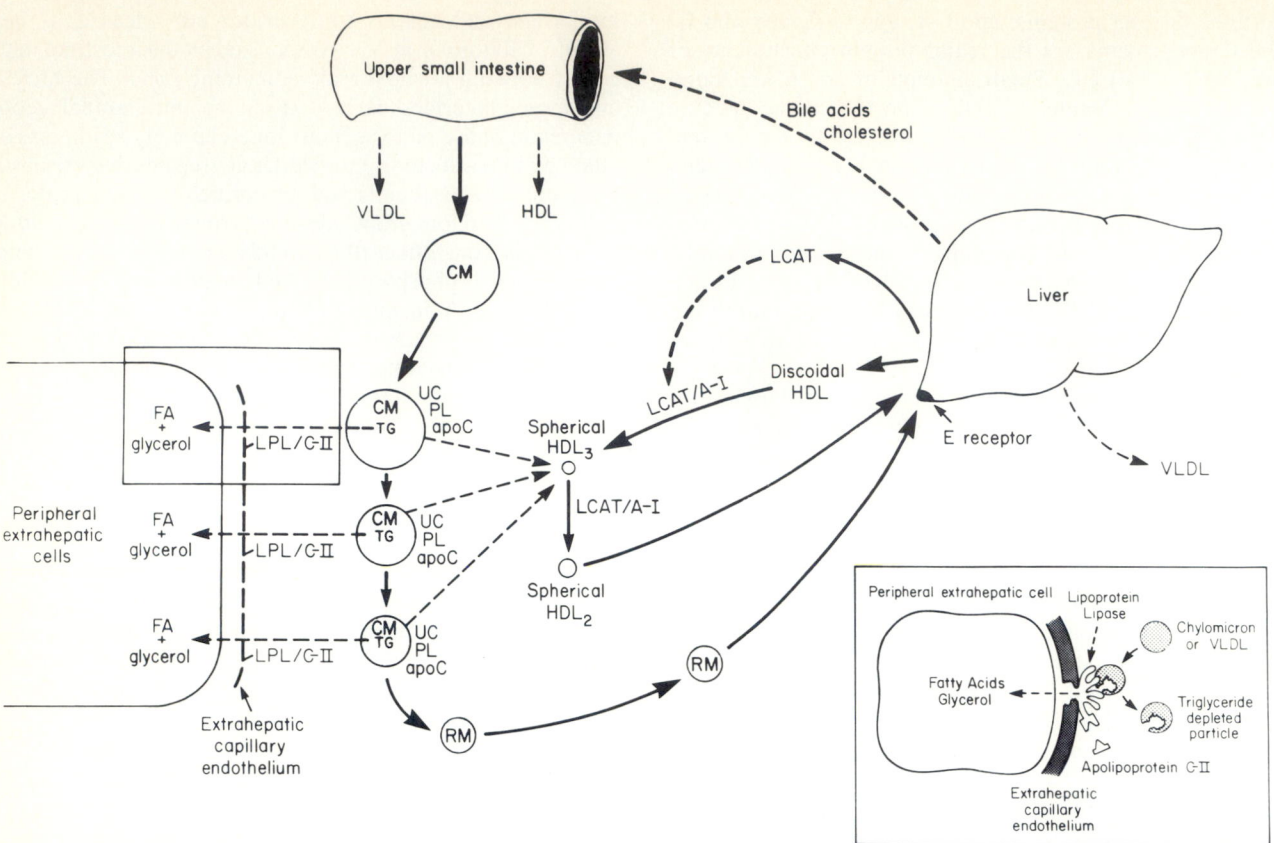

Fig. 202-1   Formation and degradation of plasma lipoproteins: exogenous pathway. After ingestion of dietary triglycerides and cholesterol, bile acids, biliary cholesterol, and pancreatic lipase enter upper intestinal lumen. Chylomicrons and, to lesser extent, VLDL and HDL, are also produced by upper intestinal mucosal cells. Chylomicrons enter bloodstream via intestinal lymphatics for transport to peripheral sites. Chylomicron triglycerides are removed in extrahepatic capillary beds, mainly of adipose tissues and muscle, after hydrolysis by LPL, activated by its apo C-II cofactor. The products of triglyceride hydrolysis are taken up by peripheral cells. During this process, lecithin phospholipids, free cholesterol, and C-apoproteins are transferred from redundant chylomicron surface to HDL₃. Lecithin phospholipids and free cholesterol interact with the enzyme LCAT activated by apo A-I to form esterified cholesterol and lysolecithins. HDL₃ undergoes conversion to HDL₂, which is removed from circulation by liver. Triglyceride-depleted remnants are removed by specific apo E receptors on hepatocyte surface membranes, internalized, and degraded. Some remnant cholesterol is excreted into biliary tract as free cholesterol and some is first oxidized to bile acids before entry into bile. Net result of exogenous pathway is delivery of exogenous triglyceride to extrahepatic sites and delivery of cholesterol to liver.

Though the triglyceride-rich lipoproteins (chylomicrons and VLDL) share similar production and removal mechanisms, a number of dissimilarities are evident. Endogenous triglyceride is generated mainly in the hepatic parenchymal cells from fatty acids that are mobilized from adipose tissue depots or synthesized de novo from carbohydrate precursors. The triglyceride cargo is packaged with apoproteins at the junctions of smooth and rough endoplasmic reticulum and secreted from intracellular Golgi vesicles into the hepatic sinusoids as VLDL. Triglyceride forms the core and major component (55% to 75% by weight) of VLDL. The surface apoproteins of VLDL consist mainly of apo B (40%) and apo C (40% to 60%). A number of factors, such as increased intake of calories and carbohydrates, excessive intake of alcohol, and elevated circulating levels of insulin, stimulate the production of VLDL. The triglyceride-laden VLDL particles secreted by the liver contain apo B-100, which differs from the apo B-48 of chylomicrons. The VLDL particles are transported to tissue capillaries, where they undergo triglyceride removal by the same apo C II–activated lipoprotein lipases that catabolize chylomicrons. Sim-

ilarly, VLDL particles are degraded via distinct and sequential extrahepatic and hepatic stages.

In the extrahepatic stage, VLDL triglycerides are hydrolyzed to fatty acids that enter extrahepatic cells (mainly in adipose tissues, muscle, and heart) for oxidation and energy production or for reesterification and energy storage. As triglycerides are progressively removed from VLDL, the surface components (phospholipids, unesterified cholesterol, and apoproteins) are transferred to HDL. Continued remodelling of the VLDL substrate facilitates continued splitting of the triglyceride core. The lecithin phospholipids and free cholesterol that are transferred to HDL interact with the LCAT enzyme after its activation by apo A-I to form esterified cholesterol and lysolecithins. HDL and LCAT, secretory products of the liver, can facilitate removal of free cholesterol from the VLDL surface and catalyze the esterification of cholesterol during its association with HDL. This newly synthesized cholesterol ester is then transferred back to the IDL particles from HDL. Intermediate density lipoprotein then undergoes a further conversion in which most of the remaining triglycerides are removed and

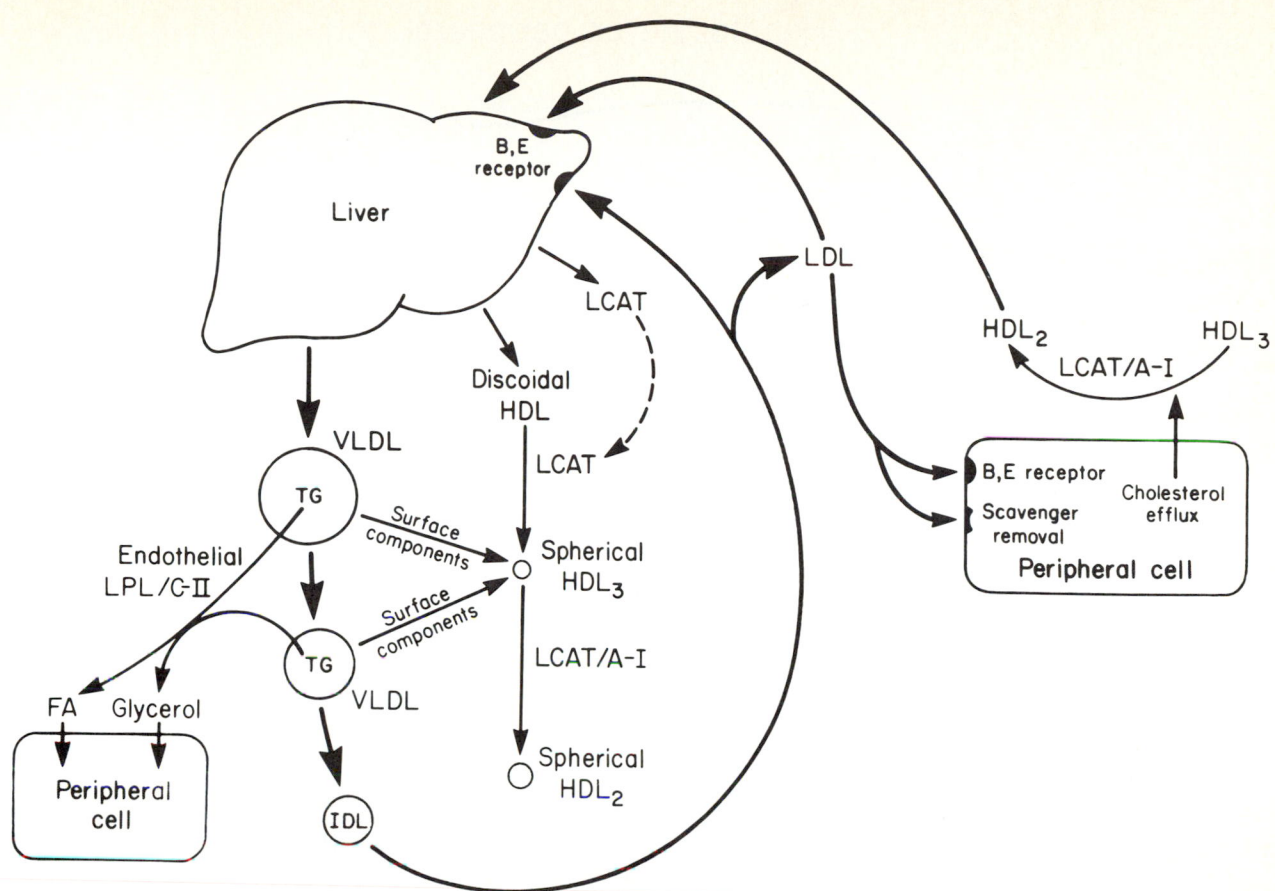

Fig. 202-2   Formation and degradation of plasma lipoproteins: endogenous pathway. VLDL and HDL are secreted into bloodstream by liver as their quantitatively major source. Extrahepatic phase of endogenous triglyceride removal from VLDL is similar to that described for chylomicrons. However, disposal of VLDL remnants or intermediate density lipoproteins (IDL) differs. A portion of IDL particles is removed by apo B, E receptors (also termed LDL receptors on hepatocyte surface). Another portion of IDL undergoes further removal of residual triglycerides and removal of all apoproteins except apo B-100 with resultant formation of LDL. In humans, about two-thirds of LDL removed from plasma occurs by LDL receptor pathway, mainly in liver but also in extrahepatic cells, while remainder is mediated by scavenger pathway that is less well understood. HDL_3 and LCAT may remove cholesterol both from surfaces of triglyceride-rich lipoproteins during hydrolysis and from cell membranes of extrahepatic tissues, thereby providing return transport system for cholesterol excretion by liver.

all apoproteins except apo B-100 are transferred to other lipoproteins. The result is the transformation of the IDL particle into the LDL particle that contains almost exclusively cholesterol ester in its core and apo B-100 over its surface.

Present evidence suggests that VLDL remnants or IDLs are removed and catabolyzed by hepatocytes after binding to the specific saturable apo B,E receptors that also bind LDL. However, at least a portion of the remnant VLDL reenters the circulation as IDL, perhaps through the action of a triglyceride lipase on the hepatocyte cell surface. In humans a relatively high fraction of IDL escapes hepatic removal and is rapidly converted to LDL. Therefore humans have relatively high circulating levels of LDL. The conversion of IDL to LDL probably occurs partially in the blood stream. The relative extent of pathways for complete hepatic degradation of the VLDL remnant versus conversion of the remnant to LDL may be an important determinant of circulating LDL levels in different animal species.

LDL arises as a catabolic end product of VLDL degradation. The apo B-100 of LDL mediates its interaction with the LDL receptor present on most nucleated cells. LDL appears to be

removed from the plasma by both hepatic and extrahepatic tissues. One function of LDL is to supply cholesterol to a variety of extrahepatic parenchymal cells, such as adrenal cortical cells, lymphocytes, muscle cells, and renal cells. After combining with the receptor, the LDL is internalized and incorporated into a lysosome leading to the hydrolysis of LDL and the liberation of free cholesterol into the cytoplasm (Fig. 202-3). Cellular free cholesterol levels are tightly regulated since the newly liberated free cholesterol inhibits the rate-limiting enzyme for its synthesis, namely hydroxymethyl glutaryl CoA reductase (HMG CoA reductase). Cellular free cholesterol also suppresses the synthesis of LDL receptors, thereby restricting further LDL uptake. In this way, intracellular cholesterol balance is maintained. About two thirds of human LDL is catabolized by this mechanism, three fourths of which occurs in the liver. The remaining one third of LDL catabolism occurs by the so-called receptor-independent or scavenger mechanisms. Cholesterol uptake mediated by this process is believed to be poorly regulated and becomes pathologically significant as LDL levels rise above concentrations that saturate the LDL receptor. Defects in the synthesis, intracellular transit, or func-

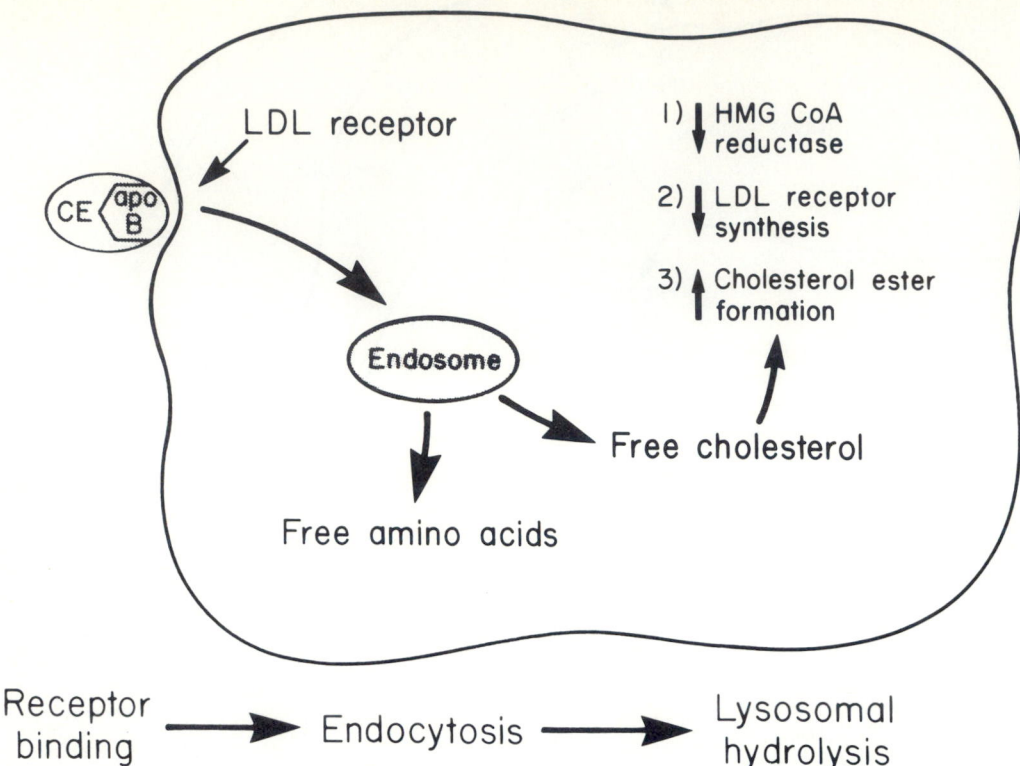

Hepatocyte or peripheral cell

Fig. 202-3   Removal of circulating LDL by LDL receptor-mediated pathway. Apo B-100 of LDL is bound to specific, saturable binding sites on surface of hepatocytes or extrahepatic cells. Receptor bound LDL is then internalized by receptor-mediated endocytosis and is digested in endosomes by lysosomal enzymes. Lysosomal acid lipases convert cholesterol esters to free cholesterol, which is used for membrane synthesis and as a precursor for other cell products. Intracellular free cholesterol, particulary in hepatocyte, regulates its own production by inhibition of enzyme HMG CoA reductase, inhibition of synthesis of LDL receptors, and stimulation of activity of cholesterol esterifying enzymes.

tion of the LDL receptor are considered to account for the striking LDL elevations and premature atherosclerosis found in patients with heritable monogenic forms of hypercholesterolemia. In addition, ingestion of a diet rich in saturated fat and cholesterol leads to accumulation of cholesterol in the liver, suppression of LDL receptor production, and elevations of LDL levels. Recent interest has surged about oxidative or other modifications of the LDL molecule that may occur in the body under certain environmental and pathologic conditions and enhance its atherogenic potential. Evidence exists that some LDL alterations may stimulate the removal of circulating LDL by scavenger cells such as macrophages and may thereby increase the hazard of a given LDL level.

Nascent HDL appears to arise from three sources: (1) direct secretion by the liver into the plasma; (2) secretion by the intestinal mucosal cells into the lymph; and (3) formation from the surface components of triglyceride-rich lipoproteins. Nascent HDL can also be formed by the association of apo A-I and phospholipids released during chylomicron metabolism. Newly secreted HDL of hepatic origin is discoidal and has a somewhat different composition than the spherical HDL found in plasma. The intestine also releases a discoidal HDL, rich in apoproteins and lecithin but poor in cholesterol. During the conversion of triglyceride-rich lipoproteins to remnants, surface components are transferred to nascent HDL, and the free cholesterol of nascent HDL is esterified by LCAT. Precursor discoidal HDL is progressively transformed into spherical HDL_3 and then to HDL_2. The cholesterol esters formed during this process can undergo transfer to IDL and then to LDL. The lysolecithin formed by the LCAT reaction is removed by binding to plasma albumin. Patients lacking LCAT have few or no cholesterol esters, and their HDL remains discoidal. HDL and LCAT may also mediate the removal of cholesterol from the cell membranes of extrahepatic tissues, thereby providing a return transport system for subsequent cholesterol excretion by the liver. HDL mediates the reverse pathway of cholesterol transport by accepting free cholesterol from cells of peripheral tissue. After esterification of the sterol by the action of LCAT, HDL directly delivers cholesterol to the liver where it can be excreted from the body. Alternatively the newly esterified cholesterol can be transferred to VLDL, IDL, or LDL before its disposal by the liver. Cholesterol ester transfer proteins are probably involved in this process.

Very little is known about the fate of circulating HDL in humans. The accumulation of cholesterol esters in the tissues of patients with HDL deficiency (Tangier disease) suggests that HDL may be required for the transport of cholesterol from peripheral tissues to removal and excretory sites in the liver. Net transfer of free cholesterol from membranes of cultivated cells has been shown to occur when the culture medium contains LCAT. HDL can also reduce the binding and uptake of LDL by cultured aortic smooth muscle cells. This finding has been postulated to explain in part the inverse relation found between plasma HDL levels and the incidence of CHD. HDL can bind to human fibroblasts in culture, but not to high-affinity binding sites. Binding is followed by uptake and degradation at rates consistent with a process of adsorptive endocytosis. Evidence suggests that the liver plays an important role in HDL removal, consistent with its function as the major site of cholesterol excretion.

Clearly the plasma lipoproteins undergo constant change because of metabolic interactions and exchanges among themselves and with the cells of the organism as they circulate. Because of lipid and apoprotein transfers, all the plasma lipoproteins are interrelated in a state of dynamic equilibrium. Both enzymatic and nonenzymatic interactions occur among the lipoprotein components, and the plasma half-lives of the apoprotein constituents of a given lipoprotein class are heterogeneous. Although increasing knowledge of the molecular events involved in lipid transport leads to improved methods for diagnosis and therapy, measurement of fasting lipid and sometimes lipoprotein levels remains the conventional approach to evaluation of the hyperlipidemias. Apolipoprotein measurements and even receptor binding and enzymatic assays of various kinds will become more feasible for diagnosis and management of patients, thereby facilitating more specifically tailored therapies.

PATHOPHYSIOLOGY OF LIPID TRANSPORT

Because of their molecular complexity and the multiplicity of steps in production and catabolism, the regulation of plasma lipoprotein levels is more complicated than that of most other plasma proteins. Rates of lipoprotein synthesis are altered by factors that influence the availability of lipids, the formation of the apoproteins, coupling of lipids to apoproteins, or secretion of the nascent lipoproteins. In addition, degradation of the plasma lipoproteins involves removal of the various apolipoproteins from the circulation by diverse tissues and rapid intermolecular exchanges among lipoprotein constituents. These intermolecular exchanges can be enzymatic or nonenzymatic in origin and may involve the mediation of lipid transfer proteins.

Hyperlipoproteinemia may result from an inherited genetic disorder of lipoprotein metabolism, other underlying diseases, or environmental factors. Fasting lipid determinations and even lipoprotein levels are of limited value in defining lipid transport abnormalities because they provide only static measurements in a dynamic system. Such measurements are not likely to detect the subtle but significant abnormalities in lipoprotein composition or homeostasis that are present in various disease states. Nonetheless, fasting lipid and lipoprotein levels have been determined in a sufficient number of subjects to define acceptable ranges for various populations.

The major pathophysiologic abnormalities that cause the various forms of hyperlipoproteinemia include overproduction of triglyceride-rich lipoproteins and defective or delayed clearance of triglyceride-rich lipoproteins, triglyceride-rich lipoprotein remnants, or LDL.

Overproduction of triglyceride-rich lipoproteins

Both in normal individuals and in those with hypertriglyceridemia, there is a postprandial rise in plasma triglyceride levels representing the transport of dietary fat as chylomicrons. These particles that transport exogenous fat normally disappear very rapidly from the circulation, with half-lives of less than 1 hour. In the postabsorptive state, fatty acids derived from depot fat or formed by hepatic lipogenesis from carbohydrate are esterified with glycerol to form triglycerides that are destined for transport as VLDL. The fate of fatty acids within the hepatocyte appears to be under hormonal control. Glucagon excess and insulin deficiency direct the partition of fatty acids from esterification to triglycerides toward mitochondrial oxidation.

Insulin appears to have a direct positive effect on hepatic triglyceride and VLDL production; considerable positive correlation in human subjects exists between circulating insulin levels, endogenous triglyceride production rates, and plasma triglyceride concentrations. In many conditions insulin resistance and consequent hyperinsulinemia are associated with VLDL overproduction. Obesity is the prime example. Other such conditions include pregnancy, therapy with estrogens or glucocorticoids, chronic renal failure with significant azotemia, and acromegaly. Implicit in this association is the hypothesis that, in the latter conditions, the liver remains sensitive to the lipogenic effects of insulin, whereas the extrahepatic tissues, particularly skeletal muscle and adipose tissues, are resistant to insulin actions. Alternatively, the hypertriglyceridemia itself may lead to peripheral insulin resistance and hyperinsulinemia.

Nephrosis and excessive intake of alcohol are other states that lead to increased endogenous VLDL production. In the nephrotic syndrome, compensatory hepatic hyperplasia in response to albumin loss can result in stimulation of VLDL generation. Excessive alcohol intake can enhance hepatic esterification, impair the hepatic oxidation of fatty acids, and increase VLDL secretion by the liver. Enhanced production of VLDL can also be a feature of familial hypertriglyceridemia—a monogenic, heritable disorder. The hypertriglyceridemia found in these patients can be markedly exacerbated by a number of factors that ordinarily have milder hyperlipidemic effects, such as obesity, uncontrolled diabetes, uremia, or intake of corticosteroids, estrogens, or alcohol. The combination of an acquired form of VLDL hypersecretion with a familial form often leads to massive hypertriglyceridemia usually complicated by hyperchylomicronemia by overloading the readily saturable removal mechanisms for triglyceride-rich lipoproteins. Affected individuals are then at risk for developing the so-called chylomicronemia syndrome, characterized by abdominal pain and acute pancreatitis.

Delayed clearance of triglyceride-rich lipoproteins

The primary destinations of the triglyceride that enters the plasma in chylomicrons and VLDL are the adipose tissues and skeletal muscles. Present in the vascular endothelium lining these tissues and in lung, heart, mammary, and other tissues is the enzyme LPL. LPL activity in adipose tissues is insulin-dependent. After ingestion of a fatty meal and the consequent increase in insulin secretion, the triglyceride cargo of chylomicrons and VLDL is hydrolyzed to fatty acids, which enter the adipocytes and become reesterified to triglyceride for energy storage. In the fasting state, diminished levels of plasma insulin activate a different enzyme the hormone-sensitive lipase of adipocytes to hydrolyze their stored triglycerides to fatty acids for energy use by most tissues of the body. Activation of the sympathetic nervous system or release of certain hormones (such as catecholamines, glucagon, growth hormone, and thyroid hormones) promote fatty acid mobilization by either direct or permissive stimulation of hormone-sensitive lipase activity.

In a variety of conditions, deficiencies in LPL activity can lead to accumulation of chylomicrons, VLDL, or both in the bloodstream. The estimated half-life of VLDL triglycerides in humans usually ranges from 2 to 4 hours. Since insulin stimulates LPL production or activity, insulin deficiency in uncontrolled diabetes mellitus can interfere with triglyceride clearance from plasma, resulting in elevated levels of chylomicrons, VLDL, or both. Replenishment with insulin corrects the LPL abnormality and usually results in a lowering of plasma triglycerides. Since LPL activity is also reduced in hypothyroid patients, plasma triglyceride levels rise despite their low circulating levels of free fatty acid (FFA). Treatment with thyroid hormone corrects the abnormality in lipoprotein clearance in this instance. In patients with chronic renal failure and uremia, the presence of one or more toxic metabolites can interfere with LPL activity and provide an additional mechanism for the hypertriglyceridemia often observed in this condition. A primary defect in LPL activity can result from an inherited absence of LPL in the adipose tissues of affected subjects. This rare genetic abnormality, inherited as an autosomal recessive condition, deserves emphasis, since patients with this disorder are afflicted with very high plasma triglyceride levels, hyperchylomicronemia, and episodic attacks of acute pancreatitis. More recently described genetic defects in LPL activity stem from abnormalities in the activation of LPL by apo C-II. A group of molecular defects in the production of apo C-II that result in its dysfunction, deficiency, or absence impairs the clearance of chylomicrons and VLDL.

Defective catabolism of triglyceride-rich lipoprotein remnants

Following partial extrahepatic removal of triglycerides, phospholipids, and C apoproteins from chylomicrons and large VLDL, partially degraded lipoprotein remnants are formed. The triglyceride-depleted remnant lipoproteins are then released back into the circulation, thus entering the second stage of lipid transport. The chylomicron remnants are taken up by the liver by means of cell surface receptors specific for the apo E present on these remnants. The VLDL remnant or IDL can also be taken up by the liver, but by a receptor known as the LDL or apo B,E receptor, which binds both apo B and apo E. Unlike the chylomicron remnant E receptor, the B,E receptor can be down-regulated so that hepatic IDL uptake may be inhibited. When the latter occurs, IDL is further catabolized to yield LDL, the end product of VLDL metabolism. When triglyceride-rich lipoprotein remnants accumulate in plasma ("remnant removal disease," "broad β disease," or type III hyperlipoproteinemia), they distribute in the density range less than 1.019, with the flotation characteristics of VLDL and LDL, and migrate on electrophoresis between the β and pre-β regions, forming a "broad β band." Patients with inherited type III hyperlipoproteinemia have an absence or deficiency of apo E-3 despite an enrichment in total apo E. Since about 1% of the population has apo E-3 deficiency and yet the great majority have unremarkable lipid levels, expression of the hyperlipidemia found in this condition seems to require an additional defect. Although hyperlipidemia is usually not expressed until early adulthood, a pediatric form of the disease has recently been discovered. Remnant accumulation in broad β disease apparently results from a defect in the later stages of chylomicron and VLDL catabolism. These remnants are very atherogenic and become readily deposited within the walls of muscular arteries throughout the body. Tissue culture studies have demonstrated brisk uptake of remnants by monolayers of fibroblasts or arterial smooth muscle cells.

Type III hyperlipoproteinemia and remnant accumulation can also be expressed when an individual homozygous for the E_2 allele develops obesity, hypothyroidism, systemic lupus erythematosus, diabetes mellitus, or liver disease. Treatment in

such forms of the condition first should be directed toward management of the exacerbating disorder.

Defective catabolism of LDL

The fate of LDL has been examined in more detail than that of the other lipoproteins. LDL, as it normally arises from the catabolism of VLDL remnants, appears to conserve the apo B entirely, even as the other apoproteins originally associated with circulating VLDL have been removed. With its rich complement of cholesterol and cholesterol esters, LDL appears to provide a circulating sterol reservoir for use in membrane biosynthesis and steroid hormone production by extrahepatic tissues. In normal human subjects, the biological half-life of LDL protein ranges from about 2.2 to 3.6 days, and the rate of LDL catabolism is an important determinant of plasma LDL levels.

Underlying the metabolic abnormalities that occur in subjects having familial hypercholesterolemia (FH) with elevated LDL levels is the defective removal of LDL from the circulation, with a consequent prolongation of the LDL half-life. Study of the mutations in the LDL receptor gene in FH patients has helped to delineate the crucial steps of receptor-mediated endocytosis. Fibroblasts from different patients with the clinical phenotype of homozygous FH show defects in the LDL receptor, but not all the defects are the same. Skin fibroblasts grown in culture from patients with autosomal dominant forms of this disorder may express one of at least 15 different mutations resulting in the absence (homozygotes), deficiency (heterozygotes), or abnormal function of receptor binding sites for LDL apo B. The LDL receptor does not have absolute specificity for apo B, since the same receptor can "recognize" and bind both IDL and HDL_c, an apo E–enriched lipoprotein devoid of apo B that is isolated from the plasma of hypercholesterolemic animals. Four major classes of mutations in the LDL receptor have been identified in FH patients: Class 1 mutations, in which no receptors are synthesized; Class 2 mutations, in which receptors are synthesized, but transported slowly from the endoplasmic reticulum to the Golgi apparatus; Class 3 mutations, in which receptors reach the cell surface, but fail to bind LDL normally; and Class 4 mutations, in which receptors fail to cluster in coated pits. Defective removal of circulating LDL by extrahepatic receptors accounts for the elevations of LDL observed in many patients with FH who have deficient or defective LDL receptors. Elevated LDL levels can also be associated with familial combined hyperlipidemia, a genetic form of hyperlipoproteinemia with apparently normal LDL receptors. In this condition, the LDL elevations may result from overproduction from VLDL resulting from increased hepatic production rates of apo B.

Alterations in circulating LDL can stem from dietary or drug interventions or can reflect other underlying conditions. Elevated LDL levels can result from diets high in cholesterol and saturated fat. Conversely, LDL levels can be lowered by institution of a diet low in cholesterol and saturated fat, but enriched with monosaturated and polyunsaturated fats. Certain plasma lipid–lowering agents, such as bile acid-binding resins, HMG CoA reductase inhibitors, and D-thyroxine, appear to lower circulating LDL levels by augmenting the rate of LDL catabolism.

Patients with hypothyroidism have increased LDL levels resulting from defective LDL removal, a defect that is corrected by the administration of thyroid hormone. Hypothyroidism can also markedly exaggerate the lipid and lipoprotein abnormalities of type III hyperlipoproteinemia. In the nephrotic syndrome, elevated LDL levels usually are associated with normal fractional catabolic rates of LDL and can be caused by hepatic

Table 202-2 Characteristics of major lipoprotein phenotypes

Lipoprotein phenotype	Lipid classes elevated	Lipoprotein classes elevated	Appearance of plasma or serum
I	Triglycerides and cholesterol (T/C > 5.0)	Chylomicrons	Creamy
IIA	Cholesterol	LDL	Clear
IIB	Cholesterol and triglycerides	LDL and VLDL	Turbid
III	Cholesterol and triglycerides (similar rises in both)	IDL and chylomicron remnants	Turbid
IV	Triglycerides	VLDL	Turbid
V	Triglycerides and cholesterol (T/C > 5.0)	Chylomicrons and VLDL	Creamy

overproduction of VLDL, the precursor of LDL. LDL elevations are frequently observed in patients with acute intermittent porphyria, anorexia nervosa, ateliotic dwarfism, and various forms of dysproteinemia, but the mechanisms for such elevations remain unclear.

Liver disease and lipoprotein metabolism

Because of the central role of the liver in lipoprotein biosynthesis and its less well-defined role in lipoprotein metabolism, changes in lipoprotein levels and composition are not unusual in various human liver diseases. Cholesterol and phospholipids are excreted in bile by the hepatic parenchymal cells. Cholesterol is also converted into bile acids, a large proportion of which undergoes enterohepatic recirculation following biliary secretion. Cholesterol for biliary disposal can be derived from the surface of triglyceride-rich lipoproteins, from lipoprotein remnants during their processing by the liver to LDL, or from LDL itself.

Obstruction of bile flow can result in an interaction between refluxed bile acid and plasma constituents, with formation of an abnormal lipoprotein termed "lipoprotein X" that is composed mainly of phospholipids, free cholesterol, albumin, and C apoproteins. In addition, various combinations of HDL and LCAT deficiency can be observed in hepatocellular diseases, presumably consequent to their decreased or defective production by the liver. The resultant declines in HDL production and abnormalities in HDL composition can lead to diminished plasma levels of cholesterol esters and to increased plasma levels of free cholesterol and phospholipids. Insufficient apo A-I is transferred to HDL in the course of reaction with LCAT, leading to abnormal electrophoretic mobility. Since HDL and LCAT are also involved in the catabolism of chylomicrons and VLDL, these triglyceride-rich lipoproteins cannot be degraded normally, and remnant lipoproteins that cannot undergo adequate hepatic clearance accumulate in the plasma. Hypertriglyceridemia results, since the triglyceride core of these particles cannot be replaced by cholesterol esters and their polar surface components cannot be depleted.

CLASSIFICATION OF HYPERLIPOPROTEINEMIA

Based on separation of plasma lipoproteins by electrophoretic methods, the hyperlipoproteinemias have been classified phenotypically into six types, each of which represents a heterogeneous group of primary and secondary abnormalities (Table 202-2). Classification by typing is solely morphologic and does not elucidate the genetic or pathophysiologic mechanisms responsible for the disorder. A single disorder may lead to different lipoprotein patterns, and a single pattern may result from a variety of mechanisms. Each type results, either singly or in combination, from an increased plasma concentration of chylomicrons, VLDL (pre-β lipoproteins), IDL (VLDL remnants), or LDL (β lipoproteins) in postabsorptive plasma (that

is, 12 to 14 hours after the last meal). The types are numbered in sequential fashion, depending on which lipoprotein class is elevated in concentration, as the electrophoretic pattern, stained with a lipid stain, is read from left to right. In type I, the presence of chylomicrons is indicated by a band at the origin. The next band on the electrophoretic medium is the β band, and an increase in its intensity leads to a type II pattern, indicating an elevated level of LDL. Type II has been further subdivided into two patterns: type IIA, in which LDL alone is elevated, and type IIB, in which both LDL and VLDL are elevated. In type III hyperlipoproteinemia a broad β band diffusely extends from the β to the pre-β region of the electrophoretic strip, indicating the presence of VLDL remnants in the plasma. An increased intensity of the pre-β band denotes the presence of increased circulating levels of VLDL and a type IV pattern. The type V pattern, in which there is stainable lipoprotein at the origin and an increased pre-β band, indicates the presence of chylomicrons and an excess of pre-β lipoproteins.

Genetic hyperlipoproteinemias resulting from single-gene mutations

The familial hyperlipoproteinemias, each apparently inherited by a single-gene mechanism, consist of six disorders.

FAMILIAL LPL DEFICIENCY. Familial LPL deficiency is an autosomal recessive condition characterized by an inability to dispose of exogenous triglyceride, resulting in massive chylomicronemia and a type I lipoprotein pattern. This rare disorder is due to the absence or marked reduction in the activity of the enzyme lipoprotein lipase. The blood appears pale and creamy and is said to be lipemic. There is a major increase in serum triglyceride levels, usually in excess of 2000 mg/dl, and the circulating triglyceride/cholesterol ratio exceeds 5:1. LPL activity in the adipose tissues of affected subjects appears to be deficient or absent, and LPL cannot be released into the plasma by injection of heparin. The manifestations are evident during childhood and include bouts of abdominal colic from acute pancreatitis, eruptive xanthomas, and hepatosplenomegaly. Eruptive xanthomas are caused by deposition of large quantities of triglycerides in cutaneous histiocytes. They appear as crops of yellowish papules, often surrounded by an erythematous base, that characteristically occur on extensor surfaces of the body when triglyceride levels are greatly elevated. Improvement occurs with limitation of dietary fat. The signs and symptoms of this disorder recede when the patient is placed on a diet containing less than 20 g of fat per day.

FAMILIAL APOPROTEIN C-II DEFICIENCY. This rare autosomal recessive disorder results from the absence of the apo C-II cofactor for LPL. Deficiency or absence of apo C-II prevents activation of LPL and produces a somewhat similar syndrome to that of LPL deficiency. Hypertriglyceridemia caused by the combined accumulation of chylomicrons and VLDL in the circulation leads to recurrent bouts of acute pancreatitis. Heterozygotes, who exhibit partial reduction of circulating apo C-II levels, may have slightly elevated triglyceride levels but do not experience pancreatitis. Treatment involves adherence to a diet restricted in fat and caloric content.

FAMILIAL HYPERCHOLESTEROLEMIA. Familial hypercholesterolemia is an autosomal dominant disorder associated with elevated plasma LDL levels and a type II lipoprotein pattern. One gene for the LDL receptor is inherited from each parent, and FH heterozygotes have about half the LDL receptor activity as normal subjects and about double the circulating levels of LDL-cholesterol. One in 500 people in the United States have heterozygous FH, and their plasma total cholesterol levels generally exceed 300 mg/dl. Affected individuals show corneal arcus, tendinous xanthomas, premature CHD, a strong family history of premature CHD, and hypercholesterolemia. Affected males usually develop CHD in their third, fourth, or fifth decades, whereas affected females often develop manifestations of CHD somewhat later in life. About 5% of patients who experience myocardial infarction before age 60 have heterozygous FH. FH homozygotes, having a double dose of the mutant gene, have plasma total cholesterol levels ranging from 600 to 1000 mg/dl and are afflicted with CHD manifestations more seriously and at earlier ages than heterozygotes. They usually show cutaneous, planar, and tuberous xanthomas in addition to tendinous xanthomas. Individuals homozygous for FH develop strikingly premature CHD that begins in childhood and usually succumb to a fatal coronary event before age 20. The basic molecular defects underlying the LDL elevations consist of deficiencies or defects in cell surface receptors involved in the catabolism of LDL.

FAMILIAL REMNANT REMOVAL DISEASE. This condition, also termed "familial dysbetalipoproteinemia," is a disorder characterized by the presence of lipoproteins of abnormal composition in the plasma. The most typical of these remnant-like particles is β-VLDL, which has a higher cholesterol/triglyceride ratio and a different apoprotein content than the normal α-VLDL. This lipoprotein is visualized on the electrophoretic strip as the broad β band or type III pattern. The mutation responsible for this disease involves the gene that encodes the structure of apo E, a normal component of chylomicron and VLDL remnants. Apo E binds with high affinity to both the apo E and the apo B,E receptors. The gene for apo E is polymorphic, with three common alleles at a single gene locus, designated E_2, E_3, and E_4. The normal apo E isoform is apo E-3. Patients having familial dysbetalipoproteinemia, or "type III hyperlipoproteinemia," are typically homozygous for the E_2 allele (genotype E_2/E_2) and therefore have apo E-2 in their triglyceride-rich lipoproteins. Because apo E-2 binds poorly to the apo E or to the apo B,E receptor, delayed clearance and the accumulation of triglyceride-rich lipoprotein remnants in plasma occur. Manifestations of this disease include premature coronary and peripheral arteriosclerosis and characteristic palmar xanthomas, usually detected in adulthood. Cholesterol and triglyceride levels are elevated to roughly the same degree. Though transmitted by a single-gene mechanism, its expression appears to require the presence of contributory environmental factors, other genetic factors, or both.

FAMILIAL HYPERTRIGLYCERIDEMIA. Familial hypertriglyceridemia is a common autosomal dominant lipoprotein disorder that results in elevated plasma VLDL levels and a type IV lipoprotein pattern. The fasting plasma triglyceride levels tend to be moderately elevated in the range of about 250 to 600 mg/dl. Affected individuals are usually detected in early adulthood and usually exhibit associated obesity, glucose in-

tolerance, hyperuricemia, and a predisposition to CHD. Hepatosplenomegaly and eruptive xanthomas may be found but only in florid cases of the disorder. Circulating triglyceride levels are always increased, whereas plasma cholesterol levels may be unremarkable or mildly raised. Patients with familial hypertriglyceridemia can undergo a change from a type IV to a type V lipoprotein pattern when their lipoprotein removal mechanisms are challenged by other factors such as estrogen or corticosteroid administration, by excessive alcohol or carbohydrate intake, or by insulin or thyroid hormone deficiency. During such exacerbations, patients develop mixed hyperlipidemia with elevations of both chylomicrons and VLDL, which can lead to formation of eruptive xanthomas and acute pancreatitis. The basic biochemical defect in this disorder remains undefined.

In some families, patients can exhibit severe mixed hyperlipidemia, even in the absence of apparent exacerbating factors. These patients are considered to have familial type V hyperlipoproteinemia. However, other members of the same families may exhibit only the milder form of the disease, with elevations of VLDL and moderate hypertriglyceridemia with a type IV lipoprotein pattern.

FAMILIAL COMBINED HYPERLIPIDEMIA. Familial combined hyperlipidemia (FCHL) is a very common familial lipoprotein disorder and appears to display autosomal dominant inheritance. Affected subjects have elevated plasma levels of VLDL, LDL, or both and can show type IIA, IIB, or IV lipoprotein patterns accompanied by elevated plasma levels of cholesterol, triglycerides, or both. Individuals with FCHL are predisposed to the premature development of CHD. At least 15% of patients below 60 years of age with clinically evident CHD are estimated to have FCHL. An abnormality that appears to be characteristic of FCHL is an increase in the apo B concentration to plasma. Although the basic biochemical defect in this condition is unknown, a consensus exists that patients with FCHL share a common underlying defect characterized by an overproduction of apo B–containing lipoproteins. This overproduction can be manifested as increased plasma levels of VLDL, IDL, LDL, apo B, or occasionally chylomicrons. The frequency of obesity, glucose intolerance, and hyperuricemia is increased, particularly in affected individuals who also have plasma triglyceride elevations. The VLDL fraction of plasma appears to contain an increased number of relatively small particles. The LDL fraction is also heterogeneous and polydisperse and generally has a predominant number of unusually dense, lipid-poor apo B-containing particles. The HDL fraction is variably affected, with some FCHL patients displaying a reduced HDL_2 subfraction of HDL. The most characteristic abnormality found in whole plasma of patients with FCHL is an increased concentration of apo B, accompanied by a decrease in the LDL cholesterol/apo B ratio (usually less than 1.25:1). The hyperlipidemia and high apo B levels in patients with FCHL often do not become manifest before adulthood.

Although patients with FCHL usually have a strong family history of premature CHD, genetic heterogeneity probably exists in various families with FCHL. Corneal arcus is commonly present, but xanthomas are uncommon in this condition. The hyperlipidemia of FCHL is worsened by concomitant illnesses such as diabetes mellitus, hypothyroidism, and alcoholism. This disorder should be suspected in individuals whose hyperlipoproteinemia is mild and variable. No consensus exists on the optimal therapeutic approach to patients with this clinical problem. But most experts recommend directing therapy at the plasma lipoprotein(s) that is elevated at the time of examination with a combination of dietary and drug therapy. More specific therapies directed at lipoprotein metabolic defects responsible for the elevations observed in FCHL are likely to become available in the near future.

PRIMARY HYPERLIPOPROTEINEMIAS OF POLYGENIC OR UNKNOWN ORIGIN
Polygenic hypercholesterolemia

The great majority of hypercholesterolemic individuals in the general population do not have a form of hyperlipoproteinemia reflective of a single mutant gene because most of the factors that place such individuals in the upper part of the bell-shaped curve for cholesterol levels are undefined. However, the hypercholesterolemia is thought to stem from a complex but subtle interplay of many genetic and environmental factors. Genetic polymorphisms are very likely to exist among proteins that govern or regulate a number of the determinants of the plasma total and LDL-cholesterol levels among individuals and populations. These polymorphisms encompass the entire range of regulatory steps and metabolic control processes concerned with cholesterol and LDL metabolism. Some of these patients have been found to have reduced fractional clearance rates for LDL resulting from reduced binding of LDL to LDL receptors, but cellular mechanisms for these and other kinds of patients with moderate elevations of plasma cholesterol remain undefined. Superimposition of various environmental conditions on these undefined, genetically-determined, metabolic alterations commonly results in plasma cholesterol elevations. Patients with polygenic hypercholesterolemia have a spectrum of disorders of lipoprotein metabolism with a variable contribution of genetic, dietary, and other environmental factors and are the most commonly observed patients with hypercholesterolemia encountered in clinical practice. These patients are generally distinguished from those with monogenic forms of hypercholesterolemia by the absence of tendinous or tuberous xanthomas and by a low incidence of hyperlipidemia in their first-degree relatives.

Hyperapobetalipoproteinemia

Hyperapobetalipoproteinemia, which occurs in patients predisposed to premature CHD, is characterized by elevated plasma levels of apo B with acceptable levels of plasma cholesterol. The relationship between hyperapobetalipoproteinemia and FCHL is unclear; they may represent one disorder or two similar disorders sharing common underlying defects. Some investigators have recommended consideration of hyperapobetalipoproteinemia as a phenotypic disorder, with patients having the familial form identified as having FCHL. Hyperapobetalipoproteinemia patients that have elevated levels of apo B and unremarkable levels of cholesterol and triglycerides can also be considered a subset of FCHL patients. Most patients with hyperapobetalipoproteinemia have overproduction of LDL apo B, but their fractional catabolic rates (FCR) are not sufficiently increased to reduce plasma LDL apo B levels. The cellular mechanisms that increase the concentrations of LDL apo B are unclear.

Sporadic hypertriglyceridemia

Another form of hypertriglyceridemia is sporadic hypertriglyceridemia, in which elevated levels of VLDL and chylomicrons occur in a heterogeneous group of individuals on a nonfamilial basis. As with patients with familial hypertriglyceridemia, individuals affected by sporadic hypertriglyceridemia display marked exacerbation of their lipid disorder complicated by the chylomicronemia syndrome when other concomitant factors are present. Such factors or conditions, which ordinarily have only a mild hyperlipidemic effect, include diabetes mellitus, chronic renal disease, excessive weight increases, or exposure to glucocorticoids, alcohol, or estrogens. Except for the absence of hyperlipidemia in first-degree relatives, these patients are clinically indistinguishable from patients with familial hypertriglyceridemia.

Familial hyperalphalipoproteinemia

A number of families in which affected individuals showed increased levels of plasma HDL and unremarkable levels of the other circulating lipoproteins on a genetic basis have been described. The modes of inheritance described have been autosomal dominant and include polygenic forms of genetic transmission. The mechanism(s) for the elevations of HDL in these individuals is unclear. However, impaired transfer of cholesterol esters from HDL to LDL has been demonstrated in one family. Familial hyperalphalipoproteinemia probably encompasses a heterogeneous group of conditions. However, the elevations in plasma HDL cholesterol levels found in these families may potentially diminish their cardiovascular risk.

EVALUATION AND MANAGEMENT OF PATIENTS

Over the past 10 years, the field of lipoprotein pathophysiology has progressed greatly. In the near future, therapy of these disorders will probably be more specifically-tailored and directed toward correction or amelioration of the underlying abnormal mechanism. In most cases the latter is due to absence or synthesis of a defective protein that impairs normal processes involved in plasma lipoprotein metabolism to a varying degree. Identification of the genetically-determined metabolic defect and the institution of therapy that includes an appropriate dietary, a pharmacologic agent, or other treatment that targets the specific metabolic dysfunction should optimize patient management and lead to improved clinical results. The use of genetic probes to identify restriction fragment length polymorphisms (RFLPs) in the DNA of individual patients should help to select patients for appropriate therapy. Advances in DNA probe technology have resulted in the development of experimental prognostic tests aimed at approximating an individual's genetic proneness to atherosclerosis. Genetic markers for predicting both high and low risk are currently undergoing clinical testing. Although current treatments remain largely empirical and are aimed at lowering elevated levels of specific lipoprotein classes, the decision-making process is similar to that used in the management of patients with other disorders. The decision to treat an individual with a disturbance of lipid transport depends on the ability of the practitioner to assess its pathophysiologic significance, the availability of an effective regimen to correct or ameliorate the metabolic disturbance, and the feasibility of implementing the treatment plan without causing adverse effects or reducing the quality of life. First, an accurate diagnosis of the condition must be made, with all factors contributing to the clinical presentation identified by careful assessment of the patient's history, physical examination, and laboratory test results. Then, the practitioner must decide on the therapeutic approach and lipid level goals to be achieved. If the decision is made to treat, then the regimen that affords the patient the most favorable risk/benefit relationship should be chosen and continually reassessed. Factors such as cost of medication and ability and willingness of the patient to comply with long-term life-style changes (including dietary modification, exercise, and avoidance of factors and conditions that exacerbate the disorder under treatment) must be considered. However, new knowledge concerning the safety and efficacy of existing drugs and the development of novel drugs that are better tolerated by patients have led to recent therapeutic improvements and exciting changes in this field.

Based upon convincing evidence that elevated blood cholesterol increases the risk of CHD and that therapies that lower plasma LDL cholesterol reduce this risk, a consensus on the need to reduce these levels has emerged. The National Heart, Lung, and Blood Institute, the American Heart Association, and other voluntary health organizations have combined their efforts in formation of the National Cholesterol Education Program (NCEP). The goal of this program is to educate physicians, other health care professionals, and the public about the need to measure blood cholesterol levels of all adult Americans and of the importance of treating hypercholesterolemia. An expert panel convened by the NCEP issued a report on the detection, evaluation, and treatment of high blood cholesterol. The panel report recommended criteria to identify candidates for medical intervention and provided detailed guidelines for their management. Two complementary approaches were utilized in a coordinated strategy aimed at lowering blood cholesterol: a population-based approach aimed at lowering the cholesterol levels of the entire population and a patient-based approach aimed at identification of individuals at high risk who would benefit from intensive intervention efforts. In the latter approach, decisions on when to lower blood cholesterol levels are based on two factors: the plasma or serum total and LDL cholesterol levels and the presence of other cardiovascular risk factors. Initial case-finding recommendations are that plasma or serum total cholesterol be measured in all adults over age 20 at least once every 5 years and that this measurement may be made in the nonfasting state. Levels below 200 mg/dl are classified as "desirable blood cholesterol"; those 200 to 239 mg/dl as "borderline-high cholesterol," and those 240 mg/dl and above as "high blood cholesterol." Along with cholesterol testing, adults should also be evaluated for the presence of other cardiovascular risk factors. High-risk status was defined as having definite CHD or at least two CHD risk factors. These other CHD risk factors identified by the panel included being male, a family history of premature CHD, cigarette smoking, hypertension, low HDL cholesterol levels (<35 mg/dl), diabetes mellitus, severe obesity, and definite cerebrovascular or peripheral vascular disease.

Panel recommendations were that those with blood cholesterol levels below 200 mg/dl be given dietary and risk reduction information and be advised to have repeat blood cholesterol testing within 5 years. Those with levels above 200 mg/dl should have a repeat test and should undergo lipoprotein analysis of a 12-hour fasted specimen if their levels exceed 240 mg/dl or if they have borderline high values and have high-risk status. Those with confirmed levels in the borderline-high range, but who are not at high risk, should receive dietary information and an annual reevaluation. The focus of attention in those requiring lipoprotein analysis should shift from total cholesterol to LDL cholesterol as the key index for clinical decision making about cholesterol-lowering therapy. LDL cholesterol levels are classified as desirable if below 130 mg/dl, borderline high if 130 to 159 mg/dl, and high if 160 mg/dl or above. The panel recommended a 3 to 6 month trial of a cholesterol-lowering diet for low-risk patients with LDL cholesterol levels above 160 mg/dl or high-risk patients with levels above 130 mg/dl. Decisions about use of cholesterol-lowering drugs were to depend on the response to diet. Those at low risk for CHD having LDL cholesterol levels above 190 mg/dl and those at high risk with levels above 160 mg/dl were to be considered as potential candidates for drug therapy. The panel emphasized that individualized clinical judgment be employed

in the implementation of these guidelines. Moreover, future modifications of these guidelines are apt to be made as new data are obtained. The imperative to manage lipoprotein disorders extends beyond these guidelines, which aimed at simplicity and the wide dissemination of sufficiently detailed information to facilitate implementation of blood cholesterol-lowering regimens on a broad scale.

There are three major reasons for treating lipoprotein disorders. The first and foremost of these is to decelerate or reverse the progression of atherosclerotic cardiovascular diseases in individuals predisposed to premature development of these conditions, thus reducing the risk of myocardial infarction and peripheral ischemic conditions. The second reason is to bring about the regression or disappearance of xanthomas (lipid deposits in the skin and tendon sheaths). The third reason is to prevent the chylomicronemia syndrome, which causes acute abdominal pain resulting from acute pancreatitis, a fulminating, sometimes life-threatening condition associated with strikingly high plasma triglyceride levels.

In the clinical evaluation of patients with elevated levels of plasma lipoproteins, appropriate assessment requires consideration of a host of variables. Diverse underlying conditions and a variety of diseases or environmental influences can produce similar lipoprotein phenotypic patterns. On the other hand, some specific underlying conditions are more commonly associated with a given abnormal lipoprotein pattern. For example, hypothyroidism is most commonly associated with a type IIA pattern. Generally, however, any of the following can cause or be associated with secondary hyperlipidemia: alcohol, estrogen, or glucocorticoid intake; pregnancy; hypothyroidism; nephrotic syndrome; chronic renal disease; obstructive or parenchymal liver disease; pancreatitis; obesity; poorly controlled diabetes mellitus; anorexia nervosa; acute intermittent porphyria; glycogen storage diseases; and dysproteinemias such as multiple myeloma or macroglobulinemia. Use of certain antihypertensive drugs such as β-blockers, thiazide diuretics, and other medications can cause changes in circulating lipids in some patients. Such underlying causal conditions can usually be diagnosed by an adequate history and physical examination and by the use of simple screening tests. Routine studies should include a urinalysis for detection of proteinuria or glycosuria, a complete blood count, and determination of serum levels of T_4, thyroid-stimulating hormone (TSH), creatinine, urea nitrogen, bilirubin, alkaline phosphatase, and hepatic transaminases. Further tests are indicated by suggestive findings obtained during the history or physical examination. A patient may have both a primary and secondary cause for hyperlipidemia, such as LPL deficiency in combination with alcoholism. A given individual may also have more than one secondary cause for hyperlipidemia, such as obesity and uncontrolled diabetes mellitus. Diagnosis and management are aimed first at detection and removal of underlying causes. Thereafter, persistence of an abnormal lipoprotein pattern or plasma lipid elevation is managed by appropriate diet and at times with adjunctive drug therapy.

The clinical clues that lead to a suspicion of hyperlipidemia include a family history of or the presence of premature coronary or peripheral arterial disease, xanthomas, and premature corneal arcus and the occurrence of frequent bouts of acute pancreatitis. The presence of any of these clearly indicates a need for determination of plasma or serum lipid levels; however, a case can be made for lipid determinations as part of any health evaluation. When the presence of hyperlipidermia is confirmed, it is important to determine the distribution of plasma cholesterol among the major lipoprotein classes by quantitation of the cholesterol content of the HDL, LDL, and VLDL fractions. Identification of an elevated HDL cholesterol level that can cause mild hypercholesterolemia does not warrant therapeutic intervention. When levels of both VLDL and LDL are increased, the relative distribution of cholesterol among both lipoprotein classes may affect the selection of therapeutic agents in a given clinical situation.

Relatives, particularly children of hyperlipidemic adults, should have a set of fasting plasma total cholesterol and triglyceride determinations, since the earlier the institution of appropriate corrective measures, the more likely the measures will be beneficial. Determination of plasma lipid concentrations should be combined with an assessment of potential cardiovascular risk. Other factors that are likely to accelerate the progression of atherosclerosis must be identified during the patient evaluation. The risk of cardiovascular event occurrence at a given plasma cholesterol level is increased by the concurrence of the CHD risk factors previously mentioned. Other CHD risk factors have been identified, such as personality factors, oral contraceptive use, and sedentary life-style, but their role in CHD causation is more controversial. Thus therapy must be directed to alteration not only of the hyperlipidemia, but also of other correctable risk factors.

In history taking, a careful dietary history should be obtained, and particular attention paid to the patient's intake of alcohol and exposure to hormones and antihypertensive medications. Although severe degrees of hyperlipidemia are invariably the result of an inherent metabolic abnormality or stem from another disease, mild elevations of plasma lipids frequently occur in subjects who ingest large quantities of calories, cholesterol, or animal fat. The hyperlipidemia in such individuals is likely to respond readily to dietary measures.

The physical examination should include a careful examination of the eye for the presence of a premature corneal arcus—a whitish, crescentic deposit of cholesterol crystals in the cornea that suggests elevations in LDL when seen in younger patients. A number of lipoprotein disorders are associated with xanthomas, observable patterns of lipid accumulation in the skin or tendons. Thickenings of the extendons of the hands or feet, particularly of the Achilles tendons, are seen in individuals with familial hypercholesterolemia. Eruptive xanthomas are crops of yellowish papules, each with a reddish base, that characteristically occur on extensor surfaces of the body when triglyceride levels are greatly elevated. They can appear and disappear within a few days as the fat content of the diet is altered and usually indicate dramatic elevations of chylomicrons, VLDL, or both. Eruptive xanthomas are common in patients with fasting hyperchylomicronemia and milky plasma (which stems from the scattering of light by these large particles).

Except for the eruptive and palpebral xanthomas, the occurrence of xanthomas usually is limited to the primary genetic forms of hyperlipoproteinemia. Tuberous xanthomas often begin as lesions that initially resemble eruptive xanthomas but have a redder base and coalesce to form larger, lipid-laden lesions. These can occur in familial hyperlipoproteinemias characterized by elevations of LDL, IDL, or VLDL. Palmar xanthomas, yellowish or whitish discolorations of the palmar or interdigital creases, occur in remnant removal abnormalities and at times in biliary cirrhosis. Xanthelasma, or xanthoma in or around the eyelids, can be associated with LDL elevations, but in many subjects with this skin lesion only, no currently definable lipoprotein disorder can be detected. Even in the absence of elevated LDL, patients with xanthelasma should undergo periodic reevaluation for lipoprotein abnormalities.

Ophthalmoscopic examination of patients with plasma triglyceride levels over about 2000 mg/dl may display lipemia retinalis, a whitish appearance of retinal arterioles and venules that results from altered reflection of light from the column of blood in these vessels. Hepatosplenomegaly in patients with hyperchylomicronemia appears to be related to engorgement with triglyceride by reticuloendothelial cells, which occurs when normal removal mechanisms become overloaded. Foam cells, or fat-laden macrophages, can be observed in bone marrow specimens from such patients. Attacks of abdominal pain are usually the result of acute pancreatitis, perhaps caused by pancreatic microinfarcts secondary to impedance of the capillary circulation by chylomicrons. Serum amylase levels may be normal in patients having pancreatitis associated with hypertriglyceridemia.

Plasma lipid and lipoprotein sampling

LDL and VLDL remnants have long been recognized as having atherogenic potential. Patients with elevations of LDL have an increased risk of accelerated coronary atherosclerosis. Whether intact VLDL is itself artherogenic remains controversial but unestablished. Premature coronary and peripheral vascular disease is often associated with elevated levels of LDL or VLDL remnants in the circulation and is related to the degree and duration of these elevations. It has been postulated that as LDL concentrations in plasma rise above levels that saturate the LDL receptor, the uptake of LDL cholesterol by vascular and other tissues occurs increasingly by receptor-independent or scavenger mechanisms. Because the latter processes are poorly regulated, cholesterol ester accumulation can occur within macrophages and smooth muscle cells and accelerate the atherogenic process. Recent studies strongly suggest that HDL confers protection against the development of premature atherosclerosis. In fact, an inverse relation has been observed between plasma HDL cholesterol levels and the incidence of myocardial infarction. HDL cholesterol can be measured in the supernatant fraction of plasma after precipitation of the lower density lipoproteins by heparin and Mn^{++} or by dextran sulfate and Ca^{++}. Unremarkable levels of HDL cholesterol in adults range from about 40 to 80 mg/dl, and the higher levels are believed to provide protection against coronary artery disease. A host of environmental influences can affect plasma HDL levels. Premenopausal females generally have higher HDL cholesterol levels than males of similar ages. Chronic renal failure, obesity, cigarette smoking, physical inactivity, excessive caloric intake, and some medications can lower circulating HDL levels. Weight reduction, smoking cessation, exercise, alcohol, and some medications can raise plasma HDL levels. Because particles with the composition of spherical HDL are formed during the catabolism of triglyceride-rich lipoproteins, elevated levels of VLDL and chylomicrons are usually associated with reduced levels of HDL. When plasma triglycerides are below about 400 mg/dl, the VLDL cholesterol level can be assumed to be one fifth of the plasma triglyceride level, and the LDL cholesterol level can be calculated by subtraction of the HDL and VLDL cholesterol levels from the total cholesterol level.

Measurements of total cholesterol and triglyceride levels in plasma or serum should be carried out after at least a 12-hour fast; the specimen should be examined visually as well. Special care should be taken to ensure that the laboratory utilized provides consistently accurate data. Patients should be maintained on their usual diet for several days before sampling but should avoid intake of alcohol for at least 3 days beforehand. Ideally patients should be ambulatory, since acute illness, trauma, and physical or emotional stress can alter plasma lipoprotein levels. The presence of turbid or lactescent serum in a fasting specimen is always abnormal and usually indicates the presence of triglyceride levels greater than 500 mg/dl. Opalescence can also occur at lower triglyceride levels, particularly if chylomicrons are present. Refrigerated plasma or serum begins to display lactescence at triglyceride levels between 200 and 250 mg/dl because chylomicrons and VLDL aggregate at lower temperatures, producing larger particles that scatter light to a greater degree. The overnight-refrigerated sample can also be tentatively used to identify the abnormal lipoprotein pattern, since chylomicrons float to the surface of the sample, whereas VLDL particles do not. Thus a floating layer of fat over clear serum is indicative of isolated chylomicronemia (type I pattern). Patients with increased VLDL levels (type IV pattern) demonstrate evenly distributed opalescence. Elevations of both chylomicrons and VLDL (type V) appear as a creamy layer superimposed over a lactescent infranatant. Remnant removal abnormalities (type III) usually have a uniformly turbid serum specimen but can on occasion reveal a floating creamy layer if chylomicron remnants are also present. Hypercholesterolemic plasma or serum without triglyceride elevations is clear. The combination of elevated cholesterol with normal triglyceride levels almost always indicates an elevation of plasma LDL (a type IIA pattern), except for rare instances of isolated HDL elevations. Measurements of cholesterol but not of triglycerides can be carried out on plasma or serum of nonfasting patients, since LDL levels do not vary greatly in relation to meals. The firm diagnosis of remnant removal disorders requires the use of ultracentrifugal flotation at serum density to demonstrate the presence of the VLDL remnant that has β-mobility on electrophoresis but pre-β density on ultracentrifugation.

Because circulating cholesterol and triglyceride levels vary among populations with differing life-styles and increase with age, ideally a subject's levels should be compared with values obtained from normal subjects from the same population in the same age range. Numerous trials investigating the use of diet, drugs, or both to lower circulating cholesterol levels have demonstrated a beneficial effect of plasma cholesterol reduction on cardiovascular morbidity and mortality. The relationship between LDL cholesterol levels and cardiovascular risk is continuous and curvilinear. The degree of risk appears to increase disproportionately as higher plasma cholesterol levels above 200 mg/dl are reached; the slope of the curve relating coronary events to plasma cholesterol levels increases more sharply as levels exceed 240 mg/dl. A recent panel conducting a National Institutes of Health (NIH)-Consensus Development Conference reviewed existing evidence and, after much discussion, issued recommendations for the population at large that targeted acceptable plasma cholesterol goal levels well below levels previously considered acceptable. The new recommendations, which are based on data from epidemiologic and intervention studies, suggest that total cholesterol levels should not exceed 180 mg/dl for adults below age 30 and should not exceed 200 mg/dl in adults above this age. Moderate- and high-risk levels were defined respectively at the 75th and 90th percentiles. Although these levels are much lower than prior recommendations in the medical literature, previous "abnormal" levels had been traditionally set at the 95th percentile of the U.S. population, at which level cardiovascular risk is increased severalfold. The Adult Treatment Panel of the NCEP expanded on the recommendations of the Consensus Development Panel with the issuance of specific, detailed guidelines for therapy.

With respect to acceptable plasma triglyceride levels, a greater degree of uncertainty and controversy exists. Hypertriglyceridemia is commonly found in patients with CHD, but there is little firm evidence of a direct causal link between the two. A panel convened in 1983 to review the state of knowledge in this area conducted a Triglyceride Consensus Conference and issued recommended guidelines that were much less stringent than those goal cholesterol levels later recommended in 1984 by the panel reviewing the host of evidence on cholesterol. The former panel concluded that although hypertriglyceridemia provides evidence for existence of a disturbance in lipid transport in a given patient, the hypertriglyceridemia may not itself impart increased cardiovascular risk. On the other hand, because of the frequent concomitance of hypertriglyceridemia and CHD, some other factor common to both conditions, such as low HDL levels, may be responsible for the association of these abnormalities. Mild to moderate hypertriglyceridemia can result from an overproduction of VLDL triglyceride without an increase in the number of VLDL particles secreted and therefore without an overproduction of VLDL apo B. This situation occurs in patients with familial hypertriglyceridemia. Further compromise of triglyceride-clearing mechanisms by saturation of the LPL system then may produce the chylomicronemia syndrome. In other clinical situations, mild to moderate plasma triglyceride elevations can result from an increased production rate of the entire VLDL particle, including apo B, such that the proportion of triglyceride to apo B in these particles does not change with the overproduction of VLDL. This form of hypertriglyceridemia is associated with an increased flux of apo B through the VLDL-IDL-LDL pathway, as in patients with familial combined hyperlipidemia, a condition known to be associated with increased cardiovascular risk. Another condition in which elevated plasma triglycerides appear to indicate accelerated atherogenesis is familial remnant removal disease. In this condition, patients have elevated levels of both triglyceride and cholesterol caused by defective removal of remnant lipoproteins from the circulation, with resultant accelerated CHD and peripheral arterial disease. From an evaluation of the available body of data on plasma triglycerides, the panel defined hypertriglyceridemia as occurring at plasma levels above 250 mg/dl and assigned potential risks at various stages above this level. Thus for most individuals an acceptable upper limit for fasting plasma triglycerides would be 200 to 250 mg/dl. Such levels should not be labeled "normal" because at present an accurate definiton of what constitutes normal levels cannot be made. Assessment of associated risk factors also influences the decision of whether a given set of plasma or serum lipid levels is acceptable for a given patient. It is easy to advocate vigorous therapy for severe degrees of hyperlipidemia, but it is difficult to apply specific rules to the management of the modest elevations of plasma lipids that are more commonly seen in clinical practice. Sound judgment and careful individual assessment are required to decide whether and how to treat. The institution of dietary or drug therapy is apt to be long-term, and interventions that do not require radical alterations in life-style are more likely to be met with patient compliance.

MANAGEMENT OF HYPERLIPIDEMIA
Dietary treatment

Dietary management, which includes both caloric restriction and limitation of saturated fat, cholesterol, and alcohol intake, remains the keystone of therapy in hyperlipidemia. The intake of a diet high in calories, saturated fat, and cholesterol is often a cause of hyperlipidemia in industrialized societies. Moreover, even when drug therapy is employed, the effects of diet and drugs are synergistic; therefore sound dietary principles must be initiated and continue to be followed. Evidence strongly indicates that a plasma cholesterol-lowering regimen coupled with a sensible exercise program and modification of other risk factors can effectively diminish cardiovascular risk. Evidence is accumulating that combined dietary and drug interventions that lower plasma levels of atherogenic lipoproteins can decelerate or even reverse coronary and peripheral atherosclerosis. However, although the great majority of hyperlipidemia patients will probably benefit to some degree from such interventions, some may not. More effective therapeutic interventions require clearer understanding of the specific abnormalities of lipoprotein metabolism present, and the development of specifically tailored therapies to reverse these metabolic abnormalities.

Diets high in cholesterol and saturated fat increase the delivery of chylomicron cholesterol to the liver, with consequent suppression of hepatic cholesterol synthesis and down-regulation of LDL receptor activity on the hepatocyte surface. These metabolic changes result in a diminished clearance of LDL from the circulation and can also lead to an accelerated rate of LDL production by diversion of IDL from hepatic uptake to increased conversion to LDL. LDL levels in plasma then rise. Although ingestion of animal fat results in increased plasma cholesterol levels, the degree of individual increments varies and both genetic and dietary factors affect the plasma levels reached. There is great individual variation in plasma cholesterol changes in response to modifications in dietary intake of cholesterol and saturated fat, and the mechanisms for these differences are poorly understood at present.

Since weight reduction alone can lower plasma lipid levels in many subjects, reduction of body weight by diminishing caloric intake should be the initial therapeutic goal for obese patients. Weight reduction alone may correct the hyperlipoproteinemia. Present evidence suggests that severe obesity probably reduces life expectancy and increases the risk of vascular complications. Reduction of body weight reduces VLDL production, lowers plasma triglycerides, and usually lowers plasma LDL cholesterol levels, while raising plasma HDL cholesterol levels. In some patients, particularly those with FCHL, plasma LDL levels may rise perhaps due to reduced LDL clearance. The addition of drug therapy then is usually warranted. In other patients whose LDL levels rise during weight reduction, continued weight loss with restriction of dietary fat and cholesterol may eventually bring about the desired reduction in LDL levels. A given therapeutic regimen with diet or drug usually requires a trial of 6 to 8 weeks to determine whether the effect is beneficial. Dietary restriction can improve most hyperlipoproteinemias, with the exception of most forms of severe hyperbetalipoproteinemia. Optimal diet alone seldom achieves greater than a 10% lowering of elevated plasma cholesterol. However, even in these patients, dietary therapy should be instituted initially, and drug therapy should be reserved for insufficiently responsive patients in the high-risk group.

The Nutrition Committee of the American Heart Association has recommended reduction of fat intake to a maximum of 30% of total caloric intake and an increase in carbohydrates, mainly complex carbohydrates, to 55% of total calories. Saturated fat should comprise not greater than 10% of total calories, and cholesterol intake should not exceed 300 mg daily. Since excessive body weight is frequently associated with high VLDL, moderately high LDL, and low HDL levels, a supervised weight reduction program of decreased caloric intake with altered distribution of calories between fat and carbohydrate,

and moderate exercise should be instituted whenever feasible. Increasing the intake of dietary fiber, particularly soluble fiber contained in oat bran, whole grain, beans, lentils, peas, and fruits can produce a mild plasma lipid–lowering effect, but may not be tolerated by some patients. Most hyperlipidemia patients, particularly those with plasma level elevations of VLDL and triglycerides, should restrict or avoid ingestion of alcohol and simple sugars.

An increased intake of omega-3 fatty acid–containing fish oils, mainly eicosapentaenoic and docosahexaenoic acids, has been shown to lower VLDL production by the liver and to decrease plasma triglyceride and to a much lesser degree, plasma cholesterol levels. In fact, patients with FCHL may actually show elevations in plasma LDL levels consequent to intake of fish oils. Dietary supplementation with fish oils may benefit some patients with hypertriglyceridemia, but a number of questions about the dosage, safety, and efficacy of these oils, particularly for diabetic patients, still are unanswered. The role of fish oils in the therapy of the hyperlipoproteinemias and the relationship of their potential antithrombotic properties in special instances to their overall therapeutic effects are currently unclear. Their use is not recommended, based on data available at present, and further studies are required to define indications for their use in patients.

If initial dietary modifications are partially effective in regulating the plasma lipids of hyperlipidemic individuals, additional restrictions of calories, saturated fat, and cholesterol may be undertaken within the limits of anticipated patient compliance. Though the effects of dietary modification often approach a plateau within 6 to 8 weeks, further plasma lipid changes may be observed if gradual weight reduction proceeds beyond this period of time. Although the panel recommends longer dietary trials of 3 to 6 months before institution of drug therapy, it often becomes necessary to consider concomitant drug therapy earlier, particularly in the more severe forms of hypercholesterolemia. There is also a consensus that earlier implementation of drug therapy should be considered in high-risk patients, particularly those with overt CHD. However, adherence to a prudent diet remains the cornerstone of therapy even when concomitant drugs must be employed to achieve LDL cholesterol level goals.

Patients with moderate to severe increases in plasma cholesterol levels tend to have monogenic or polygenic hereditary defects, which often require the addition of drug therapy after an initial trial of dietary therapy alone. However, with mild degrees of hypercholesterolemia, dietary restriction of saturated fat and cholesterol intake is often sufficient to correct the problem.

With patients having LPL deficiency or other defects in the removal of triglyceride-rich lipoproteins, the therapeutic aim should be to lower chylomicron levels sufficiently to prevent attacks of acute pancreatitis and triglyceride deposition in the skin, liver, and spleen. This goal can be achieved by simple restriction of fat intake to 25 or 30 g/day. Dietary substitution of medium-chain triglycerides for the long-chain variety can be made with commercially available preparations. When diminished LPL activity is caused by a deficiency of insulin or thyroxine, administration of the deficient hormone is indicated. When LPL activity is impaired by the intake of alcohol or high doses of estrogens or glucocorticoids, the causative agent should be discontinued.

To lower plasma cholesterol levels in patients, regardless of whether the pattern is type IIA, IIB, III, or even IV, a diet low in cholesterol and saturated fat should be instituted initially. Populations consuming diets rich in cholesterol and saturated fat generally have higher serum cholesterol levels and a higher prevalence of atherosclerosis than those on low-fat diets. Although individual variation occurs in the cholesterol levels reached in response to a given dietary intake of the sterol, these levels generally rise in a graded fashion with dietary cholesterol as intake increases in the 0 to 600 mg/day range. When dietary cholesterol intake exceeds 600 mg/day, the plasma concentration usually rises no further, probably because of inhibition of hepatic cholesterol synthesis by a negative feedback mechanism. However, even when plasma cholesterol levels reach a plateau, evidence exists that more atherogenic cholesterol-rich lipoproteins accumulate in the circulation. Therefore dietary cholesterol intake should be limited to 300 mg/day. The ingestion of saturated fat should be reduced by replacement with polyunsaturated and monounsaturated fats to achieve a polyunsaturated:monounsaturated:saturated fat ratio of 1:1:1. To follow a diet low in saturated fats and cholesterol requires limited intake of meat (especially beef, pork and lamb), egg yolks, dairy products (except soft margarine, skimmed milk, or cottage cheese), commercial pastries, candy and chocolates, and coconut or palm oil products. The ingestion of organ meats (brain, liver, kidneys, and sweetbreads) must be particularly curtailed. The diet should be supplemented with polyunsaturated oils such as sunflower, safflower, and corn oil, and monounsaturated fats such as olive oil.

The Adult Treatment Panel of the NCEP has recommended that a cholesterol-lowering diet be implemented in two stages. Step one calls for intake of saturated fat of less than 10% of total calories and of total fat of less than 30% of calories and a dietary cholesterol intake of less than 300 mg/day. Step two involves further restriction of saturated fat to 7% of total calories and limitation of dietary cholesterol to less than 200 mg/day. Referral to a registered dietician is recommended if warranted to facilitate instruction for dietary modification and monitoring.

Evidence linking plasma triglyceride elevations to premature atherogenesis is available and increasing but remains less convincing than is the case for hypercholesterolemia. Thus mild to modest rises in plasma triglyceride–caused VLDL elevations usually have been linked to premature CHD when plasma total cholesterol levels are also raised or when the total cholesterol/HDL cholesterol ratio exceeds 3.5:1. However, there is growing evidence that plasma triglyceride elevations are, in some way, related to an increased risk for CHD. Recent data from the Framingham Heart Study indicate that plasma triglyceride elevations are a highly significant independent risk factor for CHD in women and are particularly dangerous as CHD risk factors in men with HDL cholesterol levels below 40 mg/dl. Thus, measures should be instituted to lower significant elevations of plasma triglycerides, particularly when these elevations exceed 350 mg/dl. Weight reduction through caloric restriction is by far the most important therapeutic measure. Although the intake of simple refined sugars should be limited, overall restriction of complex carbohydrate as a percentage of daily dietary calories is not indicated for most hypertriglyceridemic individuals. An increase in poorly digested and unabsorbed plant polysaccharides as dietary fiber, if tolerated, may have beneficial effects on the reduction of weight and plasma lipid levels. Intake of alcohol must be severely curtailed in subjects with severe triglyceride elevations, some of whom show a greatly augmented response in plasma triglyceride increments to even minimal amounts of alcohol. In the commonly encountered patient with mild elevations in plasma triglycerides and carbohydrate intolerance, institution of the above dietary changes should bring about sufficieint declines in plasma VLDL and triglycerides.

Drug therapy

When dietary means alone fail to regulate plasma lipid and lipoprotein levels sufficiently, concomitant drug therapy can be instituted in individualized fashion. The expected therapeutic advantages from drug treatment must be carefully weighed against the potential problems of long-term intake. Factors to be considered in this decision include the goal lipid levels, the estimated cardiovascular risk, the safety, efficacy, and expense of the drug, the patient's age, and the likelihood of compliance. Only when the physician judges that the anticipated benefits of pharmacological therapy outweigh the potential difficulties and risks should such therapy be implemented.

However, the physician should encourage the patient at high risk for CHD to undergo a trial of pharmacologic therapy when dietary treatment alone gives inadequate results. It is important to provide education and encouragement to the patient and to involve other health-care professionals such as office staff and registered dieticians in this supportive effort. Because therapy with drugs is long term and often life long, the motivation and confidence of the patient in the proposed regimen is essential to attain compliance with dietary adherence, medication intake, periodic monitoring, and lifestyle modification.

The dissemination of public health and other information on cholesterol lowering by the NCEP has led to a number of articles in the lay press and to the vigorous promotion of dietary and pharmacologic products by various industries. Increased attention has been focused on the use of hypocholesterolemic and lipid-regulating drugs.

The major drugs to consider for regulation of plasma lipid levels and for lowering of LDL cholesterol levels include the bile acid sequestrants (cholestyramine and colestipol), niacin, HMG CoA reductase inhibitors (lovastatin), gemfibrozil, and probucol. The crucial importance of careful clinical judgement and individualization of patient care must be underscored in the selection and use of hypolipidemic drugs. If the response to therapy with a drug of first choice is inadequate or if the drug causes side effects, an alternative drug should be employed. Combination therapy with two or even three compatible agents should be considered. In fact, low-dose combinations of lipid-lowering drugs that have complementary or synergistic actions are often preferable to achieve long-term efficacy and avoidance of troublesome adverse effects.

The major action of the bile acid sequestrants is a lowering of LDL cholesterol levels. These agents have a long track record of safety and have the advantage that their use has reduced CHD risk in large-scale intervention trials. The sequestrants are anionic exchange resins bind bile acids in the intestine, interfere with the enterohepatic circulation of bile acids, and thereby increase the catabolism and biliary excretion of cholesterol. The resins appear to enhance the hepatic removal of circulating LDL by increasing the number of high-affinity LDL receptors in the liver. The up-regulating of LDL receptors results from the hepatic diversion of cholesterol of the sequestered bile acids. Two such resins include colestipol hydrocholoride (10 to 30 g/day) and cholestyramine resin (8 to 24 g/day), which can lower plasma LDL levels by 15% to 30%. Their major shortcoming stems from compliance difficulties. Problems encountered with their use include the inconvenience of mixing the powder with a liquid, variable palatability, frequent gastrointestinal side effects, some malabsorption of fat-soluble vitamins, and potential resin binding of other drugs. Moreover, their effectiveness, when used as monotherapy, is somewhat curtailed by the increase in hepatic cholesterol synthesis that occurs with reduction in hepatic cholesterol content during therapy. Some patients also develop some degree of hypertriglyceridemia with resin administration. The resins are effective in the therapy of the heterozygous forms of familial monogenic hypercholesterolemia, in the familial polygenic hypercholesterolemias, and in FCHL (multiple-type hyperlipproteinemia) when LDL levels are elevated.

The development of specific competitive inhibitors of cholesterol synthesis afford a novel and effective approach to the treatment of the hypercholesterolemias. Lovastatin (formerly termed "mevinolin"), a recently marketed drug that has been extensively studied in humans, has produced significant plasma cholesterol reductions (approximately 30% to 50%) at doses of 20 to 80 mg/day. Other similar inhibitors that are undergoing clinical testing include simvastin and pravastatin. Because these agents inhibit the rate-limiting enzyme for cholesterol biosynthesis, namely HMG CoA reductase, their use results in up-regulation of hepatic LDL receptors, thereby promoting the clearance of LDL from the circulation. These inhibitors are effective both in the more serious forms of familial hypercholesterolemia (except in homozygous patients) and in the various forms of moderate hypercholesterolemia. Because of their effect on cholesterol biosynthesis, their combined use with bile acid–sequestering agents counters the stimulatory actions of the resins on hepatic cholesterol formation and results in a greatly augmented hypocholesterolemic effect. Lovastatin can also produce mild increases in HDL cholesterol and mild reductions in triglyceride levels. Other HMG CoA reductase inhibitors are in different stages of new drug development. Biochemical abnormalities found in a small percentage of patients treated with lovastatin have included elevations in hepatic transaminases and creatine kinase levels in serum. Therefore careful monitoring of these enzyme levels is important. Although early concerns about cataract formation as a result of lovastatin therapy have lessened, baseline and follow-up evaluation of the lens should be carried out. Lovastatin is generally better tolerated than other plasma cholesterol-lowering drugs, but its use requires careful patient monitoring while its long-term safety profile becomes established. Therapy with these agents thus far suggests that they are well tolerated and probably safe. Provided this safety experience is established with their more widespread and long-term use, these drugs are likely to represent a major therapeutic advance potentially useful for a large target population with increased risk for CHD. Their impact on the therapy of hypercholesterolemia and on the prevention of CHD in high-risk patients could be tremendous.

Niacin (nicotine acid), a water-soluble B vitamin, lowers total and LDL cholesterol levels and triglycerides and raises HDL cholesterol levels. When used in gradually increasing doses to a maintenance level of between 3 and 6 g/day, reduces the production and plasma levels of VLDL. Nicotinic acid may impair hepatic production of VLDL at least in part by an inhibition of lipolysis in adipose tissues and consequent deficiency of fatty acid substrate for hepatic triglyceride synthesis. Niacin may have other effects on lipoprotein metabolism. Since LDL is the product of VLDL catabolism, within days LDL levels also fall. Therefore the drug is particularly useful in patients with severe hypertriglyceridemia and in patients with combined elevations of plasma triglycerides and cholesterol. Plasma HDL cholesterol levels also tend to rise during therapy with nicotinic acid. In the Coronary Drug Project Study, men with prior myocardial infarction who received niacin therapy

had a lower incidence of myocardial reinfarction than those taking placebo. Nine years after the study ended, a lower mortality rate was found in the niacin-treated group. Another placebo-controlled study that combined niacin and colestipol therapy in men with previous coronary artery bypass surgery reported less progression and more regression of atherosclerosis in both native arteries and grafts in the drug-treated group after 2 years. While niacin is very effective in lowering LDL cholesterol levels, its use requires considerable patient education. Intake of this drug is associated with pruritus and cutaneous flushing that occurs within 1 to 2 hours after intake. However, in most patients tachyphylaxis to these effects develops with continued use, and these effects can be partially mitigated to concomitant aspirin use and taking the medication with meals. More troublesome but reversible side effects include glucose intolerance, hyperuricemia, and plasma elevations of liver enzymes. The drug may also potentiate the postural hypotensive effects of some antihypertensive agents.

D-thyroxine, the dextrorotatory isomer of thyroxine, lowers circulating LDL and cholesterol levels, probably by enhancing the catabolism of LDL. The rationale for its use has been that its hypocholesterolemic action is disproportionately greater than its hypermetabolic effects, relative to the levorotatory isomer. Since this agent is potentially cardiotoxic by precipitating arrhythmias in patients with coronary atherosclerosis, D-thyroxine has an unfavorable risk/benefit ratio and its use is not generally recommended. However, D-thyroxine remains approved by the FDA for use in selected young adults with primary hypercholesterolemia who are unable to tolerate other effective cholesterol-lowering drugs.

Probucol, another agent with hypocholesterolemic activity, is structurally unrelated to other hypolipidemic agents. Probucol usually lowers plasma LDL levels by up to 15%. However, this drug also reduces plasma HDL cholesterol levels as well and has no consistent effect on triglyceride levels. The effect on plasma LDL levels is attributed to enhanced LDL clearance, perhaps by increased LDL removal from the circulation by pathways independent of high-affinity LDL receptors. The role of probucol in the therapy of hypercholesterolemia is currently unclear because evidence exists that this drug inhibits the oxidation and tissue deposition of LDL. Probucol can also cause xanthoma regression despite its lowering of HDL cholesterol levels. Further information on its effects on the course of atheroma development may be learned with completion of a currently ongoing clinical trial. When used, probucol is administered in divided doses of 0.5 to 1 g/day. Probucol is generally well-tolerated but can produce a variety of mild side effects, the most common of which are abdominal discomfort, diarrhea, nausea, and headache. Use of probucol should be currently avoided in patients with evidence of ventricular irritability or an initially prolonged QT interval, and in those taking other drugs that prolong the QT interval.

Neomycin is a poorly absorbed antibiotic; like resins, neomycin interferes with bile acid reabsorption in the intestine. In some patients an additional effect stems from neomycin's inhibition of cholesterol absorption. Neomycin is usually well tolerated and is used in divided daily doses that range from a total of 0.5 to 2 g/day. Its side effects are mainly of gastrointestinal origin and are usually mild, but this agent must be used with caution, since patients who absorb appreciable amounts of neomycin can develop ototoxicity, nephrotoxicity, or both. This drug is not approved by the FDA as a lipid-lowering agent, and no data are available on its long-term saftey in hypercholesterolemic patients.

A large number of derivatives of fibric acid have been developed that have varying properties. Their major therapeutic effect is probably secondary to a stimulation of VLDL removal from the circulation, perhaps by actions on lipoprotein lipase activity or other removal mechanisms. Inhibitory effects on hepatic production of VLDL may also contribute to the action of this class of drugs. Because of the enhanced catabolism of VLDL to LDL caused by these agents, particularly in patients with FCHL, plasma LDL levels may rise. Clofibrate was previously the agent most widely used to treat hypertriglyceridemia, but its use has been curtailed because of concerns about its long-term safety. Recently completed large scale studies have raised concerns about its potential for cardiotoxic and tumorigenic effects in humans. This drug and other fibric acid derivatives have a variety of effects on lipid and lipoprotein metabolism in the body. Fibric acid derivatives are a very effective agent in reducing plasma triglyceride levels and are particularly useful in the management of remnant removal disorders (familial dysbetalipoproteinemia). Extensive experience with clofibrate indicates that the drug increases the risk of gallstone formation in patients. Gemfibrozil, a newer fibric acid, has a more favorable safety profile than clofibrate, but its actions on plasma lipids are similar. Gemfibrozil may be less lithogenic than clofibrate, and its effects on plasma VLDL and HDL levels may be more potent. This drug was approved by the FDA for plasma triglyceride lowering to reduce the risk of acute pancreatitis. Gemfibrozil lowers circulating VLDL and triglyceride levels and can increase HDL cholesterol levels. Its effect on LDL cholesterol levels are variable, depending on the lipid disorder under treatment and on patient response. Usual doses of this drug are 600 mg to 1200 mg/day taken in two divided doses. The most common side effects observed with gemfibrozil use are gastrointestinal. The drug increases bile lithogenicity and can potentiate the effects of oral anticoagulants and produce reversible elevations of hepatic enzymes in some patients. In the Helsinki Heart Trial, treatment of a large group of middle-aged men without symptomatic CHD with gemfibrozil resulted in decreases in LDL cholesterol (10%) and triglyceride (43%) levels, and a 10% rise in HDL cholesterol levels. The overall reduction in CHD end-points in the drug-treated group averaged 34%. Fenofibrate is another fibric acid derivative effective in the treatment of the hyperlipidemias. This agent, in experimental use in the United States, has been used extensively in Europe since the mid-1970s. Effective in the lowering of plasma VLDL and triglyceride levels, this drug is also quite effective in reducing plasma total and LDL cholesterol levels. Moreover, its long-term use does not appear to be associated with hepatomegaly or increased incidence of cancer.

Nonpharmacologic forms of therapy

Because of the serious nature of familial hypercholesterolemia, unusual and somewhat daring treatments have been tried, with mixed success, in resistant cases. Some patients with this condition do not respond to vigorous treatment with diet and medications. Surgical bypass of the distal ileum to prevent bile acid recycling and to cause body cholesterol depletion has been unsuccessful in some homozygotes but has reduced plasma cholesterol levels in severely affected heterozygotes. Because of the loss of bile acid reabsorption by exclusion of the terminal ileum from the intestinal transit, an increased clearance of circulating LDL occurs by stimulation of LDL receptor activity. A second nondietary, nonpharmacologic approach to lowering plasma LDL levels in both heterozygotes and homozygotes with familial hypercholesterolemia uses plasma pheresis, plasma exchange, or the use of specific anti-LDL immobilized on columns. These procedures can be effective and cause striking reductions in plasma LDL levels regardless of levels of LDL receptor activity. End-to-side portacaval anastomosis in some homozygous patients has caused profound reductions in plasma LDL and cholesterol levels by unknown mechanisms. Other unconventional therapies that have caused rapid reduction of plasma cholesterol levels in homozygotes with familial hypercholesterolemia have included intravenous hyperalimentation and plasma exchange. The intravenous administration of high-caloric solutions that contain glucose, amino acids, and vitamins has a cholesterol-lowering action, the mechanism of which is unknown. Repeated plasma exchanges with the use of a continuous-flow blood cell separator have effectively diminished plasma cholesterol levels and have been instituted on an outpatient basis. Recently, a young girl with homozygous familial hypercholesterolemia underwent heart and liver transplantation; the resultant decline in plasma LDL and cholesterol levels was dramatic. This decline resulted from an improved clearance of circulating LDL, presumably by the introduction of functional LDL receptors present in the normal transplanted liver. Other reports have appeared concerning the successful use of transplanted livers for the therapy of FH homozygotes, and this therapeutic approach appears to hold promise for treatment of this disorder. However, it must be emphasized that the use of invasive, innovative therapies for plasma LDL lowering requires considerable expense and specialized facilities and personnel. Moreover, the relative long-term safety and efficacy of these various invasive approaches remain uncertain.

The causal associations among various specific forms of hyperlipoproteinemia and the predisposition to premature atherogenesis, episodic acute pancreatitis, and xanthoma formation have been confirmed in a variety of studies. The importance of lowering plasma lipid levels to control bouts of abdominal pain and xanthomas has been amply demonstrated. Moreover, convincing evidence for the deceleration or reversal of atherosclerosis in humans by reduction of plasma lipid and lipoprotein levels (currently the most common indicator for the treatment of hyperlipidemia) is convincing. However, the answers to several key questions remain elusive. At what age must plasma lipoproteins be lowered to prevent atherosclerosis? How vigorously should moderate degrees of hyperlipidemia be treated? How does one determine the optimal treatment approach in a specific patient given the present state of knowledge? How can one monitor the effect of therapy on the progression of the atherosclerotic process? Are fasting plasma lipid or lipoprotein measurements adequate parameters to serve as guidelines to therapy?

According to most specialists in the field, the close association between hyperlipidemia and coronary disease and the results of intervention trials justify vigorous efforts to regulate plasma lipid levels, particularly LDL cholesterol levels. However, a sensible preventive strategy still begins with the identification of all risk factors in a given patient and a concerted attempt to modify individual life-styles where indicated and feasible. First-degree relatives of patients with familial hyperlipoproteinemias or premature atherosclerosis, especially offspring, should be screened by plasma lipid and lipoprotein measurements. Such screening is particularly important in cases of familial hypercholesterolemia, which can be diagnosed in infants by sampling of umbilical cord blood. Thus dietary modification and, in selected cases drug therapy, can be initiated early when such interventions are likelier to be effective. The majority of patients with hyperlipidemia encountered in office practice have moderate plasma lipid elevations. Dietary therapy and life-style modification should suffice in these cases. Increased intake of fish, plant products, and foods containing monounsaturated and polyunsaturated fats combined with a regular exercise program are important positive measures. Decreased intake of calories, refined sugar, cholesterol, saturated fat, salt, and alcohol; elimination of cigarette smoking; avoidance of oral contraceptives; and amelioration of stress comprise a preventive regimen that can improve the quality of life for longer periods in most patients. Currently most experts in the field emphasize a much more aggressive approach to plasma LDL and cholesterol lowering in hyperlipidemic patients and even in the population at large. Studies in progress are likely to confirm the wisdom of this approach.

FAMILIAL LIPOPROTEIN DEFICIENCY DISORDERS

Among the familial dyslipoproteinemias, a number of uncommon heritable conditions exist that are characterized by low circulating lipid levels and a reduction or absence of specific apolipoproteins in the circulation. Although the particular biochemical defect underlying these abnormalities remains incompletely defined in most of these conditions, great strides have recently been made in their molecular delineation and in the correlation of clinical and biochemical findings.

Abetalipoproteinemia

Abetalipoproteinemia is inherited as an autosomal recessive trait and is considered a lipoprotein disorder characterized by the absence of measurable apo B in plasma of affected subjects. Since apo B is undetectable in the plasma of subjects with this disorder, circulating chylomicrons, VLDL, and LDL are also absent. Malabsorption of fat is present from birth, and jejunal mucosal cells are engorged with lipids, particularly triglycerides. There is severe malabsorption of the fat-soluble vitamins A, D, E, and K. Although hepatic enlargement and liver function abnormalities are usually absent, light microscopic examination reveals extensive engorgement of the hepatocytes with lipid but no gross distortion of liver architecture. Vacuolization of both mucosal and hepatic cells is thought to derive from the defective apo B secretion. Recent studies have demonstrated the presence of apo B-100 in hepatocytes and apo B-100 and apo B-48 in the intestinal mucosal cells of patients with abetalipoproteinemia. Moreover, concentrations of hepatic messenger RNA for apo B-100 are greatly increased, suggesting potential defects in apo B posttranslational processing or secretion. Because of the effects of the plasma lipoprotein abnormality on plasma membrane structure and function, the red blood cells have abnormal, notched surfaces with thorny projections. These crenated erythrocytes are termed "acanthocytes."

Levels of all the major plasma lipids are strikingly diminished in this condition. Triglyceride levels are usually below levels that can be confidently measured by conventional techniques. There is marked hypocholesterolemia, and virtually all the plasma cholesterol in abetalipoproteinemia is associated with HDL.

The neurologic manifestations of abetalipoproteinemia are devastating and involve extensive segmental demyelinization of a number of nerve pathways. The areas principally disturbed include the dorsal root ganglia, posterior columns, spinocerebellar axis, and corticospinal tracts. Thus there is loss of position and vibratory sense, with ataxia, incoordination, tremor, hypotonia, nystagmus, and abnormal reflexes. Visual difficulties caused by progressive retinal pigmentary changes lead to night blindness, a possible consequence of defective carotenoid transport. Neurologic and retinal abnormalities can

be monitored by electrophysiological and electroretinographic testing, respectively. The treatment of patients with abetalipoproteinemia involves institution of a low-fat diet and supplementation with the fat-soluble vitamins, especially vitamins E and A. Stabilization or improvement in neurophysiologic testing has been demonstrated in some patients who have been so treated.

Hypobetalipoproteinemia

Hypobetalipoproteinemia is considered to be distinct from classic abetalipoproteinemia. There is a decreased concentration rather than an absence of plasma VLDL and LDL, accompanied by low levels of circulating cholesterol and triglycerides. Evidently this condition can occur as a genetically determined abnormality but more commonly is acquired as a result of chronic debilitating diseases or severe fat malabsorptive states. In the familial form the mutations involved appear to differ from those that cause abetalipoproteinemia; apo B can be synthesized and secreted, although at a somewhat slower than normal rate. Chylomicrons can be formed and some absorption of fat occurs. The clinical manifestations of familial hypobetalipoproteinemia can simulate those found in abetalipoproteinemia but are generally much milder. Treatment with a fat-reduced diet enriched with carbohydrate and protein and supplemented with vitamins A and E is recommended for most of these patients. Since vitamin E is considered important for normal neurologic function, appropriate supplementation is advisable for all patients with chronic fat malabsorption who have low serum vitamin E levels.

Another form of familial hypobetalipoproteinemia, termed "Anderson's disease," is characterized by diarrhea, steatorrhea, failure to secrete chylomicrons after a fatty meal, and low plasma levels of apo B-100, cholesterol, triglycerides, and phospholipids. Enterocytes obtained from intestinal biopsies of patients with this abnormality show numerous fat droplets (as seen in patients with abetalipoproteinemia) and immunologic evidence of cellular apo B-48 or a fragment thereof. Additional findings include decreased LDL levels, abnormal particle size distributions of HDL_2 and HDL_3, and compositional changes in LDL and HDL. Some cases exhibit additional apolipoprotein abnormalities. Hence Anderson's disease is not solely due to failure to produce and secrete intestinal apo B, but is more complex and affects all the lipoprotein classes.

Tangier disease

Tangier disease, a rare, autosomal recessive disorder, is named after the Chesapeake Bay island home of the first discovered cases. The condition is characterized by a marked deficiency or absence of normal HDL and an accumulation of cholesterol esters, particularly in reticuloendothelial tissues but also in other body tissues. The nature of the fundamental biochemical defect in Tangier disease remains unclear. An abnormal HDL, termed HDL_T, has been described and differs in some respects from normal HDL when subjected to a variety of physicochemical measures. The small quantities of HDL in plasma differ quantitatively and qualitatively from normal HDL, particularly in apoprotein content and composition. Plasma concentrations of both apo A-I and apo A-II are greatly reduced, and the small amount of apo A-I present is recovered in a density greater than 1.21 g/ml plasma fraction. No major structural defect has been identified in Tangier apo A-I, but a rapid rate of apo A-I catabolism has been demonstrated in patients with this condition, which has been attributed to a posttranslational defect in apo A-I metabolism. Because of these alterations, cholesterol esters accumulate in tissues, especially in the liver, spleen, lymph nodes, thymus, skin, and intestinal and rectal mucosa.

The tonsils are hyperplastic and have a peculiar orange or yellowish gray discoloration, making it possible to detect the condition through examination of the oropharynx. When the tonsils have been excised, a careful examination may reveal residual tags of mucosa with the same discoloration, suggesting the diagnosis. The combination of low plasma cholesterol, with normal or elevated triglyceride levels, and enlarged, lobulated, orange-yellow tonsils and adenoids is diagnostic of this disorder. The pathognomonic color and striations of the tonsils result from stored cholesterol esters in tonsillar foam cells. Biopsy of the rectal mucosa also reveals foamy histiocytes throughout the mucosa and submucosa. Focal findings of lipid-laden cells have also been observed in kidneys, heart valves, testes, and corneas.

Besides the tonsillar findings, clinical manifestations include hepatosplenomegaly, lymphadenopathy, and a generalized, peripheral polyneuropathy that can be subtle or overt. The neurologic findings can be sensory, motor, or mixed, and transient or permanent with variable symptoms and signs. Sural nerve biopsies in patients with Tangier disease have revealed a number of histological abnormalities, including a reduced quantity of smaller myelinated and unmyelinated fibers, and abundant vacuoles in Schwann cells, endoneurial fibroblasts, macrophages, and perineurial cells. Because of the limited number of subjects with Tangier disease and their relatively normal longevity, the vascular consequences of this condition are uncertain. Whether cholesterol esters are deposited at an accelerated rate below the lining of blood vessels is unknown.

Familial LCAT deficiency

Familial deficiency of LCAT is a rare inborn error of lipoprotein metabolism that was first discovered in a Norwegian family. The primary defect results in a lack of LCAT enzyme activity in plasma. LCAT catalyzes the plasma transfer of fatty acids from the 2 position of lecithin to cholesterol, with the formation of lysolecithin and cholesterol esters. Lecithin-rich HDL is the preferred lipoprotein substrate for LCAT. Absence of this enzyme results in a number of plasma lipoprotein abnormalities. As expected, circulating lipoproteins in this condition contain relatively large amounts of lecithin and unesterified cholesterol. The absolute plasma levels of HDL, apo A-I, and cholesterol esters are very low. Greater than 10% of the circulating apo A-I is recovered in the $d > 1.21$ g/ml fraction of plasma after ultracentrifugal flotation, and the apo A-I associated with a lipid-poor HDL subfraction. The HDL particles are unusually heterogeneous, with disk-shaped and very small globular structures. Absence of LCAT action on HDL leads to accumulations of unesterified cholesterol in plasma and tissues, whereas absence of the esters causes the abnormal sizes and shapes of the HDL particles. The apo C content of circulating HDL is low, perhaps because of an accelerated rate of HDL apoproteins in this condition. VLDL migrates abnormally slowly on electrophoresis because of a low content of apo C-II and apo C-III. VLDL concentrations are usually elevated, but their content of cholesterol esters is low. The LDL particles are also abnormally large and contain mainly lecithin and unesterified cholesterol similar to the lipoprotein X isolated from patients with obstructive jaundice.

Histopathologic specimens from subjects with LCAT deficiency reveal lipid-laden foam cells in the bone marrow kidney, spleen, and arteries. Foam cells are found in the bone marrow and spleen of affected patients; those that appear light blue after Giemsa staining are termed "sea-blue histiocytes." Clin-

ical findings include proteinuria, anemia, hyperlipidemia, and corneal arcus. The proteinuria that is consistently found may be caused by lipid accumulation in the glomerular tufts, and renal involvement can progress to the point of kidney failure. The renal lesions consist of large mesangial deposits of lipid in the form of osmiophilic lamellar bodies and a sieve-like transformation of the glomerular basement membranes. The erythrocytes are abnormal in both shape and composition. They contain excessive amounts of unesterified cholesterol and lecithin and show abnormal configurations similar to those seen in patients with obstructive jaundice or Mediterranean anemia. Many of these erythrocytes are "target cells," that is, cells with a peripheral rim and a center spot of red-stained material. Anemia develops, probably from a combination of increased destruction and decreased formation of erythrocytes. Accumulation of lipid in bone marrow foam cells may interfere in some way with erythrogenesis. The important role of LCAT in the remodeling of VLDL during triglyceride removal by LPL is illustrated by the elevations of VLDL triglyceride levels observed with LCAT deficiency. Premature atherosclerotic changes occur in the large and small arteries of patients with familial LCAT deficiency. The corneal opacities reflect deposition of free cholesterol in the corneas. These clinical abnormalities support the postulated role of LCAT in the clearance of plasma triglycerides and particularly in the transport of cholesterol from the peripheral tissues to the liver.

A new concept has recently been formulated based on evidence that two different LCAT activities exist in normal plasma. Classical LCAT deficiency has been attributed to diminished activity of both α-LCAT, which primarily catalyzes esterification of HDL-cholesterol, and β-LCAT, which is more specific for VLDL and LDL, as substrates for cholesterol esterification. In a rare, related familial condition, fish eye disease, efficiency of α- but not β-LCAT activity has been observed. Patients with fish eye disease demonstrate a low relative content of cholesterol esters in their plasma HDL but a normal content of these lipids in their VLDL and LDL. These patients also have abnormalities in their plasma concentrations of various circulating isoforms of apo A-I and apo A-II.

Although the lipoprotein deficiency disorders are rare, they illustrate the multiple, far-flung consequences of a genetic abnormality leading to an absence or defective structure of a key protein involved in the complex cycle of lipoprotein formation and removal. The features of these inherited disorders also suggest that plasma lipoproteins serve other crucial physiologic needs in addition to transport of triglyceride for energy flux in the body.

BIBLIOGRAPHY

Blankenhorn DH and others: Beneficial effects of combined colestipol-niacin therapy on coronary atherosclerosis and coronary venous bypass grafts, JAMA 257:3233, 1987.

Brown MS and Goldstein JL: How LDL receptors influence cholesterol and atherosclerosis, Sci Am 251:58, 1984.

Brown MS and Goldstein JL: A receptor-mediated pathway for cholesterol homeostasis, Science 232:34, 1986.

Brown MS and Goldstein JL: Familial hypercholesterolemia. In Stanbury, JB and others, editors: The metabolic basis of inherited disease, ed 5, New York, 1983, McGraw-Hill Book Co.

Brown MS, Goldstein JL, Fredrickson DS: Familial type 3 hyperlipoproteinemia (dysbetalipoproteinemia). In Stanbury JB and others, editors: The metabolic basis of inherited disease, ed 5, New York, 1983, McGraw-Hill Book Co.

Brown MS and Goldstein JL: The hyperlipoproteinemias and other disorders of lipid metabolism. In Braunwald E and others, editors: Harrison's principles of internal medicine, ed 11, New York, 1987, McGraw-Hill Book Co.

Castelli WP: The triglyceride issue: a view from Framingham, Am Heart J 112:432, 1986.

Consensus Development Conference: Treatment of hypertriglyceridemia, JAMA 251:1196, 1984.

Consensus Development Conference: Lowering blood cholesterol to prevent heart disease, JAMA 253:2080, 1985.

Glomset JA, Norum KR, and Gjone E: Familial lecithin: cholesterol acyltransferase deficiency. In Stanbury JB and others, editors: The metabolic basis of inherited disease, ed 5 New York, 1983, McGraw-Hill Book Co.

Grundy SM and others: AHA special report: recommendations for the treatment of hyperlipidemia in adults, Arteriosclerosis 4:445A, 1984.

Grundy SM: Cholesterol and coronary heart disease: a new era, JAMA 256:2849, 1986.

Herbert PN and others: Familial lipoprotein deficiency: abetalipoproteinemia, hypobetalipoproteinemia, and Tangier disease. In Stanbury JB and others, editors: The metabolic basis of inherited disease, ed 5, New York, 1983, McGraw-Hill Book Co.

Illingworth DR: Mevinolin (lovastatin) plus colestipol in therapy for severe heterozygous familial hypercholesterolemia, Ann Int Med 101:598, 1984.

Kane JP and Havel RJ: Treatment of hypercholesterolemia, Annu Rev Med 37:427, 1986.

Lipid research clinics program: The lipid research clinics coronary primary prevention trial results. I. Reduction in the incidence of coronary heart disease, JAMA 251:351, 1984.

Lipid research clinics program: The lipid research clinics coronary primary prevention trial results. II. The relationship of reduction in incidence of coronary heart disese to cholesterol lowering, JAMA 251:365, 1984.

Nikkila EA: Familial lipoprotein lipase deficiency and related disorders of chylomicron metabolism. In Stanbury JB and others, editors: The metabolic basis of inherited disease, ed 5, New York, 1983, McGraw-Hill Book Co.

Oram JF, Chait A, and Bierman EL: Lipoprotein and cholesterol metabolism in cultured arterial smooth muscle cells. In Campbell G and Campbell J, editors: Vascular smooth muscle in culture, Boca Ratan, Fla, 1986, CRC Press.

Report of the National Cholesterol Education Program expert panel on detection, evaluation, and treatment of high blood cholesterol in adults, Arch Intern Med 148:36, 1988.

Rifai N: Lipoproteins and apolipoproteins, Arch Pathol Lab Med 110:694, 1986.

Ross R: The pathogenesis of atherosclerosis: an update, N Engl J Med 314:488, 1986.

Schaefer EJ and Levy RI: Pathogenesis and management of lipoprotein disorders, N Engl J Med 312:1300, 1985.

Steinberg D: Lipoproteins and atherosclerosis: some unanswered questions, Am Heart J 113:626, 1987.

Dental correlations

DIABETES MELLITUS

Geza T. Terezhalmy

ORAL MANIFESTATIONS. It is generally accepted that there is a direct relationship between diabetes mellitus and dental disease. The accumulation of meaningful data relative to this relationship requires oral health care professionals not only to minimize potentially serious complications by providing for optimal oral health but also to help detect the disease and monitor patient response to treatment.

The oral signs and symptoms of diabetes mellitus can range from minimal to severe and involve the complete spectrum of dental complaints. Clinical signs and symptoms can be related to salivary and dental changes, periodontal and mucosal abnormalities, opportunistic infections, acetone or diabetic breath, and altered wound healing.

A frequent complaint of the individual with uncontrolled diabetes is xerostomia. Dehydration of the oral tissues (from systemic dehydration) and neuropathy can contribute to symptoms of generalized tenderness, altered taste, and burning sensations. Dehydration may also result from alterations in salivary flow, which in turn may be caused by the altered oral flora reported in the insulin-dependent diabetic patient. The subgingival flora is composed mainly of *Capnocytophaga* and other gram-negative organisms including *Fusobacterium* and *Campylobacter* organisms and occasionally *Actinobacillus actinomycetem-comitans*. Diabetic patients may have bilateral, asymptomatic parotid gland swelling with increased salivary viscosity caused by increased fatty-acid deposition and compensatory hypertrophy resulting from a decrease in saliva production. Secondary to xerostomia, increased caries activity may be observed, especially in the cervical region, and pulpal arteritis from microangiopathies may contribute to unexplained odontalgia and percussion sensitivity (acute pulpitis).

Manifestations of the disorder in the periodontal tissues have received the most attention in dental literature. The gingival response of patients with uncontrolled diabetes to plaque accumulation is usually accentuated, resulting in hyperplastic, erythematous gingiva. Other gingival findings frequently noted include acute fulminating gingival abscesses and granular subgingival proliferations. Roentgenographic findings include widening of the periodontal ligament and excessive alveolar bone loss, resulting in extreme tooth mobility and early tooth loss.

The gingival response of healthy individuals to plaque includes a change in vascular topography and function, the accumulation of inflammatory cells, and decreased vascular permeability and exudate formation. The gingiva of the diabetic patient reveals a decreased vascular response to irritation, impaired response of inflammatory cells, and a thickened basement lamina in the gingival microvessels that can limit the permeability of these vessels.

Microvascular changes observed in other tissues, such as skeletal muscle or kidney tissue, also are found in gingival tissue. These changes include a disruption of the normally flattened endothelial wall-lining cells and the presence of varying amounts of periodic acid Schiff–positive (PAS-positive) infiltrate subendothelially as a basement membrane thickening. This material, reported to be glycogen, is not thought to be related to the degree of severity or the duration of diabetes. In the diabetic individual the altered thickness of the capillary basement lamina is thought to affect these vessels' permeability and may cause the decreased resistance to infection.

Histologic examination of oral biopsy material from diabetic and prediabetic patients shows splitting, opening of the basement membrane, and deposition of a micropolysaccharide substance in the basement membrane of small blood vessels. These result in narrowing of the lamina of gingival arterioles and degenerative changes within the vessel wall. The presence of this "obliterative endarteritis" in gingival submucosa suggests that local blood supply to the tissue is impaired, resulting in poor tissue nutrition. This may decrease the resilience of these tissues and explain the poor healing observed in diabetic patients. Almost all studies of the small blood vessels of diabetic gingiva report significant differences between diabetic and nondiabetic persons.

Significant differences in the severity of periodontal disease exist between diabetic and nondiabetic subjects, even when such variable factors as the degree of plaque, age of the patient, and brushing frequency are controlled. Oral infection, such as periapical or periodontal abscesses, and periodontal disease have been demonstrated to affect insulin requirements. Following appropriate management of active periodontal disease, diabetic patients require reduced insulin dosage. Other studies have demonstrated a positive correlation between impaired glucose tolerance and the presence of periodontal disease, as well as a decreased healing response.

Slow wound healing (including periapical lesions following endodontics) and increased susceptibility to infection are caused by reduced phagocytic activity, reduced diapedisis, delayed chemotaxis, vascular changes leading to reduced blood flow, and abnormal collagen production. Many of these are also noted in nondiabetic relatives of diabetic individuals. Impairments in chemotaxis may be due to various biochemical alterations in metabolism. For example, some diabetic persons demonstrate an increased level of free fatty acids. Palmitic acid, a saturated fatty acid, completely inhibits chemotaxis in high doses and causes a marked inhibition of chemotaxis in concentrations close to those found in diabetic subjects. This defect could cause the increased susceptibility of the diabetic individual to infection and could facilitate the development of periodontal disease in diabetic persons. A compromised immune system and the repeated use of antibiotics may further lead to opportunistic infections with *Candida albicans* and *Mucoraceae* organisms.

Microangiopathies and neuropathies can also lead to oral ulcers refractory to therapy, especially with prostheses. Neuropathies leading to decreased muscle tone can contribute to a flabby tongue with indented lateral borders. An acetone or diabetic breath is noted in some patients in a ketoacidotic state.

DENTAL MANAGEMENT. The paramount concern of the dental practitioner should be the assessment of the physical and emotional well-being of the diabetic patient. Practitioners should establish the identity of the patient's physician and the date of the last visit to that physician. The length of time the patient has had diabetes should also be determined; this information may indicate the possibility of cardiovascular or neurologic complications. The medication (type of insulin or hypoglycemic agent) taken by the patient, the incidence of hypoglycemic reactions, and frequent alterations of the therapeutic regimen should be recorded. At each appointment, it is essential to establish that the patient has taken his medication as usual and has had an adequate intake of food.

The patient whose diabetes is well controlled and who has no other associated or concurrent medical problems (for example, hypertension or coronary heart disease) may receive appropriate dental therapy without modification of accepted dental protocols. The diabetic patient who is brittle or uncontrolled or who has serious underlying organic disease should delay elective dental care or surgical procedures until blood glucose levels have been regulated. The patient's physician should be consulted and become a partner in the management of the patient during the preoperative and postoperative period.

Scheduling an appointment time is an important consideration when planning treatment for a diabetic patient. Most insulin-dependent diabetes mellitus (IDDM) patients receive an intermediate-acting insulin once a day. The insulin becomes active about 2 hours after injection, and peak activity occurs in 8 to 12 hours. Thus, provided the patient had breakfast, morning appointments are safer, since this is a time of high glucose and low insulin activity. Afternoon appointments would be a time of low glucose and high insulin activity, which may predispose the patient to a hypoglycemic reaction. Therefore it is important to know what type of and how often insulin is being taken and what the peak insulin activity is for all IDDM patients.

When the severity of diabetes or the degree of control is not known, treatment should be limited to palliation. Since infection can increase the insulin requirement, it is important to treat oral infections in conjunction with the diabetes. In urgent situations, the use of analgesics and antibiotics are appropriate palliative measures. However, certain drugs cause side effects that can directly affect the diabetic. Aspirin has been reported to decrease glucose levels in diabetics and may enhance the activity of the sulfonylurea hypoglycemic agents. Although low dosages of aspirin may be tolerated by some diabetics, acetaminophen or other agents that do not cause these effects should be considered. Corticosteroids have been shown to increase blood glucose levels, whereas sulfonamides have been shown to increase the hypoglycemic effects of sulfonylurea hypoglycemic agents.

In all diabetic patients it is important to reduce pain as much as possible. Acute stress has been shown to increase epinephrine release, increase corticosteroid release, and decrease insulin secretion, leading to increased blood levels of glucose and free fatty acids in normal patients. This is presumed to occur in diabetic individuals also. Both diabetic and nondiabetic persons exhibit an increase in urine ketones and urine volume and fluctuations in blood and urine glucose levels while under stress. However, the fluctuations seen in diabetic individuals are more severe. Stress can cause an increase in the need for insulin; when stress is reduced, lower and more stable mean daily urine glucose levels are found. Short morning appointments, informing the patient about the steps and complexity of procedures, and appropriate pharmacoanxiolytic therapy (that is, oral or intravenous benzodiazapines or barbiturates) are all valuable management options to the practitioner. These recommendations are most effective when implemented in consultation with the patient's physician.

Epinephrine has an action opposite to that of insulin. It raises glucose levels by stimulating glycogenolysis and raises free fatty acid levels by promoting lipolysis. Elevated glucose tolerance curves can be caused by stress-related epinephrine release even in nondiabetic patients. However, the minute amount of epinephrine included as a vasoconstrictor in local anesthetics represents only one fifth to one tenth of that used as part of the routine treatment of hypoglycemic coma, and this amount (five to ten times larger) only elevates the blood glucose level by 30 to 40 mg/dl. The consequences of stress-stimulated endogenous epinephrine are of much greater concern than the small amounts administered in local anesthetics, especially for the long-term or poorly controlled diabetic patient in whom cardiovascular complications are predictable sequelae. Outpatient general anesthesia should be used with caution.

Hyperglycemia has been shown to decrease phagocytosis, diapedesis, and intracellular bactericidal activity of polymorphonuclear (PMN) leukocytes. Diabetic patients have also been found to have PMN leukocytes that respond poorly to chemotactic stimuli. Impairments in chemotaxis may be due to various biochemical alterations in metabolism. This defect could be related to the increased susceptibility of the diabetic individual to infection and could facilitate the development of periodontal disease and other infectious processes. There also appears to be general agreement that patients with uncontrolled diabetes have delayed healing and are more prone to infections following oral surgical procedures. Infection may present special problems in these individuals, since fever increases the metabolic rate and decreases the effectiveness of insulin. However, well-controlled cases without evidence of infection do not require prophylatic antibiotic coverage. Excessive use of unnecessary antibiotics can lead to oral or systemic fungal infections. If an infection is present preoperatively or postoperatively, antibiotic therapy may be appropriate.

Since odontogenic and other oral infections can cause complications in the regulation and control of diabetes, it is incumbent upon the dentist to aggressively treat and eliminate oral infection. The patient must be committed to an optimal oral hygiene program and to frequent dental visits, especially because the incidence and severity of periodontal disease in these patient is so high.

Patients should eat normally and take their medications before dental appointments. Postappointment food intake is especially important if a decrease in masticatory function is anticipated. Consultation with the patient's physician for diet modifications may be indicated before treatment. A proper nutritional balance must be maintained, and since it may vary from patient to patient, it should be implemented with the physician's guidance. Hospitalization should be considered for patients whose diabetes is severe or poorly controlled if diet restriction is required following treatment.

If patients fail to eat normally but continue to take their regular insulin dosage, a hypoglycemic reaction may occur because of excess insulin (insulin shock). These patients appear weak, nervous, and confused. Their skin is moist and pale, and they exhibit excessive flow of saliva; respiration is normal to shallow, the pulse is full and pounding, and blood pressure is usually normal. Frequently, a tremor may be noted. The patient experiencing a hypoglycemic reaction should be treated in the dental office. The conscious patient who is cooperative and demonstrates clinical symptoms of hypoglycemia should be administered a high-carbohydrate beverage (such as orange juice, cola, or ginger ale) or a glucose drink (such as Glucola). A 6- or 12-oz portion of a cola soft drink contains 20 to 40 g of glucose. The patient will respond almost immediately and should be observed until vital signs are stable and all signs and symptoms of hypoglycemia have disappeared. The unconscious individual should be administered 50% dextrose in water (30 to 50 ml) intravenously at once. Within 3 to 5 minutes after injection the patient should regain consciousness. Another drug that can be administered is glucagon (1 mg intramuscularly). The patient will respond to the glucagon within 5 minutes to 2 hours after the injection. However, since 50% dextrose is faster acting, it is the treatment of choice. Any patient who has experienced periods of unconsciousness should not be permitted to leave the office but rather should be taken to a hospital for further evaluation and treatment. Management of the unconscious patient also includes airway maintenance, oxygen administration, and monitoring of vital signs.

The patient with hyperglycemia appears ill. The skin is dry and flushed; infections and fever are common; and the mouth is characteristically dry. Other frequent symptoms include excessive thirst, abdominal pain, and vomiting. Respiration rates are exaggerated, the pulse is rapid and weak, and blood pressure is low. Frequently, an acetone breath can be noted. At this stage, patients are not likely to seek help in the private office but may well be seen as patients in a hospital dental service for the management of oral complications associated with hyperglycemia. If the patient becomes unconscious, basic life support techniques should be started and the patient should be promptly transferred for definitive medical management.

In conclusion, it is imperative that the dentist ascertain a comprehensive medical history from the known or suspected diabetic patient. The severity of the disease and degree of control must be established before deciding whether dental care should be rendered at that particular time.

BIBLIOGRAPHY

Abramowicz M editor: The medical letter: adverse interactions of drugs, New Rochelle, The Medical Letter Inc., 19(2):5, 1977.

Basker RM and others: Patients with burning mouths: a clinical investigation of causative factors, including the climateric and diabetes, Br Dent J 145(1):9, 1978.

Cianciola LJ and others: Prevalence of periodontal disease in insulin-dependent diabetes mellitus (juvenile diabetes), J Am Dent Assoc 104(5):653, 1982.

Cooper G and Platt R: *Staphylococcous aureus* bacterimia in diabetic patients, Am J Med 73(5):658, 1982.

Farman AG: Cellular changes and *Candida* in diabetic outpatients having glossal papillary atrophy, J Dent Assoc S Africa 33(8)425, 1978.

Fisher EB JR and others: Psychological factors in diabetes and its treatment, J Consult Clin Psychol 50(6)993, 1982.

Gilbert JP and others. Report of the Committee for the Assessment of Biometric Aspects of Controlled Trials of Hypoglycemic Agents, JAMA 231(6):583, 1975.

Grupper C and Avril J: Lichen erosif buccal diabete et hypertension (syndrome de Grinspan), Bull Soc Fr Dermatol Syphiligr 72(5):721, 1965.

Hinkle LE Jr and Wolf S: Importance of life stress in course and management of diabetes mellitus, JAMA 148(7):513, 1952.

Hussar DA: Interactions involving drugs used in dental practice, J Am Dent Assoc 87(2):349, 1973.

Kolterman OG and others: The acute and chronic effects of sulfonylurea therapy in type II diabetes subjects, Diabetes 33(4):346, 1984.

Lustman P and others: Acute stress and metabolism in diabetes, Diabetes Care 4(6):658, 1981.

Manouchehr-Pour M and Bissada NF: Periodontal disease in juvenile and adult diabetic patients: a review of the literature, J Am Dent Assoc 107(5):766, 1983.

McKinney RV and Singh BB: Oral manifestations not well recognized as early signs of diabetes mellitus, J Ga Dent Assoc 47(4):19, 1974.

Motegi K and others: Clinical studies on diabetes mellitus and diseases of the oral region, Bull Tokyo Med Dent Univ 22(3):243, 1975.

Munroe CE: The dental patient and diabetes mellitus, Dent Clin North Am 27(2):329, 1983.

Peterson CM and others: Bioavailability of glipizide and its effect on blood glucose and insulin levels in patients with non-insulin-dependent diabetes, Diabetes Care 5(5):497, 1982.

Reiner A: Oral implications of diabetes, Ann Dent 36(2):46, 1977.

Roland JM and Bhanji S: Anorexia nervosa occuring in patients with diabetes mellitus, Postgrad Med J 58(680):354, 1982.

Rose MI and others: The effects of anxiety management training on the control of juvenile diabetes mellitus, J Behav Med 6(4):381, 1983.

Rothwell BR and Richard EL: Diabetes mellitus: medical and dental considerations, Spec Care Dent 4(2):58, 1984.

Russotto SB: Asymptomatic parotid gland enlargement in diabetes mellitus, Oral Surg 56(6):594, 1981.

Ryan DE and Bronstein SL: Dentistry and the diabetic patient, Dent Clin North Am 26(1):105, 1982.

Smith MJA: Oral lichen planus and diabetes mellitus: a possible association, J Oral Med 32(4):110, 1977.

Stege P and others: Anorexia nervosa: a review including oral and dental manifestations, J Am Dent Assoc 104(5):648, 1982.

Szmukler GI and Russell GFM: Diabetes mellitus, anorexia nervosa, and bulimia, Br J Psychiatry 142(1):305, 1983.

Tasch EG and others: Dental management of the diabetic patient, Q Natl Dent Assoc 36(3):107, 1978.

Tullman MJ and Redding SW, editors: Systemic disease in dental treatment, New York, 1982, Appleton-Century-Croft.

DISORDERS OF LIPOPROTEIN METABOLISM
Barbara J. Steinberg *and* **Barry H. Hendler**

Fabry-Anderson syndrome

ORAL MANIFESTATIONS. Angiokeratomas, which are small blood-filled cavities, occur in the oral mucosa. They are maroon or blue-black, flat or slightly elevated, and a few millimeters in diameter. The lips (most prominently the lower lip) are involved near the mucosa-skin junction. Although rare, the mucosa near the soft palate, the buccal mucosa, the gingiva, and the facial skin can also be affected. The tongue, however, is not an observed site for these vascularities. The histologic picture reveals variable dilation of superficial mucosal and cutaneous blood vessels.

DENTAL MANAGEMENT. The dentist should exercise caution whenever manipulating affected oral tissues in order to minimize hemorrhage. In the event that hemorrhage cannot be avoided, accessible angiokeratomas respond well to electrocoagulation and to topical application of 50% trichloroacetic acid.

Since the renal, cardiovascular, and nervous systems can be affected by this disease, referral to these sections of this text is suggested for effective dental management.

Gaucher's disease

ORAL MANIFESTATIONS. Yellow pigmentation occurring on the face, lips, conjunctivae, and oral mucosa is an important sign. Additional changes occur in the jaws, where the radiograph may reverse irregular osteoporotic defects with gradual expansion, thinning of the cortex, and resorption of dental roots, especially in the molar region.

DENTAL MANAGEMENT. Since extraction of teeth from affected regions of the jaws can result in hemorrhage, and since any oral peridontal surgical procedure can be further complicated by the attendant pancytopenia, the dentist must be prepared to employ precautionary measures for hemostasis. These include a complete blood count, prothrombin time (PT), partial thromboplastin time (PTT), bleeding time, and platelet count preoperatively, as well as a consultation with the patient's physician.

Urbach-Wiethe disease

ORAL MANIFESTATIONS. Granular or nodular deposits in the skin and mucous membranes are pathognomonic of Urbach-Wiethe disease. In the head and neck region lesions may be found in the facial skin, larynx, oral mucous membranes, and pharynx. When the yellow waxy nodules that occur on the face become confluent, fissuring may occur, especially around the eyes and lips, giving the face an appearance that is typical of the disease. Laryngeal involvement produces hoarseness and dysphasia that are noted in even early childhood. Lesions of the oral mucosa vary in appearance from solitary dots to confluent plaques and from whitish to yellowish white, according to the age of the patient. In general, the older the patient, the more indurated the plaques. The lower lip assumes a cobblestone appearance and the tongue may become firm and lose its papillae. There is also evidence of macroglossia, and the tongue seems to be bound to the floor of the mouth, probably secondary to infiltration of the lingual frenum. When the buccal mucosa is involved stenosis of the parotid ducts can occur with subsequent parotitis. Teeth may fail to develop or they may be hypoplastic. The skin papules and mucosal plaques contain abundant lipids, especially cholesterol (66%) and phospholipids (27%).

Type V hyperlipoproteinemia

ORAL MANIFESTATIONS. Patients with type V hyperlipoproteinemia have a chief complaint of xerostomia. Salivary scans indicate that focal inflammatory, infiltrative, or obstructive lesions of the major salivary glands may be present.

DENTAL MANAGEMENT. Parotid biopsy confirms the diagnosis of type V hyperlipoproteinemia. Patients complaining of xerostomia should be given a salivary stimulating agent to provide symptomatic relief.

ALCOHOLISM

Barry H. Hendler and **Barbara J. Steinberg**

ORAL MANIFESTATIONS. Oral abnormalities secondary to alcoholism generally occur from neglect of oral hygiene, from fatty infiltration of the salivary glands, and from moderate to severe nutritional deficiencies. Alcoholic individuals also have an increased risk of developing carcinoma of the oral cavity, pharynx, larynx, and esophagus.

As a result of poor oral hygiene, alcoholic patients frequently have a coated tongue and gross deposits of plaque and calculus on the teeth. They have an increased rate of chronic, advanced, generalized periodontitis with inflamed gingival tissues, as evidenced by loss of gingival stippling; punched-out, interdental papillae, and deep periodontal pockets with advanced loss of alveolar bone. Alcoholics tend to have more missing teeth than nonalcoholic, age-matched control groups, although the decayed, missing, or filled (DMF) profile of alcoholics as a whole is similar to that of the general population. It is postulated that alcohol stimulates the brainstem reticular activating system, causing masseter muscle contractions and nocturnal bruxism during periods of rapid eye movement (REM) sleep. This predisposes alcoholics to problems such as dental attrition and temporomandibular joint (TMJ) dysfunction.

Some chronic alcoholics have enlargement of the major salivary glands, especially the parotid glands. This asymptomatic swelling usually occurs bilaterally. Salivary flow can increase or remain unaffected. Histologically, fatty deposits infiltrate the salivary glands as a result of generalized disturbance in lipid metabolism.

Nutritional deficiencies, which are often encountered in the alcoholic patient, also cause significant oral change. The most common deficiencies involve the B-complex vitamins, specifically thiamin, niacin, riboflavin, pyridoxine, and folic acid. Thiamin deficiency produces hyperesthesia of the oral mucosa, burning tongue, and loss or diminuition of taste perception. Niacin deficiency causes an inflamed and erythematous tongue with papilliary atrophy, hyperemia of the buccal mucosa, and generalized oral erosions. A deficiency in riboflavin causes macerated lesions at the corners of the mouth (angular cheilosis), which can become infected with bacteria or *Candida* organisms, (angular cheilitis). Riboflavin deficiency can also result in glossitis and generalized erythema of the oral mucosa, redness of the conjunctiva, and burning and excessive dryness of the eyes. Pyridoxine deficiency is evidenced by nasolabial seborrhea and glossitis. The patient who is deficient in folic acid has extreme pallor of the skin and complains of burning of the tongue and oral mucosa. The tongue appears red and swollen, with enlarged papillae and numerous small vesicular lesions. Angular cheilosis, gingivitis, and diffuse painful ulcerations, particularly of the palate, tongue, and buccal mucosa, are also common findings.

DENTAL MANAGEMENT. The alcoholic patient presents challenges in almost every aspect of dental treatment, including hematologic complications, increased susceptibility to infection, impaired wound healing, alcohol-drug interactions and psychologic disturbances.

Dentists should be vigilant in identifying the alcoholic patient. Reliance on the routine medical history alone is often inadequate. People tend to underreport socially unacceptable or stigmatizing conditions like alcoholism. When directly questioned, many alcoholics deny or minimize their alcohol consumption and alcohol-related problems. An empathic, trusting dentist-patient relationship, in which the patient understands the dentist's need to have accurate information, helps improve the quality of information gathered. Questioning should always be neutral and nonjudgmental. It should never imply that a particular response is expected, is acceptable, or is nonacceptable.

The orofacial examination can be helpful in identifying the alcoholic patient, even when the obtained history is negative. Alcohol on the breath, other signs of intoxication, or withdrawal in a patient coming for a scheduled appointment should always suggest the diagnosis of alcoholism.

Table 1 Drug interactions with alcohol

Drug	Interaction	Prevention
Anticoagulants oral (coumarin derivatives)	Inhibited anticoagulant effect with chronic alcohol use; enhanced anticoagulant effect with acute intoxication	Restrict alcohol intake to small amounts
Antihistamines	Enhanced CNS depression	Prohibit or sharply curtail alcohol use
Aspirin or another salicylate	Gastrointestinal bleeding	Prohibit alcohol use in patients taking salicylates regularly
Barbiturates	Enhanced activity of each drug with acute intoxication; sedative effect diminished with chronic alcohol use	Prohibit or sharply curtail alcohol use during administration
Chloral betaine (Beta-Chlor), chloral hydrate (Kessodrate, Noctec, Somnos)	CNS depression; tachycardia; vasodilation	Prohibit or sharply curtail alcohol use during administration; cardiac patients on long-term therapy should not take alcohol
Chlordiazepoxide (Libritabs), or chlordiazeposide HCl (A-poxide, Librium, Sk-Lygen, Tenax)	In some patients, enhanced CNS depression	Inform patients of this effect, especially regarding operation of hazardous equipment or motor vehicles
Cyclobenzaprine HCl (Flexeril)	Enhanced effects of alcohol	Inform patients of this effect, especially regarding operation of hazardous equipment or motor vehicles
Diazepam (Valium)	Increased diazepam-induced sedation with high blood levels of alcohol	Instruct patients concerning excessive alcohol use while taking diazepam
Guanethidine sulfate (Ismelin)	Enhanced orthostatic hypotension from alcohol's vasodilating effect	Warn patients about this effect; limit alcohol intake in patients prone to orthostatic hypotension
Hypnotics (nonbarbiturate)	Enhanced CNS depression	Prohibit alcohol use
Insulin	Hypoglycemia (dose related)	If necessary, reduce insulin dosage during periods of substantial intake
Lorazepam (Ativan)	Potentiated CNS depressant effects	Inform patients of this effect, especially regarding operation of hazardous equipment or motor vehicles
MAO inhibitors	Sedation; with tyramine-containing alcoholic beverages, hypertensive crisis	If patient becomes sedated, prohibit alcohol; tyramine-containing alcoholic beverages must not be taken
Meprobamate (Equanil, Kesso-Bamate, Meprospan, Miltown, SK-Bamate)	Enhanced CNS depression; impairment of motor skills	Warn patients that meprobamate may increase alcohol's intoxicating effects
Metronidazole (Flagyl)	Acute alcohol intolerance (contradictory information in literature)	Prohibit alcohol use until true significance of interaction is resolved
Narcotics	Enhanced CNS depression	Prohibit or sharply curtail alcohol use
Nitroglycerin (Cardabid, Nitro-Bid, Nitroglyn, Nitrospan, Nitrostat)	Hypotension	Pending further evaluation of this interaction, warn patients to use alcohol with caution
Phenothiazines	CNS depression; sedation	Prohibit alcohol use
Phenytoin (Dilantin); phenytoin sodium (Dilantin)	Enhanced anticonvulsant metabolism with chronic alcohol use; seizures in epileptic persons previously controlled with phenytoin	Observe patients for decreased anticonvulsant effect; adjust dosage if necessary
Propoxyphene HCl (Darvon, Dolene SK-65); propoxyphene napsylate (Darvon-N)	Enhanced respiratory and CNS depression (dose related)	Warn patients taking therapeutic doses against excessive alcohol use
Sulfonylureas (hypoglycemics)	Enhanced hypoglycemic effect, especially in fasting patients; flushing, sweating, and tachycardia; accelerated sulfonylurea metabolism in patients who regularly consume large amounts of alcohol	Prohibit alcohol use
Tricyclic antidepressants	CNS depression and sedation	Prohibit alcohol use
Tranquilizers, minor	Enhanced CNS depression	Prohibit or sharply curtail alcohol use
Valproic acid (Depakene)	Potentiated CNS depressant effects	Prohibit or sharply curtail alcohol use during administration; inform patients of this effect, especially regarding operation of hazardous equipment or motor vehicles

Rhinophyma (red, beefy nose) and telangiectasias ("spiders") are common skin manifestations of chronic alcoholism. Facial edema and jaundiced skin or mucosa (mouth and eye) can occur in the patient with severe alcoholic liver disease. Because alcohol is second only to tobacco as a risk factor for oral carcinomas, the occurrence of dysplastic lesions (especially in nonsmokers) should suggest the possibility of alcoholism.

The acute effects of alcohol can inhibit coordination and judgement, lengthen reaction time, and decrease motor performance and sensory skills. As a result, alcoholics frequently incur trauma to the head and neck as a direct result of accidents or falls occurring while drinking. Many of these acutely injured patients require dental surgical procedures. (Since 50% of all fatal automobile accidents involve use of alcohol, facial injury is common in our society.) General cerebral functions are greatly altered in patients with acute alcohol intoxication, and it is often impossible to obtain a meaningful history from them. While in this condition, the patient's physical symptoms (such as neurologic abnormalities) may be blunted, and the recognition of pain is frequently lost. All intoxicated patients seen on an emergency basis should be carefully evaluated for the presence of craniofacial injury.

Pancytopenia, iron deficiency anemia, and abnormalities in both function and number of platelets leading to hemorrhagic diathesis can occur secondary to alcohol consumption or subsequent liver disease. From the dental perspective, the important organs that may be affected in alcoholism are the liver and the bone marrow. In order to obtain proper hemostasis, the liver must synthesize the many proteins involved in the coagulation cascade. Patients with severe alcoholic liver disease may have deficient protein levels that cause impaired clotting and increased risk of intraoperative or postoperative hemorrhage. As a direct suppressant of bone marrow, which manufactures platelets, alcohol may cause thrombocytopenia with a resultant potential for prolonged bleeding.

Certain basic diagnostic laboratory studies should be obtained. These include a complete blood count and differential, platelet count, prothrombin time, partial thromboplastin time, and bleeding time. In addition, consultation with the patient's physician is advisable before providing dental care.

Alcoholic individuals are frequently susceptible to infection resulting from suppressed immune mechanisms. The alcoholic patient with severe systemic infection of unknown origin should be examined to rule out an oral focus. Antibiotic therapy is certainly a strong consideration when performing any dental surgery.

The relationship between alcohol and abnormal wound healing should also be recognized. A dose-related increase in postoperative healing time often occurs in the alcoholic patient because of interference with the proper formation and deposition of collagen.

Alcohol-drug interactions are of particular importance in dental therapy. For example, alcohol combined with salicylates can predispose the patient to delayed clot formation and possible postoperative hemorrhage. The dentist should inform the alcoholic patient when alcohol is inadvisable with the prescribed drugs and should make every effort to select drugs with minimal interaction potential.

Because they have an increased tolerance to a variety of depressant drugs, patients with alcohol in their systems require a greater amount of sleep-inducing anesthetic, including nitrous oxide and fluorinated anesthetics. After the induction of anesthesia, however, the presence of alcohol results in a supraadditive interaction. This leads to the development of a deeper narcosis, an increase in sleeping time, and a lowering of the concentration of anesthetic needed to produce death. Williamson and Davis reported that for most oral surgery patients having a long history of chronic alcoholism, the amount of local anesthetic needed is significantly higher, and the onset, profoundness, and duration of the anesthetic agent is noticeably decreased. Patients who are known or suspected alcoholics should be completely detoxified before any elective dental surgery is performed because the stress of the procedure can precipitate severe, life-threatening withdrawal symptoms. During the period of detoxification, electrolyte imbalances, blood disorders, and liver disease should be evaluated and treated. Patients undergoing therapy for delirium tremens may have depressed gag and cough reflexes, rendering them more likely to aspirate oral and gastric secretions.

Alcoholism presents a variety of psychosocial, nutritional, and clinical problems. Lack of motivation to maintain good oral hygiene severely limits the long-term efficacy of caries control, advanced restorative dentistry, and periodontal therapy in alcoholic patients. In addition to the necessary dental care, the dental practitioner can provide nutritional counseling and encouragement to the alcoholic patient. Optimized dietary intake will have a remarkable impact on

Table 2 Drug recommendations for the patient with acute intermittent porphyria

Indicated	Contraindicated
Salicylates	All barbiturates
Morphine and related opiates	Diazepam (Valium)
Phenothiazines	Chlordiazepoxide HCl (Librium)
Diphenhydramine	Phenytoin sodium (Dilantin)
Guanethidine	Sulfonamides
Reserpine	Estrogen
Atropine	Some oral contraceptives
Neostigmine	Methyldopa (Aldomet)
Procaine	Alcohol
Succinylcholine	Pentazocine (Talwin)
Nitrous oxide	Lidocaine
Penicillin	Mepivacaine

*Clinical judgment on risk versus benefit may have to be used on many of these medications, but barbiturates are absolutely contraindicated.

the alcoholic's health, and an awareness of the psychosocial factors affecting the patient's perception of dental treatment will permit a more effective approach to the patient and his illness.

Porphyria
Barbara J. Steinberg and **Barry H. Hendler**

ORAL MANIFESTATIONS. In patients with congenital erythropoietic porphyria, there may be calcium phosphate deposits in the dentin and enamel. This imparts a reddish brown or pink color to the deciduous and permanent teeth (erythrodontin). The porphyrin deposits can occur in discrete bands, which are evidence of exacerbations of the disease during tooth formation. Affected teeth fluoresce bright scarlet under ultraviolet light. In addition, advanced local periodontal changes and atrophic cheilitis can occur. In the erythropoietic form of porphyria, painful bullous lesions can erupt following oral manipulation. These oral lesions are histologically similar to the cutaneous lesions that appear in individuals with this disorder.

DENTAL MANAGEMENT. The dentist should exercise great care in manipulating oral tissues to prevent the occurrence of bullous lesions in patients with congenital erythropoietic porphyria. Drugs known to cause acute exacerbations of acute intermittent porphyria must be avoided (Table 2). For example, no barbiturates (either oral or intravenous) and no barbiturate-based anesthetics should be administered to such patients; to do so could precipitate a serious crisis with lower motor neuron paralysis that may not appear for some days after the administration of the drug. Patients with acute intermittent porphyria who are advised by their physician to ingest large amounts of carbohydrates should simultaneously be advised of the detrimental effects the diet will have on the oral cavity. These patients should be referred to a dental practitioner for proper education in oral hygiene and preventive techniques. Frequent follow-up examinations are recommended. Prevention of oral disease is one of the most important services a dental professional can offer to patients with this disease, because even a simple restoration can be life-threatening if a contraindicated local anesthetic is used.

BIBLIOGRAPHY

Aznar J and others: Study of the lipids in the skin lesions in Urbach-Wiethe disease, Short Communication, Amsterdam, 1977, Elsevier/North-Holland Biomedical Press.

Becker CE: Review of pharmacologic and toxicologic effects of alcohol, J Am Dent Assoc 99:494, 1979.

Bergenholtz A, Hofer PA, and Ohman J: Oral, pharyngeal and laryngeal manifestations in Urbach-Wiethe disease, Ann Clin Res 9:1, 1977.

Browne WG: Oral pigmentation and root resorption in Gaucher's disease, J Oral Surg Oncol 35:153, 1977.

Gorlin RJ and Sedano HO: Stomatologic aspects of cutaneous diseases, J Dermatol Surg Oncol 5(3):180, 1979.

Green JB and Trowbridge AA: Hematologic and oncologic implications of alcoholism, Postgrad Med 61(5):149, 1977.

Hillman RW and Kissin B: Oralcytologic patterns and nutritional status: some relationships in alcoholic subjects, Oral Surg, 38:34, 1980.

Reinertsen JL and others: Sicca-like syndrome in type V hyperlipoproteinemia, Arthritis Rheum 23(1):114, 1980.

Ritter FN: Salivary gland involvement in systemic diseases, Otolaryngol Clin N Am 10(2):371, 1977.

Schuckit MA: Overview of alcoholism, J Am Dent Assoc 99:489, 1979.

Smith KG: Alcoholism—a nutritional approach, Dent Hyg 50:263, 1976.

Young WG, Pihlstrom BL, and Sauk JJ, Jr: Granulomatous gingivitis in Anderson-Fabry disease, J Periodontol 51:95, 1980.

INDEX

A

Abdomen
- distention of, in digestive system disorders, 866
- in patient evaluation, 10

Abdominal paracentesis in peritoneal disease, 930

Abdominal reflex in patient evaluation, 11

Abdominal ultrasonography for digestive system disorders, 873-874

Aberrant conduction versus ventricular ectopy, 482

Abetalipoproteinemia, 708-709, 1151
- malabsorption in, 898

Abortion
- septic, mycoplasmal, 190
- spontaneous, genital mycoplasma and, 190

Abscess(es)
- appendiceal, 909-910
- brain, 166-167
- epidural, 168-169
- intraabdominal, 933
  - ultrasonic diagnosis of, 873-874
- liver, amebic, 955-956
- lung, 615-616
- pancreatic, complicating acute pancreatitis, 939
- perinephric, 172
- of spleen, 345

Abuse, drug, dental correlations with, 756-757

Acanthamoeba, infections from, 246

Acetaminophen, liver disease induced by, 956

Achalasia, 878

Acid, poisoning with, 661

Acid-base balance, 525-527
- in chronic renal failure, 558-559

Acid-base homeostasis, kidney in, 519

Acid infusion test, esophageal, for gastroesophageal reflux disease, 881

Acid maltase deficiency, myopathy in, 753

Acid-peptic diseases, 884-893
- gastritis as, 891-892
- peptic ulcer disease as, 884-889; *see also* Peptic ulcer disease
- stress erosions as, 891
- Zolliner-Ellison syndromes as, 889-891

Acid perfusion test for esophageal disorders, 877

Acid reflux recordings for esophageal disorders, 877

Acidemia
- methylmalonic, 1096
- propionic, 1096

Acidosis
- lactic, ketoacidosis and, in diabetes, 1126
- metabolic, 525-526
- renal tubular, 544-545
  - distal, normocalcemic hypercalciuric stone formation in, 571-572
- respiratory, 525-527

Acoustic neurinomas, vertigo in, 698

Acquired immunodeficiency syndrome (AIDS), 130-132
- clinical manifestations of, 130-131

Acquired immunodeficiency syndrome (AIDS)—cont'd
- course of, 131
- definition of, 130
- dementia related to, 680
- diagnosis of, 131
- epidemiology of, 130
- etiology of, 130
- management of, 131-132
- pathogenesis of, 130
- prognosis of, 131
- renal lesions in, 540
- skin lesions of, 832-834

Acquired immunodeficiency syndrome (AIDS)–dementia complex, 726

Acral lentiginous melanoma in situ, 816-817

Acrocentric chromosomes, 1082

Acrochordon, 814

Acrodermatitis enteropathica, cutaneous lesions in, 790-791

Acromegaly, 991-992
- dental correlations with, 1066
- skin changes in, 783-784

Acrosclerosis, cutaneous lesions in, 802

ACTH stimulation test for Cushing's syndrome, 1024-1025

Actinic keratoses, 816

Actinomyces israelii, actinomycosis from, 214-215

Actinomycosis, 214-215
- dental correlations with, 269

Acute disseminated encephalomyelitis (ADEM), 703-704, 726

Acute intermittent porphyria (AIP), 1105-1106

Acute necrotizing encephalomyelitis (ANE), 703-704

Acute necrotizing ulcerative gingivitis (ANUG), 265

Acute renal failure (ARF), 551-555
- definition of, 551
- etiology of, 551
- intrinsic, 552
- from nephrotoxins, 547, 552-553
- pathogenesis of, 551
- in renal ischemia, 552

Acute tubular necrosis (ATN), 551-555

Acyanotic heart lesions
- with left-to-right shunts, 446-448
- with obstructive lesions, 448-449

Acycloguanosine for viral diseases, 135

Acyclovir for viral diseases, 135

Addison's disease, 1021, 1022-1023
- dental correlations with, 1068-1069
- skin changes in, 784

Adenine arabinoside for viral diseases, 135

Adenocarcinoma
- colorectal, 927-928
- dental correlations with, 970-971
- of esophagus, 923
- renal, 579-580
- of small bowel, 925
- of stomach, 923-924
  - dental correlations with, 970

Adenoma(s)
- adrenal, management of, 1025
- bronchial, 652
- hepatic, 963

Adenoma(s)—cont'd
- sebaceous, internal malignancy and, 813
- thyroid, 1017
- thyrotropin-secreting, 992

Adenoma sebaceum, 776-777
- dental correlations with, 764

Adenosine deaminase deficiency, 1098

Adenovirus (es)
- exanthems from, 127-128
- gastroenteritis from, 129
- respiratory infection from, 123-124

Adhesive capsulitis, 85

Adiposogenital dystrophy, hypopituitarism differentiated from, 995-996

Adolescent, hyperthyroidism in, 1014

Adrenal adenomas, management of, 1025

Adrenal cortex, 1019-1028
- congenital hyperplasias of, 1027
- failure of, 1021-1023
- glucocorticoid deficiency syndrome of, 1021-1023
- glucocorticoid excess syndrome and, 1023-1025
- mineralocorticoid deficiency syndrome and, 1025
- mineralocorticoid excess syndrome and, 1025-1026
- structure and function of, 1019-1021; *see also* Steroid hormones

Adrenal Cushing's syndrome, 1023

Adrenal disease, skin changes in, 784

Adrenal enzyme deficiency syndrome, 1035

Adrenal gland
- disorders of, dental correlations with, 1068-1069
- function of, in liver disease, 945

Adrenal hyperplasias, 1026-1028

Adrenergic agents for asthma, 621

Adrenergic agonists for chronic bronchitis, 610

β-Adrenergic blocking agents
- for hypertension, 418, 419*t*
- for pheochromocytoma, 1032

α-Adrenergic blocking agents for pheochromocytoma, 1031-1032

Adrenocortical hyperplasia, skin changes in, 784

Adrenocorticotropic hormone (ACTH), 990
- deficiency of, 993-994
- production of, ectopic, 1023

Adrenoleukodystrophy, 705

Adult respiratory distress syndrome (ARDS), hypoxemic respiratory failure in, 623

Adventitious sounds in lung examination, 8

Affect, 670

Afibrinogenemia, dental correlations with, 373

Afterload
- in congestive heart failure, 408
- in myocardial function, 403

Agammaglobulinemia
- acquired, 29
- x-linked, 28

Age
- coronary artery disease and, 464
- of expression, 1082

Agnogenic myeloid metaplasia, 325-327

Agnosia
- definition of, 676
- from parietal lobe lesions, 666
- visual, lesions causing, 677